10TH EDITION

MANUAL OF CLINICAL MICROBIOLOGY

10TH EDITION

MANUAL OF CLINICAL MICROBIOLOGY

EDITOR IN CHIEF

JAMES VERSALOVIC

Department of Pathology, Texas Children's Hospital, and Department of Pathology
and Immunology, Baylor College of Medicine, Houston, Texas

EDITORS

KAREN C. CARROLL

Division of Medical Microbiology
Department of Pathology
The Johns Hopkins University School of Medicine
Baltimore, Maryland

GUIDO FUNKE

Department of Medical Microbiology and Hygiene
Gärtner & Colleagues Laboratories
Ravensburg, Germany

JAMES H. JORGENSEN

Department of Pathology
University of Texas Health Science Center
San Antonio, Texas

MARIE LOUISE LANDRY

Department of Laboratory Medicine
Yale University School of Medicine
New Haven, Connecticut

DAVID W. WARNOCK

National Center for Emerging and
Zoonotic Infectious Diseases
Centers for Disease Control and Prevention
Atlanta, Georgia

Volume **1**

ASM
PRESS
Washington, DC

Address editorial correspondence to ASM Press, 1752 N St. NW,
Washington, DC 20036-2904, USA

Send orders to ASM Press, P.O. Box 605, Herndon, VA 20172, USA
Phone: (800) 546-2416 or (703) 661-1593
Fax: (703) 661-1501
E-mail: books@asmusa.org
Online: estore.asm.org

Library of Congress Cataloging-in-Publication Data
Manual of clinical microbiology / editor in chief, James Versalovic ; editors, Karen C. Carroll ...
[et al.].—10th ed.
p. ; cm.
Clinical microbiology
Includes bibliographical references and indexes.
ISBN 978-1-55581-463-2 (hardcover)
1. Medical microbiology—Handbooks, manuals, etc. 2. Diagnostic microbiology—Handbooks,
manuals, etc. I. Versalovic, James. II. American Society for Microbiology. III. Title: Clinical
microbiology.
[DNLM: 1. Microbiology. 2. Microbiological Techniques. QW 4]
QR46.M425 2011
616.9'041—dc22
2010035191

10 9 8 7 6 5 4 3 2 1

ISBN 978-1-55581-463-2 (print edition), 978-1-55581-678-0 (print/e-book bundle)

CONTENTS

CURVED AND SPIRAL-SHAPED GRAM-NEGATIVE RODS

MYCOPLASMAS AND OBLIGATE INTRACELLULAR BACTERIA

section III

ANTIBACTERIAL AGENTS AND SUSCEPTIBILITY TEST METHODS / 1041

VOLUME EDITOR: JAMES H. JORGENSEN
SECTION EDITOR: JEAN B. PATEL

Volume 2

section IV
VIROLOGY / 1262

VOLUME EDITOR: MARIE LOUISE LANDRY
SECTION EDITORS: ANGELA M. CALIENDO,
CHRISTINE C. GINOCCHIO, YI-WEI TANG, AND
ALEXANDRA VALSAMAKIS

GENERAL

RNA VIRUSES

DNA VIRUSES

Editorial Board

CONTRIBUTORS

SHARON L. ABBOTT
Microbial Diseases Laboratory, California Department of
Public Health, 850 Marina Bay Parkway, E-164,
Richmond, CA 94804

STEPHAN W. ABERLE
Department of Virology, Medical University of Vienna,
Kinderspitalgasse 15, A-1095 Vienna, Austria

ADRIANO AGUZZI
Institute of Neuropathology, University Hospital Zürich,
Schmelzbergstrasse 12, CH-8091 Zürich, Switzerland

ABDALLA O. A. AHMED
Department of Medical Microbiology, Faculty of Medicine,
Umm Al-Qura University, P.O. Box 7607, 21955 Makkah Al
Mukarramah, Saudi Arabia

AFSAR ALI
Emerging Pathogens Institute, University of Florida at
Gainesville, Gainesville, FL 32610

DAVID A. ANDERSON
Macfarlane Burnet Institute for Medical Research and Public
Health, AMREP, 85 Commercial Road, Melbourne,
Victoria 3004, Australia

GEORGE F. ARAJ
Department of Pathology and Laboratory Medicine, American
University of Beirut Medical Center, PO Box 11-0236,
Beirut 1107-2020, Lebanon

MAX Q. ARENS
Department of Pediatrics, Washington University School of
Medicine, 660 S. Euclid Avenue, Box 8237,
St. Louis, MO 63110

RONALD M. ATLAS
Department of Biology, University of Louisville,
Louisville, KY 40202

ROBERT L. ATMAR
Department of Medicine and Department of Molecular
Virology and Microbiology, Baylor College of Medicine,
1 Baylor Plaza, MS BCM280, Houston, TX 77030

S. ARUNMOZHI BALAJEE
Mycotic Diseases Branch, Division of Foodborne, Waterborne,
and Environmental Diseases, National Center for Emerging
and Zoonotic Infectious Diseases, Centers for Disease
Control and Prevention, Atlanta, GA 30333

ELLEN JO BARON
Department of Pathology, Stanford University School of
Medicine, Stanford, CA 94305, and Cepheid, 904 Caribbean
Drive, Sunnyvale, CA 94089

KARSTEN BECKER
Institute of Medical Microbiology, University Hospital of
Münster, 48149 Münster, Germany

WILLIAM J. BELLINI
Measles, Mumps, Rubella, and Herpesvirus Branch, Division
of Viral Diseases, National Center for Immunization and
Respiratory Diseases, Centers for Disease Control and
Prevention, Atlanta, GA 30333

ANJA BERGER
Bayerisches Landesamt für Gesundheit und
Lebensmittelsicherheit, Dienststelle Oberschleißheim,
Veterinärstraße 2, D-85764 Oberschleißheim, Germany

KATHRYN A. BERNARD
National Microbiology Laboratory, Public Health Agency of
Canada, Winnipeg, Manitoba R3E 3R2, Canada

BEVERLEY-ANN BIGGS
Victorian Infectious Diseases Service, Royal Melbourne
Hospital, Parkville, Victoria 3050, and Department of
Medicine, University of Melbourne, Parkville, Victoria 3050,
Australia

ROBERT A. BONOMO
Medical Service, Louis Stokes Cleveland VA Medical Center, and Department of Medicine, Case Western Reserve University, Cleveland, OH 44106

CHERYL A. BOPP
Enteric Diseases Laboratory Branch, Division of Foodborne, Waterborne, and Environmental Diseases, National Center for Emerging and Zoonotic Infectious Diseases, Centers for Disease Control and Prevention, Atlanta, GA 30333

DONALD H. BOUYER
Department of Pathology, University of Texas Medical Branch, Galveston, TX 77555-0609

MICHAEL D. BOWEN
Gastroenteritis and Respiratory Viruses Laboratory Branch, Division of Viral Diseases, National Center for Immunization and Respiratory Diseases, Centers for Disease Control and Prevention, Atlanta, GA 30333

CLAUDIA BRANDT
Institute of Medical Microbiology, Johann Wolfgang Goethe University, Paul Ehrlich Strasse 40, 60596 Frankfurt, Germany

MARY E. BRANDT
Mycotic Diseases Branch, Division of Foodborne, Waterborne, and Environmental Diseases, National Center for Emerging and Zoonotic Infectious Diseases, Centers for Disease Control and Prevention, Atlanta, GA 30333

EDWARD B. BREITSCHWERDT
Department of Clinical Sciences and Center for Comparative Medicine and Translational Research, College of Veterinary Medicine, North Carolina State University, Raleigh, NC 27606

BARBARA A. BROWN-ELLIOTT
Department of Microbiology, University of Texas Health Center at Tyler, Tyler, TX 75708

DAVID A. BRUCKNER
Department of Pathology and Laboratory Medicine, David Geffen School of Medicine at UCLA, P.O. Box 951713, Los Angeles, CA 90095-1713

AMY E. BRYANT
Infectious Diseases Section, VA Medical Center, 500 W. Fort Street (Building 45), Boise, ID 83702-7221

RICHARD S. BULLER
Department of Pediatrics, Washington University School of Medicine, St. Louis, MO 63110

ANGELA M. CALIENDO
Department of Pathology and Laboratory Medicine, Emory University School of Medicine, Atlanta, GA 30322

VITALIANO CAMA
Division of Parasitic Diseases, Centers for Disease Control and Prevention, Atlanta, GA 30341

SHELDON CAMPBELL
Department of Laboratory Medicine, Yale University School of Medicine, New Haven, CT 06520, and VA Connecticut Healthcare System, West Haven, CT 06516

A. BETTS CARPENTER
Molecular Microbiology and Cytology Laboratories, LabCorp, Charleston, WV 25312, and Department of Pathology, Joan C. Edwards School of Medicine, Marshall University, Huntington, WV 25704

KAREN C. CARROLL
Division of Medical Microbiology, Department of Pathology, The Johns Hopkins University School of Medicine, Baltimore, MD 21287

MARIA da GLÓRIA SIQUEIRA CARVALHO
Respiratory Diseases Branch, National Center for Immunization and Respiratory Diseases, Centers for Disease Control and Prevention, Atlanta, GA 30333

BRUNO B. CHOMEL
Department of Population Health and Reproduction, School of Veterinary Medicine, University of California, Davis, CA 95616

SUNWEN CHOU
Department of Medicine, Oregon Health and Sciences University, Portland, OR 97239

DIANE M. CITRON
R. M. Alden Research Laboratory, Culver City, CA 90230

TOM COENYE
Laboratory of Pharmaceutical Microbiology, Ghent University, B-9000 Gent, Belgium

PATRICIA S. CONVILLE
Microbiology Service, Department of Laboratory Medicine, Warren Grant Magnuson Clinical Center, National Institutes of Health, 10 Center Drive, MSC 1508, Bethesda, MD 20892-1508

NATALIE A. COUNIHAN
Section of Microbial Pathogenesis, Yale University School of Medicine, 295 Congress Avenue, New Haven, CT 06519-1418

ELLIOT P. COWAN
Center for Biologics Evaluation and Research, U.S. Food and Drug Administration, Rockville, MD 20852

DAVID L. COX
Laboratory Reference and Research Branch, Division of STD Prevention, National Center for HIV/AIDS, Viral Hepatitis, STD and TB Prevention, Centers for Disease Control and Prevention, Atlanta, GA 30333

FRANCIS E. G. COX
Department of Infectious and Tropical Diseases, London School of Hygiene and Tropical Medicine, London WC1E 7HT, United Kingdom

JAMES E. CROWE, JR.
Department of Pediatrics and Department of Microbiology and Immunology, Vanderbilt University School of Medicine, Nashville, TN 37232

BART J. CURRIE
Menzies School of Health Research and Northern Territory Clinical School, Royal Darwin Hospital, Darwin, Northern Territory 0811, Australia

MELANIE T. CUSHION
Division of Infectious Diseases, Department of Internal Medicine, University of Cincinnati College of Medicine, Cincinnati, OH 45267-0560

INGER K. DAMON
Poxvirus and Rabies Branch, Division of High-Consequence Pathogens and Pathology, National Center for Emerging and Zoonotic Infectious Diseases, Centers for Disease Control and Prevention, Atlanta, GA 30333

ERIC DANNAOUI
Unité Mycologie Moléculaire, CNRS URA3012, Centre National de Référence Mycologie et Antifongiques, Institut Pasteur, 75724 Paris Cedex 15, France

G. SYBREN de HOOG
Centraalbureau voor Schimmelcultures, P.O. Box 85167, NL-3508 AD Utrecht, The Netherlands

PETER DEPLAZES
Institute of Parasitology, University of Zurich, Winterthurerstrasse 266a, CH-8057 Zurich, Switzerland

EDWARD P. DESMOND
Mycobacteriology and Mycology Section, Microbial Diseases Laboratory, California Department of Public Health, 850 Marina Bay Parkway, Richmond, CA 94804

CHARLENE S. DEZZUTTI
Department of Obstetrics, Gynecology, and Reproductive Sciences, Magee-Womens Research Institute, University of Pittsburgh, Pittsburgh, PA 15213

DANIEL J. DIEKEMA
Division of Infectious Diseases, Department of Internal Medicine, and Division of Medical Microbiology, Department of Pathology, University of Iowa College of Medicine, Iowa City, IA 52242

LENIE DIJKSHOORN
Department of Infectious Diseases, Leiden University Medical Center, 2300 RC Leiden, The Netherlands

GARY V. DOERN
Department of Pathology, University of Iowa Carver College of Medicine, Iowa City, IA 52242

FRANÇOISE DROMER
Unité Mycologie Moléculaire, CNRS URA3012, Centre National de Référence Mycologie et Antifongiques, Institut Pasteur, 75724 Paris Cedex 15, France

J. STEPHEN DUMLER
Division of Medical Microbiology, Department of Pathology, The Johns Hopkins University School of Medicine, 720 Rutland Avenue, Ross 624, Baltimore, MD 21205

MARCELA ECHAVARRIA
Clinical Virology Laboratory, Center for Medical Education and Clinical Research, University Hospital, Buenos Aires C1431FWO, Argentina

PAUL H. EDELSTEIN
University of Pennsylvania Medical Center, Philadelphia, PA 19104-4283

JOHANNES ELIAS
Institute for Hygiene and Microbiology, University of Würzburg, 97080 Würzburg, Germany

HERMES ESCALANTE
Department of Microbiology, School of Biological Sciences, Universidad Nacional de Trujillo, Avenida Juan Pablo II S/N, Ciudad Universitaria, Trujillo, Peru

ANA V. ESPINEL-INGROFF
Medical Mycology Research Laboratory, Infectious Diseases/ Internal Medicine, Virginia Commonwealth University, Richmond, VA 23298-0049

ANDREAS ESSIG
Institute of Medical Microbiology and Hygiene, University of Ulm, Albert-Einstein Allee 23, D-89079 Ulm, Germany

RICHARD R. FACKLAM (RETIRED)
Respiratory Diseases Branch, National Center for Immunization and Respiratory Diseases, Centers for Disease Control and Prevention, Atlanta, GA 30333

J. J. FARMER III (RETIRED)
United States Public Health Service, Stone Mountain, GA 30087

MARY JANE FERRARO
Clinical Microbiology Laboratory, Massachusetts General Hospital and Harvard Medical School, Boston, MA 02114

PATRICIA I. FIELDS
Enteric Diseases Laboratory Branch, Division of Foodborne, Waterborne, and Environmental Diseases, National Center for Emerging and Zoonotic Infectious Diseases, Centers for Disease Control and Prevention, Atlanta, GA 30333

SYDNEY M. FINEGOLD
Infectious Diseases Section, VA Medical Center, and Department of Medicine and Department of Microbiology, Immunology, and Molecular Genetics, University of California at Los Angeles School of Medicine, Los Angeles, CA 90073

DORAN L. FINK
Laboratory of Parasitic Diseases, National Institute of Allergy and Infectious Diseases, National Institutes of Health, Bethesda, MD 20892

COLLETTE FITZGERALD
Enteric Diseases Laboratory Branch, Division of Foodborne, Waterborne, and Environmental Diseases, National Center for Emerging and Zoonotic Infectious Diseases, Centers for Disease Control and Prevention, Atlanta, GA 30333

MICHAEL S. FORMAN
Division of Medical Microbiology, Department of Pathology, The Johns Hopkins Medical Institutions, Baltimore, MD 21287

JULIE D. FOX
Provincial Laboratory for Public Health and Department of Microbiology and Infectious Diseases, University of Calgary, 3030 Hospital Drive NW, Calgary, Alberta T2N 4W4, Canada

RENO FREI
Clinical Microbiology, University Hospital Basel, 4031 Basel, Switzerland

MATTHIAS FROSCH
Institute for Hygiene and Microbiology, University of Würzburg, 97080 Würzburg, Germany

CHARLES F. FULHORST
Department of Pathology and Department of Microbiology and Immunology, University of Texas Medical Branch, 301 University Boulevard, Route 0609, Galveston, TX 77555-0609

GUIDO FUNKE
Department of Medical Microbiology and Hygiene, Gärtner & Colleagues Laboratories, D-88212 Ravensburg, Germany

HECTOR H. GARCIA
Department of Microbiology, Universidad Peruana Cayetano Heredia, and Cysticercosis Unit, Instituto de Ciencias Neurológicas, Lima, Peru

LYNNE S. GARCIA
LSG & Associates, 512 12th Street, Santa Monica, CA 90402-2908

DEA GARCIA-HERMOSO
Unité Mycologie Moléculaire, CNRS URA3012, Centre National de Référence Mycologie et Antifongiques, Institut Pasteur, 75724 Paris Cedex 15, France

BARBARA C. GÄRTNER
Institute for Virology, University of the Saarland, D-66421 Homburg/Saar, Germany

CHARLOTTE A. GAYDOS
Division of Infectious Diseases, Department of Medicine, Johns Hopkins University, 530 Rangos Building, 855 North Wolfe Street, Baltimore, MD 21205

ANNE M. GAYNOR
Department of Molecular Microbiology, Washington University School of Medicine, St. Louis, MO 63110

PETER GERNER-SMIDT
Enteric Diseases Laboratory Branch, Division of Foodborne, Waterborne, and Environmental Diseases, National Center for Emerging and Zoonotic Infectious Diseases, Centers for Disease Control and Prevention, Atlanta, GA 30333

ANTOINE GESSAIN
EPVO Unit, Department of Virology, Institut Pasteur, 75015 Paris, France

MAHMOUD A. GHANNOUM
Center for Medical Mycology, Department of Dermatology, University Hospitals/Case Western Reserve University, 11100 Euclid Avenue, Cleveland, OH 44106

CHRISTINE C. GINOCCHIO
Department of Pathology and Laboratory Medicine, North Shore-LIJ Health System Laboratories, and Department of Molecular Medicine, The Feinstein Institute for Medical Research, Hofstra North Shore-LIJ School of Medicine, Lake Success, NY 11042

MARKUS GLATZEL
Institute of Neuropathology, Universitätsklinikum Hamburg-Eppendorf, Martinistraβe 52, D-20246 Hamburg, Germany

BEATRIZ L. GOMEZ
Corporación para Investigaciones Biológicas, Medellín, Colombia

STEPHEN R. GRAVES
Hunter Area Pathology Service and Australian Rickettsial Reference Laboratory, Locked Bag 1, Hunter Region Mail Centre, NSW 2310, Australia

PATTI E. GRAVITT
Department of Epidemiology and Department of Molecular Microbiology and Immunology, Johns Hopkins Bloomberg School of Public Health, Baltimore, MD 21205

BRIGITTE P. GRIFFITH
Department of Laboratory Medicine, Yale University School of Medicine, New Haven, CT 06520

FELIX GRIMM
Institute of Parasitology, University of Zurich, Winterthurerstrasse 266a, CH-8057 Zurich, Switzerland

JOSEP GUARRO
Facultat de Medicina, Universitat Rovira i Virgili, Sant Llorenç, 21, 43201 Reus, Spain

WILLIAM J. HALSALL
Center for Medical Mycology, Department of Dermatology, University Hospitals/Case Western Reserve University, 11100 Euclid Avenue, Cleveland, OH 44106

PATRICIA C. HARRIS
Quidel Corporation—Diagnostic Hybrids, 1055 E. State Street, Suite 100, Athens, OH 45701

KEVIN C. HAZEN
Clinical Microbiology and Molecular Diagnostics (Infectious Diseases), Department of Pathology, University of Virginia Health System, Charlottesville, VA 22908-0904

DAVID W. HECHT
Department of Medicine, Loyola University Medical Center, Maywood, IL 60153

DEBORAH A. HENRY
University of British Columbia, Vancouver, British Columbia, Canada

SARAH K. HIGHLANDER
Department of Molecular Virology and Microbiology and Human Genome Sequencing Center, Baylor College of Medicine, Houston, TX 77030

JANET A. HINDLER
Department of Pathology and Laboratory Medicine, UCLA Medical Center, Los Angeles, CA 90095-1713

RICHARD L. HODINKA
Departments of Pediatrics and Pathology and Clinical Virology Laboratory, Children's Hospital of Philadelphia and University of Pennsylvania School of Medicine, Philadelphia, PA 19104

ALEX R. HOFFMASTER
Bacterial Special Pathogens Branch, Division of High-Consequence Pathogens and Pathology, National Center for Emerging and Zoonotic Infectious Diseases, Centers for Disease Control and Prevention, Atlanta, GA 30333

SAMANTHA J. HOOT
Seattle Biomedical Research Institute and Program in Pathobiology, Department of Global Health, University of Washington, Seattle, WA 98109-5219

AMY J. HORNEMAN
Pathology and Laboratory Service, VA Maryland Health Care System, Baltimore, MD 21201

REBECCA T. HORVAT
Department of Pathology and Laboratory Medicine, University of Kansas School of Medicine, Kansas City, KS 66160

SUSAN A. HOWELL
Mycology, St. Johns Institute of Dermatology, GSTS Pathology, London SE1 7EH, United Kingdom

EIJA HYYTIÄ-TREES
Enteric Diseases Laboratory Branch, Division of Foodborne, Waterborne, and Environmental Diseases, National Center for Emerging and Zoonotic Infectious Diseases, Centers for Disease Control and Prevention, Atlanta, GA 30333

JOSEPH P. ICENOGLE
Measles, Mumps, Rubella, and Herpesvirus Branch, Division of Viral Diseases, National Center for Immunization and Respiratory Diseases, Centers for Disease Control and Prevention, Atlanta, GA 30333

NANCY C. ISHAM
Center for Medical Mycology, Department of Dermatology, University Hospitals/Case Western Reserve University, 11100 Euclid Avenue, Cleveland, OH 44106

J. MICHAEL JANDA
Microbial Diseases Laboratory, California Department of Public Health, 850 Marina Bay Parkway, E-164, Richmond, CA 94804

KEITH R. JEROME
Department of Laboratory Medicine, University of Washington, and Vaccine and Infectious Disease Division, Fred Hutchinson Cancer Research Center, 1100 Fairview Avenue N., D3-100, Seattle, WA 98109

XI JIANG
Cincinnati Children's Hospital Medical Center, University of Cincinnati College of Medicine, Cincinnati, OH 45229-3039

JUAN A. JIMENEZ
Cysticercosis Unit, Instituto de Ciencias Neurológicas, Lima, Peru

ELIZABETH M. JOHNSON
Mycology Reference Laboratory, Health Protection Agency, South West Laboratory, Myrtle Road, Kingsdown, Bristol BS2 8EL, United Kingdom

JEFFREY L. JONES
Parasitic Diseases Branch, Division of Parasitic Diseases and Malaria, Center for Global Health, Centers for Disease Control and Prevention, Atlanta, GA 30333

MALCOLM K. JONES
School of Veterinary Sciences, The University of Queensland, Brisbane, Queensland 4072, and Queensland Institute of Medical Research, 300 Herston Road, Herston, Queensland 4006, Australia

TIMOTHY F. JONES
Communicable and Environmental Disease Services, Tennessee Department of Health, Nashville, TN 37243

JEANNE A. JORDAN
Epidemiology and Biostatistics, School of Public Health and Health Services, The George Washington University, 231 Ross Hall, 2300 I Street NW, Washington, DC 20037

JAMES H. JORGENSEN
Department of Pathology, The University of Texas Health Science Center, 7703 Floyd Curl Drive, San Antonio, TX 78229-3700

PETER KÄMPFER
Institut für Angewandte Mikrobiologie, Justus-Liebig-Universität Giessen, D-35392 Giessen, Germany

JAMES B. KAPER
Department of Microbiology and Immunology, University of Maryland School of Medicine, Baltimore, MD 21201

WILLIAM E. KEENE
Oregon Public Health Division, Portland, OR 97232-2162

JENNIFER KEISER
Department of Medical Parasitology and Infection Biology, Swiss Tropical and Public Health Institute, CH-4002 Basel, Switzerland

VOLKHARD A. J. KEMPF
Institute for Medical Microbiology and Infection Control, University Hospital of the Johann Wolfgang Goethe University, Paul Ehrlich-Strasse 40, D-60596 Frankfurt am Main, Germany

EIJA KÖNÖNEN
Institute of Dentistry, University of Turku, FI-20520 Turku, and Department of Infectious Disease Surveillance and Control, National Institute for Health and Welfare (THL), FI-00271 Helsinki, Finland

THOMAS G. KSIAZEK
Galveston National Laboratory, Pathology Department, University of Texas Medical Branch, Galveston, TX 77555

JAIME A. LABARCA
Department of Medicine, Facultad de Medicina, Pontificia Universidad Católica de Chile, Lira 63, Santiago, Chile

RENU B. LAL
Viral Surveillance and Diagnostic Branch, Influenza Division, National Center for Immunization and Respiratory Diseases, Centers for Disease Control and Prevention, Atlanta, GA 30333

DARYL M. LAMSON
Division of Infectious Diseases, Wadsworth Center, Albany, NY 12201

ROBERT S. LANCIOTTI
Arboviral Diseases Branch, Division of Vector-Borne Diseases, National Center for Emerging and Zoonotic Infectious Diseases, Centers for Disease Control and Prevention, Fort Collins, CO 80521

MARIE LOUISE LANDRY
Department of Laboratory Medicine, Yale University School of Medicine, New Haven, CT 06520-8035

MARK T. LaROCCO
St. Luke's Episcopal Hospital, 6720 Bertner Avenue, Houston, TX 77030

ANDREW J. LAWSON
Gastrointestinal, Emerging and Zoonotic Infections Department, Health Protection Agency, Centre for Infections, London NW9 5HT, United Kingdom

AMY L. LEBER
Clinical/Molecular Microbiology, Virology, Immunoserology, Department of Laboratory Medicine, Nationwide Children's Hospital, Building C, Room 1868, 700 Children's Drive, Columbus, OH 43205

JACQUES LE BRAS
Laboratoire de Parasitologie, Hôpital Bichat and Université Paris Descartes, 46 rue Henri Huchard, 75018 Paris, France

NATHAN A. LEDEBOER
Clinical Microbiology and Molecular Diagnostics, Dynacare Laboratories and Froedtert Memorial Lutheran Hospital, and Department of Pathology, Medical College of Wisconsin, Milwaukee, WI 53226

KARIN LEDER
Infectious Disease Epidemiology Unit, Department of Epidemiology and Preventive Medicine, Monash University, Prahran, Victoria 3181, Australia

ELLIOT J. LEFKOWITZ
Department of Microbiology, The University of Alabama at Birmingham, Birmingham, AL 35294

DIANE S. LELAND
Department of Pathology and Laboratory Medicine, Indiana University School of Medicine, Indianapolis, IN 46202

PAUL N. LEVETT
Saskatchewan Disease Control Laboratory, Regina, Saskatchewan, Canada

SHOU-YEAN GRACE LIN
Mycobacteriology and Mycology Section, Microbial Diseases Laboratory, California Department of Public Health, 850 Marina Bay Parkway, Richmond, CA 94804

DAVID S. LINDSAY
Center for Molecular Medicine and Infectious Diseases, Department of Biomedical Sciences and Pathobiology, Virginia-Maryland Regional College of Veterinary Medicine, Virginia Tech, 1410 Prices Fork Road, Blacksburg, VA 24061-0342

STEPHEN E. LINDSTROM
Viral Surveillance and Diagnostic Branch, Influenza Division, National Center for Immunization and Respiratory Diseases, Centers for Disease Control and Prevention, Atlanta, GA 30333

ANDREA J. LINSCOTT
Department of Pathology, Ochsner Medical Center, 1514 Jefferson Highway, New Orleans, LA 70121

JOHN J. LiPUMA
Department of Pediatrics and Communicable Diseases, University of Michigan Medical School, Ann Arbor, MI 48109

MIKE LOEFFELHOLZ
Department of Pathology, University of Texas Medical Branch, 301 University Blvd., Galveston, TX 77555

NIALL A. LOGAN
Department of Biological and Biomedical Sciences, School of Life Sciences, Glasgow Caledonian University, Cowcaddens Road, Glasgow G4 0BA, United Kingdom

OLIVIER LORTHOLARY
Unité Mycologie Moléculaire, CNRS URA3012, Centre
National de Référence Mycologie et Antifongiques, Institut
Pasteur, 75724 Paris Cedex 15, France

NELL S. LURAIN
Department of Immunology/Microbiology, Rush University
Medical Center, Chicago, IL 60612

RICARDO G. MAGGI
Department of Clinical Sciences and Center for Comparative
Medicine and Translational Research, College of Veterinary
Medicine, North Carolina State University, Raleigh,
NC 27606

THOMAS MARTH
Division of Internal Medicine, Krankenhaus Maria Hilf, Maria
Hilf Strasse 2, 54550 Daun, Germany

ROBERT F. MASSUNG
Rickettsial Zoonoses Branch, Division of Vector-Borne
Diseases, National Center for Emerging and Zoonotic
Infectious Diseases, Centers for Disease Control and
Prevention, Atlanta, GA 30333

ALEXANDER MATHIS
Institute of Parasitology, University of Zurich, CH-8057
Zurich, Switzerland

JAMES B. McAULEY
Rush University Medical Center, 1653 W. Congress Parkway,
Chicago, IL 60612

KARIN L. McGOWAN
Clinical Microbiology Laboratory, Children's Hospital of
Philadelphia, Departments of Pathology and Laboratory
Medicine, Pediatrics, and Microbiology, University of
Pennsylvania School of Medicine, Philadelphia, PA 19104

DONALD P. McMANUS
Queensland Institute of Medical Research, 300 Herston Road,
Herston, Queensland 4006, Australia

LEONEL MENDOZA
Biomedical Laboratory Diagnostics and Department of
Microbiology and Molecular Genetics, Michigan State
University, East Lansing, MI 48824-1031

ROBERT C. MOELLERING, JR.
Department of Medicine, Beth Israel Deaconess Medical
Center and Harvard Medical School, 110 Francis Street, Suite
6A, Boston, MA 02215

RHODA ASHLEY MORROW
Department of Laboratory Medicine, University of Washington,
1616 Eastlake Avenue E., Room 5186, Seattle, WA 98109

IRVING NACHAMKIN
Department of Pathology and Laboratory Medicine,
University of Pennsylvania School of Medicine, 3400 Spruce
Street, Philadelphia, PA 19104-4283

ISABEL NAJERA
Department of Medicine, Stanford University, Stanford, CA,
94305, and Roche Palo Alto LLC, 3431 Hillview Avenue,
Palo Alto, CA 94304

JAMES P. NATARO
Department of Pediatrics, University of Virginia School of
Medicine, Charlottesville, VA 22908

RONALD C. NEAFIE
Parasitic Infections Branch, Armed Forces Institute of
Pathology, 6825 16th Street NW, Washington, DC 20306

ALEXANDR NEMEC
Laboratory for Bacterial Genetics, National Institute of Public
Health, 10042 Prague, Czech Republic

STUART T. NICHOL
Viral Special Pathogens Branch, Division of High-
Consequence Pathogens and Pathology, National Center
for Emerging and Zoonotic Infectious Diseases, Centers for
Disease Control and Prevention, Atlanta, GA 30333

MICHAEL A. NOBLE
Department of Pathology and Laboratory Medicine,
University of British Columbia, Room 366, 2733 Heather
Street, Vancouver, British Columbia V5Z 1M9, Canada

FREDERICK S. NOLTE
Department of Pathology and Laboratory Medicine, Medical
University of South Carolina, Charleston, SC 29425

SUSAN NOVAK-WEEKLEY
SCPMG Regional Reference Laboratories, 1668 Sherman
Way, North Hollywood, CA 91605

THOMAS B. NUTMAN
Laboratory of Parasitic Diseases, National Institute of Allergy
and Infectious Diseases, National Institutes of Health,
Bethesda, MD 20892

LILLIAN A. ORCIARI
Poxvirus and Rabies Branch, Division of High-Consequence
Pathogens and Pathology, National Center for Emerging and
Zoonotic Infectious Diseases, Centers for Disease Control and
Prevention, Atlanta, GA 30333

S. MICHELE OWEN
Laboratory Branch, Division of HIV/AIDS Prevention,
National Center for HIV/AIDS, Viral Hepatitis, STD and
TB Prevention, Centers for Disease Control and Prevention,
Atlanta, GA 30333

KANTI PABBARAJU
Provincial Laboratory for Public Health, 3030 Hospital Drive
NW, Calgary, Alberta T2N 4W4, Canada

FRANTISKA PALICOVA
Department of Medical Microbiology, Center for Laboratory
Medicine, Kantonsspital Luzern, CH-6000 Lucerne 16,
Switzerland

GRAEME P. PALTRIDGE
Bacteriology and Parasitology Laboratory, Canterbury Health Laboratories, Christchurch, New Zealand

XIAOLI PANG
Provincial Laboratory for Public Health and Department of Laboratory Medicine and Pathology, University of Alberta, Edmonton, Alberta T6G 2J2, Canada

JEAN B. PATEL
Clinical and Environmental Microbiology Branch, Division of Healthcare Quality Promotion, National Center for Emerging and Zoonotic Infectious Diseases, Centers for Disease Control and Prevention, Atlanta, GA 30333

SHARON J. PEACOCK
Department of Medicine, University of Cambridge, Addenbrooke's Hospital, Cambridge CB2 0QQ, United Kingdom

PHILIP E. PELLETT
Department of Immunology and Microbiology, Wayne State University School of Medicine, Detroit, MI 48201

JEANNINE M. PETERSEN
Bacterial Diseases Branch, Division of Vector-Borne Diseases, National Center for Emerging and Zoonotic Infectious Diseases, Centers for Disease Control and Prevention, Fort Collins, CO 80521

JOSEPH F. PETROSINO
Department of Molecular Virology and Microbiology and Human Genome Sequencing Center, Baylor College of Medicine, Houston, TX 77030

CATHY A. PETTI
Department of Medicine, Stanford University School of Medicine, Stanford, CA 94305

MICHAEL A. PFALLER
Department of Pathology, University of Iowa College of Medicine, 200 Hawkins Drive, Iowa City, IA 52242-1009

GABY E. PFYFFER
Department of Medical Microbiology, Center for Laboratory Medicine, Kantonsspital Luzern, CH-6000 Lucerne 16, Switzerland

ALLAN PILLAY
Laboratory Reference and Research Branch, Division of STD Prevention, National Center for HIV/AIDS, Viral Hepatitis, STD and TB Prevention, Centers for Disease Control and Prevention, Atlanta, GA 30333

GARY W. PROCOP
Department of Molecular Pathology, Pathology and Laboratory Medicine Institute/L11, Cleveland Clinic, 9500 Euclid Avenue, Cleveland, OH 44195

ELISABETH PUCHHAMMER-STÖCKL
Department of Virology, Medical University of Vienna, Kinderspitalgasse 15, A-1095 Vienna, Austria

JUSTIN D. RADOLF
Departments of Medicine and of Genetics and Developmental Biology, University of Connecticut Health Center, Farmington, CT 06030

J. KAMILE RASHEED
Clinical and Environmental Microbiology Branch, Division of Healthcare Quality Promotion, National Center for Emerging and Zoonotic Infectious Diseases, Centers for Disease Control and Prevention, Atlanta, GA 30333

MEGAN E. RELLER
Division of Medical Microbiology, Department of Pathology, The Johns Hopkins University School of Medicine, 720 Rutland Avenue, Ross 628, Baltimore, MD 21205

LOUIS B. RICE
Department of Medicine, Alpert Medical School, Brown University, Providence, RI 02903

ELVIRA RICHTER
National Reference Center for Mycobacteria, Research Center Borstel, 23845 Borstel, Germany

SANDRA S. RICHTER
Department of Clinical Pathology, Cleveland Clinic, 9500 Euclid Avenue, L40, Cleveland, OH 44195

MARION RIFFELMANN
HELIOS Klinikum Krefeld, D-47805 Krefeld, Germany

CHRISTINE ROBINSON
Department of Pathology, The Children's Hospital, Aurora, CO 80045

WILLIAM O. ROGERS
Naval Medical Research Unit 2, Phnom Penh, Cambodia

PIERRE E. ROLLIN
Viral Special Pathogens Branch, Division of High-Consequence Pathogens and Pathology, National Center for Emerging and Zoonotic Infectious Diseases, Centers for Disease Control and Prevention, Atlanta, GA 30333

JOSÉ R. ROMERO
Pediatrics, Arkansas Children's Hospital, Little Rock, AR 72202-3591

PAUL A. ROTA
Measles, Mumps, Rubella, and Herpesvirus Branch, Division of Viral Diseases, National Center for Immunization and Respiratory Diseases, Centers for Disease Control and Prevention, Atlanta, GA 30333

KATHRYN L. RUOFF
Department of Pathology, Dartmouth Hitchcock Medical Center, Lebanon, NH 03756

CHARLES E. RUPPRECHT
Poxvirus and Rabies Branch, Division of High-Consequence Pathogens and Pathology, National Center for Emerging and Zoonotic Infectious Diseases, Centers for Disease Control and Prevention, Atlanta, GA 30333

MARTIN E. SCHRIEFER
Bacterial Diseases Branch, Division of Vector-Borne Diseases, National Center for Emerging and Zoonotic Infectious Diseases, Centers for Disease Control and Prevention, Fort Collins, CO 80521

W. EVAN SECOR
Parasitic Diseases Branch, Division of Parasitic Diseases and Malaria, Center for Global Health, Centers for Disease Control and Prevention, Atlanta, GA 30333

SEAN V. SHADOMY
Bacterial Special Pathogens Branch, Division of High-Consequence Pathogens and Pathology, National Center for Emerging and Zoonotic Infectious Diseases, Centers for Disease Control and Prevention, Atlanta, GA 30333

ROBERT W. SHAFER
Departments of Medicine and Pathology, Stanford University, Stanford, CA 94305

SUSAN E. SHARP
Kaiser Permanente and Oregon Health Sciences University, Portland, OR 97230

YVONNE R. SHEA
Microbiology Service, Department of Laboratory Medicine, Clinical Center, National Institutes of Health, Building 10, Room 2C325, 10 Center Drive, MSC 1508, Bethesda, MD 20892

HARSHA SHEOREY
Department of Microbiology, St. Vincent's Hospital Melbourne, Fitzroy, Victoria 3065, Australia

PATRICIA LYNN SHEWMAKER
Respiratory Diseases Branch, National Center for Immunization and Respiratory Diseases, Centers for Disease Control and Prevention, Atlanta, GA 30333

ROBYN Y. SHIMIZU
Department of Pathology and Laboratory Medicine, UCLA Health System, Los Angeles, CA 90095-1713

KAMALJIT SINGH
Rush University Medical Center, 1653 W. Congress Parkway, Chicago, IL 60612

JAMES W. SNYDER
Department of Pathology and Laboratory Medicine, University of Louisville School of Medicine and Hospital, 530 S. Jackson Street, Louisville, KY 40202

YULI SONG
Oral Care, R&D, Procter & Gamble, Mason, OH 45040

DAVID P. SPEERT
University of British Columbia, Vancouver, British Columbia, Canada

BARBARA SPELLERBERG
Institute of Medical Microbiology and Hygiene, University of Ulm, Albert Einstein Allee 11, 89081 Ulm, Germany

KENDRA E. STAUFFER
Bacterial Special Pathogens Branch, Division of High-Consequence Pathogens and Pathology, National Center for Emerging and Zoonotic Infectious Diseases, Centers for Disease Control and Prevention, Atlanta, GA 30333

KATHLEEN A. STELLRECHT
Department of Pathology and Laboratory Medicine, Albany Medical Center, Albany, NY 12208

DENNIS L. STEVENS
Infectious Diseases Section, VA Medical Center, 500 W. Fort Street (Building 45), Boise, ID 83702-7221

NANCY A. STROCKBINE
Enteric Diseases Laboratory Branch, Division of Foodborne, Waterborne, and Environmental Diseases, National Center for Emerging and Zoonotic Infectious Diseases, Centers for Disease Control and Prevention, Atlanta, GA 30333

RICHARD C. SUMMERBELL
Sporometrics Inc. and Dalla Lana School of Public Health, University of Toronto, Toronto, Ontario, Canada

DEANNA A. SUTTON
Department of Pathology, University of Texas Health Science Center at San Antonio, San Antonio, TX 78229-3900

JANA M. SWENSON
Clinical and Environmental Microbiology Branch, Division of Healthcare Quality Promotion, National Center for Emerging and Zoonotic Infectious Diseases, Centers for Disease Control and Prevention, Atlanta, GA 30333

ELLA M. SWIERKOSZ
Department of Pathology, Saint Louis University School of Medicine, St. Louis, MO 63104

YI-WEI TANG
Department of Pathology and Department of Medicine, Vanderbilt University School of Medicine, Nashville, TN 37232

DAVID TAYLOR-ROBINSON
Department of Medicine, Imperial College London, St. Mary's Campus, London, United Kingdom

GARY E. TEGTMEIER
Community Blood Center of Greater Kansas City, Kansas City, MO 64111

LÚCIA MARTINS TEIXEIRA
Instituto de Microbiologia, Universidade Federal do Rio de Janeiro, Rio de Janeiro, RJ 21941, Brazil

SAM R. TELFORD III
Cummings School of Veterinary Medicine, Tufts University, 200 Westboro Road, North Grafton, MA 01536

FRED C. TENOVER
Cepheid, 904 Caribbean Drive, Sunnyvale, CA 94089

KENNETH D. THOMPSON
Department of Pathology, The University of Chicago Medical Center, Chicago, IL 60637

RICHARD B. THOMSON, JR.
Clinical Microbiology Laboratories, Department of Pathology and Laboratory Medicine, Evanston Hospital and NorthShore University HealthSystem, 2650 Ridge Avenue, Evanston, IL 60201

GRAHAM TIPPLES
National Microbiology Laboratory, Public Health Agency of Canada, 1015 Arlington Street, Winnipeg, Manitoba R3E 3R2, Canada

PETER TRAYNOR
Oxoid Australia Pty Limited, Thermo Fisher Scientific, Adelaide, South Australia 5031, Australia

THEODORE F. TSAI
Novartis Vaccines, 350 Massachusetts Avenue, Cambridge, MA 02139

JOHN D. TURNIDGE
SA Pathology at Women's and Children's Hospital, 72 King William Road, North Adelaide, South Australia 5006, Australia

STEVE J. UPTON
Division of Biology, Ackert Hall, Kansas State University, Manhattan, KS 66506-4901

ALEXANDRA VALSAMAKIS
Division of Medical Microbiology, Department of Pathology, The Johns Hopkins Medical Institutions, Baltimore, MD 21287

PETER A. R. VANDAMME
Laboratorium voor Microbiologie, Faculteit Wetenschappen, Universiteit Gent, Ledeganckstraat 35, B-9000 Gent, Belgium

MARIO VANEECHOUTTE
Laboratory Bacteriology Research, Department of Clinical Chemistry, Microbiology, and Immunology, University of Ghent, B-9000 Ghent, Belgium

JAMES VERSALOVIC
Department of Pathology, Texas Children's Hospital, Feigin Center, Suite 830, 1102 Bates Avenue, and Department of Pathology and Immunology, Baylor College of Medicine, Houston, TX 77030

RAQUEL VILELA
Biomedical Laboratory Diagnostics, Michigan State University, East Lansing, MI 48824-1031

GOVINDA S. VISVESVARA
Waterborne Diseases Prevention Branch, Division of Foodborne, Waterborne, and Environmental Diseases, National Center for Emerging and Zoonotic Infectious Diseases, Centers for Disease Control and Prevention, Atlanta, GA 30333

ULRICH VOGEL
Institute for Hygiene and Microbiology, University of Würzburg, 97080 Würzburg, Germany

CHRISTOPH von EICHEL-STREIBER
Institut für Medizinische Mikrobiologie und Hygiene, Johannes Gutenberg-Universität Mainz, Hochhaus am Augustaplatz, D-55131 Mainz, Germany

CHRISTOF von EIFF
Pfizer Pharma GmbH, 10785 Berlin, Germany

ALEXANDER von GRAEVENITZ
Institute of Medical Microbiology, University of Zurich, Gloriastrasse 32, CH-8006 Zurich, Switzerland

WILLIAM G. WADE
Department of Microbiology, King's College London, Guy's Campus, London SE1 9RT, United Kingdom

KEN B. WAITES
Department of Pathology, University of Alabama at Birmingham, Birmingham, AL 35249

DAVID H. WALKER
Department of Pathology and Center for Biodefense and Emerging Infectious Diseases, University of Texas Medical Branch, Galveston, TX 77555-0609

RICHARD J. WALLACE, JR.
Department of Microbiology, University of Texas Health Center at Tyler, Tyler, TX 75708

DAVID WANG
Department of Molecular Microbiology and Department of Pathology and Immunology, Washington University School of Medicine, St. Louis, MO 63110

DAVID W. WARNOCK
National Center for Emerging and Zoonotic Infectious Diseases, Centers for Disease Control and Prevention, Atlanta, GA 30333

GEORGES WAUTERS
Department of Microbiology, Université catholique de Louvain, B-1200 Brussels, Belgium

RAINER WEBER
Division of Infectious Diseases and Hospital Epidemiology, Department of Internal Medicine, University Hospital, CH-8091 Zurich, Switzerland

MELVIN P. WEINSTEIN
Departments of Medicine and Pathology, Robert Wood
Johnson Medical School, 1 Robert Wood Johnson Place,
MEB 364, New Brunswick, NJ 08903-0019

LOUIS M. WEISS
Albert Einstein College of Medicine, 1300 Morris Park
Avenue, Room 504 Forchheimer Building, Bronx, NY 10461

PETER F. WELLER
Department of Medicine, Harvard Medical School, and
Division of Infectious Diseases and Allergy and Inflammation
Division, Beth Israel Deaconess Medical Center, Boston,
MA 02215

NELE WELLINGHAUSEN
Department of Medical Microbiology and Hygiene, Gärtner &
Colleagues Laboratories, D-88212 Ravensburg, Germany

THEODORE C. WHITE
Seattle Biomedical Research Institute and Program in
Pathobiology, Department of Global Health, University of
Washington, Seattle, WA 98109-5219

ANDREAS F. WIDMER
Infection Control and Hospital Epidemiology, University
Hospital Basel, 4031 Basel, Switzerland

DANNY L. WIEDBRAUK
Virology and Molecular Biology, Warde Medical Laboratory,
300 W. Textile Road, Ann Arbor, MI 48108

CARL-HEINZ WIRSING von KÖNIG
HELIOS Klinikum Krefeld, D-47805 Krefeld, Germany

FRANK G. WITEBSKY
Microbiology Service, Department of Laboratory Medicine,
Warren Grant Magnuson Clinical Center, National Institutes
of Health, 10 Center Drive, MSC 1508, Bethesda,
MD 20892-1508

GAIL L. WOODS
Pathology and Laboratory Medicine Service (LR/113),
Central Arkansas Veterans Healthcare System, 4300 W. 7th
Street, Little Rock, AR 72205-5484

LIHUA XIAO
Waterborne Diseases Prevention Branch, Division of
Foodborne, Waterborne, and Environmental Diseases,
National Center for Emerging and Zoonotic Infectious
Diseases, Centers for Disease Control and Prevention,
Atlanta, GA 30333

JOSEPH D. C. YAO
Division of Clinical Microbiology, Department of Laboratory
Medicine and Pathology, College of Medicine, Mayo Clinic,
Rochester, MN 55905

SHERIF ZAKI
Infectious Diseases Pathology Branch, Division of High-
Consequence Pathogens and Pathology, National Center
for Emerging and Zoonotic Infectious Diseases, Centers for
Disease Control and Prevention, Atlanta, GA 30333

REINHARD ZBINDEN
Institute of Medical Microbiology, University of Zurich,
Gloriastrasse 32, CH-8006 Zurich, Switzerland

Acknowledgment of Previous Contributors
The *Manual of Clinical Microbiology* is by its nature a continuously revised work which
refines and extends the contributions of previous editions. Since its first edition in
1970, many eminent scientists have contributed to this important reference work. The
American Society for Microbiology and its Publications Board gratefully acknowledge the
contributions of all of these generous authors over the life of this *Manual*.

PREFACE

The *Manual of Clinical Microbiology* (MCM) is the most authoritative reference in the field of diagnostic microbiology, and a team of 22 editors and 267 authors worked closely together with a group of several individuals at ASM Press (including eight freelance copy editors) to deliver the 10th edition in its prescribed 4-year publication cycle. As a profession, we are proud members of the American Society for Microbiology, and its book publishing arm, ASM Press, remains steadfastly committed to the utmost quality that the MCM readership has come to expect. As a new editor in chief, a chapter author, and a former section editor, I am proud that this commitment to excellence by everyone associated with the production of the *Manual* has always been apparent.

As in so many professional endeavors, our work rests on the shoulders of giants who preceded us. I must thank Patrick Murray, who initially asked me to succeed him as the fourth editor in chief of the *Manual*. Clearly, I had extremely large shoes to fill, as Pat had elevated the *Manual* to an unprecedented level in terms of scope and quality. My job was made immensely easier by Pat's guidance and his generosity in sharing his cumulative experience from past editions. No editor in chief could ask for more support than I received from Pat. Another prior editor of the *Manual*, Ellen Jo Baron, who served as a volume editor for several editions, provided many lessons on the "how" of editing as well as inspiration in aiming for superior quality with every chapter of the *Manual*. As a section editor working under Ellen, I immersed myself in the *Manual* and grasped its essence. In this spirit of appreciation, I must also convey a special thanks to the team at ASM Press. Ken April has served as an extremely capable and committed production editor, as we both navigated role transitions. His predecessor, Susan Birch, was a pillar working closely with Pat Murray on multiple prior editions of the *Manual*, and her expertise benefited this edition when we requested her advice. Ken kept us on track with a tight production timeline while juggling several other book projects for ASM Press in parallel. With a deep sense of gratitude, I thank Jeff Holtmeier, director of ASM Press throughout much of the planning and publication process of MCM10, who believed in me and gave me the opportunity to serve as editor in chief of the 10th edition. I know that Jeff viewed this editorship as a keystone position at ASM Press, and I am profoundly grateful for the privilege of guiding the *Manual* through the publication of the current edition.

This edition of the *Manual* will be the first to have a full-scale, Web-based HTML electronic edition. In addition to the complete contents of the printed edition, the electronic edition will contain an image library consisting of all the figures from the printed edition and more than 400 supplementary figures generously contributed by Pat Murray from his laboratory collection and the collections of a few chapter authors.

In conclusion, I want to make a few comments about our profession. Clinical microbiology will be challenged by new developments in molecular diagnostics, microbial genomics, and metagenomics. Novel viruses may require the development of targeted assays relying on newly generated nucleic acid sequencing data. The recently emerging field of human microbiome research is already upsetting the apple cart and challenging notions of single-agent or polymicrobial infections. Can microbial communities or dysbiosis predispose to or result in infectious diseases? In spite of all of the rapid changes in molecular microbiology and metagenomics, the field of clinical microbiology must sustain its core practices of culture, microscopic visualization, direct antigen detection, serology, biochemical or phenotypic characterization, and antimicrobial susceptibility testing. The *Manual of Clinical Microbiology* continues to represent the glue that binds clinical microbiology by describing its core practices and approaches while disseminating old and new knowledge to generations of practitioners around the globe.

JAMES VERSALOVIC

AUTHOR AND EDITOR CONFLICTS OF INTEREST

The authors and editors of this *Manual* have disclosed any potentially relevant conflicts of interest below, including relationships that might detract from an author's objectivity in presentation of information and interests whose value would be enhanced by the data presented.

David A. Anderson (chapter 88) is a coinventor of reagents licensed from the Burnet Institute to MP Biomedicals Asia Pacific for use in hepatitis E virus diagnostics (HEV IgM ELISA 3.0, HEV sandwich ELISA 4.0, and Assure rapid HEV IgM).

Ellen Jo Baron (chapters 16 and 47) is an employee of Cepheid, a molecular diagnostics company. She has received royalties, honoraria, or consulting income from OpGen, bioMérieux, Merck, MorphDesign, Hardy Diagnostics, and Elsevier. She is a member of product/scientific advisory boards of MicroPhage, Key Scientific Products, NanoMR, OpGen, and Immunosciences, Inc.

Karsten Becker (chapter 19) is a member of advisory boards and has received travel and research grant support and lecture fees from several companies in the pharmaceutical and diagnostic industry.

Edward B. Breitschwerdt (chapter 46) holds U.S. patent 7,115,385 (Media and Methods for Cultivation of Cultivation of Microorganisms, issued 3 October 2006) in conjunction with Sushama Sontakke and North Carolina State University. He is the chief scientific officer of Galaxy Diagnostics, a company that provides diagnostic testing for the detection of *Bartonella* species infection in animals and in human patient samples.

Angela M. Caliendo (section editor; coauthor of chapters 4, 78, and 79) has served on the scientific advisory boards of Roche Diagnostics, Idaho Technologies, Quidel, Abbott Molecular, and GenProbe; has participated in clinical trials with Roche and Qiagen; and has been a consultant to DiaSorin/Biotrin.

Karen C. Carroll (volume editor; coauthor of chapters 3 and 9) has served on the scientific advisory boards of OpGen, Inc., NanoMR, and Quidel Corp. She has received research support from Akonni Biosystems, BD Diagnostics, Great Basin Scientific, Ibis Biosciences, MicroPhage, Inc., and ProDesse, Inc.

David L. Cox (chapter 57) has worked with four companies to evaluate their tests: SpanSpirolipin, ChemBio DPP Syphilis, Bio-Rad BioPlex, and DiaSorin Liaison. He has published papers on the first two assays, the Bio-Rad manuscript is "in progress," and the DiaSorin project is in its final stages.

Mary Jane Ferraro (chapters 67 and 69) has been a member of the Becton Dickinson Worldwide Microbiology Advisory Committee and the bioMérieux Microbiology Advisory Committee.

Barbara Gärtner (chapter 99) has received lecture fees from DiaSorin, Biotest, Roche, GlaxoSmithKline, Siemens, and Merz in the past. She has also conducted research sponsored by DiaSorin, Virion, Medac, Abbott, Roche, Novitech, Bio-Rad, Kenta-Biotech, Genzyme-Virotech, Euroimmun, Wyeth, and Dako.

Christine C. Ginocchio (section editor; coauthor of chapters 77, 78, and 102) has received research funding from, is a member of the scientific advisory boards of, and has participated in clinical trials sponsored by Gen-Probe and Luminex Molecular Diagnostics. She has received consulting fees from Abbott and Nanosphere and research funding from Hologic and Diagnostic Hybrids (Quidel), and she has received honoraria from and participated in clinical trials sponsored by bioMérieux and BD Diagnostics.

Patti E. Gravitt (chapter 102) is a member of the Women's Health Scientific Advisory Board of Qiagen Corp. and has consulted for Roche.

Janet A. Hindler (chapter 71) has received speaker's honoraria from BD Diagnostics, bioMérieux, and Siemens Healthcare Diagnostics. She is on the advisory board of Forest Laboratories.

Keith R. Jerome (chapter 96) has served on an advisory panel for EraGen Biosciences.

Elizabeth M. Johnson (section editor; coauthor of chapter 128) is a member of the advisory boards of Astellas, Gilead, Merck, Pfizer, Schering-Plough, and Zeneus and the speakers' bureaus of Astellas, Gilead, Merck, Neutec, Pfizer, Schering-Plough, and Zeneus. She has received grants from AB Biodisk, Gilead, Pfizer, Schering-Plough, and Vicuron.

James H. Jorgensen (volume editor; coauthor of chapters 67, 68, 70, and 71) is on the advisory boards of BD Diagnostics and RibX Pharmaceuticals. He has received research support from BD Diagnostics, bioMérieux, Merck, and Pfizer.

Stephen E. Lindstrom (chapter 81) is included in a patent on technology associated with CDC real-time RT-PCR assays that has been licensed from the CDC and from which he receives royalties.

Ricardo G. Maggi (chapter 46) is the scientific technical advisor and laboratory director of Galaxy Diagnostics, a company that provides diagnostic testing for the detection of *Bartonella* species infection in animals and in human patient samples.

Rhoda Ashley Morrow (chapter 96) has received laboratory service contracts, honoraria, or consulting fees from Abbott Laboratories, GlaxoSmithKline, DiaSorin, and Roche Diagnostics during the past 3 years.

Philip E. Pellett (chapter 100) receives royalties related to sales of a monoclonal antibody that is specific for human herpesvirus 6B and is mentioned in Table 4 of chapter 100.

Michael A. Pfaller (chapter 128) is a member of the advisory boards of Astellas, Gilead, Merck, Schering-Plough, Esai, MethylGene, and Becton Dickinson and the speakers' bureaus of Astellas, Merck, Pfizer, and Schering-Plough. He has received grants from AB Biodisk, Astellas, bioMérieux, Merck, Pfizer, Schering-Plough, Esai, and MethylGene.

Justin D. Radolf (chapter 57) has royalty agreements via UT Southwestern Medical Center with Biokit, SA, relating to enzyme immunoassays using recombinant *Treponema pallidum* antigens. Via the University of Connecticut Health Center, he has also executed contracts for the purchase of recombinant *T. pallidum* antigens that might be used in commercialized syphilis serodiagnostic tests.

Marion Riffelmann (chapter 43) has received support for epidemiological studies from manufacturers of pertussis vaccines (Aventis Pasteur MSD and GlaxoSmithKline) and has given talks about pertussis immunization.

José R. Romero (chapter 85) has participated in clinical studies sponsored by bioMérieux.

Sandra S. Richter (section editor; coauthor of chapter 69) has received research support from BD Diagnostics.

Yi-Wei Tang (section editor; coauthor of chapters 78 and 83) has been a consultant to Ibis Biosciences, has served on the scientific advisory board of BioHelix, and has participated in clinical trials with Abbott Molecular.

Theodore F. Tsai (chapter 93) is a full-time employee of Novartis Vaccines.

John D. Turnidge (chapters 67 and 68) is a member of the advisory boards of Janssen-Cilag Australia, Pfizer Australia, and Novartis Australia.

Alexandra Valsamakis (section editor; coauthor of chapters 76, 78, and 89) has received research support from Gen-Probe, Qiagen, and Roche Diagnostics. She has served on scientific advisory panels for Abbott Molecular, Gen-Probe, Qiagen, Siemens, and Roche Diagnostics.

Carl-Heinz Wirsing von König (chapter 43) has received support for epidemiological studies from manufacturers of pertussis vaccines (Aventis Pasteur MSD and GlaxoSmithKline) and has given talks about pertussis immunization. He is a member of the Global Pertussis Initiative, an expert body that is supported by an unrestricted grant from Aventis Pasteur.

section I

DIAGNOSTIC STRATEGIES AND GENERAL TOPICS

VOLUME EDITOR: JAMES H. JORGENSEN
SECTION EDITOR: MELVIN P. WEINSTEIN

Introduction to the 10th Edition of the *Manual of Clinical Microbiology*

JAMES VERSALOVIC

1

The 10th edition of the *Manual of Clinical Microbiology* (MCM10) marks a significant milestone in the evolution of this important work. Since its inception with the publication of the first edition in 1970, the *Manual* has been served by four editors in chief working in close cooperation with a team of editors and ASM Press. The prior editor in chief, Patrick R. Murray, established the foundation for the current system of two volumes (as of the eighth edition), a comprehensive array of content in all aspects of microbiology, and a highly committed team of volume and section editors working within a four-year publication cycle. This edition includes several changes to the editorial team, including a new editor in chief and three new volume editors. The number of volume editors was increased from four to five in order to enhance the quality of the *Manual* and reduce the average volume editor workload. Two volume editors, Marie Louise Landry and James Jorgensen, served past editions of the *Manual*. Three new volume editors, Karen Carroll, Guido Funke, and David Warnock, stepped into new roles after serving the *Manual* previously as section editors and chapter authors. Guido Funke is the first volume editor from outside the United States, highlighting the growing importance of international contributions in recent editions. Approximately 19 and 30% of section editors and chapter authors, respectively, contributed content from non-U.S. countries. Historically, the *Manual* has benefited from the continuity of participation of many leaders in medical and diagnostic microbiology. The five volume editors deserve much of the credit for bringing the 10th edition "to life." In addition, Ronald Atlas was an important addition to the section editor team, providing guidance regarding media, reagents, and stains. A total of 16 section editors (including 10 new section editors) completed the editorial team and provided direct links with nearly 270 chapter authors (including 75 new authors who did not contribute to the ninth edition).

The overall organization of the *Manual* is similar to that of the ninth edition, and the chapter formats are basically unchanged. The total number of chapters was reduced from 152 in the ninth edition to 149 chapters in the current edition. The "Natural Habitats" subheading was completely removed from this edition, and this content was absorbed into the "Description of the Agents" or "Epidemiology and Transmission" subheading in organism chapters. The table of contents and introductory topics were modified and adapted to fit the needs of a changing landscape in medical microbiology. Sections I, II, and III of the ninth edition were merged into a single section entitled "Diagnostic Strategies and General Topics." The 18 chapters that comprised these three sections in the ninth edition were condensed into 14 chapters in one section. Chapters covering laboratory management and laboratory information systems were deleted because this content is covered well in general textbooks of laboratory medicine. The chapter on specimen collection and handling in Section I of the ninth edition was replaced by more-specific chapters on this topic in the bacteriology, virology, mycology, and parasitology sections. Chapters were added to address relatively new areas of pathogen discovery, microbial genomics, and metagenomics (chapters 13 and 14). The Human Microbiome Project is described in chapter 13, an entirely new chapter covering rapid advances in technology and significant implications for the future of medical microbiology. In chapter 14, microarrays and sequencing technologies are described as tools for discovery of novel human pathogens.

In the bacteriology section, some of the "Algorithms" chapters were reformulated as "General Approaches" chapters, and these chapters were moved to each subsection in the bacteriology section. The MCM9 chapter on *Enterobacteriaceae* was removed, while the chapter on *Escherichia*, *Shigella*, and *Salmonella* was retained. The *Bordetella* chapter was expanded and renamed "*Bordetella* and Related Genera." In Section III (Antibacterial Agents and Susceptibility Test Methods), one chapter covering testing instrumentation and computerized expert systems was moved from the MCM9 section on diagnostic technologies. In Section IV (Virology), the H1N1 pandemic challenged our authors and editors to expand and update the chapter on influenza viruses, and the chapter describing enteric viruses was renamed "Gastroenteritis Viruses." In Section VI (Mycology), the chapters describing fungi were restructured and renamed to keep up with changes in taxonomy. The chapter describing *Aspergillus*, *Fusarium*, and other fungi was divided into one chapter describing *Aspergillus* and *Penicillium* and a separate chapter covering *Fusarium* and hyaline fungi; the word "moniliaceous" was removed from the title. The term "dematiaceous fungi" was replaced with "melanized fungi" in the chapter describing *Bipolaris* and related organisms. The parasitology section of the 10th edition (Section VIII) is unchanged from that of the ninth edition. The virology and parasitology sections were substantially reorganized in the ninth edition, and therefore these sections did not require significant changes in the current edition.

Now entering its fifth decade, the *Manual* strives to continue to be the leading, most authoritative reference for the "real-world" practice of clinical microbiology. In order to create and assemble each edition, this publication builds on the content of past editions, and the process requires about 3 years of careful planning, design, writing, and review of chapters before the final phases of copyediting, composition, printing, and binding. In the intervening 1 to 2 years from the time of chapter acceptances until printing, new diagnostic trends, technologies, pathogens, and patterns of infectious diseases may emerge or change in ways that affect the timeliness and relevance of this comprehensive reference. This sobering reality simply "goes with the territory" of compiling any authoritative body of work. Hopefully the *Manual* continues to provide a highly respected benchmark and authoritative reference for the entire field of clinical microbiology. In the era of mass collaboration and rapid communication, our team at the *Manual* trusts that our readership, each of you, will contribute to the future of this field by pointing out errors, issues, and trends that serve to strengthen the *Manual* and its next edition. The work never stops, and the knowledge base keeps growing. So let us all continue to enhance the practice and contribute to the evolution of our cherished profession of clinical microbiology.

Microscopy

DANNY L. WIEDBRAUK

2

The history of microscopy is closely linked to the history of microbiology. Early microscopists, including Hooke, Divini, Kircher, and van Leeuwenhoek, were among the first individuals to describe microscopic life forms (16). Robert Hooke, in his landmark 1665 book *Micrographica,* included many illustrations of microscopic forms. In observation XVIII, Hooke first used the term "cell" to describe the microscopic architecture of thin pieces of cork (16, 22). Hooke's *Micrographica* was a best seller of its time, inspiring many scientists to discover the microbiological world (16). In his 1678 letters to the Royal Society in London, Antony van Leeuwenhoek provided detailed descriptions of protozoa. His descriptions of "very small animalcules" included drawings of basic organism shapes and descriptions of their movement. In an effort to observe the microscopic world in ever greater detail, van Leeuwenhoek built simple microscopes of increasing power. Some of these microscopes were capable of ×200 magnification. Van Leeuwenhoek's 1683 letters to the Royal Society included the first ever description of living bacteria from dental plaque sampled from between his teeth (17). Microscopy continued to play an important role in the study of biology and medicine, and almost two centuries later, the only scientific equipment Charles Darwin took with him on the voyage of the *Beagle* was a simple microscope (6). Today, light microscopy is used not only in biological sciences such as microbiology, botany, forensics, pathology, and cell biology but also in metallurgy, engraving, chemistry, mineralogy, gemology, computer chip design, and microsurgical applications. This chapter will attempt to describe the basic concepts of light microscopy as they are practiced in the microbiology laboratory.

TECHNICAL BACKGROUND AND DEFINITION OF TERMS

Aberration

Aberrations are unwanted artifacts in the microscopic image that are caused by elements in the optical path. Aberration can be caused by physical objects such as dust or oils on the optical surfaces, by alterations in the light path caused by improper alignment or aperture settings, and by imperfections in the lens systems. Two main types of optical aberrations can occur when white light passes through a convex lens: spherical aberration and chromatic aberration.

Spherical aberration is hallmarked by images that appear to be in focus in the center of the field and out of focus at the periphery (5). Chromatic aberration occurs because shorter light wavelengths are refracted to a greater extent than longer wavelengths (5). This wavelength separation (also called dispersion) produces color fringes within the image field. Chromatic aberration can be reduced or eliminated in optical systems by combining two lenses with different color dispersion characteristics (5).

Contrast

Contrast is a measure of the differences in image luminance that provides gray scale or color information. Contrast is expressed as the ratio of the difference in luminance between two points divided by the average luminance in the field (1). Under optimum conditions, the human eye can detect the presence of 2% contrast (1).

Depth of Field and Depth of Focus

Depth of field is a subjective measure of the vertical distance between the nearest and farthest objects in the specimen that appear to be in sharp focus. Depth of field decreases as the numerical aperture (NA) of the lens increases (3). Depth of focus is the area around the image plane where the image will appear to be sharply focused. The image plane is formed within the microscope tube at or near the level of the ocular lenses. Microscopes with greater depth of focus allow the user to employ ocular lenses with different working distances, magnification factors, and visual compensation systems without losing image sharpness. Like depth of field, depth of focus depends upon the NA of the objective. However, depth of focus increases as the NA increases (3).

Immersion Fluid (Immersion Oil)

Immersion fluid is a term used to describe any liquid that occupies the space between the object and microscope objective lens. Immersion fluids are usually required for objectives that have working distances of 3 mm or less (5). Many microscopy applications employ immersion fluids that possess the same refractive index as the glass slide (refractive index = 1.515) (3, 5). This procedure produces a homogeneous optical path which minimizes light refraction and maximizes the effective NA of the objective lens. Immersion fluids are also used between the condenser and the microscope slide in transmitted light fluorescence microscopy and in dark-field microscopy to minimize refraction, increase the NA of the objective, and improve optical resolution (3, 5).

Köhler Illumination

Köhler illumination was first introduced in 1893 by August Köhler of the Carl Zeiss Corporation as a method of providing the optimum specimen illumination (5). In this procedure, the collector lens projects an enlarged and focused image of the lamp filament onto the plane of the aperture diaphragm. Because the light source is not focused at the specimen, the specimen is bathed in a uniformly bright, glare-free light that is not seriously affected by dust and imperfections on the glass surfaces of the condenser. Köhler illumination is required to produce maximum optical resolution and high-quality photomicrographs (4, 5).

Mechanical Tube Length

Mechanical tube length describes the light path distance within the microscope body tube. Tube length is measured from the objective opening in the nosepiece to the top edge of the observation tube. Tube length is usually inscribed on the barrel of the objective as the length in millimeters (e.g., 160, 170, 210, etc.) for fixed lengths or the infinity symbol (∞) for infinity-corrected tube lengths (Fig. 1). Many of the newer objectives are infinity corrected, while older objectives will be corrected for 160-mm (Nikon, Olympus, and Zeiss) or 170-mm (Leica) tube lengths (5). Differences in mechanical tube length are among the major reasons why objectives from one manufacturer cannot be used on a different manufacturer's microscope.

Numerical Aperture

NA is a measure of the light-gathering capability of a lens or condenser. Higher-NA objectives have better resolving power and brighter images than lower-NA objectives. Higher-NA objectives also have shallower depths of field. The equation for determining NA is given by $NA = n \cdot \sin \theta$, where n is the refractive index of the imaging medium between the objective and the specimen and θ is one-half the angular aperture of the objective (Fig. 2) (3, 5, 9, 15). For visible light microscopy using standard immersion oils, the theoretical maximum for NA is about 1.52. In practice, however, a lens cannot accept a 180° cone of light, so θ has to be slightly less. This results in a maximum practical NA of about 1.40 (6).

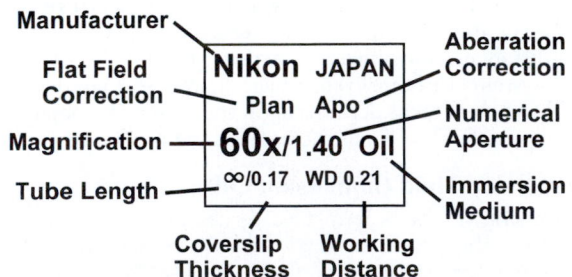

FIGURE 1 Objective lens labeling. Objective lenses are labeled with information on the manufacturer, correction factors, NA, tube length, coverslip thickness, working distance (WD), and expected immersion medium. Objectives without a listed aberration correction are considered achromats. Objectives without a listed immersion medium (Oil, Oel, W, Gly) are considered dry objectives and are meant to operate with air between the lens and the specimen.

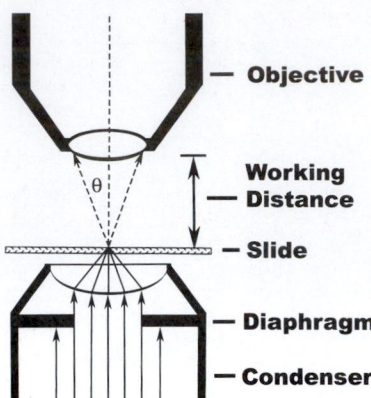

FIGURE 2 Typical configuration for bright-field microscopy. The column of light generated by the field lens and the field diaphragm enters the bottom of the condenser and is focused on the slide by the condenser lens. The condenser diaphragm controls the angle of the light, the NA of the condenser, and the amount of contrast in the image. The working distance is the vertical distance from the top of the specimen to the leading edge of the objective lens. The semiangle of the objective aperture (θ) is used to calculate NA. Modified from reference 9.

Refractive Index (Index of Refraction)

The index of refraction is the ratio of the velocity of light in a vacuum to its velocity in a transparent or translucent medium (3, 5, 9, 14, 15). As the refractive index of a material increases, light beams entering or leaving a material are deflected (refracted) to a greater extent. The refractive index of a medium depends upon the wavelength of light passing through it. Light beams containing multiple wavelengths (e.g., white light) are dispersed when they move into a different medium because each wavelength in the beam is refracted to a slightly different degree. Light dispersion causes chromatic aberration in microscope objectives (5). Refractive index is also an important variable in calculating NA (see "Numerical Aperture" above). Moving from a high-dry microscope objective that uses air as the imaging medium (refractive index of air = 1.003) to an oil immersion objective of the same power (refractive index of immersion oil = 1.515) increases the maximum theoretical NA of a given lens from 1.0 to 1.5, producing a 50% increase in light-gathering capability (3, 5).

Resolution (Resolving Power)

The resolution of an optical microscope is defined as the shortest distance between two points that can be distinguished by the observer or camera system as separate entities (3, 9, 15). The resolving power of a microscope is the most important feature of the optical system because it defines our ability to distinguish fine details in a specimen. The theoretical limit of resolution for a given lens is defined mathematically as $r = \kappa/(2NA)$, where r is the resolution, κ is the imaging wavelength, and NA is the numerical aperture of the lens (3, 9, 15). From this equation, it is obvious that only the light wavelength and NA directly affect the resolving power. Thus, a 40× oil objective with an NA of 1.30 can have the same resolving power as a 100× oil objective (Table 1). In the same manner, the resolving power of a 100× oil objective is higher when using UV wavelengths than it is when using visible light (Table 1).

TABLE 1 Resolving power of selected lenses with different NA

Lens system	NA	Light color	Avg wavelength (nm)	Medium	Resolution (μm)
Eye		White	550	Air	700
Hand magnifier	0.03	White	550	Air	10
10× objective	0.30	White	550	Air	0.92
40× objective	0.75	White	550	Air	0.37
40× objective (oil)	1.30	White	550	Oil	0.21
100× objective	1.30	White	550	Oil	0.21
100× objective	1.30	UV	400	Oil	0.15

Working Distance

Working distance is the distance between the objective front lens and the top of the cover glass when the specimen is in focus (Fig. 2). The working distance of an objective generally decreases as magnification increases (3). The working distance of an objective may not be inscribed on the barrel of older objectives, but newer objectives often contain the working distance in millimeters (Fig. 1). Longer-working-distance objectives are important when examining the inside surface of glass tubes (tube cultures) and cell culture flasks.

SIMPLE MICROSCOPES

Common objects such as jewelers' loupes, handheld photographic slide viewers, and simple magnifying or reading glasses are all examples of simple microscopes in routine use today. A simple microscope is composed of a single biconvex magnifying lens which is thicker in the center than at the periphery. In contrast with compound microscopes, simple microscopes produce a magnified image that is in the same orientation as the original object. Because of their low NA, simple microscopes have limited resolution and magnifying power. Most commercial magnifiers are able to produce a ×2 to ×30 magnification, and the better lenses will have a resolution of about 10 μm. Simple magnifiers are useful for dissection, examination of bacterial colonies, and interpretation of agglutination reactions.

COMPOUND MICROSCOPES

The first compound microscopes were constructed around 1590 by Dutch spectacle makers, Zaccharias Janssen and Hans Janssen. The Janssen microscope consisted of an object lens (objective) that was placed close to the specimen and the eye, or ocular, lens that was placed close to the eye. The lenses were separated by a body tube. In this microscope, the objective lens projected a magnified image into the body tube and the eyepiece magnified the projected image, thereby producing a two-stage magnification. Modern compound microscopes still use this general design and have two separate lens systems mounted at opposite ends of a body tube.

The stereoscopic microscope combines two compound microscopes which produce separate images for each eye. Stereoscopic microscopes may have one or two separate objectives, and many have a zoom magnification function. These microscopes are used for reflected or transmitted illumination, but the absence of a substage condenser limits their NA and resolution. Stereomicroscopes are useful in examining colonial morphology of bacteria, fungi, and cell cultures (15).

The modern light microscope is composed of optical and mechanical components that, together with the mounted specimen, make up the optical train. The optical train of a typical bright-field microscope consists of an illuminator (light source and collector lens), a substage condenser, specimen, objective, eyepiece, and a detector. The detector can be a camera or the observer's eye.

Specimen illumination is one of the most critical elements in optical microscopy. Inadequate or improper sample illumination can reduce contrast in the specimen and significantly decrease the resolving power of any microscope. There are numerous commercially available illuminators for microscopes, but 50- or 100-watt tungsten halogen lamp systems are frequently used due to their low cost and long life. Light generated by the light source is passed through a collector and a field lens (Fig. 3) before being directed into the substage condenser and onto the specimen. Image-forming light rays are captured by the microscope objective and passed into the eyepieces or a camera port. Alignment of the optical components of a microscope is critical to produce a good image (35).

Field Diaphragm

The field diaphragm is located in the light path between the light source and the substage condenser (Fig. 3). This iris-like mechanism controls the width of the light beam that enters the substage condenser. The field diaphragm does not affect the optical resolution, NA, or intensity of illumination. However, the field diaphragm should be

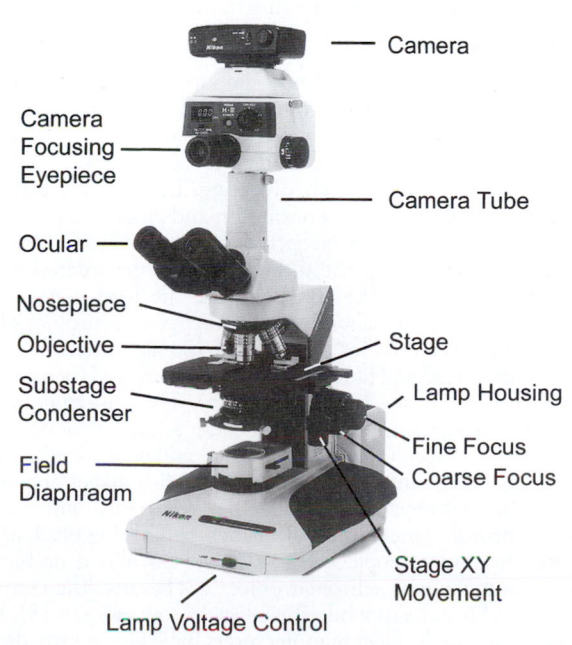

FIGURE 3 Anatomy of a typical clinical microscope with an integral camera.

centered in the optical path and opened far enough that it just overfills the field of view. This adjustment is important for preventing glare and loss of contrast in the observed image. When the field diaphragm is opened too far, scattered light and reflections can degrade image quality.

Substage Condenser

The substage condenser is typically mounted beneath the microscope stage in a bracket that can be raised or lowered independently of the stage (Fig. 3). The substage condenser gathers light from the field diaphragm and concentrates it into a cone of light that illuminates the specimen with uniform intensity over the entire field of view. Adjustment of the substage condenser is probably the most critical element for achieving proper illumination, and it is the main source of image degradation and poor quality photomicrography. The condenser light cone must be properly adjusted to optimize the intensity and angle of light entering the objective. Because each objective has different light-gathering capabilities (NA), the substage condenser should be adjusted to provide a light cone that matches the NA of the new objective. This is done by adjusting the aperture (or condenser) diaphragm control. Substage condensers on newer microscopes have a scale embossed on the condenser and an index mark on the aperture control that allows the user to quickly switch from one NA range to another. Many manufacturers are now synchronizing the NA gradations to correspond with the approximate NA of the objectives.

In clinical laboratory practice, the condenser aperture is often made smaller to improve the contrast of wet mounts and some stained preparations (9). The condenser is sometimes moved downward for the same purpose. These practices are effective for a few applications, but they will result in decreased optical resolution (1, 9). Specimen illumination intensity should not be adjusted by opening and closing the condenser diaphragm or by moving the condenser laterally in the light path. Illumination intensity should be controlled through the use of neutral density filters placed into the light path or by reducing the lamp voltage. Reducing the voltage, however, will also alter the color of the incoming light, and voltage changes are not recommended for photomicroscopy (4).

Objectives

The objective lens is the most important single determinant of the quality of the image produced by a particular microscope (15). When choosing a microscope, the purchaser must select the magnification factor, NA, and the level of correction for each objective. Lenses with higher NA values will have higher resolution and produce a brighter field of view. The level of optical correction in the objective will depend upon the ultimate use of the microscope. Achromatic (achromat) objectives are the least expensive objectives found on laboratory microscopes. Achromat objectives are corrected for axial chromatic aberration in two wavelengths (red and blue), and they are corrected for spherical aberration in one color (green) (5). The limited correction of achromatic objectives can cause a number of optical artifacts when specimens are examined and photographed in color (e.g., green images often have a reddish-magenta halo) (5). Achromat objectives produce the best results with light passed through a green filter and when performing black and white photomicroscopy. Flatness of field is also a problem when using straight achromat objectives because the center of the field is in focus while the edges are out of focus (5). In the past few years, most manufacturers have begun providing flat-field corrections for achromat objectives. These objectives are called plan-achromats.

The next higher level of correction and cost is found in objectives called fluorites or semiapochromats. Fluorite objectives are produced from advanced glass formulations that allow for greatly improved correction of optical aberration. Like the achromat objectives, the fluorite objectives are corrected chromatically for red and blue light (5). Unlike achromats, fluorites are corrected spherically for two or three colors instead of a single color (5). The superior correction of fluorite objectives compared to achromats enables these objectives to be made with a higher NA. Fluorite lenses therefore produce brighter images than achromats. Fluorite objectives have better resolving power than achromats and provide a higher degree of contrast, making them better suited for color photomicrography in white light (3, 5).

Apochromats

Apochromats are the most highly corrected microscope lenses and the most costly. Apochromats are corrected chromatically for three colors (red, green, and blue), almost eliminating chromatic aberration, and are corrected spherically for either two or three wavelengths (5). Apochromat objectives are the best choice for color photomicrography in white light. Because of their high level of correction, apochromat objectives usually have, for a given magnification, higher NAs than do achromats or fluorites (3, 5).

Fluorescence Objectives

Fluorescence objectives are designed with quartz and other special glasses that have high transmission rates for UV, visible, and infrared light. These objectives are extremely low in autofluorescence, and they use specialized optical cements and antireflection coatings that protect the lens and allow it to operate with a wide variety of excitation wavelengths. Correction for optical aberration and NA values in UV fluor objectives usually approaches that of apochromats, which contributes to image brightness and enhanced image resolution (2, 5). The primary drawback of high-performance fluorescence objectives is that many are not corrected for field curvature and produce images that do not have uniform focus throughout the entire field of view. This is not a large problem when performing direct or indirect fluorescent antibody testing, but it can be troublesome if you have to use the same objectives for bright-field or phase-contrast microscopy.

Microscope objectives that use air as the medium between the coverslip and the objective lens are considered dry objectives. The maximum working NA of a dry objective system is limited to 0.95. Higher NA values can only be achieved using optics designed for immersion media. Immersion media have the same refractive index and dispersion values as glass (refractive index = 1.51). The use of immersion media produces a homogeneous light path from the coverslip to the lens so that light is not refracted away from the objective. The use of immersion fluids and immersion lenses significantly increases the NA and the optical resolution of the system. In addition to "oil" lenses, specially corrected objective lenses designed for glycerin and water immersion are commercially available. The proper immersion fluid type is always stamped on the side of the objective. The advantages of oil immersion objectives are severely compromised if the wrong immersion fluid is utilized. Microscope manufacturers produce immersion objectives with tight refractive index and dispersion tolerances (5). It is therefore advisable to use only the immersion fluid recommended by the objective manufacturer. Mixing of immersion fluids from different manufacturers should be avoided because mixing can produce unexpected crystallization artifacts or phase separations that compromise image quality.

Many high-power (NA, ≥0.8) dry objectives are engineered to operate through 0.17-mm coverslips (designated as number 1½). In practice, however, the total thickness of the specimen-coverslip sandwich can be greater or less than 0.17 mm due to variations in coverslip and/or mounting fluid thickness (3, 5). Under these conditions, there will be noticeable spherical aberration in the microscopic image (3, 5). A 0.2-mm deviation in coverslip thickness will produce an 8% decrease in image intensity when using a 0.79 NA objective and 57% with a 0.85 NA high-dry objective (5). Therefore, some of the more advanced dry objectives are engineered with a coverslip correction collar that adjusts the objective lens elements to compensate for coverslip thickness variations. Objectives with a coverslip correction collar are labeled Corr, w/Corr, or CR. However, this labeling is usually unnecessary because the objective has a distinctive knurled ring and graduated scale on the side. The expected coverslip thickness for an objective is etched on the barrel of the objective (Fig. 1).

Eyepiece or Ocular Objective

The eyepiece or ocular objective contains the final lens system in the optical train. The purpose of the ocular objective is to magnify and focus the projected image onto the eye of the viewer. Ocular lenses generally have a magnification factor of ×10 to ×20, and the total magnification of the microscope is the product of the objective magnification and the ocular magnification (5, 9, 14, 15). Thus, a microscope with a 40× objective and a 10× ocular lens would have a magnification value of ×400. Many eyepieces have a shelf at the level of the fixed eyepiece diaphragm that allows for the insertion of ocular micrometers, pointers, or crosshairs. This shelf is located at the focal plane of the image projected by the objective lens so that the inserted element is in focus when the specimen image is in focus.

DARK-FIELD MICROSCOPY

Dark-field microscopy is a specialized illumination technique that is used in the clinical laboratory to detect thin organisms such as spirochetes and *Leptospira* (see chapters 55 and 57). High-resolution dark-field microscopy utilizes a specialized high-NA cardioid dark-field condenser that blocks the central light path light and produces a hollow cone of illumination that is directed away from the objective lens at an oblique angle (Fig. 4). Bacteria on the slide

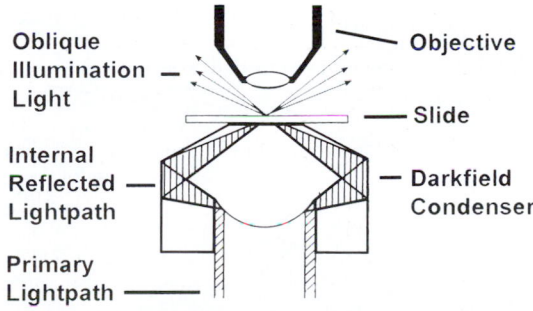

FIGURE 4 Dark-field illumination. The central light path interacts with the silvered dome located at the bottom of the condenser and is reflected away from the specimen. Peripheral light is reflected into the condenser and is reflected again by the internal condenser surfaces to produce a cone of light that is directed obliquely away from the objective.

have a slightly different refractive index than the surrounding medium, and light rays passing through the organism are refracted into the objective lens. Light rays that do not pass through an organism do not enter the lens. This type of illumination produces bright organism profiles against a dark background. Dark-field microscopy requires careful alignment of the condenser and the placement of immersion oil between the slide and the substage condenser. Dark-field microscopy, when done correctly, increases the resolution of the microscope to 0.1 μm or less (1, 9). The resolution of bright-field microscopy is 0.2 μm (9, 15).

PHASE-CONTRAST MICROSCOPY

In the early 1930s, the Dutch physicist F. Zernike introduced a new method for testing optical systems which he called phase contrast. Originally designed as a macroscopic testing system, the use of phase-contrast techniques in microscopic systems allowed the user to examine unstained biological specimens that were virtually transparent when observed under bright-field illumination. Zernike was awarded the Nobel Prize in 1953 for his contributions to microscopy.

Phase contrast is essentially an interference method wherein a ring annulus is placed directly under the lower lens of the condenser to produce a hollow cylinder of light. This light is essentially unchanged as it passes into the objective, and it arrives at the rear focal plane of the objective in the shape of a ring. Light that goes through the specimen is refracted and slowed slightly so that it is out of phase by about one-quarter wavelength from the unchanged light. This out-of-phase light is spread over the entire focal plane. Light passing through the rear focal plane of the objective interacts with a separate ring-shaped phase plate that alters the direct light path by another one-quarter wavelength (1). When the direct light and the refracted light arrive at the image plane, they are out of phase by one-half wavelength. This out-of-phase light interacts destructively so that specimen details appear as dark areas against a lighter background (1). Because the phase-shifting calculations are based on a one-quarter wavelength of green light, the phase image has the best resolution when a green filter is placed in the light path (1). Green filters also allow the microscopist to use less-expensive achromat lenses that are spherically corrected for green light. Phase microscopy is an important tool for examining living and/or unstained material in wet mounts and cell cultures. However, phase-contrast microscopy has lower resolution than bright-field microscopy of stained specimens (1). In addition, viewed objects are often surrounded by halos that can obscure boundary details. Phase-contrast microscopy does not work well with thick specimens because the phase shift may be greater than the expected one-quarter wavelength. In phase-contrast microscopy, structures within living cells appear as hills or craters, depending upon their optical thickness. This pseudo-three-dimensional effect can greatly enhance image contrast in unstained specimens.

FLUORESCENCE MICROSCOPY

The fluorescence microscope was developed in the early 1900s, and many of the initial microscopic studies involved identification and localization of compounds that autofluoresced when irradiated with UV light. In the 1930s, a number of investigators began using fluorescent compounds to identify specific tissue components and infectious agents that did not autofluoresce (2). These stains are not organism specific, but rather, they bind to and stain specific structures within the organism. Examples of this type of staining include acridine orange, auramine-rhodamine, calcofluor white, Evans blue, and Hoechst 33258.

The use of fluorochrome-antibody conjugates (immunofluorescence) was first described in the 1940s when Coons et al. (11, 12) used fluorescein-labeled antibodies to detect pneumococcal polysaccharide antigens in tissue sections of infected mice. Fluorescent antibody staining expanded significantly with the development of fluorescein isocyanate in 1950 (13) and the more stable fluorescein isothiocyanate (FITC) derivative in 1958 (19, 21, 30, 33). Today, fluorescence microscopy is also used in conjunction with nucleic acid hybridization to visualize the location of fluorescent in situ hybridization and multicolor fluorescent in situ hybridization probes (32, 38).

Fluorescence microscopy is dependent upon the ability of fluorescent substances to absorb light of a certain wavelength and emit light at a longer wavelength. Fluorescence microscopes used for clinical microbiology most often utilize fluorochromes that absorb near-UV light energy and reemit that light at a lower, green or yellow wavelength (2, 10). To work properly, the fluorescence microscope must irradiate the specimen with UV excitation light and separate the much weaker emitted light from the brighter excitation light so that only the emitted light reaches the eye. The resulting image consists of brightly shining areas against a dark background (2). Older fluorescent microscopes are configured for dark-field illumination. In these instruments, UV excitation light enters a dark-field condenser and the light is directed onto the specimen at an oblique angle (Fig. 4). Fluorescent compounds in the specimen absorb the excitation light, and the emitted light is collected by the objective lens. The emitted light then passes through a barrier filter to remove any excitation light that may enter the objective. These microscopes are difficult to use for routine diagnostics because the condenser and the objective must be carefully oiled. The dark-field condenser also reduces the effective NA of the objectives, thereby producing dim images that lack resolution (2). Most modern fluorescence microscopes use reflected light (epifluorescence). In these instruments, the excitation light is directed downward through the objective and onto the specimen. The emitted light and the reflected excitation light are collected by the objective, and they pass through a dichoric mirror which removes the excitation light and allows the longer-wavelength emitted light to form an image. With epifluorescence, the objective acts as a condenser and the alignment and oiling issues associated with a dark-field condenser are eliminated (2). The visual field is brighter with epifluorescence, the resolution is higher, and fluorescence quenching only occurs in the field of view (2).

Fluorescence microscopy requires high levels of illumination because the quantum yield of most fluorochromes is low. The most common lamps are mercury vapor (HBO) lamps, ranging in wattage from 50 to 200 watts, or xenon vapor (XBO) lamps, which range from 75 to 200 watts. It should be noted that lamp wattage is not necessarily a measure of usable brightness in a fluorescence lamp. The HBO 100-watt lamp is 4 times brighter than the 200-watt HBO lamp and 11 times brighter than the XBO 150-watt lamp (2). When purchasing a fluorescence microscope, it is also important to determine whether the emission spectrum of the lamp is compatible with the fluorochromes used in the laboratory. HBO and XBO lamps are under high pressure, and care must be taken to prevent the lamps from exploding. One should never touch these lamps with bare hands because oils on the fingers can etch or discolor the glass.

Fluorochromes must be excited by specific light wavelengths to generate the maximum amount of emitted light. Therefore, specific exciter and barrier filter combinations are used to maximize the quantum yield of the fluorophore. Exciter filters are used to select the required light wavelengths from the spectrum of light generated by the lamp (2). Excitation filters are provided in narrow, medium, and wide band-pass configurations that pass a narrower and wider range of light frequencies, respectively. Barrier filters block shorter light wavelengths and allow longer wavelengths to pass through the filter. Barrier filters are important because they remove the high-intensity excitation light that could overwhelm the low-intensity emitted light. Barrier filters also prevent UV light from entering the eye where it can cause cataracts and retinal damage. Wide band-pass barrier filters generally produce brighter images, but care must be taken to prevent the introduction of background light that could overwhelm the emitted light. Epifluorescence microscopes also have a dichromatic mirror (beam splitter) that reflects the incoming excitation light to the objective and allows the emitted light to pass to the barrier filter and onto the objectives. In most modern epifluorescence microscopes, the barrier filter, excitation mirror, and beam splitter are housed in removable optical blocks, and several of these blocks can be installed in the microscope at one time. This configuration allows the user to quickly change the excitation and barrier filters to accommodate different fluorochromes. Care must be exercised when selecting optical blocks. The excitation filter should match the excitation wavelength of the fluorophore (Table 2), and

TABLE 2 Excitation and emission wavelengths of commonly used fluorochromes[a]

Fluorescent compound	Excitation wavelength (nm)	Emission wavelength (nm)
Acridine orange (single-stranded nucleic acid)	500	526
Acridine orange (double-stranded nucleic acid)	460	640
Auramine O	460	550
Calcofluor white	440	500–520
Ethidium bromide	545	605
Evans blue	550	610
FITC	490	525
Hoechst 33258	352	461
Rhodamine B	540	625
TRITC[b]	555	580

[a]Excitation and emission wavelengths can vary depending upon the solvent and the pH of the solution.
[b]TRITC, tetramethylrhodamine isothiocyanate.

the emission barrier should allow the emitted light to pass through. For example, direct fluorescent antibody testing for viral antigens in cell smears typically employs FITC-labeled antibodies and an Evans blue counterstain. Choosing an optical block with a 450- to 490-nm-pore-size excitation filter and a 515-nm-pore-size wide band-pass barrier filter will produce a bright field of view, and the counterstained cells will appear orange-red. By selecting a more restricted band-pass barrier filter (520- to 560-nm pore size), the field of view will be darker and the red emitted light from the Evans blue counterstain will not be visible. The images produced by this optical block will have more contrast because the background is darker. Both filter combinations are appropriate for this task, but the final choice will depend upon user preference.

One of the major problems in the use and examination of fluorescent microscopic images is the tendency of fluorophores to lose fluorescence when exposed to excitation light for several minutes. This loss of fluorescence is caused by two mechanisms: photobleaching and quenching. Photobleaching (fading) is a permanent loss of fluorescence that is caused by chemical damage to the fluorophore (2). Quenching is caused by the presence of free radicals, salts of heavy metals, or halogen compounds (2). Quenching can also be caused by transfer of emission light energy to other fluorescent molecules in close proximity to the fluorophore in a process called fluorescent resonance energy transfer. To lessen the effect of quenching, slides should be stored in the dark at 2 to 8°C. In addition, the user should block the excitation light path when not viewing or photographing the specimen. Most epifluorescence microscopes have a shutter in the light path for this purpose. Quenching can be a significant problem when photographing fluorescent images because the shutter may be open for a minute or more. Quenching can be reduced somewhat by the addition of free radical scavengers such as p-phenylenediamine (24), 1,4-diazabicyclo(2,2,2)-octane (DABCO) (25), or n-propylgallate (20) to the mounting fluid. p-Phenylenediamine and n-propylgallate can be used to reduce quenching in FITC and rhodamine. DABCO is slightly less effective than p-phenylenediamine for FITC fluorescence, but unlike p-phenylenediamine, DABCO does not darken when exposed to light and it is safer to use. Quench-resistant mounting media are also available from Vector Laboratories (Burlingame, CA), Molecular Probes, Inc. (Carlsbad, CA), and Bio-Rad Laboratories (Hercules, CA).

LINEAR MEASUREMENTS (MICROMETRY)

The first reported micrometric procedures were credited to Antony van Leeuwenhoek, who used fine grains of sand as a gauge to determine the size of human erythrocytes. Since then, a variety of methods have been used to determine the dimensions of microscopic organisms. The crudest method for determining size in the clinical laboratory involves comparing the object size to the measured or calculated view field size. Other micrometric techniques include the addition of polystyrene beads of known size into the specimen. Comparative measurements are then performed utilizing a photomicrograph or digital image. The accuracy of this method is variable and depends on the homogeneity of the comparison objects. Direct measurement of microorganisms can be done by placing them on calibrated microscope slides or counting chambers. The accuracy of this method depends on the separation distance between ruled lines but averages between 10 and 50 micrometers. The most common procedure used in the clinical laboratory

utilizes a graduated scale (reticle) located within one of the eyepieces (29). Reticles must be calibrated against a stage micrometer for each objective (29). The accuracy of this type of measurement is approximately 2 to 10 micrometers (3 to 5%), depending on magnification and the resolution of the stage micrometer (29).

PHOTOMICROSCOPY

Microscopists began capturing microscopic images on film shortly after the photographic process was invented (4). Micrographic images have long been used for investigations of morphology, in scientific publications and lectures, and in teaching. Modern film technologies have high resolution and clarity, but the use of photomicrographs in day-to-day microscopy has been hampered by long turnaround times associated with film development and printing. Reacquiring fluorescence images is a particular concern because the fluorescence can fade (2). The availability of high-quality digital cameras has significantly changed how photomicrographs are used in the microbiology laboratory. Today, it is not unusual for digital photomicrographs to be shared with experts via the Internet. This process significantly extends the capabilities of the on-site microbiologist and can enhance patient care. Microscope-based digital cameras and video systems are also used to perform "plate rounds" in remote hospitals and clinics within a multihospital system. Newer Internet technologies involving robotic microscopes and high-resolution video systems now allow microbiologists to change the focus and change slide positioning of a microscope located anywhere in the world and view the resulting images on a monitor in their office. The availability of digital photomicroscopy has significantly enhanced the microbial identification process, and it has helped to standardize microbe identification.

A wide variety of microscopes are currently available that have integrated camera systems and sophisticated light metering and exposure controls. Accessory cameras are also available from a large number of aftermarket manufacturers. The performance and optical characteristics of these systems are too diverse to discuss in a single chapter, and the camera specifications necessary for digital microscopy will depend upon the type of images that will be captured. Light sensitivity is a key element in any digital camera, and camera manufacturers utilize the film-equivalent International Organization for Standardization (ISO) numbers to rate the light sensitivity of image sensors in digital cameras. ISO numbers range from 80 to 3200, and the higher the ISO value, the more sensitive the image sensor. Some digital cameras have manual or automatic sensitivity adjustments that can alter the image sensor so that the camera can be used in low-light conditions. Unfortunately, this increased sensitivity is usually achieved by amplifying the signal from the image sensor. This type of signal amplification also increases the background levels and decreases image quality (34). The "heart" of the digital camera is the image sensor, a silicon chip that measures and captures light. Presently, there are two types of image sensors, the complementary metal-oxide semiconductor (CMOS) and the charge-coupled device (CCD) sensor. Consumer cameras typically use CMOS chips because they are easier to manufacture. Many CMOS cameras can be used to capture images generated during bright-field microscopy (7, 23). CMOS cameras tend to be smaller and less expensive than CCD cameras. In addition, CMOS cameras use less power, and they have faster frame rates, fewer artifacts (smear and blooming) caused by charge transfer between adjacent pixels, and the ability to include "higher-level" camera functions such as image stabilization and wireless control (34). The major disadvantage of the CMOS camera is its lower light sensitivity. CCD and slow-scan CCD cameras, which were first developed for astronomy, are the current cameras of choice for low-light-level fluorescence microscopy (18, 34). However, these cameras are much more expensive than CMOS cameras.

Photographs are a stern judge of microscopic quality (4), and the purchase of an expensive camera system does not automatically confer the ability to produce high-quality images. Optics, optical train alignment, and proper illumination are the most important factors in the acquisition of high-quality photomicrographs (4, 7, 23). Optical image deficiencies as evidenced by chromatic variance and poor image clarity are more noticeable when using a digital camera than when using 35-mm film (23). Color photography can be especially demanding because specimens may appear yellow or blue under tungsten halogen (3,200-K color temperature) light depending upon whether the lamp voltage is above or below the recommended 9-volt setting. Photographs will also appear blue if the daylight blue filter is not removed from the light path. Photographs can also appear yellow when tungsten halogen (3,200-K) illumination is used in conjunction with daylight (5,500-K) film or digital cameras designed for daylight photography. Under these conditions, a Kodak 80A (3,200-K to 5,500-K) color conversion filter should be placed in the light path to achieve the proper 5,500-K color temperature (4).

Not all microbiologists can afford a microscope with an integrated camera system. Simple eyepiece cameras can also be used to capture bright-field images. The simplest configuration for eyepiece photography involves the use of a point-and-shoot digital camera. Some improvisation may be necessary with this method because few adapters are available for coupling a fixed-lens camera to the microscope eyepiece. Instead, the microscopist can use a camera tripod or some other support bracket to hold the camera in its proper position. Entry of stray light can be minimized by using a piece of black polyvinyl chloride (PVC) pipe with an appropriate diameter and a black camera cloth. During photography, the camera lens system should be set to infinity focus (the default in fixed lens cameras), and the lens should be positioned so that it is at the eyepoint (focal point) of the eyepiece. The location of the eyepoint can be determined by holding a piece of white paper just above the objective with the microscope turned on and focused (4). A bright circle of light will be projected onto the paper. The eyepoint is the position where the light circle is smallest (4). Photographs produced under these conditions are often acceptable, but they may be dark. Cameras with adjustable aperture settings should be set to the largest aperture value (smallest f-stop number) to maximize the amount of light entering the camera. This method will also produce some chromatic aberration (due to different lens correction factors) and vignetting (pipe view effect).

Another method for photomicroscopy is to use the camera port on microscopes fitted with a trinocular head. Olympus and Nikon have introduced adapters that allow their digital cameras to attach to the camera tube of their microscopes. In addition, camera tube and eyepiece adaptors for a number of digital cameras are available from Microscope Depot (Tracy, CA). Photography under these conditions is best done using a camera with through-the-lens exposure metering. These devices work well if the exposure is not longer than several seconds or shorter than one-third of a second (4). Many of these cameras have built-in flashes that should be turned off during photomicroscopy. These cameras may have problems with fluorescence microscopy due to the extreme contrast of fluorescent images and the tendency of metering systems to average exposure values over the entire field (4).

CARE AND USE OF THE MICROSCOPE

Proper care and maintenance of the microscope will prolong the usable life of the instrument and allow for more accurate interpretation of microbiological images. The microscope should be kept in a low-vibration, low-dust environment to facilitate viewing and decrease damage to the optical systems. The optical elements should be kept completely free of dust, dirt, oil, solvents, and any other contaminants (29). Ideally, the microscope should be covered and the lamp should be turned off when the microscope is not in use. Do not touch the optical surfaces with your fingers (29). Keep the lenses clean and be sure to remove oil or mounting fluid from the objectives, condenser, and mechanical stage after each session. Avoid dragging the high-dry objective through oil or fluorescence mounting fluid. One way to avoid accidental contact with these fluids is to place the high-dry objective and the oil immersion objective in the nosepiece on opposite sides of the low-power objective (4). Lenses should be dusted with residue-free compressed air and cleaned with lens paper and a commercial lens cleaner that is approved by the microscope manufacturer. Organic solvents such as alcohols and acetone should not be used on the lenses because the solvent may dissolve the optical mounting cement (9). Unused spaces in the nosepiece (Fig. 3) should be plugged and the eyepieces should remain installed at all times to prevent introduction of dust into the body tube. The stage should be cleaned regularly, and any spilled immersion oil must be removed or slides will stick when they are moved across the stage. Spilled immersion oil also collects dust and grit that can damage the optical and mechanical parts. Microscopists should not attempt to remove or dissemble the objectives, as this increases the potential for damage (9, 29). This is a job that is best left to professionals (29). The gears and rackwork should be cleaned and treated with new grease at intervals specified by the manufacturer. Do not use light oil on the gears or bearing surfaces because this may cause the condenser and stage to sink from their own weight (29). Periodic cleaning and adjustment by a professional microscope repair person also help to extend the usable life of the microscope.

ERGONOMICS

Peering into a microscope eyepiece for long periods is not an activity for which the body is well adapted. Microscope work requires the head and arms to be locked in a forward position and inclined toward the microscope with rounded shoulders. This unusual positioning is further exaggerated when the feet are placed on the ring-style footrests that are common to many laboratory stools. Poor posture and awkward positioning during microscopy can cause pain or injury to the neck, wrists, back, shoulders, and arms. In one regional survey of cytotechnologists, Kalavar and Hunting (26) found that 70.5% of respondents reported neck, shoulder, or upper back pain during microscopy and 56% had an increased prevalence of hand or wrist symptoms. Eyestrain and leg and foot discomfort have also been documented with long-term microscope use (8). When using older microscopes, users often have their heads inclined up to 45° from vertical and their upper backs may be inclined by as much as 30°. Even 30° inclinations of the head can produce significant muscle contractions, fatigue, and pain (8). For this reason, microscopists should be taught to sit upright and hold their heads in neutral positions (37).

During microscopy, the laboratorian should sit erect and maintain the natural curve of the spine (37). The lower back and shoulder blades should be supported by the chair, and a lumbar support cushion should be used if necessary. The legs and feet should rest firmly on the floor or a footrest. The chair should have a pneumatic height adjustment (29), and the seat should have a sloping front edge to prevent undue pressure on the thighs. The backrest should be adjustable for both height and angle, and the chair should have a five-pointed star base with caster wheels. Knee spaces, which are often used for laboratory storage, should be free from obstructions, and there should be a minimum of 2 inches of clearance between the thigh and the bottom of the desk or counter (26). Obstructions that prevent the microscopist from holding his or her shoulders perpendicular to the ocular axis of the microscope should be removed (29). The upper arms should be perpendicular to the floor, with the elbows close to the body. The forearms should be parallel with the floor, and the wrists should be straight. The head should be upright, and the neck should bend as little as possible, preferably no more than 10 to 15°. The eyepieces should be just below the eyes, and the eyes should look downward at a 30 to 45° angle. The use of tilting microscope heads can significantly improve the comfort of the microscopist (26, 27, 39). Repetitive motions of the hands and the contact stress of arms resting on (the edge of) a hard surface can cause pain and nerve injury, leading to repetitive stress injuries and/or carpal tunnel syndrome. The use of padded arm rests can moderate some of these problems. In addition, to prevent stiffening of the muscles during microscopy, microscopes should not be placed under an air vent.

Most laboratory microscopes are used by multiple individuals, and it is often a challenge to find conditions or microscope configurations that satisfy everyone. Some laboratories place microscopes on books or heavy blocks of wood to accommodate taller microscopists (29). This configuration creates a number of problems. If the microscope is raised to a sufficient height to prevent neck flexion, users may be forced to bend their wrists into an unnatural position. If the microscope is lowered to allow the forearms to remain parallel to the floor, the neck is forced to bend. Lowering the chair to its lowest position causes leg discomfort. Individuals of short stature may have to raise the chair to a level where their feet no longer touch the floor. Foot rests can ameliorate this problem, but some individuals may have insufficient space under the bench top to accommodate their legs. In practice, most laboratories will elect to use a suboptimum, but workable, microscope configuration that all users can employ. Under these conditions, microscopists can reduce stress and fatigue by taking 1-minute "microbreaks" every 10 to 15 minutes where they can stand, stretch, and allow the eyes to focus at a distance. More expensive solutions, including the use of ergonomic microscope tables (28, 36) that can be raised and lowered electrically (31), have been employed in some laboratories.

Eye fatigue can be a major problem for microscope users, especially if they have poor vision. The diopter adjustment provided on most microscope eyepieces can be adjusted to compensate for minor near- and farsightedness, thereby allowing users to remove their glasses during microscope use. The diopter adjustments do not adjust for astigmatism, and users with moderate to severe astigmatism should wear glasses when using the microscope. Most microscope manufacturers now produce high-eyepoint eyepieces that move the visual observation point further from the eyepiece, thereby facilitating the use of glasses during microscopy. Ensuring that the microscope images are as bright, sharp, and crisp as possible will also help to reduce eye fatigue and associated headaches. The importance of proper alignment of the microscope and optical components cannot be overstressed. Proper optical alignment and the use of newer objectives with higher NA values will produce brighter images and better resolution, which eases the strain of searching for tiny specimen details. The use of a neutral blue (daylight) filter during bright-field microscopy can also help to lessen eyestrain when examining microbiological specimens. In the future, many new microscopes will display the specimen image on a computer monitor. This innovation could alleviate many of the eyestrain problems that develop during extended microscope use (39).

Microscopes are as different as the people who use them, and the previous comments should not be construed as a prescription for alleviating strain or repetitive motion injuries in every situation. When purchasing a microscope, every effort should be made to allow microscopists to evaluate the new microscope under their normal working conditions. Some microscopes will be comfortable for some users and uncomfortable for others. In the long run, the feel and fit of the microscope are just as important as the optical characteristics.

CONCLUSION

Advances in the design, resolution, and ergonomics of modern microscopes have greatly enhanced our ability to study and identify microorganisms. Microscopy still has a central role in the detection of infectious agents despite highly publicized advances in DNA and RNA detection systems. Microscopic examination of clinical specimens provides a rapid and inexpensive "first pass" in the detection and identification of infectious agents. Thus, clinical microscopy will continue to be a core competency in clinical microbiology laboratories for the foreseeable future.

REFERENCES

1. **Abramowitz, M.** 1988. *Contrast Methods in Microscopy: Transmitted Light*, vol. 2. Olympus America, Inc., Melville, NY.
2. **Abramowitz, M.** 1993. *Fluorescence Microscopy: the Essentials*, vol. 4. Olympus America, Inc., Melville, NY.
3. **Abramowitz, M.** 1994. *Optics: a Primer*. Olympus America, Inc., Melville, NY.
4. **Abramowitz, M.** 1998. *Photomicrography: a Practical Guide*, vol. 5. Olympus America, Inc., Melville, NY.
5. **Abramowitz, M.** 2003. *Microscope: Basics and Beyond*, vol. 1. Olympus America, Inc., Melville, NY.
6. **Barer, R.** 1974. Microscopes, microscopy, and microbiology. *Annu. Rev. Microbiol.* **28:**371–389.
7. **Berland, K., K. Jacobson, T. French, and Z. Rajfur.** 2003. Electronic cameras for low-light microscopy. *Methods Cell Biol.* **72:**103–132.
8. **Chaffin, D., and G. Andersson.** 1991. *Occupational Biomechanics*. John Wiley & Sons, Inc., New York, NY.
9. **Chapin, K.** 1995. Clinical microscopy, p. 33–51. *In* P. R. Murray, E. J. Baron, M. A. Pfaller, F. C. Tenover, and R. H. Yolken (ed.), *Manual of Clinical Microbiology*, 6th ed. American Society for Microbiology, Washington, DC.
10. **Coling, D., and B. Kachar.** 2001. Theory and application of fluorescence microscopy. *Curr. Protoc. Neurosci.* **2001:**2.1.1–2.1.11.

11. **Coons, A. H., H. J. Creech, and R. N. Jones.** 1941. Immunological properties of an antibody containing a fluorescent group. *Proc. Soc. Exp. Biol. Med.* **47:**200–202.

12. **Coons, A. H., H. J. Creech, R. N. Jones. and E. Berliner.** 1942. The demonstration of a pneumococcal antigen in tissues by use of fluorescent antibody. *J. Immunol.* **45:**159–170.

13. **Coons, A. H., and M. M. Kaplan.** 1950. Localization of antigen in tissue cells. II. Improvements in a method for the detection of antigen by means of fluorescent antibody. *J. Exp. Med.* **91:**1–13.

14. **Delost, M. D.** 1997. *Introduction to Diagnostic Microbiology: a Text and Workbook*, p. 37–41. Mosby-Year Book, Inc., St. Louis, MO.

15. **Douglas, S. D.** 1985. Microscopy, p. 8–13. *In* E. H. Lennette, A. Balows, W. J. Hausler, Jr., and H. J. Shadomy (ed.), *Manual of Clinical Microbiology*, 4th ed. American Society for Microbiology, Washington, DC.

16. **Espinasse, M.** 1962. *Robert Hooke,* 2nd ed. University of California Press, Berkeley.

17. **Frischknecht, F., O. Renaud, and S. L. Shorte.** 2006. Imaging today's infectious animalcules. *Curr. Opin. Microbiol.* **9:**297–306.

18. **Fung, D. C., and J. A. Theriot.** 1998. Imaging techniques in microbiology. *Curr. Opin. Microbiol.* **1:**346–351.

19. **Gardner, P. S., and J. McQuillin.** 1974. *Rapid Virus Diagnosis: Application of Immunofluorescence,* 2nd ed. Butterworth, London, United Kingdom.

20. **Giloh, H., and J. W. Sedat.** 1982. Fluorescence microscopy: reduced photobleaching of rhodamine and fluorescein protein conjugates by n-propyl gallate. *Science* **217:**1252–1255.

21. **Goldman, M.** 1968. *Fluorescent antibody methods.* Academic Press, New York, NY.

22. **Hooke, R.** 1665. *Micrographica or Some Physiological Descriptions of Minute Bodies Made by Magnifying Glasses,* 1st ed. Royal Society of London, London, United Kingdom.

23. **Joel, F., W.-M. Leong, and A. S.-Y. Leong.** 2004. Digital imaging in pathology: theoretical and practical considerations. *Pathology* **36:**234–241.

24. **Johnson, G. D., and G. M. Nogueira Araujo.** 1981. A simple method of reducing the fading of immunofluorescence during microscopy. *J. Immunol. Methods* **43:**349–350.

25. **Johnson, G. D., R. S. Davidson, K. C. McNamee, G. Russell, D. Goodwin, and E. J. Holborow.** 1982. Fading of immunofluorescence during microscopy: a study of the phenomenon and its remedy. *J. Immunol. Methods* **55:**213–242.

26. **Kalavar, S. S., and K. L. Hunting.** 1996. Musculoskeletal symptoms among cytotechnologists. *Lab. Med.* **27:**765–769.

27. **Kofler, M., A. Kreczy, and A. Gschwendtner.** 1999. Underestimated health hazard: proposal for an ergonomic microscope workstation. *Lancet* **354:**1701–1702.

28. **Kofler, M., A. Kreczy, and A. Gschwendtner.** 2002. "Occupational backache"—surface electromyography demonstrates the advantage of an ergonomic versus a standard microscope workstation. *Eur. J. Appl. Physiol.* **86:**492–497.

29. **Murray, R. G. E.** 1994. Introduction to morphology, p. 5–20. *In* P. Gerhardt, R. G. E. Murray, W. A. Wood, and N. R. Krieg (ed.), *Methods for General and Molecular Bacteriology.* American Society for Microbiology, Washington, DC.

30. **Nairn, R. C.** 1976. *Fluorescent Protein Tracing,* 4th ed. Livingstone, London, United Kingdom.

31. **Nielen, K.** 2000. Ergonomic microscope workstation. *Lancet* **355:**502.

32. **Reid, T., A. Baldini, T. C. Rand, and D. C. Ward.** 1992. Simultaneous visualization of seven different DNA probes by *in situ* hybridization using combinatorial fluorescence and digital imaging microscopy. *Proc. Nat. Acad. Sci. USA* **89:**1388–1392.

33. **Riggs, J. L., R. J. Seiwald, J. Burckhalter, C. M. Downs, and T. G. Metcalf.** 1958. Isothiocyanate compounds as fluorescent labeling agents for immune serum. *Am. J. Pathol.* **34:**1081–1524.

34. **Riley, R. S., J. M. Ben-Ezra, D. Massey, R. L. Slyter, and G. Romagnoli.** 2004. Digital photography: a primer for pathologists. *J. Clin. Lab. Anal.* **18:**91–128.

35. **Salmon, E. D., K. von Lackum, and J. C. Canman.** 2005. Proper alignment and adjustment of the light microscope. *Curr. Protoc. Microbiol.* **2A:**1–31.

36. **Sillanpää, J., M. Nyberg, and P. Laippala.** 2003. A new table for work with a microscope, a solution to ergonomic problems. *Appl. Ergon.* **34:**621–628.

37. **Thompson, S. K., E. Mason, and S. Dukes.** 2003. Ergonomics and cytotechnologists: reported musculoskeletal discomfort. *Diagn. Cytopathol.* **29:**364–367.

38. **Tkachuk, D. C., D. Pinkel, W. L. Kuo, H. U. Weier, and J. W. Gray.** 1991. Clinical applications of fluorescence *in situ* hybridization. *Genet. Anal. Tech. Appl.* **8:**67–74.

39. **Vratney, M.** 1999. Considerations in microscope design to avoid cumulative trauma disorder in clinical laboratory applications. *Am. Clin. Lab.* **18:**8.

Systems for Detection and Identification
of Bacteria and Yeasts*

CATHY A. PETTI, MELVIN P. WEINSTEIN, AND KAREN C. CARROLL

3

Traditionally, the detection and identification of bacteria were based on conventional tube-based biochemical reactions, and their results were compared to historical charts of expected biochemical reactions. Due to the need for faster, simpler methods, manual biochemical-based testing kits and instrument-based semiautomated or automated methods were introduced. Automation in microbiology first occurred in the early 1970s with the introduction of semiautomated blood culture instruments, followed by instrumented systems for identification and susceptibility testing of bacteria. The trend toward automation accelerated with the development of automated continuous-monitoring blood culture systems (CMBCSs) and more rapid systems for antimicrobial identification and susceptibility testing. These semiautomated and automated methods rely on microorganisms' biochemical characteristics, fatty acid patterns, or other metabolic properties for their identification. Recent improvements to some automated instruments have involved the expansion of their databases and use of advanced technologies to decrease time to detection. Additionally, a few commercially available platforms have created novel decision support software that integrates identification and susceptibility test results with surveillance strategies for antimicrobial resistance and guidelines for therapy.

Nucleic acid-based platforms now have been incorporated into the routine clinical laboratory to identify microorganisms by DNA target sequencing, to detect a specific pathogen by real-time amplification techniques, or to simultaneously detect multiple pathogens by arrays. Another robust technique for microorganism identification relies on the protein composition of a bacterial cell using matrix-assisted laser desorption ionization–time-of-flight mass spectrometry (MALDI-TOF). Whether a laboratory uses manual, automated, DNA- or protein-based methods, the scientific approach to detect and identify microorganisms relies on the same fundamental principles. This chapter reviews the systems used for the detection of bacteria and yeasts from blood and provides an overview of technologies for microorganism

identification. For an expanded review and discussion of the blood culture and identification systems, the reader is referred to more detailed reviews (6, 13, 56, 75). Discussions relevant to systems for antimicrobial susceptibility testing (chapter 69), immunoassays (chapter 5), molecular diagnostics (chapter 4), and detection of mycobacteria (chapter 28) are found elsewhere in this *Manual*.

BLOOD CULTURE DETECTION SYSTEMS

The development and introduction of automated CMBCSs during the 1990s accelerated the trend away from conventional manual methods. However, the fundamental principles that provide the scientific basis for modern blood culture methods remain important, even with the new, automated technologies. The key variables are reviewed briefly. For expanded review and discussion of these issues, the reader is referred to more detailed treatises (6, 13, 66, 82, 92).

Technical Variables That Affect Blood Cultures

Volume of Blood Cultured

The volume of blood obtained for culture is one of the most important variables in the detection of bloodstream infections (BSIs) (15, 29, 67, 95). It has been well documented that BSIs in adults may be characterized by fewer than a single microorganism per 10 ml of blood. Studies have shown a direct relationship between the diagnostic yield of blood cultures and the volume of blood obtained for culture (15, 29, 78). Consensus guidelines recommend obtaining 20 to 30 ml per culture from adults (6, 13). This cannot be accomplished with the use of a single blood culture set, and laboratories that accept single sets should discourage this practice (see discussion below). The importance of volume for detecting BSIs in infants and small children has become evident in recent years as well. Isaacman et al. (37) showed that the detection rate with 6 ml of blood was double that with 2 ml of blood from the same blood sample. Kellogg et al. (38) documented that low-level bacteremia occurs in children and recommended that 4 to 4.5% of a child's blood volume be obtained for optimal detection of BSIs in this patient population. With tiny, premature infants, however, it may be impossible to obtain the volumes recommended by Kellogg et al. (38).

*This chapter contains information presented in chapter 14 by Caroline Mohr O'Hara, Melvin P. Weinstein, and J. Michael Miller in the eighth edition and chapter 15 by Melvin P. Weinstein and Karen C. Carroll in the ninth edition of this *Manual*.

Culture Medium

No one medium or commercial product is capable of optimally detecting all microorganisms. Decisions by microbiologists as to medium formulations should be based on data from well-controlled field trials in which large numbers of cultures are assessed.

Ratio of Blood to Broth

A number of substances in human blood are capable of inhibiting microbial growth, including leukocytes, complement, antibacterials, and lysozyme. Dilution of blood in broth by a ratio of at least 1:5 has been shown to enhance detection (2, 71), probably by reducing the concentrations of the natural inhibitory substances and antimicrobial agents to subinhibitory levels. Some commercial media, notably those containing resins or other additives such as activated charcoal, may have blood-to-broth ratios of less than 1:5; however, these media have been shown to have sufficiently improved recovery rates such that the suboptimal blood-to-broth ratios are overcome.

Some manufacturers have marketed "pediatric" blood culture bottles with decreased volumes of broth medium designed to maintain a blood-to-broth ratio of 1:5 to 1:10 when only small volumes of blood can be obtained from young children. The broth media in these bottles are supplemented with X and V factors to enhance the yield of *Haemophilus influenzae* and have reduced concentrations of sodium polyanethol sulfonate (SPS) for improved detection of *Neisseria* species. Although these bottles have become popular, unpublished data suggest that there is no added value in either detection of pathogens or time to positive results with pediatric bottles. Moreover, with the availability of the *H. influenzae* type b vaccine, *H. influenzae* bacteremia in children is now rare.

Anticoagulants

The yield from blood cultures may be reduced if the blood clots. Therefore, all broth-based blood culture medium formulations contain anticoagulants, the most common being SPS in concentrations of 0.025 to 0.050%. In addition to inhibiting clotting, SPS inhibits lysozyme, inactivates aminoglycoside antibiotics, and inhibits parts of the complement cascade and phagocytosis. SPS has some negative attributes, albeit fewer than some other anticoagulants used in blood culture media over the years. SPS has been shown to inhibit the growth of *Neisseria gonorrhoeae*, *Neisseria meningitidis*, *Gardnerella vaginalis*, *Streptobacillus moniliformis*, *Peptostreptococcus anaerobius*, *Francisella tularensis*, and *Moraxella catarrhalis* (25, 65, 66, 76). In general, higher concentrations of SPS have enhanced the growth of gram-positive cocci but inhibited the growth of gram-negative bacteria. Although SPS has its limitations, no other anticoagulant has been shown to be superior.

Neutralization and Inactivation of Antimicrobials

Because many patients are treated with antimicrobials before blood samples are obtained (92), potentially reducing test sensitivity, some manufacturers market media designed to bind, absorb, or inactivate these agents to enhance the yield of microorganisms. The BACTEC blood culture system (BD Diagnostics) utilizes antibiotic-binding resins on tiny glass beads, whereas the BacT/Alert blood culture system (bioMerieux, Inc., Durham, NC) uses activated charcoal. In both systems, culture media containing these additives have been shown to have improved abilities to detect microorganisms overall, especially staphylococci

and yeasts, and improved yields for patients receiving theoretically effective antimicrobial therapy (49) compared to medium formulations without the additives (19, 74, 85, 96). More coagulase-negative staphylococcal contaminants may be detected in the media containing the resins and activated charcoal than in the media without these additives (85, 96). The VersaTREK medium is said to be formulated to minimize the potential inhibitory effects of antimicrobials, and a recent study suggests that it performs well for patients on antibacterial therapy (52), although direct clinical comparisons with resin- or charcoal-supplemented media are lacking.

Atmosphere of Incubation

Traditional blood cultures have consisted of two blood culture bottles, one designed to support the growth of aerobes and facultative anaerobic bacteria and the other designed to support obligate anaerobes as well as facultative microorganisms. Aerobic blood culture bottles usually contain an ambient atmosphere in the bottle headspace to which various amounts of carbon dioxide have been added to support the growth of certain microorganisms. Anaerobic blood culture bottles usually contain carbon dioxide and nitrogen but no oxygen in the bottle. With the decrease in the proportion of bacteremias caused by obligate anaerobes in recent decades (6, 21, 46, 56), some investigators have concluded that the routine use of anaerobic blood culture bottles in a culture set is not necessary (54, 56, 99). Rather, the use of a second aerobic bottle is recommended to enhance the detection of the more common aerobic and facultative organisms and yeasts and to ensure that at least 20 ml of blood from adults will be cultured. An anaerobic bottle would be used only selectively for patients deemed at high risk for anaerobic bacteremia. However, a study using media with activated charcoal that compared two aerobic bottles with an aerobic and anaerobic pair of bottles found improved overall detection of microorganisms with the aerobic-anaerobic pair (69). A potential limitation of the study was the presence of few fungemias in the study population. Whether to use only aerobic bottles or to use a more traditional aerobic and anaerobic pair of bottles remains controversial (6, 82).

Bottle Agitation

Several studies have assessed the value of bottle agitation, documenting an enhanced yield and improved speed of detection of positive blood cultures from aerobic bottles (33, 64, 83). All of the commercially available CMBCSs agitate aerobic bottles, and most agitate anaerobic bottles as well.

Subcultures

The processing of conventional manual blood cultures includes Gram staining and blind subculturing of the aerobic culture bottles, usually after the first overnight incubation and, if the cultures remain negative, at the end of the incubation period. Subcultures are necessary for bottles that have been flagged positive by an automated instrument with a positive Gram stain. Blind subcultures of the anaerobic culture bottles in manual systems and of all bottles in instrumented systems are unnecessary (6).

Length of Incubation

In routine situations, manual blood cultures need not be incubated for more than 7 days. Five days of incubation is sufficient to detect most pathogens with CMBCSs (15, 31, 94). Some investigators have suggested that incubation periods of 4 days (18) and even 3 days (8, 30) may be sufficient for certain systems and media, but the current standard remains 5 days of incubation. With respect to patients with suspected endocarditis, a Mayo Clinic study with a CMBCS demonstrated that 99.5% of nonendocarditis BSIs and 100% of endocarditis episodes were detected within the standard 5-day incubation period (15). Similarly, with modern CMBCSs, extended incubation periods are not necessary for the detection of *Haemophilus*, *Aggregatibacter*, *Cardiobacterium*, *Eikenella*, and *Kingella* bacteria (5, 62).

Clinical Practices That Affect Blood Cultures

Skin Antisepsis and Prevention of Contamination

The probability that a positive blood culture represents infection rather than contamination is a function of the effectiveness of skin antisepsis at the time of venipuncture, or, when blood is obtained from an indwelling device, a function of the effectiveness of antisepsis of that device. For example, coagulase-negative staphylococci are common causes both of catheter-associated bacteremia and of blood culture contamination, and this medical uncertainty can confuse clinicians, leading to substantial expense (7). Thus, reducing contamination is a key issue for both the microbiology laboratory and the health care system in general. For many years, contamination rates (number of contaminated blood culture sets/total number of blood culture sets obtained) of <3% were considered the benchmark for good blood culture practices. A 1998 report from the College of American Pathologists of 640 institutions determined that the median contamination rate was 2.5% (72). In that study, the contamination rate for laboratories in the 10th percentile was 5.4% and that for laboratories in the 90th percentile was 0.9%.

The traditional recommendation for skin preparation has been the application of 70% alcohol followed by either povidone-iodine or 2% iodine tincture. Povidone-iodine preparations require 1.5 to 2 min of contact time for maximum antiseptic effect (82), whereas iodine tincture requires 0.5 min (41). Two studies have documented lower contamination rates with the use of iodine tincture rather than with an iodophor (45, 77). Recently, chlorhexidine has been recommended for use prior to venipuncture. One study demonstrated lower contamination rates with this preparation than with an iodophor (51). Another study compared chlorhexidine tincture with iodine tincture and found equivalent contamination rates (4).

Regardless of the type of skin preparation used, meticulous care and an aseptic technique are required to reduce contamination. Dedicated blood culture teams and/or phlebotomists are less likely than other health care workers to contaminate blood cultures (81). Lastly, blood samples for culture obtained by peripheral venipuncture are less likely than those obtained from indwelling catheters to grow contaminating microorganisms (11, 98).

Optimal Number of Blood Specimens for Culture

Studies with manual blood culture systems into which 20 ml of blood was inoculated for culture provided good evidence that culture of two or three blood samples will detect virtually all (≥99%) BSIs in adults (79, 91). When blood obtained from adults was inoculated into one of the CMBCSs, BSI detection rates in independent studies at different university medical centers were 96 and 97%, respectively, with culture of three 20-ml blood samples (15, 42).

Culture of a single blood sample should be discouraged. A single sample will provide insufficient blood volume for detection of many serious BSIs. Also, interpretation of a positive blood culture result can prove challenging when only a single blood culture is obtained.

Timing of Blood Cultures

Few studies have systematically addressed the timing of collection of blood for culture (68). Although bacteremia is associated with rigors, this physiological event usually precedes fever, and it is the latter that most often triggers the request for a blood culture. In a retrospective study, Li et al. (43) showed no difference in yields whether blood samples obtained during a 24-h period were drawn simultaneously or at spaced intervals. The clinician and microbiologist should be guided by the patient's clinical status and suspected diagnosis. With a septic, unstable patient, blood samples should be cultured promptly so that therapy can be instituted. Conversely, if subacute infective endocarditis is suspected in an otherwise stable patient, several blood samples can be obtained at spaced intervals.

BLOOD CULTURE SYSTEMS

Manual Systems

Only three manual blood culture systems are currently marketed in the United States: Septi-Chek (BD Diagnostics), Signal (Remel Inc., Lenexa, KS), and Isolator (Wampole Laboratories, Cranbury, NJ). Familiarity with manual blood systems is extremely important for microbiologists who serve resource-constrained regions. The Septi-Chek system originally was developed as a labor-saving alternative to conventional blood cultures, which had to be subcultured manually. It consists of a conventional aerobic broth blood culture bottle to which is attached an agar-coated paddle in a clear plastic cylinder, creating a biphasic system similar to that of the classic Castaneda bottle. After blood is inoculated into the bottle, the paddle is attached and the blood-broth mixture is inverted to flood the agar, inoculating onto the agar any microorganisms that may be present. A companion anaerobic bottle that does not use the paddle attachment, which is permeable to oxygen, can be used as well and processed manually. The bottles are incubated with or without agitation and inspected macroscopically for evidence of microbial growth once or twice daily. The agar paddle can be removed from its cylinder for better inspection. Following each examination of the agar paddle, the bottle is inverted, in effect repeating the subculture. There are several Septi-Chek broth medium formulations. The paddles contain three agars: chocolate, MacConkey, and malt. The Septi-Chek system performed well in published clinical trials (10, 63, 88–90).

The Signal is a one-bottle manual blood culture system that also was developed as a labor-saving alternative to conventional manual blood cultures. After blood is inoculated into the bottle in a conventional fashion, a clear plastic signal device is attached to the top of the bottle. An outer plastic sleeve that slides over the neck of the bottle anchors this signal device. Within the device is a long needle that extends beneath the level of the blood-broth mixture. If microbial growth occurs in the bottle, gases are produced in the bottle headspace. This creates increased atmospheric pressure, which forces some of the blood-broth mixture through the needle and into the clear plastic signal cylinder, where it can be detected visually by the microbiologist who inspects the bottles daily. Only one medium formulation has been marketed. In published controlled clinical trials done in the United States, the Signal system performed less well than its competitors (55, 83, 84, 86).

The Isolator blood culture system is unique as the only commercial system that does not utilize a broth culture medium. Rather, it is based on the principle of lysis-centrifugation. Blood is inoculated into an Isolator tube that contains a lysing solution consisting of saponin, the anticoagulant EDTA, and a fluorocarbon that acts as a cushion during the centrifugation step of blood processing. After the blood is lysed and centrifuged, the tube is placed into the Isostat system, which applies a disposable cap that penetrates the rubber stopper, permitting access to the contents of the tube. The disposable supernatant pipette is used to remove the supernatant, and the concentrate pipette is used to transfer the sediment from the tube directly to culture media that will support the growth of the pathogens of which detection is desired. The Isolator can be used for detection of routine bacterial pathogens; however, it has been reported to have a reduced ability to detect anaerobes, *Haemophilus* species, and pneumococci if specimens are not processed within 8 h (34, 35, 40, 80). The Isolator is an excellent system for detecting yeasts and dimorphic fungi, mycobacteria, and *Bartonella* species (9). The system is labor-intensive compared to the newer automated CMBCSs, especially during the initial processing of specimens in the laboratory.

Instrumented Systems

All of the commercially available CMBCSs have a number of characteristics in common. Some of the relevant information pertaining to these systems is shown in Table 1.

The CMBCSs have been adapted or modified so that they can be used to detect the growth of mycobacteria; additional information is provided in chapter 28 of this *Manual*. The CMBCSs have also been used, as have manual and earlier automated systems, to detect the growth of microorganisms from other normally sterile body fluids, for example, peritoneal fluid (28, 73).

Over two decades ago, the BacT/Alert system (bioMerieux, Inc.) was the first CMBCS to be marketed, and it currently offers robust platforms for laboratories of various sizes. At the base of each bottle is a colorimetric CO_2 sensor that is separated from the blood-broth mixture by a CO_2-semipermeable membrane that monitors the amount of CO_2 in the bottle. At the base of each bottle's holding cell in the incubator unit are light-emitting and light-sensing diodes. With microbial growth and production of CO_2, the bottle's sensor changes color, altering the amount of light reflected. The change in reflectance is measured by the instrument, and the information is transmitted to the instrument's computer. The computer has several algorithms to report the detection of a positive culture that is noted when (i) the reflectance exceeds an arbitrary threshold, (ii) the instrument recognizes a linear increase in the CO_2 level, or (iii) there is a change in the rate of CO_2 production. Several medium formulations are available: (i) standard aerobic (SA) and anaerobic (SN) media that contain 40 ml of supplemented tryptic soy broth (TSB) and accept up to 10 ml of blood; (ii) aerobic fastidious antibiotic neutralization (FAN) and anaerobic FAN media that contain 30 and 40 ml, respectively, of peptone-enriched TSB, supplemented with brain heart infusion (BHI) solids, and activated charcoal designed to inactivate or bind antimicrobial agents and other inhibitory substances in the blood; and (iii) a FAN medium with a lower volume (20 ml) of peptone-enriched TSB, supplemented with BHI solids, and activated charcoal marketed for use with pediatric patients and those elderly patients from whom it is difficult to obtain larger volumes of blood. A detailed review of published comparative clinical trials is beyond the scope of this chapter, and more comprehensive reviews can be found elsewhere (69, 87, 97). Overall, the system is equivalent to the other commercially available CMBCSs with regard to the yield and speed of detection of microorganisms (87, 97). BacT/Alert media are available in clear, shatter-resistant plastic bottles that have performance characteristics equivalent to those of glass bottles.

The BACTEC FX and 9000 series (BD Diagnostics) CMBCSs offer various instrument formats depending on the blood culture capacity needs of an individual laboratory. Similar to the BacT/Alert system, the BACTEC system features a CO_2 sensor at the base of each culture bottle, but unlike BacT/Alert, the BACTEC instrument uses a fluorescence-sensing mechanism to detect the growth of microorganisms. When the amount of CO_2 increases, the concomitant increase in fluorescence is detected by the instrument; the principal detection criteria are a linear increase in fluorescence and an increase in the rate of fluorescence. The BACTEC system has multiple medium formulations: (i) SA and SN media that contain 40 ml of soybean casein digest broth, (ii) aerobic and anaerobic Plus media that contain 25 ml of soybean casein digest broth plus antibiotic-binding resins on glass beads, (iii) an anaerobic lytic medium that contains 40 ml of soybean casein digest broth plus a lysing agent, (iv) a resin medium formulated for pediatric patients, and (v) a medium designated Myco/F-Lytic designed for improved detection of fungi and mycobacteria but which also supports the growth of bacterial pathogens. Published comparative clinical evaluations of the BACTEC 9000 system versus other CMBCSs have demonstrated that the system performs in a fashion relatively equivalent to those of its competitors in terms of both sensitivity and speed of detection of positive cultures (87).

TABLE 1 Commercially available CMBCSs

System (manufacturer)	Method for detecting growth	Type of bottles	Antibiotic inhibitor	Health care data management system	Manufacturer
BacT/ALERT 3D series	CO_2, colorimetric	Plastic	Charcoal	Yes	bioMérieux, Inc.
BACTEC FX and 9000 series	CO_2, O_2, fluorescence	Glass	Resin	Yes	BD Diagnostics
VersaTREK	Manometric	Glass	Proprietary formulation	Yes	TREK Diagnostics Systems

The VersaTREK (TREK Diagnostic Systems) blood culture system uses the same technology as its commercial predecessor, the ESP system, and differs from BacT/Alert and BACTEC 9000 in several ways. In this system, bottles are placed into the instrument and monitored with a transducer for pressure changes within the bottle headspaces as gases (oxygen, hydrogen, nitrogen, and carbon dioxide) are either produced or consumed by metabolizing microorganisms. Aerobic (REDOX 1) bottles are monitored every 12 min, and anaerobic (REDOX 2) bottles are monitored every 24 min. Pressure is plotted against time to yield growth curves, and positive cultures are signaled according to the instrument's proprietary algorithms. Aerobic bottles are agitated by vortexing of the blood-broth mixture with a small, stainless-steel stir bar within each bottle, whereas agitation is accomplished by gentle rocking in the other two systems. Anaerobic bottles are not agitated, whereas anaerobic bottles in the other two systems are agitated in the same manner as their aerobic counterparts. In the VersaTREK system, the basal culture medium is supplemented soy casein-peptone broth in the aerobic bottle and modified proteose-peptone broth in the anaerobic bottle. Overall, the VersaTREK system compared favorably with the BacT/Alert system when the BacT/Alert standard (SA/SN) media were used, with VersaTREK recovering more streptococci and enterococci as a group, and more microorganisms for patients receiving antimicrobial therapy (52).

Interpretation of Positive Blood Cultures

In most general hospitals, 8 to 14% of blood samples obtained will be positive by culture. Of the isolates in these positive blood cultures, approximately one-half will be isolates that are the causes of bacteremia or fungemia and the remainder will be contaminants or isolates of unknown clinical significance. Thus, interpretation of the clinical significance of positive blood cultures is sometimes a vexing clinical problem. Misinterpretation of positive results can be expensive for both the patient and the institution (7). Several useful criteria may assist in interpretation. These include the identity of the microorganism itself, the presence of more than a single blood culture positive for the same microorganism, and growth of the same microorganism as that found in the blood from another normally sterile site.

Microorganisms that almost always represent true infection when isolated from blood include *Staphylococcus aureus*, *Escherichia coli*, other members of the family *Enterobacteriaceae*, *Pseudomonas aeruginosa*, *Streptococcus pneumoniae*, and *Candida albicans* (92). Isolates from blood that rarely represent true bacteremia include *Corynebacterium* species, *Bacillus* species, and *Propionibacterium* species (92). Coagulase-negative staphylococci are perhaps the most problematic group with regard to interpreting clinical significance, in part because of their ubiquity and also because 12 to 15% of blood isolates are pathogens rather than contaminants (92). The number of positive culture bottles in a blood culture set is not a reliable criterion for decisions regarding the clinical significance of coagulase-negative staphylococci (53).

A useful interpretive factor is the number of culture sets that are positive relative to the number of sets obtained. If most or all sets are positive for the same microorganism(s), clinical significance is virtually assured (91). Although, ultimately, it is the physician who must make the final judgment, the microbiologist may provide important guidance regarding the clinical significance of blood isolates.

ORGANISM IDENTIFICATION SYSTEMS

Overview of Methods and Mechanisms of Identification

Historically, microorganisms were identified by what we now refer to as "conventional procedures," which include reactions in tubed media and observation of physical characteristics, such as colony morphology and odor, coupled with the results of Gram staining, agglutination tests, and antimicrobial susceptibility profiles. Over the years, identification methods simply miniaturized commonly used biochemical reactions into a more convenient format (32), and this system-dependent approach has become the industry standard. The system-dependent method relies on a set of substrates that are carefully selected for their positive and negative reactions. These patterns create metabolic profiles that are compared with established databases.

Biochemical profiles are determined by the reactions of individual organisms with each of the substrates in the system. The accuracy of the reactions is dependent upon the users' following the directions of the manufacturer regarding inoculum preparation, inoculum density, incubation conditions, and test interpretation. Most systems rely upon one or a combination of several indicators. These include (i) pH changes resulting from utilization of the substrate, (ii) enzymatic reactions that allow the release of a chromogenic or fluorogenic compound, (iii) tetrazolium-based indicators of metabolic activity in the presence of a variety of carbon sources, (iv) detection of volatile or nonvolatile acids, and (v) recognition of visible growth (Table 2). Additional tests for microbial identification that use other means of detecting a positive response for a given substrate may also be included.

Although no formal definition of "rapid" exists for describing the time required for results to be generated, most microbiologists expect rapid systems to provide usable results within 2 to 4 h of incubation. Clearly, the generation times of microbes (usually 30 min or longer) will not allow growth-dependent methods to generate detectable biochemical responses within this time. To overcome the problem of generation times, manufacturers of rapid systems use novel substrates with which preformed enzymes, produced by the organisms to be tested, may react to elicit responses detectable within 2 to 4 h.

Most recently, molecular methods that amplify particular gene targets novel enough to distinguish among genera and species and automated sequencing technology have supplanted phenotypic methods for microbial identification for difficult-to-identify microorganisms. These methods have expanded our knowledge of pathogenesis and have expanded and resolved erroneous taxonomic classifications in some cases. Where appropriate throughout this text, more detailed descriptions of molecular methods for detection and identification of pathogens are provided in discussions of particular organism groups. The future will likely see more widespread implementation of these platforms as costs decrease and technologies improve.

System Construction

Microbial identification systems are either manual or automated. Manual methods offer the advantage of using the analytical skills of the technologists for reading and interpreting the tests, whereas automated systems offer a hands-off approach, providing technologists more time for other duties. For all systems, the backbone of accuracy is the strength and utility of the database. Databases are

TABLE 2 Technologies for microorganism identification

System reactivity	Need for growth	Analyte	Indicator(s) of positive result	Example(s) of system
pH-based reactions (mostly 15–24 h)	Yes	Carbohydrate utilization	Color change due to pH indicator; carbohydrate utilization = acid pH; protein utilization or release of nitrogen-containing products = alkaline pH	API panels, Crystal panels, Vitek cards, MicroScan conventional panels, Phoenix panels, Sensititre panels
Enzyme profile (mostly 2–4 h)	No	Preformed enzymes	Color change due to chromogen or fluorogen release when colorless complex is hydrolyzed by an appropriate enzyme	MicroScan rapid panels, IDS panels, Crystal panels, Vitek cards, Phoenix panels, Sensititre panels
Carbon source utilization	Yes	Organic products	Color change as a result of metabolic activity transferring electrons to colorless tetrazolium-labeled carbon sources and converting the dye to purple	Biolog
Volatile or nonvolatile acid detection	Yes	Cellular fatty acids	Chromatographic tracing based on detection of end products, which are then compared to a library of known patterns	MIDI
Visual detection of growth	Yes	Various substrates	Turbidity due to growth of organism in the presence of a substrate	API 20C AUX panels
DNA target sequencing	No	Nucleic acid	Electropherogram or raw sequence of nucleotide bases	Laboratory developed; MicroSeq, GenBank, RDP, RIDOM, SmartGene
Mass spectrometry	No	Protein or nucleic acid	Patterns of mass signals in a spectrum	Laboratory developed; Ibis T5000, Sequenom

constructed by using known, clinically relevant strains and include the type strains of most taxa. In some cases, before an organism is added to the database, it is evaluated to confirm its relationship to other strains in the same taxon by using the likelihood fraction. This compares the biochemical characteristics of the new strain to those of a typical culture of the same species. Unusual microorganisms or common microorganisms with atypical phenotypic properties often cannot be reliably identified by commercial systems.

The number of species included in a database may vary from just a few for some manual assays to thousands for automated instruments. For most commercial systems, database maintenance is a continuous process and software upgrades incorporating major taxonomic changes are provided by the manufacturer at intervals of up to every 4 years. Some systems may allow users to make minor changes at the local workstation.

System identifications are supported by algorithm-based decision making that is generally available through a computer. Occasionally, these identifications are compiled into a preprinted index, which is used to manually convert the organism's biochemical profile number into an identification. Bayes's theorem, or modifications of it, is often the basis of algorithm construction from data matrices.

Bayes's theorem is one of the statistical methods that manufacturers use to arrive at an identification of a certain taxon based on the reaction profile produced by the unknown clinical isolate (93). Bayes's theorem considers two important issues in order to arrive at an accurate conclusion: (i) $P(t_i/R)$ is the probability that an organism exhibiting test pattern R belongs to taxon t_i, and (ii) $P(R/t_i)$ is the probability that members of taxon t_i will exhibit test

pattern R. Before testing, we make the assumption that an unknown isolate has an equal chance of being any taxon and that each test used to identify the isolate is independent of all other tests. In this case, Bayes's theorem can be written as

$$P(t_i/R) = \frac{P(R/t_i)}{\sum_i P(R/t_i)}$$

By observing reference identification charts derived by conventional biochemical tests, we know the expected pattern of the population of taxon t_i (e.g., *Escherichia coli* is indole positive and citrate negative). R in the formula is the test pattern composed of R_1, R_2, ... R_n, where R_1 is the result for test 1 and R_2 is the result for test 2, etc., for a given taxon. We can then incorporate the percentages (likelihoods that t_i will exhibit R_1, etc.) into Bayes's theorem to arrive at an accurate taxon.

Clinical microbiologists must not, however, become dependent upon these likelihoods and percentages when interpretive judgment would suggest an alternative taxonomic conclusion. Bacteria often tend to stretch the rules of nomenclature when isolated from clinical specimens, and they may not react as expected in a commercial system, even though a legitimate result is produced (e.g., lactose-positive *Salmonella* spp. or H_2S-positive *Escherichia coli*). The result from the most reliable system can be misleading. In these cases, an alternative method of identification must be used. D'Amato et al. (16) have described how the systems use the database profiles and probability matrices to arrive at an identification of an unknown taxon.

The manufacturers of commercial identification systems rely heavily on input from their customers. Laboratories are encouraged to communicate with the product manufacturer about problems such as unusual organism identifications that develop when a method or system is being used. Manufacturers depend on customer satisfaction, and most are willing to assist in problem solving or in projects that could add strength to their systems. These companies, like their users, are clearly interested in the highest quality of cost-effective patient care.

CRITERIA FOR SELECTING INSTRUMENTED SYSTEMS

Whether selecting a blood culture system or a method for identification and susceptibility testing, the laboratorian must consider several important issues. Supervisors and managers in the laboratory should make such major decisions carefully and with expert consultation. The process begins by answering key questions about the needs for a new system in the context of laboratory versus patient benefits.

Once these questions are answered, the next step is to begin the search for the right instrument or system to meet the needs of the laboratory and the medical staff. As a general rule, it is best not to be the first to purchase a new system without having seen in the peer-reviewed literature the results of evaluations performed by reputable clinical laboratories. If microbiology journals are unavailable, the manufacturer's representative can be asked to supply peer-reviewed articles about the ability of the system to correctly identify the range of isolates usually seen in the user's laboratory in the case of identification and susceptibility testing instruments or the results of well-designed, controlled comparative clinical evaluations with large numbers of observations (e.g., more than 5,000 comparisons and more than 500 positive cultures) in the case of blood culture systems. This phase requires demonstrations and conversations regarding space requirements, technical applications, manufacturer issues such as interface capabilities and service contracts, and personnel-related concerns such as sample preparation and throughput.

It is often helpful to visit other laboratories similar to one's own that are using the system under consideration to ask if they like the system, whether they would buy it again, how much downtime they have experienced, whether the service from the manufacturer has been acceptable, and whether the system has been mechanically reliable.

The laboratory should select a system that has been fully evaluated and whose accuracy exceeds 90% in its overall ability to identify common and uncommon bacteria normally seen in that particular hospital or laboratory. The system should be able to identify commonly isolated organisms with at least 95% accuracy compared with conventional methods.

The accuracy of antimicrobial susceptibility testing for combination panels is as important as the accuracy of identification, perhaps more so. Chapter 69 of this *Manual* discusses the issues involved in instrument susceptibility test methods.

EVALUATING AN INSTRUMENT OR SYSTEM

Several references provide useful information on the approach to evaluation, verification, and validation of kits, assays, and instruments in the clinical laboratory (24, 48, 50, 58, 75). When an identification system is added to the laboratory, laboratories must demonstrate that the system performs as described by the manufacturer (20, 44).

Published reports by other laboratories that have evaluated the system in a sound, scientific manner provide the first level of evidence of acceptable performance (75). Next, the purchasing laboratory must provide evidence of acceptable performance of the new identification instrument by an in-laboratory verification. Verification involves documentation of test accuracy in the laboratory where the instrument will be used (48). The Clinical Laboratory Improvement Amendments of 1988 (26) specify the conditions for systems placed into service.

Although smaller laboratories may have fewer resources than larger laboratories for verification of the accuracy of an identification system, laboratory size has no bearing on the need to ensure the accuracies of laboratory identification methods and of the work performed by a laboratory in support of patient care. The role of verification by the purchasing laboratory ensures that personnel can use the system at performance levels of accuracy already documented by the manufacturer and published in the literature. The laboratorian should expect a level of 95% agreement with the existing system or reference method and accept, in the final analysis, no less than 90% agreement. This takes into account the fact that the new system may be more accurate than the old one.

As of 1998, the Food and Drug Administration (FDA) no longer performs premarket [510(K)] evaluations to "clear" automated or manual phenotypic identification systems, nor does it receive or approve quality control protocols from these devices to meet the 1988 Clinical Laboratory Improvement Amendment requirements. Laboratorians must be aware that the identification component of the new or modified system that they are using is not cleared by the FDA because this approval is no longer required. This makes it even more important for laboratorians to search the literature for valid evaluations of their chosen instrument and to conduct their own in-house validation to make sure that the instrument meets the claims of the manufacturer regarding identification. Devices and methods incorporating probes, nucleic acid amplification, and other genetic methods, as well as the susceptibility test component of commercial instruments, will continue to be reviewed by the FDA for clearance.

LIMITATIONS OF MICROORGANISM IDENTIFICATION SYSTEMS

The databases of microbial identification systems must be revised frequently to accommodate newly named species. For example, had *Cronobacter sakazakii* (the yellow-pigmented variant of *Enterobacter cloacae*) not been added to the databases of these instruments, the clinical correlation of *C. sakazakii* with neonatal meningitis would likely be obscured if only *E. cloacae* was reported. Laboratorians must be aware that the accuracy of a system is limited to the claims of the manufacturer for the version of the database currently in the instrument and that the database may be outdated.

The laboratory procedure manual must stipulate the action to be taken when a result is questionable either because of the unusual biochemical profile of the organism or because of the appearance of an unexpected susceptibility profile. A backup method must be used to achieve an accurate identification profile. Otherwise the isolate should be sent to a reference laboratory for analysis.

The biochemical properties of closely related species may make it difficult or impossible for the algorithms of the identification process to separate these organisms accurately; however, the inability to distinguish all species within a genus does not always have a negative effect on patient outcome. For example, accurate identification of all of the newly recognized *Citrobacter* species may not be possible for some of the systems. In this case, the effect on patient outcome because of the inability of a system to recognize *Citrobacter werkmanii* may be negligible, and a simple report of "*Citrobacter* species" may provide adequate data for patient management. Such distinctions may be critical in the recognition of a potential agent of bioterrorism, and when such pathogens are suspected, laboratories should follow Laboratory Response Network protocols and not place these organisms on automated instruments. Users of automated systems should be aware of the limitations of commercial products with respect to their biopreparedness plans and substitute other tests for presumptive diagnosis per recommended guidelines (1). Microorganisms suspected of being biothreat pathogens should be referred to a public health or other reference laboratory for definitive identification.

As pathogens continue to evolve and taxonomic classifications are revised, laboratorians must pay attention to the manufacturer's communications about products, such as letters, notices, or test exclusions regarding the accuracy of their methods, as well as the published literature describing the potential problems encountered by others using these identification systems. Likewise, the user has a responsibility to report continued problems with a system or product where poor performance may lead to adverse patient outcomes.

PHENOTYPE-INDEPENDENT METHODS FOR IDENTIFICATION

Reliance on the phenotypic characteristics to identify microorganisms can be limiting, and some laboratories have embraced methods based on PCR, DNA target sequencing, antigen detection, and mass spectrometry. For a comprehensive review of these methods, please refer to chapter 4 in this *Manual*. Herein, we describe the identification of microorganisms by nonphenotypic methods from instrument-flagged blood culture bottles, and from pure culture. These methods can be more objective and faster, do not require optimal growth or even a viable microorganism, enable data exchange between centers, and may help define taxonomical relationships for microorganisms.

Instrument-Positive Blood Culture

Overall, Gram stain and subculture remain the most sensitive methods to detect most microorganisms from blood culture, but faster, culture-independent technologies have emerged to reduce the time required for identification of microorganisms from blood culture, including PCR, fluorescence in situ hybridization (FISH), and rRNA probe matrices (39, 47). FISH, an assay with peptide nucleic acid probes targeting specific 16S rRNA sequences of microorganisms, is a rapid technique for the identification of multiple clinically relevant microorganisms such as gram-positive cocci (*Staphylococcus aureus* and coagulase-negative staphylococci), gram-negative bacilli (*E. coli*, *Klebsiella pneumoniae*, and *Enterobacter cloacae*), and yeasts (*C. albicans* and *Candida tropicalis*). The sensitivity and specificity of FISH technology are reported to be between 95 and 100% (39, 59, 60). The approximate turnaround time of the FISH procedure is 2.5 to 3 h (without batch testing), compared with >18 to 24 h for identification of bacteria and yeasts by conventional methods. Of course, most laboratories usually

batch specimen testing for FISH, thereby increasing turnaround time. For instrument-positive blood cultures with compatible Gram reactions, species-specific PCR applied directly to a blood-broth aliquot has been used for the rapid detection and identification of methicillin-susceptible and methicillin-resistant *Staphylococcus aureus*, eliminating the need for an 18-h subculture. Testing for specific bacterial antigens directly from blood culture is also a technique in development.

DNA Target Sequencing

DNA target sequencing has been applied successfully to the identification of microorganisms directly from an instrument-flagged, gram-positive blood bottle and from pure culture. For a comprehensive review, refer to articles and guidelines that specifically address this topic (14, 61). The selection of DNA targets to identify bacteria and fungi relies on the concept that some genes have conserved segments flanked by variable regions. Conserved regions of gene targets are locations where PCR and DNA sequencing primers anneal. The variable regions are responsible for generating unique nucleotide base fragments or sequences that serve as the fingerprint for a particular genus and species. The gene target most commonly used for bacterial identification is 16S rRNA (16 rRNA gene or 16S ribosomal DNA), an ~1,500-bp gene that codes for a portion of the 30S ribosomal subunit. Partial (500-bp) 16S rRNA gene sequencing is used by large laboratories as a high-throughput method for accurate identification of mycobacteria, anaerobes, nonfermenting gram-negative bacilli, and most gram-positive bacteria (14). The optimal target for fungi has yet to be determined, but the internal transcribed spacer regions ITS1 and ITS2, which are variable regions located between conserved genes encoding 18S, 5.8S, and 28S rRNAs, have proven useful for identification of yeasts and medically relevant molds.

To identify the microorganism, its DNA sequence is compared to reference sequences that can be found in public and private databases. After comparing the query and reference sequences, the number of nucleotide mismatches between the two sequences is used to determine relatedness, and the final result is reported as percent identity. The acceptable degree of difference between the two sequences (i.e., percent identity) to identify a microorganism to the genus or species level is variable and depends on the DNA target and microorganism. When results from partial 16S rRNA sequencing are inconclusive, alternative DNA targets such as *rpoB* (the β-subunit of bacterial RNA polymerase), *tuf* (elongation factor Tu), *gyrA* or *gyrB* (gyrase A or B), *sodA* (manganese-dependent superoxide dismutase), or heat shock proteins often can provide better discrimination between species. Additionally, nucleotide databases must be carefully evaluated for their accuracy, quality of sequence data, frequencies of database updates, software, cost, and breadth of nucleotide entries. The Clinical and Laboratory Standards Institute published a comprehensive consensus document for identifying microorganisms to the genus and species levels by DNA target sequencing that can serve as a useful guide for laboratorians who wish to pursue or have already implemented DNA target sequencing (14). This area continues to evolve rapidly as we gain a better appreciation for the heterogeneity that exists within and between species. As bioinformatics improve and costs of sequencing decrease, genomic analysis of microorganisms by traditional Sanger sequencing, pyrosequencing, and whole-genome sequencing will become more routine for clinical laboratories and will provide invaluable information about the diversity of species, their virulence properties, and disease causation.

Mass Spectrometry

Mass spectrometry systems that are based on mass measurements of nucleic acids or proteins of bacteria have emerged as useful techniques for the detection and identification of microorganisms (27, 70). MALDI-TOF is a robust, fast, inexpensive method to detect and characterize a wide range of bacteria, including anaerobes (57), nonfermenting gram-negative bacilli (17), and staphylococci (12). The technology is based on analyzing the protein composition of a bacterial cell, with ribosomal proteins comprising most bacterial proteins being detected. Sequence variations from proteins of ribosomal origin are responsible for the various mass peaks and patterns detected with MALDI-TOF that provide a unique signature for identification at the species level. Unlike DNA target sequencing, reproducibility of protein mass patterns is affected by sample preparation, growth phase, and type of culture media. With advanced technologies and better bioinformatics, these limitations should be minimized.

Another technique to characterize bacteria is the application of electrospray ionization-mass spectrometry to analyze products of multilocus, broad-range PCR (PCR/ESI-MS) (3, 22, 23). Rather than measuring the mass of bacterial proteins, this strategy measures the masses of genomic DNA from amplification of ribosomal sequences and housekeeping genes. The masses are measured with sufficient accuracy to enable unambiguous calculation of the nucleotide compositions of the amplicons. Nucleotide compositions from multiple target sites of the microbial genome are used to identify the organisms present. This is conceptually similar to broad-range PCR followed by sequencing, except that mass spectrometry provides the base composition without knowing the order of the nucleotides. Analyzing multiple target sites on the microbial genome compensates the lower information content of nucleotide composition over sequence. The advantages are that mass spectrometry is fast, with a high throughput, and that mixed populations of microbes can be identified simultaneously. Mass spectrometry can also be used to resequence DNA using MALDI-TOF on amplified and base-specific cleavage fragments of microbial DNA. In this approach the microbial DNA is copied by PCR, followed by transcription of RNA and then enzymatic treatment. This has been used successfully for microbial genotyping of bacteria such as *Neisseria meningitidis* (36). Mass spectral cleavage products are compared to a database and pattern matching to reference sequences used to identify the strain type in a fashion similar to multilocus sequence typing. As with PCR/ESI-MS, this method also provides rapid and high-throughput analysis. For any mass spectrometry-based system, sophisticated computational tools are imperative for facile and meaningful analysis of mass spectral data.

We thank David Ecker for his thoughtful input on the mass spectrometry section.

REFERENCES

1. **American Society for Microbiology.** *Sentinel Level Clinical Laboratory Guidelines for Suspected Agents of Bioterrorism.* American Society for Microbiology, Washington, DC. http://www.asm.org/Policy/index.asp?bid=667.

2. **Auckenthaler, R., D. M. Ilstrup, and J. A. Washington II.** 1982. Comparison of recovery of organisms from blood cultures diluted 10% (volume/volume) and 20% (volume/volume). *J. Clin. Microbiol.* **15:**860–864.

3. **Baldwin, C. D., G. B. Howe, R. Sampath, L. B. Blyn, H. Matthews, V. Harpin, T. A. Hall, J. J. Drader, S. A. Hofstadler, M. W. Eshoo, K. Rudnick, K. Studarus, D. Moore, S. Abbott, J. M. Janda, and C. A. Whitehouse.** 2009. Usefulness of multilocus polymerase chain reaction followed by electrospray ionization mass spectrometry to identify a diverse panel of bacterial isolates. *Diagn. Microbiol. Infect. Dis.* **63:**403–408.

4. **Barenfanger, J., C. Drake, J. Lawhorn, and S. J. Verhulst.** 2004. Comparison of chlorhexidine and tincture of iodine for skin antisepsis in preparation for blood sample collection. *J. Clin. Microbiol.* **42:**2216–2217.

5. **Baron, E. J., J. D. Scott, and L. S. Tompkins.** 2005. Prolonged incubation and extensive subculturing do not increase recovery of clinically significant microorganisms from standard automated blood cultures. *Clin. Infect. Dis.* **41:**1677–1680.

6. **Baron, E. J., M. P. Weinstein, W. M. Dunne, Jr., P. Yagupsky, D. F. Welch, and D. M. Wilson.** 2005. *Cumitech 1C, Blood Cultures IV.* Coordinating ed., E. J. Baron. ASM Press, Washington, DC.

7. **Bates, D. W., L. Goldman, and T. H. Lee.** 1991. Contaminant blood cultures and resources utilization: the true consequences of false-positive results. *JAMA* **265:**365–369.

8. **Bourbeau, P. P., and J. K. Pohlman.** 2001. Three days of incubation may be sufficient for routine blood cultures with BacT/ALERT FAN blood culture bottles. *J. Clin. Microbiol.* **39:**2079–2082.

9. **Brenner, S. A., J. A. Rooney, P. Manzewitsch, and R. L. Regnery.** 1997. Isolation of *Bartonella (Rochalimaea) henselae*: effects of methods of blood collection and handling. *J. Clin. Microbiol.* **35:**544–547.

10. **Bryan, L. E.** 1981. Comparison of a slide blood culture system with a supplemented peptone broth culture method. *J. Clin. Microbiol.* **14:**389–392.

11. **Bryant, J. K., and C. L. Strand.** 1987. Reliability of blood cultures collected from intravascular catheter versus venipuncture. *Am. J. Clin. Pathol.* **88:**113–116.

12. **Carbonnelle, E., J. Beretti, S. Cottyn, G. Quesne, P. Berche, X. Nassif, and A. Ferroni.** 2007. Rapid identification of staphylococci isolated in clinical microbiology laboratories by matrix-assisted laser desorption ionization-time of flight mass spectrometry. *J. Clin. Microbiol.* **45:**2156–2161.

13. **Clinical and Laboratory Standards Institute.** 2007. *Principles and Procedures for Blood Cultures; Approved Guideline.* CLSI document M47-A. Clinical and Laboratory Standards Institute, Wayne, PA.

14. **Clinical and Laboratory Standards Institute.** 2008. *Interpretive Criteria for Identification of Bacteria and Fungi by DNA Target Sequencing.* CLSI document MM-18A. Clinical and Laboratory Standards Institute, Wayne, PA.

15. **Cockerill, F. R., J. W. Wilson, E. A. Vetter, K. M. Goodman, C. A. Torgerson, W. S. Harmsen, C. D. Schleck, D. M. Ilstrup, J. A. Washington II, and W. R. Wilson.** 2004. Optimal testing parameters for blood cultures. *Clin. Infect. Dis.* **38:**1724–1730.

16. **D'Amato, R. F., B. Holmes, and E. J. Bottone.** 1981. The systems approach to diagnostic microbiology. *Crit. Rev. Microbiol.* **9:**1–44.

17. **Degand, N., E. Carbonnelle, B. Dauphin, J. Beretti, M. Le Bourgeois, I. Sermet-Gaudelus, C. Segonds, P. Berche, X. Nassif, and A. Ferroni.** 2008. Matrix-assisted laser desorption ionization-time of flight mass spectrometry for identification of nonfermenting gram-negative bacilli isolated from cystic fibrosis patients. *J. Clin. Microbiol.* **46:**3361–3367.

18. **Doern, G. V., A. B. Brueggemann, W. M. Dunne, S. G. Jenkins, D. C. Halstead, and J. C. McLaughlin.** 1997. Four-day incubation period for blood culture bottles processed with the Difco ESP blood culture system. *J. Clin. Microbiol.* **35:**1290–1292.

19. **Doern, G. V., A. Barton, and S. Rao.** 1998. Controlled comparative evaluation of BacT/ALERT FAN and ESP 80A

aerobic media as means for detecting bacteremia and fungemia. *J. Clin. Microbiol.* **36:**2686–2689.

20. **Donay, J. L., D. Mathieu, P. Fernandes, C. Pregermain, P. Bruel, A. Wargnier, I. Casin, F. X. Weill, P. H. Lagrange, and J. L. Herrmann.** 2004. Evaluation of the automated Phoenix system for potential routine use in the clinical microbiology laboratory. *J. Clin. Microbiol.* **42:**1542–1546.

21. **Dorsher, C. W., J. E. Rosenblatt, W. R. Wilson, and D.M. Ilstrup.** 1991. Anaerobic bacteremia: decreasing rate over a 15 year period. *Rev. Infect. Dis.* **13:**633–636.

22. **Ecker, D. J., R. Sampath, L. B. Blyn, M. W. Eshoo, C. Ivy, J. A. Ecker, B. Libby, V. Samant, K. A. Sannes-Lowery, R. E. Melton, K. Russell, N. Freed, C. Barrozo, J. Wu, K. Rudnick, A. Desai, E. Moradi, D. J. Knize, D. W. Robbins, J. C. Hannis, P. M. Harrell, C. Massire, T. A. Hall, Y. Jiang, R. Ranken, J. J. Drader, N. White, J. A. McNeil, S. T. Crooke, and S. A. Hofstadler.** 2005. Rapid identification and strain-typing of respiratory pathogens for epidemic surveillance. *Proc. Natl. Acad. Sci. USA* **102:**8012–8017.

23. **Ecker, D. J., R. Sampath, C. Massire, L. B. Blyn, T. A. Hall, M. W. Eshoo, and S. A. Hofstadler.** 2008. Ibis T5000: a universal biosensor approach for microbiology. *Nat. Rev. Microbiol.* **6:**553–558.

24. **Edberg, S. C., and L. S. Konowe.** 1982. A systematic means to conduct a microbiology evaluation, p. 268–299. *In* V. Lorian (ed.), *Significance of Medical Microbiology in the Care of Patients,* 2nd ed. The Williams & Wilkins Co., Baltimore, MD.

25. **Eng, J.** 1975. Effect of sodium polyanethol sulfonate in blood cultures. *J. Clin. Microbiol.* **1:**119–123.

26. **Federal Register.** 1992. Clinical Laboratory Improvement Amendments of 1988, final rule. *Fed. Regist.* **57:**7164.

27 **Freiwald, A., and S. Sauer.** 2009. Phylogenetic classification and identification of bacteria by mass spectrometry. *Nat. Protocols* **4:**732–742.

28. **Fuller, D. D., and T. E. Davis.** 1997. Comparison of BACTEC Plus Aerobic/F, Anaerobic/F, Peds Plus/F, and Lytic/F media with and without fastidious organism supplement to conventional methods for culture of sterile body fluids. *Diagn. Microbiol. Infect. Dis.* **29:**219–225.

29 **Hall, M. M., D. M. Ilstrup, and J. A. Washington II.** 1976. Effect of volume of blood cultured on detection of bacteremia. *J. Clin. Microbiol.* **3:**643–645.

30. **Han, X. Y., and A. L. Truant.** 1999. The detection of positive blood cultures by the AccuMed ESP-384 system: the clinical significance of three-day testing. *Diagn. Microbiol. Infect. Dis.* **33:**1–6.

31. **Hardy, D. J., B. B. Hulbert, and P. C. Migneault.** 1992. Time to detection of positive BacT/ALERT blood cultures and lack of need for routine subculture of 5- to 7-day negative cultures. *J. Clin. Microbiol.* **30:**2743–2745.

32. **Hartman, P. A.** 1968. *Miniaturized Microbiological Methods.* Academic Press, Inc., New York, NY.

33. **Hawkins, B. L., E. M. Peterson, and L. M. de la Maza.** 1986. Improvement of positive blood culture detection by agitation. *Diagn. Microbiol. Infect. Dis.* **5:**207–213.

34. **Henry, N. K., C. M. Grewell, P. E. Van Grevenhof, D. M. Ilstrup, and J. A. Washington II.** 1984. Comparison of lysis-centrifugation with a biphasic blood culture medium for the recovery of aerobic and facultatively anaerobic bacteria. *J. Clin. Microbiol.* **20:**413–416.

35. **Henry, N. K., C. A. McLimans, A. J. Wright, R. L. Thompson, W. R. Wilson, and J. A. Washington II.** 1983. Microbiological and clinical evaluation of the Isolator lysis-centrifugation blood culture tube. *J. Clin. Microbiol.* **17:**864–869.

36. **Honisch, C., Y. Chen, C. Mortimer, C. Arnold, O. Schmidt, D. van den Boom, C. R. Cantor, H. N. Shah, and S. E. Gharbi.** 2007. Automated comparative sequence analysis by base-specific cleavage and mass spectrometry for nucleic acid-based microbial typing. *Proc. Natl. Acad. Sci. USA* **104:**10649–10654.

37. **Isaacman, D. J., R. B. Karasic, E. A. Reynolds, and S. I. Kost.** 1996. Effect of number of blood cultures and volume of blood on detection of bacteremia in children. *J. Pediatr.* **128:**190–195.

38. **Kellogg, J. A., J. P. Manzella, and D. A. Bankert.** 2000. Frequency of low-level bacteremia in children from birth to fifteen years of age. *J. Clin. Microbiol.* **38:**2181–2185.

39. **Kempf, V. A., K. Trebesius, and I. B. Autenrieth.** 2000. Fluorescent in situ hybridization allows rapid identification of microorganisms in blood cultures. *J. Clin. Microbiol.* **38:**830–838.

40. **Kiehn, T. E., B. Wong, F. F. Edwards, and D. Armstrong.** 1983. Comparative recovery of bacteria and yeasts from lysis-centrifugation and a conventional blood culture system. *J. Clin. Microbiol.* **18:**300–304.

41. **King, T. C., and P. B. Price.** 1963. An evaluation of iodophors as skin antiseptics. *Surg. Gynecol. Obstet.* **116:**361–365.

42. **Lee, A., S. Mirrett, L. B. Reller, and M. P. Weinstein.** 2007. Detection of bloodstream infections in adults: how many blood cultures are needed? *J. Clin. Microbiol.* **45:**3546–3548.

43. **Li, J., J. J. Plorde, and L. G. Carlson.** 1994. Effects of volume and periodicity on blood cultures. *J. Clin. Microbiol.* **32:**2829–2831.

44. **Linde, H. J., H. Neubauer, H. Meyer, S. Aleksic, and N. Lehn.** 1999. Identification of *Yersinia* species by the Vitek GNI card. *J. Clin. Microbiol.* **37:**211–214.

45. **Little, J. R., P. R. Murray, P. Traynor, and E. Spitznagel.** 1999. A randomized trial of povidone-iodine compared with iodine tincture for venipuncture site disinfection: effects on rates of blood culture contamination. *Am. J. Med.* **107:**119–125.

46. **Lombardi, D. P., and N. C. Engleberg.** 1992. Anaerobic bacteremia: incidence, patient characteristics, and clinical significance. *Am. J. Med.* **92:**53–60.

47. **Marlowe, E. M., J. J. Hogan, J. F. Hindler, I. Andruszkiewicz, P. Gordon, and D. A. Bruckner.** 2003. Application of an rRNA probe matrix for rapid identification of bacteria and fungi from routine blood cultures. *J. Clin. Microbiol.* **41:**5127–5133.

48. **McCurdy, B. W., B. L. Elder, S. A. Hansen, J. A. Kellogg, F. J. Marsik, and R. J. Zabransky.** 1997. *Cumitech 31, Verification and Validation of Procedures in the Clinical Microbiology Laboratory.* Coordinating ed., B. W. McCurdy. American Society for Microbiology, Washington, DC.

49. **McDonald, L. C., J. Fune, L. D. Guido, M. P. Weinstein, L. G. Reimer, T. M. Flynn, M. L. Wilson, S. Mirrett, and L. B. Reller.** 1996. Clinical importance of the increased sensitivity of BacT/Alert FAN aerobic and anaerobic blood culture bottles. *J. Clin. Microbiol.* **34:**2180–2184.

50. **Miller, J. M.** 1991. Evaluating biochemical identification systems. *J. Clin. Microbiol.* **29:**1559–1561.

51. **Mimoz, O., A. Karim, A. Mercat, M. Cosseron, B. Falissard, F. Parker, C. Richard, K. Samii, and P. Nordmann.** 1999. Chlorhexidine compared with povidone-iodine as skin preparation before blood culture: a randomized, controlled trial. *Ann. Intern. Med.* **131:**834–837.

52. **Mirrett, S., K. E. Hanson, and L. B. Reller.** 2007. Controlled clinical comparison of VersaTREK and BacT/ALERT blood culture systems. *J. Clin. Microbiol.* **45:**299–302.

53. **Mirrett, S., M. P. Weinstein, L. G. Reimer, M. L. Wilson, and L. B. Reller.** 2001. Relevance of the number of positive bottles in determining clinical significance of coagulase-negative staphylococci in blood cultures. *J. Clin. Microbiol.* **39:**3279–3281.

54. **Morris, A. J., M. L. Wilson, S. Mirrett, and L. B. Reller.** 1993. Rationale for selective use of anaerobic blood cultures. *J. Clin. Microbiol.* **31:**2110–2113.

55. **Murray, P. R., A. C. Niles, R. L. Heeren, M. M. Curren, L. E. James, and J. E. Hoppe-Bauer.** 1988. Comparative evaluation of the Oxoid Signal and Roche Septi-Chek blood culture systems. *J. Clin. Microbiol.* **26:**2526–2530.

56. **Murray, P. R., P. Traynor, and D. Hopson.** 1992. Critical assessment of blood culture techniques: analysis of recovery of obligate and facultative anaerobes, strict aerobic bacteria, and fungi in aerobic and anaerobic blood culture bottles. *J. Clin. Microbiol.* **30:**1462–1468.

57. **Nagy, E., T. Maier, E. Urban, G. Terhes, and M. Kostrzewa on behalf of the ECSMID Study Group on Antimicrobial Resistance in Anaerobic Bacteria.** 11 May 2009. Species identification of clinical isolates of *Bacteroides* by matrix-assisted

laser-desorption/ionization time-of-flight mass spectrometry. *Clin. Microbiol. Infect.* [Epub ahead of print.]

58. **NCCLS.** 2002. *Evaluation of Qualitative Test Performance; Approved Guideline.* NCCLS document EP-12A. NCCLS, Wayne, PA.

59. **Peters, R. P., P. H. M. Savelkoul, A. M. Simoons-Smit, S. A. Danner, C. M. Vandenbroucke-Grauls, and M. A. van Agtmael.** 2006. Faster identification of pathogens in positive blood cultures by fluorescence in situ hybridization in routine practice. *J. Clin. Microbiol.* **44:**119–123.

60. **Peters, R. P., M. A. van Agtmael, A. M. Simoons-Smit, S. A. Danner, C. M. Vandenbroucke-Grauls, and P. H. Savelkoul.** 2006. Rapid identification of pathogens in blood cultures with a modified fluorescence in situ hybridization assay. *J. Clin. Microbiol.* **44:**4186–4188.

61. **Petti, C. A.** 2007. Detection and identification of microorganisms by gene amplification and sequencing. *Clin. Infect. Dis.* **44:**1108–1114.

62. **Petti, C. A., H. S. Bhally, M. P. Weinstein, K. Joho, T. Wakefield, L. B. Reller, and K. C. Carroll.** 2006. Utility of extended blood culture incubation for isolation of *Haemophilus, Actinobacillus, Cardiobacterium, Eikenella,* and *Kingella* organisms: a retrospective multicenter evaluation. *J. Clin. Microbiol.* **44:**257–259.

63. **Pfaller, M. A., T. K. Sibley, L. M. Westfall, J. E. Hoppe-Bauer, M. A. Keating, and P. R. Murray.** 1982. Clinical laboratory comparison of a slide blood culture system with a conventional broth system. *J. Clin. Microbiol.* **16:**525–530.

64. **Prag, J., M. Nir, J. Jensen, and M. Arpi.** 1991. Should aerobic blood cultures be shaken intermittently or continuously? *APMIS* **99:**1078–1082.

65. **Reimer, L. G., and L. B. Reller.** 1985. Effect of sodium polyanetholesulfate on the recovery of *Gardnerella vaginalis* from blood culture media. *J. Clin. Microbiol.* **21:**686–688.

66. **Reimer, L. G., M. L. Wilson, and M. P. Weinstein.** 1997. Update on detection of bacteremia and fungemia. *Clin. Microbiol. Rev.* **10:**444–465.

67. **Reller, L. B., P. R. Murray, and J. D. MacLowry.** 1982. *Cumitech 1A, Blood Cultures II.* Coordinating ed., J. A. Washington II. American Society for Microbiology, Washington, DC.

68. **Riedel, S., P. Bourbeau, B. Swartz, S. Brecher, K. C. Carroll, P. D. Stamper, W. M. Dunne, T. McCardle, N. Walk, K. Fiebelkorn, D. Sewell, S. S. Richter, S. Beekmann, and G. V. Doern.** 2008. Timing of specimen collection of blood cultures from febrile patients with bacteremia. *J. Clin. Microbiol.* **46:**1381–1385.

69. **Riley, J. A., B. J. Heiter, and P. P. Bourbeau.** 2003. Comparison of recovery of blood culture isolates from two BacT/ALERT FAN aerobic blood culture bottles with recovery from one FAN aerobic bottle and one FAN anaerobic bottle. *J. Clin. Microbiol.* **41:**1399–1403.

70. **Russell, S. C.** 2009. Microorganism characterization by single particle mass spectrometry. *Mass Spect. Rev.* **28:**376–387.

71. **Salventi, J. F., T. A. Davies, E. L. Randall, S. Whitaker, and J. R. Waters.** 1979. Effect of blood dilution on recovery of organisms from clinical blood cultures in medium containing sodium polyanethol sulfonate. *J. Clin. Microbiol.* **9:**248–252.

72. **Schiffman, R. B., C. L. Strand, F. A. Meier, and P. J. Howantiz.** 1998. Blood culture contamination: a College of American Pathologists Q-Probes study involving 640 institutions and 497,134 specimens from adults. *Arch. Pathol. Lab. Med.* **122:**216–221.

73. **Simor, A. E., K. Scythes, H. Meaney, and M. Louie.** 2000. Evaluation of the Bac-T/ALERT microbial detection system with FAN aerobic and FAN anaerobic bottles for culturing normally sterile body fluids other than blood. *Diagn. Microbiol. Infect. Dis.* **37:**5–9.

74. **Smith, J. A., E. A. Bryce, J. H. Ngui-Yen, and F. J. Roberts.** 1995. Comparison of BACTEC 9240 and BacT/ALERT blood culture systems in an adult hospital. *J. Clin. Microbiol.* **33:**1905–1908.

75. **Stager, C. E., and J. R. Davis.** 1992. Automated systems for identification of microorganisms. *Clin. Microbiol. Rev.* **5:**302–327.

76. **Staneck, J. L., and S. Vincent.** 1981. Inhibition of *Neisseria gonorrhoeae* by sodium polyanetholesulfonate. *J. Clin. Microbiol.* **13:**463–467.

77. **Strand, C. L., R. R. Wajsbort, and K. Sturmann.** 1993. Effect of iodophor vs. iodine tincture skin preparation on blood culture contamination rate. *JAMA* **269:**1004–1006.

78. **Tenney, J. H., L. B. Reller, S. Mirrett, and W.-L. L. Wang.** 1982. Controlled evaluation of the volume of blood cultured in detection of bacteremia and fungemia. *J. Clin. Microbiol.* **15:**558–561.

79. **Washington, J. A., II.** 1975. Blood cultures: principles and techniques. *Mayo Clin. Proc.* **50:**91–98.

80. **Washington, J. A., II, and D. M. Ilstrup.** 1986. Blood cultures: issues and controversies. *Rev. Infect. Dis.* **8:**792–802.

81. **Weinbaum, F. I., S. Lavie, M. Danek, D. Sixsmith, G. F. Heinrich, and S. S. Mills.** 1997. Doing it right the first time: quality improvement and the contaminant blood culture. *J. Clin. Microbiol.* **35:**53–55.

82. **Weinstein, M. P.** 1996. Current blood culture methods and systems: clinical concepts, technology, and interpretation of results. *Clin. Infect. Dis.* **23:**40–46.

83. **Weinstein, M. P., S. Mirrett, L. G. Reimer, and L. B. Reller.** 1989. Effect of agitation and terminal subcultures on yield and speed of detection of the Oxoid Signal blood culture system versus the BACTEC radiometric system. *J. Clin. Microbiol.* **27:**427–430.

84. **Weinstein, M. P., S. Mirrett, L. G. Reimer, and L. B. Reller.** 1990. Effect of altered headspace atmosphere on yield and speed of detection of the Oxoid Signal blood culture system versus the BACTEC radiometric system. *J. Clin. Microbiol.* **28:**795–797.

85. **Weinstein, M. P., S. Mirrett, L. G. Reimer, M. L. Wilson, S. Smith-Elekes, C. R. Chuard, K. L. Joho, and L. B. Reller.** 1995. Controlled evaluation of BacT/ALERT standard aerobic and FAN aerobic blood culture bottles for detection of bacteremia and fungemia. *J. Clin. Microbiol.* **33:**978–981.

86. **Weinstein, M. P., S. Mirrett, and L. B. Reller.** 1988. Comparative evaluation of the Oxoid Signal and BACTEC radiometric blood culture systems for the detection of bacteremia and fungemia. *J. Clin. Microbiol.* **26:**962–964.

87. **Weinstein, M. P., and L. B. Reller.** 2002. Commercial blood culture systems and methods, p. 12–21. *In* A. L. Truant (ed.), *Manual of Commercial Methods in Clinical Microbiology.* ASM Press, Washington, DC.

88. **Weinstein, M. P., L. B. Reller, S. Mirrett, C. W. Stratton, L. G. Reimer, and W.-L. L. Wang.** 1986. Controlled evaluation of the agar slide and radiometric blood culture systems for the detection of bacteremia and fungemia. *J. Clin. Microbiol.* **23:**221–225.

89. **Weinstein, M. P., L. B. Reller, S. Mirrett, W.-L. L. Wang, and D. V. Alcid.** 1985. Controlled evaluation of Trypticase soy broth in agar slide and conventional blood culture systems. *J. Clin. Microbiol.* **21:**626–629.

90. **Weinstein, M. P., L. B. Reller, S. Mirrett, W.-L. L. Wang, and D. V. Alcid.** 1985. Clinical comparison of an agar slide blood culture system with Trypticase soy broth and a conventional blood culture bottle with supplemented peptone broth. *J. Clin. Microbiol.* **21:**815–818.

91. **Weinstein, M. P., L. B. Reller, J. R. Murphy, and K. A. Lichtenstein.** 1983. The clinical significance of positive blood cultures: a comprehensive analysis of 500 episodes of bacteremia and fungemia in adults. I. Laboratory and epidemiologic observations. *Rev. Infect. Dis.* **5:**35–53.

92. **Weinstein, M. P., M. L. Towns, S. M. Quartey, S. Mirrett, L. G. Reimer, G. Parmagiani, and L. B. Reller.** 1997. The clinical significance of positive blood cultures in the 1990s: a prospective comprehensive evaluation of the microbiology, epidemiology, and outcome of bacteremia and fungemia in adults. *Clin. Infect. Dis.* **24:**584–602.

93. **Willcox, W. R., S. P. Lapage, S. Bascomb, and M. A. Curtis.** 1973. Identification of bacteria by computer: theory and programming. *J. Gen. Microbiol.* **77:**317–330.

94. **Wilson, M. L., S. Mirrett, L. B. Reller, M. P. Weinstein, and L. G. Reimer.** 1993. Recovery of clinically important

microorganisms from the BacT/ALERT blood culture system does not require testing for 7 days. *Diagn. Microbiol. Infect. Dis.* **16:**31–34.

95. **Wilson, M. L., and M. P. Weinstein.** 1994. General principles in the laboratory detection of bacteremia and fungemia. *Clin. Lab. Med.* **14:**69–82.

96. **Wilson, M. L., M. P. Weinstein, S. Mirrett, L. G. Reimer, S. Smith-Elekes, C. R. Chuard, and L. B. Reller.** 1995. Controlled evaluation of BacT/ALERT standard anaerobic and FAN anaerobic blood culture bottles for the detection of bacteremia and fungemia. *J. Clin. Microbiol.* **33:**2265–2270.

97. **Wilson, M. L., M. P. Weinstein, L. G. Reimer, S. Mirrett, and L. B. Reller.** 1992. Controlled comparison of the BacT/ALERT and BACTEC 660/730 nonradiometric blood culture systems. *J. Clin. Microbiol.* **30:**323–329.

98. **Wormser, G., I. M. Onorato, T. J. Preminger, D. Culver, and W. J. Martone.** 1990. Sensitivity and specificity of blood cultures obtained through intravascular catheters. *Crit. Care Med.* **18:**152–156.

99. **Zaidi, A. K. M., A. L. Knaut, S. Mirrett, and L. B. Reller.** 1995. Value of routine anaerobic blood cultures for pediatric patients. *J. Pediatr.* **127:**263–268.

Molecular Microbiology

FREDERICK S. NOLTE AND ANGELA M. CALIENDO

4

Since the publication of the ninth edition of this *Manual*, significant changes have occurred in the practice of diagnostic molecular microbiology. Nucleic acid amplification techniques are commonly used to diagnose and manage patients with infectious diseases. The growth in the number of commercially available test kits and analyte-specific reagents (ASRs) has facilitated the use of this technology in the clinical laboratory. Technological advances in real-time PCR techniques, automation, nucleic acid sequencing, multiplex analysis, and mass spectrometry have reinvigorated the field and created new opportunities for growth.

Molecular microbiology is the leading area in molecular pathology in terms of both the numbers of tests performed and clinical relevance. This technology has reduced the dependency of the clinical microbiology laboratory on culture-based methods and created new opportunities for the clinical laboratory to affect patient care. This chapter covers amplified- and nonamplified-probe techniques, post-amplification detection and analysis, clinical applications of these techniques, and the special challenges and opportunities that these techniques provide for the clinical laboratory. Molecular methods used in epidemiological investigations are covered in chapter 8. A more comprehensive discussion of many of the topics covered in this chapter is found in *Molecular Microbiology: Diagnostic Principles and Practice*, 2nd ed. (129).

NONAMPLIFIED NUCLEIC ACID PROBES

Nucleic acid probes are segments of DNA or RNA labeled with radioisotopes, enzymes, or chemiluminescent reporter molecules that can bind to complementary nucleic acid sequences with high degrees of specificity. Although probes can range from 15 to thousands of nucleotides in size, synthetic oligonucleotides of less than 50 nucleotides are most commonly incorporated into commercial kits. The probes can be designed to identify microorganisms at any taxonomic level. A number of commercially available DNA probes have been developed for direct detection of pathogens in clinical specimens and identification of pathogens after isolation by culture.

The commonly used formats for probe hybridization include liquid-phase, solid-phase, and in situ hybridization. The leading method used in clinical microbiology laboratories is a liquid-phase hybridization protection assay (Gen-Probe, Inc., San Diego, CA). In this method, a single-stranded DNA (ssDNA) probe labeled with an acridinium ester is incubated with the target nucleic acid. Alkaline hydrolysis follows the hybridization step, and probe binding is measured in a luminometer after the addition of peroxides. For a positive sample, the acridinium ester on the bound probe is protected from hydrolysis and, upon the addition of peroxides, emits light. The hybridization protection assay can be completed in several hours and does not require removal of unbound single-stranded probe or isolation of probe-bound double-stranded sequences (3).

In solid-phase hybridization, target nucleic acids are bound to nylon or nitrocellulose and are hybridized with a probe in solution (164). The unbound probe is washed away, and the bound probe is detected by means of fluorescence, luminescence, radioactivity, or color development. Although solid-phase hybridization is a powerful research tool, the length of time required and the complexity of the procedure limit its application in clinical practice.

In situ hybridization is another type of solid-phase hybridization in which the nucleic acid is contained in tissues or cells which are affixed to microscope slides and is governed by the same basic principles as described previously (55). In most clinical applications, formalin-fixed, paraffin-embedded tissue sections are used. The sensitivity of in situ hybridization is often limited by the accessibility of the target nucleic acid in the cells.

In general, due to the poor analytical sensitivities of nonamplified-probe techniques, the application of these techniques to direct detection of pathogens in clinical specimens is limited to those situations in which the number of organisms is large. Such situations include cases of group A streptococcal pharyngitis, genital tract infections with *Neisseria gonorrhoeae* and *Chlamydia trachomatis*, and agents associated with vaginosis and vaginitis. These techniques are used most effectively in culture confirmation assays for mycobacteria and systemic dimorphic fungi. These culture confirmation tests have a positive effect on patient management by providing rapid and accurate detection of these slowly growing, often difficult-to-identify pathogens.

Nucleic acid probes for direct detection of group A streptococci, *C. trachomatis*, and *N. gonorrhoeae* are available from Gen-Probe. Probes for identification of *Blastomyces dermatitidis*, *Coccidioides immitis*, *Histoplasma capsulatum*, campylobacters, enterococci, group A streptococci, group B streptococci, *Haemophilus influenzae*, *Listeria monocytogenes*, mycobacteria, *N. gonorrhoeae*, *Staphylococcus aureus*, and *Streptococcus pneumoniae* isolated in culture are also available from Gen-Probe.

A solid-phase nucleic acid probe test for detection and identification of *Gardnerella vaginalis*, *Trichomonas vaginalis*, and *Candida albicans* in vaginal fluid from patients with vaginosis or vaginitis is available from BD Diagnostic Systems, Sparks, MD. It uses two distinct probes for each organism, a capture probe and a color development probe, in an easy-to-use format.

Peptide nucleic acid (PNA) probes are DNA mimics in which the negatively charged sugar phosphate backbone of DNA is replaced with a noncharged polyamide or "peptide" backbone. PNA probes contain the same nucleotide bases as DNA and follow standard Watson-Crick base pairing rules when hybridizing to complementary nucleic acid sequences (153). Because PNA probes are noncharged, they do not have to overcome the destabilizing electrostatic repulsion that occurs when two negatively charged DNA molecules hybridize. As a result, PNA probes bind more rapidly and tightly to nucleic acid targets. In addition, the relatively hydrophobic character of the PNA probes enables them to penetrate the hydrophobic cell membrane following preparation of a standard smear.

PNA probes have been used for identification of *S. aureus*, *Escherichia coli*, *Pseudomonas aeruginosa*, and *Candida albicans* directly from positive blood culture bottles (120, 135, 150) and direct detection of *Mycobacterium tuberculosis* in smear-positive sputum samples (154). PNA probes for rapid, direct identification of *S. aureus*, coagulase-negative staphylococci, *Enterococcus faecalis*, *Escherichia coli*, *Pseudomonas aeruginosa*, and *Candida* spp. from positive blood culture bottles and *Streptococcus agalactiae* from Lim broth cultures are available from AdvanDx, Woburn, MA (106, 145, 150).

TECHNIQUES USING AMPLIFIED NUCLEIC ACIDS

The development of the PCR by Saiki et al. (140) was a milestone in biotechnology and heralded the beginning of molecular diagnostics. PCR had its 20th birthday in 2005 and has stood the test of time. Although PCR is the best-developed and most widely used nucleic acid amplification strategy, other strategies have been developed, and several have clinical utility. These strategies are based on signal, target, or probe amplification. Examples of each category are discussed in the sections that follow. These techniques have sensitivity unparalleled in laboratory medicine, have created new opportunities for the clinical laboratory to have an effect on patient care, and have become the new "gold standards" for laboratory diagnosis of many infectious diseases.

SIGNAL AMPLIFICATION TECHNIQUES

In signal amplification methods, the concentration of the probe or target does not increase. The increased analytical sensitivity comes from increasing the concentration of labeled molecules attached to the target nucleic acid. Multiple enzymes, multiple probes, multiple layers of probes, and reduction of background noise have all been used to enhance target detection (74). Target amplification systems generally have greater analytical sensitivity than signal amplification methods, but technological developments, particularly in branched-DNA (bDNA) assays, have lowered

the limits of detection to levels that may rival those of target amplification assays in some applications (69).

Signal amplification assays have several advantages over target amplification assays. In signal amplification systems, the number of target molecules is not altered, and as a result, the signal is directly proportional to the amount of the target sequence present in the clinical specimen. This reduces concerns about false-positive results due to cross contamination and simplifies the development of quantitative assays. Since signal amplification systems are not dependent on enzymatic processes to amplify the target sequence, they are not affected by the presence of enzyme inhibitors in clinical specimens. Consequently, less cumbersome nucleic acid extraction methods may be used. Typically, signal amplification systems use either larger probes or more probes than target amplification systems and, consequently, are less susceptible to errors resulting from target sequence heterogeneity. Finally, RNA levels can be measured directly without the synthesis of a cDNA intermediate.

bDNA Assays

The bDNA signal amplification system is a solid-phase, sandwich hybridization assay incorporating multiple sets of synthetic oligonucleotide probes (114). The key to this technology is the amplifier molecule, a bDNA molecule with 15 identical branches, each of which can bind to three labeled probes.

The bDNA signal amplification system is illustrated in Fig. 1. Multiple target-specific probes are used to capture the target nucleic acid onto the surface of a microtiter well. A second set of target-specific probes also binds to the target. Preamplifier molecules bind to the second set of target probes and up to eight bDNA amplifiers. Three alkaline phosphatase-labeled probes hybridize to each branch of the amplifier. Detection of bound labeled probes is achieved by incubating the complex with dioxetane, an enzyme-triggerable substrate, and measuring the light emission in a luminometer. The resulting signal is directly proportional to the quantity of the target in the sample. The quantity of the target in the sample is determined from an external standard curve.

Nonspecific hybridization of any of the amplification probes and nontarget nucleic acids leads to amplification of the background signal. In order to reduce potential hybridization to nontarget nucleic acids, isocytidine (isoC) and isoguanosine (isoG) were incorporated into the preamplifier and labeled probes were used in the third-generation bDNA assays (23). IsoC and isoG form base pairs with each other but not with any of the four naturally occurring bases (130).

The use of isoC- and isoG-containing probes in bDNA assays increases target-specific signal amplification without a concomitant increase in the background signal, thereby greatly enhancing the detection limits without loss of specificity. The detection limit of the third-generation bDNA assay for human immunodeficiency virus type 1 (HIV-1) RNA is 75 copies/ml. bDNA assays for the quantification of hepatitis B virus (HBV) DNA, hepatitis C virus (HCV) RNA, and HIV-1 RNA are commercially available (Siemens Healthcare Diagnostics, Deerfield, IL). The System 340 and 440 analyzers for bDNA assays automate the incubation, washing, reading, and data processing steps.

Hybrid Capture Assays

The hybrid capture system is a solution hybridization-antibody capture method that uses chemiluminescence detection of the hybrid molecules. The target DNA in the

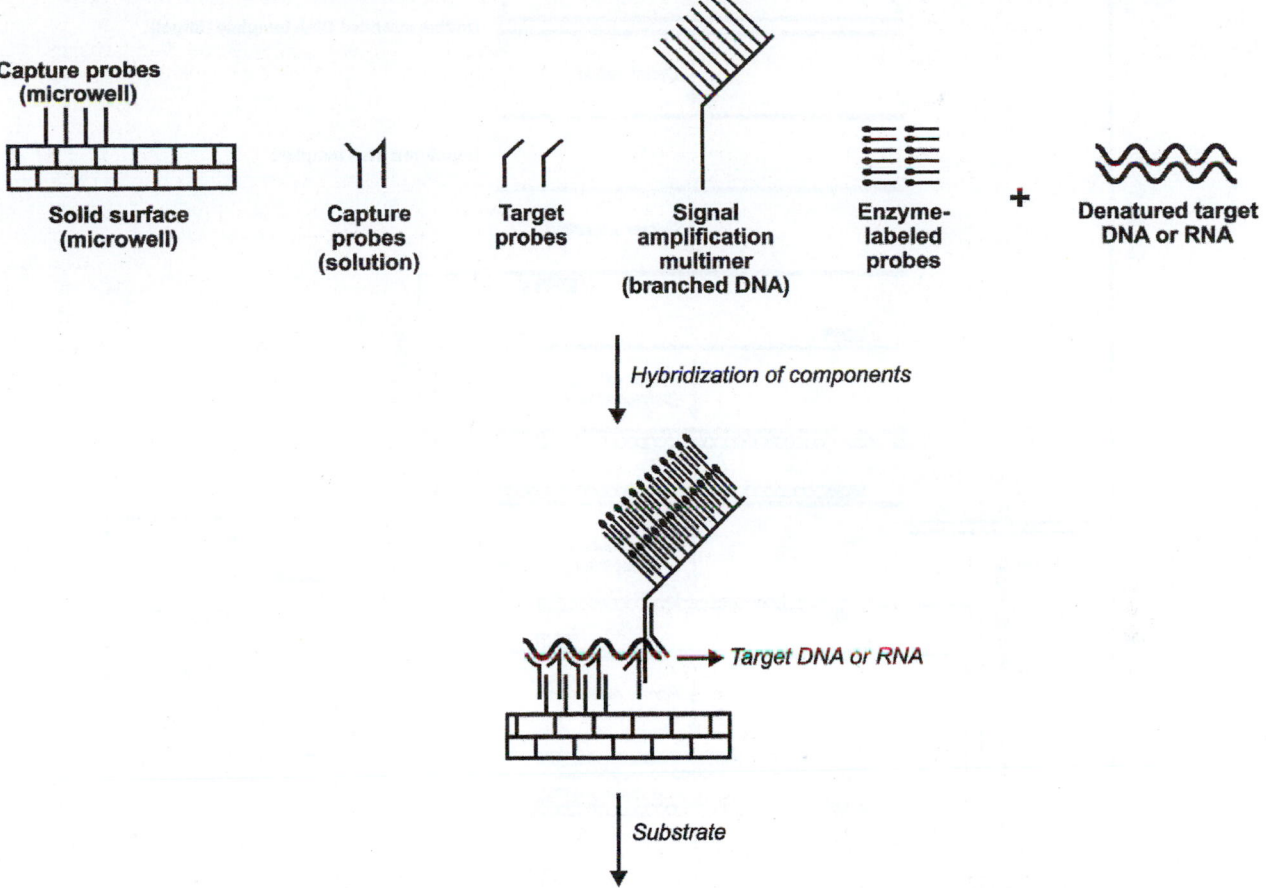

FIGURE 1 bDNA signal amplification. Reprinted with permission of Elsevier from reference 182.

specimen is denatured and then hybridized with a specific RNA probe. The DNA-RNA hybrids are captured by antihybrid antibodies that are used to coat the surface of a tube. Alkaline phosphatase-conjugated antihybrid antibodies bind to the immobilized hybrids. The bound antibody conjugate is detected with a chemiluminescent substrate, and the light emitted is measured in a luminometer. Multiple alkaline phosphatase conjugates bind to each hybrid molecule, amplifying the signal. The intensity of the emitted light is proportional to the amount of target DNA in the specimen. Hybrid capture assays for detection of *N. gonorrhoeae*, *C. trachomatis*, human papillomavirus (HPV) (25), and cytomegalovirus (CMV) (102) in clinical specimens have been developed (Qiagen, Germantown, MD).

TARGET AMPLIFICATION TECHNIQUES

All of the target amplification systems share certain fundamental characteristics. They use enzyme-mediated processes, in which a single enzyme or multiple enzymes synthesize copies of target nucleic acid. In all of these techniques, the amplification products are detected by two oligonucleotide primers that bind to complementary sequences on opposite strands of double-stranded targets. All the techniques result in the production of millions to billions of copies of the targeted sequence in a matter of hours, and in each case, the amplification products can serve as templates for subsequent rounds of amplification. Because of this, all of

the techniques are sensitive to contamination with product molecules that can lead to false-positive reactions. The potential for cross contamination is real and should be adequately addressed before any of these techniques are used in the clinical laboratory. However, the occurrence of false-positive reactions can be reduced through special laboratory design, practices, and work flow.

Polymerase Chain Reaction

PCR is a simple, in vitro, chemical reaction that permits the synthesis of essentially limitless quantities of a targeted nucleic acid sequence. This is accomplished through the action of a DNA polymerase that, under the proper conditions, can copy a DNA strand (Fig. 2). At its simplest, a PCR consists of target DNA, a molar excess of two oligonucleotide primers, a heat-stable DNA polymerase, an equimolar mixture of deoxyribonucleotide triphosphates (dNTPs; dATP, dCTP, dGTP, and dTTP), $MgCl_2$, KCl, and a Tris-HCl buffer. The two primers flank the double-stranded DNA (dsDNA) sequence to be amplified, typically <100 to several hundred bases, and are complementary to opposite strands of the target.

To initiate a PCR, the reaction mixture is heated to separate the two strands of target DNA and is then cooled to permit the primers to anneal to the target DNA in a sequence-specific manner. The DNA polymerase then initiates extension of the primers at their 3' ends toward one another. The primer extension products are dissociated from the target DNA by heating. Each extension product, as well

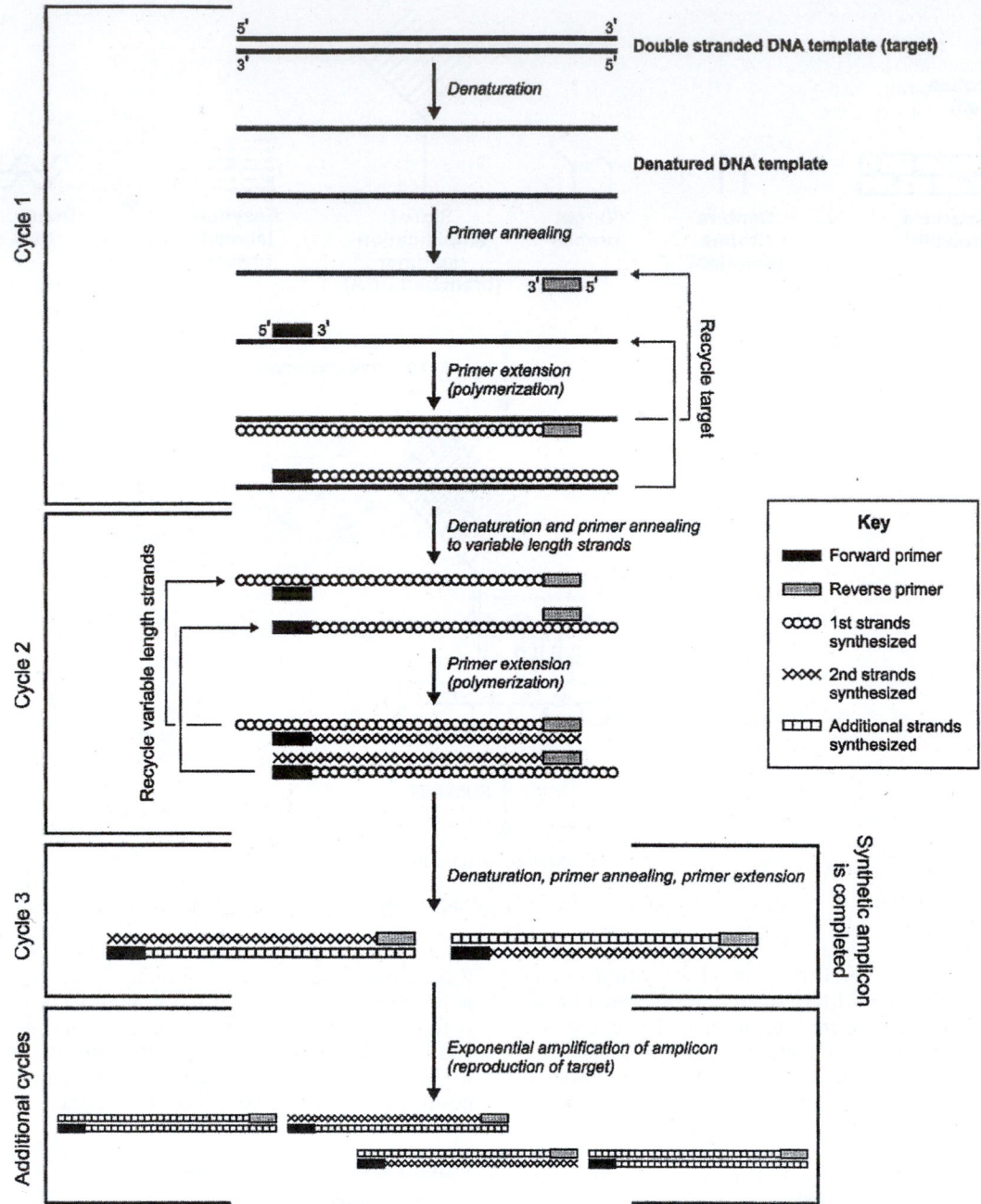

FIGURE 2 PCR target amplification. Reprinted with permission of Elsevier from reference 182.

as the original target, can serve as a template for subsequent rounds of primer annealing and extension.

At the end of each cycle, the PCR products are theoretically doubled. Thus, after n PCR cycles the target sequence can be amplified 2^n-fold. The whole procedure is carried out in a programmable thermal cycler that precisely controls the temperature at which the steps occur, the lengths of time that the reaction mixture is held at the different temperatures, and the number of cycles. Ideally, after 20 cycles of PCR a 10^6-fold amplification is achieved and after 30 cycles a 10^9-fold amplification occurs. In practice, the amplification may not be completely efficient due to failure to optimize the reaction conditions or the presence of inhibitors of the DNA polymerase. In such cases, the total amplification is best described by the expression $(1 + e)^n$, where e is the amplification efficiency ($0 \leq e \leq 1$) and n is the total number of cycles.

Reverse Transcriptase PCR

As it was originally described, PCR was a technique for DNA amplification. Reverse transcriptase PCR (RT-PCR) was developed to amplify RNA targets. In this process, cDNA is first produced from RNA targets by reverse transcription and then the cDNA is amplified by PCR. As it was originally described, RT-PCR used two enzymes: a heat-labile RT, such as avian myeloblastosis virus RT, and a thermostable DNA polymerase. Because of the temperature requirements of the heat-labile enzyme, cDNA synthesis had to occur at temperatures below the optimal annealing temperatures of the primers. This presented problems in terms of both non-specific primer annealing and inefficient primer extension due to the formation of RNA secondary structures. These problems have largely been overcome by the development of a thermostable DNA polymerase derived from *Thermus thermophilus* that under the proper conditions can function efficiently as both an RT and a DNA polymerase (109). RT-PCRs with this enzyme are more specific and efficient than previous protocols with conventional, heat-labile RT enzymes.

Nested PCR

Nested PCR was developed to increase both the sensitivity and the specificity of PCR (56). It uses two pairs of amplification primers and two rounds of PCR. Typically, one primer pair is used in the first round of PCR for 15 to 30 cycles. The products of the first round of amplification are then subjected to a second round of amplification with the second set of primers, which anneal to a sequence internal to the sequence amplified by the first primer set. The increased sensitivity arises from the high total cycle number, and the increased specificity arises from the annealing of the second primer set to sequences found only in the first-round products, thus verifying the identity of the first-round product. The major disadvantage of nested PCR is the high rates of contamination that can occur during the transfer of first-round products to the second tube for the second round of amplification. This contamination can be avoided either by physically separating the first- and second-round amplification mixtures with a layer of wax or oil or by designing single-tube amplification protocols. In practice, the enhanced sensitivity afforded by nested PCR protocols is rarely required in diagnostic applications, and the identity of an amplification product is usually confirmed by hybridization with a nucleic acid probe.

Multiplex PCR

In multiplex PCR, two or more primer sets designed for amplification of different targets are included in the same reaction mixture (13). By this technique, more than one target sequence in a clinical specimen can be coamplified in a single tube. The primers used in multiplexed reactions must be carefully selected so that they have similar annealing temperatures and lack complementarity. Multiplex PCRs have proved to be more complicated to develop and may be less sensitive than PCRs with single primer sets.

Many multiplex assays have been developed, especially for the detection of central nervous system (8, 26) and respiratory (70, 162) pathogens. Multiplex PCR assays for bacterial and viral respiratory pathogens are commercially available from Prodesse, Inc., Waukesha, WI.

A promising new platform for multiplex PCR analysis is the xMAP system (Luminex Corp., Austin, TX). The xMAP system incorporates a proprietary process to internally dye polystyrene microspheres with two spectrally distinct fluorochromes. By using precise ratios of these fluorochromes, an array is created consisting of 100 different microsphere sets with specific spectral addresses. Each microsphere set can possess a different reactant on its surface. For nucleic acid analysis, oligonucleotide probes would be covalently bound to the microsphere surface by carbodiimide coupling. Since each microsphere set can be distinguished by its spectral address, the sets can be combined, allowing up to 100 different analytes to be measured simultaneously in a single reaction vessel. A third fluorochrome coupled to a reporter molecule quantifies the biomolecular interaction that occurs at the microsphere surface.

Microspheres are interrogated individually in a rapidly flowing liquid stream as they pass by two separate lasers in the Luminex xMAP flow cytometer. High-speed digital signal processing classifies each microsphere based on its spectral address and quantifies the reaction on its surface. Thousands of microspheres are investigated per second, resulting in an analysis system capable of analyzing and reporting up to 100 different reactions in a single reaction vessel in a few seconds.

Multiplex assays run on the Luminex platform typically consist of three major steps: nucleic acid amplification by PCR, target-specific extension, and liquid bead array decoding. After PCR amplification, the amplicons are mixed with a second set of tagged primers specific for each target. If the target is present, the tagged primer will be extended through a process called target-specific extension. During this extension, a label is incorporated into the extension product. The color-coded beads are added to identify the tagged and labeled extension products. Attached to each differently colored bead is oligonucleotide complementary to the tag sequence for each target. Samples are then placed in the Luminex xMAP flow cytometer, where the beads are read by two color lasers. One laser identifies the color of the bead, and the other laser detects the presence or absence of a labeled extension product on that bead.

The technology has been adapted to a wide variety of applications in bacteriology (30), mycology (27), and virology (148, 175). Systems for the multiplex detection of respiratory viruses based on the Luminex xMAP system have been developed by Luminex Molecular Diagnostics, EraGen Biosciences (Madison, WI), and Qiagen (10, 98, 113).

Another promising technology for high-order multiplex PCR is the FilmArray, developed by Idaho Technology, Salt Lake City, UT. It is a completely automated, integrated, and self-contained lab-in-a-pouch system. The film portion of the pouch has stations for cell lysis, nucleic acid purification, reverse transcription to detect RNA targets, first-stage PCR multiplex PCR, and an array of up to 120 second-stage nested PCRs. After extracting and purifying nucleic acids from the unprocessed sample, the FilmArray performs a nested multiplex PCR that is executed in two stages. During the first-stage PCR, the FilmArray performs a single, large-volume, massively multiplexed reaction. The products from first-stage PCR are then diluted and combined with a fresh, primer-free master mix. Aliquots of this second master mix solution are then distributed to each well of the array. Each well of the array is prespotted with a single set of primers. The second-stage, small-volume PCR is performed in singleplex fashion in each well of the array. Though this assay uses nested PCR, the entire test is performed within a sealed pouch, thus eliminating concerns of carryover contamination. Using amplification and melting-curve data, the FilmArray software automatically generates a result for each target. A FilmArray for detection of 20 different respiratory pathogens is in development.

Real-Time (Homogeneous, Kinetic) PCR

The term real-time PCR refers to methods in which the target amplification and detection steps occur simultaneously in the same tube (homogeneous). These methods require special thermal cyclers with precision optics that can monitor the fluorescence emission from the sample wells. The computer software supporting the thermal cycler monitors

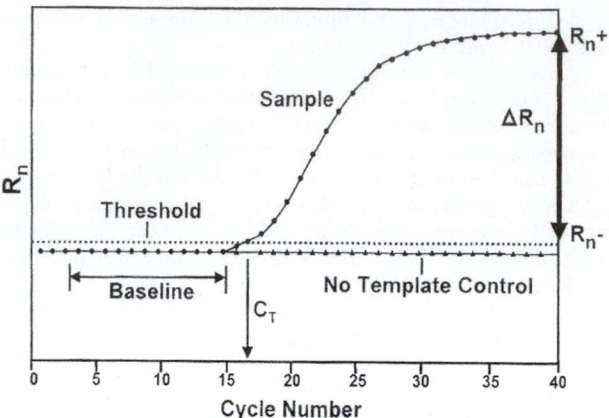

FIGURE 3 Real-time PCR amplification plot with commonly used terms and abbreviations. R_n, normalized fluorescent signal from reporter dye. From *TaqMan Universal PCR Master Mix Protocol*, p. 5–94 (Applied Biosystems, Foster City, CA, 2002). Reprinted with permission.

the data throughout the PCR at every cycle and generates an amplification plot for each reaction (kinetic).

Figure 3 shows a representative amplification plot and defines the terms used in quantitative real-time PCR. The amplification plot shows the normalized fluorescence signal from the reporter at each cycle number. In the initial cycles of PCR, there is little change in the fluorescence signal. This initial signal level defines the baseline for the plot. An increase above the baseline indicates the detection of accumulated PCR product. A fixed fluorescence threshold can be set above the baseline. The cycle threshold (C_T) is defined as the cycle number at which the fluorescence passes the fixed threshold. A plot of the log of the initial target concentration versus C_T for a set of standards is a straight line (59). The amount of the target in an unknown sample is determined by measuring the sample C_T and using a standard curve to determine the starting copy number. Alternatively, the cycle number corresponding to the maximal change in fluorescence, the second derivative maximum, has a similar relationship to the initial target concentration.

In its simplest format, the PCR product is detected as it is produced by using fluorescent dyes that preferentially bind to dsDNA. SYBR green I is one such dye that has been used in this application (107). In the dye's unbound state, the fluorescence is relatively low, but when the dye is bound to dsDNA, the fluorescence is greatly enhanced. The dye binds to both specific and nonspecific PCR products. The specificity of the detection can be improved through melting-curve analysis. As the temperature is slowly raised, the two strands of the amplicon melt apart and the amount of fluorescence decreases. The data are transformed and analyzed by plotting the first derivative of the fluorescence on the y axis and the temperature on the x axis. The specific amplified product will have a characteristic melting peak at its predicted melting temperature (T_m), whereas the primer dimers and other nonspecific products should have different T_ms or give broader peaks (136).

The specificity of real-time PCR can also be increased by including fluorescent resonance energy transfer (FRET) probes in the reaction mixture. These probes are labeled with fluorescent dyes or with combinations of fluorescent and quencher dyes. In 5′ exonuclease PCR (TaqMan) assays, the 5′- to-3′ exonuclease activity of *Taq* DNA polymerase is used

to cleave a nonextendable hybridization probe during the primer extension phase of PCR (61). This approach uses dually labeled fluorogenic hybridization probes and is illustrated in Fig. 4. One fluorescent dye serves as a reporter, and its emission spectrum is quenched by the second fluorescent dye. The nuclease degradation of the hybridization probe releases the reporter dye, resulting in an increase in the peak fluorescent emission. The increase in fluorescent emission indicates that specific PCR product has been made, and the intensity of fluorescence is related to the amount of the product (57). The specificity is increased because a signal is generated only when the primer and probe are bound to the same template strand.

The use of dual hybridization probes is another approach to real-time PCR (81). This method uses two specially designed sequence-specific oligonucleotide probes (Fig. 5). These hybridization probes are designed to hybridize within 1 to 5 nucleotides apart on the product molecule. The 3′ end of the anchor probe is labeled with a donor dye, and the 5′ end of the reporter probe is labeled with an acceptor dye. The 3′ end of the reporter probe is phosphorylated to prevent extension during PCR. The donor dye is excited by an external light source, and instead of emitting light, it transfers its energy to the acceptor dye by FRET. The excited acceptor dye emits light at a longer wavelength than the unbound donor dye, and the intensity of the acceptor dye light emission is proportional to the amount of PCR product.

Real-time detection and quantification of amplification products can also be accomplished with molecular beacons (171). Molecular beacons are hairpin-shaped oligonucleotide probes with an internally quenched fluorophore whose fluorescence is restored when the probes bind to a target nucleic acid (Fig. 6). The probes are designed in such a way that the loop portion of each probe molecule is complementary to the target sequence. The stem is formed by the annealing of complementary arm sequences on the ends of the probe. A fluorescent dye is attached to one end of one arm, and a quenching molecule is attached to the end of the other arm. The stem keeps the fluorophore and quencher in close proximity such that no light emission occurs. When the probe encounters a target molecule, it forms a hybrid that is longer and more stable than the stem and undergoes a conformational change that forces the stem apart, causing the fluorophore and the quencher to move away from each other, restoring the fluorescence.

Scorpion probes combine a PCR primer with a molecular beacon (167, 180). Intramolecular hybridization of the loop structure to a downstream portion of the amplification product separates the reporter and quencher dyes. The hybridization kinetics of Scorpion probes are generally faster than those of molecular beacons because the primer and probe are located on the same molecule.

Dark quencher probes are also used in real-time PCR applications (Epoch Biosciences, Bothell, WA). Dark quencher probes contain a fluorophore on the 5′ end and a nonfluorescent quencher molecule on the 3′ end (78). The fluorescence is quenched when the probe is a random coil and emitted when the probe anneals to the target sequence. Unlike fluorogenic 5′ nuclease probes, these probes are not degraded by the DNA polymerase during target amplification. Since the dark quencher is not fluorescent, it does not contribute to the background signal. This trait has the advantage of improving the signal-to-noise ratio for the detection system, which may improve sensitivity. These probes also incorporate a hybridization-stabilizing compound, known as a minor groove binder. It is a small, crescent-shaped molecule that is covalently linked to the 3′ end of the probe that spans about

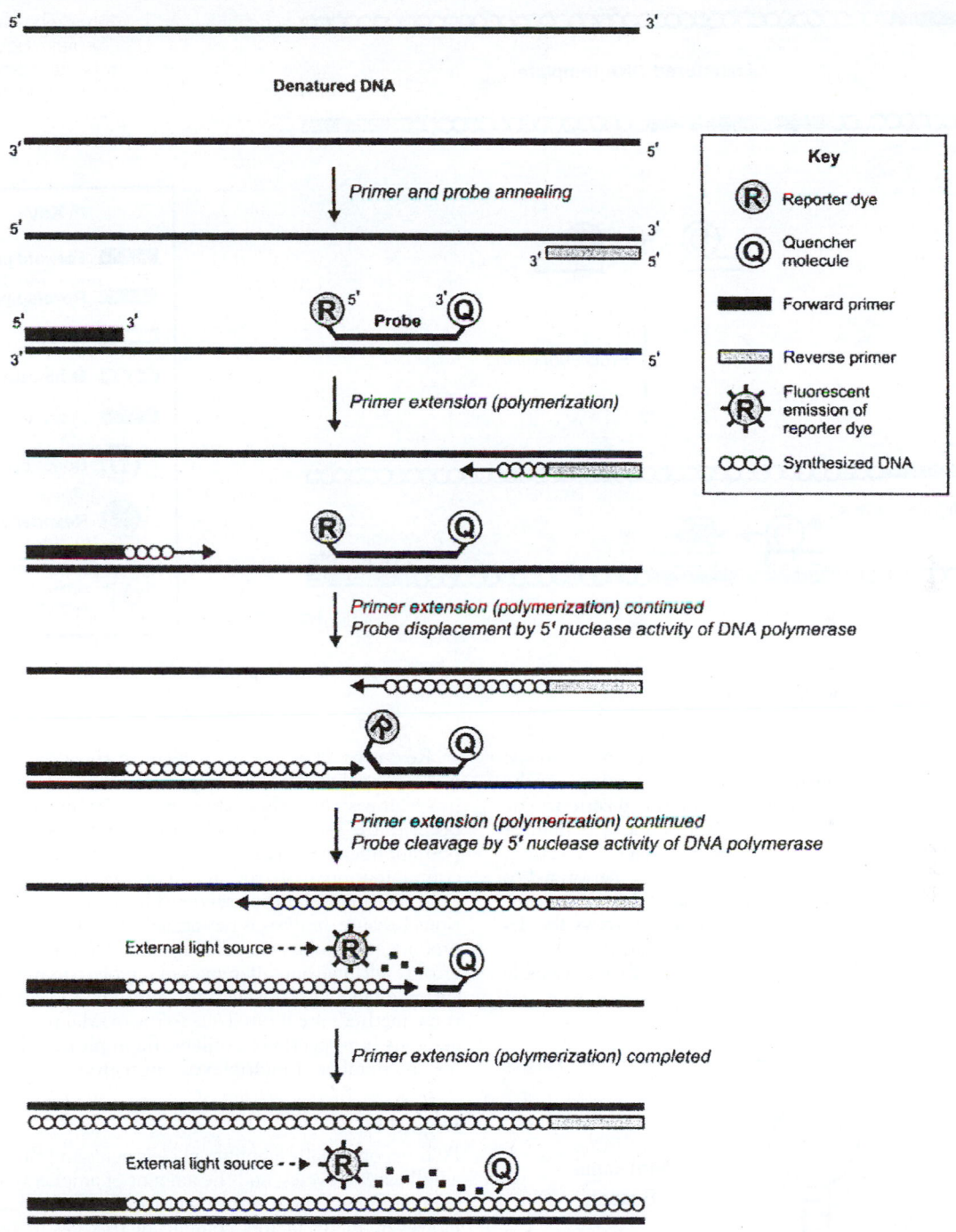

FIGURE 4 5' exonuclease chemistry for real-time PCR applications. Reprinted with permission of Elsevier from reference 182.

3 or 4 nucleotides and snugly fits into the minor groove of DNA, where it forms hydrogen bonds with the template. Minor groove binders increase the T_m of the probe. The minor groove binder allows for the use of shorter probes because of the increased T_ms and enables improved T_m leveling, which increases the specificity of the detection reaction.

Another approach to detection, characterization, and quantification of real-time PCR amplicons involves the use of a nonstandard DNA base pair constructed from isoG and isoC (108, 146, 158). These synthetic bases pair with each other, but not with the natural bases guanine and cytosine, and can be covalently coupled to a wide variety of reporter groups. In the MultiCode-RTx assays (EraGen Biosciences) the target is amplified using a forward primer with a single isoC nucleotide with fluorescent label at 5' end and an unlabeled standard base reverse primer. Amplification is performed in the presence of isoG coupled to a fluorescence quencher molecule, and site-specific incorporation by the DNA polymerase places the quencher in close proximity to the fluorophore, resulting in a decrease of fluorescence

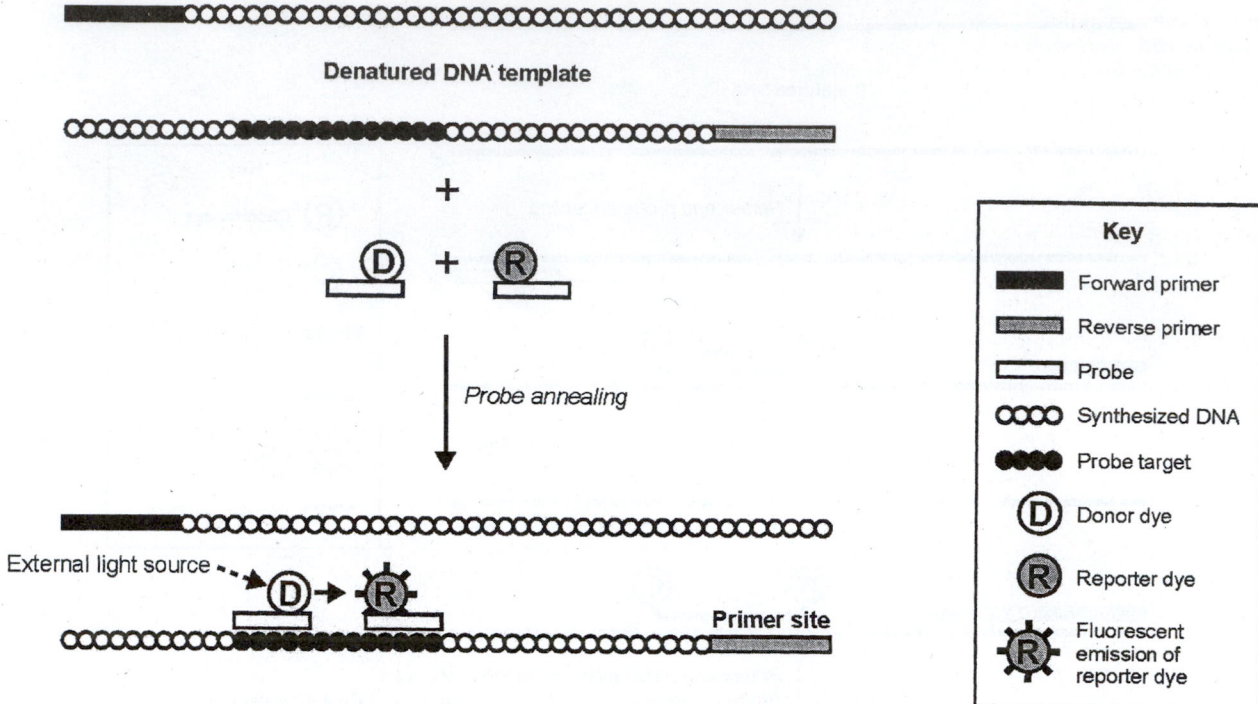

FIGURE 5 Dual hybridization probes for real-time PCR applications. Reprinted with permission of Elsevier from reference 182.

with every PCR cycle. The number of cycles in which the fluorescence change can be detected is dependent on the initial number of target molecules in the reaction. The decrease in fluorescence is easily monitored by a number of different standard real-time PCR instruments. Postreaction amplicon melting-curve analysis can be performed to confirm the identity of the amplicon and to detect sequence variants. MultiCode-RTx research-use-only assays for detection of *N. gonorrhoeae* and for quantification of CMV, Epstein-Barr virus (EBV), and BK virus (BKV) are available from EraGen.

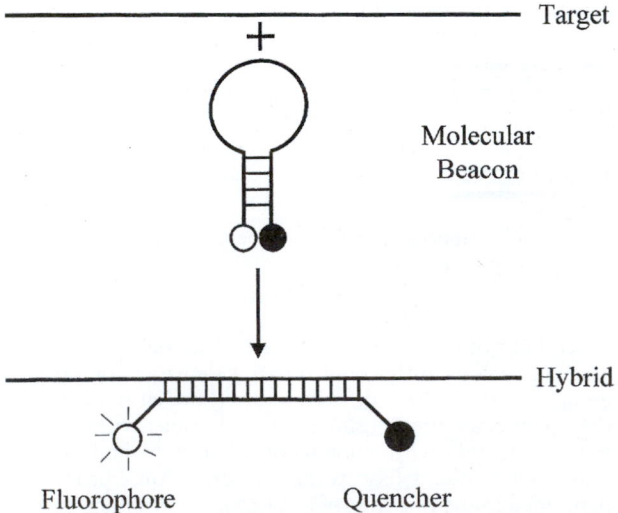

FIGURE 6 Molecular beacon probes for real-time amplification applications. Reprinted with permission of Elsevier from reference 182.

Real-time PCR methods decrease the time required to perform nucleic acid assays because there are no post-PCR processing steps. Also, since amplification and detection occur in the same closed tube, these methods eliminate the postamplification manipulations that can lead to laboratory contamination with the amplicon. In addition, real-time PCR methods lend themselves well to quantitative applications because analysis is performed early in the log phase of product accumulation, and as a result, they are less prone to error resulting from differences in sample-to-sample amplification efficiency. However, the multiplexing capabilities of these methods are limited due to the overlapping absorption and emission spectra of available fluorophores, thus restricting the number of multiplexed targets to four or five (75).

Digital PCR

PCR exponentially amplifies nucleic acids and the number of amplification cycles, and the amount of amplicon allows the computation of the starting quantity of targeted nucleic acid. However, many factors complicate this calculation, often creating uncertainties and inaccuracies, particularly when the starting concentration is low. Digital PCR attempts to overcome these difficulties by transforming the exponential data from conventional PCR to digital signals that simply indicate whether amplification occurred (68, 159, 173).

Digital PCR is accomplished by capturing or isolating each individual nucleic acid molecule present in a sample within many chambers, zones, or regions that are able to localize and concentrate the amplification product to detectable levels. After PCR amplification, a count of the areas containing PCR product is a direct measure of the absolute quantity of nucleic acid in the sample. The capture or isolation of individual nucleic acid molecules may be done in capillaries, microemulsions, or arrays of miniaturized chambers or on surfaces that bind nucleic acids. Digital PCR has many applications, including detection and quantification of low levels of pathogen sequences, rare genetic sequences, gene expression in single cells, and clonal amplification of nucleic acids for sequencing mixed nucleic acid samples. Clonal amplification enabled by digital PCR is a key element of many of the "next-generation" sequencing methods described below.

Transcription-Based Amplification Methods

Nucleic acid sequence-based amplification (NASBA) and transcription-mediated amplification (TMA) are both isothermal RNA amplification methods modeled after retroviral replication (24, 48, 79). The methods are similar in that the RNA target is reverse transcribed into cDNA and then RNA copies are synthesized with an RNA polymerase. NASBA uses avian myeloblastosis virus RT, RNase H, and T7 bacteriophage RNA polymerase, whereas TMA uses an RT enzyme with endogenous RNase H activity and T7 RNA polymerase.

Amplification involves the synthesis of cDNA from the RNA target with a primer containing the T7 RNA polymerase promoter sequence (Fig. 7). The RNase H then degrades the initial strand of target RNA in the RNA-cDNA hybrid. The second primer then binds to the cDNA and is extended by the DNA polymerase activity of the RT, resulting in the formation of dsDNA containing the T7 RNA polymerase promoter. The RNA polymerase then generates multiple copies of single-stranded, antisense RNA. These RNA product molecules reenter the cycle, with subsequent formation of more double-stranded cDNA

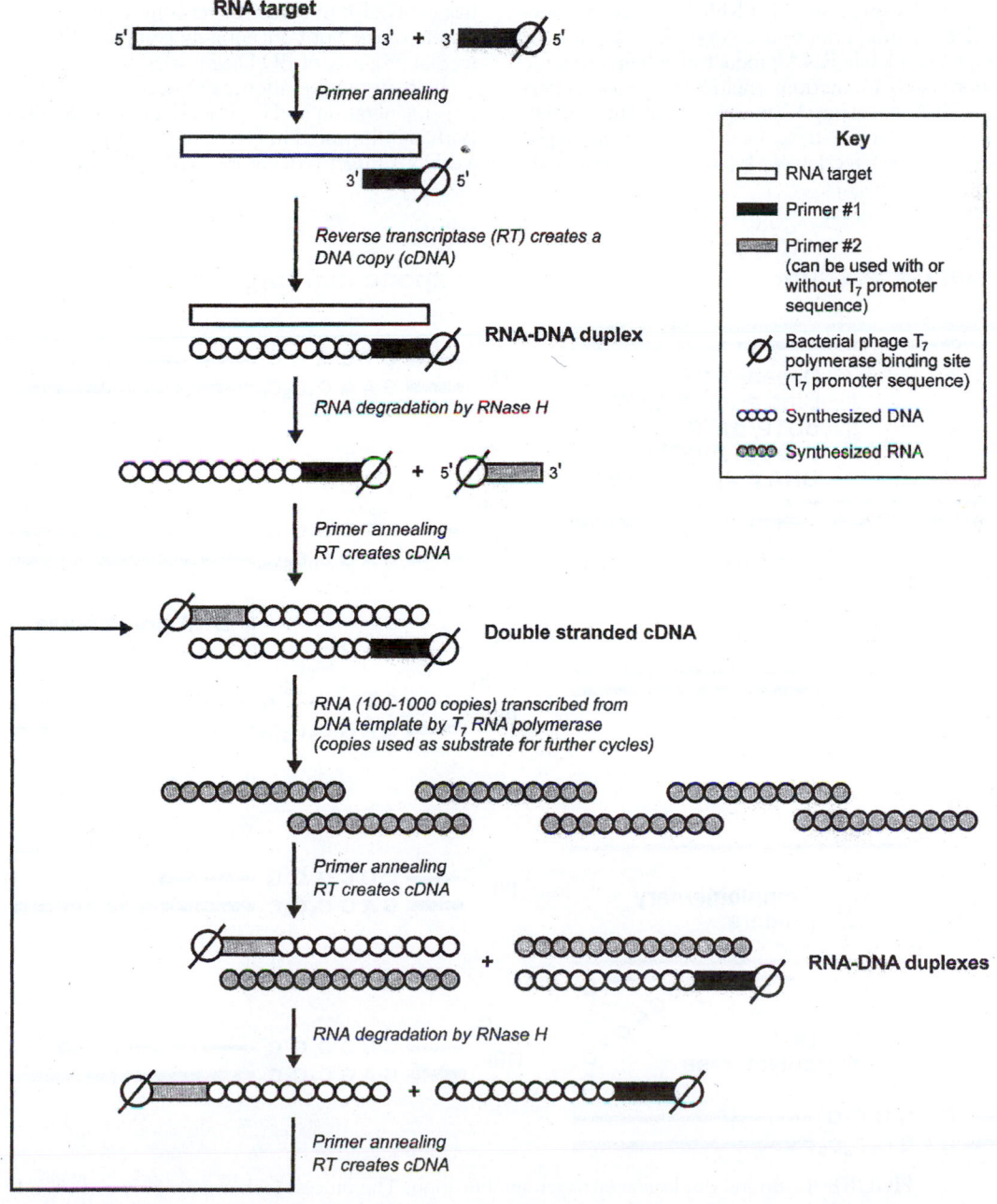

FIGURE 7 Transcription-based target amplification. NASBA and TMA are examples of transcription-based amplification systems. Reprinted with permission of Elsevier from reference 182.

molecules that can serve as templates for more RNA synthesis. A 10^9-fold amplification of the target RNA can be achieved in less than 2 h by this method.

The single-stranded RNA products of TMA in the Gen-Probe tests are detected by modification of the hybridization protection assay. Oligonucleotide probes are labeled with modified acridinium esters with either fast or slow chemiluminescence kinetics so that signals from two hybridization reactions can be analyzed simultaneously in the same tube. The NASBA products in the bioMérieux (Durham, NC) tests are detected by hybridization with probes labeled with tris(2,2′-bispyridine) ruthenium and electrochemiluminescence. NASBA has also been used with molecular beacons to create a homogeneous, kinetic amplification system similar to real-time PCR (86).

Transcription-based amplification systems have several strengths, including no requirement for a thermal cycler, rapid kinetics, and a single-stranded RNA product that does not require denaturation prior to detection. Also, single-tube clinical assays and a labile RNA product may help minimize contamination risks. Limitations include the poor performance with DNA targets and concerns about the stability of complex multienzyme systems. Gen-Probe has developed TMA-based assays for detection of *Mycobacterium tuberculosis*, *C. trachomatis*, *N. gonorrhoeae*, HCV, and HIV-1. NASBA-based kits (bioMérieux) for the detection and quantification of HIV-1 RNA and detection of enterovirus and respiratory syncytial virus RNA are commercially available. A basic NASBA kit is also available for the development of other applications defined by the user. In its latest iteration, NucliSens EasyQ, NASBA is coupled with molecular beacons for real-time amplification and detection of target nucleic acids (12).

Strand Displacement Amplification

Strand displacement amplification (SDA) is an isothermal template amplification technique that can be used to detect trace amounts of DNA or RNA of a particular sequence. SDA, as it was first described, was a conceptually straightforward amplification process with some technical limitations (174). Since its initial description, however, it has evolved into a highly versatile tool that is technically simple to use but conceptually complex. SDA is the intellectual property of BD Diagnostics.

In its current iteration, SDA occurs in two discrete phases, target generation and exponential target amplification (91). Both are illustrated in Fig. 8. In the target generation phase, a dsDNA target is denatured and hybridized to two different

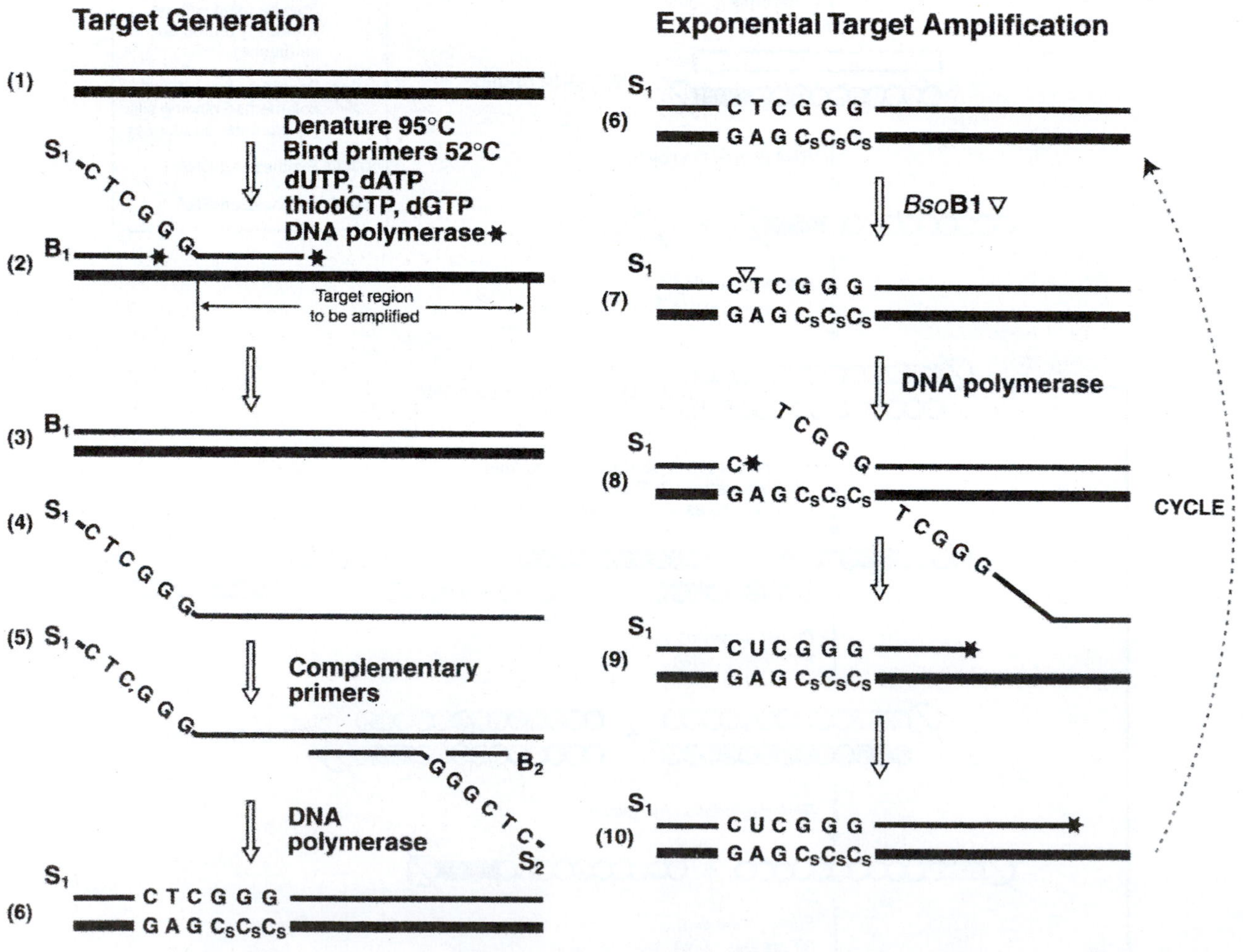

FIGURE 8 Strand displacement target amplification. The process is shown for only one strand of a dsDNA target, but amplification occurs on both strands simultaneously. B_1 and B_2, bumper primers; S_1 and S_2, amplification primers. Modified from reference 91.

primer pairs, designated as bumper and amplification primers. The amplification primers include the single-stranded restriction endonuclease enzyme sequence for BsoB1 located at the 5′ end of the target binding sequence. The bumper primers are shorter and anneal to the target DNA just upstream of the region to be amplified. In the presence of BsoB1, an exonuclease-free DNA polymerase, and a dNTP mixture consisting of dUTP, dATP, dGTP, and thiolated dCTP (C_s), simultaneous extension products of both the bumper and amplification primers are generated. This process displaces the amplification primer products, which are available for hybridization with the opposite-strand products with the opposite-strand bumper and amplification primers.

The simultaneous extension of opposite-strand primers produces strands complementary to the product formed by extension of the first amplification primer, with C_s incorporated into the BsoB1 cleavage site. This product enters the exponential target amplification phase of the reaction. The BsoB1 enzyme recognizes the double-stranded site, but because one strand contains C_s, it is nicked rather than cleaved by the enzyme. The DNA polymerase then binds to the nicked site and begins synthesis of a new strand while simultaneously displacing the downstream strand. This step re-creates the double-stranded species with the hemimodified restriction endonuclease recognition sequence, and the iterative nicking and displacement process repeats. The displaced strands are capable of binding to opposite-strand primers, which produces exponential amplification of the target sequences.

These single-stranded products also bind to detector probes for real-time detection. The detector probes are single-stranded DNA molecules with fluorescein and rhodamine labels. The region between the labels includes a stem-loop structure. The loop contains the recognition site for the BsoB1 enzyme. The target-specific sequences are located 3′ of the rhodamine label. In the absence of a specific target, the stem-loop structure is maintained with the fluorescein and rhodamine labels in close proximity. The net effect is that very little emission for the fluorescein is detected after excitation. After SDA, the probe is converted to a double-stranded species, which is cleaved by BsoB1. The cleavage causes physical separation of the fluorescein and rhodamine labels, which results in an increase in emission from the fluorescein label.

SDA has a reported sensitivity high enough to detect as few as 10 to 50 copies of a target molecule (174). By using a primer set designed to amplify a repetitive sequence with 10 copies in the *M. tuberculosis* genome, the assay is sensitive enough to detect one to five genome copies from the bacterium. SDA has also been adapted to quantify RNA by adding an RT step (RT-SDA). In this case, a primer hybridizes to the target RNA and an RT synthesizes a cDNA molecule. This cDNA can then serve as a template for primer incorporation and strand displacement. The products of this strand displacement then feed into the amplification scheme described above. RT-SDA has been used for the determination of HIV viral load (117). Food and Drug Administration (FDA)-cleared tests using SDA for the direct detection of *C. trachomatis* and *N. gonorrhoeae* in clinical specimens are available from Becton Dickinson.

The main advantage of SDA is that it is an isothermal process that, unlike PCR, can be performed at a single temperature after initial target denaturation. This eliminates the need for expensive thermal cyclers. Furthermore, samples can be subjected to SDA in a single tube, with amplification times varying from 30 min to 2 h. The main disadvantage of SDA lies in the fact that, unlike those at which PCR is performed, the relatively low temperature at which SDA is carried out (52.5°C) can result in nonspecific primer hybridization to sequences found in complex mixtures such as genomic DNA. Hence, when the target is in low abundance compared to background DNA, nonspecific amplification products can swamp the system, decreasing the sensitivity of the technique. However, the use of organic solvents to increase stringency at low temperatures and the recent introduction of more thermostable polymerases capable of strand displacement have alleviated much of this problem.

Loop-Mediated Amplification

Loop-mediated amplification (LAMP) is an isothermal method that relies on autocycling strand displacement DNA synthesis by *Bst* DNA polymerase and a set of four to six primers (116). Two inner and two outer primers define the target sequence, and an additional set of loop primers are added to increase the sensitivity of the reaction. The final products of the LAMP reaction are DNA molecules with a cauliflower-like structure of multiple loops consisting of repeats of the target sequence. The products can be analyzed in real time by monitoring of the turbidity in the reaction tube resulting from production of magnesium pyrophosphate precipitate during the DNA amplification. Amplification products can also be visualized in agarose gels after electrophoresis and staining with ethidium bromide or SYBR green.

LAMP has been used successfully in a number of laboratory-developed assays to detect DNA and RNA viruses (64, 119, 166, 186), differentiate viral subtypes (110, 126), and diagnose mycobacterial infections (66). Since LAMP is an isothermal process and positive reactions can be detected by simple turbidity measurements or visualized directly with the naked eye, it requires no expensive equipment. These attributes make it an attractive technology for resource-poor settings and field use (87). However, primer design for LAMP is more complex than for PCR, with specialized training and software required for their design. Meridian Bioscience, Inc. (Cincinnati, OH), has licensed LAMP technology from Eiken Chemical Company, Ltd., Tokyo, Japan, for the development of infectious-disease diagnostics in the United States.

Helicase-Dependent Amplification

Helicase-dependent amplification (HDA) is an isothermal process developed by BioHelix, Beverly, MA, that uses helicase to separate dsDNA and generate single-stranded templates for primer hybridization and subsequent extension by a DNA polymerase (172). As the helicase unwinds dsDNA enzymatically, the initial heat denaturation and subsequent thermocycling steps required by PCR can all be omitted. In HDA, strands of dsDNA are separated by the DNA helicase and the ssDNA-coated ssDNA-binding proteins. Two sequence-specific primers hybridize to each border of the target sequence, and a DNA polymerase extends the primers annealed to the target sequence to produce dsDNA. The two newly synthesized products are used as substrates by the helicase in the next round of amplification. Thus, a simultaneous chain reaction proceeds, resulting in exponential amplification of the selected target sequence.

HDA is compatible with multiple detection technologies, including qualitative and quantitative fluorescence technologies and with instruments designed for real-time PCR (169). Furthermore, HDA has shown potential for the development of simple, portable DNA diagnostic devices to be used in the field or at the point of care (17, 46).

PROBE AMPLIFICATION TECHNIQUES

Probe amplification methods differ from target amplification methods in that the amplification products contain only a sequence present in the initial probes. Ligase chain reaction (185), cycling probe technology (37), and cleavase-invader technology (96) are all examples of probe amplification methods for which diagnostic applications have been developed. However, diagnostic tests based on ligase chain reaction and cycling probe technology are no longer available in the United States.

Cleavase-Invader Technology

Invader assays (Hologic, Bedford, MA) are based on a probe amplification method that relies upon the specific recognition and cleavage of particular DNA structures by cleavase, a member of the FEN-1 family of DNA polymerases. These polymerases cleave the 5′ single-stranded flap of a branched base-paired duplex. This enzymatic activity likely plays an essential role in the elimination of the complex nucleic acid structures that arise during DNA replication and repair. Since these structures may occur anywhere in a replicating genome, the enzyme recognizes the molecular structure of the substrate without regard to the sequence of the nucleic acids making up the DNA complex (88).

In the invader assays, two primers are designed which hybridize to the target sequence in an overlapping fashion (Fig. 9). Under the proper annealing conditions, the probe oligonucleotide binds to the target sequence. The invader oligonucleotide is designed such that it hybridizes upstream of the probe, with a region of overlap between the 3′ end of the invader and the 5′ end of the probe. Cleavase cleaves the 5′ end of the probe and releases it. It is in this way that the target sequence acts as a scaffold upon which the proper DNA structure can form. Since the DNA structure necessary to serve as a cleavase substrate occurs only in the presence of the target sequence, the generation of cleavage products indicates the presence of the target. Use of a thermostable cleavase enzyme allows reactions to be run at temperatures high enough for a primer exchange equilibrium to exist. This allows multiple cleavase products to form off of a single target molecule.

FRET probes and a second invasive cleavage reaction are used to detect the target-specific products. Invader technology can be used for genotyping, detection of mutations, and viral load testing. FDA-cleared assays for detection of pools of high-risk genotypes and types 16 and 18 of HPV in cervical samples are available from Hologic (45).

The invader assay has several inherent advantages. Because the overlap in the invader probe need be only 1 bp, this technology can easily be adapted to detect point mutations of interest by designing the overlap region to encompass the mutation to be detected (97). The detection of these point mutations would not require postreaction restriction digestion, since the primers would be differentially cleaved on the basis of the presence or the absence of the mutation in question. This feature could be exploited to track mutations in pathogens associated with drug resistance or virulence.

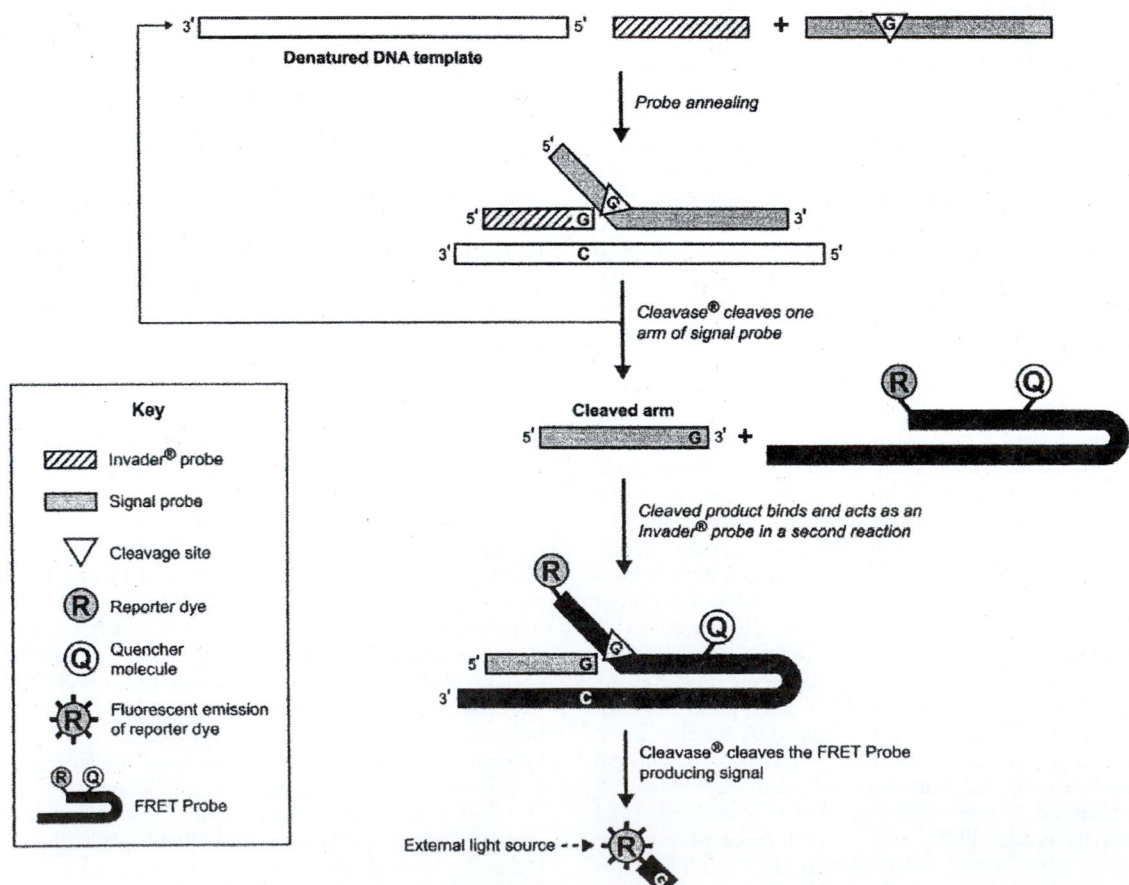

FIGURE 9 Cleavase-invader probe-based amplification. Reprinted with permission of Elsevier from reference 182.

In addition, unlike amplification techniques such as PCR, SDA, and TMA, in which the target sequence itself is amplified, the invader assay does not increase the amount of the target sequence. As a consequence, invader assays are less prone to problems of false-positive results due to amplicon cross contamination.

POSTAMPLIFICATION DETECTION AND ANALYSIS

Gel Analysis

Visualization of amplification products in agarose gels after electrophoresis and ethidium bromide staining was the earliest detection method. After gel electrophoresis, DNA is often transferred onto a nitrocellulose or nylon membrane and hybridized to a specific probe to increase both the sensitivity and the specificity of detection. Membranes with bound radiolabeled probes are placed in proximity to X-ray film, and the hybrids are visualized as dark bands. Enzyme-labeled probes can be visualized through either light or color production after the addition of the appropriate chemiluminescent or chromogenic substrates. Many of these nonisotopic approaches are at least as sensitive as isotopic methods and are faster. In addition, the enzyme-labeled probes are more stable. Although gel electrophoresis and blotting remain important research tools, these techniques are being replaced by faster and simpler methods in the clinical laboratory.

Single-strand conformation polymorphism (SSCP) analysis and restriction fragment length polymorphism (RFLP) analysis have been used to ascertain information about the base compositions of the amplification products visualized in a gel. In SSCP analysis, the PCR product is denatured and then subjected to electrophoresis in a nondenaturing gel (122). Variations in the physical conformations of the PCR products are related to the base compositions and are detected by differential gel migration. This technique has successfully been used to detect mutations causing rifampin resistance in M. tuberculosis (161).

RFLP analysis uses restriction endonucleases to cleave amplification products at specific recognition sites. The fragments are separated by electrophoresis, and the resulting banding pattern provides information about the nucleic acid sequence. When coupled with a hybridization reaction, RFLP analysis can also provide information about the location and number of loci homologous to the probe. Both SSCP analysis and RFLP analysis of short products have largely been replaced by direct DNA sequencing as this technology has improved and the costs have decreased.

Capillary Electrophoresis

Capillary electrophoresis allows for accurate size discrimination of fluorescently labeled nucleic acids from 50 to 1,000 bases with single base precision. PCR and capillary electrophoresis have been functionally integrated to produce highly multiplexed assays that can simultaneously detect dozens of targets whose identities are defined by the specific size of the corresponding amplicons (40).

PrimeraDx (Mansfield, MA) has developed a multiplexed assay for the simultaneous quantification of CMV, herpes simplex virus (HSV), BKV, human herpesvirus 6 (HHV-6), and HHV-7 viral loads that integrates PCR and capillary electrophoresis. In this assay, amplification of the nucleic acid targets is monitored by sampling the PCR during sequential cycles and separating and quantifying the PCR products by capillary electrophoresis. These data are used to construct amplification curves. Similar to the case with real-time PCR amplification, a cycle threshold is determined from the amplification curve for each of the targets in the exponential phase of amplification. Unlike real-time PCR, where standards in a separate reaction are used, the PrimeraDx assay uses multiple internal standards in each reaction to generate calibration curves for each individual assay in the multiplex reaction.

Seegene, Inc. (Seoul, South Korea), has developed a wide variety of multiplexed infectious-disease assays, including sexually transmitted disease, HPV genotyping, mycobacterial, and respiratory pathogen panels (71). The targets of these multiplexed assays are designed to be discriminated by size and are compatible with several different microfluidic and capillary electrophoresis systems, including the Agilent (Santa Clara, CA) 2100 Bioanalyzer and Applied Biosystems (Foster City, CA) sequencers.

Colorimetric Microtiter Plate Systems

Colorimetric microtiter plate (CMP) systems are convenient alternatives to traditional gel and blotting techniques for detection of amplified products. In these systems, the amplified product is captured in microtiter plate wells by specific oligonucleotide probes coating the plastic surface. Bound product is detected by a color change that takes place after addition of an enzyme conjugate and the appropriate substrate. These systems resemble enzyme immunoassays and use microtiter plate washers and readers commonly found in clinical laboratories. CMP systems are more practical and faster than the traditional membrane hybridization techniques described above.

Several variations of CMP systems are commercially available. In one popular approach, biotinylated primers are used to amplify the target, and the biotin-containing PCR product is denatured and added to the microtiter well. After hybridization with a capture probe, the bound product is detected with a streptavidin-enzyme conjugate and a chromogenic substrate (94). Enzyme-conjugated antibodies directed against dsDNA have also been used to detect PCR products in CMP systems (100). Another approach uses digoxigenin-dUTP to label the PCR product and enzyme-conjugated antidigoxigenin antibodies to detect the captured product (131).

Allele-Specific Hybridization

Line probe assays are manufactured by Innogenetics (Ghent, Belgium) for genotyping of HCV, HPV, and HBV; identification of mycobacteria; and analysis for drug resistance mutations in HIV-1, HBV, M. tuberculosis, and Helicobacter pylori (138, 156, 157). The HCV line probe assays are distributed by Siemens. In these assays, a series of probes with poly(T) tails are attached to nitrocellulose strips. Biotin-labeled PCR product is then hybridized to the immobilized probes on the strip. The labeled PCR product hybridizes only to the probes that give a perfect sequence match under the stringent hybridization conditions used. After hybridization, streptavidin labeled with alkaline phosphatase is added and binds to the biotinylated hybrids. Incubation with a chromogen results in a purple precipitate. The pattern of hybridization provides information about the nucleic acid sequence of the amplicon. This method is capable of detecting single-nucleotide polymorphisms.

A line probe for identification of 37 HPV genotypes is available from Roche (152). The method employs multiplex PCR with biotinylated primers targeted to the L1 region of the HPV genome and a linear array of L1 sequence-specific probes fixed to a nitrocellulose strip. The pattern of hybridization provides the genotype and is determined as described above.

Direct Sequencing

The combination of PCR and Sanger dideoxynucleotide chain termination methods can be used to determine DNA sequences in clinical samples (65). The use of fluorescent dye terminator chemistry and laser scanning in a polyacrylamide gel electrophoresis format has been the standard in electrophoretic separation technology. However, the recent application of capillary electrophoresis techniques to the separation of PCR and dideoxy chain termination products has streamlined the sequencing process by eliminating some of the labor-intensive steps, which makes the technology a better fit for diagnostic applications (36). The Clinical and Laboratory Standards Institute (CLSI) has developed guidelines for nucleic acid sequencing in clinical laboratories (21, 112).

CLIP, a coupled amplification and sequencing method, uses oligonucleotide primers labeled with different fluorescent dyes, standard dideoxynucleotide termination reagents, and PCR to produce extension products that end with a chain-terminating nucleotide. The nucleic acid sequence is deduced from the electrophoretic mobilities of the different extension products from a set of four reactions, each product containing a different chain-terminating nucleotide. A unique feature of CLIP sequencing is that one reaction produces sequence information for both nucleic acid strands. CLIP sequencing serves as the basis for commercially available assays for HIV-1 drug resistance (Siemens Healthcare Diagnostics).

The ViroSeq HIV-1 genotyping assays (Celera Diagnostics, Alameda, CA; distributed by Abbott Molecular Diagnostics, Des Plaines, IL) also use dideoxy chain-terminating sequencing, but each dideoxynucleotide is labeled with a different fluorescent dye. Each reaction mixture contains one primer but all four uniquely labeled dideoxynucleotides. Separation of the terminated PCR products is done by capillary electrophoresis.

Although direct sequencing of PCR products by electrophoresis is a powerful research tool, its routine use in the clinical laboratory depends upon the development of high-throughput systems with integrated databases and data analysis software. Such systems are available for HIV-1 and HCV genotyping and for identification of bacteria and fungi by rRNA gene sequence analysis.

Pyrosequencing (Qiagen, Hilden, Germany) represents an alternative approach to conventional sequencing and is useful for genotyping and short-read-length sequencing (29). Pyrosequencing is based on the luminometric detection of pyrophosphate that is generated during DNA synthesis.

A sequencing primer is hybridized to a single-stranded PCR amplicon and incubated with the enzymes DNA polymerase, ATP sulfurylase, luciferase, and apyrase and the substrates adenosine 5′-phosphosulfate and luciferin. The first of four dNTPs is added to the reaction mixture. DNA polymerase catalyzes the incorporation of the dNTP into the DNA strand. Each incorporation event is accompanied by release of pyrophosphate (PP_i) in a quantity equimolar to the amount of incorporated nucleotide. The ATP sulfurylase quantitatively converts PP_i to ATP in the presence of adenosine 5′-phosphosulfate. This ATP drives the luciferase-mediated conversion of luciferin to oxyluciferin, which generates light in amounts that are proportional to the amount of ATP. The light produced in the reaction is detected by a charge-coupled device camera. A program is produced in which the height of each peak is proportional to the number of nucleotides incorporated. Apyrase, a nucleotide-degrading enzyme, continuously degrades ATP and unincorporated dNTPs. This degradation switches off the light and regenerates the reaction solution. The next dNTP is added, and the process is repeated.

Pyrosequencing has been used in microbiology to detect drug resistance mutations and to identify and type bacteria, viruses, and fungi (2, 44, 49, 121). Unlike conventional sequencing strategies, pyrosequencing provides reliable data for sequences adjacent to the sequencing primer termini. Pyrosequencing provides a simple-to-use and robust platform for short-read-length sequencing.

Multiple new sequencing technology platforms have emerged since 2005 and have greatly surpassed conventional dideoxynucleotide chain termination methods in terms of increased total sequence production and decreased cost. Collectively, these new sequencing methods are referred to as next-generation sequencing, and they have considerable potential for clinical diagnostics (163). The three major next-generation sequencing platforms as of this writing are the Roche 454 GS-FLX (454, Branford, CT), the Illumina (San Diego, CA) Genome Analyzer, and the ABI SOLiD (Applied Biosystems). The sequencing methods, read lengths, run times, and total bases per run for each of these methods are compared with those of Sanger sequencing in Table 1. These new approaches to sequencing are all based on cyclic stepwise sequencing of massive numbers of templates in parallel in a flow cell and share similar sample preparation steps, including target DNA fragmentation, ligation to adaptor sequences, and clonal amplification of targets.

The Roche 454 platform, using pyrosequencing technology described earlier to carry out hundreds of thousands of sequencing reactions simultaneously on independent beads, works as follows. Target DNA is first randomly sheared into fragments and then ligated to adaptors. Single-stranded template DNA is isolated, mixed with beads, and then subjected to emulsion PCR to clonally amplify the template on each bead. The beads are then distributed into a "picotiter plate" that contains millions of tiny wells. Within each well that receives an individual bead, an isolated environment is created for the sequencing of each template, resulting in massively parallel sequencing of different templates simultaneously.

TABLE 1 Comparison of next-generation and Sanger sequencing platforms

Parameter	Roche 454 GS-FLX	Illumina Genome Analyzer	ABI SOLiD	Sanger
Sequencing method	Pyrosequencing	Reversible dye terminators	Ligation with two-color space coding	Dye terminators
Read length	400 bases	36–50 bases	35–50 bases	800 bases
Sequencing run time	10 h	2.5 days	3.5 days	3 h
Total bases per run	500 Mb	1.5 Gb	5 Gb	800 bases

DNA templates sequenced with the Illumina Genome Analyzer are ligated to adaptor sequences which serve as priming sites for PCR and sequencing, and to attach complementary templates to a solid surface through a mechanism called bridge amplification. Bridge amplification generates clusters of amplified template on the solid surface, where each cluster represents a different template. It uses a unique sequencing chemistry that incorporates fluorescently labeled, reversible terminator nucleotides. These nucleotides are labeled with different color fluorophores so that all four nucleotides can be added to the reactions simultaneously. Only one terminator nucleotide can be incorporated into each sequence during one sequencing cycle, and the color of the fluorescent label incorporated into the sequences of each cluster is recorded. Removal of the terminator group on the nucleotide just added enables incorporation of the next complementary nucleotide, and the cycle is repeated.

The ABI SOLiD System chemistry starts with emulsion PCR of adaptor-modified ssDNA molecules. After PCR, the templates are denatured and bead enrichment is performed to select beads with extended templates. The template on the selected beads undergoes a 3′ modification to allow covalent binding to a glass slide. The modified beads are deposited randomly on the slide. The sequencing occurs by ligation. Primers hybridize to the adaptor sequence within the library template. A set of four fluorescently labeled di-base probes compete for ligation to the sequencing primer. Specificity of the di-base probe is achieved by interrogating every first and second base in each ligation reaction. Multiple cycles of ligation, detection, and cleavage are performed, with the number of cycles determining the eventual read length. Following a series of cycles, the extension product is removed and the template is reset with a primer complementary to the $n-1$ position for a second round of ligation cycles. Five rounds of primer resets are completed for each sequencing tag. Consequently, each base is interrogated in two independent ligation reactions by two different primers. This dual interrogation provides highly accurate sequences.

Next-generation sequencing will have a major impact on genomics research. In the field of medical microbiology, applications are evolving in the areas of metagenomics, microbial identification, and detection of rare mutations. Ultradeep sequencing using the Roche 454 system can detect rare viral variants consisting of as little as 1% of the population, levels far deeper than those achievable with traditional sequencing methods, and the detection of these low-abundance drug resistance mutations may significantly impact treatment outcomes in HIV-1 infections (147, 177).

Hybridization Arrays

High-Density Arrays
High-density DNA hybridization arrays are produced by attaching or synthesizing hundreds or thousands of oligonucleotides on a solid support in precise patterns. A labeled amplification product is hybridized to the probes, and hybridization signals are mapped to various positions within the array. If the number of probes is sufficiently large, the sequence of the PCR product can be deduced from the pattern of hybridization (resequencing arrays). A number of manufacturers have developed high-density DNA microarrays and the instrumentation required to acquire and analyze the data. Hybridization arrays have a number of applications in microbiology, including microbial and host gene expression profiling and diagnostic sequencing. The CLSI has published a guideline for the use of diagnostic nucleic acid microarrays (20).

One of the most developed approaches brings together advances in synthetic nucleic acid chemistry with photolithography, a process used in the manufacture of semiconductors for the computer industry (Affymetrix, Santa Clara, CA). This approach uses light to direct the synthesis of short oligonucleotides on a silica wafer (127). On a 15-mm-square chip, thousands of individual sites or features can be established. At each feature, specific oligonucleotides are assembled one nucleotide at a time by light-activated chemistry.

There are a variety of sample preparation methods for the different array types, but all share a few fundamental characteristics. All methods start with extraction of total RNA, poly(A), or genomic DNA that is then converted to either cDNA or cRNA by enzymatic methods that modestly amplify the sample with tagging or incorporating biotinylated or fluoresceinated nucleotides. In expression applications, the amplification must maintain the relative abundance levels of the different transcripts present, whereas for resequencing applications, the relative abundance of information is rarely important. The DNA chip is hybridized in a flow cell with the sample for 2 to 12 h. After hybridization, a scanning laser confocal microscope evaluates the surface fluorescence intensity of the chip. Automated scanning by the microscope takes only a few minutes to acquire an image of the entire surface of the chip, and computer software analyzes the fluorescent image and determines the nucleic acid sequence or gene expression profile of the sample.

Another method of producing DNA hybridization arrays involves the precise micropipetting of premade dsDNA probes (typically 200 to 2,000 bp in length) onto glass slides with a robotic device (144). These arrays are not suitable for mutation detection due to the size and density of the arrayed DNA probes but have facilitated gene expression profiling. DNA arrays of this type can be used to determine the activation states (mRNA levels) of thousands of genes simultaneously. Gene expression profiling of pathogens by use of arrays may provide new insights into pathogenic mechanisms and help identify new therapeutic and vaccine targets.

High-density microarrays coupled with sequence-independent PCR have also been used in the discovery and characterization of pathogens and have the potential to provide rapid, unbiased, differential diagnoses of infectious diseases. Wang et al. described the first microarray designed to detect large numbers of viruses (178). The microarray consisted of 1,600 70-mer oligonucleotides derived from 140 different virus species, with an average of 10 oligonucleotides per virus species. They demonstrated that a wide variety of viruses could be detected by the microarray with sensitivities and specificities similar to those of individual virus-specific PCR assays (14). In addition, this approach has facilitated the discovery of a number of novel viruses from humans and animals, including the severe acute respiratory syndrome coronavirus (179). The field of diagnostic microarrays is rapidly developing, with multiple broad-range microarrays described (73, 90, 123, 183).

High-density microarrays hold much promise for molecular diagnostics. However, the complexity of fabricating the arrays, limited availability, and high test costs are obstacles to their routine use in clinical laboratories.

Low- to Moderate-Density Arrays
Recent developments of new detection techniques and simplified methodologies have facilitated the transition from expensive high-density arrays to cost-effective, low- to medium-density systems for clinical diagnostics. The three microarray systems described in the following paragraphs

all are FDA-cleared platforms for human genetic and pharmacogenetic applications. Each of the manufacturers has infectious-disease applications under development.

The INFINITI analyzer (Autogenomics, Carlsbad, CA) is a fully automated, multiplexing platform that uses novel BioFilmChip microarrays for a wide range of molecular diagnostic applications. Fluorescence-labeled PCR amplicons are hybridized to probes immobilized on a BioFilmChip microarray. The microarray is film-based microarray, which consists of multiple layers of thin hydrogel matrices on a polyester solid support. Each spot on the array is scanned with a built-in confocal microscope. The system has integrated controls for all steps and automatically processes and analyzes data. Infectious-disease applications under development include microarrays for detection of drug resistance in M. *tuberculosis*, respiratory viruses, sexually transmitted disease agents, and nontuberculous mycobacteria.

The Verigene system (Nanosphere, Inc., Northbrook, IL) uses gold nanoparticle-labeled probes to detect target nucleic acid hybridized to capture oligonucleotides arrayed on a glass slide. Silver signal amplification is then performed on the gold nanoparticle probes that are hybridized to the captured DNA targets of interest. The Verigene Reader optically scans the slide for silver signal, processes the data, and produces a qualitative result. A respiratory virus panel for the Verigene system that detects influenza A and B viruses and respiratory syncytial virus has been cleared by the FDA.

The eSensor system (Osmetech Molecular Diagnostics, Pasadena, CA) uses electrochemical-detection-based DNA microarrays (93). These microarrays are composed of a printed circuit board consisting of an array of 76 gold-plated electrodes. Each electrode is modified with a multicomponent, self-assembled monolayer that includes presynthesized oligonucleotide capture probes. Nucleic acid detection is based on a sandwich assay principle. Signal and capture probes are designed with sequences complementary to immediately adjacent regions on the corresponding target DNA sequence. A three-member complex is formed between capture probe, target sequence, and signal probe based on sequence-specific hybridization. This process brings the 5′ end of the signal probe containing electrochemically active ferrocene labels into close proximity to the electrode surface.

The ferrous ion in each ferrocene group undergoes cyclic oxidation and reduction, leading to loss or gain of an electron, which is measured as current at the electrode surface using alternating-current voltammetry. Higher-order harmonic signal analysis also facilitates discrimination of ferrocene-dependent faradic current from background capacitive current.

The eSensor cartridge consists of a printed circuit board, a cover, and a microfluidic component. The microfluidic component includes a diaphragm pump and check valves in line with a serpentine channel that forms the hybridization channel above the array of electrodes. The eSensor instrument consists of a base module and up to three cartridge-processing towers, each with eight slots for cartridges. The cartridge slots operate independently of each other. The throughput of a three-tower system can reach 300 tests in 8 h. A respiratory pathogen panel for the eSensor system is currently under development.

Mass Spectrometry

One of the most exciting developments in molecular microbiology is the application of mass spectrometry to identification and characterization of pathogens. Mass spectrometry is remarkably sensitive and accurate, with a throughput exceeding one sample per minute. Mass spectrometers are now common in clinical laboratories, and the advent of smaller, lower-cost instruments could facilitate wider use. Fully integrated systems for infectious-disease applications are available from Ibis Biosciences (Carlsbad, CA), a subsidiary of Abbott Molecular, and Sequenom (San Diego, CA).

Mass tag PCR uses a library of 64 distinct MassCode tags (Qiagen) to code different gene targets in multiplex PCRs. Target nucleic acids are amplified by multiplex PCR using primers labeled by a photocleavable link to molecular tags of different molecular weights. After removing the unincorporated primers, tags are released by UV irradiation and analyzed in a single quadropole mass spectrometer. The identity of the gene target in the clinical samples is determined by the size of its cognate tags. This approach was used to develop a rapid, sensitive, multiplex assay for the detection of 22 different respiratory pathogens in clinical samples (9).

The T5000 Universal Biosensor (Ibis) is a commercially available system capable of identification and characterization of a broad range of pathogens (31). In this system all nucleic acids present in a clinical sample are extracted and aliquoted into wells of a microtiter plate that each contain one or more pairs of broad-range primers for PCR. The primers are designed to amplify a product from a selected group of microorganisms, for example, all bacteria, specific species, or individual strains. The PCRs produce a mixture of products reflecting the complexity of the original mixture of microorganisms present in the clinical sample.

The PCR products are desalted and sequentially electrosprayed into a mass spectrometer for analysis. The spectral signals are processed to determine the masses of each of the PCR products present with sufficient accuracy that the base composition of each amplicon can be unambiguously deduced. Using the combined base compositions from multiple PCRs, the identities of the pathogens and their relative concentrations in the sample can be determined. Although it is not immediately intuitive, nucleic acid composition (i.e., the numbers of A's, G's, C's, and T's) in specific regions of the genome is equally as informative as the nucleic acid sequence. Mass spectrometry is remarkably sensitive and can measure the weight and determine the base composition from small quantities of nucleic acids in complex mixtures essentially instantaneously. A key element of the Ibis system is a curated database of genomics that associates base counts with primer pairs for thousands of organisms. Broad-range PCRs are capable of producing products from groups of organisms rather than single species. That, coupled with the ability of the mass spectrometer to rapidly and accurately derive base compositions from PCR amplicons, provides high information content and eliminates the need to anticipate which pathogen is present in the sample. The Ibis system has been used for the rapid identification and strain typing of a variety of bacteria, viruses, fungi, and protozoa (32, 141, 142).

Sequenom developed comparative sequencing by base-specific cleavage and matrix-assisted laser desorption ionization–time-of-flight (MALDI-TOF) mass spectrometry for automated, high-throughput microbial DNA sequence analysis (62). In this innovative genotyping method, PCR-amplified signature sequences are subjected to in vitro transcription and base-specific RNA cleavage by RNase A. Mass signal patterns of the resulting cleavage products, a mixture of RNA fragments known as compomers, are acquired and provide a fingerprint of the microorganism. Each RNA compomer is defined by its nucleotide composition with the cleavage base terminating its 3′ end and thus by its mass in the resulting mass spectrum.

The list of detected experimental compomer masses is compared with a calculated list of molecular weights derived from an in silico digest of a set of reference sequences in the system database. The simulated patterns of the reference set are used to identify the microorganism by its best match to a reference sequence. Small differences between the best-matching reference and sample sequences show up as a difference between the in silico and detected sample spectra. They can be used to identify and localize sequence differences down to a single base change and identify novel sequences. Depending on the gene target, MALDI-TOF mass spectrometry can provide high-level discrimination of individual microbial taxa or be used to identify lineages within a species (84, 92, 149, 155).

QUANTITATIVE METHODS

Many of the methods discussed above can be used to quantify the amount of RNA or DNA in a clinical sample. The most commonly used methods include PCR and RT-PCR, transcription-based amplification, and bDNA assays. The principle of quantitative molecular methods is that there is a linear relationship between the quantity of the input template and the amount of the product or signal generated. Competitive PCR (cPCR) is a reliable and robust method that was the basis of the first generation of viral load assays for HIV-1 and HCV (Roche Amplicor Monitor System) that were commonly used in clinical laboratories. These assays, based on conventional standard PCR, are still in use by clinical laboratories but are rapidly being replaced by real-time amplification methods. The basic concept behind cPCR is the coamplification in the same reaction tube of target and calibrator templates with equal or similar lengths and with the same primer binding sequences (18). Since the templates are amplified with the same primer pair, identical thermodynamics and amplification efficiencies are ensured. The amount of the calibrator must be known, and after amplification, products from the templates must be distinguishable from each other. Different types of calibrators have been used in cPCR, but in general those calibrators similar in size and base composition to the target work most effectively. RNA competitors should be used in quantitative RT-PCRs to address the problem of variable RT efficiency. This competitive amplification approach has also been used effectively with transcription-based amplification methods using RNA targets and RNA calibrators.

For cPCR, the concentration of the target template in the clinical sample can be determined by a simple calculation. The yield of the PCR product is described by the equation $Y = I(1 + e)^n$, where Y is the quantity of the PCR product, I is the quantity of the template at the beginning of the reaction, e is the efficiency of the reaction, and n is the number of cycles. In cPCR, this equation is written for both templates, as follows: competitor, $Y_c = I_c (1 + e)^n$; target, $Y_t = I_t (1 + e)^n$. Since e and n are the same for both the competitor and the target, the relative product ratio, Y_c/Y_t, directly depends on the initial concentration ratio, I_c/I_t, and the function, $Y_c/Y_t = I_c/I_t$, is linear.

Real-time amplification and detection methods are particularly well suited for quantification of nucleic acid because the amount of the fluorescent signal generated is proportional to the concentration of the target DNA or RNA in the original sample. Real-time PCR and transcription-based amplification methods are the most commonly used quantitative methods. For real-time PCR, the fluorescent signal is measured during the exponential phase of amplification, which is where the amplification plot crosses the threshold (Fig. 3). This is in contrast to standard PCR methods that measure the end point signal. There are advantages to measuring the fluorescent signal during the exponential phase of amplification; the reaction components are not limiting, and the assay is less sensitive to the effects of inhibitors. As a result, real-time PCR assays are more reproducible than standard PCR assays. Both internal and external calibrators can be used with real-time assays, but the improved precision of real-time assays allows more reliable results to be obtained with an external calibration curve than would be obtained with standard PCR. When external calibrators are used, a calibration curve is generated by plotting the $\log_{10}$ concentration of the external calibrator versus the C_T, and this plot is used to calculate the concentration of nucleic acid in the sample. The concentration of nucleic acid in the sample is inversely related to the C_T: the higher the concentration of the nucleic acid, the lower the C_T (59). In general, quantitative real-time PCR assays are not more sensitive than standard PCR assays; however, they have a much broader linear range, typically 6 to 7 orders of magnitude.

The CLSI has published guidelines for quantitative molecular methods for infectious diseases that address the development and application of quantitative PCR assays and other nucleic acid amplification methods (111).

AUTOMATION AND INSTRUMENTATION

Molecular assays consist of three major steps: specimen processing, nucleic acid amplification, and product detection. Sample processing is usually the most labor-intensive step and has represented the biggest challenge for manufacturers of automated test systems. However, in the past several years there have been considerable advances in this area with the availability of both semiautomated and fully automated systems. Automation of the nucleic acid extraction process offers laboratories several advantages, including ease of use, limited handling of the sample, improved reproducibility, reduced opportunity for cross contamination, and, for some systems, postelution functions such as adding samples into the master mix. These advantages need to be weighed against the costs of automated systems, the inflexibility of batch size, and the large sizes of many of the automated instruments. The systems vary in the types of nucleic acid extraction methods that they provide and include total nucleic acid, DNA-only, and RNA-only protocols. Other features of automated extraction systems to consider are the availability of protocols for various specimen types and volumes, variable elution volumes, the availability of target-specific and/or generic target extraction methods, and specimen throughput. The available automated systems range from fully automated high-throughput systems such as the MagNA Pure system (Roche) and m2000 generic extractor (Abbott) to those designed for a small number of specimens with random-access capabilities, such as BioRobot EZ1 (Qiagen).

There are a few automated systems available for the conventional amplification methods, such the COBAS system (Roche) for PCR and the System 340 and 440 platforms for bDNA assays (Siemens). Considerable advances in automation have been made with the availability of real-time amplification and detection systems.

Several instruments are commercially available for real-time PCR testing. These instruments vary as to speed, capacity of samples per test run, reaction volume, optics, and support for different fluorescence probe types. The time required for analysis depends to a great extent on the time required for thermocycling, and the speed of thermocycling depends on how quickly the instrument can change temperature over time. For example, some instruments can change the temperature at 20°C per s, permitting instrument analysis of up to 32 samples in as little as 30 min. Capacity may offset thermocycling speed. Although a higher-capacity instrument may have a longer thermocycling time than a lower-capacity instrument, potentially more samples may be analyzed by the high-capacity instrument in a specific time period than by the low-capacity instrument.

The reaction mixture volume assayed may also vary from one system to another. If target nucleic acid is present in extremely small amounts in a sample, an instrument that permits higher-volume analysis may be preferred.

Real-time PCR instruments utilize a variety of optics for fluorescence detection. A tungsten source lamp for excitation and selectable filters for excitation and emission wavelength detection are used in a number of instruments. Light-emitting diodes or laser excitation devices coupled with emission wavelength detection may also be used. The new real-time PCR instruments allow up to six different fluorogenic dyes to be used simultaneously in one reaction. Until recently, real-time PCR instruments were designed for research applications. The Prism series of sequence detection systems (Applied Biosystems), LightCycler (Roche), SmartCycler (Cepheid, Sunnyvale, CA), and Rotor-Gene (Qiagen) are examples of research instruments that find widespread use in molecular diagnostics laboratories. The COBAS TaqMan analyzer (Roche) and the m2000 system (Abbott) are the first real-time instruments designed specifically for use in clinical laboratories (4).

Many manufacturers are coupling automated nucleic acid extraction instruments with amplification and detection systems to create high-throughput, fully automated nucleic acid analyzers. The TIGRIS system (Gen-Probe), the AmpliPrep-COBAS TaqMan system (Roche), the m2000 system (Abbott), and the Viper System (BD Diagnostics) are examples of fully automated and integrated systems designed to perform sample processing, nucleic acid amplification, and product detection. The GeneXpert system (Cepheid) represents the other end of the automation spectrum, in which a single sample is added to a disposable fluidic cartridge that fully automates and integrates sample preparation, amplification, and real-time detection. The instrument is a random-access design, amendable to on-demand molecular diagnostic testing.

CURRENT APPLICATIONS

Molecular methods have created new opportunities for the clinical microbiology laboratory to affect patient care in the areas of initial diagnosis, disease prognosis, and monitoring of response to therapy. Over time the methods have become more automated, the cost of testing has decreased, and clinical utility has been proven for the diagnosis and management of a variety of infectious diseases. As a result, molecular testing is now routinely performed in many clinical microbiology laboratories, and clinical applications will continue to expand in the future.

Initial Diagnosis

With the development of molecular methods, the clinical microbiology laboratory is no longer reliant solely on the traditional culture methods for detection of pathogens in clinical specimens. Culture-based methods have long been the gold standard for infectious-disease diagnosis, but for several diseases, nucleic acid-based tests have replaced culture as the gold standard. HCV infection, enteroviral meningitis, pertussis, HSV encephalitis, and genital infections due to C. trachomatis are some examples of infectious diseases in which nucleic acid-based tests are the new gold standards for diagnosis. This technology has been used to best advantage in situations in which traditional methods are slow, insensitive, expensive, or not available. These techniques work particularly well with fragile or fastidious microorganisms that may die in transit or be overgrown by contaminating biota when cultured. N. gonorrhoeae is an example for which the nucleic acid can be detected under circumstances in which the organism cannot be cultured. The use of improper collection media, inappropriate transport conditions, or delays in transport can reduce the viability of the pathogen but may leave the nucleic acid still detectable. It is beyond the scope of this chapter to review all of the possible applications or to provide a compendium of methods for detection of various pathogens. The reader is directed to another excellent resource for this information (129).

Opportunities to actually replace culture for bacterial pathogens in routine practice are limited by the need to isolate the organisms for antibiotic susceptibility testing. In those applications in which culture has actually been replaced by nucleic acid testing, the pathogens are of predictable susceptibilities and consequently, routine susceptibility testing is not performed, or the genetics of resistance are well defined and simple to detect, such as methicillin resistance in S. aureus.

Molecular methods have had the biggest impact in clinical virology, in which the molecular approaches are often faster, more sensitive, and more cost-effective than the traditional methods. The diagnoses of enteroviral meningitis, HSV encephalitis, and CMV infections in immunocompromised patients are examples of clinically relevant and cost-effective applications of nucleic acid-based tests. There are greater opportunities to replace the conventional methods in virology than in bacteriology because the culture-based methods are costly and antiviral susceptibility testing is not routinely performed. In those situations in which antiviral susceptibility testing is required, such as identification of ganciclovir-resistant CMV, molecular methods (i.e., sequencing) are the method of choice for rapid identification of mutations. The diagnostic role of molecular tests has been further expanded with the FDA approval of the AP-TIMA HIV-1 RNA qualitative test (Gen-Probe). The diagnosis of HIV-1 infection has traditionally been performed with screening serologic tests and Western blotting as the confirmatory test. The APTIMA test can now be used for the diagnosis of acute HIV-1, to resolve indeterminate Western blot results, and to confirm the screening serologic result. A limitation of molecular tests for viral diagnostics is the clinical need for simultaneous identification of multiple pathogens, for example, respiratory viruses. Recently, multiplex PCR tests have been developed and some FDA cleared that allow for the detection of several respiratory viruses in a single test. Real-time PCR tests utilize multiple primer pairs and probes with different fluorescent dyes to detect influenza A and B viruses and respiratory syncytial virus, as well as an internal control (85). Using this approach, multiple tests will be needed to detect the common respiratory viruses that are now identified using fluorescent-antibody testing and culture. A second approach is to perform a conventional multiplex PCR utilizing primer pairs targeting a larger number of viruses and coupling this with the Luminex bead detection system described above (98, 113).

This allows for the detection of many respiratory viruses in a single test but requires postamplification manipulation of the sample, which introduces the possibility of false-positive results due to carryover contamination. It is likely that both of these multiplex approaches will be applied for other groups of pathogens, such as those causing central nervous system infections and diarrheal diseases.

Perhaps the greatest impact of molecular methods has been in the discovery of previously unrecognized or uncultivable pathogens. During the past 20 years, a number of infectious agents were first identified directly from clinical material by using molecular methods. HCV, the principal etiologic agent of what was once known as non-A, non-B hepatitis, was discovered in 1989 through the application of molecular cloning techniques by investigators from the Centers for Disease Control and the Chiron Corporation (16). Cloning and analysis of the HCV genome led to production of viral antigens that now serve as the basis of the specific serologic tests used to screen the blood supply and to diagnose hepatitis C. To date, HCV has resisted all attempts at sustained in vitro propagation. As a result, RT-PCR is used to detect, quantify, and genotype HCV in infected individuals.

Tropheryma whipplei, the causative agent of Whipple's disease, is another example of an uncultivable microorganism which was initially identified by molecular methods (134). It was discovered by the use of broad-range PCR, in which primers are directed against conserved sequences in the bacterial 16S rRNA gene. Sequence analysis of the PCR product and comparison with known 16S rRNA gene sequences were used to characterize the organism and establish its disease association. This approach provides a new paradigm for discovery of unrecognized pathogens that is of value in other diseases with features that suggest an infectious etiology.

Molecular methods are very powerful tools for the identification of emerging pathogens. RT-PCR with consensus primers was used to rapidly identify the etiologic agent of severe acute respiratory syndrome as a coronavirus (76, 128). Within a few months of the recognized outbreak, the virus was identified and sequenced and the molecular assays were developed that played an essential role in diagnosing the infection and defining the epidemiology of the infection. Similarly, high-throughput sequencing has been used to identify a novel polyomavirus, WU virus, from a nasopharyngeal aspirate from a 3-year-old with pneumonia (42). Using a specifically designed real-time PCR assay, this virus has been shown to be present in 0.7 to 3.0% of patients with acute respiratory infections; the majority of patients were coinfected with other respiratory viruses (42, 82).

Identification of Bacteria and Fungi by Nucleic Acid Sequencing

Nucleotide sequence analysis of the 16S bacterial rRNA gene has expanded our knowledge of the phylogenetic relationships among bacteria and is the new standard for bacterial identification. rRNA contains several functionally different regions, with some regions having highly conserved and others having highly varied nucleic acid sequences (181). The sequence of the 16S rRNA gene is a stable genotypic signature that can be used to identify an organism at the genus or species level. The 16S gene sequence can be determined rapidly and provides objective results independent of phenotypic characteristics. As discussed in the preceding section, it can also be used to characterize previously unrecognized species. A similar approach that targets

the nuclear large subunit of the rRNA gene can be used for the identification of fungi (77). This gene is found in all fungi and contains sufficient variation to identify most fungi accurately to the species level.

The DNA sequencing approach to microbial identification involves extraction of the nucleic acids, amplification of the target sequence by PCR, sequence determination, and a computer software-aided search of an appropriate sequence database. The major limitations of this approach to microbial identification include the high cost of automated nucleic acid sequencers, the lack of appropriate analysis software, and limited databases.

Applied Biosystems has developed ribosomal gene sequencing kits for bacteria and fungi. A sequence from an unknown bacterium is compared with either full or partial 16S rRNA sequences from over 1,000 type strains by using the MicroSeq analysis software (160). The software analysis provides percent base pair differences between the unknown bacterium and the 20 most closely related bacteria, alignment tools to show differences between the related sequences, and phylogenetic tree tools to verify that the unknown bacterium actually clusters with the 20 closest bacteria in the database. The MicroSeq fungal identification system is similar to the bacterial identification system but targets D2 large-subunit rRNA (52, 53). Continued improvements in automation, refinements of analysis software, and decreases in cost should lead to more widespread use of nucleic acid sequence-based approaches to microbial identification.

More recently, pyrosequencing, or sequencing by synthesis, has been used for the identification of infectious pathogens. Since the length of high-quality sequence generated is limited to 50 to 100 bp, it is very useful for single-nucleotide polymorphism analysis, but it has also been applied to taxonomic categorization of microorganisms. This approach requires identifying a variable region that contains a unique sequence for the different microorganisms within the group. Pyrosequencing has been successfully used to classify mycobacteria and nocardiae into clinically important groups and to identify yeasts and filamentous fungi (132, 170).

Disease Prognosis

Molecular techniques have created opportunities for the laboratory to provide important information that may predict disease progression. Probably the best example is HIV-1 viral load as a predictor of progression to AIDS and death in infected individuals. This predictive value was first demonstrated in 1996 as part of a multicenter AIDS cohort study (103). The investigators showed that the risk of progression to AIDS and death was directly related to the magnitude of the viral load in plasma at study entry. The viral load in plasma was a better predictor of disease progression than the number of $CD4^+$ lymphocytes. Subsequent studies have confirmed that baseline viral load critically influences disease progression.

Subtyping of certain viruses by molecular methods may also have prognostic value. Subtyping of respiratory syncytial viruses may provide information about the severity of infection in hospitalized infants, with those infected with group A viruses having poorer outcomes (176). HPV causes dysplasia, intraepithelial neoplasia, and carcinoma of the cervix in women. HPV types 16 and 18 are associated with a high risk of progression to neoplasia, and types 6 and 11 are associated with a low risk of progression (133). The clinical utility of molecular testing for high-risk HPV DNA has been established for managing women with the cervical cytologic diagnosis of atypical squamous cells of undetermined significance. Women with this condition can be referred for colposcopy based on the detection of high-risk HPV DNA (151). HPV DNA testing is approved by the FDA for use as an adjunct to cytology for cervical cancer screening in women aged 30 years or more (184).

CMV viral load testing has recently been shown to be useful for deciding when to initiate preemptive therapy in organ transplant recipients and distinguishing active disease from asymptomatic infection. Studies have shown that the level of CMV DNA can predict the development of active CMV disease (33, 63), with higher viral load values increasing the risk of symptomatic disease. It is likely that quantitative assays will be also useful in distinguishing disease from infection with other herpesviruses such as Epstein-Barr virus and HHV-6.

Duration of and Response to Therapy

Molecular methods have been developed to detect the genes responsible for resistance to single antibiotics or classes of antibiotics in bacteria and in many cases are superior to the phenotypic, growth-based methods. The detection of methicillin resistance in staphylococci, vancomycin resistance in enterococci, and rifampin resistance in M. *tuberculosis* provides examples of where molecular methods are used to supplement the growth-based methods (165). However, it is difficult to imagine, given our current state of knowledge of the molecular genetics of antimicrobial resistance and the technological limitations, that a genotypic approach to routine antimicrobial susceptibility testing of bacteria could rival the phenotypic methods in terms of information content and cost.

Molecular techniques are playing an increasing role in predicting and monitoring patient response to antiviral therapy. The laboratory may have a role in predicting response to therapy by detecting specific drug resistance mutations, determining viral load, and genotyping. Both viral load and genotype are independent predictors of response to combination therapy with pegylated interferon and ribavirin in chronic HCV infections, although genotype is the main predictor of response (38, 50, 99, 187). Those patients with high pretreatment viral loads ($\geq$2 million copies/ml or 600,000 IU/ml) or genotype 1 infections have lower sustained response rates than do those with genotype 2 and 3 infections (38, 50, 99). Genotype is also used to determine the duration of therapy, with genotype 1 infections requiring a longer course of therapy than genotype 2 or 3 infections (28, 187). Recent studies have more closely defined duration of therapy based on the extent of the viral response. Patients that do not reach a $\geq$2-log$_{10}$ drop in viral load at 12 weeks after initiating therapy are very unlikely to respond to pegylated interferon and ribavirin (41). Moreover, patients with a rapid virologic response (HCV RNA level of <50 IU/ml 4 weeks after initiating therapy) may require a shorter duration of therapy, provided they have a low baseline HCV RNA level ($\leq$400,000 IU/ml) and minimal hepatic fibrosis (187).

Quantitative tests for HIV-1 RNA are the standard of practice for guiding clinicians in initiating, monitoring, and changing antiretroviral therapy. Several commercially available HIV-1 viral load assays have been FDA approved, and guidelines for their use in clinical practice have been published (54; DHHS Panel on Antiretroviral Guidelines, http://AIDSinfo.nih.gov). Viral load assays have also been used in monitoring response to therapy in patients chronically infected with HBV (89) and in predicting the risk for developing BKV-associated nephropathy in renal

transplant recipients (60). In organ transplant recipients, the persistence of CMV viral load after several weeks of antiviral therapy is associated with the development of resistant virus (11).

LABORATORY PRACTICE

The unparalleled analytical sensitivity of nucleic acid amplification techniques coupled with their susceptibility to cross contamination presents unique challenges to the routine application of these techniques in the clinical laboratory. There are special concerns in the areas of specimen processing, work flow, quality assurance, and interpretation of test results. Additional information can be found in CLSI documents MM3-A2, *Molecular Diagnostic Methods for Infectious Diseases; Approved Guideline*, 2nd ed. (22); MM6-A, *Quantitative Molecular Methods for Infectious Diseases; Approved Guideline* (111); and MM13-A, *Collection, Transport, Preparation, and Storage of Specimens and Samples for Molecular Methods; Approved Guideline* (19).

Specimen Collection, Transport, and Processing

Proper collection, transport, and processing of clinical specimens are essential to ensure reliable results from molecular assays. Nucleic acid integrity must be maintained throughout these processes. Important issues to consider in specimen collection are the timing of specimen collection in relationship to disease state and the proper specimen type. Other factors that come into play include the use of the proper anticoagulant, transport and storage temperatures, and time to processing of the specimen. HIV-1 viral load testing is an example in which the proper conditions for specimen collection, transport, and processing have been well described and has provided insight into the importance of these factors. For HIV-1 viral load testing, the plasma needs to be separated from the cells within 6 h of collection to minimize degradation of RNA. Once the plasma has been separated, it can be stored at 4°C for several days, but −70°C is recommended for long-term storage (139). Most types of specimens are best stored at −20 to −70°C prior to processing.

Molecular methods have several advantages over conventional culture with regard to specimen collection. It may be easier to maintain the integrity of nucleic acid than the viability of an organism. Molecular tests for the detection of C. *trachomatis* and N. *gonorrhoeae* are an example in which DNA is stable on dry cervical swabs for a week at room temperature or refrigeration temperatures, which is in stark contrast to the conditions required to maintain organism viability for culture. Nucleic acid persists in specimens after initiation of treatment (41, 83), thus allowing detection of a pathogen even though the organism can no longer be cultured. Also, due to the increased sensitivity of molecular assays, it may be possible to test a smaller volume of specimen or use a specimen that is collected using a less invasive method.

The major goals of specimen processing are to release nucleic acid from the organism, maintain the integrity of the nucleic acid, render the sample noninfectious, remove inhibiting substances, and, in some instances, concentrate the specimen. These processes need to be balanced with minimizing manipulation of the specimen. Complex specimen processing methods are time-consuming and may lead to the loss of target nucleic acid or result in contamination between specimens. Care must be taken to avoid carrying over inhibitory substances, such as phenol or alcohol, from the nucleic acid isolation step to the amplification reaction.

There are several general methods for nucleic acid extraction. Different methods may be used depending on whether the desire is to purify RNA or DNA or both. Another factor to consider when deciding on a nucleic acid extraction method is the type of pathogen sought. Some pathogens, such as viruses, can be very easy to lyse, while mycobacteria, staphylococci, and fungi can be very difficult to lyse. Enzyme digestion, harsh lysis conditions, or mechanical disruption may be required to disrupt the cell walls of these organisms.

DNA isolation methods often use detergents to solubilize the cell wall or membranes, a proteolytic enzyme (such as proteinase K) to digest proteins, and EDTA to chelate divalent cations needed for nuclease activity (6, 47). The lysate can be used directly in amplification assays, or additional steps may follow to purify the nucleic acid. These additional steps remove proteins and traces of organic solvents and concentrate the specimen. In order to successfully use a crude lysate, the target DNA must be present in a relatively high concentration and there must be minimal inhibitors of amplification in the sample. If these criteria are not met, additional purification steps should be used.

Another commonly used method of nucleic acid isolation involves disruption of cells or organisms with the chaotropic agent guanidinium thiocyanate and a detergent (15). After a short incubation, the nucleic acid can be precipitated with isopropanol. Guanidinium thiocyanate denatures proteins and is also a strong inhibitor of ribonucleases, making it a very useful tool for RNA isolation, although it is also used for purification of DNA. The Boom extraction method is also based on the lysing and nuclease-inactivating properties of guanidinium thiocyanate but utilizes the acid-binding properties of silica or glass particles to purify nucleic acid (7). Over the past several years, various manufacturers have developed commercially available reagents using one of these basic methods or a modification of these methods. Many of these methods rely on the use of spin column technology, are easy to use, and provide a rapid, reproducible method for purification of nucleic acid from a wide variety of clinical specimens. In recent years, further advances have been made with the introduction of magnetic silica particles which are coupled with instruments providing various degrees of automation, thus further simplifying nucleic acid extraction and purification. These reagents tend to be expensive, but the additional cost can be offset by labor savings. Laboratories are increasingly using automated systems for nucleic acid extraction, as they require less hands-on time, may reduce the risk of cross contamination between specimens, and provide more consistent yields. There are now many automated systems available for use in clinical laboratories; they should be thoroughly evaluated because not all isolate nucleic acids with the same efficiency and purity. The quality of the nucleic acid can have a significant impact on the performance of a molecular test.

Tissue samples need to be disrupted prior to the nucleic acid extraction process. This can be accomplished by cutting the tissue into small pieces or mechanically homogenizing the tissue prior to proceeding with one of the above-described extraction methods. Preserved tissue specimens require removal of the paraffin with solvents and slicing into fine sections prior to processing.

Removing inhibitors of amplification is a key function of the nucleic acid extraction process. Simple methods of nucleic acid extraction that involve boiling of the specimen have been used for relatively acellular specimens such as cerebrospinal fluid (CSF). Though the boiling method is fast and easy, there are problems with inhibitors of amplification in CSF that are not inactivated by boiling (104). The inhibition rate can be reduced to <1% by using a silica-based extraction method. Similarly, crude lysates of urine and cervical swab specimens are commonly used for the detection of *C. trachomatis* and *N. gonorrhoeae*. Specimens containing amplification inhibitors have been reported to range from 1 to 5% for urine to as much as 20% for cervical swabs (137). Common inhibitory substances include hemoglobin, crystals, β-human chorionic gonadotropin, and nitrates. Blood samples are used commonly for detection and/or quantification of a variety of viral pathogens, including HIV-1, HCV, and CMV. HIV-1 viral load testing is an example in which the effects of different anticoagulants have been well studied. HIV-1 viral RNA is most stable when collected in EDTA, and heparin has been shown to be inhibitory to amplification and should be avoided (5, 67). In addition, very small volumes of whole blood (1%) can be inhibitory to *Taq* DNA polymerase (58). Other compounds such as acidic polysaccharides, which are components of glycoproteins present in sputum and cervical specimens and bile salts found in stool, can also inhibit polymerase (39). Human DNA, when present in the sample in high quantities, for example, tissue or blood, may also interfere with the detection of a low concentration of pathogen nucleic acid. With the recognition of such a wide array of inhibitors of amplification and the availability of simple, reliable, semiautomated and automated nucleic acid extraction methods, the use of crude lysates for testing becomes more difficult to justify. Regardless of the nucleic acid extraction method employed, the laboratory should monitor inhibition rates for different specimen types and nucleic acid extraction methods (see "Quality Control and Assurance" below).

Contamination Control

Several types of contamination can occur with molecular testing: cross contamination of specimens during the nucleic acid extraction step, contamination of specimens with positive control material, and carryover contamination of amplified products. Contamination with amplified products can occur with DNA or RNA target amplification and with probe amplification methods. It does not occur with signal amplification assays, since nucleic acid molecules are not synthesized with these methods. Cross contamination that occurs during specimen processing or handling of positive control material can occur with all amplification methods. The approach to the control of contamination due to amplified products has changed dramatically with the widespread use of real-time amplification and detection methods. Since the reaction tube is not opened after amplification, there is minimal risk of contamination from the amplified product. Many laboratories using real-time methods continue to use a variety of good laboratory practices to control for contamination, but the focus is on minimizing cross contamination between specimens rather than contamination from the amplified product. Refer to CLSI document MM3-A2, *Molecular Diagnostic Methods for Infectious Diseases; Approved Guideline*, 2nd ed. (22), and *Molecular Microbiology: Diagnostic Principles and Practice*, 2nd ed. (105), for detailed descriptions of good laboratory practices to minimize contamination.

Clinical microbiologists have long been concerned about minimizing contamination between samples with microorganisms during specimen processing. Molecular methods have raised the level of concern considerably, and for good reason, as current methods can detect a few molecules. The previously undetected low levels of contamination that occurred in processing specimens for routine culture can lead to false-positive results in molecular assays. Prevention of contamination due to target DNA or RNA is best done by careful handling of specimens to avoid splashing, opening only one specimen tube at a time, pulse-spinning tubes prior to opening, using screw-top tubes rather than snap-cap tubes to minimize aerosolization, bleaching work surfaces, and using plugged pipette tips. Some of these approaches can be difficult for high-volume laboratories, which is why automated extraction systems can be very useful. Care must be taken with these systems to ensure that there is no cross contamination during the automated process. This is often done by alternating negative and high-titer specimens in a checkerboard arrangement and monitoring for carryover of sample into the negative specimens. These experiments should be designed with an understanding of the concentration of the organism in the clinical specimen. For example, the concentration of HSV in CSF from patients with meningitis is quite low compared to the concentration of BKV in the urine of a patient with nephropathy.

Preventing contamination of the laboratory with DNA from a clinical specimen or positive control material is very important, because eliminating contamination with target DNA once it occurs can be very difficult. This is why care should be taken to use a positive control at the lowest concentration that consistently amplifies. The enzymatic and photochemical inactivation methods used to control carryover contamination of amplified products are not effective in preventing contamination with target DNA.

Enzymatic inactivation of amplified product can be accomplished with uracil-N-glycosylase (UNG), a DNA repair enzyme found in a variety of bacterial species. During the PCR, dTTP is replaced with dUTP so that dUTP is incorporated into the newly synthesized DNA products. This allows for a distinction between starting template DNA and amplified products; only newly synthesized PCR products will contain deoxyuracil. If UTP-containing amplification products are present as contaminants, the addition of UNG to the reaction mixture will result in the cleavage of deoxyuracil residues, thus destroying the contaminating DNA (95). The use of UNG increases the amount of carryover DNA needed to contaminate the reaction mixture by several orders of magnitude (124). When UNG is used, it is important to keep the annealing temperature above 55°C so that the UNG remains inactive, thus avoiding degradation of newly synthesized product. For the same reason, after completion of amplification, the reaction mixture should be held at 72°C (168). UNG can be inactivated at 94°C, but prolonged inactivation at 94°C may also affect the activity of the polymerase enzyme. UNG will not remove uracil from RNA molecules and is therefore ineffective in controlling contamination in RNA amplification assays, such as TMA and NASBA.

When UTP and UNG are used, the PCR conditions should be reoptimized, as the magnesium requirement may increase. The efficiency of amplification may be reduced when UTP is substituted for TTP. This can be overcome by adding a mixture of dUTP and dTTP into the master mix. The efficiency of inactivation using UNG depends on the size of the amplified product and its G+C content. Inactivation may not be effective with amplified products of fewer than 100 bp, as maximum UNG efficiency requires the DNA molecule to be 150 bp (34).

Contamination of laboratory work surfaces, equipment, reagents, and clothing of laboratory personnel with previously amplified nucleic acid products is of particular concern for clinical laboratories, since these products can accumulate over time with routine testing and can be inadvertently transferred to subsequent assay reactions, resulting in false-positive test results. To minimize the potential for such amplicon contamination and false-positive results, laboratories performing molecular tests with target amplification methods were designed traditionally to have physical separation of preamplification (i.e., reagent preparation and sample processing), amplification-detection, and postamplification (i.e., DNA sequencing) areas with separate ventilation systems. In addition to the use of dedicated rooms, biological cabinets, and dead-air boxes for various processes involved in specimen testing, laboratories have also typically employed a unidirectional work flow for the movement of specimens, supplies, and personnel from preamplification to postamplification areas through each phase of testing. The physical separation of pre- and postamplification activities and a unidirectional work flow are particularly important for those laboratories performing postamplification analyses in which the reaction vessel is opened and the amplicon transferred to another vessel or device (e.g., sequencing or liquid bead microarrays). The strict separation of pre- and postamplification areas is less important for laboratories using real-time amplification methods, particularly those using fully automated systems that perform nucleic acid extraction, amplification, and detection.

Quality Control and Assurance

Verification and validation are terms that are often used interchangeably; however, they are different processes. Verification is the process by which assay performance is determined; parameters such as sensitivity, specificity, positive and negative predictive values, and accuracy are established. The verification of an assay is completed before the assay is used for patient testing. Validation is the ongoing process of proving that the assay is performing as expected and achieves the intended result or intended use.

The analytical verification of an assay provides information on the performance characteristics of the assay, including the limit of detection, linear and measuring ranges (quantitative tests), trueness, precision, and specificity, while the clinical verification determines the clinical utility of the assay. The analytical performance characteristics of a test should be well understood prior to determining the clinical utility of a test, and any analytical limitations need to be considered when determining clinical uses. For example, a qualitative HSV DNA test may have adequate sensitivity to detect cases of HSV encephalitis but have inadequate sensitivity to detect the lower levels of DNA found in cases of HSV meningitis.

Determining the clinical utility of a molecular assay can be difficult when the molecular assay is more sensitive than the gold standard. This situation was seen with the commercial assays designed to detect *C. trachomatis* in genital specimens. Molecular assays proved to be much more sensitive than the gold standard method of culture. An insensitive gold standard can make a molecular assay appear to have a falsely low specificity. In this situation, an expanded gold standard can be used. For *C. trachomatis*, this included direct fluorescent-antibody testing and/or another molecular method (41, 83, 143). There are additional challenges in determining the clinical utility of molecular assays that detect rare pathogens. These assays are usually laboratory developed, and any given medical center may see very few cases of the disease, making clinical verification difficult. Moreover, standards and control material can be difficult to obtain for rare pathogens. Several companies now provide control material for the more common molecular assays, such as those for C. trachomatis, N. gonorrhoeae, HIV-1, HCV, and CMV. A complete list of reference materials for molecular microbiology tests is maintained by the Genetic Testing Reference Material Coordination Program, Centers for Disease Control and Prevention, and can be accessed at http://wwwn.cdc.gov/dls/genetics/rmmaterials/default.aspx. The availability of calibrators that are made based on a consensus standard (such as the WHO standards for HIV-1 and HCV) are very important in establishing the clinical utility of viral load tests. The lack of such calibrators makes standardization of laboratory-developed tests very difficult. This has been particularly problematic for CMV and EBV, for which the presence of latent infection and asymptomatic reactivation leading to low levels of viral replication underscores the need to establish clinical cutoffs for initiating therapy or reducing immunosuppression. With the lack of an international standard, there is poor agreement of viral load values between laboratory-developed tests (125), so clinically important cutoffs to predict the development of disease need to be determined by the individual laboratory. The National Institute of Standards and Technology and National Institute for Biological Standards and Controls are working to establish standards for CMV and EBV. Once available, these standards should improve the agreement of viral load values among laboratory-developed tests, which will facilitate the establishment of clinically relevant cutoffs.

A positive control is designed to ensure that the test can consistently detect a concentration of target nucleic acid at or near the limit of detection of the assay. The positive control should be at the lowest concentration that can be reproducibly amplified. A positive control that is significantly greater than the cutoff of the assay may not detect small decreases in amplification efficiency. In addition, use of large amounts of target DNA can increase problems with contamination in the laboratory. For a quantitative test, two levels of positive control are required: a low positive control near the lower limit of quantification and a high positive control near the upper limit of quantification. For real-time methods that have an upper limit of quantification of 10^7 or 10^8 copies/ml, it may not be possible to find adequate amounts of control material, so a sample in the range of 10^5 copies/ml is often used. Depending on the availability of material, the positive control may be purified nucleic acid or lysed or intact organisms. An extraction control tests the ability of the nucleic acid extraction or purification method to successfully release nucleic acid from the organism. The extraction control, which should be intact organisms, can also serve as a positive control if it is used at the appropriate concentration.

Monitoring for the presence of inhibitors in a specimen is important, particularly for complex specimens such as blood or sputum. Several methods can be used to control for inhibition. One method is to amplify two aliquots of a clinical specimen, one directly and the second spiked with an aliquot of positive control DNA. For a specimen to be considered negative for the target analyte, testing results for the direct specimen must be negative and those for the spiked specimen must be positive. If an inhibitor of amplification was present, the spiked specimen would be negative. The concentration of positive control used for the spike must be near the limit of detection of the assay to ensure that low-level inhibition of amplification is detected.

Another approach to monitoring for inhibition of amplification is adding an internal control to the clinical specimen prior to nucleic acid extraction. As discussed in "Quantitative Methods" above, the internal control molecule may be designed with the same primer binding sites as the target molecule but modified in some manner so as to allow detection separate from the target based on size or sequence. An internal control may be designed that does not share the same primer binding sites as the target molecular; in this situation a separate set of primers is needed for amplification. An internal control is an effective way to monitor for inhibition, but it may decrease the sensitivity of the assay due to competition for assay components. Amplification of a human housekeeping gene such as the β-globin gene may also be used as an internal control, but the gene should not be present in vast excess of the target molecule or inhibition of amplification of the target molecule can occur without evidence of inhibition of the housekeeping gene. Inhibition controls should be included in assays that use a new specimen extraction method or specimen type. A cost-effective approach is to discontinue these controls once the inhibition rate is determined to be less than 1%. However, discontinuing the use of an internal control limits the ability to detect inhibition due to preanalytical factors, such as collection of the specimen in a tube containing heparin rather than EDTA.

Under certain conditions, there may be a need to determine if there is adequate nucleic acid in a specimen, for example, when using paraffin-embedded tissue or when evaluating the quality of a specimen. In these situations, amplification of housekeeping genes can be used to determine if the specimen contains human DNA. The absence of amplifiable human DNA from the specimen raises concern about whether the specimen quality is adequate.

Negative controls should be included in all assays and processed in a manner similar to the processing of the clinical specimens. The negative control should be taken through all steps of the assay, including the nucleic acid extraction process. However, the absence of amplification in the negative control does not ensure that there is not contamination in the run, as contamination is often low level and sporadic. Including multiple negative controls in the run may provide additional assurance that there is no contamination, but this approach may be cost prohibitive. Ideally, the negative control should be a clinical specimen that does not contain the analyte of interest. These types of controls may be difficult to obtain, so water or buffer is often substituted.

Currently, the College of American Pathologists (CAP) is the only Centers for Medicare and Medicaid Services (CMS)-approved proficiency program for molecular testing for infectious diseases. The CAP provides proficiency testing for many common pathogens for which routine testing is done in the clinical laboratory. The Quality Control for Molecular Diagnostics proficiency program, which is jointly sponsored by the European Society for Clinical Virology and the European Society for Clinical Microbiology and Infectious Diseases (Glasgow, Scotland, United Kingdom), also provides testing for a variety of pathogens. When formal external proficiency testing programs are not available, laboratories may split samples with other laboratories, split samples between a new method and an established laboratory-developed method, or clinically validate the test result by clinical diagnosis. When exchanging specimens between laboratories for proficiency testing, it is important that the two laboratories use the same method, particularly for quantitative methods, as viral loads will differ substantially among the various assays.

Reporting and Interpretation of Results

The interpretation of molecular assays requires a basic understanding of the strengths and limitations of these technologies. There are unique problems in interpreting molecular testing results that are not routinely encountered with traditional microbiological assays, such as culture and serology. Some of the problems that may occur in interpreting molecular assays include recognizing false-positive results, distinguishing viable from nonviable organisms, and correlating nucleic acid detection with the presence of disease.

For interpretation of a positive test result, the issues that need to be considered are assay specificity and contamination. The specificities of most molecular assays are established by the primers and probes used during amplification and detection steps; if they cross-react with other pathogens, then false-positive results are possible. For example, primers designed to detect M. tuberculosis from respiratory specimens must not cross-react with organisms that are part of the normal oral biota or other common respiratory pathogens, such as Streptococcus pneumoniae. Although uncommon, problems with primer specificity do occur; the primers designed to amplify the 5′ untranslated region of enteroviruses have been reported to cross-react with rhinoviruses. This would not be a problem for testing of CSF specimens but would preclude using the assay on respiratory specimens. Problems with primer specificity have also been reported for a commercially available PCR assay designed to detect N. gonorrhoeae. The primers used in this assay cross-react with Neisseria subflava, a nonpathogenic organism found in the oropharynx (35). False-positive results can also be due to contamination, which may occur during specimen processing or as a result of carryover contamination with previously amplified products.

The interpretation of a negative result requires consideration of assay sensitivity, specimen quality, nucleic acid extraction efficacy, and amplification efficiency. Problems with any of these factors can lead to a false-negative result, which is why measures to control for each of these parameters should be included in assays whenever feasible. Another source of false-negative results is sequence variation, which may prevent binding of either primers or probes. To minimize this problem, one should perform a thorough search of known sequences before designing the assay and occasionally reexamine the available databases after the assay is put into clinical use. False-negative results may also occur when the specimen type is not optimal (throat swab versus nasopharyngeal aspirate for the detection of respiratory pathogens), or when the specimen is collected at an inappropriate time in the disease course.

Molecular assays detect pathogen nucleic acid but cannot determine whether that nucleic acid is found in a viable or nonviable organism. Pathogen nucleic acid can be detected for long periods after appropriate treatment is initiated. For example, C. trachomatis DNA can be found in the urine of patients for up to 3 weeks after completion of a course of therapy (41). Similar results have been reported for the detection of HSV DNA in the CSF of patients with encephalitis. DNA can persist for 2 weeks or longer after the initiation of acyclovir therapy (80). Due to the persistence of pathogen DNA after initiation of therapy, qualitative molecular assays should not be used to monitor response to therapy. One notable exception is the use of an HCV RNA RT-PCR assay to monitor the response to therapy with pegylated interferon and ribavirin. In this instance, the absence of detectable viral RNA from plasma is used to define treatment response (50, 99).

The detection of pathogen nucleic acid does not ensure that the organism is the cause of disease. The organism may be present as part of the normal microbiota, as a colonizer of a particular area, or as a cause of infection. Distinguishing between colonization and infection may be more difficult when molecular techniques that are more sensitive than culture are used. Organisms present in very low concentrations, which may have gone undetected by routine culture methods, may be detected by using molecular techniques.

Distinguishing colonization from infection is easier when testing a specimen from a normally sterile site such as CSF or blood; however, this factor alone does not ensure that the organism is a true pathogen. This distinction is a concern with the detection of herpesviruses, which cause lifelong latent infections. An important example of distinguishing these two states is monitoring transplant recipients for CMV disease using molecular methods. Initial studies used very sensitive qualitative PCR assays (43, 115), and it was clear that CMV DNA could be detected in the blood of patients that never went on to develop symptomatic disease. Quantitative molecular tests have been useful in stratifying the risk of active disease; the higher the viral load result, the higher the risk of active CMV disease (33, 63). Similar data are emerging for S. pneumoniae infections; early studies showed that qualitative tests of respiratory specimens could not distinguish pneumonia from asymptomatic colonization of the respiratory tract. The clinical utility of quantitative tests to differentiate infection from colonization is under investigation (72).

Reporting the results of a qualitative molecular assay is usually straightforward; results are often reported as DNA detected or not detected. Several key parameters that may also be reported are the limit of detection of the assay, data pertaining to the rate of inhibition for a given sample type, the gene target, and the amplification method used for testing. Reporting results from quantitative assays is more complex and requires consideration of several parameters, including measuring range, units, and precision. Results of quantitative assays can be expressed as copies, weight (nanograms or picograms), or international units of the target nucleic acid in a defined volume, such as milliliters of plasma or blood, grams of tissue, or number of leukocytes. Viral loads are reported as integers, in scientific notation, or as $\log_{10}$ transformed data. Ideally, $\log_{10}$ transformed results should be reported, as this better reflects biologically relevant changes in load of microorganisms that usually replicate exponentially, and because most assays exponentially amplify the target. Moreover, clinicians may be less likely to overinterpret insignificant changes in viral loads when results are reported as $\log_{10}$ transformed values. Since patients and clinicians may not be as familiar with $\log_{10}$ transformed results, laboratories may choose to report both integers and $\log_{10}$ transformed numbers. For quantitative tests, the number of significant digits reported for viral loads should be limited due to the precision of the test. Integers should be rounded to 10s or 100s (734 copies/ml to 730 copies/ml; 52,321 copies/ml to 52,300 copies/ml), and $\log_{10}$ transformed values should be limited to two decimal places.

When the results of quantitative assays are reported, the precision of the assays needs to be considered. For the currently available HIV-1 viral load assays, the intra-assay and biological variability are approximately 0.5 $\log_{10}$ (139).

Therefore, changes in viral load must exceed 0.5 log_{10} (threefold) in order to represent a biologically significant change in viral replication. For HCV, the intra-assay variability is about 0.1 to 0.2 log_{10} copy/ml, while the biological variation is 0.75 log_{10} copy/ml (51). So, a biologically important change in viral load is closer to 1.0 log_{10} copy/ml. Quantitative assays have a defined linear or measurement range. Values below the lower limit of quantification should be reported as less than the lower limit of the linear range, rather than as negative. Values above the upper limit of quantification should be reported as greater than the upper limit of the linear range. For values above the limit of detection but below the limit of quantification, results may be reported as detectable, less than the lower limit of the linear range. For example, if the lower limit of quantification of an HIV-1 viral load assay is 40 copies/ml, a value of 25 copies/ml could be reported as detectable, <40 copies/ml. Inclusion of the amplification method and specimen type in the report is particularly important for quantitative assays, as values from different assay types are not always comparable.

Regulatory and Reimbursement Issues

The medical needs for new molecular microbiology tests have exceeded the capacity of the diagnostic industry to provide FDA-cleared test kits to fill these needs. Table 2 lists the FDA-cleared/approved nucleic acid-based tests for infectious diseases (refer to http://www.amp.org for updates to FDA-cleared/approved tests). Notably absent from the list are tests that have become a standard of care in a variety of diseases, such as HSV encephalitis, CMV infection, and pertusis. Many laboratories have developed tests to fill these unmet needs. These laboratory-developed tests must be appropriately verified and validated as specified in the CMS final rule for laboratory requirements, 42 CFR part 493 (118). Such tests are eligible for reimbursement by Medicare and other payers if they are determined to be part of a standard of care or to be of proven clinical benefit.

Laboratory-developed tests often utilize a combination of reagents from different manufacturers, some of which are ASRs. ASRs are chemical substances, for example, antibodies or nucleic acid sequences, that are used in diagnostic tests to detect another specific substance in a specimen and are purchased from manufacturers under this label. The value of ASRs is that they ensure the quality of reagents used in laboratory-developed tests. ASRs do not include a protocol for use or information on analytical performance or clinical indication. The FDA requires a disclaimer on reports for laboratory-developed tests using ASRs, and it reads as follows: "This test result was developed and its performance characteristics determined by [laboratory name]. It has not been cleared or approved by the U.S. Food and Drug Administration." This disclaimer was not intended to cover laboratory-developed tests not using ASRs or the off-label uses of FDA-cleared products.

A laboratory may want to include clarifying statements in the reports of results from laboratory-developed tests employing ASRs. These statements may point out that FDA clearance is not necessary for these tests and that they are used for clinical purposes. Additional information may include that the laboratory is certified under the Clinical Laboratory Improvement Amendments of 1988 to perform high-complexity testing and that pursuant to the requirements of the amendments, the laboratory has established and verified the test's accuracy and precision.

Correct current procedural terminology (CPT) coding of molecular microbiology tests is essential to coverage and reimbursement by payers. In 1998, many analyte-specific codes for tests using direct probes, amplified probes, and amplified probes with quantification were established in the microbiology section of the CPT coding manual, and this list of available codes continues to expand (1). However, codes are lacking for some analytes that are commonly detected by molecular methods, such as respiratory viruses. Prior to 1998, molecular microbiology tests were billed using multiple-component CPT codes selected from the molecular pathology section of the manual. The introduction of analyte-specific codes has simplified the coding process and in many cases increased the reimbursement for molecular microbiology procedures, although there continues to be considerable regional variation in reimbursement rates for the codes. The analyte-specific codes cover all aspects of testing, including the interpretation of the test result, and the use of these specific codes precludes the use of the component codes.

Credentials

Staffing a molecular diagnostics laboratory with individuals who have an appropriate knowledge base and skill set remains a challenge. Until recently, molecular diagnostics was not part of the core curriculum in medical technology programs. However, the situation is changing, and the acquisition of credentials in this area is now available for medical technologists and technicians from the American Board of Bioanalysts, the National Credentialing Agency, and the American Society for Clinical Pathology. The National Credentialing Agency and the American Society for Clinical Pathology merged their credentialing activities in July 2009. Laboratory directors may receive credentials in molecular diagnostics through the American Board of Bioanalysts (physicians and clinical laboratory scientists) and the American Board of Clinical Chemistry (physicians and clinical laboratory scientists) and jointly through the American Boards of Pathology and Medical Genetics (physicians only).

FUTURE DIRECTIONS

Nucleic acid testing will continue to be one of the leading growth areas in laboratory medicine. The number of applications of this technology in diagnostic microbiology will continue to increase, and the technology will increasingly be incorporated into routine clinical microbiology laboratories as it becomes less technically complex and more accessible. More clinical and financial outcome data will be needed to justify the use of this expensive technology in an era of declining reimbursement and increased cost consciousness.

The clinical utility of molecular testing is now well established, but the availability of FDA-cleared/approved tests seriously lags behind the clinical need. The recent clarification of the ASR rule has had the unintended consequence of limiting the availability of reagents for clinical laboratories, but in the long term it should increase the number of FDA-cleared/approved tests. In the interim, laboratories continue to develop tests to satisfy medical needs not met by the diagnostic test industry. There are other important unmet needs, including the availability of international standards and traceable and commutable calibrators that can be used for assay verification and validation. These materials, when widely available, should improve agreement of viral loads between tests and aid in the establishment of the clinical utility of molecular tests. Another need is the continued development of effective proficiency testing

TABLE 2 FDA-cleared or -approved molecular diagnostic tests for infectious diseases as of 10 December 2009[a]

Test objective	Manufacturer (distributor)	Test name	Method
Bacillus anthracis detection	Idaho Technology, Inc., Salt Lake City, UT	JBAIDS anthrax detection kit	Real-time PCR
Candida albicans and *Candida* detection	AdVanDx, Woburn, MA	*C. albicans* PNA FISH	PNA FISH
	AdVanDx	Yeast Traffic Light PNA FISH[b]	PNA FISH
Clostridium difficile detection	BD Diagnostics—GeneOhm, San Diego, CA	GeneOhm Cdiff assay	Real-time PCR
	Prodesse, Waukesha, WI	GeneOhm Cdiff assay	Real-time PCR
	Cepheid, Sunnyvale, CA	Xpert *C. difficile*	Real-time PCR
Chlamydia trachomatis detection (single organism)	BD Diagnostic Systems, Sparks, MD	BD ProbeTec *Chlamydia trachomatis* (CT) Q^x Amplified DNA assay	SDA
	Gen-Probe, Inc., San Diego, CA	APTIMA CT assay	TMA
	Gen-Probe	PACE 2 CT and PACE 2 CT probe competition assay	HPA
	Qiagen, Germantown, MD	HC2 CT ID	HC
	Roche Molecular Diagnostics, Pleasanton, CA	AMPLICOR CT/NG test for *Chlamydia trachomatis*	PCR
	Roche Molecular Diagnostics	COBAS AMPLICOR CT/NG test for *Chlamydia trachomatis*	PCR
Neisseria gonorrhoeae detection (single organism)	BD Diagnostic Systems	BD ProbeTec *Neisseria gonorrhoeae* (GC) Q^x amplified DNA assay	SDA
	Gen-Probe	APTIMA GC Assay	TMA
	Gen-Probe	PACE 2 GC	HPA
		PACE 2 GC probe competition assay	
	Qiagen	HC2 GC ID	HC
	Roche Molecular Diagnostics	AMPLICOR CT/NG test for *Neisseria gonorrhoeae*	PCR
	Roche Molecular Diagnostics	COBAS AMPLICOR CT/NG test for *Neisseria gonorrhoeae*	PCR
C. trachomatis and *N. gonorrhoeae* detection	Abbott Molecular, Inc., Des Plaines, IL	Abbott Real-time CT/NG	Real-time PCR
	BD Diagnostics—GeneOhm	BD ProbeTec ET *C. trachomatis* and *N. gonorrhoeae* amplified DNA assay	SDA
	Gen-Probe	PACE 2C CT/GC	HPA
	Gen-Probe	APTIMA Combo 2 assay	TMA
	Qiagen	HC2 CT/GC Combo test	HC
	Roche Molecular Diagnostics	AMPLICOR CT/NG test	PCR
	Roche Molecular Diagnostics	COBAS AMPLICOR CT/NG test	PCR
Enterococcus faecalis detection	AdVanDx	*Enterococcus faecalis* PNA FISH	PNA FISH
Escherichia coli and *Pseudomonas aeruginosa* detection	AdVanDx	*E. coli*/*P. aeruginosa* PNA FISH	PNA FISH
Escherichia coli, *Klebsiella pneumonia*, and *Pseudomonas aeruginosa* detection	AdVanDx	EK/*P. aeruginosa* PNA FISH	PNA FISH
Francisella tularensis detection	Idaho Technology, Inc.	JBAIDS tularemia detection kit	Real-time PCR
Gardnerella, *Trichomonas vaginalis*, and *Candida* detection	BD Diagnostics—GeneOhm	BD Affirm VPIII microbial identification test	Hybridization
Group A *Streptococcus* detection	Gen-Probe	GASDirect	HPA
Group B *Streptococcus* detection	AdVanDx	GBS PNA FISH	PNA FISH
	BD Diagnostics—GeneOhm	IDI-Strep B assay	Real-time PCR
	Cepheid, Sunnyvale, CA	Smart GBS	Real-time PCR
	Cepheid	Xpert GBS	Real-time PCR
	Gen-Probe	Group B AccuProbe	HPA
MRSA for *Staphylococcus aureus*—screening assay	BD Diagnostics—GeneOhm	IDI-MRSA assay	Real-time PCR
	Cepheid	Xpert MRSA	Real-time PCR
	BD Diagnostics—GeneOhm	GeneOhm StaphSR	Real-time PCR
Diagnostic assay for positive blood cultures	Cepheid	Xpert MRSA/SA blood culture assay	Real-time PCR
MRSA for *Staphylococcus aureus*—diagnostic assay for SSTI	Cepheid	Xpert MRSA/SA SSTI test	Real-time PCR
Mycobacterium tuberculosis detection	Gen-Probe	AMPLIFIED MTD test	TMA
	Roche Molecular Diagnostics	AMPLICOR *Mycobacterium tuberculosis* test	PCR
Detection of *Mycobacterium* spp. and various fungi and bacterial culture confirmation[c]	Gen-Probe	AccuProbe culture identification test	HPA
Staphylococcus aureus detection	AdvanDx	*S. aureus* PNA FISH	PNA FISH
Avian influenza virus detection	Centers for Disease Control and Prevention	Influenza A/H5	Real-time RT-PCR
CMV detection	bioMérieux, Inc., Durham, NC	CMV pp67 mRNA	NASBA
	Gentech Diagnostics Pvt. Ltd., New Delhi, India	Hybrid Capture CMV DNA test	HC
	Qiagen	HC1 CMV DNA test	HC

(*Continued on next page*)

TABLE 2 (*Continued*)

Test objective	Manufacturer (distributor)	Test name	Method
Enterovirus detection	bioMérieux	NucliSENS EasyQ Enterovirus	Real-time NASBA
	Cepheid	Xpert EV	Real-time PCR
HBV quantification	Roche Molecular Diagnostics	COBAS TaqMan HBV test, for use with the HighPure System	Real-time PCR
HCV detection	Gen-Probe (distributed by Siemens Healthcare Diagnostics, Deerfield, IL)	VERSANT HCV RNA	TMA
	Roche Molecular Diagnostics	AMPLICOR HCV test, version 2.0	RT-PCR
	Roche Molecular Diagnostics	COBAS AMPLICOR HCV test, version 2.0	RT-PCR
HCV quantification	Roche Molecular Diagnostics	COBAS AmpliPrep/COBAS TaqMan HCV test	Real-time RT-PCR
	Siemens Healthcare Diagnostics	VERSANT HCV RNA 3.0 bDNA assay	bDNA
HIV-1 drug resistance detection	Celera Diagnostics, Alameda, CA (distributed by Abbott Laboratories, Abbott Park, IL)	ViroSeq HIV-1 genotyping system	Sequencing
	Siemens Healthcare Diagnostics	TruGene HIV-1 genotyping and open Gene DNA sequencing system	Sequencing
HIV-1 quantification	Abbott Molecular	Abbott real-time HIV-1	Real-time RT-PCR
	bioMérieux	NucliSens HIV-1 QT	NASBA
	Roche Molecular Diagnostics	AMPLICOR HIV-1 MONITOR test, version 1.5	RT-PCR
	Roche Molecular Diagnostics	COBAS AMPLICOR HIV-1 MONITOR test, version 1.5	RT-PCR
	Roche Molecular Diagnostics	COBAS AmpliPrep/COBAS TaqMan HIV-1 test	Real-time RT-PCR
	Siemens Healthcare Diagnostics	VERSANT HIV-1 RNA 3.0 bDNA assay	bDNA
HBV, HCV, and HIV-1 for blood, blood component, and tissue donations	BioLife Plasma Services, L.P., Deerfield, IL	HCV RT-PCR assay	RT-PCR
	BioLife Plasma Services	HIV-1 PCR assay	RT-PCR
	Gen-Probe (distributed by Chiron)	Procleix HIV-1/HCV assay	TC, TMA, HPA
	Gen-Probe (distributed by Chiron)	Procleix ULTRIO assay (HIV-1, HCV, HBV)	TC, TMA, HPA
	National Genetics Institute, Los Angeles, CA	UltraQual HCV RT-PCR assay	RT-PCR
	National Genetics Institute	UltraQual HIV-1 RT-PCR assay	RT-PCR
	Roche Molecular Diagnostics	COBAS AmpliScreen HBV test	PCR
	Roche Molecular Diagnostics	COBAS AmpliScreen HCV test, version 2.0	RT-PCR
	Roche Molecular Diagnostics	COBAS AmpliScreen HIV-1 test, version 1.5	RT-PCR
	Roche Molecular Diagnostics	COBAS TaqScreen MPX	Multiplex real-time PCR and RT-PCR
Human metapneumovirus detection	Prodesse	Pro hMPV+ assay	Multiplex real-time PCR
HPV detection	Hologic, Inc. (Third Wave Technologies), Bedford, MA	Cervista HPV HR	Invader chemistry
	Hologic (Third Wave Technologies)	Cervista HPV HR 16/18	Invader chemistry
	Qiagen	HC2 HR and LR	HC
	Qiagen	HC2 HPV HR	HC
	Qiagen	HC2 DNA with Pap	HC
Influenza virus panel	Centers for Disease Control and Prevention	Human influenza virus real-time RT-PCR detection and characterization panel	Real-time RT-PCR
	Focus Diagnostics, Inc. (Cypress, CA)	Influenza A H1N1 (2009) real-time PCR kit (emergency use authorization)	Real-time RT-PCR
Respiratory virus panel	Luminex Molecular Diagnostics, Toronto, Canada	xTag respiratory viral panel[d]	PCR, ASPE, Tag sorting
	Prodesse	ProFlu+ assay[e]	Multiplex real-time RT-PCR
	Nanosphere, Inc.	Verigene respiratory virus nucleic acid test and Verigene respiratory virus test-SP[f]	Multiplex gold nanoparticle Probes
West Nile virus for blood donation	Gen-Probe	Procleix WNV assay	Real-time RT-PCR
	Roche Molecular Diagnostics	COBAS TaqScreen WNV	Real-time RT-PCR

[a]Modified from http://www.amp.org.

Abbreviations: ASPE, allele-specific primer extension; HC, hybrid capture; HPA, hybridization protection assay; HR, high risk; JBAIDS, Joint Biological Agent Identification and Diagnostic System; PNA FISH, peptide nucleic acid fluorescent *in situ* hybridization; SSTI, skin and soft tissue infection; TC, target capture.

[b]Five *Candida* species directly from positive blood cultures, including *C. albicans* and/or *C. parapsilosis*, *C. tropicalis*, and *C. glabrata* and/or *C. krusei*.

[c]Mycobacteria include M. *avium*, M. *intracellulare*, M. *avium* complex, M. *gordonae*, M. *kansasii*, and M. *tuberculosis* complex. Fungi include *Blastomyces dermatitidis*, *Coccidioides immitis*, *Cryptococcus neoformans*, and *Histoplasma capsulatum*. Bacteria include *Campylobacter* spp., *Enterococcus* spp., group A *Streptococcus*, group B *Streptococcus*, *H. influenzae*, *L. monocytogenes*, *N. gonorrhoeae*, *S. pneumoniae*, and *S. aureus*.

[d]Viruses include influenza A (H1, H3) virus; influenza B virus; adenovirus; respiratory syncytial viruses A and B; metapneumovirus; parainfluenza virus types 1, 2, and 3; and rhinovirus.

[e]Viruses include influenza A and B viruses and respiratory syncytial virus.

[f]Viruses include influenza A and B viruses and respiratory syncytial virus.

programs that will help ensure that the results of molecular tests are reliable and reproducible among laboratories.

To a great extent, the future of molecular microbiology depends on automation. Many of the available tests are labor-intensive, with much of the labor devoted to tedious sample processing methods. Recently, fully automated systems for molecular diagnostics have been developed, and these primarily focus on high-volume, high-throughput testing. If there is continued menu expansion, these systems will offer solutions for high- and mid-volume laboratories. Despite these important advances over the past decade, molecular diagnostics is still not performed in many clinical microbiology laboratories. To increase access to molecular tests, simple, affordable, fully automated, random-access platforms with broad test menus are needed, particularly for laboratories that perform low- or mid-volume testing.

The use of multiplex nucleic acid-based assays to screen at-risk patients for panels of probable pathogens remains a goal for molecular microbiology. Although several such tests are available, success to date has been limited by technical difficulties. The development of newer technologies is key to providing molecular tests with the broad diagnostic range provided by culture and other conventional methods.

Advances in human genomics will be exploited in the future to develop tests for host immunogenetic factors that may influence the risk of becoming infected with certain pathogens or the progression of disease. Human gene expression profiling with microarrays may be important in defining patterns of host gene expression associated with different pathogens or disease states. Better understanding of pathogen genomics, gene expression, and proteomics will lead to the discovery of new diagnostic and therapeutic targets.

REFERENCES

1. **American Medical Association.** 2009. *CPT 2009, Current Procedural Terminology.* AMA Press, Chicago, IL.
2. **Arnold, C., L. Westland, G. Mowat, A. Underwood, J. Magee, and S. Gharbia.** 2005. Single-nucleotide polymorphism-based differentiation and drug resistance detection in *Mycobacterium tuberculosis* from isolates or directly from sputum. *Clin. Microbiol. Infect.* **11:**122–130.
3. **Arnold, L. J., Jr., P. W. Hammond, W. A. Wiese, and N. C. Nelson.** 1989. Assay formats involving acridinium ester-labeled DNA probes. *Clin. Chem.* **35:**1588–1594.
4. **Barbeau, J. M., J. Goforth, A. M. Caliendo, and F. S. Nolte.** 2004. Performance characteristics of a quantitative *TaqMan* hepatitis C virus RNA analyte-specific reagent. *J. Clin. Microbiol.* **42:**3739–3746.
5. **Beutler, E., T. Gelbart, and W. Kuhl.** 1990. Interference of heparin with the polymerase chain reaction. *BioTechniques* **9:**166.
6. **Blin, N., and D. W. Stafford.** 1976. A general method for isolation of high molecular weight DNA from eukaryotes. *Nucleic Acids Res.* **3:**2303–2308.
7. **Boom, R., C. Sol, M. Salimans, C. Jansen, P. M. Wertheim-van Dillen, and J. van der Noordaa.** 1990. Rapid and simple method for purification of nucleic acids. *J. Clin. Microbiol.* **28:**495–503.
8. **Boriskin, Y. S., P. S. Rice, R. A. Stabler, J. Hinds, H. Al-Ghusein, K. Vass, and P. D. Butcher.** 2004. DNA microarrays for virus detection in cases of central nervous system infection. *J. Clin. Microbiol.* **42:**5811–5818.
9. **Briese, T., G. Palacios, M. Kokoris, O. Jabado, Z. Liu, and N. Renwick.** 2005. Diagnostic system for rapid and sensitive differential detection of pathogens. *Emerg. Infect. Dis.* **11:**310–313.
10. **Brunstein, J. D., C. L. Cline, S. McKinney, and E. Thomas.** 2008. Evidence from multiplex molecular assays for complex multipathogen interactions in acute respiratory infections. *J. Clin. Microbiol.* **46:**97–102.
11. **Caliendo, A. M., K. St. George, S. Y. Kao, J. Allega, B. H. Tan, R. LaFontaine, L. Bui, and C. R. Rinaldo.** 2000. Comparison of quantitative cytomegalovirus (CMV) PCR in plasma and CMV antigenemia assay: clinical utility of the prototype AMPLICOR CMV MONITOR test in transplant recipients. *J. Clin. Microbiol.* **38:**2122–2127.
12. **Capaul, S. E., and M. Georgievski-Hirsoho.** 2005. Detection of enterovirus RNA in cerebrospinal fluid (CSF) using NuclioSens Easy Q Enterovirus assay. *J. Clin. Virol.* **32:**236–240.
13. **Chamberlain, J. S., R. A. Gibbs, J. E. Rainer, P. N. Nguyen, and C. T. Caskey.** 1988. Deletion screening of the Duchenne muscular dystrophy locus via multiplex DNA amplification. *Nucleic Acids Res.* **16:**11141–11156.
14. **Chin, C. Y., A. Urisman, S. Grenhow, S. Rouskin, S. Yagi, D. Schnurr, C. Wright, W. L. Drew, D. Wang, P. S. Weintrub, J. L. Derisi, and D. Ganem.** 2008. Utility of DNA microarrays for detection of viruses in acute respiratory tract infections in children. *J. Pediatr.* **153:**76–83.
15. **Chomczynski, P., and N. Sacchi.** 1987. Single-step method of RNA isolation by acid guanidinium thiocyanate-phenol-chloroform extraction. *Anal. Biochem.* **62:**156–159.
16. **Choo, Q. L., G. Kuo, A. J. Weiner, L. R. Overby, D. W. Bradley, and M. Houghton.** 1989. Isolation of a cDNA clone derived from a blood-borne non-A, non-B viral hepatitis genome. *Science* **244:**359–362.
17. **Chow, W. H. A., C. McCloskey, Y. Tong, L. Hu, Q. You, C. P. Kelly, H. Kong, Y. Tang, and W. Tang.** 2008. Application of isothermal helicase-dependent amplification with a disposable detection device in a simple sensitive stool test for toxigenic Clostridium difficile. *J. Mol. Diagn.* **10:**452–458.
18. **Clementi, M., S. Menzo, P. Bagnarelli, A. Manzin, A. Valenza, and P. E. Varaldo.** 1993. Quantitative PCR and RT-PCR in virology. *PCR Methods Appl.* **2:**191–196.
19. **Clinical and Laboratory Standards Institute.** 2006. *Collection, Transport, Preparation, and Storage of Specimens and Samples for Molecular Methods; Approved Guideline.* CLSI document MM13-A. Clinical and Laboratory Standards Institute, Wayne, PA.
20. **Clinical and Laboratory Standards Institute.** 2005. *Diagnostic Nucleic Acid Microarrays; Proposed Guideline.* CLSI document MMP12-P. Clinical and Laboratory Standards Institute, Wayne, PA.
21. **Clinical and Laboratory Standards Institute.** 2006. *Genotyping for Infectious Diseases: Identification and Characterizations; Approved Guideline.* CLSI document MM10-A. Clinical and Laboratory Standards Institute, Wayne, PA.
22. **Clinical and Laboratory Standards Institute.** 2006. *Molecular Diagnostic Methods for Infectious Diseases; Approved Guideline,* 2nd ed. CLSI document MM3-A2. Clinical and Laboratory Standards Institute, Wayne, PA.
23. **Collins, M. L., C. Zayati, J. J. Detmer, B. Daly, J. A. Kolberg, T. Cha, B. D. Irvine, J. Tucker, and M. S. Urdea.** 1995. Preparation and characterization of RNA standards for use in quantitative branched-DNA hybridization assays. *Anal. Biochem.* **226:**120–129.
24. **Compton, J.** 1991. Nucleic acid sequence-based amplification. *Nature* **350:**91–92.
25. **Cope, J. J., A. Hildesheim, M. H. Schiffman, M. M. Manos, A. T. Lorincz, R. D. Burk, A. G. Glass, C. Greer, J. Burkland, K. Helgesen, D. R. Scott, M. E. Sherman, R. J. Kurman, and K. L. Liaw.** 1997. Comparison of the hybrid capture tube test and PCR for detection of human papillomavirus DNA in cervical specimens. *J. Clin. Microbiol.* **35:**2262–2265.
26. **Corless, C. E., M. Guiver, R. Borrow, V. Edwards-Jones, A. J. Fox, and E. B. Kaczmarski.** 2001. Simultaneous detection of *Neisseria meningitidis, Haemophilus influenzae,* and *Streptococcus pneumoniae* in suspected cases of meningitis and septicemia using real-time PCR. *J. Clin. Microbiol.* **39:**1553–1558.
27. **Diaz, M. R., and J. W. Fell.** 2004. High-throughput detection of pathogenic yeasts of the genus *Trichosporon. J. Clin. Microbiol.* **42:**3696–3706.
28. **Dienstag, J. L., and J. G. Hutchinson.** 2006. American Gastroenterological Association Medical Position Statement on the management of hepatitis C. *Gastroenterology* **130:**225–230.

29. Diggle, M. A., and S. C. Clarke. 2004. Pyrosequencing: sequence typing at the speed of light. *Mol. Biotechnol.* **28:**129–137.

30. Dunbar, S. A., C. A. Vander Zee, K. G. Oliver, K. L. Karem, and J. W. Jacobson. 2003. Quantitative, multiplexed detection of bacterial pathogens: DNA and protein applications of the Luminex LabMAP system. *J. Microbiol. Methods* **53:**245–252.

31. Ecker, D., J. J. Drader, J. Gutierrez, A. Gutierrez, J. C. Hannis, A. Schink, R. Sampath, L. B. Blyn, M. W. Eshoo, T. A. Hall, M. Tobarmosquera, Y. Jiang, K. A. Sannes-Lowery, L. L. Cummins, B. Libby, D. J. Walcott, C. Massire, R. Ranken, S. Manalili, C. Ivy, R. Melton, H. Levene, V. Harpin, F. Li, N. White, M. Pear, J. A. Ecker, V. Samant, D. Knize, D. Robbins, K. Rudnick, F. Hajjar, and S. A. Hofstadler. 2006. The Ibis T5000 Universal Biosensor: an automated platform for pathogen identification and strain typing. *J. Assoc. Lab. Automation* **11:**341–351.

32. Ecker, D. J., R. Sampath, L. B. Blyn, M. W. Eshoo, C. Ivy, J. A. Ecker, B. Libby, V. Samant, K. A. Sannes-Lowery, R. E. Melton, K. Russel, N. Freed, C. Barrozo, J. Wu, K. Rudnick, A. Desai, E. Moradi, D. J. Knize, D. W. Robbins, J. C. Hannis, P. M. Harrell, C. Massire, T. A. Hall, Y. Jiang, R. Rankin, J. J. Drader, N. White, J. A. McNeil, S. T. Crooke, and S. A. Hoftadler. 2005. Rapid identification and strain-typing of respiratory pathogens for epidemic surveillance. *Proc. Natl. Acad. Sci. USA* **102:**8012–8017.

33. Emery, V. C., C. A. Sabin, A. V. Cope, D. Gor, A. F. Hassan-Walker, and P. D. Griffiths. 2000. Application of viral-load kinetics to identify patients who develop cytomegalovirus disease after transplantation. *Lancet* **355:**2032–2036.

34. Espy, M. J., T. F. Smith, and D. H. Persing. 1993. Dependence of polymerase chain reaction product inactivation protocols on amplicon length and sequence composition. *J. Clin. Microbiol.* **31:**2361–2365.

35. Farrell, D. J. 1999. Evaluation of AMPLICOR *Neisseria gonorrhoeae* PCR using *cppB* nested PCR and 16S rRNA PCR. *J. Clin. Microbiol.* **37:**386–390.

36. Felmlee, T. A., R. P. Oda, D. A. Persing, and J. P. Landers. 1995. Capillary electrophoresis of DNA potential utility for clinical diagnoses. *J. Chromatogr.* **A717:**127–137.

37. Fong, W. K., Z. Modrusan, J. P. McNevin, J. Marostenmaki, B. Zin, and F. Bekkaoui. 2000. Rapid solid-phase immunoassay for detection of methicillin-resistant *Staphylococcus aureus* using cycling probe technology. *J. Clin. Microbiol.* **38:**2525–2529.

38. Fried, M. W., M. L. Shiffman, K. R. Reddy, C. Smith, G. Marinos, F. L. Goncales, Jr., D. Haussinger, M. Diago, G. Carosi, D. Dhumeaux, A. Craxi, A. Lin, J. Hoffman, and J. Yu. 2002. Peginterferon alfa-2a plus ribavirin for chronic hepatitis C virus infection. *N. Engl. J. Med.* **347:**975–982.

39. Furukawa, K., and V. P. Bhavanandan. 1983. Influences of anionic polysaccharides on DNA synthesis in isolated nuclei and by DNA polymerase alpha: correlation of observed effects with properties of the polysaccharides. *Biochim. Biophys. Acta* **740:**466–475.

40. Garcia, E. P., L. A. Dowding, L. W. Stanton, and V. I. Slepnev. 2005. Scalable transcriptional analysis routine-multiplexed quantitative real-time polymerase chain reaction platform for gene expression analysis and molecular diagnostics. *J. Mol. Diagn.* **7:**444–454.

41. Gaydos, C. A., K. A. Crotchfelt, M. R. Howell, S. Kralian, P. Hauptman, and T. C. Quinn. 1998. Molecular amplification assays to detect chlamydial infections in urine specimens from high school female students and to monitor the persistence of chlamydial DNA after therapy. *J. Infect. Dis.* **177:**417–424.

42. Gaynor, A. M., M. D. Nissenz, D. M. Whiley, I. M. Mackay, S. B. Lambert, G. Wu, D. C. Brennan, G. A. Storch, T. P. Sloots, and D. Wang. 2007. Identification of a novel polyomavirus from patients with acute repiratory tract infections. *PLOS Pathog.* **3:**595–604.

43. Gerna, G., D. Zipeto, M. Parea, M. G. Revello, E. Silini, E. Percivalle, M. Zavattoni, P. Grossi, and G. Milanesi. 1991. Monitoring of human cytomegalovirus infections and ganciclovir treatment in heart transplant recipients by determination of viremia, antigenemia, and DNAemia. *J. Infect. Dis.* **164:**488–498.

44. Gharizadeh, B., E. Norberg, J. Loffler, S. Jalal, J. Tollemar, H. Einsele, L. Klingspor, and P. Nyren. 2004. Identification of medically important fungi by the Pyrosequencing technology. *Mycoses* **47:**29–33.

45. Ginocchio, C. C., D. Barth, and F. Zhang. 2008. Comparison of the Third Wave Invader human papillomavirus (HPV) assay and the Digene HPV Hybrid Capture 2 assay for detection of high-risk HPV DNA. *J. Clin. Microbiol.* **46:**1641–1646.

46. Goldmeyer, J., H. Li, M. McCormac, S. Cook, C. Stratton, B. Lemieux, H. Kong, W. Tang, and Y. Tang. 2008. Identification of *Staphylococcus aureus* and determination of methicillin resistance directly from positive blood cultures by isothermal amplification and a disposable detection device. *J. Clin. Microbiol.* **46:**1534–1536.

47. Gross-Bellard, M., P. Oudet, and P. Chambon. 1973. Isolation of high-molecular-weight DNA from mammalian cells. *Eur. J. Biochem.* **36:**32–38.

48. Guatelli, J. C., K. M. Whitfield, D. Y. Kwoh, K. J. Barringer, D. D. Richman, and T. R. Gingeras. 1990. Isothermal *in vitro* amplification of nucleic acids by multi-enzyme reaction modeled after retroviral replication. *Proc. Natl. Acad. Sci. USA* **87:**1874–1878.

49. Haanpera, M., P. Huovinen, and J. Jalava. 2005. Detection and quantification of macrolide resistance mutations at positions 2058 and 2059 of the 23S rRNA gene by pyrosequencing. *Antimicrob. Agents Chemother.* **49:**457–460.

50. Hadiyannis, S. J., H. Sette, Jr., T. R. Morgan, V. Balan, M. Diago, P. Marcellin, G. Ramdori, H. Bodenheimer, Jr., D. Bernstein, M. Rizzetto, S. Zeuzem, P. J. Pockros, A. Lin, and A. M. Ackrill for the PEGASYS International Study Group. 2004. Peginterferon-α2a and ribavirin combination therapy in chronic hepatitis C: a randomized study of treatment duration and ribavirin dose. *Ann. Intern. Med.* **140:**346–355.

51. Halfon, P., M. Bourlière, G. Halimi, H. Khiri, P. Bertezene, I. Portal, D. Botta-Fridlund, A. P. Gauthier, M. Jullien, J. M. Feryn, V. Gerolami, and G. Cartouzou. 1998. Assessment of spontaneous fluctuations of viral load in utreated patient with chonic hepatitis C with two standardized quatitation methods: branched DNA and Amplicor Monitor. *J. Clin. Microbiol.* **36:**2073–2075.

52. Hall, L., S. Wohlfiel, and G. D. Roberts. 2003. Experience with the MicroSeq D2 large-subunit ribosomal DNA sequencing kit for identification of commonly encountered, clinically important yeast species. *J. Clin. Microbiol.* **41:**5099–5102.

53. Hall, L., S. Wohlfiel, and G. D. Roberts. 2004. Experience with the MicroSeq D2 large-subunit ribosomal DNA sequencing kit for identification of filamentous fungi encountered in the clinical laboratory. *J. Clin. Microbiol.* **42:**622–626.

54. Hammer, S. M., J. J. Eron, P. Reiss, R. T. Schooley, M. A. Thompson, S. Walmsley, P. Cahn, M. A. Fischl, J. M. Gatel, M. S. Hirsch, D. M. Jacobsen, J. S. G. Montaner, D. D. Richman, P. G. Yeni, and P. A. Volberding. 2008. Antiretroviral treatment of adult HIV infection. Recommendations of the International AIDS Society-USA panel. *JAMA* **300:**555–570.

55. Hankin, R. C. 1992. In situ hybridization: principles and applications. *Lab. Med.* **23:**764–770.

56. Haqqi, T. M., G. Sarkar, C. S. David, and S. S. Sommer. 1988. Specific amplification with PCR of a refractory segment of genomic DNA. *Nucleic Acids Res.* **16:**11844.

57. Heid, C., J. Stevens, K. J. Livak, and P. M. Williams. 1996. Real time quantitative PCR. *Genome Res.* **6:**986–994.

58. Higuchi, R. 1989. *Simple and Rapid Preparation of Samples for PCR.* Stockton Press, New York, NY.

59. Higuchi, R., C. Fockler, G. Dollinger, and R. Watson. 1993. Kinetic PCR analysis: real-time monitoring of DNA amplification reactions. *Bio/Technology* **11:**1026–1030.

60. Hirsch, H. H., D. C. Brennan, C. B. Drachenberg, F. Ginevri, J. Gordon, A. P. Limaye, M. J. Mihatsch, V. Nickeleit, E. Ramos, P. Randhawa, E. Shapiro, J. Steiger, M. J. Suthanthiran, and J. Trofe. 2005. Polyomarvirus-associated nephropathy in renal transplantation: interdisciplinary analyses and recommendations. *Transplantation* **79:**1277–1286.

61. **Holland, P. M., R. D. Abramson, R. Watson, and D. H. Gelfand.** 1991. Detection of specific polymerase chain reaction product by utilizing the 5′→3′ exonuclease activity of *Thermus aquaticus* DNA polymerase. *Proc. Natl. Acad. Sci. USA* **88:**7276–7280.

62. **Honish, C., Y. Chen, C. Moritmer, C. Arnold, O. Schmidt, D. van den Boom, C. R. Cantor, H. N. Shah, and S. E. Gharbia.** 2007. Automated comparative sequence analysis by base-specific cleavage and mass spectrometry for nucleic acid-based microbial typing. *Proc. Natl. Acad. Sci. USA* **104:**10649–10654.

63. **Humar, A., D. Gregson, A. M. Caliendo, A. McGeer, G. Malkan, M. Krajden, P. Corey, P. Greig, S. Walmsley, G. Levy, and T. Mazzulli.** 1999. Clinical utility of quantitative cytomegalovirus viral load determination for predicting cytomegalovirus disease in liver transplant recipients. *Transplantation* **68:**1305–1311.

64. **Ihira, M., T. Yoshikawa, Y. Enomoto, S. Akimoto, M. Ohashi, S. Suga, N. Nishimura, T. Ozaki, Y. Nishiyama, T. Notomi, Y. Ohta, and Y. Asano.** 2004. Rapid diagnosis of human herpesvirus 6 infection by a novel DNA amplification method, loop-mediated isothermal amplification. *J. Clin. Microbiol.* **42:**140–145.

65. **Innis, M. A., K. B. Myambo, D. H. Gelfand, and M. A. Brow.** 1998. DNA sequencing with *Thermus aquaticus* DNA polymerase and direct sequencing of polymerase chain reaction-amplified DNA. *Proc. Natl. Acad. Sci. USA* **85:**9436–9440.

66. **Iwamoto, T., T. Sonobe, and K. Hayashi.** 2003. Loop-mediated isothermal amplification for direct detection of *Mycobacterium tuberculosis* complex, *M. avium*, and *M. intracellulare* in sputum samples. *J. Clin. Microbiol.* **41:**2616–2622.

67. **Izreli, S., C. Pfleiderer, and T. Lion.** 1991. Detection of gene expression by PCR amplification of RNA derived from frozen heparinized whole blood. *Nucleic Acids Res.* **19:**6051.

68. **Kalinina, O., J. Brown, and J. Silver.** 1997. Nanoliter scale PCR with TaqMan detection. *Nucleic Acids Res.* **25:**1999–2004.

69. **Kern, D., M. Collins, T. Fultz, J. Detmer, S. Hamren, J. J. Peterkin, P. Sheridan, M. Urdea, R. White, T. Yeghiazarian, and J. Todd.** 1996. An enhanced-sensitivity branched-DNA assay for quantification of human immunodeficiency virus type 1 RNA in plasma. *J. Clin. Microbiol.* **34:**3196–3202.

70. **Khanna, M., J. Fan, K. Pehler-Harrington, C. Waters, P. Douglass, J. Stallock, S. Kehl, and K. J. Henrickson.** 2005. The Pneumoplex assays, a multiplex PCR-enzyme hybridization assay that allows simultaneous detection of five organisms, *Mycoplasma pneumoniae, Chlamydia (Chlamydophila) pneumoniae, Legionella pneumophila, Legionella micdadei,* and *Bordetella pertussis,* and its real-time counterpart. *J. Clin. Microbiol.* **43:**565–571.

71. **Kim, S. R., C. Ki, and N. Y. Lee.** 2009. Rapid detection and identification of 12 respiratory viruses using a dual priming oligonucleotide system-based multiplex PCR assay. *J. Virol. Methods* **156:**111–116.

72. **Klugman, K. P., S. A. Madhi, and W. C. Albrich** 2008. Novel approaches to the identification of *Steptococcus pneumoniae* as the cause of community-acquired pneumonia. *Clin. Infect. Dis.* **47:**202–206.

73. **Korimbocus, J., N. Scaramozzino, B. Lecroix, J. M. Crance, D. Garin, and G. Vermet.** 2005. DNA probe array for the simultaneous identification of herpesviruses, enteroviruses, and flaviviruses. *J. Clin. Microbiol.* **43:**3779–3787.

74. **Kricka, L. J.** 1999. Nucleic acid detection technologies—labels, strategies, and formats. *Clin. Chem.* **45:**453–458.

75. **Kricka, L. J.** 2002. Stains, labels and detection strategies for nucleic acids assays. *Ann. Clin. Biochem.* **39:**114–129.

76. **Ksiazek, T. G., D. Erdman, C. S. Goldsmith, S. R. Zaki, T. Peret, S. Emery, S. Tong, C. Urbani, J. A. Comer, W. Lim, P. E. Rollin, S. F. Dowell, A. E. Ling, C. D. Humphrey, W. J. Shieh, J. Guarner, C. D. Paddock, P. Rota, B. Fields, J. DeRisi, J. Y. Yang, N. Cox, J. M. Hughes, J. W. LeDuc, W. J. Bellini, L. J. Anderson, and the SARS Working Group.** 2003. A novel coronavirus associated with severe acute respiratory syndrome. *N. Engl. J. Med.* **348:**1953–1966.

77. **Kurtzman, C. P., and C. J. Robnett.** 1997. Identification of clinically important ascomycetous yeasts based on nucleotide divergence in the 5′ end of the large-subunit (26S) ribosomal DNA gene. *J. Clin. Microbiol.* **35:**1216–1223.

78. **Kutyavin, I. V., I. A. Afonina, A. Mills, V. V. Gorn, E. A. Lukhtanov, E. S. Belousov, M. J. Singer, D. K. Walburger, S. G. Lokhov, A. A. Gall, R. Dempcy, M. W. Reed, R. B. Meyer, and J. Hedgpeth.** 2000. 3′-Minor groove binder-DNA probes increase sequence specificity at PCR extension temperatures. *Nucleic Acids Res.* **28:**655–661.

79. **Kwoh, D. Y., G. R. David, K. M. Whitfield, H. L. Chapelle, L. J. DiMichele, and T. R. Gingeras.** 1989. Transcription-based amplification system and detection of amplified human immunodeficiency virus type 1 with a bead-based sandwich hybridization format. *Proc. Natl. Acad. Sci. USA* **86:**1173–1177.

80. **Lakeman, F. D., R. J. Whitley, and the National Institute of Allergy and Infectious Diseases Collaborative Antiviral Study Group.** 1995. Diagnosis of herpes simplex encephalitis: application of polymerase chain reaction to cerebrospinal fluid from brain-biopsied patients and correlation with disease. *J. Infect. Dis.* **171:**857–863.

81. **Lay, M. J., and C. T. Wittwer.** 1997. Real-time fluorescence genotyping of factor V Leiden during rapid cycle PCR. *Clin. Chem.* **43:**2262–2267.

82. **Le, B. M., L. M. Demertzis, G. Wu, R. J. Tibbits, R. Buller, M. Q. Arens, A. M. Gaynor, G. A. Storch, and D. Wang.** 2007. Clinical and epidemiologic characterization of WU polyomavirus infection, St. Louis, Missouri. *Emerg. Infect. Dis.* **13:**1936–1938.

83. **Lee, H. H., M. A. Chernesky, J. Schachter, J. D. Burczak, W. W. Andrews, S. Muldoon, G. Leckie, and W. E. Stamm.** 1995. Diagnosis of *Chlamydia trachomatis* genitourinary infection in women by ligase chain reaction assay of urine. *Lancet* **345:**213–216.

84. **Lefmann, M., C. Honisch, S. Böcker, N. Storm, F. van Wintzingerode, C. Schlötelberg, A. Moter, D. van den Boom, and U. B. Göbel.** 2004. Novel mass spectrometry-based tool for genotypic identification of mycobacteria. *J. Clin. Microbiol.* **42:**339–346.

85. **LeGoff, J., R. Kara, F. Moulin, A. Si-Mohammed, A. Krivine, L. Bélec, and P. Lebon.** 2008. Evaluation of the one-step multiplex real-time reverse transcription-PCR ProFlu-1 assay for detection of influenza A and B viruses and respiratory syncytial viruses in children. *J. Clin. Microbiol.* **46:**789–791.

86. **Leone, G., H. Van Schijndel, B. Van Gemen, F. R. Kramer, and C. D. Schoen.** 1998. Molecular beacon probes combined with amplification by NASBA enable homogeneous, real-time detection of RNA. *Nucleic Acids Res.* **26:**2150–2155.

87. **LeRoux, C. A., T. Kubo, A. A. Grobbelaar, P. J. van Vuren, J. Weyer, L. H. Nel, R. Swanepoel, K. Morita, and J. T. Paweska.** 2009. Development and evaluation of a real-time reverse transcription-loop-mediated isothermal amplification assay for rapid detection of Rift Valley fever virus in clinical specimens. *J. Clin. Microbiol.* **47:**645–651.

88. **Lieber, M. R.** 1997. The FEN-1 family of structure-specific nucleases in eukaryotic DNA replication, recombination and repair. *Bioessays* **19:**233–240.

89. **Lim, S. G., T. M. Ng, N. Kung, Z. Krastev, M. Volfova, P. Husa, S. S. Lee, S. Chan, M. L. Shiffman, M. K. Washington, A. Rigney, J. Anderson, E. Mondou, A. Snow, J. Sorbel, R. Guan, and F. Rosseau for the Emtricitabine FTCB-301 Study Group.** 2006. A double-blind placebo-controlled study of emtricitabine in chronic hepatitis B. *Arch. Intern. Med.* **166:**49–56.

90. **Lin, B., Z. Wang, G. J. Vora, J. A. Thornton, J. M. Schnur, D. C. Thach, K. M. Blaney, A. G. Ligler, A. P. Malanoski, J. Santiago, E. A. Walter, B. K. Agan, D. Metzgar, D. Seto, L. T. Daum, R. Kruzelock, R. K. Rowley, E. H. Hanson, C. Tibbetts, and D. A. Stenger.** 2006. Broad-spectrum respiratory tract pathogen identification using resequencing DNA microarrays. *Genome Res.* **16:**527–535.

91. **Little, M. C., J. Andrews, R. Moore, S. Bustos, L. Jones, C. Embres, G. Durmowicz, J. Harris, D. Berger, K. Yanson, C. Rostkowski, D. Yursis, J. Price, T. Fort, A. Walters, M. Collis, O. Llorin, J. Wood, F. Failing, C. O'Keefe, B. Scrivens, B. Pope, T. Hansen, K. Marino, and K. Williams.** 1999. Strand displacement amplification and homogeneous real-time detection incorporated in a second-generation DNA probe system, BDProbeTecET. *Clin. Chem.* **45:**777–784.

92. **Liu, J., S. L. Lim, Y. Ruan, A. E. Ling, F. P. Ng, C. Dosten, E. T. Liu, L. W. Stanton, and M. L. Hibberd.** 2005. SARS transmission pattern in Singapore reassessed by viral sequence variation analysis. *PLoS Med.* **2:**43.

93. **Liu, R. H., W. A. Coty, M. Reed, and G. Gust.** 2008. Electrochemical detection-based DNA microarrays. *IVD Technol.* **14:**31–38.

94. **Loeffelholz, M. J., C. A. Lewinski, S. R. Silver, A. Purohit, S. A. Herman, D. A. Buonagurio, and E. A. Dragon.** 1992. Detection of *Chlamydia trachomatis* in endocervical specimens by polymerase chain reaction. *J. Clin. Microbiol.* **30:**2847–2851.

95. **Longo, M. C., M. S. Berninger, and J. L. Hartley.** 1990. Use of uracil DNA glycosylase to control carry-over contamination in polymerase chain reactions. *Gene* **93:**125–128.

96. **Lyamichev, V., A. Mast, J. G. Hall, J. R. Prudent, M. W. Kaiser, T. Takova, R. K. Kwiatkowski, T. J. Sander, M. de Arruda, D. Arco, B. P. Weri, and M. A. D. Brow.** 1999. Polymorphism identification and quantitative detection from genomic DNA by invasive cleavage of oligonucleotide probes. *Nat. Biotechnol.* **17:**292–296.

97. **Lyamichev, V., and B. Neri.** 2003. Invader assay for SNP genotyping. *Methods Mol. Biol.* **212:**229–240.

98. **Mahony, J., S. Chong, F. Merante, S. Yaghoubian, T. Sinha, C. Lisle, and R. Janeczko.** 2007. Development of a respiratory virus panel test for detection of twenty human respiratory viruses by use of multiplex PCR and a fluid microbead-based assay. *J. Clin. Microbiol.* **45:**2965–2970.

99. **Manns, M. P., J. G. McHutchison, S. C. Gordon, V. K. Rutsgi, M. Shiffman, R. Reindollar, Z. D. Goodman, K. Koury, M. H. Ling, J. K. Albrecht, and the International Hepatitis Interventional Therapy Group.** 2001. Peginterferon alfa-2b plus ribavirin compared with interferon alfa-2b plus ribavirin for initial treatment of chronic hepatitis C: a randomised trial. *Lancet* **358:**958–965.

100. **Mantero, G., A. Zonaro, A. Albertini, P. Bertolo, and D. Primi.** 1991. DNA enzyme immunoassay: general method for detecting products of polymerase chain reaction. *Clin. Chem.* **37:**422–429.

101. **Mardis, E. R.** 2008. Next-generation DNA sequencing methods. *Annu. Rev. Genomics Hum. Genet.* **9:**387–402.

102. **Mazzulli, T., L. W. Drew, B. Yen-Lieberman, D. Jekic-McMullen, D. J. Kohn, C. Isada, G. Moussa, R. Chua, and S. Walmsley.** 1999. Multicenter comparison of the Digene Hybrid Capture CMV DNA Assay (version 2.0), the pp65 antigenemia assay, and cell culture for detection of cytomegalovirus viremia. *J. Clin. Microbiol.* **37:**958–963.

103. **Mellors, J. W., C. R. Rinaldo, Jr., P. Gupta, R. M. White, J. A. Todd, and L. A. Kingsley.** 1996. Prognosis in HIV-1 infection predicted by the quantity of virus in plasma. *Science* **272:**1167–1170.

104. **Mitchell, P. S., M. J. Espy, T. F. Smith, D. R. Toal, P. N. Rys, E. F. Berbari, D. R. Osmon, and D. H. Persing.** 1997. Laboratory diagnosis of central nervous system infections with herpes simplex virus by PCR performed with cerebrospinal fluid specimens. *J. Clin. Microbiol.* **35:**2873–2877.

105. **Mitchell, P. S., J. J. Germer, and J. D. C. Yao.** 2011. Laboratory design and operations, p. 127–141. *In* D. H. Persing, F. C. Tenover, Y.-W. Tang, F. S. Nolte, R. T. Hayden, and A. van Belkum (ed.), *Molecular Microbiology: Diagnostic Principles and Practice*, 2nd ed. ASM Press, Washington, DC.

106. **Montague, N. S., T. J. Cleary, O. V. Martines, and G. W. Procop.** 2008. Detection of group B streptococci in Lim broth by use of group B *Streptococcus* peptide nucleic acid fluorescent in situ hybridization and selective and nonselective agars. *J. Clin. Microbiol.* **46:**3470–3472.

107. **Morrison, T., J. J. Weiss, and C. T. Wittwer.** 1998. Quantification of low copy transcripts by continuous SYBR green I dye monitoring during amplification. *BioTechniques* **24:**954–958.

108. **Mulligan, E. K., J. J. Germer, M. Q. Arens, K. L. D'Amore, A. D. Bisceglie, N. A. Ledboer, M. J. Moser, A. C. Newman, A. K. O'Guin, P. D. Olivo, D. S. Podzorski, K. A. Vaughan, J. D. Yao, S. A. Elagin, and S. C.** Johnson. 2009. Detection of quantification of hepatitis C virus (HCV) by MultiCode-RTx PCR targeting the HCV 3′ untranslated region. *J. Clin. Microbiol.* **47:**2635–2638.

109. **Myers, T. W., and D. H. Gelfand.** 1991. Reverse transcription and DNA amplification by a *Thermus thermophilus* DNA polymerase. *Biochemistry* **30:**7661–7666.

110. **Nakagawa, N., and M. Ito.** 2006. Rapid subtyping of influenza A virus by loop-mediated isothermal amplification: two cases of influenza patients who returned from Thailand. *Jpn. Infect. Dis.* **59:**200–201.

111. **NCCLS.** 2001. *Quantitative Molecular Methods for Infectious Diseases.* NCCLS document MM6-A. NCCLS, Wayne, PA.

112. **NCCLS.** 2004. *Nucleic Acid Sequencing Methods in Diagnostic Laboratory Medicine.* NCCLS document MM9-A. NCCLS, Wayne, PA.

113. **Nolte, F. S., D. J. Marshall, C. Rasberry, S. Schievelbein, G. G. Banks, G. A. Storch, M. Q. Arens, R. S. Buller, and J. R. Prudent.** 2007. MultiCode-PLx system for multiplexed detection of seventeen respiratory viruses. *J. Clin. Microbiol.* **45:**2779–2786.

114. **Nolte, F. S.** 1999. Branched DNA signal amplification for direct quantitation of nucleic acid sequences in clinical specimens. *Adv. Clin. Chem.* **33:**201–235.

115. **Nolte, F. S., R. K. Emmens, C. Thurmond, P. S. Mitchell, C. Pascuzzi, S. M. Devine, R. Saral, and J. R. Wingard.** 1995. Early detection of human cytomegalovirus viremia in bone marrow transplant recipients by DNA amplification. *J. Clin. Microbiol.* **33:**1263–1266.

116. **Notomi, T., H. Okayama, H. Masubuchi, T. Yonekawa, K. Wananabe, N. Amino, and T. Hase.** 2000. Loop-mediated isothermal amplification of DNA. *Nucleic Acids Res.* **28:**63.

117. **Nycz, C. M., C. H. Dean, P. D. Haaland, C. A. Spargo, and G. T. Walker.** 1998. Quantitative reverse transcription strand displacement amplification; quantitation of nucleic acids using an isothermal amplification technique. *Anal. Biochem.* **259:**226–234.

118. **Office of the Federal Register.** 2004. *Code of Federal Regulations. Clinical Laboratory Improvement Act Regulations*, part 493, subpart K, section 1253. U.S. Government Printing Office and Office of the Federal Register, Washington, DC. http://www.phppo.cdc.gov/ clia/regs/subpart_k.aspx.

119. **Okamoto, S., T. Yoshikawa, M. Ihira, K. Suszuki, K. Shimokata, Y. Nishiyama, and Y. Asano.** 2004. Rapid detection of varicella-zoster virus infection by a loop-mediated isothermal amplification method. *J. Med. Virol.* **74:**677–682.

120. **Oliveira, K., S. M. Brecher, A. Durbin, D. S. Shapiro, D. R. Schwartz, P. C. De Girolami, J. Dakos, G. W. Procop, D. Wilson, C. S. Hanna, G. Haase, H. Peltroche-Llacsahuanga, K. C. Chapin, M. C. Musgnug, M. H. Levi, C. Shoemaker, and H. Stender.** 2003. Direct identification of *Staphylococcus aureus* from positive blood culture bottles. *J. Clin. Microbiol.* **41:**889–891.

121. **O'Meara, D., K. Wilbe, T. Leitner, B. Hejdeman, J. Albert, and J. Lundeberg.** 2001. Monitoring resistance to human immunodeficiency virus type 1 protease inhibitors by pyrosequencing. *J. Clin. Microbiol.* **39:**464–473.

122. **Orita, M., H. Iwahana, H. Kanazawa, K. Hayashi, and T. Sekiya.** 1989. Detection of polymorphism of human DNA by gel electrophoresis as single-strand conformation polymorphisms. *Proc. Natl. Acad. Sci. USA* **86:**2766–2770.

123. **Palacios, G., P. Quan, O. J. Jabado, S. Conlan, D. L. Hirschberg, Y. Liu, J. Zhai, N. Renwick, J. Hui, H. Hegy, A. Grolla, J. E. Strong, J. S. Towner, T. W. Geisbert, P. B. Jahrling, C. Büchen-Osmond, H. Ellerbrok, M. P. Sanchez-Seco, Y. Lussier, P. Formenty, S. T. Nichol, H. Feldman, T. Briese, and W. Lipkin.** 2007. Panmicrobial oligonucleotide array for diagnosis of infectious diseases. *Emerg. Infect. Dis.* **13:**73–81.

124. **Pang, J., J. Modlin, and R. Yolken.** 1992. Use of modified nucleotides and uracil-DNA glycosylase (UNG) for the control of contamination in the PCR-based amplification of RNA. *Mol. Cell. Probes* **6:**251–256.

125. **Pang, X. L., J. D. Fox, J. M. Fenton, G. G. Miller, A. M. Caliendo, and J. K. Preiksaitis.** 2009. Interlaboratory comparison of cytomegalovirus viral load assays. *Am. J. Transplant.* **9:**258–268.

126. Parida, M., K. Horioke, H. Ishida, P. K. Dash, P. Saxena, A. M. Jana, S. Islam, N. Inoue, N. Hosaka, and K. Morita. 2005. Rapid detection and differentiation of dengue virus serotypes by a real-time reverse transcription-loop-mediated isothermal amplification assay. *J. Clin. Microbiol.* **43:**2895–2903.

127. Pease, A. C., D. Solas, E. J. Sullivan, M. T. Cronin, C. P. Holmes, and S. P. Fodor. 1994. Light-generated oligonucleotide arrays for rapid DNA sequence analysis. *Proc. Natl. Acad. Sci. USA* **91:**5022–5026.

128. Peiris, J. S. M., S. T. Lai, L. L. M. Poon, Y. Guan, L. Y. C. Yam, W. Lim, J. Nicholls, W. K. S. Yee, W. W. Yan, M. T. Cheung, V. C. C. Cheng, K. H. Chan, D. N. C. Tsang, R. W. H. Yung, T. K. Ng, K. Y. Yuen, and members of the SARS study group. 2003. Coronavirus as a possible cause of severe acute respiratory syndrome. *Lancet* **361:**1319–1325.

129. Persing, D. H., F. C. Tenover, Y.-W. Tang, F. S. Nolte, R. T. Hayden, and A. van Belkum (ed.). 2011. *Molecular Microbiology: Diagnostic Principles and Practice*, 2nd ed. ASM Press, Washington, DC.

130. Piccirilli, J. A., T. Krauch, S. E. Moroney, and S. A. Benner. 1990. Enzymatic incorporation of a new base pair into DNA and RNA extends the genetic alphabet. *Nature* **343:**33–37.

131. Poljak, M., and K. Seme. 1996. Rapid detection and typing of human papillomaviruses by consensus polymerase chain reaction and enzyme-linked immunosorbent assay. *J. Virol. Methods* **56:**231–238.

132. Procop, G. W. 2007.Molecular diagnostics for the detection and characterization of microbial pathogens. *Clin. Infect. Dis.* **45:**99–111.

133. Reid, R., M. Greenberg, A. B. Jensen, M. Husain, J. Willett, Y. Daoud, G. Temple, C. R. Stanhope, A. Sherman, and D. G. Phibbs. 1987. Sexually transmitted papillomaviral infections. I. The anatomic distribution and pathologic grade of neoplastic lesions associated with different viral types. *Am. J. Obstet. Gynecol.* **156:**212–222.

134. Relman, D. A., T. M. Schmidt, R. P. MacDermott, and S. Falkow. 1992. Identification of the uncultured bacillus of Whipple's disease. *N. Engl. J. Med.* **327:**293–301.

135. Rigby, S., G. W. Procop, G. Haase, D. Wilson, G. Hall, C. Kurtzman, K. Oliveira, S. Von Oy, J. J. Hyldig-Nielsen, J. Coull, and H. Stender. 2002. Fluorescence in situ hybridization with peptide nucleic acid probes for rapid identification of *Candida albicans* directly from blood culture bottles. *J. Clin. Microbiol.* **40:**2182–2186.

136. Ririe, K., R. P. Rasmussen, and C. T. Wittwer. 1997. Product differentiation by analysis of DNA melting curves during the polymerase chain reaction. *Anal. Biochem.* **245:**154–160.

137. Rosenstraus, M., Z. Wang, S.Y. Chang, D. DeBonville, and J. P. Spadoro. 1998. An internal control for routine diagnostic PCR: design, properties, and effect on clinical performance. *J. Clin. Microbiol.* **36:**191–197.

138. Rossau, R., H. Traore, H. De Beenhouwer, W. Mijs, G. Jannes, P. De Rijk, and F. Portaels. 1997. Evaluation of the INNO-LiPA Rif. TB assay, a reverse hybridization assay for the simultaneous detection of *Mycobacterium tuberculosis* complex and its resistance to rifampin. *Antimicrob. Agents Chemother.* **41:**2093–2098.

139. Saag, M. S., M. Holodniy, D. R. Kuritzkes, W. A. O'Brien, R. Coombs, M. E. Poscher, D. M. Jacobsen, G. M. Shaw, D. D. Richman, and P. A. Volberding. 1996. HIV viral load markers in clinical practice. *Nat. Med.* **2:**625–629.

140. Saiki, R. K., D. H. Gelfand, S. Stoffel, S. J. Scharf, R. Higuchi, K. B. Mullis, G. Horn, and H. A. Ehrlich. 1988. Primer-directed enzymatic amplification of DNA with a thermostable DNA polymerase. *Science* **239:**487–491.

141. Sampath, R., T. A. Hall, C. Massire, L. Feng, L. B. Blyn, M. W. Eshoo, S. A. Hofstadler, and D. J. Ecker. 2007. Rapid identification of emerging infectious agents using PCR and electrospray ionization mass spectrometry. *Ann. N. Y. Acad. Sci.* **1102:**109–120.

142. Sampath, R., K. L. Russell, C. Massiere, M. W. Eshoo, V. Harpin, L. B. Blyn, R. Melton, C. Ivy, T. Pennella, F. Li., H. Levene, T. A. Hall, B. Libby, N. Fan, D. J. Walcott, R. Ranken, M. Pear, A. Schink, J. Gutierrez, J. Drader, D. Moore, D. Metzgar, L. Addington, R. Rothman, C. A. Gaydos, S. Yang, K. St. George, M. E. Fuschino, A. B. Dean, D. E. Stallknecht, G. Goekjian, S. Yingst, M. Montevelle, M. D. Saad, C. A. Whitehouse, C. Baldwin, K. H. Rudnick, S. A. Hofstadler, S. M. Lemon, and D. J. Ecker. 2007. Global surveillance of emerging influenza virus genotypes by mass spectrometry. *PLoS ONE* **5:**489.

143. Schachter, J., W. E. Stamm, T. C. Quinn, W. W. Andrews, J. D. Burczak, and H. H. Lee. 1994. Ligase chain reaction to detect *Chlamydia trachomatis* infection of the cervix. *J. Clin. Microbiol.* **32:**2540–2543.

144. Schena, M., D. Shalon, R. Heller, A. Chai, P. O. Brown, and R. W. Davis. 1996. Parallel human genome analysis: microarray-based expression monitoring of 1000 genes. *Proc. Natl. Acad. Sci. USA* **93:**10614–10619.

145. Shepard, J. R., R. M. Addison, B. D. Alexander, P. Della-Latta, M. Gherna, G. Haase, G. Hall, J. K. Johnson, W. G. Merz, H. Peltroche-Llacsahuanga, H. Stender, R. A. Venezia, D. Wilson, G. W. Procop, F. Wu, and M. J. Fiandaca. 2008. Multicenter evaluation of the *Candida albicans/Candida glabrata* peptide nucleic acid fluorescent in situ hybridization method for simultaneous dual-color identification of *C. albicans* and *C. glabrata* directly from blood culture bottles. *J. Clin. Microbiol.* **46:**50–55.

146. Sherrill, C. B., D. J. Marshall, M. J. Moser, C. A. Larsen, L. Daude-Snow, and J. R. Prudent. 2004. Nucleic acid analysis using an expanded genetic alphabet to quench fluorescence. *J. Am. Chem. Soc.* **126:**4550–4556.

147. Simen, B. B., J. F. Simons, K. H. Hullsiek, R. M. Novak, R. D. Macarther, J. D. Baxter, C. Hugan, C. Lubeski, G. S. Turenchalk, M. S. Braverman, B. Desany, J. M. Rothberg, M. Egholm, M. J. Kozai, and Terry Beirn Community Programs for Clinical Research on AIDS. 2009. Low-abundance drug-resistant viral variants in chronically HIV-infected, antiretroviral treatment-naïve patients significantly impact treatment outcomes. *J. Infect. Dis.* **199:**610–612.

148. Smith, P. L., C. R. Walker Peach, R. J. Fulton, and D. B. DuBois. 1998. A rapid, sensitive, multiplexed assay for detection of viral nucleic acids using the FlowMetrix system. *Clin. Chem.* **44:**2054–2056.

149. Söderlund-Strand, A., J. Dillner, and J. Carlson. 2008. High-throughput genotyping of oncogenic human papilloma viruses with MALDI-TOF mass spectrometry. *Clin. Chem.* **54:**86–92.

150. Sogaard, M., H. Stender, and H. C. Schonheyder. 2005. Direct identification of major blood culture pathogens, including *Pseudomonas aeruginosa* and *Escherichia coli*, by a panel of fluorescence in situ hybridization assays using peptide nucleic acid probes. *J. Clin. Microbiol.* **43:**1947–1949.

151. Solomon, D., M. Schiffman, R. Tarone, et al. 2001. Comparison of three management strategies for patients with atypical squamous cells of undetermined significance: baseline results from a randomized trial. *J. Natl. Cancer Inst.* **93:**293–299.

152. Steinau, M., D. C. Swan, and E. R. Unger. 2008. Type-specific reproducibility of the Roche linear array HPV genotyping test. *J. Clin. Virol.* **42:**412–414.

153. Stender, H., M. Fiandaca, J. J. Hyldig-Nielsen, and J. Coull. 2002. PNA for rapid microbiology. *J. Microbiol. Methods* **48:**1–17.

154. Stender, H., T. A. Mollerup, K. Lund, K. H. Petersen, P. Hongmanee, and S. E. Godtfredsen. 1999. Direct detection and identification of Mycobacterium tuberculosis in smear-positive sputum samples by fluorescence in situ hybridization (FISH) using peptide nucleic acid (PNA) probes. *Int. J. Tuberc. Lung Dis.* **3:**830–837.

155. Stürenburg, E., N. Storm, I. Sobottka, M. A. Horstkotte, S. Scherpe, M. Aepfelbacher, and S. Müller. 2006. Detection and genotyping of SHV β-lactamase variants by mass spectrometry after base-specific cleavage of in vitro-generated RNA transcripts. *J. Clin. Microbiol.* **44:**909–915.

156. Stuyver, L., A. Wyseur, A. Rombout, J. Louwagie, T. Scarcez, C. Verhofstede, D. Rimland, R. F. Schinazi, and R. Rossau. 1997. Line probe assay for rapid detection of drug-selected mutations in the human immunodeficiency virus type 1 reverse transcriptase gene. *Antimicrob. Agents Chemother.* **41:**284–291.

157. Stuyver, L., A. Wyseur, W. van Arnhem, F. Hernandez, and G. Maertens. 1996. Second-generation line probe assay for hepatitis C virus genotyping. *J. Clin. Microbiol.* **34:**2259–2266.

158. Svarovskaia, E. S., M. J. Moser, A. S. Bae, J. R. Prudent, M. D. Miller, and K. Borroto-Esoda. 2006. MultiCode-RTx real-time PCR system for detection of subpopulations of K65R human immunodeficiency virus type 1 reverse transcriptase mutant viruses in clinical samples. *J. Clin. Microbiol.* **44:**4237–4241.

159. Sykes, P. J., S. H. Neoh, M. J. Brisco, E. Hughes, J. Condon, and A. A. Morley. 1992. Quantitation of targets for PCR by use of limiting dilution. *BioTechniques* **13:**444–449.

160. Tang, Y. W., N. M. Ellis, M. K. Hopkins, D. H. Smith, D. E. Dodge, and D. H. Persing. 1998. Comparison of phenotypic and genotypic techniques for identification of unusual aerobic pathogenic gram-negative bacilli. *J. Clin. Microbiol.* **36:**3674–3679.

161. Telenti, A., P. Imboden, F. Marchesi, T. Schmidheini, and T. Bodmer. 1993. Direct, automated detection of rifampin-resistant *Mycobacterium tuberculosis* by polymerase chain reaction and single-strand conformation polymorphism analysis. *Antimicrob. Agents Chemother.* **37:**2054–2058.

162. Templeton, K. E., S. A. Scheltinga, M. F. Beersma, A. C. Kroes, and E. C. Claas. 2004. Rapid and sensitive method using multiplex real-time PCR for diagnosis of infections by influenza A and influenza B viruses, respiratory syncytial virus, and parainfluenza viruses 1, 2, 3, and 4. *J. Clin. Microbiol.* **42:**1564–1569.

163. ten Bosch, J. R., and W. W. Grody. 2008. Keeping up with the next generation: massively parallel sequencing in clinical diagnostics. *J. Mol. Diagn.* **10:**484–492.

164. Tenover, F. C. 1988. Diagnostic deoxyribonucleic acid probes for infectious diseases. *Clin. Microbiol. Rev.* **1:**82–101.

165. Tenover, F. C., and J. K. Rasheed. 2011. Detection of antimicrobial resistance genes and mutations associated with antimicrobial resistance in bacteria, p. 507–524. *In* D. H. Persing, F. C. Tenover, Y.-W. Tang, F. S. Nolte, R. T. Hayden, and A. van Belkum (ed.), *Molecular Microbiology: Diagnostic Principles and Practice,* 2nd ed. ASM Press, Washington, DC.

166. Thai, H .T. C., M. Q. Le, C. D. Vuong, M. Parida, H. Minekawa, T. Notomi, F. Hasebe, and K. Morita. 2004. Development and evaluation of a novel loop-mediated isothermal amplification method for rapid detection of severe acute respiratory syndrome coronavirus. *J. Clin. Microbiol.* **42:**1956–1961.

167. Thelwell, N., S. Millington, A. Solinas, J. Booth, and T. Brown. 2000. Mode of action and application of Scorpion primers to mutation detection. *Nucleic Acids Res.* **28:**3752–3761.

168. Thornton, C. G., J. L. Hartley, and A. Rashtchian. 1992. Utilizing uracil DNA glycosylase to control carryover contamination in PCR: characterization of residual UDG activity following thermal cycling. *BioTechniques* **13:**180–184.

169. Tong, Y., W. Tang, H. Kim, X. Pan, T.A. Ranall, and T. Kong. 2008. Development of isothermal TaqMan assays for detection of biothreat organisms. *BioTechniques* **45:**543–557.

170. Touhy, M. J., G. S. Hall, M. Sholtis, and G. W. Procop. 2005. Pyrosequencing™ as a tool for the identification of common isolates of *Mycobacterium*. *Diagn. Microbiol. Infect. Dis.* **51:**245–250.

171. Tyagi, S., D. P. Bratu, and F. R. Kramer. 1998. Multicolor molecular beacons for allele discrimination. *Nat. Biotechnol.* **16:**49–53.

172. Vincent, M., Y. Xu, and H. Kong. 2004. Helicase-dependent isothermal DNA amplification. *EMBO Rep.* **5:**795–800.

173. Vogelstein, B., and K. W. Kinzler. 1999. Digital PCR. *Proc. Natl. Acad. Sci. USA* **96:**9236–9241.

174. Walker, G. T., M. S. Fraiser, J. L. Schram, M. C. Little, J. G. Nadeau, and D. P. Malinowski. 1992. Strand displacement amplification—an isothermal, *in vitro* DNA amplification technique. *Nucleic Acids Res.* **20:**1691–1696.

175. Wallace, J., B. A. Woda, and G. Pihan. 2005. Facile, comprehensive, high-throughput genotyping of human genital papillomaviruses using spectrally addressable liquid bead microarrays. *J. Mol. Diagn.* **7:**72–80.

176. Walsh, E. E., K. M. McConnochie, C. E. Long, and C. B. Hall. 1997. Severity of respiratory syncytial virus infection is related to virus strain. *J. Infect. Dis.* **175:**814–820.

177. Wang, C., Y. Mitsuya, and B. Gharizadeh. 2007. Characterization of mutation spectra with ultra-deep pyrosequencing: application to HIV-1 drug resistance. *Genome Res.* **17:**1195–1201.

178. Wang, D., L. Coscoy, M. Zylberberg, P.C. Avila, H. A. Boushey, D. Ganem, and J. L. DeRisi. 2002. Microarray-based detection and genotyping of viral pathogens. *Proc. Natl. Acad. Sci. USA* **99:**15687–15692.

179. Wang, D., A. Urisman, Y. T. Liu, M. Springer, T. G. Ksiazek, D. D. Erdman, E. R. Mardis, M. M. Hickenbotham, V. Magrini, J. Eldred, J. P. Latreille, R. K. Wilson, D. Ganem, and J. L. DeRisi. 2003. Viral discovery and sequence recovery using DNA microarrays. *PLOS Biol.* **1:**2.

180. Whitcombe, D., J. Theaker, S. P. Guy, T. Brown, and S. Little. 1999. Detection of PCR products using self-probing amplicons and fluorescence. *Nat. Biotechnol.* **17:**804–807.

181. Woese, C. R. 1987. Bacterial evolution. *Microbiol. Rev.* **51:**221–271.

182. Wolk, D., S. Mitchell, and R. Patel. 2001. Principles of molecular microbiology testing methods. *Infect. Dis. Clin. N. Am.* **15:**1157–1204.

183. Wong, C. W., C. L. Heng, L. Wan Yee, S. W. Soh, C. B. Kartasasmita, E. A. Simoes, M. L. Hibberd, W. K. Sung, and L. D. Miller. 2007. Optimization and clinical validation of a pathogen detection microarray. *Genome Biol.* **8:**93.

184. Wright, T. C., Jr., M. Schiffman, D. Solomon, J. T. Cox, F. Garcia, S. Goldie, K. Hatch, K. L. Noller, N. Roach, C. Runowicz, and D. Saslow. 2004. Interim guidance for the use of human papillomavirus DNA testing as an adjunct to cervical cytology for screening. *Obstet. Gynecol.* **103:**304–309.

185. Wu, D. Y., and R. B. Wallace. 1989. The ligation amplification reaction (LAR)—amplification of specific DNA sequences using sequential rounds of template-dependent ligation. *Genomics* **4:**560–569.

186. Yoda, T., Y. Suzuki, K. Yamazaki, N. Sakon, M. Kanki, I. Aoyama, and T. Tsukamoto. 2007. Evaluation and application of reverse transcription loop-mediated isothermal amplification for detection of noroviruses. *J. Med. Virol.* **79:**326–334.

187. Zeuzem, S., M. Rizzetto, P. Ferenci, and M. L. Shiffman. 2009. Management of hepatitis C virus genotype 2 or 3 infection: treatment optimization on the basis of virological response. *Antivir. Ther.* **14:**143–154.

Immunoassays for the Diagnosis of Infectious Diseases*

A. BETTS CARPENTER

5

Immunoassays are laboratory tests that employ antibodies as analytical reagents (10, 25, 27, 32, 33, 54). They have become increasingly used in the diagnosis of infectious diseases either as a primary means of diagnosis or for confirmation of culture results. Overall, immunoassays are specific, sensitive, and relatively inexpensive. They are used in all parts of the clinical laboratory. Due to the high specificity of the antigen-antibody reaction and the ease of use, immunoassays are leading the way for an increasing number of laboratory tests that are available at the patient bedside (point-of-care testing), in doctors' offices, and even for at-home testing. This chapter summarizes the variety of different assays available and their particular application in the field of infectious disease. The discussion emphasizes general assay design, with important caveats relevant to test interpretation and development. Relevant examples are given as they relate to testing for particular infectious disease agents; however, for in-depth discussions, the reader is directed to the particular chapters on the specific agents.

HISTORY OF DEVELOPMENT OF IMMUNOASSAYS

Immunoassays have changed significantly over time, with improvements in the types of antibodies and antigens available as well as in detection systems (10, 25, 27, 30, 33, 54). With immunoassays, any analyte can be measured if an antibody can be raised to it or if an antigenic form is available. The first immunoassays available measured milligram to microgram quantities of antibodies and relied primarily upon precipitation reactions between antigen and antibody. In the 1960s, the advent of radioimmunoassay (RIA) heralded techniques with greater sensitivity and greatly expanded the repertoire of analytes available for testing. By use of RIA, previously undetectable analytes were now easily available for testing in the clinical laboratory. The discovery of monoclonal antibodies led to assays with greater specificities and further expanded the repertoire of analytes available for measurement. Concerns about utilization of radioactivity and the desire for greater sensitivities led to the development of chemiluminescence (CL) immunoassays

and use of the avidin-biotin detection system. Increasing automation of laboratory testing has expanded into the area of immunoassays, with many tests requiring only limited technologist input. As immunoassays have evolved, there has been increased utilization of various solid-phase matrices for adherence of either antigens or antibodies. Initially, polypropylene test tubes were used. This has evolved to microtiter plates, and with the increased use of automated systems, smaller solid phases such as tiny disks or spheres are being increasingly used. Thus, immunoassays have significantly advanced in both the level of sensitivity detected and the breadth of their utilization, so they are now some of the most popular and most widely used of all laboratory tests.

DEFINITION OF TERMS

The array of terms used for immunoassays can be a confusing alphabet soup. This chapter discusses some widely used conventions in terminology; however, the reader may find some references in which the terms are used differently. Overall, most assays utilize "immuno" coupled with a second term which describes the type of assay or label used. For example, immunoprecipitation is an immunoassay utilizing a precipitation reaction. RIA is an immunoassay that utilizes radioactivity as the label. "Enzyme immunoassay" (EIA) is a more general term that can be applied to any immunoassay which uses an enzyme label, although often EIA is used to refer to reagent-limited competitive-type assays. The term enzyme-linked immunosorbent assay (ELISA) can also be used as a general term for any assay utilizing an enzyme label; however, it is most often used to refer to assays in which the antigen or antibody is adsorbed to a solid-phase matrix, often then employing a second enzyme-labeled antibody, the so-called "sandwich" assay format. "Immunometric" is an additional term used and generally refers to any reagent excess assay. For the purposes of this chapter, the term EIA is used to refer to any assay using an enzyme, while the term ELISA refers only to solid-phase sandwich-type assays.

GENERAL CONCEPTS OF ASSAY DESIGN

There are a number of ways to characterize immunoassays. One useful classification scheme looks at the amounts of label and reagent available (21). There are three major groups of immunoassays: label free, reagent excess, and reagent

---

*This chapter contains information presented in chapter 16 by Niel T. Constantine and Dolores P. Lana in the eighth edition of this *Manual*.

limited. The assays which are label free rely upon the ability of antigen and antibodies to bind and form detectable agglutination or precipitation. There are many classic agglutination assays used in the diagnosis of infectious diseases, such as the Widal test for typhoid fever. The reagent excess methods require an excess of labeled antigen or antibody, use either one or two sites, and include immunoblotting and solid-phase ELISA. These are commonly employed immunoassays in microbiology today. Reagent-limited assays are competitive tests and employ a limited amount of either antigen or antibody and either require separation or are separation free. These include classic RIA and EIA and are less often used in diagnosis of infectious diseases.

Another commonly used classification scheme looks at immunoassays as either heterogeneous (solid phase) or homogeneous (free-solution assays) (10, 27). Heterogeneous assays are ones in which the bound and free components must be separated, whereas homogeneous assays do not require a separation step. In addition, heterogeneous assays involve some type of solid phase to which the immunoreactants are attached. Homogeneous assays generally are free-solution methods. While this is a useful and commonly employed classification scheme, there are assays that do not strictly fit into this classification scheme. For example, agglutination assays and particle-enhanced light-scattering methods are considered homogeneous assays; however, the antibody is bound to a solid phase, and there is no required separation of the bound from the free components.

ASSAY INTERPRETATION

When choosing an assay for the laboratory and in-patient diagnosis, it is critical to understand the concepts of sensitivity, specificity, and predictive values (54). Sensitivity is the proportion of individuals *with* a disease that are correctly identified with a particular test. Sensitivity defines the true positives (TP), which are the patients with disease identified by the assay. Conversely, false negatives (FN) are the patients with disease who are not identified by the test. The formula for sensitivity is as follows: sensitivity = [TP/(TP + FN)] × 100. Specificity is the proportion of those *without* the disease that are correctly classified. Specificity is a measure of the true negatives (TN), which are the patients without disease not identified by the assay. False positives (FP) are the patients without disease who test positive. The formula for specificity is as follows: specificity = [TN/(TN + FP)] × 100. With a highly sensitive test, the majority of diseased individuals are picked up, and thus the number of false-negative results is very low. In contrast, with a highly specific test, the majority of individuals without the disease test negative, so the number of false-positive results is very low. When an assay is developed, the diagnostic cutoffs can be modified to alter both the sensitivity and the specificity. For example, if one moves the cutoff to a lower level, the assay sensitivity is increased, with a resulting decrease in specificity. The optimal balance of these two components must be evaluated for each laboratory test and depends on multiple factors, such as the utility of the test and the prevalence of the disease in the population.

The probability of having the disease, given the results of a test, is called the predictive value of the test. Positive predictive value (PPV) determines the percentage of patients with positive results who are diseased: PPV = [TP/(TP + FP)] × 100. The negative predictive value (NPV) calculates the percentage of patients with negative test results who do not have the disease: NPV = [TN/(TN + FN)] × 100. The predictive value of a test combines the prevalence of disease in a particular population with the sensitivity and specificity. Positive and negative predictive values are important because they assess the ability of a test to predict the presence or absence of disease in a patient from a particular population. In this context, the disease prevalence is a critical component. Prevalence is the proportion of the population with the disease in question. If a disease state has a low prevalence in the target population, a positive result will most likely be a false-positive result, whereas the opposite is true in a high-prevalence population. A potential use of a high negative predictive value is that a negative test can exclude disease. In addition to the values discussed above, there are a variety of other statistical methods that can be used to evaluate laboratory tests, such as odds ratio, receiver-operator curve analysis, and likelihood ratios. It is beyond the scope of this chapter to discuss these, and the reader is referred to other sources for a more complete discussion (49).

SCREENING VERSUS DIAGNOSTIC ASSAYS

An important component of assay design is based upon the ultimate use of the test, i.e., whether it will be used as a screening or diagnostic test (40, 51). Screening tests are designed to pick up disease in asymptomatic individuals who may have early disease or precursors of disease, whereas diagnostic tests are performed for persons with specific indications of possible disease. However, the screening procedure itself does not diagnose the illness; those individuals with a positive result from the screening test need further evaluation with additional diagnostic tests. If the individual has a previous positive screening test, the diagnostic test acts as a confirmatory test. The ideal screening test should be both highly specific and sensitive; however, this may be difficult to achieve. As there is such a variety of screening tests available, there is not a particular sensitivity target value which is suggested; nevertheless, the sensitivity should be as high as possible without sacrificing specificity. It is not advisable to use a test with low specificity as a screening test, since many people without the disease will screen positive and potentially receive unnecessary diagnostic procedures. Moreover, for an effective screening test, the prevalence of disease in the population should be high; if the prevalence of the disease is low, then a positive test will most likely be a false positive, leading to further unnecessary testing. Other considerations with regard to screening tests include weighing the cost of the test versus the impact of early detection. Overall, good screening tests should be easy to perform, inexpensive, and performed in high-disease-prevalence populations. In addition, early detection of disease should have a measurable impact on patient outcomes.

SEROLOGIC ASSAYS

Traditionally, serologic assays referred to the use of serum or plasma samples for the detection of antibodies to a variety of antigens. This concept has been broadened to refer to a variety of patient samples, such as cerebrospinal fluid, urine, and other body fluids. In addition, it refers to the detection of both antibodies and antigen. There are a variety of clinical scenarios in which serologic assessment is the test of choice. For the identification of organisms for which culture is difficult or requires prolonged incubation, the determination of antibody titers or antigen detection can often give a quick answer. Although molecular techniques have sometimes supplanted serology in these situations, often cost issues make serology a more viable technique. There are frequent clinical situations where it is unnecessary to perform a culture if an antigen test is positive. One of the most common situations is the diagnosis of group A beta-hemolytic streptococcal throat infection. A rapid immunoassay for the detection of the group A streptococcal antigen is performed. If this is positive, then treatment can be instituted. Only when this quick test is negative is it necessary to perform a culture.

Basic Immunologic Reactions

In order to facilitate understanding of antibody titers, a brief review of basic immunologic reactions is provided (1, 2). Upon initial exposure to an infectious disease (primary antibody response), there are four phases in the response: an initial lag (or window) phase, when there is no antibody detected; a log phase, when the antibody titer increases in a logarithmic fashion; a plateau phase, in which the amount of antibody stabilizes; and a decline phase, during which the antibody is cleared or catabolized. The actual time course and ultimate maximum antibody titer depend on the antigen and the host. In the primary response, the initial antibody response is the production of immunoglobulin M (IgM), which usually appears after 10 days. The period after initial exposure, but before antibody is produced or is at sufficient levels to be detected, is called the window period. This can vary, depending on the infectious agent, from as short as 10 days to as long as 6 months. IgG antibody production usually begins 10 days after exposure but is much less than the IgM response. As the IgM antibody level decreases, the IgG level increases, so that usually by the end of the first month, only IgG antibody is detectable. If there is a repeat infection with the same infectious agent, the kinetics of the response are different, with a lag phase of only 1 to 3 days, and IgG antibody is the primary isotype produced. In the months following antigen exposure, the IgG level reaches a plateau, and the antibody may remain detectable for life, even if there is no further exposure to the antigen. B lymphocytes utilize membrane-bound antibodies to recognize a wide array of antigens. In the case of infectious disease agents, the antigens are often expressed on the microbial surfaces. The particular parts of the expressed antigens that are bound by antibodies are referred to as epitopes; the strength of the binding of one epitope to one antibody is called the affinity. Upon repeated infection with a microbe, there is an increase in the strength of the antigen-antibody binding, a phenomenon called affinity maturation. However, depending upon the immunoglobulin molecule present, there is more than one antigen-binding site on each immunoglobulin (IgG, 2 sites; polymerized IgA, 4 sites; and IgM, 10 sites); therefore, the total strength of the antigen-antibody binding is much greater than the affinity of a single interaction. This is called the avidity. Just as with affinity maturation, there is an increase in avidity with additional exposure to an antigen. Upon initial exposure to an antigen, the avidity of the IgG is low; upon secondary exposure, there is an increase in IgG avidity. Although there is exquisite specificity in the antigen-antibody reaction, there can be a spectrum of antibodies produced in response to a particular antigen; they can have differing affinities and avidities with a particular antigen and thus can be responsible for cross-reactions. Recognizing cross-reacting antibodies can be critical to assay specificity. Often, initial screening assays are set up with crude antigen preparations in which false-positive reactions can occur. Secondary confirmatory or diagnostic assays utilize purified and more expensive antigen preparations which confer greater specificity. Recognition of cross-reactivity is critical in tests used in infectious disease, because often organisms within the same genus and species share multiple antigenic determinants, making cross-reactivity a common problem. Although assays are designed to obviate these problems, laboratorians and clinicians should just be cognizant of the potential for cross-reactions.

Caveats in Serologic Interpretation

In general, a positive IgG titer means only that an individual has been exposed to a particular infectious agent and thus is "immune." For each infectious agent, the laboratory result is usually set up so that a positive result is the minimum amount of IgG antibody present which makes the individual immune. For purposes of this discussion, the term immune is used; however, this does not necessarily mean that the level of antibody is protective against reinfection. The actual amount of antigen-specific antibody present in the serum of a particular individual is host determined and is controlled by immune response genes which are part of the human histocompatibility system. The IgG titer from a single serum sample to a particular infectious agent may not be used to determine if the infection is recent or remote. For example, person A may be a high responder to certain antigens and a low responder to others. Therefore, if a high titer of IgG is obtained for an individual, it may be tempting to think that this may represent a more recent exposure; however, this may indicate only that the individual is a high responder to that particular antigen. Therefore, a positive IgG titer establishes only that the individual has been exposed to a particular agent at some time in the past and has detectable IgG. In addition, the nature of the antigen is important, as some antigens are more effective than others in stimulating the immune system. Moreover, the ability of the immune system to respond to antigens can be affected by a variety of factors, such as age. For example, the very young may be unable to respond to certain types of antigens (e.g., carbohydrates) (1, 2).

Using serologic methods, there are several ways to determine if the infection is recent. The most useful and frequently used method is assessment of IgM antibody to a particular infectious disease agent. In general, a positive IgM titer to a particular organism is evidence of an active (i.e., recently acquired) infection with that agent. However, there are several considerations to keep in mind in the interpretation of this test. First of all, a positive IgM titer does not always mean that the infection is recent. There have been reports of persistent elevations of IgM antibody for a year or more. This has been seen with multiple organisms, including cytomegalovirus, *Mycoplasma pneumoniae*, hepatitis A virus, and *Toxoplasma gondii*, among others (11, 36, 51). Conversely, a negative IgM titer does not exclude a recent exposure. The amount of IgM may have been small and resolved quickly; thus, it was not detected at the time of the assay. The second way to establish a primary infection is to determine acute- and convalescent-phase titers. This requires drawing two sets of samples for antibody titer determination: one set early in the exposure to the infectious agent and a second set 2 to 3 weeks later. Evidence of an acute infection can be confirmed if there is a fourfold increase in antibody titer between the first and second sets.

While this can sometimes provide information on the pathogenesis of a disease state, it requires at least 2 to 3 weeks for definitive results, thus obviating its use for early clinical management. Also, a false-negative reaction is not uncommon due to the fact that it requires drawing the specimen at a point low enough on the log part of the antibody response curve to obtain the required fourfold increase in antibody titer. Therefore, the lack of a fourfold increase does not rule out a primary infection.

At present, many assays report results as absorbance values or international units, making it problematic to apply the concept of a fourfold increase in titer. While it is possible to develop an approximate equivalency between titers and absorbance values, this has to be individually developed for each assay. One method to do this involves collecting multiple pairs of acute- and convalescent-phase sera to use as reference sera. They must demonstrate a fourfold increase in titer on traditional assays. They are then run on the EIA for the agent in question, and reference ranges are reported in optical density units. Assuming that the EIA provides distinctly different absorbance ranges to adequately separate acute- and convalescent-phase sera, pairs of test sera can then be run on the EIA, and the values can be compared to the reference ranges. While this can theoretically provide an adequate way to evaluate acute- and convalescent-phase titers by using the newer assay formats, it can have multiple problems. First of all, establishment of the reference range has to be performed separately on assays for each infectious agent, which can be expensive and time-consuming. Secondly, the lab has to have multiple sets of positive acute- and convalescent-phase paired sera for each organism tested, which can be quite difficult to obtain. In addition, depending on the EIA used and the range of the standard curve, titers may not be easily converted into equivalent and meaningful absorbance values. Considering the cost and difficulties associated with this type of analysis, it is not generally recommended. Instead, it is preferable to test for the presence of an acute infection by using an IgM assay or an IgG avidity test (see below) or to directly test for the organism by using one of the increasingly available molecular techniques.

An IgG avidity test (31, 36, 41) can address some of the concerns with IgM testing and acute- and convalescent-phase titers. IgG antibodies produced early in infection have a low avidity, but a much greater avidity is seen with a secondary exposure. Using an avidity assay, in conjunction with the assessment of levels of IgG and IgM antibody to a pathogen, can provide a much clearer indication of acute infection. Avidity tests are performed with a modification of the standard IgG EIA, in which IgG antibodies are exposed to a dissociating agent (usually high concentrations of urea). The serum IgG avidity is estimated by comparing the treated sample with one left untreated. While this test can be quite useful, there are several caveats with its use. First of all, low avidity does not always mean that the infection is recent, because low-avidity antibodies can persist for months to years. In addition, there can be quality control issues in this testing, with variability in test results related to the type of assay plates used, the antigens employed, and the type of dissociating agent used. This test has special utility in testing for some of the pathogens associated with pre- and perinatal infections (toxoplasmosis, rubella, and cytomegalovirus infection) (31, 36). For example, one algorithm suggested for prenatal toxoplasmosis testing follows all positive IgG antibody assays with an avidity test. If the avidity test is high, an acute infection is ruled out; however, if the avidity test is low, an IgM test is then performed. If the IgM test is positive, then a recent IgM infection is highly suspected. However, considering the implications for pregnancy, the FDA recommends that sera with positive IgM results obtained at a nonreference laboratory then be sent to a toxoplasma reference laboratory for confirmatory testing.

TABLE 1 Sensitivities of immunoassays[a]

Technique	Approximate sensitivity (per ml)
Precipitation, tube	100 mg
Immunodiffusion	1–3 mg
Agglutination	1 µg
CF	1 µg
Hemagglutination, passive	50 ng
Particle immunoassay	30–50 ng
EIA	<1 ng

[a]Data from references 24 and 46.

SPECIFIC IMMUNOASSAYS

The spectrum of immunologic assays is discussed in detail in the following sections. Table 1 lists selected assays and provides approximate levels of detection.

Precipitation Reactions

When soluble antigens and antibodies are in equimolar concentrations, they bind and form insoluble antigen-antibody complexes which form a visible precipitate (27, 32). There are a number of laboratory tests available that utilize this reaction. Immunodiffusion is the simplest of the precipitation assays and involves putting the immunoreactants in an inert semisolid material and then viewing the visible precipitation line. There are several variants of immunodiffusion. Radial immunodiffusion is designed to provide protein quantitation, whereas double immunodiffusion (Ouchterlony analysis) allows characterization of the relationship between different antigens. Overall, immunodiffusion reactions are simple to perform, easy to evaluate, and inexpensive and can be adapted to a variety of health care settings. The drawbacks include low sensitivity, as the level of detection is microgram quantities of antibody or antigen; requirements for relatively large amounts of antigens and antibody; and long assay times. Immunodiffusion is also routinely used for determination of titers of antibody to a variety of agents, most commonly antifungal antibodies (*Coccidioides*, *Aspergillus*, and *Histoplasma*).

Agglutination Reactions

Agglutination reactions require a particulate antigen and its antibody, with the resultant visible clumping as evidence of a positive reaction (24, 27, 32, 33). A test involving the particulate antigen which agglutinates the antibody present in the patient sample is termed a direct agglutination assay. To enhance the visibility of the agglutination reaction, an indirect assay format can be used, in which the antigen is coupled with a variety of particles that serve as an inert matrix. Various materials which have been employed include gelatin, latex, erythrocytes (RBC), polypeptides, and silicates. In addition, soluble antigen can be detected in a patient sample by absorption of a specific antibody to a particle; this is termed reverse agglutination. Due to the large IgM molecule with its pentameric structure, IgM antibodies are several hundred times more efficient at agglutination than IgG and thus give more consistent and stable agglutination reactions. If the immune response involves primarily IgG antibody, the reaction may require some type of chemical enhancement or an antiglobulin reagent. Flocculation assays are another variant of agglutination assays, in which the particles are suspended. The most frequently used assays are the VDRL and rapid plasma reagin tests for syphilis.

Many agglutination assays, called hemagglutination assays, employ RBC and use either a direct or an indirect assay format. Direct agglutination of RBC is commonly used in the blood bank for ABO typing. For infectious disease diagnosis, one of the most frequently ordered direct hemagglutination assays is the Monospot test. This test detects the presence of a heterophile antibody which is produced in infectious mononucleosis and happens to spontaneously agglutinate equine RBC. The indirect hemagglutination assay is a commonly used format in which antigen is adsorbed to RBC, thus testing for the presence of specific antibody in the patient serum. Alternatively, the assay can be modified to test for antigen, in which case it is called a reverse agglutination assay. For infectious disease testing, hemagglutination (especially indirect) is a popular assay format, as it is sensitive and simple to perform and does not require sophisticated equipment. For these reasons, it has been used in many developing countries for testing of a variety of infectious disease agents, such as human immunodeficiency virus (HIV), hepatitis viruses (A, B, and C), and *Treponema pallidum*. There is a unique type of hemagglutination assay format used primarily in viral serology called hemagglutination inhibition. It is most commonly used for detection and quantitation of anti-influenza virus antibodies. It is based on the principle that some viruses have surface proteins that will agglutinate RBC, so the assay uses the ability of antiviral antibodies in the patient sample to inhibit the spontaneous agglutination of the test RBC. The titer of antiviral antibodies is reported as the last dilution of the patient serum still able to inhibit the agglutination reaction.

Specialized types of agglutination assays that require optical counting are called particle immunoassays (10, 20, 29). They involve primarily the measurement of scattered light which occurs upon the antigen-antibody reaction, and this is measured by either turbidimetry or nephelometry. They can be used for testing a wide range of proteins and analytes. Particle immunoassays are 3 orders of magnitude more sensitive than standard agglutination. One additional assay is the particle-counting immunoassay, which is used for quantitating haptens, antigens, and antibody. It is also available in a fully automated immunoassay format. In this assay, optical cell counting is employed, and there is an assessment of the decrease in agglutination following the immunoreaction. These assays are sensitive to a level of nanograms per milliliter. The patient sample is mixed with latex beads coated with antibody. As the antigen-antibody reaction occurs, the antigen particles are no longer dispersed in the solution; therefore, the antigen concentration is inversely proportional to the amount of antigen particles remaining in solution. Antibody can also be quantitated in this assay. The use of a particle-counting immunoassay has been reported for quantitation of hepatitis B virus surface antigen, along with quantitation of antibodies to hepatitis C virus, *T. pallidum*, and *T. gondii* (20, 23).

Overall, basic agglutination assays are easy to perform and inexpensive and can be done in a variety of clinical settings, such as the doctor's office, the emergency room, and the hospital bedside and in the field. They are performed either on a card, in tubes, or in microtiter plates. Often they provide only qualitative results, although an antibody or antigen titer can be obtained through serial dilutions of the sample. Direct assays continue to be performed for rare pathogens such as *Francisella* and *Brucella*. They utilize an inactivated source of the whole organism mixed with the patient sera. Although agglutination assays suffer from both limited sensitivity and limited specificity, they continue to

be utilized because they are easy to perform and relatively inexpensive. If a more quantitative assay is needed, the assay can be adapted to light-scattering equipment such as a nephelometer to provide more quantitative and sensitive results. Overall, the major drawback to direct agglutination assays is their limited sensitivity. They detect only to a level of microgram to milligram quantities of analytes per milliliter. However, greater sensitivities can be achieved with many of the variants of direct agglutination. For example, microtiter passive hemagglutination assays for infectious agents can achieve a sensitivity equivalent to that of a conventional EIA. The more sensitive hemagglutination assays for measuring antigen can measure as low as 15 to 30 μg/ml. If an agglutination assay is read visually, it is reported as a titer. While these are fairly sensitive assays, titers are always plus or minus one tube dilution, so a titer of 16 could actually represent a titer of either 8 or 32. With latex-enhanced nephelometry or turbidimetry, sensitivity ranges in the area of 30 to 50 ng/ml.

There are several problems that can affect both sensitivity and specificity. The first problem affecting sensitivity is called the prozone effect (10, 27, 32). This refers to a lack of agglutination due to an excessive amount of antibodies in the patient sample. The high concentration of antibody inhibits agglutination, giving a false-negative result. This can be easily overcome by simply diluting the sample. With regard to specificity, the major concern is false-positive reactions from IgM rheumatoid factor (RF) (10, 17, 27, 32, 35). This occurs most commonly in assays in which the latex beads are coated with IgG antibody. This has been commonly reported for the latex agglutination test for cryptococcal antigen (27, 52). IgM RF, which is specific for the Fc portion of the IgG molecule, binds and gives a false-positive reaction. RF has also been reported to bind to other serum proteins nonspecifically, also giving a false-positive reaction. It is crucial that the clinician notify the laboratory if the patient has a known RF. There are several measures that could be taken. First of all, if a false-positive reaction is suspected, the sample result can be compared to the reaction using control particles coated with normal IgG. If this indicates that there is a false-positive reaction, the sample can be treated with a reducing agent such as 2-mercaptoethanol or it can be treated with pronase. Both of these treatments have been shown to reduce the majority of false-positive reactions due to IgM RF. Alternatively, the sample could be pretreated with aggregated IgG to remove the IgM RF; however, this can result in loss of antigen or specific antibodies and give a false-negative result. Also, an alternate test method could be used for assessment of the ordered analyte. Most importantly, communication of pertinent clinical information to the laboratory is critical to ensure the most accurate diagnostic information.

CF Test

Another traditional immunoassay is the complement fixation (CF) test, which is based upon the interaction of immune complexes with complement (32). As antigen-antibody complexes form, the complement cascade is activated and complement components are "fixed" or consumed. Conversely, if there is no antigen-antibody complex formation, there will be no activation of the complement cascade. This two-step test is primarily used to determine the titer of antibodies to specific antigens. For example, to set up a CF test for anti-*Mycoplasma pneumoniae* antibodies, patient serum would be incubated with *M. pneumoniae* antigen and a defined quantity of guinea pig complement. If the patient sample contains

M. *pneumoniae* antibody, immune complexes will form and fix the complement. RBC coated with anti-RBC antibodies are then added to the tube. The final readout for the assay is the release of hemoglobin from any lysed RBC. If the patient sample is positive for M. *pneumoniae,* then there will be no complement remaining, so there will be no release of hemoglobin. The opposite will occur if the patient sample is negative for anti-M. *pneumoniae* antibody. Although CF assays are relatively sensitive and inexpensive, they can be technically demanding and time-consuming. Therefore, many of these assays have been converted to ELISA formats. However, a number of laboratories still use them as a confirmatory test for the presence of antibodies to a variety of infectious agents, such as *Coccidioides, Histoplasma capsulatum,* adenovirus, herpesvirus, influenza virus, M. *pneumoniae,* and rickettsias.

Neutralization Assays

Neutralization assays are traditional laboratory tests used to determine if an antibody which can neutralize the infectivity of a particular virus is present (32). The classic assay involves mixing patient serum antibody samples with virus and then using this mixture to inoculate either a cell line or a preparation of peripheral blood mononuclear cells. The readout involves either the assessment of viral cytopathic effect in the cell line or some other measure of viral replication, such as that obtained by a classic immunoassay of viral protein. For example, in the case of HIV testing, one can perform a p24 antigen test or reverse transcriptase assay and look for lower values. Evidence of decreased viral replication confirms the presence of neutralizing antibody. Although these assays are relatively simple, they can be expensive and can take days to complete. In addition, they can be difficult to standardize, especially when comparing results from different laboratories. To decrease the assay length, the quantitation of viral products can be assessed using PCR; however, this technique can be expensive and also difficult to standardize between laboratories. A blocking ELISA can also be performed, in which viral antigen and serum are mixed, after which a standard ELISA for virus is performed and the decrease in the amount of antibody detected is assessed. An additional traditional neutralization assay is reverse passive hemagglutination, as previously discussed. In the field of HIV vaccine development, there is interest in developing new and better assays for neutralization, since it is crucial in the assessment of vaccine efficacy to demonstrate that a putative virus can initiate antibody production to prevent infection (37).

Immunofluorescence Assays

The immunofluorescence assay (IFA) uses a histochemical technique to detect either antigen or serum antibody, utilizing a fluorescent-compound-labeled detector antibody (27, 32, 33). There are two types of IFA, direct and indirect (Fig. 1). Direct assays are used to detect the presence of antigens in tissue or body fluids. For example, to detect the presence of influenza virus in a nasal wash specimen, it is applied to a slide, and then it is overlaid with a fluorescent-compound-labeled anti-influenza virus antibody. If there is influenza virus antigen present, there is emission of fluorescent light, which is evaluated with a fluorescence microscope. Indirect assays are two-step tests used primarily for the detection of antibodies in serum or a body fluid, although they can also be used for detection of viral antigens, such as cytomegalovirus. The patient sample is applied to a slide containing the target antigen; this is allowed to incubate, and specific antibody in the patient sample forms immune

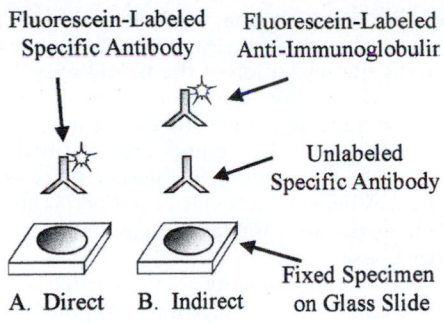

FIGURE 1   Direct and indirect IFAs.

complexes with the antigen present on the slide. Any unbound reagent is then washed away, and the slide is overlaid with a fluorescent-compound-labeled anti-immunoglobulin. Positive staining is the emission of fluorescent light. Overall, IFAs are useful tests that are relatively easy to perform and inexpensive. In addition, they allow the localization of the antibody to a specific antigen location in the tissue. For example, the IFA for antibody to Epstein-Barr virus early antigen allows visualization of a specific pattern of staining of the virus-infected cell line. The disadvantages of this assay are that it is relatively time-consuming and requires both the purchase of an expensive fluorescence microscope and the presence of trained and experienced personnel for interpretation. However, there are now available automated analyzers which perform IFA slide processing, thus freeing up hours of preparatory time (20).

Enzyme Immunoassays

EIAs are taking on increasingly more prominent roles in laboratory medicine (9, 10, 25, 27, 33, 53, 54). They are found in all areas of the clinical laboratory, in physicians' offices, and in at-home testing and are being increasingly used in molecular pathology laboratories. EIAs have taken the place of RIAs in the majority of laboratories, as they offer comparable sensitivity without the problems of disposal and the short half-life associated with radioactive materials. They are also replacing a variety of other techniques in the laboratory, such as immunofluorescence and agglutination, because EIAs provide greater objectivity, the potential to automate, and the ability to process large numbers of samples with less hands-on technician time. As a single unit of enzyme label can amplify a reaction product severalfold, many EIAs are optimized for detection at the pico- or attomole level. EIAs can be broadly classified as either homogeneous or heterogeneous assays. In homogeneous assays, the enzyme activity is altered as part of the immunologic reaction itself. In these assays, there is no requirement to separate the bound from the free immunoreactants. Although this technique is especially suited for the measurement of drugs and haptens, homogeneous assays have not achieved widespread use in microbiology laboratories. In contrast, heterogeneous immunoassays are widely used in microbiology. In these assays, the enzyme activity of the labeled immunoreactant is not directly involved in the immunologic reaction itself.

The basic principle of the heterogeneous EIA is the use of an antibody or antigen conjugated with an enzyme which, upon reacting with its substrate, forms a measurable reaction product. Often a color reaction product is produced. The color change is monitored visually or with the use of a spectrophotometer to determine the proportionality between the amount of color and the amount of analyte present. An essential component of these assays is the separation of the bound enzyme-labeled component from the free labeled reagent. Assays can be competitive or noncompetitive and can be used to measure antigens or antibodies. The presence of all antibody isotypes can be quantitated depending on the specificity of the antibodies used. Whenever antibody or antigen is absorbed to the solid phase, the assay is referred to as an ELISA and also as a sandwich assay.

EIAs can be set up primarily as competitive or noncompetitive (9). Competitive assays most commonly measure antigens and are set up with either antibody or antigen on the solid phase. They are often termed limited-reagent methods because the antigens and antibodies are used in measured and limited amounts. When the assay design uses specific antibody with which the solid phase is coated, the patient sample containing the putative antigen and the labeled antigen are added simultaneously and compete for binding to this matrix (Fig. 2). It is critical that the avidity of the antibody for both the labeled and unlabeled antigens be the same. In addition, a separate reaction is set up using enzyme-labeled antigen and buffer alone, which are added to the antibody-adsorbed solid phase. The substrate for the enzyme is added, and the color reaction is assessed. If the patient sample contains the antigen in question, it will effectively compete for binding to the solid phase, thus preventing any enzyme-labeled antigen from binding, giving no or minimal color. This reaction is compared to a reaction well to which buffer alone is substituted for the patient sample. The separation of the bound reactant from the free reactant is achieved through the washing steps. As is true with all competitive assays, the amount of labeled immunoreactant detected through the enzymatic reaction is inversely proportional to the amount of antigen present in the sample.

Antigens present in a patient sample can also be measured by using the coating of the solid phase with antigen. For this technique, the test sample containing the antigen in question is mixed with a limited amount of enzyme-labeled antibody. If the patient's sample contains the antigen, it will bind the labeled antigen, thus preventing this antibody from binding to the antigen with which the solid phase is coated. Following the washing step, the color reaction is developed, and again, no color is seen if the sample contains the antigen. This technique can be modified by using unlabeled antibody in the first step and then adding a secondary enzyme-labeled anti-immunoglobulin.

Another variant of a competitive technique uses a two-step procedure. In the first step, test antigen is preincubated with its specific antibody. Any antigen-antibody complexes that have formed are removed during a wash step. Enzyme-labeled antigen (Ag*) is then added to bind any remaining free antibody not bound by test antigen in the initial reaction. In the second step, beads coated with anti-immunoglobulin are added. These beads bind any Ag*-antibody complexes which formed in the previous step, and they can be quantitated in the pellet following centrifugation.

Competitive tests often provide more specificity and less sensitivity than do noncompetitive assays; however, this is dependent on the affinity and purity of the immunologic reagents and the design of the particular system. Competitive assays are ideal for measuring relatively small molecules which can be obtained in relative purity and in large enough amounts to be labeled with an enzyme. As they generally require small amounts of antibody, competitive assays are ideal for use in systems which have a limited amount of antibody available.

Noncompetitive ELISAs

The next major type of assay is the noncompetitive indirect solid-phase ELISA. This method is one of the most frequently employed immunoassays in the clinical laboratory. As with competitive assays, the two major variants involve using either antigen or antibody on the solid phase. When antigen is used for coating, specific antibodies in the sample bind to the solid phase and are detected with an enzyme-labeled anti-immunoglobulin secondary antibody (Fig. 3). Isotype-specific, enzyme-labeled anti-immunoglobulin antibodies can be used to determine the specific immunoglobulin class present. This type of assay is commonly used in the measurement of immune status to infectious agents and for autoantibody testing. A variety of solid-phase supports are used, including microtiter plates, nitrocellulose, and beads. One common variant, which uses nitrocellulose membranes, is the dot blot assay (17, 32, 43). In this system, the antigen or antibody is coupled to the membrane, and usually the reaction is assessed visually by a colored reaction production, providing a qualitative assay. Many of the at-home testing kits (e.g., pregnancy kits) use a variant of this technique. This assay can be modified for increased sensitivity with such variants as can be made semiquantitative by using a densitometer for reading the color reaction.

When the antibody is coupled to the solid phase, these assays are often termed capture or sandwich assays, because the antigen in the sample is captured by an antibody-coated matrix. An enzyme-labeled secondary antibody directed to a different antigenic epitope is then added, completing the sandwich. There are numerous variations of this type of assay. The antigen captured can be an immunoglobulin, a viral protein, or any antigen that has at least two epitopes.

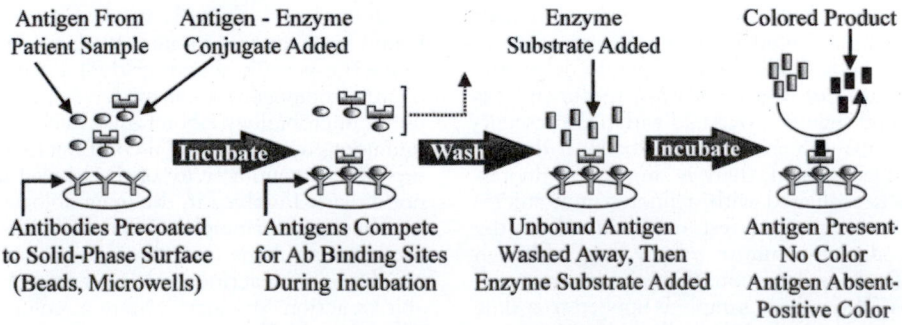

FIGURE 2 Competitive EIA. Ab, antibody.

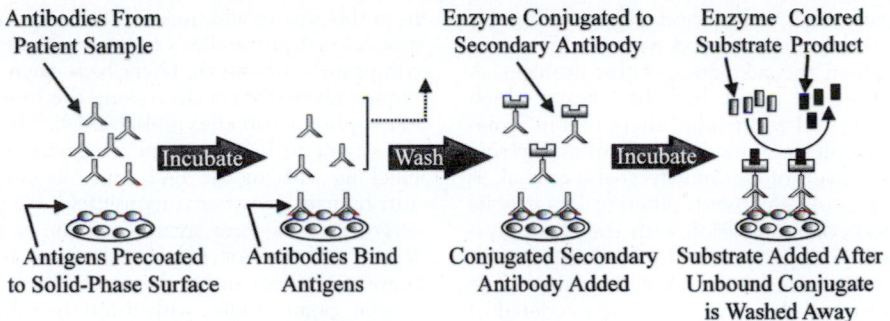

FIGURE 3 Noncompetitive indirect solid-phase ELISA.

Noncompetitive ELISAs can also be modified by incorporating additional layers of immunoreactants. This increases the sensitivity of the assay, but it also increases both the cost and time requirements. The most frequent application is the so-called avidin-biotin-peroxidase complex (ABC method), which can significantly improve the level of detectability. Biotinylated anti-immunoglobulin is generally used as the second antibody of the sandwich. This is then reacted with a preformed mixture of avidin and biotinylated peroxidase (ABC). The peroxidase can be developed with chemiluminescent reagents for increased sensitivity. Other variants include peroxidase-antiperoxidase methods and the incorporation of lectins as bridging molecules.

Microparticle EIA

The microparticle EIA is a variant of the ELISA that utilizes tiny beads (1-mm diameter or less) that can be coupled with antibody or antigens (27, 31). The small size leads to a greater surface area for binding of antibody or antigen, which results in a decrease in reaction time. The particles act as the solid phase, but the reaction can be performed in suspension. This method has been widely adapted to automate the assessment of large molecules such as hepatitis virus antigens and IgM and IgG antiviral antibodies.

Analytical Interferences and Technical Issues

As in all laboratory tests, there are always factors that can affect test validity. Overall, immunoassays are affected more than routine chemistry and microbiology assays (8, 16, 25, 34, 35, 47, 53, 54). There are various clues that should alert one to the possibility of erroneous results. These include test results that are inconsistent with the clinical findings and/or an unexplained change in a test result from a previous assessment. These findings should prompt consideration of the possibility of technical issues or some type of test interference.

Plate Variability
There are several issues to consider with solid-phase microtiter plates that are often used for reagent excess sandwich-type ELISA (9, 53, 54). First, there can be variability between readings on adjacent wells of a microtiter plate. This variability is expressed as the well coefficient of variation, which should not be greater than 3 to 5% between wells. Second, there is the "edge effect," which refers to the variability between the readings on the outer wells of a microtiter plate and the readings on the inside wells. Although manufacturing variability in the plates must be evaluated as a possible cause, this occurs primarily due to differences in temperature between outer wells and interior ones. This can

affect both the antigen-antibody and enzyme-substrate reactions. There are several ways to deal with the edge effect. One easy solution is to use smaller break-apart wells that can be placed in a larger plate. Simply being careful to protect the plate from exposure to light can also easily solve this problem. It is crucial that different plates from several manufacturers be screened for this effect when initially setting up an assay. In addition, when the lot of a plate is changed, the plates should be reevaluated to ensure that it is not necessary to modify any of the assay parameters.

Hook Effect
The hook effect refers to an unexpected fall in the amount of an analyte at the high end of the dose-response curve, resulting in a gross underestimation of the analyte (8, 16, 25, 34, 35, 47, 53, 54). This is particularly a problem in sandwich immunoassays with patient samples which contain an extremely high level of an analyte. The patient sample gives a low to moderately high result when using the standard assay dilution. However, upon further dilution of the sample, either the result is out-of-range high or, if it is diluted far enough, the sample gives an extremely elevated value. Therefore, if the laboratory ran the sample only at the routine dilution, a significant underestimation of the value would be reported.

The explanation for this phenomenon has not been completely established. Many investigators feel that it is caused by antigen excess, in which a majority of the antigen-binding sites are filled, preventing completion of the sandwich. It has also been suggested to arise from low-affinity antibody, inadequate washing, and suboptimal concentrations of labeled antibody. Tests that are especially susceptible to problems with the hook effect include ones in which there may be samples with extremely high levels of the measured substance. These include IgE, human chorionic gonadotropin, tumor markers, ferritin, infectious antigens, and antibodies.

Numerous suggestions have been made regarding ways that laboratories can deal with the hook effect. One obvious strategy is to run all patient samples at 2 dilutions to screen for this problem. If the sample provides an answer with the first dilution, while the more dilute sample is out-of-range high, then the laboratory is alerted to the possibility of the hook effect. Although this is an effective approach, many laboratories are concerned about the time, cost, and labor involved in running 2 dilutions for every sample to avoid problems with only a small minority of patients. Thus, there are other strategies which can lessen the probability of the hook effect occurring.

First, always ensure that adequate washing is performed between all steps of the ELISA, especially between the steps following the addition of each antibody. Automatic plate washers are relatively inexpensive and can simplify this task. In addition, good communication with the kit manufacturers can also lessen the frequency of this problem. A number of companies have established the level at which the hook effect occurs and will readily share this information. Also, when completing new kit evaluations, testing specimens with high levels of the analyte is also crucial, as the frequency of the hook effect with different kits may be variable. Lastly, good communication with the clinician is also important; include discussion of the hook effect with a suggestion of notifying the laboratory when patients are expected to have very high levels of the analyte ordered.

Antibody Interference

There are a number of endogenous antibodies in patients' sera that may cause either positive or negative interferences in immunoassays (8, 16, 25, 34, 35, 47, 53, 54). There are multiple types of antibody interferences; they can be caused by antibodies binding to the actual analyte (e.g., antiviral antibodies), binding to components of the detection system (e.g., anti-alkaline phosphatase), and binding to reagent antibodies (e.g., anti-immunoglobulin antibodies). The last category is the most common and involves three types of antibodies. First, there are heterophile antibodies, which are weak antibodies to immunoglobulins from multiple species with no known or obvious identifiable immunogen. Second, RF can have a known effect on a variety of immunoassays and is most often found in patients with connective tissue diseases. Third, there are various types of anti-animal antibodies; the most commonly reported are human anti-mouse antibodies (HAMA). Estimates of the prevalence of anti-mouse antibodies in normal sera vary greatly, from 0.5% to as high as 40%, depending on the sensitivity of the testing assay. There are both iatrogenic and noniatrogenic causes for the development of HAMA. With regard to iatrogenic causes, the culprit appears to be the increasing use of mouse monoclonal antibodies for therapeutic and imaging purposes. With regard to noniatrogenic causes, there are a number of suggested etiologies, including environmental exposure to mice, maternal transfer across the placenta, passage of dietary antigens across the gut wall in inflammatory conditions (such as celiac disease), and association with a number of disease states, such as cardiomyopathy (28). While human anti-mouse antibodies can affect a variety of immunoassays, they are most often reported for two-site murine monoclonal antibody assays, which often require only a small serum dilution. The presence of these antibodies can have a variable effect on immunoassays. If the analyte is present, they may cause either an over- or an underestimation. However, if the analyte is not present, a false-positive result may arise

from the anti-mouse antibody cross-linking the two mouse monoclonal antibodies of the sandwich (the coating and conjugate antibodies). There have been a number of techniques advocated for decreasing the interference caused by heterophile antibodies and HAMA. These include heating the sample to 70°C, precipitating with polyethylene glycol, blocking with mouse IgG, and blocking with solid-phase anti-human IgG or anti-mouse IgG. Caution should be observed in using heat treatment. The most popular method is the addition of nonimmune mouse immunoglobulin; however, the amount and source of the mouse serum may be crucial. Some studies with interfering anti-mouse antibodies demonstrated that the serum had to be from the same strain of mouse as the monoclonal antibody used in the assay. Therefore, it is recommended that a pool of mouse immunoglobulins from various strains be used to increase the probability of blocking as many patients' samples as possible. Most studies use approximately 10% mouse serum added to the reaction buffer; however, a few patient samples required a high concentration (>20%) of normal serum coupled with a long incubation time to correct the interference. To obviate problems with the majority of samples, laboratorians should consider routinely adding normal pooled heterologous sera to the dilution buffer of sandwich assays. In addition, special attention should be given to any sample for which the laboratory result is discordant with the clinical presentation, as this may represent a heterophile antibody resistant to the standard protocols.

Measurement of IgM

Quantitation of the IgM isotype of specific antibody poses special technical problems (9, 27, 31, 54). False positivity is common due to the presence of IgM RF in patient samples. In addition, false negativity can occur from competitive inhibition of IgM binding in the presence of high levels of specific IgG. Previously, assays for IgM used a standard indirect solid-phase ELISA with the antigen immobilized and an IgM-specific secondary antibody. However, these assays were fraught with the problems of false positivity and negativity. To obviate these problems, an IgM capture assay was developed (Fig. 4). In this procedure, a polyclonal anti-IgM antibody is bound to the solid phase. Upon incubation of the patient sample, all IgM is captured on the plate. The test antigen is then added, binding any specific IgM present on the plate. An enzyme-labeled secondary antibody is then added, and the reaction is completed. This assay obviates the problems with false-negative results due to competitive inhibition with IgM, as all the IgG in the patient sample is washed away in the first step. False-positive results, however, may still occur due to bound IgM RF reacting with either the IgG conjugate

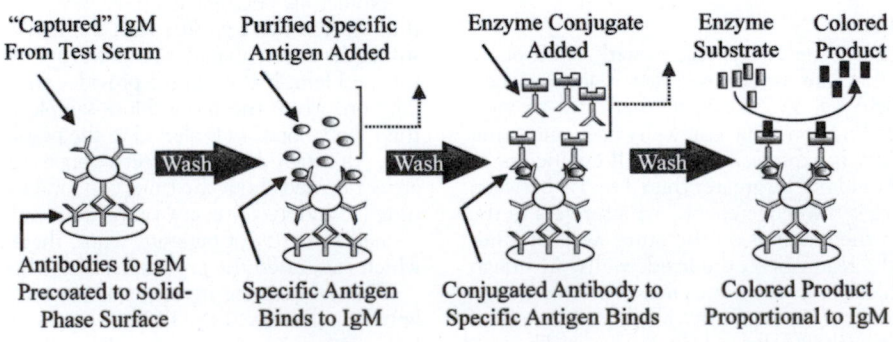

FIGURE 4 IgM capture assay.

or binding any antigen-specific IgG in the sample. One way to avoid the problem with conjugate binding is to use F(ab')₂-conjugated capture antibodies. Alternatively, the assay can be modified to a direct technique by employing enzyme-labeled antigen in the second step, thus eliminating any immunoglobulin which could bind RF. Even with these modifications, problems can still occur with borderline and low positive IgM results. For this reason, all IgM-specific antibody results should be evaluated cautiously. As mentioned above, often running an IgG avidity assay can help in the evaluation of IgM results.

Radioimmunoassay

RIA was the original immunoassay technique and ushered in the era of improved and more sensitive immunoassays. Basically, all principles of assay design for EIA were based upon the experience gleaned from RIA. Although RIA is still a viable technique, it has largely been replaced by CL and EIA in most clinical laboratories. A variety of radioisotopes are utilized, most commonly ^{125}I, ^{3}H, and ^{14}C. Both CL and EIA offer more stable reagents and are comparable to more sensitive detection limits, and they present no problems with hazardous waste disposal.

Fluorescence Immunoassays

The fluorescence immunoassay (FIA) uses fluorescence as the detection end point, and this method can be used in either homogeneous or heterogeneous assays (10, 27, 32). Fluorescence is the emission of photons of light as electrons go from an excited singlet state to the original ground state. The system requires a light source, excitation and emission filters, and a detection system utilizing photomultiplier tubes. A mercury lamp is the most frequently used light source, although xenon, halogen, and laser can also be used as excitation light. Fluorescein isothiocyanate and rhodamine are two of the most popular fluorochromes; however, there are a variety of other compounds used which have unique properties making them especially suited to a particular assay design.

There are numerous homogeneous assays which are performed in the liquid phase and do not require a separation of the bound from the free components. One popular homogeneous technique is the fluorescence polarization immunoassay. Some popular clinical analyzers utilize this methodology. This technique gives a measure of the bound/free ratio of the analyte without requiring a separation step. Polarization of light is measured by illuminating a sample with two polarizers in the same plane as the incident light and then at 90° to each other. The assay is based on an increase in light polarization which occurs when a fluorescent-tag antigen binds antibody and forms an immune complex. The labeled antigen is small and thus can rotate rapidly, causing depolarization of light. When the antigen-antibody complex forms, the increase in molecular weight causes a slower rotation and an increased emission of highly polarized light. This technique is primarily utilized for measurement of drugs and some hormones; however, it has utility for the detection of infectious disease. Its use has been described for the detection of antibodies to a variety of organisms, such as gram-negative bacteria (*Brucella* spp. and *Salmonella* spp.) and equine infectious anemia virus (23, 50). There are a number of variants of both homogeneous and heterogeneous assays; however, it is beyond the scope of this chapter to discuss these, and the reader is referred to other sources (27). FIAs have a number of advantages, including high sensitivity and speed, and they are at least as sensitive as RIA. In addition, the reagents are stable and the

assays are easily performed. For the fluorescence polarization immunoassay, one limitation is that the antigen used must be relatively small (i.e., with a molecular weight no greater than 2,000) to allow a significant difference in the polarization when it forms an immune complex. Another important drawback in the use of fluorescent assays is the problem of autofluorescent compounds both in the patient sample and in the reaction mixture. This can be a significant problem in homogeneous assays where no washing steps occur and sample components are present during the entire assay. To circumvent this problem, samples can be treated with proteolytic enzymes, oxidizing agents, or denaturing reagents which limit the amount of autofluorescence. In solid-phase assays, the majority of interfering substance is washed away.

CL Immunoassays

The CL immunoassay is a very popular technique which is widely utilized in many different assay formats (10, 27). CL is the emission of light which occurs when a substrate decays from an excited state to a ground state. In contrast to the fluorescence reaction, which utilizes incident radiation for energy, CL derives energy from the chemical reaction itself, which most often is an oxidation reaction. It is one of the most sensitive of all immunoassays, with detection limits down to the attomole (10^{-18}) or zeptomole (10^{-21}) level. CL substrates are used as the end point in both homogeneous and heterogeneous assays, in addition to their use in immunoblotting and multianalyte detection. Either CL is used as a direct label on an antigen or antibody in a reaction which is catalyzed by adding a substrate or a CL compound is used as the substrate for an enzyme-labeled immunoreactant. The acridinium ester labels most commonly employed are derivatives of isoluminol and acridinium esters. The latter is a popular label which is the most sensitive and widely used. It can be conjugated to antigen and antibody by using standard techniques. Detection is relatively simple with the addition of sodium hydroxide and hydrogen peroxide. This reaction results in a flash of light which is read using a luminometer. In addition, the light signal can be captured on photographic film.

Western Blotting and Immunoblotting

Western blotting and immunoblotting are two solid-phase assays which combine the separation of proteins, using separation by denaturing gel electrophoresis followed by transfer to a filter (Fig. 5), and the determination of reactivity of the

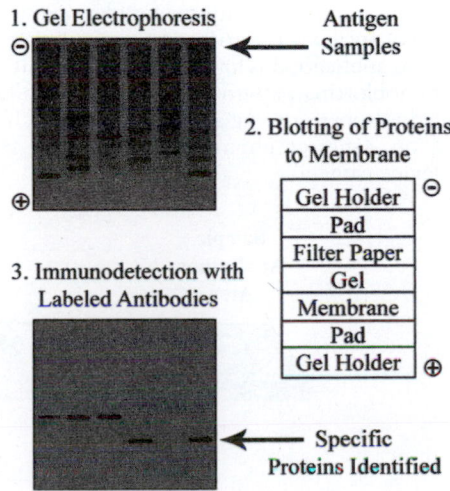

FIGURE 5   Western blot procedure.

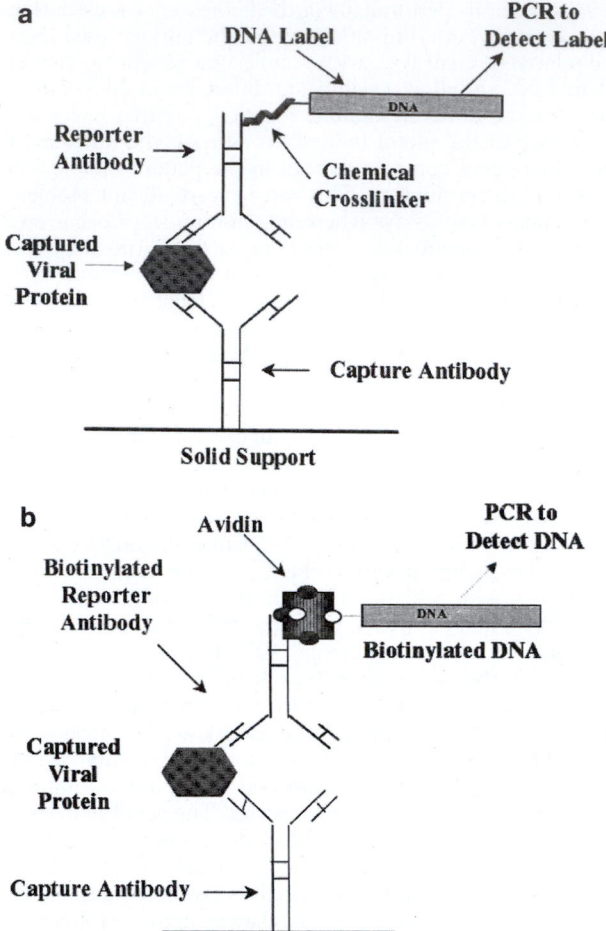

FIGURE 6 Principle of IPCR. (a) DNA directly conjugated to reporter antibody; (b) DNA conjugated via an avidin-biotin reaction.

Immuno-PCR

Immuno-PCR (IPCR) is a novel technique that combines traditional ELISA with PCR (3–5, 7, 13, 16, 19, 27, 30, 38, 44, 55). It uses antibodies labeled directly with nucleic acids (Fig. 6). It is an ultrasensitive technique which has been used for the detection of a variety of viruses. It has the advantage of being able to detect prion proteins where there is no nucleic acid present (34). A recent assay reports a detection limit corresponding to 2.3×10^2 prion epitopes (44). In addition, this technique can detect viral proteins not associated with nucleic acids. IPCR has been reported for ultrasensitive detection of a variety of infectious agents, such as *Streptococcus*, HIV, and rotavirus, and Shiga toxin 2. In the case of rotavirus, it has been reported to detect as few as 100 viral particles/ml (versus 100,000 particles detected by ELISA). IPCR is a very sensitive test for determination of HIV type 1 viral load for p24 antigen. In addition, a recent paper reports the ability to detect less than one HIV-1 virion (6). Although IPCR is a powerful technique, there can be technical issues when combining nucleic acids and proteins, and there can be problems with high assay backgrounds. An alternative approach which uses an indirect double-stranded DNA substrate for alkaline phosphatase has also been published (4). Overall, these highly sensitive methodologies represent the wave of the future, and there will be an increasing number of applications in infectious disease testing.

Rapid Immunoassays

The development of a multitude of rapid immunoassays has revolutionized diagnostic testing, for many tests that were previously available only in specialized or reference laboratories are now easily performed and can usually be completed in less than 30 min (12, 14, 18, 32, 39, 40, 42, 45, 48). There are a variety of formats utilized for these assays which can detect both antigens and antibodies along with products of nucleic acid amplification tests. One of the most popular formats is the lateral-flow immunoassay or immunochromatography. This has the advantage of being a one-step assay. One common format uses a chromatographic pad with three zones: sample application area, conjugate pad, and capture line (Fig. 7). The conjugate pad can use a variety of types of conjugates to generate a signal, including colloidal gold, dye, or latex beads. The sample is applied to the sample pad and flows laterally by capillary action. Upon reaching the conjugate pad, if the analyte is present, it binds to the conjugate, forming an immune complex. The complex then continues to flow laterally along the pad by capillary action and is captured by the second antibody or antigen impregnated in the capture line. The presence of a colored line is a positive reaction. There is a positive control line also included in the test to make sure that the test was properly performed. There are variations to this assay format with systems which require no separate venipuncture, combining collection of finger stick samples with testing in a

patient sera with the individually separated proteins, using a typical sandwich-type ELISA. Immunoblotting utilizes a solid-support membrane filter containing antigens which are identified by a specific reaction with antibody. Most commonly, this technique is utilized for identifying the specific pattern of antibody to various infectious disease agents. One common application is for confirmation of antibody to HIV. Immunoblotting patterns can be read visually, using radiolabeled isotopes or using a CL substrate which is then developed on X-ray or photographic film or a charged-coupled-device camera.

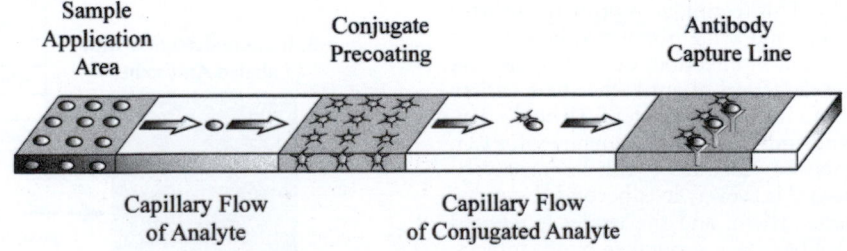

FIGURE 7 Lateral-flow immunoassay.

one-step lateral-flow assay. Another frequently used type of rapid test is the dot blot immunoassay, which has been discussed above. These rapid assay formats have been especially useful for HIV testing and have been used extensively in testing for HIV in underdeveloped countries. Overall, rapid assays are simple and easy to perform, can be used in field conditions, and can be performed by individuals with little training. While many are not as sensitive as conventional EIAs, there are reports of some with sensitivities approaching those of the traditional assays (14). Problems with rapid assays include the facts that they cannot be automated, that interpretation can be subjective, and that performance by individuals with no formal laboratory training can result in erroneous results. However, considering their overall advantages and low cost, their use will continue and be expanded as more analytes are adapted to this type of testing.

Automated Technologies

With the expansion of EIAs available, the immunoassay market of automated analyzers and the repertoire of tests available continue to dramatically increase. Recently, 62 immunoassay analyzers that can run a wide spectrum of tests important in infectious disease testing were profiled (15). The machines run the gamut of serologic assays (both antigen and antibody determinations) for infectious diseases, including HIV infection, hepatitis (A, B, and C), *T. gondii* infection, cytomegalovirus infection, rubella, and *Chlamydia trachomatis* infection, among others. Many of the systems listed are walk-away machines, requiring only limited technologist input. There are also robotic systems available which are cost-effective for even moderate-size hospital laboratories. For detailed information about each analyzer, the complete table can be downloaded from the Internet (http://www.cap.org).

An exciting new area is the development of multiplex immunoassay systems (22, 26). These are laboratory instruments which combine several technologies and allow rapid and simultaneous tests of multiple analytes in a single sample. There are many different assay designs which combine an array of technologies, including CL, FIA, flow cytometry, and molecular diagnostics (PCR and use of oligonucleotides and nanoparticles). As these assays provide rapid results and can be performed with very small sample sizes, they have wide applicability to epidemiological studies and vaccine trials. These assays are also especially suited to the assessment of multiple biological agents in a variety of samples.

With this advent of extensive tests easily performed by automated systems, the potential for both improper test utilization and incorrect interpretation of results will increase. This results in even greater pressure on laboratorians and infectious disease specialists to provide information to both their colleagues and patients about the proper use and interpretation of laboratory tests for diagnosis of infectious disease agents.

Special recognition goes to Ryan Morrison for his expertise and creativity in preparing the figures for this chapter.

REFERENCES

1. **Abbas, A. K., A. H. Lichtman, and S. Pillai.** 2007. *Cellular and Molecular Immunology*, 6th ed. Elsevier Saunders, Philadelphia, PA.
2. **Abbas, A. K., and A. H. Lichtman.** 2008. *Basic Immunology*, 3rd ed. W. B. Saunders, Philadelphia, PA.
3. **Adler, M., S. Schulz, R. Fischer, and C. M. Niemeyer.** 2005. Detection of rotavirus from stool samples using standardized immuno-PCR ("Imperacer") method with endpoint and real-time detection. *Biochem. Biophys. Res. Commun.* **12**:333.
4. **Adler, M., R. Wacker, and C. M. Niemeyer.** 2008. Sensitivity by combination: immuno-PCR and related technologies. *Analyst* **133**:702–718.
5. **Banin, S., S. M. Wilson, and C. J. Stanley.** 2004. Demonstration of an alternative approach to immuno-PCR. *Clin. Chem.* **50**:1932–1934.
6. **Barletta, J., A. Bartolome, and N. T. Constantine.** 2009. Immunomagnetic quantitative immuno-PCR for detection of less than one HIV-1 virion. *J. Virol Methods* **157**:122–132.
7. **Barletta, J. M., D. C. Edelman, and N. T. Constantine.** 2004. Lowering the detection limits of HIV-1 viral load using real-time immuno-PCR for HIV-1 p24 antigen. *Am. J. Clin. Pathol.* **122**:20–27.
8. **Bjerner, J., K. Nustaf, L. F. Norum, K. H. Olsen, and O. P. Bermer.** 2002. Immunometric assay interference. *Clin. Chem.* **48**:613–621.
9. **Carpenter, A. B.** 1997. Enzyme-linked immunoassays, p. 20–29. *In* N. R. Rose, E. Conway de Macario, J. D. Folds, H. C. Lane, and R. M. Nakamura (ed.), *Manual of Clinical Immunology*, 5th ed. ASM Press, Washington, DC.
10. **Carpenter, A. B.** 2002. Antibody-based methods, p. 20–30. *In* N. R. Rose, R. G. Hamilton, and B. Detrick (ed.), *Manual of Clinical Laboratory Immunology*, 6th ed. ASM Press, Washington, DC.
11. **Centers for Disease Control and Prevention.** 2005. Positive test results for acute hepatitis A virus infection among persons with no recent history of acute hepatitis—United States, 2002–2004. *MMWR Morb. Mortal. Wkly. Rep.* **54**:453–456.
12. **Chan, C. P., Y. C. Cheung, R. Renneberg, and M. Seydack.** 2008. New trends in immunoassays. *Adv. Biochem. Eng. Biotechnol.* **109**:123–154.
13. **Chen, L., H. Wei, Y.Guo, Z. Cui, Z. Zhang, and X. E. Zhang.** 2009. Gold nanoparticle enhanced immuno-PCR for ultrasensitive detection of Hantaan virus nucleocapsid protein. *J. Immunol. Methods* **346**:64–70.
14. **Constantine, N. T., and H. Zink.** 2005. HIV testing technologies after two decades of evolution. *Indian J. Med. Res.* **121**:519–538.
15. **Dabkowski, B.** 2009. Immunoassay: all eyes on efficiency, connectivity. *CAP Today* **23**:17–72.
16. **Demers, L. M., and J. J. Miller.** 2003. *Immunoassay Testing: Interferences, Technology and Future Direction.* [CD-ROM.] AACC Press, Washington, DC.
17. **Deodhar, L., A. Gogate, R. C. Padhi, and C. R. Desai.** 1998. Standardization of a dot blot immunoassay for antigen detection in cases of pulmonary tuberculosis and its evaluation with respect to the conventional techniques. *Indian J. Med. Res.* **108**:75–79.
18. **Duthie, M. S., G. C. Ireton, G.V. Kanaujia, W. Goto, H. Liang, A. Bhatia, J. M. Busceti, M. Macdonald, K. D. Neupane, B. R. Sapkota, M. Balagon, C. Ranjit, J. Esfandiari, D. Carter, and S. G. Reed.** 2008. Selection of antigens and development of prototype tests for point-of-care leprosy diagnosis. *Clin Vaccine Immunol.* **10**:1590–1597.
19. **Ezan, E., and J. Grassi.** 2000. Optimization, p. 187–210. *In* J. P. Gosling (ed.), *Immunoassays. Practical Approach.* Oxford University Press, Oxford, United Kingdom.
20. **Galanti, L. M., J. Dell'Omo, B. Wanet, J. L. Guarin, J. Jamart, M. G. Garrino, P. L. Masson, and C. L. Cambiaso.** 1997. Particle counting assay for anti-toxoplasma IgG antibodies. Comparison with four automated commercial enzyme-linked immunoassays. *J. Immunol. Methods* **207**:195–201.
21. **Gosling, J. P.** 2000. Analysis by specific binding, p. 1–18. *In* J. P. Gosling (ed.), *Immunoassays. Practical Approach.* Oxford University Press, Oxford, United Kingdom.
22. **Hindson, B. J., M. T. McBride, A. J. Makarewicz, B. D. Henderer, U. Setlur, S. M. Smith, D. M. Gutierrez, T. R. Metz, S. L. Nasarabadi, K. S. Venkateswaran, S. W. Farrow, B. W. Colston, Jr., and J. M. Dzenitis.** 2005. Autonomous detection of aerosolized biological agents by multiplexed immunoassay with polymerase chain reaction confirmation. *Anal. Chem.* **77**:284–289.

23. **Jolley, M. E., and M. S. Nasir.** 2003. The use of fluorescence polarization assays for the detection of infectious diseases. *Comb. Chem. High Throughput Screen.* **6:**235–244.

24. **Kasahara, Y.** 1997. Agglutination immunoassays, p. 7–12. *In* N. R. Rose, E. Conway de Macario, J. D. Folds, H. C. Lane, and R. M. Nakamura (ed.), *Manual of Clinical Laboratory Immunology,* 5th ed. ASM Press, Washington, DC.

25. **Kemeny, D. M., and S. J. Challacombe.** 1988. *ELISA and Other Solid Phase Immunoassays. Theoretical and Practical Aspects.* John Wiley & Sons, Chichester, United Kingdom.

26. **Kim, K. S., and J. K. Park.** 2005. Magnetic force-based multiplexed immunoassay using superparamagnetic nanoparticles in microfluidic channel. *Lab Chip* **5:**657–664.

27. **Kricka, L. J.** 2006. Principles of immunochemical techniques, p. 219–244. *In* C. A. Burtis, E. R. Ashwood, and D. E. Bruns (ed.), *Tietz Textbook of Clinical Chemistry and Molecular Diagnostics,* 4th ed. Elsevier Saunders, St. Louis, MO.

28. **Kricka, L. J.** 1999. Human anti-animal antibody interferences in immunological assays. *Clin. Chem.* **45:**942–956.

29. **Kudo, T., A. Kido, Y. Nishiyama, H. Koganeya, T. Okuda, M. Nabeshima, Y. Iinuma, and S. Ichiyama.** 2004. Whole-blood counting immunoassay as a short-turnaround test for detection of hepatitis B surface antigen, anti-hepatitis C virus antibodies, and anti-*Treponema pallidum* antibodies. *J. Clin. Microbiol.* **42:**4250–4252.

30. **Liang, H., S. E. Cordova, T. L. Kieft, and S. Rogelj.** 2003. A highly sensitive immuno-PCR assay for detecting group A streptococcus. *J. Immunol. Methods* **279:**101–110.

31. **Liesenfeld, O., J. G. Montoya, S. Kinney, C. Press, and J. S. Remington.** 2001. Effect of testing for IgG avidity in the diagnosis of *Toxoplasma gondii* infection in pregnant women: experience in a US reference laboratory. *J. Infect. Dis.* **183:** 1248–1253.

32. **Lowell, C.** 2001. Clinical laboratory methods for detection of antigens and antibodies, p. 215–233. *In* T. G. Parslow, D. P. Stites, A. I. Terr, and J. B. Imboden (ed.), *Medical Immunology,* 10th ed. Lange Medical Books/McGraw-Hill, New York, NY.

33. **Mahony, J. B., and M. A. Chernesky.** 1999. Immunoassays for the diagnosis of infectious diseases, p. 202–214. *In* P. R. Murray, E. J. Baron, M. A. Pfaller, F. C. Tenover, and R. H. Yolken (ed.), *Manual of Clinical Microbiology,* 7th ed. ASM Press, Washington, DC.

34. **Marks, V.** 2002. False-positive immunoassay results: a multicenter survey of erroneous immunoassay results from assays of 74 analytes in 10 donors from 66 laboratories in seven countries. *Clin. Chem.* **48:**2008–2016.

35. **Miller, J. J., and S. S. Levinson.** 1996. Interferences in immunoassays, p. 165–190. *In* E. P. Diamandis and T. K. Christopoulous (ed.), *Immunoassay.* Academic Press, San Diego, CA.

36. **Montoya, J. G., O. Liesenfeld, S. Kinney, C. Press, and J. S. Remington.** 2002. VIDAS test for avidity of *Toxoplasma*-specific immunoglobulin G for confirmatory testing of pregnant women. *J. Clin. Microbiol.* **40:**2504–2508.

37. **Nara, P. L., and G. Lin.** 2005. HIV-1: the confounding variables of virus neutralization. *Curr. Drug Targets Infect. Disord.* **5:**157–170.

38. **Niemeyer, C. M., M. Adler, and R. Wacker.** 2005. Immuno-PCR: high sensitivity detection of proteins by nucleic acid amplification. *Trends Biotechnol.* **23:**208–216.

39. **Pai, N. P., J. P. Tulsky, D. Cohan, J. M. Colford, Jr., and A. L. Reingold.** 2007. Rapid point-of-care HIV testing in pregnant women: a systematic review and meta-analysis. *Trop. Med. Int. Health* **12:**162–173.

40. **Percival, D. A.** 1996. The measurement of hormones and bacterial antigens using rapid particle-based immunoassays. *Pure Appl. Chem.* **68:**1893–1895.

41. **Prince, H. E., and A. L. Leber.** 2002. Validation of an in-house assay for cytomegalovirus immunoglobulin G (CMV IgG) avidity and relationship of avidity to CMV IgM levels. *Clin. Diagn. Lab. Immunol.* **9:**824–827.

42. **Prod'hom, G., and J. Bille.** 2008. Use of POCT (point of care tests) in the diagnosis of infectious diseases. *Rev. Med. Suisse* **4:**908–913.

43. **Reina, J., M. Munar, and I. Blanco.** 1996. Evaluation of a direct immunofluorescence assay, dot-blot enzyme immunoassay, and shell vial culture in the diagnosis of lower respiratory infections caused by influenza A virus. *Diagn. Microbiol. Infect. Dis.* **25:**143–145.

44. **Reuter, T., B. H. Gilroyed, T. W. Alexander, A. Balachandran, S. Czub, and T. A. McAllister.** 10 July 2009. Prion protein detection via direct immuno-quantitative real-time PCR. *J. Microbiol. Methods.* doi:10.1016/j.mimet.2009.07.001.

45. **Reyburn, H., H. Mbakilwa, R. Mwangi, O. Mwerinde, R. Olomi, C. Drakeley, and C. J. Whitty.** 2007. Rapid diagnostic tests compared with malaria microscopy for guiding outpatient treatment of febrile illness in Tanzania: randomised trial. *BMJ* **334:**403–410.

46. **Rodgers Channing, R. P.** 1994. Clinical laboratory methods for detection of antigens and antibodies, p. 151–194. *In* D. A. Stites, A. I. Terr, and T. G. Parslow (ed.), *Basic and Clinical Immunology,* 8th ed. Appleton and Lange, Norwalk, CT.

47. **Ryall, R. G., C. J. Story, and D. R. Turner.** 1982. Reappraisal of the causes of the "hook effect" in two site immunoradiometric assays. *Anal. Biochem.* **127:**308–315.

48. **Sabidó, M., A. S. Benzaken, E. J. de-Andrade-Rodrigues, and P. Mayaud.** 2009. Rapid point-of-care diagnostic test for syphilis in high-risk populations, Manaus, Brazil. *Emerg. Infect. Dis.* **4:**647–649.

49. **Shultz, E. K., C. Aliferis, and D. Aronsky.** 2006. Clinical evaluation of methods, p. 409–424. *In* C. A. Burtis, E. R. Ashwood, and D. E. Bruns (ed.), *Tietz Textbook of Clinical Chemistry and Molecular Diagnostics,* 4th ed. Elsevier Saunders, St. Louis, MO.

50. **Tencza, S. B., K. R. Islam, V. Kalia, M. S. Nasir, E. Jolley, and R. C. Montelaro.** 2000. Development of a fluorescence polarization-based diagnostic assay for equine infectious anemia virus. *J. Clin. Microbiol.* **38:**1854–1859.

51. **Thacker, W. L., and D. F. Talkington.** 2000. Analysis of complement fixation and commercial enzyme immunoassays for detection of antibodies to *Mycoplasma pneumoniae* in human serum. *Clin. Diagn. Lab. Immunol.* **7:**778–780.

52. **Thomson, R. B., Jr., and H. Bertram.** 2001. Laboratory diagnosis of central nervous system infections. *Infect. Dis. Clin. N. Am.* **15:**1047–1071.

53. **Tijssen, P.** 1985. *Practice and Theory of Enzyme Immunoassays.* Elsevier Science Publishers, Amsterdam, The Netherlands.

54. **Wu, J. T.** 2000. *Quantitative Immunoassay; a Practical Guide for Assay Establishment, Troubleshooting and Clinical Application.* AACC Press, Washington, DC.

55. **Zhang, W., M. Bielaszewska, M. Pulz, K. Becker, A. W. Friedrich, H. Karch, and T. Kuczius.** 2008. New immuno-PCR assay for detection of low concentrations of Shiga toxin 2 and its variants. *J. Clin. Microbiol.* **46:**1292–1297.

Infection Control Epidemiology and Clinical Microbiology

DANIEL J. DIEKEMA AND MICHAEL A. PFALLER

6

Health care-associated (or nosocomial) infections represent one of the most common complications of health care delivery, affecting approximately 2 million persons admitted to acute-care hospitals in the United States each year (14, 52). The World Health Organization has estimated that at any given time, over 1.4 million people worldwide are suffering from an infection acquired in the health care setting (31, 91). Every health care facility should therefore have an infection control program charged with monitoring, preventing, and controlling the spread of infections in the health care environment. Because infection control requires the ability to detect infections when they occur, the clinical microbiology laboratory is inextricably linked to any comprehensive infection control program. In this chapter we discuss the impact of nosocomial infections, outline the organization of the hospital infection control program, and describe the important role of the clinical microbiology laboratory in the prevention and control of health care-associated infections.

NOSOCOMIAL INFECTION

Definition

A nosocomial (or health care-associated) infection is one that is acquired in a hospital or health care facility (i.e., the infection was not present or incubating at the time of admission). For most bacterial infections, an onset of symptoms more than 48 hours after admission is evidence for nosocomial acquisition. To determine whether some infections such as legionellosis are hospital acquired, one must consider the usual incubation periods and determine whether the patient was hospitalized during that time period. Because hospital stays are getting shorter and more patients are treated in the outpatient setting, many health care-associated infections are not recognized during hospitalization. Infection control programs must therefore devise strategies for effective outpatient surveillance in order to accurately monitor nosocomial infection rates (46).

Infection Rates and Predominant Pathogens

Between 5 and 10% of patients admitted to acute care hospitals acquire an infection during hospitalization (10, 40, 61, 91). The urinary tract is the most commonly involved site, comprising 30 to 40% of all nosocomial infections.

Surgical wound and lower respiratory tract infections are the next most frequent, with each accounting for about 15 to 20% of nosocomial infections, followed by bloodstream infections (5 to 15%). The vast majority of nosocomial infections are related to devices (e.g., urinary tract catheters, endotracheal tubes in ventilated patients, and central venous catheters). For this reason, and as a way to adjust for risk when comparing rates over time or between similar units in different facilities, the Centers for Disease Control and Prevention (CDC) recommends calculating nosocomial infection rates in the intensive care unit (ICU) by using the number of device utilization days ("device-days") as the denominator (see Table 1 for definitions of common epidemiology terms).

Table 2 lists the five most common bacterial pathogens isolated from various sites of nosocomial infection in U.S. hospitals (44). From the 1970s through 2000, the spectrum of nosocomial pathogens shifted from gram-negative to gram-positive organisms, and *Candida* spp. emerged as a major problem (70). The incidence of nosocomial infections caused by staphylococci and enterococci increased as these organisms became increasingly resistant to antimicrobial agents (26, 102). More recently, multidrug-resistant gram-negative rods have become increasingly prevalent in many hospitals. For example, 2006–2007 data from the National Healthcare Safety Network (NHSN) reveals *Acinetobacter baumannii* to be the third leading cause of ventilator-associated pneumonia in U.S. hospitals (44), with over 30% of isolates resistant to the carbapenems. This represents an astonishing increase from the 1990s, when *Acinetobacter* did not even make the list of top eight causes of nosocomial pneumonia (12).

Morbidity, Mortality, and Cost

Nosocomial infections cause or contribute to thousands of deaths annually (10, 98). Because patients with the most severe underlying illness are also those most vulnerable to nosocomial infection, it is very difficult to estimate the proportion of crude or overall mortality that is directly attributable to a nosocomial infection. Studies that attempt to address this by carefully controlling for many potentially confounding variables are called attributable mortality studies. Estimates of the attributable mortality associated with nosocomial bloodstream infections have ranged from 14% for infections caused

TABLE 1 Commonly used terms in health care epidemiology[a]

Term	Definition or summary
Epidemiology	The study of the occurrence, distribution, and determinants of health and disease in a population. Hospital or health care epidemiology is the study of disease occurrence and distribution in the hospital or health care system.
Nosocomial infection	An infection acquired in a hospital or other health care facility.
Endemic infections	Infections occurring as part of the background or usual rate of infection in a specified population.
Epidemic infections	Infections occurring as part of an outbreak (or epidemic) of infection—defined as a significant increase in the usual rate of that infection in the specified population.
Incidence rate	Ratio of number of new cases of infection in a specified population at risk during a defined time period to the overall number of people in the population at risk (the denominator).
Device-associated incidence rate	Ratio of number of new cases of device-related infection in a specified population at risk during a defined time period to the number of days of device utilization in the population at risk.
Prevalence rate	Total number of cases of infection in the defined population at risk at one point in time (point prevalence) or in a given time period (period prevalence).
Observational or descriptive study	A study of the natural course of events, without an intervention in the process.
Case control study	A study frequently done as part of an outbreak investigation: a group of patients with the outcome of interest (e.g., cases of nosocomial infection) is compared to a control group of patients without the outcome. A comparison of specific factors between groups (i.e., exposures of interest) may suggest why infection occurred.
Crude or overall mortality rate	Ratio of number of patients who die to the overall number of patients in a specified population.
Attributable mortality	Ratio of number of patients who die as a direct result of the disease of interest to the overall population with the disease.

[a]Adapted from reference 62.

by coagulase-negative staphylococci (60), 31% and 37% for infections caused by vancomycin-susceptible and vancomycin-resistant enterococci (VRE) (32, 54), respectively, and 38 to 49% for infections caused by *Candida* spp. (38, 73, 100) (Table 3).

Nosocomial infections also increase hospital costs and length of stay (LOS), costing the health care system billions of dollars annually. At the University of Iowa, the median excess LOS for nosocomial bloodstream infections caused by coagulase-negative staphylococci and *Candida* spp. were 8 and 30 days, respectively (60, 100). Nosocomial bloodstream infections in the ICU were associated with an excess LOS of 24 days and excess hospital costs of $40,000 per survivor (76). Kirkland found that surgical site infections increased LOS by more than 6 days and increased hospital costs by over $3,000 per infection (50). Surgical site infections after major orthopedic surgery (e.g., hip replacement) are associated with an even greater increase in length of stay and costs (47).

The premise upon which infection control programs operate is that many of these life-threatening and costly nosocomial infections are preventable. The *Study of the Efficacy of Nosocomial Infection Control* indicated that the presence of an active surveillance and infection control program was associated with a 32% decrease in nosocomial infection rates while the absence of such a program was associated with an 18% *increase* in nosocomial infection rate (41). During the 1990s, the CDC National Nosocomial Infection Surveillance system of hospitals reported a reduction in risk-adjusted infection rates in ICUs for all monitored infection sites (urinary tract, bloodstream, and lung). The elements that were critical for reducing rates included targeted surveillance in high-risk populations (using standard definitions); adequate numbers of trained infection control professionals, who inform health care providers of their infection rates; and prevention efforts designed to address

TABLE 2 Distribution of the five most common nosocomial pathogens isolated from major infection sites, reported to the NHSN from January 2006 to October 2007[a]

Infection site and pathogens	% of total at each infection site
Central-line-associated bloodstream infection	
CoNS[b]	34.1
Enterococcus spp.	16.0
Candida spp.	11.8
Staphylococcus aureus	9.9
Klebsiella pneumoniae	4.9
Ventilator-associated pneumonia	
Staphylococcus aureus	24.4
Pseudomonas aeruginosa	16.3
Acinetobacter baumannii	8.4
Enterobacter spp.	8.4
Klebsiella pneumoniae	7.5
Catheter-associated urinary tract infection	
Escherichia coli	21.4
Candida spp.	21.0
Enterococcus spp.	14.9
Pseudomonas aeruginosa	10.0
Klebsiella pneumoniae	7.7
Surgical site infection	
Staphylococcus aureus	30.0
CoNS	13.7
Enterococcus spp.	11.2
Escherichia coli	9.6
Pseudomonas aeruginosa	5.6

[a]From reference 44.
[b]CoNS, coagulase-negative staphylococci.

TABLE 3 Attributable mortality of nosocomial bloodstream infection due to selected pathogens[a]

Organism	Mortality among cases (%)	Mortality among matched controls (%)	Attributable mortality (%)	Reference(s)
CoNS[b]	31	17	14	60
Enterococcus spp.	43	12	31	54
VRE	67	30	37	32
Candida spp.	57–61	12–19	38–49	8,100

[a]Adapted from reference 28.
[b]CoNS, coagulase-negative staphylococci.

issues identified during evaluation of infection rates (13). More recently, hospitals using combinations ("bundles") of evidence-based prevention strategies have demonstrated greater reductions in device-associated nosocomial infections than previously thought possible (5, 59, 79, 109). For example, a collaborative study involving over 100 ICUs in Michigan demonstrated a two-thirds reduction in central-line-associated bloodstream infection (CLABSI) rates, with a reduction to zero in the median CLABSI rate among participating ICUs (79). Thus, although it is not known what proportion of all nosocomial infections are truly preventable, an effective infection control program clearly improves patient care, saves lives, and decreases health care costs.

THE HOSPITAL INFECTION CONTROL PROGRAM

The hospital infection control program should include surveillance and prevention of nosocomial infections, continuing education of medical staff, control of infectious diseases outbreaks, protection of employees from infection, and advice on new products and procedures. The program is generally directed by a physician-epidemiologist and enforced by the infection control committee. Every hospital must also have a working infection control staff, comprising one or more infection preventionists (IPs). The IPs should collect data on nosocomial infections and provide the data to the infection control committee.

The Infection Control Committee

The infection control committee is responsible for reporting and evaluating nosocomial infection data and for drafting and implementing policies, procedures, and guidelines pertinent to the practice of infection control. Of note, in some hospitals the infection control program does the functions just described and the infection control committee approves the reports, policies, procedures, and guidelines. The committee should be multidisciplinary, with representatives from all departments, including clinical microbiology, and should meet every 1 to 3 months to review hospital-specific nosocomial infection data and to formulate policy. The members bring the needs and perspectives of their departments to the committee and, in turn, take back important information about infection control initiatives, policies, etc. Other responsibilities of the committee include reviewing technical information about new products, devices, or procedures pertinent to infection control, and instituting all necessary control measures in the event of an outbreak or other infection control emergency.

A clinical microbiologist must be on the infection control committee in order to provide expertise in the interpretation of culture results, advice about the appropriateness and feasibility of microbiological approaches to an infection control problem, and input regarding the laboratory resources necessary to accomplish the goals of the committee. One of the most important contributions of the clinical microbiologist is to inform the infection control committee of the strengths and limitations of methods employed to detect and characterize nosocomial pathogens. He or she should describe how changes in the methods used for detection, identification, and susceptibility testing of nosocomial pathogens would affect the infection control program. For example, if the laboratory introduces a urinary antigen detection test for diagnosis of legionellosis, the clinical microbiologist must inform the committee that the test is sensitive and specific for detecting *Legionella pneumophila* serogroup 1 only—and that culture is required to evaluate nosocomial legionellosis due to other species or serogroups. The committee should also be made aware of the budgetary and personnel constraints under which the laboratory operates, to ensure that they do not expend valuable laboratory resources unless there is a clear epidemiologic indication to do so.

Nosocomial Infection Surveillance

Active nosocomial infection surveillance programs are associated with reduced infection rates and their consequent morbidity and mortality (27, 41), and national and state accrediting agencies require hospitals to do surveillance for nosocomial infections. Thus, systematic surveillance of nosocomial infections is the infection control program's most important activity. Surveillance is also the infection control program's most costly and time-consuming activity. Surveillance allows the infection control program to monitor the frequency and types of nosocomial infection, detect outbreaks, evaluate compliance with infection control guidelines, provide data for policy development, and monitor the effect of infection control interventions on nosocomial infection rates. To accomplish the overall goal of decreasing infection rates, the infection control program must provide surveillance data to clinicians as soon as possible, accompanied by suggestions for improvement and reminders of existing infection control practices. Infection control programs that follow the CDC's advice about using device-days as the denominator for calculating rates of nosocomial infection in ICUs can compare their rates with national benchmarks compiled and reported by the CDC NHSN system (13, 33, 44). Figure 1 is a sample format for comparing infection rates in an ICU with national benchmark data. The infection control program should provide

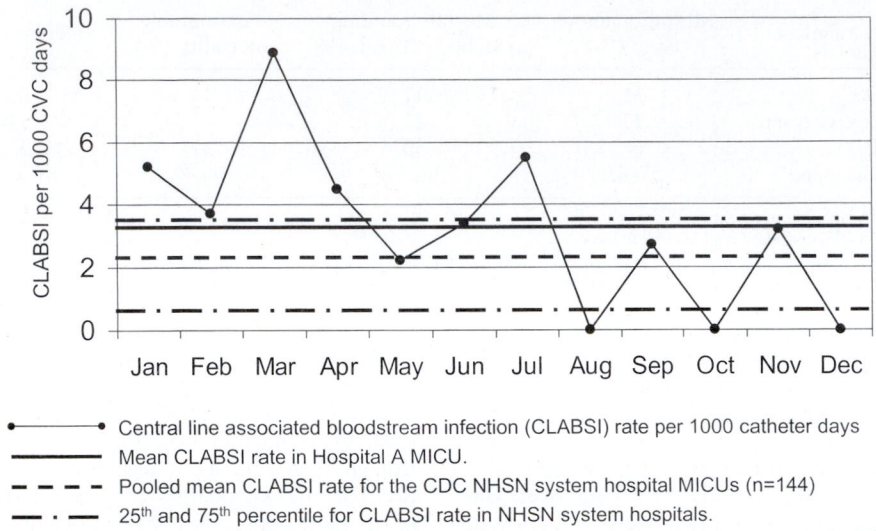

FIGURE 1 Sample chart format for reporting nosocomial infection rates in an ICU compared with CDC NHSN benchmarks. MICU, medical ICU; CVC, central venous catheter.

infection rates, recommendations for reducing rates, and assistance in implementing interventions to unit personnel such as medical directors, nurse managers, and clinicians.

The infection control program should design a surveillance system that is appropriate for the specific needs of the hospital and feasible based on the hospital's budget. For example, programs wishing to use device-days as a denominator must develop a system for counting or accurately estimating device utilization in their ICUs. Because surveillance consumes more resources than any other infection control activity (34), infection control programs must design the most efficient surveillance system possible. The most complete and accurate surveillance program would require an IP to review charts of all hospitalized patients daily, but this approach obviously is not practical in any but the smallest of hospitals. Infection control programs should focus their limited resources in the highest-risk areas (e.g., intensive care, hematology-oncology, burn, and organ transplant wards) and use various screening techniques to increase surveillance efficiency. IPs can use microbiology reports, nursing care plans, antibiotic orders, radiology reports, vital signs, and discharge diagnoses to determine which charts should be further reviewed.

Review of microbiology reports is probably the most common method for case finding, and it compares favorably in some circumstances with more comprehensive ward-based surveillance (37, 99). For example, Yokoe and colleagues reported that review of microbiology data alone was both more resource efficient than, and as effective as, applying the CDC's definition of nosocomial bloodstream infection (108). Such laboratory-based surveillance allows the IP to efficiently review large amounts of data. Moreover, medical information systems can enhance laboratory-based surveillance further by linking laboratory data with data from many other sources (9, 93), including pharmacy (antimicrobial use), radiology, billing (diagnostic codes), patient census data, and nursing notes (vital signs and care plans).

Although reviewing microbiology reports is an essential part of surveillance, these data alone may not detect all nosocomial infections or all outbreaks. The sensitivity and specificity of laboratory-based surveillance depend upon both the frequency with which clinicians obtain cultures and the quality of the culture specimens received by the lab. In addition, while laboratory-based surveillance may quickly detect outbreaks due to unusual pathogens or infections at unusual sites, outbreaks or clusters due to common pathogens at common sites (e.g., *Escherichia coli* urinary tract infection) may go undetected for longer periods of time. An optimal surveillance program includes data from more than one source (e.g., nursing care plan and microbiology reports) to help IPs determine which charts deserve further review. The University of Iowa previously validated a surveillance strategy using primarily microbiology reports and nursing care plans and found the sensitivity and specificity to be 81% and 98%, respectively (8). More recently, we introduced and validated a computer-based screening algorithm that provides each day for each IP a list of all patients on their units that had specific abnormalities in vital signs or white blood cell counts, positive cultures, a *Clostridium difficile* toxin test or a respiratory syncytial virus antigen test ordered, or one of the following combinations of tests ordered within a 24-hour period: chest radiograph and culture of respiratory secretions or cultures from two or more body sites. After reviewing this information, the IPs review the medical records of a smaller percentage of patients, thereby reducing the amount of time required for surveillance.

The overall approach to surveillance in each health care facility should be determined by the infection control committee, based on the types of patients treated, the procedures performed, the resources available for surveillance, prevailing infection rates, and other factors. This determination should be reevaluated each year during an annual "risk assessment" performed by the infection control program and approved by the infection control committee.

In addition, the infection control committee, in consultation with clinical microbiology personnel, should decide the mechanism by which the laboratory provides specific information needed for surveillance (e.g., all positive results, selected or sorted reports, etc.).

The movement toward public disclosure of nosocomial infection rates (22, 64, 97, 104) has important implications for surveillance. If interhospital comparisons of nosocomial infection rates are to have any meaning, all hospitals must use the same methods for surveillance and risk adjustment (22, 97). Unfortunately, methods for nosocomial infection surveillance vary widely among hospitals, and validated methods for risk-adjusting rates are not available (49). So although public disclosure of nosocomial infection rates is a laudable goal, is being introduced by law in many states, and is likely to be included in future health care reform legislation, much work needs to be done to ensure that such reporting improves, rather than hinders, efforts to prevent nosocomial infections (64).

Process Surveillance

Several recent studies clearly demonstrate that implementing evidence-based infection control practices, such as good hand hygiene (77) and the guidelines for placement and care of central venous catheters (5, 16), can dramatically reduce nosocomial infection rates (5, 77, 79). The obvious implication of these studies is that health care workers do not routinely adhere to the safest processes of care. For this reason, IPs must perform surveillance not only for important outcomes (infections) but also for important processes (e.g., rates of hand hygiene performance, use of maximal sterile barriers during central venous catheter placement, elevation of the head of bed to 30 degrees for ventilated patients, etc.). Process measures can help infection control personnel understand some of the variation in nosocomial infection rates. In addition, reporting compliance rates to personnel may improve practice and reduce nosocomial infection rates.

ROLE OF THE MICROBIOLOGY LABORATORY IN INFECTION CONTROL

With this overview of the structure and activities of the hospital infection control program in mind, we now focus on the most important specific roles played by the microbiology laboratory in the day-to-day practice of infection control.

Specimen Collection

Many nosocomial pathogens (e.g., coagulase-negative staphylococci) also commonly colonize patients' skin or mucous membranes and can easily contaminate cultures if specimens are not collected or handled properly. If contaminants are mistakenly considered to be infecting organisms, IPs may inadvertently count these as nosocomial infections, thereby inflating the infection rates (4, 92). Consequently, microbiologists must monitor specimen quality carefully and also set and enforce strict criteria for acceptable collection and handling of clinical specimens.

Accurate Identification and Susceptibility Testing of Nosocomial Pathogens

Commercial identification and susceptibility testing systems allow most laboratories to identify microorganisms to species level and perform antimicrobial susceptibility testing (AST). However, the expanding spectrum of organisms

that colonize and infect seriously ill patients challenges the ability of the clinical microbiology laboratory to identify and characterize nosocomial pathogens accurately (71, 72). For example, while many nosocomial pathogens are easily detected and identified by commonly used automated systems (e.g., *Staphylococcus* and the *Enterobacteriaceae*), many nonfermentative gram-negative organisms that cause nosocomial infection can be much more difficult to identify. Laboratories that identify nosocomial pathogens to the species level may find outbreaks that would otherwise have been undetected because clusters of unusual organisms or unusual clusters of common organisms may be clues to outbreaks. Thus, laboratories should establish a system for sending unusual nosocomial pathogens to a reference laboratory for definitive identification. In addition, viral, fungal and mycobacterial pathogens can cause nosocomial infections and also can be difficult to identify to a level appropriate to infection control needs.

New antimicrobial resistances continue to emerge, and existing resistances are increasing in frequency. To guard against significant AST errors for some organism-antimicrobial combinations, laboratories must supplement automated systems with additional methods. AST errors are most likely for organisms that display heteroresistance or inducible resistance mechanisms or for newly emerging resistances. For example, some systems previously underestimated oxacillin resistance among *Staphylococcus* species (105), did not adequately detect extended-spectrum beta-lactamase (ESBL) production by certain *Enterobacteriaceae* (6, 36, 89), or did not detect all enterococci or staphylococci with certain vancomycin resistance phenotypes (85, 86). More recently, investigators found that automated systems did not accurately detect carbapenemase-resistant *Klebsiella pneumoniae* (KPC producers); therefore, laboratories must use new screening methods to detect these organisms (1, 88). If the laboratory uses methods that do not accurately identify organisms or particular resistance patterns, the infection control program may not identify serious problems or even outbreaks. Conversely, infection control personnel may investigate spurious problems, thereby diverting and wasting precious resources.

Laboratories that recognize problems with commercial automated AST or organism identification systems should bring them to the manufacturers' attention so that they can improve the instrumentation, panels, or software programs to increase accuracy. This process of ongoing independent evaluation of automated systems and feedback to responsive industry representatives is extremely important. Unfortunately, in an era of shrinking laboratory resources, fewer laboratories have the ability to perform rigorous internal evaluations of new technology. The most important resistances emerging in nosocomial pathogens include ESBLs (including carbapenemases) among *Enterobacteriaceae* (1, 74, 81), glycopeptide resistance among enterococci (26) and staphylococci (15, 17, 18, 20, 24, 66, 82), methicillin resistance among *Staphylococcus aureus* strains (MRSA) (30), and multiple or pandrug resistance among nonfermenters such as *Pseudomonas aeruginosa*, *Acinetobacter* spp., and *Stenotrophomonas maltophilia* (63).

The infection control program must implement control measures to prevent the spread of important multidrug-resistant organisms (MDROs), and CDC has published a comprehensive guideline to assist in this effort (23). However, the success of any program to control MDROs depends upon the ability of the laboratory to detect these organisms. Laboratory directors must read current literature regarding automated systems' ability to detect emerging resistances, and they must implement, if necessary, additional methods to detect or confirm particular resistance patterns. The CDC website provides fact sheets summarizing current recommendations for detecting these resistances (http://www.cdc.gov/ncidod/dhqp/ar.html). They are also reviewed in chapters 69, 70, and 74 of this *Manual*.

Laboratory Information Systems

An information system that can do prospective data mining and interface with other parts of the computerized patient record could help IPs perform surveillance, monitor patient-to-patient spread of pathogens, and detect outbreaks early (9, 69, 75). Thus, persons choosing a laboratory information system must consult with both laboratory and infection control personnel before purchasing the best system for the hospital. Chapter 69 includes more complete discussions of the laboratory information system and expert systems for data analysis.

Rapid Diagnostic Testing

During the past decade, numerous rapid diagnostic tests have been developed that use molecular or immunologic methods. For example, a variety of methods are now available for rapid detection of respiratory viruses (57), *C. difficile* (90), *Mycobacterium tuberculosis* (42, 48), and *Legionella pneumophila* serogroup 1 (78). Rapid methods for detecting important antimicrobial resistances have also been developed, with most of the current focus being on rapid detection of MRSA (11, 95, 103, 107, 110) and VRE (29). A positive result from any of these tests allows clinicians to implement appropriate isolation precautions quickly in order to prevent the spread of the organisms. Of course, if clinicians order the tests indiscriminately or the laboratory has poor quality control, rapid diagnostic tests can lead to errors, including falsely positive tests that lead to inappropriate treatment and isolation of the patients. Erroneous results may also cause the infection control program to waste time investigating a pseudo-outbreak (56). The clinical microbiologist must assess the negative predictive value of any rapid tests provided by the laboratory. If the negative predictive value is not high enough, decisions to discontinue isolation precautions should not be based on the results of the rapid test.

Reporting Laboratory Data

Culture and AST results are an important data source for infection control and are usually reviewed daily by IPs. Thus, routine microbiology laboratory results should be readily accessible to IPs. In most cases, results are stored in a computer database, facilitating retrieval and analysis. The laboratory should store the following information: specimen type, date of collection, patient name, hospital number, hospital service, ward location, organisms identified, AST results, and the results of any specialized testing performed (e.g., typing). Both clinicians and IPs benefit from periodic summaries of selected microbiology results such as an antibiogram specifically for nosocomial pathogens. These results can be presented in a table that includes the antibiograms of the most common nosocomial pathogens by anatomical site and hospital service and also includes antimicrobial cost information. This information will help clinicians choose empiric antimicrobial therapy for patients with nosocomial infection. The Clinical and Laboratory Standards Institute (CLSI) has developed guidelines for antibiogram preparation (25).

Laboratory personnel should call the IP directly to report some particular results to ensure that appropriate control measures are implemented. Examples of organisms requiring immediate notification of the infection control program include *Neisseria meningitidis*, *Legionella*, acid-fast bacilli, enteric pathogens such as *Salmonella* or *Shigella*, and MDROs such as MRSA, vancomycin-intermediate and -resistant *S. aureus*, VRE, and ESBL-producing *Enterobacteriaceae*. In addition, new or unusual pathogens, or potential agents of bioterrorism (e.g., *Bacillus anthracis*, *Yersinia pestis*, and orthopoxviruses) should be reported immediately to the IP.

In addition to providing printed and verbal reports, laboratory staff should meet regularly with infection control staff to ensure that their communication is direct and clear. They can discuss areas of mutual concern, such as the status of epidemiological and microbiological investigations of clusters or outbreaks. Together they can determine whether supplementary studies such as molecular typing or environmental cultures will be necessary. If these studies are necessary, they can determine exactly what needs to be done, who will do these procedures, and when they will be done.

Outbreak Recognition and Investigation: Epidemic versus Endemic Infections

Most nosocomial infections are not associated with outbreaks; they are endemic rather than epidemic infections. If rates of nosocomial infection are consistently defined by prospective surveillance, infection control personnel may occasionally identify outbreaks of nosocomial infection—an increase in infection rate beyond that expected during a defined time period—by reviewing these rates. However, more often infection control personnel learn about potential outbreaks while interacting with personnel on the ward, in clinics, or in the laboratory.

When the infection control team detects a cluster or outbreak of nosocomial infection, they must act promptly to identify the etiologic agent if it is not known, define the extent of the outbreak, learn the mode of transmission for the pathogen, and institute appropriate control measures. The clinical microbiology laboratory must provide appropriate laboratory support during this time. Table 4 outlines recommended steps in an outbreak investigation and points out the important role of the clinical microbiology laboratory at each step.

Because the demands on the laboratory may be great during outbreaks, the laboratory staff should prepare in advance. Laboratory personnel periodically should ask IPs what types of outbreaks have occurred in the past or could be anticipated in the future and what laboratory resources would be required should similar outbreaks occur. Laboratory staff should also anticipate the extra costs associated with outbreak investigations so that they can work with hospital administrators to include funds for these efforts in annual budgets. Costs should not be borne by the laboratory or charged to individual patients involved in the outbreak.

Some problems and potential pitfalls of outbreak investigation are pertinent to the clinical microbiology laboratory and bear specific mention. Foremost among

TABLE 4 Steps in nosocomial outbreak investigation, and role of the laboratory at each step[a]

Investigative step	Role of the clinical microbiology laboratory
Recognize problem	Surveillance and early warning system—ideally part of the laboratory information system. Notify infection control personnel of infection clusters, unusual resistance patterns, possible patient-to-patient transmission.
Establish case definition	Assist and advise regarding inclusion of laboratory diagnosis in case definition.
Confirm cases........................	Perform laboratory confirmation of diagnosis.
Complete case finding.................	Characterize isolates with accuracy; store all sterile-site isolates and epidemiologically important isolates; search laboratory database for new cases.
Establish background rate of disease, compare to attack rate during suspected outbreak..................	Provide data for use in ongoing surveillance, which provide baseline rates for selected units and infection sites. Search laboratory database for all prior cases of the entity if baseline rate is not prospectively monitored.
Characterize outbreak (descriptive epidemiology)	Perform typing of involved strains, compare to previously isolated endemic strains to determine if the outbreak involves a single strain (see chapter 8). This can only be done if selected pathogens are routinely stored (see above).
Generate hypotheses about causation: reservoir, mode of spread, and vector; perform a case-control study or cohort study	Perform supplementary studies or cultures as needed, but only if justified by epidemiologic link to transmission: personnel, patients, and environment.
Institute control measures	Adjust laboratory procedures as necessary.
Ongoing surveillance to document efficacy of control measures...........	Maintain surveillance and early-warning function of the laboratory.

[a]Adapted from reference 62.

these is the problem of determining when to proceed with an outbreak investigation in the first place. The number of cases necessary to constitute an outbreak depends upon the organism, the patient population, and the institution involved. For example, while numerous cases of *Escherichia coli* urinary tract infection in a long-term-care facility may not constitute an outbreak, even a single nosocomial case of group A streptococcal surgical wound infection or vancomycin-resistant *S. aureus* infection merits an outbreak investigation. Laboratories should consider instituting a computerized program that recognizes clusters of pathogens within the hospital (39, 43). Organisms that appear to be part of a cluster could be further characterized to evaluate whether they are genetically related, which would suggest patient-to-patient spread or exposure to a contaminated common source. Investigators at Northwestern University hospital implemented such a system and noted that their rates of nosocomial infections decreased in temporal association with this intervention (39).

A second important problem is that of a pseudo-outbreak. A pseudo-outbreak has occurred when an apparent outbreak turns out not to be an outbreak after all. The usual cause of a pseudo-outbreak is either misdiagnosis (e.g., infection has not actually occurred) or misinterpretation of epidemiologic data (e.g., infections have occurred, but clustering or epidemic transmission has not). The microbiology laboratory can be the source of pseudo-outbreaks (3, 35, 45, 53, 55, 83, 94, 106). Problems in the laboratory that lead to pseudo-outbreaks include contamination of reagents for stains (45), false antimicrobial susceptibility test results (35), and contamination of culture specimens (often from construction or renovation

projects [55] or cross-contamination during specimen processing [106]). Careful attention to quality control, sterile technique in specimen processing, and preventive measures during construction and renovation projects can decrease the likelihood of pseudo-outbreaks that originate in the laboratory.

Molecular Typing To Support Infection Control Activities

Outbreaks of nosocomial infection often result when hospitalized patients are exposed to a common source or a reservoir of a pathogenic agent (e.g., water from a hot water tank colonized with *Legionella* spp.). The organisms causing such outbreaks usually derive from a single strain (i.e., they are clonally related). The infection control program may, therefore, request that the microbiology laboratory characterize isolates that may be associated with outbreaks to determine whether they are genetically related. In the appropriate clinical setting, species-level identification and AST results (antibiogram) may provide strong evidence for an epidemiologic link. However, more sensitive methods of strain delineation are often necessary. In this setting genotypic or DNA-based typing methods have replaced phenotypic typing methods (e.g., AST, biochemical profiles, and bacteriophage susceptibility patterns), which discriminate poorly among isolates (67, 80, 96).

Genotypic typing methods provide meaningful data and are cost-effective only when they are used for well-defined epidemiologic objectives. These objectives include (i) determining the source and extent of an outbreak; (ii) determining the mode of transmission of a nosocomial pathogen; (iii) evaluating the efficacy of preventative measures; and (iv) monitoring transmission of pathogens in high-risk areas (e.g., ICUs), where cross-infection is a recognized hazard.

The ideal genotypic typing system should be standardized, reproducible, stable, sensitive, broadly applicable, readily available, and inexpensive. The typing method should also have proven value in previous epidemiologic investigations. Further discussion of the relative advantages and disadvantages of the many available typing systems is beyond the scope of this chapter and has been summarized in several reviews (67, 80, 84, 87, 96) and in chapter 8 of this *Manual*.

Organism Storage

Of course, the laboratory cannot provide the infection control program with supplemental testing such as molecular typing if the appropriate isolates have not been saved. The laboratory should plan ahead and be sure to save all epidemiologically important isolates (see chapter 9). Laboratory and infection control personnel should decide which isolates should be banked and how long they should be stored based upon their epidemiological importance and the available resources. We recommend that all isolates from normally sterile sites (e.g., blood and cerebrospinal fluid), important MDROs (MRSA, VRE, and ESBL-producing *Enterobacteriaceae*) from any site, and other epidemiologically important pathogens (e.g., *M. tuberculosis*) be saved for a period of 3 to 5 years.

Surveillance Cultures of Patients, Hospital Personnel, and the Hospital Environment

The clinical microbiology laboratory is often called upon to detect potential pathogens that may be colonizers of patients, health care workers, and the hospital environment. For example, patients and health care workers increasingly are being screened for carriage of epidemiologically significant organisms. The most common organisms for which screening is performed are the MDROs (MRSA, VRE, and multidrug-resistant gram-negative rods), often as one aspect of an enhanced program for MDRO control (23). Screening for other organisms (e.g., group A streptococci) may be performed as part of a nosocomial infection or outbreak investigation. Finally, hand cultures may be performed as part of educational efforts in support of a hand hygiene campaign or to confirm the mechanism of cross-infection during an outbreak investigation (101).

For some organisms (e.g., MRSA), screening methods are standardized and well established, while for others (e.g., multidrug-resistant gram-negative rods), such methods are evolving and will continue to evolve as more complex resistance phenotypes emerge. Table 5 outlines current approaches to screening patients and health care workers for organisms of epidemiologic significance.

Laboratory and infection control personnel should weigh two important factors before deciding to culture hospital personnel during an outbreak investigation: (i) finding the outbreak strain on the hands or in the nares of a health

TABLE 5 Screening patients and health care workers for asymptomatic carriage of organisms of epidemiologic significance[a]

Organism(s)	Diagnostic procedure(s)	Turnaround time (h)	Optimum specimen(s)
Staphylococcus aureus, including MRSA	Routine aerobic culture and AST	48–96[b]	Nares swab[c]; throat, perirectal, skin, wounds
	Chromogenic agar medium	18–48[d]	Nares swab; throat, perirectal, skin, wounds
	Real-time PCR (MRSA)	1–4	Nares swab[e]
VRE	Routine aerobic culture and AST	48–72	Perirectal or stool swab
	Real-time PCR[f]	1–4	Perirectal or stool swab
Multiresistant gram-negative rods (*P. aeruginosa*, *Acinetobacter* spp, *S. maltophilia*, ESBL- and carbapenemase-producing organisms)	Routine aerobic culture and AST[g]	48–72	Perirectal or stool swab, endotracheal or sputum sample, sites of prior infection or colonization[h]
Group A *Streptococcus*	Routine aerobic culture	24–48	Rectal, vaginal, skin, and throat swabs
Various organisms carried on hands	Routine aerobic cultures: Contact agar plates Broth based (glove juice technique)	48–96	Hand cultures Direct imprint on agar plate Culture of broth after 1 min of hand immersion with agitation of broth

[a]Such cultures should only be done for the following reasons: (i) as part of an outbreak investigation, to seek carriage of an organism among patients or health care workers who are epidemiologically linked to cases; (ii) to seek carriers of MDROs as part of enhanced MDRO control strategies; (iii) to identify *S. aureus* carriers in order to proceed with a decolonization strategy to decrease risk for acquisition of *S. aureus* infection during a period of vulnerability (e.g., perioperative).

[b]The "gold standard" method includes overnight broth enrichment and confirmation of species identification and antimicrobial susceptibility, which can increase turnaround time to 96 hours. Most conventional agar-based screens (e.g., mannitol salt agar with or without oxacillin), without broth enrichment, provide a turnaround time of approximately 48 hours.

[c]The nares provides the best sensitivity and specificity of any single site for detection of *S. aureus* (including MRSA) detection (51). However, several studies have demonstrated that sampling of additional sites, including oropharynx and perirectal sites, may increase yield by 10 to 40% (2, 7, 65).

[d]Positive results for chromogenic agar medium can be reported at 18 to 24 hours, but negative results are reported at 48 hours.

[e]Currently available real-time PCR assays are FDA approved only for nares samples but have been used in some studies for oropharyngeal, skin, and perirectal samples.

[f]No real-time PCR assay for VRE detection is FDA approved at the time of this writing, but numerous "home brew" assays are in use, and commercially available assays are likely to become available soon.

[g]Several modifications of culture methods may enhance recovery by increasing medium selectivity for MDROs (e.g., addition of ceftazidime for ESBL-producing *Enterobacteriaceae*, levofloxacin for fluoroquinolone-resistant *E. coli*, etc.).

[h]Sample site choice should be guided by likely reservoirs, gastrointestinal (e.g., *E. coli*) and respiratory (e.g., *Acinetobacter*) being most common.

TABLE 6 Screening environmental sources (air, water, and surfaces) for organisms of epidemiologic significance[a]

Source and agent	Diagnostic procedure(s)	Turnaround time	Optimum specimen(s)
Air			
Fungi	Fungal cultures	48 h–7 days	Air processed with large-volume air sampler[b]
Bacteria[c]	Routine aerobic cultures	48–72 h	Air processed with large-volume air sampler
Water			
Legionella species	Culture on selective media[d]	5–10 days	500-ml–1-liter water samples[e]
			Swabs of internal surfaces of faucets, shower heads, and aerators[e]
Fungi[f]	Fungal cultures	48–96 h	500-ml–1-liter water sample[e]
			Swabs of internal surfaces of faucets, shower heads, and aerators[e]
Bacteria	Routine aerobic cultures	48–72 h	Water and dialysate samples as outlined by AAMI[g]
Surfaces			
Aerobic bacteria (including MDROs)	Routine aerobic cultures	48–72 h	Surface swab or sponge[h], contact agar plate (Rodac)
Clostridium difficile	Anaerobic cultures	48–72 h	Surface swab or sponge[h], contact agar plate (Rodac)[i]

[a]With the exception of water and dialysate cultures for monitoring of hemodialysis, and potable water cultures for *Legionella* spp., environmental cultures should be performed only when an epidemiologic investigation suggests the environment may be involved in pathogen transmission.

[b]Large-volume air samplers are preferred for air sampling for mould spores: settle plates should not be used for this purpose.

[c]There are no standards for acceptable levels of bacteria in air samples, nor is there any evidence correlating bacterial burden to infection risk. Air sampling for bacteria should be performed only rarely, either as part of an outbreak investigation or a research protocol.

[d]*Legionella* spp. will not grow on routine aerobic culture media. Buffered charcoal yeast extract agar is the most common medium used for *Legionella* isolation.

[e]The larger volume (1 liter) is preferred. If the water source is chlorinated, 0.5 ml of 0.1 N sodium thiosulfate should be added to each liter sample to neutralize the chlorine. Water samples are filter concentrated. Swabs should be immersed in 3 to 5 ml of water taken during sampling of the same site, to prevent drying.

[f]The role of waterborne fungi in infection transmission in the hospital environment remains poorly described, but cultures may be indicated as part of a search for environmental sources during an outbreak of invasive fungal infections in an immunocompromised patient population.

[g]AAMI, Association for the Advancement of Medical Instrumentation, whose standards govern microbiological monitoring of hemodialysis.

[h]The sterile swab or sponge should be moistened (e.g., with nutrient broth, sterile saline, etc.) before sample collection.

[i]For C. *difficile*, the contact agar plate should be optimized for anaerobic recovery (selective, prereduced media, promptly placed in anaerobic environment).

care worker does not establish the direction of transmission or definitively implicate a health care worker as the source or reservoir for the outbreak, and (ii) culturing hospital personnel indiscriminately can lead to confusing results and can generate ill will toward the infection control program. In general, only health care workers epidemiologically linked to cases should be cultured.

We recommend that infection control programs obtain cultures of hospital personnel only after consulting with a hospital epidemiologist experienced in outbreak investigation.

At one time, the hospital environment was felt to be the major source of nosocomial pathogens. Since then, it has been recognized that patients most often acquire infection from their own colonizing biota (19, 58). Nonetheless, the hospital environment can serve as a source of this colonizing biota, and there are specific circumstances in which environmental sampling for quality assurance or for detection of potential pathogens is necessary. Routine sampling for quality assurance should be limited to biologic monitoring of sterilization processes and monthly cultures of water and dialysate for hemodialysis. Rarely, it may be useful to perform a short-term evaluation of the effectiveness of hospital cleaning and disinfection (for example, sampling surfaces for VRE or *Clostridium difficile* after terminal room cleaning, to evaluate the effectiveness of cleaning practices). Likewise, sampling the hospital potable water for *Legionella* spp. is indicated after diagnosis of a nosocomial legionellosis case or as part of a comprehensive program to decrease risk of nosocomial legionellosis (19, 21, 68). Air

sampling for mould spores can also be an important step in identifying the source of fungal disease transmission in highly immunocompromised patients. Rarely, sampling of other inanimate objects or surfaces may be indicated, if such objects or surfaces are implicated in pathogen transmission. Table 6 outlines current approaches to screening the hospital environment for organisms of epidemiologic significance.

As a general rule, routine, undirected cultures of health care workers or the hospital environment should not be performed; such cultures are labor-intensive, nonstandardized, and difficult to interpret, and they rarely provide useful information (19). Except as previously outlined, such sampling should only be done as part of an epidemiologic investigation in consultation with the hospital epidemiologist. When such an epidemiologic investigation reveals a common organism in patient and/or environmental samples, the laboratory should also provide access to epidemiologic typing methods, as previously discussed.

CONCLUSIONS

The clinical microbiology laboratory is an essential component of any effective infection control program. The development and application of new technologies in the clinical laboratory can greatly enhance infection control efforts. A good working relationship between clinical laboratory and infection control personnel will greatly facilitate the investigation and control of health care-associated infections.

REFERENCES

1. **Anderson, K. F., D. R. Lonsway, J. K. Rasheed, J. Biddle, B. Jensen, L. K. McDougal, R. B. Carey, A. Thompson, S. Stocker, B. Limbago, and J. B. Patel.** 2007. Evaluation of methods to identify the *Klebsiella pneumoniae* carbapenemase in *Enterobacteriaceae*. *J. Clin. Microbiol.* **45:**2723–2725.

2. **Andrews, J. I., D. K. Fleener, S. A. Messer, J. S. Kroeger, and D. J. Diekema.** 2009. Screening for *Staphylococcus aureus* carriage in pregnancy: usefulness of novel sampling and culture strategies. *Am. J. Obstet. Gynecol.* **201:**396.e1–e5.

3. **Ashford, D. A., S. Kellerman, M. Yakrus, S. Brim, R. C. Good, L. Finelli, W. R. Jarvis, and M. M. McNeil.** 1997. Pseudo-outbreak of septicemia due to rapidly growing mycobacteria associated with extrinsic contamination of culture supplement. *J. Clin. Microbiol.* **35:**2040–2042.

4. **Beekmann, S. E., D. J. Diekema, and G. V. Doern.** 2005. Determining the clinical significance of coagulase-negative staphylococci isolated from blood cultures. *Infect. Control Hosp. Epidemiol.* **26:**559–566.

5. **Berenholtz, S. M., P. J. Pronovost, P. A. Lipsett, D. Hobson, K. Earsing, J. E. Farley, et al.** 2004. Eliminating catheter-related bloodstream infections in the intensive care unit. *Crit. Care Med.* **32:**2014–2020.

6. **Biedenbach, D. J., and R. N. Jones.** 1995. Interpretive errors using an automated system for the susceptibility testing of imipenem and aztreonam. *Diagn. Microbiol. Infect. Dis.* **21:**57–60.

7. **Boyce, J. M., N. L. Havill, and B. Maria.** 2005. Frequency and possible infection control implications of gastrointestinal colonization with methicillin-resistant *Staphylococcus aureus*. *J. Clin. Microbiol.* **43:**5992–5995.

8. **Broderick, A., M. Mori, M. D. Nettleman, S. A. Streed, and R. P. Wenzel.** 1990. Nosocomial infections: validation of surveillance and computer modeling to identify patients at risk. *Am. J. Epidemiol.* **131:**734–742.

9. **Brossette, S. E., D. M. Hacek, P. J. Gavin, M. A. Kamdar, K. D. Gadbois, A. G. Fisher, and L. R. Peterson.** 2006. A laboratory-based, hospital-wide, electronic marker for nosocomial infection. *Am. J. Clin. Pathol.* **125:**34–39.

10. **Burke, J. P.** 2003. Infection control—a problem for patient safety. *N. Engl. J. Med.* **348:**651–656.

11. **Carroll, K. C., R. B. Leonard, P. L. Newdomb-Gayman, and D. R. Hillyard.** 1996. Rapid detection of the staphylococcal *mecA* gene from BACTEC blood culture bottles by PCR. *Am. J. Clin. Pathol.* **106:**600–605.

12. **Centers for Disease Control and Prevention.** 1999. National Nosocomial Infections Surveillance (NNIS) report, data summary from January 1990-May 1999, issued June 1999. *Am. J. Infect. Control* **27:**520–532.

13. **Centers for Disease Control and Prevention.** 2000. Monitoring hospital-acquired infections to promote patient safety—United States, 1990–1999. *MMWR Morb. Mortal. Wkly. Rep.* **49:**149–153.

14. **Centers for Disease Control and Prevention.** 1992. Public health focus: surveillance, prevention and control of nosocomial infections. *MMWR Morb. Mortal. Wkly. Rep.* **41:**783–787.

15. **Centers for Disease Control and Prevention.** 1997. Update: *Staphylococcus aureus* with reduced susceptibility to vancomycin—United States, 1997. *MMWR Morb. Mortal. Wkly. Rep.* **46:**813–815.

16. **Centers for Disease Control and Prevention.** 2002. Guidelines for the prevention of intravascular catheter-related infections. *MMWR Recommend. Rep.* **51**(RR-10)**:**1–32.

17. **Centers for Disease Control and Prevention.** 2002. Public health dispatch: vancomycin-resistant *Staphylococcus aureus*—Pennsylvania, 2002. *MMWR Morb. Mortal. Wkly. Rep.* **51:**902.

18. **Centers for Disease Control and Prevention.** 2002. *Staphylococcus aureus* resistant to vancomycin. *MMWR Morb. Mortal. Wkly. Rep.* **51:**565–567.

19. **Centers for Disease Control and Prevention.** 2003. Guidelines for the environmental infection control in healthcare facilities. *MMWR Morb. Mortal. Wkly. Rep.* **52:**1–42.

20. **Centers for Disease Control and Prevention.** 2004. Brief report: vancomycin-resistant *Staphylococcus aureus*—New York, 2004. *MMWR Morb. Mortal. Wkly. Rep.* **53:**322–323.

21. **Centers for Disease Control and Prevention.** 2004. Guidelines for preventing health-care associated pneumonia, 2003. *MMWR Recommend. Rep.* **53**(RR-03)**:**1–36.

22. **Centers for Disease Control and Prevention.** 28 February 2005, posting date. *Guidance on Public Reporting of Healthcare-Associated Infections: Recommendations of the Healthcare Infection Control Practices Advisory Committee*. www.cdc.gov/ncidod/hip/PublicReportingGuide.pdf. Accessed 17 July 2005.

23. **Centers for Disease Control and Prevention.** 2006. *Management of Multidrug Resistant Organisms in Healthcare Settings, 2006.* http://www.cdc.gov/ncidod/dhqp/pdf/ar/mdroguideline2006.pdf. Accessed 25 July 2009.

24. **Chang, S., D. M. Sievert, J. C. Hageman, et al.** 2003. Brief report: infection with vancomycin-resistant *Staphylococcus aureus* containing the *vanA* resistance gene. *N. Engl. J. Med.* **348:**1342–1347.

25. **Clinical and Laboratory Standards Institute.** 2002. *Analysis and Presentation of Cumulative Antimicrobial Susceptibility Test Data. Document M39-A.* Clinical and Laboratory Standards Institute, Wayne, PA.

26. **Cormican, M. G., and R. N. Jones.** 1996. Emerging resistance to antimicrobial agents in gram-positive bacteria: enterococci, staphylococci, and non-pneumococcal streptococci. *Drugs* **51**(Suppl. 1)**:**6–12.

27. **Cruse, P. J. E.** 1970. Surgical wound sepsis. *Can. Med. Assoc. J.* **102:**251–258.

28. **Diekema, D. J., and M. A. Pfaller.** 2001. Role of the clinical microbiology laboratory in hospital epidemiology and infection control, p. 1247–1255. *In* K. McClatchey (ed.), *Clinical Laboratory Medicine*, 2nd ed. Lippincott Williams & Wilkins, Philadelphia, PA.

29. **Diekema, D. J., K. J. Dodgson, B. Sigurdardottir, and M. A. Pfaller.** 2004. Rapid detection of antimicrobial-resistant organism carriage: an unmet clinical need. *J. Clin. Microbiol.* **42:**2879–2883.

30. **Diekema, D. J., M. A. Pfaller, F. J. Schmitz, J. Smayevsky, J. Bell, R. N. Jones, M. L. Beach, and the SENTRY Participants Group.** 2001. Survey of infections due to *Staphylococcus* species: frequency of occurrence and antimicrobial susceptibility of isolates collected in the US, Canada and Latin America for the SENTRY program, 1997–1999. *Clin. Infect. Dis.* **32**(Suppl. 2)**:**S114–S132.

31. **Ducel, G., J. Fabry, and L. Nicolle (ed.).** 2002. *Prevention of Hospital Acquired Infections: A Practical Guide*, 2nd ed. http://www.who.int/csr/resources/publications/whocdscsreph200212.pdf. World Health Organization, Geneva, Switzerland.

32. **Edmond, M. B., J. F. Ober, J. D. Dawson, D. L. Weinbaum, and R. P. Wenzel.** 1996. Vancomycin-resistant enterococcal bacteremia: natural history and attributable mortality. *Clin. Infect. Dis.* **23:**1234–1239.

33. **Edwards, J. R., K. D. Peterson, M. L. Andrus, M. A. Dudeck, D. A. Pollock, T. C. Horan, and the National Healthcare Safety Network.** 2008. National Healthcare Safety Network Report, data summary for 2006 through 2007. *Am. J. Infect. Control* **36:**609–626.

34. **Emori, T. G., R. W. Haley, and J. S. Garner.** 1981. Technique and use of nosocomial infection surveillance in U.S. hospitals. *Am. J. Med.* **70:**933–940.

35. **Ender, P. T., S. J. Durning, W. K. Woelk, R. M. Brockett, A. Astorga, R. Reddy, and P. A. Meier.** 1999. Pseudo-outbreak of methicillin-resistant *Staphylococcus aureus*. *Mayo Clin. Proc.* **74:**885–889.

36. **Ferraro, M. J., and J. H. Jorgensen.** 1995. Instrument-based antibacterial susceptibility testing, p. 1379–1384. *In* P. R. Murray, E. J. Baron, M. A. Pfaller, F. C. Tenover, and R. H. Yolken (ed.), *Manual of Clinical Microbiology*, 6th ed. American Society for Microbiology, Washington, DC.

37. **Gross, P. A., A. Beaugard, and C. Van Antwerpen.** 1980. Surveillance for nosocomial infections: can the sources of data be reduced? *Infect. Control* **1:**233–236.

38. **Gudlaugsson, O., S. Gillespie, K. Lee, J. Vande Berg, J. Hu, S. Messer, L. Herwaldt, M. Pfaller, and D. Diekema.** 2003. Attributable mortality of nosocomial candidemia, revisited. *Clin. Infect. Dis.* **37:**1172–1177.

39. **Hacek, D. M., T. Suriano, G. A. Noskin, J. Kruszynsky, B. Reisberg, and L. R. Peterson.** 1999. Medical and economic benefit of a comprehensive infection control program that includes routine determination of microbial clonality. *Am. J. Clin. Pathol.* **111:**647–654.

40. **Haley, R. W., D. H. Culver, J. W. White, W. M. Morgan, and T. G. Emori.** 1985. The nationwide nosocomial infection rate. A new need for vital statistics. *Am. J. Epidemiol.* **121:**159–167.

41. **Haley, R. W., D. H. Culver, J. W. White, W. M. Morgan, T. G. Emori, V. P. Munn, and T. M. Hooten.** 1985. The efficacy of infection control surveillance and control programs in preventing nosocomial infections in U.S. hospitals. *Am. J. Epidemiol.* **121:**182–205.

42. **Hazbon, M. H.** 2004. Recent advances in molecular methods for early diagnosis of tuberculosis and drug-resistant tuberculosis. *Biomedica* **24:**163–164.

43. **Heisterkamp, S. H., A. L. Dekkers, and J. C. Heijne.** 2006. Automated detection of infectious disease outbreaks: hierarchical time series models. *Stat. Med.* **25:**4179–4196.

44. **Hidron, A. I., J. R. Edwards, J. Patel, T. C. Horan, D. M. Sievert, D. A. Pollock, S. K. Fridkin, and the National Healthcare Safety Network.** 2008. Antimicrobial-resistant pathogens associated with healthcare-associated infections: annual summary of data reported to the NHSN at the CDC, 2006–2007. *Infect. Control Hosp. Epidemiol.* **29:**996–1011.

45. **Hopfer, R. L., R. L. Katz, and V. Fainstein.** 1982. Pseudo-outbreak of cryptococcal meningitis. *J. Clin. Microbiol.* **15:**1141–1143.

46. **Jarvis, W. R.** 2001. Infection control and changing healthcare delivery systems. *Emerg. Infect. Dis.* **7:**170–173.

47. **Jodra, V. M., L. S. T. Soler, C. D. Perez, C. M. Requejo, and N. P. Farras.** 2006. Excess length of stay attributable to surgical site infection following hip replacement: a nested case-control study. *Infect. Control Hosp. Epidemiol.* **27:**1299–1303.

48. **Kearns, A. M., R. Freeman, M. Steward, and J. G. Magee.** 1998. A rapid PCR technique for detecting M. *tuberculosis* in a variety of clinical specimens. *J. Clin. Pathol.* **51:**922–924.

49. **Keita-Perse, O., and R. P. Gaynes.** 1996. Severity of illness scoring systems to adjust nosocomial infection rates: a review and commentary. *Am. J. Infect. Control* **24:**429–434.

50. **Kirkland, K. B., J. P. Briggs, S. L. Trivette, W. E. Wilkinson, and D. J. Sexton.** 1999. The impact of surgical-site infections in the 1990's: attributable mortality, excess length of hospitalization, and extra costs. *Infect. Control Hosp. Epidemiol.* **20:**725–730.

51. **Kluytmans, J., A. van Belkum, and H. Verbrugh.** 1997. Nasal carriage of *Staphylococcus aureus*: epidemiology, underlying mechanisms, and associated risks. *Clin. Microbiol. Rev.* **10:**505–520.

52. **Kohn, L. T., J. M. Corrigan, and M. S. Donaldson (ed.).** 2000. *To Err Is Human: Building a Safer Health System.* National Academy Press, Washington, DC.

53. **Lai, K. K., B. A. Brown, J. A. Westerling, S. A. Fontecchio, Y. Zhang, and R. J. Wallace.** 1998. Long-term laboratory contamination by *Mycobacterium abscessus* resulting in two pseudo-outbreaks: recognition with use of RAPD PCR. *Clin. Infect. Dis.* **27:**169–175.

54. **Landry, S. L., D. L. Kaiser, and R. P. Wenzel.** 1989. Hospital stay and mortality attributed to nosocomial enterococcal bacteremia: a controlled study. *Am. J. Infect. Control* **17:**323–329.

55. **Laurel, V. L., P. A. Meier, A. Astorga, D. Dolan, R. Brockett, and M. G. Rinaldi.** 1999. Pseudoepidemic of *Aspergillus niger* infections traced to specimen contamination in the microbiology laboratory. *J. Clin. Microbiol.* **37:**1612–1615.

56. **Laussucq, S., D. Schuster, W. J. Alexander, W. L. Thacker, H. W. Wilkinson, and J. S. Spika.** 1988. False-positive DNA probe test for *Legionella* species associated with a cluster of respiratory illnesses. *J. Clin. Microbiol.* **26:**1442–1444.

57. **Mahony, J. B.** 2008. Detection of respiratory viruses by molecular methods. *Clin. Microbiol. Rev.* **21:**716–747.

58. **Maki, D. G., C. J. Alvarado, C. A. Hassemer, and M. A. Zilz.** 1982. Relation of the inanimate hospital environment to endemic nosocomial infection. *N. Engl. J. Med.* **25:**1562–1566.

59. **Marra, A. R., R. G. R. Cal, C. V. Silva, R. A. Caserta, A. T. Paes, D. F. Moura, O. F. Pavao de Santos, M. B. Edmond, and M. S. Durao.** 2009. Successful prevention of ventilator-associated pneumonia in an intensive care setting. *Am. J. Infect. Control* **37:**619–625.

60. **Martin, M. A., M. A. Pfaller, and R. P. Wenzel.** 1989. Mortality and hospital stay attributable to coagulase-negative staphylococcal bacteremia. *Ann. Intern. Med.* **110:**9–16.

61. **Mayon-White, R. T., G. Ducel, T. Kereselidze, and E. Tikomirov.** 1988. An international survey of the prevalence of hospital-acquired infection. *J. Hosp. Infect.* **11**(Suppl. A)**:**43–48.

62. **McGowan, J. E., and B. G. Metchock.** 1999. Infection control epidemiology and clinical microbiology, p. 107–115. *In* P. R. Murray, E. J. Baron, M. A. Pfaller, F. C. Tenover, and R. H. Yolken (ed.), *Manual of Clinical Microbiology*, 7th ed. ASM Press, Washington, DC.

63. **McGowan, J. E.** 2006. Resistance in nonfermenting gram-negative bacteria: multidrug resistance to the maximum. *Am. J. Infect. Control* **34:**S29–S37.

64. **McKibben, L. G. Fowler, T. Horan, and P. J. Brennan.** 2006. Ensuring rational public reporting systems for healthcare-associated infections: systematic literature review and evaluation recommendations. *Am. J. Infect. Control* **34:**142–149.

65. **Mertz, D., R. Frei, N. Periat, M. Zimmerli, M. Battegay, U. Fluckiger, and A. F. Widmer.** 2009. Exclusive *Staphylococcus aureus* throat carriage: at-risk populations. *Arch. Intern. Med.* **169:**172–178.

66. **Michigan Department of Community Health.** 2005. *Bureau of Laboratory Broadcast Fax: Second Michigan VRSA case.* http://www.michigan.gov/documents/VRSA_Feb05_HAN_118391_7.pdf. Accessed 31 May 2005.

67. **Olive, D. M., and P. Bean.** 1999. Principles and applications of methods for DNA-based typing of microbial organisms. *J. Clin. Microbiol.* **37:**1661–1669.

68. **O'Neill, E., and H. Humphreys.** 2005. Surveillance of hospital water and primary prevention of nosocomial legionellosis: what is the evidence? *J. Hosp. Infect.* **59:**273–279.

69. **Peterson, L. R., and S. E. Brossette.** 2002. Hunting health care-associated infections from the clinical microbiology laboratory: passive, active, and virtual surveillance. *J. Clin. Microbiol.* **40:**1–4.

70. **Pfaller, M. A.** 1996. Nosocomial candidiasis: emerging species, reservoirs, and modes of transmission. *Clin. Infect. Dis.* **22**(S-2)**:**S89–S94.

71. **Pfaller, M. A., and L. A. Herwaldt.** 1997. The clinical microbiology laboratory and infection control: emerging pathogens, antimicrobial resistance, and new technology. *Clin. Infect. Dis.* **25:**858–870.

72. **Pfaller, M. A., and M. G. Cormican.** 1997. Microbiology: the role of the clinical laboratory, p. 95–118. *In* R. P. Wenzel (ed.), *Prevention and Control of Nosocomial Infections.* Williams & Wilkins, Baltimore, MD.

73. **Pfaller, M. A., and D. J. Diekema.** 2007. Epidemiology of invasive candidiasis: a persistent public health problem. *Clin. Microbiol. Rev.* **20:**133–163.

74. **Philippon, A., G. Arlet, and P. H. Lagrange.** 1994. Origin and impact of plasmid-mediated extended spectrum beta-lactamases. *Eur. J. Clin. Microbiol. Infect. Dis.* **13**(S1)**:**17–29.

75. **Pittet, D.** 2005. Infection control and quality health care in the new millennium. *Am. J. Infect. Control* **33:**258–267.

76. **Pittet, D., D. Tarara, and R. P. Wenzel.** 1994. Nosocomial bloodstream infection in critically ill patients: excess length of stay, extra costs, and attributable mortality. *JAMA* **271:**1598–1601.

77. **Pittet, D., S. Hugonnet, S. Harbarth, et al.** 2000. Effectiveness of a hospital-wide programme to improve compliance with hand hygiene. *Lancet* **356:**1307–1312.

78. **Plouffe, J. F., T. M. File, Jr., R. F. Breiman, B. A. Hackman, S. J. Salstrom, B. J. Marston, B. S. Fields, et al.** 1995. Re-

evaluation of the definition of Legionnaires' disease: use of the urinary antigen assay. *Clin. Infect. Dis.* **20:**1286–1291.

79. **Pronovost, P., D. Needham, S. Berenholtz, D. Sinopoli, H. Chu, S. Cosgrove, B. Sexton, R. Hyzy, R. Welsh, G. Roth, J. Bander, J. Kepros, and C. Goeschel.** 2006. An intervention to decrease catheter-related bloodstream infections in the ICU. *N. Engl. J. Med.* **26:**2725–2732.

80. **Sader, H. S., R. J. Hollis, and M. A. Pfaller.** 1995. The use of molecular techniques in the epidemiology and control of infectious diseases. *Clin. Lab. Med.* **15:**407–431.

81. **Sanders, C. C., and W. E. Sanders.** 1992. Beta-lactam resistance in gram-negative bacteria: global trends and clinical impact. *Clin. Infect. Dis.* **15:**824–839.

82. **Schwalbe, R. S., J. T. Stapleton, and P. H. Gilligan.** 1987. Emergence of vancomycin resistance in coagulase-negative staphylococci. *N. Engl. J. Med.* **316:**927–931.

83. **Segal-Maurer, S., B. N. Kreiswirth, J. M. Burns, S. Lavie, M. Lim, C. Urban, and J. J. Rahal.** 1998. *Mycobacterium tuberculosis* specimen contamination revisited: the role of laboratory environmental control in a pseudo-outbreak. *Infect. Control Hosp. Epidemiol.* **19:**101–105.

84. **Singh, A., R. V. Goering, S. Simjee, S. L. Foley, and M. J. Zervos.** 2006. Application of molecular techniques to the study of hospital infection. *Clin. Microbiol. Rev.* **19:**512–530.

85. **Tenover, F. C., and L. C. McDonald.** 2005. Vancomycin-resistant staphylococci and enterococci: epidemiology and control. *Curr. Opin. Infect. Dis.* **18:**300–305.

86. **Tenover, F. C., J. M. Swenson, C. M. O'Hara, and S. A. Stocker.** 1995. Ability of commercial and reference antimicrobial susceptibility testing methods to detect vancomycin resistance in enterococci. *J. Clin. Microbiol.* **33:**1524–1527.

87. **Tenover, F. C., R. D. Arbeit, R. V. Goering, and the Molecular Working Group of the Society for Healthcare Epidemiology of America.** 1997. How to select and interpret molecular strain typing methods for epidemiological studies of bacterial infections: a review for healthcare epidemiologists. *Infect. Control Hosp. Epidemiol.* **18:**426–439.

88. **Tenover, F. C., R. K. Kalsi, P. P. Williams, R. B. Carey, S. Stocker, D. Lonsway, J. K. Rasheed, J. W. Biddle, J. E. McGowan, Jr., and B. Hanna.** 2006. Carbapenem resistance in *Klebsiella pneumoniae* not detected by automated susceptibility testing. *Emerg. Infect. Dis.* **12:**1209–1213.

89. **Thompson, K. S., and C. C. Sanders.** 1992. Detection of extended-spectrum beta-lactamases in members of the family *Enterobacteriaceae*: comparison of the double-disk and three-dimensional tests. *Antimicrob. Agents Chemother.* **36:**1877–1882.

90. **Ticehurst, J. R., D. Z. Aird, L. M. Dam, A. P. Borek, J. T. Hargrove, and K. C. Carroll.** 2006. Effective detection of toxigenic *Clostridium difficile* by a two-step algorithm including tests for antigen and cytotoxin. *J. Clin. Microbiol.* **44:**1145–1149.

91. **Tikhomirov, E.** 1897. World Health Organization programme for the control of hospital infections. *Chemiotherapia* **3:**148–151.

92. **Tokars, J. I.** 2004. Predictive value of blood cultures positive for coagulase-negative staphylococci: implications for patient care and health care quality assurance. *Clin. Infect. Dis.* **39:**333–341.

93. **Trick, W. E., B. M. Zagorski, J. I. Tokars, et al.** 2004. Computer algorithms to detect bloodstream infections. *Emerg. Infect. Dis.* **10:**1612–1620.

94. **Tsakris, A., A. Pantazi, S. Pournaras, A. Maniatis, A. Polyzou, and D. Sofianou.** 2000. Pseudo-outbreak of imipenem-resistant *Acinetobacter baumannii* resulting from false susceptibility testing by a rapid automated system. *J. Clin. Microbiol.* **38:**3505–3507.

95. **Warren, D. K., R. S. Liao, L. R. Merz, M. Eveland, and W. M. Dunne, Jr.** 2004. Detection of methicillin-resistant *Staphylococcus aureus* directly from nasal swab specimens by a real-time PCR assay. *J. Clin. Microbiol.* **42:**5578–5581.

96. **Weber, S., M. A. Pfaller, and L. A. Herwaldt.** 1997. Role of molecular epidemiology in infection control. *Infect. Dis. Clin. N. Am.* **11:**257–278.

97. **Weinstein, R. A., J. D. Siegel, and P. J. Brennan.** 2005. Infection control report cards—securing patient safety. *N. Engl. J. Med.* **353:**225–227.

98. **Wenzel, R. P., and M. B. Edmond.** 2001. The impact of hospital-acquired bloodstream infections. *Emerg. Infect. Dis.* **7:**174–177.

99. **Wenzel, R. P., C. A. Osterman, K. J. Hunting, and J. M. Gwaltney, Jr.** 1976. Hospital-acquired infections. I. Surveillance in a university hospital. *Am. J. Epidemiol.* **103:**251–260.

100. **Wey, S. B., M. Mori, M. A. Pfaller, R. F. Woolson, and R. P. Wenzel.** 1988. Hospital acquired candidemia: attributable mortality and excess length of stay. *Arch. Intern. Med.* **148:**2642–2645.

101. **Widmer, A. F., R. P. Wenzel, A. Trilla, M. J. Bale, R. N. Jones, and B. N. Doebbeling.** 1993. Outbreak of *Pseudomonas aeruginosa* infections in a surgical intensive care unit: probable transmission via hands of a healthcare worker. *Clin. Infect. Dis.* **16:**372–376.

102. **Wisplinghoff, H., T. Bischoff, S. M. Tallent, H. Seifert, R. P. Wenzel, and M. B. Edmond.** 2004. Nosocomial bloodstream infections in US hospitals: analysis of 24,179 cases from a prospective nationwide surveillance study. *Clin. Infect. Dis.* **39:**309–317.

103. **Wolk, D. M., E. Picton, D. Johnson, T. Davis, P. Pancholi, C. C. Ginocchio, S. Finegold, D. F. Welch, M. de Boer, D. Fuller, M. C. Solomon, B. Rogers, M. S. Mehta, and L. R. Peterson.** 2009. Multicenter evaluation of the Cepheid Xpert methicillin-resistant *Staphylococcus aureus* (MRSA) test as a rapid screening method for detection of MRSA in nares. *J. Clin. Microbiol.* **47:**758–764.

104. **Wong, E. S., M. E. Rupp, L. Mermel, et al.** 2005. Public disclosure of healthcare-associated infections. *Infect. Control Hosp. Epidemiol.* **26:**210–212.

105. **Woods, G. L., D. LaTemple, and C. Cruz.** 1994. Evaluation of Microscan rapid gram-positive panels for detection of oxacillin-resistant staphylococci. *J. Clin. Microbiol.* **32:**1058–1059.

106. **Wurtz, R., P. Demarais, W. Trainor, J. McAuley, F. Kocka, L. Mosher, and S. Dietrich.** 1996. Specimen contamination in mycobacteriology laboratory detected by pseudo-outbreak of multidrug-resistant tuberculosis: analysis by routine epidemiology and confirmation by molecular technique. *J. Clin. Microbiol.* **34:**1017–1019.

107. **Yamazumi, T., S. A. Marshall, W. W. Wilke, D. J. Diekema, M. A. Pfaller, and R. N. Jones.** 2001. Comparison of the Vitek GPS 106 card and the MRSA-Screen latex agglutination test for determining oxacillin resistance in clinical bloodstream isolates of *Staphylococcus aureus*. *J. Clin. Microbiol.* **39:**53–56.

108. **Yokoe, D. S., J. Anderson, R. Chambers, M. Connor, R. Finberg, C. Hopkins, D. Lichtenberg, S. Marino, D. McGlaughlin, E. O'Rourke, M. Samore, K. Sands, J. Strymish, E. Yamplin, N. Vallonde, and R. Platt.** 1998. Simplified surveillance for nosocomial bloodstream infections. *Infect. Control Hosp. Epidemiol.* **19:**657–660.

109. **Zack, J. E., T. Garrison, E. Trovillion, D. Clinkscale, C. M. Coopersmith, V. J. Fraser, and M. H. Kollef.** 2002. Effect of an education program aimed at reducing the occurrence of ventilator-associated pneumonia. *Crit. Care Med.* **30:**2407–2412.

110. **Zheng, X., C. P. Kolbert, P. Varga-Delmore, J. Arruda, M. Lewis, J. Kolberg, F. R. Cockerill, and D. H. Persing.** 1999. Direct *mecA* detection from blood culture bottles by branched-DNA signal amplification. *J. Clin. Microbiol.* **37:**4192–4193.

Investigation of Enteric Disease Outbreaks

TIMOTHY F. JONES AND WILLIAM E. KEENE

7

The World Health Organization estimates that 1.8 million children die each year from diarrhea, and even in developed countries a third of the population experiences diarrhea each year due to pathogens commonly transmitted through food (20). In the United States, there are tens of millions of illnesses and hundreds of thousands of hospitalizations annually (15).

Most enteric illness is spread by the fecal-oral route, and the history of these diseases mirrors changes in the social, economic, and physical environments in which we live. By one estimate, nearly 90% of the global burden of diarrheal disease is attributable to unsafe water supplies (19). Improved basic sanitation, medical care, and diagnostic capabilities have helped substantially reduce both the risks for foodborne and waterborne diseases and the frequency of complications overall. That said, new problems emerge that reflect changes in both human and microbial populations—not to mention nonhuman reservoir species and the environment. For example, the population of vulnerable persons is growing as people live longer or live with immunosuppressive conditions. The rapid international movement of people and foodstuffs, shifts in food production methods and eating habits, and other factors all change patterns of food exposure and hence patterns of foodborne disease. Improved diagnostic tests identify new or newly described pathogens. Many pathogens considered important sources of morbidity today were unheard of even 40 years ago, including noroviruses, rotaviruses, *Cryptosporidium*, *Campylobacter*, and *Escherichia coli* O157:H7.

Acute gastroenteritis and other foodborne diseases can be caused by bacteria, viruses, protozoa, fungi, helminths, prions, and biological or environmental toxins. People are exposed to these pathogens or toxins in contaminated food or water, by person-to-person-contact, and by direct contact with animals. Many foodborne and waterborne diseases are self-limited and characterized by gastrointestinal symptoms such as vomiting and diarrhea. Others, however, may manifest with or progress to include systemic or neurological disease that can result in substantial morbidity and mortality, e.g., infection with *E. coli* O157:H7 (causing hemolytic-uremic syndrome), *Helicobacter pylori* (linked to gastric cancers), *Listeria* (meningitis and miscarriage), *Salmonella* (increased risk of reactive arthritis), and *Toxoplasma gondii* (birth defects).

DISEASE SURVEILLANCE

Enteric disease surveillance is generally the province of public health agencies. Surveillance includes the collection and analysis of information about disease occurrence and leads to taking considered action based upon those data. Disease surveillance often is based on mandatory reporting laws, whereby diagnostic laboratories or clinicians are required to notify public health agencies about individuals with specified conditions, e.g., salmonellosis or hepatitis A, as well as unusual clusters of illness.

While conceptually simple, disease surveillance can be a daunting logistical challenge that places demands on legal, medical, communications, transportation, scientific, and social infrastructure. Unless otherwise noted, the following discussion pertains to enteric disease surveillance and outbreak investigation in the United States.

In the United States and many other countries, public health workers collate notifiable-disease reports in search of broader patterns, often collecting additional information from patient interviews and other sources. The general public may also contact public health agencies directly with concerns about individual or apparently clustered illnesses, and these reports too must be considered for potential significance.

While definitions and usage vary, disease outbreaks in general are comprised of individual illnesses that can be connected by webs of transmission or by exposures to common sources. For example, we can refer to an outbreak of norovirus infections at a nursing home, an outbreak of cholera affecting the population of a region or country, or an outbreak of salmonellosis resulting from consumption of contaminated peanut butter. In the United States, over 95% of reported enteric illnesses are not recognized to be part of outbreaks (12). That said, outbreak-related cases play a disproportionately large role in our understanding of pathogen transmission and attempts to control it.

Since 1938, the U.S. Public Health Service has collated reports on foodborne and waterborne disease outbreaks from public health agencies (4). What was once a flow of paper has largely become an electronic reporting system. From 2004 to 2006, the CDC received ~1,200 reports of foodborne outbreaks involving at least 24,000 people annually (http://www.cdc.gov/foodborneoutbreaks/outbreak_data.htm). Examples of forms, an electronic database used for foodborne disease outbreaks, and recent data are accessible online

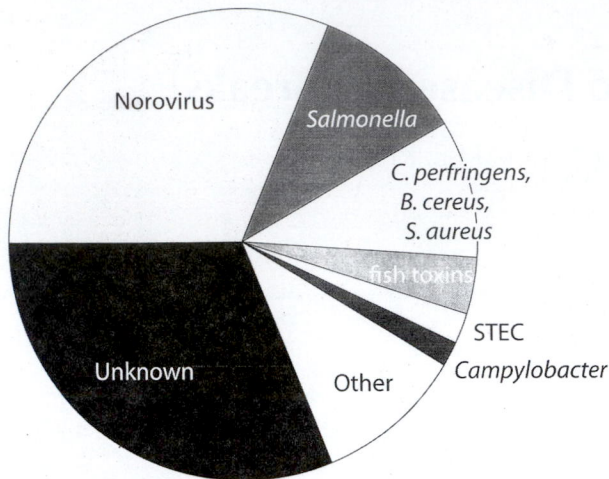

FIGURE 1 Etiology of foodborne outbreaks, United States, 2001 to 2006 (n = 7,165). Data are from reference 7.

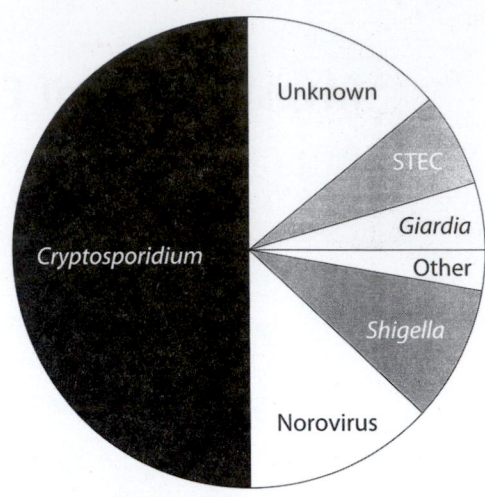

FIGURE 3 Etiology of recreational-water-associated outbreaks of gastroenteritis, United States, 2001 to 2006 (n = 108). Data are from references 9, 22, and 23.

(http://www.cdc.gov/foodborneoutbreaks/toolkit.htm). Summary information about foodborne and waterborne outbreak investigations is typically reported to the CDC, which periodically summarizes these data.

It should be emphasized that the quality of these data is highly variable, which complicates our ability to summarize them meaningfully. Most outbreaks are probably never recognized or reported, much less investigated, and those that are reported nationally are likely to be a biased sample of the whole. For example, large outbreaks or outbreaks involving more severe illnesses or deaths are much more likely to get a thorough investigation. In the United States, over half of reported foodborne disease outbreaks are associated with food eaten outside the home (6). Many investigations are inconclusive, and different people may summarize similar situations in different ways.

Pathogens most commonly identified in outbreaks reported from 2001 to 2006 are shown in Fig. 1. It is noteworthy that no etiology was identified for almost one-third of foodborne outbreaks during that period. Noroviruses were

the leading cause of half of those with a confirmed etiology, and bacteria were responsible for 38%.

While waterborne disease outbreaks are common worldwide, they are relatively uncommon in the United States. From 2001 to 2006, some 144 outbreaks of waterborne gastroenteritis were reported to the CDC, of which 36 (25%) were associated with drinking water and 108 (75%) with recreational water. Figure 2 illustrates the etiologic agents causing gastroenteritis outbreaks associated with drinking water, and Fig. 3 shows those related to recreational-water outbreaks (2, 9, 14, 22–24).

THE CONTEXT FOR OUTBREAK INVESTIGATIONS

There are many reasons to investigate outbreaks. The most obvious is to arrest an ongoing problem. Recalling a contaminated product from the marketplace or excluding a typhoid carrier from work as a food handler can prevent illness and even save lives. Given the inherent delays in disease reporting, many outbreaks are over before public health agencies learn about them; the benefits of investigating these clusters are more indirect. Investigations often reveal systemic problems that could cause illness in the future; correction of these problems reduces those risks. Examples might include substandard operation of a drinking-water treatment facility or inadequate temperature control in a peanut roasting operation. Outbreaks also provide an opportunity for public health education—education that may be targeted to the individual who manages a restaurant or to the broader community through media contacts. The identification or better characterization of the root causes of outbreaks, often assessed as aggregate data from many investigations, also helps drive the agenda of regulatory agencies, businesses, and others trying to develop more effective practices and regulations.

Public health agencies in most countries have a legal authority and responsibility to investigate certain kinds of diseases and most clusters of illness (i.e., outbreaks) (Table 1). In the United States, that legal authority rests primarily at the local and state levels, and the vast majority of outbreaks are investigated by agencies at those levels.

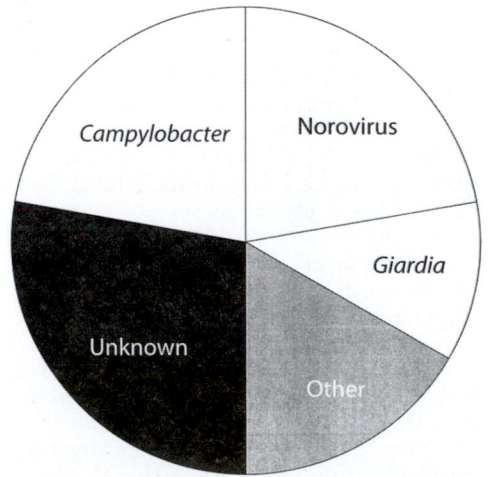

FIGURE 2 Etiology of drinking-water-associated outbreaks of gastroenteritis, United States, 2001 to 2006 (n = 36). Data are from references 2, 14, and 24.

TABLE 1 Enteric and other potential foodborne diseases and conditions designated as notifiable at the national level in the United States, 2009[a]

Bacterial diseases and conditions
    Anthrax
    Botulism
    Brucellosis
    Cholera
    Enterohemorrhagic *Escherichia coli* infection
    Hemolytic-uremic syndrome, postdiarrheal
    Listeriosis
    Salmonellosis (including typhoid)
    Shigellosis

Viral disease
    Hepatitis A

Parasitic diseases
    Cryptosporidiosis
    Cyclosporiasis
    Giardiasis
    Trichinellosis

[a]Adapted from http://www.cdc.gov/ncphi/disss/nndss/PHS/infdis.htm.

Suspected disease outbreaks must be reported to the public health department in most states, though this requirement is often unappreciated or ignored by clinicians and others.

Legal structures vary by state but typically share many general features. Federal agencies (e.g., the CDC, FDA, and U.S. Department of Agriculture [USDA]) become involved in relatively few investigations, typically those involving multiple states or industries regulated at the federal level. In some cases there is overlapping authority, and many investigations (particularly larger ones and those involving contaminated commercial products) are collaborative efforts with multiple partners. The roles of various government agencies in outbreak investigations are outlined in Table 2.

To thoroughly investigate an outbreak, epidemiologists need to collect a diverse range of information. Public health authorities have substantial legal authority to gather such data that usually goes hand in hand with state laws protecting the confidentiality of information collected in the context of an investigation. In practice, however, sweeping legal authorities are rarely invoked; epidemiological investigations typically rely on the voluntary cooperation of all parties. Regulatory agencies such as the FDA and the USDA have clearer police powers that can be utilized when circumstances demand them, but these powers typically apply only to commercial entities.

The capacity to conduct public health investigations varies with the resources, experience, and interest of the agencies involved and in practice is highly variable. Moreover, some states are hobbled by a cumbersome legal structure that makes it difficult to move quickly in a coordinated fashion. The success of many multistate investigations in the United States depends to a surprising degree on the involvement of one or more of a small number of states with expertise in outbreak investigation. Realistically, not all clusters merit a thorough investigation; resources are always finite. One must consider the severity of the disease, the community affected, and the likelihood that useful data can be obtained from an investigation. Basic laboratory testing and interviews of a limited number of ill persons may provide sufficient information to identify the source

of the outbreak and take appropriate control measures. In many cases, however, more extensive epidemiological investigation is indicated.

Outbreak Detection

A foodborne outbreak can be defined as "the occurrence of two or more cases of a similar illness resulting from ingestion of a common food" (4). There are analogous surveillance definitions for outbreaks due to drinking or recreational water (23, 24). In practice, most intrahousehold clusters are not pursued unless the disease is severe. To recognize unusual clusters of illness, public health officials must have knowledge of what "normal" or baseline rates of a disease are in the affected community. These may be available from historical surveillance data.

In general, potential outbreaks come to the attention of health authorities through one of three routes. First, people often contact public health agencies directly to report illness clusters, e.g., after a common restaurant meal or a wedding, or among persons at a nursing home, school, or prison. These reports come from physicians, infection control practitioners, institutional staff, and often from private citizens. Second, public health agencies identify clusters through review and follow-up of routinely collected surveillance information, including reports of legally notifiable diseases and subtyping of specimens submitted to public health laboratories. Third, recognition may come in response to queries from other public health agencies doing "case finding" as part of investigations in their jurisdictions.

One of the first responses to the recognition of a potential outbreak is assessing whether something "real" has actually occurred. Surveillance reports are often incomplete, misleading, or erroneous, and many "clusters" dissolve under scrutiny. Outbreak clusters are often obvious, but sometimes it is difficult to separate minor fluctuations in rates (i.e., "noise") from true increases due to a common-source outbreak ("signal").

Laboratory Investigation

The response to preventive measures and the treatment of clinical infections varies markedly depending on the etiologic agent involved. It is therefore concerning that the etiologic agents were not identified for half of foodborne disease outbreaks reported to the CDC from 2004 to 2006. While many factors can impede an investigation, laboratory testing is usually necessary to confirm an etiology. Stool specimens were not collected for laboratory testing in two-thirds of foodborne disease outbreaks of unknown etiology occurring at seven sites in 1998 and 1999 (12).

To meet most definitions of a confirmed outbreak, the etiologic agent should be isolated from the stool of two or more ill persons or from the epidemiologically implicated food (Table 3). In a few situations, such as mushroom poisoning, ciguatera fish poisoning, or other chemical intoxications, it is sufficient to document the clinical syndrome among affected persons. *Staphylococcus* can also be problematic because the organism may not be viable in stool or food samples, and most laboratories cannot test for enterotoxin. Thus, investigators must collect sufficient numbers of specimens (potentially including stool and other clinical specimens and also food, water, or environmental specimens) and handle them appropriately to ensure that laboratory testing identifies the etiologic agent. Investigators should consult early with their public health laboratory regarding appropriate collection and testing of samples.

Most private clinical laboratories currently cannot test specimens for norovirus, which is the most common cause

TABLE 2 Roles of selected government agencies in responding to possible foodborne or waterborne disease outbreaks in the United States[a]

Agency	Responsibilities	Product or situation of interest
Local and state health departments	Generally authorized under state laws to be responsible for surveillance for notifiable diseases and investigation of most foodborne and waterborne outbreaks in their jurisdiction. Often responsible for inspecting and regulating restaurants within jurisdiction. State health laboratories support outbreak investigations.	Any legally notifiable disease or outbreak of public health importance
Local and state water regulatory agencies	Generally authorized under state laws to have oversight of surface water, municipal water systems, wells, and other water supplies. Responsibility may be under the jurisdiction of different agencies, including health, agriculture, or environmental safety departments. In some areas these agencies may also regulate recreational water venues (beaches, lakes, etc.).	Regulation of drinking water supplies, often including surface water, wells, source water protection, and public water systems
State department of agriculture	Enforce state food safety laws and perform investigations associated with facilities or products they regulate.	Farms, food production facilities and warehouses, milk production facilities, water bottling facilities, grocery stores, and many retail food establishments within the state
CDC	Assists state and local authorities in outbreak investigations, by invitation. May provide extensive laboratory and epidemiology support. Frequently participates in multistate and international outbreaks.	Any disease or outbreak of public health importance
FDA	May assist local authorities in investigations associated with products they regulate, perform interstate or international product tracebacks, and provide laboratory and regulatory support	Manufacturers, processors, and distributors of human and animal foods (except meat, poultry, and processed egg products); potable water, bottled water, and dietary supplements shipped in interstate commerce
USDA, Food Safety and Inspection Service	May assist local authorities in investigations associated with products they regulate, perform interstate or international product tracebacks, and provide laboratory and regulatory support	Domestic and imported meat, poultry, and egg products, including soups, stews, pizzas, and frozen foods which contain meat or poultry
Environmental Protection Agency	Work with other agencies in responding to outbreaks associated with contaminated water or environmental contaminants	Drinking water; toxic substances and wastes to prevent their entry into the environment and food chain
Law enforcement	The Federal Bureau of Investigation has the authority to lead the investigation of any outbreak associated with terrorism. Works with other health and regulatory agencies on the investigation.	Outbreaks involving criminal actions, including acts of terrorism

[a]This table provides a general outline of typical responsibilities for different agencies involved in investigating food- and waterborne outbreaks. All states have unique food and water safety laws, policies, and organizational structures that will affect investigations, and many other agencies and organizations may play important roles in certain situations. Additional information is available at the "Gateway to Government Food Safety Information" (http://www.foodsafety.gov/) and the Environmental Protection Agency website (http://www.epa.gov/ebtpages/water.html).

of foodborne disease in the United States. Most state health department laboratories offer PCR (reverse transcriptase PCR [RT-PCR]) testing for norovirus and can help coordinate appropriate testing of specimens if this agent is suspected as the cause of an outbreak. Likewise, few private laboratories can serotype *Salmonella* isolates or definitively identify enterotoxigenic *E. coli*, non-O157:H7 Shiga-toxigenic *E. coli* strains, or staphylococcal enterotoxin.

Guidelines for collecting appropriate specimens during an outbreak investigation are listed in Table 4. It can be difficult to collect adequate specimens for laboratory testing. In general, the concentration of etiologic agents decreases with time after onset, putting a premium on prompt specimen collection, but many pathogens are sometimes detectable days or even weeks after symptoms resolve. Investigators may need to convince reluctant persons of

the social benefits of providing stool specimens and will need to arrange the necessary logistics, including distribution of collection materials, aliquoting, and transportation. Investigators should promptly contact private laboratories that may have received specimens from outbreak-associated patients to ask that the original material be held for possible additional testing.

Where applicable, samples of suspected vehicles of infection (e.g., food or water) should be collected as soon as possible after an outbreak is recognized. Actual testing is not always practical, but getting specimens preserves the option of later testing. Ideally, investigators will collect specimens from the batches or lots of food or water that patients actually ate or drank before becoming ill. If this is not possible (as is often the case), products as similar as possible are the

(Text continues on page 95)

TABLE 3 Typical characteristics of foodborne and waterborne disease outbreaks and guidelines for confirmation[a]

Etiology	Typical incubation period[c]	Clinical syndrome	Examples of vehicles[b]	Diagnostic testing	Confirmation of outbreak etiology
Bacterial					
Bacillus cereus (preformed "emetic" toxin)	1–6 h	Vomiting; some patients with diarrhea; fever uncommon	Improperly stored cooked or fried rice, meats	Clinical diagnosis; clinical laboratories do not identify; some public health laboratories can test stool and food specimens by culture and toxin identification	Isolation of organism from stool of two or more ill persons and not from stool of control patients OR Isolation of $>10^5$ organisms/g from epidemiologically implicated food, provided specimen is properly handled
Bacillus cereus (diarrheal toxin)	10–16 h	Diarrhea, abdominal cramps, and vomiting in some patients; fever uncommon	Cereal products, soups, custards, sauces, meatloaf, sausage, cooked vegetables, reconstituted dried potatoes, refried beans	No testing at private clinical laboratories; stool and food specimens may be tested at a reference laboratory for culture and toxin identification	Isolation of organism from stool of two or more ill persons and not from stool of control patients OR Isolation of $>10^5$ organisms/g from epidemiologically implicated food, provided specimen is properly handled
Brucella	7–21 days	Weakness, fever, headache, sweats, chills, arthralgia, weight loss, splenomegaly, bloody stools	Raw milk, soft cheeses made from unpasteurized milk, contaminated meats	Blood cultures and serology	Two or more ill persons and isolation of organism in culture of blood or bone marrow OR >4-fold increase in standard agglutination titer over several weeks OR Single standard agglutination titer of ≥1:160 in person who has compatible clinical symptoms and history of exposure
Campylobacter jejuni/C. coli	2–10 days; usually 2–5 days	Diarrhea (often bloody), abdominal pain, fever, vomiting	Unpasteurized milk, raw and undercooked poultry and meat, cross-contaminated produce, contaminated water; animal contact	Routine stool culture; requires special media and incubation at 42°C	Isolation of organism from clinical specimens from two or more ill persons OR Isolation of organism from epidemiologically implicated food
Clostridium botulinum (toxin)	12–72 h	Blurred vision, diplopia, dysphagia, descending muscle weakness; variable gastrointestinal symptoms, including vomiting, diarrhea, constipation	Canned low-acid foods, smoked fish, cooked potatoes in foil, garlic in oil, fish, marine mammals	Stool, serum, and food tested for toxin; stool and food cultured for organism; testing available only at public health laboratories	Detection of botulinum toxin in serum, stool, gastric contents, or implicated food OR Isolation of organism from stool or intestine
Clostridium perfringens (toxin)	8–16 h	Watery diarrhea, nausea, abdominal cramps; vomiting and fever generally very uncommon	Meats, poultry, gravy, dried or precooked foods, time- and/ or temperature-abused foods	No testing in private laboratories; tools tested for enterotoxin and cultured; because C. perfringens can normally be found in stool, quantitative cultures must be done	Isolation of $>10^6$ organisms/g from stool of two or more ill persons, provided specimen is properly handled OR Demonstration of enterotoxin in the stool of two or more ill persons OR Isolation of $>10^5$ organisms/g from epidemiologically implicated food, provided specimen is properly handled

(Continued on next page)

TABLE 3 Typical characteristics of foodborne and waterborne disease outbreaks and guidelines for confirmation[a] (Continued)

Etiology	Typical incubation period[c]	Clinical syndrome	Examples of vehicles[b]	Diagnostic testing	Confirmation of outbreak etiology
E. coli O157:H7 and other Shiga-toxin-producing E. coli isolates (also known as enterohemorrhagic E. coli)	1–8 days	Diarrhea (often bloody), abdominal pain, vomiting; fever typically moderate or absent	Fresh produce, undercooked meat, unpasteurized milk products and juice, contaminated water; animal contact; person-to-person transmission	Stool culture; Shiga toxin may be detected using commercial kits; positive isolates should be forwarded to public health laboratories for confirmation and subtyping	Isolation of E. coli O157:H7 or other Shiga-like toxin-producing E. coli isolates from clinical specimen from two or more ill persons or from epidemiologically implicated food
Enterotoxigenic E. coli	1–3 days	Watery diarrhea, abdominal cramps; vomiting and fever less common	Water or foods contaminated with human feces	Stool culture; special laboratory techniques are required for identification; if suspected, request specific testing at public health laboratory	Isolation of organism of same serotype that produces heat-stable and/or heat-labile enterotoxin from stool of two or more ill persons
Enteropathogenic E. coli	Variable	Diarrhea, fever, abdominal cramps	Water, fecal-oral contamination	Stool culture; special laboratory techniques are required for identification; if suspected, request specific testing	Isolation of organism of same enteropathogenic serotype from stool of two or more ill persons
Enteroinvasive E. coli	Variable	Diarrhea (might be bloody), fever, abdominal cramps	Salads and other foods not subsequently heated, water	Stool culture; special laboratory techniques are required for identification; if suspected, request specific testing	Isolation of same enteroinvasive serotype from stool of two or more ill persons
Listeria monocytogenes (invasive disease)	2–6 wk	Meningitis, neonatal sepsis, fever	Coleslaw, milk, soft cheese, pâté, turkey franks, processed meats	Blood or cerebrospinal fluid cultures; asymptomatic fecal carriage occurs; antibody to listerolysin O	Isolation of organism from normally sterile site
Listeria monocytogenes (diarrheal disease)	Unknown	Diarrhea, abdominal cramps, fever	Unknown. Rare examples include corn salad, chocolate milk.	Stool culture	Isolation of organism of same serotype from stool of two or more ill persons exposed to food that is epidemiologically implicated or from which organism of same serotype has been isolated
Salmonella (nontyphoidal)	1–5 days	Diarrhea, often with fever, vomiting, abdominal cramps	Poultry, eggs, meat products, raw milk or juice products, fresh produce (sprouts, melons), commercial packaged foods	Stool culture	Isolation of organism of same serotype from clinical specimens from two or more ill persons OR Isolation of organism from epidemiologically implicated food
Salmonella (typhoid and paratyphoid fever)	3–60 days; usually 7–14 days	Fever, anorexia, malaise, headache, and myalgia; sometimes diarrhea or constipation	Any food or water contaminated by an infected person; person-to-person transmission common	Stool culture, blood culture	Isolation of organism from clinical specimens from two or more ill persons OR Isolation of organism from epidemiologically implicated food
Shigella spp.	1–3 days	Diarrhea (often bloody), often accompanied by fever and abdominal cramps	Any food or water contaminated by an infected person; person-to-person transmission common	Stool culture	Isolation of organism of same serotype from clinical specimens from two or more ill persons OR Isolation of organism from epidemiologically implicated food

Etiologic agent	Incubation period	Clinical symptoms	Foods commonly implicated	Specimens/laboratory	Confirmation
Staphylococcus aureus (preformed toxin)	1–6 h	Sudden onset severe nausea and vomiting, diarrhea; fever may be present	Unrefrigerated or improperly stored meats, potato and egg salads, cream pastries	Normally a clinical diagnosis; stool, vomitus, and food can be tested for toxin	Isolation of organism of same phage type from stool or vomitus of two or more ill persons OR Detection of enterotoxin in epidemiologically implicated food OR Isolation of $>10^5$ organisms/g from epidemiologically implicated food, provided specimen is properly handled
Streptococcus, group A	1–4 days	Fever, pharyngitis, scarlet fever, upper respiratory infection	Raw milk, egg-containing salads	Throat culture, culture of food	Isolation of organism of same M or T type from throats of two or more ill persons OR Isolation of organism of same M or T type from epidemiologically implicated food
Vibrio cholerae O1 or O139	1–3 days	Profuse watery diarrhea and vomiting; dehydration and death can occur within hours	Raw fish, shellfish, crustaceans, contaminated water	Stool culture; special media required to isolate the organism; request specific testing if suspected	Isolation of toxigenic organism from stool or vomitus of two or more ill persons OR Significant rise in vibriocidal, bacterial agglutinating, or antitoxin antibodies in acute- and early convalescent-phase sera from persons not recently immunized OR Isolation of toxigenic organism from epidemiologically implicated food
Vibrio cholerae non-O1 and non-O139	1–5 days	Watery diarrhea	Shellfish, fish	Stool culture; special media required to isolate the organism; request specific testing if suspected	Isolation of organism of same serotype from stool of two or more ill persons
Vibrio parahaemolyticus	16–48 h	Watery diarrhea, cramps, nausea, vomiting	Raw oysters or other undercooked or raw seafood; cross-contaminated foods	Stool culture; special media required to isolate the organism; request specific testing if suspected	Isolation of Kanagawa-positive organism from stool of two or more ill persons OR Isolation of $>10^5$ Kanagawa-positive organisms/g from epidemiologically implicated food, provided specimen is properly handled
Yersinia enterocolitica and Yersinia pseudotuberculosis	1–2 days	Diarrhea, abdominal pain (often severe), appendicitis-like symptoms	Undercooked pork, unpasteurized milk, tofu, contaminated water, chitterlings	Stool, vomitus, or blood culture; special media required to isolate the organism; request specific testing if suspected; serology available in reference laboratories	Isolation of organism from clinical specimen from two or more ill persons OR Isolation of pathogenic strain of organism from epidemiologically implicated food
Chemical					
Marine toxins					
Ciguatera toxin	1–48 h; usually 2–8 h	Usually gastrointestinal symptoms followed by neurological symptoms (including paresthesia of lips, tongue, throat, or extremities) and reversal of hot and cold sensations	Numerous varieties of tropical fish, e.g., barracuda, grouper, red snapper, amberjack, goatfish, skipjack, parrotfish	Radioassay for toxin in fish or a consistent history	Demonstration of ciguatoxin in epidemiologically implicated fish OR Clinical syndrome among persons who have eaten a type of fish previously associated with ciguatera fish poisoning (e.g, snapper, grouper, or barracuda)

(Continued on next page)

TABLE 3 Typical characteristics of foodborne and waterborne disease outbreaks and guidelines for confirmation[a] (*Continued*)

Etiology	Typical incubation period[c]	Clinical syndrome	Examples of vehicles[b]	Diagnostic testing	Confirmation of outbreak etiology
Scombroid toxin (histamine)	Minutes to hours; usually <1 h	Flushing, dizziness, burning of mouth and throat, headache, gastrointestinal symptoms, urticaria, and generalized pruritus	Fish: tuna, mackerel, Pacific dolphin (mahimahi), bluefin, marlin, escolar	Detect histamine in food or clinical diagnosis	Demonstration of histamine in epidemiologically implicated fish OR Clinical syndrome among persons who have eaten a type of fish previously associated with histamine fish poisoning (e.g., mahimahi or fish of the order Scombroidei)
Paralytic or neurotoxic shellfish poison	30 min–3 h	Paresthesia of lips, mouth, or face, and extremities; intestinal symptoms or weakness, including respiratory difficulty	Mussels, clams, scallops	High-pressure liquid chromatography to detect toxin in food or water where fish are located	Detection of toxin in epidemiologically implicated food OR Detection of large numbers of a dinoflagellate species associated with shellfish poisoning in water from which epidemiologically implicated mollusks are gathered
Puffer fish, tetrodotoxin	Minutes to hours; usually 10–45 min	Paresthesia of lips, tongue, face, or extremities, often following numbness; loss of proprioception or floating sensations	Puffer-type fish	Toxin testing of fish	Demonstration of tetrodotoxin in epidemiologically implicated fish OR Clinical syndrome among persons who have eaten puffer fish
Heavy metals (antimony, cadmium, copper, iron, tin, zinc)	5 min–8 h; usually <1 h	Vomiting, often metallic taste	High-acid foods and beverages, metal-colored cake decorations	Testing foods	Demonstration of high concentration of metal in epidemiologically implicated food
Monosodium glutamate	Several minutes to 1 h	Burning sensation in chest, neck, abdomen, or extremities; sensation of lightness and pressure over face or heavy feeling in chest	Foods seasoned with monosodium glutamate	Clinical diagnosis; testing food	Clinical syndrome in persons who have eaten food containing monosodium glutamate
Mushroom toxins Shorter-acting toxins (muscimol, muscarine, psilocybin, *Coprinus atramentaris*, ibotenic acid)	2 h	Vomiting and diarrhea; other symptoms differ with toxin: confusion, visual disturbance, salivation, diaphoresis, hallucinations	Many species of wild mushrooms	Typical syndrome, identify mushroom, detect toxin	Clinical syndrome among persons who have eaten mushroom identified as toxic type OR Demonstration of toxin in epidemiologically implicated mushroom or food containing mushroom
Longer-acting toxins (e.g., *Amanita* spp.)	6–24 h	Diarrhea and abdominal cramps for 24 h, often followed by hepatic and renal failure	Wild mushrooms	Typical syndrome, identify mushroom, detect toxin	Clinical syndrome among persons who have eaten mushroom identified as toxic type OR Demonstration of toxin in epidemiologically implicated mushroom or food containing mushrooms

Etiologic agent	Incubation period	Clinical syndrome	Vehicles	Laboratory testing	Confirmation
Parasitic					
Cryptosporidium parvum, Cryptosporidium hominis	2–28 days; median, 7 days	Diarrhea, nausea, vomiting, fever	Water, any uncooked food or food contaminated after cooking	Request specific examination of stool, food, or water for Cryptosporidium	Demonstration of organism or antigen in stool or in small-bowel biopsy sample of two or more ill persons OR Demonstration of organism in epidemiologically implicated food
Cyclospora cayetanensis	1–11 days; median, 7 days	Fatigue, protracted diarrhea, often relapsing	Produce, including raspberries, lettuce, basil, water	Request specific examination of stool, food, or water for Cyclospora	Demonstration of organism in stool of two or more ill persons
Giardia intestinalis	3–25 days; median, 7 days	Diarrhea, gas, cramps, nausea, fatigue	Any uncooked food or food contaminated by ill food handler, water	Stool examination for ova and parasites; may require at least three specimens	Two or more ill persons and detection of antigen in stool or demonstration of organism in stool, duodenal contents, or small-bowel biopsy specimen
Trichinella spp.	1–2 days for intestinal phase; 2–4 wk for systemic phase	Fever, myalgia, periorbital edema, high eosinophil count	Meat from wild carnivores (bear, cougar, walrus), undercooked pork (rare in the United States)	Positive serology, demonstration of larvae in muscle biopsy sample, increase in eosinophils	Two or more ill persons and positive serologic test or demonstration of larvae in muscle biopsy sample OR Demonstration of larvae in epidemiologically implicated meat
Viral					
Hepatitis A virus	15–50 days; median, 28–30 days	Jaundice, dark urine, fatigue, anorexia, nausea	Any food or water contaminated by an infected person; water; uncooked shellfish; person-to-person transmission common	Increase in alanine aminotransferase, bilirubin; positive immunoglobulin M anti-hepatitis A virus antibodies	Detection of immunoglobulin M anti-hepatitis A virus in serum from two or more persons who consumed epidemiologically implicated food
Noroviruses (and other caliciviruses)	24–48 h; group median, usually 32–38 h	Vomiting, cramps, diarrhea, headache, myalgia, fever	Any food or water contaminated by an infected person; person-to-person transmission common; shellfish; water	Routine RT-PCR on fresh unpreserved stool samples; negative bacterial cultures; stool negative for white blood cells	Detection of viral RNA in stool or vomitus by RT-PCR
Astrovirus	1–2 days	Vomiting, cramps, diarrhea, headache	Ready-to-eat foods contaminated by infected food handler	Identification of virus in early acute-phase stool specimen, serology; commercial enzyme-linked immunosorbent assay kits available	Detection of virus antigen by enzyme immunoassay OR Detection of viral RNA in stool or vomitus by RT-PCR OR Visualization of viruses with characteristic surface morphology by electron microscopy

[a] Adapted from references 5, 6, and 11.

[b] Vehicles noted include examples from reported outbreaks and other commonly contaminated foods or sources.

[c] Incubation periods can vary substantially within, and sometimes outside, published "typical" ranges.

TABLE 4 Guidelines for collection and handling of stool specimens during a foodborne or waterborne disease outbreak investigation[a]

Parameter	Instructions for collecting stool specimens[b]			
	Bacterial	Parasitic[c]	Viral[d]	Chemical
When to collect	During period of active diarrhea (preferably as soon as possible after onset of illness)	Anytime after onset of illness (preferably as soon as possible)	Preferably within 48–72 h after onset of illness. Norovirus can often be detected 7–10 days after onset.	Soon after onset of illness (preferably within 48 h of exposure to contaminant)
How much to collect	Whole stools are preferred. If not available, two rectal swabs or swabs of fresh stool from 10 ill persons.	A fresh stool sample from 10 ill persons; to enhance detection, 3 stool specimens per patient can be collected >48 h apart	Whole stools are preferred (minimum of 10 ml), from at least 6 ill persons if possible	A fresh urine sample (50 ml) from 10 ill persons; samples from 10 controls also can be submitted; collect vomitus if vomiting occurs within 12 h of exposure; collect 5–10 ml of whole blood if a toxin/poison that is not excreted in urine is suspected.
Method for collection	For rectal swabs, moisten two swabs in an appropriate transport medium (e.g., Cary-Blair, Stuart, Amies; buffered glycerol-saline is suitable for E. coli, Salmonella, Shigella, and Y. enterocolitica but not for Campylobacter or Vibrio); insert swabs 1–1.5 inches into rectum and gently rotate; place the swabs in the same tube deep enough that medium covers the cotton tips; break off top portion of sticks and discard; alternatively, swab whole stools and put the swabs into Cary-Blair medium.	Collect bulk stool specimen, unmixed with urine, in a clean container; place a portion of each stool sample into 10% formalin and polyvinyl alcohol preservative at a ratio of 1 part stool to 3 parts preservative; mix well; save portion of the unpreserved stool placed into a leakproof container for antigen or PCR testing.	Place fresh stool specimens (liquid preferable), unmixed with urine, in clean, dry containers, e.g., urine specimen cups.	Collect urine, blood, or vomitus in prescreened containers[e]; if prescreened containers are not available, submit field blanks with samples[f] most analyses from blood require separation of serum from red blood cells; cyanide, lead, and mercury analyses require whole blood collected in prescreened EDTA tubes; volatile organic compounds require whole blood collected in a specially prepared gray-top tube.
Storage of specimens after collection	Refrigerate swabs in transport medium at 4°C; when possible, test within 48 h after collection; otherwise, freeze samples at −70°C. Refrigerate whole stool, process it within 2 h after collection; store portion of each stool specimen frozen at less than −15°C for antigen or PCR testing.	Store specimen in fixative at room temperature, or refrigerate unpreserved specimen at 4°C; a portion of unpreserved stool specimen may be frozen at less than −15°C for antigen or PCR testing.	Immediately refrigerate at 4°C.	Immediately refrigerate at 4°C and if possible freeze urine, serum, and vomitus specimens at less than −15°C; refrigerate whole blood for volatile organic compounds and metals at 4°C.
Transportation	For refrigeration: follow instructions for viral samples. For frozen samples: place bagged and sealed samples on dry ice. Mail in insulated box by overnight mail.	For refrigeration: follow instructions for viral samples. For room temperature samples: mail in waterproof container.	Keep refrigerated; place bagged and sealed specimens on ice or with frozen refrigerant packs in an insulated box; send by overnight mail. Send frozen specimens on dry ice for antigen or PCR testing.	Place double-bagged and sealed urine, serum, and vomitus specimens on dry ice; mail in an insulated box by overnight mail. Ship whole blood in an insulated container with prefrozen ice packs. Avoid placing specimens directly on ice packs.

[a]Adapted from reference 11.

[b]Wrap the packaged samples in sealed, waterproof containers (i.e., plastic bags). Label each specimen container in a waterproof manner. Batch the collection and send in overnight mail to arrive at the testing laboratory on a weekday during business hours unless other arrangements have been made in advance with the testing laboratory. Contact the testing laboratory before shipping, and give the testing laboratory as much advance notice as possible so that testing can begin as soon as samples arrive. When etiology is unclear and syndrome is nonspecific, consider collecting all four types of specimens.

[c]For more detailed instructions on how to collect specimens for specific parasites, please go to http://www.dpd.cdc.gov/dpdx/.

[d]For more detailed instructions on how to collect specimens for viral testing, please go to http://www.cdc.gov/mmwr/PDF/RR/RR5009.pdf.

[e]The containers have been tested for the presence of the chemical of interest before use.

[f]Unused specimen collection containers that have been brought in to the field and subjected to the same field conditions as the used containers. These containers are then tested for trace amounts of the chemical of interest.

next best thing. If investigators suspect that the source of an outbreak is contaminated packaged food, they should collect unopened packages from the implicated lot. Positive (and sometimes negative) specimens are often critical evidence in outbreaks caused by commercial products.

Laboratory subtyping is critical to many outbreak investigations, particularly those with bacterial etiologies. "Subtyping" is a generic term referring to any method that improves the specificity of the description of an etiologic agent. For example, a *Salmonella* isolate could be characterized by serotype (e.g., Enteritidis or Heidelberg), pulsed-field gel electrophoresis (PFGE) or other restriction fragment length polymorphism patterns, multilocus variable number tandem repeat analysis (MLVA) pattern, DNA sequence, or other characteristics. When methodologies are standardized, subtyping data can be shared to identify potential matches between isolates at different laboratories. PulseNet (http://pulsenetinternational.org) is an example of an international network that effectively shares such information. Specific subtyping can be invaluable: two salmonellosis reports in the same week may be normal, but two *Salmonella enterica* serovar Hvittingfoss cases in the same week in most jurisdictions would be an unlikely coincidence. On closer inspection, those matching isolates might turn out to be from the same household (or even from the same individual), but such matches are often the first indication of an outbreak. Subtype matches not only help link scattered cases but also can provide a way to exclude similar but perhaps unrelated cases (Fig. 4). Refining case definitions in this manner can greatly increase the statistical power of an analytic epidemiological study.

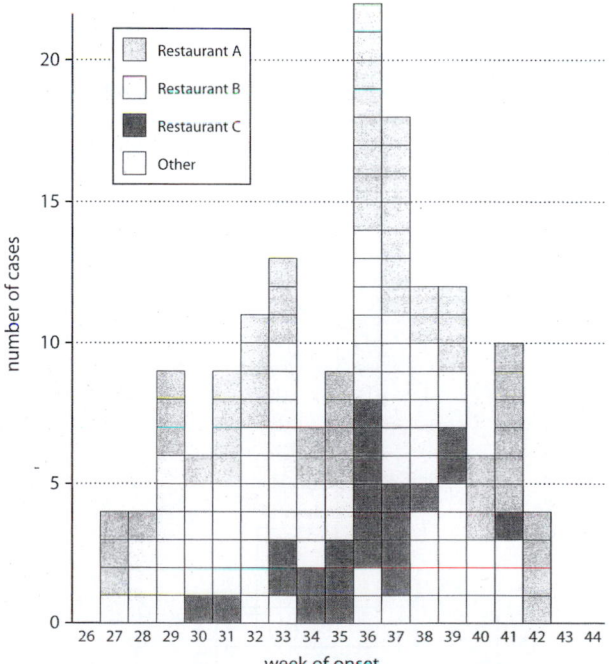

FIGURE 4 Epidemic curve of *Salmonella enterica* serovar Typhimurium by PFGE pattern, Minnesota, 1995. Molecular subtyping allowed investigators to recognize three concurrent outbreaks caused by different strains and associated with different restaurants. Adapted from reference 1.

Some outbreaks involve multiple variants of a pathogen. Investigations may start because of an increase in one PFGE pattern, but multiple patterns may eventually be recognized to be part of the same cluster, reflecting the genetic diversity or microevolution of the etiologic agent in vivo. Outbreaks that involve gross environmental contamination may even include multiple species (13, 18).

EPIDEMIOLOGICAL APPROACHES TO OUTBREAK INVESTIGATIONS

While there is much variation in practice, there is a general logic that underlies most successful outbreak investigations. These steps are outlined in Table 5. Depending on circumstances, some steps may be more implicit than explicit, and they do not necessarily occur in a neat sequence.

In any investigation, the most immediate priorities are to implement appropriate measures to control the outbreak, mitigate associated morbidity, and prevent recurrences. When outbreaks appear to be ongoing, public health officials may institute substantial and occasionally controversial control measures before the investigation is complete and before all desired data are available. Such measures may include ordering (or recommending) product recalls, confiscating products, excluding food handlers or ill persons from work, closing retail food establishments or implicated venues, and publicly notifying persons who may have been exposed. Because such interventions can have important medical, emotional, and economic implications, the larger investigative team must assimilate available data rapidly and communicate effectively with each other and the public. Such collaboration is imperative to ensure that the public health benefits are maximized while the collateral damage is minimized.

Good communication among epidemiologists, laboratorians, environmentalists, and other partners is essential to successful investigations. Most health department jurisdictions have environmental health specialists (also known as sanitarians or environmentalists) or regulatory staff with expertise in the technical aspects of food handling, inspection of food establishments, tracing of food distribution, environmental specimen collection, water safety, and other issues that are often critical to successful investigations.

Epidemiologists use case definitions to consistently include or exclude people from a cluster or study group. Case definitions typically include criteria for symptoms, time of onset, and the time and place of potential exposure, e.g., "any person reporting vomiting or diarrhea within 5 days of consuming food from restaurant A from 2 to 5 March" or "any U.S. resident with an isolate of *Salmonella enterica* serovar Rissen and PFGE pattern XYZ1234 reported in 2010."

TABLE 5 Steps of an outbreak investigation[a]

1. Establish the existence of an outbreak.
2. Verify the diagnosis.
3. Determine the population at risk.
4. Describe epidemiology.
5. Develop hypotheses.
6. Define and count cases.
7. Evaluate hypotheses.
8. Perform additional epidemiological, environmental, and laboratory studies as necessary.
9. Implement control and prevention measures.
10. Communicate findings.

[a]Adapted from references 3 and 10.

Case definitions are investigative constructs, not biological verities, and may be modified during the course of an investigation as the need arises; there can even be multiple case definitions serving different purposes.

Epidemiologists collect clinical information about potential cases, including signs and symptoms, onset time, and indices of severity such as duration of illness, hospitalization, and fatalities. Individual case data are often displayed in a spreadsheet or database layout as a "line list," and epidemiologists pore over these in search of patterns. When outbreaks manifest by matching laboratory isolates (e.g., *E. coli* O157:H7 cases with the same PFGE pattern), the pathogen is known at the outset, and there may be less interest in some clinical details. Investigations that stem from citizen reports, on the other hand, often rely on thorough symptom profiles to classify potential cases.

After confirming the existence of an outbreak, investigators interview affected persons to identify demographic characteristics of cases, the nature and timing of symptoms, and potential exposures of interest. Systematically collected information is much more useful than desultory anecdotes. Well-designed forms and questionnaires—and skilled interviewers—provide structure to that information and are essential to transforming raw reports into analyzable data. Good questionnaire design requires training, insight, and experience and can be surprisingly time-consuming. Outbreak investigations often move quickly, and template questionnaires developed in advance that can be quickly modified to fit a given situation can be very useful. The best templates allow for quick and flexible modification, deployment in multiple modes (e.g., paper and electronic) for a variety of audiences, rapid data entry, and easy abstraction of data for tabulation and statistical analyses.

A careful consideration of the cases' demographics (age, sex, race, and ethnicity) can narrow the range of plausible vehicles. For example, salmonellosis outbreaks caused by fresh produce (e.g., lettuce, spinach, and sprouts) typically manifest with disproportionate numbers of female patients in the age group from 20 to 50. Outbreaks focused among young children are less likely to be caused by vegetables. The spatial and temporal distribution of cases also is instructive. Illnesses scattered across the country are unlikely to be caused by products with local or regional distribution (e.g., milk). Products with a short shelf life (e.g., fresh produce) tend to cause shorter-lived outbreaks than processed foods with a long shelf life (e.g., peanut butter).

Different kinds of outbreaks call for different types of questionnaires. Even in a single investigation, more than one questionnaire may prove useful as things progress. The desire to be comprehensive must be balanced by practical considerations, including ease of use and acceptability to interviewees and interviewers. Complete answers to reasonably limited questions are generally preferred over incomplete answers to an unreasonable number. Questionnaire designers should be mindful of the population for which it is intended, the mode of administration, the sophistication of those collecting the data, and—often overlooked—how data will be entered and analyzed. Questionnaires can be deployed via telephone, in a face-to-face interview, or as self-administered paper or electronic forms; each choice has advantages and disadvantages. Interviewers must know how to introduce the study to participants and answer questions about it. Data collectors must also be given guidelines for obtaining data and be familiar with standard definitions so that information is elicited consistently and completely, thereby minimizing errors and potential bias.

Simple event-centric outbreaks (e.g., church suppers, wedding receptions, and many restaurant clusters) lend themselves to short questionnaires. Menus are obtained, other exposures (e.g., water) are assessed, and with a good template, questionnaire design is often straightforward. When cases are more scattered in place and time, suspicions may arise about commercially distributed food products. These can be complex, multijurisdictional investigations with large public health and economic consequences. Such investigations often evolve over weeks or even months, with different questionnaires used at different stages of the process. Broad hypothesis-generating questionnaires may be used initially to identify food items or other exposures that deserve additional scrutiny. There are several models for approaching these kinds of outbreaks that have proven effective in practice (8, 21).

Interviews with persons who were not sick (controls) are often necessary to provide a comparison group. If the population affected by the outbreak is well defined, such as attendees of a church picnic or patrons of a single restaurant within a 3-day period, a retrospective cohort study can be performed. In this situation, all members or a representative sample of the affected group (the cohort) are interviewed to assess whether they were ill and what items they consumed. Rates of illness among persons with and without certain exposures are compared with appropriate statistical methods to identify exposures associated with illness (3, 10). If the affected population is not well defined or a cohort study is not practical, a case control study may be performed. In such outbreaks, persons with the illness of interest (cases) are compared to those without it (controls). In the absence of formal control data, other information may be better than nothing in assessing case exposure data: restaurant service records (e.g., how many people got salads on Monday night), brand name market share data, or even available survey data (<3% of people drink unpasteurized milk in any given week).

To keep the investigation focused, data about cases should be regularly organized, summarized, and shared with colleagues. The occurrence of new cases over time (usually by day or week of symptom onset) can be represented graphically as an "epidemic curve" (Fig. 5 and 6),

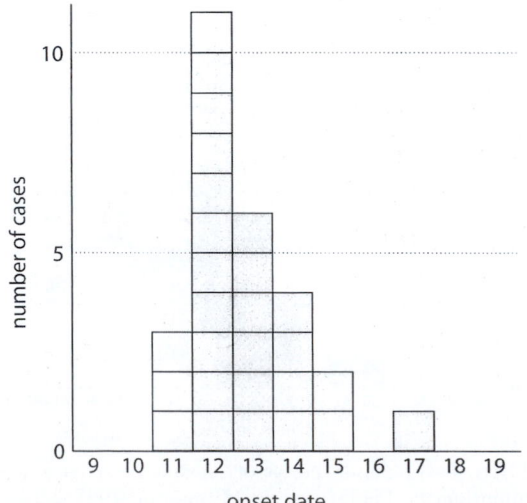

FIGURE 5 Epidemic curve of a hypothetical point source salmonellosis outbreak with onset on the 10th day of the month.

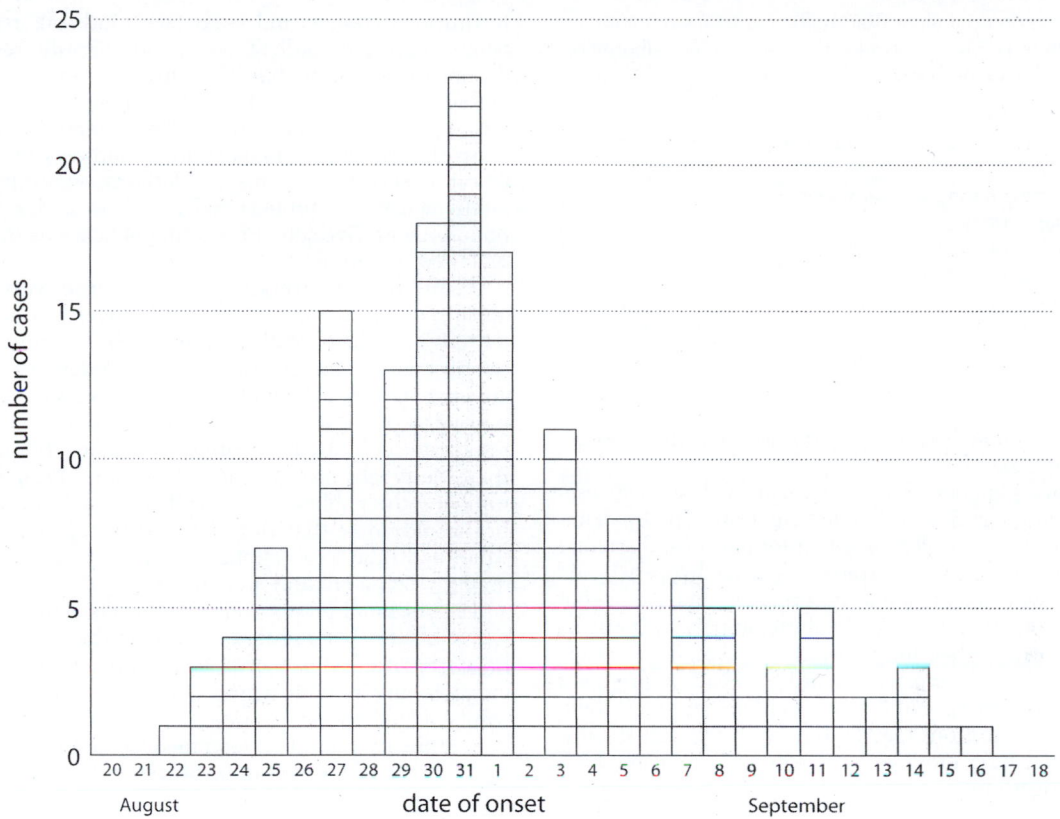

FIGURE 6 Epidemic curve of an *E. coli* O157:H7 outbreak associated with nationally distributed bagged spinach, 2006.

and the geographic distribution of cases can be plotted on a map. The line list, the epidemic curve, and the map can give the investigator clues about the source of an outbreak. Localized cases may reflect an exposure at a single time and place (a "point source" outbreak), e.g., patrons of a restaurant on a single day; such outbreaks are often associated with mishandling, undercooking, cross-contamination, or poor hygiene locally. In contrast, cases widely scattered geographically suggest the distribution of a commercial product (or a convergence at a national meeting, event, or vacation venue).

DATA ANALYSIS

Statistical analyses can help investigators summarize their findings from the epidemiological investigation and help them draw conclusions from data that may be complicated. Basic descriptive statistics include the number of ill persons, a summary of the characteristics of cases and the population at risk, the proportion of ill persons experiencing particular symptoms, mean and/or median incubation period (time between exposure and onset of symptoms), and mean and/or median duration of illness. Data from cohort studies may be used to calculate the attack rate (proportion of persons exposed to a vehicle who subsequently developed disease). Data from cohort and case control studies can be used to estimate the risk (using risk ratios [relative risks] and odds ratios, respectively) of developing disease after exposure to particular foods, water sources, or other risk factors. Basic "2 × 2" tables showing the relative risks of illness among

those exposed to and those not exposed to particular foods frequently suffice to support the most imperative decisions during an outbreak investigation. More advanced statistical techniques, such as stratified analyses, regression modeling, and sensitivity analyses, are sometimes helpful in teasing apart complicated scenarios. Detailed information on statistical methods for outbreak investigation are available from multiple sources (3, 10, 16, 17).

While statistical techniques can be powerful tools, all statistics must be interpreted cautiously and with a component of judgment. A likely cause of a foodborne or waterborne disease outbreak should not be discounted simply because its associated *P* value (a commonly cited measure of statistical significance) is >0.05, and likewise, statistical significance (particularly in larger studies) does not necessarily indicate biological plausibility or relevance in a given situation. Statistical association between an exposure and illness may reflect a causal link, but it may also reflect confounding, bias, chance, or other factors. If three food items on a questionnaire have a *P* value of <0.05, for example, it does not mean that all three (or, indeed, any of them) are implicated as a vehicle. Questionnaire data are often faulty: collected long after the fact, perhaps by proxy, and sometimes tainted by biases known and unknown. Investigators can create or compound errors during transcription, data entry, or analysis. Records are often incomplete, inconsistent, or unavailable. Absent a systematic bias, larger data sets tend to be more robust, and minor errors may be cancelled out (or ignored), but the size of the data set is often beyond one's control. Care must be taken not to

TABLE 6 Potential clues that might increase suspicion that intentional contamination is the cause of a foodborne or waterborne disease outbreak

Occurrence of a rare or novel disease
Outbreak due to a disease occurring outside its normal range of endemicity
Disease occurring during unusual season
Unusual drug resistance
Unusual epidemiological characteristics
Unusual demographic population affected
Unusual clinical presentation of disease
Widespread contamination without apparent explanation
Claims or social context suggesting intentional contamination

dismiss data simply because they do not fit with investigators' hypotheses.

Hypotheses supported by statistical evidence can usually be corroborated by other information. The epidemiologist's job is to take *all* available information and attempt to construct a coherent narrative of what happened and why. Interview questionnaires are very important but rarely yield all the answers. Analytic study data must be integrated with other information (e.g., product testing results, food handler interviews, and traceback efforts). For example, cross-referenced lists of suppliers and food items at different institutions may be hard to assess statistically, but they can help provide focus to commercial product-type investigations.

INTENTIONALLY CAUSED OUTBREAKS

Most foodborne and waterborne disease outbreaks result from unintentional contamination of food or water sources at any of innumerable points in the long food production and service chain. In recent years, however, public health officials and the public have become increasingly concerned that the food supply system is a potential target of intentional acts of contamination, sabotage, or terrorism. It is difficult to protect the myriad stages from "farm to fork"; tremendous volumes of product are rapidly distributed worldwide, and techniques for detecting intentional events are inadequate. Industry and governmental agencies associated with food safety are increasing efforts to improve security at all stages of the food supply chain (http://www .foodsafety.gov).

In general, intentional outbreaks are likely to be identified and reported in the same way as unintentional foodborne and waterborne disease outbreaks. Thus, standard surveillance and epidemiological methods remain essential to the investigations. Potential clues that might suggest bioterrorism or intentionally caused outbreaks are described in Table 6. If purposeful contamination is suspected, investigators must include law enforcement officials early in the investigation.

REPORTING

Aggregated data from many outbreaks help identify long-term trends and changing practices among both epidemiological hunters and their prey. As previously noted, summary reports on foodborne outbreaks (ideally all, but in practice only some) are prepared by local or state investigators and collated nationally.

For some investigations, a fuller narrative report is also prepared. Such reports are disseminated based on institutional policy and state law. Outbreak reports can be an important medical, legal, and scientific resource for documenting the process of an investigation, nature of an outbreak, conclusions about its causes and control, and preventive measures instituted. An example of the components that should be included in an outbreak investigation report is shown in Table 7. Outbreak investigations are often reported at professional meetings, and a small and nonrepresentative subset result in publications in the peer-reviewed literature.

Public health authorities often struggle with decisions about publicizing active outbreak investigations. When there is a product recall or other urgent warnings to make, the need is obvious, and press releases and media interviews are indicated. But do public health agencies have a duty to notify the public about every outbreak that occurs at local restaurants, child care centers, or nursing homes? When these outbreaks are over and there is no clear benefit to notifying the public—as is usually the case—most authorities would argue that the answer is no. Discussions about when and how to go public can be contentious and often do not reach a unanimous conclusion.

Only a small proportion of outbreaks generate substantial publicity, but rightly or wrongly, these outbreaks can have important effects on the development of public policies. Keeping individual outbreaks in the proper perspective can be a challenge.

Outbreaks caused by commercial product contamination or that result in serious illnesses or deaths often lead

TABLE 7 Recommended components of an outbreak investigation summary report

List of participants in the investigation and contact information for lead investigator
Timeline for outbreak and investigation
Description of process by which outbreak was recognized and reported
Description of the epidemiological steps followed in the investigation
Case definition(s) used in the investigation
Summary of total number of affected persons and description of the population exposed
Description of clinical syndrome, including proportion of persons experiencing common symptoms, summary of incubation period, duration of illness, and indices of severity, including hospitalization and death rates
Description of results from epidemiological studies, including numbers of cases or controls enrolled in cohort or case control studies and results of analyses assessing possible sources
Summary of supporting laboratory data obtained by testing clinical, food, or environmental specimens
Summary of findings of various groups contributing to the investigation, including epidemiologists, environmental health specialists regulatory agencies, institutional representatives, medical providers, or others not primarily writing report
Conclusions about the etiology, vehicle, cause, and underlying contributing factors leading to the outbreak
Lessons learned during the investigation that may benefit others in similar situations in the future
Limitations of the investigation
Specific recommendations made and control measures implemented (including dates and how and when communicated)
Results of intervention if known
Recommendations for preventing similar incidents in the future

to lawsuits. Investigative records, including epidemiological and laboratory methods and results, are often requested or subpoenaed and are made available pursuant to state law.

REFERENCES

1. Bender, J. B., C. W. Hedberg, D. J. Boxrud, J. M. Besser, J. H. Wicklund, K. E. Smith, and M. T. Osterholm. 2001. Use of molecular subtyping in surveillance for *Salmonella enterica* serotype Typhimurium. *N. Engl. J. Med.* **344:**189–195.

2. Blackburn, B. G., G. F. Craun, J. S. Yoder, et al. 2004. Surveillance for waterborne disease outbreaks associated with drinking water, United States, 2001–2002. *MMWR Surveill. Summ.* **53:**23–45.

3. Centers for Disease Control. 1992. *Principles of Epidemiology. An Introduction to Applied Epidemiology and Biostatistics.* U.S. Department of Health and Human Services, Atlanta, GA.

4. Centers for Disease Control and Prevention. 2000. Surveillance for foodborne-disease outbreaks—United States, 1993–1997. *MMWR Morb. Mortal. Wkly. Rep.* **49**(SS-1):1–62.

5. Centers for Disease Control and Prevention. 2004. Diagnosis and management of foodborne illnesses. A primer for physicians. *MMWR Morb. Mortal. Wkly. Rep.* **53:**1–33.

6. Centers for Disease Control and Prevention. 2006. Surveillance for foodborne-disease outbreaks—United States, 1998–2002. *MMWR Morb. Mortal. Wkly. Rep.* **55**(SS10):1–34.

7. Centers for Disease Control and Prevention. 2009. Surveillance for foodborne disease outbreaks—United States, 2006. *MMWR Morb. Mortal. Wkly. Rep.* **58:**609–615.

8. Council to Improve Foodborne Outbreak Response (CIFOR). 2009. *Guidelines for Foodborne Outbreak Response.* Council of State and Territorial Epidemiologists, Atlanta, GA.

9. Dziuban, E. J., J. L. Liang, G. F. Craun, et al. 2006. Surveillance for waterborne disease and outbreaks associated with recreational water—United States, 2003–2004. *MMWR Morb. Mortal. Wkly. Rep.* **55:**1–30.

10. Gregg, M. B. (ed.). 2002. *Field Epidemiology.* Oxford University Press, New York, NY.

11. International Association of Milk Food and Environmental Sanitarians, Inc. 1999. *Procedures To Investigate Foodborne Illness.* International Association of Milk Food and Environmental Sanitarians, Inc., Des Moines, IA.

12. Jones, T. F., B. Imhoff, M. Samuel, P. Mshar, K. Gibbs McCombs, M. Hawkins, V. Deneen, M. Cambridge, and S. J. Olsen. 2004. Limitations to successful investigation and reporting of foodborne outbreaks: an analysis of foodborne disease outbreaks in FoodNet catchment areas, 1998–1999. *Clin. Infect. Dis.* **38:**S297–S302.

13. Keene, W. E., J. M. McAnulty, F. C. Hoesly, L. P. Williams, Jr., K. Hedberg, G. L. Oxman, T. J. Barrett, M. A. Pfaller, and D. W. Fleming. 1994. A swimming-associated outbreak of hemorrhagic colitis caused by *Escherichia coli* O157:H7 and *Shigella sonnei. N. Engl. J. Med.* **331:**579–584.

14. Liang, J. L., E. J. Dziuban, and G. F. Craun. 2006. Surveillance for waterborne disease and outbreaks associated with drinking water and water not intended for drinking—United States, 2003–2004. *MMWR Surveill. Summ.* **55:**1–30.

15. Mead, P. S., L. Slutsker, V. Dietz, L. F. McCaig, J. S. Bresee, C. Shapiro, P. M. Griffin, and R. V. Tauxe. 1999. Food-related illness and death in the United States. *Emerg. Infect. Dis.* **5:**607–625.

16. Rothman, K. J., and K. Greenland (ed.). 1998. *Modern Epidemiology.* Lippincott-Raven, Philadelphia, PA.

17. Selvin, S. 2004. *Statistical Analysis of Epidemiologic Data.* Oxford University Press, New York, NY.

18. Vestergaard, L. S., K. E. Olsen, R. Stensvold, et al. 2007. Outbreak of severe gastroenteritis with multiple aetiologies caused by contaminated drinking water in Denmark, January 2007. *Eur. Surveill.* **12:**EO70329.

19. World Health Organization. 2005. *Burden of Disease and Cost-Effectiveness Estimates.* WHO, Geneva, Switzerland.

20. World Health Organization. 2005. *The World Health Report 2005—Making Every Child and Mother Count.* WHO, Geneva, Switzerland.

21. World Health Organization. 2008. *Foodborne Disease Outbreaks: Guidelines for Investigation and Control.* World Health Organization, Geneva, Switzerland.

22. Yoder, J. S., B. G. Blackburn, and G. F. Craun. 2004. Surveillance for waterborne disease outbreaks associated with recreational water—United States, 2001–2002. *MMWR Surveill. Summ.* **53:**1–22.

23. Yoder, J. S., M. C. Hlavsa, and G. F. Craun. 2008. Surveillance for waterborne disease and outbreaks associated with recreational water use and other aquatic facility-associated health events—United States, 2005–2006. *MMWR Surveill. Summ.* **57:**1–29.

24. Yoder, J. S., V. Roberts, and G. F. Craun. 2008. Surveillance for waterborne disease and outbreaks associated with drinking water and water not intended for drinking—United States, 2005–2006. *MMWR Surveill. Summ.* **57:**39–62.

Molecular Epidemiology

PETER GERNER-SMIDT, EIJA HYYTIÄ-TREES, AND PAUL A. ROTA

8

Most of our understanding of infectious diseases has arisen from combining observations from clinical microbiology and epidemiology. In the context of infectious diseases, epidemiology is the study of the dissemination of human pathogens, including their transmission patterns and the risk factors for, and control of, infectious disease in human populations (177). The epidemiology of infectious diseases has since the discovery of microbial pathogens been closely linked to the laboratory sciences. Until the introduction of molecular techniques in the 1970s, infectious disease epidemiology was mostly driven by discoveries in classical microbiology with the development of culture and phenotypic identification methods; subtyping techniques like biotyping, serotyping, and phage typing; and antimicrobial susceptibility testing. These methods were used for pathogen discovery and the study of their reservoirs, transmission routes, geographical distribution, infection dynamics including outbreak detection and investigations, vaccine efficacy, and other disease prevention measures.

Since the 1970s molecular methods have been introduced and are increasingly replacing the old phenotypic methods in the microbiological laboratories. These new methods have created a new discipline: molecular epidemiology. Molecular epidemiology may be defined as the application of molecular, i.e., nucleic acid-based, methods to epidemiology. With the introduction of molecular epidemiology, the epidemiology of infectious diseases has reached a new level. It is no longer a science for the few; molecular biology reagents are universally available, and almost any clinical or research laboratory has the expertise and the equipment required for performing molecular studies. We are now obtaining deeper recognition of the molecular mechanisms that form the basis of the virulence of microbial pathogens, and the subtyping methods used to trace them have become faster, more discriminatory, and therefore more powerful. The etiology of many infectious diseases may now be determined without culture in minutes or hours, thereby enabling a fast, specific therapeutic response and in some instances also a rapid public health response.

Molecular epidemiology is often confused with another related but distinct microbiology discipline: molecular taxonomy. Taxonomy is the discipline that deals with the classification, identification, and naming of microorganisms. A subdiscipline of taxonomy is phylogeny, which is the study of the evolutionary relationships of microorganisms. Before the introduction of molecular methods, phylogeny was based solely on phenotypic traits and as a result was imprecise and often yielded erroneous information. The use of nucleic acid hybridization techniques and the analysis of housekeeping gene sequences have greatly improved our understanding of microbial evolution. Compared to taxonomy and phylogeny, molecular epidemiology is the study of more recent population dynamics. In addition, taxonomy and phylogeny describe interactions between the organisms themselves, whereas epidemiology describes interaction between the organisms, their hosts, and the surrounding environment, i.e., the ecology of infectious disease. The same molecular methods may be used in both disciplines; it is their application that determines if they are used for taxonomy or epidemiology, that is, the molecular methods per se do not determine if a study is one or the other.

In molecular epidemiology, molecular methods are used for detection, identification, virulence characterization, and subtyping, i.e., to generate isolate-specific molecular fingerprints for assessment of epidemiological relatedness (177). This chapter is an introduction to molecular epidemiology and basic molecular epidemiological concepts. Some terms commonly used in molecular epidemiology are provided in Table 1.

A nonexhaustive list of subtyping methods that are commonly used now or are under development and are anticipated to supplement or replace the currently used ones is given. Subtyping method development including validation and quality control is discussed. The selection of methods appropriate in different contexts and the manner in which the choice of method and the epidemiological context influence the interpretation of data are also dealt with.

SUBTYPING METHODS

Subtyping Method Characteristics

Typeability

An ideal method should be able to produce data that can lead to the establishment of subtypes for the majority, if not all, of the strains of the pathogen being studied. In mathematical terms, typeability can be expressed as the percentage of typeable isolates among the total number of isolates subtyped. All molecular subtyping methods except plasmid profiling with some organisms show very high typeability with the organisms they target.

TABLE 1 Definitions commonly used in molecular epidemiology[a]

Term	Definition
Isolate	A population of microbial cells from a pure culture derived from a single colony on an isolation plate.
Strain	An isolate or group of isolates exhibiting phenotypic and/or genotypic traits that are distinctive from other isolates of the same species.
Clone	A group of isolates descending from a common ancestor as part of direct chain of replication and transmission from host to host or from the environment to host. The term "outbreak strain" is often used with this meaning in the context of epidemiologic subtyping.
Subtype	A specific pattern or set of markers displayed by a strain when a particular typing system is used.
Typeability	The proportion of strains for which a subtype may be generated by a given subtyping method.
Reproducibility	Also called repeatability. The ability of a subtyping method to produce the same results upon repeated testing; usually stated as the proportion of strains in a given population that display the same subtype upon repeated testing.
Stability	The ability of a subtyping method to assign the same subtype to epidemiologically related strains, e.g., as part of the same single-strain outbreak, originating from the same patient or from serial passage in vitro or in vivo, usually stated as the proportion of epidemiologically linked strains showing the same subtype.
Discriminatory power	The ability of a subtyping method to differentiate between epidemiologically unrelated strains.
Epidemiological concordance	The ability of a subtyping method to link epidemiologically related strains.
Comparative subtyping	Subtyping results generated in the same or in very few experiments in the same laboratory may be compared due to poor interexperiment reproducibility.
Definitive subtyping	Subtyping results generated in different laboratories and/or at different times may be compared and stored in a reference library.
Library subtyping	Subtyping results generated by definitive subtyping are stored in a database (library). Sometimes synonymous with definitive subtyping.
Cluster	The occurrence of clinical isolations of microbes with a particular subtype greater than would otherwise be expected in a particular time and place with no further supporting epidemiological information.
Outbreak	Epidemic. The occurrence of disease greater than would otherwise be expected in a particular time and place.
Sporadic	Antonym of epidemic. Occurring with no clear relation to an outbreak.
Endemicity	Constant presence of a disease at a significant frequency, typically restricted to, or peculiar to, a locality or region.

[a]Adapted in part from references 161 and 177.

Reproducibility and Stability

Reproducibility refers to the ability of a method to assign the same type to an isolate tested on independent occasions separated in time and/or place. It may be calculated as the percentage of strains that upon repeated testing yield the same result. This is sometimes also referred to as the repeatability. Typically, there is a direct correlation between the reproducibility and robustness of a method and the quality of the data being generated. Reproducibility may be influenced by many steps in the procedure, such as preparation of materials (growth conditions and DNA extraction), different batches of reagents, different types of instruments, and finally, bias in observing, analyzing, and interpreting results. Some methods have such a poor reproducibility that it is not possible to compare results generated in different experiments. Such methods are said to be comparative. Other methods are so reproducible that it is possible to recognize the same subtypes even though they have been generated separately in time and/or place. Such methods are considered definitive subtyping methods.

Reproducibility has both intralaboratory and interlaboratory dimensions. As is discussed later, some subtyping methods, such as amplified fragment length polymorphism (AFLP), show excellent reproducibility when performed on the same instrument in one laboratory—that is, they have a good intralaboratory reproducibility—but they may have poor or suboptimal reproducibility when testing is performed in different laboratories (poor interlaboratory reproducibility).

Reproducibility is also indirectly affected by the stability of the genetic markers being targeted by the method. The assessed markers should remain stable during outbreaks and among multiple isolates obtained from individual patients and not vary to a degree that confuses the epidemiological picture. The genetic fingerprints generated by a method should also not be affected by in vitro manipulations, such as freeze-thaw cycles and serial passages.

Discriminatory Power

Discriminatory power is defined as the ability of a method to distinguish between unrelated strains. An objective measure of discriminatory power can be obtained by calculating Simpson's index of diversity (DI) (78), which is an estimate of the probability that two epidemiologically unrelated strains will display different subtypes. The formula for calculating DI is as follows:

$$DI = 1 - \frac{1}{N(N-1)} \sum_{j=1}^{N} a_j$$

where N is the number of unrelated strains tested and a_j is the number of strains with a subtype that is indistinguishable from the jth strain. The DI is 1.0 if all strains can be differentiated from each other. A value above 0.95 is desirable for subtyping methods to be used for outbreak investigations.

The DI is a function of both the number of subtypes in the strain population (richness) and the proportion of strains with each subtype, i.e., the evenness of the distribution of the isolates among the different subtypes. It is not possible to determine the contribution of the richness or the evenness of a subtyping method to the DI from its size. This should also be taken into consideration when comparing different subtyping methods. Several other diversity indices have been devised for this purpose, among which Shannon's index (151) is the most commonly cited. However, the maximal size of this index is a direct function of the number of subtypes generated within a given strain population, and it is therefore difficult to interpret differences in the size of the index unless the populations studied generate the same number of subtypes. An easier and more comprehensible way to judge the richness of a subtyping method is to create a histogram showing the distribution of different subtypes. The results of a hypothetical experiment in subtyping the same population of 100 strains with two different methods are shown in Fig. 1. Method A has a slightly higher DI than method B. However, the difference between the methods becomes obvious when observing the histograms: method A has a greater richness than method B; the 100 strains are differentiated in 74 subtypes with all containing 5 or fewer strains by method A, whereas the six most common subtypes with method B contain one-half of the strains and overall only 43 subtypes are generated with this method.

An ideal method should have such a high discriminatory power that it is capable of discriminating all epidemiologically unrelated isolates from each other (i.e., it has a high specificity). However, the method should also be able to group together isolates that are associated with the same source (i.e., it should have a high sensitivity). In other words, a method with high sensitivity and specificity generates epidemiologically relevant data. The ability of a method to group epidemiologically related isolates together is sometimes also referred to as the epidemiological concordance.

Convenience Parameters

The convenience parameters to be considered are rapidity, cost, technical demands, accessibility of the method, and ease of data analysis. The ability of a method to generate data fast is affected by the throughput of the method, the number of steps involved, the amount of hands-on technical time required to perform the method, and whether the method is amenable for automation. Ideally, typing results should be available within a single working day. The cost of performing a method depends on numerous factors, such as the initial investment in equipment and infrastructure, the price of reagents and consumables, and the number and skill level of staff needed. Cost is usually also the most critical factor affecting the accessibility of the method to general microbiology laboratories. Ease of use encompasses technical simplicity, high throughput, and ease of scoring the results. For easy analysis, data should be objective, amenable to computerized analysis, and easily disseminated between laboratories.

Another convenience parameter rarely considered is the universal applicability of the method: may the same method be used to subtype a broad range of organisms while maintaining

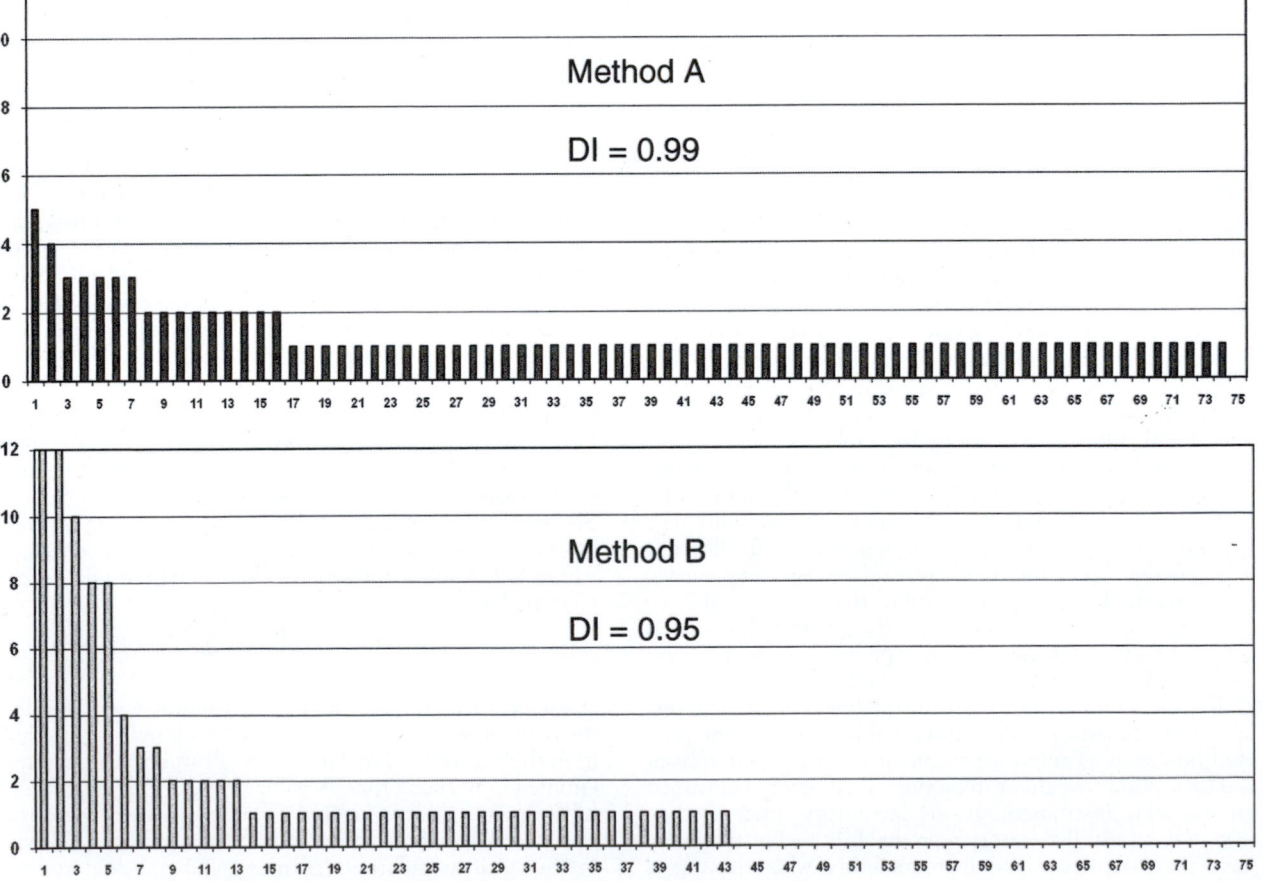

FIGURE 1 A hypothetical example of the subtype distribution of 100 epidemiologically unrelated microbial strains generated by two subtyping methods.

a universally high typeability, reproducibility, and discriminatory power? The broader the range of microbial species that can be studied, the more central the position of the method in the general typing laboratory will be.

The characteristics and applications of a number of subtyping methods are shown in Table 2.

Non-Target-Specific Methods

A short description of the principle of some non-target-specific methods is shown in Fig. 2.

Plasmid Profiling

Plasmids are circular extrachromosomal autonomous self-replicating genetic elements that are found in bacteria and some eukaryotes. Their size ranges from ~1 kb to >1 Mb. Besides genes regulating their own regulation and transmission, plasmids may carry genes conferring specific properties to the host organism, e.g., antimicrobial resistance or toxins.

Plasmid profiling was the first widely used DNA-based bacterial subtyping method to be introduced in the 1970s. The rationale for using plasmid profiling for subtyping is that bacterial strains differ in the number and size of plasmids they carry. The isolates are lysed by a method that disrupts chromosomal DNA while retaining the integrity of the plasmid, for example, alkaline lysis (84), followed by separation of the plasmids by agarose gel electrophoresis (115), staining using a fluorescent dye, such as ethidium bromide, and visualization of the plasmids under UV light.

The advantages of the method are that it is universal, i.e., it may be used to characterize any organism that contains plasmids by the same basic procedure, and that it is inexpensive, rapid, and simple with no requirements for special equipment. The typeability of the method is variable, the discriminatory power varies between organisms, and the reproducibility is in general good, but since plasmids may be lost during strain propagation in vivo and in vitro the stability is suboptimal. Additionally, if an intact plasmid is nicked or disrupted, it changes conformation from supercoiled to being relaxed or linear. These changes may happen if the purification process is performed too harshly. Two or all three conformations may be present at the same time in significant amounts and be visible as two or three bands in the gel, and since they have different migration properties in agarose, interpretation of the profiles may be difficult. In addition, large plasmids (>100 kb) are poorly separated by ordinary agarose gel electrophoresis. Unrelated plasmids of similar size may not be differentiated in an agarose gel. However, if they are digested with a restriction enzyme before electrophoresis it will often be possible to differentiate between them.

Plasmid profiling has been used in numerous epidemiological investigations of a wide range of community or nosocomially acquired infections (112) and is still used as an adjunct in investigations of outbreaks of foodborne infections in some countries (32, 138).

Plasmids may spread between different organisms and cause outbreaks of, for example, antimicrobial resistance. Plasmid profiling is the first step in the investigation of such outbreaks (56, 91).

RFLP-Based Subtyping Methods

A restriction endonuclease is an enzyme that recognizes a short specific DNA sequence and cuts it in relation to this restriction site. Genomic DNA from a single microorganism will always be cut into fragments of the same size and number if it is digested by the same restriction enzyme. The restriction fragments may be separated according to their size by electrophoresis, stained, and visualized, thereby creating a unique DNA fingerprint or restriction profile of that organism. Since different strains have different genomic content, even strains of the same species that are epidemiologically unrelated to each other usually show different restriction profiles. Subtyping methods that explore the polymorphisms of restriction profiles are called restriction fragment length polymorphism (RFLP) methods, and the process is called restriction endonuclease analysis. The method was introduced in the late1970s and the 1980s for subtyping of viruses, parasites, fungi, and bacteria (17, 85, 148, 173), using high-frequency-cutting enzymes that resulted in DNA fingerprints containing up to 500 restriction fragments ranging in size from <1 kb to 30 kb. Although the method had universal applicability, was simple, and required few resources, the resulting fragments were often difficult to resolve and the DNA fingerprints too complex to analyze accurately, especially for organisms with large genomes, e.g., bacteria, fungi, and parasites. For this reason, ways to simplify the RFLP DNA fingerprints were sought while maintaining the discriminatory power of the method. This was done by reducing the number of restriction fragments in the fingerprints by (i) reducing the number of fragments generated during the restriction reaction or (ii) reducing the number of fragments being visualized. Pulsed-field gel electrophoresis (PFGE) falls within the former category. There are numerous examples of the latter technique, among which two, ribotyping and IS6110 fingerprinting, are mentioned below.

PFGE

In PFGE, the DNA fingerprint is simplified by reducing the number of restriction fragments by using infrequently cutting restriction enzymes (macrorestriction). The resulting fragments usually range between 20 kb and >1 Mb in size. Because organisms differ in the guanine and cytosine (GC) content of their DNA, the optimal restriction enzymes for PFGE vary between organisms (61). The optimal restriction enzyme(s) generates between approximately 8 and 25 DNA fragments that are well separated and distributed evenly throughout the gel from each strain.

Large DNA fragments cannot efficiently be purified in a liquid suspension because this will cause random shearing. In order to avoid this, the genomic DNA is released and purified from cells that have been embedded in a solid agarose plug. The plug stabilizes the DNA from breaking or shearing as the cells are lysed chemically. The intact genomic DNA is then digested with an infrequent-cutting restriction enzyme. Large restriction fragments cannot be resolved with conventional agarose gel electrophoresis, which works best for separation of fragments smaller than ~30 kb. This limitation is overcome by subjecting the plug with the macrorestricted DNA to electrophoresis in a changing or pulsing electric field using an agarose gel as the separation matrix. Since the introduction of the method in 1984 (149), several different PFGE platforms have been developed (18, 19, 29). In all formats the electric field alternates in direction in a predefined manner throughout the course of the electrophoresis. During PFGE, smaller DNA fragments reorient to a directional change in the electrical field faster than larger fragments, and they therefore move more rapidly through the gel, resulting in separation of the fragments in a size-dependent manner. In some platforms, the time interval during which the electrical current is

TABLE 2 Characteristics and application of a number of subtyping methods

Characteristic	Plasmid profiling	Ribotyping	PFGE	RAPD	rep-PCR	PCR-ribotyping	AFLP	MLST	MLVA	Gene sequencing	SNP	Whole-genome sequencing
Reproducibility	Good	Good	Good	Poor	Poor	Good	Good	Good	Good	Good	Good	Good
Stability	Variable	Good	Good	Poor	Moderate	Good	Good	Good	Moderate to good	Moderate to good	Good	Moderate to good
Discriminatory power	Variable	Good	Excellent	Good	Good	Good	Excellent	Low to moderate	Excellent	Excellent	Good to excellent	Excellent
Universal applicability	Yes	Yes	Yes	Yes	Yes	Yes	Yes	No	No	No	No	Yes
Applicable for library subtyping	Yes	Yes/yes[a]	Yes	No	No/yes (in local libraries)[a]	Yes	Yes (in local libraries)	Yes	Yes	Yes	Yes	Yes
Complexity of data	Simple	Complex	Complex	Complex	Complex	Simple	Complex	Simple	Simple	Simple	Simple	Very complex
Ease of use	Simple	Labor-intensive, simple	Moderately labor-intensive	Simple	Simple/simple[a]	Simple	Moderate	Simple, moderately labor-intensive	Simple, moderately labor-intensive	Simple, moderately labor-intensive	Simple, moderately labor-intensive	Labor-intensive
Cost	Low	Moderate to high	Moderate	Low	Low to moderate	Low	Moderate	Moderate	Moderate	Moderate	Moderate	High
Suggested use of the method	Supplement to other methods	Manual ribotyping probably obsolete; automated ribotyping is a first-level, expensive screening method	Outbreak surveillance, large-scale libraries	To answer specific limited epidemiological questions, small-scale outbreak investigations	Same as RAPD	First line subtyping of C. difficile	Local outbreak surveillance, suitable for local library subtyping	Phylogenetic studies, attribution of Campylobacter, potentially forensic use	Outbreak surveillance, large-scale library subtyping if standardized, potentially good for forensic and attribution purposes	Outbreak surveillance, large-scale library subtyping, phylogenetic studies, forensic microbiology, attribution	Outbreak surveillance, large-scale library subtyping, phylogenetic studies, forensic microbiology, attribution	Outbreak investigation, (large-scale) library subtyping, phylogenetic studies, forensic microbiology, attribution
Comments			Gold standard for highly discriminatory bacterial subtyping		Semiautomated method could possibly be used for local surveillance							Method currently not feasible for large-scale studies involving prokaryotes and eukaryotes

[a]Items on left and right of slash (/) refer to manual and automated versions, respectively.

104

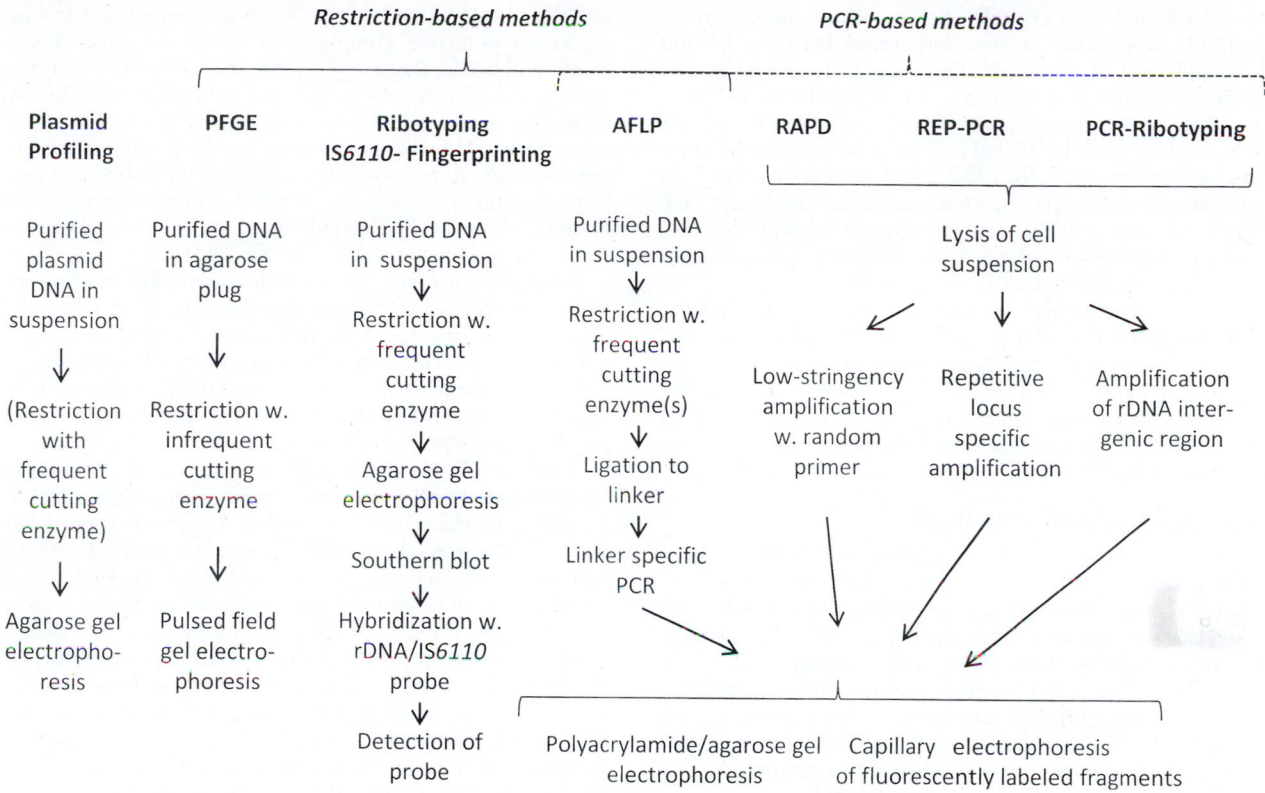

FIGURE 2   Procedural principles of some commonly used non-target-specific subtyping methods. "w." indicates "with."

applied in one direction before it switches to another direction may be changed. Usually the switch times are set to be short in the beginning of the electrophoresis and are then increased or ramped during the run.

PFGE has since the 1980s been and still remains the gold standard for bacterial molecular subtyping due to its universal applicability, virtual 100% typeability, high discriminatory power, good reproducibility, and stability. By nature all electrophoresis-based methods are comparative; i.e., only isolates investigated in the same experiment may be compared. However, this problem may be overcome by rigorous standardization of the procedure with the choice of restriction enzyme, type and brand of agarose, and electrophoresis running conditions being critical. Since 1996, PulseNet USA, the national molecular subtyping network for foodborne disease surveillance, has used PFGE as the preferred method for molecular surveillance, thereby proving its utility as a library subtyping method (166). The drawbacks of the method are that special electrophoresis equipment is required and that the procedure is rather labor-intensive. Up to 20 isolates may be subtyped within 2 working days by one person.

Ribotyping

In ribotyping, the RFLP fingerprint is simplified by visualization of the fragments that contain rRNA-encoding genes. rRNA is an essential component of all prokaryotes and eukaryotes, and its sequence is highly conserved among different organisms. Therefore, the same rRNA gene probes may be used for most organisms. The principle of the method includes whole genomic DNA restriction by high-frequency-cutting endonucleases, e.g., EcoRI or HindIII,

followed by standard agarose gel electrophoresis, transfer of the DNA fragments from the agarose gel to either a nitrocellulose or nylon membrane by Southern blotting (159), hybridization of the membrane-bound nucleic acid to labeled probes containing rRNA gene sequences, and visualization of the hybridized fragments (64). The resulting DNA fingerprint is known as the ribotype. Usually 5 to 15 fragments from each isolate are visualized. A commercially available automated ribotyping system has been developed by Qualicon-DuPont (Wilmington, DE).

Like PFGE, ribotyping is applicable to the subtyping of virtually any bacterial or fungal pathogen, its typeability is very high, and with proper standardization it is very reproducible, but the discriminatory power is somewhat less than that of PFGE. When performed manually, ribotyping is very labor-intensive. In the automated system 8 to 16 isolates may be subtyped in a working day with minimum hands-on time. However, the automated system is expensive. The workload involved with the manual procedure and the cost of the automatic one combined with the relatively low discriminatory power of the method compared to other available subtyping methods have led to a general decline in the use of ribotyping in recent years.

IS6110 Fingerprinting

Sometimes the use of a universal probe like rRNA gene sequences does not provide sufficient discrimination among strains of a clonal genus or species. This problem may be solved by using a probe that is more specific to the organism in question. An example of such a method is IS6110 fingerprinting of strains in the *Mycobacterium tuberculosis* complex (21). Only strains of M. *tuberculosis* and

Mycobacterium bovis contain this insertion sequence (60), with *M. tuberculosis* strains containing between 10 and 12 copies and *M. bovis* only between 1 and 3 copies. Because of the low number of copies of IS*6110* in *M. bovis*, the method is not optimal for subtyping of this species. The method was the first RFLP method to become standardized internationally (180), and it remains the gold standard for molecular surveillance of tuberculosis (TB). The basic principle is as in ribotyping, except that the probe is derived from the IS*6110* sequence. The preferred restriction enzyme is PvuII.

The strength of the method is that it has enabled the monitoring of the global spread of *M. tuberculosis* and tracing of outbreaks to their sources because of its high typeability, reproducibility, and discriminatory power. The drawbacks of the method are that it may only be used for surveillance of this pathogen, and like ribotyping, it is complicated and labor-intensive.

PCR-Based Subtyping Methods

Numerous subtyping methods employing PCR alone or in combination with restriction analysis have been described. Each of these techniques varies in the amplification approach and/or the genomic region it interrogates. Following amplification and restriction, if this is part of the method, the resulting fragments are separated by electrophoresis and visualized following staining with ethidium bromide. Since the fragments generated by PCR usually are small, capillary electrophoresis using a DNA sequencer may also be used to visualize the amplicons if the primers are fluorescently labeled.

RAPD/AP-PCR

In random amplification of polymorphic DNA/arbitrarily primed PCR (RAPD/AP-PCR) small genomic fragments are amplified by using short (<14-bp) primers with a random sequence under low-stringency conditions (189, 192). Because of the low-stringency PCR conditions, the primers bind not only to genomic regions with a matching sequence but also to regions with a few mismatches. The result is a number of unevenly amplified fragments of different sizes specific to each strain. The method is universally applicable, has a typeability of virtually 100%, a discriminatory power that is good but typically less than that of PFGE, and a reproducibility that is difficult to control because of the low-stringency amplification (114). The method has been used for subtyping of a broad range of prokaryotes and eukaryotes and is best suited for the comparison of a limited number of isolates subtyped under highly standardized conditions in one laboratory over a short period of time. Because of the poor reproducibility of the method, it is virtually impossible to create meaningful libraries of RAPD/AP-PCR fingerprints.

rep-PCR

Repetitive-element PCR (rep-PCR) is the common denominator for PCR-based subtyping methods in which the region between interspersed repetitive DNA elements is amplified. Repetitive elements are present in many copies in most organisms and conserved among phylogenetically related genera. If they are located close to each other in the genome, they may be amplified by PCR. Usually several amplicons are generated, and their number and size often vary between strains. Many different repetitive elements have been identified. The most commonly used are the repetitive extragenic palindromic elements, which are 33 to 40 bp in length (160, 181), the enterobacterial repetitive intergenic consensus elements, which are 124 to 127 bp in length (152, 181), and the BOX element, which is a 154-bp repetitive sequence composed of three subunits, BoxA, BoxB, and BoxC, that may be present in different combinations (111). Theoretically, it is possible to perform highly reproducible and specific rep-PCRs due to the length of the primers used. However, in practice rep-PCR suffers from the same reproducibility problems as RAPD, and when it is performed manually, results generated in different laboratories or using different PCR equipment and analysis platforms cannot be readily compared (36, 82, 142).

Recently a commercial semiautomated platform for rep-PCR, the DiversiLab System (bioMérieux, Marcy l'Etoile, France), was introduced. In this system, quality-controlled reagents are provided in a kit format with Internet-based computer-assisted analysis, reporting, and data storage (69). The company claims to have controlled the reproducibility problems encountered with manual rep-PCR this way.

Thus, rep-PCR like RAPD is a universal and simple subtyping method for most pathogens, with a high typeability and a discriminatory power that in general is good but typically less than that of PFGE. Because of the problems with the reproducibility, it is comparative and best suited for subtyping of a limited number of isolates during a short time span, but some laboratories have succeeded in creating small libraries of rep-PCR patterns. The reproducibility of the DiversiLab System seems to be better, but its applicability as a larger-scale library surveillance tool needs to be confirmed with participation of multiple laboratories. Another drawback of the DiversiLab system is that the software and database used to analyze the data are located on a server with the manufacturer and that the data cannot easily be transferred to a local database and analyzed by other commercially available image analysis software. Manual rep-PCR is inexpensive, whereas the cost of the semiautomatic system is a little higher than that of PFGE.

PCR-Ribotyping

PCR-ribotyping has little in common with the RFLP method described above. In PCR-ribotyping, the intergenic region between the genes encoding 16S and 23S rRNA is amplified. The method takes advantage of the fact that the genomes of most organisms contain more than one rRNA gene operon and that the size of the amplified intergenic region between the 16S and the 23S rRNA gene sequences often varies both within the same strain and between different strains (15). The method is rapid, simple, inexpensive, and in general universally applicable; the typeability is virtually 100%, the reproducibility is good, but the discriminatory power is moderate. Although PCR-ribotyping protocols have been described for numerous organisms, the method has gained general acceptance for the subtyping of mainly one organism, *Clostridium difficile* (10, 20).

Combined RFLP- and PCR-Based Methods

AFLP

AFLP is a patented fingerprinting technique that is based on the selective amplification of a subset of DNA fragments generated by restriction enzyme digestion (183). The method involves three steps: first, the genomic DNA is restricted with one or two restriction enzymes followed by ligation of oligonucleotide adapters to the ends of the restriction fragments; then, a subset of the fragments are amplified by PCR using primers that are complementary to the adapters, extending one to three bases into the restriction fragments, thereby reducing the number of fragments that are amplified by selection of those that are complementary to the extra (selective) bases; finally, the amplicons are separated by polyacrylamide electrophoresis or, if the primers are fluorescently labeled, in an automated DNA sequencer using capillary electrophoresis (92). Typically 50 to 100 fragments are amplified, thereby ensuring the high discriminatory power of the method. The method is universally applicable and has been used to study numerous organisms. Its typeability is very high, its discriminatory power is in general of the same magnitude as that of PFGE, and its reproducibility is good if the procedure is standardized, including using the same equipment in all experiments. However, even if the protocol is standardized, AFLP profiles may not be comparable if different detection platforms or different models of the same brand of DNA sequencer are used (53). Therefore, the intralaboratory reproducibility of the method may be excellent whereas the interlaboratory reproducibility rarely is, and the method is not suitable for creation of large-scale surveillance libraries involving multiple laboratories. Finally, the method is fairly complicated, as is the analysis of data generated by it.

Target-Specific Methods

PCR-RFLP

In PCR-RFLP, a short DNA fragment containing the whole or part of a gene or an operon is amplified followed by restriction of the amplicon with a suitable restriction enzyme. The resulting fragments are then separated and visualized in an agarose gel. In this way information about the content of the amplified fragment may be generated without sequencing it. These methods with a few exceptions do not provide much discrimination beyond the species level but may assist in the grouping of isolates at a higher level and in the identification of virulence determinants. For example, several protocols have been described for subtyping of Shiga toxin type 2 (Stx2) in Shiga-toxigenic *Escherichia coli* (STEC) (108). Toxin subtype information is useful since there seems to be a correlation between the Stx2 subtype and severity of disease (137).

Another PCR-RFLP application is amplified ribosomal DNA restriction analysis (ARDRA). In this method, the 16S rRNA gene in prokaryotes or the 18S rRNA gene in eukaryotes is the amplification target. Isolates of closely related but different bacterial and fungal species are usually differentiated, whereas the variation of the restriction patterns is low below the species level. For this reason, this method is an easy way to identify bacterial species that are difficult to differentiate phenotypically, e.g., *Acinetobacter* genomospecies (179) or mycobacteria (34).

Finally, PCR-RFLP has been used to assist in the rapid identification of *Salmonella* and STEC O157 flagellar antigens by targeting the *FljB* and/or the *FliC* genes (33, 48). Similarly, a PCR-RFLP protocol for subtyping of thermotolerant *Campylobacter* spp. has been developed. In this protocol the flagellar gene *flaA* is targeted (118). The discriminatory power of the method is good albeit less than that of PFGE (35, 123), but due to its simplicity it is useful as a screening tool and as a supplement to other methods.

Gene Sequencing

MLST and MVLST

Multilocus sequence typing (MLST) was one of the first DNA sequence-based subtyping methods. It was originally introduced by Maiden et al. (107) for the naturally transformable pathogen *Neisseria meningitidis* as a sequencing-based counterpart to the phenotypic method multilocus enzyme electrophoresis. MLST detects variation due to

mutations or recombination by direct nucleotide sequencing of 350- to 600-bp fragments typically in 5 to 10 housekeeping genes. Innovative technologies such as electrospray ionization-mass spectrometry can also be used to determine the base composition instead of direct sequencing (68). When a gene has a base pair change, the new gene sequence is considered a separate allele type. The allele types for each of the gene sequences are combined to define the multilocus sequence type (ST) to characterize the genetic relatedness of the strains. Additionally, MLST results can be analyzed using clustering techniques, such as the eBURST algorithm, which is able to divide isolates based on their STs into clonal complexes (CCs). With eBURST clustering, isolates with a high level of genetic similarity (such as sharing six of seven identical alleles) are combined as members of a CC (46). Thus, isolates in different CCs are less closely related to one another than those within the CC. Since housekeeping genes are under little selective pressure, the accumulation of changes occurring is typically slow. Because the original MLST approach often had a limited discriminatory power in many organisms for it to be an effective epidemiological tool, other, similar systems targeting more rapidly evolving genes such as virulence-associated genes or genes encoding outer membrane proteins have been developed. This use of virulence factors in an MLST scheme has been referred to as multi-virulence locus sequence typing (MVLST). The experience so far has been mixed. Noller et al. (124) used a combination of seven housekeeping genes (*arcA*, *aroE*, *dnaE*, *mdh*, *gnd*, *gapA*, and *pgm*) and two membrane protein genes (*espA* and *ompA*) to subtype a collection of STEC serotype O157:H7/H− (STEC O157) strains with highly diverse PFGE patterns. Overall, they found a striking lack of diversity in all housekeeping genes as well as in *espA* and only minimal diversity in *ompA*. In contrast, an MLST scheme developed by Zhang et al. (197) for subtyping *Listeria monocytogenes* exclusively targeted virulence genes (*prfA*, *inlV*, and *inlC*) and virulence-associated genes (*dal*, *lisR*, and *clpP*) and was able to discriminate between sporadic isolates that were indistinguishable by PFGE. An MLST assay targeting only two genes, the *por* gene encoding the outer membrane protein porin and the *tbpB* gene encoding the transferrin-binding protein subunit B, has been proven to be a highly discriminatory method for subtyping of *Neisseria gonorrhoeae* and yet being able to accurately identify sexual contact pairs (12). While MLST can be used for epidemiological surveillance for some organisms with plastic genomes, such as *Neisseria*, the key application for it in general is studying phylogeny and evolution of population lineages (191). MLST may also be used to study differences in host preference or virulence potential in human infection between clonal complexes (125).

One key advantage of MLST over gel-based techniques, such as PFGE, is that the sequence data are unambiguous regardless of the type of instrument used to generate them and can be readily compared between laboratories through curated MLST websites such as http://pubmlst.org/ and http://www.mlst.net/. MLST also has a 100% typeability and a high reproducibility. However, sequencing both directions of the DNA strands in multiple loci is rather labor-intensive and expensive compared to some other technologies, such as fragment analysis.

Other Sequencing Applications

The Lancefield M protein is an important virulence factor in group A streptococci (GAS) that is also used for serotype classification. The protein is encoded by the *emm* gene, and the M serotype may be predicted from its sequence (7). The complete set of *emm* sequences and the sequencing protocol are available at http://www.cdc.gov/ncidod/biotech/strep/M-ProteinGene_typing.htm. *emm* typing has made M serotyping available to the broader scientific community while retaining the historical and pathogenic information generated in a relatively few reference laboratories in the course of many years of research by use of the traditional method. Since there is more variation in the *emm* sequence than is apparent from the M type, *emm* typing provides additional discrimination to GAS compared to the classical M-serotyping method (45).

Similarly the capsular type is an important virulence factor for pneumococci. This capsule is encoded by the *cps* gene, and the *cps* sequences of all the pneumococcal serotypes are available at http://www.sanger.ac.uk/Projects/S_pneumoniae/CPS/. A protocol using sequential nested PCRs has been developed to identify the 29 most common pneumococcal serotypes without sequencing the whole gene (128).

Methicillin-resistant *Staphylococcus aureus* (MRSA) contains a large heterogenous mobile genetic element, the staphylococcal chromosomal cassette or SCC*mec*, carrying the *mecA* gene, the central element of methicillin resistance, and the *ccr* locus, which encodes recombinases (*ccrAB* or *ccrC*) involved in SCC*mec* mobility. SCC*mec* types are defined by combining the information on the genetic organization of the *mec* complex with *ccr* type, and so far six major types have been identified. Recent work confirmed the very close relationships among *ccrAB* alleles associated with SCC*mec* types I through IV and VI (126). It was shown that SCC*mec* types I through IV and VI can be predicted by DNA sequencing of an internal fragment of the *ccrB* gene, which enables characterization of the *ccrAB* allele present. This is epidemiologically particularly relevant since different SCC*mec* types are associated with hospital and community MRSA infections (127).

Molecular epidemiologic approaches have been used to study the transmission patterns of numerous viruses. The most common approach is to perform sequence analysis on a defined region of the viral genome that contains sufficient genetic diversity to make valid conclusions based on phylogenetic analyses. The length of these sequence "windows" varies with each viral species. Typical windows include hypervariable regions or genes that are often flanked by relatively conserved regions that make convenient PCR targets. For the purpose of molecular epidemiology, viruses are usually assigned to clades or genotypes, which are represented by established reference strains. In particular, RNA viruses have high mutation rates that increase the amount of sequence variation in the genome (38, 119).

VNTR Analysis

Many microbial genes and intergenic regions contain loci of repetitive DNA that may be variable among strains with respect to the number of repeat units present or their individual structure. These so-called variable-number tandem repeat (VNTR) regions have been identified in essentially all prokaryotic and eukaryotic species and have been successfully used for subtyping purposes (86, 175). Slipped-strand mispairing is the molecular model that best explains the variability of short sequence repeats (171). Stretches of relatively short arrays of repeat units, when being copied by DNA polymerase, may engage in illegitimate base pairing. This forces the polymerase to introduce or delete individual repeat units. The evolutionary clock speeds of different repeat loci are variable; some loci evolve very slowly and others so fast that they are too unstable to be considered as epidemiological markers. Therefore, some loci are better suited for epidemiological tracing than others (176). In the simplest form, VNTR analysis may only include a single locus (155). When multiple loci are targeted, the technology is often referred to as multiple-locus VNTR analysis or MLVA (87).

VNTR loci can be identified from a partial or complete reference genome sequence by using tandem repeat finder software, which is available free of charge on the Web (http://tandem.bu.edu/trf/trf.html). A tandem repeat database (http://minisatellites.u-psud.fr) was also developed to assist in identifying VNTRs from published sequences by using various parameters and query tools (66). A typical MLVA protocol involves a multiplex PCR amplification of VNTR targets, followed by fragment sizing using a high-resolution capillary electrophoresis (106). The use of multiple fluorescent dyes to label the forward primers facilitates multiplexing targets with overlapping fragment sizes. The observed fragment size for each VNTR defines the allele type, and the string of allele types constitutes the MLVA type.

The key application of MLVA is in the field of epidemiological surveillance, where it is used either alone or in combination with other techniques. Since MLVA targets fast-evolving repeat sequences, the discriminatory power of the method can be quite high for many highly clonal organisms that show low diversity with other methods. For example, an MLVA scheme targeting eight VNTRs was able to differentiate laboratory contaminants and non-outbreak-related strains during the 2001 anthrax outbreak in the United States (70). Other organisms that show relatively high diversity with other commonly used methods, such as PFGE, may have clonal subpopulations that can be differentiated using MLVA. This is the case for strains belonging to the *Salmonella enterica* serotype Typhimurium definitive type 104 complex, which until MLVA was introduced could be differentiated only poorly by any subtyping method (170). The downside of targeting fast-evolving genetic elements, such as VNTRs, is that patterns can evolve during an outbreak, complicating data analysis and compromising epidemiological concordance. For example, single- and even double-locus variants have been detected during STEC O157 and *S. enterica* serotype Typhimurium outbreaks (75, 80).

The advantages of MLVA are high throughput, low labor-intensiveness, and a relatively low per-sample cost. As with many other PCR-based techniques, MLVA is vulnerable to PCR artifacts, such as minus-A and stutter peaks, which can interfere with the data analysis. Robustness and reproducibility of the method can be affected by instrument- and reagent-related issues, which in turn can have an impact on the portability of the method and interlaboratory data sharing. For example, significant sizing discrepancies are known to occur between different capillary electrophoresis platforms (79). However, all these issues can be overcome by the proper assay design and optimization, strict adherence to standard operating procedures, and staff training. The overall main weakness of MLVA is that the assays are typically specific to the organism or even the serotype for which they were developed. Only few published assays have attempted to cover multiple serotypes or species (62, 105, 144). On the other hand, the specificity may also be an advantage since virtually all strains are typeable and a fingerprint can also be generated without a pure culture from a primary enrichment sample (unpublished PulseNet USA data).

DNA Microarrays

A DNA microarray is a molecular platform in which a few hundred to thousands of specific DNA oligonucleotides or short sequences (capture molecules) are bound to a matrix. The array is used to detect specific DNA sequences (target sequences) in a test sample of DNA from the organism being investigated by hybridization followed by detection of the array bound test DNA. Two types of arrays, planar and liquid, are used.

Analysis with planar microarrays is typically performed by deposition of DNA probes complementary to the genome targets of interest on a glass slide (solid matrix). Probes are typically synthetically produced oligonucleotides (9 to 100 bp) or PCR products (100 to 1,000 bp). They can target open reading frames (ORFs) amplified from the sequenced reference isolate or short intergenic oligonucleotides based on the available sequence (55). Alternatively, PCR probes may be attached to microspheres that are internally dyed with two spectrally distinct fluorophores and combined to create a suspension array (liquid matrix), such as those seen with the Luminex platform (14, 44). Overall, platforms developed may differ in a number of aspects such as probe content, density, deposition technology, and labeling and hybridization of probes, as well as sample detection and analysis. An ORF-based DNA array can detect losses of entire ORFs but does not detect minor deletions, point mutations, deletions restricted to intergenic spaces, genetic rearrangements, deletions of homologous repetitive elements, or gene insertions. Short oligonucleotide arrays are more precise at the detection of shorter nucleotide polymorphisms but require a larger number of probes, at higher cost. Such oligonucleotide arrays have been developed by companies such as Affymetrix (Santa Clara, CA), Operon (Huntsville, AL), Agilent Technologies (Santa Clara, CA), and NimbleGen (Madison, WI). Insertions of genes compared with the sequenced reference strain cannot be detected in comparative genome hybridization DNA array analysis. This problem can be alleviated by adding nonredundant amplified sequences from several closely related organisms to the array (13).

DNA microarray technology represents an attractive platform for use in bacterial identification and subtyping since it allows for rapid and accurate analysis of large numbers of different DNA molecules. Besides the remarkable resolution, DNA array analysis unveils the genetic region responsible for diversity, often allowing phenotypic predictions at the same time. In addition, due to the basic design of microarrays (i.e., detection of signal associated with sample DNA bound to fixed DNA probes), the positional variation associated with gel-based methods, such as PFGE, is eliminated and the analyses of results are easier to automate and standardize. Limitations of DNA array technology include the initial high cost for the synthesis and spotting of target-specific primers and for the fluorophores used to label the reactions. Ambiguities in the interpretation of the ratios of hybridization and cross-hybridization to analogous targets are also important limitations of the technique. Interlaboratory reproducibility of DNA array-based methods remains still unclear, since multilaboratory validation studies are largely missing. Even though planar arrays allow for the analysis of hundreds of thousands of targets at the same time, sample throughput is an obvious bottleneck of the technology. If the total number of probes can be limited to a few hundred, suspension arrays offer a higher sample throughput platform with lower cost. Currently, the Luminex xMAP system (Luminex Corp., Austin, TX) allows for up to 100 different probes to be analyzed simultaneously in a single well of a 96-well plate.

Pathogen Identification

DNA arrays provide an attractive platform for simultaneous detection of multiple pathogens. This can be accomplished by interrogating a mixture of nucleic acids that is produced from a PCR. One approach is to amplify more universal genes (e.g., 16S rRNA, 18S rRNA, and 23S rRNA) and to screen for pathogen-specific polymorphisms (43, 188). However, universal PCR can be challenging, since commercial PCR reagents are frequently contaminated with trace amounts of bacterial DNA. Additionally, since the detection is based on pathogen-specific point mutations in these genes, naturally occurring variants may not be all represented on the array, resulting in false-negative detection events. An alternative strategy for coupling PCR and DNA array detection is to use multiplex PCR to amplify a number of discreet, pathogen-specific genetic markers. The ability to construct high-density microarrays with multiple probe sequences makes it relatively trivial to include multiple markers for specific pathogens and thus permit greater validity of a positive detection event. The disadvantage of this approach is that there is a practical limit to the number of primer sets that can be included in the PCR (59). Instead of coupling PCR amplification and DNA array detection, applying a direct detection on extracted DNA or RNA is achievable when the amount of target is abundant (14). The primary goal in this case is to avoid amplification biases associated with PCR.

Several microarrays have been developed for rapid identification of viruses including the ViroChip and the GreeneChip (129, 141, 184). These arrays have the capacity to detect a large number of viral pathogens and can quickly identify the etiologic agent in outbreaks of unknown source (16, 81). In some cases, the arrays are designed to detect specific groups of viruses such as respiratory pathogens (26, 27, 104, 185, 193). The lower limit of detection for viruses in clinical samples or cell culture supernatants is approximately 10^3 to 10^4 copies of viral genomes (141). One advantage of the microarrays is that the hybridized DNA can be eluted from the array and sequenced to provide additional sequence data about the viral agent. For example, sequence information from a 1-kb fragment eluted from a microarray helped to confirm that the virus associated with severe acute respiratory syndrome (SARS) was actually a novel coronavirus (184).

Microarrays have been used not only to identify the type of virus in a clinical sample but also to provide information on the genotype or subtype of virus present. Of course, specific arrays are required for genotyping of each viral group. In many cases, sequence analysis may be the more cost-effective means for obtaining a viral genotype. However, there are numerous examples of the use of microarrays for viral genotyping including human rotavirus (28, 74), human and avian influenza viruses (77, 172), hepatitis B virus (131, 158), HIV (162), varicella-zoster virus (150), measles virus (122), human papillomavirus (47, 98), polioviruses (25), and noroviruses (16, 81).

Binary Typing

Binary typing is an alternative DNA-based typing method to MLST and is suitable for organisms with a large variation in genetic content. In binary typing, each strain is assigned a signature based on the presence or absence of a set of defined DNA sequences rather than allelic profiles. The resulting string of ones and zeros, correlating to the presence or absence of the chosen genetic regions, creates a portable "binary" type that, at least in theory, should be easily comparable across the laboratories. Either all ORFs from the sequenced genome or selected sequences can be included in the binary typing array depending on the level of discrimination desired.

Leonard et al. (100) constructed a binary typing microarray for *Campylobacter jejuni* that contained 99% of all ORFs of the sequenced reference genome. Results from the limited evaluation indicated an increased discriminatory power over other typing methods and showed that the majority of divergent genes were associated with surface modifications, which may reflect the selection of *C. jejuni* strains that survive the host immune response.

Pelludat et al. (136) used DNA fragments derived from subtractive hybridization experiments, many of them targeting noncoding regions, and sequences available on the public data banks to construct a prototype binary typing array with 83 targets for *S. enterica* serotype Typhimurium. The results indicated that arrays with a smaller number of targeted probes may be a valuable tool in discriminating closely related strains.

This is also the case in spacer oligotyping (spoligotyping) (178), a method that is routinely used for international surveillance of strains belonging to the *M. tuberculosis* complex. The target in this method is the variable spacer region between the conserved direct repeats in the clustered regularly interspaced short palindromic repeats (CRISPR) region of the *M. tuberculosis* genome. There is considerable variability in the number of repeats and therefore also the presence of spacers in this region. By detection of the spacers, a binary measure for the presence of the associated repeats is obtained. In the procedure, the whole CRISPR region is amplified by PCR, followed by hybridization and detection of the amplicons using probes specific for 43 to 51 spacers. In the earlier version of the method, the probes were bound to a membrane, but recently a DNA array-based method has been introduced (157). The method is useful for differentiating strains of *M. tuberculosis* and *M. bovis* that contain no or only a few copies of the IS6110 sequence and are therefore poorly differentiated by IS6110 fingerprinting.

SNPs

A simplified approach to sequence-based subtyping is the detection of single-nucleotide polymorphisms (SNPs). A SNP is a change in a single nucleotide in one sequence relative to another caused by nucleotide mutation, horizontal gene transfer, or intragenic recombination events. Some SNP systems have been developed as a means of simplifying MLST schemes. They offer the same phylogenetic information as the MLST schemes on which they are based but with less discrimination and are incapable of identifying new allelic types. Such SNP schemes are therefore generally not suitable for laboratory-based surveillance focusing on cluster detection (9, 73). SNP discovery can be accomplished by sequencing a number of defined target genes with a high rate of polymorphism, such as those associated with antibiotic resistance (102). A more universal approach to identify likely SNPs is to use data provided by genome-sequencing studies to generate a microarray containing probes corresponding to each of the nucleotides of potential gene SNP targets (198). Likely polymorphic loci are identified when DNAs from multiple strains are hybridized with the array. Since the mutation rate in ORFs in some highly clonal organisms is slow due to selective pressure (101), targeting intergenic regions for detection of SNPs seems to be a better strategy. For example, Hu et al. (76) identified possibly useful SNPs for subtyping *S. enterica* serotype Typhimurium by sequencing intergenic regions in 46 closely related isolates. Whether an identified SNP is indeed a novel SNP or is already contained in the National Center for Biotechnology Information dbSNP database (154) is often difficult to determine. Additionally, identifying the minimum set of SNPs that will generate epidemiologically relevant data can be difficult, since it appears that many SNPs are coinherited (108). A number of different software applications such as Haploview (5) and Seq-SNPing (24) are available on the Web free of charge to assist in these tasks. In order to obtain a set of SNPs that represents the diversity of a species in an unbiased manner, it is crucial that mutation discovery be performed on a set of strains that are representative of the breadth of diversity and the phylogenetic lineages of that species. Since the protocols developed to date are all serotype or species specific, it remains unclear whether a universal SNP typing protocol could be applied for multiple serotypes of the same species or multiple closely related species.

Even though planar microarrays are ideal SNP screening tools in the protocol development phase, suspension array technology offers a more flexible and higher-throughput platform for routine SNP subtyping protocols. Typically, genomic regions containing SNPs are amplified using multiplex PCR and the amplification products are used as templates for allele-specific primer extension reactions in which probes attached to fluorescent polystyrene microspheres serve as primers (41). Allele-specific primer extension is based on placing the probes so that the last nucleotide of the probe is placed over the SNP. A polymerase reaction can only be initiated if the probe ends with a perfect match (42). A SNP protocol can also be divided into subassays for different genetic subpopulations inside the species in question. For example, lineage-specific SNP typing protocols have been developed for the four lineages of *L. monocytogenes*, facilitating more-targeted and more-cost-effective typing of strains (41, 186).

Genome Comparison

Besides pathogen identification and genotyping, microarrays provide a rapid means for resequencing the complete genomes of viral agents (190). For these techniques, oligonucleotide probes representing the complete viral genome are synthesized in situ by using the standard resequencing array tiling strategy consisting of eight unique 25-bp probes per base position. Each 25-bp probe is varied at the central position to incorporate each possible base substitution, allowing for the detection of both known and new SNPs. In the most common strategy, large fragments of the viral genome are amplified by PCR or reverse transcriptase PCR, fragmented with DNase, labeled, and hybridized to the microarray chip. For many viruses, the PCR amplification requires viral nucleic acids that are prepared after passage of the virus in cell culture. While this technique can be rapid, the cost of designing and reproducing the sequencing chips can be significant. Resequencing arrays have been used to sequence the complete or nearly complete genomes of many viruses including the novel coronavirus associated with SARS (163, 193), HIV (174), and the 200-kb genome of poxviruses (164, 165).

Whole-Genome Sequencing

Steady advances in sequencing technology have allowed the transition from labor-intensive whole-genome sequencing of single strains to comparison of multiple strains within the same species or subtype. Sequencing projects on this scale allow the detection of novel chromosomal alterations between isolates at the single-nucleotide level, such as SNPs, repetitive elements, recombination, and insertions and deletions. Recent advances in automation and informatics have reduced the amount of time required for generation of whole-genome sequences from years to months or less. Included in these improvements are processes that eliminated the need for subcloning DNA fragments prior to sequencing (109) and detailed physical maps generated through optical scanning that serve as a guide to allow rapid sequence assembly, characterization of gaps, and validation of the finished sequence (97). In addition, completely different next-generation sequencing technologies, such as pyrosequencing (30) and resequencing microarrays (198), could reach the throughput necessary to achieve whole-genome sequencing. Some of the next-generation technologies commercially available today include the 454 GS-FLX instrument (Roche Applied Science, Basel, Switzerland), the Solexa 1 G analyzer (Illumina, Inc., San Diego, CA), and the SOLiD instrument (Applied Biosystems, Foster City, CA). The 454 technology is based on pyrosequencing on solid support and can produce read lengths of up to 300 bp (117). The Solexa and SOLiD technologies are based on sequencing by synthesis with reversible terminators and massively parallel sequencing by ligation, respectively, but can only generate read lengths of 30 to 40 bp (117). While short reads are useful for detection of substitution polymorphisms against a reference genome, they are more difficult to use for de novo assembly of a new genome, especially if the genome being investigated contains large sections of repeated sequences. However, a recent report indicated that using a mix of new sequencing technologies showed promise for producing high-quality drafts for small genomes (less than 4.0 Mb) (4). A software has also been described for assembling short reads by progressively searching a prefix tree for the longest possible overlap between any two sequences (http://www.bcgsc.ca/bioinfo/software/ssake) (187). At this time, whole-genome sequencing has limited use in the comparison of large numbers of bacterial isolates of the same species. Therefore, its utility for subtyping purposes has yet to be truly evaluated. In general, the current focus and also most likely the future focus of whole-genome sequencing of bacteria are the identification of core genetic elements and areas of variation between the strains that could then be used for more-targeted subtyping schemes (121). Continued improvements could see additional reductions in time and cost associated with whole-genome sequencing. However, interpretation of whole-genome sequencing data may present a daunting challenge to provide meaningful information for bacterial subtyping in an outbreak investigation due to the inherent instability of some genomic regions.

In contrast to the use with eukaryotes and prokaryotes, whole-genome sequencing is routinely used to answer specific epidemiological questions relating to viral infections. Advances in sequencing technology have led to a substantial increase in the number of complete viral genome sequences available on the various databases. This vast amount of information is critical to studies of viral pathogenesis and to the design of novel drugs and antiviral agents. The information can also be used to develop unique signatures that can be used to detect viruses or groups of viruses (31).

Some viruses have the capacity to recombine or reassort their genomes, and in these cases whole-genome sequencing is an important component of molecular epidemiologic studies. The live attenuated strains used in the WHO polio eradication program replicate in the human gut and can be excreted for several weeks after immunization. If the attenuating mutations in the vaccine strains revert, the vaccine may cause vaccine-associated paralytic poliomyelitis in vaccinees or result in transmissible, neurovirulent, circulating vaccine-derived poliovirus strains that have been associated with outbreaks of poliomyelitis (116, 194). The vaccine-derived polioviruses often contain mosaic genomes that result from recombination between the vaccine strains and other lineages of poliovirus or other enteroviruses (3, 194), and these variants can only be detected by full-genome sequencing.

Influenza viruses have segmented RNA genomes, and newly emergent strains can have genomes composed of gene segments derived from strains circulating in humans and animals. Analysis of the complete genomic sequence provides clues as to the origin of the new strains. A very recent example is the analysis of the complete genome of the H1N1 strain of swine origin that emerged in 2009, which showed that the virus had been circulating in humans for an extended period as the result of a single introduction. The new strain had genome segments derived from swine, human, and avian strains (57).

APPLICATIONS

Molecular Surveillance

Molecular Serotyping

Serotyping is a subtyping method in which specific antigens on the surface of microorganisms are detected by antigen-antibody reactions using diagnostic antisera. The method is definitive but only moderately discriminatory. It has nevertheless proven to be extremely useful for epidemiologic classification of a number of pathogens and has for this reason been a mainstay in the surveillance of different infectious diseases for more than 70 years. It is a cumbersome method that requires the availability of high-quality antisera and substantial expertise to perform the assay and interpret the results. More convenient, rapid, and reliable molecular alternatives to serotyping are being developed. These molecular serotyping methods are designed to generate data that are in close or complete agreement with conventional serotyping in order not to lose the connection to the historical data. In the previous sections molecular flagellin typing of *Campylobacter* (*flaA* typing), M serotyping (*emm* typing) of GAS, and capsular (*cps*) typing of pneumococci have been mentioned.

In the genus *Salmonella,* more than 2,500 serotypes are currently recognized (65). Yoshida et al. (196) recently reported a proof-of-concept study in which a planar DNA microarray was constructed to detect the top five *Salmonella* serovars in Canada (Typhimurium, Enteritidis, Heidelberg, Hadar, and Thompson). The assay targeted the *rfb* gene cluster genes directly involved in the O-antigen synthesis (*rfbJ, rfbS,* and *wbaA*) and the flagellar genes for phases 1 and 2 (*fliC* and *fljB*). Even though the high-density planar array assay can be easily expanded to include more serotypes in the future, the sample throughput and high cost may prove to be prohibitive for this assay to be widely adopted in public health laboratories. Fitzgerald et al. (50) developed a suspension array-based assay specific for *Salmonella* O groups for detection of the six most common serogroups (B, C1, C2, D, E, and O13) in the United States and serotype Paratyphi A. Depending on the serogroup, *abe*, *prt*, *wzy*, or *wzx* genes in the *rfb* gene cluster were chosen as targets. All seven targets were amplified simultaneously by multiplex PCR, and the serogroups were identified by specific probes attached to fluorescently labeled microspheres. The assay correctly and specifically identified 94% of the isolates tested in comparison to conventional serotyping and was also capable of generating serotype data for rough isolates that do not express the O antigen. Work is under way to combine this O-group identification system with DNA targets specific for H antigens to establish a comprehensive DNA-based scheme for identification of the major (top 100) *Salmonella* serotypes causing infections in humans. This typing scheme will be subdivided in multiple reactions for use in tiered fashion; i.e., the first reaction would cover the top 20 most prevalent serotypes, the second one the next 20 to 50, etc. The major advantage of the system is that it targets the genes encoding the serotype-specific antigens. Thereby, the system is compatible with the Kauffman-White scheme, which contains the phenotypic descriptions of all *Salmonella* serotypes (65), and it will be possible to identify serotypes that were not originally included in the validation of the genotyping scheme.

Cluster Detection and Outbreak Investigations

Subtyping methods that are used for community-wide routine surveillance to detect disease case clusters and to support outbreak investigations need to be rapid, highly discriminatory, reproducible, and amenable to library subtyping so trends in the occurrence of the organisms they target may be followed easily. Often subtyping results are the only information available to determine if an outbreak investigation should be initiated. In this situation, the case definition needs to be very specific; i.e., the discriminatory power of the subtyping method needs to be high, in order not to include patients that are not associated with the outbreak as cases and thereby confusing the epidemiological investigation. The molecular methods that are most suitable for this purpose are PFGE, MLVA, AFLP (when used in one center), highly discriminatory DNA array, and gene sequencing methods. These methods may be used in conjunction with less discriminatory traditional and molecular methods, e.g., biotyping, serotyping, phage typing, antibiograms, and/or plasmid profiling.

PulseNet, the national molecular subtyping network for foodborne disease surveillance, is a prime example of a network performing real-time surveillance of infectious diseases at the community level. It uses PFGE as the preferred subtyping method and considers only isolates with indistinguishable patterns for cluster detection. An outbreak of STEC O157:H7 that occurred in the summer of 2002 was caused by a strain with a pattern that differed from the most common pattern in the PulseNet database by just one band (Fig. 3A). Forty-four case patients with the outbreak pattern were identified, but during the outbreak period 41 isolates with the related most common pattern were also detected (Fig. 3B); in a case-control or in other interview studies, including these 41 patients infected with isolates displaying the common pattern as cases would have completely obscured the association with the vehicle, ground beef from one particular plant (58). As more supporting epidemiological information is gathered, it may be possible to amend the microbiological case definition. In the above-mentioned outbreak, two cases with epidemiological links

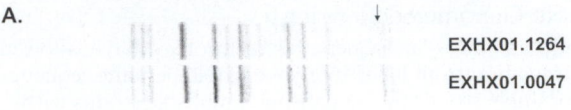

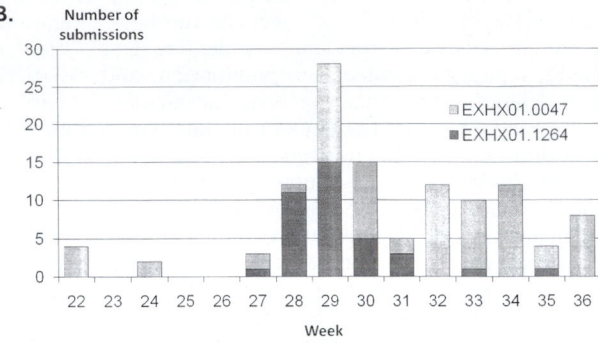

FIGURE 3 PFGE profiles of STEC O157 strains in PulseNet, showing the most common sporadic pattern EXHX01.0047 and the outbreak-associated pattern EXHX01.1264 (A) and their occurrence during the outbreak period (B).

to the outbreak were added to the list of case patients even though they were infected with a strain displaying the most common variant pattern.

The requirements for methods used for surveillance and investigation of outbreaks in hospitals and other institutions may be different from the ones used in the community: the setting is much smaller in scale, usually attended by a single laboratory, and the outbreaks are often caused by pathogens transmitted from person to person and/or by pathogens that persist in the environment. Strains that are involved in outbreaks transmitted between patients or persistently from the environment often evolve during the outbreak, and variant subtypes may be present at the same time. This was the basis for the much-cited "Tenover criteria" for interpretation of PFGE results (168); they state that strains may be related if they differ from each other by up to six restriction bands corresponding to two genetic events. Obviously these criteria do not apply to point source outbreaks. The methods that are used for community-wide surveillance may also be used for these nosocomial outbreaks, and methods that do not show good interlaboratory reproducibility may be used as long as the intralaboratory reproducibility is sufficient. AFLP has excellent intralaboratory reproducibility, and even RAPD and rep-PCR may be used for short-term surveillance and to delineate outbreaks that have been detected by other means, e.g., by phenotypic methods (51, 110, 120, 182). In local library subtyping of nosocomial pathogens, there may be a place for the semiautomated rep-PCR described in "rep-PCR" above.

The combination of molecular epidemiologic techniques and standard case classification and reporting provides a very sensitive means to describe the transmission pathways of many viruses. In particular, analysis of the sequence data can help confirm the source of virus or suggest a source for cases in which the source was unknown. The molecular data can be used to establish epidemiologic links, or lack thereof, between various cases and outbreaks. Molecular techniques have been particularly useful for the study of outbreaks of foodborne viruses such as norovirus (134). In these cases, the sequence data were used to identify the source and to trace the transport and distribution of contaminated food (39, 130).

For highly infectious viruses such as measles virus, transmission can occur anywhere. Molecular techniques have been used to identify the source of the infections when standard case investigations have failed to identify a source (146).

Source Attribution

Source attribution is the epidemiological science that studies the relative contribution of different sources to the burden of infectious diseases. Strictly speaking, outbreak investigations are source attribution analyses, but the term is more commonly used in a broader sense encompassing both outbreak-related and sporadic disease. Molecular methods may be used to study the geographic distribution or sources and spread of microbial strains, and this is discussed in "Geographic Spread" below.

Source attribution using microbiological methods is gaining increasing attention, especially in the study of foodborne disease to estimate where in the food production chain the largest public health problems originate. The decision makers use these estimates to prioritize where the control efforts can be exerted most efficiently. A subtyping method that is used for source attribution creates subtypes that are distributed unevenly among the different possible sources of human infection. When this knowledge is combined with information about the distribution of the same subtypes in sick humans and, if available, the human exposure rates to each source, it is possible to estimate the relative contribution of each source to the burden of human disease (139). Using this approach, Sheppard et al. (153) performed source attribution on *Campylobacter jejuni* and *Campylobacter coli* in Scotland, using MLST. They identified chicken meat as the principal source of the disease, with ruminants being associated with most of the remaining isolates.

The limitation of the model is that it can only attribute to sources for which there are data available; i.e., if no isolates are included from a potential major source, no estimates for this source will be generated. Subtyping methods used for source attribution do not need to be as discriminatory or reproducible as those used for outbreak investigations, as long as they clearly differentiate isolates from different sources. Choosing a subtyping method with an unnecessarily high discriminatory power will increase the complexity of the analysis of the data set. In regard to *Campylobacter*, PFGE is the gold standard for outbreak investigations whereas the less discriminatory method MLST works well for attribution. Theoretically, subtyping methods that provide phylogenetic information are more useful for source attribution than methods that do not provide this information, since the data collected from each source are likely not to be all-inclusive. Even if some subtyping information is missing, the data may still be useful since strains that are related phylogenetically to each other are more likely to originate from the same source.

Dynamics of Infectious Disease

Pathogen Evolution

Molecular techniques have made enormous contributions to our understanding of the evolution of pathogens, but a detailed description of these studies is beyond the scope of this chapter. Molecular techniques have been used to monitor the distribution of circulating strains of various pathogens, to monitor the stability of antigenic sites that are important both for diagnostics and as vaccine targets, and to assess susceptibility to antimicrobial drugs.

Improvements in computational molecular biology resources and new analytical methods such as BEAST (40) incorporate sample date and allow the evolutionary dynamics of a population to be inferred from sequence data. These approaches are called "phylodynamics" (63). With these approaches, sequence information from infectious agents can be used to infer the transmission patterns of that agent over time. Analysis of hepatitis C virus sequences from Egypt suggested an exponential increase in the number of cases in the 1930s and in 1955, when unsterile needles were used to distribute antischistosomal therapy (140). Similar studies documented the episodic transmission of HIV into London during the late 1990s (103). More recently, these methods were used to investigate the source of influenza virus A H1N1 (2009) of swine origin that was associated with the influenza pandemic in 2009 and 2010 (156).

Geographic Spread

The ability of a molecular technique to identify the source of an infectious agent can be applied on a global scale, and the information can be used to monitor the spread of the pathogen. The sensitivity of this approach depends on the level of surveillance activity and the availability of a global database of genetic information. Sequence analysis was used to identify the source of the West Nile virus that was introduced into the United States in 1999 and to track the spread of this lineage of virus across the entire country (96, 145), as well as to track the global spread of various genetic variants of HIV (95).

Sustained Transmission in Areas That Are Destined for Pathogen Elimination

Molecular surveillance for viral diseases that are prevented by vaccination is especially beneficial when it is possible to observe the change in viral genotypes over time in a particular country or region. This information, when analyzed in conjunction with standard epidemiologic data, has helped to document the interruption of transmission of endemic viruses and provides a means to measure the success of vaccination programs.

Molecular characterization of measles viruses has provided a valuable tool for measuring the effectiveness of measles control programs. In general, three patterns of measles virus genotype distribution have been described. In countries in which transmission of measles is still endemic, the majority of cases are caused by several endemic genotypes that are distributed geographically. In these cases, multiple cocirculating lineages within the endemic genotype or genotypes are present. In countries that have eliminated measles, the small numbers of cases are caused by a number of different genotypes that reflect various sources of imported virus and suggest the lack of sustained transmission of an endemic genotype or genotypes. The third pattern occurs in countries or regions that have had very good measles control but are experiencing an increase in the numbers of susceptible individuals because of failure to maintain high vaccination coverage rates. In this situation, reintroduction of measles usually results in a large outbreak associated with a single genotype of virus with nearly identical sequences (146).

Pathogen Discovery and Identification

Molecular methods are sometimes crucial for the discovery of new pathogens, especially viral pathogens, and to determine if a pathogen is truly new or has arisen from known pathogens through recombination or other genetic events.

For example, coronaviruses have the ability to recombine with other coronaviruses as well as to incorporate cellular genes into their genomes (71). The initial analysis of the complete genome sequence of the coronavirus associated with SARS confirmed that the virus was a novel coronavirus and not a recombinant between previously described coronaviruses (94, 147).

Vaccination Issues

Live attenuated vaccines are used to control a number of viral diseases. In some cases these vaccines can cause symptoms that are similar to those caused by infection with wild-type virus. When the risk of exposure to disease is very low, these vaccine reactions can be identified by temporal association with vaccination. However, when vaccination is used as part of an outbreak response, it may be difficult to distinguish vaccine reactions from symptoms caused by the wild-type virus. Since serologic techniques usually lack the sensitivity to distinguish between antibodies directed at the vaccine or the wild-type strain, genetic characterization of the viruses is usually the only means available to clearly classify the case as vaccine associated or due to a wild-type infection. Of course, this approach requires that appropriate specimens for virologic detection be collected from the suspected cases and that sequence information be available for the vaccine strains.

The availability of molecular methods that can clearly identify vaccine reactions, as described above, has contributed to our knowledge about the safety of live attenuated vaccines. In addition, molecular techniques now play an important role in the postlicensure evaluation of live attenuated viral vaccines. Here, genetic characterization is used to monitor the stability of vaccines in the field and to clearly identify vaccine reactions. In one example, PCR and RFLP were used to monitor the safety of varicella-zoster vaccine by classifying vesicular rash or zoster cases as being associated with wild-type varicella-zoster virus of the Oka vaccine strain (54).

In some cases, data from molecular surveillance of viral and bacterial pathogens are used to decide on the most appropriate formulation for vaccines. The geographic distribution of strains may affect the efficacy of the vaccines if the genetic changes are accompanied by changes in antigenicity. Therefore, for agents with variable antigenic properties (e.g., rotavirus and influenza virus), careful monitoring of the strains associated with cases in vaccinated populations is necessary (8, 132, 133).

Forensic Microbiology

Sometimes infectious disease incidents are criminally investigated if there is a suspicion that they may be the result of deliberate actions or criminal gross negligence. HIV-infected individuals have been imprisoned for spreading the virus intentionally (113) or through negligence (99), and anthrax has been spread through the mail (70, 88). Numerous outbreaks of foodborne infections occur each year, and some have been the result of intentional contamination of the food supply (169). Forensic molecular epidemiology comes into play when regulators, laymen, judges, and lawyers have to decide if an infection (or infections) is a result of criminal action. In principle, criminal microbiological investigations are not different from outbreak investigations, except that in criminal investigations the link between the infection(s) and its source(s) needs to be proven beyond reasonable doubt. In outbreak investigations, the precautionary principle is relatively often used when deciding on public

health actions since the aim of an outbreak investigation is to stop the outbreak from spreading as soon as possible. This is in contrast to criminal investigations, in which the precautionary principle is not used since an offender is presumed innocent until proven otherwise. Subtyping methods that may quantify the probability that two microbial strains are related are therefore preferred over methods that do not yield direct quantifiable information. Non-target-specific methods are therefore not ideal for criminal investigations because DNA fragments of the same size may have completely different sequence content; e.g., it is not possible to tell from the PFGE pattern if two isolates are identical, hence the use of the term "indistinguishable" for PFGE patterns that cannot be differentiated from each other. In contrast, differences observed with a target-specific method may be quantifiable if the prevalence of the detected alleles is known in the relevant microbial populations.

SUBTYPING METHOD SELECTION, VALIDATION, AND DATA INTERPRETATION

Method Selection

All too often it appears that the selection of subtyping methods is only guided by convenience criteria, in particular, the accessibility of a method to the laboratory. This has led to numerous studies in which an inappropriate method was used to study an organism (177). When selecting a subtyping method, one should first of all consider the epidemiological context it is going to be used in, i.e., determine the question that the typing data should answer. A method that is appropriate for long-term surveillance is most likely not appropriate for a short-term investigation of a nosocomial outbreak. Careful consideration should also be given for the genetic makeup of the target organisms, including the clonality, mode of transmission, and outbreak potential.

Factors That Affect the "Clonality" of a Given Population

The clonal relatedness of isolates is manifested by their display of a significantly higher level of similarity in their genotype and/or phenotype than can be expected from randomly sampled and epidemiologically unrelated isolates of the same species (177). The simplest explanation for a genetically monomorphic pathogen is that the population size of the ancestors of all extant organisms was so strongly reduced during a recent bottleneck that genetic diversity was abolished. One possibility that can result in such a bottleneck is a crucial genetic event that only happened once, such as a change in ecological niche due to the acquisition of two plasmids by the progenitor of *Yersinia pestis* (2). In the case of STEC O157, it has been suggested that clonality could be explained by source-sink evolution dynamics (101). According to this theory, mutations in microbes that reside mainly in reservoirs (the source, i.e., cattle) in which they are not pathogens confer on a small subset a phenotype that results in injury to an accidental host (the sink, i.e., humans). Alternatively, it has been argued that a strong selective advantage conferred by a mutation enabled certain strains of STEC O157 to flourish in cattle, making them more available for spillover into humans (101). On the other hand, some host-restricted pathogens, such as *S. enterica* serotype Typhi, are under relatively little selection pressure from its host or environment and therefore do not diversify through point mutations, recombination, or acquisition of new sequences (72). Finally, a sampling bias may also contribute to the appearance of population clonality. Sampling from one part of the phylogenetic tree will overlook much of the variation present in the population and collapse all isolates outside the studied population into a single type (135). In order to be able to adequately discriminate clonal organisms, subtyping methods targeting fast-evolving genetic elements, such as VNTRs or SNPs, are usually preferred (89). With some organisms, optimal results may be obtained by using multiple techniques, e.g., PFGE and VNTR analysis (80).

Method Validation

Once a proper method or approach has been selected, it must be subjected to the highest scrutiny possible to ensure that it meets the criteria discussed in "Subtyping Methods" above. This includes validation using a population of strains and isolates that originates from the epidemiological context in which the method is going to be applied. Techniques that will be applied in local investigations need to be validated on a strain collection from the same locality, whereas methods that will be used for community-wide surveillance need to be validated on a collection of strains reflecting the diversity in the whole community. When a subtyping method that has been validated for use in one given epidemiological context is to be used in a different one, it may be necessary to validate it in the new context before it is implemented. This supplementing validation may not need to be as thorough as the original validation, depending on how similar the two contexts are.

Unlike methods developed in isolation (for use by one laboratory), methods to be used in multiple laboratories for the generation of data archived in reference libraries must be particularly carefully tested, evaluated, and validated. All methods need to go through four phases of validation: initial development, internal validation, external validation, and finally postimplementation evaluation. The first two phases often overlap. Additionally, before the new method is implemented, a quality assurance and quality control (QA/QC) program needs to be established.

The goal of the initial development is to identify the optimal conditions or parameters to ensure that the protocol is robust and reproducible and generates highly discriminatory and epidemiologically concordant data on all strains. Typically, 10 to 50 isolates that represent the diversity in the study population at large are used in this phase.

During the internal validation, the method is tested by individuals not involved in the method development in order to ascertain the robustness of the protocol in the hands of laboratorians with no prior experience with it. The panel of test isolates is expanded to include the full genetic diversity of the study population and should contain both sporadic and outbreak-related isolates in order to test the true discriminatory power and the epidemiological concordance of the method. Duplicate isolates of the same strain and multiple strains from single-source outbreaks need to be included to evaluate the reproducibility and stability of the method. The test panel usually contains between 100 and 300 isolates. The isolates need to be selected from a collection of strains with a known subtype if a gold standard subtyping method exists for the organism in order to be able to evaluate the performance of the new method against this gold standard.

During the external validation, the robustness and portability of the method are further tested, typically by 5 to 10 external partner laboratories, ideally with different levels of subtyping expertise and access to different types or brands of equipment and reagents. The assay is evaluated by using 10 to 50 isolates selected by the laboratory that developed the method. The interlaboratory reproducibility of the method is also assessed during this phase. Sometimes the external validation is further expanded to include a prospective or retrospective testing of up to 50 isolates from each laboratory's own collection.

Following the successful completion of these phases, the method may be implemented. However, even after its implementation, the performance of the assay needs to be assessed on a regular basis to detect problems not identified during the initial validation and to assess emerging situations such as the impact of introduction of new brands of reagents that may have become commercially available.

Diagnostic methods also need to be validated before they are implemented, by use of a process similar to the one described in this chapter. This is described in chapter 4.

QA/QC

A QA program needs to be in place before any molecular subtyping technique is implemented to ensure consistent quality and reproducibility of the data generated. At a minimum, subtyping should be performed only by personnel trained in working with the procedure; a written standard operating procedure should be in place, and a strain with a well-established stable subtype should be included in all experiments in order to detect procedural failures. For library subtyping systems involving multiple laboratories, participation in a certification, a proficiency testing, and an external quality assessment program is mandatory.

Data Interpretation

When interpreting subtyping results, one must consider the epidemiological context and all other available data, such as associated demographic and other epidemiological information, and other subtyping information, e.g., biochemical reaction profiles, serotype, phage type, antimicrobial susceptibility profiles, and presence of virulence factors; reliance on a single parameter for characterization should be avoided whenever possible. Knowledge about the subtyping method should also be considered, including the quality of the data, the diversity of the organism, and the history of the subtypes encountered (6).

Quality of the Data

Even when a carefully standardized procedure is followed, artifacts may occur which may lead to erroneous conclusions about relationships between profiles. It is therefore important to know the nature of these artifacts in order to recognize and correct them. In this, the role of the database curator is extremely important. In PFGE, the artifacts include, among other things, ghost bands caused by incomplete restriction and subtle differences in band resolution (one thick band versus two thinner bands) (6). In PCR-based methods, such as RAPD and rep-PCR, differences in band intensities are a huge problem, and in MLVA, PCR artifacts, such as minus-A and stutter peaks, can confuse data interpretation (37). Also sequence trace files should be routinely checked for quality either manually or by using software (e.g., Phred/Phrap; http://www.phrap.org). Most major sequence databases require the submission of the raw sequence trace files from the laboratory when a new allele type is proposed (1).

Diversity of the Organism

Optimal interpretation of the differences (or lack thereof) between subtypes of two isolates depends largely on the variability of the organism being typed. Large databases should provide sufficient data to make reasonable determinations of diversity. If an organism displays little diversity, one should be cautious in assuming that closely related patterns, or even indistinguishable patterns, indicate a high likelihood that they originate from a common source. In this case, additional data from other typing methods and other available information should be considered. If the organism shows substantial diversity, one must still consider whether there are clonal subpopulations within a nonclonal organism. On the other hand, when an organism demonstrates extreme variability, any pattern matches may be significant.

Epidemiological Context

If the epidemiological setting from which the isolates are derived appears to be a point source outbreak without continued transmission, only very minor differences are likely to be observed because the outbreak strain has very little time to undergo genetic changes. In contrast, when there is ongoing transmission, such as prolonged hospital or community outbreaks, with strains being passed from person to person, more variability should be expected. Additionally, the amount of variation seen during an outbreak depends on the stability of the genetic markers targeted by the typing method. Fast-evolving genetic markers, such as VNTRs, tend to change slightly even during shorter outbreaks (80). During investigations of known outbreaks it is fairly easy and often helpful to designate patterns that differ slightly from the primary outbreak pattern as subpatterns or variants. However, when performing surveillance for cluster/outbreak detection, accepting such variations may mislead the epidemiological investigation (58), especially if one of the variants represents a common pattern as described in "Cluster Detection and Outbreak Investigations" above.

It is also important to consider how the laboratory results fit together with the epidemiologic and environmental investigations. The fact that common subtypes exist for many organisms demonstrates that indistinguishable subtypes alone do not unequivocally prove an epidemiologic connection. It is always possible that two individuals could have been infected with the same strain from different sources. On the other hand, clearly differing subtypes do not prove that isolates are epidemiologically unrelated, since multiple strains can be associated with the same outbreak and some strains contains genetic elements, e.g., prophages, that are incorporated in the genome in an unstable manner and therefore may affect the subtype of different colonies picked from the same pure culture of the organism (11).

LIBRARIES FOR MOLECULAR EPIDEMIOLOGY

International travel, migration, and food trade are the main factors that have contributed to the worldwide spread of microbes. Therefore, the need for international databases with standardized type nomenclature and information on epidemiologically relevant strains has emerged. Building such databases relies upon standardization of typing methods and on regular ring trials for all participating laboratories, to guarantee consistently comparable data.

Strain Catalogues

Strain catalogue databases are mainly public-access websites with limited-access components in some of them. Their main function is to standardize subtype nomenclature and facilitate data sharing. Most of them are curated but typically contain minimal epidemiological or demographic information about the strains and are therefore not very useful for real-time epidemiological surveillance. The laboratories that contribute data to strain catalogues use protocols that vary in the level of standardization from none (MLVA) to medium (*spa* typing).

The best-known examples of strain libraries are the two MLST databases that are hosted on Web servers located at Imperial College London (http://www.mlst.net) (1) and Oxford University (http://pubmlst.org) (83). At MLST.net, species-specific information, including limited epidemiological data, can be accessed on each of the mlst.net species websites, whereas pubmlst.org software enables multiple client databases to query a single species-specific profiles database, so that the information on isolates can be kept private for security or confidentiality reasons. Each species-specific database holds the sequences of all known alleles at each of the MLST loci and through the curator assigns new allele numbers and sequence types. The websites also provide clustering tools to explore the relationship of the query strain with other strains in the database.

SeqNet.org, coordinated by the Münster University Hospital and Robert Koch Institute in Wernigerode, Germany, is an example of a non-MLST-based strain catalogue. SeqNet is an initiative of 50 national reference laboratories and university laboratories from 27 European countries to establish a network of sequence-based typing of microbial pathogens (52). SeqNet currently only has a database for *S. aureus spa* types through the curated "SpaServer." Unlike the two MLST databases, SeqNet has a QA/QC aspect built in it in the form of a one-time certification and annual ring trials.

The *ccrB* typing tool (http://www.ccrbtyping.net) is a public online resource for storage and automatic analysis of MRSA *ccrB* sequences (127). The user's sequence is assigned to an allele based on 100% homology with an existing allele or to a new allele if a homology between 90% and 100% to any of the available alleles is found. In the case of a new allele, the most similar allele is indicated. Based on the allele assignment, a prediction of the *ccrAB* allotype and SCC*mec* type is also provided.

International databases for MLVA data have also been recently established. MLVAbank (http://mlva.u-psud.fr), hosted by University of Orsay, Orsay, France, has both public and private databases available for a handful of organisms (62). The public databases have been derived from published data, sometimes by merging publications from different groups. Since the VNTR markers used by different groups are not always the same because of the current lack of standardization, different data sets may be available for different sets of isolates. Since different sets of primers are sometimes used for the same marker by different groups and since there are sizing discrepancies between different capillary electrophoresis platforms, the data are not always directly comparable even though they are uploaded to MLVAbank as repeat copy numbers. MLVA-NET (http://www.pasteur.fr/mlva), hosted by the Pasteur Institute, tries to circumvent this problem by incorporating raw size data that are automatically translated by the system into allele numbers that have user-defined bins (67). Hence, for a given set of markers, data at least in theory can be compared across the data sets even if contributing laboratories have different preferences for bin definition or allele number assignment. In reality, however, MLVA-NET is currently not capable of normalizing sizing discrepancies seen between different capillary electrophoresis platforms.

The TB database (http://www.tbdb.org) is an integrated database for TB research that houses both annotated genome sequence data for several M. *tuberculosis* strains and microarray and reverse transcriptase PCR expression data from in vitro experiments and TB-infected tissues (143). Experimental data may be deposited into the database by any TB researcher prior to publication, providing prepublication access to tools for the analysis, annotation, visualization, and sharing of data. The data are then made public at the author's request or following publication. The database curators also actively search literature for publications containing relevant TB or host microarray data and then obtain the raw data from the researchers and load them into the database.

Surveillance Databases

Surveillance databases are restricted-access curated databases for real-time sharing of subtyping data and detailed demographic information associated with the strains. The main function of surveillance databases is to rapidly detect and define clusters of disease in order to initiate and support epidemiological investigations that are aimed at tracing the source and limiting the scope of outbreaks. Laboratories contributing data to surveillance databases typically are required to follow highly standardized protocols and comply with an extensive QA/QC program to ensure the reproducibility and the high quality of data.

PulseNet, the national and international surveillance network for foodborne disease, is the most successful example of a surveillance database. PulseNet USA was established in 1996 (166), and similar networks later followed in Canada, the Asia Pacific region, Latin America, the Middle East, and Europe (167). The participating laboratories perform PFGE on all foodborne organisms they receive from clinical and food specimens in real time. The generated patterns are analyzed locally by using highly customized software and uploaded to the central databases of each region via the Internet. The database managers confirm the quality of the patterns, name them according to a standardized scheme, and compare them against the patterns submitted to the database within the previous 60 days (120 days for *Listeria*). The epidemiologists are alerted if a new cluster of indistinguishable isolates is detected. Until now much of the work in PulseNet International has focused on establishing the infrastructure of the network, but eventually each regional network will be able to log on to the server of any other international network, query the databases for matches to pathogen subtypes of interest, and if matches are found, access the epidemiologic information on matching isolate patterns (167). Such collaboration is already taking place between PulseNet USA and PulseNet Canada.

Other PulseNet-like surveillance databases include the Salm-gene subtyping project for *Salmonella* in Europe (49), the CaliciNet network in the United States (22), and the Foodborne Viruses in Europe network (93) dealing mainly with norovirus. In addition to PFGE data, the Salm-gene network also utilizes phage typing data. The virological networks primarily use DNA sequence analysis. A number of virus-specific, curated databases have been established. These can be identified by an Internet search, though many may have restricted access.

CONCLUSIONS AND FUTURE TRENDS

Molecular methods have improved our understanding of the epidemiology of infectious diseases and the well-known, emerging, or reemerging pathogens causing them during the past 4 decades. Molecular methods have been used not only to subtype and otherwise characterize the pathogens following their culture but also to identify and detect nonculturable or slowly growing organisms (23, 90, 195). In the next decade molecular methods will bring the science of forensic microbiology and source attribution to a new level. With the rapid evolution in DNA arrays and sequencing technologies, it is to be expected that these methods will be used to an increasing extent for rapid nonculture diagnostics of infectious diseases, providing detection, virulence characterization, and subtyping of the organisms at the same time, thereby creating the potential for detection of public health events, e.g., outbreaks, in real time with no delays caused by isolating and growing the organisms as pure cultures. This in turn will create a formidable challenge to the public health informatics infrastructure to ensure that the users of the data are alerted to and know how to use the growing information flow from the clinical laboratories.

Since the DNA arrays and sequencing methods are organism specific to a very great extent, traditional methods will still be needed to detect and identify new and reemerging pathogens. Expertise in traditional microbiology will need to be maintained in national and international reference or other dedicated laboratories. Since emergence or reemergence of pathogens rarely happens, this expertise may only be achieved by ensuring a steady flow of specimens for analysis by traditional methods into these laboratories. Ensuring this will require goodwill and understanding among politicians and other public health decision makers. If this does not happen, we will lose our capability to respond quickly to public health emergencies caused by new pathogens.

REFERENCES

1. **Aanensen, D. M., and B. G. Spratt.** 2005. The multilocus sequence typing network: mlst.net. *Nucleic Acids Res.* **33:**W728–W733.
2. **Achtman, M., K. Zurth, G. Morelli, G. Torrea, A. Guiyoule, and E. Carniel.** 1999. *Yersinia pestis*, the cause of plague, is a recently emerged clone of *Yersinia pseudotuberculosis*. *Proc. Natl. Acad. Sci. USA* **96:**14043–14048.
3. **Arita, M., S. L. Zhu, H. Yoshida, T. Yoneyama, T. Miyamura, and H. Shimizu.** 2005. A Sabin 3-derived poliovirus recombinant contained a sequence homologous with indigenous human enterovirus species C in the viral polymerase coding region. *J. Virol.* **79:**12650–12657.
4. **Aury, J. M., C. Cruaud, V. Barbe, O. Rogier, S. Mangenot, G. Samson, J. Poulain, V. Anthouard, C. Scarpelli, F. Artiguenave, and P. Wincker.** 2008. High quality draft sequences for prokaryotic genomes using a mix of new sequencing technologies. *BMC Genomics* **9:**603.
5. **Barrett, J. C., B. Fry, J. Maller, and M. J. Daly.** 2005. Haploview: analysis and visualization of LD and haplotype maps. *Bioinformatics* **21:**263–265.
6. **Barrett, T. J., P. Gerner-Smidt, and B. Swaminathan.** 2006. Interpretation of pulsed-field gel electrophoresis patterns in foodborne disease investigations and surveillance. *Foodborne Pathog. Dis.* **3:**20–31.
7. **Beall, B., R. Facklam, and T. Thompson.** 1996. Sequencing *emm*-specific PCR products for routine and accurate typing of group A streptococci. *J. Clin. Microbiol.* **34:**953–958.
8. **Belongia, E. A., B. A. Kieke, J. G. Donahue, R. T. Greenlee, A. Balish, A. Foust, S. Lindstrom, and D. K. Shay.** 2009. Effectiveness of inactivated influenza vaccines varied substantially with antigenic match from the 2004–2005 season to the 2006–2007 season. *J. Infect. Dis.* **199:**159–167.
9. **Best, E. L., A. J. Fox, J. A. Frost, and F. J. Bolton.** 2005. Real-time single-nucleotide polymorphism profiling using Taqman technology for rapid recognition of *Campylobacter jejuni* clonal complexes. *J. Med. Microbiol.* **54:**919–925.

10. **Bidet, P., F. Barbut, V. Lalande, B. Burghoffer, and J. C. Petit.** 1999. Development of a new PCR-ribotyping method for *Clostridium difficile* based on ribosomal RNA gene sequencing. *FEMS Microbiol. Lett.* **175:**261–266.

11. **Bielaszewska, M., R. Prager, W. Zhang, A. W. Friedrich, A. Mellmann, H. Tschape, and H. Karch.** 2006. Chromosomal dynamism in progeny of outbreak-related sorbitol-fermenting enterohemorrhagic *Escherichia coli* O157:NM. *Appl. Environ. Microbiol.* **72:**1900–1909.

12. **Bilek, N., I. M. Martin, G. Bell, G. R. Kinghorn, C. A. Ison, and B. G. Spratt.** 2007. Concordance between *Neisseria gonorrhoeae* genotypes recovered from known sexual contacts. *J. Clin. Microbiol.* **45:**3564–3567.

13. **Borucki, M. K., S. H. Kim, D. R. Call, S. C. Smole, and F. Pagotto.** 2004. Selective discrimination of *Listeria monocytogenes* epidemic strains by a mixed-genome DNA microarray compared to discrimination by pulsed-field gel electrophoresis, ribotyping, and multilocus sequence typing. *J. Clin. Microbiol.* **42:**5270–5276.

14. **Borucki, M. K., J. Reynolds, D. R. Call, T. J. Ward, B. Page, and J. Kadushin.** 2005. Suspension microarray with dendrimer signal amplification allows direct and high-throughput subtyping of *Listeria monocytogenes* from genomic DNA. *J. Clin. Microbiol.* **43:**3255–3259.

15. **Bouchet, V., H. Huot, and R. Goldstein.** 2008. Molecular genetic basis of ribotyping. *Clin. Microbiol. Rev.* **21:**262–273.

16. **Brinkman, N. E., and G. S. Fout.** 2009. Development and evaluation of a generic tag array to detect and genotype noroviruses in water. *J. Virol. Methods* **156:**8–18.

17. **Buchman, T. G., B. Roizman, G. Adams, and B. H. Stover.** 1978. Restriction endonuclease fingerprinting of herpes simplex virus DNA: a novel epidemiological tool applied to a nosocomial outbreak. *J. Infect. Dis.* **138:**488–498.

18. **Carle, G. F., M. Frank, and M. V. Olson.** 1986. Electrophoretic separations of large DNA molecules by periodic inversion of the electric field. *Science* **232:**65–68.

19. **Carle, G. F., and M. V. Olson.** 1984. Separation of chromosomal DNA molecules from yeast by orthogonal-field-alternation gel electrophoresis. *Nucleic Acids Res.* **12:**5647–5664.

20. **Cartwright, C. P., F. Stock, S. E. Beekmann, E. C. Williams, and V. J. Gill.** 1995. PCR amplification of rRNA intergenic spacer regions as a method for epidemiologic typing of *Clostridium difficile*. *J. Clin. Microbiol.* **33:**184–187.

21. **Cave, M. D., K. D. Eisenach, P. F. McDermott, J. H. Bates, and J. T. Crawford.** 1991. IS*6110:* conservation of sequence in the *Mycobacterium tuberculosis* complex and its utilization in DNA fingerprinting. *Mol. Cell. Probes* **5:**73–80.

22. **Centers for Disease Control and Prevention.** 2003. Norovirus activity—United States, 2002. *MMWR Morb. Mortal. Wkly. Rep.* **52:**1–5.

23. **Centers for Disease Control and Prevention.** 2002. Screening tests to detect *Chlamydia trachomatis* and *Neisseria gonorrhoeae* infections—2002. *MMWR Recommend. Rep.* **51:**1–38.

24. **Chang, H. W., L. Y. Chuang, Y. H. Cheng, C. H. Ho, C. H. Wen, and C. H. Yang.** 2009. Seq-SNPing: multiple-alignment tool for SNP discovery, SNP ID identification, and RFLP genotyping. *OMICS* **13:**253–260.

25. **Cherkasova, E., M. Laassri, V. Chizhikov, E. Korotkova, E. Dragunsky, V. I. Agol, and K. Chumakov.** 2003. Microarray analysis of evolution of RNA viruses: evidence of circulation of virulent highly divergent vaccine-derived polioviruses. *Proc. Natl. Acad. Sci. USA* **100:**9398–9403.

26. **Chiu, C. Y., A. A. Alizadeh, S. Rouskin, J. D. Merker, E. Yeh, S. Yagi, D. Schnurr, B. K. Patterson, D. Ganem, and J. L. DeRisi.** 2007. Diagnosis of a critical respiratory illness caused by human metapneumovirus by use of a pan-virus microarray. *J. Clin. Microbiol.* **45:**2340–2343.

27. **Chiu, C. Y., S. Rouskin, A. Koshy, A. Urisman, K. Fischer, S. Yagi, D. Schnurr, P. B. Eckburg, L. S. Tompkins, B. G. Blackburn, J. D. Merker, B. K. Patterson, D. Ganem, and J. L. DeRisi.** 2006. Microarray detection of human parainfluenzavirus 4 infection associated with respiratory failure in an immunocompetent adult. *Clin. Infect. Dis.* **43:**e71–e76.

28. **Chizhikov, V., M. Wagner, A. Ivshina, Y. Hoshino, A. Z. Kapikian, and K. Chumakov.** 2002. Detection and genotyping of human group A rotaviruses by oligonucleotide microarray hybridization. *J. Clin. Microbiol.* **40:**2398–2407.

29. **Chu, G., D. Vollrath, and R. W. Dacis.** 1986. Separation of large DNA molecules by contour-clamped homogeneous electric fields. *Anal. Biochem.* **234:**1582–1585.

30. **Clarke, S. C.** 2005. Pyrosequencing: nucleotide sequencing technology with bacterial genotyping applications. *Expert Rev. Mol. Diagn.* **5:**947–953.

31. **Cleland, C. A., P. S. White, A. Deshpande, M. Wolinsky, J. Song, and J. P. Nolan.** 2004. Development of rationally designed nucleic acid signatures for microbial pathogens. *Expert Rev. Mol. Diagn.* **4:**303–315.

32. **Cooke, F. J., D. J. Brown, M. Fookes, D. Pickard, A. Ivens, J. Wain, M. Roberts, R. A. Kingsley, N. R. Thomson, and G. Dougan.** 2008. Characterization of the genomes of a diverse collection of *Salmonella enterica* serovar Typhimurium definitive phage type 104. *J. Bacteriol.* **190:**8155–8162.

33. **Dauga, C., A. Zabrovskaia, and P. A. D. Grimont.** 1998. Restriction fragment length polymorphism analysis of some flagellin genes of *Salmonella enterica*. *J. Clin. Microbiol.* **36:** 2835–2843.

34. **De Baere, T., R. de Mendonca, G. Claeys, G. Verschraegen, W. Mijs, R. Verhelst, S. Rottiers, L. Van Simaey, C. De Ganck, and M. Vaneechoutte.** 2002. Evaluation of amplified rDNA restriction analysis (ARDRA) for the identification of cultured mycobacteria in a diagnostic laboratory. *BMC Microbiol.* **2:**4.

35. **de Boer, P., B. Duim, A. Rigter, J. van Der Plas, W. F. Jacobs-Reitsma, and J. A. Wagenaar.** 2000. Computer-assisted analysis and epidemiological value of genotyping methods for *Campylobacter jejuni* and *Campylobacter coli*. *J. Clin. Microbiol.* **38:**1940–1946.

36. **Deplano, A., A. Schuermans, J. Van Eldere, W. Witte, H. Meugnier, J. Etienne, H. Grundmann, D. Jonas, G. T. Noordhoek, J. Dijkstra, A. van Belkum, W. van Leeuwen, P. T. Tassios, N. J. Legakis, A. van der Zee, A. Bergmans, D. S. Blanc, F. C. Tenover, B. C. Cookson, G. O'Neil, M. J. Struelens, et al.** 2000. Multicenter evaluation of epidemiological typing of methicillin-resistant *Staphylococcus aureus* strains by repetitive-element PCR analysis. *J. Clin. Microbiol.* **38:**3527–3533.

37. **de Valk, H. A., J. F. Meis, S. Bretagne, J. M. Costa, B. A. Lasker, S. A. Balajee, A. C. Pasqualotto, M. J. Anderson, L. Alcazar-Fuoli, E. Mellado, and C. H. Klaassen.** 2009. Interlaboratory reproducibility of a microsatellite-based typing assay for *Aspergillus fumigatus* through the use of allelic ladders: proof of concept. *Clin. Microbiol. Infect.* **15:**180–187.

38. **Domingo, E.** 2007. Virus evolution, p. 389–422. *In* D. M. Knipe, P. M. Howley, D. E. Griffin, R. A. Lamb, M. A. Martin, B. Roizman, and S. E. Straus (ed.), *Fields Virology*, 5th ed., vol. 1. Lippincott Williams & Wilkins, Philadelphia, PA.

39. **Dowell, S. F., C. Groves, K. B. Kirkland, H. G. Cicirello, T. Ando, Q. Jin, J. R. Gentsch, S. S. Monroe, C. D. Humphrey, C. Slemp, et al.** 1995. A multistate outbreak of oyster-associated gastroenteritis: implications for interstate tracing of contaminated shellfish. *J. Infect. Dis.* **171:**1497–1503.

40. **Drummond, A. J., and A. Rambaut.** 2007. BEAST: Bayesian evolutionary analysis by sampling trees. *BMC Evol. Biol.* **7:**214.

41. **Ducey, T. F., B. Page, T. Usgaard, M. K. Borucki, K. Pupedis, and T. J. Ward.** 2007. A single-nucleotide-polymorphism-based multilocus genotyping assay for subtyping lineage I isolates of *Listeria monocytogenes*. *Appl. Environ. Microbiol.* **73:**133–147.

42. **Dufva, M.** 2009. Introduction to microarray technology. *Methods Mol. Biol.* **529:**1–22.

43. **Dunbar, S., and J. Jacobson.** 2007. Quantitative, multiplexed detection of *Salmonella* and other pathogens by Luminex xMAP suspension array. *Methods Mol. Biol.* **394:**1–19.

44. **Dunbar, S. A.** 2006. Applications of Luminex xMAP technology for rapid, high-throughput multiplexed nucleic acid detection. *Clin. Chim. Acta* **363:**71–82.

45. Facklam, R. F., D. R. Martin, M. Lovgren, D. R. Johnson, A. Efstratiou, T. A. Thompson, S. Gowan, P. Kriz, G. J. Tyrrell, E. Kaplan, and B. Beall. 2002. Extension of the Lancefield classification for group A streptococci by addition of 22 new M protein gene sequence types from clinical isolates: emm103 to emm124. *Clin. Infect. Dis.* **34:**28–38.

46. Feil, E. J., B. C. Li, D. M. Aanensen, W. P. Hanage, and B. G. Spratt. 2004. eBURST: inferring patterns of evolutionary descent among clusters of related bacterial genotypes from multilocus sequence typing data. *J. Bacteriol.* **186:**1518–1530.

47. Feng, Q., S. Cherne, R. L. Winer, A. Balasubramanian, S. K. Lee, S. E. Hawes, N. B. Kiviat, and L. A. Koutsky. 2009. Development and evaluation of a liquid bead microarray assay for genotyping genital human papillomaviruses. *J. Clin. Microbiol.* **47:**547–553.

48. Fields, P. I., K. Blom, H. J. Hughes, L. O. Helsel, P. Feng, and B. Swaminathan. 1997. Molecular characterization of the gene encoding H antigen in *Escherichia coli* and development of a PCR-restriction fragment length polymorphism test for identification of *E. coli* O157:H7 and O157:NM. *J. Clin. Microbiol.* **35:**1066–1070.

49. Fisher, I. S., and E. J. Threlfall. 2005. The Enter-net and Salm-gene databases of foodborne bacterial pathogens that cause human infections in Europe and beyond: an international collaboration in surveillance and the development of intervention strategies. *Epidemiol. Infect.* **133:**1–7.

50. Fitzgerald, C., M. Collins, S. van Duyne, M. Mikoleit, T. Brown, and P. Fields. 2007. Multiplex, bead-based suspension array for molecular determination of common *Salmonella* serogroups. *J. Clin. Microbiol.* **45:**3323–3334.

51. Fontana, C., M. Favaro, S. Minelli, M. C. Bossa, G. P. Testore, F. Leonardis, S. Natoli, and C. Favalli. 2008. *Acinetobacter baumannii* in intensive care unit: a novel system to study clonal relationship among the isolates. *BMC Infect. Dis.* **8:**79.

52. Friedrich, A. W., W. Witte, H. de Lencastre, W. Hryniewicz, J. Scheres, and H. Westh. 2008. A European laboratory network for sequence-based typing of methicillin-resistant *Staphylococcus aureus* (MRSA) as a communication platform between human and veterinary medicine—an update on SeqNet.org. *Euro Surveill.* **13:**pii:18862.

53. Fry, N. K., B. Afshar, P. Visca, D. Jonas, J. Duncan, E. Nebuloso, A. Underwood, and T. G. Harrison. 2005. Assessment of fluorescent amplified fragment length polymorphism analysis for epidemiological genotyping of *Legionella pneumophila* serogroup 1. *Clin. Microbiol. Infect.* **11:**704–712.

54. Galea, S. A., A. Sweet, P. Beninger, S. P. Steinberg, P. S. Larussa, A. A. Gershon, and R. G. Sharrar. 2008. The safety profile of varicella vaccine: a 10-year review. *J. Infect. Dis.* **197**(Suppl. 2)**:**S165–S169.

55. Garaizar, J., A. Rementeria, and S. Porwollik. 2006. DNA microarray technology: a new tool for the epidemiological typing of bacterial pathogens? *FEMS Immunol. Med. Microbiol.* **47:**178–189.

56. Garcia, D. D. O., Y. Doi, D. Szabo, J. M. Adams-Haduch, T. M. Vaz, D. Leite, M. C. Padoveze, M. P. Freire, F. P. Silveira, and D. L. Paterson. 2008. Multiclonal outbreak of *Klebsiella pneumoniae* producing extended-spectrum beta-lactamase CTX-M-2 and novel variant CTX-M-59 in a neonatal intensive care unit in Brazil. *Antimicrob. Agents Chemother.* **52:**1790–1793.

57. Garten, R. J., C. T. Davis, C. A. Russell, B. Shu, S. Lindstrom, A. Balish, W. M. Sessions, X. Xu, E. Skepner, V. Deyde, M. Okomo-Adhiambo, L. Gubareva, J. Barnes, C. B. Smith, S. L. Emery, M. J. Hillman, P. Rivailler, J. Smagala, M. de Graaf, D. F. Burke, R. A. Fouchier, C. Pappas, C. M. Alpuche-Aranda, H. Lopez-Gatell, H. Olivera, I. Lopez, C. A. Myers, D. Faix, P. J. Blair, C. Yu, K. M. Keene, P. D. Dotson, Jr., D. Boxrud, A. R. Sambol, S. H. Abid, K. St George, T. Bannerman, A. L. Moore, D. J. Stringer, P. Blevins, G. J. Demmler-Harrison, M. Ginsberg, P. Kriner, S. Waterman, S. Smole, H. F. Guevara, E. A. Belongia, P. A. Clark, S. T. Beatrice, R. Donis, J. Katz, L. Finelli, C. B. Bridges, M. Shaw, D. B. Jernigan, T. M. Uyeki, D. J. Smith, A. I. Klimov, and N. J. Cox. 2009. Antigenic and genetic characteristics of swine-origin 2009 A(H1N1) influenza viruses circulating in humans. *Science* **325:**197–201.

58. Gerner-Smidt, P., J. Kincaid, K. Kubota, K. Hise, S. B. Hunter, M. A. Fair, D. Norton, A. Woo-Ming, T. Kurzynski, M. J. Sotir, M. Head, K. Holt, and B. Swaminathan. 2005. Molecular surveillance of Shiga toxigenic *Escherichia coli* O157 by PulseNet USA. *J. Food Prot.* **68:**1926–1931.

59. Giannino, M. L., M. Aliprandi, M. Feligini, L. Vanoni, M. Brasca, and F. Fracchetti. 2009. A DNA array-based assay for the characterization of microbial community in raw milk. *J. Microbiol. Methods* **78:**181–188.

60. Githui, W. A., S. M. Wilson, and F. A. Drobniewski. 1999. Specificity of IS6110-based DNA fingerprinting and diagnostic techniques for *Mycobacterium tuberculosis* complex. *J. Clin. Microbiol.* **37:**1224–1226.

61. Goering, R. V., E. M. Ribot, and P. Gerner-Smidt. 2011. Pulsed-field gel electrophoresis: laboratory and epidemiologic considerations for interpretation of data, p. 167–177. *In* D. H. Persing et al. (ed.), *Molecular Microbiology: Diagnostic Principles and Practice*, 2nd ed. ASM Press, Washington, DC.

62. Gorge, O., S. Lopez, V. Hilaire, O. Lisanti, V. Ramisse, and G. Vergnaud. 2008. Selection and validation of a multilocus variable-number tandem-repeat analysis panel for typing *Shigella* spp. *J. Clin. Microbiol.* **46:**1026–1036.

63. Grenfell, B. T., O. G. Pybus, J. R. Gog, J. L. Wood, J. M. Daly, J. A. Mumford, and E. C. Holmes. 2004. Unifying the epidemiological and evolutionary dynamics of pathogens. *Science* **303:**327–332.

64. Grimont, F., and P. Grimont. 1986. Ribosomal ribonucleic acid gene restriction patterns as potential taxonomic tools. *Ann. Inst. Pasteur Microbiol.* **137B:**165–175.

65. Grimont, P. A. D., and F. X. Weill. 2007. *Antigenic Formulae of the Salmonella Serovars*, 9th ed. WHO Collaborating Centre for Reference and Research on *Salmonella*, Institut Pasteur, Paris, France.

66. Grissa, I., P. Bouchon, C. Pourcel, and G. Vergnaud. 2008. On-line resources for bacterial micro-evolution studies using MLVA or CRISPR typing. *Biochimie* **90:**660–668.

67. Guigon, G., J. Cheval, R. Cahuzac, and S. Brisse. 2008. MLVA-NET—a standardised web database for bacterial genotyping and surveillance. *Euro Surveill.* **13:**pii:18863.

68. Hall, T. A., R. Sampath, L. B. Blyn, R. Ranken, C. Ivy, R. Melton, H. Matthews, N. White, F. Li, V. Harpin, D. J. Ecker, L. K. McDougal, B. Limbago, T. Ross, D. M. Wolk, V. Wysocki, and K. C. Carroll. 2009. Rapid molecular genotyping and clonal complex assignment of *Staphylococcus aureus* isolates by PCR coupled to electrospray ionization-mass spectrometry. *J. Clin. Microbiol.* **47:**1733–1741.

69. Healy, M., J. Huong, T. Bittner, M. Lising, S. Frye, S. Raza, R. Schrock, J. Manry, A. Renwick, R. Nieto, C. Woods, J. Versalovic, and J. R. Lupski. 2005. Microbial DNA typing by automated repetitive-sequence-based PCR. *J. Clin. Microbiol.* **43:**199–207.

70. Hoffmaster, A. R., C. C. Fitzgerald, E. Ribot, L. W. Mayer, and T. Popovic. 2002. Molecular subtyping of *Bacillus anthracis* and the 2001 bioterrorism-associated anthrax outbreak, United States. *Emerg. Infect. Dis.* **8:**1111–1116.

71. Holmes, E. C., and A. Rambaut. 2004. Viral evolution and the emergence of SARS coronavirus. *Philos. Trans. R. Soc. Lond. B* **359:**1059–1065.

72. Holt, K. E., J. Parkhill, C. J. Mazzoni, P. Roumagnac, F. X. Weill, I. Goodhead, R. Rance, S. Baker, D. J. Maskell, J. Wain, C. Dolecek, M. Achtman, and G. Dougan. 2008. High-throughput sequencing provides insights into genome variation and evolution in *Salmonella* Typhi. *Nat. Genet.* **40:**987–993.

73. Hommais, F., S. Pereira, C. Acquaviva, P. Escobar-Paramo, and E. Denamur. 2005. Single-nucleotide polymorphism phylotyping of *Escherichia coli*. *Appl. Environ. Microbiol.* **71:**4784–4792.

74. Honma, S., V. Chizhikov, N. Santos, M. Tatsumi, C. Timenetsky Mdo, A. C. Linhares, J. D. Mascarenhas, H. Ushijima, G. E. Armah, J. R. Gentsch, and Y. Hoshino.

2007. Development and validation of DNA microarray for genotyping group A rotavirus VP4 (P[4], P[6], P[8], P[9], and P[14]) and VP7 (G1 to G6, G8 to G10, and G12) genes. *J. Clin. Microbiol.* **45:**2641–2648.

75. **Hopkins, K. L., C. Maguire, E. Best, E. Liebana, and E. J. Threlfall.** 2007. Stability of multiple-locus variable-number tandem repeats in *Salmonella enterica* serovar Typhimurium. *J. Clin. Microbiol.* **45:**3058–3061.

76. **Hu, H., R. Lan, and P. R. Reeves.** 2006. Adaptation of multilocus sequencing for studying variation within a major clone: evolutionary relationships of *Salmonella enterica* serovar Typhimurium. *Genetics* **172:**743–750.

77. **Huang, Y., H. Tang, S. Duffy, Y. Hong, S. Norman, M. Ghosh, J. He, M. Bose, K. J. Henrickson, J. Fan, A. J. Kraft, W. G. Weisburg, and E. L. Mather.** 2009. Multiplex assay for simultaneously typing and subtyping influenza viruses by use of an electronic microarray. *J. Clin. Microbiol.* **47:**390–396.

78. **Hunter, P. R.** 1990. Reproducibility and indices of discriminatory power of microbial typing methods. *J. Clin. Microbiol.* **28:**1903–1905.

79. **Hyytia-Trees, E., P. Lafon, P. Vauterin, and E. M. Ribot.** 2009. Multilaboratory validation study of standardized multiple-locus variable-number tandem repeat analysis protocol for Shiga toxin-producing *Escherichia coli* O157: a novel approach to normalize fragment size data between capillary electrophoresis platforms. *Foodborne Pathog. Dis.* **28:**28.

80. **Hyytia-Trees, E., S. C. Smole, P. A. Fields, B. Swaminathan, and E. M. Ribot.** 2006. Second generation subtyping: a proposed PulseNet protocol for multiple-locus variable-number tandem repeat analysis of Shiga toxin-producing *Escherichia coli* O157 (STEC O157). *Foodborne Pathog. Dis.* **3:**118–131.

81. **Jaaskelainen, A. J., and L. Maunula.** 2006. Applicability of microarray technique for the detection of noro- and astroviruses. *J. Virol. Methods* **136:**210–216.

82. **Johnson, J. R., and C. Clabots.** 2000. Improved repetitive-element PCR fingerprinting of *Salmonella enterica* with the use of extremely elevated annealing temperatures. *Clin. Diagn. Lab. Immunol.* **7:**258–264.

83. **Jolley, K. A., M. S. Chan, and M. C. Maiden.** 2004. mlstdbNet - distributed multi-locus sequence typing (MLST) databases. *BMC Bioinform.* **5:**86.

84. **Kado, C. I., and S. T. Liu.** 1981. Rapid procedure for detection and isolation of large and small plasmids. *J. Bacteriol.* **145:**1365–1373.

85. **Kaper, J. B., H. B. Bradford, N. C. Roberts, and S. Falkow.** 1982. Molecular epidemiology of *Vibrio cholerae* in the U.S. Gulf Coast. *J. Clin. Microbiol.* **16:**129–134.

86. **Kashi, Y., D. King, and M. Soller.** 1997. Simple sequence repeats as a source of quantitative genetic variation. *Trends Genet.* **13:**74–78.

87. **Keim, P., L. B. Price, A. M. Klevytska, K. L. Smith, J. M. Schupp, R. Okinaka, P. J. Jackson, and M. E. Hugh-Jones.** 2000. Multiple-locus variable-number tandem repeat analysis reveals genetic relationships within *Bacillus anthracis*. *J. Bacteriol.* **182:**2928–2936.

88. **Keim, P., M. N. Van Ert, T. Pearson, A. J. Vogler, L. Y. Huynh, and D. M. Wagner.** 2004. Anthrax molecular epidemiology and forensics: using the appropriate marker for different evolutionary scales. *Infect. Genet. Evol.* **4:**205–213.

89. **Kenefic, L. J., J. Beaudry, C. Trim, R. Daly, R. Parmar, S. Zanecki, L. Huynh, M. N. Van Ert, D. M. Wagner, T. Graham, and P. Keim.** 2008. High resolution genotyping of *Bacillus anthracis* outbreak strains using four highly mutable single nucleotide repeat markers. *Lett. Appl. Microbiol.* **46:**600–603.

90. **Klingspor, L., and J. Loeffler.** 2009. *Aspergillus* PCR formidable challenges and progress. *Med. Mycol.* **47(Suppl. 1):**S241–S247.

91. **Kobayashi, S., A. Wada, S. Shibasaki, M. Annaka, H. Higuchi, K. Adachi, N. Mori, T. Ishikawa, Y. Masuda, H. Watanabe, N. Yamamoto, S. Yamaoka, and T. Inamatsu.** 2009. Spread of a large plasmid carrying the *cpe* gene and the *tcp* locus amongst *Clostridium perfringens* isolates from nosocomial outbreaks and sporadic cases of gastroenteritis in a geriatric hospital. *Epidemiol. Infect.* **137:**108–113.

92. **Koeleman, J. G., J. Stoof, D. J. Biesmans, P. H. Savelkoul, and C. M. Vandenbroucke-Grauls.** 1998. Comparison of amplified ribosomal DNA restriction analysis, random amplified polymorphic DNA analysis, and amplified fragment length polymorphism fingerprinting for identification of Acinetobacter genomic species and typing of Acinetobacter baumannii. J. Clin. Microbiol. 36:2522–2529.

93. **Koopmans, M., H. Vennema, H. Heersma, E. van Strien, Y. van Duynhoven, D. Brown, M. Reacher, and B. Lopman.** 2003. Early identification of common-source foodborne virus outbreaks in Europe. Emerg. Infect. Dis. 9:1136–1142.

94. **Ksiazek, T. G., D. Erdman, C. S. Goldsmith, S. R. Zaki, T. Peret, S. Emery, S. Tong, C. Urbani, J. A. Comer, W. Lim, P. E. Rollin, S. F. Dowell, A. E. Ling, C. D. Humphrey, W. J. Shieh, J. Guarner, C. D. Paddock, P. Rota, B. Fields, J. DeRisi, J. Y. Yang, N. Cox, J. M. Hughes, W. LeDuc, W. J. Bellini, and L. J. Anderson.** 2003. A novel coronavirus associated with severe acute respiratory syndrome. N. Engl. J. Med. 348:1953–1966.

95. **Lal, R. B., S. Chakrabarti, and C. Yang.** 2005. Impact of genetic diversity of HIV-1 on diagnosis, antiretroviral therapy and vaccine development. Indian J. Med. Res. 121:287–314.

96. **Lanciotti, R. S., G. D. Ebel, V. Deubel, A. J. Kerst, S. Murri, R. Meyer, M. Bowen, N. McKinney, W. E. Morrill, M. B. Crabtree, L. D. Kramer, and J. T. Roehrig.** 2002. Complete genome sequences and phylogenetic analysis of West Nile virus strains isolated from the United States, Europe, and the Middle East. Virology 298:96–105.

97. **Latreille, P., S. Norton, B. S. Goldman, J. Henkhaus, N. Miller, B. Barbazuk, H. B. Bode, C. Darby, Z. Du, S. Forst, S. Gaudriault, B. Goodner, H. Goodrich-Blair, and S. Slater.** 2007. Optical mapping as a routine tool for bacterial genome sequence finishing. BMC Genomics 8:321.

98. **Lee, J. K., M. K. Kim, S. H. Song, J. H. Hong, K. J. Min, J. H. Kim, E. S. Song, J. Lee, J. M. Lee, and S. Y. Hur.** 2009. Comparison of human papillomavirus detection and typing by hybrid capture 2, linear array, DNA chip, and cycle sequencing in cervical swab samples. Int. J. Gynecol. Cancer 19:266–272.

99. **Lemey, P., S. Van Dooren, K. Van Laethem, Y. Schrooten, I. Derdelinckx, P. Goubau, F. Brun-Vezinet, D. Vaira, and A. M. Vandamme.** 2005. Molecular testing of multiple HIV-1 transmissions in a criminal case. AIDS 19:1649–1658.

100. **Leonard, E. E., II, T. Takata, M. J. Blaser, S. Falkow, L. S. Tompkins, and E. C. Gaynor.** 2003. Use of an open-reading frame-specific *Campylobacter jejuni* DNA microarray as a new genotyping tool for studying epidemiologically related isolates. J. Infect. Dis. 187:691–694.

101. **Leopold, S. R., V. Magrini, N. J. Holt, N. Shaikh, E. R. Mardis, J. Cagno, Y. Ogura, A. Iguchi, T. Hayashi, A. Mellmann, H. Karch, T. E. Besser, S. A. Sawyer, T. S. Whittam, and P. I. Tarr.** 2009. A precise reconstruction of the emergence and constrained radiations of *Escherichia coli* O157 portrayed by backbone concatenomic analysis. Proc. Natl. Acad. Sci. USA 106:8713–8718.

102. **Levy, D. D., B. Sharma, and T. A. Cebula.** 2004. Single-nucleotide polymorphism mutation spectra and resistance to quinolones in *Salmonella enterica* serovar Enteritidis with a mutator phenotype. Antimicrob. Agents Chemother. 48:2355–2363.

103. **Lewis, F., G. J. Hughes, A. Rambaut, A. Pozniak, and A. J. Leigh Brown.** 2008. Episodic sexual transmission of HIV revealed by molecular phylodynamics. PLoS Med. 5:e50.

104. **Lin, B., K. M. Blaney, A. P. Malanoski, A. G. Ligler, J. M. Schnur, D. Metzgar, K. L. Russell, and D. A. Stenger.** 2007. Using a resequencing microarray as a multiple respiratory pathogen detection assay. J. Clin. Microbiol. 45:443–452.

105. **Lindstedt, B. A., L. T. Brandal, L. Aas, T. Vardund, and G. Kapperud.** 2007. Study of polymorphic variable-number of tandem repeats loci in the ECOR collection and in a set of pathogenic *Escherichia coli* and *Shigella* isolates for use in a genotyping assay. J. Microbiol. Methods 69:197–205.

106. **Lindstedt, B. A., T. Vardund, L. Aas, and G. Kapperud.** 2004. Multiple-locus variable-number tandem-repeats analysis of *Salmonella enterica* subsp. enterica serovar Typhimurium using PCR multiplexing and multicolor capillary electrophoresis. *J. Microbiol. Methods* **59:**163–172.

107. **Maiden, M. C., J. A. Bygraves, E. Feil, G. Morelli, J. E. Russell, R. Urwin, Q. Zhang, J. Zhou, K. Zurth, D. A. Caugant, I. M. Feavers, M. Achtman, and B. G. Spratt.** 1998. Multilocus sequence typing: a portable approach to the identification of clones within populations of pathogenic microorganisms. *Proc. Natl. Acad. Sci. USA* **95:**3140–3145.

108. **Manning, S. D., A. S. Motiwala, A. C. Springman, W. Qi, D. W. Lacher, L. M. Ouellette, J. M. Mladonicky, P. Somsel, J. T. Rudrik, S. E. Dietrich, W. Zhang, B. Swaminathan, D. Alland, and T. S. Whittam.** 2008. Variation in virulence among clades of *Escherichia coli* O157:H7 associated with disease outbreaks. *Proc. Natl. Acad. Sci. USA* **105:**4868–4873.

109. **Margulies, M., M. Egholm, W. E. Altman, S. Attiya, J. S. Bader, L. A. Bemben, J. Berka, M. S. Braverman, Y. J. Chen, Z. Chen, S. B. Dewell, L. Du, J. M. Fierro, X. V. Gomes, B. C. Godwin, W. He, S. Helgesen, C. H. Ho, G. P. Irzyk, S. C. Jando, M. L. Alenquer, T. P. Jarvie, K. B. Jirage, J. B. Kim, J. R. Knight, J. R. Lanza, J. H. Leamon, S. M. Lefkowitz, M. Lei, J. Li, K. L. Lohman, H. Lu, V. B. Makhijani, K. E. McDade, M. P. McKenna, E. W. Myers, E. Nickerson, J. R. Nobile, R. Plant, B. P. Puc, M. T. Ronan, G. T. Roth, G. J. Sarkis, J. F. Simons, J. W. Simpson, M. Srinivasan, K. R. Tartaro, A. Tomasz, K. A. Vogt, G. A. Volkmer, S. H. Wang, Y. Wang, M. P. Weiner, P. Yu, R. F. Begley, and J. M. Rothberg.** 2005. Genome sequencing in microfabricated high-density picolitre reactors. *Nature* **437:**376–380.

110. **Marol, S., and M. Yucesoy.** 2008. Molecular epidemiology of *Candida* species isolated from clinical specimens of intensive care unit patients. *Mycoses* **51:**40–49.

111. **Martin, B., O. Humbert, M. Camara, E. Guenzi, J. Walker, T. Mitchell, P. Andrew, M. Prudhomme, G. Alloing, R. Hakenbeck, et al.** 1992. A highly conserved repeated DNA element located in the chromosome of *Streptococcus pneumoniae. Nucleic Acids Res.* **20:**3479–3483.

112. **Mayer, L. W.** 1988. Use of plasmid profiles in epidemiologic surveillance of disease outbreaks and in tracing the transmission of antibiotic resistance. *Clin. Microbiol. Rev.* **1:**228–243.

113. **Metzker, M. L., D. P. Mindell, X. M. Liu, R. G. Ptak, R. A. Gibbs, and D. M. Hillis.** 2002. Molecular evidence of HIV-1 transmission in a criminal case. *Proc. Natl. Acad. Sci. USA* **99:**14292–14297.

114. **Meunier, J. R., and P. A. D. Grimont.** 1993. Factors affecting reproducibility of random amplified polymorphic DNA fingerprinting. *Res. Microbiol.* **144:**373–379.

115. **Meyers, J. A., D. Sanchez, L. P. Elwell, and S. Falkow.** 1976. Simple agarose gel electrophoretic method for the identification and characterization of plasmid deoxyribonucleic acid. *J. Bacteriol.* **127:**1529–1537.

116. **Minor, P.** 2009. Vaccine-derived poliovirus (VDPV): impact on poliomyelitis eradication. *Vaccine* **27:**2649–2652.

117. **Morozova, O., and M. A. Marra.** 2008. Applications of next-generation sequencing technologies in functional genomics. *Genomics* **92:**255–264.

118. **Nachamkin, I., K. Bohachick, and C. M. Patton.** 1993. Flagellin gene typing of *Campylobacter jejuni* by restriction fragment length polymorphism analysis. *J. Clin. Microbiol.* **31:**1531–1536.

119. **Nathanson, N.** 2007. Epidemiology, p. 423–443. *In* D. M. Knipe, P. M. Howley, D. E. Griffin, R. A. Lamb, M. A. Martin, B. Roizman, and S. E. Straus (ed.), *Fields Virology*, 5th ed., vol. 1. Lippincott Williams & Wilkins, Philadelphia, PA.

120. **Natoli, S., C. Fontana, M. Favaro, A. Bergamini, G. P. Testore, S. Minelli, M. C. Bossa, M. Casapulla, G. Broglio, A. Beltrame, L. Cudillo, R. Cerretti, and F. Leonardis.** 2009. Characterization of coagulase-negative staphylococcal isolates from blood with reduced susceptibility to glycopeptides and therapeutic options. *BMC Infect. Dis.* **9:**83.

121. **Nelson, K. E., D. E. Fouts, E. F. Mongodin, J. Ravel, R. T. DeBoy, J. F. Kolonay, D. A. Rasko, S. V. Angiuoli, S. R. Gill, I. T. Paulsen, J. Peterson, O. White, W. C. Nelson, W. Nierman, M. J. Beanan, L. M. Brinkac, S. C. Daugherty, R. J. Dodson, A. S. Durkin, R. Madupu, D. H. Haft, J. Selengut, S. Van Aken, H. Khouri, N. Fedorova, H. Forberger, B. Tran, S. Kathariou, L. D. Wonderling, G. A. Uhlich, D. O. Bayles, J. B. Luchansky, and C. M. Fraser.** 2004. Whole genome comparisons of serotype 4b and 1/2a strains of the food-borne pathogen *Listeria monocytogenes* reveal new insights into the core genome components of this species. *Nucleic Acids Res.* **32:**2386–2395.

122. **Neverov, A. A., M. A. Riddell, W. J. Moss, D. V. Volokhov, P. A. Rota, L. E. Lowe, D. Chibo, S. B. Smit, D. E. Griffin, K. M. Chumakov, and V. E. Chizhikov.** 2006. Genotyping of measles virus in clinical specimens on the basis of oligonucleotide microarray hybridization patterns. *J. Clin. Microbiol.* **44:**3752–3759.

123. **Nielsen, E. M., J. Engberg, V. Fussing, L. Petersen, C. H. Brogren, and S. L. On.** 2000. Evaluation of phenotypic and genotypic methods for subtyping *Campylobacter jejuni* isolates from humans, poultry, and cattle. *J. Clin. Microbiol.* **38:**3800–3810.

124. **Noller, A. C., M. C. McEllistrem, O. C. Stine, J. G. Morris, Jr., D. J. Boxrud, B. Dixon, and L. H. Harrison.** 2003. Multilocus sequence typing reveals a lack of diversity among *Escherichia coli* O157:H7 isolates that are distinct by pulsed-field gel electrophoresis. *J. Clin. Microbiol.* **41:**675–679.

125. **Odds, F. C., and M. D. Jacobsen.** 2008. Multilocus sequence typing of pathogenic *Candida* species. *Eukaryot. Cell* **7:**1075–1084.

126. **Oliveira, D. C., C. Milheirico, S. Vinga, and H. de Lencastre.** 2006. Assessment of allelic variation in the ccrAB locus in methicillin-resistant *Staphylococcus aureus* clones. *J. Antimicrob. Chemother.* **58:**23–30.

127. **Oliveira, D. C., M. Santos, C. Milheirico, J. A. Carrico, S. Vinga, A. L. Oliveira, and H. de Lencastre.** 2008. CcrB typing tool: an online resource for staphylococci *ccrB* sequence typing. *J. Antimicrob. Chemother.* **61:**959–960.

128. **Pai, R., R. E. Gertz, and B. Beall.** 2006. Sequential multiplex PCR approach for determining capsular serotypes of *Streptococcus pneumoniae* isolates. *J. Clin. Microbiol.* **44:**124–131.

129. **Palacios, G., P. L. Quan, O. J. Jabado, S. Conlan, D. L. Hirschberg, Y. Liu, J. Zhai, N. Renwick, J. Hui, H. Hegyi, A. Grolla, J. E. Strong, J. S. Towner, T. W. Geisbert, P. B. Jahrling, C. Buchen-Osmond, H. Ellerbrok, M. P. Sanchez-Seco, Y. Lussier, P. Formenty, M. S. Nichol, H. Feldmann, T. Briese, and W. I. Lipkin.** 2007. Panmicrobial oligonucleotide array for diagnosis of infectious diseases. *Emerg. Infect. Dis.* **13:**73–81.

130. **Parashar, U. D., L. Dow, R. L. Fankhauser, C. D. Humphrey, J. Miller, T. Ando, K. S. Williams, C. R. Eddy, J. S. Noel, T. Ingram, J. S. Bresee, S. S. Monroe, and R. I. Glass.** 1998. An outbreak of viral gastroenteritis associated with consumption of sandwiches: implications for the control of transmission by food handlers. *Epidemiol. Infect.* **121:**615–621.

131. **Pas, S. D., N. Tran, R. A. de Man, C. Burghoorn-Maas, G. Vernet, and H. G. Niesters.** 2008. Comparison of reverse hybridization, microarray, and sequence analysis for genotyping hepatitis B virus. *J. Clin. Microbiol.* **46:**1268–1273.

132. **Patel, M., C. Pedreira, L. H. De Oliveira, J. Tate, M. Orozco, J. Mercado, A. Gonzalez, O. Malespin, J. J. Amador, J. Umana, A. Balmaseda, M. C. Perez, J. Gentsch, T. Kerin, J. Hull, S. Mijatovic, J. Andrus, and U. Parashar.** 2009. Association between pentavalent rotavirus vaccine and severe rotavirus diarrhea among children in Nicaragua. *JAMA* **301:**2243–2251.

133. **Patel, M. M., A. D. Clark, R. I. Glass, H. Greenberg, J. Tate, M. Santosham, C. F. Sanderson, D. Steele, M. Cortese, and U. D. Parashar.** 2009. Broadening the age restriction for initiating rotavirus vaccination in regions with high rotavirus mortality: benefits of mortality reduction versus risk of fatal intussusception. *Vaccine* **27:**2916–2922.

134. **Patel, M. M., A. J. Hall, J. Vinje, and U. D. Parashar.** 2009. Noroviruses: a comprehensive review. *J. Clin. Virol.* **44:**1–8.

135. Pearson, T., J. D. Busch, J. Ravel, T. D. Read, S. D. Rhoton, J. M. U'Ren, T. S. Simonson, S. M. Kachur, R. R. Leadem, M. L. Cardon, M. N. Van Ert, L. Y. Huynh, C. M. Fraser, and P. Keim. 2004. Phylogenetic discovery bias in *Bacillus anthracis* using single-nucleotide polymorphisms from whole-genome sequencing. *Proc. Natl. Acad. Sci. USA* **101**:13536–13541.

136. Pelludat, C., R. Prager, H. Tschape, W. Rabsch, J. Schuchhardt, and W. D. Hardt. 2005. Pilot study to evaluate microarray hybridization as a tool for *Salmonella enterica* serovar Typhimurium strain differentiation. *J. Clin. Microbiol.* **43**:4092–4106.

137. Persson, S., K. E. Olsen, S. Ethelberg, and F. Scheutz. 2007. Subtyping method for *Escherichia coli* Shiga toxin (verocytotoxin) 2 variants and correlations to clinical manifestations. *J. Clin. Microbiol.* **45**:2020–2024.

138. Pezzoli, L., R. Elson, C. L. Little, H. Yip, I. Fisher, R. Yishai, E. Anis, L. Valinsky, M. Biggerstaff, N. Patel, H. Mather, D. J. Brown, J. E. Coia, W. van Pelt, E. M. Nielsen, S. Ethelberg, E. de Pinna, M. D. Hampton, T. Peters, and J. Threlfall. 2008. Packed with *Salmonella*—investigation of an international outbreak of *Salmonella* Senftenberg infection linked to contamination of prepacked basil in 2007. *Foodborne Pathog. Dis.* **5**:661–668.

139. Pires, S. M., E. G. Evers, W. van Pelt, T. Ayers, E. Scallan, F. J. Angulo, A. Havelaar, and T. Hald. 2009. Attributing the human disease burden of foodborne infections to specific sources. *Foodborne Pathog. Dis.* **6**:417–424.

140. Pybus, O. G., A. J. Drummond, T. Nakano, B. H. Robertson, and A. Rambaut. 2003. The epidemiology and iatrogenic transmission of hepatitis C virus in Egypt: a Bayesian coalescent approach. *Mol. Biol. Evol.* **20**:381–387.

141. Quan, P. L., T. Briese, G. Palacios, and W. Ian Lipkin. 2008. Rapid sequence-based diagnosis of viral infection. *Antivir. Res.* **79**:1–5.

142. Rasschaert, G., K. Houf, H. Imberechts, K. Grijspeerdt, L. De Zutter, and M. Heyndrickx. 2005. Comparison of five repetitive-sequence-based PCR typing methods for molecular discrimination of *Salmonella enterica* isolates. *J. Clin. Microbiol.* **43**:3615–3623.

143. Reddy, T. B., R. Riley, F. Wymore, P. Montgomery, D. DeCaprio, R. Engels, M. Gellesch, J. Hubble, D. Jen, H. Jin, M. Koehrsen, L. Larson, M. Mao, M. Nitzberg, P. Sisk, C. Stolte, B. Weiner, J. White, Z. K. Zachariah, G. Sherlock, J. E. Galagan, C. A. Ball, and G. K. Schoolnik. 2009. TB database: an integrated platform for tuberculosis research. *Nucleic Acids Res.* **37**:D499–D508.

144. Rees, R. K., M. Graves, N. Caton, J. M. Ely, and W. S. Probert. 2009. Single tube identification and strain typing of *Brucella melitensis* by multiplex PCR. *J. Microbiol. Methods* **78**:66–70.

145. Roehrig, J. T., M. Layton, P. Smith, G. L. Campbell, R. Nasci, and R. S. Lanciotti. 2002. The emergence of West Nile virus in North America: ecology, epidemiology, and surveillance. *Curr. Top. Microbiol. Immunol.* **267**:223–240.

146. Rota, P. A., D. A. Featherstone, and W. J. Bellini. 2009. Molecular epidemiology of measles virus. *Curr. Top. Microbiol. Immunol.* **330**:129–150.

147. Rota, P. A., M. S. Oberste, S. S. Monroe, W. A. Nix, R. Campagnoli, J. P. Icenogle, S. Penaranda, B. Bankamp, K. Maher, M. H. Chen, S. Tong, A. Tamin, L. Lowe, M. Frace, J. L. DeRisi, Q. Chen, D. Wang, D. D. Erdman, T. C. Peret, C. Burns, T. G. Ksiazek, P. E. Rollin, A. Sanchez, S. Liffick, B. Holloway, J. Limor, K. McCaustland, M. Olsen-Rasmussen, R. Fouchier, S. Gunther, A. D. Osterhaus, C. Drosten, M. A. Pallansch, L. J. Anderson, and W. J. Bellini. 2003. Characterization of a novel coronavirus associated with severe acute respiratory syndrome. *Science* **300**:1394–1399.

148. Scherer, S., and D. A. Stevens. 1987. Application of DNA typing methods to epidemiology and taxonomy of *Candida* species. *J. Clin. Microbiol.* **25**:675–679.

149. Schwartz, D. C., and C. R. Cantor. 1984. Separation of yeast chromosome-sized DNAs by pulsed field gradient gel electrophoresis. *Cell* **37**:67–75.

150. Sergeev, N., E. Rubtcova, V. Chizikov, D. S. Schmid, and V. N. Loparev. 2006. New mosaic subgenotype of varicella-zoster virus in the USA: VZV detection and genotyping by oligonucleotide-microarray. *J. Virol. Methods* **136**:8–16.

151. Shannon, C. E., and W. Weaver. 1949. *The Mathematical Theory of Communication.* University of Illinois Press, Urbana-Champaign.

152. Sharples, G. J., and R. G. Lloyd. 1990. A novel repeated DNA sequence located in the intergenic regions of bacterial chromosomes. *Nucleic Acids Res.* **18**:6503–6508.

153. Sheppard, S. K., J. F. Dallas, N. J. Strachan, M. MacRae, N. D. McCarthy, D. J. Wilson, F. J. Gormley, D. Falush, I. D. Ogden, M. C. Maiden, and K. J. Forbes. 2009. *Campylobacter* genotyping to determine the source of human infection. *Clin. Infect. Dis.* **48**:1072–1078.

154. Sherry, S. T., M. H. Ward, M. Kholodov, J. Baker, L. Phan, E. M. Smigielski, and K. Sirotkin. 2001. dbSNP: the NCBI database of genetic variation. *Nucleic Acids Res.* **29**:308–311.

155. Shopsin, B., M. Gomez, S. O. Montgomery, D. H. Smith, M. Waddington, D. E. Dodge, D. A. Bost, M. Riehman, S. Naidich, and B. N. Kreiswirth. 1999. Evaluation of protein A gene polymorphic region DNA sequencing for typing of *Staphylococcus aureus* strains. *J. Clin. Microbiol.* **37**:3556–3563.

156. Smith, G. J., D. Vijaykrishna, J. Bahl, S. J. Lycett, M. Worobey, O. G. Pybus, S. K. Ma, C. L. Cheung, J. Raghwani, S. Bhatt, J. S. Peiris, Y. Guan, and A. Rambaut. 2009. Origins and evolutionary genomics of the 2009 swine-origin H1N1 influenza A epidemic. *Nature* **459**:1122–1125.

157. Song, E. J., H. J. Jeong, S. M. Lee, C. M. Kim, E. S. Song, Y. K. Park, G. H. Bai, E. Y. Lee, and C. L. Chang. 2007. A DNA chip-based spoligotyping method for the strain identification of *Mycobacterium tuberculosis* isolates. *J. Microbiol. Methods* **68**:430–433.

158. Song, Y., E. Dai, J. Wang, H. Liu, J. Zhai, C. Chen, Z. Du, Z. Guo, and R. Yang. 2006. Genotyping of hepatitis B virus (HBV) by oligonucleotides microarray. *Mol. Cell. Probes* **20**:121–127.

159. Southern, E. 1975. Detection of specific sequences among DNA fragments separated by gel electrophoresis. *J. Mol. Biol.* **98**:503–517.

160. Stern, M. J., G. F. Ames, N. H. Smith, E. C. Robinson, and C. F. Higgins. 1984. Repetitive extragenic palindromic sequences: a major component of the bacterial genome. *Cell* **37**:1015–1026.

161. Struelens, M. J. 1996. Consensus guidelines for appropriate use and evaluation of microbial epidemiologic typing systems. *Clin. Microbiol. Infect.* **2**:2–11.

162. Sturmer, M., A. Berger, and W. Preiser. 2004. HIV-1 genotyping: comparison of two commercially available assays. *Expert Rev. Mol. Diagn.* **4**:281–291.

163. Sulaiman, I. M., X. Liu, M. Frace, N. Sulaiman, M. Olsen-Rasmussen, E. Neuhaus, P. A. Rota, and R. M. Wohlhueter. 2006. Evaluation of affymetrix severe acute respiratory syndrome resequencing GeneChips in characterization of the genomes of two strains of coronavirus infecting humans. *Appl. Environ. Microbiol.* **72**:207–211.

164. Sulaiman, I. M., S. A. Sammons, and R. M. Wohlhueter. 2008. Smallpox virus resequencing GeneChips can also rapidly ascertain species status for some zoonotic non-variola orthopoxviruses. *J. Clin. Microbiol.* **46**:1507–1509.

165. Sulaiman, I. M., K. Tang, J. Osborne, S. Sammons, and R. M. Wohlhueter. 2007. GeneChip resequencing of the smallpox virus genome can identify novel strains: a biodefense application. *J. Clin. Microbiol.* **45**:358–363.

166. Swaminathan, B., T. J. Barrett, S. B. Hunter, R. V. Tauxe, and the CDC PulseNet task force. 2001. PulseNet: the molecular subtyping network for foodborne bacterial disease surveillance, United States. *Emerg. Infect. Dis.* **7**: 382–389.

167. Swaminathan, B., P. Gerner-Smidt, L. K. Ng, S. Lukinmaa, K. M. Kam, S. Rolando, E. P. Gutierrez, and N. Binsztein. 2006. Building PulseNet International: an interconnected system of laboratory networks to facilitate timely public health recognition and response to foodborne disease outbreaks and emerging foodborne diseases. *Foodborne Pathog. Dis.* **3**:36–50.

168. Tenover, F. C., R. D. Arbeit, R. V. Goering, P. A. Mickelsen, B. E. Murray, D. H. Persing, and B. Swaminathan. 1995. Interpreting chromosomal DNA restriction patterns produced by pulsed-field gel electrophoresis: criteria for bacterial strain typing. *J. Clin. Microbiol.* **33:**2233–2239.

169. Török, T. J., R. V. Tauxe, R. P. Wise, J. R. Livengood, R. Sokolow, S. Mauvais, K. A. Birkness, M. R. Skeels, J. M. Horan, and L. R. Foster. 1997. A large community outbreak of salmonellosis caused by intentional contamination of restaurant salad bars. *JAMA* **278:**389–395.

170. Torpdahl, M., G. Sorensen, B. A. Lindstedt, and E. M. Nielsen. 2007. Tandem repeat analysis for surveillance of human *Salmonella* Typhimurium infections. *Emerg. Infect. Dis.* **13:**388–395.

171. Torres-Cruz, J., and M. W. van der Woude. 2003. Slipped-strand mispairing can function as a phase variation mechanism in *Escherichia coli. J. Bacteriol.* **185:**6990–6994.

172. Townsend, M. B., E. D. Dawson, M. Mehlmann, J. A. Smagala, D. M. Dankbar, C. L. Moore, C. B. Smith, N. J. Cox, R. D. Kuchta, and K. L. Rowlen. 2006. Experimental evaluation of the FluChip diagnostic microarray for influenza virus surveillance. *J. Clin. Microbiol.* **44:**2863–2871.

173. Tungpradabkul, S., S. Panyim, P. Wilairat, and Y. Yuthavong. 1983. Analysis of DNA from various species and strains of malaria parasites by restriction endonuclease fingerprinting. *Comp. Biochem. Physiol. B* **74:**481–485.

174. Vahey, M., M. E. Nau, S. Barrick, J. D. Cooley, R. Sawyer, A. A. Sleeker, P. Vickerman, S. Bloor, B. Larder, N. L. Michael, and S. A. Wegner. 1999. Performance of the Affymetrix GeneChip HIV PRT 440 platform for antiretroviral drug resistance genotyping of human immunodeficiency virus type 1 clades and viral isolates with length polymorphisms. *J. Clin. Microbiol.* **37:**2533–2537.

175. van Belkum, A., S. Scherer, L. van Alphen, and H. Verbrugh. 1998. Short-sequence DNA repeats in prokaryotic genomes. *Microbiol. Mol. Biol. Rev.* **62:**275–293.

176. van Belkum, A., S. Scherer, W. van Leeuwen, D. Willemse, L. van Alphen, and H. Verbrugh. 1997. Variable number of tandem repeats in clinical strains of *Haemophilus influenzae. Infect. Immun.* **65:**5017–5027.

177. van Belkum, A., P. T. Tassios, L. Dijkshoorn, S. Haeggman, B. Cookson, N. K. Fry, V. Fussing, J. Green, E. Feil, P. Gerner-Smidt, S. Brisse, and M. Struelens. 2007. Guidelines for the validation and application of typing methods for use in bacterial epidemiology. *Clin. Microbiol. Infect.* **13**(Suppl. 3):1–46.

178. van der Zanden, A. G., K. Kremer, L. M. Schouls, K. Caimi, A. Cataldi, A. Hulleman, N. J. Nagelkerke, and D. van Soolingen. 2002. Improvement of differentiation and interpretability of spoligotyping for *Mycobacterium tuberculosis* complex isolates by introduction of new spacer oligonucleotides. *J. Clin. Microbiol.* **40:**4628–4639.

179. Vaneechoutte, M., L. Dijkshoorn, I. Tjernberg, A. Elaichouni, P. de Vos, G. Claeys, and G. Verschraegen. 1995. Identification of *Acinetobacter* genomic species by amplified ribosomal DNA restriction analysis. *J. Clin. Microbiol.* **33:**11–15.

180. van Embden, J. D., M. D. Cave, J. T. Crawford, J. W. Dale, K. D. Eisenach, B. Gicquel, P. Hermans, C. Martin, R. McAdam, T. M. Shinnick, et al. 1993. Strain identification of *Mycobacterium tuberculosis* by DNA fingerprinting: recommendations for a standardized methodology. *J. Clin. Microbiol.* **31:**406–409.

181. Versalovic, J., T. Koeuth, and J. R. Lupski. 1991. Distribution of repetitive DNA sequences in eubacteria and application to fingerprinting of bacterial genomes. *Nucleic Acids Res.* **19:**6823–6831.

182. Vigil, K. J., J. A. Adachi, H. Aboufaycal, R. Y. Hachem, R. A. Reitzel, Y. Jiang, J. J. Tarrand, R. F. Chemaly, G. P. Bodey, K. V. Rolston, and I. Raad. 2009. Multidrug-resistant *Escherichia coli* bacteremia in cancer patients. *Am. J. Infect. Control* **30:**30.

183. Vos, P., R. Hogers, M. Bleeker, M. Reijans, T. van de Lee, M. Hornes, A. Frijters, J. Pot, J. Peleman, M. Kuiper, et al. 1995. AFLP: a new technique for DNA fingerprinting. *Nucleic Acids Res.* **23:**4407–4414.

184. Wang, D., A. Urisman, Y. T. Liu, M. Springer, T. G. Ksiazek, D. D. Erdman, E. R. Mardis, M. Hickenbotham, V. Magrini, J. Eldred, J. P. Latreille, R. K. Wilson, D. Ganem, and J. L. DeRisi. 2003. Viral discovery and sequence recovery using DNA microarrays. *PLoS Biol.* **1:**E2.

185. Wang, L. C., C. H. Pan, L. L. Severinghaus, L. Y. Liu, C. T. Chen, C. E. Pu, D. Huang, J. T. Lir, S. C. Chin, M. C. Cheng, S. H. Lee, and C. H. Wang. 2008. Simultaneous detection and differentiation of Newcastle disease and avian influenza viruses using oligonucleotide microarrays. *Vet. Microbiol.* **127:**217–226.

186. Ward, T. J., T. F. Ducey, T. Usgaard, K. A. Dunn, and J. P. Bielawski. 2008. Multilocus genotyping assays for single nucleotide polymorphism-based subtyping of *Listeria monocytogenes* isolates. *Appl. Environ. Microbiol.* **74:**7629–7642.

187. Warren, R. L., G. G. Sutton, S. J. Jones, and R. A. Holt. 2007. Assembling millions of short DNA sequences using SSAKE. *Bioinformatics* **23:**500–501.

188. Warsen, A. E., M. J. Krug, S. LaFrentz, D. R. Stanek, F. J. Loge, and D. R. Call. 2004. Simultaneous discrimination between 15 fish pathogens by using 16S ribosomal DNA PCR and DNA microarrays. *Appl. Environ. Microbiol.* **70:**4216–4221.

189. Welsh, J., and M. McClelland. 1990. Fingerprinting genomes using PCR with arbitrary primers. *Nucleic Acids Res.* **18:**7213–7227.

190. Wheelan, S. J., F. Martinez Murillo, and J. D. Boeke. 2008. The incredible shrinking world of DNA microarrays. *Mol. Biosyst.* **4:**726–732.

191. Wick, L. M., W. Qi, D. W. Lacher, and T. S. Whittam. 2005. Evolution of genomic content in the stepwise emergence of *Escherichia coli* O157:H7. *J. Bacteriol.* **187:**1783–1791.

192. Williams, J. G. K., A. R. Kubelik, K. J. Livak, J. A. Rafalski, and S. V. Tingey. 1990. DNA polymorphisms amplified by arbitrary primers are useful as genetic markers. *Nucleic Acids Res.* **17:**6531–6535.

193. Wong, C. W., T. J. Albert, V. B. Vega, J. E. Norton, D. J. Cutler, T. A. Richmond, L. W. Stanton, E. T. Liu, and L. D. Miller. 2004. Tracking the evolution of the SARS coronavirus using high-throughput, high-density resequencing arrays. *Genome Res.* **14:**398–405.

194. Yang, C. F., H. Y. Chen, J. Jorba, H. C. Sun, S. J. Yang, H. C. Lee, Y. C. Huang, T. Y. Lin, P. J. Chen, H. Shimizu, Y. Nishimura, A. Utama, M. Pallansch, T. Miyamura, O. Kew, and J. Y. Yang. 2005. Intratypic recombination among lineages of type 1 vaccine-derived poliovirus emerging during chronic infection of an immunodeficient patient. *J. Virol.* **79:**12623–12634.

195. Yilmaz, O., and E. Demiray. 2007. Clinical role and importance of fluorescence in situ hybridization method in diagnosis of *H. pylori* infection and determination of clarithromycin resistance in *H. pylori* eradication therapy. *World J. Gastroenterol.* **13:**671–675.

196. Yoshida, C., K. Franklin, P. Konczy, J. R. McQuiston, P. I. Fields, J. H. Nash, E. N. Taboada, and K. Rahn. 2007. Methodologies towards the development of an oligonucleotide microarray for determination of *Salmonella* serotypes. *J. Microbiol. Methods* **70:**261–271.

197. Zhang, W., B. M. Jayarao, and S. J. Knabel. 2004. Multi-virulence-locus sequence typing of *Listeria monocytogenes. Appl. Environ. Microbiol.* **70:**913–920.

198. Zhang, W., W. Qi, T. J. Albert, A. S. Motiwala, D. Alland, E. K. Hyytia-Trees, E. M. Ribot, P. I. Fields, T. S. Whittam, and B. Swaminathan. 2006. Probing genomic diversity and evolution of *Escherichia coli* O157 by single nucleotide polymorphisms. *Genome Res.* **16:**757–767.

Procedures for the Storage of Microorganisms*

CATHY A. PETTI AND KAREN C. CARROLL

9

Long- and short-term preservation of microorganisms for future study has a long tradition in microbiology. Culture collections of microorganisms are valuable resources for scientific research in microbial diversity and evolution, patient care management, epidemiological investigations, and educational purposes. Preserved individual strains of microorganisms serve as permanent records of microorganisms' unique phenotypic profiles and provide the material for further genotypic characterizations. Such reference collections can encompass rare infectious agents unique to an individual or catalog the history of disease caused by common pathogens such as those responsible for community outbreaks.

There are multiple methods for microbial preservation. Effective storage is defined by the ability to maintain an organism in a viable state free of contamination and without changes in its genotypic or phenotypic characteristics. Secondly, the organism must be easily restored to its condition prior to preservation. Microbial preservation methods have been evaluated extensively over the past 60 years, and often, optimal methods for preservation depend on a microorganism's taxonomic classification. Review articles, monographs, and books have been published that provide detailed information about the storage of various types of microorganisms (1, 15, 19, 20, 36). For clinical microbiology laboratories, simple and broadly applied methods are necessary to maintain organisms for short- and long-term recovery. This chapter presents methods that can be used for the storage of bacteria, protozoa, fungi, and viruses.

OVERVIEW OF PRESERVATION METHODS

Short-Term Preservation Methods

Direct Transfer to Subculture

The simplest method for maintaining the short-term viability of microorganisms, most often used for bacteria, is periodic subculture to fresh medium. Although simple, if microorganisms are saved for more than 1 week, this method is potentially labor-intensive, requires extensive laboratory space, and may compromise a microorganism's

phenotypic profile. Each transfer to a new subculture increases the likelihood of mutation with undesirable changes in a microorganism's characteristics.

The interval between transfers varies among organisms. Additionally, the rate of mutation is quite variable. Some organisms appear stable indefinitely with repeated transfer, and others may change phenotypic traits after as few as two or three passages. The actual rate of mutation, however, has not been studied using sequencing technology. Issues that must be addressed with direct transfer include the medium to be used, the storage conditions, and the frequency of transfer.

Maintenance Medium

The medium should support the survival of the microorganism but minimize its metabolic processes and slow its rate of growth. Extreme environments should be avoided because microorganisms have the unique ability to adapt through mutation events in order to survive in suboptimal surroundings. A medium with too high a nutrient content will induce rapid replication that requires more frequent transfers. The optimal medium for maintaining microorganisms has not been clearly defined and most likely varies from one genus to another. Media that have been used include distilled water, tryptic soy broth, and nutrient broths (e.g., from Becton Dickinson and Co. and Oxoid Ltd.), all of which may be used with or without cryopreservatives.

Storage Conditions

Many laboratories store organisms, most often bacteria, for short periods on routine agar media at the workbench. Cultures kept in this fashion are subject to drying. A better method is to transfer organisms into screw-top test tubes and to store them in an organized location away from light and significant temperature changes. To prevent drying, caps can include rubber liners, or film can be wrapped over the top of the tube before or after the cap is screwed on. Storage at lower temperatures (5 to 8°C) slows metabolic processes and maintains viability for longer periods.

Frequency of Transfer

There is no set protocol for the frequency of transfer since storage conditions, media used, and types of microorganisms vary among laboratories. Individual laboratories should conduct studies for each category of microorganism to determine acceptable intervals between transfers under their

---

*This chapter contains information presented in chapter 6 by Cathy A. Petti, Karen C. Carroll, and Larry G. Reimer in the ninth edition of this *Manual.*

conditions used for storage. Such studies would involve performing subcultures at scheduled times until the laboratory identifies an acceptable interval between transfers at which a microorganism can reliably and reproducibly be recovered. (When transfers are performed, 5 to 10 representative colonies should be used to avoid the possibility of introducing an altered genotypic or phenotypic characteristic.)

Quality Control Procedures

Although it is not necessary with each transfer, the status of the specimen should be assessed periodically. Ongoing viability, stability of phenotype, microorganism identity, and the rate of contamination of specimens should be determined and noted in a log.

Immersion in Oil

An alternative to capping tubes is to add a layer of mineral oil to the top of the specimen. Many bacteria and fungi can be stored for periods of up to 2 to 3 years by this method, and transfers are not needed as frequently. Microorganisms are still metabolically active in this environment, and mutations can still occur. Contamination of the specimen can occur if the mineral oil is not adequately sterilized.

Mineral oil should be medicinal-grade oil with a specific gravity of 0.865 to 0.890 (e.g., from Roxane Laboratories or Becton Dickinson and Co.). For sterilization, it should be heated to 170°C for 1 to 2 h in an oven (15). Autoclaving is not considered acceptable.

To prepare the specimen, an inoculum of 5 to 10 colonies of the microorganism should be placed on an agar slant or in tubed broth media. Once growth is identified, a layer of mineral oil at least 1 to 2 cm deep is added, and the agar must not be exposed to air. As with the simple transfer method, tests for viability should be performed to determine the optimal transfer schedule that will ensure microorganism recovery. Transfers will be less frequent than those of microorganisms stored without oil; however, oil is more difficult to add to vials and to clean up in the event of spills.

Freezing at −20°C

Refrigeration or freezing in ordinary freezers at −20°C may be used to preserve microorganisms for periods longer than those that can be accomplished by repeated transfers. Viability may be maintained for as long as 1 to 2 years for specific microorganisms, but overall, damage caused by ice crystal formation (20) and electrolyte fluctuations (15) results in poor long-term survival. The medium used for storage appears to be important, since preservation times vary from a few months to 2 years depending upon which medium is used (17, 20, 22). Modern self-defrosting freezers with freeze-thaw cycles must be avoided because cyclic temperature fluctuation will destroy the microorganism.

Drying

Although most microorganisms do not survive drying, molds and some spore-forming bacteria may be dried and stored for prolonged periods. Soil can be used as a storage medium if it is autoclaved and air dried. Soil should be autoclaved for several hours on two successive days. It is then transferred into sterile glass tubes. A 1-ml suspension of the microorganism is inoculated into the tube, and the tube is left open to air dry before being closed with a sterile stopper. The sample is stored in a refrigerator (15). Although potentially effective, soil is not a standardized, defined, and consistent product for use over long periods. Instead, commercial silica gel can be used in small cotton-plugged tubes after being heated in an oven to 175°C for 1.5 to 2 h (20), with moderately successful recovery of fungi. Alternatively, a suspension of 10^8 microorganisms can be inoculated onto sterile filter paper strips or disks. The paper is dried in air or under a vacuum and is placed in sterile vials. These vials can be stored in the refrigerator for up to 4 years, and then single strips or disks can be removed as needed (15). This method is commonly used for quality control organisms.

Storage in Distilled Water

Most organisms do poorly in distilled water, but some survive for prolonged periods. Many fungi and *Pseudomonas* spp. survive for several years in distilled water at room temperature (20, 27). McGinnis et al. found that with the exception of fungi that do not easily sporulate, 93% of yeasts, molds, and aerobic actinomycetes can be easily and inexpensively preserved this way (26).

Long-Term Preservation Methods

Whereas the methods described above may be used to store microorganisms for periods of up to a few years, ultralow-temperature freezing and freeze-drying (lyophilization) are recommended for long-term storage. Although the initial investment in ultralow-temperature freezers and lyophilization may be costly, these methods are less labor-intensive over time, require less laboratory space (e.g., a cryovial versus broth or agar media), and reduce the chances of mutation events. Of course, mutations may still occur, and this phenomenon was observed in *Staphylococcus aureus* strains that lost the *mecA* gene during long-term preservation at −80°C (39). Similar to those with other preservation methods, survival rates after freeze-drying vary with species. Evaluating microorganisms over a 10-year period, Miyamoto-Shinohara et al. found that survival rates after freeze-drying for *Brevibacterium* spp. and *Corynebacterium* spp. approached 80%, whereas those for *Streptococcus mutans* decreased to 20% after 10 years (27).

Ultralow-Temperature Freezing

Microorganisms can be maintained at temperatures of −70°C or lower for prolonged periods. Systems for achieving these temperatures include ultralow-temperature electric freezers and liquid nitrogen storage units. With either system, unwanted heating can occur due to the loss of electrical power or liquid nitrogen. Close observation of the system and an adequate alarm mechanism are essential, since any increase in temperature will reduce viability. In the event that the temperature does rise, restoring power and returning to the target storage temperature as quickly as possible are essential. The presence of a cryopreservative such as glycerol may reduce the risk to microorganisms upon short exposure to higher temperatures (29). If thawing does occur, there are no guidelines for rapid restoration of the storage condition. Refreezing of the sealed vials as described below may be considered.

Storage Vials

Storage vials must be able to withstand very low temperatures and maintain a seal for their contents. Plastic (polypropylene) or glass (borosilicate) tubes may be used. Plastic vials with screw tops and silicone washers are much easier to use than glass vials that must be sealed with a flame and then scored and broken open. Several commercial suppliers stock acceptable vials (e.g., Fisher Scientific

Products, VWR Scientific, Wheaton Science Products, and Becton Dickinson and Co.). Vials come in a variety of sizes. Half-dram vials are available from several suppliers and can be conveniently packaged in a 12-by-12 grid so that 144 vials are stored in one box or layer.

Cryoprotective Agents

To protect microorganisms from damage during the freezing process, during storage, and during thawing, cryoprotective agents are often added to the culture suspension. Whereas most bacteria, fungi, and viruses survive better with such additives, studies have shown that cryoprotective agents significantly damage others. The reader is referred to detailed references for specifics (Table 1) (1, 20). Rapid freezing without additives may still be acceptable for the long-term survival of protozoa, although freeze-drying may be preferred.

There are two types of cryoprotective agents: those that enter the cell and protect the intracellular environment and others that protect the external milieu of the organism. Glycerol and dimethyl sulfoxide (DMSO) are most often

used for the former; sucrose, lactose, glucose, mannitol, sorbitol, dextran, polyvinylpyrrolidone, polyglycol, and skim milk are used for the latter. Combinations of agents as well as detergents (e.g., Tween 80 and Triton WR 1339), other carbohydrates (e.g., honey), and calcium lactobionate have also been used. The most universal cryoprotectant is DMSO; however, the optimal cryoprotectant often varies with the microorganism. For example, glycerol appears to be best suited for the preservation of bacteria. A current and comprehensive review of protectant additives used in the cryopreservation of microorganisms is provided by Hubalek (21).

Glycerol is added at a concentration of 10% (vol/vol), and DMSO is added at 5% (vol/vol). Prior to use, glycerol is sterilized by autoclaving. Once prepared, it can be stocked at room temperature for months. DMSO must be filter sterilized and can be stored in open containers for only 1 month prior to use.

Of the external products, skim milk is the most often used. Dehydrated skim milk is purchased from medical product suppliers (e.g., Becton Dickinson and Co. and

TABLE 1 Common procedures for preservation of microorganisms

Organism group	Storage method	Cryopreservative	Storage temp (°C)	Storage duration (yr)
Gram-positive bacteria	Transfer	None	Room temp	0.2–0.3
	Immersion in mineral oil	None	4	0.6–2
	Freezing	Sucrose, glycerol	−20	1–3
	Ultralow-temp freezing	Skim milk, sucrose, glycerol	−70 to −196	1–30
	Lyophilization	Skim milk, sucrose	4	30
Streptococci	Freezing	Skim milk	−20	0.2
	Ultralow-temp freezing	Skim milk	−70 to −196	0.2–1
	Lyophilization	Skim milk	4	0.5–30
Mycobacteria	Freezing	Skim milk	−20	3–5
	Ultralow-temp freezing	Skim milk	−70 to −196	3–5
	Lyophilization	Skim milk	4	16–30
Gram-negative bacteria	Transfer	None	Room temp	0.1–0.3
	Immersion in mineral oil	None	4	1–2
	Freezing	Sucrose, lactose	−20	1–2
	Ultralow-temp freezing	Sucrose, lactose, glycerol	−70 to −196	2–30
	Lyophilization	Skim milk, sucrose, lactose	4	30
Spore-forming bacteria	Transfer	None	Room temp	0.2–1
	Immersion in mineral oil	None	4	1
	Drying	None	Room temp	1–2
	Freezing	Glucose	−20	1–2
	Ultralow-temp freezing	Skim milk, glycerol	−70 to −196	2–30
	Lyophilization	Skim milk, lactose	4	30
Filamentous fungi	Transfer	None	4 to 25	2–10
	Immersion in mineral oil	None	Room temp	1–40
	Storage in distilled water	None	Room temp	1–10
	Drying	Soil, silica gel	Room temp	1–4
	Ultralow-temp freezing	Glycerol, DMSO	−70 to −196	2–30
	Lyophilization (sporeformers)	Glycerol, sucrose, DMSO, skim milk	4	2–30
Yeasts	Storage in distilled water	None	Room temp	1–2
	Drying	Nutrient medium	Room temp	1–2
	Lyophilization	Nutrient medium	4	2+
Protozoa	Freezing	Blood, nutrient broth with DMSO or sucrose	−20 to −40	
	Ultralow-temp freezing	Blood, nutrient medium with DMSO or glycerol	−70 to −196	
Viruses	Transfer	Nutrient medium	4	0.5
	Ultralow-temp freezing	SPGA	−70 to −196	1–30
	Lyophilization	SPGA	4	6–10

Oxoid). It is autoclaved and used in a final concentration of 20% (wt/vol) in distilled water (1). This is double the concentration suggested by the manufacturers if the intent is to make a reconstituted equivalent of regular milk.

Preparation of Microorganisms for Freezing
Microorganisms are inoculated into a medium that adequately supports maximal growth. Cultures are allowed to mature to the late growth or stationary phase before being harvested. Broth specimens are centrifuged to create a pellet of microorganisms. The pellet is withdrawn and resuspended in 2 to 5 ml of broth with the appropriate concentration of cryoprotectant additive. For agar specimens, broth containing the cryoprotectant is placed on the surface of the agar. The surface is scraped with a pipette or sterile loop to suspend microorganisms, and then the broth mixture is pipetted directly into freezer vials. Alternatively, the agar surface can be scraped with a sterile loop. The microorganisms can then be transferred directly into the vial of cryoprotectant and emulsified into a final dense suspension. The volume of the aliquots to be frozen is typically 0.2 to 0.5 ml.

Freezing Method
The American Type Culture Collection (ATCC) recommends slow, controlled-rate freezing at a rate of 1°C per min until the vials cool to a temperature of at least −30°C, followed by more rapid cooling until the final storage temperature is achieved (1). Controlled-rate freezers are required for the initial phase of cooling. Studies in the 1970s showed that uncontrolled-rate freezing may be acceptable for most organisms and is much less expensive or labor-intensive (20). When organisms are stored in liquid nitrogen, however, it is still recommended that vials be placed initially in a −60°C freezer for 1 h and then transferred into the liquid nitrogen. When organisms are stored permanently at −60 to −70°C, the vials can be placed directly into the freezer.

Small glass beads or plastic beads (e.g., from Fisher Scientific Products or Wheaton Science Products) can also be added to storage vials before freezing. The culture suspension will coat the beads, and then individual beads can be removed from storage for reconstitution without thawing the entire sample (13).

Thawing
Damage to microorganisms occurs as they are warmed from the frozen state. Critical temperatures appear to be between −40 and −5°C. Studies suggest that rapid warming through these temperatures improves recovery rates. Stored culture vials should be warmed rapidly in a 35°C water bath until all ice has disappeared (1, 20). Once a vial is thawed, it should be opened and the organism should be transferred to an appropriate growth medium immediately. Great care must be exercised during the thawing phase, since rapid temperature changes and resulting air pressure changes inside vials can cause the vials to explode. Protective clothing and eyewear must be worn during this process.

Freeze-Drying (Lyophilization)
Freeze-drying is considered to be the most effective way to provide long-term storage of most bacteria, yeasts, sporulating molds, and viruses. Better preservation occurs with freeze-drying than with other methods because freeze-drying reduces the risk of intracellular ice crystallization, which compromises viability. Removal of water from the

specimen effectively prevents this damage. Among bacteria, the relative viability with lyophilization is greatest with gram-positive bacteria (sporeformers in particular) and decreases with gram-negative bacteria (20, 28), but overall, the viability of bacteria can be maintained for as long as 30 years. In addition, large numbers of vials of dried microorganisms can be stored with limited space, and organisms can be easily transported long distances at room temperature.

The process combines freezing and dehydration. Organisms are initially frozen and then dried by lowering the atmospheric pressure with a vacuum apparatus. Freeze-drying has been extensively reviewed in the past (19), and the required equipment includes a vacuum pump connected in line to a condenser and to the specimens. Specimens can be connected individually to the condenser (manifold method) or can be placed in a chamber where they are dehydrated in one larger air space (chamber or batch method). Alexander et al. and Heckly have both published detailed descriptions of equipment options (1, 19).

Storage Vials
Glass vials are used for all freeze-dried specimens. When freeze-drying is performed in a chamber, double glass vials are used. In the chamber method, an outer soft-glass vial is added for protection and preservation of the dehydrated specimen. Silica gel granules are placed in the bottom of the outer vial before the inner vial is inserted and cushioned with cotton. For the manifold method, a single glass vial is used. For both methods, the vial containing the actual specimen is lightly plugged with absorbent cotton. The storage vial in the manifold method or the outer vial in the chamber method must be sealed to maintain the vacuum and the dry atmospheric condition. All vials are sterilized prior to use by heating in a hot-air oven.

Cryoprotective Agents
Research concerning cryoprotective agents has been extensively reviewed (19). In general, the two most commonly used agents are skim milk and sucrose. Skim milk is used most often for chamber lyophilization, and sucrose is used most often for manifold lyophilization. Skim milk is prepared by making a 20% (vol/vol) solution of skim milk in distilled water. The solution is divided into 5-ml aliquots and autoclaved at 116°C, with care taken to prevent overheating and caramelization of the solution. The preparation is then used in smaller volumes as described above for freezing. Sucrose is prepared in an initial mixture of 24% (vol/vol) sucrose in water and added in equal volumes to the microorganism suspension in growth medium to make a final concentration of 12% (vol/vol).

Preparation of Microorganisms for Lyophilization
As with simple freezing, maximum recovery of organisms is achieved by using microorganisms in the late growth or stationary phase from the growth of an inoculum in an appropriate growth medium. High concentrations of microorganisms are considered to be important. The ATCC recommends a concentration of at least 10^8 CFU/ml (1), and Heckly suggests a concentration of 10^{10} CFU/ml or higher (20).

Freeze-Drying Methods
In the chamber method, inner vials with the microorganism suspension are placed in a single layer inside a stainless steel container. This container is placed in a low-temperature freezer at −60°C for 1 h. The container is

then transferred to a chamber containing dry ice and ethyl Cellosolve (Becton Dickinson and Co.) and covered with a sealable vacuum top, which is connected in sequence to a condenser reservoir also filled with dry ice and ethyl Cellosolve and to a vacuum pump. The vacuum is maintained at a minimum of 30 μm Hg for 18 h. At the same time, the outer vials are prepared by being heated in an oven overnight, filled with silica gel granules and cotton, and placed in a dry cabinet (with <10% relative humidity). The freeze-dried inner vials are inserted into the outer vials, and the outer vials are heat sealed. Multiple different strains or species should probably not be processed in the same batch. Cross contamination rates vary from 0.8 to 3.3% when two different microorganisms are placed on opposite sides of the same container and are as high as 8.3 to 13.3% when microorganisms are intermingled (3).

In the manifold method, a rack of individual vials is used rather than a single container. The rack is placed in a dry ice-ethyl Cellosolve bath. After the freezing process, the vials are connected by individual rubber tubes in sequence to the condenser container filled with dry ice and ethyl Cellosolve and to the vacuum pump. As in the method described above, the vacuum is maintained at 30 μm Hg for 18 h and then the individual vials are sealed.

Storage
Individual vials need to be appropriately labeled and sorted. Storage at room temperature does not maintain viability and is not recommended. Storage at 4°C in an ordinary refrigerator is acceptable, but survival rates may be improved at temperatures of −30 to −60°C (1, 19).

Reconstitution
Care must be taken when opening vials for reconstitution because of the vacuum inside the vial. Safety glasses should always be worn, and vials should be covered with gauze to prevent injury if the vial explodes when air rushes in. Reconstitution should also be conducted in a closed hood to avoid dispersal of microorganisms. The surface of the vial should be wiped with 70% alcohol, and then the top of the glass vial can be scored and broken off or punctured with a hot needle. A small amount (0.1 to 0.4 ml) of growth medium is injected into the vial with a needle and syringe or a Pasteur pipette, the contents are stirred until the specimen is dissolved, and then the entire contents are transferred with the same syringe or a pipette to appropriate broth or agar media. A purity check must be done on each specimen because of the possibility of either cross contamination or mutation during the preservation process.

Newer Technologies
The long-term preservation methods previously described are specifically designed for recovery of microorganisms for further cultivation. Culture-independent tests based on antigen or nucleic acid technologies are in widespread use and do not require viable microorganisms. In this regard, storage of microorganisms to preserve their antigens or nucleic acids is also important for clinical laboratories. The use of Whatman Flinders Technology Associates (FTA) matrix cards (Whatman International Ltd., Maidstone, United Kingdom) or other filter paper-based products is a novel approach for long-term storage of microbial DNA that is safe (microorganisms are inactivated), inexpensive, and fast (4, 33). Bacterial and/or fungal cell suspensions are applied directly to dry FTA paper. The FTA cards are impregnated with buffers, free radical trap and protein denaturants that lyse cell membranes on contact, entrap DNA, and protect DNA from degradation. This technology has been successfully applied to a variety of bacteria and fungi and serves as a reusable DNA archiving system. Although beyond the scope of this chapter, direct specimens such as blood can be preserved using a dry blood spot on filter paper or with a non-paper-based matrix for future antibody or nucleic acid testing to detect human immunodeficiency virus (5, 8, 25), hepatitis B virus (8), hepatitis C virus (8, 25), *Rickettsia typhi*, and *Orientia tsutsugamushi* (30).

Procedures for Specific Organisms
Procedures for specific organisms are described below and summarized in Table 1.

Bacteria
All of the material presented in this chapter applies primarily to the preservation of bacteria. Simple transfer, storage under mineral oil, drying, or freezing at −20°C can maintain bacteria for short periods; freezing in ultralow-temperature electric freezers at −70°C or in liquid nitrogen at −196°C or freeze-drying can provide long-term preservation. A summary of the studies of bacterial preservation has been published (20). In general, serial transfer will preserve bacteria for up to a few months, storage under mineral oil or with drying will last 1 to 2 years, freezing at −20°C will preserve bacteria for 1 to 3 years, freezing at −70°C will preserve bacteria for 1 to 10 years, and freezing in liquid nitrogen and freeze-drying will preserve bacteria for up to 30 years (15). For fastidious bacteria such as *Streptococcus pneumoniae*, *Neisseria* spp., and *Haemophilus* spp., the optimal methods are lyophilization and freezing at −70°C by using Trypticase soy broth with glycerol as a preservation medium (31, 35, 40). Stock cultures of quality control microorganisms can be maintained in a cryopreservative suspension for up to 1 year at −20°C or indefinitely at −70°C.

Protozoa
Information concerning the preservation of protozoa is limited, in keeping with the infrequent need for such a process in clinical microbiology laboratories. Variable methods for individual genera are described. In general, freezing appears to be preferred to freeze-drying. All of the following procedures are as described by the ATCC (1).

Acanthamoeba spp., *Leishmania* spp., *Naegleria* spp., *Trichomonas* spp., and *Trypanosoma* spp. can be handled as described above for ultralow-temperature freezing with 5% (vol/vol) DMSO as the cryoprotective agent. These organisms should be stored in liquid nitrogen.

Acanthamoeba spp. and *Naegleria* spp. can also be dried at room temperature onto filter paper. Aliquots of a microorganism suspension (0.3 ml) are pipetted onto the paper in a shell vial and dried in air for 14 days at room temperature and then in a vacuum desiccator for an additional week. The vials are sealed and stored in liquid nitrogen.

Entamoeba spp. are stored frozen at −40°C. Specimens should be suspended in a mixture of growth medium containing 12% (vol/vol) DMSO and 6% (vol/vol) sucrose.

Leishmania spp. may also be prepared by inoculation of the organism into an animal host. At the peak of infection, the spleen is harvested and homogenized in half the final volume of ATCC medium 811 salt solution. Freezing is completed with 10% glycerol as the cryoprotectant.

Plasmodium spp. can be stored from infected blood samples. At the height of parasitemia, blood is obtained and anticoagulated with the following preparation: 1.33 g of sodium citrate, 0.47 g of citric acid, 3.00 g of dextrose, 200 mg of heparin (sodium), and 100 ml of distilled water. The final concentration of anticoagulant added to blood is 10%. To this anticoagulated blood, 30% glycerol in 0.0667 M phosphate buffer is added to a final concentration of 10% (vol/vol) glycerol. Freezing should occur in liquid nitrogen.

Trypanosoma spp. must be harvested from an animal host. At the peak of parasitemia, blood is withdrawn into heparinized tubes and diluted 1:1 in Tyrode's solution (8.0 g of NaCl per liter, 0.02 g of KCl per liter, 0.2 g of $CaCl_2$ per liter, 0.1 g of $MgCl_2$ per liter, 0.05 g of NaH_2PO_4 per liter, 1.0 g of $NaHCO_3$ per liter, and 1.0 g of glucose per liter) with 1 to 5% phenol red added. Then 5% DMSO is added as the cryoprotectant, and the specimen is stored in liquid nitrogen.

Yeasts and Filamentous Fungi

All of the techniques described above have been applied to the storage of yeasts and fungi (7, 15, 20, 36). The individual method employed depends upon the species to be preserved and whether or not it sporulates.

Subculturing. Subculturing is the simplest method of maintaining living fungi and involves serial transfer to fresh solid or liquid media. Storage is accomplished usually at room or refrigerator temperature. Fungi may be maintained by subculturing for a number of years. Care must be taken to avoid aerosolization and contamination of the laboratory or other specimens.

Storage under oil. Whereas species of *Aspergillus* and *Penicillium* have remained viable under oil for 40 years (36), many species have shown deterioration after 1 to 2 years and must be transferred periodically. Taddei et al. also reported the successful storage and recovery of actinomycetes stored under paraffin oil for 10 to 30 years (37).

Water storage. Many fungi can be stored successfully for prolonged periods in distilled water (27, 32). A simple method is to pipette 6 to 7 ml of sterile distilled water onto 2-week-old culture slants in screw-cap tubes. The spores and fragments of hyphae are dislodged by scraping with the pipette, and the suspension is transferred to a sterile 1-g vial, which is tightly capped and stored at 25°C. Fungi are revived by subculturing 0.2 to 0.3 ml of the suspension to appropriate media (6).

An alternative method is to cut agar blocks from the growing edge of a fungal colony and place them in sterile distilled water in bottles with screw-cap lids (18). The cultures are stored at 20 to 25°C. The fungi are retrieved by removing a block and placing it mycelium side down on growth medium appropriate for that species (36). Contamination (22.8%) is a significant problem with this method (18).

Drying. Drying as described above has been used for fungi. Only 6 of 16 genera of fungi stored in this fashion survived for 4 years (2). The greatest success is reported for sporulating fungi stored in silica gel or in soil (36).

Freezing. Fungi have been successfully preserved by storage in liquid nitrogen by using glycerol or DMSO as a cryopreservative. Broth cultures containing nonpathogenic fungi are disrupted in a Waring blender and suspended in equal parts of DMSO or glycerol to achieve final concentrations of 5 or 10%, respectively. Pathogens should not be disrupted in a mechanical blender because of the potential biohazard associated with aerosolization. *Histoplasma*, *Paracoccidioides*, and *Blastomyces* species should be frozen in the yeast phase, and *Coccidioides* species should be frozen in the early mycelial phase to minimize exposure of laboratory personnel. Otherwise, procedures for freezing are as described above.

Freeze-drying. Most spore-forming fungi can be preserved by freeze-drying. Cultures to be stored by freeze-drying should be grown on agar or broth media to the point of maximum sporulation (1) and processed as described above. Survival in storage for many years has been demonstrated (11, 34), but this is true only for sporulating organisms. Young vegetative hyphae of fungi do not survive freeze-drying (36).

Viruses

Viruses tend to be more stable than other microorganisms because of their small size and simple structure and the absence of free water. Many viruses can be stored for months at refrigerator temperatures or for years by ultralow-temperature freezing or freeze-drying. Storage at −20°C is not recommended (20, 23). Larger viruses tend to be less stable than smaller ones (16).

Ultralow-temperature freezing is effective in a number of situations. In addition to cryoprotectants described above, sucrose-phosphate-glutamate containing 1% bovine albumin (SPGA) (20, 23) and hypertonic sucrose are particularly effective, the latter for storing labile viruses such as respiratory syncytial virus (24). If ultralow-temperature freezing is employed, the rate of freezing should be as high as possible, using small-volume suspensions (0.1 to 0.5 ml). In addition to freezing of pure isolates, stool specimens known to contain viral enteric pathogens have been maintained at −70 to −85°C for 6 to 10 years with reasonable recovery and no change in the morphological characteristics of astroviruses, small round structured viruses, enteric adenoviruses, rotaviruses, and caliciviruses (41).

Gallo et al. evaluated five types of media for storage of human immunodeficiency virus-infected peripheral blood lymphocytes and concluded that freezing peripheral blood lymphocytes in RPMI 1640 containing 10% fetal bovine serum and 10% DMSO and storing them at −60°C is acceptable for human immunodeficiency virus isolation (14).

Freeze-drying is probably the optimum method for preserving viruses for extended periods. A detailed review of acceptable procedures has been published (16). Virus suspensions freeze-dried in medium supported with SPGA appear to survive better (20, 38). Lyophilization of polioviruses and other enteroviruses works best when electrolytes are removed by dialysis or ultrafiltration (20).

Select Agents

In response to the Public Health Security and Bioterrorism Preparedness and Response Act of 2002, federal regulations require laboratories that store select agents to register and comply with the standards established by the act (12). A current and complete list of microorganisms considered to be select agents can be found at http://www.cdc.gov/od/sap. Regardless of the method for long-term preservation, laboratories must register with the Department of Health and Human Services and Centers for Disease Control and Prevention Select Agent Program. In order to minimize risk to public health and safety, select agents must be stored in a highly secured area with restricted access and appropriate safeguards.

Only registered individuals who have completed training for handling select agents can access and retrieve these microorganisms from storage. An accurate and current inventory of select agents held in long-term storage must be maintained.

FUTURE DIRECTIONS

The field of microbiology is rapidly evolving, especially in the era of genomics and proteomics. Scientific research in human genetics, health care epidemiology, global health, antimicrobial resistance, microbial taxonomy, and infectious diseases relies heavily upon carefully curated repositories of microorganisms. Clinical laboratories have various levels of resources for the preservation of microorganisms and their long-term storage, but we all can contribute to national or international culture collections. Additionally, we can participate in the scientific advancements of pathogen discovery, genomics, and proteomics by collecting and storing biological specimens such as human blood and urine, particularly from patients with noncultivable pathogens or ill-defined clinical syndromes. Scientific protocols have been developed to preserve the integrity of these biological specimens for long-term storage, up to 30 years (9, 10). We encourage both resource-plenty and -constrained laboratories to partner with the scientific community (e.g., regional research centers of excellence or government-sponsored projects) and to contribute to both specimen and microorganism repositories. The answers to many future questions lie in our clinical laboratories of today.

REFERENCES

1. **Alexander, M., P. M. Daggett, R. Gherna, J. Jong, and F. Simione.** 1980. *American Type Culture Collection Methods,* vol. I. *Laboratory Manual on Preservation, Freezing, and Freeze-Drying as Applied to Algae, Bacteria, Fungi and Protozoa,* p. 1–46. American Type Culture Collection, Rockville, MD.
2. **Antheunisse, J., J. W. DeBruin-Tol, and M. E. Van Der Pol-Van Soest.** 1981. Survival of microorganisms after drying and storage. *Antonie van Leeuwenhoek* **47:**539–545.
3. **Barbaree, J. M., and A. Sanchez.** 1982. Cross-contamination during lyophilization. *Cryobiology* **19:**443–447.
4. **Borman, A. M., C. J. Linton, S. J. Miles, C. K. Campbell, and E. M. Johnson.** Ultra-rapid preparation of total genomic DNA from isolates of yeast and mould using Whatman FTA filter paper technology—a reusable DNA archiving system. *Med. Mycol.* **44:**389–398.
5. **Cassol, S., T. Salas, M. J. Gill, M. Montpetit, J. Rudnik, C. T. Sy, and M. V. O'Shaughnessy.** 1992. Stability of dried blood spot specimens for detection of human immunodeficiency virus DNA by polymerase chain reaction. *J. Clin. Microbiol.* **30:**3039–3042.
6. **Castellani, A.** 1939. Viability of some pathogenic fungi in distilled water. *J. Trop. Med. Hyg.* **42:**225–226.
7. **Crespo, M. J., M. L. Abarca, and F. J. Cabanes.** 2000. Evaluation of different preservation and storage methods for *Malassezia* spp. *J. Clin. Microbiol.* **38:**3872–3875.
8. **Das, P. C., A. H. de Vries, R. L. McShine, and C. T. Sibinga.** 1996. Dried sera for confirming blood-borne virus infections (HCV, HTLV-I, HIV & HBsAg). *Transfus. Med.* **6:**319–323.
9. **DePaoli, P.** 2005. Bio-banking in microbiology: from sample collection to epidemiology, diagnosis, and research. *FEMS Microbiol. Rev.* **29:**897–910.
10. **Elliott, P., and T. C. Peakman on behalf of UK Biobank.** 2008. The UK Biobank sample handling and storage protocol for the collection, processing and archiving of human blood and urine. *Int. J. Epidemiol.* **37:**234–244.
11. **Ellis, J. J., and J. A. Roberson.** 1968. Viability of fungus cultures preserved by lyophilization. *Mycologia* **60:**399–404.
12. **Federal Register.** 2005. Possession, use, and transfer of select agents and toxins, final rule. *Fed. Regist.* **70:**13294–13325.
13. **Feltham, R. K. A., A. K. Power, P. A. Pell, and P. H. A. Sneath.** 1978. A simple method for storage of bacteria at −76°C. *J. Appl. Bacteriol.* **44:**313–316.
14. **Gallo, D., J. S. Kimpton, and P. J. Johnson.** 1989. Isolation of human immunodeficiency virus from peripheral blood lymphocytes in various transport media and frozen at −60°C. *J. Clin. Microbiol.* **27:**88–90.
15. **Gherna, R. L.** 1981. Preservation, p. 208–217. *In* P. Gerhardt, R. G. E. Murray, R. N. Costilow, E. W. Nester, W. A. Wood, N. R. Krieg, and G. B. Phillips (ed.), *Manual of Methods for General Bacteriology.* American Society for Microbiology, Washington, DC.
16. **Gould, E. A.** 1999. Methods for long-term virus preservation. *Mol. Biotechnol.* **13:**57–66.
17. **Harbec, P. S., and P. Turcotte.** 1996. Preservation of *Neisseria gonorrhoeae* at −20°C. *J. Clin. Microbiol.* **34:**1143–1146.
18. **Hartung de Capriles, C., S. Mata, and M. Middelveen.** 1989. Preservation of fungi in water (Castellani): 20 years. *Mycopathologia* **106:**73–79.
19. **Heckly, R. J.** 1961. Preservation of bacteria by lyophilization. *Adv. Appl. Microbiol.* **3:**1–76.
20. **Heckly, R. J.** 1978. Preservation of microorganisms. *Adv. Appl. Microbiol.* **24:**1–53.
21. **Hubalek, Z.** 2003. Protectants used in the cryopreservation of microorganisms. *Cryobiology* **46:**205–229.
22. **Jackson, H.** 1974. Loss of viability and metabolic injury of *Staphylococcus aureus* resulting from storage at 5°C. *J. Appl. Bacteriol.* **37:**59–64.
23. **Johnson, F. B.** 1990. Transport of viral specimens. *Clin. Microbiol. Rev.* **3:**120–131.
24. **Law, T. J., and R. N. Hull.** 1968. The stabilizing effect of sucrose upon respiratory syncytial virus infectivity. *Proc. Soc. Exp. Biol. Med.* **128:**515–518.
25. **Lloyd, R. M., D. A. Burns, J. T. Huong, R. L. Mathis, M. A. Winters, M. Tanner, A. De La Rosa, B. Yen-Lieberman, W. Armstrong, A. Taege, D. R. McClernon, J. L. Wetshtein, B. M. Friedrich, M. R. Ferguson, W. O'Brien, P. M. Feorino, and M. Holodniy.** 2009. Dried plasma transport using a novel matrix and collection system for human immunodeficiency virus and hepatitis C virus virologic testing. *J. Clin. Microbiol.* **47:**1491–1496.
26. **McGinnis, M. R., A. A. Padhye, and L. Ajello.** 1974. Storage of stock cultures of filamentous fungi, yeasts, and some aerobic actinomycetes in sterile distilled water. *Appl. Microbiol.* **28:**218–222.
27. **Miyamoto-Shinohara, Y., T. Imaizumi, J. Sukenobe, Y. Murakami, S. Kawamura, and Y. Komatsu.** 2000. Survival rate of microbes after freeze-drying and long-term storage. *Cryobiology* **41:**251–255.
28. **Miyamoto-Shinohara, Y., J. Sukenobe, T. Imaizumi, and T. Nakahara.** 2008. Survival of freeze-dried bacteria. *J. Gen. Appl. Microbiol.* **54:**9–24.
29. **Pell, P. A., and A. E. Sneath.** 1984. A note on survival of bacteria in cryoprotectant medium at temperatures above 0°C. *J. Appl. Bacteriol.* **57:**165–167.
30. **Phetsouvanh, R., S. D. Blacksell, K. Jenjaroen, N. P. Day, and P. N. Newton.** 2009. Comparison of indirect immunofluorescence assays for diagnosis of scrub typhus and murine typus using venous blood and finger prick filter paper blood spots. *Am. J. Trop. Med. Hyg.* **80:**837–840.
31. **Popovic, T., G. Ajello, and R. Facklam.** 1999. *Laboratory Manual for the Diagnosis of Meningitis Caused by* Neisseria meningitidis, Streptococcus pneumoniae, *and* Haemophilus influenzae. *World Health Organization WHO/CDS/EDC/99.7.* World Health Organization, Geneva, Switzerland.
32. **Qiangqiang, Z., W. Jiajun, and L. Li.** 1998. Storage of fungi using sterile distilled water or lyophilization: comparison after 12 years. *Mycoses* **41:**255–257.
33. **Rajendram, D., R. Ayenza, F. M. Holder, B. Moran, T. Long, and H. N. Shah.** 2006. Long-term storage and safe retrieval of DNA from microorganisms for molecular analysis using FTA matrix cards. *J. Microbiol. Methods* **67:**582–592.

34. **Rybnikar, A.** 1995. Long-term maintenance of lyophilized fungal cultures of the genera *Epidermophyton, Microsporum, Paecilomyces* and *Trichophyton. Mycoses* **39:**145–147.

35. **Siberry, G., K. N. Brahmadathan, R. Pandian, M. K. Lalitha, M. C. Steinhoff, and T. J. John.** 2001. Comparison of different culture media and storage temperatures for the long-term preservation of *Streptococcus pneumoniae* in the tropics. *Bull. W. H. O.* **79:**43–47.

36. **Smith, D., and A. H. S. Onions.** 1994. *The Preservation and Maintenance of Living Fungi,* 2nd ed., p. 1–122. CAB International, Wallingford, Oxon, United Kingdom.

37. **Taddei, A., M. M. Tremarias, and C. Hartung de Capriles.** 1998–1999. Viability studies on actinomycetes. *Mycopathologia* **143:**161–164.

38. **Tannock, G. A., J. C. Hierholzer, D. A. Bryce, C. F. Chee, and J. A. Paul.** 1987. Freeze-drying of respiratory syncytial viruses for transportation and storage. *J. Clin. Microbiol.* **25:**1769–1771.

39. **van Griethuysen, A., I. van Loo, A. van Belkum, C. Vandenbroucke-Grauls, W. Wannet, P. van Keulen, and J. Kluytmans.** 2005. Loss of the *mecA* gene during storage of methicillin-resistant *Staphylococcus aureus* strains. *J. Clin. Microbiol.* **43:**1361–1365.

40. **Votava, M., and M. Stritecka.** 2001. Preservation of *Haemophilus influenzae* and *Haemophilus parainfluenzae* at −70 degrees C. *Cryobiology* **43:**85–87.

41. **Williams, F. P., Jr.** 1989. Electron microscopy of stool-shed viruses: retention of characteristic morphologies after long-term storage at ultralow temperatures. *J. Med. Virol.* **29:**192–195.

Prevention and Control of Laboratory-Acquired Infections

MICHAEL A. NOBLE

10

Laboratory biosafety is an active, assertive process, based on evidence-based principles, to ensure safety from microbial contamination or infection or from toxic reactions for workers, the public, and the environment as a result of the active manipulations of live microorganisms or their products while pursuing academic, research, industrial, and clinical investigations (54). The goals are to prevent laboratory-acquired infections in workers and to prevent accidental releases of live agents which can potentially endanger and have severe negative impact on humans, animals, and plants. Laboratory safety involves all aspects of the laboratory cycle, starting from before microorganisms arrive in the facility and continuing through the training of personnel, the establishment and monitoring of safe working practices, the proper use of reagents, materials, and equipment, the safe storage and transport of agents, and ultimately the terminal sterilization and destruction of microorganisms.

EPIDEMIOLOGY

The characterization of a person's infection as laboratory acquired is usually retrospective and is based on the assumption that the only likely exposure occurred while the person was in a laboratory. A trivial laboratory event may be considered the possible exposure because no other circumstance outside the laboratory could account for infection (40, 44).

It is important, however, to appreciate that the total laboratory testing cycle begins well before the sample actually reaches the laboratory (the preanalytic phase of laboratory testing) and that exposures during the collection and transport of the sample should also be considered. In the past, infections acquired during the collection of some samples were included if it could be ascertained that the collection was solely for the purpose of a laboratory investigation. Infections experienced by phlebotomists as a result of needlestick injuries are now routinely considered laboratory-acquired infections (27). In contrast, phlebotomist infections (e.g., chicken pox) acquired while collecting samples in patient rooms are not included (24).

Although difficult to date precisely, the first microbiology laboratories of Pasteur and Koch were active by 1840 to 1860. The first report of a laboratory-acquired infection, Mediterranean fever, was in 1899 (7).

Various compilations of laboratory-acquired infection have been published over the past 60 years (20, 32, 33, 69, 73, 74). The first survey published, in 1953, was a survey of 5,000 American laboratories by Sulkin and Pike. They provided additional updates in 1961, 1965, and 1976. They cited 3,921 laboratory infections dating between 1930 and 1974, with a mortality of 4.1%. Of note, 2,307 (58.8%) of the infections were reported from research facilities, 677 (17.3%) were from diagnostic facilities, 134 (3.4%) were from the generation of biological products (industry), and 106 (2.7%) were from teaching facilities. The remaining 697 (17.8%) infections had an unspecified source.

Four series performed in the United Kingdom between 1971 and 1991 revealed that within clinical facilities, the majority of infections were reported from workers in the microbiology laboratory, followed by the autopsy service. Over this 20-year period, the number of infections reported dropped over 80%, from 104 to only 17. While it is tempting to conclude that laboratories are becoming safer, there are no active monitoring programs in place to capture the true number of accidents and infections.

Compiled information tends to be limited to events that are reported in the literature or in specific databases. Thus, while uncommon community infections, such as those associated with *Brucella* species (1, 36a, 49a, 50a, 55a, 73a, 76a), are commonly reported as laboratory-acquired infections, very common infections such as *Staphylococcus aureus* (including methicillin-resistant *S. aureus*) infection are rarely identified (70) as being acquired in the laboratory. It is assumed that even complete listings reflect an immeasurable minority of infections that actually occur (69).

More recently, Internet-based discussion groups have worked to create information-gathering approaches (5, 68). While these newer surveys have challenges similar to those of former retrospective compilations, they demonstrate the potential for gathering important information on laboratory safety and infection.

Two hundred cases of laboratory-acquired infections with parasites resulting from laboratory accidents, from 1929 through 1999, have been published (40, 41). While the distribution of cases changed from decade to decade, the number of cases identified in each decade (19 to 28) remained relatively constant. Sharps-related injuries (e.g., needles and glass) were common factors, often associated with manipulation of research animals and the production of blood smears for malaria.

LABORATORY SAFETY AND PERSONAL ATTRIBUTES

A matched case-control study of 33 laboratory workers who experienced a laboratory-associated injury over a 2-year period was previously described (57). No differences were noted related to age, length of employment, years of formal education, wearing of glasses, use of prescription medications, or off-the-job accidents or driving record. On the other hand, the accident-involved persons were significantly more likely to have had a laboratory accident or laboratory infection prior to the 2-year study period and were significantly more likely to have a low opinion of laboratory safety programs. When the conditions surrounding the accidents were examined, 36% occurred when the employee was working too quickly, either just before lunch or at the end of the day. In 30% of accidents, the employee acknowledged a breach in safety regulations. In summary, in this study, attitudes and work habits were important contributing factors to laboratory accidents. While this study may seem to be unduly dated, in today's circumstances, with increasing numbers of samples and increasing complexity of tests, along with an aging and shrinking workforce, rush, stress, and awareness of risk continue to be relevant issues (1a, 47).

In a study in which laboratory practices were observed directly and then related to laboratory environmental contamination with hepatitis B virus (HBV), contamination was strongly related to flawed technique and high workload. Unsafe work practices were also related, but to a lesser degree (32).

Over time, laboratorians have learned that even conventionally accepted practices can result in serious infection. Mouth pipetting, marking of blood spots, transport of samples to the laboratory in corked or sheathed sharps, recapping of needles, eating, and smoking were all practiced commonly at one time in properly run medical laboratories. All of these practices are now appreciated as risky and are prohibited.

Injuries with sharp objects continue to be identified as an area of concern (20). Examination of bacterial culture plates with an eyeglass or sniffing plates to help identify organisms is now controversial (3). Laboratory safety requires diligent review and ongoing critique of current conventional practice, as well as openness to change when new risks are identified.

RISK-BASED CLASSIFICATION OF MICROORGANISMS

As a foundation for determining environmental requirements and best laboratory practices, the international community has developed a common risk-based classification of microorganisms. Group 1 biological agents are unlikely to cause human disease. Group 2 biological agents can cause human disease and might be a hazard to workers but are unlikely to spread to the community, and there is usually effective prophylaxis or treatment available. Group 3 biological agents cause severe human disease and present a serious hazard to workers. They may present a risk of spreading to the community, but there is usually effective prophylaxis or treatment available. Group 4 biological agents cause severe human disease and are a serious hazard to workers. They may present a high risk of spreading to the community, and there is usually no effective prophylaxis or treatment available. A partial list of microorganisms by category is shown in Table 1.

While there is general consistency in classification of organisms by different countries, there are some examples where the same organism can be classified differently. This can have implications with respect to certification

TABLE 1 Risk-based classification of microorganisms[a]

Group	Bacteria	Viruses	Fungi	Parasites
1	No clinical organisms	No clinical organisms	No clinical organisms	No clinical organisms
2	Bacillus species (not Bacillus anthracis)	Adenovirus	Cryptococcus species	All clinical parasites
	Clostridium species	Calicivirus	Candida species	
	Corynebacterium diphtheriae	Coronavirus (not SARS coronavirus)	All dermatophytes	
	Escherichia coli	Herpesvirus	Aspergillus species	
	Enterobacteriaceae	Influenza virus		
	Mycobacteria other than Mycobacterium tuberculosis			
	Staphylococcus species			
	Streptococcus species			
3	Bacillus anthracis	Lymphocytic choriomeningitis virus	Coccidioides immitis	
	Brucella species	Hantaan virus	Blastomyces dermatitidis	
	Coxiella burnetii	St. Louis encephalitis virus	Histoplasma capsulatum	
	Francisella tularensis	Japanese encephalitis virus	Paracoccidioides brasiliensis	
	Mycobacterium tuberculosis	Western equine encephalitis virus		
	Mycobacterium avium	West Nile virus		
		SARS coronavirus		
		Prions		
4		Lassa virus		
		Marburg virus		
		Ebola virus		
		Herpesvirus simiae		

[a]Based on reference 39. This table is presented as a guide only. It should not be considered complete or consistent within all jurisdictions. Specific national requirements may differ from the information presented in this table.

of the laboratory or to regulations surrounding transportation of these agents. Laboratories need to be aware of both domestic and international requirements prior to transport.

Increasingly, the emphasis has been to rely less on the classification of organisms and to focus more on the level of safety with respect to containment and practices. For example, this approach allows for recommendations to contain organisms by using the requirements of biosafety level 2 but to increase the caution level by using a higher level of safety practices.

BIOSAFETY AND CLINICAL LABORATORY DESIGN

Knowledge of the classification of microorganisms flowing into a laboratory aids in the design of containment equipment and facilities. For research laboratories where the microorganism load is known, the process of matching risk and containment is straightforward. In the clinical laboratory, the content of samples is more likely to be unknown and may, in certain situations, contain microorganisms across the spectrum of classification. With that being said, most isolates recovered within clinical samples can be categorized within biosafety level 1 or 2; thus, most facilities require containment level 2 (Table 2). Laboratories that process viral cultures or investigate mycobacterial cultures should be designed to accommodate biosafety level 3. For many clinical laboratories, biosafety level 3 is considered beyond their scope of practice.

In the wake of the 2001 terrorist attacks in New York and the anthrax mail scares that happened shortly afterward, the interest in laboratory biosafety measures as a component of bioterrorism defense was brought to the fore (13a, 42a, 63a, 69a, 78a). Specific funding has been allocated for construction of new national and regional biocontainment laboratories. Laboratories with increased levels of containment and security not only provide benefits against bioterrorism and for biosecurity but also provide facilities to address potential epidemics, such as severe acute respiratory syndrome (SARS) and the current H1N1 influenza pandemic. In order to protect workers, the public, and the environment, laboratories need to ensure controlled access, controlled procedures

TABLE 2 Laboratory design requirements for biosafety level 2 laboratories[a]

---

1. Separated from public areas by lockable doors
2. Laboratory doors with appropriate signage
3. Door openings of sufficient size to allow safe passage of equipment
4. Work surfaces nonabsorptive and scratch, stain, chemical and heat resistant
5. Readily available means of waste treatment prior to disposal
6. Windows designed to prevent ingress of flying insects
7. Separate spaces for street and laboratory clothing
8. Ready access to hand-washing sinks
9. Emergency access to showers and eyewash stations
10. Biosafety cabinets and other primary containment equipment (recommended)
11. Hands-free operation of hand-wash sinks (recommended)
12. Air supply 100% outside air with no recirculation (recommended)

---

[a]Adapted from references 39 and 78.

for specimen receiving and disposal and incident reporting, emergency response plans, higher security for stored agents, and, for research facilities, accurate animal tracking and trace-back systems (49, 62, 63). Caution needs to be taken to ensure that the needs for confidentiality and information containment do not interfere with the open communications necessary for laboratory safety and public health (44).

Handling of exotic pathogens of risk group 4 requires high-containment level 4 facilities. Discussion of these facilities is beyond the scope of this chapter.

ASSESSING RISKS AND HAZARDS

Conventionally, laboratory behavior and practice are matched to the level of risk associated with expected hazards. See Table 3 for practices considered appropriate for handling samples containing group 2 agents.

Rather than treating all situations as equal, the laboratorian needs to consider biosafety a dynamic rather than static interaction. Factors that influence risk include the potential biohazardous agents to be handled, the volumes of potential samples, the most likely potential routes of exposure, workload, host factors such as health (e.g., immunosuppression or pregnancy), knowledge, and experience, and the complexity of the task required. In planning laboratory strategies, recognition of the risk factors and potential process weak points and implementation of potential solutions can be performed by using failure mode effects analysis strategies. Process weak points can often be identified through regular laboratory audits and can be amended through implementation or reactivation of established guidelines. By taking a more dynamic view, levels of safety can be augmented through appropriate and selective use of enhanced practices, such as the use of biosafety level 3 practices in biosafety level 2 containment facilities to address situations of increased risk associated with potential aerosolization of particular pathogens.

SAFETY EQUIPMENT AND THE CLINICAL LABORATORY

Splashguards

Splashguards made of clear glass or plastic represent the minimum level of equipment for protecting workers. They are more likely to protect workers from gross splashes than from aerosols. They can be an appropriate alternative to biosafety cabinets for opening vacuum blood tubes. They should be of sufficient size and should be cleanable to remove the occasional blood splatter. The effectiveness of splashguards depends on appropriate placement with respect to both work flow and worker height. It is inappropriate to obscure vision by using splashguards as a convenient location for taped memos and procedures.

Biosafety Cabinets

Biosafety cabinets can protect the laboratory worker and the laboratory environment from splashes and aerosols and can also reduce the opportunities for sample contamination (73, 75). Biosafety cabinets are enclosed units with various degrees of openness and access and with control of exhausted air. Class 1 cabinets have an open front but work under negative pressure, exhausting their air through a HEPA filter. Exhausted air usually is returned

TABLE 3 Standard microbiology practices for all laboratories (biosafety level 2 and higher)[a]

1. A documented safety manual must be available for all staff.
2. Personnel must receive training on the potential hazards associated with the work involved and the necessary precautions to prevent exposure to infectious agents.
3. Eating, drinking, smoking, storing of either food or personal belongings, or applying cosmetics is not permitted.
4. Mouth pipetting is prohibited.
5. Long hair is to be tied back or restrained.
6. Access to laboratory and support areas is limited to authorized personnel.
7. Doors to working areas in laboratories must not be left open.
8. Personnel's open wounds and cuts should be covered with waterproof dressings.
9. Laboratories are to be kept clean and tidy.
10. Properly fastened protective laboratory clothing must be worn properly by all personnel, including visitors, trainees, and others working in the laboratory. Suitable footwear requires closed toes and heels.
11. Eye and face protection must be used where there is a known or potential risk of exposure to splashes or flying objects.
12. Gloves must be worn for all procedures that might involve direct skin contact with biohazardous material. Gloves are to be removed at the completion of the laboratory task and before leaving the laboratory.
13. Protective laboratory clothing must not be worn in nonlaboratory areas.
14. If a known or suspected exposure occurs, contaminated clothing must be decontaminated before being laundered.
15. The use of needles, syringes, and other sharp objects should be strictly limited. Needles should not be bent, sheared, recapped, or removed from the syringe; they should be promptly placed in a puncture-resistant sharps container for disposal.
16. Hands must be washed with an appropriate disinfectant after gloves have been removed, before leaving the laboratory, and after handling materials known or suspected to be contaminated.
17. Work surfaces must be cleaned and decontaminated with a suitable disinfectant at the end of the day and after any spill of potentially biohazardous material.
18. Contaminated materials and equipment leaving the laboratory for servicing or disposal must be decontaminated appropriately.
19. Autoclaves used for decontamination should be monitored regularly with biological indicators.
20. All contaminated materials must be decontaminated before disposal or reuse.
21. Leakproof containers are to be used for the transport of infectious materials.
22. Spills, accidents, or exposures to infectious materials, and losses of containment must be reported immediately to the laboratory supervisor.
23. An effective rodent and insect control program must be maintained.

[a]Adapted from references 39 and 78.

to the work area. Class 2 cabinets increase the level of safety by including a HEPA-filtered downward-flow air curtain designed to increase the degree of separation between room air and interior cabinet air. Class 2 cabinets may exhaust back to room air (class 2A) or through an exhaust system to outside the building environment (class 2B). Class 2B cabinets can be subclassified further based on additional features. Class 3 cabinets are completely enclosed, providing gas-tight containment. They are accessible only through front-end glove ports. Class 3 cabinets provide the most suitable containment for working with exotic pathogens. Because class 1 and class 2A units exhaust to the laboratory air, they are unacceptable for use with volatile chemicals and reagents. Biological safety cabinets cannot be used as alternatives to chemical fume hoods.

All safety cabinets must be tested and certified by a qualified person on a regular basis to ensure that they maintain their required face velocity and negative pressure.

Even properly maintained and certified cabinets can be a hazard if equipment and materials are placed improperly inside the cabinet. Overcrowding the cabinet or stacking of equipment against either the front or back grill will disrupt the airflow, resulting in backwash out the front of the unit (46). This can result in a compound

hazard because biological safety cabinets are detrimental to worker dexterity, making for a greater potential for accidents (66).

Centrifuges

Although the safety centrifuge was first described in 1975 (37), accidental contamination of laboratory and personnel via centrifuges is regularly reported (18, 34). While other equipment may result in greater aerosol dispersal, the frequency of use of centrifuges increases their significance in accident risk assessment (6). Accidents occur because of a lack of tight seals on containers and rotors. Centrifuges can be susceptible to contamination because prolonged use without regular inspection can lead to worn O-ring container seals (38). Plastic centrifuge tubes can crack or distort and result in increased risk (34). Accidents can be avoided if centrifuges are used, cared for, and maintained in a safe manner. Lids must be closed at all times during operation. The centrifuge should not be left until full operating speed is attained and the machine is running safely without vibration. If vibration does occur, the centrifuge should be stopped immediately and the load balances checked. Swing-out buckets should be checked for clearance and support. Ideally, rotors and cups should be cleaned and disinfected with noncorrosive cleaning solutions after each use.

All spills and breakage should be reported to the laboratory safety officer and should be cleaned immediately, after giving time for aerosols to settle. In the context of quality control, a log should be maintained and should include the rotor serial number, speed (revolutions per minute), duration of spin, times of use, and operator's name.

Chemical Fume Protection

A fume hood is a mechanically ventilated, partially enclosed workspace where harmful volatile chemicals and reagents can be handled safely. The primary function of a fume hood is to contain and remove gases and vapors.

Most fume hoods use ducts and a fan to ensure that heat and airborne contaminants are captured, transported out of the work area, and eventually discharged into the atmosphere outside the building. Chemical fume hoods differ from biosafety cabinets in that they are usually ducted. They must be constructed of noncombustible materials, and they must also be explosion proof.

Nonducted, or recirculating, fume hoods are of limited use in the laboratory and should not be considered acceptable substitutes for ducted fume hoods for containment of volatile chemicals (26).

Special fume hoods are designed to protect workers from specific highly corrosive reagents or chemicals, such as perchloric acid or radioisotopes. Installation of fume hoods without consideration of airflow and balance can result in increased risk due to backwash and room contamination (26).

As with biological safety cabinets, chemical fume hoods require regular testing and recertification. It is recommended that chemical fume hoods be tested for both face velocity and containment by use of the ASHRAE 110 tracer gas test. Face velocity alone is not a valid indication of containment (26).

Protection from Sharps

Scalpels, needles, broken glass, and other sharps are commonly associated with wound injuries and laboratory-acquired infections (2). To the extent that it is possible, the use of sharps should be eliminated or safety barriers should be implemented (29, 70). Sharps may be contaminated with infectious or cytotoxic agents, or both. All sharps should be considered potentially infectious and should be discarded in safety containers. Sharps containers minimize injuries and transmission of potentially harmful agents, provided that they are readily accessible and appropriately used.

Sharps containers used in medical laboratories should be designed specifically for the containment and disposal of needles, syringes with needles, scalpel blades, clinical glass, and other items capable of causing cuts or punctures (29, 71). If containers are not resistant to penetration or compression, they pose a health risk to those involved in their handling and disposal.

The characteristics of well-designed containers are that they are leakproof and puncture resistant, do not degrade in autoclaves, either require no assembly or are easy to assemble, are appropriately labeled, and come in a variety of sizes. Within this framework, manufacturers can implement a variety of designs. Sharps containers should be stable enough to resist toppling over and durable enough to withstand being dropped onto a hard surface (13). Using locally available tin cans or other containers in lieu of designed containers is inappropriate, as they do not address important aspects of containment.

Sharps containers must have a prominently displayed universal biohazard symbol. In addition, sharps containers intended to contain sharps contaminated with cytotoxic substances must display the cytotoxic hazard symbol. The international color code is yellow for biohazardous medical sharps and red for cytotoxic medical sharps.

Containers should not be filled to more than three-quarters of their maximum capacity to avoid accidents from overfilling, and sharps should never be forced into a container. Properly designed containers have a designated fill line.

Most sharps containers are designed for a single use only. Once filled, they are securely and irreversibly closed for containment. Following autoclave treatment, the containers should be disposed of in accordance with local requirements. Containers with cytotoxic sharps or probable prion proteins should not be autoclaved but rather require incineration.

To reduce the challenges associated with disposal of single-use containers, reuse container services can provide collection and transport to an off-site location for safe, secure reopening, emptying, and decontamination prior to redistribution for reuse.

MEDICAL WASTE AS AN INFECTION HAZARD

Medical facilities generate large volumes of waste that can be hazardous to workers and the community (74). According to a recent survey, most university hospitals in the United States continue to use autoclaves to sterilize medical waste, although many do not appear to monitor autoclave effectiveness appropriately by use of biological indicators (50). Contractual arrangements with biomedical waste management organizations may be an economical or environmentally sound alternative. Alternatives such as microwave inactivation can be considered, with recognition of the necessity of required rigorous conditions (76). In some areas where economic or environmental issues are of extreme concern, solar disinfection (21) of biomedical waste may be a viable consideration. In rare circumstances in addressing zoonotic outbreaks, and more commonly in resource-limited regions, incineration of medical waste continues to be performed, even though it has been demonstrated to be harmful to health and the environment (31, 38, 50, 74a).

SAFETY AS A QUALITY MANAGEMENT INITIATIVE

There is an increasing interest in medical laboratory quality, safety, and risk, with a resulting convergence of these issues (55). International Organization for Standardization Technical Committee 212 has developed documents to improve the quality of medical laboratories, including ISO 15189:2003 (*Medical Laboratories—Particular Requirements for Quality and Competence*) and ISO 15190:2003 (*Medical Laboratories—Requirements for Safety*) (41b, 41c). In those countries where laboratories are certified or accredited to the requirements of the International Organization for Standardization, these documents are considered essential standards.

With respect to safety, ISO 15190:2003 addresses management responsibility, safety managers, safety manuals, safety programs, education, training, competence, and audit and review. It states that laboratory management is responsible for the safety of all employees and visitors to the laboratory and that ultimate responsibility rests with the laboratory director. The laboratory must identify an appropriately trained and experienced laboratory safety officer

TABLE 4 Laboratory safety audits required by ISO 15190:2003[a]

Health and safety policy
Written procedures that include safe work practices
Safety-oriented education and training of staff
Safety-oriented supervision
Use and maintenance of hazardous materials and substances
Health surveillance
First aid equipment and services
Accident and illness investigations
Health and safety committee review
Records and statistics on accidents and near misses
Review of safety program
Regular site safety inspections

[a]See reference 41c.

to assist the laboratory director and managers with safety issues. The laboratory safety officer must have the authority to stop activities that are deemed unsafe. The laboratory safety officer is responsible for designing and maintaining the laboratory safety program and is responsible for monitoring its effectiveness.

The elements of a laboratory safety program include development of the laboratory safety manual, safety audits and inspections (see Table 4 for audits required by ISO 15190:2003), risk assessments, and the maintenance of records. For further details, ISO 15190:2003 is available through the International Organization for Standardization website (www.iso.org) or the Clinical and Laboratory Standards Institute website (www.clsi.org).

SAFETY PREPAREDNESS AND THE MATERIAL SAFETY DATA SHEET

Guidelines for the protection of laboratory workers describe the preparations required in case of accidents. In the event of an accident, a prompt and appropriate response requires preparedness, rapid access to critical information, and equipment. Every laboratory should have a written and prepared plan in case of emergency. Routes for evacuation in case of fire or spill should be planned and practiced on a regular basis. Personnel trained in first aid should be readily available. Up-to-date Material Safety Data Sheets (MSDS) for all chemicals and microorganisms should be available. The locations of emergency equipment, including showers and eyewash stations, should be known to all, and equipment should be tested on a regular basis to ensure functionality at the time of need. Equipment and materials for containment of spills, including personal protective equipment, an absorbent, and a disinfectant (bleach or accelerated hydrogen peroxide), should be readily available, and their location should be known. Accident preparedness should be the subject of a regular internal safety audit program.

MSDS for chemicals should be obtained from the supplier or may be available from a variety of commercial and free Internet sites. A list of appropriately formatted MSDS for microorganisms is available through the Public Health Agency of Canada website (http://www.phac-aspc.gc.ca/msds-ftss/).

Every incident must be reported to appropriate management and required authorities. Every incident should be investigated internally for details of the accident, root causes, and steps necessary to prevent similar events. Recommendations for required changes should be the subject of safety audit to ensure that they are acted upon in a timely manner.

HAND WASHING AND THE USE OF PERSONAL PROTECTIVE EQUIPMENT

Hand Washing

Hand washing is the single most useful technique to stop the transmission of microorganisms and acquisition of infection in medical laboratories (11). Hands can be contaminated during sample collection, handling of sample containers, handling of contaminated equipment, and touching of sample storage units.

While contamination can be reduced by the use of gloves, gloves alone are not completely effective. Hand hygiene can be performed with running water and either plain or antimicrobial soaps. Nonmedicated detergent-based soap products and water alone do not disrupt the normal skin biota but can have some effect on reduction of the transient hand biota, including both bacteria and viruses (11, 72). The efficacy is directly related to the duration of hand washing. Plain soaps, similar to other products, can be associated with detrimental effects, including skin drying and irritation.

It is less clear whether soaps containing antimicrobial products are essential for the vast majority of hand-washing situations, even in the microbiology laboratory. For example, hand washing with plain soap is as efficacious as that with antiseptic soap for removing *Clostridium difficile* (36), nonenveloped viruses, and *Bacillus anthracis* (79). For short-term hand cleansing, the two product types are equally efficacious for the removal of common bacterial pathogens (9, 72).

Most laboratories will continue to see value in regular use of antiseptic soaps. Selection of an appropriate product for the laboratory depends upon both the types of organisms processed by the laboratory and issues such as fragrance, consistency, and potential for irritation and skin drying. Commonly used products contain chlorhexidine, iodophors, triclosan, or related compounds. Other ingredients, such as those including tea tree oil, may be acceptable alternatives (52).

Waterless alcohol-based products can be a rapid and convenient alternative to conventional hand washing, especially when a sink with running water is not immediately accessible (45, 72). When they are used correctly, alcohol-based hand gels are as active as traditional 70% alcohol for removing methicillin-resistant *S. aureus*, *Serratia marcescens*, and *Candida albicans* from contaminated hands (81), but alcohol-based products may have reduced efficacy if hands are contaminated with spore-forming organisms, including *C. difficile* and *B. anthracis* (79), or with nonenveloped viruses (72). Alcohol-based products should not be relied upon when hands are visibly soiled, contaminated with proteinaceous materials, or contaminated with materials that have a known high microbial load.

It is common in many laboratories to place alcohol-containing bottles by hand-washing sinks. Others have noted that health care workers are more compliant with hand care when agents are close to the site of contamination (25). Accordingly, laboratories might consider having containers of alcohol-containing hand gel closer to workstations.

Gloves

Gloves can provide an important barrier within the laboratory, provided that they are used appropriately. Clearly, gloves are essential to prevent damage when hands are exposed to heat, cold, and toxic materials. Insulated gloves are essential for taking materials out of −70°C freezers, exposure to liquid nitrogen, or removing materials from autoclaves.

General purpose utility gloves ("kitchen" or "rubber" gloves) provide ample protection for cleaning biological spills, for general cleaning, and for decontamination. Utility gloves can be cleaned and reused, although they should be examined regularly for cracks, tears, and peeling. Damaged utility gloves should be discarded. Utility gloves may be inappropriate for handling chemical solvents and should not be used. Chemical-resistant gloves should be available in all laboratories that handle chemical solvents and other toxic chemicals and dyes.

The degree of protection that gloves can provide depends upon many factors, including composition, size, fit, grip, and thickness, all of which can affect user dexterity. Latex-containing gloves may provide superior fine finger dexterity, which could be associated with fewer spills or accidents (65).

Disposable gloves of latex, vinyl, or nitrile can provide an effective barrier, especially for handling blood, body fluids, and excrement. This is especially true because open abrasions on hands can often go unnoticed (43). In specific settings, gloves of increased length, to elbow or shoulder, may be appropriate. Gloves are easily torn. In-use durability studies indicate that vinyl gloves may tear as often as 40% of the time, depending upon the presence of powder and the length of the user's fingernails (43). Latex gloves are more durable but may be associated with atopic reactions.

It is critical for the user to remember that handling equipment and materials with contaminated gloves can cause considerable environmental contamination. Gloves must be removed either at the end of the task or when the task is interrupted.

Regardless of the type of gloves and their composition, it is essential that the user always wash his or her hands as soon as gloves are removed, either with running water and soap or, in many settings, with alcohol-containing hand hygiene products.

While it has become customary for phlebotomists to wear gloves during specimen collection, this may not be essential if the risk of exposure to blood and body fluids is considered sufficiently low and gloves of an appropriate size or material are not readily available. Regardless of whether gloves are worn or not during the task of collection, hands should always be cleansed immediately after the completion of the task. Contaminated gloves often result in contamination of equipment (53) but can also contribute to transmission of serious infection (59).

Disposable gloves do not provide significant protection against needlestick injury. If sharps exposure and the risk of injury are possible, double gloving can provide some protection. Cotton undergloves may provide more protection than a second vinyl or latex glove. In the morgue, use of chain mail gloves may be appropriate.

Gloves provide an important protective barrier, but they may also be a source of harm. Use of vinyl, latex, or cotton undergloves can reduce contact irritation noted with rubber gloves. Excessive glove use can result in moisture damage to skin (12, 19, 61). Surveys of dentists wearing gloves for 6 h daily indicated that many of them, especially young women with preexisting eczema, suffered from glove intolerance (80).

IMMUNIZATION

Immunization provides protection against some laboratory-acquired infectious diseases but should be considered secondary to mental alertness and good laboratory practices. Immunization may not prevent infection but can protect against serious illness. All adults, including pregnant women, should have a complete primary immunization with tetanus and diphtheria toxoids and should receive a booster every 10 years (15).

Laboratory workers should receive annual influenza immunizations. Similarly, all staff with possible occupational exposure to human blood and body fluids should receive the hepatitis B vaccine. The value of meningococcal immunization for laboratory workers has been discussed previously (10, 14, 22). Cases of meningococcal illness possibly linked to laboratory exposure have been published, and it has been recommended that microbiologists routinely exposed to meningococci, especially aerosolized organisms, should consider meningococcal immunization. Laboratorians working with specific pathogens and in specific situations should consider additional immunizations, for example, human diploid cell rabies vaccine, typhoid vaccine, and vaccinia vaccine (48, 51).

In the past, *Mycobacterium bovis* BCG vaccination has been considered valuable for health care workers. However, it is no longer recommended as a primary tuberculosis control strategy because the protective efficacy of the vaccine in health care workers is uncertain and because immunization with BCG may cause difficulty in the interpretation of tuberculin skin test responses caused by true infections with *Mycobacterium tuberculosis*. In laboratory and other health care workers with positive tuberculin skin tests, the new gamma interferon release assays can help to differentiate likely tuberculosis exposure (positive assay) from BCG vaccination (negative assay).

LABORATORY-ACQUIRED HIV INFECTION, HEPATITIS B, AND HEPATITIS C

Laboratory workers are at risk of blood-borne infections such as hepatitis C virus (HCV), HBV, and human immunodeficiency virus (HIV) infections. However, the safeguards introduced to medical laboratories have decreased the risk to workers. According to the Division of Health Care Quality Promotion, Centers for Disease Control and Prevention (http://www.cdc.gov/ncidod/hip/BLOOD/hivpersonnel.htm), between 1978 and December 2001, only 16 clinical laboratory workers acquired HIV occupationally; 17 other persons may have been infected in the laboratory. Following a deep-tissue exposure injury (e.g., needlestick), it is recommended that workers consider postexposure prophylaxis (35), even though this prophylaxis does not always prevent HIV infection following an exposure (31).

There is less information on the prevalence of hepatitis C in health care workers, although it is estimated by the National Center for Infectious Diseases (28) that after needlestick or sharps exposure to HCV-positive blood, about 2 (1.8%) health care workers of 100 will become infected with HCV (range, 0% to 10%). Following the introduction of the hepatitis B vaccine in 1982, the incidence of HBV infection was reduced by over 95% (70).

While blood-borne infection information may be thought to be well established, recent knowledge surveys of health care workers have demonstrated that regular education sessions to update existing staff and inform new staff are required (67).

LABORATORY-ACQUIRED INFECTIONS AND EXTERNAL QUALITY ASSESSMENT

Infections acquired in the clinical laboratory are not always associated with clinical samples. Documented clusters of bacterial infections have been associated with samples sent to laboratories for proficiency testing (8). Contamination of other samples by quality control organisms has also been documented (23), although no in-laboratory infections resulted. Regardless of the source, all viable microorganisms processed in the clinical laboratory must be handled with full awareness of appropriate biosafety practices.

PRIONS

Samples from patients with Creutzfeldt-Jakob disease (CJD) may be submitted to the laboratory for investigation. To date, there are no known cases of laboratory-acquired CJD, and there is no evidence that laboratorians are at increased risk of developing CJD. With that being said, the progressive deteriorating nature of CJD raises concerns for those handling samples from patients with CJD, especially for samples of neurological origin (64). This represents a special problem in the medical laboratory because of the difficulty in inactivating the underlying prions.

Current precautions while handling tissue samples require glove use. All tissue samples must be discarded as medical waste. No special precautions are required for disposal of body fluids.

Equipment that has been exposed to CJD tissues should either be discarded or, if tolerant to heat, autoclaved at 134°C for 18 min (prevacuum sterilizer) or at 121 to 132°C for 1 h (gravity displacement sterilizer). Autoclaving in water may be more effective than autoclaving in its absence (33). Equipment may also be soaked in 1 N NaOH for 1 h (33, 42). Work surfaces should be cleaned with a 1:10 dilution of sodium hypochlorite.

Milder chemical treatments based upon combinations of enzymes, including proteinase K and pronase, in conjunction with detergents such as alkaline cleaners or sodium dodecyl sulfate, have been shown to experimentally reduce PrPSc material to levels below detection and to prevent infectivity. The advantages of these methods are that they are described as being inexpensive, noncorrosive, and nonhazardous to staff (33, 42).

SARS CORONAVIRUS INFECTION AND OTHER SEVERE VIRAL RESPIRATORY INFECTIONS

The 2002 outbreak of SARS associated with a coronavirus reinforced international health concerns about the hazards of aerosol spread of communicable viruses. While laboratory workers were at risk (56), containment was readily addressable (4), and laboratory workers were among those with the lowest rates of illness or serological conversion (56). However, microbiology and accessioning laboratory workers receiving respiratory samples, especially via vacuum tube delivery systems, were deemed to be at increased risk. Since that time, the concerns for similar events occurring with influenza viruses, including H2N2 (17), H5N1 (30), H7N7 (43), and novel H1N1 (35) viruses, have pointed out the potential gaps in biosafety protection for laboratory workers. Laboratories equipped and designed to biosafety level 2 should use practices more consistent with those for biosafety level 3, which require that all samples be opened and handled only in a biosafety cabinet (4). In addition, centrifugation of samples should be performed only by using sealed safety buckets that are opened within a cabinet. Finally, personal protective equipment, including M95 respirators, should be considered for additional protection. Frequent hand washing should be required (35), using either soap and running water or alcohol-based hand gels. While caution and reasonable practices have been demonstrated to contain outbreaks, effective influenza immunization is most likely required in conjunction for optimal protection.

SAFETY AND POINT-OF-CARE TESTING

Medical laboratories are responsible for all aspects of laboratory testing throughout the total testing cycle, even when the testing is performed outside the laboratory itself. Increasingly, medical laboratories are responsible for point-of-care testing, such as blood glucose monitoring, coagulation, and oxygenation. Despite improvements in equipment and hygiene protocols, cases of hepatitis B and C continue to be associated with point-of-care devices. Prevention of transmission requires strict adherence to infection control protocols for equipment cleaning. The international standard ISO 22870:2006 [lsqb]Point-of-Care Testing (POCT)—Requirements for Quality and Competence[rsqb] (41d) provides guidance on quality management for point-of-care testing.

TRANSPORTATION OF SAMPLES

Laboratories have a responsibility to prevent exposure of individuals to infectious agents in laboratory samples to the extent that is possible. This responsibility includes samples being transported to and from the laboratory. For local transport within a clinic or hospital, the laboratory should ensure that leakproof containers are available, are transported

TABLE 5 Electronic information sources and resources

Regulation, agency, or organization	Abbreviation	Website (source or reference)
Regulatory resources		
Occupational Safety and Health Administration	OSHA	www.osha.gov
Clinical Laboratory Improvement Amendments	CLIA	www.cms.hhs.gov/clia (U.S. Department of Health and Human Services)
Code of Federal Regulations	CFR	www.gpoaccess.gov/cfr/
Department of Transportation	DOT	www.dot.gov
Nonregulatory resources		
International Organization for Standardization	ISO	www.iso.org
Clinical and Laboratory Standards Institute	CLSI	www.clsi.org
American Biosafety Association	ABSA	www.absa.org
International Air Transport Association	IATA	www.iata.org
Public Health Agency of Canada	PHAC	www.phac-aspc.gc.ca/msds-ftss/msds12e.html (60)

in secure outer packaging such as a sealable plastic bag, and preferably are emblazoned with the international biohazard label. For transport outside the facility, especially by road, rail, ship, or air, local and federal regulations apply. Even for short distances, it is appropriate that samples be transported in secure firm outer containers with sufficient absorbent materials inside, in case of a spill. In most jurisdictions, transport of samples with infectious agents by postal services is prohibited.

Air transport is under the authority of federal regulations directed by the requirements of the International Civil Aviation Organization, as adopted by the International Air Transport Association. The International Civil Aviation Organization specifies packaging and labeling requirements, including proper shipping name, appropriate United Nations number (for samples known to contain infectious agents based on the source of the sample), and the likely pathogens contained. Every laboratory that transports samples is required to have at least one person certified as knowledgeable with respect to packaging and transport requirements, including the completion of shipping documents.

For additional information, direct reference can be made to the International Civil Aviation Organization's *Technical Instructions for the Safe Transport of Dangerous Goods by Air* (41a) or to federal requirements (58).

POSTEXPOSURE MANAGEMENT FOR ACCIDENTS INVOLVING INFECTIOUS AGENTS

It is beyond the scope of this chapter to address the specifics of medical management following accidents that involve infectious agents. However, it is important that the following steps always be undertaken or considered. Every accident or injury, including those that are seemingly trivial (40), should be reported to the appropriate safety officer or supervisor. Scratches and puncture wounds should be cleaned immediately. For some injuries, especially those involving blood exposures, time may be a critical factor (16). If it is deemed appropriate to seek medical attention, it is important to identify that the accident was laboratory acquired. If the likely or probable agent is known, bringing the microorganism MSDS can be helpful and can save time. In research or animal facilities, preparation of information sheets on specific organisms and availability of standardized investigation and treatment protocols in the event of an accident can be invaluable.

ELECTRONIC INFORMATION SOURCES AND RESOURCES

Laboratory safety is a primary focus of interest for many organizations. Some agencies carry the authority of regulation in their specific nations or areas of jurisdiction. Nonregulatory resources, including international organizations, can provide instructive materials that aid in the implementation of improved laboratory safety programs. Table 5 provides access to current important safety information.

REFERENCES

1. **al-Aska, A. K., and A. H. Chagla.** 1989. Laboratory-acquired brucellosis. *J. Hosp. Infect.* **14:**69–71.
1a. **Anonymous.** 1968. Medical laboratory manpower recommendations. *Public Health Rep.* **83:**518.
2. **Ansa, V. O., E. J. Udoma, M. S. Umoh, and M. U. Anah.** 2002. Occupational risk of infection by human immunodeficiency and hepatitis B viruses among health workers in southeastern Nigeria. *East Afr. Med. J.* **79:**254–256.
3. **Ashdown, L. R.** 1992. Melioidosis and safety in the clinical laboratory. *J. Hosp. Infect.* **21:**301–306.
4. **Barkham, T. M.** 2004. Laboratory safety aspects of SARS at biosafety level 2. *Ann. Acad. Med. Singapore* **33:**252–256.
5. **Baron, E. J., and J. M. Miller.** 2008. Bacterial and fungal infections among diagnostic laboratory workers: evaluating the risks. *Diagn. Microbiol. Infect. Dis.* **60:**241–246.
6. **Bennett, A., and S. Parks.** 2006. Microbial aerosol generation during laboratory accidents and subsequent risk assessment. *J. Appl. Microbiol.* **100:**658–663.
7. **Birt, C., and C. Lamb.** 1899. Mediterranean or Malta fever. *Lancet* **i:**701–710.
8. **Blaser, M. J., and J. P. Lofgren.** 1981. Fatal salmonellosis originating in a clinical microbiology laboratory. *J. Clin. Microbiol.* **13:**855–858.
9. **Bottone, E. J., M. Cheng, and S. Hymes.** 2004. Ineffectiveness of handwashing with lotion soap to remove nosocomial bacterial pathogens persisting on fingertips: a major link in their intrahospital spread. *Infect. Control Hosp. Epidemiol.* **25:**262–264.
10. **Boutet, R., J. M. Stuart, E. B. Kaczmarski, S. J. Gray, D. M. Jones, and N. Andrews.** 2001. Risk of laboratory-acquired meningococcal disease. *J. Hosp. Infect.* **49:**282–284.
11. **Boyce, J. M., and D. Pittet.** 2002. Guideline for hand hygiene in health-care settings. Recommendations of the Healthcare Infection Control Practices Advisory Committee and the HIPAC/SHEA/APIC/IDSA Hand Hygiene Task Force. *Am. J. Infect. Control* **30:**S1–S46.
12. **Burke, F. J., N. H. Wilson, and S. W. Cheung.** 1995. Factors associated with skin irritation of the hands experienced by general dental practitioners. *Contact Dermatitis* **32:**35–38.
13. **Canadian Standards Association.** 2002. *Evaluation of Single-Use Medical Sharps Containers for Biohazardous and Cytotoxic Waste,* vol. Z316.6-02. Canadian Standards Association, Mississauga, Ontario, Canada.
13a. **Canton, R.** 2005. Role of the microbiology laboratory in infectious disease surveillance, alert and response. *Clin. Microbiol. Infect.* **11**(Suppl. 1):3–8.
14. **Centers for Disease Control and Prevention.** 2002. Laboratory-acquired meningococcal disease—United States, 2000. *Morb. Mortal. Wkly. Rep.* **51:**141–144.
15. **Centers for Disease Control and Prevention.** 2003. Recommended adult immunization schedule—United States, 2003–2004. *Morb. Mortal. Wkly. Rep.* **52:**965–969.
16. **Centers for Disease Control and Prevention.** 2001. Updated U.S. Public Health Service guidelines for the management of occupational exposures to HBV, HCV, and HIV and recommendations for postexposure prophylaxis. *MMWR Recomm. Rep.* **50:**1–42.
17. **Centers for Disease Control and Prevention.** 2005. *Threat to Public Health from Influenza A (H2N2) Is Low.* Centers for Disease Control and Prevention, Atlanta, GA.
18. **Chang, C. L., H. H. Kim, H. C. Son, S. S. Park, M. K. Lee, S. K. Park, W. W. Park, and C. H. Jeon.** 2001. False-positive growth of *Mycobacterium tuberculosis* attributable to laboratory contamination confirmed by restriction fragment length polymorphism analysis. *Int. J. Tuberc. Lung Dis.* **5:**861–867.
19. **Checchi, L., M. R. Gatto, P. Legnani, G. A. Pelliccioni, and P. Bisbini.** 1999. Use of gloves and prevalence of glove-related reactions in a sample of general dental practitioners in Italy. *Quintessence Int.* **30:**633–636.
20. **Chen, L., M. Zhang, Y. Yan, J. Miao, Y. Lin, Y. Zhang, H. Wang, X. Du, and T. Li.** 2009. Sharp object injuries among health care workers in a Chinese province. *AAOHN J.* **57:**13–16.
21. **Chitnis, V., S. Chitnis, S. Patil, and D. Chitnis.** 2003. Solar disinfection of infectious biomedical waste: a new approach for developing countries. *Lancet* **362:**1285–1286.
22. **Christen, G., and D. Tagan.** 2004. Laboratory-acquired *Neisseria meningitidis* infection. *Med. Mal. Infect.* **34:**137–138.

23. **College of American Pathologists.** 13 April 2005, posting date. *CAP Laboratories Alerted To Destroy an Influenza A Specimen Included in Some Proficiency Testing Kits.* College of American Pathologists, Northfield, IL.

24. **Collins, C. H., and D. A. Kennedy.** 1999. *Laboratory Acquired Infections,* 4th ed. Butterworth-Heinemann, Oxford, United Kingdom.

25. **Creedon, S. A.** 2005. Healthcare workers' hand decontamination practices: compliance with recommended guidelines. *J. Adv. Nurs.* **51:**208–216.

26. **CSA.** 2004. *Fume Hoods and Associated Exhaust Systems,* vol. Z316.5. Canadian Standards Association, Toronto, Ontario, Canada.

27. **Dale, J. C., S. K. Pruett, and M. D. Maker.** 1998. Accidental needlesticks in the phlebotomy service of the Department of Laboratory Medicine and Pathology at Mayo Clinic Rochester. *Mayo Clin. Proc.* **73:**611–615.

28. **Daniels, D., S. Grytdal, and A. Wasley.** 2009. Surveillance for acute viral hepatitis—United States, 2007. *MMWR Surveill. Summ.* **58:**1–27.

29. **David, L., and P. Sewell (ed.).** 2005. *Protection of Laboratory Workers from Occupationally Acquired Infections; Approved Guideline,* 3rd ed., vol. 21. Clinical and Laboratory Standards Institute, Wayne, PA.

30. **Dinh, P. N., H. T. Long, N. T. Tien, N. T. Hien, T. Q. Mai Le, H. Phong Le, V. Tuan Le, H. Van Tan, N. B. Nguyen, P. Van Tu, and N. T. Phuong.** 2006. Risk factors for human infection with avian influenza A H5N1, Vietnam, 2004. *Emerg. Infect. Dis.* **12:**1841–1847.

31. **Do, A. N., C. A. Ciesielski, R. P. Metler, T. A. Hammett, J. Li, and P. L. Fleming.** 2003. Occupationally acquired human immunodeficiency virus (HIV) infection: national case surveillance data during 20 years of the HIV epidemic in the United States. *Infect. Control Hosp. Epidemiol.* **24:**86–96.

32. **Evans, M. R., D. K. Henderson, and J. E. Bennett.** 1990. Potential for laboratory exposures to biohazardous agents found in blood. *Am. J. Public Health* **80:**423–427.

33. **Fichet, G., E. Comoy, C. Duval, K. Antloga, C. Dehen, A. Charbonnier, G. McDonnell, P. Brown, C. I. Lasmezas, and J. P. Deslys.** 2004. Novel methods for disinfection of prion-contaminated medical devices. *Lancet* **364:**521–526.

34. **Fiori, P. L., S. Mastrandrea, P. Rappelli, and P. Cappuccinelli.** 2000. *Brucella abortus* infection acquired in microbiology laboratories. *J. Clin. Microbiol.* **38:**2005–2006.

35. **Gallaher, W. R.** 2009. Towards a sane and rational approach to management of influenza H1N1. *Virol. J.* **6:**51.

36. **Gerding, D. N., C. A. Muto, and R. C. Owens, Jr.** 2008. Measures to control and prevent *Clostridium difficile* infection. *Clin. Infect. Dis.* **46**(Suppl. 1)**:**S43–S49.

36a. **Griffith, J., M. Sullivan, J. Howell, et al.** 2008. Laboratory-acquired brucellosis—Indiana and Minnesota, 2006. *Morb. Mortal. Wkly. Rep.* **57:**39–42.

37. **Hall, C. V.** 1975. A biological safety centrifuge. *Health Lab. Sci.* **12:**104–106.

38. **Hambleton, P., and G. Dedonato.** 1992. Protecting researchers from instrument biohazards. *Biotechniques* **13:**450–453.

39. **Health Canada.** 2004. *Laboratory Biosafety Guidelines,* 3rd ed. Health Canada, Ottawa, Canada.

40. **Herwaldt, B. L.** 2001. Laboratory-acquired parasitic infections from accidental exposures. *Clin. Microbiol. Rev.* **14:**659–688.

41. **Herwaldt, B. L., and D. D. Juranek.** 1993. Laboratory-acquired malaria, leishmaniasis, trypanosomiasis, and toxoplasmosis. *Am. J. Trop. Med. Hyg.* **48:**313–323.

41a. **International Civil Aviation Organization.** 2006. *Technical Instructions for the Safe Transport of Dangerous Goods by Air.* International Civil Aviation Organization, Montreal, Canada.

41b. **International Organization for Standardization.** 2003. *Medical Laboratories—Particular Requirements for Quality and Competence.* ISO 15189:2003. International Organization for Standardization, Geneva, Switzerland.

41c. **International Organization for Standardization.** 2003. *Medical Laboratories—Requirements for Safety.* ISO 15190:2003. International Organization for Standardization, Geneva, Switzerland.

41d. **International Organization for Standardization.** 2006. *Point-of-Care Testing (POCT)—Requirements for Quality and Competence.* ISO 22870:2006. International Organization for Standardization, Geneva, Switzerland.

42. **Jackson, G. S., E. McKintosh, E. Flechsig, K. Prodromidou, P. Hirsch, J. Linehan, S. Brandner, A. R. Clarke, C. Weissmann, and J. Collinge.** 2005. An enzyme-detergent method for effective prion decontamination of surgical steel. *J. Gen. Virol.* **86:**869–878.

42a. **James, G., M. Yuen, and L. Gilbert.** 2003. Laboratory investigation of suspected bioterrorism incidents, New South Wales, October 2001 to February 2002. *NSW Publ. Health Bull.* **14:**221–223.

43. **Jungbauer, F. H., J. J. van der Harst, J. W. Groothoff, and P. J. Coenraads.** 2004. Skin protection in nursing work: promoting the use of gloves and hand alcohol. *Contact Dermatitis* **51:**135–140.

44. **Kahn, L. H.** 2004. Biodefense research: can secrecy and safety coexist? *Biosecur. Bioterror.* **2:**81–85.

45. **Kampf, G., and A. Kramer.** 2004. Epidemiologic background of hand hygiene and evaluation of the most important agents for scrubs and rubs. *Clin. Microbiol. Rev.* **17:**863–893.

46. **Kimman, T. G., E. Smit, and M. R. Klein.** 2008. Evidence-based biosafety: a review of the principles and effectiveness of microbiological containment measures. *Clin. Microbiol. Rev.* **21:**403–425.

47. **Landro, L.** 13 March 2009. Staff shortages in labs may put patients at risk. *The Wall Street Journal.*

48. **Loeb, M., I. Zando, M. C. Orvidas, A. Bialachowski, D. Groves, and J. Mahoney.** 2003. Laboratory-acquired vaccinia infection. *Can. Commun. Dis. Rep.* **29:**134–136.

49. **Logan-Henfrey, L.** 2000. Mitigation of bioterrorist threats in the 21st century. *Ann. N. Y. Acad. Sci.* **916:**121–133.

49a. **Martin-Mazuelos, E., M. C. Nogales, C. Florez, J. M. Gomez-Mateos, F. Lozano, and A. Sanchez.** 1994. Outbreak of *Brucella melitensis* among microbiology laboratory workers. *J. Clin. Microbiol.* **32:**2035–2036.

50. **Mecklem, R. L., and C. M. Neumann.** 2003. Defining and managing biohazardous waste in U.S. research-oriented universities: a survey of environmental health and safety professionals. *J. Environ. Health* **66:**17–22.

50a. **Memish, Z. A., and M. W. Mah.** 2001. Brucellosis in laboratory workers at a Saudi Arabian hospital. *Am. J. Infect. Control* **29:**48–52.

51. **Mempel, M., G. Isa, N. Klugbauer, H. Meyer, G. Wildi, J. Ring, F. Hofmann, and H. Hofmann.** 2003. Laboratory acquired infection with recombinant vaccinia virus containing an immunomodulating construct. *J. Investig. Dermatol.* **120:**356–358.

52. **Messager, S., K. A. Hammer, C. F. Carson, and T. V. Riley.** 2005. Effectiveness of hand-cleansing formulations containing tea tree oil assessed ex vivo on human skin and in vivo with volunteers using European standard EN 1499. *J. Hosp. Infect.* **59:**220–228.

53. **Neely, A. N., and D. F. Sittig.** 2002. Basic microbiologic and infection control information to reduce the potential transmission of pathogens to patients via computer hardware. *J. Am. Med. Inform. Assoc.* **9:**500–508.

54. **Noble, M.** 2005. Biological safety for the clinical laboratory, p. 760. *In* S. P. Borriello, P. R. Murray, and G. Funke (ed.), *Topley and Wilson's Microbiology and Microbial Infections,* 10th ed. *Bacteriology.* Hodder Arnold, London, United Kingdom.

55. **Noble, M. A.** 2008. Convergence of laboratory quality, safety, and risk. *Lab. Focus* **12:**1–30.

55a. **Noviello, S., R. Gallo, M. Kelly, R. J. Limberger, K. DeAngelis, L. Cain, B. Wallace, and N. Dumas.** 2004. Laboratory-acquired brucellosis. *Emerg. Infect. Dis.* **10:**1848–1850.

56. **Orellana, C.** 2004. Laboratory-acquired SARS raises worries on biosafety. *Lancet Infect. Dis.* **4:**64.

57. **Phillips, G. B.** 1986. Human factors in microbiological laboratory accidents, p. 43–48. *In* B. M. Miller (ed.), *Laboratory Safety: Principles and Practices.* American Society for Microbiology, Washington, DC.

58. **PHMSA.** 2009. *Hazardous Materials: Infectious Substances; Harmonization with the United Nations Recommendations; Final Rule.* Office of Hazardous Materials Safety, Washington, DC.

59. **Piro, S., M. Sammud, S. Badi, and L. Al Ssabi.** 2001. Hospital-acquired malaria transmitted by contaminated gloves. *J. Hosp. Infect.* **47:**156–158.

60. **Public Health Agency of Canada.** 2006. *Material Safety Data Sheets (MSDS) for Infectious Substances.* Public Health Agency of Canada, Ottawa, Canada.

61. **Ramsing, D. W., and T. Agner.** 1996. Effect of glove occlusion on human skin. I. Short-term experimental exposure. *Contact Dermatitis* **34:**1–5.

62. **Richmond, J. Y., and S. L. Nesby-O'Dell.** 2002. Laboratory security and emergency response guidance for laboratories working with select agents. *MMWR Recomm. Rep.* **51:**1–6.

63. **Robinson-Dunn, B.** 2002. The microbiology laboratory's role in response to bioterrorism. *Arch. Pathol. Lab. Med.* **126:** 291–294.

64. **Rutala, W. A., and D. J. Weber.** 2001. Creutzfeldt-Jakob disease: recommendations for disinfection and sterilization. *Clin. Infect. Dis.* **32:**1348–1356.

65. **Sawyer, J., and A. Bennett.** 2006. Comparing the level of dexterity offered by latex and nitrile SafeSkin gloves. *Ann. Occup. Hyg.* **50:**289–296.

66. **Sawyer, J., A. Bennett, V. Haines, E. Elton, K. Crago, and S. Speight.** 2007. The effect of microbiological containment systems on dexterity. *J. Occup. Environ. Hyg.* **4:**166–173.

67. **Scoular, A., A. D. Watt, M. Watson, and B. Kelly.** 2000. Knowledge and attitudes of hospital staff to occupational exposure to bloodborne viruses. *Commun. Dis. Public Health* **3:**247–249.

68. **Sejvar, J. J., D. Johnson, T. Popovic, J. M. Miller, F. Downes, P. Somsel, R. Weyant, D. S. Stephens, B. A. Perkins, and N. E. Rosenstein.** 2005. Assessing the risk of laboratory-acquired meningococcal disease. *J. Clin. Microbiol.* **43:**4811–4814.

69. **Sewell, D.** 1995. Laboratory-associated infections and biosafety. *Clin. Microbiol. Rev.* **8:**389–405.

69a. **Sewell, D. L.** 2003. Laboratory safety practices associated with potential agents of biocrime or bioterrorism. *J. Clin. Microbiol.* **41:**2801–2809.

70. **Sewell, D. L.** 2006. Laboratory-acquired infections: are microbiologists at risk? *Clin. Microbiol. Newsl.* **28:**1–6.

71. **Sewell, D. L. (ed.).** 2005. *Protection of Laboratory Workers from Occupationally Acquired Infections; Approved Guideline,* 3rd ed., vol. 21. CLSI, Wayne, PA.

72. **Sickbert-Bennett, E. E., D. J. Weber, M. F. Gergen-Teague, M. D. Sobsey, G. P. Samsa, and W. A. Rutala.** 2005. Comparative efficacy of hand hygiene agents in the reduction of bacteria and viruses. *Am. J. Infect. Control* **33:**67–77.

73. **Simhon, A., G. Rahav, M. Shapiro, and C. Block.** 2001. Skin disease presenting as an outbreak of pseudobacteremia in a laboratory worker. *J. Clin. Microbiol.* **39:**392–393.

73a. **Singh, K.** 2009. Laboratory-acquired infections. *Clin. Infect. Dis.* **49:**142–147.

74. **Tan, R., and M. A. Noble.** 1993. Sharps utilization and disposal in British Columbia physicians' offices. *Can. J. Public Health* **84:**31–34.

74a. **Thabuis, A., M. Schmitt, F. Megas, and B. Fabres.** 2007. Retrospective census of cancers between 1994 and 2002 around the municipal solid waste incinerator of Gilly-sur-Isere. *Rev. Epidemiol. Sante Publique* **55:**426–432. (In French.)

75. **Thomson, R. B., Jr., S. J. Vanzo, N. K. Henry, K. L. Guenther, and J. A. Washington II.** 1984. Contamination of cultures processed with the Isolator lysis-centrifugation blood culture tube. *J. Clin. Microbiol.* **19:**97–99.

76. **Tonuci, L. R., C. F. Paschoalatto, and R. Pisani, Jr.** 2007. Microwave inactivation of *Escherichia coli* in healthcare waste. *Waste Manag.* **28:**840–848.

76a. **Trever, R. W., L. E. Cluff, R. N. Peeler, and I. L. Bennett, Jr.** 1959. Brucellosis. I. Laboratory-acquired acute infection. *AMA Arch. Intern. Med.* **103:**381–397.

77. **U.S. Department of Health and Human Services.** 2009. *Centers for Medicare and Medicaid Services Clinical Laboratory Improvement Amendments (CLIA).* U.S. Department of Health and Human Services, Washington, DC.

78. **U.S. Department of Health and Human Services.** 1999. *Biosafety in Microbiological and Biomedical Laboratories,* 4th ed. U.S. Department of Health and Human Services, Washington, DC.

78a. **van Asten, L., M. van der Lubben, C. van den Wijngaard, W. van Pelt, R. Verheij, A. Jacobi, P. Overduin, A. Meijer, D. Luijt, E. Claas, M. Hermans, W. Melchers, J. Rossen, R. Schuurman, P. Wolffs, C. Bouchier, J. Schirm, L. Kroes, S. Leenders, J. Galama, M. Peeters, A. van Loon, E. Stobberingh, M. Schutten, and M. Koopmans.** 2009. Strengthening the diagnostic capacity to detect Bio Safety Level 3 organisms in unusual respiratory viral outbreaks. *J. Clin. Virol.* **45:**185–190.

79. **Weber, D. J., E. Sickbert-Bennett, M. F. Gergen, and W. A. Rutala.** 2003. Efficacy of selected hand hygiene agents used to remove *Bacillus atrophaeus* (a surrogate of *Bacillus anthracis*) from contaminated hands. *JAMA* **289:**1274–1277.

80. **Wrangsjo, K., L. M. Wallenhammar, U. Ortengren, L. Barregard, H. Andreasson, B. Bjorkner, S. Karlsson, and B. Meding.** 2001. Protective gloves in Swedish dentistry: use and side-effects. *Br. J. Dermatol.* **145:**32–37.

81. **Zarpellon, M. N., V. S. Soares, N. R. Albrecht, D. R. Bergamasco, L. B. Garcia, and C. L. Cardoso.** 2008. Comparison of 3 alcohol gels and 70% ethyl alcohol for hand hygiene. *Infect. Control Hosp. Epidemiol.* **29:**960–962.

Decontamination, Disinfection, and Sterilization

ANDREAS F. WIDMER AND RENO FREI

11

Decontamination, disinfection, and sterilization are basic components of any infection control program. Patients expect that any reusable instrument or device used for diagnosis or treatment has undergone a process to eliminate any risks for cross-infection. However, the infection control literature documents many reprocessing failures, including numerous reports of transmission of nosocomial pathogens from contaminated endoscopes (29, 111, 240, 248, 251). Before 1990, it was very difficult to prove a causal relationship between a contaminated device and a subsequent nosocomial infection. Today, state-of-the-art clinical epidemiology supported by molecular typing tools such as pulsed-field gel electrophoresis, PCR, and genome sequencing can enable the hospital epidemiologist to prove a causal relationship between the use of a contaminated device and a consequent infection. Molecular epidemiology has thus provided scientific tools that can identify the limitations of the available disinfection and sterilization methods and can provide the impetus to improve reprocessing technologies. Despite those advances, little research has been done that will lead to major breakthroughs in disinfection and sterilization in the near future. Thus, we believe the key issues instead will be to standardize and optimize our applications of current knowledge.

Clearly, more research is needed in this field, but resources for such work have been limited. In fact, most disinfectants were introduced to the market more than 30 years ago and little is known about their modes of action and the mechanisms of resistance. Excellent reviews on this topic are published by Block (33) and by Russell and coworkers (179, 215). In addition, few basic procedures in decontamination, disinfection, and sterilization have been tested in randomized clinical trials. In this chapter, we have tried to cite the highest level of evidence available. However, given the dearth of studies, we have often had to cite results of observational studies, animal models, in vitro tests, and expert opinion because higher levels of evidence were unavailable.

Despite the lack of resources, reprocessing techniques, disinfectants, and general infection control practice have garnered more attention recently than in the past. This is due in part to the increasing frequency of multiresistant bacterial pathogens at a time when pharmaceutical companies have shifted from developing antimicrobial agents to designing drugs for chronic diseases (281). Moreover, new pathogens, such as the viruses causing severe acute respiratory syndrome (SARS) and avian influenza (131) and swine flu (192) or the prions causing Creutzfeldt-Jakob disease (CJD) and variant CJD (vCJD), are emerging, for which there are few if any treatments. Consequently, the medical community needs better knowledge on disinfection and sterilization to prevent spread of these pathogens.

PRINCIPLES OF TERMINOLOGY, DEFINITIONS, AND CLASSIFICATION OF MEDICAL DEVICES

Background

There is no uniform terminology for disinfection and sterilization, and many problems arise as a result. Many terms are ill defined even within the United States or Europe. In addition, the testing procedures for disinfectants are not as far advanced and well defined as MIC testing based on the recommendations of the Clinical and Laboratory Standards Institute (CLSI). However, there currently are efforts to standardize and harmonize the terminology on an international level. For example, the International Organization for Standardization (ISO) norms for sterilization were published in 2004 and included in the new guidelines published in 2010 (229). In addition, manufacturers now must provide specific data on how to reprocess their medical devices. In the past, such information was frequently missing in the user's manuals.

Classification of Devices for Reprocessing

Background

The principal goal of disinfection and sterilization is to reduce the numbers of microorganisms on a device to a level that is insufficient to transmit infectious organisms, with a considerable safety margin. The most conservative approach would be to reprocess all items and devices with overkill sterilization. Obviously, not all items must undergo the most vigorous process to eliminate any microorganisms. For example, items such as blood pressure cuffs that are used at nonsterile body sites do not need to be sterilized between patients. In contrast, only sterilization will eliminate any

TABLE 1 Spaulding classification of devices

Clinical device	Definition	Example(s)	Infectious risk	Reprocessing procedure (FDA classification)
Critical device	Medical device that is intended to enter a normally sterile environment, sterile tissue, or the vasculature	Surgical instruments	High	Sterilization by steam, plasma, or ethylene oxide; liquid sterilization acceptable if no other methods feasible
Semicritical device	Medical device that is intended to come in contact with mucous membranes or minor skin breaches	Flexible endoscope	High, intermediate	Sterilization desirable; high-level disinfection acceptable
Noncritical device	Medical device that comes in contact with intact skin	Blood pressure cuff, electrocardiogram electrodes	Low	Intermediate or low-level
Medical equipment	Device or component of a device that does not typically come in direct contact with the patient	Examination table	Low	Low-level disinfection, sanitizer

risk of infection for devices used in a normally sterile body site. In some cases, the best choice may be to use disposable items instead of reusable devices, because reprocessing may be more expensive or does not provide the desired level of safety. The latter may apply to items in contact with neural tissue of a patient suffering from any form of CJD or with tonsils and other lymphatic tissues of persons with spongiform encephalopathy (bovine spongiform encephalopathy [BSE] or vCJD) (25, 70, 280). Therefore, devices must be classified to allow staff to define the appropriate method for disinfection and/or sterilization for each item. A classification system should balance the potential risks for transmission of infection (e.g., the infectious dose) and the resources available to achieve the necessary or desired level of antimicrobial killing. The most commonly used classification was proposed by Earle H. Spaulding in 1968 (249). He proposed three categories that are based on the devices' potential for transmitting infectious agents: critical, semicritical, and noncritical (Table 1). The Centers for Disease Control and Prevention (CDC) cites this classification in its *Guidelines for Handwashing and Hospital Environmental Control* (http://www.cdc.gov/mmwr/PDF/rr/rr5116.pdf), as does the U.S. Food and Drug Administration (FDA), for approval of sterilants and high-level disinfectants (see http://www. fda.gov/MedicalDevices/DeviceRegulationandGuidance/ ReprocessingofSingle-UseDevices/ucm133514.htm). Most infection control professionals worldwide use this classification as well. However, this simple classification does not work perfectly for all devices. Even the definition of sterilization as the absence of any viable microorganisms must be revised to address the prions responsible for CJD and vCJD (202).

Critical Items

Items that enter normally sterile parts of the human body, such as surgical instruments, implants, or invasive monitoring devices (Table 1), are classified as "critical items." Because items classified as critical carry the highest risk for the patient, sterilization is the preferred method for reprocessing these items. Autoclaving is the method of choice if the device is not heat labile. Alternative sterilization processes that use ethylene oxide or plasma require prolonged times, and the FDA has not approved them for use with instruments that have small dead-end lumens, which are difficult to sterilize. Liquid sterilization with a glutaraldehyde-based formulation or peracetic acid is acceptable if sterilization by one of the methods mentioned above is not feasible and the formulation and/or automated device has been cleared by the FDA.

Semicritical Items

Semicritical objects come into contact with mucous membranes or nonintact skin and should be free of microorganisms except spores. Intact mucous membranes generally resist bacterial spores but are susceptible to other microorganisms such as vegetative bacteria (e.g., *Mycobacterium tuberculosis*) or viruses (e.g., HIV and cytomegalovirus). Examples of semicritical equipment include anesthesia equipment, respiratory equipment, and endoscopes. These items should be processed with a high-level disinfectant such as glutaraldehyde, stabilized hydrogen peroxide, peracetic acid, or a chlorine compound. Chlorine compounds corrode items and, therefore, are rarely used to disinfect medical devices.

Noncritical Items

Noncritical items (bedside tables, crutches, stethoscopes, furniture, and floors) come into contact with intact skin only. Intact skin is a very effective barrier against microorganisms, and therefore, these items and devices do not need to be sterilized. Such items pose a very low risk for direct transmission of pathogens and can usually be cleaned at the bedside or at their point of use with a low-level disinfectant. For example, health care workers (HCWs) can disinfect their stethoscopes by wiping the surfaces with alcohol. However, noncritical devices can contribute to the transmission of pathogens by the indirect route. For instance, up to 60% of cultures of the environment near patients colonized or infected with vancomycin-resistant enterococci are positive for this organism (58). HCWs can contaminate their hands when they touch these surfaces. If they do not practice hand hygiene, they can spread these pathogens to devices or directly to other patients. Therefore, noncritical items must be decontaminated if they are likely to be contaminated with pathogenic organisms. The FDA also developed a classification based on safety considerations and the regulations manufacturers must meet before marketing a device. Medical products are listed as class I to III products (Table 2). Simple products (e.g., a tongue depressor) are classified as medical product class I, which must meet very simple requirements before being marketed legally. Class II products (e.g., autoclaves) require a premarket notification [510(k)] demonstrating that the device is at least as safe and effective as a legally marketed device. Class III devices are those that support or sustain human life and are of substantial importance in preventing impairment of human health (e.g., a pacemaker).

TABLE 2 Principles of medical device classification

Classification	FDA regulation	Premarket requirements by the FDA	Proposed classification by Global Harmonization Task Force[a]	Examples
Class I	Least regulated, requires fewest regulations	None	A	Band-Aid, tongue depressor
Class II	Must meet federal performance standards	Premarket notification [(510(k)]	B	Surgical gowns, drapes, scrub sponges
			C	Orthopedic implants
Class III	Implanted and life-supporting or life-sustaining devices are required to have FDA approval for safety and effectiveness	Premarket approval	D	Artificial hearts

[a] Details available at http://www.ghtf.org/sg1/inventorysg1/pd_sg1_n015r22.pdf.

Due to the level of risk associated with class III devices, the FDA requires companies (section 515 of the Federal Food, Drug and Cosmetic Act) to file a premarket approval application to obtain marketing clearance. The premarket approval application must contain sufficient valid scientific evidence documenting that the device is safe and effective for its intended use (58).

DECONTAMINATION AND CLEANING

In Europe, decontamination basically means cleaning an item to remove organic material, protein, and fat. In the United States, the term describes a cleaning step and any additional step required to eliminate any risk of infection to HCWs while they handle a device without protective attire. The CDC guideline defines cleaning as the removal of visible soil (e.g., organic and inorganic material) from objects and surfaces by using water with detergents or enzymatic products. Thorough cleaning is essential before high-level disinfection and sterilization because inorganic and organic materials that remain on the surfaces of instruments interfere with the effectiveness of these processes. Decontamination removes pathogenic microorganisms from objects so they are safe to handle, use, or discard (196). The FDA defines the *cleaning process* as including all steps necessary to remove, inactivate, or contain contamination, beginning immediately after an item has been used for clinical purposes, continuing with the steps to decontaminate, clean, and package a device up to the first step of the sterilization process and ending with quality control tests.

Regardless of regulations, cleaning is always the initial step of the decontamination process on both continents. In this chapter, we use the term "decontamination" to describe the removal of debris, blood, proteins, and most microorganisms. This process usually, but not necessarily, renders the device "safe to handle" by HCWs who are not wearing protective attire. Basic definitions are outlined in Table 3.

The first step in reprocessing used medical devices is for HCWS to prevent debris from drying on the item. Research on prion diseases demonstrated that removal of debris is seriously impaired if the debris is allowed to dry on a medical device (96). Therefore, the reprocessing cycle should start as soon as possible: the item should be kept wet if delays in reprocessing are anticipated (124, 191). Cleaning can be done physically or chemically; it can also be done manually, by sonication, or with washers. In the United States, cleaning is frequently performed manually with water and a detergent. In Europe, many countries rely

primarily on washer-disinfectors that rinse items with cold water and then with warm water plus a detergent. The cycle is completed with hot water at ≥90°C. Items such as bedpans and urinals can be cleaned and disinfected by putting the items into a machine, pushing a button, and removing them after a 2- to 5-min procedure. All sterilization techniques other than steaming have been shown to fail in 1 to 40% of sterilization cycles if residual proteins and/or salts are not removed by a proper cleaning process (11). Even steam sterilization at 134°C for 18 min, recommended by the World Health Organization (WHO) to inactivate prions, can fail to prevent cross-transmission if the device does not undergo a cleaning process beforehand (96, 124, 191).

For floors, surfaces, and noncritical items, cleaning with a detergent is sufficient in most situations, and a disinfection process adds little if any additional effect (83). In addition, disinfectants may interfere and even lose activity with residual proteins and debris that escape the cleaning process (83). Routine disinfection of environmental surfaces in patient care areas is recommended in the United States to add a step of additional safety in cases of unrecognized body fluids, but it is restricted to intensive care units and emergency rooms in Europe (243).

DISINFECTION

Disinfection is the second critical step in reprocessing medical devices. To be effective, disinfection must be preceded by thorough cleaning and must be done properly. Staff members must check the disinfectant's concentration regularly if it is diluted at the place of use, even if it is diluted with an electronically monitored dilution device. Failures of the valve or other critical parts of the device can result in an insufficient final concentration, which usually cannot be detected by checking either the appearance or the odor of the disinfectant. Many manufacturers provide test strips to check for the appropriate concentration. Of note, numerous outbreaks have occurred when staff members have not followed appropriate protocols (277). For example, *Klebsiella oxytoca* caused an outbreak after an infection control committee allowed staff members to decrease the concentration of a glutaraldehyde-based surface disinfectant because they didn't like the odor. The outbreak stopped after staff resumed using the disinfectant at the recommended concentration (205). An outbreak of 58 cases of *Mycobacterium xenopi* infection occurred when instruments used for discovertebral operations were rinsed with tap water after they were disinfected (20).

TABLE 3 Definitions and terms

Term	Standard	Technical-microbiological log CFU reduction	Comment
Sterilization	A (closely monitored) validated process used to render a product free of all forms of viable microorganisms, including all bacterial endospores	≥6 log CFU reduction of the most resistant spores for the sterilization process studied, achieved at the half-time of the regular cycle (ISO 14937)	Prions require an adapted definition because of their high resistance to any form of sterilization
Examples for standards	Sterilization method Ethylene oxide Moist heat	Industrial facility use ISO 11135 ISO 11134	Health care facility use ANSI/AAMI ST 41 ANSI/AAMI ST 46
Disinfection	Elimination of most if not all pathogenic microorganisms, excluding spores	There is not a clear-cut defined reduction level; a minimum estimate is ≥3 log CFU reduction of microorganisms, excluding spores; common reduction is 4 to 5 log for devices; these are estimates, because there is no international standardization	Some high-level disinfectants achieve microbial reduction, including spores, similar to sterilization, if long incubation times and/or temperatures of >25°C are applied; this is called liquid sterilization by sterilants
Decontamination	Reduction of pathogenic microorganisms to a level where items are "safe to handle" without protective attire	Elimination of debris and proteins by cleaning and/or disinfection/sterilization process; in Europe, it is restricted to cleaning only, which achieves a minimum of ≥1 log CFU; most cleaning processes achieve 3 to 5 log CFU reduction; these are estimates, because there is no international standardization	Manual and/or mechanical cleaning (with water and detergents or enzymes), a prerequisite before disinfection or sterilization; in Europe, this term is used for cleaning the items; in the United States, it defines an item to be "safe to handle"; it may include a cleaning process but also a disinfection or even a sterilization process; the U.S. term "decontamination" refers to the HCW's safety; in Europe, the term is used for the item only
Antisepsis	Patient related: disinfection of living tissue or skin HCW related: reduction or removal of transient microbiota	Preoperative skin preparation with an alcohol-based iodine compound Hand washing (scrub): reduction of ≥1 log CFU Hand disinfection (rub-in): reduction of ≥2.5 log CFU	Antiseptic agents are handled as drugs by the FDA

Principles and Antimicrobial Activities of Compounds

The antimicrobial spectrum of disinfectants is tested differently from that of antimicrobial agents. Microbiology laboratories that test disinfectants must know the special methods needed to accurately assess their activity. In fact, MICs are of little help because the goal of disinfection is to kill rather than inhibit the growth of microorganisms. In contrast to sterilization, but similar to antimicrobial agents, killing curves for disinfectants are not linear and the rate of log killing decreases as the inoculum concentrations decrease (i.e., as the number of CFU per milliliter decreases). Therefore, a 3-log-unit killing is more easily achieved with disinfectants if the inoculum is large, e.g., 10^8 CFU, than if the inoculum is 10^4 CFU. Most disinfectants must be inactivated before they are incubated in media or plated because bacteria do not grow in the presence of very low concentrations of a disinfectant (inhibitory effect). However, if the compound is inactivated, bacterial growth can be demonstrated. Like antimicrobial agents, some disinfectants display a postexposure effect on bacterial growth. The postexposure effect has been quantified for a variety of disinfectants. Alcohols lack a postexposure effect, but chlorhexidine, octenidine, polyhexanide, and chloramine delay regrowth after exposure for several hours (34).

Low-level disinfectants destroy lipid-enveloped viruses such as HIV and most vegetative bacteria (Fig. 1) (34), but many disinfectants, including alcohol, are ineffective against nonlipid or small viruses such as poliovirus. For example, isopropyl alcohol has little activity against poliovirus but >90% ethanol is very active (265). The FDA requires that the microbicidal efficacy of liquid chemical sterilants and high-level disinfectants be assessed in three different types of tests before they can be legally marketed in the United States.

1. Potency testing incorporates the Environmental Protection Agency's (EPA) test requirements for registration of germicides, such as the Association of Official Analytical Chemists' (AOAC) sporicidal test, tuberculocidal test, and use-dilution tests for *Staphylococcus aureus* ATCC 6538, *Salmonella enterica* serovar *choleraesuis* ATCC 10708, and *Pseudomonas aeruginosa*; EPA virucidal tests for viruses including poliovirus type 2 and herpes simplex virus; and FDA-recommended tests, such as total killing or endpoint analysis and comparing survivor and predicted curves. (Note: in Europe, disinfectants should have been tested by the methods defined by European Norms [EN] such as EN 1040 [bactericidal activity] and EN 1275 [fungicidal activity]).

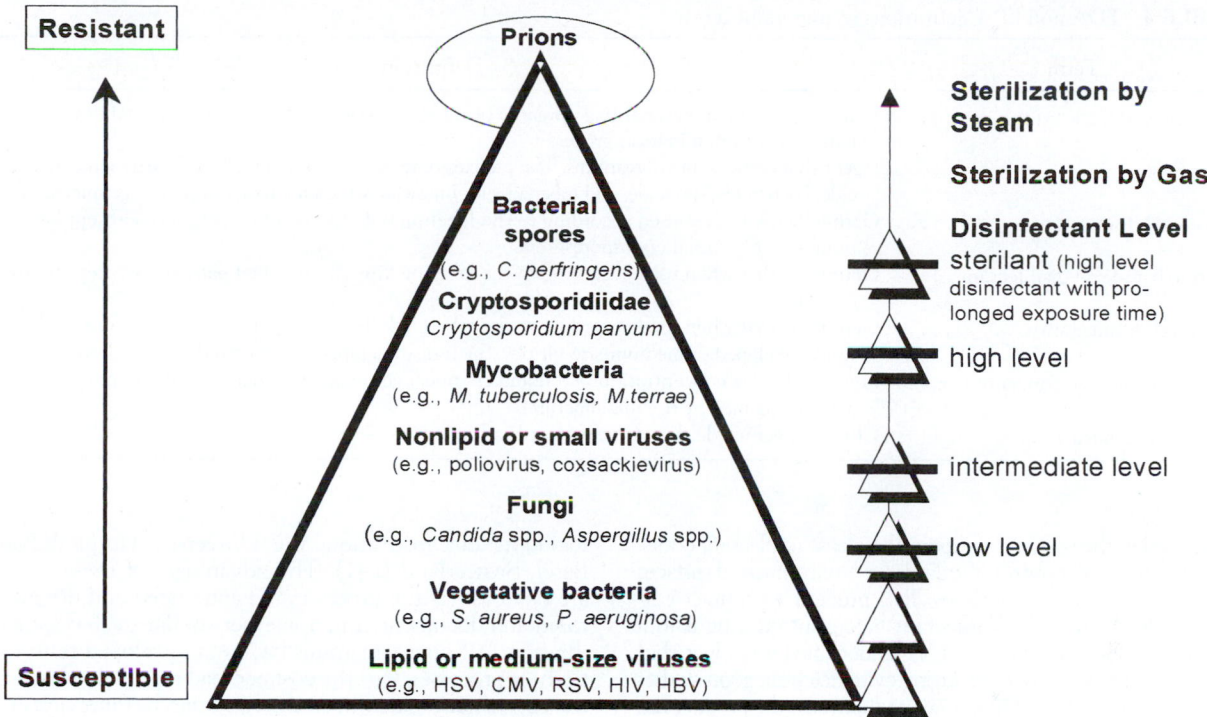

FIGURE 1 Microorganisms' resistance to disinfectants. HSV, herpes simplex virus; CMV, cytomegalovirus; RSV, respiratory syncytial virus.

2. Simulated-use testing involves testing the disinfectant under artificially created worst-case scenarios to determine how long instruments need to be in contact with the disinfectant if cleaning failed and the instruments are still contaminated with substantial organic matter and microbes. The instruments are contaminated with an organic load and appropriate test microorganisms (the organism depends on the level of disinfection being claimed), and the conditions of the artificially contaminated devices represent worst-case postcleaning conditions prior to exposure to the germicide.

3. "In-use" testing involves cleaning medical devices used for clinical purposes according to a facility's operating procedures.

As noted above, the FDA includes a tuberculocidal test in its testing procedures. This test does not account for the effect of cleaning before devices are disinfected. Devices are treated with 2% horse serum (proteinaceous load) and with 10^5 to 10^6 CFU of *Mycobacterium terrae* or equivalent nontuberculous mycobacteria. Under these conditions, a device would need to be immersed in a disinfectant (e.g., 2.4% alkaline glutaraldehyde) for ≥45 min at ≥25°C for complete tuberculocidal killing. However, Rutala and Weber demonstrated that proper cleaning eradicates at least 4 log units of microorganisms (224) and Hanson et al. showed that cleaning bronchoscopes before disinfection removed all detectable contaminants, with up to an 8-log-unit reduction in the viral load (123). Therefore, Rutala and Weber recommended that the FDA accept a standardized cleaning protocol followed by a 20-min immersion at 20°C with an FDA-approved disinfectant as adequate to kill mycobacteria (224). An updated list of low-level and intermediate-level disinfectants registered by EPA or high-level disinfectants and sterilants approved by the FDA is provided on their home pages, http://www.fda.gov/cdrh/ode/germlab.html and http://www.epa.gov/oppad001/chemregindex.htm.

Definitions and Terms (Adapted from FDA and EPA Definitions)

Since the FDA regulates the most critical part of disinfection and sterilization, FDA definitions are used throughout the chapter unless stated otherwise. The most important definitions are given in Table 4.

Guidelines for Choosing a Disinfectant

Rutala and Weber have published guidelines for the selection and use of disinfectants and recommendations on the preferred method for disinfection and sterilization of patient care items (64, 216, 217). The CDC issued guidelines for environmental infection control in health care facilities, including recommendations for cleaning and disinfection (243), and updated its recommendation in 2008 (http://www.cdc.gov/ncidod/dhqp/pdf/guidelines/Disinfection_Nov_2008.pdf) (196).

When choosing a disinfectant, individuals responsible for infection control should review its effectiveness against the expected spectrum of pathogens (Tables 4 and 5) to ensure that it is adequate for the intended purpose. In addition, staff must ensure that the disinfectant is compatible with the devices it is intended to disinfect and that devices that are immersed longer than recommended will not be damaged. The latter is important because staff might forget to remove instruments, for example, during weekends or night shifts. Prolonged exposure to a disinfectant may damage the instrument. Staff should also consider the toxicity, odor, compatibility with other compounds, and residual activity of disinfectants before choosing (Table 6). Advice from health care professionals of different institutions is very helpful to learn about their experience and to uncover problems such as interactions with detergents, unexpected coloring, odors, and, last but not least, emotions elicited. A new disinfectant used for environmental surfaces may interact with

TABLE 4 FDA and EPA definitions of important terms

Term	Definition
Cleaning (or precleaning)	Removal of foreign material (e.g., organic or inorganic contaminants) from medical devices as part of a decontamination process
Germicide	Agent that destroys microorganisms. The prefixes of terms with the suffix "-cide" (e.g., virucide, fungicide, bactericide, sporicide, and tuberculocide) indicate which microorganisms the germicide kills.
High-level disinfectant	Germicide that when used according to the labeling kills all microbial pathogens except large numbers of bacterial endospores
Intermediate-level disinfectant	Germicide that when used according to the labeling kills all microbial pathogens except bacterial endospores
Low-level disinfectant	Germicide that when used according to the labeling kills most vegetative bacteria and lipid-enveloped or medium-size viruses. Such disinfectants are regulated by the EPA.
Minimum effective concentration	Lowest effective concentration of a liquid chemical germicide that achieves the microbicidal activity claimed by the manufacturer
Sterilant (chemical)	Chemical germicide that achieves sterilization

those used in the past and temporarily release unpleasant odors. Written infection control standards for environmental surfaces help to avoid incompatibilities. It is prudent to contact colleagues already using a disinfectant before introducing it in a health care facility. Once staff have identified a product that meets a facility's needs, only strong evidence from good studies should lead to a change to a new product (e.g., the product has improved activity or works faster).

Disinfection by Heat versus Immersion in Germicides

Disinfection by heat has become much more common than in the past and has replaced disinfection with germicides for many applications in European health care facilities,

including our institution, the University Hospital Basel, Basel, Switzerland (241). The advantages of these devices are obvious: (i) the processes are automated and are monitored and documented in a manner similar to that for sterilization; (ii) microorganisms have not developed resistance to these processes; (iii) the cost per load is probably less than the cost of germicides. In addition, studies by Gurevich et al. (120) indicate that pasteurization with a germicide is more effective than pasteurization without a germicide. However, washers include a cleaning process with an average reduction of 4 log units, coupled with heat disinfection (5-log-unit killing; washer-disinfectors such as the AMSCO Reliance 430 achieve an inactivation factor of >5 log units [111, 139]) resulting in a total reduction of 8 to 9 log units. This surpasses

TABLE 5 Overview of common disinfectants[a]

Germicide	Use dilution	Level of disinfection	Bacteria	Lipophilic viruses	Fungi	Small or hydrophilic viruses	M. tuberculosis	Bacterial spores	Shelf life of >1 wk	Corrosive or deleterious effect	Residue	Inactivated by organic matter	Skin irritant	Eye irritant	Respiratory irritant	Toxic	Environmental concerns	Application in hospitals
Glutaraldehyde	2–3.2%	High/CS	+	+	+	+	+	+	+	−	+	−	+	+	+	+	−	Endoscopes
Hydrogen peroxide	3–25%	High/CS	+	+	+	+	+	±	+	±	−	±	+	+	−	+	−	Contact lenses
Chlorine	100–1,000 ppm free chlorine	High	+	+	+	+	+	±	+	+	+	+	+	+	+	+	±	Selected semicritical devices
Isopropyl alcohol	60–95%	Intermediate	+	+	+	±	+	−	+	±	−	±	±	+	−	+	−	Small area surfaces
Glucoprotamine	1.5–4%	Intermediate	+	+	+	+	+	−	+	−	−	−	+	+	−	−	−	Diagnostic instruments
Phenolic compounds	0.4–5% aqueous	Intermediate	+	+	+	±	+	−	+	−	+	−	+	+	−	+	+	Surgical instruments
Iodophors	30–50 ppm free iodine	Intermediate	+	+	+	±	+	−	+	±	+	+	±	+	−	+	−	Medical equipment
Quaternary ammonium compounds	0.4–1.6% aqueous	Low	±	+	±	−	−	−	+	−	+	+	+	+	−	+	−	Disinfection in food preparation areas and floors

[a]Data from references 33, 98, 216, 265, and 291. Abbreviations: CS, chemical sterilant; +, yes; −, no; ±, variable results. Efficacy of the disinfectants is based on an exposure time of less than 30 min at room temperature. Spores require prolonged exposure times (up to 10 h) unless used with a machine at higher temperatures.

TABLE 6 Overview of common antiseptic compounds[a]

Compound(s)	Antiseptic effect on:					Rapidity of action	Residual activity	Typical concn (%)	Affected by organic matter	Safety for humans
	Gram-positive bacteria	Gram-negative bacteria	Viruses	Fungi	M. tuberculosis					
Alcohols	+++	+++	++[b]	+++	+++	15–30 s	None	70–95	?[d]	Drying, flammable
Chlorhexidine	+++	++	++	+	++	Minutes	+++	4, 2, 0.5 in alcohol	Minimally	Ototoxicity, keratitis
Iodophors	+++	++	++	++	++	Minutes	+	10, 7.5, 2, 0.5	Yes	Skin irritation
Octenidine[c]	+++	+++	++	++	++	Minutes	+++	0.1	Minimally	Limited data
PCMX	++	+	+	+	+	Minutes	++	0.5–3.75	Minimally	Appears to be safe
Triclosan	++	++	++	±	+	Minutes	+++	0.3–1.0	Minimally	Appears to be safe

[a]Data from references 159, 204, and 283. Symbols: ±, poor; +, fair; ++, good; +++, excellent.
[b]Ethanol at >95% is highly effective against viruses; isopropanol has limited effectiveness against small or nonlipid viruses.
[c]Not available in the United States.
[d]Conflicting data.

any international requirements for high-level disinfection. Thermal disinfection has several disadvantages. First, the cost to purchase and install the equipment is much higher than for systems using a germicide. Second, considerable power is needed to heat the water. Third, some non-spore-forming microorganisms such as enterococci resist temperatures of up to 71°C for 10 min. Thus, recommendations such as those in the United Kingdom (the Department of Health requires 65°C for 10 min, 71°C for 3 min, or 80°C for 1 min) may not be adequate for these organisms (43). Medical washer-disinfectors that are intended to clean, disinfect at a low or intermediate level, and dry surgical instruments, anesthesia equipment, hollowware, and other medical devices, are exempt from the premarket notification procedures in subpart E of part 807 of the chapter subject to §880.9 (265a). The ISO provided standards for these processes in ISO norm 15883, which defines the standards for washer-disinfectors by heat with and without the addition of disinfectants. This organization has not defined a temperature at which these devices must work but rather allows manufacturers to choose a temperature in a given range at which their devices should operate. In the United States, hot-water pasteurization is generally performed at 77°C for 30 min (35), but few scientific data support use of a particular temperature. ISO 15883 introduces the A_0 concept, which is based on the fact that a defined temperature will generate a predictable lethality effect against microorganisms. Corresponding exposure temperatures and time periods that achieve high-level disinfection can be calculated assuming the presence of particularly heat-resistant microorganisms in numbers in excess of those likely to be encountered on the medical devices to be processed. ISO 15883 introduces the term A_0 for moist heat disinfection (thermal disinfection). The A_0 value of a moist heat disinfection process denotes the lethality effects expressed in terms of the equivalent time in seconds at a temperature of 80°C delivered by the process to the medical device with reference to microorganisms possessing a z value of 10. Given a predefined A_0, equivalent killing of microorganisms is achieved if the following formula is followed: $A_0 = \Delta T \sum 10^{(T-80)/z} t$, where T is the temperature in degrees Celsius, and t is time in seconds. An A_0 value of 600, which can be achieved at 80°C over 10 min, 90°C over 1 min, or 70°C over 100 min, is the minimum requirement for noncritical medical devices (297, 298). An A_0 value of at least 3,000, which can be achieved by exposure to hot water, e.g., at 90°C (the medical device must tolerate this temperature for >5 min), must be employed for medical devices contaminated with heat-resistant viruses such as rotavirus and hepatitis B virus (HBV). An A_0 value of at least 3,000 is also appropriate for high-level disinfection of all semicritical devices. The test procedure based on the A_0 concept has been highly reproducible and found to be suitable to test washer-disinfectors (297, 298).

Overview of Commonly Used Disinfectants for Devices

Glutaraldehyde

Among aldehydes that exhibit biocidal activity, including glyoxal, ortho-phthalaldehyde (OPA), succinaldehyde, and benzaldehydes, glutaraldehyde and formaldehyde are the most extensively studied aldehydes. In-depth reviews may be found elsewhere (19, 213, 216).

In commercially available products, glutaraldehyde is the predominant aldehyde. Because it has potent and broad-spectrum microbicidal activity and is compatible with many materials (including metal, rubber, and plastic), glutaraldehyde is often regarded as the high-level disinfectant and chemical sterilant of choice in many health care facilities. Glutaraldehyde-based formulations are most commonly used for high-level disinfection of medical equipment such as endoscopes, transducers, dialysis systems, and anesthesia and respiratory therapy equipment (216). The mechanism of action is complex and is related to alkylation of sulfhydryl, hydroxyl, carboxy, and amino groups in the cell wall, cell membrane, nucleic acids, enzymes, and other proteins of microorganisms. The biocidal activities of glutaraldehyde solutions are dependent on a variety of variables, such as pH, temperature, concentration at the time of use, the presence of inorganic ions, and the age of the solution (19). Aqueous solutions of glutaraldehyde are usually acidic and are not sporicidal in this form. Therefore, they need to be activated by adding an alkalinizing agent. These activated solutions, however, rapidly lose their activity because glutaraldehyde molecules polymerize at an alkaline pH. Therefore, the shelf life of such solutions is limited to 14 days unless the manufacturer recommends otherwise. To overcome this problem, some manufacturers have developed novel formulations with longer shelf lives (e.g., activated dialdehyde solutions containing 2.4 to 3.5% glutaraldehyde with a maximum reuse life of 28 days).

The activities of disinfectants increase as the temperature rises. Among eight disinfectants tested, glutaraldehyde was found to be the chemical most strongly affected by temperature (108). Some stable acid glutaraldehydes may be used at temperatures of 35 to 55°C at concentrations below 2%. Glutaraldehyde retains its activity in the presence of organic matter. A standard 2% aqueous solution of glutaraldehyde buffered to pH 7.5 to 8.5 is bactericidal, tuberculocidal, sporicidal, fungicidal, and virucidal. It rapidly kills both gram-negative and gram-positive vegetative bacteria. Longer exposure times are required to inactivate spores and mycobacteria. Spores of *Bacillus* and *Clostridium* spp. are generally destroyed by 2% glutaraldehyde in 3 h, whereas spores of *Clostridium difficile* are eliminated more rapidly (221). In contrast, *Cryptosporidium parvum* oocysts remained viable and infectious after 10 h in a 2.5% glutaraldehyde solution (290). Several investigators have questioned glutaraldehyde's ability to inactivate mycobacteria. For example, Rubbo et al. (212) demonstrated that glutaraldehyde more slowly inactivated *Mycobacterium tuberculosis* than did alcohols, formaldehyde, iodine, and phenol. Ascenzi (19) showed in the quantitative suspension test that 2% glutaraldehyde killed only 2 to 3 log units of *M. tuberculosis* in 20 min at 20°C. Similarly, Collins (69) reported that glutaraldehyde could not completely inactivate a standardized suspension of *M. tuberculosis* within 10 min. Nontuberculous mycobacteria such as *Myobacterium avium*, *Myobacterium intracellulare*, and *Myobacterium gordonae* are more resistant to inactivation than *M. tuberculosis* (68). These and other data suggest that 20 min (at 20°C) is the minimum exposure time needed to reliably inactivate tuberculous and nontuberculous mycobacteria by 2% glutaraldehyde, provided that the contaminated item has been thoroughly cleaned before disinfection (140, 216). Glutaraldehyde-resistant mycobacteria have been isolated from endoscope washer-disinfectors (116, 269; see "Endoscopes" below). The virucidal activity of glutaraldehyde extends to the nonenveloped (hydrophilic) viruses, which are generally more resistant to disinfectants than are the enveloped (lipophilic) viruses. Numerous viruses were documented to be inactivated, including HIV, hepatitis A virus (HAV), HBV, poliovirus type 1, coxsackievirus type B, yellow fever virus, and rotavirus (19, 151). The disadvantages of glutaraldehyde include the fact that it coagulates blood and can fix proteins and tissue to surfaces (177, 216). In addition, glutaraldehyde has a pungent and irritating odor and its vapor at the level of 0.2 ppm irritates the eyes, throat, and nose. HCWs exposed to glutaraldehyde can develop allergic contact dermatitis, asthma, rhinitis, and epistaxis. Measures that may minimize employee exposure include covering immersion baths with tight-fitting lids, improved ventilation, ducted exhaust hoods or ductless fume hoods with vapor absorbents, personal protective equipment, and appropriate automated machines for endoscope disinfection (12, 216). Due to dilution, glutaraldehyde concentrations commonly decline during use in manual and automatic baths used for endoscopes (177). Test strips should be used to ensure that the glutaraldehyde concentration has not fallen below 1 to 1.5%. Equipment disinfected with glutaraldehyde and rinsed inadequately has caused serious clinical complications including proctocolitis (colonoscopes), (87, 282); and keratopathy (ophthalmic instruments). Because the infectivity of prions can be stabilized when instruments are treated with formaldehyde before they are autoclaved (48), aldehydes are no longer recommended for disinfecting endoscopes in some European countries (e.g., France) (see "Bovine Spongiform Encephalopathy and Variant Creutzfeldt-Jakob Disease" below).

ortho-Phthalaldehyde

A 0.55% OPA solution has been approved as a high-level disinfectant by the FDA and by agencies in other countries. However, different countries or areas have set different exposure times for a 0.55% solution of OPA at 20°C to achieve high-level disinfection: 12 min in the United States, 10 min in Canada, and 5 min in Europe, Asia, and Latin America. Compared with glutaraldehyde, OPA has several advantages: (i) it does not require activation; (ii) it is compatible with many materials (i.e., similar to glutaraldehyde); (iii) it is more stable during storage and reuse as well as at a wide pH range of 3 to 9; (iv) it has low vapor properties; (v) its odor is barely perceptible; (vi) it is more rapidly mycobactericidal than glutaraldehyde in vitro and has good activity against glutaraldehyde-resistant strains at longer exposure times (102). However, 0.5% OPA is slowly sporicidal and does not inactivate all spores within 270 min of exposure (273). In addition, OPA stains proteins, skin, clothing, and instruments. OPA vapors may irritate the respiratory tract and eyes. At present, the effects of long-term exposure and safe exposure levels are not well defined. Therefore, OPA must be handled with appropriate safety precautions (i.e., gloves, fluid-resistant gowns, and eye protection) and it must be stored in containers with tight-fitting lids. If additional studies corroborate OPA's advantages, this compound may replace glutaraldehyde for many uses, especially endoscope disinfection. The new agent appears to be particularly useful in washer-disinfectors, where glutaraldehyde-resistant mycobacteria have emerged (269, 273).

Formaldehyde

Formaldehyde and its condensates are reviewed in depth elsewhere (207). Formaldehyde in aqueous solutions or as a gas has been used as a disinfectant and sterilant for many decades. Its use in the health care setting, however, has sharply decreased for several reasons. The irritating vapors and pungent odor produced by formaldehyde are apparent at very low levels (<1 ppm). Moreover, allergy to formaldehyde is fairly common. In addition, the Occupational Safety and Health Administration in the United States and the Health and Safety Executive of the United Kingdom indicated that formaldehyde vapors may be carcinogenic. Thus, the Occupational Safety and Health Administration limits the 8-h time-weighted average exposure in the workplace to a concentration of 0.75 ppm. Elevated levels of occupational exposures have been found among workers in dialysis units and gross anatomy laboratories (8). Consequently, formaldehyde and formaldehyde-releasing agents are used infrequently in health care institutions, despite this agent's broad-spectrum microbicidal activity. In fact, formaldehyde has been largely replaced by peracetic acid as an agent for disinfecting hemodialysis equipment and water dialysate tubing systems. Paraformaldehyde vaporized by heat is used to decontaminate biological safety cabinets.

Chlorine and Chlorine-Releasing Compounds

Due to its hazardous nature, chlorine gas is rarely used as a disinfectant. Among the large number of chlorine compounds commercially available, hypochlorites are the most widely used disinfectants. Hypochlorite has been used for more than a century and remains an important disinfectant.

Rutala and Weber published an extensive review of uses for inorganic hypochlorite in health care facilities (225), and Karol reviewed the potential hazards and significant benefits of chlorine use (148). Aqueous solutions of sodium hypochlorite are usually called household bleach. Bleach commonly contains 5.25% sodium hypochlorite or 52,500 ppm available chlorine; a 1:10 dilution of bleach provides about 300 to 600 mg of free chlorine per liter. Alternative chlorine-releasing compounds frequently used in health care facilities include chloramine-T, sodium dichloroisocyanurate tablets, and chlorine dioxide. Demand-release chlorine dioxide is an extremely reactive compound and must be prepared at the point of use. It is used primarily to chlorinate potable water, swimming pools, and wastewater. In Europe, commercial chlorine dioxide preparations are available to disinfect instruments. In aqueous solution, all chlorine compounds release hypochlorous acid, the most likely active compound. The mechanism of microbicidal action of hypochlorous acid has not been fully elucidated, but it inhibits key enzymatic reactions within cells and denatures proteins. Lowering the pH or raising the temperature or concentration increases its antimicrobial efficacy. Chlorine compounds have broad antimicrobial spectra including, at higher concentrations, bacterial spores and M. tuberculosis. Therefore, hypochlorite can be used as a high-level disinfectant for semicritical items. Concentrations of 100 ppm of available chlorine inactivate vegetative bacteria and viruses in 10 min. Suspension tests document that both enveloped and nonenveloped viruses, including HIV, HAV, HBV, herpes simplex virus types 1 and 2, poliovirus, coxsackievirus, and rotavirus are inactivated (225). In one study, a concentration of 100 ppm chlorine eliminated 99.9% of Bacillus subtilis endospores in 5 min (289). However, endospore-forming bacteria, mycobacteria, fungi, and protozoa usually are less susceptible to chlorine than other microorganisms, and high concentrations of chlorine (1,000 ppm) are required to completely destroy them. Despite this limitation, sodium hypochlorite solutions (500 ppm and 1,600 ppm) have been reported to decrease C. difficile environmental contamination and terminate outbreaks of infections caused by this organism (143). Cryptosporidium oocysts are particularly resistant to chlorine. These oocysts remain infective for several days in swimming pool water containing recommended chlorine concentrations, and because of their small size they may not be removed efficiently by conventional pool filters. Outbreaks of cryptosporidium infections have been associated with drinking water and swimming pools (54). Of note, chloramine-T and sodium dichloroisocyanurate seem to have less sporicidal action than does sodium hypochlorite. Hypochlorite is fast acting, nonstaining, nonflammable, and inexpensive. However, its use is limited because it is corrosive, inactivated by organic matter, and relatively instable. Sodium hypochlorite can injure tissue; however, this occurs rarely in health care facilities (225). Inhalation of chlorine gas may irritate the respiratory tract, resulting in cough, dyspnea, and pulmonary edema or chemical pneumonitis. The potential carcinogens trihalomethanes have been detected in chlorine-treated water, and high levels of trihalomethanes can be detected when hospitals hyperchlorinate their water systems (127).

Chlorine compounds have other important disadvantages. Blood or other organic matter substantially inactivates hypochlorites and other chlorine compounds. Consequently, items used for patient care and environmental surfaces must be cleaned before hypochlorite is used. In addition, biofilm (e.g., in the pipes of a water distribution system) also reduces the efficacy of chlorines significantly. Moreover, the free available chlorine levels in solutions can decay to 40 to 50% of the original concentration after the container has been opened for 1 month. Therefore, concentrations higher than those established in laboratory experiments should be used in practice. Loss of free chlorine can be minimized if the solutions are kept and used at room temperature, in dilution, in an alkaline pH range, and stored in closed opaque containers.

Depending on the concentrations employed, sodium hypochlorite is used in hospitals as a high-level disinfectant for selected semicritical devices (e.g., dental equipment and mannequins used for cardiopulmonary resuscitation training), as an intermediate-level disinfectant (e.g., hemodialysis equipment), and as a low-level disinfectant for environmental surfaces and hydrotherapy tanks. For example, the CDC recommends that HCWs use a 1:100 dilution (5,000 ppm) of hypochlorite to decontaminate spills of blood and certain other body fluids (55). Because chlorine can be inactivated by blood and other organic material, a full-strength solution or a 1:10 dilution will be safer unless the surface is cleaned before it is disinfected (64, 97, 276). Household bleach also can be used to disinfect tabletops, incubators, and spills in laboratories or to disinfect syringes used by drug addicts if sterile disposable syringes are not available (56). At low concentrations, chlorines (usually about 0.5 ppm free chlorine) are used to chlorinate the drinking water. Hyperchlorination of institutional water systems has controlled epidemics caused by Legionella pneumophila (127) but also corrodes the water distribution system (127). Stabilized solutions of chlorine dioxide appear to be less toxic and more efficacious than chlorine for controlling growth of legionellae (122). A growing number of municipal water treatment plants in the United States are using monochloramine as a residual disinfectant. Chloramination of drinking water has several advantages compared to the use of free chlorine, including decreasing the risk of Legionnaires' disease at the municipal level or in individual hospitals (154). However, outbreaks of Cryptosporidium infections have occurred in cities that use chloramines in their drinking water.

Hydrogen Peroxide

Hydrogen peroxide, a strong oxidizer, is used for high-level disinfection and sterilization. It produces destructive hydroxyl free radicals that attack membrane lipids, DNA, and other essential cell components. Although the catalase produced by anaerobic and some aerobic bacteria may protect cells from hydrogen peroxide, this defense is overwhelmed by the concentrations used for disinfection (164). Generally, a 3% hydrogen peroxide solution is rapidly bactericidal, but it kills organisms with high cellular catalase activity (e.g., S. aureus and Serratia marcescens) less rapidly. Surprisingly, 3% hydrogen peroxide was ineffective against vancomycin-resistant enterococci (174, 239). Spores are more resistant than vegetative bacteria to hydrogen peroxide. For example, a 3% solution of hydrogen peroxide destroyed 10^6 spores in six of seven exposure trials that were 150 min long; a 10% solution was always successful in 60 min (275). Higher concentrations of hydrogen peroxide (17.7 and 35.4%) killed Bacillus subtilis spores in 9.4 and 2.3 min, respectively (162). In a recent investigation, 10% hydrogen peroxide was the most active of the seven chemical disinfectants tested against B. subtilis spores (234). However, other investigators found that the sporicidal activity of hydrogen peroxide was lower than those of peracetic acid and chlorine (10).

Hydrogen peroxide's sporicidal activity can be enhanced by increasing the concentration or temperature or by using it in conjunction with ultrasonic energy, UV radiation, and some chemical agents such as peracetic acid (172, 180, 265). A 0.3% solution of hydrogen peroxide is able to inactivate HIV in 10 min (172), and a 3% concentration inactivates rhinovirus in 6 to 8 min at 37°C (180). However, a 6% solution was ineffective against poliovirus at 1 min (265). Hydrogen peroxide does not coagulate blood and does not fix tissues to surfaces. In fact, it may enhance removal of organic material from equipment. Hydrogen peroxide has a low toxicity for humans. It decomposes to oxygen and water, and therefore, it is environmentally safe. It is neither carcinogenic nor mutagenic. Concentrated solutions may irritate the eyes, skin, and mucous membranes. Hydrogen peroxide can be destroyed easily by heat or enzymes (catalase and peroxidases). Stabilized solutions can be used for high-level disinfection of semicritical items, considering the corrosive effects of hydrogen peroxide on copper, zinc, and brass (216). The FDA has approved commercial products containing either 7.5% hydrogen peroxide alone or combinations with peracetic acid as liquid sterilants and high-level disinfectants for processing reusable medical and dental devices (www.fda.gov) (232). Concentrations of 3 to 6% are used to disinfect ventilators, soft contact lenses (3% for 2 to 4 h) (134), and tonometer biprisms (163, 164, 216). Vaporized hydrogen peroxide is also used for plasma sterilization (see below). Despite its limited toxicity, hydrogen peroxide can damage human tissues. Patients exposed to endoscopes contaminated by residual hydrogen peroxide have developed pseudomembrane-like enterocolitis (pseudolipomatosis) (232). In addition, patients who were exposed to tonometer tips disinfected with hydrogen peroxide and rinsed improperly suffered corneal damage (163). Use of hydrogen peroxide to clean wounds and in dental regimens remains controversial (164).

Peracetic Acid

Peracetic acid (or peroxyacetic acid) is a more potent germicidal agent than hydrogen peroxide and was the most active agent in several in vitro studies (9, 235). Concentrations of ≤1% are sporicidal even at low temperatures. The mechanism of action of peracetic acid has not been fully elucidated, but its mechanism of action is likely to be similar to that of hydrogen peroxide and other oxidizing agents. Peracetic acid remains effective in the presence of organic matter. At low concentrations it is considerably less stable than hydrogen peroxide; preparations with appropriate stability have been developed and are commercially available. Peracetic acid corrodes steel, galvanized iron, copper, brass, and bronze, and it attacks natural and synthetic rubbers. In addition, concentrated solutions can seriously damage eyes and skin. Furthermore, some investigators have raised concerns about the potential toxicity of the combination of peracetic and acetic acids (126). Feldman et al. reported that mortality rates in freestanding dialysis facilities that reprocessed dialyzers with peracetic and acetic acid were higher than in facilities that discarded dialysis filters or used formaldehyde for reprocessing (94). To date, investigators have not determined whether the higher death rate was caused by the disinfectants or was associated with other practices at the facilities or with patient risk factors. Nevertheless, because peracetic acid has powerful germicidal activity and does not produce toxic residues, peracetic acid is very attractive for use in health care settings, most frequently in combination with hydrogen peroxide to disinfect

hemodialyzers. The FDA lists several commercial products containing a combination of peracetic acid and hydrogen peroxide as high-level disinfectants and chemical sterilants. The use of peracetic acid for chemical sterilization of instruments and endoscopes (Steris System 1) is discussed below.

Alcohols

For centuries, the alcohols have been appreciated for their antimicrobial properties. Alcohol is defined by the FDA as having one of the following active ingredients: ethyl alcohol, 60% to 95% by volume in an aqueous solution, or isopropyl alcohol, 50% to 91.3% by volume in an aqueous solution. Ethyl alcohol (ethanol) and isopropyl alcohol (isopropanol) are the alcoholic solutions most often used as surface disinfectants and antiseptic agents in health care institutions because they possess many qualities that make them suitable both for disinfection of equipment and for antisepsis of skin. They are fast acting, minimally toxic to the skin, nonstaining, and nonallergenic. Alcohols evaporate readily, which is advantageous for most disinfection and antisepsis procedures. The uptake of alcohol by intact skin and the lungs when alcohol is used topically is negligible. Alcohols have better wetting properties than water due to their lower surface tensions, which along with their cleansing and degreasing actions make alcohols effective skin antiseptics. Alcoholic formulations used to prepare the skin before invasive procedures should be filtered to ensure that they are free of spores, or 0.5% hydrogen peroxide should be added (208). Alcohols are also excellent products for intermediate-level and low-level disinfection of small, clean surfaces, equipment, and the environment (e.g., rubber stoppers of medication vials, stethoscopes, and medication preparation areas). Alcohols have some disadvantages. If alcoholic antiseptics are used repeatedly, they may dry and irritate the skin. Therefore, preparations for hand disinfection should contain emollients (see the discussion on hand antisepsis in "Disinfectants for Living Tissue" below). Moreover, alcohols may damage rubber, certain plastic items, and the shellac mountings of lensed instruments after prolonged and repeated use (216). Moreover, alcohols are flammable (one should consider the flash point) and thus must not be used on large surfaces, particularly in closed, poorly ventilated areas. Alcohols cannot penetrate proteinrich materials. Therefore, a spray or a wipe with alcohol may not disinfect a surface contaminated with blood or other body fluids that has not been cleaned first.

The exact mechanism by which alcohols destroy microorganisms is not fully understood. The most plausible explanation for the antimicrobial action is that alcohols coagulate (denature) proteins (e.g., enzymatic proteins), impairing specific cellular functions (160). Ethyl and isopropyl alcohols at appropriate concentrations have broad spectra of antimicrobial activity that include vegetative bacteria, fungi, and viruses. In fact, their antimicrobial efficacies are enhanced in the presence of water, with optimal alcohol concentrations being 60 to 90% by volume.

Alcohols (i.e., 70 to 80% ethyl alcohol) rapidly (i.e., within 10 to 90 s) kill vegetative bacteria, such as *S. aureus*, *Streptococcus pyogenes*, Enterobacteriaceae, and *P. aeruginosa* in suspension tests (208). Isopropyl alcohol is slightly more bactericidal than ethyl alcohol (160) and is highly effective against vancomycin-resistant enterococci (239). It also has excellent activity against fungi, such as *Candida* spp., *Cryptococcus neoformans*, *Blastomyces dermatitidis*, *Coccidioides immitis*, *Histoplasma capsulatum*, *Aspergillus niger*, and dermatophytes and mycobacteria, including M. *tuberculosis*. However, alcohols generally do not destroy bacterial spores. In fact, fatal infections due to *Clostridium* spp. occurred when alcohol was used to sterilize surgical instruments. Both ethyl and isopropyl alcohols inactivate most viruses with a lipid envelope (e.g., influenza virus, herpes simplex virus, and adenovirus). However, several investigators found that isopropyl alcohol had less virucidal activity against naked, nonenveloped viruses (216). In the experiments by Klein and DeForest, 2-propanol, even at 95%, could not inactivate the nonenveloped poliovirus type 1 and coxsackievirus type B in 10 min (151). In contrast, 70% ethanol inactivated these enteroviruses (151). Neither 70% ethanol nor 45% 2-propanol killed HAV when their activities were assessed on stainless steel disks contaminated with fecally suspended virus. Among 20 disinfectants tested, only 3 reduced the titer of HAV by greater than 99.9% in 1 min (2% glutaraldehyde, sodium hypochlorite with >5,000 ppm free chlorine, and a quaternary ammonium formulation containing 23% HCl) (176). Bond et al. (34) and Kobayashi et al. (153) demonstrated that 2-propanol (70% for 10 min) or ethanol (80% for 2 min) made human plasma contaminated with HBV at high titer noninfectious for susceptible chimpanzees (153). Both 15% ethyl alcohol and 35% isopropyl alcohol (172) readily inactivate HIV, and 70% ethanol rapidly inactivates high titers of HIV in suspension, independent of the protein load. However, the rate of inactivation decreased when virus was dried onto a glass surface and high levels of protein were present (267). In a suspension test, 40% propanol reduced the rotavirus titer by at least 4 log in 1 min (157) and both 70% propanol and 70% ethanol reduced the release of rotavirus from contaminated fingertips by 2.7 log units. In comparison, the mean reductions obtained with liquid soap and an aqueous solution of chlorhexidine gluconate were 0.9 and 0.7 log units, respectively (15).

Phenolics

Since Lister's pioneering use of phenol (carbolic acid) as an antiseptic, a large number of phenol derivatives (or phenolics) have been developed and marketed. Phenol derivatives originate when one of the hydrogen atoms on an aromatic ring is replaced by a functional group (e.g., alkyl, benzyl, phenyl, amyl, or chloro). The three phenolics most commonly used as constituents of disinfectants are o-phenylphenol, o-benzyl-p-chlorophenol, and p-tert-amylphenol. The addition of detergents to the basic formulation results in products that clean, dissolve proteins, and disinfect in one step. Phenolics at higher concentrations act as gross protoplasmic poisons, penetrating and disrupting the bacterial cell wall and precipitating the cell proteins (193). Lower concentrations of these compounds inactivate cellular enzyme systems and cause essential metabolites to leak from the cell. Phenol compounds at concentrations of 2 to 5% are generally considered bactericidal, tuberculocidal, fungicidal, and virucidal against lipophilic viruses (193). However, the manufacturers' efficacy claims have generally not been verified by independent laboratories or the EPA (216). A collaborative study by Rutala and Cole documented the fact that randomly selected EPA-registered phenolic detergents and quaternary ammonium compounds do not consistently meet the manufacturers' bactericidal label claims (218). Phenolics tested by the AOAC use-dilution method at the recommended use dilution failed to kill *P. aeruginosa* in 33 to 78% of laboratories. However, extreme variability of test results has been observed among laboratories testing identical products (218). Phenolics at in-use dilutions are not lethal to bacterial spores. Terleckyj and

Axler found that a 2% phenolic killed a wide spectrum of clinically important fungi but did not kill *Aspergillus fumigatus* (260). Although 5% phenol inactivated both lipophilic and hydrophilic viruses, Klein and DeForest found that 12% o-phenylphenol was effective only against lipophilic viruses (151). Similarly, other investigators demonstrated little or no virucidal effect of a phenolic against coxsackievirus type B4, echovirus type 11, or poliovirus type 1 (190). Martin et al. showed that a 0.5% commercial phenolic formulation (2.8% o-phenylphenol and 2.7% o-benzyl-p-chlorophenol) inactivated HIV (172), but another commercial product containing phenolics at a final concentration of 1% did not completely inactivate cell-associated HIV suspended in blood (89). A phenol-based preparation (14.7% phenol diluted 1:256 in tap water) and a bleach dilution (800 ppm available chlorine) reduced rotavirus numbers similarly and interrupted transfer of virus from disks to fingerpads (238). Phenolic compounds are relatively tolerant of anionic and organic matter. They are absorbed by rubber and plastics and leave a residual film, which may irritate skin and tissues. p-tert-Butylphenol and p-tert-amylphenol have been reported to depigment skin. Although differences between the various compounds exist, phenolics are degraded in wastewater at a lower rate than other germicides, which limits their use in Europe. Phenolic germicidal detergent solutions may be used for intermediate-level and low-level disinfection of surgical instruments and noncritical patient care items. These compounds are also appropriate for decontaminating the hospital environment, including laboratory surfaces. They should not be used to disinfect bassinets and incubators because they can cause hyperbilirubinemia in infants (216).

Quaternary Ammonium Compounds

A wide variety of quaternary ammonium compounds (quats) with antimicrobial activity have been introduced in the past decade. Some of the compounds used in health care settings are benzalkonium chloride, alkyldimethylbenzyl ammonium chloride, and didecyldimethyl ammonium chloride. Quats are cationic surface-active detergents, which appear to kill microorganisms by disrupting cell membranes, inactivating enzymes, and denaturing cell proteins (181). However, they have a limited antimicrobial spectrum. Products sold as hospital disinfectants are not sporicidal and are generally not tuberculocidal or virucidal against hydrophilic viruses. Scientific investigations using the AOAC use-dilution method have not reproduced the bactericidal and tuberculocidal claims made by the manufacturers (219). Consequently, HCWs should be suspicious of the claims on labels and of results from in-house evaluations that have not been verified by an independent laboratory. The overestimation of the germicidal activity may be related to incomplete inactivation of the compounds tested. In this case, the bacteriostatic (inhibitory) activity rather than the bactericidal activity is measured (181). The antimicrobial spectrum of quats may be improved by combining them with amines and biguanides or by using them at higher temperatures in washing machines. Several outbreaks of infections have been associated with quat solutions contaminated in use by gram-negative bacteria such as *Pseudomonas* spp. or *S. marcescens* or by *Mycobacterium abscessus* (99, 189, 262). The contaminated solutions were used as antiseptics on skin and tissue and to disinfect patient care supplies or equipment (i.e., cardiac catheters and cystoscopes). In fact, microbiology laboratories use the quat cetrimide in selective media to isolate *P. aeruginosa*. Quats have other disadvantages.

Genes conferring resistance to quats have been detected in 6 to 42% of *S. aureus* isolates collected in Japan and Europe (175). Organic matter, anionic detergents (soaps), and materials such as cotton and gauze pads can reduce the microbicidal activities of quats. Despite these limitations, quats are nonstaining, odorless, noncorrosive, and relatively nontoxic. They are excellent cleaning agents, but sticky residue may build up on surfaces. On the basis of their limited antimicrobial spectra, they should be used in hospitals only for environmental sanitation of noncritical surfaces such as floors, furniture, and walls (216).

Other Germicides of Interest

Glucoprotamine, the conversion product of L-glutamic acid and cocopropylene-1,3-diamine, possesses a broad antimicrobial spectrum that includes vegetative bacteria, mycobacteria, fungi, and enveloped viruses (85, 183). A clinical study examining used specula from a gynecologic clinic demonstrated that the product killed >6 log units of vegetative bacteria excluding spores (284). The manufacturer's data sheets indicate good compatibility of the compound with humans, the environment, and various materials. A commercial product, available in Europe, can be used to disinfect instruments and endoscopes.

Peroxygen compounds have proven efficacy against bacteria, bacterial spores, fungi, and a broad spectrum of viruses. A 1% concentration of a new commercial formulation containing peroxygen achieved a 10^5-fold killing of *B. subtilis* in 2 to 3 h in the absence of blood, but killing was poor in the presence of blood (67). Moreover, several investigators have found that peroxygen has poor mycobactericidal activity (45, 116). Besides other applications, these compounds may be suitable for disinfecting laboratory equipment and workbenches. Superoxidized water is prepared at the point of use by the electrolysis of NaCl solution, which generates hypochlorous acid and a mixture of radicals with strong oxidizing properties (185). Freshly generated solutions rapidly destroy bacteria including spores and mycobacteria, fungi, and viruses in the absence of organic loading (245). A commercial adaptation of this process (i.e., Sterilox) has been marketed in Europe since 1999 and recently was approved by the FDA (see "Endoscopes" below) (185). Because Sterilox solutions are unstable, they should be used only once for high-level disinfection. Some investigators have claimed that superoxidized water is compatible with instruments and that it does not damage the environment, irritate the respiratory tract and skin, or corrode metal. However, others have reported that superoxidized water damages flexible endoscopes. Further studies are needed to explore the use of this new disinfectant in clinical settings.

Metals such as copper and silver ions inactivate a wide variety of microorganisms (233). Although further work is required to explore their use in health care, they currently are used to disinfect water and to prevent infections associated with medical devices (e.g., intravascular catheters impregnated with silver sulfadiazine). For example, copper-silver ionization systems are successfully used to minimize legionella colonization in water systems (254). Surfacine is a new silver-based surface germicide that may be applied to inanimate or animate surfaces. Surfacine immediately eliminates microorganisms from surfaces and also has long-term residual activity (44, 227). This novel antimicrobial coating might be suitable for a wide range of applications including the preventing of microbial contamination of medical devices, if further studies confirm the promising preliminary data.

Specific Issues

Cleaning and Disinfecting Surfaces and Floors

In general, the environment is not a primary reservoir for nosocomial pathogens. However, in some cases environmental contamination may be important. Recent examples include respiratory syncytial virus (121) and the SARS coronavirus (106). The CDC's recent guidelines for environmental infection control in health care facilities recommend using an EPA-registered hospital detergent/disinfectant designed for general housekeeping purposes in patient care areas, especially in intensive care units, operating theaters, and emergency rooms, where blood, body fluids, or multidrug-resistant organisms may have contaminated surfaces (243). A one-step process is adequate in most areas, but a rinse step is necessary in nurseries and neonatal intensive care units, especially if a phenolic agent was used (294). Products with quats allow cleaning and disinfecting in one step, but residual quats on the surface may result in sticky, smeary surfaces. Other products may require a two-step approach (a cleaning step and a disinfection step), doubling the workload. "High-touch" surfaces (e.g., doorknobs, bed rails, and light switches) should be disinfected more frequently than "minimal-touch" surfaces. A simple detergent is adequate for cleaning surfaces for other patient care areas and in non-patient care areas. Cleaning with a detergent is much more important than adding a disinfectant to the solution. In fact, several studies found that adding a disinfectant did not prolong the reduction in bacterial load on surfaces (83). Routine disinfection of environmental surfaces is necessary for all areas with patients in contact isolation (e.g., patients infected with methicillin-resistant *S. aureus* [MRSA]). Twice-daily disinfection is necessary to control an outbreak with vancomycin-intermediate *S. aureus* (78, 178).

In rare situations, routine disinfection of surfaces and floors is crucial: when cases of norovirus or clusters with *C. difficile* or MRSA are detected, an immediate switch from cleaning floors and surfaces to using a highly active disinfectant is warranted. Several studies demonstrate a correlation between contaminated surfaces and clinical cases (66, 75, 150). When patients with suspected norovirus infection vomit, immediate disinfection of the vomitus with highly concentrated bleach or an oxygen-release compound is crucial. Norovirus is highly contagious; in fact, 100 virions are sufficient to induce infection, but >106 virions are shed by infected patients.

Emergence of Resistance to Biocides

Microorganisms rarely become resistant to disinfectants. However, frequent use of sublethal concentrations of disinfectants can select for resistant strains (17, 36, 271). Mechanisms of resistance include acquisition of resistance plasmids, changes in the cell membrane (e.g., chlorhexidine in *Psuedomonas stutzeri*), capsule formation (*Klebsiella* spp.), and activation of the *norA* efflux pump (*S. aureus*). A large proportion of household soaps now contain antibacterial agents (up to 45% in one study), which may increase the probability that resistant bacteria will emerge (197). Multiple outbreaks have been associated with soaps containing antibacterial agents such as chlorhexidine, hexetidine solution, or chlorxylenol (17, 36, 271). However, the concentrations of biocides used in the health care setting are much higher than the minimum biocidal concentrations in vitro. Therefore, resistance has not become a major problem in the clinical setting to date. Readers desiring more information about disinfectants and antiseptics (33, 98) and resistance to these agents should read several excellent articles (33, 98, 167, 244).

Inactivation of Emerging Pathogens and Antibiotic-Resistant Bacteria

New and emerging pathogens such as the causative agent of vCJD, noroviruses, SARS coronavirus, avian and swine influenza viruses, hypervirulent *C. difficile*, Panton-Valentine leukocidin-producing *S. aureus*, gram-negative rods producing extended-spectrum β-lactamases or metallo-β-lactamases, or *Klebsiella pneumoniae* producing carbapenemases threaten the public health. Only limited data exist regarding the susceptibility of emerging pathogens to commonly used disinfectants or sterilants. Surrogate microbes have been studied for some pathogens. Examples include feline calicivirus for noroviruses, vaccinia virus for variola virus, and *Bacillus atrophaeus* (formerly *B. subtilis*) for *B. anthracis* (278). Other infectious agents that cannot be evaluated by standard testing procedures (e.g., hepatitis C virus [HCV]) have been tested by alternative methods, such as PCR. With the exception of prions, there is no evidence that emerging pathogens are less susceptible to approved standard disinfection and sterilization procedures than are comparable classical pathogens. Standard disinfection and sterilization procedures for patient care equipment as recommended in guidelines and in this chapter are adequate to disinfect or sterilize instruments or devices contaminated with blood and other body fluids (228). Hospital disinfectants registered by the EPA, other than one peroxygen compound, do not have specific claims for activity against noroviruses. Because noroviruses are nonenveloped, most quats do not have significant activity against them. Phenolic-based preparations have been found to be active in vitro against a surrogate virus of this group. However, concentrations two- to four-fold higher than those recommended for routine use by manufacturers may be required. In the event of a norovirus outbreak, the CDC recommends using a hypochlorite solution (minimum concentration of 1,000 ppm chlorine) to decontaminate hard, nonporous, environmental surfaces (http://www.cdc.gov /ncidod/dhqp/id_norovirusFS.html). SARS coronavirus and avian influenza virus are inactivated by sodium hypochlorite and a commercially available peroxygen compound (158); phenolic compounds and quats are less effective. A sporicidal germicide is required to efficiently eliminate *C. difficile* spores. In a recent study, glutaraldehyde (2%), peracetyl ions (1.6%, equivalent to 0.26% peracetic acid), and acidified nitrite demonstrated biocidal activity against *C. difficile* spores (293). Hypochlorite-based disinfectants have been used, with some success, to disinfect environmental surfaces in areas with ongoing transmission of *C. difficile*. Recent outbreaks with virulent strains may require more focus on environmental cleaning and disinfection (95, 178). There are no data demonstrating that disinfectants used at recommended contact conditions and concentrations are less effective against antimicrobial-resistant bacteria than against antimicrobial-susceptible bacteria (228). Inactivation of prions, including those causing vCJD, is discussed below.

Decontamination in the Event of Biological Terrorism

If a biological agent is released, environmental decontamination measures may be necessary to decrease the risk of spreading of the disease. A decontamination agent should be effective against possible pathogens and readily available at reasonable cost. Therefore, sodium hypochlorite (household bleach) is usually recommended, especially if bacterial spores are involved. This agent is well suited for various decontamination procedures in the laboratory and health care setting. In addition, it may be used to decontaminate protective equipment and clothing worn by first responders and decontamination workers. Smallpox virus does not survive long in the environment but may remain viable for extended periods under favorable conditions. CDC guidelines recommend incinerating items that are not needed or cannot be decontaminated, sterilizing items in an autoclave or an ethylene oxide sterilizer, decontaminating spaces and rooms with vaporized paraformaldehyde (or use of an Amphyl fogger), and soaking equipment or wiping down surfaces with a 5% aqueous solution of a phenolic germicidal detergent (http://www.bt.cdc.gov/agent /smallpox/response-plan/index.asp#guidef). Since contaminated clothing can spread the virus to personnel, bed linens and clothes must be autoclaved or laundered in hot water supplemented with bleach (128). Other disinfectants that are used for standard hospital infection control, such as sodium hypochlorite and quaternary ammonium compounds, are also effective to decontaminate surfaces (128). Only vaccinated personnel should perform the decontamination procedures. *B. anthracis* spores are extremely stable and can remain viable for decades in the environment (138). The CDC recommends that laboratory staff use a 1:10-diluted hypochlorite solution when addressing spills, items, and surfaces contaminated with *B. anthracis* (http://www.bt.cdc .gov/agent/anthrax/infection-control/). Decontamination of a building or of large areas contaminated with anthrax spores is extremely difficult. Spotts et al. summarized the literature on inactivation of *B. anthracis* spores (250). *C. botulinum* and its spores are killed by a 1:10 dilution of sodium hypochlorite. Heat (≥85°C for 5 min) or 0.1 M sodium hydroxide (contact time, 20 min) inactivates the toxin (18). Persons with direct exposure to powder or liquid aerosols containing *Francisella tularensis* should wash their body and clothing with soapy water (79). In the circumstances of a laboratory spill or intentional release, environmental surfaces can be decontaminated with a 1:10-diluted hypochlorite solution. After 10 min, a 70% alcohol solution can be used to further clean the area and reduce the corrosive action of the bleach (79). *Yersinia pestis* does not survive long outside the host. The WHO estimated that a plague aerosol would be effective and infectious for 1 h. Thus, areas exposed to aerosols of *Y. pestis* do not need to be decontaminated (137). Equipment or environmental surfaces contaminated with the agents causing Ebola hemorrhagic fever, Marburg hemorrhagic fever (*Filoviridae*), Lassa fever, and related infections (*Arenaviridae* and *Bunyaviridae*) should be disinfected with a suitable registered hospital disinfectant or a 1:100 dilution of a hypochlorite solution. Surfaces grossly soiled with vomitus or stool should be disinfected with a 1:10 dilution. If possible, serum used for laboratory tests should be pretreated with heat inactivation at 56°C and polyethylene glycol *p-tert*-octylphenyl ether (Triton X-100). Treatment with 10 μl of 10% Triton X-100 per ml of serum for 1 h reduces the titer of hemorrhagic fever viruses in serum. If treatment with Triton X-100 is not feasible, heat inactivation alone may reduce infectivity somewhat (52). Medical, public health, and laboratory responses to the release of organisms or toxins that pose a risk to national security, i.e., variola major virus (smallpox), *Bacillus anthracis*, *Clostridium botulinum* toxin, *Francisella tularensis*, *Yersinia pestis*, and certain filoviruses and arenaviruses are discussed in chapter 10 of this *Manual* and in numerous publications (18, 79, 128, 137, 138). The CDC published guidelines for the management of patients with suspected viral hemorrhagic fever (52) and recently posted updated guidelines at www.cdc.gov/ncidod/hip/BLOOD/VHFinterimGuidance05_19_05.pdf.

Endoscopes

Reprocessing endoscopes is probably the most challenging reprocessing task in health care. Multiple reports of outbreaks associated with insufficient reprocessing techniques or defects of the endoscope have been published (Table 7). However, ample data indicate that a sufficient level of safety can be achieved even with manual disinfection of endoscopes if the guidelines are strictly followed (173). Today, endoscopes are involved in transmission of infectious diseases in less than 1 of 10^6 Mio endoscopies. Flexible endoscopes have intricate, sophisticated small parts that are difficult to clean but must be cleaned before they can be disinfected because organic material such as blood, feces, and respiratory secretions interfere with disinfection (71). Several studies have demonstrated the importance of cleaning in experimental studies with duck HBV, HIV, and *Helicobacter pylori*, (82, 292). A large study in several centers in the United States found that 23.9% of the cultures of specimens from the internal channels of 71 gastrointestinal reprocessed endoscopes grew $\geq 10^6$ CFU of bacteria and that 78% of the facilities did not sterilize all biopsy forceps (144). Other studies have documented that up to 40% of the institutions do not follow published guidelines for endoscope disinfection (12, 92, 113) and reuse of disposable endoscopic accessories is common in the United States. These items frequently are not sterilized, and reprocessing protocols are not standardized. Therefore, reused disposable items might be a source of cross-transmission (63, 71). Currently, most high-level disinfectants approved by the FDA for reprocessing endoscopes contain >2% aldehyde with or without peracetic acid (http://www.fda.gov/cdrh/ode/germlab.html). However, aldehydes should only be used after completing the cleaning cycle because they may stain prions to the instruments. Endoscopes, which are semicritical items, must be immersed in ≥2% glutaraldehyde for ≥20 min to achieve the necessary level of disinfection. These parameters are sufficient to kill ≥3 log units of mycobacteria, the most resistant vegetative bacteria. Glutaraldehyde-resistant mycobacteria have been identified (116). Several authors raised concerns that *C. difficile* may not be fully inactivated

TABLE 7 Outbreaks and pseudo-outbreaks associated with contaminated endoscopes or instruments for minimally invasive procedures

Microorganisms	No. of cases	No. of deaths	Yr of publication	Problem identified	Type of outbreak	Reference(s)
P. aeruginosa	20	0	2009	Failure of automatic endoscope reprocessor and noncompliance	Mixed	84
P. aeruginosa	7	0	2008	Failure of automatic endoscope reprocessor and noncompliance	Infections	246
P. aeruginosa	17	Not reported	2006	Inadequate processing and storage of a flexible bronchoscope	Mixed	37
K. pneumoniae, Proteus vulgaris, Morganella morganii	11	0	2005	Loose port of the bronchoscope's biopsy channel	Mixed	59
P. aeruginosa	16	0	2005	Defective biopsy forceps	Mixed	71
P. aeruginosa	3	0	2004	Probable defective endoscope	Infections	100
P. aeruginosa	39	3	2003	Loose biopsy port cap in the bronchoscope	Infections	251
P. aeruginosa	18	0	2001	Improper connection to liquid sterilization device	Mixed	247
M. xenopi	58	0	2001	Inappropriate disinfection of microsurgical instruments, tap water rinse after disinfection	Infections	20
P. aeruginosa	11	2	2000	Failure of washer-disinfector, purchased without expert advice, poor maintenance	Infections	226, 240
P. aeruginosa, mycobacteria	29	0	1999	Problems related to the use of STERIS System 1 processor	Mixed	53
HCV	2	0	1997	Cleaning, immersion	Infections	46
M. tuberculosis	2	0	1997	Cleaning, immersion	Infections	184
M. tuberculosis (multidrug resistant)	5	1	1997	Cleaning, immersion	Infections	3
P. aeruginosa	23	0	1996	Failure of washer-disinfector	Pseudo-outbreak	31
Nontuberculous mycobacteria	4	0	1992	Failure of washer-disinfector	Pseudo-outbreak	117
Multiple microorganisms	377	7	1993	Cleaning, immersion, use of tap water, poorly designed washer-disinfector	Infections	248 (review)

by standard reprocessing procedures. However, transmission of *C. difficile* by contaminated endoscopes has not been reported to date. Moreover, cryptosporidia withstand several hours of exposure to glutaraldehyde (290) but do not survive on dry surfaces (206). Therefore, drying before storing reprocessed items is part of the process and should not be cut to save time, e.g., in endoscopy units. The glutaraldehyde concentration in commercial cleaner-disinfectors can decrease by more than 50% after 2 weeks, which may promote the emergence of resistant bacteria (269). Higher concentrations of glutaraldehyde (3.2% instead of 2%) appear to be safe for endoscopes and achieve the required ≥3-log-unit killing with a higher margin of safety than achieved with the standard concentration (7). OPA and peracetic acid plus hydrogen peroxide can be used to disinfect endoscopes. Because the latter might corrode some endoscopes, reprocessing staff should ensure that the manufacturer of the endoscope approves this disinfectant for reprocessing. Automated washer-disinfectors specifically for endoscopes were developed, in part, to reduce the work needed to reprocess endoscopes and to decrease the risk of human errors during manual reprocessing. These machines rinse the endoscopes, clean them in several steps, and run a full-cycle disinfection process. The time endoscopes are exposed to disinfectants is set by the machine and cannot be shortened, as it can be by busy staff manually reprocessing endoscopes. However, endoscope washers can become contaminated with pathogenic bacteria. For example, one study found gram-negative bacteria and/or mycobacteria in 27% of cultures of specimens obtained before the final alcohol rinse and in 10% of cultures of specimens obtained thereafter. In the same study, 37 and 27% of the manually disinfected endoscopes remained contaminated at the same time points (101). In 1992, Olympus recalled (recall no. Z-039/040-2 by the FDA) its 835 model endoscope washers because the design allowed the internal tanks and tubing to become colonized by waterborne organisms such as *Pseudomonas* spp. In 1999, CDC reported three outbreaks related to the Steris System 1 (53). This device is supposed to sterilize the endoscopes, but they must first be cleaned manually (42). See Table 7 for a summary of outbreaks related to endoscopes, including those related to contaminated washer-disinfectors. Newer washer-disinfectors should continuously monitor the pressure in all channels to detect debris blocking the channels, provide adapters for all types of endoscopes, use an appropriate disinfection process with an FDA-approved disinfectant, use filtered water or sterile water for rinsing, and have a built-in automatic disinfection process. These washer-disinfectors can help staff trace problems by monitoring and documenting the disinfecting process in a manner similar to that used by autoclaves. To avoid problems, knowledgeable staff should review currently marketed machines before purchasing a washer-disinfector to ensure that the one they choose is appropriate for their needs (21). To facilitate this process, the FDA recommends that the manufacturer provide a list of all brands and models of endoscopes that are compatible with the washer-disinfector and highlight limitations associated with processing of certain brands and models of endoscopes and accessories. Preferably, the manufacturer should identify endoscopes and accessories that cannot be reliably reprocessed in the device (negative list). In addition, HCWs should be trained to use the equipment and monitored subsequently to ensure that they follow the protocol exactly. Although this is not yet mandatory, it is prudent to regularly culture

the rinse water of washer-disinfectors for pathogens such as *Pseudomonas* spp. and *Mycobacterium* spp. to identify problems before clinical cases occur. In Europe, validation of the whole procedure is necessary to ensure that it complies with the requirements of the European Standard EN ISO 15883 parts 1, 4, and 5 for automated endoscope reprocessing (23). However, outbreaks may occur despite negative routine culture results (206, 290).

If washer-disinfectors recycle water, residual glutaraldehyde may remain on the endoscopes. Manual reprocessing is more prone to leave residual glutaraldehyde on endoscopes than are automated washer-disinfectors (91). Thus, endoscopes that are manually disinfected should be thoroughly rinsed to remove any residual disinfectant, specifically glutaraldehyde. Patients exposed to residual glutaraldehyde can develop colitis (87, 282). Reprocessed endoscopes should be stored vertically (to facilitate drying) in a cabinet (to protect them from dust and secondary contamination). Drying cabinets with a heat fan, which keep the endoscope dry in a clean-air environment, are available. Reprocessed endoscopes that are stored for days or weeks before use probably should be reprocessed again, or alternatively, the channels should be rinsed with spore-filtered alcohol (70%) if this agent is compatible with the instrument. In France, reprocessing is mandatory if the reprocessed endoscope has not been used within certain time limits. However, the necessity of these precautions has not been established. Guidelines for infection prevention and control in flexible endoscopes have been updated (12) and should be consulted before choosing a method and/or disinfectant for reprocessing. The following checklist adapted from the FDA recommendations may help staff reprocessing endoscopes avoid errors (http://www.fda.gov/cdrh/safety/endoreprocess.html).

1. All staff must comply with the manufacturer's instructions for cleaning endoscopes.
2. Determine whether your endoscope is suitable for reprocessing in an automatic washer-disinfector, which is the preferred method.
3. Compare the reprocessing instructions provided by the endoscope and washer-disinfector manufacturers and resolve any conflicting recommendations.
4. Follow the instructions provided by the manufacturers of the endoscopes and the chemical germicides.
5. Consider drying endoscopes with alcohol.
6. Monitor adherence to the protocols for reprocessing endoscopes.
7. Provide comprehensive, intensive training for all staff reprocessing endoscopes; keep records of persons attending training.
8. Endoscopes sent for repairs should be labeled as "contaminated equipment for repair."
9. Implement a comprehensive quality control program.

An updated list of sterilants and high-level disinfectants approved by the FDA in a 510(k) with general claims for processing reusable medical and dental devices can be found on the FDA home page (http://www.fda.gov/cdrh/ode/germlab.html). Of note, more than 20% of all damage to endoscopes is associated with disinfecting agents. Therefore, staff members who reprocess these items must ensure that the instruments and the disinfectant are compatible (63). More detailed information is available in the new CDC guideline (http://www.cdc.gov/ncidod/dhqp/pdf/guidelines/Disinfection_Nov_2008.pdf).

Dental Equipment

Critical and semicritical dental instruments should be sterilized; if they will not be used immediately, they should be packaged before they are sterilized. All high-speed dental handheld pieces should be sterilized routinely between patients. Handheld pieces that cannot be heat sterilized should be retrofitted to attain heat tolerance; if this is not feasible, they should not be used. The adequacy of sterilization cycles should be verified by periodically (e.g., at least weekly) including a biological indicator with the load. This recommendation is rarely followed in Europe (118). In fact, 33% of British dental practices do not have a policy on general disinfection and sterilization procedures and only 3% own a vacuum autoclave (22).

Environmental contamination can be a problem in dental offices. For example, *Legionella* spp. can contaminate the air-water syringes and high-speed outlets. In one study, 25% of the water on patients infected with bloodborne pathogen can contaminate surfaces and equipment. In fact, Piazza et al. found that more than 6% of samples from workbenches, air turbine handheld pieces, holders, suction units, forceps, and dental mirrors were positive by PCR for HCV (198). Therefore, infection control issues, particularly in regard to HCV and HBV, may be more important in dentistry than has been appreciated previously. The CDC and the American Dental Association (ADA) have published guidelines for infection control in dental settings (1, 57). The ADA recommends that metal and porcelain equipment be immersed in glutaraldehyde or exposed to this disinfectant, that removable dentures and acrylic or porcelain be disinfected with iodophors or chlorine compounds, and that wax rims or bite plates be disinfected by a spray containing iodophors. Additional information can be found on the home page of the ADA (http://www.ada.org/prof/resources/positions/doc_policies.pdf).

Disinfectants for Living Tissue

Compounds that disinfect living tissue are frequently called antiseptic agents. They must meet many more requirements than compounds used to disinfect inanimate surfaces, e.g., floors. In addition, some of the agents are considered drugs and, thus, are regulated by the FDA. The antimicrobial spectra of commercially available agents are summarized in Table 6. The choice of the agent should be based not only on the desired effect but also, like antimicrobial agents, on side effects. Antiseptics rarely cause serious side effects, and most agents on the market have excellent safety profiles. Nevertheless, HCWs must remember that these agents can cause side effects such as anaphylactic shock in patients who have had contact with chlorhexidine, mainly patients originating from the Far East (90, 195).

Hygienic Hand Washing and Hand Disinfection

Hand hygiene is the single most important infection control measure (40). However, it remains difficult to motivate HCWs to perform this simple procedure faithfully (86). The CDC has published detailed guidelines on hand hygiene (40) and in 2006, the WHO launched a global effort to improve hand hygiene in health care facilities with a reference book published in 2009 (http://whqlibdoc.who.int/hq/2009/WHO_IER_PSP_2009.07_eng.pdf). In-depth reviews have been published by several authors (146, 263, 283). Microorganisms on the hands can be classified into three groups (200): (i) the transient biota, which consists of contaminants taken up from the environment; (ii) the resident biota, which consists of permanent microorganisms

on the skin (283); and (iii) the infectious biota. Resident bacteria, most of which are on the uppermost level of the stratum corneum, have low pathogenicity and infectivity, and persons with normal immune systems who do not have implants or foreign bodies rarely acquire infections with these organisms. The density of resident bacteria on the skin ranges between 10^2 and 10^3 CFU/cm^2, and these resident bacteria limit colonization with more pathogenic microorganisms (i.e., colonization resistance). During their daily work, HCWs can contaminate their hands with pathogens. If they do not practice good hand hygiene, they can transmit these organisms to susceptible patients. Several studies indicated that pathogens such as *S. aureus* (136), *Klebsiella pneumoniae* (2), *Acinetobacter* spp., *Enterobacter* spp., or *Candida* spp., can be found on the hands of >20% of HCWs. Moreover, numerous epidemics have been traced to HCWs' contaminated hands (41, 231, 237, 288, 296). The goal of hand hygiene outside the operating room is to eliminate the transient biota without altering the resident biota. Hand washing for 15 and 30 s kills 0.6 to 1.1 and 1.8 to 2.8 log units, respectively (211). However, HCWs are very busy and frequently wash their hands for less than 10 s, which is insufficient to kill the transient biota (263, 283). One major advantage of the alcohol-based hand rub is that performance with these products takes about 25% of the time required for hand washing (263, 283). Morover, compliance with hand-washing procedures does not exceed 40% even under controlled study conditions (40). However, recent studies have shown that compliance with using the alcohol-based hand rubs exceeds that of hand washing (199). Furthermore, other studies have demonstrated that rubbing one's hands with an alcohol-based hand rub kills bacteria and most viruses more effectively than hand washing with a medicated soap (26, 209). Of note, investigators have not determined whether the level of killing is associated with the efficacy of preventing nosocomial infections. Alcohol-based hand rubs have several other practical advantages for hand hygiene over washing with soap and water. Compared with sinks, dispensers for the alcohol-based products are inexpensive, and they can be installed at locations that are more convenient for HCWs. Furthermore, unlike sinks (182), the dispensers have not been associated with outbreaks. Given the numerous advantages of these products, CDC's current hand hygiene guidelines recommend that health care facilities consider introducing alcohol-based hand rubs as the primary mode of hand hygiene (40). Most U.S. institutions promote hand hygiene using an alcoholic hand rub as standard of care, driven by the guidelines issued by WHO in a draft form in 2004 and finalized in 2009. In the United States, health care facilities should consult with the fire marshall before installing dispensers because many states have laws that prohibit placing multiple containers in emergency exits and halls. However, there are no published reports of fires caused by these products in Europe and such events are also very rare in the United States (39).

Surgical Hand Washing (Scrub) or Surgical Hand Disinfection (Rub-in)

In contrast to hand hygiene outside of the operating room, the surgical hand scrub aims to eliminate both transient biota and resident biota so that if the surgeon's gloves are punctured or torn, bacteria from his or her hands do not contaminate the surgical site. Tiny holes are observed in ≥30% of surgeons' gloves after operations, even when high-quality gloves are used. Cruse and Foord found that the incidence of surgical site infection was three times higher if the surgeon's gloves were punctured than if they were intact after the procedure (5.7 and 1.7%, respectively) (74). An experimental study demonstrated that the level of bacterial leakage through pinholes ranged between 10^3 and 10^4 CFU (103). Recently, a clinical trial clearly demonstrated that the presence of holes in a surgical glove without adequate antimicrobial prophylaxis increases the risk of postoperative surgical site infections fourfold (187). Moreover, a persistent antimicrobial effect is required after washing or disinfection to limit bacterial regrowth underneath the gloves (105). Thus, antiseptic preparations intended for use as surgical hand preparation are evaluated for their ability to reduce the number of bacteria released from hands (i) immediately after scrubbing, (ii) after wearing surgical gloves for 6 h (persistent activity), and (iii) after numerous applications over 5 days (cumulative activity). Immediate and persistent activities are considered the most important. Guidelines in the United States recommend that agents used for surgical hand preparation should significantly reduce microorganisms on intact skin, contain a nonirritating antimicrobial preparation, have broad-spectrum activity, and be fast acting and persistent. Agents, such as chlorhexidine, that have a prolonged postexposure effect are preferred because of this theoretical advantage, but there are no data from controlled clinical trials proving that the incidence of surgical site infections is lower when this agent is used. The WHO has issued a guideline for surgical hand antisepsis (www.who.int) with an executive summary published (285, 287).

Alcohol-based surgical rubs have several advantages over traditional surgical scrubs. Alcoholic preparations are more effective than any medicated soap for the surgical scrub and they do not alter the skin as much as chlorhexidine washes do. Moreover, the water supply in an operating room could harbor *Pseudomonas* spp. that might contaminate the hands of surgical personnel after they perform their surgical scrub (30). Brushes, which are used during a surgical scrub, may do more harm than good, and they should be used only to clean the fingernails, not to clean the skin. Given the advantages of the alcohol-based preparations, the presurgical scrub has been replaced in many European countries by the alcohol-based surgical rubs (263) and the WHO guidelines recommend the surgical hand rubs. Alcoholic gels are frequently promoted, but most of them are significantly less effective than liquids and should not be used in the operating room (156). A very rapid protocol (1.5 min) for the surgical hand rub has been recently proposed and was rapidly accepted by surgeons at the author's institution (147). The results of this investigational study were confirmed in a clinical trial (279, 287). However, few commercially available products have been successfully tested, and quite a few failed. Therefore, a 1.5-min surgical hand antisepsis is only acceptable if the product is cleared for such a short exposure to the hands.

Of note, both routine hand hygiene and surgical hand preparations must balance removing unwanted bacteria from HCWs' hands and maintaining the integrity of the HCWs' skin because damaged skin is more likely than normal skin to become colonized with pathogenic organisms. Therefore, either hand hygiene products should contain emollients or health care facilities should provide moisturizing hand lotions that do not damage latex for their staff so that their skin does not become dry, cracked, and irritated.

Presurgical Skin Disinfection

The aim of skin disinfection is to remove and kill the skin biota at the site of a planned surgical incision rapidly. However, currently available antiseptics do not eliminate all microorganisms at the incision site. In fact, coagulase-negative staphylococci can be frequently isolated even after three applications of agents such as iodine-alcohol to the skin (107). The FDA defines a skin disinfectant as a "fast acting, broad-spectrum and persistent antiseptic-containing preparation that significantly reduces the number of microorganisms on intact skin" (14). Spore-free alcohols are well suited for this purpose, but they lack persistent activity; iodine is frequently added for this purpose (109). Polyvinylpyrrolidone (PVP) iodine (also known as povidone iodine) continuously releases free iodine, which results in a limited prolonged antimicrobial effect. Chlorhexidine, with its profound prolonged effect after application, seems to be favorable compared to PVP iodine; however, PVP excelled chlorhexidine according to a recent clinical trial (256). The very recent WHO guideline on "safe surgery" recommends PVP iodine or chlorhexidine as reasonable choices for preoperative skin preparation (http://www.who.int/patientsafety/safesurgery/en). A recent randomized controlled clinical trial indicates a preference for chlorhexidine-alcohol over iodophors (76), but the addition of alcohol may be the reason for the favorable effect rather than chlorhexidine, as shown in a similar trial favoring iodophor in alcohol (256).

Before a patient's skin is prepared for a surgical procedure, the skin should be free of gross contamination (i.e., dirt, soil, or any other debris) (170). Although preoperative showering has not been shown to reduce the incidence of surgical site infections, this practice may decrease bacterial counts and ensure that the skin is clean (210). The antiseptics used to prepare the skin should be applied using sterile supplies and gloves or by a no-touch technique, moving from the incision area to the periphery (170). The person preparing the skin should use pressure because friction increases the antibacterial effect of the antiseptic. For example, alcohol applied without friction reduces bacterial counts by 1.0 to 1.2 log CFU compared with 1.9 to 3.0 log CFU when friction is used. In comparison, alcoholic sprays have little antimicrobial effect and produce potentially explosive vapors (166).

Common Antiseptic Compounds

Alcoholic Compounds

The reader is referred to the section above on alcohols. As outlined above, alcohol is the most important skin disinfectant. Alcohols used for skin disinfection prior to invasive procedures should generally be free of spores to avoid any contamination. Although the risk of infection is minimal, the low additional cost for a spore-free product is justified. One study indicated that alcohol may result in dermal absorption of isopropyl alcohol from a commercial hand rub, which may interfere with religious beliefs of HCWs (264). However, the WHO resolved this issue in their most recent guidelines published in 2009, and Muslims, for example, are allowed to use alcoholic compounds for hand hygiene.

Chlorhexidine

Chlorhexidine gluconate, a cationic bisbiguanide, has been widely recognized as an effective and safe antiseptic for nearly 40 years (80, 204). Chlorhexidine formulations are extensively used for surgical and hygienic hand disinfection (see previous discussion). Other applications include preoperative showers (or whole-body disinfection), antisepsis in obstetrics and gynecology, management of burns, wound antisepsis, and prevention and treatment of oral disease (plaque control, pre- and postoperative mouthwash, and oral hygiene) (80, 204). When chlorhexidine is used orally, its bitter taste must be masked and it can stain the teeth. Intravenous catheters coated with chlorhexidine and silver sulfadiazine are used to prevent catheter-associated bloodstream infections (169). In fact, an infection control program to prevent catheter-associated bloodstream infections included hand hygiene, chlorhexidine site care, and full-barrier precautions in a large clinical study in intensive care units: these interventions led to an infection rate close to zero (201). Today, chlorhexidine compounds are considered the gold standard for catheter site care (186). Chlorhexidine is most commonly formulated as a 4% aqueous solution in a detergent base. However, alcoholic preparations have been demonstrated in numerous studies to have better antimicrobial activity than detergent-based formulations (161). Bactericidal concentrations destroy the bacterial cell membrane, causing cellular constituents to leak out of the cell and cell contents to coagulate (80). Chlorhexidine gluconate bactericidal activity against vegetative gram-positive and gram-negative bacteria is intermediately rapid. In addition, it provides a persistent antimicrobial action that prevents the regrowth of microorganisms for up to 6 h. This effect is desirable when a sustained reduction in the microbiota reduces infection risk (e.g., during surgical procedures). Chlorhexidine has little activity against bacterial and fungal spores except at high temperatures. Mycobacteria are inhibited but are not killed by aqueous solutions. Yeasts and dermatophytes are usually susceptible, although the fungicidal action varies with the species (79). Chlorhexidine is effective against lipophilic viruses (e.g., HIV, influenza virus, and herpes simplex virus types 1 and 2), but viruses such as poliovirus, coxsackievirus, and rotavirus are not inactivated (80). Unlike what occurs with povidone iodine, blood and other organic materials do not affect the antimicrobial activity of chlorhexidine significantly (165). However, inorganic anions and organic anions such as soaps are incompatible with chlorhexidine and its activity is reduced at extreme acidic or alkaline pH and in the presence of anionic- and nonionic-based moisturizers and detergents. Microorganisms can contaminate chlorhexidine solutions (194) and resistant isolates have been identified. For example, Stickler found chlorhexidine-resistant *Proteus mirabilis* after chlorhexidine was used extensively over a long period to prepare patients for bladder catheterization (252). The chlorhexidine resistance among vegetative bacteria was thought to be limited to certain gram-negative bacilli (such as *P. aeruginosa*, *Burkholderia* [*Pseudomonas*] *cepacia*, *P. mirabilis*, and *S. marcescens*) (253). However, genes conferring resistance to various organic cations, including chlorhexidine, have been identified in *S. aureus* clinical isolates (175, 188). Chlorhexidine has several other limitations. When absorbed onto cotton and other fabrics, it usually resists removal by washing. If a hypochlorite (bleach) is used during the washing procedure, a brown stain may develop (80). Long-term experience with the use of chlorhexidine has demonstrated that the incidence of hypersensitivity and skin irritation is low. However, severe allergic reactions including anaphylaxis have been reported (90, 295). Although cytotoxicity has been observed in exposed fibroblasts, no deleterious effects on wound healing have been demonstrated in vivo. There is no evidence that chlorhexidine gluconate is toxic if it is absorbed through the skin, but ototoxicity can occur when chlorhexidine is instilled into the middle ear during operative procedures.

High concentrations of chlorhexidine and preparations containing other compounds (e.g., alcohols and surfactants) may damage eyes (257).

Iodophors

Iodophors essentially have replaced aqueous iodine and tincture as antiseptics. Iodophors are chemical complexes of iodine bound to a carrier such as PVP or ethoxylated nonionic detergents (poloxamers). These complexes gradually release small amounts of free microbicidal iodine. The most commonly used iodophor is PVP iodine. Its preparations generally contain 1 to 10% PVP iodine, which is equivalent to 0.1 to 1.0% available iodine. The active component appears to be free molecular iodine (I_2). A paradoxical effect of dilution on the activity of PVP iodine has been observed. As the dilution increases, bactericidal activity increases up to a maximum and then falls (114). Commercial PVP iodine solutions at dilutions of 1:2 to 1:100 kill *S. aureus* and *Mycobacterium chelonae* more rapidly than do stock solutions (27). *S. aureus* can survive a 2-min exposure to full-strength PVP iodine solution but cannot survive a 15-s exposure to a 1:100 dilution of the iodophor (27). Thus, iodophors must be used at the dilution stated by the manufacturer. The exact mechanism by which iodine destroys microorganisms is not known. Iodine may react with microorganisms' amino acids and fatty acids, destroying cell structures and enzymes (114). Depending on the concentration of free iodine and other factors, iodophors exhibit a broad range of microbicidal activity. Commercial preparations are bactericidal, mycobactericidal, fungicidal, and virucidal but not sporicidal at the dilutions recommended for use. Prolonged contact times are required to inactivate certain fungi and bacterial spores (216). Despite their bactericidal activity, PVP iodine and poloxamer-iodine solutions can become contaminated with *B. (P.) cepacia* or *P. aeruginosa*, and contaminated solutions have caused outbreaks of pseudobacteremia and peritonitis (28, 72). In fact, *B. cepacia* was found to survive for up to 68 weeks in a PVP iodine antiseptic solution (13). The most likely explanation for the prolonged survival of these microorganisms in iodophor solutions is that organic or inorganic material and biofilm may mechanically protect the microorganisms. Iodophors are widely used for antisepsis of skin, mucous membranes, and wounds. A 2.5% ophthalmic solution of PVP iodine is more effective and less toxic than silver nitrate or erythromycin ointment when used as prophylaxis against neonatal conjunctivitis (ophthalmia neonatorum) (139). In some countries, PVP iodine alcoholic solutions are used extensively for skin antisepsis before invasive procedures (16). Iodophors containing higher concentrations of free iodine may be used to disinfect medical equipment. Solutions designed for use on the skin should not be used to disinfect hard surfaces because the concentrations of the antiseptic solutions are usually too low for this purpose (216). The risk of side effects, such as staining, tissue irritation, and resorption, is lower for iodophors than for aqueous iodine. Iodophors do not corrode metal surfaces (114). However, a body surface treated with an iodine or iodophor solution may absorb free iodine. Consequently, increased serum iodine levels (and serum iodide levels) have been found in patients, especially when large areas were treated for a long period (114). For this reason, hyperthyroidism and other disorders of thyroid functions are contraindications for the use of iodine-containing preparations. Likewise, iodophors should not be applied to pregnant and nursing women or to newborns and infants (50). Because severe local and systemic allergic reactions have been observed, iodophors and iodine should not be used in patients with allergies to these preparations (274). Iodophores have little if any residual effect. However, for a limited time they may have residual bactericidal activity on the skin surface, because free iodine diffuses into deep regions but also back to the skin surface (114). The antimicrobial efficacy of iodophors is reduced in the presence of organic material such as blood.

Triclosan and PCMX

Triclosan (Irgasan DP-300 or Irgacare MP) has been used for more than 30 years in a wide array of skin care products, including hand washes, surgical scrubs, and consumer products. A review of its effectiveness and safety in health care settings has been published (141). A concentration of 1% has good activity against gram-positive bacteria, including antibiotic-resistant strains, but less activity against gram-negative organisms, mycobacteria, and fungi. Limited data suggest that triclosan has a relatively broad antiviral spectrum, with high-level activity against enveloped viruses, such as HIV type 1, influenza A virus, and herpes simplex virus type 1. However, the nonenveloped viruses proved more difficult to inactivate. Clinical strains with low-level resistance to triclosan have been identified, but the clinical significance of this remains unknown (255). Triclosan is added to various soaps, lotions, deodorants, toothpastes, mouth rinses, commonly used household fabrics, plastics, and medical devices. Moreover, the mechanisms of triclosan resistance may be similar to those involved in antimicrobial resistance (6) and some of these mechanisms may account for the observed cross-resistance of laboratory isolates to antimicrobial agents (65). Consequently, concerns have been raised that widespread use of triclosan formulations in non-health care settings and products may select for biocide resistance and even cross-resistance to antibiotics. However, environmental surveys have not demonstrated an association between triclosan usage and antibiotic resistance (214). Triclosan solutions produce a sustained residual effect against resident and transient microbiotas, which is minimally affected by organic matter. Numerous studies have not identified toxic, allergenic, mutagenic, or carcinogenic potential. Triclosan formulations may help control outbreaks of MRSA when used for hand hygiene and as a bathing cleanser for patients (141). However, some MRSA isolates have reduced triclosan susceptibility. Triclosan formulations are less effective than 2 to 4% chlorhexidine gluconate when used for surgical scrub solutions; properly formulated triclosan solutions may be used for hygienic hand washing. PCMX (chloroxylenol) is an antimicrobial used in hand-washing products. It is available at concentrations of 0.5 to 3.75%. Its properties are similar to those of triclosan. Nonionic surfactants may neutralize PCMX.

Octenidine

Octenidine dihydrochloride is a novel bispyridine compound which is an effective and safe antiseptic agent. The 0.1% commercial formulation favorably compared with other antiseptics with respect to antimicrobial activity and toxicological properties. In vitro and in vivo it rapidly killed both gram-positive and gram-negative bacteria as well as fungi (110, 242). Octenidine is virucidal against HIV, HBV, and herpes simplex virus. Similar to chlorhexidine, it has a marked residual effect. No toxicological problems have been found when the 0.1% formulation was applied according to the manufacturer's recommendations. The colorless solution is a useful antiseptic for mucous membranes of the female and male genitals and the oral cavity (24), but

its bad taste limits its use orally. In a recent observational study, the 0.1% formulation was highly effective and well tolerated for the care of central venous catheter insertion sites (261). The results of this study have also been supported by a randomized controlled clinical trial (81). Octenidine is not registered for use in the United States.

STERILIZATION

Principles, Definitions, and Terms

As outlined in Table 3, sterilization is not a relative term but defines the complete absence of any viable microorganisms including spores. However, this absence cannot be proved by current microbiological techniques (142). Therefore, sterilization can be defined as a closely monitored, validated process used to render a product free of all forms of viable microorganisms, including all bacterial endospores. To test the ability of sterilization systems to meet the latter definition of sterilization, manufacturers developed a worst-case scenario that allows the process (log killing) to be quantified and estimates the probability of process failure. Large safety margins were included in this test, which is based on the assumption that items are heavily contaminated with spores, soil, and proteins. It is important to note that while these conditions are used for the testing, in clinical practice items that are heavily soiled should not be sterilized and such a scenario would represent a critical failure of the reprocessing cycle. Any device undergoing sterilization first must undergo an appropriate cleaning process. A manufacturer must demonstrate that a sterilizer is effective against a wide range of clinically important microorganisms before being approved by the FDA. In addition, proof of efficacy must be performed with organisms (usually bacterial spores) that have been shown to be the most resistant to the new technology. A validated and reliable biological indicator must be developed, and studies must establish that sterility will be consistently achieved when critical process parameters operate within a defined range. This assures the operator that as long as there is no operational error or equipment failure, sterility is achieved. Several guidelines are essential documents for staff needing to understand reprocessing and sterilization of medical devices. ISO 14937 provides general criteria for characterizing a sterilizing agent and for the development, validation, and routine control of a sterilization process for medical devices. ISO 11134 (moist heat) and ISO 11135 (ethylene oxide) documents describe the standards for use of these methods of sterilization in the industrial setting in the United States. The American National Standard Institute/Association for the Advancement of Medical Instrumentation (ANSI/AAMI) published adaptations of these standards for health care facilities: Standard 46 (moist heat) and Standard 41 (ethylene oxide) (Table 3). In Europe, EN 550, EN 554, and EN 285 define the standards for steam and ethylene oxide sterilization. ISO 14161 provides guidance that staff can use when selecting and using biological indicators and when interpreting the results of these tests. ISO 17664 specifies which information medical device manufacturers must provide so that the medical device can be processed safely and continue to function properly. Readers are referred to other publications for additional information about sterilization (33, 115, 142). Hot-air sterilization does not belong to the state-of-the-art technologies, but it is still used in many countries. However, the distribution of dry heat to the instruments requires long exposure times. Temperatures of >185°C resinify paraffin, destroying the lubricating function of instruments, and higher temperatures are corrosive, resulting in loss of hardness. Therefore, hot-air sterilization has largely been replaced by better, safer, and faster technologies.

Monitoring

Any sterilization process must be monitored by mechanical, physical, chemical, and facultatively biological methods. Before routine use, the performance of the machine should be validated with the most difficult load used at the institution to ensure safety of the process. In addition, a printout of the physical parameters (e.g., temperature and pressure) during sterilization should be kept for documentation purposes. In addition, chemical indicators placed on the tested items change color if they are exposed to adequate temperatures and exposure times. They are inexpensive and easy to use and provide a visual indication that the item has been exposed to the sterilization process. Good clinical indicators are able to identify a sterilizer failure. However, some are too sensitive, giving false-positive results (220, 223), which may cause unnecessary recalls of adequately sterilized items. Less sensitive chemical indicators do not detect small deviations in the process. In 1963 Bowie and Dick determined that if residual air remained in a sterilizer after the vacuum phase and there was only one package in the chamber, the air would concentrate in that package (38). They developed the Bowie-Dick test to determine whether steam penetration and air removal occurred successfully. This test does not provide information about the sterilization process.

Biological indicators are the best monitors of the sterilization process. If the spores in commercially available standard biological indicators do not grow during an appropriate incubation period, the results indicate that the process was able to kill $\geq 10^6$ CFU. For flash sterilization, the Attest Rapid Readout biological indicator detects the presence of a spore-associated enzyme, α-D-glucosidase, and permits staff to assess the efficacy of sterilization within 60 min (270). Staff should investigate positive biologicals because they can provide the only indication that something is wrong with the sterilization process (51).

An important question is whether a load can be distributed before the final results of the biological indicator are available (i.e., parametric release). The Joint Commission on Accreditation of Healthcare Organizations standard allows the use of appropriate chemical indicators without routine use of a biological indicator. A common approach is to use the sterilized items if the physical and chemical parameters of adequate sterilization were met without awaiting the culture results from the biological indicators. In Europe, routine use of biological indicators is not required if the sterilizer has undergone testing by a validation procedure used for industrial steam sterilization (EN 285, EN 550, EN 554, or EN 556). Most sterilizers in European hospitals probably do not meet these very strict requirements (268), and consequently, biological indicators are used regularly to ensure that they are working properly. These industrial standards for validation of steam sterilization will be implemented in health care organizations, but this change is controversial because of the associated expenses. The future is likely to involve parametric release with regular validation and/or commissions of the equipment. Legal aspects will probably determine the outcome of this discussion, and lawyers are likely to accept nothing but a zero risk. However, the goal of a zero risk for contamination in central sterilization services will probably contribute to excessive health care costs.

Therefore, standards for sterilization should exclude a risk for contamination after the reprocessing cycle but should avoid steps that are performed only for legal reasons.

Packaging, Loading, and Storage

Items that are clean and dry should be inspected and then wrapped and packaged (or put in containers) before sterilization. Wrappers should allow steam or gas to penetrate into the package but should protect the items from recontamination after sterilization. For steam sterilization, muslin as the only wrapper has limitations and handling of items made of muslin leads to contamination (286). Items should be labeled with information such as expiration date, type of sterilization, and identification code for traceability.

Steam Sterilization

The most reliable method of sterilization is one that uses saturated steam under pressure. It is inexpensive, nontoxic, and very reliable.

Steam penetrates fabrics, and its inherent safety margin is much higher than that of any other sterilization technique. Therefore, it should be used whenever possible. Obviously, other techniques must be used for heat-sensitive items. Steam irreversibly coagulates and causes denaturation of microbial enzymes and proteins. Three parameters are critical to ensure that steam sterilization is effective: the amount of time the items are exposed to steam, the temperature of the process, and moisture. Unlike time and temperature, the moisture condition in the autoclave cannot be directly determined. The D-value determines the time required to kill 10^6 CFU of the spores most resistant to the sterilization process under study. Devices or instruments must reach the desired temperature, which is not necessarily identical to the temperature displayed on the autoclave's gauge. A drop of only 1.7°C (3°F) increases the time required to sterilize an item by 48%. Without moisture, a temperature of 160°C is required for dry-heat sterilization. Dry air does not provide steam for condensation, and the heat transfer to objects is slower than when moisture is present. Pressurized steam quickly transfers energy to the sterilizer load and causes more rapid denaturation and coagulation of microbial proteins. In addition, pressurizing the steam allows one to achieve dry 100% saturated steam. Thus, there is no mist that could cause the packaging and/or the items to become wet.

Residual air in the autoclave interferes with the sterilization process. The amount of air within the sterilizer can be estimated by comparing the chamber pressure with the saturated steam pressure calculated from the average chamber temperature. A measured pressure greater than the calculated saturated pressure indicates the presence of residual air in the chamber. Such monitoring devices are common in the United Kingdom.

Several types of autoclaves are available: gravity displacement steam sterilization, prevacuum steam sterilization, and steam flash-pressure pulsing steam sterilization autoclaves. The sterilization process is less consistent in gravity displacement steam sterilizers than in the other sterilizers (73). For example, gravity displacement autoclaves are more likely than the other systems to leave residual air in the chamber before the steam is introduced. Prevacuum sterilizers resolved part of this problem and cut the cycle time in half. However, the effectiveness of sterilization still can be compromised by small leaks (1 to 10 mm Hg/min) in the sterilizer (142). The most current technology is the steam flash-pressure pulsing steam sterilization technique because air leaks do not decrease the effectiveness of the process, it nearly eliminates the problem of air in the chamber, and it reduces the thermal lag upon heating of the load to the desired exposure temperature (73).

The process of sterilization has several cycles: conditioning, exposure, and drying. Common cycles for steam sterilization in prevacuum or flash-pressure pulsing steam sterilizers are 121°C for 15 min (121°C for 30 min in a gravity displacement sterilizer) or 132°C for 4 min. EN 554 requires steam sterilizers to provide this temperature throughout the entire chamber within a narrow margin (0 to +3°C).

Flash sterilization is an emergency process used, for example, after a surgical instrument is dropped but needs to be immediately available during a procedure (168). Unwrapped devices are exposed to pressurized steam for 3 min, usually in the operating suite, sometimes without a biological indicator. The autoclaves employed are gravity displacement sterilizers that have the problems mentioned above. If HCWs are in a hurry, they may not clean the item properly, which will prevent proper sterilization. In addition, because the items are not wrapped, they can be contaminated easily when they are transported to the operating room. Even properly wrapped sterile items can become contaminated if they are transported several times (286). Moreover, some patients have been injured by items that were flash sterilized (230). Therefore, flash sterilization is controversial and several investigators have suggested that it should be used only in emergency situations when no other device is available. Flash sterilization should not replace standard sterilization protocols (93) and should not be used to save time instead of sterilizing items by the standard methods or because the health care facility does not want to purchase an extra instrument set (170). Flash sterilization also means there is a lack of any written documentation, rendering futile any tracing in cases where something went wrong.

Ethylene Oxide Gas

Temperature- and/or pressure-sensitive items have been sterilized traditionally with ethylene oxide in a standard gas. Ethylene oxide inactivates all microorganisms, including spores, probably by an alkylation process. B. subtilis bacterial spores are among the most resistant, and therefore, these are used as a biological monitor for this process. A new rapid-readout ethylene oxide biological indicator indicates an ethylene oxide sterilization process failure by producing fluorescence, which is detected in an autoreader within 4 h of incubation at 37°C, and a color change related to a change in pH of the growth media within 96 h of continued incubation (227).

The process of sterilizing items with ethylene oxide begins by adding nitrogen gas to remove air or by evacuating the chamber. Items are then exposed to ethylene oxide at 55°C (130°F). Six variable but interdependent parameters—gas concentration, vacuum, pressure, temperature, relative humidity, and time of exposure—must be controlled when ethylene oxide is used. The gas concentration cannot be measured online, limiting the extent of monitoring. Therefore, the concentration should be validated as outlined in ISO 11135.

Ethylene oxide sterilization has several disadvantages. It is useful only as a surface sterilizer because it does not reach blocked-off surfaces. In addition, ethylene oxide is flammable, explosive, and carcinogenic to laboratory animals, and it requires special safety precautions. Moreover, items sterilized by ethylene oxide must be aerated for ap-

proximately 12 h to remove any traces of the gas. Thus, the entire process takes >16 h, but modern sterilizers can run at shorter cycles. Furthermore, toxic residues can be trapped in the wrapper or the items. Polyvinyl chloride and polyurethane absorb ethylene oxide readily and require long periods to dissipate the oxide. The wrapper should be a barrier against recontamination after sterilization, but it also can prevent ethylene oxide from reaching the item. Therefore, only materials with documented ethylene oxide penetration and dissipation properties should be used as wrappers.

The future of ethylene oxide in sterilization is limited, mainly due to its toxicity. However, no currently available technology, including plasma sterilization (see below), can replace sterilization with ethylene oxide entirely. In addition, sterilization with ethylene oxide does not fail as frequently as sterilization with plasma when residual proteins and/or salts are present on the items (11).

Plasma Sterilization

The low-temperature plasma is produced in a closed chamber with deep vacuum, an electromagnetic field, and a chemical precursor (hydrogen peroxide or a mixture of hydrogen peroxide and peracetic acid). The resulting free radicals, the chemical precursors, and the UV radiation are thought to be the products that rapidly destroy vegetative microorganisms including spores.

Sterrad

The Sterrad 100 sterilizer was the first plasma sterilizer for use in health care facilities and has been on the market in Europe since 1990 and in the United States since 1993. In August 1997, the Sterrad 100 System was approved to sterilize certain surgical instruments with long lumens, such as those used in urologic, laparoscopic, and arthroscopic procedures, including instruments with single stainless steel lumens of ≥3 and <400 mm in length. The Sterrad 100S has since replaced the Sterrad 100. The Sterrad 100S adds one sterilization cycle and thereby fulfills the requirement to kill 10^6 spores halfway through the cycle. A smaller device, the Sterrad 50, has been independently tested for efficacy (222). Other sizes, e.g., the large Sterrad 200, approved by the FDA in 2003, can sterilize small lumens (single stainless steel lumens with an inside diameter of 1 mm or larger or Teflon/polyethylene lumens with an inside diameter of 6 mm or larger). The new Sterrad NX System, approved by the FDA in April 2005, is the fastest low-temperature hydrogen peroxide gas plasma sterilizer yet. This system employs a new vaporization system that removes most of the water from the hydrogen peroxide, improving diffusion of peroxide into lumens. Consequently, a broad range of instruments, including single-channel flexible endoscopes, can be processed within 38 min. In 2001, the FDA cleared biological indicators suitable for plasma sterilization.

Regardless of the model, the basic steps are the same. Medical instruments are placed in the sterilization chamber, a strong vacuum is created in the chamber, and a solution of 59% hydrogen peroxide and water is automatically injected from a cassette into the sterilization chamber. The solution vaporizes and diffuses throughout the chamber, surrounding the items to be sterilized. Radiofrequency energy is applied to create an electric field, which in turn generates the low-temperature plasma, inducing free radicals. The combination of the diffusion pretreatment and plasma phases sterilizes the item while eliminating harmful residuals. At the end of the cycle, the radiofrequency energy is turned off, the vacuum is released, and the chamber is filled with filtered air, returning it to normal atmospheric pressure.

Plasma sterilizers have several disadvantages. First, materials that absorb too much hydrogen peroxide (e.g., cellulosics and some nylons such as those from connectors, cables, and insulators), materials that catalytically decompose hydrogen peroxide (e.g., copper and nickel alloys from electrical wire, solder, and surgical instruments), and materials that react with hydrogen peroxide such as organic dyes (colored anodized aluminum) and organic sulfides of solid lubricant in endoscopic devices) cannot be sterilized in a Sterrad. Second, the cassettes required to run the device and the special nonmuslim wrapper are relatively expensive.

Low-Temperature Sterilization by Ozone

The 125L Ozone Sterilizer (TSO3, Quebec Canada) uses medical-grade oxygen, water, and electricity to generate ozone within the sterilizer to provide an efficient sterilant without producing toxic chemicals or using high temperatures. (It runs at 25 to 35°C). Ozone forms when oxygen is submitted to an intense electrical field that separates oxygen molecules into atomic oxygen (O), which in turn combines with other oxygen molecules (O_2) to form triatomic oxygen (O_3) or ozone, providing a sterility assurance level of 10^{-6} in approximately 4 h. At the end of the cycle, the oxygen and water vapor safely vent directly into the room. The sterilization chamber has a capacity of 125 liters. Processed medical instruments require no aeration at the end of the sterilization cycle. Medical devices are packaged in a TSO3 sterilization pouch or inanodized aluminum sterilization containers. The TSO3 OZO-TEST self-contained biological and chemical indicators should be used to evaluate the machine's performance. An ozone sterilizer can be installed as a free-standing unit or recessed behind a wall. These devices are used primarily in Canada. These sterilizers are approved by the FDA, but few health care facilities in the United States use them.

Liquid Sterilization

The FDA approved the Steris System 1 in 1988, but it is not considered a sterilizer in Europe (77). The machine is designed to sterilize immersible devices, including flexible endoscopes, with 35% liquid peracetic acid (an FDA-approved sterilant that is sporicidal [132, 135]), supplemented with buffering, anticorrosion, wetting, and surface-active agents. Peracetic acid is automatically diluted with sterile filtered water, and the items are exposed for 12 min. The entire sterilization process takes approximately 30 min at ca. 50°C. Items can be used immediately after the process is completed and do not need to be aerated.

Clinical studies of the Steris System 1 have been performed with bronchoscopes, hysteroscopes, colonoscopes, and rigid endoscopes (42, 272). Independent efficacy tests demonstrated some failures (42). Exposure time and temperature are monitored electronically, and conductivity is used as a surrogate marker for peracetic acid concentration. However, the machine can complete its cycle normally and print a report stating that the concentration of peracetic acid was in the normal range when it was run intentionally without peracetic acid (171). Commercially available spores can be used for monitoring sterilization (155), but false-positive test strips can occur as a result of improper use of the clip used to attach the test strips (119). Other disadvantages of this system include the high cost of purchasing and using the equipment, which is considerably greater than the cost of purchasing and using systems for high-level disinfection with glutaraldehyde (104). In addition, the device does not clean the items. Thus, the cleaning step adds to the overall time of reprocessing the items. The Steris System 1, like all other nonsteam sterilizers, cannot meet the requirements for sterilization if residual debris and/or proteins are present on the items. The system has been considerably improved over the last decade, but the changes have not yet been approved by the FDA, which has issued a letter of concern (http://www.fda.gov/ICECI/EnforcementActions/WarningLetters/2008/ucm1048303.htm).

REUSE OF SINGLE-USE DEVICES

Current FDA policy states that the responsibility for the safety and performance of reprocessed single-use devices lies with the reprocessor, not the original manufacturer. The FDA considers the hospital to be the manufacturer of a single-use device if it has been resterilized. Therefore, the reprocessor must ensure that the reprocessed items are sterile and not contaminated with toxic substances such as endotoxins or residual ethylene oxide and that the product's integrity, composition, and function are essentially identical to those of a new product. Most hospitals cannot afford to generate appropriate data on the quality and performance of reprocessed single-use items. In addition, if a manufacturer changes the product, the reprocessor would need to redo the analyses before the device could legally be marketed after reprocessing (management of change).

The FDA published a final guidance on this topic (see homepage for details: http://www.fda.gov/MedicalDevices/DeviceRegulationandGuidance/GuidanceDocuments/ucm071434.htm0.

Some institutions resterilize items that have not been used on patients but that, for instance, were dropped and/or whose package was damaged. Even this approach can be problematic. For example, the FDA published an alert documenting that the quality of an implant that was originally sterilized with ethylene oxide and resterilized with steam was impaired by the reprocessing method. In addition, the quality, product integrity, and performance of many plastic or rubber products after reprocessing are unknown. Moreover, the FDA does not allow health care facilities that send equipment and supplies to a reprocessing company to transfer full responsibility to that company (see the full text at http://www.fda.gov/MedicalDevices/DeviceRegulationandGuidance/ReprocessingofSingle-UseDevices/default.htm). Furthermore, if a hospital reprocesses a single-use device, the hospital is responsible for ensuring that the device complies with all applicable FDA labeling requirements, even if the device is exempt from the premarket requirements. If the hospital does not ensure that the device complies with FDA labeling requirements, the device is misbranded, and the hospital may be considered in violation of section 301(k) of the Act. As of 14 August 2001 and of 14 February 2002, FDA enforced premarket filing requirements for reprocessed class II devices (i.e., moderate-risk devices such as a cardiac mapping catheter used to map electrical activity of the heart).

In many countries throughout the world, health care facilities reprocess single-use items (sometimes illegally) because resources are limited and this may be the only way to provide patients with access to state-of-the-art health care. We believe that new reprocessing technologies using washer-disinfectors coupled with highly effective low-temperature sterilizers can kill all microorganisms, even in narrow lumens such as cardiac catheters. In fact, a commercial reprocessor in Germany legally has reprocessed >4 million single-use items without any published serious side effects, saving between 30 and 50% of the cost for a new item. With the expertise of an infection control professional, the health care facilities may provide the desired level of microbiological and toxicological safety. However, they probably cannot ensure that the design and function of the device are still adequate. Thus, in the United States and countries with similar regulations on quality assurance programs, reuse of single-use devices may not be cost-effective. In addition, organizations that sell used single-use devices to patients and/or insurance companies as new devices will encounter legal and ethical issues. Continuous improvements of new devices also impede reprocessing of single-use devices on a large scale. However, financial restriction may change the current beliefs; the reader should consult the FDA home page and experts in the field before considering reprocessing single-use devices.

BOVINE SPONGIFORM ENCEPHALOPATHY AND VARIANT CREUTZFELDT-JAKOB DISEASE

CJD has been identified on all continents and is thought to occur worldwide. The incidence of CJD is estimated to be about 1 case per 10^6 persons per year. Most cases of CJD are sporadic; <10% of CJD cases may be related to a genetic autosomal dominant predisposition, and few nosocomial cases are related to use of contaminated tissue or contaminated human growth hormone. The emergence of vCJD has brought about a major medical and economic crisis in Europe (49, 149, 203). As of 2006, no curative therapy is available for CJD or vCJD; however, several approaches have been investigated with limited success (112). It is generally accepted that eating BSE agent-contaminated meat is the cause of vCJD (130, 203). As of 1 January 2010, 167 cases had been reported from the United Kingdom. Cases that fulfill the new WHO case definition (21 May 2001) also have been reported from France (14 cases), Canada (1 case), Spain (1 case), Ireland (1 case), and Italy (1 case). The peak of the epidemic was in the year 2000 (28 cases in the United Kingdom), falling to 5 cases in 2005 (December 2005).

The agent causing vCJD is not a classic microorganism but an altered prion protein (5, 32, 202, 236). Its origin remains obscure, but the BSE agent from cattle is most probably responsible for the vCJD in humans. In the mid-1980s, because of the elimination several years earlier of a step in tallow extraction from rendered carcasses that allowed some tissue infected with scrapie to survive the process, the infectious agent was recycled as cattle-adapted scrapie or BSE. The animal food was no longer sterilized at 134°C for 20 to 30 min but, rather, was pasteurized before being fed to animals whose carcasses, with encased spinal cords and paraspinal ganglia, were legally processed as hot dogs, sausages, and precooked meat patties (47). Investigators postulate that a high incidence of scrapie in sheep and a large proportion of sheep in the mix of carcasses that were rendered for livestock feed may explain why the incidence of BSE in British cattle was more than 10 times higher than in cattle in any other European country.

vCJD has a different clinical presentation and occurs at a much younger age (62). The mean age at death from vCJD is 28 years; only 6 of 90 patients died at the age of 50 years or older (266). Among several hypotheses that may explain why this age group is most affected is that the incubation period is shorter in the young than in the elderly or they are more susceptible to infection. In the United Kingdom, the number of people exposed to potentially infective doses through food may be extremely high. All patients genotyped so far are homozygous for methionine on codon 129 of the prion protein gene. It is postulated that heterozygous individuals may have much longer incubation times before vCJD becomes evident. Therefore, asymptomatic carriers may pose a risk for transmission if they undergo routine surgery and instruments are not reprocessed by a prion-safe program.

Patients suffering from vCJD harbor large numbers of prions in their tonsils and spleen before they have signs, symptoms, and pathological findings of the disease. In contrast, patients with sporadic CJD suffer from spongiform encephalopathy long before the prion spreads into muscles and lymphoid tissue (129). Consequently, the United Kingdom has developed very strict precautions; for example, it was required that all tonsillectomies be performed with disposable instruments. In 2002, this practice was discontinued because serious complications arose when disposable instruments were used. However, none of the samples, including 276 samples initially reactive in one enzyme immunoassay, that were investigated by immunohistochemistry or immunoblotting was positive for the presence of CJD.

The fact that the vCJD prion agent is found in lymphoid tissue and tonsils indicates that prions are not restricted to neural tissue (112). Studies of sheep naturally infected with scrapie demonstrated that the infectious agent first appears in lymphatic tissue of the tonsils and gastrointestinal tract, suggesting the oral route may be the principal mode of transmission. In addition, numerous studies underline the importance of the B cell in transmission of the BSE agent (152). Lymphatic organs typically show early accumulation of prions, and B cells and follicular dendritic cells are required for efficient neuroinvasion. The actual entry into the central nervous system probably occurs via peripheral nerves, and the prions accumulate in neural tissue once inflammation of the lymphoid tissue is in progress (125).

Experimental evidence from animal models indicates that blood can contain prion infectivity, which suggests a potential risk for BSE transmission via proteins isolated from human plasma (133). Three cases of probable transmission by blood transfusion raise more concern about the safety of the blood supply (4). In the United States, beginning in August 1999, persons who resided in or traveled to the United Kingdom for a total of 6 months from 1980 through 1996 have been deferred from blood donation, as have persons who received bovine insulin derived from cattle in the United Kingdom. Recently, both the American Red Cross and the FDA announced new, expanded deferrals for travel and residence in the United Kingdom and other European countries (60), and they are conducting a retrospective study of persons who received potentially contaminated blood. The United Kingdom no longer collects plasma from its inhabitants and, as a further precautionary measure, has instituted leukocyte reduction (removal of white blood cells) from blood transfusions.

Previously, problems with reprocessing instruments used on patients with CJD were limited to invasive instruments that came into contact with neural tissue, predominantly instruments used in neurosurgery. However, as noted above, vCJD is highly lymphotropic, so that any instruments used on lymphoid tissues may be contaminated with prions (152). As outlined above, appropriate reprocessing of surgical items includes cleaning, disinfection, and sterilization. Aldehydes enhance the resistance of prions and abolish the inactivating effect of autoclaving (48). Therefore, aldehydes are no longer recommended for disinfecting surgical instruments in Europe before they have undergone a thorough cleaning process. In France, aldehydes are no longer used for endoscope reprocessing, despite evidence that peracetic acid may stain prions as well (145). Small resistant subpopulations of infective prions may survive autoclaving at 132 to 138°C. These resistant subpopulations are not inactivated by simply reautoclaving, and they have biological characteristics that differentiate them from the main population (258). The worst-case scenario is that the agent for vCJD might become self-replicating when it contaminates surgical instruments. Therefore, prions challenge reprocessing techniques like never before.

The minimum requirements for decontamination procedures and precautions for materials potentially contaminated with the agent that causes CJD or, still more, vCJD remain unknown. However, it is clear that dry heat (160°C for 24 h), formaldehyde sterilization, and standard steam sterilization do not sterilize prion-contaminated items (88). The scientific uncertainties and lack of data do not allow agencies like national health departments, the WHO, or the CDC to formulate guidelines that are completely evidence based, and this explains why various countries have taken different approaches to addressing issues of reprocessing instruments. In January 2001, the British government spent the equivalent of $300 million to improve reprocessing techniques in Central Sterilization Services and required the use of disposable instruments for tonsillectomies. The French Public Health Office published its recommendations on 14 March 2001. They require all surgical instruments with potential exposure to lymphatic tissue, the central nervous system, or the eyes to be soaked in sodium hypochlorite for 1 h or NaOH for 1 h and sterilized at 134°C for 18 min. If instruments do not tolerate this aggressive approach, they must be cleaned twice, treated with various chemicals such as peracetic acid, or iodophors, or 3% sodium dodecyl sulfate, or 6 M urea and autoclaved at 121°C for 30 min. Since 2002, Switzerland requires all surgical instruments to be sterilized at 134°C for 18 min. The background of the Swiss recommendation is that the usual rendering process for carcasses, which was discontinued, resulted in only a 1-log-unit reduction of the infectious particles (259). Therefore, a reduction in the number of infectious particles may suffice to stop transmission. CDC recommends that instruments exposed to potentially prion contaminated items be autoclaved for 1 to 1.5 h at 132 to 134°C, immersed in 1 N sodium hydroxide for 1 h at room temperature, or immersed in sodium hypochlorite 0.5% (at least 2% free chlorine) for 2 h at room temperature. (See the CDC website for further information: http://www.cdc.gov/ncidod/dvrd/vcjd/index.htm). However, these recommendations are not based on what is known about the agent of vCJD.

In the United States, one patient who was a former resident of the United Kingdom has been diagnosed with vCJD and the first case of BSE in cattle was identified in 2003. However, more cases may occur because 37 tons of "meals of meat or offal" that were "unfit for human consumption" was sent from the United Kingdom to the United States in 1997, well after the government banned imports of such risky meat (61).

High-risk patients are patients with suspected CJD and their family members, patients treated with pituitary extracts, and patients who received cornea transplants.

In addition, items should be considered contaminated with prions if a brain biopsy for the diagnosis of CJD is requested. Instruments used in such procedures should be discarded or placed under quarantine until the histopathological diagnosis is known. The incidence of vCJD in the United Kingdom is decreasing rapidly, indicating that current reprocessing techniques suffice. However, knowledge about this topic is increasing rapidly over time and our current understanding may be shown to be false in the future (25). In May 2005, British officials published an excellent assessment of the risk for contaminating surgical instruments with prions (http://www.dh.gov.uk/assetRoot/04/11/35/42/04113542.pdf). The key observation in this report is that on average 0.2 mg of protein remains on surgical instruments despite "standard cleaning and disinfection," which was sufficient to cause an experimental case of CJD. Therefore, more research and new methods of cleaning and disinfection are needed for surgical instruments. The reader is referred to the home pages of the CDC, the FDA, and the WHO to obtain the most recent updates on this topic. In addition, the Society for Healthcare Epidemiology of America published detailed guidelines on this topic (229). More information about prions can be found in chapter 107 of this *Manual.*

REFERENCES

1. **ADA Council on Scientific Affairs and ADA Council on Dental Practice.** 1996. Infection control recommendations for the dental office and the dental laboratory. *J. Am. Dent. Assoc.* **127:**672–680.

2. **Adams, B. G., and T. J. Marrie.** 1982. Hand carriage of aerobic gram-negative rods may not be transient. *J. Hyg. (London)* **89:**33–46.

3. **Agerton, T., S. Valway, B. Gore, C. Pozsik, B. Plikaytis, C. Woodley, and I. Onorato.** 1997. Transmission of a highly drug-resistant strain (strain W1) of *Mycobacterium tuberculosis.* Community outbreak and nosocomial transmission via a contaminated bronchoscope. *JAMA* **278:**1073–1077.

4. **Aguzzi, A., and M. Glatzel.** 2004. vCJD tissue distribution and transmission by transfusion—a worst-case scenario coming true? *Lancet* **363:**411–412.

5. **Aguzzi, A., and C. Weissmann.** 1998. Spongiform encephalopathies. The prion's perplexing persistence. *Nature* **392:**763–764.

6. **Aiello, A. E., and E. Larson.** 2003. Antibacterial cleaning and hygiene products as an emerging risk factor for antibiotic resistance in the community. *Lancet Infect. Dis.* **3:**501–506.

7. **Akamatsu, T., K. Tabata, M. Hironaga, and M. Uyeda.** 1997. Evaluation of the efficacy of a 3.2% glutaraldehyde product for disinfection of fibreoptic endoscopes with an automatic machine. *J. Hosp. Infect.* **35:**47–57.

8. **Akbar-Khanzadeh, F., M. U. Vaquerano, M. Akbar-Khanzadeh, and M. S. Bisesi.** 1994. Formaldehyde exposure, acute pulmonary response, and exposure control options in a gross anatomy laboratory. *Am. J. Ind. Med.* **26:**61–75.

9. **Alasri, A., C. Roques, G. Michel, C. Cabassud, and P. Aptel.** 1992. Bactericidal properties of peracetic acid and hydrogen peroxide, alone and in combination, and chlorine and formaldehyde against bacterial water strains. *Can. J. Microbiol.* **38:**635–642.

10. **Alasri, A., M. Valverde, C. Roques, G. Michel, C. Cabassud, and P. Aptel.** 1993. Sporocidal properties of peracetic acid and hydrogen peroxide, alone and in combination, in comparison with chlorine and formaldehyde for ultrafiltration membrane disinfection. *Can. J. Microbiol.* **39:**52–60.

11. **Alfa, M. J., P. DeGagne, and N. Olson.** 1997. Bacterial killing ability of 10% ethylene oxide plus 90% hydrochlorofluorocarbon sterilizing gas. *Infect. Control. Hosp. Epidemiol.* **18:**641–645.

12. **Alvarado, C. J., M. Reichelderfer, et al.** 2000. APIC guideline for infection prevention and control in flexible endoscopy. *Am. J. Infect. Control* **28:**138–155.

13. **Anderson, R. L., R. W. Vess, A. L. Panlilio, and M. S. Favero.** 1990. Prolonged survival of *Pseudomonas cepacia* in commercially manufactured povidone-iodine. *Appl. Environ. Microbiol.* **56:**3598–3600.

14. **Anonymous.** 1994. Tentative final monograph for health-care antiseptic drug products. *Fed. Regist* **59:**31401–31452.

15. **Ansari, S. A., S. A. Sattar, V. S. Springthorpe, G. A. Wells, and W. Tostowaryk.** 1989. In vivo protocol for testing efficacy of hand-washing agents against viruses and bacteria: experiments with rotavirus and *Escherichia coli. Appl. Environ. Microbiol.* **55:**3113–3118.

16. **Arata, T., T. Murakami, and Y. Hirai.** 1993. Evaluation of povidone-iodine alcoholic solution for operative site disinfection. *Postgrad. Med. J.* **69** (Suppl. 3)**:**S93–S96.

17. **Archibald, L. K., A. Corl, B. Shah, M. Schulte, M. J. Arduino, S. Aguero, D. J. Fisher, B. W. Stechenberg, S. N. Banerjee, and W. R. Jarvis.** 1997. *Serratia marcescens* outbreak associated with extrinsic contamination of 1% chlorxylenol soap. *Infect Control. Hosp. Epidemiol.* **18:**704–709.

18. **Arnon, S. S., R. Schechter, T. V. Inglesby, D. A. Henderson, J. G. Bartlett, M. S. Ascher, E. Eitzen, A. D. Fine, J. Hauer, M. Layton, S. Lillibridge, M. T. Osterholm, T. O'Toole, G. Parker, T. M. Perl, P. K. Russell, D. L. Swerdlow, and K. Tonat.** 2001. Botulinum toxin as a biological weapon: medical and public health management. *JAMA* **285:**1059–1070.

19. **Ascenzi, J. M.** 1996. Glutaraldehyde-based disinfectants, p. 111–132. In J. P. Ascenzi (ed.), *Handbook of Disinfectants and Antiseptics.* Marcel Dekker, Inc. New York, NY.

20. **Astagneau, P., N. Desplaces, V. Vincent, V. Chicheportiche, A. Botherel, S. Maugat, K. Lebascle, P. Leonard, J. Desenclos, J. Grosset, J. Ziza, and G. Brucker.** 2001. *Mycobacterium xenopi* spinal infections after discovertebral surgery: investigation and screening of a large outbreak. *Lancet* **358:**747–751.

21. **Axon, A., M. Jung, A. Kruse, T. Ponchon, J. F. Rey, U. Beilenhoff, D. Duforest-Rey, C. Neumann, M. Pietsch, K. Roth, A. Papoz, D. Wilson, I. Kircher-Felgenstreff, M. Stief, R. Blum, K. B. Spencer, J. Mills, E. P. Mart, B. Slowey, H. Biering, U. Lorenz, et al.** 2000. The European Society of Gastrointestinal Endoscopy (ESGE): check list for the purchase of washer-disinfectors for flexible endoscopes. *Endoscopy* **32:**914–919.

22. **Bagg, J., C. P. Sweeney, K. M. Roy, T. Sharp, and A. Smith.** 2001. Cross infection control measures and the treatment of patients at risk of Creutzfeldt Jakob disease in UK general dental practice. *Br. Dent. J.* **191:**87–90.

23. **Beilenhoff, U., C. S. Neumann, J. F. Rey, H. Biering, R. Blum, M. Cimbro, B. Kampf, M. Rogers, and V. Schmidt.** 2008. ESGE-ESGENA guideline: cleaning and disinfection in gastrointestinal endoscopy. *Endoscopy* **40:**939–957.

24. **Beiswanger, B. B., M. E. Mallatt, M. S. Mau, R. D. Jackson, and D. K. Hennon.** 1990. The clinical effects of a mouthrinse containing 0. 1% octenidine. *J. Dent. Res.* **69:**454–457.

25. **Belay, E. D., and L. B. Schonberger.** 2005. The public health impact of prion diseases. *Annu. Rev. Public Health* **26:**191–212.

26. **Bellamy, K., R. Alcock, J. R. Babb, J. G. Davies, and G. A. Ayliffe.** 1993. A test for the assessment of 'hygienic' hand disinfection using rotavirus. *J. Hosp. Infect.* **24:**201–210.

27. **Berkelman, R. L., B. W. Holland, and R. L. Anderson.** 1982. Increased bactericidal activity of dilute preparations of povidone-iodine solutions. *J. Clin. Microbiol.* **15:**635–639.

28. **Berkelman, R. L., S. Lewin, J. R. Allen, R. L. Anderson, L. D. Budnick, S. Shapiro, S. M. Friedman, P. Nicholas, R. S. Holzman, and R. W. Haley.** 1981. Pseudobacteremia attributed to contamination of povidone-iodine with *Pseudomonas cepacia. Ann. Intern. Med* **95:**32–36.

29. **Biron, F., B. Verrier, and D. Peyramond.** 1997. Transmission of the human immunodeficiency virus and the hepatitis C virus. *N. Engl. J. Med.* **337:**348–349.

30. **Blanc, D. S., I. Nahimana, C. Petignat, A. Wenger, J. Bille, and P. Francioli.** 2004. Faucets as a reservoir of endemic *Pseudomonas aeruginosa* colonization/infections in intensive care units. *Intensive Care Med.* **30:**1964–1968.

31. **Blanc, D. S., T. Parret, B. Janin, P. Raselli, and P. Francioli.** 1997. Nosocomial infections and pseudoinfections from contaminated bronchoscopes: two-year follow up using molecular markers. *Infect. Control. Hosp. Epidemiol.* **18:**134–136.

32. **Blattler, T., S. Brandner, A. J. Raeber, M. A. Klein, T. Voigtlander, C. Weissmann, and A. Aguzzi.** 1997. PrP-expressing tissue required for transfer of scrapie infectivity from spleen to brain. *Nature* **389:**69–73.

33. **Block, S. S.** 2001. *Disinfection, Sterilization, and Preservation.* Lippincott Williams & Wilkins, Philadelphia, PA.

34. **Bond, W. W., M. S. Favero, N. J. Petersen, and J. W. Ebert.** 1983. Inactivation of hepatitis B virus by intermediate-to-high-level disinfectant chemicals. *J. Clin. Microbiol.* **18:**535–538.

35 **Borchardt, M. A., P. D. Bertz, S. K. Spencer, and D. A. Battigelli.** 2003. Incidence of enteric viruses in groundwater from household wells in Wisconsin. *Appl. Environ. Microbiol.* **69:**1172–1180.

36. **Bosi, C., A. Davin-Regli, R. Charrel, B. Rocca, D. Monnet, and C. Bollet.** 1996. *Serratia marcescens* nosocomial outbreak due to contamination of hexetidine solution. *J. Hosp. Infect.* **33:**217–224.

37. **Bou, R., A. Aguilar, J. Perpinan, P. Ramos, M. Peris, L. Lorente, and A. Zuniga.** 2006. Nosocomial outbreak of *Pseudomonas aeruginosa* infections related to a flexible bronchoscope. *J. Hosp. Infect.* **64:**129–135.

38. **Bowie, J. H., M. H. Kennedy, and I. Robertson.** 1975. Improved Bowie and Dick test. *Lancet* **1:**1135.

39. **Boyce, J. M., and M. L. Pearson.** 2003. Low frequency of fires from alcohol-based hand rub dispensers in healthcare facilities. *Infect. Control Hosp. Epidemiol.* **24:**618–619.

40. **Boyce, J. M., and D. Pittet.** 2002. Guideline for hand hygiene in health-care settings: recommendations of the Health-care Infection Control Practices Advisory Committee and the HICPAC/SHEA/APIC/IDSA Hand Hygiene Task Force. *Infect. Control Hosp. Epidemiol.* **23:**S3–S40.

41. **Boyce, J. M., G. Potter-Bynoe, S. M. Opal, L. Dziobek, and A. A. Medeiros.** 1990. A common-source outbreak of *Staphylococcus epidermidis* infections among patients undergoing cardiac surgery. *J. Infect. Dis.* **161:**493–499.

42. **Bradley, C. R., J. R. Babb, and G. A. Ayliffe.** 1995. Evaluation of the Steris System 1 peracetic acid endoscope processor. *J. Hosp. Infect.* **29:**143–151.

43. **Bradley, C. R., and A. P. Fraise.** 1996. Heat and chemical resistance of enterococci. *J. Hosp. Infect.* **34:**191–196.

44. **Brady, M. J., C. M. Lisay, A. V. Yurkovetskiy, and S. P. Sawan.** 2003. Persistent silver disinfectant for the environmental control of pathogenic bacteria. *Am. J. Infect. Control* **31:**208–214.

45. **Broadley, S. J., J. R. Furr, P. A. Jenkins, and A. D. Russell.** 1993. Antimycobacterial activity of 'Virkon'. *J. Hosp. Infect.* **23:**189–197.

46. **Bronowicki, J. P., V. Venard, C. Botte, N. Monhoven, I. Gastin, L. Chone, H. Hudziak, B. Rhin, C. Delanoe, A. LeFaou, M. A. Bigard, and P. Gaucher.** 1997. Patient-to-patient transmission of hepatitis C virus during colonoscopy. *N. Engl. J. Med.* **337:**237–240.

47. **Brown, P.** 2001. Bovine spongiform encephalopathy and variant Creutzfeldt-Jakob disease. *BMJ* **322:**841–844.

48. **Brown, P., P. P. Liberski, A. Wolff, and D. C. Gajdusek.** 1990. Resistance of scrapie infectivity to steam autoclaving after formaldehyde fixation and limited survival after ashing at 360 degrees C: practical and theoretical implications. *J. Infect. Dis.* **161:**467–472.

49. **Bruce, M. E., R. G. Will, J. W. Ironside, I. McConnell, D. Drummond, A. Suttie, L. McCardle, A. Chree, J. Hope, C. Birkett, S. Cousens, H. Fraser, and C. J. Bostock.** 1997. Transmissions to mice indicate that 'new variant' CJD is caused by the BSE agent. *Nature* **389:**498–501.

50. **Bryant, W. P., and D. Zimmerman.** 1995. Iodine-induced hyperthyroidism in a newborn. *Pediatrics* **95:**434–436.

51. **Bryce, E. A., F. J. Roberts, B. Clements, and S. MacLean.** 1997. When the biological indicator is positive: investigating autoclave failures. *Infect. Control. Hosp. Epidemiol.* **18:**654–656.

52. **Centers for Disease Control.** 1995. Management of Patients with Suspected Viral Hemorrhagic Fever—United States. *MMWR. Morb. Mortal. Wkly. Rep.* **44:**475–479.

53. **Centers for Disease Control and Prevention.** 1999. Bronchoscopy-related infections and pseudoinfections—New York, 1996 and 1998. *MMWR Morb. Mortal. Wkly. Rep.* **48:**557–560.

54. **Centers for Disease Control and Prevention.** 2001. Protracted outbreaks of cryptosporidiosis associated with swimming pool use—Ohio and Nebraska, 2000. *MMWR Morb. Mortal. Wkly. Rep.* **50:**406–410.

55. **Centers for Disease Control and Prevention.** 1989. Guidelines for prevention of transmission of human immunodeficiency virus and hepatitis B virus to health-care and public-safety workers. *MMWR. Morb. Mortal. Wkly. Rep.* **38** (Suppl. 6):1–37.

56. **Centers for Disease Control and Prevention.** 1996. Community-level prevention of human immunodeficiency virus infection among high-risk populations: the AIDS community demonstration projects. *MMWR Recommend. Rep.* **45**(RR-6):1–31.

57. **Centers for Disease Control and Prevention.** 1993. Recommended infection-control practices for dentistry. *MMWR. Morb. Mortal. Wkly. Rep.* **42:**1–12.

58. **Cetinkaya, Y., P. Falk, and C. G. Mayhall.** 2000. Vancomycin-resistant enterococci. *Clin. Microbiol. Rev.* **13:**686–707.

59. **Cetre, J. C., M. C. Nicolle, H. Salord, M. Perol, S. Tigaud, G. David, M. Bourjault, and P. Vanhems.** 2005. Outbreaks of contaminated broncho-alveolar lavage related to intrinsically defective bronchoscopes. *J. Hosp. Infect.* **61:**39–45.

60. **Chamberland, M. E.** 2002. Emerging infectious agents: do they pose a risk to the safety of transfused blood and blood products? *Clin. Infect. Dis.* **34:**797–805.

61. **Charatan, F.** 2001. United States takes precautions against BSE. *West. J. Med.* **174:**235.

62. **Chazot, G., E. Broussolle, C. Lapras, T. Blattler, A. Aguzzi, and N. Kopp.** 1996. New variant of Creutzfeldt-Jakob disease in a 26-year-old French man. *Lancet* **347:**1181.

63. **Cheung, R. J., D. Ortiz, and A. J. DiMarino, Jr.** 1999. GI endoscopic reprocessing practices in the United States. *Gastrointest. Endosc.* **50:**362–368.

64. **Chitnis, V., S. Chitnis, S. Patil, and D. Chitnis.** 2004. Practical limitations of disinfection of body fluid spills with 10,000 ppm sodium hypochlorite (NaOCl). *Am. J. Infect. Control* **32:**306–308.

65. **Chuanchuen, R., K. Beinlich, T. T. Hoang, A. Becher, R. R. Karkhoff-Schweizer, and H. P. Schweizer.** 2001. Cross-resistance between triclosan and antibiotics in *Pseudomonas aeruginosa* is mediated by multidrug efflux pumps: exposure of a susceptible mutant strain to triclosan selects *nfxB* mutants overexpressing MexCD-Opr J. *Antimicrob. Agents Chemother.* **45:**428–432.

66. **Clay, S., S. Maherchandani, Y. S. Malik, and S. M. Goyal.** 2006. Survival on uncommon fomites of feline calicivirus, a surrogate of noroviruses. *Am. J. Infect. Control.* **34:**41–43.

67. **Coates, D.** 1996. Sporicidal activity of sodium dichloroisocyanurate, peroxygen and glutaraldehyde disinfectants against *Bacillus subtilis. J. Hosp. Infect.* **32:**283–294.

68. **Collins, F. M.** 1986. Bactericidal activity of alkaline glutaraldehyde solution against a number of atypical mycobacterial species. *J. Appl. Bacteriol.* **61:**247–251.

69. **Collins, F. M.** 1986. Kinetics of the tuberculocidal response by alkaline glutaraldehyde in solution and on an inert surface. *J. Appl. Bacteriol.* **61:**87–93.

70. **Collins, S. J., V. A. Lawson, and C. L. Masters.** 2004. Transmissible spongiform encephalopathies. *Lancet* **363:**51–61.

71. **Corne, P., S. Godreuil, H. Jean-Pierre, O. Jonquet, J. Campos, E. Jumas-Bilak, S. Parer, and H. Marchandin.** 2005. Unusual implication of biopsy forceps in outbreaks of *Pseudomonas aeruginosa* infections and pseudo-infections related to bronchoscopy. *J. Hosp. Infect.* **61:**20–26.

72. **Craven, D. E., B. Moody, M. G. Connolly, N. R. Kollisch, K. D. Stottmeier, and W. R. McCabe.** 1981. Pseudobacteremia caused by povidone-iodine solution contaminated with *Pseudomonas cepacia. N. Engl. J. Med.* **305:**621–623.

73. **Crow, S.** 1993. Steam sterilizers: an evolution in design. *Infect. Control. Hosp. Epidemiol.* **14:**488–490.

74. **Cruse, P. J. and R. Foord.** 1973. A five-year prospective study of 23,649 surgical wounds. *Arch. Surg.* **107:**206–210.

75. **Dancer, S. J.** 2008. Importance of the environment in meticillin-resistant *Staphylococcus aureus* acquisition: the case for hospital cleaning. *Lancet Infect. Dis.* **8:**101–113.

76. **Darouiche, R. O., M. J. Wall, Jr., K. M. Itani, M. F. Otterson, A. L. Webb, M. M. Carrick, H. J. Miller, S. S. Awad, C. T. Crosby, M. C. Mosier, A. Alsharif, and D. H. Berger.** 2010. Chlorhexidine-alcohol versus povidone-iodine for surgical-site antisepsis. *N. Engl. J. Med.* **362:**18–26.

77. **Daschner, F.** 1994. STERIS SYSTEM 1 in Germany. *Infect. Control Hosp. Epidemiol.* **15:**294, 296. (Letter and comment.)

78. **de Lassence, A., N. Hidri, J. F. Timsit, M. L. Joly-Guillou, G. Thiery, A. Boyer, P. Lable, A. Blivet, H. Kalinowski, Y. Martin, J. P. Lajonchere, and D. Dreyfuss.** 2006. Control and outcome of a large outbreak of colonization and infection with glycopeptide-intermediate *Staphylococcus aureus* in an intensive care unit. *Clin. Infect. Dis.* **42:**170–178.

79. **Dennis, D. T., T. V. Inglesby, D. A. Henderson, J. G. Bartlett, M. S. Ascher, E. Eitzen, A. D. Fine, A. M. Friedlander, J. Hauer, M. Layton, S. R. Lillibridge, J. E. McDade, M. T. Osterholm, T. O'Toole, G. Parker, T. M. Perl, P. K. Russell, and K. Tonat.** 2001. Tularemia as a biological weapon: medical and public health management. *JAMA* **285:**2763–2773.

80. **Denton, G. E.** 1991. Chlorhexidine, p. 274–289. *In* S. S. Block (ed.), *Disinfection, Sterilization and Preservation.* Lea & Febiger, Philadelphia, PA.

81. **Dettenkofer, M., C. Wilson, A. Gratwohl, C. Schmoor, H. Bertz, R. Frei, D. Heim, S. Luft, S. Schulz, and A. F. Widmer.** 2010. Skin disinfection with octenidine dihydrochloride for central venous catheter site care: a double-blind, randomized, controlled trial. *Clin. Microbiol. Infect.* **16:**600–606.

82. **Deva, A. K., K. Vickery, J. Zou, R. H. West, J. P. Harris, and Y. E. Cossart.** 1996. Establishment of an in-use testing method for evaluating disinfection of surgical instruments using the duck hepatitis B model. *J. Hosp. Infect.* **33:**119–130.

83. **Dharan, S., P. Mourouga, P. Copin, G. Bessmer, B. Tschanz, and D. Pittet.** 1999. Routine disinfection of patients' environmental surfaces. Myth or reality? *J. Hosp. Infect.* **42:**113–117.

84. **DiazGranados, C. A., M. Y. Jones, T. Kongphet-Tran, N. White, M. Shapiro, Y. F. Wang, S. M. Ray, and H. M. Blumberg.** 2009. Outbreak of *Pseudomonas aeruginosa* infection associated with contamination of a flexible bronchoscope. *Infect. Control Hosp. Epidemiol.* **30:**550–555.

85. **Disch, K.** 1994. Glucoprotamine—a new antimicrobial substance. *Zentralbl. Hyg. Umweltmed.* **195:**357–365.

86. **Doebbeling, B. N., G. L. Stanley, C. T. Sheetz, M. A. Pfaller, A. K. Houston, L. Annis, N. Li, and R. P. Wenzel.** 1992. Comparative efficacy of alternative hand-washing agents in reducing nosocomial infections in intensive care units. *N. Engl. J. Med.* **327:**88–93.

87. **Dolce, P., M. Gourdeau, N. April, and P. M. Bernard.** 1995. Outbreak of glutaraldehyde-induced proctocolitis. *Am. J. Infect. Control* **23:**34–39.

88. **Dormont, D.** 1996. How to limit the spread of Creutzfeldt-Jakob disease. *Infect. Control Hosp. Epidemiol.* **17:**521–528.

89. **Druce, J. D., D. Jardine, S. A. Locarnini, and C. J. Birch.** 1995. Susceptibility of HIV to inactivation by disinfectants and ultraviolet light. *J. Hosp. Infect.* **30:**167–180.

90. **Evans, R. J.** 1992. Acute anaphylaxis due to topical chlorhexidine acetate. *BMJ* **304:**686.

91. **Farina, A., M. H. Fievet, F. Plassart, M. C. Menet, and A. Thuillier.** 1999. Residual glutaraldehyde levels in fiberoptic endoscopes: measurement and implications for patient toxicity. *J. Hosp. Infect.* **43:**293–297.

92. **Favero, M. S.** 1991. Strategies for disinfection and sterilization of endoscopes: the gap between basic principles and actual practice. *Infect. Control Hosp. Epidemiol.* **12:**279–281.

93. **Favero, M. S., and F. A. Manian.** 1993. Is eliminating flash sterilization practical? *Infect. Control Hosp. Epidemiol.* **14:**479–480.

94. Feldman, H. I., M. Kinosian, W. B. Bilker, C. Simmons, J. H. Holmes, M. V. Pauly, and J. J. Escarce. 1996. Effect of dialyzer reuse on survival of patients treated with hemodialysis. *JAMA* **276:**1724.

95. Fenner, L., A. F. Widmer, A. Stranden, M. Conzelmann, A. Goorhuis, C. Harmanus, E. J. Kuijper, and R. Frei. 2008. First cluster of clindamycin-resistant *Clostridium difficile* PCR ribotype 027 in Switzerland. *Clin. Microbiol. Infect.* **14:**514–515.

96. Fichet, G., E. Comoy, C. Duval, K. Antloga, C. Dehen, A. Charbonnier, G. McDonnell, P. Brown, C. I. Lasmezas, and J. P. Deslys. 2004. Novel methods for disinfection of prion-contaminated medical devices. *Lancet* **364:**521–526.

97. Flynn, N., S. Jain, E. M. Keddie, J. R. Carlson, M. B. Jennings, H. W. Haverkos, N. Nassar, R. Anderson, S. Cohen, and D. Goldberg. 1994. In vitro activity of readily available household materials against HIV-1: is bleach enough? *J. Acquir. Immune. Defic. Syndr.* **7:**747–753.

98. Fraise, A. P., P. A. Lambert, and J. Y. Maillard. 2004. *Russell, Hugo and Ayliffe's Principles and Practice of Disinfection, Preservation and Sterilization.* Blackwell Publishing, Malden, MA.

99. Frank, M. J., and W. Schaffner. 1976. Contaminated aqueous benzalkonium chloride. An unnecessary hospital infection hazard. *JAMA* **236:**2418–2419.

100. Fraser, T. G., S. Reiner, M. Malczynski, P. R. Yarnold, J. Warren, and G. A. Noskin. 2004. Multidrug-resistant *Pseudomonas aeruginosa* cholangitis after endoscopic retrograde cholangiopancreatography: failure of routine endoscope cultures to prevent an outbreak. *Infect. Control Hosp. Epidemiol.* **25:**856–859.

101. Fraser, V. J., G. Zuckerman, R. E. Clouse, S. O'Rourke, M. Jones, J. Klasner, and P. Murray. 1993. A prospective randomized trial comparing manual and automated endoscope disinfection methods. *Infect. Control Hosp. Epidemiol.* **14:**383–389.

102. Fraud, S., J. Y. Maillard, and A. D. Russell. 2001. Comparison of the mycobactericidal activity of ortho-phthalaldehyde, glutaraldehyde and other dialdehydes by a quantitative suspension test. *J. Hosp. Infect.* **48:**214–221.

103. Furuhashi, M., and T. Miyamae. 1979. Effect of pre-operative hand scrubbing and influence of pinholes appearing in surgical rubber gloves during operation. *Bull. Tokyo. Med. Dent. Univ.* **26:**73–80.

104. Fuselier, H. A. J., and C. Mason. 1997. Liquid sterilization versus high level disinfection in the urologic office. *Urology.* **50:**337–340.

105. Fuursted, K., A. Hjort, and L. Knudsen. 1997. Evaluation of bactericidal activity and lag of regrowth (postantibiotic effect) of five antiseptics on nine bacterial pathogens. *J. Antimicrob. Chemother.* **40:**221–226.

106. Gamage, B., D. Moore, R. Copes, A. Yassi, and E. Bryce. 2005. Protecting HCWs from SARS and other respiratory pathogens: a review of the infection control literature. *Am. J. Infect. Control* **33:**114–121.

107. Garibaldi, R. A., D. Skolnick, T. Lerer, A. Poirot, J. Graham, E. Krisuinas, and R. Lyons. 1988. The impact of preoperative skin disinfection on preventing intraoperative wound contamination. *Infect. Control Hosp. Epidemiol.* **9:**109–113.

108. Gelinas, P., J. Goulet, G. M. Tastayre, and G. A. Picard. 1991. Effect of temperature and contact time on the activity of eight disinfectants—a classification. *J. Food Prot.* **47:**841–847.

109. Georgiade, G., R. Riefkohl, N. Georgiade, R. Georgiade, and M. F. Wildman. 1985. Efficacy of povidone-iodine in pre-operative skin preparation. *J Hosp. Infect* **6** (Suppl. A):67–71.

110. Ghannoum, M. A., K. A. Elteen, M. Ellabib, and P. A. Whittaker. 1990. Antimycotic effects of octenidine and pirtenidine. *J. Antimicrob. Chemother.* **25:**237–245.

111. Gillespie, T. G., L. Hogg, E. Budge, A. Duncan, and J. E. Coia. 2000. *Mycobacterium chelonae* isolated from rinse water within an endoscope washer-disinfector. *J. Hosp. Infect.* **45:**332–334.

112. Glatzel, M., K. Stoeck, H. Seeger, T. Luhrs, and A. Aguzzi. 2005. Human prion diseases: molecular and clinical aspects. *Arch. Neurol.* **62:**545–552.

113. Gorse, G. J., and R. L. Messner. 1991. Infection control practices in gastrointestinal endoscopy in the United States: a national survey. *Infect. Control Hosp. Epidemiol.* **12:**289–296.

114. Gottardi, W. 1991. Iodine and iodine compounds, p. 152–166. *In* S. S. Block (ed.), *Disinfection, Sterilization and Preservation.* Lea & Febiger, Philadelphia.

115. Graham, G. S. 1997. Decontamination: scientific principles, p. 1–9. *In* M. Reichert and J. H. Young (ed.), *Sterilization Technology.* Aspen Publishers, Gaithersburg, MD.

116. Griffiths, P. A., J. R. Babb, C. R. Bradley, and A. P. Fraise. 1997. Glutaraldehyde-resistant *Mycobacterium chelonae* from endoscope washer disinfectors. *J. Appl. Microbiol.* **82:**519–526.

117. Gubler, J. G., M. Salfinger, and A. von Graevenitz. 1992. Pseudoepidemic of nontuberculous mycobacteria due to a contaminated bronchoscope cleaning machine. Report of an outbreak and review of the literature. *Chest* **101:**1245–1249.

118. Gurevich, I., R. Dubin, and B. A. Cunha. 1996. Dental instrument and device sterilization and disinfection practices. *J. Hosp. Infect.* **32:**295–304.

119. Gurevich, I., S. M. Qadri, and B. A. Cunha. 1993. False-positive results of spore tests from improper clip use with the STERIS chemical sterilant system. *Am. J. Infect. Control.* **21:**42–43.

120. Gurevich, I., P. Tafuro, P. Ristuccia, J. Herrmann, A. R. Young, and B. A. Cunha. 1983. Disinfection of respirator tubing: a comparison of chemical versus hot water machine-assisted processing. *J. Hosp. Infect.* **4:**199–208.

121. Hall, C. B., and R. G. Douglas, Jr. 1981. Modes of transmission of respiratory syncytial virus. *J. Pediatr.* **99:**100–103.

122. Hamilton, E., D. V. Seal, and J. Hay. 1996. Comparison of chlorine and chlorine dioxide disinfection for control of *Legionella* in a hospital potable water supply. *J Hosp. Infect* **32:**156–160.

123. Hanson, P. J., D. Gor, J. R. Clarke, M. V. Chadwick, B. Gazzard, D. J. Jeffries, H. Gaya, and J. V. Collins. 1991. Recovery of the human immunodeficiency virus from fibre-optic bronchoscopes. *Thorax* **46:**410–412.

124. Hanson, P. J., D. J. Jeffries, and J. V. Collins. 1991. Viral transmission and fibreoptic endoscopy. *J. Hosp. Infect.* **18** (Suppl. A):136–140.

125. Heikenwalder, M., N. Zeller, H. Seeger, M. Prinz, P. C. Klohn, P. Schwarz, N. H. Ruddle, C. Weissmann, and A. Aguzzi. 2005. Chronic lymphocytic inflammation specifies the organ tropism of prions. *Science* **307:**1107–1110.

126. Held, P. J., R. A. Wolfe, D. S. Gaylin, F. K. Port, N. W. Levin, and M. N. Turenne. 1994. Analysis of the association of dialyzer reuse practices and patient outcomes. *Am. J. Kidney Dis.* **23:**692–708.

127. Helms, C. M., R. M. Massanari, R. P. Wenzel, M. A. Pfaller, N. P. Moyer, and N. Hall. 1988. Legionnaires' disease associated with a hospital water system. A five-year progress report on continuous hyperchlorination. *JAMA* **259:**2423–2427.

128. Henderson, D. A., T. V. Inglesby, J. G. Bartlett, M. S. Ascher, E. Eitzen, P. B. Jahrling, J. Hauer, M. Layton, J. McDade, M. T. Osterholm, T. O'Toole, G. Parker, T. Perl, P. K. Russell, K. Tonat, et al. 1999. Smallpox as a biological weapon: medical and public health management. *JAMA* **281:**2127–2137.

129. Herzog, C., N. Sales, N. Etchegaray, A. Charbonnier, S. Freire, D. Dormont, J. P. Deslys, and C. I. Lasmezas. 2004. Tissue distribution of bovine spongiform encephalopathy agent in primates after intravenous or oral infection. *Lancet* **363:**422–428.

130. Hill, A. F., M. Desbruslais, S. Joiner, K. C. Sidle, I. Gowland, J. Collinge, L. J. Doey, and P. Lantos. 1997. The same prion strain causes vCJD and BSE. *Nature* **389:**448–450.

131. Holmes, K. V. 2003. SARS-associated coronavirus. *N. Engl. J. Med.* **348:**1948–1951.

132. **Holton, J., and N. Shetty.** 1997. In-use stability of Nu-Cidex. *J. Hosp. Infect* **35:**245–248.

133. **Houston, F., J. D. Foster, A. Chong, N. Hunter, and C. J. Bostock.** 2000. Transmission of BSE by blood transfusion in sheep. *Lancet* **356:**999–1000.

134. **Hughes, R., and S. Kilvington.** 2001. Comparison of hydrogen peroxide contact lens disinfection systems and solutions against *Acanthamoeba polyphaga. Antimicrob. Agents Chemother.* **45:**2038–2043.

135. **Hussaini, S. N., and K. R. Ruby.** 1976. Sporicidal activity of peracetic acid against *B. anthracis* spores. *Vet. Rec.* **98:**257–259.

136. **Im, S. W., J. P. Fung, S. Y. So, and D. Y. Yu.** 1982. Unusual dissemination of pseudomonads by ventilators. *Anaesthesia* **37:**1074–1077.

137. **Inglesby, T. V., D. T. Dennis, D. A. Henderson, J. G. Bartlett, M. S. Ascher, E. Eitzen, A. D. Fine, A. M. Friedlander, J. Hauer, J. F. Koerner, M. Layton, J. McDade, M. T. Osterholm, T. O'Toole, G. Parker, T. M. Perl, P. K. Russell, M. Schoch-Spana, K. Tonat, et al.** 2000. Plague as a biological weapon: medical and public health management. *JAMA* **283:**2281–2290.

138. **Inglesby, T. V., D. A. Henderson, J. G. Bartlett, M. S. Ascher, E. Eitzen, A. M. Friedlander, J. Hauer, J. McDade, M. T. Osterholm, T. O'Toole, G. Parker, T. M. Perl, P. K. Russell, K. Tonat, et al.** 1999. Anthrax as a biological weapon: medical and public health management. *JAMA* **281:**1735–1745.

139. **Isenberg, S. J., L. Apt, and M. Wood.** 1995. A controlled trial of povidone-iodine as prophylaxis against ophthalmia neonatorum. *N. Engl. J. Med.* **332:**562–566.

140. **Jackson, J., J. E. Leggett, D. A. Wilson, and D. N. Gilbert.** 1996. *Mycobacterium gordonae* in fiberoptic bronchoscopes. *Am. J. Infect. Control.* **24:**19–23.

141. **Jones, R. D., H. B. Jampani, J. L. Newman, and A. S. Lee.** 2000. Triclosan: a review of effectiveness and safety in health care settings. *Am. J. Infect Control* **28:**184–196.

142. **Joslyn, L. J.** 1991. Sterilization by heat, p. 495–526. *In* S. S. Block (ed.), *Disinfection, Sterilization and Preservation.* Lea & Febiger, Philadelphia, PA.

143. **Kaatz, G. W., S. D. Gitlin, D. R. Schaberg, K. H. Wilson, C. A. Kauffman, S. M. Seo, and R. Fekety.** 1988. Acquisition of *Clostridium difficile* from the hospital environment. *Am. J. Epidemiol.* **127:**1289–1293.

144. **Kaczmarek, R. G., R. M. J. Moore, J. McCrohan, D. A. Goldmann, C. Reynolds, C. Caquelin, and E. Israel.** 1992. Multi-state investigation of the actual disinfection/sterilization of endoscopes in health care facilities. *Am. J. Med.* **92:**257–261.

145. **Kampf, G., R. Bloss, and H. Martiny.** 2004. Surface fixation of dried blood by glutaraldehyde and peracetic acid. *J. Hosp. Infect.* **57:**139–143.

146. **Kampf, G., and A. Kramer.** 2004. Epidemiologic background of hand hygiene and evaluation of the most important agents for scrubs and rubs. *Clin. Microbiol. Rev.* **17:**863–893.

147. **Kampf, G., C. Ostermeyer, and P. Heeg.** 2005. Surgical hand disinfection with a propanol-based hand rub: equivalence of shorter application times. *J. Hosp. Infect.* **59:**304–310.

148. **Karol, M. H.** 1995. Toxicologic principles do not support the banning of chlorine. A Society of Toxicology position paper. *Fundam. Appl. Toxicol.* **24:**1–2.

149. **Kawashima, T., H. Furukawa, K. Doh-ura, and T. Iwaki.** 1997. Diagnosis of new variant Creutzfeldt-Jakob disease by tonsil biopsy. *Lancet* **350:**68–69.

150. **Khanna, N., D. Goldenberger, P. Graber, M. Battegay, and A. F. Widmer.** 2003. Gastroenteritis outbreak with norovirus in a Swiss university hospital with a newly identified virus strain. *J. Hosp. Infect.* **55:**131–136.

151. **Klein, M., and A. DeForest.** 1963. The inactivation of viruses by germicides. *Chem. Specialists Manuf. Assoc. Proc.* **49:**116–118.

152. **Klein, M. A., R. Frigg, E. Flechsig, A. J. Raeber, U. Kalinke, H. Bluethman, F. Bootz, J. Suter, R. M. Zinkernagel, and A. Aguzzi.** 1997. A crucial role for B cells in neuroinvasive scrapie. *Nature* **390:**687.

153. **Kobayashi, H., M. Tsuzuki, K. Koshimizu, H. Toyama, N. Yoshihara, T. Shikata, K. Abe, K. Mizuno, N. Otomo, and T. Oda.** 1984. Susceptibility of hepatitis B virus to disinfectants or heat. *J. Clin. Microbiol.* **20:**214–216.

154. **Kool, J. L., J. C. Carpenter, and B. S. Fields.** 1999. Effect of monochloramine disinfection of municipal drinking water on risk of nosocomial Legionnaires' disease. *Lancet* **353:**272–277.

155. **Kralovic, R. C.** 1993. Use of biological indicators designed for steam or ethylene oxide to monitor a liquid chemical sterilization process. Infect. Control Hosp. Epidemiol. **14:**313–319.

156. **Kramer, A., P. Rudolph, G. Kampf, and D. Pittet.** 2002. Limited efficacy of alcohol-based hand gels. *Lancet* **359:**1489–1490.

157. **Kurtz, J. B., T. W. Lee, and A. J. Parsons.** 1980. The action of alcohols on rotavirus, astrovirus and enterovirus. *J. Hosp. Infect.* **1:**321–325.

158. **Lai, M. Y., P. K. Cheng, and W. W. Lim.** 2005. Survival of severe acute respiratory syndrome coronavirus. *Clin. Infect. Dis.* **41:**e67–e71.

159. **Larson, E.** 1988. Guideline for use of topical antimicrobial agents. *Am. J. Infect. Control.* **16:**253–266.

160. **Larson, E. L.** 1991. Alcohols, p. 191–203. *In* S. S. Block (ed.), *Disinfection, Sterilization and Preservation.* Lea & Febiger, Philadelphia, PA.

161. **Larson, E. L., A. M. Butz, D. L. Gullette, and B. A. Laughon.** 1990. Alcohol for surgical scrubbing? *Infect. Control. Hosp. Epidemiol.* **11:**139–143.

162. **Leaper, S.** 1984. Influence of temperature on the synergistic sporicidal effect of peracetic acid plus hydrogen peroxide in *Bacillus subtilis* SA22 (NCA 72–52). *Food Microbiol* **1:**199–203.

163. **Levenson, J. E.** 1989. Corneal damage from improperly cleaned tonometer tips. *Arch. Ophthalmol.* **107:**1117.

164. **Lever, A. M., and S. V. W. Sutton.** 1996. Antimicrobial effects of hydrogen peroxide as an antiseptic and disinfectant, p. 159–176. *In* J. P. Ascenzi (ed.), *Handbook of Disinfectants and Antiseptics.* Marcel Dekker, Inc., New York, NY.

165. **Lowbury, E. J., and H. A. Lilly.** 1974. The effect of blood on disinfection of surgeons' hands. *Br. J. Surg.* **61:**19–21.

166. **Lowbury, E. J., H. A. Lilly, and J. P. Bull.** 1964. Methods for disinfection of operation sites. *Br. Med. J.* **2:**531–533.

167. **Maillard, J. Y.** 2002. Bacterial target sites for biocide action. *J. Appl. Microbiol.* **92** (Suppl.):16S–27S.

168. **Maki, D. G., and C. A. Hassemer.** 1987. Flash sterilization: carefully measured haste. *Infect. Control* **8:**307–310.

169. **Maki, D. G., S. M. Stolz, S. Wheeler, and L. A. Mermel.** 1997. Prevention of central venous catheter-related bloodstream infection by use of an antiseptic-impregnated catheter. A randomized, controlled trial. *Ann. Intern. Med.* **127:**257–266.

170. **Mangram, A. J., T. C. Horan, M. L. Pearson, L. C. Silver, W. R. Jarvis, et al.** 1999. Guideline for prevention of surgical site infection, 1999. *Infect. Control Hosp. Epidemiol.* **20:**250–278.

171. **Mannion, P. T.** 1995. The use of peracetic acid for the reprocessing of flexible endoscopes and rigid cystoscopes and laparoscopes. *J. Hosp. Infect.* **29:**313–315.

172. **Martin, L. S., J. S. McDougal, and S. L. Loskoski.** 1985. Disinfection and inactivation of the human T lymphotropic virus type III/lymphadenopathy-associated virus. *J. Infect. Dis.* **152:**400–403.

173. **Martin, M. A., M. Reichelderfer, et al.** 1994. APIC guidelines for infection prevention and control in flexible endoscopy. *Am. J. Infect. Control.* **22:**19–38.

174. **Mathers, W. D., J. E. Sutphin, R. Folberg, P. A. Meier, R. P. Wenzel, and R. G. Elgin.** 1996. Outbreak of keratitis presumed to be caused by *Acanthamoeba. Am. J. Ophthalmol.* **121:**129–142.

175. **Mayer, S., M. Boos, A. Beyer, A. C. Fluit, and F. J. Schmitz.** 2001. Distribution of the antiseptic resistance genes qacA, qacB and qacC in 497 methicillin-resistant and -susceptible European isolates of *Staphylococcus aureus. J. Antimicrob. Chemother.* **47:**896–897.

176. **Mbithi, J. N., V. S. Springthorpe, and S. A. Sattar.** 1990. Chemical disinfection of hepatitis A virus on environmental surfaces. *Appl. Environ. Microbiol.* **56:**3601–3604.

177. **Mbithi, J. N., V. S. Springthorpe, S. A. Sattar, and M. Pacquette.** 1993. Bactericidal, virucidal, and mycobactericidal activities of reused alkaline glutaraldehyde in an endoscopy unit. *J. Clin. Microbiol.* **31:**2988–2995.

178. **McDonald, L. C., G. E. Killgore, A. Thompson, R. C. Owens, Jr., S. V. Kazakova, S. P. Sambol, S. Johnson, and D. N. Gerding.** 2005. An epidemic, toxin gene-variant strain of *Clostridium difficile*. *N. Engl. J. Med.* **353:**2433–2441.

179. **McDonnell, G., and A. D. Russell.** 1999. Antiseptics and disinfectants: activity, action, and resistance. *Clin. Microbiol. Rev.* **12:**147–179.

180. **Mentel, R., and J. Schmidt.** 1973. Investigations on rhinovirus inactivation by hydrogen peroxide. *Acta Virol.* **17:**351–354.

181. **Merianos, J. J.** 1991. Quaternary ammonium antimicrobial compounds, p. 225–255. *In* S. S. Block (ed.), *Disinfection, Sterilization and Preservation.* Lea & Febiger, Philadelphia, PA.

182. **Mermel, L. A., S. L. Josephson, J. Dempsey, S. Parenteau, C. Perry, and N. Magill.** 1997. Outbreak of *Shigella sonnei* in a clinical microbiology laboratory. *J. Clin. Microbiol.* **35:**3163–3165.

183. **Meyer, B., and C. Kluin.** 1999. Efficacy of Glucoprotamin containing disinfectants against different species of atypical mycobacteria. *J. Hosp. Infect.* **42:**151–154.

184. **Michele, T. M., W. A. Cronin, N. M. Graham, D. M. Dwyer, D. S. Pope, S. Harrington, R. E. Chaisson, and W. R. Bishai.** 1997. Transmission of *Mycobacterium tuberculosis* by a fiberoptic bronchoscope. Identification by DNA fingerprinting. *JAMA* **278:**1093–1095.

185. **Middleton, A. M., M. V. Chadwick, J. L. Sanderson, and H. Gaya.** 2000. Comparison of a solution of super-oxidized water (Sterilox) with glutaraldehyde for the disinfection of bronchoscopes, contaminated. *J. Hosp. Infect.* **45:**278–282.

186. **Milstone, A. M., C. L. Passaretti, and T. M. Perl.** 2008. Chlorhexidine: expanding the armamentarium for infection control and prevention. *Clin. Infect. Dis.* **46:**274–281.

187. **Misteli, H., W. P. Weber, S. Reck, R. Rosenthal, M. Zwahlen, P. Fueglistaler, M. K. Bolli, D. Oertli, A. F. Widmer, and W. R. Marti.** 2009. Surgical glove perforation and the risk of surgical site infection. *Arch. Surg.* **144:**553–558.

188. **Mitchell, B. A., M. H. Brown, and R. A. Skurray.** 1998. QacA multidrug efflux pump from *Staphylococcus aureus*: comparative analysis of resistance to diamidines, biguanidines, and guanylhydrazones. *Antimicrob. Agents Chemother.* **42:**475–477.

189. **Nakashima, A. K., A. K. Highsmith, and W. J. Martone.** 1987. Survival of *Serratia marcescens* in benzalkonium chloride and in multiple-dose medication vials: relationship to epidemic septic arthritis. *J. Clin. Microbiol.* **25:**1019–1021.

190. **Narang, H. K., and A. A. Codd.** 1983. Action of commonly used disinfectants against enteroviruses. *J Hosp. Infect* **4:**209–212.

191. **Nelson, D. B., W. R. Jarvis, W. A. Rutala, A. E. Foxx-Orenstein, G. Isenberg, G. R. Dash, C. J. Alvarado, M. Ball, J. Griffin-Sobel, C. Petersen, K. A. Ball, J. Henderson, R. L. Stricof, et al.** 2003. Multi-society guideline for reprocessing flexible gastrointestinal endoscopes. *Infect. Control Hosp. Epidemiol.* **24:**532–537.

192. **Neumann, G., T. Noda, and Y. Kawaoka.** 2009. Emergence and pandemic potential of swine-origin H1N1 influenza virus. *Nature.* **459:**931–939.

193. **O'Connor, D. O., and J. R. Rubino.** 1991. Phenolic compounds, p. 204–224. *In* S. S. Block (ed.), *Disinfection, Sterilization and Preservation.* Lea & Febiger, Philadelphia, PA.

194. **Oie, S., and A. Kamiya.** 1996. Microbial contamination of antiseptics and disinfectants. *Am. J. Infect. Control.* **24:**389–395.

195. **Parker, F., and S. Foran.** 1995. Chlorhexidine catheter lubricant anaphylaxis. *Anaesth. Intensive Care* **23:**126.

196. **Patterson, P.** 2009. CDC sterilization, disinfection guideline. *OR Manager* **25:**14–16.

197. **Perencevich, E. N., M. T. Wong, and A. D. Harris.** 2001. National and regional assessment of the antibacterial soap market: a step toward determining the impact of prevalent antibacterial soaps. *Am. J. Infect. Control* **29:**281–283.

198. **Piazza, M., G. Borgia, L. Picciotto, S. Nappa, S. Cicciarello, and R. Orlando.** 1995. Detection of hepatitis C virus-RNA by polymerase chain reaction in dental surgeries. *J. Med. Virol.* **45:**40–42.

199. **Pittet, D., S. Hugonnet, S. Harbarth, P. Mourouga, V. Sauvan, S. Touveneau, and T. V. Perneger.** 2000. Effectiveness of a hospital-wide programme to improve compliance with hand hygiene. *Lancet* **356:**1307–1312.

200. **Price, P. B.** 1938. The bacteriology of normal skin; a new quantitative test applied to a study of the bacterial biota and the disinfectant action of mechanical cleansing. *J. Infect. Dis.* **63:**301–318.

201. **Pronovost, P., D. Needham, S. Berenholtz, D. Sinopoli, H. Chu, S. Cosgrove, B. Sexton, R. Hyzy, R. Welsh, G. Roth, J. Bander, J. Kepros, and C. Goeschel.** 2006. An intervention to decrease catheter-related bloodstream infections in the ICU. *N. Engl. J. Med.* **355:**2725–2732.

202. **Prusiner, S. B.** 1982. Novel proteinaceous infectious particles cause scrapie. *Science* **216:**136–144.

203. **Prusiner, S. B.** 1997. Prion diseases and the BSE crisis. *Science* **278:**245–251.

204. **Ranganathan, N. S.** 1996. Chlorhexidine, p. 235–264. *In* J. P. Ascenzi (ed.), *Handbook of Disinfectants and Antiseptics.* Marcel Dekker, Inc., New York, NY.

205. **Reiss, I., A. Borkhardt, R. Fussle, A. Sziegoleit, and L. Gortner.** 2000. Disinfectant contaminated with *Klebsiella oxytoca* as a source of sepsis in babies. *Lancet* **356:**310.

206. **Robertson, L. J., A. T. Campbell, and H. V. Smith.** 1992. Survival of *Cryptosporidium parvum* oocysts under various environmental pressures. *Appl. Environ. Microbiol.* **58:**3494–3500.

207. **Rossmoore, H. W., and M. Sondossi.** 1988. Applications and mode of action of formaldehyde condensate biocides. *Adv. Appl. Microbiol.* **33:**223–277.

208. **Rotter, M. A.** 1996. Alcohols for antisepsis of hands and skin, p. 177–234. *In* J. P. Ascenzi (ed.), *Handbook of Disinfectants and Antiseptics.* Marcel Dekker, Inc., New York, NY.

209. **Rotter, M. L., W. Koller, G. Wewalka, H. P. Werner, G. A. Ayliffe, and J. R. Babb.** 1986. Evaluation of procedures for hygienic hand-disinfection: controlled parallel experiments on the Vienna test model. *J. Hyg.* (London) **96:**27–37.

210. **Rotter, M. L., S. O. Larsen, E. M. Cooke, J. Dankert, F. Daschner, D. Greco, P. Gronross, O. B. Jepsen, A. Lystad, B. Nystrom, et al.** 1988. A comparison of the effects of preoperative whole-body bathing with detergent alone and with detergent containing chlorhexidine gluconate on the frequency of wound infections after clean surgery. *J. Hosp. Infect.* **11:**310–320.

211. **Rotter, M. L., R. A. Simpson, and W. Koller.** 1998. Surgical hand disinfection with alcohols at various concentrations: parallel experiments using the new proposed European standards method. *Infect. Control Hosp. Epidemiol.* **19:**778–781.

212. **Rubbo, S. D., J. F. Gardner, and R. L. Webb.** 1967. Biocidal activities of glutaraldehyde and related compounds. *J. Appl. Bacteriol.* **30:**78–87.

213. **Russell, A. D.** 1994. Glutaraldehyde: current status and uses. *Infect. Control Hosp. Epidemiol.* **15:**724–733.

214. **Russell, A. D.** 2004. Whither triclosan? *J. Antimicrob. Chemother.* **53:**693–695.

215. **Russell, A. D., W. B. Hugo, and G. A. J. Ayliffe.** 1992. *Principles and Practice of Disinfection, Preservation and Sterilization.* Blackwell Scientific Publications, London, United Kingdom.

216. **Rutala, W. A, et al.** 1996. APIC guideline for selection and use of disinfectants. *Am. J. Infect. Control.* **24:**313–342.

217. **Rutala, W. A.** 1996. Disinfection and sterilization of patient-care items. *Infect. Control Hosp. Epidemiol.* **17:**377–384.

218. **Rutala, W. A., and E. C. Cole.** 1987. Ineffectiveness of hospital disinfectants against bacteria: a collaborative study. *Infect. Control* **8:**501–506.

219. **Rutala, W. A., E. C. Cole, N. S. Wannamaker, and D. J. Weber.** 1991. Inactivation of *Mycobacterium tuberculosis* and *Mycobacterium bovis* by 14 hospital disinfectants. *Am. J Med.* **91:**267S–271S.

220. **Rutala, W. A., M. F. Gergen, and D. J. Weber.** 1993. Evaluation of a rapid readout biological indicator for flash sterilization with three biological indicators and three chemical indicators. *Infect. Control. Hosp. Epidemiol.* **14:**390–394.

221. **Rutala, W. A., M. F. Gergen, and D. J. Weber.** 1993. Inactivation of *Clostridium difficile* spores by disinfectants. *Infect Control Hosp. Epidemiol.* **14:**36–39.

222. **Rutala, W. A., M. F. Gergen, and D. J. Weber.** 1999. Sporicidal activity of a new low-temperature sterilization technology: the Sterrad 50 sterilizer. *Infect. Control Hosp. Epidemiol.* **20:**514–516.

223. **Rutala, W. A., S. M. Jones, and D. J. Weber.** 1996. Comparison of a rapid readout biological indicator for steam sterilization with four conventional biological indicators and five chemical indicators. *Infect. Control Hosp. Epidemiol.* **17:**423–428.

224. **Rutala, W. A., and D. J. Weber.** 1995. FDA labeling requirements for disinfection of endoscopes: a counterpoint. *Infect. Control Hosp. Epidemiol.* **16:**231–235.

225. **Rutala, W. A., and D. J. Weber.** 1997. Uses of inorganic hypochlorite (bleach) in health-care facilities. *Clin. Microbiol. Rev.* **10:**597–610.

226. **Rutala, W. A., and D. J. Weber.** 1999. Disinfection of endoscopes: review of new chemical sterilants used for high-level disinfection. *Infect. Control Hosp. Epidemiol.* **20:**69–76.

227. **Rutala, W. A., and D. J. Weber.** 2001. New disinfection and sterilization methods. *Emerg. Infect. Dis.* **7:**348–353.

228. **Rutala, W. A., and D. J. Weber.** 2004. Disinfection and sterilization in health care facilities: what clinicians need to know. *Clin. Infect. Dis.* **39:**702–709.

229. **Rutala, W. A., and D. J. Weber.** 2010. Guideline for disinfection and sterilization of prion-contaminated medical instruments. *Infect. Control Hosp. Epidemiol.* **31:**107–117.

230. **Rutala, W. A., D. J. Weber, and K. J. Chappell.** 1999. Patient injury from flash-sterilized instruments. *Infect. Control Hosp. Epidemiol.* **20:**458.

231. **Rutala, W. A., D. J. Weber, C. A. Thomann, J. F. John, S. M. Saviteer, and F. A. Sarubbi.** 1988. An outbreak of *Pseudomonas cepacia* bacteremia associated with a contaminated intra-aortic balloon pump. *J. Thorac. Cardiovasc. Surg.* **96:**157–161.

232. **Ryan, C. K., and G. D. Potter.** 1995. Disinfectant colitis. Rinse as well as you wash. *J. Clin. Gastroenterol.* **21:**6–9.

233. **Sagripanti, J. L.** 1992. Metal-based formulations with high microbicidal activity. *Appl. Environ. Microbiol.* **58:**3157–3162.

234. **Sagripanti, J. L., and A. Bonifacino.** 1996. Comparative sporicidal effect of liquid chemical germicides on three medical devices contaminated with spores of *Bacillus subtilis. Am. J. Infect. Control* **24:**364–371.

235. **Sagripanti, J. L., C. A. Eklund, P. A. Trost, K. C. Jinneman, C. J. Abeyta, C. A. Kaysner, and W. E. Hill.** 1997. Comparative sensitivity of 13 species of pathogenic bacteria to seven chemical germicides. *Am. J. Infect. Control* **25:**335–339.

236. **Sailer, A., H. Bueler, M. Fischer, A. Aguzzi, and C. Weissmann.** 1994. No propagation of prions in mice devoid of PrP. *Cell* **77:**967–968.

237. **Samore, M. H., L. Venkataraman, P. C. DeGirolami, R. D. Arbeit, and A. W. Karchmer.** 1996. Clinical and molecular epidemiology of sporadic and clustered cases of nosocomial *Clostridium difficile* diarrhea. *Am. J. Med.* **100:**32–40.

238. **Sattar, S. A., H. Jacobsen, H. Rahman, T. M. Cusack, and J. R. Rubino.** 1994. Interruption of rotavirus spread through chemical disinfection. *Infect. Control. Hosp. Epidemiol.* **15:**751–756.

239. **Saurina, G., D. Landman, and J. M. Quale.** 1997. Activity of disinfectants against vancomycin-resistant *Enterococcus faecium. Infect. Control Hosp. Epidemiol.* **18:**345–347.

240. **Schelenz, S., and G. French.** 2000. An outbreak of multidrug-resistant *Pseudomonas aeruginosa* infection associated with contamination of bronchoscopes and an endoscope washer-disinfector. *J. Hosp. Infect.* **46:**23–30.

241. **Scherrer, M., and K. Kümmerer.** 1997. Manual and automated processing of medical instruments. Environmental and economic aspects. *Central Service* **5:**183–194.

242. **Sedlock, D. M., and D. M. Bailey.** 1985. Microbicidal activity of octenidine hydrochloride, a new alkanediylbis[pyridine] germicidal agent. *Antimicrob. Agents Chemother.* **28:**786–790.

243. **Sehulster, L., and R. Y. Chinn.** 2003. Guidelines for environmental infection control in health-care facilities. Recommendations of CDC and the Healthcare Infection Control Practices Advisory Committee (HICPAC). *MMWR Recommend. Rep.* **52:**1–42.

244. **Sheldon, A. T., Jr.** 2005. Antiseptic "resistance": real or perceived threat? *Clin. Infect. Dis.* **40:**1650–1656.

245. **Shetty, N., S. Srinivasan, J. Holton, and G. L. Ridgway.** 1999. Evaluation of microbicidal activity of a new disinfectant: Sterilox 2500 against *Clostridium difficile* spores, *Helicobacter pylori*, vancomycin resistant Enterococcus species, *Candida albicans* and several Mycobacterium species. *J. Hosp. Infect.* **41:**101–105.

246. **Shimono, N., T. Takuma, N. Tsuchimochi, A. Shiose, M. Murata, Y. Kanamoto, Y. Uchida, S. Morita, H. Matsumoto, and J. Hayashi.** 2008. An outbreak of *Pseudomonas aeruginosa* infections following thoracic surgeries occurring via the contamination of bronchoscopes and an automatic endoscope reprocessor. *J. Infect. Chemother.* **14:**418–423.

247. **Sorin, M., S. Segal-Maurer, N. Mariano, C. Urban, A. Combest, and J. J. Rahal.** 2001. Nosocomial transmission of imipenem-resistant *Pseudomonas aeruginosa* following bronchoscopy associated with improper connection to the Steris System 1 processor. *Infect. Control Hosp. Epidemiol.* **22:**409–413.

248. **Spach, D. H., F. E. Silverstein, and W. E. Stamm.** 1993. Transmission of infection by gastrointestinal endoscopy and bronchoscopy. *Ann. Intern. Med.* **118:**117–128.

249. **Spaulding, E. H.** 1968. Chemical disinfection of medical and surgical materials, p. 517–531. *In* S. Block (ed.), *Disinfection, Sterilization and Preservation.* Lean & Febiger, Philadelphia, PA.

250. **Spotts Whitney, E. A., M. E. Beatty, T. H. Taylor, Jr., R. Weyant, J. Sobel, M. J. Arduino, and D. A. Ashford.** 2003. Inactivation of *Bacillus anthracis* spores. *Emerg. Infect. Dis.* **9:**623–627.

251. **Srinivasan, A., L. L. Wolfenden, X. Song, K. Mackie, T. L. Hartsell, H. D. Jones, G. B. Diette, J. B. Orens, R. C. Yung, T. L. Ross, W. Merz, P. J. Scheel, E. F. Haponik, and T. M. Perl.** 2003. An outbreak of *Pseudomonas aeruginosa* infections associated with flexible bronchoscopes. *N. Engl. J. Med.* **348:**221–227.

252. **Stickler, D. J.** 1974. Chlorhexidine resistance in *Proteus mirabilis. J. Clin. Pathol.* **27:**284–287.

253. **Stickler, D. J., and B. Thomas.** 1980. Antiseptic and antibiotic resistance in Gram-negative bacteria causing urinary tract infection. *J. Clin. Pathol.* **33:**288–296.

254. **Stout, J. E., Y. S. Lin, A. M. Goetz, and R. R. Muder.** 1998. Controlling *Legionella* in hospital water systems: experience with the superheat-and-flush method and copper-silver ionization. *Infect. Control Hosp. Epidemiol.* **19:**911–914.

255. **Suller, M. T., and A. D. Russell.** 2000. Triclosan and antibiotic resistance in *Staphylococcus aureus. J. Antimicrob. Chemother.* **46:**11–18.

256. **Swenson, B. R., T. L. Hedrick, R. Metzger, H. Bonatti, T. L. Pruett, and R. G. Sawyer.** 2009. Effects of preoperative skin preparation on postoperative wound infection rates: a prospective study of 3 skin preparation protocols. *Infect. Control Hosp. Epidemiol.* **30:**964–971.

257. **Tabor, E., D. C. Bostwick, and C. C. Evans.** 1989. Corneal damage due to eye contact with chlorhexidine gluconate. *JAMA* **261:**557–558.

258. **Taylor, D. M.** 1999. Inactivation of prions by physical and chemical means. *J. Hosp. Infect.* **43** (Suppl.):S69–S76.

259. **Taylor, D. M., S. L. Woodgate, A. J. Fleetwood, and R. J. Cawthorne.** 1997. Effect of rendering procedures on the scrapie agent. *Vet. Rec.* **141:**643–649.

260. Terleckyj, B., and D. A. Axler. 1987. Quantitative neutralization assay of fungicidal activity of disinfectants. *Antimicrob. Agents Chemother.* **31**:794–798.

261. Tietz, A., R. Frei, M. Dangel, D. Bolliger, J. R. Passweg, A. Gratwohl, and A. E. Widmer. 2005. Octenidine hydrochloride for the care of central venous catheter insertion sites in severely immunocompromised patients. *Infect. Control Hosp. Epidemiol.* **26**:703–707.

262. Tiwari, T. S., B. Ray, K. C. Jost, Jr., M. K. Rathod, Y. Zhang, B. A. Brown-Elliott, K. Hendricks, and R. J. Wallace, Jr. 2003. Forty years of disinfectant failure: outbreak of postinjection *Mycobacterium abscessus* infection caused by contamination of benzalkonium chloride. *Clin. Infect. Dis.* **36**:954–962.

263. Trampuz, A., and A. F. Widmer. 2004. Hand hygiene: a frequently missed lifesaving opportunity during patient care. *Mayo Clin. Proc.* **79**:109–116.

264. Turner, P., B. Saeed, and M. C. Kelsey. 2004. Dermal absorption of isopropyl alcohol from a commercial hand rub: implications for its use in hand decontamination. *J. Hosp. Infect.* **56**:287–290.

265. Tyler, R., G. A. Ayliffe, and C. Bradley. 1990. Virucidal activity of disinfectants: studies with the poliovirus. *J. Hosp. Infect.* **15**:339–345.

265a. U.S. Food and Drug Administration. 2002. Medical devices: classification for medical washer and medical washer disinfector. *Fed. Regist.* **67**:69119–69121.

266. Valleron, A. J., P. Y. Boelle, R. Will, and J. Y. Cesbron. 2001. Estimation of epidemic size and incubation time based on age characteristics of vCJD in the United Kingdom. *Science* **294**:1726–1728.

267. van Bueren, J., D. P. Larkin, and R. A. Simpson. 1994. Inactivation of human immunodeficiency virus type 1 by alcohols. *J. Hosp. Infect.* **28**:137–148.

268. van Doornmalen, J. P., and J. Dankert. 2005. A validation survey of 197 hospital steam sterilizers in The Netherlands in 2001 and 2002. *J. Hosp. Infect.* **59**:126–130.

269. Van Klingeren, B., and W. Pullen. 1993. Glutaraldehyde resistant mycobacteria from endoscope washers. *J. Hosp. Infect.* **25**:147–149.

270. Vesley, D., M. A. Nellis, and P. B. Allwood. 1995. Evaluation of a rapid readout biological indicator for 121 degrees C gravity and 132 degrees C vacuum-assisted steam sterilization cycles. *Infect. Control Hosp. Epidemiol.* **16**:281–286.

271. Vigeant, P., V. G. Loo, C. Bertrand, C. Dixon, R. Hollis, M. A. Pfaller, A. P. McLean, D. J. Briedis, T. M. Perl, and H. G. Robson. 1998. An outbreak of *Serratia marcescens* infections related to contaminated chlorhexidine. *Infect. Control Hosp. Epidemiol.* **19**:791–794.

272. Wallace, J., P. M. Agee, and D. M. Demicco. 1995. Liquid chemical sterilization using peracetic acid. An alternative approach to endoscope processing. *ASAIO J.* **41**:151–154.

273. Walsh, S. E., J. Y. Maillard, and A. D. Russell. 1999. Ortho-phthalaldehyde: a possible alternative to glutaraldehyde for high level disinfection. *J. Appl. Microbiol.* **86**:1039–1046.

274. Waran, K. D., and R. A. Munsick. 1995. Anaphylaxis from povidone-iodine. *Lancet.* **345**:1506.

275. Wardle, M. D., and G. M. Renninger. 1975. Bactericidal effect of hydrogen peroxide on spacecraft isolates. *Appl. Microbiol.* **30**:710–711.

276. Weber, D. J., S. L. Barbee, M. D. Sobsey, and W. A. Rutala. 1999. The effect of blood on the antiviral activity of sodium hypochlorite, a phenolic, and a quaternary ammonium compound. *Infect. Control Hosp. Epidemiol.* **20**:821–827.

277. Weber, D. J., W. A. Rutala, and E. E. Sickbert-Bennett. 2007. Outbreaks associated with contaminated antiseptics and disinfectants. *Antimicrob. Agents Chemother.* **51**:4217–4224.

278. Weber, D. J., E. Sickbert-Bennett, M. F. Gergen, and W. A. Rutala. 2003. Efficacy of selected hand hygiene agents used to remove *Bacillus atrophaeus* (a surrogate of *Bacillus anthracis*) from contaminated hands. *JAMA* **289**:1274–1277.

279. Weber, W. P., S. Reck, U. Neff, R. Saccilotto, M. Dangel, M. L. Rotter, R. Frei, D. Oertli, W. R. Marti, and A. F. Widmer. 2009. Surgical hand antisepsis with alcohol-based hand rub: comparison of effectiveness after 1. 5 and 3 minutes of application. *Infect. Control Hosp. Epidemiol.* **30**:420–426.

280. Weissmann, C. 2005. Birth of a prion: spontaneous generation revisited. *Cell* **122**:165–168.

281. Wenzel, R. P. 2004. The antibiotic pipeline—challenges, costs, and values. *N. Engl. J. Med.* **351**:523–526.

282. West, A. B., S. F. Kuan, M. Bennick, and S. Lagarde. 1995. Glutaraldehyde colitis following endoscopy: clinical and pathological features and investigation of an outbreak. *Gastroenterology* **108**:1250–1255.

283. Widmer, A. F. 2000. Replace hand washing with use of a waterless alcohol hand rub? *Clin. Infect. Dis.* **31**:136–143.

284. Widmer, A. F. 2003. Sterilization of skin and catheters before drawing blood cultures. *J. Clin. Microbiol.* **41**:4910.

285. Widmer, A. F. 2009. Surgical hand antisepsis, p. 54–60. In World Health Organization (ed.), *WHO Guidelines on Hand Hygiene in Health Care*. World Health Organization, Geneva, Switzerland.

286. Widmer, A. F., A. Houston, E. Bollinger, and R. P. Wenzel. 1992. A new standard for sterility testing for autoclaved surgical trays. *J. Hosp. Infect.* **21**:253–260.

287. Widmer, A. F., M. Rotter, A. Voss, P. Nthumba, B. Allegranzi, J. Boyce, and D. Pittet. 2009. Surgical hand preparation: state-of-the-art. *J. Hosp. Infect.* **74**:112–122.

288. Widmer, A. F., R. P. Wenzel, A. Trilla, M. J. Bale, R. N. Jones, and B. N. Doebbeling. 1993. Outbreak of *Pseudomonas aeruginosa* infections in a surgical intensive care unit: probable transmission via hands of a health care worker. *Clin. Infect. Dis.* **16**:372–376.

289. Williams, N. D., and A. D. Russell. 1991. The effects of some halogen-containing compounds on *Bacillus subtilis* endospores. *J. Appl. Bacteriol.* **70**:427–436.

290. Wilson, J. A., and A. B. Margolin. 1999. The efficacy of three common hospital liquid germicides to inactivate *Cryptosporidium parvum* oocysts. *J. Hosp. Infect.* **42**:231–237.

291. World Health Organization. 1983. *Laboratory Safety Manual*. World Health Organization, Geneva, Switzerland.

292. Wu, M. S., J. T. Wang, J. C. Yang, H. H. Wang, J. C. Sheu, D. S. Chen, and T. H. Wang. 1996. Effective reduction of *Helicobacter pylori* infection after upper gastrointestinal endoscopy by mechanical washing of the endoscope. *Hepatogastroenterology* **43**:1660–1664.

293. Wullt, M., I. Odenholt, and M. Walder. 2003. Activity of three disinfectants and acidified nitrite against *Clostridium difficile* spores. *Infect. Control Hosp. Epidemiol.* **24**:765–768.

294. Wysowski, D. K., J. W. J. Flynt, M. Goldfield, R. Altman, and A. T. Davis. 1978. Epidemic neonatal hyperbilirubinemia and use of a phenolic disinfectant detergent. *Pediatrics* **61**:165–170.

295. Yong, D., F. C. Parker, and S. M. Foran. 1995. Severe allergic reactions and intra-urethral chlorhexidine gluconate. *Med. J. Aust.* **162**:257–258.

296. Zaidi, M., J. Sifuentes, M. Bobadilla, D. Moncada, and S. Ponce de León. 1989. Epidemic of *Serratia marcescens* bacteremia and meningitis in a neonatal unit in Mexico City. *Infect. Control Hosp. Epidemiol.* **10**:14–20.

297. Zuhlsdorf, B., G. Kampf, H. Floss, and H. Martiny. 2005. Suitability of the German test method for cleaning efficacy in washer-disinfectors for flexible endoscopes according to prEN ISO 15883. *J. Hosp. Infect.* **61**:46–52.

298. Zuhlsdorf, B., and H. Martiny. 2005. Intralaboratory reproducibility of the German test method of prEN ISO 15883–1 for determination of the cleaning efficacy of washer-disinfectors for flexible endoscopes. *J. Hosp. Infect.* **59**:286–291.

Biothreat Agents

SUSAN E. SHARP AND MIKE LOEFFELHOLZ

12

INTRODUCTION

The ideal qualities for a successful biothreat agent are a high rate of illness in exposed persons/animals, a high case fatality rate, a short incubation period, and a paucity of immunity in the targeted population. Success is also influenced by the availability of treatment, the ability of the agent to transmit from person to person, and the ease with which the agent can be produced and disseminated; in addition, a disease that is, at least initially, difficult to recognize clinically or diagnose contributes to the success of the agent. The Centers for Disease Control and Prevention (CDC) has classified these agents into categories depending on the basis of their threat to national security, with those organisms belonging to category A being the most serious threats (Table 1).

General clues that one could be dealing with an unrecognized bioterror event include a large outbreak of illness with a high death rate, a recognized case(s) of an uncommon disease, disease in a region of the world where the disease is not endemic, disease out of its usual seasonality, simultaneous outbreaks of the same disease in various parts of the country or world, and sick and dying animals.

Due to their unique features in causing mass destructive diseases, the priority biological agents for use in bioterror events include anthrax, brucellosis, Q fever, tularemia, plague, hemorrhagic fever viruses, and toxins (botulinum, staphylococcal enterotoxins, and T-2 mycotoxins). Each of these is discussed with regard to its significance as a biothreat agent, its epidemiology and natural routes of transmission, and appropriate specimens to submit for laboratory diagnosis (Table 2).

The LRN

In 1999, the CDC, together with the Association of Public Health Laboratories (APHL) and the Federal Bureau of Investigation, formed a network to facilitate the recognition and identification of possible biothreat agents. The Laboratory Response Network (LRN) currently includes all levels of clinical laboratories which perform patient testing, as well as food-testing laboratories, diagnostic veterinary laboratories, and environmental-testing laboratories (Fig. 1). LRN sentinel laboratories generally consist of clinical diagnostic laboratories associated with hospitals and other health-providing entities, while LRN reference laboratories consist primarily of county and state public health laboratories. The two laboratories considered LRN national laboratories are the CDC and the United States Army Medical Research Institute of Infectious Diseases (USAMRIID). These two laboratories function to perform susceptibility testing on biothreat agents when necessary and can also safely handle highly infectious viral agents. The function of the LRN sentinel laboratories is to recognize possible biothreat agents and submit them to an LRN reference laboratory as soon as possible for definitive identification. The LRN reference laboratory then refers the identified agents to the LRN national laboratory for further characterization and storage. LRN sentinel laboratories are not allowed to evaluate environmental and animal specimens but should instead refer them to the closest appropriate LRN reference laboratory.

Sentinel Laboratory Protocols

The American Society for Microbiology (ASM), the APHL, and the CDC have jointly developed protocols for LRN sentinel laboratories that will allow clinical laboratories to rapidly rule out organisms as biothreat agents or to refer suspected biothreat agents to the appropriate LRN reference laboratory. For more information regarding these and other sentinel laboratory protocols, refer to the ASM website http://www.asm.org/index.php/policy/sentinel-level-clinical-microbiology-laboratory-guidelines.html.

The Select Agent Program

Through its Select Agent Program, the CDC regulates the possession, use, and transfer of select agents and toxins that have the potential to pose a severe threat to public health and safety. This program oversees the above activities and registers all laboratories and entities in the United States that possess, use, or transfer a select agent or toxin.

The U.S. Departments of Health and Human Services (HHS) and Agriculture (USDA) set forth final rules for the possession, use, and transfer of select agents and toxins in the Federal Register (36a), which were effective on 18 April 2005. The website http://www.cdc.gov/od/sap// contains additional information regarding application packages, current regulations regarding select agents, and additional resource information.

TABLE 1 Critical biological agents for public health preparedness

Category A	Category B	Category C
Variola major (smallpox)	Coxiella burnetii (Q fever)	Nipah virus
Bacillus anthracis (anthrax)	Brucella spp. (brucellosis)	Hantaviruses
Yersinia pestis (plague)	Burkholderia mallei (glanders)	Tick-borne hemorrhagic fever
Clostridium botulinum	Alphaviruses (i.e., Venezuelan,	viruses
neurotoxins (botulism)	Eastern, and Western equine	Tick-borne encephalitis viruses
Francisella tularensis (tularemia)	encephalitis viruses)	Yellow fever virus
Filoviruses (e.g., Ebola and	Ricin from Ricinus communis	Multidrug-resistant
Marburg) and arenaviruses	(ricin intoxication)	Mycobacterium tuberculosis
(e.g., Lassa and Junin)	Epsilon toxin of Clostridium	
(hemorrhagic fever)	perfringens	
	Staphylococcal enterotoxin B	
	Food- and waterborne agents	
	(e.g., Salmonella spp., Shigella	
	dysenteriae, Escherichia coli	
	O157:H7, Vibrio cholerae,	
	Cryptosporidium parvum)	

BIOTHREAT AGENTS AND INFECTIONS

Anthrax (Bacillus anthracis)

Significance

The bioterror threat associated with the inhalation of spores from *Bacillus anthracis* has been known for decades, and the organism had been developed as a potential military weapon by many countries, including the United States (23, 56). Throughout the 1990s, envelopes containing powders said to contain anthrax spores (which they did not) were sent to various institutions in the United States (56). Then in 2001, envelopes containing confirmed anthrax were mailed to southern Florida, New York City, and Washington, DC. Exposure from these events caused 22 persons to develop anthrax (11 inhalational cases, with five deaths, and 11 cases of cutaneous anthrax) (56). Prior to 2001, 18 cases of inhalational anthrax (16 deaths) were reported in the United States, none of which were due to bioterrorism (8).

Natural Transmission and Epidemiology

Bacillus anthracis is a large, aerobic or facultatively anaerobic, spore-forming, gram-positive bacillus that naturally inhabits the soil. Natural transmission to humans usually occurs by direct contact with the organism from infected or contaminated animal products. Four forms of the disease can occur: cutaneous (>95% of all human anthrax cases), inhalational, and gastrointestinal anthrax and meningitis. The inhalational form (acquired through inhalation of organism spores) is associated primarily with bioterror attacks and causes pulmonary anthrax. In addition, anthrax meningitis can occur as a result of a bioterror event. Any case of inhalational or meningeal anthrax should prompt suspicion for possible bioterrorism. Human-to-human transmission of anthrax has not been reported.

Anthrax is considered hyperendemic in parts of Asia, Africa, and the Middle East, and endemic in parts of Latin and South America and Europe (57). Additionally, anthrax sporadically occurs in many other parts of the world. A map with areas of anthrax endemicity can be found at the WHO website (http://www.vetmed.lsu.edu/whocc/mp_world.htm). Additional information regarding *B. anthracis* can be found in chapter 24.

Brucellosis (Brucella Species)

Significance

Brucella suis was the first biological agent to be utilized in the biological warfare program of the United States during the mid-1950s. The very low pulmonary infective dose (as low as 10 bacteria) for this organism makes it an extremely good bioweapon if infection is acquired through the inhalational route (1a, 45).

Natural Transmission and Epidemiology

Brucella organisms are small, aerobic, gram-negative coccobacilli that grow slowly (2 to 3 days for initial isolation) on blood and chocolate agars. Natural transmission is zoonotic and can occur with any of the *Brucella* species. Humans usually are infected by occupational exposure to infected animals, consumption of unpasteurized dairy products from infected animals, or inhalation of infectious aerosols from animals. Brucellosis is a disease of nonspecific symptoms which can last for months and relapse after discontinuation of therapy (106).

Fewer than 150 cases of brucellosis have been reported annually in the United States since the mid-1980s, and most were reported in California, Florida, Texas, and Virginia (17). However, brucellosis in humans and animals is increasing in certain parts of the world, especially in developing areas of the Mediterranean region, Middle East, western Asia, and parts of Africa and Latin America (Medilinks Brucellosis Fact Sheet, http://medilinkz.org/HealthTopics/Diseases/zoonoses/brucellosis.htm). Of note, brucellosis is among the most commonly reported laboratory-acquired bacterial infections (79). Additional information regarding *Brucella* spp. can be found in chapter 44.

Q Fever (Coxiella burnetii)

Significance

Coxiella burnetii has a very low infective dose and is resistant to the effects of drying and heat. Humans are very susceptible to infection with this organism, and a single organism is capable of causing disease in a susceptible person (for Q fever information from the CDC, see http://www.cdc.gov/ncidod/dvrd/qfever/index.htm). These characteristics

TABLE 2 Diagnosis of biothreat agents

Agent(s)	Specimen(s)	Gram stain characteristics	Culture/notes	BSL[a]
Bacillus anthracis	Blood cultures, lower respiratory secretions	Large gram-positive bacilli	Organisms grow aerobically on sheep blood and chocolate agars and other nonselective media as tenacious colonies that are large and grainy or look like ground glass.	2
Brucella species	Blood cultures, bone marrow, spleen, liver, joint, and abscess material	Small gram-negative coccobacilli	Organisms grow aerobically on sheep blood and chocolate agars and other nonselective media as slow-growing, small colonies that are oxidase and catalase positive and rapidly urea positive.	3
Coxiella burnetii	Tissue and body fluids, serum for serological diagnosis		No growth on standard laboratory media.	3
Fransicella tularensis	Blood cultures, aspirates or scrapings of ulcers or lymph nodes, lower respiratory secretions	Small gram-negative coccobacilli	Organisms grow aerobically on chocolate agar (may initially grow on sheep blood agar) as slow-growing, small colonies that are oxidase negative and weakly catalase and β-lactamase positive.	2
Yersinia pestis	Sputum, bronchial wash/lavage specimens, blood cultures, specimens from aspiration/ biopsy of involved tissue (liver, spleen, bone marrow, lymph node, lung)	Enteric-organism-like, gram-negative bacilli	Organisms grow on all routine media as non-lactose-fermenting colonies that are catalase and indole positive, oxidase negative, and urea negative.	
Smallpox virus		Not applicable	Contact your public health laboratory if suspected.	
Hemorrhagic fever viruses	Serum, heparinized plasma, whole blood, throat washings, tissue, urine		No testing in the routine laboratory. Contact your public health laboratory. Caution: these viruses may grow in nonhuman primate and human cell lines such as Vero and MRC-5 cells.	
Botulism toxin	Feces, gastric aspirate, vomitus, tissue, exudates, serum, food samples		No testing in the routine laboratory. Contact your public health laboratory.	
Staphylococcal enterotoxin B	Nasal swabs, induced respiratory specimens, urine, stool, gastric aspirates, intestinal contents, serum, suspected isolates		No testing in the routine laboratory. Contact your public health laboratory.	
T-2 mycotoxins	Blood, tissue, environmental samples		No testing in the routine laboratory. Contact your public health laboratory.	

[a]BSL, biosafety level.

make this organism a likely candidate for development as a bioterror weapon (http://www.cdc.gov/ncidod/dvrd/qfever/index.htm). In the 1960s, the U.S. military considered *Coxiella* an excellent "incapacitating" agent, as the disease is debilitating but rarely lethal, and envisioned using this agent to cripple enemy forces. The Russians, and possibly the Iraqis, have developed and tested the Q fever agent as a bioweapon, and the cult Aum Shinrikyo obtained C. *burnetii* but was unsuccessful in weaponizing it (for Q fever bioterrorism agent profiles for health care workers, see http://www.azdhs.gov/phs/edc/edrp/pdf/qfeverset.pdf [Arizona Department of Health Services]).

Natural Transmission and Epidemiology

C. burnetii is a pleomorphic, gram-negative, intracellular coccobacillus that cannot be cultured on routine bacteriologic media. Diagnosis is made primarily through serological

investigation. The extracellular sporelike form is extremely resistant to the effects of the environment (http://www.pbs.org/wgbh/nova/bioterror/agen_qfever.html [NOVA, "Agents of Bioterror"]). Transmission is from inhalation of this sporelike form through aerosolized dust particles or, less commonly, through ingestion of contaminated milk products (1b). Q fever is a zoonotic disease seen primarily in parturient goats, sheep, and cattle. Only occasionally is this organism seen in domestic cats. Q fever has been identified in at least 51 countries, and recent naturally occurring outbreaks have occurred in Switzerland and Great Britain (60). There are three presentations of this infection: atypical pneumonia, progressive pneumonia (of a rapid nature), and pneumonia as an incidental finding in patients with fever, with the last description being the most common form of the disease (60). Additional information regarding *C. burnetii* can be found in chapter 63.

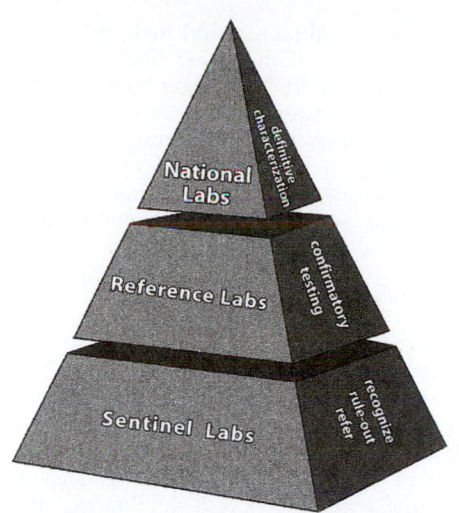

FIGURE 1 The LRN is charged with the task of maintaining an integrated network of state and local public health, federal, military, and international laboratories that can respond to bioterrorism, chemical terrorism, and other public health emergencies.

Tularemia (*Francisella tularensis*)

Significance

The highly infectious nature of this organism due to low inhalation inocula and a very susceptible human population, as well as its substantial morbidity and mortality in untreated patients, makes this bacterium a useful agent of bioterrorism (67). A WHO committee estimated that if approximately 100 pounds of a virulent strain of this organism were sprayed over a city of 5 million, it could incapacitate approximately 250,000 people and kill approximately 20,000 (http://www.pbs.org/wgbh/nova/bioterror/agen_tularemia.html [NOVA, "Agents of Bioterror"]). The Japanese began experiments on human prisoners for use of this agent as a military weapon in the early 1930s, and in 1955 the United States used volunteers and military personnel to test the effects of inhaled organisms (67). In the 1990s, Russia developed antibiotic- and vaccine-resistant strains of *F. tularensis* (http://www.pbs.org/wgbh/nova/bioterror/agen_tularemia.html [Nova, "Agents of Bioterror"]).

Natural Transmission and Epidemiology

F. tularensis is an extremely small, fastidious, pleomorphic, gram-negative coccobacillus. Tularemia is a disease of wild animals that can infect humans; ticks, mosquitoes, and biting flies have been implicated in its transmission (20a). Aerosolized particles containing the organism (moving contaminated hay and landscaping have been implicated in outbreaks of pulmonary disease) account for the acquisition of pneumonic tularemia; however, patients inhaling aerosolized organisms may present with other forms of tularemia, as discussed below (12a, 67). Respiratory failure or shock causes most fatalities with pneumonic disease (http://www.pbs.org/wgbh/nova/bioterror/agen_tularemia.html [Nova, "Agents of Bioterror"]). Other forms of tularemia are ulceroglandular, glandular, oculoglandular, pharyngeal, and typhoidal. The type of disease is determined largely by the disease manifestations in patients (77). A total of 1,368 cases of tularemia were reported to the CDC from 44 states during the 1990s. Four states accounted for 56% of all reported cases: Arkansas, Missouri, South Dakota,

and Oklahoma (13). Additional information regarding *F. tularensis* can be found in chapter 44.

Plague (*Yersinia pestis*)

Significance

The first reported use of *Y. pestis* as a bioweapon was in the 1300s as the Tartars, invading the city of Kaffa (now Feodosiya, Ukraine), catapulted bodies of plague victims over the city walls, resulting in an epidemic (30). Many countries have developed this agent as a bioweapon, including the former Soviet Union and Japan (7). An incident involving a white supremacist who fraudulently obtained cultures of *Y. pestis* from the American Type Culture Collection prompted the U.S. Congress to pass a 1996 regulation governing the acquisition, transfer, and use of agents that could be used for bioterrorism purposes (98). Plague is considered a bioweapon threat for several reasons, including the wide availability of the organism, its potential for mass production and aerosolization, its contagious nature, and its potential to cause high fatality rates (7).

Natural Transmission and Epidemiology

Y. pestis is a slow-growing (optimal growth is at 28°C), plump, gram-negative coccobacillus/bacillus and is part of the *Enterobacteriaceae* family (1c, 11). Plague is a worldwide zoonotic disease that is transmitted between animals by infected fleas. Recent outbreaks have occurred in India and southeastern Africa (1c, 11). In the United States, a majority of the cases occur in New Mexico, Arizona, Colorado, and California (11). There are three forms of plague: bubonic, septicemic, and pneumonic. The pneumonic form would be the most likely disease manifestation seen in the event of a bioterror attack. Additional information regarding *Yersinia pestis* can be found in chapter 36.

Smallpox

Significance

An excellent overview of smallpox and its historical use as a bioterror weapon is given by Rotz et al. (84). Briefly, one of the first possibilities of smallpox's use as a bioterror weapon dates back to the 1600s, when the Spanish supplied the natives of South America with smallpox-contaminated clothing in an effort to gain control of their lands. Then in the 1760s, the North American British forces gave smallpox-contaminated blankets to the native Indians in an effort to reduce their populations and gain control of land. In more recent times, the Soviet agency Biopreparat worked with many potential biothreat agents, including smallpox, for use in intercontinental missiles (28). Today, concern still exists regarding illegitimate stores of the smallpox agent and their potential use in bioterrorism, especially as routine vaccination has not been in place for decades, leading to a susceptible populace.

Natural Transmission and Epidemiology

As there is no known disease associated with smallpox in the world, even one case would prompt the suspicion of a bioterror incident. Smallpox could make a successful bioterror weapon due to its high infectivity and lethality, person-to-person transmissibility, ease of large-scale production, and lack of medical treatments/prevention (84). Human transmission occurs primarily by inhalation of airborne particles containing the virus, but transmission may occur via fomites (contaminated bedding, clothing) as well (40). The incubation period is normally 2 weeks, and then come symptoms of malaise, fever, chills, vomiting, headache, and backache. After an additional 2 to 3 days, a papular rash forms on the face, hands, and arms, later spreading to the legs and, lastly, the trunk. The mortality due to smallpox in an unvaccinated population is approximately 30% (40).

Diseases Caused by Hemorrhagic Fever Viruses

Significance
Hemorrhagic fever viruses (HFVs) were developed as biological weapons by both the United States and the Soviet Union. The United States stopped this program and destroyed all weapons in the late 1960s. These agents, if produced as small-particle aerosols, would be extremely dangerous as bioweapons. Most of these viruses can be found in their natural reservoirs or collected from infected patients (78).

Natural Transmission and Epidemiology
The HFVs comprise four families: the *Arenaviridae*, *Bunyaviridae*, *Filoviridae*, and *Flaviviridae*. Many of the HFVs are naturally transmitted to humans via the respiratory route by aerosols or are acquired from insect (mosquito or tick) bites. The epidemiology varies with the type of HFV. The reader is referred to reference 78 for the geography associated with each of the viruses.

The clinical course following exposure varies with the virus causing the infection, but typically patients have symptoms of fever, myalgia, and malaise for a few days. This is followed by exacerbation of symptoms and development of prostration and hemorrhage with central nervous system depression. Patients who develop shock with extensive hemorrhage and central nervous system damage generally have poor outcomes (78). Additional information regarding the HFVs can be found in chapters 93 to 95.

BIOLOGICAL TOXINS

Botulism

Significance
Clostridial toxins are among the most powerful neurotoxins known. Botulinum toxin acts at the neuromuscular junction and at the peripheral autonomic synapses, resulting in neuromuscular weakness and autonomic dysfunction (5). A bioterror attack using botulinum toxin could result from ingestion or inhalation of the toxin after contamination of a food or air supply. Many countries, including Japan, the United States, the former Soviet Union, and Iraq, have, at some point, developed botulinum toxin for biological warfare (5).

Natural Transmission and Epidemiology
Clostridium botulinum is an anaerobic, spore-forming, gram-positive bacillus that is found naturally in the environment (soil and water). Approximately 100 cases of botulism are reported in the United States each year. Western states (California, Washington, Oregon, Colorado, and Alaska) seem to have the majority of the cases (1d). The organisms primarily associated with human disease produce toxin types A, B, and E (1d). Botulism is naturally acquired from contaminated food products processed by methods that do not destroy spores. This allows bacteria contained in the food to become vegetative and toxins to be produced. The clinical presentation associated with a bioter-

ror attack with botulinum would include gastrointestinal symptoms (nausea, vomiting, and diarrhea), followed by neurological signs of dry mouth and blurred and/or double vision. In severe disease, symptoms continue, producing difficulty swallowing, voice impairment, and peripheral-muscle weakness. If the muscles of the respiratory tract are involved, respiratory failure and death may result. Additional information regarding *C. botulinum* can be found in chapter 50.

Staphylococcal Enterotoxins

Significance
Staphylococcus enterotoxin B (SEB) was part of the United States' bioweapons program until the early 1970s. SEB was thought to be useful as a weapon due to its ease of aerosolization, its stability, and its ability to produce death if inhaled in large amounts. Even if inhaled in smaller amounts, this toxin produces a debilitating disease that requires up to 2 weeks for recovery (1e).

Natural Transmission and Epidemiology
SEB is one of several enterotoxins produced by *Staphylococcus aureus*. It is also a potent superantigen, capable of massive overstimulation of the immune system, resulting in an overwhelming inflammatory response and an endotoxin-like shock which can result in multiorgan failure and death (68). SEB is the enterotoxin that classically causes staphylococcus-associated heat-stable food poisoning. It is normally acquired from contaminated food or beverages. Normally acquired disease results in malaise, nausea, vomiting, abdominal pain, and diarrhea 2 to 6 hours after ingestion of contaminated food or drink. These symptoms do not persist and usually resolve over 6 to 12 h. *S. aureus* strains containing SEB are found worldwide. Additional information regarding staphylococcal enterotoxins can be found in chapter 19.

T-2 Mycotoxins

Significance
When their civilians ate bread baked from flour contaminated with a *Fusarium* mold, the Russian military discovered the use of trichothecene mycotoxins as biological toxins. Some of these victims developed a protracted lethal illness characterized by initial symptoms of abdominal pain, diarrhea, vomiting, and exhaustion, followed within days by fever, chills, muscular pain, and infections. According to the United Nations Special Commission, Iraq researched trichothecene mycotoxins, including T-2 (100). T-2 mycotoxins can be delivered via food or water sources, as well as via droplets, aerosols, or smoke, from various dispersal systems. These properties make T-2 mycotoxin a potentially viable biological warfare agent.

Natural Transmission and Epidemiology
Trichothecene mycotoxins are low-molecular-weight, nonvolatile, pathogenic compounds produced by more than 350 species of fungi. T-2 mycotoxin is the most extensively studied of the trichothecenes. These toxins are well absorbed topically, orally, and by inhalational routes, causing systemic toxicity and clinical symptoms within seconds of exposure. Upon skin contact, T-2 mycotoxins produce painful erythema, blistering, and bullous lesions which lead to desquamation. Respiratory effects include nose and throat pain, nasal discharge, itching, sneezing, coughing, wheezing, dyspnea, chest pain, and hemoptysis. Nausea,

vomiting, anorexia, and watery diarrhea with abdominal cramping occur after ingestion. Severe dizziness, blurred vision, ataxia, prostration, tachycardia, hypothermia, vascular collapse, and death can result from systemic exposure (32, 76a). Trichothecene mycotoxins are extremely stable and are resistant to heat and UV light inactivation. Exposures in the United States have largely been due to accidental ingestion of contaminated foods.

EMERGING PATHOGENS

In a 2004 review, Morens et al. listed 30 recent emerging and reemerging infectious diseases (69). At least a dozen additional diseases or agents could be added since the publication of this review. In spite of predictions in the mid-20th century that infectious diseases in man would be defeated, they continue to emerge and reemerge at an alarming rate, due in large part to human behavior and environmental factors. These include climate change, changes in insect vectors or reservoir hosts, human demographics, regional and international travel, poverty, technology, and microbial change through genetic mutation or recombination (69). The inevitable outcome is contact between infectious agents and immunologically naïve humans, and diseases range from outbreaks (e.g., monkeypox and *Cryptococcus gattii*) to ongoing epidemics (e.g. AIDS, tuberculosis, and dengue). Comprehensive reviews of emerging agents are available (74). This section focuses on 16 recently emergent pathogens—some well recognized, others less so—and provides contemporary knowledge, with emphasis on epidemiology and factors responsible for emergence.

Bacteria

Clostridium difficile BI/NAP1/027

Significance
Clostridium difficile is one of the most important health care-associated pathogens, causing diarrhea and pseudomembranous colitis in hospitalized patients and residents of long-term care facilities. It is also increasingly recognized as a cause of community-onset diarrhea (4). An epidemic strain of *C. difficile* (restriction endonuclease analysis group BI/North American pulsed-field type 1 [NAP1]/ribotype 027), producing unusually large amounts of toxins A and B, emerged as a cause of outbreaks of severe disease in Canada and the United States in 2000 to 2002 (62, 102). Increased virulence is attributed to production of a binary toxin, over-expression of toxins A and B as a result of an 18-base-pair deletion in *tcdC* (25, 62, 102), and novel *tcdB* sequences that may affect binding capacity (94).

Natural Transmission and Epidemiology
Since emerging as a cause of outbreaks in North America, *C. difficile* BI/NAP1/027 has spread rapidly and become predominant in some locations (63, 66). This hypertoxin-producing strain is also a cause of outbreaks in the United Kingdom (102). In Quebec, Canada, *C. difficile* BI/NAP1/027 represented about 2% of recovered isolates during a preepidemic period and 80% of isolates in the following 2-year period (2003 to 2005) (52). Surveillance in Ontario showed high prevalence (34% of all *C. difficile* isolates) and wide distribution (61).
Potential factors for emergence of *C. difficile* BI/NAP1/027 include increased sporulation, which could enhance survival in the environment and spread of the organism (1), and

selective antibiotic pressure, resulting in the shift of *C. difficile* ribotypes and the replacement of previous predominant ribotypes (52). Strain BI/NAP1/027 has been detected in cases of community-associated *C. difficile* infection in the United States (16).

Clinical Significance
C. difficile BI/NAP1/027 is associated with increased morbidity and mortality relative to other *C. difficile* strains. Patients infected with strain BI/NAP1/027 were twice as likely to die within 30 days of diagnosis as were patients infected with strains of other ribotypes (52). Infections caused by strain BI/NAP1/027 showed a lower rate of response to metronidazole (63). Subtypes of *C. difficile* BI/NAP1/027 have been identified using highly discriminatory molecular methods, but it is unknown if clinical outcomes are related to subtype (36). Additional information regarding *C. difficile* BI/NAP1/027 can be found in chapter 50.

Non-O157 Shiga Toxin-Producing *Escherichia coli*

Significance
Shiga toxin-producing *Escherichia coli* (STEC) strains are important causes of bacterial gastroenteritis and are the etiologic agents of hemolytic uremic syndrome (HUS). While strains of serotype O157:H7 are responsible for the majority of reported HUS cases, strains of non-O157 serotypes are emerging as important etiologic agents of gastroenteritis and HUS. In the United States and Europe, between one-third and two-thirds of human STEC isolates are of non-O157 serotypes (9, 35, 47).

Natural Transmission and Epidemiology
Ruminants are the main reservoir of STEC isolates, including those of non-O157 serotypes. Most human infections are associated with consumption of beef or direct contact with animals and animal feces. Wild ruminants (deer and goats) also harbor non-O157 STEC, although the most common serotypes found during a study in Spain (85) did not correspond with the most predominant serotypes of strains isolated from human specimens in Europe (64). Non-O157 STEC isolates were responsible for 27% of HUS cases among children in a French surveillance study (34). One-third of HUS-associated *E. coli* isolates in a German study were caused by strains of non-O157 serotypes. Nearly 80% of these were represented by four serotypes: O26:H11 (43%), O145:H8 (19%), O111:H8 (8%), and O103:H2 (8%) (64). In a large U.S. study, strains of serotype O111 were the most common cause of HUS among isolates of non-O157 serotypes (9). Among all human STEC infections, serotype O26 is consistently the most common non-O157 serotype found (9, 35). In addition to O26 and O111, frequently found serotypes are O103 (47), O121, O45, and O145 (9, 64).
The frequency of reported non-O157 infections has increased recently at a much higher rate than that of O157-associated infections (47). Perhaps the greatest contributors to the identification of the emergence of non-O157 STEC are improved surveillance systems and the availability of laboratory diagnostics. In 2002, the Council of State and Territorial Epidemiologists requested that public health departments report STEC infections to the CDC's National Notifiable Diseases Surveillance System. In the late 1990s, enzyme immunoassay-based tests for detection of Shiga toxin became commercially available. These events resulted in a substantial increase in the number of human non-O157 STEC isolates submitted to

the CDC (9). Non-O157 STEC isolates show considerable genetic diversity, perhaps reflecting their adaptation to different environmental niches and selective pressures (47). To what extent this diversity is a cause of emergence or a result is unknown.

Clinical Significance

Non-O157 STEC infections range from mild gastroenteritis to bloody diarrhea to HUS. In the United States, isolates of serotype O111 account for most cases of HUS, after isolates of serotype O157 (9). In Denmark, 20 food-borne cases were associated with an outbreak caused by a strain of serotype O26:H11; one case involved bloody diarrhea, and none progressed to HUS (35). Some non-O157 STEC strains are nonpathogenic. Isolates expressing Shiga toxin 2 (*stx2*) are more likely to cause HUS than those that do not (9). Additional information regarding non-O157 STEC can be found in chapter 35.

Viruses

Novel Influenza A Virus Subtypes

Significance

New influenza A virus subtypes emerge as the result of reassortment of genes between two distinct strains, referred to as antigenic shift. If the reassortant virus is readily transmitted among a highly susceptible human population, the likely result is an influenza pandemic. During the 20th century, influenza pandemics occurred in 1918, 1957, and 1968. Recently, viruses of the novel subtypes H5N1 (105), H9N2 (55), H7N7 (51), and swine-origin H1N1 (73) have emerged and caused infection in humans. Of these recent novel-subtype viruses, only the swine-origin influenza A (H1N1) virus (2009 novel H1N1) has resulted in pandemic spread among humans. Influenza A virus subtype H5N1 is unique among novel avian strains of influenza A virus in its wide geographical distribution in avian species, its ability to cross normal species barriers and directly infect humans, and the number and severity of the human infections it causes (105).

Natural Transmission and Epidemiology

Novel avian influenza A viruses of subtypes H5N1, H7N7, and H9N2 have bypassed the classical epidemiologic cycle of influenza A virus and are capable of being transmitted directly from poultry to humans. Because these viruses are of completely bird-adapted subtypes, human-to-human transmission is relatively inefficient. Subtype H7N7 and H9N2 viruses have resulted in a limited number of human cases (51, 55). However, since the identification of influenza A virus H5N1 in China in 1996, this subtype has since spread rapidly among poultry and a variety of wild migratory bird species to the continents of Asia, Europe, and Africa. Human H5N1 virus infections are the result of exposure to high viral titers in infected birds or feces. There is evidence of human-to-human transmission, yet secondary cases are very limited due to the avian host specificity of H5N1 (99). To date, over 400 confirmed human cases of avian influenza H5N1 virus have been reported to the World Health Organization, with a mortality rate of 60% (among confirmed human cases of avian influenza A [H5N1] reported on the World Health Organization website http://www.who.int/csr/disease/avian_influenza/country/en/, accessed 5 August 2009). Most recently (2009), a novel H1N1 virus has emerged in humans (73). Unlike with the novel subtypes of purely avian origin, the presence of a unique combination

of genes from human, swine, and avian influenza A viruses in the 2009 novel H1N1 virus has resulted in its efficient transmission among humans and the first influenza pandemic in several decades.

Clinical Significance

Morbidity and mortality of H5N1 infections are severe in previously healthy, young, and middle-aged persons. The innate immune response is in part responsible for pathogenesis, causing fluid accumulation in the lungs. While influenza caused by H5N1 virus is notable for its aggressive course, evidence indicates that mild disease and asymptomatic infections occur. Symptomatic cases are characterized by high fever, cough, and lower respiratory tract symptoms in virtually 100% of patients. Diarrhea occurs more frequently than from influenza caused by viruses of human-adapted subtypes (105). Over 60% of reported H5N1 influenza cases have been fatal, with death primarily due to respiratory or multiorgan failure. The clinical features of 2009 novel H1N1 infection are similar to those of seasonal influenza, including fever and cough in over 90% of patients (73). Neurological complications have been reported (19). Severe and fatal cases of 2009 novel H1N1 virus have been reported for patients who are obese (20) and pregnant (see "Pandemic influenza in pregnant women" at the World Health Organization's website http://www.who.int/csr/disease/swineflu/notes/h1n1_pregnancy_20090731/en/index.html [accessed 5 August 2009]). Additional information regarding novel subtypes of influenza A virus can be found in chapter 81.

Chikungunya Virus

Significance

Chikungunya virus is an alphavirus of the family *Togaviridae*. It is an arthropod-borne virus transmitted by *Aedes* mosquitoes. Chikungunya is endemic in Africa and Asia, and recent explosive outbreaks have occurred in India and Indian Ocean islands. In 2007, an outbreak of autochthonous cases occurred in Italy, representing a significant expansion of the range of this virus.

Natural Transmission and Epidemiology

Chikungunya virus is endemic in Africa, India, the Indian Ocean islands, and Southeast Asia, with periodic outbreaks. There are two genotypes of chikungunya virus: Central/East African (responsible for recent outbreaks in India and the Indian Ocean islands) and Asian (91). Both genotypes are increasing in range throughout Asia (91). The strain responsible for the 2004–2007 epidemic in the Indian Ocean islands originated in Africa and is related to the Central/East African clade (48). Chikungunya virus is transmitted by *Aedes albopictus* and *Aedes aegypti* vectors. Peridomestic containers may support breeding and transmission (49). Dispersion of mosquito vectors can contribute to the spread and emergence of arboviruses such as chikungunya virus. *A. albopictus* has become established and widespread across a number of industrialized countries, including Italy (83), creating both a risk and the reality of introduction and emergence of arboviral diseases.

Recent outbreaks of chikungunya in India and the Indian Ocean islands are noteworthy in their magnitude, with attack rates of 33 to 45% (97) and mortality rates of over 10% (31). The evolution of chikungunya virus has played a role in its emergence. Several mutations in the outbreak strain are believed to have facilitated transmission and contributed to the epidemic among the Indian Ocean islands (88). Islands in the southwest Indian Ocean are popular vacation spots for Europeans, and several European countries have reported imported cases of chikungunya ("Chikungunya and dengue in the south west Indian Ocean," at http://www.who.int/csr/don/2006_03_17/en/print.html [accessed 8 March 2009]). The introduction of chikungunya virus in Italy in 2007, similar to the introduction of West Nile virus in the United States in 1999, highlights the roles of international travel and human-assisted spread of vectors in the emergence of arboviral diseases. Chikungunya virus was introduced into Italy by an individual who had recently traveled to India. A total of 205 autochthonous cases of chikungunya were reported in a small geographic area of northeastern Italy during the summer of 2007 (83). It has been suggested that the chikungunya virus variant possessed high virus-vector fitness, enabling introduction and rapid spread within this geographical region. Another key factor was the high density of A. *albopictus* in the area (83).

Clinical Significance

Chikungunya is characterized by a high attack rate (49, 93). Symptoms are similar to those of dengue fever and include fever, headache, nausea, vomiting, joint pain, lower back pain, and rash. In the Italy outbreak, 100% of cases presented with fever (mandatory in the case definition), and over 90% presented with joint pain and fatigue (83). Unique clinical features have been reported for neonates (82). Unusual features of infection include cutaneous ulcerations (33), persistent arthralgia (6), acute flaccid paralysis (92), and severe central nervous system illness requiring hospitalization (31, 53). While mortality rates of over 10% have been reported from outbreaks in the region of endemicity (31), the case fatality rate in the Italian outbreak was less than 0.5% (83). Additional information regarding chikungunya virus can be found in chapter 93.

Dengue Viruses

Significance

Dengue viruses are the most geographically widespread of the clinically significant arboviruses. Approximately 40% of the world's population is at risk of infection. There are an estimated 50 million dengue virus infections worldwide annually (see "Dengue and dengue hemorrhagic fever" at http://www.who.int/mediacentre/factsheets/fs117/en/print.html [accessed 8 March 2009]). Dengue is the only arboviral disease in which humans are the primary carriers and multipliers of the virus, which does not require an enzootic cycle for maintenance. There are four dengue virus serotypes, 1 to 4. Infection with one serotype does not provide immunity against the others. Both dengue viruses and the mosquito vectors have increased in range.

Natural Transmission and Epidemiology

Humans are the reservoir hosts for the vector of dengue, *Aedes aegypti,* a city-adapted mosquito. Additional epidemiologic cycles in Asia and Africa involving nonhuman primates and *Aedes* species may be a source of reemergence of dengue (101). In Asia and the Americas, A. *aegypti* breeds primarily in man-made peridomestic containers. A. *albopictus,* a secondary vector of dengue in Asia, has rapidly become established in the United States, South America, Africa, and Europe as a result of international trade in used tires (see "Dengue and dengue hemorrhagic fever" at http://www.who.int/mediacentre/factsheets/fs117/en/print.html) and ornamental plants (87).

Dengue occurs in tropical and subtropical climates worldwide, primarily in urban and semiurban environments. Dengue is endemic in more than 100 countries in Africa, the Americas, the eastern Mediterranean, Southeast Asia, and the western Pacific. There were nearly 900,000 reported cases of dengue in the Americas in 2007, of which 26,000 cases were dengue hemorrhagic fever (see "Dengue and dengue hemorrhagic fever" at http://www.who.int/mediacentre/factsheets/fs117/en/print.html). Emergence and reemergence is global. The A. *aegypti* vector has expanded rapidly and dramatically worldwide in tropical areas, followed by all four dengue virus serotypes. In Sri Lanka, new genotypes and clades of dengue virus 3 have replaced older clades, coinciding with an increase in severe disease (46). Worldwide, outbreaks and epidemics have increased in number, size, and severity (proportions of dengue hemorrhagic fever have also increased among all cases).

Causes of the emergence of dengue include lack of mosquito control programs, increased urbanization with concurrent poor sanitation, population growth in urban locations in tropical countries, and international travel (103) both of infected humans and breeding habitats such as used tires and ornamental plants (44). Another potential cause of emergence is serotype shift. In 2008, dengue virus 2 appeared and circulated in Brazil for several years, during which dengue virus 3 was the predominant serotype (see "Dengue/dengue hemorrhagic fever in Brazil" at http://www.who.int/csr/don/2008_04_10/en/print.html [accessed 8 March 2009]). There is also evidence of rapid evolution of the virus between outbreaks over a period as short as less than 1 year (22).

Clinical Significance

Evidence that the morbidity and mortality associated with dengue are becoming more severe is the growing proportion of cases of hemorrhagic fever (22). Dengue is among the most contagious of infectious diseases, with infection rates among immune naïve individuals during epidemics usually being 40 to 50% (see "Dengue and dengue hemorrhagic fever" at http://www.who.int/mediacentre/factsheets/fs117/en/print.html [accessed 8 March 2009]). Additional information regarding dengue viruses can be found in chapter 93.

Japanese Encephalitis Virus

Significance

Japanese encephalitis virus (JEV) is endemic in East and Southeast Asia, where it is the most important cause of mosquito-borne encephalitis. Additionally, JEV has emerged in new geographical areas, including regions of India, Pakistan, and Northern Australia (75, 76, 80). As many as 50,000 cases of severe central nervous system infection due to JEV are reported annually (see "Vector-borne viral infections" at http://www.who.int/vaccine_research/diseases/vector/en/print.html [accessed 8 March 2009]).

Natural Transmission and Epidemiology

JEV is a flavivirus, and strains are grouped into five genotypes (71). JEV is maintained in a zoonotic cycle involving wading birds, pigs, and *Culex* mosquitoes. Pigs serve as amplifying hosts. The virus spills over into humans when populations of infected mosquitoes increase dramatically. Humans are dead-end hosts for JEV and do not contribute significantly to the spread of natural infection. Causes of emergence of JEV include spread by infected birds and wind-blown mosquitoes, increased intensity and expansion of rice production and irrigation programs, and increased contact between humans and pigs (71, 75) (see "Vector-borne viral infections" at http://www.who .int/vaccine_research/diseases/vector/en/print.html). Conversely, efforts to eliminate Japanese encephalitis (by means of vaccination programs, decreasing areas of irrigation fields, and segregation of pigs from residential areas) have resulted in the marked decrease in cases in Japan (2). Viral genotype shift or introduction of new genotypes (most likely through bird migration) has possibly contributed to the emergence of JEV. The recent shift from genotype 3 to genotype 1 has been reported in Thailand (72) and in Japan and Vietnam (71). In northern Australia, where previously all JEV isolates belonged to genotype 2, genotype 1 appeared suddenly in 2000 (80). Recent outbreaks of JEV are notable not only in the appearance of a new genotype within a geographic region but also in the overall expansion of the range of JEV (71, 75).

Clinical Significance

JEV is a significant cause of encephalitis among children and adults in Asia. In Vietnam, it is the etiology of 67% of cases of acute encephalitis in children (71). Most JEV infections are asymptomatic or result in mild febrile illness. Among patients with severe central nervous system infection, the mortality is as high as 35%, and about half of survivors suffer from permanent neurologic sequelae. While the majority of cases occur in adults (2), morbidity and mortality are most severe in children. A recent review of 361 cases of Japanese encephalitis reported between 1981 and 2004 showed an overall case fatality rate of 18%. Half of the cases recovered with neurologic sequelae. Incidence peaked in the young (less than 5 years of age) and in the elderly (greater than 60 years of age) (2). Additional information regarding JEV can be found in chapter 93.

Parasites

Leishmania Species

Significance

Leishmaniasis is a disease transmitted by the bite of female phlebotomine sand flies. Over 20 species of *Leishmania* are pathogenic for humans, causing cutaneous, mucocutaneous, and visceral forms of disease. As many as 350 million people are at risk for *Leishmania* infections, an estimated 12 million people are infected worldwide, and 2 million new infections occur each year (see "Leishmaniasis: the global trend" at http://www.who.int/neglected_diseases/ integrated_media_leishmaniasis/en/print.html [accessed 8 March 2009]).

Natural Transmission and Epidemiology

According to the World Health Organization, leishmaniasis is endemic in 88 countries in East and Central Asia, the Middle East, North Africa, southern Europe, and Central and South America. Cases are concentrated in four geographical areas, South America, the Middle East, South Asia, and Sudan, Africa: 90% of cutaneous leishmaniasis cases occur in Afghanistan, Saudi Arabia, Syria, Brazil, and Peru; 90% of mucocutaneous cases occur in Brazil, Bolivia, and Peru; and 90% of visceral cases occur in Bangladesh, India, Nepal, Sudan, and Brazil ("Leishmaniasis: the global trend" at http://www.who.int/neglected_diseases/ integrated_media_leishmaniasis/en/print.html). Although very rare in the United States, cutaneous leishmaniasis is endemic in Texas (104).

The vector of *Leishmania* spp., the sand fly, is found throughout the intertropical and temperate regions of the world. Dogs, wild rodents, and other mammals are reservoir hosts. Dogs play an important role in the maintenance of leishmaniasis in densely populated suburban settlements in Brazil (see "Leishmaniasis: the global trend" at http://www .who.int/neglected_diseases/integrated_media_leishmaniasis/ en/print.html). However, in Sri Lanka, where incidence is increasing, surveillance of pet dogs and rodents from areas where human cases were diagnosed failed to incriminate either as reservoirs (70). The causes of the emergence of leishmaniasis are human behavior (international travel, urbanization of and migration to areas of endemicity, deforestation, and construction of dams and irrigation projects), increased awareness and surveillance, and the global human immunodeficiency virus (HIV) epidemic. Movement of humans, without existing infrastructure and sanitation, has fueled outbreaks of visceral and cutaneous leishmaniasis in Sudan, Afghanistan, and Brazil. In Sudan, extreme malnutrition has contributed to a sharp increase in the visceral form of disease (see "Leishmaniasis: the global trend" at http://www .who.int/neglected_diseases/integrated_media_leishmaniasis/ en/print.html). Additionally, environmental factors may contribute to the emergence of the disease in certain parts of the world. An association between the El Niño cycle and incidence of visceral leishmaniasis has been reported in Brazil (38). International travel, including deployment of military personnel, and immigration are contributing to emergence. The number of imported cases has risen substantially in Europe (89). A review of 20 imported cases in Australia showed that 7 originated in South America (all caused by *Leishmania mexicana* or *Leishmania braziliensis*), and 10 originated in Afghanistan or Pakistan (all caused by *Leishmania tropica* or *Leishmania major*). Cutaneous leishmaniasis was the predominant presentation (95). The global HIV epidemic is also contributing to the emergence of leishmaniasis. Coinfection with HIV and *Leishmania* spp. has been reported in 34 countries in Africa, Asia, Europe, and South American (see "Leishmaniasis: the global trend" at http://www.who .int/neglected_diseases/integrated_media_leishmaniasis/ en/print.html). The geographic range of *Leishmania* spp. is expanding. Locally acquired visceral leishmaniasis was reported in Thailand, a country considered an area where leishmaniasis is not endemic (59). *L. tropica* is now established in areas of Afghanistan and Pakistan that were previously free of *Leishmania* (95). Although very rare, cutaneous leishmaniasis has long been recognized as endemic in south-central Texas (41, 90). Of potential significance is a recent report suggesting that the range of autochthonous cases of cutaneous leishmaniasis in Texas is expanding northward (104).

Clinical Significance

Leishmaniasis exists in three forms: cutaneous, mucocutaneous, and visceral (kala azar). Cutaneous leishmaniasis is the most common form of disease. Multiple ulcers can occur on the face, arms, and legs, although presentation with a single lesion is common (95). HIV coinfection is associated with poorer clinical outcomes. HIV-infected individuals have a greater risk of developing visceral disease, and leishmaniasis stimulates replication of HIV and accelerates the onset of AIDS (26). In southern Europe, 70% of adults with visceral leishmaniasis are coinfected with HIV, and in Ethiopia, 35% of all leishmaniasis cases are coinfected with HIV (see "Leishmaniasis: the global trend" at http://www.who.int/neglected_ diseases/integrated_media_leishmaniasis/en/print.html).

Additional information regarding *Leishmania* can be found in chapter 134.

Trypanosoma cruzi

Significance

Trypanosoma cruzi is the etiologic agent of Chagas disease (American trypanosomiasis), a generalized acute disease that can manifest as chronic fatal cardiomyopathy. Chagas disease is endemic throughout Central and South America. Cases are increasing within the epidemic region, and there is risk for emergence in the United States.

Natural Transmission and Epidemiology

T. cruzi is most commonly spread when the feces of the vector *Triatoma* (kissing or reduviid bug) is rubbed into an insect bite, wounds, or the eyes or mucous membranes. Animal reservoirs include domestic dogs and various wild mammal species. Although the parasite is considered to be restricted to the continental Americas, it was recently reported that trypanosomes of the cruzi clade were detected in African terrestrial mammals (43). An estimated 8 million to 11 million people in Central and South America are infected (15).

International travel and immigration are largely responsible for the emergence of Chagas disease in countries where it is not endemic. Most reported cases of Chagas disease in the United States are acquired in countries where it is not endemic. It has been estimated that between 100,000 and nearly 700,000 persons infected with *T. cruzi* immigrated legally to the United States between 1981 and 2005 (65). Triatomine bugs are present in the United States, and various animal species are infected, including dogs, raccoons, and armadillos. Serological surveys conducted primarily in southern U.S states have found infection rates of over 60%, which are equal to or greater than those found in the same animal species in Argentina, where Chagas disease is endemic in humans (65). However, autochthonous transmission of *T. cruzi* remains very rare in the United States. The most likely explanation is lack of contact of humans with the triatomine vector. The type of homes that facilitate contact—built with porous materials such as mud, adobe, or straw—is virtually nonexistent in the United States. However, the potential for the emergence of vector-borne transmission in the United States exists in areas with deteriorating housing and ample populations of the triatomine vector, if conditions cause the parasite to spill over from the natural animal reservoirs.

In addition to being transmitted by vector, *T. cruzi* has been transmitted within the United States via organ transplantation (14), via blood transfusion (15), and possibly congenitally (10). The increase in reported cases of Chagas disease in some Latin American countries is due in part to improved recognition through surveillance and laboratory diagnostic capability. Environmental factors could also contribute to the emergence of Chagas disease. After a hurricane on the Yucatan Peninsula of Mexico, there was an increase in the number of triatomine vectors (42).

Clinical Significance

Chagas disease consists of three stages: acute, indeterminate, and chronic. The acute stage is characterized by fever, lymphadenopathy, and malaise. Acute infection in immunocompromised persons can be serious. During the indeterminate phase, the patient is asymptomatic but seropositive. While most patients are asymptomatic during the chronic stage, the lifetime risk of severe heart disease is approximately 30%. Myocardial damage is irreversible. Other forms of chronic disease involve the intestinal tract and alimentary canal (megacolon and megaesophagus). HIV coinfection can lead to reactivation of *T. cruzi* infection, potentially resulting in severe meningoencephalitis (24). Additional information regarding *T. cruzi* can be found in chapter 134.

Fungi

Coccidioides posadasii

Significance

Coccidioides posadasii was described as a species genetically distinct from *Coccidioides immitis* in 2002 (37). *C. posadasii* and *C. immitis* have different geographical ranges; *C. posadasii* is now recognized as the most common cause of coccidioidomycosis acquired outside California, including cases from Central and South America. Reported cases of coccidioidomycosis have increased recently in the United States (18, 86).

Natural Transmission and Epidemiology

Coccidioides spp. are found in the Western Hemisphere, within arid and semiarid regions of endemicity. *C. immitis* and *C. posadasii* have separate and distinct regions of endemicity; *C. immitis* is endemic to the San Joaquin Valley of central California, while *C. posadasii* is endemic to southern Arizona and New Mexico, western Texas, Mexico, and regions of Central and South America (86). A review of patients in Brazil showed that all were young males from a semiarid region of the country and that armadillo hunting was a risk behavior (29). Coccidioidomycosis is a growing threat in the United States. Reported cases in Arizona tripled from 1999 to 2006 (18). The emergence of *C. posadasii* is a result of the recognition of the organism as a separate species, environmental factors (climate change, wildfires), and human activity (travel, dramatic growth of an immunologically naïve population in the southwestern United States, construction activity) (86). This emergence is often reported in states in which the disease is not endemic, to which residents return following vacations in the southwestern United States (81). Wildfires and construction activity (both increasing in frequency or scope) result in the disruption of the soil and aerosolization of infectious arthroconidia.

Clinical Significance

While genetically distinct, *C. posadasii* and *C. immitis* share many phenotypic characteristics, including morphology, clinical disease, and susceptibility to antifungal agents (3, 81). Sixty percent of infections are asymptomatic. Features of symptomatic infections range from mild (fever and headache) to severe (pneumonia and disseminated infection). Additional information regarding *C. posadasii* can be found in chapter 120.

Cryptococcus gattii

Significance

Cryptococcus gattii (formerly *Cryptococcus neoformans* var. *gattii*) was identified as the cause of a 1999 outbreak of human and animal cryptococcosis on Vancouver Island, British Columbia, Canada (96). The sudden emergence of this organism in a temperate region, previously thought to be restricted to tropical and subtropical climates, was unexpected. More recently, *C. gattii* has been detected in the environment and in human and animal specimens from mainland British Columbia and the states of Washington and Oregon.

Natural Transmission and Epidemiology

C. gattii is endemic in tropical and subtropical regions of the world, where it is associated with various ecologic niches, including eucalyptus trees. In 2001, British Columbia public health authorities were notified of increasing cases of cryptococcosis among companion animals (primarily dogs and cats) and humans. The etiologic agent was identified as *C. neoformans gattii* (96). Studies of archived materials have identified the Vancouver Island strain of *C. gattii* among North American isolates dating as far back as the 1970s (27). It has been suggested that *C. gattii* was introduced to Vancouver Island via exported trees, soil on transported vehicles, or wooden pallets or crates (50), where it encountered defined environmental niches favorable for its survival and maintenance. The requirement for particular environmental niches is exemplified by the near total confinement to climatic zones located along the east coast of Vancouver Island and later to similar zones throughout the Pacific Northwest (58). The 1999 outbreak was not likely the result of recent introduction of the organism. Rather, human activities are believed to be largely responsible for the proliferation and dispersal of infectious propagules such that levels are sufficiently high to cause disease. Environmental niches in the Pacific Northwest include trees of various species, soil, and water (50). *C. gattii* concentration in environmental samples (58) and the percentage of environmental samples positive for *C. gattii* (21) correlate with incidence rates. Additional causes for emergence in the Pacific Northwest include human activities (travel, soil contamination of vehicle tires and human footwear, deforestation, production of wood chips, landscaping, and construction activity) (50) and climate change (27). It has also been proposed that cryptic same-sex reproduction of *C. gattii* may have resulted in a more virulent strain and one better able to adapt and propagate in the Vancouver Island environment (39).

Following the 1999 outbreak on Vancouver Island, *C. gattii* emerged on the British Columbia mainland and in limited locations in Washington and Oregon in 2004 (58). Since 2006, *C. gattii* has continued to spread with increased incidence of human disease in Washington and Oregon (12, 27). A previously unrecognized genotype, VGIIa, was predominant on Vancouver Island and mainland British Columbia. This same strain is also common among more recent cases in the United States, but in addition a new strain has emerged in Oregon (12). Climatic zones outside Vancouver Island may be suboptimal for long-term maintenance of *C. gattii*, as demonstrated by the failure to detect the organism in environmental samples from mainland British Columbia in 2005 (58). Colonization of environments outside Vancouver Island may be transient or at levels below the limit of detection (58).

Clinical Significance

C. gattii infection is a result of inhalation of propagules (yeast or spores). Pulmonary infections can disseminate to the central nervous system. To date, over 200 cases have been reported since 1999 in the Pacific Northwest of North America (and many more in companion animals), with an estimated case fatality rate of 4.5% (27).

Cases associated with Vancouver Island were most common in males over 60 years of age. Symptoms included shortness of breath, cough, chills, night sweats, and weight loss (58). The incubation period is long (median, 6 to 7 months), and meningitis has presented as late as 11 months after exposure (54). Additional information regarding *C. gattii* can be found in chapter 115.

REFERENCES

1. **Akerlund, T., I. Persson, M. Unemo, T. Noren, B. Svenungsson, M. Wullt, and L. G. Burman.** 2008. Increased sporulation rate of epidemic *Clostridium difficile* type 027/NAP1. *J. Clin. Microbiol.* **46:**1530–1533.
1a. **American Society for Microbiology.** 2004. Sentinel laboratory guidelines for suspected agents of bioterrorism. *Brucella* species. ASM, Washington, DC. http://www.asm.org/images/pdf/Brucella101504.pdf.
1b. **American Society for Microbiology.** 2003. Sentinel laboratory guidelines for suspected agents of bioterrorism. *Coxiella burnetii.* American Society for Microbiology, Washington, DC. http://www.asm.org/images/pdf/CoxiellaBurnetti.pdf.
1c. **American Society for Microbiology.** 2010. Sentinel level clinical laboratory guidelines for suspected agents of bioterrorism and emerging infectious diseases. *Yersinia pestis.* American Society for Microbiology, Washington, DC. http://www.asm.org/images/pdf/Clinical/ypestisrevised6-11-10.pdf.
1d. **American Society for Microbiology.** 2004. Sentinel laboratory guidelines for suspected agents of bioterrorism. Botulinum toxin. ASM, Washington, DC. http://www.asm.org/images/pdf/Botulism.pdf.
1e. **American Society for Microbiology.** 2003. Sentinel laboratory guidelines for suspected agents of bioterrorism. Staphylococcal enterotoxin B. ASM, Washington, DC. http://www.asm.org/images/pdf/SEBrevised.pdf.
2. **Arai, S., Y. Matsunaga, T. Takasaki, K. Tanaka-Taya, K. Taniguchi, N. Okabe, I. Kurane, and the Vaccine Preventable Diseases Surveillance Program of Japan.** 2008. Japanese encephalitis: surveillance and elimination effort in Japan from 1982 to 2004. *Jpn. J. Infect. Dis.* **61:**333–338.
3. **Barker, B. M., K. A. Jewell, S. Kroken, and M. J. Orbach.** 2007. The population biology of *Coccidioides*—epidemiologic implications for disease outbreaks. *Ann. N. Y. Acad. Sci.* **1111:**147–163.
4. **Bauer, M. P., A. Goorhuis, T. Koster, S. C. Numan-Ruberg, E. C. Hagen, S. B. Debast, E. J. Kuijper, and J. T. van Dissel.** 2008. Community-onset *Clostridium difficile*-associated diarrhea not associated with antibiotic usage—two case reports with review of the changing epidemiology of *Clostridium difficile*-associated diarrhea. *Neth. J. Med.* **66:**207–211.
5. **Bleck, T. P.** 2005. Botulinum toxin as a biological weapon, p. 3624–3625. *In* G. L. Mandell, J. E. Bennett, and R. Dolin (ed.), *Principles and Practices of Infectious Diseases,* 6th ed. Elsevier Churchill Livingstone, Philadelphia, PA.
6. **Borgherini, G., P. Poubeau, A. Jossaume, A. Gouix, L. Cotte, A. Michault, C. Arvin-Berod, and F. Paganin.** 2008. Persistent arthralgia associated with chikungunya virus: a study of 88 adult patients on Reunion Island. *Clin. Infect. Dis.* **47:**469–475.
7. **Borio, L. L.** 2005. Plague as an agent of bioterrorism, p. 3601–3605. *In* G. L. Mandell, J. E. Bennett, and R. Dolin (ed.), *Principles and Practices of Infectious Diseases,* 6th ed. Elsevier Churchill Livingstone, Philadelphia, PA.
8. **Brachman, P. S.** 1980. Inhalational anthrax. *Ann. N. Y. Acad. Sci.* **353:**83–93.
9. **Brooks, J. T., E. G. Sowers, J. G. Wells, K. D. Greene, P. M. Griffin, R. M. Hoekstra, and N. A. Strockbine.** 2005. Non-O157 Shiga toxin-producing *Escherichia coli* infections in the United States, 1983–2002. *J. Infect. Dis.* **192:**1422–1429.
10. **Buekens, P., O. Almendares, Y. Carlier, E. Dumonteil, M. Eberhard, R. Gamboa-Leon, M. James, N. Padilla, D. Wesson, and X. Xiong.** 2007. Mother-to-child transmission of Chagas' disease in North American: why don't we do more? *Matern. Child Health J.* **12:**283–286.

11. **Butler, T., and D. T. Dennis.** 2005. Yersinia species, including plague, p. 2691–2701. *In* G. L. Mandell, J. E. Bennett, and R. Dolin (ed.), *Principles and Practices of Infectious Diseases,* 6th ed. Elsevier Churchill Livingstone, Philadelphia, PA.

12. **Byrnes, E. J., R. J. Bildfell, S. A. Frank, T. G. Mitchell, K. A. Marr, and J. Heitman.** 2009. Molecular evidence that the range of the Vancouver Island outbreak of *Cryptococcus gattii* infection has expanded into the Pacific Northwest in the United States. *J. Infect. Dis.* **199:**1081–1086.

13. **Centers for Disease Control and Prevention.** 2002. Tularemia—United States, 1990–2000. *MMWR Morb. Mortal. Wkly. Rep.* **51:**182–184.

14. **Centers for Disease Control and Prevention.** 2006. Chagas disease after organ transplantation—Los Angeles, California, 2006. *MMWR Morb. Mortal. Wkly. Rep.* **55:**798–800.

15. **Centers for Disease Control and Prevention.** 2007. Blood donor screening for Chagas disease—United States, 2006–2007. *MMWR Morb. Mortal. Wkly. Rep.* **56:**141–143.

16. **Centers for Disease Control and Prevention.** 2008. Surveillance for community-associated *Clostridium difficile*—Connecticut, 2006. *MMWR Morb. Mortal. Wkly. Rep.* **57:**340–343.

17. **Centers for Disease Control and Prevention.** 2008. Laboratory-acquired brucellosis—Indiana and Minnesota, 2006. *MMWR Morb. Mortal. Wkly. Rep.* **57:**39–42.

18. **Centers for Disease Control and Prevention.** 2009. Increase in coccidioidomycosis—California, 2000–2007. *MMWR Morb. Mortal. Wkly. Rep.* **58:**105–109.

19. **Centers for Disease Control and Prevention.** 2009. Neurologic complications associated with novel influenza A (H1N1) virus infection in children—Dallas, Texas, May 2009. *MMWR Morb. Mortal. Wkly. Rep.* **58:**773–778.

20. **Centers for Disease Control and Prevention.** 2009. Intensive-care patients with severe novel influenza A (H1N1) virus infection—Michigan, June 2009. *MMWR Morb. Mortal. Wkly. Rep.* **58:**749–752.

20a. **Centers for Disease Control and Prevention, American Society for Microbiology, and the Association of Public Health Laboratories.** 2001. Basic protocols for level A laboratories for the presumptive identification of *Francisella tularensis.* American Society for Microbiology, Washington, DC. http://www.asm.org/images/pdf/tularemiaprotocol.pdf.

21. **Chambers, C., L. MacDougall, M. Li, and E. Galanis.** 2008. Tourism and specific risk areas for *Cryptococcus gattii,* Vancouver Island, Canada. *Emerg. Infect. Dis.* **14:**1781–1783.

22. **Chen, H. L., S. R. Lin, H. F. Liu, C. C. King, S. C. Hsieh, and W. K. Wang.** 2008. Evolution of dengue virus type 2 during two consecutive outbreaks with an increase in severity in southern Taiwan in 2001–2002. *Am. J. Trop. Med. Hyg.* **79:**495–505.

23. **Christopher, G. W., T. J. Cieslak, J. A. Pavlin, and E. M. Litzen.** 1997. Biological warfare: a historical perspective. *JAMA* **278:**412–417.

24. **Cordova, E., A. Boschi, and J. Ambrosioni.** 2008. Reactivation of Chagas disease with central nervous system involvement in HIV-infected patients in Argentina, 1992–2007. *Int. J. Infect. Dis.* **12:**587–592.

25. **Curry, S. R., J. W. Marsh, C. A. Muto, M. M. O'Leary, A. W. Pasculle, and L. H. Harrison.** 2007. tcdC genotypes associated with severe TcdC truncation in an epidemic clone and other strains of *Clostridium difficile. J. Clin. Microbiol.* **45:**21–221.

26. **Daher, E. D., P. P. Fonseca, E. S. Gerhard, T. D. Silva Leitao, and G. B. Silva.** 2008. Clinical and epidemiological features of visceral leishmaniasis and HIV co-infection in 15 patients from Brazil. *J. Parasitol.* **2:**1. (Epub ahead of print.)

27. **Datta, K., K. H. Bartlett, and K. A. Marr.** 2009. *Cryptococcus gattii*: emergence in western North America: exploitation of a novel ecological niche. *Interdiscip. Perspect. Infect. Dis.* **2009:**176532. (Epub 15 January 2009.)

28. **Davis, C. J.** 1999. Nuclear blindness: an overview of the biological weapons programs of the former Soviet Union and Iraq. *Emerg. Infect. Dis.* **5:**509–512.

29. **de Aguiar Cordeiro, R., R. S. N. Brilhante, M. F. G. Rocha, S. P. Bandeira, M. A. B. Fechine, Z. P. de Camargo, and J. J. C. Sidrim.** 2008. Twelve years of coccidioidomycosis in Ceara State, northeast Brazil: epidemiologic and diagnostic aspects. *Diagn. Microbiol. Infect. Dis.* **66:**65–72.

30. **Derbes, V. J.** 1966. De Mussis and the great plague of 1348. A forgotten episode of bacteriological warfare. *JAMA* **196:**59–62.

31. **Economopoulou, A., M. Dominguez, B. Helynck, D. Sissoko, O. Wichmann, P. Quenel, P. Germonneau, and I. Quatresous.** 2008. Atypical Chikungunya virus infections: clinical manifestations, mortality and risk factors for severe disease during the 2005–2008 outbreak on Reunion. *Epidemiol. Infect.* **11:**1–8.

32. **Eitzem, E., J. Pavlin, T. Cieslak, G. Christopher, and R. Culpepper.** 1998. *Medical Management of Biological Casualties Handbook,* 3rd ed., p. 107–109. U.S. Army Medical Research Institute of Infectious Diseases, Fort Detrick, Frederick, MD.

33. **El Sayed, F., and R. Dhaybi.** 2008. Chikungunya associated with cutaneous ulcerations. *Clin. Exp. Dermatol.* **33:**463–464.

34. **Espie, E., F. Grimont, P. Mariani-Kurkdjian, P. Bouvet, S. Haeghebaert, I. Filliol, C. Loirat, B. Decludt, N. N. Minh, V. Vaillant, and H. de Valk.** 2008. Surveillance of hemolytic uremic syndrome in children less than 15 years of age, a system to monitor O157 and non-O157 Shiga toxin-producing *Escherichia coli* infections in France, 1996–2006. *Pediatr. Infect. Dis. J.* **27:**595–601.

35. **Ethelberg, S., B. Smith, M. Torpdahl, M. Lisby, J. Boel, T. Jensen, E. Moller Nielsen, and K. Molbak.** 2009. Outbreak of non-O157 Shiga toxin-producing *Escherichia coli* infection from consumption of beef sausage. *Clin. Infect. Dis.* **48:**e78–e81.

36. **Fawley, W. N., J. Freeman, C. Smith, C. Harmanus, R. J. van den Berg, E. J. Kuijper, and M. H. Wilcox.** 2008. Use of highly discriminatory fingerprinting to analyze clusters of *Clostridium difficile* infection cases due to epidemic ribotype 027 strains. *J. Clin. Microbiol.* **46:**954–960.

36a. **Federal Register.** 2009. HHS and USDA select agents and toxins. 7 CFR Part 331, 9 CFR Part 121, and 42 CFR Part 73. Department of Health and Human Services, Washington, DC.

37. **Fisher, M. C., G. L. Koenig, T. J. White, and J. W. Taylor.** 2002. Molecular and phenotypic description of *Coccidioides posadasii* sp. nov., previously recognized as the non-California population of *Coccidioides immitis. Mycologia* **94:**73–84.

38. **Franke, C. R., M. Ziller, C. Staubach, and M. Latif.** 2002. Impact of the El Nino/southern oscillation on visceral leishmaniasis, Brazil. *Emerg. Infect. Dis.* **8:**914–917.

39. **Fraser, J. A., S. S. Giles, E. C. Wenink, S. G. Geunes-Boyer, J. R. Wright, S. Diezmann, A. Allen, J. E. Stajich, F. S. Dietrich, J. R. Perfect, and J. Heitman.** 2005. Same-sex mating and the origin of the Vancouver Island *Cryptococcus gattii* outbreak. *Nature* **437:**1360–1364.

40. **Gilchrist, M. J. R., W. P. McKinney, J. M. Miller, and J. W. Snyder.** 2000. Cumitech 33. Laboratory safety, management, and diagnosis of biological agents associated with bioterrorism. Coord. ed., J. W. Snyder. ASM Press, Washington, DC.

41. **Gustafson, T. L., C. M. Reed, P. B. McGreevy, M. G. Pappas, J. C. Fox, and P. G. Lawyer.** 1985. Human cutaneous leishmaniasis acquired in Texas. *Am. J. Trop. Med. Hyg.* **34:**58–63.

42. **Guzman-Tapia, Y., M. J. Ramirez-Sierra, J. Escobedo-Ortegon, and E. Dumonteil.** 2005. Effect of hurricane Isidore on triatoma dimidiate distribution and Chagas disease transmission risk in the Yucatan peninsula of Mexico. *Am. J. Trop. Med. Hyg.* **73:**1019–1025.

43. **Hamilton, P. B., E. R. Adams, F. Njiokou, W. C. Gibson, G. Cuny, and S. Herder.** 2009. Phylogenetic analysis reveals the presence of the Trypanosoma cruzi clade in African terrestrial mammals. *Infect. Genet. Evol.* **9:**81–86.

44. **Hofhuis, A., J. Reimerink, C. Reusken, E. J. Scholte, A. D. Boer, W. Takken, and M. Koopmans.** 2009. The hidden passenger of lucky bamboo: do imported *Aedes albopictus* mosquitoes cause dengue virus transmission in the Netherlands? *Vector Borne Zoonotic Dis.* **9:**217–220. (Epub ahead of print 30 October 2008.)

45. **Kamboj, D. V., A. K. Goel, and L. Singh.** 2006. Biological warfare agents. *Defense Sci. J.* **56:**495–506.

46. **Kanakaratne, N., W. M. P. B. Wahala, W. B. Messer, H. A. Tissera, A. Shahani, N. Abeysinghe, A. M. de Silva, and M. Gunasekera.** 2009. Severe dengue epidemics in Sri Lanka, 2003–2006. *Emerg. Infect. Dis.* **15:**192–199.

47. **Karama, M., R. P. Johnson, R. Holtslander, and C. L. Gyles.** 2008. Phenotypic and genotypic characteristics of verotoxin-producing *Escherichia coli* O103:H2 isolates from cattle and humans. *J. Clin. Microbiol.* **46:**3569–3575.

48. **Kariuki Njenga, M., L. Nderitu, J. P. Ledermann, A. Ndirangu, C. H. Logue, C. H. Kelly, R. Sang, K. Sergon, R. Breiman, and A. M. Powers.** 2008. Tracking epidemic Chikungunya virus into the Indian Ocean from East Africa. *J. Gen. Virol.* **89:**2754–2760.

49. **Kaur, P., M. Punish, M. V. Moorhead, V. Ramachandran, R. Ramachandran, H. K. Raju, V. Perumal, A. C. Mishra, and M. D. Gupte.** 2008. Chikungunya outbreak, South India, 2006. *Emerg. Infect. Dis.* **14:**1623–1625.

50. **Kidd, S. E., P. J. Bach, A. O. Hingston, S. Mak, Y. Chow, L. MacDougall, J. W. Kronstad, and K. H. Bartlett.** 2007. Cryptococcus gattii dispersal mechanisms, British Columbia, Canada. *Emerg. Infect. Dis.* **13:**51–57.

51. **Koopmans, M., B. Wilbrink, M. Conyn, G. Natrop, H. van der Nat, H. Vennema, A. Meijer, J. van Steenbergen, R. Fouchier, A. Osterhaus, and A. Bosman.** 2004. Transmission of H7N7 avian influenza A virus to human beings during a large outbreak in commercial poultry farms in the Netherlands. *Lancet* **363:**587–593.

52. **Labbe, A. C., L. Poirier, D. Maccannell, T. Louie, M. Savoie, C. Beliveau, M. Laverdiere, and J. Pepin.** 2008. *Clostridium difficile* infections in a Canadian tertiary care hospital before and during a regional epidemic associated with the BI/NAP1/027 strain. *Antimicrob. Agents Chemother.* **52:**3180–3187.

53. **Lemant, J., V. Boisson, A. Winer, L. Thibault, H. Andre, F. Tixier, M. Lemercier, E. Antok, M. P. Cresta, P. Grivard, M. Besnard, O. Rollot, F. Favier, M. Huerre, J. L. Campinos, and A. Michault.** 2008. Serious acute chikungunya virus infection requiring intensive care during the Reunion Island outbreak in 2005–2006. *Crit. Care Med.* **36:**2536–2541.

54. **Levy, R., J. Pitout, P. Long, and M. J. Gill.** 2007. Late presentation of *Cryptococcus gattii* meningitis in a traveler to Vancouver Island: a case report. *Can. J. Infect. Dis. Med. Microbiol.* **18:**197–199.

55. **Lin, Y. P., M. Shaw, V. Gregory, K. Cameron, W. Lim, A. Klimov, K. Subbarao, Y. Guan, S. Krauss, K. Shortridge, R. Webster, N. Cox, and A. Hay.** 2000. Avian-to-human transmission of H9N2 subtype influenza A viruses: relationship between H9N2 and H5N1 human isolates. *Proc. Natl. Acad. Sci. USA* **97:**9654–9658.

56. **Lucey, D.** 2005. Anthrax, p. 3618. *In* G. L. Mandell, J. E. Bennett, and R. Dolin (ed.), *Principles and Practices of Infectious Diseases*, 6th ed. Elsevier Churchill Livingstone, Philadelphia, PA.

57. **Lucey, D.** 2005. Bacillus anthracis (anthrax), p. 2486. *In* G. L. Mandell, J. E. Bennett, and R. Dolin (ed.), *Principles and Practices of Infectious Diseases*, 6th ed. Elsevier Churchill Livingstone, Philadelphia, PA.

58. **MacDougall, L., S. E. Kidd, E. Galanis, S. Mak, M. J. Leslie, P. R. Cieslak, J. W. Kronstad, M. G. Morshed, and K. H. Bartlett.** 2007. Spread of *Cryptococcus gattii* in British Columbia, Canada, and detection in the Pacific Northwest, USA. *Emerg. Infect. Dis.* **13:**42–50.

59. **Maharom, P., S. Siripattanapipong, M. Mungthin, T. Naaglor, R. Sukkawee, R. Pudkorn, W. Wattana, D. Wanachiwanawin, D. Areechokchai, and S. Leelayoova.** 2008. Visceral leishmaniasis caused by *Leishmania infantum* in Thailand. *Southeast Asian J. Trop. Med. Public Health* **39:**988–990.

60. **Marrie, T. J., and D. Roult.** 2005. Coxiella burnetii (Q fever), p. 2296–2303. *In* G. L. Mandell, J. E. Bennett, and R. Dolin (ed.), *Principles and Practices of Infectious Diseases*, 6th ed. Elsevier Churchill Livingstone, Philadelphia, PA.

61. **Martin, H., B. Willey, D. E. Low, H. R. Staempfli, A. McGeer, P. Boerlin, M. Mulvey, and J. S. Weese.** 2008. Characterization of *Clostridium difficile* strains isolated from patients in Ontario, Canada, from 2004 to 2006. *J. Clin. Microbiol.* **46:**2999–3004.

62. **McDonald, L. C., G. E. Killgore, A. Thompson, R. C. Owens, S. V. Kazakova, S. P. Sambol, S. Johnson, and D. N. Gerding.** 2005. An epidemic, toxin gene-variant strain of *Clostridium difficile*. *N. Engl. J. Med.* **353:**2433–2441.

63. **McFarland, L. V.** 2009. Renewed interest in a difficult disease: *Clostridium difficile* infections—epidemiology and current treatment strategies. *Curr. Opin. Gastroenterol.* **25:**24–35.

64. **Mellmann, A., M. Bielaszewska, R. Kock, A. W. Friedrich, A. Fruth, B. Middendorf, D. Harmsen, M. A. Schmidt, and H. Karch.** 2008. Analysis of collection of hemolytic uremic syndrome-associated enterohemorrhagic *Escherichia coli*. *Emerg. Infect. Dis.* **14:**1287–1290.

65. **Milei, J., R. A. Guerri-Guttenberg, D. R. Grana, and R. Storino.** 2009. Prognostic impact of Chagas disease in the United States. *Am. Heart J.* **157:**22–29.

66. **Missaghi, B., A. J. Valenti, and R. C. Owens.** 2008. *Clostridium difficile* infection: a critical review. *Curr. Infect. Dis. Rep.* **10:**165–173.

67. **Mitchell, C. L., and R. L. Penn.** 2005. *Francisella tularensis* (tularemia) as an agent of bioterrorism, p. 3607–3612. *In* G. L. Mandell, J. E. Bennett, and R. Dolin (ed.), *Principles and Practices of Infectious Diseases*, 6th ed. Elsevier Churchill Livingstone, Philadelphia, PA.

68. **Moreillon, P., Y. Que, and M. P. Glauser.** 2005. *Staphylococcus aureus* (including staphylococcal toxin shock), p. 2330–2332. *In* G. L. Mandell, J. E. Bennett, and R. Dolin (ed.), *Principles and Practices of Infectious Diseases*, 6th ed. Elsevier Churchill Livingstone, Philadelphia, PA.

69. **Morens, D. M., G. K. Folkers, and A. S. Fauci.** 2004. The challenge of emerging and re-emerging infectious diseases. *Nature* **430:**242–249.

70. **Nawaratna, S. S., D. J. Weilgama, and K. Rajapaksha.** 2009. Cutaneous leishmaniasis in Sri Lanka: a study of possible animal reservoirs. *Int. J. Infect. Dis.* **13:**513–517. (Epub ahead of print 16 December 2008.)

71. **Nga, P. T., M. del Carmen Parquet, V. D. Cuong, S.-P. Ma, F. Hasebe, S. Inoue, Y. Makino, M. Takagi, V. S. Nam, and K. Morita.** 2004. Shift in Japanese encephalitis virus (JEV) genotype circulating in northern Vietnam: implications for frequent introductions of JEV from Southeast Asia to East Asia. *J. Gen. Virol.* **85:**1625–1631.

72. **Nitatpattana, N., A. Dubot-Peres, M. A. Gouilh, M. Souris, P. Barbazan, S. Yoksan, X. de Lamballerie, and J. P. Gonzalez.** 2008. Change in Japanese encephalitis virus distribution, Thailand. *Emerg. Infect. Dis.* **14:**1762–1765.

73. **Novel Swine-Origin Influenza A (H1N1) Virus Investigation Team.** 2009. Emergence of a novel swine-origin influenza A (H1N1) virus in humans. *N. Engl. J. Med.* **360:**2605–2615. (Erratum, **360:**102-a.)

74. **Olano, J. P., and D. H. Walker.** 2009. Agents of emerging infectious diseases, p. 3–20. *In* A. D. Barrett and L. R. Stanberry (ed.), *Vaccines for Biodefense and Emerging and Neglected Diseases.* Elsevier, London, United Kingdom.

75. **Oya, A., and I. Kurane.** 2007. Japanese encephalitis for a reference to international travelers. *Int. Soc. Travel Med.* **14:**259–268.

76. **Parida, M., P. K. Dash, N. K. Tripathi, Ambuj, S. Sannaran-gaiah, P. Saxena, S. Agarwal, A. K. Sahni, S. P. Singh, A. K. Rathi, R. Bhargava, A. Abhyankar, S. K. Verma, P. V. Lakshmana Rao, and K. Sekhar.** 2006. Japanese encephalitis outbreak, India, 2005. *Emerg. Infect. Dis.* **12:**1427–1430.

76a. **Park, C. W., M. R. Melia, L. F. Littlejohn, and T. M. Stein.** 2008. CBRNE - T-2 mycotoxins. Emedicine from WebMD. http://emedicine.medscape.com/article/830892-overview.

77. **Penn, R. L.** 2005. *Francisella tularensis* (tularemia), p. 2674–2685. *In* G. L. Mandell, J. E. Bennett, and R. Dolin (ed.), *Principles and Practices of Infectious Diseases*, 6th ed. Elsevier Churchill Livingstone, Philadelphia, PA.

78. **Peters, C. J.** 2005. Bioterrorism: viral hemorrhagic fevers, p. 3626–3629. *In* G. L. Mandell, J. E. Bennett, and R. Dolin (ed.), *Principles and Practices of Infectious Diseases*, 6th ed. Elsevier Churchill Livingstone, Philadelphia, PA.

79. **Pike, R. M.** 1976. Laboratory-associated infections: summary and analysis of 3921 cases. *Health Lab. Sci.* **13:**105–114.

80. **Pyke, A. T., D. T. Williams, D. J. Nisbet, A. F. van den Hurk, C. T. Taylor, C. A. Johansen, J. MacDonald, R. A. Hall, R. J. Simmons, R. J. V. Mason, J. M. Lee, S. A. Ritchie, G. A. Smith, and J. S. Mackenzie.** 2001. The appearance of a second genotype of Japanese encephalitis virus in the Australasian region. *Am. J. Trop. Med. Hyg.* **65:**747–753.

81. **Ramani, R., and V. Chaturvedi.** 2007. Antifungal susceptibility profiles of *Coccidioides immitis* and *Coccidioides posadasii* from endemic and non-endemic areas. *Mycopathologia* **163:**315–319.

82. **Rao, G., Y. Z. Khan, and D. S. Chitins.** 2008. Chikungunya infection in neonates. *Indian Pediatr.* **45:**240–242.

83. **Rezza, G., L. Nicoletti, R. Angelini, R. Romi, A. C. Finarelli, M. Panning, P. Cordioli, C. Fortuna, S. Boros, F. Magurano, G. Silvi, P. Angelini, M. Dottori, M. G. Ciufolini, G. C. Majori, A. Cassone, for the CHIKV Study Group.** 2007. Infection with chikungunya virus in Italy: an outbreak in a temperate region. *Lancet* **370:**1840–1846.

84. **Rotz, L. D., J. Cono, and I. Damon.** 2005. Smallpox and bioterrorism, p. 3612–3617. *In* G. L. Mandell, J. E. Bennett, and R. Dolin (ed.), *Principles and Practices of Infectious Diseases*, 6th ed. Elsevier Churchill Livingstone, Philadelphia, PA.

85. **Sanchez, S. A. Garcia-Sanchez, R. Martinez, J. Blanco, J. E. Blanco, M. Blanco, G. Dahbi, A. Mora, J. Hermoso de Mendoza, J. M. Alonso, and J. Rey.** 2009. Detection and characterization of Shiga toxin-producing *Escherichia coli* other than *Escherichia coli* O157:H7 in wild ruminants. *Vet. J.* **180:**384–388.

86. **Saubolle, M. A., P. P. McKellar, and D. Sussland.** 2007. Epidemiologic, clinical, and diagnostic aspects of coccidioidomycosis. *J. Clin. Microbiol.* **45:**26–30.

87. **Scholte E. J., Dijkstra, E. H. Blok, A. De Vries, W. Takken, A. Hofhuis, M. Koopmans, A. De Boer, and C. B. Reusken.** 2008. Accidental importation of the mosquito *Aedes albopictus* into the Netherlands: a survey of mosquito distribution and the presence of dengue virus. *Med. Vet. Entomol.* **22:**352–358.

88. **Schuffenecker, I., I. Iteman, A. Michault, S. Murri, L. Frangeul, M. C. Vaney, R. Lavenir, N. Pardigon, J. M. Reynes, F. Pettinelli, L Biscornet, L. Diancourt, S. Michel, S. Duquerroy, G. Guigon, M. P. Frenkiel, A. C. Brehin, N. Cubito, P. Despres, F. Kunst, F. A. Rey, H. Zeller, and S. Brisse.** 2006. Genome microevolution of chikungunya viruses causing the Indian Ocean outbreak. *PLoS Med.* **3:**e263.

89. **Schwartz, E., C. Hatz, and J. Blum.** 2006. New world cutaneous leishmaniasis in travelers. *Lancet Infect. Dis.* **6:**342–349.

90. **Shaw, P. K., L. T. Quigg, D. S. Allain, D. D. Juranek, and G. R. Healy.** 1976. Autochthonous dermal leishmaniasis in Texas. *Am. J. Trop. Med. Hyg.* **25:**788–796.

91. **Shu, P.-Y., C.-F. Yang, C.-L. Su, C.-Y. Chen, S.-F. Chang, K.-H. Tsai, C.-H. Cheng, and J.-H. Huang.** 2008. Two imported chikungunya cases, Taiwan. *Emerg. Infect. Dis.* **14:**1325–1326.

92. **Singh, S. S., S. P. Manimunda, A. P. Sugunan, Sahina, and P. Vijayachari.** 2008. Four cases of acute flaccid paralysis associated with chikungunya virus infection. *Epidemiol. Infect.* **136:**1277–1280.

93. **Sissoko, D., D. Malvy, C. Giry, G. Delmas, C. Paquet, P. Gabrie, F. Pettinelli, M. A. Sanquer, and V. Pierre.** 2008. Outbreak of Chikungunya fever in Mayotte, Comoros archipelago, 2005–2006. *Trans. R. Soc. Trop. Med. Hyg.* **102:**780–786.

94. **Stabler, R. A., L. F. Dawson, L. T. Phua, and B. W. Wren.** 2008. Comparative analysis of BI/NAP1/027 hypervirulent strains reveals novel toxin B encoding gene (*tcdB*) sequences. *J. Med. Microbiol.* **57:**771–775.

95. **Stark, D., S. van Hal, R. Lee, D. Marriott, and J. Harkness.** 2008. Leishmaniasis, and emerging imported infection: report of 20 cases from Australia. *J. Travel Med.* **15:**351–354.

96. **Stephen, C., S. Lester, W. Black, M. Fyfe, and S. Raverty.** 2002. Multispecies outbreak of cryptococcosis on southern Vancouver Island, British Columbia. *Can. Vet. J.* **43:**792–794.

97. **Townson, H., and M. B. Nathan.** 2008. Resurgence of chikungunya. *Trans. R. Soc. Trop. Med. Hyg.* **102:**308–309.

98. **Tucker, J. B.** 2000. Toxic terror. BCSIA studies in international security. MIT Press, Cambridge, MA.

99. **Ungchusak K., P. Auewarakul, S. F. Dowell, R. Kitphati, W. Auwanit, P. Puthavathana, M. Uiprasertkul, K. Boonnak, C. Pittayawonganon, N. J. Cox, S. R. Zaki, P. Thawatsupha, M. Chittaganpitch, R. Khontong, J. M. Simmerman, and S. Chunsutthiwat.** 2005. Probable person-to-person transmission of avian influenza A (H5N1). *N. Eng. J. Med.* **352:**333–340.

100. **United Nations, Department of Public Information.** 1996. The United Nations and the Iraq-Kuwait conflict, 1990–1996, p. 784. United Nations Blue Book Series, vol. IX. United Nations, Department of Public Information, New York, NY.

101. **Vasilakis, N., and S. C. Weaver.** 2008. The history and evolution of human dengue emergence. *Adv. Virus Res.* **72:**1–76.

102. **Warny, M., J. Pepin, A. Fang, G. Killgore, A. Thompson, J. Brazier, E. Frost, and L. C. McDonald.** 2005. Toxin production by an emerging strain of *Clostridium difficile* associated with outbreaks of severe disease in North American and Europe. *Lancet* **366:**1079–1084.

103. **Wilder-Smith, A., and D. J. Gubler.** 2008. Geographic expansion of dengue: the impact of international travel. *Med. Clin. North Am.* **92:**1377–1390.

104. **Wright, N. A., L. E. Davis, K. S. Aftergut, C. A. Parrish, and C. J. Cockerell.** 2008. Cutaneous leishmaniasis in Texas: a northern spread of endemic areas. *J. Am. Acad. Dermatol.* **58:**650–652.

105. **Writing Committee of the Second World Health Organization (WHO) Consultation on Clinical Aspects of Human Infection with Avian Influenza A (H5N1) Virus.** 2008. Update on avian influenza A (H5N1) virus infection in humans. *N. Engl. J. Med.* **358:**261–273.

106. **Young, E. J.** 2005. Brucella species, p. 2669–2674. *In* G. L. Mandell, J. E. Bennett, and R. Dolin (ed.), *Principles and Practices of Infectious Diseases*, 6th ed. Elsevier Churchill Livingstone, Philadelphia, PA.

The Human Microbiome

SARAH K. HIGHLANDER, JAMES VERSALOVIC, AND JOSEPH F. PETROSINO

13

The total number of bacteria in the human body is at least 10 times greater than the number of human cells (97), yet the identity and distribution of the microorganisms that constitute these populations are not well understood. More importantly, how these bacteria contribute to, and are affected by, human health is also relatively understudied, not because of an underappreciation of the impact that these organisms may have but because the strategies and tools necessary to study these populations have not been available until recently. Some progress in cataloging and characterizing these organisms and genes has been made in recent years, but most studies have focused on a single body site. Recent advances in DNA sequencing technologies have enabled more comprehensive analyses of the human microbiota and its role in human health, and it has been proposed that a concerted effort leveraging these technologies would increase the understanding of the microbial communities ("microbiomes" as coined by Lederberg in 1958 [52]) that inhabit various niches within the human body. The newest DNA sequencing platforms make it possible to sequence the DNA of the collective genome (or metagenome) of entire communities of microbes from all body sites, effectively enabling the characterization of the "human microbiome."

INTRODUCTION TO THE HUMAN MICROBIOME PROJECT

In 2007, an NIH Roadmap for Medical Research Project called the Human Microbiome Project (HMP) was initiated (http://nihroadmap.nih.gov/hmp/). The overarching goal of the HMP is to develop tools and resources for characterization of the human microbiota and to relate this microbiota to human health and disease. The HMP is leveraging the constantly advancing sequencing and bioinformatics technologies to address the following broad goals:

- Determining whether individuals share a core human microbiome.
- Understanding whether changes in the human microbiome can be correlated with changes in human health and disease.
- Developing the new technological and bioinformatics tools needed to support these goals.
- Addressing the ethical, legal, and social implications raised by human microbiome research.

The HMP is a multiphase project that began with a "jumpstart phase" that involved four genome sequencing centers: the Baylor College of Medicine Human Genome Sequencing Center, the Broad Institute, the J. Craig Venter Institute, and the Genome Center at Washington University. The goals of the jumpstart phase have been to sequence 900 reference genomes to provide a catalog of genomes for metagenomic studies, to sample at least 300 healthy adults between 18 and 40 years of age at five body sites, and to develop sequencing and analysis protocols for the samples derived from human subjects (88). The second phase of the HMP includes human microbiome studies that target particular disease states. While the human microbiome includes bacteria, viruses, and small eukaryotes, such as fungi, this chapter focuses on the bacterial members of the microbiome.

TECHNIQUES FOR THE STUDY OF THE HUMAN MICROBIOME

Early studies of the human microbiome relied on culture-dependent methods; however, it is now known that the majority of microorganisms from the human body cannot be cultured in vitro. Most current techniques for characterization of a metagenomic sample are polymerase chain reaction (PCR) based and target the highly conserved bacterial 16S ribosomal small subunit RNA. Portions of the gene can be amplified and fingerprinted by using electrophoretic techniques, such as terminal restriction fragment length polymorphism (TRFLP) and denaturing gradient gel electrophoresis. Full-length 16S rRNA genes or segments of these genes can be amplified prior to microarray analyses or DNA sequencing studies. 16S rRNA gene sequences that are ≥97% identical are considered to be within the same species, while those that are ≥95% identical are within the same genus. Currently, metagenomic samples are most often analyzed by sequencing of 16S rRNA gene or gene fragment amplicons by direct whole-genome shotgun (WGS) sequencing (5, 27, 33).

Culture-dependent and culture-independent surveys have shown that the human body is home to only four predominant phyla (Table 1). The *Firmicutes* and *Actinobacteria* are the most highly represented phyla when all body sites are considered. In a recent study, four phyla comprised 92.3% of bacterial DNA sequences analyzed from multiple

TABLE 1 Predominant phyla by body site

Body site	Predominant phylum or phyla[a]	Reference(s)
Oral cavity	*Firmicutes, Actinobacteria*	82
Esophagus	*Firmicutes, Bacteroidetes, Actinobacteria*	84
Stomach	*Proteobacteria, Firmicutes, Actinobacteria*	5, 11
Small intestine	*Firmicutes*	97, 111
Colon (stool)	*Firmicutes, Actinobacteria, Bacteroidetes*	5, 29, 39, 105
Genitourinary tract	*Firmicutes, Actinobacteria, Fusobacteria*	15, 112
Upper respiratory tract	*Firmicutes, Proteobacteria*	53
Skin, sebaceous	*Actinobacteria, Firmicutes, Proteobacteria*	42
Skin, moist	*Actinobacteria, Proteobacteria, Firmicutes, Bacteroidetes*	42
Skin, dry	*Proteobacteria, Actinobacteria, Bacteroidetes*	42

[a]Phyla are listed in order of predominance inferred from the reference(s) cited.

human sources, including hair, oral cavity, skin, and gastrointestinal tract (21). The predominant phyla vary by anatomical site, and presumably the host milieu has a crucial role in shaping the composition of microbial communities at each site. Recent efforts have been aimed at expanding the DNA sequence representation within each phylum so that more comprehensive phylogenetic assessments can be performed in the future (109).

HUMAN MICROBIOME STUDIES

The Oral Microbiome
The oral cavity includes various ecologic niches, such as saliva, gingival crevices, the tongue surfaces, and the posterior pharynx, and is colonized with hundreds of species of bacteria. Estimates range from 500 to 700 or more different species (82, 83). The dental plaque biofilm found on the surface of the teeth and in the subgingival pocket represents a complex assemblage of microbes (1, 82), and such structured microbial communities reside in intimate contact with host tissues. Health-associated microbial communities may protect against infection, but the oral cavity also harbors organisms that are implicated in both local and systemic diseases, including periodontal diseases (92), endocarditis (10), and aspiration pneumonia (98). The relative preponderance of health- or disease-associated microbes combined with human genetic susceptibilities may ultimately account for different disease phenotypes.

Periodontal disease includes conditions of oral inflammation and oral infections that may be associated with the composition of tooth-borne microbiomes in adults. It is a condition with various degrees of inflammation and is considered to be an infectious disease. Socransky et al. have proposed that periodontitis is the result of complexes or consortia of pathogens (100). The so-called red complex, containing *Porphyromonas gingivalis, Tannerella forsythia,* and *Treponema denticola,* is the pathogenic group that

seems to be most strongly associated with disease (49, 100). Periodontitis is associated with systemic disease, such as coronary heart and cerebrovascular diseases (26). Antibody responses to oral bacteria suggest that immune responses to specific microbial components may contribute to conditions of chronic inflammation (8, 9). Progressive periodontitis in pregnant women has been reported to increase the risk of severely adverse pregnancy outcomes (40, 80). These associations underscore the significance of the oral microbiome to systemic health status and predisposition to specific diseases.

16S rDNA sequencing and other techniques have been used to evaluate the oral microbiome. These methods include denaturing gradient gel electrophoresis (63, 64, 91), TRFLP (50, 51, 94, 95), and checkerboard DNA-DNA hybridization, where 45 DNA samples can be queried against 30 to 40 DNA probes (101). The last technique was used by Socransky and coworkers to examine microbial communities in supragingival (44) and subgingival (100) plaque. In both studies, distinct complexes were identified by principal component and correspondence analyses and were assigned to color groups. The supragingival plaque samples from 187 subjects (4,475 samples total) clustered into six groups (Fig. 1), including the aforementioned pathogen-associated red complex. In the subgingival study, a similar clustering was revealed, though the blue complex, composed of *Actinomyces* species, was not observed in these samples.

Paster et al. performed a 16S rDNA survey of subgingival plaque by analyzing 2,522 full-length clones (82). They compared healthy subjects and those with disease. Unlike most other 16S rDNA surveys that use only "universal" primers, they used three different primer sets to capture a more diverse group of bacteria, including spirochetes and *Bacteroidetes.* Sixty percent of the clones represented 132 known species, while the remaining 40% of the species were unknown. Some particular organisms were proposed as pathogens because of their association with samples from subjects with oral diseases. Overall, a

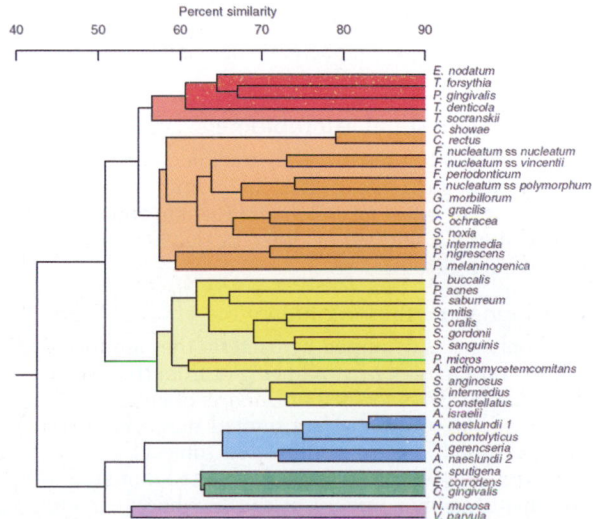

FIGURE 1 Dendrogram showing results of cluster analysis of 40 taxa from subgingival plaque from 4,475 samples collected from 187 subjects. Distinct red, orange, yellow, blue, green, and purple clusters are highlighted. Reprinted with permission from *Oral Microbiology and Immunology* (44).

total of 347 species were detected, and rarefaction analyses predicted a total of 415 species in the subgingiva. Thus, these methods appear to be quite robust, as a majority of detectable species were amplified and sequenced.

In another study, Aas et al. (1) examined nine oral sites: tongue dorsum, tongue lateral sides, buccal epithelium, hard palate, soft palate, supragingival plaque, subgingival plaque, maxillary anterior vestibule, and tonsils. These sites are similar to the sites being sampled as part of the jumpstart phase of the HMP. A total of 2,589 16S rDNA clones from five subjects were evaluated; this resulted in 141 predominant species and 13 new phylotypes. All sites contained *Gemella*, *Granulicatella*, *Streptococcus*, and *Veillonella* genera, and some sites had specific genera not found in others. The tonsils were found to have the most diversity and varied significantly among subjects. Organisms implicated in bacterial endocarditis, such as *Streptococcus mitis*, *Streptococcus oralis* (28), and *Granulicatella adiacens* (108), were found in each healthy subject, which supports the concept that such organisms could potentially seed cardiac valves after dental manipulations and entrance into the bloodstream.

A Human Oral Microbe Identification Microarray (mim.forsyth.org) that contains 16S rDNA oligonucleotide probes that represent approximately 300 oral bacterial species has been previously described. This microarray was used to compare the microbial compositions in subgingival plaques of subjects with refractory periodontitis, treatable periodontitis, or periodontal health (20). While key differences were seen among the different groups, such as the presence of more periodontal pathogens in the diseased subjects, the main conclusion from the study was that the increased microbial diversity was associated with the presence of diseased subgingivae.

The salivary microbiome has also been studied (78, 79). Samples from 120 healthy subjects from 12 worldwide locations were first analyzed by Sanger sequencing of the V4 to V6 regions of the 16S rDNA gene (14,115 sequences). A total of 101 genera were identified, and the number per subject ranged from 6 to 30. The most prevalent genus was *Streptococcus* (23.7%). Geographic variance was not observed—indeed, only a 13.5% variance among individuals was observed. The same group compared the results of Sanger sequencing to amplicon sequencing by 454 technology and obtained concordant results (79).

The Gastrointestinal Microbiome

The human gastrointestinal (GI) tract encompasses numerous different anatomical sites, including the esophagus, stomach, small intestine, colon and rectum, and anus. Each of these sites is colonized by different numbers and populations of microbes.

The Esophagus Microbiome

The esophagus is colonized by bacteria that are introduced from the oropharynx by swallowing or from the stomach by reflux. Early studies focused on surveys of culturable bacteria (30, 35, 58, 69, 81). Very limited numbers of bacteria were examined, and in nondiseased subjects, aerobic and anaerobic gram-positive organisms predominated. Only three metagenomic surveys of the esophageal microbiota have been reported. A study by Pei et al. (84) showed that the distal esophageal microbiomes of four adults had compositions similar to that of the oropharynx, with the exception that no spirochetes were found in the esophagus. These sequences were categorized in six phyla or groups: *Firmicutes* (70%), *Bacteroidetes* (20%), *Actinobacteria* (4%),

Proteobacteria (2%), *Fusobacteria* (2%), and TM7 (1%). This highlights the preponderance of *Firmicutes* and *Bacteroidetes* in the GI tract. Thirty-six new species were discovered, and Chao 1 (17) analysis estimated that the esophageal community contains about 140 species-level operational taxonomic units (OTUs). The same group examined the differences in the esophageal microbial communities in patients with esophagitis or Barrett's esophagus (intestinal metaplasia) (85, 110). Two distinct microbiomes were seen in the healthy and diseased subjects (Fig. 2). The individuals with healthy esophagi had microbiomes that were predominantly composed of streptococci, while the diseased patients' microbiomes had greater numbers of gram-negative anaerobes and increased bacterial diversity (110). A similar shift away from the normal esophageal microbiota was reported in a study of esophageal carcinomas (58).

The Gastric Microbiome

The low pH and rapid peristalsis in the stomach suppress persistent colonization by many bacteria. The stomach and small intestine each are thought to contain about 100 culturable organisms per milliliter, but the organismal counts can increase to 10^5 per ml following a meal (66). The best-studied and most dominant member of the stomach microbiota is *Helicobacter pylori* (22). Culture-dependent methods have revealed other genera, such as *Lactobacillus*, *Streptococcus*, and *Staphylococcus*, as well as members of the *Enterobacteriaceae*, in the stomach (2, 103), although a metagenomic analysis of gastric biopsy specimens revealed far more diversity (128 phylotypes) than had been appreciated previously by culture-based approaches (11).

The Small Intestine Microbiome

Like the stomach, the small intestine is colonized by relatively low numbers of bacteria, especially in proximal regions, such as the duodenum and jejunum. Bile in the small intestine inhibits bacterial colonization. The organisms found in the small intestine are usually lactobacilli, enterococci, other gram-positive aerobes, and facultative anaerobes (97, 111). This portion of the GI tract has been assessed mainly by culture-dependent methods; no metagenomics studies of the small intestine have been reported. A recent quantitative-PCR-based study described the differences in

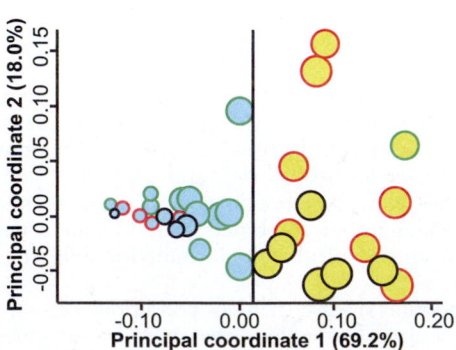

FIGURE 2 Plot of double principal coordinate analysis of esophageal samples showing a distinction of type I (blue fill, healthy) and type II (yellow fill, diseased) microbiomes. Edge colors indicate host phenotype (green, normal; red, esophagitis; black, Barrett's esophagus). Adapted with permission from *Gastroenterology* (110).

microbial composition between ileostomy specimens and intact small intestinal tissue (45). More distally in the ileum, the microbial composition becomes more complex and approaches that of the colon in terms of species richness and the nature of predominant bacterial genera.

The Colon Microbiome

The human colon is colonized by 10^{11} to 10^{12} bacteria per gram; this number represents at least 800 bacterial species and nine phyla (and one archaeal phylum), the majority of which are obligate anaerobes of the *Bacteroidetes* and *Firmicutes* (7, 29). Some studies have suggested that 15,000 to 36,000 species are present in the intestine (32, 87).

Bacteria from the distal gut are critical to host nutrition and may play key roles in health and disease. Microbe-derived carbohydrate fermentation by-products, such as short-chain fatty acids (SCFAs) like butyrate, acetate, and propionate, provide 10% or more of the body's metabolic requirements (65). Butyrate, produced by the clostridial clusters IV and XIVa, is the primary energy source of the colonic epithelium, and this SCFA has been reported to possess anticancer features (6, 47, 73). SCFAs also may play a role in preventing ulcerative colitis (19, 76) and infection by pathogens such as *Salmonella enterica* serovar Typhimurium (59). Colonic bacteria further contribute to nutrition by synthesizing amino acids (74) and vitamins (e.g., K, B_{12}, biotin, folic acid, and pantothenate) (3, 46).

Studies in germfree mice have indicated that the gut microbiota is important for the maturation and function of the mucosal immunity (72). Intestinal epithelial cells are in direct contact with the lumen and are involved in signaling to host innate and adaptive mucosal immune responses. Interactions between commensal ligands and the Toll-like receptors are critical for maintenance of epithelial homeostasis in the gut (90). The microbiota directs production of pathogen-specific mucosal immunoglobulin A (67). *Bacteroides fragilis* produces a polysaccharide that can correct T-cell deficiencies and T helper 1 and T helper 2 imbalances that lead to immune maturation (72). Some *Lactobacillus* species reduce cytokine responses to lipopolysaccharide, resulting in decreased inflammation (86).

Several groundbreaking gut microbiome studies have been reported in the literature during the past several years. Eckburg et al. sampled six sites within the colon of three individuals and performed 16S rDNA analysis of these samples plus fecal samples (29). Most of the sequences represented uncultured or novel microorganisms. Of the sequences that could be characterized, the majority were members of the *Firmicutes* and *Bacteroidetes*, with 95% of the *Firmicutes* belonging to the class *Clostridia*. The compositions of the six mucosal sites clustered together, but the mucosal microbiomes differed in composition from those found in stool specimens. Since the fecal microbiome overlaps that of the colonic lumen but is not identical, the authors suggested that the stool bacterial population is composed of a combination of mucosa-associated bacteria and a nonadherent luminal population (29). The distinction between microbiomes intimately associated with the intestinal mucosa and those associated with fecal specimens is important to consider, because many studies rely on fecal samples alone.

In another deep sequencing study, both 16S rDNA gene and WGS reads from fecal samples of two individuals were analyzed (39). The communities represented only *Firmicutes* and *Actinobacteria* plus one archaeon, *Methanobacter smithii*. No *Bacteroidetes* were observed, in contrast to other studies.

This key difference may be due to the individuals sampled (e.g., diet or genotypes) or methodological details (e.g., the PCR primers used). More than 50,000 open reading frames were predicted and examined for enrichment of COG (clusters of orthologous groups) and KEGG (Kyoto Encyclopedia of Genes and Genomes) pathways. Analysis of these pathways revealed enzymes required for degradation of plant polysaccharides, production of SCFAs, vitamin biosynthesis, methanogenesis, and degradation of toxic plant phenolics. These results are consistent with premicrobiome studies examining the metabolic capabilities of the gut microbiota.

Tap et al. identified 66 OTUs that are common to 50% or more of fecal samples from 17 healthy adult donors (105). This "core" microbiome was dominated by seven species (Fig. 3). Fifty-seven of the OTUs belonged to the *Firmicutes* phylum, and seven belonged to the *Bacteroidetes*. Forty-two percent of the OTUs could not be assigned to a species. The authors also compared these OTUs to those discovered in other published gut metagenomics analyses (29, 39, 62, 68). All 66 OTUs were detected at least once in each of the other studies (Fig. 3, inset). The authors concluded that the core human intestinal microbiome is composed of approximately 50 bacterial species.

The composition of the gut microbiome has been shown to differ in genetically obese versus lean mice (60). Turnbaugh et al. have used metagenomics to show that the metabolic potential of obese mice is increased (106). The ratio of *Firmicutes* to *Bacteroidetes* was increased in the obese mice, and more archaea were found in these animals. The microbiome of obese mice was enriched for genes encoding polysaccharolytic enzymes and production of SCFAs. Transplantation of the microbiome of obese mice into lean germfree mice caused the lean mice to gain more body fat than the control mice given the same diet. Ley et al. compared the microbiomes from stool samples of obese human subjects placed on fat-restricted and carbohydrate-restricted diets (60). Regardless of the diet type, the percentage of *Bacteroidetes* increased with weight loss, while the percentage of *Firmicutes* decreased. All of these studies point to the importance of the gut microbiota in obesity.

The gut microbiota may play a role in development of type I diabetes. In nonobese diabetic (NOD) mice reared under specific-pathogen-free conditions, the progression to type I diabetes occurs more rapidly than for mice grown conventionally (4). Thus, it is inferred that the presence of gut microbiota can provide some protection against development of disease. Wen et al. showed that germfree NOD mice lacking the Toll-like receptor adaptor protein MyD88 do not develop type 1 diabetes (107a), and further, that depletion of the microbiota with an antibiotic leads to an increased susceptibility to type I diabetes. Cecal contents of MyD88-positive and -negative NOD mice showed a predominance of *Firmicutes* and *Bacteroidetes* in both groups, but the ratio of *Firmicutes* to *Bacteroidetes* was lower in the MyD88 knockout mice. These studies strongly suggest that the microbiota in the gut may be required for activation of signaling pathways required for the development of human diseases such as diabetes.

Metagenomics studies aimed at understanding the microbial contributions to inflammatory bowel disease (IBD) have been reported. IBDs are thought to be multifactorial in pathogenesis, with factors including host genetics and immune responses as well as environment and gut bacteria (96). Crohn's disease and ulcerative colitis are associated with diminished fecal diversity. A PCR-based survey indicated that IBD biopsy samples were depleted of commensal bacteria of the *Firmicutes* and *Bacteroidetes* phyla (31).

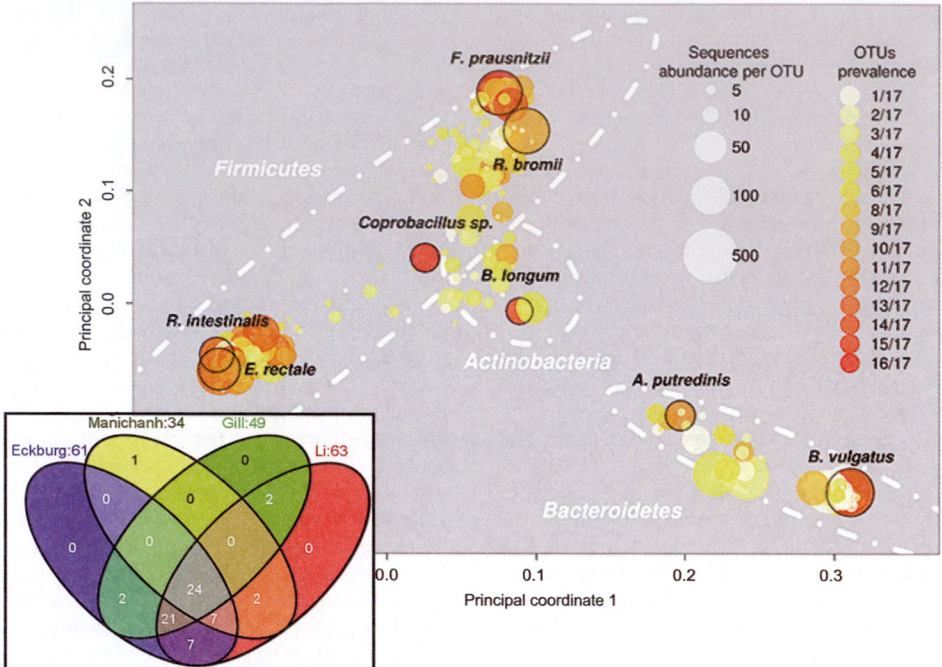

FIGURE 3 Principal coordinate plot of OTUs from the stools of 17 healthy subjects. The size of the circle corresponds to the number of sequences per OTU, and the color indicates the prevalence of OTUs among the 17 subjects. Inset: Venn diagram summarizing four studies of fecal microbiota from healthy donors compared with the core data set of 66 OTUs generated by Tap et al. (105). The four studies are Eckburg et al. (29), Manichanh et al. (68), Gill et al. (39), and Li et al. (62). Numbers above the ovals indicate the number of core OTUs observed in the study. Numbers within the ovals indicate the number of OTUs that overlap with the core set of 66. Reprinted with permission from *Environmental Microbiology* (105).

In particular, there was a depletion of the *Clostridiales*, many in clostridial cluster XIVa, which contains butyrate-producing organisms. Conversely, there was an expansion of *Proteobacteria* and *Actinobacteria* in the IBD samples. The expansion of *Proteobacteria* is consistent with reports of increased numbers of adherent and invasive *Escherichia coli* in biopsies from Crohn's disease patients (23). Other studies have revealed low levels of *Faecalibacterium prausnitzii* in patients with IBD (31, 70, 71). Sokol et al. have shown that a secreted product or products of *F. prausnitzii* yielded potent anti-inflammatory effects in vitro and suppressed mortality in a mouse model of acute chemical-induced colitis (102). The nature of the anti-inflammatory molecule(s) has not been determined, but these studies have generated a conceptual framework regarding potential microbial deficiency syndromes and human disease susceptibilities.

The Genitourinary Microbiome

The Vaginal Microbiome

The vaginal microbiota plays an important role in preventing genital and urinary tract infections. It is known that the composition of the vaginal microbiota varies with age, pH, and hormonal levels (37). Lactobacilli are usually considered to be the most prevalent organisms in healthy premenopausal women (57) and are considered protective for the host by virtue of their presumed role in suppression of pathogen colonization. Such effects may result from mucus adherence by lactobacilli, production of organic acids and reduction

of vaginal pH, and production of antimicrobial compounds that prevent pathogen proliferation (12). In addition to the lactobacilli, the predominant culturable vaginal microbes are *Mobiluncus* spp., *Gardnerella vaginalis*, *Bacteroides* spp., *Prevotella* spp., and *Mycoplasma hominis* (48).

Most 16S rDNA-based metagenomics studies have demonstrated that the vaginal microbiota are highly variable, and differences presumably depend on differences in sexual and hygienic practices in addition to host genetics. *Lactobacillus* is the predominant member of the vaginal community in most individuals, but in some cases, vaginal lactobacilli may be undetectable. The microbiotas of eight healthy women with three different "grades" of vaginosis were examined by sequencing the V1 to V3 16S region by the Sanger method (107). The biotas associated with each of these grades were quite distinct: grade one individuals (healthy) were almost exclusively colonized by *Lactobacillus crispatus*, *Lactobacillus gasseri*, and *Lactobacillus jensenii*; grade two subjects had *Lactobacillus iners*, *Atopobium vaginae*, *Prevotella bivia*, and *Sneathia sanguinegens*; and grade three subjects were predominantly colonized with *A. vaginae* or *Peptostreptococcus anaerobius*. Several studies have also associated altered vaginal microbiota with an increased risk for viral coinfection (55, 77, 99).

In 2007, the Forney group published the results of a 16S rDNA survey of the midvaginal microbiota from five healthy Caucasian women (112). The authors targeted the V1 to V5 region of the 16S rRNA gene and classified ca. 1,200 clones. The number and distribution of phylotypes differed among the five subjects. Two females had exclusively or nearly exclusively *L. crispatus*, one had *L. iners* as the predominant species, and one was predominantly colonized by *A. vaginae*. The fifth subject had seven phylotypes, predominantly *L. iners* but also significant amounts of *A. vaginae*, *Megasphaera*, and *Leptotrichia*. Like lactobacilli, *Leptotrichia* and *Atopobium* are lactic acid producers. This suggests that different microbial communities may manifest shared functions. A study of the vulval microbiota of four of the five women from the prior study was published by the same group (15). While the communities in the labia majora were more diverse than those from the vaginal samples, the general trend of *Lactobacillus* predominance was reported for four of the five women. The overall conclusion was that the vaginal and vulval microbiotas are highly variable. These results have in general been confirmed by another group that sequenced full-length 16S rDNA clones (2,000 reads per each of 20 healthy subjects) (54).

The Microbiome of the Upper Respiratory Tract

The healthy nares and nasopharynx contain streptococci, staphylococci, corynebacteria, *Moraxella* spp., *Neisseria* spp. (including *N. meningitidis*), and *Haemophilus* (53). Viridans streptococci predominate, and organisms associated with inner ear infections of children are also found (e.g., *Streptococcus pneumoniae*, *Haemophilus influenzae*, and *Moraxella catarrhalis*), though the numbers of these organisms vary significantly with age (56). The carriage rate for *Staphylococcus aureus* has been estimated to be ca. 30%, with methicillin-resistant *S. aureus* representing 1.5% of the strains isolated (41). The paranasal sinuses are normally sterile, but they can become infected because of their close proximity to other sites that are colonized by bacteria.

The Skin Microbiome

Most skin microbes are gram-positive organisms, such as staphylococci, micrococci, brevibacteria, propionibacteria, and corynebacteria (61, 93). Colonization by gram-negative organisms was previously thought to be extremely rare (18), although *Acinetobacter* spp. could sometimes be cultured. Metagenomics studies have changed these views. The skin microbiota generally protects individuals against colonization by pathogens, but under certain circumstances the microbiota may be pathogenic if these organisms can penetrate the skin in a susceptible host. For example, *Staphylococcus epidermidis* is a common skin colonizer. However, this species may cause infections in immunocompromised patients or those with indwelling devices. Conversely, *Pseudomonas fluorescens* is thought to be a protective skin organism, because it produces the polyketide antibiotic mupirocin (34), which is active against gram-positive bacteria, including methicillin-resistant *S. aureus* (104).

A 16S rDNA survey of samples from the human volar forearm (six healthy subjects; 1,221 16S rDNA clones total) revealed that 94.6% of the sequences fell into three phyla—*Actinobacteria*, *Firmicutes*, and *Proteobacteria*—yet the total diversity represented 182 species-level OTUs (36). Chao estimation suggested that the communities were composed of ca. 250 OTUs, and the results indicated that communities varied substantially between subjects. Samples from the antecubital fossae of five healthy subjects (ca. 200 clones per subject) revealed 113 OTUs belonging to six bacterial divisions and a predicted community size of 130 OTUs (43). In contrast to the study by Gao et al. (36), this study revealed that the *Proteobacteria* predominate the antecubital fossae of the subjects tested.

It was proposed that the differences might be representative of the different environments of the two sites: the volar forearm is dry and hairy, while the antecubital fossa is sweaty and hairless.

The differences in the composition of the skin microbiome based on microenvironment were underscored in a 2009 report by Grice et al. (42). Twenty sites on 10 healthy volunteers were sampled, and full-length 16S amplicons were sequenced. The skin sites included sebaceous, moist, and dry sites. While a significant amount of variability was observed between subjects, clustering was apparent by site type (Fig. 4). The sebaceous sites were dominated by propionibacteria and staphylococci and the moist sites by corynebacteria, while the dry sites contained a mixed population of bacteria. The volar forearm had the greatest number of OTUs (44 OTUs), while the retroauricular crease was the least rich with 15. Overall, the sebaceous sites were the least complex, and intrapersonal variation was generally less than interpersonal variation. Temporal intrapersonal variation, based on a second sampling of five subjects 4 to 6 months after the primary sampling, revealed similarities for samples from the external auditory canal, inguinal crease, alar crease, and naris. In contrast, considerable variation was observed during this time period for samples taken from the popliteal fossa, volar forearm, and buttock.

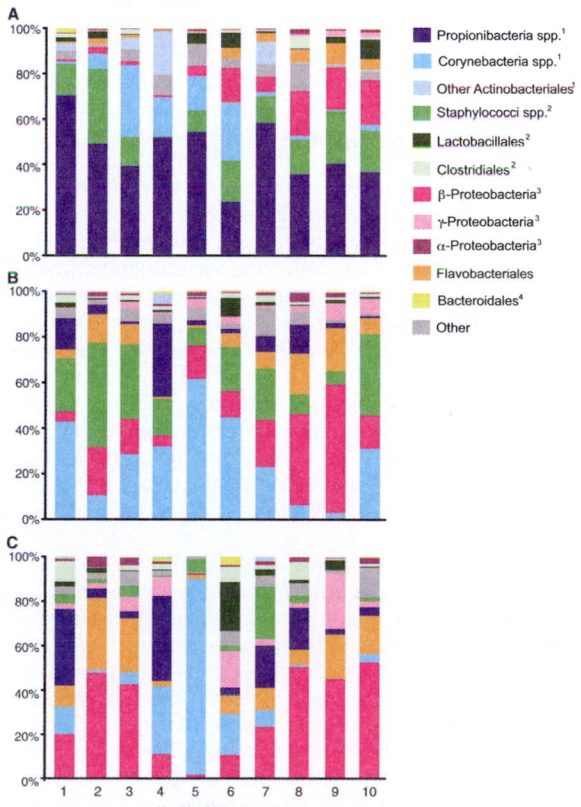

FIGURE 4 Abundance plot of bacterial groups from four phyla in skin samples from 10 healthy volunteers. (A) Sebaceous skin sites; (B) moist skin sites; (C) dry skin sites. Superscripts indicate the following phyla: 1, *Actinobacteria*; 2, *Firmicutes*; 3, *Proteobacteria*; and 4, *Bacteroidetes*. Reprinted with permission from *Science* (42).

A CATALOG OF REFERENCE STRAIN GENOMES FOR THE HMP

An important component of the HMP is creation of a catalog of reference genomes to serve as a data set for metagenomics analyses. Before the project began, less than 10% of the completed bacterial and archaeal genomes in GenBank could be considered to be human commensal organisms. At the time of this writing, sequencing of over 900 reference strains is in progress. DNA is prepared by a variety of methods and is subjected to long-tag paired-end sequencing on a 454 Life Sciences GS FLX instrument. Four organisms are sequenced per run, yielding ca. 400 Mb of sequence or about 30- to 40-fold coverage. Sequences are assembled using the 454 Newbler assembler. This generally results in an assembly of hundreds of contigs and tens of scaffolds that constitute >95% genome coverage and a scaffold N50 of 0.5 to 1 Mb. About 15% of strains are selected for gold standard finishing (16). Finishing involves automated efforts using Autofinish and targeted PCR as well as manual curation. Most genomes are autoannotated using a set of tools developed at the J. Craig Venter Institute and implemented by the HMP jumpstart centers. All data are deposited in the NCBI Short Read Archive and in GenBank.

STATUS OF HMP JUMPSTART HUMAN SAMPLING AND ANALYSIS

One primary goal of the HMP is to provide an unmatched collection of human specimens from five primary body sites—mouth, skin, GI tract, urogenital tract, and nasal cavity—of healthy individuals so that definitive insights can be made as to the composition of the microbiota of healthy humans. During the HMP jumpstart phase, samples were taken from 300 subjects at 18 subsites (15 in males and 18 in females) within the primary sites listed above. Samples were collected at least twice so that temporal relationships in the human microbiome can be further examined. The monumental task of collecting samples and extracting DNA from diverse sites is being achieved by teams of clinicians, nurses, and researchers at the Baylor College of Medicine, St. Louis University, Washington University, and the National Institutes of Health. The study protocol, informed consent documents, and subject recruitment materials have all been subjected to institutional review board approval and follow good clinical practice guidelines. At the time this chapter was being finalized, all 300 subjects had been sampled once, and more than 250 individuals had been sampled twice.

One of the initial considerations that needed to be addressed in terms of clinical sampling for the HMP was the parameters that qualified an individual as healthy or "normal." Potential HMP subjects are screened thoroughly (including blood and urine collections for viral markers and pregnancy determination, a dental exam, a skin exam, and a gynecological exam) to ensure that the subject and specific sampling sites are within normal health parameters. To assess the impact of ethnicity and gender on the human microbiota, the study targets equal numbers of males and females to be sampled, and approximately 20% of the recruited subjects belong to a minority group.

Samples from each HMP subject are cataloged, and microbial genomic DNA is isolated by using a single protocol for all samples. A variety of DNA isolation protocols were vetted for HMP use. A series of benchmarking steps utilizing a mock community of bacterial cells and other clinical samples was performed to ensure that no detectable bias was introduced at the sample collection or DNA isolation step.

The HMP evolved into an NIH Roadmap project, in part because of the revolutionary advances in DNA sequencing technologies as a means to detect and quantify the microbes in a given population. As described in the beginning of this chapter, definition of the bacterial composition of metagenomic samples often relies upon characterization of the 16S rDNA sequences in the genomes within the sample. Many of the microbiome studies to date (and many of those described above) rely upon Sanger sequencing of whole or partial 16S rDNA sequences amplified from a metagenomic sample. Capturing the entire 16S rDNA sequence is considered the gold standard for any subsequent metagenomic analysis, as the full-length gene logically encodes the greatest amount of information for subsequent sequence-based phylogenetic assignment. Unfortunately, Sanger deep sequencing of metagenomic samples is cost prohibitive, but next-generation sequencing (NextGen) methods provide options to survey these samples more thoroughly.

The first NextGen platform used for metagenomic sequencing is the Roche 454 pyrosequencing platform, which currently features over 1 million reads per run with an average read length of over 400 bases (on the newest GS FLX Titanium platform). The Titanium platform currently produces the longest reads among the NextGen options, which enables the most information to be captured from each 16S rDNA read. While a 454 read cannot cover the sequence of a full-length 16S rRNA gene, up to four of the nine V regions within the 16S gene may be sequenced in a single read. The ideal V regions to target for metagenomic analyses are still under debate; however, it is apparent that some V regions demonstrate greater variability for certain families of bacteria, and metagenomic sequencing of these V regions can lead to better resolution of genus and species for these particular families. As a result, the ideal V regions used to analyze samples from individual body sites may differ depending on the microbial composition of the sample being studied and the desired resolution. The use of multiplex identifier tags, or molecular barcodes, enables many metagenomic samples to be multiplexed in a single sequencing run. For example, initial 454 sequencing of HMP samples incorporated 96 barcodes, thus enabling the sequencing of 96 samples in a single run and generating an average of approximately 10,000 reads per sample.

In addition to the inability to sequence entire 16S genes, NextGen platforms, including 454, have not yet matched the low sequencing error rates that are typically associated with Sanger data (less than 1 error per 1,000 bases). High confidence sequence data from NextGen projects normally rely on high coverage to establish high confidence at each base position in an assembled sequence. However, the nature of metagenomic templates often results in a large number of reads generated for abundant members of a bacterial community and a relatively low number of reads for rarer members of the community. This low coverage, combined with an error rate of between 1 in 100 or 1 in 1,000 bases, can lead to the generation of sequences that impact downstream analyses in the form of false OTUs (i.e., the perceived presence of an organism that does not actually exist in the sample). Extensive efforts are being made to reduce the number of false OTUs from downstream analyses. These efforts include removal of sequences found only once or twice in a given sample and development of software to remove errors from 454 data to reduce false OTUs; such software has shown promise as an effective tool to reduce noise in 454 metagenomic data (89).

Metagenomic DNA sequencing was benchmarked at the four HMP jumpstart centers by using a mock community of 22 microbial genomic DNAs diluted in specific ratios and with DNA from shared clinical samples to ascertain each sequencing center's ability to detect and enumerate the relative numbers of organisms in a given population by using a common sequencing protocol. The questions of the HMP jumpstart phase (e.g., Is there a core microbiome? If so, what organisms belong to the core microbiome at each body site? How do gender and ethnicity impact the microbiome?) will initially be addressed by performing low-coverage 454 16S rDNA sequencing (approximately 10,000 reads per sample) on each sample to determine the general bacterial membership and to differentiate (or bin) each sample. Not all organisms are expected to be detected at this level of coverage, so a representative subset of samples will be explored further by more in-depth genomic analyses using WGS. WGS of metagenomic samples entails direct sequencing of the genomic DNA harvested from a particular sample and provides deep coverage over the total genomic content of a sample. Both 454 and Illumina (Solexa) platforms have the ability to query metagenomic samples deeply at the whole-genome level. Analyses examining both 16S rRNA gene content and overall gene content will provide abundant information regarding the microbial composition and total gene content and will provide insights into the various metabolic and pathogenic capacities of a particular sample.

Other methods to deeply survey microbial communities within the HMP include the use of a DNA microarray (PhyloChip) that is able to identify multiple bacterial and archaeal organisms from complex microbial samples (24). Like 16S rRNA gene amplicon sequencing, the PhyloChip probes sample the 16S rRNA gene; through its design, PhyloChip has the ability to classify unknown organisms based on their similarities to known microbes. The utility of PhyloChip-based classification approaches has been demonstrated in multiple studies (13, 14, 75) and has been used as a validation tool for the mock microbial DNA community used to benchmark the jumpstart centers' sequencing pipelines.

SUMMARY AND CONCLUSIONS

The human microbiome includes a diverse collection of human-associated microbes that represent a small fraction of the total microbial "universe" in other animals, life forms, and the environment. This human microbiome can be defined due to the rapid development of advanced DNA sequencing technologies coupled with bioinformatics strategies. The informatics tools include augmented phylogenetic sequence databases, annotation and genome assembly tools, and refined functional approaches to aggregate sequence data. Metagenomics strategies are being applied to a variety of anatomical sites to provide glimpses into the tremendous variation at different body locations and among different individuals.

Future approaches in medical microbiology will be shaped in part by developments in the fields of metagenomics and human microbiome research. The identification of single agents of infection will be supplemented by techniques exploring the relative composition of microbiomes in the context of different infections and other diseases.

Differences in microbial composition that are associated with noninfectious immune-mediated disorders may extend the "reach" of the medical microbiology laboratory into other areas of human medicine in the future. Finally, pathogen discovery efforts will be enhanced by new metagenomics strategies, and these studies may uncover single etiologic agents of infections as well as relative shifts in groups of bacterial pathogens that may contribute to human disease.

REFERENCES

1. Aas, J. A., B. J. Paster, L. N. Stokes, I. Olsen, and F. E. Dewhirst. 2005. Defining the normal bacterial flora of the oral cavity. *J. Clin. Microbiol.* **43:**5721–5732.
2. Adamsson, I., C. E. Nord, P. Lundquist, S. Sjostedt, and C. Edlund. 1999. Comparative effects of omeprazole, amoxycillin plus metronidazole versus omeprazole, clarithromycin plus metronidazole on the oral, gastric and intestinal microflora in *Helicobacter pylori*-infected patients. *J. Antimicrob. Chemother.* **44:**629–640.
3. Albert, M. J., V. I. Mathan, and S. J. Baker. 1980. Vitamin B12 synthesis by human small intestinal bacteria. *Nature* **283:**781–782.
4. Anderson, M. S., and J. A. Bluestone. 2005. The NOD mouse: a model of immune dysregulation. *Annu. Rev. Immunol.* **23:**447–485.
5. Andersson, A. F., M. Lindberg, H. Jakobsson, F. Backhed, P. Nyren, and L. Engstrand. 2008. Comparative analysis of human gut microbiota by barcoded pyrosequencing. *PLoS ONE* **3:**e2836.
6. Archer, S. Y., S. Meng, A. Shei, and R. A. Hodin. 1998. p21(WAF1) is required for butyrate-mediated growth inhibition of human colon cancer cells. *Proc. Natl. Acad. Sci. USA* **95:**6791–6796.
7. Bäckhed, F., R. E. Ley, J. L. Sonnenburg, D. A. Peterson, and J. I. Gordon. 2005. Host-bacterial mutualism in the human intestine. *Science* **307:**1915–1920.
8. Beck, J. D., P. Eke, G. Heiss, P. Madianos, D. Couper, D. Lin, K. Moss, J. Elter, and S. Offenbacher. 2005. Periodontal disease and coronary heart disease: a reappraisal of the exposure. *Circulation* **112:**19–24.
9. Beck, J. D., P. Eke, D. Lin, P. Madianos, D. Couper, K. Moss, J. Elter, G. Heiss, and S. Offenbacher. 2005. Associations between IgG antibody to oral organisms and carotid intima-medial thickness in community-dwelling adults. *Atherosclerosis* **183:**342–348.
10. Berbari, E. F., F. R. Cockerill III, and J. M. Steckelberg. 1997. Infective endocarditis due to unusual or fastidious microorganisms. *Mayo Clin. Proc.* **72:**532–542.
11. Bik, E. M., P. B. Eckburg, S. R. Gill, K. E. Nelson, E. A. Purdom, F. Francois, G. Perez-Perez, M. J. Blaser, and D. A. Relman. 2006. Molecular analysis of the bacterial microbiota in the human stomach. *Proc. Natl. Acad. Sci. USA* **103:**732–737.
12. Boris, S., and C. Barbés. 2000. Role played by lactobacilli in controlling the population of vaginal pathogens. *Microb. Infect.* **2:**543–546.
13. Brodie, E. L., T. Z. Desantis, D. C. Joyner, S. M. Baek, J. T. Larsen, G. L. Andersen, T. C. Hazen, P. M. Richardson, D. J. Herman, T. K. Tokunaga, J. M. Wan, and M. K. Firestone. 2006. Application of a high-density oligonucleotide microarray approach to study bacterial population dynamics during uranium reduction and reoxidation. *Appl. Environ. Microbiol.* **72:**6288–6298.
14. Brodie, E. L., T. Z. DeSantis, J. P. Parker, I. X. Zubietta, Y. M. Piceno, and G. L. Andersen. 2007. Urban aerosols harbor diverse and dynamic bacterial populations. *Proc. Natl. Acad. Sci. USA* **104:**299–304.
15. Brown, C. J., M. Wong, C. C. Davis, A. Kanti, X. Zhou, and L. J. Forney. 2007. Preliminary characterization of the normal microbiota of the human vulva using cultivation-independent methods. *J. Med. Microbiol.* **56:**271–276.

16. Chain, P. S., D. V. Grafham, R. S. Fulton, M. G. Fitzgerald, J. Hostetler, D. Muzny, J. Ali, B. Birren, D. C. Bruce, C. Buhay, J. R. Cole, Y. Ding, S. Dugan, D. Field, G. M. Garrity, R. Gibbs, T. Graves, C. S. Han, S. H. Harrison, S. Highlander, P. Hugenholtz, H. M. Khouri, C. D. Kodira, E. Kolker, N. C. Kyrpides, D. Lang, A. Lapidus, S. A. Malfatti, V. Markowitz, T. Metha, K. E. Nelson, J. Parkhill, S. Pitluck, X. Qin, T. D. Read, J. Schmutz, S. Sozhamannan, P. Sterk, R. L. Strausberg, G. Sutton, N. R. Thomson, J. M. Tiedje, G. Weinstock, A. Wollam, and J. C. Detter. 2009. Genomics. Genome project standards in a new era of sequencing. *Science* **326:**236–237.

17. Chao, A. 1987. Estimating the population size for capture-recapture data with unequal catchability. *Biometrics* **43:**783–791.

18. Chiller, K., B. A. Selkin, and G. J. Murakawa. 2001. Skin microflora and bacterial infections of the skin. *J. Investig. Dermatol. Symp. Proc.* **6:**170–174.

19. Clausen, M. R., and P. B. Mortensen. 1995. Kinetic studies on colonocyte metabolism of short chain fatty acids and glucose in ulcerative colitis. *Gut* **37:**684–689.

20. Colombo, A. P., S. K. Boches, S. L. Cotton, J. M. Goodson, R. Kent, A. D. Haffajee, S. S. Socransky, H. Hasturk, T. E. Van Dyke, F. Dewhirst, and B. J. Paster. 2009. Comparisons of subgingival microbial profiles of refractory periodontitis, severe periodontitis, and periodontal health using the human oral microbe identification microarray. *J. Periodontol.* **80:**1421–1432.

21. Costello, E. K., C. L. Lauber, M. Hamady, N. Fierer, J. I. Gordon, and R. Knight. 2009. Bacterial community variation in human body habitats across space and time. *Science* **326:**1694–1697.

22. Cover, T. L., and M. J. Blaser. 2009. Helicobacter pylori in health and disease. *Gastroenterology* **136:**1863–1873.

23. Darfeuille-Michaud, A., J. Boudeau, P. Bulois, C. Neut, A. L. Glasser, N. Barnich, M. A. Bringer, A. Swidsinski, L. Beaugerie, and J. F. Colombel. 2004. High prevalence of adherent-invasive *Escherichia coli* associated with ileal mucosa in Crohn's disease. *Gastroenterology* **127:**412–421.

24. DeSantis, T. Z., E. L. Brodie, J. P. Moberg, I. X. Zubieta, Y. M. Piceno, and G. L. Andersen. 2007. High-density universal 16S rRNA microarray analysis reveals broader diversity than typical clone library when sampling the environment. *Microb. Ecol.* **53:**371–383.

25. Reference deleted.

26. DeStefano, F., R. F. Anda, H. S. Kahn, D. F. Williamson, and C. M. Russell. 1993. Dental disease and risk of coronary heart disease and mortality. *BMJ* **306:**688–691.

27. Dethlefsen, L., S. Huse, M. L. Sogin, and D. A. Relman. 2008. The pervasive effects of an antibiotic on the human gut microbiota, as revealed by deep 16S rRNA sequencing. *PLoS Biol.* **6:**e280.

28. Douglas, C. W., J. Heath, K. K. Hampton, and F. E. Preston. 1993. Identity of viridans streptococci isolated from cases of infective endocarditis. *J. Med. Microbiol.* **39:**179–182.

29. Eckburg, P. B., E. M. Bik, C. N. Bernstein, E. Purdom, L. Dethlefsen, M. Sargent, S. R. Gill, K. E. Nelson, and D. A. Relman. 2005. Diversity of the human intestinal microbial flora. *Science* **308:**1635–1638.

30. Finlay, I. G., P. A. Wright, T. Menzies, and C. S. McArdle. 1982. Microbial flora in carcinoma of oesophagus. *Thorax* **37:**181–184.

31. Frank, D. N., A. L. St Amand, R. A. Feldman, E. C. Boedeker, N. Harpaz, and N. R. Pace. 2007. Molecular-phylogenetic characterization of microbial community imbalances in human inflammatory bowel diseases. *Proc. Natl. Acad. Sci. USA* **104:**13780–13785.

32. Frank, J. A., C. I. Reich, S. Sharma, J. S. Weisbaum, B. A. Wilson, and G. J. Olsen. 2008. Critical evaluation of two primers commonly used for amplification of bacterial 16S rRNA genes. *Appl. Environ. Microbiol.* **74:**2461–2470.

33. Frias-Lopez, J., Y. Shi, G. W. Tyson, M. L. Coleman, S. C. Schuster, S. W. Chisholm, and E. F. Delong. 2008. Microbial community gene expression in ocean surface waters. *Proc. Natl. Acad. Sci. USA* **105:**3805–3810.

34. Fuller, A. T., G. Mellows, M. Woolford, G. T. Banks, K. D. Barrow, and E. B. Chain. 1971. Pseudomonic acid: an antibiotic produced by *Pseudomonas fluorescens*. *Nature* **234:**416–417.

35. Gagliardi, D., S. Makihara, P. R. Corsi, T. Viana Ade, M. V. Wiczer, S. Nakakubo, and L. M. Mimica. 1998. Microbial flora of the normal esophagus. *Dis. Esophagus* **11:** 248–250.

36. Gao, Z., C. H. Tseng, Z. Pei, and M. J. Blaser. 2007. Molecular analysis of human forearm superficial skin bacterial biota. *Proc. Natl. Acad. Sci. USA* **104:**2927–2932.

37. Garcia-Closas, M., R. Herrero, C. Bratti, A. Hildesheim, M. E. Sherman, L. A. Morera, and M. Schiffman. 1999. Epidemiologic determinants of vaginal pH. *Am. J. Obstet. Gynecol.* **180:**1060–1066.

38. Reference deleted.

39. Gill, S. R., M. Pop, R. T. Deboy, P. B. Eckburg, P. J. Turnbaugh, B. S. Samuel, J. I. Gordon, D. A. Relman, C. M. Fraser-Liggett, and K. E. Nelson. 2006. Metagenomic analysis of the human distal gut microbiome. *Science* **312:**1355–1359.

40. Goepfert, A. R., M. K. Jeffcoat, W. W. Andrews, O. Faye-Petersen, S. P. Cliver, R. L. Goldenberg, and J. C. Hauth. 2004. Periodontal disease and upper genital tract inflammation in early spontaneous preterm birth. *Obstet. Gynecol.* **104:**777–783.

41. Gorwitz, R. J., D. Kruszon-Moran, S. K. McAllister, G. McQuillan, L. K. McDougal, G. E. Fosheim, B. J. Jensen, G. Killgore, F. C. Tenover, and M. J. Kuehnert. 2008. Changes in the prevalence of nasal colonization with *Staphylococcus aureus* in the United States, 2001–2004. *J. Infect. Dis.* **197:**1226–1234.

42. Grice, E. A., H. H. Kong, S. Conlan, C. B. Deming, J. Davis, A. C. Young, G. G. Bouffard, R. W. Blakesley, P. R. Murray, E. D. Green, M. L. Turner, and J. A. Segre. 2009. Topographical and temporal diversity of the human skin microbiome. *Science* **324:**1190–1192.

43. Grice, E. A., H. H. Kong, G. Renaud, A. C. Young, G. G. Bouffard, R. W. Blakesley, T. G. Wolfsberg, M. L. Turner, and J. A. Segre. 2008. A diversity profile of the human skin microbiota. *Genome Res.* **18:**1043–1050.

44. Haffajee, A. D., S. S. Socransky, M. R. Patel, and X. Song. 2008. Microbial complexes in supragingival plaque. *Oral Microbiol. Immunol.* **23:**196–205.

45. Hartman, A. L., D. M. Lough, D. K. Barupal, O. Fiehn, T. Fishbein, M. Zasloff, and J. A. Eisen. 2009. Human gut microbiome adopts an alternative state following small bowel transplantation. *Proc. Natl. Acad. Sci. USA* **106:**17187–17192.

46. Hill, M. J. 1997. Intestinal flora and endogenous vitamin synthesis. *Eur. J. Cancer Prev.* **6**(Suppl. 1)**:**S43–S45.

47. Hinnebusch, B. F., S. Meng, J. T. Wu, S. Y. Archer, and R. A. Hodin. 2002. The effects of short-chain fatty acids on human colon cancer cell phenotype are associated with histone hyperacetylation. *J. Nutr.* **132:**1012–1017.

48. Holst, E., B. Wathne, B. Hovelius, and P. A. Mardh. 1987. Bacterial vaginosis: microbiological and clinical findings. *Eur. J. Clin. Microbiol.* **6:**536–541.

49. Holt, S. C., and J. L. Ebersole. 2005. *Porphyromonas gingivalis*, *Treponema denticola*, and *Tannerella forsythia*: the "red complex", a prototype polybacterial pathogenic consortium in periodontitis. *Periodontol. 2000* **38:**72–122.

50. Hommez, G. M., R. Verhelst, G. Claeys, M. Vaneechoutte, and R. J. De Moor. 2004. Investigation of the effect of the coronal restoration quality on the composition of the root canal microflora in teeth with apical periodontitis by means of T-RFLP analysis. *Int. Endod. J.* **37:**819–827.

51. Hommez, G. M., R. Verhelst, M. Vaneechoutte, G. Claeys, and R. J. De Moor. 2008. Terminal restriction fragment length polymorphism analysis of the microflora in necrotic teeth of patients irradiated in the head and neck region. *J. Endod.* **34:**1048–1051.

52. Hooper, L. V., and J. I. Gordon. 2001. Commensal host-bacterial relationships in the gut. *Science* **292:**1115–1118.

53. **Hull, M. W., and A. W. Chow.** 2007. Indigenous microflora and innate immunity of the head and neck. *Infect. Dis. Clin. N. Am.* **21:**265–282.

54. **Hyman, R. W., M. Fukushima, L. Diamond, J. Kumm, L. C. Giudice, and R. W. Davis.** 2005. Microbes on the human vaginal epithelium. *Proc. Natl. Acad. Sci. USA* **102:**7952–7957.

55. **Kaul, R., N. J. Nagelkerke, J. Kimani, E. Ngugi, J. J. Bwayo, K. S. Macdonald, A. Rebbaprgada, K. Fonck, M. Temmerman, A. R. Ronald, and S. Moses.** 2007. Prevalent herpes simplex virus type 2 infection is associated with altered vaginal flora and an increased susceptibility to multiple sexually transmitted infections. *J. Infect. Dis.* **196:**1692–1697.

56. **Konno, M., S. Baba, H. Mikawa, K. Hara, F. Matsumoto, K. Kaga, T. Nishimura, T. Kobayashi, N. Furuya, H. Moriyama, Y. Okamoto, M. Furukawa, N. Yamanaka, T. Matsushima, Y. Yoshizawa, S. Kohno, K. Kobayashi, A. Morikawa, S. Koizumi, K. Sunakawa, M. Inoue, and K. Ubukata.** 2006. Study of nasopharyngeal bacterial flora. Second report. Variations in nasopharyngeal bacterial flora in children aged 6 years or younger when administered antimicrobial agents. Part 2. *J. Infect. Chemother.* **12:**305–330.

57. **Larsen, B.** 1993. Vaginal flora in health and disease. *Clin. Obstet. Gynecol.* **36:**107–121.

58. **Lau, W. F., J. Wong, K. H. Lam, and G. B. Ong.** 1981. Oesophageal microbial flora in carcinoma of the oesophagus. *Aust. N. Z. J. Surg.* **51:**52–55.

59. **Lawhon, S. D., R. Maurer, M. Suyemoto, and C. Altier.** 2002. Intestinal short-chain fatty acids alter Salmonella typhimurium invasion gene expression and virulence through BarA/SirA. *Mol. Microbiol.* **46:**1451–1464.

60. **Ley, R. E., P. J. Turnbaugh, S. Klein, and J. I. Gordon.** 2006. Microbial ecology: human gut microbes associated with obesity. *Nature* **444:**1022–1023.

61. **Leyden, J. J., K. J. McGinley, K. M. Nordstrom, and G. F. Webster.** 1987. Skin microflora. *J. Investig. Dermatol.* **88:**65s–72s.

62. **Li, M., B. Wang, M. Zhang, M. Rantalainen, S. Wang, H. Zhou, Y. Zhang, J. Shen, X. Pang, M. Zhang, H. Wei, Y. Chen, H. Lu, J. Zuo, M. Su, Y. Qiu, W. Jia, C. Xiao, L. M. Smith, S. Yang, E. Holmes, H. Tang, G. Zhao, J. K. Nicholson, L. Li, and L. Zhao.** 2008. Symbiotic gut microbes modulate human metabolic phenotypes. *Proc. Natl. Acad. Sci. USA* **105:**2117–2122.

63. **Li, Y., C. Y. Ku, J. Xu, D. Saxena, and P. W. Caufield.** 2005. Survey of oral microbial diversity using PCR-based denaturing gradient gel electrophoresis. *J. Dent. Res.* **84:**559–564.

64. **Li, Y., D. Saxena, V. M. Barnes, H. M. Trivedi, Y. Ge, and T. Xu.** 2006. Polymerase chain reaction-based denaturing gradient gel electrophoresis in the evaluation of oral microbiota. *Oral Microbiol. Immunol.* **21:**333–339.

65. **Macfarlane, G. T., and J. H. Cummings.** 1991. The colonic flora, fermentation, and large bowel digestive function, p. 51–92. *In* S. Phillips, J. Pemberton, and R. Shorter (ed.), *The Large Intestine: Physiology, Pathophysiology and Disease.* Raven Press, New York, NY.

66. **Macfarlane, S., and G. T. Macfarlane.** 2004. Bacterial diversity in the human gut. *Adv. Appl. Microbiol.* **54:**261–289.

67. **Macpherson, A., and T. Uhr.** 2004. Induction of protective IgA by intestinal dendritic cells carrying commensal bacteria. *Science* **303:**1662–1665.

68. **Manichanh, C., L. Rigottier-Gois, E. Bonnaud, K. Gloux, E. Pelletier, L. Frangeul, R. Nalin, C. Jarrin, P. Chardon, P. Marteau, J. Roca, and J. Dore.** 2006. Reduced diversity of faecal microbiota in Crohn's disease revealed by a metagenomic approach. *Gut* **55:**205–211.

69. **Mannell, A., M. Plant, and J. Frolich.** 1983. The microflora of the oesophagus. *Ann. R. Coll. Surg. Engl.* **65:**152–154.

70. **Mariat, D., O. Firmesse, F. Levenez, V. Guimaraes, H. Sokol, J. Dore, G. Corthier, and J. P. Furet.** 2009. The Firmicutes/Bacteroidetes ratio of the human microbiota changes with age. *BMC Microbiol.* **9:**123.

71. **Martinez-Medina, M., X. Aldeguer, F. Gonzalez-Huix, D. Acero, and L. J. Garcia-Gil.** 2006. Abnormal microbiota composition in the ileocolonic mucosa of Crohn's disease patients as revealed by polymerase chain reaction-denaturing gradient gel electrophoresis. *Inflamm. Bowel Dis.* **12:**1136–1145.

72. **Mazmanian, S. K., C. H. Liu, A. O. Tzianabos, and D. L. Kasper.** 2005. An immunomodulatory molecule of symbiotic bacteria directs maturation of the host immune system. *Cell* **122:**107–118.

73. **McIntyre, A., P. R. Gibson, and G. P. Young.** 1993. Butyrate production from dietary fibre and protection against large bowel cancer in a rat model. *Gut* **34:**386–391.

74. **Metges, C. C.** 2000. Contribution of microbial amino acids to amino acid homeostasis of the host. *J. Nutr.* **130:**1857S–1864S.

75. **Moissl, C., S. Osman, M. T. La Duc, A. Dekas, E. Brodie, T. DeSantis, and K. Venkateswaran.** 2007. Molecular bacterial community analysis of clean rooms where spacecraft are assembled. *FEMS Microbiol. Ecol.* **61:**509–521.

76. **Mortensen, P. B., and M. R. Clausen.** 1996. Short-chain fatty acids in the human colon: relation to gastrointestinal health and disease. *Scand. J. Gastroenterol. Suppl.* **216:**132–148.

77. **Myer, L., L. Denny, R. Telerant, M. Souza, T. C. Wright, Jr., and L. Kuhn.** 2005. Bacterial vaginosis and susceptibility to HIV infection in South African women: a nested case-control study. *J. Infect. Dis.* **192:**1372–1380.

78. **Nasidze, I., J. Li, D. Quinque, K. Tang, and M. Stoneking.** 2009. Global diversity in the human salivary microbiome. *Genome Res.* **19:**636–643.

79. **Nasidze, I., D. Quinque, J. Li, M. Li, K. Tang, and M. Stoneking.** 2009. Comparative analysis of human saliva microbiome diversity by barcoded pyrosequencing and cloning approaches. *Anal. Biochem.* **391:**64–68.

80. **Offenbacher, S., K. A. Boggess, A. P. Murtha, H. L. Jared, S. Lieff, R. G. McKaig, S. M. Mauriello, K. L. Moss, and J. D. Beck.** 2006. Progressive periodontal disease and risk of very preterm delivery. *Obstet. Gynecol.* **107:**29–36.

81. **Pajecki, D., B. Zilberstein, M. A. dos Santos, J. A. Ubriaco, A. G. Quintanilha, I. Cecconello, and J. Gama-Rodrigues.** 2002. Megaesophagus microbiota: a qualitative and quantitative analysis. *J. Gastrointest. Surg.* **6:**723–729.

82. **Paster, B. J., S. K. Boches, J. L. Galvin, R. E. Ericson, C. N. Lau, V. A. Levanos, A. Sahasrabudhe, and F. E. Dewhirst.** 2001. Bacterial diversity in human subgingival plaque. *J. Bacteriol.* **183:**3770–3783.

83. **Paster, B. J., I. Olsen, J. A. Aas, and F. E. Dewhirst.** 2006. The breadth of bacterial diversity in the human periodontal pocket and other oral sites. *Periodontol. 2000* **42:**80–87.

84. **Pei, Z., E. J. Bini, L. Yang, M. Zhou, F. Francois, and M. J. Blaser.** 2004. Bacterial biota in the human distal esophagus. *Proc. Natl. Acad. Sci. USA* **101:**4250–4255.

85. **Pei, Z., L. Yang, R. M. Peek, S. M. Levine, Jr., D. T. Pride, and M. J. Blaser.** 2005. Bacterial biota in reflux esophagitis and Barrett's esophagus. *World J. Gastroenterol.* **11:**7277–7283.

86. **Peña, J., and J. Versalovic.** 2003. *Lactobacillus rhamnosus* GG decreases TNF-alpha production in lipopolysaccharide-activated murine macrophages by a contact-independent mechanism. *Cell. Microbiol.* **5:**277–285.

87. **Peterson, D. A., D. N. Frank, N. R. Pace, and J. I. Gordon.** 2008. Metagenomic approaches for defining the pathogenesis of inflammatory bowel diseases. *Cell Host Microbe* **3:**417–427.

88. **Peterson, J., S. Garges, M. Giovanni, P. McInnes, L. Wang, J. A. Schloss, V. Bonazzi, J. E. McEwen, K. A. Wetterstrand, C. Deal, C. C. Baker, V. Di Francesco, T. K. Howcroft, R. W. Karp, R. D. Lunsford, C. R. Wellington, T. Belachew, M. Wright, C. Giblin, H. David, M. Mills, R. Salomon, C. Mullins, B. Akolkar, L. Begg, C. Davis, L. Grandison, M. Humble, J. Khalsa, A. R. Little, H. Peavy, C. Pontzer, M. Portnoy, M. H. Sayre, P. Starke-Reed, S. Zakhari, J. Read, B. Watson, and M. Guyer.** 2009. The NIH Human Microbiome Project. *Genome Res.* **19:**2317–2323.

89. Quince, C., A. Lanzen, T. P. Curtis, R. J. Davenport, N. Hall, I. M. Head, L. F. Read, and W. T. Sloan. 2009. Accurate determination of microbial diversity from 454 pyrosequencing data. *Nat. Methods* **6:**639–641.

90. Rakoff-Nahoum, S., J. Paglino, F. Eslami-Varzaneh, S. Edberg, and R. Medzhitov. 2004. Recognition of commensal microflora by toll-like receptors is required for intestinal homeostasis. *Cell* **118:**229–241.

91. Rasiah, I. A., L. Wong, S. A. Anderson, and C. H. Sissons. 2005. Variation in bacterial DGGE patterns from human saliva: over time, between individuals and in corresponding dental plaque microcosms. *Arch. Oral Biol.* **50:**779–787.

92. Rocas, I. N., J. C. Baumgartner, T. Xia, and J. F. Siqueira, Jr. 2006. Prevalence of selected bacterial named species and uncultivated phylotypes in endodontic abscesses from two geographic locations. *J. Endod.* **32:**1135–1138.

93. Roth, R. R., and W. D. James. 1988. Microbial ecology of the skin. *Annu. Rev. Microbiol.* **42:**441–464.

94. Sakamoto, M., Y. Huang, M. Ohnishi, M. Umeda, I. Ishikawa, and Y. Benno. 2004. Changes in oral microbial profiles after periodontal treatment as determined by molecular analysis of 16S rRNA genes. *J. Med. Microbiol.* **53:**563–571.

95. Sakamoto, M., Y. Takeuchi, M. Umeda, I. Ishikawa, and Y. Benno. 2003. Application of terminal RFLP analysis to characterize oral bacterial flora in saliva of healthy subjects and patients with periodontitis. *J. Med. Microbiol.* **52:**79–89.

96. Sartor, R. B. 2006. Mechanisms of disease: pathogenesis of Crohn's disease and ulcerative colitis. *Nat. Clin. Pract. Gastroenterol. Hepatol.* **3:**390–407.

97. Savage, D. C. 1977. Microbial ecology of the gastrointestinal tract. *Annu. Rev. Microbiol.* **31:**107–133.

98. Scannapieco, F. A. 1999. Role of oral bacteria in respiratory infection. *J. Periodontol.* **70:**793–802.

99. Schwebke, J. R. 2005. Abnormal vaginal flora as a biological risk factor for acquisition of HIV infection and sexually transmitted diseases. *J. Infect. Dis.* **192:**1315–1317.

100. Socransky, S. S., A. D. Haffajee, M. A. Cugini, C. Smith, and R. L. Kent, Jr. 1998. Microbial complexes in subgingival plaque. *J. Clin. Periodontol.* **25:**134–144.

101. Socransky, S. S., C. Smith, L. Martin, B. J. Paster, F. E. Dewhirst, and A. E. Levin. 1994. "Checkerboard" DNA-DNA hybridization. *BioTechniques* **17:**788–792.

102. Sokol, H., B. Pigneur, L. Watterlot, O. Lakhdari, L. G. Bermudez-Humaran, J. J. Gratadoux, S. Blugeon, C. Bridonneau, J. P. Furet, G. Corthier, C. Grangette, N. Vasquez, P. Pochart, G. Trugnan, G. Thomas, H. M. Blottiere, J. Dore, P. Marteau, P. Seksik, and P. Langella. 2008. *Faecalibacterium prausnitzii* is an anti-inflammatory commensal bacterium identified by gut microbiota analysis of Crohn disease patients. *Proc. Natl. Acad. Sci. USA* **105:**16731–16736.

103. Stark, C. A., I. Adamsson, C. Edlund, S. Sjosted, R. Seensalu, B. Wikstrom, and C. E. Nord. 1996. Effects of omeprazole and amoxycillin on the human oral and gastrointestinal microflora in patients with *Helicobacter pylori* infection. *J. Antimicrob. Chemother.* **38:**927–939.

104. Sutherland, R., R. J. Boon, K. E. Griffin, P. J. Masters, B. Slocombe, and A. R. White. 1985. Antibacterial activity of mupirocin (pseudomonic acid), a new antibiotic for topical use. *Antimicrob. Agents Chemother.* **27:**495–498.

105. Tap, J., S. Mondot, F. Levenez, E. Pelletier, C. Caron, J.-P. Furet, E. Ugarte, R. Muñoz-Tamayo, D. L. E. Paslier, R. Nalin, J. Dore, and M. Leclerc. 2009. Towards the human intestinal microbiota phylogenetic core. *Environ. Microbiol.* **11:**2574–2584.

106. Turnbaugh, P. J., R. E. Ley, M. A. Mahowald, V. Magrini, E. R. Mardis, and J. I. Gordon. 2006. An obesity-associated gut microbiome with increased capacity for energy harvest. *Nature* **444:**1027–1031.

107. Verhelst, R., H. Verstraelen, G. Claeys, G. Verschraegen, J. Delanghe, L. Van Simaey, C. De Ganck, M. Temmerman, and M. Vaneechoutte. 2004. Cloning of 16S rRNA genes amplified from normal and disturbed vaginal microflora suggests a strong association between *Atopobium vaginae*, *Gardnerella vaginalis* and bacterial vaginosis. *BMC Microbiol.* **4:**16.

107a. Wen, L., R. E. Ley, P. Y. Volchkov, P. B. Stranges, L. Avanesyan, A. C. Stonebraker, C. Hu, F. S. Wong, G. L. Szot, J. A. Bluestone, J. I. Gordon, and A. V. Chervonsky. Innate immunity and intestinal microbiota in the development of type 1 diabetes. *Nature* **455:**1109–1113.

108. Woo, P. C., A. M. Fung, S. K. Lau, B. Y. Chan, S. K. Chiu, J. L. Teng, T. L. Que, R. W. Yung, and K. Y. Yuen. 2003. *Granulicatella adiacens* and *Abiotrophia defectiva* bacteraemia characterized by 16S rRNA gene sequencing. *J. Med. Microbiol.* **52:**137–140.

109. Wu, D., A. Hartman, N. Ward, and J. A. Eisen. 2008. An automated phylogenetic tree-based small subunit rRNA taxonomy and alignment pipeline (STAP). *PLoS ONE* **3:**e2566.

110. Yang, L., X. Lu, C. W. Nossa, F. Francois, R. M. Peek, and Z. Pei. 2009. Inflammation and intestinal metaplasia of the distal esophagus are associated with alterations in the microbiome. *Gastroenterology* **137:**588–597.

111. Zaidel, O., and H. C. Lin. 2003. Uninvited guests: the impact of small intestinal bacterial overgrowth on nutritional status. *Pract. Gastroenterol.* **27:**27–34.

112. Zhou, X., C. J. Brown, Z. Abdo, C. C. Davis, M. A. Hansmann, P. Joyce, J. A. Foster, and L. J. Forney. 2007. Differences in the composition of vaginal microbial communities found in healthy Caucasian and black women. *ISME J.* **1:**121–133.

Microbial Genomics and Pathogen Discovery

ANNE M. GAYNOR AND DAVID WANG

14

OVERVIEW

In the past several decades, our understanding of the diversity of microbes present in the world has grown tremendously as many previously unidentified bacterial, archaeal, and viral species have been discovered and sequenced. Further geometric growth in defining microbial diversity is currently underway, driven in large part by advances in genomic technologies. As more and more microbes are identified, the potential role of these microbes as pathogens, as well as the broader concept of how microbes can cause disease, must be reevaluated. In the 21st century, the concepts of microbial genomics and pathogen discovery have become intricately linked, and they are discussed in this review. We begin with an overview of traditional efforts, followed by a brief description of the evolution of sequencing technologies; finally, we illustrate how these two fields began to intersect in the first few years of the 21st century.

INTRODUCTION

Our ability to "see" the microbes that surround us first arose in the 17th century when Anton van Leeuwenhoek created a microscope, which provided the first physical evidence of the diversity and ubiquity of microbes in the world. Another giant leap occurred in the 19th century when Koch first demonstrated that bacteria could be grown in pure culture, beginning with the analysis of blood from cows infected with the anthrax agent. He subsequently became most widely known for the postulates regarding microbial disease causation that bear his name. For decades following, a combination of culture and microscopy was the only tool available to see microbes. In the last decade of the 20th century, however, consensus ribosomal PCR revealed that a much greater diversity of bacteria exists beyond what could be cultured, and that cultured bacteria represented only ~1% of all bacterial species. Today, sequencing technology has evolved to the point that it is feasible to comprehensively define the collection of microbes present in humans (i.e., the human "microbiome") or any other ecological niche in a fashion that is completely independent of culture or microscopy.

A BRIEF HISTORY OF PATHOGEN DISCOVERY

Classic Methods

Classic methods of microbial discovery have relied heavily on the ability to readily cultivate or passage the organism in question. Clinical material associated with a disease thought to be of infectious origin is used to inoculate diverse growth media to cultivate the microbe(s) present in the sample. In the case of suspected bacterial agents, selective or nonselective growth media can be utilized, while primary or immortal cell lines are inoculated for suspected viruses. In addition, the clinical specimens could also be used to infect animal models. If a microbe could be cultivated, attempts to identify it would follow. For bacterial identification, differential stains and growth conditions are used to categorize and ascertain the genus or species present. Viral identification is similarly based on differential growth in various cell types as well as serological reactions to a variety of specific antisera. The use of microscopic techniques, including light and electron microscopy, is also extremely important in the process of identification. These classic tools have been incredibly useful and resulted in the discovery of many currently accepted human pathogens, for example, *Bacillus anthracis*, *Mycobacterium tuberculosis*, *Yellow fever virus*, and *Poliovirus*. However, there are two fundamental limitations to this approach: (i) these methods are dependent on the ability of the microbe to grow in the substrate provided, and (ii) even if the microbe can be cultivated, that fact alone will not necessarily lead to unambiguous identification of the unknown agent.

Molecular Approaches: Candidate Dependent

In the late 1980s, with the advent of PCR, scientists could now easily use molecular approaches to detect microbes present in a given clinical sample if there was existing sequence for the microbe(s) to be targeted. The recognition that selecting PCR primers designed to highly conserved regions in a set of sequences (e.g., multiple bacteria or several viruses from a common taxonomic group) could enable the detection of previously unsequenced or unidentified microbes provided a novel approach for the identification of microbes. These types of approaches are referred to interchangeably as broad-range or consensus PCR methods. One of the broadest applications of this technique has been the design of primers to the 16S rRNA gene, which enables the detection of nearly all members of the bacterial domain. Alternatively, more specific primers can be selected that are conserved within a given taxon (family, genus, or species) to identify a more targeted set of microbes. The ability to design highly conserved primers is, of course, predicated on the existence of sufficient sequence data to identify the appropriate conserved regions. There are a large number of microbes that have been discovered by using PCR in conjunction with the classical methods of microbial detection and discovery.

Two pioneering papers by Relman and coworkers describe the first examples of using consensus PCR primers to identify the causative agents of specific human diseases. Bacillary angiomatosis was commonly thought to be of infectious origin, but for many years no specific microbial agent could be identified. A putative agent could be visualized in tissue sections following staining, but efforts to culture the organism had failed. Sequencing of amplicons generated by PCR using 16S rRNA gene consensus primers demonstrated that a previously uncharacterized rickettsia-like bacterium was present in tissue samples of patients with bacillary angiomatosis (67). The bacterium was later identified as a member of the genus *Bartonella*. A similar approach was subsequently applied to address the etiology of Whipple's disease. Whipple's disease was first described in 1907 as a rare systemic disorder that primarily caused malabsorption but could affect any part of the body. Consensus PCR using primers targeting the bacterial 16S ribosomal gene resulted in the identification of an uncharacterized actinomycete, which would later be classified as *Tropheryma whipplei* (68). These two cases demonstrated the power of molecular pathogen discovery methods.

The use of conserved PCR primers has also been applied to the discovery of viruses. However, since no universally conserved sequence akin to the 16S rRNA sequences in bacteria is present in all viruses, consensus sequences must be identified and consensus primers designed for each given viral taxon of interest. A seminal example of using consensus PCR to identify a viral pathogen occurred during the emergence of hantavirus pulmonary syndrome in 1993 (61). In the course of investigating an unusual outbreak of a lethal pulmonary disease in otherwise healthy young adults in the southwestern United States, extensive testing by classic microbiological methods ruled out most of the likely candidates known to cause severe respiratory disease. Serological tests revealed that patient sera were cross-reactive with known hantaviruses. From this lead, PCR primers were designed to conserved regions of known hantavirus sequences, which were then used to amplify nucleic acids extracted from tissue samples isolated from dying patients. Sequencing of the amplicon generated by the primers resulted in the identification of a novel member of this family, which was ultimately named *Sin Nombre virus*.

Since these seminal applications of consensus PCR for the identification of bacterial and viral pathogens, there have been many instances of microbial identification using this strategy. Consensus PCR, either alone or in conjunction with classic culture and antigen detection methods, continues to be of great utility in the discovery of novel microbes, as illustrated by the recent discoveries of a new phylogenetic group of rhinoviruses (47, 49, 51, 52, 59), a spate of parechoviruses (4, 7, 8, 23, 40, 55, 78), the

arenavirus *Chapare virus* (19), and Bundibugyo ebolavirus (70). However, what is not documented in the literature is the number of times that broad-range PCR strategies were applied but failed to identify an agent. It should also be evident that in order for this approach to be useful and successful, the list of potential candidates must be relatively short. In these successful examples described above, the authors had a strong hypothesis regarding the nature of the microbe (i.e., bacterium versus virus) present or which specific candidate viral taxon might be present. However, in many situations, there may not be a leading candidate(s), thus limiting the feasibility of using consensus PCR approaches, especially for viral identification. Thus, despite these successes, there has been significant impetus for the development of pathogen discovery strategies that are broad range and not candidate dependent.

Molecular Approaches: Candidate Independent

The discoveries of *Hepatitis C virus* (HCV) and *Human herpesvirus 8* (HHV-8), also called Kaposi's sarcoma-associated herpesvirus (KSHV), represented two breakthroughs in the application of candidate-independent molecular methods for pathogen discovery. In 1989, the identification of HCV in patients with non-A, non-B (NANB) hepatitis relied upon a library immunoscreening strategy (17). A randomly primed cDNA library was made from material from infected animals and screened using patient serum from NANB hepatitis patients with the goal of identifying cDNA clones that generated peptide sequences recognized by the patient sera. From over a million clones that were screened, a single clone reacted specifically with NANB hepatitis patient sera. From this initial cDNA clone fragment, the HCV genome was eventually sequenced. Today, HCV is recognized as being responsible for the vast majority of cases of NANB hepatitis. In 1994, human herpesvirus 8 was discovered in the lesions of AIDS-associated Kaposi's sarcoma (13). The identification of Kaposi's sarcoma-associated herpesvirus relied on representational difference analysis, a subtractive hybridization-based method, to enrich for and then identify unique sequences present in Kaposi's sarcoma lesions but not in healthy tissue controls. While these two examples demonstrate the potential of these methods, there have been few subsequent success stories using either of these two methods, most likely due to technical challenges associated with both of these strategies. Thus, there remained a clear need for further improved strategies for pathogen discovery.

By the end of the 20th century, the classic culture-based methods for microbial discovery had been augmented by multiple molecular approaches, such as consensus PCR, library immunoscreening, and representational difference analysis. In parallel, targeted sequencing of specific microbes was starting to become feasible, thus setting the stage for the convergence of pathogen discovery efforts and microbial sequencing efforts.

MICROBIAL GENOMICS HISTORY

Microbe sequencing in the 20th century relied exclusively upon Sanger dideoxy sequencing, the dominant sequencing strategy since its invention in 1977. From its initial incarnation using slab gels as a readout, incremental advances in sequencing capacity evolved as the readout transitioned to capillary electrophoresis, and then from single capillaries to simultaneous analysis of 96 capillaries, which is still used today.

Formally, the era of microbial genomics began with the complete sequencing of the *Haemophilus influenzae* genome in 1995. However, it was recognized almost two decades earlier that an organism's genomic sequence, as the ultimate marker of evolution, could serve to classify and define the relatedness of both prokaryotic and eukaryotic organisms (80). rRNA was a molecule with an appropriately broad distribution which mutated slowly over time, permitting the detection of relatedness. With the advent of Sanger sequencing, entire 16S rRNA genes could be sequenced, including the *Escherichia coli* 16S rRNA gene in 1978 (11). Sequencing at the time and in the ensuing decades was time-consuming and expensive and was performed to obtain the minimum amount of data that was needed.

When the *H. influenzae* genome was sequenced, this bacterium became the first free-living organism to have its genome sequenced in its entirety (31). This was a landmark achievement, notable also because of the use of a "shotgun" strategy to assemble the complete genome. "Shotgun" refers to the random fragmentation and cloning of DNA fragments followed by computational assembly of the overlapping regions to generate a complete genome sequence. Based on this proof of principle, genomes of larger microbes and eukaryotic organisms were subsequently sequenced in this fashion. The following year, *Saccharomyces cerevisiae* was the first eukaryotic organism to be fully sequenced (35), and then in 1998, the first multicellular eukaryotic genome to be sequenced, that of *Caenorhabditis elegans*, was published (12). Since then, the complete genomes of many human and animal pathogens have been sequenced, including notable pathogens such as *Mycobacterium tuberculosis* (2001), *Yersinia pestis* (2001), and *Plasmodium falciparum* (2002). In 2004, the complete 1.2-Mb genome of mimivirus, the largest known virus, was published (65).

The human genome project was first proposed in 1990, and initial sequencing began in 1995. By 2001 two drafts of the human genome had been published (50, 75). During the course of this massive project, many technological refinements in the efficiency of Sanger sequencing itself, as well as novel tools for the downstream computational analysis, were implemented. These developments could naturally be applied to sequencing of much smaller microbial genomes and therefore contributed substantially to the rapid increase in the rate of microbial sequencing.

Over the past 5 years, a number of new sequencing modalities that together have been termed the next generation, or NextGen, of sequencing have been developed. The three major platforms in current use are 454 (Roche Titanium), Solexa (Illumina), and SOLiD (ABI). Key characteristics of these platforms include the fact that all of them have geometrically increased the raw sequence generation capacity and decreased the cost per base pair 10- to 100-fold relative to Sanger sequencing. Although each of these new platforms utilizes a fundamentally different sequencing modality, in all cases, clonal amplification of the template DNA has been moved from bacteria (thereby eliminating the need for plasmid cloning and propagation) to an in vitro setting. In the 454 technology, approximately 1 million sequence reads averaging 400 bp, or about 400 Mb of total sequence, is generated per run. Clearly, in terms of microbes such as bacteria, one sequencing run of a 454 instrument is sufficient to generate greater than 100 times the coverage of the average 3-Mb bacterial genome. By comparison, the Illumina platform currently produces ~20 Gb of sequence with read lengths up to 100 bp, while the SOLiD can generate ~30 Gb with an average read length

of 35 bp. For a more detailed description of each of these platforms and capabilities, see reference 58.

With these increases in sequencing capacity, the sequencing of microbial genomes has become routine. In fact, there are currently ambitious projects that have been conceived to comprehensively sequence the microbial diversity of the human microbiome and the viral diversity, "the virome," present in humans (see chapter 13). These efforts will vastly expand the world of sequenced microbes far beyond the current 5,900 species of bacteria, fungi, parasites, and viruses that have been completely sequenced and whose sequences have been deposited in GenBank (GenBank Genome Records 11.12.09; http://www.ncbi.nlm.nih.gov/sites/entrez?db=genom).

THE MERGING OF PATHOGEN DISCOVERY AND MICROBIAL GENOMICS

The onset of the 21st century has seen the convergence of the fields of pathogen discovery and microbial genomics (Fig. 1). The goals of systematically defining the microbes present in a given clinical sample dovetail with the goals of "pathogen discovery," namely, to identify one or more microbes present in a clinical sample that are responsible for a disease phenotype. Two new molecular approaches for massively parallel analysis have recently emerged that are capable of defining the spectrum of microbes present in clinical specimens: microarray and sequencing-based detection. Both of these strategies have benefited greatly from the increased focus on human and microbial sequencing. The vast database of nucleic acid sequences provides the substrate from which consensus PCR primers (described above) and probes for microarrays (described below) have been designed. Naturally, sequencing-based approaches have evolved along with the sequencing capacity of new platforms. In the first half of this decade, Sanger method-based sequencing dominated these efforts, and due to the costs and limited throughput, experimental strategies were devised to minimize the extent of sequencing necessary to identify microbial agents. As the decade progressed, and more robust sequencing methods evolved, the need to enrich for microbial sequences diminished and more brute force strategies have come to the forefront. For all the sequencing-based methods, a critical component of the process is the bioinformatic analysis of the sequences generated. Typically, computational pipelines have been established that compare the resulting sequences against various public sequence databases to determine the origin of each sequence read. The "discovery" of a novel microbial sequence results when a sequence with only limited similarity to existing microbial sequences is encountered.

Microarray-Based Approaches

Microarrays were initially developed in the early 1990s to analyze gene expression patterns of a single organism in a highly parallel fashion. For example, early studies analyzed every gene present in the yeast *Saccharomyces cerevisiae* (20). Since then, a wide variety of microarray platforms have evolved. Regardless of the technical format, the fundamental principle driving all microarrays is that of nucleic acid hybridization. If a given sample contains sequences that are complementary to those represented on the array, hybridization should occur. Thus, the target sequences to be detected by a given microarray are limited only by the availability of DNA sequences from which probes can be designed. As DNA microarray technology evolved in

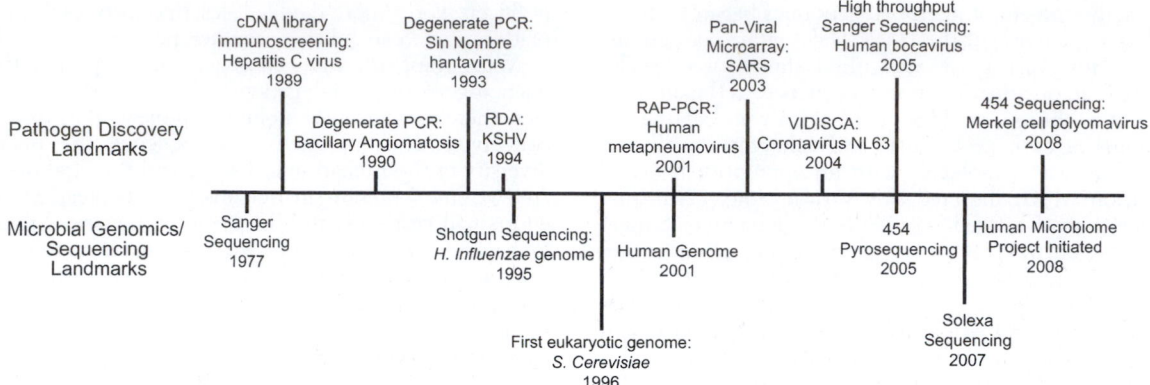

FIGURE 1 Major landmarks in pathogen discovery and microbial genomics. RDA, representational difference analysis; RAP-PCR, random arbitrarily primed PCR; VIDISCA, virus discovery cDNA-AFLP (amplified restriction fragment length polymorphism).

the late 1990s, it became clear at a theoretical level that microarrays might make excellent microbial diagnostic tools. The inherently highly parallel nature of microarrays, coupled to the increasing availability of microbial sequence data generated by targeted efforts to sequence microbes as discussed earlier, made it possible to design microarrays with the capacity to simultaneously detect a wide range of microbes, including novel microbes.

The first significant effort to develop a microarray for broad-range pathogen identification focused on detecting all known respiratory viruses (76). This microarray contained ~1,600 oligonucleotides representing ~140 viruses from all virus families with members known to cause respiratory disease. Soon thereafter, a second, more comprehensive array, the ViroChip, was designed using 70-mer oligonucleotides derived from every fully sequenced viral genome in GenBank at the time (77). The oligonucleotide probes selected were the most highly conserved 70-mers from each viral taxon and were chosen to increase the possibility of detecting known, unknown, and unsequenced family members through cross-hybridization. Sample preparation for the array includes standard nucleic acid extraction and then random amplification using a primer comprised of a fixed linker sequence at the 5' end and a random 5- to 9-mer at the 3' end. The use of a random PCR step eliminates the need for prior knowledge of the infectious agent, and thus, identification is limited only by the spectrum of viral probes present on the array. Following the random amplification, samples are labeled with fluorescent dyes (typically Cy3 or Cy5). The resulting hybridization patterns on the array must then be interpreted to infer the presence or absence of known or novel viruses. A variety of approaches have been developed for this purpose, including visual inspection, hierarchical clustering (25), and several customized bioinformatic programs, such as E-predict (71), Dectiviv (79), Phylodetect (66), and VIPR (3a).

The first example wherein a DNA microarray was used to identify a novel virus arose during the severe acute respiratory syndrome (SARS) outbreak in 2003 (48, 69, 77). At that time, a mysterious outbreak of highly lethal respiratory disease that tested negative for all known respiratory pathogens was emerging from southeast China. An unknown virus was cultured from the respiratory swab of a SARS patient. Total nucleic acid was extracted from this virus

culture and then amplified and hybridized to the ViroChip. The resulting hybridization pattern demonstrated that a divergent member of the family *Coronaviridae* was present in the sample. To further characterize the nature of this putative new coronavirus, fragments of the unknown virus were physically recovered from the oligonucleotide spots on the microarray surface (77). Sequencing of these eluted fragments confirmed that the sequences were derived from a novel coronavirus with only 33% amino acid identity to murine hepatitis virus, a murine coronavirus. Koch's postulates were fulfilled when cultured SARS coronavirus was used to infect nonhuman primates, which then developed signs of respiratory diseases (32).

The ViroChip was also utilized to examine a subset of hereditary prostate cancers that harbor loss-of-function mutations in *RNASEL*, a known antiviral factor. Given this linkage, it was hypothesized that such cells might be more susceptible to viral infections. RNA from prostate tumors with wild-type *RNASEL* alleles and homozygous mutant R462Q alleles were extracted and hybridized to the ViroChip. In 7 of 11 (63.4%) tumors from patients homozygous for the mutation, a hybridization pattern characteristic of a murine retrovirus was observed (72). The complete genome was recovered from the tumors following cloning and sequencing which revealed that the novel virus was most closely related to xenotropic murine retroviruses in the genus *Gammaretrovirus;* the virus was named *Xenotropic murine leukemia virus-related virus* (XMRV). Subsequent screening identified additional tumors that demonstrated a strong association of XMRV with prostate cancers homozygous for R462Q. Other studies have confirmed the association of XMRV with prostate cancer, but the role of the RNase L mutation was ambiguous (46). Most recently, a statistical association between the presence of XMRV in the blood cells of patients with chronic fatigue syndrome has been reported (57).

Other broad-range DNA microarrays aside from the ViroChip have been described (6), including the GreeneChip, a pan-microbial microarray that contains probes for viruses, bacteria, and parasites (62), which, along with the ViroChip, has been successfully used in a variety of diagnostic scenarios to detect known or unexpected viruses (14, 16, 56, 64, 81). However, none of these other platforms has been applied explicitly in the discovery of novel viruses to date.

On the bacterial front, microarrays with probes targeted towards detection of 16S rRNA sequences have been developed to define the bacterial diversity present in a given sample. While early efforts focused on detecting specific targeted bacterial taxa, in 2007 two separate groups published broad-range universal arrays. The PhyloChip, a high-density 16S rRNA microarray containing ~300,000 probes, was used to examine the microbial diversity in three environmental samples, including urban aerosol, subsurface soil, and subsurface water (21). This study demonstrated that the array could reveal broader diversity than classical cloning and sequencing of the same sample. A second array containing 10,500 probes, including 9,000 taxonomically specific probes targeting the 16S rRNA gene, was used to perform a detailed, systematic, and quantitative study of the bacterial colonization of the infant gastrointestinal tract (63). The results of the array were compared to those of sequencing-based techniques, and the results were in good concordance, demonstrating the utility of the array.

DNA microarrays aimed at microbial diagnostics have benefited immensely from the genomic era, which has spawned a wealth of microbial sequence available in public databases. As more diverse microbe sequences become available, the diagnostic potential of microarrays will undoubtedly improve even further. The ability to simultaneously screen in a relatively unbiased fashion for many target microbes makes microarrays powerful tools for microbial detection. As demonstrated by the successful examples using the ViroChip, it can also be a robust platform for discovery of novel viruses. There is, however, a clear limitation of all hybridization-based strategies for pathogen discovery, including DNA microarrays: the novel microbe must have significant levels of nucleotide identity within the probe region in order to be detected. Thus, highly divergent microbes that have little similarity to known microbes at the nucleotide level are unlikely to be detected. Hence, sequencing-based approaches, which enable the analysis of sequence similarity at the amino acid level, have the potential to detect microbes that have diverged to a greater extent from currently sequenced microbes.

Sequencing-Based Approaches

The discovery of *Human metapneumovirus* (HMPV) in 2001 combined classic viral culture with a molecular strategy termed random arbitrarily primed PCR (73). Efforts to culture respiratory secretions from children suffering respiratory tract infections led to the identification of a putative unidentified virus that could be passaged in tertiary monkey kidney (tMK) cells, Vero cells, and, to a lesser extent, A549 cells. In order to identify the virus present, random, arbitrary primers were used to generate PCR amplicons. Differentially represented amplicons present in infected cells but absent from control cells were identified by gel electrophoresis and selectively sequenced. Multiple fragments having limited sequence identity to avian pneumoviruses were detected, indicating that a novel virus, now known as HMPV, was present in the infected cells. Seroprevalence studies indicated that by the age of 5 to 10 years, most individuals were antibody positive, suggesting that this virus is a common infection acquired in childhood. HMPV can cause severe respiratory infections, including pneumonia and bronchiolitis, and is responsible for 5 to 10% of hospitalizations of patients with respiratory tract infection (18). The presentation and case severity are very similar to those of respiratory syncytial virus (18).

In the same year, a candidate independent sequencing strategy for identification of novel viruses termed DNase-SISPA was described (2). The experimental strategy relied upon sequence-independent single primer amplification (SISPA), wherein an adaptor containing a primer binding sequence is ligated to both ends of a cDNA fragment and a single primer is then used for PCR. To enrich specifically for viral nucleic acids present in virions, the clinical sample is first subjected to ultracentrifugation to pellet the virions and is then treated with DNase to degrade any cellular nucleic acids that are not protected within the viral capsids. Following this enrichment, the sample is then extracted for DNA or RNA and amplified using SISPA. The enrichment steps in this protocol are necessary to increase the chances of sequencing a virus-derived sequence, given the labor and costs of performing extensive Sanger sequencing on the unenriched sample. In this proof-of-concept study, two novel bovine parvoviruses were identified (2).

A variation of the DNase-SISPA strategy, called virus discovery cDNA-AFLP (amplified restriction fragment length polymorphism), was utilized in 2004 to identify a novel virus from the family *Coronaviridae*, human coronavirus NL63 (HCoV-NL63), from a child with bronchiolitis (74). In this protocol, following the standard ultracentrifugation, DNase treatment, nucleic acid purification, restriction digestion, linker ligation, and PCR amplification, a second set of PCRs was performed to identify differentially expressed bands present only in the putatively infected sample. There were 16 such bands that were cloned and sequenced. Of these, 13 had limited sequence similarity to known coronaviruses. Once completely sequenced, genome analysis demonstrated that HCoV-NL63 is most closely related to HCoV-229, a known respiratory pathogen, with 65% nucleotide identity. Subsequent studies have associated HCoV-NL63 with croup, and infection rates approaching 80% by the age of 6 as defined by serology have been reported (22). Of note, a third novel coronavirus, coronavirus HKU1, was identified using consensus PCR from a patient with pneumonia (82).

Application of DNase-SISPA to examine plasma samples from patients with febrile illness resulted in the identification of sequences with only limited identity to known members of the family *Parvoviridae* and the *Anellovirus* genus in 2005 (41). The entire sequence was obtained for the novel parvovirus, *Parvovirus 4* (PARV4), and phylogenetic analysis revealed that the greatest similarity was only 24 to 29% identity to open reading frame 1 (ORF1) of *Adeno-associated virus* and *Avian parvovirus*. PARV4 has been detected in blood, bone marrow, and lymphoid tissue from patients with either HCV or human immunodeficiency virus/AIDS and in plasma of kidney transplant patients, and high frequencies of exposure have been reported for hemophiliacs and injection drug users. Two novel anelloviruses, SA1 and SA2, were also identified in this study. Notably, these viruses were highly divergent from known viruses and shared only 32 to 35% similarity to TT virus (TTV). TTVs and TTV-related viruses have been ubiquitously found to infect humans, but there has been no direct causal evidence to link these viruses to any specific disease. The findings of these three novel viruses with very low amino acid similarity to known viruses highlights the importance of sequencing over methods that require nucleic acid homology for detection, as these viruses would likely have been missed by those methods.

A similar method was also used to identify several novel sequences with similarity to anelloviruses in the blood of healthy donors (9). Blood samples were subjected to density centrifugation followed by chloroform and DNase treatment before nucleic acid extraction. The nucleic acids were amplified using a polymerase with strand displacement activity, randomly sheared, ligated to linkers, and then PCR amplified before cloning and sequencing. Using this technique, seven sequences with limited similarity to known members of the genus *Anellovirus* were identified. Detailed analysis of two of these sequences demonstrated that one shared 35% amino acid identity to SA2, which had just been discovered only months earlier, while the second sequence shared 63% amino acid identity to SEN virus, another known anellovirus. As discussed previously, the role of anelloviruses in the causation of disease has not been established.

The discovery of *Human bocavirus* (HBoV) in 2005 relied on yet another slight variation of the DNase-SISPA strategy (3). Pooled respiratory secretions from multiple patients with unexplained respiratory illness were ultracentrifuged to concentrate viral particles and DNase treated. Following nucleic acid extraction, a random-primer-linker-based amplification (similar to that used for the previously described DNA microarray studies) was used. Amplicons of 600 to 1,500 bp were cloned and sequenced using high-throughput Sanger sequencing (one 384-well plate). Sequences were identified with amino acid similarity to known *Parvoviridae* family members, *Bovine parvovirus* and *Canine minute virus*. The original sample was identified from the pool, and the complete genome was obtained. Phylogenetic analysis demonstrated that this novel genome is a previously uncharacterized species of the genus *Bocavirus*, HBoV. Subsequent studies of this virus have demonstrated that HBoV is frequently detected in children with respiratory tract infection, children with asthma exacerbation, and children with acute gastroenteritis. Seroepidemiology studies have confirmed infection in a Japanese cohort, with 71.1% overall prevalence with exposure by age 6 (26), while a second study in Sweden reported a lower rate, 33%, in a cohort of children with acute wheezing (43).

Using the exact same method on pooled respiratory secretions, a novel member of the family *Polyomaviridae*, KI polyomavirus (KIV), was identified in 2007 (1). A single sequence read of 363 bp was identified that had limited similarity to the simian virus 40 (SV40) VP1 protein, and using primers to span the circular genome resulted in the completion of the genome of 5,040 bp. KIV has approximately 36 to 48% amino acid identity to the BK virus, JC virus, and SV40 T antigens, the most conserved proteins of the family. As described in the initial publication and subsequent publications, KIV has been identified in both respiratory secretions and feces. Although no clear disease association has been demonstrated to date, seroprevalence rates ranging from 55 to 90% (60) have been described, indicating that KIV infection is relatively ubiquitous.

The discovery of the *WU polyomavirus* (WUV) utilized a similar strategy of high-throughput Sanger sequencing analysis of respiratory secretions, although in this instance, individual samples rather than a pool were analyzed (34). Total nucleic acid of the respiratory secretions of a child with pneumonia was randomly amplified, and 384 clones were sequenced. The library contained six sequence reads that shared 35 to 50% amino acid identity to JC virus and SV40. The genome of WUV followed the canonical organization of the family *Polyomaviridae* and was 5,229 bp. Initial experiments as well as numerous subsequent publications

have identified WUV in respiratory secretions. It has also been found in feces, blood (whole, plasma, and serum), cerebrospinal fluid, and lymphoid tissue. Using seroprevalence as a measure, infection rates with WUV range from 69 to 98% (60), but no disease association has been established to date.

Saffold virus, a novel member of the *Cardiovirus* genus, was discovered using DNase-SISPA on a virus cultured from a patient stool sample (42). The following year, Saffold-like viruses were found in patients with acute enteritis and in respiratory secretions from three countries (24). In parallel, a series of related cardioviruses were identified using the ViroChip and subsequent PCR screening (15). To date, there has been one study examining the seroepidemiology of Saffold virus. Using a virus neutralization assay to Saffold virus 3, a seropositivity rate of 75% was observed by 24 months, which increased to ~90% in older children and adults (83).

The first application of high-throughput sequencing to identify viruses in diarrhea patients by shotgun sequencing resulted in the identification of a novel species in the family *Astroviridae*, *Astrovirus MLB1* (28). The methodology used was essentially identical to that used in the discovery of WUV except that a filtration step was implemented to minimize the recovery and amplification of bacterial sequences. Sequencing of a stool sample from a 3-year-old child from Australia with acute diarrhea resulted in the identification of seven sequences with 67% or less amino acid identity to known astroviruses. Phylogenetic analysis of the complete genome demonstrated that it was a highly divergent astrovirus. Subsequent studies have described astrovirus MLB1 in 4 out of 254 additional stool samples of children with diarrhea (29). To date, no case control studies have been described.

A novel genus, *Cosavirus*, of the family *Picornaviridae* was first proposed in 2008 following the identification of a handful of novel viruses with limited similarity to other picornaviruses. The first isolate, human cosavirus A1 (HCoSV-A1), was identified from a stool sample of a child with nonpolio acute flaccid paralysis from Pakistan (45). Analysis of the complete genome of 7,634 bp established that this virus shared 33 to 49% amino acid identity to its closest known relative, *Seneca Valley virus* (37), a member of the genus *Cardiovirus*. Subsequent PCR screening of a cohort composed of 57 symptomatic patients and 9 healthy contacts resulted in 34 positives that could be classified into four distinct genetic groups (A to D) based on sequence analysis and phylogeny. A proposed genetic group E has also been described following its identification from a child with acute diarrhea in Australia (38).

Two independent groups using similar Sanger sequencing-based screening of stool samples described *Human bocavirus 2* (HBoV2), a putative new species of the *Parvoviridae* family (5, 44). In a similar cohort of patients with acute flaccid paralysis from which human cosaviruses A to D were discovered, Kapoor et. al. identified HBoV2 from two consecutive stool samples of a child with acute flaccid paralysis. The entire genome was sequenced; it shares 67 to 80% similarity to the corresponding HBoV proteins (44). In parallel, HBoV2 was also identified in an Australian cohort of children with acute gastroenteritis. In this study, analysis of cases and controls revealed a statistically significant association between infection with HBoV2 and acute gastroenteritis (5). In subsequent PCR-based screens to define the prevalence of HBoV2, yet another divergent bocavirus, HBoV3, was identified (5).

These discoveries demonstrate that sequence-independent amplification followed by limited Sanger capillary sequencing (typically ≤384 clones) is a robust method for identification of novel viruses present in clinical specimens. With the advent of next-generation sequencing technology, samples could be sequenced in much greater depth, allowing for detection of microbes present at lower titers as well as facilitating the generation of complete genomes of novel microbes.

The discovery in 2008 of *Merkel cell polyomavirus* (MCPyV) was the first study describing identification of a novel virus using a next-generation sequencing platform (Roche/454 FLX platform) to identify a novel virus (27). In this instance, cDNA libraries were made from Merkel cell carcinoma (MCC) tumors and then sequenced using the 454 FLX platform. From ~382,000 high-quality sequence reads generated, one fragment had detectable sequence similarity to a known polyomavirus. Further analysis demonstrated that a highly divergent polyomavirus genome, that of MCPyV, was present in the majority of the MCC tumors examined. Subsequent studies have corroborated this finding, and mapping of integration sites demonstrated that in several instances the virus was clonally integrated in the respective tumors. Given the very low abundance of MCPyV mRNA sequences in these samples, the detection of viral transcripts would not have been possible without the use of the next-generation platform, which enabled the samples to be sequenced deeply in a cost-effective fashion. If the same study had been attempted with Sanger sequencing to the same depth, the effort would have been prohibitively expensive.

Next-generation sequencing played a pivotal role in defining the etiology of a mysterious case cluster of five patients with undiagnosed hemorrhagic fever (10). RNAs from two postmortem liver biopsy samples and one serum sample were randomly amplified and sequenced with 454. Analysis of the approximately 300,000 sequences generated yielded nine fragments with limited sequence similarity to viruses in the genus *Arenavirus*. Phylogenetic analysis of the novel virus Lujo virus demonstrated that it branched from the Old World arenavirus complex and had the greatest identity to Mobala virus, Lassa fever virus, and *Tamiami virus* with 67 to 74% amino acid identity in the nucleoprotein. Further examination of the receptor-binding portion of G1 demonstrated that Lujo virus is equally distant from the Old World and New World arenaviruses.

The identification of *Human klassevirus 1*, a novel picornavirus, also utilized 454 sequencing. This virus was most similar to members of the genus *Kobuvirus* and has been detected in both human stool specimens and raw sewage (36, 39). Greninger et al. were able to sequence the complete genome of 7,889 bp [excluding the poly(A) tail] from an infant with gastroenteritis of unknown etiology. Subsequent screening of 751 stool samples identified a second positive sample, which turned out to be from the twin sibling of the index case. Holtz et al. identified a similar virus in an acute diarrheal sample collected in 1984 from a child in Australia. Reverse transcriptase PCR (RT-PCR) screening for klassevirus 1 resulted in the identification of two slightly divergent isolates, one from raw sewage collected in Barcelona, Spain, and one from a pediatric patient with acute diarrhea (out of 340 pediatric stool specimens tested). Given the low homology of human klassevirus 1 to Aichi virus at 34.8 to 43.3% amino acid identity in the P1, P2, and P3 coding regions, a novel genus, *Klassevirus*, has been proposed.

In an unexplained outbreak of gastrointestinal illness, a novel astrovirus, *Astrovirus VA1*, was identified by simultaneous Sanger and 454 mass sequencing efforts (30). The complete genome of 6,586 bp was sequenced using a combination of Sanger shotgun sequencing and targeted RT-PCR and rapid amplification of cDNA ends. In parallel, 454 sequencing alone generated a contig of 6,581 bp, demonstrating again the benefits of the next-generation platforms. In the most conserved region, ORF1B, VA1 shared 61% amino acid identity to mink astrovirus and 62% amino acid identity to ovine astrovirus. RT-PCR screening of the six samples from the outbreak demonstrated that three samples were unequivocally positive, with high copy numbers. While these initial results support a potential role for VA1 in this outbreak, further studies are necessary to explicitly define the relationship between VA1 and human diarrhea.

ASSESSING THE ROLE OF PATHOGENICITY

From the above examples, it has become increasingly clear that tremendous microbial diversity is being uncovered and many more microbes remain to be discovered. The pace at which new microbes (and viruses in particular) in clinical samples from humans are being discovered is growing geometrically. The challenge that now faces the scientific community is how best to define the relevance of the growing list of new microbes to human disease. This has long been a challenge in the study of infectious diseases. In 1890, Robert Koch published a set of postulates in an attempt to standardize the evidence needed to demonstrate a causal role for a microbe in a disease. Koch's postulates are well known to this day and, despite being over 100 years old, still serve as guidelines for proof of causality. They are as follows.

1. The parasite occurs in every case of the disease in question and under circumstances which can account for the pathological chances and clinical course of the disease.
2. The parasite occurs in no other disease as a fortuitous and nonpathogenic parasite.
3. After being fully isolated from the body and repeatedly grown in pure culture, the parasite can induce disease anew.

A major challenge in the fulfillment of Koch's postulates, especially in a molecular era, is that many microbes cannot be grown in pure culture. Another limitation is that microbes that have either a carrier state or can cause subclinical infections, such as *Neisseria meningitidis* and *Mycobacterium tuberculosis*, violate Koch's postulates. Other scenarios that limit the applicability of Koch's postulates include cases in which coinfection with more than one microbe causes disease, or situations in which the host genetic background contributes to the disease state.

Over the years, various incarnations of Koch's postulates have been formulated. Bradford Hill (1965) and Alfred Evans (1976) proposed broader criteria for causation, including epidemiological and immunological data. Most recently, a guide for disease causality that accounts for molecular methods of microbial detection has been proposed by Fredericks and Relman (33). These revisions of Koch's postulates have remained focused on the traditional concept that disease arises from the presence of a foreign microbe (and the biological consequences of its presence). However, in the genomic era, the concept of a "pathogen" and how it causes disease must be reimagined in the 21st century. With the increasing recognition that humans (and animals) are hosts to large communities of bacteria and viruses, more complex models of human disease, such as those resulting from imbalances or alterations in the endogenous community of microbes, must be entertained. For example, researchers have begun to elucidate the complex role of microbial communities in obesity by analysis of the microbiomes of animal models of human disease, as well as humans themselves.

In a genetic model of obesity, sequencing of 16S ribosomal DNA (rDNA) of the distal gut of genetically obese (ob/ob) mice and their lean (ob/+) and wild-type (+/+) siblings demonstrated that the microbial composition in the ob/ob mice differed in the relative abundance of *Bacteroidetes* and *Firmicutes* (53). Specifically, ob/ob animals have a 50% reduction in the number of *Bacteroidetes* and a proportional increase in *Firmicutes* compared to lean (ob/+) mice. Similar results were obtained in human studies in which 12 obese humans were assigned to either a fat- or carbohydrate-restricted diet, and their gut composition was analyzed throughout the year by monitoring of 16S rDNA sequencing (54). Obese humans have fewer *Bacteroidetes* than *Firmicutes* in comparison with lean controls. Whether this imbalance is the cause of disease or whether the imbalance is a consequence of the disease is currently unclear. Regardless, these observations demonstrate that a "pathogenic state," in this case obesity, can be associated with the makeup of a microbial population rather than the presence or absence of a specific, singular, "causal microbe." Thus, in efforts to define the role of the newly identified microbes in human disease, we must not limit ourselves to the traditional one-microbe, one-disease definition of a pathogen.

CONCLUSION

Comprehensive sequencing of individual or pooled samples has now become feasible, making it possible to systematically define the microbial nucleic acid content present in any sample of interest. The ability to "discover" novel microbes has become increasingly robust, largely due to a revolution in sequencing technology. The challenge facing the scientific community for the remainder of this century is to develop commensurate approaches to defining the biological relevance of this multitude of novel microbes to human disease and, in the course of these studies, to come to a more nuanced and sophisticated understanding of the role of microbes in human health and disease.

REFERENCES

1. **Allander, T., K. Andreasson, S. Gupta, A. Bjerkner, G. Bogdanovic, M. A. A. Persson, T. Dalianis, T. Ramqvist, and B. Andersson.** 2007. Identification of a third human polyomavirus. *J. Virol.* **81:**4130–4136.
2. **Allander, T., S. U. Emerson, R. E. Engle, R. H. Purcell, and J. Bukh.** 2001. A virus discovery method incorporating DNase treatment and its application to the identification of two bovine parvovirus species. *Proc. Natl. Acad. Sci. USA* **98:**11609–11614.
3. **Allander, T., M. T. Tammi, M. Eriksson, A. Bjerkner, A. Tiveljung-Lindell, and B. Andersson.** 2005. Cloning of a human parvovirus by molecular screening of respiratory tract samples. *Proc. Natl. Acad. Sci. USA* **102:**12891–12896.
3a. **Allred, A. F., G. Wu, T. Wulan, K. F. Fischer, M. R. Holbrook, R. B. Tesh, and D. Wang.** 2010. VIPR: a probabilistic algorithm for analysis of microbial detection bioarrays. *BMC Bioinformatics* **11:**384.
4. **Al-Sunaidi, M., C. H. Williams, P. J. Hughes, D. P. Schnurr, and G. Stanway.** 2007. Analysis of a new human

5. **Arthur, J. L., G. D. Higgins, G. P. Davidson, R. C. Givney, and R. M. Ratcliff.** 2009. A novel bocavirus associated with acute gastroenteritis in Australian children. *PLoS Pathog.* **5:**e1000391.
6. **Barrette, R. W., S. A. Metwally, J. M. Rowland, L. Xu, S. R. Zaki, S. T. Nichol, P. E. Rollin, J. S. Towner, W. J. Shieh, B. Batten, T. K. Sealy, C. Carrillo, K. E. Moran, A. J. Bracht, G. A. Mayr, M. Sirios-Cruz, D. P. Catbagan, E. A. Lautner, T. G. Ksiazek, W. R. White, and M. T. McIntosh.** 2009. Discovery of swine as a host for the Reston ebolavirus. *Science* **325:**204–206.
7. **Baumgarte, S., L. K. de Souza Luna, K. Grywna, M. Panning, J. F. Drexler, C. Karsten, H. I. Huppertz, and C. Drosten.** 2008. Prevalence, types, and RNA concentrations of human parechoviruses, including a sixth parechovirus type, in stool samples from patients with acute enteritis. *J. Clin. Microbiol.* **46:**242–248.
8. **Benschop, K. S., J. Schinkel, M. E. Luken, P. J. van den Broek, M. F. Beersma, N. Menelik, H. W. van Eijk, H. L. Zaaijer, C. M. VandenBroucke-Grauls, M. G. Beld, and K. C. Wolthers.** 2006. Fourth human parechovirus serotype. *Emerg. Infect. Dis.* **12:**1572–1575.
9. **Breitbart, M., and F. Rohwer.** 2005. Method for discovering novel DNA viruses in blood using viral particle selection and shotgun sequencing. *BioTechniques* **39:**729–736.
10. **Briese, T., J. T. Paweska, L. K. McMullan, S. K. Hutchison, C. Street, G. Palacios, M. L. Khristova, J. Weyer, R. Swanepoel, M. Egholm, S. T. Nichol, and W. I. Lipkin.** 2009. Genetic detection and characterization of Lujo virus, a new hemorrhagic fever-associated arenavirus from southern Africa. *PLoS Pathog.* **5:**e1000455.
11. **Brosius, J., M. L. Palmer, P. J. Kennedy, and H. F. Noller.** 1978. Complete nucleotide sequence of a 16S ribosomal RNA gene from Escherichia coli. *Proc. Natl. Acad. Sci. USA* **75:**4801–4805.
12. **The C. elegans Sequencing Consortium.** 1998. Genome sequence of the nematode C. elegans: a platform for investigating biology. *Science* **282:**2012–2018.
13. **Chang, Y., E. Cesarman, M. S. Pessin, F. Lee, J. Culpepper, D. M. Knowles, and P. S. Moore.** 1994. Identification of herpesvirus-like DNA sequences in AIDS-associated Kaposi's sarcoma. *Science* **266:**1865–1869.
14. **Chiu, C. Y., A. A. Alizadeh, S. Rouskin, J. D. Merker, E. Yeh, S. Yagi, D. Schnurr, B. K. Patterson, D. Ganem, and J. L. DeRisi.** 2007. Diagnosis of a critical respiratory illness caused by human metapneumovirus by use of a pan-virus microarray. *J. Clin. Microbiol.* **45:**2340–2343.
15. **Chiu, C. Y., A. L. Greninger, K. Kanada, T. Kwok, K. F. Fischer, C. Runckel, J. K. Louie, C. A. Glaser, S. Yagi, D. P. Schnurr, T. D. Haggerty, J. Parsonnet, D. Ganem, and J. L. Derisi.** 2008. Identification of cardioviruses related to Theiler's murine encephalomyelitis virus in human infections. *Proc. Natl. Acad. Sci. USA* **105:**14124–14129.
16. **Chiu, C. Y., S. Rouskin, A. Koshy, A. Urisman, K. Fischer, S. Yagi, D. Schnurr, P. B. Eckburg, L. S. Tompkins, B. G. Blackburn, J. D. Merker, B. K. Patterson, D. Ganem, and J. L. DeRisi.** 2006. Microarray detection of human parainfluenzavirus 4 infection associated with respiratory failure in an immunocompetent adult. *Clin. Infect. Dis.* **43:**e71–e76.
17. **Choo, Q. L., G. Kuo, A. J. Weiner, L. R. Overby, D. W. Bradley, and M. Houghton.** 1989. Isolation of a cDNA clone derived from a blood-borne non-A, non-B viral hepatitis genome. *Science* **244:**359–362.
18. **Deffrasnes, C., M. E. Hamelin, and G. Boivin.** 2007. Human metapneumovirus. *Semin. Respir. Crit. Care Med.* **28:**213–221.
19. **Delgado, S., B. R. Erickson, R. Agudo, P. J. Blair, E. Vallejo, C. G. Albarino, J. Vargas, J. A. Comer, P. E. Rollin, T. G. Ksiazek, J. G. Olson, and S. T. Nichol.** 2008. Chapare virus, a newly discovered arenavirus isolated

from a fatal hemorrhagic fever case in Bolivia. *PLoS Pathog.* **4**:e1000047.

20. **DeRisi, J. L., V. R. Iyer, and P. O. Brown.** 1997. Exploring the metabolic and genetic control of gene expression on a genomic scale. *Science* **278**:680–686.

21. **DeSantis, T. Z., E. L. Brodie, J. P. Moberg, I. X. Zubieta, Y. M. Piceno, and G. L. Andersen.** 2007. High-density universal 16S rRNA microarray analysis reveals broader diversity than typical clone library when sampling the environment. *Microb. Ecol.* **53**:371–383.

22. **Dijkman, R., M. F. Jebbink, N. B. El Idrissi, K. Pyrc, M. A. Muller, T. W. Kuijpers, H. L. Zaaijer, and L. van der Hoek.** 2008. Human coronavirus NL63 and 229E seroconversion in children. *J. Clin. Microbiol.* **46**:2368–2373.

23. **Drexler, J. F., K. Grywna, A. Stöcker, P. S. Almeida, T. C. Medrado Ribeiro, M. Eschbach-Bludau, N. Petersen, H. da Costa Ribeiro, Jr., and C. Drosten.** 2009. Novel human parechovirus from Brazil. *Emerg. Infect. Dis.* **15**:310–313.

24. **Drexler, J. F., L. K. Luna, A. Stöcker, P. S. Almeida, T. C. Medrado Ribeiro, N. Petersen, P. Herzog, C. Pedroso, H. I. Huppertz, H. da Costa Ribeiro, Jr., S. Baumgarte, and C. Drosten.** 2008. Circulation of 3 lineages of a novel Saffold cardiovirus in humans. *Emerg. Infect. Dis.* **14**:1398–1405.

25. **Eisen, M. B., P. T. Spellman, P. O. Brown, and D. Botstein.** 1998. Cluster analysis and display of genome-wide expression patterns. *Proc. Natl. Acad. Sci. USA* **95**:14863–14868.

26. **Endo, R., N. Ishiguro, H. Kikuta, S. Teramoto, R. Shirkoohi, X. Ma, T. Ebihara, H. Ishiko, and T. Ariga.** 2007. Seroepidemiology of human bocavirus in Hokkaido prefecture, Japan. *J. Clin. Microbiol.* **45**:3218–3223.

27. **Feng, H., M. Shuda, Y. Chang, and P. S. Moore.** 2008. Clonal integration of a polyomavirus in human Merkel cell carcinoma. *Science* **319**:1096–1100.

28. **Finkbeiner, S. R., C. D. Kirkwood, and D. Wang.** 2008. Complete genome sequence of a highly divergent astrovirus isolated from a child with acute diarrhea. *Virol. J.* **5**:117.

29. **Finkbeiner, S. R., B. M. Le, L. R. Holtz, G. A. Storch, and D. Wang.** 2009. Detection of newly described astrovirus MLB1 in stool samples from children. *Emerg. Infect. Dis.* **15**:441–444.

30. **Finkbeiner, S. R., Y. Li, S. Ruone, C. Conrardy, N. Gregoricus, D. Toney, H. W. Virgin, L. J. Anderson, J. Vinje, D. Wang, and S. Tong.** 2009. Identification of a novel astrovirus (astrovirus VA1) associated with an outbreak of acute gastroenteritis. *J. Virol.* **83**:10836–10839.

31. **Fleischmann, R. D., M. D. Adams, O. White, R. A. Clayton, E. F. Kirkness, A. R. Kerlavage, C. J. Bult, J. F. Tomb, B. A. Dougherty, J. M. Merrick, et al.** 1995. Whole-genome random sequencing and assembly of Haemophilus influenzae Rd. *Science* **269**:496–512.

32. **Fouchier, R. A., V. Munster, A. Wallensten, T. M. Bestebroer, S. Herfst, D. Smith, G. F. Rimmelzwaan, B. Olsen, and A. D. Osterhaus.** 2005. Characterization of a novel influenza A virus hemagglutinin subtype (H16) obtained from black-headed gulls. *J. Virol.* **79**:2814–2822.

33. **Fredericks, D. N., and D. A. Relman.** 1996. Sequence-based identification of microbial pathogens: a reconsideration of Koch's postulates. *Clin. Microbiol. Rev.* **9**:18–33.

34. **Gaynor, A. M., M. D. Nissen, D. M. Whiley, I. M. Mackay, S. B. Lambert, G. Wu, D. C. Brennan, G. A. Storch, T. P. Sloots, and D. Wang.** 2007. Identification of a novel polyomavirus from patients with acute respiratory tract infections. *PLoS Pathog.* **3**:e64.

35. **Goffeau, A., B. G. Barrell, H. Bussey, R. W. Davis, B. Dujon, H. Feldmann, F. Galibert, J. D. Hoheisel, C. Jacq, M. Johnston, E. J. Louis, H. W. Mewes, Y. Murakami, P. Philippsen, H. Tettelin, and S. G. Oliver.** 1996. Life with 6000 genes. *Science* **274**:546, 563–567.

36. **Greninger, A. L., C. Runckel, C. Y. Chiu, T. Haggerty, J. Parsonnet, D. Ganem, and J. L. DeRisi.** 2009. The complete genome of klassevirus—a novel picornavirus in pediatric stool. *Virol. J.* **6**:82.

37. **Hales, L. M., N. J. Knowles, P. S. Reddy, L. Xu, C. Hay, and P. L. Hallenbeck.** 2008. Complete genome sequence analysis of Seneca Valley virus-001, a novel oncolytic picornavirus. *J. Gen. Virol.* **89**:1265–1275.

38. **Holtz, L. R., S. R. Finkbeiner, C. D. Kirkwood, and D. Wang.** 2008. Identification of a novel picornavirus related to cosaviruses in a child with acute diarrhea. *Virol. J.* **5**:159.

39. **Holtz, L. R., S. R. Finkbeiner, G. Zhao, C. D. Kirkwood, R. Girones, J. M. Pipas, and D. Wang.** 2009. Klassevirus 1, a previously undescribed member of the family Picornaviridae, is globally widespread. *Virol. J.* **6**:86.

40. **Ito, M., T. Yamashita, H. Tsuzuki, N. Takeda, and K. Sakae.** 2004. Isolation and identification of a novel human parechovirus. *J. Gen. Virol.* **85**:391–398.

41. **Jones, M. S., A. Kapoor, V. V. Lukashov, P. Simmonds, F. Hecht, and E. Delwart.** 2005. New DNA viruses identified in patients with acute viral infection syndrome. *J. Virol.* **79**:8230–8236.

42. **Jones, M. S., V. V. Lukashov, R. D. Ganac, and D. P. Schnurr.** 2007. Discovery of a novel human picornavirus in a stool sample from a pediatric patient presenting with fever of unknown origin. *J. Clin. Microbiol.* **45**:2144–2150.

43. **Kantola, K., L. Hedman, T. Allander, T. Jartti, P. Lehtinen, O. Ruuskanen, K. Hedman, and M. Soderlund-Venermo.** 2008. Serodiagnosis of human bocavirus infection. *Clin. Infect. Dis.* **46**:540–546.

44. **Kapoor, A., E. Slikas, P. Simmonds, T. Chieochansin, A. Naeem, S. Shaukat, M. M. Alam, S. Sharif, M. Angez, S. Zaidi, and E. Delwart.** 2009. A newly identified bocavirus species in human stool. *J. Infect. Dis.* **199**:196–200.

45. **Kapoor, A., J. Victoria, P. Simmonds, E. Slikas, T. Chieochansin, A. Naeem, S. Shaukat, S. Sharif, M. M. Alam, M. Angez, C. Wang, R. W. Shafer, S. Zaidi, and E. Delwart.** 2008. A highly prevalent and genetically diversified Picornaviridae genus in South Asian children. *Proc. Natl. Acad. Sci. USA* **105**:20482–20487.

46. **Kim, S., N. Kim, B. Dong, D. Boren, S. A. Lee, J. Das Gupta, C. Gaughan, E. A. Klein, C. Lee, R. H. Silverman, and S. A. Chow.** 2008. Integration site preference of xenotropic murine leukemia virus-related virus, a new human retrovirus associated with prostate cancer. *J. Virol.* **82**:9964–9977.

47. **Kistler, A., P. C. Avila, S. Rouskin, D. Wang, T. Ward, S. Yagi, D. Schnurr, D. Ganem, J. L. Derisi, and H. A. Boushey.** 2007. Pan-viral screening of respiratory tract infections in adults with and without asthma reveals unexpected human coronavirus and human rhinovirus diversity. *J. Infect. Dis.* **196**:817–825.

48. **Ksiazek, T. G., D. Erdman, C. S. Goldsmith, S. R. Zaki, T. Peret, S. Emery, S. Tong, C. Urbani, J. A. Comer, W. Lim, P. E. Rollin, S. F. Dowell, A. E. Ling, C. D. Humphrey, W. J. Shieh, J. Guarner, C. D. Paddock, P. Rota, B. Fields, J. DeRisi, J. Y. Yang, N. Cox, J. M. Hughes, J. W. LeDuc, W. J. Bellini, and L. J. Anderson.** 2003. A novel coronavirus associated with severe acute respiratory syndrome. *N. Engl. J. Med.* **348**:1953–1966.

49. **Lamson, D., N. Renwick, V. Kapoor, Z. Liu, G. Palacios, J. Ju, A. Dean, K. St. George, T. Briese, and W. I. Lipkin.** 2006. MassTag polymerase-chain-reaction detection of respiratory pathogens, including a new rhinovirus genotype, that caused influenza-like illness in New York State during 2004–2005. *J. Infect. Dis.* **194**:1398–1402.

50. **Lander, E. S., L. M. Linton, B. Birren, C. Nusbaum, M. C. Zody, J. Baldwin, K. Devon, K. Dewar, M. Doyle, W. FitzHugh, R. Funke, D. Gage, K. Harris, A. Heaford, J. Howland, L. Kann, J. Lehoczky, R. LeVine, P. McEwan, K. McKernan, J. Meldrim, J. P. Mesirov, C. Miranda, W. Morris, J. Naylor, C. Raymond, M. Rosetti, R. Santos, A. Sheridan, C. Sougnez, N. Stange-Thomann, N. Stojanovic, A. Subramanian, D. Wyman, J. Rogers, J. Sulston, R. Ainscough, S. Beck, D. Bentley, J. Burton, C. Clee, N. Carter, A. Coulson, R. Deadman, P. Deloukas, A. Dunham, I. Dunham, R. Durbin, L. French, D. Grafham, S. Gregory, T. Hubbard, S. Humphray, A. Hunt, M. Jones, C. Lloyd, A. McMurray, L. Matthews, S. Mercer, S. Milne, J. C. Mullikin, A. Mungall, R. Plumb, M. Ross, R. Shownkeen, S. Sims, R. H. Waterston,**

R. K. Wilson, L. W. Hillier, J. D. McPherson, M. A. Marra, E. R. Mardis, L. A. Fulton, A. T. Chinwalla, K. H. Pepin, W. R. Gish, S. L. Chissoe, M. C. Wendl, K. D. Delehaunty, T. L. Miner, A. Delehaunty, J. B. Kramer, L. L. Cook, R. S. Fulton, D. L. Johnson, P. J. Minx, S. W. Clifton, T. Hawkins, E. Branscomb, P. Predki, P. Richardson, S. Wenning, T. Slezak, N. Doggett, J. F. Cheng, A. Olsen, S. Lucas, C. Elkin, E. Uberbacher, M. Frazier, et al. 2001. Initial sequencing and analysis of the human genome. *Nature* **409:**860–921.

51. Lau, S. K., C. C. Yip, H. W. Tsoi, R. A. Lee, L. Y. So, Y. L. Lau, K. H. Chan, P. C. Woo, and K. Y. Yuen. 2007. Clinical features and complete genome characterization of a distinct human rhinovirus (HRV) genetic cluster, probably representing a previously undetected HRV species, HRV-C, associated with acute respiratory illness in children. *J. Clin. Microbiol.* **45:**3655–3664.

52. Lee, W. M., C. Kiesner, T. Pappas, I. Lee, K. Grindle, T. Jartti, B. Jakiela, R. F. Lemanske, Jr., P. A. Shult, and J. E. Gern. 2007. A diverse group of previously unrecognized human rhinoviruses are common causes of respiratory illnesses in infants. *PLoS ONE* **2:**e966.

53. Ley, R. E., F. Backhed, P. Turnbaugh, C. A. Lozupone, R. D. Knight, and J. I. Gordon. 2005. Obesity alters gut microbial ecology. *Proc. Natl. Acad. Sci. USA* **102:**11070–11075.

54. Ley, R. E., P. J. Turnbaugh, S. Klein, and J. I. Gordon. 2006. Microbial ecology: human gut microbes associated with obesity. *Nature* **444:**1022–1023.

55. Li, L., J. Victoria, A. Kapoor, A. Naeem, S. Shaukat, S. Sharif, M. M. Alam, M. Angez, S. Z. Zaidi, and E. Delwart. 2009. Genomic characterization of novel human parechovirus type. *Emerg. Infect. Dis.* **15:**288–291.

56. Lin, B., A. P. Malanoski, Z. Wang, K. M. Blaney, A. G. Ligler, R. K. Rowley, E. H. Hanson, E. von Rosenvinge, F. S. Ligler, A. W. Kusterbeck, D. Metzgar, C. P. Barrozo, K. L. Russell, C. Tibbetts, J. M. Schnur, and D. A. Stenger. 2007. Application of broad-spectrum, sequence-based pathogen identification in an urban population. *PLoS ONE* **2:**e419.

57. Lombardi, V. C., F. W. Ruscetti, J. Das Gupta, M. A. Pfost, K. S. Hagen, D. L. Peterson, S. K. Ruscetti, R. K. Bagni, C. Petrow-Sadowski, B. Gold, M. Dean, R. H. Silverman, and J. A. Mikovits. 2009. Detection of an infectious retrovirus, XMRV, in blood cells of patients with chronic fatigue syndrome. *Science* **326:**585–589.

58. Mardis, E. R. 2008. Next-generation DNA sequencing methods. *Annu. Rev. Genomics Hum. Genet.* **9:**387–402.

59. McErlean, P., L. A. Shackelton, S. B. Lambert, M. D. Nissen, T. P. Sloots, and I. M. Mackay. 2007. Characterisation of a newly identified human rhinovirus, HRV-QPM, discovered in infants with bronchiolitis. *J. Clin. Virol.* **39:**67–75.

60. Nguyen, N. L., B. M. Le, and D. Wang. 2009. Serologic evidence of frequent human infection with WU and KI polyomaviruses. *Emerg Infect Dis.* **15:**1199–1205.

61. Nichol, S. T., C. F. Spiropoulou, S. Morzunov, P. E. Rollin, T. G. Ksiazek, H. Feldmann, A. Sanchez, J. Childs, S. Zaki, and C. J. Peters. 1993. Genetic identification of a hantavirus associated with an outbreak of acute respiratory illness. *Science* **262:**914–917.

62. Palacios, G., P. L. Quan, O. J. Jabado, S. Conlan, D. L. Hirschberg, Y. Liu, J. Zhai, N. Renwick, J. Hui, H. Hegyi, A. Grolla, J. E. Strong, J. S. Towner, T. W. Geisbert, P. B. Jahrling, C. Buchen-Osmond, H. Ellerbrok, M. P. Sanchez-Seco, Y. Lussier, P. Formenty, M. S. Nichol, H. Feldmann, T. Briese, and W. I. Lipkin. 2007. Panmicrobial oligonucleotide array for diagnosis of infectious diseases. *Emerg. Infect. Dis.* **13:**73–81.

63. Palmer, C., E. M. Bik, D. B. DiGiulio, D. A. Relman, and P. O. Brown. 2007. Development of the human infant intestinal microbiota. *PLoS Biol.* **5:**e177.

64. Quan, P. L., G. Palacios, O. J. Jabado, S. Conlan, D. L. Hirschberg, F. Pozo, P. J. Jack, D. Cisterna, N. Renwick, J. Hui, A. Drysdale, R. Amos-Ritchie, E. Baumeister, V. Savy, K. M. Lager, J. A. Richt, D. B. Boyle, A. Garcia-Sastre, I. Casas, P. Perez-Brena, T. Briese, and W. I. Lipkin. 2007. Detection of respiratory viruses and subtype identification of influenza A viruses by GreeneChipResp oligonucleotide microarray. *J. Clin. Microbiol.* **45:**2359–2364.

65. Raoult, D., S. Audic, C. Robert, C. Abergel, P. Renesto, H. Ogata, B. La Scola, M. Suzan, and J. M. Claverie. 2004. The 1.2-megabase genome sequence of Mimivirus. *Science* **306:**1344–1350.

66. Rehrauer, H., S. Schonmann, L. Eberl, and R. Schlapbach. 2008. PhyloDetect: a likelihood-based strategy for detecting microorganisms with diagnostic microarrays. *Bioinformatics* **24:**i83–i89.

67. Relman, D. A., J. S. Loutit, T. M. Schmidt, S. Falkow, and L. S. Tompkins. 1990. The agent of bacillary angiomatosis. An approach to the identification of uncultured pathogens. *N. Engl. J. Med.* **323:**1573–1580.

68. Relman, D. A., T. M. Schmidt, R. P. MacDermott, and S. Falkow. 1992. Identification of the uncultured bacillus of Whipple's disease. *N. Engl. J. Med.* **327:**293–301.

69. Rota, P. A., M. S. Oberste, S. S. Monroe, W. A. Nix, R. Campagnoli, J. P. Icenogle, S. Penaranda, B. Bankamp, K. Maher, M. H. Chen, S. Tong, A. Tamin, L. Lowe, M. Frace, J. L. DeRisi, Q. Chen, D. Wang, D. D. Erdman, T. C. Peret, C. Burns, T. G. Ksiazek, P. E. Rollin, A. Sanchez, S. Liffick, B. Holloway, J. Limor, K. McCaustland, M. Olsen-Rasmussen, R. Fouchier, S. Gunther, A. D. Osterhaus, C. Drosten, M. A. Pallansch, L. J. Anderson, and W. J. Bellini. 2003. Characterization of a novel coronavirus associated with severe acute respiratory syndrome. *Science* **300:**1394–1399.

70. Towner, J. S., T. K. Sealy, M. L. Khristova, C. G. Albarino, S. Conlan, S. A. Reeder, P. L. Quan, W. I. Lipkin, R. Downing, J. W. Tappero, S. Okware, J. Lutwama, B. Bakamutumaho, J. Kayiwa, J. A. Comer, P. E. Rollin, T. G. Ksiazek, and S. T. Nichol. 2008. Newly discovered Ebola virus associated with hemorrhagic fever outbreak in Uganda. *PLoS Pathog.* **4:**e1000212.

71. Urisman, A., K. F. Fischer, C. Y. Chiu, A. L. Kistler, S. Beck, D. Wang, and J. L. DeRisi. 2005. E-Predict: a computational strategy for species identification based on observed DNA microarray hybridization patterns. *Genome Biol.* **6:**R78.

72. Urisman, A., R. J. Molinaro, N. Fischer, S. J. Plummer, G. Casey, E. A. Klein, K. Malathi, C. Magi-Galluzzi, R. R. Tubbs, D. Ganem, R. H. Silverman, and J. L. DeRisi. 2006. Identification of a novel Gammaretrovirus in prostate tumors of patients homozygous for R462Q RNASEL variant. *PLoS Pathog.* **2:**e25.

73. van den Hoogen, B. G., J. C. de Jong, J. Groen, T. Kuiken, R. de Groot, R. A. Fouchier, and A. D. Osterhaus. 2001. A newly discovered human pneumovirus isolated from young children with respiratory tract disease. *Nat. Med.* **7:**719–724.

74. van der Hoek, L., K. Pyrc, M. F. Jebbink, W. Vermeulen-Oost, R. J. Berkhout, K. C. Wolthers, P. M. Wertheim-van Dillen, J. Kaandorp, J. Spaargaren, and B. Berkhout. 2004. Identification of a new human coronavirus. *Nat. Med.* **10:**368–373.

75. Venter, J. C., M. D. Adams, E. W. Myers, P. W. Li, R. J. Mural, G. G. Sutton, H. O. Smith, M. Yandell, C. A. Evans, R. A. Holt, J. D. Gocayne, P. Amanatides, R. M. Ballew, D. H. Huson, J. R. Wortman, Q. Zhang, C. D. Kodira, X. H. Zheng, L. Chen, M. Skupski, G. Subramanian, P. D. Thomas, J. Zhang, G. L. Gabor Miklos, C. Nelson, S. Broder, A. G. Clark, J. Nadeau, V. A. McKusick, N. Zinder, A. J. Levine, R. J. Roberts, M. Simon, C. Slayman, M. Hunkapiller, R. Bolanos, A. Delcher, I. Dew, D. Fasulo, M. Flanigan, L. Florea, A. Halpern, S. Hannenhalli, S. Kravitz, S. Levy, C. Mobarry, K. Reinert, K. Remington, J. Abu-Threideh, E. Beasley, K. Biddick, V. Bonazzi, R. Brandon, M. Cargill, I. Chandramouliswaran, R. Charlab, K. Chaturvedi, Z. Deng, V. Di Francesco, P. Dunn, K. Eilbeck, C. Evangelista, A. E. Gabrielian, W. Gan, W. Ge, F. Gong, Z. Gu, P. Guan, T. J. Heiman, M. E. Higgins, R. R. Ji, Z. Ke, K. A. Ketchum, Z. Lai, Y. Lei, Z. Li, J. Li, Y. Liang, X. Lin, F. Lu, G. V. Merkulov, N. Milshina, H. M.

Moore, A. K. Naik, V. A. Narayan, B. Neelam, D. Nussk-ern, D. B. Rusch, S. Salzberg, W. Shao, B. Shue, J. Sun, Z. Wang, A. Wang, X. Wang, J. Wang, M. Wei, R. Wides, C. Xiao, C. Yan, et al. 2001. The sequence of the human genome. *Science* **291:**1304–1351.

76. Wang, D., L. Coscoy, M. Zylberberg, P. C. Avila, H. A. Boushey, D. Ganem, and J. L. DeRisi. 2002. Microarray-based detection and genotyping of viral pathogens. *Proc. Natl. Acad. Sci. USA* **99:**15687–15692.

77. Wang, D., A. Urisman, Y. T. Liu, M. Springer, T. G. Ksiazek, D. D. Erdman, E. R. Mardis, M. Hickenbotham, V. Magrini, J. Eldred, J. P. Latreille, R. K. Wilson, D. Ganem, and J. L. DeRisi. 2003. Viral discovery and sequence recovery using DNA microarrays. *PLoS Biol.* **1:**e2.

78. Watanabe, K., M. Oie, M. Higuchi, M. Nishikawa, and M. Fujii. 2007. Isolation and characterization of novel human parechovirus from clinical samples. *Emerg. Infect. Dis.* **13:**889–895.

79. Watson, M., J. Dukes, A. B. Abu-Median, D. P. King, and P. Britton. 2007. DetectiV: visualization, normalization and significance testing for pathogen-detection microarray data. *Genome Biol.* **8:**R190.

80. Woese, C. R., and G. E. Fox. 1977. Phylogenetic structure of the prokaryotic domain: the primary kingdoms. *Proc. Natl. Acad. Sci. USA* **74:**5088–5090.

81. Wong, C. W., C. L. Heng, L. Wan Yee, S. W. Soh, C. B. Kartasasmita, E. A. Simoes, M. L. Hibberd, W. K. Sung, and L. D. Miller. 2007. Optimization and clinical validation of a pathogen detection microarray. *Genome Biol.* **8:**R93.

82. Woo, P. C., S. K. Lau, C. M. Chu, K. H. Chan, H. W. Tsoi, Y. Huang, B. H. Wong, R. W. Poon, J. J. Cai, W. K. Luk, L. L. Poon, S. S. Wong, Y. Guan, J. S. Peiris, and K. Y. Yuen. 2005. Characterization and complete genome sequence of a novel coronavirus, coronavirus HKU1, from patients with pneumonia. *J. Virol.* **79:**884–895.

83. Zoll, J., S. Erkens Hulshof, K. Lanke, F. Verduyn Lunel, W. J. Melchers, E. Schoondermark-van de Ven, M. Roivainen, J. M. Galama, and F. J. van Kuppeveld. 2009. Saffold virus, a human Theiler's-like cardiovirus, is ubiquitous and causes infection early in life. *PLoS Pathog.* **5:**e1000416.

BACTERIOLOGY

VOLUME EDITORS: KAREN C. CARROLL AND GUIDO FUNKE

SECTION EDITORS: KATHRYN A. BERNARD, J. STEPHEN DUMLER, CATHY A. PETTI, SANDRA S. RICHTER, AND PETER A. R. VANDAMME section **II**

(continued)

Taxonomy and Classification of Bacteria

PETER A. R. VANDAMME

15

Taxonomy is written by taxonomists for taxonomists; in this form the subject is so dull that few, if any, non-taxonomists are tempted to read it and presumably even fewer try their hand at it. It is the most subjective branch of any biological discipline, and in many ways is more of an art than a science.

With these words, S. T. Cowan introduced a sparkling essay on the sense and nonsense in bacterial taxonomy in 1971 (19). His contributions to the practice of bacterial taxonomy, written in the 1960s and 1970s (17–19), should be read by everyone interested in this field, also now that genomics have moved the species concept from obscurity into the spotlight of microbiology's highest-impact journals (34, 36, 64, 65, 91). Taxonomy is generally considered a synonym of systematics and is traditionally divided into classification (the orderly arrangement of organisms into taxonomic groups on the basis of similarity), nomenclature (the labeling of the units), and identification (the process of determining whether an unknown belongs to one of the units defined). It is generally accepted that bacterial classification should reflect as much as possible the natural relationships among bacteria, which are considered the phylogenetic relationships as encoded in highly conserved macromolecules such as 16S or 23S rRNA genes (129). Nowadays, whole-genome comparisons offer new and exciting opportunities for the study of these natural relationships. Boundaries are nevertheless made by humans, and every classification of bacteria is artificial. However, classification serves very practical purposes, i.e., recognition of organisms that were encountered previously and categorization of new ones into a logical and tractable system. In this era of whole-genome sequence analysis, it is more than ever obvious that the genomes of microbes undergo change, sometimes considerably. Although the extent of lateral gene transfer is controversial, it does not alter our need to identify organisms, particularly in the context of epidemiological studies and surveillance, as identification yields a tremendous amount of accompanying information. Science indeed has a way of making itself useful, and the useful application of classification is identification (17).

CLASSIFICATION OF BACTERIA

The process of species delineation in bacterial systematics underwent drastic modifications as the species concept evolved in parallel with technical progress. Early classifica-

tion systems used mainly morphological and biochemical criteria to delineate the species of bacteria. This type of classification was monothetic, as it was based on a unique set of characteristics necessary and sufficient to delineate groups. This early classification concept was replaced by theories of so-called natural concepts, which were the phenetic and phylogenetic classifications (40). In the former, relationships between bacteria were based on the overall similarity of phenotypic and genotypic characteristics. Phenetic classifications demonstrate the relationships among organisms, as they exist without reference to ancestry or evolution. In phylogenetic classifications, relationships are described by ancestry, not according to their present properties.

Special-purpose and general-purpose classification systems are the main categories of classification systems. Special-purpose classification systems are objectively determined and do not fit a preconceived idea. For instance, the separation between the very closely related species *Escherichia coli* and *Shigella dysenteriae* or between *Bordetella pertussis* and *Bordetella bronchiseptica* does not conform to the general ideas of present-day species delineation but fits primarily a practical and historical purpose (40). Yet, nowadays, most taxonomists favor a general-purpose classification system that is stable, objective, and predictive and that can be applied to all bacteria. The classifications obtained with a general-purpose classification system do not fit a single purpose but attempt to reflect the natural diversity among bacteria. The best way to generate such general-purpose classifications is by combining the strengths of both phenetic and phylogenetic studies, a practice nowadays often referred to as polyphasic taxonomy (15, 118).

Criteria for Species Delineation

The criteria used to delineate species have developed in parallel with technology. The early classifications were based on morphology and biochemical data. When evaluated by means of our present views, many of these early phenotype-based classifications generated extremely heterogeneous assemblages of bacteria. Individual species were characterized by a common set of phenotypic characters and differed from other species in one or a few characters which were considered important. The introduction of computer technology allowed comparison of large sets of characteristics for large numbers of strains, forming the basis for phenetic taxonomy (100). Such numerical analyses of phenotypic characters yielded superior classifications in terms of objectivity and stability. Gradually, chemotaxonomic and genotypic methods were introduced into classification systems. Numerous different chemical compounds were extracted from bacterial cells, and their suitability for use in the classification of bacteria and the definition of species has been analyzed.

In 1987, the Ad Hoc Committee on Reconciliation of Approaches to Bacterial Systematics (123) stated that taxonomy should be determined phylogenetically and that the complete genome sequence should therefore be the standard for species delineation. Whole-genome DNA-DNA hybridization analysis was the best approach to the sequence standard for several decades and represented the best applicable procedure. A bacterial species was defined as a group of strains, including the type strain, that share 70% or greater DNA-DNA relatedness, with a ΔT_m of 5°C or less (T_m is the melting temperature of the hybrid, as determined by stepwise denaturation; ΔT_m is the difference in T_m [in degrees Celsius] between the homologous hybrid and the heterologous hybrid formed under standard conditions) (123). This species definition was based on a large amount of empirical data, including both DNA-DNA hybridization data and other characteristics. The designated type strain of a species serves as the name bearer of the species and as the reference specimen. It was also recommended that phenotypic and chemotaxonomic features agree with this definition. Preferentially, several simple and straightforward tests should endorse the species delineation based on DNA-DNA hybridization values. Groups of strains which were delineated by means of DNA-DNA hybridization studies as distinct species but which could not be distinguished by phenotypic characteristics should not be named. The term "genomovar" was subsequently introduced for such phenotypically similar genomic species (111); however, this term may be somewhat misleading, as these taxa are given an infraspecific rank, whereas by definition they are to be considered species that cannot be reliably differentiated by phenotypic tests.

The level of DNA-DNA hybridization thus plays a key role in our present species concept as defined by Wayne et al. (123). Although that seems to suggest that the species definition has become less vague, the practice of DNA-DNA hybridization is complex (see below).

The Polyphasic Species Concept

A wide variety of cellular components have been used to study relationships among bacteria and to design classifications. The information present at the DNA level has been analyzed by estimations of the DNA base composition and the genome size, whole-genome DNA-DNA hybridization, restriction enzyme analysis, and, increasingly more often, direct sequence analysis of various genes. rRNA fractions have been studied intensively, particularly because they serve as phylogenetic markers (123, 129). Various chemical compounds, including fatty acids, mycolic acids, polar lipids, polysaccharides, sugars, polyamines, and respiratory quinones, as well as, again, a tremendous number of expressed features (data derived from, e.g., morphologic, serologic, and enzymologic studies), were all used to characterize bacteria. Several of these approaches have been applied to taxonomic analyses of virtually all bacteria. Others, such as amino acid sequencing, were performed with a limited number of organisms because they are laborious,

time-consuming, or technically demanding or because they were relevant only for a particular group.

The term "polyphasic taxonomy" was coined by Colwell (15) in 1970 and described the integration of all available genotypic, phenotypic, and phylogenetic information into a consensus type of general-purpose classification. It departs from the assumption that the overall biological diversity cannot be encoded in a single molecule and that the variability of characters is group dependent; it integrates several generally accepted ideas for the classification and reclassification of bacteria. Polyphasic taxonomy is phylogeny based and uses sequence analysis and signature features of rRNA for the deduction of a phylogenetic framework for the classification of bacteria (118, 129). The next step in the process of classification is the delineation of individual species—and other taxa—within these phylogenetic branches. Despite its drawbacks, DNA-DNA hybridization forms the cornerstone of species delineation. However, the threshold value for species delineation should be allowed considerable variation. This polyphasic approach is pragmatic; for instance, B. pertussis, Bordetella parapertussis, and B. bronchiseptica, which share DNA-DNA hybridization levels of over 80%, are considered three distinct species because they differ in many phenotypic and chemotaxonomic aspects (115). In other genera which are phenotypically more homogeneous, such as Acidovorax (128), species have been defined as groups of strains that have DNA-DNA hybridization levels of at least 40%. It is essential that the boundaries of species demarcation be flexible in order to achieve a classification scheme that facilitates identification.

The application of numerous other types of analyses of genotypic, chemotaxonomic, and phenotypic characteristics of bacteria to the delineation of bacteria at various hierarchical levels represents the third component of polyphasic taxonomy (118). The goal is to collect as much information as possible and to evaluate all results in relation to each other in order to draw useful conclusions. An additional advantage is that, once the taxonomic resolution of these approaches has been established for a particular group of bacteria through the analysis of taxonomically well-characterized strains, they may be used as alternative tools to identify new isolates at different taxonomic levels. It should be noted that the resolution of these alternative methods is often group dependent. For instance, cellular fatty acid analysis is useful for the accurate identification of strains of many bacterial species to the species level. In certain bacterial groups, however, the cellular fatty acid profile may be indicative of the genus or a group of phylogenetically related genera but not of a particular species within one of these genera (118).

The contours of a polyphasic bacterial species are obviously less clear than the ones defined by Wayne et al. (123), and this lack of a rigid definition has been contested, as it allows too many interpretations (134). Polyphasic classification is empirical and contains elements from both phenetic and phylogenetic classifications. There are no strict rules or guidelines, and the approach integrates any significant information on the organisms, resulting in a consensus type of classification. In this respect, its main weakness is indeed that it relies on common sense to draw its conclusions. The bacterial species appears as a group of isolates in which a steady generation of genetic diversity resulted in clones characterized by a certain degree of phenotypic consistency, by a significant degree of DNA-DNA hybridization, and by a high level of 16S rRNA sequence similarity (118). In the colloquium report *Reconciling Microbial Systematics and Genomics* (3), this taxonomic practice was referred to as somewhat functional but inadequate because of the conflicts between phenotypic and phylogenetic classifications, limited means for classifying uncultured microbes, and the lack of cohesiveness in the current species. From a practical point of view and in light of the immense microbial diversity that awaits formal description, its lack of throughput capacity is also critical.

The species is the most important and, at the same time, the central element of bacterial taxonomy. There are at present no rules for the delineation of higher hierarchical ranks such as genus, family, and order. Although there is an expectation that at the generic level, taxa should be supported by phenotypic descriptions (78, 102), in practice, higher ranks are delineated mostly on the basis of 16S rRNA sequence comparison and stability analyses of the clusters that are obtained. Undoubtedly, the latter has weakened the emphasis on phenotypic descriptions of taxa (134).

Toward a New Species Concept

In 2002, a new ad hoc committee for the reevaluation of the species definition in bacteriology made various recommendations regarding the species definition in light of developments in methodologies available to systematists (102). As stated by the ad hoc committee, the introduction of innovative methods is providing new opportunities for prokaryotic systematics. The particularly interesting developments include multilocus sequence analysis (MLSA) and whole-genome sequence analysis. In contrast with multilocus sequence typing, a specific tool designed for molecular epidemiology and for defining strains within named species by which similarities and differences are usually measured as differences in allelic profiles, MLSA employs phylogenetic procedures based on the nucleotide sequences of the alleles to reveal similarities between strains representing different species and genera (34, 36, 48). Many examples of such studies have recently been published, and in general the clusters delineated correlate well with species demarcated by DNA-DNA hybridization experiments (34). Especially for depicting relationships within and between closely related species, this approach thus has a resolution superior to that of traditional 16S rRNA gene sequence analysis. The deduced phylogenetic trees not only provide a phylogenetic backbone but also reveal intraspecies relationships at a level where comparative 16S rRNA sequence analysis is no longer discriminatory. It is, for instance, noteworthy that the DNA-DNA hybridization results which demonstrated that *Yersinia pestis* and *Yersinia pseudotuberculosis* represented single species each were mirrored in the MLSA tree where *Y. pestis* clusters among *Y. pseudotuberculosis* strains; the same observation was made for *Burkholderia mallei* and *Burkholderia pseudomallei* (38, 66).

Two studies of complete genomes have suggested a universal set of protein-coding genes that may be useful for a phylogenomic species concept in microbial taxonomy (93, 137). Housekeeping genes are preferentially used because they evolve relatively slowly and most of the variation that accumulates in these genes is considered selectively neutral. The number and lengths of gene fragments to be used have not been systematically studied, although typically six to eight genes are analyzed (48). Analyses based on this number of genes revealed that MLSA phylogenies of closely related organisms correspond accurately to phylogenies based on state-of-the-art analysis of their whole-genome sequences (63). In addition, almost all core genes, regardless of their functions and positions in the genome, offered robust phylogenetic reconstruction among closely related strains, and three was considered the minimum number of genes to use for phylogenetic analyses to anticipate recognition of horizontal gene transfer or recombination events. However, there is no universal cutoff or descriptor of clusters that characterizes species, nor are ecological features consistently available to distinguish natural clusters which could be used to define species. Most importantly, sequence diversity often precludes the development of primer sets that can be used for studying multiple genera or even species. Although very appealing for its resolution, portability, and throughput capacity, MLSA suffers from the difficulty of developing widely applicable schemes.

For more than 2 decades, bacterial taxonomists consider whole-genome information the standard for determining taxonomy. The number of whole-genome sequences is increasing rapidly and allows assessment of genome-level variation within and between species. It has become clear that, in addition to nucleotide substitutions, other genetic forces, such as gene loss, gene duplication, horizontal gene transfer, and chromosomal rearrangements, shape the genome and that considerable fractions of the genome of any particular strain may be unique to that strain (10, 65). There is a growing interest in using these genome sequence data to assess evolutionary relationships among prokaryotic species, and a range of novel approaches for determining taxonomic relationships within and between closely related species has become available. These novel approaches include analysis of gene content and gene order, comparative sequence analysis of conserved and other macromolecules or of complete genomes, presence-absence analyses, nucleotide signature composition analyses, and even metabolic pathway reaction content analyses (10). Despite the documented strain-to-strain variation in genome content, these novel taxonomic analytical tools generally substantiate the idea that bacterial species delineated by DNA-DNA hybridization experiments and ordered along a phylogenetic backbone through comparative 16S rRNA gene sequence analysis represent coherent biological entities, although, in terms of population genetics, they still encompass considerable ecological and genetic heterogeneity (12, 34).

Studies by Konstantinidis and Tiedje (65) and Goris et al. (42) revealed the average nucleotide identity (ANI) of the genes shared by two strains to be a robust means of comparing levels of genetic relatedness. ANI values of approximately 95% corresponded to the traditional 70% DNA-DNA reassociation standard of the current species definition. At the 95% ANI cutoff, current species include only moderately homogeneous strains, apparently as a result of the strains having evolved in different ecological settings. A large fraction of the differences in gene content within species was associated with bacteriophage and transposase elements, revealing an important role of these elements during bacterial speciation. These findings were consistent with a definition for species that would include a more homogeneous set of strains than that provided by the current definition and one that considers the ecology of the strains in addition to their evolutionary distance (12). Goris et al. (42) also demonstrated that the 70% DNA-DNA reassociation threshold corresponded with 69%-conserved DNA or, when the analysis was restricted to the protein-coding portion of the genome, 85%-conserved genes.

ANI values detect the DNA conservation of the core genome, whereas conserved DNA calculates the proportion of DNA shared by two genomes. Both estimates of intraspecies similarity therefore do not necessarily correlate, and for that reason, Deloger et al. (22) introduced maximal unique match index (MUMi) values, which take into account both criteria of diversity. MUMi values represent a calculation for genomic distances that is based on the number of maximal unique and exact matches of a given minimal length shared by the two genomes being compared. MUMi values correlate better with the ANI than with the DNA content and group strains in a way that is congruent with MLSA trees.

Major Groups of Bacteria

The tree of life, based on comparative small-subunit rRNA studies, comprises three lines of descent that are nowadays referred to as the domains *Bacteria, Archaea,* and *Eucarya* (129). The *Bacteria* have been grouped into 27 formally named phyla, which are further subdivided into numerous taxa (http://www.ncbi.nlm.nih.gov/Taxonomy/tax.html/). However, a large number of uncultured bacteria represent additional phylogenetic lineages awaiting formal classification, and alternative phylogenetic classification systems (and thus alternative nomenclatures) have been proposed in which, for instance, more-comprehensive data sets, including multiple molecular sequences and cell envelope and ultrastructural characteristics, rather then reliance solely on rRNA sequence similarity, define the units of classification (4).

In the traditional (rRNA gene sequence-based) view of higher-order taxonomy and phylogeny, three phyla, the *Proteobacteria,* the *Firmicutes* (gram-positive organisms with low G+C contents, including *Bacillus, Clostridium, Staphylococcus, Mycoplasma,* and the classical lactic acid bacteria, such as *Enterococcus, Streptococcus,* and *Lactobacillus*), and the *Actinobacteria* (gram-positive organisms with high G+C contents, including *Bifidobacterium, Mycobacterium,* and *Corynebacterium*), comprise the large majority of clinically relevant species. The *Bacteroidetes* (*Bacteroides,* flavobacteria, and sphingobacteria), the *Spirochaetes* (spirochetes and leptospiras), and the *Chlamydiae* (chlamydias) represent some of the other phyla. A detailed overview is given by Krieg and Garrity (67) and Ludwig and Klenk (72) in their introductory chapters to the second edition of *Bergey's Manual of Systematic Bacteriology.* That edition is structured in an order based on the topology of the 16S rRNA phylogenetic tree.

The largest phylum by far is the *Proteobacteria,* which contains five main clusters (classes) of genera that are referred to with the Greek letters alpha, beta, gamma, delta, and epsilon (72). The *Proteobacteria* comprise the majority of the known gram-negative bacteria of medical, industrial, and agricultural significance. This phylum includes *Brucella, Ehrlichia,* and *Rickettsia* (*Alphaproteobacteria*); *Burkholderia, Bordetella,* and *Neisseria* (*Betaproteobacteria*); *Aeromonas, Legionella, Vibrio,* and the family *Enterobacteriaceae* (*Gammaproteobacteria*); and *Campylobacter* and *Helicobacter* (*Epsilonproteobacteria*). The *Deltaproteobacteria* comprise a variety mainly of sulfate-reducing bacteria that have little clinical relevance.

Uncultured Bacteria

The classification and naming of uncultured bacteria that are only minimally characterized by morphological characteristics or by differences in molecular sequence (79) are outstanding challenges in bacterial classification. The members of the International Committee on Systematic Bacteriology have agreed to recognize a category that formally classifies incompletely described prokaryotes (80). "*Candidatus*" is considered a taxonomic status for uncultured "candidate" species for which relatedness has been determined (for instance, for which phylogenetic relatedness has been determined by amplification and sequence analysis of prokaryotic RNA genes by use of universal prokaryotic primers) and whose authenticity has been verified by in situ probing or a similar technique for cell identification. In addition, it is also mandatory that information concerning phenotypic, metabolic, or physiological features be made available. Physiological features may serve as a starting point for further investigation and eventual description and naming. A detailed list of items for inclusion in the codified record of a "*Candidatus*" taxon has been provided (80). With the advent of genomics, these original concerns may appear trivial now that we have the technical means to study large genomic fragments of uncultured microbes by shotgun cloning and sequencing of bulk DNA extracted from mixed communities (90, 110) or by DNA amplification from single cells (88) by multiple displacement amplification, enabling sequencing from uncultured microorganisms from the environment (69). In particular, the metagenomics field is opening a fascinating new window for studying the uncultured microbial diversity in a range of ecosystems, including those of the human body (see chapter 13). Exploring the diversity of such ecosystems by comparative rRNA sequence analysis is based on identification of so-called species-level phylogenetic types, i.e., phylotypes, which are defined as groups of 16S rRNA gene sequences with a certain level of similarity. The cutoff values of rRNA sequence similarity that are used for phylotype definition are not consistent. In studies of the diversity of microbes in the human gastrointestinal tract, these values vary between 97 and 99% (139). The higher the cutoff value, the higher is the number of distinct phylotypes and thus estimated species richness. However, regardless of the cutoff value used, the resulting diversity estimates should be considered rough indicators of the microbial diversity present, as bacteria with rRNA sequences that are 99% similar may still encompass multiple species and considerable ecological and genomic heterogeneity (34).

IDENTIFICATION

Identification is part of taxonomy. It is the process whereby an organism is recognized as belonging to a known taxon (species, genus) and designated accordingly. It relies on a comparison of the characters of an unknown with those of established units in order to name it appropriately. This implies that identification depends on adequate characterization.

As part of identification strategies, dichotomous keys based on morphological and biochemical characteristics have only partly been replaced by other methods. Taxonomic studies provide an impressive array of alternative techniques derived from analytical biochemistry and molecular biology for examination of numerous cellular compounds (40, 41). Molecular diagnostics and immunoassays will be discussed in chapters 4 and 5, respectively. Each of these techniques is useful for characterization and hence identification of bacteria. Databases of rRNA sequences, whole-cell fatty acid components, ribotyping profiles, matrix-assisted laser desorption ionization–time-of-flight (MALDI-TOF) mass spectra and Fourier transform infrared (FTIR) spectra, or miniaturized series of phenotypic characteristics may allow identification of many isolates. Yet, the success of these databases also depends on the exactness of the methods and how carefully the individual entries have been delineated.

CLASSIFICATION AND IDENTIFICATION METHODS

In principle, all genotypic, phenotypic, and phylogenetic information can be used to classify bacteria. Genotypic information is derived from the nucleic acids present in the cell, whereas phenotypic information is derived from proteins and their functions, different chemotaxonomic markers, and a wide range of other expressed features. In the present polyphasic-species concept, a minimal taxonomic study consists of sequence analysis to determine the phylogenetic position of the unknown species (the 16S rRNA gene is most commonly used), DNA-DNA hybridizations to determine its precise level of relatedness toward its nearest phylogenetic neighbors, and biochemical characterization to distinguish the new taxon from the established ones. Typical for the process of polyphasic taxonomy is that information from other approaches is used to classify bacteria at different taxonomic levels. When working one's way through lists of methods, it is of primary interest to understand at which level these methods carry information and to realize their technical complexity, i.e., the amount of time and work required to analyze a certain number of isolates. The validation of a new classification or identification tool involves a determination of its taxonomic resolution by means of well-characterized reference strains. As a proof of concept, such validation studies mostly start with the analysis of type strains only, but because of the genotypic variability of bacterial species (both in gene content and in gene sequences), the true value of new classification or identification tools can appropriately be assessed only through the analysis of multiple well-characterized reference strains and subsequent validation using new isolates. The list of methods given below is not meant to be complete or to describe all of their aspects. It comprises the major categories of taxonomic techniques required to classify and identify bacteria and focuses on novel developments.

DNA-DNA Hybridization Studies

Although contested for its technical difficulties and for the inability to build cumulative databases, at present, DNA-DNA hybridization is still acknowledged as the reference method to establish relationships within and between species. Different DNA-DNA hybridization procedures have been described; the hydroxyapatite method, the optical renaturation method, and the S1 nuclease method have mostly been used (45, 118). These classical techniques, however, need considerable amounts of DNA and are time-consuming. New, quick methods that consume less DNA have been described (8, 29, 43, 54) and have partially replaced the classical methodologies.

Many DNA-DNA hybridization protocols have been described, and it is often not clear if hybridizations were performed under optimal, stringent, or suboptimal conditions. The stringency of the reaction is determined by the salt and formamide concentrations, by the temperature, and by the molar percentages of G+C of the DNAs used. DNA-DNA hybridizations are often performed under standard conditions that are not necessarily optimal or stringent for all bacterial DNAs. As a standard, optimal conditions for hybridizations should be preferred because the optimal

temperature curve for hybridization is rather broad (about 5°C) (118).

Quantitative comparisons of DNA hybridization values generated with different techniques should be handled with caution. When different methodologies are used, it is safer to distinguish categories of DNA-DNA relatedness, such as "high DNA-DNA relatedness" (denoting relationships between strains of a single species), "low-but-significant DNA-DNA relatedness" (comprising the significant hybridization levels below the cutoff for a separate species; the depth of this range depends primarily on the technique used), and, finally, "nonsignificant DNA-DNA relatedness" (denoting that the degree of DNA hybridization is too low to be measured by the method used).

rRNA Studies

rRNA is the best single target for studying phylogenetic relationships because it is present in all bacteria, it is functionally constant, and it is composed of highly conserved as well as more variable domains (67, 72, 103, 129). The components of the ribosome (rRNA and ribosomal proteins) have been the subjects of phylogenetic studies for several decades. The gradual development of molecular techniques enabled microbiologists to focus on the comparative study of the rRNA molecules, and direct sequencing of parts of or nearly entire 16S or 23S rRNA molecules by the PCR technique with a selection of appropriate primers has become common practice. These sequences provide a phylogenetic framework that serves as the backbone for modern microbial taxonomy (67, 72). The larger the conserved elements examined, the more information they bear and the more reliable the conclusions become. International databases comprising published and unpublished partial or complete sequences have been constructed (13, 85) but have also accumulated poor-quality sequences and sequences that are not accurately or even not correctly labeled. For these and other reasons, several initiatives for providing the scientific community with curated 16S rRNA databases have been undertaken (e.g., see references 7, 13, and 133). The All-Species Living Tree project (133; http://www.arb-silva.de/projects/living-tree/) aims to reconstruct a single 16S rRNA tree harboring all sequenced type strains of the hitherto-classified species of *Archaea* and *Bacteria*. Sequences are selected manually due to a high error rate in the names and information fields provided for the publicly deposited entries. A most useful tool for tracking the identities of strains for which sequences are deposited is the StrainInfo bioportal (20; http://www.straininfo.net/), which brings together the biological material kept at multiple biological resource centers into a single portal interface, with direct pointers to the relevant information at the culture collections' websites. This information is automatically linked to related sequences in the public domain and refers to all known scientific publications that deal with the organism. To support the taxonomic depth of the information provided by the StrainInfo bioportal, all taxonomic names appearing in the bioportal are fully integrated with and linked out to key taxonomic information sources.

rRNA sequence analysis not only is used to determine relationships among genera, families, and other higher ranks but often replaces DNA-DNA hybridization studies for the delineation of species in taxonomic practice. Such application of rRNA similarity data is often not appropriate. In 1992, Fox et al. (33) reported that 16S rRNA sequence identity is not always sufficient to guarantee species identity. Indeed, three phenotypically similar *Bacillus* strains exhibited more than 99.5% rRNA sequence similarity, while DNA-DNA hybridization experiments indicated that they belonged to two distinct species. Stackebrandt and Goebel (103) reported on the place for 16S rRNA gene sequence analysis and DNA-DNA reassociation in the present species definition in bacteriology. Their extensive literature review revealed that organisms sharing more than 98.5% rRNA similarity may or may not belong to a single species and that the resolution of 16S rRNA sequence analysis for determination of the degree of relatedness between closely related organisms is generally low. There is no threshold value of 16S rRNA similarity for species recognition (103). However, they reported that organisms with less than 97% 16S rRNA sequence similarity do not give a DNA-DNA reassociation level of more than 60%, no matter which DNA-DNA hybridization method is used. In fact, rRNA sequence analysis seemed to rightfully replace DNA-DNA hybridization studies in the description of new species, provided that the rRNA similarity level was below 97% and provided that rRNA sequence data for all relevant taxa were available for comparison. Subsequent studies revealed that for the majority of organisms, the 97% cutoff value could be raised to 98.7 to 99% (101). Nevertheless, other studies extended the observations on intraspecies 16S rRNA divergence considerably, as differences in 16S rRNA gene sequences of up to 4.5% were reported among strains of several species belonging to the *Epsilonproteobacteria* (49, 117). Studies by Jaspers and Overmann (57) and Gonzalez-Escalona et al. (39) provided compelling examples of diversity among 16S rRNA genes within single organisms and sequence identity in bacteria with highly divergent genomes and ecophysiologies.

In spite of its limitations, rRNA sequence analysis is now commonly used for the identification of bacteria. In routine diagnostic laboratories, the majority of isolates are identified using classical biochemical tests and a combination of intuition and stepwise analysis of results that are obtained. However, if an organism is not readily identified in a minimal length of time and at minimal expense, it often remains unidentified. Comparison of (nearly) entire 16S rRNA gene sequences is arguably the most powerful tool for establishment of the phylogenetic neighborhood of an unknown organism, and commercial identification systems based on analysis of rRNA gene sequences are available (e.g., MicroSeq 500 and a bacterial 16S rRNA gene sequencing kit [Perkin-Elmer Applied Biosystems, Foster City, CA]). A fraction of the 5′-terminal region of the 16S rRNA gene (positions 60 to 110 of the *Escherichia coli* numbering system) is one of the most informative or discriminatory regions for closely related organisms (72). Similar variable regions (flanked by highly conserved regions) occur in the 23S rRNA gene (114). A review by Clarridge covered this topic in detail (9) but struggled with the rRNA sequence similarity level as a limit for species delineation. As outlined above, use of the DNA-DNA hybridization level as a threshold for species delineation is more than a mere "proposal" (9) and is now supported by results of whole-genome studies. Comparison of 16S rRNA gene sequences in many bacterial genera will lead to correct identification to the species level, but it is equally true that many taxonomic studies have revealed that comparative rRNA sequence analysis is often not sensitive enough to identify strains to the species level. There is a lack of knowledge not only of the strain-to-strain variation within a species but also of the interoperon variation within a single strain. Therefore, concluding that an unidentified isolate belongs to a particular species because it shares a high percentage of its 16S rRNA gene sequence with particular species or concluding that it represents a novel species because it occupies a unique position in the phylogenetic tree supported by a high bootstrap value or because it shares only 97% of its 16S rRNA sequence with its closest neighbor is premature in the absence of appropriate complementary data. This is even more true for partial sequence data, as partial rRNA gene sequences carry only limited information of the molecule, and different parts of the gene may carry information for different taxonomic levels (60, 72). Nevertheless, erroneous claims that 16S rRNA gene sequencing represents the general "gold standard" for identification of new isolates appear regularly in medical (and other) microbiological literature (e.g., reference 31).

The interesting taxonomic properties of rRNA or rRNA gene molecules have been exploited in many ways (6, 44, 46, 50, 99, 125). Although highly conserved, the rRNA genes also consist of variable domains which are particularly useful for diagnostic purposes (5, 135). Amplification of part of the rRNA operon by means of PCR assays, followed by digestion of the amplicon by means of restriction enzymes and the electrophoretic separation of the resulting array of DNA fragments, is referred to as amplified rRNA restriction analysis or rRNA restriction fragment length polymorphism analysis (46). Depending on the target selected, the banding pattern is useful for species-level discrimination (for target sequences that are highly conserved) or for strain typing (for target sequences that are variable).

Another rRNA-based approach for the identification and classification of bacteria is ribotyping (44). By this procedure, genomic DNA is digested with a restriction enzyme (or with a set of restriction enzymes). The digest is separated by electrophoresis, and the bands are transferred to a membrane and hybridized with a labeled rRNA probe. This probe may be based on 16S rRNA, 23S rRNA, or both, with or without the spacer region, or on a conserved fragment of one of the rRNA genes. Although designed and mostly used to determine interstrain relationships (44), a fully automated procedure for identification of bacteria to the species level is commercially available (RiboPrinter; Dupont Qualicon Inc., Wilmington, DE).

Terminal restriction fragment length polymorphism analysis of 16S rRNA genes and denaturing gradient gel electrophoresis of variable rRNA domains have been used in several studies for the characterization of microbial diversity in natural specimens and for identification of the members therein (71, 81, 89). The former technique employs a PCR assay in which one of the two primers used is fluorescently labeled at the 5′ end and is used to amplify a selected region of bacterial genes encoding 16S rRNA from total community DNA. The PCR product is digested with restriction enzymes, and the fluorescently labeled terminal restriction fragment is precisely measured by using an automated DNA sequencer. Computer-simulated analysis of terminal restriction fragment length polymorphisms for 1,002 bacterial sequences showed that with proper selection of PCR primers and restriction enzymes, 686 sequences could be PCR amplified and classified into 233 unique terminal restriction fragment lengths or "ribotypes" (71). Denaturing gradient gel electrophoresis of variable rRNA domains relies on the sequence-based separation of a mixture of equally sized amplicons generated from a common target gene on a polyacrylamide gel containing a linear gradient of denaturing components. Sequence-based separation is the result of differences in melting behavior which depend mainly on

G+C content and nucleotide sequence, rather than on amplicon size. Bands can subsequently be excised, purified, and sequenced, thus resulting in a tentative identification.

New technologies, exploiting the universal characteristics of the rRNA genes and their potential for species identification emerge regularly. A growing number of studies report on the use of pyrosequencing (Biotage, Uppsala, Sweden), which provides rapid, short-read sequencing of 30 bases in approximately 30 min to classify, identify, and subtype bacteria, yeasts, and fungi (47, 52, 58). Most of these pyrosequencing applications test purified isolates; others use clinical specimens, such as sputum samples of cystic fibrosis patients (62), specimens obtained from orthopedic surgeries (61), or blood cultures (58). Turenne et al. (109) used single-stranded conformation polymorphism analysis of PCR amplicons to distinguish between organisms, and Yang et al. (131) used high-resolution melt analysis to characterize PCR products generated from three hypervariable regions of the 16S rRNA gene of clinically relevant bacterial pathogens and concluded that it allowed highly specific species identification. Still other approaches combine the diagnostic potential of 16S rRNA genes with the speed and discriminatory power of mass spectrometric analyses (see below).

Sequence Analysis of Protein-Encoding Genes

As an alternative to the 16S rRNA gene sequence analysis, numerous other macromolecules have been examined for their potential as microbiological clocks. Among others, various ribosomal proteins (84), the beta subunit of ATPase (72, 73), elongation factor Tu (72, 73), chaperonin (121), RNA polymerases (1, 60, 138), RecA (28), and manganese-dependent superoxide dismutase (35) were shown to be valuable molecular chronometers in bacterial systematics. These alternative macromolecules should be widely or universally distributed among bacteria, they should not be transmitted horizontally, and their molecular evolution rate should be comparable to or somewhat higher than that of 16S rRNA, which would render them more suitable for differentiation of closely related organisms (for example, see reference 35). Potential pitfalls of overreliance on a single phylogenetic marker are illustrated in the taxonomic studies of species of the *Streptococcus bovis* group. *Streptococcus infantarius* subsp. *coli* was reclassified as the novel species *Streptococcus lutetiensis*, and another group of streptococci was proposed as the novel species *Streptococcus pasteurianus*, primarily on the basis of manganese-dependent superoxide dismutase gene sequences (87). Subsequent studies by Schlegel et al. (94) demonstrated that neither *S. lutetiensis* nor *S. pasteurianus* represented novel species.

As discussed above, the analysis of multiple protein-encoding genes (not necessarily the most conserved ones) allows us to depict relationships within and between closely related species with a resolution superior to that of traditional 16S rRNA gene sequence analysis (34), and it buffers the distorting effects of horizontal gene transfer or recombination events (63). There is a growing body of literature providing multilocus sequence typing and MLSA schemes for the identification and typing of a large number of bacteria (see also http://pubmlst.org/).

Other Genotypic Methods for Bacterial Classification

A range of different genotypic techniques has been used to characterize bacteria at various taxonomic levels. The molar percentage of guanosine plus cytosine (the DNA base ratio or percent G+C value) is one of the classical genotypic characteristics and is part of the standard description of bacterial taxa. Generally, the range in G+C content observed among the strains of a species should not be more than 3%, and among the species of a genus, it should not be more than 10%, with few exceptions, such as the genus *Campylobacter* (118). In general, in the bacterial world the G+C content varies between 24 and 76%.

During the past decade, a tremendous number of molecular diagnostic methods, most of which are PCR based, have been developed. Most of these generate arrays of DNA fragments that are separated and detected in various ways, and appropriate software has been developed for pattern recognition and analysis and for database construction.

One of these DNA fingerprinting methods, amplified fragment length polymorphism (AFLP) analysis (136), is useful for the classification of strains at the species and genus levels. The basic principle of AFLP analysis is restriction fragment length polymorphism analysis, modified by using PCR-mediated amplification to select particular DNA fragments from the pool of restriction fragments. AFLP analysis screens for AFLPs by selective amplification of restriction fragments. The restriction is performed with two restriction enzymes, which yield DNA fragments with two different types of sticky ends that are randomly combined. To these ends, short oligonucleotides (adapters) are ligated to form templates for the PCR. The selective amplification reaction is performed by using two different primers that contain the same sequence as the adapters but whose sequences are extended to include one or more selective bases next to the restriction site of the primer. Only those fragments that completely match the primer sequence are amplified. The amplification process results in an array of about 30 to 40 DNA fragments, some of which are species (or even genus) specific, while others are strain specific (56).

PCR-based typing methods that use random or repetitive elements as primers have been applied to strain characterization of a wide variety of bacteria (53, 113, 125). In several of these studies, species-specific DNA fragments or patterns have been generated (e.g., for species belonging to the genera *Campylobacter*, *Capnocytophaga*, *Enterococcus*, and *Naegleria* [23, 37]). These specific DNA fragments may be useful as probes to rapidly screen and identify other isolates. Although primarily applied for infraspecies strain comparisons, these techniques are useful in classification as well.

Phenotypic Methods

Phenotypic methods comprise all those that are not directed toward DNA or RNA and therefore also include the chemical or chemotaxonomic techniques. As the introduction of chemotaxonomy is generally considered one of the essential milestones in the development of modern bacterial classification, it is often treated as a separate unit in taxonomic reviews. The classical phenotypic tests traditionally constituted the basis for the formal description of bacterial species, subspecies, genera, and families. While genotypic data are used to allocate taxa to a phylogenetic tree and to draw the major borderlines in classification systems, phenotypic consistency is required to generate useful classification systems and may therefore influence the depth of a hierarchical line (102, 118, 123). The paucity or variability of phenotypic characteristics for certain bacterial groups regularly causes problems in describing or differentiating taxa. For such bacteria, alternative chemotaxonomic or genotypic methods are often required to reliably characterize strains.

The classical phenotypic characteristics of bacteria comprise morphological, physiological, and biochemical features. Individually, many of these characteristics are poor parameters for genetic relatedness, yet as a whole, they provide descriptive information for the recognition of taxa. The morphology of a bacterium comprises both cellular (shape; the presence of an endospore, flagella, and inclusion bodies; and Gram staining characteristics) and colonial (color, dimensions, and form) characteristics. The physiological and biochemical features comprise data on growth at different temperatures; growth in the presence of different pH values, salt concentrations, or atmospheric conditions; growth in the presence of various substances, such as antimicrobial agents; and data on the presence or activities of various enzymes and utilization of compounds, etc. Very often, highly standardized procedures are required to obtain reproducible results within and between laboratories.

Phenotypic data were the first to be analyzed by means of computer-assisted numerical comparison. In the 1950s, numerical taxonomy arose in parallel with the development of computers (100) and allowed comparison of large numbers of phenotypic traits for large numbers of strains. Data matrices showing the degree of similarity between each pair of strains and cluster analyses resulting in dendrograms revealed a general picture of the phenotypic consistency of a particular group of strains. Because such large numbers of characteristics reflect a considerable amount of genotypic information, it soon became evident that numerical analysis of large numbers of phenotypic characteristics was indeed taxonomically relevant.

A large number of miniaturized semiautomated phenotypic test systems are commercially available and partially replace classical phenotypic analyses. These microtest galleries can be used for both classification and identification. It should be noted that the outcomes of a particular test obtained with a commercial system and by a classical procedure may be different. This, however, may occur with two classical procedures of the same test as well.

In taxonomic practice, phenotypic characterization became compromised and sometimes more of a burden than a useful taxonomic activity. Frequently, phenotypic data are compared with literature data obtained using other conditions or methods. The need for continued phenotypic characterization at every taxonomic level not only to delineate taxa and appreciate their phenotypic coherence but also to evaluate their physiological and ecological functions cannot be denied. A minimal phenotypic description is not only the identity card of a taxon but also a key to its biology. Although accepted as necessary, differential phenotypic characters are often hard to find with a reasonable amount of effort and time.

Chemical Methods

The term "chemotaxonomy" refers to the application of analytical methods to the collection of information on various chemical constituents of the cell to classify bacteria. As with the other phenotypic and the genotypic techniques, some of the chemotaxonomic methods have been widely applied to vast numbers of bacteria, whereas others were so specific that their application was restricted to particular taxa. The markers studied include whole-cell protein profiles, isoprenoid quinones, cytochromes, polyamines, pigments, particular enzymes, sterols, and hopanoids (14, 16, 41, 105, 106). Very often, analytical difficulties have been the main restrictions to their wide-scale application.

Cell Wall Composition

The distinction between gram-negative and gram-positive types of bacteria is still one of the characteristics that are first analyzed in order to guide subsequent characterization and identification steps. The determination of the cell wall composition has traditionally been important for gram-positive bacteria. The peptidoglycan type of cell wall of gram-negative bacteria is rather uniform and provides little information. The cell walls of gram-positive bacteria, in contrast, contain various peptidoglycan types which may be genus or species specific (95, 105). The most valuable information is derived from the type and composition of the peptide cross-link between adjacent chains in the polymer network. A variable that received little attention is the degree of N and O acetylation of the amino sugars of the glycan chain. The analytical procedure is time-consuming, although a rapid screening method has been proposed. Membrane-bound teichoic acid is present in all gram-positive species, but cell wall-bound teichoic acid is present in only some gram-positive species. Teichoic acids can easily be extracted and purified and can be analyzed by gas-liquid chromatography (30).

Cellular Fatty Acid Analysis

Over 300 fatty acids and related compounds are present in bacterial cells. Polar lipids are the constituents of the lipid bilayer of bacterial membranes and have frequently been studied for classification and identification purposes. Other types of lipids, such as sphingophospholipids, occur in only a restricted number of taxa and were shown to have taxonomic value within these groups (105). Fatty acids are the major constituents of lipids and lipopolysaccharides and have been used extensively for taxonomic purposes. Variations in chain lengths, double-bond positions, and substituent groups are very useful for the characterization of bacterial taxa (105, 124). Mostly, the total cellular fatty acid fraction is extracted, but particular fractions, such as the polar lipids, have also been analyzed. The cellular fatty acid methyl ester composition is a stable parameter, provided highly standardized culture conditions are used. The methylated fatty acids are typically separated by gas-liquid chromatography, and both the occurrence and the relative amounts of methylated fatty acids characterize bacterial fatty acid profiles.

Cellular fatty acid analysis offers many advantages over other phenotype-based identification systems; however, it has several limitations as well. First, the result of the analysis is culture dependent. Strains must be grown under identical conditions so that their fatty acid compositions can be compared. Although the conditions recommended by the manufacturer allow cultivation of a large number of bacteria, different sets of conditions and databases are used for different groups of bacteria (e.g., the aerobic bacteria, anaerobic bacteria, and mycobacteria). In addition, the level of resolution is organism dependent. Many bacteria may be adequately characterized and identified at the species level by means of their cellular fatty acid profiles. However, others are not, and often species of the same genus or even different genera have highly similar fatty acid compositions. In the framework of polyphasic taxonomy, cellular fatty acid analysis is often very useful as a rapid and fairly inexpensive screening method. The method allows the comparison and clustering of large numbers of strains with minimal effort and cost and yields descriptive information to characterize the organisms.

MALDI-TOF and Other Mass Spectrometric Methods

The first reports involving the use of MALDI-TOF mass spectrometry (MS) were published in the late 1980s, and its application increased exponentially during the past 15 years. The two main research areas are the field of proteomics, where it is used as an instrument to identify proteins, and the detection of biomarkers of several diseases. In MALDI-TOF MS, the sample is mixed with a matrix that is chosen such that it specifically absorbs a laser beam. The resulting high-energy impact is followed by the formation of ions that are extracted through an electric field and that are subsequently focused and detected as an m/z (mass/charge) spectrum. Typically, high-abundance peptides, like those derived from ribosomal protein fractions, that are of low mass and ionize readily are observed in the spectra (32, 76). The simplicity and speed of analysis represent part of its strength, and the whole process can be highly automated. These features make the approach particularly attractive to research laboratories that routinely deal with the analysis and identification of large numbers of bacterial isolates. In microbiology, MALDI-TOF MS has different applications. Although the method was used to distinguish antimicrobial-resistant isolates from susceptible ones and to differentiate strains within a single species, the method is not generally suitable as a typing technique in epidemiological studies (112). The most challenging diagnostic problem, i.e., the differentiation of closely related species through the analysis of an appropriate number of reference strains of multiple closely related species, is gradually being explored, and special-purpose identification databases are being constructed (25, 26). Among other techniques, MALDI-TOF MS was succesfully used for the rapid identification of nonfermenting gram-negative bacilli (21, 76, 120) and anaerobic bacteria (104).

The potential of MALDI-TOF MS for bacterial identification has also been used in a number of alternative ways. These include the fast and accurate differentiation of PCR products according to their lengths and rapid analysis of PCR products and restriction fragment length polymorphism patterns of microbial samples for size determination of double-stranded amplicons and restriction fragments (51, 107). Because of limitations of these approaches by length heterogeneities of specific marker genes which diminish their discriminatory power, von Wintzingerode et al. (122) combined base-specific cleavage of amplified 16S rRNA genes with MALDI-TOF MS. In this process, 16S rRNA gene signature sequences are amplified in the presence of dUTP instead of dTTP, followed by strand separation and uracil-DNA-glycosylase-mediated cleavage at each T-specific site. Fragment pattern detection was performed by MALDI-TOF MS and proved useful for the identification of several bacteria, including *Bordetella* and *Mycobacterium* strains (70, 122).

Other studies report on the use of surface-enhanced laser desorption ionization-TOF MS for the identification of bacteria (74, 96, 132). Surface-enhanced laser desorption ionization is distinguished from MALDI in its use of an active sample probe (the ProteinChip array) which has an adsorptive surface that allows bacterial lysates to be subjected directly, without prior treatments, to on-chip sample preparation steps, such as selective washing and desalting. This procedure minimizes sample losses, while speeding up and simplifying sample preparation, compared to that of the standard methods normally employed prior to the use of MALDI. Furthermore, the active capture of the proteins by the protein chip array ensures nondiscriminatory binding of

target proteins, which in turn improves the reproducibility and allows both peak mass-to-charge (m/z) ratios and intensity to be used in sample characterization.

Finally, the Ibis T5000 biosensor technology (Bruker Daltonics Inc., Billerica, MA) uses broad-range PCR primers that target conserved regions of bacterial genomes, such as ribosomal sequences and conserved elements from essential protein-coding genes (i.e., housekeeping genes) and is designed to rapidly detect and identify a variety of pathogens without prior knowledge of the pathogen's nucleic acid sequence (2). The use of such broad-range priming targets across the widest possible grouping of organisms enables amplification of most species within a group. The T5000 biosensor uses electrospray ionization MS to analyze the products of broad-range PCR, which allows for the precise determination of the molecular mass of the PCR products. These high-precision mass measurements are then used to unambiguously derive base compositions of the PCR products, which are compared to a database for identifying the organism. This technology allows for a multilocus identification of bacteria in samples with significantly less time and effort than sequencing and performs well with samples from a variety of clinical and environmental matrices, including blood, serum, various tissues, and even mosquito homogenates (27).

FTIR Spectroscopy

FTIR spectroscopy is used for the identification of substances in chemical analyses. In general, the wave number, the reciprocal of the wavelength, is used as the physical unit. FTIR spectroscopy involves the observation of vibrations of molecules that are excited by an infrared beam. Molecules are able to absorb the energy of distinct light quanta and start a rocking or rotation movement. The FTIR spectrum uses only vibrations that lead to a change in the dipole moment. An infrared spectrum represents a fingerprint which is characteristic for any chemical substance. The composition of biological material and, thus, of its FTIR spectrum, is exceedingly complex, representing a characteristic fingerprint. Naumann and coworkers suggested identifying microorganisms by FTIR spectroscopy (82). In principle, a reference spectrum library is assembled based on well-characterized strains and species. The FTIR spectrum of any unidentified isolate is then measured under the same conditions as those used for the reference spectra and is compared to spectra in the reference spectrum library. The application of FTIR spectroscopy is reported for a growing number of bacteria and yeasts (55, 68, 83, 92, 127).

Conclusions

At present, the scientifically and economically ideal identification technique remains beyond reach. Cowan's (17) intuitive approach (which is used when the identity of the unknown is anticipated) and stepwise method (which involves the use of dichotomous keys) suffice for numerous isolates and require only simple, rapid, and inexpensive biochemical tests. Cowan's views are easily adapted to modern methodology. If this first-line approach fails, alternative procedures are required and available. For several reasons, including the comprehensiveness of the public databases, complete 16S rRNA gene sequence analysis is the most straightforward and obvious choice for establishing a rough identity for an isolate, although it often fails to differentiate closely related species. Much of its superiority is based on its robust capacity to reveal the phylogenetic neighborhood of the organism studied, which is information not provided by any of the other current identification protocols. This information will direct the additional analyses required for final identification to the species level. Accurate species-level identification is thus very often a two-step process in which an unknown is first assigned to a particular group, after which it can be accurately identified at the species level. The former can be achieved through sequence analysis of 16S rRNA genes using near-universal primers, the latter through an appropriate selection of housekeeping genes and specific primers once the tentative identity of an unknown is established.

NOMENCLATURE

Valid Publication of Bacterial Names

The *International Code of Nomenclature of Bacteria* (98) includes rules on how to name bacteria at different taxonomic ranks. The aim of nomenclature is to ensure that an organism is tagged with a unique name that carries valuable information. Prior to 1980, a proposal of a new bacterial taxon could be validly published in any microbiological book or journal, and the authors of the relevant sections of the successive editions of *Bergey's Manual of Determinative Bacteriology* had to attempt to give a complete list of the members of any particular genus or group of genera. The unavailability of type strains and the fact that microbiologists from different disciplines were not always familiar with one another's work caused great difficulty. All too often a worker would discover several years later that "his" or "her" organism had in fact been described earlier under a different name.

To overcome such problems and others, 1 January 1980 was chosen as a new starting date for bacterial nomenclature. At that time, the Approved Lists of Bacterial Names were published on behalf of the Judicial Commission of the International Committee on Systematic Bacteriology (97). Only those names included on these lists had standing in bacterial nomenclature, and names of taxa were to be included only if they were adequately described and if a type strain was available. From then onwards, all new names were validly published only in the *International Journal of Systematic Bacteriology* (now the *International Journal of Systematic and Evolutionary Microbiology*). Names could effectively be published in other journals and then validated subsequently by announcement in the Validation Lists in the *International Journal of Systematic and Evolutionary Microbiology*. A number of organisms were involuntarily omitted from the Approved Lists and were revived later. After 1980, several updates of these lists were published in the form of Validation Lists, and in 1989, an update of all names validly published between 1 January 1980 and 1 January 1989 was published (77). Nowadays, complete overviews of validly published names can easily be obtained through Internet sites such as http://www.bacterio.cict.fr/ and http://www.dsmz.de/microorganisms/bacterial_nomenclature.php. Proposals of new taxa can be made in any journal, but their names are validated only the moment that they are included in one of the Validation Lists, published regularly in the *International Journal of Systematic and Evolutionary Microbiology*. One of the conditions for valid publication of names is that type strains of novel species must be deposited in two public culture collections in different countries. In case different names for the same organism are validly published, nomenclatural priority goes to the name that was validated first. As a result of this practice, all valid species

in any particular group can easily be traced and reference strains are available.

Why Do Names Change?

There are more important causes for the modification of bacterial names than the occasional detection of synonymy. As described above, our present view of bacterial classification is phylogeny based. With the advent of rRNA-DNA hybridization in the 1970s and, subsequently, the various rRNA gene-sequencing methods, taxonomists had a new framework in which they could revise classification schemes. The classical—and extreme—example is the revision of the taxonomy and nomenclature of the genus *Pseudomonas*, which has been proceeding painstakingly slowly during the past 3 decades. The most important reason for this slow progress is that, through the work of De Vos and De Ley (24), it became clear not only that the genus *Pseudomonas* consisted of five major species clusters but also that these clusters formed a polyphyletic part of a major group of bacteria now known as the *Proteobacteria*. Revision of the taxonomy of the pseudomonads had to consider the relationships of the various subbranches toward their numerous respective neighbors (59).

The modification of our view of classification is by far the most important reason for name changes. However, various forms of poor taxonomic practice also invoke a lot of changes, and hence irritation. As observed long ago (19), nomenclature often is "the generator of heat, bad temper, and ill-will among taxonomists and every kind of microbiologists." The classification (and identification) of *Helicobacter* species represents a fine example of the difficulties encountered in our present-day view of taxonomy. Although often challenged, the level of DNA-DNA hybridization and not the level of 16S rRNA gene sequence similarity is the most critical parameter for species delineation. Relatively few laboratories have the experience required to perform DNA-DNA hybridization experiments in a highly standardized way. Yet, because of the tremendous clinical relevance of these bacteria, numerous investigators study all sorts of *Helicobacter*-like organisms from human and animal hosts. The biodiversity within *Helicobacter* is very high, and there is a need for many DNA-DNA hybridization data to delineate the species. Regrettably, helicobacters are mostly fastidious organisms, and many are difficult (and some nearly impossible) to culture in vitro; in addition, the preparation of sufficient DNA for the hybridization experiments is a hardy, if not impossible, task. In practice, new species have often been described on the basis of 16S rRNA gene sequence data and a limited number of differential phenotypic characteristics. A recent study that involved various taxonomic approaches, including DNA-DNA hybridization experiments, demonstrated that comparison of nearly complete 16S rRNA gene sequences combined with minimal biochemical characterization does not provide conclusive evidence for identification to the species level and may prove highly misleading (117).

Another example is the ongoing revision of the classification and nomenclature of group II pseudomonads. In 1992, Yabuuchi et al. (130) reclassified several rRNA group II pseudomonads as *Burkholderia* species. In that study, only some of the rRNA group II pseudomonads were examined, and the conclusions were based on data for only a limited set of strains. As a consequence, several additional rounds of name changes were required to reclassify the remaining rRNA group II pseudomonads as *Burkholderia* species (11). This group of bacteria also serves as an example to illustrate other causes for name changes: (i) the lack of criteria for genus delineation (two of the *Burkholderia* species [*B. solanacearum* and *B. pickettii*] were—again—reclassified into the new genus *Ralstonia* [11], and some of the *Ralstonia* species were then further reclassified into the novel genus *Wautersia* [119]) and (ii) the intrinsically inadequate description of species that comprise only a single isolate. The lack of precise guidelines for genus-level delineation was discussed recently by Young (134), who argued strongly that phenotypic coherence at the genus level should have priority over phylogenetic information.

The *Ralstonia* example also illustrates a tedious problem raised by Clarridge (9), namely, the challenges in the nomenclature for organisms named before their phylogeny was revealed by 16S rRNA gene sequence comparisons. Shortly after the reclassification of several *Ralstonia* species into the novel genus *Wautersia* (119), it became clear that *Wautersia eutropha*, the type species of the genus *Wautersia*, is a junior synonym of *Cupriavidus necator*, the type (and only) species of the genus *Cupriavidus*, which was validly named in 1987, i.e., long before 16S rRNA gene sequence studies were performed routinely (75, 116). The only possible consequence—if one does not decide to bend the rules each time they turn out to be inconvenient—was to replace the name *Wautersia* by *Cupriavidus* and to consider all species of the genus *Wautersia* species of the genus *Cupriavidus*. While renaming and subsequent further renaming of bacterial species causes confusion and, not least, irritation in the wider microbiological community, adhering to the rules of nomenclature is essential for establishing a truly systematic taxonomy.

The so-called "one-strain taxa" (species [or genera] that are proposed on the basis of data for only one strain) have probably caused more problems than they have solved, and this is definitely the case in the context of diagnostic microbiology. It is not possible to estimate the variability of the phenotype in the case of a species with one strain or in the case of a genus with one species and one strain, for which many recent examples exist. The question of whether such strains can be validly named has been the subject of many debates. There are different views, each with advantages and disadvantages. In diagnostic microbiology, it is well known that a species is characterized by a certain degree of variability. This variability can be measured by both phenotypic and genotypic criteria and may be revealed by simple biochemical testing or sophisticated genomic-fingerprinting techniques. In the absence of sufficient strains for quantitation of the range of divergence within a species, it will be difficult or impossible to identify new isolates of this species without DNA-DNA hybridization experiments. A classification based on results obtained with a single strain cannot be stable. Indeed, already the detection of a second strain will inevitably necessitate revision of the original species description.

Clearly, some of the instances of nomenclatural modifications described above could have been avoided, and that is an important reason why they jeopardize the credibility of taxonomists in the microbiology community. As a concluding remark, it should be mentioned that there is no "undo" function in bacterial nomenclature. A name that was validly published remains valid regardless of the number of modifications it undergoes thereafter. For instance, the changes of the name *Pseudomonas maltophilia* to *Xanthomonas maltophilia* and finally to *Stenotrophomonas maltophilia* (86) or the changes of the name *Pseudomonas acidovorans* to *Comamonas acidovorans* and finally to *Delftia acidovorans* (126) may be reasonable to some taxonomists, but the changes, particularly the most recent, have been refuted by many clinical microbiologists. As these six names were all proposed according to the rules of bacterial nomenclature, they were all validated, and the use of each of them is correct and valid. Use of the original *Pseudomonas* names could imply that the user disagrees with the phylogenetic rationale for present-day genus-level classification. Use of the names *X. maltophilia* or *C. acidovorans* may simply indicate that one disagrees with the most recent modification, whether the reason is scientific or practical, or it may be a simple statement of discord with successive and excessive name changes.

CONCLUSIONS

A much broader range of taxonomic studies of bacteria has gradually replaced the former reliance upon morphological, physiological, and biochemical characterization. This polyphasic taxonomy takes into account all available phenotypic and genotypic information and integrates it into a consensus type of classification, framed in a general phylogeny derived from 16S rRNA gene sequence analysis. The bacterial species appears as a group of isolates which originated from a common ancestor population in which a steady generation of genetic diversity resulted in clones that had different degrees of recombination and that were characterized by a certain degree of phenotypic consistency, a significant degree of DNA-DNA hybridization, and a high degree of 16S rRNA gene sequence similarity (118). In its turn, this polyphasic-species concept is nowadays challenged using information from whole-genome sequencing studies which reveal that bacterial species genomes consist of core genes that are shared by all (or nearly all) strains of that species and accessory genes that are not. These studies also revealed that the DNA-DNA hybridization species threshold correlates with the degree of ANI of the core genes and with maximal unique and exact matches of a given minimal length shared by the genomes being compared, the so-called MUMi value. In addition, MLSA of a rapidly growing number of bacteria offers superior taxonomic resolution compared to the traditional 16S rRNA gene sequence analysis, and in general the clusters delineated correlate well with species demarcated by DNA-DNA hybridization experiments.

The majority of bacteria in routine diagnostic laboratories will continue to be identified by classical methods, as these methods are adequate, inexpensive, readily available, and easy to handle. In the case of new or atypical isolates, or for many research groups in which, for example, bacteria are isolated from new sources, a straightforward means of identification of microorganisms by a single method is often not possible, and several methods are needed. The most direct approach is first to allocate such isolates in the phylogenetic framework and then to determine the finer relationships by means of an appropriate approach, which may be polyphasic. This tendency of identification to become polyphasic is an unavoidable reality.

In some cases, the consensus classification is a compromise that contains a minimum of contradictions. It is often thought that the more information that becomes available in the future, the more classification will gain stability. Yet, whole-genome and MLSA studies too are being confronted with microbial diversity, as the percentages of genes belonging to the core genomes and their degree of sequence diversity vary strongly between bacterial lineages (34, 108). Undoubtedly, there is a huge amount of biodiversity, which can be handled in a practical manner only if it is arrayed in an ordered structure, artificial or not, with appropriate terms for communication.

Our present view of classification reflects the best science of this time. The same was true in the past, when only data from morphological and biochemical analyses were available. The main perspective in bacterial taxonomy is that technological progress will dominate and drastically influence methodology, as it always has. More whole-genome sequences will become available, more bacteria will be detected (whether they can be cultivated or not), there will be more automation, and bioinformatics will have to address the combination and linking of databases. The future bacterial species definitions may be based on whole-genome sequences, on a shared core of genes, on a certain type of genes, such as housekeeping or informational genes, or on a well-balanced selection of genes included in an MLSA type of analysis (3, 10, 36). It will be a formidable challenge to translate such information into pragmatic classification and identification schemes and to evaluate classifications that have been carefully designed.

REFERENCES

1. Adékambi, T., M. Drancourt, and D. Raoult. 2009. The rpoB gene as a tool for clinical microbiologists. *Trends Microbiol.* **17:**37–45.

2. Baldwin, C. D., G. B. Howe, R. Sampath, L. B. Blyn, H. Matthews, V. Harpin, T. A. Hall, J. J. Drader, S. A. Hofstadler, M. W. Eshoo, K. Rudnick, K. Studarus, D. Moore, S. Abbott, J. M. Janda, and C. A. Whitehouse. 2009. Usefulness of multilocus polymerase chain reaction followed by electrospray ionization mass spectrometry to identify a diverse panel of bacterial isolates. *Diagn. Microbiol. Infect. Dis.* **63:**403–408.

3. Buckley, M., and R. Roberts. 2006. *Reconciling Microbial Systematics and Genomics.* American Academy of Microbiology, Washington, DC. http://academy.asm.org/index.php?option =com_content&task=view&id=60&Itemid=57.

4. Cavalier-Smith, T. 2003. The excavate protozoan phyla Metamonada Grassé emend. (Anaeromonadea, Parabasalia, Carpediemonas, Eopharyngia) and Loukozoa emend. (Jakobea, Malawimonas): their evolutionary affinities and new higher taxa. *Int. J. Syst. Evol. Microbiol.* **53:**1741–1758.

5. Chakravorty, S., D. Helb, M. Burday, N. Connell, and D. Alland. 2007. A detailed analysis of 16S ribosomal RNA gene segments for the diagnosis of pathogenic bacteria. *J. Microbiol. Methods* **69:**330–339.

6. Chen, C. C., L. J. Teng, S. Kaiung, and T. C. Chang. 2005. Identification of clinically relevant viridans streptococci by an oligonucleotide array. *J. Clin. Microbiol.* **43:**1515–1521.

7. Chun, J., J.-H. Lee, Y. Jung, M. Kim, S. Kim, B. Kwon Kim, and Y.-W. Lim. 2007. EzTaxon: a web-based tool for the identification of prokaryotes based on 16S ribosomal RNA gene sequences. *Int. J. Syst. Evol. Microbiol.* **57:**2259–2261.

8. Christensen, H., O. Angen, R. Mutters, J. E. Olsen, and M. Bisgaard. 2000. DNA-DNA hybridization determined in micro-wells using covalent attachment of DNA. *Int. J. Syst. Evol. Microbiol.* **50:**1095–1102.

9. Clarridge, J. E. 2004. Impact of 16S rRNA gene sequence analysis for identification of bacteria on clinical microbiology and infectious diseases. *Clin. Microbiol. Rev.* **17:**840–862.

10. Coenye, T., D. Gevers, Y. Van de Peer, P. Vandamme, and J. Swings. 2005. Towards a prokaryotic genomic taxonomy. *FEMS Microbiol. Rev.* **29:**147–167.

11. Coenye, T., P. Vandamme, J. R. W. Govan, and J. J. LiPuma. 2001. Taxonomy and identification of the Burkholderia cepacia complex. *J. Clin. Microbiol.* **39:**3427–3436.

12. Cohan, F. M. 2002. What are bacterial species? *Annu. Rev. Microbiol.* **56:**457–487.

13. Cole, J. R., Q. Wang, E. Cardenas, J. Fish, B. Chai, R. J. Farris, A. S. Kulam-Syed-Mohideen, D. M. McGarrell, T. Marsh, G. M. Garrity, and J. M. Tiedje. 2009. The Ribosomal Database Project: improved alignments and new tools for rRNA analysis. *Nucleic Acids Res.* **37:**D141–D145.

14. Collins, M. D. 1994. Isoprenoid quinones, p. 265–311. *In* M. Goodfellow and A. G. O'Donnell (ed.), *Modern Microbial Methods. Chemical Methods in Prokaryotic Systematics.* J. Wiley and Sons, Chichester, United Kingdom.

15. Colwell, R. R. 1970. Polyphasic taxonomy of the genus *Vibrio:* numerical taxonomy of *Vibrio cholerae*, *Vibrio parahaemolyticus*, and related *Vibrio* species. *J. Bacteriol.* **104:**410–433.

16. Costas, M. 1992. Classification, identification, and typing of bacteria by the analysis of their one-dimensional polyacrylamide gel electrophoretic protein patterns, p. 351–408. *In* A. Chambrach, M. J. Dunn, and B. J. Radola (ed.), *Advances in Electrophoresis*, vol. 5. VCH Verlagsgesellschaft, Weinheim, Germany.

17. Cowan, S. T. 1965. Principles and practice of bacterial taxonomy—a forward look. *J. Gen. Microbiol.* **39:**143–153.

18. Cowan, S. T. 1970. Heretical taxonomy for bacteriologists. *J. Gen. Microbiol.* **61:**145–154.

19. Cowan, S. T. 1971. Sense and nonsense in bacterial taxonomy. *J. Gen. Microbiol.* **67:**1–8

20. Dawyndt, P., M. Vancanneyt, H. De Meyer, and J. Swings. 2005. Knowledge accumulation and resolution of data inconsistencies during the integration of microbial information sources. *IEEE Trans. Knowl. Data Eng.* **17:**1111–1126.

21. Degand, N., E. Carbonnelle, B. Dauphin, J. L. Beretti, M. Le Bourgeois, I. Sermet-Gaudelus, C. Segonds, P. Berche, X. Nassif, and A. Ferroni. 2008. Matrix-assisted laser desorption ionization-time of flight mass spectrometry for identification of nonfermenting gram-negative bacilli isolated from cystic fibrosis patients. *J. Clin. Microbiol.* **46:**3361–3367.

22. Deloger, M., M. El Karoui, and M. A. Petit. 2009. A genomic distance based on MUM indicates discontinuity between most bacterial species and genera. *J. Bacteriol.* **191:**91–99.

23. Descheemaeker, P., C. Lammens, B. Pot, P. Vandamme, and H. Goossens. 1997. Evaluation of arbitrarily primed PCR analysis and pulsed-field gel electrophoresis of large genomic DNA fragments for identification of enterococci important in human medicine. *Int. J. Syst. Bacteriol.* **47:**555–561.

24. De Vos, P., and J. De Ley. 1983. Intra- and intergeneric similarities of *Pseudomonas* and *Xanthomonas* ribosomal ribonucleic acid cistrons. *Int. J. Syst. Bacteriol.* **33:**487–509.

25. Dickinson, D. N., M. T. La Duc, M. Satomi, J. D. Winefordner, D. H. Powell, and K. Venkateswaran. 2004. MALDI-TOF MS compared with other polyphasic taxonomy approaches for the identification and classification of *Bacillus pumilus* spores. *J. Microbiol. Methods* **58:**1–12.

26. Dieckmann, R., R. Helmuth, M. Erhard, and B. Malorny. 2008 Rapid classification and identification of salmonellae at the species and subspecies levels by whole-cell matrix-assisted laser desorption ionization-time of flight mass spectrometry. *Appl. Environ. Microbiol.* **74:**7767–7778.

27. Ecker, D. J., R. Sampath, C. Massire, L. B. Blyn, T. A. Hall, M. W. Eshoo, and S. A. Hofstadler. 2008. Ibis T5000: a universal biosensor approach for microbiology. *Nat. Rev. Microbiol.* **6:**553–558.

28. Eisen, J. A. 1995. The RecA protein as a model molecule for systematic studies bacteria: comparison of trees of RecAs and 16S rRNAs from the same species. *J. Mol. Evol.* **41:**1105–1123.

29. Ezaki, T., Y. Hashimoto, and E. Yabuuchi. 1989. Fluorometric deoxyribonucleic acid-deoxyribonucleic acid hybridization in microdilution wells as an alternative to membrane filter hybridization in which radioisotopes are used to determine genetic relatedness among bacterial strains. *Int. J. Syst. Bacteriol.* **39:**224–229.

30. Fischer, W., P. Rösel, and H. U. Koch. 1981. Effect of alanine ester substitution and other structural features of lipoteichoic acids on their inhibitory activity against autolysins of *Staphylococcus aureus*. *J. Bacteriol.* **146:**467–475.

31. Fontana, C., M. Favaro, M. Pelliccioni, E. S. Pistoia, and C. Favalli. 2005. Use of the MicroSeq 500 16S rRNA gene-based sequencing for identification of bacterial isolates that

commercial automated systems failed to identify correctly. *J. Clin. Microbiol.* **43:**615–619.

32. **Fox, A.** 2006. Mass spectrometry for species and strain identification after culture or without culture: past, present, and future. *J. Clin. Microbiol.* **44:**2677–2680.

33. **Fox, G. E., J. D. Wisotzkey, and P. Jurtshuk.** 1992. How close is close: 16S rRNA sequence identity may not be sufficient to guarantee species identity. *Int. J. Syst. Bacteriol.* **42:**166–170.

34. **Fraser, C., E. J. Alm, M. F. Polz, B. G. Spratt, and W. P. Hanage.** 2009. The bacterial species challenge: making sense of genetic and ecological diversity. *Science* **323:**741–746.

35. **Gautier, A.-L., D. Dubois, F. Escande, J.-L. Avril, P. Trieu-Cuot, and O. Gaillot.** 2005. Rapid and accurate identification of human isolates of *Pasteurella* and related species by sequencing the *sodA* gene. *J. Clin. Microbiol.* **43:**2307–2314.

36. **Gevers, D., F. M. Cohan, J. G. Lawrence, B. G. Spratt, T. Coenye, E. J. Feil, E. Stackebrandt, Y. Van de Peer, P. Vandamme, F. L. Thompson, and J. Swings.** 2005. Re-evaluating prokaryotic species. *Nat. Rev. Microbiol.* **3:**733–779.

37. **Giesendorf, B. A. J., W. G. V. Quint, P. Vandamme, and A. Van Belkum.** 1996. Generation of DNA probes for detection of microorganisms by polymerase chain reaction fingerprinting. *Zentbl. Bakteriol.* **283:**417–430.

38. **Godoy, D., G. Randle, A. J. Simpson, D. M. Aanensen, T. L. Pitt, R. Kinoshita, and B. G. Spratt.** 2003. Multilocus sequence typing and evolutionary relationships among the causative agents of melioidosis and glanders, *Burkholderia pseudomallei* and *Burkholderia mallei*. *J. Clin. Microbiol.* **41:**2068–2079.

39. **Gonzalez-Escalona, N., J. Romero, and R. T. Espejo.** 2005. Polymorphism and gene conversion of the 16S rRNA genes in the multiple rRNA operons of *Vibrio parahaemolyticus*. *FEMS Microbiol. Lett.* **246:**213–219.

40. **Goodfellow, M., and A. G. O'Donnell.** 1993. *Handbook of New Bacterial Systematics.* Academic Press, London, United Kingdom.

41. **Goodfellow, M., and A. G. O'Donnell.** 1994. *Modern Microbial Methods. Chemical Methods in Prokaryotic Systematics.* J. Wiley and Sons, Ltd., Chichester, United Kingdom.

42. **Goris, J., K. T. Konstantinidis, J. A. Klappenbach, T. Coenye, P. Vandamme, and J. M. Tiedje.** 2007. DNA-DNA hybridization values and their relationship to whole genome sequence similarities. *Int. J. Syst. Evol. Microbiol.* **57:**81–91.

43. **Goris, J., K. Suzuki, P. De Vos, T. Nakase, and K. Kersters.** 1998. Evaluation of a microplate DNA-DNA hybridization method compared with the initial renaturation method. *Can. J. Microbiol.* **44:**1148–1153.

44. **Grimont, F., and P. Grimont.** 1986. Ribosomal ribonucleic acid gene restriction patterns as possible taxonomic tools. *Ann. Inst. Pasteur Microbiol.* (Paris) **137B:**165–175.

45. **Grimont, P. A. D., M. Y. Popoff, F. Grimont, C. Coynault, and M. Lemelin.** 1980. Reproducibility and correlation study of three deoxyribonucleic acid hybridization procedures. *Curr. Microbiol.* **4:**325–330.

46. **Gürtler, V., and V. A. Stanisich.** 1996. New approaches to typing and identification of bacteria using the 16S-23S rDNA spacer region. *Microbiology* **142:**3–16.

47. **Haanperä, M., J. Jalava, P. Huovinen, O. Meurman, and K. Rantakokko-Jalava.** 2007. Identification of alpha-hemolytic streptococci by pyrosequencing the 16S rRNA gene and by use of VITEK 2. *J. Clin. Microbiol.* **45:**762–770.

48. **Hanage, W. P., C. Fraser, and B. G. Spratt.** 2006. Sequences, sequence clusters and bacterial species. *Philos. Trans. R. Soc. Lond. B* **361:**1917–1927.

49. **Harrington, C. S., and S. L. W. On.** 1999. Extensive 16S ribosomal RNA gene sequence diversity in *Campylobacter hyointestinalis* strains: taxonomic and applied implications. *Int. J. Syst. Bacteriol.* **49:**1171–1175.

50. **Höfle, M. G.** 1990. Transfer RNAs as genotypic fingerprints of eubacteria. *Arch. Microbiol.* **153:**299–304.

51. **Hurst, G. B., K. Weaver, M. J. Doktycz, M. V. Buchanan, A. M. Costello, and M. E. Lidstrom.** 1998. MALDI-TOF analysis of polymerase chain reaction products from methanotrophic bacteria. *Anal. Chem.* **70:**2693–2698.

52. **Innings, A., M. Krabbe, M. Ullberg, and B. Herrmann.** 2005. Identification of 43 *Streptococcus* species by pyrosequencing analysis of the *rnpB* gene. *J. Clin. Microbiol.* **43:**5983–5991.

53. **Ishii, S., and M. J. Sadowski.** 2009. Applications of the rep-PCR DNA fingerprinting technique to study microbial diversity, ecology and evolution. *Environ. Microbiol.* **11:**733–740.

54. **Jahnke, K.-D.** 1994. A modified method of quantitative colorimetric DNA-DNA hybridization on membrane filters for bacterial identification. *J. Microbiol. Methods* **20:**273–288.

55. **Janbu, A. O., T. Møretrø, D. Bertrand, and A. Kohler.** 2008. FT-IR microspectroscopy: a promising method for the rapid identification of *Listeria* species. *FEMS Microbiol. Lett.* **278:**164–170.

56. **Janssen, P., R. Coopman, G. Huys, J. Swings, M. Bleeker, P. Vos, M. Zabeau, and K. Kersters.** 1996. Evaluation of the DNA fingerprinting method AFLP as a new tool in bacterial taxonomy. *Microbiology* **142:**1881–1893.

57. **Jaspers, E., and J. Overmann.** 2004. Ecological significance of microdiversity: identical 16S rRNA gene sequences can be found in bacteria with highly divergent genomes and ecophysiologies. *Appl. Environ. Microbiol.* **70:**4831–4839.

58. **Jordan, J. A., J. Jones-Laughner, and M. B. Durso.** 2009. Utility of pyrosequencing in identifying bacteria directly from positive blood culture bottles. *J. Clin. Microbiol.* **47:**368–372.

59. **Kersters, K., W. Ludwig, M. Vancanneyt, P. De Vos, M. Gillis, and K.-H. Schleifer.** 1996. Recent changes in the classification of the pseudomonads: an overview. *Syst. Appl. Microbiol.* **19:**465–477.

60. **Khamis, A., D. Raoult, and B. La Scola.** 2005. Comparison between *rpoB* and 16S rRNA gene sequencing for molecular identification of 168 clinical isolates of *Corynebacterium*. *J. Clin. Microbiol.* **43:**1934–1936.

61. **Kobayashi, N., T. W. Bauer, M. J. Tuohy, I. H. Lieberman, V. Krebs, D. Togawa, T. Fujishiro, and G. W. Procop.** 2006. The comparison of pyrosequencing molecular Gram stain, culture, and conventional Gram stain for diagnosing orthopaedic infections. *J. Orthop. Res.* **24:**1641–1649.

62. **Kolak, M., F. Karpati, H. J. Monstein, and J. Jonasson.** 2003. Molecular typing of the bacterial flora in sputum of cystic fibrosis patients. *Int. J. Med. Microbiol.* **293:**309–317.

63. **Konstantinidis, K. T., A. Ramette, and J. M. Tiedje.** 2006. Toward a more robust assessment of intraspecies diversity, using fewer genetic markers. *Appl. Environ. Microbiol.* **72:**7286–7293.

64. **Konstantinidis, K. T., A. Ramette, and J. M. Tiedje.** 2006. The bacterial species definition in the genomic era. *Philos. Trans. R. Soc. Lond. B* **361:**1929–1940.

65. **Konstantinidis, K. T., and J. M. Tiedje.** 2005 Genomic insights that advance the species definition for prokaryotes. *Proc. Natl. Acad. Sci. USA* **102:**2567–2572.

66. **Kotetishvili, M., A. Kreger, G. Wauters, J. G. Morris, Jr., A. Sulakvelidze, and O. C. Stine.** 2005. Multilocus sequence typing for studying genetic relationships among *Yersinia* species. *J. Clin. Microbiol.* **43:**2674–2684.

67. **Krieg, N. R., and G. M. Garrity.** 2001. On using the manual, p. 15–19. *In* D. R. Boone, R. W. Castenholz, and G. M. Garrity (ed.), *Bergey's Manual of Systematic Bacteriology,* vol. 2. Springer-Verlag, New York, NY.

68. **Kümmerle, M., S. Scherer, and H. Seiler.** 1998. Rapid and reliable identification of food-borne yeasts by Fourier-transform infrared spectroscopy. *Appl. Environ. Microbiol.* **64:**2207–2214.

69. **Kvist, T., B. K. Ahring, R. S. Lasken, and P. Westermann.** 2007. Specific single-cell isolation and genomic amplification of uncultured microorganisms. *Appl. Microbiol. Biotechnol.* **74:**926–935.

70. **Lefmann, M., C. Honisch, S. Böcker, N. Storm, F. von Wintzingerode, C. Schlötelburg, A. Moter, D. van den Boom, and U. B. Göbel.** 2004. Novel mass spectrometry-based tool for genotypic identification of mycobacteria. *J. Clin. Microbiol.* **42:**339–346.

71. **Liu, W., T. L. Marsh, H. Cheng, and L. J. Forney.** 1997. Characterization of microbial diversity by determining terminal

restriction fragment length polymorphism of genes encoding 16S rRNA. *Appl. Environ. Microbiol.* **63:**4516–4522.

72. **Ludwig, J., and H.-P. Klenk.** 2001. Overview: a phylogenetic backbone and taxonomic framework for procaryotic systematics, p. 49–65. *In* D. R. Boone, R. W. Castenholz, and G. M. Garrity (ed.), *Bergey's Manual of Systematic Bacteriology,* vol. 2. Springer-Verlag, New York, NY.

73. **Ludwig, J., W. Neumann, N. Klugbauer, E. Brockmann, C. Roller, S. Jilg, K. Reetz, I. Schchtner, A. Ludvigsen, G. Wallner, M. Bachleitner, U. Fisher, and K. H. Schleifer.** 1993. Phylogenetic relationships of bacteria based on comparative sequence analysis of elongation factor Tu and ATP-synthase beta subunit genes. *Antonie van Leeuwenhoek J. Microbiol. Serol.* **64:**285–305.

74. **Lundquist, M., M. B. Caspersen, P. Wikström, and M. Forsman.** 2005. Discrimination of *Francisella tularensis* subspecies using surface enhanced laser desorption ionization mass spectrometry and multivariate data analysis. *FEMS Microbiol. Lett.* **243:**303–310.

75. **Makkar, N. S., and L. E. Casida.** 1987. *Cupriavidus necator* gen. nov., sp. nov.: a nonobligate bacterial predator of bacteria in soil. *Int. J. Syst. Bacteriol.* **37:**323–326.

76. **Mellmann, A., J. Cloud, T. Maier, U. Keckevoet, I. Ramminger, P. Iwen, J. Dunn, G. Hall, D. Wilson, P. Lasala, M. Kostrzewa, and D. Harmsen.** 2008. Evaluation of matrix-assisted laser desorption ionization–time-of-flight mass spectrometry in comparison to 16S rRNA gene sequencing for species identification of nonfermenting bacteria. *J. Clin. Microbiol.* **46:**1946–1954.

77. **Moore, W. E. C., and L. V. H. Moore (ed.).** 1989. *Index of the Bacterial and Yeast Nomenclatural Changes Published in the* International Journal of Systematic Bacteriology *Since the 1980 Approved Lists of Bacterial Names (1 January 1980 to 1 January 1989).* American Society for Microbiology, Washington, DC.

78. **Murray, R. G. E., D. J. Brenner, R. R. Colwell, P. De Vos, M. Goodfellow, P. A. D. Grimont, N. Pfennig, E. Stackebrandt, and G. A. Zavarzin.** 1990. Report of the Ad Hoc Committee on Approaches to Taxonomy within the *Proteobacteria. Int. J. Syst. Bacteriol.* **40:**213–215.

79. **Murray, R. G. E., and K. H. Schleifer.** 1994. Taxonomic notes: a proposal for recording the properties of putative taxa of procaryotes. *Int. J. Syst. Bacteriol.* **44:**174–176.

80. **Murray, R. G. E., and E. Stackebrandt.** 1995. Taxonomic note: implementation of the provisional status *Candidatus* for incompletely described procaryotes. *Int. J. Syst. Bacteriol.* **45:**186–187.

81. **Muyzer, G., E. C. de Waal, and A. G. Uitterlinden.** 1993. Profiling of complex microbial populations by denaturing gradient gel electrophoresis analysis of polymerase chain reaction-amplified genes coding for 16S rRNA. *Appl. Environ. Microbiol.* **59:**695–700.

82. **Naumann, D., D. Helm, and H. Labischinski.** 1991. Microbiological characterizations by FT-IR spectroscopy. *Nature* **351:**81–82.

83. **Oberreuter, H., H. Seiler, and S. Scherer.** 2002. Identification of coryneform bacteria and related taxa by Fourier-transform infrared (FT-IR) spectroscopy. *Int. J. Syst. Evol. Microbiol.* **52:**91–100.

84. **Ochi, K.** 1995. Comparative ribosomal protein sequence analyses of a phylogenetically defined genus, *Pseudomonas,* and its relatives. *Int. J. Syst. Bacteriol.* **45:**268–273.

85. **Olsen, G. J., G. Larsen, and C. R. Woese.** 1991. The ribosomal RNA database project. *Nucleic Acids Res.* **19**(Suppl.):2017–2021.

86. **Palleroni, N. J., and J. F. Bradbury.** 1993. *Stenotrophomonas,* a new bacterial genus for *Xanthomonas maltophilia* (Hugh 1980) Swings et al. 1983. *Int. J. Syst. Bacteriol.* **43:**606–609.

87. **Poyart, C., G. Quesne, and P. Trieu-Cuot.** 2002. Taxonomic dissection of the *Streptococcus bovis* group by analysis of manganese-dependent superoxide dismutase gene (*sodA*) sequences: reclassification of 'Streptococcus infantarius subsp. coli' as *Streptococcus lutetiensis* sp. nov. and of *Streptococcus bovis* biotype 11.2 as *Streptococcus pasteurianus* sp. nov. *Int. J. Syst. Evol. Microbiol.* **52:**1247–1255.

88. **Raghunathan, A., H. R. Ferguson, C. J. Bornarth, W. M. Song, M. Driscoll, and R. S. Lasken.** 2005. Genomic DNA amplification from a single bacterium. *Appl. Environ. Microbiol.* **71:**3342–3347.

89. **Rogers, G. B., M. P. Carroll, D. J. Serisier, P. M. Hockey, G. Jones, and K. D. Bruce.** 2004. Characterization of bacterial community diversity in cystic fibrosis lung infections by use of 16S ribosomal DNA terminal restriction fragment length polymorphism profiling. *J. Clin. Microbiol.* **42:**5176–5183.

90. **Rondon, M. R., P. R. August, A. D. Bettermann, S. F. Brady, T. H. Grossman, M. R. Liles, K. A. Loiacono, B. A. Lynch, I. A. MacNeil, C. Minor, C. L. Tiong, M. Gilman, M. S. Osburne, J. Clardy, J. Handelsman, and R. M. Goodman.** 2000. Cloning the soil metagenome: a strategy for accessing the genetic and functional diversity of uncultured microorganisms. *Appl. Environ. Microbiol.* **66:**2541–2547.

91. **Rossello-Mora, R., and R. Amann.** 2001. The species concept for prokaryotes. *FEMS Microbiol. Rev.* **25:**39–67.

92. **Sandt, C., C. Madoulet, A. Kohler, P. Allouch, C. De Champs, M. Manfait, and G. D. Sockalingum.** 2006. FT-IR microspectroscopy for early identification of some clinically relevant pathogens. *J. Appl. Microbiol.* **101:**785–797.

93. **Santos, S. R., and H. Ochman.** 2004 Identification and phylogenetic sorting of bacterial lineages with universally conserved genes and proteins. *Environ. Microbiol.* **6:**754–759.

94. **Schlegel, L., F. Grimont, E. Ageron, P. A. D. Grimont, and A. Bouvet.** 2003. Reappraisal of the taxonomy of the *Streptococcus bovis/Streptococcus equinus* complex and related species: description of *Streptococcus gallolyticus* subsp. *gallolyticus* subsp. nov., *S. gallolyticus* subsp. *macedonicus* subsp. nov. and *S. gallolyticus* subsp. *pasteurianus* subsp. nov. *Int. J. Syst. Evol. Microbiol.* **53:**631–645.

95. **Schleifer, K. H., and O. Kandler.** 1972. Peptidoglycan types of bacterial cell walls and their taxonomic implications. *Bacteriol. Rev.* **36:**407–477.

96. **Schmid, O., G. Ball, L. Lancashire, R. Culak, and H. Shah.** 2005. New approaches to identification of bacterial pathogens by surface enhanced laser desorption/ionization time of flight mass spectrometry in concert with artificial neural networks, with special reference to *Neisseria gonorrhoeae. J. Med. Microbiol.* **54:**1205–1211.

97. **Skerman, V. B. D., V. McGowan, and P. H. A. Sneath (ed.).** 1980. Approved lists of bacterial names. *Int. J. Syst. Bacteriol.* **30:**225–420.

98. **Sneath, P. H. A. (ed.).** 1992. *International Code of Nomenclature of Bacteria,* 1990 revision. American Society for Microbiology, Washington, DC.

99. **Sogin, M. L., H. G. Morrison, J. A. Huber, D. M. Welch, S. M. Huse, P. R. Neal, J. M. Arrieta, and G. J. Herndl.** 2006. Microbial diversity in the deep sea and the underexplored "rare biosphere." *Proc. Natl. Acad. Sci. USA* **103:**12115–12120.

100. **Sokal, R. R., and P. H. A. Sneath.** 1963. *Principles of Numerical Taxonomy.* W. H. Freeman and Co., San Francisco, CA.

101. **Stackebrandt, E., and J. Ebers.** 2006. Taxonomic parameters revisited: tarnished golden standards. *Microbiol. Today* **33:**152–155.

102. **Stackebrandt, E., W. Frederiksen, G. M. Garrity, P. A. Grimont, P. Kampfer, M. C. Maiden, X. Nesme, R. Rossello-Mora, J. Swings, H. G. Truper, L. Vauterin, A. C. Ward, and W. B. Whitman.** 2002. Report of the Ad Hoc Committee for the Re-evaluation of the Species Definition in Bacteriology. *Int. J. Syst. Evol. Microbiol.* **52:**1043–1047.

103. **Stackebrandt, E., and B. M. Goebel.** 1994. Taxonomic note: a place for DNA-DNA reassociation and 16S rRNA sequence analysis in the present species definition in bacteriology. *Int. J. Syst. Bacteriol.* **44:**846–849.

104. **Stîngu, C. S., A. C. Rodloff, H. Jentsch, R. Schaumann, and K. Eschrich.** 2008. Rapid identification of oral anaerobic bacteria cultivated from subgingival biofilm by MALDI-TOF-MS. *Oral Microbiol. Immunol.* **23:**372–376.

105. **Suzuki, K., M. Goodfellow, and A. G. O'Donnell.** 1993. Cell envelopes and classification, p. 195–250. *In* M. Goodfellow and A. G. O'Donnell (ed.), *Handbook of New Bacterial Systematics.* Academic Press, London, United Kingdom.

106. **Tabor, C. W., and H. Tabor.** 1985. Polyamines in microorganisms. *Microbiol. Rev.* **49:**81–99.

107. **Taranenko, N. I., R. Hurt, J. Z. Zhou, N. R. Isola, H. Huang, S. H. Lee, and C. H. Chen.** 2002. Laser desorption mass spectrometry for microbial DNA analysis. *J. Microbiol. Methods* **48:**101–106.

108. **Tettelin, H., D. Riley, C. Cattuto, and D. Medini.** 2008. Comparative genomics: the bacterial pan-genome. *Curr. Opin. Microbiol.* **11:**472–477.

109. **Turenne, C. Y., E. Witwicki, D. J. Hoban, J. A. Karlowsky, and A. M. Kabani.** 2000. Rapid identification of bacteria from positive blood cultures by fluorescence-based PCR-single-strand conformation polymorphism analysis of the 16S rRNA gene. *J. Clin. Microbiol.* **38:**513–520.

110. **Tyson, G. W., J. Chapman, P. Hugenholtz, E. E. Allen, R. J. Ram, P. M. Richardson, V. V. Solovyev, E. M. Rubin, D. S. Rokhsar, and J. F. Banfield.** 2004. Community structure and metabolism through reconstruction of microbial genomes from the environment. *Nature* **428:**37–43.

111. **Ursing, J. B., R. A. Rossello-Mora, E. Garcia-Valdes, and J. Lalucat.** 1995. Taxonomic note: a pragmatic approach to the nomenclature of phenotypically similar genomic groups. *Int. J. Syst. Bacteriol.* **45:**604.

112. **van Baar, B. L.** 2000. Characterisation of bacteria by matrix-assisted laser desorption/ionisation and electrospray mass spectrometry. *FEMS Microbiol. Rev.* **24:**193–219.

113. **Van Belkum, A.** 1994. DNA fingerprinting of medically important microorganisms by use of PCR. *Clin. Microbiol. Rev.* **7:**174–184.

114. **Van Camp, G., S. Chapelle, and R. De Wachter.** 1993. Amplification and sequencing of variable regions in bacterial 23S ribosomal RNA genes with conserved primer sequences. *Curr. Microbiol.* **27:**147–151.

115. **Vancanneyt, M., P. Vandamme, and K. Kersters.** 1995. Differentiation of *Bordetella pertussis, B. parapertussis,* and *B. bronchiseptica* by whole-cell protein electrophoresis and fatty acid analysis. *Int. J. Syst. Bacteriol.* **45:**843–847.

116. **Vandamme, P., and T. Coenye.** 2004. Taxonomy of the genus *Cupriavidus*: a tale of lost and found. *Int. J. Syst. Evol. Microbiol.* **54:**2285–2289.

117. **Vandamme, P., C. S. Harrington, K. Jalava, and S. L. W. On.** 2000. Misidentifying helicobacters: the *Helicobacter cinaedi* example. *J. Clin. Microbiol.* **38:**2261–2266.

118. **Vandamme, P., B. Pot, M. Gillis, P. De Vos, K. Kersters, and J. Swings.** 1996. Polyphasic taxonomy, a consensus approach to bacterial classification. *Microbiol. Rev.* **60:**407–438.

119. **Vaneechoutte, M., P. Kaempfer, T. De Baere, E. Falsen, and G. Verschraegen.** 2004. *Wautersia* gen. nov., a novel genus accommodating the phylogenetic lineage including *Ralstonia eutropha* and related species, and proposal of *Ralstonia* [*Pseudomonas*] *syzygii* (Roberts et al. 1990) comb. nov. *Int. J. Syst. Evol. Microbiol.* **54:**317–327.

120. **Vanlaere, E., K. Sergeant, P. Dawyndt, W. Kallow, M. Erhard, H. Sutton, D. Dare, B. Devreese, B. Samyn, and P. Vandamme.** 2008. Matrix-assisted laser desorption-ionisation-time of flight mass spectrometry of intact cells allows rapid identification of *Burkholderia cepacia* complex. *J. Microbiol. Methods* **75:**279–286.

121. **Viale, A. M., A. K. Arakaki, F. C. Soncini, and R. G. Ferreyra.** 1994. Evolutionary relationships among eubacterial groups as inferred from GroEL (chaperonin) sequence comparisons. *Int. J. Syst. Bacteriol.* **44:**527–533.

122. **von Wintzingerode, F., S. Böcker, C. Schlötelburg, N. H. L. Chiu, N. Storm, C. Jurinke, C. R. Cantor, U. B. Göbel, and D. van den Boom.** 2002. Base-specific fragmentation of amplified 16S rRNA genes analyzed by mass spectrometry: a tool for rapid bacterial identification. *Proc. Natl. Acad. Sci. U. S. A.* **99:**7039–7044.

123. **Wayne, L. G., D. J. Brenner, R. R. Colwell, P. A. D. Grimont, P. Kandler, M. I. Krichevsky, L. H. Moore, W. E. C. Moore, R. G. E. Murray, E. Stackebrandt, M. P. Starr, and H. G. Trüper.** 1987. Report of the ad hoc committee on reconciliation of approaches to bacterial systematics. *Int. J. Syst. Bacteriol.* **37:**463–464.

124. **Welch, D. F.** 1991. Applications of cellular fatty acid analysis. *Clin. Microbiol. Rev.* **4:**422–438.

125. **Welsh, J., and M. McClelland.** 1992. PCR-amplified length polymorphisms in tRNA intergenic spacers for categorizing staphylococci. *Mol. Microbiol.* **6:**1673–1680.

126. **Wen, A., M. Fegan, C. Hayward, S. Chakraborty, and L. I. Sly.** 1999. Phylogenetic relationships among members of the *Comamonadaceae*, and description of *Delftia acidovorans* (den Dooren de Jong 1926 and Tamaoka *et al.* 1987) gen. nov., comb. nov. *Int. J. Syst. Bacteriol.* **49:**567–576.

127. **Wenning, M. H. Seiler, and S. Scherer.** 2002. Fourier-transform infrared microspectroscopy, a novel and rapid tool for identification of yeasts. *Appl. Environ. Microbiol.* **68:**4717–4721.

128. **Willems, A., E. Falsen, B. Pot, E. Jantzen, B. Hoste, P. Vandamme, M. Gillis, K. Kersters, and J. De Ley.** 1990. *Acidovorax*, a new genus for *Pseudomonas facilis, Pseudomonas delafieldii*, E. Falsen (EF) group 13, EF group 16, and several clinical isolates, with the species *Acidovorax facilis* comb. nov., *Acidovorax delafieldii* comb. nov., and *Acidovorax temperans* sp. nov. *Int. J. Syst. Bacteriol.* **40:**384–398.

129. **Woese, C. R.** 1987. Bacterial evolution. *Microbiol. Rev.* **51:**221–271.

130. **Yabuuchi, E., Y. Kosako, I. Oyaizu, I. Yano, H. Hotta, Y. Hashimoto, T. Ezaki, and M. Arakawa.** 1992. Proposal of *Burkholderia* gen. nov. and transfer of seven species of the genus *Pseudomonas* homology group II to the new genus, with the type species *Burkholderia cepacia* (Palleroni and Holmes 1981) comb. nov. *Microbiol. Immunol.* **36:**1251–1275.

131. **Yang, S., P. Ramachandran, R. Rothman, Y. H. Hsieh, A. Hardick, H. Won, A. Kecojevic, J. Jackman, and C. Gaydos.** 2009. Rapid identification of biothreat and other clinically relevant bacterial species by use of universal PCR coupled with high-resolution melting analysis. *J. Clin. Microbiol.* **47:**2252–2255.

132. **Yang, Y. C., H. Yu, D. W. Xiao, H. Liu, Q. Hu, B. Huang, W. J. Liao, and W. F. Huang.** 2009. Rapid identification of *Staphylococcus aureus* by surface enhanced laser desorption and ionization time of flight mass spectrometry. *J. Microbiol. Methods* **77:**202–206.

133. **Yarza, P., M. Richter, J. Peplies, J. Euzeby, R. Amann, K. H. Schleifer, W. Ludwig, F. O. Glöckner, and R. Rossello-Mora.** 2008. The All-Species Living Tree project: a 16S rRNA-based phylogenetic tree of all sequenced type strains. *Syst. Appl. Microbiol* **31:**241–250.

134. **Young, J. M.** 2001. Implications of alternative classifications and horizontal gene transfer for bacterial taxonomy. *Int. J. Syst. Evol. Microbiol.* **51:**945–953.

135. **Yu, Z. T., and M. Morrison.** 2004. Comparisons of different hypervariable regions of *rrs* genes for use in fingerprinting of microbial communities by PCR-denaturing gradient gel electrophoresis. *Appl. Environ. Microbiol.* **70:**4800–4806.

136. **Zabeau, M., and P. Vos.** 1993. Selective restriction fragment amplification: a general method for DNA fingerprinting. European Patent Office publication 0534858 A1.

137. **Zeigler, D. R.** 2003. Gene sequences useful for predicting relatedness of whole genomes in bacteria. *Int. J. Syst. Evol. Microbiol.* **53:**1893–1900.

138. **Zillig, W., H.-P. Klenk, P. Palm, G. Pühler, F. Gropp, R. A. Garret, and H. Leffers.** 1989. The phylogenetic relations of DNA-dependent RNA polymerases of archaebacteria, eukaryotes, and eubacteria. *Can. J. Microbiol.* **35:**73–80.

139. **Zoetendal, E. G., M. Rajilic-Stojanovic, and W. M. De Vos.** 2008. High-throughput diversity and functionality analysis of the gastrointestinal tract microbiota. *Gut* **57:**1605–1615.

Specimen Collection, Transport, and Processing: Bacteriology

ELLEN JO BARON AND RICHARD B. THOMSON, JR.

16

One of the key principles of good specimen collection is to avoid introduction of colonizing bacteria surrounding the site of infection or on the skin or mucous membranes near the infectious site. This is done by disinfecting the surface skin and aspirating material, by using sheathed collection devices, or by collecting samples during surgical procedures. For sites naturally colonized by more than one species, selective methods are used to detect specific pathogens and prevent contamination with nonpathogenic commensals.

Specimens for bacteriologic culture should be collected as soon as possible after the onset of disease and before the initiation of antimicrobial therapy or as soon after the start of therapy as possible. A second specimen may be necessary because of poor specimen quality or inadequate transport conditions that affected the first specimen, but is otherwise rarely required for diagnosis of an acute infectious disease. Exceptions include the collection of multiple blood specimens for culture, and those obtained for additional studies other than those originally requested.

Microbiologists must help caregivers to choose, collect, and transport the specimen in a manner that optimizes the laboratory's diagnostic testing activities. A common mechanism today is to provide a written or online laboratory specimen collection guide (20); an example can be found at http://www.stanfordlab.com.

GENERAL PRINCIPLES OF SPECIMEN COLLECTION AND TRANSPORT

The Specimen Must Represent the Infected Site

The choice of specimen to be collected for laboratory diagnosis is based on the site of the infection and the nature of the suspected bacteria. Table 1 lists anatomic sites with appropriate and inappropriate clinical specimens (225, 252). General specimen selection and collection guidelines include proper labeling of the sample to include two patient identifiers, the source of the sample, and information on who collected the sample.

Suspected Agent of Bioterrorism or Intentional Release of Biological Agent

Specimens from suspected acts of terrorism are important legally, and a chain of custody must be employed. See the ASM Biodefense Resources website (http://www.asm.org/policy/index.asp?bid=52) and chapter 12 for more in-depth information.

Use of the Best Collection Method (Table 2)

Swabs

Swabs are appropriate when a large volume of sample is not necessary, such as from surface wounds (where the organism load is high) or oropharyngeal samples (where the presence of even one colony of Streptococcus pyogenes is clinically relevant) and where there will be a limited number of media to inoculate. Swabs should be collected carefully to avoid touching noninvolved surfaces or mucosae, which harbor contaminating bacteria, and they should be rolled or rubbed vigorously over the infected surface to maximize adsorption of the infecting agent.

A relatively recently introduced type of swab, the flocked swab, has proved to be superior to fiber swabs for collection of nasopharyngeal samples for detection of respiratory viruses, but there were no significant differences between flocked and rayon swabs when throat cultures were evaluated (46, 83). In one evaluation using seeded samples, flocked swabs in a transport medium even preserved several anaerobic bacteria when refrigerated for up to 24 h (237). Further testing on actual patient samples should be performed to determine if flocked swabs are advantageous for bacterial cultures.

Swabs may be transported dry (with desiccant to enhance survival) for recovery of Corynebacterium diphtheriae and S. pyogenes only (113, 184).

Swabs should not be used when more than one type of culture (routine bacterial and fungal, for example) is ordered. Swabs are also not recommended for anaerobic cultures (Table 3) (too little material, likely to be aerated, and can pick up contaminants) or fungal cultures (hyphal elements are not picked up). Swabs may be used to collect material from surface lesions for detection of mycobacteria, such as Mycobacterium marinum, but if there is fluid or tissue, that material should be obtained for culture, not a swab of the fluid.

Swabs from the surface of decubitus ulcers should not be accepted for culture, as they are more likely to yield colonizing bacteria that have superinfected the surface than to

TABLE 1 Selection of common clinical specimens for bacterial culture[a]

Anatomic site	Clinical specimen	
	Appropriate	Inappropriate
Lower respiratory tract	Freshly expectorated mucus and inflammatory cells (pus), sputum Bronchoalveolar lavage fluids Endotracheal aspirates	Saliva, oropharyngeal secretions, sinus drainage from nasopharynx; bronchial washes
Sinus	Secretions collected by direct sinus aspiration, or washes, curettage, and biopsy material collected during endoscopy	Nasal or nasopharyngeal swab, nasopharyngeal secretions, sputum, and saliva
Urinary tract	Midstream urine, urine collected by "straight" catheterization, urine collected by suprapubic aspiration, urine collected during cystoscopy or other surgical procedure	Urine from Foley catheter collection bag, "bagged" urine from infants
Superficial wound	Aspirations of pus or local irrigation fluid (nonbacteriostatic saline), swab of purulence originating from beneath the dermis	Swab of surface material or specimen contaminated with surface material, irrigation with saline-containing preservative
Deep wound	Purulence, necrosis, or tissue from deep subcutaneous site	Specimen contaminated with surface material
Gastrointestinal tract	Freshly passed stool, washes, or feces collected during endoscopy; rectal swab (in selected cases)	Rectal swab, specimen for bacterial culture if diarrhea developed after patient in hospital for >3 days
Venous blood	Two to four blood specimens collected from separate venipunctures before initiation of antibiotics, each containing approximately 20 ml of blood for patients >90 lb (see Table 9 for pediatric volumes); antisepsis with iodine-containing compound or chlorhexidine	Clotted blood; one or more than four blood specimens collected within a 24-h period; volume of blood <20 ml per culture (i.e., per venipuncture); antisepsis with alcohol only (adults)

[a]Reprinted from reference 225 with permission.

yield the true pathogen affecting the underlying tissue (35). Swabs collected through the nose for diagnosis of sinusitis are other specimens of dubious value. If the swabs have been endoscopically obtained, they may be free of nasal mucosal contamination and reveal infecting bacteria, but they will not recover fungi, which are the etiological agents of chronic sinusitis in approximately 25% of cases (239).

Aspirates

For abscess contents, body fluids, and other fluid collections below the skin, aspirates obtained through disinfected intact skin are preferred over swabs. The skin should be thoroughly cleaned with 70% alcohol, followed by disinfection with tincture of iodine or chlorhexidine, which must be completely dry before inserting the needle. An angel wing type of device can be used to safely inject the fluid in the syringe into a transport container. If anaerobes are being considered, the transport container must be free of air. Anaerobic transport vials with a nitrogen atmosphere above a gel containing oxygen-scavenging components are commercially available. Special small anaerobic transport vials containing specific anaerobic transport media for endodontal samples are also available. Only laboratories with expertise in diagnosis of dental infection should attempt to culture this type of specimen.

Normally sterile fluids are aspirated, but in addition to placing some of the fluid into a sterile tube or a citrated or EDTA tube (to prevent clot formation) for immediate Gram stain evaluation, a quantity (preferably 10 ml) should be injected either into an aerobic blood culture bottle or a Wampole Isolator (Inverness Medical, Waltham, MA) tube directly at the patient's bedside (195, 259).

Complications occur in the clinical setting of intestinal tract perforation when microorganisms other than the expected Enterobacteriaceae, anaerobes, and enterococci are involved. New standards include recommendations for when and how cultures from intra-abdominal sites should be handled (16a, 213). Standard empirical therapy may not adequately treat Staphylococcus aureus, Pseudomonas aeruginosa, Candida spp., or multidrug-resistant bacteria. Laboratory policies on the extent of identification of isolates based on an arbitrary number (such as 3 or fewer) should be modified with appropriate clinician justification and discussion.

Tissues

Biopsied tissue should be obtained by the surgeon using aseptic technique. Surface skin should be disinfected with chlorhexidine before the skin is cut. Once the first incision is made, which may inadvertently cut through a subsurface microcolony of bacteria (Propionibacterium acnes and Staphylococcus epidermidis), surgeons should switch to a fresh, sterile scalpel. Tissue should be placed into an anaerobic transport vial. If anaerobes are not considered, tissue may be placed into a sterile tube or cup with a tight lid. Tissue from draining sinus lesions should be obtained by curetting deep within the interior of the tract after thorough surface skin disinfection. Swabs from the drainage are likely to harbor surface bacteria that may not be associated with the underlying infection. Bone biopsy samples to diagnose osteomyelitis should be obtained directly from the bone itself after debridement of the overlying, usually superinfected tissue (35). Infected bone is soft enough to easily be removed by curetting or sometimes by aspiration with a large-bore needle.

TABLE 2 Collection, transport, and storage guidelines for microbiological laboratory diagnostic studies[a]

Specimen type	Collection guideline(s)	Transport[b] device and/or minimum vol	Transport time	Storage time and temp	Replica limits	Comment(s)
Abscess						
General	Remove surface exudate by wiping with sterile saline or 70% alcohol.					Tissue or aspirate is always superior to a swab specimen. If swabs must be used (aerobic culture only), collect two, one for culture and one for Gram staining. Preserve material on swab by placing in Stuart's or Amies medium.
Open	Aspirate if possible or pass a swab deep into the lesion to firmly sample the lesion's "fresh border."	Swab transport system	≤2 h, RT	≤24 h, RT	1/day/source	A sample of the base of the lesion and one of the abscess wall are most productive.
Closed	Aspirate abscess material with needle and syringe. Aseptically transfer *all* material into anaerobic transport device.	Anaerobic transport system, ≥1 ml	≤2 h, RT	≤24 h, RT	1/day/source	Contamination with surface material will introduce colonizing bacteria not involved in the infectious process. Do not use syringe for transport.
Bite wound	See Abscess					Do not culture animal bite wounds ≤12 h old (agents are usually not recovered) unless signs of infection are present.
Blood	Disinfect culture bottle; apply 70% isopropyl alcohol or chlorhexidine to rubber stoppers and wait 1 min. Palpate vein before disinfection of venipuncture site. Disinfection of venipuncture site: 1. Cleanse site with 70% alcohol. 2. Swab concentrically, starting at the center, with tincture of iodine or chlorhexidine. 3. Allow the disinfectant to dry. 4. *Do not palpate vein at this point without sterile glove.* 5. Collect blood. 6. After venipuncture, remove iodine from the skin with alcohol.	Blood culture bottles for bacteria; adult, 20 ml/set[c] (higher vol most productive); infant and child, 1–20 ml/set depending on weight of patient (see Table 9)	≤2 h, RT	≤2 h, RT or per instructions	Four sets in 24 h	Acute febrile episode: two sets[c] from separate sites, all within 10 min (before antimicrobials) Nonacute disease: antimicrobials will not be started or changed immediately: two to four sets from separate sites, all within 24 h at intervals no closer than 3 h (before antimicrobials) Endocarditis, acute: three sets from three separate sites, within 1–2 h, before antimicrobials if possible. Fever of unknown origin: two to four sets from separate sites. If negative at 24–48 h, obtain two or three more sets. Pediatric: collect immediately; rarely necessary to document continuous bacteremia with hours between cultures
Bone marrow aspirate	Prepare puncture site as for surgical incision.	Inoculate blood culture bottle or a 1.5-ml lysis-centrifugation tube.	≤24 h, RT if in culture bottle or tube	≤24 h, RT	1/day	Small volumes of bone marrow may be inoculated directly onto culture media. Routine bacterial culture of bone marrow is rarely useful.

Specimen	Collection	Container	Transport	Storage	No.	Comments
Burn	Cleanse and debride the burn.	Tissue is placed into a sterile screw-cap container. Aspirate or swab exudates should be transported in sterile container or swab transport system.	≤24 h, RT	≤24 h, RT	1/day/source	A 3- to 4-mm punch biopsy specimen is optimum when quantitative cultures are ordered. Process for aerobic culture only. Quantitative culture may or may not be valuable. Cultures of surface samples of burns may be misleading.
Catheter						
Intravenous	1. Cleanse the skin around the catheter site with alcohol. 2. Aseptically remove catheter and clip 5 cm of distal tip directly into a sterile tube. Some elect to culture the 5-cm intracutaneous portion to evaluate for soft tissue infection. 3. Transport immediately to microbiology laboratory to prevent drying.	Sterile screw-cap tube or cup	≤15 min, RT	≤2 h, 4°C	None	Controversial whether culture of catheter tips is clinically relevant. Acceptable intravenous catheters for semiquantitative culture (Maki roll method): central, CVP, Hickman, Broviac, peripheral, arterial, umbilical, hyperalimentation, Swan-Ganz
Foley	Do not culture, since growth represents distal urethral biota.					Not acceptable for culture
Cellulitis, aspirate from area of	1. Cleanse site by wiping with sterile saline or 70% alcohol. 2. Aspirate the area of maximum inflammation (commonly the center rather than the leading edge) with a needle and syringe. Irrigation with a small amount of sterile saline may be necessary. 3. Aspirate saline into syringe and expel into sterile screw-cap tube.	Sterile tube (syringe transport not recommended)	≤15 min, RT	≤24 h, RT	None	Yield of potential pathogens in minority of specimens cultured
CSF	1. Disinfect site with iodine or chlorhexidine preparation. 2. Insert a needle with stylet at L3-L4, L4-L5, or L5-S1 interspace. 3. Upon reaching the subarachnoid space, remove the stylet and collect 1–5 ml of fluid into each of three leakproof tubes.	Sterile screw-cap tubes. Minimum amt required: bacteria, ≥1 ml; acid fast, ≥5 ml.	Bacteria: never refrigerate; ≤15 min, RT	≤24 h, RT	None	Obtain blood for culture also. If only one tube of CSF is collected, it should be submitted to microbiology first; otherwise, submit tube 2 to microbiology. Aspirate of brain abscess or a biopsy may be necessary to detect anaerobic bacteria or parasites.

(Continued on next page)

TABLE 2 Collection, transport, and storage guidelines for microbiological laboratory diagnostic studies[a] (*Continued*)

Specimen type	Collection guideline(s)	Transport[b] device and/or minimum vol	Transport time	Storage time and temp	Replica limits	Comment(s)
Decubitus ulcer	A swab is not the specimen of choice. 1. Cleanse surface with sterile saline. 2. If a biopsy sample is not available, aspirate inflammatory material from the base of the ulcer.	Sterile tube/container (aerobic) or anaerobic system (for tissue)	≤2 h, RT	≤24 h, RT	1/day/source	Since a swab specimen of a decubitus ulcer provides no clinical information, it should not be submitted. A tissue biopsy sample or needle aspirate is the specimen of choice.
Dental culture: gingival, periodontal, periapical, Vincent's stomatitis	1. Carefully cleanse gingival margin and supragingival tooth surface to remove saliva, debris, and plaque. 2. Using a periodontal scaler, carefully remove subgingival lesion material and transfer it to an anaerobic transport system. 3. Prepare smear for staining with specimen collected in the same fashion.	Anaerobic transport system	≤2 h, RT	≤24 h, RT	1/day	Periodontal lesions should be processed only by laboratories equipped to provide specialized techniques for the detection and enumeration of recognized pathogens.
Ear Inner	Tympanocentesis reserved for complicated, recurrent, or chronic persistent otitis media 1. For intact ear drum, clean ear canal with soap solution and collect fluid via syringe aspiration technique (tympanocentesis). 2. For ruptured ear drum, collect fluid on flexible shaft swab via an auditory speculum (aerobic culture only).	Sterile tube, swab transport medium, or anaerobic system	≤2 h, RT	≤24 h, RT	1/day/source	Results of throat or nasopharyngeal swab cultures are not predictive of agents responsible for otitis media and should not be submitted for that purpose.
Outer	1. Use a moistened swab to remove any debris or crust from the ear canal. 2. Obtain a sample by firmly rotating swab in the outer canal.	Swab transport	≤2 h, RT	≤24 h, 4°C	1/day/source	For otitis externa, *vigorous* swabbing is required since surface swabbing may miss streptococcal cellulitis.
Eye Conjunctiva	1. Sample both eyes with separate swabs (premoistened with sterile saline) by rolling over each conjunctiva. 2. Medium may be inoculated at time of collection. 3. Smear may be prepared at time of collection. Roll swab over 1- to 2-cm area of slide.	Direct culture inoculation: BAP and CHOC Laboratory inoculation: swab transport	Plates: ≤15 min, RT Swabs: ≤2 h, RT	≤24 h, RT	None	If possible, sample both conjunctivae, even if only one is infected, to determine indigenous microbiota. The uninfected eye can serve as a control with which to compare the agents isolated from the infected eye. If cost prohibits this approach, rely on the Gram stain to assist in interpretation of culture.

Specimen	Collection	Device	Transport (unpreserved)	Transport (preserved/temp)	Frequency	Comments
Corneal scrapings	1. Specimen is collected by an ophthalmologist. 2. Using a sterile spatula, scrape ulcers or lesions, and inoculate scraping onto medium. 3. Prepare two smears by rubbing material from spatula onto 1- to 2-cm area of slide.	Direct culture inoculations: BHI with 10% sheep blood, CHOC, and inhibitory mold agar	≤15 min, RT	≤24 h, RT	None	If conjunctival specimen is collected, do so before anesthetic application, which may inhibit some bacteria. Corneal scrapings are obtained after anesthesia. Include fungal media. Scrapings for virus isolation and ameba detection should be submitted in a sterile container.
Vitreous fluid aspirates	Prepare eye for needle aspiration of fluid.	Sterile screw-cap tube or direct inoculation of small amount of fluid onto media	≤15 min, RT	≤24 h, RT	1/day	Include fungal media. Anesthetics may be inhibitory to some etiological agents.
Feces Routine culture	Pass specimen directly into a clean, dry container. Transport to microbiology laboratory within 1 h of collection or transfer to Cary-Blair holding medium.	Clean, leakproof, widemouthed container or use Cary-Blair holding medium (>2 g)	Unpreserved: ≤1 h, RT Holding medium: ≤24 h, RT	≤24 h, 4°C ≤48 h, RT or 4°C	1/day	Do not perform routine stool cultures for patients whose length of hospital stay is >3 days and the admitting diagnosis was not gastroenteritis without consultation with physician. Tests for *Clostridium difficile* should be considered for these patients. Swabs for routine pathogens are not recommended except for infants (see Rectal swab).
C. difficile	Pass liquid or soft stool directly into a clean, dry container. Soft stool is defined as stool assuming the shape of its container. Swab specimens are not recommended for toxin testing.	Sterile, leakproof, widemouthed container, >5 ml	≤1 h, RT 1–24 h, 4°C >24 h, −20°C or colder	2 days, 4°C, for culture 3 days, 4°C or longer at −70°C for toxin test	EIA not recommended; 1/wk for NAAT	Patients should be passing ≥5 liquid or soft stools per 24 h. Testing of formed or hard stool is not acceptable except for toxic megacolon. Freezing at −20°C or above results in rapid loss of cytotoxin activity.
E. coli (O157:H7) and other Shiga toxin-producing serotypes	Pass liquid or bloody stool into a clean, dry container.	Sterile, leakproof, widemouthed container, or Cary-Blair holding medium (>2 g)	Unpreserved: ≤1 h, RT Swab transport system: ≤24 h, RT or 4°C	≤24 h, 4°C ≤24 h, RT	1/day	Bloody or liquid stools collected within 6 days of onset from patients with abdominal cramps have the highest yield. Shiga toxin assay for all EHEC serotypes is better than sorbitol-MacConkey or chromogenic agar culture for O157:H7 only.
Leukocyte detection	Send in clean, dry container.	For direct methylene blue smear, no transport medium.	For direct smear, <2 h For lactoferrin tests, <48 h	For lactoferrin, 2–8°C		Controversial: some authors believe that this procedure provides results of little clinical value

(Continued on next page)

TABLE 2 Collection, transport, and storage guidelines for microbiological laboratory diagnostic studies[a] (Continued)

Specimen type	Collection guideline(s)	Transport[b] device and/or minimum vol	Transport time	Storage time and temp	Replica limits	Comment(s)
Rectal swab	1. Carefully insert a swab approx. 1 in. beyond the anal sphincter. 2. Gently rotate the swab to sample the anal crypts. 3. Feces should be visible on the swab for detection of diarrheal pathogens.	Swab transport	≤ 2 h, RT	≤ 24 h, RT	1/day	Reserved for detecting *Neisseria gonorrhoeae*, *Shigella*, *Campylobacter*, herpes simplex virus, and anal carriage of group B *Streptococcus* and other beta-hemolytic streptococci, or for patients (usually children) unable to pass a specimen.
Fistulas	See Abscess					
Fluids: abdominal, amniotic, ascites, bile, joint, pericardial, peritoneal, pleural, synovial	1. Disinfect overlying skin with iodine or chlorhexidine preparation. 2. Obtain specimen via percutaneous needle aspiration or surgery. 3. Always submit as much fluid as possible; *never* submit a swab dipped in fluid.	Anaerobic transport system, sterile screw-cap tube, or blood culture bottle for bacteria. Transport immediately to laboratory. Bacteria, >1 ml.	≤15 min, RT	≤24 h, RT Pericardial fluid and fluids for fungal cultures, ≤24 h, 4°C	None	Amniotic and culdocentesis fluids should be transported in an anaerobic system and need not be centrifuged prior to Gram staining. Other fluids are best examined by Gram staining of a cytocentrifuged preparation. One aerobic blood culture bottle inoculated at bedside is highly recommended.
Gangrenous tissue	See Abscess					Discourage sampling of surface or superficial tissue. Tissue biopsy samples or aspirates should be collected.
Gastric Wash or lavage for mycobacteria	Collect in early morning before patients eat and while they are still in bed. 1. Introduce a nasogastric tube into the stomach. 2. Perform lavage with 25–50 ml of chilled sterile, distilled water. 3. Recover sample and place in a leakproof, sterile container.	Sterile, leakproof container	≤15 min, RT, or neutralize within 1 h of collection	≤24 h, 4°C	1/day	The specimen must be processed promptly, since mycobacteria die rapidly in gastric washings. Neutralize when holding for >1 h with sodium bicarbonate.
Biopsy sample for *H. pylori*	Collected by gastroenterologist during endoscopy	Sterile tube with transport medium	<1 h, RT	≤24 h, 4°C	None	Culture may be needed for antimicrobial testing.
Genital: female Amniotic fluid	Aspirate *via* amniocentesis, or collect during cesarean delivery.	Anaerobic transport system, ≥1 ml	≤2 h, RT	≤24 h, RT	None	Swabbing or aspiration of vaginal secretions is *not* acceptable because of the potential for contamination with commensal members of the vaginal biota.

Specimen	Collection instructions	Transport system				Comments
Bartholin gland secretions	1. Disinfect skin with iodine preparation. 2. Aspirate fluid from ducts.	Anaerobic transport system, ≥1 ml	≤2 h, RT	≤24 h, RT	1/day	
Cervical secretions	1. Visualize the cervix using a speculum without lubricant. 2. Remove mucus and secretions from the cervical os with swab and discard the swab. 3. Firmly yet gently sample the endocervical canal with a new sterile swab.	Swab transport	≤2 h, RT	≤24 h, RT	1/day	See text for collection and transport needs for *C. trachomatis* and *N. gonorrhoeae.*
Cul-de-sac fluid	Submit aspirate or fluid.	Anaerobic transport system, >1 ml	≤2 h, RT	≤24 h, RT	1/day	
Endometrial tissue and secretions	1. Collect transcervical aspirate via a telescoping catheter. 2. Transfer entire amount to anaerobic transport system.	Anaerobic transport system, ≥1 ml	≤2 h, RT	≤24 h, RT	1/day	
Products of conception	1. Submit a portion of tissue in a sterile container. 2. If obtained by cesarean delivery, immediately transfer to an anaerobic transport system.	Sterile tube or anaerobic transport system	≤2 h, RT	≤24 h, RT	1/day	Do not process lochia, culture of which may give misleading results.
Urethral secretions	Collect at least 1 h after patient has urinated. 1. Remove old exudate from the urethral orifice. 2. Collect discharge material on a swab by massaging the urethra against the pubic symphysis through the vagina.	Swab transport	≤2 h, RT	≤24 h, RT	1/day	If no discharge can be obtained, wash the periurethral area with Betadine soap and rinse with water. Insert a small swab 2 to 4 cm into the urethra, rotate swab, and leave swab in place for at least 2 s to facilitate absorption.
Vaginal secretions	1. Wipe away old secretions/discharge. 2. Obtain secretions from the mucosal membrane of the vaginal wall with a sterile swab or pipette. 3. If a smear is also needed, use a second swab.	Swab transport	≤2 h, RT	≤24 h, RT	1/day	For IUD, place entire device into a sterile container and submit at RT. Gram stain, not culture, is recommended for the diagnosis of BV.

(Continued on next page)

TABLE 2 Collection, transport, and storage guidelines for microbiological laboratory diagnostic studies[a] (*Continued*)

Specimen type	Collection guideline(s)	Transport[b] device and/or minimum vol	Transport time	Storage time and temp	Replica limits	Comment(s)
Genital: female or male lesion	1. Clean with sterile saline and remove lesion's surface with a sterile scalpel blade. 2. Allow transudate to accumulate. 3. While pressing the base of the lesion, firmly rub base with a sterile swab to collect fluid.	Swab transport	≤2 h, RT	≤24 h, RT	1/day	For dark-field examination to detect *T. pallidum*, touch a glass slide to the transudate, add coverslip, and transport immediately to the laboratory in a humidified chamber (petri dish with moist gauze). *T. pallidum* cannot be cultured on artificial media.
Pilonidal cyst	See Abscess					
Genital: male						
Prostate	1. Cleanse the urethral meatus with soap and water. 2. Massage the prostate through the rectum. 3. Collect fluid expressed from the urethra on a sterile swab.	Swab transport or sterile tube for >1 ml of specimen	≤2 h, RT	≤24 h, RT	1/day	Pathogens in prostatic secretions may be identified by quantitative culture of urine before and after massage. Ejaculate may also be cultured.
Urethra	Insert a small swab 2–4 cm into the urethral lumen, rotate swab, and leave it in place for at least 2 s to facilitate absorption.	Swab transport	≤2 h, RT	≤24 h, RT	1/day	
Respiratory, lower						
Bronchoalveolar lavage, fluid, brush sample or washing, endotracheal aspirate	1. Collect washing or aspirate in a sputum trap. 2. Place brush in sterile container with 1 ml of saline	Sterile container, >1 ml	≤2 h, RT	≤24 h, 4°C	1/day	A total of 40–80 ml of fluid is needed for quantitative analysis. For quantitative analysis of brushings, place brush into 1.0 ml of saline (aerobic only).
Sputum, expectorated	1. Collect specimen under the direct supervision of a nurse or physician. 2. Have patient rinse or gargle with water to remove excess members of the oral biota. 3. Instruct patient to cough deeply to produce a lower respiratory specimen (not postnasal fluid). 4. Collect in a sterile container.	Sterile container, >1 ml Minimum amount: bacteria, >1 ml	≤2 h, RT	≤24 h, 4°C	1/day	For pediatric patients unable to produce a sputum specimen, a respiratory therapist should collect a specimen via suction. The best specimen from all patients should have ≤10 squamous cells/100 × field (10× objective and 10× ocular).

Specimen	Collection	Transport device/container	Transport time/temp	Storage	Frequency	Comments
Sputum, induced	1. Have patient rinse mouth with water after brushing gums and tongue. 2. With the aid of a nebulizer, have patients inhale approx 25 ml of 3–10% sterile saline. 3. Collect in a sterile container.	Sterile container, >1 ml	≤2 h, RT	≤24 h, RT	1/day	Same as above for sputum, expectorated.
Respiratory, upper — Oral	1. Remove oral secretions and debris from the surface of the lesion with a swab. Discard this swab. 2. Using a second swab, vigorously sample the lesion, avoiding any areas of normal tissue.	Swab transport	≤2 h, RT	≤24 h, RT	1/day	Discourage sampling of superficial tissue for bacterial evaluation. Tissue biopsy specimens or needle aspirates are the specimens of choice.
Nasal	1. Insert a swab, premoistened with sterile saline, approx 1–2 cm into the nares. 2. Rotate the swab against the nasal mucosa.	Swab transport	≤2 h, RT	≤24 h, RT	1/day	Anterior nose cultures are reserved for identifying staphylococcal carriers or for nasal lesions.
Nasopharynx	1. Gently insert a small swab (e.g., calcium alginate) into the posterior nasopharynx via the nose. 2. Rotate swab slowly for 5 s to absorb secretions.	Direct medium inoculation at bedside or examination table, swab transport	Plates: ≤15 min, RT Swabs: ≤2 h, RT	≤24 h, RT	1/day	
Throat or pharynx	1. Depress tongue with a tongue depressor. 2. Sample the posterior pharynx, tonsils, and inflamed areas with a sterile swab.	Swab transport (dry swab with or without silica gel is good for *S. pyogenes* and *C. diphtheriae*)	≤2 h, RT	≤24 h, RT	1/day	Throat swab cultures are contraindicated for patients with epiglottitis. Swabs for *Neisseria gonorrhoeae* should be placed in charcoal-containing transport medium and plated ≤12 h after collection. JEMBEC, Bio-Bags, and the GonoPak are better for transport at RT.
Tissue	Collected during surgery or cutaneous biopsy procedure	Anaerobic transport system or sterile, screw-cap container. Add several drops of sterile saline to keep small pieces of tissue moist.	≤15 min, RT	≤24 h, RT	None	Always submit as much tissue as possible. If there is excess tissue, save a portion of surgical tissue at −70°C in case further studies are needed. Never submit a swab that has been rubbed over the surface of a tissue. For quantitative study, a sample of 1 cm^3 is appropriate.

(Continued on next page)

TABLE 2 Collection, transport, and storage guidelines for microbiological laboratory diagnostic studies[a] (*Continued*)

Specimen type	Collection guideline(s)	Transport[b] device and/or minimum vol	Transport time	Storage time and temp	Replica limits	Comment(s)
Urine Female, midstream	1. While holding the labia apart, begin voiding. 2. After several milliliters has passed, collect a midstream portion without stopping the flow of urine. 3. The midstream portion is used for bacterial culture.	Sterile, widemouthed container, ≥1 ml, or urine transport tube with boric acid preservative	Unpreserved: ≤2 h, RT Preserved: ≤24 h, RT	≤24 h, 4°C	1/day	Chlamydial DNA detection in urine from women is less sensitive than in urine from men. Urine is toxic to cell lines and is therefore not the specimen of choice for chlamydial culture. Cleansing before voiding does not improve urine specimen quality; i.e., midstream urines samples are equivalent to clean-catch midstream urines samples.
Male, midstream	1. While holding the foreskin retracted, begin voiding. 2. After several milliliters has passed, collect a midstream portion without stopping the flow of urine. 3. The midstream portion is used for culture.	Sterile, widemouthed container, ≥1 ml, or urine transport tube with boric acid preservative.	Unpreserved: ≤2 h, RT	≤24 h, 4°C	1/day	The first part of the urine stream is used for probe and DNA amplification tests for *Chlamydia*. Collect urine for probe and DNA amplification tests at least 2 h after previous urination.
Straight catheter	1. Thoroughly cleanse the urethral opening with soap and water. 2. Rinse area with wet gauze pads. 3. Aseptically, insert catheter into the bladder. 4. After allowing approx 15 ml to pass, collect urine to be submitted in a sterile container.	Sterile, leakproof container or urine transport tube with boric acid preservative	Unpreserved: ≤2 h, RT Preserved: ≤24 h, RT	≤24 h, 4°C	1/day	Catheterization may introduce members of the urethral biota into the bladder and increase the risk of iatrogenic infection.
Indwelling catheter	1. Disinfect the catheter collection port with 70% alcohol. Clamp catheter below port and allow urine to collect in tubing for 10–20 min. 2. Use needle and syringe to aseptically collect 5–10 ml of urine. 3. Transfer to a sterile tube or container.	Sterile leakproof container or urine transport tube with boric acid preservative	Unpreserved: ≤2 h, RT Preserved: ≤24 h, RT	≤24 h, 4°C	1/day	Patients with indwelling catheters always have bacteria in their bladders. Do not collect urine from these patients unless they are symptomatic.
Wound	See Abscess					

[a] Abbreviations: AFB, acid-fast bacilli; BAP, blood agar plate; BHI, brain heart infusion; CHOC, chocolate agar; CVP, central venous pressure; EHEC, enterohemorrhagic *E. coli*; NAAT, nucleic acid amplification test; RT, room temperature.

[b] All specimen containers are to be transported in leakproof plastic bags having a separate compartment for the requisition.

[c] One set usually refers to one culture with both aerobic and anaerobic broths.

TABLE 3 Suitability of various specimens for anaerobic culture

Acceptable material (method of collection)	Unacceptable material
Aspirate (by needle and syringe)	Bronchoalveolar lavage washing
Bartholin's gland inflammation/secretions	Cervical secretions
Blood (venipuncture)	Endotracheal secretions (aspirate)
Bone marrow (aspirate)	Lochia secretions
Bronchoscopic secretions (protected specimen brush)	Nasopharyngeal swab
Culdocentesis fluid (aspirate)	Perineal swab
Fallopian tube fluid or tissue (aspirate/biopsy sample)	Prostatic or seminal fluid
IUD for *Actinomyces* spp.	Sinus washings or swabs
Nasal sinus (aspirate)	Sputum (expectorated or induced)
Placenta tissue (via cesarean delivery)	Stool or rectal swab samples
Stool for *Clostridium difficile*	Tracheostomy secretions
Surgical site (aspirate, tissue)	Urethral secretions
Transtracheal aspirate	Urine (voided or from catheter)
Urine (suprapubic aspirate)	Vaginal or vulvar secretions (swab)

Sputum

Expectorated sputum is the best sample for diagnosis of pneumonia, a disease of the distal lung alveolar spaces. Endotracheal aspirates are more likely to contain upper respiratory microbes and saliva from the upper tract and may not represent the bacteria causing the pneumonia (153). For these reasons, respiratory tract secretions from patients other than those with cystic fibrosis should be evaluated microscopically for the presence of squamous epithelial cells and bacteria (159). Sufficiently hydrated patients with pneumonia should be able to produce a good sputum specimen if properly coached by the collecting staff. The patient should be sitting up, should rinse out his mouth with water, and should be encouraged to bring up a deep cough from the lungs. Sometimes mild percussion on the chest can help dislodge deep phlegm. If a patient cannot produce an acceptable sputum sample the first time, it is very unlikely that a repeat collection will yield a good specimen, and it is probably better to call respiratory therapy to try to obtain a specimen. For some respiratory diseases, such as pneumococcal pneumonia and Legionnaires' disease, the inability to obtain reliable sputum has spurred the development of urinary antigen tests with very good sensitivity (52, 212).

Urine

Urine can be collected by midstream collection, catheterization (straight/in-out or indwelling), cystoscopic collection, or suprapubic aspiration. Foley catheter tips should not be submitted or accepted for culture, since they are always contaminated with members of the urethral microbiota and quantitation is not possible. A first-voided morning urine is optimal, since in most cases bacteria have been multiplying in the bladder for a number of hours. Cleansing of the periurethral areas has not been shown to improve the quality of urine culture, but midstream collection is still recommended (126).

Feces (Stool)

Stool is always superior to a rectal swab for bacterial testing, but if a swab is the only sample available, the swab should be inserted deep enough into the rectum to encounter some stool (appear brown). Swabs should always be submitted in transport media to preserve viability of pathogens. Some pathogens, especially *Shigella*, are labile in stool, so stool not submitted in appropriate transport medium should be inoculated to media without delay. Testing more than one stool for bacterial pathogens is usually not productive. Fresh stool should be examined visually, and the areas showing blood, pus, or mucus should be sampled preferentially. Diarrheal stool is loose and takes the shape of the container. Although formed stool may be tested for some pathogens, it is less productive, and for *Clostridium difficile* in particular, testing formed stool can lead to recovery of organisms that are colonizers and not causing disease except in patients with toxic megacolon.

Volume of Sample

In general, the more material available for testing, the better. This is true especially when more than one type of culture is requested. However, receiving more than the volume necessary to accommodate all requests could be problematic, particularly if less-trained staff choose the best section to use for microbiological studies. Caregivers should not be allowed to send large bags of fluids, or very large pieces of tissue, as that requires more manipulation in the laboratory than necessary and could introduce contaminants or result in a less productive part of the sample being tested. Since a drop of material (approximately 0.05 ml) is the minimum amount necessary to inoculate an agar plate or an enrichment broth, at least 1 drop per medium used should be received in the laboratory. As a general rule, at least 0.5 ml or 0.5 g of material should be received for routine bacterial culture, and more is necessary for additional studies. If the volume received is not sufficient to perform all requests or inoculate all the usual media, the physician should be contacted to prioritize the requests. This not only helps the microbiologist to perform the appropriate test but also alerts the physician that the sample was problematic and could serve as a motivator for more adequate specimens in the future. Problems with volume often occur when fine-needle biopsy samples from interventional radiology are sent for microbiological studies, as further discussed below.

A recent series of studies at the Mayo Clinic have shown that sonication of a complete joint prosthesis may allow recovery of organisms from the biofilm on the device that would not be detected if only tissue or fluid were cultured (179, 230). Other studies have shown that sonication at 22°C for 7 min yields the best results (147). This method may become the laboratory standard for testing removed prosthetic devices in the future.

Specimen Maintenance during Transport

The type of test to be performed determines the nature of the transport system. The ability of various swab types and transport media should be validated prior to implementation. Manufacturers are required to do this, and laboratories often perform limited validations. For example, nonviable bacteria in transport media may be seen in initial Gram stains, so microbiologists may wish to sample several lots of the product to ascertain a low burden of dead but stainable organisms. The Clinical and Laboratory Standards Institute has developed standards for evaluating transport devices (160). Table 2 summarizes transport recommendations for routine bacteriology.

1. Transport specimens to the laboratory as soon as possible after collection. If transport will require more than 2 h (some organisms require a shorter period), either a specific transport medium or refrigeration is required (Table 2). For samples to be tested by molecular methods only, refrigeration or even freezing (the lower the temperature, the better; $-80°C$ is best) is acceptable. One study found that a molecular test for group A streptococci performed better with dry swabs than with those sent in transport media (26).

2. Inoculate bacterial culture media within 24 h even if appropriate holding medium or refrigeration is maintained.

3. Small volumes of fluid (<1 ml) or tissue (<1 cm³) should be submitted within 15 to 30 min to avoid evaporation, drying, and exposure to ambient conditions. Larger volumes and those specimens in holding medium may be stored for as long as 24 h.

4. Bacteria that are especially sensitive to ambient conditions include *Shigella* spp., *Neisseria gonorrhoeae*, *Neisseria meningitidis*, *Haemophilus influenzae*, *Streptococcus pneumoniae*, and anaerobes. Reliable detection of these species requires immediate processing. Delays of up to 6 h result in some loss of CFU when transport media are used (189). Longer delays, even with the use of transport media, result in significant loss of organisms. For delays beyond 6 h, refrigeration improves recovery; however, specimens containing anaerobes should be stored at ambient temperatures (8, 58).

5. Moving clinical specimens and infectious substances from one laboratory to another, regardless of the distance and vehicle used, requires adherence to specimen packaging and labeling instructions mandated by the federal government. Materials for transport must be labeled properly, packaged so as to be able to absorb and contain any liquid released during a break or spill, and protected during transport. Refer to the Centers for Disease Control and Prevention (CDC) website (http://www.cdc.gov/od/ohs/biosfty/shipdir.htm) for a complete description of packaging and shipping regulations mandated by the U.S. Department of Transportation.

6. Some fastidious microbes or special testing protocols have more unusual transport requirements (Table 4). The laboratory test guide or manual should include clear instructions for special transport methods (54). If specimens are to be shipped to a distant reference laboratory, the reference laboratory's conditions and requests must be met, and in many instances the laboratory provides transport devices

TABLE 4 Specimen management for infrequently encountered organisms[a]

Organism	Specimen(s) of choice	Transport issues	Comment(s)
Bartonella spp. (cat scratch fever)	Blood, tissue, lymph node aspirate	1 wk at 4°C; indefinitely at −70°C	May see organisms in or on erythrocytes with Giemsa stain. Use Warthin-Starry silver stain for tissue. SPS is toxic.
Borrelia burgdorferi (Lyme disease)	Skin biopsy sample at lesion periphery, blood, CSF	Keep tissue moist and sterile; hand carry to laboratory if possible	Consider PCR in addition to culture. Culture yield is low. Warthin-Starry silver stain for tissue. AO, Giemsa for blood and CSF.
Borrelia spp. (relapsing fever)	Blood smear (blood)	Hand carry to laboratory if possible	Use direct wet mount in saline for dark-field microscopy. Stain with Wright's or Giemsa stain. Blood culture is unreliable.
Coxiella (Q fever),[b] *Rickettsia* (spotted fevers, typhus)	Serum, tissue (blood)	Blood and tissue are frozen at −70°C until shipped	Refer isolation to reference laboratory. Serological diagnosis is preferred.
Ehrlichia spp.	Blood smear, skin biopsy, blood (with heparin or EDTA anticoagulant), CSF, serum	Material for culture sent on ice; keep tissue moist and sterile; hold at 4–20°C until tested or at −70°C for shipment; transport on ice or frozen for PCR	Serological diagnosis preferred. Fix smear in methanol. Tissue stained with FA or Gimenez stain. Refer isolation to reference laboratory. CSF for direct examination and PCR.
Francisella spp. (tularemia)[b]	Lymph node aspirate, scrapings, lesion biopsy sample, blood, sputum	Rapid transport to laboratory or freeze; ship on dry ice	Send to reference laboratory. Serology helpful. Gram stain of tissue is not productive. IFA available. Culture effective 10% of the time.
Leptospira spp.	Serum, blood (citrate-containing anticoagulants should not be used), CSF (1st wk), urine (after 1st wk)	Blood, <1 h; urine, <1 h or dilute 1:10 in 1% bovine serum albumin and store at 4–20°C	Serology most helpful. Acidic urine is detrimental. Dark-field microscopy and direct FA available. Warthin-Starry silver stain for tissue.
Streptobacillus spp. (rat-bite fever, Haverhill fever)	Blood, aspirates of joint fluid	High-volume bottle preferred	Do not refrigerate. Requires blood, serum, or ascitic fluid for growth. SPS is inhibitory. AO staining is helpful.

[a] Abbreviations: AO, acridine orange; FA, fluorescent antibody; IFA, indirect fluorescent antibody.
[b] Laboratory safety hazard. Class II biological safety cabinet required. Also see chapter 10.

to users. Continuous dialogue with physicians and other caregivers ensures that the appropriate information on collection and transport is accessed before specimen collection begins.

LABORATORY SAFETY ISSUES REGARDING BACTERIAL PATHOGENS

Workers should always maintain a level of suspicion that any specimen could harbor an infectious agent. Physicians may fail to alert the laboratory when they suspect the possibility of any dangerous pathogen, including *Coccidioides immitis*, *Brucella*, etc. Some bacteria, such as *Mycobacterium tuberculosis*, and potential bioweapons on the list of select agents, such as *Francisella tularensis*, pose a threat to health care workers. Some precautions can be taken even before laboratory activities occur. These include obtaining proper vaccines, such as those for *Neisseria meningitidis* and more unusual agents if the laboratory is expected to encounter them. It is prudent to obtain baseline serum from each worker and store it in an ultralow-temperature freezer to have a basis for comparison in the event of a future exposure. Workers with conditions that place them at higher risk for some infections (immunocompromised persons and those in certain ethnic groups) may wish to avoid those tasks or laboratory assignments that could place them at risk. Any laboratorians who handle specimens or who might have to enter an environment where aerosols are possible must be fit tested for an N95 mask or similar protective face shield respirator. These masks should be worn in any situation where aerosols are possible. The Occupational Safety and Health Administration mandates the Respiratory Protection Standard specifically for potential tuberculosis or severe acute respiratory syndrome virus exposures, but the standard is extended to other respiratory hazards by other regulatory agencies and most employers (69a). One guideline on the safety of various agents is *Biosafety in Microbiological and Biomedical Laboratories*, 5th ed. (144a). Chapter 10 of this *Manual* contains a more in-depth discussion of biosafety in the laboratory.

Engineering Controls

Laboratory environments should be designed to protect workers from biohazards inherent in the nature of the work. Ready access to properly maintained and certified biosafety level 2 (BSL 2) laminar-flow biological cabinets and good training in the proper use of such equipment are important and should be encouraged, even in resource-poor laboratory settings. The laboratory environment should have good lighting over work surfaces and sufficient air exchanges to decrease exposure for workers (12 exchanges per hour has been recommended). When BSL 2 cabinets are not available, all manipulations that may result in aerosol formation, and those involving samples containing blood or body fluids (such as blood culture bottles), should be performed behind a Plexiglas or other clear shield. As many devices as possible to prevent contamination or acquisition of pathogens should be employed, including showers, eyewashes, and hands-free faucets at all hand washing sinks. Specimen containers should be carried within the laboratory in trays with solid sides and bottoms to prevent spillage if dropped accidentally. Staff should try to avoid carrying bottles or groups of tubes in their hands. Counters should be solid with backstops, and in BSL 2 or 3 rooms, the ceiling and walls should be smooth and waterproof and the floor should be smooth, with coved edges. See chapter 10 for more information.

Personal Protective Equipment

Workers should be allowed to wear gloves on the bench if they wish, and gloves should be changed often. Gloves should always be worn when handling original patient samples. Whether gloved or not, workers must wash their hands with alcohol gel or soap and water before leaving the laboratory, after removing gloves, and often at other times during normal work tasks. If splattering or aerosol is possible, face shields or goggles should be freely provided by the employer.

Education and a Culture of Safety

Supervisors, managers, and directors should create an atmosphere where workers maintain an environment of safe working habits and are constantly reminded of their responsibilities in this area. Everyone should know what to do in the event of a spill or accidental release in the laboratory, and drills should be conducted periodically to reinforce proper responses.

HANDLING OF SPECIMENS IN THE LABORATORY

Documentation of Arrival, Condition, and Appropriate Sample for Test Ordered

Upon arrival of specimens in the laboratory, the time and date of receipt should be recorded. Subsequently, the time of plating, which may differ substantially from the time of receipt, should be recorded. At the time of receipt, all specimens and requisitions should be carefully inspected. Specimens must be labeled and accompanied by a requisition reflecting the physician's order. The requisition must include the following information: patient name, age, sex, identifying number (such as social security number or unique registration/billing number), and location (hospital room, physician's office address, etc.); ordering physician's name; specimen source; date and time of collection; and test ordered. If the information is incomplete, laboratory personnel must call the collecting location and request the missing information. If a specimen is mislabeled or no patient name is provided, another specimen should be collected. Relabeling of a specimen is allowed only if another specimen cannot be collected, such as for tissue collected during a surgical procedure. Laboratory procedures must clearly state the exceptions that are allowed, the steps needed to verify and document exceptions, and the individuals responsible for relabeling. When relabeling has occurred, the course of events must be outlined in the laboratory report so that the physician interpreting the results is aware of potential errors. Speedy initial inspection of incoming samples can allow re-collection or notification of problems in an actionable time frame.

Laws governing specimen labeling can be reviewed at the Clinical Laboratory Improvement Amendments website (http://wwwn.cdc.gov/clia/regs/subpart_k.asp). Specimens from outpatient facilities require additional information for Medicare and Medicaid billing. Patient diagnosis, in the form of an International Classification of Diseases, 9th revision, code, is needed to confirm the justification for a particular test. If a test is not deemed necessary for a specific diagnosis, the patient must sign an advanced beneficiary notice documenting that the test is not considered necessary and that if it is performed, the patient will be required to pay the test charge. Medicare and Medicaid compliance rules also can be reviewed at the Centers for Medicare and Medicaid Services website (http://www.cms.hhs.gov).

Specimen Rejection

In spite of acceptable labeling, some specimen collection sites, transport containers, or transport conditions render the specimen unacceptable for processing (144). Table 2 lists acceptable criteria for specimen management based on collection or transport conditions and times. When specimens fall outside these limits (too long in transit, incorrect temperature, not in proper transport medium, wrong site for requested test, etc.), new specimens should be collected whenever possible. To protect the safety of laboratory workers, specimens that leaked or those that are grossly contaminated on the outside of the container should also be rejected. In addition, specimens may be rejected because of poor quality of specimen material collected or because it is the wrong specimen type for the test requested, rather than the conditions of transport (Tables 3 and 5). Specimen quality is evaluated by examining the quantity and cellular composition. Although the quantity of many specimens is limited by the collection method or physical size of the infected area, some specimens, such as urine, stool, and sputum, are available in abundance. If another specimen can be collected easily with a larger volume, it is appropriate and necessary to request new or additional material. If the specimen volume is less than needed for essential tests, small volumes of liquid specimens can be extended by adding 0.5 to 1 ml of sterile saline or a nutrient broth. It is important to add just enough liquid to provide specimen for all tests requested. A comment such as "Specimen has been diluted to allow performance of requested tests" should be added to the results documenting this action. In some cases, too much sample should also be considered for rejection. For example, if >20 ml of urine is received for *Chlamydia trachomatis* molecular testing, the dilution

of rare infectious particles may yield false-negative results. When blood culture bottles are overfilled, the excess blood volume may overwhelm the ability of sodium polyanethol sulfonate (SPS) to adequately anticoagulate the blood or remove inhibitors.

Specimens determined to have gross bacterial contamination from members of the normal microbiota, indicated by an abundance of squamous epithelial cells visualized on the initial Gram stain, should be rejected. Specimens are rejected by contacting the patient's caregiver, explaining the reason for rejection, and requesting a replacement specimen of acceptable quality. Timely notification and collection of replacement are necessary, especially in instances where antimicrobial therapy has been initiated. Regardless of the reason for rejection, it may be more politically palatable to state that the specimen cannot be accepted due to inability to correctly interpret the results, rather than to use the word "rejected" (N. Cornish, personal communication). Specimen rejection criteria should be reviewed by appropriate laboratory and medical staff representatives before becoming policy. Examples of acceptable and unacceptable specimens based on screening criteria are listed in Table 5.

Handling Samples That Are To Be Processed at a Remote Site

Transport and processing time limits suitable for laboratories near the specimen collection site are not appropriate for remote laboratories. Specimens must be handled in the same manner as if they are to be transported via public or private mail service. See the CDC Office of Health and Safety site (http://www.cdc.gov/od/ohs/biosfty/shipdir.ht) for the latest guidelines. The Infectious Disease Society of America, recognizing the problem, has suggested guidelines for providing

TABLE 5 Screening specimens requested for routine bacterial culture to ensure quality[a]

Specimen	Screening method	Results of screen	
		Acceptable for culture	No further testing; request another sample
Sputum (206)	Microscopic examination of Gram-stained smear	<10 SEC[b]/average 10× field	>10 SEC/average 10× field
Endotracheal aspirate (153)	Microscopic examination of Gram-stained smear	<10 SEC/average 10× field and bacteria seen in at least 1 of 20 oil immersion fields	>10 SEC/average 10× field and no bacteria seen in 20 oil immersion fields
Bronchoalveolar lavage fluid (181, 228)	Microscopic examination of Gram-stained smear	<1% of cells present are SEC	>1% of cells present are SEC
Superficial wound (207)	Microscopic examination of Gram-stained smear	<2+ SEC, polymorphonuclear leukocytes present	>2+ SEC and no polymorphonuclear neutrophils
Stool for bacterial pathogens	Days in hospital	≤3 days	>3 days (exception: physician provides good rationale)
Urine (204, 233)	Urinalysis, Gram stain of urine sediment	Positive dipstick leukocyte esterase test result or seeing >10 polymorphonuclear leukocytes/mm³ is an indicator of possible infection, but no method has yet proved truly reliable. One bacterium per oil power field corresponds to 10,000 CFU/ml in the urine.	Growth of three or more potential pathogens usually indicates biofilm on indwelling catheter or fecal contamination. Mixed fecal morphologies on Gram stain may indicate fistula into bladder from gastrointestinal tract.

[a]Modified from reference 225 with permission.
[b]SEC, squamous epithelial cells.

the best patient care under less-than-ideal circumstances (174). Managing movement of specimens using temperature-controlled boxes, reliable courier service, and good tracking systems is a challenge facing many providers today.

Prioritization

For busy laboratories that receive many samples over a short period, it is helpful to use a priority list to assist accessioning staff to determine in which order samples should be processed. Specimens ordered for STAT tests, such as Gram stains on specimens from patients still in the operating rooms, should receive the highest priority. A sample priority list is shown in Table 6.

Initial Sample Handling

1. Swabs that will be inoculated onto only one or two plates can be rolled directly onto the agar surface, inoculating the least inhibitory medium first. If a Gram stain is requested or if numerous media must be inoculated, the swab can be vortexed in 0.8 to 1.0 ml of sterile saline or Trypticase soy broth and drops of the suspension can be used to prepare the slide and inoculate media. Swabs should also be used to dip into stool, but usually not for sputum unless the sample is uniformly viscous without visible saliva. Sputum is best picked up from the container with wooden sticks, which do not adsorb the fluid sections but stick to the more purulent portions, where the pathogens are likely to be.

2. Clear fluids other than urine should be concentrated on a slide using a cytocentrifuge. If a cytocentrifuge is not available, samples of >1 ml should be centrifuged (1,500 to 2,500 × g) and the supernatant removed with a pipette down to 1.0 ml. This sediment is mixed thoroughly (vortex or pipette) and used for testing. Only if the material is thick, bloody, or frank pus can it be placed onto the slide without concentration, and it should be smeared thinly, similar to making a thin blood film.

3. Tissue and bone should be minced (using two sterile scalpels), and if fungus cultures are requested, a small piece of intact tissue should be inoculated into the surface of each

agar medium (see chapter 112) in addition to the standard inoculum. Tissue and bone for bacteriology cultures should also be ground up with a mortar and pestle, or tissue may be dispersed in an automated stomacher (Seward Limited, Worthing, West Sussex, United Kingdom) or grinder (208). A drop of this suspension should be streaked to obtain isolated colonies.

4. A Gram stain should be examined for all fluids and tissues and some swabs, such as those received for diagnosis of bacterial vaginosis (BV). Gram stains can deliver rapid, actionable results to clinicians, can determine if a specimen is acceptable for culture based on cellularity, and should be used to aid the microbiologist in interpretation of the culture (165). Table 7 suggests specimen types appropriate for Gram stain. Infection gives rise to purulence (abundant polymorphonuclear cells), blood, necrosis, and mucus (mucous membrane specimens). In general, gross examination of the specimen should identify yellow to tan purulence, red to rust-colored blood, clear and tenacious mucus, and brown to black discoloration of necrotic tissue. Portions for smear and culture should be taken from these areas. It may be beneficial to ask the assistance of a surgical pathologist when choosing the best portion of excised tissue for examination (224). Two smears of thick material such as sputum or tissue can be prepared by placing sufficient material between two glass slides and pressing the slides together while sliding them back and forth lengthwise to spread the material evenly one cell layer thick and to break up mucous strands. Ideally, microscopic examination of smears, using a 10× microscope objective, should demonstrate many polymorphonuclear cells and few or no squamous epithelial cells that would suggest cutaneous or mucocutaneous contamination with members of the normal bacterial microbiota. Specimens in which tissue necrosis is present also may show elastin fibers (Fig. 1) in stained smears. Lower respiratory tract specimens are likely to show alveolar macrophages and Curschmann's spirals (Fig. 2), indicating that secretions have originated from the distal airways. Curschmann's spirals are casts of bronchioles found in patients with chronic lung disease caused most commonly by asthma and cigarette smoking. Although elastin fibers are present in noninfected surgical wounds and specimens from areas of tissue damage, they are also found in infected tissue where necrosis has occurred.

5. Based on the site of the sample and the physician's request, each specimen should be inoculated to an appropriate medium chosen to recover suspected pathogens (Table 7). In this era of diminishing resources, two relatively recent innovations improve this process: chromogenic agars and automated plate inoculators. Chromogenic agars produce colonies that can be identified to genus or sometimes even species level directly from the appearance of the colonies without any further testing. Not only are they available for urinary tract pathogens (101) and some stool pathogens (235), but also they are used widely for screening samples for resistant bacteria, such as methicillin-resistant *Staphylococcus aureus* (MRSA) (158). These special media are discussed further in chapters covering organisms for which chromogenic media are available. In most cases, they are cost-effective by reducing both time and reagents used to identify the organisms in the conventional manner (60).

At least four automated medium inoculators are available, and all have been reported to perform at least as well as manual plating and to reduce workload for short-staffed laboratories (81). Some require that the sample be inoculated onto the plate (Isoplater; Vista Technology, Edmonton, Alberta, Canada); others handle the container

TABLE 6 Suggested priority list for accessioning samples received for bacteriology studies[a]

1. STAT requests (in order: operating room, pediatric intensive care units, emergency department)
2. CSF for routine culture and Gram stain
3. Rapid antigen detection tests (group A *Streptococcus*, *Campylobacter*, others)
4. Endotracheal aspirates in Lukens trap (patients on transplant and neonatal and pediatric intensive care units only)
5. Acid-fast specimens (if arrive near the processing cutoff time)
6. Bronchoalveolar lavage samples
7. Tissues from operating room
8. Body fluids (not CSF)
9. Blood cultures
10. Tissues and aspirates (not from operating room)
11. Fresh stools not in transport media (place into transport medium)
12. Sputa, other tracheal aspirates
13. Swabs in transport tubes
14. Urine samples
15. Stools in transport medium, including Cary-Blair

[a]Virology, mycology, and molecular test specimens may also need to be included in the list depending on the laboratory's policies and sample handling personnel distribution).

TABLE 7 Recommendations for Gram stain and plating media for bacteriology specimens or organisms

Specimen or organism	Gram stain	Aerobic media[a]	Anaerobic media[a,b]	Comments
Body cavity fluids	x (separate fluid specimen needed)			Blood culture bottles should be used to incubate large volumes of specimens for all body cavity fluids, following manufacturers' recommendations regarding supplements, etc.
CSF (routine)	x	B, C		
CSF (shunt)	x	B, C, Th		
Pericardial	x	B, C	BBA	
Pleural	x	B, C	BBA	
Peritoneal	x	B, C, Mac, CNA	BBA, LKV, BBE	
CAPD	x	B, C, Th	BBA	
Synovial	x	B, C		
Bone marrow	x	B, C	BBA	
Catheter tip		B		
Ear external fluid/swab	x	B, C, Mac		
Ear internal fluid	x	B, C	BBA	
Eye	x	B, C		
Gastrointestinal tract				
Feces		B, Mac, HE, Ca, EB (optional); sorbitol-Mac/chromogenic agar/ Shiga toxin testing		*C. jejuni/coli* in 5% O_2–10% CO_2–85% N_2 at 42°C for all gastrointestinal tract specimens
Rectal swab		B, Mac, HE, Ca, EB		
Genitourinary tract				
Vaginal/cervix	x	B, TM		Gram stain is method of choice for diagnosis of BV
Urethra/penis	x	TM		
Other	x	B, C, Mac, TM, CNA	BBA, LKV, BBE	
Group B streptococcal screen (vaginal/anal screen)		Selective broth, subculture to B		
Lower respiratory tract				
Sputum	x	B, C, Mac (PC OFPBL for cystic fibrosis)		
Tracheal aspirate	x	B, C, Mac		
Bronchoalveolar lavage fluid	x	B, C, Mac, CNA	BBA, LKV	Protected bronchoscopic brushing (in anaerobic transport) required for anaerobic culture
Bronchoalveolar brushing, washing	x	B, C, Mac		
Tissue	x	B, C, Mac, CNA, Th	BBA, LKV, BBE	
Upper respiratory tract				
Nasopharynx		B, C		
Nose		B, chromogenic agar		
Throat		B or SSA		
Urine		B, Mac or chromogenic agar		
Wound or abscess				
Swab	x	B, C, Mac, CNA	BBA, LKV, BBE	
Aspirate	x	B, C, Mac, CNA	BBA, LKV, BBE	
Bordetella pertussis and *B. parapertussis*		Regan-Lowe		
Brucella spp.		B, C		
Corynebacterium diphtheriae		Cystine-tellurite or Loeffler's serum		
Clostridium difficile		CCFA		
E. coli O157:H7 (EHEC, STEC)		Sorbitol-Mac chromogenic agar		Shiga toxin EIA more sensitive

(Continued on next page)

TABLE 7 Recommendations for Gram stain and plating media for bacteriology specimens or organisms (*Continued*)

Specimen or organism	Gram stain	Aerobic media[a]	Anaerobic media[a,b]	Comments
Francisella tularensis		C or BCYE		
Haemophilus ducreyi		C + vancomycin (3 µg/ml)		Gram stain resembling "school of fish"
Helicobacter pylori	x	B		Campylobacter gaseous atmosphere at 35–37°C
Legionella		BCYE		
Leptospira		Fletcher's medium or EMJH		30°C for up to 13 wk
Neisseria gonorrhoeae		TM		
Vibrio		TCBS		
Yersinia		CIN		

[a]B, blood agar; C, chocolate blood agar; Mac, MacConkey agar; Th, thioglycolate broth; Ca, campylobacter agar; HE, Hektoen enteric agar; EB, enrichment broth; SSA, group A *Streptococcus* selective agar; TM, Thayer-Martin agar; TCBS, thiosulfate-citrate-bile salts-sucrose agar; CIN, cefsulodin-Irgasan-novobiocin agar; BBA, brucella blood agar; LKV, laked blood agar with kanamycin and vancomycin; BBE, *Bacteroides* bile esculin agar; CNA, colistin-nalidixic acid agar; CCFA, cycloserine-cefoxitin-fructose agar; EMJH, Ellinghausen-McCullough-Johnson-Harris medium; CAPD, fluid from chronic ambulatory peritoneal dialysis; EHEC, enterohemorrhagic *E. coli*; PC, *Pseudomonas cepacia* agar; OFPBL, oxidative-fermentative polymyxin B-bacitracin-lactose agar.

[b]Set up anaerobic culture upon request, if specimen is collected and transported appropriately. Call physician if appropriate specimen does not have request for anaerobic culture.

containing any liquid specimen (MicroStreak [LBT Innovations, Adelaide, South Australia, Australia] and Inoculab [Dynacon, Mississauga, Ontario, Canada]). Streaking patterns vary from spiral to quadrant. A recent instrument even manages to handle swabs submitted in the new swab devices that contain liquid transport media (Walk Away Specimen Processor; Copan Inc., Murrieta, CA) (28). The estimated return on investment for one of the instruments ranged from 76 to 100% depending on whether technicians or technologists performed manual streaking and whether disposable or wire loops were used for the manual streaking comparison (http://www.vistatechnology .com/vistapayback.htm). These instruments will be important labor-saving devices as laboratory staffing becomes even leaner in the future.

The use of enrichment broth is controversial (154), but it should be conservative. Table 7 presents our recommendations. For many samples, such as swabs, broth cultures are more likely to yield contaminating members of the skin microbiota than pathogens (154). When fastidious species or organisms that may be present in small numbers are clinically important, enrichment broths make sense. When simultaneously inoculated plates yield growth, it is rarely useful or efficient to continue to work with the broth. When initial plates do not show growth in the face of a sample with polymorphonuclear leukocytes or other suggestions of an infectious process, the broth should be held for at least 5 days, and sometimes up to 14 days (looking for *Actinomyces* in eye samples or *Propionibacterium acnes* in prosthetic joint infection fluids, for example). Broths inoculated with cerebrospinal fluid (CSF) samples obtained from patients with indwelling shunts, joint fluids (should be injected directly into blood culture bottles), pericardial effusions, and other important fluids should be held for 14 days. Growth of skin organisms, such as coagulase-negative *Staphylococcus* and *Propionibacterium* species, must be evaluated in concert with clinical criteria to avoid overinterpretation (263, 264). In fact, for clean orthopedic surgeries, culture is not indicated (21). Once inoculated to the appropriate media based on the laboratory's protocols (Table 7), plates and broths are incubated in the appropriate atmosphere before they are examined for growth. Chocolate plates are always incubated in 5% CO_2, blood may be incubated in either air or CO_2 (depending on the requirements of the organisms to be recovered), and selective agar plates are best incubated

in air, although MacConkey agar colonies appear virtually the same whether incubated in CO_2 or air. Special incubation atmospheres are mentioned in the chapters covering those species and in this chapter. Lighting a candle in an enclosed jar or metal box and allowing it to burn out naturally creates an excellent CO_2 atmosphere for good recovery of microaerophilic, capnophilic (requiring higher CO_2 concentration than air) bacteria. Unless otherwise noted, temperatures for bacterial growth are 35 to 37°C.

Specimens for anaerobic culture should be processed as soon as possible after arrival in the laboratory. Usual media include an anaerobic blood agar plate (CDC blood agar or brucella blood agar), a medium that inhibits gram-positive and facultative gram-negative bacilli such as KV blood agar (kanamycin-vancomycin), a differential or selective medium such as *Bacteroides* bile esculin, a gram-positive selective medium (colistin-nalidixic acid blood agar or phenylethyl alcohol blood agar), and an enrichment broth such as chopped meat carbohydrate or thioglycolate (Table 7). Media should be incubated in an anaerobic environment immediately after inoculation. Incubation in anaerobic containers, such as GasPak jars (Becton Dickinson Microbiology Systems, Cockeysville, MD), AnaeroPack (Mitsubishi Gas Chemical America, Inc., New York, NY), or Bio-Bag Anaerobic Culture Set (Becton Dickinson Microbiology Systems) or in an anaerobic chamber is acceptable (49, 53). Anaerobes grow more slowly than aerobic or facultative bacteria. Jars or boxes should not be opened in air until after 48 h so that organisms in growth phase are not killed by exposure to oxygen (106). Anaerobic cultures should be held for at least 5 days before being reported as negative. Longer incubation (usually 14 days) of the broth is necessary for isolation of *Actinomyces*, *Propionibacterium* species from prosthetic joint infections, and some other fastidious anaerobes (263). See chapter 47 for further discussion.

6. For many reasons, it is best to retain specimens, or even empty containers if the entire specimen was used. Sometimes additional tests are requested later after other results, such as histopathology, become available. Sometimes there is an error during laboratory processing and the original aliquot must be resampled. Other reasons include checking the label on the specimen, preparing a second smear if there is a question on interpretation of the first one, or examining the gross appearance of

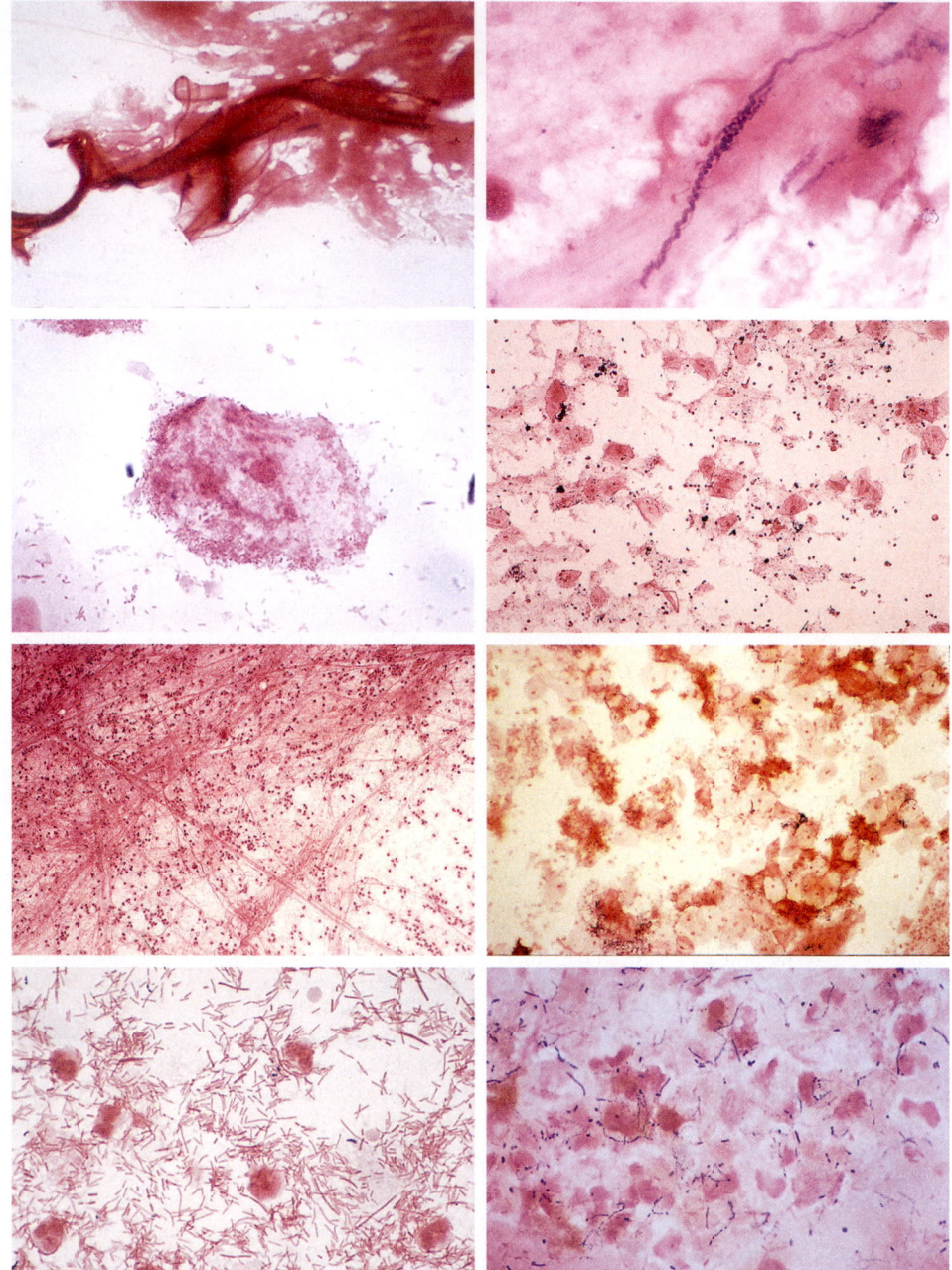

FIGURE 1 (row 1, left)   Gram stain (×100) of surgical wound showing elastin fibers.
FIGURE 2 (row 1, right)   Gram stain (×1,000) of sputum showing Curschman's spirals.
FIGURE 3 (row 2, left)   Gram stain (×1,000) of vaginal secretions showing clue cells.
FIGURE 4 (row 2, right)   Gram stain (×100) of unacceptable sputum specimen (grossly contaminated with members of the oropharyngeal microbiota) showing >10 squamous epithelial cells per low-power field.
FIGURE 5 (row 3, left)   Gram stain (×100) of acceptable sputum specimen showing <10 squamous epithelial cells per low-power field.
FIGURE 6 (row 3, right)   Gram stain (×100) of urine showing 4+ squamous epithelial cells, indicating gross contamination with vaginal or periurethral secretions and bacteria.
FIGURE 7 (row 4, left)   Gram stain (×1,000) of urine showing polymorphonuclear leukocytes and 4+ gram-negative bacilli.
FIGURE 8 (row 4, right)   Gram stain (×1,000) of a wound showing polymorphonuclear leukocytes, mixed bacterial morphotypes suggesting aerobic and anaerobic bacteria, and both intra- and extracellular bacteria. This appearance suggests a mixed aerobic and anaerobic abscess or closed-space infection.

the sample. If possible, specimens should be stored in a refrigerator or ultracold freezer. A minimum of 5 days is recommended.

Culture Examination and Interpretation

Once colonies have grown on agar culture plates, microbiologists must differentiate potential pathogens requiring identification and antimicrobial testing from contaminants that represent members of the normal microbiota. Aids to interpretation are the relative quantities of each isolate, correlating culture results with Gram-stained smear results, and recognizing usual contaminants and pathogens from respective specimen sites. In general, when examining cultures of specimens from sites adjacent to normally colonized mucosae (e.g., sputum, urine, or superficial wounds), potential pathogens should outnumber indigenous members of the microbiota and should be seen in the direct Gram stain (207). When examining cultures of specimens from presumably sterile sites (e.g., CSF, joint fluids, other body fluids, and deep tissue), potential pathogens occur in any quantity and may or may not be seen in the direct Gram-stained smear. Specific criteria for identifying potentially significant isolates and contaminating members of the normal microbiota are addressed in the following sections of this chapter. It is a useful policy to save culture plates with significant growth for 1 week, allowing caregivers the opportunity to call to request further identification or additional antimicrobial testing when clinically indicated.

Specimens Received for Molecular Detection of Bacteria

Although blood has not yet been used widely for detection of bacteria using nucleic acid amplification (NAA) tests or hybridization, such tests are in development. Whole blood can be collected in EDTA tubes, in specially formulated acid-citrate vacuum tubes, or in other specialized tubes developed for NAA tests. In cases in which plasma is the specimen for testing, removal of the liquid component from the red blood cells as quickly as possible will enhance test results.

Tissue should be collected aseptically and submitted in a sterile container. Tissue is usually treated in some way to dissolve the matrix and release the nucleic acid contents of the microbe being sought; often this is done on an automated extraction instrument. If >24 h will pass before the test can be performed, tissue should be frozen at −70°C and transported to the laboratory on dry ice to prevent thawing. For some samples, such as nasopharyngeal swabs and aspirates for *Bordetella pertussis* or oropharyngeal swabs for *Mycoplasma pneumoniae*, transport on ice is recommended. Special swabs with proprietary transport media or regular urine (the first 20 ml) are often sent for molecular detection of *Neisseria gonorrhoeae* and *Chlamydia trachomatis*. The transport system should be specific for the type of test. Recommended procedures and transport systems vary widely depending on the laboratory and the test system employed.

Reporting Results

"No growth"- and "normal microbiota"-type reports can be safely entered into a laboratory information system for routine reporting to be seen by the caregiver whenever the caregiver chooses to look. But reports that are important enough to result in a possible change of management or complex enough to require person-to-person discussion should be telephoned directly to a caregiver. In the case of acid-fast and fungal cultures, reports are often available days or weeks after the sample was received. Since the physician may no longer be actively following the case, it is especially important to telephone those results. Critical values, those that are immediately life threatening, require the recipient of the call to write the result down and read it back to the caller. Each institution must develop its own critical-call procedure. Examples of critical values in bacteriology might include a positive CSF Gram stain, results suggestive of gas gangrene, a bioterrorism-related isolate, or a positive blood culture. Many microbiology results, including detection of a sexually transmitted infectious agent, detection of M. *tuberculosis*, or detection of a multidrug-resistant bacterium, should also be called to infection control personnel and/or local public health officials.

SPECIAL CONSIDERATIONS BASED ON SPECIFIC SPECIMEN TYPES (ALSO SEE TABLE 8)

Tissue Biopsy Samples

Tissue from a sterile site is usually obtained during a surgical procedure. Because this is among the most difficult and important specimens to get, it should be handled with utmost care and the surgeon should obtain a sufficient volume for all possible tests, including histopathology and various microbiological studies. A 1-cm^3 piece should suffice for any microbiology requests. This is difficult with fine-needle aspirates and biopsy samples, which usually are minuscule. Tissue should be transported in a sterile container that maintains moisture. To avoid drying, small pieces of tissue can be moistened with a few drops of sterile, nonbacteriostatic saline. Alternatively, very small pieces of tissue can be placed on a square of moistened sterile gauze. This serves to maintain moisture and allow easy identification by those receiving and processing the specimen. Large pieces of tissue, approximately 1 cm^3 or greater, maintain a reduced atmosphere in spite of brief aerobic transport. Oxygen-free transport may not be necessary in this circumstance, and the absence of anaerobic transport should not disqualify large pieces of tissue from anaerobic culture.

The laboratory may require the caregiver to prioritize the tests, as the volume will not be enough if several tests are ordered. The material can be emulsified and diluted in saline or broth, but that will compromise the sensitivity of any studies. Tissue is presumed to be uncontaminated by external or luminal microbes, but this is not always the case. Coagulase-negative staphylococci and *P. acnes* are particularly problematic in orthopedics, because they can cause slow, chronic infections in prosthetic joints and bones, sometimes manifesting years after placement of the prosthesis. A method to help the laboratory differentiate between contamination and true infection, especially useful for orthopedic joint prosthesis revision surgeries, is to collect as many as five separate pieces of tissue from different areas within the same surgical site. The laboratory should perform minimal processing of all five samples sufficient to detect staphylococci and propionibacteria in addition to complete processing of one sample as ordered by the physician. If three or more samples from the same general surgical field yield the same organism in culture, the organism is likely to be an etiological agent in that joint and not a contaminant (10, 149, 243). If anaerobic cultures are requested, the tissue must be transported in an anaerobic transport tube or vial, some versions of which maintain anaerobes extremely well even during overnight shipping (17). The same tissue can also be used for all other

TABLE 8   Usual etiologies of selected infectious disease syndromes

Disease	Etiologies
Central nervous system infection	
Acute meningitis, neutrophilic pleocytosis	*Streptococcus pneumoniae, Neisseria meningitidis, Listeria monocytogenes, Streptococcus agalactiae, Haemophilus influenzae, Staphylococcus aureus,* gram-negative rods,[a] *Bacillus anthracis*
Acute meningitis, CSF shunt related	Coagulase-negative staphylococci, *Staphylococcus aureus, Propionibacterium* spp., gram-negative enteric rods (e.g., *E. coli* and *Klebsiella* spp.), gram-negative nonfermenting rods (e.g., *P. aeruginosa* and *Acinetobacter* spp.)
Chronic meningitis, predominantly lymphocytic pleocytosis	*Nocardia* species, *Brucella* species, *Leptospira interrogans, Mycobacterium tuberculosis, Treponema pallidum, Borrelia burgdorferi*
Gastrointestinal tract infection	
Infectious diarrhea[b]	*Salmonella* serotypes; *Shigella* spp.; *Campylobacter jejuni; Campylobacter coli;* other *Campylobacter* spp.; *C. difficile; Vibrio* spp.; *Aeromonas* spp.; *Plesiomonas shigelloides; Y. enterocolitica; E. coli* toxigenic, invasive, and effacing strains; *Listeria monocytogenes* (possibly); *C. perfringens; B. cereus*
Ingestion of preformed toxin[c]	*S. aureus, B. cereus, C. botulinum*
Gastritis, gastric and duodenal ulcers	*Helicobacter pylori*
Genital tract infection	
Ulcers	*T. pallidum, H. ducreyi, C. trachomatis* (LGV), *Klebsiella granulomatis*
Urethritis	*N. gonorrhoeae, C. trachomatis*
Vulvovaginitis	*N. gonorrhoeae* and *C. trachomatis* in prepubescent girls
BV	Overgrowth of the vaginal biota with anaerobic bacteria and *Gardnerella vaginalis*
Cervicitis	*N. gonorrhoeae, C. trachomatis*
Endometritis	*Enterobacteriaceae,* streptococci (groups A and B), enterococci, mixed anaerobic genera
Salpingitis, oophoritis	*N. gonorrhoeae, C. trachomatis,* mixed aerobic and anaerobic microbiotas
Pelvic abscess	Mixed aerobic and anaerobic microbiotas
Epididymitis	*N. gonorrhoeae, C. trachomatis, Enterobacteriaceae, P. aeruginosa,* various gram-positive cocci
Ocular infections	
Conjunctivitis	*S. pneumoniae, S. aureus, H. influenzae, N. meningitidis, N. gonorrhoeae, C. trachomatis* (inclusion conjunctivitis), *C. trachomatis* (trachoma), others[d]
Keratitis	*S. aureus, S. pneumoniae, P. aeruginosa,* enterococci, *S. pyogenes* (group A), *Enterobacteriaceae, Pasteurella multocida,* coagulase-negative staphylococci (postsurgery), *Propionibacterium acnes* (especially postsurgery), others[e]
Endophthalmitis	*S. aureus, P. aeruginosa, P. acnes, S. pneumoniae, N. meningitidis, Nocardia* spp.
Periorbital cellulitis	*S. aureus, S. pyogenes* (group A), *S. pneumoniae, H. influenzae, Clostridium* spp.
Otitis	
Otitis externa	*S. aureus, S. pyogenes* (group A), *P. aeruginosa, Vibrio alginolyticus*
Otitis media	*S. pneumoniae, H. influenzae, Moraxella catarrhalis, S. aureus,* rare pathogens: gram-negative rods, anaerobes, aerobic actinomycetes
Respiratory tract infection	
Tracheitis, intubated patient	*Enterobacteriaceae, S. aureus, P. aeruginosa,* other nonfermenting gram-negative rods
Bronchitis, community acquired	*S. pneumoniae, H. influenzae* (rarely, other *Haemophilus* species), *M. catarrhalis, S. aureus, Chlamydophila pneumoniae, M. pneumoniae, B. pertussis, S. pyogenes* (group A); less commonly, same as hospital acquired
Bronchitis, hospital acquired	*Enterobacteriaceae, S. aureus, P. aeruginosa,* other nonfermenting gram-negative rods; less commonly, same as community acquired
Pneumonia, community acquired	*S. pneumoniae, H. influenzae, M. catarrhalis, Chlamydophila pneumoniae, M. pneumoniae, L. pneumophila, Nocardia* spp., *P. multocida,* aspiration (anaerobes); less commonly, same as hospital acquired
Pneumonia, hospital acquired	*Enterobacteriaceae, S. aureus, P. aeruginosa, L. pneumophila,* other nonfermenting gram-negative rods; aspiration (anaerobes); less commonly, same as community acquired
Lung abscess	*S. aureus, Klebsiella pneumoniae, P. aeruginosa, S. pyogenes* (group A), anaerobes (aspiration pneumonia), *Nocardia* spp.
Empyema	*S. pneumoniae;* anaerobes; viridans group streptococci, especially *Streptococcus anginosus* group; *S. aureus; S. pyogenes* (group A); gram-negative rods
Osteomyelitis	*Staphylococcus aureus, Mycobacterium tuberculosis, Pseudomonas aeruginosa,* other organisms depending on site

(Continued on next page)

TABLE 8 Usual etiologies of selected infectious disease syndromes (*Continued*)

Disease	Etiologies
Urinary tract infection	
Prostatitis	*Enterobacteriaceae*, *P. aeruginosa*, enterococci
Urethral syndrome	Same as cystitis, but in lower numbers; *C. trachomatis/N. gonorrhoeae*; unknown, negative culture (about 15% of this disease group)
Cystitis	*Enterobacteriaceae*, especially *E. coli*; enterococci; *Staphylococcus saprophyticus* (women of childbearing age); nonfermenting gram-negative rods; *Corynebacterium urealyticum* (patients with underlying urinary tract pathology)
Pyelonephritis	*Enterobacteriaceae*; enterococci; agents of bacteremia (descending infection), e.g., *S. aureus*

[a] Gram-negative rods, including *Enterobacteriaceae*, *P. aeruginosa*, other nonfermenting gram-negative rods.
[b] Disease caused by ingestion of bacteria followed by tissue invasion, toxin production, or other pathogenic mechanism.
[c] Disease caused by ingestion of preformed toxin.
[d] *C. diphtheriae*, *M. tuberculosis*, *F. tularensis*, *T. pallidum*, *B. henselae* (cat scratch), *P. multocida*, *Bacillus thuringiensis*, *Moraxella lacunata*.
[e] *T. pallidum*, *N. gonorrhoeae*, *Moraxella* spp., *C. diphtheriae*, *Bacillus* spp., anaerobes, nontuberculous mycobacteria.

microbiological assays, as anaerobic transport vials are universal transport devices.

Cultures growing small numbers of bacteria not commonly associated with infection, such as coagulase-negative staphylococci, corynebacteria, propionibacteria, and saprophytic *Neisseria* spp., may represent contamination rather than true pathogens. One or two bacterial colonies growing on a single plate, of multiple plates inoculated, and not growing in broth culture, if used, generally represent contamination. Growth of one or two bacterial colonies on agar media not in the area of specimen inoculation or on streak lines in the second through fourth plate quadrants also is likely to represent contamination. In addition, bacteria considered contaminants are not detected in original Gram-stained smears. On the other hand, detection of the bacteria listed above as unlikely pathogens should always be reported when seen in the original Gram-stained smear, when present in quantities above a few colonies, and when detected on or in multiple media (56).

Bone Marrow Transport and Culture

Bone marrow aspirates can be submitted for culture in lysis centrifugation tubes (Wampole Isolator; Inverness Medical, Princeton, NJ). The "pediatric" tube holds a maximum of 1.5 ml of specimen. One or more of the 1.5-ml tubes can be used. Aspirates may also be submitted in a sterile container containing anticoagulant. Sterile tubes with anticoagulant are less desirable since they use heparin, sodium citrate, or EDTA as an anticoagulant, all of which are more inhibitory than SPS (67, 192). Although SPS inhibits meningococci, gonococci, *Gardnerella vaginalis*, anaerobic cocci, and *Streptobacillus moniliformis*, these bacteria are unlikely to be detected in bone marrow aspirate specimens (185).

Although bone marrow aspirate cultures may be helpful in identifying disseminated fungal and mycobacterial diseases, they are unlikely to assist in the identification of usual bacterial diseases (241). It is policy in some laboratories to consult with the ordering physician and suggest that routine bacterial culture is not necessary. In most cases, blood or other organ system culture is preferred for the identification of disseminated bacterial infections. Even if bone marrow culture is performed, direct Gram stain of bone marrow aspirates is not helpful and should not be a routine component of bacterial culture.

Lymph Nodes

Aspirates and biopsy samples from lymph nodes are usually sent to the laboratory for detection of nonbacterial infectious agents. However, studies of lymph nodes from patients with cat scratch disease, plague (*Yersinia pestis*), brucellosis, or tularemia (*Francisella tularensis*) can be fruitful. Initial handling of the tissue itself and of the culture plates, whether showing growth or not, should be done with extreme care and employing all safety practices. Plates should be taped on both sides to allow circulation of atmosphere but not allow accidental opening. Manipulations of any colonies should be done with full biosafety standards employed until a highly virulent pathogen has been ruled out (also see chapter 12).

Necrotizing Fasciitis

Necrotizing fasciitis and gas gangrene (myonecrosis) are medical emergencies requiring immediate diagnosis and therapy that may include antimicrobials, surgical debridement, and the use of immunoglobulin and immunomediators to combat the fatal complications of severe septic shock (50, 161). Necrotizing fasciitis and gas gangrene are caused most commonly by toxin-producing *S. pyogenes*, other beta-hemolytic streptococci, *S. aureus*, *Clostridium* spp., and mixed aerobic and anaerobic bacteria (66, 219). Gram-stained smears generally show proteinaceous fluid, necrotic cell debris, rare or few polymorphonuclear leukocytes (because of cell lysis), and the bacterial etiology. Culture should confirm the etiology and provide antimicrobial testing results where appropriate.

Cellulitis

Several studies have shown that aspirates from the leading edge of areas of cellulitis are not particularly fruitful. Injection of nonbacteriostatic saline and subsequent aspiration may be necessary to obtain enough material to culture (30, 131). Under the best of conditions, these specimens are unlikely to be positive (84). Blood cultures from patients with cellulitis also are unlikely to be positive (172). Tissue biopsy may be required if microbiological testing is deemed crucial for a rapidly progressing lesion.

Uncultivable Bacteria in Tissues

Some bacterial infections in tissue cannot be cultivated in vitro using standard microbiological media. These include tissue stages of syphilis caused by *Treponema pallidum*, donovanosis caused by *Klebsiella* (formerly *Calymmatobacterium*) *granulomatis*, rat-bite fever caused by *Spirillum minus*, and others. The organisms may be visualized by histopathological stains. Newer molecular technologies are proving to be most reliable, especially for organisms causing genital ulcer disease (34, 132). The use of universal primer PCR to identify bacteria seen in tissue sections by histology, including *Tropheryma whipplei*, *Coxiella burnetii*, and *Bartonella henselae*, is gaining widespread favor (123). Additional discussion can be found in chapter 46.

Placenta for Agents of BV

Placentas are sent to microbiology to determine the etiology of a preterm birth or if the obstetrician suspects an infection. A piece of tissue from the chorionic layer below the amnion should be obtained in an anaerobic transport vial. If the intact placenta is received in the laboratory, the top layer (amnion) of the placenta is cut using sterile scissors, and sterile forceps are used to pull it away from the underlying chorionic layer. Sterile scalpel or another sterile scissors is used to cut a small piece of the freshly exposed chorionic tissue for aerobic and anaerobic culture, and occasionally a piece can be placed into 2SP or SP4 transport medium for *Mycoplasma* or *Ureaplasma* culture. Molecular methods have not been productive (167). Chapter 59 has more information on detection of mycoplasmas.

Quantitative Culture

Tissue from traumatic wound or burn injury may be submitted for quantitative culture, with results of $\geq 10^5$ CFU/ml being used to predict the likelihood of development of wound-related sepsis (140, 233). Limitations include the lack of reproducible results and the low predictive value compared to histologic examination of tissue (256). Swab cultures have been shown to correlate poorly with the biopsy culture results. Full-thickness punch biopsy samples should be collected for this process. To perform a quantitative culture, a portion of the specimen is weighed and homogenized in saline. The saline suspension is used to prepare serial dilutions for culture. Detailed procedures for quantitative tissue culture are given elsewhere (262).

Blood Cultures

Detection of bacteria and fungi circulating in the bloodstream is a major function of the microbiology laboratory (18, 253). Key factors in obtaining optimal samples are thorough disinfection of the skin surface or the catheter port through which the blood will be obtained, an adequate volume of blood removed, and the appropriate timing of when to draw the blood. Blood obtained through an indwelling intravenous line is twice as likely to contain a surface organism contaminant, leading to a false-positive culture result, as is blood obtained through a peripheral skin site (68). It is important to recognize potential contaminants that grow, since treating contaminants as significant isolates is associated with unnecessary expense and dangers of antimicrobial misuse (68, 200, 247). Common contaminants include coagulase-negative staphylococci, corynebacteria, *Bacillus* spp., and propionibacteria. In general, single cultures positive for these bacteria represent contamination. Multiple, separate cultures growing one of these isolates are more likely to indicate a clinically significant bacteremia (18). Careful site preparation using 70% ethanol and chlorhexidine is critical to avoiding drawing up those contaminants, primarily coagulase-negative staphylococci (200, 231). For patients for whom chlorhexidine is contraindicated, either tincture of iodine or betadine can be used after alcohol disinfection (231). All skin disinfectants are activated as they go from wet to dry on the skin surface, so a waiting period of 30 s (chlorhexidine) to 1 min (betadine) is necessary after application before the needle is inserted. Contamination rates of less than 2 to 3% are desired (200). Higher rates should be investigated and corrected by educational efforts (186).

Another factor that aids the laboratory in interpreting blood culture results is obtaining two separate blood culture sets from two separate sites (18). Especially if one set of samples has been obtained via a central or peripheral intravenous line, the second set should be drawn through well-prepared intact skin. Skin organisms involved in true sepsis should be recovered from both sites. Some hospital laboratories have a standard policy that blood culture orders always involve obtaining blood from two separate sites and injecting at least two separate bottles. Recovery of all organisms is enhanced if two types of media are used. Most often, laboratories choose one aerobic and one anaerobic broth and atmosphere formulation (97). Even though the numbers of septicemias caused by strictly anaerobic bacteria are relatively low, the anaerobic medium can improve recovery of other facultative anaerobic bacteria as well and provides another opportunity to recover a greater range of bacteria. In addition, failure to detect an anaerobe can have serious consequences, as empirical therapy may not be adequate (23).

Culture of intravascular catheter tips is controversial for determining the source of a bacteremia because by the time the culture result is obtained, the catheter (if it was the source) has already been removed. These cultures should be performed by special request only, and only when concurrent blood cultures are obtained. The most common technique used to culture the exterior of the intravascular portion of a catheter is the semiquantitative method in which the 5-cm distal portion of the catheter is rolled across a blood agar plate four times (133). The catheter tip is discarded. Growth of more than 15 colonies is considered to be significant, i.e., implicating the catheter tip as the likely source of a bacteremia caused by the same organism as simultaneously isolated from blood cultures. Interpretation of clinical importance is not possible without an accompanying positive blood culture. Soft tissue infections around a catheter insertion site should be cultured as a wound specimen using freshly expressed purulence that can be aspirated.

Recently, some laboratories have adopted a method for determining if the indwelling intravenous (usually central) line is the source of a bacteremia that takes into account the relative numbers of organisms obtained in an identical volume of blood from first the peripheral site and then another blood culture set obtained immediately through the line (182). Because many intravenous lines are removed unnecessarily, this method can preserve those lines not considered colonized, as determined by a higher ratio of organisms recovered in the blood obtained through the line than that obtained peripherally. The organisms can be counted directly using Wampole Isolator tubes, a lysis-centrifugation system that allows plating of the sediment of lysed blood containing all the organisms so that actual CFU can be counted and the original CFU per milliliter of blood can be calculated (202). Alternatively, the time to positivity can be determined in an automated blood culture system, with the assumption that a faster time to a positive flag in the instrument, more than 2 h before the peripheral blood culture flags positive, relates to a higher original number of organisms in the culture and thus a colonized line requiring removal (202).

The Isolator system is additionally utilized to recover fastidious organisms or those that do not multiply well in standard blood culture broth formulations or atmospheres. If specialized broth/atmospheres available for recovery of fungi and mycobacteria are not used routinely, laboratories should stock a supply of Isolator tubes and the centrifuge and capping instruments required to use the Isolator tubes. Because the white blood cells are lysed, intracellular organisms are released and better able to grow in cultures. The sediment containing the organisms can be inoculated onto any number of specialized media to enhance recovery. Infectious agents best recovered by the Isolator system include filamentous or dimorphic fungi (*Fusarium* and *Histoplasma capsulatum* are examples), *Legionella*, some yeasts (*Cryptococcus* and yeasts from patients on antifungal therapy), *Bartonella* species, some *N. meningitidis* strains, *N. gonorrhoeae*, and other fastidious organisms that fail to grow in routine blood culture media or that fail to produce sufficient metabolites to trigger the detection system of an automated blood culture instrument. The Isolator system does not perform as well as other systems when recovering *Streptococcus pneumoniae*, other streptococci, *Pseudomonas aeruginosa*, and anaerobes (246). Advantages of the Isolator system are the ability to inoculate the pellet to specific agar media when attempting to detect unusual etiologies of bacteremia, such as those caused by *Legionella pneumophila*, *Franciscella tularensis*, and *Bartonella* spp., and to provide colony counts, reported as CFU per milliliter of blood (40, 246). Disadvantages of the system are the labor involved with initial processing and the potential for increased contamination that accompanies manipulation during processing (227).

Total volume of blood cultured is the major factor for identifying true positive patients. For an adult, the most sensitive recovery requires at least 40 ml of blood (42, 97). This is a small percentage of total blood volume. Yields from 20 and 30 ml of blood were 29.8 and 47.2% greater, respectively, than those from 10 ml of blood; yields from 40 ml were 7.2% greater than from 30 ml (42). In fact, more blood can and should be obtained from all patients than is currently practiced. Table 9 shows recommended blood culture volumes based on the weight of the patient and the corresponding percentage of the patient's total blood volume (108). Blood should be collected as quickly as possible after the culture is ordered and before antibiotics are given, if possible, and all the blood can be obtained at the same time (from different sites) (42, 118, 125).

For automated blood culture systems, the standard 5-day protocol is sufficient to recover all the usual pathogens, and holding bottles for additional incubation time only increases the numbers of contaminants recovered (16, 178).

For patients with suspected bloodstream infections that fail to yield a pathogen with standard blood culture protocols, either the Isolator tube should be employed for culture or serological or molecular methods (which may not be available) must be attempted (18). However, blind subculture may be needed if the patient is receiving antimicrobials at the time of blood collection, particularly for recovery of yeasts (16, 178).

In most cases, timing of the blood culture with respect to the maximum temperature recorded for the patient during a febrile episode is less important than the total volume cultured. This has been reinforced by results of a multicenter study (187). Although there was a slight benefit for patients <30 years old for blood cultures to be obtained >1 h after the maximum temperature, this was not seen with other age groups, and in general, only 10% of positive blood cultures were actually drawn at the time of the patient's peak temperature.

Semiautomated blood culture systems are present in nearly every clinical laboratory. Refer to chapter 3 for a complete discussion of manual and automated blood culture systems. The anticoagulant used in all blood culture systems is SPS and is known to be inhibitory to meningococci, gonococci, *Peptostreptococcus anaerobius*, *Streptobacillus moniliformis*, and *Gardnerella vaginalis* (185), for which other methods of detection should be employed.

Positive blood culture bottles are evaluated initially by examining a Gram-stained smear of the broth. The report should include a description of the bacterial morphology and the Gram reaction. If a presumptive identification of the microorganism can be made, it may be added to the report. For example, a blood culture Gram stain report might state "gram-positive cocci in clusters suggesting staphylococci." Specimens in positive blood culture bottles should be subcultured to media based on the organism seen in the Gram-stained smear. In addition, since 5 to 10% of all bacteremias are polymicrobial (contain more than one bacterial type), additional media are recommended. Anaerobic media and culture conditions should be used if the morphology of the organism seen in the Gram-stained smear is suggestive of an anaerobic bacterium or if the organism is recovered from an anaerobic culture bottle only. If a positively flagged bottle shows no organisms on Gram stain, a second smear should be prepared and stained using acridine orange, a DNA stain (93). If organisms are present, even if they have damaged or no cell walls, they will stain bright orange and can be recognized more easily (103).

Occasionally, direct staining of blood collected by venipuncture can provide rapid, nearly immediate detection of bacteria in blood (190). Gram staining a smear of peripheral

TABLE 9 Recommended blood volumes to obtain for blood cultures[a]

Patient wt (lb)	Recommended blood vol per culture (ml)	Total blood vol for two cultures (ml)	Vol of blood equal to 1% of patient's total blood vol (ml)[b]
<18	1	2	2
18–30	3	6	6–10
30–60	5	10	10–20
60–90	10	20	20–30
90–120	15	30	30–40
>120	20	40	>40

[a]Data from reference 108.
[b]Blood volume calculated by assuming 85 ml/kg in newborns and 73 ml/kg in other patients. Two 20-ml blood specimens collected from an 80-kg adult (40 ml total) represent approximately 0.7% of the patient's total blood volume.

blood or buffy coat layer may detect bacterial cells in the blood of patients with meningococcemia, S. pneumoniae infection, or overwhelming sepsis caused by other bacteria when the bacterial concentration in blood is very high (approaching 10,000 bacterial cells per ml of blood). In spite of published reports documenting the occasional use of direct staining of blood, the likelihood of results affecting patient management does not warrant use as a routine laboratory procedure.

Diagnosis of leptospirosis may prompt a special blood culture request (see below). Recent studies used 0.1 ml of heparinized whole blood or 0.2 ml from high-speed-centrifuged plasma sediment inoculated into Ellinghausen-McCullough-Johnson-Harris medium and incubated from a minimum of 1 month to up to 3 months (258).

Cerebrospinal Fluid

CSF is collected for the diagnosis of meningitis (87). Bacterial meningitis can be divided into acute and chronic clinical presentations (226). Acute meningitis with onset of symptoms within the previous 24 h is usually caused by pyogenic bacteria. Specific etiologies are related to age of the patient and whether the disease is community or nosocomially acquired. Chronic meningitis, with symptoms lasting at least 4 weeks, can have a wide variety of causes (Table 8). As with all clinical specimens, even those collected from a presumably sterile site, growth of contaminants occasionally does occur. The first tube collected by lumbar puncture, most likely to have a few skin organisms introduced during the procedure, should be used for chemistry tests; the second or third tube, less likely to contain the rare contaminant, should be used for microbiology studies.

CSF is usually obtained by lumbar puncture. Although bacterial stain and culture can be performed with as little as 0.5 ml of fluid, larger volumes are preferred since culture methods are more sensitive when low numbers of bacteria are concentrated by centrifugation before culture. A minimum of 5.0 ml and high-speed (3,000 × g) centrifugation are recommended for recovery of Mycobacterium tuberculosis, although the yield may still be low (14). Filtration through a 0.45-μm-pore-size filter results in better concentration of M. tuberculosis in CSF. Specimens should be transported to the laboratory immediately in a sterile container maintained at room temperature. All smears should be prepared by cytocentrifugation (173), and cultures should be inoculated with 0.5 ml of CSF or sediment resuspended in 0.5 ml of CSF following centrifugation (1,500 × g for 15 min) when >1 ml of fluid is received. Media are inoculated in accordance with recommendations in Table 7. Broth enrichment should not be used routinely. PCR has not been widely used for the diagnosis of tuberculous meningitis (168, 229); however, a commercially available probe amplification technology has been reported to be sensitive and specific (39). Anaerobes are rarely found in CSF, even in cases of mixed anaerobic abscess of brain tissue. However, anaerobic incubation of CSF is necessary to recover microaerophilic streptococci that cause infection after trigeminal nerve injection. Propionibacterium acnes may be the cause of infection in patients with indwelling CSF shunts, hence the recommendation to inoculate an anaerobic broth such as thioglycolate or chopped meat carbohydrate with an aliquot of shunt fluid (142, 220).

Smears should be Gram stained and results reported to the physician immediately. Results should include a description and semiquantitative enumeration of polymorphonuclear inflammatory cells and bacterial morphology. If the results are suggestive of a bacterial group, this, too, can be communicated. Because of low sensitivity and lack of effect on the care and management of patients, and because the cost of antigen testing is much higher than the cost of the Gram stain, direct antigen tests should be considered only when direct communication with the clinical service documents a specific need, such as prior antimicrobial therapy (141, 171). Direct NAA of panbacterial DNA from CSF will likely completely replace the residual antigen tests very soon. Leptospires can be detected in CSF during the first 10 days of acute illness. CSF should be collected before initiation of antimicrobial therapy and while the patient is febrile. Direct detection of leptospires by dark-field examination of CSF is not recommended. CSF should be inoculated into Ellinghausen-McCullough-Johnson-Harris medium. An inoculum of 0.5 ml is recommended. Cultures should be incubated at room temperature for up to 13 weeks (54) (see chapter 55).

Eyes

Several types of specimens may be collected for the microbiological analysis of eye infections, including conjunctival scrapings obtained with a swab or sterile spatula for the diagnosis of conjunctivitis, corneal scrapings collected with a sterile spatula for the diagnosis of keratitis, vitreous fluid collected by aspiration for the diagnosis of endophthalmitis, and fluid material collected by aspiration or tissue biopsy for the diagnosis of periorbital cellulitis (250). Pathogenic bacteria potentially present in these anatomic sites are listed in Table 8 (88). Because the volume of specimen collected from corneal scrapings and vitreous fluid aspiration is very small, direct inoculation of agar culture plates and preparation of smears in the clinic or at the bedside is recommended (250). A close working association is needed between the laboratory and ophthalmologist to ensure a supply of appropriate culture media, correct technique for inoculation of media, and rapid transport of plates and smears to the laboratory. Media should be inoculated by rubbing the specimen onto a small area of the agar plates (swab) or wiping the material from the scraping off the spatula gently onto the agar surface, sometimes in the shapes of little C's. Plates are placed directly into the incubator without cross-streaking by laboratory personnel. This allows the plate reader to detect more easily airborne contaminants that settle on the plate during inoculation procedures that occur outside controlled laboratory conditions.

Media needed for the detection of usual pathogens should include chocolate agar for fastidious bacteria (Table 7). Media for other microorganisms (fungi, viruses, mycobacteria, etc.) should be inoculated if deemed appropriate by the ophthalmologist and microbiologist and specifically ordered. Incubation at 35 to 37°C in 3 to 5% CO_2 is necessary.

Chlamydia trachomatis in Eyes

Examination of conjunctival smears using direct fluorescent antibody (DFA) staining with fluorescein-conjugated monoclonal antibodies and detection of chlamydial nucleic acid (NAA) in conjunctival scrapings are useful in the diagnosis of inclusion conjunctivitis or trachoma (115, 261). A less sensitive but readily available method is examination of Giemsa-stained conjunctival smears for intracytoplasmic, perinuclear inclusions within epithelial cells (155). Cell culture for the isolation of C. trachomatis is sensitive but more time-consuming and technically demanding than DFA or NAA (211). Conjunctival scrapings and secretions for culture should be transported in 2SP medium (sucrose phosphate or sucrose phosphate glutamate) with bovine serum and antimicrobials (usually gentamicin, vancomycin, and nystatin or amphotericin B). Swabs with wooden shafts should be avoided, since constituents of the wood are toxic to chlamydiae. Specimens for culture should be refrigerated during short delays or stored at −70°C for delays longer than 48 h. Molecular probes and PCR methods are available for the detection of *C. trachomatis* but are not FDA cleared at this time for eye specimens (115, 261).

Ears

Nasopharyngeal cultures have poor predictability for detection of middle ear pathogens and should not be used for that purpose (64). Two types of ear specimens are received most commonly by the laboratory: swab specimens for the diagnosis of otitis externa and middle ear fluid specimens for the diagnosis of otitis media (Table 8). Potential pathogens at these two sites differ (197). Since anaerobic bacteria may be involved in middle ear infections (albeit rarely), anaerobic culture should be performed on properly collected aspirates that are transported in anaerobic transport vials. Direct examination of Gram-stained smears of middle ear fluid is helpful and is recommended with all culture requests.

External ear specimens may be contaminated with normal members of the microbiota of the skin or ear canal. Isolates of coagulase-negative staphylococci, diphtheroids, and viridans group streptococci may be listed as presumptive identifications without including results of antimicrobial testing. Even *Staphylococcus aureus* is often recovered from patients without infection, so the presence of inflammation should be used to help guide the extent of workup. It is a useful policy to save the culture plates for 1 week, allowing physicians the opportunity to call to request further identification or antimicrobial testing when clinically indicated. Middle ear fluid is less likely to be contaminated. All isolates should be reported and, if requested, antimicrobial testing performed on strains with unpredictable susceptibility to antimicrobials.

Genital Discharge, Exudates, and Lesions

Bacterial infections of genital tract sites produce various clinical syndromes, including vulvovaginitis, BV, genital ulcers, urethritis, cervicitis, endometritis, salpingitis, and ovarian abscess in females and urethritis, epididymitis, prostatitis, and genital ulcers in males. These diseases and their etiologies are listed in Table 8.

Many specimens are contaminated with members of the normal microbiota of the skin or mucous membrane. Pathogens such as *Haemophilus ducreyi*, *Neisseria gonorrhoeae*, *Trichomonas vaginalis*, *Treponema pallidum*, and *Chlamydia trachomatis* are always significant. Other organisms such as *S. aureus*, beta-hemolytic streptococci, *Enterobacteriaceae*, and anaerobes are pathogenic only in certain clinical situations. The specimen source, relative quantity of potential pathogen compared to members of the normal microbiota, and Gram stain interpretation help the technologist determine which isolates require identification and antimicrobial testing. At a minimum, isolates from presumably sterile specimens and pure or predominant potential pathogens from specimens likely to be contaminated with members of the normal microbiota and containing polymorphonuclear neutrophils should be identified and reported. Mixtures of anaerobes do not require individual identification and listing in most cases. Laboratories should avoid isolating, identifying, and

performing antimicrobial testing on every bacterial isolate from all specimens (15). In addition to the excessive cost of this approach, unnecessary reporting of bacterial species contributes to excessive treatment of patients. Exact protocols for workup and reporting may require discussion and mutual agreement with knowledgeable clinicians in each practice environment.

Detection of *N. gonorrhoeae* and *C. trachomatis*

NAA methods are the state of the art for detection of *N. gonorrhoeae* and *C. trachomatis* in endocervical, urethral, and urine specimens. Users must pay close attention to the types of specimens approved for use with each kit. Specimens should be collected and transported using the procedures and devices recommended by the manufacturer. In addition, false-positive and false-negative reactions have been reported with some kits, particularly when nonvalidated sample types are tested, necessitating confirmation of positive results for those test systems that do not include an internal validation. Aptima 2 does include an internal validation (Gen-Probe, San Diego, CA) (122, 137).

Although eye, rectal, oropharyngeal, and abscess specimens are not FDA cleared for testing in the commercial amplification systems, molecular amplification is still the best method (199). In fact, self-collected swabs submitted by both men and women perform at least as well as those collected by health care workers in the molecular tests for *Chlamydia* and *N. gonorrhoeae* (205). At this time, culture is still the only acceptable diagnostic procedure in some jurisdictions for medical-legal cases, but that should be changing soon (22).

Culture for *N. gonorrhoeae* is optimal when the specimen is directly inoculated to a selective medium, such as modified Thayer-Martin medium, and incubated immediately (8). Swab specimens (cotton swabs should be avoided because they may be toxic) should be placed in a transport system containing Stuart's or Amies medium and delivered to the laboratory as quickly as possible. Some newer products have shown good ability to retain the viability of *N. gonorrhoeae* (189, 237). Specimens for *N. gonorrhoeae* culture should be held at refrigeration temperature during transport (8, 189). As transport time increases, recovery by culture decreases. Specimens requiring more than 24 h for transport are unacceptable. Recent publications have shown that for specimens from ocular, pharyngeal, or anal sites, molecular methods are far superior to culture (199, 261). In fact, one system outperformed other methods. Molecular tests are replacing culture even for genital samples (38).

BV and Vaginitis

BV occurs when conditions result in overgrowth of the usual vaginal microbiota with various anaerobic genera, including *Mobiluncus* and *Bacteroides* (214). Although not characterized by a polymorphonuclear response, BV results in an increase in vaginal secretions that are relatively alkaline (pH > 4.5) compared to normal, the usual predominant microbiota of lactobacilli being replaced by anaerobes, and the presence of aromatic amines, which are detected by adding 10% potassium hydroxide and noting a pungent, fishy odor. In addition, excessive growth of a facultative bacterium called *Gardnerella vaginalis* generally coincides with BV. Although G. *vaginalis* commonly is a member of the normal vaginal microbiota, the presence of increased concentrations that adhere to vaginal squamous

TABLE 10 Diagnosis of BV using a Gram-stained smear of vaginal secretions, by the Vaginal Infection and Prematurity Study Group criteria[a]

Morphotype	No. of morphotypes seen per oil power field					Score
	None	≤1	1–5	5–30	>30	
Lactobacillus	4	3	2	1	0	_____
Gardnerella/Bacteroides	0	1	2	3	4	_____
Curved gram-variable rods (*Mobiluncus*)	0	1	2	3	4	_____
Total score						_____

[a]Adapted from reference 165. A total score of 0 to 3 is considered normal, 4 to 6 is intermediate, and 7 to 10 indicates BV.

epithelial cells, called clue cells, is characteristic of BV. Clue cells are squamous epithelial cells peppered with G. *vaginalis* bacteria, frequently showing heavier adherence toward the periphery of the cell and appearing like a doughnut (Fig. 3). New studies are showing that the bulk of bacteria actually associated with BV are identified only by molecular analysis, which at this time is beyond the scope of routine diagnostic laboratories (214). Thus, BV is diagnosed best without culture (55, 116). Gram-stained smears should be examined and interpreted according to Table 10. In summary, BV should be diagnosed by performing a bedside pH and KOH "whiff test," and a laboratory Gram stain (138).

A combination probe assay (Affirm VPIII identification test; Becton Dickinson, Sparks, MD) is commercially available for the simultaneous detection of *Candida* spp., G. *vaginalis*, and T. *vaginalis* in vaginal secretions (32).

Screening for Group B *Streptococcus*

Pregnant women colonized vaginally or rectally with group B streptococci prior to delivery are at increased risk of infecting their newborns during delivery. Such women need intrapartum prophylaxis; currently 25% of all women receive antibiotics during labor in the United States, although the incidence of neonatal disease is only 0.3% (236). Current recommendations are for collecting vaginal and rectal swabs at 35 to 37 weeks of gestation for culture in a single enrichment broth such as LIM broth. This broth is incubated at 35°C overnight and subcultured to a blood agar plate the following day. Recent studies have shown that this approach misses approximately 10% of women who become colonized after their screening test, and a substantial number of women convert to negative and would not require prophylaxis (48, 260). Real-time PCR performed on overnight enrichment broth culture has been used to improve sensitivity, but this approach still requires at least a 24-h turnaround time, not enough to allow timely use of intrapartum chemoprophylaxis for prevention of disease (27, 251). Newer PCR tests allow high sensitivity and specificity and rapid turnaround time, and some products can be performed by non-laboratory personnel at the time of delivery (48, 65). New recommendations are likely to include use of such tests for women who have not been screened previously or those with negative screening culture results (236).

Dark-Field Examination for *Treponema pallidum*

Dark-field examination of tissues, tissue exudates, and material collected from chancres can be used to confirm the diagnosis of syphilis. For dark-field microscopy, the specimen should be examined within 20 min of collection to ensure motility of treponemes and should not be exposed to temperature extremes during transport to a dark-field microscope. The test requires a microscope equipped with a dark-field condenser and experienced personnel who are able to recognize T. *pallidum* spirochetes based on the tightness and regularity of the spirals and on its characteristic corkscrew movement (120). Only a few laboratories perform this test anymore. A DFA stain can be used and is performed on air-dried smears. The stability of the smear during transport and the easily identified, fluorescing treponemes make the DFA an attractive alternative to dark-field microscopy (105, 120). Unfortunately, reagents for the DFA test are not commercially or widely available; it may be performed at some public health laboratories.

Haemophilus ducreyi

If infection with H. *ducreyi* is suspected, material from the base of the ulcer is collected and held at room temperature until needed for processing (124). One swab is used to prepare a smear for Gram staining. The presence of many small, pleomorphic, gram-negative bacilli and coccobacilli arranged in chains and groups ("school of fish") suggests H. *ducreyi* but is rarely seen (see chapter 34). Recovery of the organisms by culturing on an enriched medium such as GC agar containing 3 µg of vancomycin/ml, 1% hemoglobin, 5% fetal bovine serum, and 1% IsoVitaleX or Mueller-Hinton agar with 5% horse blood, 1% IsoVitaleX, and 3 µg of vancomycin/ml is necessary to confirm the diagnosis; culturing at 33°C yields better recovery than does culturing at 35°C (see chapter 34). Genital ulcer disease is much better diagnosed with molecular methods (132).

Actinomyces spp.

Actinomyces spp. may cause pelvic inflammatory disease in women who use intrauterine contraceptive devices (IUD) (127). An IUD submitted for culture should be placed in a sterile liquid medium (preferably reduced, such as thioglycolate) and vortexed, and the liquid medium should be used to inoculate aerobic and anaerobic culture media. Inflammatory debris and tissue attached to the IUD should be removed and cultured aerobically and anaerobically. Mixed infections with *Aggregatibacter actinomycetemcomitans* involving *Actinomyces*, sometimes mistaken for malignancy, involve bone or other tissue sites (78). *Actinomyces* spp. produce small knots of intertwined bacterial filaments, called grains or granules, which may be 1 mm or more in diameter. These grains should be crushed on a slide for staining (Gram stain is acceptable) and transferred to medium for culture. The presence of branching gram-positive filaments suggests *Actinomyces*; culture confirms the diagnosis.

Lower Respiratory Tract

Specimens from the lower respiratory tract are submitted to determine the etiology of airway disease (tracheitis and bronchitis), pneumonia, lung abscess, and empyema (134, 206, 210). Table 8 gives a list of lower respiratory tract diseases and their common etiologies. Usual specimens submitted consist of expectorated sputum; induced sputum; endotracheal tube aspirations (intubated patients); bronchial brushings, washes, or alveolar lavages collected during bronchoscopy; and pleural fluid (223). Specimens should be delivered to the laboratory promptly and processed without delay (within 1 h of collection). If delays are unavoidable, the specimen should be refrigerated. *Streptococcus pneumoniae*, the most common etiology of bacterial pneumonia, is very susceptible to conditions outside the body and may be missed by culture when the sample is not plated immediately. A urinary antigen test for *S. pneumoniae* may be more sensitive in such cases (51, 104, 212).

Lower respiratory tract secretions containing pathogens usually contain acute inflammatory cells (polymorphonuclear leukocytes). Frequently, pathogenic bacteria are present within the polymorphonuclear leukocytes. With the exception of aspiration pneumonia, characterized by mixed morphologies of bacteria including anaerobic species, pneumonia is caused by one or two organisms, and they should be predominant on Gram stain and culture. Endotracheal aspirates and sputum with numerous squamous epithelial cells are contaminated with upper respiratory tract organisms and cannot be used to determine the agent of the pneumonia. Most bacterial lower respiratory tract disease is caused by inapparent aspiration of oropharyngeal contents. It follows that oropharyngeal microbiotas include the bacteria that cause lower respiratory tract disease. Detection of a potential pathogen in a grossly contaminated specimen may represent contamination with an oropharyngeal microbiota. The lack of usefulness of data from contaminated specimens has resulted in policies for screening and rejecting grossly contaminated respiratory tract specimens. There are many ways to assess the quality of respiratory tact specimens. A simple screening method involves assessment of squamous epithelial cells only (152, 153). Squamous epithelial cells are found in the oropharynx but not in the lower respiratory tract. Increased numbers (defined as >10 per 10× objective microscopic field) indicate gross contamination with oropharyngeal contents, which includes usual members of the oral bacterial microbiota (Fig. 4). Acceptable sputum samples usually show numerous polymorphonuclear neutrophils and rare squamous epithelial cells and often have mucous strands (Fig. 5). Table 5 lists respiratory tract specimens and usual screening policies. Respiratory tract specimens for the detection of M. *pneumoniae*, *Legionella* spp., and M. *tuberculosis* should not be screened for adequacy. All specimens are considered acceptable for the detection of these microorganisms (45).

Bacteria should be reported when detected in Gram-stained smears if they are potential pathogens. Bacteria not in sufficient quantity or not representative of morphotypes resembling potential pathogens should be lumped together and reported as members of the normal respiratory microbiota. It is important to differentiate contaminating members of the respiratory microbiota from members of the respiratory microbiota causing aspiration pneumonia. Aspiration of relatively large amounts of oropharyngeal contents following loss of consciousness, paralysis of muscles involved with swallowing and breathing, or medical procedures such as intubation can result in infection of the airways with mixed members of the respiratory microbiota, leading to lung abscess and empyema (135). Gram stain of sputum from patients with aspiration pneumonia can be highly suggestive of the diagnosis. Stained smears show many polymorphonuclear leukocytes and many mixed respiratory microbiota morphotypes, especially those suggesting streptococci and anaerobes. Much of the microbiota is intracellular. Aspiration pneumonia can be detected in hospitalized patients and those admitted directly from the community (5, 134).

Cultures of respiratory tract material should include a selective gram-negative medium, such as MacConkey's agar, sheep blood agar, and chocolate agar for the detection of *Haemophilus* spp. (Table 7). Culture plates should be incubated at 35°C in 3 to 5% CO_2 for 48 h before being reported as negative. Cultures are interpreted by examining the relative numbers and types of bacteria that grow and correlating these results to the Gram stain. Table 11 summarizes interpretative criteria used with respiratory tract specimens.

Special Considerations for Lower Respiratory Tract Specimens

Specimens Collected during Bronchoscopy

Bronchoalveolar lavage fluid and bronchial brush specimens from patients with suspected pneumonia should be cultured quantitatively to evaluate the significance of potential pathogens recovered (11, 228). Bronchial brush specimens, which contain approximately 0.01 to 0.001 ml of secretions,

---

TABLE 11 Interpretation of bacterial lower respiratory tract culture results[a]

Specimen	Likely to be significant	Not likely to be significant	Additional data suggesting that isolate is significant
Sputum—coughed or induced	Predominant potential pathogen in Gram stain and culture. Neutrophils abundant.	Potential pathogen not present in Gram stain and only 1–2+ growth in culture. Neutrophils not abundant in Gram stain.	Potential pathogen within neutrophils (intracellular bacteria).
Endotracheal tube aspirate (136)	Predominant potential pathogen in Gram stain and culture. Neutrophils abundant.	Potential pathogen only 1–2+ growth in culture. Neutrophils not abundant in Gram stain.	Potential pathogen in quantities >10^6 CFU/ml. Potential pathogen within neutrophils (intracellular bacteria).
Bronchoalveolar lavage fluid	Predominant potential pathogen seen in every 100× field of Gram stain. Quantitative culture detects >10^5 CFU of potential pathogen/ml.	Potential pathogen not seen in Gram stain. Quantitative culture detects <10^4 CFU of potential pathogen/ml.	Potential pathogen within neutrophils (intracellular bacteria).

[a]Reprinted from reference 225 with permission.

should be placed in 1 ml of sterile nonbacteriostatic saline after collection. If anaerobes are to be cultured, the broth must be chopped meat or freshly boiled thioglycolate. The specimen should be delivered to the laboratory immediately. In the laboratory, the specimen is agitated on a vortex mixer, a smear is prepared by cytocentrifugation for staining with the Gram stain, and 0.01 ml of specimen is inoculated to appropriate medium by using a pipette or calibrated loop. Any growth of >10 colonies per plate of potential pathogens (corresponding to 10^6 CFU/ml of original specimen) appears to correlate with disease. Bronchoalveolar lavage results in collection of 50 ml or more of saline from a larger lung volume. In the laboratory, a smear is prepared by cytocentrifugation and Gram stained (181). The Gram stain report should include a comment about the presence of squamous epithelial cells and intracellular bacteria. Grossly contaminated fluid (>1% of all cells are squamous epithelial cells) may have falsely elevated counts of potential pathogens. Intracellular bacteria are more likely to be potential pathogens. A 0.01- or 0.001-ml aliquot of bronchoalveolar fluid should be inoculated to agar media (Table 7). The recovery of <10,000 bacteria/ml suggests contamination. The recovery of >100,000 bacteria/ml suggests that the isolate is a potential pathogen. Detection of 10,000 to 100,000 bacteria per ml represents a "gray" zone (228). Counts of pathogens may be reduced by prior antimicrobial therapy or variations in "return" of lavage fluid during the bronchoscopy procedure (Table 11).

Legionella spp.

Legionella spp., especially L. pneumophila, are important causes of community- and hospital-acquired pneumonia (70) (also see chapter 45). Legionellosis can be diagnosed by culture, DFA staining of smears of respiratory secretions, detection of antigens in urine, or serological testing. Culture is preferred because, unlike other methods, it is not limited to detection of certain species or serotypes. The urinary antigen tests for L. pneumophila serotype 1 are 74% sensitive overall (209). However, the immunochromatographic product used most commonly (BinaxNOW Legionella; Inverness Medical) was 95% sensitive with frozen urine samples (product insert) and 100% sensitive in a recent outbreak investigation in Germany (242). Antigen tests for other serotypes are not widely available. Before culture, respiratory samples should be diluted 10-fold in a bacteriologic broth, such as tryptic soy, or sterile water to dilute inhibitory substances that may be present in the specimen. Because legionellae grow slowly, optimal isolation from highly contaminated specimens, such as sputum, is achieved by decontaminating the specimens with acid before plating (244). The specimen is diluted 1:10 in KCl-HCl buffer (pH 2.2) and incubated for 4 min at room temperature. It is important not to incubate the specimen for longer than 4 min because legionellae may themselves be killed by acid exposure. Specimens are inoculated onto buffered charcoal yeast extract (BCYE) agar with and without antimicrobial agents (e.g., vancomycin, polymyxin B, and anisomycin). The cultures are incubated in humidified air at 35°C for a minimum of 5 days. Using a dissecting microscope, small colonies with a ground glass appearance, typical of Legionella spp., can be detected after 3 days of incubation.

Mycoplasma pneumoniae

Mycoplasma pneumoniae is a common cause of pneumonia, referred to as primary atypical pneumonia. Because M. pneumoniae is fastidious and grows very slowly, a definitive

diagnosis is often based on the results of serological or molecular detection tests. When culture is required, the specimen of choice is a throat swab; however, sputum or other respiratory specimens are also acceptable. The specimen should be placed immediately into a transport medium containing protein, such as albumin, and penicillin to reduce the growth of contaminating bacteria. Specimens may be stored in the transport medium for up to 48 h at 4°C or frozen for longer periods at −70°C. PCR methods have been used successfully to detect M. pneumoniae directly in respiratory tract specimens. Molecular detection by PCR or a related technique is the most sensitive method for the detection of M. pneumoniae, but there are still cases not detected by PCR (183).

Specimens from Patients with Cystic Fibrosis (Also See Chapters 40 and 41)

Respiratory samples (sputum, aspirates, or "gag sputa" [deep throat swabs found to reliably recover important pathogens in these patients]) from cystic fibrosis patients require additional media and a tremendous extra effort to detect the important pathogens found in these patients (107, 128). Burkholderia cepacia organisms, particularly some genomospecies, are especially important (3, 157). B. cepacia grows well on routine media; however, selective media such as B. cepacia selective agar, Pseudomonas cepacia agar, and oxidative-fermentative polymyxin B-bacitracin-lactose agar are useful for optimal recovery from respiratory secretions (98). Comparative studies show B. cepacia selective agar to be superior (also see chapter 41) (98). Haemophilus influenzae, Staphylococcus aureus (often difficult-to-recognize small-colony variants), and mucoid Pseudomonas aeruginosa are also important to identify. Many laboratories now use selective agar or chromogenic agar for S. aureus detection in cystic fibrosis patient samples (59, 73). Molecular methods are proving useful for detecting important organisms in cystic fibrosis patients (31, 47).

Chlamydia and Chlamydophila spp.

Chlamydiae are important causes of respiratory illnesses in children and adults (99, 222). Chlamydia trachomatis can cause serious respiratory disease in newborn infants. Chlamydophila pneumoniae causes illness in all age groups, but most disease occurs in adolescents and young adults (also see chapter 60). Chlamydophila psittaci is primarily an animal pathogen but occasionally causes disease in humans exposed to sick animals. Lower respiratory tract secretions, in addition to nasopharyngeal washes, for the detection of chlamydiae are collected and transported to the laboratory immediately in a medium containing antimicrobial agents (e.g., gentamicin and nystatin). If delays in transport or processing occur, the specimens should be stored at 4°C for up to 48 h. Longer storage should be at −70°C or colder. Chlamydiae are detected by rapid cell culture techniques (shell vial) using McCoy cells for C. trachomatis and C. psittaci and HEp-2 cells for C. pneumoniae. Most laboratories do not perform these types of cultures. As with M. pneumoniae, PCR may prove to be the most sensitive method for the detection of respiratory chlamydiae (99, 145).

Nocardia spp.

Respiratory specimens for the detection of Nocardia spp. should be transported to the laboratory as soon as they are collected. For short delays, storage at 4°C is acceptable. Direct examination of a Gram-stained smear containing a Nocardia species shows thin, beaded gram-positive branching filaments. The filaments are also partially acid fast when stained by the modified Kinyoun method (chapters 2, 17, and 27). Although *Nocardia* spp. grow readily on many common media such as sheep blood and chocolate agar plates, Sabouraud agar for fungi, and Lowenstein-Jensen medium for mycobacteria, better recovery may be seen on BCYE agar for *Legionella* and modified Thayer-Martin medium. Mycobacterial decontamination procedures reduce the recovery of *Nocardia*. Selective BCYE agar is optimal for culture from contaminated specimens (240). Although *Nocardia* spp. are detected commonly following 1 week of incubation, cultures are incubated for a total of 3 weeks at 35°C.

Upper Respiratory Tract

Upper respiratory tract specimens include the external nares, nasopharynx, throat, oral ulcerations, and inflammatory material from the nasal sinuses. Although few serious diseases involve these areas, many pathogens colonize or persist in these sites while causing symptomatic infection in deeper, less accessible sites (177).

Throat specimens are collected to diagnose pharyngitis. The most common etiological agent is *Streptococcus pyogenes*; however, other beta-hemolytic streptococci, *Arcanobacterium haemolyticum*, *Neisseria gonorrhoeae*, *Corynebacterium diphtheriae*, mycoplasmas, chlamydophilas, and *Fusobacterium necrophorum* may also occasionally cause pharyngitis. Special requests are required for most of these agents, although routine throat cultures reveal beta-hemolytic streptococci and *A. haemolyticum*. New data on *F. necrophorum* suggest that it should be sought (by anaerobic culture) for patients with chronic sore throat and that the standard swab is sufficient for recovery (4, 6, 19). Swab specimens should be placed in a standard transport carrier containing Amies or modified Stuart's medium. If only group A streptococci are to be detected, the swab can be sent dry with desiccant. Refrigeration is preferred if transport requires more than a few hours. Many rapid direct tests for group A streptococci are commercially available, including enzyme immunoassay (EIA), immunochromatographic assays, and nucleic acid-based probe assays (221). Rapid tests still lack sufficient sensitivity to be used without culture backup for negative results in the pediatric population (257). When a rapid test is requested, two throat swabs should be collected. If only one swab is received, the culture plate should be inoculated first. Material remaining on the swab is used for the direct test. If the rapid test is positive the second swab can be discarded, but if the rapid test is negative the second swab must be used for culture to confirm the negative direct test. The nucleic acid-based probe test is considered sensitive and specific enough by many to eliminate the need for confirmatory culture (96). A position paper by representatives of the American Academy of Family Physicians, the American College of Physicians-American Society of Internal Medicine, and the CDC states that rapid tests do not require confirmatory culture when used with adult patients (43).

To culture group A streptococci, either horse or sheep blood agar or selective blood agar may be used. Selective agar makes the organism easier to visualize by inhibiting accompanying members of the microbiota but may delay the appearance of colonies of *S. pyogenes*. Cultures should be incubated for 48 h at 35°C in an environment of reduced oxygen achieved by incubating anaerobically, in 5% CO_2, or in air with multiple "stabs" through the agar surface. Stabbing the agar surface with the inoculating loop pushes inoculum containing streptococci below the surface, where the oxygen

concentration is reduced compared to the ambient (33, 111). These culture conditions allow the recovery of group C and G streptococci, organisms which may cause pharyngitis but do not cause the serious sequelae associated with group A streptococci (265). Reports from such cultures may state "beta-hemolytic streptococci, not group A, isolated." Although relative numbers of colonies are usually reported (1+, 2+, etc.), this number may only reflect the quality of the sample and should not contribute to therapy decisions.

Throat specimens also are used to identify patients infected with *Neisseria gonorrhoeae*. For best results, the specimen should be inoculated immediately to a selective medium, such as modified Thayer-Martin agar. Cultures are incubated at 35°C in the presence of 5% CO_2 for 72 h. *A. haemolyticum* is usually recognized on the second day, when its characteristic hemolysis manifests (see chapter 26).

The external nares can be cultured to identify carriers of *Staphylococcus aureus* by using a single swab inserted only as far as the tip to collect secretions from both the left and right nares. The nose should be gently pressed inward during collection to maximize contact of the swab. The usual carrier systems used for swab transport containing Amies or Stuart's medium are acceptable. In the laboratory, the specimen can be inoculated to a sheep blood agar plate; however, use of selective media such as colistin-nalidixic acid agar, or a selective and differential medium such as BBL CHROMagar Staph aureus (BD Diagnostics, Sparks, MD), BBL CHROMagar MRSA (BD Diagnostics), MRSA-Select (Bio-Rad, Hercules, CA), or Spectra MRSA (Remel, Lenexa, KS), is helpful in differentiating *S. aureus* or MRSA from other members of the microbiota and useful when interpreting large numbers of specimens (59, 72, 73). Mannitol salt is not as sensitive as the chromogenic media. Cultures should be incubated at 35°C for 1 to 2 days per product insert. Molecular testing by PCR for the detection of *S. aureus* in swabs from the external nares has been shown to be as sensitive as culture but much more rapid (169, 193, 255). Commercially available, FDA-approved molecular tests (GeneOhm [BD, Franklin Lakes, NJ] and GeneXpert MRSA, Cepheid, Sunnyvale, CA) for the detection of MRSA in nasal swabs are more sensitive than culture, and results are available much faster (169, 193, 255).

Specimens for the recovery of *B. pertussis*, *Bordetella parapertussis*, and *Bordetella holmesii* should be collected with a small-tipped Dacron swab. Cotton may be toxic to the organism. Swabs should be transported to the laboratory in special media. For delays of up to 24 h, Amies medium with charcoal can be used. If the transport time will exceed 24 h, Regan-Lowe transport medium should be used (150). Culture, DFA staining, and PCR have been used for detection, but PCR is the most sensitive for detecting *B. pertussis*, *B. parapertussis*, and *B. holmesii* (Dacron swabs are preferred for PCR) (7, 76). Culture, primarily for epidemiological studies, is performed using Regan-Lowe charcoal agar containing 10% horse blood and cephalexin. Because a few strains of *B. pertussis* do not grow in the presence of cephalexin, the use of Regan-Lowe medium with and without cephalexin is recommended for optimal recovery (95). Cultures are incubated at 35°C for 5 to 7 days in a humid atmosphere. The DFA test can yield rapid results for *Bordetella* but should probably be discontinued in favor of PCR methods (130). Depending on the reagents used, either *B. pertussis* or *B. parapertussis* is detected.

Nasopharyngeal swab specimens are used to identify carriers of *N. meningitidis*. Transport in a swab container with Amies or Stuart's medium is acceptable. Specimens should be inoculated as quickly as possible to sheep blood or chocolate agar; however, selective agars for pathogenic *Neisseria* spp., such as modified Thayer-Martin, are necessary if interference by normal members of the microbiota is expected. Culture plates are incubated for 72 h in a humidified atmosphere at 35°C in the presence of 5% CO_2.

Vincent's angina is an oral infection characterized by pharyngitis, membranous exudate, fetid breath, and oral ulcerations. Sometimes referred to as fusospirochetal disease or necrotizing ulcerative gingivitis, it is caused by *Fusobacterium* spp., *Borrelia* spp., and other anaerobes. Diagnosis is made by direct examination of a smear of a swab specimen collected from the ulcerated lesions and stained with the Gram stain (177). The presence of many spirochetes, fusiform bacilli, and polymorphonuclear leukocytes is presumptive evidence of this disease. Culture for *F. necrophorum* may also be attempted (6). It should be noted that canker sores do not have a known bacterial etiology and should not be cultured.

Inflammatory material from the nasal sinuses should be cultured to detect the etiologies of sinusitis. Nearly all cases of bacterial sinusitis follow a primary, upper respiratory tract viral infection. Bacteria are trapped in the sinus as a result of damage to the epithelial lining cells of the sinus, and inflammation and swelling narrow or close the nasal ostium, preventing normal drainage (91, 196). Specimens collected during endoscopic procedures by physicians specializing in otorhinolaryngology are optimal since they are sampled directly from the infected sinus, avoiding contamination by normal members of the microbiota in the nasal passages. Aspirates, washes, scrapings/debridements, and biopsy material should be kept moist and sent in a sterile container to the laboratory (82, 91). Examination of Gram-stained smears can provide a rapid, presumptive identification of likely pathogens. Aerobic culture is needed in all cases; anaerobic transport and culture may be needed in cases of chronic sinusitis. Ventilator-associated sinusitis occurs in less than 10% of patients with nasotracheal intubation. Members of the nosocomial microbiota are implicated. Endoscopic inspection is needed to obtain acceptable specimens for culture (249). Although swabs obtained with endoscopic guidance correlate well with aspirates for recovery of bacteria, they do a poor job of recovering fungi, which are the etiological agents of approximately 23% of sinusitis cases (61, 239).

Special Considerations for Upper Respiratory Tract Specimens

Arcanobacterium haemolyticum

A. haemolyticum can cause pharyngitis and peritonsillar abscess (109). The organism can be recovered on media used to detect *S. pyogenes*. Colonies of *A. haemolyticum* are beta-hemolytic and easily confused with those of beta-hemolytic streptococci. Rapid differentiation can be accomplished with the Gram stain. *A. haemolyticum* is a diphtheroid-shaped gram-positive rod (see chapter 26). Incubation of plates at 35°C for up to 72 h may be required for optimal detection.

Corynebacterium diphtheriae

Cultures of both throat and nasopharyngeal specimens are used in the diagnosis of diphtheria. When specimens are processed for culture without delay, no special transport medium or conditions are required. For transport to a reference laboratory, specimens should be sent dry in a container with desiccant (63). Alternatively, specimens collected on swabs may be placed in Stuart's or Amies medium for transport to the laboratory. Smears of specimens for *C. diphtheriae* can be stained with the Gram stain and examined for pleomorphic (diphtheroid morphology) gram-positive rods. In addition, smears can be stained with Loeffler's methylene blue stain and examined for pleomorphic, beaded rods with swollen (club-shaped) ends and reddish purple metachromatic granules. Bacteria with these characteristics are suggestive but not specific for *C. diphtheriae*. Specimens should be inoculated to Loeffler's serum and potassium tellurite media for the recovery of *C. diphtheriae*. Cultures are incubated for 2 days at 35°C in 5% CO_2 before being reported as negative. See chapter 26 for more information.

Epiglottitis

A throat swab specimen may be helpful in determining the etiology of epiglottitis, a rapidly progressing cellulitis of the epiglottis and adjacent structures with the potential for swollen tissues to cause airway obstruction. Epiglottitis is almost always caused by *H. influenzae* serotype b but occasionally by other bacteria such as *S. pneumoniae* and *S. pyogenes* (232). The specimen should be collected by a physician only in a setting where emergency intubation can be performed immediately to secure a patent airway. Specimens should be inoculated onto enriched medium, such as chocolate agar, and incubated at 35°C in an atmosphere of 5% CO_2 for 72 h. Nearly 100% of patients with epiglottitis caused by *H. influenzae* have a blood culture positive for the same bacterium, so blood cultures should be ordered as part of differential diagnostic testing.

Gastrointestinal Tract

Feces and in some cases rectal swab specimens are submitted to the microbiology laboratory to determine the etiological agent of infectious diarrhea or food poisoning. In fact, most diarrhea is caused not by bacteria but by viruses, parasites, immune-related disease, or other factors. Occasional requests for quantitative culture are received to help with diagnosis of small bowel bacterial overgrowth syndrome, in which the numbers of organisms in the jejunum increases to resemble the numbers in the colon ($>10^5$/ml) (75). Feces should be collected in a clean container with a tight lid and should not be contaminated with urine, barium, or toilet paper. Because intestinal pathogens can be killed by the metabolism of other fecal bacteria rapidly acidifying the specimen, specimens should be transferred to Cary-Blair transport medium soon after collection. *Shigella* is the most labile, often becoming nondetectable within 30 min of collection. For *Vibrio cholerae*, other transport media such as alkaline peptone water are preferred (see chapter 39). Rectal swabs should be placed in a transport system containing an all-purpose medium such as Stuart's.

It should be standard practice in all laboratories to evaluate the appropriateness of stool culture requests. It is well established that hospitalized patients who did not enter the hospital with diarrhea are unlikely to develop bacterial enterocolitis caused by bacterial agents other than *Clostridium difficile* (90, 151). For this reason, stool from patients who have been hospitalized for more than 3 days should not be processed for enteric pathogens without consultation with and justification by the patient's physician or caregiver. A simple policy of rejecting stool for routine bacterial culture from patients hospitalized for more than 3 days and offering *C. difficile* testing for health care-acquired diarrhea is recommended. On the other hand, *C. difficile* infection is rapidly expanding as a community-acquired disease, sometimes following hospital discharge or the use of outpatient antimicrobial therapy, and sometimes in patients with no previous risk factors. Therefore, requests for *C. difficile* infection testing should not be rejected when ordered for outpatients (36, 117, 166).

Fecal leukocyte examinations have been recommended for the differentiation of inflammatory diarrheas (fecal leukocyte positive) from secretory diarrheas (fecal leukocyte negative). Infectious, inflammatory diarrheas are caused by invasive bacteria, while secretory diarrheas result from toxin-producing bacteria, viruses, and protozoan pathogens (90, 198, 218). Unfortunately, fecal leukocytes degrade in feces, making accurate recognition and quantification difficult. A lactoferrin test can serve as a surrogate marker for fecal leukocytes (EZ Leuko Vue; TechLab, Blacksburg, VA) since lactoferrin is not degraded during normal transport and processing times. Lactoferrin-positive stool specimens are considered positive for fecal leukocytes. However, invasive pathogens may result in fecal leukocytes being intermittently present or unevenly distributed in stool specimens, and fecal leukocytes may not be present in severe *C. difficile* infection. Numerous studies have shown either fecal white blood cells or lactoferrin to be not useful for differentiating inflammatory from noninflammatory diarrhea (9, 37, 198). For these reasons, use of any tests for fecal leukocytes should not be relied on to rule in or rule out acute, infectious diarrhea (90). The lactoferrin assay can be used in the evaluation of patients with inflammatory bowel disease (71).

Usual gastrointestinal pathogens are listed in Table 8 (79). Inclusion of less frequently encountered pathogens should be considered when epidemiological factors suggest an increased likelihood. This may require periodic surveys of one's community to establish which pathogens are most common, especially when considering the addition of selective media or toxin assay for the routine detection of campylobacters other than *Campylobacter jejuni* or *C. coli*, *Vibrio* spp., and *Yersinia enterocolitica*.

Selective and differential media are used to detect *Salmonella* and *Shigella* spp. (Table 7). These should include one that is differential but not selective for these pathogens, such as MacConkey agar, and one that is a mildly selective medium, such as Hektoen enteric or xylose-lysine desoxycholate agar. In some settings, a highly selective medium such as salmonella-shigella agar is also included. In addition, enrichment broth, such as gram-negative broth or Selenite F broth, may increase detection of *Salmonella* and is recommended for testing samples from sensitive populations such as food handlers. *Shigella* is generally not enriched. Subculture of gram-negative and Selenite F broths to a mildly selective and differential medium after 6 to 8 h and 12 to 18 h of incubation, respectively, is necessary to prevent overgrowth of normal members of the microbiota and decreased usefulness of the broth (79). All agar plates should be incubated in air at 35 to 37°C for 2 days before being reported as negative. The decision whether to use a highly selective agar medium and an enrichment broth varies from one laboratory to another. Optimally, additional media are used for a trial period to determine their value, which is measured by the detection of strains not present on the two standard media. In settings where such a trial is not possible, the use of MacConkey, Hektoen enteric, or xylose-lysine desoxycholate agar and an enrichment broth is recommended (79). Routine culture of all stools on a selective medium and use of an EIA on an enriched broth

(either gram-negative or MacConkey broth) culture for detection of Shiga toxin-producing *Escherichia coli* (STEC) have been recommended by the CDC (37). Either sorbitol-MacConkey agar, cefixime-tellurite-sorbitol-MacConkey agar, or a chromogenic agar can be used to detect O157 serotype strains.

Campylobacter jejuni and *C. coli* are detected in culture with a medium such as campylobacter agar with 10% sheep blood and selective antimicrobial agents (Table 7). Media are incubated at 42°C in a microaerophilic atmosphere of nitrogen (85%), carbon dioxide (10%), and oxygen (5%) for up to 3 days. Special enrichment broths do not increase the number of campylobacter-positive cultures significantly (1). Detection of other *Campylobacter* species may require media without antibiotics and 37°C incubation (44). EIA methods for detection of surface antigens of some *Campylobacter* species have been evaluated and shown to be relatively sensitive and specific (100, 110). New molecular methods will probably replace culture for enteric pathogens, including *Campylobacter*, in the near future (85, 201). See chapter 53 for more information on methods of detection of fecal campylobacters.

Special Considerations for Gastrointestinal Tract Specimens

Other Enteric Pathogens
A physician order for *Vibrio* spp., *Y. enterocolitica*, *Aeromonas* spp., and *Plesiomonas shigelloides* may be needed in some geographic locations or epidemiological situations, since incidence is so low in most parts of the United States that the routine use of selective media is not justified. Media used for these enteric pathogens include thiosulfate-citrate-bile salts-sucrose agar for vibrios, cefsulodin-Irgasan-novobiocin agar for *Y. enterocolitica*, and blood agar or selective blood agar to demonstrate hemolysis and provide a medium for oxidase testing for *Aeromonas* spp. and *P. shigelloides* (both oxidase positive) (79). All of these enteric pathogens grow on usual media, but detection is enhanced and simplified using specific selective media.

STEC
The prevalence of STEC varies in different parts of the United States and the rest of the world. In addition to *E. coli* O157:H7, many other serotypes are implicated. In fact, in the United States approximately 50% of STEC organisms, those capable of causing hemorrhagic colitis and hemolytic-uremic syndrome, are not serotype O157:H7 (12, 94). Shiga toxin EIAs and PCR assays detect all serotypes (89). Some Shiga toxin-producing strains may not harbor all the mechanisms needed to be fully pathogenic in humans. The CDC's recommendations for universal STEC testing contain strategies for referral of non-O157 strains for further testing by public health laboratories (37).

Clostridium difficile
C. difficile infection is diagnosed by detecting the organism or its toxins in stool, in conjunction with clinical criteria (139). The "gold standard" test for disease is the toxigenic culture, which requires direct plating on enrichment agar containing taurocholate, or alcohol or heat treatment to enrich for spores, followed by culture in broth and/or solid media (25, 77) (also see chapter 50). Colonies must then be tested by a cell culture cytotoxin assay for toxin production (216). Because toxins are labile, molecular testing for the gene encoding toxin B, the major virulence

factor, is becoming the standard test (13, 102, 164, 175). Cell culture cytotoxicity assay for the detection of toxin B, EIA for the detection of toxins A and B, and latex agglutination or EIA for the detection of glutamate dehydrogenase (an antigen associated with C. difficile and occasionally other bacterial species) are all methods that have been used for diagnosis (139, 176). EIAs are now known to have low sensitivity and specificity (2, 146).

C. difficile-associated gastrointestinal disease is now appearing in patients without any risk factors, even in patients who had no antibiotic exposure (117, 194). Testing should not be performed on formed stool, or as a follow-up to therapy to confirm cure. Repeat testing is only appropriate if symptoms persist or recur more than 7 days after an initial intervention (176). Since 2002, outbreaks of severe C. difficile disease in North America and Europe have been reported due to an epidemic strain, BI/NAP-1/027 (166). This strain is also now widely acknowledged to cause more quickly progressing and serious disease, so aggressive diagnosis and treatment are important. In the future, other strains may also be associated with varying severity of disease.

Staphylococcus aureus, MRSA, and Bacillus cereus

Stool specimens or gastric contents collected from persons with short-incubation food poisoning (2 to 6 h) can be evaluated for S. aureus and B. cereus (also see chapters 19 and 24). In general, investigation is beneficial for general public health, rather than a sick individual who recovers quickly, and is best performed by public health laboratories rather than hospital clinical microbiology laboratories. Specimens should be examined by Gram stain, and because both of these organisms may be present normally in food, quantitative cultures must be performed. A series of dilutions (10^{-1} to 10^{-5}) of the specimen are prepared in buffered gelatin diluent, and 0.1-ml samples of the undiluted specimen and each of the dilutions are plated onto colistin-nalidixic acid or phenylethyl alcohol blood agar. The presence of 10^5 CFU or more of S. aureus or B. cereus per g of specimen is of potential significance (57).

MRSA may be a cause of nosocomial antibiotic-associated diarrhea (29, 129). The overall incidence is unknown. Gram stain of smears of nonformed stool showing sheets of staphylococcal clusters in combination with appropriate clinical findings suggests the diagnosis. Diagnosis consists of the detection of heavy growth of MRSA in combination with the detection of staphylococcal enterotoxin in stool, available from some national reference laboratories and numerous public health laboratories (because Staphylococcus enterotoxin B is a category B bioterrorism agent). Greater recognition of this disease should confirm its significance and result in rapid diagnostic methods and appropriate treatment.

Clostridium botulinum

The clinical diagnosis of foodborne and infant botulism may be confirmed by detecting botulinum toxin, C. botulinum, or both in feces (143) (also see chapter 50). Optimally, 25 to 50 g of stool, 15 to 20 ml of serum, and a sample of suspect food should be collected (57). Most clinical laboratories are not properly equipped to process specimens from persons with suspected botulism. In the United States when a case of botulism is suspected, investigators at the CDC should be notified, usually through a local public health laboratory, to ensure appropriate diagnosis, treatment, and investigation of the potential outbreak.

Botulinum toxin could be used as a biological weapon (see chapter 12). Unexpected numbers of cases or unusual presentations should be investigated.

Helicobacter pylori

Helicobacter pylori is an important cause of gastritis and peptic ulcer disease (148, 203). The organism can be observed in tissue sections by using hematoxylin and eosin, Giemsa, or Warthin-Starry silver staining. In addition, organisms can be visualized in touch preparations of dissected tissue stained with the Gram stain. As discussed above, the presence of H. pylori in stomach or small bowel lesions can be confirmed by culture, antigen detection, urease detection, or detection of exhaled bacterial metabolite (H. pylori breath test) (24, 80, 203). Tissue biopsy specimens collected during endoscopy are used for culture and urease detection. Specimens for culture should be placed in transport medium (a medium such as brucella broth containing 20% glycerol is best for transport and storage) and transported to the laboratory immediately, or refrigerated during delays (92). Lightly minced tissue is inoculated to freshly prepared blood agar and incubated in a humid, microaerophilic atmosphere (5 to 10% carbon dioxide, 80 to 90% nitrogen, and 5 to 10% oxygen) at 37°C for 7 days (Table 7). The addition of 5% hydrogen should improve the yield of H. pylori. Tissue for urease detection is placed as soon as possible into the detection system and processed as specified by the manufacturer. Stool for antigen detection should be collected and handled according to instructions from the manufacturer. Antigen tests are still useful, but PCR methods are being developed, especially for posttreatment testing (24, 69, 80, 203). In some clinical situations serological testing for H. pylori antibody may be necessary (see chapter 54). Serum should be collected and stored at refrigeration temperature for short periods (up to 1 week) or frozen at −70°C for longer periods, as for other antibody tests.

Screening for VRE or Beta-Hemolytic Streptococci

Identifying carriers of vancomycin-resistant enterococci (VRE) for infection control purposes and group A streptococci during investigations of outbreaks of necrotizing fasciitis or streptococcal toxic shock requires collection of a rectal swab specimen. Carriers of VRE can be identified by culturing rectal swab or perirectal swabbed material (245). Specimens are inoculated to selective enrichment broth, such as Enterococcosel broth with 6 μg of vancomycin/ml, or agar media such as colistin-nalidixic acid blood agar containing 6 μg of vancomycin/ml (see chapter 21). Culture methods detect both vanA- and vanB-containing strains, but further testing is required to differentiate them. The fact that vanB is also present in nonenterococci in the bowel complicates the use of new molecular tests for surveillance of VRE (217). Carriers of group A streptococci can be identified by culturing rectal swab specimens on sheep blood agar or selective streptococcal agars used to identify patients with streptococcal pharyngitis.

Small Bowel Bacterial Overgrowth Syndrome

At this time, it is unclear which method best aids in diagnosis of the small bowel bacterial overgrowth syndrome (112). Laboratories receive jejunal aspirate material in a sterile container. Because the test requested is to determine whether the number of CFU in the sample is above or below the threshold of 10^5 CFU/ml, a simple method such as thorough vortexing of the sample and inoculation of a blood agar plate using a 0.001-ml calibrated loop can be used. Counting colonies in the same manner as for urine cultures is sufficient.

Urinary Tract

Diseases of the urinary tract include prostatitis, urethral syndrome, cystitis, and pyelonephritis. Etiologies are summarized in Table 8. Urine, prostatic secretion, or urethral cell/secretion specimens are needed to diagnose these diseases. Urine can be collected by midstream collection, catheterization (straight/in-out or indwelling), cystoscopic collection, or suprapubic aspiration. Foley catheter tips should not be submitted or accepted for culture since they are always contaminated with members of the urethral microbiota and quantitation is not possible. A first-voided morning urine is optimal, since in most cases bacteria have been multiplying in the bladder for a number of hours. Clean-catch urine, implying cleansing of periurethral areas, has not been shown to improve the quality of urine culture and is not recommended (126, 180).

Urine specimens should be transported to the laboratory immediately and processed within 2 h of collection. If a delay occurs, specimens may be refrigerated for up to 24 h. Transport tubes containing boric acid are available to stabilize the bacterial population at room temperature for 24 h, if refrigeration is not available (162, 248). Boric acid-preserved urine samples are acceptable for dipstick leukocyte esterase testing (248).

Urine culture is the most common test performed by most microbiology laboratories, and most urine cultures are negative; i.e., no specific potential pathogen is detected. Screening methods are available that attempt to rapidly separate those specimens containing significant counts of bacteria from negative specimens. In general, screening methods compare well with specimens containing 10^5 CFU/ml or greater of bacteria but perform poorly when colony counts are lower. Screening urine specimens by staining with the Gram stain is rapid and economical with regard to reagents but is labor-intensive and requires a trained technologist. The presence of 1 or 2 bacteria of similar morphotype, or more, in each oil immersion field (100× objective lens) correlates with a count of 100,000 or greater by culture (188, 254). Commercially available dipstick tests that detect leukocyte esterase (an enzyme produced by neutrophils) and nitrite (the result of bacterial nitrate reductase acting on nitrate in the urine) are rapid, inexpensive, and simple to perform, but their sensitivity is low in some patient populations (204). False-negative dipstick screening occurs because frequent voiding dilutes the concentrations of leukocyte esterase and nitrite in urine, enterococci and other less common urinary tract pathogens do not produce nitrate reductase, and many patients with asymptomatic bacteriuria do not have significant numbers of leukocytes in urine. In spite of this, outpatient screening algorithms have been proposed that incorporate enzyme screening in a "reflexive" urine test: i.e., urinalysis is performed; if positive for leukocyte esterase or nitrate reductase, a culture will be set up, and if negative, a culture will not be done (41). Such screening works best for symptomatic patients, diabetics, and women older than 60 years (170, 204). Active research continues for an accurate, cost-effective, sensitive, and specific automated urine screening system that eliminates the need to culture urine samples that are not indicative of urinary tract infection (UTI). After decades, this goal has not been reached.

The standard for quantitative bacterial culture of urine is the inoculation of 0.01 or 0.001 ml of specimen using a calibrated plastic or wire loop to appropriate medium,

usually sheep blood and MacConkey agars or cystine–lactose–electrolyte-deficient (CLED) agar. The loop is dipped vertically into the well-mixed urine, just far enough to cover the loop, and the loopful of urine is spread over the surface of the agar plate by streaking from top to bottom in a vertical line and again from top to bottom perpendicular to this line in a back-and-forth fashion. Prior to plate inoculation, it is necessary to ensure that a film of urine fills the loop with no bubbles to alter the calibrated volume. The inoculum of urine is spread over the entire agar surface to simplify counting of colonies after growth. Urine cultures are incubated at 35°C for 24 to 48 h. Although most urinary tract pathogens grow readily on usual agar media, slowly growing pathogens and those inhibited by the presence of antimicrobials in the patient specimen may not appear after overnight incubation (16 h). One approach uses the results of the leukocyte esterase and nitrite tests to determine which cultures get incubated for a full 48 h. Urine cultures that are negative after overnight incubation but had one or both positive enzyme tests are incubated for an additional day. Those that had negative enzyme tests are reported as "no growth" in a final report (156).

Contamination of urine, defined as growth of colonizing skin, vaginal, or fecal microbes in the absence of UTI, is detected in approximately 5 to 40% of cultures. Contamination is not reduced by the use of central processing areas, refrigeration, urine screening systems, specimen preservatives, or insulated specimen transport (234). Using a minicatheter to collect urine directly from the bladder can circumvent some of these contaminating bacteria, and collecting a suprapubic urine sample with a transcutaneous needle aspiration guarantees an even more representative urine sample. Urine collected by attaching a plastic bag to a baby's perineal region (bagged urine) is never suitable for culture. Either catheter-obtained urine or a suprapubic aspirate of urine must be submitted to avoid a contaminated specimen from babies. Suprapubic aspirates should be handled in the same manner as sterile body fluids and may be cultured anaerobically.

Agar paddles are available for urine culture in settings where inoculation and incubation of conventional agar plates are not convenient or possible (191). A standard film of urine is distributed over the agar-covered paddle, usually by dipping the paddle into a jar of urine. The paddle is then reinserted into its plastic container for incubation. Following incubation, the density of growth is estimated by comparison to photographs or drawings. A preliminary identification of gram positive or gram negative can be determined by colony color and morphology, and when appropriate, the entire paddle can be forwarded to a reference laboratory for complete identification and antimicrobial testing of the isolate. Agar paddle culture of urine with approximate colony counts compares favorably with standard culture (191).

The urinary tract above the urethra is sterile in healthy humans, but the urethra is colonized normally with many different bacteria from the vagina, skin, or feces. Because of this, voided urine often becomes contaminated during passage. Commensal bacteria are differentiated from potential pathogens by quantitative culture. Bacterial counts indicating "significant" bacteriuria (isolate is a likely pathogen) vary with the host and type of infection. Table 12 summarizes significant counts for common clinical situations (41, 215).

Severe UTI generally involves the kidneys (pyelonephritis) and results in bacteremia. Rapid diagnosis and

TABLE 12 Interpretation of urine culture results[a]

Urine specimen and patient	Likely to be significant	Not likely to be significant	Additional data suggesting that isolate is significant
Midstream, female with cystitis	>10^2 CFU of potential pathogen/ml, urine LE[b] is positive	Quantity of potential pathogen ≤ quantity of contaminating members of the biota	
Midstream, female with pyelonephritis	>10^5 CFU of potential pathogen/ml, urine LE is positive	Quantity of potential pathogen ≤ quantity of contaminating members of the biota	Gram stain demonstrates potential pathogen in neutrophils and/or casts.
Midstream, asymptomatic bacteriuria	>10^5 CFU of potential pathogen/ml, LE is usually negative	<10^5 CFU/ml of potential pathogen; quantity of potential pathogen ≤ quantity of contaminating members of the biota	Confirm by repeating urine when clinically indicated.
Midstream, male with UTI	>10^3 CFU of potential pathogen/ml, urine LE is positive	<10^3 CFU/ml of potential pathogen; quantity of potential pathogen ≤ quantity of contaminating members of the biota	Gram stain demonstrates potential pathogen in neutrophils and/or casts.
Straight catheter, all patients	>10^2 CFU of potential pathogen/ml, urine LE positive for symptomatic patients	<10^2 CFU/ml of potential pathogen, urine LE is negative	Gram stain demonstrates potential pathogen in neutrophils and/or casts.
Indwelling catheter, all patients	>10^3 CFU of potential pathogens/ml (multiple pathogens may be present)	Bacteriuria detected in asymptomatic patients, urine LE is positive or negative	No reason to culture unless patient is symptomatic.

[a]Reprinted from reference 225 with permission.
[b]LE, leukocyte esterase.

administration of appropriate antimicrobial therapy are necessary. In this clinical setting, blood cultures are needed and a STAT Gram stain of the urine can be useful. The Gram stain provides an immediate indication of the quality of the urine and a preliminary identification of the likely pathogen. Specimens containing high numbers of squamous epithelial cells are likely to be grossly contaminated with members of the periurethral or vaginal microbiota and should be re-collected immediately, before antimicrobials inhibit growth of the true pathogen (Fig. 6) (225). Gram stain identification of a potential pathogen (usually gram-negative rods such as in Fig. 7) confirms that empirical therapy is correct or may suggest a change based on an unexpected pathogen such as *S. aureus*.

Infectious prostatitis can be a difficult diagnosis. Prostatic secretions may be submitted for culture, but interpreting results when cultures yield low numbers of potential pathogens or mixed cultures is not clear-cut. Culture results should be correlated with Gram stain results. Organisms not recovered from routine cultures, such as mycoplasmas, may be etiological agents in prostatitis. New molecular methods will likely provide assistance in the future (121).

Special Considerations for Urine Specimens

Leptospires

Leptospira interrogans can be recovered from blood and CSF during the acute stages of disease and from urine after the first week of illness and for several months thereafter. Urine should be processed as soon as possible after collection, because the acidity of urine harms the organisms. If a delay in processing is expected, urine should be neutralized with sodium bicarbonate, centrifuged (1,500 × *g* for 30 min), and resuspended in buffered saline before being used to inoculate media (see chapter 55). Alternatively, the urine may be diluted 1:10 in 1% bovine serum albumin and stored at 5 to 20°C. Undiluted urine and urine diluted 1:10, 1:100, and 1:1,000 in sterile buffered saline should be inoculated to Ellinghausen-McCullough-Johnson-Harris or equivalent medium, with and without neomycin (54). Cultures should be incubated at 30°C for at least 13 weeks (Table 7). Many clinicians also collect serum for serological tests for leptospirosis.

Bacterial Antigen Testing

Bacterial antigen testing kits, for the purpose of diagnosing bacterial meningitis, should not be used with urine specimens due to lack of a strong correlation with meningitis. In particular, the FDA issued a product alert specifically cautioning against the use of the group B *Streptococcus* antigen kits with urine specimens because of the risk of both false-positive and false-negative results (74).

Wounds

Superficial wound exudates and pus may be submitted on swabs, but these are inferior to biopsy samples or aspirates. Newer swab designs do allow better sample collection (46, 83, 238). It is helpful to perform a Gram stain on all possible specimens to help determine how to interpret the culture, but with only one swab, this is difficult. The swab can be vortexed in <1.0 ml of sterile saline or broth and squeezed to express any moisture and the suspension used to inoculate the plates and make a smear for Gram stain, but this is a labor-intensive activity. Therefore, two swabs should be requested for samples collected on swabs. Examination of a Gram-stained smear reveals bacterial morphotypes, acute inflammatory cells (polymorphonuclear neutrophils), intracellular bacteria, cell necrosis, and elastin fibers resulting from tissue necrosis (Fig. 8). The quality of wound specimen can be evaluated by noting the relative number of polymorphonuclear cells and squamous epithelial cells (Table 5). Excess numbers of squamous epithelial cells suggest gross contamination with members of the cutaneous microbiota. It is acceptable to limit workup of bacterial isolates when the specimen shows gross contamination. An example of a limited workup would be to list by Gram stain morphology the isolates encountered, with a comment explaining that the physician must call if a replacement specimen cannot be collected and further identification and antimicrobial testing is clinically warranted. If swabs of ulcers or decubiti are received for culture, despite the laboratory's attempts to discourage such samples, a limited workup of the organisms most likely to cause an underlying osteomyelitis should be performed (35, 86). The bacteria of importance include beta-hemolytic streptococci, *S. aureus*, *P. aeruginosa*, *Proteus* spp., *E. coli*, and *Klebsiella* spp.

Autopsy Samples

Microbiology testing as a component of the autopsy examination has been and continues to be controversial (32a). Postmortem and agonal invasion of sterile tissues confuses the significance of positive culture results, prompting some to argue against microbiology testing. Others have found that the postmortem examination continues to uncover a significant number of infectious diagnoses, whether in the community or university hospital setting, which were missed by modern high-technology medicine (119). The value of autopsy microbiology is further enhanced by its use to identify emerging diseases, etiologies of biological warfare, community outbreaks, nosocomial infections, and antimicrobial resistance and uncover the cause of death in organ transplant patients and others with immunocompromising conditions. Safety precautions designed to protect the pathologist and dissection assistants during autopsy procedures have been thoroughly reviewed (163).

To minimize contamination of postmortem specimens, the body should be moved to a refrigerated locker (4 to 6°C) as soon as possible after death. Limited movement of the body has been shown to decrease the incidence of false-positive postmortem cultures (62). Although it has been shown that cultures collected within 48 h of death from a refrigerated cadaver did not show an increase in false-positive results, tissue and fluid specimens, as a rule, should be taken from refrigerated bodies within 15 h of death (114). This serves to diminish the likelihood of postmortem overgrowth of contaminants and improve detection of true pathogens.

Specimens should be obtained by sterilizing the surface of the organ with a hot spatula or iron surface until the surface is thoroughly dry (62). Body fluids, including blood, should be collected first. For blood collection, the wall of the heart and large vessel should be seared and a sterile needle (18 to 20 gauge) inserted. A 20-ml volume, or as close to 20 ml as possible, should be collected and injected directly into aerobic and anaerobic blood culture bottles. Blood culture results obtained before opening the chest cavity by percutaneous subxyphoid aspiration have been shown to have greater interpretive value (less contamination but detection of relevant organisms). Most conclude that postmortem blood cultures rarely provide information that is not already known. Solid viscera should be sampled by immediately cutting blocks of tissue from the center of the seared area. Samples should be submitted to microbiology with a requisition providing a full explanation of the studies needed. Postmortem cultures can be very useful for detecting pathogens that are not considered members of the normal human microbiota, such as *M. tuberculosis*, *Brucella* spp., *B. pertussis*, some systemic fungi (*H. capsulatum*, *C. immitis*, etc.), parasitic helminths, and agents of biological warfare. Tissue samples should be transported to the microbiology laboratory immediately in sterile tubes. The use of transport media and laboratory processing methods should follow recommendations for premortem specimens. An efficient way to avoid unnecessary workup of contaminating microorganisms is to issue a preliminary report to the pathologist who performed the autopsy listing organisms detected by colony or Gram stain morphology, such as "lactose-fermenting gram-negative rod" or "gram-positive cocci in clusters." This is accompanied with a notation that further identification and antimicrobial testing will not be performed unless there is consultation with the laboratory director or technologist conducting the culture investigation. Plates can be held for 1 week and discarded if no additional information is requested.

REFERENCES

1. **Agulla, A., F. J. Merino, P. A. Villasante, J. V. Saz, A. Diaz, and A. C. Velasco.** 1987. Evaluation of four enrichment media for isolation of *Campylobacter jejuni. J. Clin. Microbiol.* **25:**174–175.
2. **Aichinger, E., C. D. Schleck, W. S. Harmsen, L. M. Nyre, and R. Patel.** 2008. Nonutility of repeat laboratory testing for detection of *Clostridium difficile* by use of PCR or enzyme immunoassay. *J. Clin. Microbiol.* **46:**3795–3797.
3. **Alexander, B. D., E. W. Petzold, L. B. Reller, S. M. Palmer, R. D. Davis, C. W. Woods, and J. J. LiPuma.** 2008. Survival after lung transplantation of cystic fibrosis patients infected with *Burkholderia cepacia* complex. *Am. J. Transplant.* **8:**1025–1030.
4. **Aliyu, S. H., R. K. Marriott, M. D. Curran, S. Parmar, N. Bentley, N. M. Brown, J. S. Brazier, and H. Ludlam.** 2004. Real-time PCR investigation into the importance of *Fusobacterium necrophorum* as a cause of acute pharyngitis in general practice. *J. Med. Microbiol.* **53:**1029–1035.
5. **American Thoracic Society and Infectious Diseases Society of America.** 2005. Guidelines for the management of adults with hospital-acquired, ventilator-associated, and healthcare-associated pneumonia. *Am. J. Respir. Crit. Care Med.* **171:**388–416.
6. **Amess, J. A., W. O'Neill, C. N. Giollariabhaigh, and J. K. Dytrych.** 2007. A six-month audit of the isolation of *Fusobacterium necrophorum* from patients with sore throat in a district general hospital. *Br. J. Biomed. Sci.* **64:**63–65.
7. **Andre, P., V. Caro, E. Njamkepo, A. M. Wendelboe, A. Van Rie, and N. Guiso.** 2008. Comparison of serological and real-time PCR assays to diagnose *Bordetella pertussis* infection in 2007. *J. Clin. Microbiol.* **46:**1672–1677.
8. **Arbique, J. C., K. R. Forward, and J. LeBlanc.** 2000. Evaluation of four commercial transport media for the survival of *Neisseria gonorrhoeae. Diagn. Microbiol. Infect. Dis.* **36:**163–168.
9. **Ashraf, H., J. Beltinger, N. H. Alam, P. K. Bardhan, A. S. Faruque, J. Akter, M. A. Salam, and N. Gyr.** 2007. Evaluation of faecal occult blood test and lactoferrin latex agglutination test in screening hospitalized patients for diagnosing inflammatory and non-inflammatory diarrhoea in Dhaka, Bangladesh. *Digestion* **76:**256–261.
10. **Atkins, B. L., N. Athanasou, J. J. Deeks, D. W. Crook, H. Simpson, T. E. Peto, P. Lardy-Smith, A. R. Berendt, and The OSIRIS Collaborative Study Group.** 1998. Prospective evaluation of criteria for microbiological diagnosis of prosthetic-joint infection at revision arthroplasty. *J. Clin. Microbiol.* **36:**2932–2939.
11. **Aucar, J. A., M. Bongera, J. O. Phillips, R. Kamath, and M. H. Metzler.** 2003. Quantitative tracheal lavage versus bronchoscopic protected specimen brush for the diagnosis of nosocomial pneumonia in mechanically ventilated patients. *Am. J. Surg.* **186:**591–596.
12. **Banatvala, N., P. M. Griffin, K. D. Greene, T. J. Barrett, W. F. Bibb, J. H. Green, and J. G. Wells.** 2001. The United States National Prospective Hemolytic Uremic Syndrome Study: microbiologic, serologic, clinical, and epidemiologic findings. *J. Infect. Dis.* **183:**1063–1070.

13. **Barbut, F., M. Braun, B. Burghoffer, V. Lalande, and C. Eckert.** 2009. Rapid detection of toxigenic strains of *Clostridium difficile* in diarrheal stools by real-time PCR. *J. Clin. Microbiol.* **47:**1276–1277.

14. **Baron, E. J., and K. C. Carroll.** 2005. Rapid diagnosis of tuberculous meningitis: what is the optimal method? *Infect. Med.* **22:**633–637.

15. **Baron, E. J., G. H. Cassell, L. B. Duffy, D. A. Eschenbach, J. R. Greenwood, S. M. Harvey, N. E. Madinger, E. M. Peterson, and K. B. Waites.** 1993. *Cumitech 17A, Laboratory Diagnosis of Female Genital Tract Infections.* Coordinating ed., E. J. Baron. American Society for Microbiology, Washington, DC.

16. **Baron, E. J., J. D. Scott, and L. S. Tompkins.** 2005. Prolonged incubation and extensive subculturing do not increase recovery of clinically significant microorganisms from standard automated blood cultures. *Clin. Infect. Dis.* **41:**1677–1680.

16a. **Baron, E. J., and S. E. Sharp.** 2010. Clarification on specimen collection and transportation for intra-abdominal infections. *Clin. Infect. Dis.* **51:**759.

17. **Baron, E. J., M. L. Vaisanen, M. McTeague, C. A. Strong, D. Norman, and S. M. Finegold.** 1993. Comparison of the Accu-CulShure system and a swab placed in a B-D Port-a-Cul tube for specimen collection and transport. *Clin. Infect. Dis.* **16**(Suppl. 4)**:**S325–S327.

18. **Baron, E. J., M. P. Weinstein, W. M. Dunne, P. Yagupsky, D. F. Welch, and D. M. Wilson.** 2005. *Cumitech 1C, Blood Cultures IV.* Coordinating ed., E. J. Baron. ASM Press, Washington, DC.

19. **Batty, A., and M. W. Wren.** 2005. Prevalence of *Fusobacterium necrophorum* and other upper respiratory tract pathogens isolated from throat swabs. *Br. J. Biomed. Sci.* **62:**66–70.

20. **Bennett, S. T., and D. A. Kern.** 2002. Automated production of an on-line laboratory reference manual from a laboratory information system. *J. Med. Syst.* **26:**145–149.

21. **Bernard, L., C. Sadowski, D. Monin, R. Stern, B. Wyssa, P. Rohner, D. Lew, and P. Hoffmeyer.** 2004. The value of bacterial culture during clean orthopedic surgery: a prospective study of 1,036 patients. *Infect. Control Hosp. Epidemiol.* **25:**512–514.

22. **Black, C. M., E. M. Driebe, L. A. Howard, N. N. Fajman, M. K. Sawyer, R. G. Girardet, R. L. Sautter, E. Greenwald, C. M. Beck-Sague, E. R. Unger, J. U. Igietseme, and M. R. Hammerschlag.** 2009. Multicenter study of nucleic acid amplification tests for detection of *Chlamydia trachomatis* and *Neisseria gonorrhoeae* in children being evaluated for sexual abuse. *Pediatr. Infect. Dis. J.* **28:**608–613.

23. **Blairon, L., Y. De Gheldre, B. Delaere, A. Sonet, A. Bosly, and Y. Glupczynski.** 2006. A 62-month retrospective epidemiological survey of anaerobic bacteraemia in a university hospital. *Clin. Microbiol. Infect.* **12:**527–532.

24. **Blanco, S., M. Forne, A. Lacoma, C. Prat, M. A. Cuesta, I. Latorre, J. M. Viver, G. Fernandez, S. Molinos, and J. Dominguez.** 2008. Comparison of stool antigen immunoassay methods for detecting *Helicobacter pylori* infection before and after eradication treatment. *Diagn. Microbiol. Infect. Dis.* **61:**150–155.

25. **Bliss, D. Z., S. Johnson, C. R. Clabots, K. Savik, and D. N. Gerding.** 1997. Comparison of cycloserine-cefoxitin-fructose agar (CCFA) and taurocholate-CCFA for recovery of *Clostridium difficile* during surveillance of hospitalized patients. *Diagn. Microbiol. Infect. Dis.* **29:**1–4.

26. **Bourbeau, P. P., and B. J. Heiter.** 2004. Use of swabs without transport media for the Gen-Probe Group A Strep Direct Test. *J. Clin. Microbiol.* **42:**3207–3211.

27. **Bourbeau, P. P., B. J. Heiter, and M. Figdore.** 1997. Use of Gen-Probe AccuProbe Group B streptococcus test to detect group B streptococci in broth cultures of vaginal-anorectal specimens from pregnant women: comparison with traditional culture method. *J. Clin. Microbiol.* **35:**144–147.

28. **Bourbeau, P. P., and B. L. Swartz.** 2009. First evaluation of the WASP, a new automated microbiology plating instrument. *J. Clin. Microbiol.* **47:**1101–1106.

29. **Boyce, J. M., and N. L. Havill.** 2005. Nosocomial antibiotic-associated diarrhea associated with enterotoxin-producing strains of methicillin-resistant *Staphylococcus aureus.* *Am. J. Gastroenterol.* **100:**1828–1834.

30. **Brook, I.** 1998. Microbiology of perianal cellulitis in children: comparison of skin swabs and needle aspiration. *Int. J. Dermatol.* **37:**922–924.

31. **Brown, A. R., and J. R. Govan.** 2007. Assessment of fluorescent in situ hybridization and PCR-based methods for rapid identification of *Burkholderia cepacia* complex organisms directly from sputum samples. *J. Clin. Microbiol.* **45:**1920–1926.

32. **Brown, H. L., D. D. Fuller, L. T. Jasper, T. E. Davis, and J. D. Wright.** 2004. Clinical evaluation of Affirm VPIII in the detection and identification of *Trichomonas vaginalis, Gardnerella vaginalis,* and *Candida* species in vaginitis/vaginosis. *Infect. Dis. Obstet. Gynecol.* **12:**17–21.

32a. **Caplan, M. J., and F. P. Koontz.** 2001. *Cumitech 35, Postmortem Microbiology.* Coordinating ed., B. W. McCurdy. ASM Press, Washington, DC.

33. **Carroll, K., and L. Reimer.** 1996. Microbiology and laboratory diagnosis of upper respiratory tract infections. *Clin. Infect. Dis.* **23:**442–448.

34. **Carter, J. S., and D. J. Kemp.** 2000. A colorimetric detection system for *Calymmatobacterium granulomatis.* *Sex. Transm. Infect.* **76:**134–136.

35. **Cavanagh, P. R., B. A. Lipsky, A. W. Bradbury, and G. Botek.** 2005. Treatment for diabetic foot ulcers. *Lancet* **366:**1725–1735.

36. **Centers for Disease Control and Prevention.** 2005. Severe *Clostridium difficile*-associated disease in populations previously at low risk. *MMWR Morb. Mortal. Wkly. Rep.* **54:**1201–1205.

37. **Centers for Disease Control and Prevention.** 2009. Recommendations for diagnosis of Shiga toxin-producing *Escherichia coli* infections by clinical laboratories. *MMWR Morb. Mortal. Wkly. Rep.* **58:**1–14.

38. **Chapin, K. C.** 2006. Molecular tests for detection of the sexually-transmitted pathogens *Neisseria gonorrhoeae* and *Chlamydia trachomatis.* *Med. Health R. I.* **89:**202–204.

39. **Chedore, P., and F. B. Jamieson.** 2002. Rapid molecular diagnosis of tuberculous meningitis using the Gen-Probe Amplified Mycobacterium Tuberculosis direct test in a large Canadian public health laboratory. *Int. J. Tuberc. Lung Dis.* **6:**913–919.

40. **Cirillo, D. M., E. J. Baron, and G. Marchiaro.** 2000. *Legionella pneumophila* fails to multiply in blood culture broths but can be recovered from Isolator tubes, p. 189. *Abstr. 100th Annu. Meet. Am. Soc. Microbiol.*

41. **Clarridge, J. E., M. T. Pezzlo, and K. L. Vosti.** 1987. *Cumitech 2A, Laboratory Diagnosis of Urinary Tract Infections.* Coordinating ed., A. S. Weissfeld. American Society for Microbiology, Washington, DC.

42. **Cockerill, F. R., III, J. W. Wilson, E. A. Vetter, K. M. Goodman, C. A. Torgerson, W. S. Harmsen, C. D. Schleck, D. M. Ilstrup, J. A. Washington, and W. R. Wilson.** 2004. Optimal testing parameters for blood cultures. *Clin. Infect. Dis.* **38:**1724–1730.

43. **Cooper, R. J., J. R. Hoffman, J. G. Bartlett, R. E. Besser, R. Gonzales, J. M. Hickner, and M. A. Sande.** 2001. Principles of appropriate antibiotic use for acute pharyngitis in adults: background. *Ann. Emerg. Med.* **37:**711–719.

44. **Cornick, N. A., and S. L. Gorbach.** 1988. Campylobacter. *Infect. Dis. Clin. N. Am.* **2:**643–654.

45. **Curione, C. J., Jr., G. S. Kaneko, J. L. Voss, F. Hesse, and R. F. Smith.** 1977. Gram stain evaluation of the quality of sputum specimens for mycobacterial culture. *J. Clin. Microbiol.* **5:**381–382.

46. **Daley, P., S. Castriciano, M. Chernesky, and M. Smieja.** 2006. Comparison of flocked and rayon swabs for collection of respiratory epithelial cells from uninfected volunteers and symptomatic patients. *J. Clin. Microbiol.* **44:**2265–2267.

47. **da Silva Filho, L. V., A. F. Tateno, L. F. Velloso, J. E. Levi, S. Fernandes, C. N. Bento, J. C. Rodrigues, and S. R. Ramos.** 2004. Identification of *Pseudomonas aeruginosa, Burkholderia cepacia* complex, and *Stenotrophomonas maltophilia*

in respiratory samples from cystic fibrosis patients using multiplex PCR. *Pediatr. Pulmonol.* **37:**537–547.

48. **Davies, H. D., M. A. Miller, S. Faro, D. Gregson, S. C. Kehl, and J. A. Jordan.** 2004. Multicenter study of a rapid molecular-based assay for the diagnosis of group B *Streptococcus* colonization in pregnant women. *Clin. Infect. Dis.* **39:**1129–1135.

49. **Delaney, M. L., and A. B. Onderdonk.** 1997. Evaluation of the AnaeroPack system for growth of clinically significant anaerobes. *J. Clin. Microbiol.* **35:**558–562.

50. **Dellinger, R. P., M. M. Levy, J. M. Carlet, J. Bion, M. M. Parker, R. Jaeschke, K. Reinhart, D. C. Angus, C. Brun-Buisson, R. Beale, T. Calandra, J. F. Dhainaut, H. Gerlach, M. Harvey, J. J. Marini, J. Marshall, M. Ranieri, G. Ramsay, J. Sevransky, B. T. Thompson, S. Townsend, J. S. Vender, J. L. Zimmerman, and J. L. Vincent.** 2008. Surviving Sepsis Campaign: international guidelines for management of severe sepsis and septic shock: 2008. *Intensive Care Med.* **34:**17–60.

51. **Diederen, B. M., and M. F. Peeters.** 2007. Rapid diagnosis of pneumococcal pneumonia in adults using the Binax NOW *Streptococcus pneumoniae* urinary antigen test. *Int. J. Infect. Dis.* **11:**284–285.

52. **Diederen, B. M., and M. F. Peeters.** 2007. Evaluation of the SAS Legionella Test, a new immunochromatographic assay for the detection of *Legionella pneumophila* serogroup 1 antigen in urine. *Clin. Microbiol. Infect.* **13:**86–88.

53. **Doan, N., A. Contreras, J. Flynn, J. Morrison, and J. Slots.** 1999. Proficiencies of three anaerobic culture systems for recovering periodontal pathogenic bacteria. *J. Clin. Microbiol.* **37:**171–174.

54. **Doern, G. V.** 2000. Detection of selected fastidious bacteria. *Clin. Infect. Dis.* **30:**166–173.

55. **Donders, G. G.** 1999. Microscopy of the bacterial flora on fresh vaginal smears. *Infect. Dis. Obstet. Gynecol.* **7:**177–179.

56. **Dow, G., A. Browne, and R. G. Sibbald.** 1999. Infection in chronic wounds: controversies in diagnosis and treatment. *Ostomy Wound Manag.* **45:**23–40.

57. **Downes, F. P., and K. Ito.** 2001. *Compendium of Methods for the Microbiological Examination of Foods.* American Public Health Association, Washington, DC.

58. **Drake, C., J. Barenfanger, J. Lawhorn, and S. Verhulst.** 2005. Comparison of Easy-Flow Copan Liquid Stuart's and Starplex swab transport systems for recovery of fastidious aerobic bacteria. *J. Clin. Microbiol.* **43:**1301–1303.

59. **D'Souza, H. A., and E. J. Baron.** 2005. BBL CHROMagar Staph aureus is superior to mannitol salt for detection of *Staphylococcus aureus* in complex mixed infections. *Am. J. Clin. Pathol.* **123:**806–808.

60. **D'Souza, H. A., M. Campbell, and E. J. Baron.** 2004. Practical bench comparison of BBL CHROMagar Orientation and standard two-plate media for urine cultures. *J. Clin. Microbiol.* **42:**60–64.

61. **Dubin, M. G., C. S. Ebert, C. S. Coffey, C. T. Melroy, R. E. Sonnenburg, and B. A. Senior.** 2005. Concordance of middle meatal swab and maxillary sinus aspirate in acute and chronic sinusitis: a meta-analysis. *Am. J. Rhinol.* **19:**462–470.

62. **du Moulin, G. C., and W. Love.** 1988. The value of autopsy microbiology. *Clin. Microbiol. Newsl.* **10:**165–167.

63. **Efstratiou, A., K. H. Engler, I. K. Mazurova, T. Glushkevich, J. Vuopio-Varkila, and T. Popovic.** 2000. Current approaches to the laboratory diagnosis of diphtheria. *J. Infect. Dis.* **181**(Suppl. 1):S138–S145.

64. **Eldan, M., E. Leibovitz, L. Piglansky, S. Raiz, J. Press, P. Yagupsky, A. Leiberman, and R. Dagan.** 2000. Predictive value of pneumococcal nasopharyngeal cultures for the assessment of nonresponsive acute otitis media in children. *Pediatr. Infect. Dis. J.* **19:**298–303.

65. **El-Helali, N., J. C. Nguyen, A. Ly, Y. Giovangrandi, and L. Trinquart.** 2009. Diagnostic accuracy of a rapid real-time polymerase chain reaction assay for universal intrapartum group B streptococcus screening. *Clin. Infect. Dis.* **49:**417–423.

66. **Elliott, D., J. A. Kufera, and R. A. Myers.** 2000. The microbiology of necrotizing soft tissue infections. *Am. J. Surg.* **179:**361–366.

67. **Evans, G. L., T. Cekoric, Jr., and R. L. Searcy.** 1968. Comparative effects of anticoagulants on bacterial growth in experimental blood cultures. *Am. J. Med. Technol.* **34:**103–112.

68. **Everts, R. J., E. N. Vinson, P. O. Adholla, and L. B. Reller.** 2001. Contamination of catheter-drawn blood cultures. *J. Clin. Microbiol.* **39:**3393–3394.

69. **Falsafi, T., R. Favaedi, F. Mahjoub, and M. Najafi.** 2009. Application of stool-PCR test for diagnosis of *Helicobacter pylori* infection in children. *World J. Gastroenterol.* **15:**484–488.

69a. **Federal Register.** 2006. Assigned protection factors; final rule. 29 CFR parts 1910, 1915, and 1926. *Fed. Regist.* **71:**50121–50192. http://www.osha.gov/pls/oshaweb/owadisp.show_document?p_table=FEDERAL_REGISTER&p_id=18846.

70. **File, T. M.** 2000. The epidemiology of respiratory tract infections. *Semin. Respir. Infect.* **15:**184–194.

71. **Fine, K. D., F. Ogunji, J. George, M. D. Niehaus, and R. L. Guerrant.** 1998. Utility of a rapid fecal latex agglutination test detecting the neutrophil protein, lactoferrin, for diagnosing inflammatory causes of chronic diarrhea. *Am. J. Gastroenterol.* **93:**1300–1305.

72. **Flayhart, D., J. F. Hindler, D. A. Bruckner, G. Hall, R. K. Shrestha, S. A. Vogel, S. S. Richter, W. Howard, R. Walther, and K. C. Carroll.** 2005. Multicenter evaluation of BBL CHROMagar MRSA medium for direct detection of methicillin-resistant *Staphylococcus aureus* from surveillance cultures of the anterior nares. *J. Clin. Microbiol.* **43:**5536–5540.

73. **Flayhart, D., C. Lema, A. Borek, and K. C. Carroll.** 2004. Comparison of the BBL CHROMagar Staph aureus agar medium to conventional media for detection of *Staphylococcus aureus* in respiratory samples. *J. Clin. Microbiol.* **42:**3566–3569.

74. **Food and Drug Administration.** 1997. *FDA Safety Alert: Risks of Devices for Direct Detection of Group B Streptococcal Antigen.* Food and Drug Administration, Washington, DC.

75. **Ford, A. C., B. M. Spiegel, N. J. Talley, and P. Moayyedi.** 2009. Small intestinal bacterial overgrowth in irritable bowel syndrome: systematic review and meta-analysis. *Clin. Gastroenterol. Hepatol.* **7:**1279–1286.

76. **Fry, N. K., J. Duncan, K. Wagner, O. Tzivra, N. Doshi, D. J. Litt, N. Crowcroft, E. Miller, R. C. George, and T. G. Harrison.** 2009. Role of PCR in the diagnosis of pertussis infection in infants: 5 years' experience of provision of a same-day real-time PCR service in England and Wales from 2002 to 2007. *J. Med. Microbiol.* **58:**1023–1029.

77. **Gerding, D. N., and J. S. Brazier.** 1993. Optimal methods for identifying *Clostridium difficile* infections. *Clin. Infect. Dis.* **16**(Suppl. 4):S439–S442.

78. **Ghafghaichi, L., S. Troy, I. Budvytiene, N. Banaei, and E. J. Baron.** 2010. Mixed infection involving *Actinomyces, Aggregatibacter,* and *Fusobacterium* species presenting as perispinal tumor. *Anaerobe* **16:**174–178.

79. **Gilligan, P. H., J. M. Janda, M. A. Karmali, and J. M. Miller.** 1992. *Cumitech 12A, Laboratory Diagnosis of Bacterial Diarrhea.* Coordinating ed., F. S. Nolte. American Society for Microbiology, Washington, DC.

80. **Gisbert, J. P., F. de la Morena, and V. Abraira.** 2006. Accuracy of monoclonal stool antigen test for the diagnosis of *H. pylori* infection: a systematic review and meta-analysis. *Am. J. Gastroenterol.* **101:**1921–1930.

81. **Glasson, J. H., L. H. Guthrie, D. J. Nielsen, and F. A. Bethell.** 2008. Evaluation of an automated instrument for inoculating and spreading samples onto agar plates. *J. Clin. Microbiol.* **46:**1281–1284.

82. **Gold, S. M., and T. A. Tami.** 1997. Role of middle meatus aspiration culture in the diagnosis of chronic sinusitis. *Laryngoscope* **107:**1586–1589.

83. **Goldfarb, D. M., R. Slinger, R. K. Tam, N. Barrowman, and F. Chan.** 2009. Assessment of flocked swabs for use in identification of streptococcal pharyngitis. *J. Clin. Microbiol.* **47:**3029–3030.

84. **Goldgeier, M. H.** 1983. The microbial evaluation of acute cellulitis. *Cutis* **31:**649–650, 653–654, 656.

85. **Gomez-Duarte, O. G., J. Bai, and E. Newell.** 2009. Detection of *Escherichia coli, Salmonella* spp., *Shigella* spp., *Yersinia enterocolitica, Vibrio cholerae,* and *Campylobacter* spp. enteropathogens by 3-reaction multiplex polymerase chain reaction. *Diagn. Microbiol. Infect. Dis.* **63:**1–9.

86. **Gradon, J., and C. Adamson.** 1995. Infections of pressure ulcers: management and controversies. *Infect. Dis. Clin. Pract.* **4:**11–16.

87. **Gray, L. D., and D. P. Fedorko.** 1992. Laboratory diagnosis of bacterial meningitis. *Clin. Microbiol. Rev.* **5:**130–145.

88. **Green, M., A. Apel, and F. Stapleton.** 2008. Risk factors and causative organisms in microbial keratitis. *Cornea* **27:**22–27.

89. **Grys, T. E., L. M. Sloan, J. E. Rosenblatt, and R. Patel.** 2009. Rapid and sensitive detection of Shiga toxin-producing *Escherichia coli* from nonenriched stool specimens by real-time PCR in comparison to enzyme immunoassay and culture. *J. Clin. Microbiol.* **47:**2008–2012.

90. **Guerrant, R. L., T. Van Gilder, T. S. Steiner, N. M. Thielman, L. Slutsker, R. V. Tauxe, T. Hennessy, P. M. Griffin, H. DuPont, R. B. Sack, P. Tarr, M. Neill, I. Nachamkin, L. B. Reller, M. T. Osterholm, M. L. Bennish, and L. K. Pickering.** 2001. Practice guidelines for the management of infectious diarrhea. *Clin. Infect. Dis.* **32:**331–351.

91. **Gwaltney, J. M., Jr.** 1996. Acute community-acquired sinusitis. *Clin. Infect. Dis.* **23:**1209–1223.

92. **Han, S. W., R. Flamm, C. Y. Hachem, H. Y. Kim, J. E. Clarridge, D. G. Evans, J. Beyer, J. Drnec, and D. Y. Graham.** 1995. Transport and storage of *Helicobacter pylori* from gastric mucosal biopsies and clinical isolates. *Eur. J. Clin. Microbiol. Infect. Dis.* **14:**349–352.

93. **Harrell, L. J., S. Mirrett, and L. B. Reller.** 1994. Subcultures of BACTEC-positive but gram or acridine orange stain-negative NR 6A and 7A blood culture bottles are unnecessary. *Diagn. Microbiol. Infect. Dis.* **20:**121–125.

94. **Hedican, E. B., C. Medus, J. M. Besser, B. A. Juni, B. Koziol, C. Taylor, and K. E. Smith.** 2009. Characteristics of O157 versus non-O157 Shiga toxin-producing *Escherichia coli* infections in Minnesota, 2000–2006. *Clin. Infect. Dis.* **49:**358–364.

95. **Heininger, U., G. Schmidt-Schlapfer, J. D. Cherry, and K. Stehr.** 2000. Clinical validation of a polymerase chain reaction assay for the diagnosis of pertussis by comparison with serology, culture, and symptoms during a large pertussis vaccine efficacy trial. *Pediatrics* **105:**E31.

96. **Heiter, B. J., and P. P. Bourbeau.** 1993. Comparison of the Gen-Probe Group A Streptococcus Direct Test with culture and a rapid streptococcal antigen detection assay for diagnosis of streptococcal pharyngitis. *J. Clin. Microbiol.* **31:**2070–2073.

97. **Hellinger, W. C., J. J. Cawley, S. Alvarez, S. F. Hogan, W. S. Harmesen, D. M. Ilstrup, and F. R. Cockerill III.** 1996. Assessment of routine use of an anaerobic bottle in a three-component, high-volume blood culture system. *J. Clin. Microbiol.* **34:**2544–2547.

98. **Henry, D., M. Campbell, C. McGimpsey, A. Clarke, L. Louden, J. L. Burns, M. H. Roe, P. Vandamme, and D. Speert.** 1999. Comparison of isolation media for recovery of *Burkholderia cepacia* complex from respiratory secretions of patients with cystic fibrosis. *J. Clin. Microbiol.* **37:**1004–1007.

99. **Higgins, R. R., E. Lombos, P. Tang, K. Rohoman, A. Maki, S. Brown, F. Jamieson, and S. J. Drews.** 2009. Verification of the ProPneumo-1 assay for the simultaneous detection of *Mycoplasma pneumoniae* and *Chlamydophila pneumoniae* in clinical respiratory specimens. *Ann. Clin. Microbiol. Antimicrob.* **8:**10.

100. **Hindiyeh, M., S. Jense, S. Hohmann, H. Benett, C. Edwards, W. Aldeen, A. Croft, J. Daly, S. Mottice, and K. C. Carroll.** 2000. Rapid detection of *Campylobacter jejuni* in stool specimens by an enzyme immunoassay and surveillance for *Campylobacter upsaliensis* in the greater Salt Lake City area. *J. Clin. Microbiol.* **38:**3076–3079.

101. **Houang, E. T., P. C. Tam, S. L. Lui, and A. F. Cheng.** 1999. The use of CHROMagar Orientation as a primary isolation medium with presumptive identification for the routine screening of urine specimens. *APMIS* **107:**859–862.

102. **Huang, H., A. Weintraub, H. Fang, and C. E. Nord.** 2009. Comparison of a commercial multiplex real-time PCR to the cell cytotoxicity neutralization assay for diagnosis of *Clostridium difficile* infections. *J. Clin. Microbiol.* **47:**3729–3731.

103. **Hunter, J. S.** 1993. Acridine orange staining as a replacement for subculturing of false-positive blood cultures with the BACTEC NR 660. *J. Clin. Microbiol.* **31:**465–466.

104. **Ishida, T., T. Hashimoto, M. Arita, Y. Tojo, H. Tachibana, and M. Jinnai.** 2004. A 3-year prospective study of a urinary antigen-detection test for *Streptococcus pneumoniae* in community-acquired pneumonia: utility and clinical impact on the reported etiology. *J. Infect. Chemother.* **10:**359–363.

105. **Ito, F., R. W. George, E. F. Hunter, S. A. Larsen, and V. Pope.** 1992. Specific immunofluorescent staining of pathogenic treponemes with a monoclonal antibody. *J. Clin. Microbiol.* **30:**831–838.

106. **Jousimies-Somer, H., P. Summanen, D. M. Citron, E. J. Baron, H. Wexler, and S. M. Finegold.** 2002. *Wadsworth-KTL Anaerobic Bacteriology Manual.* Star Publishing Co., Belmont, CA.

107. **Kabra, S. K., A. Alok, A. Kapil, G. Aggarwal, M. Kabra, R. Lodha, R. M. Pandey, K. Sridevi, and J. Mathews.** 2004. Can throat swab after physiotherapy replace sputum for identification of microbial pathogens in children with cystic fibrosis? *Indian J. Pediatr.* **71:**21–23.

108. **Kaditis, A. G., A. S. O'Marcaigh, K. H. Rhodes, A. L. Weaver, and N. K. Henry.** 1996. Yield of positive blood cultures in pediatric oncology patients by a new method of blood culture collection. *Pediatr. Infect. Dis. J.* **15:**615–620.

109. **Kain, K. C., M. A. Noble, R. L. Barteluk, and R. H. Tubbesing.** 1991. *Arcanobacterium haemolyticum* infection: confused with scarlet fever and diphtheria. *J. Emerg. Med.* **9:**33–35.

110. **Kawatsu, K., Y. Kumeda, M. Taguchi, W. Yamazaki-Matsune, M. Kanki, and K. Inoue.** 2008. Development and evaluation of immunochromatographic assay for simple and rapid detection of *Campylobacter jejuni* and *Campylobacter coli* in human stool specimens. *J. Clin. Microbiol.* **46:** 1226–1231.

111. **Kellogg, J. A.** 1990. Suitability of throat culture procedures for detection of group A streptococci and as reference standards for evaluation of streptococcal antigen detection kits. *J. Clin. Microbiol.* **28:**165–169.

112. **Khoshini, R., S. C. Dai, S. Lezcano, and M. Pimentel.** 2008. A systematic review of diagnostic tests for small intestinal bacterial overgrowth. *Dig. Dis. Sci.* **53:**1443–1454.

113. **Kim-Farley, R. J., T. I. Soewarso, S. Rejeki, S. Soeharto, A. Karyadi, and S. Nurhayati.** 1987. Silica gel as transport medium for *Corynebacterium diphtheriae* under tropical conditions (Indonesia). *J. Clin. Microbiol.* **25:**964–965.

114. **Koneman, E. W., T. M. Minckler, D. B. Shires, and D. S. De Jongh.** 1971. Postmortem bacteriology. II. Selection of cases for culture. *Am. J. Clin. Pathol.* **55:**17–23.

115. **Kowalski, R. P., P. P. Thompson, P. R. Kinchington, and Y. J. Gordon.** 2006. Evaluation of the SmartCycler II system for real-time detection of viruses and *Chlamydia* from ocular specimens. *Arch. Ophthalmol.* **124:**1135–1139.

116. **Krohn, M. A., S. L. Hillier, and D. A. Eschenbach.** 1989. Comparison of methods for diagnosing bacterial vaginosis in pregnant women. *J. Clin. Microbiol.* **27:**1266–1271.

117. **Kutty, P. K., S. R. Benoit, C. W. Woods, A. C. Sena, S. Naggie, J. Frederick, J. Engemann, S. Evans, B. C. Pien, S. N. Banerjee, J. Engel, and L. C. McDonald.** 2008. Assessment of *Clostridium difficile*-associated disease surveillance definitions, North Carolina, 2005. *Infect. Control Hosp. Epidemiol.* **29:**197–202.

118. **Lamy, B., P. Roy, G. Carret, J. P. Flandrois, and M. L. Ignette-Muller.** 2002. What is the relevance of obtaining multiple blood samples for culture? A comprehensive model

to optimize the strategy for diagnosing bacteremia. *Clin. Infect. Dis.* **35**:842–850.

119. **Landefeld, C. S., M. M. Chren, A. Myers, R. Geller, S. Robbins, and L. Goldman.** 1988. Diagnostic yield of the autopsy in a university hospital and a community hospital. *N. Engl. J. Med.* **318**:1249–1254.

120. **Larsen, S. A.** 1989. Syphilis. *Clin. Lab. Med.* **9**:545–557.

121. **Lee, S. R., J. M. Chung, and Y. G. Kim.** 2007. Rapid one step detection of pathogenic bacteria in urine with sexually transmitted disease (STD) and prostatitis patient by multiplex PCR assay (mPCR). *J. Microbiol.* **45**:453–459.

122. **Levett, P. N., K. Brandt, K. Olenius, C. Brown, K. Montgomery, and G. B. Horsman.** 2008. Evaluation of three automated nucleic acid amplification systems for detection of *Chlamydia trachomatis* and *Neisseria gonorrhoeae* in first-void urine specimens. *J. Clin. Microbiol.* **46**:2109–2111.

123. **Levy, P. Y., P. E. Fournier, R. Charrel, D. Metras, G. Habib, and D. Raoult.** 2006. Molecular analysis of pericardial fluid: a 7-year experience. *Eur. Heart J.* **27**:1942–1946.

124. **Lewis, D. A.** 2000. Diagnostic tests for chancroid. *Sex. Transm. Infect.* **76**:137–141.

125. **Li, J., J. J. Plorde, and L. G. Carlson.** 1994. Effects of volume and periodicity on blood cultures. *J. Clin. Microbiol.* **32**:2829–2831.

126. **Lifshitz, E., and L. Kramer.** 2000. Outpatient urine culture: does collection technique matter? *Arch. Intern. Med.* **160**:2537–2540.

127. **Lippes, J.** 1999. Pelvic actinomycosis: a review and preliminary look at prevalence. *Am.J.Obstet.Gynecol.* **180**:265–269.

128. **LiPuma, J. J.** 2003. *Burkholderia* and emerging pathogens in cystic fibrosis. *Semin. Respir. Crit. Care Med.* **24**:681–692.

129. **Lo, T. S., and S. M. Borchardt.** 2009. Antibiotic-associated diarrhea due to methicillin-resistant *Staphylococcus aureus*. *Diagn. Microbiol. Infect. Dis.* **63**:388–389.

130. **Loeffelholz, M. J., C. J. Thompson, K. S. Long, and M. J. Gilchrist.** 1999. Comparison of PCR, culture, and direct fluorescent-antibody testing for detection of *Bordetella pertussis*. *J. Clin. Microbiol.* **37**:2872–2876.

131. **Lutomski, D. M., A. T. Trott, J. M. Runyon, C. I. Miyagawa, J. L. Staneck, and J. O. Rivera.** 1988. Microbiology of adult cellulitis. *J. Fam. Pract.* **26**:45–48.

132. **Mackay, I. M., G. Harnett, N. Jeoffreys, I. Bastian, K. S. Sriprakash, D. Siebert, and T. P. Sloots.** 2006. Detection and discrimination of herpes simplex viruses, *Haemophilus ducreyi*, *Treponema pallidum*, and *Calymmatobacterium (Klebsiella) granulomatis* from genital ulcers. *Clin. Infect. Dis.* **42**:1431–1438.

133. **Maki, D. G., C. E. Weise, and H. W. Sarafin.** 1977. A semiquantitative culture method for identifying intravenous-catheter-related infection. *N. Engl. J. Med.* **296**:1305–1309.

134. **Mandell, L. A., R. G. Wunderink, A. Anzueto, J. G. Bartlett, G. D. Campbell, N. C. Dean, S. F. Dowell, T. M. File, Jr., D. M. Musher, M. S. Niederman, A. Torres, and C. G. Whitney.** 2007. Infectious Diseases Society of America/American Thoracic Society consensus guidelines on the management of community-acquired pneumonia in adults. *Clin. Infect. Dis.* **44**(Suppl. 2):S27–S72.

135. **Marik, P. E.** 2001. Aspiration pneumonitis and aspiration pneumonia. *N. Engl. J. Med.* **344**:665–671.

136. **Marquette, C. H., H. Georges, F. Wallet, P. Ramon, F. Saulnier, R. Neviere, D. Mathieu, A. Rime, and A. B. Tonnel.** 1993. Diagnostic efficiency of endotracheal aspirates with quantitative bacterial cultures in intubated patients with suspected pneumonia. Comparison with the protected specimen brush. *Am. Rev. Respir. Dis.* **148**:138–144.

137. **Masek, B. J., N. Arora, N. Quinn, B. Aumakhan, J. Holden, A. Hardick, P. Agreda, M. Barnes, and C. A. Gaydos.** 2009. Performance of three nucleic acid amplification tests for detection of *Chlamydia trachomatis* and *Neisseria gonorrhoeae* by use of self-collected vaginal swabs obtained via an Internet-based screening program. *J. Clin. Microbiol.* **47**:1663–1667.

138. **Mazzulli, T., A. E. Simor, and D. E. Low.** 1990. Reproducibility of interpretation of gram-stained vaginal smears for the diagnosis of bacterial vaginosis. *J. Clin. Microbiol.* **28**:1506–1508.

139. **McFarland, L. V.** 2009. Renewed interest in a difficult disease: *Clostridium difficile* infections—epidemiology and current treatment strategies. *Curr. Opin. Gastroenterol.* **25**:24–35.

140. **McManus, A. T., S. H. Kim, W. F. McManus, A. D. Mason, Jr., and B. A. Pruitt, Jr.** 1987. Comparison of quantitative microbiology and histopathology in divided burn-wound biopsy specimens. *Arch. Surg.* **122**:74–76.

141. **Mein, J., and G. Lum.** 1999. CSF bacterial antigen detection tests offer no advantage over Gram's stain in the diagnosis of bacterial meningitis. *Pathology* **31**:67–69.

142. **Meredith, F. T., H. K. Phillips, and L. B. Reller.** 1997. Clinical utility of broth cultures of cerebrospinal fluid from patients at risk for shunt infections. *J. Clin. Microbiol.* **35**:3109–3111.

143. **Midura, T. F.** 1996. Update: infant botulism. *Clin. Microbiol. Rev.* **9**:119–125.

144. **Miller, J. M.** 1998. *A Guide to Specimen Management in Clinical Microbiology*, 2nd ed. ASM Press, Washington, DC.

144a. **Miller, J. M. (ed.).** *Guidelines for Safe Work Practices in Human and Animal Clinical Diagnostic Laboratories.* In review for publication in MMWR Morb. Mortal. Wkly. Rep. http://www.asm.org/images/pdf/CDCCompleteSafetyDocument.pdf.

145. **Miyashita, N., Y. Obase, M. Fukuda, H. Shouji, K. Yoshida, K. Ouchi, and M. Oka.** 2007. Evaluation of the diagnostic usefulness of real-time PCR for detection of *Chlamydophila pneumoniae* in acute respiratory infections. *J. Infect. Chemother.* **13**:183–187.

146. **Mohan, S. S., B. P. McDermott, S. Parchuri, and B. A. Cunha.** 2006. Lack of value of repeat stool testing for *Clostridium difficile* toxin. *Am. J. Med.* **119**:356–358.

147. **Monsen, T., E. Lovgren, M. Widerstrom, and L. Wallinder.** 2009. In vitro effect of ultrasound on bacteria and suggested protocol for sonication and diagnosis of prosthetic infections. *J. Clin. Microbiol.* **47**:2496–2501.

148. **Monteiro, L., M. Oleastro, P. Lehours, and F. Megraud.** 2009. Diagnosis of *Helicobacter pylori* infection. *Helicobacter* **14**(Suppl. 1):8–14.

149. **Moran, E., S. Masters, A. R. Berendt, P. Lardy-Smith, I. Byren, and B. L. Atkins.** 2007. Guiding empirical antibiotic therapy in orthopaedics: the microbiology of prosthetic joint infection managed by debridement, irrigation and prosthesis retention. *J. Infect.* **55**:1–7.

150. **Morrill, W. E., J. M. Barbaree, B. S. Fields, G. N. Sanden, and W. T. Martin.** 1988. Effects of transport temperature and medium on recovery of *Bordetella pertussis* from nasopharyngeal swabs. *J. Clin. Microbiol.* **26**:1814–1817.

151. **Morris, A. J., P. R. Murray, and L. B. Reller.** 1996. Contemporary testing for enteric pathogens: the potential for cost, time, and health care savings. *J. Clin. Microbiol.* **34**:1776–1778.

152. **Morris, A. J., L. K. Smith, S. Mirrett, and L. B. Reller.** 1996. Cost and time savings following introduction of rejection criteria for clinical specimens. *J. Clin. Microbiol.* **34**:355–357.

153. **Morris, A. J., D. C. Tanner, and L. B. Reller.** 1993. Rejection criteria for endotracheal aspirates from adults. *J. Clin. Microbiol.* **31**:1027–1029.

154. **Morris, A. J., S. J. Wilson, C. E. Marx, M. L. Wilson, S. Mirrett, and L. B. Reller.** 1995. Clinical impact of bacteria and fungi recovered only from broth cultures. *J. Clin. Microbiol.* **33**:161–165.

155. **Munday, P. E., A. P. Johnson, B. J. Thomas, and D. Taylor-Robinson.** 1980. A comparison of immunofluorescence and Giemsa for staining *Chlamydia trachomatis* inclusions in cycloheximide-treated McCoy cells. *J. Clin. Pathol.* **33**:177–179.

156. **Murray, P., P. Traynor, and D. Hopson.** 1992. Evaluation of microbiological processing of urine specimens: comparison of overnight versus two-day incubation. *J. Clin. Microbiol.* **30**:1600–1601.

157. **Murray, S., J. Charbeneau, B. C. Marshall, and J. J. LiPuma.** 2008. Impact of *Burkholderia* infection on lung transplantation in cystic fibrosis. *Am. J. Respir. Crit. Care Med.* **178**:363–371.

158. Nahimana, I., P. Francioli, and D. S. Blanc. 2006. Evaluation of three chromogenic media (MRSA-ID, MRSA-Select and CHROMagar MRSA) and ORSAB for surveillance cultures of methicillin-resistant *Staphylococcus aureus*. *Clin. Microbiol. Infect.* **12**:1168–1174.

159. Nair, B., J. Stapp, L. Stapp, L. Bugni, J. Van Dalfsen, and J. L. Burns. 2002. Utility of Gram staining for evaluation of the quality of cystic fibrosis sputum samples. *J. Clin. Microbiol.* **40**:2791–2794.

160. National Committee for Clinical Laboratory Standards/ CLSI. 2003. *Quality Control of Microbiological Transport Systems; Approved Standard.* NCCLS document M40-A. National Committee for Clinical Laboratory Standards, Wayne, PA.

161. Nguyen, H. B., E. P. Rivers, F. M. Abrahamian, G. J. Moran, E. Abraham, S. Trzeciak, D. T. Huang, T. Osborn, D. Stevens, and D. A. Talan. 2006. Severe sepsis and septic shock: review of the literature and emergency department management guidelines. *Ann. Emerg. Med.* **48**:28–54.

162. Nickander, K. K., C. J. Shanholtzer, and L. R. Peterson. 1982. Urine culture transport tubes: effect of sample volume on bacterial toxicity of the preservative. *J. Clin. Microbiol.* **15**:593–595.

163. Nolte, K. B., D. G. Taylor, and J. Y. Richmond. 2002. Biosafety considerations for autopsy. *Am. J. Forensic Med. Pathol.* **23**:107–122.

164. Novak-Weekley, S. M., E. M. Marlowe, J. M. Miller, J. Cumpio, J. H. Nomura, P. H. Vance, and A. Weissfeld. 2010. *Clostridium difficile* testing in the clinical laboratory by use of multiple testing algorithms. *J. Clin. Microbiol.* **48**:889–893.

165. Nugent, R. P., M. A. Krohn, and S. L. Hillier. 1991. Reliability of diagnosing bacterial vaginosis is improved by a standardized method of Gram stain interpretation. *J. Clin. Microbiol.* **29**:297–301.

166. O'Connor, J. R., S. Johnson, and D. N. Gerding. 2009. *Clostridium difficile* infection caused by the epidemic BI/ NAP1/027 strain. *Gastroenterology* **136**:1913–1924.

167. Onderdonk, A. B., M. L. Delaney, A. M. DuBois, E. N. Allred, and A. Leviton. 2008. Detection of bacteria in placental tissues obtained from extremely low gestational age neonates. *Am. J. Obstet. Gynecol.* **198**:110–117.

168. Pai, M., L. L. Flores, N. Pai, A. Hubbard, L. W. Riley, and J. M. Colford, Jr. 2003. Diagnostic accuracy of nucleic acid amplification tests for tuberculous meningitis: a systematic review and meta-analysis. *Lancet Infect. Dis.* **3**:633–643.

169. Paule, S. M., M. Mehta, D. M. Hacek, T.-M. Gonzalzles, A. Robicsek, and L. R. Peterson. 2009. Chromogenic media vs real-time PCR for nasal surveillance of methicillin-resistant *Staphylococcus aureus*: impact on detection of MRSA-positive persons. *Am. J. Clin. Pathol.* **131**:532–539.

170. Pels, R. J., D. H. Bor, S. Woolhandler, D. U. Himmelstein, and R. S. Lawrence. 1989. Dipstick urinalysis screening of asymptomatic adults for urinary tract disorders. II. Bacteriuria. *JAMA* **262**:1221–1224.

171. Perkins, M. D., S. Mirrett, and L. B. Reller. 1995. Rapid bacterial antigen detection is not clinically useful. *J. Clin. Microbiol.* **33**:1486–1491.

172. Perl, B., N. P. Gottehrer, D. Raveh, Y. Schlesinger, B. Rudensky, and A. M. Yinnon. 1999. Cost-effectiveness of blood cultures for adult patients with cellulitis. *Clin. Infect. Dis.* **29**:1483–1488.

173. Perry, J. L. 1995. Utility of cytocentrifugation for direct examination of clinical specimens. *Clin. Microbiol. Newsl.* **17**:29–32.

174. Peterson, L. R., J. D. Hamilton, E. J. Baron, L. S. Tompkins, J. M. Miller, C. M. Wilfert, F. C. Tenover, and J. R. Thomson, Jr. 2001. Role of clinical microbiology laboratories in the management and control of infectious diseases and the delivery of health care. *Clin. Infect. Dis.* **32**:605–611.

175. Peterson, L. R., R. U. Manson, S. M. Paule, D. M. Hacek, A. Robicsek, R. B. Thomson, Jr., and K. L. Kaul. 2007. Detection of toxigenic *Clostridium difficile* in stool samples by real-time polymerase chain reaction for the diagnosis of *C. difficile*-associated diarrhea. *Clin. Infect. Dis.* **45**:1152–1160.

176. Peterson, L. R., and A. Robicsek. 2009. Does my patient have *Clostridium difficile* infection? *Ann. Intern. Med.* **151**:176–179.

177. Peterson, L. R., and R. B. Thomson, Jr. 1999. Use of the clinical microbiology laboratory for the diagnosis and management of infectious diseases related to the oral cavity. *Infect. Dis. Clin. N. Am.* **13**:775–795.

178. Petti, C. A., H. S. Bhally, M. P. Weinstein, K. Joho, T. Wakefield, L. B. Reller, and K. C. Carroll. 2006. Utility of extended blood culture incubation for isolation of *Haemophilus*, *Actinobacillus*, *Cardiobacterium*, *Eikenella*, and *Kingella* organisms: a retrospective multicenter evaluation. *J. Clin. Microbiol.* **44**:257–259.

179. Piper, K. E., M. J. Jacobson, R. H. Cofield, J. W. Sperling, J. Sanchez-Sotelo, D. R. Osmon, A. McDowell, S. Patrick, J. M. Steckelberg, J. N. Mandrekar, S. M. Fernandez, and R. Patel. 2009. Microbiologic diagnosis of prosthetic shoulder infection by use of implant sonication. *J. Clin. Microbiol.* **47**:1878–1884.

180. Prandoni, D., M. H. Boone, E. Larson, C. G. Blane, and H. Fitzpatrick. 1996. Assessment of urine collection technique for microbial culture. *Am. J. Infect. Control* **24**:219–221.

181. Prekates, A., S. Nanas, A. Argyropoulou, G. Margariti, T. Kyprianou, E. Papagalos, O. Paniara, and C. Roussos. 1998. The diagnostic value of Gram stain of bronchoalveolar lavage samples in patients with suspected ventilator-associated pneumonia. *Scand. J. Infect. Dis.* **30**:43–47.

182. Raad, I., H. A. Hanna, B. Alakech, I. Chatzinikolaou, M. M. Johnson, and J. Tarrand. 2004. Differential time to positivity: a useful method for diagnosing catheter-related bloodstream infections. *Ann. Intern. Med.* **140**:18–25.

183. Ramirez, J. A., S. Ahkee, A. Tolentino, R. D. Miller, and J. T. Summersgill. 1996. Diagnosis of *Legionella pneumophila*, *Mycoplasma pneumoniae*, or *Chlamydia pneumoniae* lower respiratory infection using the polymerase chain reaction on a single throat swab specimen. *Diagn. Microbiol. Infect. Dis.* **24**:7–14.

184. Redys, J. J., E. W. Hibbard, and E. K. Borman. 1968. Improved dry-swab transportation for streptococcal specimens. *Public Health Rep.* **83**:143–149.

185. Reimer, L. G., and L. B. Reller. 1985. Effect of sodium polyanetholesulfonate and gelatin on the recovery of *Gardnerella vaginalis* from blood culture media. *J. Clin. Microbiol.* **21**:686–688.

186. Richter, S. S., S. E. Beekmann, J. L. Croco, D. J. Diekema, F. P. Koontz, M. A. Pfaller, and G. V. Doern. 2002. Minimizing the workup of blood culture contaminants: implementation and evaluation of a laboratory-based algorithm. *J. Clin. Microbiol.* **40**:2437–2444.

187. Riedel, S., P. Bourbeau, B. Swartz, S. Brecher, K. C. Carroll, P. D. Stamper, W. M. Dunne, T. McCardle, N. Walk, K. Fiebelkorn, D. Sewell, S. S. Richter, S. Beekmann, and G. V. Doern. 2008. Timing of specimen collection for blood cultures from febrile patients with bacteremia. *J. Clin. Microbiol.* **46**:1381–1385.

188. Rippin, K. P., W. C. Stinson, J. Eisenstadt, and J. A. Washington. 1995. Clinical evaluation of the slide centrifuge (cytospin) Gram's stained smear for the detection of bacteriuria and comparison with the FiltraCheck-UTI and UTIscreen. *Am. J. Clin. Pathol.* **103**:316–319.

189. Rishmawi, N., R. Ghneim, R. Kattan, R. Ghneim, M. Zoughbi, A. Abu-Diab, S. Turkuman, R. Dauodi, I. Shomali, A. Issa, I. Siriani, H. Marzouka, I. Schmid, and M. Y. Hindiyeh. 2007. Survival of fastidious and nonfastidious aerobic bacteria in three bacterial transport swab systems. *J. Clin. Microbiol.* **45**:1278–1283.

190. Ristuccia, P. A., R. A. Hoeffner, M. Gamon-Beltran, and B. A. Cunha. 1987. Detection of bacteremia by buffy coat smears. *Scand. J. Infect. Dis.* **19**:215–217.

191. Rosenberg, M., S. A. Berger, M. Barki, S. Goldberg, A. Fink, and A. Miskin. 1992. Initial testing of a novel urine culture device. *J. Clin. Microbiol.* **30**:2686–2691.

192. **Rosett, W., and G. R. Hodges.** 1980. Antimicrobial activity of heparin. *J. Clin. Microbiol.* **11:**30–34.

193. **Rossney, A. S., C. M. Herra, G. I. Brennan, P. M. Morgan, and B. O'Connell.** 2008. Evaluation of the Xpert methicillin-resistant *Staphylococcus aureus* (MRSA) assay using the Gen-eXpert real-time PCR platform for rapid detection of MRSA from screening specimens. *J. Clin. Microbiol.* **46:**3285–3290.

194. **Rouphael, N. G., J. A. O'Donnell, J. Bhatnagar, F. Lewis, P. M. Polgreen, S. Beekmann, J. Guarner, G. E. Killgore, B. Coffman, J. Campbell, S. R. Zaki, and L. C. McDonald.** 2008. *Clostridium difficile*-associated diarrhea: an emerging threat to pregnant women. *Am. J. Obstet. Gynecol.* **198:**635–636.

195. **Runyon, B. A., M. R. Antillon, E. A. Akriviadis, and J. G. McHutchison.** 1990. Bedside inoculation of blood culture bottles with ascitic fluid is superior to delayed inoculation in the detection of spontaneous bacterial peritonitis. *J. Clin. Microbiol.* **28:**2811–2812.

196. **Sande, M. A., and J. M. Gwaltney.** 2004. Acute community-acquired bacterial sinusitis: continuing challenges and current management. *Clin. Infect. Dis.* **39**(Suppl. 3)**:**S151–S158.

197. **Sander, R.** 2001. Otitis externa: a practical guide to treatment and prevention. *Am. Fam. Physician* **63:**927–937.

198. **Savola, K. L., E. J. Baron, L. S. Tompkins, and D. J. Passaro.** 2001. Fecal leukocyte stain has diagnostic value for outpatients but not inpatients. *J. Clin. Microbiol.* **39:**266–269.

199. **Schachter, J., J. Moncada, S. Liska, C. Shayevich, and J. D. Klausner.** 2008. Nucleic acid amplification tests in the diagnosis of chlamydial and gonococcal infections of the oropharynx and rectum in men who have sex with men. *Sex. Transm. Dis.* **35:**637–642.

200. **Schifman, R. B., C. L. Strand, F. A. Meier, and P. J. Howanitz.** 1998. Blood culture contamination: a College of American Pathologists Q-Probes study involving 640 institutions and 497134 specimens from adult patients. *Arch. Pathol. Lab. Med.* **122:**216–221.

201. **Schuurman, T., R. F. de Boer, E. Van Zanten, K. R. van Slochteren, H. R. Scheper, B. G. Dijk-Alberts, A. V. M. Möller, and A. M. D. Kooistra-Smid.** 2007. Feasibility of a molecular screening method for detection of *Salmonella enterica* and *Campylobacter jejuni* in a routine community-based clinical microbiology laboratory. *J. Clin. Microbiol.* **45:**3692–3700.

202. **Seifert, H., O. Cornely, K. Seggewiss, M. Decker, D. Stefanik, H. Wisplinghoff, and G. Fatkenheuer.** 2003. Bloodstream infection in neutropenic cancer patients related to short-term nontunnelled catheters determined by quantitative blood cultures, differential time to positivity, and molecular epidemiological typing with pulsed-field gel electrophoresis. *J. Clin. Microbiol.* **41:**118–123.

203. **Selgrad, M., A. Kandulski, and P. Malfertheiner.** 2009. *Helicobacter pylori*: diagnosis and treatment. *Curr. Opin. Gastroenterol.* **25:**549–556.

204. **Semeniuk, H., and D. Church.** 1999. Evaluation of the leukocyte esterase and nitrite urine dipstick screening tests for detection of bacteriuria in women with suspected uncomplicated urinary tract infections. *J. Clin. Microbiol.* **37:**3051–3052.

205. **Shafer, M. A., J. Moncada, C. B. Boyer, K. Betsinger, S. D. Flinn, and J. Schachter.** 2003. Comparing first-void urine specimens, self-collected vaginal swabs, and endocervical specimens to detect *Chlamydia trachomatis* and *Neisseria gonorrhoeae* by a nucleic acid amplification test. *J. Clin. Microbiol.* **41:**4395–4399.

206. **Sharp, S. E., A. Robinson, M. Saubolle, M. Santa Cruz, K. Carroll, and V. Baselski.** 2004. *Cumitech 7B, Lower Respiratory Tract Infections*. Coordinating ed., S. E. Sharp. ASM Press, Washington, DC.

207. **Sharp, S. E.** 1999. Algorithms for wound specimens. *Clin. Microbiol. Newsl.* **21:**118–120.

208. **Sharpe, A. N., and A. K. Jackson.** 1972. Stomaching: a new concept in bacteriological sample preparation. *Appl. Microbiol.* **24:**175–178.

209. **Shimada, T., Y. Noguchi, J. L. Jackson, J. Miyashita, Y. Hayashino, T. Kamiya, S. Yamazaki, T. Matsumura, and S. Fukuhara.** 2009. Systematic review and metaanalysis: urinary antigen tests for legionellosis. *Chest* **136:**1576–1585.

210. **Shorr, A. F., and R. C. Owens, Jr.** 2009. Guidelines and quality for community-acquired pneumonia: measures from the Joint Commission and the Centers for Medicare and Medicaid Services. *Am. J. Health Syst. Pharm.* **66:**S2–S7.

211. **Skulnick, M., G. W. Small, A. E. Simor, D. E. Low, H. Khosid, S. Fraser, and R. Chua.** 1991. Comparison of Clearview Chlamydia test, Chlamydiazyme, and cell culture for detection of *Chlamydia trachomatis* in women with a low prevalence of infection. *J. Clin. Microbiol.* **29:**2086–2088.

212. **Smith, M. D., C. L. Sheppard, A. Hogan, T. G. Harrison, D. A. Dance, P. Derrington, and R. C. George.** 2009. Diagnosis of *Streptococcus pneumoniae* infections in adults with bacteremia and community-acquired pneumonia: clinical comparison of pneumococcal PCR and urinary antigen detection. *J. Clin. Microbiol.* **47:**1046–1049.

213. **Solomkin, J. S., J. E. Mazuski, J. S. Bradley, K. A. Rodvold, E. J. Goldstein, E. J. Baron, P. J. O'Neill, A. W. Chow, E. P. Dellinger, S. R. Eachempati, S. Gorbach, M. Hilfiker, A. K. May, A. B. Nathens, R. G. Sawyer, and J. G. Bartlett.** 2010. Diagnosis and management of complicated intra-abdominal infection in adults and children: guidelines by the Surgical Infection Society and the Infectious Diseases Society of America. *Clin. Infect. Dis.* **50:**133–164.

214. **Srinivasan, S., and D. N. Fredricks.** 2008. The human vaginal bacterial biota and bacterial vaginosis. *Interdiscip. Perspect. Infect. Dis.* **2008:**750479.

215. **Stamm, W. E., and T. M. Hooton.** 1993. Management of urinary tract infections in adults. *N. Engl. J. Med.* **329:**1328–1334.

216. **Stamper, P. D., R. Alcabasa, D. Aird, W. Babiker, J. Wehrlin, I. Ikpeama, and K. C. Carroll.** 2009. Comparison of a commercial real-time PCR assay for *tcdB* detection to a cell culture cytotoxicity assay and toxigenic culture for direct detection of toxin-producing *Clostridium difficile* in clinical samples. *J. Clin. Microbiol.* **47:**373–378.

217. **Stamper, P. D., M. Cai, C. Lema, K. Eskey, and K. C. Carroll.** 2007. Comparison of the BD GeneOhm VanR assay to culture for identification of vancomycin-resistant enterococci in rectal and stool specimens. *J. Clin. Microbiol.* **45:**3360–3365.

218. **Stephen, J.** 2001. Pathogenesis of infectious diarrhea. *Can. J. Gastroenterol.* **15:**669–683.

219. **Stevens, D. L.** 2000. Streptococcal toxic shock syndrome associated with necrotizing fasciitis. *Annu. Rev. Med.* **51:**271–288.

220. **Sturgis, C. D., L. R. Peterson, and J. R. Warren.** 1997. Cerebrospinal fluid broth culture isolates: their significance for antibiotic treatment. *Am. J. Clin. Pathol.* **108:**217–221.

221. **Tanz, R. R., M. A. Gerber, W. Kabat, J. Rippe, R. Seshadri, and S. T. Shulman.** 2009. Performance of a rapid antigen-detection test and throat culture in community pediatric offices: implications for management of pharyngitis. *Pediatrics* **123:**437–444.

222. **Teig, N., A. Anders, C. Schmidt, C. Rieger, and S. Gatermann.** 2005. *Chlamydophila pneumoniae* and *Mycoplasma pneumoniae* in respiratory specimens of children with chronic lung diseases. *Thorax* **60:**962–966.

223. **Thomson, J. R., Jr., and L. Peterson.** 2009. Microbiology laboratory diagnosis of pulmonary infections, p. 541–559. *In* M. S. Niederman, G. A. Sarosi, and J. Glassroth (ed.), *Respiratory Infections*. Lippincott Williams & Wilkins, Philadelphia, PA.

224. **Thomson, R. B., Jr., and R. Clarke.** 1988. Interaction between the clinical microbiology and anatomic pathology services. *Clin. Microbiol. Newsl.* **10:**45–47.

225. **Thomson, R. B., Jr.** 2002. Use of microbiology laboratory tests in the diagnosis of infectious diseases, p. 1–41. *In* J. S. Tan (ed.), *Expert Guide to Infectious Diseases*. American College of Physicians, Philadelphia, PA.

226. **Thomson, R. B., Jr., and H. Bertram.** 2001. Laboratory diagnosis of central nervous system infections. *Infect. Dis. Clin. N. Am.* **15**:1047–1071.

227. **Thomson, R. B., Jr., S. J. Vanzo, N. K. Henry, K. L. Guenther, and J. A. Washington II.** 1984. Contamination of cultures processed with the Isolator lysis-centrifugation blood culture tube. *J. Clin. Microbiol.* **19**:97–99.

228. **Thorpe, J. E., R. P. Baughman, P. T. Frame, T. A. Wesseler, and J. L. Staneck.** 1987. Bronchoalveolar lavage for diagnosing acute bacterial pneumonia. *J. Infect. Dis.* **155**:855–861.

229. **Thwaites, G. E., M. Caws, T. T. Chau, N. T. Dung, J. I. Campbell, N. H. Phu, T. T. Hien, N. J. White, and J. J. Farrar.** 2004. Comparison of conventional bacteriology with nucleic acid amplification (amplified mycobacterium direct test) for diagnosis of tuberculous meningitis before and after inception of antituberculosis chemotherapy. *J. Clin. Microbiol.* **42**:996–1002.

230. **Trampuz, A., K. E. Piper, M. J. Jacobson, A. D. Hanssen, K. K. Unni, D. R. Osmon, J. N. Mandrekar, F. R. Cockerill, J. M. Steckelberg, J. F. Greenleaf, and R. Patel.** 2007. Sonication of removed hip and knee prostheses for diagnosis of infection. *N. Engl. J. Med.* **357**:654–663.

231. **Trautner, B. W., J. E. Clarridge, and R. O. Darouiche.** 2002. Skin antisepsis kits containing alcohol and chlorhexidine gluconate or tincture of iodine are associated with low rates of blood culture contamination. *Infect. Control Hosp. Epidemiol.* **23**:397–401.

232. **Trollfors, B., O. Nylen, C. Carenfelt, M. Fogle-Hansson, A. Freijd, A. Geterud, S. Hugosson, K. Prellner, E. Neovius, H. Nordell, A. Backman, B. Kaijser, T. Lagergard, M. Leinonen, P. Olcen, and J. Pilichowska-Paszkiet.** 1998. Aetiology of acute epiglottitis in adults. *Scand. J. Infect. Dis.* **30**:49–51.

233. **Uppal, S. K., S. Ram, B. Kwatra, S. Garg, and R. Gupta.** 2007. Comparative evaluation of surface swab and quantitative full thickness wound biopsy culture in burn patients. *Burns* **33**:460–463.

234. **Valenstein, P., and F. Meier.** 1998. Urine culture contamination: a College of American Pathologists Q-Probes study of contaminated urine cultures in 906 institutions. *Arch. Pathol. Lab. Med.* **122**:123–129.

235. **van Dijk, S., M. J. Bruins, and G. J. H. M. Ruijs.** 2009. Evaluation and implementation of a chromogenic agar medium for *Salmonella* detection in stool in routine laboratory diagnostics. *J. Clin. Microbiol.* **47**:456–458.

236. **Van Dyke, M. K., C. R. Phares, R. Lynfield, A. R. Thomas, K. E. Arnold, A. S. Craig, J. Mohle-Boetani, K. Gershman, W. Schaffner, S. Petit, S. M. Zansky, C. A. Morin, N. L. Spina, K. Wymore, L. H. Harrison, K. A. Shutt, J. Bareta, S. N. Bulens, E. R. Zell, A. Schuchat, and S. J. Schrag.** 2009. Evaluation of universal antenatal screening for group B streptococcus. *N. Engl. J. Med.* **360**:2626–2636.

237. **Van Horn, K. G., C. D. Audette, D. Sebeck, and K. A. Tucker.** 2008. Comparison of the Copan ESwab system with two Amies agar swab transport systems for maintenance of microorganism viability. *J. Clin. Microbiol.* **46**:1655–1658.

238. **Van Horn, K. G., C. D. Audette, K. A. Tucker, and D. Sebeck.** 2008. Comparison of 3 swab transport systems for direct release and recovery of aerobic and anaerobic bacteria. *Diagn. Microbiol. Infect. Dis.* **62**:471–473.

239. **Vaughan, W. C., and G. Carvalho.** 2002. Use of nebulized antibiotics for acute infections in chronic sinusitis. *Otolaryngol. Head Neck Surg.* **127**:558–568.

240. **Vickers, R. M., J. D. Rihs, and V. L. Yu.** 1992. Clinical demonstration of isolation of *Nocardia asteroides* on buffered charcoal-yeast extract media. *J. Clin. Microbiol.* **30**:227–228.

241. **Volk, E. E., M. L. Miller, B. A. Kirkley, and J. A. Washington.** 1998. The diagnostic usefulness of bone marrow cultures in patients with fever of unknown origin. *Am. J. Clin. Pathol.* **110**:150–153.

242. **von Baum, H., G. Harter, A. Essig, C. Luck, T. Gonser, A. Embacher, and S. Brochmann.** 2010. Rapid communications:

preliminary report: outbreak of Legionnaires' disease in the cities of Ulm and Neu-Ulm in Germany, December 2009–January 2010. *Eurosurveillance* **15**(4):pii=19472.

243. **Wadey, V. M., J. I. Huddleston, S. B. Goodman, D. J. Schurman, W. J. Maloney, and E. J. Baron.** 2010. Use and cost-effectiveness of intraoperative acid-fast bacilli and fungal cultures in assessing infection of joint arthroplasties. *J. Arthroplasty* **25**:1231–1234.

244. **Ward, K. W.** 1992. Processing and interpretation of specimens for *Legionella* spp. Part 1. *Legionella* specimen processing, p. 1.12.1–1.12.8. *In* H. D. Isenberg (ed.), *Clinical Microbiology Procedures Handbook.* American Society for Microbiology, Washington, DC.

245. **Weinstein, J. W., S. Tallapragada, P. Farrel, and L. M. Dembry.** 1996. Comparison of rectal and perirectal swabs for detection of colonization with vancomycin-resistant enterococci. *J. Clin. Microbiol.* **34**:210–212.

246. **Weinstein, M. P.** 1996. Current blood culture methods and systems: clinical concepts, technology, and interpretation of results. *Clin. Infect. Dis.* **23**:40–46.

247. **Weinstein, M. P.** 2003. Blood culture contamination: persisting problems and partial progress. *J. Clin. Microbiol.* **41**:2275–2278.

248. **Weinstein, M. P.** 1985. Clinical evaluation of a urine transport kit with lyophilized preservative for culture, urinalysis, and sediment microscopy. *Diagn. Microbiol. Infect. Dis.* **3**:501–508.

249. **Westergren, V., L. Lundblad, H. B. Hellquist, and U. Forsum.** 1998. Ventilator-associated sinusitis: a review. *Clin. Infect. Dis.* **27**:851–864.

250. **Wilhelmus, K. R., T. J. Liesegang, M. S. Osato, and D. B. Jones.** 1994. *Cumitech 13A, Laboratory Diagnosis of Ocular Infections.* Coordinating ed., S. C. Specter. ASM Press, Washington, DC.

251. **Williams-Bouyer, N., B. S. Reisner, and G. L. Woods.** 2000. Comparison of Gen-Probe AccuProbe group B streptococcus culture identification test with conventional culture for the detection of group B streptococci in broth cultures of vaginal-anorectal specimens from pregnant women. *Diagn. Microbiol. Infect. Dis.* **36**:159–162.

252. **Wilson, M. L.** 1997. Clinically relevant, cost-effective clinical microbiology. Strategies to decrease unnecessary testing. *Am. J. Clin. Pathol.* **107**:154–167.

253. **Wilson, M. L., M. Mitchell, A. J. Morris, et al.** 2007. *Principles and Procedures for Blood Cultures; Approved Guideline.* CLSI document M47-A. Clinical and Laboratory Standards Institute, Wayne, PA.

254. **Winquist, A. G., M. A. Orrico, and L. R. Peterson.** 1997. Evaluation of the cytocentrifuge Gram stain as a screening test for bacteriuria in specimens from specific patient populations. *Am. J. Clin. Pathol.* **108**:515–524.

255. **Wolk, D. M., E. Picton, D. Johnson, T. Davis, P. Pancholi, C. C. Ginocchio, S. Finegold, D. F. Welch, M. de Boer, D. Fuller, M. C. Solomon, B. Rogers, M. S. Mehta, and L. R. Peterson.** 2009. Multicenter evaluation of the Cepheid Xpert methicillin-resistant *Staphylococcus aureus* (MRSA) test as a rapid screening method for detection of MRSA in nares. *J. Clin. Microbiol.* **47**:758–764.

256. **Woolfrey, B. F., J. M. Fox, and C. O. Quall.** 1981. An evaluation of burn wound quantitative microbiology. I. Quantitative eschar cultures. *Am. J. Clin. Pathol.* **75**:532–537.

257. **Wright, M., G. Williams, and L. Ludeman.** 2007. Comparison of two rapid tests for detecting group A streptococcal pharyngitis in the pediatric population at Wright-Patterson Air Force Base. *Mil. Med.* **172**:644–646.

258. **Wuthiekanun, V., W. Chierakul, D. Limmathurotsakul, L. D. Smythe, M. L. Symonds, M. F. Dohnt, A. T. Slack, R. Limpaiboon, Y. Suputtamongkol, N. J. White, N. P. Day, and S. J. Peacock.** 2007. Optimization of culture of *Leptospira* from humans with leptospirosis. *J. Clin. Microbiol.* **45**:1363–1365.

259. **Yagupsky, P., and J. Press.** 1997. Use of the Isolator 1.5 microbial tube for culture of synovial fluid from patients with septic arthritis. *J. Clin. Microbiol.* **35**:2410–2412.

260. **Yancey, M. K., T. Armer, P. Clark, and P. Duff.** 1992. Assessment of rapid identification tests for genital carriage of group B streptococci. *Obstet. Gynecol.* **80:**1038–1047.

261. **Yang, J. L., K. C. Hong, J. Schachter, J. Moncada, T. Lekew, J. I. House, Z. Zhou, M. D. Neuwelt, T. Rutar, C. Halfpenny, N. Shah, J. P. Whitcher, and T. M. Lietman.** 2009. Detection of *Chlamydia trachomatis* ocular infection in trachoma-endemic communities by rRNA amplification. *Investig. Ophthalmol. Vis. Sci.* **50:**90–94.

262. **York, M. K.** 2004. Quantitative cultures of wound tissues, p. 3.13.2.1–3.13.2.4. *In* H. D. Isenberg (ed.), *Clinical Microbiology Procedures Handbook*, 2nd ed. ASM Press, Washington, DC.

263. **Zappe, B., S. Graf, P. E. Ochsner, W. Zimmerli, and P. Sendi.** 2008. *Propionibacterium* spp. in prosthetic joint infections: a diagnostic challenge. *Arch. Orthop. Trauma Surg.* **128:**1039–1046.

264. **Zeller, V., A. Ghorbani, C. Strady, P. Leonard, P. Mamoudy, and N. Desplaces.** 2007. *Propionibacterium acnes:* an agent of prosthetic joint infection and colonization. *J. Infect.* **55:**119–124.

265. **Zwart, S., G. J. Ruijs, A. P. Sachs, W. J. van Leeuwen, J. W. Gubbels, and R. A. de Melker.** 2000. Beta-haemolytic streptococci isolated from acute sore-throat patients: cause or coincidence? A case-control study in general practice. *Scand. J. Infect. Dis.* **32:**377–384.

Reagents, Stains, and Media: Bacteriology*

RONALD M. ATLAS AND JAMES W. SNYDER

17

REAGENTS

A number of classical and rapid tests are used for the identification of medically important bacteria. Below are brief descriptions of commonly performed tests and reagents used in clinical microbiology. See references 5, 13, 27, and 38 for more detailed descriptions of these tests and the reagents they use.

Biochemical Tests

■ Acetamide hydrolysis test (Nessler reagent)

Nessler reagent is used in the determination of acetamide hydrolysis. This test is useful in differentiating some gram-negative bacteria. Acetamide agar or broth is inoculated. After incubation at 35 to 37°C until colonies or turbidity develops, 1 drop of Nessler reagent is added to 1 ml of broth or directly to the plate. A positive reaction is indicated by the formation of a red-brown sediment. Nessler reagent is prepared by dissolving 1 g of mercuric chloride in 6 ml of distilled water and then adding 2 or 3 drops of concentrated hydrochloric acid to dissolve the sediment. Separately, 2.5 g of potassium iodide is dissolved in 6 ml of distilled water and then added to the mercuric chloride solution. Then 6 g of potassium hydroxide is dissolved in 6 ml of distilled water and added to the mercuric chloride-iodide solution along with an additional 13 ml of distilled water. The solution is filtered using a sintered glass funnel (not a Nalgene filter). The Nessler reagent is stored in the dark and should be useful for several weeks. The solution should be checked for decomposition prior to use (any color change other than yellow indicates decomposition, and a fresh solution should be prepared). Nessler reagent is toxic if swallowed, inhaled, or absorbed through the skin. It presents a neurological hazard, may act as a carcinogen, and may be a reproductive hazard. It is corrosive and causes burns.

■ Alkaline phosphatase

Alkaline phosphatase is detected by the hydrolysis of a colorless phosphate-containing compound to a colored product, e.g., p-nitrophenol phosphate to p-nitrophenol, which is yellow; phenolphthalein phosphate to phenolthalein, which is red under alkaline conditions; or indolyl phosphate to indigo, which is blue. This test is useful in the differentiation of *Staphylococcus* species and non-glucose-fermenting gram-negative rods, and it is incorporated in several commercial identification systems.

■ Arginine arylamidase (L-arginine-4-methoxy-β-naphthylamide)

Arginine arylamidase (trypsin) is included as a diagnostic test in some commercial systems, e.g., the API test system of bioMérieux. The substrate for this test is L-arginine-4-methoxy-β-naphthylamide. A negative test is colorless, and a positive test produces an orange color. This test is useful in differentiating staphylococcal species and various other bacteria.

■ Benzidine test (benzidine hydrochloride)

The benzidine test is useful for differentiating coagulase-negative *Staphylococcus* species. This test is included in several commercial systems. It is based upon the presence of iron-porphyrin compounds. Addition of a solution of 1 g of benzidine hydrochloride dissolved in 20 ml of glacial acetic acid, 30 ml of water, and 50 ml of 95% ethanol followed by addition of a 5% solution of hydrogen peroxide (H_2O_2) results in the formation of a blue-green to deep blue color for positive organisms.

■ Bile solubility test (deoxycholate)

The bile solubility test is used in the presumptive identification of *Streptococcus pneumoniae*. The key reagent in this test is sodium deoxycholate, which is a surface-active bile salt. The test may be run in a tube or on agar plates. The test is performed on alpha-hemolytic streptococcal colonies. A few drops of a 10% solution of sodium deoxycholate can be applied directly to the surface of a colony. The plate is then incubated for 30 min at 35°C. Pneumococcal colonies are lysed, whereas viridans group streptococci are not lysed. Alternatively, a heavy suspension of cells can be added to physiological saline solution (pH 7.0) and divided into two tubes. The 10% sodium deoxycholate solution is added to one tube, and sterile physiological saline is added to the other. The tubes are incubated at 35°C and are visually compared. If the organism is bile soluble, the tube

*This chapter contains information presented in chapter 21 by Kimberle C. Chapin and Tsai-Ling Lauderdale in the ninth edition of this *Manual*. In particular, Tables 2 and 3 and the section on medium additives have been taken directly from that chapter. Descriptions of a number of stains and reagents also were based on material in that chapter.

containing the deoxycholate will exhibit reduced turbidity within 15 min and show an increase in viscosity along with clearing of the solution.

■ CAMP test (beta-lysin)

The CAMP factor test is used to identify group B beta-hemolytic streptococci based on their formation of a substance (CAMP factor) that enlarges the area of hemolysis formed by beta-hemolysin. Hardy Diagnostics CAMP Spot Test Reagent is used as a rapid CAMP test method. The reagent, containing staphylococcal beta-lysin (also called beta-toxin, beta-hemolysin, or beta-staphylolysin), acts directly with the CAMP factor that is diffused into the medium around the suspect colony. The beta-lysin has a synergistic effect in the presence of CAMP factor, producing enhanced hemolysis of sheep erythrocytes. Enhanced hemolysis is visible within 30 min to 1 h of placing a drop of CAMP Spot Test Reagent next to an isolated beta-hemolytic *Streptococcus* colony.

■ Catalase test (H₂O₂)

H_2O_2 is used to detect bacterial production of catalase. A concentration of 15% is used for the differentiation of anaerobes, which do not produce catalase. A 30% peroxide concentration is used to test *Neisseria* species. Cells from a colony are transferred to a clean glass slide, and a drop of hydrogen peroxide is added. Production of bubbles indicates a positive reaction. Blood must be avoided, as erythrocytes produce catalase and can cause a false-positive reaction. It is also possible to add a drop of hydrogen peroxide directly to a colony or slant as long as the medium does not contain blood. Immediate bubbling indicates a positive reaction.

■ Coagulase test (rabbit plasma)

Dehydrated rabbit plasma with EDTA is used to detect free or bound (clumping factor) coagulase produced by *Staphylococcus* species. Human plasma is preferred for the detection of bound coagulase produced by *Staphylococcus lugdunensis* and *Staphylococcus schleiferi* but is not routinely used because it may contain antibodies against staphylococci. A heavy suspension of cells is added to a clean glass slide and mixed with a drop of distilled water. If agglutination does not occur spontaneously, the procedure can be performed by adding a drop of rabbit plasma to the suspension and mixing with a circular motion. The formation of visible white clumps indicates the presence of bound coagulase. Positive and negative controls should be run. The test can also be run in a test tube which detects both free and bound coagulase. For this test, 0.5 ml of rabbit plasma is added to a sterile tube. The tube is inoculated with a loopful of the test organism and incubated at 35°C for 4 h. Observations for clotting should be made within the first 4 h since some staphylococci produce fibrolysin, which can dissolve the clot. If no clotting is observed, however, the tube should be incubated overnight at room temperature and again observed for delayed clotting.

■ Decarboxylase tests (Moeller broth, bromcresol purple)

Moeller broth, which contains bromcresol purple and cresol red, is used to detect the pH change due to decarboxylation of either of the amino acids lysine and ornithine. Decarboxylase tests are useful for differentiating the *Enterobacteriaceae*. The broth at neutral or slightly acidic pH containing an individual amino acid being tested is inoculated for at least 24 h in most cases. The test may also be run after growth

on other broths by adding a solution of bromcresol purple to a drop of the medium to determine if the pH is alkaline. Moeller broth can be used to this purpose. A rapid test has been described omitting glucose from the medium and using a starting pH of 5.5 (17). In a positive result, the increased pH is indicated by a change in color of bromcresol purple from yellow to purple.

■ Esculin hydrolysis (ferric ammonium citrate)

The hydrolysis of esculin to esculetin is detected using a 1% solution of ferric ammonium citrate. After incubation in esculin-containing medium for 1 to 2 days, a few drops of ferric ammonium citrate is added. The immediate formation of a brown-black color indicates a positive reaction. Esculin hydrolysis can also be determined using esculin agar without bile, which contains iron; using this preferred medium, esculin hydrolysis is indicated by blackening after overnight incubation.

■ β-Galactosidase (o-nitrophenyl-β-D-galactopyranoside [ONPG])

ONPG at a concentration of 4 mg/ml is used to detect β-galactosidase activity. This enzyme facilitates growth on a carbon source like lactose by cleaving it into a molecule of glucose and a molecule of galactose which the cells can catabolize and on which the cells can grow. The substrate ONPG is used in place of lactose. When the β-galactosidase cleaves ONPG, o-nitrophenol is released. This compound has a yellow color. This test is especially useful for identification of members of the family *Enterobacteriaceae*. ONPG-impregnated tablets can be used for this test. In API ZYM, 2-naphthyl-β-galactopyranoside is used as the substrate.

■ Gelatin hydrolysis (gelatin)

Gelatin hydrolysis, sometimes referred to as gelatin liquefaction, is performed to determine the presence of the proteolytic enzyme gelatinase, which liquefies/hydrolyzes gelatin. Following inoculation of semisolid nutrient gelatin medium with the test organism, the medium, which is commercially available, is incubated at 35 to 37°C for up to 1 week, depending on the organism being tested. The culture is then placed at 4°C for a minimum of 15 min. A positive test is denoted by the observation of a completely liquid medium indicative of the hydrolysis (liquefaction) of the gelatin; in a negative test the medium is solid at 4°C.

Gelatin hydrolysis can also be assessed by using a plate method, which tends to give superior results for gram-negative nonfermenting bacteria. A plate with nutrient agar plus 0.4% gelatin is inoculated with a spot or a streak and incubated until luxuriant growth is obtained. When the isolate is gelatin hydrolysis positive, visual clearing of the agar is usually obvious. If not, a HgCl₂ solution (12 g of HgCl₂, 16 ml of 35% HCl, and 80 ml of distilled water) can be added to enhance the observation of clearing. Because of the high toxicity of HgCl₂, it often is better to use the test tube method; it also is possible to replace it with sulfosalicylic acid to avoid exposure to mercuric chloride.

■ β-Glucuronidase (p-nitrophenyl-β-D-glucopyranoside, 4-methylumbelliferyl-β-D-glucuronide [MUG])

Detection of β-glucuronidase activity can be accomplished using either a colorimetric substrate (p-nitrophenyl-β-D-glucopyranoside) or a fluorometric substrate (MUG). This test is useful for the rapid identification of *Escherichia coli*, members of the *Streptococcus anginosus* group, and other bacteria. For the colorimetric test, a solution of 0.1% (wt/vol) *p*-nitrophenyl-β-D-glucopyranoside (colorimetric substrate) in 0.067 M Sorensen phosphate buffer (pH 8.0) is prepared. Tubes containing 0.5 ml of the substrate solution are inoculated with a loopful of bacteria from an overnight culture. The tubes are incubated at 35°C and examined after 4 h for the appearance of a yellow color (liberated *p*-nitrophenol). In the fluorometric test the substrate MUG yields the product 4-methylumbelliferyl, which fluoresces blue under long-wave UV light. The MUG test is normally used for the presumptive identification of *E. coli* and more recently for streptococcal strains. To prepare MUG for the fluorescent test, dissolve 50 mg of MUG in 10 ml of 0.05 M Sorensen phosphate buffer, pH 7.5. Dilute 1:16 of the stock MUG and add 1.25 ml to a vial containing 50 sterile paper disks. Allow the disks to be thoroughly saturated until no liquid remains in the vial. Spread the saturated disks out and allow to dry completely. The disks can be stored in a dark bottle at −20°C for 1 year or at 4°C for 1 month. Wet the disk with 1 drop of sterile water. Apply the organism to the disk using a wooden stick or loop and then incubate the disk for up to 2 h at 35°C. Shine a long-wave UV light on the disk. A positive reaction is indicated by blue fluorescence.

■ Hippurate hydrolysis (ninhydrin reagent) (ferric chloride)

Hippurate hydrolysis to benzoic acid and glycine is useful in the identification of group B streptococci (GBS), some *Listeria* spp., *Gardnerella vaginalis*, *Campylobacter jejuni*, and *Legionella pneumophila*. Ninhydrin reagent can be used to detect the production of glycine. Ninhydrin reagent (3.5%) is prepared by adding 3.5 g of ninhydrin to 50.0 ml of acetone and 50.0 ml of 1-butanol. The ninhydrin reagent is stored in the dark at room temperature. A 1% (wt/vol) solution of sodium hippurate is prepared in 0.067 M Sorensen phosphate buffer (pH 6.4). Tubes containing 0.5 ml of this solution are inoculated and incubated at 35°C for 2 h, after which 0.2 ml of the ninhydrin reagent is added. Development of a deep blue-purple color within 5 min indicates a positive reaction. For *L. pneumophila*, 0.5 ml of 1% sodium hippurate solution is inoculated with a loopful of organism and incubated at 35°C in ambient air for 18 to 20 h, after which 0.2 ml of ninhydrin reagent is added. The cells and ninhydrin are mixed and incubated for an additional 10 min at 35°C. The mixture is observed for 20 min for blue-purple color development, which is indicative of a positive reaction. Ferric chloride can also be used to detect hippurate hydrolysis. Ferric chloride reagent (12 g of FeCl₃ 6H₂O in 100.0 ml of 2% HCl) is added to inoculated broth (e.g., heart infusion broth or Todd-Hewitt broth) supplemented with hippurate. An insoluble brown ferric benzoate precipitate indicates a positive hydrolysis reaction.

■ Indole test (Ehrlich reagent, Kovács reagent, *p*-dimethylaminocinnamaldehyde [DMACA])

The indole test is used for the determination of production of indole from deamination of tryptophan by tryptophanase. This reaction can be detected using Ehrlich reagent, Kovács reagent, or dimethylaminocinnamaldehyde (DMACA). Kovács reagent is added directly to the medium; an extraction phase using xylene is required before adding Ehrlich reagent. To prepare Ehrlich reagent, add 1 g of *p*-dimethylaminobenzaldehyde to 95 ml of 95% ethyl alcohol. Then slowly add 10 ml of concentrated hydrochloric acid. Using Ehrlich reagent, first extract the indole

by adding 1 ml of xylene to a 48-h-old tryptone broth or other tryptophan-containing broth medium. Shake the tube vigorously for 20 s and let stand for 1 to 2 min to allow the xylene extract to come to the top of the broth. Gently add 0.5 ml of the Ehrlich reagent down the side of the tube. Do not shake the tube. A red ring at the interface of the medium and the reagent phase within 5 min represents a positive test. Ehrlich reagent is preferred for organisms that produce small amounts of indole, such as nonfermenters and anaerobes. To prepare Kovács indole reagent, add 10 g of *p*-dimethylaminobenzaldehyde to 150 ml of either amyl or isoamyl alcohol. Then add 50 ml of concentrated hydrochloric acid. Add 5 drops of Kovács reagent to either 48-h-old 2% tryptone broth or an 18- to 24-h-old tryptophan broth culture. Do not shake the tube after the addition of reagent. A red color at the surface of the medium indicates a positive test. For the spot indole test, add 2 ml of concentrated HCl to 18 ml of distilled water. Allow the mixture to cool. Then add 200 mg of DMACA. Moisten a piece of Whatman no. 3 paper with a couple of drops of the reagent. Remove a well-isolated colony from an 18- to 24-h-old culture onto a blood agar plate with a sterile inoculating loop or a wooden stick and smear it onto the moistened filter paper. Observe for a blue to blue-green color within 2 min, which indicates a positive reaction. No color change or a pinkish tinge is considered negative. This test should be used only on colonies from media containing sufficient tryptophan and no glucose (blood agar). Colonies from media containing dyes (e.g., MacConkey or eosin-methylene blue [EMB] agar) may cause misleading results and should not be used. Colonies from mixed cultures should not be used, as indole-positive colonies can cause indole-negative colonies to appear weakly positive. The test can also be run using a heavy bacterial suspension in 0.3% tryptophan solution and revelation with Kovács reagent after 4 h.

■ LAP test (leucine naphthylamide)

The LAP test detects the presence of leucine aminopeptidase (LAP). The substrate leucine naphthylamide is hydrolyzed by LAP to leucine and free naphthylamine. The LAP test is helpful in the presumptive characterization of catalase-negative, gram-positive cocci (streptococci, enterococci, and streptococcus-like organisms). *S. pneumoniae*, *Streptococcus pyogenes*, *Pediococcus*, *Lactococcus*, and *Enterococcus* species are all LAP positive, while other beta-hemolytic streptococci are LAP negative. Disks are impregnated with leucine-β-naphthylamide or leucine-α-naphthylamide, which is hydrolyzed by the enzyme LAP, produced by LAP-positive organisms. This test is performed by inoculating several colonies from overnight growth of the test organism to a moistened LAP disk aseptically placed in a sterile petri disk at room temperature. One drop of DMACA reagent is added. After 1 min, enzymatic activity results in the release of β-naphthylamine, which couples with DMACA reagent to form a highly visible red color indicating a positive test.

■ Lysozyme test (lysozyme)

The lysozyme test measures the ability of organisms, such as *Nocardia*, to grow in the presence of lysozyme. A solution of 50 mg of lysozyme in 50 ml of 0.01 N HCl is used for this test. The solution is filter sterilized and can be stored refrigerated for up to a week. For the lysozyme test, add 5 ml of lysozyme solution to 95 ml of basal glycerol broth (peptone, 1 g; beef extract, 0.6 g; glycerol, 14.0 ml; distilled water, 200 ml). Dispense in 5-ml aliquots and keep refrigerated. Growth of the test organism in the lysozyme-supplemented glycerol broth is compared with growth in the unsupplemented glycerol broth.

■ Nitrate reduction test (*N,N*-dimethyl-naphthylamine and sulfanilic acid)

The nitrate reduction test is used to determine the ability to reduce nitrate to nitrite or free nitrogen gas. This test involves the use of two Griess reagents. Griess reagent A (0.8 g of sulfanilic acid in 100 ml of 5 N [i.e., 30%] acetic acid) reacts with nitrite to produce diazonium salt, which, after addition of Griess reagent B (0.5 g of α-naphthylamine or 0.6 g of *N,N*-dimethyl-naphthylamine in 100 ml of 5 N acetic acid), will react to produce *para*-sulfobenzene-azo-naphthylamine (prontosil), the red end product of this reaction. The reagents may be stored in the dark under refrigeration. To perform the test, add 0.05 ml of reagent A to 10 drops of an overnight growth from the nitrate broth culture and incubate for 5 to 10 min. Then add 0.05 ml of reagent B and incubate for an additional 5 to 10 min. Incubation should be in the dark. (Note: reagents A and B may be mixed and added together as indicated in the previous edition of this *Manual*, but this lowers the sensitivity of the test since Griess reagent B reacts with the product formed by the reaction of Griess reagent A with nitrite.) An organism may be reported as nitrate positive if a red or purple-magenta color develops in the medium within a few minutes after nitrate reagents A and B are added to the medium, indicating that the organism has reduced nitrate to nitrite. The absence of a red-purple color after the addition of both reagents does not automatically mean that the organism is unable to reduce nitrate. Strains may have reduced the nitrate to nitrite and then reduced the nitrite completely to nitrogenous gases which are not detected when nitrate reagents A and B are added to the medium. If the medium does not change color after the addition of sulfanilic acid and α-naphthylamine, a small amount ("knife point") of zinc dust is added to the incubated medium. The zinc dust will catalyze the reduction of nitrate to nitrite chemically. Thus, if the nitrate has not been reduced by the organisms, i.e., they are nitrate negative, it will be reduced by the zinc dust and a red color will develop in the incubated medium within 15 min. If no color develops in the incubated medium after the addition of zinc dust, the organisms not only have reduced nitrate to nitrite but also have reduced nitrite to nitrogenous gases; these organisms are also nitrate positive. See Table 1 for nitrate and nitrite reduction reactions.

■ Oxidase test (TMPD/DMPD)

The oxidase test is a test used in microbiology to determine if a bacterium produces certain cytochrome oxidases (16). It uses disks impregnated with a reagent such as *N,N,N',N'*-tetramethyl-*p*-phenylenediamine dihydrochloride (TMPD) or *N,N*-dimethyl-*p*-phenylenediamine dihydrochloride (DMPD), which is also a redox indicator. TMPD is more sensitive than DMPD and therefore generally the preferred reagent. The reagent is a dark blue to maroon color when oxidized and colorless when reduced. A modified oxidase test is used for the differentiation of *Micrococcus* and related organisms from most other aerobic gram-positive cocci. Six percent TMPD (the same chemical used in Kovács oxidase reagent) dissolved in dimethyl sulfoxide is used as the reagent. Keep the reagent away from light because light degrades it. Commercially available strips (Merck) containing the dimethyl compound are much more stable. A loopful of colonies from blood agar plates is smeared onto filter paper, and the reagent is dropped onto the bacterial growth. Development of a blue to purple-blue color in 2 min indicates a positive reaction.

■ Phenylalanine deaminase test (ferric chloride)

Phenylalanine deaminase activity can be determined on 1% of DL-phenylalanine agar media or agar slants, which are flooded with a 12% $FeCl_3$ solution in 2% HCl after 1 to 2 days of incubation. The hydrochloric acid is prepared by adding 5.4 ml of concentrated HCl (37%) to 94.6 ml of distilled water. To perform the phenylalanine deaminase test, 4 or 5 drops of ferric chloride reagent are added to a culture grown overnight on phenylalanine agar or broth. The development of a green to brown color, due to the reaction of phenylpyruvic acid with Fe in the medium or on the slant, indicates a positive reaction.

■ Pyrrolidonyl aminopeptidase activity (PYR test)

Pyrrolidonyl aminopeptidase (pyrrolidonyl arylamidase) or PYR is a rapid colorimetric method for presumptive identification of certain groups of bacteria based on the activity of the enzyme pyrrolidonyl arylamidase. This test is used in the identification of gram-positive cocci and nonfermentative gram-negative bacteria. The reaction involves addition of DMACA, which can be suspended in a solution of 2.5 ml of sodium dodecyl sulfate, 2.5 ml of glacial acetic acid, 5.0 ml of 2-methoxyethanol, and 90 ml of distilled water (stored at 4°C in a dark container). There also is a commercial kit in which L-pyroglutamic acid β-naphthylamide is impregnated into the test disk and serves as the substrate for the detection of pyrrolidonyl arylamidase. Hydrolysis of the substrate yields β-naphthylamide, which combines with the PYR reagent (DMACA) to form a bright pink to cherry red color. A positive PYR tests allows for the presumptive identification of group A streptococci (*Streptococcus pyogenes*) and group D enterococci.

TABLE 1 Nitrite and nitrate reductase activities[a]

Biochemical reactivity of isolate	KNO$_3$ + Griess/Zn[b]	NaNO$_2$ + Griess
Nitrate reductase p, nitrite reductase n	Red	Red
Nitrate reductase p, nitrite reductase p[c]	Red	Colorless
Nitrate reductase p, nitrite reductase pp[c]	Colorless/colorless	Colorless
Nitrate reductase n, nitrite reductase p	Colorless/red	Colorless
Nitrate reductase n, nitrite reductase n	Colorless	Red

[a]Courtesy of Georges Wauters and Mario Vaneechoutte.
[b]Addition of Zn is necessary only when both broths remain colorless. It can then differentiate between situations 3 and 4.
[c]In case of normal nitrite reductase positivity (p), as in situation 2, nitrite is still present. In the case of very strong positive nitrite reductase activity (pp), as in situation 3, all nitrite is further reduced quickly, resulting in a false-negative nitrate reductase reaction upon addition of Griess reagents to the nitrate broth. In that case, addition of Zn is needed to confirm that nitrate is no longer present.

■ Tributyrin esterase (tributyrate glycerol, bromo-chloro-indolyl butyrate)

Tributyrin esterase activity is used in the differentiation of nonfermenting gram-negative bacteria and for the identifcation of *Moraxella catarrhalis*. Tributyrin esterase activity can be detected using disks containing tributyrate glycerol and phenol red, which are available from Rosco, or strips (TRIBU strips) that are available from Sigma. Tributyrin esterase activity frees butyric acid, resulting in the formation of a yellow color due to acidification. Tributyrin esterase can also be detected using disks impregnated with bromo-chloro-indolyl butyrate (CatScreen) from Hardy Diagnostics. Hydrolysis of this substrate by the butyrate esterase yields a chromogenic compound which appears blue to blue-violet. For this test a heavy inoculum from a 24- to 72-h-old culture is smeared onto a disk that has been wet with sterile distilled water and incubated for 5 min. Longer incubation can yield false positives.

■ Tween 80 (polysorbitol) hydrolysis (Tween 80)

The formation of a precipitate around colonies after growth on Trypticase soy agar containing 1% Tween 80 and 0.01% calcium chloride indicates Tween 80 hydrolysis due to esterase activity. This method is used for differentiation of nonfermenting gram-negative bacteria and identification of *Moraxella catarrhalis*. Esterase activity can also be detected using a medium containing Tween 80 and neutral red; the neutral red binds to the Tween 80, producing an amber color. When Tween 80 is hydrolyzed by esterase activity, a red color develops due to the release of oleic acid. This method has been used for identifcation of mycobacteria.

■ Urease test (phenol red)

The urease test is used to determine the ability of an organism to split urea through the production of the enzyme urease. Ammonia is produced, which causes a rise in pH that is detected by a change in color of the indicator phenol red to pink under alkaline conditions (pH 8.4). Bacteria are cultured on a medium containing urea, e.g., Christensen urea agar. While many enteric bacteria can hydrolyze urea, only a few "rapid urease-positive" organisms, e.g., *Proteus* species, can degrade urea quickly (less than 4 h). Urea broth is formulated to test for rapid urease-positive organisms. The restrictive amount of nutrients, coupled with the use of pH buffers, prevents all but rapid urease-positive organisms from producing enough ammonia to turn phenol red to pink. The rapid urease test also is used for the diagnosis of *Helicobacter pylori*. To detect *H. pylori*, this test is performed on stomach lining cells collected by biopsy at the time of endoscopy. A basic broth for performing the urease test can be made by adding 10.4 ml of a 20% (wt/vol) aqueous solution of urea to a solution containing 0.1 g of KH_2PO_4, 0.1 g of K_2HPO_4, and 0.5 ml of 1:500 phenol red, adjusted to pH 6.8 in 100 ml. To make 1:500 phenol red, dissolve 0.2 g of phenol red in NaOH and add distilled water to 100 ml. This solution not only is easier to prepare than Christensen agar but also is more sensitive for assessing urease activity by nonfermenters when a dense inoculum is used. Red color developing within 4 h after inoculation indicates urease activity.

■ Voges-Proskauer (VP) test (α-naphthol/KOH)

The VP test is used to detect acetoin (acetyl-methylcarbinol), which is produced by certain bacteria during growth in a buffered peptone-glucose broth (methyl red VP [MR-VP] broth). The VP test is commonly used to aid in differentiation between genera (such as *E. coli* from the *Klebsiella* and *Enterobacter*

species) and among species of the *Enterobacteriaceae* family. The test can be used as a differential test for other organism groups (viridans group streptococci). The test uses 5% α-naphthol, which is prepared by dissolving 5 g of α-naphthol in 100 ml of absolute ethanol, and 40% KOH, which is prepared by dissolving 40 g of potassium hydroxide in 100 ml of distilled water. To perform the test, MR-VP broth is inoculated and incubated until good growth is obtained. Then 0.6 ml of the α-naphthol solution and 0.2 ml of the 40% KOH are added to 2.5 ml of culture broth. A positive reaction is indicated by the formation of a pink-red product within 5 min. However, allow 15 min for color development before considering the test negative.

Buffers

■ Bovine albumin fraction V

A 0.2% solution of bovine albumin fraction V is used to buffer mycobacterial specimens following decontamination with N-acetyl-L-cysteine-sodium hydroxide (NALC-NaOH). The solution is prepared by mixing 40.0 ml of 5% bovine albumin with 8.5 g of NaCl and 960.0 ml of distilled water. The pH is adjusted to 6.8 using 4% NaOH. The solution is filter sterilized and stored refrigerated. Before addition to the buffer, samples are decontaminated with NALC-NaOH and concentrated by centrifugation. The sedimented sample is suspended in 1 to 2 ml of the sterile 0.2% bovine albumin solution. The preserved cells can then be examined microscopically or inoculated into a culture medium.

■ Glycine-buffered saline

Glycine-buffered saline (0.043 M glycine, 0.15 M NaCl [pH 9.0]) is used in some serological procedures and is also used as a transport medium for enteric organisms. It is prepared by dissolving 3.22 g of glycine and 8.77 g of NaCl in 1 liter of distilled water.

■ Phosphate-buffered saline

Phosphate-buffered saline solutions are made by mixing various amounts of 0.1 N mono- and dibasic phosphates, depending upon the pH desired, with 0.85% NaCl. These are prepared as 10× stock solutions. For 0.1 M NaH_2PO_4 (sodium phosphate, monobasic), dissolve 13.9 g of NaH_2PO_4 in 1 liter of deionized water; for 0.1 M Na_2HPO_4 (sodium phosphate, dibasic), dissolve 26.8 g of $Na_2HPO_4·7H_2O$ in 1 liter of deionized water; and for 8.5% NaCl (sodium chloride), dissolve 85.0 g of NaCl in 1 liter of deionized water. Sterilize by autoclaving for 20 min or by filtration. Store refrigerated. For the working phosphate-buffered saline, combine the appropriate amounts of the 10× stock solutions of the mono- and dibasic phosphate solutions that are combined with 100 ml of 8.5% NaCl and bring the volume to 1 liter with distilled or deionized water. See the ninth edition of this *Manual* (8a) for the appropriate amounts of the mono- and dibasic phosphate solutions needed to achieve specific pH values.

■ Sorensen pH buffers

Sorensen pH buffers are prepared by mixing appropriate amounts of 0.067 M dibasic sodium phosphate and 0.067 M monobasic potassium phosphate. To prepare 0.067 M dibasic sodium phosphate, dissolve 9.464 g of anhydrous Na_2HPO_4 in 1 liter of distilled water. To prepare 0.067 M monobasic potassium phosphate, dissolve 9.073 g of anhydrous KH_2PO_4 in 1 liter of distilled water. See the ninth edition of this *Manual* (8a) for appropriate amounts of dibasic and monobasic phosphate solutions to achieve specific pH values.

Decontamination Agents

■ NALC-NaOH

NALC (mucolytic agent)-NaOH (decontamination agent) is used in the processing of mycobacterial specimens. The reagent consists of 50.0 ml of sterile 4% NaOH, 50.0 ml of 2.9% sodium citrate, and 0.5 g of NALC. The sodium citrate is included to stabilize the acetylcysteine. This reagent should be used within 24 h of preparation.

■ Cetylpuridium chloride-sodium chloride (CPC-NaCl)

CPC-NaCl is used for decontamination of transported sputum specimens for culturing mycobacteria. It is prepared by dissolving 1 g of CPC and 2 g of NaCl in 100 ml of distilled water. It can be stored in a sealed brown bottle at room temperature. If crystals form, the solution should be gently heated before use. An equal amount of sputum and CPC-NaCl is mixed until the specimen is liquefied, and then the specimen can be shipped to the testing site. Specimens treated with CPC-NaCl must be cultured on egg-based media or else residual CPC will inhibit mycobacterial growth.

■ Oxalic acid

Oxalic acid is used as a decontamination agent for specimens that contain *Pseudomonas* spp. when culturing for mycobacteria. The reagent is especially helpful when processing respiratory specimens from cystic fibrosis patients. To prepare the solution, 50 g of oxalic acid is added to 1.0 liter of distilled water. The solution is autoclaved at 121°C for 15 min. It can be stored at room temperature for up to a year.

Dyes and Indicators

A variety of dyes and indicators are used to detect specific reactions such as pH and oxygen production. Commonly used dyes and pH indicators are shown in Table 2.

Preservatives

■ Skim milk

Skim milk is used to stabilize bacterial suspensions, particularly those containing anaerobes, for freezing. The skim milk is prepared by adding 20 g of skim milk powder to 100 ml of distilled water. After the skim milk is dissolved in the water, the solution is dispensed as 0.25- to 0.5-ml aliquots into 2-ml vials. The skim milk is autoclaved at 110°C for 10 min. The vials can be refrigerated for up to 6 months.

McFarland Standards

McFarland standards are used as a reference to adjust the turbidity of bacterial suspensions so that the number of bacteria will be within a given range. These standards can be prepared using $BaCl_2$. They also are available using latex beads. To prepare McFarland standards, mix the designated amounts of 1% anhydrous barium chloride ($BaCl_2$) and 1% (vol/vol) cold pure sulfuric acid (H_2SO_4) in screw-cap tubes as shown in Table 3. Tightly seal the tubes. When the barium sulfate is shaken up well, the density in each tube corresponds approximately to the bacterial suspension listed in Table 3. Store the prepared standard tubes in the dark at room temperature. The absorbance of the 0.5 McFarland standard should be 0.08 to 0.10 at 625 nm using a spectrophotometer with a 1-cm light path. Standards are checked regularly using a densitometer. No policy exists regarding the frequency of monitoring. However, when placed in the densitometer and it fails to read in the defined optical range, it should be considered unusable. Companies that produce automated identification/antibiotic susceptibility testing systems provide guidelines with the instrument. The manufacturer is responsible for the accuracy and reliability of the McFarland standards and should supply a quality control record with each production lot.

TABLE 2 Dyes and pH indicators

Indicator	pH and color
Acid fuchsin (Andrade's)	5.0, pink
	8.0, pale yellow
Bromcresol green	3.8, yellow
	5.4, blue
Bromcresol purple	5.2, yellow
	6.8, purple
Bromphenol blue	3.0, yellow
	4.6, blue
Bromthymol blue	6.0, yellow
	7.6, dark blue
Chlorcresol green	4.0, yellow
	5.6, blue
Chlorphenol red	5.0, yellow
	6.6, red
Cresolphthalein	8.2, colorless
	9.8, red
m-Cresol purple	7.4, yellow
	9.0, purple
Cresol red	7.2, yellow
	8.8, red
Methyl red	4.4, red
	6.2, yellow
Neutral red	6.8, red
	8.0, yellow
Phenolphthalein	8.3, colorless
	10.0, red
Phenol red	6.8, yellow
	8.4, red
Resazurin	Oxidized: blue, nonfluorescent
	Reduced: red, fluorescent
Thymol blue	8.0, yellow
	9.6, blue
Triphenyltetrazolium chloride	Oxidized: colorless
	Reduced: red

TABLE 3 McFarland standards protocol

Standard	Vol (ml)		Corresponding bacterial suspension (10^8 CFU/ml)
	1% $BaCl_2$	1% H_2SO_4	
0.5	0.05	9.95	1.5
1	0.1	9.9	3
2	0.2	9.8	6
3	0.3	9.7	9
4	0.4	9.6	12
5	0.5	9.5	15
6	0.6	9.4	18
7	0.7	9.3	21
8	0.8	9.2	24
9	0.9	9.1	27
10	1.0	9.0	30

STAINS

Microscopic examination is useful in the identification of clinically important specimens. Smears can be made from relevant tissues and body fluids. If there are sufficient quantities of cells, the smear may be prepared by direct contact with a tissue sample or by applying a drop of body fluid, e.g., sputum, to a clean glass slide. Cytocentrifugation may be used to concentrate cells (9, 20, 31). Samples are fixed to the slides with either heat or methanol. Methanol fixation is preferred since heating may produce artifacts, may create aerosols, and may not adhere the specimen adequately to the slide. A variety of stains can then be used to help visualize and differentiate bacteria from the specimen. The following are some of the commonly used staining procedures.

■ Acid-fast stain

Acid-fast staining is useful for the identification of *Mycobacterium*, *Nocardia*, *Rhodococcus*, *Tsukamurella*, *Gordonia*, and *Legionella micdadei*. These bacteria have long-chain fatty acids (mycolic acids) that make them difficult to stain with crystal violet and other basic dyes.

Mycobacteria often appear as slender, slightly curved rods and may show darker granules that give the impression of beading. *Mycobacterium tuberculosis* can appear as beaded rods arranged in parallel strands or "cords"; *Mycobacterium kansasii* may form long, often broad and banded cells; and *Mycobacterium avium* complex cells appear as short, uniformly staining coccobacilli. *Nocardia* spp. often branch and almost always show a speckled appearance. A number of staining procedures have been developed for acid-fast staining.

In the Ziehl-Neelsen (Z-N) procedure, the slide is heat fixed for 2 h at 70°C. The slide is then flooded with carbol fuchsin (0.3 g of basic fuchsin is dissolved in 10 ml of 95% ethanol, 5 ml of phenol, and 95 ml of water; the solution is filtered before use). The slide is slowly heated to steaming and maintained for 3 to 5 min at 60°C. After cooling, the slide is washed with water and decolorized with acid-alcohol (97 ml of 95% ethanol in 3 ml of HCl). The slide is counterstained for 20 to 30 s with methylene blue (0.3 g of dye in 100 ml of water). An acid-fast organism will stain red, and the background of cellular elements and other bacteria will be blue, the color of the counterstain.

In the Kinyoun modification of the Z-N staining procedure, heating during staining with carbol fuchsin is eliminated and a higher concentration of phenol is used in the primary stain. The primary stain consists of 4 g of basic fuchsin in 20 ml of 95% alcohol, 8 g of phenol, and 100 ml of distilled water. The Z-N and Kinyoun stains have the same sensitivity and specificity; however, the Kinyoun (cold) staining procedure is less time-consuming and is easier to perform.

Another modification of the acid-fast staining procedure has been the use of a weaker decolorizing agent (0.5 to 1.0% sulfuric acid) in place of the 3% acid-alcohol. This particular stain helps differentiate those organisms known to be partially or weakly acid-fast, particularly *Nocardia*, *Rhodococcus*, *Tsukamurella*, *Gordonia*, and *Dietzia*. These organisms do not stain well with the Z-N or Kinyoun stain.

Factors such as age, exposure to drugs, and a particular acid-fast organism itself may vary the acid-fast presentation. For example, while M. *tuberculosis* is consistently acid fast (with the Z-N or Kinyoun stain), rapidly growing mycobacteria and *Nocardia* are not. Therefore, use of the modified Kinyoun stain may be necessary for these organisms. Other modifications used in tissue preparations, such as the Fite-Faraco stain and Pottz stain, may be preferred for unusual isolates such as *Mycobacterium leprae*.

Detection of small numbers of acid-fast organisms in clinical specimens is generally significant. However, the use of acid-fast stains for gastric aspirates in the interpretation of pulmonary disease in adults or for stool specimens from human immunodeficiency virus-positive patients in diagnosing *Mycobacterium avium-Mycobacterium intracellulare* infection yields very poor specificity (false-positive smears with saprophytic organisms) as well as poor sensitivity. In addition, patients receiving adequate therapy may still have positive smears without positive cultures for a number of weeks.

■ Acridine orange stain

Acridine orange is a fluorochrome that can be intercalated into nucleic acid in both the native and the denatured states. Acridine orange is useful in a number of miscellaneous infections, such as *Acanthamoeba* infections, infectious keratitis, and *Helicobacter pylori* gastritis (26). In the acridine orange staining procedure, the slide is flooded with acridine orange solution (stock solution, 1 g of dye in 100 ml of water; working solution, 0.5 ml of stock added to 5 ml of 0.2 M acetate buffer [pH 4.0]). The slide is then examined by UV fluorescence microscopy.

■ Auramine-rhodamine stain

Auramine and rhodamine are nonspecific fluorochromes that bind to mycolic acids and that are resistant to decolorization with acid-alcohol. Staining procedures with these fluorochromes are thus equivalent to the fuchsin-based acid-fast procedures (34). Acid-fast organisms fluoresce orange-yellow in a black background. If the secondary stain is not used, the organisms will fluoresce a yellow-green color. In this procedure, the slide is heat fixed at 65°C for at least 2 h. It is then stained for 15 min with auramine-rhodamine solution (1.5 g of auramine O, 0.75 g of rhodamine B, 75 ml of glycerol, 10 ml of phenol, and 50 ml of H$_2$O) and rinsed with water, followed by decolorization for 2 to 3 min with 0.5% HCl in 70% ethanol. After being rinsed, the slide is counterstained with 0.5% potassium permanganate for 2 to 4 min. The slide is rinsed, dried, and examined under UV fluorescence microscopy.

■ Gimenez stain

The Gimenez stain is used for the visualization of *Rickettsia* and *Coxiella* from cell cultures and *L. pneumophila*. Carbol fuchsin is the primary stain, and fast green and malachite green are the counterstains, allowing greater contrast with the organisms and background for easier visualization of the organisms. The stain must be heated 48 h prior to use and filtered.

■ Gram stain

Gram staining is the differential staining procedure most commonly used for microscopic examination of bacteria. The procedure was first described by Hans Christian Joachim Gram. Based upon the staining reaction, bacteria are classified as gram-positive organisms, which retain the primary crystal violet dye and appear deep blue or purple, and gram-negative organisms, which can be decolorized, thereby losing the primary stain and subsequently taking up the counterstain safranin and appearing red or pink. The staining reaction reflects underlying differences in cell wall structure which are relevant for antibiotic susceptibility as well as identification. The Gram stain reaction works well with most bacteria but is not useful for bacteria that are too small or lack a cell wall, i.e., *Treponema*, *Mycoplasma*, *Chlamydia*, and *Rickettsia* (18). Mycobacteria are generally not seen by Gram staining; however, in smears illustrating heavy infections, the organisms may give a beaded appearance that is somewhat similar to that of *Nocardia* spp. or may exhibit organism "ghosts" (18). Anaerobic bacteria, older cultures, and organisms that are exhibiting the effects of antibiotics may be especially difficult to interpret.

In the conventional Gram stain procedure used in most clinical laboratories, the slide is first flooded with a primary stain of crystal violet (10 g of 90% dye in 500 ml of absolute methanol). After at least 15 s, the slide is washed with water and flooded with the mordant Gram's iodine (6 g of I_2 and 12 g of KI in 1,800 ml of H_2O), which increases the affinity of the primary stain to the bacterial cell. The slide is washed with water after 15 s with the decolorizing agent acetone-alcohol (400 ml of acetone in 1,200 ml of 95% ethanol). The decolorizing agent will remove the primary stain from a gram-negative cell. Gram-positive bacterial cells retain the primary stain. The slide is washed immediately and counterstained for at least 15 s with safranin (10 g of dye in 1 liter of distilled or deionized water). This slide is then washed, blotted dry, and examined by light microscopy at ×1,000 magnification.

Gram stain confirmation

The Gram stain reaction, which can be difficult to properly interpret for some gram-variable bacteria, can be confirmed using APNA K915 disks (L-alanine-*p*-nitroanilide in Tris buffer) from Key Scientific products or by using Gram-Sure (L-alanine 7-amido-4-methycoumarin) from Remel as reagent-impregnated disks. These reagents detect the presence of cell wall aminopeptidase, which is present in the cell walls of gram-negative bacteria. Each lot of disks should be tested prior to use with organisms whose Gram reactions are known. A pure colony of overnight growth is inoculated into demineralized water and then inoculated onto the disk. The Gram-Sure disk is incubated at room temperature for 5 to 10 min. The APNA K915 disk is incubated at 37°C for 5 to 20 min. The aminopeptidase in the cell walls of gram-negative organisms will hydrolyze the L-alanine-7-amido-4-methycoumarin in the Gram-Sure disk from a nonfluorescent substrate to a blue fluorescent compound that can be observed under long-wave UV light. Blue fluorescence is indicative of gram-negative bacteria, and the absence of blue fluorescence is indicative of gram-positive bacteria. The APNA K915 disk will yield a yellow color for a positive test for gram-negative bacteria; no color change from the white/cream colored disk indicates that the organism is gram positive. Obligate anaerobes and some microaerophiles may fail to give expected results (29).

Immunofluorescent antibody stain

Immunofluorescent staining consists of labeling antibodies with a fluorescent dye, allowing the labeled antibodies to react with their specific antigens, and observing the stained bacterial cells under a fluorescence microscope (14). This method allows the identification of specific bacterial species and subtypes based upon the specificity of the antibody reaction, e.g., for *Legionella* spp. They are used in bacteriology primarily for culture confirmation, as other methods for direct specimen testing, such as enzyme immunoassays and nucleic acid amplification tests, have supplanted them.

Methylene blue stain

Staining with methylene blue is used to show bacterial cell shape. This is useful for revealing the morphology of fusiform bacteria and spirochetes from oral infections (Vincent's angina). It may also establish the intracellular location of microorganisms such as *Neisseria*. Methylene blue is the stain of choice for identification of the metachromatic granules of diphtheria; however, one should be careful about overstaining, because this will lessen the contrast between the bacteria and the granules. Methylene blue stains organisms or leukocytes a deep blue against a light gray background. *Corynebacterium diphtheriae* appears as a blue bacillus with prominent darker blue metachromatic granules. For methylene blue staining, a 0.5 to 1.0% aqueous solution of methylene blue is applied for 30 to 60 s and up to 10 min for possible *C. diphtheriae* granules. The slide is rinsed with water, blotted dry, and examined by light microscopy at magnifications of ×100 to ×1,000.

M'Fadyean stain

The M'Fadyean stain is a modification of the methylene blue stain developed for detecting *Bacillus anthracis* in clinical specimens. The stain is prepared by dissolving 0.05 mg of methylene blue per ml in 20 mM potassium phosphate adjusted to pH 7.3. Slides are stained for 1 min and then washed. As a safety precaution, washing of the slide is performed using a 10% hypochlorite solution. The dried slide is examined by light microscopy. Virulent *B. anthracis* rods will be surrounded by a clearly demarcated zone giving the appearance of a reddish pink capsule (M'Fadyean reaction).

Spore stain

The Wirtz-Conklin spore stain is a differential stain for detection of spores. This is very useful for the identification of *Bacillus* and *Clostridium* species. Using this procedure, spores stain green while the rest of the cell stains pink. Non-spore-forming bacteria are pink. In this procedure the slide is flooded with 5 to 10% aqueous malachite green. The stain is left on the slide for 45 min. Alternatively, the slide can be heated gently to steaming for 3 to 6 min. Heating to steaming enhances the uptake of the stain into the spores. The slide is then rinsed with water. Aqueous safranin (0.5%) is used as a counterstain for 30 s. The slide is then washed, blotted dry, and examined by light microscopy at ×1,000 magnification.

Wayson stain

The Wayson stain can be used to demonstrate bipolar staining characteristics of *Yersinia pestis* but is not commonly used in clinical microbiology laboratories. It is no longer used for screening cerebrospinal fluid for bacteria due to the rarity of *Haemophilus influenzae* infections. The staining reagents are prepared by dissolving 0.2 g of basic fuchsin in 10 ml of 95% ethyl alcohol and 0.75 g of methylene blue in 10 ml of 95% ethyl alcohol. The two solutions are added together slowly into 200 ml of 5% phenol in distilled water. The stain is then filtered and stored in an opaque bottle at room temperature. The stain is applied for 1 min. The slide is then washed, blotted dry, and examined by light microscopy at ×1,000 magnification.

CULTURE MEDIA

Laboratory cultivation of pathogenic microorganisms has been central to the laboratory diagnosis of infectious diseases caused by bacteria. Louis Pasteur in 1860 was the first to use culture media for growing bacteria in the laboratory. Pasteur's first medium consisted of sugar, ammonium salts, and yeast ash. It met the basic growth requirements of many bacteria, namely, a carbon source in the form of sugar that could be metabolized for energy and growth, a nitrogen source needed by bacteria to synthesize proteins and nucleic acids, and growth factors, including vitamins and minerals from the yeast ash.

Almost immediately, additional media began to be developed by Robert Koch and his colleagues, who used animal and plant tissues as sources of nutrients to support bacterial growth. One of the major discoveries of Fanny Hesse, who was the wife of one of the workers in Koch's laboratory, was that agar could be used to form solidified culture media on which microorganisms would grow. Using solid media permits the isolation of pure cultures of bacteria. Extracts of plants and animal tissues were prepared as broths or mixed with agar to form a variety of solid culture media. Virtually any plant, animal, or animal organ was considered for use in preparing media. Infusions were prepared from beef heart, calf brains, and beef liver, as a few examples. From the earliest development of media, there was a balance between scientific design and chance findings regarding which media would support the growth of specific pathogens. By the early 1900s, many media were available to aid in diagnostic activities. These classic infusions still form the primary components of many media that are widely used today in clinical microbiology laboratories, such as brain heart infusion agar.

Each medium has a specific use. See Table 4 for a guide to media used in the clinical laboratory for the enrichment, isolation, and culture of pathogenic bacteria. Often there are pros and cons to the choice of a specific medium—the advantages and disadvantages of each must be considered and the results obtained in the clinical laboratory must be evaluated in light of the limitations of a given medium. Articles frequently appear comparing media (e.g., see references 4, 19, 33, and 37).

Several comprehensive volumes have been compiled describing in detail the formulations of these media for the culture of bacteria (1–4, 7, 8, 22, 23, 36). Additionally, the major commercial producers of microbiological culture media maintain websites that provide important information about the composition, preparation, and use of the specific culture media they supply (Becton, Dickinson and Company, http://www.bd.com/; Gibco Invitrogen Cell Culture Products, http://www.invitrogen.com/site/us/en/home/Applications/Cell-Culture.html?cid=invggl123000000000095s&; Hardy Diagnostics, http://www.hardydiagnostics.com/?gclid=CMifuc62t JsCFR7yDAodZlWRQg; HiMedia, http://www.himedialabs.com/; and Oxoid Ltd., http://www.oxoid.com/uk/blue/index.as). The inserts available with commercial media also provide critical information about their proper use.

Composition of Media

Agar is the most common solidifying agent used in microbiological media (24). Agar is a polysaccharide extract from marine algae. It melts at 84°C and solidifies at 38°C. Agar concentrations of 15.0 g/liter typically are used to form solid media. Lower concentrations, 7.5 to 10.0 g/liter, are used to produce soft agars or semisolid media.

Many media contain peptones as the source of nitrogen. Peptones are hydrolyzed proteins formed by enzymatic or acidic digestion. Casein most often is used as the protein substrate for forming peptones, but other substances, such as soybean meal, also are commonly employed.

Meat and plant infusions are aqueous extracts that are commonly used as sources of nutrients for the cultivation of microorganisms. Such infusions contain amino acids and low-molecular-weight peptides, carbohydrates, vitamins, minerals, and trace metals. Extracts of animal tissues contain relatively high concentrations of water-soluble protein components and glycogen. Extracts of plant tissues contain relatively high concentrations of carbohydrates.

The pH generally is maintained within a few tenths of a pH unit. For this reason, buffers are key components of many media. Some pathogens are anaerobic, and factors such as thioglycolate are included in some media to reduce the availability of molecular oxygen so that anaerobes may be cultured. The use of specialized media for the culture of anaerobes is important for clinical microbiology (25).

Many microorganisms have specific growth factor requirements that must be included in media for their successful cultivation. The incorporation of key growth factors began in the 1930s. Gradually new formulations were developed that incorporated vitamins, amino acids, fatty acids, trace metals, and blood components to meet the growth factor requirements of specific pathogens. Most often, mixtures of growth factors are used in microbiological media. Acid hydrolysates of casein commonly are used as sources of amino acids. Extracts of yeast cells also are employed as sources of amino acids and vitamins for the cultivation of microorganisms. Many of the media used in the clinical laboratory contain blood or blood components that serve as essential nutrients for fastidious microorganisms.

Many media contain selective components that inhibit the growth of nontarget bacteria. Selective media are especially useful in the isolation of specific pathogens from mixed populations. Selective toxic compounds are also frequently used to select for the cultivation of particular microbial species. The isolation of a pathogen from a stool specimen, for example, where there is a high abundance of nonpathogenic organisms in the normal microbiota, requires selective media. Often, antimicrobials or other selectively toxic compounds are incorporated into media to suppress the growth of the background microbiota while permitting the cultivation of the organism of interest. Bile salts, selenite, tetrathionate, tellurite, azide, phenylethanol, sodium lauryl sulfate, high sodium chloride concentrations, and various dyes—such as eosin, crystal violet, and methylene blue—are used as selective toxic chemicals. Antimicrobial agents used to suppress specific types of microorganisms include ampicillin, chloramphenicol, colistin, cycloheximide, gentamicin, kanamycin, nalidixic acid, sulfadiazine, and vancomycin. Various combinations of antimicrobials are effective in suppressing classes of microorganisms, such as enteric bacteria.

Some media contain components that permit the differentiation of specific pathogens based upon key metabolic reactions. These include production of acid from various carbohydrates and other carbon sources or the decarboxylation of amino acids. Some media include indicators that permit the visual detection of changes in pH resulting from such metabolic reactions. A number of media also include chromogenic dyes that change color when specific

TABLE 4 Culture media for enrichment, isolation, and cultivation of pathogenic bacteria

Pathogen(s)	Culture medium			
	Enrichment	Isolation/nonselective	Isolation/selective	Cultivation
Blood specimens				
Bacillus anthracis	Columbia broth base	Columbia agar base with 1% agar	PLET agar base	Columbia agar base with 1% agar
Clostridium spp.	Brain heart infusion broth	Clostridial agar	Clostridial agar	Anaerobic agar
	Cooked meat medium	McClung-Toabe agar base	Forget-Fredette agar	
			Perfringens agar base	
			Wilkins-Chalgren anaerobic agar	
			Tryptose-sulfite-cycloserine agar	
Brucella spp.			Brucella agar base	Brucella agar base
	Eugonic LT100 broth base without Tween 80		Columbia blood agar base	Eugonic LT100 medium base without Tween 80
	Schaedler broth		Columbia blood agar base with 1% agar	
Francisella tularensis	Blood agar base	Cystine heart agar		
	Brain heart infusion agar	Eugonic LT100 medium base without Tween 80		
	Tryptose agar			
		Tryptose blood agar base		
Staphylococcus spp.	Mannitol salt broth	Blood agar base	Azide blood agar base	Azide blood agar base
		Columbia blood agar base	Coagulase mannitol agar base	Blood agar base
		Columbia blood agar base with 1% agar	Columbia CNA agar	Brain heart infusion agar
			Mannitol salt agar	Columbia blood agar base with 1% agar
			Phenylethyl alcohol agar	
MRSA			MeReSA with methicillin	
Streptococcus spp.	Brain heart infusion broth	Blood agar base	Blood agar base no. 2	Azide blood agar base
		Columbia blood agar base with 1% agar	Columbia CNA agar	Brain heart infusion agar
	Columbia broth base	Tryptose blood agar base	Differential agar for group D streptococci	Columbia blood agar base with 1% agar
	Pike streptococcal broth		*Streptococcus* selection agar	
	SF broth		Kanamycin-esculin-azide agar	
Legionella spp.		Feeley-Gorman agar	Buffered charcoal-yeast extract agar base	Buffered charcoal-yeast extract agar base
			Differential buffered charcoal-yeast extract agar base	Feeley-Gorman agar
Salmonella spp.	Selenite broth	Salmonella-shigella agar	Brilliance *Salmonella* agar	BPL agar
	Tetrathionate broth		Brilliant green agar	
			XLT-4 agar	
			Xylose sodium	
Ear culture				
Corynebacteria	Hartley's digest broth	Columbia blood agar base	Diphtheria virulence agar base	Loeffler serum medium
	Hoyle medium base	Cystine-tellurite agar base	Hoyle medium base	Tellurite blood agar base
		Loeffler medium base	Mueller tellurite agar base	CTA agar
			Tinsdale agar base	
Proteus spp.		EMB agar	Hektoen enteric agar base	DCLS agar
Pseudomonas spp.	Cetrimide broth		Cetrimide agar base	Acetamide agar
Staphylococcus spp.	Mannitol salt broth	Columbia blood agar base	Azide blood agar base	Azide blood agar base
		Blood agar base	Phenylethyl alcohol agar	Blood agar base

(Continued on next page)

TABLE 4 Culture media for enrichment, isolation, and cultivation of pathogenic bacteria *(Continued)*

Pathogen(s)	Culture medium			
	Enrichment	Isolation/nonselective	Isolation/selective	Cultivation
Eye culture				
Streptococci, staphylococci, *Haemophilus* spp.	Pike streptococcal broth	Columbia blood agar base	Azide blood agar base	Azide blood agar base
		Columbia blood agar base with 1% agar	Blood agar base	Blood agar base
			Columbia CNA agar	Brain heart infusion agar
			Chocolate agar base	Columbia blood agar base with 1% agar
			GC agar base	
			Mannitol salt agar	
			Phenylethyl alcohol agar	Agar
Proteus spp.		Blood agar base	EMB agar	
			Hektoen enteric agar base	
			MacConkey agar	
Pseudomonas spp.	Cetrimide broth		Cetrimide agar base	
			Pseudomonas agar base	
Corynebacteria	Hartley's digest broth		Diphtheria virulence agar base	Loeffler medium base
			Hoyle medium base	
			Mueller tellurite agar base	
			Tinsdale agar base	
Feces and rectal swabs				
Vibrio spp.		*Vibrio parahaemolyticus* medium		TCBS agar
		STT agar		*Vibrio* agar
		Vibrio parahaemolyticus agar		Heart infusion agar
Campylobacter spp.		*Campylobacter* thioglycolate medium	Blood agar base no. 2	Brucella agar base
		Campylobacter agar, blaser	*Campylobacter* selective medium, Blaser-Wang	Brucella agar base, modified
				Columbia blood agar base
				Columbia blood agar base with 1% agar
Shigella spp., salmonellae	Fluid selenite cystine broth	Bismuth sulfite agar, modified	Brilliant green agar, modified	Tergitol-7 agar base
	Mannitol selenite broth	Hektoen enteric agar	Deoxycholate-citrate agar	Xylose-lysine-deoxycholate agar
			Deoxycholate-citrate agar modified	Acetate differential agar
			Hektoen enteric agar	BCP DCLS
				MLCB agar
	Selenite broth	MacConkey agars	GN broth	
	Selenite cystine broth base	Önöz *Salmonella* agar		
Proteus spp. *Escherichia coli*	Brilliant green bile broth, 2%	Endo agar	MacConkey agar	EMB agar
		EMB agar	Tergitol-7 agar base	
E. coli O157:H7		MacConkey agar with sorbitol		Sorbitol MacConkey agar with BCIG
Yersinia enterocolitica		CRBHO medium	Bile esculin agar	
			Yersinia selective agar base	
			CIN agar	
Staphylococci		Columbia blood agar base	Azide blood agar base	Azide blood agar base
		Coagulase-mannitol agar base	Columbia CNA agar	Blood agar base
			Mannitol salt agar	Brain heart infusion agar
			Phenylethyl alcohol agar	Columbia blood agar base
			KRANEP agar base	
			Vogel-Johnson agar base	

(Continued on next page)

TABLE 4 *(Continued)*

Pathogen(s)	Culture medium			
	Enrichment	Isolation/nonselective	Isolation/selective	Cultivation
Streptococci, enterococci	Pike streptococcal broth	Blood agar base	Arabinose agar base	Casman agar
	SF broth base	Columbia blood agar base with 1% agar	Differential agar for group D streptococci	Columbia blood agar base with 1% agar
		Anaerobic CNA agar	Kanamycin-esculin-azide agar	Bile esculin agar
			Streptococcus selection agar	TTC agar
			Bile esculin azide agar	
VRE		Enterococcosel agar with vancomycin	VRE agar	
Bacillus cereus		Heart infusion agar		Mannitol-egg yolk-polymyxin agar
Clostridium difficile			Cycloserine-cefoxitin-egg yolk-fructose agar	
Spinal and joint fluids				
Neisseria spp.	Brain heart infusion broth	Blood agar base no. 2	Chocolate no. 2 agar base	Blood agar base
	Columbia broth base	Blood agar base	GC agar base	Brain heart infusion agar
	Heart infusion agar	Chocolate agar base	Modified Thayer-Martin medium base	Columbia blood agar base
		Columbia blood agar base	GC Lect agar	Thayer-Martin medium
		Columbia blood agar base with 1% agar	Martin-Lewis agar	
		Heart infusion agar	*Neisseria meningitidis* medium	
		Mueller-Hinton agar		
		New York City medium		
Mycobacterium spp.		Middlebrook media	Middlebrook media	Lowenstein-Jensen medium
		Lowenstein-Jensen medium	Mycobactosel agar	
			ATS	
Haemophilus spp.	Blood agar base	Chocolate agar base	*Haemophilus* test agar base	Chocolate agar base
		Eugonic LT100 medium base without Tween 80		GC agar base
		GC agar base		
		CAL agar		
Bacteroides	Wilkins-Chalgren anaerobic agar		*Bacteroides* bile esculin agar	Blood agar base
			Wilkins-Chalgren anaerobic agar	*Bacteroides* bile esculin agar
			Bile esculin agar with kanamycin	Lombard-Dowell agar
Pasteurella	Blood agar base			Blood agar base
	Tryptose blood agar base			Tryptose blood agar base
Throat, nose				
Corynebacteria	Hartley's digest broth	Columbia blood agar base	Tinsdale blood agar base	Loeffler medium base
	Hoyle's medium base			Loeffler medium base
Bordetella spp.		Bordet-Gengou agar base	*Bordetella pertussis* selective medium	Charcoal agar base with niacin
Erysipelothrix spp.		Bordet-Gengou agar base with agar 1.6%	Bordet-Gengou agar	Charcoal agar base
		Charcoal agar base with niacin	Regan-Lowe medium	
Listeria spp.		LPM agar base	Gum *Listeria* medium	*L. monocytogenes* confirmatory agar
Streptococcus spp.	Pike streptococcal broth	Columbia blood agar base	SXT blood agar	Columbia blood agar base with 1% agar
	Streptococcus enrichment broth	Columbia blood agar base with 1% agar	Kanamycin-esculin-azide agar	*Streptococcus* selection broth
		Islam GBS agar	Anaerobic blood agar with neomycin	Hartley's digest broth
		Strep B carrot broth	Streptosel agar	Todd-Hewitt broth

(Continued on next page)

TABLE 4 Culture media for enrichment, isolation, and cultivation of pathogenic bacteria (*Continued*)

Pathogen(s)	Culture medium			
	Enrichment	Isolation/nonselective	Isolation/selective	Cultivation
Staphylococcus		Anaerobic neomycin blood agar SK agar		Vogel-Johnson agar
Sputum				
Haemophilus spp.		Charcoal agar base with niacin Columbia blood agar base with 1% agar	Chocolate no. 2 agar base Columbia CNA agar	Charcoal agar base with niacin GC agar base
Streptococci		Charcoal agar base with niacin Columbia blood agar base with 1% agar GC agar base	Chocolate no. 2 agar base Columbia CNA agar Modified bile esculin azide agar	Charcoal agar base with niacin GC agar base
Mycobacterium spp.		Lowenstein-Jensen medium	Middlebrook media Dubos broth base Kirschner medium base, modified	Lowenstein-Jensen medium Lowenstein-Gruft medium Middlebrook media
Mycoplasma	*Mycoplasma* broth base with crystal violet *Mycoplasma* broth base without crystal violet	*Mycoplasma* agar base	*Mycoplasma* agar base with crystal violet	Buffered yeast extract agar *Mycoplasma* agar base
Burkholderia cepacia	*Burkholderia cepacia* agar	*Burkholderia cepacia* selective agar	Ashdown's medium	
Urine, urethral swabs				
Coliforms, including *E. coli* and *Klebsiella*		Endo agar EMB agar-Levine	Tergitol-7 agar base Tergitol-7 agar H	BCPD agar
Proteus			Columbia CNA agar	Azide blood agar base Blood agar base
Gardnerella vaginalis			Columbia blood agar base	V agar
Leptospires				Ellinghausen-McCullough medium
Ureaplasma	A7 and A8 agars	A7 and A8 agars	Urogenital *Mycoplasma* broth	A7 and A8 agars
Neisseria gonorrhoeae			PPNG selective medium	Thayer-Martin medium
Wound cultures				
Clostridium spp.	Anaerobic thioglycolate medium base Brewer thioglycolate medium	Clostridial agar	Clostridial agar Forget-Fredette agar Perfringens agar base Wilkins-Chalgren anaerobic agar	Perfringens agar base Anaerobic egg agar base
Corynebacterium spp.	Hartley's digest broth Hoyle medium base	Columbia blood agar base Cystine-tellurite agar base	Mueller-tellurite agar Tinsdale agar base	
Pseudomonas spp.	Cetrimide broth		Cetrimide agar base MacConkey agar Pseudomonas agar base Acetamide agar	Acetamide agar
Staphylococcus spp.	Columbia broth base Mannitol salt broth	Blood agar base Coagulase mannitol agar base Mannitol salt agar Phenylethyl alcohol agar *Staphylococcus-Streptococcus* selection agar	Azide blood agar base Phenylethyl alcohol agar Vogel-Johnson agar base	Azide blood agar base Blood agar base Brain heart infusion agar

[a]BPL, brilliant green-phenol red-lactose agar; KRANEP, potassium thiocyanate–Acti-Dione–sodium azide–egg yolk–pyruvate; CAL, cellobiose arginine lysine.

TABLE 5 Commercial sources of chromogenic agar media for bacteria

Organism(s)	Medium	Manufacturer
E. coli	CHROMagar E. coli	CHROMagar
	CHROMagar ECC	CHROMagar
	Chromocult coliform agar ES	Merck
	Brilliance UTI agar	Oxoid
	Brilliance UTI Clarity agar	Oxoid
E. coli O157:H7	CHROMagar O157	CHROMagar
	BBL CHROMagar O157	BD[a]
	Rainbow agar O157	BIOLOG[b]
	O157:H7 ID agar	bioMérieux
Enteric bacteria in urine	Brilliance UTI agar	Oxoid
	Brilliance UTI Clarity agar	Oxoid
	CHROMagar Orientation	CHROMagar
	CHROMagar Rambach	CHROMagar
	HiCrome UTI agar	HiMedia
Listeria	CHROMagar Listeria	CHROMagar
	BBL CHROMagar Listeria	BD
	Listeria HiCrome agar base, modified	HiMedia
MRSA	CHROMagar MRSA	CHROMagar
	BBL CHROMagar MRSA	BD
	Brilliance MRSA agar	Oxoid
	HiCrome MeRaSa agar with methicillin	HiMedia
	Spectra MRSA	Remel
	MRSA Select	Bio-Rad
Enterococcus	CHROMagar Orientation	CHROMagar
	BBL CHROMagar Orientation	BD
Pseudomonas	CHROMagar Pseudomonas	CHROMagar
	HiFluoro Pseudomonas agar	HiMedia
Salmonella	CHROMagar Salmonella	CHROMagar
	BBL CHROMagar Salmonella	BD
	Rainbow agar Salmonella	BIOLOG
	CHROMagar Salmonella PLUS	CHROMagar
	Brilliance Salmonella agar	Oxoid
	Salmonella chromogenic agar	Oxoid
	HiCrome RajHans agar	HiMedia
Staphylococcus	CHROMagar Staphylococcus	CHROMagar
	BBL CHROMagar Staph aureus	BD
	S. aureus ID	bioMérieux
	Staphylococcus aureus agar, HiCrome	HiMedia
GBS	CHROMagar StrepB	CHROMagar
Vibrio	CHROMagar Vibrio	CHROMagar
VRE	CHROMagar VRE	CHROMagar

[a]Becton Dickinson (BD) licensing agreement with CHROMagar (Paris, France).
[b]Licensing agreement with FocusBiotech Sdn. Bhd.

enzymatic reactions occur. See Table 5 for descriptions of chromogenic media.

Some media contain components that are toxic or carcinogenic. Appropriate safety precautions must be taken when using media with such components. Basic fuchsin and acid fuchsin are carcinogens, and caution must be used in handling media with these compounds to avoid dangerous exposures.

Thallium salts, sodium azide, sodium biselenite, and cyanide are among the toxic components found in some media. These compounds are poisonous, and steps must be taken to avoid ingestion, inhalation, or skin contact. Azides also react with many metals, especially copper, to form explosive metal azides. The disposal of azides must avoid contact with copper or achieve sufficient dilution to avoid the formation of such hazardous explosive compounds. Cycloheximide is toxic. Avoid skin contact or aerosol formation and inhalation. Proper handling and disposal procedures must be followed with blood-containing media as well as other media that are used to cultivate microorganisms (see chapter 10).

Preparation of Media

It is important to follow the manufacturers' instructions in preparing media. The ingredients in a medium are usually dissolved, and the medium is then sterilized. When agar is used as a solidifying agent, the medium must be heated gently, usually to boiling, to dissolve the agar. In some cases where interactions of components, such as metals, would cause precipitates, solutions must be prepared and occasionally sterilized separately before the various solutions are mixed to prepare the complete medium. The pH often is adjusted prior to sterilization, but in some cases sterile acid or base is used to adjust the pH of the medium following sterilization. Many media are sterilized by exposure to elevated temperatures. The most common method is to autoclave the medium. Different sterilization procedures are employed when heat-labile compounds are included in the formulation of the medium.

Autoclaving uses exposure to steam, generally under pressure, to kill microorganisms. Exposure for 15 min to steam at 15 lb/in^2 at 121°C is most commonly used. Such exposure kills vegetative bacterial cells and bacterial endospores. However, some substances do not tolerate such exposures, and lower temperatures and different exposure times are sometimes employed. Media containing carbohydrates often are sterilized at 116 to 118°C in order to prevent the decomposition of the carbohydrate and the formation of toxic compounds that would inhibit microbial growth.

The proper preparation of media is critical for performance. For this reason, as well as because of personnel costs, many clinical laboratories purchase prepared media. Quality control is essential regardless of whether the medium is prepared in the laboratory or purchased as a preprepared medium (6, 12). Quality control test cultures are used to periodically check the performance of the media. For general-purpose media, sufficient, characteristic growth and typical colony morphology should be obtained with all test strains. For selective media, growth of designated organisms should be inhibited and adequate growth of desired organisms must be obtained. Differential characteristics of the medium for specific bacterial strains, e.g., color and hemolytic reactions, must be met. Media must not be used past expiration dates. The Clinical and Laboratory Standards Institute issues standards for quality assurance of commercially prepared microbiological culture media (12).

Bacteriological Media

Below are descriptions of some of the media used in clinical microbiology.

■ A7 agar (Shepard's differential agar)

A7 agar is used for cultivation and differentiation of *Ureaplasma urealyticum* from urine based on its ability to produce ammonia from urea. The medium contains digests of casein and soybeans plus growth factors, including cysteine, NAD, cocarboxylase, vitamins, yeast extract, and penicillin as a selective factor. Manganous sulfide is included as a nutritional factor. Urea is a key component which allows the detection of *Ureaplasma* species. Bacteria that produce ammonia from the hydrolysis of urea appear as golden to dark brown colonies.

■ A8 agar

This agar is used for cultivation and differentiation of *U. urealyticum* from urine based on its ability to produce ammonia from urea. This medium also supports the growth of *Mycoplasma hominis*. The medium contains digests of casein and soybeans plus growth factors, including cysteine, NAD, cocarboxylase, vitamins, yeast extract, and penicillin as a selective factor. Manganous sulfide, calcium chloride, and putrescine dihydrochloride are included as nutritional factors. Amphotericin B and penicillin G are added as selective factors. Urea is a key component which allows the detection of *Ureaplasma* species. *U. urealyticum* can be differentiated from other genital mycoplasmas on this medium due to manganous sulfate in the medium, which combines with the urease to form a golden brown pigment.

■ Acetamide agar

Acetamide agar is used for differentiation of nonfermentative gram-negative bacteria, especially *Pseudomonas aeruginosa* (21, 30). Acetamide is the key component that supports growth and forms the basis for differentiation. Most bacteria are unable to grow on acetamide as the sole source of carbon and nitrogen. Bacteria that deamidate acetamide turn the medium blue if bromthymol blue is included as the indicator or red if the medium contains phenol red. The color change is due to the liberation of ammonia from the utilization of acetamide.

■ Acetate differential agar (Simmons' citrate agar, modified)

This agar is used for differentiation of *Shigella* species from *E. coli* and also for differentiation of nonfermenting gram-negative bacteria (35). The medium contains acetate as the sole source of carbon. Bacteria that can utilize acetate as the sole carbon source turn the medium blue due to the increase in pH as the acidic acetate is utilized.

■ Alkaline peptone salt broth

This broth is used for cultivation of *Vibrio cholerae* and other *Vibrio* species from stool specimens. Peptone is the growth substrate. A salt concentration of 3% is selective for *Vibrio* species.

■ Alkaline peptone water

This medium is used for cultivation and transport of *Vibrio cholerae* and *Aeromonas hydrophila*. Peptone is the growth substrate. The salt concentration is 1%.

■ American Trudeau Society (ATS) medium

ATS medium is used for isolation and cultivation of *Mycobacterium* species other than *Mycobacterium leprae*. It is especially useful for the detection of *M. tuberculosis* from clinical specimens such as cerebrospinal fluid, pleural fluid, and tissues. The medium contains eggs, which supply the fatty acids needed for growth by mycobacteria. Potatoes are also included as a source of carbon. Malachite green is a selective factor included in the medium.

■ Amies transport medium with charcoal

This medium is used for transport of swab specimens to prolong the survival of microorganisms between collection and culturing. The phosphate buffer and calcium and magnesium ions in the medium help protect cells against lysis. The addition of charcoal to this medium neutralizes metabolic products that may be toxic to *Neisseria gonorrhoeae*.

■ Amies transport medium without charcoal

This medium is used for transport of swab specimens to prolong the survival of microorganisms. This medium contains phosphate buffer and calcium and magnesium ions to protect cells against lysis.

■ Anaerobe neomycin-5% sheep blood agar

This medium, used for isolation of anaerobes, employs Trypticase soy agar supplemented with additional agar, yeast extract, vitamin K_1, hemin, cystine, and 5% sheep blood. Neomycin inhibits the growth of most staphylococci and *Enterobacteriaceae*.

■ Anaerobic blood agar base with blood and neomycin

This medium is used for isolation and cultivation of group A and group B streptococci from throat cultures and other clinical samples. It contains digests of casein and soybeans plus growth factors. Blood is included and allows differentiation based upon hemolysis reactions. Neomycin sulfate is a selective factor in the medium.

■ Anaerobic colistin-nalidixic acid (CNA) agar

This agar is used for selective isolation of anaerobic streptococci. Digests of casein and animal tissue along with yeast extract, beef extract, and glucose supply the carbon and nitrogen for growth. Dithiothreitol and cysteine help create anaerobic conditions. The medium contains colistin and nalidixic acid as selective factors. Blood is added to support the growth of fastidious strains and also to permit differentiation based upon hemolytic reactions.

■ Ashdown medium

Ashdown medium is used for selective isolation and characterization of *Burkholderia pseudomallei* from clinical specimens such as sputum. The medium contains crystal violet and gentamicin as selective factors. It is enriched with glycerol and contains neutral red. *Burkholderia pseudomallei* produces flat, wrinkled, purple colonies on this medium. Both Ashdown agar and Ashdown broth can be modified by the addition of antimicrobials for the selective culture of *B. pseudomallei*. Modified Ashdown broth remains the standard for isolation of *B. pseudomallei* from throat swabs in patients with suspected melioidosis (10).

■ Azide blood agar

This agar is used for isolation and differentiation of streptococci and staphylococci from specimens containing mixed biotas. The medium contains digests of casein and animal tissue, beef extract, sodium azide, and blood.

■ *Bacteroides* bile esculin (BBE) agar

BBE agar is used for selection and presumptive identification of the *Bacteriodes fragilis* group and for differentiation of *Bacteroides* species based on the hydrolysis of esculin and presence of catalase (27). The medium contains digests of casein and soybeans. Hemin, vitamin K_1, oxgall, and gentamicin are included in the medium as selective factors. Esculin is a key component for differentiation of *Bacteroides* species. *Bacteroides* colonies appear as gray, circular, raised colonies larger than 1.0 mm. Esculin hydrolysis is indicated by the presence of a blackened zone around the colonies.

■ Baird-Parker agar base with egg yolk-tellurite enrichment

This broth is used for selective isolation of coagulase-positive staphylococci. The medium contains glycine, pyruvate, digest of casein, and yeast extract. The medium is enriched with egg yolks and tellurite, which support the growth and differentiation of *Staphylococcus aureus*. Lithium chloride is included as a selective factor. Reduction of tellurite produces black colonies, and lecithinase activity results in a clear zone around the colony. *S. aureus* produces black-brown colonies surrounded by a zone of clearing on this medium. The inclusion of sulfamethazine suppresses swarming by *Proteus* species.

■ Barbour-Stoenner-Kelly medium

This medium is used for cultivation of a wide variety of microorganisms in a chemically defined medium, including *Borrelia* and *Spirochaeta* species. This is a complex medium containing numerous vitamins and growth factors. It also contains gelatin, glucose, pyruvate, peptone, albumin, and serum.

■ Bile esculin agar

This medium is used for differentiation between group D streptococci and non-group D streptococci; for differentiation of members of the *Enterobacteriaceae*, particularly *Klebsiella*, *Enterobacter*, and *Serratia*, from other enteric bacteria; and for differentiation of *Listeria monocytogenes*. Bile tolerance and esculin hydrolysis (seen as a dark brown to black complex) are presumptive for enterococci (group D streptococci). Vancomycin can be added to identify vancomycin-resistant enterococci (VRE).

■ Bile esculin agar with kanamycin

This medium is used for selective isolation and/or presumptive identification of bacteria of the *Bacteroides fragilis* group from specimens containing a mixed biota. The medium contains beef extract and esculin. It also contains hemin and vitamin K_1 as growth factors. When examined with long-wave UV light, pigmented colonies of the *Bacteroides* group fluoresce red-orange. Oxgall and kanamycin are selective factors in the medium. Growth on this medium with blackening of the medium is presumptive for members of the *Bacteroides fragilis* group.

■ Bile esculin azide agar

This medium is used for isolation and presumptive identification of group D streptococci. The medium contains digest of casein, proteose peptone, iron, esculin, and yeast extract. Oxgall (bile) and sodium azide are included as selective factors. The hydrolysis of esculin in the presence of ferric citrate results in the formation of a black-brown color. *Streptococcus bovis* group organisms and *Enterococcus faecalis* produce black zones around colonies as a result of this reaction.

■ Blood agar

This medium is used for isolation and detection of hemolytic activity of streptococci and other fastidious microorganisms. The base medium contains beef extract and peptone. Sheep blood is added to complete the medium.

■ Bordet-Gengou agar

This medium is used for detection and isolation of *Bordetella pertussis* and *Bordetella parapertussis* from clinical specimens. The medium is rendered selective by the addition of methicillin. The medium contains digest of casein and animal tissue plus glycerol, potato infusion, and rabbit blood. *Bordetella pertussis* appears as small (<1-mm), smooth, pearl-like colonies surrounded by a narrow zone of hemolysis. *Bordetella parapertussis* appears as brown, nonshiny colonies with a green-black coloration on the reverse side. *Bordetella bronchiseptica* appears as brown, nonshiny, moderately sized colonies with a roughly pitted surface.

■ *Bordetella pertussis* selective medium

This medium is used for selective isolation and presumptive identification of *Bordetella pertussis* and *Bordetella parapertussis*. The medium contains Bordet-Gengou agar base, which includes digest of casein and animal tissue. It also contains blood and cephalexin. *Bordetella pertussis* appears as small, nearly transparent, "bisected pearl-like" colonies.

■ *Bordetella pertussis* selective medium with charcoal agar base

This medium is used for selective isolation and presumptive identification of *Bordetella pertussis* and *Bordetella parapertussis*. The medium contains charcoal agar base, which includes digest of casein and animal tissue, beef extract, nicotinic acid, starch, and charcoal. It also contains blood and cephalexin. *Bordetella pertussis* appears as small, pale, shiny colonies.

■ Bovine albumin Tween 80 medium, Ellinghausen and McCullough, modified (albumin fatty acid broth, *Leptospira* medium)

This medium is used for cultivation of *Leptospira* species. The medium contains glycerol, pyruvate, thiamine, and an albumin fatty acid supplement.

■ Brain heart infusion

This medium is used for cultivation of fastidious and nonfastidious microorganisms, including aerobic and anaerobic bacteria, from a variety of clinical specimens. The medium contains digests of gelatin and animal tissue plus glucose and brain heart infusion. The medium is particularly useful for culturing streptococci, pneumococci, and meningococci. Vancomycin can be added for the detection of VRE.

■ Brain heart infusion agar, 0.7%

This medium is used for detection of staphylococcal enterotoxin. The medium contains peptone, glucose, and infusions from beef heart and calf brains.

■ Brilliant green agar

This medium is used for selective isolation of salmonellae other than *Salmonella enterica* serovar Typhi from feces and other clinical specimens. The medium contains lactose, sucrose, and digests of casein and animal tissue plus phenol red and brilliant green. *Salmonella* species other than serovar Typhi appear as red, pink, or white colonies surrounded by a zone of red in the agar, indicating nonfermentation of lactose and sucrose. *Proteus* or *Pseudomonas* species may appear as small red colonies. Lactose- or sucrose-fermenting bacteria appear as yellow-green colonies surrounded by a zone of yellow-green in the agar.

■ Bromcresol purple-deoxycholate (BCPD) agar

This medium is used for isolation and differentiation of gram-negative enteric bacilli from clinical specimens, especially from fecal specimens. The medium contains lactose, sucrose, and sodium deoxycholate, which form the basis for differentiation. The medium also contains peptones, yeast extract, and citrate. Non-lactose- and non-sucrose-fermenting microorganisms appear as colorless or blue colonies. Lactose- and sucrose-fermenting microorganisms, such as coliform bacteria, appear as yellow-opaque white colonies surrounded by a zone of precipitated deoxycholate.

■ Bromcresol purple-deoxycholate-citrate-lactose-sucrose (BCP DCLS) agar

This medium is used for differential isolation of gram-negative enteric bacilli (*Salmonella*, *Shigella*, and other non-lactose- and non-sucrose-fermenting microorganisms) from clinical specimens, especially from fecal specimens. Non-lactose- and non-sucrose-fermenting microorganisms appear as colorless or blue colonies. The medium also contains peptones, yeast extract, meat extract, sodium thiosulfate, and a high level of citrate. Lactose- and sucrose-fermenting microorganisms, such as coliform bacteria, appear as yellow-opaque white colonies surrounded by a zone of precipitated deoxycholate.

■ Brucella agar

This medium is used for cultivation of *Brucella* species and for isolation of both nonfastidious and fastidious microorganisms from a variety of clinical specimens. The medium contains digests of casein and animal tissue plus sodium sulfite, yeast extract, glucose, and blood. The medium can be supplemented with hemin and vitamin K$_1$ to improve growth. Blood can also be added for the detection of hemolytic reactions of *Streptococcus* and *Haemophilus* species.

■ Brucella agar base campylobacter medium

This medium is used for selective isolation and cultivation of *Campylobacter jejuni* from fecal specimens or rectal swabs. It contains digests of casein and animal tissue, yeast extract, glucose, pyruvate, sodium sulfite, and ferrous sulfate. It also includes cycloheximide, sodium cefazolin, novobiocin, bacitracin, and colistin sulfate as selective factors.

■ Brucella agar base with blood and selective supplement

This medium is used for cultivation and maintenance of *Brucella* species and for isolation and cultivation of nonfastidious and fastidious microorganisms from a variety of clinical specimens. This medium contains hydrolysate of casein, peptone, yeast extract, glucose, sodium sulfite, and blood. Cycloheximide, nalidixic acid, vancomycin, bacitracin, and polymyxin B are included as selective supplements.

■ Brucella blood culture broth

This medium is used for isolation and cultivation of microorganisms from blood. The medium is especially useful for the cultivation of anaerobes. It contains digests of casein and animal tissue plus sodium sulfite, yeast extract, sucrose, glucose, hemin, vitamin K$_1$, and blood. The medium can be supplemented with hemin.

■ Brucella laked sheep blood agar with kanamycin and vancomycin

This medium is used for selective isolation of fastidious and slow-growing, obligately anaerobic bacteria from the same specimen. The medium contains peptones, dextrose, yeast extract, sheep blood, hemin, and vitamin K$_1$. Kanamycin and vancomycin are included as selective factors. The laked blood improves pigmentation of the *Prevotella melaninogenica-Porphyromonas asaccharolytica* group.

■ Buffered charcoal-yeast extract agar with cysteine (BCYE alpha base)

This medium is used for isolation of *L. pneumophila* and other *Legionella* species from clinical specimens. The medium contains cysteine, α-ketoglutarate, iron, yeast extract, *N*-(2-acetamido)-2-aminoethanesulfonic acid (ACES) buffer, and activated charcoal. The iron and cysteine are specific growth factors required by *Legionella* species for growth. The charcoal removes toxic metabolites. Antibiotics such as polymyxin B, anisomycin, and either vancomycin or cefamandole are typically included as selective factors. *L. pneumophila* produces light blue colonies with a pale green tint on this medium (see chapter 45).

■ Buffered charcoal-yeast extract differential agar

This medium is used for isolation, cultivation, and maintenance of *L. pneumophila* and other *Legionella* species from clinical specimens. The medium contains charcoal to reduce toxicity from metabolites. It also includes cysteine and iron, which are required growth factors for *Legionella*. Vancomycin and polymyxin B are included as selective factors.

■ *Burkholderia cepacia* agar

This medium is used for selective isolation of *Burkholderia cepacia* from the respiratory secretions of patients with cystic fibrosis. Slow-growing *B. cepacia* can be missed on conventional media such as blood or MacConkey agar due to overgrowth caused by other faster-growing organisms found in the respiratory tract of cystic fibrosis patients, such as mucoid *Klebsiella* species, *P. aeruginosa*, and *Staphylococcus* species. This may lead to the infection being missed or wrongly diagnosed. The medium contains bile salts, gentamicin, ticarcillin, and polymyxin B as selective factors. It also contains pyruvate, peptone, and yeast extract.

■ *Burkholderia cepacia* selective agar

This medium is used for selective isolation of *B. cepacia*. The medium contains digests of casein, yeast extract, sucrose, and lactose. It also contains polymyxin B, gentamicin, vancomycin, and crystal violet as selective factors.

■ *Burkholderia pseudomallei* selective agar

This medium is used for selective isolation of *Burkholderia pseudomallei*. The medium is an improvement over Ashdown selective agar for clinical specimens from nonsterile sites. The medium contains standard agar, maltose, and neutral red.

■ *Campylobacter* agar, Blaser's

This medium is used for selective isolation of *Campylobacter jejuni* from fecal specimens. The medium contains cephalothin, vancomycin, trimethoprim, amphotericin B, and polymyxin B as selective factors. It also contains peptone, yeast extract, and liver digest.

■ *Campylobacter* agar, Skirrow's

This medium is used for selective isolation of *Campylobacter jejuni* from fecal specimens. The medium contains vancomycin, trimethoprim, and polymyxin B as selective factors. It also contains peptone, yeast extract, and liver digest.

■ *Campylobacter* blood agar

This medium is used for isolation of *Campylobacter jejuni* from clinical specimens. It contains peptone, glucose, yeast extract, and blood. It also contains cephalothin, vancomycin, trimethoprim, amphotericin B, and polymyxin B as selective factors.

■ *Campylobacter* selective medium, Blaser-Wang

This medium is used for selective isolation of *Campylobacter* species. The medium contains vancomycin, trimethoprim, and polymyxin B as selective factors. It also includes peptone, starch, and blood.

■ *Campylobacter* thioglycolate medium

This medium is used for maintenance—as a holding or transport medium—of *Campylobacter* species isolated from clinical specimens on swabs. The medium contains cephalothin, vancomycin, trimethoprim, amphotericin B, and polymyxin B as selective factors to prevent unwanted growth of contaminating organisms. It contains sodium sulfite and sodium thioglycolate to protect the cells against damage.

■ *Campylobacter* thioglycolate medium with five antimicrobials

This medium is used for maintenance—as a holding or transport medium—of fecal specimens or swabs suspected of containing *Campylobacter jejuni* or other *Campylobacter* species when immediate inoculation of *Campylobacter* growth medium is unavailable. The medium contains cephalothin, vancomycin, trimethoprim, amphotericin B, and polymyxin B as selective factors. It also contains sodium thiosulfate, sodium sulfite, glucose, and digests of casein and animal tissue.

■ Cary-Blair transport medium

This medium is used primarily for maintenance—as a holding or transport medium—of clinical specimens, especially enteric pathogens, following collection or shipment. The medium contains sodium thioglycolate and calcium chloride to protect cells.

■ CDC anaerobe 5% sheep blood agar

This medium is used for isolation and cultivation of fastidious and slow-growing, obligately anaerobic bacteria from a variety of clinical materials. The medium employs Trypticase soy agar supplemented with additional agar, yeast extract, vitamin K_1, hemin, cystine, and 5% sheep blood. Improved growth of *Prevotella melaninogenica*, *Fusobacterium necrophorum*, and *Clostridium haemolyticum*, as well as certain strains of *Actinomyces israelii* and *Bacteroides thetaiotaomicron*, has been demonstrated on this medium.

■ Cefsulodin-Irgasan-novobiocin (CIN) agar

This medium is used for selective isolation and differentiation of *Yersinia enterocolitica* based on mannitol fermentation. The medium contains strontium chloride, cefsulodin, novobiocin, crystal violet, neutral red, Irgasan, magnesium sulfate, mannitol, peptone, yeast extract, and pyruvate. *Yersinia enterocolitica* appears as "bull's eye" colonies with deep red centers surrounded by a transparent periphery.

■ Cetrimide agar, non-USP

This medium is used for selective isolation, cultivation, and identification of *P. aeruginosa* and other gram-negative, nonfermentative bacteria. The medium contains tryptose, cetrimide, and infusion from beef heart.

■ Cetrimide agar, USP (Pseudosel agar)

This medium is used for selective isolation, cultivation, and identification of *P. aeruginosa* and other gram-negative, nonfermentative bacteria. The medium contains glycerol, digest of gelatin, cetrimide, potassium sulfate, and magnesium chloride.

■ Charcoal agar

This medium is used for cultivation and isolation of various bacteria. The medium contains peptone, beef extract, starch, nicotinic acid, and charcoal. With the addition of blood, this medium is used for the cultivation of fastidious bacteria.

■ Chocolate agar

This medium is used for isolation and cultivation of a variety of fastidious microorganisms. The medium contains cephalothin, vancomycin, trimethoprim, amphotericin B, and polymyxin B as selective factors. It also contains peptone, starch, digest of beef heart, and blood.

■ Chocolate agar, enriched

This medium is used for cultivation of fastidious microorganisms, especially *Neisseria* species. The medium contains cephalothin, vancomycin, trimethoprim, amphotericin B, and polymyxin B as selective factors. It also contains peptone, starch, digest of beef heart, and blood. The medium is enriched by the addition of hemoglobin.

■ Chocolate II agar (chocolate no. 2 agar base with hemoglobin)

This medium is used for isolation of *Neisseria* and *Haemophilus* species from a variety of clinical specimens. The medium contains cephalothin, vancomycin, trimethoprim, amphotericin B, and polymyxin B as selective factors. It also contains peptone, starch, digest of casein, vitamin B_{12}, and blood. The medium is enriched by the addition of hemoglobin. Yeast autolysate can also be added to improve the isolation of *N. gonorrhoeae* from chronic and acute cases of gonococcal infections.

■ Chocolate tellurite agar (tellurite blood agar)

This medium is used for selective isolation of *Corynebacterium* species. The medium contains extensive growth factors, including amino acids, vitamins, iron, NAD, and cocarboxylase. It also contains digests of casein and meat cornstarch, and tellurite. *Corynebacterium diphtheriae* appears as gray-black colonies.

■ Cholera medium (thiosulfate-citrate-bile salts-sucrose [TCBS] agar)

This medium is used for isolation of pathogenic vibrios, especially *Vibrio cholerae*. The medium is suitable for the growth of *Vibrio cholerae*, *Vibrio parahaemolyticus*, and most other vibrios. Most of the *Enterobacteriaceae* encountered in feces are totally suppressed for at least 24 h. Slight growth of *Proteus* species and *E. faecalis* may occur, but the colonies are easily distinguished from vibrio colonies. While inhibiting nonvibrios, it promotes rapid growth of pathogenic vibrios after overnight incubation at 35°C. The following species form yellow colonies: *Vibrio cholerae* El Tor biotype, *V. alginolyticus*, *V. metschnikovii*, *V. fluvialis*, *Enterococcus* spp., and some strains of *Aeromonas hydrophila*. *Vibrio parahaemolyticus*, *V. vulnificus*, *V. mimicus*, and *Pseudomonas* spp. form blue-green colonies. *Proteus* species form yellow-green colonies. *Plesiomonas shigelloides* does not usually grow well on this medium. This medium contains sucrose, peptone sodium thiosulfate, ox bile, ferric citrate, bromthymol blue, and thymol blue.

■ Chopped meat broth

This medium is used for cultivation of various anaerobes. The medium contains digest of casein, yeast extract, and meat. It also contains cysteine to protect against oxygen exposure.

■ Chopped meat broth with carbohydrates

This medium is used for cultivation of numerous anaerobes. The medium contains starch, glucose, cellobiose, maltose, digest of casein, yeast extract, and meat. It also contains cysteine to protect against oxygen exposure.

■ Chopped meat broth with formate and fumarate

This medium is used for cultivation of various *Clostridium* spp. The medium contains digest of casein, yeast extract, and meat. It is enriched with formate and fumarate to test the ability of bacterial strains to convert fumarate and formate to succinic acid. It also contains cysteine to protect against oxygen exposure.

■ Chopped meat broth with vitamin K₁

This medium is used for cultivation of various *Clostridium* spp. The medium contains digest of casein, yeast extract, and meat. It is enriched with vitamin K_1. It also contains cysteine to protect against oxygen exposure.

■ Christensen agar

See Urea agar.

■ Clostridial agar

This medium is used for selective isolation of pathogenic clostridia from mixed biotas. The medium contains digests of casein and soybean meal, glucose, sodium thioglycolate, sodium formaldehyde sulfoxylate, cysteine, sodium azide, and neomycin.

■ Coagulase-mannitol agar

This medium is used for differentiation of *S. aureus* from other *Staphylococcus* species based on coagulase production and mannitol fermentation. The medium contains digest of casein, mannitol, brain heart infusion, digest of soybean meal, plasma, and bromcresol purple.

■ Coliform agar ES, Chromocult (Chromocult enhanced selectivity agar)

This medium is used for detection of *E. coli* and total coliforms. The combination of suitable peptones and buffering using morpholinepropanesulfonic acid (MOPS) allow rapid growth of coliforms and an optimal transformation of the chromogenic substrates. The amounts of bile salts and propionate largely inhibit growth of gram-positive and gram-negative accompanying microbiotas. The simultaneous detection of total coliforms and *E. coli* is achieved using the combination of two chromogrenic substrates. The substrate salmon-β-D-galactosidase (β-D-Gal) is split by β-D-Gal, characteristic for coliforms, resulting in a salmon to red coloration of coliform colonies. The detection of the β-D-glucuronidase, characteristic for *E. coli*, is cleaved via the substrate X-β-D-glucuronide, causing a blue coloration of positive colonies. As *E. coli* splits salmon-β-D-Gal as well as X-β-D-glucuronide, the colonies turn to a dark violet color and can be easily differentiated from the other coliforms, which are salmon red.

■ Colistin-oxolinic acid-blood agar

This medium is used for isolation and cultivation of streptococci from mixed biotas in clinical specimens. The medium contains colistin sulfate and oxolinic acid as selective factors. It also contains starch, beef extract, yeast extract, and digests of animal tissue and casein plus blood.

■ Columbia blood agar

This medium is used for cultivation of *Corynebacterium* spp., *Actinomyces* spp., *S. pneumoniae*, *Staphylococcus* spp., and a variety of fastidious microorganisms. The medium contains starch, peptone, and blood (usually sheep blood at 5%).

■ Columbia CNA agar

This medium is used for selective isolation, cultivation, and differentiation of gram-positive cocci from clinical specimens. The medium contains starch, peptone, and blood. It also contains colistin and nalidixic acid as selective factors.

■ Congo red-brain heart infusion-agarose medium (CRBHO medium)

This medium is used for isolation and detection of virulent strains of *Yersinia enterocolitica*. The medium contains digest of gelatin, agarose (instead of agar), digest of animal tissue, infusion from brain heart, glucose, magnesium chloride, and Congo red.

■ Cooked meat medium

This medium is used for cultivation of anaerobes, especially pathogenic clostridia. The medium contains heart tissue, glucose, and digest of animal tissue.

■ Cycloserine-cefoxitin-egg yolk-fructose agar (*Clostridium difficile* agar)

This medium is used for selective isolation and cultivation of *Clostridium difficile* from feces. The medium contains peptone, fructose, hemin, neutral red, and egg yolk emulsion. It also contains cycloserine and cefoxitin as selective factors.

■ Cysteine albumin broth

This medium is used for transport and storage of biopsy samples for the detection of *H. pylori*. The medium contains cysteine, albumin, and glycerol.

■ Cystine heart agar (cystine-glucose-blood agar)

This medium is used for cultivation and maintenance of *Francisella tularensis*. The medium contains glucose, peptone, and infusion from beef heart. It also contains hemoglobin and cystine. Without the hemoglobin enrichment, it supports excellent growth of gram-negative cocci and other pathogenic microorganisms.

■ Cystine-tellurite-blood agar

This medium is used for isolation, differentiation, and cultivation of *C. diphtheriae*. The medium contains infusion from beef heart, tryptose, yeast extract, cystine, blood, and potassium tellurite. *C. diphtheriae* appears as dark gray to black colonies.

■ Cystine tryptic agar (CTA)

This medium is used for cultivation and maintenance of a variety of fastidious microorganisms, including *C. diphtheriae*. It is also used for carbohydrate fermentation tests in the differentiation of *Neisseria* species. The medium contains sodium sulfite, cystine, and digest of casein plus phenol red indicator.

■ DeMan-Rogosa-Sharpe (MRS) agar (*Lactobacillus MRS agar*)

This medium is used for isolation and cultivation of *Lactobacillus* spp. from clinical specimens. The medium contains digest of gelatin, beef extract, yeast extract, sodium acetate, ammonium citrate, and Tween 80.

■ Deoxycholate agar

This medium is used for selective isolation and differentiation of gram-negative enteric microorganisms from a variety of clinical specimens. The medium contains lactose, digests of casein and animal tissue, ferric citrate, sodium citrate, sodium deoxycholate, and neutral red. *E. coli* appears as large, flat, rose red colonies. *Enterobacter* and *Klebsiella* species appear as large, mucoid, pale colonies with a pink center. *Proteus* and *Salmonella* species appear as large, colorless to tan colonies. *Shigella* species appear as colorless to pink colonies. *Pseudomonas* species appear as irregular colorless to brown colonies.

■ Deoxycholate-citrate agar

This medium is used for selective isolation and cultivation of enteric pathogens, especially *Salmonella* and *Shigella* species. The medium contains citrate, lactose, digest of animal tissue, infusion of meat, deoxycholate, ferric citrate, and neutral red.

■ Deoxycholate-citrate agar, Hynes

This medium is used for selective isolation and differentiation of enteric pathogens, especially *Salmonella* and *Shigella* species. The medium contains lactose, citrate, peptone, beef extract, deoxycholate, ferric citrate, and neutral red. Lactose-fermenting bacteria appear as pink colonies that may or may not be surrounded by a zone of precipitated deoxycholate. Non-lactose-fermenting bacteria appear as colorless colonies that are surrounded by a clear orange-yellow zone.

■ Deoxycholate-citrate-lactose-sucrose (DCLS) agar

This medium is used for selective isolation of *Salmonella* species, *Shigella* species, and *Vibrio* species from fecal specimens. The medium contains citrate, lactose, sucrose, thiosulfate, beef extract, deoxycholate, digests of casein and animal tissue, and neutral red.

■ DCLS agar, Hajna

This medium is used for selective isolation of *Salmonella* species, *Shigella* species, and *Vibrio* species from fecal specimens. The medium contains citrate, lactose, sucrose, thiosulfate, beef extract, deoxycholate, digests of casein and animal tissue, and bromcresol purple.

■ Differential agar for group D streptococci

This medium is used for differentiation and identification of group D streptococci. The medium contains digests of casein and animal tissue, glucose, infusion from brain heart, and bromcresol purple.

■ Diphtheria virulence agar base with tellurite and diphtheria virulence supplement

This medium is used for detection of diphtheria toxin-producing strains of *C. diphtheriae* and for testing the toxigenicity of *C. diphtheriae*. The reaction of antitoxin forms the actual basis for the detection of the diphtheria toxin. The medium contains peptone, tellurite, horse serum, and a filter paper strip saturated with potent diphtheria antitoxin.

■ DNase test agar with toluidine blue

This medium is used for differentiation of microorganisms, especially *Staphylococcus* species and *Serratia marcescens*, based on their production of DNase. The medium contains digests of casein and animal tissue, DNA, and toluidine blue.

■ Egg yolk agar

This medium is used for isolation and differentiation of *Clostridium* species and some other anaerobic bacteria. The medium contains peptone, glucose, hemin, and egg yolk emulsion.

■ Ellinghausen-McCullough-Johnson-Harris medium

This medium is used for isolation and cultivation of *Leptospira* species. Albumin and Tween 80 are included to provide lipids. Lysed erythrocytes also are included in the medium to provide iron. The medium can be rendered selective by the addition of 5-fluorouracil.

■ EMB agar, Levine

This medium is used for isolation, cultivation, and differentiation of gram-negative enteric bacteria based on lactose fermentation. The medium contains digest of casein, lactose, sucrose, eosin, dipotassium phosphate, and methylene blue. Bacteria that ferment lactose, especially the coliform bacterium *E. coli*, appear as colonies with a green metallic sheen or blue-black to brown color. Bacteria that do not ferment lactose appear as colorless or transparent, light purple colonies.

■ EMB agar, modified, Holt-Harris and Teague

This medium is used for isolation, cultivation, and differentiation of gram-negative enteric bacteria based on lactose fermentation. The medium contains digest of casein, lactose, sucrose, eosin, dipotassium phosphate and methylene blue. Bacteria that ferment lactose, especially the coliform bacterium *E. coli*, appear as colonies with a green metallic sheen or blue-black to brown color. Bacteria that do not ferment lactose appear as colorless or transparent, light purple colonies.

■ Endo agar

This medium is used for selective isolation, cultivation, and differentiation of coliform and other enteric microorganisms based on their ability to ferment lactose. The medium contains lactose, digest of animal tissue, and basic fuchsin. Lactose-fermenting bacteria appear as dark red colonies with a gold metallic sheen. Non-lactose-fermenting bacteria appear as colorless or translucent colonies.

■ Enterococcosel agar

This medium is used for rapid, selective isolation of fecal group D streptococci (enterococci). It is also used for the cultivation of staphylococci and *L. monocytogenes*. The medium contains digest of casein, proteose peptone, iron, esculin, and yeast extract. Oxgall (bile) and sodium azide are included as selective factors. The hydrolysis of esculin in the presence of ferric citrate results in the formation of a black-brown color.

■ Enterococcosel agar with vancomycin

This medium is used for detection of VRE, particularly for primary screening of asymptomatic gastrointestinal carriage of VRE. The medium contains digest of casein, proteose peptone, iron, esculin, and yeast extract. Oxgall (bile), sodium azide, and vancomycin (8.0 mg/liter) are included as selective factors.

■ Enterococcosel broth

This medium is used for differentiation of group D streptococci (enterococci). The medium contains digest of casein, proteose peptone, iron, esculin, and yeast extract. Oxgall (bile) and sodium azide are included as selective factors.

■ *E. coli* O157:H7 MUG agar

This medium is used for isolation and differentiation of enterohemorrhagic *E. coli* O157:H7 strains from clinical specimens. The medium contains peptone, sorbitol, meat extract, thiosulfate, deoxycholate, yeast extract, ammonium ferric citrate, MUG, and bromthymol blue.

■ Esculin azide broth

This medium is used for cultivation of enterococci from feces. The medium contains digest of animal tissue, bile salts, yeast extract, esculin, sodium citrate, ferric ammonium citrate, and sodium azide.

■ ESP Myco medium

This medium is used with ESP Culture System II (TREK Diagnostic Systems) for detection of mycobacterial growth. The medium is a Middlebrook 7H9 broth enriched with glycerol, Casitone, and cellulose sponge disks. Oleic acid-albumin-dextrose-catalase (OADC) enrichment is added before use.

■ Eugonic LT100 medium base without Tween 80

This medium is used for cultivation of fastidious microorganisms such as *Haemophilus*, *Neisseria*, *Pasteurella*, *Brucella*, and *Lactobacillus* species.

■ Feeley-Gorman agar

This medium is used for isolation and cultivation of *L. pneumophila*. The medium contains acid hydrolyzed casein, beef extract, starch, cysteine, and ferric pyrophosphate (see chapter 45).

■ Fildes enrichment agar

This medium is used for isolation of *Haemophilus influenzae*. The medium contains peptone, beef extract, pepsin, and blood.

■ Fletcher medium

This medium is used for isolation of *Leptospira* species. The medium contains peptone, beef extract, pepsin, and blood. It can be supplemented with 5-fluorouracil to render it selective.

■ Forget-Fredette agar

This medium is used for selective isolation of *Clostridium* species and other anaerobic bacteria. The medium contains digests of casein and soybean meal, glucose, and sodium azide.

■ **GC agar**

This medium is used for isolation of *Neisseria* and *Haemophilus* species from clinical specimens. The medium contains digest of casein and starch and may be enriched by the addition of hemin and NAD. Cysteine and antibiotics can also be added to make the medium selective.

■ **GC II agar**

This medium is used for isolation of fastidious microorganisms, especially *Neisseria* and *Haemophilus* species, from clinical specimens. The medium contains digest of casein, meat peptone, and starch.

■ **GC-Lect agar**

This medium is used for isolation and cultivation of *N. gonorrhoeae* from clinical specimens. The medium contains digest of casein, meat peptone, starch, hemoglobin, a selective supplement of numerous growth factors, and a proprietary selective supplement. The medium is described in the *Difco & BBL Manual: Dehydrated Culture Media and Reagents for Microbiology* (8). GC-Lect agar is used in the Miles Laboratory JEMBEC system, which consists of a John E. Martin Biological Environmental Chamber-style plate, a carbon dioxide tablet, and resealable plastic bag.

■ **Gum *Listeria* medium (gum base-nalidixic acid medium)**

This medium is used for isolation of *Listeria monocytogenes* from clinical specimens. The medium contains gellan gum, digests of casein and soybean meal, glucose, and nalidixic acid.

■ **H broth**

This medium is used for preparation of the H agglutination antigen used in the differentiation and identification of *Salmonella* species types and subtypes. The medium contains digest of casein, peptone, beef extract, and glucose.

■ ***Haemophilus* test medium**

This medium is used for antibiotic susceptibility testing of *Haemophilus* species. The medium contains digests of casein and animal tissue, yeast extract, hematin, NAD, and growth factors.

■ **Hartley's digest broth**

This medium is used for isolation and cultivation of actinomycetes. The medium contains ox heart, pancreatin, sodium carbonate, and hydrochloric acid.

■ **Heart infusion agar**

This medium is used for isolation and cultivation of a wide variety of microorganisms, including *Bacillus cereus*, *S. aureus*, *Vibrio vulnificus*, and *Vibrio cholerae*. The medium contains tryptose and infusion from beef heart. It can be used as a base for the preparation of blood agar in determining hemolytic reactions.

■ **Hektoen enteric agar**

This medium is used for isolation and cultivation of gram-negative enteric microorganisms from a variety of clinical specimens based on lactose or sucrose fermentation and H_2S production. Bacteria that ferment lactose or sucrose appear as yellow to orange colonies. Bacteria that produce H_2S appear as colonies with black centers. The medium contains lactose, digest of animal tissue, sucrose, bile salts, thiosulfate, yeast extract, salicin ferric ammonium citrate, acid fuchsin, and bromthymol blue.

■ **Hemo ID Quad Plate with growth factors (*Haemophilus* identification quadrant plate with growth factors)**

This medium is used for differentiation and presumptive identification of *Haemophilus* species. The Hemo ID Quad Plate from BD Diagnostics is a four-sectored plate, each sector with a different medium. Quadrant 1 contains X factor (hemin) only, quadrant 2 contains V factor (NAD) only, quadrant 3 contains both X and V factors, and quadrant 4 contains 5% defibrinated horse blood.

■ **Hoyle medium**

This medium permits very rapid growth of all types of *C. diphtheriae*, so that diagnosis is possible after 18 hours' incubation. The medium contains peptone, Lab-Lemco powder, tellurite, and laked blood.

■ **Islam GBS agar (GBS agar)**

This medium is used for isolation and detection of GBS in clinical specimens. The medium contains peptone, starch, and serum. The medium is designed to exploit the ability of most GBS to produce orange-red-pigmented colonies when incubated under anaerobic conditions. There is a pigment-enhancing effect around a sulfonamide disk; the enhanced pigment effect can be seen over a radius of 10 to 20 mm. Non-group B organisms able to grow on this medium do not produce the orange-red pigment.

■ **Iso-Sensitest agar**

This medium is used for antimicrobial susceptibility testing. The medium contains a complex mixture of growth factors, including nucleotides, vitamins, and amino acids.

■ **Iso-Sensitest broth**

This medium is used for antimicrobial susceptibility testing. The medium contains a complex mixture of growth factors, including nucleotides, vitamins, and amino acids.

■ **Kanamycin-esculin-azide agar**

This medium is used for isolation of enterococci. The medium contains digest of casein, yeast extract, esculin, sodium citrate, ferric ammonium citrate, sodium azide, and kanamycin.

■ **Lim broth**

This medium is a modification of Todd-Hewitt broth and is an enriched selective liquid medium used for the isolation and cultivation of *Streptococcus agalactiae*. Peptones, salts, and dextrose provide the nutritive base. Yeast extract provides B vitamins and additional enrichment. The antibiotics colistin and nalidixic acid inhibit gram-negative bacteria. The effectiveness of this medium has been evaluated by Elsayed et al. (15).

■ ***Listeria monocytogenes* confirmatory agar base**

This medium is used for selective and differential isolation of *L. monocytogenes* from clinical specimens. The medium contains peptone, lithium chloride, yeast extract, α-methyl-D-mannoside, phosphatidylinositol, polymyxin B, ceftazidime, nalidixic acid, and amphotericin B. The multiple antimicrobials make this a highly selective medium.

■ *Listeria* Oxford medium base with antibiotic inhibitor

This medium is used for isolation and cultivation of *L. monocytogenes* from specimens containing a mixed bacterial biota, including from pathological specimens. The medium contains peptone, lithium chloride, starch, esculin, and ammonium ferric citrate. It also includes cycloheximide, colistin sulfate, fosfomycin, acriflavine, and cefotetan as selective factors.

■ *Listeria* transport enrichment medium

This medium is used for maintenance—as a transport medium—and enrichment of *Listeria* spp. The medium contains sodium glycerophosphate, sodium thioglycolate, nalidixic acid, and acridine.

■ Lithium chloride-phenylethanol-moxalactam plating (LPM) agar

This medium is used for isolation and cultivation of *L. monocytogenes*. The medium contains potassium thiocyanate, glycine, lithium chloride, digests of casein and animal tissue, beef extract, phenylethyl alcohol, and moxalactam.

■ Loeffler medium

This medium is used for detection of C. *diphtheriae*. The medium contains beef serum, eggs, infusion from heart muscle, glucose, and digest of animal tissue.

■ Lombard-Dowell agar

This medium is used for identification of a variety of obligate anaerobic bacteria, including *Bacteroides* spp., *Fusobacterium* spp., *Clostridium* spp., and non-spore-forming gram-positive anaerobes. The medium contains digest of casein, yeast extract, cystine, tryptophan, sodium sulfite, hemin, and vitamin K_1.

■ Lombard-Dowell egg yolk agar

This medium is used for cultivation and differentiation of a wide variety of anaerobic bacteria based on lecithinase production, lipase production, and proteolytic ability. The medium contains digest of casein, yeast extract, cystine, tryptophan, sodium sulfite, egg yolk emulsion, hemin, and vitamin K_1. Bacteria that produce lecithinase appear as colonies surrounded by a zone of insoluble precipitate. Bacteria that produce lipase appear as colonies with a pearly iridescent sheen. Bacteria that produce proteolytic activity appear as colonies surrounded by a clear zone.

■ Lowenstein-Gruft medium

This medium is used for cultivation and differentiation of *Mycobacterium* spp. The medium contains starch, asparagine, magnesium citrate, malachite green, nalidixic acid, RNA, eggs, glycerol, and penicillin. M. *tuberculosis* appears as granular, rough, dry colonies. *Mycobacterium kansasii* appears as smooth to rough photochromogenic colonies. *Mycobacterium gordonae* appears as smooth yellow-orange colonies. *Mycobacterium avium* appears as smooth, colorless colonies. *Mycobacterium smegmatis* appears as wrinkled, creamy white colonies.

■ Lowenstein-Jensen medium

This medium is used for cultivation and differentiation of *Mycobacterium* spp. The medium contains starch, asparagine, magnesium citrate, malachite green, eggs, and glycerol. M. *tuberculosis* appears as granular, rough, dry colonies. *Mycobacterium kansasii* appears as smooth to rough photochromogenic colonies. *Mycobacterium gordonae* appears as smooth yellow-orange colonies. *Mycobacterium avium* appears as smooth, colorless colonies. *Mycobacterium smegmatis* appears as wrinkled, creamy white colonies.

■ MacConkey agar

This medium is used for selective isolation and differentiation of coliforms and enteric pathogens based on the ability to ferment lactose. The medium contains digest of gelatin, lactose, bile salts, digests of casein and animal tissue, neutral red, and crystal violet. Lactose-fermenting organisms appear as red to pink colonies. Non-lactose-fermenting organisms appear as colorless or transparent colonies.

■ MacConkey agar, Fluorocult

This medium is used for isolation of *Salmonella*, *Shigella*, and coliform bacteria, in particular *E. coli*, from various specimens. The medium contains digest of gelatin, lactose, bile salts, digests of casein and animal tissue, neutral red, crystal violet, and MUG. The bile salts and crystal violet largely inhibit the growth of gram-positive microbial biotas. Lactose and the pH indicator neutral red are used to detect lactose-positive colonies, and *E. coli* can be seen among these because of fluorescence under UV light.

■ MacConkey agar with sorbitol

This medium is used for selective isolation and differentiation of *E. coli* O157:H7. The medium contains digest of gelatin, bile salts, digests of casein and animal tissue, neutral red, crystal violet, and sorbitol. Some Shiga toxin-producing strains of *E. coli* do not ferment sorbitol and appear as colorless colonies. Sorbitol-fermenting strains appear as pink colonies.

■ Mannitol-egg yolk-polymyxin agar

This medium is used for cultivation and enumeration of *Bacillus cereus* from clinical specimens. The medium contains mannitol, peptone, beef extract, phenol red, polymyxin B, and egg yolk emulsion.

■ Mannitol-lysine crystal violet-brilliant green (MLCB) agar

This medium is used for selective isolation and cultivation of *Salmonella* spp. from fecal material. The medium contains peptone, yeast extract, lysine, sodium thiosulfate, mannitol, beef extract, ferric ammonium citrate, crystal violet, and brilliant green.

■ Mannitol salt agar

This medium is used for selective isolation, cultivation, and enumeration of staphylococci from clinical specimens. The medium contains mannitol, digests of casein and animal tissue, beef extract, and phenol red. Mannitol-utilizing organisms turn the medium yellow.

■ Mannitol salt broth

This medium is used for selective isolation of presumptive pathogenic staphylococci. The medium contains peptone, mannitol, beef extract, and phenol red.

■ Mannitol selenite broth (selenite mannitol broth)

This medium is used for selective enrichment of *Salmonella* spp. from clinical specimens. The medium contains digest of animal tissue, mannitol, and sodium selenite.

■ Martin-Lewis agar

This medium is used for isolation and cultivation of pathogenic *Neisseria* from specimens containing mixed biotas. The medium contains hemoglobin, digest of casein, meat peptone, and starch. It also contains a complex growth supplement solution with amino acids, nucleotides, and vitamins. Colistin, trimethoprim, lactate, vancomycin, and anisomycin are included as selective factors.

■ McBride *Listeria* agar

This medium is used for selective isolation of *L. monocytogenes* from clinical specimens containing mixed biotas. The medium contains glycine, digests of casein and animal tissue, beef extract, phenylethyl alcohol, and lithium chloride.

■ McClung-Toabe agar base with egg yolk

This medium is used for isolation and cultivation of *Clostridium perfringens*. The medium contains peptone, glucose, and egg yolk emulsion.

■ MeReSa agar base with methicillin (methicillin-resistant Staphylococcus aureus [MRSA] agar)

This medium is used for isolation and cultivation of methicillin-resistant *S. aureus* (MRSA). The medium contains casein enzymatic hydrolysate, glycine, mannitol, sodium pyruvate, lithium chloride, beef extract, an indicator mix, and methicillin.

■ Methyl red VP medium

This medium is used for differentiation of bacteria based on acid production (methyl red test) and acetoin production (VP reaction). The medium contains glucose, peptone, and phosphate buffer.

■ Middlebrook albumin-dextrose-catalase (ADC) enrichment

This medium is used as a supplement to other Middlebrook media for isolation, cultivation, and maintenance of *Mycobacterium* spp. It is also used as a supplement to other Middlebrook media for determining the antimicrobial susceptibility of mycobacteria. This enrichment supplement contains bovine albumin fraction V, glucose, and catalase.

■ Middlebrook 7H9 broth with Middlebrook ADC enrichment

This medium is used for isolation of *Mycobacterium* spp., including *M. tuberculosis*, and also for determining the antimicrobial susceptibility of mycobacteria. The medium contains glutamate, citrate, ferric ammonium citrate, pyridoxine, biotin, glycerol, and Middlebrook ADC enrichment.

■ Middlebrook 7H10 agar with Middlebrook ADC enrichment

This medium is used for isolation, cultivation, and maintenance of *Mycobacterium* spp., including *M. tuberculosis*. It is also used for determining the antimicrobial susceptibility of mycobacteria. The medium contains glutamate, citrate, ferric ammonium citrate, pyridoxine, biotin, glycerol, malachite green, and Middlebrook ADC enrichment.

■ Middlebrook 7H11 agar with Middlebrook ADC enrichment (mycobacteria 7H11 agar with Middlebrook ADC enrichment)

This medium is used for cultivation of drug-resistant (isoniazid) strains of *M. tuberculosis*, and particularly for cultivation of fastidious strains of tubercle bacilli that occur following treatment of tuberculosis patients with secondary antitubercular drugs. Generally, these strains fail to grow on 7H10 medium. The medium contains glutamate, citrate, ferric ammonium citrate, pyridoxine, biotin, glycerol, malachite green, and Middlebrook ADC enrichment.

■ Middlebrook OADC enrichment

This medium is used as a supplement to other Middlebrook media for isolation, cultivation, and maintenance of *Mycobacterium* spp. It is also used as a supplement to other Middlebrook media for determining the antimicrobial susceptibility of mycobacteria. This enrichment supplement contains bovine albumin fraction V, glucose, oleic acid, and catalase.

■ Moeller decarboxylase broth

This medium is used for differentiation of gram-negative enteric bacteria based on the production of arginine dihydrolase, lysine decarboxylase, or ornithine decarboxylase. The medium contains beef extract, peptone, glucose, the amino acid being tested, cresol red, bromcresol purple, and pyridoxal phosphate.

■ Mueller-Hinton agar

This medium is used for antimicrobial susceptibility testing of a variety of bacterial species. The medium contains infusion from beef, acid hydrolysate of casein, and starch.

■ Mueller-Hinton broth

This medium is used for antimicrobial susceptibility testing. The medium contains infusion from beef, acid hydrolysate of casein, and starch.

■ Mueller-Hinton chocolate agar

This medium is used for cultivation of *N. gonorrhoeae* and *Neisseria meningitidis* and for antimicrobial susceptibility testing of fastidious microorganisms. The medium contains infusion from beef, acid hydrolysate of casein, starch, and blood.

■ Mueller-Hinton II agar

This medium is used for antimicrobial disk diffusion susceptibility testing of a variety of bacteria by the Bauer-Kirby method. The medium contains acid hydrolysate of casein and starch. This medium, supplemented with 5% sheep blood, is recommended for use in antimicrobial susceptibility testing of *S. pneumoniae* and *Haemophilus influenzae*.

■ Mueller tellurite medium

This medium is used for isolation, cultivation, and differentiation of *C. diphtheriae*. The medium contains casein, Casamino Acids, tryptophan, serum, sodium lactate, ethyl alcohol, calcium pantothenate, and tellurite.

■ Mycobactosel agar

This medium is used for selective isolation of mycobacteria from specimens containing mixed biotas. The medium contains digest of casein, albumin, glutamate, biotin, glycerol, oleic acid, catalase, and malachite green. It also contains cycloheximide, nalidixic acid, and lincomycin as selective factors.

■ Mycobactosel L-J medium

This medium is used for isolation and cultivation of *Mycobacterium* spp. from clinical specimens. The medium contains potato flour, asparagine, citrate, glycerol, malachite green, and eggs. It also contains cycloheximide, nalidixic acid, and lincomycin as selective factors. Mycobactosel L-J medium is Lowenstein-Jensen medium plus cycloheximide, lincomycin, and nalidixic acid for use with specimens likely to contain many contaminating organisms.

■ *Mycoplasma* agar base (PPLO agar base)

This medium is used for preparation of media for cultivation of *Mycoplasma* spp. The medium contains digest of casein, beef extract, yeast extract, infusion from beef heart, horse serum, and fresh yeast extract solution.

■ *Mycoplasma* broth base without crystal violet and with ascitic fluid (PPLO broth base without crystal violet)

This medium is used for enrichment of pleuropneumonia-like organisms (PPLOs) and *Mycoplasma* spp. from clinical specimens. The medium contains peptone, infusion from beef, and ascitic fluid.

■ NaCl agar

This medium is used for differentiation of gram-positive cocci, especially *Staphylococcus* spp., based on salt tolerance. The medium contains various concentrations of NaCl (e.g., 6.5 or 12%) and digests of casein and soybean meal. It can be supplemented with glucose and sheep blood.

■ *Neisseria meningitidis* medium

This medium is used for selective isolation and cultivation of *Neisseria meningitidis*. The medium contains acid hydroxylate of casein and starch. It also contains vancomycin, colistin, and nystatin as selective factors.

■ New York City medium

This medium is used for isolation and cultivation of pathogenic *Neisseria* spp. It is also used as a transport medium for urogenital and other clinical specimens and for isolation and presumptive identification of *Mycoplasmatales*, including large-colony species (*Mycoplasma pneumoniae*) and T-mycoplasmas from urogenital specimens. The medium contains starch, peptone, glucose, plasma, and blood. It also contains colistin, trimethoprim, and vancomycin as selective factors.

■ Nitrate broth

This medium is used for differentiation of aerobic and facultative gram-negative microorganisms based on their ability to reduce nitrate. The medium contains digest of gelatin and potassium nitrate. The test for nitrates uses sulfanilic acid and α-naphthylamine reagents. Bacteria that reduce nitrate to nitrite turn the reagents red or pink.

■ Nutrient agar, 1.5%, HiVeg with ascitic fluid

This medium is used for enrichment of PPLOs and *Mycoplasma* spp. from clinical specimens. The medium contains peptones and ascitic fluid.

■ Nutrient gelatin

This medium is used for detection of gelatin liquefaction. The medium contains peptone, beef extract, and gelatin.

■ N-Z amine A-glycerol agar

This medium is used for isolation and cultivation of *Actinomadura* species. The medium contains N-Z amine A, beef extract, and glycerol.

■ Önöz *Salmonella* agar

This medium is used for isolation and cultivation of *Salmonella* from feces. The medium contains sucrose, lactose, sodium citrate, meat peptone, beef extract, phenylalanine, thiosulfate, bile salts, yeast extract, ferric citrate, metachrome yellow, aniline blue, neutral red, and brilliant green.

■ Oxford agar (*Listeria* selective sgar, Oxford)

This medium is used for isolation and cultivation of *L. monocytogenes* from specimens containing a mixed bacterial biota. The medium contains peptone, starch, esculin, ferric ammonium citrate, lithium chloride, and the antimicrobials cycloheximide, colistin, fosfomycin, acriflavine, and cefotetan.

■ Oxford agar, modified (*Listeria* selective agar, modified Oxford agar)

This medium is used for isolation of *L. monocytogenes* from specimens containing a mixed bacterial biota. The medium contains peptone, lithium chloride, starch, esculin, ferric ammonium citrate, and the antimicrobials moxalactam and colistin sulfate.

■ Oxidation-fermentation medium, Hugh-Leifson's

This medium is used for differentiating gram-negative bacteria, such as *Vibrio* species, based upon determining the oxidative and fermentative metabolism of carbohydrates. The medium contains peptone, a carbohydrate substrate, and bromthymol blue. Bacteria that ferment the carbohydrate turn the medium yellow.

■ Oxidation-fermentation medium, King's

This medium is used for differentiating bacteria based upon determining the oxidative and fermentative metabolism of carbohydrates. The medium contains digest of casein, a carbohydrate substrate, and phenol red. Bacteria that ferment the carbohydrate turn the medium yellow.

■ Oxidation-reduction indicator agar

This medium is used as an indicator of oxygen-free conditions in anaerobic culture chambers. The medium contains sodium glycerol phosphate, sodium thioglycolate, calcium chloride, and methylene blue.

■ P agar

This medium is used for cultivation of *Staphylococcus* spp. The medium contains peptone, NaCl, yeast extract, and glucose.

■ *Pasteurella haemolytica* selective medium

This medium is used for selective cultivation of *Pasteurella haemolytica*. The medium contains digest of casein, digest of animal tissue, glucose, peptic digest of blood, and the antimicrobials cycloheximide, novobiocin, and neomycin.

■ Penicillinase-producing *Neisseria gonorrhoeae* medium (PPNG selective medium)

This medium is used for differentiation and presumptive identification of penicillinase-producing strains of *N. gonorrhoeae*. PPNG selective medium is a two-sectored plate, each containing a different Martin-Lewis agar.

■ Peptone iron agar

This medium is used for cultivation and differentiation of microorganisms based on their ability to produce H_2S. The medium contains peptones, sodium glycerophosphate, ferric ammonium citrate, and sodium thiosulfate. Microorganisms that produce H_2S turn the medium black.

■ Perfringens agar (Shahidi-Ferguson perfringens agar)

This medium is used for isolation and enumeration of *Clostridium perfringens* organisms, which appear as black colonies surrounded by a precipitate. The medium contains tryptose, digest of soybean meal, yeast extract, ferric ammonium citrate, sodium sulfite, egg yolk emulsion, kanamycin, and polymyxin sulfate.

■ Petragnani medium

This medium is used for isolation and cultivation of *Mycobacterium* spp. from clinical specimens, particularly for cultivation and maintenance of *Mycobacterium smegmatis*. The medium contains milk, potato flour, asparagine, digest of casein, eggs, glycerol, and malachite green.

■ Phenethyl alcohol agar (phenylethanol agar, phenylethyl alcohol agar)

This medium is used for selective isolation of gram-positive bacteria, particularly gram-positive cocci, from specimens with a mixed biota. The medium should not be used for observation of hemolytic reactions. The medium contains digests of casein and soybean meal, blood, and phenethyl alcohol. Moxalactam and lithium chloride can be added as selective factors.

■ Phenol red agar

This medium is used for determination of fermentation reactions. The medium contains peptone, beef extract, a carbohydrate substrate, and phenol red. Bacteria that can ferment the added carbohydrate turn the medium yellow.

■ Phenol red tartrate broth

This medium is used for differentiation of gram-negative bacteria of the enteric groups, particularly members of the *Salmonella* (paratyphoid) group, based on their ability to ferment tartrate. The medium contains digest of casein, tartrate, and phenol red.

■ Pike streptococcal broth

This medium is used for isolation and enrichment of hemolytic streptococci from throat swabs and other clinical specimens. The medium contains digest of casein, tryptose, yeast extract, glucose, sodium azide, blood, and crystal violet. After incubation of bacteria for 18 to 24 h in this medium, they may be isolated by streaking the culture onto blood agar plates.

■ PPLO agar

This medium is used for isolation and cultivation of *Mycoplasma* spp. (PPLOs). The medium contains infusion from beef heart, peptone, and serum.

■ Polymyxin B-lysozyme-EDTA-thallous acetate (PLET) agar

This medium is used for selective isolation and cultivation of *Bacillus anthracis*. The medium contains infusion from beef heart, tryptose, EDTA, thallous acetate, lysozyme, and polymyxin B.

■ Potassium tellurite agar

This medium is used for differentiation of *E. faecalis*. The medium contains infusion from beef heart, tryptose, blood, and potassium tellurite. *E. faecalis* appears as black colonies.

■ *Pseudomonas* isolation agar base with glycerol

This medium is used for selective isolation and identification of *P. aeruginosa* from clinical specimens. The medium contains peptone, Irgasan, and glycerol.

■ Rapid fermentation medium

This medium is used for differentiation of *Neisseria* spp. isolated from clinical specimens. The medium contains digest of casein, cystine, sodium sulfite, and phenol red.

■ Regan-Lowe charcoal agar (Regan-Lowe medium)

This medium is used for selective isolation of *Bordetella pertussis* and *Bordetella parapertussis* from clinical specimens. The medium contains beef extract, digest of gelatin, starch, charcoal, niacin, blood, and cephalexin.

■ Regan-Lowe semisolid transport medium

This medium is used for transport of *Bordetella pertussis* and *Bordetella parapertussis* isolated from clinical specimens. The medium contains beef extract, digest of gelatin, starch, charcoal, niacin, blood, and cephalexin.

■ Salmonella-shigella agar (SS agar)

This medium is used for selective isolation and differentiation of pathogenic enteric bacilli, especially those belonging to the genus *Salmonella*. The medium is not recommended for primary isolation of *Shigella* spp. The medium contains lactose, bile salts, thiosulfate, citrate, beef extract, digests of casein and animal tissue, ferric citrate, neutral red, and brilliant green. Lactose-fermenting bacteria such as *E. coli* or *Klebsiella pneumoniae* appear as small pink or red colonies. Non-lactose-fermenting bacteria—such as *Salmonella* spp., *Proteus* spp., and *Shigella* spp.—appear as colorless colonies. Production of H_2S by *Salmonella* spp. turns the center of the colonies black.

■ **Salt tolerance medium**

This medium is used for cultivation of salt-tolerant *Streptococcus* spp. and other salt-tolerant gram-positive cocci. It is also used for differentiation of gram-positive cocci, especially *Staphylococcus* spp., based on salt tolerance. This medium contain 6.5% NaCl, infusion from beef heart, tryptose, glucose, and bromcresol purple.

■ **Schaedler agar (Schaedler anaerobic agar)**

This medium is used for isolation of anaerobic and aerobic microorganisms. The medium contains glucose digests of casein and soybean meal, peptone, yeast extract, Tris buffer, cystine, and hemin.

■ **Schaedler CNA agar with vitamin K₁ and sheep blood**

This medium is used for selective isolation of anaerobic gram-positive cocci. The medium contains digests of casein, animal tissue, and soybean meal; glucose; yeast extract; cystine; hemin; colistin; nalidixic acid; blood; and vitamin K₁.

■ **Schleifer-Krämer agar (SK agar)**

This medium is used for isolation and cultivation of *Staphylococcus* spp. The medium contains glycerol, pyruvate, digest of casein, beef extract, yeast extract, potassium isothiocyanate, lithium chloride, glycine, and sodium azide.

■ **Selenite broth (Selenite-F broth)**

This medium is used for isolation and enrichment of *Salmonella* spp. from clinical specimens. The medium contains digest of casein, lactose, and sodium biselenite.

■ **Selenite broth base, mannitol**

This medium is used for isolation and cultivation of *Salmonella enterica* serovars Typhi and Paratyphi. The medium contains peptone, mannitol, and sodium selenite.

■ **Selenite cystine broth**

This medium is used for isolation and cultivation of *Salmonella* spp. from feces. The medium contains digest of casein, lactose, cystine, and sodium selenite.

■ **Sensitest agar**

This medium is used for performance of antibiotic susceptibility assays. The medium contains digest of casein, peptone, glucose, starch, nucleotides, thiamine, and buffer salts.

■ **Serum tellurite agar**

This medium is used for isolation and cultivation of *Corynebacterium* spp., especially in the laboratory diagnosis of diphtheria. The medium contains digests of casein and animal tissue, glucose, lamb serum, and tellurite.

■ **Simmons' citrate agar (citrate agar)**

This medium is used for differentiation of gram-negative bacteria on the basis of citrate utilization. The medium contains citrate, phosphate buffer, and bromthymol blue. Bacteria that can utilize citrate as a sole carbon source turn the medium blue. The medium is yellow at pH 6.0, green at pH 6.9, and blue at pH 7.6.

■ **Skirrow brucella medium**

This medium is used for selective isolation and cultivation of *Campylobacter* spp. The medium contains peptone, yeast extract, liver digest, and blood. It also contains vancomycin, trimethoprim, and polymyxin B as selective factors.

■ **Snyder test agar (BCG glucose agar)**

This medium is used for cultivation and enumeration of lactobacilli in saliva, an indication of dental caries activity. The medium contains glucose, peptone, and bromcresol green. The procedure employing this medium for the amount of acid produced in the oral cavity by bacteria has been described by Snyder (32).

■ **Sodium hippurate broth (hippurate broth)**

This medium is used for identification and differentiation of beta-hemolytic streptococci based on hippurate hydrolysis. The medium contains infusion from beef heart, tryptose, and sodium hippurate. After inoculation and incubation, tubes are treated with $FeCl_3$ reagent. A heavy precipitate remaining after 10 to 15 min indicates that hippurate has been hydrolyzed.

■ **Sorbitol-MacConkey agar with 5-bromo-4-chloro-3-indolyl-β-D-glucuronide (BCIG)**

This agar is used as a selective and differential medium for detection of *E. coli* O157:H7 incorporating the chromogen BCIG. The medium combines two different screening mechanisms for detection of *E. coli* O157:H7, the failure to ferment sorbitol and the absence of β-glucuronidase activity. The non-sorbitol-fermenting and β-glucuronidase-negative *E. coli* O157:H7 will appear as straw-colored colonies. Organisms with β-glucuronidase activity will cleave the substrate, leading to a distinct blue-green coloration of the colonies.

■ **Soybean medium with 0.1% agar (tryptone soya HiVeg broth with 0.1% agar)**

This medium is used for cultivation of anaerobes from root canals, blood, and other clinical specimens. The medium contains 0.1% agar, casein hydrolysate, and digest of soybean meal.

■ **Special infusion broth with blood**

This medium is used for propagation of pathogenic cocci and other fastidious organisms associated with blood culture work and allied pathological investigations. The medium contains infusion from animal tissues, peptones, glucose, and blood.

■ **Specimen preservative medium**

This medium is used for preservation and transport of viable microorganisms in stool specimens. The medium contains glycerol, citrate, yeast extract, and deoxycholate.

■ **Standard fluid medium 10B (Shepard's M10 medium)**

This medium is used for isolation and cultivation of *U. urealyticum* from clinical specimens. The medium contains numerous growth factors, including serum yeast extract, glucose, amino acids, cocarboxylase, NAD, vitamins, and serum. It also contains infusion from beef heart, peptone, and phenol red. Penicillin is included as a selective factor.

■ **Staphylococcus-Streptococcus selective medium**
This medium is used for selective isolation of *S. aureus* and streptococci from clinical specimens. The medium contains peptone, starch, and blood. It also contains nalidixic acid and colistin sulfate as selective factors.

■ **StrepB carrot broth**
This is a proprietary broth that is used for detecting the presence of group B *Streptococcus* (GBS) infections in pregnant women. This medium contains peptone, starch, MOPS, glucose, pyruvate, growth factors, and selective factors. It is a modification of Granada medium consisting of a one-step method for screening pregnant women for the presence of GBS. Tubes show an orange-to-red color change, typical of GBS. The production of orange, red, or brick red pigment is a unique characteristic of hemolytic GBS due to reaction with substrates such as starch, proteose peptone, serum, and folate pathway inhibitors. Church et al. reported that StrepB carrot broth compared favorably with Lim broth and was less labor-intensive (11).

■ **Streptococcus faecalis (SF) broth**
This medium is used for cultivation and differentiation of group D enterococci ("*Streptococcus*" *faecalis* and "*Streptococcus*" *faecium*) from group D nonenterococci and from other *Streptococcus* spp. Group D enterococci turn the medium turbid and yellow-brown.

■ **Streptococcus selective medium**
This medium is used for selective isolation of streptococci from clinical specimens. The medium contains peptone, starch, and blood. It also contains colistin sulfate and oxolinic acid as selective factors.

■ **Streptosel agar**
This medium is used for selective isolation, cultivation, and enumeration of streptococci from specimens containing a mixed biota. The medium contains digest of casein, glucose, digest of soybean meal, sodium citrate, cystine, sodium azide, sodium sulfite, and crystal violet.

■ **Stuart transport medium, modified**
This medium is used for preservation of *Neisseria* spp. and other fastidious organisms during their transport from clinic to laboratory. The medium contains sodium glycerophosphate, cysteine, sodium thioglycolate, and methylene blue.

■ **Sucrose-Teepol-tellurite (STT) agar**
This medium is used for selective isolation and differentiation of *Vibrio* spp. based on their ability to ferment sucrose. The medium contains beef extract, peptone, sucrose, Teepol, tellurite, and bromthymol blue. *Vibrio cholerae* appears as flat yellow colonies. *Vibrio parahaemolyticus* appears as elevated green-yellow mucoid colonies.

■ **Sulfide-indole-motility (SIM) medium**
This medium is used for differentiation of members of the *Enterobacteriaceae* based on H_2S production, indole production, and motility. This medium contains peptone, beef extract, peptonized iron, and sodium thiosulfate.

■ **Susceptibility test medium with blood serum**
This medium is used for antimicrobial susceptibility testing of sulfonamides and other antimicrobials. The medium contains glucose, infusion from veal, peptone, acetate, guanine, uracil, xanthine, adenine, and blood.

■ **Sulfamethoxazole-trimethoprim (SXT) blood agar**
This medium is used for selective isolation of Lancefield group A and group B streptococci from throat cultures and other clinical specimens. The medium contains digests of casein and soybean meal, sulfamethoxazole, trimethoprim, blood, and growth factors.

■ **Tergitol-7 agar H**
This medium is used for selective isolation and differentiation of enteric bacteria from urine. The medium contains lactose, peptone, yeast extract, ferric ammonium citrate, thiosulfate, Tergitol, and bromthymol blue.

■ **Tetrathionate broth, Hajna**
This medium is used for isolation of *Salmonella* species, except serovars Typhi and Arizonae, from fecal specimens and urine. This medium contains thiosulfate, peptones, mannitol, yeast extract, glucose, sodium deoxycholate, brilliant green, and iodine.

■ **Tetrazolium tolerance (TTC) agar**
This medium is used for differentiation of bacteria based upon the ability to tolerate and grow in the presence of tetrazolium. The medium contains digests of casein and soybean meal plus triphenyltetrazolium chloride. *E. faecalis* rapidly reduces tetrazolium.

■ **Thayer-Martin medium**
This medium is used for isolation and cultivation of fastidious microorganisms, especially *Neisseria* spp. The medium contains peptone starch, hemoglobin, and a complex mixture of amino acids, glucose, nucleotides, iron, and vitamins.

■ **Thayer-Martin medium, modified**
This medium is used for isolation and cultivation of fastidious microorganisms, especially *Neisseria* spp. The medium contains peptone starch, hemoglobin, and a complex mixture of amino acids, glucose, nucleotides, iron, and vitamins. The glucose and agar concentrations are lower than in the original formulation, which improves growth. The medium also contains trimethoprim.

■ **Thioglycolate bile broth**
This medium is used for cultivation of *Bacteroides fragilis* and *Clostridium perfringens* from clinical specimens. The medium contains digest of casein, glucose, yeast extract, cystine, sodium thioglycolate, and bile.

■ **Thioglycolate medium, enriched (thioglycolate medium with vitamin K$_1$ and hemin, anaerobic thioglycolate medium)**
This medium is used for isolation, cultivation, and identification of a wide variety of obligate anaerobic bacteria. The medium contains digest of casein, glucose, yeast extract, cystine, sodium thioglycolate, bile, hemin, and vitamin K$_1$.

■ **Thiophene-2-carboxylic acid hydrazide (TCH) medium**
This medium is used for differentiation of *Mycobacterium* spp. based on sensitivity to TCH. This medium contains TCH plus Middlebrook 7H10 agar base with Middlebrook

OADC enrichment. *Mycobacterium bovis* is inhibited by TCH. *M. tuberculosis* and other mycobacteria are generally resistant to low concentrations of TCH. This distinguishes *Mycobacterium bovis* from other nonchromogenic, slow-growing mycobacteria.

■ TCBS agar
This medium is used for selective isolation of *Vibrio cholerae* and *Vibrio parahaemolyticus* from a variety of clinical specimens. The medium contains sucrose, citrate, thiosulfate, yeast extract, digests of casein and animal tissue, oxgall (bile), sodium cholate, ferric citrate, thymol blue, and bromthymol blue (see chapter 39).

■ Tinsdale agar
This medium is used for primary isolation and identification of *C. diphtheriae*. The medium contains peptone, yeast extract, cystine, sodium sulfite, and potassium tellurite.

■ Todd-Hewitt broth
This medium is used for cultivation of group A streptococci used in serological typing and for cultivation of a variety of pathogenic microorganisms. The medium contains infusion from beef heart, neopeptone, and glucose. Gentamicin and nalidixic acid may be added to render the medium selective.

■ Transport medium, Stuart
This medium is used for transportation of swab specimens for the recovery of a wide variety of microorganisms, including *N. gonorrhoeae*. The medium contains sodium glycerophosphate, sodium thioglycolate, and methylene blue.

■ Tryptic soy blood agar (tryptose blood agar, TSA blood agar)
This medium is used for cultivation of a wide variety of fastidious microorganisms. It is also used for the observation of hemolytic reactions of a variety of bacteria. It may be used to perform the CAMP test for presumptive identification of GBS (*Streptococcus agalactiae*). The medium contains digests of casein and soybean meal and blood.

■ Trypticase soy agar (tryptic soy agar, soybean-casein digest medium)
This medium is used as a base for general culture of numerous bacteria or, when supplemented, for cultivation of fastidious microorganisms. The medium contains digests of casein and soybean meal. It can be supplemented with glucose, various amino acids (e.g., glutamine), and vitamins. It can also be supplemented with various antimicrobials as selective factors. When supplemented with sheep blood, this medium is useful for observation of hemolytic reactions of a variety of bacteria.

■ Trypticase soy agar with sheep blood and gentamicin (TSA II with sheep blood and gentamicin)
This medium is used for isolation of *S. pneumoniae* from a variety of clinical specimens. The medium contains digests of casein and soybean meal, growth factors, blood, and gentamicin.

■ Trypticase soy agar with sheep blood, sucrose, and tetracycline
This medium is used for isolation of *S. pneumoniae* from a variety of clinical specimens. The medium contains digests of casein and soybean meal, growth factors, sucrose, blood, and tetracycline.

■ Trypticase soy agar with sheep blood and vancomycin
This medium is used for isolation of VRE from a variety of clinical specimens. The medium contains digests of casein and soybean meal, blood, and vancomycin.

■ Trypticase tellurite agar base
This medium is used for selective isolation of microorganisms from clinical specimens, especially from the nose, throat, and vagina. The medium contains digests of casein and soybean meal, blood, glucose, serum, and tellurite.

■ Tryptose-sulfite-cycloserine agar with polymyxin and kanamycin
This medium is used for isolation and enumeration of *Clostridium perfringens* from clinical specimens. The medium contains tryptose, beef extract, digest of soybean meal, yeast extract, ferric ammonium citrate, and ferric ammonium sulfate. It also includes cycloserine, polymyxin B, and kanamycin as selective factors.

■ U9B broth
This medium is used for isolation and identification of T-strain mycoplasmas from clinical specimens, especially *U. urealyticum*. T-mycoplasmas are the only members of the *Mycoplasma* group known to contain urease. Bacteria with urease activity turn the medium dark pink. The medium contains digests of casein and soybean meal, glucose, cysteine, penicillin, phenol red, and urea.

■ Urea agar (urease test agar; urea agar base, Christensen)
This medium is used for detection of *Proteus* spp. based on rapid urease activity and for identification of other members of the *Enterobacteriaceae* based on urease activity. Urease-positive bacteria turn the medium pink. The medium contains urea, peptone, glucose, and phenol red.

■ Urogenital *Mycoplasma* broth base
This medium is used for selective culture of *Mycoplasma hominis* and *Ureaplasma urealyticum*. The medium contains heart infusion, digest of casein, yeast extract, arginine, cysteine, phenol red, serum, vitamins, and urea. It also contains penicillin and amphotericin B as selective factors.

■ V agar
This medium is used for isolation and differentiation of *Gardnerella vaginalis* from clinical specimens. The medium contains digests of casein and animal tissue, peptone, beef extract, yeast extract, starch, and blood. Plates are incubated under an atmosphere with 3 to 10% CO_2. *Gardnerella vaginalis* appears as small white colonies with diffuse beta-hemolysis (see chapter 26).

■ VRE agar
This medium is used for isolation of VRE and high-level-aminoglycoside-resistant enterococci from clinical samples. Nonresistant enterococci containing the *vanC* genes will not grow on this medium. The medium contains tryptone, yeast extract, citrate, esculin, ferric ammonium citrate,

sodium azide, and a selective supplement of meropenem and vancomycin. The selective supplement suppresses growth of gram-negative bacteria and *Enterococcus gallinarum*. The medium contains an indicator system to detect the growth of esculin-hydrolyzing organisms. Enterococci produce black zones around the colonies from the formation of black iron phenolic compounds derived from esculin hydrolyis products and ferrous iron.

■ *Vibrio parahaemolyticus* agar
This medium is used for isolation, cultivation, enumeration, and presumptive identification of *Vibrio parahaemolyticus*. Sucrose-fermenting bacteria appear as yellow colonies with pale yellow peripheries. Non-sucrose-fermenting bacteria appear as mucoid, green colonies with a dark green center. The medium contains sucrose, citrate, thiosulfate, peptone, sodium taurocholate, yeast extract sodium lauryl sulfate, bromthymol blue, and thymol blue.

■ *Vibrio parahaemolyticus* sucrose agar
This medium is used for isolation, cultivation, and differentiation of *Vibrio parahaemolyticus*. *Vibrio parahaemolyticus* and *Vibrio vulnificus* appear as blue to green colonies. Other *Vibrio* spp. appear as yellow colonies (sucrose positive). The medium contains sucrose, yeast extract, tryptose, digest of casein, bile salts, and bromthymol blue.

■ Vogel and Johnson agar
This medium is used for detection of coagulase-positive *S. aureus*. The medium contains digest of casein, mannitol, glycine, yeast extract, lithium chloride, phenol red, and tellurite.

■ Wilkins-Chalgren anaerobe broth (anaerobe broth, MIC)
This medium is used for cultivation and antimicrobial susceptibility (MIC) testing of anaerobic bacteria. The medium contains digest of casein, gelatin, peptone, yeast extract, glucose, arginine, sodium pyruvate, hemin, and menadione.

■ Xylose-lysine-deoxycholate agar
This medium is used for isolation and differentiation of enteric pathogens, especially *Shigella* and *Providencia* spp. The medium contains lactose, sucrose, thioglycolate, lysine, xylose, sodium deoxycholate, ferric ammonium citrate, and phenol red. Bacteria which do not ferment xylose, lactose, or sucrose appear as red colonies. Xylose-fermenting, lysine-decarboxylating bacteria appear as red colonies. Xylose-fermenting, non-lysine-decarboxylating bacteria appear as opaque yellow colonies. Lactose- or sucrose-fermenting bacteria appear as yellow colonies.

■ Xylose-lactose-Tergitol 4 (XLT-4)
This medium is used for isolation and identification of salmonellae from clinical samples. The medium contains lactose, sucrose, thioglycolate, lysine, xylose, yeast extract, peptone, phenol red, and a selective supplement containing Tergitol. The presence of the selective agent, Tergitol 4, in this medium inhibits many organisms that can be problematic on other plating media. In addition, biochemical and pH changes within the medium allow *Salmonella* spp. (black colonies) to be differentiated from organisms such as *E. coli* (yellow colonies) and *Shigella* spp. (red colonies). The

enhanced selectivity of XLT-4 agar reduces the need for further identification procedures, saving time and money, and results in fewer false presumptive positive colonies than do other *Salmonella* plating media.

■ Xylose-sodium deoxycholate-citrate agar
This medium is used for cultivation of *Salmonella* spp. and some *Shigella* spp. The medium contains xylose, citrate, thiosulfate, beef extract, peptone, ferric ammonium citrate, deoxycholate, and neutral red.

■ *Yersinia* selective agar base
This medium is used for isolation and enumeration of *Yersinia enterocolitica* from clinical specimens. The medium contains mannitol, peptones, yeast extract, sodium pyruvate, deoxycholate, neutral red, and crystal violet. It also contains cefsulodin, Irgasan, novobiocin, and selective factors.

APPENDIX
Medium Additives

Many media contain additives that have specific functions ranging from selection to differentiation to protection of certain bacterial species. Below are descriptions of some of the commonly used medium additives.

ACES: allows optimal pH buffering capacity without inhibition of bacteria as seen with other inorganic buffers

Acriflavine: selective agent; suppresses gram-positive organisms

ADC enrichment: a supplement added to mycobacteriology media that includes albumin, dextrose, catalase, and sodium chloride; catalase destroys peroxides that may be in the medium

Agar used in broth medium (0.05 to 0.1%): used to reduce O_2 tension

Albumin: protects against toxic by-products in medium; binds free fatty acids

Antibiotics: one or many may be added to make a medium selective; inhibitory capacity may vary depending on the concentration used

Bicarbonate-citric acid pellet: used to generate CO_2 gas within closed environment after exposure to moisture: used in transport devices for isolating *N. gonorrhoeae*

Bismuth sulfite: heavy metal that is inhibitory to commensal organisms

Carbohydrates: energy source; used to make medium differential when combined with an indicator

Cetrimide: acts as a quaternary ammonium cationic detergent that causes nitrogen and phosphorus to be released from bacterial cells other than *P. aeruginosa*

Charcoal: detoxifying agent, surface tension modifier, scavenger of radicals and peroxides

Cornstarch: works as a detoxifying agent; may provide additional nutrients as an energy source

Dent's supplement (Oxoid): vancomycin, trimethoprim, cefsulodin, and amphotericin B added to Columbia blood agar and laked horse blood for isolation of *Helicobacter*

Dextrose (glucose): makes medium hypertonic; energy source

Egg yolk: used to demonstrate lecithinase, lipase, and proteolytic activities and fatty acids

Ferric ammonium citrate: iron salt used in combination with other agents (esculin and sodium thiosulfate) to make medium differential by producing a black precipitate

Fildes enrichment: peptic digest of sheep blood that provides a rich source of nutrients, including X (hemin) and V (NAD) factors; X originally stood for unknown and V originally stood for vitamin

Glycerol: a purified alcohol and an abundant source of carbon; used in culture, transport, and storage medium and reagent preparation

Glycine: a selective agent that is inhibitory to organisms

Horse serum: an enrichment used in growth media for such organisms as *Mycoplasma* and *Ureaplasma*

IsoVitaleX (BBL): provides V factor (NAD) and additional nutritive ingredients, such as vitamins, amino acids, ferric ion, and dextrose, to stimulate growth of fastidious organisms

Laked blood or laked horse blood: created by freeze-thaw cycles of blood; enhances pigment production of anaerobes and used in susceptibility testing of fastidious organisms

Lithium chloride: a selective agent that inhibits organisms

Malachite green: a dye that partially inhibits bacteria

NAD (V factor): necessary for growth of some fastidious organisms

OADC enrichment: a supplement added to mycobacteriology media that includes oleic acid, albumin, dextrose, catalase, and sodium chloride; the oleic acid provides fatty acids utilized by mycobacteria, and the catalase destroys peroxides that may be in medium

Oxgall (bile): inhibits specific organisms; allows medium to be selective

Peptones: carbohydrate-free source of nutrients

Phenylethyl alcohol: reversibly inhibits DNA synthesis; results in inhibition of facultative anaerobic gram-negative organisms

Pyridoxal phosphate: liquid supplement added to media for isolation of fastidious organisms; also comes in the form of a disk to be used in satelliting tests

Rabbit blood: enhances pigment production of anaerobes; hemolytic reactions of streptococci are "correct"; additive to heart infusion agar for isolation of *Bartonella* spp.

Serum: albumin, fatty acids

Sheep blood and human blood: provide hemin and other nutrients; allow true hemolytic reactions of streptococci; NADase enzyme inactivates the NAD in the sheep blood and is not available for organisms

Skirrow's supplement: vancomycin, trimethoprim, and polymyxin B added to Columbia agar and laked horse blood for isolation of *Helicobacter*

Sodium azide: a selective agent that inhibits gram-negative organisms

Sodium bicarbonate: neutralization agent used with gastric wash or lavage specimens for recovery of acid-fast organisms

Sodium bisulfite: disinfectant, antioxidant, or reducing agent

Sodium chloride: maintains osmotic equilibrium; when added at a high concentration, it may be a selective agent

Sodium citrate: a selective agent inhibitory to organisms

Sodium deoxycholate: a salt of bile acid and a selective agent that inhibits gram-positive and spore-forming organisms

Sodium polyanethole sulfonate: a polyanionic anticoagulant that inactivates aminoglycosides and interferes with the complement cascade, lysozyme activity, and phagocytic activity inherent in blood. May be inhibitory to *Neisseria*, *Gardnerella*, *Streptobacillus*, *Peptostreptococcus*, *Francisella*, and *Moraxella* spp.

Sodium pyruvate: growth stimulant

Sodium selenite: a selective agent that inhibits coliforms

Sodium thioglycolate: a reducing agent

Starch: a polysaccharide and detoxifying agent incorporated into some media as a differential agent

Tellurite: is toxic to egg-clearing strains of bacteria; imparts black color to colony

Tween 80 (polysorbate 80): an oleic acid ester that stimulates growth and provides fatty acids as well as acts as a dispersal agent

Vitamin K: ingredient required for optimal growth of certain obligate anaerobes, such as the *Bacteroides* group

Vitox (Oxoid): provides V factor (NAD) and other essential growth factors to stimulate growth of fastidious organisms; see IsoVitaleX

Yeast extract: water-soluble product that provides B vitamins and protein

REFERENCES

1. **AOAC International.** 2006. *Best Practices in Microbiological Methodology.* AOAC International, Gaithersburg, MD. http://www.fda.gov/Food/ScienceResearch/LaboratoryMethods/ucm124900.htm.

2. **Atlas, R. M.** 2010. *Handbook of Microbiological Media,* 4th ed. Taylor and Francis, Boca Raton, FL.

3. **Atlas, R. M., and J. Snyder.** 2006. *Handbook of Media for Clinical Microbiology,* 2nd ed. CRC Press, Boca Raton, FL.

4. **Baird, R. M., and W. H. Lee.** 1995. Media used in the detection and enumeration of *Staphylococcus aureus. Int. J. Food Microbiol.* **26:**15–24.

5. **Barrow, G. I., and R. K. A. Feltham (ed.).** 1993. *Cowan and Steel's Manual for the Identification of Medical Bacteria,* 3rd ed. Cambridge University Press, Cambridge, United Kingdom.

6. **Basu, S., A. Pal, and P. K. Desai.** 2005. Quality control of culture media in a microbiology laboratory. *Indian J. Med. Microbiol.* **23:**159–163.

7. **BD Diagnostics.** 2003. *Difco & BBL Manual: Dehydrated Culture Media and Reagents for Microbiology.* Becton, Dickinson and Co., Sparks, MD. http://www.bd.com/ds/technicalCenter/inserts/difcoBblManual.asp.

8. **Bridson, E. Y. (ed.).** 1998. *The Oxoid Manual.* Unipath Ltd., Basingstoke, Hampshire, United Kingdom. http://www.oxoid.com/UK/blue/catbrowse/catbrowse.asp.

8a. **Chapin, K. C., and T.-L. Lauderdale.** 2007. Reagents, stains, and media: bacteriology, p. 334–364. *In* P. R. Murray, E. J. Baron, J. H. Jorgensen, M. L. Landry, and M. A. Pfaller (ed.), *Manual of Clinical Microbiology,* 9th ed. ASM Press, Washington, DC.

9. **Chapin-Robertson, K., S. E. Dahlberg, and S. C. Edberg.** 1992. Clinical and laboratory analyses of cytospin-prepared Gram stains for recovery and diagnosis of bacteria from sterile body fluids. *J. Clin. Microbiol.* **30:**377–380.

10. **Cheng, A. C., V. Wuthiekanun, D. Limmathurosakul, G. Wongsuvan, N. P. J. Day, and S. J. Peacock.** 2006. Role of selective and nonselective media for isolation of *Burkholderia pseudomallei* from throat swabs of patients with melioidosis. *J. Clin. Microbiol.* **44:**2316.

11. **Church, D. L., H. Baxter, T. Lloyd, B. Miller, and S. Elsayed.** 2008. Evaluation of StrepB carrot broth versus Lim broth for detection of group B *Streptococcus* colonization status of near-term pregnant women. *J. Clin. Microbiol.* **46:**2780–2782.

12. **Clinical and Laboratory Standards Institute/NCCLS.** 2004. *Quality Assurance for Commercially Prepared Microbiological Culture Media.* Standard M22-A3. NCCLS, Wayne, PA.

13. **Collins, C. H., P. M. Lyne, J. M. Grange, and J. O. Falkinham (ed.).** 2004. *Collins and Lyne's Microbiological Methods,* 8th ed. Arnold, London, United Kingdom.

14. **Coons, A. H.** 1959. The diagnostic application of fluorescent antibodies. *Schweiz. Z. Pathol. Bakteriol.* **22:**700–723.

15. **Elsayed, S., D. Gregson, and D. Church.** 2003. Comparison of direct selective versus nonselective agar media plus LIM broth enrichment for determination of group B *Streptococcus* colonization status in pregnant women. *Arch. Pathol. Lab. Med.* **127:**718–720.

16. **Faller, A., and K.-H. Schleifer.** 1981. Modified oxidase and benzidine tests for separation of staphylococci from micrococci. *J. Clin. Microbiol.* **13:**1031–1035.

17. **Fay, G. D., and A. L. Barry.** 1972. Rapid ornithine decarboxylase test for the identification of *Enterobacteriaceae. Appl. Microbiol.* **23:**710–713.

18. **Fisher, J. F., M. Ganapathy, B. H. Edwards, and C. L. Newman.** 1990. Utility of Gram's and Giemsa stains in the diagnosis of pulmonary tuberculosis. *Am. Rev. Respir. Dis.* **141:**511–513.

19. **Froud, S. J.** 1999. The development, benefits and disadvantages of serum-free media. *Dev. Biol. Stand.* **99:**157–166.
20. **Gill, V. J., N. A. Nelson, F. Stock, and G. Evans.** 1988. Optimal use of the cytocentrifuge for recovery and diagnosis of *Pneumocystis jiroveci* in bronchoalveolar lavage and sputum specimens. *J. Clin. Microbiol.* **26:**1641–1644.
21. **Hedberg, M.** 1969. Acetamide agar medium selective for *Pseudomonas aeruginosa. Appl. Microbiol.* **17:**481.
22. **HiMedia.** 2009. *The HiMedia Manual.* HiMedia Laboratories Pvt. Limited, Mumbai, India.
23. **HiMedia.** 2006. *The HiVeg Manual.* HiMedia Laboratories Pvt. Limited, Mumbai, India.
24. **Hitchens, A. P., and M. C. Leikind.** 1939. The introduction of agar-agar into bacteriology. *J. Bacteriol.* **37:**485–493.
25. **Jousimies-Somer, H., P. E. Summanen, D. M. Citron, E. J. Baron, H. M. Wexler, and S. M. Finegold.** 2002. *Anaerobic Bacteriology Manual,* 6th ed. Star Publishing Co., Belmont, CA.
26. **Lauer, B. A., L. B. Reller, and S. Mirrett.** 1981. Comparison of acridine orange and Gram stains for detection of microorganisms in cerebrospinal fluid and other clinical specimens. *J. Clin. Microbiol.* **14:**201–205.
27. **Livingston, S. J., S. D. Kominos, and R. B. Yee.** 1978. New medium for selection and presumptive identification of the *Bacteroides fragilis* group. *J. Clin. Microbiol.* **7:**448–453.
28. Reference deleted.
29. **Manafi, M., and W. Kneifel.** 1990. Rapid methods for differentiating gram-positive from gram-negative aerobic and facultative anaerobic bacteria. *J. Appl. Bacteriol.* **69:**822–827.
30. **Oberhofer, T. R., and J. W. Rowen.** 1974. Acetamide agar for differentiation of nonfermentative bacteria. *Appl. Microbiol.* **28:**720–721.
31. **Shanholtzer, C. J., P. J. Schaper, and L. R. Peterson.** 1982. Concentrated Gram stain smears prepared with a cytospin centrifuge. *J. Clin. Microbiol.* **16:**1052–1056.
32. **Snyder, M. L.** 1941. Simple colorimetric method for diagnosis of caries activity. *J. Am. Dent. Assoc.* **28:**44–49.
33. **Stoakes, L., R. Reyes, J. Daniel, G. Lennox, M. A. John, R. Lannigan, and Z. Hussain.** 2006. Prospective comparison of a new chromogenic medium, MRSA*Select*, to CHROMagar MRSA and mannitol-salt medium supplemented with oxacillin or cefoxitin for detection of methicillin-resistant *Staphylococcus aureus. J. Clin. Microbiol.* **44:**637–639.
34. **Strumpf, I. J., A. Y. Tsang, M. A. Schork, and J. G. Weg.** 1976. The reliability of gastric smears by auramine-rhodamine staining technique for the diagnosis of tuberculosis. *Am. Rev. Respir. Dis.* **114:**971–976.
35. **Trabulsi, L. R., and W. H. Ewing.** 1962. Sodium acetate medium for the differentiation of *Shigella* and *Escherichia* cultures. *Public Health Lab.* **20:**137–140.
36. **U.S. Food and Drug Administration.** 2000. *Bacteriological Analytical Manual.* U.S. Food and Drug Administration, Silver Spring, MD. http://www.fda.gov/Food/ScienceResearch/LaboratoryMethods/BacteriologicalAnalyticalManualBAM/default.htm.
37. **Vimont, A., C. Vernozy-Rozand, and M. L. Delignette-Muller.** 2006. Isolation of *E. coli* O157:H7 and non-O157 STEC in different matrices: review of the most commonly used enrichment protocols. *Lett. Appl. Microbiol.* **42:**102–108.
38. **Wentworth, B. B., et al. (ed.).** 1987. *Diagnostic Procedures for Bacterial Infections,* 7th ed. American Public Health Association, Washington, DC.

General Approaches to Identification of Aerobic Gram-Positive Cocci

KATHRYN L. RUOFF

18

The majority of aerobic, or facultatively aerobic, gram-positive cocci isolated from clinical specimens are distributed among the genera *Staphylococcus*, *Streptococcus*, and *Enterococcus*. Molecular taxonomic studies of this group of bacteria have revealed additional genera and species that are phenotypically similar to the commonly encountered organisms but are infrequently isolated from clinical specimens. Tables 1 and 2 and chapters 19 to 22 describe basic phenotypic tests that can be used to distinguish these infrequent isolates from staphylococci, streptococci, and enterococci. It should be noted that the reactions listed in Tables 1 and 2 represent those of the majority of strains in each group; isolates with variant reactions may be encountered. Each of the tables contains organisms with similar cellular morphologies, either "streptococcal," consisting of gram-positive cocci or coccobacilli arranged primarily in pairs and/or chains, or "staphylococcal," signifying that cells appear as cocci arranged in pairs, tetrads, clusters, and irregular groups. No taxonomic kinship is implied by division of these bacteria into two groups based on cellular morphology.

The commonly isolated aerobic gram-positive cocci (staphylococci, streptococci, enterococci) can usually be

TABLE 1. Characteristics of catalase-negative gram-positive cocci that grow aerobically and form cells arranged in pairs and chains[a]

PYR	LAP	6.5% NaCl	BE	Motility	45°C	Probe	HIP	Satellitism	10°C	Vancomycin resistance	Organism (chapter)
+	+	+	+	+	+	NA	NA	NA	NA	NA	*Enterococcus* (21)
+	+	+	+	+	−	NA	NA	NA	NA	NA	*Vagococcus* (22)
+	+	+	+	−	NA	+	NA	NA	NA	NA	*Enterococcus* (21)
+	+	+	+	−	NA	−	NA	NA	NA	NA	*Lactococcus* (22)
+	+	+	−	NA	NA	NA	+	−	NA	NA	*Facklamia* spp.[b] (22)
+	+	+	−	NA	NA	NA	−	V	NA	NA	*Ignavigranum* (22)
+	+	−	+	+	NA	NA	NA	NA	NA	NA	*Vagococcus* (22)
+	+	−	+	−	NA	NA	NA	NA	NA	NA	*Lactococcus* (22)
+	+	−	−	NA	NA	NA	NA	+	NA	NA	*Abiotrophia, Granulicatella* (22)
+	+	−	−	NA	NA	NA	NA	−	NA	NA	*Gemella* spp.[c] (22)
+	−	+	NA	NA	NA	NA	NA	NA	NA	NA	*Globicatella* (22)
+	−	−	NA	NA	NA	NA	NA	NA	NA	NA	*Dolosicoccus* (22)
−	−	NA	NA	NA	NA	NA	NA	NA	NA	+	*Leuconostoc*[d] (22)
−	−	NA	NA	NA	NA	NA	NA	NA	NA	−	*Globicatella* (22)
−	+	NA	NA	NA	NA	NA	NA	NA	+	NA	*Lactococcus* (22)
−	+	NA	NA	NA	NA	NA	NA	NA	−	NA	*Streptococcus*[e] (20)

[a]See chapters 17 and 20 to 22 for methods for tests referred to in this table. Reactions shown are typical, but exceptions may occur. Abbreviations and symbols: PYR, production of pyrrolidonyl arylamidase; LAP, production of leucine aminopeptidase; 6.5% NaCl, growth in 6.5% NaCl; BE, hydrolysis of esculin in the presence of 40% bile; 45°C, growth at 45°C; probe, reaction with commercially available nucleic acid probe for the genus *Enterococcus*; HIP, hydrolysis of hippurate; satellitism, satellite growth behavior; 10°C, growth at 10°C; +, most strains positive; −, most strains negative; V, variable reactions are observed; NA, not applicable.

[b]The reactions in this table are typical for *F. hominis*, *F. sourekii*, and *F. ignava*. *F. languida* cells tend to be arranged in clusters, and isolates are hippurate hydrolysis negative (Table 2).

[c]*G. morbillorum*, *G. bergeri*, and *G. sanguinis* cells tend to be arranged in pairs and chains, in contrast to the cells of *G. haemolysans*, which are arranged in pairs, tetrads, and clusters (Table 2).

[d]*Leuconostoc* is distinguished from the other catalase-negative organisms in Table 1 by its ability to produce gas as an end product of glucose metabolism and intrinsic resistance to vancomycin. The phenotypically similar genus *Weissella* contains organisms formerly classified as leuconostocs and the species formerly named *Lactobacillus confusus* (see chapter 22).

[e]Most streptococci are PYR negative, with the exception of *Streptococcus pyogenes* isolates and some strains of *Streptococcus pneumoniae*, which are PYR positive.

TABLE 2. Differentiating features of gram-positive cocci that grow aerobically and form cells arranged in clusters or irregular groups[a]

Catalase	Obligate aerobe	Oxidase	PYR	LAP	NaCl	ESC	Hemolysis	Vancomycin	BGUR	Organism (chapter)
+	+	+	NA	NA	+[b]	NA	NA	NA	NA	*Micrococcus*[c] spp. (19)
+	+	−	NA	NA	+[d]	NA	NA	NA	NA	*Alloiococcus* spp. (19)
+	−	−	NA	NA	+[b]	NA	NA	NA	NA	*Staphylococcus* (19)
+	−	−	NA	NA	−[b]	NA	NA	NA	NA	*Rothia mucilaginosa*[e] (19, 26)
−	−	NA	+	+	+[d]	+	NA	NA	−	*Dolosigranulum* (22)
−	−	NA	+	+	+[d]	+	NA	NA	+	*Aerococcus sanguinicola* (22)
−	−	NA	+	+	+[d]	−	NA	NA	−	*Facklamia languida*[f] (22)
−	−	NA	+	+	−[d]	+	NA	NA	NA	*Rothia mucilaginosa*[e] (19, 26)
−	−	NA	+	+	−[d]	−	NA	NA	NA	*Gemella haemolysans*[g] (22)
−	−	NA	+	−	NA	NA	α	NA	NA	*Aerococcus viridans*[h] (22)
−	−	NA	+	−	NA	NA	γ	NA	NA	*Helcococcus kunzii*[h] (22)
−	−	NA	−	+	NA	NA	NA	R	NA	*Pediococcus*[i] (22)
−	−	NA	−	+	NA	NA	NA	S	+	*Aerococcus urinae* (22)
−	−	NA	−	−	NA	NA	NA	NA	+	*Aerococcus urinaehominis* (22)
−	−	NA	−	−	NA	NA	NA	NA	−	*Aerococcus christensenii* (22)

[a]See chapters 17, 19, and 22 for methods for performing the phenotypic tests referred to in this table. Reactions shown are typical; exceptions may occur. Abbreviations: PYR, production of pyrrolidonyl arylamidase; LAP, production of leucine aminopeptidase; NaCl, growth in the presence of either 5% or 6.5% NaCl (see footnotes b and d); ESC, esculin hydrolysis; BGUR, production of β-glucuronidase; +, most strains positive; −, most strains negative; V, variable reactions are observed; NA, not applicable; α, alpha-hemolysis on sheep blood agar; γ, nonhemolytic reaction on sheep blood agar; S, susceptible; R, resistant.

[b]Growth in the presence of 5% sodium chloride.

[c]*Kocuria*, a related genus infrequently isolated from clinical specimens, is distinguished from *Micrococcus* by its ability to produce acid aerobically from D-glucose and glycerol (see chapter 19).

[d]Growth in the presence of 6.5% sodium chloride.

[e]*Rothia mucilaginosa* isolates are usually catalase negative or weakly positive but may be strongly catalase positive.

[f]*Ignavigranum ruoffiae* (Table 1) exhibits reactions identical to those of *F. languida* in the PYR, ESC, and NaCl tests. However, *I. ruoffiae* cells are arranged primarily in chains, while *F. languida* cells usually form clusters. Other *Facklamia* species form cells arranged in pairs and chains (Table 1).

[g]*G. haemolysans* cells tend to be arranged in pairs, tetrads, and groups, in contrast to the cells of other *Gemella* species, which usually occur in pairs and short chains (Table 1).

[h]*H. kunzii* strains form tiny pinpoint nonhemolytic colonies on blood agar after 24 h of aerobic incubation at 35°C, while *A. viridans* isolates form larger alpha-hemolytic colonies under similar incubation conditions. In contrast to *H. kunzii*, *A. viridans* prefers aerobic incubation atmospheres. Two additional species of *Helcococcus* isolated from human sources have been described, each based on a single isolate. In contrast to *H. kunzii*, the new species *Helcococcus sueciensis* and the proposed species "*Helcococcus pyogenes*" are PYR negative (see chapter 22).

[i]The genera *Pediococcus* and *Tetragenococcus* have similar phenotypic characteristics, except that tetragenococci are vancomycin susceptible. The bile esculin test can differentiate between tetragenococci (positive) and *Aerococcus urinae* (negative) (see chapter 22).

accurately identified by determining a few basic phenotypic traits (cellular morphology, catalase reaction, and production of pyrrolidonyl arylamidase [PYR], etc. [see reference 5, Tables 1 and 2 herein, and chapters 19 to 22). Reliance on a single or only a few phenotypic tests can, however, lead to misidentification. For example, optochin-resistant *Streptococcus pneumoniae* strains (19) might be incorrectly identified as alpha-hemolytic (viridans) streptococci (chapter 20). Clumping factor (slide coagulase)-positive *Staphylococcus lugdunensis*, a coagulase-negative species, could be misidentified as *Staphylococcus aureus* (see reference 9 and chapter 19). PYR-positive *Lactococcus* isolates might be incorrectly identified as members of the genus *Enterococcus* (see reference 8 and chapter 22).

As new genera and species of aerobic gram-positive cocci are described and characterized, it becomes increasingly difficult to identify some of the less frequently isolated organisms solely on the basis of phenotypic traits. A variety of automated and manual systems have proven to be fairly accurate for identification of commonly encountered staphylococcal, streptococcal, and enterococcal species (see the "Identification" sections in chapters 19 to 22 and references 3, 4, 6, and 10 to 12). These systems are less effective for identification of infrequently isolated aerobic gram-positive cocci (see chapter 22). The less commonly isolated organisms may not be identified by these systems or may be misidentified as other genera or species. Basic phenotypic tests can usually suggest a possible identity for strains of infrequently encountered aerobic gram-positive cocci, but evaluation with a larger battery of phenotypic tests or molecular identification methods is often valuable, if not indispensible, for accurate identification.

Nucleic acid probe tests and amplification methods for identification of some of the commonly isolated aerobic gram-positive cocci are commercially available and designed for use in medium- to large-volume clinical microbiology laboratories. These methods may also be useful for ruling out enterococcal, streptococcal, or staphylococcal strains when attempting to identify phenotypically similar, infrequently isolated organisms. One of the most useful methods for molecular characterization of the aerobic gram-positive cocci of clinical interest is comparison of 16S rRNA gene sequences (1, 2), although sequence comparison of other genes may also be helpful for identification. Genes that have been examined for this purpose include the *rpoB*, *tuf*, and *sodA* genes of staphylococci (14, 15, 18), the *rpoB* gene of streptococci (7), the *atpA* gene of enterococci (16), and the *sodA* gene of lactococci (8). Other identification methods, such as multilocus sequence analysis of enterococci (*rpoA* and *pheS* genes) (17) and melting curve analysis of restriction fragments obtained from amplified regions of the *sodA* gene and the 16S–23S intergenic spacer region (enterococci) (13), have also been reported. More information on the use of molecular methods for identification of this group of organisms can be found in chapters 3 and 19 to 22.

Each microbiology laboratory needs to establish criteria for the extent of identification of routinely isolated aerobic gram-positive cocci. Efforts should be made to recognize and report organisms described as pathogens in various clinical scenarios or organisms with well-known susceptibility patterns, since identification should, in these cases, play an important role in guiding patient treatment. For example, in one scenario, all staphylococcal isolates could be fully identified to the species level with an automated system; alternatively, in a different setting, staphylococci might be examined initially with the coagulase test to identify *S. aureus*. Coagulase-negative strains could then be subjected to a few simple screening tests and be identified simply as coagulase-negative staphylococci, presumptively as *Staphylococcus saprophyticus*, or presumptively as *Staphylococcus lugdunensis*. An identification of "viridans streptococcus" might be sufficient when these organisms are isolated in mixed culture, but species identification of important isolates can offer clinically relevant information (e.g., *Streptococcus bovis* in endocarditis cases or "*Streptococcus anginosus* group" ["*milleri*" group] in cases of brain or hepatic abscess). Procedures for identification should reflect laboratory resources, workflow, the composition of patient populations served by the laboratory, and the clinical utility of results for the laboratory's users.

REFERENCES

1. **Becker, K., D. Harmsen, A. Mellmann, C. Meier, P. Schumann, G. Peters, and C. von Eiff.** 2004. Development and evaluation of a quality-controlled ribosomal sequence database for 16S ribosomal DNA-based identification of *Staphylococcus* species. *J. Clin. Microbiol.* **42:**4988–4995.

2. **Bosshard, P. P., S. Abels, M. Altwegg, E. C. Bottger, and R. Zbinden.** 2004. Comparison of conventional and molecular methods for identification of aerobic catalase-negative gram-positive cocci in the clinical laboratory. *J. Clin. Microbiol.* **42:**2065–2073.

3. **Brigante, G., F. Luzzaro, A. Bettaccini, G. Lombardi, F. Meacci, B. Pini, S. Stefani, and A. Toniolo.** 2006. Use of the Phoenix automated system for identification of *Streptococcus* and *Enterococcus* spp. *J. Clin. Microbiol.* **44:**3263–3267.

4. **Carroll, K. C., A. P. Borek, C. Burger, B. Glanz, H. Bhally, S. Henciak, and D. C. Flayhart.** 2006. Evaluation of the BD Phoenix automated microbiology system for identification and antimicrobial susceptibility testing of staphylococci and enterococci. *J. Clin. Microbiol.* **44:**2072–2077.

5. **Clinical and Laboratory Standards Institute.** 2008. Abbreviated identification of bacteria and yeast. Approved guideline M35-A2, 2nd ed. Clinical and Laboratory Standards Institute, Wayne, PA.

6. **Delmas, J., J. P. Chacornac, F. Robin, P. Giammarinaro, R. Talon, and R. Bonnet.** 2008. Evaluation of the Vitek 2 system with a variety of *Staphylococcus* species. *J. Clin. Microbiol.* **46:**311–313.

7. **Drancourt, M., V. Roux, P.-E. Fournier, and D. Raoult.** 2004. *rpoB* gene sequence-based identification of aerobic gram-positive cocci of the genera *Streptococcus*, *Enterococcus*, *Gemella*, *Abiotrophia*, and *Granulicatella*. *J. Clin. Microbiol.* **42:**497–504.

8. **Fihman, V., L. Raskine, Z Barrou, C. Kiffel, J. Riahi, B. Bercot, and M.-J. Sanson-Le Pors.** 2006. *Lactococcus garvieae* endocarditis: identification by 16S rRNA and *sodA* sequence analysis. *J. Infect.* **52:**e3–e6.

9. **Frank, K. L., J. L. del Pozo, and R. Patel.** 2008. From clinical microbiology to infection pathogenesis: how daring to be different works for *Staphylococcus lugdunensis*. *Clin. Microbiol. Rev.* **21:**111–133.

10. **Funke, G., and P. Funke-Kissling.** 2005. Performance of the new VITEK 2 GP card for identification of medically relevant gram-positive cocci in a routine clinical laboratory. *J. Clin. Microbiol.* **43:**84–88.

11. **Kim, M., S. R. Heo, S. H. Choi, H. Kwon, J. S. Park, M.-W. Seong, D.-H. Lee, K. U. Park, J. Song, and E.-C. Kim.** 2008. Comparison of the MicroScan, VITEK 2 and Crystal GP with 16S rRNA sequencing and MicroSeq 500 v2.0 analysis for coagulase-negative staphylococci. *BMC Microbiol.* **8:**233.

12. **Layer, F., B. Ghebremedhin, K.-A. Moder, W. König, and B. König.** 2006. Comparative study using various methods for identification of *Staphylococcus* species in clinical specimens. *J. Clin. Microbiol.* **44:**2824–2830.

13. **Martín, B., M. Garriga, and T. Aymerich.** 2008. Identification of *Enterococcus* species by melting curve analysis of restriction fragments. *J. Microbiol. Methods* **75:**145–147.

14. **Martineau, F., F. J. Picard, D. Ke, S. Paradis, P. H. Roy, M. Ouellette, and M. G. Bergeron.** 2001. Development of a PCR assay for identification of staphylococci at genus and species levels. *J. Clin. Microbiol.* **39:**2541–2547.

15. **Mellmann, A., K. Becker, C. von Eiff, U. Keckevoet, P. Schumann, and D. Harmsen.** 2006. Sequencing and staphylococci identification. *Emerg. Infect. Dis.* **12:**333–336.

16. **Naser, S., F. L. Thompson, B. Hoste, D. Gevers, K. Vandemeulebroecke, I. Cleenwerck, C. C. Thompson, M. Vancanneyt, and J. Swings.** 2005. Phylogeny and identification of enterococci by *atpA* gene sequence analysis. *J. Clin. Microbiol.* **43:**2224–2230.

17. **Naser, S. M., F. L. Thompson, B. Hoste, D. Gevers, P. Dawyndt, M. Vancanneyt, and J. Swings.** 2005. Application of multilocus sequence analysis (MLSA) for rapid identification of *Enterococcus* species based on *rpoA* and *pheS* genes. *Microbiology* **151:**2141–2150.

18. **Poyart, C., G. Quesne, C. Boumaila, and P. Trieu-Cuot.** 2001. Rapid and accurate species-level identification of coagulase-negative staphylococci by using the *sodA* gene as a target. *J. Clin. Microbiol.* **39:**4296–4301.

19. **Richter, S. S., K. P. Heilmann, C. L. Dohrn, F. Riahi, S. E. Beekmann, and G. V. Doern.** 2008. Accuracy of phenotypic methods for identification of *Streptococcus pneumoniae* isolates included in surveillance programs. *J. Clin. Microbiol.* **46:**2184–2188.

Staphylococcus, Micrococcus, and Other Catalase-Positive Cocci*

KARSTEN BECKER AND CHRISTOF von EIFF

19

TAXONOMY

Historically, the genera *Staphylococcus* and *Micrococcus* were placed together with the genera *Stomatococcus* and *Planococcus* in the family *Micrococcaceae* containing gram-positive, catalase-positive cocci. Molecular phylogenetic and chemotaxonomic analyses have revealed that staphylococci and "micrococci" are not closely related (175). Staphylococci belong to the *Bacillus-Lactobacillus-Streptococcus* cluster, which consists of gram-positive bacteria with DNA of a low G+C content. In the taxonomic outline (2004) of the 2nd edition of *Bergey's Manual of Systematic Bacteriology* (68), a classification of the *Staphylococcus* genus together with the genera *Jeotgalicoccus, Macrococcus, Salinicoccus,* and *Gemella* was outlined in a newly established family, *Staphylococcaceae,* meanwhile supplemented by *Nosocomiicoccus* and diminished by *Gemella* (now *Bacillales* Family XI. Incertae Sedis) (117). The *Staphylococcaceae* combined with *Bacillaceae, Planococcaceae, Listeriaceae,* and other families are now part of the order *Bacillales* of the suggested class *Bacilli* (117).

In addition to the sustained *Micrococcus* genus, certain micrococcal species previously belonging to this genus were reclassified into the newly established genera *Kocuria, Nesterenkonia, Kytococcus,* and *Dermacoccus.* These genera were rearranged into two families, the redefined *Micrococcaceae* and the newly established *Dermacoccaceae,* both consisting of gram-positive cocci with high G+C content DNA (174, 176). Both families belong to the suborder *Micrococcineae* (class *Actinobacteria*) (175). The type genus *Micrococcus* and the genera *Kocuria* and *Nesterenkonia* as well as the genera *Acaricomes, Arthrobacter, Citricoccus, Renibacterium, Rothia,* and *Zhihengliuella* now constitute the *Micrococcaceae* family. The only species of the former genus *Stomatococcus, S. mucilaginosus,* was reclassified as *Rothia mucilaginosa* (40). The other family of the *Micrococcineae* containing also previous *Micrococcus* species, designated *Dermacoccaceae,* contains the type genus *Dermacoccus* as well as the genera *Demetria, Kytococcus, Luteipulveratus,* and *Yimella.*

An unrelated species of gram-positive cocci exhibiting positive catalase reaction and occurring in human specimens is *Alloiococcus otitis,* the only species of this genus,

which is a member of the *Carnobacteriaceae* family belonging to the order *Lactobacillales* (class *Bacilli*) (117).

For further taxonomic details and references, see the taxonomic outline of the 2nd edition of *Bergey's Manual of Systematic Bacteriology* (68) and the *List of Prokaryotic Names with Standing in Nomenclature* (http://www.bacterio.cict.fr/).

DESCRIPTION OF THE GENERA

Staphylococcus and Related Genera

Staphylococci are characterized by gram-positive, nonmotile, non-spore-forming, spherical cells of 0.5 to 1.5 µm in diameter, occurring as single cocci, in pairs, tetrads, or short chains, which characteristically divide in more than one plane, thereby forming irregular clusters like a bunch of grapes. With the exception of the anaerobic species *S. saccharolyticus* (formerly *Peptococcus saccharolyticus*) and *S. aureus* subsp. *anaerobius,* the staphylococci are facultative anaerobes (Table 1). Although staphylococci are usually catalase positive, rare catalase-negative strains have been reported (137). Most staphylococcal species are oxidase negative in the modified oxidase test, with the exception of *S. fleurettii, S. lentus, S. sciuri,* and *S. vitulinus.* They grow in the presence of 10% NaCl between 18°C and 40°C. The metabolism is respiratory and fermentative. Their cell wall contains peptidoglycan and teichoic acid. Staphylococci are susceptible to lysostaphin.

The major genotypic criterion of the members of the genus *Staphylococcus* is the G+C content of 30 to 39 mol%. Whole-genome sequencing has been performed for an increasing number of *S. aureus* strains (e.g., COL, Mu3, Mu50, MW2, N315, NCTC8325, Newman, and USA300-FPR3757). The genome is composed of a single chromosome ranging in size from approximately 2.8 to 2.9 Mbp with a highly conserved core genome of ca. 75%. A wide range of mobile DNA elements have been identified. Most naturally occurring staphylococcal strains contain small multicopy and/or large (conjugative) multiresistance plasmids (classes I to III). For more details and other staphylococcal species, see the NCBI Genome database (http://www.ncbi.nlm.nih.gov/sites/entrez?db=genome).

As of October 2009, 39 species including 21 subspecies are recognized in the genus *Staphylococcus* (Table 2). Another species, "*S. pseudolugdunensis,*" closely related to the latest validly

---

*This chapter contains information presented in chapter 28 by Tammy L. Bannerman and Sharon J. Peacock in the ninth edition of this *Manual.*

TABLE 1 Differentiation of members of the genus *Staphylococcus* from other gram-positive cocci[a]

Genus and exceptional species	G+C content (molecular %) of DNA	Strict aerobe	Facultative anaerobe or microaerophile	Strict anaerobe	Tetrad cell arrangement	Strong adherence on agar	Motility	Growth on: 5% NaCl agar	6.5% NaCl agar	12% NaCl agar	P agar in 18 h[b]	Schleifer-Kramer agar[c]	Catalase reaction result[d]	Benzidine test result[e]	Modified oxidase test result[f]	Anaerobic acid production from glucose[g]	Aerobic acid production from glycerol	Resistance to: Lysostaphin (200 µg/ml)	Erythromycin (0.4 µg/ml)	Bacitracin (0.04 U)[h]	Furazolidone (100 µg)[i]
Staphylococcus spp.	30–39	−	d	−	d	−[j]	−	+	+	d	+	+	+	+	−	d	+	−	+	+	−
S. aureus subsp. anaerobius		−	±	±				+	+	d	−	ND	+	−		+	+	−	+	ND	
S. saccharolyticus		−	±	±	+			+	+	±	−	ND	−	±		+	+	−	+	ND	
S. hominis		+[k]	±	−	+			+	+	±	+	+	+	+	−	+	+	−	+	+	
S. auricularis		−	+	−	+			+	+	±	−	ND	+	+	−	−	+	−	+	+	
S. saprophyticus, S. cohnii, S. xylosus		d	d	−	−			+	+	±	+	+	+	+	−	−	+	−	+	+	
S. kloosii, S. equorum, S. arlettae		±	±	−	−	−	−	+	+	±	d	+	+	+	−	−	+	−	+	+	
S. intermedius		−	+	−	−	−	−	+	+	+	+	±	+	+	−	+	+	−	+	+	
S. sciuri, S. lentus, S. vitulinus		±	±	−	d	−	−	+	+	d	d	+	+	+	+	−	+	−	+	+	−
Macrococcus[l]	38–45	±	±	−	d	−	−	+	+	±	d	ND	+	+	+	−	d	−	+	+	
Enterococcus	34–42	−	+	−	−	−	d	+	+	(±)	±	(±)	−	−	−	+	d	+	+	+	−
Streptococcus	34–46	−	+	d	−	−	−	d	d	−	−	−	−	−	−	+	d	+	−	d	
Aerococcus	35–40	−	+	d	+	−	−	+	+	+		ND	−	−	−	(+)	ND	+	ND	−	−
Planococcus	39–52	+	−	−	d	−	+	+	+	+		ND	+	+	ND	−	−	+	ND	ND	−
Alloiococcus	44–45	+	−	−	−	−	−	+	+	ND	ND	ND	±	−	−	ND	−	ND	ND	ND	ND
R. mucilaginosa	56–60	−	+	−	d	+	−	−	−	−	−	ND	±	−	−	+	d	+	ND	−	d
Micrococcus	66–75	+	−	−	+	−	−	+	+	d	−	−	+	+	+	−	−	+	−[m]	−	+
Kocuria kristinae	67	±	±	−	+	−	−	+	+	±	−	(±)	+	+	+	(+)	+	+	−	−	+

[a]Symbols and abbreviations: +, 90% or more species or strains positive; ±, 90% or more species or strains weakly positive; −, 90% or more species or strains negative; d, 11 to 89% of species or strains positive; ND, not determined. Parentheses indicate a delayed reaction.

[b]Growth on P agar is under aerobic conditions at 35 to 37°C. Positive growth is indicated for detectable formation of colonies of at least 1 mm in diameter; ± indicates detectable formation of colonies of between 0.5 and 1 mm in diameter. Growth on sheep or bovine blood agar is slightly greater but less discriminative between staphylococci and other genera.

[c]Growth is under aerobic conditions at 35 to 37°C for 24 to 48 h. Positive growth is indicated for a number of CFU on selective medium comparable to that on plate count agar and a colony of 0.5 mm in diameter; ± indicates a significant reduction in the number of CFU on the selective medium compared to that on plate count agar, and parentheses indicate a colony of pinpoint size to 0.5 mm in diameter.

[d]Sometimes a weak catalase or pseudocatalase reaction can be observed with certain strains of species designated as catalase negative. In some species, catalase activity may be activated by hemin supplementation.

[e]Detects the presence of cytochromes. Some strains of benzidine test-negative species can synthesize cytochromes on aerobic media supplemented with hemin (59).

[f]Determined by the modified oxidase test using tetramethyl-*p*-phenylenediamine dihydrochloride-impregnated disks or strips to detect the presence of cytochrome c (59).

[g]Standard oxidation/fermentation test.

[h]A disk is used. Positive indicates resistance and no zone of inhibition. *Micrococcus, Kocuria, Kytococcus, Stomatococcus,* and *Aerococcus* spp. are susceptible and have an inhibition zone of 10 to 25 mm in diameter.

[i]A disk is used. Positive indicates resistance and no zone of inhibition or a zone of up to 9 mm in diameter. Susceptible species have an inhibition zone of 15 to 35 mm in diameter.

[j]Some strains of *S. epidermidis* adhere tenaciously to the surface of agar, and this property is correlated with heavy slime production.

[k]*S. hominis* does not demonstrate growth in the anaerobic portion of a thioglycolate medium within 24 h and may produce only very poor growth in this portion following 3 to 5 days of incubation. However, it grows and ferments glucose anaerobically (standard oxidation-fermentation test). Failure to grow anaerobically in thioglycolate may be due in part to inhibition by the ingredien... .

[l]*Macrococcus* species can also be differentiated from *Staphylococcus* species on the basis of their generally larger Gram-stained cell size (≥2 µm) and larger number of chromosome fragments produced by digestion with NotI (12 to 36 fragments).

[m]A few *Micrococcus* strains demonstrate high-level (MIC, ≥50 µg/ml) erythromycin resistance.

TABLE 2 Differentiation of *Staphylococcus* species

Species	Large colonies[b]	Colony pigmentation[c]	Anaerobic growth[d]	Aerobic growth[e]	Coagulase test result	Clumping factor[f]	Heat-stable nuclease	Hemolysins[g]	Catalase[h]	Oxidase[i]	Alkaline phosphatase	Arginine arylamidase	Pyrrolidonyl arylamidase[j]	Ornithine decarboxylase	Urease[j]	β-Glucosidase[j]	β-Glucuronidase[j]	β-Galactosidase[j]	Arginine utilization[j]	Acetoin production	Nitrate reduction	Esculin hydrolysis	Novobiocin resistance[k]	Polymyxin B resistance[l]	D-Trehalose	D-Mannitol	D-Mannose	D-Turanose	D-Xylose	D-Cellobiose	L-Arabinose	Maltose	α-Lactose	Sucrose	N-Acetylglucosamine	Raffinose
S. arlettae	d	+	−	+	−	−	−	−	+	−	(+)	−	ND	ND	−	ND	+	d	−	ND	−	−	+	ND	+	+	+	+	+	−	+	+	+	+	−	+
S. aureus subsp. *anaerobius*	−	−	(+)	(±)	+	+	+	+	−	−	+	ND	ND	ND	ND	−	−	−	ND	−	−	−	+	ND	−	ND	−	ND	−	−	+	+	+	+	−	−
S. aureus subsp. *aureus*	+	+	+	+	+	+	+	+	+	−	+	−	−	−	d	+	−	−	+	+	+	−	−	+	+	+	+	+	+	−	−	+	+	+	+	−
S. auricularis	−	−	(±)	(+)	−	−	−	(d)	+	−	−	+	d	−	−	−	−	(d)	d	−	(d)	−	−	−	(+)	−	+	(d)	−	−	−	(+)	−	d	−	−
S. capitis subsp. *capitis*	−	−	(±)	+	−	−	−	(d)	+	−	−	−	−	−	+	−	−	−	d	d	d	−	−	−	−	+	+	−	−	−	−	+	−	(+)	−	−
S. capitis subsp. *urealyticus*	−	(d)	(+)	+	−	−	−	(d)	+	−	−	−	(d)	−	+	−	−	−	+	d	+	−	−	ND	−	+	+	−	−	−	−	+	−	+	−	−
S. caprae	d	−	(+)	+	−	−	−	(d)	+	−	(+)	−	−	−	+	−	−	−	+	+	+	−	−	−	(±)	d	+	−	−	−	−	(d)	d	+	ND	−
S. carnosus subsp. *carnosus*	+	−	+	+	−	−	−	−	+	−	+	−	+	−	−	−	−	+	+	+	+	−	+	−	+	+	+	−	ND	−	−	+	+	+	ND	−
S. carnosus subsp. *utilis*	−	−	d	+	−	ND	ND	ND	+	ND	−	ND	ND	ND	−	ND	−	ND	+	ND	d	ND	ND	ND	d	d	−	d	ND	−	−	d	d	−	ND	−
S. cohnii subsp. *cohnii*	d	−	(+)	+	−	−	−	(d)	+	−	+	−	d	−	+	−	−	+	+	d	−	d	+	+	+	(+)	(d)	ND	ND	ND	−	(d)	d	+	ND	−
S. cohnii subsp. *urealyticus*	+	d	+	+	−	−	−	−	+	ND	+	−	−	−	+	−	−	−	−	−	−	−	+	+	+	−	+	d	+	(d)	+	+	d	+	d	ND
S. chromogenes	+	+	+	+	−	ND	−	−	+	−	+	ND	ND	ND	+	p	−	+	+	ND	+	ND	−	ND	+	d	+	p	−	−	−	+	+	+	d	−
S. condimenti	ND	d	(+)	+	−	−	ND	ND	+	−	+	ND	ND	ND	+	ND	ND	ND	+	ND	+	ND	ND	ND	+	+	+	ND	ND	ND	−	+	d	±	ND	ND
S. delphini	+	−	(+)	+	−	−	+	+	+	−	+m	ND	ND	(d)	+	(d)	ND	−	d	d	+	d	−	+	+	d	+	(d)	−	(d)	−	+	d	+	ND	−
S. epidermidis	−	−	+	+	−	−	−	(d)	+	−	(+)	ND	−	ND	+	ND	+	−	+	+	+	ND	−	ND	+	−	(+)	p	−	−	−	+	d	+	−	−
S. equorum subsp. *equorum*	−	−	−	(+)	−	−	−	−	+	−	d	ND	−	−	+	ND	+	d	ND	d	d	d	+	ND	+	ND	+	d	d	−	d	+	d	−	ND	ND
S. equorum subsp. *linens*	ND	−	−	+	−	ND	−	(d)	+	−	p	ND	−	−	+	ND	−	−	ND	d	+	ND	+	ND	−	ND	+	±	+	−	+	+	−	−	ND	ND
S. felis	+	−	+	+	−	−	+	(d)	+	−	d	ND	+	ND	−	+	+	−	+	d	+	d	−	ND	+	+	+	+	−	−	+	+	−	+	+	−
S. fleurettii	+	−	(+)	+	−	−	+	(+)	+	+	(+)	ND	−	−	+	+	+	d	+	d	+	d	+	−	+	d	+	+	−	(d)	−	+	−	+	+	+
S. gallinarum	+	d	+	+	−	−	−	−	+	−	−	−	−	−	+	−	−	−	+	+	+	+	+	−	+	d	+	+	−	−	+	+	−	+	+	+
S. haemolyticus	+	d	+	+	−	−	−	(d)	+	−	−	−	−	−	−	−	−	−	+	−	+	−	−	−	+	+	+	(d)	−	−	−	+	d	(+)	+	−
S. hominis subsp. *hominis*	+	d	(+)	+	−	d	−	−	+	−	−	−	−	−	+	p	d	d	d	d	d	p	−	−	+	d	+	ND	−	−	−	+	d	+	+	−
S. hominis subsp. *novobiosepticus*[n]	−	−	−	+	−	−	−	−	+	−	−	ND	−	−	+	−	−	−	−	−	−	−	+	−	−	−	+	−	−	−	−	+	−	(±)	d	−
S. hyicus	+	−	(+)	+	d	d	d	d	+	−	+	−	d	−	+	p	d	d	d	d	+	p	−	+	+	(d)	+	d	−	−	d	(±)	d	+	+	−
S. intermedius	+	−	(±)	+	+	+	+	p	+	−	+	ND	−	−	+	p	+	+	+	−	+	d	+	−	+	+	+	d	−	−	d	d	d	(±)	+	−
S. kloosii	d	d	(±)	+	−	−	d	(d)	+	−	+	ND	d	−	+	p	−	+	d	d	+	d	+	−	+	+	+	±	(d)	−	d	d	d	(±)	+	−
S. lentus	−	d	(±)	(+)	−	−	−	−	+	+	(±)	ND	−	−	−	+	d	d	−	−	−	+	+	−	+	+	(+)	(±)	(±)	+	d	(±)	d	(±)	d	+

310

Table (rotated 90°). Row labels (species):

- S. lugdunensis
- S. lutrae
- S. muscae
- S. nepalensis
- S. pasteuri
- S. pettenkoferi
- S. piscifermentans
- S. pseudintermedius
- S. saccharolyticus
- S. saprophyticus subsp. bovis
- S. saprophyticus subsp. saprophyticus
- S. schleiferi subsp. coagulans
- S. schleiferi subsp. schleiferi
- S. sciuri subsp. carnaticus
- S. sciuri subsp. rodentium
- S. sciuri subsp. sciuri
- S. simiae
- S. simulans
- S. succinus subsp. casei
- S. succinus subsp. succinus
- S. warneri
- S. xylosus

[a] Symbols and abbreviations (unless otherwise indicated): +, 90% or more strains positive; −, 90% or more strains negative; d, 11 to 89% of strains positive; ND, not determined. Parentheses indicate a delayed reaction.

[b] Positive is defined as a colony diameter of ≥6 mm after incubation on P agar at 34 to 35°C for 3 days and at room temperature (ca. 25°C) for an additional 2 days; exceptions are S. succinus (4 to 6 mm on tryptic soy agar) and S. fleurettii (8 to 12 mm on tryptic soy agar).

[c] Positive is defined by the visual detection of carotenoid pigments (e.g., yellow, yellow-orange, or orange) during colony development at normal incubation or room temperatures. Pigments may be enhanced by the addition of milk, fat, glycerol monoacetate, or soaps to P agar.

[d] Growth is in a semisolid thioglycolate medium. Symbols: +, moderate or heavy growth down the tube within 18 to 24 h; ±, heavier growth in the upper portion of the tube and weaker growth in the lower, anaerobic portion of tube; −, no visible growth within 48 h but very weak diffuse growth or a few scattered, small colonies may be observed in the lower portion of the tube by 72 to 96 h. Parentheses indicate delayed growth appearing within 24 to 72 h, sometimes noted as large, discrete colonies in the lower portion of the tube.

[e] Growth is on P agar or bovine, sheep, or human blood agar at 34 to 37°C. The subspecies of S. equorum and S. succinus grow slowly at 35 to 37°C; the optimum growth temperatures of S. equorum subsp. equorum and S. equorum subsp. linens are 30°C and 32°C, respectively, and those of S. succinus subsp. succinus and S. succinus subsp. casei are 28°C and 32°C, respectively. Anaerobic species S. saccharolyticus and S. aureus subsp. anaerobius grow very slowly in the presence of air. S. aureus subsp. anaerobius requires the addition of blood, serum, or egg yolk for growth on primary isolation medium. S. auricularis, S. lentus, and S. vitulus produce just-detectable colonies on P agar in 24 to 36 h, and these colonies remain very small (1 to 2 mm in diameter).

[f] The slide agglutination test using rabbit or human plasma detects the expression of clumping factor. Use human plasma for S. lugdunensis and S. schleiferi. Latex agglutination is less reliable for the detection of clumping factor for S. lugdunensis.

[g] Hemolysis on bovine blood agar. Symbols and abbreviations: +, wide zone of hemolysis within 24 to 36 h; (+) delayed moderate to wide zone of hemolysis within 48 to 72 h; (d), no or delayed hemolysis; −, no or only very narrow (1-mm) zone of hemolysis within 72 h. Some strains designated as negative may produce a slight greening or browning of blood agar. Analysis of hemolysis for both S. succinus subspecies was performed on Wilkins-Chalgren anaerobe agar plates containing 5% sheep blood.

[h] Catalase and cytochrome synthesis cannot be induced in S. aureus subsp. anaerobius by the addition of H_2O_2 or hemin to the culture medium. Catalase activity can be induced in S. saccharolyticus by hemin supplementation. In this species, cytochromes a and b are present in small quantities.

[i] Determined by the modified oxidase test to detect the presence of cytochrome c (59).

[j] Determined primarily by commercial rapid identification tests (see the text).

[k] Positive (resistant) is defined by an MIC of ≥1.6 µg/ml or a growth inhibition zone diameter of ≤16 mm with a 5-µg novobiocin disk.

[l] Positive is defined by a growth inhibition zone diameter of <10 mm with a 300-U polymyxin B disk.

[m] Approximately 6 to 15% of strains of S. epidermidis are negative for alkaline phosphatase activity, depending on the population sampled. A low but significant number of clinical isolates are phosphatase negative.

[n] All strains tested are also resistant to penicillin G, methicillin, oxacillin, gentamicin, and streptomycin.

[o] Positive with the STAPH-ZYM tests, but negative with the API STAPH tests (48).

[p] Positive reactions are with the Staph latex agglutination test (Remel) that detects clumping factor and/or protein A.

described species, *S. pettenkoferi*, was proposed in 2008 (181, 187). In 1925, the differentiation into coagulase-positive ("*S. aureus* group") and coagulase-negative staphylococci (CoNS) based on the detection of the plasma coagulase was introduced (193). This was later followed by a further subclassification of the CoNS into novobiocin-susceptible ("*S. epidermidis* group") and novobiocin-resistant ("*S. saprophyticus* group") species (14, 127). The "*S. epidermidis* group" comprises, besides the eponym, historically *S. capitis*, *S. haemolyticus*, *S. hominis* subsp. *hominis*, *S. lugdunensis*, *S. saccharolyticus*, and *S. warneri*; however, many other species are also novobiocin susceptible (Table 2). In addition to both *S. saprophyticus* subspecies, numerous other CoNS species are novobiocin resistant (e.g., *S. cohnii*, *S. kloosii*, and *S. xylosus*) (Table 2). Despite limitations, coagulase activity and novobiocin susceptibility are still used for presumptive identification of clinical isolates.

The genus *Macrococcus* was established by delimiting the genus *Staphylococcus* through description of *Macrococcus caseolyticus*, the former *Staphylococcus* (*Micrococcus*) *caseolyticus*, and the description of novel species. The macrococcal cells are similar to those of staphylococci with the exception of the larger cell diameter, reaching 2.5 μm in some species, hence their genus name. Recently, *Macrococcus* was considered to reflect the genome of ancestral bacteria before the speciation of staphylococcal species (12). As shown for the fully sequenced strain JCSC5402, *M. caseolyticus* has a G+C content of 36.9 mol% (12). In contrast to other macrococci, the cell wall of *M. caseolyticus* contains teichoic acid. With the exception of *Nosocomiicoccus*, the other genera, *Salinicoccus* and *Jeotgalicoccus*, have a G+C content that is generally higher than those of staphylococci. Whereas salinicocci are strictly aerobes, the other genera comprise facultative anaerobes.

Micrococcaceae and Dermacoccaceae

Most species of the gram-positive, non-spore-forming families *Micrococcaceae* and *Dermacoccaceae* are characterized by nonmotile and spherical cells of 0.5 to 1.8 μm in diameter arranged in tetrads and clusters. Deviating from this, rod-shaped species are found in some genera. *Arthrobacter* and *Rothia* species may display coccoid forms. Except for *Rothia mucilaginosa*, both genera are discussed in chapter 26. Members of the *Micrococcaceae* and *Dermacoccaceae* have G+C contents within the range of 52 to 75%.

Of the mostly strictly aerobic and mesophilic members of the *Micrococcaceae* family, the genus *Micrococcus* contains the classical micrococcal species *M. luteus* and *M. lylae*. Other former *Micrococcus* members are now part of the *Kocuria* genus such as *K.* (*Micrococcus*) *kristinae*, *K.* (*Micrococcus*) *varians*, and *K. rosea* (formerly *Micrococcus roseus*, now united with former *Pelczaria aurantia*) (174). The former *Micrococcus halobius* was transferred into the novel genus *Nesterenkonia* as *N. halobia*. For all these genera, several novel species have been described. In this chapter, the term "micrococci" in quotes is used to indicate the members of the genus *Micrococcus* as understood before the emendation, reflecting most of the clinically relevant species (174).

Two of the former "micrococcal" species are now assigned to the *Dermacoccaceae* family, either to the genus *Dermacoccus* containing *D.* (*Micrococcus*) *nishinomiyaensis* and other species or to the genus *Kytococcus* comprising, besides *K.* (*Micrococcus*) *sedentarius*, the recently described species *K. schroeteri* and *K. aerolatus*.

Alloiococcus

The name of the only species of the genus *Alloiococcus* still standing in nomenclature is *A. otitis* [sic]; however, the proposed emended name, *A. otitidis*, is frequently used in the literature. This slow-growing species is characterized by gram-positive ovoid cocci, occurring mostly in clusters and pairs. Alloiococci show aerobic atmospheric requirements, but they are able to grow sparsely in the candle jar atmosphere (126). The G+C content is 44 to 45%.

EPIDEMIOLOGY AND TRANSMISSION

Staphylococcus and Related Genera

The major habitats of most staphylococcal species are the skin and mucous membranes of mammals and birds. *S. aureus* subsp. *aureus* is considered to be the most important human pathogen among staphylococci, followed by *S. epidermidis*, *S. haemolyticus*, and *S. saprophyticus* subsp. *saprophyticus*. *S. auricularis*, *S. capitis* subsp. *capitis* and *urealyticus*, *S. caprae*, *S. cohnii* subsp. *cohnii* and *urealyticus*, *S. hominis* subsp. *hominis* and *novobiosepticus*, *S. lugdunensis*, *S. pasteuri*, *S. pettenkoferi*, *S. saccharolyticus*, *S. schleiferi* subsp. *schleiferi*, *S. simiae*, *S. simulans*, *S. warneri*, and *S. xylosus* are also encountered in human specimens (164). These species are found mainly as part of the resident microbiota. For references concerning species description, see "*List of Prokaryotic Names with Standing in Nomenclature*" (http://www.bacterio.cict.fr/).

S. aureus and Other Coagulase-Positive Species

As determined in longitudinal studies, three types of *S. aureus* nasal carriers have been historically distinguished: persistent carriers (10 to 35%, carrying one strain over time), intermittent carriers (20 to 75%, carrying different strains), and noncarriers (5 to 50%) (203). Since intermittent carriers and noncarriers share similar *S. aureus* nasal elimination kinetics, it was recently proposed that there are only two types of nasal carriers: persistent carriers and others (189). From the vestibulum nasi, *S. aureus* can be transferred to skin and other body areas. Health care workers have a high *S. aureus* nasal carriage rate (50% to 90%) as do patients with insulin-dependent diabetes mellitus, patients receiving long-term hemodialysis, and users of illegal intravenous drugs (37). The vaginal carriage rate in adult premenopausal women is about 10% (119). The intertriginous skin folds, the axillae, and the perineum are also found to be regularly colonized. Of particular interest, nasal colonization plays a crucial role as a source of invasive infections (107, 195, 202).

The population of *S. aureus* presents a highly clonal structure dominated by approximately a dozen major clonal complexes comprising hundreds of clonal lineages or sequence types (58). The *S. aureus* populations are also divided into four distinct groups based on *agr* (accessory gene regulator system) allelic variation (135).

Within health care facilities, *S. aureus* strains are transmitted from patient to patient primarily via hand carriage of medical personnel. This is of utmost importance for the transmission of methicillin-resistant *S. aureus* (MRSA) strains (MRSA strains are further discussed in "Antimicrobial Susceptibilities" below). The role of the external environment is less important, except for certain areas such as intensive care units and burn units. Colonized or infected health care workers may act as a reservoir (2). MRSA strains circulating in livestock and found in meat production differ from companion animal strains. For companion animals, MRSA acquisition is primarily a humanosis, in contrast to the newly emerging livestock-associated MRSA and methicillin-susceptible *S. aureus* (MSSA) strains such as ST398, presenting a genuine zoonotic risk (130).

Staphylococcus aureus subsp. *anaerobius* has been recovered from subcutaneous abscesses of sheep (45). So far, it has not been isolated from human clinical specimens. *S. intermedius*, the recently delineated species *S. pseudintermedius*, and two clusters of *S. delphini* are closely related coagulase-positive species commonly recovered from carnivores, other mammals (e.g., horses and cats), and birds. Since it is very difficult to differentiate among these species, it is very likely that previously reported *S. intermedius* isolates with variant biotypes might have included *S. delphini* and, in particular, *S. pseudintermedius* (163). *S. pseudintermedius* might be the predominant coagulase-positive *Staphylococcus* species recovered from normal and infected canine skin (48). Further coagulase-positive animal-adapted staphylococci are *S. schleiferi* subsp. *coagulans*, *S. felis*, and *S. lutrae*.

Coagulase-Negative Staphylococci

In humans, *S. epidermidis* is the most frequently recovered staphylococcal species colonizing the body surface, where it is particularly prevalent on moist areas such as the axillae, inguinal and perineal area, anterior nares, and toe webs. *S. auricularis* is part of the healthy human external auditory canal microbiota colonizing exclusively this region; *S. capitis* is found surrounding the sebaceous glands on the forehead and scalp following puberty; *S. haemolyticus* and *S. hominis* are preferentially isolated from axillae and pubic areas high in apocrine glands; and *S. saprophyticus* subsp. *saprophyticus* is frequently colonizing the rectum and the genitourinary tract of young women (106, 159, 164). *S. lugdunensis* is frequently found on the lower extremities and on the groin (28). However, these species may be found occasionally on other body sites.

S. sciuri and *S. xylosus* are commensals of the skin and the mucous membranes of many animals and, occasionally, of humans. Both species are also found in food; *S. xylosus* represents one of the major starter cultures used for meat fermentation. *S. sciuri* subsp. *carnaticus* is recovered mainly from bovine hosts, and subsp. *rodentium* is found mainly in rodents. *S. kloosii*, *S. equorum* subsp. *equorum*, and *S. gallinarum* are found on several mammals and food products. *S. chromogenes*, *S. hyicus*, and *S. lentus* are common residents of cloven-hoofed animals and, in addition, may be isolated from their food products. *S. vitulinus* (syn. *S. pulvereri*) is found preferentially on horses and whales. *S. arlettae* is found on mammals and birds; *S. nepalensis* has been isolated from Himalayan goats; *S. muscae* is described on flies. *S. carnosus* subsp. *carnosus* and *utilis*, *S. condimenti*, *S. equorum* subsp. *linens*, *S. fleurettii*, *S. piscifermentans*, and *S. succinus* subsp. *casei* have been associated with fermented food and dairy products; and *S. succinus* subsp. *succinus* was isolated from an amber fragment. However, the complete and/or true natural habitat for many of these species is still unclear.

Macrococcus, Salinicoccus, Jeotgalicoccus, and Nosocomiicoccus

The *Macrococcus* genus comprises four hoofed-animal-adapted species including *M. caseolyticus*, first described as *S. caseolyticus* (102). This species is found on food such as sausages and meat products. The halotolerant/halophilic *Jeotgalicoccus* and *Salinicoccus* species are recovered from fermented seafood and salted fish or found in saline and desert soil or salt mines. Thus far, the only reported recovery of *Nosocomiicoccus ampullae* has been isolation from surfaces of bottles of saline solution used in wound cleansing (4).

Micrococcaceae and Dermacoccaceae

The skin of humans and other mammals is the primary habitat for most *Micrococcaceae* and *Dermacoccaceae* isolated from clinical specimens. Cutaneous populations of micrococci are carried by most people (ca. 96%) with *M. luteus* as the most frequent species followed by *K. varians* (104). *R. mucilaginosa* is probably a normal inhabitant of the mouth and upper respiratory tract. Animal and dairy products may be considered secondary sources of micrococci. Many of the recently discovered members of the *Micrococcaceae* and *Dermacoccaceae* are associated with different environmental habitats.

Alloiococcus

Recently, a high incidence of *A. otitis* in the outer ear canal of healthy persons was demonstrated, suggesting that alloiococci are part of the normal bacterial microbiota (182).

CLINICAL SIGNIFICANCE

Staphylococcus

Many staphylococcal species are classical opportunists colonizing skin and mucous membranes but may become pathogenic in a species- and strain-dependent manner following breaks in the cutaneous epithelial barrier through trauma or medical interventions. The recovery of a staphylococcal isolate always requires assessment of clinical significance to determine whether it is a contaminant, colonizer, or pathogen.

S. aureus is the clinically most important species, capable of causing a wide range of human and animal diseases. *S. aureus* possesses an extensive, often redundant and overlapping arsenal of virulence factors, such as adhesins, enzymes, and toxins, and has various strategies to evade the host immune response. In addition, the pathogen has become resistant to many of the therapeutic agents available. National Nosocomial Infection Surveillance and National Healthcare Safety Network data indicate that *S. aureus* is the most common cause of nosocomial pneumonia and skin and soft tissue infections. *S. aureus* is second only to CoNS as a cause of primary bacteremia in hospitals (84, 205).

Disease entities caused by *S. aureus* can be broadly divided into toxin-mediated diseases and suppurative infections comprising skin and soft tissue infections (SSTIs), organic and systemic infections, and foreign-body-related infections (FBRIs). The spectrum of SSTIs ranges from superficial (impetigo, folliculitis, furuncles/carbuncles, hydradenitis suppurativa, pyoderma, and wound infections) to deep entities (abscesses, mastitis, cellulitis, and pyomyositis) to life-threatening necrotizing fasciitis and myositis. SSTIs are the most frequent infections associated with community-acquired MRSA (CA-MRSA) with a single clone (pulsed-field gel electrophoresis [PFGE] type USA 300; multilocus sequence typing [MLST] type ST-8) being most prevalent (99). Infection of other sites may involve any body compartments and organ systems resulting in empyemas, osteomyelitis, arthritis, endocarditis, pneumonia, otitis media, sinusitis, mastoiditis, and parotitis. Any localized *S. aureus* infection can become invasive and lead to bacteremia. Systemic infections comprise primary and secondary bacteremia, meningitis, and endocarditis. Bacteremia may be complicated by metastatic foci (e.g., vertebral osteomyelitis). Congenital or acquired defects in host defense and the presence of foreign bodies may predispose patients to serious infections.

Besides an acute aggressive course, *S. aureus* may also cause chronic, persistent, and relapsing infections often due to a phenotypic subpopulation designated small-colony variants (SCVs) (147). SCVs of *S. aureus* and other staphylococcal species (e.g., *S. epidermidis* and *S. lugdunensis*) have been isolated from patients with chronic osteomyelitis, abscesses, and FBRIs as well as from cystic fibrosis patients with chronic airway infection (96, 167, 196).

Classical toxin-mediated diseases due to *S. aureus* include the staphylococcal toxic shock syndrome (TSS), staphylococcal food poisoning, and staphylococcal scalded skin syndrome (SSSS). TSS is associated with colonization by or infection with an isolate of *S. aureus* that is positive for TSS toxin-1 (TSST-1) or, less frequently, for other members of the staphylococcal pyrogenic toxin superantigen (PTSAg) family (primarily staphylococcal enterotoxin B or C). TSS is diagnosed on clinical grounds characterized by high fever, rapid-onset hypotension, a diffuse erythematous rash that becomes desquamating 1 to 2 weeks after onset, and involvement of three or more organ systems. After its initial description in children, it was associated with menstruating women who were using highly absorbent tampons. While the incidence of menstrual TSS decreased due to changes of the tampons' absorbency and chemical composition, the frequency of nonmenstrual TSS entities has remained constant (78). Although commonly no source of infection is confirmed, nonmenstrual TSS is usually associated with focal postoperative wound or soft tissue infections.

Staphylococcal food poisoning is caused by consumption of food contaminated with one or more preformed, relatively heat-stable enterotoxins. Nausea, vomiting, abdominal cramps, and diarrhea occur 2 to 6 hours after food ingestion. Symptoms usually subside 8 to 12 hours later.

SSSS is a type of bullous exfoliative dermatitis caused by exfoliative (epidermolytic) toxins (ETA and ETB) (112). The syndrome is typically found in neonates and young children. In addition to severe exfoliation affecting up to 90% or more of the entire body surface ("Ritter's disease"), a localized form (pemphigus neonatorum) with a few blisters is known. Diagnosis is made on the basis of clinical features, including Nikolsky's sign, in which the skin wrinkles on gentle pressure.

The other coagulase-positive or -variable staphylococci are members of the skin microbiota of various animal species and occasionally cause infections in their hosts. The members of the *S. intermedius/pseudintermedius/delphini* cluster are the most common etiologic agents of the canine pyoderma. *S. hyicus* is predominantly associated with the exudative epidermitis (greasy pig syndrome) in pigs, *S. schleiferi* subsp. *coagulans* is found in dogs suffering from external otitis, and *S. aureus* subsp. *anaerobius* is the etiological agent of abscess disease, a specific lymphadenitis of sheep and goats. In humans, *S. intermedius/S. pseudintermedius* appears to be occasionally responsible for canine-inflicted wound infections, FBRIs, food poisoning, and invasive infections in immunocompromised patients (19, 180). Only a few reports are known for human infections due to *S. schleiferi* subsp. *coagulans* and *S. hyicus*.

Since 1980, CoNS have been increasingly recognized as nosocomial pathogens, especially *S. epidermidis*. CoNS cause nosocomial infections in patients with predisposing factors such as immunodeficiency and/or indwelling or implanted foreign polymer bodies (84, 156, 194, 198). CoNS are less often implicated as the cause of infections of natural tissue. CoNS are the most common cause of nosocomial bloodstream infection typically associated with central and peripheral intravascular catheters (205). Most important in the pathogenesis of FBRIs is the ability of CoNS to colonize the surface of the device by the formation of a thick, multilayered biofilm (142). *S. epidermidis* is the predominant cause of infections associated with prosthetic vascular grafts, prosthetic orthopedic devices, and cerebrospinal fluid shunts. CoNS are

frequently isolated causative agents of prosthetic-valve endocarditis; rarely they are involved in infections of (previously damaged) native valves (ca. 5%) (113). A right-sided native valve endocarditis is observed in intravenous drug abusers. Virtually any other surgically inserted materials and devices may become infected by CoNS. They account for 45 to 75% of all late-onset bloodstream infections in preterm and low-birth-weight neonates in neonatal intensive care units (43).

In addition to prosthetic-valve endocarditis, unusually fulminant cases of native-valve endocarditis may be caused by *S. lugdunensis*, characterized by an aggressive clinical course with high mortality (8). Thus, patients with *S. lugdunensis* bacteremia should be carefully examined for signs of endocarditis. Besides other invasive infections, this organism is also a common pathogen involved in FBRIs (167). *S. lugdunensis* infections resemble those caused by *S. aureus* rather than those caused by other CoNS.

Based on special urotropic and ecologic characteristics, *S. saprophyticus* subsp. *saprophyticus* is a well-documented causative agent of acute, commonly recurrent, urinary tract infections in young, otherwise healthy, sexually active women and, less frequently, in young men or boys. This pathogen is the second most common (after *Escherichia coli*) cause of uncomplicated cystitis among young women. While colony counts of ≥100,000 CFU/ml in two or more cultures of midstream urine usually indicate significant bacteriuria, lower counts may be significant in the symptomatic patient. Infections due to the recently described subspecies *S. saprophyticus* subsp. *bovis* have not been reported.

Since human infections due to *Macrococcus*, *Jeotgalicoccus*, *Nosocomiicoccus*, and *Salinicoccus* have not been described, these genera are not discussed further in this chapter.

Micrococcaceae and *Dermacoccaceae*

While "micrococci" are generally acknowledged as harmless saprophytes, they can also act as opportunistic pathogens. *Micrococcus*, *Kocuria*, and *Kytococcus* species have been found to cause infections such as endocarditis, pneumonia, and sepsis or FBRIs predominantly in immunocompromised patients (3, 25, 166). Recovery of the more recently described micrococcal species associated primarily with the environment must be assessed for clinical significance as reported for *K. rhizophila* (23).

R. mucilaginosa has been implicated in cases of bacteremia, endocarditis, endophthalmitis, intravascular catheter-related and central nervous system infections, pneumonia, peritonitis, septicemia, and cervical necrotizing fasciitis (75, 76, 116).

Since human infections due to *Acaricomes*, *Citricoccus*, *Luteipulveratus*, *Nesterenkonia*, *Renibacterium*, *Sinomonas*, *Yimella*, and *Zhihengliuella* have not been reported, these genera are not discussed further in this chapter.

Alloiococcus

A. otitis has been associated with infections of the middle ear (114). While immunostimulatory capacity suggests that *A. otitis* has pathogenic potential (80), other studies revealed that *A. otitis* may be a commensal rather than a cause of otitis media (182).

COLLECTION, TRANSPORT, AND STORAGE

The general principles of collection, transport, and storage of specimens as given in chapters 9 and 16 of this *Manual* are applicable to the microorganisms listed in this chapter. No special methods or precautions are usually required for these organisms because they are easily obtained from clinical material of most infection sites and are relatively resistant to drying and to moderate temperature changes. While some staphylococcal species may require anaerobic conditions or CO_2 supplementation for satisfactory growth, they survive transport and limited storage in air.

DIRECT EXAMINATION

The direct microscopic examination of normally sterile fluids such as cerebrospinal fluid and joint aspirates may be helpful. Direct examination of nonsterile fluids may also be useful, if the presence of inflammatory cells versus epithelial cells is taken into consideration. As the result of direct microscopic examination, only a presumptive report of "gram-positive cocci resembling staphylococci" should be made. Cells of microorganisms discussed here are gram-positive, nonmotile, non-spore-forming cocci that are arranged mostly in pairs and tetrads but occur also singly, in irregular (grape-like) clusters or in short chains (three or four cells). However, within the Micrococcaceae and Dermacoccaceae, some species exhibit rod-shaped cells and have been shown to be motile.

Rapid PCR-based approaches have been introduced for detection of MRSA directly from surveillance swabs. The multiple-locus approach, detecting the mecA gene and additionally an S. aureus-specific target (see "Species Identification by Nucleic Acid-Based and Spectroscopic Approaches" below), may be influenced by the coexistence of MSSA and MR-CoNS in the patient's physiological microbiota and thus may lead to false-positive MRSA findings (21). Nevertheless, the fundamental advantage of this approach is the direct detection of the methicillin resistance-encoding mecA gene. Tests applying this principle, such as hyplex StaphyloResist (plus) (BAG Health Care, Lich, Germany) and StaphPlex Panel (Qiagen), are commercially available.

The alternative single-locus amplification strategy overcomes the MSSA/MR-CoNS coexistence drawback by using oligonucleotide primers binding on the staphylococcal cassette chromosome (SCCmec) right extremity and on the neighboring orfX region of the S. aureus chromosome, amplifying both a taxonomic marker and a resistance marker in one step (89). This principle is the basis for several rapid test systems (e.g., BD GeneOhm MRSA assay; BD, Franklin Lakes, NJ; GenoType MRSA Direct and GenoQuick MRSA; Hain Lifescience; Xpert MRSA; Cepheid, Sunnyvale, CA; and LightCycler MRSA Advanced Test; Roche, Basel, Switzerland). However, the use of the surrogate marker SCCmec region instead of mecA as target may lead to false-positive or false-negative results, e.g., due to the exchange of the mecA gene by other genes, partial excision of the cassette, and variability of the cassette primer binding sites (53). Overall, the amplification-based rapid MRSA screening assays are characterized by very good negative predictive values (approximately 97 to 99%) and are hampered by moderate positive predictive values (approximately 65 to 95%). To date, MRSA cultures remain essential for confirming the molecular results, for typing purposes, and for determination of the complete susceptibility profile.

ISOLATION PROCEDURES

Considering the widespread distribution of staphylococci and "micrococci" on the skin and mucous membranes, careful procedures should be used to isolate organisms from the presumed focus of infection without collecting surrounding microbiota. The basic procedures for culture and isolation described in chapter 16 of this Manual should be followed.

The primary culture plate used for the isolation of staphylococci from clinical specimens is Columbia blood agar containing 5% defibrinated sheep blood (see also chapter 17). Abundant growth of most staphylococcal species occurs within 18 to 24 h. The simultaneous use of an enrichment broth (e.g., dextrose broth) streaked after 24 and 48 h on Columbia blood agar may enhance the recovery rate of S. aureus and other staphylococci.

The use of selective agars for S. aureus such as mannitol salt agar, egg yolk-tellurite pyruvate containing Baird-Parker medium, Columbia colistin-nalidixic acid agar, lipase-salt-mannitol agar (Remel, Lenexa, KS), and phenylethyl alcohol agar may be appropriate for specimens from heavily contaminated sources such as feces. It is mandatory to confirm putative S. aureus isolates recovered on these media.

Novel selective agars using chromogenic enzyme substrates specifically for S. aureus, such as CHROMagar Staph aureus (CHROMagar, Paris, France), BBL CHROMagar Staph aureus (BD Diagnostics, Sparks, MD), and S. aureus ID (bioMérieux, La Balme Les Grottes, France), have been launched on the market with chromogen-dependent coloration of the colonies. In particular for screening purposes, the chromogenic agars have been proven to be suitably sensitive and specific, allowing a presumptive but not final identification (141). Chromogenic agars designed for MRSA detection are discussed in "Antimicrobial Susceptibilities" below.

The diagnosis of catheter-related bloodstream infections by CoNS and other organisms remains a major challenge. One of the most frequently studied diagnostic techniques is represented by the semiquantitative roll-plate catheter culture. Here, the distal segment of the central venous catheter is cut and rolled across the surface of a Columbia blood agar plate at least four times followed by overnight incubation. A colony count of 15 CFU/ml or more may indicate catheter colonization (118). Examination of paired quantitative blood cultures drawn simultaneously from the catheter and a peripheral vein enhanced by the analysis of differential time to positivity represents an example of an approach that does not require catheter removal (148) (see also "Evaluation, Interpretation, and Reporting of Results" below).

Cultivation of "micrococci" and R. mucilaginosa should be performed as described for staphylococci on Columbia blood agar at 35°C to 37°C under aerobic conditions. However, abundant growth of Micrococcaceae and Dermacoccaceae needs consistent incubation times of 36 to 48 h.

Because of the slow growth rate, it is difficult to isolate A. otitis by conventional nonselective culture methods (29). Blood agar plates with 6% NaCl were shown to be useful.

IDENTIFICATION

The basic criteria distinguishing catalase-positive gram-positive cocci and their relatives among themselves and from other microbial taxa are given in "Description of the Genera" above and in Table 1. Misidentification is likely to occur if automated test system results are accepted without critical review by skilled lab personnel. In specialized settings, species can be identified by chemotaxonomic procedures and molecular methods.

Staphylococcus and Related Genera

Staphylococcus species can be identified phenotypically on the basis of a variety of conventional characteristics (Tables 1 to 3). The most clinically significant species in human and veterinary medicine can be identified on the

TABLE 3 Key tests for identification of the most clinically significant *Staphylococcus* species

Species	Colony pigmentation[b]	Staphylocoagulase	Clumping factor[b]	Heat-stable nuclease	Alkaline phosphatase	Pyrrolidonyl arylamidase[b]	Ornithine decarboxylase	Urease[b]	β-Galactosidase[b]	Acetoin production	Novobiocin resistance[b]	Polymyxin B resistance[b]	D-Trehalose	D-Mannitol	D-Mannose	D-Turanose	D-Xylose	D-Cellobiose	Maltose	Sucrose
S. aureus subsp. aureus	+	+	+	+	+	−	−	d	−	+	−	+	+	+	+	+	−	−	+	+
S. epidermidis	−	−	−	−	+	−	(d)	+	−	+	−	+	−	−	(+)	(d)	−	−	+	+
S. haemolyticus	d	−	−	−	−	+	−	−	−	+	−	−	+	d	−	(d)	−	−	+	+
S. hyicus (veterinary)	−	d	−	+	+	−	−	d	−	−	−	+	+	−	+	−	−	−	−	+
S. intermedius (veterinary)	−	+	d	+	+	+	−	+	+	−	−	−	+	(d)	+	d	−	−	(±)	+
S. lugdunensis	d	−	(+)	−	−	+	+	d	−	+	−	d	+	−	+	(d)	−	−	+	+
S. pseudintermedius (veterinary)	−	+	−	ND	+[c]	+	ND	+	+	+	−	+	+	(±)	+	(±)	−	−	+	+
S. schleiferi subsp. schleiferi	−	−	+	+	+	+	−	−	(+)	+	−	−	d	−	+	−	−	−	−	−
S. saprophyticus subsp. saprophyticus	d	−	−	−	−	−	−	+	+	+	+	−	+	d	−	+	−	−	+	+

[a]Symbols and abbreviations (unless otherwise indicated): +, 90% or more strains positive; ±, 90% or more strains weakly positive; −, 90% or more strains negative; d, 11 to 89% of strains positive; ND, not determined. Parentheses indicate a delayed reaction.
[b]Descriptions are the same as those in Table 2.
[c]Alkaline phosphatase reactions tested positive in the STAPH-ZYM gallery but negative in the API STAPH gallery.

basis of several key characteristics (Table 3). The application of the extensive scheme originally published by Kloos and Schleifer in 1975 (105) has been mostly replaced by the use of commercial identification systems.

Colony Morphology

Most staphylococcal colonies are 1 to 3 mm in diameter within 24 h and 3 to 8 mm in diameter after 72 h of incubation in air at 34 to 37°C. Exceptions are *S. aureus* subsp. *anaerobius*, *S. saccharolyticus*, *S. auricularis*, *S. equorum*, *S. vitulinus*, and *S. lentus*, which grow more slowly and usually require 24 to 36 h for detectable colony development. Further incubation of agar plates for a period of up to 48 to 72 hours (optimally followed by 2-day incubation at room temperature) enhances morphologic differences.

On routine blood agar, the typical *S. aureus* colony is pigmented (cream yellow to orange), smooth, entire, slightly raised, and hemolytic (Fig. 1). Mucoid colonies due to highly encapsulated strains are rarely encountered. A number of isolates of *S. aureus* as well as some CoNS species (e.g., *S. haemolyticus* and *S. lugdunensis*) may have a hazy or distinct zone of beta-hemolysis around the colonies ranging from weak to strong. SCVs of *S. aureus* or other staphylococcal species are characterized by pinpoint colonies (1/10 the size of the wild type), mostly nonpigmented and nonhemolytic after 24 to 72 hours of incubation (Fig. 1) (147, 192). They are often mixed with colonies displaying the normal phenotype, thus giving the appearance of a mixed culture. Upon subculture they may remain stable or revert to the wild type. Depending on their auxotrophy, normal growth may be restored if the isolate is grown in the presence of hemin, menadione, or thymidine and/or CO_2 supplementation (147).

The typical colony appearance of CoNS species is nonpigmented, smooth, entire, glistening, and opaque. Rare strong slime producers display mucoid colony morphology. Colony diameter reaches 3 to 6 mm after 3 days of incubation. Colonies of *S. chromogenes*, *S. lugdunensis*, *S. sciuri*, *S. warneri*, and *S. xylosus* are found to be more or less regularly yellow-orange pigmented. Other CoNS species may show pigmentation that usually has a yellowish tint (Table 2).

Coagulase Production

A widely used criterion for the identification of *S. aureus* in the clinical laboratory is the clotting of plasma proven by two different tests: (i) detection of the extracellular free coagulase by the tube test due to staphylococcal coagulase that converts fibrinogen to fibrin and (ii) detection of the cell wall bound "coagulase" (i.e., the clumping factor) by the slide agglutination test (see below).

The tube coagulase test is performed by transferring a large, well-isolated colony from a noninhibitory agar into 0.5 ml of reconstituted rabbit plasma. It is crucial to incubate the tube at 37°C for 4 h and to observe the tube for clot formation by slowly tilting the tube 90° from the vertical. Any degree of clotting represents a positive test. A flocculent

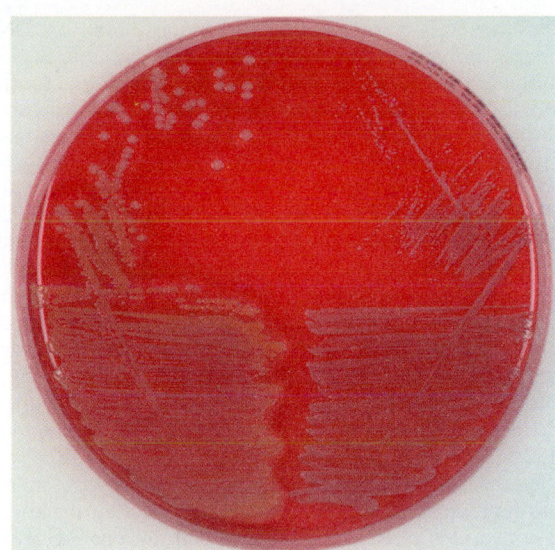

FIGURE 1 Columbia blood agar plate with 5% sheep blood showing *S. aureus* subsp. *aureus* after 24 h of incubation displaying the typical shapes of the normal phenotype with golden yellow-pigmented colonies surrounded by a hemolysis zone (left) and of the small-colony phenotype characterized by tiny, nonhemolytic, and nonpigmented colonies (right).

or fibrous precipitate is not a true clot and should be recorded as negative. If no clot is formed by 4 h, the tube should be read again after 18 h of incubation. False-negative results may occur for some strains producing staphylokinase, which may lyse the clot after formation (usually after prolonged incubation). Inaccurate results may occur if nonsterile plasma is used or the colony tested is not pure.

Particularly in veterinary microbiological laboratories, the other coagulase-positive or -variable species (Table 1) must not be disregarded. The detection of free coagulase in staphylococci obtained from human specimens is usually equated with the species identification of *S. aureus*. However, for animal-inflicted wounds, additional testing should be performed to provide identification beyond "coagulase-positive staphylococci."

Agglutination Assays

The classical slide agglutination test detects bacterial aggregation of *S. aureus* and other clumping factor-positive staphylococcal species in the presence of rabbit plasma through the action of clumping factor A, a cell wall-associated adhesin for fibrinogen. The detection of this factor expressed by non-*aureus* species (Table 1) may require the application of human plasma. While this test is very quick to perform (less than 1 minute), several limitations concerning sensitivity and specificity (e.g., masking of the factor by capsular polysaccharides and autoagglutination by picking colonies from media with high salt concentrations) have to be noted.

To overcome the disadvantages of the slide coagulase test (low sensitivity) and of the tube coagulase test (long incubation time), rapid latex and hemagglutination assays allowing presumptive identification of *S. aureus* have been developed. Besides detecting protein A and clumping factor A, recent third-generation assays include monoclonal antibodies recognizing the clinically most prevalent capsular polysaccharide serotypes 5 and 8 or other structures (e.g., Pastorex Staph-Plus [Bio-Rad Laboratories, Hercules, CA]; Slidex Staph Plus

[bioMérieux, Marcy l'Etoile, France]; and Staphaurex Plus and Staphytect Plus [Oxoid, Cambridge, United Kingdom]). The higher sensitivity (>98 to 100%) of the third-generation tests has reduced their specificity (72 to 99%). False-positive reactions occur with some CoNS strains (*S. haemolyticus* and *S. hominis*) possessing type 8 capsular polysaccharide or owning a cell wall hemagglutinin (*S. saprophyticus*). When an isolate is suspected to be *S. aureus*, negative slide tests should be confirmed by the tube coagulase test.

Identification of Species by Susceptibility Tests

Novobiocin resistance is intrinsic to *S. saprophyticus* and other CoNS species (Table 2) but is uncommon in the other clinically important CoNS species of the "*S. epidermidis* group." A disk diffusion test for estimating novobiocin susceptibility can be performed using a 5-μg novobiocin disk on Mueller-Hinton agar or tryptic soy sheep blood agar. With an inoculum suspension equivalent in turbidity to a 0.5 McFarland opacity standard and incubation at 35 to 37°C overnight or up to 24 h, novobiocin resistance is indicated by an inhibition zone diameter of ≤16 mm with any of these media.

Polymyxin B resistance is usually observed for isolates of *S. aureus*, *S. epidermidis*, *S. hyicus*, *S. chromogenes*, and to a lesser extent, for some strains of *S. lugdunensis*. A disk diffusion test may be performed using a 300-U polymyxin B disk on tryptic soy sheep blood agar with the same test conditions as those described for novobiocin. Polymyxin B resistance is indicated by an inhibition zone diameter of <10 mm.

Identification of Species by Biochemical Procedures

For speed, standardization, cost reduction, and convenience, the classical tests for fermentation, oxidation, degradation, and hydrolysis of various substrates (details are available in chapter 17) have been incorporated into commercial manual and automated biochemical test systems (see below and chapter 3). They are often complemented by simultaneously performed antimicrobial susceptibility testing, an advanced expert system, and an interface to the laboratory informatics software. Results with conventional tests (Tables 2 and 3) may be slightly different from those obtained with rapid biochemical test systems due to the use of other, more sensitive indicators. Commercial identification systems identify the staphylococci (and some other aerobic gram-positive cocci) of clinical importance with an accuracy of 70 to >90%. For some systems, reliability depends on additional testing as suggested by the manufacturer. Uncommon strains or phenotypic variants (e.g., SCVs) may have altered patterns of biochemical reactions requiring molecular testing for identification.

The API Staph (bioMérieux) strip represents an overnight method for manual identification of primarily staphylococci for health care and product safety applications. Necessitating the same incubation time and also fashioned in the strip format, the ID32 Staph (bioMérieux) may be read manually as well as automatically by the bioMérieux ATB system. The databases of both systems comprise more than 20 staphylococcal species with clinical significance, some "micrococcal" species, and *R. mucilaginosa*. A rapid version allowing 2-h identification of *S. aureus*, *S. epidermidis*, and *S. saprophyticus* is provided by the same manufacturer (Rapidec Staph). The Vitek 2 (bioMérieux) system is a fully automated platform that performs bacterial identification and antibiotic susceptibility testing. The VITEK 2 gram-positive identification card encompasses a total of more than 100 species, including 26 staphylococcal species, a small spectrum of "micrococci," and *R. mucilaginosa*; identification of CoNS usually requires 10 h.

The MicroScan product Pos ID family (Siemens Healthcare Diagnostics, Deerfield, IL) includes "Conventional" (overnight identification time), "Rapid" (2.5-h identification time), and "Synergies plus" (2- to 2.5-h identification time, with key antimicrobial results in as little as 4.5 hours) panels in a microtiter format. Identification of 19 clinical staphylococcal species, some "micrococcal" species, and *R. mucilaginosa* is available with either manual or automated processing on the autoSCAN-4 and WalkAway systems.

The BD BBL Crystal identification systems' Rapid Gram-Positive ID kit (BD Diagnostic Systems, Sparks, MD) is a three-row panel that may be read manually or with the BBL Crystal AutoReader requiring a 4-hour incubation period. Besides 14 staphylococcal species, the database encompasses a total of 88 taxa including *M. caseolyticus*, *R. mucilaginosa*, and several "micrococci." The BBL Crystal Gram-Positive ID system represents the overnight incubation (18-h) version with an extended taxa profile of 121 gram-positive organisms. A further enhanced taxa profile (covering about 200 taxa) is covered by the automated nephelometry-based BD Phoenix Automated Microbiology System using one combination panel with the identification substrates on one side and the antimicrobial agents on the other side of the panel. For staphylococci, about 10 to 15.5 hours are required for complete results (identification and antimicrobial susceptibility testing) (56).

The gram-positive aerobic bacteria database (339 taxa) of the Biolog Systems family (Biolog, Hayward, CA) comprises 34 staphylococcal and 4 macrococcal (sub-)species and many members of the *Micrococcaceae* and *Dermacoccaceae* families not found in other commercial phenotype-based systems. The system's redox chemistry based on the utilization of a wide variety of carbon sources is used to generate a "metabolic fingerprint" providing results in 4 hours or less and is available with different automation levels.

The Sherlock Microbial Identification System (MIDI, Newark, DE) represents an identification system that automates microbial identification by combining cellular fatty acid analysis with computerized high-resolution gas chromatography. In addition to a multitude of other species, 30 staphylococcal species, *M. caseolyticus*, and several "micrococci" are listed in the fatty acid-based database. A new sample preparation method (Instant FAME) allows for rapid identification from pure cultures in less than 15 minutes.

Most systems are fairly successful in differentiating *S. aureus*, *S. epidermidis*, and *S. saprophyticus*, while the accurate identification of less common species is more variable (152). Systems may fail in distinguishing commonly encountered staphylococcal species, in particular if phenotypic variants or isolates recovered from livestock and food are tested (18, 210). A verification of the identification result by a second, independent approach is recommended for isolates with presumptive identification as *S. aureus*, particularly for oxacillin-resistant strains. Additional tests should be performed on clinically significant isolates with questionable identification results that impact patient management.

Species Identification by Nucleic Acid-Based and Spectroscopic Approaches

Extraction of staphylococcal nucleic acids may be challenging due to the gram-positive nature requiring special conditions for lysis of the cell wall. For this purpose, lysostaphin, lysozyme, proteinase K, and achromopeptidase have been described.

Besides PCR fingerprinting techniques based on DNA sequence polymorphisms, species-specific variable regions of universal genes or genes unique for *S. aureus* or other staphylococcal species may serve as targets for identification and differentiation of staphylococcal isolates. Assays based on the specific amplification of fragments of the universal 16S and 23S rRNA genes and of their spacer sequences have been published (18, 41, 55, 92, 124, 173, 178). The 16S rRNA gene is also used as target for the in situ detection and identification of *S. aureus* and *S. epidermidis* (111). Other universal DNA targets shown to be useful for identification of staphylococci include the elongation factor gene (*tuf*), the gyrase gene (*gyrA*), the manganese-dependent superoxide dismutase gene (*sodA*), the glyceraldehyde-3-phosphate dehydrogenase-encoding gene (*gap*), and a 60-kDa heat shock protein (HSP60/GroE) (73, 74, 120, 144, 211).

Sequencing of selected universal phylogenetic marker genes represents the ultimate approach to identify known and not yet described staphylococcal species. For 16S rRNA gene sequencing, the regions between bp 70 to 300, 420 to 500, 1,000 to 1050, and 1,250 to1,290 (corresponding to nucleotides of the *Escherichia coli* 16S rRNA gene) are useful to determine sequence differences among the staphylococcal species. For differentiation of staphylococcal subspecies, sequencing of partial *rpoB* gene sequences seems to be superior to partial 16S rRNA gene sequencing (123). The recognized limitations of currently available public sequence databases apply to sequencing of staphylococcal isolates (18).

The most popular and well-studied specific target for *S. aureus* identification is the *nuc* gene that encodes thermostable nuclease (thermonuclease or TNase) (31, 204). PCR methods targeting the *nuc* gene are highly specific for *S. aureus*. A specific PCR for the *S. intermedius nuc* gene has also been described (24). Further specific targets used for identification of *S. aureus* include the genes encoding clumping factor (*clfA*), coagulase (*coa*), manganese-dependent superoxide dismutase (*sodM*, absent in CoNS), the factors essential for the expression of methicillin resistance (*femA* and *B*), and for MRSA only, the staphylococcal insertion element *431* (108, 122, 188, 191, 211). Misidentification using the *fem* factors may occur due to *fem*-negative *S. aureus* strains and CoNS with a gene structurally related to *femA*.

For molecular identification of *S. aureus* and some other staphylococcal species isolated from culture, several commercial tests (e.g., GenoType Staphylococcus [Hain Lifescience, Nehren, Germany]; StaphPlex Panel [Qiagen, Germantown, MD]; AccuProbe [Gen-Probe, San Diego, CA]; and *S. aureus* Evigene [AdvanDx, Woburn, MA]) are available. Some assays also detect resistance genes (see below) and/or toxin genes. The GeneXpert (Cepheid) and BD GeneOhm (BD Diagnostics) instruments offer assays to detect MSSA and MRSA directly from positive blood cultures. The RiboPrinter microbial characterization system (DuPont Qualicon, Wilmington, DE) utilizes ribotype pattern analysis for the differentiation of staphylococcal species with patterns in the database.

The *S. aureus* PNA FISH (bioMérieux) is a qualitative nucleic acid hybridization assay targeting rRNA sequences based on peptide nucleic acid (PNA) fluorescence in situ hybridization (FISH). The assay is intended for rapid identification of *S. aureus* in a smear prepared from a positive blood culture. The *S. aureus*/CNS PNA FISH is expanded to identify simultaneously several CoNS species that commonly cause bacteremia (83). Diagnostic DNA oligonucleotide microarrays that identify the genus *Staphylococcus*, clinically important staphylococcal species, other pathogens, drug resistance genes, and toxin genes have been designed and tested on clinical isolates (66, 129).

Alternative high-throughput approaches involving mass spectral analysis of surface-associated proteins of intact staphylococcal cells are represented by the matrix-assisted laser desorption ionization–time of flight and related methods (32, 150, 206). Here, the quality of the database and the standardization of variable parameters are crucial to achieve reproducible results. Nondestructive techniques such as Fourier transform infrared (FT-IR) and Raman spectroscopy are currently being developed as alternative methods for the rapid identification of staphylococci (6). This approach also allows discrimination between the SCV and the normal *S. aureus* phenotype (20).

Diagnosis of Toxin-Mediated Staphylococcal Syndromes

The diagnosis of TSS and SSSS is based on clinical signs supplemented by serologic tests and the detection of the toxin production by staphylococcal isolates (*S. aureus*, rarely other species). While the skin manifestations are mostly culture negative, isolates are usually recovered from the suspected site of infection. Blood cultures are positive in fewer than 5% of cases of staphylococcal TSS. In patients with TSS, protective antibodies against causative PTSAgs are absent or present at very low levels. However, seroconversion after onset of the disease and during convalescence may be observed. The same phenomenon holds true for exfoliatin antibodies in patients with SSSS. Currently available immunoassays for antibody detection are for research use only. Beyond the recognition of the characteristic rapid onset and the clinical signs, staphylococcal food poisoning is difficult to verify because the incriminated food source may not contain cultivable staphylococcal cells and requires detection of staphylococcal enterotoxin.

Traditional immunological procedures may be used to measure the toxin in culture supernatants of isolated strains, in contaminated food extracts, or in patient specimens. Kits for the detection of strains producing TSST-1 (TST-RPLA [Oxoid, Cambridge, United Kingdom]; TST-RPLA "Seiken" [Denka Seiken, Tokyo, Japan]; and TSST-1 Evigene [AdvanDx, Woburn, MA]), staphylococcal enterotoxins (Rida Screen set A, B, C, D, E [R-Biopharm, Darmstadt, Germany]; SET-RPLA "Seiken" [Denka Seiken]; SET-RPLA Kit toxin detection kit [Oxoid]), and ETA/ETB (EXT-RPLA "Seiken" [Denka Seiken]) are offered. A quantitative real-time immuno-PCR was recently described for the detection of small amounts of enterotoxins (61). An adaptation of a flow cytometry-assisted multiplex immunoassay (Bio-Plex system; Bio-Rad, Hercules, CA) for the detection of ETA and ETB has been recently reported (94). Since phenotypic methods may be hampered by low sensitivity and specificity (cross-reactivity between PTSAgs) and in vitro expression of PTSAgs might be negatively influenced by various factors, detection of PTSAg/ET-encoding sequences by nucleic acid-based methods has come into favor (17, 22, 128, 209).

Due to renewed interest in Panton-Valentine leukocidin (PVL), PCR procedures targeting leukocidal (synergohymenotropic) pore-forming toxins produced by *S. aureus* were established (115). The detection of PVL-encoding genes is included in the GenoType Staphylococcus and MRSA test systems (Hain Lifescience) and offered by the PVL EVIGENE kit (AdvanDx, Woburn, MA).

Micrococcaceae and *Dermacoccaceae*

Micrococci and staphylococci might be easily confused with one another on the basis of similar cellular morphologies, Gram stain appearance, and positive catalase activities. The exact species affiliation of "micrococci" may be frequently misjudged. The frequent pigmentation of micrococcal colonies with high convex profile leads to their presumptive identification as members of the *Micrococcaceae* and *Dermacoccaceae* families. Colonies of M. *luteus*, K. *varians*, and the kytococcal species are characterized by yellowish tints. K. *kristinae* and D. *nishinomiyaensis* appear orange-like, and K. *rosea* shows pink to red colonies. Some species (e.g., M. *lylae*) or strains of the usually pigmented species are nonpigmented. On routine blood agar, R. *mucilaginosa* colonies are mucoid or sticky, transparent to white, and nonhemolytic and in the majority of cases adhere to the agar (differentiation from streptococci). This organism may be distinguished from other similar organisms by its weak catalase reaction and its inability to grow in the presence of 5% NaCl.

In the clinical laboratory, "micrococcal" species can be preliminarily distinguished from staphylococci by their resistance to furazolidone (100 µg/disk; resistance is indicated by a ≤9-mm zone diameter) and lysostaphin (200 µg/disk; resistance, no zone) and susceptibility to bacitracin (0.04 U/disk; susceptibility, ≥10-mm zone diameter) in contrast to members of the *Staphylococcus* genus, which show inverse susceptibility patterns (zone diameters: furazolidone, ≥15mm; lysostaphin, 10 to 16 mm; bacitracin, no zone) (Table 1). Details are available in previous editions of this *Manual*. In contrast to most staphylococci, micrococci are positive by the modified oxidase test (59). Regarded as a reference method to distinguish "micrococcal" species from staphylococci, the fermentation of glucose in a manner similar to the oxidation-fermentation test for nonfermenters requires a specific oxidation-fermentation medium and prolonged incubation. In contrast to staphylococci, "micrococci" are characterized by the lack of acid production from glucose under anaerobic conditions.

Key features for differentiation of species reported to occur in human specimens are given in Table 4. Data concerning the applicability of manual and automated identification systems for members of *Micrococcaceae* and *Dermacoccaceae* are given in the respective *Staphylococcus* section; however, their use is limited to a small spectrum of the clinical "micrococcal" species. In cases of doubt and extraordinary clinical relevance, the use of sequencing-based approaches is recommended for definite species recognition.

Alloiococcus

After 48 h of incubation at 37°C, alloiococci form small alpha-hemolytic colonies on blood agar. Colonies formed on brain heart infusion agar with 5% rabbit blood are small, moist, and slightly yellow at 72 h, and the blood is partially hemolyzed. Growth occurs in the presence of 6.5% NaCl and on bile esculin agar. No growth occurs at 10°C or 45°C. A. *otitis* can be distinguished from similar organisms by its positive catalase and negative oxidase activities, its obligate aerobic nature, and its inability to produce acid from glucose or other carbohydrates (Table 1). Arginine dihydrolase is not produced. Pyrrolidonyl arylamidase, leucine aminopeptidase, and P-galactose are produced. Starch and esculin are not hydrolyzed; hippurate is mostly hydrolyzed (29). A. *otitis* is included in the database of the API Strep gallery (bioMérieux).

As the bacterium is quite inert biochemically, molecular methods are often necessary to confirm the identification. For the molecular verification of suspected colonies,

TABLE 4 Key tests for the identification of *Micrococcaceae* and *Dermacoccaceae* found in clinical specimens

Species	Colony pigmentation	Nitrate reduction	β-Galactosidase	β-Glucuronidase	α-D-Glucosidase	Arginine dihydrolase	Urease	Gelatin hydrolysis	Tween 80 hydrolysis	D-Mannose	Lactose	Sucrose	D-Trehalose	D-Xylose	D-Mannitol
Kocuria carniphila	Yellow	+	+	+	ND	−	−	−	−	−	+	±	−	−	−
Kocuria kristinae	Pale cream to pale orange	d	−	−	ND	−	d	±	−	+	d	+	+	−	−
Kocuria rhizophila	Yellow	−	−	−		−	−	+	+	+	−	−	−	−	−
Kocuria rosea	Pastel or orange-red	+	−	−	ND	−	−	−	−	−	−	−	−	+	+
Kocuria varians	Different shades of (dark) yellow	+	+	−	−	−	+	±	−	−	d	d	−	+	−
Micrococcus luteus	Different shades of yellow, yellowish green, or cream white	−	ND	ND	+	−	d	+	−	d	−	d			
Micrococcus lylae	Unpigmented or cream white	−	ND	ND	ND	−	−	+	d	−	−	−	+	−	−
Dermacoccus nishinomiyaensis	Bright orange pigment	d	ND	ND	ND	−	+	+	d	−	−	d	ND	−	ND
Kytococcus schroeteri	Muddy yellow	−	−	ND	−	+	−	+	+	−	ND	d	+	−	−
Kytococcus sedentarius	Cream white to deep buttercup yellow	−	ND	ND	+	+	−	+	−	d	−	d	+	−	ND
Rothia mucilaginosa	Transparent or whitish	+	ND	ND	+	−	−	+	−	+	−	+	+	−	−

[a]Symbols and abbreviations: +, 90% or more strains positive; ±, 90% or more strains weakly positive; −, 90% or more strains negative; d, 11 to 89% of strains positive; ND, not determined. Parentheses indicate a delayed reaction.

an *A. otitis*-specific PCR assay has been described (1). A PCR assay for direct detection of this microorganism in clinical specimens has been reported as part of a multiplex approach targeting pathogens that cause otitis media with effusion (82).

TYPING SYSTEMS

Traditional phenotyping techniques such as phage typing, capsule serotyping, antibiotic susceptibility pattern analysis, and other biotyping methods have been replaced by molecular band-based and sequence-based typing methods (179). The reference method for defining the core genetic population structure of *S. aureus* is MLST. In a standardized manner, the allelic polymorphism of seven housekeeping genes is indexed. A web-based database is available (http://saureus.mlst.net/). MLST has limited discriminatory power and low throughput capacity in the context of MRSA outbreak investigation and surveillance. In the case of common ancestry but assumed distinct epidemiological origin of MRSA isolates, subtyping of SCC*mec* may provide additional information (155).

For local MRSA outbreak investigation as well as for long-term MRSA surveillance, SmaI macrorestriction pattern analysis by PFGE represents a highly discriminatory "gold standard" tool with detailed performance and interpretation guidelines (133, 183). However, PFGE is technically demanding with low throughput, limited portability, problems with intercenter reproducibility, and different national nomenclatures. The emerging livestock-associated ST398 isolates are mostly nontypeable by standard PFGE protocols (88). Attribution of PFGE clusters to genetic lineages may be problematic (179).

The number of polymorphisms and the sequence of tandem repeat elements of the hypervariable X region of the *S. aureus* protein A (*spa*) gene are the basis of a single-locus sequence typing approach that has become one of the primary genotyping methods for MRSA surveillance (65, 170). Beside total reproducibility, other advantages include low costs, high throughput, a standardized nomenclature, and complete portability of data transferable into an international database (http://spaserver.ridom.de/) curated by SeqNet.org (http://www.seqnet.org/) (81). For particular genetic lineages, misclassification may occur, necessitating the use of additional tests for reliable inference.

Other molecular typing techniques used for typing of staphylococci include several other band-based molecular fingerprinting approaches, ribotyping, and more recently, multiple-locus variable-number tandem-repeat analysis and microarray-based approaches (110, 160, 185). Modern approaches based on phenotype structures applied for staphylococci include the matrix-assisted laser desorption ionization–time of flight/mass spectrometry and whole-cell fingerprinting techniques, such as the FT-IR spectroscopy (7).

While many typing systems have been developed and evaluated for *S. aureus*, fewer applications are available for CoNS. These include antibiotic resistance analysis, phage typing, slime production, and some modern genotyping procedures (PFGE and ribotyping) (69, 190).

For "micrococcal" species, phage typing and PFGE approaches applying phage sets and restriction enzymes, respectively, different from those used for staphylococci (132) have been described. A restriction fragment length polymorphism approach has been described for *Alloiococcus* (29).

SEROLOGIC TESTS

Because serological testing for antistaphylococcal antibodies lacks specificity and predictive accuracy, it plays no role for the diagnosis of most staphylococcal diseases. The one exception is the determination of protective antibodies in the case of toxin-mediated syndromes such as TSS and SSSS (see above). For the other microorganisms discussed in this chapter, detection of antibodies is not clinically useful.

ANTIMICROBIAL SUSCEPTIBILITIES

Staphylococcus and Related Genera

Genetic Basis and Prevalence of Antimicrobial Susceptibilities

Methicillin resistance mediated by the *mecA* gene has the greatest impact on patient management by excluding all traditional β-lactam antibiotics from the antibiotic armamentarium. Since the early 1980s, the prevalence of health care-associated MRSA (HA-MRSA) has increased in many regions. In some areas of the United States, the prevalence of MRSA is >50% (50, 101). In Europe, with the low-prevalence exception of The Netherlands and the Scandinavian countries, approximately 20% or more of *S. aureus* isolates are methicillin resistant (177). In Asia, Australia, and Africa, high MRSA rates (approximately 20 to 80%) have also been noted (158, 169, 212). The worldwide burden of infections caused by MRSA is increasing due to the advent of CA-MRSA in the past decade and, most recently, by livestock-associated *S. aureus* infections (85, 109). A number of studies and reviews describing antimicrobial and biocide susceptibilities of clinically important staphylococcal species have been published (51, 64, 87). Networks have also been established that provide online or published resistance data for staphylococci: the National Nosocomial Infections Surveillance System (http://www.cdc.gov/ncidod/dhqp/), the European Antimicrobial Resistance Surveillance System (http://www.rivm.nl/earss/), and the International Nosocomial Infection Control Consortium (http://www.inicc.org/).

The *mecA* gene is acquired by *S. aureus* and other staphylococcal species on a foreign, mobile DNA element (SCC*mec*) and encodes an additional penicillin-binding protein (PBP), PBP2a. Seven major variants of SCC*mec*, types I to VII, and many subtypes have been recognized (27, 44, 90, 91, 136). SCC*mec* types I, II, III, and VI are predominantly associated with HA-MRSA (47).

Multidrug resistance is regularly observed in HA-MRSA and usually includes resistance to aminoglycosides, fosfomycin, fusidic acid, glycopeptides, ketolides, lincosamides, macrolides, quinolones, rifampin, tetracyclines, and trimethoprim-sulfamethoxazole (51, 62, 87). There are rare reports of *S. aureus* and CoNS isolates resistant to new agents such as linezolid, daptomycin, and tigecycline (54, 143, 171). In contrast to HA-MRSA, CA-MRSA strains are more susceptible to non-β-lactam antibiotic classes and harbor different SCC*mec* (mostly types IVa, V, and VII) (13, 27, 44, 91). CA-MRSA isolates are more likely to carry PVL, a pore-forming toxin with potent cytolytic and inflammatory activities (72). Whereas in Europe an array of diverse CA-MRSA clones (mainly the "European" ST-80, *spa* type t044) have been reported, the PFGE type USA300 (ST-8, *spa* types t008 and t024) predominates in the United States followed by USA400 (47, 101). Populations at increased risk for CA-MRSA infections include children in day care centers, athletes, military recruits, jailed inmates, and men who have sex with men (52, 97, 138). CA-MRSA causes superficial skin and soft tissue infections and can also be associated with necrotizing fasciitis and myositis, necrotizing pneumonia, and other severe entities (115). Infections by PVL-positive *S. aureus* in young, otherwise healthy children following a respiratory viral infection (most frequently influenza) can be a devastating disease (72). However, some of the distinctions between HA-MRSA and CA-MRSA strains may disappear since CA-MRSA is now becoming endemic in hospitals and acquiring additional resistances (52, 162, 168).

Since 1996, vancomycin-intermediate *S. aureus* (VISA) isolates (MIC of 4 to 8 µg/ml) (39) and their putative precursors, termed heterogeneous VISA (hVISA) strains, have been identified first in Japan followed by detection in the United States and other regions (33, 86, 154). Reduced susceptibility is thought to be caused by cell wall alterations resulting in reorganization and thickening (30, 42). In 2002, the first of multiple vancomycin-resistant *S. aureus* (VRSA) strains containing the *vanA* gene were reported in the United States (34). *S. aureus* isolates currently defined as vancomycin-resistant exhibit MICs of ≥16 µg/ml (39). Since most VISAs are also resistant to teicoplanin, the acronym GISA (glycopeptide-intermediate *S. aureus*) is preferred by some authors. A few clinical isolates that are resistant to teicoplanin but fully susceptible to vancomycin have been reported (57).

More than 90% of all of nosocomial CoNS (mainly *S. epidermidis* and *S. haemolyticus*) are resistant to penicillin due to β-lactamase production, and approximately 60 to 80% are resistant to methicillin and other agents (51, 93, 121). Rare acquisition of *mecA*-encoded methicillin-resistance in *S. intermedius*/*S. pseudintermedius* has been reported (15).

Determination of Antimicrobial Susceptibilities

Antimicrobial susceptibility testing of staphylococci may be performed conventionally by Clinical and Laboratory Standards Institute (CLSI) reference methods (38) or commercial systems as described in chapters 67 to 70 of this *Manual*. Direct detection of MRSA is discussed in "Direct Examination" above. For SCVs, no approved method has been developed to determine the susceptibility (146, 192).

Detection of MRSA represents the most important task in determining the antimicrobial susceptibilities of staphylococci. To distinguish MRSA from MSSA, traditional methods may have reduced sensitivity and specificity due to heteroresistance and borderline oxacillin-resistant *S. aureus* characterized by β-lactamase hyperproduction. In the case of heterogeneous PBP2a expression, only a small fraction of the bacterial cell population (10^{-8} to 10^{-4}) expresses the resistance phenotype under in vitro test conditions. The resistant subpopulation may be overlooked because it usually grows more slowly than the susceptible population. The successful detection of heteroresistant strains is favored by cooler incubation temperatures (30 to 35°C), the presence of NaCl (2 to 4%), and prolonged incubation time (up to 48 h). Cefoxitin (30 µg) disk diffusion tests correlate better with the presence of *mecA* than do the oxacillin disks used previously. The cefoxitin disk diffusion method may be used for testing *S. aureus* and *S. lugdunensis* (resistance is indicated by a zone diameter of ≤21 mm) as well as other CoNS (resistance, ≤24 mm) for *mecA*-mediated resistance (60, 172). For broth microdilution testing, oxacillin or cefoxitin may be used to detect *mecA*-mediated resistance in *S. aureus* and *S. lugdunensis* (resistance: cefoxitin, MIC ≥ 8 µg/ml; oxacillin, MIC ≥ 4 µg/ml). For other CoNS isolates, the presence of *mecA* is predicted by applying lower oxacillin MIC breakpoints (resistance: oxacillin, MIC ≥ 0.5 μg/ml). Cefoxitin has also improved the detection of MRSA by automated susceptibility testing systems (157). The slow growth rate of SCVs prevents the use of disk diffusion and automated methods to determine the susceptibility of these strains (147).

An alternative method for detection of methicillin resistance is the use of anti-PBP2a monoclonal antibodies available as a latex agglutination assay that may be performed on isolated colonies from a pure culture (MRSA Screen; Denka Seiken, Tokyo, Japan) (134). If the latex test is used for SCVs, then the number of colonies must be increased 100-fold (100).

For heterogeneous methicillin-resistant staphylococci, strains displaying growth-impaired phenotype (SCVs) or borderline oxacillin-resistant *S. aureus* strains, the methicillin resistance of cultivated staphylococcal isolates may be determined by detection of the *mecA* gene (131). For the genetic verification of MRSA isolates, the occurrence of both the *mecA* gene and a species-specific marker (see above) has to be proven. The use of pure colony material is a vital premise for this approach.

For MRSA screening to detect colonization (preferentially nasal, also pharyngeal), selective media (e.g., mannitol salt agar) supplemented with oxacillin are widely used. Inclusion of a broth enrichment step prior to plating enhances sensitivity but delays results. Media containing chromogenic enzyme substrates (e.g., MRSA ID [bioMérieux]; BBL CHROMagar MRSA [BD]; and Brilliance MRSA agar [Oxoid]) have better specificity; however, confirmation of MRSA with a coagulase test is recommended for some products (36, 49, 140).

Detection of VISA is unreliable and probably underreported by routine susceptibility testing methods, including automated methods (9). According to current CLSI recommendations, *S. aureus* isolates with vancomycin MICs of 4 to 8 μg/ml are classified as VISA (39). These vancomycin MIC breakpoints were lowered for *S. aureus* (the intermediate category remained defined as 8 to 16 μg/ml for CoNS) in order to better detect hVISA strains that are potentially associated with vancomycin clinical failure (35, 184). Detection of hVISA requires a "modified population analysis profile–area under the curve" method or a macroEtest method (201, 207). Recently, FT-IR spectroscopy has been successfully applied for rapid and accurate identification of VISA and hVISA among isolates of MRSA (5). VRSA strains (MIC, ≥16 μg/ml) are reliably detected by the broth microdilution reference method, most FDA-cleared automated systems, or a brain heart infusion vancomycin (6 μg/ml) agar screen plate (39). In 2009, the European Union Committee on Antimicrobial Susceptibility Testing reduced the glycopeptide MIC breakpoints (resistance: vancomycin, >2 μg/ml for *S. aureus* and CoNS; teicoplanin, >2 μg/ml for *S. aureus* and >4 μg/ml for CoNS) to avoid reporting VISA isolates as "intermediate" (http://www.srga .org/eucastwt/MICTAB/MICglycopeptides_v2.html).

Additional information on the determination of antimicrobial susceptibilities is contained in chapters 67 to 70 of this *Manual*. There are no CLSI methods for susceptibility testing of "micrococci" and alloiococci.

Treatment

For additional and annually updated information regarding treatment, the reader should consult the current edition of *The Sanford Guide to Antimicrobial Therapy* (71) or other guidelines. Effective treatment of focal infections such as empyema and abscesses requires incision and drainage. Penicillin G is the most effective compound for the treatment of the uncommon penicillin-susceptible *S. aureus* strain. In general, penicillin-resistant, oxacillin-susceptible staphylococcal strains should be treated with penicillinase-stable penicillins, β-lactam/β-lactamase inhibitor combinations, and cephalosporins (151). For patients with penicillin allergy or chronic renal failure, clindamycin or vancomycin may be an option in the case of MSSA. However, the use of vancomycin, known to be poorly bactericidal against staphylococci, is not recommended for severe infections due to MSSA as it is inferior to β-lactams in terms of mortality and bacteriological outcome.

Strains that are oxacillin- or cefoxitin-resistant (MRSA) should be considered resistant to all β-lactams including penicillins, carbapenems, and cephalosporins (except for the new "fifth-generation" cephalosporins [ceftobiprole and ceftaroline] with anti-MRSA activity) (77). Vancomycin and the newer agents such as linezolid, daptomycin, dalbavancin, and tigecycline are suitable options for empiric therapy of MRSA infections (note the different spectra and the approved indications of these compounds) (63, 161, 208). Occasionally, trimethoprim-sulfamethoxazole (SXT) may be helpful, but it should be used with caution (145). In particular in terms of "collateral damage," quinolones should be avoided for the therapy of staphylococcal infections (139).

While there are only a few, partly uncorroborated studies and case reports available supporting combination therapy for treatment of severe staphylococcal infections, aminoglycosides, rifampin, fosfomycin, co-trimoxazole, and fusidic acid in combination with glycopeptides and β-lactams have been recommended (70). A careful risk-benefit assessment concerning drug-drug interactions and side effects should be performed. Since resistance towards rifampin, fusidic acid, and fosfomycin develops rapidly, these compounds must not be administered alone.

Since the majority of clinically recovered CoNS strains are methicillin resistant, most infections by CoNS require treatment with vancomycin or, where appropriate, the new agents described above. Replacement of these by β-lactamase-resistant penicillins is advisable for methicillin-susceptible isolates. When used simultaneously, antibiotics with cell wall activity (β-lactams and vancomycin) combined with rifampin were shown to act synergistically; however, this combination is not recommended for catheter-related bloodstream infections (125). FBRIs remain a therapeutic challenge and frequently require removal of the device (125, 198).

Prospective studies on the most appropriate treatment for patients infected with staphylococcal SCVs are unavailable. A reduced susceptibility to aminoglycosides can be expected (16). Resistance to trimethoprim-sulfamethoxazole is observed in thymidine-auxotrophic SCVs (96). Due to the fact that SCVs may persist intracellularly, a combined treatment regimen of rifampin (intracellular activity) with either β-lactam antibiotics or vancomycin (for methicillin-resistant SCVs) may be effective.

Micrococcaceae and *Dermacoccaceae*

Systematic data on susceptibilities of the two families *Micrococcaceae* and *Dermacoccaceae* are rare, and the real species affiliation in older reports is often unclear. Members of the genera *Micrococcus* and *Kocuria* appear to be susceptible to β-lactams, macrolides, tetracycline, linezolid, rifampin, and the glycopeptides; however, clinical isolates resistant to these agents have been reported (25, 95, 197).

While most kytococcal isolates have been susceptible to carbapenems, gentamicin, ciprofloxacin, tetracycline, rifampin, and glycopeptides, kytococci are usually resistant to penicillin G, cephalosporins, and oxacillin (not *mecA*-based) (25, 95, 174). An antibiotic regimen that has been suggested for the treatment of infection by members of both families is a combination of vancomycin with rifampin and gentamicin (199). *R. mucilaginosa* appears to be variable in its antimicrobial susceptibility (197, 200). The observation that *R. mucilaginosa* exhibits poor to no growth on Mueller-Hinton agar makes susceptibility testing a challenge for clinical laboratories. A supplementation with 5% sheep blood and incubation in 6% CO_2 may enhance susceptibility testing (197, 200).

Alloiococcus

A. otitis has been reported as susceptible to ampicillin, cefotaxime, tetracycline, and vancomycin but resistant to macrolides, azithromycin, and co-trimoxazole (10, 29, 46). In addition to gentamicin-resistant isolates, some *A. otitis* isolates with intermediate levels of resistance to β-lactams have been reported, although they are β-lactamase negative.

EVALUATION, INTERPRETATION, AND REPORTING OF RESULTS

Distinguishing contaminants and colonizers from staphylococcal and "micrococcal" isolates causing infection continues to be an important challenge for laboratorians and clinicians. It is imperative to have an appreciation of the quality of the specimen under consideration. Clinical features and the results of other investigations should be taken into account during the interpretative process. There is no replacement for good communication between laboratory staff and primary physicians.

Cultivation and identification of the causative pathogen to the species level represent the "gold standard" for the diagnosis of staphylococcal infections. The most critical step when interpreting a culture that is suspect for staphylococci is to distinguish between *S. aureus* and other species. Due to the importance of the report of "*S. aureus*" and, in particular, of "MRSA" for prognosis, therapy, hospital hygiene, and infection control, any uncertainty regarding the species identification or the susceptibility to oxacillin (cefoxitin) should be investigated via a second independent method. Considering costs and rapidity, applicable routine proceedings may comprise the use of respective latex agglutination assays combined with the use of automated systems for identification and susceptibility testing. In case of doubt, further tests, preferentially nucleic acid-based approaches, should be applied. However, the need for additional procedures must be weighed against delay in informing the physician concerning a preliminary *S. aureus* identification as the putative causative agent.

Species-level identification of CoNS associated with infection should be considered, though it is still a matter for debate because species-level identification of CoNS rarely leads to an intervention or to changes in therapy. To rule out *S. saprophyticus* for urine isolates, the novobiocin test could be used. Isolates from deep-tissue infections and blood cultures of patients with suspected endocarditis should be differentiated to the species level, since the identification of *S. lugdunensis* raises the index of suspicion for aggressive disease. To rule out *S. lugdunensis* for invasive and sterile-site isolates, its positivity for pyrrolidonase and ornithine decarboxylase could be considered (Tables 2 and 3). Other CoNS have also been increasingly described as causative

pathogens of severe infection. Ribotyping and/or PFGE should be used when determination of genetic relatedness is required. Contaminants and colonizing CoNS do not require susceptibility testing or identification. Several reports suggest that cultures of colonially indistinguishable CoNS may contain multiple different strains (67). Extending the incubation period of the initial cultures to 72 h may enable different colony types to be more readily identified.

Unless there is strong evidence to the contrary, isolation of *S. aureus* from a sterile-site culture (such as aspirated pus, blood, or cerebrospinal fluid) should be considered clinically significant. Contamination of high-quality samples by *S. aureus* is rare, and further samples should be taken if there is clinical doubt. Interpreting the isolation of *S. aureus* from specimens contaminated with elements of a normal microbiota requires consideration of setting, clinical features, and recent interventions. Quantitative culture may be helpful, for example, when interpreting a bronchoalveolar lavage or urine sample. In persons with *S. aureus* endocarditis, bacteremia is continuous and associated with higher loads, while in cases with transient bacteremia (e.g., manipulations with mucous membrane trauma) bacteremia is associated with lower loads and typically has a short duration. Because quantitative blood cultures are not routinely performed, the time between incubation onset and growth detection (defined as the time to positivity) may provide additional information in continuous blood culture-monitoring systems. Rapid growth of *S. aureus* (within 14 h after the initiation of incubation) has been associated with a high likelihood of endovascular infection, delayed clearance, and complications (98). Isolation of *S. aureus* from surgical wounds and other sites such as ulcers may represent infection or colonization, and the clinician's response to the culture report should be guided by a bedside assessment of signs and symptoms of infection. Colonization alone is an insufficient reason to treat, unless the patient is colonized by MRSA and decolonization is undertaken as part of a specific infection control policy.

Compared to *S. aureus*, interpreting the significance of cultures that are positive for CoNS is more challenging. CoNS are an important cause of nosocomial bloodstream infections, but they are also the most common contaminants of blood cultures (79). It is obvious that samples taken from colonized sites will contain members of these species. Blood samples or biopsy specimens taken without careful skin cleaning and disinfection will become contaminated with the microbiota of the skin or mucous membranes. However, even careful attention to collection techniques will not prevent all episodes of contamination. Interpretation of blood cultures positive for CoNS requires knowledge of the presence of prosthetic material in the intravascular compartment, risk factors for true CoNS sepsis such as prematurity or the presence of an impaired immune system, and clinical features of sepsis. Factors helpful in distinguishing between true positive and contaminated cultures taken from a patient with clinical features of infection include (i) isolation of a strain in pure culture from the infected site or body fluid and (ii) the repeated isolation of the same strain or combination of strains over the course of the infection (103, 186). An algorithm to reduce misclassification of nosocomial bloodstream infections due to CoNS was defined as at least two blood cultures positive for CoNS within 5 days or one positive blood culture plus clinical evidence of infection (26).

The presence of the same CoNS strain on an intravenous catheter tip and in a blood culture is supportive evidence for intravascular catheter-associated bacteremia. Measurement of differential time to positivity between blood cultures drawn through the central venous catheter and those drawn from the peripheral vein was reported as highly sensitive and specific for the in situ diagnosis of catheter-related bloodstream infection in patients with short- and long-term catheters; however, other studies did not show that this method was of major diagnostic value (149, 153, 165). Isolation of CoNS from peritoneal dialysis fluid or cerebrospinal fluid taken from ventricular shunts in a patient suspected of having infection is usually significant. While most contaminated clinical specimens produce mixed cultures of different strains and/or species, some infections may be attributable to more than one strain or species (67).

For patients with complicated cases, who probably have a true CoNS infection, it is advisable to develop a sampling strategy. This is particularly pertinent when dealing with patients with low-grade infection associated with implanted prosthetic material such as a joint replacement or vascular graft. Samples should include those from each anatomical layer or region, and fresh instruments should be used to gather deep-site samples (11).

Susceptibility testing, and in particular the detection of methicillin resistance, should always be carried out following the identification of *S. aureus*. For surveillance cultures to detect MRSA colonization, susceptibility testing beyond the determination of methicillin resistance may only be needed for patients undergoing decolonization to predict the success of mupirocin therapy. All CoNS associated with true infection require susceptibility testing.

The considerations of clinical significance discussed for CoNS are also appropriate for members of the *Micrococcaceae* and *Dermacoccaceae* families; however, the criteria used for distinguishing etiologically relevant isolates from contaminants and colonizers, respectively, should be applied much more strictly. Since species of the *Kytococcus* genus are resistant to some β-lactams, they should be (if clinically relevant) carefully distinguished from other "micrococci" that are usually susceptible.

REFERENCES

1. Aguirre, M., and M. D. Collins. 1992. Development of a polymerase chain reaction-probe test for identification of *Alloiococcus otitis*. *J. Clin. Microbiol.* **30**:2177–2180.
2. Albrich, W. C., and S. Harbarth. 2008. Health-care workers: source, vector, or victim of MRSA? *Lancet Infect. Dis.* **8**:289–301.
3. Altuntas, F., O. Yildiz, B. Eser, K. Gundogan, B. Sumerkan, and M. Cetin. 2004. Catheter-related bacteremia due to *Kocuria rosea* in a patient undergoing peripheral blood stem cell transplantation. *BMC Infect. Dis.* **4**:62.
4. Alves, M., C. Nogueira, A. de Magalhães-Sant'Ana, A. P. Chung, P. V. Morais, and M. S. da Costa. 2008. *Nosocomiicoccus ampullae* gen. nov., sp. nov., isolated from the surface of bottles of saline solution used in wound cleansing. *Int. J. Syst. Evol. Microbiol.* **58**:2939–2944.
5. Amiali, N. M., M. R. Mulvey, B. Berger-Bächi, J. Sedman, A. E. Simor, and A. A. Ismail. 2008. Evaluation of Fourier transform infrared spectroscopy for the rapid identification of glycopeptide-intermediate *Staphylococcus aureus*. *J. Antimicrob. Chemother.* **61**:95–102.
6. Amiali, N. M., M. R. Mulvey, J. Sedman, M. Louie, A. E. Simor, and A. A. Ismail. 2007. Rapid identification of coagulase-negative staphylococci by Fourier transform infrared spectroscopy. *J. Microbiol. Methods* **68**:236–242.
7. Amiali, N. M., M. R. Mulvey, J. Sedman, A. E. Simor, and A. A. Ismail. 2007. Epidemiological typing of methicillin-resistant *Staphylococcus aureus* strains by Fourier transform infrared spectroscopy. *J. Microbiol. Methods* **69**:146–153.
8. Anguera, I., A. Del Río, J. M. Miró, X. Matínez-Lacasa, F. Marco, J. R. Gumá, G. Quaglio, X. Claramonte, A. Moreno, C. A. Mestres, M. Azqueta, N. Benito, C. García-de la Maria, M. Almela, M. J. Jiménez-Expósito, O. Sued, E. De Lazzari, and J. M. Gatell. 2005. *Staphylococcus lugdunensis* infective endocarditis: description of 10 cases and analysis of native valve, prosthetic valve, and pacemaker lead endocarditis clinical profiles. *Heart* **91**:e10.
9. Appelbaum, P. C. 2007. Reduced glycopeptide susceptibility in methicillin-resistant *Staphylococcus aureus* (MRSA). *Int. J. Antimicrob. Agents* **30**:398–408.
10. Ashhurst-Smith, C., S. T. Hall, P. Walker, J. Stuart, P. M. Hansbro, and C. C. Blackwell. 2007. Isolation of *Alloiococcus otitidis* from Indigenous and non-Indigenous Australian children with chronic otitis media with effusion. *FEMS Immunol. Med. Microbiol.* **51**:163–170.
11. Atkins, B. L., N. Athanasou, J. J. Deeks, D. W. Crook, H. Simpson, T. E. Peto, P. McLardy-Smith, A. R. Berendt, et al. 1998. Prospective evaluation of criteria for microbiological diagnosis of prosthetic-joint infection at revision arthroplasty. *J. Clin. Microbiol.* **36**:2932–2939.
12. Baba, T., K. Kuwahara-Arai, I. Uchiyama, F. Takeuchi, T. Ito, and K. Hiramatsu. 2009. Complete genome sequence of *Macrococcus caseolyticus* strain JCSCS5402, reflecting the ancestral genome of the human-pathogenic staphylococci. *J. Bacteriol.* **191**:1180–1190.
13. Baba, T., F. Takeuchi, M. Kuroda, H. Yuzawa, K. Aoki, A. Oguchi, Y. Nagai, N. Iwama, K. Asano, T. Naimi, H. Kuroda, L. Cui, K. Yamamoto, and K. Hiramatsu. 2002. Genome and virulence determinants of high virulence community-acquired MRSA. *Lancet* **359**:1819–1827.
14. Baird-Parker, A. C. 1963. A classification of micrococci and staphylococci based on physiological and chemical tests. *J. Gen. Microbiol.* **30**:409–427.
15. Bannoehr, J., N. L. Ben Zakour, A. S. Waller, L. Guardabassi, K. L. Thoday, A. H. van den Broek, and J. R. Fitzgerald. 2007. Population genetic structure of the *Staphylococcus intermedius* group: insights into *agr* diversification and the emergence of methicillin-resistant strains. *J. Bacteriol.* **189**:8685–8692.
16. Baumert, N., C. von Eiff, F. Schaaff, G. Peters, R. A. Proctor, and H. G. Sahl. 2002. Physiology and antibiotic susceptibility of *Staphylococcus aureus* small colony variants. *Microb. Drug Resist.* **8**:253–260.
17. Becker, K., A. W. Friedrich, G. Lubritz, M. Weilert, G. Peters, and C. von Eiff. 2003. Prevalence of genes encoding pyrogenic toxin superantigens and exfoliative toxins among strains of *Staphylococcus aureus* isolated from blood and nasal specimens. *J. Clin. Microbiol.* **41**:1434–1439.
18. Becker, K., D. Harmsen, A. Mellmann, C. Meier, P. Schumann, G. Peters, and C. von Eiff. 2004. Development and evaluation of a quality-controlled ribosomal sequence database for 16S ribosomal DNA-based identification of *Staphylococcus* species. *J. Clin. Microbiol.* **42**:4988–4995.
19. Becker, K., B. Keller, C. von Eiff, M. Brück, G. Lubritz, J. Etienne, and G. Peters. 2001. Enterotoxigenic potential of *Staphylococcus intermedius*. *Appl. Environ. Microbiol.* **67**:5551–5557.
20. Becker, K., N. A. Laham, W. Fegeler, R. A. Proctor, G. Peters, and C. von Eiff. 2006. Fourier-transform infrared spectroscopic analysis is a powerful tool for studying the dynamic changes in *Staphylococcus aureus* small-colony variants. *J. Clin. Microbiol.* **44**:3274–3278.
21. Becker, K., I. Pagnier, B. Schuhen, F. Wenzelburger, A. W. Friedrich, F. Kipp, G. Peters, and C. von Eiff. 2006. Does nasal cocolonization by methicillin-resistant coagulase-negative staphylococci and methicillin-susceptible *Staphylococcus aureus* strains occur frequently enough to represent a risk of false-positive methicillin-resistant *S. aureus* determinations by molecular methods? *J. Clin. Microbiol.* **44**:229–231.
22. Becker, K., R. Roth, and G. Peters. 1998. Rapid and specific detection of toxigenic *Staphylococcus aureus*: use of two multiplex PCR enzyme immunoassays for amplification and hybridization of staphylococcal enterotoxin genes, exfoliative toxin genes, and toxic shock syndrome toxin 1 gene. *J. Clin. Microbiol.* **36**:2548–2553.

23. **Becker, K., F. Rutsch, A. Uekötter, F. Kipp, J. König, T. Marquardt, G. Peters, and C. von Eiff.** 2008. *Kocuria rhizophila* adds to the emerging spectrum of micrococcal species involved in human infections. *J. Clin. Microbiol.* **46:**3537–3539.

24. **Becker, K., C. von Eiff, B. Keller, M. Brück, J. Etienne, and G. Peters.** 2005. Thermonuclease gene as a target for specific identification of *Staphylococcus intermedius* isolates: use of a PCR-DNA enzyme immunoassay. *Diagn. Microbiol. Infect. Dis.* **51:**237–244.

25. **Becker, K., J. Wüllenweber, H. J. Odenthal, M. Moeller, P. Schumann, G. Peters, and C. von Eiff.** 2003. Prosthetic valve endocarditis due to *Kytococcus schroeteri. Emerg. Infect. Dis.* **9:**1493–1495.

26. **Beekmann, S. E., D. J. Diekema, and G. V. Doern.** 2005. Determining the clinical significance of coagulase-negative staphylococci isolated from blood cultures. *Infect. Control Hosp. Epidemiol.* **26:**559–566.

27. **Berglund, C., T. Ito, M. Ikeda, X. X. Ma, B. Söderquist, and K. Hiramatsu.** 2008. Novel type of staphylococcal cassette chromosome *mec* in a methicillin-resistant *Staphylococcus aureus* strain isolated in Sweden. *Antimicrob. Agents Chemother.* **52:**3512–3516.

28. **Bieber, L., and G. Kahlmeter.** 2009. *Staphylococcus lugdunensis* in several niches of the normal skin flora. *Clin. Microbiol. Infect.* **16:**385–388.

29. **Bosley, G. S., A. M. Whitney, J. M. Pruckler, C. W. Moss, M. Daneshvar, T. Sih, and D. F. Talkington.** 1995. Characterization of ear fluid isolates of *Alloiococcus otitidis* from patients with recurrent otitis media. *J. Clin. Microbiol.* **33:**2876–2880.

30. **Boyle-Vavra, S., H. Labischinski, C. C. Ebert, K. Ehlert, and R. S. Daum.** 2001. A spectrum of changes occurs in peptidoglycan composition of glycopeptide-intermediate clinical *Staphylococcus aureus* isolates. *Antimicrob. Agents Chemother.* **45:**280–287.

31. **Brakstad, O. G., K. Aasbakk, and J. A. Maeland.** 1992. Detection of *Staphylococcus aureus* by polymerase chain reaction amplification of the *nuc* gene. *J. Clin. Microbiol.* **30:**1654–1660.

32. **Carbonnelle, E., J. L. Beretti, S. Cottyn, G. Quesne, P. Berche, X. Nassif, and A. Ferroni.** 2007. Rapid identification of staphylococci isolated in clinical microbiology laboratories by matrix-assisted laser desorption ionization-time of flight mass spectrometry. *J. Clin. Microbiol.* **45:**2156–2161.

33. **Centers for Disease Control and Prevention.** 1997. *Staphylococcus aureus* with reduced susceptibility to vancomycin—United States, 1997. *MMWR Morb. Mortal. Wkly. Rep.* **46:**765–766.

34. **Centers for Disease Control and Prevention.** 2002. *Staphylococcus aureus* resistant to vancomycin—United States, 2002. *MMWR Morb. Mortal. Wkly. Rep.* **51:**565–567.

35. **Charles, P. G., P. B. Ward, P. D. Johnson, B. P. Howden, and M. L. Grayson.** 2004. Clinical features associated with bacteremia due to heterogeneous vancomycin-intermediate *Staphylococcus aureus. Clin. Infect. Dis.* **38:**448–451.

36. **Cherkaoui, A., G. Renzi, P. Francois, and J. Schrenzel.** 2007. Comparison of four chromogenic media for culture-based screening of meticillin-resistant *Staphylococcus aureus. J. Med. Microbiol.* **56:**500–503.

37. **Chow, J. W., and V. L. Yu.** 1989. *Staphylococcus aureus* nasal carriage in hemodialysis patients. Its role in infection and approaches to prophylaxis. *Arch. Intern. Med.* **149:**1258–1262.

38. **Clinical and Laboratory Standards Institute.** 2009. *Methods for Dilution Antimicrobial Susceptibility Testing for Bacteria That Grow Aerobically; Approved Standard—Eighth ed.* CLSI document M07-A8. Clinical and Laboratory Standards Institute, Wayne, PA.

39. **Clinical and Laboratory Standards Institute.** 2010. *Performance Standards for Antimicrobial Susceptibility Testing; Twentieth Informational Supplement.* CLSI document M100-S20. Clinical and Laboratory Standards Institute, Wayne, PA.

40. **Collins, M. D., R. A. Hutson, V. Baverud, and E. Falsen.** 2000. Characterization of a *Rothia*-like organism from a mouse: description of *Rothia nasimurium* sp. nov. and reclassification of *Stomatococcus mucilaginosus* as *Rothia mucilaginosa* comb. nov. *Int. J. Syst. Evol. Microbiol.* **50:**1247–1251.

41. **Couto, I., S. Pereira, M. Miragaia, I. S. Sanches, and H. de Lencastre.** 2001. Identification of clinical staphylococcal isolates from humans by internal transcribed spacer PCR. *J. Clin. Microbiol.* **39:**3099–3103.

42. **Cui, L., X. Ma, K. Sato, K. Okuma, F. C. Tenover, E. M. Mamizuka, C. G. Gemmell, M. N. Kim, M. C. Ploy, N. El-Solh, V. Ferraz, and K. Hiramatsu.** 2003. Cell wall thickening is a common feature of vancomycin resistance in *Staphylococcus aureus. J. Clin. Microbiol.* **41:**5–14.

43. **Curtis, C., and N. Shetty.** 2008. Recent trends and prevention of infection in the neonatal intensive care unit. *Curr. Opin. Infect. Dis.* **21:**350–356.

44. **Daum, R. S., T. Ito, K. Hiramatsu, F. Hussain, K. Mongkolrattanothai, M. Jamklang, and S. Boyle-Vavra.** 2002. A novel methicillin-resistance cassette in community-acquired methicillin-resistant *Staphylococcus aureus* isolates of diverse genetic backgrounds. *J. Infect. Dis.* **186:**1344–1347.

45. **de la Fuente, R., G. Suarez, and K. H. Schleifer.** 1985. *Staphylococcus aureus* subsp. *anaerobius* subsp. nov., the causal agent of abscess disease of sheep. *Int. J. Syst. Bacteriol.* **35:**99–102.

46. **de Miguel Martínez, I., and A. R. Macías.** 2008. Serous otitis media in children: implication of *Alloiococcus otitidis. Otol. Neurotol.* **29:**526–530.

47. **Deurenberg, R. H., and E. E. Stobberingh.** 2009. The molecular evolution of hospital- and community-associated methicillin-resistant *Staphylococcus aureus. Curr. Mol. Med.* **9:**100–115.

48. **Devriese, L. A., M. Vancanneyt, M. Baele, M. Vaneechoutte, E. De Graef, C. Snauwaert, I. Cleenwerck, P. Dawyndt, J. Swings, A. Decostere, and F. Haesebrouck.** 2005. *Staphylococcus pseudintermedius* sp. nov., a coagulase-positive species from animals. *Int. J. Syst. Evol. Microbiol.* **55:**1569–1573.

49. **Diederen, B., I. van Duijn, A. van Belkum, P. Willemse, P. Van Keulen, and J. Kluytmans.** 2005. Performance of CHROMagar MRSA medium for detection of methicillin-resistant *Staphylococcus aureus. J. Clin. Microbiol.* **43:**1925–1927.

50. **Diekema, D. J., B. J. BootsMiller, T. E. Vaughn, R. F. Woolson, J. W. Yankey, E. J. Ernst, S. D. Flach, M. M. Ward, C. L. Franciscus, M. A. Pfaller, and B. N. Doebbeling.** 2004. Antimicrobial resistance trends and outbreak frequency in United States hospitals. *Clin. Infect. Dis.* **38:**78–85.

51. **Diekema, D. J., M. A. Pfaller, F. J. Schmitz, J. Smayevsky, J. Bell, R. N. Jones, and M. Beach.** 2001. Survey of infections due to *Staphylococcus* species: frequency of occurrence and antimicrobial susceptibility of isolates collected in the United States, Canada, Latin America, Europe, and the Western Pacific region for the SENTRY Antimicrobial Surveillance Program, 1997–1999. *Clin. Infect. Dis.* **32**(Suppl. 2):S114–S132.

52. **Diep, B. A., H. F. Chambers, C. J. Graber, J. D. Szumowski, L. G. Miller, L. L. Han, J. H. Chen, F. Lin, J. Lin, T. H. Phan, H. A. Carleton, L. K. McDougal, F. C. Tenover, D. E. Cohen, K. H. Mayer, G. F. Sensabaugh, and F. Perdreau-Remington.** 2008. Emergence of multidrug-resistant, community-associated, methicillin-resistant *Staphylococcus aureus* clone USA300 in men who have sex with men. *Ann. Intern. Med.* **148:**249–257.

53. **Donnio, P. Y., D. C. Oliveira, N. A. Faria, N. Wilhelm, A. Le Coustumier, and H. de Lencastre.** 2005. Partial excision of the chromosomal cassette containing the methicillin resistance determinant results in methicillin-susceptible *Staphylococcus aureus. J. Clin. Microbiol.* **43:**4191–4193.

54. **Draghi, D. C., S. Tench, M. J. Dowzicky, and D. F. Sahm.** 2008. Baseline in vitro activity of tigecycline among key bacterial pathogens exhibiting multidrug resistance. *Chemotherapy* **54:**91–100.

55. **Edwards, K. J., M. E. Kaufmann, and N. A. Saunders.** 2001. Rapid and accurate identification of coagulase-negative staphylococci by real-time PCR. *J. Clin. Microbiol.* **39:**3047–3051.

56. **Eigner, U., A. Schmid, U. Wild, D. Bertsch, and A. M. Fahr.** 2005. Analysis of the comparative workflow and performance characteristics of the VITEK 2 and Phoenix systems. *J. Clin. Microbiol.* **43:**3829–3834.

57. el Solh, N., M. Davi, A. Morvan, H. A. Damon, and N. Marty. 2003. Characteristics of French methicillin-resistant *Staphylococcus aureus* isolates with decreased susceptibility or resistance to glycopeptides. *J. Antimicrob. Chemother.* **52:**691–694.

58. Enright, M. C., N. P. Day, C. E. Davies, S. J. Peacock, and B. G. Spratt. 2000. Multilocus sequence typing for characterization of methicillin-resistant and methicillin-susceptible clones of *Staphylococcus aureus. J. Clin. Microbiol.* **38:**1008–1015.

59. Faller, A., and K. H. Schleifer. 1981. Modified oxidase and benzidine tests for separation of staphylococci from micrococci. *J. Clin. Microbiol.* **13:**1031–1035.

60. Felten, A., B. Grandry, P. H. Lagrange, and I. Casin. 2002. Evaluation of three techniques for detection of low-level methicillin-resistant *Staphylococcus aureus* (MRSA): a disk diffusion method with cefoxitin and moxalactam, the Vitek 2 system, and the MRSA-screen latex agglutination test. *J. Clin. Microbiol.* **40:**2766–2771.

61. Fischer, A., C. von Eiff, T. Kuczius, K. Omoe, G. Peters, and K. Becker. 2007. A quantitative real-time immuno-PCR approach for detection of staphylococcal enterotoxins. *J. Mol. Med.* **85:**461–469.

62. Fluit, A. C., C. L. Wielders, J. Verhoef, and F. J. Schmitz. 2001. Epidemiology and susceptibility of 3,051 *Staphylococcus aureus* isolates from 25 university hospitals participating in the European SENTRY study. *J. Clin. Microbiol.* **39:**3727–3732.

63. Fowler, V. G., Jr., H. W. Boucher, G. R. Corey, E. Abrutyn, A. W. Karchmer, M. E. Rupp, D. P. Levine, H. F. Chambers, F. P. Tally, G. A. Vigliani, C. H. Cabell, A. S. Link, I. DeMeyer, S. G. Filler, M. Zervos, P. Cook, J. Parsonnet, J. M. Bernstein, C. S. Price, G. N. Forrest, G. Fätkenheuer, M. Gareca, S. J. Rehm, H. R. Brodt, A. Tice, and S. E. Cosgrove. 2006. Daptomycin versus standard therapy for bacteremia and endocarditis caused by *Staphylococcus aureus. N. Engl. J. Med.* **355:**653–665.

64. Fraise, A. P. 2002. Susceptibility of antibiotic-resistant cocci to biocides. *J. Appl. Microbiol.* **92**(Suppl.):158S–162S.

65. Frénay, H. M., A. E. Bunschoten, L. M. Schouls, W. J. van Leeuwen, G. C. Vandenbroucke, J. Verhoef, and F. R. Mooi. 1996. Molecular typing of methicillin-resistant *Staphylococcus aureus* on the basis of protein A gene polymorphism. *Eur. J. Clin. Microbiol. Infect. Dis.* **15:**60–64.

66. Frye, J. G., T. Jesse, F. Long, G. Rondeau, S. Porwollik, M. McClelland, C. R. Jackson, M. Englen, and P. J. Fedorka-Cray. 2006. DNA microarray detection of antimicrobial resistance genes in diverse bacteria. *Int. J. Antimicrob. Agents* **27:**138–151.

67. García de Viedma, D., P. Martín Rabadán, M. Díaz, E. Cercenado, and E. Bouza. 2000. Heterogeneous antimicrobial resistance patterns in polyclonal populations of coagulase-negative staphylococci isolated from catheters. *J. Clin. Microbiol.* **38:**1359–1363.

68. Garrity, G. M., K. L. Johnson, J. Bell, and D. B. Searles. 2004. *Taxonomic Outline of the Procaryotes. Bergey's Manual of Systematic Bacteriology*, 2nd ed., release 5.0. Springer-Verlag, New York, NY.

69. Geary, C., J. Z. Jordens, J. F. Richardson, D. M. Hawcroft, and C. J. Mitchell. 1997. Epidemiological typing of coagulase-negative staphylococci from nosocomial infections. *J. Med. Microbiol.* **46:**195–203.

70. Gemmell, C. G., D. I. Edwards, A. P. Fraise, F. K. Gould, G. L. Ridgway, and R. E. Warren. 2006. Guidelines for the prophylaxis and treatment of methicillin-resistant *Staphylococcus aureus* (MRSA) infections in the UK. *J. Antimicrob. Chemother.* **57:**589–608.

71. Gilbert, D. N., R. C. Moellering, Jr., G. M. Eliopoulos, H. F. Chambers, and M. S. Saag. 2009. *The Sanford Guide to Antimicrobial Therapy.* Antimicrobial Therapy, Sperryville, VA.

72. Gillet, Y., B. Issartel, P. Vanhems, J. C. Fournet, G. Lina, M. Bes, F. Vandenesch, Y. Piemont, N. Brousse, D. Floret, and J. Etienne. 2002. Association between *Staphylococcus aureus* strains carrying gene for Panton-Valentine leukocidin and highly lethal necrotising pneumonia in young immunocompetent patients. *Lancet* **359:**753–759.

73. Goh, S. H., S. Potter, J. O. Wood, S. M. Hemmingsen, R. P. Reynolds, and A. W. Chow. 1996. HSP60 gene sequences as universal targets for microbial species identification: studies with coagulase-negative staphylococci. *J. Clin. Microbiol.* **34:**818–823.

74. Goh, S. H., Z. Santucci, W. E. Kloos, M. Faltyn, C. G. George, D. Driedger, and S. M. Hemmingsen. 1997. Identification of *Staphylococcus* species and subspecies by the chaperonin 60 gene identification method and reverse checkerboard hybridization. *J. Clin. Microbiol.* **35:**3116–3121.

75. Goldman, M., U. B. Chaudhary, A. Greist, and C. A. Fausel. 1998. Central nervous system infections due to *Stomatococcus mucilaginosus* in immunocompromised hosts. *Clin. Infect. Dis.* **27:**1241–1246.

76. Granlund, M., M. Linderholm, M. Norgren, C. Olofsson, A. Wahlin, and S. E. Holm. 1996. *Stomatococcus mucilaginosus* septicemia in leukemic patients. *Clin. Microbiol. Infect.* **2:**179–185.

77. Guignard, B., J. M. Entenza, and P. Moreillon. 2005. Beta-lactams against methicillin-resistant *Staphylococcus aureus. Curr. Opin. Pharmacol.* **5:**479–489.

78. Hajjeh, R. A., A. Reingold, A. Weil, K. Shutt, A. Schuchat, and B. A. Perkins. 1999. Toxic shock syndrome in the United States: surveillance update, 1979–1996. *Emerg. Infect. Dis.* **5:**807–810.

79. Hall, K. K., and J. A. Lyman. 2006. Updated review of blood culture contamination. *Clin. Microbiol. Rev.* **19:**788–802.

80. Harimaya, A., N. Fujii, and T. Himi. 2009. Preliminary study of proinflammatory cytokines and chemokines in the middle ear of acute otitis media due to *Alloiococcus otitidis. Int. J. Pediatr. Otorhinolaryngol.* **73:**677–680.

81. Harmsen, D., H. Claus, W. Witte, J. Rothgänger, H. Claus, D. Turnwald, and U. Vogel. 2003. Typing of methicillin-resistant *Staphylococcus aureus* in a university hospital setting by using novel software for *spa* repeat determination and database management. *J. Clin. Microbiol.* **41:**5442–5448.

82. Hendolin, P. H., A. Markkanen, J. Ylikoski, and J. J. Wahlfors. 1997. Use of multiplex PCR for simultaneous detection of four bacterial species in middle ear effusions. *J. Clin. Microbiol.* **35:**2854–2858.

83. Hensley, D. M., R. Tapia, and Y. Encina. 2009. An evaluation of the advandx Staphylococcus aureus/CNS PNA FISH assay. *Clin. Lab. Sci.* **22:**30–33.

84. Hidron, A. I., J. R. Edwards, J. Patel, T. C. Horan, D. M. Sievert, D. A. Pollock, and S. K. Fridkin. 2008. NHSN annual update: antimicrobial-resistant pathogens associated with healthcare-associated infections: annual summary of data reported to the National Healthcare Safety Network at the Centers for Disease Control and Prevention, 2006–2007. *Infect. Control Hosp. Epidemiol.* **29:**996–1011.

85. Hidron, A. I., C. E. Low, E. G. Honig, and H. M. Blumberg. 2009. Emergence of community-acquired meticillin-resistant *Staphylococcus aureus* strain USA300 as a cause of necrotising community-onset pneumonia. *Lancet Infect. Dis.* **9:**384–392.

86. Hiramatsu, K., N. Aritaka, H. Hanaki, S. Kawasaki, Y. Hosoda, S. Hori, Y. Fukuchi, and I. Kobayashi. 1997. Dissemination in Japanese hospitals of strains of *Staphylococcus aureus* heterogeneously resistant to vancomycin. *Lancet* **350:**1670–1673.

87. Hope, R., D. M. Livermore, G. Brick, M. Lillie, and R. Reynolds. 2008. Non-susceptibility trends among staphylococci from bacteraemias in the UK and Ireland, 2001–06. *J. Antimicrob. Chemother.* **62**(Suppl. 2):ii65–ii74.

88. Huijsdens, X. W., B. J. van Dijke, E. Spalburg, M. G. van Santen-Verheuvel, M. E. Heck, G. N. Pluister, A. Voss, W. J. Wannet, and A. J. de Neeling. 2006. Community-acquired MRSA and pig-farming. *Ann. Clin. Microbiol. Antimicrob.* **5:**26.

89. Huletsky, A., R. Giroux, V. Rossbach, M. Gagnon, M. Vaillancourt, M. Bernier, F. Gagnon, K. Truchon, M. Bastien, F. J. Picard, A. van Belkum, M. Ouellette, P. H. Roy, and M. G. Bergeron. 2004. New real-time PCR assay for rapid detection of methicillin-resistant *Staphylococcus aureus* directly from specimens containing a mixture of staphylococci. *J. Clin. Microbiol.* **42:**1875–1884.

90. **Ito, T., Y. Katayama, K. Asada, N. Mori, K. Tsutsumimoto, C. Tiensasitorn, and K. Hiramatsu.** 2001. Structural comparison of three types of staphylococcal cassette chromosome *mec* integrated in the chromosome in methicillin-resistant *Staphylococcus aureus. Antimicrob. Agents Chemother.* **45:**1323–1336.

91. **Ito, T., X. X. Ma, F. Takeuchi, K. Okuma, H. Yuzawa, and K. Hiramatsu.** 2004. Novel type V staphylococcal cassette chromosome *mec* driven by a novel cassette chromosome recombinase, *ccrC. Antimicrob. Agents Chemother.* **48:**2637–2651.

92. **Jensen, M. A., J. A. Webster, and N. Straus.** 1993. Rapid identification of bacteria on the basis of polymerase chain reaction-amplified ribosomal DNA spacer polymorphisms. *Appl. Environ. Microbiol.* **59:**945–952.

93. **John, J. F., and A. M. Harvin.** 2007. History and evolution of antibiotic resistance in coagulase-negative staphylococci: susceptibility profiles of new anti-staphylococcal agents. *Ther. Clin. Risk Manag.* **3:**1143–1152.

94. **Joubert, O., D. Keller, A. Pinck, H. Monteil, and G. Prevost.** 2005. Sensitive and specific detection of staphylococcal epidermolysins A and B in broth cultures by flow cytometry-assisted multiplex immunoassay. *J. Clin. Microbiol.* **43:**1076–1080.

95. **Jourdain, S., D. Miendje, V. K. Musampa, G. Wauters, O. Denis, P. Lepage, and A. Vergison.** 2009. *Kytococcus schroeteri* infection of a ventriculoperitoneal shunt in a child. *Int. J. Infect. Dis.* **13:**e153–e155.

96. **Kahl, B., M. Herrmann, A. S. Everding, H. G. Koch, K. Becker, E. Harms, R. A. Proctor, and G. Peters.** 1998. Persistent infection with small colony variant strains of *Staphylococcus aureus* in patients with cystic fibrosis. *J. Infect. Dis.* **177:**1023–1029.

97. **Kazakova, S. V., J. C. Hageman, M. Matava, A. Srinivasan, L. Phelan, B. Garfinkel, T. Boo, S. McAllister, J. Anderson, B. Jensen, D. Dodson, D. Lonsway, L. K. McDougal, M. Arduino, V. J. Fraser, G. Killgore, F. C. Tenover, S. Cody, and D. B. Jernigan.** 2005. A clone of methicillin-resistant *Staphylococcus aureus* among professional football players. *N. Engl. J. Med.* **352:**468–475.

98. **Khatib, R., K. Riederer, S. Saeed, L. B. Johnson, M. G. Fakih, M. Sharma, M. S. Tabriz, and A. Khosrovaneh.** 2005. Time to positivity in *Staphylococcus aureus* bacteremia: possible correlation with the source and outcome of infection. *Clin. Infect. Dis.* **41:**594–598.

99. **King, M. D., B. J. Humphrey, Y. F. Wang, E. V. Kourbatova, S. M. Ray, and H. M. Blumberg.** 2006. Emergence of community-acquired methicillin-resistant *Staphylococcus aureus* USA 300 clone as the predominant cause of skin and soft-tissue infections. *Ann. Intern. Med.* **144:**309–317.

100. **Kipp, F., K. Becker, G. Peters, and C. von Eiff.** 2004. Evaluation of different methods to detect methicillin resistance in small-colony variants of *Staphylococcus aureus. J. Clin. Microbiol.* **42:**1277–1279.

101. **Klevens, R. M., M. A. Morrison, J. Nadle, S. Petit, K. Gershman, S. Ray, L. H. Harrison, R. Lynfield, G. Dumyati, J. M. Townes, A. S. Craig, E. R. Zell, G. E. Fosheim, L. K. McDougal, R. B. Carey, and S. K. Fridkin.** 2007. Invasive methicillin-resistant *Staphylococcus aureus* infections in the United States. *JAMA* **298:**1763–1771.

102. **Kloos, W. E., D. N. Ballard, C. G. George, J. A. Webster, R. J. Hubner, W. Ludwig, K. H. Schleifer, F. Fiedler, and K. Schubert.** 1998. Delimiting the genus *Staphylococcus* through description of *Macrococcus caseolyticus* gen. nov., comb. nov. and *Macrococcus equipercicus* sp. nov., and *Macrococcus bovicus* sp. no. and *Macrococcus carouselicus* sp. nov. *Int. J. Syst. Bacteriol.* **48:**859–877.

103. **Kloos, W. E., and T. L. Bannerman.** 1994. Update on clinical significance of coagulase-negative staphylococci. *Clin. Microbiol. Rev.* **7:**117–140.

104. **Kloos, W. E., and M. S. Musselwhite.** 1975. Distribution and persistence of *Staphylococcus* and *Micrococcus* species and other aerobic bacteria on human skin. *Appl. Microbiol.* **30:**381–385.

105. **Kloos, W. E., and K. H. Schleifer.** 1975. Simplified scheme for routine identification of human *Staphylococcus* species. *J. Clin. Microbiol.* **1:**82–88.

106. **Kloos, W. E., and K. H. Schleifer.** 1983. *Staphylococcus auricularis* sp. nov.: an inhabitant of the human external ear. *Int. J. Syst. Bacteriol.* **33:**9–14.

107. **Kluytmans, J. A., J. W. Mouton, E. P. Ijzerman, C. M. Vandenbroucke-Grauls, A. W. Maat, J. H. Wagenvoort, and H. A. Verbrugh.** 1995. Nasal carriage of *Staphylococcus aureus* as a major risk factor for wound infections after cardiac surgery. *J. Infect. Dis.* **171:**216–219.

108. **Kobayashi, N., M. Alam, and S. Urasawa.** 2001. Analysis on distribution of insertion sequence IS*431* in clinical isolates of staphylococci. *Diagn. Microbiol. Infect. Dis.* **39:**61–64.

109. **Köck, R., J. Harlizius, N. Bressan, R. Laerberg, L. H. Wieler, W. Witte, R. H. Deurenberg, A. Voss, K. Becker, and A. W. Friedrich.** 2009. Prevalence and molecular characteristics of methicillin-resistant *Staphylococcus aureus* (MRSA) among pigs on German farms and import of livestock-related MRSA into hospitals. *Eur. J. Clin. Microbiol. Infect. Dis.* **28:**1375–1382.

110. **Koessler, T., P. Francois, Y. Charbonnier, A. Huyghe, M. Bento, S. Dharan, G. Renzi, D. Lew, S. Harbarth, D. Pittet, and J. Schrenzel.** 2006. Use of oligoarrays for characterization of community-onset methicillin-resistant *Staphylococcus aureus. J. Clin. Microbiol.* **44:**1040–1048.

111. **Krimmer, V., H. Merkert, C. von Eiff, M. Frosch, J. Eulert, J. F. Löhr, J. Hacker, and W. Ziebuhr.** 1999. Detection of *Staphylococcus aureus* and *Staphylococcus epidermidis* in clinical samples by 16S rRNA-directed in situ hybridization. *J. Clin. Microbiol.* **37:**2667–2673.

112. **Ladhani, S., C. L. Joannou, D. P. Lochrie, R. W. Evans, and S. M. Poston.** 1999. Clinical, microbial, and biochemical aspects of the exfoliative toxins causing staphylococcal scalded-skin syndrome. *Clin. Microbiol. Rev.* **12:**224–242.

113. **Lalani, T., Z. A. Kanafani, V. H. Chu, L. Moore, G. R. Corey, P. Pappas, C. W. Woods, C. H. Cabell, B. Hoen, C. Selton-Suty, T. Doco-Lecompte, C. Chirouze, D. Raoult, J. M. Miro, C. A. Mestres, L. Olaison, S. Eykyn, E. Abrutyn, and V. G. Fowler, Jr.** 2006. Prosthetic valve endocarditis due to coagulase-negative staphylococci: findings from the International Collaboration on Endocarditis Merged Database. *Eur. J. Clin. Microbiol. Infect. Dis.* **25:**365–368.

114. **Leskinen, K., P. Hendolin, A. Virolainen-Julkunen, J. Ylikoski, and J. Jero.** 2002. The clinical role of *Alloiococcus otitidis* in otitis media with effusion. *Int. J. Pediatr. Otorhinolaryngol.* **66:**41–48.

115. **Lina, G., Y. Piémont, F. Godail-Gamot, M. Bes, M.-O. Peter, V. Gauduchon, F. Vandenesch, and J. Etienne.** 1999. Involvement of Panton-Valentine leukocidin-producing *Staphylococcus aureus* in primary skin infections and pneumonia. *Clin. Infect. Dis.* **29:**1128–1132.

116. **Lowry, T. R., and J. A. Brennan.** 2005. *Stomatococcus mucilaginosis* infection leading to early cervical necrotizing fasciitis. *Otolaryngol. Head Neck Surg.* **132:**658–660.

117. **Ludwig, W., K. H. Schleifer, and W. B. Whitman.** 2009. Class I. *Bacilli* class nov., p. 19–20. *In* P. De Vos, G. M. Garrity, D. Jones, N. R. Krieg, W. Ludwig, F. A. Rainey, K. H. Schleifer, and W. B. Whitman (ed.), *Bergey's Manual of Systematic Bacteriology*, 2nd ed., vol. 3. *The Firmicutes.* Springer, New York, NY.

118. **Maki, D. G., C. E. Weise, and H. W. Sarafin.** 1977. A semiquantitative culture method for identifying intravenous-catheter-related infection. *N. Engl. J. Med.* **296:**1305–1309.

119. **Martin, R. R., V. Buttram, P. Besch, J. J. Kirkland, and G. P. Petty.** 1982. Nasal and vaginal *Staphylococcus aureus* in young women: quantitative studies. *Ann. Intern. Med.* **96:**951–953.

120. **Martineau, F., F. J. Picard, D. Ke, S. Paradis, P. H. Roy, M. Ouellette, and M. G. Bergeron.** 2001. Development of a PCR assay for identification of staphylococci at genus and species levels. *J. Clin. Microbiol.* **39:**2541–2547.

121. **Martins, A., and M. de Lourdes R. S. Cunha.** 2007. Methicillin resistance in *Staphylococcus aureus* and coagulase-negative staphylococci: epidemiological and molecular aspects. *Microbiol. Immunol.* **51**:787–795.

122. **Mason, W. J., J. S. Blevins, K. Beenken, N. Wibowo, N. Ojha, and M. S. Smeltzer.** 2001. Multiplex PCR protocol for the diagnosis of staphylococcal infection. *J. Clin. Microbiol.* **39**:3332–3338.

123. **Mellmann, A., K. Becker, C. von Eiff, U. Keckevoet, P. Schumann, and D. Harmsen.** 2006. Sequencing and staphylococci identification. *Emerg. Infect. Dis.* **12**:333–336.

124. **Mendoza, M., H. Meugnier, M. Bes, J. Etienne, and J. Freney.** 1998. Identification of *Staphylococcus* species by 16S-23S rDNA intergenic spacer PCR analysis. *Int. J. Syst. Bacteriol.* **48**:1049–1055.

125. **Mermel, L. A., B. M. Farr, R. J. Sherertz, I. I. Raad, N. O'Grady, J. S. Harris, and D. E. Craven.** 2001. Guidelines for the management of intravascular catheter-related infections. *Clin. Infect. Dis.* **32**:1249–1272.

126. **Miller, P. H., R. R. Facklam, and J. M. Miller.** 1996. Atmospheric growth requirements for *Alloiococcus species* and related gram-positive cocci. *J. Clin. Microbiol.* **34**:1027–1028.

127. **Mitchell, R. G., and A. C. Baird-Parker.** 1967. Novobiocin resistance and the classification of staphylococci and micrococci. *J. Appl. Bacteriol.* **30**:251–254.

128. **Monday, S. R., and G. A. Bohach.** 1999. Use of multiplex PCR to detect classical and newly described pyrogenic toxin genes in staphylococcal isolates. *J. Clin. Microbiol.* **37**:3411–3414.

129. **Monecke, S., and R. Ehricht.** 2005. Rapid genotyping of methicillin-resistant *Staphylococcus aureus* (MRSA) isolates using miniaturised oligonucleotide arrays. *Clin. Microbiol. Infect.* **11**:825–833.

130. **Morgan, M.** 2008. Methicillin-resistant *Staphylococcus aureus* and animals: zoonosis or humanosis? *J. Antimicrob. Chemother.* **62**:1181–1187.

131. **Murakami, K., W. Minamide, K. Wada, E. Nakamura, H. Teraoka, and S. Watanabe.** 1991. Identification of methicillin-resistant strains of staphylococci by polymerase chain reaction. *J. Clin. Microbiol.* **29**:2240–2244.

132. **Murayama, O., M. Matsuda, and J. E. Moore.** 2003. Studies on the genomic heterogeneity of *Micrococcus luteus* strains by macro-restriction analysis using pulsed-field gel electrophoresis. *J. Basic Microbiol.* **43**:337–340.

133. **Murchan, S., M. E. Kaufmann, A. Deplano, R. De Ryck, M. Struelens, C. E. Zinn, V. Fussing, S. Salmenlinna, J. Vuopio-Varkila, N. el Solh, C. Cuny, W. Witte, P. T. Tassios, N. Legakis, W. van Leeuwen, A. van Belkum, A. Vindel, I. Laconcha, J. Garaizar, S. Haeggman, B. Olsson-Liljequist, U. Ransjo, G. Coombes, and B. Cookson.** 2003. Harmonization of pulsed-field gel electrophoresis protocols for epidemiological typing of strains of methicillin-resistant *Staphylococcus aureus*: a single approach developed by consensus in 10 European laboratories and its application for tracing the spread of related strains. *J. Clin. Microbiol.* **41**:1574–1585.

134. **Nakatomi, Y., and J. Sugiyama.** 1998. A rapid latex agglutination assay for the detection of penicillin-binding protein 2'. *Microbiol. Immunol.* **42**:739–743.

135. **Novick, R. P., S. J. Projan, J. Kornblum, H. F. Ross, G. Ji, B. Kreiswirth, F. Vandenesch, and S. Moghazeh.** 1995. The agr P2 operon: an autocatalytic sensory transduction system in *Staphylococcus aureus*. *Mol. Gen. Genet.* **248**:446–458.

136. **Oliveira, D. C., C. Milheiriço, and H. de Lencastre.** 2006. Redefining a structural variant of staphylococcal cassette chromosome *mec*, SCC*mec* type VI. *Antimicrob. Agents Chemother.* **50**:3457–3459.

137. **Över, U., Y. Tüc, and G. Söyletir.** 2000. Catalase-negative *Staphylococcus aureus*: a rare isolate of human infection. *Clin. Microbiol. Infect.* **6**:681–682.

138. **Pan, E. S., B. A. Diep, H. A. Carleton, E. D. Charlebois, G. F. Sensabaugh, B. L. Haller, and F. Perdreau-Remington.** 2003. Increasing prevalence of methicillin-resistant *Staphylococcus aureus* infection in California jails. *Clin. Infect. Dis.* **37**:1384–1388.

139. **Paterson, D. L.** 2004. "Collateral damage" from cephalosporin or quinolone antibiotic therapy. *Clin. Infect. Dis.* **38**(Suppl. 4):S341–S345.

140. **Perry, J. D., A. Davies, L. A. Butterworth, A. L. Hopley, A. Nicholson, and F. K. Gould.** 2004. Development and evaluation of a chromogenic agar medium for methicillin-resistant *Staphylococcus aureus*. *J. Clin. Microbiol.* **42**:4519–4523.

141. **Perry, J. D., C. Rennison, L. A. Butterworth, A. L. Hopley, and F. K. Gould.** 2003. Evaluation of S. aureus ID, a new chromogenic agar medium for detection of *Staphylococcus aureus*. *J. Clin. Microbiol.* **41**:5695–5698.

142. **Peters, G., R. Locci, and G. Pulverer.** 1981. Microbial colonization of prosthetic devices. II. Scanning electron microscopy of naturally infected intravenous catheters. *Zentralbl. Bakteriol. Mikrobiol. Hyg. B* **173**:293–299.

143. **Potoski, B. A., J. Adams, L. Clarke, K. Shutt, P. K. Linden, C. Baxter, A. W. Pasculle, B. Capitano, A. Y. Peleg, D. Szabo, and D. L. Paterson.** 2006. Epidemiological profile of linezolid-resistant coagulase-negative staphylococci. *Clin. Infect. Dis.* **43**:165–171.

144. **Poyart, C., G. Quesne, C. Boumaila, and P. Trieu-Cuot.** 2001. Rapid and accurate species-level identification of coagulase-negative staphylococci by using the *sodA* gene as a target. *J. Clin. Microbiol.* **39**:4296–4301.

145. **Proctor, R. A.** 2008. Role of folate antagonists in the treatment of methicillin-resistant *Staphylococcus aureus* infection. *Clin. Infect. Dis.* **46**:584–593.

146. **Proctor, R. A., B. Kahl, C. von Eiff, P. E. Vaudaux, D. P. Lew, and G. Peters.** 1998. Staphylococcal small colony variants have novel mechanisms for antibiotic resistance. *Clin. Infect. Dis.* **27**(Suppl. 1):S68–S74.

147. **Proctor, R. A., C. von Eiff, B. C. Kahl, K. Becker, P. McNamara, M. Herrmann, and G. Peters.** 2006. Small colony variants: a pathogenic form of bacteria that facilitates persistent and recurrent infections. *Nat. Rev. Microbiol.* **4**:295–305.

148. **Raad, I., H. Hanna, and D. Maki.** 2007. Intravascular catheter-related infections: advances in diagnosis, prevention, and management. *Lancet Infect. Dis.* **7**:645–657.

149. **Raad, I., H. A. Hanna, B. Alakech, I. Chatzinikolaou, M. M. Johnson, and J. Tarrand.** 2004. Differential time to positivity: a useful method for diagnosing catheter-related bloodstream infections. *Ann. Intern. Med.* **140**:18–25.

150. **Rajakaruna, L., G. Hallas, L. Molenaar, D. Dare, H. Sutton, V. Encheva, R. Culak, I. Innes, G. Ball, A. M. Sefton, M. Eydmann, A. M. Kearns, and H. N. Shah.** 2009. High throughput identification of clinical isolates of *Staphylococcus aureus* using MALDI-TOF-MS of intact cells. *Infect. Genet. Evol.* **9**:507–513.

151. **Rayner, C., and W. J. Munckhof.** 2005. Antibiotics currently used in the treatment of infections caused by *Staphylococcus aureus*. *Intern. Med. J.* **35**(Suppl. 2):S3–16.

152. **Renneberg, J., K. Rieneck, and E. Gutschik.** 1995. Evaluation of Staph ID 32 system and Staph-Zym system for identification of coagulase-negative staphylococci. *J. Clin. Microbiol.* **33**:1150–1153.

153. **Rijnders, B. J., C. Verwaest, W. E. Peetermans, A. Wilmer, S. Vandecasteele, E. J. Van, and W. E. Van.** 2001. Difference in time to positivity of hub-blood versus nonhub-blood cultures is not useful for the diagnosis of catheter-related bloodstream infection in critically ill patients. *Crit. Care Med.* **29**:1399–1403.

154. **Robert, J., R. Bismuth, and V. Jarlier.** 2006. Decreased susceptibility to glycopeptides in methicillin-resistant *Staphylococcus aureus*: a 20 year study in a large French teaching hospital, 1983–2002. *J. Antimicrob. Chemother.* **57**:506–510.

155. **Robinson, D. A., and M. C. Enright.** 2004. Multilocus sequence typing and the evolution of methicillin-resistant *Staphylococcus aureus*. *Clin. Microbiol. Infect.* **10**:92–97.

156. **Rogers, K. L., P. D. Fey, and M. E. Rupp.** 2009. Coagulase-negative staphylococcal infections. *Infect. Dis. Clin. N. Am.* **23**:73–98.

157. **Roisin, S., C. Nonhoff, O. Denis, and M. J. Struelens.** 2008. Evaluation of new Vitek 2 card and disk diffusion method for determining susceptibility of *Staphylococcus aureus* to oxacillin. *J. Clin. Microbiol.* **46**:2525–2528.

158. Rosenthal, V. D., D. G. Maki, A. Mehta, C. Álvarez-Moreno, H. Leblebicioglu, F. Higuera, L. E. Cuellar, N. Madani, Z. Mitrev, L. Dueñas, J. A. Navoa-Ng, H. G. Garcell, L. Raka, R. F. Hidalgo, E. A. Medeiros, S. S. Kanj, S. Abubakar, P. Nercelles, and R. D. Pratesi. 2008. International Nosocomial Infection Control Consortium report, data summary for 2002–2007, issued January 2008. *Am. J. Infect. Control* **36**:627–637.

159. Rupp, M. E., D. E. Soper, and G. L. Archer. 1992. Colonization of the female genital tract with *Staphylococcus saprophyticus. J. Clin. Microbiol.* **30**:2975–2979.

160. Sabat, A., J. Krzyszton-Russjan, W. Strzalka, R. Filipek, K. Kosowska, W. Hryniewicz, J. Travis, and J. Potempa. 2003. New method for typing *Staphylococcus aureus* strains: multiple-locus variable-number tandem repeat analysis of polymorphism and genetic relationships of clinical isolates. *J. Clin. Microbiol.* **41**:1801–1804.

161. Sacchidanand, S., R. L. Penn, J. M. Embil, M. E. Campos, D. Curcio, E. Ellis-Grosse, E. Loh, and G. Rose. 2005. Efficacy and safety of tigecycline monotherapy compared with vancomycin plus aztreonam in patients with complicated skin and skin structure infections: results from a phase 3, randomized, double-blind trial. *Int. J. Infect. Dis.* **9**:251–261.

162. Saiman, L., M. O'Keefe, P. L. Graham III, F. Wu, B. Said-Salim, B. Kreiswirth, A. LaSala, P. M. Schlievert, and P. Della-Latta. 2003. Hospital transmission of community-acquired methicillin-resistant *Staphylococcus aureus* among postpartum women. *Clin. Infect. Dis.* **37**:1313–1319.

163. Sasaki, T., K. Kikuchi, Y. Tanaka, N. Takahashi, S. Kamata, and K. Hiramatsu. 2007. Reclassification of phenotypically identified *Staphylococcus intermedius* strains. *J. Clin. Microbiol.* **45**:2770–2778.

164. Schleifer, K. H., and W. E. Kloos. 1975. Isolation and characterization of staphylococci from human skin. I. Amended descriptions of *Staphylococcus epidermidis* and *Staphylococcus saprophyticus* and descriptions of three new species: *Staphylococcus cohnii, Staphylococcus haemolyticus,* and *Staphylococcus xylosus. Int. J. Syst. Bacteriol.* **25**:50–61.

165. Seifert, H., O. Cornely, K. Seggewiss, M. Decker, D. Stefanik, H. Wisplinghoff, and G. Fätkenheuer. 2003. Bloodstream infection in neutropenic cancer patients related to short-term nontunnelled catheters determined by quantitative blood cultures, differential time to positivity, and molecular epidemiological typing with pulsed-field gel electrophoresis. *J. Clin. Microbiol.* **41**:118–123.

166. Seifert, H., M. Kaltheuner, and F. Perdreau-Remington. 1995. *Micrococcus luteus* endocarditis: case report and review of the literature. *Zentralbl. Bakteriol.* **282**:431–435.

167. Seifert, H., D. Oltmanns, K. Becker, H. Wisplinghoff, and C. von Eiff. 2005. *Staphylococcus lugdunensis* pacemaker-related infection. *Emerg. Infect. Dis.* **11**:1283–1286.

168. Seybold, U., E. V. Kourbatova, J. G. Johnson, S. J. Halvosa, Y. F. Wang, M. D. King, S. M. Ray, and H. M. Blumberg. 2006. Emergence of community-associated methicillin-resistant *Staphylococcus aureus* USA300 genotype as a major cause of health care-associated blood stream infections. *Clin. Infect. Dis.* **42**:647–656.

169. Shittu, A. O., and J. Lin. 2006. Antimicrobial susceptibility patterns and characterization of clinical isolates of *Staphylococcus aureus* in KwaZulu-Natal province, South Africa. *BMC Infect. Dis.* **6**:125.

170. Shopsin, B., M. Gomez, S. O. Montgomery, D. H. Smith, M. Waddington, D. E. Dodge, D. A. Bost, M. Riehman, S. Naidich, and B. N. Kreiswirth. 1999. Evaluation of protein A gene polymorphic region DNA sequencing for typing of *Staphylococcus aureus* strains. *J. Clin. Microbiol.* **37**:3556–3563.

171. Skiest, D. J. 2006. Treatment failure resulting from resistance of *Staphylococcus aureus* to daptomycin. *J. Clin. Microbiol.* **44**:655–656.

172. Skov, R., R. Smyth, A. R. Larsen, A. Bolmstrom, A. Karlsson, K. Mills, N. Frimodt-Moller, and G. Kahlmeter. 2006. Phenotypic detection of methicillin resistance in *Staphylococcus aureus* by disk diffusion testing and Etest on Mueller-Hinton agar. *J. Clin. Microbiol.* **44**:4395–4399.

173. Skow, A., K. A. Mangold, M. Tajuddin, A. Huntington, B. Fritz, R. B. Thomson, Jr., and K. L. Kaul. 2005. Species-level identification of staphylococcal isolates by real-time PCR and melt curve analysis. *J. Clin. Microbiol.* **43**:2876–2880.

174. Stackebrandt, E., C. Koch, O. Gvozdiak, and P. Schumann. 1995. Taxonomic dissection of the genus *Micrococcus*: *Kocuria* gen. nov., *Nesterenkonia* gen. nov., *Kytococcus* gen. nov., *Dermacoccus* gen. nov., and *Micrococcus* Cohn 1872 gen. emend. *Int. J. Syst. Bacteriol.* **45**:682–692.

175. Stackebrandt, E., F. A. Rainey, and N. L. Ward-Rainey. 1997. Proposal for a new hierarchic classification system, *Actinobacteria* classis nov. *Int. J. Syst. Bacteriol.* **47**:479–491.

176. Stackebrandt, E., and P. Schumann. 2000. Description of *Bogoriellaceae* fam. nov., *Dermacoccaceae* fam. nov., *Rarobacteraceae* fam. nov. and *Sanguibacteraceae* fam. nov. and emendation of some families of the suborder *Micrococcineae. Int. J. Syst. Evol. Microbiol.* **50**:1279–1285.

177. Stefani, S., and P. E. Varaldo. 2003. Epidemiology of methicillin-resistant staphylococci in Europe. *Clin. Microbiol. Infect.* **9**:1179–1186.

178. Straub, J. A., C. Hertel, and W. P. Hammes. 1999. A 23S rDNA-targeted polymerase chain reaction-based system for detection of *Staphylococcus aureus* in meat starter cultures and dairy products. *J. Food Prot.* **62**:1150–1156.

179. Struelens, M. J., P. M. Hawkey, G. L. French, W. Witte, and E. Tacconelli. 2009. Laboratory tools and strategies for methicillin-resistant *Staphylococcus aureus* screening, surveillance and typing: state of the art and unmet needs. *Clin. Microbiol. Infect.* **15**:112–119.

180. Talan, D. A., D. Staatz, A. Staatz, E. J. Goldstein, K. Singer, and G. D. Overturf. 1989. *Staphylococcus intermedius* in canine gingiva and canine-inflicted human wound infections: laboratory characterization of a newly recognized zoonotic pathogen. *J. Clin. Microbiol.* **27**:78–81.

181. Tang, Y. W., J. Han, M. A. McCormac, H. Li, and C. W. Stratton. 2008. *Staphylococcus pseudolugdunensis* sp. nov., a pyrrolidonyl arylamidase/ornithine decarboxylase-positive bacterium isolated from blood cultures. *Diagn. Microbiol. Infect. Dis.* **60**:351–359.

182. Tano, K., R. von Essen, P. O. Eriksson, and A. Sjöstedt. 2008. *Alloiococcus otitidis*—otitis media pathogen or normal bacterial flora? *APMIS* **116**:785–790.

183. Tenover, F. C., R. D. Arbeit, R. V. Goering, P. A. Mickelsen, B. E. Murray, D. H. Persing, and B. Swaminathan. 1995. Interpreting chromosomal DNA restriction patterns produced by pulsed-field gel electrophoresis: criteria for bacterial strain typing. *J. Clin. Microbiol.* **33**:2233–2239.

184. Tenover, F. C., and R. C. Moellering, Jr. 2007. The rationale for revising the Clinical and Laboratory Standards Institute vancomycin minimal inhibitory concentration interpretive criteria for *Staphylococcus aureus. Clin. Infect. Dis.* **44**:1208–1215.

185. Thomson-Carter, F. M., P. E. Carter, and T. H. Pennington. 1989. Differentiation of staphylococcal species and strains by ribosomal RNA gene restriction patterns. *J. Gen. Microbiol.* **135**:2093–2097.

186. Tokars, J. I. 2004. Predictive value of blood cultures positive for coagulase-negative staphylococci: implications for patient care and health care quality assurance. *Clin. Infect. Dis.* **39**:333–341.

187. Trülzsch, K., B. Grabein, P. Schumann, A. Mellmann, U. Antonenka, J. Heesemann, and K. Becker. 2007. *Staphylococcus pettenkoferi* sp. nov., a novel coagulase-negative staphylococcal species isolated from human clinical specimens. *Int. J. Syst. Evol. Microbiol.* **57**:1543–1548.

188. Valderas, M. W., J. W. Gatson, N. Wreyford, and M. E. Hart. 2002. The superoxide dismutase gene *sodM* is unique to *Staphylococcus aureus*: absence of *sodM* in coagulase-negative staphylococci. *J. Bacteriol.* **184**:2465–2472.

189. van Belkum, A., N. J. Verkaik, C. P. de Vogel, H. A. Boelens, J. Verveer, J. L. Nouwen, H. A. Verbrugh, and H. F. Wertheim. 2009. Reclassification of *Staphylococcus aureus* nasal carriage types. *J. Infect. Dis.* **199**:1820–1826.

190. Vandenesch, F., B. Lina, C. Lebeau, T. B. Greenland, and J. Etienne. 1993. Epidemiological markers of coagulase-negative staphylococci. *Intensive Care Med.* **19**:311–315.

191. **Vannuffel, P., J. Gigi, H. Ezzedine, B. Vandercam, M. Delmee, G. Wauters, and J. L. Gala.** 1995. Specific detection of methicillin-resistant *Staphylococcus species* by multiplex PCR. *J. Clin. Microbiol.* **33:**2864–2867.

192. **Vaudaux, P., W. L. Kelley, and D. P. Lew.** 2006. *Staphylococcus aureus* small colony variants: difficult to diagnose and difficult to treat. *Clin. Infect. Dis.* **43:**968–970.

193. **von Darányi, J.** 1925. Qualitative Untersuchungen der Luftbakterien. *Arch. Hyg.* (Berlin) **96:**182.

194. **von Eiff, C., C. R. Arciola, L. Montanaro, K. Becker, and D. Campoccia.** 2006. Emerging *Staphylococcus* species as new pathogens in implant infections. *Int. J. Artif. Organs* **29:**360–367.

195. **von Eiff, C., K. Becker, K. Machka, H. Stammer, and G. Peters.** 2001. Nasal carriage as a source of *Staphylococcus aureus* bacteremia. *N. Engl. J. Med.* **344:**11–16.

196. **von Eiff, C., D. Bettin, R. A. Proctor, B. Rolauffs, N. Lindner, W. Winkelmann, and G. Peters.** 1997. Recovery of small colony variants of *Staphylococcus aureus* following gentamicin bead placement for osteomyelitis. *Clin. Infect. Dis.* **25:**1250–1251.

197. **von Eiff, C., M. Herrmann, and G. Peters.** 1995. Antimicrobial susceptibilities of *Stomatococcus mucilaginosus* and of *Micrococcus* spp. *Antimicrob. Agents Chemother.* **39:**268–270.

198. **von Eiff, C., B. Jansen, W. Kohnen, and K. Becker.** 2005. Infections associated with medical devices: pathogenesis, management and prophylaxis. *Drugs* **65:**179–214.

199. **von Eiff, C., N. Kuhn, M. Herrmann, S. Weber, and G. Peters.** 1996. *Micrococcus luteus* as a cause of recurrent bacteremia. *Pediatr. Infect. Dis. J.* **15:**711–713.

200. **von Eiff, C., and G. Peters.** 1998. In vitro activity of ciprofloxacin, ofloxacin, and levofloxacin against *Micrococcus* species and *Stomatococcus mucilaginosus* isolated from healthy subjects and neutropenic patients. *Eur. J. Clin. Microbiol. Infect. Dis.* **17:**890–892.

201. **Walsh, T. R., A. Bolmstrom, A. Qwarnstrom, P. Ho, M. Wootton, R. A. Howe, A. P. MacGowan, and D. Diekema.** 2001. Evaluation of current methods for detection of staphylococci with reduced susceptibility to glycopeptides. *J. Clin. Microbiol.* **39:**2439–2444.

202. **Wenzel, R. P., and T. M. Perl.** 1995. The significance of nasal carriage of *Staphylococcus aureus* and the incidence of postoperative wound infection. *J. Hosp. Infect.* **31:**13–24.

203. **Williams, R. E.** 1963. Healthy carriage of *Staphylococcus aureus*: its prevalence and importance. *Bacteriol. Rev.* **27:**56–71.

204. **Wilson, I. G., J. E. Cooper, and A. Gilmour.** 1991. Detection of enterotoxigenic *Staphylococcus aureus* in dried skimmed milk: use of the polymerase chain reaction for amplification and detection of staphylococcal enterotoxin genes *entB* and *entC1* and the thermonuclease gene *nuc*. *Appl. Environ. Microbiol.* **57:**1793–1798.

205. **Wisplinghoff, H., T. Bischoff, S. M. Tallent, H. Seifert, R. P. Wenzel, and M. B. Edmond.** 2004. Nosocomial bloodstream infections in US hospitals: analysis of 24,179 cases from a prospective nationwide surveillance study. *Clin. Infect. Dis.* **39:**309–317.

206. **Wolk, D. M., L. B. Blyn, T. A. Hall, R. Sampath, R. Ranken, C. Ivy, R. Melton, H. Matthews, N. White, F. Li, V. Harpin, D. J. Ecker, B. Limbago, L. K. McDougal, V. H. Wysocki, M. Cai, and K. C. Carroll.** 2009. Pathogen profiling: rapid molecular characterization of *Staphylococcus aureus* by PCR/ electrospray ionization-mass spectrometry and correlation with phenotype. *J. Clin. Microbiol.* **47:**3129–3137.

207. **Wootton, M., R. A. Howe, R. Hillman, T. R. Walsh, P. M. Bennett, and A. P. MacGowan.** 2001. A modified population analysis profile (PAP) method to detect heteroresistance to vancomycin in *Staphylococcus aureus* in a UK hospital. *J. Antimicrob. Chemother.* **47:**399–403.

208. **Wunderink, R. G., J. Rello, S. K. Cammarata, R. V. Croos-Dabrera, and M. H. Kollef.** 2003. Linezolid vs vancomycin: analysis of two double-blind studies of patients with methicillin-resistant *Staphylococcus aureus* nosocomial pneumonia. *Chest* **124:**1789–1797.

209. **Yamaguchi, T., K. Nishifuji, M. Sasaki, Y. Fudaba, M. Aepfelbacher, T. Takata, M. Ohara, H. Komatsuzawa, M. Amagai, and M. Sugai.** 2002. Identification of the *Staphylococcus aureus etd* pathogenicity island which encodes a novel exfoliative toxin, ETD, and EDIN-B. *Infect. Immun.* **70:**5835–5845.

210. **Zadoks, R. N., and J. L. Watts.** 2009. Species identification of coagulase-negative staphylococci: genotyping is superior to phenotyping. *Vet. Microbiol.* **134:**20–28.

211. **Zambardi, G., M. E. Reverdy, S. Bland, M. Bes, J. Freney, and J. Fleurette.** 1994. Laboratory diagnosis of oxacillin resistance in *Staphylococcus aureus* by a multiplex-polymerase chain reaction assay. *Diagn. Microbiol. Infect. Dis.* **19:**25–31.

212. **Zinn, C. S., H. Westh, and V. T. Rosdahl.** 2004. An international multicenter study of antimicrobial resistance and typing of hospital *Staphylococcus aureus* isolates from 21 laboratories in 19 countries or states. *Microb. Drug Resist.* **10:**160–168.

Streptococcus

BARBARA SPELLERBERG AND CLAUDIA BRANDT

20

TAXONOMY

The taxonomy of streptococci has experienced a number of changes in recent years due to the application of DNA-DNA reassociation studies and 16S rRNA gene sequencing. Streptococci are firmicutes of the order *Lactobacillales* and belong to the family *Streptococcaceae*. Among the currently established 17 different genera of catalase-negative gram-positive cocci are several genera that were split off from the genus *Streptococcus* some time ago, such as *Enterococcus* and *Lactococcus*, or more recently *Abiotrophia*, *Granulicatella*, *Facklamia*, and *Globicatella*. For excellent reviews on the topic, see references 36 and 70. Streptococcal species designation based solely on the hemolysis reaction, colony size, and the presence of Lancefield antigens does not always correspond well with the molecular analysis of the 16S rRNA gene sequence. However, the traditional streptococcal classification system is well established and still of value to the clinical microbiologist and health care provider. It correlates with clinical syndromes caused by different species and enables a first distinction of broad categories of streptococci that is useful for the choice of further tests and guidance of empirical treatments. The information and the identification schemes presented in this chapter therefore adhere in many aspects to the phenotypic classification system.

The classical differentiation of streptococci separates the group of beta-hemolytic streptococci from the group of non-beta-hemolytic streptococcal species. Beta-hemolytic streptococci, also referred to as pyogenic streptococci, include the human pathogenic species *Streptococcus pyogenes*, *S. agalactiae*, *S. dysgalactiae* subsp. *equisimilis*, and a number of primarily veterinary pathogens. The designation "pyogenic streptococci" is more precise, since the group includes species that are non-beta-hemolytic like *S. dysgalactiae* subsp. *dysgalactiae* and the term excludes beta-hemolytic strains of the *S. anginosus* group, which belong to the viridans streptococcal group. The small colony size of streptococci from the anginosus group (≤0.5 mm) helps to distinguish them from the large-colony-forming (>0.5 mm) streptococci of the pyogenic group. Species from the pyogenic or beta-hemolytic group are further characterized by the presence of Lancefield antigens, which correlate to some extent with the proper streptococcal species designations. While the B antigen appears to be limited to *S. agalactiae*, the Lancefield group A antigen has been detected not only in *S. pyogenes* but also in *S. dysgalactiae* subsp. *equisimilis* isolates (16) and in species from the *S. anginosus* group (Table 1). Correlation with the other Lancefield antigens is even more complicated, and molecular taxonomic studies led to novel species designations, presented below and in Table 1.

The group of nonpyogenic streptococci includes mostly alpha-hemolytic as well as nonhemolytic and even beta-hemolytic streptococcal species from the large category of viridans group streptococci. In a study of the genus *Streptococcus* based on sequence comparisons of small-subunit (16S) rRNA genes, five species groups of viridans group streptococci were demonstrated (59) in addition to the pyogenic group (beta-hemolytic, large-colony formers). These nonpyogenic groups were designated the *S. mitis* group, the *S. anginosus* group, the *S. mutans* group, the *S. salivarius* group, and the *S. bovis* group. Several streptococcal species were not unequivocally assigned and remain ungrouped (36, 70). Among alpha-hemolytic streptococci, *S. pneumoniae* can be separated from other streptococci of the viridans group through bile solubility and optochin susceptibility. However, phenotypic characterization and taxonomic considerations place *S. pneumoniae* into the *S. mitis* group (59). The relationship of *S. pneumoniae* to other species of the *S. mitis* group is so close that 16S rRNA gene analysis reveals greater than 99% identity to the nucleotide sequences of *S. mitis* and *S. oralis* and the current concept of separate species in this group has been challenged (66). A novel, closely related species, *S. pseudopneumoniae*, has recently been split off from *S. pneumoniae*, following DNA-DNA hybridization studies and phenotypic characterization (1). Strains are nonencapsulated, insoluble in bile, and optochin susceptible only when incubated in ambient air and may be associated with chronic obstructive pulmonary disease (61).

S. mitis, *S. sanguinis*, *S. parasanguinis*, *S. gordonii*, *S. cristatus*, *S. oralis*, *S. infantis*, *S. peroris* (60), *S. australis* (131), *S. oligofermentans* (118), *S. massiliensis* (46), *S. sinensis*, *S. orisratti*, *S. pseudopneumoniae*, and *S. pneumoniae* are members of the *S. mitis* group. These species form a group whose classification and nomenclature have been a source of considerable confusion in the past. Among the changes that were made are the reclassification of the original *S. mitis* type strain as an *S. gordonii* strain and the subsequent replacement by a new *S. mitis* type strain (NCTC12261^T) (65). Based on

TABLE 1 Phenotypic characteristics of beta-hemolytic streptococci[a]

Species	Lancefield group(s)	Colony size[e]	Hosts[i]	Bacitracin susceptibility	PYR[f]	CAMP[g]	VP[h]	Hippurate hydrolysis	Trehalose	Sorbitol
S. pyogenes	A	Large	Humans	+	+	−	−	−	+	−
S. agalactiae	B	Large	Humans, cows	−	−	+	−	+	v	−
S. dysgalactiae subsp. dysgalactiae[b]	C	Large	Animals	−	−	−	−	−	+	v
S. dysgalactiae subsp. equisimilis	A, C, G, L	Large	Humans (animals)	−	−	−	−	−	+	−
S. equi subsp. equi	C	Large	Animals	−	−	−	−	−	−	−
S. equi subsp. zooepidemicus[c]	C	Large	Animals (humans)	−	−	−	−	−	−	+
S. canis[c]	G	Large	Dogs (humans)	−	−	+	−	−	v	−
S. anginosus group[d]	A, C, G, F, none	Small	Humans	−	−	−	+	−	+	−
S. porcinus[c]	E, P, U, V, none	Large	Swine (humans)	−	+	+	+	v	+	+

[a]Symbols and abbreviations: +, positive; −, negative; v, variable.
[b]S. dysgalactiae subsp. dysgalactiae is alpha-hemolytic on sheep blood agar plates.
[c]S. equi subsp. zooepidemicus, S. canis, and S. porcinus are primarily animal pathogens that are only rarely isolated from humans.
[d]Species included in the S. anginosus group can be beta-hemolytic, alpha-hemolytic, or nonhemolytic on sheep blood agar plates.
[e]Large colony size refers to colonies >0.5 mm after 24 h of incubation, whereas small colony size is <0.5 mm.
[f]Presence of the enzyme pyrrolidonyl aminopeptidase.
[g]CAMP factor reaction (cohemolysis in the presence of the Staphylococcus aureus beta-hemolysin)
[h]Voges-Proskauer test (formation of acetoin from glucose fermentation).
[i]Parenthetical entries indicate hosts from which the organism is rarely isolated.

phenotypic reactions (especially arginine hydrolysis and the esculin test), the S. mitis group can be further subdivided into the S. sanguinis and the S. mitis groups (36), but based on 16S rRNA analysis, these two groups appear to belong together (59). Since correlation of the renamed streptococcal species with human infections is still difficult, we chose to present these species as part of the S. mitis group until further information becomes available.

The small-colony-forming S. anginosus group consists of the three distinct species S. anginosus, S. constellatus, and S. intermedius (128). It includes streptococcal species previously referred to as Lancefield group F streptococci, "S. milleri" group or "S. milleri," but "S. milleri" has no standing taxonomically. The S. mutans group comprises the species S. mutans, S. sobrinus, S. criceti, S. ratti, S. downei, and numerous species that have only been identified from animals thus far (S. ferus, S. macacae, S. hyovaginalis, and S. devriesei).

The human species S. salivarius, S. vestibularis, and S. thermophilus, which is found in dairy products, belong to the S. salivarius group. The whole S. salivarius group is closely related to the S. bovis group. Some streptococcal species that are currently part of the S. bovis group (S. infantarius and S. alactolyticus) (103) were formerly part of the S. salivarius group (36).

The S. bovis group has experienced extensive taxonomic changes (30, 103, 104). These changes were made because DNA-DNA reassociation studies revealed considerable heterogeneity among the human isolates described as S. bovis biotypes. Four DNA clusters are currently recognized. DNA cluster I consists of animal strains of S. bovis and S. equinus, which were shown to belong to a single species.

The earlier species name S. equinus has been formally adopted. DNA cluster II consists of S. gallolyticus, with three subspecies: subsp. gallolyticus (formerly S. bovis biotype I), subsp. pasteurianus (formerly S. bovis biotype II.2), and subsp. macedonicus. DNA cluster III consists of S. infantarius (formerly S. bovis biotype II.1), with two subspecies: subsp. infantarius and subsp. coli (formerly called S. lutetiensis). DNA cluster IV consists of S. alactolyticus.

DESCRIPTION OF THE GENUS

Bacterial species belonging to the genus Streptococcus are catalase-negative, gram-positive cocci of less than 2 μm that tend to grow in chains in liquid media. Most species of the genus Streptococcus have a low G+C content of DNA ranging between 34 and 46%. The cell wall composition is typical for gram-positive bacteria and consists mainly of peptidoglycan with glucosamine and muramic acid as amino sugars and galactosamine as a variable component. A variety of carbohydrates, surface protein antigens, and teichoic acid are attached to the cell wall and are, among other characteristics, responsible for intra- and interspecies differences among streptococci. Streptococci are facultative anaerobic bacteria. Due to a lack of heme compounds, streptococci are incapable of respiratory metabolism. Some species of the viridans streptococcal group and S. pneumoniae require 5% CO_2 levels for adequate growth, and the growth of many streptococcal species is enhanced in the presence of 5% CO_2. The optimum temperature for growth of most streptococci is around 37°C, while some species like S. uberis also grow at temperatures as low as 10°C. The complex nutritional requirements of streptococci are usually provided by the addition of blood or serum to the growth medium. Glucose and other carbohydrates are metabolized fermentatively with lactic acid as the major metabolic end product. The addition of glucose or other carbohydrates to liquid medium enhances growth but lowers the pH, resulting in growth inhibition unless the medium is highly buffered (e.g., Todd-Hewitt broth [THB]). Leucine aminopeptidase (LAP) is produced by all streptococci and enterococci but can also be found in lactococci, pediococci, and other catalase-negative gram-positive cocci. It helps to distinguish these species from the LAP-negative *Aerococcus* species and *Leuconostoc*. All streptococci are catalase negative upon exposure to 3% hydrogen peroxide with the exception of *S. didelphis*, a veterinary pathogen (102). False-positive catalase reactions may occur if bacteria are grown on blood-containing media.

EPIDEMIOLOGY AND TRANSMISSION

Streptococci can cause infections in humans and in many different animal species including mammals and fish. Different species of streptococci are frequently found as commensal bacteria on mucous membranes. Occasionally streptococci are present as transient skin microbiota. Several species exhibit a high virulence potential, but even the highly pathogenic streptococcal species are frequently found as colonizing strains. *S. pneumoniae* was responsible for approximately 42,000 invasive infections in the United States in 2007, leading to an estimated 4,500 deaths (http://www.cdc.gov/abcs), and was found as a colonizing bacterial species in many asymptomatic carriers. The asymptomatic carriage rate for *S. pneumoniae* differs considerably between children and adults. Detection rates of 30 to 70% have been reported for young children, depending on the sampling method, while carriage rates among healthy adults are often reported to be below 5% (48, 97). Significantly higher colonization rates for adults living in households with preschool children suggests the occurrence of household transmission between parents and their children (53).

Due to active bacterial surveillance in the emerging infections program network (107), reliable epidemiologic data on invasive infections due to *S. pneumoniae* (described above), *S. pyogenes* (group A), and *S. agalactiae* (group B) have been obtained for a population of almost 30 million people in the United States during 2007. National estimates are that *S. pyogenes* caused 11,400 cases of invasive disease and 1,350 deaths, with the peak of infections in people older than 65 years. Invasive infections due to *S. agalactiae* were second to those due to *S. pneumoniae*, with an estimated 20,000 cases and 1,475 deaths in 2007. Reflecting the ongoing changes in the epidemiology of group B streptococcal disease, the highest attack rates were observed in patients less than 1 year and adults greater than 65 years of age. Apart from causing invasive infections, pyogenic streptococci are frequently encountered as colonizing strains. While asymptomatic pharyngeal colonization with *S. pyogenes* occurs in less than 5% of the adult population, *S. agalactiae* colonization rates of the urogenital and gastrointestinal tracts can be demonstrated in 10 to 30% of the female as well as the male population. No significant differences are observed in the colonization rates of pregnant and nonpregnant women.

Transmission of streptococcal infections can occur by different routes. Pathogenic species like *S. pyogenes* and *S. pneumoniae* are primarily transmitted through droplets or direct contact. Transmission can first lead to colonization, with the potential for the development of a subsequent infection. Transmission from mother to child is typical for neonatal invasive *S. agalactiae* infections. Newborns acquire the bacteria usually during delivery, although transmissions, shortly after birth, from the mother or health care personnel to infants have been documented, especially in late-onset neonatal infections. Endogenous infections most often occur by viridans group streptococci as part of the oral microbiota. The tooth decay-causing species *S. mutans* is also transmitted from mother to child during early infancy, most probably through oral secretions.

Streptococcal infections do not represent classical zoonoses, although most species have a preferred host. While occasional animal-to-human transmissions do occur, as in the case of *Streptococcus suis*, genotypic and phenotypic analyses of animal and human strains demonstrated that most strains causing human infections were distinct from the strains causing animal infections. For large-colony-forming group C and G streptococci, such an analysis led to an important change in species designations (120, 122). Currently all beta-hemolytic group C and L and human group G streptococci are defined as *S. dysgalactiae* subsp. *equisimilis*, while alpha-hemolytic group C streptococcal animal isolates are classified as *S. dysgalactiae* subsp. *dysgalactiae* and animal group G streptococcal strains as *S. canis* (17). Other closely related veterinary species are *S. equi* subsp. *equi* and *S. equi* subsp. *zooepidemicus*. The predominant reservoir for *S. dysgalactiae* subsp. *equisimilis* strains is the human host, and transmission usually occurs among humans.

CLINICAL SIGNIFICANCE

Streptococcus pyogenes (Group A Streptococci)

S. pyogenes colonizes the human throat and skin and has developed complex virulence mechanisms to avoid host defenses (23, 33). The upper respiratory tract and skin lesions serve as primary focal sites of infections and principal reservoirs of transmission. *S. pyogenes* can cause superficial or deep infections due to toxin-mediated and immunologically mediated mechanisms of disease. *S. pyogenes* is the most common cause of bacterial pharyngitis and impetigo. In the past, *S. pyogenes* was a common cause of childbed fever or puerperal sepsis. *S. pyogenes* is responsible for deep or invasive infections, especially bacteremia, sepsis, deep soft tissue infections, such as erysipelas, cellulitis, and necrotizing fasciitis. Less common presentations include myositis, osteomyelitis, septic arthritis, pneumonia, meningitis, endocarditis, pericarditis, and severe neonatal infections following intrapartum transmission. One or more erythrogenic exotoxins produced by *S. pyogenes* may cause a confluent erythemathous sandpaper-like rash characteristic of scarlet fever. While systemic toxic effects occur rarely with scarlet fever, severe clinical manifestations in streptococcal toxic shock syndrome (STSS) may result from massive superantigen-induced cytokine and lymphokine production. Nonsuppurative complications include poststreptococcal glomerulonephritis (GN) and acute rheumatic fever (ARF). While either of these conditions may follow pharyngitis, only GN is linked with skin infections due to *S. pyogenes*. *S. pyogenes* has also been associated with pediatric autoimmune neuropsychiatric disorders (114).

The causes of the emergence of STSS, frequently accompanied by necrotizing fasciitis, and the resurgence of invasive *S. pyogenes* infections since the mid-1980s are mostly unexplained (112). *S. pyogenes* remains exquisitely sensitive to penicillin. Despite the continuous exposure and subsequent type-specific immunity, the most prevalent M types associated with STSS continue to be M1 and M3, together accounting for approximately 50% of invasive infections. Since identical strains have accounted for less serious infections (86), host factors and comorbid conditions account for different diseases. The incidence of STSS seems to be highest among young children, particularly those with varicella, and the elderly. Other persons at risk include those with diabetes mellitus, chronic cardiac or pulmonary diseases, HIV infection, and intravenous drug or alcohol abuse. The risk for severe invasive infection in contacts has been estimated to be 200 times greater than for the general population, but most contacts are asymptomatically colonized (26).

Streptococcus agalactiae (GBS)

S. agalactiae was first identified as the cause of bovine mastitis at the end of the 19th century. Since the 1970s it has been reported as the cause of invasive neonatal infections. Neonatal infections present as two different clinical entities: early-onset neonatal disease, characterized by sepsis and pneumonia within the first 7 days of life; and late-onset disease with meningitis and sepsis between day 7 and 3 months of age. The most important risk factor for the development of invasive neonatal disease is the colonization of the maternal urogenital or gastrointestinal tract by S. agalactiae, which is found in 10 to 30% of pregnant women. Prevention of early-onset neonatal infections can be achieved in the majority of cases by administration of intrapartum antibiotic prophylaxis starting at least 4 hours before delivery. Official CDC recommendations for the prevention of neonatal S. agalactiae infections were first issued in 1996, were revised in 2002 (105), and resulted in a substantial decline of early-onset neonatal group B streptococcus (GBS) disease (106). Invasive S. agalactiae infections of adult patients may be observed as postpartum infections or in immunocompromised adult patients with alcoholism, diabetes mellitus, cancer, or HIV infection (41). The spectrum of infections in adult patients includes pneumonia, bacteremia, meningitis, endocarditis, urinary tract infections, skin and soft tissue infections, and osteomyelitis.

Streptococcus dysgalactiae subsp. equisimilis (Human Group C and G Streptococci)

Human isolates of large-colony-forming beta-hemolytic streptococci harboring the Lancefield group C or group G antigens belong to this novel species (120, 122). While most isolates of this species possess either the Lancefield group C or the group G antigen, strains harboring the Lancefield group L as well as the group A antigen (16) have been described. The clinical spectrum of disease caused by S. dysgalactiae subsp. equisimilis resembles infections caused by S. pyogenes (17). The responsible strains harbor genes similar to virulence factor genes of S. pyogenes, such as emm-like genes, and can be isolated from upper respiratory tract infections, skin infections, soft tissue infections, and invasive infections such as necrotizing fasciitis, STSS, bacteremia, and endocarditis. However, convincing reports of scarlet fever due to S. dysgalactiae subsp. equisimilis have so far not been published. Similar to what is observed with S. pyogenes, cases of GN and ARF have been reported (4, 52) following S. equi subsp. zooepidemicus (GN) and S. dysgalactiae subsp. equisimilis infections (GN and ARF).

Streptococcus pneumoniae

S. pneumoniae is described separately in this section due to its clinical features that distinguish it from other species of the S. mitis group. S. pneumoniae is the most frequently isolated respiratory pathogen in community-acquired pneumonia. In as many as 30% of community-acquired pneumonia cases, S. pneumoniae can be found in blood cultures of patients. S. pneumoniae is also a major cause of meningitis, leading to high morbidity and mortality in pediatric and adult patients. The most frequently observed infection due to S. pneumoniae is otitis media, with an estimate of one infection for every child up to the age of 6 years in the United States. Other infections due to S. pneumoniae include sinusitis, peritonitis, and rare cases of endocarditis. S. pneumoniae colonizes the upper respiratory tract, especially in children, without evidence of infection. Prevention of pneumococcal infections can be achieved by immunization with a 23-valent capsular polysaccharide vaccine in adults or the 7-valent conjugate vaccine in children. Conjugate vaccines for children including a larger number of serotypes have recently been released in Europe. Widespread use of these vaccines has resulted in a reduction of invasive pneumococcal infections during the past several years but also in changes of the serotypes responsible for invasive and noninvasive infections (20, 62, 99).

Streptococcus mitis Group

S. mitis, S. sanguinis, S. parasanguinis, S. gordonii, S. cristatus, S. oralis, S. infantis, S. peroris, S. australis, S. sinensis, S. orisratti, S. oligofermentans, S. massiliensis, S. pseudopneumoniae, and S. pneumoniae are members of this group. Members of the S. mitis group are regular commensals of the oral cavity, the gastrointestinal tract, and the female genital tract. The S. mitis group can be found as a transient microbiota of the normal skin and may represent contaminants when isolated from blood cultures. At the same time, these species are the most frequently isolated bacteria in bacterial endocarditis in native valve and, less frequently, in prosthetic valve infections. Careful evaluation of the clinical situation is therefore crucial to correctly interpret the clinical significance of blood culture isolates from the S. mitis group. In neutropenic patients, streptococcal species from the S. mitis group are often responsible for life-threatening sepsis and pneumonia cases following immunosuppression by chemotherapy (15). Treatment of these infections is further complicated by high penicillin resistance rates.

Streptococcus anginosus Group

Species from the S. anginosus group (S. anginosus, S. constellatus, and S. intermedius) are often harmless commensals of the oropharyngeal, urogenital, and gastrointestinal microbiota. However, these organisms are strongly associated with abscess formation in the brain, oropharynx, or peritoneal cavity. A subspecies of S. constellatus, S. constellatus subsp. pharyngis, has also been described and associated with pharyngitis (130). All species of this group are small-colony-forming bacteria (colony size, ≤0.5 mm) that can display variable patterns of hemolysis (alpha, beta, or gamma). Since they can also harbor the Lancefield group antigen A, C, F, or G (or none at all), it is especially important to reliably distinguish them from large-colony-forming (>0.5 mm) beta-hemolytic streptococci of the pyogenic group. Association of certain species with specific isolation sites has been reported. While S. anginosus is frequently found in specimens from the urogenital or gastrointestinal tracts, *S. constellatus* is commonly isolated from the respiratory tract, and *S. intermedius* is most often identified in abscesses of the brain or liver.

Streptococcus salivarius Group

Streptococcal species that belong to the *S. salivarius* group include *S. salivarius* and *S. vestibularis*. They have been primarily isolated from the oral cavity and blood. Another species of this group, *S. thermophilus*, is found only in dairy products. *S. salivarius* has been repeatedly reported as a cause of bacteremia, endocarditis, and meningitis (sometimes iatrogenic), while *S. vestibularis* has not been clearly associated with human infection. Isolation of *S. salivarius* from blood cultures does correlate to some extent with intestinal neoplasia (101).

Streptococcus mutans Group

S. mutans and *S. sobrinus* belong to the *S. mutans* group. They are the most commonly isolated species of the group that originate from human clinical specimens, usually obtained from the oral cavity. *S. criceti*, *S. ratti*, and *S. downei* have occasionally been identified from human sources, while the other streptococcal species of the *S. mutans* group (*S. ferus*, *S. macacae*, *S. hyovaginalis*, and *S. devriesei*) have only been identified in animals. *S. mutans* is the primary etiologic agent of dental caries, and infection is transmissible. By 18 years of age, 85% of the population have at least one caries lesion (111). Permanent colonization with *S. mutans* occurs under normal living conditions in the Western world between the second and the end of the third year of life (111). Molecular analysis of mother and infant isolates reveals that strains are usually acquired from the mother and that the colonization rate of infants depends on the bacterial load of the mother (19). Analyses of streptococcal blood culture isolates show that *S. mutans* is the most frequently isolated species of this group in cases of bacteremia (36).

Streptococcus bovis Group

Extensive taxonomic changes have occurred in the *S. bovis* group, and strains formerly known as human *S. bovis* isolates are designated as different species (see "Taxonomy" above). The group now includes *S. equinus*, *S. gallolyticus*, *S. infantarius*, and *S. alactolyticus*. Species from this group are frequently encountered in blood cultures of patients with bacteremia, sepsis, and endocarditis. The clinical significance of blood cultures growing streptococci from the *S. bovis* group lies in the association of *S. gallolyticus* subsp. *gallolyticus* with gastrointestinal disorders including colon cancer and chronic liver disease and *S. gallolyticus* subsp. *pasteurianus* with meningitis (6, 43, 69, 88).

Other Streptococci Infrequently Isolated from Human Specimens

Streptococcal species that are primarily animal pathogens are sometimes isolated from human hosts, in most cases from humans that are in close contact with animals. *S. suis*, *S. porcinus*, and *S. iniae* belong to this category. *S. suis* is a swine pathogen that has occasionally been isolated from cases of human meningitis and bacteremia. *S. suis* is encapsulated and appears to be alpha-hemolytic on sheep blood agar plates, although some strains are beta-hemolytic on horse blood agar. *S. suis* strains are positive for the Lancefield group antigen R, S, or T, which helps to distinguish them from the phenotypically similar species *S. gordonii*, *S. ...guinis*, and *S. parasanguinis*. Similar to *S. suis*, *S. porcinus* (Lancefield groups E, P, U, and V) is primarily a swine pathogen. Beta-hemolytic *S. porcinus* strains have rarely been isolated from human sources

such as peripheral blood, wounds, and the female genital tract (37). A recent molecular study of *S. porcinus* isolates from the female genital tract, however, indicates that these isolates belong to a novel species designated *S. pseudoporcinus* (8). *S. porcinus* can be misidentified as *S. agalactiae* due to its isolation from the female genital tract, false-positive reactions with commercially available group B antisera, and a positive CAMP test reaction. *S. porcinus* and *S. pseudoporcinus* can be L-pyrrolidonyl-β-naphthylamide (PYR) positive and do not hydrolyze hippurate, in contrast to *S. agalactiae*. *S. iniae* is a fish pathogen that is beta-hemolytic but does not possess any Lancefield group antigens. It has been isolated from soft tissue infections, bacteremia, endocarditis, and meningitis in people handling fish (38, 125). *S. iniae* isolates resemble *S. pyogenes* strains due to the fact that both are PYR positive. Beta-hemolysis of the species can be observed only around agar stabs or under anaerobic culture conditions. Commercial identification systems do not correctly identify the species; the failure to react with Lancefield group antisera is important to notice, since it is rare among beta-hemolytic streptococci.

COLLECTION, TRANSPORT, AND STORAGE OF SPECIMENS

Specimens suspected of harboring streptococci should be collected by methods outlined elsewhere in this *Manual* (chapter 16). Since many streptococcal species lose viability fairly quickly, it is best to place swabs in an appropriate moist transport medium and process specimens rapidly. If transport time is below 1 to 2 hours, a special transport system is not absolutely necessary. *S. pyogenes* can safely be transported on dry swabs; desiccation enhances recovery from mixed cultures by suppression of the accompanying microbiota (77). Detailed recommendations for collection and storage of swabs from pregnant women to detect *S. agalactiae* colonization have been issued by the U.S. Centers for Disease Control and Prevention. These recommendations are summarized below under "Special Procedures for *Streptococcus agalactiae* Screening."

DIRECT EXAMINATION

Microscopy

Microscopic examination shows streptococci as gram-positive bacteria growing in chains of varying length. *S. pneumoniae* organisms most often present as gram-positive diplococci with an elongated appearance, but a reliable microscopic distinction of *S. pneumoniae* from enterococci and other streptococci is not possible. In blood culture specimens, *S. pneumoniae* tends to form chains of varying length, similar to other streptococci. Direct identification of streptococci by microscopic methods is most helpful in the case of clinical specimens from sterile body sites, such as cerebrospinal fluid (CSF). Tiny, irregular cocci in clumps of chains seen in abscess- or peritonitis-associated aspirates are suggestive of the *S. anginosus* group. Interpretation of Gram stain results from nonsterile body sites is difficult, due to the residential microbiota that frequently includes streptococci. Thus, for example, throat swabs should not be examined by Gram stain for diagnosis of "strep throat."

Direct Antigen Detection of *S. pyogenes* from Throat Specimens

S. pyogenes is the most common cause of acute pharyngitis and accounts for 15 to 30% of cases of acute pharyngitis in children and 5 to 10% of cases in adults. If diagnosis can be provided rapidly, antibiotic therapy can be initiated promptly to relieve symptoms, to avoid sequelae, and to reduce transmission. Numerous assays for direct detection of the group A-specific carbohydrate antigen in throat swabs by agglutination methods or immunoassays (enzyme, liposome, or optical), also referred to as "rapid antigen assays," have become commercially available during the past 2 decades. A list of FDA-cleared tests is accessible via the Internet (http://www.accessdata.fda.gov/scripts/cdrh/devicesatfda/index.cfm?Search_Term=866.3740). Although these tests provide rapid results and allow early treatment decisions, the throat culture remains the gold standard. Sensitivities of rapid antigen tests range from 58% to 96% and have never equalled that of culture (40, 119). Negative rapid antigen test results should therefore be confirmed by culture in children and adolescents, when typical clinical signs are present (13). The specificity, however, is generally high, even though false-positive antigen results are seen from patients previously diagnosed and/or treated for *S. pyogenes* infection (21). Moreover, the low positive predictive value of rapid group A antigen tests in the adult population frequently results in the prescribing of unnecessary antimicrobial therapy (89).

Antigen Detection of *S. agalactiae* in Urogenital Tract Samples

Several different commercially available antigen detection tests have been developed for the identification of *S. agalactiae* in samples from the urogenital tract. Independent from the technique involved (latex agglutination, enzyme immunoassay, or optical immunoassay), all of the currently available tests lack sufficient sensitivities to detect bacterial colonization with *S. agalactiae* (115). They are not recommended by the CDC for screening of pregnant women. Even though modified protocols with an incubation of the samples in selective broth prior to antigen testing appear to increase assay sensitivities, the current CDC recommendations rely on selective broth culture performed at 35 to 37 weeks of gestation for this purpose (see "Special Procedures for *Streptococcus agalactiae* Screening" under "Isolation Procedures" below).

Antigen Detection of *S. pneumoniae* in Urine Samples

An immunochromatographic membrane test relying on the detection of the cell wall-associated polysaccharide that is common to all *S. pneumoniae* serotypes (C-polysaccharide antigen) (Binax NOW; Binax Inc., Portland, ME) has proven helpful for the identification of *S. pneumoniae* infections in adult patients, especially in patients that already received antibiotic treatment. Compared to conventional diagnostic methods, reported sensitivities of antigen detection in urine samples range between 50 and 80% and specificities are approximately 90% (49, 83). Due to the fact that the test is also positive in *S. pneumoniae* carriage without infection, as is often observed among infants (32), it is of limited value in pediatric patients. The test should not be used for children below the age of 6 years (32), and comprehensive studies on schoolchildren with lower colonization rates have not been performed. It can currently only be recommended in adults as an addition to conventional diagnostic culture techniques for *S. pneumoniae* (75) and is probably most helpful for patients who received antimicrobial treatment before cultures were obtained.

Streptococcal Antigen Detection in CSF

Commercially available antigen detection tests for the diagnosis of pathogenic microorganisms in CSF samples include reagents for the detection of *S. agalactiae* and *S. pneumoniae*. These tests have also been used on positive blood culture specimens. The tests are not recommended for routine use, as the results should not be used to change decisions about empiric therapy based on clinical and laboratory criteria (116). It has also been shown that the sensitivity of direct antigen detection in CSF is low (<30%) and offers no advantage over a conventional cytospun Gram stain (78). However, very promising results have been published for the use of the *S. pneumoniae* urinary antigen test on CSF samples (81).

Nucleic Acid Detection Techniques

S. pyogenes

A rapid method for the detection of *S. pyogenes* in pharyngeal specimens is based on a single-stranded chemiluminescent nucleic acid probe assay to identify specific rRNA sequences (Group A Streptococcus Direct Test; Gen-Probe, Inc., San Diego, CA). This test performed well in comparative studies with the culture technique. Sensitivity and specificity for the probe test ranged from 89% to 95% and 98% to 100%, respectively, compared to the results of the culture technique with a sensitivity of 98% to 99% (21, 92). These data suggest that the probe test may be suitable as a primary test or as a backup test to negative antigen tests, particularly for batch screening of throat cultures. Moreover, a real-time PCR assay (LightCycler Strep A assay; Roche Diagnostics, Indianapolis, IN) has been recently developed for the detection of *S. pyogenes* in throat swabs (119). Real-time PCR proved to be more sensitive than the standard culture method (119), and it appears to be unnecessary to perform cultures when results of the real-time PCR are negative. Real-time PCR allows the detection of beta-hemolytic species *S. pyogenes* and *S. dysgalactiae* subsp. *equisimilis*.

S. agalactiae

A rapid method for the detection of *S. agalactiae* colonization in pregnant women at the time of the delivery has recently been developed and evaluated (11). The test is based on the detection of the *S. agalactiae cfb* gene (91) by a fluorogenic real-time PCR assay (BD GeneOhm StrepB; Becton Dickinson, Sparks, MD), and results can be obtained in a few hours with a reported sensitivity of 94% and specificity of 95.9% (27). The test has been evaluated and approved by the FDA for rectal/vaginal swabs. It is commercially available and performed well in a multicenter evaluation study (27). A novel FDA-cleared automated test for PCR detection is the GBS GeneXpert test from Cepheid (Sunnyvale, CA), which proved to be highly sensitive but not very specific (less than 65%) in clinical evaluation (44). Both tests are performed directly on clinical samples. While the costs are exceedingly higher than selective culture, a major advantage is that results may be available within a short time frame, and vaginal colonization status can be assessed at the time of delivery. In comparison with the gold standard of antenatal selective broth culture, as recommended by the CDC, the tests may offer alternatives for the future. Nevertheless, it has to be kept in mind that PCR tests performed at the time of delivery have the major problem that despite rapid performance time, time to delivery is often too short to allow effective administration of peripartum antibiotics, if needed.

S. pneumoniae

Several different PCR assays have been developed for the identification of S. pneumoniae from culture isolates. Tests are based on the detection of the genes for autolysin lytA, the pneumococcal surface antigen psaA, and the pneumolysin gene ply. Comparison of the ability to distinguish difficult-to-identify S. pneumoniae strains and closely related atypical streptococci revealed that the lytA-based PCR was the most specific method (79). A novel and improved PCR for the detection of lytA has recently been evaluated, confirming these results (18). While results based on the detection of psaA are also acceptable, the different pneumolysin-targeted methods appear to be relatively nonspecific. So far these assays are not commercially available and have to be established as "in-house" PCRs. Nucleic acid probes for the detection of cultured isolates of S. pneumoniae are commercially available (AccuProbe; GenProbe, San Diego, CA) (28). Detection relies on hybridization of a specific probe to 16S rRNA sequences but fails to distinguish S. pseudopneumoniae from S. pneumoniae. These tests are not routinely performed for standard identification procedures but can aid in the identification of atypical S. pneumoniae isolates with unusual patterns of bile solubility and optochin susceptibility.

ISOLATION PROCEDURES

General Procedures

Streptococci are usually grown on blood agar media because the assessment of the hemolytic reaction is important for identification. Growth of streptococci is often enhanced in the presence of an exogenous catalase source. Streptococcal species with low or absent hydrogen peroxide production, such as S. agalactiae, can be grown on other commonly used nonselective media without blood.

Agar media selective for gram-positive bacteria (e.g., phenylethyl alcohol-containing agar or Columbia agar with colistin and nalidixic acid) support the growth of streptococci. The optimal incubation temperature range for most streptococcal species lies between 35°C and 37°C. Supplemental carbon dioxide (5% CO_2) or anaerobic conditions enhance the growth of many streptococcal species since streptococci are facultative anaerobes. Although some streptococci grow well in ambient air, incubation in 5% CO_2 is recommended for the culture of S. pneumoniae and other streptococcal species of the viridans group.

Special Procedures for Streptococcus pyogenes Throat Cultures

A properly performed and interpreted throat culture on a 5% sheep agar with trypticase soy base incubated in air remains the gold standard for the diagnosis of S. pyogenes acute pharyngitis (85). The isolation of only a few colonies of S. pyogenes does not allow the differentiation between a carrier and an acutely infected individual and may reflect inadequate specimen collection (12). Lack of hemolysis, overgrowth, and production of toxic bacterial metabolites by nonpathogenic organisms of the upper respiratory tract microbiota or depletion of substrates often leads to false-negative results or delays caused by labor-intensive reisolation steps. In order to enhance S. pyogenes isolation, numerous studies analyzed incubation conditions in anaerobic or CO_2-enriched atmosphere as well as different media selective for beta-hemolytic streptococci (63, 72, 126). Due to cost restraints and an uncertain benefit, these additional efforts are not generally recommended. After 18 to 24 h of incubation, culture plates should be examined for growth of beta-hemolytic colonies. Negative cultures should be reexamined after an additional 24-h incubation period. Presumptive identification of S. pyogenes can be achieved by susceptibility to bacitracin or testing for PYR activity. Other beta-hemolytic streptococci are occasionally positive in one of these tests, but not in both. Definitive diagnosis includes the demonstration of the Lancefield group A antigen by immunoassay. Although other species may rarely possess the group A antigen (Table 1), they lack PYR activity (36).

Special Procedures for Streptococcus agalactiae Screening

Early-onset neonatal GBS (S. agalactiae) infections can be prevented by administration of antibiotic prophylaxis during delivery (105). An essential requirement for efficient prophylaxis is the reliable detection of colonization with S. agalactiae in pregnant women before delivery. Screening should be performed between weeks 35 and 37 of pregnancy. A lower vaginal and a rectal swab (i.e., insertion of a swab through the anal sphincter) should be obtained either with one or two different swabs and placed in appropriate transport medium (Amies or Stuart's medium without charcoal; see chapter 16). While culture counts decline to some extent, viability of S. agalactiae is preserved in transport medium kept at room temperature or 4°C for up to 4 days. To reduce costs, vaginal and rectal swabs can be placed in a single transport medium tube and cultured together. Swabs should be cultured in selective broth medium for 18 to 24 hours at 35 to 37°C in ambient air or 5% CO_2 and subsequently plated on tryptic soy agar (TSA) blood agar plates or S. agalactiae selective agar medium. Selective broth medium is commercially available (Trans-Vag broth supplemented with 5% sheep blood [Remel Inc., Lenexa, KS] or LIM broth [BBL Microbiology Systems, Cockeysville, MD]). Selective broth can also be prepared by supplementation of THB with nalidixic acid (15 μg/ml) and colistin (10 μg/ml) or by supplementation of THB with nalidixic acid (15 μg/ml) and gentamicin (8 μg/ml). TSA blood agar plates should be checked for typical colonies (narrow zone of beta-hemolysis) of S. agalactiae after 24 and 48 hours of incubation at 35 to 37°C. Identification of S. agalactiae is then achieved by standard techniques as described below. Selective media relying on the detection of the orange S. agalactiae pigment (Granada medium or StrepB Carrot broth [Hardy Diagnostics, Santa Maria, CA] or GBS broth [Northeast Laboratory Services, Waterville, ME]) are highly specific and sensitive (100, 123). Subculture of enrichment broth on Granada medium enhances sensitivity and obviates the need for further identification steps due to excellent specificity, but nonhemolytic strains cannot be detected with pigment-dependent selective media. PCR-based detection of S. agalactiae following overnight enrichment broth increases sensitivity and detection time in comparison to conventional selective culture (14). For the identification of questionable cultured strains as S. agalactiae, a 16S RNA-based nucleic acid detection test (AccuProbe; GenProbe, San Diego, CA) can be helpful. However, all of the nucleic acid-based detection techniques are more expensive than conventional enrichment culture.

IDENTIFICATION

Description of Colonies

Colonies of streptococci usually appear gray or almost white with moist or glistening features. Dry colonies are rarely encountered. Colony size varies among the different beta-hemolytic species and helps to distinguish groups of streptococci. Beta-hemolytic streptococci of the pyogenic group (S. pyogenes, S. agalactiae, and S. dysgalactiae subsp. equisimilis) form colonies of >0.5 mm after 24 hours of incubation, in contrast to the beta-hemolytic strains of the S. anginosus group (formerly called "S. milleri" group), which present with pinpoint colonies of ≤0.5 mm after the same incubation time (Fig. 1). Members of the S. anginosus group emit a distinct odor resembling butterscotch or caramel,

presumably due to the production of diacetyl by the species belonging to this group. Among the beta-hemolytic species of the pyogenic group, S. agalactiae produces the largest colonies with a relatively small zone of hemolysis. Nonhemolytic S. agalactiae strains do occur and resemble enterococci.

Within the group of alpha-hemolytic streptococci, S. pneumoniae has a colony morphology that helps to distinguish pneumococcal isolates from other streptococci of the viridans group. Due to the production of capsular polysaccharide, colonies glisten and appear moist. Colonies may be large and mucoid if large amounts of capsular polysaccharide are made, a feature often encountered in serotype 3 strains. This phenotype is usually typical for S. pneumoniae but can also occasionally be observed in S. pyogenes. Another characteristic feature of

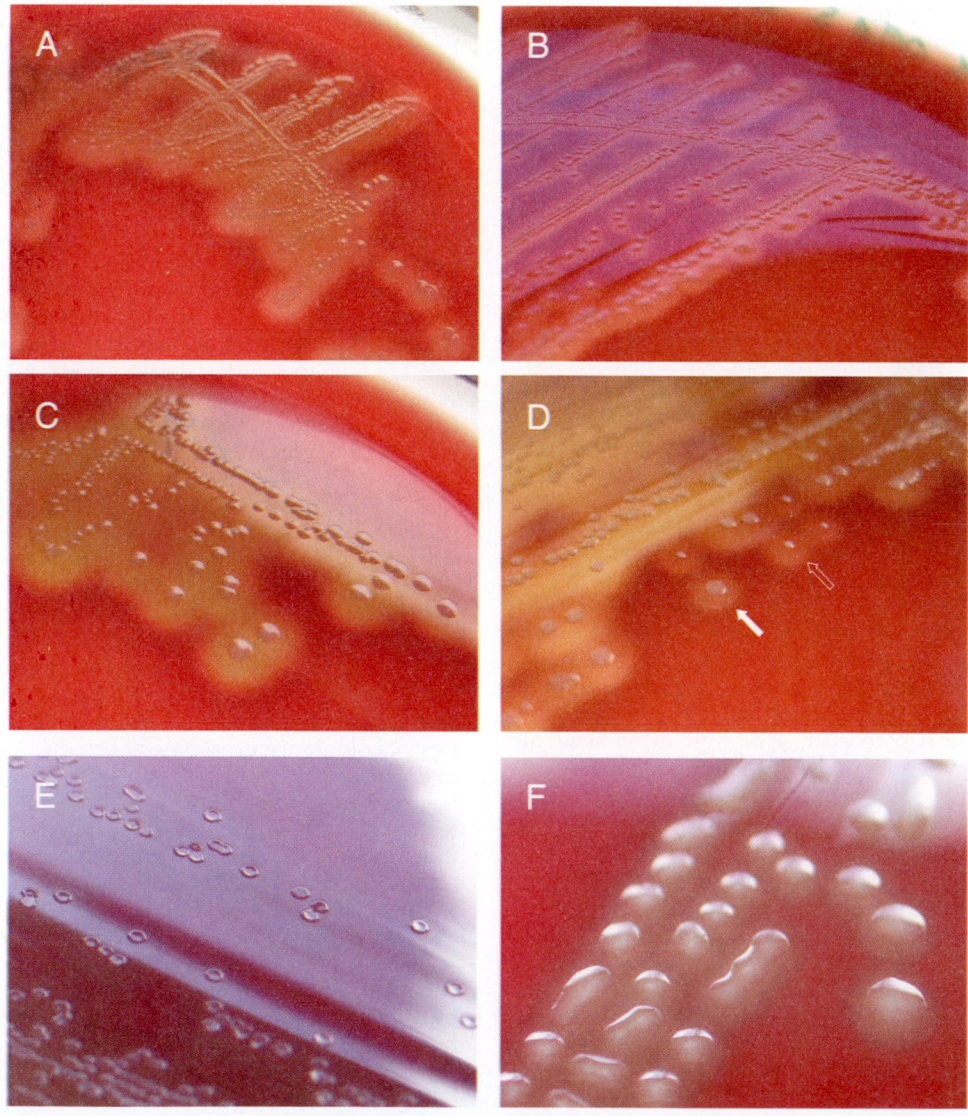

FIGURE 1 Colony morphology of selected streptococci. (A) S. pyogenes strain ATCC12344; (B) clinical isolate of S. agalactiae; (C) clinical isolate of S. dysgalactiae subsp. equisimilis (Lancefield group G); (D) mixed culture of S. anginosus (ATCC12395, open arrow) and clinical isolate of S. dysgalactiae subsp. equisimilis (closed arrow) (note the difference in colony size); (E) clinical isolate of S. pneumoniae (note the central depression of the colonies); (F) clinical isolate of S. pneumoniae (note the mucoid appearance of colonies).

S. pneumoniae is the central navel-like depression of the colonies that is caused by the pneumococcal autolysin. Other viridans group streptococci lack this feature and have a dome-like appearance; however, up to 20% of *S. pneumoniae* strains display a phenotype that is indistinguishable from that of viridans group streptococci (98). Nonhemolytic gray colonies are typical for species of the *S. bovis* and *S. salivarius* groups. Typical streptococcal colony morphologies are presented in Fig. 1.

Identification of Beta-Hemolytic Streptococci by Lancefield Antigen Immunoassays

Commercially available Lancefield antigen grouping sera are primarily used for the differentiation of beta-hemolytic streptococci. Products for rapid antigen extraction and subsequent agglutination can be obtained from many different suppliers. The presence of the Lancefield group B antigen in beta-hemolytic isolates from human clinical specimens correlates with the species *S. agalactiae*. Similarly, the detection of the Lancefield group F antigen in small-colony-forming streptococci from human clinical material allows a fairly reliable identification of a strain as a member of the *S. anginosus* group. The presence of Lancefield group A, C, or G antigens necessitates further testing (Table 1). Beta-hemolytic streptococcal strains not reacting with any of the Lancefield antisera are rare and should be further identified by phenotypic tests or nucleic acid detection techniques.

Identification of Beta-Hemolytic Streptococci by Phenotypic Tests

A number of streptococcal identification products incorporating batteries of physiologic tests are commercially available (see chapters 3 and 17). In general, these products perform well with commonly isolated pathogenic streptococci but may lack accuracy for identifying streptococci of the viridans group. For the bulk of pathogenic streptococci isolated in clinical laboratories (e.g., *S. pyogenes*, *S. agalactiae*, and *S. pneumoniae*), serologic or presumptive physiologic tests (as described below) offer an acceptable alternative to commercially available identification systems.

PYR Test

The presence of the enzyme PYR is often tested to distinguish *S. pyogenes* from other beta-hemolytic streptococci. Hydrolysis of L-pyrrolidonyl-β-naphthylamide by the enzyme to β-naphthylamide produces a red color with the addition of cinnamaldehyde reagent (chapter 17). The beta-hemolytic streptococcal species *S. iniae* and *S. porcinus* can be PYR positive but are only rarely identified in human clinical specimens, since they are primarily animal-associated species. PYR spot tests are commercially available. It is important to distinguish *Streptococcus* from *Enterococcus* prior to PYR testing, and strains of other related genera may be PYR positive (including the genera *Abiotrophia*, *Aerococcus*, *Enterococcus*, *Gemella*, and *Lactococcus*). However, PYR-positive beta-hemolytic enterococcal isolates typically present with a different colonial morphology (smaller zone of beta-hemolysis and bigger colony size) and when combined with other phenotypic characteristics (see chapter 21) may be distinguished from streptococci. To avoid false-positive reactions caused by other PYR-positive bacterial species (for example, staphylococci), the test should be performed on pure cultures only.

Bacitracin Susceptibility

With rare exceptions, *S. pyogenes* displays bacitracin susceptibility, in contrast to other human beta-hemolytic streptococci.

Together with Lancefield antigen determination, it can be used for the identification of *S. pyogenes* since beta-hemolytic strains of other streptococcal species that may contain the group A antigen are bacitracin resistant. The test can also be used to distinguish *S. pyogenes* from other PYR-positive beta-hemolytic streptococci (*S. iniae* and *S. porcinus*). A bacitracin disk (0.04 U) is applied to a sheep blood agar plate that has been heavily inoculated with three or four colonies of a pure culture of the strain to be tested. It is important to perform the test from a subculture on sheep blood agar, since placement of bacitracin disks on primary plates is not sensitive enough. After overnight incubation at 35°C in 5% CO$_2$, any zone of inhibition around the disk is interpreted as indicating susceptibility. Importantly, bacitracin-resistant *S. pyogenes* isolates have been reported, and clusters of bacitracin-resistant strains were observed in several European countries (74, 80, 90).

VP Test

The Voges-Proskauer (VP) test detects the formation of acetoin from glucose fermentation. It is performed on streptococci as a modification of the classical VP reaction that is used for the differentiation of enteric bacteria. Small-colony-forming beta-hemolytic streptococci of the *S. anginosus* group that are VP positive may be distinguished from large colony-forming beta-hemolytic streptococci harboring identical Lancefield antigens (A, C, or G). Streptococci of the *S. mitis* group are VP negative. For the modified VP reaction described by Facklam and Washington in the fifth edition of this *Manual* (40a), the culture growth of an entire agar plate is used to inoculate 2 ml of VP broth and incubated at 35°C for 6 hours. Following the addition of 5% α-naphthol and 40% KOH, the tube is shaken vigorously for a few seconds and incubated at room temperature for 30 min. A positive test yields a pink-red color that results from the reaction of diacetyl with guanidine.

BGUR Test

Detection of β-glucuronidase (BGUR) activity distinguishes *S. dysgalactiae* subsp. *equisimilis* strains containing Lancefield group antigens C or G from BGUR-negative, small-colony-forming streptococci of the *S. anginosus* group with the same Lancefield group antigens. Rapid methods for the BGUR test are commercially available. Alternatively, a rapid fluorogenic assay with methylumbelliferyl-β-D-glucuronide (MUG)-containing MacConkey agar, often used for *Escherichia coli*, has been described (68).

CAMP Test

The CAMP factor reaction was first described in 1944 by Christie, Atkins, and Munch-Petersen and refers to the synergistic lysis of erythrocytes by the beta-hemolysin of *Staphylococcus aureus* and the extracellular CFB protein of *S. agalactiae*. The gene and its expression can be demonstrated in the vast majority (>98%) of *S. agalactiae* isolates, but CAMP-negative mutants do occur. The strain to be tested and a *Staphylococcus aureus* strain (ATCC 25923) are streaked onto a sheep blood agar plate at a 90° angle. Plates are incubated in ambient air overnight at 36 ± 1°C. A positive reaction can be detected by the presence of a triangular zone of enhanced beta-hemolysis in the diffusion zone of the beta-hemolysin of *S. aureus* and the CAMP factor (Fig. 2). CAMP factor-positive strains can also be detected by a method using beta-lysin containing disks (Remel) or by a rapid CAMP factor spot method (96). Despite the fact that close homologs of the CAMP factor gene are present in many *S. pyogenes* strains, most beta-hemolytic streptococci other

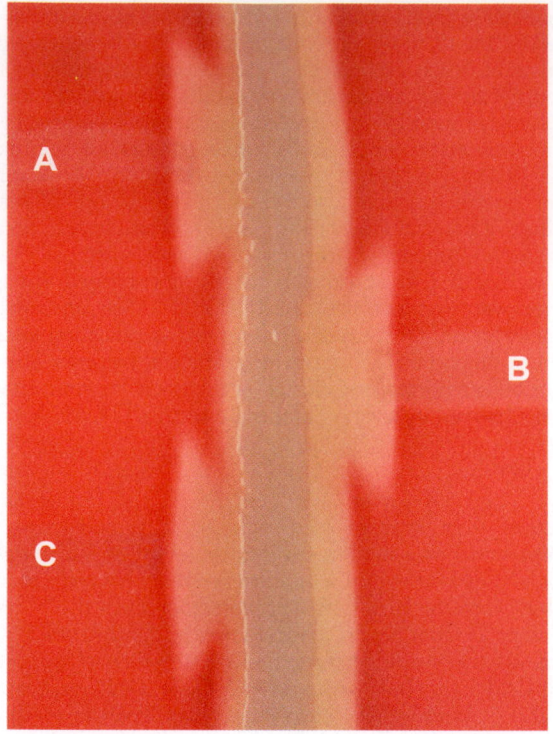

FIGURE 2 CAMP factor test. An arrowhead-shaped zone of hemolysis in the zone of the *S. aureus* beta-hemolysin is shown. (A) Clinical isolate of a weakly beta-hemolytic *S. agalactiae* strain. (B) Beta-hemolytic *S. agalactiae* strain O90R. (C) Nonhemolytic *S. agalactiae* strain R268.

than *S. agalactiae* are negative in the above-described CAMP factor test, except for the rare human isolates of *S. iniae*, *S. porcinus*, and *S. pseudoporcinus*. Several gram-positive rods including corynebacteria and *Listeria monocytogenes* strains may also be CAMP factor positive.

Hippurate Hydrolysis Test

The ability to hydrolyze hippurate is an alternative test for the presumptive identification of *S. agalactiae*. A rapid version of the test, as it is used for campylobacters, can be performed by incubating a turbid suspension of bacterial cells in 0.5 ml of 1% aqueous sodium hippurate for 2 h at 35°C. Glycine formed as an end product of hippurate hydrolysis is detected by adding ninhydrin reagent and observing the development of a deep purple color, signifying a positive test (chapter 17) (55). Streptococci other than *S. agalactiae* may also be hippurate hydrolysis positive, especially viridans group streptococci.

Identification of *S. pneumoniae* and Viridans Group Streptococci

The correct species identification of viridans group streptococci other than *S. pneumoniae* is challenging. Recent taxonomic changes and identification of novel streptococcal species have further complicated matters. The number of recognized species in this group is now greater than 30. The viridans group includes alpha-hemolytic, nonhemolytic (*S. salivarius* group and *S. bovis* group), and beta-hemolytic (*S. anginosus* group) streptococcal strains. All of the viridans group streptococci are LAP positive and PYR negative. Conventional microbiologic tests are limited with respect to species identification but are helpful in placing isolates into the correct streptococcal groups (Table 2). Beighton et al. described an identification scheme based on phenotypic tests that allowed the differentiation and correct species identification of the majority of viridans group species (7). The scheme requires the evaluation of enzymatic reactions performed by in-house fluorogenic tests that are not commercially available. Importantly, most clinical laboratories must strive for group, instead of species, classifications with current phenotypic test panels.

The API tests (bioMerieux, Marcy l'Etoile, France) offer species identification of viridans group streptococci. While many species from this group are identified with acceptable accuracy, several species have not been included in the database. Comparisons of molecular species identification by DNA reassociation studies with the results of the API Rapid ID 32 Strep system showed that more than 85% of 156 strains from streptococcal species included in the database were correctly identified (64). However, in the same study, more than 50% of six species not included in the database were incorrectly identified by the test (64). Evaluation studies performed under routine clinical conditions appear to yield less favorable results (47). In a recent evaluation of the Vitek 2 (bioMerieux) automated phenotypic identification

TABLE 2 Phenotypic characteristics of major streptococcal groups[a]

Streptococcal group	Arginine hydrolysis	Esculin	Mannitol	Sorbitol	Urea hydrolysis	VP
S. mitis[b]	v	v	−	v	−	−
S. anginosus[c]	+	+	−	−	−	+
S. mutans[d]	−	+	+	+	−	+
S. salivarius[e]	−	v	−	−	v	+
S. bovis[f]	−	v	v	−	−	+

[a]Symbols and abbreviations: +, positive; −, negative; v, variable.
[b]This group comprises the species *S. mitis*, *S. sanguinis*, *S. parasanguinis*, *S. gordonii*, *S. cristatus*, *S. oralis*, *S. infantis*, *S. peroris*, *S. australis*, *S. sinensis*, *S. orisratti*, *S. oligofermentans*, *S. massiliensis*. *S. sanguinis*, *S. parasanguinis*, *S. gordonii*, and *S. cristatus* are arginine hydrolysis positive; other species from the *S. mitis* group are arginine hydrolysis negative.
[c]*S. anginosus*, *S. constellatus*, and *S. intermedius* belong to the *S. anginosus* group.
[d]The *S. mutans* group includes *S. mutans*, *S. sobrinus*, and the following species rarely isolated from humans: *S. criceti*, *S. ratti*, and *S. downei*.
[e]The *S. salivarius* group contains *S. salivarius*, *S. vestibularis*, and *S. thermophilus*. *S. salivarius* is variable, *S. vestibularis* is positive, and *S. thermophilus* is negative for urea hydrolysis.
[f]The *S. bovis* group now includes *S. equinus*, *S. gallolyticus*, *S. infantarius*, and *S. alactolyticus*. *S. gallolyticus* subsp. *gallolyticus* is positive for the acidification of mannitol; the other species from the *S. bovis* group are negative.

system, streptococcal group assignment for 75% of isolates was concordant with 16S rRNA gene sequencing data (51). In conclusion, phenotypic identification of viridans group streptococci remains difficult and acceptable results can currently be achieved at the group level only.

Molecular methods may offer alternative approaches to conventional phenotypic identification schemes. The most common molecular identification method, 16S rRNA gene sequencing, does not yield reliable species identification for several species including *S. mitis*, *S. oralis*, and *S. pneumoniae*. The 16S rRNA gene sequences are more than 99% identical (59). Whole-cell protein analyses were unable to yield good correlation with species identification by other methods. Sequence determination of the manganese-dependent superoxide dismutase gene *sodA* appears promising (94). In contrast to 16S rRNA sequencing, it allows the differentiation of *S. mitis*, *S. oralis*, and *S. pneumoniae* and the correct identification of almost 30 different streptococcal species including 16 species from the viridans group.

Descriptions of the species belonging to the nonpyogenic groups are given below. Physiological traits of the groups are shown in Table 2.

S. mitis Group

The large number of different streptococcal species belonging to the *S. mitis* group has been mentioned earlier. This group of predominantly alpha-hemolytic streptococci includes several species of known clinical significance together with others for which few or no clinical data have been collected. Among the phenotypic characteristics of the species in this group, extracellular polysaccharide production is negative for *S. mitis* strains but a variable characteristic of *S. oralis* isolates. This feature correlates with the smooth colony surface of many *S. oralis* strains and the rough and dry appearance of *S. mitis* colonies.

S. anginosus Group

The small-colony-forming species *S. anginosus*, *S. constellatus*, and *S. intermedius* belong to the *S. anginosus* group. Strains of the *S. anginosus* group may be non-, alpha-, or beta-hemolytic on blood agar plates with some variations among the species. While *S. constellatus* is frequently beta-hemolytic, most isolates of *S. intermedius* are nonhemolytic. For many strains, growth is enhanced in the presence of CO_2, with some strains requiring anaerobic conditions. *S. anginosus* and *S. constellatus* strains may possess Lancefield group antigens A, C, F, or G. Most *S. constellatus* or *S. intermedius* strains react with antisera against Lancefield group F antigen or are nongroupable.

The species *S. constellatus* has been further subdivided into two subspecies, *S. constellatus* subsp. *constellatus* and *S. constellatus* subsp. *pharyngis* (130). *S. constellatus* subsp. *constellatus* is phenotypically different from *S. constellatus* subsp. *pharyngis*, which usually possesses the Lancefield group antigen C, is beta-hemolytic, and has been associated with pharyngitis. Detailed phenotypic characteristics of the *S. anginosus* group are shown in Table 3 (36, 113, 129).

S. mutans Group

The *S. mutans* group includes *S. mutans*, *S. sobrinus*, *S. criceti*, *S. ratti*, *S. downei*, *S. ferus*, *S. hyovaginalis*, *S. devriesei*, and *S. macacae*. *S. mutans* and *S. sobrinus* are frequently found in human hosts, while the other species are only rarely encountered in humans or represent animal pathogens. The species of the *S. mutans* group are characterized by the production of extracellular polysaccharides from sucrose, which can be tested by culturing the bacteria on sucrose-containing agar and by the ability to produce acid from a relatively wide range of carbohydrates. *S. mutans* strains may present with an atypical morphology for streptococci, forming short rods on solid media or in broth culture under acidic conditions. On blood agar, colonies are often hard, adherent, and usually alpha-hemolytic. Under anaerobic growth conditions, some strains are beta-hemolytic. *S. sobrinus* strains are mostly nonhemolytic or occasionally alpha-hemolytic. On sucrose-containing agar, species from this group form colonies that are rough (frosted glass appearance), heaped, and surrounded by liquid-containing glucan.

TABLE 3 Phenotypic characteristics of streptococcal species of the *S. anginosus* group[a]

Test	*S. anginosus*	*S. constellatus*[b]	*S. intermedius*
β-D-Fucosidase	−	−	+
β-N-Acetylglucosaminidase	−	−	+
β-N-Acetylgalactosaminidase	−	−	+
Neuraminidase	−	−	+
α-D-Glucosidase	v	+	+
β-D-Glucosidase	+	−	v
β-D-Galactosidase	v	−	+
Amygdalin (acidification)	+	v	v
Mannitol (acidification)	v	−	−
Sorbitol (acidification)	−	−	−
Lactose (acidification)	+	v	+
Arginine hydrolysis	+	+	+
Esculin hydrolysis	+	v	+
VP[c]	+	+	+
Urease	−	−	−

[a]Symbols and abbreviations: +, positive; −, negative; v, variable. Data are from Summanen et al. (113), Facklam (36), and Whiley et al. (129).
[b]The species *S. constellatus* subsp. *pharyngis* is β-D-fucosidase, β-D-acetylglucosaminidase, β-D-acetylgalactosaminidase, and β-D-glucosidase positive, in contrast to *S. constellatus* subsp. *constellatus*, which is negative for these activities.
[c]Voges-Proskauer test (formation of acetoin from glucose fermentation).

S. salivarius Group

Streptococcal species in the *S. salivarius* group are *S. salivarius*, *S. vestibularis*, and *S. thermophilus*. *S. salivarius* strains are usually non- or alpha-hemolytic on blood agar. On sucrose-containing agar, strains form large mucoid or hard colonies due to the production of extracellular polysaccharides. A high proportion of *S. salivarius* strains react with the Lancefield group K antiserum. Species in this group may also react with the streptococcal group D antiserum. It is unclear if these strains truly possess the group D antigen or yield a nonspecific cross-reaction. *S. vestibularis* is alpha-hemolytic, and the failure of this species to produce extracellular polysaccharides on sucrose-containing agar is helpful in distinguishing *S. vestibularis* from *S. salivarius* strains. *S. thermophilus* is found in dairy products but has not been isolated from clinical specimens.

S. bovis Group

The species belonging to the *S. bovis* group (*S. equinus*, *S. gallolyticus*, *S. infantarius*, and *S. alactolyticus*) are nonenterococcal group D streptococci that are PYR negative. Most strains grow on bile esculin agar and are unable to grow in 6.5% NaCl. On blood agar, strains are either non-hemolytic or alpha-hemolytic. Strains of the *S. bovis* group share phenotypic characteristics with *S. mutans* strains, such as production of glucan, fermentation of mannitol, and growth on bile esculin agar. However, the *S. bovis* group does not ferment sorbitol. *S. gallolyticus* subsp. *gallolyticus* and *S. infantarius* subsp. *coli* typically ferment starch or glycogen and give a Lancefield group D reaction, in contrast to *S. gallolyticus* subsp. *pasteurianus*. A detailed phenotypic characterization and emended description of the different subspecies have recently been published (6). For the identification of species in this group, testing of BGUR, α- and β-galactosidase, β-mannosidase, acid production from starch, glycogen, inulin, and mannitol is helpful. As described earlier, strains formerly known as *S. bovis* currently belong to several species of the *S. bovis* group.

Physiologic Tests

Optochin Test

Most *S. pneumoniae* isolates are optochin susceptible. Before application of the optochin disk, several colonies of a pure culture are streaked onto a sheep blood agar plate. Optochin testing should be performed on plates that are incubated at 35 to 36°C overnight in 5% CO_2 because up to 8% of strains will not grow under ambient conditions. *S. pneumoniae* isolates show zones of inhibition of ≥14 mm with a 6-mm-diameter disk (containing 5 μg of optochin) and zones of inhibition of ≥16 mm with a 10-mm-diameter disk. Incubation in 5% CO_2 yielded increased specificity (1, 98). Optochin-resistant *S. pneumoniae* strains have been reported as well as optochin-susceptible *S. mitis* isolates (especially when tested under ambient conditions). Since optochin testing may miss between 4% and 11% of bile-soluble *S. pneumoniae* isolates (1, 98), strains displaying a smaller zone of inhibition (9 to 13 mm for the 6-mm-diameter disk) should be subjected to additional testing (e.g., bile solubility and genetic testing) to confirm species identification.

Application of an optochin disk onto the primary culture medium may facilitate a rapid presumptive identification but may miss pneumococcal isolates in a mixed culture. The optochin susceptibility test should be repeated with a pure culture in cases of mixed cultures, or additional tests should be performed (e.g., bile solubility).

Bile Solubility Test

Bile solubility can be performed either in a test tube or by direct application of the reagent to an agar plate. For the test tube method, a saline suspension of a pure culture is adjusted to a McFarland standard of 0.5 to 1.0, and 0.5 ml of the suspension is added to a small tube. The bacterial suspension is mixed with 0.5 ml of 10% sodium deoxycholate (bile) and incubated at 35°C. A control containing 0.5 ml of bacterial suspension with 0.5 ml of saline should be prepared for each strain tested. A positive result is characterized by clearing of the bile suspension within 3 hours. Clearing can start as early as 5 to 15 min after inoculation and allows the identification of a strain as *S. pneumoniae*. For the plate method, one drop of 10% sodium deoxycholate is placed directly onto a colony of the strain in question and incubated at 35°C for 15 to 30 min in ambient air. It is important to keep the plates in a horizontal position in order to prevent the reagent from washing away the colony. Colonies of *S. pneumoniae* will disappear or demonstrate a flattened colony morphology, while other viridans group streptococci will appear unchanged. In contrast to optochin susceptibility, bile solubility testing demonstrated excellent sensitivity and specificity in a recent comprehensive evaluation (98).

Bile Esculin Test

Bile esculin medium (available from commercial sources) in either plates or slants should be inoculated with one to three colonies of the organism to be tested and incubated at 35°C in ambient air for up to 48 h. Optimal results can be achieved by using media supplemented with 4% oxgall (equivalent of 40% bile) (Remel, Lenexa, KS) and a standardized inoculum of 10^6 CFU (22). A definitive blackening of plated media or blackening of at least one-half of an agar slant is considered a positive test, indicative of species belonging to the *S. bovis* group or enterococci. Occasional other viridans group streptococci are positive with this test or display weakly positive reactions that are difficult to interpret. Isolates from patients with serious infections (e.g., endocarditis) should be more completely characterized.

Arginine Hydrolysis

Arginine hydrolysis is a key reaction for the identification of viridans group streptococci. Discrepancies can occur among test methods (127). Two commonly used methods are detailed here. Moeller's decarboxylase broth containing arginine (Becton Dickinson, Sparks, MD, and other sources) should be inoculated with the test organism, overlaid with mineral oil, and incubated at 35 to 37°C for up to 7 days. Degradation of arginine results in elevated pH, indicated by development of a purple color. Negative results are indicated by a yellow color, which is due to acid accumulation from metabolism of glucose only. For the microtiter plate method (7), three drops of the arginine-containing reagent are inoculated with 1 drop of an overnight THB culture and incubated for 24 h at 37°C anaerobically. Production of ammonia is detected by the appearance of an orange color following addition of 1 drop of Nessler's reagent.

Urea Hydrolysis

Christensen urea agar (Becton Dickinson and other sources) is inoculated and incubated aerobically at 35°C for up to 7 days. Development of a pink color indicates a positive reaction. An alternative format is to dispense Christensen's medium without agar into a microtiter tray well and, after inoculation, overlay it with mineral oil prior to incubation.

VP Test

The VP test can be performed as described above for the identification of beta-hemolytic streptococci. A standard method for performing the VP test, requiring extended incubation, is described in chapter 17.

Esculin Hydrolysis

Esculin agar slants (Becton Dickinson and other sources) are inoculated and incubated for up to 1 week. A positive reaction appears as a blackening of the medium; no change in color indicates a negative esculin hydrolysis test.

Hyaluronidase Production

Hyaluronidase activity can be detected on brain heart infusion agar plates supplemented with 2 mg/liter of sodium hyaluronate (Sigma-Aldrich, St. Louis, MO). The strains to be tested are inoculated by stabbing into the agar, and plates are incubated anaerobically at 37°C overnight. After the plate is flooded with 2 M acetic acid, hyaluronidase activity is indicated by the appearance of a clear zone around the stab. A quantitative method for determining hyaluronidase activity can be performed in microtiter trays (54).

Production of Extracellular Polysaccharide

Strains may be isolated as single colonies on sucrose-containing agar. The two most commonly used media are (i) mitis-salivarius agar containing 0.001% (wt/vol) potassium tellurite (Becton Dickinson) and (ii) tryptone-yeast-cystine agar (Lab M, Bury, United Kingdom). Incubation may require up to 5 days at 37°C under anaerobic incubation conditions.

TYPING SYSTEMS

In the majority of cases, typing of streptococci has no immediate clinical or therapeutic consequences. It is most often performed by reference laboratories for the purposes of epidemiologic studies and the evaluation of vaccine efficacy. Although classical antibody-dependent typing systems for capsular serotypes and surface proteins have been used for years, molecular methods have become attractive, since they do not require special techniques or the maintenance of rarely used reagents such as a large antibody panel. Another advantage is the independence of DNA sequences from culture conditions and gene expression. For the differentiation of distinct clones, pulsed-field gel electrophoresis (PFGE) and multilocus sequence typing (MLST) systems have been established for many streptococcal species (34).

S. pneumoniae comprises more than 90 antigenically distinct capsular serotypes that can be detected by the Neufeld test (Quellung reaction), which is still regarded as the gold standard for epidemiologic studies. Pure cultures of pneumococci are grown on a freshly prepared 5% sheep blood agar plate or a 10% horse blood agar plate at 35°C to 37°C and 5% CO_2 for 18 to 24 hours. A small amount of bacterial growth (less than a 10-μl loop) is resuspended in a droplet of phosphate-buffered or physiological saline (McFarland standard of approximately 0.5). A few microliters of the saline suspension is mixed with an equal amount of specific pneumococcal rabbit antisera on a glass slide. The specimen is subsequently evaluated for capsular swelling (a clear area surrounding the bacterial cells) by phase-contrast microscopy (×1,000 magnification; oil immersion) (2). The reaction is stable for approximately 30 min. Best results are achieved when 10 to 50 bacterial cells are visible per high-power (×1,000) microscopic field. To increase visibility

of the result, it is possible to add 0.3% aqueous methylene blue in the same amount as the antiserum to the mixture. Following the same principle, commercially available kits (Pneumotest Statens Serum Institut, Copenhagen, Denmark) allow rapid testing of S. pneumoniae serotypes with pooled antisera by a checkerboard method. A rapid antigen detection test using pooled antisera coupled to latex beads (Statens Serum Institut) has been developed (110). Due to strain discrepancies, confirmation by Neufeld Quellung reaction is recommended. For the distinction of single clones, PFGE (73) or MLST typing schemes (34) have been used in pneumococcal investigations.

Ten different antibody-defined capsular polysaccharides have been described for S. agalactiae (Ia, Ib, and II through IX). The percentage of nontypeable strains can be minimized by optimization of capsular expression (10). In addition to antibody detection of capsular serotypes, PCR- and DNA sequencing-based techniques allow the detection of capsular serotypes (71, 95). Individual clones of S. agalactiae have been detected either by MLST (57) or by PFGE (9).

Conventional typing of S. pyogenes is based upon the antigenic specificity of the surface-expressed T and M proteins (56). The trypsin-resistant T protein is part of the recently discovered pilus structures (82). The T type can be identified by agglutination with commercially available serologic assays utilizing approximately 20 accepted anti-T sera. M proteins are major antiphagocytic virulence factors of S. pyogenes (42). N-terminal sequence variation in genes encoding these highly protective antigens is the basis of the S. pyogenes precipitation typing system. At present, 83 M serotypes are unequivocally validated and internationally recognized to be serologically unique and are designated M1 to M93 in the Lancefield classification (39). M serotypes that are not included are from non-S. pyogenes organisms or correspond to an existing M serotype.

A molecular typing system is based on the nucleotide sequences encoding the amino termini of M proteins. The emm gene sequences encode M proteins and have been correlated with Lancefield M serotypes. This methodology allows assignment to a validated M protein gene sequence (emm1 through emm124) and the identification of new emm sequence types and has evolved into the gold standard of S. pyogenes typing (39). A large database of approximately 350 emm gene sequences from strains originally used for Lancefield serotyping and including emm sequences from beta-hemolytic groups C, G, and L streptococci is maintained at the CDC (http://www.cdc.gov/ncidod/biotech/infotech_hp.html). Recently, MLST has been developed for S. pyogenes. Population genetic studies demonstrated stable associations between emm type and MLST among isolates obtained decades apart and/or from different continents (35).

In outbreak situations that include S. pyogenes, restriction enzyme-mediated digestion of emm amplicons is a valuable tool for rapid identification of isolates containing similar emm genes (5). For clusters of isolates sharing the same emm type, PFGE profiles may be helpful for distinguishing similar strains (87).

SEROLOGIC TESTS

Determination of streptococcal antibodies is indicated for the diagnosis of poststreptococcal disease, such as ARF or GN (108). A fourfold rise in antibody titer is regarded as definitive proof of an antecedent streptococcal infection. Multiple variables, including site of infection, time since the onset of infection, age, the background prevalence of streptococcal infections (3), antimicrobial therapy, and other comorbidities, influence antibody levels. The most widely used antibodies are anti-streptolysin O and anti-DNase B.

Antibodies against streptolysin O (ASO) reach a maximum at 3 to 6 weeks after infection. While ASO responses following streptococcal upper respiratory tract infections are usually elevated, pyoderma caused by *S. pyogenes* does not elicit a strong ASO response. *Streptococcus dysgalactiae* subsp. *equisimilis* can also produce streptolysin O, and thus elevated ASO titers are not specific for *S. pyogenes* infections.

Among the four streptococcal DNases produced, the host response is most consistent against DNase B. Anti-DNase B titers may not reach maximum titers for 6 to 8 weeks but remain elevated longer than ASO titers and are more reliable than ASO for the confirmation of a preceding streptococcal skin infection. Moreover, since only 80 to 85% of patients with rheumatic fever have elevated ASO titers, additional anti-DNase B titers may be helpful.

Due to frequent exposure to *S. pyogenes*, ASO and anti-DNase B titers are higher in children in the United States from 2 to 12 years of age. Geometric mean values are 89 Todd units for ASO and 112 Todd units for anti-DNase B, while the upper limits of normal values are 240 Todd units (ASO) and 640 Todd units (anti-DNAse B) (58). Prompt antibiotic therapy of streptococcal infections can reduce the titer but does not abolish antibody production. Streptococcal carriers do not experience a rise in streptococcal antibody titers.

The hemagglutination-based streptozyme test (Streptozyme; Carter-Wallace, Inc., Cranbury, NJ) was developed to detect antibodies against multiple extracellular streptococcal products. However, variabilities in test standardization and inconsistent specificities have been reported (45). Assays for antibody detection against other *S. pyogenes* proteins (hyaluronidase, streptokinase, and NAD glycohydrolase) are technically difficult to perform and are not commercially available.

ANTIMICROBIAL SUSCEPTIBILITIES

Beta-Hemolytic Streptococci

Penicillin remains the drug of choice for the empirical treatment of streptococcal infections due to *S. pyogenes*, because in contrast to *S. pneumoniae* and other alpha-hemolytic streptococci, *S. pyogenes* remains uniformly susceptible to penicillin. Reports about reduced penicillin susceptibility in strains of *S. pyogenes* have not been confirmed by reference laboratories. This is, however, no longer true for *S. agalactiae*. Recent reports show the emergence of diminished susceptibility to penicillin G caused by a mutation of the penicillin binding proteins Pbp2x in isolated strains in Asia and the United States (24, 67). Due to suspected or confirmed penicillin allergies in more than 10% of patients, macrolides are often given as an alternative treatment. Macrolide resistance rates among isolates of *S. pyogenes* and *S. agalactiae* have been increasing in North America as well as in Europe (29). Resistance rates correlate with the use of macrolides in clinical practice, and geographic differences in resistance rates are often due to differences in macrolide use. In the United States, the rate of macrolide resistance among *S. agalactiae* rose from 12 to 20% from 1990 to 2000 (84) and has recently been reported as 38% (50). Beta-hemolytic streptococcal isolates with a reduced susceptibility to glycopeptides have not been reported. Due to the uniform susceptibility of *S. pyogenes* to penicillin, resistance

testing for penicillins or other beta-lactams approved for treatment of *S. pyogenes* and *S. agalactiae* is not necessary for clinical purposes. So far the existence of rare isolates of *S. agalactiae* with reduced susceptibility to penicillin has not resulted in a change of this recommendation, which may of course change if increasing numbers of such strains are encountered. Susceptibility testing for macrolides should be performed by using erythromycin, since resistance and susceptibility of azithromycin, clarithromycin, and dirithromycin can be predicted by testing erythromycin.

S. pneumoniae and Viridans Group Streptococci

In view of the development of penicillin resistance in *S. pneumoniae* and other alpha-hemolytic streptococci, penicillin can no longer be recommended as the empirical treatment of choice in many countries. Penicillin is considered a preferred antimicrobial agent for only *S. pneumoniae* and other alpha-hemolytic streptococci with demonstrated susceptibilities to penicillin. Penicillin resistance in *S. pneumoniae* is caused by altered penicillin-binding proteins. Approximately 25% of *S. pneumoniae* isolates from the United States were not fully susceptible to penicillin in 2007 (http://www.cdc.gov/abcs). But the recent changes of *S. pneumoniae* breakpoints in nonmeningeal isolates (susceptibility, ≤2 µg/ml; intermediate resistance, 4 µg/ml; resistance, ≥8 µg/ml) for penicillin in CLSI definitions caused this value to drop to less than 10% (124). Susceptibility to penicillin can be determined by a disk diffusion test with 1 µg of oxacillin. According to the current CLSI guidelines, in all cases where oxacillin zone sizes (≤19 mm) indicate a reduced susceptibility to penicillin, MIC determinations for penicillin should be performed. For susceptibility testing of all other β-lactams in *S. pneumoniae*, MIC determinations are recommended. *S. pneumoniae* infections should be treated according to current guidelines (76). Depending on the clinical situation, treatment options include penicillin, extended-spectrum cephalosporins, macrolides, fluoroquinolones, and vancomycin. In addition, more than one-third of blood culture isolates of the viridans group collected in the late 1990s in the United States were not susceptible to penicillin (31). Elevated percentages of penicillin-resistant strains can be found among *S. mitis* and *S. salivarius* isolates. *S. pneumoniae* was uniformly susceptible to macrolides until the late 1980s in the United States, but macrolide resistance is now evident in about 25% of *S. pneumoniae* strains (117).

The increased use of fluoroquinolones to treat *S. pneumoniae* infections has been accompanied by a rise in fluoroquinolone-resistant *S. pneumoniae* strains. Resistance occurs in a stepwise fashion and is due to mutations in DNA topoisomerase IV or a subunit of DNA gyrase. While the overall prevalence of fluoroquinolone resistance is below 1% according to the CDC's Active Bacterial Core surveillance data (http://www.cdc.gov/abcs), the increase in resistant strains during recent years emphasizes the need for close monitoring. Clinical failures of levofloxacin therapy due to resistance have been reported (25). Vancomycin-resistant *S. pneumoniae* isolates have not been described. However, the isolation of a vancomycin-resistant *S. bovis* isolate has been reported (93).

EVALUATION, INTERPRETATION, AND REPORTING OF RESULTS

Streptococci from the pyogenic group are important human pathogens. Timely identification of these species in clinical specimens is therefore crucial to treat infections adequately and to reduce transmission. Tonsillopharyngitis caused by *S. pyogenes* remains a substantial health problem in childhood and adolescence. Diagnosis by either rapid antigen tests or bacteriological culture minimizes unjustified antibiotic treatment of viral pharyngitis. Serologic tests are usually applied in cases of suspected poststreptococcal sequelae. Proper identification and reporting, however, should not be limited to *S. pyogenes*, since *S. dysgalactiae* subsp. *equisimilis* (human group C and G streptococci) has been documented as an agent of pharyngitis including cases complicated by nonsuppurative sequelae. In this context it is important to correctly differentiate these pathogens from the small-colony-forming beta-hemolytic species of the *S. anginosus* group that make up part of the oropharyngeal microbiota. While invasive neonatal *S. agalactiae* infections are declining due to improved prenatal screening and peripartal antibiotic prophylaxis, increased detection of *S. agalactiae* from adult patients has been reported (109). Thorough identification and reporting of this organism should therefore not be confined to screening swabs during pregnancy or in newborns.

Despite the fact that *S. pneumoniae* is often found as a colonizer in respiratory samples, it should always be clearly distinguished from viridans group streptococci and reported. Cultural methods remain the mainstay in pneumococcal pneumonia and sepsis as well as meningitis. To enable the initiation of adequate antibiotic treatment, resistance testing should be performed for all isolates. Special care should be taken to ensure the reporting of the correct β-lactam breakpoints for non-CSF and CSF *S. pneumoniae* isolates, which have just recently been changed. If antibiotic treatment was started before microbiological samples were obtained, the urinary antigen test or nucleic acid detection techniques may help to properly identify the causative agent, especially in invasive infections.

The correct identification of viridans group streptococci and the distinction of strains causing infections from isolates of the physiological microbiota remain a major challenge. Identification to the group or species level should be confined to strains causing abscesses, endocarditis, and serious infections in neutropenic patients. Many *S. mitis* isolates are no longer penicillin susceptible, and special attention has to be paid to susceptibility testing. Due to the association of *S. gallolyticus* subsp. *gallolyticus* with malignancies of the gastrointestinal tract and in view of the recent taxonomic changes within the *S. bovis* group, reports of novel species designations should include the information that the species belongs to the *S. bovis* group (121).

REFERENCES

1. **Arbique, J. C., C. Poyart, P. Trieu-Cuot, G. Quesne, M. D. G. S. Carvalho, A. G. Steigerwalt, R. E. Morey, D. Jackson, R. J. Davidson, and R. R. Facklam.** 2004. Accuracy of phenotypic and genotypic testing for identification of *Streptococcus pneumoniae* and description of *Streptococcus pseudopneumoniae* sp. nov. *J. Clin. Microbiol.* **42:**4686–4696.
2. **Austrian, R.** 1976. The quellung reaction, a neglected microbiologic technique. *Mt. Sinai J. Med.* **43:**699–709.
3. **Ayoub, E. M., B. Nelson, S. T. Shulman, D. J. Barrett, J. D. Campbell, G. Armstrong, J. Lovejoy, G. H. Angoff, and S. Rockenmacher.** 2003. Group A streptococcal antibodies in subjects with or without rheumatic fever in areas with high or low incidences of rheumatic fever. *Clin. Diagn. Lab. Immunol.* **10:**886–890.
4. **Barnham, M., T. J. Thornton, and K. Lange.** 1983. Nephritis caused by Streptococcus zooepidemicus (Lancefield group C). *Lancet* **i:**945–948.
5. **Beall, B., R. R. Facklam, J. A. Elliott, A. R. Franklin, T. Hoenes, D. Jackson, L. Laclaire, T. Thompson, and R. Viswanathan.** 1998. Streptococcal emm types associated with T-agglutination types and the use of conserved emm gene restriction fragment patterns for subtyping group A streptococci. *J. Med. Microbiol.* **47:**893–898.
6. **Beck, M., R. Frodl, and G. Funke.** 2008. Comprehensive study of strains previously designated *Streptococcus bovis* consecutively isolated from human blood cultures and emended description of *Streptococcus gallolyticus* and *Streptococcus infantarius* subsp. *coli. J. Clin. Microbiol.* **46:**2966–2972.
7. **Beighton, D., J. M. Hardie, and R. A. Whiley.** 1991. A scheme for the identification of viridans streptococci. *J. Med. Microbiol.* **35:**367–372.
8. **Bekal, S., C. Gaudreau, R. A. Laurence, E. Simoneau, and L. Raynal.** 2006. *Streptococcus pseudoporcinus* sp. nov., a novel species isolated from the genitourinary tract of women. *J. Clin. Microbiol.* **44:**2584–2586.
9. **Benson, J. A., and P. Ferrieri.** 2001. Rapid pulsed-field gel electrophoresis method for group B streptococcus isolates. *J. Clin. Microbiol.* **39:**3006–3008.
10. **Benson, J. A., A. E. Flores, C. J. Baker, S. L. Hillier, and P. Ferrieri.** 2002. Improved methods for typing nontypeable isolates of group B streptococci. *Int. J. Med. Microbiol.* **292:**37–42.
11. **Bergeron, M. G., D. Ke, C. Menard, F. J. Picard, M. Gagnon, M. Bernier, M. Ouellette, P. H. Roy, S. Marcoux, and W. D. Fraser.** 2000. Rapid detection of group B streptococci in pregnant women at delivery. *N. Engl. J. Med.* **343:**175–179.
12. **Bisno, A. L.** 2001. Acute pharyngitis. *N. Engl. J. Med.* **344:**205–211.
13. **Bisno, A. L., M. A. Gerber, J. M. Gwaltney, Jr., E. L. Kaplan, R. H. Schwartz, et al.** 2002. Practice guidelines for the diagnosis and management of group A streptococcal pharyngitis. *Clin. Infect. Dis.* **35:**113–125.
14. **Block, T., E. Munson, A. Culver, K. Vaughan, and J. E. Hryciuk.** 2008. Comparison of carrot broth- and selective Todd-Hewitt broth-enhanced PCR protocols for real-time detection of *Streptococcus agalactiae* in prenatal vaginal/anorectal specimens. *J. Clin. Microbiol.* **46:**3615–3620.
15. **Bochud, P. Y., T. Calandra, and P. Francioli.** 1994. Bacteremia due to viridans streptococci in neutropenic patients: a review. *Am. J. Med.* **97:**256–264.
16. **Brandt, C. M., G. Haase, N. Schnitzler, R. Zbinden, and R. Lutticken.** 1999. Characterization of blood culture isolates of *Streptococcus dysgalactiae* subsp. *equisimilis* possessing Lancefield's group A antigen. *J. Clin. Microbiol.* **37:**4194–4197.
17. **Brandt, C. M., and B. Spellerberg.** 2009. Human infections due to Streptococcus dysgalactiae subspecies equisimilis. *Clin. Infect. Dis.* **49:**766–772.
18. **Carvalho Mda, G., M. L. Tondella, K. McCaustland, L. Weidlich, L. McGee, L. W. Mayer, A. Steigerwalt, M. Whaley, R. R. Facklam, B. Fields, G. Carlone, E. W. Ades, R. Dagan, and J. S. Sampson.** 2007. Evaluation and improvement of real-time PCR assays targeting lytA, ply, and psaA genes for detection of pneumococcal DNA. *J. Clin. Microbiol.* **45:**2460–2466.
19. **Caufield, P. W., G. R. Cutter, and A. P. Dasanayake.** 1993. Initial acquisition of mutans streptococci by infants: evidence for a discrete window of infectivity. *J. Dent. Res.* **72:**37–45.
20. **Centers for Disease Control and Prevention.** 2008. Invasive pneumococcal disease in children 5 years after conjugate vaccine introduction—eight states, 1998–2005. *MMWR Morb. Mortal. Wkly. Rep.* **57:**144–148.
21. **Chapin, K. C., P. Blake, and C. D. Wilson.** 2002. Performance characteristics and utilization of rapid antigen test, DNA probe, and culture for detection of group A streptococci in an acute care clinic. *J. Clin. Microbiol.* **40:**4207–4210.
22. **Chuard, C., and L. B. Reller.** 1998. Bile-esculin test for presumptive identification of enterococci and streptococci: effects of bile concentration, inoculation technique, and incubation time. *J. Clin. Microbiol.* **36:**1135–1136.

23. **Cunningham, M. W.** 2000. Pathogenesis of group A streptococcal infections. *Clin. Microbiol. Rev.* **13:**470–511.

24. **Dahesh, S., M. E. Hensler, N. M. Van Sorge, R. E. Gertz, Jr., S. Schrag, V. Nizet, and B. W. Beall.** 2008. Point mutation in the group B streptococcal *pbp2x* gene conferring decreased susceptibility to beta-lactam antibiotics. *Antimicrob. Agents Chemother.* **52:**2915–2918.

25. **Davidson, R., R. Cavalcanti, J. L. Brunton, D. J. Bast, J. C. de Azavedo, P. Kibsey, C. Fleming, and D. E. Low.** 2002. Resistance to levofloxacin and failure of treatment of pneumococcal pneumonia. *N. Engl. J. Med.* **346:**747–750.

26. **Davies, H. D., A. McGeer, B. Schwartz, K. Green, D. Cann, A. E. Simor, D. E. Low, et al.** 1996. Invasive group A streptococcal infections in Ontario, Canada. *N. Engl. J. Med.* **335:**547–554.

27. **Davies, H. D., M. A. Miller, S. Faro, D. Gregson, S. C. Kehl, and J. A. Jordan.** 2004. Multicenter study of a rapid molecular-based assay for the diagnosis of group B Streptococcus colonization in pregnant women. *Clin. Infect. Dis.* **39:**1129–1135.

28. **Denys, G. A., and R. B. Carey.** 1992. Identification of *Streptococcus pneumoniae* with a DNA probe. *J. Clin. Microbiol.* **30:**2725–2727.

29. **Desjardins, M., K. L. Delgaty, K. Ramotar, C. Seetaram, and B. Toye.** 2004. Prevalence and mechanisms of erythromycin resistance in group A and group B *Streptococcus*: implications for reporting susceptibility results. *J. Clin. Microbiol.* **42:**5620–5623.

30. **Devriese, L. A., P. Vandamme, B. Pot, M. Vanrobaeys, K. Kersters, and F. Haesebrouck.** 1998. Differentiation between *Streptococcus gallolyticus* strains of human clinical and veterinary origins and *Streptococcus bovis* strains from the intestinal tracts of ruminants. *J. Clin. Microbiol.* **36:**3520–3523.

31. **Doern, G. V., M. J. Ferraro, A. B. Brueggemann, and K. L. Ruoff.** 1996. Emergence of high rates of antimicrobial resistance among viridans group streptococci in the United States. *Antimicrob. Agents Chemother.* **40:**891–894.

32. **Dowell, S. F., R. L. Garman, G. Liu, O. S. Levine, and Y. H. Yang.** 2001. Evaluation of Binax NOW, an assay for the detection of pneumococcal antigen in urine samples, performed among pediatric patients. *Clin. Infect. Dis.* **32:**824–825.

33. **Efstratiou, A.** 2000. Group A streptococci in the 1990s. *J. Antimicrob. Chemother.* **45**(Suppl.):3–12.

34. **Enright, M. C., and B. G. Spratt.** 1999. Multilocus sequence typing. *Trends Microbiol.* **7:**482–487.

35. **Enright, M. C., B. G. Spratt, A. Kalia, J. H. Cross, and D. E. Bessen.** 2001. Multilocus sequence typing of *Streptococcus pyogenes* and the relationships between *emm* type and clone. *Infect. Immun.* **69:**2416–2427.

36. **Facklam, R.** 2002. What happened to the streptococci: overview of taxonomic and nomenclature changes. *Clin. Microbiol. Rev.* **15:**613–630.

37. **Facklam, R., J. Elliott, N. Pigott, and A. R. Franklin.** 1995. Identification of *Streptococcus porcinus* from human sources. *J. Clin. Microbiol.* **33:**385–388.

38. **Facklam, R., J. Elliott, L. Shewmaker, and A. Reingold.** 2005. Identification and characterization of sporadic isolates of *Streptococcus iniae* isolated from humans. *J. Clin. Microbiol.* **43:**933–937.

39. **Facklam, R. R., D. R. Martin, M. Lovgren, D. R. Johnson, A. Efstratiou, T. A. Thompson, S. Gowan, P. Kriz, G. J. Tyrrell, E. Kaplan, and B. Beall.** 2002. Extension of the Lancefield classification for group A streptococci by addition of 22 new M protein gene sequence types from clinical isolates: emm103 to emm124. *Clin. Infect. Dis.* **34:**28–38.

40. **Facklam, R. R.** 1987. Specificity study of kits for detection of group A streptococci directly from throat swabs. *J. Clin. Microbiol.* **25:**504–508.

40a. **Facklam, R. R., and J. A. Washington II.** 1991. *Streptococcus* and related catalase-negative gram-positive cocci, p. 238–257. *In* A. Balows, W. J. Hausler, Jr., K. L. Herrmann, H. D. Isenberg, and H. J. Shadomy (ed.), *Manual of Clinical Microbiology*, 5th ed. American Society for Microbiology, Washington, DC.

41. **Farley, M.** 1995. Group B streptococcal infection in older patients. Spectrum of disease and management strategies. *Drugs Aging* **6:**293–300.

42. **Fischetti, V. A.** 1989. Streptococcal M protein: molecular design and biological behavior. *Clin. Microbiol. Rev.* **2:**285–314.

43. **Gavin, P. J., R. B. Thomson, Jr., S. J. Horng, and R. Yogev.** 2003. Neonatal sepsis caused by *Streptococcus bovis* variant (biotype II/2): report of a case and review. *J. Clin. Microbiol.* **41:**3433–3435.

44. **Gavino, M., and E. Wang.** 2007. A comparison of a new rapid real-time polymerase chain reaction system to traditional culture in determining group B streptococcus colonization. *Am. J. Obstet. Gynecol.* **197:**388.e1–4.

45. **Gerber, M. A., L. L. Wright, and M. F. Randolph.** 1987. Streptozyme test for antibodies to group A streptococcal antigens. *Pediatr. Infect. Dis. J.* **6:**36–40.

46. **Glazunova, O. O., D. Raoult, and V. Roux.** 2006. Streptococcus massiliensis sp. nov., isolated from a patient blood culture. *Int. J. Syst. Evol. Microbiol.* **56:**1127–1131.

47. **Gorm Jensen, T., H. Bossen Konradsen, and B. Bruun.** 1999. Evaluation of the Rapid ID 32 Strep system. *Clin. Microbiol. Infect.* **5:**417–423.

48. **Greenberg, D., A. Broides, I. Blancovich, N. Peled, N. Givon-Lavi, and R. Dagan.** 2004. Relative importance of nasopharyngeal versus oropharyngeal sampling for isolation of *Streptococcus pneumoniae* and *Haemophilus influenzae* from healthy and sick individuals varies with age. *J. Clin. Microbiol.* **42:**4604–4609.

49. **Gutierrez, F., M. Masia, J. C. Rodriguez, A. Ayelo, L. Cebrian, C. Mirete, G. Royo, and A. M. Hidalgo.** 2003. Evaluation of the immunochromatographic Binax NOW assay for detection of Streptococcus pneumoniae urinary antigen in a prospective study of community-acquired pneumonia in Spain. *Clin. Infect. Dis.* **36:**286–292.

50. **Gygax, S. E., J. A. Schuyler, L. E. Kimmel, J. P. Trama, E. Mordechai, and M. E. Adelson.** 2006. Erythromycin and clindamycin resistance in group B streptococcal clinical isolates. *Antimicrob. Agents Chemother.* **50:**1875–1877.

51. **Haanpera, M., J. Jalava, P. Huovinen, O. Meurman, and K. Rantakokko-Jalava.** 2007. Identification of alpha-hemolytic streptococci by pyrosequencing the 16S rRNA gene and by use of VITEK 2. *J. Clin. Microbiol.* **45:**762–770.

52. **Haidan, A., S. R. Talay, M. Rohde, K. S. Sriprakash, B. J. Currie, and G. S. Chhatwal.** 2000. Pharyngeal carriage of group C and group G streptococci and acute rheumatic fever in an Aboriginal population. *Lancet* **356:**1167–1169.

53. **Hendley, J. O., M. A. Sande, P. M. Stewart, and J. M. Gwaltney, Jr.** 1975. Spread of Streptococcus pneumoniae in families. I. Carriage rates and distribution of types. *J. Infect. Dis.* **132:**55–61.

54. **Homer, K. A., L. Denbow, R. A. Whiley, and D. Beighton.** 1993. Chondroitin sulfate depolymerase and hyaluronidase activities of viridans streptococci determined by a sensitive spectrophotometric assay. *J. Clin. Microbiol.* **31:**1648–1651.

55. **Hwang, M. N., and G. M. Ederer.** 1975. Rapid hippurate hydrolysis method for presumptive identification of group B streptococci. *J. Clin. Microbiol.* **1:**114–115.

56. **Johnson, D. R., and E. L. Kaplan.** 1993. A review of the correlation of T-agglutination patterns and M-protein typing and opacity factor production in the identification of group A streptococci. *J. Med. Microbiol.* **38:**311–315.

57. **Jones, N., J. F. Bohnsack, S. Takahashi, K. A. Oliver, M. S. Chan, F. Kunst, P. Glaser, C. Rusniok, D. W. Crook, R. M. Harding, N. Bisharat, and B. G. Spratt.** 2003. Multilocus sequence typing system for group B streptococcus. *J. Clin. Microbiol.* **41:**2530–2536.

58. **Kaplan, E. L., C. D. Rothermel, and D. R. Johnson.** 1998. Antistreptolysin O and anti-deoxyribonuclease B titers: normal values for children ages 2 to 12 in the United States. *Pediatrics* **101:**86–88.

59. **Kawamura, Y., X. G. Hou, F. Sultana, H. Miura, and T. Ezaki.** 1995. Determination of 16S rRNA sequences of *Streptococcus mitis* and *Streptococcus gordonii* and phylogenetic

relationships among members of the genus *Streptococcus*. *Int. J. Syst. Bacteriol.* **45**:406–408.

60. **Kawamura, Y., X. G. Hou, Y. Todome, F. Sultana, K. Hirose, S. E. Shu, T. Ezaki, and H. Ohkuni.** 1998. Streptococcus peroris sp. nov. and Streptococcus infantis sp. nov., new members of the Streptococcus mitis group, isolated from human clinical specimens. *Int. J. Syst. Bacteriol.* **48**(Pt. 3):921–927.

61. **Keith, E. R., R. G. Podmore, T. P. Anderson, and D. R. Murdoch.** 2006. Characteristics of *Streptococcus pseudopneumoniae* isolated from purulent sputum samples. *J. Clin. Microbiol.* **44**:923–927.

62. **Kellner, J. D., O. G. Vanderkooi, J. MacDonald, D. L. Church, G. J. Tyrrell, and D. W. Scheifele.** 2009. Changing epidemiology of invasive pneumococcal disease in Canada, 1998–2007: update from the Calgary-area Streptococcus pneumoniae research (CASPER) study. *Clin. Infect. Dis.* **49**:205–212.

63. **Kellogg, J. A.** 1990. Suitability of throat culture procedures for detection of group A streptococci and as reference standards for evaluation of streptococcal antigen detection kits. *J. Clin. Microbiol.* **28**:165–169.

64. **Kikuchi, K., T. Enari, K. Totsuka, and K. Shimizu.** 1995. Comparison of phenotypic characteristics, DNA-DNA hybridization results, and results with a commercial rapid biochemical and enzymatic reaction system for identification of viridans group streptococci. *J. Clin. Microbiol.* **33**:1215–1222.

65. **Kilian, M., L. Mikkelsen, and J. Henrichsen.** 1989. Taxonomic study of viridans streptococci: description of Streptococcus gordonii sp. nov. and emended descriptions of Streptococcus sanguis (White and Niven 1946), Streptococcus oralis (Bridge and Sneath 1982), and Streptococcus mitis (Andrews and Horder 1906). *Int. J. Syst. Bacteriol.* **39**:471–484.

66. **Kilian, M., K. Poulsen, T. Blomqvist, L. S. Havarstein, M. Bek-Thomsen, H. Tettelin, and U. B. Sorensen.** 2008. Evolution of Streptococcus pneumoniae and its close commensal relatives. *PLoS One* **3**:e2683.

67. **Kimura, K., S. Suzuki, J. Wachino, H. Kurokawa, K. Yamane, N. Shibata, N. Nagano, H. Kato, K. Shibayama, and Y. Arakawa.** 2008. First molecular characterization of group B streptococci with reduced penicillin susceptibility. *Antimicrob. Agents Chemother.* **52**:2890–2897.

68. **Kirby, R., and K. L. Ruoff.** 1995. Cost-effective, clinically relevant method for rapid identification of beta-hemolytic streptococci and enterococci. *J. Clin. Microbiol.* **33**:1154–1157.

69. **Klein, R. S., R. A. Recco, M. T. Catalano, S. C. Edberg, J. I. Casey, and N. H. Steigbigel.** 1977. Association of Streptococcus bovis with carcinoma of the colon. *N. Engl. J. Med.* **297**:800–802.

70. **Kohler, W.** 2007. The present state of species within the genera Streptococcus and Enterococcus. *Int. J. Med. Microbiol.* **297**:133–150.

71. **Kong, F., S. Gowan, D. Martin, G. James, and G. L. Gilbert.** 2002. Serotype identification of group B streptococci by PCR and sequencing. *J. Clin. Microbiol.* **40**:216–226.

72. **Kurzynski, T. A., and C. K. Meise.** 1979. Evaluation of sulfamethoxazole-trimethoprim blood agar plates for recovery of group A streptococci from throat cultures. *J. Clin. Microbiol.* **9**:189–193.

73. **Lefevre, J. C., G. Faucon, A. M. Sicard, and A. M. Gasc.** 1993. DNA fingerprinting of *Streptococcus pneumoniae* strains by pulsed-field gel electrophoresis. *J. Clin. Microbiol.* **31**:2724–2728.

74. **Malhotra-Kumar, S., S. Wang, C. Lammens, S. Chapelle, and H. Goossens.** 2003. Bacitracin-resistant clone of *Streptococcus pyogenes* isolated from pharyngitis patients in Belgium. *J. Clin. Microbiol.* **41**:5282–5284.

75. **Mandell, L. A., J. G. Bartlett, S. F. Dowell, T. M. File, Jr., D. M. Musher, and C. Whitney.** 2003. Update of practice guidelines for the management of community-acquired pneumonia in immunocompetent adults. *Clin. Infect. Dis.* **37**:1405–1433.

76. **Mandell, L. A., R. G. Wunderink, A. Anzueto, J. G. Bartlett, G. D. Campbell, N. C. Dean, S. F. Dowell, T. M. File, Jr., D. M. Musher, M. S. Niederman, A. Torres, and C. G. Whitney.** 2007. Infectious Diseases Society of America/American Thoracic Society consensus guidelines on the management of community-acquired pneumonia in adults. *Clin. Infect. Dis.* **44**(Suppl. 2):S27–S72.

77. **Martin, D. R., J. M. Stanhope, and L. A. Finch.** 1977. Delayed culture of group-A streptococci: an evaluation of variables in methods of examining throat swabs. *J. Med. Microbiol.* **10**:249–253.

78. **Mein, J., and G. Lum.** 1999. CSF bacterial antigen detection tests offer no advantage over Gram's stain in the diagnosis of bacterial meningitis. *Pathology* **31**:67–69.

79. **Messmer, T. O., J. S. Sampson, A. Stinson, B. Wong, G. M. Carlone, and R. R. Facklam.** 2004. Comparison of four polymerase chain reaction assays for specificity in the identification of Streptococcus pneumoniae. *Diagn. Microbiol. Infect. Dis.* **49**:249–254.

80. **Mihaila-Amrouche, L., A. Bouvet, and J. Loubinoux.** 2004. Clonal spread of *emm* type 28 isolates of *Streptococcus pyogenes* that are multiresistant to antibiotics. *J. Clin. Microbiol.* **42**:3844–3846.

81. **Moisi, J. C., S. K. Saha, A. G. Falade, B. M. Njanpop-Lafourcade, J. Oundo, A. K. Zaidi, S. Afroj, R. A. Bakare, J. K. Buss, R. Lasi, J. Mueller, A. A. Odekanmi, L. Sangare, J. A. Scott, M. D. Knoll, O. S. Levine, and B. D. Gessner.** 2009. Enhanced diagnosis of pneumococcal meningitis with use of the Binax NOW immunochromatographic test of *Streptococcus pneumoniae* antigen: a multisite study. *Clin. Infect. Dis.* **48**(Suppl. 2):S49–S56.

82. **Mora, M., G. Bensi, S. Capo, F. Falugi, C. Zingaretti, A. G. Manetti, T. Maggi, A. R. Taddei, G. Grandi, and J. L. Telford.** 2005. Group A Streptococcus produce pilus-like structures containing protective antigens and Lancefield T antigens. *Proc. Natl. Acad. Sci. USA* **102**:15641–15646.

83. **Murdoch, D. R., R. T. Laing, G. D. Mills, N. C. Karalus, G. I. Town, S. Mirrett, and L. B. Reller.** 2001. Evaluation of a rapid immunochromatographic test for detection of *Streptococcus pneumoniae* antigen in urine samples from adults with community-acquired pneumonia. *J. Clin. Microbiol.* **39**:3495–3498.

84. **Murdoch, D. R., and L. B. Reller.** 2001. Antimicrobial susceptibilities of group B streptococci isolated from patients with invasive disease: 10-year perspective. *Antimicrob. Agents Chemother.* **45**:3623–3624.

85. **Murray, P. R., A. D. Wold, C. A. Schreck, and J. A. Washington II.** 1976. Effects of selective media and atmosphere of incubation on the isolation of group A streptococci. *J. Clin. Microbiol.* **4**:54–56.

86. **Musser, J. M., B. M. Gray, P. M. Schlievert, and M. E. Pichichero.** 1992. *Streptococcus pyogenes* pharyngitis: characterization of strains by multilocus enzyme genotype, M and T protein serotype, and pyrogenic exotoxin gene probing. *J. Clin. Microbiol.* **30**:600–603.

87. **Musser, J. M., V. Kapur, J. Szeto, X. Pan, D. S. Swanson, and D. R. Martin.** 1995. Genetic diversity and relationships among *Streptococcus pyogenes* strains expressing serotype M1 protein: recent intercontinental spread of a subclone causing episodes of invasive disease. *Infect. Immun.* **63**:994–1003.

88. **Pergola, V., G. Di Salvo, G. Habib, J. F. Avierinos, E. Philip, J. M. Vailloud, F. Thuny, J. P. Casalta, P. Ambrosi, M. Lambert, A. Riberi, A. Ferracci, T. Mesana, D. Metras, J. R. Harle, P. J. Weiller, D. Raoult, and R. Luccioni.** 2001. Comparison of clinical and echocardiographic characteristics of Streptococcus bovis endocarditis with that caused by other pathogens. *Am. J. Cardiol.* **88**:871–875.

89. **Peterson, L. R., and R. B. Thomson, Jr.** 1999. Use of the clinical microbiology laboratory for the diagnosis and management of infectious diseases related to the oral cavity. *Infect. Dis. Clin. N. Am.* **13**:775–795.

90. **Pires, R., D. Rolo, R. Mato, J. Feio de Almeida, C. Johansson, B. Henriques-Normark, A. Morais, A. Brito-Avo, J. Goncalo-Marques, and I. Santos-Sanches.**

2009. Resistance to bacitracin in Streptococcus pyogenes from oropharyngeal colonization and noninvasive infections in Portugal was caused by two clones of distinct virulence genotypes. FEMS Microbiol. Lett. **296:**235–240.

91. **Podbielski, A., O. Blankenstein, and R. Lutticken.** 1994. Molecular characterization of the cfb gene encoding group B streptococcal CAMP-factor. Med. Microbiol. Immunol. (Berlin) **183:**239–256.

92. **Pokorski, S. J., E. A. Vetter, P. C. Wollan, and F. R. Cockerill III.** 1994. Comparison of Gen-Probe Group A streptococcus Direct Test with culture for diagnosing streptococcal pharyngitis. J. Clin. Microbiol. **32:**1440–1443.

93. **Poyart, C., C. Pierre, G. Quesne, B. Pron, P. Berche, and P. Trieu-Cuot.** 1997. Emergence of vancomycin resistance in the genus Streptococcus: characterization of a vanB transferable determinant in Streptococcus bovis. Antimicrob. Agents Chemother. **41:**24–29.

94. **Poyart, C., G. Quesne, S. Coulon, P. Berche, and P. Trieu-Cuot.** 1998. Identification of streptococci to species level by sequencing the gene encoding the manganese-dependent superoxide dismutase. J. Clin. Microbiol. **36:**41–47.

95. **Poyart, C., A. Tazi, H. Reglier-Poupet, A. Billoet, N. Tavares, J. Raymond, and P. Trieu-Cuot.** 2007. Multiplex PCR assay for rapid and accurate capsular typing of group B streptococci. J. Clin. Microbiol. **45:**1985–1988.

96. **Ratner, H. B., L. S. Weeks, and C. W. Stratton.** 1986. Evaluation of spot CAMP test for identification of group B streptococci. J. Clin. Microbiol. **24:**296–297.

97. **Regev-Yochay, G., M. Raz, R. Dagan, N. Porat, B. Shainberg, E. Pinco, N. Keller, and E. Rubinstein.** 2004. Nasopharyngeal carriage of Streptococcus pneumoniae by adults and children in community and family settings. Clin. Infect. Dis. **38:**632–639.

98. **Richter, S. S., K. P. Heilmann, C. L. Dohrn, F. Riahi, S. E. Beekmann, and G. V. Doern.** 2008. Accuracy of phenotypic methods for identification of Streptococcus pneumoniae isolates included in surveillance programs. J. Clin. Microbiol. **46:**2184–2188.

99. **Richter, S. S., K. P. Heilmann, C. L. Dohrn, F. Riahi, S. E. Beekmann, and G. V. Doern.** 2009. Changing epidemiology of antimicrobial-resistant Streptococcus pneumoniae in the United States, 2004–2005. Clin. Infect. Dis. **48:**e23–e33.

100. **Rosa-Fraile, M., J. Rodriguez-Granger, M. Cueto-Lopez, A. Sampedro, E. B. Gaye, J. M. Haro, and A. Andreu.** 1999. Use of Granada medium to detect group B streptococcal colonization in pregnant women. J. Clin. Microbiol. **37:**2674–2677.

101. **Ruoff, K. L., S. I. Miller, C. V. Garner, M. J. Ferraro, and S. B. Calderwood.** 1989. Bacteremia with Streptococcus bovis and Streptococcus salivarius: clinical correlates of more accurate identification of isolates. J. Clin. Microbiol. **27:**305–308.

102. **Rurangirwa, F. R., C. A. Teitzel, J. Cui, D. M. French, P. L. McDonough, and T. Besser.** 2000. Streptococcus didelphis sp. nov., a streptococcus with marked catalase activity isolated from opossums (Didelphis virginiana) with suppurative dermatitis and liver fibrosis. Int. J. Syst. Evol. Microbiol. **50(Pt. 2):**759–765.

103. **Schlegel, L., F. Grimont, E. Ageron, P. A. Grimont, and A. Bouvet.** 2003. Reappraisal of the taxonomy of the Streptococcus bovis/Streptococcus equinus complex and related species: description of Streptococcus gallolyticus subsp. gallolyticus subsp. nov., S. gallolyticus subsp. macedonicus subsp. nov. and S. gallolyticus subsp. pasteurianus subsp. nov. Int. J. Syst. Evol. Microbiol. **53:**631–645.

104. **Schlegel, L., F. Grimont, M. D. Collins, B. Regnault, P. A. Grimont, and A. Bouvet.** 2000. Streptococcus infantarius sp. nov., Streptococcus infantarius subsp. infantarius subsp. nov. and Streptococcus infantarius subsp. coli subsp. nov., isolated from humans and food. Int. J. Syst. Evol. Microbiol. **50(Pt. 4):**1425–1434.

105. **Schrag, S., R. Gorwitz, K. Fultz-Butts, and A. Schuchat.** 2002. Prevention of perinatal group B streptococcal disease.

Revised guidelines from CDC. MMWR Recommend. Rep. **51:**1–22.

106. **Schrag, S. J., S. Zywicki, M. M. Farley, A. L. Reingold, L. H. Harrison, L. B. Lefkowitz, J. L. Hadler, R. Danila, P. R. Cieslak, and A. Schuchat.** 2000. Group B streptococcal disease in the era of intrapartum antibiotic prophylaxis. N. Engl. J. Med. **342:**15–20.

107. **Schuchat, A., T. Hilger, E. Zell, M. M. Farley, A. Reingold, L. Harrison, L. Lefkowitz, R. Danila, K. Stefonek, N. Barrett, D. Morse, and R. Pinner.** 2001. Active bacterial core surveillance of the emerging infections program network. Emerg. Infect. Dis. **7:**92–99.

108. **Shet, A., and E. L. Kaplan.** 2002. Clinical use and interpretation of group A streptococcal antibody tests: a practical approach for the pediatrician or primary care physician. Pediatr. Infect. Dis. J. **21:**42–46, 427–430.

109. **Skoff, T. H., M. M. Farley, S. Petit, A. S. Craig, W. Schaffner, K. Gershman, L. H. Harrison, R. Lynfield, J. Mohle-Boetani, S. Zansky, B. A. Albanese, K. Stefonek, E. R. Zell, D. Jackson, T. Thompson, and S. J. Schrag.** 2009. Increasing burden of invasive group B streptococcal disease in nonpregnant adults, 1990–2007. Clin. Infect. Dis. **49:**85–92.

110. **Slotved, H. C., M. Kaltoft, I. C. Skovsted, M. B. Kerrn, and F. Espersen.** 2004. Simple, rapid latex agglutination test for serotyping of pneumococci (Pneumotest-Latex). J. Clin. Microbiol. **42:**2518–2522.

111. **Smith, D. J.** 2002. Dental caries vaccines: prospects and concerns. Crit. Rev. Oral Biol. Med. **13:**335–349.

112. **Stevens, D. L.** 2001. Invasive streptococcal infections. J. Infect. Chemother. **7:**69–80.

113. **Summanen, P. H., M. C. Rowlinson, J. Wooton, and S. M. Finegold.** 2009. Evaluation of genotypic and phenotypic methods for differentiation of the members of the Anginosus group streptococci. Eur. J. Clin. Microbiol. Infect. Dis. **28:**1123–1128.

114. **Swedo, S. E., H. L. Leonard, B. B. Mittleman, A. J. Allen, J. L. Rapoport, S. P. Dow, M. E. Kanter, F. Chapman, and J. Zabriskie.** 1997. Identification of children with pediatric autoimmune neuropsychiatric disorders associated with streptococcal infections by a marker associated with rheumatic fever. Am. J. Psychiatry **154:**110–112.

115. **Thinkhamrop, J., S. Limpongsanurak, M. R. Festin, S. Daly, A. Schuchat, P. Lumbiganon, E. Zell, T. Chipato, A. A. Win, M. J. Perilla, J. E. Tolosa, and C. G. Whitney.** 2003. Infections in international pregnancy study: performance of the optical immunoassay test for detection of group B streptococcus. J. Clin. Microbiol. **41:**5288–5290.

116. **Thomas, J. G.** 1994. Routine CSF antigen detection for agents associated with bacterial meningitis: another point of view. Clin. Microbiol. Newsl. **16:**89–95.

117. **Thornsberry, C., D. F. Sahm, L. J. Kelly, I. A. Critchley, M. E. Jones, A. T. Evangelista, and J. A. Karlowsky.** 2002. Regional trends in antimicrobial resistance among clinical isolates of Streptococcus pneumoniae, Haemophilus influenzae, and Moraxella catarrhalis in the United States: results from the TRUST Surveillance Program, 1999–2000. Clin. Infect. Dis. **34(Suppl. 1):**S4–S16.

118. **Tong, H., X. Gao, and X. Dong.** 2003. Streptococcus oligofermentans sp. nov., a novel oral isolate from caries-free humans. Int. J. Syst. Evol. Microbiol. **53:**1101–1104.

119. **Uhl, J. R., S. C. Adamson, E. A. Vetter, C. D. Schleck, W. S. Harmsen, L. K. Iverson, P. J. Santrach, N. K. Henry, and F. R. Cockerill.** 2003. Comparison of LightCycler PCR, rapid antigen immunoassay, and culture for detection of group A streptococci from throat swabs. J. Clin. Microbiol. **41:**242–249.

120. **Vandamme, P., B. Pot, E. Falsen, K. Kersters, and L. A. Devriese.** 1996. Taxonomic study of Lancefield streptococcal groups C, G, and L (Streptococcus dysgalactiae) and proposal of S. dysgalactiae subsp. equisimilis subsp. nov. Int. J. Syst. Bacteriol. **46:**774–781.

121. **van't Wout, J. W., and H. A. Bijlmer.** 2005. Bacteremia due to Streptococcus gallolyticus, or the perils of revised nomenclature in bacteriology. Clin. Infect. Dis. **40:**1070–1071.

122. **Vieira, V., L. Teixeira, V. Zahner, H. Momen, R. Facklam, A. Steigerwalt, D. Brenner, and A. Castro.** 1998. Genetic relationships among the different phenotypes of Streptococcus dysgalactiae strains. *Int. J. Syst. Bacteriol.* **48:**1231–1243.

123. **Votava, M., M. Tejkalova, M. Drabkova, V. Unzeitig, and I. Braveny.** 2001. Use of GBS media for rapid detection of group B streptococci in vaginal and rectal swabs from women in labor. *Eur. J. Clin. Microbiol. Infect. Dis.* **20:**120–122.

124. **Weinstein, M. P., K. P. Klugman, and R. N. Jones.** 2009. Rationale for revised penicillin susceptibility breakpoints versus Streptococcus pneumoniae: coping with antimicrobial susceptibility in an era of resistance. *Clin. Infect. Dis.* **48:**1596–1600.

125. **Weinstein, M. R., M. Litt, D. A. Kertesz, P. Wyper, D. Rose, M. Coulter, A. McGeer, R. Facklam, C. Ostach, B. M. Willey, A. Borczyk, D. E. Low, et al.** 1997. Invasive infections due to a fish pathogen, Streptococcus iniae. *N. Engl. J. Med.* **337:**589–594.

126. **Welch, D. F., D. Hensel, D. Pickett, and S. Johnson.** 1991. Comparative evaluation of selective and nonselective culture techniques for isolation of group A beta-hemolytic streptococci. *Am. J. Clin. Pathol.* **95:**587–590.

127. **West, P. W., H. A. Foster, Q. Electricwala, and A. Alex.** 1996. Comparison of five methods for the determination of arginine hydrolysis by viridans streptococci. *J. Med. Microbiol.* **45:**501–504.

128. **Whiley, R. A., and D. Beighton.** 1991. Emended descriptions and recognition of Streptococcus constellatus, Streptococcus intermedius, and Streptococcus anginosus as distinct species. *Int. J. Syst. Bacteriol.* **41:**1–5.

129. **Whiley, R. A., H. Fraser, J. M. Hardie, and D. Beighton.** 1990. Phenotypic differentiation of *Streptococcus intermedius*, *Streptococcus constellatus*, and *Streptococcus anginosus* strains within the "Streptococcus milleri group." *J. Clin. Microbiol.* **28:**1497–1501.

130. **Whiley, R. A., L. M. Hall, J. M. Hardie, and D. Beighton.** 1999. A study of small-colony, beta-haemolytic, Lancefield group C streptococci within the anginosus group: description of Streptococcus constellatus subsp. pharyngis subsp. nov., associated with the human throat and pharyngitis. *Int. J. Syst. Bacteriol.* **49:**1443–1449.

131. **Willcox, M. D., H. Zhu, and K. W. Knox.** 2001. Streptococcus australis sp. nov., a novel oral streptococcus. *Int. J. Syst. Evol. Microbiol.* **51:**1277–1281.

Enterococcus

LÚCIA MARTINS TEIXEIRA, MARIA ᴅᴀ GLÓRIA SIQUEIRA CARVALHO,
PATRICIA LYNN SHEWMAKER, AND RICHARD R. FACKLAM

21

TAXONOMY

Early documentation on the microorganisms that are now included in the genus *Enterococcus* is mainly related to the "streptococci of fecal origin" or "enterococci" (see reference 31 for a brief historical overview). For a long time, they were considered a major category within the genus *Streptococcus,* distinguished by their higher resistance to chemical and physical agents and accommodating most of the serological group D streptococci. After the introduction of molecular methods for studying these microorganisms, however, the enterococci have undergone considerable changes in taxonomy, which started with the splitting of the genus *Streptococcus,* and the recognition of *Enterococcus* as a separate genus, in 1984 (87). *Streptococcus faecalis* and *Streptococcus faecium* were the first species to be transferred to the new genus as *Enterococcus faecalis* (the type species) and *Enterococcus faecium,* respectively. Subsequently, other earlier streptococcal species and subspecies were transferred and received new denominations as species of the genus *Enterococcus* (18). Since then, several new species have been described and proposed for inclusion in the genus *Enterococcus* (30, 31).

The enterococci belong to the low-guanine-plus-cytosine-content (G+C <50 mol%) branch of the phylum *Firmicutes.* Phylogenetic analysis based on the comparison of the 16S rRNA gene sequences showed that members of the genus *Enterococcus* are more closely related to those included in the genera *Vagococcus, Tetragenococcus,* and *Carnobacterium* than they are to *Streptococcus* and *Lactococcus,* genera to which they have been phenotypically associated (25, 31).

Current criteria for inclusion in the genus *Enterococcus* and for the description of new enterococcal species encompass a polyphasic approach resulting from a combination of different molecular techniques (frequently involving DNA-DNA reassociation experiments, 16S rRNA gene sequencing, and whole-cell protein profiling analysis) and phenotypic tests. Partial or nearly entire sequencing of the 16S rDNA is nowadays considered a practical and powerful tool in aiding the identification of enterococcal species, and it has been performed for all recognized species of *Enterococcus.* Figure 1 shows the phylogenetic relationships among the species of *Enterococcus* based on the analysis of 16S rRNA gene sequences, which are available from the GenBank database. Several other molecular methods, mostly nucleic acid-based assays, have been used as additional tools to assess the phylogenetic relationships among enterococcal species and to formulate the description of new species, but their use is still limited.

DESCRIPTION OF THE GENUS

The members of the genus *Enterococcus* are gram-positive, catalase-negative cocci that occur singly or are arranged in pairs or as short chains. Cells are sometimes coccobacillary when Gram stains are prepared from growth on solid medium but tend to be ovoid and in chains when grown in liquid media, such as thioglycolate broth. After growth on blood agar media for 24 h, colonies are usually between 1 and 2 mm in diameter, although some variants may appear smaller. Some (about one-third) cultures of *E. faecalis* may be β-hemolytic on agar containing rabbit, horse, or human blood but nonhemolytic on agar containing sheep blood. Some cultures of *E. faecalis* and *Enterococcus durans* may be β-hemolytic regardless of the type of blood used. All other species are usually α-hemolytic or nonhemolytic. Enterococci are facultative anaerobes with a homofermentative metabolism that results in the production of ʟ-(+)-lactic acid as the major end product of glucose fermentation. Because of their ability to ferment a wide range of carbohydrates to lactic acid, the enterococci are referred to as typical lactic acid bacteria. Gas is not produced. These microorganisms are usually able to grow at temperatures ranging from 10 to 45°C, with optimum growth at 35 to 37°C. The majority of the species grow in broth containing 6.5% NaCl, and they hydrolyze esculin in the presence of bile salts (bile-esculin [BE] test). They also hydrolyze leucine-β-naphthylamide by producing leucine aminopeptidase (LAP). Most enterococci, apart from *Enterococcus cecorum, Enterococcus columbae, Enterococcus pallens, Enterococcus saccharolyticus,* and some strains of the recently described species *Enterococcus canintestini, Enterococcus devriesei, Enterococcus moraviensis,* and *Enterococcus termitis,* hydrolyze ʟ-pyrrolidonyl-β-naphthylamide (PYR) by producing pyrrolidonyl arylamidase (pyrrolidonase). Results for both LAP and PYR testing, especially for some of the more recently described species, may vary according to the methodology, including the test format and media used to grow the

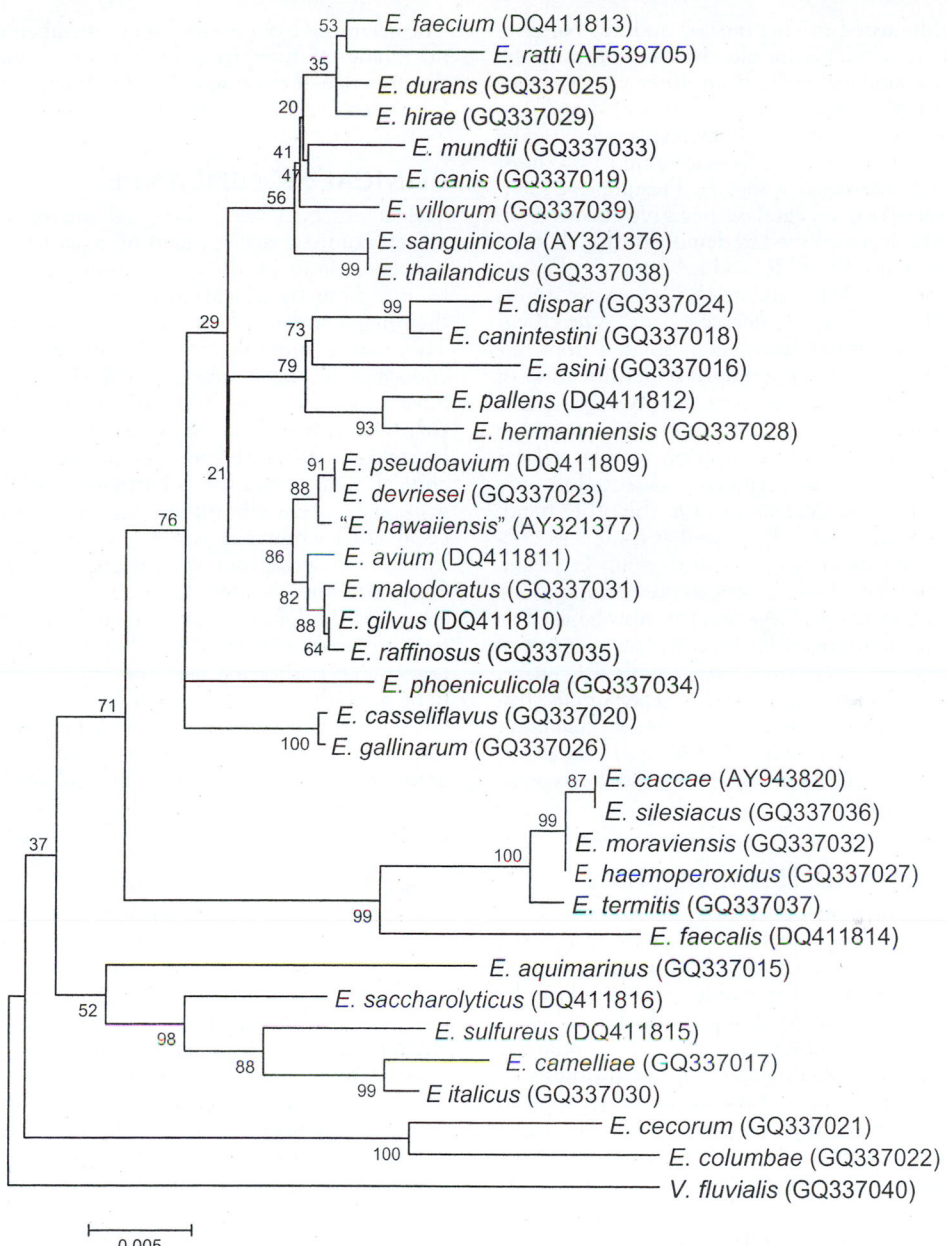

FIGURE 1 Phylogenetic tree based on comparative analysis of the 16S rDNA sequences, showing the relationships among the type strains of species of *Enterococcus*. *Vagococcus fluvialis* was used as an outgroup, and bootstrap values at the nodes are displayed as percentages.

bacterial cells. A few species are motile (*Enterococcus casseliflavus* and *Enterococcus gallinarum*), and some are pigmented (*E. casseliflavus*, *Enterococcus gilvus*, *Enterococcus mundtii*, *E. pallens*, and *Enterococcus sulfureus*) (25, 31, 46). Methods used for detection of enterococcal motility have to be selected carefully, as differences in motility due to the composition of the medium have been demonstrated (108). Enterococci are not able to synthesize porphyrins and therefore do not produce cytochrome enzymes (46). However, cytochrome activity is sometimes expressed when strains of *E. faecalis* are grown on blood-containing media, and a weak effervescence is observed in the catalase test. Positive catalase testing has also been reported for strains of

Enterococcus haemoperoxidus (94) and *Enterococcus silesiacus* (95) when cultivated on blood-containing agar media. Most enterococcal strains produce a cell wall-associated glycerol teichoic acid that is identified as Lancefield's serological group D antigen. The G+C content of the DNA ranges from 32 to 44 mol%. The genome size is in the range of approximately 2.0 to 3.5 Mb (5, 78, 89). Genome sequencing of *E. faecalis* V583 (80), the first vancomycin-resistant clinical isolate in the United States, has opened many lines of investigation to improve our understanding about the genus *Enterococcus*.

The other genera of catalase-negative gram-positive cocci and the characteristics that distinguish them from the enterococci are discussed in chapters 20 and 22. No phenotypic criteria are available for clearly distinguishing the genus *Enterococcus* unequivocally from other genera, since there are no particular characteristics that are common to all enterococci. However, certain characteristics are usually found in the majority of the strains belonging to the most frequently isolated enterococcal species. Presumptive identification of a gram-positive, catalase-negative coccus as an *Enterococcus* can be accomplished by demonstrating that the strain is positive for the BE, PYR, and LAP tests and grows in the presence of 6.5% NaCl and at 45°C. Because strains of *Lactococcus*, *Leuconostoc*, *Pediococcus*, and *Vagococcus* with phenotypic similarities have been isolated from human infections (33, 98), the presumptive identification of enterococci based only on BE reaction and growth in 6.5% NaCl broth can be erroneous. Demonstrating the presence of group D antigen by serological reaction may be helpful in identification, although this antigen is detected in only about 80% of the enterococcal strains. On the other hand, pediococci and leuconostocs (33), as well as some vagococcal strains (98), can also react with anti-group D serum. Reactivity with the AccuProbe *Enterococcus* genetic probe (GenProbe, Inc., San Diego, CA) test can also be used to confirm an unknown strain as an *Enterococcus*. Strains of most known species of *Enterococcus* react with this probe, except for the type strains of *Enterococcus aquimarinus*, *Enterococcus asini*, *Enterococcus canis*, *E. cecorum*, *E. columbae*, *E. haemoperoxidus*, *E. moraviensis*, *E. pallens*, *E. saccharolyticus*, *E. silesiacus*, and *E. termitis*. However, *Vagococcus* strains may also react (98).

EPIDEMIOLOGY AND TRANSMISSION

Several intrinsic characteristics of the enterococci allow them to grow and survive in harsh conditions and persist almost everywhere, colonizing several ecological niches. These microorganisms are widespread in nature and can be found in soil, plants, water, food, and animals, including mammals, birds, insects, and reptiles (25, 97). In humans, they are predominantly inhabitants of the gastrointestinal tract and are less commonly found in other sites, such as in the genitourinary tract, the oral cavity, and skin, especially in the perineal area (25, 97). The prevalence of the different enterococcal species appears to vary according to the host and is also influenced by age, diet, and other factors that may be related to changes in physiologic conditions, such as underlying diseases and prior antimicrobial therapy. Enterococci are considered the most abundant gram-positive cocci colonizing the intestine, with *E. faecalis* being one of the most common bacteria isolated from this site (25, 97). Other species, such as *E. faecium*, *E. casseliflavus*, *E. durans*, and *E. gallinarum*, are also found in variable proportions in the gastrointestinal tract of humans. Since the enterococci are opportunistic pathogens, the incidence of each species found in human infections probably reflects the distribution of the different species of *Enterococcus* in the human gastrointestinal tract. This site is believed to represent an important reservoir for strains associated with disease; from this location they may migrate to cause infections and can also disseminate to other hosts and to the environment. On the other hand, the occurrence of high numbers of enterococci in the feces, as well as their ability to resist different chemical and physical conditions and to survive in the environment, implies that the enterococci can be used as indicators of fecal contamination and of the hygienic quality of food, milk, and drinking water (36).

The occurrence of enterococci as members of the intestinal microbiota of humans (97) and the relationship between the presence of enterococci in foods and human safety (36) have been extensively reviewed.

CLINICAL SIGNIFICANCE

The enterococci are commensal microorganisms that act as opportunistic agents, causing a variety of infections in humans. Many of these infections have been suggested to arise from translocation of the enterococcal cells from their major site of colonization in the gastrointestinal tract. They most commonly infect the urinary tract, bloodstream, endocardium, burn and surgical site wounds, abdomen, biliary tract, catheters, and other implanted medical devices (62, 69, 71, 84). The ubiquitous presence of enterococci, however, requires the use of caution in establishing the clinical significance of a particular isolate. Unnecessary work and potentially misleading laboratory reports should be avoided whenever possible, especially with respect to in vitro susceptibility testing decisions (see "Antimicrobial Susceptibilities" below). Over the last decades, they have emerged from long being considered virtually harmless bacteria to medically important multiple-antibiotic-resistant nosocomial pathogens that contribute significantly to patient morbidity and mortality, as well as healthcare costs. Changes in the dynamics of the host-commensal relationship, such as those promoted by the use of broad-spectrum antibiotics, host injury, or diminished host immunity, could allow these bacteria to gain access to extraintestinal host sites and cause infection. Therefore, elderly patients with serious underlying diseases and other severely ill immunocompromised patients who have been hospitalized for prolonged periods, treated with invasive devices, and/or received broad-spectrum antimicrobial therapy are at higher risk to acquire enterococcal infections (2, 62, 71).

The pathogenesis of enterococcal infections is still poorly understood. Although a debate subsists over whether serious enterococcal infections arise from one's own indigenous biota or from exogenously acquired strains, epidemiological studies show the existence of clonal relationships among outbreak isolates and support the notion that a subset of virulent lineages with greater propensity to cause disease exist and are often responsible for infections of epidemic proportions (57, 100, 105, 114). Several potential virulence factors were identified in enterococcal isolates and have been suggested to play a role in the pathogenesis of enterococcal infections; these include the surface adhesins Esp (enterococcal surface protein) and aggregation substance, the secreted toxin cytolysin/hemolysin, the secreted proteases gelatinase and serine protease, MSCRAMM Ace (adhesin to collagen of *E. faecalis*), *E. faecalis* antigen A, enterococcal capsule, cell wall polysaccharides, and extracellular superoxide (47, 83, 100). Nevertheless, none has been established as having a major contribution to enterococcal virulence in humans. One mechanism by which the enterococci can deviate from their commensal behavior is through the acquisition of new traits that allow the bacterium to overcome host defenses and colonize new niches, as suggested by the identification of the *E. faecalis* pathogenicity island, which highlights genetic differences between infection-derived and commensal strains (64, 88, 100). In this context, acquired antimicrobial resistance is considered one of the many traits that virulent enterococci possess compared with commensal isolates, as it may be fundamental to allow members of this genus to survive for extended periods of time in the host or environment, leading to their persistence and role as prominent nosocomial pathogens (47, 88, 100). In addition, enterococci can transfer resistance determinants to other bacteria, for example, staphylococci, which further increases the clinical importance of the enterococci. The ability to form biofilms has recently been listed among the most prominent virulence properties of these microorganisms, allowing colonization of inert and biological surfaces while protecting against antimicrobial substances and mediating adhesion and invasion of host cells (2, 28). Biofilm formation may be of particular importance in the development of endocarditis, endodontic and urinary infections, and implant- as well as other medical device-associated infections (2, 117).

The variety of infections associated with the enterococci has been thoroughly reviewed and summarized (62, 71). Although the spectrum of infections has remained relatively unchanged since the extensive review by Murray (71), trends to increasing prevalence of these organisms as nosocomial pathogens have been frequently observed. Enterococci have become the second or third leading cause of nosocomial urinary tract infections (UTIs), wound infections (mostly surgical, decubitus ulcers, and burn wounds), and bacteremia in the United States (4, 53, 62, 71, 73, 74). UTIs are the most common of the enterococcal infections: enterococci have been implicated in approximately 10% of all UTIs and in up to approximately 16% of nosocomial UTIs. Enterococcal bacteremia is frequently associated with metastatic abscesses in multiple organs and high mortality rates. Enterococci have also been considered an important cause of endocarditis; they are estimated to account for about 20% of the cases of native valve bacterial endocarditis and for about 6 to 7% of prosthetic valve endocarditis. Endocarditis remains among the most difficult-to-treat enterococcal infections because of limitations on bactericidal antimicrobial therapy for enterococcal infections, especially when caused by vancomycin-resistant enterococci (VRE). Intra-abdominal and pelvic infections are also commonly associated with enterococci. However, cultures from patients with peritonitis, intra-abdominal or pelvic abscesses, biliary tract infections, surgical site infections, and endomyometritis are frequently polymicrobial, and the role of enterococci in these settings remains controversial. The significance of isolates from some of these sites, then, should be carefully evaluated before clinical decisions are made. There is also a growing concern about the role of the enterococci in endodontic and implant- and medical device-associated infections (2, 117). Infections of the respiratory tract or the central nervous system, as well as otitis, sinusitis, septic arthritis, and endophthalmitis, may occur but are rare.

E. faecalis is usually the enterococcal species most frequently isolated from human clinical specimens, representing 80 to 90% of the isolates, followed by *E. faecium*, which is found in 5 to 10% of enterococcal infections (8, 32, 40, 70). However, the ratios of isolation of the different enterococcal species can vary according to each setting and can be affected by a number of aspects, including the increasing dissemination of outbreak-related strains, such as vancomycin-resistant *E. faecium* (42, 49, 53, 105). A trend for a progressive decline in the ratio of *E. faecalis* to *E. faecium* seems to be particularly evident among bloodstream isolates (42, 49, 53). The other enterococcal species are identified less frequently, even though clusters of infections associated with *E. casseliflavus* (75), *E. gallinarum* (19, 67, 76), and *E. raffinosus* (55, 113) have been reported. Several of the other enterococcal

species, including *E. avium*, *E. caccae*, *E. cecorum*, *E. dispar*, *E. durans*, *E. gallinarum*, *E. gilvus*, "*E. hawaiiensis*," *E. hirae*, *E. italicus*, *E. malodoratus*, *E. mundtii*, *E. pallens*, *E. pseudoavium*, and *E. sanguinicola*, have also been isolated from human sources.

Although the enterococci can cause human infections in the community and in the hospital, these microorganisms began to be recognized with increasing frequency as common causes of hospital-acquired infections in the late 1970s, paralleling the increasing resistance to most currently used antimicrobial agents. A major impact on the incidence and epidemiology of enterococcal infections was noted after the first reports on the occurrence and epidemic increase of VRE in hospitals in the United States. By 1993, the rates of VRE had already increased 34-fold in intensive care units of U.S. hospitals (12). The percentage of VRE isolates reported by U.S. hospitals increased from 0.3% in 1989 to over 25% of all isolates in 1999 (73). Since then, the enterococci have usually been listed as the second or third most frequent nosocomial pathogen isolated from intensive care unit patients in the United States, depending on the type of infection (42, 74, 84). In the 2006–2007 report from the National Healthcare Safety Network at the Centers for Disease Control and Prevention (CDC), the enterococci were listed as the third most common antimicrobial-resistant pathogen associated with healthcare-associated infections, accounting for 12% of the them (42). Considering both the Surveillance and Control of Pathogens of Epidemiological Importance (SCOPE) and the Antimicrobial Resistance Surveillance Program (SENTRY) databases, about 2% of *E. faecalis* and 60% of *E. faecium* isolates recovered from the bloodstream were resistant to vancomycin (4). The occurrence and spread of VRE have now reached a more global dimension. According to the European Antimicrobial Resistance Surveillance System (www.earss.rivm.nl) data, the prevalence of VRE in nosocomial enterococcal bacteremia is already ranging from 5 to 30% in several European countries (112). VRE are also encountered at different rates in several other parts of the world, including South America, Asia, and Australia, illustrating the pandemic spread of hospital-associated VRE (114).

Hospitalized patients with gastrointestinal carriage of VRE appear to be the major reservoir of the organism, and once colonized, the patients remain so for weeks or months. Thus, as colonized patients leave the hospital, the possibility that transmission might occur in the community cannot be discounted. VRE can be disseminated by direct patient-to-patient contact or indirectly via transient carriage on healthcare workers' hands; contaminated medical instruments, such as glucose meters, blood pressure cuffs, electronic thermometers, and electrocardiogram monitors and wires; and environmental surfaces, such as patient gowns and linens, beds, bedside rails, overbed tables, floors, door knobs, and wash basins (56, 118).

As a response to the rising rates of VRE colonization and infection in U.S. hospitals, the CDC's Hospital Infection Control Practices Advisory Committee established guidelines with recommendations for preventing the spread of VRE (44). These include prudent vancomycin use, implementation of surveillance procedures for early detection of VRE, and infection control procedures to limit cross-contamination, such as isolation precautions, hand washing, and education about transmission of VRE.

Although only a small percentage of colonized patients develop serious systemic enterococcal infections, intestinal colonization with VRE has been clearly associated with subsequent VRE infections. However, in certain specific clinical situations, such as liver transplant recipients, patients on chronic hemodialysis, and oncology patients, particularly those with hematological malignancies, VRE-colonized patients appear to be at increased risk for developing serious enterococcal infections (2, 16, 118). This underscores the importance of active surveillance in high-risk patient groups to prevent transmission and outbreaks.

COLLECTION, TRANSPORT, AND STORAGE OF SPECIMENS

The standard methods for collecting blood, urine, wound secretions, and other secretions or swab specimens suspected of harboring enterococci are adequate (see chapter 16). No special methods or procedures are usually necessary for transport and storage of clinical specimens containing enterococci because these microorganisms are easily recovered and are relatively resistant to environmental changes and adverse conditions. Transport can be performed on almost any transport medium or on swabs that are kept dry. Like most clinical samples, the material should be cultured as soon as possible.

Enterococcal strains can be stored indefinitely when lyophilized. In our experience, cultures frozen at −70°C or less can be stored for several years as heavy cell suspensions made directly in defibrinated sheep or rabbit blood or in a skim milk (10%) solution containing glycerol (10%). These are the preferable methods for preservation of enterococcal strains. Cultures can also be preserved for many years at −20°C in other cryopreservative media commonly used for maintenance of bacteria. Most strains of enterococci can survive for several months at 4°C on agar slants prepared with ordinary agar bases, such as brain heart infusion agar and Trypticase soy agar. Certain of the less well known species, however, are not as resistant to adverse conditions and may not survive long if more adequate preservation procedures are not used.

DIRECT EXAMINATION

The direct microscopic examination of Gram-stained smears of normally sterile clinical specimens, such as blood, may be useful for the diagnosis of enterococcal infections. Direct examination of certain nonsterile specimens may also be informative but should not be overemphasized. In any case, only a presumptive report of the "presence of gram-positive cocci" should be made, as microscopy by itself cannot differentiate the enterococci from most of the other gram-positive cocci. Culture and appropriate identification techniques should be performed for confirmation.

As the occurrence of VRE continues to represent an important problem worldwide, hospitals are encouraged to implement surveillance programs for VRE detection. In an attempt to overcome the inherent limitations of the culture-based methods of detection (discussed in "Isolation Procedures" below), conventional PCR and real-time PCR-based methods have been developed and evaluated for direct detection of these microorganisms in clinical and surveillance specimens (3, 29, 63, 79, 86, 90, 92, 116). Commercially available molecular tests that have been approved by the U.S. Food and Drug Administration (FDA) for VRE screening directly from rectal swabs include the BD GeneOhm VanR assay (BD GeneOhm, San Diego, CA)

(92) and the Xpert vanA assay (Cepheid, Sunnyvale, CA). The LightCycler vanA/vanB detection assay (Roche Diagnostics, Basel, Switzerland) has also been evaluated (29, 90, 116), but it has not been licensed for use in the United States yet. Different investigators have developed assays independently (3, 86). All of these studies have reported improved detection of VRE in rectal swabs and fecal specimens over conventional culture techniques. It is important to note that most systems use different primers for detection of the *van* genes and that sensitivities may vary (3, 63, 116). Specificity is also a potential problem unless PCR controls for genus and/or species identification are included, because *van* genes may be found in bacteria other than enterococci (3, 63, 116).

Assays for detection and identification of enterococci directly in blood samples have been reported. An in-house real-time PCR assay for quantitative detection of *E. faecalis* DNA in blood samples without prior cultivation has been proposed for the diagnosis of bacteremia (82). The LightCycler SeptiFast Test (Roche Molecular Systems, Branchburg, NJ) is, to date, the only multiplex real-time PCR assay licensed for use in the United States for the rapid detection and identification of major pathogens involved in nosocomial bacteremia, including *E. faecalis* and *E. faecium*, directly from whole blood (11). As the technology evolves, these molecular methods may become widely available for the rapid and precise detection of enterococci directly in clinical samples. However, further evaluation is needed to determine the real impact of their use on laboratory diagnosis of invasive enterococcal infections and on patient management.

ISOLATION PROCEDURES

The source of clinical specimens to be tested for the presence of enterococci influences the type of medium needed for primary isolation. Clinical specimens from normally sterile body sites can be plated directly onto a nonselective medium, such as Trypticase soy agar, brain heart infusion agar, or other blood agar base containing 5% sheep, horse, or rabbit blood. In general, strains of the most clinically relevant species grow well at 35 to 37°C and do not require an atmosphere containing increased levels of CO_2, although some strains grow better in this atmosphere. Samples for blood culture can be inoculated into conventional blood culture systems. For clinical specimens obtained from nonsterile sites, especially those heavily contaminated with gram-negative bacteria, use of selective media is a good option for primary isolation. Many different media have been devised for selective isolation of enterococci, but none has been proven to be specific. Furthermore, not all enterococcal species grow on these selective media. Most of these media contain sodium azide, bile salts, and/or antibiotics as selective components and esculin or tetrazolium as indicator substances. Some of these media are supplied under different designations by various manufacturers. The diversity of media used for the isolation of enterococci from various sources has been reviewed (26). Consideration must also be given to whether or not an enrichment broth should be employed when rectal or fecal samples are tested. The use of a broth enrichment step in the primary isolation delays identification but increases the recovery rates of enterococci (23, 77). Enrichment procedures are applied mainly to detect VRE present in low numbers (48).

The increasing incidence of vancomycin resistance among the enterococci has raised the importance of selective isolation of VRE. Early identification of infection or colonization by VRE is recommended to prevent the spread of these microorganisms (44, 110). Current recommendations for hospital infection control include VRE fecal surveillance cultures, but the optimal methods for obtaining these cultures are still unclear. Different selective agar and/or broth media formulations and several procedures have been employed for the isolation of VRE from sources containing normal biota, such as stool samples and rectal or perianal swab specimens (21, 26, 45, 77, 79, 86). Most of them are variations of selective media differing with regard to the antimicrobial agents or the antimicrobial concentrations used. However, no consensus has been established for medium base, vancomycin concentration, or method of use. Although there is not a single generally accepted screening method for isolation at this point, the use of a selective enrichment broth to enhance the recovery of VRE seems to be a highly effective procedure. Enterococcosel broth (a bile-esculin azide [BEA] medium supplied by Becton Dickinson Microbiology Systems) has been used in a number of studies as the base medium supplemented with different concentrations of vancomycin, with 6 μg/ml being the most common concentration. A commercially available medium, labeled BEAV and containing 6 μg/ml vancomycin (distributed by Remel Inc., Lenexa, KS), has also been evaluated (59).

Media containing chromogenic substrates have also been proposed for the isolation and presumptive identification of enterococci. The first of these media, CHROMagar orientation (from Becton Dickinson Microbiology Systems), was promoted as an isolation and identification medium for enterococci from urine (66). Another chromogenic medium, CPS ID3 (bioMérieux, Marcy l'Etoile, France), has been made available (14) to do the same. Several studies have employed another new chromogenic agar medium, ChromID VRE (bioMérieux), on which *E. faecium* colonies appear purple and *E. faecalis* colonies appear blue or blue-green (21, 23, 41, 59, 63). Thus, the two most common species of VRE are identified on this chromogenic primary isolation medium. Results obtained by using ChromID VRE medium have been considered more rapid (41) and more specific than those obtained with BEA or BEAV-based media (21).

Culture-based screening methods for VRE may be especially demanding and can take several days to complete, besides having variable degrees of sensitivity, which affects the timely implementation of infection control procedures. Therefore, some microbiology laboratories have recently considered the introduction of molecular techniques to detect VRE to facilitate the rapid and accurate identification of these organisms and to improve sensitivity for detecting this pathogen. However, most of the current approaches still require bacterial growth in culture prior to detection, requiring 24 h or more to complete. The application of methods for a more rapid detection of VRE directly from clinical samples is still an area of major interest (see "Direct Examination" above).

IDENTIFICATION OF *ENTEROCOCCUS* SPECIES

Identification by Conventional Physiological Testing

Once it is established that an unknown catalase-negative gram-positive coccus is an *Enterococcus* or closely related genus (see "Description of the Genus" above), the tests (see reference 33 and chapters 3, 17, and 18) listed in Table 1

can be used to identify the species. The data presented in Table 1 for the phenotypic characteristics are derived from conventional testing (except for β-galactosidase) performed at the CDC *Streptococcus* laboratory (see http://www.cdc.gov/ncidod/biotech/strep/strep-doc/index.htm). Most of the information presented in Table 1 for the most frequent species is related to the phenotypic characteristics of isolates obtained from humans. Isolates from nonhuman sources, even those belonging to well-known species, may have different results for some tests. Species that have not been recovered from humans to date are also included in Table 1 due to the possibility that they will be isolated from human sources in the future.

Enterococcal species can be initially separated into five physiological groups of species based on acid formation from mannitol and sorbose and hydrolysis of arginine (Table 1). Identification of enterococcal species by conventional tests is not rapid and may require incubation of the tests for up to 10 days. However, the majority of the isolates recovered from human sources can be identified after 2 days of incubation.

Group I includes nine species (see Table 1 for details). "*E. hawaiiensis*" is a denomination that has been proposed for the new species previously designated *Enterococcus* sp. nov. CDC PNS-E3 (10). *E. avium* and *E. raffinosus* are the most relevant species in this group, considering the association with human clinical sources. Group II comprises eight species. The majority of the isolates recovered from human sources belong to species included in this group. Atypical strains that do not hydrolyze arginine or do not form acid from mannitol have been documented. *Lactococcus* sp. is also listed in this group because the phenotypic characteristics of some strains can lead to misidentification as an *Enterococcus*. If nonmotile variants of *E. casseliflavus* and *E. gallinarum* are encountered, production of acid from methyl-α-D-glucopyranoside can be used to help in the identification of these species. *E. sanguinicola* is the denomination proposed for the species provisionally designated *Enterococcus* sp. nov. CDC PNS-E2 (9, 10). Group III consists of six species. Three of these species (*E. durans*, *E. ratti*, and *E. villorum*) have very similar phenotypic profiles in the tests listed in Table 1. Reactions in litmus milk and hydrolysis of hippurate, in addition to the reactions listed in Table 1, may also be used to help differentiate the species. In litmus milk, *E. durans* forms acid and clot, *E. villorum* forms acid but no clot, and *E. ratti* does not form acid or clot. *E. durans* hydrolyzes hippurate, while *E. villorum* does not. *E. ratti* is variable in the hippurate hydrolysis test. The other members of this group are easily identified by the reactions shown in Table 1. Uncommon mannitol-negative variant strains of *E. faecalis* and *E. faecium* resemble species in this group. However, *E. faecalis* strains are positive in the pyruvate test but not for acid formation from arabinose, raffinose, or sucrose, and *E. faecium* variant strains form acid from arabinose. Group IV includes eight species. *E. caccae* and *E. cecorum* are the only species in this group that have been isolated from human sources to date. Group V comprises six species. Variant strains of *E. casseliflavus*, *E. gallinarum*, and *E. faecalis* that fail to hydrolyze arginine resemble the microorganisms included in this group. However, these variant strains have characteristics similar to the strains that hydrolyze arginine and can be differentiated by the same phenotypic tests. *Vagococcus fluvialis* is listed here because the phenotypic characteristics of this species are very similar to those of the genus *Enterococcus*, and some strains may be identified as enterococci (98). *E. italicus*

TABLE 1 Phenotypic characteristics used for the identification of *Enterococcus* species and some physiologically related species of other gram-positive cocci

Group and species	Phenotypic characteristic[a]														
	MAN	SOR	ARG	ARA	SBL	RAF	TEL	MOT	PIG	SUC	PYU	MGP	TRE	XYL	GAL
Group I															
E. avium	+	+	−	+	+	−	−	−	−	+	+	V	+	−	V
E. raffinosus	+	+	−	+	+	+	−	−	−	+	+	V	+	−	−
E. gilvus	+	+	−	−	+	+	−	−	+	+	+	−	+	−	−
E. pallens	+	+	−	−	+	+	−	−	+	+	−	+	+	−	−
E. saccharolyticus[b]	+	+	−	−	+	+	−	−	−	+	−	+	+	−	+
E. malodoratus	+	+	−	−	+	+	−	−	−	+	+	V	+	V	+
E. pseudoavium	+	+	−	−	+	−	−	−	−	+	+	+	+	V	V
E. devriesei[b]	+	+	−	−	+	−	−	−	−	+	−	−	+	−	−
"E. hawaiiensis"	+	+	−	−	+	−	−	−	−	+	−	−	+	−	−
Group II															
E. faecium	+[d]	−	+	+	V	V	−	−	−	+[d]	−	−	+	−[d]	V
E. casseliflavus	+	−	+[d]	+	V	+	−[d]	+[d]	+[d]	+	V	+	+	+	+
E. gallinarum	+	−	+[d]	+	−	+	−	+[d]	−	+	−	+	+	+	+
E. mundtii	+	−	+	+	V	+	−	−	+	+	−	−	+	+	V
E. faecalis	+[d]	−	+[d]	−	+	−	+	−	−	+[d]	+	−	+	−[d]	−
E. haemoperoxidus[b]	+[c]	−	+[c]	−	−	−	−	−	−	+	−	+	+	−	−
E. sanguinicola	+	−	+	−	−	−	V[e]	−	−	+	−	−	+	−	−
E. thailandicus[b]	+	−	+	−	−	−	−	−	−	+	−	−	+	−	−
Lactococcus sp.	+	−	+	−	−	−	−	−	−	V	−	−	+	−	−
Group III															
E. dispar	−	−	+	−	−	+	−	−	−	+	+	+	+[e]	−	+
E. canintestini[b]	−	−	+	−	−	+	−	−	−	+	+	+	+	−	−
E. hirae	−	−	+	−	−	+	−	−	−	+	−	−	+	−	V
E. durans	−	−	+	−	−	−	−	−	−	−	−	−	−[d]	−	V
E. ratti	−	−	+	−	−	−	−	−	−	−	−	−	V	−	−
E. villorum	−	−	+	−	−	−	−	−	−	−	−	−	+	+	+
Group IV															
E. aquimarinus[b]	−	−	−	+	−	+	−	−	−	+	−	+	+	+	+
E. phoeniculicola[b]	−	−	−	+	−	+	−	−	−	+	−	+	+	+	+
E. cecorum[b]	−	−	−	−	−	+	−	−	−	+	+	−	+	−	+
E. sulfureus	−	−	−	−	−	+	−	−	+	+	−	+	+	−	+
E. asini[b]	−	−	−	−	−	−	−	−	−	+	−	−	+	+	+
E. caccae	−	−	−	−	−	−	−	−	−	+	+	+[c]	+	−	−
E. silesiacus[b]	−	−	−	−	−	−	−	−	−	+	−	+[c]	+	+	−
E. termitis[b]	−	−	−	−	−	−	−	−	−	+	+	+	+	+	−
Group V															
E. canis[b]	+	−	−	+	−	−	−	−	−	+	+	+	+	+	−
E. columbae[b]	+	−	−	+	+	+	−	−	−	+	+	−	+	+	−
E. moraviensis[b]	+	−	−	+	−	−	−	−	−	+	+	+	+	−	+
E. camelliae[b]	+	−	−	−	−	−	−	−	−	+	+	+	+	−	−
E. hermanniensis	+	−	−	−	−	−	−	−	−	−	−	−	+	−	−
E. italicus	V	−	−	−	V	−	−	−	−	+	+	+	+	−	−
Vagococcus fluvialis	+	−	−	−	+	−	−	+	−	+	−	+	+	−	−

[a] Abbreviations and symbols: MAN, mannitol; SOR, sorbose; ARG, arginine; ARA, arabinose; SBL, sorbitol; RAF, raffinose; TEL, 0.04% tellurite; MOT, motility; PIG, pigment; SUC, sucrose; PYU, pyruvate; MGP, methyl-α-D-glucopyranoside; TRE, trehalose; XYL, xylose; GAL, 2-naphthyl-β-D-galactopyranoside; +, 90% or more of the strains are positive; −, 90% or more of the strains are negative; V, variable (11 to 89% of the strains are positive).

[b] Phenotypic characteristics are based on data from type strains.

[c] Late positive (3 days' incubation or longer).

[d] Occasional exceptions occur (<3% of strains show atypical reactions).

[e] w, weak reaction.

corresponds to the new species previously designated *Enterococcus* sp. nov. CDC PNS-E1 (9, 10, 35). Among this group, only a single strain of *E. italicus* has been isolated from human sources (9).

Identification by Commercial Systems

There are several commercially available miniaturized, manual, semiautomated, and automated identification systems that may be an alternative to conventional testing for the phenotypic identification of enterococcal species in routine diagnostic laboratories. Since their introduction, these systems have been updated to improve their performance characteristics and expand their identification capabilities as investigators have become more aware of inaccuracies (22, 38, 50, 113). In general, these systems are reliable for the identification of the most common species: *E. faecalis* and, to a lesser extent, *E. faecium*. Precise identification of other species by most systems depends on additional testing, although improvements have been observed with updated formats and databases. Commercial systems available for the identification of enterococcal species include the API 20S and the API Rapid ID32 STREP systems (bioMérieux Vitek, Inc., Hazelwood, MO), the Crystal Gram-Positive and the Crystal Rapid Gram-Positive identification systems (Becton Dickinson Microbiology Systems, Sparks, MD), the Gram Positive Identification Card of the Vitek system (bioMérieux), the Gram-Positive Identification panel of the MicroScan Walk/Away system (Dade MicroScan, West Sacramento, CA), and the BD Phoenix Automated Microbiology system (Becton Dickinson Microbiology Systems). Overall, a large proportion of enterococcal isolates recovered from human sources can be accurately identified by most of the commercial systems now available; however, the accuracy is dependent on the distribution of species found in each specific setting. Difficulties in the identification of a variety of enterococcal species, including *E. faecalis* and *E. faecium*, are still being reported (7, 50, 81). Strict adherence to the instructions provided by the manufacturer, including the base of the media used to grow strains for testing, is of paramount importance. Our own unpublished experimental results indicate that differences in growth conditions can lead to variation in the results of some tests, interfering with the accuracy of the identification. Identification of an unusual enterococcal species by a commercial system should be confirmed by a reference method before being reported.

Identification by Molecular Methods

Molecular methods, such as DNA-DNA hybridization and sequencing of the 16S rRNA genes, have been used primarily for taxonomic purposes in reference or research laboratories. In the past 2 decades, however, the application of molecular techniques for the rapid identification of *Enterococcus* species has expanded dramatically for use in clinical microbiology laboratories.

A variety of molecular procedures have been proposed for the identification of enterococcal species, as previously reviewed and summarized (27, 31). Many of these molecular procedures have been performed in only a few laboratories and have not been evaluated for all of the species of *Enterococcus*. Most of them are potentially applicable to all enterococcal species, and others are species specific. Several of these methods deserve consideration for expanded testing and future improvements, as they represent promising adjunct tools for a more rapid and precise identification of enterococcal species.

Among the molecular techniques proposed to identify the different enterococcal species, sodium dodecyl sulfate-polyacrylamide gel electrophoresis analysis of whole-cell protein (WCP) profiles and sequencing of the 16S rRNA genes have been more extensively evaluated in reference laboratories. Sodium dodecyl sulfate-polyacrylamide gel electrophoresis analysis of WCP profiles was shown to be a reliable tool for the differentiation and identification of typical and atypical *Enterococcus* strains, since WCP profiles are species specific (10, 31, 68, 99). Table 1, which depicts the phenotypic characteristics of the *Enterococcus* species discussed in this chapter, is based on correlations between the WCP profiles and the phenotypic tests, in conjunction with DNA-DNA reassociation experiments and 16S DNA sequencing. Sequencing of the 16S rRNA gene is currently the most frequently used among the nucleic acid-based methods for identification of enterococcal species. It has been performed for all species of enterococci, and the sequences are available for comparison purposes via public databanks of nucleotide sequences, such as GenBank. Comparisons can be made by using one of several sequence-comparing software packages, many of which are available for public access. Figure 1 depicts a dendrogram generated by comparison of 16S rDNA sequences of the type strains of the species included in the genus *Enterococcus*. However, clear-cut differentiation is not always obtained for all enterococcal species, since some of them differ by only 2 or 3 bases over the approximately 1,500-base span of the 16S rRNA gene. Therefore, this procedure should not be used alone, but together with phenotypic characterization and other alternative molecular methods, it can be an important tool to establish enterococcal species identity.

PCR-based techniques have also been a focus of major interest for rapid and accurate enterococcal identification. Schemes for amplification of the *ddl* (24, 50) or *sodA* (50) genes have already been designed for several enterococcal species and constitute convenient alternative approaches for rapid routine identification.

The use of molecular methods for the rapid identification of enterococci directly in routine blood cultures has been investigated. The usefulness of the commercially available DNA probe kit AccuProbe (Gen-Probe, Inc.) for the identification of enterococci directly in blood cultures has been demonstrated (61), although this test has been validated by the manufacturer only with the use of fresh growth from solid medium or from broth cultures. In addition, fluorescence in situ hybridization (FISH) techniques have been developed and evaluated for the identification of enterococci from positive blood culture bottles (34, 39). One of these assays, the *E. faecalis*/other *Enterococcus* species PNA FISH (AdvanDx, Woburn, MA), is a peptide nucleic acid FISH test that is FDA cleared (34). This assay has been considered relatively easy to implement, leading to earlier identification of *Enterococcus* species in comparison with conventional microbiological methods (34).

TYPING SYSTEMS

The increasing documentation of *Enterococcus* as a leading nosocomial pathogen frequently resistant to several antimicrobial agents, as well as the evidence supporting the concept of exogenous acquisition of enterococcal infections, has generated demand for strain typing and epidemiological studies. Classic phenotypic methods used to investigate the diversity among isolates of a given enterococcal species have frequently failed to adequately discriminate among strains, and they have limited value in epidemiological studies. However, phenotypic information in association with molecular data can constitute valuable information (27, 31).

The introduction of molecular techniques has substantially improved the ability to discriminate enterococcal isolates and has provided critical insights into the epidemiology of the enterococci. By using molecular typing approaches, it was possible to demonstrate the exogenous acquisition of enterococcal strains by direct and indirect contact among patients, breaking the traditional conception that enterococcal infections were endogenous in nature. Intrahospital transmission and interhospital spread have been extensively documented for antimicrobial-resistant enterococci, especially VRE (31, 37, 62, 107). In addition to epidemiological investigations, some of the molecular typing techniques are now used to trace the dissemination of enterococci in different environments and hosts and the evolution of multidrug-resistant strains, greatly expanding our understanding of enterococcal epidemiology, population structure, antimicrobial resistance, and virulence. Emergence and global dispersion of certain epidemic enterococcal clonal complexes have been identified (57, 64, 91, 105, 114, 115).

Several molecular methods have been proposed to type enterococcal isolates, as previously reviewed (27, 31). In addition to differences in complexity and costs, these methods vary in their reproducibility and discriminatory power. Overall, there is not a single definitive typing technique for enterococci, so a strong match among the results of different typing techniques, particularly those based on different genomic polymorphisms, should be used as indicative of high relatedness. Among these techniques, analysis of chromosomal DNA restriction profiles by pulsed-field gel electrophoresis (PFGE) has been extensively evaluated for epidemiological characterization of enterococcal outbreaks, showing improved discrimination and allowing the identification of clonal complexes that predominate among multidrug-resistant enterococci, mainly high-level resistance (HLR) to aminoglycosides and VRE (31, 37, 40, 72). SmaI is the restriction enzyme most frequently used to digest enterococcal DNA, although the usefulness of others, such as ApaI and SfiI, has also been reported (31). PFGE is possibly the typing method most commonly used in clinical microbiology settings, and it is considered by many investigators to be the gold standard for the epidemiological analysis of enterococcal outbreaks. Several protocols for performing PFGE typing of enterococcal strains have been published. However, the development of standardized protocols for execution, interpretation, and nomenclature as a result of collaborative studies is still needed in order to allow for interlaboratory data exchange and comparisons. On the other hand, although PFGE is quite discriminatory, epidemiological interpretation of PFGE profiles is not always clear-cut. The occurrence of genetic events can be associated with substantial changes in the PFGE profiles, leading to problems in clonality assessment (54). Due to the possibility of such inconsistencies in DNA banding patterns of enterococci, PFGE is recommended mostly for the purpose of evaluating the genetic relatedness and tracing the transmission of strains that are associated in time and location, as usefulness for long-term epidemiological studies may be limited. The use of PFGE in conjunction with at least one additional typing technique, or independent PFGE analysis using different restriction enzymes, is highly recommended to help in clarifying epidemiological interpretation. General principles proposed for the interpretation of molecular typing data based on fragment differences are usually applied to interpret PFGE profiles obtained for enterococcal strains (31, 101). Well-characterized control strains should be evaluated along with unknown isolates. For that purpose, two reference strains, E. faecalis OG1RF (ATCC 47077) and E. faecium GE1 (ATCC 51558), have been proposed (101).

Two other robust molecular techniques became available more recently, named multilocus sequence typing (MLST) and multiple-locus variable-number tandem repeat analysis (MLVA). These techniques circumvent the difficulties in data exchange between different laboratories by generating information that is suitable for the development of Web-based databases. MLST is based on identifying alleles after sequencing of internal fragments of a number of selected housekeeping genes, resulting in a numeric allelic profile. Each profile is assigned a sequence type. Internet sites with the possibility for data exchange (www.mlst.net and www.pubMLST.org), which contain MLST schemes for E. faecium (43) and E. faecalis (85), have been developed. Application of MLST has revealed the occurrence of host-specific genogroups of E. faecium and allowed the recognition of a hospital-adapted E. faecium subpopulation (initially named the C1 lineage) that seems to predominate in several geographic areas (57, 64, 105, 107, 115). This hospital-adapted lineage was later renamed clonal complex 17 (CC17) and classified as an example of the so-called high-risk enterococcal complexes. Major clonal complexes have also been identified among E. faecalis isolates (37, 64, 85) by using MLST. Two simultaneously published studies described the development of MLVA typing schemes for E. faecalis (102) and E. faecium (104). MLVA is based on variation in variable-number tandem repeat loci dispersed over the enterococcal genome. For each variable-number tandem repeat locus, the number of repeats is determined by PCR using primers based on the conserved flanking regions of the tandem repeats. PCR products are separated on agarose gels, and the band size is determined by the number of repeats. These numbers together result in an MLVA profile, and each profile is assigned an MLVA type. An internet site has been developed (www.mlva.umcutrecht.nl) to serve as a database and also for the submission of MLVA profiles to assign MLVA types. Comparative studies indicate that both techniques can achieve high degrees of discrimination between isolates and have comparable discriminatory power (103) that appears to be similar to that of PFGE-based typing (37, 85, 104). In contrast to the overt advantages (being reproducible, portable, highly discriminatory, and unambiguous), MLST is time-consuming, expensive, and still limited to laboratories that have facilities for both PCR and sequencing, while MLVA requires PCR and basic electrophoresis facilities. Thus, MLVA may be a quicker and less expensive alternative to MLST for clinical laboratory settings.

SEROLOGIC TESTS

Serologic tests for detecting antibody responses to different enterococcal antigens have been proposed (15, 93). However, their usefulness in the clinical laboratory setting for the diagnosis of enterococcal infections has not been demonstrated.

ANTIMICROBIAL SUSCEPTIBILITIES

Resistance to several commonly used antimicrobial agents is a remarkable characteristic of most enterococcal species.

Moreover, most of the information about this is based on studies with *E. faecalis* and *E. faecium*, the two species that are more frequently associated with human infections. Antimicrobial resistance can be classified as either intrinsic or acquired. Intrinsic resistance is related to inherent or natural chromosomally encoded characteristics present in all or most of the enterococci. Furthermore, certain specific mechanisms of intrinsic resistance to some antimicrobial agents are typically associated with a particular enterococcal species or groups of species. In contrast, the occurrence of acquired resistance is more variable, resulting from either mutations in existing DNA or acquisition of new genetic determinants carried in plasmids or transposons (20, 47, 51, 58, 71). Enterococcal intrinsic resistance involves several antimicrobial agents, particularly two major groups: the aminoglycosides and the β-lactams. Because of the poor activity of several antimicrobial agents against enterococci due to intrinsic resistance, the recommended therapy for serious infections (i.e., endocarditis, meningitis, and other systemic infections), especially in immunocompromised patients, includes a combination of a cell wall-active agent, such as a β-lactam (usually penicillin or ampicillin) or vancomycin, and an aminoglycoside (usually gentamicin or streptomycin). These combinations overcome the intrinsic resistance exhibited by the enterococci, and a synergistic bactericidal effect is generally achieved, since the intracellular penetration of the aminoglycoside is facilitated by the cell wall-active agent.

In addition to the intrinsic resistance traits, enterococci have acquired different genetic determinants that confer resistance to several classes of antimicrobial agents, including chloramphenicol, tetracyclines, macrolides, lincosamides and streptogramins, aminoglycosides, β-lactams, glycopeptides, quinolones, and even some of the more recently available drugs, such as linezolid, daptomycin, and quinupristin-dalfopristin (51, 60, 118). During the past several decades, the occurrence of acquired antimicrobial resistance among enterococci, especially HLR to aminoglycosides and β-lactams and resistance to glycopeptides (especially vancomycin), has been increasingly reported. Isolates that are resistant to the cell wall-active agent or have HLR to aminoglycosides are resistant to the synergistic effects of combination therapy and constitute a problem of peculiar importance. Therefore, the detection of resistance to these groups of antimicrobial agents is critical in order to predict the likelihood of synergy by using antimicrobial combinations as a therapeutic strategy. Enterococcal isolates exhibiting HLR to aminoglycosides have been described with increasing frequencies (40, 47, 51, 70, 71) and are now present in large proportions in several geographic areas. Such strains frequently have MICs of >2,000 μg/ml and cannot be detected by diffusion tests with conventional disks. Special tests using high-content gentamicin and streptomycin disks, as well as a single dilution method, were developed to screen for this type of resistance (see references 17 and 31 and chapters 68 and 70). Strains exhibiting HLR to penicillin and ampicillin due to altered penicillin-binding proteins have also disseminated widely (47, 51, 71), while strains producing β-lactamase have been rarely identified (40, 71). Results of susceptibility testing with ampicillin may be used to predict susceptibility to amoxicillin, amoxicillin-clavulanate, ampicillin-sulbactam, piperacillin, and piperacillin-tazobactam among non-β-lactamase-producing enterococci. Ampicillin susceptibility can also be used to predict imipenem susceptibility, providing the species is *E. faecalis* (17, 111). However, enterococcal susceptibility to

penicillin cannot be predicted on the basis of ampicillin testing results. If penicillin results are needed, testing of penicillin is required. On the other hand, enterococci susceptible to penicillin are predictably susceptible to ampicillin and the other β-lactams mentioned above. Penicillin and ampicillin resistance due to β-lactamase production is not reliably detected by routine disk or dilution methods but is detected by using a nitrocefin-based β-lactamase test (17, 31).

The emergence of vancomycin resistance as a therapeutic problem in enterococcal strains was first documented in western Europe and in the United States (52, 58, 106). Thereafter, the isolation of VRE has been continuously reported, showing epidemic proportions in diverse geographic locations (13, 47, 51). VRE strains have been classified according to phenotypic and genotypic features (Table 2). Seven types of glycopeptide resistance have already been described among enterococci. Each type is associated with different genetic elements, some of which, in turn, can be divided into subtypes. Three of them are the most common: the VanA phenotype, encoded by the *vanA* gene, with inducible HLR to vancomycin as well as to teicoplanin; the VanB phenotype, encoded by the *vanB* genes, with variable (moderate to high) levels of inducible resistance to vancomycin only; and the VanC phenotype, encoded by the *vanC* genes, conferring constitutive low-level resistance to vancomycin. VanA and VanB are considered the most clinically relevant phenotypes and are usually associated with *E. faecium* and *E. faecalis* isolates, while VanC resistance is an intrinsic characteristic of *E. gallinarum* (*vanC1* genotype) and *E. casseliflavus* (*vanC2* to *vanC4* genotypes) (13, 16, 20, 47, 109). The additional types of glycopeptide resistance encoded by the *vanD*, *vanE*, *vanG*, and *vanL* (6, 20, 65) genes seem to occur rarely among enterococci. Furthermore, the isolation of vancomycin-dependent (96) and of vancomycin-heteroresistant (1) enterococcal strains from clinically significant infections, although sporadically reported, may also represent additional serious threats for the treatment and control of enterococcal infections.

While in vitro methods for detecting vancomycin resistance are discussed in detail in references 17 and 31, as well as in chapters 67 and 68, some aspects regarding *vanC*-containing species (i.e., *E. gallinarum* and *E. casseliflavus*) need to be emphasized. Resistance associated with *vanC* genotypes is not usually detected by disk diffusion, but VanC strains frequently grow on vancomycin agar screen tests. Because of the low clinical significance of the VanC resistance, the implications of susceptibility testing for patient management may be unclear. However, the need to differentiate VanA or VanB strains from VanC strains is quite evident for therapeutic, infection control, and surveillance reasons. Because growth on vancomycin agar screening fails to help with this important distinction, species identification is necessary. VanC resistance is yet to be described in *E. faecalis* or *E. faecium*, so that growth on the vancomycin screening agar test by either of these species is likely due to the presence of the *vanA* or *vanB* genes. Although rare, the occurrence of the other kinds of vancomycin resistance may also be considered. Additionally, simultaneous occurrence of the *vanA* gene has been increasingly reported for *vanC*-carrying species, especially *E. gallinarum*, so that identification of a species that usually harbors only VanC resistance does not completely rule out moderate to high levels of vancomycin resistance (8, 62, 76). In this regard, determining vancomycin MICs is useful, as VanC resistance frequently results in MICs <32 μg/ml, whereas VanA and VanB usually result in MICs >32 μg/ml. In such cases, determination of the genetic

TABLE 2 Types of resistance to glycopeptides among members of the genus *Enterococcus*

Characteristic	Characterization by type of resistance to glycopeptides						
	VanA	VanB	VanC	VanD	VanE	VanG	VanL
MIC (μg/ml)[a] of:							
Vancomycin	64–1,000 (R)	8–1,000 (I/R)	2–32 (S/R)	64–128 (R)	8–32 (I)	16 (I)	8 (I)
Teicoplanin	16–512 (R)	0.5–1 (S)	0.5–1 (S)	4–64 (S/R)	0.5 (S)	0.5 (S)	0.5 (S)
Classification (level)	High	Variable	Low	Moderate	Low	Low	Low
Genotype	*vanA*	*vanB*[b]	*vanC*[b]	*vanD*[b]	*vanE*	*vanG*[b]	*vanL*
Mobile element	Tn*1546*	Tn*1547* or Tn*1549*-Tn*5382*	Unknown	Unknown	Unknown	Unknown	Unknown
Occurrence of conjugation	+	+	−	−	−	+	Unknown
Location of *van* genes	Plasmid, chromosome	Plasmid, chromosome	Chromosome	Chromosome	Chromosome	Chromosome	Unknown
Type of expression	Inducible	Inducible	Constitutive	Constitutive	Inducible	Inducible	Unknown
Gene product[c] (modified target)	D-Ala–D-Lac	D-Ala–D-Lac	D-Ala–D-Ser	D-Ala–D-Lac	D-Ala–D-Ser	D-Ala–D-Ser	D-Ala–D-Ser
Distribution among species	*E. faecalis, E. faecium, E. avium, E. casseliflavus, E. durans, E. gallinarum, E. hirae, E. mundtii, E. raffinosus, E. sanguinicola*	*E. faecalis, E. faecium, E. durans, E. gallinarum*	*E. casseliflavus, E. gallinarum*	*E. faecium, E. faecalis, E. avium, E. gallinarum, E. raffinosus*	*E. faecalis*	*E. faecalis*	*E. faecalis*

[a]R, resistant; S, susceptible; I, intermediate.
[b]Subtypes exist: *vanB1-3; vanC1-4; vanD1-5;* and *vanG1-2.*
[c]D-Ala-D-Lac, D-alanine–D-lactate; D-Ala-D-Ser, D-alanine–D-serine.

elements associated with vancomycin resistance has important epidemiological and infection control implications. Also, resistance to other agents such as ampicillin and aminoglycosides is uncommon among VanC isolates. Because of limited alternatives, chloramphenicol, erythromycin, tetracycline (or doxycycline or minocycline), and rifampin may be tested for VRE. Testing of quinupristin-dalfopristin, linezolid, and daptomycin is recommended when reporting on vancomycin-resistant *E. faecium.*

Molecular methods (see chapter 74) have been used to detect specific antimicrobial resistance genes and have substantially contributed to the understanding of the spread of acquired resistance among enterococci, especially resistance to vancomycin. However, because of their high specificity, molecular methods do not detect antimicrobial resistance due to mechanisms not targeted by the testing, including emerging resistance mechanisms.

EVALUATION, INTERPRETATION, AND REPORTING OF RESULTS

The diversity and species specificity of acquired antimicrobial resistance traits among enterococcal isolates created an additional need for accurate identification at the species level and for in vitro evaluation of susceptibility to antimicrobial agents. The significance of a particular enterococcal isolate is a major factor in determining when

antimicrobial testing should be done. Once the need to test a particular isolate has been established, selection of the appropriate antimicrobial agents for testing must be considered on the basis of the site of infection. Testing of antimicrobial agents to which enterococci are intrinsically resistant is contraindicated. The drugs that should not be reported include aminoglycosides at standard concentrations, cephalosporins, clindamycin, and trimethoprim-sulfamethoxazole: they may appear active for enterococci in vitro but are not effective clinically, and isolates should not be reported as susceptible. Updated guidelines (17) for the selection of antimicrobial agents should be followed for routine testing and reporting. The in vitro methods for detecting antimicrobial resistance in enterococcal isolates were reviewed and summarized (31) and are also discussed in chapters 68 and 70.

As already mentioned, synergy testing should be done with any enterococcal isolate implicated in infections for which combination therapy is indicated, e.g., from systemic infections. Enterococci are also frequently encountered in polymicrobial infections associated with the gastrointestinal tract or superficial wounds of hospitalized patients. Their pathogenic significance in such settings is uncertain, but susceptibility testing is warranted when predominant or heavy growth is observed (69). Testing of *E. faecalis* isolates from lower urinary tract infections is optional, as these infections usually respond to therapy with ampicillin or nitrofurantoin. However, many hospital infection control programs require routine testing as part of surveillance programs for VRE. For those instances when testing a urinary tract isolate is appropriate, ciprofloxacin, fosfomycin, levofloxacin, norfloxacin, and tetracycline could be selected, in addition to nitrofurantoin and ampicillin (17, 47, 60, 62). In cases of treatment failure, testing is always warranted.

REFERENCES

1. **Alam, M. R., S. Donabedian, W. Brown, J. Gordon, J. W. Chow, M. J. Zervos, and E. Hershberger.** 2001. Heteroresistance to vancomycin in *Enterococcus faecium*. *J. Clin. Microbiol.* **39:**3379–3381.

2. **Baldassarri, L., R. Creti, L. Montanaro, G. Orefici, and C. R. Arciola.** 2005. Pathogenesis of implant infections by enterococci. *Int. J. Artif. Organs* **28:**1101–1109.

3. **Ballard, S. A., F. A. Grabsch, P. D. R. Johnson, and M. L. Grayson.** 2006. Comparison of three PCR primer sets for identification of *vanB* gene carriage in feces and correlation with carriage of vancomycin-resistant enterococci: interference by *vanB*-containing anaerobic bacilli. *Antimicrob. Agents Chemother.* **49:**77–81.

4. **Bearman, G. M. L., and R. P. Wenzel.** 2005. Bacteraemias: a leading cause of death. *Arch. Med. Res.* **36:**646–659.

5. **Bourgogne, A., D. A. Garsin, X. Qin, K. V. Singh, J. Sillanpaa, S. Yerrapragada, Y. Ding, S. Dugan-Rocha, C. Buhay, H. Shen, G. Chen, G. Williams, D. Muzny, A. Maadani, K. A. Fox, J. Gioia, L. Chen, Y. Shang, C. A. Arias, S. R. Nallapareddy, M. Zhao, V. P. Prakash, S. Chowdhury, H. Jiang, R. A. Gibbs, B. E. Murray, S. K. Highlander, and G. M. Weinstock.** 2008. Large scale variation in *Enterococcus faecalis* illustrated by the genome analysis of strain OG1RF. *Genome Biol.* **9:**R110.

6. **Boyd, D. A., B. M. Willey, D. Fawcett, N. Gillani, and M. R. Mulvey.** 2008. Molecular characterization of *Enterococcus faecalis* N06-0364 with low-level vancomycin resistance harboring a novel D-Ala-D-Ser gene cluster, *vanL. Antimicrob. Agents Chemother.* **52:**2667–2672.

7. **Brigante, G., F. Luzzaro, A. Bettaccini, G. Lombarda, F. Meacci, B. Pini, S. Stefani, and A. Toniolo.** 2006. Use of the Phoenix automated system for identification of *Streptococcus* and *Enterococcus* spp. *J. Clin. Microbiol.* **44:**3263–3267.

8. **Buschelman, B. J., M. J. Bale, and R. N. Jones.** 1993. Species identification and determination of high-level aminoglycoside resistance among enterococci. Comparison study of sterile body fluid isolates, 1985–1991. *Diagn. Microbiol. Infect. Dis.* **16:**119–122.

9. **Carvalho, M. G., A. G. Steigerwalt, R. E. Morey, P. L. Shewmaker, E. Falsen, R. R. Facklam, and L. M. Teixeira.** 2008. Designation of the provisional new *Enterococcus* species CDC PNS-E2 as *Enterococcus sanguinicola* sp. nov., isolated from human blood, and identification of a strain previously named *Enterococcus* CDC PNS-E1 as *Enterococcus italicus* Fortina, Ricci, Mora, and Manachini 2004. *J. Clin. Microbiol.* **46:**3473–3476.

10. **Carvalho, M. G. S., A. G. Steigerwalt, R. E. Morey, P. L. Shewmaker, L. M. Teixeira, and R. R. Facklam.** 2004. Characterization of three new enterococcal species, *Enterococcus* sp. nov. CDC PNS-E1, *Enterococcus* sp. nov. CDC PNS-E2, and *Enterococcus* sp. nov. CDC PNS-E3, isolated from human clinical specimens. *J. Clin. Microbiol.* **42:**1192–1198.

11. **Casalta, J. P., F. Gouriet, V. Roux, F. Thuny, G. Habib, and D. Raoult.** 2009. Evaluation of the LightCycler® Septi-Fast test in the rapid etiologic diagnostic of infectious endocarditis. *Eur. J. Clin. Microbiol. Infect. Dis.* **28:**569–573.

12. **Centers for Disease Control and Prevention.** 1993. Nosocomial enterococci resistant to vancomycin—United States, 1989–1993. *MMWR Morb. Mortal. Wkly. Rep.* **42:**597–599.

13. **Cetinkaya, Y., P. Falk, and C. G. Mayhall.** 2000. Vancomycin-resistant enterococci. *Clin. Microbiol. Rev.* **13:**686–707.

14. **Chang, J. C., M. L. Chien, H. M. Chen, J. J. Yan, and J. J. Wu.** 2008. Comparison of CPS ID 3 and CHROMagar Orientation chromogenic agars with standard biplate technique for culture of clinical urine samples. *J. Microbiol. Immunol. Infect.* **41:**422–427.

15. **Cho, Y. S., H. S. Lee, J. M. Kim, M. H. Lee, H. S. Yoo, Y. H. Park, and P. D. Ryu.** 2008. Immunogenic proteins in the cell envelope and cytoplasm of vancomycin-resistant enterococci. *J. Immunoassay Immunochem.* **29:**319–331.

16. **Clark, N. C., L. M. Teixeira, R. R. Facklam, and F. C. Tenover.** 1998. Detection and differentiation of the *vanC-1*, *vanC-2*, and *vanC-3* glycopeptide resistance genes in enterococci. *J. Clin. Microbiol.* **36:**2294–2297.

17. **Clinical and Laboratory Standards Institute.** 2010. *Performance Standards for Antimicrobial Susceptibility: Twentieth Informational Supplement.* CLSI document M100-S20. Clinical and Laboratory Standards Institute, Wayne, PA.

18. **Collins, M. D., D. Jones, J. A. E. Farrow, R. Kilpper-Balz, and K. H. Schleifer.** 1984. *Enterococcus avium* nom. rev., comb. nov.; *E. casseliflavus* nom. rev., comb. nov.; *E. durans* nom. rev., comb. nov.; *E. gallinarum* comb. nov.; and *E. malodoratus* sp. nov. *Int. J. Syst. Bacteriol.* **34:**220–223.

19. **Contreras, G. A., C. A. DiazGranados, L. Cortes, J. Reyes, S. Vanegas, D. Panesso, S. Rincón, L. Díaz, G. Prada, B. E. Murray, and C. A. Arias.** 2008. Nosocomial outbreak of *Enteroccocus gallinarum*: untaming of rare species of enterococci. *J. Hosp. Infect.* **70:**346–352.

20. **Courvalin, P.** 2006. Vancomycin resistance in gram-positive cocci. *Clin. Infect. Dis.* **42:**S25–S34.

21. **Cuzon, G., T. Naas, N. Fortineau, and P. Nordmann.** 2008. Novel chromogenic medium for detection of vancomycin-resistant *Enterococcus faecium* and *Enterococcus faecalis*. *J. Clin. Microbiol.* **46:**2442–2444.

22. **d'Azevedo, P. A., C. A. G. Dias, A. L. S. Goncalves, F. Rowe, and L. M. Teixeira.** 2001. Evaluation of an automated system for the identification and antimicrobial susceptibility testing of enterococci. *Diagn. Microbiol. Infect. Dis.* **42:**157–161.

23. **Delmas, J., F. Robin, C. Schweitzer, O. Lesens, and R. Bonnet.** 2007. Evaluation of a new chromogenic medium, chromID VRE, for detection of vancomycin-resistant enterococci in stool samples and rectal swabs. *J. Clin. Microbiol.* **45:**2731–2733.

24. **Depardieu, F., B. Perichon, and P. Courvalin.** 2004. Detection of the *van* alphabet and identification of enterococci and staphylococci at the species level by multiplex PCR. *J. Clin. Microbiol.* **42:**5857–5860.

25. **Devriese, L., M. Baele, and P. Butaye.** 2006. The genus *Enterococcus*: taxonomy, p. 163–174. *In* M. Dworkin, S. Falkow, E. Rosenberg, K.-H. Schleifer, and E. Stackebrandt (ed.), *The Prokaryotes: a Handbook on the Biology of Bacteria*, 3rd ed., vol 4. Springer, New York, NY.

26. **Domig, K. J., H. K. Mayer, and W. Kneifel.** 2003. Methods used for the isolation, enumeration, characterisation and identification of *Enterococcus* spp. 1. Media for isolation and enumeration. *Int. J. Food Microbiol.* **88:**147–164.

27. **Domig, K. J., H. K. Mayer, and W. Kneifel.** 2003. Methods used for the isolation, enumeration, characterisation and identification of *Enterococcus* spp. 2. Pheno- and genotypic criteria. *Int. J. Food Microbiol.* **88:**165–188.

28. **Donelli, G., and E. Guaglianone.** 2004. Emerging role of *Enterococcus* spp in catheter-related infections: biofilm formation and novel mechanisms of antibiotic resistance. *J. Vasc. Access* **5:**3–9.

29. **Drews, S. J., G. Johnson, F. Gharabaghi, M. Roscoe, A. Matlow, R. Tellier, and S. E. Richardson.** 2006. A 24-hour screening protocol for identification of vancomycin-resistant *Enterococcus faecium*. *J. Clin. Microbiol.* **44:**1578–1580.

30. **Euzéby, J. P.** 1997. List of bacterial names with standing in nomenclature: a folder available on the internet. *Int. J. Syst. Bacteriol.* **47:**590–592. (*List of Prokaryotic Names with Standing in Nomenclature.* [Online.] http://www.bacterio.cict.fr. Last full update 5 August 2010.)

31. **Facklam, R. R., M. G. S. Carvalho, and L. M. Teixeira.** 2002. History, taxonomy, biochemical characteristics, and antibiotic susceptibility testing of enterococci, p. 1–54. *In* M. S. Gilmore, D. B. Clewell, P. Courvalin, G. M. Dunny, B. E. Murray, and L. B. Rice (ed.), *The Enterococci: Pathogenesis, Molecular Biology, and Antibiotic Resistance.* ASM Press, Washington, DC.

32. **Facklam, R. R., and M. D. Collins.** 1989. Identification of *Enterococcus* species isolated from human infections by a conventional test scheme. *J. Clin. Microbiol.* **27:**731–734.

33. **Facklam, R. R., and J. A. Elliott.** 1995. Identification, classification, and clinical relevance of catalase-negative, grampositive cocci, excluding the streptococci and enterococci. *Clin. Microbiol. Rev.* **8:**479–495.

34. **Forrest, G. N., M. C. Roghmann, L. S. Toombs, J. K. Johnson, E. Weekes, D. P. Lincalis, and R. A. Venezia.** 2008. Peptide nucleic acid fluorescent in situ hybridization for hospital-acquired enterococcal bacteremia: delivering earlier effective antimicrobial therapy. *Antimicrob. Agents Chemother.* **52:**3558–3563.

35. **Fortina, M. G., G. Ricci, D. Mora, and P. L. Manachini.** 2004. Molecular analysis of artisanal Italian cheeses reveals *Enterococcus italicus* sp. nov. *Int. J. Syst. Evol. Microbiol.* **54:**1717–1721.

36. **Franz, C. M., M. E. Stiles, K. H. Schleifer, and W. H. Holzapfel.** 2003. Enterococci in foods—a conundrum for food safety. *Int. J. Food Microbiol.* **88:**105–122.

37. **Freitas, A. R., C. Novais, P. Ruiz-Garbajosa, T. M. Coque, and L. Peixe.** 2009. Clonal expansion within clonal complex 2 and spread of vancomycin-resistant plasmids among different genetic lineages of *Enterococcus faecalis* from Portugal. *J. Antimicrob. Chemother.* **63:**1104–1111.

38. **Garcia-Garrote, F., E. Cercenado, and E. Bouza.** 2000. Evaluation of a new system, VITEK 2, for identification and antimicrobial susceptibility testing of enterococci. *J. Clin. Microbiol.* **38:**2108–2111.

39. **Gescher, D. M., D. Kovaecevic, D. Schmiedel, S. Siemoneit, C. Mallmann, E. Halle, U. B. Gobel, and A. Moter.** 2008. Fluorescence in situ hybridisation (FISH) accelerates identification of Gram-positive cocci in positive blood cultures. *Int. J. Antimicrob. Agents* **32**(Suppl.)**:**S51–S59.

40. **Gordon, S., J. S. Swenson, B. C. Hill, N. E. Pigott, R. R. Facklam, R. C. Cooksey, C. Thornsberry, the Enterococcal Study Group, W. R. Jarvis, and F. C. Tenover.** 1992. Antimicrobial susceptibility patterns of common and unusual species of enterococci causing infections in the United States. *J. Clin. Microbiol.* **30:**2373–2378.

41. **Grabsch, E. A., S. Ghaly-Derias, W. Gao, and B. P. Howden.** 2008. Comparative study of selective chromogenic (chromID VRE) and bile esculin agars for isolation and identification of *vanB*-containing vancomycin-resistant enterococci from feces and rectal swabs. *J. Clin. Microbiol.* **46:**4034–4036.

42. **Hidron, A. I., J. R. Edwards, J. Patel, T. C. Horan, D. M. Sievert, D. A. Pollock, and S. K. Fridkin for the National Healthcare Safety Network Team and Participating National Healthcare Safety Network Facilities.** 2008. Antimicrobial-resistant pathogens associated with healthcare-associated infections: annual summary of data reported to the National Healthcare Safety Network at the Centers for Disease Control and Prevention, 2006–2007. *Infect. Control Hosp. Epidemiol.* **29:**996–1011.

43. **Homan, W. L., D. Tribe, S. Poznanski, M. Li, G. Hogg, E. Spalburg, J. D. Van Embden, and R. J. Willems.** 2002. Multilocus sequence typing scheme for *Enterococcus faecium.* *J. Clin. Microbiol.* **40:**1963–1971.

44. **Hospital Infection Control Practices Advisory Committee.** 1995. Recommendations for preventing the spread of vancomycin resistance. *Infect. Control Hosp. Epidemiol.* **16:**105–113.

45. **Huckabee, C. M., W. C. Huskins, and P. R. Murray.** 2009. Predicting clearance of colonization with vancomycin-resistant enterococci and methicillin-resistant *Staphylococcus aureus* by use of weekly surveillance cultures. *J. Clin. Microbiol.* **47:**1229–1230.

46. **Huycke, M. M.** 2002. Physiology of enterococci, p. 133–175. *In* M. S. Gilmore, D. B. Clewell, P. Courvalin, G. M. Dunny, B. E. Murray, and L. B. Rice (ed.), *The Enterococci: Pathogenesis, Molecular Biology, and Antibiotic Resistance.* ASM Press, Washington, DC.

47. **Huycke, M. M., D. F. Sahm, and M. S. Gilmore.** 1998. Multiple-resistant enterococci: the nature of the problem and an agenda for the future. *Emerg. Infect. Dis.* **4:**239–249.

48. **Ieven, M., E. Vercauteren, P. Descheemacker, F. van Laer, and H. Goossens.** 1999. Comparison of direct plating and broth enrichment culture for detection of intestinal colonization by glycopeptide-resistant enterococci among hospitalized patients. *J. Clin. Microbiol.* **37:**1436–1440.

49. **Iwen, P. C., D. M. Kelly, J. Linder, S. H. Hinrichs, E. A. Dominguez, M. E. Rupp, and K. D. Patil.** 1997. Change in prevalence and antibiotic resistance of *Enterococcus* species isolated from blood cultures over an 8-year period. *Antimicrob. Agents Chemother.* **41:**494–495.

50. **Jackson, C. R., P. J. Fedorka-Cray, and J. B. Barrett.** 2004. Use of a genus- and species-specific multiplex PCR for identification of enterococci. *J. Clin. Microbiol.* **42:**3558–3565.

51. **Kak, V., and J. W. Chow.** 2002. Acquired antibiotic resistances in enterococci, p. 355–383. *In* M. S. Gilmore, D. B. Clewell, P. Courvalin, G. M. Dunny, B. E. Murray, and L. B. Rice (ed.), *The Enterococci: Pathogenesis, Molecular Biology, and Antibiotic Resistance.* ASM Press, Washington, DC.

52. **Kaplan, A. H., P. H. Gilligan, and R. R. Facklam.** 1988. Recovery of resistant enterococci during vancomycin prophylaxis. *J. Clin. Microbiol.* **26:**1216–1218.

53. **Karlowsky, J. A., M. E. Jones, D. C. Draghi, C. Thornsberry, D. F. Sahm, and G. A. Volturo.** 2004. Prevalence and antimicrobial susceptibilities of bacteria isolated from blood cultures of hospitalized patients in the United States in 2002. *Ann. Clin. Microbiol. Antimicrob.* **10:**3–7.

54. **Kawalec, M., M. Gniadkowski, and W. Hryniewicz.** 2000. Outbreak of vancomycin-resistant enterococci in a hospital in Gdansk, Poland, due to horizontal transfer of different Tn*1546*-like transposon variants and clonal spread of several strains. *J. Clin. Microbiol.* **38:**3317–3322.

55. **Kawalec, M., J. Kedzierska, A. Gajda, E. Sadowy, J. Wegrzyn, S. Naser, A. B. Skotnicki, M. Gniadkowski, and W. Hryniewicz.** 2007. Hospital outbreak of vancomycin-resistant enterococci caused by a single clone of *Enterococcus raffinosus* and several clones of *Enterococcus faecium.* *Clin. Microbiol. Infect.* **13:**893–901.

56. **Kramer, A., I. Schwebke, and G. Kampf.** 2006. How long do nosocomial pathogens persist on inanimate surfaces? A systematic review. *BMC Infect. Dis.* **6:**130–137.

57. **Leavis, H. L., M. J. Bonten, and R. J. Willems.** 2006. Identification of high-risk enterococcal clonal complexes: global dispersion and antibiotic resistance. *Curr. Opin. Microbiol.* **9:**454–460.

58. **Leclercq, R., E. Derlot. J. Duval, and P. Courvalin.** 1988. Plasmid-mediated resistance to vancomycin and teicoplanin in *Enterococcus faecium. N. Engl. J. Med.* **319:**157–161.

59. **Ledeboer, N. A., R. J. Tibbetts, and W. M. Dunne.** 2007. A new chromogenic agar medium, chromID VRE, to screen for vancomycin-resistant *Enterococcus faecium* and *Enterococcus faecalis. Diagn. Microbiol. Infect. Dis.* **59:**477–479.

60. **Linden, P. K.** 2007. Optimizing therapy for vancomycin-resistant enterococci (VRE). *Semin. Respir. Crit. Care Med.* **28:**632–645.

61. **Lindholm, L., and H. Sarkkinen.** 2004. Direct identification of gram-positive cocci from routine blood cultures by using AccuProbe tests. *J. Clin. Microbiol.* **42:**5609–5613.

62. **Malani, P. N., C. A. Kauffman, and M. J. Zervos.** 2002. Enterococcal disease, epidemiology, and treatment, p. 385–408. *In* M. S. Gilmore, D. B. Clewell, P. Courvalin, G. M. Dunny, B. E. Murray, and L. B. Rice (ed.), *The Enterococci: Pathogenesis, Molecular Biology, and Antibiotic Resistance.* ASM Press, Washington, DC.

63. Malhotra-Kumar, S., K. Haccuria, M. Michiels, M. Ieven, C. Poyart, W. Hryniewicz, and H. Goossens on behalf of the MOSAR WP2 Study Team. 2008. Current trends in rapid diagnostics for methicillin-resistant *Staphylococcus aureus* and glycopeptide-resistant *Enterococcus* species. *J. Clin. Microbiol.* **46**:1577–1587.

64. McBride, S. M., V. A. Fischetti, D. J. Leblanc, R. C. Moellering, Jr., and M. S. Gilmore. 2007. Genetic diversity among *Enterococcus faecalis*. *PLoS ONE* **2**:e582.

65. McKessar, S. J., A. M. Berry, J. M. Bell, J. D. Turnidge, and J. C. Paton. 2000. Genetic characterization of *vanG*, a novel vancomycin resistance locus of *Enterococcus faecalis*. *Antimicrob. Agents Chemother.* **44**:3224–3228.

66. Merlino, J., S. Siarakas, G. J. Robertson, G. R. Funnell, T. Gottieb, and R. Bradbury. 1996. Evaluation of CHROMagar Orientation for differentiation and presumptive identification of gram-negative bacilli and *Enterococcus* species. *J. Clin. Microbiol.* **34**:1788–1793.

67. Merquior, V. L., F. P. G. Neves, R. I. Ribeiro, R. S. Duarte, E. A. Marques, and L. M. Teixeira. 2008. Bacteraemia associated with a vancomycin-resistant *Enterococcus gallinarum* strain harboring both the *vanA* and *vanC1* genes. *J. Med. Microbiol.* **57**:244–245.

68. Merquior, V. L. C., J. M. Peralta, R. R. Facklam, and L. M. Teixeira. 1994. Analysis of electrophoretic whole-cell protein profiles as a tool for characterization of *Enterococcus* species. *Curr. Microbiol.* **28**:149–153.

69. Moellering, R. C., Jr. 1992. Emergence of *Enterococcus* as a significant pathogen. *Clin. Infect. Dis.* **14**:1173–1178.

70. Mondino, S. S. B., A. C. D. Castro, P. J. J. Mondino, M. G. S. Carvalho, K. M. F. Silva, and L. M. Teixeira. 2003. Phenotypic and genotypic characterization of clinical and intestinal enterococci isolated from inpatients and outpatients in two Brazilian hospitals. *Microb. Drug Resist.* **9**:167–174.

71. Murray, B. E. 1990. The life and times of the *Enterococcus*. *Clin. Microbiol. Rev.* **3**:46–65.

72. Murray, B. E., K. V. Singh, J. D. Heath, B. R. Sharma, and G. M. Weinstock. 1990. Comparison of genomic DNAs of different enterococcal isolates using restriction endonucleases with infrequent recognition sites. *J. Clin. Microbiol.* **28**:2059–2063.

73. National Nosocomial Infections Surveillance System. 2000. National Nosocomial Infections Surveillance (NNIS) system report, data summary from January 1992–April 2000, issued June 2000. *Am. J. Infect. Control* **28**:429–448.

74. National Nosocomial Infections Surveillance System. 2004. National Nosocomial Infections Surveillance (NNIS) system report, data summary from January 1992 through June 2004, issued October 2004. *Am. J. Infect. Control* **32**:470–485.

75. Nauschuetz, W. F., S. B. Trevino, L. S. Harrison, R. N. Longfield, L. Fletcher, and W. G. Wortham. 1993. *Enterococcus casseliflavus* as an agent of nosocomial bloodstream infections. *Med. Microbiol. Lett.* **2**:102–108.

76. Neves, F. P., R. I. Ribeiro, R. S. Duarte, L. M. Teixeira, and V. L. Merquior. 2009. Emergence of the *vanA* genotype among *Enterococcus gallinarum* isolates colonising the intestinal tract of patients in a university hospital in Rio de Janeiro, Brazil. *Int. J. Antimicrob. Agents* **33**:211–215.

77. Novicki, T. J., J. M. Schapiro, B. K. Ulness, A. Sebeste, L. Busse-Johnston, K. M. Swanson, S. R. Swanzy, W. Leisenring, and A. P. Limaye. 2004. Convenient selective differential broth for isolation of vancomycin-resistant *Enterococcus* from fecal material. *J. Clin. Microbiol.* **42**:1637–1640.

78. Oana, K., Y. Okimura, Y. Kawakami, N. Hayashida, M. Shimosaka, M. Okazaki, T. Hayashi, and M. Ohnishi. 2002. Physical and genetic map of *Enterococcus faecium* ATCC19434 and demonstration of intra- and interspecific genomic diversity in enterococci. *FEMS Microbiol. Lett.* **207**:133–139.

79. Palladino, S., I. D. Kay, J. P. Flexman, I. Boehm, A. M. G. Costa, E. J. Lambert, and K. J. Christiansen. 2003. Rapid detection of *vanA* and *vanB* genes directly from clinical specimens and enrichment broths by real-time multiplex PCR assay. *J. Clin. Microbiol.* **41**:2483–2486.

80. Paulsen, I. T., L. Banerjei, G. S. Myers, K. E. Nelson, R. Seshadri, T. D. Read, D. E. Fouts, J. A. Eisen, S. R. Gill, J. F. Heidelberg, H. Tettelin, R. J. Dodson, L. Umayam, L. Brinkac, M. Beanan, S. Daugherty, R. T. DeBoy, S. Durkin, J. Kolonay, R. Madupu, W. Nelson, J. Vamathevan, B. Tran, J. Upton, T. Hansen, J. Shetty, H. Khouri, T. Utterback, D. Radune, K. A. Ketchum, B. A. Dougherty, and C. M. Fraser. 2003. Role of mobile DNA in the evolution of vancomycin-resistant *Enterococcus faecalis*. *Science* **299**:2071–2074.

81. Pendle, S., P. Jelfs, T. Olma, Y. Su, N. Gilroy, and G. L. Gilbert. 2008. Difficulties in detection and identification of *Enterococcus faecium* with low-level inducible resistance to vancomycin, during a hospital outbreak. *Clin. Microbiol. Infect.* **14**:853–857.

82. Peters, R. P., M. A. van Agtmael, S. Gierveld, S. A. Danner, A. B. Groeneveld, C. M. Vandenbroucke-Grauls, and P. H. Savelkoul. 2007. Quantitative detection of *Staphylococcus aureus* and *Enterococcus faecalis* DNA in blood to diagnose bacteremia in patients in the intensive care unit. *J. Clin. Microbiol.* **45**:3641–3646.

83. Pillar, C. M., and M. S. Gilmore. 2004. Enterococcal virulence-pathogenicity island of *E. faecalis*. *Front. Biosci.* **9**:2335–2346.

84. Richards, M. J., J. R. Edwards, D. H. Culver, and R. P. Gaynes. 2000. Nosocomial infections in combined medical-surgical intensive care units in the United States. *Infect. Control Hosp. Epidemiol.* **21**:510–515.

85. Ruiz-Garbajosa, P., M. J. M. Bonten, D. A. Robinson, J. Top, S. R. Nallapareddy, C. Torres, T. M. C. Coque, R. Canton, F. Baquero, B. E. Murray, R. del Campo, and R. J. Willems. 2006. A multilocus sequence typing scheme for *Enterococcus faecalis* reveals hospital-adapted genetic complexes in a background of high rates of recombination. *J. Clin. Microbiol.* **44**:2220–2228.

86. Satake, S., N. Clark, D. Rimland, F. S. Nolte, and F. C. Tenover. 1997. Detection of vancomycin-resistant enterococci in fecal samples by PCR. *J. Clin. Microbiol.* **35**:2325–2330.

87. Schleifer, K. H., and R. Kilpper-Balz. 1984. Transfer of *Streptococcus faecalis* and *Streptococcus faecium* to the genus *Enterococcus* nom. rev. as *Enterococcus faecalis* comb. nov. and *Enterococcus faecium* comb. nov. *Int. J. Syst. Bacteriol.* **34**:31–34.

88. Shankar, N., A. S. Baghdayan, and M. S. Gilmore. 2002. Modulation of virulence within a pathogenicity island in vancomycin resistant *Enterococcus faecalis*. *Nature* **417**:746–750.

89. Singh, K. V., and B. E. Murray. 1994. Revised estimates of enterococcal chromosomal sizes. *DNA Cell Biol.* **13**:1145–1146.

90. Sloan, L. M., J. R. Uhl, E. A. Better, C. D. Schleck, W. W. Harmsen, J. Manahan, R. L. Thompson, J. E. Rosenblatt, and F. R. Cockerill III. 2004. Comparison of the Roche LightCycler *vanA/vanB* detection assay and culture for detection of vancomycin-resistant enterococci from perianal swabs. *J. Clin. Microbiol.* **42**:2636–2643.

91. Solheim, M., A. Aakra, L. G. Snipen, D. A. Brede, and I. F. Nes. 2009. Comparative genomics of *Enterococcus faecalis* from healthy Norwegian infants. *BMC Genomics* **10**:194.

92. Stamper, P. D., M. Cai, C. Lema, K. Eskey, and K. C. Carroll. 2007. Comparison of the BD GeneOhm VanR assay to culture for identification of vancomycin-resistant enterococci in rectal and stool specimens. *J. Clin. Microbiol.* **45**:3360–3365.

93. Sulaiman, A., R. M. Rakita, R. C. Arduino, J. E. Patterson, J. M. Steckelberg, K. V. Singh, and B. E. Murray. 1996. Serological investigation of enterococcal infections using western blot. *Eur. J. Clin. Microbiol. Infect. Dis.* **15**:826–829.

94. Švec, P., L. A. Devriese, I. Sedlacek, M. Baele, M. Vancanneyt, F. Haesbrouck, J. Swings, and J. Doskar. 2001. *Enterococcus haemoperoxidus* sp. nov. and *Enterococcus moraviensis* sp. nov., isolated from water. *Int. J. Syst. Evol. Microbiol.* **51**:1567–1574.

95. Švec, P., M. Vancanneyt, I. Sedlácek, S. M. Naser, C. Snauwaert, K. Lefebvre, B. Hoste, and J. Swings. 2006. *Enterococcus silesiacus* sp. nov. and *Enterococcus termitis* sp. nov. *Int. J. Syst. Evol. Microbiol.* **56**:577–581.

96. **Tambyah, P. A., J. A. Marx, and D. G. Maki.** 2004. Nosocomial infection with vancomycin-dependent enterococci. *Emerg. Infect. Dis.* **10:**1277–1281.

97. **Tannock, G. W., and G. Cook.** 2002. Enterococci as members of the intestinal microflora of humans, p. 101–132. *In* M. S. Gilmore, D. B. Clewell, P. Courvalin, G. M. Dunny, B. E. Murray, and L. B. Rice (ed.), *The Enterococci: Pathogenesis, Molecular Biology, and Antibiotic Resistance.* ASM Press, Washington, DC.

98. **Teixeira, L. M., M. G. S. Carvalho, V. L. Merquior, A. G. Steigerwalt, D. J. Brenner, and R. R. Facklam.** 1997. Phenotypic and genotypic characterization of *Vagococcus fluvialis,* including strains isolated from human sources. *J. Clin. Microbiol.* **35:**2778–2781.

99. **Teixeira, L. M., R. R. Facklam, A. G. Steigerwalt, N. E. Pigott, V. L. C. Merquior, and D. J. Brenner.** 1995. Correlation between phenotypic characteristics and DNA relatedness with *Enterococcus faecium* strains. *J. Clin. Microbiol.* **33:**1520–1523.

100. **Tendolkar, P. M., A. S. Baghdayan, and N. Shankar.** 2003. Pathogenic enterococci: new developments in the 21st century. *Cell. Mol. Life Sci.* **60:**2622–2636.

101. **Tenover, F. C., R. D. Arbeit, R. V. Goering, P. A. Mickelsen, B. E. Murray, D. H. Persing, and B. Swaminathan.** 1995. Interpreting chromosomal DNA restriction patterns produced by pulsed-field gel electrophoresis: criteria for bacterial strain typing. *J. Clin. Microbiol.* **33:**2233–2239.

102. **Titze-de-Almeida, R., R. J. L. Willems, J. Top, I. P. Rodrigues, R. F. Ferreira II, H. Boelens, M. C. C. Brandileone, R. C. Zanella, M. S. S. Felipe, and A. van Belkum.** 2004. Multilocus variable-number tandem-repeat polymorphism among Brazilian *Enterococcus faecalis* strains. *J. Clin. Microbiol.* **42:**4879–4881.

103. **Top, J., N. M. Banga, R. Hayes, R. J. Willems, M. J. Bonten, and M. K. Hayden.** 2008. Comparison of multiple-locus variable-number tandem repeat analysis and pulsed-field gel electrophoresis in a setting of polyclonal endemicity of vancomycin-resistant *Enterococcus faecium.* *Clin. Microbiol. Infect.* **14:**363–369.

104. **Top, J., L. M. Schouls, M. J. Bonten, and R. J. Willems.** 2004. Multiple-locus variable-number tandem repeat analysis, a novel typing scheme to study the genetic relatedness and epidemiology of *Enterococcus faecium* isolates. *J. Clin. Microbiol.* **42:**4503–4511.

105. **Top, J., R. Willems, H. Blok, M. de Regt, K. Jalink, A. Troelstra, B. Goorhuis, and M. Bonten.** 2007. Ecological replacement of *Enterococcus faecalis* by multiresistant clonal complex 17 *Enterococcus faecium.* *Clin. Microbiol. Infect.* **13:**316–319.

106. **Uttley, A. H. C., C. H. Collins, J. Naidoo, and R. C. George.** 1988. Vancomycin-resistant enterococci. *Lancet* **1:**57–58.

107. **Valdezate, S., C. Labayru, A. Navarro, M. A. Mantecón, M. Ortega, T. M. Coque, M. García, and J. A. Saéz-Nieto.** 2009. Large clonal outbreak of multidrug-resistant CC17 ST17 *Enterococcus faecium* containing Tn5382 in a Spanish hospital. *J. Antimicrob. Chemother.* **63:**17–20.

108. **Van Horn, K., C. Tóth, R. Kariyama, R. Mitsuhata, and H. Kumon.** 2002. Evaluation of 15 motility media and a direct microscopic method for detection of motility in enterococci. *J. Clin. Microbiol.* **40:**2476–2479.

109. **Watanabe, S., N. Kobayashi, D. Quiñones, S. Hayakawa, S. Nagashima, N. Uehara, and N. Watanabe.** 2009. Genetic diversity of the low-level vancomycin resistance gene *vanC-2/vanC-3* and identification of a novel *vanC* subtype (*vanC-4*) in *Enterococcus casseliflavus.* *Microb. Drug Resist.* **15:**1–9.

110. **Weber, S. G., S. S. Huang, S. Oriola, W. C. Huskins, G. A. Noskin, K. Harriman, R. N. Olmsted, M. Bonten, T. Lundstrom, M. W. Climo, M. C. Roghmann, C. L. Murphy, and T. B. Karchmer.** 2007. Legislative mandates for use of active surveillance cultures to screen for methicillin-resistant *Staphylococcus aureus* and vancomycin-resistant enterococci: position statement from the joint SHEA and APIC task force. *Infect. Control Hosp. Epidemiol.* **28:**249–260.

111. **Weinstein, M. P.** 2001. Comparative evaluation of penicillin, ampicillin, and imipenem MICs and susceptibility breakpoints for vancomycin-susceptible and vancomycin-resistant *Enterococcus faecalis* and *Enterococcus faecium.* *J. Clin. Microbiol.* **39:**2729–2731.

112. **Werner, G., T. M. Coque, A. M. Hammerum, R. Hope, W. Hryniewicz, A. Johnson, I. Klare, K. G. Kristinsson, R. Leclercq, C. H. Lester, M. Lillie, C. Novais, B. Olsson-Liljequist, L. V. Peixe, E. Sadowy, G. S. Simonsen, J. Top, J. Vuopio-Varkila, R. J. Willems, W. Witte, and N. Woodford.** 2008. Emergence and spread of vancomycin resistance among enterococci in Europe. *Euro Surveill.* **13:**1–11.

113. **Wilke, W. W., S. A. Marshall, S. L. Coffman, M. A. Pfaller, M. B. Edmund, R. P. Wenzel, and R. N. Jones.** 1997. Vancomycin-resistant *Enterococcus raffinosus:* molecular epidemiology, species identification error, and frequency of occurrence in national resistance surveillance program. *Diagn. Microbiol. Infect. Dis.* **28:**43–49.

114. **Willems, R. J., and M. J. Bonten.** 2007. Glycopeptide-resistant enterococci: deciphering virulence, resistance and epidemicity. *Curr. Opin. Infect. Dis.* **20:**384–390.

115. **Willems, R. J., J. Top, M. van Santen, D. A. Robinson, T. M. Coque, F. Baquero, H. Grundmann, and M. J. Bonten.** 2005. Global spread of vancomycin-resistant *Enterococcus faecium* from distinct nosocomial genetic complex. *Emerg. Infect. Dis.* **11:**821–828.

116. **Young, H. L., S. A. Ballard, P. Roffey, and M. L. Grayson.** 2007. Direct detection of *vanB2* using the Roche LightCycler *vanA/B* detection assay to indicate vancomycin-resistant enterococcal carriage—sensitive but not specific. *J. Antimicrob. Chemother.* **58:**809–810.

117. **Zehnder, M., and B. Guggenheim.** 2009. The mysterious appearance of enterococci in filled root canals. *Int. Endod. J.* **42:**277–287.

118. **Zirakzadeh, A., and R. Patel.** 2006. Vancomycin-resistant enterococci: colonization, infection, detection, and treatment. *Mayo Clin. Proc.* **81:**529–536.

Aerococcus, Abiotrophia, and Other Aerobic Catalase-Negative, Gram-Positive Cocci

KATHRYN L. RUOFF

22

TAXONOMY

The catalase-negative, gram-positive cocci included in this chapter form a taxonomically diverse group of bacteria that are isolated infrequently as opportunistic agents of infection. Most of these organisms resemble other more well-known clinical isolates (i.e., streptococci and enterococci) and consequently may be mistaken for members of those genera. Although probably misidentified or overlooked in clinical cultures in the past, these organisms may represent emerging pathogens in immunocompromised patient populations. Table 1 lists the organisms included here, along with some of their basic characteristics. The bacteria discussed in this chapter are members of the phylum *Firmicutes* (low-G+C, gram-positive bacteria). *Helcococcus* is the only genus in the group to reside in the class "*Clostridia*," while the remaining genera are classified in the class "*Bacilli*" (W. Ludwig, K.-H. Schleifer, and W. B. Whitman, *Bergey's Taxonomic Outlines*, vol. 3 [http://www.bergeys.org/outlines .html]). The reader is referred to chapter 19 for information on *Rothia mucilaginosa*, another infrequently isolated gram-positive coccus that may be catalase negative.

The genus *Lactococcus* is composed of organisms formerly classified as Lancefield group N streptococci (122). The species *Lactococcus lactis* and *Lactococcus garvieae* have been documented to be associated with human infections. Motile *Lactococcus*-like organisms with Lancefield's group N antigen (a teichoic acid antigen) are classified in the genus *Vagococcus* (29, 141). The vagococci also resemble the enterococci, and Facklam and Elliott (55) reported that *Vagococcus fluvialis* (the principal species described to occur in human clinical specimens to date) isolates examined at the CDC gave positive reactions in a commercially available nucleic acid probe test for enterococci.

The genera *Abiotrophia* and *Granulicatella* accommodate organisms previously known as nutritionally variant or satelliting streptococci (37, 80). These bacteria were originally thought to be nutritional mutants of viridans group streptococcal strains, most notably of the species *Streptococcus mitis*. Bouvet and colleagues (15) suggested that this group of organisms were really members of two novel streptococcal species given the names *Streptococcus defectivus* and *Streptococcus adjacens*. A comparative analysis of 16S rRNA sequences led Kawamura and coworkers to propose the creation of a new genus, *Abiotrophia*, containing two species, *Abiotrophia*

defectiva and *Abiotrophia adiacens*, to accommodate these bacteria (80). A third species from human sources, *Abiotrophia elegans*, was described in 1998 (119). Kanamoto et al. noted the heterogeneity among *Abiotrophia* strains and proposed a fourth species, *Abiotrophia para-adiacens* (78). In 2000 Collins and Lawson proposed a new genus, *Granulicatella*, with *Granulicatella adiacens* and *Granulicatella elegans* representing strains formerly called *A. adiacens* and *A. elegans*. *A. defectiva* remains as the sole *Abiotrophia* species (37).

Among the intrinsically vancomycin-resistant catalase-negative, gram-positive cocci, a number of *Leuconostoc* species have been noted in human infection (*Leuconostoc mesenteroides*, *Leuconostoc lactis*, *Leuconostoc pseudomesenteroides*, and *Leuconostoc citreum* [50]). In 1993, the former *Leuconostoc paramesenteroides* and related species were placed into a novel genus, *Weissella* (41). *Pediococcus acidilactici* and *Pediococcus pentosaceus* are the most common clinical isolates of pediococci (11). The vancomycin-susceptible species formerly named *Pediococcus halophilus* was reclassified in the genus *Tetragenococcus* (42). The organism formerly called *Enterococcus solitarius* has also been transferred to the *Tetragenococcus* genus as *Tetragenococcus solitarius* (52). Little is known about the role of the tetragenococci in human infection.

The organism we now know as *Gemella morbillorum* was described in 1917 by Tunnicliff (134) as an isolate from the blood of patients with measles. *G. morbillorum* was originally named *Diplococcus rubeolae* and was also called *Diplococcus morbillorum*, *Peptostreptococcus morbillorum*, and *Streptococcus morbillorum* until a proposal to include it in the genus *Gemella* as *Gemella morbillorum* was made in 1988 (83). A second species, *Gemella haemolysans*, was originally classified as a *Neisseria* species, due to its gram-variable or even gram-negative nature and its cellular morphology (diplococci with flattened adjacent sides). Collins and coworkers described two additional *Gemella* species isolated from human sources, *Gemella bergeri* (originally named *Gemella bergeriae* [34]) and *Gemella sanguinis* (35). The genus *Dolosigranulum* shows phenotypic similarities to *Gemella*, although it is not phylogenetically closely related to *Gemella* strains (2, 87).

Aerococcus urinae, described in 1992, is negative for pyrrolidonyl arylamidase production (PYR) and positive for leucine aminopeptidase production (LAP), showing

TABLE 1 Possible identities of catalase-negative, gram-positive cocci based on certain phenotypic reactions and cellular morphology[a]

Phenotypic reaction			Cellular morphology	
PYR	LAP	NaCl	Pairs, chains	Clusters, tetrads, irregular groups
+	+	+	Enterococcus,[b,c,d] Vagococcus,[c,e] Lactococcus,[d] Facklamia spp. other than F. languida, Ignavigranum[f]	Facklamia languida, Dolosigranulum, Aerococcus sanguinicola
+	+	−	Abiotrophia,[g] Granulicatella,[g] Gemella spp. other than G. haemolysans	G. haemolysans (cells arranged primarily in pairs, with adjacent sides flattened)
+	−	+	Globicatella	Aerococcus viridans,[h] Helcococcus kunzii[h,i]
+	−	−	Dolosicoccus	
−	+	+		Aerococcus urinae, Pediococcus,[j] Tetragenococcus
−	+	−	Viridans group streptococci[k]	
−	−	+	Leuconostoc,[j] Weissella[j]	

[a]Abbreviations and symbols: NaCl, growth in 6.5% NaCl; +, ≥90% of strains positive; −, ≤10% of strains positive.

[b]Some strains may display vancomycin resistance, and some strains are motile.

[c]Most enterococcal strains are capable of growth at 45°C, differentiating them from vagococci, which may be phenotypically similar. Strains of vagococci have been reported as testing positive with a commercially available nucleic acid probe for members of the genus Enterococcus.

[d]Phenotypically similar strains of enterococci and lactococci can be differentiated with a commercially available nucleic acid probe for members of the genus Enterococcus.

[e]Motile.

[f]Some strains display satelliting growth; some strains are urease positive.

[g]Members of this genus display satelliting growth.

[h]Although H. kunzii shares some phenotypic traits with A. viridans, it is facultative and usually nonhemolytic, in contrast to A. viridans, which prefers an aerobic growth atmosphere and is alpha-hemolytic.

[i]Two additional species of Helcococcus (H. sueciensis and "H. pyogenes") have been proposed (31, 107, 108), both based on the isolation of a single strain. These new species display negative reactions in the PYR test, in contrast to H. kunzii.

[j]Vancomycin resistant.

[k]Viridans group streptococci include streptococci of the anginosus, mitis, mutans, salivarius, and bovis species groups. Some strains of Streptococcus pneumoniae (a member of the mitis species group) may produce positive reactions in the PYR test.

opposite reactions of Aerococcus viridans in these important identification tests (1). In spite of these phenotypic differences, molecular taxonomic studies suggest that A. urinae should remain in the Aerococcus genus. Organisms currently included in the A. urinae species are fairly heterogeneous and can probably be subdivided into at least two subspecies (24). Aerococcus christensenii, isolated from the human genitourinary tract, was described by Collins and coworkers in 1999 (36) and was joined by the species Aerococcus sanguinicola (originally named Aerococcus sanguicola [56, 94]) and Aerococcus urinaehominis (93) in 2001.

Globicatella, Facklamia, Ignavigranum, and Dolosicoccus are related genera that are isolated infrequently from clinical specimens. Globicatella sanguinis, initially named Globicatella sanguis, was described in 1992 (28). Facklamia currently contains four species isolated from human sources: Facklamia hominis (32), Facklamia sourekii (33), Facklamia ignava (38), and Facklamia languida (92). The genus Ignavigranum, currently consisting of a single species, Ignavigranum ruoffiae, was described by Collins and coworkers (39), along with the genus Dolosicoccus and its single species, Dolosicoccus paucivorans (40).

The genus Helcococcus, originally composed of the single species Helcococcus kunzii (30), came to include a new species isolated from humans, Helcococcus sueciensis, in 2004 (31). A third human species, "Helcococcus pyogenes," has been proposed, but to date it has not received official taxonomic standing (107, 108). Helcococcus ovis, isolated from infections in animals, displays satelliting growth, unlike the human Helcococcus species (86).

DESCRIPTION OF THE GENERA

The organisms included in this chapter form gram-positive coccoid cells, but G. haemolysans may appear gram variable or gram negative due to the ease with which its cells are decolorized. Cell shape and arrangement can be used to divide these organisms into two broad groups: those with a "streptococcal-like" Gram stain (coccobacilli in pairs and chains) or those with a "staphylococcal-like" Gram stain (more spherical cocci in pairs, tetrads, clusters, or irregular groups). Abiotrophia and Granulicatella isolates (formerly the nutritionally variant streptococci) form coccobacilli arranged in pairs and chains, but these organisms may also appear pleomorphic, especially when grown under suboptimal nutritional conditions (22). Dividing these diverse bacteria into two groups based on cellular shape and arrangement serves only as an aid in identification; no relatedness of organisms is implied by this grouping. With the exception of the infrequently isolated vagococci, these bacteria are all nonmotile.

Most of the genera described here are catalase-negative facultative anaerobes, but A. viridans is classified as a microaerophile that grows poorly, if at all, under anaerobic conditions. Some strains of Aerococcus may exhibit weakly positive catalase reactions due to nonheme catalase activity. None of the genera are beta-hemolytic on routinely employed blood agars, but strains of G. haemolysans, G. bergeri, and G. sanguinis have been described as beta-hemolytic on agars supplemented with horse blood (34, 35, 114).

EPIDEMIOLOGY AND TRANSMISSION

The organisms discussed in this chapter are opportunistic pathogens. Some of the genera have been characterized as constituents of the normal microbiota of the human oral cavity or upper respiratory tract (Gemella, Abiotrophia, and Granulicatella) and skin (Helcococcus). Lactococci, pediococci, and leuconostocs can be isolated from foods and vegetation (60, 61) and may also be found as part of the normal microbiota of the alimentary tract. Aerococci are environmental isolates that can also be found on human skin. Although they have been isolated from human clinical cultures, the natural habitats of many of the organisms mentioned here are not well characterized.

The bacteria examined here seem to be of low virulence and are usually pathogenic only in immunocompromised hosts. Infection often occurs in previously damaged tissues (e.g., heart valves) or may be nosocomial and associated with prolonged hospitalization, antibiotic treatment, invasive procedures, and the presence of foreign bodies.

CLINICAL SIGNIFICANCE

The bacteria described in this chapter may be present as contaminants in clinical cultures, but they are also isolated infrequently as opportunistic pathogens. Blood, cerebrospinal fluid, urine, and wound specimens are likely to yield significant isolates of these bacteria. Details on reported infections due to each of the genera follow.

Lactococcus

Due to their phenotypic similarities with streptococci and enterococci, clinical isolates of lactococci have probably been misidentified in the past, accounting at least in part for the paucity of reports concerning the clinical role of these bacteria. Elliott and coworkers (49) studied the phenotypic characteristics of a number of lactococcal strains isolated from blood, urinary tract infections, and an eye wound culture. Lactococci have been associated with prosthetic valve endocarditis (49, 59). Other reports have documented cases of lactococcal native valve endocarditis (58, 101, 111, 140, 148), septicemia in an immunosuppressed patient (103), osteomyelitis (74), peritonitis (65), and liver abscess (8, 66). *Lactococcus garvieae* is a known pathogen of aquacultured fish, and human infections have been linked to fish consumption (143).

Vagococcus

To date, only a handful of *Vagococcus* isolates from human sources have been reported in the literature. Teixeira and coworkers (133) described strains isolated from blood, peritoneal fluid, and a wound. Al-Ahmad and colleagues reported isolation of *Vagococcus fluvialis* from an infected root canal system (3). Vagococci are motile organisms that, like lactococci, elaborate Lancefield's group N antigen (55). Difficulties encountered in identifying vagococci may partially account for their infrequent recognition in clinical cultures.

Abiotrophia and Granulicatella

Organisms in the genera *Abiotrophia* and *Granulicatella* (formally known as nutritionally variant streptococci) are normal residents of the oral cavity and are recognized as agents of endocarditis involving both native and prosthetic valves (6, 21, 71, 75). These organisms have also been isolated from other types of infection, including ophthalmic infections (104, 106), central nervous system infections (19, 149), peritonitis in patients undergoing continuous ambulatory peritoneal dialysis (9), musculoskeletal infection (144), septic arthritis (132), and a breast implant-associated infection (45).

Leuconostoc, Pediococcus, and Weissella

The vancomycin-resistant genera *Leuconostoc* and *Pediococcus* were first recognized in clinical specimens in the mid-1980s. Handwerger and colleagues (69) observed that host defense impairment, invasive procedures breaching the integument, gastrointestinal symptoms, and prior antibiotic treatment were common features among adult patients with *Leuconostoc* infection. They also noted a predisposition to *Leuconostoc* bacteremia among neonates, suggesting that infants may become colonized during delivery by leuconostocs inhabiting the maternal genital tract. Leuconostocs have been isolated from blood, cerebrospinal fluid, peritoneal dialysate fluid, and wounds. Case reports have implicated leuconostocs as agents of infection in osteomyelitis (147), ventriculitis (47), brain abscess (4), and postsurgical endophthalmitis (85).

Pediococcus strains have been isolated from bacteremia and cases of sepsis and hepatic abscess in compromised patients (11, 12, 63, 102, 128). Barros and coworkers (11) noted that *Pediococcus acidilactici* was isolated from clinical specimens more frequently than *Pediococcus pentosaceus* and was also more commonly isolated from cases of bacteremia. Barton and coworkers noted the role of *Pediococcus* in bacteremia in infants with gastrointestinal malformations requiring surgical correction (12).

Weissella confusa, formerly classified as *Lactobacillus confusus*, has been reported infrequently as an agent of bacteremia and endocarditis (126).

Gemella

G. haemolysans has been isolated from cases of endocarditis (82), meningitis (7), brain abscess (96), and ocular infection (77, 113, 117) and a total knee arthroplasty (48). *G. morbillorum* has been implicated in cases of endocarditis (5, 62), empyema and lung abscess (136), septic shock (139), brain abscess (130), osteomyelitis (138), septic arthritis (118), and peritonitis (90). The clinical significance of *G. bergeri* and *G. sanguinis* is not well described, but strains of these species have been isolated from blood cultures, and they may also be causative agents of endocarditis (34, 35, 100).

Dolosigranulum

Dolosigranulum, a genus phenotypically similar, but not closely related, to *Gemella* (2), has been documented to occur in blood, eye, and respiratory specimens (87). The single species of the genus, *Dolosigranulum pigrum*, has been associated with nosocomial pneumonia and septicemia (95), synovitis (68), and acute cholecystitis accompanied by acute pancreatitis (99).

Aerococcus

A. viridans has been noted as a contaminant in clinical cultures and infrequently as a clinically significant isolate from cases of endocarditis and bacteremia and a case of spondylodiscitis (43, 81, 105, 109). Four additional *Aerococcus* species isolated from humans have been described since the early 1990s. *A. urinae* (1, 64) has been implicated as a urinary tract pathogen in patients predisposed to infection (23, 127) and as an agent of endocarditis (79, 84), lymphadenitis (121), and peritonitis (27). *A. sanguinicola* has been isolated from blood and urine specimens (56, 94) and cases of urosepsis and endocarditis (73). Little is currently known about the clinical significance of *A. christensenii* (isolated from vaginal specimens [36]) and *A. urinaehominis* (isolated from urine [93]).

Globicatella

G. sanguinis, isolated from human clinical specimens, has been implicated in cases of bacteremia, urinary tract infection, and meningitis (28, 91, 124). A second species in the genus, *Globicatella sulfidifaciens*, has been isolated from purulent infections in domestic mammals (137).

Facklamia

The *Facklamia* genus is closely related to, but phenotypically and phylogenetically distinct from, *Globicatella* (32). Strains of the four *Facklamia* species isolated from humans have been recovered from blood, wound, and genitourinary sites (32, 33, 38, 92) and a case of chorioamnionitis (70).

Ignavigranum

A limited number of isolates of *I. ruoffiae*, the sole species of *Ignavigranum*, have been described to date. Sites of isolation include a wound and an ear abscess (39).

Dolosicoccus

The single species of the genus *Dolosicoccus*, *D. paucivorans*, has been isolated from blood cultures (40, 54).

Helcococcus

Helcococcus kunzii can be isolated from intact skin of the lower extremities (67) as well as from mixed cultures of wounds, notably foot infections (30, 97). In such scenarios the clinical significance of this organism is difficult to interpret, since it may be present merely as a colonizer of the wound site. The ability of *H. kunzii* to function as an opportunist is, however, suggested by its isolation as the sole or predominant organism from an infected sebaceous cyst (110), a breast abscess (20), a postsurgical foot abscess (116), and cases of bacteremia and empyema in intravenous drug users (146). Two additional species isolated from humans, *H. sueciensis* and "*H. pyogenes*," are based on single isolates from a wound and a prosthetic joint infection, respectively (31, 107, 108).

COLLECTION, TRANSPORT, AND STORAGE OF SPECIMENS

No special requirements for collection and transport of specimens for isolation of the organisms discussed in this chapter have been described. Routine procedures for collection, transport, and storage of specimens for aerobic culture allow for the isolation of these bacteria, since the majority are facultative anaerobes or microaerophiles. With the exception of some *Aerococcus* strains that require an aerobic atmosphere for good growth, these organisms should also be recovered from specimens that have been collected and transported under anaerobic conditions (see chapter 16).

DIRECT EXAMINATION

The organisms described in this chapter can be visualized in direct Gram stains of clinical material but have no outstanding morphological characteristics that distinguish them from commonly isolated gram-positive cocci (streptococci and staphylococci). Although *Abiotrophia* and *Granulicatella* isolates may appear pleomorphic in direct Gram stains, they form gram-positive cocci in pairs and chains when grown on nutritionally adequate media. Direct detection of these genera by antigenic methods has not been described, but some authors have employed amplification of 16S rRNA genes for direct detection in clinical specimens (71).

ISOLATION PROCEDURES

Generally, there are no special requirements for isolation of the group of bacteria discussed here; general recommendations for the culture of blood, body fluids, and other specimens should be followed (see chapter 16). These organisms are likely to be isolated on rich, nonselective media (e.g., blood or chocolate agar and thioglycolate broth) since they are nutritionally fastidious. If selective isolation of the vancomycin-resistant genera *Leuconostoc* and *Pediococcus* is desired, Thayer-Martin medium may be used to inhibit normal microbiota or other contaminating microorganisms (120). Some of the genera (e.g., *Helcococcus*) grow slowly, forming tiny colonies that may not be visible unless extended incubation (48 to 72 h) is employed. The recovery of many of the genera included in this chapter may be enhanced by CO_2 enrichment of the incubation atmosphere.

Members of the genera *Abiotrophia* and *Granulicatella* usually grow on chocolate agar, on brucella agar with 5% horse blood, and in thioglycolate broth, but not on Trypticase soy agar with 5% sheep blood. These organisms can be cultured on nonsupportive media that have been appropriately supplemented (see "Procedures for Phenotypic Differentiation, *Abiotrophia* and *Granulicatella*," below).

IDENTIFICATION

Procedures for Phenotypic Differentiation

While molecular characterization may be required for accurate species-level identification of the aerobic, catalase-negative, gram-positive cocci encountered infrequently in clinical laboratories, phenotypic methods can be helpful in characterization of these bacteria to the genus level. Gram stain morphology has been employed as a major decision point in the identification protocols in Fig. 1 and 2 and Table 1, with two general categories: morphology resembling that of streptococci, meaning cocci or coccobacilli in pairs and chains versus staphylococcal morphology, consisting of coccoid cells arranged in pairs, clusters, tetrads, or irregular groups. Broth-grown cells (thioglycolate broth is suitable) should be used for making accurate morphological determinations. Note that *Gemella* and *Facklamia* strains may display either type of cellular morphology, depending on the species. Figures 1 and 2 display phenotypic tests used to differentiate the genera of bacteria discussed in this chapter. Descriptions of tests for catalase, PYR, LAP, beta-glucuronidase, and hippurate hydrolysis, as well as bile esculin agar and lactobacillus MRS (deMan, Rogosa, Sharpe) broth media, can be found in chapter 17 and reference 55. Additional phenotypic tests are described below in the discussion of identification criteria for each genus.

Lactococcus and *Vagococcus*

The members of the genera *Lactococcus* and *Vagococcus* are usually PYR and LAP positive, grow in the presence of 6.5% NaCl, and can be confused with enterococci or streptococci. For the salt tolerance test, heart infusion broth supplemented with 6.0% NaCl (producing a final NaCl concentration of 6.5%), with or without the acid-base indicator bromcresol purple, is inoculated with two or three colonies and incubated at 35°C for up to 72 h. Turbidity with or without a color change from purple to yellow indicates growth (55, 57). Facklam and colleagues (55, 57) recommended growth temperature tests for distinguishing lactococci from streptococci and enterococci. Consult Fig. 1 for growth temperature characteristics of each of the genera. For growth temperature tests, broths (heart infusion broth containing 1% glucose and bromcresol purple indicator) are inoculated with a single colony or drop of broth culture of the test strain and incubated at 35°C for up to 7 days. A water bath is recommended for incubation

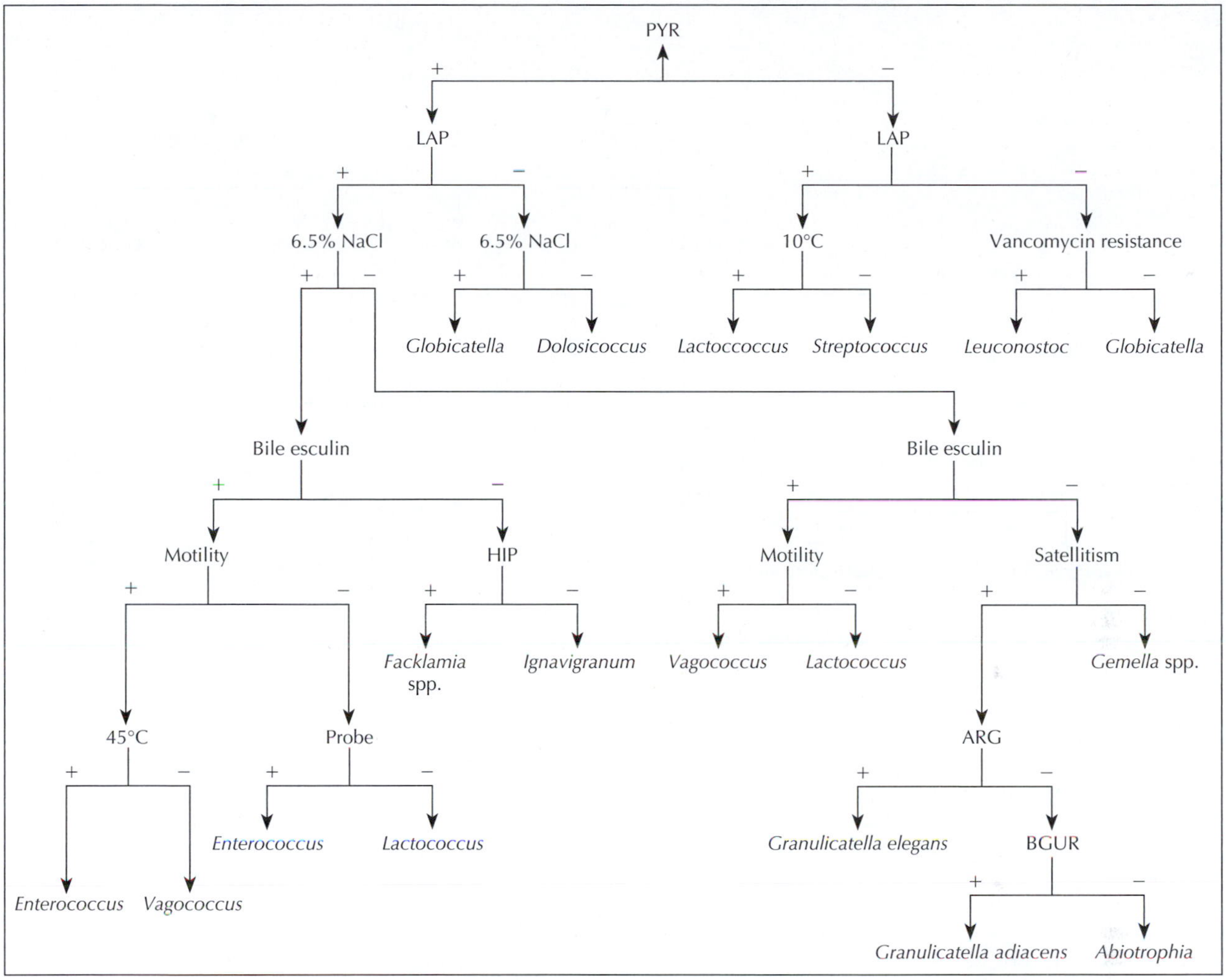

FIGURE 1 Identification of catalase-negative gram-positive cocci that grow aerobically with cells arranged in pairs and chains. Abbreviations: 6.5% NaCl, growth in broth containing 6.5% NaCl; bile esculin, hydrolysis of esculin in the presence of 40% bile; motility, motility in motility test medium; 45°C, growth at 45°C; 10°C, growth at 10°C; probe, reaction with commercially available nucleic acid probe for the genus *Enterococcus*; HIP, hydrolysis of hippurate; satellitism, satelliting growth behavior; ARG, arginine hydrolysis activity; BGUR, beta-glucuronidase activity.

of cultures at 45°C. Turbidity with or without a change in the broth's indicator to yellow indicates a positive test. The motile vagococci can be distinguished from lactococci with modified motility test medium, stab-inoculated and incubated at 30°C for up to 48 h, according to the method of Facklam and Elliott (55). Further information on the phenotypic traits of *Lactococcus* and *Vagococcus* isolates may be found in references 49, 51, 122, and 133.

Abiotrophia and Granulicatella

A test for satelliting behavior is important for identification of these two genera. The strain to be examined is streaked for confluent growth on a medium that does not support growth or supports only weak growth (e.g., sheep blood agar). A single cross streak of *Staphylococcus aureus* (ATCC 25923 or another suitable strain) is applied to the inoculated area. After incubation at 35°C in an atmosphere containing elevated CO$_2$, strains of *Abiotrophia* or *Granulicatella* grow only in the vicinity of the staphylococcal growth. Some

strains of *Ignavigranum* may also show satelliting behavior (39). Alternatively, media can be supplemented with pyridoxal. An aqueous stock solution of filter-sterilized 0.01% pyridoxal hydrochloride (which can be stored frozen) should be added to media to achieve a final concentration of 0.001%. Pyridoxal disks (Remel, Lenexa, KS) may also be used in the satellite test.

Detailed phenotypic information for the PYR- and LAP-positive *Abiotrophia* and *Granulicatella* species can be found in references 13, 16, 22, and 37. Davis and Peel (44) reported that the API 20 Strep system (bioMérieux, Durham, NC) was superior to the Rapid ID32 Strep system (bioMérieux) for identification of these organisms.

Leuconostoc, Pediococcus, and Weissella

Members of the PYR-negative, vancomycin-resistant genera *Leuconostoc*, *Pediococcus*, and *Weissella* produce small, alpha-hemolytic or nonhemolytic colonies on blood agar. Vancomycin resistance can be tested by streaking several colonies

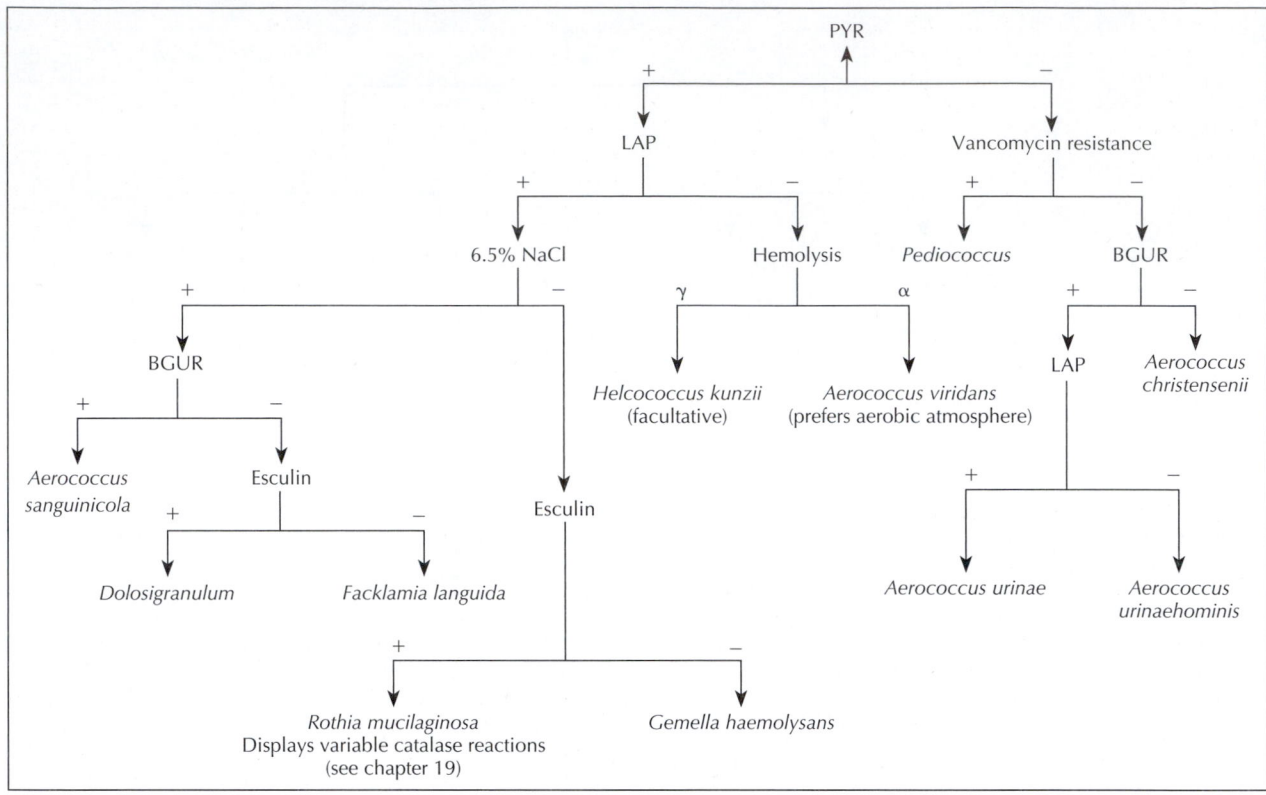

FIGURE 2 Identification of catalase-negative gram-positive cocci that grow aerobically with cells arranged in pairs, tetrads, clusters, or irregular groups. Abbreviations: 6.5% NaCl, growth in broth containing 6.5% NaCl; esculin, hydrolysis of esculin; BGUR, beta-glucuronidase activity.

over half of a Trypticase soy agar with 5% sheep blood plate. After placing a 30-μg vancomycin disk in the center of the inoculated area, the plate is incubated overnight in a CO$_2$-enriched atmosphere at 35°C. Any zone of inhibition indicates susceptibility, while resistant strains exhibit no inhibition zone (55, 57). In addition to differing cellular morphologies (Table 1), these vancomycin-resistant genera, along with vancomycin-resistant strains of lactobacilli that form short coccoid cells, can be differentiated by tests for gas production from glucose and arginine hydrolysis. Leuconostocs produce gas and are always arginine negative. Lactobacilli are variable in both tests, but a positive arginine test for a gas-producing strain would rule out identity of the organism as a leuconostoc. Pediococci are gas production negative and show variable reactions in the arginine test, although *P. acidilactici* and *Pediococcus pentosaceus*, the two species commonly found in clinical material, are arginine positive. *Weissella* strains may be misidentified as leuconostocs or lactobacilli. These organisms produce gas from glucose. The few clinical isolates reported in the literature have been described as positive for hydrolysis of arginine (41, 126).

MRS broth (BD Diagnostic Systems, Franklin Lakes, NJ; Hardy Diagnostics, Santa Maria, CA; see chapter 17), sealed with melted petrolatum and incubated for up to 7 days at 35°C, is used to test for gas production, indicated by displacement of the petrolatum plug (55, 57). The arginine hydrolysis test can be performed with Moeller's decarboxylase broth containing arginine (55). Lancefield group D antigen can be detected in pediococci (57). References 10, 11, 50, 55, 57, and 115 should be consulted for further information on identification of *Leuconostoc* and *Pediococcus* to the species level.

Gemella

On sheep blood agar media, members of the *Gemella* genus (usually PYR positive) form small colonies that are similar in appearance to those of viridans group streptococci. Slow growth of some *Gemella* strains may lead to confusion of these organisms with *Abiotrophia* or *Granulicatella* (formerly called nutritionally variant streptococci). A test for satelliting behavior separates these two groups of bacteria (57). Cells of *G. haemolysans* are easily decolorized and resemble those of neisserias, since they occur in pairs with the adjacent sides flattened. *G. haemolysans* prefers an aerobic growth atmosphere. The esculin hydrolysis test for differentiation of *G. haemolysans* and *Rothia mucilaginosa* in Fig. 2 is performed with esculin agar slants (heart infusion agar containing 0.1% esculin and 0.5% ferric citrate) that are inoculated and incubated at 35°C for up to 7 days. Partial or complete blackening of the agar indicates a positive reaction (55). *G. morbillorum* cells are gram positive and arranged in pairs and short chains; individual cells in a given pair may be of unequal sizes. Only a small number of strains of *G. bergeri* and *G. sanguinis* have been reported on to date. Information on phenotypic characteristics of these *Gemella* species can be found in references 34 and 35.

Aerococcus

The PYR-positive, LAP-negative member of the genus, A. *viridans*, is characterized by displaying weak or no growth when incubated in an anaerobic atmosphere (53). This trait can be tested by incubating duplicate blood agar plate cultures of the organism in question in anaerobic and aerobic atmospheres and comparing growth after 24 to 48 h. *A. viridans* forms alpha-hemolytic colonies that could be confused with those of either viridans group streptococci or enterococci. *A. sanguinicola* is positive in the PYR and LAP tests, while *A. urinaehominis* is negative in both. The PYR-negative, LAP-positive species, *A. urinae* and *A. christensenii*, are differentiated by production of beta-glucuronidase (*A. christensenii* is negative and *A. urinae* is positive). *A. urinae* forms small (0.5 mm in diameter after 24 h of incubation) alpha-hemolytic, convex, shiny, transparent colonies on blood agar media. Additional information on the identifying characteristics of *A. urinae* can be found in reference 23, and a second biotype (esculin hydrolysis positive) of this species is described in reference 24. Additional information on phenotypic traits of the species *A. christensenii*, *A. sanguinicola*, and *A. urinaehominis* can be found in Table 1, Fig. 2, and references 36, 56, 93, and 94.

Dolosigranulum

D. pigrum, the sole species of *Dolosigranulum* described to date, displays positive PYR and LAP reactions and was initially described as phenotypically similar, though not closely related, to members of the genus *Gemella* (2). *D. pigrum* is distinguished from *Gemella* species by its abilities to hydrolyze arginine and to grow in the presence of 6.5% NaCl.

Globicatella and Related Genera (Facklamia, Dolosicoccus, and Ignavigranum)

Globicatella and the related genera *Facklamia*, *Dolosicoccus*, and *Ignavigranum* are all PYR positive. *Facklamia* and *Ignavigranum* are also LAP positive and salt tolerant. *Globicatella* is LAP negative and salt tolerant, while *Dolosicoccus* is LAP negative and salt intolerant. *Dolosicoccus* strains are also hippurate hydrolysis negative, which further distinguishes them from strains of *Facklamia* and *Globicatella* (hippurate hydrolysis positive). Strains of *Facklamia hominis* and *Ignavigranum* may produce urease. *Ignavigranum* strains may exhibit satelliting behavior. Further details of phenotypic traits of these organisms can be found in references 32, 33, 38–40, 89, and 92.

Helcococcus

Colonial morphology (tiny gray, usually slightly alpha-hemolytic colonies), good growth under anaerobic conditions, and stimulation of growth by addition of 1% horse serum or 0.1% Tween 80 to the medium differentiate *H. kunzii* from aerococci (30). Isolates of *H. kunzii* are PYR positive, and most produce an API 20 Strep (bioMérieux) profile of 4100413. Additional *Helcococcus* species isolated from humans (*H. sueciensis* and the proposed "*H. pyogenes*") are negative in the PYR test. Detailed phenotypic data on these organisms can be found in references 30, 31, 107, and 108.

Commercially Available Kits and Automated Methods Based on Phenotypic Traits

There have been no comprehensive evaluations of the ability of commercially available products to identify the diverse and infrequently isolated bacteria described in this chapter. Phenotypic variation among isolates classified in the same species, the relative metabolic inactivity of some organisms, and a relatively small number of strains available for inclusion in databases have challenged the capabilities of

these products for accurate identification. Manual methods for performance of some of the basic differentiation tests (e.g., PYR and LAP) are available (e.g., BactiCard Strep [Remel]). Commercially available identification kits or systems offering a more comprehensive array of phenotypic tests are improving in their ability to identify many of the organisms discussed in this chapter (14, 56, 89, 142, 145). These products include manual methods (e.g., API 20 Strep [bioMérieux] and RapID Strep [Remel]) and automated systems (e.g., Vitek 2 [bioMérieux], MicroScan [Siemens Healthcare Diagnostics, Inc., Deerfield, IL], and Phoenix [BD Diagnostics, Sparks, MD]). In the absence of an accurate genus or species level identification, these systems will at least provide additional phenotypic information that can be used to augment results of the basic tests mentioned above.

Molecular Methods

16S rRNA gene sequencing-based identification methods appear to be more accurate than phenotypic methods, either manual or automated, for identifying many of the infrequently isolated aerobic catalase-negative, gram-positive cocci (14, 145). Bosshard and colleagues (14) observed that this method produced more species or genus level identifications than a commercially available phenotypic method (API 20 Strep), and identifications based on phenotypic traits often disagreed with those determined by 16S rRNA gene sequencing. *Abiotrophia*, *Aerococcus*, and *Gemella* strains were included in their study. Woo and coworkers (145) examined strains of *Abiotrophia*, *Granulicatella*, *Gemella*, and *Helcococcus* in their evaluation of a commercially available rRNA gene sequence-based identification system (MicroSeq 500 [Perkin-Elmer Applied Biosystems Division, Foster City, CA]). They noted disagreement in identifications obtained with commercially available phenotypic test systems (API 20 Strep and Vitek) and the commercially available sequence-based identification system compared with conventional 16S rRNA gene sequencing. The authors stressed the importance of adequate databases for accurate rRNA gene sequence-based identification. The use of alternative sequencing targets for identification of the organisms discussed in this chapter has not been extensively investigated, but Drancourt and colleagues demonstrated the utility of *rpoB* gene sequencing for identification of strains of *Abiotrophia*, *Granulicatella*, and *Gemella* (46).

TYPING SYSTEMS

Little information exists on typing methods for the genera of infrequently isolated gram-positive cocci included in this chapter. Typing is not routinely used for characterizing these organisms.

SEROLOGIC TESTS

Serologic response to the organisms described in this chapter has not been extensively investigated. No clinically useful tests have been described.

ANTIMICROBIAL SUSCEPTIBILITIES

Antimicrobial susceptibility studies on the organisms mentioned in this chapter have generally employed dilution testing methods. Little or no data exist on the utility of disk diffusion or the correlation of Etest results with those of broth or agar dilution methods. Standardized dilution methods and interpretive criteria for observed MICs have been described for only four of the genera (*Abiotrophia, Granulicatella, Leuconostoc,* and *Pediococcus* [reference 25 and chapter 71]). The lack of standardized methods and interpretive criteria and the relatively small collections of isolates for some of the genera discussed in this chapter make it difficult to accurately assess antimicrobial susceptibility patterns. With the exception of *Leuconostoc, Pediococcus,* and *Weissella,* all of the genera display susceptibility to vancomycin. While many of the genera are susceptible to beta-lactams and other antimicrobials, observed strain variations suggest that MICs of antimicrobials used for treatment should be determined for individual isolates. When susceptibility testing is requested for isolates for which no guidelines exist, dilution methods may be used to generate MICs which can be reported without interpretation. Since many of the bacteria dealt with here are fairly fastidious, investigators have often employed blood-supplemented Mueller-Hinton media and, if necessary for good growth, incubation in a CO_2-enriched atmosphere for susceptibility testing. Pyridoxal hydrochloride (final concentration of 0.001%) should also be added to blood-supplemented media for testing strains of *Abiotrophia* and *Granulicatella* (25, 26). Details of published susceptibility testing studies for each of the genera appear below.

Information on the in vitro antimicrobial susceptibility of *Lactococcus lactis* and *Lactococcus garvieae* strains isolated from humans suggests that *L. garvieae* isolates are less susceptible to penicillin and cephalothin than are strains of *L. lactis.* The uniform resistance of *L. garvieae* versus the uniform susceptibility to clindamycin of the *L. lactis* strains examined by Elliott and Facklam (51) led them to propose a test for clindamycin susceptibility as an aid in differentiation of these two species. In clinical practice, cases of lactococcal endocarditis have been successfully treated either with penicillin alone or with penicillin and gentamicin (101, 111).

Teixeira and colleagues observed that a collection of *Vagococcus* isolates were all susceptible to ampicillin, cefotaxime, and trimethoprim-sulfamethoxazole. All strains were resistant to clindamycin, lomefloxacin, and ofloxacin. Variable results were observed with other antimicrobial agents (133).

The vancomycin-resistant genera *Leuconostoc* and *Pediococcus* are considered penicillin susceptible when MICs are interpreted using criteria adapted from those for *Enterococcus* spp. (25, 131). They are usually susceptible to chloramphenicol, tetracyclines, and aminoglycosides. Carbapenem and cephalosporin resistance has been noted in some strains of *Leuconostoc* (25). Huang and colleagues (72) noted MIC ranges of 0.5 to 8 µg/ml for linezolid and 0.06 to 2 µg/ml for daptomycin in 68 strains of *Leuconostoc* tested and ranges of 1 to 4 µg/ml for linezolid and 0.06 to 0.5 µg/ml for daptomycin in 13 *Pediococcus* isolates.

Abiotrophia and *Granulicatella* isolates display a range of penicillin MICs, with authors reporting reduced penicillin susceptibility in 33 to 65% of isolates (76, 98, 135). Susceptibility to aminoglycosides is also variable, but no cases of high-level resistance have been reported. A synergistic effect between beta-lactam agents and aminoglycosides has been demonstrated for isolates of *Abiotrophia,* and combination therapy with penicillin and gentamicin is the currently recommended treatment for endocarditis caused by *Abiotrophia* and *Granulicatella.* High relapse rates have been reported, even with appropriate therapy (76). Tuohy and colleagues (135) examined a collection of 27 *G. adiacens* and 12 *A. defectiva* strains, noting susceptibility of all isolates to clindamycin, rifampin, levofloxacin, ofloxacin,

and quinupristin-dalfopristin. These authors noted that the susceptibilities of *G. adiacens* and *A. defective,* respectively, to other agents tested were as follows: penicillin, 55 and 8%; amoxicillin, 81 and 92%; ceftriaxone, 63 and 83%; and meropenem, 96 and 100% (135). Zheng and coworkers reported high rates of beta-lactam and macrolide resistance in a collection of pediatric *Abiotrophia* and *Granulicatella* isolates (150). A daptomycin MIC range of ≤0.125 to 2 µg/ml was observed for 10 strains of this group of bacteria (112).

A. viridans and *G. haemolysans* appear to be susceptible to penicillin and display a low level of resistance to aminoglycosides (17, 18). Resistance to tetracycline and macrolides has been described to occur in *Gemella* isolates (151), as well as a synergistic effect for penicillin and gentamicin (18). Piper and colleagues (112) noted daptomycin MICs of ≤0.125 µg/ml for four strains of *G. morbillorum.* Buu-Hoi and colleagues (17) noted that while *A. viridans* seems to be naturally susceptible to macrolides, tetracyclines, and chloramphenicol, resistance to these agents has been observed. *A. urinae* has been described as susceptible to penicillin, amoxicillin, piperacillin, cefepime, rifampin, and nitrofurantoin but resistant to sulfonamides and netilmicin. Isolates displayed variable susceptibilities to trimethoprim and co-trimoxazole (23, 123, 129). *A. sanguinicola* isolates display susceptibility to penicillin, amoxicillin, cefotaxime, cefuroxime, erythromycin, chloramphenicol, quinupristin-dalfopristin, rifampin, linezolid, and tetracycline (56).

Clinical isolates of *D. pigrum* studied by LaClaire and Facklam (87) were all susceptible to penicillin, amoxicillin, cefotaxime, cefuroxime, clindamycin, levofloxacin, meropenem, quinupristin-dalfopristin, rifampin, and tetracycline. Variable susceptibility to erythromycin was noted, and 1 of the 27 strains examined was resistant to trimethoprim-sulfamethoxazole. The small number of *Helcococcus* isolates examined displayed susceptibility to penicillin and clindamycin, and most strains were resistant to erythromycin (20, 110). Woo and coworkers described an *H. kunzii* strain with *ermA*-mediated erythromycin and clindamycin resistance (146). Strains of *Facklamia* exhibit variable MICs for a variety of antibiotics (88). A study of 27 strains of *G. sanguinis* reported susceptibility of all isolates to amoxicillin but various levels of resistance to other antimicrobials tested (125).

EVALUATION, INTERPRETATION, AND REPORTING OF RESULTS

Efforts to identify the gram-positive cocci included in this chapter should be made only when isolates are considered to be clinically significant (i.e., isolated repeatedly, in pure culture, or from normally sterile sites), since these organisms may also appear in clinical cultures as contaminants or constituents of the normal microbiota. Communication with clinicians should guide the microbiology laboratory in evaluating the significance of these infrequently isolated organisms. The phenotypic tests mentioned in Table 1 and Fig. 1 and 2 facilitate presumptive identification of the infrequently isolated catalase-negative, gram-positive cocci. More extensive phenotypic testing using commercially available identification systems and molecular methods should be employed for definitive identification. Currently there are susceptibility testing guidelines for only four of the genera mentioned in this chapter. The MICs generated with dilution methods can be reported without interpretation when susceptibility testing is requested for significant isolates for which no guidelines exist.

Abiotrophia, *Granulicatella*, and *Gemella* species are well-documented agents of endocarditis. The satelliting behavior of *Abiotrophia* and *Granulicatella* and the positive PYR reactions of all three genera are useful for distinguishing them from viridans group streptococci. CLSI guidelines should be employed for susceptibility testing and interpretation of results for *Abiotrophia* and *Granulicatella*. The vancomycin-resistant genera *Leuconostoc*, *Pediococcus*, and *Weissella* are infrequent clinical isolates, but they have been described as agents of bacteremia and central nervous system and other infections in compromised hosts. Phenotypic testing for vancomycin resistance (see "Identification" above) is important for identifying these genera and also helps guide antimicrobial therapy. Guidelines for antimicrobial susceptibility testing and interpretation of results are available for *Leuconostoc* and *Pediococcus* (25). Among the aerococci, *A. urinae* is a well-documented urinary tract pathogen and should be reported when isolated in significant amounts as the predominant organism in urine cultures. Phenotypic tests mentioned in this chapter presumptively identify *A. urinae*, which has been described as susceptible to beta-lactam agents and nitrofurantoin (23, 123, 129).

REFERENCES

1. **Aguirre, M., and M. D. Collins.** 1992. Phylogenetic analysis of some *Aerococcus*-like organisms from urinary tract infections: description of *Aerococcus urinae* sp. nov. *J. Gen. Microbiol.* **138:**401–405.

2. **Aguirre, M., D. Morrison, B. D. Cookson, F. W. Gay, and M. D. Collins.** 1993. Phenotypic and phylogenetic characterization of some *Gemella*-like organisms from human infections: description of *Dolosigranulum pigrum* gen. nov., sp. nov. *J. Appl. Bacteriol.* **75:**608–612.

3. **Al-Ahmad, A., K. Pelz, J. F. Schirrmeister, E. Hellwid, and R. Pukall.** 2008. Characterization of the first oral *Vagococcus* isolate from a root-filled tooth with periradicular lesions. *Curr. Microbiol.* **57:**235–238.

4. **Albanese, A., T. Spanu, M. Sali, F. Novegno, T. D'Inzeo, R. Santangelo, A. Mangiola, C. Anile, and G. Fadda.** 2006. Molecular identification of *Leuconostoc mesenteroides* as a cause of brain abscess in an immunocompromised patient. *J. Clin. Microbiol.* **44:**3044–3045.

5. **Al-Hujailan, G., and P. Lagace-Wiens.** 2007. Mechanical valve endocarditis caused by *Gemella morbillorum*. *J. Med. Microbiol.* **56:**1689–1691.

6. **Al-Tawfiq, J. A., G. Kiwan, and H. Murrar.** 2007. *Granulicatella elegans* native valve infective endocarditis: case report and review. *Diagn. Microbiol. Infect. Dis.* **57:**439–441.

7. **Anil, M., N. Ozkalay, M. Helvaci, N. Agus, O. Guler, A. Dikerler, and B. Kanar.** 2007. Meningitis due to *Gemella haemolysans* in a pediatric case. *J. Clin. Microbiol.* **45:**2337–2339.

8. **Antolin, J., R. Ciguenza, I. Saluena, E. Vazquez, J. Hernandez, and D. Espinos.** 2004. Liver abscess caused by *Lactococcus lactis cremoris*: a new pathogen. *Scand. J. Infect. Dis.* **36:**490–491.

9. **Atlay, M., H. Akay, E. Yildiz, and M. Duranay.** 2008. A novel agent of peritoneal dialysis-related peritonitis: *Granulicatella adiacens*. *Peritoneal Dialysis Int.* **28:**96–101.

10. **Barreau, C., and G. Wagener.** 1990. Characterization of *Leuconostoc lactis* strains from human sources. *J. Clin. Microbiol.* **28:**1728–1733.

11. **Barros, R. R., M. D. Carvalho, J. M. Peralta, R. R. Facklam, and L. M. Teixeira.** 2001. Phenotypic and genotypic characterization of *Pediococcus* strains isolated from human clinical sources. *J. Clin. Microbiol.* **39:**1241–1246.

12. **Barton, L. L., E. D. Rider, and R. W. Coen.** 2001. Bacteremic infection with *Pediococcus*: vancomycin-resistant opportunist. *Pediatrics* **107:**775–776.

13. **Beighton, D., K. A. Homer, A. Bouvet, and A. R. Storey.** 1995. Analysis of enzymatic activities for differentiation of two species of nutritionally variant streptococci, *Streptococcus defectivus* and *Streptococcus adjacens*. *J. Clin. Microbiol.* **33:**1584–1587.

14. **Bosshard, P. P., S. Abels, M. Altwegg, E. C. Bottger, and R. Zbinden.** 2004. Comparison of conventional and molecular methods for identification of aerobic catalase-negative gram-positive cocci in the clinical laboratory. *J. Clin. Microbiol.* **42:**2065–2073.

15. **Bouvet, A., F. Grimont, and P. A. D. Grimont.** 1989. *Streptococcus defectivus* sp. nov. and *Streptococcus adjacens* sp. nov., nutritionally variant streptococci from human clinical specimens. *Int. J. Syst. Bacteriol.* **39:**290–294.

16. **Bouvet, A., F. Villeroy, F. Cheng, C. Lamesch, R. Williamson, and L. Gutmann.** 1985. Characterization of nutritionally variant streptococci by biochemical tests and penicillin-binding proteins. *J. Clin. Microbiol.* **22:**1030–1034.

17. **Buu-Hoi, A., C. LeBouguenec, and T. Horaud.** 1989. Genetic basis of antibiotic resistance in *Aerococcus viridans*. *Antimicrob. Agents Chemother.* **33:**529–534.

18. **Buu-Hoi, A., A. Sapoetra, C. Branger, and J. F. Acar.** 1982. Antimicrobial susceptibility of *Gemella haemolysans* isolated from patients with subacute endocarditis. *Eur. J. Clin. Microbiol.* **1:**102–106.

19. **Cerceo, E., J. D. Christie, I. Nachamkin, and E. Lautenbach.** 2004. Central nervous system infections due to *Abiotrophia* and *Granulicatella* species: an emerging challenge? *Diagn. Microbiol. Infect. Dis.* **48:**161–165.

20. **Chagla, A. H., A. A. Borczyk, R. R. Facklam, and M. Lovgren.** 1998. Breast abscess associated with *Helcococcus kunzii*. *J. Clin. Microbiol.* **36:**2377–2379.

21. **Chang, S.-H., C.-C. Lee, S.-Y. Chen, I.-C. Chen, M.-R. Hsieh, and S.-C. Chen.** 2008. Infectious intracranial aneurysms caused by *Granulicatella adiacens*. *Diagn. Microbiol. Infect. Dis.* **60:**201–204.

22. **Christensen, J. J., and R. R. Facklam.** 2001. *Granulicatella* and *Abiotrophia* species from human clinical specimens. *J. Clin. Microbiol.* **39:**3520–3523.

23. **Christensen, J. J., H. Vibits, J. Ursing, and B. Korner.** 1991. *Aerococcus*-like organism, a newly recognized potential urinary tract pathogen. *J. Clin. Microbiol.* **29:**1049–1053.

24. **Christensen, J. J., A. M. Whitney, L. M. Teixeira, A. G. Steigerwalt, R. R. Facklam, B. Korner, and D. J. Brenner.** 1997. *Aerococcus urinae*: intraspecies genetic and phenotypic relatedness. *Int. J. Syst. Bacteriol.* **47:**28–32.

25. **Clinical and Laboratory Standards Institute.** 2006. *Methods for Antimicrobial Dilution and Disk Susceptibility Testing of Infrequently Isolated or Fastidious Bacteria; Approved Guideline M45-A.* Clinical and Laboratory Standards Institute, Wayne, PA.

26. **Clinical and Laboratory Standards Institute.** 2009. *Methods for Dilution Antimicrobial Susceptibility Tests for Bacteria That Grow Aerobically; Approved Standard—Eighth ed., M07-A8.* Clinical and Laboratory Standards Institute, Wayne, PA.

27. **Colakoglu, S., T. Turunc, M. Taskoparan, H. Aliskan, E. Kizilkilic, Y. Z. Demiroglu, and H. Arslan.** 2008. Three cases of serious infection caused by *Aerococcus urinae*: a patient with spontaneous bacterial peritonitis and two patients with bacteremia. *Infection* **36:**288–290.

28. **Collins, M. D., M. Aguirre, R. R. Facklam, J. Shallcross, and A. M. Williams.** 1992. *Globicatella sanguis* gen. nov., sp. nov., a new Gram-positive catalase negative bacterium from human sources. *J. Appl. Bacteriol.* **73:**433–437.

29. **Collins, M. D., C. Ash, J. A. E. Farrow, S. Wallbanks, and A. M. Williams.** 1989. 16S ribosomal ribonucleic acid sequence analyses of lactococci and related taxa. Description of *Vagococcus fluvialis* gen. nov., sp. nov. *J. Appl. Bacteriol.* **67:**453–460.

30. **Collins, M. D., R. R. Facklam, U. M. Rodrigues, and K. L. Ruoff.** 1993. Phylogenetic analysis of some *Aerococcus*-like organisms from clinical sources: description of *Helcococcus kunzii* gen. nov., sp. nov. *Int. J. Syst. Bacteriol.* **43:**425–429.

31. Collins, M. D., E. Falsen, K. Brownlee, and P. A. Lawson. 2004. *Helcococcus sueciensis* sp. nov., isolated from a human wound. *Int. J. Syst. Evol. Microbiol.* **54**:1557–1560.

32. Collins, M. D., E. Falsen, J. Lemozy, E. Åkervall, B. Sjödén, and P. A. Lawson. 1997. Phenotypic and phylogenetic characterization of some *Globicatella*-like organisms from human sources: description of *Facklamia hominis* gen. nov., sp. nov. *Int. J. Syst. Bacteriol.* **47**:880–882.

33. Collins, M. D., R. A. Hutson, E. Falsen, and B. Sjoden. 1999. *Facklamia sourekii* sp. nov., isolated from human sources. *Int. J. Syst. Bacteriol.* **49**:635–638.

34. Collins, M. D., R. A. Hutson, E. Falsen, B. Sjoden, and R. R. Facklam. 1998. *Gemella bergeriae* sp. nov., isolated from human clinical specimens. *J. Clin. Microbiol.* **36**:1290–1293.

35. Collins, M. D., R. A. Hutson, E. Falsen, B. Sjoden, and R. R. Facklam. 1998. Description of *Gemella sanguinis* sp. nov., isolated from human clinical specimens. *J. Clin. Microbiol.* **36**:3090–3093.

36. Collins, M. D., M. R. Jovita, R. A. Hutson, M. Ohlen, and E. Falsen. 1999. *Aerococcus christensenii* sp. nov., from the human vagina. *Int. J. Syst. Bacteriol.* **49**:1125–1128.

37. Collins, M. D., and P. A. Lawson. 2000. The genus *Abiotrophia* (Kawamura et al.) is not monophyletic: proposal of *Granulicatella* gen. nov., *Granulicatella adiacens* comb. nov., *Granulicatella elegans* comb. nov., and *Granulicatella balaenopterae* comb. nov. *Int. J. Syst. Evol. Microbiol.* **50**:365–369.

38. Collins, M. D., P. A. Lawson, R. Monasterio, E. Falsen, B. Sjoden, and R. R. Facklam. 1998. *Facklamia ignava* sp. nov., isolated from human clinical specimens. *J. Clin. Microbiol.* **36**:2146–2148.

39. Collins, M. D., P. A. Lawson, R. Monasterio, E. Falsen, B. Sjoden, and R. R. Facklam. 1999. *Ignavigranum ruoffiae* sp. nov., isolated from human clinical specimens. *Int. J. Syst. Bacteriol.* **49**:97–101.

40. Collins, M. D., M. Rodriguez Jovita, R. A. Hutson, E. Falsen, B. Sjoden, and R. R. Facklam. 1999. *Dolosicoccus paucivorans* gen. nov., sp. nov., isolated from human blood. *Int. J. Syst. Bacteriol.* **49**:1439–1442.

41. Collins, M. D., J. Samelis, J. Metaxopoulos, and S. Wallbanks. 1993. Taxonomic studies on some leuconostoc-like organisms from fermented sausages: description of a new genus *Weissella* for the *Leuconostoc paramesenteroides* group of species. *J. Appl. Bacteriol.* **75**:595–603.

42. Collins, M. D., A. M. Williams, and S. Wallbanks. 1990. The phylogeny of *Aerococcus* and *Pediococcus* as determined by 16S rRNA sequence analysis: description of *Tetragenococcus* gen. nov. *FEMS Microbiol. Lett.* **70**:255–262.

43. Colman, G. 1967. *Aerococcus*-like organisms isolated from human infections. *J. Clin. Pathol.* **20**:294–297.

44. Davis, J. M., and M. M. Peel. 1994. Identification of ten clinical isolates of nutritionally variant streptococci by commercial streptococcal identification systems. *Aust. J. Med. Sci.* **15**:52–55.

45. delPozo, J. L., E. Garcia-Quetglas, S. Hernaez, A. Serrera, M. Alonso, L. Pina, J. Leiva, and J. R. Azanza. 2008. *Granulicatella adiacens* breast implant-associated infection. *Diagn. Microbiol. Infect. Dis.* **61**:58–60.

46. Drancourt, M., V. Roux, P.-E. Fournier, and D. Raoult. 2004. *rpoB* gene sequence-based identification of aerobic gram-positive cocci of the genera *Streptococcus*, *Enterococcus*, *Gemella*, *Abiotrophia*, and *Granulicatella*. *J. Clin. Microbiol.* **42**:497–504.

47. Dye, G., J. Lewis, J. Patterson, and J. Jorgensen. 2003. A case of *Leuconostoc* ventriculitis with resistance to carbapenem antibiotics. *Clin. Infect. Dis.* **37**:869–870.

48. Eggelmeijer, F., P. Petit, and B. A. C. Dijkmans. 1992. Total knee arthroplasty infection due to *Gemella haemolysans*. *Br. J. Rheumatol.* **31**:67–69.

49. Elliott, J. A., M. D. Collins, N. E. Pigott, and R. R. Facklam. 1991. Differentiation of *Lactococcus lactis* and *Lactococcus garvieae* from humans by comparison of whole-cell protein patterns. *J. Clin. Microbiol.* **29**:2731–2734.

50. Elliott, J. A., and R. R. Facklam. 1993. Identification of *Leuconostoc* spp. by analysis of soluble whole-cell protein patterns. *J. Clin. Microbiol.* **31**:1030–1033.

51. Elliott, J. A., and R. R. Facklam. 1996. Antimicrobial susceptibilities of *Lactococcus lactis* and *Lactococcus garvieae* and a proposed method to discriminate between them. *J. Clin. Microbiol.* **34**:1296–1298.

52. Ennahar, S., and Y. Cai. 2005. Biochemical and genetic evidence for the transfer of *Enterococcus solitarius* Collins et al. 1989 to the genus *Tetragenococcus* as *Tetragenococcus solitarius* comb. nov. *Int. J. Syst. Evol. Microbiol.* **55**:589–592.

53. Evans, J. B. 1986. Genus *Aerococcus* Williams, Hirch and Cowan 1953, 475[AL], p. 1080. *In* P. H. A. Sneath, N. S. Mair, M. E. Sharpe, and J. G. Holt (ed.), *Bergey's Manual of Systematic Bacteriology*, vol. 2. Williams and Wilkins, Baltimore, MD.

54. Facklam, R. 2002. What happened to the streptococci: overview of taxonomic and nomenclature changes. *Clin. Microbiol. Rev.* **15**:613–630.

55. Facklam, R., and J. A. Elliott. 1995. Identification, classification, and clinical relevance of catalase-negative, gram-positive cocci, excluding the streptococci and enterococci. *Clin. Microbiol. Rev.* **8**:479–495.

56. Facklam, R., M. Lovgren, P. L. Shewmaker, and G. Tyrrell. 2003. Phenotypic description and antimicrobial susceptibilities of *Aerococcus sanguinicola* isolates from human clinical samples. *J. Clin. Microbiol.* **41**:2587–2592.

57. Facklam, R. R., and J. A. Washington II. 1991. *Streptococcus* and related catalase-negative Gram-positive cocci, p. 238–257. *In* A. Balows, W. J. Hausler, Jr., K. L. Herrmann, H. D. Isenberg, and H. J. Shadomy (ed.), *Manual of Clinical Microbiology*, 5th ed. American Society for Microbiology, Washington, DC.

58. Fefer, J. J., K. R. Ratzan, S. E. Sharp, and E. Saiz. 1998. *Lactococcus garvieae* endocarditis: report of a case and review of the literature. *Diagn. Microbiol. Infect. Dis.* **32**:127–130.

59. Fihman, V., L. Raskine, Z. Barrou, C. Kiffel, J. Riahi, B. Bercot, and M.-J. Sanson-Le Pors. 2006. *Lactococcus garvieae* endocarditis: identification by 16S rRNA and *sodA* sequence analysis. *J. Infect.* **52**:e3–e6.

60. Garvie, E. I. 1986. Genus *Leuconostoc* van Tieghem 1878, 198[AL] emend mut. char. Hucker and Pederson 1930, 66[AL], p. 1071–1075. *In* P. H. A. Sneath, N. S. Mair, M. E. Sharpe, and J. G. Holt (ed.), *Bergey's Manual of Systematic Bacteriology*, vol. 2. Williams and Wilkins, Baltimore, MD.

61. Garvie, E. I. 1986. Genus *Pediococcus* Claussen 1903, 68[AL], p. 1075–1079. *In* P. H. A. Sneath, N. S. Mair, M. E. Sharpe, and J. G. Holt (ed.), *Bergey's Manual of Systematic Bacteriology*, vol. 2. Williams and Wilkins, Baltimore, MD.

62. Gimigliano, F., M. Carletti, G. Carducci, F. Iodice, and L. Ballerini. 2005. *Gemella morbillorum* endocarditis in a child. *Pediatr. Infect. Dis. J.* **24**:190.

63. Golledge, C. L., N. Stingemore, M. Aravena, and K. Joske. 1990. Septicemia caused by vancomycin-resistant *Pediococcus acidilactici*. *J. Clin. Microbiol.* **28**:1678–1679.

64. Grude, N., A. Jenkins, Y. Tveten, and B.-E. Kristiansen. 2003. Identification of *Aerococcus urinae* in urine samples. *Clin. Microbiol. Infect.* **9**:976–979.

65. Guz, G., B. Colak, K. Hizel, E. Suyani, and S. Sindel. 2006. Peritonitis due to *Lactococcus lactis* in a CAPD patient. *Scand. J. Infect. Dis.* **38**:698–699.

66. Guz, G., Z. A. Yegin, I. Dogan, K. Hizel, M. Bali, and S. Sindel. 2006. Portal vein thrombosis and liver abscess due to *Lactococcus lactis*. *Turk. J. Gastroenterol.* **17**:144–147.

67. Haas, J., S. L. Jernick, R. J. Scardina, J. Teruya, A. M. Caliendo, and K. L. Ruoff. 1997. Colonization of skin by *Helcococcus kunzii*. *J. Clin. Microbiol.* **35**:2759–2761.

68. Hall, G. S., S. Gordon, S Schroeder, K. Smith, K. Anthony, and G. W. Procop. 2001. Case of synovitis potentially caused by *Dolosigranulum pigrum*. *J. Clin. Microbiol.* **39**:1202–1203.

69. Handwerger, S., H. Horowitz, K. Coburn, A. Kolokathis, and G. P. Wormser. 1990. Infection due to *Leuconostoc* species: six cases and review. *Rev. Infect. Dis.* **12**:602–610.

70. Healy, B., R. W. Beukenholt, D. Tuthill, and C. D. Ribeiro. 2005. *Facklamia hominis* causing chorioamnionitis and puerperal bacteraemia. *J. Infect.* **50**:353–355.

71. Houpikian, P., and D. Raoult. 2005. Blood culture-negative endocarditis in a reference center: etiologic diagnosis of 348 cases. *Medicine* **84**:162–173.

72. Huang, Y.-T., C.-H. Liao, L.-J. Teng, and P.-R. Hsueh. 2007. Daptomycin susceptibility of unusual gram-positive bacteria: comparison of results obtained by the Etest and the broth microdilution method. *Antimicrob. Agents Chemother.* **51:**1570–1572.

73. Ibler, K., K. Truberg Jensen, C. Ostergaard, U. Wolff Sonksen, B. Bruun, H. C. Schonheyder, M. Kemp, R. Dargis, K. Andresen, and J. J. Christensen. 2008. Six cases of *Aerococcus sanguinicola* infection: clinical relevance and bacterial identification. *Scand. J. Infect. Dis.* **40:**761–765.

74. James, P. R., S. M. Hardman, and D. L. Patterson. 2000. Osteomyelitis and possible endocarditis secondary to *Lactococcus garvieae*: a first case report. *Postgrad. Med. J.* **76:**301–303.

75. Jeng, A., J. Chen, and T. Katsivas. 2005. Prosthetic valve endocarditis from *Granulicatella adiacens* (nutritionally variant streptococci). *J. Infect.* **51:**e125–e129.

76. Johnson, C. C., and A. R. Tunkel. 2005. Viridans streptococci and groups C and G streptococci, p. 2435–2440. In G. L. Mandell, J. E. Bennett, and R. Dolin (ed.), *Mandell, Douglas and Bennett's Principles and Practice of Infectious Diseases*, 6th ed. Churchill Livingstone, New York, NY.

77. Kailasanathan, A., and D. Anderson. 2009. Infectious crystalline keratopathy caused by *Gemella haemolysans*. *Cornea* **26:**643–644.

78. Kanamoto, T., S. Sato, and M. Inoue. 2000. Genetic heterogeneities and phenotypic characteristics of strains of the genus *Abiotrophia* and proposal of *Abiotrophia para-adiacens* sp. nov. *J. Clin. Microbiol.* **38:**492–498.

79. Kass, M., B. Toye, and J. P. Veinot. 2008. Fatal infective endocarditis due to *Aerococcus urinae*—case report and review of literature. *Cardiovascular Pathol.* **17:**410–412.

80. Kawamura, Y., X. Hou, F. Sultana, S. Liu, H. Yamamoto, and T. Ezaki. 1995. Transfer of *Streptococcus adjacens* and *Streptococcus defectivus* to *Abiotrophia* gen. nov. as *Abiotrophia adiacens* comb. nov. and *Abiotrophia defectiva* comb. nov., respectively. *Int. J. Syst. Bacteriol.* **45:**798–803.

81. Kern, W., and E. Vanek. 1987. *Aerococcus* bacteremia associated with granulocytopenia. *Eur. J. Clin. Microbiol.* **6:**670–673.

82. Khan, R., C. Urbin, D. Rubin, and S. Segal-Maurer. 2004. Subacute endocarditis caused by *Gemella haemolysans* and a review of the literature. *Scand. J. Infect. Dis.* **36:**885–888.

83. Kilpper-Balz, R., and K. H. Schleifer. 1988. Transfer of *Streptococcus morbillorum* to the genus *Gemella* as *Gemella morbillorum* comb. nov. *Int. J. Syst. Bacteriol.* **38:**442–443.

84. Kristensen, B., and G. Nielsen. 1995. Endocarditis caused by *Aerococcus urinae*, a newly recognized pathogen. *Eur. J. Clin. Microbiol. Infect. Dis.* **14:**49–51.

85. Kumudhan, D., and S. Mars. 2004. *Leuconostoc mesenteroids* [sic] as a cause of post-operative endophthalmitis—a case report. *Eye* **18:**1023–1024.

86. Kutzer, P., C. Schulze, A. Engelhardt, L.H. Wieler, and M. Nordhoff. 2008. *Helcococcus ovis*, an emerging pathogen in bovine valvular endocarditis. *J. Clin. Microbiol.* **46:**3291–3295.

87. LaClaire, L., and R. Facklam. 2000. Antimicrobial susceptibility and clinical sources of *Dolosigranulum pigrum* cultures. *Antimicrob. Agents Chemother.* **44:**2001–2003.

88. LaClaire, L., and R. Facklam. 2000. Antimicrobial susceptibilities and clinical sources of *Facklamia* species. *Antimicrob. Agents Chemother.* **44:**2130–2132.

89. LaClaire, L. L., and R. R. Facklam. 2000. Comparison of three commercial rapid identification systems for the unusual gram-positive cocci *Dolosigranulum pigrum*, *Ignavigranum ruoffiae*, and *Facklamia* species. *J. Clin. Microbiol.* **38:**2037–2042.

90. Lai, C.-C., C.-H. Wu, J.-T. Chen, and P.-R. Hsueh. 2008. Peritoneal dialysis-related peritonitis caused by *Gemella morbillorum* in a patient with systemic lupus erythematosus receiving steroid therapy. *J. Microbiol. Immunol. Infect.* **41:**272–274.

91. Lau, S. K. P., P. C. Y. Woo, N. K. H. Li, J. L. L. Teng, D.-W. Leung, K. H. L. Ng, T.-L. Que, and K.-Y. Yuen. 2006. *Globicatella* bacteraemia identified by 16S ribosomal RNA gene sequencing. *J. Clin. Pathol.* **59:**303–307.

92. Lawson, P. A., M. D. Collins, E. Falsen, B. Sjoden, and R. R. Facklam. 1999. *Facklamia languida* sp. nov., isolated from human clinical specimens. *J. Clin. Microbiol.* **37:**1161–1164.

93. Lawson, P. A., E. Falsen, M. Ohlen, and M. D. Collins. 2001. *Aerococcus urinaehominis* sp. nov., isolated from human urine. *Int. J. Syst. Evol. Microbiol.* **51:**683–686.

94. Lawson, P. A., E. Falsen, K. Truberg-Jensen, and M. D. Collins. 2001. *Aerococcus sanguicola* sp. nov., isolated from a human clinical source. *Int. J. Syst. Evol. Microbiol.* **51:**475–479.

95. Lecuyer, H., J. Audibert, A. Bobigny, C. Eckert, C. Janniere-Nartey, A. Buu-Hoi, J.-L. Mainardi, and I. Podglajen. 2007. *Dolosigranulum pigrum* causing nosocomial pneumonia and septicemia. *J. Clin. Microbiol.* **45:**3474–3475.

96. Lee, M. R., S.-O. Lee, S.-Y. Kim, S. M. Yang, Y.-H. Seo, and Y. K. Cho. 2004. Brain abscess due to *Gemella haemolysans*. *J. Clin. Microbiol.* **42:**2338–2340.

97. Lemaitre, N., D. Huvent, C. Loiez, F. Wallet, and R. J. Courcol. 2008. Isolation of *Helcococcus kunzii* from plantar phlegmon in a vascular patient. *J. Med. Microbiol.* **57:**907–908.

98. Liao, C.-H., L.-J. Teng, P.-R. Hsueh, Y.-C. Chen, L.-M. Huang, S.-C. Chang, and S.-W. Ho. 2004. Nutritionally variant streptococcal infections at a university hospital in Taiwan: disease emergence and high prevalence of beta-lactam and macrolide resistance. *Clin. Infect. Dis.* **38:**452–455.

99. Lin, J.-C., S.-J. Hou, L.-U. Huang, J.-R. Sun, W.-K. Chang, and J.-J. Lu. 2006. Acute cholecystitis accompanied by acute pancreatitis potentially caused by *Dolosigranulum pigrum*. *J. Clin. Microbiol.* **44:**2298–2299.

100. Logan, L. K., X. Zheng, and S. T. Shulman. 2008. *Gemella bergeriae* endocarditis in a boy. *Pediatr. Infect. Dis.* **27:**184–186.

101. Mannion, P. T., and M. M. Rothburn. 1990. Diagnosis of bacterial endocarditis caused by *Streptococcus lactis*. *J. Infect.* **21:**317–318.

102. Mastro, T. D., J. S. Spika, P. Lozano, J. Appel, and R. R. Facklam. 1990. Vancomycin-resistant *Pediococcus acidilactici*: nine cases of bacteremia. *J. Infect. Dis.* **161:**956–960.

103. Mofredj, A., D. Baraka, G. Kloeti, and J. L. Dumont. 2000. *Lactococcus garvieae* septicemia with liver abscess in an immunosuppressed patient. *Am. J. Med.* **109:**513–514.

104. Namdari, H., K. Kintner, B. A. Jackson, S. Namdari, J. L. Hughes, R. R. Peairs, and D. J. Savage. 1999. *Abiotrophia* species as a cause of endophthalmitis following cataract extraction. *J. Clin. Microbiol.* **37:**1564–1566.

105. Nasoodi, A., A. G. Ali, W. J. Gray, and D. A. Hedderwick. 2008. Spondylodiscitis due to *Aerococcus viridans*. *J. Med. Microbiol.* **57:**532–533.

106. Ormerod, L. D., K. L. Ruoff, D. M. Meisler, P. J. Wasson, J. C. Kinter, S. P. Dunn, J. H. Lass, and I. Van de Rijn. 1991. Infectious crystalline keratopathy. Role of nutritionally variant streptococci and other bacterial factors. *Ophthalmology* **98:**159–169.

107. Panackal, A. A., Y. B. Houze, J. Prentice, S. S. Leopold, B. T. Cookson, W. C. Liles, and A. P. Limaye. 2004. Prosthetic joint infection due to "*Helcococcus pyogenica*." *J. Clin. Microbiol.* **42:**2872–2874.

108. Panackal, A. A., Y. B. Houze, J. Prentice, S. S. Leopold, B. T. Cookson, W. C. Liles, and A. P. Limaye. 2004. Prosthetic joint infection due to "*Helcococcus pyogenes*." *J. Clin. Microbiol.* **42:**5966. (Author's correction.)

109. Parker, M. T., and L. C. Ball. 1976. Streptococci and aerococci associated with systemic infection in man. *J. Med. Microbiol.* **9:**275–302.

110. Peel, M. M., J. M. Davis, K. J. Griffin, and D. L. Freedman. 1997. *Helcococcus kunzii* as sole isolate from an infected sebaceous cyst. *J. Clin. Microbiol.* **35:**328–329.

111. Pellizzer, G., P. Benedetti, F. Biavasco, V. Manfrin, M. Franzetti, M. Scagnelli, C. Scarparo, and F. de Lalla. 1996. Bacterial endocarditis due to *Lactococcus lactis* subsp. *cremoris*: case report. *Clin. Microbiol. Infect.* **2:**230–232.

112. Piper, K. E., J. M. Steckelberg, and R. Patel. 2005. In vitro activity of daptomycin against clinical isolates of gram-positive bacteria. *J. Infect. Chemother.* **11:**207–209.

113. Raman, S. V., N. Evans, T. J. Freegard, and R. Cunningham. *Gemella haemolysans* acute postoperative endophthalmitis. *Br. J. Ophthalmol.* **87:**1192–1193.

114. **Reyn, A.** 1986. Genus *Gemella* Berger 1960, 253[AL], p. 1081–1082. *In* P. H. A. Sneath, N. S. Mair, M. E. Sharpe, and J. G. Holt (ed.), *Bergey's Manual of Systematic Bacteriology*, vol. 2. Williams and Wilkins, Baltimore, MD.

115. **Riebel, W. J., and J. A. Washington.** 1990. Clinical and microbiologic characteristics of pediococci. *J. Clin. Microbiol.* **28:**1348–1355.

116. **Riegel, P., and J.-P. Lepargneur.** 2003. Isolation of *Helcococcus kunzii* from a post-surgical foot abscess. *Int. J. Med. Microbiol.* **293:**437–439.

117. **Ritterband, D., M. Shah, M. Kresloff, M. Intal, U. Shabto, and J. Seedor.** 2002. *Gemella haemolysans* keratitis and consecutive endophthalmitis. *Am. J. Ophthalmol.* **133:**268–269.

118. **Roche, M., and E. Smyth.** 2005. A case of septic arthritis due to infection with *Gemella morbillorum*. *J. Infect.* **51:**e187–e189.

119. **Roggenkamp, A., M. Abele-Horn, K-H. Trebesius, U. Tretter, I. B. Autenrieth, and J. Heesemann.** 1998. *Abiotrophia elegans* sp. nov., a possible pathogen in patients with culture-negative endocarditis. *J. Clin. Microbiol.* **36:**100–104.

120. **Ruoff, K. L., D. R. Kuritzkes, J. S. Wolfson, and M. J. Ferraro.** 1988. Vancomycin-resistant Gram-positive bacteria isolated from human sources. *J. Clin. Microbiol.* **26:**2064–2068.

121. **Santos, R., E. Santos, S. Goncalves, A. Marques, J. Sequeira, P. Abecasis, and M. Cadete.** 2003. Lymphadenitis caused by *Aerococcus urinae* infection. *Scand. J. Infect. Dis.* **35:**353–354.

122. **Schleifer, K. H., J. Kraus, C. Dvorak, R. Kilpper-Balz, M. D. Collins, and W. Fischer.** 1985. Transfer of *Streptococcus lactis* and related streptococci to the genus *Lactococcus* gen. nov. *Syst. Appl. Microbiol.* **6:**183–195.

123. **Schurr, P. M. H., M. E. E. van Kasteren, L. Sabbe, M. C. Vos, M. M. P. C. Janssens, and A. G. M. Buiting.** 1997. Urinary tract infections with *Aerococcus urinae* in the south of the Netherlands. *Eur. J. Clin. Microbiol. Infect. Dis.* **16:**871–875.

124. **Seegmuller, I., M. van der Linden, C. Heeg, and R. R. Reinert.** 2007. *Globicatella sanguis* is an etiological agent of ventriculoperitoneal shunt-associated meningitis. *J. Clin. Microbiol.* **45:**666–667.

125. **Shewmaker, P. L., A. G. Steigerwalt, L. Shealey, R. Weyant, and R. R. Facklam.** 2001. DNA relatedness, phenotypic characteristics, and antimicrobial susceptibilities of *Globicatella sanguinis* strains. *J. Clin. Microbiol.* **39:**4052–4057.

126. **Shin, J. H., D. I. Kim, H. R. Kim, D. S. Kim, J.-K. Kook, and J. N. Lee.** 2007. Severe infective endocarditis of native valves caused by *Weissella confusa* detected incidentally on echocardiography. *J. Infect.* **54:**e149–e151.

127. **Sierra-Hoffman, M., K. Watkins, C. Jinadatha, R. Fader, and J. L. Carpenter.** 2005. Clinical significance of *Aerococcus urinae*: a retrospective review. *Diagn. Microbiol. Infect. Dis.* **53:**289–292.

128. **Sire, J. M., P. Y. Donnio, R. Mensard, P. Pouedras, and J. L. Avril.** 1992. Septicemia and hepatic abscess caused by *Pediococcus acidilactici*. *Eur. J. Clin. Microbiol. Infect. Dis.* **11:**623–625.

129. **Skov, R., J. J. Christensen, B. Korner, N. Frimodt-Moeller, and F. Espersen.** 2001. *In vitro* antimicrobial susceptibility of *Aerococcus urinae* to 14 antibiotics, and time-kill curves for penicillin, gentamicin and vancomycin. *J. Antimicrob. Chemother.* **48:**653–658.

130. **Spagnoli, D., L. Innocenti, M. L. Ranzi, G. Tomei, and R. M. Villani.** 2003. Cerebral abscess due to *Gemella morbillorum*. *Eur. J. Clin. Microbiol. Infect. Dis.* **22:**515–517.

131. **Swenson, J. M., R. R. Facklam, and C. Thornsberry.** 1990. Antimicrobial susceptibility of vancomycin-resistant *Leuconostoc*, *Pediococcus*, and *Lactobacillus* species. *Antimicrob. Agents Chemother.* **34:**543–549.

132. **Taylor, C. E., and M. A. Fang.** 2006. Septic arthritis caused by *Abiotrophia defectiva*. *Arthritis Rheum.* **55:**976–977.

133. **Teixeira, L. M., M. G. Carvalho, V. L. Merquior, A. G. Steigerwalt, D. J. Brenner, and R. R. Facklam.** 1997. Phenotypic and genotypic characterization of *Vagococcus fluvialis*, including strains isolated from human sources. *J. Clin. Microbiol.* **35:**2778–2781.

134. **Tunnicliff, R.** 1917. The cultivation of a micrococcus from blood in pre-eruptive and eruptive stages of measles. *JAMA* **68:**1028–1030.

135. **Tuohy, M. J., G. W. Procop, and J. A. Washington.** 2000. Antimicrobial susceptibility of *Abiotrophia adiacens* and *Abiotrophia defectiva*. *Diagn. Microbiol. Infect. Dis.* **38:**189–191.

136. **Valipour, A., H. Koller, U. Setinek, and O. C. Burghuber.** 2005. Pleural empyema associated with *Gemella morbillorum*: report of a case and review of the literature. *Scand. J. Infect. Dis.* **37:**378–381.

137. **Vandamme, P.** 2001. *Globicatella sulfidifaciens* sp. nov., isolated from purulent infections in domestic animals. *Int. J. Syst. Evol. Microbiol.* **51:**1745–1749.

138. **van Dijk, M., B. J. van Royen, P. I. Wuisman, T. A. Hekker, and C. van Guldener.** 1999. Trochanter osteomyelitis and ipsilateral arthritis due to *Gemella morbillorum*. *Eur. J. Clin. Microbiol. Infect. Dis.* **18:**600–602.

139. **Vasishtha, S., H. D. Isenberg, and S. K. Sood.** 1996. *Gemella morbillorum* as a cause of septic shock. *Clin. Infect. Dis.* **22:**1084–1086.

140. **Vinh, D. C., K. A. Nichol, F. Rand, and J. M. Embil.** 2006. Native-valve endocarditis caused by *Lactococcus garvieae*. *Diagn. Microbiol. Infect. Dis.* **56:**91–94.

141. **Wallbanks, S., A. J. Martinez-Murcia, J. L. Fryer, B. A. Phillips, and M. D. Collins.** 1990. 16S rRNA sequence determination for members of the genus *Carnobacterium* and related lactic acid bacteria and description of *Vagococcus salmoninarum* sp. nov. *Int. J. Syst. Bacteriol.* **40:**224–230.

142. **Wallet, F., C. Loiez, E. Renaux, N. Lemaitre, and R. J. Courcol.** 2005. Performances of VITEK 2 colorimetric cards for identification of gram-positive and gram-negative bacteria. *J. Clin. Microbiol.* **43:**4402–4406.

143. **Wang, C.-Y. C., H.-S. Shie, S.-C. Chen, J.-P. Chen, J.-P. Huang, I.-C. Hsieh, M.-S. Wen, F.-C. Lin, and D. Wu.** 2007. *Lactococcus garvieae* infections in humans: possible associations with aquaculture outbreaks. *Int. J. Clin. Pract.* **61:**68–73.

144. **Wilhelm, N., S. Sire, A. Le Coustumier, J. Loubinoux, M. Beljerd, and A. Bouvet.** 2005. First case of multiple discitis and sacroiliitis due to *Abiotrophia defectiva*. *Eur. J. Clin. Microbiol. Infect. Dis.* **24:**76–78.

145. **Woo, P. C. Y., K. H. L. Ng, S. K. P. Lau, K. Yip, A. M. Y. Fung, K. Leung, D. M. W. Tam, T. Que, and K. Yuen.** 2003. Usefulness of the MicroSeq 500 16S ribosomal DNA-based bacterial identification system for identification of clinically significant bacterial isolates with ambiguous biochemical profiles. *J. Clin. Microbiol.* **41:**1996–2001.

146. **Woo, P. C. Y., H. Tse, S. S. Y. Wong, C. W. S. Tse, A. M. Y. Fung, D. M. W. Tam, S. K. P. Lau, and K. Yuen.** 2005. Life-threatening invasive *Helcococcus kunzii* infections in intravenous-drug users and *ermA*-mediated erythromycin resistance. *J. Clin. Microbiol.* **43:**6205–6208.

147. **Zaoui, A., C. Brousse, O. Bletry, L.W. Augouard, and B. Boisaubert.** 2005. *Leuconostoc* osteomyelitis. *Joint Bone Spine* **72:**79–81.

148. **Zechini, B., P. Cipriani, S. Papadopoulou, G. DiNucci, A. Petrucca, and A. Teggi.** 2006. Endocarditis caused by *Lactococcus lactis* subsp. *lactis* in a patient with atrial myxoma: a case report. *Diagn. Microbiol. Infect. Dis.* **56:**325–328.

149. **Zenone, T., and D. V. Durand.** 2004. Brain abscesses caused by *Abiotrophia defectiva*: complication of immunosuppressive therapy in a patient with connective-tissue disease. *Scand. J. Infect. Dis.* **36:**497–499.

150. **Zheng, X., A. F. Freeman, J. Villafranca, D. Shortridge, J. Beyer, W. Kabat, K. Dembkowski, and S. T. Shulman.** 2004. Antimicrobial susceptibilities of invasive pediatric *Abiotrophia* and *Granulicatella* isolates. *J. Clin. Microbiol.* **42:**4323–4326.

151. **Zolezzi, P. C., P. G. Cepero, J. Ruiz, L. M. Laplana, C. R. Calvo, and R. Gomez-Lus.** 2007. Molecular epidemiology of macrolide and tetracycline resistances in commensal *Gemella* sp. isolates. *Antimicrob. Agents Chemother.* **51:**1487–1490.

General Approaches to the Identification of Aerobic Gram-Positive Rods

KATHRYN A. BERNARD

23

The purpose of this algorithm for the identification of aerobic gram-positive rods is to assist the reader in finding the appropriate chapter of this *Manual* for further information. The algorithm emphasizes that the Gram stain (performed on 24- to 48-h-old colonies from rich media) and macroscopic morphologies are initial key features for the differentiation of aerobic gram-positive rods. All strains of aerobic gram-positive rods (except the non-rapidly growing mycobacteria) are initially grown on blood agar plates.

Gram-positive organisms demonstrating "regular" rods are those with cells whose longitudinal edges are usually not curved but are parallel. If spore formation is not observed initially, it can be tested for on a nutritionally depleted medium. Catalase activity should be tested with colonies grown on media lacking heme groups. Type of metabolism can be evaluated using oxidative-fermentative media or in cystine Trypticase agar (CTA) medium. "Irregular" rods are those organisms with cells whose longitudinal edges are curved and not parallel. Diagnostic end products of glucose metabolism are detected by chromatographic methods. Slight beta-hemolysis is best observed when cells are incubated in a CO_2-enriched atmosphere. Organisms which have yellow- or orange-pigmented colonies are usually composed of irregular rods. Some genera that stain partially acid-fast (e.g., *Gordonia* and *Rhodococcus*) may also show a yellow-orange pigment (see chapter 27). Rods exhibiting vegetative substrate filaments may show branched-type hyphae, which either form spores or reproduce by fragmentation. It is obvious that vegetative substrate filaments might not be present initially (i.e., within 48 h), and so these organisms are prone to being misidentified.

For yellow-orange-pigmented genera (e.g., *Microbacterium*, *Curtobacterium*, and *Leifsonia*; see chapter 26), as well as for those rods exhibiting vegetative substrate filaments, chemotaxonomic or molecular genetic methods may be required for definitive identification to the genus level; partially acid-fast bacteria may be identified to the genus level by analysis of mycolic acids or genetically.

Genera which contain strictly anaerobic gram-positive rods may also contain species, or strains within a species, which grow reasonably well aerotolerantly or aerobically. This is particularly true for the genera *Actinomyces* and *Actinobaculum*, some *Propionibacterium* spp. (see chapter 49), and *Clostridium tertium* (a strong gas producer) as well as other aerotolerant *Clostridium* spp. (see chapter 50). Some aerobic gram-positive cocci, e.g., *Leuconostoc* spp. (see chapter 22) and *Streptococcus mutans* (see chapter 20), might initially be misidentified as gram-positive rods because of their initial Gram stain appearance after growth on plate agar rather than from a broth. Some gram-positive rods (e.g., *Rhodococcus* spp. [see chapter 27] or *Dermabacter* [see chapter 26]) might be initially misidentified as gram-positive cocci because of their initial Gram stain appearance. After preliminary examination of the pathogen, the microbiologist should refer to Table 1, where a wide variety of genera of gram-positive rods are cross-referenced, with respect to relevant chapters in this *Manual*.

Molecular approaches to characterize or subtype pathogens described in this section, as adjuncts to conventional phenotypic or chemotaxonomic assays, are described briefly in each chapter of this *Manual*, as well as in overview in chapters 4, 8, and 14. Use of 16S rRNA gene sequencing as a means to characterize an isolate has become an established tool in many microbiology laboratories. However, interpretation of this work must be done by personnel with a good working knowledge of current approaches for taxonomy and systematics (see chapter 15). Readers using this method must be aware of instances where 16S rRNA gene sequence analysis cannot be used as the sole characterization method, particularly where two or more validly named taxon groups have ≥98.7% identity to each other, a cutoff value described by Stackebrandt and Ebers as being suggestive of members of the same species (6). In such cases, sequencing of secondary or additional gene targets is recommended (2); see recommendations for individual taxa by chapter in this *Manual*. Additional reviews describing some of these pathogens are found in references 1 and 3 to 5.

TABLE 1 Algorithm for identification of gram-positive rods[a]

Cellular morphology	Pigmented	Vegetative substrate filaments	Spore-former	Catalase	Metabolism	Unusual Gram stain features	Acid fast	Partially/ weakly acid fast	Aerial vegetative filaments	Motility	Genus or genera (chapter) and major fermentation products if relevant	Additional comment
Regular	-	-	+	V	O or F	Often large cells	-	-	-	V	Bacillus, Paenibacillus, Aneurinibacillus, Virgibacillus, occasionally other genera in family Bacillaceae (24)	Bacillus anthracis, also chapter 12
	-	-	-	+	F	-	-	-	-	+	Listeria (25)	Motility better observed at 20–25°C
	-	-	-	-	F	-	-	-	-	-	Erysipelothrix (25)	H₂S produced in TSI
	-	-	-	-	F	-	-	-	-	-	Lactobacillus (49) Lactic acid	Some strains weakly catalase +
Irregular	-, also Y or B-G	-	-	+	O or F	Club shaped; rarely, some unusual forms, e.g., "whip handles" or "bulges"	-	-	-	-	Corynebacterium (26), succinic, lactic, propionic species specific	
	-	-	-	+	O	Long slim rods	-	-	-	-	Turicella (26)	
	-	-	-	+	F	Coccoid Short rods	-	-	-	-	Dermabacter (26)	
		-	-	+	F		-	-	-	-	Helcobacillus (26)	
	-, also Y	-	-	+	O	Shorter rods	-	-	-	-	Brevibacterium (26)	
	-	-	-	+	F	May show branching or short rods	-	-	-	-	Actinomyces (49), succinic, lactic; Propionibacterium (49), propionic	Actinomyces radicidentis, coccoid
	-, also B-G	-	-	+	F	Pleomorphic	-	-	-	-	Rothia (19 and 26)	Some strains catalase –
	-	-	-	-	F	Gram variable, coccoidal	-	-	-	-	Gardnerella (26)	Beta-hemolysis on vaginalis agar
	-	-	-	-	F	Some Actinomyces spp. branching	-	-	-	-	Arcanobacterium (26) and Actinomyces (49), succinic, lactic; Actinobaculum (49), acetic	Some species with slight beta-hemolysis

Organism					Morphology	Metabolism				Pigment	Comments
Bifidobacterium and genera formerly Bifidobacterium[b] (49), acetic	−	−	−	−	Pleomorphic, "bifidoforms"	F	−	−	−	−	
Oerskovia (26); Cellulosimicrobium (26)	V	−	−	−		O or F; O or F	+	−	+	Y, Y-O	
Curtobacterium (26)	V	−	−	−		O	+	−	−	Y, Y-O	
Microbacterium (26), Leifsonia (26)	V / +	−	−	−		O or F; O	+	−	−	Y, Y-O	Some Microbacterium spp. catalase −
Cellulomonas, Exiguobacterium (26 for both)	V / +	−	−	−		F	+	−	−	Y, Y-O	
Mycobacterium (28, 29 and 30)	−	−	−	+		O	+	−	+	−	
Segniliparus (27)	−	−	−	+		O	+	−	+	−	No growth on MacConkey agar
Nocardia (27)	−	+	+	−		O	+	−	+	−	
Tsukamurella, Gordonia, Rhodococcus, Dietzia, Williamsia (27 for all)	−	−	+ or −	−		O	+	−	+	−, Y, P-C	Dietzia generally not considered acid fast
Dermatophilus (27)	+	−	−	−	Dense aggregates of rounded cells	O	+	−	+	−	Beta-hemolysis
Actinomadura, Streptomyces, Amycolatopsis, Nocardiopsis, occasionally other genera among Pseudonocardiaceae (27 for all)	−	+	−	−		O	+	−	+	−, Y	Some strains lack aerial filaments
Saccharomonospora, Saccharopolyspora, Thermoactinomyces (27 for all)	−	+	−	−		O	+	−	+	−	All grow at 50°C

[a] +, all or nearly all strains positive; −, all or nearly all strains negative; V, feature variable; O, oxidative metabolism; F, fermentative metabolism. "Pigment" implies that colonies have pigment other than gray-white or white colony; yellow or yellowish (Y) or yellow-orange (Y-O) pigment is typical, blackish-gray (B-G) pigment is occasionally seen, and pinkish coral (P-C) is seen for some Rhodococcus and Williamsia spp. Table excludes extremely infrequently isolated genera described in chapter 26, e.g., Brachybacterium, Knoellia, Janibacter.

[b] Strains of the genus Alloscardovia in particular can be aerotolerant.

REFERENCES

1. **Bernard, K. A.** 2005. *Corynebacterium* species and coryneforms: an update on taxonomy and diseases attributed to these taxa. *Clin. Microbiol. Newsl.* **27:**9–18.
2. **Clinical and Laboratory Standards Institute.** 2008. *Interpretive Criteria for Identification of Bacteria and Fungi by DNA Target Sequencing; Approved Guideline.* CLSI document MM18-A. Clinical and Laboratory Standards Institute, Wayne, PA.
3. **Funke, G., A. von Graevenitz, J. E. Clarridge III, and K. A. Bernard.** 1997. Clinical microbiology of coryneform bacteria. *Clin. Microbiol. Rev.* **10:**125–159.
4. **Gneiding, K., R. Frodl, and G. Funke.** 2008. Identities of *Microbacterium* spp. encountered in human clinical specimens. *J. Clin. Microbiol.* **46:**3646–3652.
5. **Mages, I. S., R. Frodl, K. A. Bernard, and G. Funke.** 2008. Identities of *Arthrobacter* spp. and *Arthrobacter*-like bacteria encountered in human clinical specimens. *J. Clin. Microbiol.* **46:**2980–2986.
6. **Stackebrandt, E., and J. Ebers.** 2006. Taxonomic parameters revisited: tarnished gold standards. *Microbiol. Today* **33:**152–155.

Bacillus and Other Aerobic Endospore-Forming Bacteria*

NIALL A. LOGAN, ALEX R. HOFFMASTER,
SEAN V. SHADOMY, AND KENDRA E. STAUFFER

24

TAXONOMY

Bacillus was defined in 1920 as a genus of gram-positive, aerobic sporeformers, but since 1995 three strictly anaerobic and seven asporogenous *Bacillus* species have been proposed. This undermining of the definition has occurred because 16S rRNA gene sequence analysis has permitted the recognition of genus boundaries, whereas genera were previously defined phenotypically, as pragmatic collections of species sharing key (i.e., diagnostic) features. Many new species have been delineated largely on the basis of 16S rRNA gene sequence similarity and DNA-DNA relatedness—phenotypic descriptions may be brief, and routine phenotypic characters for distinguishing some species are very few and of little practical value.

With the accumulation of 16S rRNA gene sequence data, *Bacillus* has been divided; 14 new genera containing species originally allocated to *Bacillus* have been published since 1990, and together with *Bacillus* itself the species in these genera now number 388. In addition, 38 genera containing aerobic endospore formers not originally allocated to *Bacillus* have been described. *Sporosarcina* was proposed in 1936, but the other 37 genera have been proposed since 1990, and together they contain 109 species. Following some mergers, there are now 53 genera of aerobic endospore formers overall, and over 520 species. Although seven named families containing aerobic endospore formers now lie within the order *Bacillales* of the class "*Bacilli*," in the phylum *Firmicutes*, only the families *Bacillaceae* and *Paenibacillaceae* contain species that may be of clinical interest.

The clinical bacteriologist need not, therefore, be greatly concerned at this taxonomic expansion, because for the medically relevant species it does not represent taxonomic upheaval. *Bacillus* is still the largest genus, with 162 species (90), and it continues to accommodate most of the best-known names such as *Bacillus subtilis* (the type species), *B. anthracis*, *B. cereus*, *B. licheniformis*, *B. megaterium*, *B. pumilus*, and *B. thuringiensis*. Relatively few other familiar names, some of which are of potential clinical interest, have been transferred to newer genera: *Brevibacillus brevis* (91), *Geobacillus stearothermophilus* (92; important as a thermophilic contaminant and autoclave

test organism), *Lysinibacillus sphaericus* (2), and *Paenibacillus polymyxa* and *Paenibacillus macerans*. However, several new *Bacillus* and *Paenibacillus* species have been proposed on the basis of single isolates of unknown significance from clinical sources: *B. idriensis* and *B. infantis* from neonatal sepsis (82); *P. konsidensis*, *P. massiliensis*, *P. sanguinis*, and *P. timonensis* from blood cultures (83, 116); *B. massiliensis* and *P. provencensis* isolated from cerebrospinal fluid (CSF) (56, 117); *P. turicensis* from a CSF shunt (14); and *P. urinalis* from urine (117). "*Paenibacillus hongkongensis*," now classified in a new genus of aerobic endospore formers, as *Cohnella hongkongensis* (74), was isolated from a case of pseudobacteremia in a boy with neutropenic fever.

DESCRIPTION OF THE GENERA

Notwithstanding the handful of strictly anaerobic and asporogenous members of *Bacillus*, those species likely to be isolated in a clinical laboratory are rod-shaped, endospore-forming organisms that may be aerobic or facultatively anaerobic, and young cultures are usually gram positive but sometimes gram variable or clearly gram negative. They are mostly catalase positive and may be motile by means of peritrichous flagella. Most species are mesophilic, but there are some thermophilic and psychrophilic species. A large number of the other, newer genera comprise small numbers of species that are unlikely to be encountered in a clinical laboratory, as many of them are from exotic and extreme environments.

EPIDEMIOLOGY AND TRANSMISSION

Most aerobic endospore formers are saprophytic organisms living in the natural environment, and many species are very widely distributed. Some species, however, are opportunistic or obligate pathogens of animals, including humans, other mammals, and insects. The main habitats are soils of all kinds, ranging from acid to alkaline, nonsaline to highly saline, hot to cold, and fertile to desert, and the water columns and bottom deposits of fresh and marine waters. They have been isolated from air at high altitude, from subterranean waters, and from volcanic and permafrost soils. Endospores readily survive distribution in soils, dusts, and aerosols from natural environments to a wide variety of other habitats such as man-made environments, and they may be carried across the globe by wind. The resistance of the spores to

---

*This chapter contains information presented in chapter 32 by Niall A. Logan, Tanja Popovic, and Alex R. Hoffmaster in the ninth edition of this *Manual*.

heat, radiation, disinfectants, and desiccation also results in aerobic endospore formers being frequent contaminants in the operating room, on surgical dressings, in pharmaceutical products, and in foods. Dried foods such as spices, milk powders, and farinaceous products are often quite heavily contaminated with spores, and when water becomes available during food preparation these spores may germinate, leading to spoilage or food poisoning. *B. anthracis* is, to all intents and purposes, an obligate pathogen of animals and humans. Its close relative *B. cereus* is well established as an opportunistic pathogen, and other aerobic endospore formers can also be opportunistic pathogens occasionally. Three members of the *B. cereus* group—*B. anthracis*, *B. cereus*, and *B. thuringiensis*—are regarded by many as pathovars of a single species, and there is evidence of extensive horizontal gene transfer within the *B. cereus* group (18).

Anthrax was the first example of an infection of humans and animals proven as caused by a bacterium, and this disease remains the most widely recognized clinical condition caused by a *Bacillus* species. It is primarily a disease of domestic or wild animals, and prior to the availability of an effective veterinary vaccine in the late 1930s, anthrax was one of the foremost causes worldwide of mortality in cattle, sheep, goats, and horses. Humans almost invariably contract anthrax directly or indirectly from animals. Over the past half century there has been a marked decline in the incidence of anthrax in both animals and humans; the use of veterinary and human vaccines, improvements in factory hygiene, sterilization procedures for imported animal products, and the increased use of man-made alternatives to animal hides or hair have all contributed to this. Nevertheless, the disease continues to be endemic in many countries, particularly those that lack efficient vaccination policies. It is still common in several sub-Saharan African countries, western China, some Mediterranean countries, small pockets in Canada and the United States, and certain countries of central Asia and central and South America. National vaccination programs have led to a progressive global reduction in livestock cases over the last 30 years, but there are concomitant problems of diminishing veterinary experience and a public ignorance of the disease; the former problem may lead to individual outbreaks taking longer to recognize and control, and the latter to the sale and slaughter of affected animals (140). Direct animal-to-animal transmission (i.e., excluding scavengers feeding on carcasses of animals with anthrax) is very rare. Because *B. anthracis* spores remain viable in soil for many years and their persistence does not depend on animal reservoirs, *B. anthracis* is exceedingly difficult to eradicate from an area of endemicity, and regions of nonendemicity must be constantly on the alert for the arrival of *B. anthracis* in imported animal products. Anthrax is not contagious, and transmission to humans is usually restricted to direct contact with infected animals, or products from infected animals; however, there have been reports of person-to-person transmission of cutaneous anthrax, including a case of a mother with a cutaneous lesion on her finger infecting her 1-year-old child, and a case of transmission of cutaneous abdominal lesions from one brother to another brother who shared a bed (146). Contaminated fomites, including such oddities as a communal loofah, or infection of an injection site by contamination of the skin or by syringe have also rarely been implicated (86), as has person-to-person, nosocomial spread from an umbilical infection (151).

The continued existence of *B. anthracis* in the ecosystem appears to depend on a periodic multiplication phase within an animal host, and so it is generally regarded as an obligate pathogen. Its environmental presence thus reflects contamination from an animal source at some time and persistence of spores, rather than replication within the soil. However, some authorities believe that self-maintenance may occur within certain soils, and germination of *B. anthracis* spores and genetic exchange between vegetative cells growing in grass rhizosphere have been demonstrated (119). In human and animal specimens the organism is usually sought only when the case history suggests that it is reasonable to suspect anthrax.

B. anthracis has been subjected to military research, development, and occasional deployment in several different countries over many years, following attacks on livestock during World War I, and it has remained high on the list of agents that could be used in biological warfare or bioterrorism. Few reports of laboratory-acquired infections exist, but a major outbreak occurred in April 1979 in the city of Sverdlovsk, USSR (now Yekaterinburg, Russia), in the Urals as a result of the accidental release of spores from a military production facility. Although the natural disease is readily controllable, the 2001 bioterrorism-related anthrax outbreak in the United States increased the public concern about this disease (see chapter 12).

CLINICAL SIGNIFICANCE

The majority of aerobic endospore-forming species apparently have little or no pathogenic potential and are rarely associated with disease. The principal exceptions to this are *B. anthracis*, the agent of anthrax, and *B. cereus*, but a number of other species, particularly *B. licheniformis* and *B. pumilus*, have been implicated in food poisoning and other human and animal infections.

Bacillus anthracis

Human anthrax has traditionally been classified as either (i) nonindustrial, resulting from close contact with infected animals or their carcasses after death from the disease, or (ii) industrial, as acquired by those employed in processing wool, hair, hides, bones, or other animal products. Dependent on the route of infection, there are three major clinical forms of anthrax: cutaneous, inhalation, and ingestion or oral-route anthrax. Anthrax meningitis can develop as a complication of any of these forms, or occasionally in the absence of any of them (57, 121).

Cutaneous anthrax accounts for about 99% of naturally acquired human anthrax cases worldwide; an estimated 2,000 cases are reported annually. Infection typically occurs when spores are inoculated through a break in the skin, although case reports and animal studies suggest that preexisting lesions are not necessary for infection (60); infections following insect bites have been reported. Following an incubation period of usually 2 to 6 days (but with extremes of a few hours to 3 weeks) a small papule appears, progressing over the next 24 h to a ring of vesicles, with subsequent ulceration and formation of a characteristic blackened eschar. Subsequent eschar formation may become thick and surrounded by extensive edema. Fever, pus, and pain at the site are normally absent; their presence probably indicates secondary bacterial infection. Before the availability of antimicrobial therapy, 10 to 20% of untreated cases of cutaneous anthrax were fatal. Less than 1% of cases are fatal today, and they are mainly due to obstruction of the airways by the edema that accompanies lesions on the face or neck or as a result of progression of the cutaneous disease into systemic infection. Eschars take several days to evolve, and even with effective antimicrobial therapy they may take several weeks to resolve.

Ingestion anthrax is not uncommon in regions of endemicity worldwide where socioeconomic conditions are poor and people eat raw or undercooked meat of anthrax-infected animals that have died suddenly; asymptomatic infections and symptomatic infections with recovery may not be uncommon (124). It takes two forms: oral or oropharyngeal infection, in which the lesion is in the buccal cavity or on the tongue, tonsils, or posterior pharyngeal wall, and gastrointestinal anthrax, in which ulcerations develop anywhere within the tract, but primarily in the mucosae of the terminal ileum or cecum. Oropharyngeal symptoms include sore throat, dysphagia, and regional lymphadenopathy, followed by severe edema of neck and chest. Intestinal anthrax causes nausea, vomiting, anorexia, abdominal pain, mild diarrhea, and fever; this can progress to bloody diarrhea, hematemesis, and massive ascites (140). Mortality rates range widely, owing to the nonspecific nature of the early symptoms and late initiation of antimicrobial therapy.

Between 1900 and 2001, only 18 cases of naturally acquired inhalation anthrax were recorded in the United States, with 16 (89%) being fatal (16), and figures in the United Kingdom show a similar picture. Recently, however, anthrax has occurred in persons using contaminated imported animal hides for drum making. A case of inhalation anthrax in an African drum maker in 2006 was the first naturally occurring case of inhalation anthrax in the United States since 1976; the hides from west Africa were contaminated with *B. anthracis* spores. Two cases of cutaneous anthrax, in a drum maker and a family member, occurred in the United States in 2007 (23), and there was a fatal case of inhalation anthrax in a drum maker in the United Kingdom in 2008 (3). Both cutaneous and inhalation anthrax have also been associated with the handling or playing of goatskin drums contaminated with spores of *B. anthracis* (40). Among the 22 cases of the anthrax outbreak in the United States in late 2001, in which spores were delivered in mailed letters, early recognition and treatment of the 11 patients with confirmed inhalation anthrax resulted in a 65% survival rate (9).

The inhaled spores are ingested by macrophages, but the role of macrophages thereafter is unclear, as they may be bactericidal towards germinated spores but also be crippled by lethal and/or edema toxin and so allow bacterial outgrowth (31). The replacement of the older name for this form of the disease, "pulmonary anthrax," with the newer name "inhalation anthrax" is a reflection of the fact that active infection occurs in the lymph nodes rather than the lungs themselves. Analysis of 10 of the cases associated with the bioterrorism events of 2001 (71) revealed a median incubation period of 4 days (range, 4 to 6 days). All of the patients with inhalation anthrax had severe illness and were hospitalized. Their clinical presentation included fever or chills, fatigue or malaise, minimal or nonproductive cough, dyspnea, and nausea or vomiting; some had chest pain and sweats. All patients had abnormal chest radiographic images, with pleural effusion, infiltrates, or mediastinal widening.

Regardless of the form of the disease, the generalized symptoms that may initially be mild (fatigue, malaise, fever, and/or gastrointestinal symptoms) can rapidly develop into a fulminant state following lymphohematogenous spread from a primary lesion, with symptoms of dyspnea, cyanosis, severe pyrexia, and disorientation, followed by circulatory failure, shock, coma, and death (71). Depending on the host, there is a rapid buildup of the bacteria in the blood over the last few hours to terminal levels of 10^7 to 10^9/ml in the most susceptible species. Enhanced clinical and laboratory expertise and conducting prospective surveillance are critical components of rapid anthrax diagnosis and for response preparedness, should *B. anthracis* be used in bioterrorist attacks (52).

Bacillus cereus Group

Bacillus cereus is a ubiquitous organism, and clinical isolates are phylogenetically diverse (68); it is a wide-ranging opportunistic pathogen of humans and other animals and an important cause of foodborne illness. *B. cereus* caused 21 (2%) mean annual total foodborne outbreaks and 160 (1%) mean annual total foodborne illnesses between 2001 and 2005 in the United States as reported through the Foodborne Diseases Active Surveillance Network (FoodNet) of the Centers for Disease Control and Prevention's (CDC's) Emerging Infections Program. However, this probably underrepresents the true burden of illness, since outbreaks involving less commonly identified pathogens, such as *B. cereus*, are less likely to have a confirmed etiology because these organisms are not always considered in clinical, epidemiological, and laboratory investigations of foodborne disease outbreaks (24).

B. cereus is the etiological agent of two distinct food poisoning syndromes. The diarrheal type is characterized by abdominal pain and diarrhea 8 to 16 h after ingestion of contaminated food; it is associated with a wide diversity of foods, from meats and vegetable dishes to pastas, desserts, cakes, sauces, and milk. The emetic type is characterized by nausea and vomiting 1 to 5 h after eating the offending food; oriental rice dishes are predominant sources, although occasionally other foods such as pasteurized cream, milk pudding, pastas, and reconstituted formulas have been implicated. One emetic outbreak followed the mere handling of contaminated rice in a children's craft activity, and fulminant liver failure associated with the emetic toxin has been reported (94). *B. cereus* spores are very adherent to surfaces and are widespread in food preparation environments, and they can survive many cleaning and normal cooking procedures. These are key factors for both syndromes; under conditions of improper food storage after cooking, the spores germinate and the vegetative cells multiply.

The toxigenic basis of *B. cereus* food poisonings and other *B. cereus* infections have been much elucidated over the last three decades. In diarrheal illness, one or more enterotoxins are produced by vegetative cells in the small intestine, following the ingestion of spores or vegetative cells; the toxins are believed to cause diarrhea by damaging the integrity of ileal epithelial cell membranes. *B. cereus* produces a range of protein toxins, of which three have been implicated in diarrheal illness: hemolysin BL (Hbl) and nonhemolytic enterotoxin (Nhe), both of which are three-component toxins restricted to the *B. cereus* group, and the single-component β-barrel, pore-forming cytotoxin K (CytK). These toxins may act synergistically, but there is evidence that Nhe is the most dominant in diarrheal illness (128). The emetic illness is an intoxication caused by a highly heat-, proteolysis-, and acid-resistant toxin preformed in the food—hence its rapid onset. The toxin, cereulide, is a small ring-formed dodecadepsipeptide produced at the end of logarithmic growth, and its genetic determinants are borne on a plasmid related to the pXO1 virulence plasmid of *B. anthracis* (41). Cereulide production by *B. cereus* has not been demonstrated at temperatures below 12°C, but the related and psychrotolerant species *Bacillus weihenstephanensis* may produce detectable cereulide at 8°C (135). Gherlardi et al. (53) used PCR amplification of toxin genes in conjunction with randomly amplified polymorphic DNA (RAPD)-PCR and multiplex RAPD-PCR to trace the source of two outbreaks of food poisoning.

Bacillus cereus is an important ocular pathogen, causing a rapidly progressive endophthalmitis that is refractory to treatment. Cases are, fortunately, infrequent; they usually occur after penetrating trauma of the eye but sometimes follow hematogenous spread or, occasionally, eye surgery. Significant loss of vision, and often loss of the eye itself, can occur within 24 to 48 h (101). *B. cereus* keratitis associated with contact lens wear has also been reported (109). Other *B. cereus* infections occur mainly, though not exclusively, in persons predisposed by neoplastic disease, immunosuppression, alcoholism and other drug abuse (including cases associated with contaminated heroin), the presence of catheters (65) or implants such as fluid shunts, or some other underlying condition such as diabetes, and fatalities occasionally result. Reported conditions include bacteremia, septicemia, fulminant sepsis with hemolysis, meningitis (following allogenic stem cell transplants in two cases) (58), brain hemorrhage, ocular infections including panophthalmitis, ventricular shunt infections, endocarditis (1), pneumonia (47), pseudomembranous tracheobronchitis, exacerbation of bronchiectasis, empyema, pleurisy, peritonitis in a dialysis patient, lung abscess, brain abscess, liver abscess, osteomyelitis, salpingitis, urinary tract infection, and primary cutaneous infections. El Saleeby et al. (42) found an association between tea drinking and invasive *B. cereus* infection in immunocompromised children. Ko et al. (84) reported the emergence of a β-lactam-dependent strain associated with prolonged administration of β-lactams via an indwelling catheter in a neutropenic patient. Strains of *B. cereus* have been isolated in association with periodontitis (63). Wound infections, often of open fractures (38), and mostly in otherwise healthy persons, have been reported following surgery (associated, in one report, with contaminated incontinence pads), road traffic and other accidents, scalds, burns, plaster fixation, drug injection, and close-range gunshot and nail bomb injuries; some became necrotic and gangrenous (32). Fatal neonatal meningitis was caused by a blank firearm injury; blank cartridge propellants are commonly contaminated with the organism. Neonates also appear to be particularly susceptible to *B. cereus*, especially with umbilical stump infections, and cases of meningitis have been associated with the use of catheters and manual ventilation balloons (44). Respiratory tract infections have also been associated with contaminated ventilation systems among neonates and in a pediatric intensive care unit (73). Several cases of *B. cereus* pneumonia in metal workers and welders have been reported, including fatal infections (67). Infection of these metal workers may be related to welding-fume exposure, demonstrated to suppress pulmonary defenses in animal studies. Interestingly, the isolate from one of these cases was found to harbor a plasmid (pBCXO1) that was 99.6% similar to the pXO1 virulence plasmid of *B. anthracis*, while other isolates were also found to harbor either pXO1 virulence genes or both pXO1 and pXO2 virulence genes (67); the role of these pXO1 or pXO2 plasmid genes, if any, in the virulence of these isolates is not known. Additional atypical *B. cereus* strains, originally identified as *B. anthracis* due to the presence of pXO1 and pXO2 plasmids, have also been isolated in association with fatal infections of chimpanzees and a gorilla in Ivory Coast and Cameroon (79, 85). A nosocomial outbreak of *B. cereus* infection related to catheter use was associated with reused towels (35), and a hospital pseudo-outbreak was associated with contaminated ethanol used as a skin disinfectant. *B. cereus* also causes infections in domestic animals. It is a well-recognized agent of mastitis and abortion in cattle, particularly when animals are in winter housing, and can cause these conditions in other livestock.

Strains of *B. thuringiensis* commonly carry genes for *B. cereus* enterotoxins, and assays have demonstrated that enterotoxin production occurs, but the cereulide synthetase gene has not been detected in this species (6, 105). *B. thuringiensis* is well known as an insect pathogen, preparations of certain strains are widely used as biopesticides, and transgenic crop plants that express the insecticidal crystal toxin genes have been developed, but there is as yet no evidence of infections directly associated with the use of this organism as an insecticide. Occupational exposure to the organism has been connected with presence of the organism in feces but without gastrointestinal symptoms. A review of the safety of using *B. thuringiensis* as a biopesticide on crop plants found that the main pesticide strains assayed produced low titers of enterotoxin (13). There have been few reports of gastroenteritis outbreaks in which *B. thuringiensis* was implicated (98, 128). However, cases of such illness caused by *B. thuringiensis* may have been attributed to *B. cereus*, as the former may not produce its characteristic insecticidal toxin crystals when incubated at 37°C, owing to the loss of the plasmids carrying the relevant genes. There have been reports of wound, burn, and ocular infections with *B. thuringiensis*, and in a fatal case of pulmonary disease and bacteremia in a neutropenic patient, there was evidence that membrane-damaging toxins contributed to the infection (54). Experimental *B. thuringiensis* endophthalmitis has been achieved in rabbits (17).

Other Species

Reports of infections with non-*B. cereus* group species are comparatively rare but very diverse, and there have been several hospital pseudoepidemics associated with contaminated blood culture systems. *B. licheniformis* has been reported from prosthetic-valve endocarditis, pacemaker wire infection, ventriculitis following the removal of a meningioma, brain abscesses, septicemia following arteriography, bacteremia associated with indwelling central venous catheters, bacteremia during pregnancy with eclampsia and acute fibrinolysis, peritonitis in patients undergoing continuous ambulatory peritoneal dialysis (CAPD) and in a patient with volvulus and small-bowel perforation, ophthalmitis, and corneal ulcer after trauma. An outbreak of bacteremia among patients with blood malignancies was related to nonsterile cotton wool used during skin disinfection (106). *B. licheniformis* bacteremia has been reported for an immunocompetent man and has twice been reported in association with Munchausen's syndrome: one case followed self-inoculation with organic drain cleaner (61), and in another case following self-inoculation with soil, *B. pumilus* and *Paenibacillus polymyxa* were also isolated (51). *B. licheniformis* can cause foodborne diarrheal illness, and in a case associated with an infant fatality, lichenilysin A, a heat-stable cyclic lipopeptide, has been implicated (99). This organism is frequently associated with bovine abortion and has been shown to have a tropism for the bovine placenta; it has also been associated with abortion in water buffalo and occasionally with bovine mastitis. As with such *B. cereus* infections, these types of *B. licheniformis* infection are associated with wet and dirty conditions during winter housing, particularly when the animals lie in spilled silage, and in one outbreak a water tank contaminated with *B. licheniformis* was implicated.

The name *B. subtilis* was often used in the past for any clinical isolate, but since 1970 there have been reports of infection in which this species appears to have been identified accurately. They include cases of pneumonia, bacteremia, and septicemia associated with neoplastic disease;

breast prosthesis and ventriculo-atrial shunt infections; isolations from surgical wound drainage sites; endocarditis in a drug abuser; meningitis following a head injury; bacteremia associated with trauma; bacteremia in cancer patients; cholangitis associated with kidney and liver disease; and isolation from dermatolymphangioadenitis associated with filarial lymphedema. Two cases of severe hepatotoxicity followed the ingestion of nutritional supplements contaminated with *B. subtilis* (130). Administration of an oral probiotic preparation marketed for the treatment or prevention of intestinal disorders, and allegedly containing *B. subtilis*, led to a fatal septicemia in an immunocompromised patient; subsequently, the organism concerned was identified as *Bacillus clausii* (127). These authors reported another *B. clausii* infection, cholangitis in polycystic kidney disease, in a 15-year-old French boy who had undergone a renal transplant, but the source of the organism was unclear. *B. subtilis* has also been associated with cases of bovine mastitis and ovine abortion. *B. subtilis* has been implicated in foodborne illness: vomiting has been the commonest symptom, but with accompanying diarrhea frequently reported, the onset periods have been short (ranging from 10 min to 14 h; median, 2.5 h), the bacterial loads of the organism were high (10^5 to 10^9 CFU/g), and the implicated foods were often prepared dishes in which meat or fish was served with cereal-based components such as bread, pastry, rice, or stuffing. *Bacillus amyloliquefaciens*, a close relative of *B. subtilis*, is widely used industrially for enzyme and amino acid production, but human consumption of L-tryptophan manufactured in an organism genetically engineered from a strain of this species was associated with a large epidemic of eosinophilia-myalgia syndrome with 37 deaths; the causative agent has not been identified with certainty (100). Environmental strains of this species producing a heat-stable, nonprotein toxin have been isolated in association with building-related health problems (100).

Organisms identified as *B. circulans* have been isolated from cases of bacteremia in cancer patients, meningitis, CSF shunt infections, endocarditis, a wound infection in a cancer patient, a bite wound, endophthalmitis, peritonitis in a patient undergoing CAPD (12), and epidemic endophthalmitis associated with a contaminated product used during cataract surgery. It must be noted, however, that many isolates previously regarded as *B. circulans* might have been wrongly identified (see comments on *B. circulans* below). *B. coagulans* has been isolated from corneal infection, bacteremia, and bovine abortion. *B. pumilus* has been found in cases of cutaneous, pustule, and rectal fistula infections, central venous catheter infection in an immunocompetent child (10), bacteremias in immunosuppressed patients (106), bacteremia in a patient with Munchausen's syndrome (51), and repeated contamination of a blood platelet screening procedure; it has also been found in association with bovine mastitis. Toxigenic strains of *B. pumilus* have been isolated in association with foodborne illness and from clinical and environmental specimens, and a heat-stable cyclic lipopeptide, pumilacidin, was implicated in a rice-associated food poisoning outbreak (50). *Lysinibacillus sphaericus* has been implicated in a fatal lung pseudotumor, bacteremia, and meningitis. *B. megaterium* (eight isolates), *B. pumilus* (six), *Brevibacillus brevis* (five), *B. licheniformis* (two), and *B. subtilis* (one) isolated from chewing tobacco were found to produce potent exogenous virulence factors that caused plasma exudation and tissue dysfunction in an animal model (118). *B. megaterium* caused a delayed-onset lamellar keratitis following laser-assisted eye surgery (114).

Bacillus brevis has been isolated from corneal infection and implicated in several incidents of food poisoning; since those reports, the species was split (see "Taxonomy" above) and transferred to the new genus *Brevibacillus*. Strains of one of the newer species, *Brevibacillus agri*, were isolated in association with an outbreak of waterborne illness in Sweden; *Brevibacillus centrosporus* was isolated from a bronchoalveolar lavage fluid sample, *Brevibacillus parabrevis* was found in a breast abscess, and both species have been isolated from human blood (93). *Brevibacillus laterosporus* has been reported in association with a severe case of endophthalmitis.

Paenibacillus alvei has been isolated from cases of meningitis, endophthalmitis, a prosthetic hip infection in a patient with sickle cell anemia, wound infections, and, in association with *Clostridium perfringens*, a case of gas gangrene. *P. macerans* has been isolated from a wound infection following removal of a malignant melanoma, from a brain abscess following penetrating periorbital injury, from a catheter-associated infection in a leukemic patient, and from bovine abortion, and *P. polymyxa* has been isolated from bacteremia in a patient with cerebral infarction, a bacteremic case of Munchausen's syndrome (51), and ovine abortion. *Paenibacillus popilliae* has been reported from endocarditis, and *Paenibacillus larvae* has been reported from infection of a CSF shunt system.

Single isolations of several new *Bacillus* and *Paenibacillus* species from clinical specimens, but of unknown significance, are mentioned in "Taxonomy" above.

COLLECTION, TRANSPORT, AND STORAGE OF SPECIMENS

Bacillus species normally survive transport in freshly collected specimens or in a standard transport medium. Local transport of specimens (for no longer than a few hours) can be done at room temperature or at 2 to 8°C for most specimens, including serum. Generally, if specimens such as stool, sputum, pleural fluid, blood, and material on swabs are to be shipped overnight or longer, they should be sent at 2 to 8°C, while fresh tissue and serum samples should be shipped frozen. Formalin-fixed tissues can be sent at room temperature primarily for detection using immunohistochemistry and (although they are much less suitable) PCR. For blood specimens with which PCR will be used to detect *B. anthracis* DNA, collection tubes containing EDTA or citrate as an anticoagulant are preferable to those containing heparin.

All the clinically significant isolates reported to date are of species that grow, and often sporulate, on routine laboratory media at 37°C. It seems unlikely that many clinically important but more fastidious strains are being missed for the want of special media or growth conditions. Maintenance is simple if spores can be obtained, but it is a mistake to assume that a primary culture or subculture on blood agar will automatically yield spores if it is stored on the bench or in the incubator. It is best to grow the organism on nutrient agar (or Trypticase soy agar) containing 5 mg/liter manganese sulfate for a few days, and refrigerate when microscopy shows that most cells have sporulated. For most species, sporulated cultures on slants of this medium, sealed after incubation, can survive in a refrigerator for years. Alternatively, cultures (preferably sporulated) can be frozen or lyophilized.

Safety Aspects

Clinical specimens for isolation of *Bacillus* species other than *B. anthracis* can be handled safely on the open bench without special precautions. Efforts should be made to avoid methods that produce aerosols. Any procedures that have the potential to generate aerosols should be done in a microbiological safety cabinet. Biosafety level 2 practices, containment equipment, and facilities are recommended for activities using clinical materials and diagnostic quantities of infectious cultures.

Isolation and presumptive identification of *B. anthracis* can be performed safely in the routine clinical microbiology laboratory, provided that normal good laboratory practice is observed. Preexposure vaccination is not recommended for laboratory personnel doing routine processing of clinical or environmental specimens in general diagnostic laboratories (26); however, biosafety level 3 facilities are recommended for all such work (140). When working with pure cultures of *B. anthracis*, direct and indirect contact of broken skin with cultures and contaminated laboratory surfaces, accidental parenteral inoculation, and, rarely, exposure to infectious aerosols are the primary hazards to laboratory personnel. Laboratories that frequently centrifuge *B. anthracis* suspensions should use an aerosol-tight rotor that can be repeatedly autoclaved (26).

Human infectious doses have not been established for *B. anthracis*; the U.S. Department of Defense estimates that a 50% lethal dose for humans is 8,000 to 10,000 spores, but this is largely based on data from nonhuman primate studies. When collecting clinical specimens for suspected anthrax, appropriate personal protective equipment should be used, such as disposable gloves, disposable apron or overalls, and boots which can be disinfected after use; for dusty samples that might contain many spores, the use of a face shield and/or a respirator should be considered. Full details of personal protective equipment and of disinfection and decontamination are given in Annexes 1 and 3 of the WHO *Anthrax in Humans and Animals* guidelines (140). It should be noted that although hand washing with soap and water or with chlorhexidine gluconate, and the use of hypochlorite-releasing towels, may reduce endospore contamination of the skin, waterless rubs containing ethanol are ineffective at removing endospores. Preexposure vaccination recommendations by Advisory Committee on Immunization Practices (ACIP) for laboratory exposures are addressed in "Vaccination" below.

Bacillus anthracis is defined as a select agent and is included on both the Department of Health and Human Services/CDC and U.S. Department of Agriculture/APHIS select agent lists. Thus, possession of the agent in the United States requires registration of the laboratory with either the CDC or APHIS. When *B. anthracis* is identified by a laboratory, the identification of this agent must be reported to the CDC or APHIS immediately and a APHIS/CDC Form 4 (Report of the Identification of a Select Agent or Toxin) submitted within 7 days. Other authorities should be notified as required by federal, state, or local laws. When *B. anthracis* is isolated in an unregistered laboratory, the organism must either be destroyed on-site by a recognized sterilization or inactivation process or be transferred to a registered laboratory within 7 days. Shipping of this agent requires completion of the APHIS/CDC Form 2 (Request to Transfer Select Agents and Toxins) and prior approval from either the CDC or APHIS (see http://www.cdc.gov/od/sap/final_rule.htm or http://www.selectagents.gov/formsOverview.htm for additional information of select agent regulation in the United States).

Specimens from Patients Suspected To Have Anthrax

In all cases, specimens from possible sources of infection (carcass, hides, hair, bones, etc.) should be sought in addition to patient specimens. Leakproof containers, to be placed in secondary containers for "double-bagging," and then secure, outer containers for carriage are needed. A blood smear may reveal the capsulated rods or, if treatment has started, capsule "ghosts." Postmortem blood collected by venipuncture (a characteristic of anthrax is nonclotting blood at death) should be examined by smear (for capsule) and culture.

Guidelines for clinical evaluation of persons with possible anthrax can be found at http://www.cdc.gov/mmwr/preview/mmwrhtml/mm5043a1.htm.

Cutaneous Anthrax

The edge of an eschar should be lifted and two specimens of vesicular fluid collected (preferably prior to initiation of antimicrobial therapy) by rotating swabs beneath it; one is for a smear for visualizing the capsule, Gram stain, and culture, and the other is for PCR. For immunohistochemical (IHC) analysis of cutaneous lesions, a full-thickness punch biopsy specimen fixed in 10% buffered formalin from a papule or vesicle lesion and including adjacent skin should be taken. Biopsies should also be taken from both vesicle and eschar if present (122).

Inhalation Anthrax

Anthrax will be suspected only if the patient's history suggests it. Chest radiographs and chest computed tomography scans are recommended. In addition to imaging studies, obtain blood cultures prior to antimicrobial therapy. Pleural fluid, if present, should be obtained for Gram stain, culture, and PCR. Serology is also useful for the diagnosis of cases when culture fails owing to previous treatment. Collect acute- and convalescent-phase serum samples 2 to 4 weeks apart for serologic testing. Pleural and/or bronchial biopsy samples can be tested by immunohistochemistry. Postmortem, the approach given for ingestion anthrax should be followed (see below).

Ingestion Anthrax

As with the inhalation form, anthrax is suspected only if an adequate history of the patient is known. Specimens from oral lesions may be collected in the same way as for the cutaneous disease (140). Premortem, obtain blood cultures before antimicrobial therapy. Ascites fluid, if present, should be collected for Gram stain, culture, and PCR. A stool or rectal swab, and material from any oropharyngeal lesions, should also be collected for Gram stain, culture, and PCR. Acute- and convalescent-phase serum samples, with the first obtained within 7 days of onset and the convalescent-phase sample obtained 2 to 3 weeks later, should be collected for serologic testing. Postmortem blood collected by venipuncture should be examined by smear (for observation of capsule) and culture. Any hemorrhagic fluid from the nose, mouth, or anus should be cultured. If these are positive, no further specimens are needed. Again, if negative, specimens of peritoneal or ascitic fluid, spleen, and/or mesenteric lymph nodes, aspirated by techniques avoiding spillage of fluids, may be collected for smear and culture.

Anthrax Meningitis

Collect CSF and blood specimens for cultivation, capsule staining, and PCR; specimens should also be subjected to antigen detection testing, if available.

Specimens from Animals Suspected To Have Died of Anthrax

Although the organism is rapidly destroyed by putrefaction in the intact carcass, the carcass of an animal that died of anthrax still generally yields positive cultures from appropriate specimens, such as blood from a peripheral vein, or from snips of tissue such as from the tip of an ear, as sporulation will still occur in some tissues; however, hemorrhagic exudate is preferred to aspirated blood or tissue specimens for direct demonstration of the capsulated organism using Gram, Giemsa, or polychrome methylene blue (M'Fadyean) staining.

DIRECT EXAMINATION

The first examination of smears and cultures in many clinical laboratories is done with the Gram stain. In the past, it was regarded as of limited value in anthrax diagnosis, because the capsule is not seen. Notwithstanding this, if large numbers of gram-positive bacteria are observed in a patient's blood at death, then *B. anthracis* should be suspected. As in the 2001 bioterrorism incident in the United States, such preparations can be very useful (Fig. 1a). In other circumstances and in animals in particular, the blood or other specimen may not be collected soon after death and before putrefactive organisms appear; *B. anthracis* may then be indistinguishable without the use of the proper capsule stain.

The M'Fadyean polychrome methylene blue staining test dates from 1903 and has proved a remarkably successful rapid diagnostic test over the decades. Satisfactory polychrome methylene blue is now hard to obtain, but the slow, natural ripening process that produces it may be hastened by adding 1% K_2CO_3 to Loeffler's alkaline methylene blue. For putrefied specimens, Giemsa-type stains may be better. For more information on capsule staining, see reference 140.

In addition to culturing *B. anthracis*, there are molecular and antigen-based detection methods available for direct detection in clinical and environmental samples. These detection methods may provide additional information. Several methods, including a *B. anthracis*-specific Laboratory Response Network (LRN) PCR assay, IHC assays, and serology, were useful for confirmation of cases during the 2001 bioterrorism-associated outbreak and more recent cases associated with drum making using *B. anthracis*-contaminated hides (23, 66, 112, 113, 122).

The IHC assay, as performed at the CDC, uses the same antibodies as the direct fluorescent-antibody (DFA) assay (specific to cell wall antigen or the capsule) to detect *B. anthracis* in formalin-fixed, paraffin-embedded tissues. This method was particularly useful in the diagnosis of cutaneous cases during the 2001 bioterrorism-associated outbreak. Skin biopsy samples from cutaneous lesions from 8 of 10 patients were positive for both the capsule and cell wall antigens (122). The most widely used and available detection

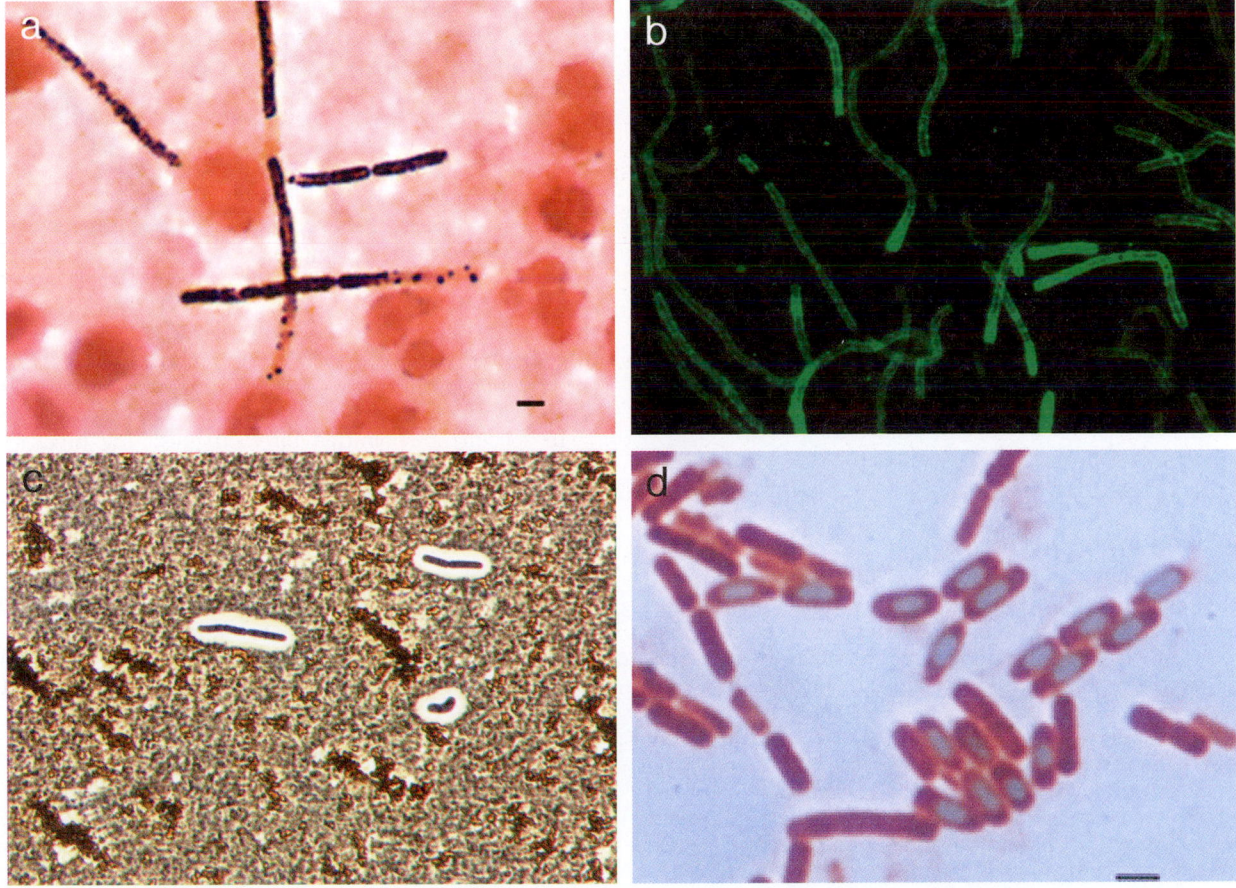

FIGURE 1 (a) Gram stain of *B. anthracis*, associated with a bioterrorism attack, showing gram-positive rods in peripheral blood buffy coat following admission of patient; bar marker represents 3 μm. (Courtesy of H. Masur.) (b) DFA-stained preparation of *B. anthracis* using an antibody specific for the poly-γ-D-glutamic acid capsule. (c) India ink stain of *B. anthracis* incubated in horse blood. Clear zones surrounding the rods are due to the exclusion of the India ink by the capsule. (d) Spore-stained preparation of *Bacillus cereus* sporangia, viewed by bright-field microscopy. Spores are stained green, and vegetative cells are counterstained red. Bar marker represents 2 μm. (Photograph kindly provided by M. Rodríguez-Díaz.)

method in the U.S. public health system is the LRN PCR (66). In addition to being widely used in 2001, this assay and the IHC assay were used in 2007 to diagnose two cutaneous anthrax cases in a drum maker and his child (23).

At the CDC, a positive PCR result on any clinical specimen from a patient collected from a normally sterile site (such as blood or CSF) or a lesion of other affected tissue (skin, pulmonary, reticuloendothelial, or gastrointestinal) is regarded as a supportive or presumptive diagnostic test. It is considered sufficient to provide a probable diagnosis but is not confirmatory in itself. The principal reason for such stringent guidelines on the use of PCR approaches and the value of their results towards providing a confirmatory diagnosis is based on the possibility that environmental contamination of a non-anthrax-related lesion could result in a positive result; this is especially the case with the use of some previously published PCR primers for capsule and chromosomal genes that can produce false positives with reactions to soil microbiota. This is quite similar to the recommendations that are included in the 2008 WHO guidelines (140), in which PCR can be used for identification of an isolate but is not recommended for testing of specimens.

There are numerous reports on the use of alternative technologies for the detection of *B. anthracis*, such as mass spectrometry, flow cytometry, time-resolved fluorescent assays, high-performance liquid chromatography, and even the use of engineered B cells to detect *B. anthracis* (5, 69, 115, 149, 152). Two recent studies focused on detecting the anthrax toxins, which are highly expressed during infection, in specimens instead of directly detecting the bacilli (15, 133). One reported on an immunoassay using highly fluorescent europium nanoparticles to detect protective antigen (PA), while the other reported detection of lethal factor (LF) by taking advantage of its metalloprotease activity, which cleaves specific peptides. The LF protein was captured by monoclonal antibodies and then incubated with a synthetic peptide substrate whose cleavage products were detected by matrix-assisted laser desorption ionization–time of flight (MALDI-TOF) mass spectrometry (15). These and other novel approaches may allow for detection of *B. anthracis* infection earlier in the course of the disease and thus allow for more successful treatment.

ISOLATION

Isolation from Human Specimens

Fresh specimens from patients should be inoculated onto plates of blood agar in the normal way. Enrichment procedures are generally inappropriate for isolations from clinical specimens. However, when seeking *B. cereus* in stools several days after a food poisoning episode, nutrient or tryptic soy broth with polymyxin (100,000 U/liter) may be added to a heat-treated specimen. Heat treatments at 70°C for 30 min or 80°C for 10 min are widely used for aerobic endospore formers in general, but 62 to 65°C for 15 to 20 min is more suitable for *B. anthracis*; temperatures above 70°C are not recommended for this species (142). There is no effective enrichment method for *B. anthracis* in old animal specimens or environmental samples, and isolation from these is best attempted using polymyxin-lysozyme EDTA-thallous acetate (PLET) agar (80; see also chapter 17). Aliquots (0.1 ml) of the undiluted suspension and 1:10 and 1:100 dilutions of a heat-treated suspension of the specimen are spread across PLET plates, which are read after incubation for 36 to 40 h at 37°C. Creamy white, domed, circular colonies, 1 to 3 mm, are subcultured onto (i) blood agar plates to

test for gamma phage and for hemolysis and (ii) directly or subsequently in blood to look for capsule production using either the M'Fadyean stain or India ink negative stain (the latter is less reliable, because the ink coagulates the blood and makes interpretation difficult); 2.5 ml of blood (preferably defibrinated horse blood, but horse or fetal calf serum is satisfactory) is inoculated with a pinhead quantity of growth from the suspect colony, incubated statically for 6 to 18 h at 37°C, and then stained. A differential/selective chromogenic medium is marketed by R&F Laboratories, Downers Grove, IL (R&F *Anthracis* chromogenic agar), and it has undergone some independent evaluation (72), but another study (97) found PLET to be more sensitive and selective.

Several media have been designed for the isolation, identification, and enumeration of *B. cereus* organisms. They exploit the organism's egg yolk reaction (phospholipase C) positivity and acid-from-mannitol negativity; pyruvate and polymyxin may be included for selectivity. Three satisfactory formulations are MEYP or MYP (mannitol, egg yolk, polymyxin B agar; MEYP, Oxoid, Basingstoke, United Kingdom; MYP, Difco, BD, Franklin Lakes, NJ), PEMBA (polymyxin B, egg yolk, mannitol, bromthymol blue agar; Oxoid), and BCM (*Bacillus cereus* medium; LabM, Bury, United Kingdom) (see chapter 17). There are more recent formulations that reveal phospholipase C positivity using specific chromogenic substrates rather than natural egg yolk: *Bacillus cereus* group plating medium (Biosynth Chemistry and Biology, Staad, Switzerland, also available as Cereus-Ident-Agar from Heipha, Eppelheim, Germany) and *Bacillus cereus/Bacillus thuringiensis* chromogenic plating medium (R&F Laboratories).

There are no selective media for other *Bacillus* species, but spores can be selected for by heat treating part of the specimen as described above; however, this is not appropriate for fresh clinical specimens, where spores are usually sparse or absent. Vegetative cells of both sporeformers and non-sporeformers are killed by heat treatment, but the heat-resistant spores not only survive but also may be heat shocked into subsequent germination; another part of the specimen is cultivated without heat treatment in case spores are very heat sensitive or absent.

In specimens submitted for food poisoning investigations, or for isolation of *B. anthracis* from old carcasses, animal products, or environmental specimens, the organisms will mostly be present as spores. Heat treatment, as described above, will both heat shock the spores and effectively destroy non-spore-forming contaminants. A variety of approaches are used to process dry or solid samples prior to heat treatment. Direct plate cultures are then made on blood, nutrient, or selective agars, as appropriate, by spreading up to 0.1-ml volumes from undiluted sample and 10- and 100-fold dilutions of the treated sample.

Isolation from Animals Suspected To Have Died of Anthrax

Anthrax should be considered as the possible cause of death in herbivorous animals that have died suddenly and unexpectedly, especially if hemorrhage from the nose, mouth, or anus has occurred, and if death has taken place at a site with a history of anthrax—perhaps even several decades before. PCR-based approaches are becoming more widely used for direct detection of *B. anthracis* in veterinary specimens.

Carcasses 1 to 2 Days Old

Due to the nonclotting nature of blood in animals that have died of anthrax infection, it is usually possible to aspirate a few drops of blood from a peripheral vein for (i) a M'Fadyean-stained smear and (ii) direct plate culture on blood agar.

In pigs, the enormous terminal bacteremia seen in herbivores may not develop, and the capsulated rods may not be visible in blood smears. When cervical edema is present, smears and cultures should be made of fluid aspirated from the enlarged mandibular and suprapharyngeal lymph nodes. Intestinal anthrax of pigs may be obvious only at necropsy, when rods are usually visible in stained smears made from mesenteric lymph nodes.

Older Putrefying Carcasses

The organism may not be visible in smears 2 to 3 days following death, as it competes poorly with putrefactive organisms; culture is then necessary for diagnostic confirmation. Sections of tissue, or any blood-stained material, should be collected, and spleen or lymph node specimens should be taken if the animal has been opened. With putrefied and very old carcasses, swabs of the nostrils, nasal turbinates, and eye sockets are likely to yield *B. anthracis*, but the best specimens may be samples of contaminated soil taken from beneath the head and tail.

Isolation of *B. anthracis* from Bioterrorism-Related Specimens

In 1999, an LRN was established in the United States by the CDC in partnership with the Association of Public Health Laboratories, Federal Bureau of Investigation, and Department of Defense to provide the public health laboratory response to acts of bioterrorism (103). This network links local (sentinel) laboratories to laboratories with more specialized testing and increased biosafety capacity at the state (reference) and federal (national) levels. There are reference level laboratories in all 50 states able to detect agents, including *B. anthracis*, rapidly. State public health laboratories are part of the LRN and are able to provide guidance, or the LRN can be accessed using the Internet (http://www.bt.cdc.gov/lrn/). If unable to reach the state public health laboratory during nonbusiness hours, LRN consultations may be requested by calling the CDC Emergency Operations Center at 770-488-7100. State and territorial public health laboratory contact information and sentinel laboratory guidelines are also available on the American Society for Microbiology website at http://www.asm.org. For general questions there is a 24-h hotline number, 800-CDC-INFO (800-232-4636), and an e-mail address, cdcinfo@cdc.gov. Although initially limited to the United States, there are now over 150 national and international locations, including laboratories within Canada, Australia, Germany (U.S. military base), Japan (U.S. military base), South Korea (U.S. military base), and the United Kingdom, capable of providing a rapid response to acts of biological terrorism, emerging infectious diseases, and other public health threats and emergencies.

Isolation of *B. anthracis* from Environmental and Animal Product Specimens

Tests for the presence of *B. anthracis* may be requested for diverse specimens, such as animal products (e.g., wool, hides, hair, and bonemeal) from regions of endemicity, soil or other materials from old burial sites or tannery or laboratory sites due for redevelopment, or other environmental materials associated with outbreaks (e.g., sewage sludge). Detection in such specimens may mean searching for rather few spores of *B. anthracis* among those of many other species,

especially other members of the *B. cereus* group. Some environmental specimens may contain substances that inhibit germination and growth of *B. anthracis* (140). At present, there is no enrichment method for *B. anthracis*, and culture by the selective agar techniques described above is the best approach. PCR-based methods are being used increasingly for the direct detection of *B. anthracis* in clinical and environmental samples (125), but it is still advisable to confirm positive results by conventional methods.

IDENTIFICATION

Remember that these organisms do not always stain gram positive; some are gram variable, gram positivity is readily lost in older cultures, and some species or strains are frankly gram negative. Before attempting to identify to the species level, it is important to establish that the isolate really is an aerobic endospore former and that other inclusions are not being mistaken for spores. Phase contrast (at a magnification of ×1,000) should be used if available, as it is superior to spore staining and more convenient. Spores are larger, more phase bright, and more regular in shape, size, and position than other kinds of inclusions such as polyhydroxybutyrate (PHB) granules (Fig. 2d), and sporangial appearance is valuable in identification (Fig. 2). For spore staining, flood a heat-fixed smear with 10% aqueous malachite green for up to 45 min (without heating), followed by washing and counterstaining with 0.5% aqueous safranin for 30 s; spores are green within pink-red cells at a magnification of ×1,000 (Fig. 1d). A Gram-stained smear showing cells with unstained areas suggestive of spores can be stripped of oil with acetone-alcohol, washed, and then stained for spores.

Isolates have often been submitted to reference laboratories as *Bacillus* species because they were large, aerobic gram-positive rods, even though sporulation had not been observed, or because PHB granules or other storage inclusions had been mistaken for spores. Members of the *B. cereus* group and *B. megaterium* produce large amounts of storage material when grown on carbohydrate media, but on routine media this vacuolate or foamy appearance is rarely sufficiently pronounced to cause confusion.

Bacillus and related genera contain facultative anaerobes as well as strict aerobes, which can be a valuable characteristic in identification. For example, *B. licheniformis* and *B. subtilis*, which have very similar colonial (Fig. 3j) and microscopic (Fig. 2e) morphologies, are facultatively anaerobic and strictly aerobic, respectively. Likewise, the two large-celled species *B. cereus* and *B. megaterium* (Fig. 2b and d) are facultatively anaerobic and strictly aerobic, respectively.

The most widely used diagnostic schemes use traditional phenotypic tests, or miniaturized tests of the API 20E and 50CHB kits used together (90) (bioMérieux, Marcy l'Etoile, France). The API 20E and 50CHB kits can be used for the presumptive distinction of *B. anthracis* from other members of the *B. cereus* group within 48 h. bioMérieux also offers identification cards for *Bacillus* and related genera for the VITEK and VITEK Compact automated identification systems. As many new species have been proposed since these schemes were established, updated API and VITEK databases have been prepared. Biolog Inc. (Hayward, CA) also offers a *Bacillus* database. The effectiveness of such kits can vary with the genera and species of aerobic endospore formers concerned, but they are improving with continuing development and enlarged databases. The many proposals for new species, often on the basis of single isolates, make the satisfactory expansion of such databases problematic; for a database to be

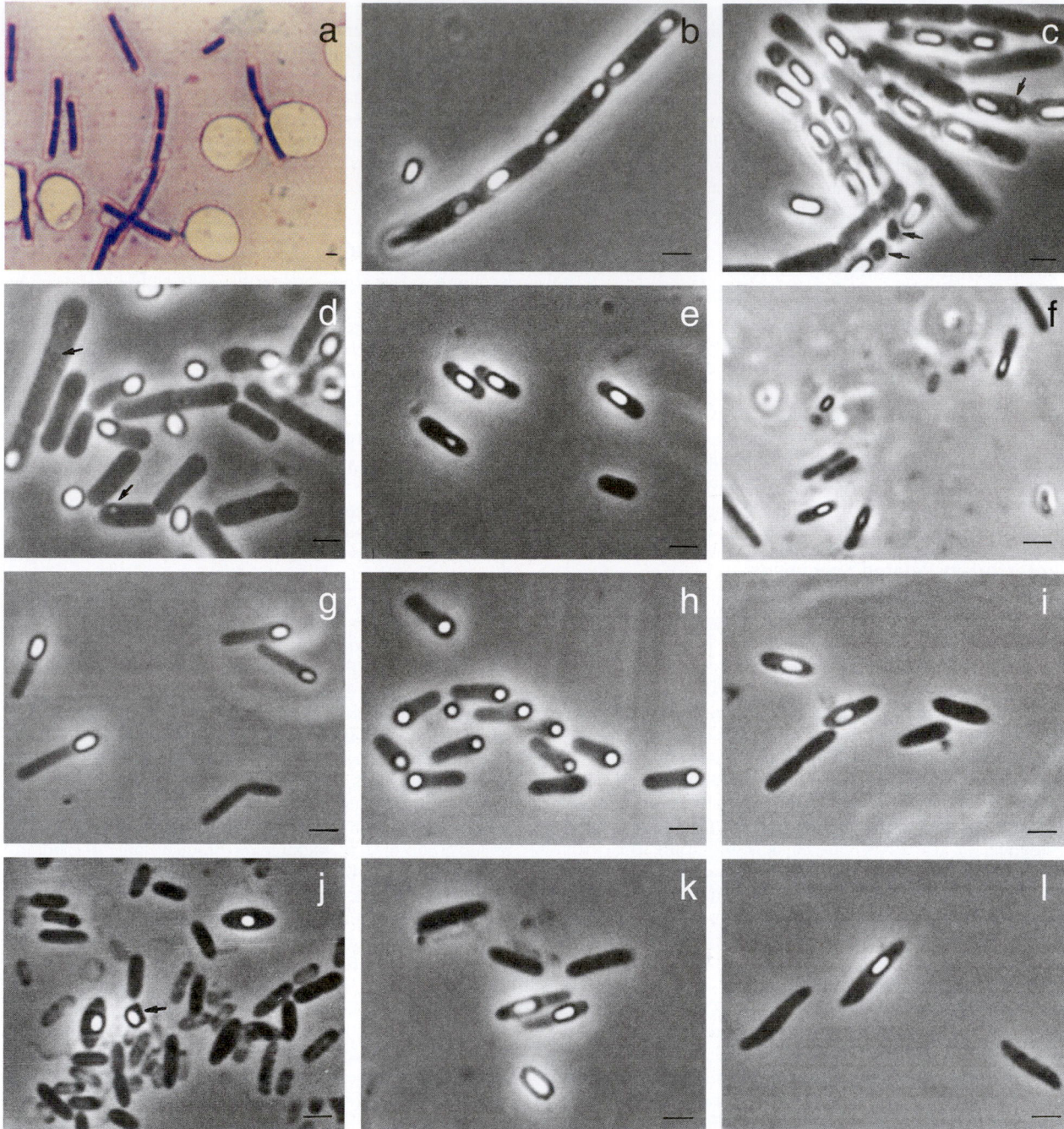

FIGURE 2 Photomicrographs of endospore-forming bacteria viewed by bright-field microscopy (a) and phase-contrast microscopy (b to l). Bar markers represent 2 μm. (a) *B. anthracis*, M'Fadyean stain showing capsulate rods in guinea pig blood smear; (b) *B. cereus*, broad cells with ellipsoidal, subterminal spores, not swelling the sporangia; (c) *B. thuringiensis*, broad cells with ellipsoidal, subterminal spores, not swelling the sporangia, and showing parasporal crystals of insecticidal toxin (arrows); (d) *B. megaterium*, broad cells with ellipsoidal and spherical, subterminal and terminal spores, not swelling the sporangia, and showing PHB inclusions (arrows); (e) *B. subtilis*, ellipsoidal, central and subterminal spores, not swelling the sporangia; (f) *B. pumilus*, slender cells with cylindrical, subterminal spores, not swelling the sporangia; (g) *B. circulans*, ellipsoidal, subterminal spores, swelling the sporangia; (h) *Lysinibacillus sphaericus*, spherical, terminal spores, swelling the sporangia; (i) *Brevibacillus brevis*, ellipsoidal, subterminal spores, one swelling its sporangium slightly; (j) *Brevibacillus laterosporus*, ellipsoidal, central spores with thickened rims on one side (arrow), swelling the sporangia; (k) *Paenibacillus polymyxa*, ellipsoidal, paracentral to subterminal spores, swelling the sporangia slightly; (l) *Paenibacillus alvei*, cells with tapered ends, ellipsoidal, paracentral to subterminal spores, not swelling the sporangium.

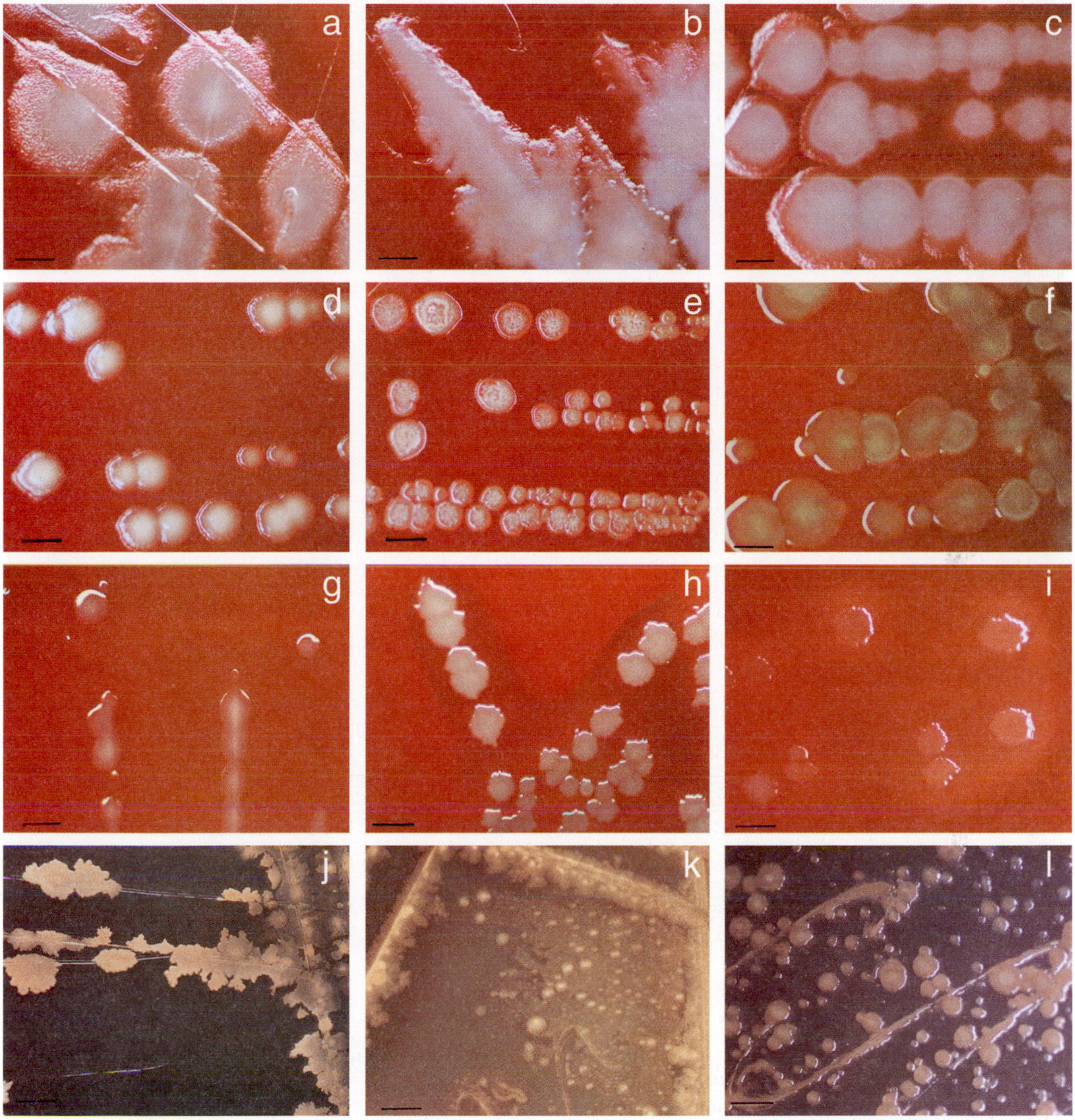

FIGURE 3   Colonies of endospore-forming bacteria on blood agar (a to i) and nutrient agar (j to l) after 24 to 36 h at 37°C. Bar markers represent 2 mm. (a) *B. anthracis;* (b) *B. cereus;* (c) *B. thuringiensis;* (d) *B. megaterium;* (e) *B. pumilus;* (f) *Lysinibacillus sphaericus;* (g) *Brevibacillus brevis;* (h) *Brevibacillus laterosporus;* (i) *Paenibacillus polymyxa;* (j) *B. subtilis;* (k) *B. circulans;* (l) *Paenibacillus alvei.*

effective in identifying a particular species, its entry for that species needs to reflect the characterization of at least 10 authentic strains from a range of sources, but this requirement can be very difficult, even impossible, to fulfill. It is stressed that the use of these kits should always be preceded by the basic characterization tests described below.

Other approaches include chemotaxonomic fingerprinting by fatty acid methyl ester profiling, pyrolysis mass spectrometry, and Fourier transform infrared spectroscopy. All these approaches have been successfully applied either across the genera or to small groups. As with genotypic profiling

methods, large databases of authentic strains are necessary; some of these are commercially available, such as the Microbial Identification System software (Microbial ID Inc., Newark, DE) database for fatty acid methyl ester analysis.

For diagnostic purposes, the aerobic endospore formers comprise two groups: the reactive ones, which give positive results in various routine biochemical tests and which are therefore easier to identify, and the nonreactive ones, which give few, if any, positive results in such tests. Nonreactive isolates tend to dominate the identification requests sent to reference laboratories. Table 1 shows reactions for some

TABLE 1 Characters for differentiating some species of *Bacillus*, *Geobacillus*, *Paenibacillus*, and *Virgibacillus*[a]

Character[b]	Bacillus								B. megaterium
	B. subtilis group				B. cereus group				
	B. subtilis	B. amyloliquefaciens	B. licheniformis	B. pumilus	B. cereus[c]	B. anthracis	B. thuringiensis	B. mycoides	
Rod mean diam. (μm)	0.8	0.8	0.8	0.7	1.2	1.2	1.2	1.2	1.4
Chains of cells	(−)	(+)	(+)	−	+	+	+	+	+
Motility	+	+	+	+	+	−	+	−	+
Sporangia[d]									
Spore shape	E	E	E (C)	C, E	E (C) [E]	E	E (C)	E	E, S
Spore position	S, C	S, C	S, C	S, C	S, C	S	S	S (C)	S, C
Sporangium swollen	−	−	−	−	−	−	−	−	−
Parasporal crystals	−	−	−	−	−	−	+	−	−
Anaerobic growth	−	−	+	−	+	+	+	+	
Growth at:									
50°C	v	v	+	v	−	−	−	−	v
65°C	−	−	−	−	−	−	−	−	−
Egg yolk reaction	−	−	−	−	+	+	+	+	−
Casein hydrolysis	+	+	+	+	+	+	+	+	+
Starch hydrolysis	+	+	+		+	+	+	+	+
Arginine dihydrolase	−	−	(+)	−	v [(−)]	−	+	v	−
Indole production	−	−	−	−	−				
Gelatin hydrolysis	+	+	+	+	+	+	+	+	+
Nitrate reduction	+	+	+	−	(+) [+]	+	+	(+)	v
Gas from carbohydrates	−	−	−	−	−	−	−	−	−
Acid from:									
D-Arabinose	−	−	−	−	−	−	−	−	−
Glycerol	+	+	+	+	+ [v]	−	+	+	+
Glycogen	+	+	+	−	+ [−]	+	+	+	+
Inulin	(+)	−	v	−	−	−	−	−	+
Mannitol	+	+	+	+	−	−	−	−	+
Salicin	+	+	+	+	+ [−]	−	(+)	(+)	+
D-Trehalose	+	+	+	+	+	+	+	+	+

[a] Symbols and abbreviations: +, ≥85% positive; +/w, positive or weakly positive; w, weakly positive; (+), 75 to 84% positive; v, variable (26 to 74% positive); (−), 16 to 25% positive; −, 0 to 15% positive; −/w, negative or weakly positive.

[b] Arginine dihydrolase, indole production, gelatin hydrolysis, and nitrate reduction reactions was determined using tests in the API 20E strip (bioMérieux). Acid from carbohydrate reactions was determined using the API 50CHB System (bioMérieux).

species belonging to the former group, and the phenotypic test scheme outlined above may be used in conjunction with it.

Identification and Detection of *B. anthracis*

It is generally easy to distinguish virulent *B. anthracis* from other members of the *B. cereus* group. *B. anthracis* isolates are characterized by typical microscopic appearance (Fig. 1b and 2a) and colonial morphology (Fig. 3a): colonies are white or gray, nonhemolytic or only weakly hemolytic, susceptible to the diagnostic gamma phage (inquiries about gamma phage should be addressed to the Diagnostics Systems Division, USAMRIID, Fort Detrick, Frederick, MD), generally susceptible to penicillin, nonmotile, and able to produce the characteristic capsule as shown by M'Fadyean staining (Fig. 2a) or India ink staining (Fig. 1b). As an alternative to culture in blood, the capsule of virulent *B. anthracis* can be demonstrated on nutrient agar containing 0.7% sodium bicarbonate, incubated overnight under 5 to 7% CO$_2$ (candle jars perform well). Colonies of the capsulated organism appear mucoid, and the capsule can be visualized by M'Fadyean or India ink staining of smears or by DFA staining (Fig. 1c; see below).

In addition to phenotypic analysis, molecular and antigenic detection assays are available for the rapid identification of *B. anthracis*. The LRN PCR (restricted to LRN laboratories; see above) targets three distinct loci on the *B. anthracis* chromosome, pXO1 virulence plasmid, and pXO2 virulence plasmid. Using several loci increases specificity and allows for the detection of avirulent strains (lacking pXO1 or pXO2). The anthrax toxin genes (*pagA*, *lef*, and *cya*) are located on pXO1, while the genes required for capsule biosynthesis (*capBCA*) are located on pXO2. Isolates lacking pXO2 or both plasmids are mostly found in the environment and are frequently mistaken for *B. cereus*, due to the lack of a capsule, and discarded. These genes have been widely used as *B. anthracis*-specific gene targets; however, there have been recent reports of these genes in species other than *B. anthracis* (8, 55, 67). Recently several laboratories have developed specific PCR assays for *B. anthracis* that target chromosomal genes such as *rpoB*, *gyrA*, and *plcR* (39, 70, 111).

A two-component DFA assay has been and is currently used to identify encapsulated vegetative cells of *B. anthracis* (33, 45). This assay uses two different monoclonal

| *Bacillus* | | | | *Geobacillus* | | *Paenibacillus* | | | | *Virgibacillus pantothenticus* |
| B. circulans group | | | | | | | | | | |
B. circulans	B. firmus	B. lentus	B. coagulans	G. stearothermophilus	G. thermodenitrificans	P. polymyxa	P. alvei	P. macerans	P. validus	
0.8	0.8	0.8	0.8	0.9	0.8	0.9	0.8	0.7	0.8	0.6
−	(+)	(+)	v	v	v	−	(−)	−	−	+
+	+	+	+	+	+	+	+	+	+	+
E S, T	E (C) S, C	E S, C	E (S) S, C, T	E S, T	E S, T	E S (C)	E S, C	E S (T)	E S, T	E, S T (S)
+	v	v	+	v	−	+	+	+	+	+
−	−	−	−	−	−	−	−	−	−	−
+	+	−	+	−/w	+	+	+	+	−	+
+	v	−	+	+	+	−	−	v	+	v
−	−	−	−	+	+	−	−	−	−	−
−	−	−	−	−	−	−	−	−	−	−
w	w	−	−	+/w	−	+	+	−	−	+
+	+	+	+	+	+/w	+	+	+	+	+
−	−	−	v	−	−	−	−	−	−	(−)
−	−	−	−	−	−	−	+	−	−	−
v	+	−	v	+	v	+	+	v	−	+
v	+	+	v	v	v	+	−	v	v	v
−	−	−	−	−	−	−	−	+	−	+
+	v	−	+	w	−	+	+	+	+	+
+	v	−	−	+	−	+	v	+	v	−
+	−	−	−	v	−	+	−	+	v	−
+	+	+/w	−	−	w	+	−	+	+	−
+	−	+/w	v	−	v	+	v	+	−	+
+	v	+	+	+	+	+	v	+	+	+

^{c} Reactions shown in brackets are for the biotype isolated particularly in connection with outbreaks of emetic-type food poisoning and for strains of serovars 1, 3, 5, and 8, which are commonly associated with such outbreaks.

^{d} Spore shape: C, cylindrical; E, ellipsoidal; S, spherical. Spore position: C, central or paracentral; S, subterminal; T, terminal. The commonest shapes and positions are listed first, and those shown in parentheses are infrequently observed.

antibodies specific for a *B. anthracis* cell wall antigen and the *B. anthracis* capsule (Fig. 1c). Neither antigen is 100% specific for *B. anthracis*; however, only *B. anthracis* has been found to be positive for both antigens, and thus, the assay is 100% specific when both cell wall and capsule components are used together. It was heavily used at the CDC during the 2001 bioterrorism-associated outbreak for the rapid (<4-h) identification of isolates (33).

Tetracore Inc. (Gaithersburg, MD) has produced a rapid (yielding a result within 15 min) immunochromatographic test (RedLine Alert) utilizing an antibody specific for one of the *B. anthracis* S-layer proteins. This assay has been approved by the Food and Drug Administration (FDA) for use on nonhemolytic *Bacillus* species colonies cultured on sheep blood agar plates. Manufacturer's data suggest that the test was 98.6% sensitive when tested on 145 *B. anthracis* isolates and 45 nonhemolytic, non-*B. anthracis* isolates; however, such identification of *B. anthracis* is only considered presumptive, and this test should not be used as a stand-alone test.

An immunochromatographic field assay has been developed by the U.S. Naval Medical Research Center (NMRC),

Silver Spring, MD, to detect PA in samples of blood or tissue exudates (*Bacillus anthracis* immunochromatographic field assay). Inquiries from veterinary and public health authorities should be directed to the NMRC by calling 301-319-7409 or in writing to the Naval Medical Research Center, 503 Robert Grant Ave., Silver Spring, MD 20910 (J. Czarnecki, NMRC, personal communication, 2007). The assay has been used to detect *B. anthracis* in animals, even several days after death. The assay has a high sensitivity for the detection of *B. anthracis* in an infected animal and has a high specificity (regarded as 100%; 95% confidence interval, 98.5 to 100%) for detection of the organism in cattle (104). Among 10 recently vaccinated bovines in one study, the assay yielded no false-positive reactions.

Identification of *Bacillus cereus* and *B. thuringiensis*

Colonies of *B. cereus* and relatives are very variable but readily recognized (Fig. 3a to c): they are characteristically large (2 to 7 mm in diameter) and vary in shape from circular to irregular, with entire to undulate, crenate or fimbriate edges; they have matte or granular textures. Smooth and moist colonies are not uncommon, however.

The optimum growth temperature is about 37°C, with minima and maxima of 15 to 20°C and 40 to 45°C, respectively. Although colonies of *B. anthracis* and *B. cereus* can be similar in appearance, those of the former are generally smaller and nonhemolytic, may show more spiking or tailing along the lines of inoculation streaks, and are very tenacious compared with the usually more butyrous consistency of *B. cereus* and *B. thuringiensis* colonies, so that they may be pulled into standing peaks with a loop. *Bacillus mycoides* produces characteristic rhizoid or hairy-looking, adherent colonies which readily cover the whole agar surface.

The key characteristics for recognizing and distinguishing the *B. cereus* group are colonial morphology (Fig. 3a to c); large cells often in chains, producing ellipsoidal spores not swelling the sporangia (Fig. 2b and c), usually within 48 h and often apparent after 24 h; facultative anaerobes; and positive egg yolk reaction (i.e., lecithinase). Negative or very weak hemolysis and lack of motility distinguish *B. anthracis* and *B. mycoides* from *B. cereus* and *B. thuringiensis*. *Bacillus cereus*, *B. mycoides*, *B. thuringiensis*, and, to a lesser extent, *B. anthracis* synthesize lecithinases, forming opaque zones of precipitation around colonies on egg yolk agar as the colonies grow (i.e., usually after overnight or perhaps 24 h of incubation). Recognition of *B. thuringiensis* is largely dependent on observation of its cuboid or diamond-shaped parasporal crystals in sporulated cultures (after 2 to 5 days) by phase-contrast microscopy (Fig. 2c), or by staining with malachite green counterstained with carbol fuchsin or safranin.

Toxin Detection

The enterotoxin complex responsible for the diarrheal type of *B. cereus* food poisoning has been increasingly well characterized (128). Two commercial kits are available for its detection in foods and feces, the Oxoid BCET-RPLA (Oxoid Ltd.) and the TECRA VIA (TECRA Diagnostics, Roseville, New South Wales, Australia). However, these kits detect different antigens, and there is some controversy about their reliabilities. Other assays, based on tissue culture, have also been developed. The emetic toxin of *B. cereus*, cereulide, has been identified as a dodecadepsipeptide, and it may be nonspecifically assayed in food extracts or culture filtrates using HEp-2 cells (46), boar semen (4), and rat mitochondria (75). Specific detection requires high-performance liquid chromatography-mass spectrometry (59), and the synthetic apparatus may be detected by real-time PCR (49).

Other Species

Other species show a very wide range of colonial morphologies, both within and between species after 24 to 48 h (Fig. 3). They vary from moist and glossy (Fig. 3f and i) through granular to wrinkled (Fig. 3e); shape varies from round to irregular (Fig. 3d to i), sometimes spreading (Fig. 3k and l), with entire through undulate or crenate to fimbriate edges (Fig. 3d to j). Sizes range from 1 to 5 mm; color commonly ranges from buff or creamy gray to off-white, but some strains may produce orange pigment. Hemolysis may be absent, slight or marked, partial, or complete (Fig. 3h); elevations range from effuse through raised to convex. Consistency is usually butyrous, but mucoid and dry, adherent colonies are not uncommon. Despite this diversity, *Bacillus* colonies are not generally difficult to recognize, and some species have characteristic yet seemingly infinitely variable colonial morphologies, as does the *B. cereus* group (Fig. 3a to c).

Bacillus subtilis and *B. licheniformis* produce similar colonies which are exceptionally variable in appearance and often appear to be mixed cultures (Fig. 3j); colonies are irregular in shape and of moderate (2 to 4 mm) diameter and range from moist and butyrous or mucoid, with margins varying from undulate to fimbriate through membranous with an underlying mucoid matrix, with or without mucoid beading at the surface, to rough and crusty as they dry. The "licheniform" colonies of *B. licheniformis* tend to be quite adherent.

Rotating and migrating microcolonies, which may show spreading growth (Fig. 3k), have been observed macroscopically in about 13% of strains received as *B. circulans*, but this very heterogeneous species continues to undergo radical taxonomic revision, and such spreading strains are now assigned to *Paenibacillus* species (Fig. 3l).

Other species that have been encountered in the clinical laboratory include *B. coagulans*, *B. megaterium*, *B. pumilus*, and *B. sphaericus*; *B. brevis* and *B. laterosporus* (now both in *Brevibacillus*); and *B. macerans* and *B. polymyxa* (now both in *Paenibacillus*), and they do not produce particularly distinctive growth (Fig. 3d to i).

Microscopic morphologies, particularly of sporangia (Fig. 2), are much more helpful for distinguishing between species. Vegetative cells are usually round ended, but those of *P. alvei* may be tapered (Fig. 2l). The large cells of *B. megaterium* may accumulate PHB (Fig. 2d) and appear vacuolate or foamy when grown on glucose nutrient agar. Overall, cell widths vary from about 0.5 to 1.5 mm and lengths from 1.5 to 8 mm. Most strains of these species are motile. Spore shapes vary from cylindrical (Fig. 2f) through ellipsoidal (Fig. 2b, c to e, g, and i to l) to spherical (Fig. 2d and h); bean- or kidney-shaped, curved-cylindrical, and pear-shaped spores are also seen occasionally. Spores may be terminally (Fig. 2h), subterminally (Fig. 2b, c, f, g, and i), or centrally (Fig. 2e and j) positioned within sporangia and may distend them (Fig. 2g and k). Despite within-species and within-strain variation, sporangial morphologies tend to be characteristic of species and may allow tentative identification by the experienced worker. One species, *Brevibacillus laterosporus*, produces very distinctive ellipsoidal spores that have thickened rims on one side, so that they appear to be laterally displaced in the sporangia (Fig. 2j).

All these species are mesophilic and grow well between 30 and 37°C. Minimum growth temperatures lie mostly between 5 and 20°C and maxima mostly between 35 and 50°C. Strains of *B. coagulans* may show slight thermophily and grow up to 55 to 60°C.

TYPING SYSTEMS

Genotyping of *B. anthracis*

B. anthracis is a genetically monomorphic species and has been shown to be clonal by multilocus sequence typing (MLST). The first method described that could differentiate strains with any useful resolution was a multiple-locus variable-number tandem-repeat analysis (MLVA) assay targeting eight loci, MLVA-8 (76). This method was relied on during the 2001 bioterrorism-associated outbreak in the United States, which implicated the Ames strain, and continues to be useful today (76, 132). There are now multiple MLVA schemes available for the genotyping of *B. anthracis*, including expanded versions of the original MLVA-8. These include schemes which employ agarose electrophoresis, capillary electrophoresis, or mass spectrometry for fragment analysis (76, 87, 89, 143). An online database, MLVAbank, is also now available at http://minisatellites.u-psud.fr/MLVAnet/, which can accept data entry for 25 variable-number tandem repeats. There are also several reports on the analysis of single nucleotide repeats to differentiate very closely related isolates (77, 78, 87, 89, 131).

The sequencing of multiple *B. anthracis* genomes has also led to additional approaches to the genotyping of *B. anthracis*, such as the use of single nucleotide polymorphisms and DNA microarrays. Single nucleotide polymorphisms have been identified and used for the differentiation of *B. anthracis* lineages and for detection of specific strains such as the Ames strain (144, 145). This approach may continue to become more powerful as more genome data become available and are analyzed. Microarrays have also been used for strain characterization and comparisons (36, 153). However, they have not been widely used and seem to be less attractive now that newer de novo sequencing technologies have become more affordable and allow for the rapid generation of complete or almost complete genome sequence data. As technologies continue to improve and the costs decrease, the complete genomic sequence will increasingly be used for isolate characterization.

Genotyping of Other Species

The majority of work on molecular typing (i.e., genotyping) of *Bacillus* spp. has focused on members of the *B. cereus* group due to their clinical importance and the value of genotyping for molecular epidemiology. In the past, this group was differentiated into serovars based on flagellar antigen variations; however, this is not commonly used today and has largely been replaced by molecular methods. Numerous molecular methods have been attempted to some degree for the differentiation of *Bacillus* isolates. Recently, MLST, which compares the partial sequences of seven housekeeping genes to differentiate strains, has become the favored approach due to decreasing costs, portability of data, and availability of public databases on the World Wide Web. Several MLST schemes targeting different sets of genes have been reported and generally show similar clusters of isolates into three distinct clades (64, 81, 110, 126, 136). Pathogenic isolates are distributed throughout clades 1 and 2, while no clinical isolates have been identified as belonging in clade 3 (34, 68). With the exception of *B. anthracis* and emetic isolates of *B. cereus*, which are largely clonal, *B. cereus* group isolates are represented by a large number of distinct sequence types, and clustering does not correlate with classic microbiological species identification. Simpson's index of diversity (measure of the likelihood of two isolates from epidemiologically distinct events having the same sequence type) was calculated to be 0.989 (1.0 is absolute discrimination) in one study of clinical isolates, which suggests that in addition to being a powerful phylogenetic tool, it may be useful for molecular epidemiology (68). The most powerful aspect of MLST is the availability of online databases for several of the MLST schemes, which allows for worldwide access to view and deposit isolate data. The Priest scheme is available at http://pubmlst.org/bcereus/, and an optimized version of the Tourasse scheme, including a multischeme database (SuperCAT), is available at http://mlstoslo.uio.no/ (110, 136, 137).

SEROLOGIC TESTS

Serologic assays for the detection of antibody response against the anthrax toxin protein, PA, have been used in combination with PCR or IHC assay results to confirm anthrax cases when culture failed. A quantitative human anti-PA immunoglobulin G (IgG) enzyme-linked immunosorbent assay was performed at the CDC during the 2001 outbreak and was positive only with sera from individuals with anthrax or vaccinated with anthrax vaccine adsorbed (AVA; see "Vaccines" below) (112). An FDA-approved, qualitative kit (QuickELISA Anthrax-PA kit) from Immunetics (Boston, MA) is not currently available, but production could be initiated if needed for the detection of anti-PA IgG and IgM antibodies in human serum. Serologic assays aided in the effort to confirm cases in the 2001 attack, particularly cutaneous ones; however, the time to seroconversion after infection limits the usefulness of this approach, given the rapid diagnosis necessary for treatment and public health response.

The three protein components of anthrax toxin (PA, LF, and edema factor [EF]), and antibodies to them, can be used in enzyme immunoassay systems. For routine confirmation of anthrax infection or for monitoring response to anthrax vaccines, antibodies against PA alone appear to be satisfactory; they have proved useful for epidemiological investigations with humans and animals. In human anthrax, however, early treatment sometimes prevents development of a detectable rise in antibody titer (113). PA, LF, and EF are available commercially from List Biological Laboratories, Inc., Campbell, CA (http://www.listlabs.com).

In countries of the former USSR, a skin test utilizing anthraxin, a heat-stable extract from a noncapsulate strain of *B. anthracis* that has been licensed for human and animal use since 1962, is widely acclaimed for retrospective diagnosis (123). The delayed-type hypersensitivity is interpreted as indicating cell-mediated immunity to anthrax and can be used to evaluate the vaccine-induced immune status after periods of several years, as well as to diagnose anthrax retrospectively. Anthraxin does not contain highly specific anthrax antigens and relies on the fact that the only *Bacillus* species likely to proliferate within and throughout an animal is *B. anthracis*. This is also true of the Ascoli test, which, dating from 1911, must be one of the oldest antigen detection tests in microbiology. It is a precipitin test using hyperimmune serum raised to *B. anthracis* whole-cell antigen to provide rapid retrospective evidence of anthrax infection in an animal from which the material being tested was derived. The test is still in use in Eastern Europe and central Asia.

ANTIMICROBIAL SUSCEPTIBILITIES

Bacillus anthracis

Most strains of *B. anthracis* remain susceptible to penicillin (30, 102, 141). Of 25 genetically diverse isolates from around the world, three strains were resistant to penicillin but were negative for β-lactamase production. Most strains give variable susceptibility results for cephalosporins; in vitro results, even if susceptible, may not predict clinical efficacy, particularly for expanded- and broad-spectrum cephalosporins (30). In a study of 50 historical isolates from humans and animals and 15 clinical isolates from the 2001 bioterrorism attack in the United States, the majority of strains could be regarded as not susceptible to the broad-spectrum cephalosporin ceftriaxone, and 3 were resistant to penicillin (102). Tetracyclines, fluoroquinolones, and chloramphenicol are suitable for the treatment of patients allergic to penicillin; most strains in the previously mentioned study showed only intermediate susceptibility to erythromycin (102). Ciprofloxacin and the newer quinolone gatifloxacin had good in vitro activities against 40 Turkish isolates, but for another new quinolone, levofloxacin, it was observed that MICs were high for 10 strains (43). Other in vitro studies have shown novel fluoroquinolones and a ketolide to be of potential therapeutic value (37, 48). Standards for antimicrobial susceptibility testing of *B. anthracis* have been recently adopted (28), and a DNA microarray for detecting antimicrobial resistance determinants in *B. anthracis* and *B. cereus* has been developed (7).

Postexposure prophylaxis (PEP) is needed for the prevention of inhalation anthrax following exposure to aerosols containing *B. anthracis* spores; the recommended regimen is 60 days of antimicrobial therapy and three doses of AVA (17), and recommended antimicrobial agents include ciprofloxacin, doxycycline, and levofloxacin. PEP was, for example, recommended for four persons who had been in the unventilated work space during procedures that generated aerosols from untreated animal hides used for making drums. Amoxicillin is recommended as an option in cases where the *B. anthracis* strain has been demonstrated to be susceptible to penicillins, and when other antimicrobial agents are not considered safe, as in the treatment of children and pregnant or lactating women (20, 21). The use of penicillins for PEP or for treatment of inhalation anthrax following the use of *B. anthracis* as a bioweapon gives cause for concern, owing to the presence of β-lactamases in *B. anthracis* isolates and the poor penetration of β-lactams into macrophages, the site of spore germination (9). Combination intravenous antimicrobial therapy with two or more antimicrobial agents, begun early, such as with ciprofloxacin and one or more other antimicrobial agents to which the organism is sensitive, appeared to improve survival rates during treatment of cases in the 2001 event in the United States (71). Following that event, the recommendation for initial treatment of inhalation anthrax is intravenous ciprofloxacin or doxycycline along with one or more agents to which the organism is normally susceptible (19); ciprofloxacin is favored over doxycycline as the primary antimicrobial agent due to its bactericidal action and central nervous system penetration in the event of meningeal involvement (129). A mouse aerosol challenge model has been developed for determining antimicrobial agent efficacy in the treatment of inhalation anthrax (62). In a case of inhalation anthrax that was naturally acquired when processing untreated animal hides for drum construction, the patient's therapy included adjunctive use of human anthrax immunoglobulin (147); however, the use of anthrax immunoglobulin in the treatment of a subsequent inhalation anthrax case in 2008 did not prevent a fatal outcome (3).

Bacillus cereus

There have been rather few studies of the antimicrobial susceptibility of *Bacillus cereus*, and most information has to be gleaned from reports of individual cases or outbreaks. *Bacillus cereus* and *B. thuringiensis* produce a broad-spectrum β-lactamase and are thus resistant to aminopenicillins and cephalosporins; they are also resistant to trimethoprim. An in vitro study of 54 isolates from blood cultures by disk diffusion assay found that all strains were susceptible to imipenem and vancomycin and that most were sensitive to chloramphenicol, ciprofloxacin, erythromycin, and gentamicin (but a small number of strains showed moderate or intermediate susceptibility), while 22 and 37% of strains showed only moderate or intermediate susceptibilities to clindamycin and tetracycline, respectively (148). Although strains are almost always susceptible to clindamycin, erythromycin, chloramphenicol, vancomycin, and the aminoglycosides, and are usually sensitive to tetracycline and sulfonamides, there have been several reports of treatment failures with some of these drugs: a fulminant meningitis which did not respond to chloramphenicol (96); a fulminant infection in a neonate which was refractory to treatment that included vancomycin, gentamicin, imipenem, clindamycin, and ciprofloxacin (139); failure of vancomycin to eliminate the organism from CSF in association with a fluid shunt infection (11); vancomycin resistance in strains from respiratory specimens from pediatric intensive care patients (73); and persistent bacteremias with strains showing resistance to vancomycin in two hemodialysis patients (A. von Gottberg and W. van Nierop, personal communication). Oral ciprofloxacin has been used successfully in the treatment of *B. cereus* wound infections, bacteremia, and pulmonary infection, and in vitro activity has been shown for daptomycin (27). Clindamycin with gentamicin, given early, appears to be the best treatment for ophthalmic infections caused by *B. cereus*, and experiments with rabbits suggest that intravitreal corticosteroids and antimicrobials may be effective in such cases. CLSI document M45-A (29) tabulates antimicrobial breakpoints for aerobic, endospore-forming species.

Other Species

Information is sparse on treatment of infections with other species. Gentamicin was effective in treating a case of *B. licheniformis* ophthalmitis, vancomycin was successful in cases of *B. licheniformis* peritonitis in a CAPD patient (107) and a pacemaker wire infection, meropenem succeeded in a case of brain abscess, and cephalozin was effective against *B. licheniformis* prosthetic aortic valve endocarditis. Resistance to macrolides appears to occur naturally in *B. licheniformis*. *B. subtilis* endocarditis in a drug abuser was successfully treated with a cephalosporin, and gentamicin was successful against *B. subtilis* septicemia. A *B. pumilus* central venous catheter infection treated with several drugs, including flucloxacillin, clindamycin, and vancomycin, failed to clear, and the catheter had to be replaced with a new one (10). Two cases of cutaneous infections with *B. pumilus* initially diagnosed as anthrax were treated successfully with amoxicillin-clavulanate, while a third such case was treated with ciprofloxacin (134). Daptomycin and ciprofloxacin show in vitro activity against strains of *B. pumilus*, *B. subtilis*, and some other species (27). Penicillin, or its derivatives, or cephalosporins probably have long been the first choices for treatment of infections attributed to other *Bacillus* species. However, in a study by Weber et al. (148), over 95% of isolates of *B. megaterium*, *B. pumilus*, *B. subtilis*, *B. circulans*, *B. amyloliquefaciens*, and *B. licheniformis*, along with strains of *B. (now Paenibacillus) polymyxa* and three unidentified strains from blood cultures, were susceptible to imipenem, ciprofloxacin, and vancomycin, and only between 75 and 90% were susceptible to penicillins, cephalosporins, and chloramphenicol. Isolates of "*B. polymyxa*" and *B. circulans* were more likely to be resistant to the penicillins and cephalosporins than strains of the other species—it is probable that some or all of the strains identified as *B. circulans* might now be accommodated in *Paenibacillus*, along with "*B. polymyxa*." An infection of a human bite wound with an organism identified as *B. circulans* did not respond to treatment with amoxicillin and flucloxacillin but was resolved with clindamycin, while peritonitis in a CAPD patient was resolved with vancomycin. However, a strain identified as *B. circulans* and showing vancomycin resistance has been isolated from an Italian clinical specimen (88). Vancomycin resistance has been reported for *P. popilliae*, a biopesticide, and isolates of this species have been shown to carry genes resembling those responsible for high-level vancomycin resistance in enterococci (108). Of two South African vancomycin-resistant clinical isolates, one was identified as *Paenibacillus thiaminolyticus* and the other was unidentified but considered to be related to *Bacillus lentus*. The latter was isolated from a case of neonatal sepsis and has been shown to have inducible resistance to vancomycin and teicoplanin; this is in contrast to the *B. circulans* and *P. thiaminolyticus* isolates mentioned above, in which expression of resistance was found to be constitutive (von Gottberg and van Nierop, personal communication).

VACCINATION

AVA, the current human vaccine in the United States, is a cell-free filtrate (formalin treated), in an aluminum hydroxide-adsorbed gel, from a noncapsulated, nonproteolytic derivative of strain V770-NP1_R grown under microaerobic conditions. The FDA has approved a new route and schedule for preexposure immunization with AVA, which calls for a series of five intramuscular injections administered at 0 and 4 weeks and at 6, 12, and 18 months (95). To maintain immunity, an annual booster injection is recommended. Anthrax vaccine precipitated, the current human vaccine in the United Kingdom, is an alum-precipitated cell-free filtrate of Sterne strain (34F2) cultured, under static batch conditions, with activated charcoal to increase PA production. Both anthrax vaccine precipitated (150) and AVA contain PA as well as trace amounts of LF, EF, and cell wall proteins. In October 2008 the ACIP voted to accept provisional recommendations for the pre-event use of anthrax vaccine among persons considered to be at risk for exposure to aerosolized *B. anthracis* spores; these provisional recommendations included new language to address emergency responders, in addition to the previously approved recommended occupational and laboratory populations. The ACIP recommends routine preexposure vaccination with AVA for persons engaged in work involving (i) production of high concentrations or pure cultures of *B. anthracis* spores, (ii) activities with a high potential for production of aerosolized spores, (iii) handling of environmental samples associated with anthrax investigations (especially powders) and performance of confirmatory testing for *B. anthracis* in the U.S. LRN for bioterrorism level B laboratories or above, (iv) making repeated entries into known *B. anthracis* spore-contaminated areas or settings in which repeated exposure to aerosolized *B. anthracis* spores might occur, and (v) engaging in environmental investigations or remediation efforts of spore-contaminated areas or other settings with aerosol exposure. Immunization is not routinely recommended for emergency and other responders but may be offered on a voluntary basis as part of a comprehensive occupational health and safety program. Laboratory workers using standard biosafety level 2 practices in the routine processing of clinical or environmental specimens in general diagnostic laboratories are not at increased risk for exposure to *B. anthracis* spores (22, 25). The development of anthrax vaccines, including second- and third-generation products, and that of several human monoclonal and polyclonal antibody products currently in their early development and testing phases are the subjects of recent reviews (120, 138).

EVALUATION, INTERPRETATION, AND REPORTING OF RESULTS

While, of course, the isolation of *B. anthracis* is always significant and requires urgent reporting, the majority of other aerobic endospore-forming species are environmental organisms, and so they are frequent laboratory contaminants. Therefore, isolation from a single clinical specimen is generally not a sufficient basis for incriminating one of these organisms as the etiological agent; however, any such organism should be considered of potential clinical significance if it is isolated in pure culture or at least apparently dominating the microbiota, or if it is isolated in large numbers or isolated more than once. Opportunistic infections with *Bacillus* species other than *B. anthracis* have been reported since the late 19th century, and in the last 30 years the clinical importance of aerobic endospore formers (most, but not all, of them *Bacillus* species) has become widely accepted. It is most important to assess any clinical isolation of such an organism in the light of any other species cultured and the clinical context and to be wary of dismissing it as a mere contaminant. Moderate or heavy growth of aerobic endospore formers from wounds is usually significant, and *B. cereus* infections of the eye are serious emergencies that should always be reported to the physician immediately.

Low-level contamination of foodstuffs by aerobic endospore formers is commonplace, as is asymptomatic transient fecal carriage. Therefore, in foodborne illness investigations, qualitative isolation tests are insufficient. The ideal criteria for establishing that an aerobic endospore former is the etiological agent are (i) isolation of significant numbers ($>10^5$ CFU/g) of the organism from the epidemiologically incriminated food (and, in the case of suspected *B. cereus* food poisoning, detection of emetic toxin and/or enterotoxin) and (ii) recovery of the same strain (biovar, plasmid type, etc.) in significant numbers from acute-phase specimens (feces or vomitus) from the patients but not from healthy controls.

REFERENCES

1. Abusin, S., A. Bhimaraj, and S. Khadra. 2008. *Bacillus cereus* endocarditis in a permanent pacemaker: a case report. *Cases J.* 1:95.
2. Ahmed, I., A. Yokota, A. Yamazoe, and T. Fujiwara. 2007. Proposal of *Lysinibacillus boronitolerans* gen. nov. sp. nov., and transfer of *Bacillus fusiformis* to *Lysinibacillus fusiformis* comb. nov. and *Bacillus sphaericus* to *Lysinibacillus sphaericus* comb. nov. *Int. J. Syst. Evol. Microbiol.* 57:1117–1125.
3. Anaraki, S., S. Addiman, G. Nixon, D. Krahé, R. Ghosh, T. Brooks, G. Lloyd, R. Spencer, A. Walsh, B. McCloskey, and N. Lightfoot. 2008. Investigations and control measures following a case of inhalation anthrax in East London in a drum maker and drummer, October 2008. *Eurosurveillance* 13:1–3.
4. Andersson, M. A., R. Mikkola, J. Helin, M. C. Andersson, and M. Salkinoja-Salonen. 1998. A novel sensitive bioassay for detection of *Bacillus cereus* emetic toxin and related depsipeptide ionophores. *Appl. Environ. Microbiol.* 64:1338–1343.
5. Andreotti, P. E., G. V. Ludwig, A. H. Peruski, J. J. Tuite, S. S. Morse, and L. F. Peruski. 2003. Immunoassay of infectious agents. *BioTechniques* 35:850–859.
6. Ankolekar, C., T. Rahmati, and R. G. Labbe. 2009. Detection of toxigenic *Bacillus cereus* and *Bacillus thuringiensis* spores in U.S. rice. *Int. J. Food Microbiol.* 128:460–466.
7. Antwerpen, M. H., M. Schellhase, E. Ehrentreich-Förster, F. Bier, W. Witte, and U. Nübel. 2007. DNA microarray for detection of antimicrobial resistance determinants in *Bacillus anthracis* and closely related *Bacillus cereus*. *Mol. Cell. Probes* 21:152–160.
8. Bell, C. A., J. R. Uhl, T. L. Hadfield, J. C. David, R. F. Meyer, T. F. Smith, and F. R. Cockerill. 2002. Detection of

Bacillus anthracis DNA by LightCycler PCR. *J. Clin. Microbiol.* **40:**2897–2902.

9. **Bell, D. M., S. Blank, P. E. Kozarsky, and D. S. Stephens.** 2002. Clinical issues in the prophylaxis, diagnosis, and treatment of anthrax. *Emerg. Infect. Dis.* **8:**222–225.

10. **Bentur, H. N., A. M. Dalzell, and F. A. I. Riordan.** 2007. Central venous catheter infection with *Bacillus pumilus* in an immunocompetent child: a case report. *Ann. Clin. Microbiol. Antimicrobials* **6:**12.

11. **Berne, R., F. Heinen, K. Pelz, V. van Velthoven, M. Sauer, and R. Korinthenberg.** 1997. Ventricular shunt infection and meningitis due to *Bacillus cereus. Neuropediatrics* **28:**333–334.

12. **Berry, N. I. Hassan, S. Majumdar, A. Vardhan, A. McEwen, and R. Gokal.** 2004. *Bacillus circulans* peritonitis in a patient treated with CAPD. *Peritoneal Dial. Int.* **24:**488–489.

13. **Bishop, A. H.** 2002. *Bacillus thuringiensis* insecticides, p. 160–175. *In* R. C. W. Berkeley, M. Heyndrickx, N. A. Logan, and P. De Vos (ed.), *Applications and Systematics of Bacillus and Relatives.* Blackwell Science, Oxford, United Kingdom.

14. **Bosshard, P. P., R. Zbinden, and M. Altwegg.** 2002. *Paenibacillus turicensis* sp. nov., a novel bacterium harbouring heterogeneities between 16S rRNA genes. *Int. J. Syst. Evol. Microbiol.* **52:**2241–2249.

15. **Boyer, A. E., C. P. Quinn, A. R. Woolfitt, J. L. Pirkle, L. G. McWilliams, K. L. Stamey, D. A. Bagarozzi, J. C. Hart, Jr., and J. R. Barr.** 2007. Detection and quantification of anthrax lethal factor in serum by mass spectrometry. *Anal. Chem.* **79:**8463–8470.

16. **Brachman, P., and A. Kaufmann.** 1998. Anthrax, p. 95–107. *In* A.Evans and P. Brachman (ed.), *Bacterial Infections of Humans.* Plenum Medical Book Company, New York, NY.

17. **Callegan, M. C., S. T. Kane, D. C. Cochran, B. Novosad, M. S. Gilmore, M. Gominet, and D. Lereclus.** 2005. *Bacillus* endophthalmitis: roles of bacterial toxins and motility during infection. *Investig. Ophthalmol. Vis. Sci.* **46:**3233–3238.

18. **Cardazzo, B., E. Negrisolo, L. Carraro, L. Alberghini, T. Patarnello, and V. Giaccone.** 2008. Multiple-locus sequence typing and analysis of toxin genes in *Bacillus cereus* food-borne isolates. *Appl. Environ. Microbiol.* **74:**850–860.

19. **Centers for Disease Control and Prevention.** 2001. Update: investigation of bioterrorism-related anthrax and interim guidelines for exposure management and antimicrobial therapy. *MMWR Morb. Mortal. Wkly. Rep.* **50:**909.

20. **Centers for Disease Control and Prevention.** 2001. Updated recommendations for antimicrobial prophylaxis among asymptomatic pregnant women after exposure to *Bacillus anthracis. MMWR Morb. Mortal. Wkly. Rep.* **50:**960.

21. **Centers for Disease Control and Prevention.** 2001. Interim recommendations for antimicrobial prophylaxis for children and breastfeeding mothers and treatment of children with anthrax. *MMWR Morb. Mortal. Wkly. Rep.* **50:**1014–1016.

22. **Centers for Disease Control and Prevention.** 2002. Notice to readers: use of anthrax vaccine in response to terrorism: supplemental recommendations of the Advisory Committee on Immunization Practices. *MMWR Morb. Mortal. Wkly. Rep.* **51:**1024–1026.

23. **Centers for Disease Control and Prevention.** 2008. Cutaneous anthrax associated with drum making using goat hides from West Africa—Connecticut, 2007. *MMWR Morb. Mortal. Wkly. Rep.* **57:**628–631.

24. **Centers for Disease Control and Prevention.** 2009. Surveillance for foodborne disease outbreaks—United States, 2006. *MMWR Morb. Mortal. Wkly. Rep.* **58:**609–615.

25. **Centers for Disease Control and Prevention.** 2009. *Advisory Committee on Immunization Practices (ACIP) Provisional Recommendations for Use of Anthrax Vaccine Adsorbed.* Centers for Disease Control and Prevention, Atlanta, GA. http://www.cdc.gov/vaccines/recs/provisional/downloads/anthrax-vax-oct2009-508.pdf.

26. **Centers for Disease Control and Prevention and National Institutes of Health.** 2007. *Biosafety in Microbiological and Biomedical Laboratories,* 5th ed. U.S. Government Printing Office, Washington, DC.

27. **Citron, D. M., and M. D. Appleman.** 2006. In vitro activities of daptomycin, ciprofloxacin, and other antimicrobial agents against the cells and spores of clinical isolates of *Bacillus* species. *J. Clin. Microbiol.* **44:**3814–3818.

28. **Clinical and Laboratory Standards Institute.** 2005. *Performance Standards for Antimicrobial Susceptibility Testing: 15th Informational Supplement.* CLSI document M100-S15. Clinical and Laboratory Standards Institute, Wayne, PA.

29. **Clinical and Laboratory Standards Institute.** 2006. *Methods for Antimicrobial Dilution and Disk Susceptibility Testing of Infrequently Isolated or Fastidious Bacteria.* CLSI/NCCLS Approved Guideline M45-A. Clinical and Laboratory Standards Institute, Wayne, PA.

30. **Coker, P. R., K. L. Smith, and M. E. Hugh-Jones.** 2002. Antimicrobial susceptibilities of diverse *Bacillus anthracis* isolates. *Antimicrob. Agents Chemother.* **46:**3843–3845.

31. **Cote, C. K., T. L. DiMezzo, D. J. Banks, B. France, K. A. Bradley, and S. L. Welkos.** 2008. Early interactions between fully virulent *Bacillus anthracis* and macrophages that influence the balance between spore clearance and development of a lethal infection. *Microb. Infect. Inst. Pasteur* **10:**613–619.

32. **Darbar, A., I. A. Harris, and I. B. Gosbell.** 2005. Necrotizing infection due to *Bacillus cereus* mimicking gas gangrene following penetrating trauma. *J. Orthop. Trauma* **19:**353–355.

33. **De, B. K., S. L. Bragg, G. N. Sanden, K. E. Wilson, L. A. Diem, C. K. Marston, A. R. Hoffmaster, G. A. Barnett, R. S. Weyant, T. G. Abshire, J. W. Ezzell, and T. Popovic.** 2002. Two-component direct fluorescent-antibody assay for rapid identification of *Bacillus anthracis. Emerg. Infect. Dis.* **8:**1060–1065.

34. **Didelot, X., M. Barker, D. Falush, and F. G. Priest.** 2009. Evolution of pathogenicity in the *Bacillus cereus* group. *Syst. Appl. Microbiol.* **32:**81–90.

35. **Dohmae, S., T. Okubo, W. Higuchi, T. Takano, H. Isobe, T. Baranovich, S. Kobayashi, M. Uchiyama, Y. Tanabe, M. Itoh, and T. Yamamoto.** 2008. *Bacillus cereus* nosocomial infection from reused towels in Japan. *J. Hosp. Infect.* **69:**361–367.

36. **Doran, M., D. S. Raicu, J. D. Furst, R. Settimi, M. Schipma, and D. P. Chandler.** 2007. Oligonucleotide microarray identification of *Bacillus anthracis* strains using support vector machines. *Bioinformatics* **23:**487–492.

37. **Drago, L., E., De Vecchi, A. Lombardi, L. Incola, M. Valli, and M. R. Gismondo.** 2002. Bactericidal activity of levofloxacin, gatifloxacin, penicillin, meropenem and rokitamycin against *Bacillus anthracis* clinical isolates. *J. Antimicrob. Chemother.* **50:**1059–1063.

38. **Dubouix, A., E. Bonnet, M. Alvarez, H. Bensafi, M. Archambaud, B. Chaminade, G. Chabanon, and N. Marty.** 2005. *Bacillus cereus* infections in traumatology-orthopaedics department: retrospective investigation and improvement of healthcare practices. *J. Infect.* **50:**22–30.

39. **Easterday, W. R., M. N. Van Ert, S. Zanecki, and P. Keim.** 2005. Specific detection of *Bacillus anthracis* using a TaqMan mismatch amplification mutation assay. *BioTechniques* **38:**731–735.

40. **Editorial team.** 2006. Probable human anthrax death in Scotland. *Eurosurveillance* **11:**pii=3025.

41. **Ehling-Schulz, M., M. Fricker, H. Grallert, P. Rieck, M. Wagner, and S. Scherer.** 2006. Cereulide synthetase gene cluster from emetic *Bacillus cereus*: structure and location on a mega virulence plasmid related to *Bacillus anthracis* toxin plasmid pXO1. *BMC Microbiol.* **6:**20.

42. **El Saleeby, C. M., S. C. Howard, R. T. Hayden, and J. A. McCullers.** 2004. Association between tea ingestion and invasive *Bacillus cereus* infection among children with cancer. *Clin. Infect. Dis.* **39:**1536–1539.

43. **Esel, D., M. Doganay, and B. Sumerkan.** 2003. Antimicrobial susceptibilities of 40 isolates of *Bacillus anthracis* isolated in Turkey. *Int. J. Antimicrob. Agents* **22:**70–72.

44. **Evreux, F., B. Delaporte, N. Leret, C. Buffet-Janvresse, and A. Morel.** 2007. A case of fatal neonatal *Bacillus cereus* meningitis. *Arch. Pediatr.* **14:**365–368. (In French.)

45. **Ezzell, J. W., Jr., T. G. Abshire, S. F. Little, B. C. Lidgerding, and C. Brown.** 1990. Identification of *Bacillus anthracis* by using monoclonal antibody to cell wall galactose-*N*-acetylglucosamine polysaccharide. *J. Clin. Microbiol.* **28:**223–231.

46. **Finlay, W. J. J., N. A. Logan, and A. D. Sutherland.** 1999. Semiautomated metabolic staining assay for *Bacillus cereus* emetic toxin. *Appl. Environ. Microbiol.* **65:**1811–1812.

47. **Frankard, J., R. Li, F. Taccone, M. J. Struelens, F. Jacobs, and A. Kentos.** 2004. *Bacillus cereus* pneumonia in a patient with acute lymphoblastic leukemia. *Eur. J. Clin. Microbiol. Infect. Dis.* **23:**725–728.

48. **Frean, J., K. P. Klugman, L. Arntzen, and S. Bukofzer.** 2003. Susceptibility of *Bacillus anthracis* to eleven antimicrobial agents including novel fluoroquinolones and a ketolide. *J. Antimicrob. Chemother.* **52:**297–299.

49. **Fricker, M., U. Messelhäusser, U. Busch, S. Scherer, and M. Ehling-Schulz.** 2007. Diagnostic real-time PCR assays for the detection of emetic *Bacillus cereus* strains in foods and recent food-borne outbreaks. *Appl. Environ. Microbiol.* **73:**1892–1898.

50. **From, C., V. Hormazabal, and P. E. Granum.** 2007. Food poisoning associated with pumilacidin-producing *Bacillus pumilus* in rice. *Int. J. Food Microbiol.* **115:**319–324.

51. **Galanos, J., S. Perera, H. Smith, D. O'Neal, H. Sheorey, and M. J. Waters.** 2003. Bacteremia due to three *Bacillus* species in a case of Munchausen's syndrome. *J. Clin. Microbiol.* **41:**2247–2248.

52. **Gerberding, J. L., J. M. Hughes, and J. P. Koplan.** 2002. Bioterrorism preparedness and response: clinicians and public health agencies as essential partners. *JAMA* **287:**898–900.

53. **Ghelardi, E., F. Celandroni, S. Salvetti, C. Barsotti, A. Baggiani, and S. Senesi.** 2002. Identification and characterization of toxigenic *Bacillus cereus* isolates responsible for two food-poisoning outbreaks. *FEMS Microbiol. Lett.* **208:**129–134.

54. **Ghelardi, E., F. Celandroni, S. Salvetti, E. Fiscarelli, and S. Senesi.** 2007. *Bacillus thuringiensis* pulmonary infection: critical role for bacterial membrane-damaging toxins and host neutrophils. *Microbes Infect.* **9:**591–598.

55. **Gill, S. R., D. E. Fouts, G. L. Archer, E. F. Mongodin, R. T. Deboy, J. Ravel, I. T. Paulsen, J. F. Kolonay, L. Brinkac, M. Beanan, R. J. Dodson, S. C. Daugherty, R. Madupu, S. V. Angiuoli, A. S. Durkin, D. H. Haft, J. Vamathevan, H. Khouri, T. Utterback, C. Lee, G. Dimitrov, L. Jiang, H. Qin, J. Weidman, K. Tran, K. Kang, I. R. Hance, K. E. Nelson, and C. M. Fraser.** 2005. Insights on evolution of virulence and resistance from the complete genome analysis of an early methicillin-resistant *Staphylococcus aureus* strain and a biofilm-producing methicillin-resistant *Staphylococcus epidermidis* strain. *J. Bacteriol.* **187:**2426–2438.

56. **Glazunova, O. O., D. Raoult, and V. Roux.** 2006. *Bacillus massiliensis* sp. nov., isolated from cerebrospinal fluid. *Int. J. Syst. Evol. Microbiol.* **56:**1485–1488.

57. **Gürcan, S., F. Akata, F. Kuloğlu, S. Erdoğan, and M. Tuğrul.** 2005. Meningitis due to *Bacillus anthracis*. *Yonsei Med. J.* **46:**159–160.

58. **Haase, R., H. Sauer, U. Dagwadordsch, J. Foell, and U. Lieser.** 2005. Successful treatment of *Bacillus cereus* meningitis following allogenic stem cell transplantation. *Pediatr. Transplant.* **9:**338–341.

59. **Häggblom, M. M., C. Apetroaie, M. A. Andersson, and M. S. Salkinoja-Salonen.** 2002. Quantitative analysis of cereulide, the emetic toxin of *Bacillus cereus*, produced under various conditions. *Appl. Environ. Microbiol.* **68:**2479–2483.

60. **Hahn, B. L., S. Sharma, and P. G. Sohnle.** 2005. Analysis of epidermal entry in experimental cutaneous *Bacillus anthracis* infections in mice. *J. Lab. Clin. Med.* **146:**95–102.

61. **Hannah, W., and P. T. Ender.** 1999. Persistent *Bacillus licheniformis* bacteraemia associated with an intentional injection of organic drain cleaner. *Clin. Infect. Dis.* **29:**659–661.

62. **Heine, H. S., J. Bassett, L. Miller, J. M. Hartings, B. E. Ivins, M. L. Pitt, D. Fritz, S. L. Norris, and W. R. Byrne.** 2007. Determination of antibiotic efficacy against *Bacillus anthracis* in a mouse aerosol challenge model. *Antimicrob. Agents Chemother.* **51:**1373–1379.

63. **Helgason, E., D. A. Caugant, I. Olsen, and A.-B. Kolstø.** 2000. Genetic structure of population of *Bacillus cereus* and *B. thuringiensis* isolates associated with periodontitis and other human infections. *J. Clin. Microbiol.* **38:**1615–1622.

64. **Helgason, E., N. J. Tourasse, R. Meisal, D. A. Caugant, and A. B. Kolstø.** 2004. Multilocus sequence typing scheme for bacteria of the *Bacillus cereus* group. *Appl. Environ. Microbiol.* **70:**191–201.

65. **Hernaiz, C., A. Picardo, J. I. Alos, and J. L. Gomez-Garces.** 2003. Nosocomial bacteremia and catheter infection by *Bacillus cereus* in an immunocompetent patient. *Clin. Microbiol. Infect.* **9:**973–975.

66. **Hoffmaster, A. R., R. F. Meyer, M. D. Bowen, C. K. Marston, R. S. Weyant, K. Thurman, S. L. Messenger, E. E. Minor, J. M. Winchell, M. V. Rassmussen, B. R. Newton, J. T. Parker, W. E. Morrill, N. McKinney, G. A. Barnett, J. J. Sejvar, J. A. Jernigan, B. A. Perkins, and T. Popovic.** 2002. Evaluation and validation of a real-time polymerase chain reaction assay for rapid identification of *Bacillus anthracis*. *Emerg. Infect. Dis.* **8:**1178–1182.

67. **Hoffmaster, A. R., K. K. Hill, J. E. Gee, C. K. Marston, B. K. De, T. Popovic, D. Sue, P. P. Wilkins, S. B. Avashia, R. Drumgoole, C. H. Helma, L. O. Ticknor, R. T. Okinaka, and P. J. Jackson.** 2006. Characterization of *Bacillus cereus* isolates associated with fatal pneumonias: isolates are closely related to *Bacillus anthracis* and harbor *B. anthracis* virulence genes. *J. Clin. Microbiol.* **44:**3352–3360.

68. **Hoffmaster, A. R., R. T. Novak, C. K. Marston, J. E. Gee, L. Helsel, J. M. Pruckler, and P. P. Wilkins.** 2008. Genetic diversity of clinical isolates of *Bacillus cereus* using multilocus sequence typing. *BMC Microbiol.* **8:**191.

69. **Hurtle, W., E. Bode, R. S. Kaplan, J. Garrison, B. Kearney, D. Shoemaker, E. Henchal, and D. Norwood.** 2003. Use of denaturing high-performance liquid chromatography to identify *Bacillus anthracis* by analysis of the 16S-23S rRNA interspacer region and *gyrA* gene. *J. Clin. Microbiol.* **41:**4758–4766.

70. **Hurtle, W., E. Bode, D. A. Kulesh, R. S. Kaplan, J. Garrison, D. Bridge, M. House, M. S. Frye, B. Loveless, and D. Norwood.** 2004. Detection of the *Bacillus anthracis gyrA* gene by using a minor groove binder probe. *J. Clin. Microbiol.* **42:**179–185.

71. **Jernigan, J. A., D. S. Stephens, D. A. Ashford, C. Omenaca, M. S. Topiel, M. Galbraith, M. Tapper, T. L. Fisk, S. Zaki, T. Popovic, R. F. Meyer, C. P. Quinn, S. A. Harper, S. K. Fridkin, J. J. Sejvar, C. W. Shepard, M. McConnell, J. Guarner, W.-J. Shieh, J. M. Malecki, J. L. Gerberding, J. M. Hughes, and B. A. Perkins.** 2002. Anthrax bioterrorism investigation. Bioterrorism-related inhalational anthrax: the first 10 cases reported in the United States. *Emerg. Infect. Dis.* **7:**933–944.

72. **Juergensmeyer, M. A., B. A. Gingras, L. Restaino, and E. W. Frampton.** 2006. A selective chromogenic agar that distinguishes *Bacillus anthracis* from *Bacillus cereus* and *Bacillus thuringiensis*. *J. Food. Prot.* **69:**2002–2006.

73. **Kalpoe, J. S., K. Hogenbirk, N. M. van Maarseveen, B. J. Gesink-Van der Veer, M. E. M. Kraakman, J. J. Maarleveld, T. J. K. van der Reyden, L. Dijkshoorn, and A. T. Bernards.** 2008. Dissemination of *Bacillus cereus* in a paediatric intensive care unit traced to insufficient disinfection of reusable ventilator air-flow sensors. *J. Hosp. Infect.* **68:**341–347.

74. **Kämpfer, P., R. Rosselló-Mora, E. Falsen, H.-J. Busse, and B. J. Tindall.** 2006. Cohnella thermotolerans gen. nov., sp. nov., and classification of 'Paenibacillus hongkongensis' as Cohnella hongkongensis sp. nov. *Int. J. Syst. Evol. Microbiol.* **56:**781–786.

75. **Kawamura-Sato, K., Y. Hirama, N. Agata, M. Ito, K. Torii, A. Takeno, T. Hasegawa, Y. Shimomura, and M. Ohta.** 2005. Quantitative analysis of cereulide, an emetic toxin of *Bacillus cereus*, by using rat liver mitochondria. *Microbiol. Immunol.* **49:**25–30.

76. **Keim, P., L. B. Price, A. M. Klevytska, K. L. Smith, J. M. Schupp, R. Okinaka, P. J. Jackson, and M. E. Hugh-Jones.** 2000. Multiple-locus variable-number tandem repeat analysis

reveals genetic relationships within *Bacillus anthracis*. *J. Bacteriol.* **182**:2928–2936.

77. **Kenefic, L. J., J. Beaudry, C. Trim, R. Daly, R. Parmar, S. Zanecki, L. Huynh, M. N. Van Ert, D. M. Wagner, T. Graham, and P. Keim.** 2008. High resolution genotyping of *Bacillus anthracis* outbreak strains using four highly mutable single nucleotide repeat markers. *Lett. Appl. Microbiol.* **46**:600–603.

78. **Kenefic, L. J., J. Beaudry, C. Trim, L. Huynh, S. Zanecki, M. Matthews, J. Schupp, M. Van Ert, and P. Keim.** 2008. A high resolution four-locus multiplex single nucleotide repeat (SNR) genotyping system in *Bacillus anthracis*. *J. Microbiol. Methods* **73**:269–272.

79. **Klee, S. R., M. Ozel, B. Appel, C. Boesch, H. Ellerbrok, D. Jacob, G. Holland, F. H. Leendertz, G. Pauli, R. Grunow, and H. Nattermann.** 2006. Characterization of *Bacillus anthracis*-like bacteria isolated from wild great apes from Côte d'Ivoire and Cameroon. *J. Bacteriol.* **188**:5333–5344.

80. **Knisely, R. F.** 1966. Selective medium for *Bacillus anthracis*. *J. Bacteriol.* **92**:784–786.

81. **Ko, K. S., J. W. Kim, J. M. Kim, W. Kim, S. I. Chung, I. J. Kim, and Y. H. Kook.** 2004. Population structure of the *Bacillus cereus* group as determined by sequence analysis of six housekeeping genes and the *plcR* gene. *Infect. Immun.* **72**:5253–5261.

82. **Ko, K. S., W. S. Oh, M. Y. Lee, J. H. Lee, H. Lee, K. R. Peck, N. Y. Lee, and J.-H. Song.** 2006. *Bacillus infantis* sp. nov. and *Bacillus idriensis* sp. nov., isolated from a patient with neonatal sepsis. *Int. J. Syst. Evol. Microbiol.* **56**:2541–2544.

83. **Ko, K. S., Y.-S. Kim, M. Y. Lee, S. Y. Shin, D. S. Jung, K. R. Peck, and J.-H. Song.** 2008. *Paenibacillus konsidensis* sp. nov., isolated from a patient. *Int. J. Syst. Evol. Microbiol.* **58**:2164–2168.

84. **Ko, S.-Y., H. J. Chung, H.-S. Sung, and M.-N. Kim.** 2007. Emergence of beta-lactam-dependent *Bacillus cereus* associated with prolonged treatment with cefepime in a neutropenic patient. *Korean J. Lab. Med.* **27**:216–220. (In Korean.)

85. **Kolstø, A.-B., N. J. Tourasse, and O. A. Økstad.** 2009. What sets *Bacillus anthracis* apart from other *Bacillus* species? *Annu. Rev. Microbiol.* **63**:451–476.

86. **Lalitha, M. K., V. Anandi, N. Walter, J. O. Devadatta, and B. M. Pulimood.** 1988. Primary anthrax presenting as an injection "abscess." *Indian J. Pathol. Microbiol.* **31**:254–256.

87. **Le Fleche, P., Y. Hauck, L. Onteniente, A. Prieur, F. Denoeud, V. Ramisse, P. Sylvestre, G. Benson, F. Ramisse, and G. Vergnaud.** 2001. A tandem repeats database for bacterial genomes: application to the genotyping of *Yersinia pestis* and *Bacillus anthracis*. *BMC Microbiol.* **1**:2.

88. **Ligozzi, M., G. L. Cascio, and R. Fontana.** 1998. *vanA* gene cluster in a vancomycin-resistant clinical isolate of *Bacillus circulans*. *Antimicrob. Agents Chemother.* **42**:2055–2059.

89. **Lista, F., G. Faggioni, S. Valjevac, A. Ciammaruconi, J. Vaissaire, C. le Doujet, O. Gorge, R. De Santis, A. Carattoli, A. Ciervo, A. Fasanella, F. Orsini, R. D'Amelio, C. Pourcel, A. Cassone, and G. Vergnaud.** 2006. Genotyping of Bacillus anthracis strains based on automated capillary 25-loci multiple locus variable-number tandem repeats analysis. *BMC Microbiol.* **6**:33.

90. **Logan, N. A., and P. De Vos.** 2009. *Bacillus*, p. 21–128. *In* P. De Vos, G. M. Garrity, D. Jones, N. R. Krieg, W. Ludwig, F. R. Rainey, K.-H. Schleifer, and W. B. Whitman (ed.), *Bergey's Manual of Systematic Bacteriology*, 2nd ed., vol. 3. Springer, New York, NY.

91. **Logan, N. A., and P. De Vos.** 2009. *Brevibacillus*, p. 305–316. *In* P. De Vos, G. M. Garrity, D. Jones, N. R. Krieg, W. Ludwig, F. R. Rainey, K.-H. Schleifer, and W. B. Whitman (ed.), *Bergey's Manual of Systematic Bacteriology*, 2nd ed., vol. 3. Springer, New York, NY.

92. **Logan, N. A., P. De Vos, and A. E. Dinsdale.** 2009. *Geobacillus*, p. 144–160. *In* P. De Vos, G. M. Garrity, D. Jones, N. R. Krieg, W. Ludwig, F. R. Rainey, K.-H. Schleifer, and W. B. Whitman (ed.), *Bergey's Manual of Systematic Bacteriology*, 2nd ed., vol. 3. Springer, New York, NY.

93. **Logan, N. A., G. Forsyth, L. Lebbe, J. Goris, M. Heyndrickx, A. Balcaen, A. Verhelst, E. Falsen, Å. Ljungh, H. B. Hansson, and P. De Vos.** 2002. Polyphasic identification of *Bacillus* and *Brevibacillus* strains from clinical, dairy, and industrial specimens and proposal of *Brevibacillus invocatus* sp. nov. *Int. J. Syst. Evol. Microbiol.* **52**:953–966.

94. **Mahler, H., A. Pasi, J. M. Kramer, P. Schulte, A. C. Scoging, W. Bär, and S. Krähenbühl.** 1997. Fulminant liver failure in association with the emetic toxin of *Bacillus cereus*. *N. Engl. J. Med.* **336**:1142–1148.

95. **Marano, N., B. D. Plikaytis, S. W. Martin, C. Rose, V. A. Semenova, S. K. Martin, A. E. Freeman, H. Li, M. J. Mulligan, S. D. Parker, J. Babcock, W. Keitel, H. El Sahly, G. A. Poland, R. M. Jacobson, H. L. Keyserling, S. D. Soroka, S. P. Fox, J. L. Stamper, M. M. McNeil, B. A. Perkins, N. Messonnier, and C. P. Quinn.** 2008. Effects of a reduced dose schedule and intramuscular administration of anthrax vaccine adsorbed on immunogenicity and safety at 7 months: a randomized trial. *JAMA* **300**:1532–1543.

96. **Marshman, L. A. G., C. Hardwidge, and P. M. W. Donaldson.** 2000. *Bacillus cereus* meningitis complicating cerebrospinal fluid fistula repair and spinal drainage. *Br. J. Neurosurg.* **14**:580–582.

97. **Marston, C. K., C. Beesley, L. Helsel, and A. R. Hoffmaster.** 2008. Evaluation of two selective media for the isolation of *Bacillus anthracis*. *Lett. Appl. Microbiol.* **47**:25–30.

98. **McIntyre, L., K. Bernard, D. Beniac, J. L. Isaac-Renton, and D. C. Naseby.** 2008. Identification of *Bacillus cereus* group species associated with food poisoning outbreaks in British Columbia, Canada. *Appl. Environ. Microbiol.* **74**:7451–7453.

99. **Mikkola, R., M. Kolari, M. A. Andersson, J. Helin, and M. S. Salkinoja-Salonen.** 2000. Toxic lactonic lipopeptide from food poisoning isolates of *Bacillus licheniformis*. *Eur. J. Biochem.* **267**:4068–4074.

100. **Mikkola, R., M. A. Andersson, P. Grigoriev, V. V. Teplova, N.-E. L. Saris, F. A. Rainey, and M. S. Salkinoja-Salonen.** 2004. Toxic lactonic lipopeptide from food poisoning isolates of *Bacillus amyloliquefaciens* strains isolated from moisture-damaged buildings produced surfactin and a substance toxic to mammalian cells. *Arch. Microbiol.* **181**:314–323.

101. **Miller, J. J., I. U. Scott, H. W. Flynn, W. E. Smiddy, T. G. Murray, A. Berrocal, and D. Miller.** 2008. Endophthalmitis caused by *Bacillus* species. *Am. J. Ophthalmol.* **145**:883–888.

102. **Mohammed, M. J., C. H. Marston, T. Popovic, R. S. Weyant, and F. C. Tenover.** 2002. Antimicrobial susceptibility testing of *Bacillus anthracis*: comparison of results obtained by using the National Committee for Clinical Laboratory Standards broth microdilution reference and Etest agar gradient diffusion methods. *J. Clin. Microbiol.* **40**:1902–1907.

103. **Morse, S. A., R. B. Kellogg, S. Perry, R. F. Meyer, D. Bray, D. Nichelson, and J. M. Miller.** 2003. Detecting biothreat agents: the Laboratory Response Network. *ASM News* **69**:433–437.

104. **Muller, J. D., C. R. Wilks, K. J. O'Riley, R. J. Condron, R. Bull, and A. Mateczun.** 2004. Specificity of an immunochromatographic test for anthrax. *Aust. Vet. J.* **82**:220–222.

105. **Ngamwongsatit, P., W. Buasri, P. Pianariyanon, C. Pulsrikarn, M. Ohba, A. Assavanig, and W. Panbangred.** 2008. Broad distribution of enterotoxin genes (hblCDA, nheABC, cytK, and entFM) among *Bacillus thuringiensis* and *Bacillus cereus* as shown by novel primers. *Int. J. Food Microbiol.* **121**:352–356.

106. **Ozkocaman, V., T. Ozcelik, R. Ali, F. Ozkalemkas, A. Ozkan, C. Ozakin, H. Akalin, A. Ursavas, F. Coskun, and B. Ener.** 2006. *Bacillus* spp. among hospitalized patients with haematological malignancies: clinical features, epidemics and outcomes. *J. Hosp. Infect.* **64**:169–176.

107. **Park, D. J., J. C. Yun, J. E. Baek, E. Y. Jung, D. W. Lee, M.-A. Kim, and S.-H. Chang.** 2006. Relapsing *Bacillus licheniformis* peritonitis in a continuous ambulatory peritoneal dialysis patient. *Nephrology* (Carlton) **11:**21–22.

108. **Patel, R., K. Piper, F. R. Cockerill, J. M. Steckelberg, and A. A. Yousten.** 2000. The biopesticide *Paenibacillus popilliae* has a vancomycin resistance gene cluster homologous to the enterococcal VanA vancomycin gene cluster. *Antimicrob. Agents Chemother.* **44:**705–709.

109. **Pinna, A., L. A. Sechi, S. Zanetti, D. Esai, G. Delogu, P. Cappuccinelli, and F. Carta.** 2001. *Bacillus cereus* keratitis associated with contact lens wear. *Ophthalmology* **108:**1830–1834.

110. **Priest, F. G., M. Barker, L. W. Baillie, E. C. Holmes, and M. C. Maiden.** 2004. Population structure and evolution of the *Bacillus cereus* group. *J. Bacteriol.* **186:**7959–7970.

111. **Qi, Y., G. Patra, X. Liang, L. E. Williams, S. Rose, R. J. Redkar, and V. G. DelVecchio.** 2001. Utilization of the *rpoB* gene as a specific chromosomal marker for real-time PCR detection of *Bacillus anthracis*. *Appl. Environ. Microbiol.* **67:**3720–3727.

112. **Quinn, C. P., V. A. Semenova, C. M. Elie, S. Romero-Steiner, C. Greene, H. Li, K. Stamey, E. Steward-Clark, D. S. Schmidt, E. Mothershed, J. Pruckler, S. Schwartz, R. F. Benson, L. O. Helsel, P. F. Holder, S. E. Johnson, M. Kellum, T. Messmer, W. L. Thacker, L. Besser, B. D. Plikaytis, T. H. Taylor, Jr., A. E. Freeman, K. J. Wallace, P. Dull, J. Sejvar, E. Bruce, R. Moreno, A. Schuchat, J. R. Lingappa, S. K. Martin, J. Walls, M. Bronsdon, G. M. Carlone, M. Bajani-Ari, D. A. Ashford, D. S. Stephens, and B. A. Perkins.** 2002. Specific, sensitive, and quantitative enzyme-linked immunosorbent assay for human immunoglobulin G antibodies to anthrax toxin protective antigen. *Emerg. Infect. Dis.* **8:**1103–1110.

113. **Quinn, C. P., P. M. Dull, V. Semenova, H. Li, S. Crotty, T. H. Taylor, E. Steward-Clark, K. L. Stamey, D. S. Schmidt, K. W. Stinson, A. E. Freeman, C. M. Elie, S. K. Martin, C. Greene, R. D. Aubert, J. Glidewell, B. A. Perkins, R. Ahmed, and D. S. Stephens.** 2004. Immune responses to *Bacillus anthracis* protective antigen in patients with bioterrorism-related cutaneous or inhalation anthrax. *J. Infect. Dis.* **190:**1228–1236.

114. **Ramos-Esteban, J. C., J. J. Servat, S. Tauber, and F. Bia.** 2006. *Bacillus megaterium* delayed onset lamellar keratitis after LASIK. *J. Refract. Surg.* **22:**309–312.

115. **Rider, T. H., M. S. Petrovick, F. E. Nargi, J. D. Harper, E. D. Schwoebel, R. H. Mathews, D. J. Blanchard, L. T. Bortolin, A. M. Young, J. Chen, and M. A. Hollis.** 2003. A B cell-based sensor for rapid identification of pathogens. *Science* **301:**213–215.

116. **Roux, V., and D. Raoult.** 2004. *Paenibacillus massiliensis* sp. nov., *Paenibacillus sanguinis* sp. nov. and *Paenibacillus timonensis* sp. nov., isolated from blood cultures. *Int. J. Syst. Evol. Microbiol.* **54:**1049–1054.

117. **Roux, V., L. Fenner, and D. Raoult.** 2008. *Paenibacillus provencensis* sp. nov., isolated from human cerebrospinal fluid, and *Paenibacillus urinalis* sp. nov., isolated from human urine. *Int. J. Syst. Evol. Microbiol.* **58:**682–687.

118. **Rubinstein, I., and G. W. Pedersen.** 2002. *Bacillus* species are present in chewing tobacco sold in the United States and evoke plasma exudation from the oral mucosa. *Clin. Diagn. Lab. Immunol.* **9:**1057–1060.

119. **Saile, E., and T. M. Koehler.** 2006. *Bacillus anthracis* multiplication, persistence, and genetic exchange in the rhizosphere of grass plants. *Appl. Environ. Microbiol.* **72:**3168–3174.

120. **Schneemann, A., and M. Manchester.** 2009. Anti-toxin antibodies in prophylaxis and treatment of inhalation anthrax. *Future Microbiol.* **4:**35–43.

121. **Sejvar, J. J., F. C. Tenover, and D. S. Stephens.** 2005. Management of anthrax meningitis. *Lancet Infect. Dis.* **5:**287–295.

122. **Shieh, W. J., J. Guarner, C. Paddock, P. Greer, K. Tatti, M. Fischer, M. Layton, M. Philips, E. Bresnitz, C. P. Quinn, T. Popovic, B. A. Perkins, S. R. Zaki, and the Anthrax Bioterrorism Investigation Team.** 2003. The critical role of pathology in the investigation of bioterrorism-related cutaneous anthrax. *Am. J. Pathol.* **163:**1901–1910.

123. **Shlyakhov, E., and E. Rubinstein.** 1994. Human live anthrax vaccine in the former USSR. *Vaccine* **12:**727–730.

124. **Sirisanthana, T., and A. E. Brown.** 2002. Anthrax of the gastrointestinal tract. *Emerg. Infect. Dis.* **8:**649–651.

125. **Sohni, Y., S. Kanjilal, and V. Kapur.** 2008. Performance evaluation of five commercial real-time PCR reagent systems using TaqMan assays for *B. anthracis* detection. *Clin. Biochem.* **41:**640–644.

126. **Sorokin, A., B. Candelon, K. Guilloux, N. Galleron, N. Wackerow-Kouzova, S. D. Ehrlich, D. Bourguet, and V. Sanchis.** 2006. Multiple-locus sequence typing analysis of *Bacillus cereus* and *Bacillus thuringiensis* reveals separate clustering and a distinct population structure of psychrotrophic strains. *Appl. Environ. Microbiol.* **72:**1569–1578.

127. **Spinosa, M. R., F. Wallet, R. J. Courcol, and M. R. Oggioni.** 2000. The trouble in tracing opportunistic pathogens: cholangitis due to *Bacillus* in a French hospital caused by a strain related to an Italian product? *Microb. Ecol. Health. Dis.* **12:**99–101.

128. **Stenfors Arnesen, L. P., A. Fagerlund, and P. E. Granum.** 2008. From soil to gut: *Bacillus cereus* and its food poisoning toxins. *FEMS Microbiol. Rev.* **32:**579–606.

129. **Stern, E. J., K. B. Uhde, S. V. Shadomy, and N. Messonnier.** 2008. Conference report on public health and clinical guidelines for anthrax. *Emerg. Infect. Dis.* **14:**e1.

130. **Stickel, F., S. Droz, E. Patsenker, K. Bögli-Stuber, B. Aebi, and S. Leib.** 2009. Severe hepatotoxicity following ingestion of Herbalife nutritional supplements contaminated with *Bacillus subtilis*. *J. Hepatol.* **50:**111–117.

131. **Stratilo, C. W., C. T. Lewis, L. Bryden, M. R. Mulvey, and D. Bader.** 2006. Single-nucleotide repeat analysis for subtyping *Bacillus anthracis* isolates. *J. Clin. Microbiol.* **44:**777–782.

132. **Sue, D., C. K. Marston, A. R. Hoffmaster, and P. P. Wilkins.** 2007. Genetic diversity in a *Bacillus anthracis* historical collection (1954 to 1988). *J. Clin. Microbiol.* **45:**1777–1782.

133. **Tang, S., M. Moayeri, Z. Chen, H. Harma, J. Zhao, H. Hu, R. H. Purcell, S. H. Leppla, and I. K. Hewlett.** 2009. Detection of anthrax toxin by an ultrasensitive immunoassay using europium nanoparticles. *Clin. Vaccine Immunol.* **16:**408–413.

134. **Tena, D., J. A. Martinez-Torres, M. T. Perez-Pomata, J. A. Sáez-Nieto, V. Rubio, and J. Bisquert.** 2007. Cutaneous infection due to Bacillus pumilus: report of 3 cases. Clin. Infect. Dis. **44:**40–42.

135. **Thorsen, L., B. M. Hansen, K. F. Nielsen, N. B. Hendriksen, R. K. Phipps, and B. B. Budde.** 2006. Characterization of emetic *Bacillus weihenstephanensis*, a new cereulide-producing bacterium. *Appl, Environ. Microbiol.* **72:**5118–5121.

136. **Tourasse, N. J., E. Helgason, O. A. Okstad, I. K. Hegna, and A. B. Kolsto.** 2006. The *Bacillus cereus* group: novel aspects of population structure and genome dynamics. *J. Appl. Microbiol.* **101:**579–593.

137. **Tourasse, N. J., and A.-B. Kolstø.** 2008. SuperCAT: a supertree database for combined and integrative multilocus sequence typing analysis of the *Bacillus cereus* group of bacteria (including *B. cereus*, *B. anthracis* and *B. thuringiensis*). *Nucleic Acids Res.* **36:**D461–D468.

138. **Tournier, J. N., R. G. Ulrich, A. Quesnel-Hellmann, M. Mohamadzadeh, and B. G. Stiles.** 2009. Anthrax, toxins and vaccines: a 125-year journey targeting *Bacillus anthracis*. *Expert Rev. Anti-Infect. Ther.* **7:**219–236.

139. **Tuladhar, R., S. K. Patole, T. H. Koh, R. Norton, and J. S. Whitehall.** 2000. Refractory *Bacillus cereus* infection in a neonate. *Int. J. Clin. Pract.* **54:**345–347.

140. **Turnbull, P. C. B. (ed.).** 2008. *Anthrax in Humans and Animals*, 4th ed. World Health Organization, Geneva, Switzerland. http://www.who.int/csr/resources/publications/AnthraxGuidelines2008

141. **Turnbull, P. C. B., N. M. Sirianni, C. I. LeBron, M. N. Samaan, F. N. Sutton, A. E. Reyes, and L. F. Peruski.** 2004. MICs of selected antibiotics for *Bacillus anthracis*, *Bacillus cereus*, *Bacillus thuringiensis*, and *Bacillus mycoides* from a range of clinical and environmental sources as determined by the Etest. *J. Clin. Microbiol.* **42:**3626–3634.

142. **Turnbull, P. C. B., D. A. Frawley, and R. L. Bull.** 2007. Heat activation/shock temperatures for *Bacillus anthracis* spores and the issue of spore plate counts versus true numbers of spores. *J. Microbiol. Methods* **68:**353–357.

143. **Van Ert, M. N., S. A. Hofstadler, Y. Jiang, J. D. Busch, D. M. Wagner, J. J. Drader, D. J. Ecker, J. C. Hannis, L. Y. Huynh, J. M. Schupp, T. S. Simonson, and P. Keim.** 2004. Mass spectrometry provides accurate characterization of two genetic marker types in *Bacillus anthracis*. *BioTechniques* **37:**642–644, 646, 648 passim.

144. **Van Ert, M. N., W. R. Easterday, L. Y. Huynh, R. T. Okinaka, M. E. Hugh-Jones, J. Ravel, S. R. Zanecki, T. Pearson, T. S. Simonson, J. M. U'Ren, S. M. Kachur, R. R. Leadem-Dougherty, S. D. Rhoton, G. Zinser, J. Farlow, P. R. Coker, K. L. Smith, B. Wang, L. J. Kenefic, C. M. Fraser-Liggett, D. M. Wagner, and P. Keim.** 2007. Global genetic population structure of *Bacillus anthracis*. *PLoS ONE* **2:**e461.

145. **Van Ert, M. N., W. R. Easterday, T. S. Simonson, J. M. U'Ren, T. Pearson, L. J. Kenefic, J. D. Busch, L. Y. Huynh, M. Dukerich, C. B. Trim, J. Beaudry, A. Welty-Bernard, T. Read, C. M. Fraser, J. Ravel, and P. Keim.** 2007. Strain-specific single-nucleotide polymorphism assays for the *Bacillus anthracis* Ames strain. *J. Clin. Microbiol.* **45:**47–53.

146. **Vijaikumar, M., D. M. Thappa, and K. Karthikeyan.** 2002 Cutaneous anthrax: an endemic outbreak in South India. *J. Trop. Pediatr.* **48:**225–226.

147. **Walsh, J., J. N. Pesik, C. P. Quinn, V. Urdaneta, C. A. Dykewicz, A. E. Boyer, J. Guarner, P. Wilkins, K. J. Norville, J. R. Barr, S. R. Zaki, J. B. Patel, S. P. Reagan, J. L. Pirkle, T. A. Treadwell, N. Rosenstein Messonnier, L. D. Rotz, R. F. Meyer, and D. S. Stephens.** 2007. A case of naturally acquired inhalation anthrax: clinical care and analyses of anti-protective antigen immunoglobulin G and lethal factor. *Clin. Infect. Dis.* **44:**968–971.

148. **Weber, D. J., S. M. Saviteer, W. A. Rutala, and C. A. Thomann.** 1988. In vitro susceptibility of *Bacillus* spp. to selected antimicrobial agents. *Antimicrob. Agents Chemother.* **32:**642–645.

149. **Whiteaker, J., J. Karns, C. Fenselau, and M. L. Perdue.** 2004. Analysis of *Bacillus anthracis* spores in milk using mass spectrometry. *Foodborne Pathog. Dis.* **1:**185–194.

150. **Whiting, G. C., S. Rijpkema, T. Adams, and M. J. Corbel.** 2004. Characterization of adsorbed anthrax vaccine by two-dimensional gel electrophoresis. *Vaccine* **22:**4245–4251.

151. **Yakupogullari, Y., and M. Koroglu.** 2007. Nosocomial spread of *Bacillus anthracis*. *J. Hosp. Infect.* **66:**401–402.

152. **Zahavy, E., M. Fisher, A. Bromberg, and U. Olshevsky.** 2003. Detection of frequency resonance energy transfer pair on double-labeled microsphere and *Bacillus anthracis* spores by flow cytometry. *Appl. Environ. Microbiol.* **69:**2330–2339.

153. **Zwick, M. E., F. McAfee, D. J. Cutler, T. D. Read, J. Ravel, G. R. Bowman, D. R. Galloway, and A. Mateczun.** 2005. Microarray-based resequencing of multiple *Bacillus anthracis* isolates. *Genome Biol.* **6:**R10.

Listeria and Erysipelothrix*

NELE WELLINGHAUSEN

25

LISTERIA

Taxonomy

The genus *Listeria* consists of gram-positive, non-spore-forming, facultative anaerobic, regular rod-shaped bacteria with a low G+C content of 36 to 42 mol%. While early phylogenetic studies suggested a close relation between *Listeria* and the *Lactobacillaceae*, comparisons of 16S rRNA gene sequences have shown that *Listeria* is most closely related to *Staphylococcus* and *Bacillus*. Together with *Brochothrix, Listeria* is provisionally assigned to the family "*Listeriaceae*" within the order *Bacillales*. Synthesis of menaquinones and major amounts of branched-chain fatty acids confirms the taxonomic separation of *Listeria* from the *Lactobacillaceae* (29, 51).

Until recently, the genus *Listeria* comprised six validated species including *Listeria monocytogenes* as the type species in the genus, *L. grayi, L. innocua, L. ivanovii, L. seeligeri*, and *L. welshimeri*. Within *L. ivanovii* two subspecies, *L. ivanovii* subsp. *ivanovii* and *L. ivanovii* subsp. *londoniensis*, are differentiated (8). Recently, a seventh *Listeria* species, *L. marthii*, has been described from the natural environment and is most closely related to *L. monocytogenes* (38).

Based on the results of multilocus enzyme electrophoresis, DNA-DNA hybridization, and 16S rRNA gene sequencing, the species of *Listeria* are divided into two closely related but distinct lines of descent: (i) the *L. monocytogenes* group of species, including *L. innocua, L. ivanovii, L. marthii, L. monocytogenes, L. seeligeri*, and *L. welshimeri*; and (ii) *L. grayi* (8, 16, 38). Of the seven species within the genus *Listeria*, only *L. monocytogenes* and *L. ivanovii* are pathogenic for humans and animals.

Description of the Agent

Members of the genus *Listeria* are gram-positive, facultative anaerobic, non-spore-forming, nonbranching, regular, short (0.5 to 2 by 0.4 to 0.5 μm) rods that occur singly or in short chains. Filaments of 6 to 20 μm in length may occur in older or rough cultures. Temperature-regulated expression of flagellin results in a characteristic tumbling motility at 20 to 28°C by means of one to six peritrichous flagella. At 37°C the organisms are much less motile. Colonies are small (1 to 2 mm in diameter after 1 or 2 days of incubation at 37°C), smooth, and blue-gray on nutrient agar when examined with obliquely transmitted light. *Listeria* spp. show an exceptionally large growth temperature range from 0 to 50°C. The optimum growth temperature is between 30 and 37°C, but at 4°C growth is also observed within a few days. Catalase is typically produced, but catalase-negative strains causing disease in humans have been described (13, 25). The oxidase test is negative. Acid is produced from D-glucose and other sugars. The Voges-Proskauer and methyl red tests are positive. Esculin is hydrolyzed in a few hours. Urea and gelatin are not hydrolyzed. Neither indole nor H_2S is produced. The cell wall contains a directly cross-linked peptidoglycan based on *meso*-diaminopimelic acid, as well as lipoteichoic acid, but no mycolic acids. The two predominant cellular fatty acids are $C_{ai15:0}$ and $C_{ai17:0}$ (branched-chain type) (6).

Epidemiology and Transmission

The primary habitat of *Listeria* species is the environment, where they exhibit a saprophytic lifestyle. *L. monocytogenes* has been isolated from various animals, like mammals, birds, fish, and crustaceans. Infected animals can asymptomatically pass the organism or develop clinical disease. Due to its widespread distribution, *L. monocytogenes* has many opportunities to enter human food production, resulting in contamination of fresh and processed poultry, meat, and vegetables; raw milk; cheese; smoked salmon; etc. (27). Numbers of organisms exceeding 10^3 CFU/g were detected in food products (27). Infection of humans ingesting colonized food is potentiated by the ability of the organism to multiply at 4°C. The intestinal tract of adults is consistently colonized with nonpathogenic *Listeria* species and, to a lesser extent (1 to 5%), with pathogenic *L. monocytogenes* (41). Cervicovaginal carriage in women has not been reported. Apart from food-related infections, a few nosocomial outbreaks, mainly in neonatal wards, have been described (28, 69). The number of sporadic cases of listeriosis in countries that report the illness is typically in the range of 0.1 to 0.9 cases per 100,000 persons (37, 89). While the number of cases and the mortality in the United States have decreased (incidence, 0.4 per 100,000 per year) in recent years (89), the incidence of sporadic listeriosis has increased in several European countries, reaching numbers from 0.4 up to 1.0 per 100,000 per year (12, 37).

---

*This chapter contains information presented in chapter 33 by Jacques Bille in the ninth edition of this *Manual*.

Clinical Significance

The majority of cases of listeriosis occur in individuals who have an underlying condition that leads to suppression of their cell-mediated immunity. However, infections in immunocompetent individuals are increasingly reported. About one-half of the cases of listeriosis occur in individuals older than 60 years and younger than 1 month. In adults, *L. monocytogenes* causes primarily septicemia, meningitis, and encephalitis with a mortality reaching up to 50%. Focal infections with *Listeria* spp. have been infrequently described and include endocarditis, arthritis, osteomyelitis, intra-abdominal abscesses, endophthalmitis, (sclero-)keratitis, peritonitis, and intravenous catheter and pleuropulmonary infections (19). Among veterinarians and abattoir workers, primary cutaneous listeriosis with or without bacteremia has been reported (53).

In pregnant women, *L. monocytogenes* often causes a mild, self-limited influenzalike illness. Transient bacteremia can result in placentitis and/or amnionitis, and since *Listeria* is able to cross the placenta (49), it can infect the fetus, causing abortion, stillbirth, or, most commonly, preterm labor. In neonates, an early-onset form and a late-onset form of listeriosis occur. The early form is presumably caused by intrauterine infection and manifests as granulomatosis infantisepticum. The organism is widely disseminated in the body, including the central nervous system. The source of the organism in the late-onset cases, which manifest at a mean of 14 days after birth, is unclear and may comprise the mother's genital tract or environmental sources.

The infectious dose and the incubation period for human listeriosis have not been firmly established, and reported incubation periods vary from a few days to 2 to 3 months. Doses of 10^5 CFU or greater have been reported to cause gastroenteritis in outbreak situations (2). A dose-response model using rhesus monkeys as a surrogate for pregnant women recently indicated that oral exposure to 10^7 CFU of *L. monocytogenes* results in about 50% stillbirths (71). Thus, it may be much less than the extrapolated estimate of 10^{13} CFU from the FDA-U.S. Department of Agriculture-CDC risk assessment based on mouse data (32).

Most cases of *Listeria* gastroenteritis are linked to foodborne outbreaks. Typically, patients with *Listeria* gastroenteritis have no known predisposing risk factors for listeriosis, illness occurs about 24 h after ingestion of a food item that is contaminated with a large number of bacteria (10^5 to 10^9 CFU/g or ml), and illness lasts about 2 days. Apart from gastroenteritis, fever, headache, and pain in joints and muscles are frequently seen (59).

After ingestion of *L. monocytogenes*, pathogen and host factors as well as the number of pathogens ingested determine whether invasive infection develops. Immunity to listeriosis is effected primarily via the cell-mediated immune system. Penetration of the epithelial barrier in the gut by *L. monocytogenes* is facilitated by its ability to escape from the host cell vacuole, intracytoplasmic multiplication, movement via bacterially induced polymerization of host cell actin, and spread to neighboring cells through pseudopodlike extensions of the host cell membrane. Virulence genes are clustered on an 8.2-kb pathogenicity island and include genes coding for internalin A and B and listeriolysin, a hemolysin (65). Interaction between internalin and E-cadherin, a receptor of the trophoblast, facilitates the spread of the organism to the fetus (49).

L. ivanovii is primarily a pathogen of ruminants. Systemic infections in human immunodeficiency virus-infected and nonimmunosuppressed patients have, however, been described (17, 72).

Collection, Transport, and Storage of Specimens

Suitable specimens for detection of listeriosis include blood and cerebrospinal fluid (CSF). In neonates with suspicion of listeriosis, investigation of blood, CSF, amniotic fluid, respiratory secretions, placental or cutaneous swabs, gastric aspirates, or meconium can facilitate detection of the organism. For epidemiologic purposes or rare causes of gastroenteritis, stool specimens are preferred to rectal swabs. In general, specimens for detection of *Listeria* do not need special handling during collection.

Clinical specimens for culture of *L. monocytogenes* should be processed as soon as possible or stored and transported at room temperature or 4°C for up to 48 h. At 4°C even longer storage times may be tolerated due to the specific cold resistance of the organism, but multiplication of *Listeria* has to be regarded (15). Stool samples (1 g each) can be inoculated into 100 ml of a selective University of Vermont or polymyxin-acriflavin-lithium chloride-ceftazidime esculin-mannitol (PALCAM) enrichment broth and then shipped overnight at room temperature. To avoid overgrowth of *L. monocytogenes* by contaminating microbiota during longer periods of storage, nonsterile-site specimens should be stored at 4°C for 24 to 48 h or frozen at −20°C.

Food samples should include a minimum of 100 g of a sample and should be collected aseptically in sterile containers. Food packaged in original containers should always be preferred. Samples should be shipped overnight frozen. Although *L. monocytogenes* is relatively resistant to freezing, repeated freezing and thawing should be avoided.

Cultures of *Listeria* spp. should be frozen at −20 to −70°C for long-time storage. They can be shipped on a non-glucose-containing agar slant and packaged and declared according to the respective national and international requirements.

Because *L. monocytogenes* can infect the fetus, leading to stillbirths and abortions while causing only mild symptoms in the mother, pregnant women should be particularly careful when working in a laboratory where *L. monocytogenes* is propagated or handled.

Direct Examination

Direct microscopy should be performed in CSF, positive blood cultures, and if available, tissue samples. Detection of gram-positive, regular short rods in CSF or blood cultures should lead to the suspicion of listeriosis. Nevertheless, *L. monocytogenes* may be confused with members of the coryneform rods (especially in direct slides from positive blood cultures), since the cells may be arranged in V forms or palisades. Commercial tests licensed for antigen detection in clinical specimens other than nucleic acid-based tests are not available.

Sensitive and specific in-house PCR assays have been described for detection of *L. monocytogenes* in CSF, stool, or lung tissue (10, 34, 93) and may be particularly useful for specimens from patients with prior antimicrobial therapy. Regarding commercial assays, the Probelia *Listeria monocytogenes* assay (Bio-Rad, Hercules, CA) has been evaluated in clinical stool specimens (41) while other commercial assays (e.g., LightCycler PCR, Roche Diagnostics, Indianapolis, IN) have been validated only for food specimens.

Isolation Procedures

Clinical specimens from normally sterile sites should be plated onto tryptic soy agar containing 5% sheep, horse, or rabbit blood. Plates should be incubated at 35 to 37°C under room air with 5% CO_2 for a minimum of 48 h. Blood samples should be inoculated into conventional blood culture media. Clinical specimens obtained from nonsterile sites, like stool samples, as well as food and environmental specimens should be plated on *Listeria* spp. selective agars. In addition, enrichment by inoculation into selective broth for *Listeria* spp. (see above) should be done before plating.

Selective agars for culture of *Listeria* spp. include lithium chloride-phenylethanol-moxalactam (LPM) (50), Oxford, modified Oxford, and PALCAM agars (34). On LPM agar, colonies have to be examined under a stereomicroscope with Henry illumination (magnification, ×15 to ×25, with oblique lighting directed to the microscope stage by a concave mirror positioned at a 45° angle to the incident light). *Listeria* colonies appear blue, and colonies of other bacteria appear yellowish or orange. Oxford and PALCAM agars contain selective substances that eliminate the need for examination under oblique lighting (84). On Oxford and modified Oxford agars, *Listeria* colonies appear black due to esculin hydrolysis, are 1 to 3 mm in diameter, and are surrounded by a black halo after 24 to 48 h of incubation at 35 to 37°C. On PALCAM agar, *Listeria* colonies appear gray-green, are approximately 2 mm in diameter, and have black sunken centers.

For the detection of *Listeria* spp. in food samples, enrichment methods have to be used. The most widely used reference methods for food and environmental samples are the Food and Drug Administration (FDA) *Bacteriological and Analytical Manual* (BAM) (83) and the U.S. Department of Agriculture (USDA) method (82) in the United States and the International Organization of Standards (ISO) 11290 method in Europe (34). All methods require enrichment of the samples in a selective broth (*Listeria* enrichment broth, FDA BAM formulation, or University of Vermont broth in the FDA BAM and USDA methods; and Fraser broth in the ISO method) prior to plating onto selective agar and

biochemical identification of typical colonies (18). A detailed comparison of methods is given in reference 18.

New chromogenic media allow selective isolation of *Listeria* species (34, 62). Several media identify *L. monocytogenes* by the production of a phosphatidylinositol-specific phospholipase C. Media include ALOAgar (Biolife, Milan, Italy) (88), BCM *L. monocytogenes* (Biosynth, Staad, Switzerland) (64), LIMONO-Ident-Agar (Heipha, Eppelheim, Germany), and BBL CHROMagar (BD, Sparks, MD) (43). However, none of these agars differentiate between *L. monocytogenes* and *L. ivanovii*. Specific detection of *L. monocytogenes* is facilitated on RAPID *L.mono* agar (Bio-Rad, Hercules, CA) (4). Chromogenic media showed sensitivities comparable to those of Oxford and PALCAM agar (4, 43, 62).

Identification

A simplified identification is based on the following tests: Gram staining, observation of tumbling motility in a wet mount, and tests for a positive catalase reaction and esculin hydrolysis. Acid production from D-glucose and positive Voges-Proskauer test are confirmatory results.

Listeria spp. may be confused with other gram-positive bacteria due to similar morphologic or biochemical characteristics. *Streptococcus* and *Enterococcus* spp. can be differentiated from *Listeria* spp. on the basis of Gram stain morphology, motility, and catalase reaction. *Erysipelothrix* spp. differ from *Listeria* spp. in motility, catalase reaction, and ability to grow at 4°C (*Erysipelothrix* spp. do not grow at that temperature). *Lactobacillus* spp. are usually nonmotile and catalase negative.

Identification of *Listeria* isolates to the species level is crucial, because all species can contaminate foods but only *L. monocytogenes* is of public health concern. A scheme for identification of *Listeria* species based on morphological and biochemical characteristics is shown in Table 1. Among

TABLE 1 Biochemical differentiation of species in the genus *Listeria*[a]

Characteristic	L. grayi	L. innocua	L. ivanovii subsp. ivanovii	L. ivanovii subsp. londoniensis	L. marthii	L. monocytogenes	L. seeligeri	L. welshimeri
Beta-hemolysis	−	−	++[b]	++	−	+	+	−
CAMP[c] test reaction								
S. aureus	−	−	−	−	ND	+	+	−
R. equi	−	−	+	+	ND	V	−	−
Acid production from:								
Mannitol	+	−	−	−	−	−	−	−
α-Methyl-D-mannoside	+	−	−	−	ND	+	−	+
L-Rhamnose	V	V	−	−	−	+	−	V
Soluble starch	+	−	−	−	ND	−	ND	ND
D-Xylose	−	−	+	+	−	−	+	+
Ribose	V	−	+	−	ND	−	−	−
N-Acetyl-β-D-mannosamine	ND	ND	V	+	ND	ND	ND	ND
Hippurate hydrolysis	−	+	+	+	ND	+	ND	ND
Reduction of nitrate	V	−	−	−	−	−	ND	ND
Associated serovar(s)	S	4ab, US, 6a, 6b	5	5	ND	1/2a, 1/2b, 1/2c, 3a, 3b, 3c, 4a, 4ab, 4b, 4c, 4d, 4e, 7	1/2a, 1/2b, 1/2c, 4a, US, 4b, 4d, 6b	1/2b, 4c, 6a, 6b, US

[a]Symbols and abbreviations: +, ≥90% of strains are positive; −, ≥90% of strains are negative; ND, not determined; V, variable; US, undesignated serotype; S, specific.
[b]++, usually a wide zone or multiple zones.
[c]See text and Fig. 2.

these markers, hemolysis is essential for differentiating between *L. monocytogenes* and the most frequently isolated nonpathogenic species, *L. innocua*.

Production of hemolysin is regarded as a key virulence factor of *L. monocytogenes* and is visible on sheep blood agar plates as a narrow zone of hemolysis that frequently does not extend much beyond the edges of the colonies (Fig. 1). Like *L. monocytogenes*, *L. ivanovii* is also hemolytic, but hemolysis alone cannot be used to discriminate pathogenic and nonpathogenic species since *L. seeligeri* is, besides rare exceptions (90), hemolytic and since hemolytic strains of *L. innocua* have been described as well (47).

The CAMP (Christie, Atkins, Munch-Petersen) test can be used to differentiate among hemolytic *Listeria* species. The test is carried out by streaking a beta-hemolysis-producing *Staphylococcus aureus* strain and *Rhodococcus equi* parallel to each other on a blood agar plate. Suspect cultures are streaked at right angles in between (but not touching) the two streaks. Hemolysis by *L. monocytogenes* and to a lesser degree *L. seeligeri* is enhanced in the vicinity of *S. aureus*, and hemolysis by *L. ivanovii* is enhanced in the vicinity of the *R. equi* streak (Fig. 2). However, the reliability of the CAMP test is limited (85). As recommended in the USDA method (82), commercially available β-lysis disks (Remel, Lenexa, KS) may be used instead.

L. monocytogenes is, apart from rare atypical strains, L-rhamnose and α-methyl-D-mannoside positive and D-xylose negative. Incubation of test tubes for up to 7 days (37°C, aerobically) may be necessary.

Commercially available miniaturized tests considerably speed up biochemical identification of *Listeria* spp. The API *Coryne* and *Listeria* (bioMérieux, Durham, NC), Micro-ID *Listeria* (Remel), BBL Crystal Gram-Pos ID (BD, Franklin Lakes, NJ), and Microbact Listeria 12L (Oxoid) reliably identify *Listeria* isolates to the genus and species level (7, 33).

Identification of *L. monocytogenes* is possible with the Vitek2 (bioMérieux), MicroScan WalkAway (Siemens Healthcare, Malvern, PA), Micronaut (Merlin, Bornheim-Hesel, Germany), Phoenix (BD), and Biolog (Biolog Inc., Hayward, CA) systems. All systems allow reliable species identification, while Vitek1 (bioMérieux) facilitates identification of *Listeria* isolates to the genus level only (57).

A chemiluminescence DNA probe assay (AccuProbe, BioMérieux) (56) is available for rapid identification of *L. monocytogenes* from primary isolation plates. However, false-positive results were observed with the new species *L. marthii* (38).

The matrix-assisted laser desorption ionization–time of flight (mass spectrometry) (MALDI-TOF [MS]) technique has recently been introduced and allowed discrimination of the *Listeria* species by use of the respective software (MALDI Biotyper, Bruker Daltonics, Billerica, MA; AnagnosTec, Shimadzu, Duisburg, Germany) (3).

Typing Systems

Subtyping of *L. monocytogenes* is crucial for the workup of disease acquired from foodborne agents. Based on somatic "O" and flagellar "H" antigens, 13 serovars of *L. monocytogenes* are known (1/2a, 1/2b, 1/2c, 3a, 3b, 3c, 4a, 4ab, 4b/4bX, 4c, 4d, 4e, and 7). Since the vast majority of *L. monocytogenes* strains that cause sporadic infections or outbreaks belong to the same serotypes, i.e., 1/2a, 1/2b, and 4b, and since serotyping antigens are shared among *L. monocytogenes*, *L. innocua*, *L. seeligeri*, and *L. welshimeri*, reliable discrimination below the level of serotype is necessary. Thus, serotyping is only useful as a first-level discriminator or for the selection of further typing methods in suspected outbreaks. Antisera are commercially available from Difco (Difco Laboratories/BD, Sparks, MD) and Denka Seiken (Tokyo, Japan). A multiplex PCR has been described for identification of the four major serovars of *L. monocytogenes* (1/2a, 1/2b, 1/2c, and 4b) and has been validated by interlaboratory comparison (20, 21).

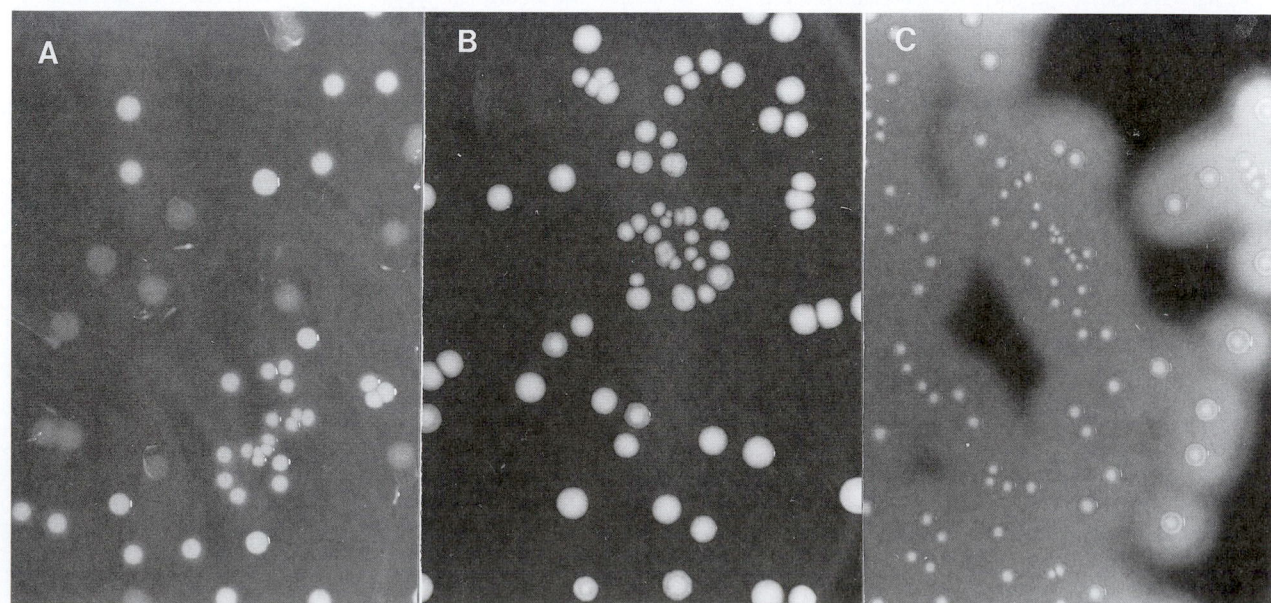

FIGURE 1   Macroscopic view of colonies on 5% human blood agar plates after 24 h of incubation. (A) *L. monocytogenes*: discrete zone of beta-hemolysis under the removed colonies. (B) *L. innocua*: no hemolysis. (C) *L. ivanovii*: wide zone of beta-hemolysis around the colonies.

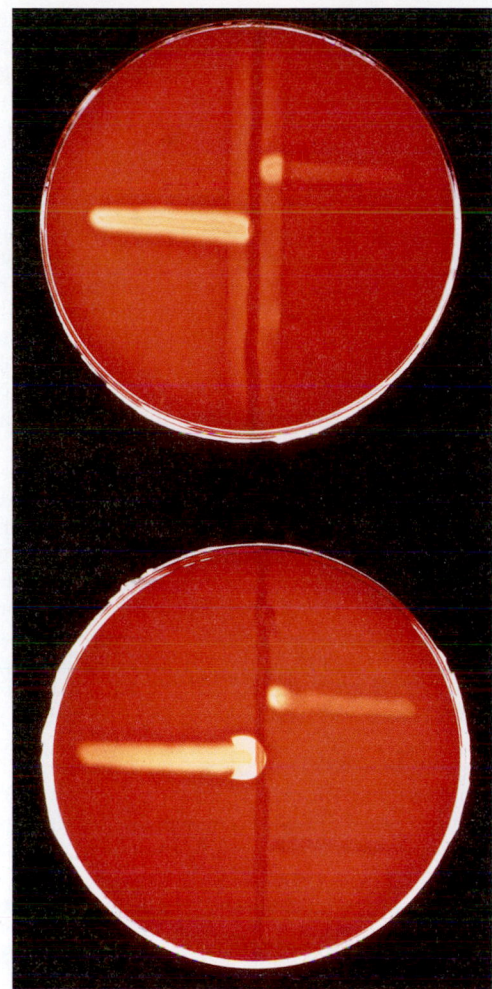

FIGURE 2 CAMP test done with *S. aureus* CIP 5710 (top plate) and *R. equi* CIP 5869 (bottom plate) after 24 h of incubation. Upper right, *L. monocytogenes*; lower right, *L. innocua*; middle left, *L. ivanovii*.

Pulsed-field gel electrophoresis (PFGE) is considered to be the standard typing method for *L. monocytogenes*. Its discriminatory power and reproducibility of results have been confirmed in a World Health Organization multicenter international typing study (11) as well as in a large number of other studies. PFGE is particularly useful for subtyping of serovar 4b isolates. Since interlaboratory comparison of results is difficult, considerable efforts have been undertaken for standardization of the method.

In the mid 1990s, a network (PulseNet) of public health and food regulatory laboratories that routinely subtype foodborne pathogenic bacteria in order to rapidly detect foodborne disease outbreaks was established by the Centers for Disease Control and Prevention in the United States.

In order to improve quality and interlaboratory comparability of PFGE, standardized laboratory protocols, including a 1-day protocol, were developed and rapid comparison of PFGE patterns from different locations is possible via the Internet (39). According to the standardized protocol, restriction endonucleases ApaI and AscI are used. In the last years, PulseNet networks have been established in other continents as well, linking laboratories from all over the world (http://www.pulsenetinternational.or) and facilitating rapid detection and comparison of strains (35, 52). Recently, PulseNet surveillance provided definitive linkages between ready-to-eat-meats and human cases in a large Canadian outbreak of listeriosis, resulting in 22 deaths and 57 confirmed cases (http://www.phac-aspc.gc.ca/alert-alerte/listeria/listeria_2009-eng.ph).

In the recent past, faster and simpler molecular subtyping methods, like multilocus variable-number tandem-repeat analysis and multilocus sequence typing, have evolved, and their application for subtyping of *L. monocytogenes* is supported by PulseNet. Both methods showed a discriminatory power comparable to that of PFGE (54, 67, 73, 94). Recently, a single-nucleotide-polymorphism-based multilocus genotyping assay that has a very high discriminatory power for all lineages of *L. monocytogenes* has been developed (23, 91). In addition, typing of *L. monocytogenes* isolates with a mixed-genome DNA microarray has been established (9, 22) and compared to PFGE, ribotyping, and multilocus sequence typing. Subtyping results were comparable to those obtained with PFGE (9).

Sequence-based molecular methods may further improve subtyping of *L. monocytogenes* and allow easier data comparison via the Internet. They may further replace typing methods with high discriminatory power but lacking interlaboratory standardization, like random amplification of polymorphic DNA (RAPD) (31), amplified fragment length polymorphism (31), multilocus single-strand conformation polymorphism (76), and ribotyping (46, 75).

As a new technique, MALDI-TOF (MS) has been recently introduced for rapid typing of *L. monocytogenes*. It allowed clear discrimination of all lineages and serotypes of *L. monocytogenes* (3). Reproducibility, speed, and simplicity are major advantages of the method.

Serologic Tests

Antibodies directed against listeriolysin-O have been detected in listeriosis patients by blotting techniques with sensitivities from 50 to 96%, but the sensitivity was markedly lower with complement fixation or O-agglutination tests (5, 63). A test based on the detection of antibodies against recombinant truncated forms of listeriolysin O may be more specific (36). Serologic tests cannot be recommended for the detection of past or acute listeriosis.

Antimicrobial Susceptibilities

Treatment with an aminopenicillin (ampicillin or amoxicillin) plus gentamicin is still regarded as the most effective therapeutic regimen for listeriosis, and in vitro resistance to ampicillin has not been described. Aminoglycosides exhibit a synergistic effect on penicillin and aminopenicillins. Trimethoprim-sulfamethoxazole is recommended for patients who are allergic to penicillin, and moxifloxacin may be a valuable alternative since it shows bactericidal efficacy comparable to that of amoxicillin in vitro (40). *L. monocytogenes* is intrinsically resistant to cephalosporins, fosfomycin, and fusidic acid, and even when in vitro susceptibility may be determined, cephalosporins should not be used for therapy. Isolated resistance against tetracycline has been noted (87) as well as multiresistance to chloramphenicol, macrolides, and tetracyclines due to the presence of resistance plasmids (42). Newer substances against gram-positive pathogens, like linezolid and daptomycin, elicited high susceptibility in vitro (44, 66, 74). In addition, *L. monocytogenes* is generally susceptible in vitro to erythromycin and vancomycin (81, 87). Antimicrobial susceptibility testing should be performed in cases of suspected treatment failures, severe disease, and patients with penicillin allergy. A CLSI guideline (M45-A2) for broth microdilution antimicrobial susceptibility testing of *L. monocytogenes* including interpretive breakpoints for penicillin, ampicillin, and trimethoprim-sulfamethoxazole is available (14).

Evaluation, Interpretation, and Reporting of Results

The diagnosis of listeriosis can be made by isolation of *L. monocytogenes* from blood, CSF, or specimens from other normally sterile sites. Species identification is necessary to differentiate *L. monocytogenes* from nonpathogenic *Listeria* species. Especially for patients with underlying immunosuppression and for individuals older than 60 years and younger than 1 month, direct microscopic detection of gram-positive, regular, short rods in the above-mentioned specimens should raise suspicion of listeriosis and should promptly be communicated to the clinician in order to ensure eradication of *L. monocytogenes* by antimicrobial therapy. While the presence of *L. monocytogenes* in specimens from normally sterile sites indicates infection and should always be reported, detection of *Listeria* species in stool samples likely represents colonization. Routine screening of stool samples for *Listeria* remains unwarranted, although sporadic cases of *L. monocytogenes* gastroenteritis have been reported (68).

Standard antimicrobial therapy of meningitis with cefotaxime or ceftriaxone is not active against *L. monocytogenes*. Antimicrobial susceptibility testing should be performed in cases of suspected treatment failures, severe disease, and patients with penicillin allergy. Cultures from blood and CSF that were obtained after the initiation of antimicrobial therapy may be negative. In these cases, detection of *Listeria* DNA may be useful. Commercial kits for PCR-based detection of *L. monocytogenes* in CSF specimens are not yet available, but in-house protocols and multiplex PCR formats are promising (10).

ERYSIPELOTHRIX

Taxonomy

The genus *Erysipelothrix* is taxonomically classified within the *Erysipelotrichaceae*, distinct from the order *Bacillales* (86). The genus *Erysipelothrix* has three validly published species, *E. rhusiopathiae*, *E. tonsillarum*, and the more recently described *E. inopinata* (51). Only *E. rhusiopathiae* has been detected as a pathogen of humans. Based on peptidoglycan antigens of the cell wall, several serovars can be distinguished in *E. rhusiopathiae* (serovars 1a, 1b, 2a, 2b, 3, 4, 5, 6, 8, 9, 11, 12, 15, 16, 17, 19, 21, and N) and *E. tonsillarum* (serovars 3, 7, 10, 14, 15, 16, 20, 22, and 23) (77). The vast majority of infections in humans are caused by serovars 1 and 2.

Description of the Agent

Erysipelothrix organisms are facultatively anaerobic, non-spore-forming, non-acid-fast, gram-positive bacteria that appear microscopically as short rods (0.2 to 0.5 μm by 0.8 to 2.5 μm) with rounded ends and occur singly, in short chains, or in long, nonbranching filaments (60 μm or more in length). Some cells stain unevenly. They are nonmotile and grow in complex media at a wide range of temperatures (5 to 42°C; optimum, 30 to 37°C) and at alkaline pH (pH 6.7 to 9.2; optimum, pH 7.2 to 7.6). Like *Listeria* organisms, they can grow in the presence of high concentrations of sodium chloride (up to 8.5%). *Erysipelothrix* organisms are catalase negative and oxidase negative, do not hydrolyze esculin, and weakly ferment glucose without the production of gas. They are methyl red and Voges-Proskauer negative and do not produce indole or hydrolyze urea but distinctively produce H_2S in triple sugar iron agar. Key fatty acids are $C_{16:0}$ and $C_{18:cis9}$ (6).

Epidemiology and Transmission

E. rhusiopathiae is distributed worldwide in nature and is remarkably stable under varying environmental conditions. The organism is carried by a variety of animals, like mammals, birds, and fish, in their digestive tract or tonsils but is most frequently associated with pigs. Other domestic animals that are frequently infected include sheep, rabbits, cattle, and turkeys. Infected animals, both sick and asymptomatic, pass the organism by urine and feces, leading to contamination of water and soil.

Infection in animals is most likely acquired by ingestion of contaminated matter. Human infection with *E. rhusiopathiae* is a zoonosis. Most cases are related to occupational exposure, occurring most frequently among fish handlers, veterinarians, and butchers. The disease is contracted through direct contact via skin abrasions, injuries, or animal bites (61).

E. tonsillarum has been recovered from tonsils of healthy pigs and cattle, water, and seafood. *E. inopinata* has been isolated once from a vegetable-based peptone broth.

Clinical Significance

E. rhusiopathiae has been recognized for more than 100 years as the agent of swine erysipelas, an acute or chronic disease. In humans, *E. rhusiopathiae* causes erysipeloid, a localized cellulitis developing within 2 to 7 days around the inoculation site. The infected area is swollen, and the mostly painful lesion consists of a well-defined, slightly elevated, violaceous zone which spreads peripherally as discoloration of the central area fades. Vesicles may be present, but suppuration does not occur. Regional lymphangitis is present in one-third of patients, and low-grade fever and arthralgias occur in about 10% of patients. Healing of erysipeloids usually takes 2 to 4 weeks and sometimes months, and relapses are frequently seen. Dissemination of the organism can occur and manifests in most of the cases as endocarditis with a poor prognosis (61). Uncommon manifestations of infection with *E. rhusiopathiae* include peritonitis, endophthalmitis, osteomyelitis, intracranial abscesses, and prosthetic joint arthritis (26, 80).

Progress has been made in the understanding of *E. rhusiopathiae* pathogenesis, although data are still scarce. *E. rhusiopathiae* has a capsule consisting of polysaccharide antigen that confers increased resistance to phagocytosis. Neuraminidase plays a significant role in bacterial attachment and subsequent invasion into host cells. The 69-kDa surface antigens SpaA, SpaB, and SpaC appear to be the major protective antigens of *E. rhusiopathiae*, and recombinant SpaA and SpaC elicit a protective immune response in pigs and mice, making them potential candidates for a new vaccine against erysipelas (70, 79).

Collection, Transport, and Storage of Specimens

Biopsy specimens from erysipeloid lesions are the best source of *E. rhusiopathiae*. Care should be taken to cleanse and disinfect the skin before sampling. The organisms typically are located deep in the subcutaneous layer of the leading edge of the lesion; hence, a biopsy of the entire thickness of the dermis at the periphery of the lesion should be taken for

Gram staining and culture. Swabs from the surface of the skin are not useful. In disseminated disease, the organism can be cultured in standard blood cultures or from aspirates of the respective infected location. For transport and storage of specimens standard procedures should be applied.

Direct Examination

Direct microscopy should be performed in aspirates, biopsy specimens, and positive blood cultures. Gram stain morphology of *E. rhusiopathiae* includes short rods and very long filaments and thus is not distinctive. However, the presence of long, slender, gram-positive rods in tissue from an individual with a known exposure is suggestive of erysipeloid. It has to be noted that the organism may appear gram negative in stains from cultures (see below).

PCR assays for specific detection of *E. rhusiopathiae* in animal tissue as well as for discrimination of *E. rhusiopathiae* from *E. tonsillarum* have been described (78, 92), but their application to human samples has not been evaluated yet.

Isolation Procedures

Tissue or biopsy specimens should be processed as described in chapter 16 and plated onto blood agar or chocolate blood agar, placed in tryptic soy, Schaedler, or thioglycolate broth, and incubated at 35 to 37°C aerobically or in 5% CO_2 for 7 days. Special pretreatment of samples is not necessary, but inoculation of an enrichment broth significantly increases the detection rate. Blood from patients with septicemia or endocarditis can be inoculated into commercial blood culture systems. *E. rhusiopathiae* colonies generally develop in 1 to 3 days, appearing as pinpoints (<0.1 to 0.5 mm in diameter) on blood agar plates after 24 h of incubation; at 48 h, two distinct colony types can be observed. The smaller, smooth colonies are 0.3 to 1.5 mm in diameter, transparent, convex, and circular with entire edges. Larger, rough colonies are flatter and more opaque and have a matte surface and an irregular, fimbriated edge. While a temperature of 37°C favors rough colonies, smooth colonies are favored at 30°C. A zone of greenish discoloration frequently develops underneath the colonies on blood agar plates after 2 days of incubation (48).

Identification

Cells stain gram positive, but especially those from rough colonies can decolorize and appear gram negative, sometimes with a beaded morphology. Cells from smooth colonies appear as rods or coccobacilli, sometimes in short chains. Cells from rough colonies appear as long filaments, often more than 60 μm in length.

E. rhusiopathiae is catalase negative; it also tests negative for nitrate, urease, esculin, gelatin, xylose, mannose, maltose, and sucrose but positive for glucose, lactose, and H_2S. The extent of H_2S production is influenced by the culture medium, and the strongest reaction is found on triple sugar iron agar. Vitek2 and Phoenix automated systems, as well as the API system (API Coryne, API ID 32 Strep), identify *E. rhusiopathiae* reliably. *E. tonsillarum* differs biochemically from *E. rhusiopathiae* by being sucrose positive.

Human-pathogenic genera that have morphological and physiological characteristics in common with *Erysipelothrix* include mainly *Lactobacillus* and *Listeria* (24). They are regular nonpigmented, non-spore-forming, gram-positive rods. A major discriminatory characteristic is that *E. rhusiopathiae* produces H_2S in triple sugar iron, whereas species of the other genera do not. Exceptions include some *Bacillus* strains, but they are easily differentiated from *E. rhusiopathiae* by cellular morphology,

spore formation, and catalase reaction. *Listeria* species are catalase positive, motile, esculin positive, and not alpha-hemolytic. Corynebacteria and streptococci also can be confused with *E. rhusiopathiae*, but careful examination of cell morphology should facilitate the distinction. An additional trait highly characteristic of *E. rhusiopathiae* is its "pipe cleaner" pattern of growth in gelatin stab cultures incubated at 22°C (48).

Typing Systems

Serotyping schemes are available for routine use in clinical laboratories but are of limited value since most clinical isolates belong to serovar 1 or 2. RAPD and ribotyping methods have proved useful for epidemiological analysis of *Erysipelothrix* strains (1, 58). PFGE using SmaI was superior to RAPD and ribotyping in discriminating *E. rhusiopathiae* isolates (58). Recently, nucleotide sequence analysis of a hypervariable region in the *spaA* gene has been introduced allowing discrimination of certain serovars of *E. rhusiopathiae* (55, 79).

Serologic Tests

Serologic tests for detection of antibodies to *E. rhusiopathiae* in humans are not available. Vaccines for active immunization of animals are available, and protective antibodies can be measured by enzyme immunoassay (45).

Antimicrobial Susceptibilities

Penicillin or ampicillin is the treatment of choice for both localized and systemic infections. Broad-spectrum cephalosporins or fluoroquinolones are suitable alternatives, since no resistance has been described yet. *E. rhusiopathiae* is also usually in vitro susceptible to clindamycin, erythromycin, daptomycin, imipenem, and tetracycline (30, 60). Of note, *E. rhusiopathiae* is intrinsically resistant to vancomycin and usually also to aminoglycosides and sulfonamides. Although antimicrobial susceptibility testing of isolates is not routinely required, testing of erythromycin and clindamycin, or further substances, may be warranted for patients with penicillin allergy. A CLSI guideline (M45-A2) for broth microdilution antimicrobial susceptibility testing of *Erysipelothrix* including interpretative breakpoints for penicillin, ampicillin, cefepime, cefotaxime, ceftriaxone, imipenem, meropenem, erythromycin, ciprofloxacin, gatifloxacin, levofloxacin, and clindamycin has been published (14).

Evaluation, Interpretation, and Reporting of Results

Since human infection is rare and clinical knowledge about the disease is scarce, diagnosis of erysipeloid is usually made accidentally by culture of *E. rhusiopathiae* from tissue biopsy specimens or blood. If there is no clinical suspicion, identification of *E. rhusiopathiae* in the clinical laboratory may be challenging. Detection of gram-positive and gram-variable rods, including decolorized, beaded cells and the presence of coccobacilli and very long filaments in direct microscopy of the specimens, gives a hint to this organism. A major discriminatory biochemical characteristic of *E. rhusiopathiae* is the production of H_2S.

Detection of *E. rhusiopathiae* in clinical samples should always be reported. Occurrence of this species in wound or tissue specimen indicates erysipeloid rather than contamination. Species identification is essential in order to ensure adequate antimicrobial therapy. While penicillin and ampicillin are generally active and recommended as first-line therapy, intrinsic resistance to vancomycin has to be noted.

REFERENCES

1. **Ahrne, S., I. M. Stenstrom, N. E. Jensen, B. Pettersson, M. Uhlen, and G. Molin.** 1995. Classification of *Erysipelothrix* strains on the basis of restriction fragment length polymorphisms. *Int. J. Syst. Bacteriol.* **45:**382–385.

2. **Aureli, P., G. C. Fiorucci, D. Caroli, G. Marchiaro, O. Novara, L. Leone, and S. Salmaso.** 2000. An outbreak of febrile gastroenteritis associated with corn contaminated by *Listeria monocytogenes.* *N. Engl. J. Med.* **342:**1236–1241.

3. **Barbuddhe, S. B., T. Maier, G. Schwarz, M. Kostrzewa, H. Hof, E. Domann, T. Chakraborty, and T. Hain.** 2008. Rapid identification and typing of *Listeria* species by matrix-assisted laser desorption ionization–time of flight mass spectrometry. *Appl. Environ. Microbiol.* **74:**5402–5407.

4. **Becker, B., S. Schuler, M. Lohneis, A. Sabrowski, G. D. Curtis, and W. H. Holzapfel.** 2006. Comparison of two chromogenic media for the detection of *Listeria monocytogenes* with the plating media recommended by EN/DIN 11290-1. *Int. J. Food Microbiol.* **109:**127–131.

5. **Berche, P., K. A. Reich, M. Bonnichon, J. L. Beretti, C. Geoffroy, J. Raveneau, P. Cossart, J. L. Gaillard, P. Geslin, and H. Kreis.** 1990. Detection of anti-listeriolysin O for serodiagnosis of human listeriosis. *Lancet* **335:**624–627.

6. **Bernard, K. A., M. Bellefeuille, and E. P. Ewan.** 1991. Cellular fatty acid composition as an adjunct to the identification of asporogenous, aerobic gram-positive rods. *J. Clin. Microbiol.* **29:**83–89.

7. **Bille, J., B. Catimel, E. Bannerman, C. Jacquet, M. N. Yersin, I. Caniaux, D. Monget, and J. Rocourt.** 1992. API *Listeria*, a new and promising one-day system to identify *Listeria* isolates. *Appl. Environ. Microbiol.* **58:**1857–1860.

8. **Boerlin, P., J. Rocourt, F. Grimont, P. A. D. Grimont, C. Jacquet, and J. C. Piffaretti.** 1992. *Listeria ivanovii* subsp. *londoniensis* subsp. nov. *Int. J. Syst. Bacteriol.* **42:**69–73.

9. **Borucki, M. K., S. H. Kim, D. R. Call, S. C. Smole, and F. Pagotto.** 2004. Selective discrimination of *Listeria monocytogenes* epidemic strains by a mixed-genome DNA microarray compared to discrimination by pulsed-field gel electrophoresis, ribotyping, and multilocus sequence typing. *J. Clin. Microbiol.* **42:**5270–5276.

10. **Boving, M. K., L. N. Pedersen, and J. K. Moller.** 2009. Eight-plex PCR and liquid array detection of bacterial and viral pathogens in cerebrospinal fluid from patients with suspected meningitis. *J. Clin. Microbiol.* **47:**908–913.

11. **Brosch, R., M. Brett, B. Catimel, J. B. Luchansky, B. Ojeniyi, and J. Rocourt.** 1996. Genomic fingerprinting of 80 strains from the WHO multicenter international typing study of *Listeria monocytogenes* via pulsed-field gel electrophoresis (PFGE). *Int. J. Food Microbiol.* **32:**343–355.

12. **Cairns, B. J., and R. J. Payne.** 2009. Sudden increases in listeriosis rates in England and Wales, 2001 and 2003. *Emerg. Infect. Dis.* **15:**465–468.

13. **Cepeda, J. A., M. Millar, E. A. Sheridan, S. Warwick, M. Raftery, D. C. Bean, and D. W. Wareham.** 2006. Listeriosis due to infection with a catalase-negative strain of *Listeria monocytogenes.* *J. Clin. Microbiol.* **44:**1917–1918.

14. **Clinical and Laboratory Standards Institute (CLSI).** 2010. *Methods for Antimicrobial Dilution and Disk Susceptibility Testing of Infrequently Isolated and Fastidious Bacteria. Approved Guideline M45-A2.* Clinical and Laboratory Standards Institute, Wayne, PA.

15. **Cole, M. B., M. V. Jones, and C. Holyoak.** 1990. The effect of pH, salt concentration and temperature on the survival and growth of *Listeria monocytogenes.* *J. Appl. Bacteriol.* **69:**63–72.

16. **Collins, M. D., S. Wallbanks, D. J. Lane, J. Shah, R. Nietupski, J. Smida, M. Dorsch, and E. Stackebrandt.** 1991. Phylogenetic analysis of the genus *Listeria* based on reverse transcriptase sequencing of 16S rRNA. *Int. J. Syst. Bacteriol.* **41:**240–246.

17. **Cummins, A. J., A. K. Fielding, and J. McLauchlin.** 1994. *Listeria ivanovii* infection in a patient with AIDS. *J. Infect.* **28:**89–91.

18. **Dever, F. P., D. W. Schaffner, and P. J. Slade.** 1993. Methods for the detection of foodborne *Listeria monocytogenes* in the U.S. *J. Food Saf.* **13:**263–292.

19. **Doganay, M.** 2003. Listeriosis: clinical presentation. *FEMS Immunol. Med. Microbiol.* **35:**173–175.

20. **Doumith, M., C. Buchrieser, P. Glaser, C. Jacquet, and P. Martin.** 2004. Differentiation of the major *Listeria monocytogenes* serovars by multiplex PCR. *J. Clin. Microbiol.* **42:**3819–3822.

21. **Doumith, M., C. Jacquet, P. Gerner-Smidt, L. M. Graves, S. Loncarevic, T. Mathisen, A. Morvan, C. Salcedo, M. Torpdahl, J. A. Vazquez, and P. Martin.** 2005. Multicenter validation of a multiplex PCR assay for differentiating the major *Listeria monocytogenes* serovars 1/2a, 1/2b, 1/2c, and 4b: toward an international standard. *J. Food Prot.* **68:**2648–2650.

22. **Doumith, M., C. Jacquet, V. Goulet, C. Oggioni, L. F. Van, C. Buchrieser, and P. Martin.** 2006. Use of DNA arrays for the analysis of outbreak-related strains of *Listeria monocytogenes.* *Int. J. Med. Microbiol.* **296:**559–562.

23. **Ducey, T. F., B. Page, T. Usgaard, M. K. Borucki, K. Pupedis, and T. J. Ward.** 2007. A single-nucleotide-polymorphism-based multilocus genotyping assay for subtyping lineage I isolates of *Listeria monocytogenes.* *Appl. Environ. Microbiol.* **73:**133–147.

24. **Dunbar, S. A., and J. E. Clarridge III.** 2000. Potential errors in recognition of *Erysipelothrix rhusiopathiae.* *J. Clin. Microbiol.* **38:**1302–1304.

25. **Elsner, H. A., I. Sobottka, A. Bubert, H. Albrecht, R. Laufs, and D. Mack.** 1996. Catalase-negative *Listeria monocytogenes* causing lethal sepsis and meningitis in an adult hematologic patient. *Eur. J. Clin. Microbiol. Infect. Dis.* **15:**965–967.

26. **Elvy, J., I. Hanspal, and P. Simcock.** 2008. A case of *Erysipelothrix rhusiopathiae* causing bilateral endogenous endophthalmitis. *J. Clin. Pathol.* **61:**1223–1224.

27. **Farber, J. M., and P. I. Peterkin.** 1991. *Listeria monocytogenes,* a food-borne pathogen. *Microbiol. Rev.* **55:**476–511.

28. **Farber, J. M., P. I. Peterkin, A. O. Carter, P. V. Varughese, F. E. Ashton, and E. P. Ewan.** 1991. Neonatal listeriosis due to cross-infection confirmed by isoenzyme typing and DNA fingerprinting. *J. Infect. Dis.* **163:**927–928.

29. **Feresu, S. B., and D. Jones.** 1988. Taxonomic studies on *Brochothrix, Erysipelothrix, Listeria* and atypical lactobacilli. *J. Gen. Microbiol.* **134:**1165–1183.

30. **Fidalgo, S. G., C. J. Longbottom, and T. V. Rjley.** 2002. Susceptibility of *Erysipelothrix rhusiopathiae* to antimicrobial agents and home disinfectants. *Pathology* **34:**462–465.

31. **Fonnesbech, V. B., V. Fussing, B. Ojeniyi, L. Gram, and P. Ahrens.** 2004. High-resolution genotyping of *Listeria monocytogenes* by fluorescent amplified fragment length polymorphism analysis compared to pulsed-field gel electrophoresis, random amplified polymorphic DNA analysis, ribotyping, and PCR-restriction fragment length polymorphism analysis. *J. Food Prot.* **67:**1656–1665.

32. **Food and Drug Administration, U.S. Department of Agriculture, and Centers for Disease Control and Prevention.** 2003. Quantitative assessment of relative risk to public health from foodborne *Listeria monocytogenes* among selected categories of ready-to-eat food. http://www.cfsan.fda.gov.

33. **Funke, G., F. N. Renaud, J. Freney, and P. Riegel.** 1997. Multicenter evaluation of the updated and extended API (RAPID) *Coryne* database 2.0. *J. Clin. Microbiol.* **35:**3122–3126.

34. **Gasanov, U., D. Hughes, and P. M. Hansbro.** 2005. Methods for the isolation and identification of *Listeria* spp. and *Listeria monocytogenes:* a review. *FEMS Microbiol. Rev.* **29:**851–875.

35. **Gerner-Smidt, P., K. Hise, J. Kincaid, S. Hunter, S. Rolando, E. Hyytia-Trees, E. M. Ribot, and B. Swaminathan.** 2006. PulseNet USA: a five-year update. *Foodborne Pathog. Dis.* **3:**9–19.

36. **Gholizadeh, Y., C. Poyart, M. Juvin, J. L. Beretti, J. Croize, P. Berche, and J. L. Gaillard.** 1996. Serodiagnosis of listeriosis based upon detection of antibodies against recombinant

truncated forms of listeriolysin O. *J. Clin. Microbiol.* **34:** 1391–1395.

37. **Goulet, V., C. Hedberg, A. Le Monnier, and H. de Valk.** 2008. Increasing incidence of listeriosis in France and other European countries. *Emerg. Infect. Dis.* **14:**734–740.

38. **Graves, L. M., L. O. Helsel, A. G. Steigerwalt, R. E. Morey, M. I. Daneshvar, S. E. Roof, R. H. Orsi, E. D. Fortes, S. R. Millilo, H. C. den Bakker, M. Wiedmann, B. Swaminathan, and B. D. Sauders.** 2010. *Listeria marthii* sp. nov., isolated from the natural environment, Finger Lakes National Forest. *Int. J. Syst. Evol. Microbiol.* **60:** 1280–1288.

39. **Graves, L. M., and B. Swaminathan.** 2001. PulseNet standardized protocol for subtyping *Listeria monocytogenes* by macrorestriction and pulsed-field gel electrophoresis. *Int. J. Food Microbiol.* **65:**55–62.

40. **Grayo, S., O. Join-Lambert, M. C. Desroches, and M. A. Le.** 2008. Comparison of the in vitro efficacies of moxifloxacin and amoxicillin against *Listeria monocytogenes. Antimicrob. Agents Chemother.* **52:**1697–1702.

41. **Grif, K., G. Patscheider, M. P. Dierich, and F. Allerberger.** 2003. Incidence of fecal carriage of *Listeria monocytogenes* in three healthy volunteers: a one-year prospective stool survey. *Eur. J. Clin. Microbiol. Infect. Dis.* **22:**16–20.

42. **Hadorn, K., H. Hachler, A. Schaffner, and F. H. Kayser.** 1993. Genetic characterization of plasmid-encoded multiple antibiotic resistance in a strain of *Listeria monocytogenes* causing endocarditis. *Eur. J. Clin. Microbiol. Infect. Dis.* **12:** 928–937.

43. **Hegde, V., C. G. Leon-Velarde, C. M. Stam, L. A. Jaykus, and J. A. Odumeru.** 2007. Evaluation of BBL CHROMagar *Listeria* agar for the isolation and identification of *Listeria monocytogenes* from food and environmental samples. *J. Microbiol. Methods* **68:**82–87.

44. **Hof, H.** 2004. An update on the medical management of listeriosis. *Expert Opin. Pharmacother.* **5:**1727–1735.

45. **Imada, Y., Y. Mori, M. Daizoh, K. Kudoh, and T. Sakano.** 2003. Enzyme-linked immunosorbent assay employing a recombinant antigen for detection of protective antibody against swine erysipelas. *J. Clin. Microbiol.* **41:** 5015–5021.

46. **Jacquet, C., J. Bille, and J. Rocourt.** 1992. Typing of *Listeria monocytogenes* by restriction polymorphism of the ribosomal ribonucleic acid gene region. *Zentralbl. Bakteriol.* **276:**356–365.

47. **Johnson, J., K. Jinneman, G. Stelma, B. G. Smith, D. Lye, J. Messer, J. Ulaszek, L. Evsen, S. Gendel, R. W. Bennett, B. Swaminathan, J. Pruckler, A. Steigerwalt, S. Kathariou, S. Yildirim, D. Volokhov, A. Rasooly, V. Chizhikov, M. Wiedmann, E. Fortes, R. E. Duvall, and A. D. Hitchins.** 2004. Natural atypical *Listeria innocua* strains with *Listeria monocytogenes* pathogenicity island 1 genes. *Appl. Environ. Microbiol.* **70:**4256–4266.

48. **Jones, D.** 1986. Genus *Erysipelothrix* Rosenbach 1909, p. 1245–1249. *In* P. H. A. Sneath, N. S. Mair, M. E. Shape, and J. G. Holt (ed.), *Bergey's Manual of Systematic Bacteriology,* vol. 2. Williams & Wilkins, Baltimore, MD.

49. **Lecuit, M., D. M. Nelson, S. D. Smith, H. Khun, M. Huerre, M. C. Vacher-Lavenu, J. I. Gordon, and P. Cossart.** 2004. Targeting and crossing of the human maternofetal barrier by *Listeria monocytogenes*: role of internalin interaction with trophoblast E-cadherin. *Proc. Natl. Acad. Sci. USA* **101:** 6152–6157.

50. **Lee, W. H., and D. McClain.** 1986. Improved *Listeria monocytogenes* selective agar. *Appl. Environ. Microbiol.* **52:** 1215–1217.

51. **Ludwig, W., K.-H. Schleifer, and W. B. Whitman.** 2009. Revised road map to the phylum Firmicutes. *In* P. De Vos et al. (ed.), *Bergey's Manual of Systematic Bacteriology,* 2nd ed., vol. 3. *The Firmicutes.* Springer-Verlag, New York, NY.

52. **Martin, P., C. Jacquet, V. Goulet, V. Vaillant, and V. H. De.** 2006. Pulsed-field gel electrophoresis of *Listeria monocytogenes* strains: the PulseNet Europe Feasibility Study. *Foodborne Pathog. Dis.* **3:**303–308.

53. **McLauchlin, J., and J. C. Low.** 1994. Primary cutaneous listeriosis in adults: an occupational disease of veterinarians and farmers. *Vet. Rec.* **135:**615–617.

54. **Murphy, M., D. Corcoran, J. F. Buckley, M. O'Mahony, P. Whyte, and S. Fanning.** 2007. Development and application of multiple-locus variable number of tandem repeat analysis (MLVA) to subtype a collection of *Listeria monocytogenes. Int. J. Food Microbiol.* **115:**187–194.

55. **Nagai, S., H. To, and A. Kanda.** 2008. Differentiation of *Erysipelothrix rhusiopathiae* strains by nucleotide sequence analysis of a hypervariable region in the spaA gene: discrimination of a live vaccine strain from field isolates. *J. Vet. Diagn. Investig.* **20:**336–342.

56. **Ninet, B., E. Bannerman, and J. Bille.** 1992. Assessment of the Accuprobe *Listeria monocytogenes* culture identification reagent kit for rapid colony confirmation and its application in various enrichment broths. *Appl. Environ. Microbiol.* **58:**4055–4059.

57. **Odumeru, J. A., M. Steele, L. Fruhner, C. Larkin, J. Jiang, E. Mann, and W. B. McNab.** 1999. Evaluation of accuracy and repeatability of identification of food-borne pathogens by automated bacterial identification systems. *J. Clin. Microbiol.* **37:**944–949.

58. **Okatani, T. A., M. Ishikawa, S. Yoshida, M. Sekiguchi, K. Tanno, M. Ogawa, T. Horikita, T. Horisaka, T. Taniguchi, Y. Kato, and H. Hayashidani.** 2004. Automated ribotyping, a rapid typing method for analysis of *Erysipelothrix* spp. strains. *J. Vet. Med. Sci.* **66:**729–733.

59. **Ooi, S. T., and B. Lorber.** 2005. Gastroenteritis due to *Listeria monocytogenes. Clin. Infect. Dis.* **40:**1327–1332.

60. **Piper, K. E., J. M. Steckelberg, and R. Patel.** 2005. In vitro activity of daptomycin against clinical isolates of Gram-positive bacteria. *J. Infect. Chemother.* **11:**207–209.

61. **Reboli, A. C., and W. E. Farrar.** 1989. *Erysipelothrix rhusiopathiae*: an occupational pathogen. *Clin. Microbiol. Rev.* **2:**354–359.

62. **Reissbrodt, R.** 2004. New chromogenic plating media for detection and enumeration of pathogenic *Listeria* spp.—an overview. *Int. J. Food Microbiol.* **95:**1–9.

63. **Renneberg, J., K. Persson, and P. Christensen.** 1990. Western blot analysis of the antibody response in patients with *Listeria monocytogenes* meningitis and septicemia. *Eur. J. Clin. Microbiol. Infect. Dis.* **9:**659–663.

64. **Restaino, L., E. W. Frampton, R. M. Irbe, G. Schabert, and H. Spitz.** 1999. Isolation and detection of *Listeria monocytogenes* using fluorogenic and chromogenic substrates for phosphatidylinositol-specific phospholipase C. *J. Food Prot.* **62:**244–251.

65. **Roberts, A. J., and M. Wiedmann.** 2003. Pathogen, host and environmental factors contributing to the pathogenesis of listeriosis. *Cell. Mol. Life Sci.* **60:**904–918.

66. **Salas, C., J. Calvo, and L. Martinez-Martinez.** 2008. Activity of tigecycline against coryneform bacteria of clinical interest and *Listeria monocytogenes. Antimicrob. Agents Chemother.* **52:**1503–1505.

67. **Salcedo, C., L. Arreaza, B. Alcala, L. de la Fuente, and J. A. Vazquez.** 2003. Development of a multilocus sequence typing method for analysis of *Listeria monocytogenes* clones. *J. Clin. Microbiol.* **41:**757–762.

68. **Schlech, W. F., III, P. M. Lavigne, R. A. Bortolussi, A. C. Allen, E. V. Haldane, A. J. Wort, A. W. Hightower, S. E. Johnson, S. H. King, E. S. Nicholls, and C. V. Broome.** 1983. Epidemic listeriosis—evidence for transmission by food. *N. Engl. J. Med.* **308:**203–206.

69. **Schuchat, A., C. Lizano, C. V. Broome, B. Swaminathan, C. Kim, and K. Winn.** 1991. Outbreak of neonatal listeriosis associated with mineral oil. *Pediatr. Infect. Dis. J.* **10:**183–189.

70. **Shimoji, Y.** 2000. Pathogenicity of *Erysipelothrix rhusiopathiae*: virulence factors and protective immunity. *Microbes Infect.* **2:**965–972.

71. **Smith, M. A., K. Takeuchi, G. Anderson, G. O. Ware, H. M. McClure, R. B. Raybourne, N. Mytle, and M. P. Doyle.** 2008. Dose-response model for *Listeria monocytogenes*-induced stillbirths in nonhuman primates. *Infect. Immun.* **76:**726–731.

72. **Snapir, Y. M., E. Vaisbein, and F. Nassar.** 2006. Low virulence but potentially fatal outcome-*Listeria ivanovii*. *Eur. J. Intern. Med.* **17:**286–287.

73. **Sperry, K. E., S. Kathariou, J. S. Edwards, and L. A. Wolf.** 2008. Multiple-locus variable-number tandem-repeat analysis as a tool for subtyping *Listeria monocytogenes* strains. *J. Clin. Microbiol.* **46:**1435–1450.

74. **Streit, J. M., R. N. Jones, and H. S. Sader.** 2004. Daptomycin activity and spectrum: a worldwide sample of 6737 clinical Gram-positive organisms. *J. Antimicrob. Chemother.* **53:**669–674.

75. **Swaminathan, B., S. B. Hunter, P. M. Desmarchelier, P. Gerner-Smidt, L. M. Graves, S. Harlander, R. Hubner, C. Jacquet, B. Pedersen, K. Reineccius, A. Ridley, N. A. Saunders, and J. A. Webster.** 1996. WHO-sponsored international collaborative study to evaluate methods for subtyping *Listeria monocytogenes*: restriction fragment length polymorphism (RFLP) analysis using ribotyping and Southern hybridization with two probes derived from *L. monocytogenes* chromosome. *Int. J. Food Microbiol.* **32:**263–278.

76. **Takahashi, H., S. Handa-Miya, B. Kimura, M. Sato, A. Yokoi, S. Goto, I. Watanabe, T. Koda, K. Hisa, and T. Fujii.** 2007. Development of multilocus single strand conformation polymorphism (MLSSCP) analysis of virulence genes of *Listeria monocytogenes* and comparison with existing DNA typing methods. *Int. J. Food Microbiol.* **118:**274–284.

77. **Takahashi, T., T. Fujisawa, A. Umeno, T. Kozasa, K. Yamamoto, and T. Sawada.** 2008. A taxonomic study on *Erysipelothrix* by DNA-DNA hybridization experiments with numerous strains isolated from extensive origins. *Microbiol. Immunol.* **52:**469–478.

78. **Takeshi, K., S. Makino, T. Ikeda, N. Takada, A. Nakashiro, K. Nakanishi, K. Oguma, Y. Katoh, H. Sunagawa, and T. Ohyama.** 1999. Direct and rapid detection by PCR of *Erysipelothrix* sp. DNAs prepared from bacterial strains and animal tissues. *J. Clin. Microbiol.* **37:**4093–4098.

79. **To, H., and S. Nagai.** 2007. Genetic and antigenic diversity of the surface protective antigen proteins of *Erysipelothrix rhusiopathiae*. *Clin. Vaccine Immunol.* **14:**813–820.

80. **Traer, E. A., M. R. Williams, and J. N. Keenan.** 2008. *Erysipelothrix rhusiopathiae* infection of a total knee arthroplasty an occupational hazard. *J. Arthroplasty* **23:**609–611.

81. **Troxler, R., A. vonGraevenitz, G. Funke, B. Wiedemann, and I. Stock.** 2000. Natural antibiotic susceptibility of *Listeria* species: *L. grayi, L. innocua, L. ivanovii, L. monocytogenes, L. seeligeri* and *L. welshimeri* strains. *Clin. Microbiol. Infect.* **6:**525–535.

82. **U.S. Department of Agriculture.** 2008. *Microbiology Laboratory Guidebook* (online), Chapter 8.06, 19.02.2008. http://www.fsis.usda.gov/Science/Microbiological_Lab_Guidebook/index.asp.

83. **U.S. Food and Drug Administration.** 2003. *Bacteriological Analytical Manual: Listeria monocytogenes*. http://www.fda.gov/Food/ScienceResearch/LaboratoryMethods/BacteriologicalAnalyticalManualBAM/default.htm.

84. **van Netten, P., I. Perales, A. van de Moosdijk, G. D. Curtis, and D. A. Mossel.** 1989. Liquid and solid selective differential media for the detection and enumeration of *L. monocytogenes* and other *Listeria* spp. *Int. J. Food Microbiol.* **8:**299–316.

85. **Vazquez-Boland, J. A., L. Dominguez, J. F. Fernandez, E. F. Rodriguez-Ferri, V. Briones, M. Blanco, and G. Suarez.** 1990. Revision of the validity of CAMP tests for *Listeria* identification. Proposal of an alternative method for the determination of haemolytic activity by *Listeria* strains. *Acta Microbiol. Hung.* **37:**201–206.

86. **Verbarg, S., H. Rheims, S. Emus, A. Fruhling, R. M. Kroppenstedt, E. Stackebrandt, and P. Schumann.** 2004. *Erysipelothrix inopinata* sp. nov., isolated in the course of sterile filtration of vegetable peptone broth, and description of *Erysipelotrichaceae* fam. nov. *Int. J. Syst. Evol. Microbiol.* **54:**221–225.

87. **Vitas, A. I., R. M. Sanchez, V. Aguado, and I. Garcia-Jalon.** 2007. Antimicrobial susceptibility of *Listeria monocytogenes* isolated from food and clinical cases in Navarra, Spain. *J. Food Prot.* **70:**2402–2406.

88. **Vlaemynck, G., V. Lafarge, and S. Scotter.** 2000. Improvement of the detection of *Listeria monocytogenes* by the application of ALOA, a diagnostic, chromogenic isolation medium. *J. Appl. Microbiol.* **88:**430–441.

89. **Voetsch, A. C., F. J. Angulo, T. F. Jones, M. R. Moore, C. Nadon, P. McCarthy, B. Shiferaw, M. B. Megginson, S. Hurd, B. J. Anderson, A. Cronquist, D. J. Vugia, C. Medus, S. Segler, L. M. Graves, R. M. Hoekstra, and P. M. Griffin.** 2007. Reduction in the incidence of invasive listeriosis in foodborne diseases active surveillance network sites, 1996–2003. *Clin. Infect. Dis.* **44:**513–520.

90. **Volokhov, D., J. George, C. Anderson, R. E. Duvall, and A. D. Hitchins.** 2006. Discovery of natural atypical non-hemolytic *Listeria seeligeri* isolates. *Appl. Environ. Microbiol.* **72:**2439–2448.

91. **Ward, T. J., T. F. Ducey, T. Usgaard, K. A. Dunn, and J. P. Bielawski.** 2008. Multilocus genotyping assays for single nucleotide polymorphism-based subtyping of *Listeria monocytogenes* isolates. *Appl. Environ. Microbiol.* **74:** 7629–7642.

92. **Yamazaki, Y.** 2006. A multiplex polymerase chain reaction for discriminating *Erysipelothrix rhusiopathiae* from *Erysipelothrix tonsillarum*. *J. Vet. Diagn. Investig.* **18:**384–387.

93. **You, Y., C. Fu, X. Zeng, D. Fang, X. Yan, B. Sun, D. Xiao, and J. Zhang.** 2008. A novel DNA microarray for rapid diagnosis of enteropathogenic bacteria in stool specimens of patients with diarrhea. *J. Microbiol. Methods* **75:** 566–571.

94. **Zhang, W., B. M. Jayarao, and S. J. Knabel.** 2004. Multi-virulence-locus sequence typing of *Listeria monocytogenes*. *Appl. Environ. Microbiol.* **70:**913–920.

Coryneform Gram-Positive Rods

GUIDO FUNKE AND KATHRYN A. BERNARD

26

This chapter deals with aerobically growing, asporogenous, irregularly shaped, non-partially acid-fast, gram-positive rods generally called "coryneforms." The term "coryneform" is actually somewhat misleading since only true *Corynebacterium* spp. exhibit a typical club-shaped ("coryne," meaning "club" in ancient Greek) morphology, whereas all the other bacteria discussed in this chapter show an irregular morphology. However, in our experience, the term "coryneforms" is a common and convenient expression used by many clinical microbiologists, and therefore, the term will be used in this chapter.

The coryneform bacteria which were, for didactical reasons, not included in this chapter comprise *Actinomyces* spp. (in particular, the most frequently encountered species on aerobic plates, *A. europaeus, A. neuii, A. radingae,* and *A. turicensis), Actinobaculum* spp., *Propionibacterium* spp., and *Propioniferax* sp. (see chapter 49 in this *Manual),* whereas *Arcanobacterium* spp. and *Gardnerella* are included. Regularly shaped aerobically growing gram-positive rods (*Bacillus, Listeria* and *Erysipelothrix, Lactobacillus,* and *Clostridium tertium)* are covered in chapters 24, 25, 49, and 50, respectively. Taxa which might initially be misidentified as coryneform bacteria also include partially acid-fast bacteria and other aerobic actinomycetes (see chapter 27) as well as rapidly growing mycobacteria (see chapter 30).

TAXONOMY

The bacteria discussed in this chapter all belong to the class *Actinobacteria,* the genera of which are characterized by specific 16S rRNA gene signature nucleotides (144, 168) belonging to the lineage of gram-positive bacteria with high guanine-plus-cytosine (G+C) contents, with the exception of the genus *Exiguobacterium,* which belongs to the class *Firmicutes,* the members of which have low G+C contents. The coryneform bacteria are most diverse and are differentiated by chemotaxonomic features (Table 1). Phylogenetic investigations, in particular, 16S rRNA gene sequencing, have in general confirmed the framework set by chemotaxonomic investigations. The 16S rRNA gene sequencing data demonstrate that the genera *Corynebacterium* and *Turicella* are more closely related to the partially acid-fast bacteria and to the genus *Mycobacterium* than to the other coryneform organisms covered in this chapter (71, 108, 133). The genus *Arthrobacter,* which contains rods, is phylogenetically intermixed with the genus *Micrococcus*

(and genera formerly called *Micrococcus),* which contains cocci (see chapter 19) (54, 84). The genus *Rothia* contains both rod-forming organisms, represented by *Rothia dentocariosa,* and a coccus-forming species, *Rothia mucilaginosa,* formerly *Stomatococcus mucilaginosus* (24). Other genera which are phylogenetically closely related include *Oerskovia, Cellulosimicrobium,* and *Cellulomonas* (14, 64, 137, 143), as well as *Arcanobacterium* and *Actinomyces* (109).

DESCRIPTIONS OF THE GENERA

Genus *Corynebacterium*

The number of species belonging to the genus *Corynebacterium* has dramatically increased from 22 in 1990 to 81 species (and one taxon group) at the time of writing, 50 of which (and one taxon group) are medically relevant. Clinically relevant *Corynebacterium* species validly described since the last edition of this *Manual* include *C. canis* (50), *C. freiburgense* (53), *C. hansenii* (119), *C. massiliense* (96), *C. pilbarense* (3), *C. pyruviciproducens* (151), *C. sputi* (164), *C. stationis* (9), *C. timonense* (96), and *C. ureicelerivorans* (163).

The cell walls of corynebacteria contain *meso*-diaminopimelic acid (*m*-DAP) as the diamino acid as well as short-chain mycolic acids with 22 to 36 carbon atoms (22). The medically relevant *Corynebacterium* species *C. amycolatum, C. atypicum,* and *C. kroppenstedtii* as well as *C. caspium* (from seals) and *C. ciconiae* (from storks) lack mycolates (21, 23, 77). The corynebacterial cell wall contains arabinose and galactose (22). Palmitic ($C_{16:0}$), oleic ($C_{18:1\omega9c}$), and stearic ($C_{18:0}$) acids are the main cellular fatty acids (CFAs) in all corynebacteria, and tuberculostearic acid (TBSA) can be detected in some medically relevant *Corynebacterium* species (e.g., *C. urealyticum, C. kroppenstedtii, C. confusum, C. appendicis,* and *C. minutissimum)* (7, 23, 61, 165). The G+C contents of *Corynebacterium* spp. vary from 46 to 74 mol%, indicating the enormous diversity within this genus. The phylogenetic relationships within the genus *Corynebacterium* have been outlined previously (108, 133), creating an extensive and reliable database for future comparative 16S rRNA gene studies, e.g., for the delineation of new species. Complete genome sequences for *Corynebacterium diphtheriae* (17), *Corynebacterium jeikeium* (148), *C. urealyticum* (150), and *C. kroppenstedtii* (149) have been described previously.

TABLE 1 Some chemotaxonomic features of the bacteria covered in this chapter

Genus	Major CFAs	Mycolic acids	Peptidoglycan diamino acid[a]	Acyl type[c]
Corynebacterium	18:1ω9c, 16:0, 18:0	+[b]	m-DAP	Acetyl
Turicella	18:1ω9c, 16:0, 18:0	−	m-DAP	Glycolyl
Arthrobacter	15:0ai, 17:0ai, 15:0i	−	LYS	Acetyl
Brevibacterium	15:0ai, 17:0ai, 15:0i	−	m-DAP	Acetyl
Dermabacter	17:0ai, 15:0ai, 16:0i	−	m-DAP	ND
Helcobacillus	17:0ai, 15:0ai, 16:0i	−	m-DAP	ND
Rothia	15:0ai, 17:0ai, 16:0i	−	LYS	ND
Exiguobacterium	17:0ai, 15:0ai, 16:0, 13:0i	−	LYS	ND
Oerskovia	15:0ai, 15:0i, 17:0ai	−	LYS	Acetyl
Cellulomonas	15:0ai, 16:0, 17:0ai	−	ORN	Acetyl
Cellulosimicrobium	15:0ai, 15:0i, 17:0ai	−	LYS	Acetyl
Microbacterium	15:0ai, 17:0ai, 16:0i	−	LYS, ORN	Glycolyl
Curtobacterium	15:0ai, 17:0ai, 16:0i	−	ORN	Acetyl
Leifsonia	17:0ai, 15:0ai, 16:0i	−	DAB	ND
Janibacter	17:1, 16:0i, 17:0	−	m-DAP	Acetyl
Pseudoclavibacter	15:0ai, 17:0ai, 16:0i, 16:0	−	DAB	Acetyl
Brachybacterium	15:0ai, 16:0i, 17:0ai	−	m-DAP	Acetyl
Knoellia	17:1i, 15:0i, 16:0i, 17:0i	−	m-DAP	Acetyl
Arcanobacterium	18:1ω9c, 16:0, 18:0	−	LYS	ND
Gardnerella	16:0, 18:1ω9c, 14:0	−	LYS	ND

[a]m-DAP, *meso*-diaminopimelic acid; LYS, lysine; ORN, ornithine; DAB, diaminobutyric acid.
[b]Exceptions: *C. amycolatum*, *C. atypicum*, and *C. kroppenstedtii*.
[c]ND, no data.

Gram staining of corynebacteria shows slightly curved, gram-positive rods with sides not parallel and sometimes slightly wider ends, giving some of the bacteria a typical club shape (Fig. 1a). Corynebacteria whose morphologies differ from this morphology include *C. canis*, *C. durum*, *C. matruchotii*, and *C. sundsvallense* (see below under each species' name). Cells generally stain evenly. If *Corynebacterium* cells are taken from fluid media, they are arranged as single cells, in pairs, in V forms, in palisades, or in clusters with a so-called Chinese-letter appearance. It is again emphasized that the club-shaped form of the rods is observed only for true *Corynebacterium* spp.

All medically relevant taxa in the genus *Corynebacterium* are catalase positive and nonmotile. The genus *Corynebacterium* includes both fermenting and nonfermenting species.

Genus *Turicella*

The genus *Turicella* is phylogenetically closely related to the genus *Corynebacterium* but contains *Turicella otitidis* as the only species. The cell wall contains *m*-DAP, but mycolic acids are not present (71). The main CFAs for *T. otitidis* are the same as those for *Corynebacterium* spp., but all *T. otitidis* strains also contain significant amounts of TBSA (2 to 10% of all CFAs) (71). *T. otitidis* is the only coryneform bacterium that has a polar lipid profile without glycolipids. The G+C content varies between 65 and 72 mol% (71). Gram staining shows relatively long gram-positive rods (Fig. 1b). *T. otitidis* is catalase positive, nonmotile, and an oxidizer.

Genus *Arthrobacter*

The genera *Arthrobacter* and *Micrococcus* are so closely related phylogenetically that it has been stated that micrococci are, in fact, arthrobacters which are unable to express rod forms (84). Presently, the genus *Arthrobacter* contains over 50 species, of which only a few have been recovered from human clinical specimens (92). Lysine is the diamino

acid of the cell wall, and C[15:0ai] is the overall dominating CFA; it represents more than 50% of all CFAs in most *Arthrobacter* species. The G+C contents vary between 59 and 70 mol%, indicating the diversity within this genus.

Gram staining may demonstrate a rod-coccus cycle (i.e., rod forms in younger cultures and cocci in older colonies) when cells are grown on rich media (e.g., Columbia base agar). Jointed rods (i.e., rods in a rectangular form that contributed to the designation of this genus as "arthros," which means "joint" in ancient Greek) may also be observed in younger cultures (i.e., at 24 h) but may not be demonstrable for every species. Arthrobacters are catalase positive, their motility is variable, and they are always oxidizers.

Genus *Brevibacterium*

The genus *Brevibacterium* presently comprises 22 species, of which 9 species are medically relevant. *m*-DAP is the diamino acid type found in the cell wall. C[15:0ai] and C[17:0ai] usually represent more than 75% of all CFAs (48). The G+C contents vary between 60 and 70 mol%.

Gram staining demonstrates relatively short rods, which may develop into cocci when cultures become older (after 3 days). Brevibacteria are catalase positive, nonmotile, and oxidizers.

Genus *Dermabacter*

The genus *Dermabacter* presently comprises only one species, *D. hominis*. *m*-DAP is the diamino acid of the cell wall, and C[15:0ai] and C[17:0ai] usually account for 40 to 60% of all CFAs. The G+C content range is between 60 and 62 mol% (81). Gram staining shows very short rods (Fig. 1c), which are often initially misinterpreted as cocci. *D. hominis* strains are catalase positive, nonmotile, and glucose fermenters.

Genus *Helcobacillus*

The genus *Helcobacillus*, part of the family *Dermabacteraceae*, has been described for an isolate recovered from

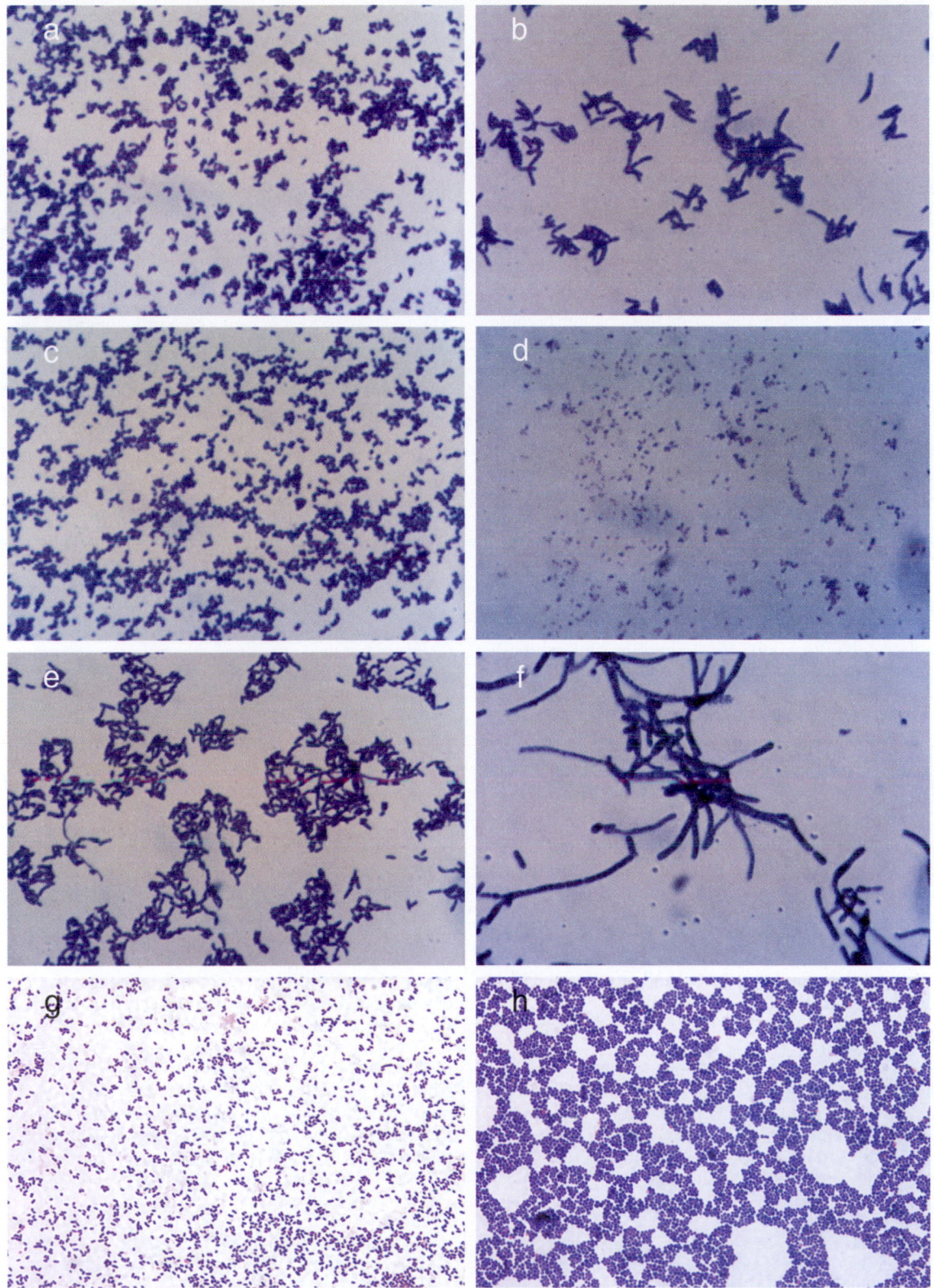

FIGURE 1 Gram stain morphologies of *Corynebacterium diphtheriae* ATCC 14779 after 48 h of incubation (a), *Turicella otitidis* DSM 8821 (48 h) (b), *Dermabacter hominis* ATCC 51325 (48 h) (c), *Gardnerella vaginalis* ATCC 14018 (48 h) (d), *Corynebacterium durum* DMMZ 2544 (72 h) (e), and *Corynebacterium matruchotii* ATCC 14266 (24 h) (f), *Corynebacterium aurimucosum* HC-NML 91-0032 (24 h) (g), and black-pigmented *Rothia dentocariosa* HC-NML 77-0298 (24 h) (h).

a patient with a cutaneous discharge presenting with an erythrasma. Interestingly, phenotypic features of the bacterium were initially thought to be suggestive of *C. minutissimum* but later, by a polyphasic approach, of *D. hominis*. The Gram stain shows gram-positive, straight, short (0.7 to 1.0 μm in length by 0.4 to 0.7 μm in diameter), irregular rods. Colonies are apigmented. The type strain is catalase positive, nonmotile, and a glucose fermenter. This taxon is amycolated, with a G+C content of 68.6 mol%; *m*-DAP is the cell wall diamino acid, with the CFAs $C_{15:0ai}$, $C_{17:0ai}$, and $C_{16:0i}$ (together, ~70% of the total) predominating (122).

Genus *Rothia*

The genus *Rothia* is also included in this chapter because some species are rod-like. The genus *Rothia* belongs to the family *Micrococcaceae*. Collins and colleagues reclassified *Stomatococcus mucilaginosus* as *Rothia mucilaginosa* (24). Since *Rothia mucilaginosa* exhibits coccoid forms in Gram stains, the genus *Rothia* is also covered in chapter 19 (on the catalase-positive gram-positive cocci). However, the species *Rothia dentocariosa* clearly exhibits mainly rod forms and is, therefore, covered in this chapter on coryneform bacteria.

Lysine is the diamino acid of the cell wall, and $C_{15:0ai}$ and $C_{17:0ai}$ usually represent 40 to 60% of all CFAs. The G+C contents range between 47 and 56 mol%. *Rothia* strains can be quite pleomorphic by Gram staining, but filamentous forms are normally not observed. They have a variable catalase reaction, are nonmotile, and exhibit a fermentative metabolism.

Genus *Exiguobacterium*

The genus *Exiguobacterium* is phylogenetically related to the so-called "group 2 bacilli" (39). Presently, 13 species are included in this genus, of which only *E. acetylicum* and *E. aurantiacum* have been mentioned in publications as being isolated from human clinical material. Lysine is the diamino acid of the cell wall, and $C_{15:0ai}$ and $C_{17:0ai}$ comprise only about 30 to 40% of the total CFAs. *E. acetylicum* contains significant amounts of $C_{13:0}$ and $C_{13:0ai}$, which are not found in any other coryneform taxon (7). The G+C content is about 47 mol%.

Exiguobacteria present as relatively short rods in young cultures. Strains are catalase positive and motile and have a fermentative metabolism.

Genus *Oerskovia*

In older textbooks, oerskoviae were assigned to the nocardioform group of organisms due to their morphological features. This includes branching vegetative substrate hyphae and penetration into agar but no aerial hyphae. However, there is now phylogenetic and chemotaxonomic evidence that *Oerskovia*, including the reclassified genus *Promicromonospora* (143), is more closely related to genera like *Cellulomonas* than to the mycolic acid-containing genera like *Nocardia*. Representatives of the type species, *Oerskovia turbata*, were recovered from soil, but human pathogens originally identified as *O. turbata* have now been placed in *Cellulosimicrobium funkei* (14). Lysine is the diamino acid of the cell wall, and $C_{15:0ai}$ is the main CFA in oerskoviae. The G+C content is 70 to 75 mol%.

Gram staining shows coccoid-to-rod-shaped bacteria which originate from the breaking up of mycelia. *Oerskovia* strains are catalase positive, their motility is variable, and they are fermentative.

Genus *Cellulomonas*

The genus *Cellulomonas* presently comprises 17 species, of which only *C. hominis* and *C. denverensis* have been described as being isolated from humans (13, 64, 105). Ornithine is the diamino acid of the cell wall, and $C_{15:0ai}$ and $C_{16:0}$ are the main CFAs. The G+C content is 71 to 76 mol%.

Gram staining shows small, thin rods. All *Cellulomonas* spp., except *C. fermentans* and *C. humilata*, are catalase positive, their motility is variable, the environmental *Cellulomonas* strains are cellulolytic (whereas *C. hominis* did not hydrolyze cellulose in the test system used) (64), and they have a fermentative metabolism.

Genus *Cellulosimicrobium*

The *Cellulosimicrobium* genus presently comprises three species. The medically relevant species *C. cellulans* had been designated *Cellulomonas cellulans* or *Oerskovia xanthineolytica* in the past (137). The reason for removing *C. cellulans* from the genus *Cellulomonas* was that the topology of the 16S rRNA gene dendrogram indicated that the branching point of this taxon was outside *Cellulomonas* proper. In addition, the chemotaxonomic characteristic of lysine as diamino acid supported reclassification. Predominant CFAs include $C_{15:0ai}$, $C_{15:0i}$, $C_{16:0i}$, and $C_{16:0}$. The major menaquinone (MK) is MK-9(H_4), and the G+C content is 74 mol%. It should be noted that the genus *Cellulosimicrobium* is related to the genus *Oerskovia* but is nevertheless distinct.

In young cultures, a mycelium that fragments later into irregular, curved, and club-shaped rods is produced. Catalase activity is detected, and strains are nonmotile. All strains have a fermentative metabolism.

Genus *Microbacterium*

It has been known since the mid-1990s that the genera *Microbacterium* and *Aureobacterium* are phylogenetically intermixed (114), and the diamino acid in the third position of the tetrapeptide of the peptidoglycan was considered a most important chemotaxonomical marker. L-Lysine is present in microbacteria and D-ornithine in the former aureobacteria, a phenomenon noted for some genera (e.g., *Propionibacterium* and *Bifidobacterium*), where there is not a good correlation between the type of the diamino acid in the peptidoglycan layer and their phylogenetic positioning. Because a set of signature nucleotides within the 16S rRNA genes of both microbacteria and aureobacteria could be demonstrated, it was proposed that both genera be unified in a redefined genus, *Microbacterium* (145).

Now, over 50 *Microbacterium* species have been validly named, but only a minority of them has been demonstrated to be of clinical importance (74). Microbacteria are most frequently encountered in environmental specimens (e.g., soil). $C_{15:0ai}$ and $C_{17:0ai}$ are the two main CFAs, often representing up to 75% of the total CFAs (51, 73, 145). The G+C content of *Microbacterium* spp. is 65 to 76 mol%, indicating the diversity within the genus.

Gram staining often shows thin or short rods with no branching. Catalase activity and motility are variable. Microbacteria can be either fermenters or oxidizers.

Genus *Curtobacterium*

Curtobacterium spp., like microbacteria, belong to the peptidoglycan type B actinomycetes (i.e., cross-linkage exists between positions 2 and 4 of the two peptide subunits). Ornithine is the diamino acid and the only amino acid composing the interpeptide bridge. Curtobacteria have an acetyl peptidoglycan acyl type and MK-9 as the major MK, whereas microbacteria possess a glycolyl type and MK-11,12 (Table 1). For most curtobacteria, $C_{15:0ai}$ and $C_{17:0ai}$ represent more than 75% of all CFAs (46). The G+C contents range from 68 to 75 mol%. Presently, nine *Curtobacterium* species are validly described.

Gram staining shows small and short rods with no branching. Catalase activity is positive, motility is observed in most strains, and all strains show a respiratory metabolism which proceeds slowly in oxidizing carbohydrates.

Genus *Leifsonia*

The former "*Corynebacterium aquaticum*" was transferred into the genus *Leifsonia* as *Leifsonia aquatica* in 2000 (38) and is the only medically relevant species in this genus. *L. aquatica* strains belong to the peptidoglycan B-type actinomycetes and, therefore, cannot be true corynebacteria, which actually possess an A-type peptidoglycan (i.e., cross-linkage exists between positions 3 and 4 of the two peptide subunits). Diaminobutyric acid is the diamino acid of the cell wall peptidoglycan, and $C_{15:0ai}$ and $C_{17:0ai}$ are the main CFAs, as with microbacteria, but represent <75% of all CFAs (73). The G+C content is about 70 mol%.

Gram staining shows thin rods. The strains are catalase and oxidase positive (the latter feature is atypical for coryneform bacteria), always motile, and oxidizers.

Other Unusual Coryneforms

Recent examination of coryneform bacteria using primarily sequence-based identification approaches have shown that additional genera can be recovered from human clinical materials. These are briefly mentioned below.

Genus *Janibacter*

Strains of the genus *Janibacter* (94), the first medically relevant coryneform reported from the family *Intrasporangiaceae*, were found to be associated with bacteremia (36, 91; K. A. Bernard, unpublished observation). *Janibacter* strains can have Gram stain-variable or gram-positive coccoidal-to-rod-like forms in singles, pairs, or irregular clumps. Their DNA base composition is 69 to 73 mol% G+C, with an unusual CFA profile consisting of significant volumes of the CFAs $C_{16:0i}$, $C_{17:1}$, and $C_{17:0}$. These bacteria are described as oxidizers, with white, creamy, or yellowish pigments. They are nonmotile, and optimal growth may occur at 25 to 30°C.

Genus *Pseudoclavibacter*

The *Pseudoclavibacter* genus was first described in 2004 to accommodate the misidentified type strain of "*Brevibacterium helvolum*" (93). Shortly afterwards, the novel genus *Zimmermannella* was proposed but was found to be an illegitimate, later, homotypic synonym of *Pseudoclavibacter* (http://www.bacterio.cict.fr/xz/zimmermannella.html).

Pseudoclavibacter alba strains were recovered from urine, and *Pseudoclavibacter bifida* strains were recovered from blood cultures and wounds. By Gram staining, these species were short or medium-length gram-positive rods, with *P. bifida* demonstrating some rudimentary branching. Their DNA base composition is 62 to 68 mol% G+C. Major CFAs are $C_{15:0ai}$, $C_{16:0}$, $C_{16:0i}$, and $C_{17:0ai}$. These strains are oxidizers, with white or yellowish colonies (93). Optimal growth occurs at 30°C.

Genera *Brachybacterium* and *Knoellia*

Isolates from the genus *Brachybacterium* and one strain from the genus *Knoellia*, all recovered from blood cultures, have been characterized (K. A. Bernard, unpublished observations). There are currently 12 species in the genus *Brachybacterium*, which is part of the family *Dermabacteraceae*, and so they are most closely related to the genus *Dermabacter*. Members of this genus grow at 37°C, exhibit gram-positive coccoidal and rod-like forms, and have a G+C content of 68 to 73 mol%. The *Brachybacterium* blood culture isolates are metabolically fermentative and have branched-chain-type CFAs. The genus *Knoellia*, like that of the genus *Janibacter*, is a member of the family *Intrasporangiaceae*. Cells are irregular gram-positive rods or cocci with major CFAs of the branched-chain type, and their G+C content is 68 to 69 mol%. The single *Knoellia* blood culture isolate is capnophilic, growing best in 5% CO_2 at 37°C.

Genus *Arcanobacterium*

The *Arcanobacterium* genus presently contains nine species, of which *A. haemolyticum*, *A. bernardiae*, and *A. pyogenes* have been recovered from human clinical specimens. Lysine is the diamino acid of the cell wall, whereas in the phylogenetically closely related *Actinomyces* spp., lysine or ornithine is found. Arcanobacteria contain MKs of the MK-9(H_4) type, whereas the *Actinomyces* spp. examined so far have MK-10(H_4). The main CFAs of arcanobacteria are $C_{16:0}$, $C_{18:1\omega9c}$, and $C_{18:0}$ (as in *Corynebacterium* spp. and *T. otitidis*), but unlike with corynebacteria, significant amounts of $C_{10:0}$, $C_{12:0}$, and $C_{14:0}$ may also be detected (7). The G+C content is 48 to 52 mol%.

Gram staining of arcanobacteria shows irregular, gram-positive rods. All clinically relevant arcanobacteria are catalase negative; they are nonmotile and fermenters.

Genus *Gardnerella*

The genus *Gardnerella* does not have a particular phylogenetic relationship to any of the established genera described in this chapter. It is remotely related to the genus *Bifidobacterium* (97), and these genera share some important features, such as production of acetic and lactic acids as fermentation products. *G. vaginalis* is the only species belonging to the genus *Gardnerella*. Studies of the ultrastructure of the cell wall of *G. vaginalis* have demonstrated that it has a cell wall similar to but much thinner than the cell walls of other gram-positive bacteria (i.e., there is a smaller peptidoglycan layer) (134). Lysine is the diamino acid of the cell wall, and CFAs are similar to those detected in *Actinomyces* spp., *Arcanobacterium* spp., and *Corynebacterium* spp., with $C_{16:0}$ and $C_{18:1\omega9c}$ predominating. The G+C content of 42 to 44 mol% is lower than that of every other genus described in this chapter.

Gram stains show thin Gram stain-variable rods or coccobacilli (Fig. 1d). Catalase is not produced, and cells are nonmotile and have a slow fermentative metabolism.

EPIDEMIOLOGY AND TRANSMISSION

Many species of the corynebacteria are part of the normal biota of the skin and mucous membranes in humans and other mammals. The habitat for some medically irrelevant corynebacteria (e.g., *C. terpenotabidum* and *C. halotolerans*) is the environment. It is noteworthy that not all corynebacteria are equally distributed over skin and mucous membranes; many of them occupy a specific niche. *C. diphtheriae* can be isolated from the nasopharynx as well as from skin lesions, which actually represent a reservoir for the spread of diphtheria. Important opportunistic pathogens like *C. amycolatum*, *Corynebacterium striatum*, and *D. hominis* are part of the normal human skin biota but have thus far not been recovered from throat swabs from healthy individuals (158). Coryneform bacteria prominent in the oropharynx include *Corynebacterium durum* and *R. dentocariosa* (158). *Corynebacterium auris* and *T. otitidis* seem to have an almost exclusive preference for the external auditory canal. In nearly every instance that *Corynebacterium macginleyi* has been isolated, eye specimens have been the source (62). Another *Corynebacterium* species with a distinctive niche is *Corynebacterium glucuronolyticum*, which is almost exclusively isolated from genitourinary specimens from humans (47) and from animals (28). *C. urealyticum*, another genitourinary pathogen, has, like *C. jeikeium*, been cultured from inanimate hospital environments.

The natural habitat of arcanobacteria is not fully understood, but *A. haemolyticum* is recovered from throat as well as from wound swabs, whereas *A. bernardiae* has been found mainly in abscesses adjacent to skin (G. Funke and K. Bernard, unpublished observations). It is unclear whether the two species are part of the normal skin and/or the gastrointestinal biota. *A. pyogenes* is found on mucous membranes of cattle, sheep, and swine. Brevibacteria can be found on dairy products (e.g., cheese) but are also inhabitants of the human skin (48). Arthrobacters are some of the most frequently isolated bacteria when soil samples are cultured, but at least *Arthrobacter cumminsii* also seems to be present on human skin (63, 92). Members of the genera *Exiguobacterium*, *Oerskovia*, *Cellulomonas*, *Cellulosimicrobium*, and *Microbacterium* have their habitats in the inanimate environment (e.g., soil and activated sludge). *Microbacterium* spp. have also been recovered from hospital environments (51). Curtobacteria are primarily plant pathogens (46).

G. vaginalis can be found in the anorectal biota of healthy adults of both sexes as well as in that of children (16). It is also part of the endogenous vaginal biota in women of reproductive age. The optimal pH for the growth of *G. vaginalis* is between 6 and 7, i.e., at elevated pH in the vagina. The organism can also be recovered from the urethras of the male partners of women with bacterial vaginosis (BV) (16).

CLINICAL SIGNIFICANCE

Estimating the clinical significance of coryneform bacteria isolated from clinical specimens is often confusing for clinical microbiologists. This is in part due to the natural habitat of coryneform bacteria, which may lead to their recovery if specimens were not taken correctly. The reader is referred to the guidelines on minimal microbiological requirements in publications on disease associations of coryneform bacteria (72).

Coryneform bacteria should be identified to the species level if they are isolated (i) from normally sterile body sites, e.g., blood (but not if only one of multiple specimens becomes positive), (ii) from adequately collected clinical material if they are the predominant organisms, and (iii) from urine specimens if they are the only bacteria encountered and the bacterial count is >10⁴/ml or if they are the predominant organisms and the total bacterial count is >10⁵/ml.

The clinical significance of coryneform bacteria is strengthened by the following findings: (i) multiple specimens are positive for the same coryneform bacteria; (ii) coryneform bacteria are seen in direct Gram stains, and a strong leukocyte reaction is also observed; and (iii) other organisms recovered from the same material are of low pathogenicity.

For a comprehensive summary of case reports on individual coryneform bacteria, the reader is referred to review articles (6, 72). The most frequently reported coryneforms as well as their established disease associations are listed in Table 2.

Historically, diphtheria caused by *C. diphtheriae* (or *Corynebacterium ulcerans*) has been the most prominent infectious disease for which coryneform bacteria are responsible. Therefore, special attention is given to that disease in this chapter. Due to immunization programs, the disease has nearly disappeared in countries with high socioeconomic standards. However, the disease is still endemic in some subtropical and tropical countries as well as among individuals of certain ethnic groups (e.g., indigenous peoples in the Americas and Australia). In the 1990s, diphtheria reemerged in the states of the former Soviet Union. However, despite increased global travel activities, only a few imported cases have been reported by countries with well-developed health care systems.

The main manifestation of diphtheria is an upper respiratory tract illness accompanied by a sore throat, dysphagia, lymphadenitis, low-grade fever, malaise, and headache. A nasopharynx-adherent membrane which may occasionally lead to obstruction is characteristic. The severe systemic effects of diphtheria include myocarditis, neuritis, and kidney damage caused by the *C. diphtheriae* exotoxin, which is encoded by a bacteriophage carrying the *tox* gene. *C. diphtheriae* may also cause cutaneous diphtheria or endocarditis (with either toxin-positive or toxin-negative strains). Some people with poor hygienic standards (e.g., drug and alcohol abusers) are prone to colonization (on the skin more often than in the pharynx) by *C. diphtheriae* strains, which are often nontoxigenic.

G. vaginalis is associated with BV. Its causative role in the syndrome is controversial (141, 142), as it is certainly not the sole cause; other bacteria, like *Atopobium vaginae*, *Leptotrichia/Sneathia* species, and *Megasphaera*-like bacteria are also involved in BV (44, 155). Recurrent BV is due to reinfection rather than to relapse (i.e., overgrowth of the previously colonizing biotype). In pregnant women, BV may lead to preterm birth, premature rupture of membranes, and chorioamnionitis (16). *G. vaginalis* may also be recovered from cultures of blood from patients with postpartum or postabortal fevers and may also cause infections in newborns. Although it might be recovered from the urethras of males, its disease association in males is usually questionable. Cases involving serious infections (septicemia, wound infections) in sites other than those associated with the genital tract or obstetrics are rare but have been reported, including in men (87).

COLLECTION, TRANSPORT, AND STORAGE OF SPECIMENS

In general, coryneform bacteria do not need special handling when samples are collected. The general principles outlined in chapters 9 and 16 in this *Manual* apply to this group of organisms as well.

C. diphtheriae

The diagnosis of diphtheria is primarily a clinical one. The physician should notify the receiving laboratory immediately of suspected diphtheria. In case of respiratory diphtheria, material for culture should be obtained on a swab (either a cotton- or a polyester-tipped swab) from the inflamed areas in the nasopharynx. Multisite sampling (nasopharynx) is

TABLE 2 Most frequently reported disease associations of coryneform bacteria in humans

Taxon	Disease(s) or disease association(s)	Reference(s)[a]
C. amycolatum	Wound infections, foreign-body infections, bacteremia, sepsis, urinary tract infections, respiratory tract infections	56, 161, 170
C. aurimucosum	Genitourinary tract infections (mainly in females)	26
CDC group F-1	Urinary tract infections	
C. diphtheriae (toxigenic)	Throat diphtheria, cutaneous diphtheria	33, 34
C. diphtheriae	Endocarditis, foreign-body infections, pharyngitis (nontoxigenic)	45, 116, 131
C. glucuronolyticum	Genitourinary tract infections (mainly in males)	47
C. jeikeium	Endocarditis, bacteremia, foreign-body infections, wound infections	124
C. kroppenstedtii	Granulomatous lobular mastitis	110
C. macginleyi	Eye infections	35, 62
C. minutissimum	Wound infections, urinary tract infections, respiratory tract infections	
C. pseudodiphtheriticum	Respiratory tract infections, endocarditis	
C. pseudotuberculosis	Lymphadenitis (occupational)	
C. resistens	Bacteremia	106
C. riegelii	Urinary tract infections (females)	59
C. striatum	Wound infections, respiratory tract infections, foreign-body infections	10
C. tuberculostearicum	Catheter infections, bacteremia, endocarditis, wound infections, eye infections	43
C. ulcerans (toxigenic)	Respiratory diphtheria	
C. urealyticum	Urinary tract infections, bacteremia, wound infections	140
Arthrobacter spp.	Bacteremia, foreign-body infections, urinary tract infections	54, 63, 92, 160
Brevibacterium spp.	Bacteremia, foreign-body infections, malodorous feet	48
Dermabacter hominis	Wound infections, bacteremia	70
Helcobacillus sp.	Cutaneous infection with erythrasma	122
Rothia spp.	Endocarditis, bacteremia, respiratory tract infections	156
Cellulomonas spp.	Bacteremia, wound infections, cholecystitis	13, 64, 105
Cellulosimicrobium sp.	Foreign-body infections, bacteremia	14
Microbacterium spp.	Bacteremia, foreign-body infections, wound infections	51, 74, 86
A. bernardiae	Abscess formation (together with mixed anaerobic biota)	66
A. haemolyticum	Pharyngitis in older children/young adults, wound and tissue infections	
A. pyogenes	Abscess formation, wound and soft tissue infections	
G. vaginalis	Bacterial vaginosis, endometritis, postpartum sepsis	16

[a]Taxa shown without references are from our observations or from references 6 and 72.

thought to increase sensitivity. If membranes are present and can be removed (swabs from beneath the membrane are most valuable), they should also be sent to the microbiology laboratory (although C. diphtheriae might not be culturable from those in every instance). Nasopharyngeal swabs should be obtained from suspected carriers. It is preferable that the swabs are immediately transferred to the microbiology laboratory for culturing. If the swabs must be sent to the laboratory, semisolid transport media (e.g., Amies) ensure the maintenance of the bacteria. All coryneform bacteria are relatively resistant to drying and moderate temperature changes. Material from patients with suspected cases of wound diphtheria can be obtained by swab or aspiration.

Vaginal and extravaginal specimens for culturing G. vaginalis can be collected with cotton-tipped swabs. It is best to take one swab for direct examination and to take another swab for culture if necessary, such as for epidemiologic studies. If culture media cannot be directly inoculated, then the swab should be placed in a transport medium (e.g., Amies) and culture should be done within 24 h. It is noteworthy that G. vaginalis is susceptible to sodium polyanethol sulfonate (SPS), so an SPS-free medium (or an SPS medium supplemented with gelatin) should be used in order to achieve optimal recovery of G. vaginalis from blood culture systems whenever G. vaginalis is suspected.

Long-term preservation in skim milk at −70°C is applicable to all coryneform bacteria. Except with samples containing lipophilic corynebacteria, the same skim milk tube can be repeatedly thawed and frozen (G. Funke, unpublished observation). For nonlipophilic coryneforms, good results were also observed with Microbank tubes (Pro Lab Diagnostics, Austin, TX) (G. Funke, unpublished observation). The advantage of using these tubes is that individual beads can be taken out of the tube. Coryneform bacteria can also be stored for decades when they are kept lyophilized in an appropriate medium (e.g., 0.9% NaCl containing 2% bovine serum albumin).

DIRECT EXAMINATION

After the appropriate isolation media have been inoculated (see below under "Isolation Procedures"), the swabs taken from diphtheritic membranes may be subjected to Neisser or Loeffler methylene blue staining. A positive stain is characterized by metachromatic granules (polar bodies). However, it is noteworthy that the sensitivity of the microscopic examination is limited. Antigen assays for the direct detection of coryneform bacteria are not recommended.

As described previously, C. diphtheriae, C. ulcerans, and C. pseudotuberculosis are the only species able to harbor the bacteriophage which carries the diphtheria tox gene and potentially produce diphtheria toxin (72). PCR-based, direct-detection systems for the diphtheria tox gene have been described, using methods to detect fragment A and/or the entire *tox* gene (32, 107) or fragment A and B subunits of the *tox* gene (101). The system described by Nakao and Popovic had the highest sensitivity when Dacron polyester-tipped swabs were used and when silica gel packages were stored at 4°C rather than at room temperature (101). Conventional PCR detection of the regulatory *dtxR* gene has been evaluated (111). Detection of the *tox* gene using a real-time platform has been outlined (15, 99, 136). Real-time detection using primers targeting the *C. diphtheriae tox* gene for *C. ulcerans* strains have required modifications (15, 135, 136). Direct detection of the diphtheria *tox* or *dtxR* gene as the sole test of clinical specimens has not been recommended, as expression of diphtheria toxin must be demonstrated (some strains may harbor but not express the gene), and so microbiological culture is essential for confirming diphtheria (33).

The "gold standard" for the diagnosis of BV is direct examination of vaginal secretions and not the culture of *G. vaginalis*, since *G. vaginalis* can also be recovered from healthy women. A bedside test for BV is examination of the vaginal discharge to detect the typical "fishy" trimethylamine odor, which is enhanced after alkalinization with 10% KOH (but *G. vaginalis* is not responsible for the amine production). The typical smear of vaginal discharge from BV patients shows "clue cells" (bacteria covering epithelial cell margins) together with a mixed biota consisting of large numbers of small gram-negative (predominantly *Prevotella* and *Porphyromonas* spp.) and gram-variable (*G. vaginalis*) rods and coccobacilli, whereas lactobacilli are almost always absent. It is recommended that a standardized Gram staining interpretative scheme be used in order to improve the reproducibility of this method (104, 142). Although not recommended for routine laboratory procedures, the isolation of *G. vaginalis* can support the diagnosis of BV.

ISOLATION PROCEDURES

Coryneform bacteria, including *C. diphtheriae*, can be readily isolated from a 5% sheep blood agar (SBA)-based selective medium containing 100 μg of fosfomycin per ml (plus 12.5 μg of glucose-6-phosphate per ml), since nearly all coryneforms (except *Actinomyces* spp. and *D. hominis*) are highly resistant to this compound (152). It is also possible to put disks containing 50 μg of fosfomycin (plus 50 μg of glucose-6-phosphate [already incorporated in the disk]) (BD Diagnostics, Sparks, MD) on an SBA plate and then examine the colonies which grow around the disk. Selective media for coryneform bacteria containing 50 to 100 μg/ml furazolidone (Sigma, St. Louis, MO) have also been described. If lipophilic corynebacteria like *C. jeikeium* or *C. urealyticum* are sought, then 0.1 to 1.0% Tween 80 (Merck, Darmstadt, Germany) could be added to an SBA plate (add Tween 80 before pouring the medium). Additional methods to demonstrate lipophilia are described below. Medically relevant coryneforms described to date do not grow on MacConkey agar. However, if "coryneform" bacteria are recovered from this medium, they should be examined carefully to rule out rapidly growing mycobacteria.

With very few exceptions (some arthrobacters, microbacteria, and curtobacteria, which have optimal growth temperatures of between 30 and 35°C), the medically relevant coryneform bacteria grow at 37°C. It is desirable to culture specimens for coryneform bacteria in a CO_2-enriched atmosphere since some taxa, e.g., *Rothia* and *Arcanobacterium* spp., grow much better under those conditions. Nearly all medically relevant coryneform bacteria

grow within 48 h, so that primary culture plates should not be incubated longer than that. However, if liquid media are used (e.g., for specimens from normally sterile body sites), specimens should be held for 5 days before the culture is declared negative. Final Gram staining and subculture should be performed only with turbid broths.

It is recommended that urine specimens be incubated for longer than 24 h to check for the presence of *C. urealyticum* but only when patients are symptomatic or have alkaline urine or struvite crystals in their urine sediment.

C. diphtheriae

The primary plating media for the cultivation of *C. diphtheriae* should be SBA plus one selective medium (e.g., cystine-tellurite blood agar [CTBA] or freshly prepared Tinsdale medium) (33, 34). If silica gel is used as a transport medium, the desiccated swabs need to be additionally incubated overnight in broth (supplemented with either plasma or blood), which should then be streaked onto the primary plating medium. The plates are read after 18 to 24 h of incubation at 37°C, preferably in a 5% CO_2-enriched atmosphere. Tellurite inhibits the growth of many noncoryneform bacteria, but even a few *C. diphtheriae* strains are sensitive to potassium tellurite and will therefore not grow on CTBA but may grow on SBA. It is noteworthy that growth on CTBA and tellurite reduction are not specific for *C. diphtheriae*, since many other coryneforms may also produce black (albeit smaller) colonies. The best medium for direct culturing of *C. diphtheriae* is Tinsdale medium (34). However, the limitations of Tinsdale medium are its relatively short shelf life (<4 weeks) and the necessity to add horse serum to it. On Tinsdale plates, both tellurite reductase activity (as shown by black colonies) and cystinase activity (as shown by a brown halo around the colonies) can be observed. If neither CTBA nor Tinsdale medium is available, colistin-nalidixic acid blood agar plates are recommended for the isolation of *C. diphtheriae* or any other coryneform bacterium. It is necessary to pick multiple colonies from colistin-nalidixic acid blood agar plates to rule out *C. diphtheriae* (first by Gram staining and then by subculturing, with subsequent biochemical testing). Nonselective Loeffler serum slants are no longer recommended for the primary isolation of *C. diphtheriae* because of overgrowth by other bacteria.

G. vaginalis

Vaginal swabs are cultured on vaginalis agar (see chapter 17 in this *Manual* for the preparation) and should be semiquantitatively streaked out with a loop. Incubation is at 35 to 37°C in a 5% CO_2-enriched atmosphere or in a candle jar. Slight beta-hemolysis is observed on human or rabbit blood-containing media but not on SBA (on which *G. vaginalis* can also grow, exhibiting alpha-hemolysis). Plates may be checked for the growth of diffuse beta-hemolytic colonies of <0.5 mm in diameter after 24 h, but very often *G. vaginalis* is best observed after 48 h. Gram staining of the suspected colonies confirms the diagnosis of *G. vaginalis*.

IDENTIFICATION

Basic tests available in every microbiology laboratory are of great value for the identification of coryneform bacteria. The Gram staining morphology of the cells can exclude the assignment to many genera and may even lead to the assignment to the correct genus (e.g., to the genus *Corynebacterium*, *Turicella*, or *Dermabacter*) (Fig. 1). Morphology, size, pigment, odor, and hemolysis of colonies are also valuable criteria in the differential diagnosis of coryneform bacteria.

von Graevenitz and Funke (157) outlined a biochemical identification system for coryneform bacteria which was based on previous results from the Centers for Disease Control and Prevention's (CDC's) Special Bacteriology Reference Laboratory (79). This system includes testing for catalase; fermentation or oxidation (which is best observed in semisolid cystine-Trypticase agar medium rather than on triple sugar iron or oxidation-fermentation media, with fermentation indicated by acid or alkali production in the entire tube and oxidation found at the surface of the tube); motility; nitrate reduction (24 h of incubation); urea hydrolysis (24 h of incubation); esculin hydrolysis (up to 48 h of incubation); acid production from glucose, maltose, sucrose, mannitol, and xylose (48 h of incubation); CAMP reaction (24 h of incubation) with a beta-hemolysin-producing strain of *Staphylococcus aureus* (e.g., strain ATCC 25923), i.e., with a positive reaction indicated by an augmentation of the effect of *S. aureus* beta-hemolysin on erythrocytes, resulting in a complete hemolysis in an arrowhead configuration (Fig. 2); and lipophilia (24 h of incubation), the test for which is performed only for catalase-positive

colonies of <0.5 mm in diameter. For the test for lipophilia, colonies are subcultured onto ordinary SBA and onto a 0.1%- to 1%-Tween 80-containing SBA plate. Lipophilic corynebacteria develop colonies up to 2 mm in diameter after 24 h on Tween 80-supplemented agar. It has also been suggested that levels of growth in brain heart infusion broth with and without supplementation of 1% (vol/vol) sterile Tween 80 be compared and that strains which grow only in the supplemented broth can be called lipophilic. The identification protocols given in this chapter are, in principle, based on the identification system of von Graevenitz and Funke (157) (Tables 3 and 4).

Manually performed identification panels include the API (formerly RapID) Coryne system (bioMérieux, Marcy l'Etoile, France) and the RapID CB Plus system (Remel, Lenexa, KS), which are widely used. The API Coryne system contains 50 taxa in its present database (version 3.0), and comparison to an online database, APIWEB, is available (https://apiweb.biomerieux.com). In a comprehensive multicenter study, it was found that 90.5% of the strains belonging to the taxa included were correctly identified, with additional tests needed for correct identification for 55.1% of all strains tested (69). Reproducible results are best obtained if the manufacturer's recommendations for use are rigorously followed. It was concluded that the system is a useful tool for the identification of the diverse group of coryneform bacteria encountered in routine clinical laboratories. The RapID CB Plus system correctly identified 80.9% of the strains to the genus and species levels and an additional 12.2% to the genus level, but with less accurate species designations; it was also concluded that this system may perform well under the conditions of a routine clinical laboratory (67). An updated version of a panel for the automated Vitek system (bioMérieux) has been described (120). However, it is always important to question critically the identifications provided by any commercial identification system and to correlate the results with simple basic characteristics, such as macroscopic morphology and Gram staining results. Furthermore, it is important to note that for both commercially available manual identification systems, the databases have not been updated since the end of the1990s, and therefore, the recently described taxa are not covered.

For some identifications, the commercial API 50CH system (bioMérieux) has been found to be useful. For example, when the AUX medium (usually attached to the kit for gram-negative nonfermenters [bioMérieux]) is applied to the API 50CH system, utilization reactions which allow the differentiation of *Brevibacterium* spp. or some *Arthrobacter* spp. can be observed (48, 54).

A reference laboratory also uses chromatographic techniques for further characterization of coryneform bacteria. The presence of mycolic acids and their chain lengths can be detected by thin-layer chromatography (TLC), gas chromatography, and mass spectrometry or high-performance liquid chromatography (27). These methods can be useful for the differentiation of *Corynebacterium* spp. (mycolic acids of 22 to 36 carbon atoms) from the partially acid-fast bacteria (mycolic acids of 30 to 78 carbon atoms) but may also provide evidence that a coryneform bacterium is not a *Corynebacterium* (exceptions include *C. amycolatum*, *C. atypicum*, and *C. kroppenstedtii*) if mycolic acids are not detected. The detection of the diamino acid of the peptidoglycan by one-dimensional TLC is of certain value for determining the genus to which a particular strain belongs (Table 1). In some cases, partial hydrolysates of

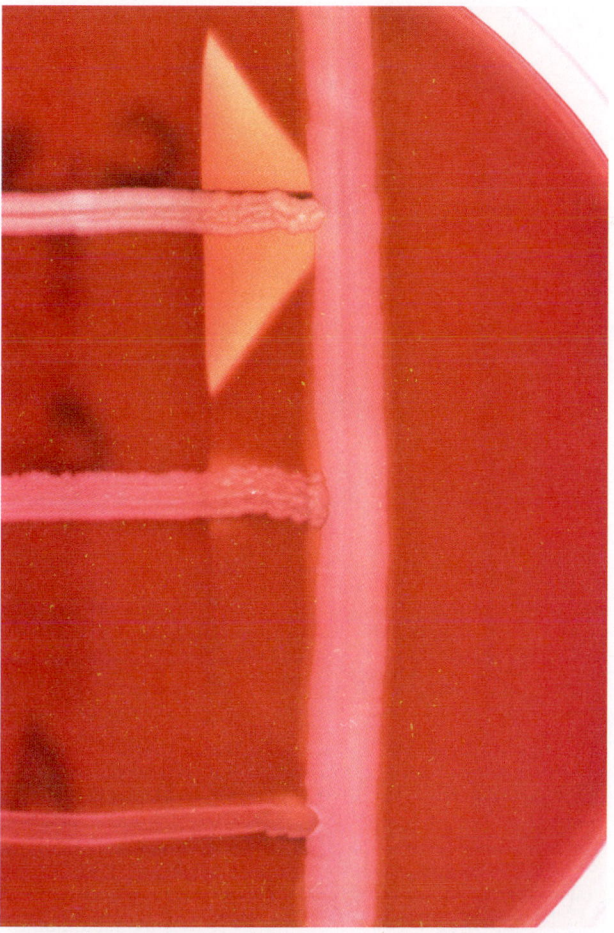

FIGURE 2 CAMP reactions of different coryneform bacteria after 24 h. (Top) *C. glucuronolyticum* DMMZ 891 (positive reaction); (middle) *C. diphtheriae* ATCC 14779 (negative reaction); (bottom) *A. haemolyticum* ATCC 9345 (CAMP inhibition reaction). The vertical streak is *S. aureus* ATCC 25923.

TABLE 3 Identification of medically relevant *Corynebacterium* spp.[a]

Species	Fermentation/oxidation	Lipophilism	Nitrate reduction	Urease	Esculin hydrolysis	Pyrazinamidase	Alkaline phosphatase	Acid production from:					CAMP reaction	Other trait(s)
								Glucose	Maltose	Sucrose	Mannitol	Xylose		
C. accolens	F	+	+	−	−	V	−	+	−	V	V	−	−	
C. afermentans subsp. afermentans	O	−	−	−	−	+	+	−	−	−	−	−	V	
C. afermentans subsp. lipophilum	O	+	−	−	−	+	+	−	−	−	−	−	V	
C. amycolatum	F	−	V	V	−	+	+	+	V	V	−	−	−	Most O/129 resistant, propionic acid detected
C. appendicis	F	+	−	+	−	+	+	+	+	−	−	−	ND	Large volume of TBSA present
C. argentoratense	F	−	−	−	−	+	V	+	−	−	−	−	−	Chymotrypsin may be positive; propionic acid detected[b]
C. atypicum	F	−	−	−	−	−	−	+	+	+	−	−	ND	Pinpoint-sized colonies, β-glucuronidase positive
C. aurimucosum	F	−	−	−	V	+	+	+	+	+	−	−	ND	Most strains yellowish, some exhibit blackish-gray pigment or pit agar
C. auris	O	−	−	−	−	+	+	−	−	−	−	−	+	Slightly adherent to agar, cleaved mycolic acids
C. bovis[c]	F	+	−	−	−	−	+	+	−	−	−	−	−	TBSA positive; fructose positive
C. canis	F	−	+	−	+	+	+	+	+	+	−	−	−	Long rods, α-glucosidase positive, trypsin positive
C. confusum	F	−	+	−	−	+	+	(+)	−	−	−	−	−	Tyrosine negative, TBSA positive; propionic acid detected
C. coyleae	F	−	−	−	−	+	+	(+)	−	−	−	−	+	
CDC group F-1	F	+	V	+	−	+	−	+	+	+	−	−	−	
C. diphtheriae biotype gravis	F	−	+	−	−	−	−	+	+	−	−	−	−	Glycogen positive, propionic acid detected
C. diphtheriae biotype intermedius	F	+	+	−	−	−	−	+	+	−	−	−	−	Propionic acid detected
C. diphtheriae biotypes mitis and belfanti	F	−	+/−[d]	−	−	−	−	+	+	−	−	−	−	Glycogen negative, propionic acid detected
C. durum	F	−	+	(V)	(V)	+	−	+	+	+	V	−	−	Adherent to agar, propionic acid detected
C. falsenii	F	−	−	(+)	−	(+)	+	(+)	V	−	−	−	−	Yellowish
C. freiburgense	F	−	+	−	+	−	ND	+	+	+	−	−	−	β-Galactosidase positive, spoked-wheel colonies, strongly adherent to agar
C. freneyi	F	−	V	−	−	+	+	+	+	+	−	−	ND	α-Glucosidase positive, grows at 20°C and 42°C
C. glucuronolyticum	F	−	V	V	V	+	V	+	V	+	−	V	+	β-Glucuronidase positive, propionic acid detected
C. hansenii	F	−	−	−	−	+	−	+	+	+	−	−	ND	Yellow, dry
C. imitans	F	−	−	−	−	(+)	+	+	+	(+)	−	−	+	Tyrosine negative, O/129 resistant

(Continued on next page)

TABLE 3 (*Continued*)

Species	Fermentation/ oxidation	Lipophilism	Nitrate reduction	Urease	Esculin hydrolysis	Pyrazinamidase	Alkaline phosphatase	Acid production from:					CAMP reaction	Other trait(s)
								Glucose	Maltose	Sucrose	Mannitol	Xylose		
C. jeikeium	O	+	−	−	−	+	+	+	V	−	−	−	−	Fructose negative, anaerobic growth negative
C. kroppenstedtii	F	+	−	−	+	+	−	+	V^c	+	−	−	−	Lacks mycolates, propionic acid detected
C. lipophiloflavum	(F)	+/−	−	(+)	−	+	+	(+)	−	−	−	−	V	Yellow, cleaved mycolics
C. macginleyi	F	+	+	−	−	−	+	+	−	+	V	−	−	
C. massiliense	F	−	−	−	−	(+)	(+)	−	−	−	−	−	ND	TBSA positive
C. matruchotii	F	−	+	−	V	+	−	+	+	+	−	−	−	"Whip handle" (upon Gram staining); propionic acid detected
C. minutissimum	F	−	−	−	−	+	+	+	+	V	V	−	−	Tyrosine positive
C. mucifaciens	O	−	−	−	−	+	+	+	−	V	−	−	−	Very mucoid yellowish colonies
C. pilbarense	F	−	−	−	−	+	+	+	−	+	−	−	ND	
C. propinquum	O	−	+	−	−	V	V	−	−	−	−	−	−	Tyrosine positive
C. pseudodiphtheriticum	O	−	+	+	−	+	V	−	−	−	−	−	−	
C. pseudotuberculosis	F	−	V	+	−	−	V	+	+	V	−	−	REV	Propionic acid detected
C. pyruviciproducens	F	+	−	−	−	+	+	+	+	+	−	−	+	β-Glucuronidase positive; pyruvic acid detected
C. resistens	F	+	−	−	−	−	+	+	−	−	−	−	−	Slow growth in anaerobic atmosphere
C. riegelii	F	−	−	+	−	V	V	−	(+)	−	−	−	−	
C. simulans^e	F	−	+	−	−	V	+	+	−	+	−	−	−	Reduces nitrite
C. singulare	F	−	−	+	−	+	+	+	+	+	−	−	−	Tyrosine positive
C. sputi	F	−	−	+	−	+	−	+	−	−	−	−	ND	α-Glucosidase positive, TBSA positive
C. stationis	F	−	+	+	−	(+)	−	(+)	−	−	−	−	−	Citrate alkalinized; ribose, fructose positive
C. striatum	F	−	+	−	−	+	+	+	−	V	−	−	V	Tyrosine positive
C. sundsvallense	F	−	−	+	−	V	V	+	+	+	−	−	−	Sticky colonies
C. thomssenii	F	−	−	+	−	+	+	+	+	+	−	−	−	N-Acetyl-β-glucosaminidase positive, sticky colonies
C. timonense	F	−	−	−	(+)	+	+	+	−	−	−	−	ND	Yellow
C. tuberculostearicum	F	+	V	−	−	+	V	+	V	V	−	−	−	
C. tuscaniense	O	−	−	−	−	+	+	+	+	−	−	−	−	Hippurate positive, tyrosine negative
C. ulcerans	F	−	−	+	−	−	+	+	+	−	−	−	REV	Glycogen positive, propionic acid detected
C. urealyticum	O	+	−	+	−	+	V	−	−	−	−	−	−	
C. ureicelerivorans	F	+	−	+	−	+	+	+	−	−	−	(+)	ND	Very strong, rapid urease reaction; TBSA detected; hippurate positive
C. xerosis	F	−	V	−	−	+	+	+	+	+	−	−	−	O/129 susceptible, propionic acid not detected

^{a}Abbreviations and symbols: F, fermentation; O, oxidation; +, positive, −, negative, V, variable; ( ), delayed or weak reaction; ND, no data; REV, CAMP inhibition reaction; TBSA, tuberculostearic acid.

^{b}Propionic acid as a glucose fermentation product.

^{c}A blood culture isolate (8) was also O-nitrophenyl-β-D-galactopyranoside positive, oxidase positive, and weakly maltose positive but negative by the API Coryne system; propionic acid was not detected; β-galactosidase was not observed using two methods (API Coryne and API Zym systems); the API Coryne system code obtained is 0101104.

^{d}C. diphtheriae biotype mitis is nitrate reductase positive, and C. diphtheriae biotype belfanti is nitrate reductase negative.

^{e}C. simulans (159) is a strong nitrite reducer at low and high concentrations; nitrate reduction may appear to be negative unless further tested using zinc dust; one strain was catalase negative (8).

TABLE 4 Identification of medically relevant coryneform bacteria other than *Corynebacterium* spp.[a]

Taxon	Catalase	Fermentation/ oxidation	Motility	Nitrate reduction	Urease	Esculin hydrolysis	Acid production from:					Other trait(s)
							Glucose	Maltose	Sucrose	Mannitol	Xylose	
Turicella otitidis	+	O	−	−	−	−	−	−	−	−	−	CAMP reaction positive, long rods
Arthrobacter spp.	+	O	v	v	v	v	v	v	v	−	−	
Brevibacterium spp.	+	O	−	v	−	−	v	v	v	−	−	Cheese-like odor
Dermabacter hominis	+	F	−	−	−	+	+	+	+	−	v	Small rods
Helcobacillus sp.	+	F	−	+	−	−	+	+	+	+	+	Gelatin, starch hydrolyzed
Rothia dentocariosa	v	F	−	+	−	+	+	+	+	−	−	Some strains adherent, grayish-black-pigmented strains exist
Exiguobacterium acetylicum	+	F	+	v	−	+	+	+	+	+	−	Golden-yellow pigment
Oerskovia turbata	+	F	v	+	−	+	+	+	+	−	+	Xanthine not hydrolyzed
Cellulomonas spp.	+	F	v	+	−	+	+	+	+	v	+	
Cellulosimicrobium spp.	+	F	v	v	v	+	+	+	+	−	+	Hydrolysis of xanthine
Microbacterium spp.	v	F/O	v	v	v	v	+	+	v	v	v	
Curtobacterium spp.	+	O	v	−	−	+	+	v	v	v	+	
Leifsonia aquatica	+	O	+	v	−	v	+	v	v	+	+	
Arcanobacterium haemolyticum	−	F	−	−	−	−	+	+	v	−	−	CAMP inhibition reaction
Arcanobacterium pyogenes	−	F	−	−	−	v	+	v	v	v	+	
Arcanobacterium bernardiae	−	F	−	−	−	−	+	+	−	−	−	Glycogen positive
Gardnerella vaginalis	−	F	−	−	−	−	+	+	v	−	−	Decolorized cells in Gram stain

[a]Abbreviations and symbols: +, positive reaction; −, negative reaction; v, variable reaction; O, oxidation; F, fermentation. See also references 6, 72, and 122.

the peptidoglycan are separated by two-dimensional TLC to reveal the interpeptide bridge of the peptidoglycan in order to distinguish between genera having the same diamino acid in the peptide moiety. For example, some of the yellow-pigmented microbacteria and all curtobacteria have ornithine as their diamino acids, but microbacteria have (glycine)-ornithine as the interpeptide bridge, whereas curtobacteria possess ornithine only.

The analysis of CFAs by means of gas-liquid chromatography with the Sherlock system (MIDI Inc., Newark, DE) is a useful method for the identification of coryneform bacteria. This system is, in general, able to correctly identify coryneform bacteria to the genus level, but identification to the species level is, in most cases, impossible, although the commercial database suggests that it is possible. This is due to the very closely similar CFA profiles obtained for coryneform bacteria belonging to the same genus (7) and because the quantitative profiles observed strongly depend on the incubation conditions. When a laboratory creates an individual database based on its own entries, species identification becomes more likely (K. A. Bernard, unpublished observation). The mycolic acids of some corynebacteria (e.g., *C. auris*) are cleaved at the temperature (300°C) produced in the injection port of the system, resulting in peaks being misidentified as fatty acids, e.g., $C_{17:1\omega6c}$ to $C_{\omega9c}$, by the Sherlock system (7, 57).

Molecular genetics-based identification systems for coryneform bacteria have been outlined in recent years. Restriction fragment length polymorphism analysis of the partly amplified and digested 16S rRNA gene has been demonstrated to be of use for the identification of species, e.g., within the genus *Corynebacterium* (154). Some corynebacteria may also be identified to the species level by examination of the length of the 16S-23S rRNA intergenic spacer region (4). A very useful approach for the identification of true corynebacteria is the sequencing of a 434- to 452-bp fragment of the *rpoB* gene (using primers designated C2700F and C3130R), since this particular region of the gene displays a high degree of polymorphism within the genus *Corynebacterium* (82, 83). A divergence of >5% within this particular part of the *rpoB* genes of two compared strains suggests that they belong to two different species. For more definitive taxonomic investigations of coryneforms, and in cases of the growth of coryneform bacteria from difficult-to-obtain clinical material (132), full-length 16S rRNA gene sequencing might be indicated. Determination of the complete 16S rRNA gene sequence is a rational approach for identifying corynebacteria, since most established species exhibit 3% or greater divergence, except for *C. afermentans*, *C. coyleae*, *C. mucifaciens* (<2% divergent); *C. aurimucosum*, *C. minutissimum*, and *C. singulare* (<2%); *C. sundsvallense* and *C. thomssenii* (<1.5%); *C. ulcerans* and *C. pseudotuberculosis* (<1% divergent from each other and both <2% divergent from *C. diphtheriae*); *C. propinquum* and *C. pseudodiphtheriticum* (<2%); *C. xerosis*, *C. freneyi*, and *C. hansenii* (<2%); and *C. macginleyi* and *C. accolens* (<2%).

In very few selected cases (i.e., if the divergence of the 16S rRNA genes is ≤1.3%), quantitative DNA-DNA hybridizations might be necessary, with sequencing of the complete *rpoB* gene recently being suggested as a substitute for that approach (2). Because of the ever-growing number of coryneform taxa encountered in clinical specimens, it has become difficult to readily differentiate these taxa by biochemical means alone, so sequencing studies are likely to replace some of the biochemical testing in the near future. It is emphasized that unidentifiable, clinically significant coryneform bacteria should be sent to an established reference laboratory experienced in corynebacterial identification for characterization which includes sequence-based analyses.

IDENTIFICATION: DESCRIPTIONS OF GENERA AND SPECIES

Genus *Corynebacterium*

C. accolens

C. accolens (103) is found in specimens from the eyes, ears, nose, and oropharynx. Endocarditis of native aortic and mitral valves due to this agent has been described. Colonies are, as for all other lipophilic corynebacteria, convex, smooth, and <0.5 mm in diameter on SBA. *C. accolens* strains had initially been described to exhibit satellitism in the vicinity of *S. aureus* strains, attributable to its lipophilism (for the method recommended to demonstrate lipophilism, see above under "Identification"). *C. accolens* has a variable pyrazinamidase reaction but is negative for alkaline phosphatase, which differentiates it from the morphologically and biochemically closely related species *C. tuberculostearicum* (Table 3). The API Coryne and RapID CB Plus systems correctly identify *C. accolens* (67, 69). *C. accolens* strains are susceptible to a broad spectrum of antibiotics.

C. afermentans subsp. afermentans

C. afermentans subsp. *afermentans* (125) is part of the normal human skin biota and has so far been isolated mainly from blood cultures. Colonies are whitish, convex with regular edges, creamy, and about 1 to 1.5 mm in diameter after 24 h of incubation. *C. afermentans* subsp. *afermentans* has an oxidative metabolism. The API Coryne system provides the numerical code 2100004 for this species. About 60% of all strains of this taxon are CAMP reaction positive. *C. afermentans* subsp. *afermentans* can be differentiated from *C. auris* and *T. otitidis* (both of which give the same API Coryne numerical code) by the consistency of its colonies (*C. auris* is slightly adherent to agar) and morphology upon Gram staining (*T. otitidis* has longer cells). By chemotaxonomic means, both *C. afermentans* subspecies and *C. auris* contain mycolates, whereas *T. otitidis* lacks them, but this technique is not applicable in routine clinical laboratories. *C. afermentans* subsp. *afermentans* is generally susceptible to β-lactam antibiotics, but resistance to erythromycin, clarithromycin, azithromycin, and clindamycin have been reported (42).

C. afermentans subsp. lipophilum

Strains belonging to the species *C. afermentans* subsp. *lipophilum* (125) have been isolated mainly from blood cultures but also from superficial wounds. Colonies are, typically for lipophilic corynebacteria, convex, smooth, and <0.5 mm in diameter after 24 h. *C. afermentans* subsp. *lipophilum* has an oxidative metabolism and does not produce acid from any of the carbohydrates usually tested (Table 3). It is the only species of nonfermenting, lipophilic corynebacteria which may exhibit a positive CAMP reaction. *C. afermentans* subsp. *lipophilum* is not included in the API Coryne database. The numerical profile observed for the species is 2100004 and so by that method cannot be discerned from more robustly growing *C. afermentans* subsp. *afermentans*, *C. auris*, or *T. otitidis*, which have the same code as well. Strains are usually susceptible to β-lactam antibiotics.

C. amycolatum

C. amycolatum is part of the normal human skin biota but was not recovered from throat swabs from healthy persons (158). *C. amycolatum* is the most frequently encountered *Corynebacterium* species in human clinical material (56). It is also the most frequently isolated nonlipophilic *Corynebacterium* in dairy cows with mastitis (80). *C. amycolatum* strains are nearly always multidrug resistant (68). Colonies are very typically dry, waxy, and grayish white with irregular edges and are 1 to 2 mm in diameter after 24 h of incubation (Fig. 3a). *C. amycolatum* actually has a fermentative metabolism, but when cystine-Trypticase agar media are used for the observation of acid production from carbohydrates, *C. amycolatum* appears to resemble an oxidizer (i.e., to have main acid production at the surface of the medium). Strains of *C. amycolatum* are remarkable for their variability in basic biochemical reactions (Table 3) and are often misidentified as the biochemically similar species *C. xerosis*, *C. striatum*, or *C. minutissimum* (56, 161, 170). These species can be differentiated by the following means. *C. amycolatum* and *C. minutissimum* do not grow at 20°C, but *C. xerosis* and *C. striatum* do; in addition, *C. xerosis* does not ferment glucose at 42°C, whereas the other three species do; and *C. minutissimum* and *C. striatum* produce alkali from formate but *C. amycolatum* and *C. xerosis* do not (161). When tested on Mueller-Hinton agar supplemented with 5% sheep blood, nearly all *C. amycolatum* strains were resistant to the vibriocidal compound O/129 (150-μg disks) (Oxoid, Basingstoke, United Kingdom), as indicated by there being no zone of inhibition around the disk (56). In contrast, only 4% of all *C. amycolatum* strains were resistant to O/129 when tested on Mueller-Hinton agar with 5% horse blood (80). The API Coryne system identifies this species well, but in every case additional reactions must be carried out in order to confirm the identification of *C. amycolatum* (69). All *C. amycolatum* strains produce propionic acid as the major end product of glucose metabolism. In contrast to many other corynebacteria, *C. amycolatum* exhibits only weak or no leucine arylamidase activity. The identification may also be suggested by the absence of mycolic acids. In addition, it may be shown that acyl phosphatidylglycerol is a major phospholipid in *C. amycolatum*, unlike in other *Corynebacterium* spp., in which other phospholipids are predominant (153).

C. appendicis

The one strain of *C. appendicis* described in the literature was isolated from a patient with appendicitis accompanied with abscess formation (165). This lipophilic species contains large amounts of TBSA (up to 50% of all CFAs), which is not seen in any other *Corynebacterium* species. It is differentiated from CDC coryneform group F-1 bacteria by a positive alkaline phosphatase reaction but negative reactions for nitrate reduction and sucrose fermentation.

C. argentoratense

C. argentoratense (127) has been isolated from the human throat and was once recovered from a blood culture (8). Colonies are cream colored, nonhemolytic, slightly rough, and 2 mm in diameter after 48 h of incubation. Phenotypically, *C. argentoratense* may appear to be very similar to (rare) ribose-negative strains of *C. coyleae*. However, glucose fermentation by *C. argentoratense* is quite rapid, compared to that of the slowly fermenting species *C. coyleae*. In addition, CAMP reaction-negative *C. argentoratense* produces propionic acid as a fermentation product, but CAMP reaction-positive *C. coyleae* does not (8). *C. argentoratense* is the only medically relevant *Corynebacterium* species expressing α-chymotrypsin activity, which can be observed in the API ZYM (bioMérieux) system; however, the blood culture isolate was not observed to produce that enzyme (8).

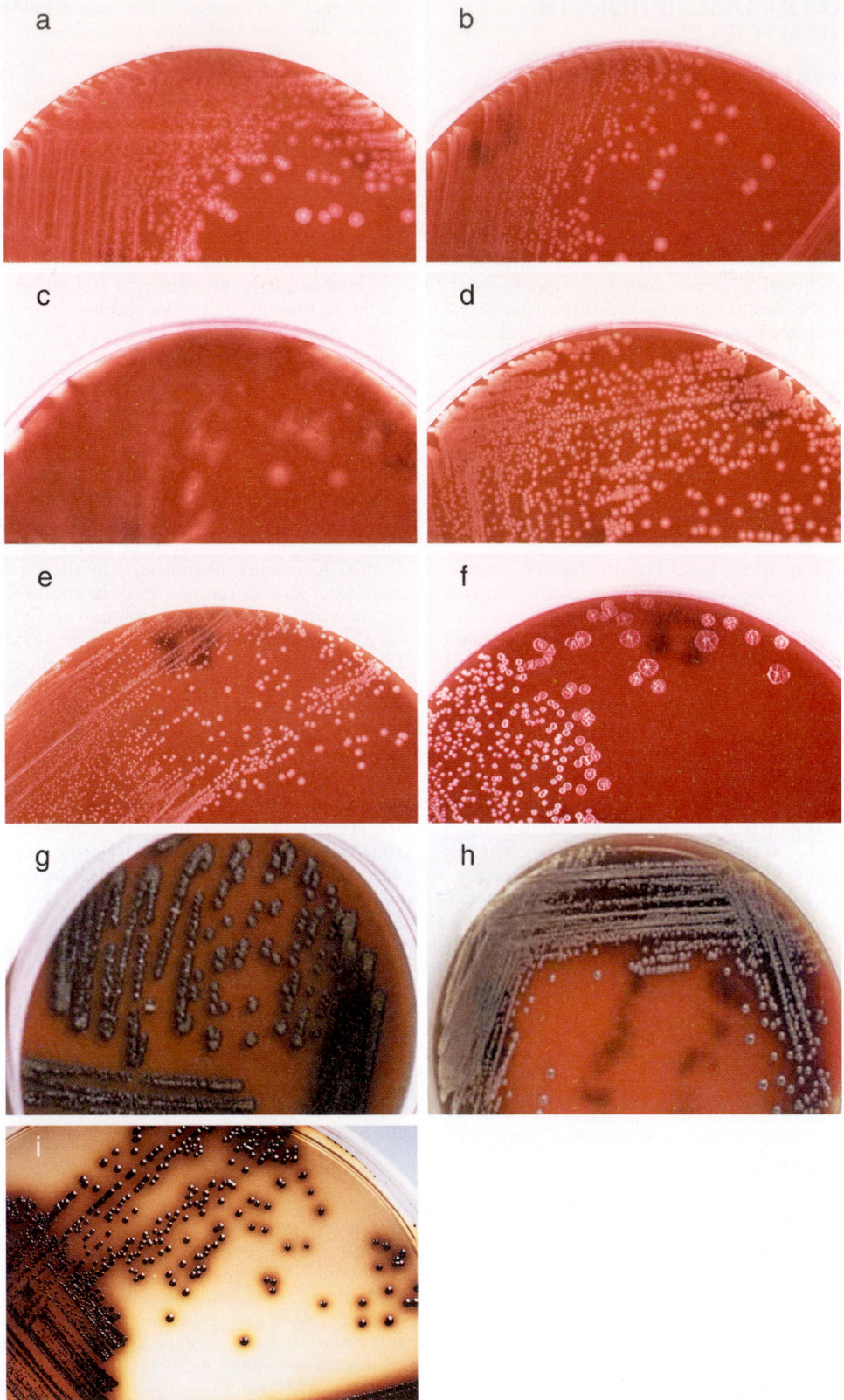

FIGURE 3 Colony morphologies of different coryneform bacteria after 48 h of incubation on SBA. (a) *C. amycolatum* LCDC 91-0077; (b) *C. diphtheriae* ATCC 14779; (c) *C. mucifaciens* LCDC 97-0202; (d) *C. striatum* ATCC 6940; (e) *D. hominis* ATCC 51325; (f) *R. dentocariosa* LCDC 95-0154; (g) *C. aurimucosum* HC-NML 91-0032 (after 96 h); (h) black-pigmented *Rothia dentocariosa* HC-NML 77-0298 (after 96 h); (i) *C. diphtheriae* biotype gravis colonies on a Tinsdale agar plate. The last photo was kindly provided by C. Hinnebusch and M. Cohen, UCLA School of Medicine, Los Angeles, CA.

Although *C. argentoratense* is phylogenetically closely related to *C. diphtheriae*, it does not harbor the *tox* gene, coding for the diphtheria toxin.

C. atypicum

Although *C. atypicum* clearly belongs to the genus *Corynebacterium*, corynomycolic acids, as in *C. amycolatum* and *C. kroppenstedtii*, are not detected (77). *C. atypicum* is not lipophilic but shows only pinpoint-sized colonies after 48 h of incubation. It is the only medically relevant *Corynebacterium* not expressing pyrazinamidase but expressing β-glucuronidase activity.

C. aurimucosum

The initial description of *C. aurimucosum* was based on a single strain which exhibited slightly yellow and sticky colonies on 5% SBA plates but had colorless and slimy colonies on Trypticase soy agar without blood (166). Biochemically, this particular *C. aurimucosum* strain was similar to *C. minutissimum*. The number of *C. aurimucosum* strains was significantly enhanced when it was demonstrated that some former CDC coryneform group 4 bacteria actually belong to *C. aurimucosum* (26). It is important to note that strains of *C. aurimucosum* exhibit a grayish-black pigment which is not seen in any other true *Corynebacterium*. Strains originally designated "*Corynebacterium nigricans*" were later shown to be *C. aurimucosum* (26). Some strains of *R. dentocariosa* can also exhibit a charcoal-black pigment (26); these strains are differentiated from *C. aurimucosum* by being constantly nitrate reductase positive, having a possibly negative catalase reaction, and having branched-chained CFAs, as opposed to straight-chain-type CFAs in *C. aurimucosum*. API Coryne codes for pigmented *C. aurimucosum* strains include 0000125, 2000125, and 2100327. Phylogenetically, *C. aurimucosum* is closely related (>98.8% identity) to both *C. singulare* and *C. minutissimum* by 16S rRNA gene sequencing but can readily be discerned by partial *rpoB* gene sequence analysis.

C. auris

C. auris (57) has almost exclusively been isolated from the ear region. Colonies are dryish and slightly adherent to agar but do not penetrate agar; they become slightly yellowish with time, and they have diameters ranging from 1 to 2 mm after 48 h of incubation. *C. auris* does not produce acid from any carbohydrates usually tested. All *C. auris* strains are strongly CAMP test positive. The API Coryne system provides the numerical code 2100004 for this species. Abundant degradation products of mycolic acids are indirectly observed when CFA patterns are determined with the Sherlock system (57). It is noteworthy that the MICs of β-lactam antibiotics for *C. auris* strains are elevated, but the molecular mechanism for this is not known at present (68).

C. bovis

Occasionally, human infections have been attributed to the lipophilic bovine species *C. bovis*. Characterization of lipophilic corynebacteria solely on the basis of the results of phenotypic tests, in the absence of modern polyphasic methods or identification schemes, was probably incorrect (Table 3). This species had not been definitively recovered for many years from human clinical material (72). Recently, an oxidase-positive, human blood culture isolate of *C. bovis* was identified based on a polyphasic approach, with an API Coryne code of 0101104 (8), as was an isolate from a prosthetic joint infection (1).

C. canis

This nonlipophilic *Corynebacterium* was isolated from a wound infection after a dog bite (50). It has some unusual microscopic features in that it exhibits very filamentous rods (>15 μm in length), and some cells even show branching. *C. canis* is esculinase and α-glucosidase positive and is the only *Corynebacterium* expressing trypsin activity.

C. confusum

C. confusum has been isolated from patients with foot infections, a blood culture (61), and a breast abscess (8). Colonies are whitish, glistening, convex, creamy, and up to 1.5 mm in diameter after 48 h. Acid from glucose is produced only very weakly, becoming visible in the API Coryne or the API 50CH gallery only after 48 to 72 h. Weak growth under anaerobic conditions corresponds to slow fermentative acid production. It is advisable to incubate the API Coryne system after 24 h for another day in those cases in which the results for acid production are ambiguous (i.e., with only a slight change in the color of the indicator). After 48 h of incubation, the API Coryne system provides the numerical code 3100304 for this species; the breast abscess strain had a code of 3100104. Interestingly, the breast abscess strain was also CAMP reaction positive, making it potentially more difficult to discern from *C. coyleae* isolates (8). *C. confusum* is correctly identified by the RapID CB Plus system (67). If glucose fermentation is judged to be negative, *C. confusum* strains can be misidentified as *C. propinquum*. However, in contrast to that species, *C. confusum* does not hydrolyze tyrosine and contains small amounts of TBSA (1 to 3%), whereas *C. propinquum* hydrolyzes tyrosine but does not contain TBSA. *C. confusum* is differentiated from *C. coyleae* and *C. argentoratense* by its ability to reduce nitrate.

C. coyleae

C. coyleae (65) has been isolated mainly from cultures of blood and other normally sterile body fluids, but it may also be recovered from a variety of sterile body fluids, abscesses, and urogenital specimens (8, 40). Colonies are whitish and slightly glistening, with entire edges, and are about 1 mm in diameter after 24 h. The consistency of the colonies is either creamy or sticky. A slow fermentative acid production from glucose and a strongly positive CAMP reaction are the most significant phenotypic characteristics. *C. coyleae* is positive for cystine arylamidase, which is not observed for many other corynebacteria. Various API Coryne numerical codes have been observed, especially 2100304 and 6100304. *C. coyleae* is always positive for ribose fermentation, whereas the biochemically similar species *C. argentoratense* varies in this reaction. The API Coryne database lists only 6% of glucose-fermenting *C. coyleae* strains, and therefore, when applying this commercial identification system, the clinical microbiologist may not receive a correct identification (69). However, the two numerical profiles given above combined with a positive CAMP reaction are highly indicative of *C. coyleae*. This species is correctly identified by the RapID CB Plus system (67). Macrolide resistance has been reported (42).

CDC Group F-1 Bacteria

The lipophilic CDC group F-1 bacteria (128) have not been given a species name. Although genetically distinct, no distinguishing phenotypic markers which clearly allow their separation from other defined *Corynebacterium* spp. have been found. The characteristics of the CDC group

F-1 bacteria are consistent with the definition of the genus *Corynebacterium* in all respects. Of note is the negative alkaline phosphatase reaction (Table 3). CDC group F-1 strains are usually susceptible to penicillin but are often resistant to macrolides.

C. diphtheriae

In 2003, the complete genome sequence of a *Corynebacterium diphtheriae* strain representative of the diphtheria outbreak in the former Soviet Union states in the 1990s was determined (17). The genome consists of a single circular chromosome of 2,488,635 bp with no plasmids. A complete set of enzymes for the glycolysis, gluconeogenesis, and pentose-phosphate pathways is present, as are all the de novo amino acid biosynthesis pathways. Fimbrial and fimbria-related genes, sialidase (neuraminidase) genes, and iron uptake systems have been detected as pathogenicity factors.

C. diphtheriae is commonly divided into four biotypes, gravis, mitis, belfanti, and intermedius; biotype differentiation is recommended by the WHO (33, 34), although biotypes cannot be assigned separate subspecies status, and biotyping is not satisfactory for epidemiologic tracking. Initially, these biotypes were defined by differences in colony morphology and biochemical reactions (Table 3). However, only C. diphtheriae biotype intermedius can be identified on the basis of colonial morphology (small, gray, or translucent lipophilic colonies) as well as positivity for dextrin fermentation. Other C. diphtheriae biotypes produce larger (up to 2 mm after 24 h) white or opaque colonies (Fig. 3b) which are indistinguishable from each other. The lipophilic C. diphtheriae biotype intermedius occurs only rarely in clinical infections, and C. diphtheriae biotype belfanti strains rarely express diphtheria toxin.

Presumptive identification of C. diphtheriae (as well as of C. pseudotuberculosis and C. ulcerans) may be made by testing suspicious gram-positive rods for the presence of cystinase (as detected by using freshly prepared Tinsdale medium or diagnostic tablets [Rosco, Taastrup, Denmark]) and the absence of pyrazinamidase (diagnostic tablets are available from Key Scientific Products, Stamford, TX). The API Coryne system identifies C. diphtheriae strains, but additional tests are needed for the differentiation of C. diphtheriae biotype mitis, C. diphtheriae biotype belfanti, and C. diphtheriae biotype intermedius (69). Usually, C. diphtheriae strains do not ferment sucrose, but in Brazil, sucrose-positive strains have been described. Large amounts of propionic acid are produced as the end product of glucose metabolism. C. diphtheriae strains are distinct from all other coryneform bacteria (except C. pseudotuberculosis and C. ulcerans) in their CFA patterns by the presence of a large volume of $C_{16:1\omega7c}$ (7).

Diphtheria Toxin Testing

It is recommended that at least 10 colonies of C. diphtheriae and related species be tested for diphtheria toxin by the Elek method, modified as described by Engler et al. (37), in a laboratory with skill in performing the test and in interpreting the test results. The modified Elek method as described by the WHO Diphtheria Reference Unit was initially used to characterize strains from the epidemic in the 1990s in Russia and Ukraine and was found to be faster and less technically problematic than the original version. Antitoxin from various suppliers (Berna Biotech AG [Switzerland], Mikrogen [Russia], Biomed [Russia], Pasteur Mérieux/Aventis Pasteur [France], BulBio-NCIPD

[Bulgaria], Instituto Butantan [Brazil], or Refik Saydam National Hygiene Centre [Turkey]) (102) applied to blank filter disks at 10 IU/disk have been successfully used with the modified Elek test.

PCR-based methods for the detection of the diphtheria toxin gene (*tox*) in isolated bacteria have been developed and validated (32, 78, 107). Conventional PCR detection of the regulatory *dtxR* gene has been evaluated (111). Detection of the *tox* gene using a real-time platform has been described (15, 99, 136). Primers targeting the C. diphtheriae *tox* gene for C. ulcerans strains perform better with modifications (15, 135, 136). *tox* PCR assays applied directly to clinical specimens are acceptable, particularly because isolation is not always possible for patients already receiving antibiotics. However, a PCR-positive patient from whom bacteria are not isolated or who lacks a histopathologic diagnosis and an epidemiologic linkage to a patient with a laboratory-confirmed case of diphtheria should be classified as a "probable case" of diphtheria, since to date there are insufficient data to conclude that a PCR-positive result always infers diphtheria. Also, detection of the toxin gene in samples by PCR cannot automatically be attributed to one species because C. diphtheriae as well as C. ulcerans and C. pseudotuberculosis may harbor the bacteriophage which carries the diphtheria toxin gene. Furthermore, *tox*-containing, nontoxigenic isolates have been described and characterized further. Difficulties in identifying C. diphtheriae and in correctly performing toxigenicity tests have recently been demonstrated by an external quality control program observing 23 national diphtheria reference centers in Europe; in these centers, 21% of specimens were misidentified and 13% of toxigenicity reports were determined to be unacceptable (102).

Nontoxigenic strains of C. diphtheriae, i.e., those which do not express toxin in the Elek test or those which lack a detectable diphtheria toxin gene by PCR, have also caused serious disease, such as cases or outbreaks of skin disease, endocarditis, and occasional mortality among homeless people, alcoholics, and intravenous drug abusers (45, 116, 131). For nontoxigenic C. diphtheriae strains circulating in the United Kingdom, it has been shown that the diphtheria toxin repressor (*dtxR*) genes are functional, so that if these strains are lysogenized by a bacteriophage, they could represent a reservoir for toxigenic C. diphtheriae (29).

Antibiotic treatment, with antibiotics of choice being penicillins or macrolides, is required to eliminate C. diphtheriae and prevent its spread; however, it is not a substitute for antitoxin prevention. Sporadic isolates of C. diphtheriae resistant to erythromycin or rifampin have been reported.

C. durum

C. durum (126) was originally described as being exclusively isolated from respiratory tract specimens. Well-characterized isolates have now been recovered from additional sites, including the gingiva, blood cultures, and abscesses (115). C. durum strains were originally isolated after 2 to 3 days from nonselective buffered charcoal-yeast extract plates inoculated with sputa or bronchial washings, but isolates grow well on other standard laboratory media. C. durum is the most frequent *Corynebacterium* isolated from throat swabs of healthy persons (158). Its pathogenic potential remains unclear. C. durum is a peculiar nonlipophilic organism that forms colonies of only 0.5 to 1 mm in diameter after aerobic incubation for 72 h. The original description of this bacterium cited beige and rough colonies with convolutions, an irregular margin, and strong adherence to agar if grown under aerobic conditions (126). However, strains were later described to be sometimes smoother and not necessarily adherent to agar (115). Gram staining of aerobic cultures shows long and filamentous rods, with occasional "bulges," but true *C. durum* isolates do not have *C. matruchotii*-like "whip handles" (Fig. 1e and f). Long forms are not otherwise found among other *Corynebacterium* species (except *C. canis*), nor are they observed for *C. durum* when cells are grown in a 10% CO$_2$-enriched atmosphere (126). Strains grow only weakly under anaerobic conditions. They always reduce nitrate, and some may exhibit weak and delayed urease and esculinase activities. The majority (but not all) of *C. durum* strains ferment mannitol, which is another very unusual feature for true corynebacteria (Table 3). API Coryne codes observed for *C. durum* include 3000135, 3001135, 3040135, 3400115, 3400135, 3400305, 3400325, and 3400335 (126), as well as 3040325, 3040335, 3440335, and 3441335 (115). This suggests that most strains are negative for alkaline phosphatase, and all appear to be negative for pyrrolidonyl arylamidase. Only a small number of *C. durum* strains have been tested with the RapID CB Plus system, and all were correctly identified (67). It is most likely that some strains identified as *C. matruchotii* in the past may actually have been *C. durum* strains and that differentiation can be difficult if phenotypic methods alone are used. Both species produce propionic acid as a fermentation product (6). *C. durum* usually ferments galactose and very often mannitol, whereas *C. matruchotii* is usually negative for those sugars. The *C. matruchotii* type strain exhibits α-glucosidase activity, which is not observed in *C. durum* (126). It has been shown that some *C. durum* strains also express β-galactosidase activity and ferment ribose (158).

C. falsenii

C. falsenii strains (139) have been isolated mainly from sterile body fluids. Colonies are whitish, glistening, and smooth, with entire edges, and are 1 to 2 mm in diameter after 24 h. After 72 h, most strains described to date exhibit a yellowish pigment which becomes even more intense after 120 h. The most characteristic biochemical features of *C. falsenii* are a slow but fermentative acid production from glucose, a weak pyrazinamidase reaction, and a weak urease activity which becomes visible in either Christensen's urea broth or the API Coryne system after overnight incubation only. API Coryne codes observed for *C. falsenii* have been 2101104 and 2101304 (8, 139).

C. freiburgense

This nonlipophilic species has probably been transmitted to a human by a dog bite (53). The 5-day-old colonies exhibit a very peculiar "spoked-wheel" macroscopic morphology not observed in other true corynebacteria but observed in some *R. dentocariosa* strains. Colonies are also strongly adherent to blood agar. Distinct biochemical features are the lack of pyrazinamidase activity and a positive β-galactosidase reaction.

C. freneyi

This species was initially outlined on the basis of a study of three strains (117) which came from skin-related material. There is now evidence that *C. freneyi* is also isolated from genitourinary specimens (52) and bacteremic patients (5). *C. freneyi* is phylogenetically closely related to *C. xerosis*. Colonies are typically wrinkled, whitish, dry, and rough, have irregular edges, and are 0.5 to 1 mm in diameter after 48 h incubation, but *C. freneyi* strains are nonlipophilic.

The basic biochemical profile (Table 3) is similar to that of *C. xerosis*. All *C. freneyi* strains studied so far exhibit α-glucosidase activity, which is not frequently observed in other *Corynebacterium* species (very few *C. amycolatum* and all *C. xerosis* strains express this enzyme). *C. freneyi* can be furthermore differentiated from *C. xerosis* by glucose fermentation at 42°C and growth at 20°C, whereas *C. xerosis* is negative for these two reactions. This species is also closely related to *C. hansenii*.

C. glucuronolyticum

C. seminale is a later synonym of *C. glucuronolyticum* (28, 47). This species is probably part of the normal genitourinary biota of males, while its presence in females is uncertain. Recoveries from blood cultures have been documented (8). Colonies are whitish yellow, convex, and creamy, and they are 1 to 1.5 mm in diameter after 24 h. The fermentative species *C. glucuronolyticum* is remarkable for its variability in basic biochemical reactions (Table 3). It is the only medically relevant, large-colony *Corynebacterium* species exhibiting β-glucuronidase activity. When urease activity is present, it is abundant in Christensen's urea broth, becoming positive after only 5 min of incubation at room temperature (47). *C. glucuronolyticum* is also one of the very few corynebacteria which are able to hydrolyze esculin. All *C. glucuronolyticum* strains are CAMP reaction positive (Fig. 2). The API Coryne strip identifies *C. glucuronolyticum* well but not strains which are alkaline phosphatase positive (69), although profiles obtained from human strains may differ from those of animal isolates (28). Propionic acid is one of the major end products of glucose metabolism. *C. glucuronolyticum* strains are often tetracycline resistant and may also exhibit resistance to macrolides and lincosamides (68). 16S rRNA gene sequences derived from fluids of patients with prostatitis have been found to be homologous with sequences derived for this species, indicating that *C. glucuronolyticum* might be involved in selected cases of prostatitis (146).

C. hansenii

This nonlipophilic species exhibits yellow and dry colonies (119). Biochemical identification reactions are similar to those of *C. freneyi* and *C. xerosis*. However, *C. hansenii* can be distinguished from these species by being negative for alkaline phosphatase and α-glucosidase reactions. These three species are not well discerned by either 16S rRNA or partial *rpoB* gene sequencing but were found to represent different taxa by DNA-DNA hybridization (119).

C. imitans

C. imitans was originally isolated from a nasopharyngeal specimen of a child suspected of having throat diphtheria, as well as from three adult contacts (49). This was the first well-documented case of the person-to-person transmission of a *Corynebacterium* species other than *C. diphtheriae* in a nonhospital setting. Additional strains of *C. imitans* have been recovered from blood cultures (8). Colonies are creamy, whitish gray, and glistening, with entire edges, and they are 1 to 2 mm in diameter. The strain does not produce a brown halo on Tinsdale medium but is tellurite reductase positive. Interestingly, it is positive for polar bodies by Neisser staining. Pyrazinamidase activity is only weak, as is fermentation of sucrose, which may lead to an initial misidentification as an atypical *C. diphtheriae* strain. It is possible that *C. imitans* may have been misidentified as *C. minutissimum* in the past, since the biochemical reactions of both taxa are similar (Table 3). However, *C. imitans* is CAMP reaction positive and does not hydrolyze tyrosine, whereas the opposite reactions are observed for *C. minutissimum*. The API Coryne system provided the numerical codes 1100325, 2100324, and 3100325 for *C. imitans*, indicating a negative α-glucosidase reaction, whereas all *C. diphtheriae* strains express this enzyme. *C. imitans* strains do not produce propionic acid as a fermentation product, unlike *C. diphtheriae* (8), and the CFA composition profiles for the species qualitatively differ, as *C. diphtheriae* and closely related species have a unique pattern among *Corynebacterium* species. Diphtheria toxin assessment by Elek testing or by assaying for the *tox* gene by PCR are negative for *C. imitans* strains (8, 49). *C. imitans* is resistant to O/129, while *C. diphtheriae* is not.

C. jeikeium

C. jeikeium is a frequently encountered *Corynebacterium* in clinical specimens (72). Nosocomial transmission has been described. The complete genome sequence of a *C. jeikeium* strain has been determined (147, 148), indicating that the lipophilic phenotype of *C. jeikeium* originates from the absence of fatty acid synthase. *C. jeikeium* is often resistant to multiple antibiotics (including penicillin and gentamicin) (42, 75), but this cannot be used as a taxonomic characteristic because the phenotypically closely related *C. tuberculostearicum* may also demonstrate multidrug resistance. Quantitative DNA-DNA hybridization experiments have shown that *C. jeikeium* includes two genomospecies for which penicillin and gentamicin MICs are low, but as they could not otherwise be differentiated phenotypically from the resistant *C. jeikeium* strains, they were not proposed as independent species (124). Colonies of *C. jeikeium* are tiny, low, entire, and grayish white. *C. jeikeium* is a strict aerobe which may oxidatively produce acid from glucose and sometimes from maltose but not from fructose (*C. tuberculostearicum* is positive for acid production from fructose). The RapID CB Plus system correctly identifies *C. jeikeium*, as does the API Coryne system if ancillary tests are used (67, 69).

C. kroppenstedtii

C. kroppenstedtii (23), a rather rarely recovered species, was originally recovered from the sputum of a patient with pulmonary disease. Additional strains have been isolated from lung biopsy specimens, sputum, a breast abscess, and patients with granulomatous lobular mastitis (8, 110). Colonies are grayish, translucent, slightly dry, and less than 0.5 mm in diameter after 24 h of incubation at 37°C. *C. kroppenstedtii* is lipophilic and is one of the few medically relevant *Corynebacterium* species exhibiting esculinase activity. Other biochemical characteristics are given in Table 3. API Codes of *C. kroppenstedtii* include 0101104, 2040104, and 2040105 (8). It can be separated from *C. durum*, *C. matruchotii*, and *C. glucuronolyticum* by colony and Gram stain morphologies and from *C. glucuronolyticum* by its negative CAMP reaction. The determination of the whole-genome sequence revealed that lipophilism is the dominant feature involved in the pathogenicity of *C. kroppenstedtii* (149).

C. lipophiloflavum

Initially, *C. lipophiloflavum* (55) was represented by a single strain which had been isolated from vaginal discharge from a patient with BV. Additional strains have now been described from blood cultures (G. Funke, R. Frodl, E. Falsen, C. Spröer, H.-P. Klenk, and S. Stenger, submitted for publication). This species contains lipophilic strains, but the majority of strains are nonlipophilic (Funke et al., submitted). The lipophilic strains have the same biochemical screening pattern as *C. urealyticum*, except that they exhibit a strong yellow pigment and weaker urease activity and slowly produce acid from glucose (Table 3). In contrast to most *C. urealyticum* strains, the *C. lipophiloflavum* strains isolated were not multidrug resistant. The nonlipophilic strains have a biochemical profile similar to that of *C. falsenii* but do not ferment galactose and trehalose (Funke et al., submitted).

C. macginleyi

C. macginleyi (128) has almost exclusively been isolated from eye specimens, whether from diseased (62) or healthy conjunctiva. Colonies are typical for lipophilic corynebacteria (see above). When grown on Tween 80-SBA plates (better growth is usually found on plates supplemented with 0.1% Tween 80 than on those supplemented with 1.0% Tween 80), some *C. macginleyi* strains exhibit a rose pigment which is not seen for any other lipophilic *Corynebacterium* species. *C. macginleyi* is one of the very few *Corynebacterium* species not expressing pyrazinamidase activity (Table 3). Most strains ferment mannitol, while the majority of other corynebacteria are unable to do so. The API Coryne system correctly identifies *C. macginleyi* (69). Strains belonging to this species are susceptible to a broad spectrum of antibiotics (62), but high-level fluoroquinolone resistance has been reported (35).

C. massiliense

This species was isolated from synovial fluid (96). It does not produce acid from any of the carbohydrates tested in the differentiation of true corynebacteria (Table 3), but its cell wall contains TBSA.

C. mastitidis-Like Organism

Bacteria recovered from ocular specimens (patients with cataracts, diabetic retinopathy, or dry eyes) were by 16S rRNA gene sequencing found to be closest (98.2% identity) to *C. mastitidis*, which to date has otherwise been found to cause sheep mastitis. In contrast to *C. macginleyi*, these strains are susceptible to the fluoroquinolones, but no other information about these strains is extant (35).

C. matruchotii

C. matruchotii is thought to be a natural inhabitant of the oral cavity, particularly on calculus and plaque deposits, and so has been much studied by oral microbiologists (115). Otherwise, it is a very rare human pathogen. Microcolonies appear flat, filamentous, and spider-like, but macrocolonies have a variable appearance (19). *C. matruchotii* demonstrates a very unusual appearance by Gram staining in that so-called whip handles (i.e., filamentous bacteria with a single short bacillus adjacent to the end of the filament that creates the illusion of a whip) are observed (Fig. 1f). This microscopic presentation is consistent even when isolates that have been preserved for many years in a culture collection are stained. It has been demonstrated that heterogeneity exists among *C. matruchotii* strains obtained from international culture collections and that some strains represented were misidentified *C. durum* isolates (115). *C. matruchotii* strains are consistently negative for galactose, whereas *C. durum* strains can be positive. The API Coryne system database does not contain *C. matruchotii*; the numerical codes observed for *C. matruchotii* include 7000325, 7010325, and 7050325.

C. matruchotii-Like Strain

A C. matruchotii-like strain is represented by a single strain, ATCC 43833 (115). It was deposited in the ATCC as C. matruchotii, but it is a distinct species, as revealed by dot blot hybridization and 16S rRNA gene sequencing data (GenBank accession no. AF260434). Colonies are the size of pinpoints to 0.1 mm in diameter and grayish white, with a smooth, nonadherent texture. Biochemical screening reactions are similar to those of C. minutissimum except that strain ATCC 43833 exhibits esculinase activity in the API Coryne system, with an API Coryne code of 2140325.

C. minutissimum

C. minutissimum is part of the normal human skin biota, and its historical association with erythrasma is highly questionable (72). Colonies of C. minutissimum are whitish gray, shiny, moist, convex, and circular; they have entire edges and are about 1 to 1.5 mm in diameter after 24 h. Most of the colonies are creamy, but some may also have a sticky consistency. C. minutissimum strains have a fermentative metabolism and produce acid from sucrose variably. Very few C. minutissimum strains are also able to produce acid from mannitol. The API Coryne system identifies C. minutissimum, with additional tests being necessary for most strains (69). Many C. minutissimum strains are pyrrolidonyl arylamidase positive. C. minutissimum strains exhibit DNase activity, nearly all strains hydrolyze tyrosine, and a very few strains exhibit a positive CAMP reaction. Lactic and succinic acids are major end products of glucose metabolism. Some isolates possess TBSA in their cell membranes. Nearly all C. minutissimum strains are susceptible to O/129 (150-μg disk); i.e., they exhibit an inhibition zone around the disk (usually between 20 and 35 mm in diameter). Phylogenetically, C. minutissimum is closely related (>98.8% identity) to both C. singulare and C. aurimucosum by 16S rRNA gene sequencing, but these are readily discerned by partial rpoB gene sequence analysis.

C. mucifaciens

C. mucifaciens (58) has been isolated mainly from blood cultures and other sterile body fluids but has also been recovered from abscesses, soft tissue, and dialysate (8). Colonies are very distinct because they are slightly to overtly yellow and very mucoid (Fig. 3c) (very few strains are not mucoid [G. Funke, unpublished observation]). C. mucifaciens is the only presently known Corynebacterium species exhibiting such mucoid colonies; this characteristic strongly reminds bacteriologists of Rhodococcus equi colonies. An extracellular substance (probably polysaccharides) causing connective filaments between the cells has been demonstrated as the ultrastructural correlate of the mucoid colonies. Colonies are about 1 to 1.5 mm after 24 h of incubation and have entire edges. They appear less mucoid after extended incubation for 96 h. C. mucifaciens has an oxidative metabolism. It consistently produces acid from glucose, but acid production from sucrose is variable. The API Coryne numerical codes 2000004, 2000104, 2000105, 2100104, 2100105, 6000004, 6100104, and 6100105 have been observed for C. mucifaciens, suggesting that occasionally glucose oxidation may be too slow to be observed by that method. C. mucifaciens is enzymatically less active than R. equi, which exhibits α- and β-glucosidase activities not observed for C. mucifaciens. In addition, C. mucifaciens produces acid from fructose and may produce acid from glycerol and mannose, but acid production from these sugars is not seen in R. equi strains. TBSA can be detected in amounts of

1 to 2% of the total CFAs. β-Lactam antibiotics and aminoglycosides show very good activities against C. mucifaciens.

C. pilbarense

This nonlipophilic species was isolated from an ankle aspirate of a male thought to be suffering from gout (3). It can be differentiated from C. striatum and C. simulans by being nitrate reduction negative and from C. minutissimum by not fermenting maltose. Phylogenetically, it is closest (98.7 to 99.0% identity) to C. ureicelerivorans, C. coyleae, C afermentans, and C. mucifaciens but was distinguished from those species by DNA-DNA hybridization and biochemically (Table 3) (3).

C. propinquum

C. propinquum is the closest phylogenetic relative of C. pseudodiphtheriticum (108, 133) and shares the same niche (i.e., the oropharynx) as C. pseudodiphtheriticum. Colonies are whitish and somewhat dryish, with entire edges, and are 1 to 2 mm in diameter after 24 h of incubation. This species reduces nitrate and hydrolyzes tyrosine but does not hydrolyze urea (Table 3). The API Coryne system and the RapID CB Plus system correctly identify C. propinquum strains (67, 69).

C. pseudodiphtheriticum

C. pseudodiphtheriticum is part of the normal oropharyngeal biota. As described in Table 2, this species has been well documented to cause pneumonia in various patient populations. Colonies are whitish and slightly dry, with entire edges, and they are 1 to 2 mm in diameter after 48 h of incubation. This nonfermenting species reduces nitrate and hydrolyzes urea but does not produce acid from any of the commonly tested carbohydrates (Table 3). Some strains hydrolyze tyrosine. The API Coryne and the RapID CB Plus systems correctly identify C. pseudodiphtheriticum strains (67, 69). Imperfectly cleaved mycolic acids coelute with CFAs (7). C. pseudodiphtheriticum strains are susceptible to β-lactam antibiotics, but resistance to macrolides and lincosamides has been observed.

C. pseudotuberculosis

C. pseudotuberculosis is phylogenetically closest to C. ulcerans and to C. diphtheriae (108, 133); like those species, it may harbor the diphtheria toxin gene and produce propionic acid as a fermentation product, and its cell wall contains large amounts of the CFA $C_{16:1\omega7c}$ (7). Colonies are yellowish white, opaque, convex, and about 1 mm in diameter after 24 h. Like C. ulcerans, C. pseudotuberculosis is positive for urease and positive by the CAMP inhibition test. In this test, complete inhibition of the effect of S. aureus beta-hemolysin on sheep erythrocytes is achieved by streaking the presumed C. pseudotuberculosis strain in a right angle toward S. aureus and incubating overnight; a beta-hemolysin inhibition zone in the form of a triangle is observed, as is true for A. haemolyticum (Fig. 2). C. pseudotuberculosis is not susceptible to O/129, whereas C. ulcerans strains are. C. pseudotuberculosis has varied results for both nitrate reduction and sucrose fermentation. The API Coryne system and the RapID CB Plus panel correctly identify this species (67, 69). Human disease to date has been acquired by handling of infected sheep.

C. pyruviciproducens

This species was independently isolated from a groin abscess (151) and a urethral swab (G. Funke, unpublished observation) and was initially believed to be a lipophilic variant of *C. glucuronolyticum*, which was β-glucuronidase and CAMP test positive. However, 16S rRNA gene sequence analysis, quantitative DNA-DNA hybridization, and partial *rpoB* gene sequence analysis clearly demonstrated that this species is distinct from *C. glucuronolyticum* (151).

C. resistens

This species has entire, grayish-white, and glistening colonies and is lipophilic. It is unusual in having a negative pyrazinamidase reaction, which separates it from the phenotypically related *C. jeikeium* or *C. tuberculostearicum*. In addition, *C. resistens* grows slowly under anaerobic conditions, whereas *C. jeikeium* is unable to do so. The *C. resistens* strains reported in the literature are resistant to penicillin, cephalosporins, aminoglycosides, clindamycin, and ciprofloxacin but remain susceptible to glycopeptides (106). It is presently unknown whether true *C. resistens* strains are often misidentified as *C. jeikeium* in routine laboratories.

C. riegelii

C. riegelii strains were originally described as being isolated from females with urinary tract infections (59), but additional strains have been recovered from blood cultures, including cord blood (8). Colonies are whitish, glistening, and convex, with entire margins, and are up to 1.5 mm in diameter after 48 h of incubation. Some colonies are of a creamy consistency, whereas others are sticky. *C. riegelii* strains exhibit a very strong urease activity with Christensen's urea broth, becoming positive within 5 min at room temperature after inoculation. A very peculiar characteristic of *C. riegelii* is the slow fermentation of maltose but not glucose. No other defined *Corynebacterium* species exhibits this feature (Table 3). The weak anaerobic growth of *C. riegelii* corresponds to the weak fermentative metabolism. API Coryne system codes observed for *C. riegelii* include 0101224, 2001224, and 2101224.

C. simulans

This species was originally delineated from some *C. striatum*-like strains (159). The three strains described in the original publication came from skin-related specimens (foot abscess, lymph node biopsy specimen, and boil). Two additional strains have been characterized, one from bile and one from a blood culture (8). Colonies of *C. simulans* (grayish white, glistening, creamy, 1 to 2 mm in diameter) are very similar to those of *C. minutissimum*, *C. singulare*, and *C. striatum*, its closest phylogenetic neighbors. *C. simulans* is the only valid *Corynebacterium* species described to date which reduces nitrite. Further characteristics which separate *C. simulans* from the closely related nonlipophilic, fermentative corynebacteria are an inability to acidify ethylene glycol and to grow at 20°C (unlike *C. striatum*). API Coryne profiles include 0100305, 2100105, 2100301, 2100305, and 3000125 (including a falsely negative nitrate reduction reaction because of the strong nitrite reduction).

C. singulare

C. singulare colonies are circular and slightly convex, with entire margins, and are of a creamy consistency, as observed for *C. minutissimum* and *C. striatum* (130). Key biochemical reactions are like those for *C. minutissimum* except that urease activity is observed (Table 3). The numerical API Coryne system profile is 6101125, which indicates that pyrrolidonyl arylamidase activity is present. Like *C. minutissimum* and *C. striatum*, *C. singulare* hydrolyzes tyrosine. *C. singulare* does not produce propionic acid as a fermentation

product, differentiating it from *C. amycolatum*. Phylogenetically, this species is closely related (>98.8% identity) to both *C. aurimucosum* and *C. minutissimum* by 16S rRNA gene sequencing but can readily be discerned by partial *rpoB* gene sequence analysis.

C. sputi

This species is the only true *Corynebacterium* that expresses α-glucosidase activity and is positive for TBSA (164). It can be differentiated from *C. ulcerans* by being positive for pyrazinamidase activity but negative for alkaline phosphatase and maltose fermentation. Unlike *C. ulcerans*, this species cannot harbor the bacteriophage which bears the diphtheria *tox* gene.

C. stationis

This species, originally called *Brevibacterium stationis*, has recently been reassigned to the genus *Corynebacterium* (9). *B. stationis* ATCC 14403^T was originally recovered from sea water, but subsequent studies found that two human blood culture isolates plus "*C. ammoniagenes*" ATCC 6872, recovered from an infant's stools, formed a single taxon group now designated *C. stationis* comb. nov. Strains of both *C. stationis* and *C. ammoniagenes* sensu stricto demonstrate the ability to alkalinize citrate, using either Simmon's citrate or a heavy (not light) inoculum in the citrate reaction chamber found in an API 20E strip, a feature not previously associated with members of the genus *Corynebacterium*. Colonies of *C. stationis* grow well in 24 h (that is, they are not lipophilic), are yellow or yellowish, and ferment glucose, fructose, ribose, and mannose. All are positive for the alkalinization of citrate, produce urease, reduce nitrate, and hydrolyze tyrosine (other features are shown in Table 3). API Coryne codes generated were 1001304 and 3001304 (that is, the enzyme PYZ is variably detected). Strains of this species are susceptible to all antimicrobials; however, one blood culture isolate was shown to be resistant to erythromycin.

C. striatum

C. striatum is part of the normal human skin biota. Nosocomial transmission of *C. striatum* has been documented (89, 121). Colonies are convex, circular, shiny, moist, and creamy, with entire edges, and are about 1 to 1.5 mm in diameter after 24 h of incubation. Some investigators have described *C. striatum* colonies as being somewhat like those of small coagulase-negative staphylococci. *C. striatum* has a fermentative metabolism, and acid production from sucrose is variable. The API Coryne system identifies *C. striatum*, but additional tests are needed in most cases (69). All *C. striatum* strains hydrolyze tyrosine, and some strains are CAMP reaction positive; however, the CAMP reaction of *C. striatum* strains is usually not as strong as that of other CAMP test-positive species (e.g., *C. auris* or *C. glucuronolyticum*). Lactic and succinic acids are the major end products of glucose metabolism. All *C. striatum* strains are susceptible to O/129. Resistance to macrolides and lincosamides due to the presence of an rRNA methylase has been described. *C. striatum* may also be resistant to quinolones and tetracyclines (42, 75), which has led to a renewed interest in this agent as an emerging pathogen (10).

C. sundsvallense

C. sundsvallense (8, 20) has been isolated from blood cultures, a vaginal swab, and a sinus drainage specimen from an infected groin. Colonies of this nonlipophilic species are buff or slightly yellowish, they adhere to agar, and they have a sticky consistency. Gram staining shows bulges or knobs at the ends of some rods, and these are not seen in any other corynebacteria. Fermentation of glucose, lactose, and sucrose is slow (Table 3). *C. sundsvallense* can be separated from *C. durum* by its positive α-glucosidase reaction and its inability to ferment galactose. It is differentiated from *C. matruchotii* by expressing urease but not nitrate reductase activity and by not producing propionic acid as an end product of glucose metabolism (8, 20).

C. thomssenii

C. thomssenii (169) is a rarely found species. It was originally repeatedly isolated from a patient with pleural effusion, and a second strain was recovered from the environment in Canada (8). This species is fastidious and grows slowly, resulting in colonies of <0.5 mm after 48 h, but it is not lipophilic. After 96 h, colonies are molar-tooth-like, very sticky, and slightly adherent to agar. The clinical strain of *C. thomssenii* is the only *Corynebacterium* species expressing *N*-acetyl-β-glucosaminidase activity, which can be observed in either the API Coryne or the API ZYM system. Acid is slowly and fermentatively produced from glucose, maltose, and sucrose, and the resulting API Coryne code for *C. thomssenii* is 2121125.

C. timonense

This species was isolated from blood cultures of a patient with endocarditis. Its most peculiar feature is a weakly positive esculinase reaction. It can be differentiated from other esculinase-positive corynebacteria by having negative reactions for maltose and sucrose fermentation as well as a negative CAMP reaction (96).

C. tuberculostearicum

This species was revived for a never validly published taxon and also includes a strain of the nonvalidated species "*C. pseudogenitalium*" (43). Nearly all "CDC group G" bacteria can be assigned to *C. tuberculostearicum* (K. A. Bernard and G. Funke, unpublished observation). Unfortunately, the effective publication on *C. tuberculostearicum* did not include any strains of CDC group G bacteria (43). *C. tuberculostearicum* has some variable biochemical key reactions and can be differentiated from *C. accolens* if TBSA is detected as one of its CFAs. It can be separated from *C. jeikeium* by anaerobic growth and fermentative acid production from fructose. *C. tuberculostearicum* can be multidrug resistant, but the most frequently observed resistance is to macrolides and lincosamides.

C. tuscaniense

This species has been isolated from blood cultures of a patient suffering from endocarditis. *C. tuscaniense* does not grow under anaerobic conditions, which distinguishes this species from the phenotypically similar *C. minutissimum*. In addition, *C. tuscaniense* hydrolyzes hippurate but not tyrosine, whereas *C. minutissimum* has opposite reactions (Table 3). *C. tuscaniense* colonies are rounded and regular, in contrast to the biochemically similar species *C. amycolatum*, whose colonies exhibit irregular edges (123).

C. ulcerans

Phylogenetically, *C. ulcerans* (129) is closely related to *C. pseudotuberculosis*, and both species are the closest relatives to *C. diphtheriae* (108, 133). Its cell membrane contains significant amounts of the CFA $C_{16:1\omega7c}$. As described previously, *C. ulcerans* can harbor the diphtheria toxin gene,

but differences in the receptor-binding and translocation domains have been described, so a *C. ulcerans* diphtheria toxin-specific PCR has been developed for conventional PCR (138) or real-time PCR (15, 135, 136). Disease associated with this bacterium is rare, but if it is recovered from pseudomembranous material, it must be treated like a case of diphtheria (33, 34). Recent reports have described the transmission of *C. ulcerans* from companion pets to humans (11, 31, 88), and so expanded national cases of diphtheria-like diseases that include cases involving toxigenic strains of *C. ulcerans* or *C. pseudotuberculosis* have formally been defined in some countries (K. Bernard, unpublished observation) (11). *C. ulcerans* colonies are somewhat dry, waxy, and grayish white, with light hemolysis; they are 1 to 2 mm in diameter after 24 h. *C. ulcerans* may be differentiated from *C. diphtheriae* by urease activity and a CAMP inhibition reaction and from *C. pseudotuberculosis* by source, biochemically, and by partial *rpoB* gene but not 16S rRNA gene sequencing. Strains of *C. ulcerans* are positive for glycogen, starch, and trehalose fermentation. The API Coryne system and the RapID CB Plus identification strip correctly identify *C. ulcerans* (67, 69).

C. urealyticum

C. urealyticum is one of the relatively frequently isolated clinically significant corynebacteria in clinical specimens (72). *C. urealyticum* is strongly associated with urinary tract infections. Recovery of this bacterium is often associated with urine with an alkaline pH, resulting in struvite crystals. As for all other lipophilic corynebacteria, colonies are the size of a pinpoint, convex, smooth, and whitish gray on regular SBA. *C. urealyticum* is a strict aerobe and has very strong urease activity (Table 3). Commercial identification systems correctly identify *C. urealyticum*. *C. urealyticum* is almost always multidrug resistant (42, 72, 140). Sequencing of the whole *C. urealyticum* genome indicated that the multidrug resistance is mediated by transposable elements (150).

C. ureicelerivorans

Lipophilic *C. ureicelerivorans*, first described from a blood culture, has very strong and rapidly detected (~60 s) urease activity as its most prominent feature (163). Subsequently, recovery of this organism from ascites fluid and multiple blood cultures from immunocompromised patients or those with digestive disorders has been described (41). It can be differentiated from CDC group F-1 bacteria by a positive alkaline phosphatase reaction and by a negative reaction for acid production from maltose and sucrose. By 16S rRNA and partial *rpoB* gene sequencing, this species is closest to *C. mucifaciens*; *C. ureicelerivorans* can readily be discerned from that species by its smooth rather than mucoid yellowish colonies as well as by observation of rapid urease activity.

C. xerosis

C. xerosis colonies are dry, granular, and yellowish, with irregular edges, and are 1 to 1.5 mm in diameter after 24 h. It must be emphasized that nearly all "*C. xerosis*" strains which have been described in the literature before 1996 may have been misidentified *C. amycolatum* strains (56). *C. striatum* strains were also misidentified as *C. xerosis* in the past. *C. xerosis* has a fermentative metabolism and has variable results for the presence of nitrate reductase but always expresses α-glucosidase as well as leucine arylamidase activity. Because *C. xerosis* was thought to be rarely encountered in clinical specimens, it was not included in the API Coryne system version 3.0 database. The numerical profiles observed for *C. xerosis* strains, such as 2110325 and 3110325, provide API Web responses that include "*C. striatum/C. amycolatum.*" The RapID CB Plus system correctly identifies *C. xerosis* (67). Lactic acid is the major end product of glucose metabolism, and strains are susceptible to O/129. As described previously, *C. xerosis* is closely phylogenetically related to *C. freneyi* and *C. hansenii* (119), and so if definitive identification is required, characterization must include genetic testing.

Genus *Turicella*

T. otitidis is almost exclusively isolated from clinical specimens from the ear region, but it does not cause otitis media with effusion in children. Colonies are whitish, convex, and creamy, with entire edges, and are 1 to 1.5 mm in diameter after 48 h of incubation. Some young colonies show a greenish appearance when taken away from the plates with a swab. The distinctive Gram stain morphology of *T. otitidis* is given in Fig. 1b. Differentiation from *C. auris* and *C. afermentans* subsp. *afermentans* is readily achieved by morphologic features, but utilization reactions may also assist in the differentiation of these taxa (Tables 3 and 4) (57, 118). All *T. otitidis* strains are strongly CAMP reaction positive and give the numerical code 2100004 in the API Coryne system. The MICs of β-lactam antibiotics for many strains are very low; some strains might be resistant to macrolides and clindamycin (68, 75). The mechanism of resistance to macrolides appears to be due in part to mutations in the 23S rRNA (*rrl*) gene (12).

Genus *Arthrobacter*

Arthrobacter spp. might be part of the indigenous normal human biota, but their main habitat is soil. *A. cumminsii* seems to be a normal commensal in humans and appears to be the most frequently isolated *Arthrobacter* species in human clinical specimens (63, 92), and *A. oxydans* is the second-most-frequently encountered species (92). *Arthrobacter* colonies are usually whitish gray, slightly glistening, creamy, and 2 mm or greater in diameter after 24 h. *A. cumminsii* is slightly smaller than the other arthrobacters and may also exhibit a sticky consistency (63). *Arthrobacter* spp. usually do not oxidize any of the carbohydrates routinely tested and do not emit a cheese-like smell, as is often found for the phenotypically closely related brevibacteria. Some arthrobacters are motile, whereas brevibacteria are always nonmotile. Like brevibacteria, *Arthrobacter* spp. express DNase and have gelatinase activity (54). The identification of arthrobacters to the species level might be achieved by carbohydrate utilization tests, but this is recommended for reference laboratories only. *A. albus* (160) is phylogenetically most closely related to *A. cumminsii* but might be differentiated phenotypically by being resistant to desferrioxamine, whereas *A. cumminsii* is susceptible. *A. cumminsii* has a distinctive CFA pattern, with $C_{14:0i}$ and $C_{14:0}$ each representing 2 to 4% of all CFAs (54). Penicillin MICs for most *Arthrobacter* strains are low, with quinolones showing only weak activities against *Arthrobacter* spp. (54, 92).

Genus *Brevibacterium*

Some *Brevibacterium* spp. are part of the normal human skin biota. Colonies are whitish gray (or yellowish like *B. luteolum*), convex, mostly creamy, and 2 mm or greater in diameter after 24 h. *B. mcbrellneri* colonies have a more granular appearance and are dryer than those of other brevibacteria. Some brevibacteria may develop a yellowish or greenish pigment after prolonged incubation. Many *Brevibacterium* strains isolated from human clinical material give off a distinctive cheese-like odor. Brevibacteria are nonmotile, are halotolerant (6.5% NaCl), and form methanethiol from methionine, but this test is specific for brevibacteria only when it is read within 2 h (48). Brevibacteria can be identified to the species level by carbohydrate utilization tests. More than 90% of all clinical *Brevibacterium* isolates are *B. casei* (48). *Brevibacterium sanguinis* is very similar to *B. casei* and can be differentiated from this species by susceptibility to thallium acetate. The MICs of β-lactam antibiotics for brevibacteria are often elevated (68).

Genus *Dermabacter*

D. hominis strains are part of the normal skin biota. Colonies are whitish, convex, of a creamy or sticky consistency, and 1 to 1.5 mm in diameter after 48 h (Fig. 3e). *D. hominis* strains are sometimes mistaken for small-colony coagulase-negative staphylococci. The Gram staining result is distinctive, with coccobacillary or coccoidal forms (Fig. 1c). The key biochemical reactions are given in Table 4. *D. hominis* is one of the few coryneform bacteria with a variable reaction for xylose fermentation. It is the only catalase-positive coryneform bacterium (except *Actinomyces neuii*) that is able to decarboxylate lysine and ornithine (70). The API Coryne system and the RapID CB Plus panel correctly identify this species (67, 69). *D. hominis* strains may be resistant to aminoglycosides (68, 152).

Genus *Helcobacillus*

The genus *Helcobacillus* contains one species, *H. massiliensis*, and by phenotypic testing resembles *D. hominis*. However, when substrates found in the API Coryne or API 50CH panel are used, *H. massiliensis* can be differentiated from *D. hominis* by several key reactions, including the abilities to ferment erythritol, arabinose, xylose, inositol, and mannitol and reduce nitrate (122).

Genus *Rothia*

The *Rothia* genus presently comprises six validly named species, two of which are deemed to be clinically relevant: *R. mucilaginosa* (formerly designated *Stomatococcus mucilaginosus*) (24) and *R. dentocariosa*, as emended by Daneshvar et al. (26). A taxon group provisionally called *R. dentocariosa* genomovar II (85) has been found to be consistent with *Rothia aeria* (90), and occasional isolates most closely related to *R. aeria*, recovered from respiratory specimens and blood cultures, have been characterized (K. Bernard, unpublished observation). Morphologically, biochemically, and by CFA composition analysis, these were very similar to *R. dentocariosa*, as described by Kronvall for genomospecies II, but were readily discerned by 16S rRNA gene sequencing.

Some strains formerly designated CDC coryneform group 4 (Fig. 3h) have been shown to be representatives of *R. dentocariosa* (26). These grayish-black-pigmented strains were isolated primarily from respiratory materials, pus, or blood cultures, in contrast to black-pigmented *C. aurimucosum* strains derived from the female urogenital tract.

Colonies of *R. dentocariosa* are typically whitish (or, more rarely, grayish black), raised, and smooth or rough or have a spoked-wheel form (Fig. 3f), and they are up to 2 mm in diameter after 48 h. *Rothia* strains usually grow slightly better in a CO_2-enriched atmosphere. The biochemical features of *R. dentocariosa* are given in Table 4. The API Coryne system correctly identifies *R. dentocariosa* (69).

Its CFA composition is of the branched-chain type (7), which allows differentiation from the biochemically similar species C. durum, C. matruchotii, and Actinomyces viscosus (see chapter 49 in this Manual), all of which also occupy the oropharynx. R. dentocariosa may also be confused with D. hominis and Propionibacterium avidum (see chapter 49) (156), both of which, in contrast, always exhibit smooth colonies. As shown in a study on the pharyngeal bacterial biota of healthy adults, one-third of all R. dentocariosa strains isolated were negative for the key biochemical reaction, catalase (158). The MICs of aminoglycosides for some R. dentocariosa strains are elevated, whereas penicillins usually show good in vitro activities against Rothia strains.

Genus Exiguobacterium

It is not known whether exiguobacteria are part of the indigenous bacterial biota of humans. Colonies of E. acetylicum are smooth, golden-yellow to orange, and up to 2 mm in diameter after 24 h of incubation. It is positive for oxidase, and acid from carbohydrates, except xylose, is rapidly produced by fermentative metabolism. Exiguobacteria are motile. They might be confused with microbacteria, but CFA and phylogenetic analyses provide a clear-cut distinction between the two genera (Table 1). The pathogenic potential of E. acetylicum seems to be rather low; this species has been isolated from different sources (e.g., skin, wounds, and cerebrospinal fluid [79]). Cases of pseudobacteremia due to E. acetylicum have been observed. Six E. aurantiacum strains isolated from blood cultures had been received by a national reference center over a 10-year period; these strains, although biochemically similar to E. acetylicum, are oxidase negative and positive or variably positive for DNase and xylose, with strains being susceptible to all drug classes as tested by the Etest (bioMérieux) (112).

Genus Oerskovia

Oerskovia turbata, a very rare human pathogen, is usually acquired from the environment (e.g., soil). Colonies are pale yellow to phosphorous yellow, convex, and creamy; they penetrate into agar ("substrate hyphae") and are approximately 1 to 2 mm in diameter after 24 h. O. turbata rapidly produces acid from sugars by fermentation; it also exhibits a very strong esculin reaction. The genus is identified by the API Coryne system (69). O. turbata liquefies gelatin but does not hydrolyze xanthine or hypoxanthine. In contrast, the related Cellulomonas cellulans (see below) does not liquefy gelatin but is able to hydrolyze xanthine and hypoxanthine (14).

Genus Cellulomonas

Cellulomonas strains are usually acquired from the environment. Colonies are at first whitish or pale or bright yellow, but after 7 days, nearly all Cellulomonas strains are somewhat yellow. Colonies vary between 0.5 and 1.5 mm in diameter after 24 h, they are convex and creamy, and they have entire edges but do not demonstrate substrate hyphae (13). Cellulomonas spp. are variable for the fermentation of mannitol. Other key biochemical reactions are given in Table 4. The majority of Cellulomonas strains express cellulase activity, as was demonstrated by incubating a heavy bacterial suspension (McFarland no. 6 standard) with a piece of sterile copy paper in a 0.9% NaCl solution for 10 days, resulting in dissolution of the paper (64). The medically relevant species C. denverensis can be differentiated from C. hominis by its positive reaction for D-sorbitol fermentation (13, 105).

Genus Cellulosimicrobium

Colonies of C. cellulans are similar to O. turbata (see above) and also pit the agar. In addition, C. cellulans exhibits a biochemical screening profile which is very similar to that of O. turbata (Table 4). However, C. cellulans hydrolyzes either xanthine or hypoxanthine, whereas O. turbata does not, and O. turbata strains might be motile, whereas C. cellulans strains are not (143). C. funkei strains can be differentiated from C. cellulans (formerly Oerskovia xanthineolytica) by their negative inulin and raffinose fermentation reactions (14); in addition, C. funkei strains are motile, but C. cellulans strains are not.

Genus Microbacterium

Microbacteria account for the majority of yellow-pigmented coryneform bacteria isolated from clinical specimens. All shades of yellow pigment are observed, ranging from pale yellow to bright yellow and orange. Most of the strains are catalase positive, but catalase-negative strains might be observed. Some microbacteria grow under anaerobic conditions but only weakly. Some microbacteria are nitrate reductase negative, which separates them from the phenotypically closely related genus Cellulomonas, of which all presently defined species are nitrate reductase positive (Table 4). Microbacteria may ferment mannitol and xylose. In contrast, no Cellulomonas strain was observed to ferment mannitol and all fermented xylose.

Species identification is almost impossible since the type strain is the only representative for many defined Microbacterium species, preventing the creation of a comprehensive database. Final identification to the species level is best achieved by molecular investigations (e.g., using 16S rRNA gene sequencing). The most frequently isolated, validated microbacteria in clinical specimens include M. oxydans, M. paraoxydans, and M. foliorum (74, 86).

Microbacteria are usually susceptible to meropenem, linezolid, doxycycline, and vancomycin (except M. resistens, which is resistant to vancomycin but susceptible to teicoplanin [60]). Susceptibility to other antimicrobial agents is unpredictable, and therefore, individual clinically significant strains must be tested (74).

Genus Curtobacterium

Curtobacteria are very infrequently isolated yellow- or yellow-orange-pigmented oxidative coryneform bacteria. In contrast to most microbacteria, they produce acid from carbohydrates very slowly (within 4 to 7 days) (46). Curtobacteria are usually nitrate reductase negative but strongly hydrolyze esculin (Table 4). Curtobacterium pusillum and related strains have a very unusual CFA composition which is not observed in any other coryneform bacteria, with an ω-cyclohexyl fatty acid identified as feature 7 ($C_{18:1\omega7c/\omega9c/\omega12t}$) representing more than 50% of all CFAs (46). Again, the differentiation of curtobacteria is very difficult and should be performed only in a reference laboratory. The MICs of macrolides and rifampin for curtobacteria are very low.

Genus Leifsonia

Leifsonia aquatica is very rarely encountered in clinical specimens. It is always motile, does not hydrolyze either gelatin or casein, and has a stronger DNase activity than most microbacteria (73). L. aquatica is the only species within the genus Leifsonia which is able to grow in broth enriched with 5% NaCl (38). Its yellow pigment develops relatively slowly, within 3 to 4 days. The MICs of vancomycin for some L. aquatica strains were shown to be elevated (8 μg/ml) (73), but the precise mechanism of this resistance is not known.

Genera *Janibacter, Pseudoclavibacter (Zimmermannella), Brachybacterium,* and *Knoellia*

Strains belonging to the *Janibacter, Pseudoclavibacter (Zimmermannella), Brachybacterium,* and *Knoellia* genera have been derived from the environment, foods, or animals but have also been recovered recently from clinical materials and characterized using 16S rRNA gene sequencing. These taxa were described as having white, creamy, or yellowish pigment, and all were nonmotile. *Janibacter, Pseudoclavibacter* (later synonym, *Zimmermannella*), and *Knoellia* were oxidative, and *Brachybacterium* strains were fermentative. All strains tested so far were susceptible to vancomycin. Since no comprehensive biochemical data based on a large number of strains are available at present, these genera were not included in Table 4.

Genus *Arcanobacterium*

The genus *Arcanobacterium* comprises nine species. The three medically relevant species, *A. haemolyticum, A. pyogenes,* and *A. bernardiae,* are all catalase negative and exhibit β-hemolysis on SBA. All species show a fermentative glucose metabolism, with succinic and lactic acids as their major end products. All arcanobacteria grow and express hemolysis best in a CO_2-enriched atmosphere.

The colonies of the type species, *A. haemolyticum,* are 0.5 mm in diameter after 48 h of incubation at 37°C, and two morphotypes have been described: one rough type isolated mainly from the respiratory tract and one smooth type isolated mainly from wounds. The biochemical reactions of *A. haemolyticum* are given in Table 4. Of major value for the identification of *A. haemolyticum* is the so-called CAMP inhibition test (see the description of the CAMP inhibition test in the section on *C. pseudotuberculosis*) (Fig. 2). The protein responsible for this phenomenon is a phospholipase D excreted by *A. haemolyticum,* and this protein is genetically and functionally similar to the ones expressed by *C. ulcerans* and *C. pseudotuberculosis. A. haemolyticum* as well as the two other medically relevant arcanobacteria are correctly identified by the API Coryne system (69).

A. pyogenes colonies are the largest of all arcanobacteria colonies, with diameters of up to 1 mm after 48 h of incubation. Of all the arcanobacteria, this species also shows the sharpest zone of β-hemolysis on SBA. The protein responsible for hemolysis, named pyolysin, is also an important virulence factor in vivo. Gram stains may show some branching rods. *A. pyogenes* is the only *Arcanobacterium* species of medical relevance that expresses β-glucuronidase activity and that is capable of fermenting xylose.

A. bernardiae (66, 109) shows glassy, whitish colonies of <0.5 mm in diameter after 48 h. Some colonies have a creamy consistency, whereas others are sticky. Gram staining shows relatively short rods without branching. Most *A. bernardiae* strains belong to the very few coryneform bacteria that are able to ferment glycogen. Another peculiar feature of *A. bernardiae* strains is their ability to produce acid faster from maltose than from glucose.

The MICs of all β-lactams, rifampin, and tetracycline for arcanobacteria are very low, whereas aminoglycosides and quinolones have reduced activities against arcanobacteria (G. Funke, unpublished observation). Macrolides also exhibit excellent activities against arcanobacteria and are an alternative to β-lactam antibiotics for the treatment of infections. Treatment failures with β-lactam antibiotics have been reported due to the inability of β-lactam antibiotics to act intracellularly.

Genus *Gardnerella*

G. vaginalis strains are consistently α-glucosidase, starch hydrolysis, and proline aminopeptidase positive, but only 90% of all *G. vaginalis* strains hydrolyze hippurate. Both the API Strep and API Coryne systems identify *G. vaginalis* well (69). Confirmation of the identification of *G. vaginalis* can also be achieved by antimicrobial agent disk inhibition tests with 50 μg of metronidazole (inhibition present), 5 μg of trimethoprim (inhibition present), and 1 mg of sulfonamide (inhibition absent).

TYPING SYSTEMS

Outbreaks of *C. diphtheriae* in the states of the former Soviet Union and other locations have been studied by whole-cell peptide analysis, whole-genome restriction fragment length polymorphism analysis, ribotyping, pulsed-field gel electrophoresis, PCR–single-strand conformation polymorphism analysis, analysis of *tox* and *dtxR* as well as of the 16S-23S rRNA spacer region, amplified fragment length polymorphism analysis, random amplification of polymorphic DNA, and multilocus enzyme electrophoresis (30, 113). An international database for *C. diphtheriae* ribotypes using the endonuclease BstEII has been established (76). Ribotyping is regarded as being highly discriminatory and, based on a comprehensive comparison of methods, was found to be a preferred typing method for *C. diphtheriae* (30). Other methods, including a spoligotyping system (similar to the spacer oligonucleotide typing for *Mycobacterium tuberculosis*), have been described (98). Sequencing studies with *C. diphtheriae* strains from the epidemic in the former Soviet Union have shown that point mutations within the *tox* gene were silent mutations and that multiple point mutations (which even led to amino acid substitutions) were observed for the *dtxR* gene, corresponding to the heterogeneity of outbreak strains as revealed by PCR–single-strand conformation polymorphism analysis (100). Isolates derived from specific populations in the United States and Canada and characterized by multilocus enzyme electrophoresis, ribotyping, and random amplification of polymorphic DNA were found to be members of persistent endemic strains, rather than being imported from other countries where diphtheria is endemic. More recently, a standardized multilocus sequence typing method based on analysis of short sequences derived from seven housekeeping alleles has been under development, with which concatenated sequence data, sent by the Internet to the curator (initially the University of Warwick and then the Institut Pasteur, Paris [relocation in 2009]), are compared to a large database and given an existing or new sequence type (25). Due to the technical simplicity of this approach and the ease of comparison of strain data internationally, this is being touted as a typing method for the future. Multilocus sequence typing has also been effectively applied to an outbreak investigation involving *C. macginleyi* and *C mastitidis*-like isolates (35).

SEROLOGIC TESTS

Detection of antibodies directed against diphtheria toxin is the only established serologic test for coryneform bacteria. Toxin neutralization assays using a Vero cell culture system have been replaced mainly by enzyme immunoassays. Levels of ≥0.1 IU/ml serum are thought to confer protection, whereas levels of <0.01 IU/ml indicate a susceptible host and levels of 0.01 to 0.1 IU/ml indicate partially immune individuals. It is believed that between 20 and 60% of adults in the United States lack protective antibodies to diphtheria toxin due to declining antibody titers in immunized persons and in those persons who did not receive the primary immunization series. This could pose a potentially significant public health risk and could result in the reemergence of this disease. Booster doses of toxoid should be administered at 10-year intervals.

ANTIMICROBIAL SUSCEPTIBILITIES

The susceptibility patterns for each taxon were given with the descriptions of each taxon (see above). Since the antimicrobial susceptibility of coryneform bacteria is not predictable in every case, susceptibility testing should always be performed with clinically significant isolates (see "Clinical Significance" above). Due to the emergence of vancomycin-resistant gram-positive organisms, it has become inappropriate to recommend glycopeptides as first-line drugs for the treatment of infections caused by coryneform bacteria. It is also noteworthy that some coryneform bacteria (e.g., *Microbacterium resistens*) are intrinsically vancomycin resistant.

The Clinical and Laboratory Standards Institute has published testing conditions and interpretive criteria for susceptibility testing of coryneform bacteria using a broth microdilution method (18). Direct colony suspensions equivalent to a 0.5 McFarland standard are prepared and strains are incubated in cation-adjusted Mueller-Hinton broth with 2 to 5% (vol/vol) lysed horse blood at 35°C in ambient air for up to 48 h. Interpretative categories for the MICs obtained are presently available for 16 antimicrobial agents. In summary, using the broth microdilution method, it has recently been established that multidrug resistance was found for 4 or more drug classes (out of 16 classes tested) for some or most strains of *C. amycolatum*, *C. jeikeium*, *C. urealyticum*, *C. resistens*, *C. tuberculostearicum*, and *C. striatum*, as well as representatives of *C. afermentans* and *C. aurimucosum* found in one national culture collection (C. Singh, T. Burdz, and K. Bernard, unpublished observations). Very few studies have been performed comparing broth microdilution and disk diffusion results for susceptibility testing of coryneform bacteria (162).

In the past, MICs were determined by either the Etest or the agar dilution or broth microdilution method. The results of the Etest have been shown to correlate reasonably well with those of both the broth microdilution and the agar dilution method for *Corynebacterium* spp. (95, 167). The Etest should be carried out on Mueller-Hinton agar supplemented with 5% sheep blood. The same medium is used for the agar dilution method (68), but this method is not applicable in routine laboratories and, rather, should be used in studies with individual antimicrobial agents.

Metronidazole is the drug of choice both for local therapy of BV and for systemic therapy of extravaginal infections caused by BV-associated biota. Systemic infections due to *G. vaginalis* alone can be treated with ampicillin or amoxicillin, since β-lactamase-producing *G. vaginalis* strains have not been observed so far. Susceptibility testing for *G. vaginalis* is not recommended.

EVALUATION, INTERPRETATION, AND REPORTING OF RESULTS

The guidelines related to when coryneform bacteria should be identified to the species level (see "Clinical Significance" above) are also applicable for evaluating and interpreting culture results; i.e., whenever coryneform bacteria are identified to the species level, the results should be reported.

In the rare case of microscopically suspected *C. diphtheriae* (i.e., a positive Neisser staining result), the physician in charge of the patient should be notified immediately, although culture results and toxin testing results become available only later.

It is evident that repeated isolation of a predominant strain of a coryneform bacterium or a coryneform bacterium growing in pure culture suggests an etiological relationship to the patient's disease. If coryneform bacteria are present in blood cultures, the physician in charge should be notified immediately, and it should be emphasized when reporting that the clinical significance of the coryneform bacteria must be carefully examined by cooperation between the microbiology laboratory and the physician. In our experience, one positive blood culture out of two or three aerobically and anaerobically incubated pairs of blood cultures is hardly ever clinically significant (except in cases of treated endocarditis). Care must be taken in the interpretation of the results for those patients for whom half or more of the blood specimens taken for culture become positive for coryneform bacteria, in particular when lipophilic corynebacteria are cultured, since not all blood samples taken from patients with endocarditis due to lipophilic corynebacteria may eventually become positive.

On the other hand, coryneform bacteria should be reported as "normal flora" when they are grown from nonsterile sites together with other resident biota in equal or smaller numbers. It is suggested that the primary isolation plates be retained for at least 72 h before they are discarded in order to have the opportunity to assess the bacterial population retrospectively.

REFERENCES

1. **Achermann, Y., A. Trampuz, F. Moro, J. Wüst, and M. Vogt.** 2009. *Corynebacterium bovis* shoulder prosthetic joint infection: the first reported case. *Diagn. Microbiol. Infect. Dis.* **64:**213–215.
2. **Adekambi, T., T. M. Shinnick, D. Raoult, and M. Drancourt.** 2008. Complete *rpoB* gene sequencing as a suitable supplement to DNA-DNA hybridization for bacterial species and genus delineation. *Int. J. Syst. Evol. Microbiol.* **58:**1807–1814.
3. **Aravena-Roman, M., C. Spröer, B. Sträubler, T. Inglis, and A. F. Yassin.** 2010. *Corynebacterium pilbarense* sp. nov., a non-lipophilic corynebacterium isolated from a human ankle aspirate. *Int. J. Syst. Evol. Microbiol.* **60:**1484–1487.
4. **Aubel, D., F. N. R. Renaud, and J. Freney.** 1997. Genomic diversity of several *Corynebacterium* species identified by amplification of the 16S-23S rRNA gene spacer regions. *Int. J. Syst. Bacteriol.* **47:**767–772.
5. **Auzias, A., C. Bollet, R. Ayari, M. Drancourt, and D. Raoult.** 2003. *Corynebacterium freneyi* bacteremia. *J. Clin. Microbiol.* **41:**2777–2778.
6. **Bernard, K. A.** 2005. *Corynebacterium* species and coryneforms: an update on taxonomy and diseases attributed to these taxa. *Clin. Microbiol. Newsl.* **27:**9–18.
7. **Bernard, K. A., M. Bellefeuille, and E. P. Ewan.** 1991. Cellular fatty acid composition as an adjunct to the identification of asporogenous, aerobic gram-positive rods. *J. Clin. Microbiol.* **29:**83–89.
8. **Bernard, K. A., C. Munro, D. Wiebe, and E. Ongsansoy.** 2002. Characteristics of rare or recently described *Corynebacterium* species recovered from human clinical material in Canada. *J. Clin. Microbiol.* **40:**4375–4381.
9. **Bernard, K. A., D. Wiebe, T. Burdz, A. Reimer, B. Ng, C. Singh, S. Schindle, and A. L. Pacheco.** 2009. Assignment of *Brevibacterium stationis* (ZoBell and Upham 1994) Breed 1953 to the genus *Corynebacterium* as *Corynebacterium stationis* comb. nov. and emended description of the genus *Corynebacterium* to include isolates which can alkalinize citrate. *Int. J. Syst. Evol. Microbiol.* **60:**874–879.

10. **Boltin, D., M. Katzir, V. Bugoslavsky, I. Yalashvili, T. Brosh-Nissimov, M. Fried, and O. Elkayam.** 2009. *Corynebacterium striatum*—a classic pathogen eluding diagnosis. *Eur. J. Intern. Med.* **20:**e49–e52.

11. **Bonmarin, I., N. Guiso, A. Le Flèche-Matéos, O. Patey, A. D. Patrick, and D. Levy-Bruhl.** 2009. Diphtheria: a zoonotic disease in France? *Vaccine* **27:**4196–4200.

12. **Boumghar-Bourtchai, L., H. Chardon, B. Malbruny, S. Mezghani, R. Leclercq, and A. Dhalluin.** 2009. Resistance to macrolides by ribosomal mutation in clinical isolates of *Turicella otitidis*. *Int. J. Antimicrob. Agents* **34:**274–277.

13. **Brown, J. M., R. P. Frazier, R. E. Morey, A. G. Steigerwalt, G. J. Pellegrini, M. I. Daneshvar, D. G. Hollis, and M. M. McNeil.** 2005. Phenotypic and genetic characterization of clinical isolates of CDC coryneform group A-3: proposal of a new species of *Cellulomonas, Cellulomonas denverensis* sp. nov. *J. Clin. Microbiol.* **43:**1732–1737.

14. **Brown, J. M., A. G. Steigerwalt, R. E. Morey, M. I. Daneshvar, L. J. Romero, and M. M. McNeil.** 2006. Characterization of clinical isolates previously identified as *Oerskovia turbata*: proposal of *Cellulosimicrobium funkei* sp. nov. and emended description of the genus *Cellulosimicrobium*. *Int. J. Syst. Evol. Microbiol.* **56:**801–804.

15. **Cassiday, P. K., L. C. Pawloski, T. Tiwari, G. N. Sanden, and P. P. Wilkins.** 2008. Analysis of toxigenic *Corynebacterium ulcerans* strains revealing potential for false-negative real-time PCR results. *J. Clin. Microbiol.* **46:**331–333.

16. **Catlin, B. W.** 1992. *Gardnerella vaginalis*: characteristics, clinical considerations, and controversies. *Clin. Microbiol. Rev.* **5:**213–237.

17. **Cerdeno-Tarraga, A. M., A. Efstratiou, L. G. Dover, M. T. G. Holden, M. Pallen, S. D. Bentley, G. S. Besra, C. Churcher, K. D. James, A. De Zoysa, T. Chillingworth, A. Cronin, L. Dowd, T. Feltwell, N. Hamlin, S. Holroyd, K. Jagels, K. Moule, M. A. Quail, E. Rabbinowitsch, K. M. Rutherford, N. R. Thomson, L. Unwin, S. Whitehead, B. G. Barrell, and J. Parkhill.** 2003. The complete genome sequence and analysis of *Corynebacterium diphtheriae* NCTC 13129. *Nucleic Acid Res.* **31:**6516–6523.

18. **Clinical and Laboratory Standards Institute.** 2010. Methods for antimicrobial dilution and disk susceptibility testing of infrequently isolated or fastidious bacteria. Document M45-A2. Clinical and Laboratory Standards Institute, Wayne, PA.

19. **Collins, M. D.** 1982. Reclassification of *Bacterionema matruchotii* (Mendel) in the genus *Corynebacterium*, as *Corynebacterium matruchotii* comb. nov. *Zentralbl. Bakteriol. Mikrobiol. Hyg. Abt. 1 Orig.* **C3:**364–367.

20. **Collins, M. D., K. A. Bernard, R. A. Hutson, B. Sjöden, A. Nyberg, and E. Falsen.** 1999. *Corynebacterium sundsvallense* sp. nov., from human clinical specimens. *Int. J. Syst. Bacteriol.* **49:**361–366.

21. **Collins, M. D., R. A. Burton, and D. Jones.** 1988. *Corynebacterium amycolatum* sp. nov., a new mycolic acid-less *Corynebacterium* species from human skin. *FEMS Microbiol. Lett.* **49:**349–352.

22. **Collins, M. D., and C. S. Cummins.** 1986. Genus *Corynebacterium*, p. 1266–1276. *In* P. H. A. Sneath, N. S. Mair, M. E. Sharpe, and J. G. Holt (ed.), *Bergey's Manual of Systematic Bacteriology*, vol. 2. The Williams & Wilkins Co., Baltimore, MD.

23. **Collins, M. D., E. Falsen, E. Akervall, B. Sjöden, and A. Alvarez.** 1998. *Corynebacterium kroppenstedtii* sp. nov., a novel corynebacterium that does not contain mycolic acids. *Int. J. Syst. Bacteriol.* **48:**1449–1454.

24. **Collins, M. D., R. A. Hutson, V. Baverud, and E. Falsen.** 2000. Characterization of a *Rothia*-like organism from a mouse: description of *Rothia nasimurium* sp. nov. and reclassification of *Stomatococcus mucilaginosus* as *Rothia mucilaginosa* comb. nov. *Int. J. Syst. Evol. Microbiol.* **50:**1247–1251.

25. **Dallman, T., S. Neal, J. Green, and A. Efstratiou.** 2008. Development of an online database for diphtheria molecular epidemiology under the remit of the DIPNET project. *Euro Surveill.* **13:**18865.

26. **Daneshvar, M. I., D. G. Hollis, R. S. Weyant, J. G. Jordan, J. P. MacGregor, R. E. Morey, A. M. Whitney, D. J. Brenner, A. G. Steigerwalt, L. O. Helsel, P. M. Raney, J. B. Patel, P. N. Levett, and J. M. Brown.** 2004. Identification of some charcoal-black-pigmented CDC fermentative coryneform group 4 isolates as *Rothia dentocariosa* and some as *Corynebacterium aurimucosum*: proposal of *Rothia dentocariosa* emend. Georg and Brown 1967, *Corynebacterium aurimucosum* emend. Yassin et al. 2002, and *Corynebacterium nigricans* Shukla et al. 2003 pro synon. *Corynebacterium aurimucosum*. *J. Clin. Microbiol.* **42:**4189–4198.

27. **De Briel, D., F. Couderc, P. Riegel, F. Jehl, and R. Minck.** 1992. High-performance liquid chromatography of corynomycolic acids as a tool in identification of *Corynebacterium* species and related organisms. *J. Clin. Microbiol.* **30:**1407–1417.

28. **Devriese, L. A., P. Riegel, J. Hommez, M. Vaneechoutte, T. de Baere, and F. Haesebrouck.** 2000. Identification of *Corynebacterium glucuronolyticum* strains from the urogenital tract of humans and pigs. *J. Clin. Microbiol.* **38:**4657–4659.

29. **De Zoysa, A., A. Efstratiou, and P. M. Hawkey.** 2005. Molecular characterization of diphtheria toxin repressor (*dtxR*) genes present in nontoxigenic *Corynebacterium diphtheriae* strains isolated in the United Kingdom. *J. Clin. Microbiol.* **43:**223–228.

30. **De Zoysa, A., P. Hawkey, A. Charlett, and A. Efstratiou.** 2008. Comparison of four molecular typing methods for characterization of *Corynebacterium diphtheriae*: transcontinental spread of *C. diphtheriae* based on BstEII rRNA gene profiles. *J. Clin. Microbiol.* **46:**3626–3635.

31. **De Zoysa, A., P. M. Hawkey, K. Engler, R. George, G. Mann, W. Reilly, D. Taylor, and A. Efstratiou.** 2005. Characterization of toxigenic *Corynebacterium ulcerans* strains isolated from humans and domestic cats in the United Kingdom. *J. Clin. Microbiol.* **43:**4377–4381.

32. **Efstratiou, A., K. H. Engler, C. S. Dawes, and D. Sesardic.** 1998. Comparison of phenotypic and genotypic methods for detection of diphtheria toxin among isolates of pathogenic corynebacteria. *J. Clin. Microbiol.* **36:**3173–3177.

33. **Efstratiou, A., K. H. Engler, I. K. Mazurova, T. Glushkevich, J. Vuopio-Varkila, and T. Popovic.** 2000. Current approaches to the laboratory diagnosis of diphtheria. *J. Infect. Dis.* **181**(Suppl. 1):S138–S145.

34. **Efstratiou, A., and R. C. George.** 1999. Laboratory guidelines for the diagnosis of infections caused by *Corynebacterium diphtheriae* and *C. ulcerans*. *WHO Commun. Dis. Public Health* **2:**250–257.

35. **Eguchi, H., T. Kuwahara, T. Miyamoto, H. Nakayama-Imaohji, M. Ichimura, T. Hayashi, and H. Shiota.** 2008. High-level fluoroquinolone resistance in ophthalmic clinical isolates belonging to the species *Corynebacterium macginleyi*. *J. Clin. Microbiol.* **46:**527–532.

36. **Elsayed, S., and K. Zhang.** 2005. Bacteremia caused by *Janibacter melonis*. *J. Clin. Microbiol.* **43:**3537–3539.

37. **Engler, K. H., T. Glushkevich, I. K. Mazarova, R. C. George, and A. Efstratiou.** 1997. A modified Elek test for detection of toxigenic corynebacteria in the diagnostic laboratory. *J. Clin. Microbiol.* **35:**495–498.

38. **Evtushenko, L. I., L. V. Dorofeeva, S. A. Subbotin, J. R. Cole, and J. M. Tiedje.** 2000. *Leifsonia poae* gen. nov., sp. nov., isolated from nematode gall on *Poa annua*, and reclassification of 'Corynebacterium aquaticum' Leifson 1962 as *Leifsonia aquatica* (ex Leifson 1962) gen. nov., nom. rev., comb. nov. and *Clavibacter xyli* Davis et al. 1984 with two subspecies as *Leifsonia xyli* (Davis et al. 1984) gen. nov., comb. nov. *Int. J. Syst. Evol. Microbiol.* **50:**371–380.

39. **Farrow, J. A. E., S. Wallbanks, and M. D. Collins.** 1994. Phylogenetic interrelationships of round-spore-forming bacilli containing cell walls based on lysine and the non-spore-forming genera *Caryophanon, Exiguobacterium, Kurthia*, and *Planococcus*. *Int. J. Syst. Bacteriol.* **44:**74–82.

40. **Fernández-Natal, M. I., J. A. Sáez-Nieto, R. Fernández-Roblas, M. Asencio, S. Valdezate, S. Lapeña, R. H. Rodríguez-Pollán, J. M. Guerra, J. Blanco, F. Cachón, and F. Soriano.** 2008. The isolation of *Corynebacterium coyleae* from clinical samples: clinical and microbiological data. *Eur. J. Clin. Microbiol. Infect. Dis.* **27:**177–184.

41. Fernández-Natal, M. I., J. A. Sáez-Nieto, S. Valdezate, R. H. Rodríguez-Pollán, S. Lapeña, F. Cachón, and F. Soriano. 2009. Isolation of *Corynebacterium ureicelerivorans* from normally sterile sites in humans. *Eur. J. Clin. Microbiol. Infect. Dis.* **28:**677–681.

42. Fernandez-Roblas, R., H. Adames, N. Z. Martín-de-Hijas, D. G. Almeida, I. Gadea, and J. Esteban. 2009. In vitro activity of tigecycline and 10 other antimicrobials against clinical isolates of the genus *Corynebacterium. Int. J. Antimicrob. Agents* **33:**453–455.

43. Feurer, C., D. Clermont, F. Bimet, A. Candrea, M. Jackson, P. Glaser, C. Bizet, and C. Dauga. 2004. Taxonomic characterization of nine strains isolated from clinical and environmental specimens, and proposal of *Corynebacterium tuberculostearicum* sp. nov. *Int. J. Syst. Evol. Microbiol.* **54:**1055–1061.

44. Fredricks, D. N., T. L. Fiedler, K. K. Thomas, B. B. Oakley, and J. M. Marrazzo. 2007. Targeted PCR for detection of vaginal bacteria associated with bacterial vaginosis. *J. Clin. Microbiol.* **45:**3270–3276.

45. Funke, G., M. Altwegg, L. Frommelt, and A. von Graevenitz. 1999. Emergence of related nontoxigenic *C. diphtheriae* biotype *mitis* strains in Western Europe. *Emerg. Infect. Dis.* **5:**477–480.

46. Funke, G., M. Aravena-Roman, and R. Frodl. 2005. First description of *Curtobacterium* spp. isolated from human clinical specimens. *J. Clin. Microbiol.* **43:**1032–1036.

47. Funke, G., K. A. Bernard, C. Bucher, G. E. Pfyffer, and M. D. Collins. 1995. *Corynebacterium glucuronolyticum* sp. nov. isolated from male patients with genitourinary infections. *Med. Microbiol. Lett.* **4:**204–215.

48. Funke, G., and A. Carlotti. 1994. Differentiation of *Brevibacterium* spp. encountered in clinical specimens. *J. Clin. Microbiol.* **32:**1729–1732.

49. Funke, G., A. Efstratiou, D. Kuklinska, R. A. Hutson, A. De Zoysa, K. H. Engler, and M. D. Collins. 1997. *Corynebacterium imitans* sp. nov. isolated from patients with suspected diphtheria. *J. Clin. Microbiol.* **35:**1978–1983.

50. Funke, G., R. Englert, R. Frodl, K. A. Bernard, and S. Stenger. 2010. *Corynebacterium canis* sp. nov., isolated from a wound infection caused by a dog bite. *Int. J. Syst. Evol. Microbiol.* **60:**2544–2547.

51. Funke, G., E. Falsen, and C. Barreau. 1995. Primary identification of *Microbacterium* spp. encountered in clinical specimens as CDC coryneform group A-4 and A-5 bacteria. *J. Clin. Microbiol.* **33:**188–192.

52. Funke, G., and R. Frodl. 2008. Comprehensive study of *Corynebacterium freneyi* strains and extended and emended description of *Corynebacterium freneyi* Renaud, Aubel, Riegel, Meugnier, and Bollet 2001. *J. Clin. Microbiol.* **46:**638–643.

53. Funke, G., R. Frodl, K. A. Bernard, and R. Englert. 2009. *Corynebacterium freiburgense* sp. nov., isolated from a wound from a dog bite. *Int. J. Syst. Evol. Microbiol.* **59:**2054–2057.

54. Funke, G., R. A. Hutson, K. A. Bernard, G. E. Pfyffer, K. Weiss, M. D. Collins, and G. Wauters. 1996. Isolation of *Arthrobacter* spp. from clinical specimens and description of *Arthrobacter cumminsii* sp. nov. and *Arthrobacter woluwensis* sp. nov. *J. Clin. Microbiol.* **34:**2356–2363.

55. Funke, G., R. A. Hutson, M. Hilleringmann, W. R. Heizmann, and M. D. Collins. 1997. *Corynebacterium lipophiloflavum* sp. nov. isolated from a patient with bacterial vaginosis. *FEMS Microbiol. Lett.* **150:**219–224.

56. Funke, G., P. A. Lawson, K. A. Bernard, and M. D. Collins. 1996. Most *Corynebacterium xerosis* strains identified in the routine clinical laboratory correspond to *Corynebacterium amycolatum. J. Clin. Microbiol.* **34:**1124–1128.

57. Funke, G., P. A. Lawson, and M. D. Collins. 1995. Heterogeneity within Centers for Disease Control and Prevention coryneform group ANF-1-like bacteria and description of *Corynebacterium auris* sp. nov. *Int. J. Syst. Bacteriol.* **45:**735–739.

58. Funke, G., P. A. Lawson, and M. D. Collins. 1997. *Corynebacterium mucifaciens* sp. nov., an unusual species from human clinical material. *Int. J. Syst. Bacteriol.* **47:**952–957.

59. Funke, G., P. A. Lawson, and M. D. Collins. 1998. *Corynebacterium riegelii* sp. nov., an unusual species isolated from female patients with urinary tract infections. *J. Clin. Microbiol.* **36:**624–627.

60. Funke, G., P. A. Lawson, F. S. Nolte, N. Weiss, and M. D. Collins. 1998. *Aureobacterium resistens* sp. nov. exhibiting vancomycin resistance and teicoplanin susceptibility. *FEMS Microbiol. Lett.* **158:**89–93.

61. Funke, G., C. R. Osorio, R. Frei, P. Riegel, and M. D. Collins. 1998. *Corynebacterium confusum* sp. nov., isolated from human clinical specimens. *Int. J. Syst. Bacteriol.* **48:**1291–1296.

62. Funke, G., M. Pagano-Niederer, and W. Bernauer. 1998. *Corynebacterium macginleyi* has to date been isolated exclusively from conjunctival swabs. *J. Clin. Microbiol.* **36:**3670–3673.

63. Funke, G., M. Pagano-Niederer, B. Sjöden, and E. Falsen. 1998. Characteristics of *Arthrobacter cumminsii*, the most frequently encountered *Arthrobacter* species in human clinical specimens. *J. Clin. Microbiol.* **36:**1539–1543.

64. Funke, G., C. Pascual Ramos, and M. D. Collins. 1995. Identification of some clinical strains of CDC coryneform group A-3 and group A-4 bacteria as *Cellulomonas* species and proposal of *Cellulomonas hominis* sp. nov. for some group A-3 strains. *J. Clin. Microbiol.* **33:**2091–2097.

65. Funke, G., C. Pascual Ramos, and M. D. Collins. 1997. *Corynebacterium coyleae* sp. nov., isolated from human clinical specimens. *Int. J. Syst. Bacteriol.* **47:**92–96.

66. Funke, G., C. Pascual Ramos, J. F. Fernandez-Garayzabal, N. Weiss, and M. D. Collins. 1995. Description of human-derived Centers for Disease Control coryneform group 2 bacteria as *Actinomyces bernardiae* sp. nov. *Int. J. Syst. Bacteriol.* **45:**57–60.

67. Funke, G., K. Peters, and M. Aravena-Roman. 1998. Evaluation of the RapID CB Plus system for identification of coryneform bacteria and *Listeria* spp. *J. Clin. Microbiol.* **36:**2439–2442.

68. Funke, G., V. Pünter, and A. von Graevenitz. 1996. Antimicrobial susceptibility patterns of some recently established coryneform bacteria. *Antimicrob. Agents Chemother.* **40:**2874–2878.

69. Funke, G., F. N. R. Renaud, J. Freney, and P. Riegel. 1997. Multicenter evaluation of the updated and extended API (RAPID) Coryne database 2.0. *J. Clin. Microbiol.* **35:**3122–3126.

70. Funke, G., S. Stubbs, G. E. Pfyffer, M. Marchiani, and M. D. Collins. 1994. Characteristics of CDC group 3 and group 5 coryneform bacteria isolated from clinical specimens and assignment to the genus *Dermabacter. J. Clin. Microbiol.* **32:**1223–1228.

71. Funke, G., S. Stubbs, G. E. Pfyffer, M. Marchiani, and M. D. Collins. 1994. *Turicella otitidis* gen. nov., sp. nov., a coryneform bacterium isolated from patients with otitis media. *Int. J. Syst. Bacteriol.* **44:**270–273.

72. Funke, G., A. von Graevenitz, J. Clarridge III, and K. A. Bernard. 1997. Clinical microbiology of coryneform bacteria. *Clin. Microbiol. Rev.* **10:**125–159.

73. Funke, G., A. von Graevenitz, and N. Weiss. 1994. Primary identification of *Aureobacterium* spp. isolated from clinical specimens as "*Corynebacterium aquaticum.*" *J. Clin. Microbiol.* **32:**2686–2691.

74. Gneiding, K., R. Frodl, and G. Funke. 2008. Identities of *Microbacterium* spp. encountered in human clinical specimens. *J. Clin. Microbiol.* **46:**3646–3652.

75. Gomez-Garces, J. L., J. I. Alos, and J. Tamayo. 2007. In vitro activity of linezolid and 12 other antimicrobials against coryneform bacteria. *Int. J. Antimicrob. Agents* **29:**688–692.

76. Grimont, P. A. D., F. Grimont, A. Efstratiou, A. De Zoysa, I. Mazurova, C. Ruckly, M. Lejay-Collin, S. Martin-Delautre, B. Regnault, and members of the European Laboratory Working Group on Diphtheria. 2004. International nomenclature for *Corynebacterium diphtheriae* ribotypes. *Res. Microbiol.* **155:**162–166.

77. Hall, V., M. D. Collins, R. A. Hutson, P. A. Lawson, E. Falsen, and B. Duerden. 2003. *Corynebacterium atypicum* sp. nov., from a human clinical source, does not contain corynomycolic acids. *Int. J. Syst. Evol. Microbiol.* **53:**1065–1068.

78. Hauser, D., M. R. Popoff, M. Kiredjian, P. Boquet, and F. Bimet. 1993. Polymerase chain assay for diagnosis of potentially toxigenic *Corynebacterium diphtheriae* strains: correlation with ADP-ribosylation activity assay. *J. Clin. Microbiol.* **31:**2720–2723.

79. Hollis, D. G., and R. E. Weaver. 1981. Gram-positive organisms: a guide to identification. Special Bacteriology Section, Centers for Disease Control, Atlanta, GA.

80. Hommez, J., L. A. Devriese, M. Vaneechoutte, P. Riegel, P. Butaye, and F. Haesebrouck. 1999. Identification of nonlipophilic corynebacteria isolated from dairy cows with mastitis. *J. Clin. Microbiol.* **37:**954–957.

81. Jones, D., and M. D. Collins. 1988. Taxonomic studies on some human cutaneous coryneform bacteria: description of *Dermabacter hominis* gen. nov., sp. nov. *FEMS Microbiol. Lett.* **51:**51–56.

82. Khamis, A., D. Raoult, and B. La Scola. 2004. *rpoB* gene sequencing for identification of *Corynebacterium* species. *J. Clin. Microbiol.* **42:**3925–3931.

83. Khamis, A., D. Raoult, and B. La Scola. 2005. Comparison between *rpoB* and 16S rRNA gene sequencing for molecular identification of 168 clinical isolates of *Corynebacterium*. *J. Clin. Microbiol.* **43:**1934–1936.

84. Koch, C., F. A. Rainey, and E. Stackebrandt. 1994. 16S rDNA studies on members of *Arthrobacter* and *Micrococcus*: an aid for their future taxonomic restructuring. *FEMS Microbiol. Lett.* **123:**167–172.

85. Kronvall, G., M. Lanner-Sjoberg, L. V. von Stedingk, H. S. Hanson, B. Pettersson, and E. Falsen. 1998. Whole cell protein and partial 16S rRNA gene sequence analysis suggest the existence of a second *Rothia* species. *Clin. Microbiol. Infect.* **4:**255–263.

86. Laffineur, K., V. Avesani, G. Cornu, J. Charlier, M. Janssens, G. Wauters, and M. Delmee. 2003. Bacteremia due to a novel *Microbacterium* species in a patient with leukemia and description of *Microbacterium paraoxydans* sp. nov. *J. Clin. Microbiol.* **41:**2242–2246.

87. Lagace-Wiens, P. R., B. Ng, A. Reimer, T. Burdz, D. Wiebe, and K. Bernard. 2008. *Gardnerella vaginalis* bacteremia in a previously healthy man: case report and characterization of the isolate. *J. Clin. Microbiol.* **46:**804–806.

88. Lartigue, M. F., X. Monnet, A. Le Flèche, P. A. Grimont, J. J. Benet, A. Durrbach, M. Fabre, and P. Nordmann. 2005. *Corynebacterium ulcerans* in an immunocompromised patient with diphtheria and her dog. *J. Clin. Microbiol.* **43:**999–1001.

89. Leonard, R. B., D. J. Nowowiejski, J. J. Warren, D. J. Finn, and M. B. Coyle. 1994. Molecular evidence of person-to-person transmission of a pigmented strain of *Corynebacterium striatum* in intensive care units. *J. Clin. Microbiol.* **32:**164–169.

90. Li, Y., Y. Kawamura, N. Fujiwara, T. Naka, H. Liu, X. Huang, K. Kobayashi, and T. Ezaki. 2004. *Rothia aeria* sp. nov., *Rhodococcus baikonurensis* sp. nov. and *Arthrobacter russicus* sp. nov., isolated from air in the Russian space laboratory Mir. *Int. J. Syst. Evol. Microbiol.* **54:**827–835.

91. Loubinoux, J., B. Rio, L. Mihaila, E. Fois, A. Le Flèche, P. A. D. Grimont, J.-P. Marie, and A. Bouvet. 2005. Bacteremia caused by an undescribed species of *Janibacter*. *J. Clin. Microbiol.* **43:**3564–3566.

92. Mages, I. S., R. Frodl, K. A. Bernard, and G. Funke. 2008. Identities of *Arthrobacter* spp. and *Arthrobacter*-like bacteria encountered in human clinical specimens. *J. Clin. Microbiol.* **46:**2980–2986.

93. Manaia, C. M., B. Nogales, N. Weiss, and O. C. Nunes. 2004. *Gulosibacter molinativorax* gen. nov., sp. nov., a molinate degrading bacterium, and classification of "*Brevibacterium helvolum*" DSM 20419 as *Pseudoclavibacter helvolus* gen. nov., sp. nov. *Int. J. Syst. Evol. Microbiol.* **54:**783–789.

94. Martin, K., P. Schumann, F. A. Rainey, B. Schuetze, and I. Groth. 1997. *Janibacter limosus* gen. nov., sp. nov., a new actinomycete with *meso*-diaminopimelic acid in the cell wall. *Int. J. Syst. Bacteriol.* **47:**529–534.

95. Martinez-Martinez, L., M. C. Ortega, and A. I. Suarez. 1995. Comparison of E-test with broth microdilution and disk diffusion for susceptibility testing of coryneform bacteria. *J. Clin. Microbiol.* **33:**1318–1321.

96. Merhej, V., E. Falsen, D. Raoult, and V. Roux. 2009. *Corynebacterium timonense* and *Corynebacterium massiliense* sp. nov., isolated from human blood and human articular hip liquid. *Int. J. Syst. Evol. Microbiol.* **59:**1953–1959.

97. Miyake, T., K. Watanabe, T. Watanabe, and H. Oyaizu. 1998. Phylogenetic analysis of the genus *Bifidobacterium* and related genera based on 16S rDNA sequences. *Microbiol. Immun.* **42:**661–667.

98. Mokrousov, I., O. Narvskaya, E. Limeschenko, and A. Vyazovaya. 2005. Efficient discrimination within a *Corynebacterium diphtheriae* epidemic clonal group by a novel macroarray-based method. *J. Clin. Microbiol.* **43:**1662–1668.

99. Mothershed, E. A., P. K. Cassiday, K. Pierson, L. W. Mayer, and T. Popovic. 2002. Development of a real-time fluorescence PCR assay for rapid detection of the diphtheria toxin gene. *J. Clin. Microbiol.* **40:**4713–4719.

100. Nakao, H., I. K. Mazarova, T. Glushkevich, and T. Popovic. 1997. Analysis of heterogeneity of *Corynebacterium diphtheriae* toxin gene, *tox*, and its regulatory element, *dtxR*, by direct sequencing. *Res. Microbiol.* **148:**45–54.

101. Nakao, H., and T. Popovic. 1997. Development of a direct PCR assay for detection of the diphtheria toxin gene. *J. Clin. Microbiol.* **35:**1651–1655.

102. Neal, S. E., A. Efstratiou, on behalf of DIPNET and international diphtheria reference laboratories. 2010. International external quality assurance for the laboratory diagnosis of diphtheria. *J. Clin. Microbiol.* **47:**4037–4042.

103. Neubauer, M., J. Sourek, M. Ryc, J. Bohacek, M. Mara, and J. Mnukova. 1991. *Corynebacterium accolens* sp. nov., a gram-positive rod exhibiting satellitism, from clinical material. *Syst. Appl. Microbiol.* **14:**46–51.

104. Nugent, R. P., M. A. Krohn, and S. L. Hillier. 1991. Reliability of diagnosing bacterial vaginosis is improved by a standardized method of Gram stain interpretation. *J. Clin. Microbiol.* **29:**297–301.

105. Ohtaki, H., K. Ohkusu, H. Sawamura, H. Ohta, R. Inoue, J. Iwasa, H. Ito, N. Murakami, T. Ezaki, H. Moriwaki, and M. Seishima. 2009. First case report of acute cholecystitis with sepsis caused by *Cellulomonas denverensis*. *J. Clin. Microbiol.* **47:**3391–3393.

106. Otsuka, Y., Y. Kawamura, T. Koyama, H. Iihara, K. Ohkusu, and T. Ezaki. 2005. *Corynebacterium resistens* sp. nov., a new multidrug-resistant coryneform bacterium isolated from human infections. *J. Clin. Microbiol.* **43:**3713–3717.

107. Pallen, M. J., A. J. Hay, L. H. Puckey, and A. Efstratiou. 1994. Polymerase chain reaction for screening clinical isolates of corynebacteria for the production of diphtheria toxin. *J. Clin. Pathol.* **47:**353–356.

108. Pascual, C., P. A. Lawson, J. A. E. Farrow, M. Navarro Gimenez, and M. D. Collins. 1995. Phylogenetic analysis of the genus *Corynebacterium* based on 16S rRNA gene sequences. *Int. J. Syst. Bacteriol.* **45:**724–728.

109. Pascual Ramos, C., G. Foster, and M. D. Collins. 1997. Phylogenetic analysis of the genus *Actinomyces* based on 16S rRNA gene sequences: description of *Arcanobacterium phocae* sp. nov., *Arcanobacterium bernardiae* comb. nov., and *Arcanobacterium pyogenes* comb. nov. *Int. J. Syst. Bacteriol.* **47:**46–53.

110. Paviour, S., S. Musaad, S. Roberts, G. Taylor, S. Taylor, K. Shore, S. Lang, and D. Holland. 2002. *Corynebacterium* species isolated from patients with mastitis. *Clin. Infect. Dis.* **35:**1434–1440.

111. Pimenta, F. P., G. A. Matias, G. A. Pereira, T. C. Camello, G. B. Alves, A. C. Rosa, R. Hirata, Jr., and A. L. Mattos-Guaraldi. 2008. A PCR for *dtxR* gene: application to diagnosis of non-toxigenic and toxigenic *Corynebacterium diphtheriae*. *Mol. Cell. Probes* **22:**189–192.

112. Pitt, T. L., H. Malnick, J. Shah, M. A. Chattaway, C. J. Keys, F. J. Cooke, and H. N. Shah. 2007. Characterisation of *Exiguobacterium aurantiacum* isolates from blood cultures of six patients. *Clin. Microbiol. Infect.* **13:**946–948.

113. Popovic, T., I. K. Mazurova, A. Efstratiou, J. Vuopio-Varkila, M. Reeves, A. De Zoysa, T. Glushkevich, and P. A. D. Grimont. 2000. Molecular epidemiology of diphtheria. *J. Infect. Dis.* **181:**S168–S177.

114. Rainey, F. A., N. Weiss, H. Prauser, and E. Stackebrandt. 1994. Further evidence for the phylogenetic coherence of actinomycetes with group B-peptidoglycan and evidence for the phylogenetic intermixing of the genera *Microbacterium* and *Aureobacterium* as determined by 16S rDNA analysis. *FEMS Microbiol. Lett.* **118:**135–140.

115. Rassoulian-Barrett, S. L., B. T. Cookson, L. C. Carlson, K. A. Bernard, and M. B. Coyle. 2001. Diversity within reference strains of *Corynebacterium matruchotii* includes *Corynebacterium durum* and a novel organism. *J. Clin. Microbiol.* **39:**943–948.

116. Reacher, M., M. Ramsay, J. White, A. De Zoysa, A. Efstratiou, G. Mann, A. Mackay, and R. C. George. 2000. Nontoxigenic *Corynebacterium diphtheriae:* an emerging pathogen in England and Wales? *Emerg. Infect. Dis.* **6:**640–645.

117. Renaud, F. N., D. Aubel, P. Riegel, H. Meugnier, and C. Bollet. 2001. *Corynebacterium freneyi* sp. nov., alpha-glucosidase-positive strains related to *Corynebacterium xerosis. Int. J. Syst. Evol. Microbiol.* **51:**1723–1728.

118. Renaud, F. N. R., A. Gregory, C. Barreau, D. Aubel, and J. Freney. 1996. Identification of *Turicella otitidis* isolated from a patient with otorrhea associated with surgery: differentiation from *Corynebacterium afermentans* and *Corynebacterium auris. J. Clin. Microbiol.* **34:**2625–2627.

119. Renaud, F. N. R., A. L. Coustumier, N. Wilhem, D. Aubel, P. Riegel, C. Bollet, and J. Freney. 2007. *Corynebacterium hansenii* sp. nov., an alpha-glucosidase-negative bacterium related to *Corynebacterium xerosis. Int. J. Syst. Evol. Microbiol.* **57:**1113–1116.

120. Rennie, R. P., C. Brosnikoff, L. Turnbull, L. B. Reller, S. Mirrett, W. Janda, K. Ristow, and A. Krilcich. 2008. Multicenter evaluation of the Vitek 2 anaerobe and *Corynebacterium* identification card. *J. Clin. Microbiol.* **46:**2646–2651.

121. Renom, F., M. Garau, M. Rubi, F. Ramis, A. Galmes, and J. B. Soriano. 2007. Nosocomial outbreak of *Corynebacterium striatum* infection in patients with chronic obstructive pulmonary disease. *J. Clin. Microbiol.* **45:**2064–2067.

122. Renvoise, A., N. Aldrovandi, D. Raoult, and V. Roux. 2009. *Helcobacillus massiliensis* gen. nov., sp. nov., a novel representative of the family *Dermabacteraceae* isolated from a patient with a cutaneous discharge. *Int. J. Syst. Evol. Microbiol.* **59:**2346–2351.

123. Riegel, P., R. Creti, R. Mattei, A. Nieri, and C. von Hunolstein. 2006. Isolation of *Corynebacterium tuscaniae* sp. nov. from blood cultures of a patient suffering from endocarditis. *J. Clin. Microbiol.* **44:**307–312.

124. Riegel, P., D. de Briel, G. Prevost, F. Jehl, and H. Monteil. 1994. Genomic diversity among *Corynebacterium jeikeium* strains and comparison with biochemical characteristics. *J. Clin. Microbiol.* **32:**1860–1865.

125. Riegel, P., D. de Briel, G. Prevost, F. Jehl, H. Monteil, and R. Minck. 1993. Taxonomic study of *Corynebacterium* group ANF-1 strains: proposal of *Corynebacterium afermentans* sp. nov. containing the subspecies C. *afermentans* subsp. *afermentans* subsp. nov. and C. *afermentans* subsp. *lipophilum* subsp. nov. *Int. J. Syst. Bacteriol.* **43:**287–292.

126. Riegel, P., R. Heller, G. Prevost, F. Jehl, and H. Monteil. 1997. *Corynebacterium durum* sp. nov., from human clinical specimens. *Int. J. Syst. Bacteriol.* **47:**1107–1111.

127. Riegel, P., R. Ruimy, D. de Briel, G. Prevost, F. Jehl, F. Bimet, R. Christen, and H. Monteil. 1995. *Corynebacterium argentoratense* sp. nov., from human throat. *Int. J. Syst. Bacteriol.* **45:**533–537.

128. Riegel, P., R. Ruimy, D. de Briel, G. Prevost, F. Jehl, R. Christen, and H. Monteil. 1995. Genomic diversity and phylogenetic relationships among lipid-requiring diphtheroids from humans and characterization of *Corynebacterium macginleyi* sp. nov. *Int. J. Syst. Bacteriol.* **45:**128–133.

129. Riegel, P., R. Ruimy, D. de Briel, G. Prevost, F. Jehl, R. Christen, and H. Monteil. 1995. Taxonomy of *Corynebacterium diphtheriae* and related taxa, with the recognition of *Corynebacterium ulcerans* sp. nov., nom. rev. *FEMS Microbiol. Lett.* **126:**271–276.

130. Riegel, P., R. Ruimy, F. N. R. Renaud, J. Freney, G. Prevost, F. Jehl, R. Christen, and H. Monteil. 1997. *Corynebacterium singulare* sp. nov., a new species for urease-positive strains related to *Corynebacterium minutissimum. Int. J. Syst. Bacteriol.* **47:**1092–1096.

131. Romney, M. G., D. L. Roscoe, K. Bernard, S. Lai, A. Efstratiou, and A. M. Clarke. 2006. Emergence of an invasive clone of nontoxigenic *Corynebacterium diphtheriae* in the urban poor population of Vancouver, Canada. *J. Clin. Microbiol.* **44:**1625–1629.

132. Roux, V., M. Drancourt, A. Stein, P. Riegel, D. Raoult, and B. La Scola. 2004. *Corynebacterium* species isolated from bone and joint infections identified by 16S rRNA gene sequence analysis. *J. Clin. Microbiol.* **42:**2231–2233.

133. Ruimy, R., P. Riegel, P. Boiron, H. Monteil, and R. Christen. 1995. Phylogeny of the genus *Corynebacterium* deduced from analysis of small-subunit ribosomal DNA sequences. *Int. J. Syst. Bacteriol.* **45:**740–746.

134. Sadhu, K., P. A. G. Domingue, A. W. Chow, J. Nelligan, N. Cheng, and J. W. Costerton. 1989. *Gardnerella vaginalis* has a gram-positive cell-wall ultrastructure and lacks classical cell-wall lipopolysaccharide. *J. Med. Microbiol.* **29:**229–235.

135. Schuhegger, R., R. Kugler, and A. Sing. 2008. Pitfalls with diphtheria-like illness due to toxigenic *Corynebacterium ulcerans. Clin. Infect. Dis.* **47:**288.

136. Schuhegger, R., M. Lindermayer, R. Kugler, J. Heesemann, U. Busch, and A. Sing. 2008. Detection of toxigenic *Corynebacterium diphtheriae* and *Corynebacterium ulcerans* strains by a novel real-time PCR. *J. Clin. Microbiol.* **46:**2822–2823.

137. Schumann, P., N. Weiss, and E. Stackebrandt. 2001. Reclassification of *Cellulomonas cellulans* (Stackebrandt and Keddie 1986) as *Cellulosimicrobium cellulans* gen. nov., comb. nov. *Int. J. Syst. Evol. Microbiol.* **51:**1007–1010.

138. Sing, A., M. Hogardt, S. Bierschenk, and J. Heesemann. 2003. Detection of differences in the nucleotide and amino acid sequences of diphtheria toxin from *Corynebacterium diphtheriae* and *Corynebacterium ulcerans* causing extrapharyngeal infections. *J. Clin. Microbiol.* **41:**4848–4851.

139. Sjödén, B., G. Funke, A. Izquierdo, E. Akervall, and M. D. Collins. 1998. Description of some coryneform bacteria isolated from human clinical specimens as *Corynebacterium falsenii* sp. nov. *Int. J. Syst. Bacteriol.* **48:**69–74.

140. Soriano, F., J. M. Aguado, C. Ponte, R. Fernandez-Roblas, and J. L. Rodriguez-Tudela. 1990. Urinary tract infection caused by *Corynebacterium* group D2: report of 82 cases and review. *Rev. Infect. Dis.* **12:**1019–1034.

141. Spiegel, C. A. 1991. Bacterial vaginosis. *Clin. Microbiol. Rev.* **4:**485–502.

142. Spiegel, C. A. 1999. Bacterial vaginosis: changes in laboratory practice. *Clin. Microbiol. Newsl.* **21:**33–37.

143. Stackebrandt, E., S. Breymann, U. Steiner, H. Prauser, N. Weiss, and P. Schumann. 2002. Re-evaluation of the status of the genus *Oerskovia*, reclassification of *Promicromonospora enterophila* (Jager et al. 1983) as *Oerskovia enterophila* comb. nov. and description of *Oerskovia jenensis* sp. nov. and *Oerskovia paurometabola* sp. nov. *Int. J. Syst. Evol. Microbiol.* **52:**1105–1111.

144. Stackebrandt, E., F. A. Rainey, and N. L. Ward-Rainey. 1997. Proposal for a new hierarchic classification system, *Actinobacteria* classis nov. *Int. J. Syst. Bacteriol.* **47:**479–491.

145. Takeuchi, M., and K. Hatano. 1998. Union of the genera *Microbacterium* Orla-Jensen and *Aureobacterium* Collins et al. in a redefined genus *Microbacterium. Int. J. Syst. Bacteriol.* **48:**739–747.

146. Tanner, M. A., D. Shoskes, A. Shahed, and N. R. Pace. 1999. Prevalence of corynebacterial 16S rRNA sequences in patients with bacterial and "nonbacterial" prostatitis. *J. Clin. Microbiol.* **37:**1863–1870.

147. **Tauch, A., N. Bischoff, A. Pühler, and J. Kalinowski.** 2004. Comparative genomics identified two conserved DNA modules in a corynebacterial plasmid family present in clinical isolates of the opportunistic human pathogen *Corynebacterium jeikeium. Plasmid* **52:**102–118

148. **Tauch, A., O. Kaiser, T. Hain, A. Goesmann, B. Weisshaar, A. Albersmeier, T. Bekel, N. Bischoff, I. Brune, T. Chakraborty, J. Kalinowski, F. Meyer, O. Rupp, S. Schneiker, P. Viehoever, and A. Pühler.** 2005. Complete genome sequence and analysis of the multiresistant nosocomial pathogen *Corynebacterium jeikeium* K411, a lipid-requiring bacterium of the human skin flora. *J. Bacteriol.* **187:**4671–4682.

149. **Tauch, A., J. Schneider, R. Szczepanowski, A. Tilker, P. Viehoever, K. H. Gartemann, W. Arnold, J. Blom, K. Brinkrolf, I. Brune, S. Gotker, B. Weisshaar, A. Goesmann, M. Droge, and A. Pühler.** 2008. Ultrafast pyrosequencing of *Corynebacterium kroppenstedtii* DSM44385 revealed insights into the physiology of a lipophilic corynebacterium that lacks mycolic acids. *J. Biotechnol.* **136:**22–30.

150. **Tauch, A., E. Trost, A. Tilker, U. Ludewig, S. Schneiker, A. Goesmann, W. Arnold, T. Bekel, K. Brinkrolf, I. Brune, S. Gotker, J. Kalinowski, P. B. Kamp, F. P. Lobo, P. Viehoever, B. Weisshaar, F. Soriano, M. Droge, and A. Pühler.** 2008. The lifestyle of *Corynebacterium urealyticum* derived from its complete genome sequence established by pyrosequencing. *J. Biotechnol.* **136:**11–21.

151. **Tong, J., C. Liu, P. Summanen, H. Xu, and S. M. Finegold.** 2010. *Corynebacterium pyruviciproducens* sp. nov., producing pyruvic acid. *Int. J. Syst. Evol. Microbiol.* **60:**1135–1140.

152. **Troxler, R., G. Funke, A. von Graevenitz, and I. Stock.** 2001. Natural antibiotic susceptibility of recently established coryneform bacteria. *Eur. J. Clin. Microbiol. Infect. Dis.* **20:**315–323.

153. **Valero-Guillen, P. L., G. Yague, and M. Segovia.** 2005. Characterization of acyl-phosphatidylinositol from the opportunistic pathogen *Corynebacterium amycolatum. Chem. Phys. Lipids* **133:**17–26.

154. **Vaneechoutte, M., P. Riegel, D. de Briel, H. Monteil, G. Verschraegen, A. De Rouck, and G. Claeys.** 1995. Evaluation of the applicability of amplified rDNA-restriction analysis (ARDRA) to identification of species of the genus *Corynebacterium. Res. Microbiol.* **146:**633–641.

155. **Verhelst, R., H. Verstraelen, G. Claeys, G. Verschraegen, J. Delanghe, L. Van Simaey, C. De Ganck, M. Temmerman, and M. Vaneechoutte.** 2004. Cloning of 16S rRNA genes amplified from normal and disturbed vaginal microflora suggests a strong association between *Atopobium vaginae, Gardnerella vaginalis* and bacterial vaginosis. *BMC Microbiol.* **4:**16.

156. **von Graevenitz, A.** 2004. *Rothia dentocariosa:* taxonomy and differential diagnosis. *Clin. Microbiol. Infect.* **10:**399–402.

157. **von Graevenitz, A., and G. Funke.** 1996. An identification scheme for rapidly and aerobically growing gram-positive rods. *Zentral. Bakteriol. Parasitenkd. Infektionskr. Hyg. Abt. 1 Orig.* **284:**246–254.

158. **von Graevenitz, A., V. Pünter-Streit, P. Riegel, and G. Funke.** 1998. Coryneform bacteria in throat cultures of healthy individuals. *J. Clin. Microbiol.* **36:**2087–2088.

159. **Wattiau, P., M. Janssens, and G. Wauters.** 2000. *Corynebacterium simulans* sp. nov., a non-lipophilic, fermentative *Corynebacterium. Int. J. Syst. Evol. Microbiol.* **50:**347–353.

160. **Wauters, G., J. Charlier, M. Janssens, and M. Delmee.** 2000. Identification of *Arthrobacter oxydans, Arthrobacter luteolus* sp. nov., and *Arthrobacter albus* sp. nov., isolated from human clinical specimens. *J. Clin. Microbiol.* **38:**2412–2415.

161. **Wauters, G., B. van Bosterhaut, M. Janssens, and J. Verhaegen.** 1998. Identification of *Corynebacterium amycolatum* and other nonlipophilic fermentative corynebacteria of human origin. *J. Clin. Microbiol.* **36:**1430–1432.

162. **Weiss, K., M. Laverdiere, and R. Rivest.** 1996. Comparison of antimicrobial susceptibilities of *Corynebacterium* species by broth microdilution and disk diffusion methods. *Antimicrob. Agents Chemother.* **40:**930–933.

163. **Yassin, A. F.** 2007. *Corynebacterium ureicelerivorans* sp. nov., a lipophilic bacterium isolated from blood culture. *Int. J. Syst. Evol. Microbiol.* **57:**1200–1203.

164. **Yassin, A. F., and C. Siering.** 2008. *Corynebacterium sputi* sp. nov., isolated from the sputum of a patient with pneumonia. *Int. J. Syst. Evol. Microbiol.* **58:**2876–2879.

165. **Yassin, A. F., U. Steiner, and W. Ludwig.** 2002. *Corynebacterium appendicis* sp. nov. *Int. J. Syst. Evol. Microbiol.* **52:**1165–1169.

166. **Yassin, A. F., U. Steiner, and W. Ludwig.** 2002. *Corynebacterium aurimucosum* sp. nov. and emended description of *Corynebacterium minutissimum* Collins and Jones (1983). *Int. J. Syst. Evol. Microbiol.* **52:**1001–1005.

167. **Zapardiel, J., E. Nieto, M. I. Gegundez, I. Gadea, and F. Soriano.** 1994. Problems in minimum inhibitory concentration determinations in coryneform organisms—comparison of an agar dilution and the Etest. *Diagn. Microbiol. Infect. Dis.* **19:**171–173.

168. **Zhi, X., W. Li, and E. Stackebrandt.** 2009. An update of the structure and 16S rRNA gene sequence-based definition of higher ranks of the class *Actinobacteria,* with the proposal of two new suborders and four new families and emended descriptions of the existing higher taxa. *Int. J. Syst. Evol. Microbiol.* **59:**589–608.

169. **Zimmermann, O., C. Spröer, R. M. Kroppenstedt, E. Fuchs, E. G. Köchel, and G. Funke.** 1998. *Corynebacterium thomssenii* sp. nov., a *Corynebacterium* with N-acetyl-β-glucosaminidase activity from human clinical specimens. *Int. J. Syst. Bacteriol.* **48:**489–494.

170. **Zinkernagel, A. S., A. von Graevenitz, and G. Funke.** 1996. Heterogeneity within *Corynebacterium minutissimum* strains is explained by misidentified *Corynebacterium amycolatum* strains. *Am. J. Clin. Pathol.* **106:**378–383.

Nocardia, Rhodococcus, Gordonia, Actinomadura, Streptomyces, and Other Aerobic Actinomycetes

PATRICIA S. CONVILLE AND FRANK G. WITEBSKY

27

TAXONOMY

The word "actinomycete" is derived from two Greek roots (actino- and -mycete) meaning "ray" (and hence also "rod") and "fungus," respectively. The anaerobic organisms now in the genus *Actinomyces* and the aerobic organisms grouped together as the "aerobic actinomycetes" were previously presumed to be related to one another on the basis of shared features of organismal and colonial morphology. The aerobic actinomycetes, a group for which no agreed-upon operational definition currently exists, are now known to be an evolutionarily heterogeneous assemblage of genera. At some stage they all form gram-positive rods, and most of the more commonly isolated species exhibit at least rudimentary branching under certain growth conditions; all grow better under aerobic than anaerobic conditions, a feature distinguishing them from most organisms in the genus *Actinomyces*. Figure 1 shows the current classification of genera included in this chapter according to J. P. Euzéby (List of Prokaryotic Names with Standing in Nomenclature [LPSN; www.bacterio.cict.fr]).

The organisms containing mycolic acids in their cell walls (included in the genera *Dietzia, Gordonia, Nocardia, Rhodococcus, Segniliparus, Tsukamurella,* and *Williamsia*) are rather closely related on the basis of molecular genetic studies (36, 191); these mycolic-acid-containing genera appear phylogenetically more closely related to the genera *Corynebacterium* and *Mycobacterium* (both of which are sometimes considered aerobic actinomycetes) than to the other non-mycolic-acid-containing genera usually also included with the aerobic actinomycetes. According to a recent classification scheme, these 7 genera of actinomycetes, along with the genera *Corynebacterium* and *Mycobacterium*, are classified together in the suborder *Corynebacterineae* (LPSN). Note in Fig. 1 that the genera *Corynebacterium, Williamsia,* and possibly *Dietzia* are the only genera in the suborder *Corynebacterineae* that are not at least weakly acid-fast.

The number of recognized pathogenic species of aerobic actinomycetes has been rising rapidly. Only genera containing species of clinical significance are dealt with in this chapter. Unfortunately, the increasingly fine discrimination of species has made it increasingly difficult to delineate important species-specific differences in geographic distribution, pathogenic and other biological mechanisms, disease associations, and antimicrobial susceptibility patterns. This enormous proliferation of distinct species for which association with human disease has been claimed presents several problems for the clinical microbiologist. First, phenotypic testing has been rendered virtually useless for accurate discrimination among species. Particularly for the aerobic actinomycetes, the number of phenotypic tests available in the clinical laboratory (and in most research laboratories) is far too small for accurate differentiation among so many species, and often, information on the percent positivity for a specific reaction in a given species is not known. Furthermore, precisely the same biochemical testing format has generally not been employed with isolates of all the species, making the usefulness of multistudy comparisons uncertain. Second, some types of testing, such as analysis of cell wall constituents and of whole-cell sugars, are available in only a few research settings and are rarely of use for species-level identification. Some general information regarding these features is provided herein, but the references should be consulted for performance procedures and additional details. Third, only gene sequencing is currently adequately discriminatory, reproducible, and sufficiently available to be useful for precise species identifications in clinical laboratories. Fourth, because of the growing problems with accurate species determinations, the clinical literature is rife with erroneous identifications; nowhere is this problem more apparent than with organisms in the genus *Nocardia*. Additionally, as some species have been described on the basis of only a single isolate, and for others only a handful of reports exist, little if any meaningful clinical information can be associated with many species names. Particularly when molecular methods are not available, precise identification of isolates may be impossible—and is also frequently not of immediate clinical utility.

There are a few terminological issues that, while they pertain to all bacteria, seem to cause confusion particularly frequently with regard to the aerobic actinomycetes. First, for every bacterial species, there is only one "type strain," the strain on which the original description of the species was based. Other strains contained in culture collections that are thought to belong to the same species as a given type strain could be referred to as "reference strains," but they are not type strains. Second, the term "sensu stricto" means "in the strict sense." The term, when used with a species name, should be restricted to mean organisms

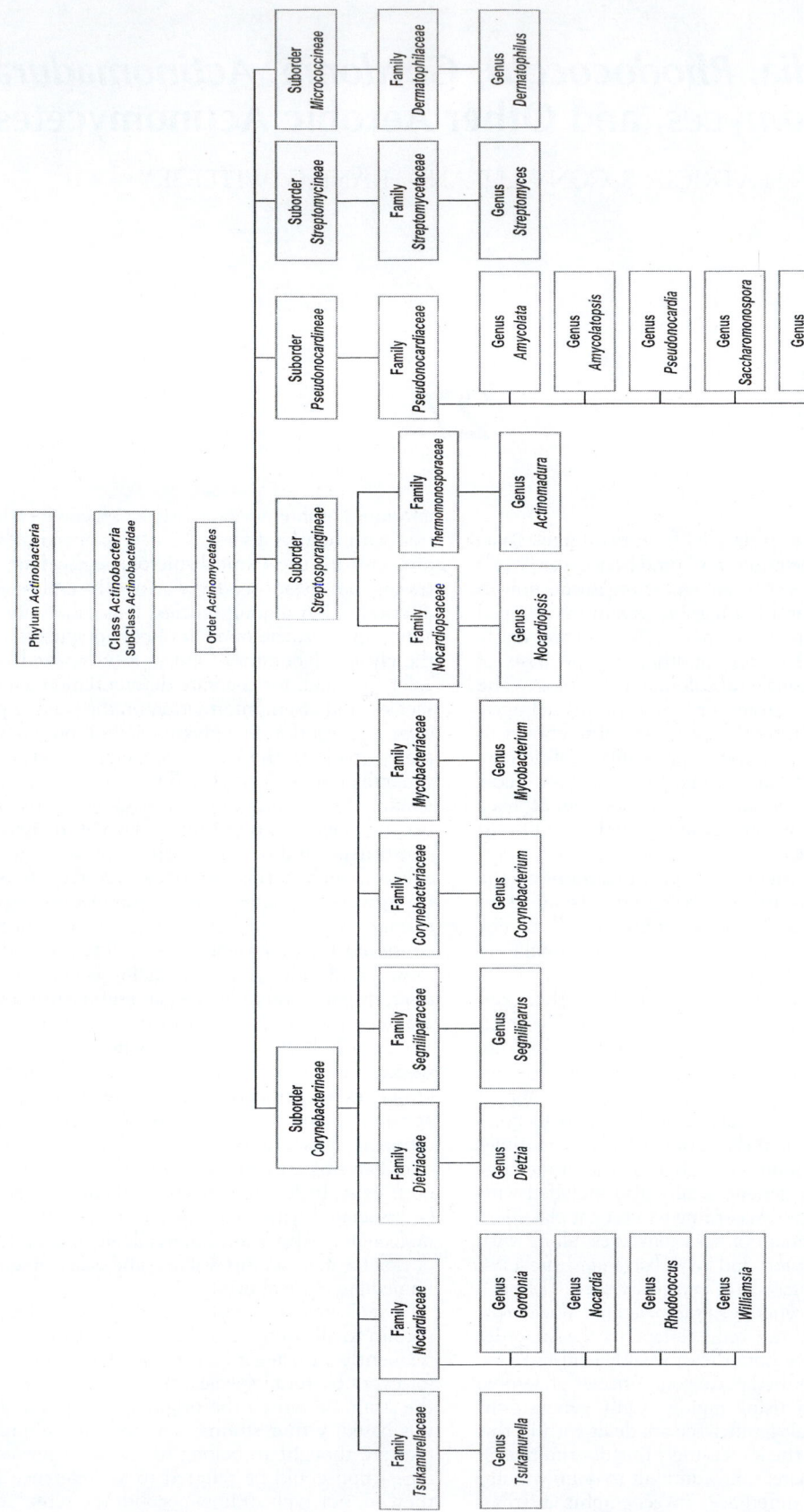

FIGURE 1 Classification of genera of aerobic actinomycetes considered to be human pathogens. Information from J. P. Euzéby (LPSN; www.bacterio.cict.fr).

belonging to that particular species, as determined by the best available methods. So, to refer to isolates that are "*Nocardia asteroides* sensu stricto" should mean isolates that by gene sequencing are identical to the type strain of *N. asteroides* (ATCC 19247^T).

DESCRIPTION OF THE GENERA

Basic information about specific microscopic and colonial morphologies of the following genera is presented in Table 1; additional information is included in the text below for some genera. See Table 2 for a comparison of the chemotaxonomic characteristics and lysozyme resistance that distinguish these genera. In the listings that follow, enumeration of species within a genus is taken from LPSN.

Actinomadura

The microscopic and colonial morphology of organisms in the genus *Actinomadura*, which contains approximately 67 validly named species or subspecies, is very similar to those in the genus *Streptomyces* (Fig. 2A and B and 3A). The color of the colonies may vary considerably among different species. Cell walls contain the sugar madurose, a feature shared only with organisms in the genus *Dermatophilus*.

Amycolata and Amycolatopsis

The genera *Amycolata* and *Amycolatopsis* were proposed by Lechevalier et al. for *Nocardia*-like organisms that were gram positive and modified acid-fast negative but lacked mycolic acids (128) (Fig. 2F and 3B). Among the species transferred to the genus *Amycolatopsis* was *Nocardia orientalis*, two isolates of which were reported from clinical specimens (80). A study based on 16S rRNA gene sequences recommended combining the genera *Amycolata* and *Pseudonocardia* into an emended genus, *Pseudonocardia* (214). Currently, there are 4 validly named species in the genus *Amycolata* and approximately 44 validly named species or subspecies in the genus *Amycolatopsis*.

Dermatophilus

The two species currently making up the genus *Dermatophilus* are probably not closely related to most of the other organisms considered in this chapter. Aerial mycelium may be produced by colonies if the organism is grown in an atmosphere of increased CO_2; the organisms are facultatively anaerobic (77). The microscopic morphology is unusual and striking; this branching organism develops both longitudinal and transverse septa (Fig. 3D). The resulting chains of coccoid cells may occur in as many as eight parallel rows (232). The coccoid cells may develop into motile zoospores under favorable environmental conditions.

Dietzia

The species *Dietzia maris* was removed from the genus *Rhodococcus* because of chemotaxonomic and 16S rRNA gene sequence differences from *Rhodococcus* species (174). Seven additional species have since been included in the genus. These organisms apparently rarely, if ever, branch, but like organisms in the genus *Rhodococcus*, they may show coccal and rod forms.

Gordonia

The biology of the genus *Gordonia* has been recently reviewed (5). On Gram stain, *Gordonia* species appear coryneform and could easily be mistaken for a component of the normal oral biota in sputum specimens (Fig. 3C).

The genus "*Gordona*" (now *Gordonia*), originally described by Tsukamura, was revived in 1988 by Stackebrandt et al. (192) to contain species with mycolic acids of approximately 46 to 66 carbon atoms in length (73) and a predominant menaquinone of nine isoprene units. *Gordonia* and *Rhodococcus* were also found to be separable on the basis of their 16S rRNA gene sequences. There are approximately 29 validly named species in the genus (Fig. 2I and 3C).

Nocardia

The most commonly isolated aerobic actinomycete human pathogens belong to the genus *Nocardia*. In direct Gram smears, organisms generally appear as very long, obviously branching, thin, and finely beaded gram-positive rods (Fig. 3E and K). Unlike the individual cells composing a streptococcal chain, the beads generally do not abut one another (Fig. 3H and O). Particularly when prepared from cultures, smears may show streptococcus-like chains or small branching filaments, probably as a result of the fragile nocardial mycelium breaking during smear preparation (157, 158) (Fig. 3E, F, G, K, and L).

Colonial morphology varies from species to species and frequently varies from isolate to isolate within a species (Fig. 2D, E, G, and L). Colony color may best be seen on the reverse when colonies are grown on translucent media such as Sabouraud agar, as color may become obscured on the surface by the powdery aerial hyphae typically produced.

A brief account of the nomenclatural history of the designation "*Nocardia asteroides*" is necessary to clarify a confusing and widely unappreciated taxonomic issue. In 1888, Edmond Nocard obtained an isolate of an organism thought to be the causative agent of bovine farcy. This organism was given the name *Nocardia farcinica* by Trevisan in 1889, and thereupon, it became the type strain for both the genus and species. Gordon and Mihm (79) found, using their battery of phenotypic tests, that *N. farcinica* could not be distinguished from isolates to which the name *Nocardia asteroides* had been applied. Because of some uncertainty relating to the isolate obtained by Nocard and what was presumed to be the conspecificity of the organisms then known as *N. farcinica* and *N. asteroides*, an appeal was made to the Judicial Commission to have the type species of the genus changed to *N. asteroides*, with strain ATCC 19247^T selected as the type strain of the species. The appeal was accepted, but the isolate of *N. farcinica* was retained as the type strain for that particular species, as not all were convinced that the two species were truly identical.

Nocardiopsis

The genus *Nocardiopsis* was originally described by Meyer to accommodate an organism that at the time was called *Actinomadura dassonvillei* but differed chemotaxonomically and in certain colonial morphologic features from other organisms in the genus *Actinomadura* (147). The cell wall of this organism does not contain madurose. The substrate mycelium fragments into coccal forms, and the aerial hyphae fragment into variable-sized spores (147). Currently, there are approximately 41 validly named species or subspecies in the genus.

Pseudonocardia

Pseudonocardia are characterized by the microscopic morphology of their aerial hyphae that are segmented as a result of elongation by budding. Aerial and substrate hyphae are often zigzag shaped (91). Currently, there are approximately 31 validly published species names in the genus.

TABLE 1 Morphologic characteristics of genera of aerobic actinomycetes[a]

Genus (reference[s])	Aerial hyphae	Modified acid fast	Microscopic morphology	Figure(s)	Colonial morphology[b]	Figure(s)
Actinomadura (145)	V	Neg	Thin, short branching filaments	3A	Powdery aerial hyphae may be blue, brown, cream, gray, green, pink, white, violet, or yellow. Colonies are wrinkled and may have a leathery or cartilaginous appearance when aerial mycelium is absent.	2A, 2B
Amycolata (128)	V	Neg	Best distinguished by slide culture	3B	When present, aerial hyphae may be white, yellow, or cream. Colonies can be off-white, yellow, gold, or brown	
Amycolatopsis (128)	V	Neg	Best distinguished by slide culture		White, beige, yellow, olive, or brown; may have soluble brown pigment	2F
Corynebacterium[c] (63)	Neg	Neg	Straight or slightly curved rods arranged singly or in pairs, often in V formation or in palisades of several parallel cells; may be coccobacillary; may be beaded or club shaped		Varies by species (see chapter 26)	
Dermatophilus (77, 232)	Pos[d]	Neg	Branching, septate hyphae, 0.6–1.0 μm in diam; mycelial elements consist of coccoid cells arranged longitudinally in a single row or up to 8 parallel rows (see text)	3D	Colonies gray-white to yellow or orange on prolonged incubation; rough, heaped, opaque, granular colonies with beta hemolysis; colonies may be adherent to the agar	
Dietzia (174)	Neg	Neg[e]	Coccobaccili to rods, often in V formation		Smooth, yellow	
Gordonia (114, 192)	Neg[f]	W	Short coryneform rods; no branching	3C	Rough, wrinkled, brownish, pink, or orange to red colonies	2I
Mycobacterium[c] (165)	V	Pos	Straight or slightly curved rods, may appear as thin, beaded rods or negative images by Gram stain.		Varies by species (see chapters 29 and 30)	
Nocardia (75)	Pos[g]	W	Thin, filamentous branching rods, 0.5–1.0 μm in diam; beading generally apparent (see text)	3E, 3F, 3G, 3K, 3L	Chalky, matte or velvety, powdery (usually), irregular, wrinkled, heaped, or smooth on surface; may be brown, tan, pink, orange, red, purple, gray, yellow, peach, or white on reverse; smooth or granular; soluble brown or yellow pigments may be produced (see text)	2D, 2E, 2G, 2L
Nocardiopsis (146, 147)	Pos	Neg	Best distinguished by slide culture (see text)		Aerial mycelium can be sparse to abundant and blue, white, cream, yellow, gray, or green; zigzag arrangement of developing spores on aerial hyphae; colonies are coarsely wrinkled or folded; greenish-yellow or brown soluble pigment may be present	
Pseudonocardia (91)	V	Neg	Best distinguished by slide culture		White aerial hyphae; yellow colonies	
Rhodococcus (72)	Neg[h]	W	Coccoid to bacillary forms (see text)	3I, 3J	Rough, smooth, or mucoid; buff, cream, yellow, orange, or red; colorless variants occur; may become increasingly pigmented and rough with age	2H
Saccharomonospora (26, 138)	Pos	Neg	Best distinguished by slide culture		Leathery; aerial mycelium is initially white, becoming gray-green, dark green, or bluish; yellow, green, or brown soluble pigment	
Saccharopolyspora (119)	Pos	Neg	Best distinguished by slide culture		Thin, raised or convex colorless colonies, slightly wrinkled, and mucoid or gelatinous with sparse aerial mycelium; may have yellow soluble pigment	

(Continued on next page)

TABLE 1 *(Continued)*

Genus (reference[s])	Aerial hyphae	Modified acid fast	Microscopic morphology	Figure(s)	Colonial morphology[b]	Figure(s)
Segniliparus (32)	Neg	Strongly Pos	Rod shaped with occasional V forms; no branching; size varies by species	3M, 3N	Smooth and domed to wrinkled and rough, varies by species; nonpigmented colonies; may produce a soluble pigment.	2M
Streptomyces (219)	Pos	Neg	Filamentous branching rods, 0.5–2.0 μm in diam; filaments may fragment into short rods; may stain more solidly gram positive than *Nocardia*; may show beading		Colonies are discrete and lichenoid, leathery, or butyrous; variety of pigments; aerial hyphae may appear floccose, granular, powdery, or velvety; may produce a colored soluble pigment	2C
Thermoactinomyces (116, 120)	V	NF	May become gram negative with age		Slowly growing, white, yellow, or colorless colonies; aerial hyphae may be sparse	
Tsukamurella (41)	Neg	W	Straight to slightly curved long rods; occur singly, in pairs, or in masses; very short rods may be seen; no apparent branching	3J	White/creamy to orange; small with convex elevation; dry	2J, 2K
Williamsia (105)	Neg	Neg	Short rods or coccobacilli (see text)	3O	Smooth, yellow, orange to orange-red colonies	2N, 2O

[a]Abbreviations: V, variable; Neg, negative; Pos, positive; NF, test result not found; W, weak positive.
[b]Colonial morphology descriptions are from various references, the authors of which used a variety of different media; see reference for more information.
[c]Included for completeness; some consider *Corynebacterium* and *Mycobacterium* to be aerobic actinomycetes.
[d]Aerial hyphae may be produced in an increased CO_2 atmosphere.
[e]Original description was Pos.
[f]Sparse aerial hyphae may be produced by G. *amarae*.
[g]Occasionally no aerial hyphae produced.
[h]Occasional rudimentary aerial hyphae seen.

TABLE 2 Chemotaxonomic and lysozyme growth characteristics of genera of aerobic actinomycetes[a]

Genus (reference[s])	Cell wall type[b]	Mycolic acids	No. of carbon atoms in mycolic acid	Growth in lysozyme	Menaquinone
Actinomadura (26, 145)	III	Neg	NA	V	MK-9($H_4H_6H_8$)
Amycolatopsis (128)	IV	Neg	NA	V	MK-9(H_2H_4)
Corynebacterium[c] (63, 75)	IV	Pos	22–38	NT	MK-8(H_2) or MK-9(H_2)
Dermatophilus (26, 77)	III	Neg	NA	NF	NF
Dietzia (174)	IV	Pos	34–38	NF	MK-8(H_2)
Gordonia (114, 192)	IV	Pos	48–66	V	MK-9(H_2)
Mycobacterium[c] (26, 75, 165)	IV	Pos	60–90	Pos	MK-9(H_2)
Nocardia (75)	IV	Pos	44–64	Pos	MK-8(H_4) or MK-9(H_2)
Nocardiopsis (146, 147)	III	Neg	NA	Neg	MK-10($H_2H_4H_6$)
Pseudonocardia (91)	IV	Neg	NA	NF	MK-9(H_4)
Rhodococcus (72)	IV	Pos	34–64	Neg	MK-8(H_2) or MK-9(H_2)
Saccharomonospora (138)	IV	Neg	NA	Neg	MK-9(H_4)
Saccharopolyspora (119)	IV	Neg	NA	Neg	MK-9(H_4)
Segniliparus (32)	meso-DAP[d]	Pos	70–90	V	NF
Streptomyces (219)	I	Neg	NA	V	MK-9(H_6H_8)
Thermoactinomyces (116, 120)	III	NF	NF	Pos	MK-7, MK-9
Tsukamurella (41)	IV	Pos	62–78	Pos	MK-9
Williamsia (105)	IV	Pos	50–56	NF	MK-9

[a]Abbreviations: V, variable; Neg, negative; NA, not applicable; Pos, positive; NF, test result not found.
[b]Cell wall types: I, L-DAP, no sugars; III, meso-DAP, madurose or no sugars; IV, meso-DAP, arabinose, and galactose.
[c]Included for completeness; some consider *Corynebacterium* and *Mycobacterium* to be aerobic actinomycetes.
[d]Cell wall contains meso-DAP; no data regarding cell wall sugars found.

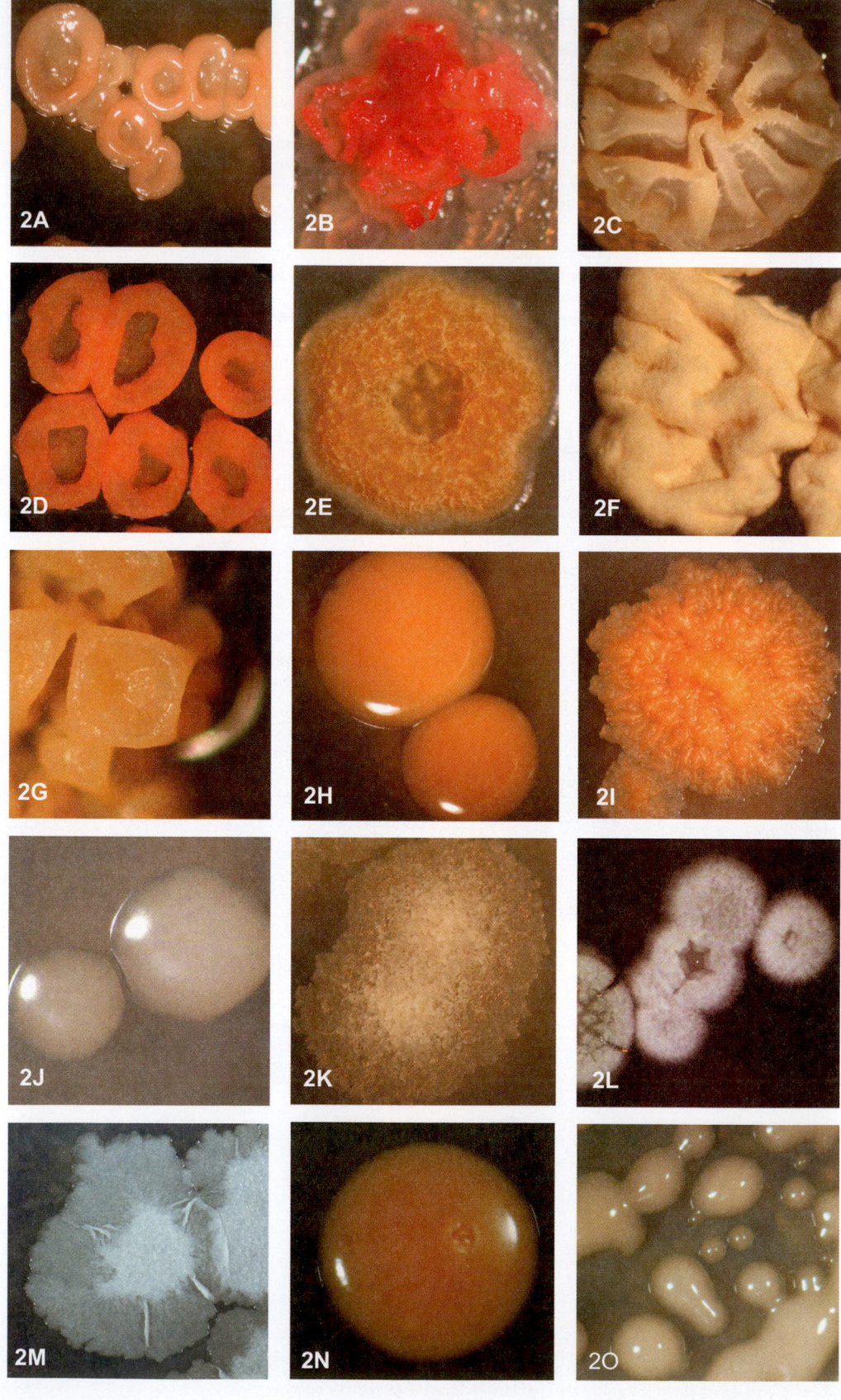

Rhodococcus

The microscopic morphology of rhodococci can range from coccoid to bacillary depending on species and specimen type and on the stage of growth of the organism (52). The organisms exhibit a rod-coccus growth cycle. Rod forms are best visualized by growing isolates in a liquid medium, and under such conditions some branching of individual cells may be found. Generally, however, the organisms appear as gram-positive, beaded to solidly staining coccobacilli (Fig. 3H). The modified acid-fast stain must be performed and interpreted with particular care when dealing with isolates that may belong to this genus, as only a tiny fraction of the cells may retain the stain (Fig. 3I). Modified acid-fast smears prepared from isolates growing on trypticase soy agar with 5% sheep blood or chocolate agar may appear to be acid-fast negative (60). Rhodococcus species can easily be dismissed as "diphtheroids" because of their Gram stain morphology (Fig. 3H) and their frequent failure to develop obvious pigmentation during the first few days of growth. At 37°C, colonies may be only about 1 mm in diameter after 24 h of incubation. An aerial mycelium is generally not macroscopically visible but may occasionally be seen microscopically (72). Rhodococcus has been the subject of several recent reviews (13, 74, 83). Some data suggest that it may be justifiable to separate the genus into several additional genera (83). There are approximately 34 validly named species in the genus.

Saccharomonospora

The approximately eight validly described species of the genus Saccharomonospora are characterized by the presence of single spores tightly packed on aerial hyphae. The organisms are commonly found in soil, lake sediment, peat, compost, and manure. They are moderately thermophilic, with optimum growth occurring at 35 to 50°C (138).

Saccharopolyspora

Species in the genus Saccharopolyspora were initially thought to be related to Nocardia and Streptomyces by biochemical characteristics but are phylogenetically distinct from those genera. The organism was originally isolated from sugar cane and has a microscopic morphology similar to species in the genus Nocardiopsis. It is so named because of the presence of beadlike chains of sheath-enclosed spores formed by segmentation of the aerial hyphae. The organism grows in temperatures between 25 and 50°C, with optimum growth at 37 to 40°C (119). There are approximately 16 validly described species in the genus.

Segniliparus

The presence of unique high-pressure liquid chromatography mycolic acid patterns in 4 clinical isolates thought to belong to the genus Mycobacterium initiated an investigation into the characteristics of this recently described genus. By 16S rRNA gene sequence, the genus is most closely related to members of the genus Rhodococcus, and cell wall chemistry places it in the suborder Corynebacterineae with Rhodococcus and other related genera (31). Segniliparus is the only aerobic actinomycete (besides Mycobacterium) that is strongly acid-fast (Fig. 2M and 3M and N).

Streptomyces

The genus- and species-level taxonomy of this huge group, which contains approximately 597 validly named species or subspecies, remains problematic (3, 141). Many of these species have been patented because of the commercially useful products they synthesize (3) (Fig. 2C).

Thermoactinomycetes

The approximately eight species of the genus Thermoactinomycetes are characterized by their production of abundant endospores that are resistant to heat and easily become airborne. Organisms are found in soil, moldy and decaying plant materials, and composts. By 16S rRNA gene sequence and G+C content, members of this genus are more closely related to the genus Bacillus than they are to the other genera considered aerobic actinomycetes, but they are considered with this group because of their similar morphologic features. Optimum growth temperatures vary by species, but most species grow between 35 and 58°C (120).

Tsukamurella

The genus Tsukamurella was created to accommodate organisms with a specific cell wall chemistry that separated it from other aerobic actinomycetes (41). The type species of the genus, T. paurometabola (corrected from T. paurometabolum), was previously known as Corynebacterium paurometabolum. There are approximately 11 validly named species in the genus. The taxonomy of the genus remains confusing; see below for additional details (Fig. 2J and K and 3J).

Williamsia

The genus Williamsia was recently established to include environmental organisms that resembled those in genera belonging to the family Nocardiaceae but which had an unusual cell morphology. When examined by electron microscopy, cells of Williamsia show hairy structures distributed over the whole surface of the cell. These structures are not visible in negative-stained preparations (105). The genus contains approximately five species (Fig. 2N and O and 3O).

FIGURE 2 Colonial morphology of type strains of various aerobic actinomycetes grown on Sabouraud dextrose agar (Emmons modification) unless otherwise noted. While appearances are typical for the species illustrated, the extent of possible colonial variation within a given species is not known. (A) *Actinomadura latina* at 21 days; smooth umbilicate colonies with no aerial hyphae. (B) *Actinomadura pelletieri* at 10 days; ropy but smooth-surfaced colony with no aerial hyphae. (C) *Streptomyces griseus* at 10 days; rugose colony with some aerial hyphae. (D) *Nocardia brasiliensis* at 10 days; umbilicate colonies; sparse aerial hyphae present, but visible only on microscopic inspection of colonies. (E) *Nocardia carnea* at 25 days; aerial hyphae present. (F) *Amycolatopsis orientalis* at 21 days; aerial hyphae present. (G) *Nocardia otitidiscaviarum* at 7 days; rugose colony; sparse aerial hyphae present, visible only on careful microscopic inspection. (H) *Rhodococcus equi* at 10 days; smooth colonies with no aerial hyphae. (I) *Gordonia bronchialis* at 10 days; irregular but smooth surface with no aerial hyphae. (J) *Tsukamurella pulmonis* at 10 days; smooth colonies with no aerial hyphae. (K) *Tsukamurella strandjordii* at 10 days; rough colonies with no aerial hyphae. (L) *Nocardia cyriacigeorgica* at 10 days; dense powdery aerial hyphae cover most or all the surface of the colonies. (M) *Segniliparus rugosus* at 15 days on Middlebrook agar; rough colonies with no aerial hyphae. (N) *Williamsia deligens* at 15 days; smooth colonies with no aerial hyphae. (O) *Williamsia muralis* at 15 days; mucoid colonies.

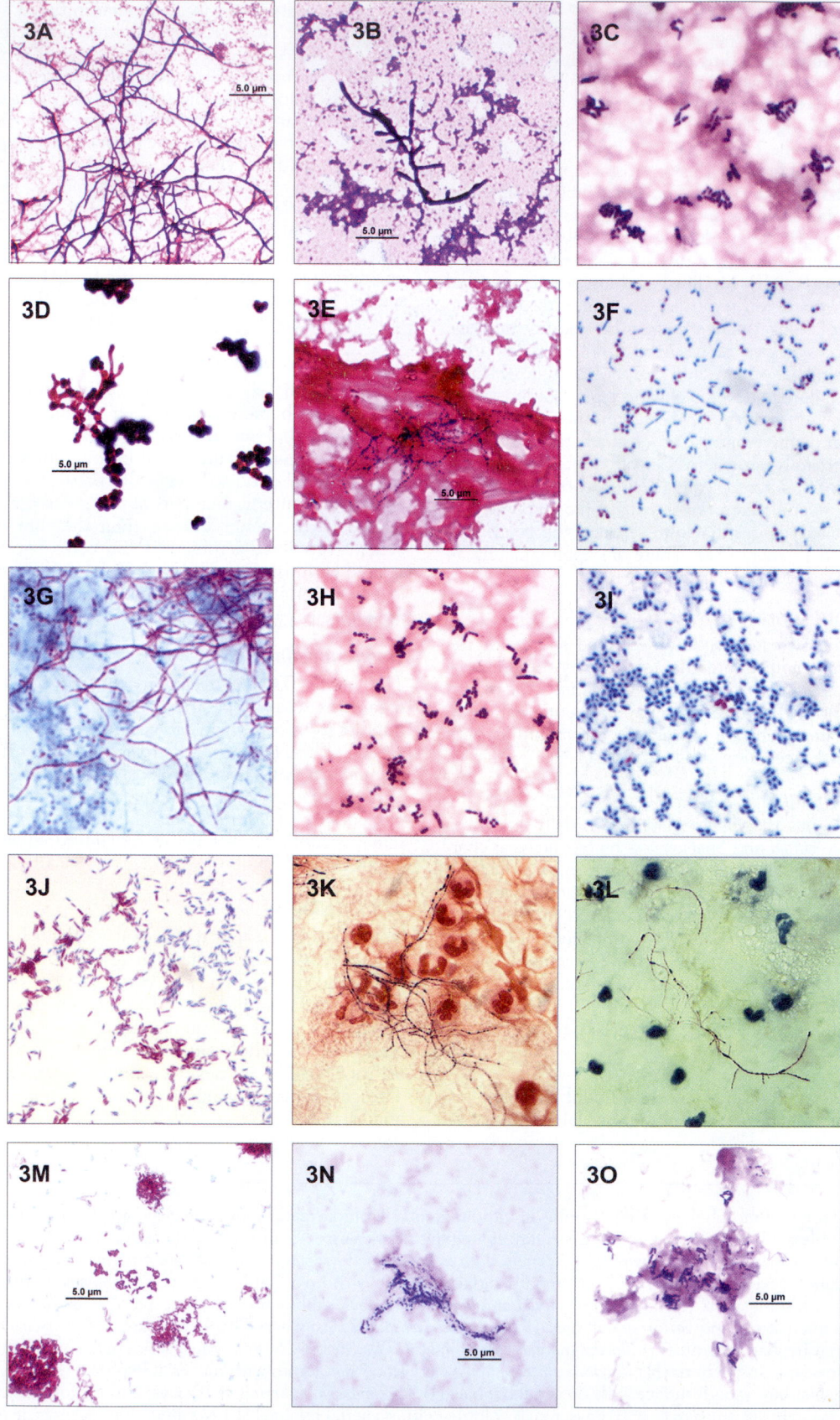

EPIDEMIOLOGY AND TRANSMISSION

While the aerobic actinomycetes are widely distributed in the environment, the extent to which particular species are geographically restricted is not well known. Their primary ecological niche is probably the decomposition of plant material (141).

The majority of infections caused by aerobic actinomycetes stem from environmental sources, and even most nosocomial infections appear attributable to an environmental source such as dust from construction work (18). There has not yet been a documented case of direct patient-to-patient spread of an aerobic actinomycete infection without the intermediation of another human agent or of environmental contamination.

Most of the reports of outbreaks and pseudo-outbreaks of infection have been attributed to *Nocardia* species. For a brief discussion of these outbreaks, see the *Manual of Clinical Microbiology*, 9th ed. (48)

A seven-patient outbreak of *Gordonia bronchialis* sternal wound infections was traced to a nurse from whose hands and other body sites the organism was isolated; it was also isolated from two of the nurse's dogs (176).

Two pseudo-outbreaks of infection with *N. asteroides* associated with the use of the BACTEC 460 TB system and inadequate needle sterilization have been reported (132, 161).

An outbreak of pseudoinfection attributed to *T. paurometabola*, involving specimens from 10 different patients and attributed to a common source somewhere in the laboratory, has also been reported (8).

CLINICAL SIGNIFICANCE

While the number of recognized species of aerobic actinomycetes is rapidly increasing, assessment of the clinical significance of many species is becoming increasingly difficult. In some cases, a new species is described on the basis of a single isolate, and while careful attention is paid to its molecular features, little or no information may be provided to document that the isolate was actually a cause of disease in the patient from whom it was isolated. On the other hand, reports continue to be published regarding organisms that, while unquestionably the cause of disease, have been misidentified because of failure to use molecular methods; in other cases, even when molecular methods have been used, the accuracy of the reported identifications may be in doubt because of the provision of inadequate detail regarding the

TABLE 3 Species of aerobic actinomycetes other than *Nocardia* species more frequently reported as human pathogens and GenBank[a] accession number of the type strain sequence

Genus and species	GenBank accession no. of type strain sequence
Actinomadura madurae	NR_026343
Actinomadura pelletieri	AJ293710
Dermatophilus congolensis	AJ243918
Dietzia maris	FJ468333
Gordonia bronchialis	NR_027594
Gordonia terrae	X79286[b]
Nocardiopsis dassonvillei	NR_029314
Rhodococcus equi	FJ468344
Streptomyces somaliensis	AJ007403
Tsukamurella paurometabola	AF283281

[a]GenBank sequences available at http://www.ncbi.nlm.nih.gov/.
[b]Best sequence available for the *G. terrae* type strain.

molecular technique used and the methods of interpretation used. Furthermore, many identifications reported in the older literature would be considered incorrect by currently accepted species criteria; perhaps the most glaring example is that of *Nocardia asteroides*, which to the best of the authors' knowledge, has never been documented to be a human pathogen using currently accepted taxonomy.

Unfortunately, all these factors hinder the accurate association of clinically useful information with a given species. There is perhaps a growing tendency to assemble species into "groups" on the basis of certain features such as antimicrobial susceptibility, as was originally done by Wallace et al. for what were considered antibiogram types of *N. asteroides* but which are now all divided into different species. While currently "species" are delineated and identified primarily, if not entirely, on the basis of molecular features, possibly a separate but more relevant clinically based taxonomy may emerge, based not only on molecular features but on such aspects as pathogenicity, antimicrobial susceptibility, and type of disease produced—all of which presumably do have a basis in the fundamental molecular features of the organism.

Tables 3 and 4 list species of aerobic actinomycetes other than those in the genus *Nocardia* and those in the genus *Nocardia*, respectively, that are considered relatively frequent human pathogens or, in a few cases,

FIGURE 3 Microscopic morphology of various aerobic actinomycetes. All photomicrographs taken at ×1,000 magnification. (A) *Actinomadura latina*; Gram stain from Tween-albumin broth (TAB) at 4 days; long, branching, relatively solidly staining rods. (B) *Amycolata autotrophica*; Gram stain from TAB at 4 days; long beaded rods with some branching. (C) *Gordonia bronchialis*; Gram stain from TAB at 4 days; coryneform rods with no obvious branching. (D) *Dermatophilus congolensis*; Gram stain from Sabouraud dextrose agar at 14 days in CO_2; dense aggregates of cells of varying sizes; note the chains of longitudinally and transversely dividing cells near the top. (E) *Nocardia abscessus*; Gram stain from TAB at 10 days; long, beaded, branching rods; note that the beads generally do not abut one another. (F) *Nocardia farcinica*; modified acid-fast stain from horse blood agar at 2 to 3 days; many coccal forms are present; it is mostly these that are staining modified acid-fast positive. (G) *N. veterana*; modified acid-fast stain from TAB at 25 days; some long, branching forms are staining modified acid-fast positive. (H) *Rhodococcus equi*; Gram stain from TAB at 4 days; coccobacilli and short coryneform rods without obvious branching. (I) *Rhodococcus equi*; modifed acid-fast stain from charcoal yeast extract (CYE) agar at 10 days; only a small percentage of the cells stain positive. (J) *Tsukamurella pulmonis*; modified acid-fast stain from Lowenstein-Jensen medium at 4 days; thin rods, many of which stain positive. (K) Direct Gram stain of sputum that grew a *Nocardia* species; note the lacy network of long, thin, branching, beaded rods (courtesy of Daniel P. Fedorko). (L) Direct modified acid-fast stain of the same specimen as in panel K; the beads are purplish, but the intervening areas of the organism stain positive (courtesy of Daniel P. Fedorko). (M) *Segniliparus rotundus*; Kinyoun stain from Middlebrook at 12 days. (N) *Segniliparus rugosus*; Gram stain from TAB at 7 days. (O) *Williamsia deligens*; Gram stain from TAB at 5 days.

TABLE 4 Species of *Nocardia* more frequently reported as human pathogens and GenBank accession number of the type strain sequence

Species	GenBank accession no. of the type strain sequence
N. abscessus	AF430018
N. brasiliensis	AF430038
N. cyriacigeorgica	GQ376180
N. farcinica	AF430033
N. nova	AF430028
N. otitidiscaviarum	AF430067
N. paucivorans	GQ376188
N. pseudobrasiliensis	AF430042
N. transvalensis	AF430047
N. veterana	AY171039
N. wallacei	GQ853074

are clearly established pathogens but probably have been previously unrecognized as separate species. Tables 5 and 6 list species of aerobic actinomycetes other than those in the genus *Nocardia* and those in the genus *Nocardia*, respectively, that have only rarely (often only once) been reported as human isolates, whose actual causative role in human disease does not seem well established or for which there are no recent reports. Tables 5 and 6 should by no means be considered exhaustive. Whenever a laboratory isolates an aerobic actinomycete for which sequencing indicates that the organism belongs to a species that has been rarely isolated, the circumstances surrounding the isolation of the organism should be carefully evaluated to assess its potential clinical significance. A search of the current literature may be conducted to determine what is already established regarding that species, including its known pathogenicity and antibiotic susceptibilities. For such searches, LPSN and PubMed (www.pubmed.gov) may be good starting points; current nomenclature and taxonomic standing should be followed as stated in LPSN.

Actinomadura

A useful clue to the identification of organisms in the genus *Actinomadura* is the nature of the lesion from which an isolate originates. Most commonly, this organism causes a mycetoma, a chronic, invasive, slowly progressive infection usually occurring in the foot (Madura foot) and nearby anatomic structures and nearly always resulting from traumatic implantation of the organism. Draining sinuses are typically present in a mycetoma; macroscopically visible grains (organism aggregates or microcolonies) may be visible in the discharge from the lesions. There are not adequate data available to allow using grain color for species or even genus level discrimination of the etiologic agent. The infection occurs most frequently in tropical regions, where people are more likely to walk barefoot. The word "mycetoma" is used only to describe the clinical nature of the infection, not the etiologic agent. Actinomycotic mycetomas are caused by aerobic actinomycetes; eumycotic mycetomas are caused by true fungi. Organisms in this genus have very rarely been implicated in other types of infection. *Actinomadura madurae* and *A. pelletieri* have been the two species most frequently reported as pathogens. In many reports mentioning the species causing mycetomas, identification has been made solely on the basis of the

TABLE 5 Species of aerobic actinomycetes other than *Nocardia* species infrequently reported or poorly documented as human pathogens and GenBank accession number of the type strain sequence

Species	GenBank accession no. of the type strain[a] sequence
Actinomadura chibensis	AB264086
Actinomadura cremea	AF134067
Actinomadura latina	AY035998
Actinomadura nitritigenes	AY035999
Actinomadura vinacea	AF134070
Amycolatopsis benzoatilytica	AY957506
Amycolatopsis orientalis	AJ400711
Amycolatopsis palatopharyngis	AF479268
Dietzia cinnamea	AJ920289
Gordonia araii	AB162800
Gordonia effusa	AB162799
Gordonia otitidis	AB122026
Gordonia polyisoprenivorans	NR_026500
Gordonia rubripertincta	X80632
Gordonia sputi	X80634
Rhodococcus corynebacterioides[b]	AF430066
Rhodococcus erythropolis	X79289[c]
Rhodococcus fascians[d]	X79186
Rhodococcus globerulus	NR_026184
Rhodococcus gordoniae	AY233201
Rhodococcus rhodochrous	FJ468342
Segniliparus rotundus	AY608918
Segniliparus rugosus	AY608920
Streptomyces albus	AJ621602
Streptomyces bikiniensis	X79851
Streptomyces cinereoruber	AY999771
Streptomyces griseus	AY207604[e]
Streptomyces sudanensis[f]	EF515876
Streptomyces thermovulgaris	Z68094
Tsukamurella inchonensis	AF283281
Tsukamurella pulmonis	X92981
Tsukamurella strandjordii	AF283283
Tsukamurella tyrosinosolvens	AY238514
Williamsia deligens	AJ920290
Williamsia muralis	Y17384[g]

[a]From J. P. Euzéby (LSPN; www.bacterio.cict.fr); sequences submitted prior to 2000 replaced when possible with similar, more recent sequences.
[b]Previously *Nocardia corynebacterioides*.
[c]GenBank record X79289 lists the name for this species as *R. erythreus* strain DSM 43066, the type strain of *R. erythropolis*.
[d]Later synonym *R. luteus*; best sequence found for the type strain of *R. fascians*.
[e]GenBank record is for strain KACC 20084.
[f]See reference 173.
[g]Best sequence found for the type strain of *W. muralis*.

histological appearance of the grains, on the basis of a small number of phenotypic tests, or in ways not specified in any detail (34, 113, 133, 134). As with virtually all the aerobic actinomycetes, molecular methods are the only accurate procedures to use for definitive species level identification of organisms in this genus.

Amycolata and Amycolatopsis

There are no recent reports documenting human infection caused by species in either the genus *Amycolata* or *Amycolatopsis*. Three species in the genus *Amycolatopsis* and several other aerobic actinomycete species may be causative agents of equine placental infection and abortion (118).

TABLE 6 Species of *Nocardia* infrequently reported or poorly documented as human pathogens and GenBank accession number of the type strain sequence

Species	GenBank accession no. of the type strain sequence
N. africana	AF430054
N. anaemiae	GQ376192
N. aobensis	GQ376159
N. araoensis	GQ376160
N. arthritidis	GQ217494
N. asiatica	GQ217495
N. asteroides	DQ659898
N. beijingensis	GQ217493
N. blacklockiae	GQ376162
N. brevicatena	AF430040
N. carnea	AF430035
N. concava[a]	EF177464
N. corynebacterioides[b]	AF430066
N. elegans	GQ376166
N. exalbida	GQ376167
N. higoensis	GQ376169
N. ignorata[a]	DQ659907
N. inohanensis	DQ6599908
N. kruczakiae	DQ659909
N. mexicana	GQ376178
N. neocaledoniensis	GQ853080
N. niigatensis	GQ853079
N. ninae	GQ853078
N. niwae[c]	FJ765056
N. pneumoniae	GQ853075
N. puris	GQ217500
N. shimofusensis	NR_028650
N. sienata	AB516654
N. takedensis	GQ376185
N. terpenica	GQ376183
N. testacea	AB192415
N. thailandica	AB126874
N. vermiculata	GQ853068
N. vinacea	DQ659919
N. yamanashiensis[a]	DQ659920

[a]Type strains of these species are known to contain multiple differing copies of the 16S rRNA gene (see text).

[b]Later synonym *Rhodococcus corynebacterioides*.

[c]B. D. Moser, B. A. Lasker, A. G. Steigerwalt, H. P. Hinrikson, and J. M. Brown, *Abstr. 109th Gen. Meet. Am. Soc. Microbiol.*, 2009, abstr.Y-019.

Dermatophilus

D. congolensis causes dermatitis in a wide variety of animals worldwide, including cattle, horses, goats, and sheep, but has only rarely been noted as a cause of human infection (198). In humans, the organism has been reported to cause a variety of cutaneous manifestations, including scaling and exudative lesions, pustules, pitted keratolysis (69), and hairy leukoplakia of the tongue (30). Filamentous and coccoid forms of the organism may be visualized directly in tissue specimens. Optimal therapy has not been defined, but infections may be self-limiting. *Dermatophilus chelonae* has been reported to cause disease in several species of animals (137, 217).

Dietzia

Dietzia maris is the species in this genus most frequently associated with human infection (Table 5). In one reported case, the organism was isolated from blood and from an intravascular catheter. Biochemical and chemotaxonomic

studies of the isolate were performed (14), but the isolate was noted to be modified Kinyoun stain negative, although from the description of the species, *D. maris* would be expected to be modified acid-fast positive. The other reported case involved infection of a hip prosthesis; a variety of identification techniques were employed, including 16S rRNA sequencing. The closest match was with the *D. maris* type strain with a sequence similarity of only 98% (166). The patient responded to treatment with teicoplanin. A case of aortic dissection associated with this organism has also been reported (175).

Gordonia

There have been relatively few reports of infections attributed to species in the genus *Gordonia*. However, an unknown number of *Gordonia* infections may be missed, either because the isolate is considered an insignificant coryneform gram-positive rod or the isolate is misidentified as belonging to another genus such as *Nocardia* or *Rhodococcus* (17). In 5 patients with catheter-related *Gordonia* species infection, the organism was correctly identified to the genus level in only one case until 16S rRNA gene sequencing was employed (17). In three of these five patients, *Gordonia terrae* was the infecting organism, one was G. *bronchialis*, and one was G. *otitidis*. Recently, there has been a review published on medical device-associated *Gordonia* infections in connection with a report of infection of an orthopedic device caused by G. *araii*; most of the infections reviewed were attributed to G. *terrae* (99). One of the very few clusters of infection attributable to any aerobic actinomycete involved seven patients who developed sternal wound infections following coronary artery bypass surgery (176). The organism involved, *Gordonia bronchialis* (then called *Rhodococcus bronchialis*), was identified by biochemical testing and cell wall mycolic acid analysis only. Immunocompromise and/or the presence of foreign bodies appear to have been contributing factors in many of the infections caused by *Gordonia* species.

Nocardia

Nocardia infections generally result either from trauma-related introduction of the organism or, particularly in immunocompromised patients, from inhalation and the resulting establishment of a pulmonary focus. The brain is one of the most common secondary sites of infection (158). An initial advance in the clinically useful categorization of pathogenic nocardial isolates was provided by Wallace and his coworkers (211). They divided organisms phenotypically resembling *N. asteroides* into six different drug pattern types and one additional miscellaneous group. With more recent work, numerous different species have been described within this set of organisms, which came to be known as the *Nocardia asteroides* complex. These include *N. abscessus* (drug pattern I), *N. cyriacigeorgica* (drug pattern VI), *N. farcinica* (drug pattern V), *N. nova* (drug pattern III), *N. wallacei* (drug pattern IV), and isolates of drug pattern II. Other new *Nocardia* species are continually being described, and undoubtedly, by current species definition criteria, many more will be described in the future.

Given the current state of the literature, it is possible to make only the most tentative statements regarding geographic distribution and disease correlates of different species. While accurate species assignment allows one to make some predictions regarding likely antimicrobial susceptibility patterns, such a species assignment today requires the use of molecular methods (38). Nonetheless, susceptibility testing of all clinically significant isolates is recommended, whether or not molecular techniques have been used for their identification. Typical susceptibility patterns of different species can be found in Table 7.

TABLE 7 Typical in vitro antimicrobial susceptibility patterns of various Nocardia species[a]

Drug	N. abscessus	N. brasiliensis	N. brevicatena and N. paucivorans	N. cyriacigeorgica	N. farcinica	N. nova complex[b]	N. otitidiscaviarum	N. pseudobrasiliensis	N. transvalensis complex[c]
AMC[d]	S	S	S	R	—	R	R	R	—
Amikacin	S	—	S	S	S	S[e]	S	—	R
Ceftriaxone	S	—	S	S	R	S	R	—	S
Ciprofloxacin	R	R	S	R	S	—	S	S	S
Clarithromycin	R	R	R[f]	R	R	S	—	S	R
Gentamicin	R[f]	—	R	—	R	S[e]	S	—	R
Imipenem	S	—	S	S	R	S	R	—	S
Linezolid	S	S	S	S	S	S	S	S	S
Minocycline	—	S	—	—	—	—	—	R	—
Sulfamethoxazole[g]	—	S	—	—	R	—	S	S	—
Tobramycin	—	—	—	—	R	—	—	—	R

[a]From reference 28. Based on interpretation of MICs, using CLSI breakpoints. Abbreviations: S, susceptible; R, resistant; —, no consistent result.
[b]Includes N. nova sensu stricto, N. africana, N. kruczakiae, and N. veterana.
[c]Includes N. transvalensis sensu stricto and N. wallacei.
[d]AMC, amoxicillin-clavulanic acid.
[e]MICs of this drug are very low.
[f]Most strains exhibit this pattern.
[g]Interpretation of the 80% inhibition endpoint may be difficult to determine (38).

Of the 88 species of *Nocardia* currently recognized, 46 have been reported as human isolates, and several others have been reported as pathogens of animals. Importantly, isolates in many reports of infection, even in the recent literature, are incorrectly identified because of failure to use optimal identification methods.

Nocardia abscessus

Nocardia abscessus was formally named in 2000 by Yassin et al. (228). ATCC strain 23824, the reference strain of *N. asteroides* drug pattern type I (195), was one of the isolates found to be *N. abscessus* on the basis of 16S rRNA sequencing and DNA-DNA hybridization. In their description in 1988 of the antimicrobial susceptibility patterns of 78 clinical isolates of *Nocardia* from various sources, Wallace et al. noted that 20% of the isolates had this drug pattern type (211). Several of the strains in the report naming the species were from abscesses; a subsequent report from Japan reported several isolates from pulmonary sources and one from a brain abscess (103). Two isolates have been reported from Germany, one from pericardial fluid (218) and the other from a posttraumatic wound (94). More recent cases have included a report of disseminated infection in an AIDS patient (56).

Nocardia asteroides and the "N. asteroides Complex"

There are innumerable reports of human infection attributed to *N. asteroides* (48); it has probably been considered the most commonly isolated human pathogenic *Nocardia* species. However, molecular analyses of the pathogenic isolates attributed to this species that have been conducted thus far have indicated that all belong to some other named or as-yet-unnamed species. It is currently believed that *N. asteroides* sensu stricto is rarely, if ever, pathogenic.

The term "*N. asteroides* complex" has been used for organisms phenotypically resembling the *N. asteroides* type strain. However, several distinct species have now been described within that complex, and precisely what the complex is intended to designate is usually unclear. Given the current ability to identify *Nocardia* isolates molecularly, the phrase "*N. asteroides* complex" should be avoided. The term "complex" is best restricted to groups of species that are related on a molecular basis and have similar phenotypic features. Such groups would include the "*N. nova* complex" and the "*N. transvalensis* complex." Whenever the term "complex" is used, it is best to state initially precisely which species are intended to be included in the complex.

Nocardia brasiliensis

N. brasiliensis appears to be the most common cause of actinomycotic mycetoma (see "*Actinomadura*" above) in the Western Hemisphere, especially in Mexico (33, 34). The organism probably occurs worldwide; there are reports of infection from Australia (68), West Bengal (134), and Europe (135) and many from North America (189). A variety of cutaneous manifestations in addition to mycetoma have been reported, including cellulites, abscesses, and lymphocutaneous infection. Nearly all cases are a result of trauma, including that caused by thorns (135), cat scratch (21), and insect bite (159). Most of the trauma-related infections have occurred in immunocompetent individuals. Disseminated infection, usually originating from a pulmonary focus, has also been reported (189); such infections are more likely to occur in immunocompromised patients (115). Some cases, such as one of a brain abscess resulting from dissemination from a pulmonary focus (154), do occur in patients who appear to be immunocompetent. However, most of the cases of invasive disease, as well as some of the cases of cutaneous infection, attributed to *N. brasiliensis* (prior to 1995) almost certainly have been caused by *N. pseudobrasiliensis* (see below).

Nocardia brevicatena

In 1982, Goodfellow and Pirouz examined 108 phenotypic characteristics of sporoactinomycetes that contained meso-diaminopimelic acid in their cell walls. Results showed that one species they examined, *Micropolyspora brevicatena*, shared many characteristics with *Nocardia* isolates included in the study. The authors recommended that this organism be transferred to the genus *Nocardia* as *Nocardia brevicatena* (76). Brown et al. suggested in 1997 that *Nocardia* isolates sharing both an unusual drug susceptibility pattern and one or another of three different RFLP patterns of an amplified portion of the 65-kDa heat shock protein (HSP) gene should be considered to form the *Nocardia brevicatena* complex (B. A. Brown, R. W. Wilson, V. A. Steingrube, Z. Blacklock, and R. J. Wallace, Jr., *Abstr. 97th Gen. Meet. Am. Soc. Microbiol. 1997*, abstr. C-65, p. 131, 1997). These organisms included 19 clinical isolates from the United States, 10 clinical isolates from Australia, and three ATCC reference strains of *N. brevicatena*. There have been no subsequent reports of clinical isolates or taxonomic studies of these organisms. Given the different restriction fragment length polymorphism (RFLP) patterns involved, several different species may be included in this complex, one of which may be *Nocardia paucivorans* (see below).

Nocardia cyriacigeorgica

N. cyriacigeorgica (spelling corrected from the original *N. cyriacigeorgici*) was described on the basis of an isolate obtained from the sputum of a patient with chronic bronchitis (229). Subsequent isolates were obtained from brain abscesses in an immunocompromised patient (66) and from a patient with pneumonia following a near-drowning incident, from whom *N. farcinica* and several other pathogens were also isolated (203). Isolates of this species were reported to constitute 13 of 96 (14%) clinical isolates of *Nocardia* from Thailand (169) and 13 of 86 (15%) such isolates from Belgium (215). The 16S rRNA sequence of the type strain of this species (1,400 bp) was found to be identical to that of the reference strain of "*N. asteroides* drug pattern type VI" (ATCC 14759) (179, 195). DNA-DNA hybridization studies subsequently established that this drug pattern type VI reference strain and *N. cyriacigeorgica* belong to the same species (49). In the original work describing the different *N. asteroides* drug pattern types, type VI was the most commonly isolated strain (35%) (211). *N. cyriacigeorgica* is probably the most frequent human nocardial pathogen, at least in areas where actinomycotic mycetomas are relatively rare. While the species *N. cyriacigeorgica* has been designated an emerging pathogen (183), it is actually a relatively common and long-recognized pathogen that has recently acquired a valid name. In fact, many isolates previously reported as "*N. asteroides*" almost certainly belong to this species. Note that the designation "*N. asteroides* drug pattern type VI" is not a valid species name.

Nocardia farcinica

The organisms initially described by Wallace et al. as belonging to the group "*N. asteroides* drug pattern type V" (211) were subsequently found to belong to *N. farcinica* (212). Isolates of this species are perhaps the most resistant of all *Nocardia* isolates (Table 7). *N. farcinica* isolates that showed in vitro resistance to trimethoprim-sulfamethoxazole have been reported to respond to meropenem alone (92) and to the combination of linezolid and minocycline (130). This species may have a particular propensity for causing disseminated disease; Wallace et al. reported that among 30 patients for which disease extent was known, 57% had disseminated disease and one-third had central nervous system (CNS) involvement (212). Most patients infected by this species, especially those with disseminated disease, have some type of immunocompromise (212), but cutaneous and other infections have been reported to occur in the apparently immunocompetent as well (182). The lung is a common site of involvement, affecting 43% of patients according to one review (196). As verified by molecular analysis, *N. farcinica* has been isolated from brain abscesses (122, 148, 190), blood (35, 122), cases of keratitis (57), and an infected cochlear implant (123). *N. farcinica* has also been isolated from the bronchoalveolar wash fluid of a cystic fibrosis patient (163). Isolates of this species were reported to make up 34 of 96 (35%) clinical isolates of *Nocardia* from Thailand (169) and 38 of 86 (44%) such isolates from Belgium (215).

Nocardia nova

N. nova was described by Tsukamura in 1982 and was distinguished from *N. asteroides* by several phenotypic tests (199) and confirmed to be a separate and distinct species by DNA-DNA hybridization (224). Wallace et al. found that 18% of 78 clinical isolates fell into their type III drug susceptibility pattern, characterized by susceptibility to ampicillin and erythromycin and resistance to carbenicillin (211). In a subsequent study of 223 clinical isolates, employing both biochemical and susceptibility testing procedures, 17% of the isolates, as well as the type strain of *N. nova*, had similar characteristics, including the type III drug pattern; these isolates were all then considered members of *N. nova* (210). Of the patients for whom clinical information was available, 35% were thought to have disseminated disease; organisms were obtained from many sites, including blood, lung, CNS, skin and soft tissue, joints, and cornea. An upper extremity sporotrichoid form of nocardiosis attributed to *N. nova* in a human immunodeficiency virus (HIV)-positive patient who sustained a thumb injury while working in a field has been reported (96). Hamad et al. reported the isolation of *N. nova* identified by 16S rRNA gene sequencing from a case of spondylodiscitis and psoas abscess (86).

Recent investigations have revealed that the organisms identified as *N. nova* by phenotypic testing, including antibiogram, as well as by the RFLP patterns obtainable from the *hsp65* gene, actually may belong to other species in addition to *N. nova*, including *N. africana*, *N. kruczakiae*, and *N. veterana* (43). These species can be distinguished from one another and from *N. nova* sensu stricto only by gene sequencing. Phylogenetic analysis using sequence data of the HSP and *secA1* genes consistently place these species in the same clade as *N. nova* sensu strict, indicating the close relationship among these species (P. S. Conville and F. G. Witebsky, unpublished data). Phylogenetic analysis of the 16S rRNA, HSP, and *secA1* genes also place *Nocardia aobensis* and *N. elegans* in the *N. nova* complex clade; no phenotypic characteristics of these two species have been examined to determine their similarity to other species in the complex. All species included in the *N. nova* complex (including *N. aobensis* and *N. elegans*) have been isolated from humans or implicated in human disease. Isolates identified only by phenotypic testing as belonging to one or another of these species are probably best reported as members of the "*N. nova* complex."

Nocardia otitidiscaviarum

The initial isolate of the species *N. otitidiscaviarum*, described by Snijders in 1924, was obtained from the infected middle ear of a guinea pig; for a time this species was known as *N. caviae* (78). This species is a relatively infrequent cause of human infection. Clark et al. reviewed 28 cases of cutaneous infection, including several of mycetoma, attributed to this species; many of those for which information was available were considered trauma related (37). There are a few reports of infection at other sites, including brain abscess (90), pyothorax (231), catheter-related infection (129), and disseminated infection (162, 164, 186). This species is relatively reliably identified on the basis of its decomposition reactions; it decomposes xanthine and hypoxanthine but not casein or tyrosine. In a recent molecular study of numerous clinical isolates, several different sequences were obtained from nine different strains that had been phenotypically identified as *N. otitidiscaviarum* (160). These results were interpreted as suggesting the presence of several different species within this group, but some of the results also suggested that individual isolates might contain two or more differing copies of the 16S rRNA gene.

Nocardia paucivorans

The species *N. paucivorans* was described by Yassin et al. in 2000 on the basis of a respiratory isolate from a patient with chronic lung disease (227). By 16S rRNA gene sequence, this organism showed 99.6% sequence similarity to *N. brevicatena*; results of DNA-DNA hybridization indicated that they were distinct species. *N. paucivorans* and *N. brevicatena*, along with isolates belonging to the unnamed group *N. asteroides* drug pattern II (211), are sometimes considered to belong to the "*N. paucivorans*/*N. brevicatena* complex" based on similar phenotypic characteristics and antibiograms (28).

N. paucivorans has been recovered from cerebrospinal fluid in a case of cerebral nocardiosis in an immunocompromised individual (58), an intracerebral abscess in an immunocompetent patient (112), and a mitral valve (24). Two of 86 (2.3%) clinical isolates from Belgium were identified as belonging to this species (215). Gray at al. reported that in a retrospective study of *Nocardia* isolates recovered from Australian patients over a 20-year period, 32 isolates were identified as *N. paucivorans* by 16S rRNA gene sequence. No indication of the identification criteria used for species assignment was presented. These isolates were recovered from a variety of sources including skin, lung, blood, brain, pleural fluid, and lymph node (81).

Nocardia pseudobrasiliensis

In 1995, Wallace et al. (209) reported on a subset of organisms that had been identified as *N. brasiliensis* that were sometimes isolated from cutaneous infections but were predominantly associated with noncutaneous invasive disease. This subset of isolates appeared to belong to another taxon, formally named *N. pseudobrasiliensis* the following year (180). Most infections have occurred in immunocompromised patients; cases have been reported from North and South America, Japan, and Australia (25, 101, 209).

Unlike true *N. brasiliensis* isolates, most *N. pseudobrasiliensis* isolates hydrolyze adenine, are susceptible to ciprofloxacin

and clarithromycin, and are resistant to minocycline. The two species also differ in their mycolic acid patterns and 16S rRNA, HSP, and *secA1* gene sequences. Most cases of infectious disease of a nonmycetomatous nature previously attributed to *N. brasiliensis* have probably been caused by this species (see "*Nocardia brasiliensis*" above).

Nocardia transvalensis and the N. transvalensis Complex

N. transvalensis was originally described in 1927 on the basis of an isolate from an African patient with a mycetoma (168). In 1997, Wilson et al. published a study of 58 clinical isolates from the United States and Australia that showed resistance to amikacin (220). Using biochemical and molecular methods, these authors were able to separate the isolates into four distinct groups. One group comprised 53% of the isolates studied, were all recovered from patients in the United States, and were similar to isolates classified as *N. asteroides* drug pattern type IV as defined by Wallace et al. (211). Isolates belonging to this group were later officially designated *Nocardia wallacei* (42) (see below). Another group (17% of isolates) included organisms similar to the type strain of *N. transvalensis*. Two additional groups, new taxon 1 (14% of isolates) and new taxon 2 (16% of isolates), were also defined. Australian isolates belonged to the *N. transvalensis* sensu stricto group and to new taxon 1. Isolates belonging to new taxon 1 have been given the species designation *N. blacklockiae* (42). Because of their similar phenotypic and molecular characteristics, Wilson proposed that these three species and the unnamed new taxon 2 be considered to belong to the "*N. transvalensis* complex."

There have been numerous reports in the literature describing the isolation of *N. transvalensis* from clinical specimens; many of these reports base the identification of the isolate on a small number of phenotypic tests. It is unclear if these reports represent accurate species assignments, given the similarity of related species as described above. McNeil et al. reported on 16 patients from whom isolates attributed to this species had been obtained (142). The isolates from 10 of the patients were considered clinically significant; the other isolates were considered colonizers or of uncertain significance. A variety of sites of infection were involved, some of the infections were disseminated, and several patients were known to be immunocompromised. There are a few other case reports of molecularly characterized disseminated infection attributed to the *N. transvalensis* complex, including a brain abscess in a cancer patient (230), brain and cutaneous infection in a heart transplant patient (131), and pulmonary infection and subcutaneous abscess in a patient with histiocytosis X (2). Three clinical isolates assigned to this species complex have been reported from Japan (102).

Nocardia veterana

N. veterana was first described on the basis of an isolate obtained from the bronchial lavage fluid of a patient with pulmonary lesions, but that isolate was thought not to be clinically significant (84). Subsequently, *N. veterana* has been implicated as the causative agent in cases of mycetomas (108), three patients with pulmonary disease (170), ascitic fluid infection in an HIV patient (70), and bloodstream infection in a cancer patient (4). In a report of three additional clinical isolates, two of which were shown to have been causative agents of pulmonary disease, it was noted that the isolates had an antimicrobial susceptibility pattern essentially identical to the patterns of *N. africana* and *N. nova* (44), demonstrating that species identification could not be definitively established by susceptibility testing alone. It was also noted that the isolates of this species that were studied showed 16S rRNA gene similarities to the type strains of *N. africana* and *N. nova* of 99.0 and 97.7%, respectively. *N. veterana* is one of the species included in the "*N. nova* complex" (see "*Nocardia nova*" above). HSP, *secA1*, and 16S rRNA gene sequencing place *N. veterana* in a clade with other members of the complex.

N. wallacei

Officially described in 2008, *N. wallacei* is the most commonly isolated member of the *N. transvalensis* complex (42). 16S rRNA, HSP, and *secA1* gene sequencing showed ≥99.8% sequence similarity among five clinical isolates obtained from sputum samples; one of these was also recovered from pleural fluid. This species was initially designated as *N. asteroides* drug pattern IV by Wallace et al. and comprised 5% of 78 isolates identified as "*N. asteroides*" by phenotypic methods but unique in their resistance to amikacin (211).

Nocardiopsis

Nearly all of the very few infections attributed to organisms in the genus *Nocardiopsis* have been attributed to *N. dassonvillei*. In a letter to the editor regarding a case of actinomycetoma attributed to this species, it was stated that *N. dassonvillei* was "regularly encountered" at the Centers for Disease Control and Prevention, with 21 isolates having been identified from 1981 through 1986; no clinical details were provided (1). In the case of a blood isolate, a variety of methods, including 16S rRNA gene sequencing, was used to identify the isolate; the same report provided references to a number of other cases of infection, including mycetomas and cutaneous infections, attributed to this species (11).

Rhodococcus

The most commonly isolated pathogen in the genus *Rhodococcus* is *Rhodococcus equi*. While other species have occasionally been reported to cause disease, in most but not all of these reports, gene sequencing was not used, and it is impossible to obtain reliable species-level identifications without this technique (13, 74). There is some evidence that *R. equi* itself may be a complex of several different species (139). Infections caused by *R. equi* have been the subject of several reviews (6, 52, 110, 197). The organism has long been known as a significant pulmonary pathogen in horses (hence the species name) (171). The initial report of human disease caused by the organism (reported as *Corynebacterium equi*) involved a patient on high-dose steroids with a pulmonary abscess; he had worked briefly in stockyards contaminated with animal feces shortly before the onset of his illness (71). Herbivore manure provides an ideal growth medium for the organism, and inhalation of the organism is presumed to be the major mode of infection in horses (171) and is probably also the principal mechanism for human infections. Direct inoculation and oral ingestion are other possible routes of infection (216). Most patients who develop *R. equi* infection are immunocompromised, and at least until recently, approximately two-thirds of infected patients were also HIV infected (216). Essentially any body site can be involved, but the lung is a site of involvement in approximately 80% of immunocompromised patients and at least 40% of immunocompetent patients. Bacteremia has been reported in >80% of immunocompromised patients and approximately 30% of immunocompetent patients (216). Pulmonary

cavitation is a frequent finding. Malacoplakia, an aggregation of histiocytes containing concentrically layered basophilic structures known as Michaelis-Gutmann bodies, has been noted as a histopathologic finding in several studies (82, 197). Two virulence-associated antigens (VapA and VapB) encoded by plasmids have been identified. Isolates producing the VapA antigen are the predominant, possibly the sole, cause of disease in horses, but isolates producing the VapA antigen, the VapB antigen, or neither antigen have been isolated from human cases of infection (156). A combination of antimicrobials is generally used for the treatment of infections. Agents used include aminoglycosides, erythromycin, imipenem, quinolones, rifampin, and vancomycin. Linezolid may also be efficacious (216); in an in vitro study of 102 *R. equi* isolates obtained from humans and animals, the linezolid MIC ranged from 0.5 to 2.0 μg/ml (23). Some rifampin-resistant strains with *rpoB* gene mutations have been reported (7). Without careful assessment, *R. equi* isolates can easily be mistaken for coryneform bacteria and dismissed as insignificant (Fig. 2H). A recent report describes two patients who died of overwhelming *R. equi* infection; for both patients, isolates from multiple positive blood cultures were initially misidentified as a *Corynebacterium* species (201).

Segniliparus

Although the two species that make up this genus (*S. rotundus* and *S. rugosus*) were originally recovered from clinical material, no information was provided concerning the significance of these isolates except that they were from "nonsterile human sources" (31). Published reports of the recovery of *S. rugosus* seem to indicate the predilection of this organism for patients with cystic fibrosis. A report of the recovery of *S. rugosus* from the bronchoalveolar lavage fluid or induced sputum of three cystic fibrosis patients emphasized the microscopic and colonial similarities of this species with those of rapidly growing mycobacteria (Fig. 2M and 3M and N). All 3 isolates were initially identified phenotypically as either *Mycobacterium abscessus* or *Mycobacterium chelonae*; sequence analysis of the first 500 bases of the 16S rRNA gene of two of the isolates (from each of two siblings) showed 100% sequence similarity to the type strain of *S. rugosus* (32). Drug susceptibility testing on these isolates was problematic because of insufficient growth in cation-adjusted Mueller-Hinton broth; Middlebrook 7H9 broth was necessary to achieve adequate growth. Using breakpoints recommended for *Nocardia* and for rapidly growing mycobacteria (38), results indicated that the *S. rugosus* isolates were susceptible to imipenem, rifabutin, sulfamethoxazole, and trimethoprim-sulfamethoxazole and resistant or intermediate to amikacin, amoxicillin-clavulanate, ceftriaxone, ciprofloxacin, clarithromycin, linezolid, minocycline, and tobramycin. Using bacterial breakpoints, the isolates were susceptible to moxifloxacin. In a subsequent report from Australia, *S. rugosus* was isolated from the mycobacterial culture of sputum from a cystic fibrosis patient; the sputum had undergone a standard mycobacterial decontamination process. PCR of a region of the 16S rRNA gene used to identify mycobacteria was negative, but sequence analysis of a 1,250-bp region of the 16S rRNA gene showed 100% similarity to the type strain of *S. rugosus* (87).

Streptomyces

The most common type of infection attributed to species in the genus *Streptomyces* is mycetoma (see "*Actinomadura*" above), and the most commonly mentioned etiologic agent is *Streptomyces somaliensis*, although in many reports the identification procedures employed could not have ensured that other species were not involved. There are a few reports implicating other species in the genus as occasional pathogens. In case reports of bacteremias attributed to *Streptomyces bikiniensis* (150) and *Streptomyces thermovulgaris* (59), molecular methods were used in identifying the isolates, and such methods were described in detail in a case report of a mycetoma attributed to *Streptomyces albus* (136). While the majority of isolates from nonmycetomatous lesions probably represent either contamination or colonization, these organisms are capable of occasionally causing disease other than mycetoma. Recently, six cases of invasive *Streptomyces* infections have been reported, along with a literature review of such infections (107). Because of the huge number of validly described species of *Streptomyces* and the lack of information about clinical significance of many of these species, identification to the genus level is probably sufficient in most cases. In a study of the susceptibility of 92 *Streptomyces* species from clinical specimens, 100% of those tested were found to be susceptible to amikacin and linezolid, 77% to minocycline, 67% to imipenem, and 51% to clarithromycin and amoxicillin-clavulanate (178).

Tsukamurella

Tsukamurella infections have been most commonly reported in connection with a foreign body, such as an intravenous catheter (22), but have also been reported even in apparently immunologically normal patients in the absence of any foreign body (188). The literature on catheter-related infections caused by *Tsukamurella* species has recently been reviewed in connection with two additional reports of such infection (22); several other of the relatively few infections reportedly caused by *Tsukamurella* species are also briefly mentioned in that review. *Rhodococcus aurantiacus* ATCC 25938 (the initial type strain of the species), which has had a convoluted taxonomic history, has been placed in the species *T. paurometabola* (41). In the older literature, there are a few reports of infection attributed to *R. aurantiacus*, such as pulmonary infection, meningitis, peritonitis, and subcutaneous abscesses (200). Organisms isolated from clinical material have generally been found to resemble strain ATCC 25938. An outbreak of pseudoinfection (8) was also attributed to *T. paurometabola*.

Williamsia

The first clinical isolate of the genus *Williamsia* was recovered from a protected bronchial brush sample of a patient with bilateral alveolar infiltrates following aortic valve replacement. Gram stain of the sample showed numerous gram-positive rods, and culture of the fluid grew >1,000 CFU/ml of an organism identified by 16S rRNA gene sequencing as *Williamsia muralis* (99.9% sequence similarity). Using breakpoints established for *Nocardia* spp., susceptibility testing of the *W. muralis* isolate indicated that the isolate was susceptible to amoxicillin-clavulanate, cefotaxime, imipenem, ciprofloxacin, tobramycin, gentamicin, and trimethoprim-sulfamethoxazole (55). The recovery of *W. muralis* was also reported from a case of endophthalmitis. The isolate showed only 98.4% 16S rRNA gene similarity, but 100% DNA-DNA hybridization, with the type strain of *W. muralis* (153). Two isolates of *W. deligens* have been reported from human blood, but no clinical information was provided (226).

Other Genera

Some other genera of aerobic actinomycetes do have roles in human diseases but are unlikely to be encountered in the clinical laboratory. Organisms in three genera of thermophilic aerobic actinomycetes, *Saccharomonospora*, *Saccharopolyspora*, and *Thermoactinomyces*, have been implicated in the etiology of hypersensitivity pneumonitis. Spores of these organisms may be encountered when performing air sampling; molecular methods are helpful for species-level identification when needed (89, 222).

COLLECTION, TRANSPORT, AND STORAGE

In temperate climates, the respiratory tract is the most frequent portal of entry for the aerobic actinomycetes and therefore the primary site of nocardial infections in the immunocompromised host. Sputum is the most easily obtained pulmonary specimen, and examination of several fresh early-morning samples collected on separate days (213) may maximize the chances of organism recovery; isolation of an aerobic actinomycete from multiple samples may help to establish the clinical significance of the isolated organism (73, 117). *Nocardia* species may, however, be difficult to recover from sputum even in documented cases of pulmonary infection (158), either because of low numbers of organisms present in the sample or because contaminating bacteria in the sample may overgrow the more slowly growing aerobic actinomycetes. More invasive procedures, such as bronchoalveolar lavage or fine needle or open lung biopsy, may be required to obtain a definitive diagnosis (158). These more invasive procedures may be necessary for diagnosis of as many as 44% of primary pulmonary infections (68); macrophage-rich samples may be necessary to maximize recovery of organisms such as rhodococci, which tend to localize within these cells (52).

Exudates from abscesses or mycetomas should be delivered to the laboratory in a sterile container for macroscopic and microscopic examination for characteristic granules and for smear and culture. In the case of disseminated cutaneous lesions or small lesions secondary to trauma, a skin biopsy can be useful. The use of swabs is not recommended, as fibers can make smear interpretation difficult (213). To optimize isolation of *Dermatophilus*, scabs or crusty lesions should be removed and soaked in sterile distilled water, and the fluid should be inoculated onto blood agar plates (232).

In immunocompromised patients, the aerobic actinomycetes, especially *Nocardia*, can disseminate to almost any organ. A biopsy sample or aspirate, when obtainable, may be the best specimen to evaluate for the presence of such organisms. Normally sterile body fluids should be collected in a sterile container and sent immediately to the laboratory. *Nocardia* isolates are infrequently recovered from cerebrospinal fluid, even if numerous brain lesions are present, because the organisms may be confined to the brain abscess itself. Blood should be inoculated directly into blood culture media; many commercially available blood culture systems as well as lysis centrifugation methodologies have been shown to support the growth of *Nocardia* species. Various aerobic actinomycetes have been implicated as the cause of catheter-related bacteremia; potentially infected catheter tips should be transported to the laboratory in a sterile container and cultured by appropriate methods.

In all cases where infection with an aerobic actinomycete is suspected, it is of utmost importance that the laboratory be notified of the suspected diagnosis. This will ensure that samples will receive appropriate handling, that the correct direct smears will be prepared, and that the sample will be inoculated onto the appropriate media and incubated for an extended period of time (a minimum of 2 weeks, preferably for up to 3 weeks) at the appropriate temperature.

All samples should be transported promptly to the laboratory following the specimen collection and handling procedures outlined in chapter 16.

DIRECT EXAMINATION

Microscopy

Careful microscopic examination of clinical specimens suspected of containing aerobic actinomycetes is extremely important. The observation of organisms characteristic of *Nocardia* and other aerobic actinomycetes should alert laboratory personnel to inoculate appropriate media and to extend incubation at the appropriate temperature. In addition, the detection of organisms directly in the patient specimen may assist in the interpretation of culture results; smears of such specimens may show more diagnostic morphologies of organisms than smears from colonial growth.

Smears can be made directly from sputum, drainages, and aspirates; however, liquid specimens such as bronchoalveolar lavage or normally sterile body fluids that are not excessively cellular should be concentrated before smear preparation and medium inoculation. For example, a 5-ml aliquot of the sample can be centrifuged for 10 minutes at $2,800 \times g$ and the pellet can be used for smears and medium inoculation. Alternatively, smears can be prepared using a cytocentrifuge. For tissue samples, smears can be made from ground material and from touch preps. Two important stains that should be used in the clinical laboratory for direct samples are the Gram stain and the modified acid-fast stain. Histopathologic examination of fixed tissue by use of special stains (including Fite stain and Grocott-Gomori methenamine silver stain) may also reveal the presence of organisms belonging to these genera (221).

Gram stain morphologies of the aerobic actinomycetes vary by genus; organisms appear as gram-positive rods ranging in shape from coccoid to bacillary. Filamentous and branching forms may be present, depending on the species involved and the stage of growth in infected tissues (Fig. 3). See Table 1 for a summary of the microscopic morphologies of the aerobic actinomycetes.

The modified acid-fast stain used on direct specimens may more accurately reflect the true partially acid-fast nature of the organisms than do modified acid-fast stains prepared from colonial growth. The modified acid-fast stain uses a weaker decolorizer (1% H_2SO_4) than does the mycobacterial stain (3% HCl). See chapters 17 and 28 for details on reagent preparation and staining methodology. Because of the difficulty of standardizing this technique, it is imperative that positive and negative controls be run simultaneously with patient smears. The control slides can be made from growing suspensions of *Streptomyces* species (negative control) and *Nocardia* species (positive control). Smears should be evaluated by experienced laboratory personnel, and the quality of the stain itself should be evaluated before results are reported. *Gordonia, Nocardia, Rhodococcus,* and *Tsukamurella* (and possibly *Dietzia*) are known to be partially acid-fast with this stain; *Segniliparus* is strongly acid-fast.

Careful attention should be paid to the cellular material present in the sample (Fig. 3K and L). *Nocardia* is frequently seen in association with polymorphonuclear leukocytes (28). Phagocytized gram-positive or acid-fast organisms can sometimes be seen within macrophages and mononuclear cells; in the modified acid-fast smear these may appear as "beaded" cells with strongly acid-fast granules within nonacid-fast or weakly acid-fast rods (52, 157).

In cases of suspected actinomycetoma, aspirated material should be examined grossly for the presence of granules by spreading the sample in a sterile petri dish. Granules found should be washed and crushed. Smears should be prepared from the crushed material, and appropriate media should be inoculated. Granules are most often seen in infections caused by *N. brasiliensis* or *Actinomyces* species but can also be seen in infections caused by other species of *Nocardia* (28).

Nucleic Acid Detection

Several authors have reported the use of molecular methodologies for the detection of *Nocardia* directly from clinical specimens. Targets include the 65-kDa HSP gene (172), the 16S rRNA gene (53, 208), and the *secA1* gene (G. Fahle, personal communication). These techniques have the potential to provide rapid diagnosis of nocardiosis from samples exhibiting bacterial morphologies suggestive of this genus. Further assessment of these techniques will be needed to assess their clinical utility.

R. equi chromosomal DNA and *vapA* plasmid DNA (a gene that codes for, and mediates expression of, a virulence-associated protein on the cell wall surface) have been directly detected from tracheal wash fluid and other specimens of potentially infected foals. PCR with amplicon detection by gel electrophoresis (185) and real-time PCR (88) have been shown to be highly specific and more sensitive than culture or serologic testing for the diagnosis of *R. equi* infection.

ISOLATION PROCEDURES

Blood agar, chocolate agar, brain heart infusion agar, Sabouraud dextrose agar, and Lowenstein-Jensen medium support the growth of most aerobic actinomycetes; *Dermatophilus congolensis* may not grow on Sabouraud dextrose agar or Lowenstein-Jensen medium (232). Buffered charcoal yeast extract agar (BCYE) is particularly useful for the recovery of *Nocardia* species. Specimens from sterile sites or concentrated sterile body fluids can be inoculated directly onto these media. Specimens from respiratory sites, skin, and other potentially contaminated sites, such as mycetomas, should additionally be inoculated onto selective media, such as modified Thayer-Martin agar (152) and selective BCYE (containing polymyxin B, anisomycin, and either vancomycin or cefamandole) (206). Sabouraud agar with added chloramphenicol may not be useful, as it may also suppress the growth of some *Nocardia* species (85). A specialized medium for the recovery of *R. equi* using a Mueller-Hinton agar-based medium with added ceftazidime and novobiocin has been described (207).

Cultures for aerobic actinomycetes should be handled as fungal cultures, thus ensuring that the cultures will be incubated and regularly examined over an extended period. Two BCYE plates (for samples from sterile sites) or selective BCYE plates (for respiratory or other potentially contaminated sites) should be inoculated. One BCYE or selective BCYE plate should be incubated at 30°C and the other at 35°C, both in ambient air. It should be noted, however, that *Streptomyces* species may show best growth at 25°C and that *Dermatophilus congolensis* grows better and shows enhanced production of aerial hyphae in increased CO_2 (232). For all cultures, plates should be held for a minimum of 2 weeks, preferably for up to 3 weeks, and should be sealed to prevent dehydration.

A low-pH decontamination procedure has been successfully used for pretreatment of heavily contaminated specimens suspected of harboring *Nocardia* species. The sample is diluted 1:10 in 0.2 M HCl–0.2 M KCl at pH 2.2, mixed, and allowed to stand for 3 to 5 minutes, after which it is inoculated onto selective and nonselective media (20, 206). Murray et al. reported a drop in viability of *Nocardia* species after 30-min exposures to *N*-acetyl-L-cysteine (NALC), NaOH-NALC, or Zephiran-trisodium phosphate (151). The key to improved recovery of *Nocardia* from NaOH-NALC-treated specimens may be a shorter exposure to the decontaminating reagents (15 min), as is in fact also recommended for recovery of mycobacteria (111).

Aerobic actinomycetes have been recovered from blood using a variety of commercially available blood culture systems, including conventional 2-bottle systems, biphasic bottles, systems using radiometric and nonradiometric detection, and lysis-centrifugation systems. Using various blood culture systems, aerobic actinomycetes have been recovered after 3 to 19 days of incubation, which in some cases included the incubation times of terminal subcultures (150, 205). Studies employing newer blood culture systems have resulted in recommendations that extended incubation is no longer necessary (9); however, such studies have not established that such shorter incubation would generally be adequate for the isolation of aerobic actinomycetes. If the possibility of bacteremia with a member of one of these genera is anticipated, it would be advisable to perform fungal blood cultures (for the expanded incubation period, at least 3 weeks) or to perform terminal subcultures if the incubation period of routine blood cultures cannot be extended.

Cultures from all sources should be examined daily for the first week of incubation and then weekly thereafter, preferably using a dissecting microscope, which will allow detection of tiny colonies. Such microscopic examination is particularly important for specimens that contain contaminating flora, as an aerobic actinomycete can be quickly overgrown by more rapidly growing organisms. Care should also be exercised when Lowenstein-Jensen or Middlebrook media are examined for mycobacteria or when BCYE plates are examined for *Legionella* species, as *Nocardia* and other aerobic actinomycetes can grow on these media.

IDENTIFICATION

Microscopic Morphology

Evaluation of Gram stain morphology of a suspected aerobic actinomycete should be the initial step in organism identification, as microscopic morphology can vary among the genera (Table 1 and Fig. 3). A sufficient number of fields should be reviewed to allow determination of the most prevalent morphology and to detect the sometimes-rare branching forms. Care should be taken not to confuse perpendicular aligning of the organisms with true branching. Smears made from colonial growth of filamentous isolates may fragment and appear as bacillary or coccoid forms (28).

A properly prepared and carefully interpreted modified acid-fast smear can assist in the preliminary identification of the organism (Fig. 3F, G, I, J, and L). Quality control slides should be stained along with stains of colonies from cultures. With the modified acid-fast stain, the background should be blue; slides that have a pink background may be inadequately decolorized and should be repeated. The smear should be scanned for areas where individual cells can be seen or areas where single layers of cells allow clear differentiation of cell borders. The acid-fast reaction of tightly packed clumps of organisms may not represent the true partially acid-fast nature of the cells; be wary of large clumps of cells which all appear to be acid-fast positive. Acid-fast cells will be clearly red; cells that stain purple or light pink may or may not be truly acid-fast. A stain that shows an unambiguous acid-fast positive reaction may frequently show only a few clearly red cells, with a majority of blue cells. Frequently, only the beads appear acid-fast positive. If modified acid-fast stain results are ambiguous, transfer of the organism to a lipid-rich medium, such as Lowenstein-Jensen medium or Middlebrook 7H11 agar, and repeat staining may give a more clear-cut stain result. Acid-fastness may become more evident as colonies age; the acid-fast reaction has been reported to be most reliable when performed from colonies after 1 to 4 weeks of growth (202). Occasionally, coccoid forms of *Streptomyces* may appear partially acid-fast; hyphae, however, are acid-fast negative. Because of the difficulties of interpretation of the modified acid-fast smear, results of this stain should be considered preliminary and must be used only in conjunction with results from other tests.

Slide Cultures

Slide cultures may be used to evaluate the microscopic morphology of actively growing cultures and are probably the best way to evaluate the morphology of some genera, such as *Amycolata*, *Amycolatopsis*, and *Nocardiopsis*. Small blocks of a minimal agar (such as tap water agar) are inoculated on the side with the organism of interest, and a coverslip is placed on the top of the block. The slide culture is incubated in a humid environment at 25°C for 2 to 3 weeks and examined regularly for the characteristic features of the various genera. Vegetative mycelia (also called substrate hyphae) that grow beneath the surface of the agar and aerial hyphae show various morphologies and degrees of branching based on the organism being tested (26, 93). Differences among the genera of aerobic actinomycetes in the growth characteristics seen on slide culture may be subtle; experience in recognizing these morphologic differences is required for correct interpretation of these tests.

Colonial Morphology

The colonial appearance of members of the aerobic actinomycetes is extremely variable among genera and even between isolates of the same species (Fig. 2). Environmental factors such as growth medium, incubation temperature, air circulation, presence of CO_2, and age of culture can affect the size and consistency of the colonies and the production of aerial hyphae (15). Some species produce a diffusible pigment that can vary from strain to strain. See Table 1 for information on specific colonial morphologies.

Aerial Hyphae

Aerial hyphae project away from the surface of the colony into the air but may not be apparent until 7 to 14 days for some species that form such hyphae. *Nocardia* and *Streptomyces* usually produce abundant aerial hyphae that give the colonies their characteristic powdery or velvety appearance (Fig. 2C, E, and L); rare strains of *Nocardia* produce sparse or no aerial hyphae (Fig. 2D and G). Of the genera that are partially acid-fast, only *Nocardia* species regularly produce aerial hyphae. The presence of spores and their relative number and arrangement on the aerial hyphae can also give some clue to genus identification (93).

Genus Assignment

To determine the genus of an unknown isolate, observation of microscopic and colonial morphology is especially important

(Table 1 and Fig. 2 and 3). In assessing the characteristics of colonial growth, the presence or absence of aerial hyphae should be determined. *Nocardia* and *Streptomyces* generally produce aerial hyphae, with other less commonly isolated genera also showing this morphologic trait (Table 1). Positive results of a carefully prepared and interpreted modified acid-fast smear combined with the presence of aerial hyphae help to distinguish *Nocardia* from the other genera.

The lysozyme test may also assist in initial genus assignment. Lysozyme catalyzes the hydrolysis of certain polysaccharides in the cell wall, resulting in a weakening of the cell wall (15). *Nocardia* and *Tsukamurella* (both modified acid-fast-positive organisms) are resistant to lysozyme and show good growth in lysozyme broth; of these, only *Nocardia* species show aerial hyphae. *Gordonia* shows variable growth in lysozyme broth but does not show aerial hyphae (15). Berd recommends the use of a very small inoculum into glycerol broth with 0.005% lysozyme (see chapter 17), and a second similarly inoculated glycerol broth without lysozyme as a control. After 4 weeks of incubation, results are interpreted by comparing organism growth in the broths with and without lysozyme. All *Nocardia* isolates in one study (Brown et al., *Abstr. 97th Gen. Meet. Am. Soc. Microbiol.*, abstr. C-65, p. 131, 1997) were resistant to lysozyme, except for 10 lysozyme-susceptible isolates that belonged to the *N. brevicatena* complex.

Laurent et al. describe a PCR-based method that allows differentiation of members of the genus *Nocardia* from other genera of aerobic actinomycetes (127). It is not known if this method allows discrimination of newly described *Nocardia* species.

Species Assignment

Limitations

Given the increasing number of species of aerobic actinomycetes, the use of phenotypic or biochemical tests to obtain exact species or even genus-level identification has become impossible. In addition, phenotypic attributes may be unstable based on environmental and procedural variation. Among the *Nocardia*, most species are nonreactive in most commercially available biochemicals, precluding the definitive identification of these isolates. For laboratories without molecular capabilities, assignment to the genus level should be attempted.

When a precise identification is required for a significant patient isolate, molecular testing is strongly recommended.

Some new species have been described based on a single isolate; such species present problems for laboratories attempting to make identification decisions phenotypically, as characteristics described may not reflect the typical reactions of the species that would be determined if more isolates were analyzed (98).

Biochemicals

Because of the increasing number of described species and the low discrimination power and small number of commercially available phenotypic tests, biochemical testing is not recommended for definitive identification of these organisms. For laboratories without molecular capabilities, the use of antibiotic susceptibility patterns and basic biochemical results may provide preliminary identifications of frequently isolated *Nocardia* species or complexes obtained from clinical specimens. Most (but not all) of the isolates of a given species show the results listed in Table 8. When biochemical tests are performed, it is extremely important to include appropriate positive and negative controls to ensure that tests are inoculated, incubated, and interpreted correctly. See "Evaluation, Interpretation, and Reporting of Results" below for recommendations on reporting preliminary identifications obtained using these methods.

The biochemical tests that may be useful for the preliminary identification of *Nocardia* species include arylsulfatase; acid production from carbohydrates; utilization of carbohydrates or other compounds as sole carbon sources; hydrolysis of acetamide, esculin, gelatin, and urease; nitrate reduction; decomposition of adenine, xanthine, hypoxanthine, and casein; and temperature studies. See reference 48 for a discussion of the action and performance of these tests.

Susceptibility Testing

For *Nocardia* species, basic biochemical testing may be paired with susceptibility testing to achieve preliminary identifications. Some species or species complexes have predictable susceptibility patterns that may assist in isolate characterization (28) (Table 7). These patterns should not be used exclusively as identification techniques, as many newly described species have not been tested for their antibiotic susceptibilities.

TABLE 8 Phenotypic characteristics of commonly isolated *Nocardia* species known to cause human disease[a]

| Species | Growth at 45°C | Production of: | | | Hydrolysis of: | | | | | | Utilization of: | | | |
		Arylsulfatase (14 days)	Nitrate reductase	Urease	Adenine	Casein	Esculin	Hypoxanthine	Tyrosine	Xanthine	Acetamide[b]	Citrate[c]	L-Rhamnose[c]	D-Sorbitol[c]
N. abscessus	−	−	+	+	−	−	−	−	−	−	−	+	−	−
N. brasiliensis	−	−	+	+	−	+	+	+	+	−	−	+	−	−
N. cyriacigeorgica	−	NA	+	−	−	−	−	−	−	−	+	−	−	−
N. farcinica[d]	−	−	−	+	−	−	−	−	+	−	+	−	+	−
N. nova	−	+	+	+	−	−	−	−	−	−	−	−	−	−
N. otitidiscaviarum	V	NA	−	+	−	−	+	+	−	−	−	−	−	−
N. pseudobrasiliensis	−	−	−	+	+	+	+	−	+	−	NA	+	−	−
N. wallacei	+	−	NA	+	−	−	+	+	−	−	−	+	−	−

[a]Adapted from reference 48. Symbols and abbreviations: −, negative; +, positive; NA, not available; V, variable; W, weak.
[b]Utilization as sole source of carbon and nitrogen.
[c]Utilization as sole source of carbon.
[d]*N. farcinica* may show opacification of Middlebrook 7H10 or 7H11 agar within 2 to 10 days of incubation at 28 or 35°C (62).

Test Systems

Several studies investigating the use of commercial panels for the identification of *Nocardia* and other aerobic actinomycetes have been published. Test systems studied include the API Zym panels (bioMérieux, Durham, NC) (19), Rapid Anaerobe ID and Haemophilus/Neisseria ID panels (Siemens Healthcare Diagnostics, Deerfield, IL) (16), the API (Rapid) Coryne panel (with an extended database) (bioMérieux) (65), and the RapID CB Plus System (Remel, Lenexa, KS) (64). To date, there is insufficient evidence to establish the utility of any of these tests for the identification of the increasing number of described species.

Cell Wall and Cell Membrane Analysis

Analysis of the cell wall chemistry of the aerobic actinomycetes can aid in the identification of isolates to the genus level (Table 2). While these organisms have distinct cell walls that are characteristic for each genus, methodologies for the investigation of these chemical structures are generally only available in research or reference laboratories. Cell wall analysis is not useful for species level identification.

Analysis of whole-cell hydrolysates has been used to identify various forms of diaminopimelic acid (DAP) and sugars present in the peptidoglycan layer of the cell walls. The form of DAP combined with the type of sugars present in the cell wall allows classification of the various genera into cell wall types (54, 193) (Table 2).

Members of the aerobic actinomycetes and related genera contain elevated levels of cell wall lipids; analysis of the variations in chain length, degree of saturation, and the presence of various functional groups on cell wall lipids has been evaluated for identification to the genus or species level (204). McNabb et al. used gas-liquid chromatography and the Microbial Identification System (MIDI, Inc., Newark, DE) to analyze the fatty acids of aerobic actinomycetes. Their results showed distinct clustering of the genera included in the aerobic actinomycetes into two groups based on the presence or absence of branching of the cell wall fatty acids (140).

Mycolic acids, high-molecular-weight fatty acids with an α-branched, β-hydroxy structure are present in the cell walls of some genera of aerobic actinomycetes. Mycolic acids are thought to contribute to the staining characteristics and pathogenicity of these organisms (10). The aerobic actinomycetes containing mycolic acids can be differentiated based on the number of carbon atoms of their constituent mycolic acids (Table 2). It should be noted that the number of carbon atoms making up the mycolic acids of some genera varies from one report to another.

Menaquinones, the type of isoprenoid quinone present in the cell membranes of the aerobic actinomycetes, vary among genera in the number of isoprene units and in the degree of unsaturation of the C_3 isoprenyl side chain (40, 225) (Table 2). Menaquinone analysis has been particularly useful for distinguishing *Nocardia* species from other mycolic acid-containing aerobic actinomycetes (Table 2).

Molecular Identification

Molecular techniques, particularly gene sequencing, are currently the only methods that can provide definitive identification of most isolates of aerobic actinomycetes. These methods have the added benefit of providing identifications in a fraction of the time needed for biochemical tests.

PCR with Amplicon Detection

The use of PCR and amplicon detection by gel electrophoresis, with genus- or species-specific primers, enables the identification of aerobic actinomycetes that have unique gene regions. Regions of the 16S rRNA gene have been targeted for the genus-level identification of *Nocardia* (127), *Pseudonocardia* and *Saccharopolyspora* (149), *Gordonia* (187), and *Nocardiopsis* (181). PCR assays of the 16S rRNA gene have also been used for the species-level identification of *Rhodococcus* spp. (12). Other gene targets for PCR and gel analysis include the *choE* gene for *Rhodococcus* (121) and a putative nonribosomal peptide synthetase gene for *N. farcinica* (27).

PCR with REA

PCR paired with restriction endonuclease analysis (REA) has been used for the identification of commonly isolated *Nocardia* species. The procedure takes advantage of the presence of restriction endonuclease recognition sites within the variable regions of an organism's gene sequence (48). With REA of a portion of the HSP gene, Steingrube et al. were able to differentiate among 12 taxonomic groups of *Nocardia*, in addition to species of *Actinomadura*, *Gordonia*, *Rhodococcus*, *Streptomyces*, and *Tsukamurella* (194). In 2000, an REA technique utilizing a portion of the 16S rRNA gene allowing differentiation of 10 species of *Nocardia* was described (45). This study compared REA results for both the HSP and 16S rRNA genes and found that identification discrepancies between the two methods assisted in the recognition of previously undescribed species.

Recently, Rodríguez-Nava et al. challenged the HSP REA procedure of Steingrube with 44 species of *Nocardia* (some currently recognized human pathogens were not tested) and, using in silico analysis, determined that this technique is no longer reliable for the identification of the expanding number of described *Nocardia* species. Their results showed that while some species did give unique RFLP patterns, many species, including the most commonly isolated species from clinical specimens, fell into clusters that could not be discriminated from one another. In silico analysis of over 550 additional restriction endonucleases, tested singly and in combination, showed that no combination of endonucleases was able to discriminate among all the species of *Nocardia* (177).

Because of the increasing number of recognized *Nocardia* species, and because these REA methodologies are only able to detect alterations within the relatively short restriction endonuclease recognition sequence, the usefulness of these techniques is limited to the identification of only a few species. Recent reports of *Nocardia* isolates with multiple differing copies of the 16S rRNA gene indicate that REAs of this gene in such organisms may result in excess RFLP bands that in total exceed the size of the original PCR product (47). Identification of these isolates would be impossible with this technique. If a laboratory decides to use REA of any gene as an identification tool, the RFLP patterns for the specific gene and endonuclease combinations for each newly described species must be determined (experimentally or by in silico analysis) to prevent misidentifications. This will ensure that the pattern obtained from a newly described species is different from that obtained from all other species. For information on which species can be presumptively identified using REA of the HSP gene, see the report by Rodríguez-Nava et al. (177). Presumptive identification of *N. abscessus*, *N. brasiliensis*, *N. cyriacigeorgica*, and *N. otitidiscaviarum* can be achieved using REA of the 16S rRNA gene; see the previous edition of the *Manual of Clinical Microbiology* (48) for information on this technique.

In addition to its use for the identification of *Nocardia* species, REA has been used for differentiation among numerous genera of aerobic actinomycetes and identification of some species of thermophilic actinomycetes (51, 89). It is likely that the usefulness of these procedures, too, will be limited as the number of recognized species within these genera increases.

Gene Sequencing

Gene sequencing has become a powerful and, currently, a necessary tool for the identification of isolates within this complex group of organisms. Sequence analysis of the 16S rRNA gene has been used for the species-level identification of members of nearly all genera of the aerobic actinomycetes (5, 11, 95, 105, 109, 136, 155, 174, 179, 222).

Several genes have been shown to discriminate adequately among *Nocardia* species. By far, the most sequence information is available for the 16S rRNA gene sequences of members of this genus. See chapter 15 for a discussion of the phylogenetic attributes of this gene. The presence of a variable sequence region, located near the 5′ terminus of the gene (45), has made partial 16S rRNA sequencing of a 500-bp region of the gene a useful method for the identification of many *Nocardia* species. Cloud et al. (39) compared identifications obtained with the MicroSeq 500 system (Applied BioSystems, Foster City, CA) with results obtained using phenotypic identifications and with sequencing results from a 999-bp region of the same gene. The 500-bp-based identification of 94 clinical isolates representing 10 species showed 72% agreement with identification obtained by phenotypic methods and 90% agreement with those obtained by sequencing a larger portion of the gene. Patel et al. (160) used the MicroSeq 500 system to determine the 16S rRNA gene sequences of 28 reference strains and 71 clinical isolates and found significant sequence heterogeneity among isolates identified as *N. asteroides* drug pattern type II, *N. nova*, *N. otitidiscaviarum*, and *N. transvalensis*, indicating that these species may actually be species complexes. Species complexes of *N. nova* and *N. transvalensis* have been described (see above) (42, 43, 220). At present, the MicroSeq 500 system is capable of distinguishing among the more commonly isolated *Nocardia* species. However, as the number of described species increases, the number of species that can be unambiguously identified using 500-bp sequences will almost inevitably decrease. The MicroSeq method was also shown to be useful for the identification of *Gordonia*, *Rhodococcus*, *Streptomyces*, and *Tsukamurella* isolates to the genus level (160).

Sequencing a larger region of the 16S rRNA gene is necessary for the separation of some species that have identical or nearly identical sequences within the 500-bp region (for example, *N. abscessus*, *N. asiatica*, and *N. arthritidis*; *N. elegans* and *N. veterana*; and *N. higoensis* and *N. shimofusensis*). These species are clearly distinguished with sequence analysis of 1,300 bases.

There is no consensus on how similar 16S rRNA gene sequences must be to consider isolates of *Nocardia* to belong to the same species. It is well known that the interspecies heterogeneity of closely related *Nocardia* species can be quite low, making unambiguous identification of some isolates difficult, if not impossible. The species pairs *N. brevicatena*/*N. paucivorans* and *N. kruczakiae*/*N. veterana* show 99.5% (1,352 bp) and 99.8% (1,379 bp) 16S rRNA gene sequence similarity, respectively (43, 227). *N. testacea* and *N. sienata* differ in their 16S rRNA gene sequence by only 2 bases. These species pairs were all shown to be

distinct by DNA-DNA hybridization studies. Considering these high levels of species similarity, it may be that, at least for *Nocardia* species, sequence similarity of >99.8% is necessary for the unambiguous identification of clinical isolates. Roth et al. (179) noted significant microheterogeneity among isolates known to be members of the same *Nocardia* species (1 to 5 base differences). Sequence information from longer regions of the 16S rRNA gene, or sequence data from alternate gene targets, may provide better discrimination of closely related isolates.

The presence of multiple copies of the 16S rRNA gene in some isolates of *Nocardia* has recently been reported (46, 47). The presence of up to five gene copies per organism was noted, and in some isolates, the various copies showed different base sequences. Sequence chromatograms from such isolates show multiple overlapping peaks at a particular position, especially within variable regions of the gene. These multiple peaks remain unresolved with repeat testing; only cloning and sequence analysis of the resulting clones allow clear definition of the gene sequences in these regions. If the various copies of a particular gene are different, it is impossible to determine by sequencing which genes are functional, and therefore, identification using sequencing of this gene is not possible. In addition, several type strains have been described that contain multiple copies of the 16S rRNA gene (46); the sequences initially deposited in GenBank at the time the species were described do not reflect the presence of these multiple copies. If these sequences are compared to the sequences of unknown isolates, misidentification could occur. Furthermore, it is unclear how sequencing of a given gene could be used to establish the conspecificity of an unknown isolate with a species of which the type strain had multiple differing copies of that gene.

Other gene targets have been examined for their ability to discriminate among closely related *Nocardia* species. Rodríguez-Nava et al. evaluated a 441-bp region of the HSP gene for its discriminatory ability for the identification of 44 *Nocardia* species (177). They found this gene to have more variable sequence regions than found in the 16S rRNA gene, resulting in more sequence dissimilarity among species. This level of sequence heterogeneity will allow discrimination of some species that are very similar by 16S rRNA gene sequence.

The *secA1* gene is a housekeeping gene that codes for the SecA1 protein. This protein is essential for the export of proteins across the bacterial cytoplasmic membrane (184). Sequence analysis of a 468-bp region of the *secA1* gene has been shown to give good discrimination among *Nocardia* species (50). In a study of 30 type or reference strains of clinical significance, clear differentiation of all species was obtained. In addition, alignment of the deduced amino acid sequence (156 amino acid residues) showed good separation of all type and reference strains and eliminated some within-species microheterogeneities seen in the gene sequences. The deduced amino acid sequences of 38 of 40 clinical isolates tested were identical to that of the type strain of the species to which that isolate was assigned. Kang et al. reported that the analysis of the *gyrB* gene and the *secA1* gene sequences of *Gordonia* spp. allow greater discrimination among species than does the 16S rRNA gene (106).

While there are *rpoB* gene sequences for *Nocardia* species in the GenBank database, we are not aware of any publication documenting the usefulness of this gene for identification.

An additional benefit of these alternate gene targets is that sequence analysis involves a shorter region than that required for complete 16S rRNA gene sequencing, which could result in cost and time savings for such molecular analysis.

For some genera, such as *Nocardia*, sequence analysis of more than one gene may be useful for unambiguous identification of a clinical isolate and for the recognition of an unusual species. Rodríguez-Nava et al. (177) noted that a combined analysis using both the 16S rRNA and the HSP gene resolved identification inconsistencies of some *Nocardia* isolates. Multilocus sequencing may also help clarify taxonomic relationships of other members of the aerobic actinomycetes.

An important component of identification of isolates by gene sequencing is the quality of the database used for sequence comparison. Users of any sequence database should be aware of the limitations inherent in that database. The public database GenBank (http://www.ncbi.nlm.nih.gov/) includes the most extensive collection of sequences from many gene targets. The drawback to its use is that entries are not curated, and comparison of an unknown sequence with some poor-quality entries may result in an erroneous identification. See Tables 3 through 6 for GenBank type strain sequences deemed to be reliable for the identification of *Nocardia* and other aerobic actinomycetes. For organisms not listed, laboratories may want to obtain specific type strains and determine the sequence of that isolate to use as a comparison for unknown patient isolates. The proprietary 16S rRNA gene database used with the MicroSeq system (Applied BioSystems) for the identification of *Nocardia* species is limited in the number of species represented and in the number of sequences of each species included. Cloud et al. expanded this database with additional entries to obtain more reliable matches for query organisms (39). The Ribosomal Differentiation of Medical Microorganisms (RIDOM) is a quality-controlled 16S rRNA gene database (144), but the portion pertaining to *Nocardia* is not available for public use. Other useful databases include the Ribosomal Database Project (http://rdp.cme.msu.edu/) for 16S rRNA gene sequences, BiBi (http://pbil.univ-lyon1.fr/bibi/), which includes sequences from a variety of gene targets, and the commercially available SmartGene (IDNS, Lausanne, Switzerland), which includes curated 16S rRNA and *rpoB* gene sequences.

Other Molecular Methods

Ribotyping (see chapter 8) has been used to identify isolates of *N. farcinica* (143) and to discriminate among four members of the "*N. asteroides* complex" (125). Ribotyping of *Rhodococcus* species has shown specific patterns for all rhodococcal type strains and heterogeneous patterns for members of *R. equi* and *R. rhodochrous* (100, 124), possibly indicating that these are species complexes and require a more in-depth analysis.

The use of the PCR-randomly amplified polymorphic DNA (RAPD) technique (see chapter 8) has shown species-specific patterns for some species of *Nocardia*; Isik and Goodfellow reported that *N. nova*, *N. pseudobrasiliensis*, *N. transvalensis*, and isolates identified as *N. asteroides* show a variety of patterns (97); it is not clear if the variations reported by these authors represent the presence of additional unrecognized species, within-species variation, or both.

Pyrosequencing provides sequence information for short regions of a DNA target and takes advantage of variable regions of otherwise conserved genes. Pyrosequencing has been used for the identification of commonly isolated species of *Nocardia*, using a 30-bp sequence through an area of variable bases as the target sequencing region (M. J. Tuohy, J. J. Farrell, B. A. Brown-Elliott, L. Mann, R. W. Wilson, R. J. Wallace, G. S. Hall, and G. W. Procop, *Abstr. 104th Gen. Meet. Am. Soc. Microbiol.*, 2004, abstr. C-017). Tuohy et al. have also reported on the use of pyrosequencing for the identification of some rhodococci to the species level and genus-level identification of *Tsukamurella*, *Gordonia*, and *Dietzia* (M. J. Tuohy, J. L. Cloud, G. W. Procop, G. S. Hall. *Abstr. 109th Gen. Meet. Am. Soc. Microbiol.*, 2009, abstr. C-115). Galor et al. reported on the use of pyrosequencing to identify a *Nocardia* isolate causing keratitis; the authors were only able to determine that the isolate belonged to the group consisting of *N. abscessus*, *N. arthritidis*, and *N. asiatica* (67). The usefulness of pyrosequencing is limited due to the short region sequenced, the inability of this technique to easily distinguish among some closely related species, and the increasing number of recognized species.

Proteomics

Matrix-assisted laser desorption ionization–time of flight (MALDI-TOF) mass spectrometry, based on proteomic profiling by mass spectral analysis, has been used successfully for the identification of mycobacterial species (167) and has been preliminarily shown to be useful for the identification of some species of *Nocardia* (L. Stevenson, S. Drake, P. Conville, and P. Murray, *Abstr. 109th Gen. Meet. Am. Soc. Microbiol.*, 2009, abstr. C-126).

TYPING SYSTEMS

Among the aerobic actinomycetes, reports on various strain typing methodologies are limited to studies on *Rhodococcus* spp. and *Nocardia* spp. For *Nocardia*, there is no consensus on the best method for performing strain typing. Lack of reproducibility and/or insufficient differences among strains are common difficulties seen with most methods. In addition, interpretive criteria for the various methods are undefined.

Ribotyping has been reported to discriminate among 20 species of *Rhodococcus* and showed strain variation among isolates of *R. equi* and *R. rhodochrous* (100, 124).

Among *Nocardia* species, *N. farcinica* is most frequently implicated in infection outbreaks. Strains of *N. farcinica* were compared utilizing RAPD; methodologies vary in the primers used and results obtained when compared to other methods (61, 104). There are several reports of strain typing of *N. asteroides* using this method, but it is unclear if results reflect differences in strains or genetic differences inherent in members of the "*N. asteroides* complex." Laurent et al. reported that isolates of "*N. asteroides*" suspected to be related had identical banding patterns using this method (126).

Similarly, results of pulsed-field gel electrophoresis (PFGE) vary by report; clear differentiation of *N. farcinica* strains from postoperative wound infections in a surgical ward was reported by Blümel et al. (18). Kalpoe et al. (104) obtained unsatisfactory results using PFGE to identify *N. farcinica* strains in an outbreak in a renal transplant unit.

Yamamura et al. reported on the use of repetitive extragenic palindromic-PCR fingerprinting to be useful for the strain distinction of "*N. asteroides*" from clinical and environmental sources (223). Again, it is unclear if results obtained reflect strain differences or species differences among members of the *N. asteroides* complex.

Kalpoe et al. (104) reported on the use of amplified fragment length polymorphism (AFLP) analysis for an investigation of a possible outbreak of *N. farcinica*. They found AFLP results to be more reliable than those obtained from RAPD or PFGE. See chapter 8 for a description of the AFLP technique.

SEROLOGIC METHODS

There have been no recent publications (since 1988) describing serologic methods for the diagnosis of infections caused by aerobic actinomycetes. Older reports in the literature describe methodologies that are specific to a particular *Nocardia* species, frequently *N. asteroides*. It is unlikely that any of these methods would be considered useful or reliable to detect antibodies in patients who have diminished immunologic responses, and these are the very ones who are most prone to infections caused by aerobic actinomycetes.

ANTIMICROBIAL SUSCEPTIBILITIES

The Clinical Laboratory Standards Institute (CLSI, formerly NCCLS) has published an approved standard for susceptibility testing of both mycobacteria and aerobic actinomycetes (38). The recommended procedure for *Nocardia* and the other aerobic actinomycetes is broth microdilution; panels containing the appropriate dilutions of antimicrobials specifically active against these genera are commercially available (Trek Diagnostics, Westlake, OH). Custom-made panels may be available from other companies (such as PML Microbiologicals, Wilsonville, OR). The applicability of the procedure to the genera other than *Nocardia*, such as *Rhodococcus*, is currently under discussion. The CLSI document outlines methods for correct panel inoculation, incubation, and interpretation. Panels are read after incubation for 3 to 5 days, with the length of time depending on the particular species being tested. Both an MIC and an interpretation of the MIC result should be provided in the report to the physician. Currently, the interpretive breakpoints of three drugs, amikacin, minocycline, and sulfamethoxazole, differ from the breakpoints recommended for rapidly growing aerobic bacteria.

Susceptibility testing should be performed on all isolates of *Nocardia* and other aerobic actinomycetes thought to be of possible clinical significance and especially for isolates from patients for whom a sulfonamide cannot be used. Because significant expertise is required for accurate performance and interpretation of susceptibility tests, it is recommended that laboratories not performing such testing on a regular basis send isolates to an experienced reference laboratory. Antimicrobial agents recommended for primary susceptibility testing of all of these genera are amikacin, amoxicillin-clavulanic acid, ceftriaxone, ciprofloxacin, clarithromycin, imipenem, linezolid, minocycline, sulfamethoxazole or trimethoprim-sulfamethoxazole, and tobramycin. Agents to be considered for secondary testing include cefepime, cefotaxime, doxycycline, moxifloxacin, and gentamicin. In addition, rifampin and vancomycin should be tested for isolates of *Rhodococcus equi*. A few drugs with trailing endpoints, such as the sulfonamides and linezolid, may present interpretive problems. Most isolates of *Nocardia* species are susceptible to trimethoprim-sulfamethoxazole; one should be careful not to assume too readily that an isolate is resistant to this combination of drugs. Additionally, most, if not all, isolates of *Nocardia* species are susceptible in vitro to linezolid (29).

Sulfonamides or trimethoprim-sulfamethoxazole may not be adequate in certain circumstances, such as patients with CNS nocardiosis, disseminated disease, or concurrent HIV infection (28).

Table 7 shows the typical susceptibility patterns for the different *Nocardia* species for which adequate data are available.

EVALUATION, INTERPRETATION, AND REPORTING OF RESULTS

The aerobic actinomycetes are widespread in the environment. Therefore, particularly when an aerobic actinomycete is isolated in culture in small amounts without having been visualized in the direct patient specimen, it may be impossible for the laboratory to know if the isolate is the result of specimen or laboratory contamination, patient colonization, or actual infection. Some indication of the quantity of organism present should be given for any isolate of an aerobic actinomycete. Discussion between the clinical and laboratory staff is extremely useful for selection of additional patient specimens and laboratory procedures for determination of the clinical significance of an isolate from a given patient. See the "Clinical Significance" section of this chapter for information on species known to cause human disease. Additionally, see Tables 3 through 6 for information on the frequency of isolation of species known to be clinically significant. Identification of an organism to the genus level may help determine its significance. However, even for accurate genus assignment, molecular methods may need to be employed. In some cases, genus-level identification (if possible) suffices.

When an isolate is reported to the species level, the laboratory should be certain that clinicians are aware of the reliability of the identification method used. Reports should indicate how the isolate was identified. It may be possible to preliminarily identify the more commonly encountered aerobic actinomycetes, particularly *Nocardia* species, to the species level using phenotypic methods (Table 8) (215), but some are inevitably misidentified by such procedures. Precise identification can only be achieved by gene sequencing; if identification is obtained by other methods, the report should indicate that the identification is presumptive. Susceptibility results should be reported for isolates considered to be clinically significant. For accurate determination of both identification and susceptibility patterns, referral to a laboratory with expertise in working with these organisms may be necessary.

Whenever a laboratory isolates an aerobic actinomycete for which sequencing indicates that the organism has been rarely isolated, the circumstances surrounding the isolation of the organism should be carefully evaluated to assess its potential clinical significance, and a search of recent literature may be conducted to determine what is already established regarding pathogenicity and antibiotic susceptibility for that species. For such searches, LPSN and Pub Med may be good starting points; care should be taken to consider current nomenclature and taxonomy as stated by Euzéby. The report of a rare or unusual species should be accompanied by a brief summary of whatever is known regarding its clinical significance.

We gratefully acknowledge the assistance of Yvonne R. Shea in the preparation of the colony photographs and Patrick R. Murray for critically reviewing the manuscript.

REFERENCES

1. **Ajello, L., and J. Brown.** 1987. Actinomycetoma caused by *Nocardiopsis dassonvillei. Arch. Dermatol.* **123:**426.
2. **Alp, E., O. Yildiz, B. Aygen, B. Sumerkan, I. Sari, K. Koc, A. Couble, F. Laurent, P. Boiron, and M. Doganay.** 2006. Disseminated nocardiosis due to unusual species: two case reports. *Scand. J. Infect. Dis.* **38:**545–548.

3. **Anderson, A. S., and E. M. H. Wellington.** 2001. The taxonomy of *Streptomyces* and related genera. *Int. J. Syst. Evol. Microbiol.* **51:**797–814.

4. **Ansari, S. R., A. Safdar, X. Y. Han, and S. O'Brien.** 2006. *Nocardia veterana* bloodstream infection in a patient with cancer and a summary of reported cases. *Int. J. Infect. Dis.* **10:**483–486.

5. **Arenskötter, M., D. Bröker, and A. Steinbücher.** 2004. Biology of the metabolically diverse genus *Gordonia*. *Appl. Environ. Microbiol.* **70:**3195–3204.

6. **Arya, B., S. Hussian, and S. Hariharan.** 2004. *Rhodococcus equi* pneumonia in a renal transplant patient: a case report and review of literature. *Clin. Transplant.* **18:**748–752.

7. **Asoh, N., H. Watanabe, M. Fines-Guyon, K. Watanabe, K. Oishi, W. Kositsakulchai, T. Sanchai, K. Kunsuikmengrai, S. Kahintapong, B. Khantawa, P. Tharavichitkul, T. Sirisanthana, and T. Nagatake.** 2003. Emergence of rifampin-resistant *Rhodococcus equi* with several types of mutations in the *rpoB* gene among AIDS patients in northern Thailand. *J. Clin. Microbiol.* **41:**2337–2340.

8. **Auerbach, S. B., M. M. McNeil, J. M. Brown, B. A. Lasker, and W. R. Jarvis.** 1992. Outbreak of pseudoinfection with *Tsukamurella paurometabolum* traced to laboratory contamination: efficacy of joint epidemiological and laboratory investigation. *Clin. Infect. Dis.* **14:**1015–1022.

9. **Baron, E. J., J. D. Scott, and L. S. Tompkins.** 2005. Prolonged incubation and extensive subculturing do not increase recovery of clinically significant microorganisms from standard automated blood cultures. *Clin. Infect. Dis.* **41:**1677–1680.

10. **Beaman, B. L., and L. Beaman.** 1994. *Nocardia* species: host-parasite relationships. *Clin. Microbiol. Rev.* **7:**213–264.

11. **Beau, F., C. Bollet, T. Coton, E. Garnotel, and M. Drancourt.** 1999. Molecular identification of a *Nocardiopsis dassonvillei* blood isolate. *J. Clin. Microbiol.* **37:**3366–3368.

12. **Bell, K. S., J. C. Philip, N. Christofi, and D. W. J. Aw.** 1996. Identification of *Rhodococcus equi* using the polymerase chain reaction. *Lett. Appl. Microbiol.* **23:**72–74.

13. **Bell, K. S., J. C. Philp, D. W. J. Aw, and N. Christofi.** 1998. The genus *Rhodococcus*. *J. Appl. Microbiol.* **85:**195–210.

14. **Bemer-Melchior, P., A. Haloun, P. Riegel, and H. B. Drugeon.** 1999. Bacteremia due to *Dietzia maris* in an immunocompromised patient. *Clin. Infect. Dis.* **29:**1338–1340.

15. **Berd, D.** 1973. Laboratory identification of clinically important aerobic actinomycetes. *Appl. Microbiol.* **25:**665–681.

16. **Biehle, J. R., S. J. Cavalieri, T. Felland, and B. L. Zimmer.** 1996. Novel method for rapid identification of *Nocardia* species by detection of preformed enzymes. *J. Clin. Microbiol.* **34:**103–107.

17. **Blaschke, A. J., J. Bender, C. L. Byington, K. Korgenski, J. Daly, C. A. Petti, A. T. Pavia, and K. Ampofo.** 2007. *Gordonia* species: emerging pathogens in pediatric patients that are identified by 16S ribosomal RNA gene sequencing. *Clin. Infect. Dis.* **45:**483–486.

18. **Blümel, J., E. Blümel, A. F. Yassin, H. Schmidt-Rotte, and K. P. Schaal.** 1998. Typing of *Nocardia farcinica* by pulsed-field gel electrophoresis reveals an endemic strain as source of hospital infections. *J. Clin. Microbiol.* **36:**118–122.

19. **Boiron, P., and F. Provost.** 1990. Enzymatic characterization of *Nocardia* spp. and related bacteria by API ZYM profile. *Mycopathologia* **110:**51–56.

20. **Bopp, C. A., J. W. Sumner, G. K. Morris, and J. G. Wells.** 1981. Isolation of *Legionella* spp. from environmental water samples by low-pH treatment and use of a selective medium. *J. Clin. Microbiol.* **13:**714–719.

21. **Bottei, E., J. P. Flaherty, L. J. Kaplan, and L. Duffee-Kerr.** 1994. Lymphocutaneous *Nocardia brasiliensis* infection transmitted via a cat scratch: a second case. *Clin. Infect. Dis.* **18:**649–650.

22. **Bouza, E., A. Pérez-Parra, M. Rosal, P. Martín-Rabadán, M. Rodriguez-Créixems, and M. Marín.** 2009. *Tsukamurella*: a cause of catheter-related bloodstream infections. *Eur. J. Clin. Microbiol. Infect. Dis.* **28:**203–210.

23. **Bowersock, T. L., S. A. Salmon, E. S. Portis, P. J. F, D. A. Robinson, C. W. Ford, and J. Watts.** 2000. MICs of oxazolidinones for *Rhodococcus equi* strains isolated from humans and animals. *Antimicrob. Agents Chemother.* **44:**1367–1369.

24. **Breitkopf, C., D. Hammel, H. H. Scheld, G. Peters, and K. Becker.** 2005. Impact of a molecular approach to improve the microbiological diagnosis of infective heart valve endocarditis. *Circulation* **111:**1415–1421.

25. **Brown, B. A., J. O. Lopes, R. W. Wilson, J. M. Costa, A. C. deVargas, S. H. Alves, C. Klock, G. O. Onyi, and R. J. Wallace, Jr.** 1999. Disseminated *Nocardia pseudobrasiliensis* infection in a patient with AIDS in Brasil. *Clin. Infect. Dis.* **28:**144–145.

26. **Brown, J. M., and M. M. McNeil.** 2003. *Nocardia, Rhodococcus, Gordonia, Actinomadura, Streptomyces*, and other aerobic actinomycetes, p. 502–531. *In* P. R. Murray et al. (ed.), *Manual of Clinical Microbiology*, 8th ed. ASM Press, Washington, DC.

27. **Brown, J. M., K. N. Pham, M. M. McNeil, and B. A. Lasker.** 2004. Rapid identification of *Nocardia farcinica* clinical isolates by a PCR assay targeting a 314-base-pair species-specific DNA fragment. *J. Clin. Microbiol.* **42:**3655–3660.

28. **Brown-Elliott, B. A., J. M. Brown, P. S. Conville, and R. J. Wallace, Jr.** 2006. Clinical and laboratory features of the *Nocardia* spp. based on current molecular taxonomy. *Clin. Microbiol. Rev.* **19:**259–282.

29. **Brown-Elliott, B. A., S. C. Ward, C. J. Crist, L. B. Mann, R. W. Wilson, and R. J. Wallace, Jr.** 2001. In vitro activities of linezolid against multiple *Nocardia* species. *Antimicrob. Agents Chemother.* **45:**1295–1297.

30. **Bunker, M. L., L. Chewning, S. E. Wang, and M. A. Gordon.** 1988. *Dermatophilus congolensis* and "hairy" leukoplakia. *Am. J. Clin. Pathol.* **89:**683–687.

31. **Butler, W. R., M. M. Floyd, J. M. Brown, S. R. Toney, M. I. Daneshvar, R. C. Cooksey, J. Carr, A. G. Steigerwalt, and N. Charles.** 2005. Novel mycolic acid-containing bacteria in the family *Segniliparaceae* fam. nov., including the genus *Segniliparus rotundus* gen. nov. with descriptions of *Segniliparus rotundus* sp. nov. and *Segniliparus rugosus* sp. nov. *Int. J. Syst. Evol. Microbiol.* **55:**1615–1624.

32. **Butler, W. R., C. Sheils, B. A. Brown-Elliott, N. Charles, A. A. Colin, M. J. Gant, J. Goodill, D. Hindman, S. R. Toney, R. J. Wallace, Jr, and M. A. Yakrus.** 2007. First isolations of *Segniliparus rugosus* from patients with cystic fibrosis. *J. Clin. Microbiol.* **45:**3449–3452.

33. **Castro, L. G. M., W. Belda, Jr, A. Salebian, and L. C. Cucé.** 1993. Mycetoma: a retrospective study of 41 cases seen in São Paulo, Brazil, from 1978 to 1989. *Mycoses* **36:**89–95.

34. **Chávez, G., R. Estrada, and A. Bonifaz.** 2002. Perianal actinomycetoma experience of 20 cases. *Int. J. Dermatol.* **41:**491–493.

35. **Christidou, A., S. Maraki, E. Scoulica, E. Mantadakis, S. Agelaki, and G. Samonis.** 2004. Fatal *Nocardia farcinica* bacteremia in a patient with lung cancer. *Diagn. Microbiol. Infect. Dis.* **50:**135–139.

36. **Chun, J., S.-O. Kang, Y. C. Hah, and M. Goodfellow.** 1996. Phylogeny of mycolic acid-containing actinomycetes. *J. Ind. Microbiol.* **17:**205–213.

37. **Clark, N. M., D. K. Braun, A. Pasternak, and C. E. Chenoweth.** 1995. Primary cutaneous *Nocardia otitidiscaviarum* infection: case report and review. *Clin. Infect. Dis.* **20:**1266–1270.

38. **Clinical and Laboratory Standards Institute/NCCLS.** 2003. *Susceptibility Testing of Mycobacteria, Nocardiae and Other Aerobic Actinomycetes. Approved Standard M24-A.* National Committee for Clinical Laboratory Standards, Wayne, PA.

39. **Cloud, J. L., P. S. Conville, A. Croft, D. Harmsen, F. G. Witebsky, and K. C. Carroll.** 2004. Evaluation of partial 16S ribosomal DNA sequencing for identification of *Nocardia* species by using the MicroSeq 500 system with an expanded database. *J. Clin. Microbiol.* **42:**578–584.

40. **Collins, M. D., M. Goodfellow, D. E. Minnikin, and G. Alderson.** 1985. Menaquinone composition of mycolic acid-containing actinomycetes and some sporoactinomycetes. *J. Appl. Bacteriol.* **58:**77–86.

41. **Collins, M. D., J. Smida, M. Dorsch, and E. Stackebrandt.** 1988. *Tsukamurella* gen. nov. harboring *Corynebacterium*

paurometabolum and *Rhodococcus aurantiacus*. *Int. J. Syst. Bacteriol.* **38**:385–391.

42. Conville, P. S., J. M. Brown, A. G. Steigerwalt, B. A. Brown-Elliott, and F. G. Witebsky. 2008. *Nocardia wallacei* sp. nov. and *Nocardia blacklockiae* sp. nov., human pathogens and members of the "*Nocardia transvalensis* complex." *J. Clin. Microbiol.* **46**:1178–1184.

43. Conville, P. S., J. M. Brown, A. G. Steigerwalt, J. W. Lee, V. L. Anderson, J. T. Fishbain, S. M. Holland, and F. G. Witebsky. 2004. *Nocardia kruczakiae* sp. nov., a pathogen in immunocompromised patients and a member of the "*N. nova* complex." *J. Clin. Microbiol.* **42**:5139–5145.

44. Conville, P. S., J. M. Brown, A. G. Steigerwalt, J. W. Lee, D. E. Byrer, V. L. Anderson, S. E. Dorman, S. M. Holland, B. Cahill, K. C. Carroll, and F. G. Witebsky. 2003. *Nocardia veterana* as a pathogen in North American patients. *J. Clin. Microbiol.* **41**:2560–2568.

45. Conville, P. S., S. H. Fischer, C. P. Cartwright, and F. G. Witebsky. 2000. Identification of *Nocardia* species by restriction endonuclease analysis of an amplified portion of the 16S rRNA gene. *J. Clin. Microbiol.* **38**:158–164.

46. Conville, P. S., and F. G. Witebsky. 2007. Analysis of multiple differing copies of the 16S rRNA gene in five clinical isolates and three type strains of *Nocardia* species, and implications for species assignment. *J. Clin. Microbiol.* **45**:1146–1151.

47. Conville, P. S., and F. G. Witebsky. 2005. Multiple copies of the 16S rRNA gene in *Nocardia nova* isolates and implications for sequence-based identification procedures. *J. Clin. Microbiol.* **43**:2881–2885.

48. Conville, P. S., and F. G. Witebsky. 2007. *Nocardia, Rhodococcus, Gordonia, Actinomadura, Streptomyces*, and other aerobic actinomycetes, p. 515–542. *In* P. R. Murray, E. J. Baron, J. H. Jorgensen, M. L. Landry, and M. A. Pfaller (ed.), *Manual of Clinical Microbiology*, 9th ed, vol. 1. ASM Press, Washington, DC.

49. Conville, P. S., and F. G. Witebsky. 2007. Organisms designated as *Nocardia asteroides* drug pattern type VI are members of the species *Nocardia cyriacigeorgica*. *J. Clin. Microbiol.* **45**:2257–2259.

50. Conville, P. S., A. M. Zelazny, and F. G. Witebsky. 2006. Analysis of *secA1* gene sequences for identification of *Nocardia* species. *J. Clin. Microbiol.* **44**:2760–2766.

51. Cook, A. E., and P. R. Meyers. 2003. Rapid identification of filamentous actinomycetes to the genus level using genus-specific 16S rRNA gene restriction fragment patterns. *Int. J. Syst. Evol. Microbiol.* **53**:1907–1915.

52. Cornish, N., and J. A. Washington. 1999. *Rhodococcus equi* infections: clinical features and laboratory diagnosis. *Curr. Clin. Top. Infect. Dis.* **19**:198–215.

53. Couble, A., V. Rodríguez-Nava, M. P. de Montclos, P. Boiron, and F. Laurent. 2005. Direct detection of *Nocardia* spp. in clinical samples by a rapid molecular method. *J. Clin. Microbiol.* **43**:1921–1924.

54. Cummins, C. S. 1962. Chemical composition and antigenic structure of cell walls of *Corynebacterium, Mycobacterium, Nocardia, Actinomyces* and *Arthrobacter*. *J. Gen. Microbiol.* **28**:35–50.

55. del Mar Tomas, M., R. Moure, J. A. S. Nieto, S. Fojon, A. Fernandez, M. Diaz, R. Villanueva, and G. Bou. 2005. *Williamsia muralis* pulmonary infection. *Emerg. Infect. Dis.* **11**:1324–1325.

56. Diego, C., J. C. Ambrosioni, G. Abel, B. Fernando, O. Tomás, N. Ricardo, and B. Jorge. 2005. Disseminated nocardiosis caused by *Nocardia abscessus* in an HIV-infected patient: first reported case. *AIDS* **19**:1330–1331.

57. Eggink, C. A., P. Wesseling, P. Boiron, and J. F. G. M. Meis. 1997. Severe keratitis due to *Nocardia farcinica*. *J. Clin. Microbiol.* **35**:999–1001.

58. Eisenblätter, M., U. Disko, G. Stoltenburg-Didinger, H. Scherübl, K. P. Schaal, A. Roth, R. Ignatius, M. Zeitz, H. Hahn, and J. Wagner. 2002. Isolation of *Nocardia paucivorans* from the cerebrospinal fluid of a patient with relapse of cerebral nocardiosis. *J. Clin. Microbiol.* **40**:3532–3534.

59. Ekkelenkamp, M. B., W. de Jong, W. Hustinx, and S. Thijsen. 2004. *Streptomyces thermovulgaris* bacteremia in Crohn's disease patient. *Emerg. Infect. Dis.* **10**:1883–1885.

60. Emmons, W., B. Reichwein, and D. L. Winslow. 1991. *Rhodococcus equi* infection in the patient with AIDS: literature review and report of an unusual case. *Rev. Infect. Dis.* **13**:91–96.

61. Exmelin, L., B. Malbruny, M. Vergnaud, F. Provost, P. Boiron, and C. Morel. 1996. Molecular study of nosocomial nocardiosis outbreak involving heart transplant recipients. *J. Clin. Microbiol.* **34**:1014–1016.

62. Flores, M., and E. P. Desmond. 1993. Opacification of Middlebrook agar as an aid in identification of *Nocardia farcinica*. *J. Clin. Microbiol.* **31**:3040–3041.

63. Funke, G., and K. Bernard. 2007. Coryneform gram-positive rods, p. 485–514. *In* P. R. Murray (ed.), *Manual of Clinical Microbiology*, vol. 9. ASM Press, Washington, DC.

64. Funke, G., K. Peters, and M. Aravena-Roman. 1998. Evaluation of the RapID CB Plus system for identification of coryneform bacteria and *Listeria* spp. *J. Clin. Microbiol.* **36**:2439–2442.

65. Funke, G., F. N. R. Renaud, J. Freney, and P. Riegel. 1997. Multicenter evaluation of the updated and extended API (RAPID) Coryne Database 2.0. *J. Clin. Microbiol.* **35**:3122–3126.

66. Fux, C., T. Bodmer, H. R. Ziswiler, and S. L. Leib. 2003. *Nocardia cyriacigeorgici*: first report of invasive human infection. *Dtsch. Med. Wochenschr.* **128**:1038–1041.

67. Galor, A., G. S. Hall, G. W. Procop, M. Tuohy, and B. Jeng. 2006. Rapid species determination of *Nocardia* keratitis using pyrosequencing technology. *Am. J. Ophthalmol.* **143**:182–183.

68. Georghiou, P. R., and Z. M. Blacklock. 1992. Infection with *Nocardia* species in Queensland. *Med. J. Aust.* **156**:692–697.

69. Gillum, R. L., S. M. H. Qadri, M. N. Al-Ahdal, D. H. Connor, and A. J. Strano. 1988. Pitted keratolysis: a manifestation of human dermatophilosis. *Dermatologica* **177**:305–308.

70. Godreuil, S., M.-N. Didelot, C. Perez, A. Leflèche, P. Boiron, J. Reynes, F. Laurent, H. Jean-Pierre, and H. Marchandin. 2003. *Nocardia veterana* isolated from ascitic fluid of a patient with human immunodeficiency virus infection. *J. Clin. Microbiol.* **41**:2768–2773.

71. Golub, B., G. Falk, and W. Spink. 1967. Lung abscess due to *Corynebacterium equi*. *Ann. Intern. Med.* **66**:1174–1177.

72. Goodfellow, M. 1989. Genus *Rhodococcus* Zopf 1891, 28, p. 2362–2371. *In* S. T. Williams, M. E. Sharpe, and J. G. Holt (ed.), *Bergey's Manual of Systematic Bacteriology*, vol. 4. Williams & Wilkins, Baltimore, MD.

73. Goodfellow, M. 1998. *Nocardia* and related genera, p. 463–489. *In* L. Collier, A. Balows, and M. Sussman (ed.), *Topley and Wilson's Microbiology and Microbial Infections*, vol. 2. Arnold, London, United Kingdom.

74. Goodfellow, M., G. Alderson, and J. Chun. 1998. Rhodococcal systematics: problems and developments. *Antonie van Leeuwenhoek* **74**:3–20.

75. Goodfellow, M., and M. P. Lechevalier. 1989. Genus *Nocardia* Trevisan 1889, 9, p. 2350–2361. *In* S. T. Williams, M. E. Sharpe, and J. G. Holt (ed.), *Bergey's Manual of Systematic Bacteriology*, vol. 4. Williams & Wilkins, Baltimore, MD.

76. Goodfellow, M., and T. Pirouz. 1982. Numerical classification of sporoactinomycetes containing *meso*-diaminopimelic acid in the cell wall. *J. Med. Microbiol.* **128**:503–527.

77. Gordon, M. A. 1989. Genus *Dermatophilus* Van Saceghem 1915, 357, emend. mut. char. Gordon 1964, 521, p. 2409–2410. *In* S. T. Williams, M. E. Sharpe, and J. G. Holt (ed.), *Bergey's Manual of Systematic Bacteriology*, vol. 4. Williams & Wilkins, Baltimore, MD.

78. Gordon, R. E., and J. M. Mihm. 1962. Identification of *Nocardia caviae* (Erikson) nov. comb. *Ann. N. Y. Acad. Sci.* **98**:628–636.

79. Gordon, R. E., and J. M. Mihm. 1962. The type species of the genus *Nocardia*. *J. Gen. Microbiol.* **27**:1–10.

80. Gordon, R. E., S. K. Mishra, and D. A. Barnett. 1978. Some bits and pieces of the genus *Nocardia*: *N. carnea, N. vaccinii, N. transvalensis, N. orientalis* and *N. aerocolonigenes*. *J. Gen. Microbiol.* **109**:69–78.

81. Gray, T. J., D. J. Serisier, C. M. Gilpin, C. Coultr, S. J. Bowler, and J. G. McCormack. 2007. *Nocardia paucivorans* - a cause of disseminated nocardiosis. *J. Infect.* **54**:e95–e98.

82. Guerrero, M. F., J. M. Ramos, G. Renedo, I. Gadea, and A. Alix. 1999. Pulmonary malacoplakia associated with *Rhodococcus equi* infection in patients with AIDS: case report and review. *Clin. Infect. Dis.* **28**:1334–1336.

83. Gürtler, V., B. C. Mayall, and R. Seviour. 2004. Can whole genome analysis refine the taxonomy of the genus *Rhodococcus?* *FEMS Microbiol. Rev.* **28**:377–403.

84. Gürtler, V., R. Smith, B. C. Mayall, G. Pötter-Reinemann, E. Stackebrandt, and R. M. Kroppenstedt. 2001. *Nocardia veterana* sp. nov., isolated from human bronchial lavage. *Int. J. Syst. Evol. Microbiol.* **51**:933–936.

85. Gutmann, L., F. W. Goldstein, M. D. Kitzis, B. Hautefort, C. Darmon, and J. F. Acar. 1983. Susceptibility of *Nocardia asteroides* to 46 antibiotics, including 22 B-Lactams. *Antimicrob. Agents Chemother.* **23**:248–251.

86. Hamdad, F., B. Vidal, Y. Douadi, G. Laurans, B. Canarelli, G. Choukroun, V. Rodriguez-Nava, P. Boiron, B. Beaman, and F. Eb. 2007. *Nocardia nova* as the causative agent in spondylodiscitis and psoas abscess. *J. Clin. Microbiol.* **45**:262–265.

87. Hansen, T., J. Van Kerckhof, P. Jelfs, C. Wainwright, P. Ryan, and C. Coulter. 2009. *Segniliparus rugosus* infection, Australia. *Emerg. Infect. Dis.* **15**:611–613.

88. Harrington, J. R., M. C. Golding, R. J. Martens, N. D. Halbert, and N. D. Cohen. 2005. Evaluation of a real-time polymerase chain reaction assay for detection and quantitation of virulent *Rhodococcus equi*. *Am. J. Vet. Res.* **66**:755–761.

89. Harvey, I., Y. Cormier, C. Beaulieu, V. N. Akimov, A. Mériaux, and C. Duchaine. 2001. Random amplified ribosomal DNA restriction analysis for rapid identification of thermophilic actinomycete-like bacteria involved in hypersensitivity pneumonitis. *Syst. Appl. Microbiol.* **24**:277–284.

90. Hemmersbach-Miller, M., A. C. Martel, A. Bordes Benítez, and A. O. Sosa. 2004. Brain abscess due to *Nocardia otitidiscaviarum*: report of a case and review. *Scand. J. Infect. Dis.* **36**:381–383.

91. Henssen, A. 1989. Genus *Pseudonocardia* Henssen 1957, 408, p. 2376–2378. *In* S. T. Williams, M. E. Sharpe, and J. G. Holt (ed.), *Bergey's Manual of Systematic Bacteriology*, vol. 4. Williams & Wilkins, Baltimore, MD.

92. Hitti, W., and M. Wolff. 2005. Two cases of multidrug resistant *Nocardia farcinica* infection in immunosuppressed patients and implications for empiric therapy. *Eur. J. Clin. Microbiol. Infect. Dis.* **24**:142–144.

93. Holt, J. G., N. R. Krieg, P. H. A. Sneath, J. T. Staley, and S. T. Williams (ed.). 1994. *Bergey's Manual of Determinative Bacteriology*, 9th ed., p. 605–618. Williams & Wilkins, Baltimore, MD.

94. Horré, R., G. Schumacher, G. Marklein, H. Stratmann, E. Wardelmann, S. Gilges, G. S. de Hoog, and K. P. Schaal. 2002. Mycetoma due to *Pseudallescheria boydii* and co-isolation of *Nocardia abscessus* in a patient injured in road accident. *Med. Mycol.* **40**:525–527.

95. Huang, Y., M. Pasciak, Z. Liu, Q. Xie, and A. Gamian. 2004. *Amycolatopsis palatopharyngis* sp. nov., a potentially pathogenic actinomycete isolated from a human clinical source. *Int. J. Syst. Evol. Microbiol.* **54**:359–363.

96. Inamadar, A. C., A. Palit, B. V. Peerapur, and S. D. Rao. 2004. Sporotrichoid nocardiosis caused by *Nocardia nova* in a patient infected with human immunodeficiency virus. *Int. J. Dermatol.* **43**:824–826.

97. Isik, K., and M. Goodfellow. 2002. Differentiation of *Nocardia* species by PCR-randomly amplified polymorphic DNA fingerprinting. *Syst. Appl. Microbiol.* **25**:60–67.

98. Janda, J. M., and S. L. Abbott. 2002. Bacterial identification for publication: when is enough enough? *J. Clin. Microbiol.* **40**:1887–1891.

99. Jannat-Khah, D. P., E. S. Halsey, B. A. Lasker, A. G. Steigerwalt, H. P. Hinrikson, and J. M. Brown. 2009. *Gordonia araii* infection of an orthopedic device and review of the literature on medical device-associated *Gordonia* infections. *J. Clin. Microbiol.* **47**:499–502.

100. Jorks, S. 1996. Differentiation of *Rhodococcus* species by ribotyping. *J. Basic Microbiol.* **36**:399–406.

101. Kageyama, A., H. Sato, M. Nagata, K. Yazawa, M. Katsu, Y. Mikami, K. Kamei, and K. Nishimura. 2002. First human case of nocardiosis caused by *Nocardia pseudobrasiliensis* in Japan. *Mycopathologia* **156**:187–192.

102. Kageyama, A., K. Yazawa, J. Ishikawa, K. Hotta, K. Nishimura, and Y. Mikami. 2004. Nocardial infections in Japan from 1992 to 2001, including the first report of infection by *Nocardia transvalensis*. *Eur. J. Epidemiol.* **19**:383–389.

103. Kageyama, A., K. Yazawa, T. Kudo, K. Nishimura, and Y. Mikami. 2004. First isolates of *Nocardia abscessus* from humans and soil in Japan. *Jpn. J. Med. Mycol.* **45**:17–21.

104. Kalpoe, J. S., K. E. Templeton, A. M. Horrevorts, H. P. Endtz, E. J. Kuijper, A. T. Bernards, and C. H. W. Klaassen. 2007. Molecular typing of a suspected cluster of *Nocardia farcinica* infections by use of randomly amplified polymorphic DNA, pulsed-field gel electrophoresis, and amplified fragment length polymorphism analyses. *J. Clin. Microbiol.* **45**:4048–4050.

105. Kämpfer, P., M. A. Andersson, F. A. Rainey, R. M. Kroppenstedt, and M. Salkinoja-Salonen. 1999. *Williamsia muralis* gen. nov., sp. nov., isolated from the indoor environment of a children's day care center. *Int. J. Syst. Evol. Microbiol.* **49**:681–687.

106. Kang, Y., K. Takeda, K. Yazawa, and Y. Mikami. 2009. Phylogenetic studies of *Gordonia* species based on *gyrB* and *secA1* gene analysis. *Mycopathologia* **167**:95–105.

107. Kapadia, M., K. V. I. Rolston, and X. Y. Han. 2007. Invasive *Streptomyces* infections: six cases and literature review. *Am. J. Clin. Pathol.* **127**:619–624.

108. Kashima, M., R. Kano, H. Takahama, Y. Mikami, M. Ito, A. Hasegawa, and M. Mizoguchi. 2005. A successfully treated case of mycetoma due to *Nocardia veterana*. *Br. J. Dermatol.* **152**:1349–1352.

109. Kattar, M. M., B. T. Cookson, L. C. Carlson, S. K. Stiglich, M. A. Schwartz, T. T. Nguyen, R. Daza, C. K. Wallis, S. L. Yarfitz, and M. B. Coyle. 2001. *Tsukamurella standjordae* sp. nov., a proposed new species causing sepsis. *J. Clin. Microbiol.* **39**:1467–1476.

110. Kedlaya, I., M. B. Ing, and S. S. Wong. 2001. *Rhodococcus equi* infections in immunocompetent hosts: case report and review. *Clin. Infect. Dis.* **32**:e39–e47.

111. Kent, P. T., and G. P. Kubica. 1985. *Public Health Mycobacteriology. A Guide for the Level III Laboratory*. U.S. Department of Health and Human Services, Centers for Disease Control, Atlanta, GA.

112. Khan, S.-N. H., S. E. Sanche, C. A. Robinson, and F. Pirouzmand. 2006. *N. paucivorans* infection presenting as a brain abscess. *Can. J. Neurol. Sci.* **33**:426–427.

113. Khatri, M. L., H. M. Al-Halali, M. F. Khalid, S. A. Saif, and M. C. R. Vyas. 2002. Mycetoma in Yemen: clinicoepidemiologic and histopathologic study. *Int. J. Dermatol.* **41**:586–593.

114. Klatte, S., F. A. Rainey, and R. M. Kroppenstedt. 1994. Transfer of *Rhodococcus aichiensis* Tsukamura 1982 and *Nocardia amarae* Lechevalier and Lechevalier 1974 to the genus *Gordona* as *Gordona aichiensis* comb. nov. and *Gordona amarae* comb. nov. *Int. J. Syst. Bacteriol.* **44**:769–773.

115. Koll, B. S., A. E. Brown, T. E. Kiehn, and D. Armstrong. 1992. Disseminated *Nocardia brasiliensis* infection with septic arthritis. *Clin. Infect. Dis.* **15**:469–472.

116. Kurup, V. P., J. J. Barboriak, J. N. Fink, and M. P. Lechevalier. 1975. *Thermoactinomyces candidus*, a new species of thermophilic actinomycetes. *Int. J. Syst. Bacteriol.* **25**:150–154.

117. Kurup, V. P., and J. N. Fink. 1975. A scheme for the identification of thermophilic actinomycetes associated with hypersensitivity pneumonitis. *J. Clin. Microbiol.* **2**:55–61.

118. Labeda, D. P., J. M. Donahue, N. M. Williams, S. F. Sells, and M. M. Henton. 2003. *Amycolatopsis kentuckyensis* sp. nov., *Amycolatopsis lexingtonensis* sp. nov. and *Amycolatopsis pretoriensis* sp. nov., isolated from equine placentas. *Int. J. Syst. Evol. Microbiol.* **53**:1601–1605.

119. **Lacey, J.** 1989. Genus *Saccharopolyspora* Lacey and Goodfellow 1975, 77, p. 2382–2386. *In* S. T. Williams, M. E. Sharpe, and J. G. Holt (ed.), *Bergey's Manual of Systematic Bacteriology*, vol. 4. Williams & Wilkins, Baltimore, MD.

120. **Lacey, J., and T. Cross.** 1989. Genus *Thermoactinomyces* Tsiklinsky 1899, 501, p. 2573–2585. *In* S. T. Williams, M. E. Sharpe, and J. G. Holt (ed.), *Bergey's Manual of Systematic Bacteriology*, vol. 4. Williams & Wilkins, Baltimore, MD.

121. **Ladrón, N., M. Fernández, J. Agüero, B. G. Zörn, J. A. Vásques-Boland, and J. Navas.** 2003. Rapid identification of *Rhodococcus equi* by a PCR assay targeting the choE gene. *J. Clin. Microbiol.* **41:**3241–3245.

122. **Lai, C.-C., L.-N. Lee, L.-J. Teng, M. S. Wu, J.-C. Tsai, and P.-R. Hseuh.** 2005. Disseminated *Nocardia farcinica* infection in a uraemia patient with idiopathic thrombocytopenia purpura receiving steroid therapy. *J. Med. Microbiol.* **54:**1107–1110.

123. **Lanotte, P., S. Watt, R. Ruimy, P. Boiron, A. Robier, and R. Quentin.** 2001. *Nocardia farcinica* infection of a cochlear implant in an immunocompetent boy. *Eur. J. Clin. Microbiol. Infect. Dis.* **20:**880–882.

124. **Lasker, B. A., J. M. Brown, and M. M. McNeil.** 1992. Identification and epidemiological typing of clinical and environmental isolates of the genus *Rhodococcus* with use of a digoxigenin-labeled rDNA gene probe. *Clin. Infect. Dis.* **15:**223–233.

125. **Laurent, F., A. Carlotti, P. Boiron, J. Villard, and J. Freney.** 1996. Ribotyping: a tool for taxonomy and identification of the *Nocardia asteroides* complex species. *J. Clin. Microbiol.* **34:**1079–1082.

126. **Laurent, F., F. Provost, A. Couble, E. Casoli, and P. Boiron.** 2000. Genetic relatedness analysis of *Nocardia* strains by random amplification polymorphic DNA: validation and applications. *Res. Microbiol.* **151:**263–270.

127. **Laurent, F. J., F. Provost, and P. Boiron.** 1999. Rapid identification of clinically relevant *Nocardia* species to genus level by 16S rRNA gene PCR. *J. Clin. Microbiol.* **37:**99–102.

128. **Lechevalier, M. P., H. Prauser, D. P. Labeda, and J.-S. Ruan.** 1986. Two new genera of nocardioform actinomycetes: *Amycolata* gen. nov. and *Amycolatopsis* gen. nov. *Int. J. Syst. Bacteriol.* **36:**29–37.

129. **Lee, A. C. W., K. Y. Yuen, and Y. L. Lau.** 1994. Catheter-associated nocardiosis. *Pediatr. Infect. Dis. J.* **13:**1023–1024.

130. **Lewis, K. E., P. Ebden, S. L. Wooster, J. Rees, and G. A. J. Harrison.** 2003. Multi-system infection with *Nocardia farcinica*—therapy with linezolid and minocycline. *J. Infect.* **46:**199–202.

131. **Lopez, F. A., F. Johnson, D. M. Novosad, B. L. Beaman, and M. Holodniy.** 2003. Successful management of disseminated *Nocardia transvalensis* infection in a heart transplant recipient after development of sulfonamide resistance: case report and review. *J. Heart Lung Transplant.* **22:**492–497.

132. **Louie, L., M. Louie, and A. E. Simor.** 1997. Investigation of a pseudo-outbreak of *Nocardia asteroides* infection by pulsed-field gel electrophoresis and randomly amplified polymorphic DNA PCR. *J. Clin. Microbiol.* **35:**1582–1584.

133. **Mahe, A., M. Develoux, C. Lienhardt, S. Keita, and P. Bobin.** 1996. Mycetomas in Mali: causative agents and geographic distribution. *Am. J. Trop. Med. Hyg.* **54:**77–79.

134. **Maiti, P. K., A. Ray, and S. Bandyopadhyay.** 2002. Epidemiological aspects of mycetoma from a retrospective study of 264 cases in West Bengal. *Trop. Med. Int. Health* **7:**788–792.

135. **Maraki, S., E. Scoulica, K. Alpantaki, M. Dialynas, and Y. Tselentis.** 2003. Lymphocutaneous nocardiosis due to *Nocardia brasiliensis*. *Diagn. Microbiol. Infect. Dis.* **47:**341–344.

136. **Martín, M. C., A. Manteca, M. Castillo, F. Vázquez, and F. J. Méndez.** 2004. *Streptomyces albus* isolated from a human actinomycetoma and characterized by molecular techniques. *J. Clin. Microbiol.* **42:**5957–5960.

137. **Masters, A. M., T. M. Ellis, J. M. Carson, S. S. Sutherland, and A. R. Gregory.** 1995. *Dermatophilus chelonae* sp. nov., isolated from chelonids in Australia. *Int. J. Syst. Bacteriol.* **45:**50–56.

138. **McCarthy, A. J.** 1989. Genus *Saccharomonospora* Nonomura and Ohara 1971c, 889, p. 2402–2404. *In* S. T. Williams, M. E. Sharpe, and J. G. Holt (ed.), *Bergey's Manual of Systematic Bacteriology*, vol. 4. Williams & Wilkins, Baltimore, MD.

139. **McMinn, E. J., G. Alderson, H. I. Dodson, M. Goodfellow, and A. C. Ward.** 2000. Genomic and phenomic differentiation of *Rhodococcus equi* and related strains. *Antonie van Leeuwenhoek* **78:**331–340.

140. **McNabb, A., R. Shuttleworth, R. Behme, and W. D. Colby.** 1997. Fatty acid characterization of rapidly growing pathogenic aerobic actinomycetes as a means of identification. *J. Clin. Microbiol.* **35:**1361–1368.

141. **McNeil, M. M., and J. M. Brown.** 1994. The medically important aerobic actinomycetes: epidemiology and microbiology. *Clin. Microbiol. Rev.* **7:**357–417.

142. **McNeil, M. M., J. M. Brown, C. H. Magruder, K. T. Shearlock, R. A. Saul, D. P. Allred, and L. Ajello.** 1992. Disseminated *Nocardia transvalensis* infection: an unusual opportunistic pathogen in severely immunocompromised patients. *J. Infect. Dis.* **165:**175–178.

143. **McNeil, M. M., S. Ray, P. E. Kozarsky, and J. M. Brown.** 1997. *Nocardia farcinica* pneumonia in a previously healthy woman: species characterization with use of a digoxigenin-labeled cDNA probe. *Clin. Infect. Dis.* **25:**933–934.

144. **Mellmann, A., J. L. Cloud, S. Andrees, K. Blackwood, K. C. Carroll, A. Kabani, A. Roth, and D. Harmsen.** 2003. Evaluation of RIDDOM, MicroSeq, and GenBank services in the molecular identification of *Nocardia* species. *Int. J. Med. Microbiol.* **293:**359–370.

145. **Meyer, J.** 1989. Genus *Actinomadura* Lechevalier and Lechevalier 1970a, 400, p. 2511–2526. *In* S. T. Williams, M. E. Sharpe, and J. G. Holt (ed.), *Bergey's Manual of Systematic Bacteriology*, vol. 4. Williams & Wilkins, Baltimore, MD.

146. **Meyer, J.** 1989. Genus *Nocardiopsis* Meyer 1976, 487, p. 2562–2568. *In* S. T. Williams, M. E. Sharpe, and J. G. Holt (ed.), *Bergey's Manual of Systematic Bacteriology*, vol. 4. Williams & Wilkins, Baltimore, MD.

147. **Meyer, J.** 1976. *Nocardiopsis*, a new genus of the order *Actinomycetales*. *Int. J. Syst. Bacteriol.* **26:**487–493.

148. **Miksits, K., G. Stoltenburg, H. Neumayer, H. Spiegal, K. P. Schaal, J. Cervós-Navarro, A. Distler, H. Stein, and H. Hahn.** 1991. Disseminated infection of the central nervous system caused by *Nocardia farcinica*. *Nephrol. Dial. Transplant.* **6:**209–214.

149. **Morón, R., I. González, and O. Genilloud.** 1999. New genus-specific primers for the PCR identification of members of the genera *Pseudonocardia* and *Saccharopolyspora*. *Int. J. Syst. Evol. Microbiol.* **49:**149–162.

150. **Moss, W. J., J. A. Sager, J. D. Dick, and A. Ruff.** 2003. *Streptomyces bikiniensis* bacteremia. *Emerg. Infect. Dis.* **9:**273–274.

151. **Murray, P. R., R. L. Heeren, and A. C. Niles.** 1987. Effect of decontamination procedures on recovery of *Nocardia* spp. *J. Clin. Microbiol.* **25:**2010–2011.

152. **Murray, P. R., A. C. Niles, and R. L. Heeren.** 1988. Modified Thayer-Martin medium for recovery of *Nocardia* species from contaminated specimens. *J. Clin. Microbiol.* **26:**1219–1220.

153. **Murray, R. J., M. Aravena-Román, and P. Kämpfer.** 2007. Endophthalmitis due to *Williamsia muralis*. *J. Med. Microbiol.* **56:**1410–1412.

154. **Naguib, M. T., and D. P. Fine.** 1995. Brain abscess due to *Nocardia brasiliensis* hematogenously spread from a pulmonary infection. *Clin. Infect. Dis.* **21:**459–460.

155. **Napoleão, F., P. V. Damasco, T. C. F. Camello, M. D. do Vale, A. F. B. de Andrade, R. Hirata, Jr, and A. L. de Mattos-Guaraldi.** 2005. Pyogenic liver abscess due to *Rhodococcus equi* in an immunocompetent host. *J. Clin. Microbiol.* **43:**1002–1004.

156. **Oldfield, C., H. Bonella, L. Renwick, H. I. Dodson, G. Alderson, and M. Goodfellow.** 2004. Rapid determination of vapA/vapB genotype in *Rhodococcus equi* using a differential polymerase chain reaction method. *Antonie van Leeuwenhoek* **85:**317–326.

157. Osoagbaka, O. U., and A. N. U. Njoku-Obi. 1987. Presumptive diagnosis of pulmonary nocardiosis: value of sputum microscopy. *J. Appl. Bacteriol.* **63:**27–38.

158. Palmer, D. L., R. L. Harvey, and J. K. Wheeler. 1974. Diagnostic and therapeutic considerations in *Nocardia asteroides* infection. *Medicine* (Baltimore) **53:**391–401.

159. Paredes, B. E., R. E. Hunger, L. R. Braathen, and C. U. Brand. 1998. Cutaneous nocardiosis caused by *Nocardia brasiliensis* after an insect bite. *Dermatology* **198:**159–161.

160. Patel, J. B., R. J. Wallace, Jr, B. A. Brown-Elliott, T. Taylor, C. Imperatrice, D. G. B. Leonard, R. W. Wilson, L. Mann, K. C. Jost, and I. Nachamkin. 2004. Sequence-based identification of aerobic actinomycetes. *J. Clin. Microbiol.* **42:**2530–2540.

161. Patterson, J. E., K. Chapin-Robertson, S. Waycott, P. Farrel, A. McGeer, M. M. McNeil, and S. Edberg. 1992. Pseudoepidemic of *Nocardia asteroides* associated with a mycobacterial culture system. *J. Clin. Microbiol.* **30:**1357–1360.

162. Pelaez, A. I., M. D. M. Garcia-Suarez, A. Manteca, O. Melon, C. Aranaz, R. Cimadevilla, F. J. Mendez, and F. Vazquez. 2009. A fatal case of *Nocardia otitidiscaviarum* pulmonary infection and brain abscess: taxonomic characterization by molecular methods. *Ann. Clin. Microbiol. Antimicrob.* **8:**11. http://www.ann-clinmicrob.com/content/8/1/11.

163. Peterson, B. E., S. G. Jenkins, S. Yuan, C. Lamm, and A. H. Szporn. 2007. *Nocardia farcinica* isolated from bronchoalveolar lavage fluid of a child with cystic fibrosis. *Pediatr. Infect. Dis. J.* **26:**858–859.

164. Peterson, D. L., L. D. Hudson, and K. Sullivan. 1978. Disseminated *Nocardia caviae* with positive blood cultures. *Arch. Intern. Med.* **138:**1164–1165.

165. Pfyffer, G. 2007. Mycobacterium: general characteristics, laboratory detection, and staining properties, p. 543–572. *In* P. R. Murray (ed.), *Manual of Clinical Microbiology*, vol. 9. ASM Press, Washington, DC.

166. Pidoux, O., J.-N. Argenson, V. Jacomo, and M. Drancourt. 2001. Molecular identification of a *Dietzia maris* hip prosthesis infection isolate. *J. Clin. Microbiol.* **39:**2634–2636.

167. Pigone, M., K. M. Greth, J. Cooper, D. Emerson, and J. Tang. 2006. Identification of mycobacteria by matrix-assisted laser desorption ionization-time-of-flight mass spectrometry. *J. Clin. Microbiol.* **44:**1963–1970.

168. Pijper, A., and B. D. Pullinger. 1927. South African Nocardiases. *J. Trop. Med. Hyg.* **30:**153–156.

169. Poonwan, N., N. Mekha, K. Yazawa, S. Thunyaharn, A. Yamanaka, and Y. Mikami. 2005. Characterization of clinical isolates of pathogenic *Nocardia* strains and related actinomycetes in Thailand from 1996 to 2003. *Mycopathologia* **159:**361–368.

170. Pottumarthy, S., A. P. Limaye, J. L. Prentice, Y. B. Houze, S. R. Swanzy, and B. T. Cookson. 2003. *Nocardia veterana*, a new emerging pathogen. *J. Clin. Microbiol.* **41:**1705–1709.

171. Prescott, J. F. 1991. *Rhodococcus equi*: an animal and human pathogen. *Clin. Microbiol. Rev.* **4:**20–34.

172. Qasem, J. A., Z. U. Khan, and A. S. Mustafa. 2001. Diagnosis of nocardiosis by polymerase chain reaction: an experimental study in mice. *Microbiol. Res.* **156:**317–322.

173. Quintana, E. T., K. Wierzbicka, P. Mackiewicz, A. Osman, A. H. Fahal, M. E. Hamid, J. Zakrzewska-Czerwinska, L. A. Maldonado, and M. Goodfellow. 2008. *Streptomyces sudanensis* sp. nov., a new pathogen isolated from patients with actinomycetoma. *Antonie van Leeuwenhoek* **93:**305–313.

174. Rainey, F. A., S. Klatte, R. M. Kroppenstedt, and E. Stackebrandt. 1995. *Dietzia*, a new genus including *Dietzia maris* comb. nov., formerly *Rhodococcus maris*. *Int. J. Syst. Bacteriol.* **45:**32–36.

175. Reyes, G., J.-L. Navarro, C. Gamallo, and M.-C. de las Cuevas. 2006. Type A aortic dissection associated with *Dietzia maris*. *Interact. Cardiovasc. Thorac. Surg.* **5:**666–668.

176. Richet, H. M., P. C. Craven, J. M. Brown, B. A. Lasker, C. D. Cox, M. M. McNeil, A. D. Tice, W. R. Jarvis, and O. C. Tablan. 1991. A cluster of *Rhodococcus* (*Gordona*) *bronchialis* sternal-wound infections after coronary-artery bypass surgery. *N. Engl. J. Med.* **324:**104–109.

177. Rodríguez-Nava, V., A. Couble, G. Devulder, J.-P. Flandrois, P. Boiron, and F. Laurent. 2006. Use of PCR-restriction enzyme pattern analysis and sequencing database for *hsp65* gene-based identification of *Nocardia* species. *J. Clin. Microbiol.* **44:**536–546.

178. Rose, C. E. I., J. M. Brown, and J. F. Fisher. 2008. Brain abscess caused by *Streptomyces* infection following penetration trauma: case report and results of susceptibility analysis of 92 isolates of *Streptomyces* species submitted to the CDC from 2000 to 2004. *J. Clin. Microbiol.* **46:**821–823.

179. Roth, A., S. Andrees, R. M. Kroppenstedt, D. Harmsen, and H. Mauch. 2003. Phylogeny of the genus *Nocardia* based on reassessed 16S rRNA gene sequences reveals underspeciation and division of strains classified as *Nocardia asteroides* into three established species and two unnamed taxons. *J. Clin. Microbiol.* **41:**851–856.

180. Ruimy, R., P. Riegel, A. Carlotti, P. Boiron, G. Bernardin, H. Monteil, R. J. Wallace, Jr., and R. Christen. 1996. *Nocardia pseudobrasiliensis* sp. nov., a new species of Nocardia which groups bacterial strains previously identified as *Nocardia brasiliensis* and associated with invasive diseases. *Int. J. Syst. Bacteriol.* **46:**259–264.

181. Salazar, O., I. González, and O. Genilloud. 2002. New genus-specific primers for the PCR identification of novel isolates of the genera *Nocardiopsis* and *Saccharothrix*. *Int. J. Syst. Evol. Microbiol.* **52:**1411–1421.

182. Schiff, T. A., M. M. McNeil, and J. M. Brown. 1993. Cutaneous *Nocardia farcinica* infection in a nonimmunocompromised patient: case report and review. *Clin. Infect. Dis.* **16:**756–760.

183. Schlaberg, R., R. C. Huard, and P. Della-Latta. 2008. *Nocardia cyriacigeorgica*, an emerging pathogen in the United States. *J. Clin. Microbiol.* **46:**265–273.

184. Schmidt, M. G., and K. B. Kiser. 1999. SecA: the ubiquitous component of preprotein translocase in prokaryotes. *Microbes Infect.* **1:**993–1004.

185. Sellon, D. C., T. E. Besser, S. L. Vivrette, and R. S. McConnico. 2001. Comparison of nucleic acid amplification, serology and microbiologic culture for diagnosis of *Rhodococcus equi* pneumonia in foals. *J. Clin. Microbiol.* **39:**1289–1293.

186. Sharma, M., B. C. Gilbert, R. L. Benz, and J. Santoro. 2007. Disseminated *Nocardia otitidiscaviarum* infection in a woman with sickle cell anemia and end-stage renal disease. *Am. J. Med. Sci.* **333:**372–375.

187. Shen, F.-T., and C.-C. Young. 2005. Rapid detection and identification of the metabolically diverse genus *Gordonia* by 16S rRNA-gene-targeted genus-specific primers. *FEMS Microbiol. Lett.* **250:**221–227.

188. Sheng, W.-H., Y.-T. Huang, S.-C. Chang, and P.-R. Hsueh. 2009. Brain abscess caused by *Tsukamurella tyrosinosolvens* in an immunocompetent patient. *J. Clin. Microbiol.* **47:**1602–1604.

189. Smego, R. A., and H. A. Gallis. 1984. The clinical spectrum of *Nocardia brasiliensis* infection in the United States. *Rev. Infect. Dis.* **6:**164–180.

190. Sonesson, A., B. Öqvist, P. Hagstam, I. M. Björkman-Burtscher, H. Miörner, and A. C. Petersson. 2004. An immunosupressed patient with systemic vasculitis suffering from cerebral abscesses due to Nocardia farcinica identified by 16S rRNA gene universal PCR. *Nephrol. Dial. Transplant.* **19:**2896–2900.

191. Stackebrandt, E., F. A. Rainey, and N. L. Ward-Rainey. 1997. Proposal for a new hierarchic classification system, Actinobacteria classis nov. *Int. J. Syst. Bacteriol.* **47:**479–491.

192. Stackebrandt, E., J. Smida, and M. D. Collins. 1988. Evidence of phylogenetic heterogeneity within the genus *Rhodococcus*: revival of the genus *Gordona* (Tsukamura). *J. Gen. Appl. Microbiol.* **34:**341–348.

193. Staneck, J. L., and G. D. Roberts. 1974. Simplified approach to identification of aerobic actinomycetes by thin-layer chromatography. *Appl. Microbiol.* **28:**226–231.

194. Steingrube, V. A., B. A. Brown, J. L. Gibson, R. W. Wilson, J. Brown, Z. Blacklock, K. Jost, S. Locke, R. F. Ulrich, and R. J. Wallace, Jr. 1995. DNA amplification and restriction endonuclease analysis for differentiation of

12 species and taxa of *Nocardia*, including recognition of four new taxa within the *Nocardia asteroides* complex. *J. Clin. Microbiol.* **33**:3096–3101.

195. **Steingrube, V. A., R. W. Wilson, B. A. Brown, K. C. Jost, Jr, Z. Blacklock, J. L. Gibson, and R. J. Wallace, Jr.** 1997. Rapid identification of clinically significant species and taxa of aerobic actinomycetes, including *Actinomadura*, *Gordona*, *Nocardia*, *Rhodococcus*, *Streptomyces*, and *Tsukamurella* isolates, by DNA amplification and restriction endonuclease analysis. *J. Clin. Microbiol.* **35**:817–822.

196. **Torres, O. H., P. Domingo, R. Pericas, P. Boiron, J. A. Montiel, and G. Vázquez.** 2000. Infection caused by *Nocardia farcinica*: case report and review. *Eur. J. Clin. Microbiol. Infect. Dis.* **19**:205–212.

197. **Torres-Tortosa, M., J. Arrizabalaga, J. L. Villanueva, J. Gálvez, M. Leyes, M. E. Valencia, J. Flores, J. M. Peña, E. Pérez-Cecilia, and C. Quereda.** 2003. Prognosis and clinical evaluation of infection caused by *Rhodococcus equi* in HIV-infected patients. *Chest* **123**:1970–1976.

198. **Towersey, L., E. S. Martins, A. T. Londero, R. J. Hay, P. J. S. Filho, C. M. Takiya, C. C. Martins, and O. F. Gompertz.** 1993. *Dermatophilus congolensis* human infection. *J. Am. Acad. Dermatol.* **29**:351–354.

199. **Tsukamura, M.** 1982. Numerical analysis of the taxonomy of nocardiae and rhodococci. *Microbiol. Immunol.* **26**:1101–1119.

200. **Tsukamura, M., K. Hikosaka, K. Nishimura, and S. Hara.** 1988. Severe progressive subcutaneous abscesses and necrotizing tenosynovitis caused by *Rhodococcus aurantiacus*. *J. Clin. Microbiol.* **26**:201–205.

201. **Tuon, F. F., R. F. Siciliano, T. Al-Musawi, F. Rossi, V. L. Capelozzi, R. C. Gryschek, and E. A. S. Medeiros.** 2007. *Rhodococcus equi* bacteremia with lung abscess misdiagnosed as Corynebacterium. A report of 2 cases. *Clinics* **62**:795–798.

202. **Uesaka, I., and N. M. McClung.** 1961. On the morphology of *Nocardia*, especially on its acid-fastness. *Jpn. J. Tuberc.* **8**:116–117.

203. **van Dam, A. P., M. T. C. Pruijm, B. I. J. Harinck, L. B. S. Gelinck, and E. J. Kuijper.** 2005. Pneumonia involving *Aspergillus* and *Rhizopus* spp. after a near-drowning incident with subsequent *Nocardia cyriacigeorgici* and *N. farcinica* coinfection as a late complication. *Eur. J. Clin. Microbiol. Infect. Dis.* **24**:61–64.

204. **Vandamme, P., B. Pot, M. Gillis, K. De Vos, K. Kersters, and J. Swings.** 1996. Polyphasic taxonomy, a consensus approach to bacterial systematics. *Microbiol. Rev.* **60**:407–438.

205. **Vannier, A. M., B. H. Ackerman, and L. F. Hutchins.** 1992. Disseminated *Nocardia asteroides* diagnosed by blood culture in a patient with disseminated histoplasmosis. *Arch. Pathol. Lab. Med.* **116**:537–539.

206. **Vickers, R. M., J. D. Rihs, and V. L. Yu.** 1992. Clinical demonstration of isolation of *Nocardia asteroides* on buffered charcoal-yeast extract media. *J. Clin. Microbiol.* **30**:227–228.

207. **von Graevenitz, A., and V. Pünter-Streit.** 1995. Development of a new selective plating medium for *Rhodococcus equi*. *Microbiol. Immunol.* **39**:283–284.

208. **Wada, R., C. Itabashi, Y. Nakayama, Y. Ono, C. Murakami, and S. Yagihashi.** 2003. Chronic granulomatous pleuritis caused by nocardia: PCR based diagnosis by nocardial 16S rDNA in pathological specimens. *J. Clin. Pathol.* **56**:966–969.

209. **Wallace, R. J., Jr., B. A. Brown, Z. Blacklock, R. Ulrich, K. Jost, J. M. Brown, M. M. McNeil, G. Onyi, V. A. Steingrube, and J. Gibson.** 1995. New *Nocardia* taxon among isolates of *Nocardia brasiliensis* associated with invasive disease. *J. Clin. Microbiol.* **33**:1528–1533.

210. **Wallace, R. J., Jr., B. A. Brown, M. Tsukamura, J. M. Brown, and G. O. Onyi.** 1991. Clinical and laboratory features of *Nocardia nova*. *J. Clin. Microbiol.* **29**:2407–2411.

211. **Wallace, R. J., Jr., L. C. Steele, G. Sumter, and J. M. Smith.** 1988. Antimicrobial susceptibility patterns of *Nocardia asteroides*. *Antimicrob. Agents Chemother.* **32**:1776–1779.

212. **Wallace, R. J., Jr., M. Tsukamura, B. A. Brown, J. Brown, V. A. Steingrube, Y. Zhang, and D. R. Nash.** 1990. Cefotaxime-resistant *Nocardia asteroides* strains are isolates of the controversial species *Nocardia farcinica*. *J. Clin. Microbiol.* **28**:2726–2732.

213. **Warren, N. G.** 1996. Actinomycosis, nocardiosis, and actinomycetoma. *Dermatol. Clin.* **14**:85–95.

214. **Warwick, S., T. Bowen, H. McVeigh, and T. M. Embley.** 1994. A phylogenetic analysis of the family *Pseudonocardiaceae* and the genera *Actinokineospora* and *Saccharothrix* with 16S rRNA sequences and a proposal to combine the genera *Amycolata* and *Pseudonocardia* in an emended genus *Pseudonocardia*. *Int. J. Syst. Bacteriol.* **44**:293–299.

215. **Wauters, G., V. Avesani, J. Charlier, M. Janssens, M. Vaneechoutte, and M. Delmée.** 2005. Distribution of *Nocardia* species in clinical samples and their routine rapid identification in the laboratory. *J. Clin. Microbiol.* **43**:2624–2628.

216. **Weinstock, D. M., and A. E. Brown.** 2002. *Rhodococcus equi*: an emerging pathogen. *Clin. Infect. Dis.* **34**:1379–1385.

217. **Wellehan, J. F. X., C. Turenne, D. J. Heard, C. J. Detrisac, and J. J. O'Kelley.** 2004. *Dermatophilus chelonae* in a king cobra (*Ophiophagus hannah*). *J. Zoo Wildl. Med.* **35**:553–556.

218. **Wellinghausen, N., T. Pietzcker, W. Kern, A. Essig, and R. Marre.** 2002. Expanded spectrum of *Nocardia* species causing clinical nocardiosis detected by molecular methods. *Int. J. Med. Microbiol.* **292**:277–282.

219. **Williams, S. T., M. Goodfellow, and G. Alderson.** 1989. Genus *Streptomyces* Waksman and Henrici 1943, 339, p. 2452–2492. *In* S. T. Williams, M. E. Sharpe, and J. G. Holt (ed.), *Bergey's Manual of Systematic Bacteriology*, vol. 4. Williams & Wilkins, Baltimore, MD.

220. **Wilson, R. W., V. A. Steingrube, B. A. Brown, Z. Blacklock, K. C. Jost, Jr, A. McNabb, W. D. Colby, J. R. Biehle, J. L. Gibson, and R. J. Wallace, Jr.** 1997. Recognition of a *Nocardia transvalensis* complex by resistance to aminoglycosides, including amikacin, and PCR-restriction fragment length polymorphism analysis. *J. Clin. Microbiol.* **35**:2235–2242.

221. **Woods, G. L., and D. H. Walker.** 1996. Detection of infection or infectious agents by use of cytologic and histologic stains. *Clin. Microbiol. Rev.* **9**:382–404.

222. **Xu, J., J. R. Rao, B. C. Millar, J. S. Elborn, J. Evans, J. G. Barr, and J. E. Moore.** 2002. Improved molecular identification of *Thermoactinomyces* spp. associated with mushroom worker's lung by 16S rDNA sequence typing. *J. Med. Microbiol.* **51**:1117–1127.

223. **Yamamura, H., M. Hayakawa, Y. Nakagawa, and Y. Iimura.** 2004. Characterization of *Nocardia asteroides* isolates from different ecological habitats on the basis of repetitive extragenic palindromic-PCR fingerprinting. *Appl. Environ. Microbiol.* **70**:3149–3151.

224. **Yano, I., T. Imaeda, and M. Tsukamura.** 1990. Characterization of *Nocardia nova*. *Int. J. Syst. Bacteriol.* **40**:170–174.

225. **Yassin, A. F., H. Brzezinka, K. P. Schaal, H. G. Trüper, and G. Pulverer.** 1988. Menaquinone composition in the classification and identification of aerobic actinomycetes. *Zentralbl. Bakteriol. Mikrobiol. Hyg. A* **267**:339–356.

226. **Yassin, A. F., and H. Hupfer.** 2006. *Williamsia deligens* sp. nov., isolated from human blood. *Int. J. Syst. Evol. Microbiol.* **56**:193–197.

227. **Yassin, A. F., F. A. Rainey, J. Burghardt, H. Brzezinka, M. Mauch, and K. P. Schaal.** 2000. *Nocardia paucivorans* sp. nov. *Int. J. Syst. Evol. Microbiol.* **50**:803–809.

228. **Yassin, A. F., F. A. Rainey, U. Mendrock, H. Brzezinka, and K. P. Schaal.** 2000. *Nocardia abscessus* sp. nov. *Int. J. Syst. Evol. Microbiol.* **50**:1487–1493.

229. **Yassin, A. F., F. A. Rainey, and U. Steiner.** 2001. *Nocardia cyriacigeorgici* sp. nov. *Int. J. Syst. Evol. Microbiol.* **51**:1419–1423.

230. **Yorke, R. F., and E. Rouah.** 2003. Nocardiosis with brain abscess due to an unusual species, *Nocardia transvalensis*. *Arch. Pathol. Lab. Med.* **127**:224–226.

231. **Yoshida, K., S. Bandoh, J. Fujita, M. Tokuda, K. Negayama, and T. Ishida.** 2004. Pyothorax caused by *Nocardia otitidiscaviarum* in a patient with rheumatoid vasculitis. *Intern. Med.* **43**:615–619.

232. **Zaria, L. T.** 1993. *Dermatophilus congolensis* infection (dermatophilosis) in animals and man! An update. *Comp. Immun. Microbiol. Infect. Dis.* **16**:179–222.

Mycobacterium: General Characteristics, Laboratory Detection, and Staining Procedures*

GABY E. PFYFFER AND FRANTISKA PALICOVA

28

Many species within the genus *Mycobacterium* are prominent pathogens, above all the members of *Mycobacterium tuberculosis* complex as well as *M. leprae* and *M. ulcerans*. In addition, numerous species of environmental mycobacteria, called nontuberculous mycobacteria (NTM), are responsible for various kinds of mycobacterioses.

Tuberculosis remains a major global public health problem. Based on the recent survey data of the World Health Organization (WHO) the actual global prevalence of *M. tuberculosis* infection is 33%, corresponding to approximately 2.2 billion people. It is estimated that 9.27 million new cases of tuberculosis occurred in 2007 (139 per 100,000 population). Of these, approximately 44%, or 4.1 million (61 per 100,000), were smear positive and hence highly infectious cases. In 2007, an estimated 1.8 million people died of tuberculosis (237). Reducing the burden of tuberculosis largely depends on how rapidly DOTS (directly observed therapy, short course) programs can be implemented. Among the prime obstacles for DOTS expansion are shortages of trained staff, lack of political commitment, and poor laboratory services, together with inadequate patient management. Of particular concern is the increasing number of multidrug-resistant tuberculosis cases (0.5 million in 2007) and extensively drug-resistant tuberculosis cases (92) as well as the problem of people coinfected with human immunodeficiency virus (HIV). According to the WHO, one of four TB deaths is HIV related. In 2007, there were 456,000 deaths and an estimated 1.37 million new tuberculosis cases among HIV-infected individuals. The total number of global tuberculosis cases is still increasing in absolute terms as a result of population growth. Nevertheless, the number of incident cases per capita is falling globally in all WHO regions. In the Western hemisphere, the number of reported cases is steadily decreasing (approximate case rate, 6.8/100,000), reflecting the effectiveness of prevention strategies and control measures implemented by the health authorities, among them the use of more rapid and efficient laboratory algorithms to detect *M. tuberculosis* and susceptibility testing against anti-TB drugs. In this context, the clinical mycobacteriology laboratory plays a pivotal role.

Apart from *M. tuberculosis* complex, there is a growing number of NTM species, some of which are sources of important diseases in humans (4, 52, 163, 195). Thus, rapid and reliable identification of NTM is mandatory. The level of service and the choice of methods applied in the clinical mycobacteriology laboratory should be determined by the patient population served and by the resources available.

TAXONOMY AND DESCRIPTION OF THE GENUS

The genus *Mycobacterium* is the only genus in the family *Mycobacteriaceae* (224) and is related to other mycolic acid-containing genera. The high G+C content of the DNA of *Mycobacterium* species (61 to 71 mol% for all species except *M. leprae* [55%]) is within the range of the other mycolic acid-containing genera, i.e., *Gordonia* (63 to 69 mol%), *Tsukamurella* (68 to 74 mol%), *Nocardia* (64 to 72 mol%), and *Rhodococcus* (63 to 73 mol%) (34).

Mycobacteria are aerobic (though some species are able to grow under a reduced O_2 atmosphere), non-spore-forming (except *M. marinum* [66]), nonmotile, slightly curved or straight rods, 0.2 to 0.6 μm by 1.0 to 10 μm, which may branch. Colony morphology varies among the species, ranging from smooth to rough and from nonpigmented (nonphotochromogens) to pigmented. Colonies of the latter are regularly or variably yellow, orange, or, rarely, pink, usually due to carotenoid pigments. Some species require light to form pigment (photochromogens), while other species form pigment in either the light or the dark (scotochromogens). Aerial filaments are very rarely formed and never visible without magnification. Filamentous or mycelium-like growth may sometimes occur but on slight disturbance easily fragments into rods or coccoid elements (154).

The cell wall peptidoglycolipid contains *meso*-diaminopimelic acid, alanine, glutamic acid, glucosamine, muramic acid, arabinose, and galactose. Mycolic acids (number of carbon atoms ranging from 70 to 90), together with free lipids (e.g., trehalose-6,6′-dimycolate), provide for a hydrophobic permeability barrier (105, 112). Other important fatty acids are waxes, phospholipids, mycoserosic, and phthienoic acids. Various patterns of cellular fatty acids (number of carbon atoms ranging from 10 to 20) are found as well, among which is tuberculostearic (10-*R*-methyloctadecanoic) acid, a unique cell component for a number of aerobic actinomycetes (105).

---

*This chapter contains information (Safety and Transport Issues) presented in chapter 36 by Barbara A. Brown-Elliott and Richard J. Wallace, Jr., and in chapter 37 by Véronique Vincent, Barbara A. Brown-Elliott, Kenneth C. Jost, Jr., and Richard J. Wallace, Jr., in the eighth edition of this *Manual*.

The high content of complex lipids of the cell wall prevents access of common aniline dyes. Although not readily stained by Gram's method, mycobacteria are usually considered gram positive. When stained with special procedures (e.g., Ziehl-Neelsen staining) mycobacteria are not easily decolorized, even with acid-alcohol; i.e., they are acid fast. However, acid fastness can be partly or completely lost at some stage of growth by a proportion of the cells of some species, particularly the rapidly growing ones.

Compared to other bacteria, the growth of most mycobacterial species is slow, with generation times of up to ~20 h (for M. ulcerans, up to 36 h) on commonly used media. A natural division exists between slowly and rapidly growing species of mycobacteria. Slow growers require more than 7 days to produce colonies on solid media from a dilute inoculum under ideal culture conditions. Rapid growers, by definition, require less than 7 days when subcultured on Löwenstein-Jensen (L-J) medium but may also take several weeks to appear on primary culture from clinical specimens.

NUTRITIONAL REQUIREMENTS AND GROWTH

Most species adapt readily to growth on relatively simple substrates, using ammonia or amino acids as nitrogen sources and glycerol as a carbon source in the presence of mineral salts. A few species (e.g., M. haemophilum and M. genavense) are fastidious and require supplements such as mycobactin, hemin, or other iron compounds. To date, M. leprae has not been cultured outside living cells. Growth of mycobacteria is stimulated by carbon dioxide and by fatty acids, which may be provided in the form of egg yolk or oleic acid, even though the latter is toxic in higher concentrations ($\geq$1%) and has to be neutralized by albumin. Optimum temperatures for growth vary widely among species (from <30 to 45°C).

With the genomes of several mycobacterial species deciphered, functional genomics provide new insights into their physiological and metabolic regulation and relation to virulence (226).

SUSCEPTIBILITY TO PHYSICAL AND CHEMICAL AGENTS

Mycobacteria are able to survive for weeks to months on inanimate objects if protected from sunlight. M. tuberculosis complex, for instance, survives for several months on surfaces or in soil or cow dung from which other animals may be infected (127). Mycobacteria are easily killed by heat (>65°C for at least 30 min) and by UV (sun) light, but not by freezing or desiccation. They are more resistant to acids, alkali, and some chemical disinfectants than most other non-spore-forming bacteria. Quaternary ammonium compounds, hexachlorophene, and chlorhexidine are bacteriostatic at best. The concentration of malachite green in standard acid-fast media (e.g., L-J) was selected to maximize growth of mycobacteria while inhibiting other microorganisms. Other commonly used agents, such as ethylene oxide and formaldehyde vapor, as well as disinfectants such as chlorine compounds, 70% ethanol, 2% alkaline glutaraldehyde, peracetic acid, and stabilized hydrogen peroxide are effective in killing M. tuberculosis. However, agents that are inactivated in the presence of organic matter (e.g., alcohols) cannot be relied upon to disinfect sputum and other protein-containing materials.

With iodophors, the bactericidal effect depends on the content of available iodine as well as on the presence of organic matter (14). In their guidelines, the Centers for Disease Control and Prevention (CDC) and National Institutes of Health (NIH) suggest intermediate-level disinfectants (25; see also chapter 11).

EPIDEMIOLOGY AND TRANSMISSION

The genus Mycobacterium includes obligate pathogens, opportunistic pathogens, and saprophytes. Incapable of replication in the inanimate environment, the major ecological niche for M. leprae and M. tuberculosis complex are tissues of humans and warm-blooded animals. M. tuberculosis is carried in airborne particles (droplet nuclei) generated when patients with pulmonary tuberculosis cough. These particles, 1 to 5 μm in size, are kept "suspended" by normal air currents. Infection occurs when a susceptible person inhales the droplet nuclei. Once in the alveoli, the organisms are engulfed by alveolar macrophages. Usually, the host cell-mediated immune response limits multiplication and spread of M. tuberculosis. However, some bacilli can remain viable but dormant for many years after initial infection. Patients latently infected with M. tuberculosis are asymptomatic and not infectious but usually have a positive tuberculin skin test (TST) or a positive result with one of the commercially available interferon gamma (IFN-γ) release assays (IGRAs). In general, persons with a latent infection have a 10% risk during their lifetime for development of active tuberculosis, whereas patients with HIV infection have a 10 to 15% risk per year for progression to manifest disease (2).

In contrast, the NTM are free-living mycobacteria, usually found in association with watery habitats such as lakes, rivers, wet soil, etc. For some human pathogenic NTM species, e.g., M. ulcerans, M. haemophilum, or M. szulgai, the reservoir has not yet been defined (4). M. avium complex (MAC), M. genavense, M. kansasii, M. xenopi, M. simiae, M. gordonae, and some rapidly growing mycobacteria have been recovered from tap water. Some of them can play a role in nosocomial disease and/or pseudo-outbreaks (4, 81, 221). A well-known set of other sources for positive cultures are bronchoscopes and related devices. Organisms isolated representing pseudoinfections include M. tuberculosis (179) and M. xenopi (11) as well as other NTM. Although not components of the microbiota of humans or animals, NTM may be isolated as "bystanders" from the skin, upper respiratory tract, intestinal tract, and genital tract in asymptomatic individuals (52). Due to their ubiquitous nature, the question of their clinical significance is therefore important but often difficult to answer (4).

CLINICAL SIGNIFICANCE AND DESCRIPTION OF SPECIES

With the advent of molecular techniques for appropriate identification, close to 200 mycobacterial species have now been described, and their number is increasing steadily. This chapter focuses on the slowly growing mycobacteria only; rapidly growing mycobacteria are described in chapter 30.

M. tuberculosis Complex

The M. tuberculosis complex includes M. tuberculosis, M. bovis, M. bovis BCG, M. africanum, M. caprae, M. microti, "M. canettii," and M. pinnipedii. Although the members of M. tuberculosis complex are characterized by different phenotypes and mammalian host ranges, they display a most extreme genetic homogeneity, with ~0.01 to 0.03% synonymous nucleotide variation only and no significant trace of genetic exchange among them (18, 63, 71). Identification to the species level is not merely an academic exercise but is justified for epidemiologic, public health, and therapeutic reasons.

M. tuberculosis

In the industrialized world, a higher prevalence of tuberculosis occurs in the medically underserved ethnic minorities, the urban poor, homeless persons, prison inmates, alcoholics, intravenous drug users, the elderly in general, foreign-born persons from areas of high prevalence, and contacts of persons with active tuberculosis. The greatest known risk factor for progression of latent infection to active tuberculosis is HIV infection. Combined HIV and tuberculosis infections, especially in combination with drug resistance, have caused outbreaks in the past with extremely high mortality rates. In addition, the recent emergence of extensively drug-resistant tuberculosis exerts a dramatic impact on the changing patterns of global tuberculosis (64). Groups with a higher likelihood of progression also include individuals with underlying medical conditions, persons who have been infected within the past 2 years, children ≤4 years old, and persons with fibrotic and cancerous lesions on chest X rays.

Tuberculosis in adults is a slowly progressive process characterized by chronic inflammation and caseation and formation of cavities. These foci may rupture into the bronchi, allowing very large numbers of organisms to spread to other areas of the lungs and to be aerosolized by coughing, hence infecting other persons. The clinical features of pulmonary tuberculosis are cough, weight loss, night sweat, low-grade fever, dyspnea, and chest pain. Extrapulmonary manifestations of M. tuberculosis infection include cervical lymphadenitis, pleuritis, pericarditis, synovitis, meningitis, and infections of the skin, joints, bones, and internal organs (85). Unlike the ordinary clinical picture of tuberculosis, pulmonary disease in AIDS patients often differs in radiologic findings and is usually rapidly progressing. In these patients, extrapulmonary manifestation and disseminated disease, sometimes even without the formation of granulomas, are seen more frequently (85).

In culture, colonies of M. tuberculosis are off-white and rough on solid medium (Fig. 1), although on moist media they may tend to be smoother. The genome of M. tuberculosis (4,411,529 bp) was deciphered more than 10 years ago (32). Newer studies have shown that M. tuberculosis has an extremely low level of genetic variation, suggesting that the entire population of M. tuberculosis resulted from clonal expansion after an evolutionary bottleneck some 35,000 years ago; i.e., today's strains constitute just the visible tip of a much broader progenitor species. Based on very recent molecular data, the M. tuberculosis genome appears to be a composite assembly resulting from horizontal gene transfer events predating clonal expansion. The amount of synonymous nucleotide variation in housekeeping genes suggests that tuberculosis bacilli were contemporaneous with early hominids in East Africa and coevolved with their human host much longer than previously thought (71).

M. bovis

M. bovis causes tuberculosis in warm-blooded animals, such as cattle, dogs, cats, pigs, parrots, badgers, deer, some birds of prey, and also in primates and humans. While M. bovis

caused as much as 25% of cases of human tuberculosis in developed countries in the late 19th century, the number of cases has dropped to 1 to 2% today (144). Human disease is very similar to that caused by M. tuberculosis and treated accordingly, except that pyrazinamide is ineffective due to inherent resistance of M. bovis. Colonies on egg-based media are small and rounded, with irregular edges and a granular surface; on agar media colonies are small and flat (224). The genome of M. bovis has a size of 4,345,492 bp with a G+C content of 65.6%. The sequence is >99.95% identical to that of M. tuberculosis. There are some deletions in the genome which led to a reduced genome size (65).

M. bovis BCG

In many parts of the world, bacillus Calmette-Guérin (BCG) is still used for vaccine purposes. The strain was distributed by Calmette in 1924 to laboratories around the world and has been maintained in vitro by serial passages. Today, there exists a genetically heterogeneous conglomerate of BCG strains (Fig. 2) (10, 189; www.bcgatlas.org) that predominantly conform to the properties described for M. bovis, except that they are more attenuated in virulence. The 4,374,522-bp genome contains nearly 4,000 protein-coding genes, 58 of which are present in two copies as a result of two independent tandem duplications, DU1 and DU2. Recently, lesions in genes encoding σ-factors and pleiotrophic transcription regulators, like PhoRn and Crp, were uncovered in various BCG strains. Together with gene amplification, these lesions affect gene expression levels, immunogenicity, and possibly protection against tuberculosis, suggesting that early BCG vaccines may be superior to the later ones, which are more widely used (17). In rare instances, BCG may disseminate as a complication of intravesical BCG immunostimulation against bladder cancer (1).

M. africanum

M. africanum causes human tuberculosis in tropical Africa but has also been reported from other continents such as the United States, mainly in patients who had lived in Africa (42). The colonies of M. africanum resemble those of M. tuberculosis, and the physiological and biochemical properties position the organism between M. tuberculosis and M. bovis. Prior to molecular genetics, the definition of M. africanum was difficult and its validity was questioned by some authors. Recent genotypic analyses based on variable numbers of tandem repeats (VNTRs) and other molecular characteristics have set M. africanum clearly apart from other members of the complex (60, 218). Likewise, Mostowy et al. (134) and Niemann et al. (139) consider M. africanum to be a unique species within M. tuberculosis complex. Brosch et al. (18) had reported that isolates of M. tuberculosis do not have the deletion of chromosomal region 9 (RD 9), in contrast to M. bovis, M. microti, and M. africanum. The distribution of deleted sequences suggests that M. africanum subtype II isolates are situated among strains of "modern" M. tuberculosis, while subtype I isolates are heterogenous and constitute two distinct evolutionary branches within the M. tuberculosis complex. Currently, the genome (4,389,314 bp) with a G+C content of 65.6% is being sequenced (www.sanger.ac.uk).

M. caprae

M. caprae, formerly called M. tuberculosis subsp. caprae (5) and M. bovis subsp. caprae (106), was originally described as preferring goats to cattle as hosts. M. caprae not only is seen

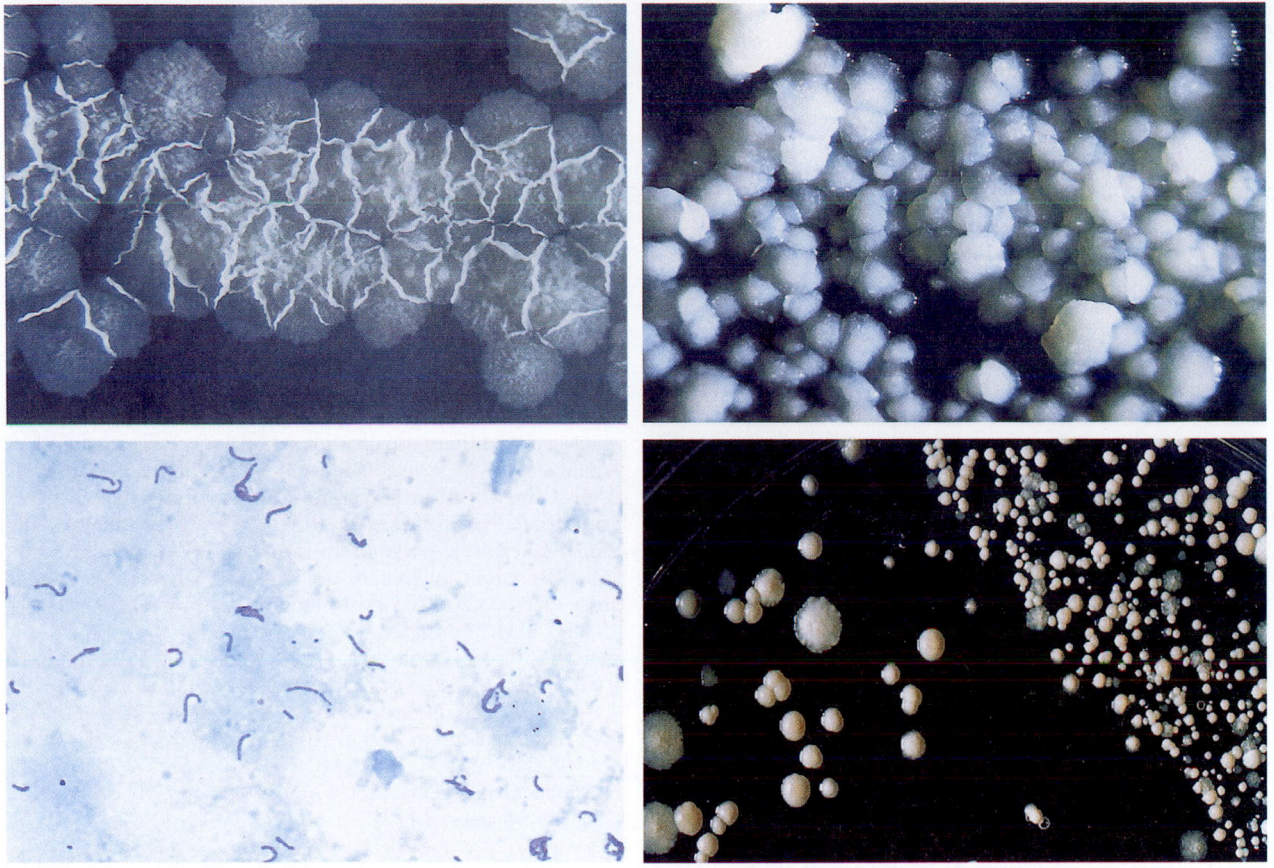

FIGURE 1 (top left)   *Mycobacterium tuberculosis* on Middlebrook 7H10 agar. Note the dry and rough colonies with sometimes a nodular or wrinkled surface.

FIGURE 2 (top right)   *Mycobacterium bovis* BCG on Middlebrook 7H10 agar. Colonies may be flat as well as round with irregular edges.

FIGURE 3 (bottom left)   Acid-fast staining (Ziehl-Neelsen) of *Mycobacterium microti*. Note the characteristic curved ("croissant-like") microscopic morphology.

FIGURE 4 (bottom right)   *Mycobacterium canettii* on Middlebrook 7H10 agar. Note the heterogeneous colony morphology consisting of some flat and smooth but predominantly domed and glossy colonies (photograph kindly provided by D. van Soolingen).

in cattle but also accounted for 31% of human tuberculosis cases, mostly as pulmonary manifestation, in Germany between 1999 and 2001 (106). Easily recognized by its susceptibility to pyrazinamide, *M. caprae* thus adds to the agents of human tuberculosis contracted from animals. Based on mycobacterial interspersed repetitive unit genotyping, it was demonstrated that *M. caprae* is closely related to the branches of classical *M. bovis*, *M. pinnipedii*, *M. microti*, and ancestral *M. tuberculosis* but stands apart from modern *M. tuberculosis* (164).

M. microti

Originally isolated from rodents such as voles and shrews, *M. microti* causes naturally acquired tuberculosis in guinea pigs, rabbits, llamas (142), cats, and other warm-blooded animals. It has recently been identified as the causative agent of tuberculosis in both immunocompetent and immunosuppressed humans (49, 216). Usually revealing a characteristic "croissant"-like morphology in stained smears (Fig. 3), the organism normally fails to grow in culture. At least the vole type of *M. microti* can easily be recognized

upon spacer oligotyping (see chapter 29), since it contains an exceptionally short genomic direct repeat region resulting in identical two-spacer sequence reactions (216). Compared to *M. tuberculosis*, numerous deletions have been discovered (59), and the whole genome is currently being sequenced (www.sanger.ac.uk).

M. canettii

This organism was first collected by Georges Canetti in 1969. van Soolingen et al. (215) and Pfyffer et al. (153) reported *M. canettii* causing lymphadenitis in a child and generalized tuberculosis in an HIV-positive patient, respectively. Although its natural reservoir is unknown, the facts that both patients were exposed in Africa and more cases of cervical lymphadenitis have been reported from Djibouti (51) supported the hypothesis that *M. canettii* might be more abundant on the African continent. In 2002, pulmonary manifestation of *M. canettii* was reported in Africa (126), and in 2009, the first case of *M. canettii* meningitis recognized in a Sudanese refugee living in the United States was reported (184).

With its smooth, round, and glossy colonies (Fig. 4), M. canettii differs considerably from all other members of M. tuberculosis complex and can even be mistaken for an NTM. However, it has to be stressed that M. canettii may also exist as a stable rough morphotype (69), mimicking M. tuberculosis. As a consequence, adequate molecular techniques have to be applied to identify the organism at the species level (e.g., line probe assay [Hain Lifescience, Nehren, Germany], or 65-kDa hsp PCR restriction enzyme analysis). Studies by Brosch et al. (18) and Marmiesse et al. (116) of 20 regions where insertion-deletion events took place in the genome of M. tuberculosis suggested that M. canettii diverged first from the rest of M. tuberculosis complex. Based on VNTR genotyping and analysis of hsp65 gene polymorphism in 44 strains of M. canettii Fabre et al. (51) confirmed that M. canettii is the most probable source species of M. tuberculosis complex rather than just another branch of the taxon. In fact, it is assumed that M. canettii appeared some 2.8 million years ago and may, therefore, be the ancestor of all members of the present-day M. tuberculosis complex (71).

M. pinnipedii sp. nov.

On the basis of host preference, phenotypic, and genotypic characteristics, M. pinnipedii, a new member of the M. tuberculosis complex, was defined by Cousins et al. in 2003 (36). Pinnipeds appear to be the natural host, but the organism is also pathogenic for guinea pigs, rabbits, and possibly cattle. The organism also affects animals in zoological gardens, e.g., camels (Camelus bactrianus) and tapirs (Tapirus indicus [133]). Transmission of M. pinnipedii infection from sea lions to humans was recently demonstrated by TST and IGRAs (99). Infections with the "seal bacillus" manifest with granulomatous lesions in lymph nodes, lungs, pleura, and spleen and are able to disseminate.

M. leprae

As a result of rigorous control programs in many areas of endemicity such as South and Southeast Asia, Africa, and Latin America, the number of new cases of leprosy (Hansen's disease) has declined steadily. At the beginning of 2008, the registered prevalence of leprosy was 212,802 compared to >763,000 in 2001 (236). Access to diagnosis and treatment with multidrug therapy (dapsone, rifampin, and clofazimine [234]) remain key elements in the strategy to eliminate the disease. While most countries where the disease was previously endemic have now reached elimination (defined as a registered prevalence rate of <1 case/10,000 population), Brazil, Nepal, and Timor-Leste accounted for about 23% of registered cases at the beginning of 2008 (236). In the past centuries, leprosy occurred on a large scale also in Europe, in particular in Norway.

Leprosy is a chronic, granulomatous, and debilitating disease (77). Its principal manifestations include anesthetic skin lesions and peripheral neuropathy with nerve thickening. Leprosy illustrates a continuous spectrum of disease with very few demonstrable bacilli (tuberculoid leprosy) to a progressive, widespread, and most severe form of the disease with massive numbers of organisms due to the absence of cell-mediated immunity (lepromatous leprosy). The majority of leprosy patients show manifestations between these two polar forms and are clinically unstable. Medical complications arise from nerve damage and immune reactions (77).

Shedding from the nose, rather than from skin lesions, is important for transmission, which results most likely from prolonged and intimate contact with a person with multibacillary disease. The natural reservoir for M. leprae is not well established, but naturally occurring infections in the nine-banded armadillo (Dasypus novemcinctus) have been documented in the southern United States with a prevalence of 0 to 10% in the animal (111).

Together with M. lepraemurium, M. leprae differs from all other mycobacteria in that it cannot be cultured in vitro. By tradition, the diagnosis of leprosy is essentially a clinical one, based on finding one or more signs of disease which are supported by the presence of acid-fast bacilli (AFB) on slit skin smears or in skin biopsy specimens. Since leprosy bacilli are much less acid and alcohol fast than M. tuberculosis, 10% sulfuric acid is preferentially used as a decolorizer in place of an acid/alcohol solution (Fite-Faraco stain [57]). In the case of lepromatous disease, nodules and plaques are the preferred sites for biopsies, which will reveal numerous AFB. Conversely, in patients with tuberculoid leprosy, the rims of lesions should be biopsied, and there usually only a few or no AFB are found. A number of PCR assays have been established to conclusively detect the organism (171) and to characterize the M. leprae genotypes. For instance, multiple-locus VNTR analysis and single-nucleotide polymorphism typing (175) have been applied to search for leprosy transmission. The complete gene sequence is 3,268,203 bp in length with a G+C content of 57.8% (33). Similar to what is observed with M. bovis, the genome of M. leprae has lost >1.1 Mb and accumulated >1,100 pseudogenes during reductive evolution (33).

Unique clinicopathologic features of two cases of diffuse lepromatous leprosy and phylogenetic analyses of the genes of 16S rRNA, rpoB, and hsp65 led to the discovery of a new mycobacterial species, for which the name M. lepromatosis has been proposed (72).

Nontuberculous Mycobacteria Frequently Involved in Human Disease

The American Thoracic Society (ATS) and the Infectious Diseases Society of America have recently revised the guidelines for the diagnosis, treatment, and prevention of NTM disease in HIV-positive and HIV-negative individuals (4).

Slowly Growing Species

M. avium Complex

MAC organisms have been isolated from water, soil, plants, animals, indoor water systems, hot tubs, and pools. They are important pathogens of poultry and swine but were not recognized as a cause of human disease until the 1940s. Generally, these organisms are of low pathogenicity. Single positive specimens with low numbers of AFB are not infrequently observed in individuals without apparent disease. This complicates the interpretation of culture results, particularly from specimens of the respiratory tract (4, 52).

Before the advent of AIDS, the most common presentation of MAC infection was pulmonary disease showing several different clinical patterns, i.e., tuberculosis-like infiltrates, nodular bronchiectasis, and solitary nodules, as well as diffuse infiltrates in immunocompromised patients (222). Tuberculosis-like upper lobe fibrocavitary disease due to MAC typically occurs in white men 45 to 60 years of age who are heavy smokers, many of whom abuse alcohol, and some of whom have preexisting lung disease. The clinical presentation is similar to that of tuberculosis. In women, nodular bronchiectasis usually occurs in elderly nonsmoking individuals with no predisposing disorders of the lungs or immune system other than associated bronchiectasis ("Lady Windermere Syndrome" [44]). These patients usually present with persistent cough only; this disease tends to have a much slower progression than cavitary disease. Less frequent are thoracic infections in otherwise healthy children (55). MAC is also the leading cause of localized mycobacterial lymphadenitis in children, which is usually unilateral and involves lymph nodes in the submandibular, submaxillary, or periauricular areas (229). Generalized MAC infections in non-AIDS patients are extremely rare (87).

In patients (n = 385) with cystic fibrosis, overall prevalence of NTM was 8%, with the most prominent species being M. *abscessus* (39%), MAC (21%), and M. *gordonae* (18%) (158). While M. *abscessus* was isolated at all ages (study population, 1 to 24 years), MAC was not recovered before 15 years.

In conjunction with HIV infection MAC has become the most common environmental NTM causing disease in humans. Patients with AIDS may present with disseminated or focal infections (86, 87), mostly when the CD4 count is below 100 cells/mm^3. Bacteremia occurs in nearly all those patients, its magnitude ranging from <1 to 10^2 CFU/ml. The organism is found predominantly in circulating monocytes. Almost any organ (e.g., lungs or intestines) may be involved, with levels of mycobacteria as high as 10^{10} CFU/g of tissue. Focal infections commonly involve the lungs or the gastrointestinal tract, occasionally also peripheral lymph nodes (89).

MAC organisms are well known for their heterogeneous colony morphology. Glossy, whitish colonies may often occur together with smaller translucent colonies. A third, less frequent morphology resembles the dry and flat colonies of M. *tuberculosis*. Some MAC strains may develop a yellowish pigment with age.

MAC is a very heterogeneous group of AFB comprised of, by classical definition, the two taxa M. *avium* and M. *intracellulare*. Clinically, the former seems to be the more important pathogen in disseminated disease, while the latter is more often seen in respiratory disease. As more sophisticated molecular tools have become available in the laboratory, the taxonomy of MAC has become increasingly complex. New species have been proposed, and new subspecies have been discovered (206). At present, the species M. *avium* consists of three subspecies, i.e., subsp. *avium*, subsp. *silvaticum*, and subsp. *paratuberculosis* (194). The latter is an obligate pathogen of ruminants (Johne's disease), while in humans, the association of the organism with Crohn's disease seems to be specific. However, its role in the etiology of the disease remains to be defined (54). Since M. *avium* subsp. *paratuberculosis* is one of the slowest growing mycobacterial species, primary isolation can take several months, and the medium needs special supplements (206).

Additional strains that are similar to the classical MAC have been described. There are several important differences at the genetic level that distinguish a newer MAC organism, M. *avium* subsp. *hominissuis*, from M. *avium* subsp. *avium* (206). By using IS*1245*-based restriction fragment length polymorphism (RFLP), M. *avium* isolates from birds have been identified as M. *avium* subsp. *avium*. Since highly variable RFLP patterns were found among the M. *avium* isolates that all belonged to the M. *avium* subsp. *hominissuis*, a relation to pet birds in the etiology of lymphadenitis could not be established, i.e., the source of infection may be environmental (19, 125).

Genetically closely related to MAC organisms, but not typically considered part of the MAC is M. *lepraemurium*, the agent of rodent leprosy. This organism cannot be cultured and is identified by sequencing techniques only (206).

There are other taxa very closely related to MAC that could not be assigned to one or the other classical species of MAC. For instance, Tortoli et al. (199) proposed to elevate a genetic variant of MAC (MAC-A) to species rank as M. *chimaera* sp. nov. (see also reference 180), the former MAC-X sequevar gave rise to the species M. *colombiense* (137, 220), and the scotochromogenic sequevar MAC-Q is now also considered a species, named M. *vulneris* (212). Finally, Ben Salah et al. (12) have found clinical MAC isolates that appear to represent three other new species: M. *marseillense*, M. *timonense*, and M. *bouchedurhonense*.

M. genavense

M. *genavense* is a slowly growing NTM that was isolated in 1991 from the blood of an AIDS patient in Geneva, Switzerland, and was subsequently found in the United States and in several European countries (37, 52, 196). It has been associated with enteritis, genital and soft tissue infections, and lymphadenitis in HIV-positive and in HIV-negative immunocompromised individuals. M. *genavense* causes up to 12.8% of all NTM infections in AIDS patients (40). These infections are similar to those caused by MAC, except that stool specimens are more often smear positive in M. *genavense* infections (145). M. *genavense* is also the most common cause of mycobacterial disease in a variety of pet birds, including parrots and parakeets (84, 113).

Analysis of the 16S rRNA gene sequence indicates that this species is most closely related to M. *simiae*.

M. haemophilum

M. *haemophilum* was first isolated in 1978 from a subcutaneous lesion in a patient with Hodgkin's disease (178). Approximately 50% of infections have been in patients with AIDS, with a relatively large number reported from New York City. The other cases have been in other immunosuppressed individuals (96, 178), but also in immunocompetent pediatric patients with localized cervical lymphadenopathy (20, 31) or with a pulmonary nodule (227). The classical clinical presentation is that of multiple skin nodules in clusters or without a definite pattern, commonly involving the extremities, and occasionally associated with abscesses, draining fistulas, cellulitis, endophthalmitis, and osteomyelitis (52, 178).

M. kansasii

In the United States and many other countries, M. *kansasii* is second to MAC as a cause of NTM lung disease (4, 52). The organism has been cultured from its major reservoir, tap water, in municipalities around the world where clinical disease occurs. It is common in mine workers in both the United Kingdom and South Africa (35) and differs from that due to MAC in that the response to chemotherapy is much better (4).

Chronic pulmonary disease resembling classical tuberculosis is the most common manifestation of M. *kansasii* (183). Extrapulmonary infections are uncommon and include cervical lymphadenitis in children, cutaneous and soft tissue infections, and musculoskeletal disease. M. *kansasii* rarely disseminates, except in patients with severely impaired cellular immunity (e.g., due to organ transplants or AIDS [4]).

M. *kansasii* is a photochromogenic species. Studies of the base sequences of the 16S rRNA gene suggest that phylogenetically, it is closely related to the slowly growing, nonpigmented species M. *gastri*. Molecular studies have defined up to seven genotypes of M. *kansasii*, with subtypes I and II being the predominant subspecies responsible for human infection (4, 190).

M. malmoense

The species name M. malmoense is derived from the city of Malmö in Sweden, where the first strains were isolated from patients in 1977. Disease due to this organism was later found in other European countries (4) with increasing incidence in Scandinavia (83). It remains rare in the United States, Canada, and other areas of the world. However, in these countries M. malmoense infection may be more common than suspected, because it may require 8 to 12 weeks to isolate some strains, which is longer than many laboratories in North America hold mycobacterial cultures.

M. malmoense isolates are clinically significant in 70 to 80% of patients (83). Patients with M. malmoense infection are usually adults with chronic, difficult-to-treat pulmonary disease, mostly middle-aged men with previously documented pneumoconiosis or young children with cervical lymphadenitis (4, 52). Other extrapulmonary and disseminated infections have rarely been reported.

M. marinum

M. marinum causes cutaneous infections as a result of trauma to the skin and subsequent exposure to contaminated freshwater fish tanks ("fish tank granuloma") or salt water (109). The disease occurs worldwide. In the United States, it is most common in southern coastal states. The typical presentation is a single papulonodular lesion confined to one extremity, usually involving the elbow, knee, foot, toe, or finger. It appears 2 to 3 weeks after inoculation and, with time, may become verrucous or ulcerated (4, 52). A second type resembles cutaneous sporotrichosis, in which the primary inoculation is followed by spread along the lymphatics. More severe complications include tenosynovitis, arthritis, bursitis, and osteomyelitis. Disseminated infections, including infections in patients with AIDS or persons under systemic steroid therapy, have been rare (4).

M. marinum is photochromogenic and requires temperatures of 28 to 30°C for primary isolation. Israeli M. marinum isolates from humans and fish were compared by direct sequencing of the 16S rRNA and hsp65 genes and restriction mapping and amplified fragment length polymorphism analysis. Surprisingly, significant molecular differences separated all clinical isolates from the piscine isolates (207). Ghosh et al. (66) observed spores in old cultures of M. marinum, which upon exposure to fresh medium germinated into vegetative cells and reappeared again in the stationary phase with endospore formation. With its genome comprising ~6,636,827 bp (G+C content, 65.8%), M. marinum is genetically very closely related to M. ulcerans but also to M. tuberculosis, the latter having undergone genome downsizing and external lateral gene transfer to become a specialized pathogen of humans and other mammals (188).

M. simiae

M. simiae was first isolated in 1965 from rhesus macaques. More than 400 cases have been reported from a few geographic areas, including the southwestern United States, Israel, and the Caribbean (4, 172). The environmental niche is assumed to be aquatic. The majority of cases relate to HIV-positive patients, involving primarily the lungs and the reticuloendothelial system. In non-HIV patients, pulmonary manifestations are common, but lymphadenopathy, skin lesions, genitourinary tract infections, and uveitis also occur (4, 114, 183, 211). In Israeli cystic fibrosis patients, M. simiae was the organism seen most often (40.5%), followed by M. abscessus (31%) and MAC (14.3%) (108). M. simiae is one of the very few NTM synthesizing niacin.

Unless tested for pigment production under the influence of light, it may be misidentified as M. tuberculosis by inexperienced observers.

M. szulgai

M. szulgai was first described as a distinct species in 1972 and is rarely recovered from the environment. Therefore, isolation of this organism is almost always considered clinically significant. Patients were mainly middle-aged men presenting with chronic pulmonary disease indistinguishable from tuberculosis (4). The remaining presentations included rare cases of bursitis, cervical adenitis, tenosynovitis, cutaneous infections, and osteomyelitis (4, 52). Cases of M. szulgai infection in AIDS patients and disseminated disease in an immunocompetent patient have been reported as well. Although M. szulgai is closely related to M. malmoense based on the 16S rRNA gene sequences, phenotypic distinction between the two species is easy. M. szulgai is scotochromogenic at 37°C and photochromogenic at 25°C (98).

M. ulcerans

The frequency of M. ulcerans infection has long been underestimated due to difficulties in isolating the pathogen. Today, it is the third most frequent mycobacterial disease in humans after tuberculosis and leprosy. In Africa the disease is known as Buruli ulcer and in Australia as Bairnsdale ulcer (4, 52, 162, 235). Cases of Buruli ulcer have also become evident in Peru in the most recent past (70). Closely associated with tropical wetlands, M. ulcerans most likely proliferates in mud beneath stagnant waters. Evidence for a role of insects in transmission of this pathogen is growing.

All ages and both sexes are affected, among them many children under 15 years. Manifestation typically begins as a painless lump under the skin at the site of previous trauma on the lower extremities. After a few weeks, a shallow ulcer develops at the site of the lump. M. ulcerans produces a cytotoxin (mycolactone) with immunomodulating properties that causes necrosis (208). The type of disease ranges from a localized nodule or ulcer to widespread ulcerative or nonulcerative disease including osteomyelitis. If untreated, severe limb deformities with contractures and scarring are common. There is growing evidence that M. ulcerans also produces disease in wild animals such as lizards, opossums, koala bears, armadillos, rats, mice, and cattle (161).

Failure to cultivate this organism in the past was due to its fastidious, heat-sensitive nature (temperature optimum, 30°C) as well as to an excessively long generation time (up to 36 h). The organism often requires several months of incubation to achieve isolation in primary culture. Molecular techniques that may provide a more rapid result have been developed (62, 157). Comparative genomic analysis has revealed that M. ulcerans arose from M. marinum by horizontal gene transfer of a virulence plasmid that carries a cluster of genes for mycolactone production, followed by reductive evolution (41).

M. xenopi

M. xenopi was first isolated in 1957 from skin lesions on an African toad (Xenopus laevis), but it was not recognized as a human pathogen until 1965. In some areas such as Canada and Southeast England, it is second only to MAC as an NTM clinical isolate (4). Increased isolation of M. xenopi from clinical specimens may also be due to improved laboratory techniques. With an optimum growth temperature of 45°C, it seems to frequently occur in hot water systems.

Nosocomial infection and pseudoinfection via water storage tanks in hospitals have also been described.

Most M. *xenopi* infections occur in the lungs, usually in male adult patients with underlying lung disease such as chronic obstructive pulmonary disease or bronchiectasis. Extrapulmonary infections such as septic arthritis, spondylitis, and disseminated disease have also been described in immunocompromised individuals (4). Skin and soft tissue manifestations as well as a recent case report of M. *xenopi* spondylodiscitis in an AIDS patient not only highlight its potential pathogenic role but also point to the uncertainties in therapeutic management (124).

Nontuberculous Slowly Growing Mycobacteria That Are Rarely Recovered or Rarely Cause Human Disease

Several species of slowly growing mycobacteria including M. *gordonae*, M. *scrofulaceum*, and M. *terrae* complex are frequently recovered but are rarely associated with human disease. Some of the case reports of infections attributable to these mycobacteria, especially from the era before the introduction of molecular laboratory techniques, lack sufficient documentation of identification or disease association. Other species (such as M. *asiaticum* or M. *shimoidei*) are so rarely recovered that most laboratories will never see them.

M. asiaticum

M. *asiaticum* was not recognized as a distinct species until 1971. The photochromogenic organism has since very infrequently been isolated from patients with respiratory disease in Australia, the United States, and elsewhere (193). Cases of bursitis and tenosynovitis have been described as well.

M. celatum

First described in 1993, M. *celatum* has been isolated from diverse geographic areas (throughout the United States as well as in Finland and Somalia), mostly from respiratory tract specimens but also from stool and blood. In one series, 32% of the patients from whom M. *celatum* was isolated were infected with HIV. M. *celatum* has also been isolated from immunocompetent patients (a child with lymphadenitis and an elderly patient with a fatal pulmonary infection [195]).

M. *celatum* shares phenotypical characteristics with MAC, M. *malmoense*, and M. *shimoidei* and thus cannot be identified with conventional tests. Within the bacterial chromosome, M. *celatum* has two copies of the 16S rRNA gene. Several subtypes (1 to 3) have been identified by 16S rRNA gene sequencing or RFLP of the gene encoding the 65-kDa *hsp*. Due to high similarities of the 16S rRNA gene sequence with that of M. *tuberculosis* a few strains have been misidentified as M. *tuberculosis* complex by a commercially available DNA probe or as M. *xenopi* on account of similar biochemical and cultural features (195).

M. gordonae

M. *gordonae* is the most commonly encountered "nonpathogenic" species in clinical mycobacteriology laboratories. This scotochromogenic species is widely distributed in soil and water. A pseudo-outbreak associated with drinking water in a French hospital underlined the necessity for proper maintenance of water supply equipment (107). Convincing evidence that M. *gordonae* plays a role in disease is difficult to find (4). There are a few reports of peritonitis in patients undergoing continuous ambulatory peritoneal dialysis and in renal transplant patients (160). Eckburg et al. (47) have reviewed clinical and chest radiographic findings among persons with sputum culture positive for M. *gordonae* and concluded that it is a nonpathogenic colonizing organism, even among persons with local or general immune suppression and abnormal chest X-ray findings.

M. scrofulaceum

The name of this species was derived from scrofula, a historical term used to describe mycobacterial infections of the cervical lymph glands. Until the 1980s, M. *scrofulaceum* was the most common cause of mycobacterial cervical lymphadenitis in children. Since then it has been replaced primarily by MAC (229). Other types of clinical disease are rare. They include pulmonary disease, conjunctivitis, osteomyelitis, meningitis, granulomatous hepatitis, and disseminated disease (4, 52). M. *scrofulaceum* accounted for 14% of the isolates tested in respiratory specimens collected from South African miners (35) and for ~2% of the mycobacterial infections in AIDS patients (4).

M. shimoidei

M. *shimoidei* was first described in 1988 in a case of a Japanese patient with chronic cavitary lung disease. Only a few clinical cases have been reported since, mainly in Japan and Finland (120). It is a thermophilic organism growing well at 45°C. Biochemically, the organism is similar to M. *terrae* complex, but it can be distinguished by catalase and β-galactosidase tests. The unique sequence of the 16S rRNA gene and the 16S-23S rRNA gene spacer region allow unambiguous identification of the organism (104).

M. terrae complex

M. *terrae* complex consists of three species, M. *terrae*, M. *nonchromogenicum*, and M. *triviale*. Clinical disease due to M. *terrae* is generally limited to tenosynovitis of the hand following local trauma and pulmonary disease (4). M. *nonchromogenicum*, ubiquitous in the aquatic environment, has been the cause of bacteremia in an AIDS patient (4). Separation of the members of the complex, especially M. *terrae* from M. *nonchromogenicum*, requires molecular methods.

New Species of Nontuberculous Mycobacteria

Most of these species have been described within the past 10 years (195). As a consequence of more sophisticated molecular technologies applied in the clinical mycobacteriology laboratory, the number of new species is rapidly increasing (Table 1). However, much less is known about these species and their clinical relevance remains to be elucidated.

SAFETY, TRANSPORT, AND COLLECTION OF SPECIMENS

Laboratory Safety Procedures

Nosocomial transmission of M. *tuberculosis* from patients or specimens is of major concern to health care workers and laboratory personnel. Because of the low infective dose of M. *tuberculosis* for humans (50% infective dose, <10 AFB), specimens from suspected or known cases of tuberculosis must be considered to be potentially infectious and handled with appropriate precautions (25, 58). Risk assessment and the use of appropriate biosafety practices are of prime importance. Control of aerosol production and other forms of mycobacterial contamination requires the use of

TABLE 1 Recently discovered NTM species associated with human disease[a]

Species	Clinical manifestation or origin of specimen	Remarks	Yr detected (reference[s])
M. arosiense	Osteomyelitis	Scotochromogenic	2008 (9)
M. arupense	Tenosynovitis	Former "MCRO 6," genetically close to M. nonchromogenicum	2006 (118, 203)
M. bohemicum	Lymphadenitis, respiratory tract, skin	Scotochromogenic, HPLC and GLC profiles overlapping with MAC and M. scrofulaceum	1998 (88, 195)
M. branderi	Ulcerative tenosynovitis, respiratory tract	Photochromogen, genotypically most closely related to M. celatum	1995 (195)
M. conspicuum	Respiratory tract	Pale yellow, coccobacillary, temperature optimum 22–31°C, grows at 37°C in liquid media only, closely related to M. asiaticum and M. gordonae; a few clinical cases only	1995 (195, 213)
M. doricum	CSF	Scotochromogenic, pathogenic potential unclear	2001 (198)
M. florentinum	Lymphadenitis, respiratory tract	Close to M. triplex and M. lentiflavum	2005 (200)
M. heckeshornense	Cavitary lung disease, lymphadenitis, tenosynovitis	Scotochromogenic, grows poorly on solid media, colonies resemble M. xenopi	2000 (68, 93, 122, 195, 209)
M. heidelbergense	Lymphadenitis, pulmonary disease	Nonpigmented, grows poorly on egg-based medium, biochemically indistinguishable from M. malmoense, genetically closely related to M. simiae	1997 (195)
M. interjectum	Lymphadenitis, chronic lung disease, polyangitis	Scotochromogenic as well as nonpigmented, coccobacillary, genetically related to M. simiae	1993 (59, 61, 168, 195)
M. intermedium	Chronic bronchitis, dermatitis	Photochromogenic and scotochromogenic, coccobacillary	1993 (48, 195)
M. kubicae	Respiratory tract	Scotochromogenic, domed colonies, cells rod shaped, frequently bent, genetically related to M. simiae, pathogenic potential questionable	2000 (195)
M. kumamotonense	Respiratory tract	Nonchromogenic, related to M. xenopi complex	2006 (118)
M. kyorinense	Lymphadenitis, respiratory tract	Closely related to M. celatum	2009 (143)
M. lacus	Bursitis with caseating granulomas after trauma	Large bacilli with prominent beading, nonpigmented, genetically related to M. malmoense and M. marinum	2002 (195)
M. lentiflavum	Lymphadenitis, cavitary pulmonary disease, chronic pulmonary disease, spondylodiscitis, disseminated disease; skin, pleural effusion	Scotochromogenic, coccobacillary, colonies pale yellow, tiny, genetically related to M. simiae	1996 (195, 197)
M. mantenii	Lymphadenitis, pulmonary disease	Scotochromogenic, closely related to M. scrofulaceum	2009 (214)
M. nebraskense	Pulmonary	Photochromogenic, close to MAC, M. scrofulaceum, M. malmoense, and M. kansasii	2004 (129)
M. palustre	Lymphadenitis	Scotochromogenic, genetically related to M. simiae group and M. kubicae, single case reported	2002 (195)
M. parascrofulaceum	Cervix, respiratory tract	Scotochromogenic, formerly "MCRO," phenotypically close to M. scrofulaceum, genetically close to M. simiae	2004 (204)
M. parmense	Lymphadenitis	Scotochromogenic	2004 (53)
M. riyadhense	Maxillary sinusitis	Nonchromogenic	2009 (210)
M. sherrisii	"Type strains" from various clinical sources	Previously considered "M. simiae serotype 2"	2004 (181)
M. saskatchewanense	Sputum, pleural fluid	Scotochromogenic, former "MCRO 8," genetically close to M. interjectum	2004 (205)
M. senuense	Respiratory tract	Nonchromogenic, belongs to M. terrae subclade	2008 (136)
M. seoulense	Respiratory tract	Scotochromogenic, close to M. nebraskense and M. scrofulaceum	2007 (135)
M. tilburgii	Dysuria, hematuria, intestinal lesions, pulmonary nodules, disseminated disease	Not cultivable	2006 (149)
M. triplex	Lymphadenitis, pulmonary disease, disseminated disease	Nonphotochromogenic, closely related to M. genavense and M. simiae	1996 (195)
M. tusciae	Lymphadenitis, respiratory tract (cystic fibrosis)	Scotochromogenic, rough colonies, role as a pathogen unclear	1999 (195)

[a]CSF, cerebrospinal fluid; HPLC, high-performance liquid chromatography; GLC, gas liquid chromatography.

properly functioning biosafety cabinets (BSCs), centrifuges with safety carriers, and meticulous processing techniques (29, 58; see also chapter 10).

The most recent CDC *Guidelines on Biosafety in Microbiological and Biomedical Laboratories* (25) have given more restrictive recommendations for working with M. *tuberculosis* complex. In the light of the three-times-higher incidence of tuberculosis in laboratory personnel working with M. *tuberculosis* complex than that of those not working with these agents, the low infective dose of tubercle bacilli, and the rapid spread by infecting aerosols, biosafety level 2 practices are not ideal. Therefore, the CDC suggests biosafety level 2 practices and procedures, containment equipment, and facilities only for non-aerosol-producing manipulations of clinical specimens such as preparation of AFB smears. All aerosol-generating activities must be conducted in a BSC class II. Efforts should be made to apply rigorous biosafety level 3 practices and containment equipment and to provide biosafety level 3 facilities for laboratories associated with higher risk, i.e., those involved in the manipulation of cultures (identification and susceptibility testing) of M. *tuberculosis* complex. Such practices require that laboratory access be restricted, that directional airflow be used to maintain the laboratory under negative pressure, and that workers wear special laboratory clothing and gloves, etc. (25, 29). The changes by the CDC may, in the future, invite more laboratories to abandon mycobacterial culture, if biosafety level 3 facilities cannot be afforded.

All respiratory protective devices (respirators) used in the workplace should be certified by the National Institute for Occupational Safety and Health (NIOSH) (94). Respirators that contain a NIOSH-certified N-series filter with a 95% efficiency (N-95) rating are appropriate for use. They meet the recommendations from the CDC for selection of respirators for protection against M. *tuberculosis*, i.e., (i) the unloaded filter must filter particles 0.3 μm in size with an efficiency of 95% at flow rates up to 50 liters/min; (ii) the respirator must be qualitatively or quantitatively fit tested to obtain a face seal leakage rate of no more than 10%; (iii) it must fit different facial sizes and characteristics, which is attained by making the respirators available in at least three sizes; and (iv) it must be checked for face piece fit by the person wearing the respirator each time it is worn in accordance with the Occupational Safety and Health Administration (OSHA) standards. Surgical masks are not NIOSH-certified respirators and must not be worn to provide respiratory protection.

The decision regarding when and if to use respiratory protective devices in the laboratory should be based on risk assessment. A respirator program should be implemented by the laboratory and include a written protocol describing when respirator use is necessary and procedures addressing the following: (i) selection of the appropriate respirator; (ii) how to conduct fit testing; and (iii) training of personnel in the use, fit checking, and storage of the respirator.

All work involving specimens or cultures, such as making smears, inoculating media, adding reagents to biochemical tests, opening centrifuge cups, and sonication, must be performed in a BSC. The handling of all specimens suspected of containing mycobacteria (including specimens processed for other microorganisms), with the exception of centrifugation for concentration purposes, must be done within the BSC. Specimens that are to be taken out of the BSC should be covered before transport. All work surfaces, including benchtops and the inside of the BSC, should be cleaned with an appropriate disinfectant before and after work. Effective disinfectants include Amphyl (Reckitt Benckiser North America, Wayne, NJ) or other phenol-soap mixtures, and 0.05% to 0.5% sodium hypochlorite (the concentration varies according to the nature of the contaminated surface). Five percent phenol is no longer recommended as a surface disinfectant due to the documented toxicity of this compound to personnel. UV light is a useful adjunct for surface decontamination and may be used to radiate the work area when it is not in use. Centrifuges should be used with aerosol-free safety carriers to contain debris in the event that tubes break. Use of electric incinerators rather than open flames is recommended. The excess inoculum from inoculating loops, wire, or spades may be removed by dipping the tool into a container of 95% ethanol in washed sand prior to insertion in an incinerator. Disposable inoculating loops are recommended, as are syringes with permanently attached needles if needles are required. An autoclave should be available in an easily accessible area and used to decontaminate infectious waste before removal to disposal areas.

Personnel should be regularly monitored with either the TST or one of the IGRAs, annually or more often if a conversion in the laboratory/institution has been documented. Those with positive TST or positive IGRAs should be evaluated for active tuberculosis with a chest X ray and clinical evaluation. Physical examinations should be obtained when necessary. New converters should be referred to the employee health and infection control departments for epidemiological evaluation. Laboratories should have written protocols describing procedures for handling laboratory accidents. In case of a laboratory accident with possible formation of aerosols, personnel should hold their breath as much as possible, make sure BSCs are on and centrifuges are turned off, and then leave the area to get protection as soon as possible, with the door closed for at least 30 minutes (the amount of time depends on the type of accident and the amount of risk). Using appropriate respiratory protection devices, personnel can return to the accident area to clean the spill. After such an incident, TST-negative personnel or IGRA-negative personnel should be monitored and retested. Persons who are pregnant or immunocompromised should be discouraged from working in the mycobacteriology laboratory. (See also chapter 10.)

Transportation and Transfer of Biological Agents

Mycobacteria are on the list of infectious agents being regulated for shipping and transfer. Stringent regulations on the transportation of biological agents have been enacted in the United States (for instance, M. *tuberculosis* cultures are no longer accepted by the U.S. Postal Services) as well as in other countries to ensure that the public and workers in the transportation chain are protected from exposure to any infectious agents. Protection is achieved through (i) the requirements of rigorous packaging that will withstand rough handling and contain all liquid material within the package without leakage to the outside; (ii) appropriate labeling of the package with the biohazard symbol and other labels to alert the workers in the transportation chain to the hazardous contents of the package; (iii) documentation of hazardous contents of the package, should such information be necessary in an emergency situation; and (iv) training of workers in the transportation chain to familiarize them with the hazardous contents in order to be able to respond to emergency situations. Transport of specimens within and outside a facility are well described in a document published by the CLSI (29).

Readers are referred to the regulatory documents of their respective countries. For the United States further information is available in the following documents.

Public Health Service. 42 CFR Part 72. *Interstate Transportation of Etiologic Agents*. This regulation is in revision to harmonize it with the other U.S. and international regulations. http://www.cdc.gov/od/ohs/biosfty/shipregs.htm

Department of Transportation. 49 CFR Parts 171–180. *Hazardous Materials Regulations*. Applies to the shipment of infectious substances in commercial transportation within the United States. http://www.hazmat.dot.gov.

U.S. Postal Service. 39 CFR Part 20. *International Postal Service (International Mail Manual)*. 39 CFR Part 111. *General Information on Postal Service (Domestic Mail Manual)*. Regulations on transporting infectious substances through the U.S. Postal Services are codified in Section 601.10.17 of the *Domestic Mail Manual* and Section 135 of the *International Mail Manual*. A copy of the *Domestic Mail Manual* may be obtained from the Government Printing Office by calling 1-202-512-1800 or 866-512-1800 (toll free). http://bookstore.gpo.gov or http://pe.usps.gov.

OSHA. 29 CFR Part 1910.1030. *Occupational Exposure to Bloodborne Pathogens*. Provides minimal packaging and labeling requirements for transport of blood and body fluids. Information may be obtained from your local OSHA office. http://www.osha.gov/pls/oshaweb/owadisp.show_document?p_table=STANDARDS&p_id=10051.

Technical Instructions for the Safe Transport of Dangerous Goods by Air. International Civil Aviation Organization (ICAO). Applies to the shipment of infectious substances by air and is recognized in the United States and by most countries worldwide. A copy of these regulations may be obtained from the ICAO Document Sales Unit at 514-954-8022. http://www.icao.org.

International Air Transport Association. *Dangerous Goods Regulations*. These regulations are issued by an airline association, are based on the ICAO Technical Instructions, and are followed by most airline carriers. A copy of the DGR may be obtained by calling 1-800-716-6326 (for the United States and Canada) or +41-22-770-2751 (for Europe, Africa, and the Middle East). http://www.iata.org/index.htm or http://www.who.int/en/.

There is also a Saf-T-Pak CD available including updates, which is available at http://www.saftpak.com/stpcdrom.asp.

Permits *must* be obtained for importation and exportation of biological and infectious agents. These are obtained by contacting the Centers for Disease Control and Prevention, Atlanta, GA (http://www.cdc.gov).

Collection and Storage of Specimens

General Rules

Many different types of clinical specimens may be collected for mycobacteriological analyses (90, 98). The majority originate from the respiratory tract (sputum, tracheal and bronchial aspirates, and bronchoalveolar lavage specimens), but urine, gastric aspirates, tissues, biopsy specimens, and normally sterile body fluids such as cerebrospinal fluid and pleural and pericardial aspirates are other commonly submitted specimens. Blood and fecal specimens are usually submitted from immunocompromised patients only.

Specimens should always be collected and submitted in sterile, leakproof, disposable, appropriately labeled laboratory-approved containers without any fixatives. Generally, transport media or preservatives are not necessary owing to the robust nature of mycobacteria. Minute biopsy material (e.g., fine-needle aspirates) may be immersed in a small amount of sterile physiological saline. Collection should bypass areas of possible contamination as much as possible, e.g., tap water, since the presence of environmental mycobacteria may result in false-positive smear and/or culture results (221). In general, swabs are not optimal for the recovery of AFB since they provide limited material and the hydrophobicity of the mycobacterial cell envelope often compromises a transfer from swabs to solid or broth media. If transport to the laboratory is delayed more than 1 h, specimens (except blood) should be refrigerated at 4°C. Likewise, upon arrival in the laboratory, specimens should be refrigerated until processed (see chapters 9 and 16 for additional information on specimen collection).

Sputum

Sputum, expectorated or induced, is the principal specimen obtained for the diagnosis of pulmonary tuberculosis. Major guidelines recommend that an early-morning specimen should be collected on three consecutive days (3, 29). The number of specimens has, however, been questioned for quite some time. Recent meta-analyses confirmed the low yield of the third specimen in the classical spot-morning-spot strategy (119, 128), inasmuch as the average incremental yield and/or the increase in sensitivity of examining a third specimen ranged between 2% and 5% only. Similarly, Monkongdee et al. (130) and Noeske et al. (140) concluded that a third sputum smear added little to the diagnosis of tuberculosis, even in populations with high HIV prevalence. Pooled sputum specimens are unacceptable for mycobacterial processing because of increased contamination (98). Follow-up cultures should be considered because it is culture (and not smear) that yields a definite answer as to whether chemotherapy has been effective. Children may have difficulties producing sputum. In this age group, a gastric aspirate is usually the specimen of choice for the diagnosis of pulmonary tuberculosis.

Bronchial Aspirates, Bronchoalveolar Lavage Specimens, Fine-Needle Aspirates, and Lung Biopsies

For some patients unable to produce sputum, invasive collection techniques such as bronchoscopy may be necessary to diagnose pulmonary tuberculosis or mycobacteriosis. Special care is imperative for cleansing the bronchoscope to avoid cross-contamination with AFB from a preceding patient who underwent bronchoscopy. Also, the bronchoscope should not be in contact with tap water, which may contain environmental mycobacteria. Specimens collected by other invasive techniques such as fine-needle aspiration and open-lung biopsy may be submitted in difficult-to-diagnose cases.

Gastric Lavage Fluids

Aspiration of swallowed sputum from the stomach by gastric lavage may be necessary for infants, young children, and the obtunded. Fasting, early-morning specimens are recommended in order to obtain sputum swallowed during sleep. Samples of 5 to 10 ml, adjusted to neutral pH, should be collected on three consecutive days. If they cannot be processed within 4 h, the laboratory should provide sterile disposable containers with 100 mg of sodium carbonate for collection. Nonneutralized specimens are not acceptable because long-term exposure to acid is detrimental to mycobacteria.

Urine

The first morning specimen should be collected on three consecutive days by midstream (clean catch) into a sterile container. The first morning specimen provides the best results because organisms accumulate in the bladder overnight. A minimum of 40 ml of urine is usually required for culture. Twenty-four-hour pooled specimens and small-volume specimens (unless a larger volume is not obtainable) are unacceptable. Catheterization should be used only if a midstream sample cannot be obtained.

Body Fluids

As much body fluid as possible (e.g., cerebrospinal, pleural, peritoneal, pericardial, or synovial [joint] fluid) is aseptically collected by aspiration or during surgical procedures. Bloody specimens may be anticoagulated with sodium polyanethol sulfonate. Certain body fluids (such as cerebrospinal fluid and peritoneal dialysis effluent) may contain very small numbers of mycobacteria. It is advisable to submit larger specimen volumes (e.g., >5 ml for cerebrospinal fluid) to increase culture yields and the chance to detect mycobacterial organisms. Never submit a swab dipped in fluid.

Tissues (Lymph Node, Skin, and Other Biopsy Material), Abscess Contents, Aspirated Pus, and Wounds

Specimens submitted in formalin are unacceptable for smear and culture. As much material as possible should be aspirated aseptically into a sterile container. Tissues must not be immersed in saline or other liquid or wrapped in gauze. For cutaneous ulcers, biopsy material should be collected from the periphery of the lesion. Minute biopsy material may be moistened with a small amount of sterile saline. It is advisable to incubate a second set of cultures at 30°C since one of the organisms with a lower temperature optimum (*M. haemophilum*, *M. marinum*, and *M. ulcerans*) may be the infectious agent. Swabs are strongly discouraged, unless they are the only specimens available.

Blood

The majority of disseminated mycobacterial infections are due to MAC. Therefore, if this organism is isolated from blood, it is always associated with clinical disease. If blood has to be transported before inoculation of the medium, sodium polyanethol sulfate, heparin, or citrate may be used as anticoagulants. Blood collected in EDTA or in conventional blood culture bottles and coagulated blood are not acceptable. Direct inoculation of blood onto a solid medium is not recommended either.

For many years, the Isolator system (Wampole Laboratories, Cranbury, NJ) and the radiometric BACTEC 13A blood culture bottle (Becton Dickinson Microbiology Systems, Sparks, MD) were the only reliable and recommended systems for mycobacterial blood cultures (6). Since the BACTEC 13A medium is no longer available, cultures from blood and bone marrow specimens have to be obtained by alternative media, e.g., the MYCO/F LYTIC bottles (Becton Dickinson) (6, 102) or the BacT/Alert MB Blood medium (Biomérieux, Marcy-L'Etoile/France) (75).

Stool Specimens

Generally, cultures from feces (>1 g) for mycobacteria are not encouraged, except for patients with AIDS to detect MAC. Past recommendations have been that stool be cultured for mycobacteria only if the direct smear of unprocessed stool is positive for AFB. The sensitivity of the stool smear, however, is only 32 to 34% (131), suggesting that its results should not determine whether a culture for mycobacteria be performed. Screening with smears is, therefore, not an effective way to identify patients at risk for developing disseminated MAC infection (78).

Inadequate Specimens

Processing of inappropriate clinical specimens for mycobacteria is a waste of both financial and personnel resources. There are quite a few reasons why a specimen should not be accepted (and the clinician should be notified), e.g., (i) too small an amount submitted; (ii) specimens consisting of saliva; (iii) dried swabs (biopsy preferable); (iv) pooled sputum or urine; (v) broken sample containers; (vi) too long an interval (>7 days) between specimen collection and processing (29). Clinical staff must be properly trained to prevent submission of unacceptable specimens.

For additional information regarding the collection and storage of specimens the reader is referred to the new document of the CLSI (29).

ISOLATION AND STAINING PROCEDURES

Because mycobacteria are usually slowly growing and require long incubation times, a variety of microorganisms other than mycobacteria can overgrow cultures of specimens obtained from nonsterile sites. Appropriate pretreatment and processing procedures (homogenization, decontamination, concentration, culture media, and conditions of incubation) must be selected to facilitate optimum recovery of mycobacteria (29, 90, 98). In particular, pretreatment of specimens has to be done carefully, i.e., by eliminating contaminants as much as possible while not seriously affecting the viability of mycobacteria.

Processing of Specimens

Decontamination of a specimen should be attempted only if it is thought to be contaminated. Tissues or body fluids collected aseptically usually do not require pretreatment. If the need to decontaminate a specimen is not clear, the specimen may be refrigerated until routine bacteriologic cultures are checked the next day. It may, however, be easier to initially inoculate a chocolate agar plate to check for sterility overnight before a sample is processed for mycobacteria.

Normally Sterile Specimens

Normally sterile tissue samples may be ground in sterile 0.85% saline or 0.2% bovine albumin and then inoculated directly to the media. Because body fluids commonly contain only small numbers of mycobacteria, they should be concentrated to maximize the yield of mycobacteria before inoculation of media, i.e., centrifuged at ≥3,000 × *g* for 15 min prior to inoculating the sediment. If the volume of fluid submitted for culture is small and cannot be obtained again, it may be added directly to liquid media.

Contaminated Specimens

The majority of specimens submitted for mycobacterial culture consists of a complex organic matrix contaminated with a variety of organisms. Mucin may trap mycobacterial cells and protect contaminating bacteria from the action of decontaminating agents. Thus, mycobacteria are recovered optimally from clinical specimens through the use of procedures which reduce or eliminate contaminating bacteria while releasing mycobacteria trapped in mucin and cells. Liquefaction of certain specimens, particularly sputum, is often necessary. Mycobacteria are then concentrated to enhance detection in stained smears and by culture.

Digestion and Decontamination Methods

Sodium hydroxide (NaOH), the most commonly used decontaminant, also serves as a mucolytic agent but must be used cautiously because it is only slightly less harmful to tubercle bacilli than to the contaminating organisms. The stronger the alkali, the higher its temperature during the time it acts on the specimen, and the longer it is allowed to act, the greater will be the killing action on both contaminants and mycobacteria. Harsh decontamination can kill 20 to 90% of the mycobacteria in a clinical specimen (29, 90, 98). Homogenization should occur by centrifugal swirling, and this swirling should not be vigorous enough to allow material to rise to the cap. After agitation, there should be at least a 15-min delay before opening the tube to allow any fine aerosol droplets formed during the mixing to settle. All such procedures should be carried out in a class II BSC.

Most commonly, a combination liquefaction-decontamination mixture is used. N-Acetyl-L-cysteine (NALC), dithiothreitol, and several enzymes effectively liquefy sputum. These agents have no direct inhibitory effect on bacterial cells; however, their use permits treatment with lower concentrations of NaOH, thereby indirectly improving the recovery of mycobacteria. The appropriate concentration of NaOH is dependent on the observed contamination rate for the individual laboratory. If specimens are heavily contaminated, NaOH may be increased (not exceeding 5 to 6%). The most widely used digestion-decontamination method is the NALC-2% NaOH method (29, 90, 98; see Appendix 1 below). Pretreatment of clinical specimens with sodium dodecyl (lauryl) sulfate-NaOH is, by contrast, not suitable for the Mycobacteria Growth Indicator Tube (MGIT) cultivation method (155) since it results in poor recovery of mycobacteria and a delayed mean time to detection of AFB. When C_{18}-carboxypropylbetaine was utilized, culture and smear sensitivity significantly improved compared to the NALC-NaOH procedure. However, the contamination rate was extremely high (20.8%) (146). Pretreatment of sputum from cystic fibrosis patients with chlorhexidine has yielded twice as many NTM-positive cultures compared to specimens treated with NALC-NaOH. This option is interesting, taking into account that recovery of NTM is hampered by the presence of *Pseudomonas aeruginosa* in the respiratory tract of 80% of these patients (56).

Addition of cetylpyridinium chloride (CPC) (see Appendix 1) to specimens mailed from remote collection stations to a central processing station has yielded a good recovery of *M. tuberculosis* without overgrowth by contaminating bacteria, but based on the authors' experience, this agent may seriously compromise culture, e.g., in the BACTEC 460TB System.

In addition to CPC, use of sodium carbonate and sodium borate has been recommended for rural areas, allowing *M. tuberculosis* to remain viable for 5 to 18 days (16). Under field conditions liquefaction and concentration of sputum for acid-fast staining may also be conducted by treating the specimens with an equal volume of 5% sodium hypochlorite solution (undiluted household bleach) and waiting 15 min before centrifugation (98). Such treated specimens, however, cannot be cultured because the chemical seriously affects viability of AFB. The major limitation, therefore, is that a second specimen must be collected for culture. The method is very useful, however, only for rapid smear preparation and interpretation in laboratories that do not process specimens for culture or that do not have a BSC. Finally, a universal sample-processing method utilizing guanidium isothiocyanate did not provide any significant advantage over the standard NALC method in a recent field study performed in Uganda (22).

Many conventional decontamination protocols used in mycobacteriology interfere with the viability of *M. ulcerans*. Oxalic acid, NaOH, and to a lesser extent mild HCl have a detrimental impact on the viability of *M. ulcerans* (150). However, treatment with *mild* hydrochloric acid (final concentration, 0.03 N) (150) or oxalic acid (239) as a decontamination agent provides best results. A mixture of polymyxin B, amphotericin B, nalidixic acid, trimethoprim, and azlocillin (PANTA) may control secondary contamination.

No one method of digestion and decontamination is ideal for all clinical specimens, for all laboratories, and under all circumstances. The laboratorian must be aware of the inherent limitations of the various methods used. Even under the best of conditions, all currently available procedures are toxic for mycobacteria to some extent. Thus, the best yield of mycobacteria may be expected to result from the use of the mildest decontamination procedure that sufficiently controls contaminants. Strict adherence to specimen processing is mandatory to ensure survival of the maximal number of mycobacteria.

Commonly used digestion-decontamination methods are described with step-by-step instructions in references 29, 90, and 98 and in Appendix 1 of this chapter. In general, the specimen is diluted with an equal volume of digestant and allowed to incubate for some time. A neutralizing buffer is added, and the specimen is centrifuged in order to sediment any AFB present. Centrifugation should be carried out at ≥3,000 × g for 15 min to get maximum recovery. The sediment is then inoculated onto the appropriate liquid and solid media.

Whatever method is used, care must be taken to prevent laboratory cross-contamination of patient specimens during processing due to aerosols (7, 21, 29). A single false-positive culture for *M. tuberculosis* could easily be the basis of a diagnosis of tuberculosis, with profound consequences for the patient, clinical management, epidemiologic investigations, and public health control measures.

Optimizing Decontamination Procedures

While no contamination or very low rates of contamination indicate that the pretreatment conditions were too harsh and eliminated not only bacteria and fungi but also mycobacteria, a rate exceeding 5% of all digested and decontaminated specimens cultured is generally defined as excessive contamination. A high contamination rate suggests either too weak decontamination or incomplete digestion. One or a combination of several of the following measures may be used to help decrease the contamination rate.

1. Cautiously and slightly increase the strength of the alkali treatment. Be aware that >4% NaOH affects the viability of tubercle bacilli.

2. Use a selective medium (one containing antibiotics) in addition to a nonselective primary culture medium to inhibit the growth of bacterial and fungal contaminants.

Selective 7H11 agar (Mitchison medium), Mycobactosel agar (BBL Microbiology Systems, Cockeysville, MD), or the Gruft modification of L-J medium should be considered. The most useful media for recovering MAC from stool specimens have been Mitchison's selective 7H11 agar and Mycobactosel L-J medium (238).

3. Make sure specimens are completely digested; partially digested specimens may not be completely decontaminated. Increase the NALC concentration to digest thick, mucoid specimens.

4. Use an alternative digestion-decontamination procedure for problem specimen types. Respiratory secretions from patients with cystic fibrosis, often overgrown with pseudomonads, can successfully be decontaminated with NALC-NaOH followed by addition of 5% oxalic acid to the concentrated sediment.

To determine the decontaminating capabilities of each new batch of reagents, the laboratory may wish to inoculate blood agar plates with four to six decontaminated sputum specimens in addition to inoculating mycobacterial media. The number of contaminants that grow after 48 h of incubation at 35°C should be minimal to none (29, 90, 98).

Acid-Fast Stain Procedures

Smear microscopy, the most rapid and inexpensive way to diagnose TB, is preferentially done from pretreated and concentrated specimens. In parallel, it is a rapid means to identify the most contagious patients. Normally, its predictive value for M. *tuberculosis* in expectorated sputum is >90% (110).

The common Gram stain is not suitable for mycobacteria. They may be Gram invisible, may appear as clear zones or "ghosts," or may appear as beaded gram-positive rods, particularly rapidly growing mycobacteria (202). Special acid-fast staining procedures are necessary to promote the uptake of dyes. Although the exact nature of the acid-fast staining reaction is not completely understood, phenol allows penetration of the stain which is facilitated by higher temperatures as applied, for instance, with Ziehl-Neelsen staining. Mycobacteria are able to form stable complexes with certain arylmethane dyes such as fuchsin. The cell wall mycolic acid residues retain the primary stain even after exposure to acid-alcohol or strong mineral acids. This resistance to decolorization is required for an organism to be termed acid fast. Certain staining protocols include a counterstain to highlight the stained organisms for easier microscopic recognition.

Alternatively, mycobacteria can be stained by fluorescent dyes (auramine O alone or in combination with rhodamine B). In contrast to carbol fuchsin, auramine O fluorescence is enhanced on binding to both DNA and RNA. The advantages of fluorescence microscopy over conventional light microscopy outweigh the higher cost for the microscope for the following reasons: (i) there is a much shorter observation time than with Ziehl-Neelsen; (ii) there is no requirement for heating the smear; and (iii) the fluorochrome protocol is no more complex than the carbol fuchsin staining (76). Using high-intensive light-emitting diodes to retrofit transmitted light microscopes to fluorescence microscopes may be an attractive option for resource-poor settings in the future (74, 115, 182). Information about specific staining procedures is given in chapter 17 as well as references 29, 90, and 98.

Because acid-fast artifacts may be present in a smear, it is necessary to view the cell morphology carefully. AFB are approximately 1 to 10 μm long and typically are slender rods, 0.2 to 0.6 μm wide, that may appear curved or bent. Individual bacilli may display heavily stained areas and areas of alternating stain, producing a beaded appearance. Assessing AFB morphology for presumptive identification of mycobacterial species has to be done with caution and needs ample training and experience of the laboratory personnel. In liquid medium M. *tuberculosis* often exhibits serpentine cording, but cords are also seen with some NTM species such as MAC, M. *gordonae*, M. *chelonae*, and M. *marinum* (132). NTM may be pleomorphic, appearing as long filaments or coccoid forms, with uniform staining properties. M. *kansasii* organisms can often be suspected in stained sputum smears by their large size and cross-banding appearance (8). Cells of rapidly growing mycobacteria may be <10% acid fast and may not stain with the fluorochrome stain (95). If the presence of a rapid grower is suspected and acid-fast stains, in particular fluorochrome stains, are negative, it may be worthwhile to stain the smear with carbol fuchsin and a weaker decolorizing process. Organisms that are truly acid fast are difficult to overdecolorize. The laboratory must be aware that there are nonmycobacterial organisms with various degrees of acid fastness such as *Rhodococcus* species, *Nocardia* species, *Legionella micdadei*, as well as the cysts of *Cryptosporidium*, *Isospora*, *Cyclospora*, and *Microsporidium* spores. Kinyoun's cold carbol fuchsin method appears to be inferior to both the Ziehl-Neelsen and fluorochrome methods (185).

Each slide made from a clinical specimen should be thoroughly examined for the presence of AFB. When a carbol fuchsin-stained smear is read, a minimum of 300 fields should be examined (magnification, ×1,000) before the smear is reported as negative (29, 90, 98). The fluorochrome stain is read at a lower power (×250) than the carbol fuchsin stain; therefore, more material can be examined in a given period. At the lower magnification, a minimum of 30 fields of view should be examined. This requires as little as 90 seconds. This ease of detection of AFB with the fluorochrome stain makes it the preferred staining method for clinical specimens, although an inexperienced observer may misinterpret fluorescent debris as bacilli.

All smears in which no AFB have been seen should be reported as negative. Conversely, when acid-fast organisms are detected on a smear, the smear should be reported as AFB positive and the staining method specified. It is best to confirm positive smears by having them reviewed by another experienced reader. Ideally, all positive fluorochrome-stained smears should be confirmed by a carbol fuchsin-based staining method, e.g., Ziehl-Neelsen, and slides should be stored for future reference (29, 90, 98). The widely accepted practice of confirming positive fluorochrome stains may be challenged in the future. Murray et al. (138) have demonstrated that stain applied to a liquefied (dithiothreitol), concentrated sample and examined before the decontamination process (NaOH) was the most effective method for the detection of AFB.

Information about the quantity of AFB observed on the smear should be provided. The recommended interpretations and reporting of smear results are given in Table 2 (see also reference 29). If only one or two organisms are seen on an entire smear, this should be noted but not reported. Confirmation of this finding should be attempted by preparation of additional smears from the same specimen, or, if possible, smears should be prepared from a new specimen. Observations made with the fluorochrome smears should be converted to a format that equates these observations with those made with a 100× oil immersion objective.

TABLE 2 Acid-fast smear evaluation and reporting[a]

Report	No. of AFB seen by staining method and magnification		
	Fuchsin stain, ×1,000	Fluorochrome stain	
		×250	×450
No AFB seen	0	0	0
Doubtful; repeat	1–2/300 F[b] (3 sweeps)[c]	1–2/30 F (1 sweep)	1–2/70 F (1.5 sweeps)
1+	1–9/100 F (1 sweep)	1–9/10 F	2–18/50 F (1 sweep)
2+	1–9/10 F	1–9/F	4–36/10 F
3+	1–9/F	10–90/F	4–36/F
4+	>9/F	>90/F	>36/F

[a] Adapted from reference 98.
[b] F, microscope fields.
[c] In all cases, one full sweep refers to scanning the full length (2 cm) of a smear 1 cm wide by 2 cm long.

The reliability of smear microscopy is highly dependent not only on the experience of the laboratory technician but also on the number of AFB present in the specimen. While 10^6 AFB/ml of specimen usually result in a positive smear, only 60% of the smears are positive if 10^4 AFB/ml are present (50). The overall sensitivity of the smear has been reported to range from 22 to 80% (110). An important factor influencing sensitivity is the minimum amount of sputum submitted to the laboratory. In a long-term study, the sensitivity of a concentrated smear from >5 ml of sputum was significantly greater than the sensitivity of a smear processed regardless of volume (223). Other factors influencing smear sensitivity include the type of specimens examined, staining techniques, experience of the reader, the patient population being evaluated, and whether the smear has been done with or without pretreatment (indirect versus direct smear). Respiratory specimens yield the highest smear positivity rate (110). In practice, the fluorochrome stain is more sensitive than the carbol fuchsin stain, even when read at lower magnification, probably because the fluorochrome-stained smears are easier to read.

The specificity of the smear for the detection of mycobacteria is very high. Prolonged or very harsh specimen decontamination and short incubation of cultures may account for smear-positive but culture-negative results. Patients with pulmonary tuberculosis may have positive smears with negative cultures (for 2 to 10 weeks on average) during a course of appropriate treatment (101).

Cytocentrifugation of sputum has resulted in controversial results concerning sensitivity of smear microscopy (173, 232). Concentration of sputum by centrifugation after liquefaction with 5% sodium hypochlorite is a possible means of increasing smear sensitivity, in particular, in developing countries.

The diagnostic yield of acid-fast stains of body fluids is less than for respiratory specimens because the number of mycobacteria is usually lower. A variety of techniques have been used to concentrate mycobacteria from cerebrospinal and other body fluids, but comparative data are lacking. Centrifugation is not an effective way to concentrate mycobacteria in body fluids; since mycobacteria have a buoyant density of approximately 1, many organisms remain in the supernatant.

With each new batch of staining reagents good laboratory practice includes the preparation of a positive and a negative smear for internal quality assessment (29). Smears containing *M. tuberculosis* or an NTM (positive control) and a gram-positive organism, preferentially a *Nocardia* sp. strain that is not totally acid fast (negative control) may be prepared in advance. Cross-contamination of slides during the staining process and the use of water contaminated with NTM during staining procedures are potential sources of false-positive results (221). Staining jars or dishes should not be used. Transfer of AFB in the oil used for microscopy may also occur. Troubleshooting protocols to prevent false-positive and false-negative smear results are available (7, 29).

Culture

In detecting as few as 10^1 to 10^2 viable organisms/ml, specimen culture is more effective than smear. Media available for the recovery of mycobacteria include nonselective and selective ones (29, 90, 98), the latter containing one or more antibiotics to prevent overgrowth by contaminating bacteria or fungi. Broth media are preferred for a rapid initial isolation of mycobacteria.

Solid Media

Egg-Based Media

Egg-based media contain whole eggs or egg yolk, potato flour, salts, and glycerol and are solidified by inspissation. These media have a good buffer capacity and a long shelf life (several months when refrigerated) and support good growth of most mycobacteria. Also, materials in the inoculum or medium toxic to mycobacteria are neutralized. Disadvantages of these media include variations from batch to batch depending on the quality of the eggs used, difficulties in discerning colonies from debris, and the inability to achieve accurate and consistent drug concentrations for susceptibility testing. When egg-based media become contaminated, they may liquefy.

Of the egg-based media, L-J medium is most commonly used in clinical laboratories. In general, it recovers *M. tuberculosis* well but is not as reliable for the recovery of other species. *M. bovis*, for instance, grows poorly on L-J medium, but growth is stimulated if glycerol is replaced by pyruvate. In contrast to most members of the *M. tuberculosis* complex, *M. bovis* is able to grow in a reduced O_2 atmosphere. *M. genavense* fails to grow on L-J. Good recovery of *M. ulcerans* is obtained on L-J medium with glycerol (239). Petragnani medium contains about twice as much malachite green as does L-J medium and is most commonly used for recovery of mycobacteria from heavily contaminated specimens. American Trudeau Society medium contains a lower concentration of malachite green than L-J medium and is, therefore, more easily overgrown by contaminants; however, growth of mycobacteria is less inhibited, resulting in earlier growth of larger colonies.

Agar-Based Media

In contrast to egg-containing media, agar-based media are chemically better defined. Agar-based media are transparent and provide a ready means for detecting early growth of microscopic colonies easily distinguished from inoculum debris. Colonies may be observed in 10 to 12 days, in contrast to 18 to 24 days with egg-based media. Microscopic examination can be performed by simply turning over the plate and examining it by focusing on the agar surface through the bottom of the plate at ×10 to ×100 magnification. This may provide both earlier detection of growth than unaided visual examination and presumptive identification of the species of mycobacteria present. The use of thinly poured 7H11 agar plates (10 by 90 mm; Remel, Lenexa, KS) facilitates this process, as microcolonies are visible after 11 days (225). This method is an alternative to broth cultures for some laboratories. Agar-based media can be used for susceptibility testing. They do not readily support growth of contaminants; however, the plates are expensive to prepare and their shelf life is relatively short (1 month in the refrigerator). Care should be exercised in preparation, incubation, and storage of the media, because excessive heat or light exposure may result in deterioration and in the release of formaldehyde, which is toxic to mycobacteria.

Middlebrook medium contains 2% glycerol, which enhances growth of MAC. Nonantibiotic supplements may be helpful for recovery of other mycobacteria and in special situations. Addition of 0.2% pyruvic acid is recommended if M. *bovis* is suspected, and 0.25% L-asparagine or 0.1% potassium aspartate added to 7H10 agar maximizes production of niacin. Addition of 0.1% enzymatic hydrolysate of casein to the Middlebrook 7H11 formulation (the only difference from 7H10) improves the recovery of isoniazid-resistant strains of M. *tuberculosis*. M. *genavense* fails to grow on 7H11 agar as well. However, Middlebrook 7H11 agar supplemented with mycobactin J (Allied Monitor, Fayette, MO) supports growth of this organism (37), as do microaerophilic conditions (167), the radiometric BACTEC 7H12 PZA test medium (201), or addition of blood and charcoal to acidified Middlebrook agar (166).

Selective Media

The addition of antimicrobial agents may be helpful in eliminating growth of contaminating organisms. If a selective medium is used for a particular specimen, it should not be used alone but in conjunction with a nonselective agar- or egg-based medium. Egg-based selective media include L-J Gruft with penicillin and nalidixic acid and Mycobactosel L-J medium with cycloheximide, lincomycin, and nalidixic acid. Mitchison selective 7H11 (7H11S) medium and its modifications contain carbenicillin (especially useful for inhibiting pseudomonads), polymyxin B, trimethoprim lactate, and amphotericin B.

Heme-Containing Medium for the Growth of M. *haemophilum*

M. *haemophilum* grows on egg- or agar-based media only if they are supplemented with hemin, hemoglobin, or ferric ammonium citrate (178). Thus, specimens from skin lesions, joints, or bone should be inoculated either on chocolate agar or on media with supplements (e.g., Middlebrook 7H10 agar with hemolyzed sheep erythrocytes, hemin, or a factor X disk, or on L-J medium containing 1% ferric ammonium citrate) to enhance recovery of this organism. Broth media should be similarly supplemented. M. *haemophilum* can also be isolated

from radiometric BACTEC 12B medium, from MB Redox broth (177), as well as from MGIT (174), whereas the MB/BacT ALERT 3D System has been found to be less optimal for this organism (159). As a whole, M. *haemophilum* infections may be underrecognized because of the predilection of this organism for a low incubation temperature (30°C) and its unique nutritional requirements.

Biphasic Media

The Septi-Chek System (Becton Dickinson Microbiology Systems) is a mycobacterial culture system consisting of a capped bottle containing 20 ml of modified 7H9 broth in an enhanced (20%) CO_2 atmosphere, and a paddle containing three types of solid media, i.e., modified L-J, Middlebrook 7H11 agar, and chocolate agar, encased in a plastic tube. Bacterial contamination is detected on the chocolate agar. Cultures are inoculated by removing the bottle cap, adding the processed specimen, and then attaching the paddle to the bottle. Solid media are inoculated after 24 h of incubation in an upright position by inverting the bottles. A supplement containing glucose, glycerol, oleic acid, pyridoxal HCl, catalase, albumin, and antibiotics (PANTA) is added to the culture bottle before inoculation. During the incubation period, the bottles are periodically tipped to reinoculate the solid media as cultures are being read. The sensitivity of this system is comparable to that of the BACTEC 460TB System (91). Although the average time to detection of growth is longer than with the BACTEC systems, it is shorter than with conventional media.

Liquid Media

Broth media may be used for both primary isolation and subculturing of mycobacteria. Cultures based on liquid media yield significantly more rapid results than solid medium-based cultures. Also, isolation rates for mycobacteria are higher. Middlebrook 7H9 and Dubos Tween albumin broths are commonly used for subculturing stock strains of mycobacteria and preparing the inoculum for drug susceptibility tests and other in vitro tests. 7H9 broth is used as the basal medium for several biochemical tests. Tween 80 can be added to liquid media and acts as a surfactant, which allows the dispersal of clumps of mycobacteria, resulting in a more homogeneous growth.

At present, a number of elaborate commercially available culture systems marketed for the isolation of mycobacteria range from simple bottles and tubes such as MGIT (Becton Dickinson Microbiology Systems) and MB Redox (Heipha Diagnostica Biotest, Eppelheim, Germany) to semiautomated systems (BACTEC 460TB system; Becton Dickinson) and fully automated systems (e.g., BACTEC MGIT 960 [Becton Dickinson]; ESP Culture System II and versaTREK Culture System II [Trek Diagnostic Systems, Cleveland, OH]; and MB/BacT ALERT 3D system [bioMérieux]).

MB Redox

MB Redox (Heipha Diagnostica Biotest) is a nonradiometric medium based on a modified Kirchner medium enriched with growth-promoting additives, antibiotic compounds, and a colorless tetrazolium salt as a redox indicator which is reduced to colored formazan by actively growing mycobacteria. With the naked eye, AFB are detected in the medium as pink to purple pinhead-sized particles. Recovery rates are similar to those observed by using other liquid systems (80, 186). Overall, it is a cost-efficient alternative, with the disadvantage that it requires much handling during visual reading.

MGIT

The MGIT (Becton Dickinson Microbiology Systems) contains a modified Middlebrook 7H9 broth in conjunction with a fluorescence-quenching-based oxygen sensor (silicon rubber impregnated with a ruthenium pentahydrate) to detect growth of mycobacteria. The large amount of oxygen initially present in the medium quenches the fluorescence of the sensor. Growth of mycobacteria or other microorganisms in the broth depletes the oxygen, and the indicator fluoresces brightly when the tubes are illuminated with UV light at 365 nm. For the manual version, a Wood's lamp or a transilluminator can be used as the UV light source, while in the automated BACTEC MGIT 960 System (see below) tubes are continuously monitored by the instrument. Prior to use, the 7H9 broth is supplemented with oleic acid-albumin-dextrose to promote growth of mycobacteria and with PANTA to suppress growth of contaminants.

Overall, sensitivity and time to growth detection of the MGIT system are similar to those of the BACTEC 460TB system and have been superior to those obtained with solid media in clinical evaluations (156). However, contamination rates for the MGIT system are slightly higher than for the BACTEC 460TB system, probably owing to the enrichments added to the MGIT broth, which enhance the growth of both mycobacteria and nonmycobacterial organisms.

The principal advantages of the manual MGIT system over the BACTEC 460TB system include reduced opportunity for cross-contamination of cultures, no need for needle inoculation, no radioisotopes, and no need for special instrumentation other than the UV light source. Its limitations include higher contamination rates, masking of fluorescence by blood or grossly bloody specimens, and lack of compatibility with some methods of digestion and decontamination of specimens (155).

BACTEC 460TB System

The BACTEC 460TB system was introduced more than 25 years ago. Although still widely used, it is slowly vanishing from clinical mycobacteriology laboratories due to its well-known limitations (see below). The BACTEC 460TB service agreement continues to be supported by the manufacturer (Becton Dickinson Microbiology Systems), but new instruments and some parts are no longer available. ^{14}C-labeled palmitic acid as a carbon source in the medium is metabolized by microorganisms to $^{14}CO_2$ which is monitored by the instrument. The amount of $^{14}CO_2$ and the rate at which the gas is produced are directly proportional to the growth rate of the organism in the medium.

An antimicrobial mixture/growth-promoting supplement, PANTA (see above), is added to BACTEC 12B medium inoculated with decontaminated specimens in order to suppress residual contaminants. To potentially sterile specimens polyoxyethylene stearate is added to enhance mycobacterial growth. For pretreatment of nonsterile specimens, the NALC-NaOH protocol is the method of choice, although some other procedures such as the sodium dodecyl sulfate-NaOH method are compatible with the BACTEC 460TB system as well (176). Specimens processed by the Zephiran-trisodium phosphate, benzalkonium chloride, or cetylpyridinium chloride method, however, cannot be used with the BACTEC 460TB system because residual quantities of these substances in the inoculum inhibit mycobacterial growth. The use of the BACTEC 460TB method has significantly improved recovery rates and times of mycobacterial isolation from respiratory secretions and other specimens (170).

Smear-positive specimens usually grow within a few days. The average detection time is 9 to 14 days for M. *tuberculosis* and <7 days for NTM. This is also obvious with smear-negative specimens and specimens from treated patients. It is good laboratory practice to confirm acid fastness and to subculture positive BACTEC vials to a chocolate agar to check for potential contaminants or, if suspected, for mixed cultures. The limitations of the BACTEC 460TB system include inability to observe colony morphology, difficulty in recognizing mixed cultures, overgrowth by contaminants, cost, radioisotope disposal, and extensive use of syringes with its potential for needle punctures among laboratory technicians. Since it is only semiautomated, vials have to be transferred to the incubator once the growth index has been read by the instrument.

The BACTEC 460TB system allows efficient antimicrobial susceptibility testing as well (see chapter 73). Generally, the initial positive vial can be used directly for identification and drug susceptibility testing.

Automated Continuously Monitoring Systems

Several automated continuously monitoring systems have been developed for growth and detection of mycobacteria, i.e., the recently discontinued BACTEC 9000 MB (Becton Dickinson), the BACTEC MGIT 960 (Becton Dickinson), the ESP Culture System II (Trek Diagnostic Systems), and the MB/BacT ALERT 3D (bioMérieux). All have in common that they are no longer based on the use of radioisotopes. The BACTEC 9000 MB system used the same fluorescence-quenching-based oxygen sensor as the MGIT system to detect growth. The technology used in the ESP Culture System II is based on detection of pressure changes in the headspace above the broth medium in a sealed bottle resulting from gas production or consumption due to growth of microorganisms. The MB/BacT ALERT 3D system, finally, employs a colorimetric carbon dioxide sensor in each bottle to detect growth of mycobacteria. Each of the systems includes a broth similar to 7H9 supplemented with a variety of growth factors and antimicrobial agents.

These systems have similar performance and operational characteristics. In clinical evaluations, recovery rates were similar to those of the BACTEC 460TB system and superior to those of conventional solid media (BACTEC MGIT 960 [73, 228]; ESP Culture System II [230]; MB/BacT ALERT 3D [159, 228]). In a meta-analysis of 10 published studies encompassing 1,381 strains from 14,745 clinical specimens, the BACTEC MGIT 960 and BACTEC 460TB systems revealed sensitivity and specificity in detecting mycobacteria of 81.5 and 99.6% and 85.8 and 99.9%, respectively. Combined with solid media the sensitivities of the two systems increased to 87.7 and 89.7%, respectively (38). For some systems, time to detection of mycobacteria is similar to that obtained with the radiometric BACTEC 460TB technique. Very recently, Parrish et al. (151) demonstrated for the BACTEC MGIT 960 system a shorter time to detection (13.5 versus 25.2 days) and a greater sensitivity (100% versus 66.6%) for recovery of M. *tuberculosis* complex than the MB BacT/ALERT system. For blood specimens, the continuously monitored systems (BACTEC MYCO/F LYTIC and MB BacT/Alert) were as sensitive as, and faster than, the Isolator system and the radiometric BACTEC 13A medium for the detection of MAC bacteremia (39).

Throughout, contamination rates reported have been higher with these new systems than with the BACTEC 460TB System (82). However, all of them share the advantages over the radiometric broth system of having no potential for cross-contamination by the instrument, being less labor-intensive, having continuous monitoring, using no radioisotopes, addressing safety more appropriately, and offering electronic data management. Since these systems are monitoring continuously, bottles are incubated in the instruments for their entire life in the laboratory. As a consequence, these systems are both instrument and space intensive. Some automated systems also lack the versatility of the BACTEC 460TB system, in that inoculation of blood is not possible, and therefore, additional instruments, e.g., BACTEC 9050 with BACTEC MYCO/F Lytic medium, have to be used for this purpose. The same holds for the incubation of cultures harboring mycobacteria with a lower temperature optimum such as M. *chelonae*, M. *haemophilum*, M. *marinum*, or M. *ulcerans*. Susceptibility testing applications for the primary and second-line antituberculosis drugs are available for the BACTEC MGIT 960 and ESP Culture System II (30; see also chapter 73).

Medium Selection

Medium selection for the isolation of mycobacteria and culture reading schedules are usually based on personal preferences and/or laboratory tradition. Both should be optimized for the most rapid detection of positive cultures and identification of mycobacterial isolates. The variety of media and methods available today is sufficient to permit laboratories to develop an algorithm that is optimal for their patient population and administrative needs. Workload, financial resources, and in particular, the limited amounts of processed sediments are, however, restraining factors in working with too many different types of media. Thus, cultivation of mycobacteria always involves a compromise.

Today, it is generally accepted that the use of a liquid medium in combination with at least one solid medium is essential for good laboratory practice in the isolation of mycobacteria (29). Addition of a solid medium is advantageous for those strains that occasionally do not grow in liquid medium, aids in the detection of mixed mycobacterial infections, and can serve as a backup for broth with its higher contamination rate. All positive cultures, even if identified directly from the broth, must be subcultured to solid media to detect mixed cultures and to correlate direct identification results with colony morphology. The Septi-Chek system can be used as a stand-alone system. In contrast, the radiometric BACTEC 460TB system and the nonradiometric growth systems cannot serve as stand-alone culture systems for mycobacteria for the reasons stated above.

Detection of colonies on solid medium certainly offers several advantages over detection of growth in broth, because colonial morphology can provide clues to identification and facilitate the selection of confirmatory tests. However, smears from broth-based systems can sometimes provide microscopic clues such as cord formation (see above), although the reliability for presumptive identification of M. *tuberculosis* should be applied with caution since the phenomenon is also being observed with some NTM species (8, 131).

Incubation

Temperature

The optimum incubation temperature for most cultures is 35 to 37°C. Exceptions to this include cultures obtained from skin and soft tissue suspected to contain M. *marinum*, M. *ulcerans*, M. *chelonae*, or M. *haemophilum*, which have a lower optimum temperature. For such specimens, a second set of media have to be inoculated and incubated at 25 to 33°C. BACTEC 460TB vials should be incubated at 36 to 38°C because optimum metabolism of the radiolabeled substrate occurs at 37 to 37.5°C for most species. Lower temperatures increase detection time. The newer liquid-medium-based culture automated systems do not offer the possibility to incubate at temperatures lower than $36 \pm 1°C$.

Atmosphere

Five to 10% CO_2 in air stimulates growth of mycobacteria in primary isolation cultures using conventional media. Middlebrook agar requires CO_2 atmosphere to ensure growth, while it is necessary to incubate egg media under CO_2 for only the first 7 to 10 days after inoculation, i.e., the log phase of growth. Subsequently, L-J cultures can be removed to ambient-air incubators if space is limited. In the absence of CO_2 incubators, plates may be incubated in commercially available bags with CO_2-generating tablets. Candle extinction jars are unacceptable for use in the mycobacteriology laboratory because the oxygen tension is less than that required for growth of mycobacteria. Broth systems usually do not require incubation at increased CO_2 concentrations.

Time

Mycobacterial cultures on solid and in liquid media are generally held for 6 to 8 weeks before being discarded as negative. Specimens with positive smears that are culture negative should be held for an additional 4 weeks. The same should be done for culture-negative specimens that were positive for mycobacteria by one of the nucleic acid-based amplification assays or for cases with a persisting suspicion of TB. Plates should be incubated with the medium side down until the entire inoculum has been absorbed. Once this has happened, media should be incubated inverted in CO_2-permeable polyethylene bags or sealed with CO_2-permeable shrink-seal bands to prevent them from drying up during the incubation period. Tubed media should be incubated in a slanted position with the screw caps loose for at least a week until the inoculum has been absorbed; they can then be incubated upright if space is at a premium. Caps on the tubes should be tightened at 2 to 3 weeks to prevent desiccation of the media. Specimens from skin lesions should be incubated for 8 to 12 weeks if M. *ulcerans* is suspected.

Reading Schedule

Since many mycobacteria are slowly growing organisms, cultures can be examined less frequently than routine bacteriologic cultures. All solid media should be examined within 3 to 5 days after inoculation to permit early detection of rapidly growing mycobacteria and to enable prompt removal of contaminated cultures. Young cultures (up to 4 weeks of age) should be examined twice a week, whereas older cultures could be examined at weekly intervals. Use of a hand lens for opaque media and a microscope for agar media will facilitate early detection of microcolonies.

Septi-Chek and the manual MGIT may be inspected for growth daily for the first 1 to 2 weeks; Septi-Chek bottles should be inverted for reinoculation of the agar medium if growth is not observed. Afterwards, these systems are inspected twice weekly or weekly for growth.

For BACTEC 460TB vials the reading schedule varies according to the laboratory workload. Low-volume laboratories may read cultures three times a week for the first 2 or

3 weeks and weekly thereafter for a total of 6 weeks, while high-volume laboratories may read cultures twice a week for the first 2 weeks and weekly thereafter. Readings of negative cultures in 12B medium usually remain below a growth index (GI) of 10; a GI of 10 or more is considered presumptively positive. At this point, the vials should be separated and tested daily. An acid-fast stain is performed when the GI is >50 to determine whether the culture contains mycobacteria. In addition, a smear of the broth from the vial may be Gram stained and/or the broth may be subcultured onto a sheep blood agar or chocolate agar plate to determine whether contamination is present. When the GI is 500 or more, BACTEC 460TB antimicrobial susceptibility testing can be performed (see below).

When using one of the nonradiometric continuously monitoring systems, technicians are automatically alerted by the instrument if a specimen turns positive. Irrespective of the system used, the acid fastness of the organism has to be confirmed by smear staining. Also, it is highly advisable to subculture the broth on a sheep blood or chocolate agar plate to rule out contaminants. Once growth of AFB is detected, susceptibility testing can be performed, always following the instructions specified by the manufacturers.

Storage of Positive Cultures

Positive cultures may be kept at room temperature for several weeks. If subcultured, they may be saved at room temperature for several months. Solid cultures have to be sealed to avoid dehydration of the medium. CLSI (29) recommends that cultures that may be needed for possible follow-up in the future be frozen at −70°C (a minimum of 1 year is recommended).

IMMUNODIAGNOSTIC TESTS FOR TUBERCULOSIS

Historically, the first immunodiagnostic test for tuberculosis was the TST. The shortcomings of this test are well known and include the inability to distinguish active tuberculosis disease from past sensitization by BCG, unknown predictive values, and cross-reaction with NTM.

Over time, much effort has been devoted to the development of serological tests for the diagnosis of tuberculosis, but no test has found widespread clinical use. The sensitivity and specificity of serological tests with crude antigen preparations are too low for clinical application.

In contrast, the commercially available whole-blood IGRAs have become a more promising, though not perfect, tool to detect tuberculosis infection, particularly if TST remains equivocal. The two test systems, the T-SPOT.TB (Oxford Immunotec, Oxford, United Kingdom) and the QuantiFERON Gold In-Tube (QFNG-IT; Cellestis, Chadstone, Victoria, Australia), are not affected by BCG vaccination, do not cross-react with the majority of NTM, and are less prone to variability and subjectivity associated with placing and reading of the TST. Also, individuals to be tested have to see the doctor or the health care personnel only once. However, IGRAs are more costly than a simple TST.

Although both tests measure T-cell IFN-γ responses to two or three *M. tuberculosis*-specific antigens (ESAT-6, CFP-10, and TB 7.7) over a 16- to 24-h incubation period, they are based on different technologies. The T-SPOT.TB assay is based on the enzyme-linked immunospot assay methodology and requires the isolation and incubation of peripheral blood mononuclear cells (PBMC) and the standardization of 250,000 PBMC in each of its test wells.

The assay requires, overall, two working days and may be more laborious than the QFNG-IT. Nevertheless, the use of a standardized number of washed PBMC may represent another advantage. In contrast, the QFNG-IT has technical advantages over the T-SPOT.TB assay, since the stimulation of T-cell IFN-γ response in whole blood is performed in tubes precoated with the *M. tuberculosis* antigens. Also, the enzyme-linked immunosorbent assay is simple to perform and requires one working day. Since background noise may occur, a "Nil" control is required to adjust for this background as well as for heterophile antibody effects, and nonspecific IFN-γ in blood samples. Reproducibility of QFNG-IT in duplicate tests is excellent (43).

It is important to stress that neither of these new tests distinguishes between latent and active infection. To date, there are several guidelines available, among them one for the United States (121). A large number of publications focus on the performance characteristics of each test compared to TST. As a whole, IGRAs are better correlated with the intensity of TB exposure than TST (241).

There are few published head-to-head comparisons of the QFNG-IT and the T-SPOT.TB assays specifying their feasibility in different patient cohorts. In a recent systematic review of the literature Pai et al. (148) concluded that QFNG-IT has a specificity of 99% (T-SPOT.TB specificity, 96%) among non-BCG-vaccinated participants and a specificity of 96% (T-SPOT.TB specificity, 93%) among BCG-vaccinated participants, while the T-SPOT.TB appears to be more sensitive than QFNG-IT and TST. Diel et al. (45) compared the two IGRAs in TST-positive persons recently exposed to pulmonary tuberculosis cases. In this study, factors independently influencing the risk of *M. tuberculosis* infection and their interactions with each other were evaluated by multivariate analysis. There were five variables that significantly predicted a positive IGRA result, i.e., age, AFB positivity of the source case, cough, cumulative exposure time, and foreign origin of the patient. There was excellent agreement between the two assays (93.9%, kappa = 0.85), with QFNG-IT finding 30.2% of contacts positive and T-SPOT.TB finding 28.7% of them. Again, the IGRAs were more accurate indicators of the presence of latent tuberculosis than the TST (45).

In HIV-positive asymptomatic individuals (*n* = 286) both QFNG-IT and T-SPOT.TB assay were more sensitive than TST (20.0% and 25.2%, respectively, compared with 12.8% for TST), but seemed, as a whole, to be less sensitive than in immunocompetent patients (187). The current information about the performance of the TST and the IGRAs in the detection of latent tuberculosis infection in patients with rheumatic diseases (who are treated with monoclonal antibodies directed against tumor necrosis factor alpha) strongly suggests a clinically relevant advantage of the IGRAs (219).

The performance of IGRAs in children is less understood. Without the inconveniences and complications associated with TST, IGRAs are acceptable substitutes for TST. The sensitivity and specificity of IGRAs are, however, not significantly higher than the values observed for the TST (192). In latent tuberculosis the agreement between QFNG-IT and T-SPOT.TB assay was very good (92%) in children, with moderate agreement betweeen TST and QFNG-IT (77%) and TST and T-SPOT.TB (75%) (97). For culture-confirmed active tuberculosis, however, the same authors stated that the sensitivity of the TST was 83%, compared to 80% for the QFNG-IT and 58% for the T-SPOT.TB.

Basically, the problem of indeterminate results occurs with both IFN-γ release assays. In HIV-infected individuals, T-SPOT.TB yielded more indeterminate results than the QFNG-IT (8/256 versus 1/256; $P < 0.01$ [187]), similar to what has been confirmed by others (14% versus 1.8% [191]). Indeterminate results appear to be dependent on the number of CD4 cells inasmuch as patients with a CD4 count of ≤200 cells/ml were significantly more likely to have an indeterminate result (187, 191). In children <4 years of age indeterminate results were more often seen when using the QFNG-IT than the T-SPOT.TB (13). When the T-SPOT.TB assay was applied after indeterminate results had been obtained from the QFNG-IT test, 65% of the 40 patients yielded a valid result (103).

Since the experience with IGRAs is still limited, longitudinal studies are needed to define their predictive values, especially in children and high-risk populations (240). A large meta-analysis has pointed out very clearly areas of uncertainty and recommendations for research (123). Other problems concern altered performance characteristics of the assays in conjunction with ethnicity (26) and the phenomena of conversions, reversions, and nonspecific variations in serial testing (147). Assessment of within-subject IGRA variability is important in establishing thresholds for conversions and reversions. With the QFNG-IT Detjen et al. (43) observed considerable intraindividual variability in serial analyses within 3 days. van Zyl-Smit et al. (217) concluded from their study that a three-spot or 80% IFN-γ response variation on either side of the baseline values explains 95% of the short-term variability and may be useful for interpreting conversions, reversions, and values close to the cut point. Therefore, these authors have proposed a borderline or uncertainty zone for both tests (four to eight spots [inclusive] for the T-SPOT.TB assay and 0.2 to 0.7 IU/ml for the QFNG-IT instead of strictly adhering to the manufacturer-defined cutoff value (T-SPOT.TB assay, >6 spots; QFNG-IT test, >0.35 IU/ml).

The optimal strategy for the diagnosis of latent *M. tuberculosis* infection is controversial. Adoption of a two-step strategy (TST followed by an IGRA) may be limited by TST-mediated boosting of subsequent IGRA responses. van Zyl-Smit et al. (217) have demonstrated that it appears safe to perform a QFNG-IT or T-SPOT.TB assay within 3 days of performing the TST.

From the present state of knowledge it is obvious that the applications of the IGRAs for *M. tuberculosis* infection in different high-risk groups have to be tailored. Also, caution has to be exerted in their current use in immunosuppressed patients.

CROSS-CONTAMINATION

With the advent of molecular techniques designed for molecular epidemiology, cross-contamination either linked to laboratory procedures (46, 117) or, more rarely, to contaminated bronchoscopes can easily be proven (27, 67, 179). False-positive results may be generated at any step between specimen collection and reading of cultures (29). Laboratory personnel should be alerted for a possible laboratory error if (i) the culture result is not compatible with the clinical picture; (ii) there is a late-appearing cluster of cultures that have scanty growth (<10 colonies on solid medium) or a significant delay in recovering mycobacteria from a liquid system; (iii) there is a large number of isolates of a particular species that is usually rare in the laboratory or of an organism that is normally considered an environmental contaminant;

or (iv) there is only one positive culture from multiple specimens submitted from a single patient. Practices that can lead to false-positive culture results are numerous and include inadequate sterilization of instruments or equipment (such as bronchoscopes), use of contaminated water for specimen collection or for laboratory procedures, transfer of organisms from one specimen to another through direct contact or via common reagents or equipment, mix-up of testing samples or lids of specimen containers, failure to take precautions to minimize the production of aerosols, etc. Laboratory aspects of cross-contamination are addressed in more detail in the following section.

QUALITY ASSURANCE

General Aspects

Quality control (QC) is vital for monitoring a laboratory's effectiveness in detecting and isolating mycobacteria. This includes standard components of laboratory quality assurance, such as personnel competency, procedure manuals, external proficiency testing, and quality control of media, tests, and reagents. Laboratories performing mycobacterial testing should follow QC recommendations in the scientific literature and in ad hoc publications (7, 29, 30, 90, 231). The Centers for Medicare and Medicaid Services has reported recently that applications of a principal sanction against laboratories for a proficiency test violation were rare during a 14-year period of study (100).

The Public Health Service introduced the "levels of service concept" for mycobacteriology laboratories in 1967. In this scheme, laboratories define the level of service which best fits the needs of the patient population they serve, the experience of their personnel, their laboratory facilities, and the number of specimens they receive, always keeping the biosafety risk in mind. Levels of service were promulgated by the CDC, the ATS, and the College of American Pathologists and are based on workload, personal experience, and cost-effectiveness (79). Personnel working in the clinical mycobacteriology laboratory must have proper training and certification in the specific functions that they perform. In the United States, all laboratories performing mycobacteriology testing must be enrolled in an external proficiency test program approved by federal and state regulatory agencies. Level I (acid-fast smear) must prepare at least 15 specimens per week, level II (smear, culture, identification, and susceptibility testing of *M. tuberculosis* complex) must process at least 15 specimens per week. Level III performs the same activities as level II and in addition identifies all NTM (including susceptibility testing, where applicable).

Multiple test parameters are monitored by adherence to the quality assurance guidelines described in the recent CLSI standard documents (29, 30). Acceptable results derived from testing QC reference strains do not guarantee accurate results with all clinical isolates. If inconsistent results are seen with clinical isolates, the test should be repeated in an attempt to ensure accuracy. Each laboratory should put its own policies into effect regarding the verification of atypical test results.

The laboratory must maintain a collection of well-characterized mycobacterial strains that are used for QC of test systems. These controls may be obtained from the American Type Culture Collection (ATCC) and proficiency testing programs. Frequently used stock cultures can be maintained on L-J slants or in 7H9 broth at 37°C or room temperature if subcultured monthly. Cultures on L-J slants may be held for up to 1 year if stored at 4°C. Such maintenance is not recommended for strains with drug resistance. Freezing of organisms suspended in skim milk or broth medium and storage at −20 to −70°C is the best option for long-term maintenance of stock cultures (29, 30).

QC of Smear, Culture, and Molecular Tests

Apart from the external QC the laboratory should make every possible effort to perform internal QC tests, e.g., with each new lot of media commercially obtained or prepared in-house. Detailed procedures to monitor the many different working steps in the clinical mycobacteriology laboratory are outlined in references 29 and 90.

Ideally, positive-control slides should be prepared from a concentrated sputum sample obtained from a patient with active tuberculosis. In practice, many laboratories use suspensions of stock cultures or seeded negative sputa as positive controls for acid-fast staining procedures. Control slides are also commercially available (BBL AFB QC Slides; Becton Dickinson Diagnostic Systems, Sparks, MD). An increase in the percentage of smear-positive but culture-negative specimens of >2%, which cannot be attributed to a response to mycobacterial therapy or the presence of AFB in the negative controls, suggests that water or reagents used in the pretreatment or staining procedures were contaminated with NTM. M. *gordonae* or M. *terrae* complex is most often involved. AFB may also be carried over from one slide to another if slides are not set properly apart from each other during the staining process. AFB may also be found in the oil used with the immersion lens after a positive slide is examined. The sensitivity of the AFB smear is directly related to the relative centrifugal force (RCF) (*g* force) attained during centrifugation. Thus, laboratories should calculate the RCF of their centrifuge and periodically monitor and document that they are reaching sufficient RCF by checking the revolutions per minute with a tachometer (98).

Laboratories should also monitor contamination rates (percentage of specimens producing contaminating growth on culture media) for decontaminated specimens. Contamination rates of 3 to 5% are generally considered acceptable. Rates below 3% usually indicate that the decontamination procedure is too harsh and the procedure needs to be modified to minimize the lethal effect on mycobacteria. Contamination rates above 5% often indicate a too weak decontamination, which could compromise mycobacterial cultures due to overgrowth of contaminants. It should be emphasized that the widespread use of liquid media increases the generation of aerosols; as a consequence, the risk of contamination between samples also increases. Laboratories that handle large numbers of isolates of MAC, M. *abscessus*, or specimens from patients with cystic fibrosis will probably have much higher contamination rates due to the high incidence of colonization of the sputum with gram-negative bacteria, especially *Pseudomonas aeruginosa*.

Culturing mycobacteria is naturally prone to errors because of the multiple steps involved in processing cultures, the viability of mycobacteria for long periods in the laboratory environment, and the large number of mycobacteria present in some specimens (21). False-positive cultures may result from mislabeling, specimen switching during handling, specimen carryover (including proficiency testing specimens), contaminated reagents, or cross-contamination between culture tubes or vials (21, 24, 29). Inclusion of a "positive control" (e.g., a suspension of M. *tuberculosis*) in the processing of patient specimens is discouraged due to the risk of cross-contamination. Cross-contamination of culture vials

in the BACTEC 460 TB system due to inadequately sterilized sample needles has been documented (15). Standardized laboratory procedures that minimize the potential for errors leading to false-positive cultures should be followed, and mechanisms should be in place to rapidly recognize their occurrence. Transfers or inoculation of cultures must be accomplished by using individual transfer pipettes, single-delivery diluent tubes, or disposable labware. The order in which specimens are processed and media are inoculated should be recorded. A negative-control specimen following processing of patient specimens with the same digestion or decontamination solution can be used for detecting possible specimen contamination of the solutions (7). Alternatively, processing solutions may be cultured directly. Laboratories should prospectively track positivity rates. The significance of an isolate may be determined by reviewing the order in which specimens were handled for all manipulations (e.g., initial processing, liquid media readings, and subculturing), the direct-smear results, the time to positivity, and the clinical history. Since the introduction of molecular fingerprinting of M. *tuberculosis* strains, false-positive cultures have been demonstrated to occur more frequently than previously assumed, from 1 to more than 10% (165). The deleterious impact of these undesirable events may be minimized if the evidence of false positivity is established in a timely manner and a rapid molecular method of fingerprinting is available. It has been suggested that single positive cultures of M. *tuberculosis* strains grown from AFB smear-negative specimens should be analyzed by a PCR-derived typing technique to rule out laboratory contamination (165). Strains with identical fingerprints isolated within a 1-week period from different patients should be considered probably false positive.

The CDC and others have recommended that AFB smear results be available and positive results be reported within 24 h of specimen receipt (7). The time required for identification and susceptibility testing of M. *tuberculosis* should average 14 to 21 days and 15 to 30 days from time of specimen receipt, respectively (7, 233). Pascopella et al. (152) have evaluated laboratory reporting of tuberculosis test results and patient treatment initiation in California.

Nucleic acid amplification (NAA)-based assays require several levels of controls (e.g., to detect amplification inhibition as well as contamination between specimens), in addition to positive or negative controls (28). When used as approved by the FDA, NAA tests for M. *tuberculosis* diagnosis do not replace any previously recommended tests (23). Laboratories that test patient specimens by using research or "home-brew" methods or commercially available NAA assays for nonapproved or off-label indications and report their results must validate the assays and establish their performance characteristics prior to diagnostic use. The information available is often insufficient to guide test interpretation. Approved guidelines for molecular diagnostic methods in clinical microbiology are available from the CLSI; in these documents, the development, validation, quality assurance, and routine use of NAA assays are addressed in detail (28). However, basing the identification of M. *tuberculosis* on a sole positive home-brew PCR result is not recommended because the results of such assays vary considerably (7).

Potential probes and/or primers must be selected for sensitivity by using multiple clinical and reference strains of the target organism. Additionally, specificity must be evaluated by testing for cross-hybridization with other organisms that may be present in patient samples (28).

Several types of validation tests are used to evaluate the presence of a target nucleic acid in the sample and to determine that it was isolated in a manner whereby the target has not been introduced. Testing to assess amplification should include positive and negative controls and controls for detection of the presence of inhibitors, such as endogenous nucleic acid. Other QC measures include those referring to assays of restriction enzymes, reagents, inspection of equipment, and laboratory design (i.e., separate areas for processing, amplification, and detection steps [28]). Excellent proficiency testing schemes to assess laboratory performance of NAA tests are currently available both in the United States (169) and in Europe (141).

EVALUATION, INTERPRETATION, AND REPORTING OF RESULTS

Adequate funding and focused training are critical in maintaining state-of-the-art mycobacteriology laboratories (28, 29, 231). Laboratories play a pivotal role in the diagnosis and control of tuberculosis, and every effort should be made to implement sensitive and rapid methods for the detection, identification, and susceptibility testing of the M. tuberculosis complex as well as other mycobacterial species. Specifically, these include (i) the use of fluorochrome stain for mycobacteria in smears; (ii) a broth-based or microcolony method for culture; (iii) the use of rapid identification methods (e.g., molecular assays); and (iv) direct susceptibility testing of smear-positive specimen concentrates.

The 24-h turnaround time for AFB smear results presents a challenge for most laboratories. The daily processing of specimens required to meet this goal adds considerable expense to the laboratory budget.

NAA assays offer the promise of same-day detection and identification of M. tuberculosis. Implementation of these new technologies presents several new challenges. Although the performance characteristics of many of these assays are quite good for smear-positive respiratory specimens, limited information exists on the use of these tests for diagnosis of paucibacillary pulmonary or extrapulmonary disease. The new technologies have been shown to supplement rather than replace culture. Culture will still be required to obtain organisms for susceptibility testing and detect mycobacteria other than M. tuberculosis.

The significance of the isolation of NTM may be difficult to assess since many species are opportunistic pathogens, and the reader is referred to the criteria suggested by the ATS for the evaluation (4). In addition to these criteria, accurate identification of NTM will prevent rarely encountered pathogens from being mistaken for nonpathogenic species.

Thus, accurate and timely reporting of the results of AFB microscopy, culture, identification, and drug susceptibility tests is essential to the effective management of individual patients and to the appropriate implementation of public health and infection control measures (29).

APPENDIX
Commonly Used Digestion-Decontamination Methods

Refer to references 29, 90, and 98 for details.

NALC-NaOH Method
Reagents

Digestant: For each 100 ml, combine 50 ml of sterile 0.1 M (2.94%) trisodium citrate with 50 ml of 4% NaOH. The NaOH and citrate mixtures can be mixed, sterilized, and stored for future use. To this solution, add 0.5 g of powdered NALC just before use. Use within 24 h of addition of the NALC because the mucolytic action of NALC is inactivated on exposure to air.

Phosphate buffer: The buffer is 0.067 M and pH 6.8. Mix 50 ml of solution A (0.067 M Na_2HPO_4; 9.47 g of anhydrous Na_2HPO_4 in 1 liter of distilled water) and 50 ml of solution B (0.067 M KH_2PO_4; 9.07 g of KH_2PO_4 in 1 liter of distilled water). If the final buffer requires pH adjustment, add solution A to raise the pH or solution B to lower it.

BSA (optional): Use sterile 0.2% bovine serum albumin (BSA) fraction V (pH 6.8).

Procedure

1. Transfer up to 10 ml of specimen to a sterile, graduated, 50-ml plastic centrifuge tube labeled with appropriate identification. The tube should have a leakproof, aerosol-free screw cap. Add an equal volume of the NALC-NaOH solution. The final concentration of NaOH in the tube is 1%.

2. Tighten the cap completely. Invert the tube so that the NALC-NaOH solution contacts all the inside surfaces of the tube and cap, and then mix the contents for approximately 5 to 20 s with a Vortex mixer. If liquefaction is not complete during this time, agitate the solution at intervals during the following decontamination period.

3. Allow the mixture to stand for 15 min at room temperature with occasional gentle shaking by hand. Avoid movement that causes aeration of the specimen. A small pinch of crystalline NALC may be added to viscous specimens for better liquefaction. Specimens should remain in contact with the decontaminating agent for only 15 min, since overprocessing results in reduced recovery of mycobacteria. If more-active decontamination is needed, slightly increase the concentration of NaOH.

4. Add phosphate buffer (pH 6.8) up to the 50-ml mark on the tube.

5. Centrifuge the solution for at least 15 min at ≥3,000 × g.

6. Decant the supernatant fluid into a splashproof discard container containing a suitable disinfectant. Do not touch the lip of the tube to the discard container. Wipe the lip of each tube with disinfectant-soaked gauze (separate piece for each tube) to absorb drips, and recap.

7. Using a separate sterile pipette for each tube, add to the sediment 1 to 2 ml of sterile, 0.2% BSA fraction V (pH 6.8) or 1 to 2 ml of phosphate buffer (pH 6.8), and resuspend the sediment with the pipette or by shaking the tube gently by hand. BSA may have a buffering and detoxifying effect on the sediment and increases the adhesion of the specimen to solid media. However, BSA may lengthen detection times (for instance, in the BACTEC 460TB system).

8. Inoculate the specimens onto appropriate solid culture media and into broth media. Use a separate disposable capillary pipette for each specimen to deliver 3 drops to solid medium.

9. Prepare a smear for acid-fast staining. Use a sterile disposable pipette to place 1 drop of the sediment onto a clean, properly labeled microscope slide covering an area approximately 1 by 2 cm. Place the smears on an electric slide warmer at 65 to 75°C for 2 h to dry and fix them. Alternatively, air dry the smears and fix them by passing the slide three or four times through the blue cone of a flame (heat fixing does not always kill mycobacteria, and the slides are potentially infectious).

10. Refrigerate (4°C) the remaining sediment for later use if needed (direct susceptibility testing, further treatment if specimen is contaminated, etc.).

The NALC-NaOH method can be used to process gastric lavage specimens, tissues, stool, urine, and other body fluids. For neutralized gastric lavage specimens and other body fluids (≥10 ml), centrifuge at ×3,000 × g for 30 min in sterile screw-cap 50-ml centrifuge tubes, decant the supernatants, resuspend the sediments in 2 to 5 ml of sterile distilled water, and proceed as for sputum. If a gastric lavage specimen is mucopurulent, add 50 mg of NALC powder per 50 ml of lavage fluid and vortex before centrifugation. Tissue that is not collected aseptically can be ground, placed in a tube, homogenized by vortexing, and processed as for sputum. For stool specimens, place approximately 1 g of a formed specimen or 1 to 5 ml of a liquid specimen in a total volume of 10 ml of 7H9 broth, sterile water, or sterile saline; vortex vigorously for 30 s; and then allow large particles to settle to the bottom of the tube for 15 min. Remove 7 to

8 ml of supernatant, place into a 50-ml centrifuge tube, and process as for sputum.

Sodium Hydroxide Method

Reagents

Digestant: NaOH solution (2 to 4%). Sterilize by autoclaving.
2 N HCl: Dilute 33 ml of concentrated HCl to 200 ml with water. Sterilize by autoclaving.
Phenol red indicator: Combine 20 ml of phenol red solution (0.4% in 4% NaOH) and 85 ml of concentrated HCl with distilled water to make 1,000 ml.
Phosphate buffer: The buffer is 0.067 M and pH 6.8. See the NALC-NaOH procedure for buffer preparation.

Procedure

Follow the steps described for the NALC-NaOH method, substituting 2% NaOH for the NALC-alkali digestant.

1. Transfer a maximum volume of 10 ml of specimen to a sterile 50-ml screw-cap plastic centrifuge tube. Add an equal volume of NaOH.
2. With the cap tightened, invert the tube and then agitate the mixture vigorously for 15 min on a mechanical mixer, or vortex vigorously and let stand for exactly 15 min. If it is necessary to reduce excessive contamination, the NaOH concentration can be increased to 3 or 4%.
3. Add phosphate buffer (pH 6.8) up to the 50-ml mark on the tube. Recap the tube, and swirl by hand to mix well.
4. Centrifuge the specimen at $\geq$3,000 $\times$ g for 15 min, decant the supernatant, and add a few drops of phenol red indicator to the sediment. Neutralize the sediment with HCl. Thoroughly mix the contents of the tube. Stop acid addition when the solution is persistently yellow.
5. Resuspend the sediment in 1 to 2 ml of phosphate buffer or sterile 0.1% BSA fraction V.
6. Inoculate the resuspended sediment to appropriate culture media, and prepare a smear.

Zephiran-Trisodium Phosphate Method

Principle

This system can be used when the laboratory cannot monitor the exposure time to the decontaminating agent, since the timing of this digestion-decontamination process is not critical. Benzalkonium chloride (Zephiran), a quaternary ammonium compound, together with trisodium phosphate selectively destroys many contaminants with little activity on tubercle bacilli. Zephiran is bacteriostatic to mycobacteria, and so the digested, centrifuged sediment must be neutralized with buffer before being inoculated onto agar medium. The phospholipids of egg medium neutralize this compound. It is incompatible with the BACTEC 460TB system.

Reagents

Zephiran-trisodium phosphate digestant: Dissolve 1 kg of trisodium phosphate ($Na_3PO_4 \cdot 12H_2O$) in 4 liters of hot distilled water. Add 7.5 ml of Zephiran concentrate (17% benzalkonium chloride [Winthrop Laboratories, New York, NY]), and mix. Store at room temperature.
Neutralizing buffer: Neutralizing buffer has a pH of 6.6. Add 37.5 ml of 0.067 M disodium phosphate to 62.5 ml of 0.067 M monopotassium phosphate (for preparation of buffer solutions, see the NALC-NaOH procedure).

Procedure

1. Transfer a maximum volume of 10 ml of specimen to a sterile, 50-ml screw-cap plastic centrifuge tube. Add an equal volume of the Zephiran-trisodium phosphate digestant.
2. Tighten the cap, invert the tube, and then agitate the mixture vigorously for 30 min on a mechanical shaker. Permit the material to stand, without shaking, for an additional 20 to 30 min at room temperature.
3. Centrifuge the specimen at $\geq$3,000 $\times$ g for 15 min, decant the supernatant, and add 20 ml of neutralizing buffer. Vortex for 30 s to thoroughly suspend the sediment in the buffer (the neutralizing

buffer serves to inactivate traces of Zephiran in the sediment, which is critical if inoculation of an agar-based medium is intended).
4. Centrifuge the specimen again for 15 min.
5. Decant the supernatant, retaining some fluid to resuspend the sediment.
6. Inoculate egg-based medium, and make a smear. The phospholipids of egg medium provide neutralization for this quaternary compound.

Oxalic Acid Method

Principle

The oxalic acid method is superior to alkali methods for processing specimens consistently contaminated with *Pseudomonas* species and certain other contaminants. Specimens processed by this method may be used with the BACTEC 460TB system. It can also be used to decontaminate a previously processed sediment when cultures are contaminated with *Pseudomonas*.

Reagents

5% oxalic acid
Physiological saline (0.85%)
4% NaOH
Phenol red indicator or pH paper

Procedure

1. Add an equal volume of 5% oxalic acid to 10 ml, or less, of specimen in a 50-ml centrifuge tube (vol/vol, 1/1).
2. Vortex the solution, and then allow it to stand at room temperature for 30 min with occasional shaking.
3. Add sterile saline to the 50-ml mark on the centrifuge tube. Recap the tube, and invert it several times to mix the contents.
4. Centrifuge for 15 min at $\geq$3,000 $\times$ g, decant the supernatant fluid, and add a few drops of phenol red indicator to the sediment. Alternatively, use pH paper.
5. Neutralize with 4% NaOH.
6. Resuspend the sediment, inoculate it to media, and make a smear.

CPC Method

Principle

Cetylpyridinium chloride (CPC), a quaternary ammonium compound, is used to decontaminate specimens, while sodium chloride effects liquefaction. CPC is bacteriostatic for mycobacteria inoculated onto agar-based media. This effect is not neutralized in the digestion process, and thus sediments from specimens treated with CPC should be inoculated only on egg-based media. This method is incompatible with the BACTEC 460TB system.

This method is a means of digesting and decontaminating specimens in transit (>24 h). Mycobacteria remain viable for 8 days in the solution.

Reagents

CPC digestant-decontaminant: Dissolve 10 g of CPC and 20 g of NaCl in 1,000 ml of distilled water. The solution is self-sterilizing and remains stable if protected from light, extreme heat, and evaporation. Dissolve with gentle heat any crystals that might form in the working solution. Other reagents used in processing include sterile water and sterile saline or 0.2% sterile BSA fraction V.

Procedure

1. Collect 10 ml or less of sputum in a 50-ml screw-cap centrifuge tube.
2. Inside a BSC, add an equal volume of CPC-NaCl, cap securely, and shake by hand until the specimen liquefies.
3. Package the specimen appropriately as specified by current postal regulations, and send it to a processing laboratory.
4. Upon receipt in the processing laboratory (allow at least 24 h for digestion-decontamination to be completed), dilute the digested-decontaminated specimen to the 50-ml mark with sterile distilled water and recap securely. Invert the tube several times to mix the contents.

5. Centrifuge at ≥3,000 × *g* for 15 min, decant the supernatant fluid, and suspend the sediment in 1 to 2 ml of sterile water, saline, or 0.2% BSA fraction V.

6. Inoculate the resuspended sediment onto egg medium, and make a smear.

Sulfuric Acid Method

Principle

The sulfuric acid method may be useful for urine and other body fluids that yield contaminated cultures when processed by one of the alkaline digestants.

Reagents

4% sulfuric acid
4% sodium hydroxide
Sterile distilled water
Phenol red indicator

Procedure

1. Centrifuge the entire specimen for 30 min at ≥3,000 × *g*. This may require several tubes.

2. Decant the supernatant fluids; pool the sediments if several tubes were used for a single specimen.

3. Add an equal volume of 4% sulfuric acid to the sediment.

4. Vortex, and let stand for 15 min at room temperature.

5. Fill the tube to the 50-ml mark with sterile water.

6. Centrifuge at ≥3,000 × *g* for 15 min and decant the supernatant.

7. Add 1 drop of phenol red indicator, and neutralize with 4% NaOH until a persistent pale pink color forms.

8. Inoculate the media, and make a smear.

REFERENCES

1. **Abramowsky, C., B. Gonzalez, and R. U. Sorensen.** 1993. Disseminated Bacillus Calmette-Guérin infections in patients with primary immunodeficiencies. *Am. J. Clin. Pathol.* **100:**52–56.

2. **Allen, S., J. Batungwanayo, K. Kerlikowske, A. R. Lifson, W. Wolf, R. Granich, H. Taelman, P. van de Perre, A. Serufilira, J. Bogaerts, et al.** 1993. Two-year incidence of tuberculosis in cohorts of HIV-infected and uninfected urban Rwandan women. *Am. Respir. Dis.* **146:**1439–1444.

3. **American Thoracic Society.** 2000. Diagnostic standards and classification of tuberculosis in adults and children. *Am. J. Respir. Crit. Care Med.* **161:**1376–1395.

4. **American Thoracic Society.** 2007. Diagnosis, treatment, and prevention of nontuberculous mycobacterial diseases. *Am. J. Respir. Crit. Care Med.* **175:**367–416.

5. **Aranaz, A., E. Liebana, E. Gomez-Mampaso, J. C. Galan, D. Cousins, A. Ortega, J. Blazquez, F. Baquero, A. Mateos, G. Suarez, and L. Dominguez.** 1999. *Mycobacterium tuberculosis* subsp. *caprae* subsp. nov.: a taxonomic study of the *Mycobacterium tuberculosis* complex isolated from goats in Spain. *Int. J. Syst. Bacteriol.* **49:**1263–1273.

6. **Archibald, L. K., L. C. McDonald, R. M. Addison, C. McKnight, T. Byrne, H. Dobbie, O. Nwanyanwu, P. Kezembe, L. B. Reller, and W. R. Jarvis.** 2000. Comparison of BACTEC MYCO/F LYTIC and WAMPOLE ISOLATOR 10 (lysis-centrifugation) systems for detection of bacteremia, mycobacteremia, and fungemia in a developing country. *J. Clin. Microbiol.* **38:**2994–2997.

7. **Association of State and Territorial Public Health Laboratory Directors and Centers for Disease Control and Prevention.** 1997. *Recognition and Prevention of False-Positive Test Results in Mycobacteriology. A Laboratory Training Program.* Centers for Disease Control and Prevention, Atlanta, GA.

8. **Attorri, S., S. Dunbar, and J. E. Clarridge III.** 2000. Assessment of morphology for rapid presumptive identification of *Mycobacterium tuberculosis* and *Mycobacterium kansasii*. *J. Clin. Microbiol.* **38:**1426–1429.

9. **Bang, D., T. Herlin, M. Stegger, A. B. Andersen, P. Torkko, E. Tortoli, and V. O. Thomsen.** 2008. *Mycobacterium arosiense* sp. nov., a slowly growing, scotochromogenic species causing osteomyelitis in an immunocompromised child. *Int. J. Syst. Evol. Microbiol.* **58:**2398–2402.

10. **Behr, M. A., and P. M. Small.** 1999. A historical and molecular phylogeny of BCG strains. *Vaccine* **17:**915–922.

11. **Bennett, S. N., D. E. Peterson, D. R. Johnson, W. N. Hall, B. Robinson-Dunn, and S. Dietrich.** 1994. Bronchoscopy-associated *Mycobacterium xenopi* pseudoinfections. *Am. J. Respir. Crit. Care Med.* **150:**245–250.

12. **Ben Salah, I., C. Cayrou, D. Raoult, and M. Drancourt.** 2009. *Mycobacterium marseillense* sp. nov., *Mycobacterium timonense* sp. nov. and *Mycobacterium bouchedurhonense* sp. nov., novel species in the *Mycobacterium avium* complex. *Int. J. Syst. Evol. Microbiol.* **59:**2803–2808.

13. **Bergamini, B. M., M. Losi, F. Valenti, R. D'Amico, B. Meccugni, M. Meacci, D. de Giovanni, F. Rumianesi, L. M. Fabbri, F. Balli, and L. Richeldi.** 2009. Performance of commercial blood tests for the diagnosis of latent tuberculosis infection in children and adolescents. *Pediatrics* **123:**e419–e424.

14. **Best, M., S. A. Sattar, V. S. Springthorpe, and M. E. Kennedy.** 1990. Efficacies of selected disinfectants against *Mycobacterium tuberculosis*. *J. Clin. Microbiol.* **28:**2234–2239.

15. **Bignardi, G. E., S. P. Barrett, R. Hinkins, P. A. Jenkins, and M. P. Rebec.** 1994. False-positive *Mycobacterium avium-intracellulare* cultures with the BACTEC 460 TB system. *J. Hosp. Infect.* **26:**203–210.

16. **Bobadilla-del-Valle, M., A. Ponce-de-Leon, M. Kato-Maeda, A. Hernandez-Cruz, J. J. Calva-Mercado, B. Chavez-Mazari, B. A. Caballero-Rivera, J. C. Nolasco-Garcia, and J. Sifuentes-Osornio.** 2003. Comparison of sodium bicarbonate, cetyl-pyridinium chloride, and sodium borate for preservation of sputa for culture of *Mycobacterium tuberculosis*. *J. Clin. Microbiol.* **41:**487–4488.

17. **Brosch, R., S. V. Gordon, T. Garnier, K. Eiglmeier, W. Frigui, P. Valenti, S. Dos Santos, S. Duthoy, S. Lacroix, C. Garcia-Pelayo, J. K. Inwald, et al.** 2007. Genome plasticity of BCG and impact on vaccine efficacy. *Proc. Natl. Acad. Sci. USA* **104:**5596–5601.

18. **Brosch, R., S. V. Gordon, M. Marmiesse, P. Brodin, C. Buchrieser, K. Eiglmeier, T. Garnier, C. Gutierrez, G. Hewinson, K. Kremer, L. M. Parsons, et al.** 2002. A new evolutionary scenario for the *Mycobacterium tuberculosis* complex. *Proc. Natl. Acad. Sci. USA* **99:**3684–3689.

19. **Bruijnesteijn van Coppenraet, L. E. S., P. E. W. de Haas, J. A. Lindeboom, E. J. Kuijper, and D. van Soolingen.** 2008. Lymphadenitis in children is caused by *Mycobacterium avium hominissuis* and not related to "bird tuberculosis." *Eur. J. Clin. Microbiol. Infect. Dis.* **27:**293–299.

20. **Bruijnesteijn van Coppenraet, L. E. S., E. J. Kuijper, J. A. Lindeboom, J. M. Prins, and E. C. Class.** 2005. *Mycobacterium haemophilum* in immunocompromised patients. *Clin. Infect. Dis.* **33:**330–337.

21. **Burman, W. J., and R. R. Reves.** 2000. Review of false-positive cultures for *Mycobacterium tuberculosis* and recommendations for avoiding unnecessary treatment. *Clin. Infect. Dis.* **31:**1390–1395.

22. **Cattamanchi, A., J. L. Davis, W. Worodria, S. Yoo, J. Matovu, J. Kiidha, F. Nankya, R. Kyeyune, A. Andama, M. Joloba, D. Osmond, et al.** 2008. Poor performance of universal sample processing method for diagnosis of pulmonary tuberculosis by smear microscopy and culture in Uganda. *J. Clin. Microbiol.* **46:**3325–3329.

23. **Centers for Disease Control and Prevention.** 1996. Nucleic acid amplification tests for tuberculosis. *MMWR Morb. Mortal. Wkly. Rep.* **45:**950–952.

24. **Centers for Disease Control and Prevention.** 1997. Multiple misdiagnoses of tuberculosis resulting from laboratory error—Wisconsin 1996. *MMWR Morb. Mortal. Wkly. Rep.* **46:**797–801.

25. **Centers for Disease Control and Prevention—National Institutes of Health.** 2007. *Biosafety in Microbiological and Biomedical Laboratories*, 5th ed. L. C. Chosewood and D. E.

Wilson (ed.). U. S. Government Printing Office, Washington, DC. http://www.cdc.gov/od/ohs.

26. **Chee, C. B. E., S. H. Gan, K. W. KhinMar, T. M. Barkham, C. K. Koh, S. Liang, and Y. T. Wang.** 2008. Comparison of sensitivities of two commercial gamma interferon release assays for pulmonary tuberculosis. *J. Clin. Microbiol.* **46:**1935–1940.

27. **Chroneou, A., S. K. Zimmerman, S. Cook, S. Willey, J. Eyre-Kelly, N. Zias, D. S. Shapiro, J. F. Beamis, Jr., and D. E. Craven.** 2008. Molecular typing of *Mycobacterium chelonae* isolates from a pseudo-outbreak involving an automated bronchoscope washer. *Infect. Contr. Hosp. Epidemiol.* **29:**1088–1090.

28. **Clinical and Laboratory Standards Institute.** 2006. *Molecular Diagnostic Methods for Infectious Diseases.* Document MM03-A2. CLSI, Wayne, PA.

29. **Clinical and Laboratory Standards Institute.** 2008. *Laboratory Detection and Identification of Mycobacteria.* Document M48-A. CLSI, Wayne, PA.

30. **Clinical and Laboratory Standards Institute.** 2009. *Susceptibility Testing of Mycobacteria, Nocardiae, and Other Aerobic Actinomycetes.* Document M24-A2. CLSI, Wayne, PA.

31. **Cohen, Y. H., A. Jacob, S. Ashkenazi, T. Edlitz-Markus, Z. Samra, L. Kaufmann, and A. Zeharia.** 2008. *Mycobacterium haemophilum* and lymphadenitis in immunocompetent children, Israel. *Emerg. Infect. Dis.* **14:**1437–1439.

32. **Cole, S. T., R. Brosch, J. Parkhill, T. Garnier, C. Churcher, D. Harris, S. V. Gordon, K. Eiglmeier, S. Gas, C. E. Barry III, F. Tekaia, et al.** 1998. Deciphering the biology of *Mycobacterium tuberculosis* from the complete genome sequence. *Nature* **393:**537–544.

33. **Cole, S. T., K. Eiglmeier, J. Parkhill, K. D. James, N. R. Thomson, P. R. Wheeler, N. Honoré, T. Garnier, C. Churcher, D. Harris, K. Mungall, et al.** 2001. Massive gene decay in the leprosy bacillus. *Nature* **409:**1007–1011.

34. **Conville, P. S., and F. G. Witebsky.** 2005. *Nocardia* and other aerobic actinomycetes, p. 1137–1180. *In* S. P. Borriello, P. R. Murray, and G. Funke (ed.), *Topley & Wilson's Microbiology and Microbial Infections, Bacteriology,* 10th ed., vol. 2. Hodder Arnold, London, England.

35. **Corbett, E. L., M. Hay, G. J. Churchyard, T. Clayton, B. G. Williams, D. Hayes, D. Mulder, and K. M. de Cock.** 1999. *Mycobacterium kansasii* and M. *scrofulaceum* isolates from HIV-negative South African gold miners: incidence, clinical significance and radiology. *Int. J. Tuberc. Lung Dis.* **3:**501–507.

36. **Cousins, D. V., R. Bastida, A. Cataldi, V. Quse, S. Redrobe, S. Dow, P. Duignan, A. Murray, C. Dupont, N. Ahmed, D. M. Collins, et al.** 2003. Tuberculosis in seals caused by a novel member of the *Mycobacterium tuberculosis* complex: *Mycobacterium pinnipedii* sp. nov. *Int. J. Syst. Evol. Microbiol.* **53:**1305–1314.

37. **Coyle, M. B., L. Carlson, C. Wallis, R. Leonard, V. Raisys, J. Kilburn, M. Samadpour, and E. Böttger.** 1992. Laboratory aspects of *Mycobacterium genavense,* a proposed species isolated from AIDS patients. *J. Clin. Microbiol.* **30:**3206–3212.

38. **Cruciani, M., C. Scarpaio, M. Malena, O. Bosco, G. Serpelloni, and C. Mengoli.** 2004. Meta-analysis of BACTEC MGIT 960 and BACTEC 460 TB, with or without solid media, for detection of mycobacteria. *J. Clin. Microbiol.* **42:**2321–2325.

39. **Crump, J. A., D. C. Tanner, S. Mirrett, C. M. McKnight, and L. B. Reller.** 2003. Controlled comparison of BACTEC 13A, MYCO/F LYTIC, BacT/ALERT MB, and ISOLATOR 10 systems for detection of mycobacteremia. *J. Clin. Microbiol.* **41:**1987–1990.

40. **de Lastours, V., R. Guillemain, J.-L. Mainardi, A. Aubert, P. Chevalier, A. Lefort, and I. Podglajen.** 2008. Early diagnosis of disseminated *Mycobacterium genavense* infection. *Emerg. Infect. Dis.* **14:**346–347.

41. **Demangel, C., T. P. Stinear, and S. T. Cole.** 2009. Buruli ulcer: reductive evolution enhances pathogenicity of *Mycobacterium ulcerans. Nat. Rev. Microbiol.* **7:**50–60.

42. **Desmond, E., A. T. Ahmed, W. S. Probert, J. Ely, Y. Jang, C. A. Sanders, S.-Y. Lin, and J. Flood.** 2004. *Mycobacterium africanum* cases, California. *Emerg. Infect. Dis.* **10:**921–923.

43. **Detjen, A. K., L. Loebenberg, H. M. Grewal, K. Stanley, A. Gutschmidt, C. Kruger, N. Du Plessis, M. Kidd, N. Beyers, G. Walzl, and A. C. Hesseling.** 2009. Short-term reproducibility of a commercial interferon gamma release assay. *Clin. Vaccine Immunol.* **16:**1170–1175.

44. **Dhillon, S. S., and C. Watanakunakorn.** 2000. Lady Windermere syndrome: middle lobe bronchiectasis and *Mycobacterium avium* complex infection due to voluntary cough suppression. *Clin. Infect. Dis.* **30:**572–575.

45. **Diel, R., R. Loddenkemper, K. Meywald-Walter, R. Gottschalk, and A. Nienhaus.** 2009. Comparative performance of tuberculin test, QuantiFERON-TB-Gold In Tube assay, and T-Spot.TB test in contact investigations for tuberculosis. *Chest* **135:**1010–1018.

46. **Djelouadji, Z., J. Orehek, and M. Drancourt.** 2009. Rapid detection of laboratory cross-contamination with *Mycobacterium tuberculosis* using multispacer sequence typing. *BMC Microbiol.* **9:**47–51.

47. **Eckburg, P. B., E. O. Buadu, P. Stark, P. S. A. Sarinas, R. K. Chitkara, and W. G. Kuschner.** 2000. Clinical and chest radiographic findings among persons with sputum culture positive for *Mycobacterium gordonae. Chest* **117:**96–102.

48. **Edson, R. S., C. L. Terrell, W. M. Brutinel, and N. L. Wengenack.** 2006. *Mycobacterium intermedium* granulomatous dermatitis from hot tub exposure. *Emerg. Infect. Dis.* **12:**821–823.

49. **Emmanuel, F. X., A.-L. Seagar, C. Doig, A. Rayner, P. Claxton, and I. Laurenson.** 2007. Human and animal infections with *Mycobacterium microti,* Scotland. *Emerg. Infect. Dis.* **13:**1924–1927.

50. **European Society of Mycobacteriology.** 1991. *Diagnostic Public Health Mycobacteriology,* p. 57–64. M. D. Yates, and D. G. Groothuis (ed.). Bureau of Hygiene and Tropical Disease, London, United Kingdom.

51. **Fabre, M., J.-L. Koeck, P. Le Flèche, F. Simon, V. Hervé, G. Vergnaud, and C. Pourcel.** 2004. High genetic diversity revealed by variable-number tandem repeat genotyping and analysis of *hsp65* gene polymorphism in a large collection of "*Mycobacterium canettii*" strains indicates that the M. *tuberculosis* complex is a recently emerged clone of "M. *canettii.*" *J. Clin. Microbiol.* **42:**3248–3255.

52. **Falkinham, J. O.** 1996. Epidemiology of infection by nontuberculous mycobacteria. *Clin. Microbiol. Rev.* **9:**178–215.

53. **Fanti, F., E. Tortoli, L. Hall, G. D. Roberts, R. M. Kroppenstedt, I. Dodi, S. Conti, L. Polonelli, and C. Chezzi.** 2004. *Mycobacterium parmense* sp. nov. *Int. J. Syst. Evol. Microbiol.* **54:**1123–1127.

54. **Feller, M., K. Huwiler, R. Stephan, E. Altpeter, A. Shang, H. Furrer, G. E. Pfyffer, T. Jemmi, A. Baumgartner, and M. Egger.** 2007. *Mycobacterium avium* subspecies *paratuberculosis* and Crohn's disease: a systematic review and meta-analysis. *Lancet Infect. Dis.* **7:**607–613.

55. **Fergie, J. E., T. W. Milligan, B. M. Henderson, and W. W. Stafford.** 1997. Intrathoracic *Mycobacterium avium* complex infection in immunocompetent children: case report and review. *J. Infect. Dis.* **24:**250–253.

56. **Ferroni, A., H. Vu-Thien, P. Lanotte, M. Le Bourgeois, I. Sermet-Gaudelus, B. Fauroux, S. Marchand, F. Varaigne, P. Berche, J.-L. Gaillard, and C. Offredo.** 2006. Value of the chlorhexidine decontamination method for recovery of nontuberculous mycobacteria from sputum samples of patients with cystic fibrosis. *J. Clin. Microbiol.* **44:**2237–2239.

57. **Fite, G. L., F. J. Cambre, and M. H. Hunt.** 1947. Procedures for demonstrating lepra bacilli in paraffin sections. *Arch. Pathol.* **43:**624–625.

58. **Fleming, D. O., and D. L. Hunt.** 2006. *Biological Safety: Principles and Practices,* 4th ed. American Society for Microbiology, Washington, DC.

59. **Frota, C. C., D. M. Hunt, R. S. Buxton, L. Rickman, J. Hinds, K. Kremer, R. van Soolingen, and M. J. Colston.** 2004. Genome structure in the vole bacillus, *Mycobacterium microti,* a member of the *Mycobacterium tuberculosis* complex with a low virulence for humans. *Microbiology* **15:**1519–1527.

60. **Frothingham, R., P. L. Strickland, G. Bretzel, S. Ramaswamy, J. M. Musser, and D. L. Williams.** 1999. Phenotypic and genotypic characterization of *Mycobacterium africanum* isolates from West Africa. *J. Clin. Microbiol.* **37:**1921–1926.

61. **Fukuoka, M., Y. Matsumura, S. Kore-eda, Y. Iinuma, and Y. Miyachi.** 2008. Cutaneous infection due to *Mycobacterium interjectum* in an immunosuppressed patient with microscopic polyangitis. *Br. J. Dermatol.* **159:**1382–1384.

62. **Fyfe, J. A., C. J. Lavender, P. D. Johnson, M. Globan, A. Sievers, J. Azuolas, and T. P. Stinear.** 2007. Development and application of two multiplex real-time PCR assays for the detection of *Mycobacterium ulcerans* in clinical and environmental samples. *Appl. Environ. Microbiol.* **73:**4733–4740.

63. **Gagneux, S., K. DeRiemer, T. Van, M. Kato-Maeda, B. C. de Jong, S. Narayanan, M. Nicol, S. Niemann, K. Kremer, M. C. Gutierrez, M. Hilty, et al.** 2006. Variable host-pathogen compatibility in *Mycobacterium tuberculosis*. *Proc. Natl. Acad. Sci. USA* **103:**2869–2873.

64. **Gandhi, N. R., A. Moll, A. W. Sturm, R. Pawinski, T. Govender, U. Lalloo, K. Zeller, J. Andrews, and G. Friedland.** 2006. Extensively drug-resistant tuberculosis as a cause of death in patients co-infected with tuberculosis and HIV in a rural area of South Africa. *Lancet* **368:**1575–1580.

65. **Garnier, T., K. Eigelmeier, J.-C. Camus, N. Medina, H. Mansoor, M. Pryor, S. Duthoy, S. Grondlin, C. Lacroix, C. Monsempe, S. Simon, et al.** 2003. The complete genome sequence of *Mycobacterium bovis*. *Proc. Natl. Acad. Sci. USA* **100:**7877–7882.

66. **Ghosh, J., P. Larsson, B. Singh, B. M. Pettersson, N. M. Islam, S. N. Sarkar, S. Dasgupta, and L. A. Kirsebom.** 2009. Sporulation in mycobacteria. *Proc. Natl. Acad. Sci. USA* **106:**10781–10786.

67. **Gillespie, E. E., D. Kotsanas, and R. L. Stuart.** 2008. Microbiological monitoring of endoscopes: 5-year review. *J. Gastroenterol. Hepatol.* **23:**1069–1074.

68. **Godreuil, S., H. Marchandin, D. Terru, V. Le Moing, M. Chammas, V. Vincent, E. Jumas-Bilak, P. van de Perre, and C. Carriere.** 2006. *Mycobacterium heckeshornense* tenosynovitis. *Scand. J. Infect. Dis.* **38:**1098–1101.

69. **Goh, K. S., E. Legrand, C. Sola, and N. Rastogi.** 2001. Rapid differentiation of "*Mycobacterium canettii*" from other *Mycobacterium tuberculosis* complex organisms by PCR-restriction analysis of the *hsp65* gene. *J. Clin. Microbiol.* **39:**3705–3708.

70. **Guerra, H., J. C. Palomino, E. Falconi, F. Bravo, N. Donaires, E. van Marck, and F. Portaels.** 2008. *Mycobacterium ulcerans* disease, Peru. *Emerg. Infect. Dis.* **14:**373–377.

71. **Gutierrez, M. C., S. Brisse, R. Brosch, M. Fabre, B. Omaïs, M. Marmiesse, P. Supply, and V. Vincent.** 2005. Ancient origin and gene mosaicism of the progenitor of *Mycobacterium tuberculosis*. *PLoS Pathog.* **1:**e5.

72. **Han, X. Y., Y. H. Seo, K. C. Sizer, T. Schoberle, G. S. May, J. S. Spencer, W. Li, and R. G. Nair.** 2008. A new *Mycobacterium* species causing diffuse lepromatous leprosy. *Am. Clin. Pathol.* **130:**856–864.

73. **Hanna, B. A., A. Ebrahimzadeh, L. B. Elliott, M. A. Morgan, S. M. Novak, S. Rüsch-Gerdes, M. Acio, D. F. Dunbar, T. M. Holmes, C. H. Rexer, C. Savthyakumar, et al.** 1999. Multicenter evaluation of the BACTEC MGIT 960 System for recovery of mycobacteria. *J. Clin. Microbiol.* **37:**748–752.

74. **Hänscheid, T.** 2008. The future looks bright: low-cost fluorescent microscopes for detection of *Mycobacterium tuberculosis* and Coccidiae. *Trans. R. Soc. Trop. Med. Hyg.* **102:**520–521.

75. **Hänscheid, T., C. Monteiro, J. Melo Cristino, L. Marques Lito, and M. J. Salgano.** 2005. Growth of *Mycobacterium tuberculosis* in conventional BacT/ALERT FA blood culture bottles allows reliable diagnosis of mycobacteremia. *J. Clin. Microbiol.* **43:**890–891.

76. **Hänscheid, T., C. M. Ribeiro, H. M. Shapiro, and N. G. Perlmutter.** 2007. Fluorescence microscopy for tuberculosis diagnosis. *Lancet Infect. Dis.* **6:**570–581.

77. **Hastings, R. C., T. P. Gillis, J. L. Krahenbuhl, and S. G. Franzblau.** 1988. Leprosy. *Clin. Microbiol. Rev.* **1:**330–348.

78. **Havlik, J. A., B. Metchock, S. E. Thompson III, K. Barrett, D. Rimland, and C. R. Horsburgh, Jr.** 1993. A prospective evaluation of *Mycobacterium avium* complex colonization of the respiratory and gastrointestinal tracts of persons with human immunodeficiency virus infection. *J. Infect. Dis.* **168:**1045–1048.

79. **Hawkins, J. E., R. C. Good, G. P. Kubica, P. R. J. Gangadharam, H. M. Gruft, K. D. Stottmeier, H. M. Sommers, and L. G. Wayne.** 1983. Levels of laboratory services for mycobacterial diseases: official statement of the American Thoracic Society. *Am. Rev. Respir. Dis.* **128:**213.

80. **Heifets, L., T. Linder, T. Sanchez, D. Spencer, and J. Brennan.** 2000. Two liquid medium systems, Mycobacteria Growth Indicator Tube and MB Redox Tube, for *Mycobacterium tuberculosis* isolation from sputum specimens. *J. Clin. Microbiol.* **38:**1227–1230.

81. **Hillebrand-Haverkort, M. E., A. H. Kolk, L. F. Kox, J. J. ten Velden, and J. H. ten Veen.** 1999. Generalized *Mycobacterium genavense* infection in HIV-infected patients: detection of the mycobacterium in hospital tap water. *Scand. J. Infect. Dis.* **31:**63–68.

82. **Hines, N., J. B. Payeur, and L. J. Hoffman.** 2006. Comparison of the recovery of *Mycobacterium bovis* isolates using the BACTEC MGIT 960 System, BACTEC 460 System, and Middlebrook7H10 and 7H11 solid media. *J. Vet. Diagn. Investig.* **18:**243–250.

83. **Hoefsloot, W., M. J. Boeree, J. van Ingen, S. Bendien, C. Magis, W. de Lange, P. N. Dekhuijzen, and D. van Soolingen.** 2008. The rising incidence and clinical relevance of *Mycobacterium malmoense*: a review of the literature. *Int. J. Tuberc. Lung Dis.* **12:**987–993.

84. **Hoop, R. K., E. C. Böttger, and G. E. Pfyffer.** 1996. Etiological agents of mycobacterioses in pet birds between 1986 and 1995. *J. Clin. Microbiol.* **34:**991–992.

85. **Hopewell, P. C., and R. M. Jasmer.** 2005. Overview of clinical tuberculosis, p. 15–31. In S. T. Cole, K. D. Eisenach, D. N. McMurray, and W. R. Jacobs, Jr. (ed.), *Tuberculosis and the Tubercle Bacillus*. ASM Press, Washington, DC.

86. **Horsburgh, C., B. Metchock, J. McGowan, Jr., and S. Thompson.** 1992. Clinical implications of recovery of *Mycobacterium avium* complex from the stool or respiratory tract of HIV-infected individuals. *AIDS* **6:**512–514.

87. **Horsburgh, C. R., Jr., U. G. Mason III, D. C. Farhi, and M. D. Iseman.** 1985. Disseminated infection with *Mycobacterium avium-intracellulare*. A report of 13 cases and review of the literature. *Medicine* **64:**36–48.

88. **Huber, J., E. Richter, L. Binder, M. Maass, R. Eberl, and W. Zenz.** 2008. *Mycobacterium bohemicum* and cervical lymphadenitis. *Emerg. Infect. Dis.* **14:**1158–1159.

89. **Inderlied, C., C. Kempler, and L. Bermudez.** 1993. The *Mycobacterium avium* complex. *Clin. Microbiol. Rev.* **6:**266–310.

90. **Isenberg, H. D.** 2004. *Clinical Microbiology Procedures Handbook*, 2nd ed. American Society for Microbiology, Washington, DC.

91. **Isenberg, H. D., R. F. D'Amato, L. Heifets, P. R. Murray, M. Scardamaglia, M. C. Jacobs, P. Alperstein, and A. Niles.** 1991. Collaborative feasibility study of a biphasic system (Roche Septi-Chek AFB) for rapid detection and isolation of mycobacteria. *J. Clin. Microbiol.* **29:**1719–1722.

92. **Jassal, M., and W. R. Bishai.** 2009. Extensively drug-resistant tuberculosis. *Lancet Infect. Dis.* **9:**19–30.

93. **Jauréguy, F., V. Ioos, P. Arzouk, M. Hornstein, B. Picard, M. C. Gutierrez, and D. Valeyre.** 2007. *Mycobacterium heckeshornense*: an emerging pathogen responsible for a recurrent lung infection. *J. Infect.* **54:**e33–e35.

94. **Jensen, P. A., L. A. Lamber, M. F. Iademarco, and R. Rizon.** 2005. Guidelines for preventing transmission of *Mycobacterium tuberculosis* in health care settings. *MMWR Recommend. Rep.* **54**(RR-17):1–139.

95. **Joseph, S., E. Vaichulis, and V. Houk.** 1967. Lack of auramine-rhodamine fluorescence of Runyon group IV mycobacteria. *Am. Rev. Respir. Dis.* **95:**114–115.

96. **Kamboj, M., E. Louie, T. Kiehn, G. Papanicolaou, M. Glickman, and K. Sepkowitz.** 2008. *Mycobacterium haemophilum* infection after alemtuzumab treatment. *Emerg. Infect. Dis.* **14:**1821–1823.

97. **Kampmann, B., E. Whittaker, A. Williams, S. Walters, A. Gordon, N. Martinez-Alier, B. Williams, A. M. Crook, A. M. Hutton, and S. T. Anderson.** 2009. Interferon-gamma release assays do not identify more children with active TB than TST. *Eur. Respir. J.* **33:**1374–1382.

98. **Kent, P. T., and G. P. Kubica.** 1985. *Public Health Mycobacteriology: a Guide for the Level III Laboratory.* U.S. Department of Health and Human Services, Centers for Disease Control, Atlanta, GA.

99. **Kiers, A., A. Klarenbeek, B. Mendelts, D. van Soolingen, and G. Koëter.** 2008. Transmission of *Mycobacterium pinnipedii* to humans in a zoo with marine mammals. *Int. J. Tuberc. Lung Dis.* **12:**1469–1473.

100. **Killeen, A. A.** 2009. Laboratory sanctions for proficiency testing sample referral and result communication: a review of actions from 1993–2006. *Arch. Pathol. Lab. Med.* **133:**979–982.

101. **Kim, T. C., R. S. Blackman, K. M. Heatwole, T. Kim, and D. F. Rochester.** 1984. Acid-fast bacilli in sputum smears of patients with pulmonary tuberculosis. Prevalence and significance of negative smears pretreatment and positive smears post-treatment. *Am. Rev. Respir. Dis.* **129:**264–268.

102. **Kirby, J. E., M. Delaney, Q. Qian, and H. S. Gold.** 2009. Optimal use of Myco/F Lytic and standard BACTEC blood culture bottles for detection of yeast and mycobacteria. *Arch. Pathol. Lab. Med.* **133:**93–96.

103. **Kobashi, Y., T. Sugiu, H. Shimizu, Y. Ohue, K. Mouri, Y. Obase, N. Miyashita, and M. Oka.** 2009. Clinical evaluation of the T-SPOT.TB Test for patients with indeterminate results on the QuantiFERON TB-2G Test. *Intern. Med.* **48:**137–142.

104. **Koukila-Kähkölä, P., L. Paulin, E. Brander, E. Jantzen, M. Eho-Remes, and M. L. Katila.** 2000. Characterization of a new isolate of *Mycobacterium shimoidei* from Finland. *J. Med. Microbiol.* **49:**937–940.

105. **Kremer, L., and G. S. Besra.** 2005. A waxy tale, by *Mycobacterium tuberculosis*, p. 287–305. *In* S. T. Cole, K. D. Eisenach, D. N. McMurray, and W. R. Jacobs, Jr. (ed.), *Tuberculosis and the Tubercle Bacillus.* ASM Press, Washington, DC.

106. **Kubica, T., S. Rüsch-Gerdes, and S. Niemann.** 2003. *Mycobacterium bovis* subsp. *caprae* caused one-third of human *M. bovis*-associated tuberculosis cases reported in Germany between 1999 and 2001. *J. Clin. Microbiol.* **41:**3070–3077.

107. **Lalande, V., F. Barbut, A. Vernerot, M. Febvre, D. Nesa, S. Wadel, V. Vincent, and J. C. Petit.** 2001. Pseudo-outbreak of *Mycobacterium gordonae* associated with water from refrigerated fountains. *J. Hosp. Infect.* **48:**76–79.

108. **Levy, I., G. Grisaru-Soen, L. Lerner-Geva, E. Kerem, H. Blau, M. Bentur, M. Aviram, J. Rivlin, E. Picard, A. Lavy, Y. Yahav, et al.** 2008. Multicenter cross-sectional study of nontuberculous mycobacterial infections among cystic fibrosis patients, Israel. *Emerg. Infect. Dis.* **14:**378–384.

109. **Lewis, M. T., B. J. Marsh, and C. Fordham von Reyn.** 2003. Fish tank exposure and cutaneous infections due to *Mycobacterium marinum*: tuberculin skin testing, treatment, and prevention. *Clin. Infect. Dis.* **37:**390–397.

110. **Lipsky, B. A., J. Gates, F. C. Tenover, and J. J. Plorde.** 1984. Factors affecting the clinical value of microscopy for acid-fast bacilli. *Rev. Infect. Dis.* **6:**214–222.

111. **Loughry, W. J., R. W. Trumman, C. M. McDonough, M. K. Tilak, S. Garnier, and F. Delsuc.** 2009. Is leprosy spreading among nine-banded armadillos in the southeastern United States? *J. Wildl. Dis.* **45:**144–152.

112. **Mahapatra, S., J. Basu, P. J. Brennan, and D. C. Crick.** 2005. Structure, biosynthesis, and genetics of the mycolic acid-arabinogalactan-peptidoglycan complex, p. 275–285. *In* S. T. Cole, K. D. Eisenach, D. N. McMurray, and W. R. Jacobs, Jr. (ed.), *Tuberculosis and the Tubercle Bacillus.* ASM Press, Washington, DC.

113. **Manarolla, G., E. Liandris, G. Pisoni, D. Sassera, G. Grilli, D. Gallazzi, G. Sironi, P. Moroni, R. Piccinini, and T. Rampin.** 2008. Avian mycobacteriosis in companion birds: 20-year survey. *Vet. Microbiol.* **133:**323–327.

114. **Maoz, C., D. Shitrit, Z. Samra, N. Peled, L. Kaufman, M. R. Kramer, and J. Bishara.** 2008. Pulmonary *Mycobacterium simiae* infection: comparison with pulmonary tuberculosis. *Eur. J. Clin. Microbiol. Infect. Dis.* **27:**945–950.

115. **Marais, B. J., W. Brittle, K. Painczyk, A. C. Hesseling, N. Beyers, E. Wasserman, D. van Soolingen, and R. M. Warren.** 2008. Use of light-emitting diode fluorescence microscopy to detect acid-fast bacilli in sputum. *Clin. Infect. Dis.* **47:**203–207.

116. **Marmiesse, M., P. Brodin, C. Buchrieser, C. Gutierrez, N. Simoes, V. Vincent, P. Glaser, S. T. Cole, and R. Brosch.** 2004. Macro-array and bioinformatics analyses reveal mycobacterial "core" genes, variation in the ESAT-6 gene family and new phylogenetic markers for the *Mycobacterium tuberculosis* complex. *Microbiology* **150:**483–496.

117. **Martin, A., M. Herranz, M. M. Lirola, R. F. Fernandez, INDAL-TB Group, E. Bouza, and D. Garcia de Viedma.** 2008. Optimized molecular resolution of cross-contamination alerts in clinical mycobacteriology laboratories. *BMC Microbiol.* **8:**30–34.

118. **Masaki, T., K. Ohkusu, H. Hata, N. Fujiwara, H. Iihara, M. Yamada-Noda, P. H. Nhung, M. Hayashi, Y. Asano, Y. Kawamura, and T. Ezaki.** 2006. *Mycobacterium kumamotonense* sp. nov., recovered from clinical specimen and the first isolation report of *Mycobacterium arupense* in Japan: novel slowly growing, non-chromogenic clinical isolates related to *Mycobacterium terrae* complex. *Microbiol. Immunol.* **50:**889–897.

119. **Mase, S. R., A. Ramsay, V. Ng, M. Henry, P. C. Hopewell, J. Cunningham, R. Urbanczik, M. D. Perkins, M. A. Aziz, and M. Pai.** 2007. Yield of serial sputum specimen examinations in the diagnosis of tuberculosis: a systematic review. *Int. J. Tuberc. Lung Dis.* **11:**485–495.

120. **Mayall, B., V. Gurtler, L. Irving, A. Marzec, and D. Leslie.** 1999. Identification of *Mycobacterium shimoidei* by molecular techniques: case report and summary of the literature. *Int. J. Tuberc. Lung Dis.* **3:**169–173.

121. **Mazurek, G. H., J. Jerab, P. Lobue, M. F. Iademarco, B. Metchock, and A. Vernon.** 2005. Guidelines for using the QuantiFERON-TB Gold test for detecting *Mycobacterium tuberculosis* infection, United States. Centers for Disease Control and Prevention. *MMWR Recommend. Rep.* **54(RR-15):**49–55.

122. **McBride, S. J., S. L. Taylor, S. K. Pandey, and D. J. Holland.** 2009. First case of *Mycobacterium heckeshornense* lymphadenitis. *J. Clin. Microbiol.* **47:**268–270.

123. **Menzies, D., M. Pai, and G. Comstock.** 2007. Meta-analysis: new tests for the diagnosis of latent tuberculosis infection: areas of uncertainty and recommendations for research. *Ann. Intern. Med.* **146:**340–354.

124. **Meybeck, A., C. Fortin, S. Abgrall, H. Adle-Biassette, G. Hayem, R. Ruimy, and P. Yeni.** 2005. Spondylitis due to *Mycobacterium xenopi* in a human immunodeficiency virus type 1-infected patient: case report and review of the literature. *J. Clin. Microbiol.* **43:**1465–1466.

125. **Mijs, W., P. de Haas, R. Rossau, T. van der Laan, L. Rigouts, F. Portaels, and D. van Soolingen.** 2002. Molecular evidence to support a proposal to reserve the designation *Mycobacterium avium* subsp. *avium* for the bird-type isolates and *M. avium* subsp. *hominissuis* for the human/porcine type of *M. avium. Int. J. Syst. Evol. Microbiol.* **52:**1505–1518.

126. **Miltgen, J., M. Morillon, J. L. Koeck, A. Varnerot, J. F. Briant, G. Nguyen, D. Verrot, D. Bonnet, and V. Vincent.** 2002. Two cases of pulmonary tuberculosis caused by *Mycobacterium tuberculosis* subsp. *canettii. Emerg. Infect. Dis.* **8:**1350–1352.

127. **Mitscherlich, E., and E. H. Marth.** 1984. *Microbial Survival in the Environment,* p. 232–266. Springer Verlag, New York, NY.

128. **Mixides, G., V. Shende, L. D. Teeter, R. Awe, J. M. Musser, and E. A. Graviss.** 2005. Number of negative acid-fast smears needed to adequately assess infectivity of patients with pulmonary tuberculosis. *Chest* **128:**108–115.

129. **Mohamed, A. M., P. C. Iwen, S. Tarantolo, and S. H. Hinrichs.** 2004. *Mycobacterium nebraskense* sp. nov., a novel slowly growing scotochromogenic species. *Int. J. Syst. Evol. Microbiol.* **54:**2057–2060.

130. **Monkongdee, P., K. D. McCarthy, K. P. Cain, T. Tasaneepayan, N. H. Dung, N. T. Lan, N. T. Yen, N. Teeratakulpisarn, N. Udomsantisuk, C. Heilig, and J. K. Varma.** 2009. Yield of acid-fast smear and mycobacterial culture for tuberculosis diagnosis in people with human immunodeficiency virus. *Am. J. Respir. Crit. Care Med.* **180:**903–908.

131. **Morris, A., L. B. Reller, M. Salfinger, K. Jackson, A. Sievers, and B. Dwyer.** 1993. Mycobacteria in stool specimens: the nonvalue of smears for predicting culture results. *J. Clin. Microbiol.* **31:**1385–1387.

132. **Morris, A. J., and L. B. Reller.** 1993. Reliability of cord formation in BACTEC media for presumptive identification of mycobacteria. *J. Clin. Microbiol.* **31:**2533–2534.

133. **Moser, I., W. M. Prodinger, H. Hotzel, R. Greenwald, K. P. Lyashchenko, D. Bakker, D. Gomis, T. Seidler, C. Ellenberger, U. Hetzel, K. Wuennemann, et al.** 2008. *Mycobacterium pinnipedii*: transmission from South American sea lion (*Otaria byronia*) to Bactrian camel (*Camelus bactrianus bactrianus*) and Malayan tapirs (*Tapirus indicus*). *Vet. Microbiol.* **127:**399–406.

134. **Mostowy, S., A. Onipede, S. Gagneux, S. Niemann, K. Kremer, E. P. Desmond, M. Kato-Maeda, and M. Behr.** 2004. Genomic analysis distinguishes *Mycobacterium africanum*. *J. Clin. Microbiol.* **42:**3594–3599.

135. **Mun, H. S., H. J. Kim, E. J. Oh, H. Kim, G. H. Bai, H. K. Yu, Y. G.Park, C. Y. Cha, Y. H. Kook, and B. J. Kim.** 2007. *Mycobacterium seoulense* sp. nov., a slowly growing scotochromogenic species. *Int. J. Syst. Evol. Microbiol.* **57:**594–599.

136. **Mun, H. S., J. H. Park, H. Kim, H. K. Yu, Y. G. Park, C. Y. Cha, Y. H. Kook, and B. J. Kim.** 2008. *Mycobacterium senuense* sp. nov., a slowly growing, nonchromogenic species closely related to the *Mycobacterium terrae* complex. *Int. J. Syst. Evol. Microbiol.* **58:**641–646.

137. **Murcia, M. I., E. Tortoli, M. C. Menendez, E. Palenque, and M. J. Garcia.** 2006. *Mycobacterium colombiense* sp. nov., a novel member of the *Mycobacterium avium* complex and description of MAC-X as a new ITS genetic variant. *Int. J. Syst. Evol. Microbiol.* **56:**2049–2054.

138. **Murray, S. J., A. Barrett, J. G. Magee, and R. Freeman.** 2003. Optimisation of acid-fast smears for the direct detection of mycobacteria in clinical samples. *J. Clin. Pathol.* **56:**613–615.

139. **Niemann, S., T. Kubica, F. C. Bange, O. Adjei, E. N. Browne, M. A. Chinbuah, R. Diel, J. Gyapong, R. D. Horstmann, M. L. Joloba, C. G. Meyer, et al.** 2004. The species *Mycobacterium africanum* in the light of new molecular markers. *J. Clin. Microbiol.* **42:**3958–3962.

140. **Noeske, J., E. Dopico, G. Torrea, H. Wang, and A. van Deun.** 2009. Two vs. three sputum samples for microscopic detection of tuberculosis in a high HIV prevalence population. *Int. J. Tuberc. Lung Dis.* **13:**842–847.

141. **Noordhoek, G. T., S. Mulder, P. Wallace, and A. M. van Loon.** 2004. Multicentre quality control study for detection of *Mycobacterium tuberculosis* in clinical samples by nucleic amplification methods. *Clin. Microbiol. Infect.* **10:**295–301.

142. **Oevermann, A., G. E. Pfyffer, P. Zanolari, M. Meylan, and N. Robert.** 2004. Generalized tuberculosis in llamas (*Lama glama*) due to *Mycobacterium microti*. *J. Clin. Microbiol.* **42:**1818–1821.

143. **Okazaki, M., K. Ohkusu, H. Hata, H. Ohnisi, K. Sugahara, C. Kawamura, N. Fujiwara, S. Matsumoto, Y. Nishiuchi, K. Toyoda, H. Saito, et al.** 2009. *Mycobacterium kyorinense* sp. nov., a novel slow-growing species, related to *Mycobacterium celatum*, isolated from human clinical specimens. *Int. J. Syst. Evol. Microbiol.* **59:**1336–1341.

144. **O'Reilly, L. M., and C. J. Daborn.** 1995. The epidemiology of *Mycobacterium bovis* infections in animals and man: a review. *Tuberc. Lung Dis.* **76**(Suppl. 1):S1–46.

145. **Ostergaard Thompson, V., U. B. Dragsted, J. Bauer, K. Fuursted, and J. Lundgren.** 1999. Disseminated infection with *Mycobacterium genavense*: a challenge to physicians and mycobacteriologists. *J. Clin. Microbiol.* **37:**3901–3905.

146. **Padilla, E., J. M. Manterola, V. Gonzalez, C. G. Thornton, M. D. Quesada, M. D. Sanchez, M. Perez, and V. Ausina.** 2005. Comparison of the sodium hydroxide specimen processing method with the C_{18}-carboxypropylbetaine specimen processing method using independent specimens with auramine smear, the MB/BacT liquid culture system, and the COBAS AMPLICOR MTB Test. *J. Clin. Microbiol.* **43:**6091–6097.

147. **Pai, M., and R. O'Brien.** 2007. Serial testing for tuberculosis: can we make sense of T cell assay conversions and reversions? *PLOS Med.* **4:**980–983.

148. **Pai, M., A. Zwerling, and D. Menzies.** 2008. Systematic review: T-cell-based assays for the diagnosis of latent tuberculosis infection: an update. *Ann. Intern. Med.* **149:**177–184.

149. **Palmore, T. N., Y. R. Shea, P. S. Conville, F. G. Witebsky, V. L. Anderson, I. P. Rupp Hodge, and S. M. Holland.** 2009. "*Mycobacterium tilburgii*," a newly described, uncultivated opportunistic pathogen. *J. Clin. Microbiol.* **47:**1585–1587.

150. **Palomino, J. C., and F. Portaels.** 1998. Effects of decontamination methods and culture conditions on viability of *Mycobacterium ulcerans* in the BACTEC system. *J. Clin. Microbiol.* **36:**402–408.

151. **Parrish, N., K. Dionne, A. Sweeney, A. Hedgepeth, and K. Carroll.** 2009. Differences in time to detection and recovery of *Mycobacterium* spp. between the MGIT 960 and the BacT/ALERT MB automated culture systems. *Diagn. Microbiol. Infect. Dis.* **63:**342–345.

152. **Pascopella, L., S. Kellam, J. Ridderhof, D. P. Chin, A. Reingold, E. Desmond, J. Flood, and S. Royce.** 2004. Laboratory reporting of tuberculosis test results and patient treatment initiation in California. *J. Clin. Microbiol.* **42:**4209–4213.

153. **Pfyffer, G. E., R. Auckenthaler, J. D. A. van Embden, and D. van Soolingen.** 1998. *Mycobacterium canettii*, the smooth variant of M. *tuberculosis*, isolated from a Swiss patient exposed in Africa. *Emerg. Infect. Dis.* **4:**631–634.

154. **Pfyffer, G. E., and V. Vincent.** 2005. *Mycobacterium tuberculosis* complex, *Mycobacterium leprae*, and other slowly growing mycobacteria, p. 1181–1235. *In* S. P. Boriello, P. R. Murray, and G. Funke (ed.), *Topley & Wilson's Microbiology and Microbial Infections, Bacteriology*, 10th ed., vol. 2. Hodder Arnold, London, England.

155. **Pfyffer, G. E., H. M. Welscher, and P. Kissling.** 1997. Pretreatment of clinical specimens with sodium dodecyl (lauryl) sulfate is not suitable for the Mycobacteria Growth Indicator Tube cultivation method. *J. Clin. Microbiol.* **35:**2142–2144.

156. **Pfyffer, G. E., H. M. Welscher, P. Kissling, C. Cieslak, M. J. Casal, J. Gutierrez, and S. Rüsch-Gerdes.** 1997. Comparison of the Mycobacteria Growth Indicator Tube (MGIT) with radiometric and solid culture for recovery of acid-fast bacilli. *J. Clin. Microbiol.* **35:**364–368.

157. **Phillips, R. O., F. S. Sarfo, F. Osei-Sarpong, A. Oateng, I. Tetteh, A. Lartey, E. Adentwe, W. Opare, K. B. Asiedu, and M. Wansbrough-Jones.** 2009. Sensitivity of PCR targeting *Mycobacterium ulcerans* by use of fine-needle aspirates for diagnosis of Buruli ulcer. *J. Clin. Microbiol.* **47:**924–926.

158. **Pierre-Audigier, C., A. Ferroni, I. Sermet-Gaudelus, M. Le Bourgeois, C. Offredo, H. Vu-Thien, B. Fauroux, P. Mariani, A. Munck, E. Bingen, D. Guillemot, et al.** 2005. Age-related prevalence and distribution of nontuberculous mycobacterial species among patients with cystic fibrosis. *J. Clin. Microbiol.* **43:**3467–3470.

159. **Piersimoni, C., C. Scarparo, A. Callegaro, C. Passerini Tosi, D. Nista, S. Bornigia, M. Scagnelli, A. Rigon, G. Ruggiero, and A. Goglio.** 2001. Comparison of MB/BacT ALERT 3D System with radiometric BACTEC System and Löwenstein-Jensen medium for recovery and identification of mycobacteria from clinical specimen: a multicenter study. *J. Clin. Microbiol.* **39:**651–657.

160. Pinho, L., J. Santos, G. Oliveira, and M. Pestana. 2009. *Mycobacterium gordonae* urinary infection in a renal transplant recipient. *Transpl. Infect. Dis.* **11**:253–256.

161. Portaels, F., K. Chemlal, P. Elsen, P. D. R. Johnson, J. A. Hayman, J. Hibble, R. Kirkwood, and W. M. Meyers. 2001. *Mycobacterium ulcerans* in wild animals. *Rev. Sci. Tech. Off. Int. Epizoot.* **20**:252–264.

162. Portaels, F., M. T. Silva, and W. M. Meyers. 2009. Buruli ulcer. *Clin. Dermatol.* **27**:291–305.

163. Primm, T. P., C. A. Lucero, and J. O. Falkinham III. 2004. Health impacts of environmental mycobacteria. *Clin. Microbiol. Rev.* **17**:98–106.

164. Prodinger, W. M., A. Brandstätter, L. Naumann, M. Pacciarini, T. Kubica, M. L. Boschiroli, A. Aranaz, G. Nagy, Z. Cvetnic, M. Ocepek, A. Skrypnyk, et al. 2005. Characterization of *Mycobacterium caprae* isolates from Europe by mycobacterial interspersed repetitive unit genotyping. *J. Clin. Microbiol.* **43**:4984–4992.

165. Ramos, M., H. Soini, G. C. Roscanni, M. Jaques, M. C. Villares, and J. M. Musser. 1999. Extensive cross-contamination of specimens with *Mycobacterium tuberculosis* in a reference laboratory. *J. Clin. Microbiol.* **37**:916–919.

166. Realini, L., K. de Ridder, B. Hirschel, and F. Portaels. 1999. Blood and charcoal added to acidified agar media promote growth of *Mycobacterium genavense*. *Diagn. Microbiol. Infect. Dis.* **34**:45–50.

167. Realini, L., K. de Ridder, J. Palomino, B. Hirschel, and F. Portaels. 1998. Microaerophilic conditions promote growth of *Mycobacterium genavense*. *J. Clin. Microbiol.* **36**:2565–2570.

168. Remacha, M. A., A. Esteban, M. I. Parra, and M. S. Jiménez. 2007. Cervical lymphadenitis due to *Mycobacterium interjectum*. *Pediatr. Pulmonol.* **42**:398–399.

169. Ridderhof, J. C., L. O. Williams, S. Legois, P. A. Shult, B. Metchock, L. N. Kubista, J. H. Handsfield, R. J. Fehd, and P. H. Robinson. 2003. Assessment of laboratory performance of nucleic acid amplification tests for detection of *Mycobacterium tuberculosis*. *J. Clin. Microbiol.* **41**:5258–5261.

170. Roberts, G. D., N. L. Goodman, L. Heifets, H. W. Larsh, T. H. Lindner, J. K. McClatchy, M. R. McGinnis, S. H. Siddiqi, and P. Wright. 1983. Evaluation of the BACTEC radiometric method for recovery of mycobacteria and drug susceptibility testing of *Mycobacterium tuberculosis* from acid-fast smear-positive specimens. *J. Clin. Microbiol.* **18**:689–696.

171. Rudeeaneskin, J., S. Srisungngam, P. Sawanpanyalert, T. Sittiwakin, S. Likanonsakul, S. Pasadorn, P. Palittapongarnpim, P. J. Brennan, and B. Phetsuksiri. 2008. Light-Cycler real-time PCR for rapid detection and quantitation of *Mycobacterium leprae* in skin specimens. *FEMS Immunol. Med. Microbiol.* **54**:263–270.

172. Rynkiewicz, D. L., G. D. Cage, W. R. Butler, and N. M. Ampel. 1998. Clinical and microbiological assessment of *Mycobacterium simiae* isolates from a single laboratory in southern Arizona. *Clin. Infect. Dis.* **26**:625–630.

173. Saceanu, C., N. Pfeiffer, and T. McLean. 1993. Evaluation of sputum smears concentrated by cytocentrifugation for detection of acid-fast bacilli. *J. Clin. Microbiol.* **31**:2371–2374.

174. Saito, H., K. Toda, I. Matsumoto, K. Matsuo, K. Nakanaga, and N. Ishii. 2004. Bacteriological features of *Mycobacterium haemophilum* isolated from skin lesions in an immunodeficient patient. *Kansenshogaku Zasshi* **78**:389–397.

175. Sakamuri, R. M., M. Kimura, W. Li, H. C. Kim, H. Lee, K. Madanahally, W. C. Blackiv IV, M. Balagon, R. Gelber, S. N. Cho, P. J. Brennan, et al. 2009. Population-based molecular epidemiology of leprosy in Cebu, Philippines. *J. Clin. Microbiol.* **47**:2844–2854.

176. Salfinger, M., and F. Kafader. 1987. Comparison of two pretreatment methods for the detection of mycobacteria of BACTEC and Löwenstein-Jensen slants. *J. Microbiol. Methods* **6**:315–321.

177. Samra, Z., L. Kaufman, J. Bechor, and J. Bahar. 2000. Comparative study of three culture systems for optimal recovery of mycobacteria from different clinical specimens. *Eur. J. Clin. Microbiol. Infect. Dis.* **19**:750–754.

178. Saubolle, M. A., T. E. Kiehn, M. H. White, M. F. Rudinsky, and D. Armstrong. 1996. *Mycobacterium haemophilum*: microbiology and expanding clinical and geographic spectra of diseases in humans. *Clin. Microbiol. Rev.* **9**:435–447.

179. Schoch, O. D., G. E. Pfyffer, D. Buhl, and A. Paky. 2003. False-positive *Mycobacterium tuberculosis* culture revealed by restriction fragment length polymorphism analysis. *Infection* **31**:189–191.

180. Schweickert, B., O. Goldenberg, E. Richter, U. B. Göbel, A. Petrich, P. Buchholz, and A. Moter. 2008. Occurrence and clinical relevance of *Mycobacterium chimaera* sp. nov., Germany. *Emerg. Infect. Dis.* **14**:1443–1446.

181. Selvarangan, R., W.-K. Wu, T. T. Nguyen, L. D. C. Carlson, C. K. Wallis, S. K. Stiglich, Y.-C. Chen, K. C. Jost, Jr., J. L. Prentice, R. J. Wallace, Jr., S. L. Rassoulian Barrett, et al. 2004. Characterization of a novel group of mycobacteria and proposal of *Mycobacterium sherrisii* sp. nov. *J. Clin. Microbiol.* **42**:52–59.

182. Shapiro, H. M., and N. G. Perlmutter. 2007. Killer applications: toward affordable rapid cell-based diagnostics for malaria and tuberculosis. *Cytometry B* **74**(Suppl. 1):S152–S164.

183. Shirit, D., N. Peled, J. Bishara, R. Priess, S. Pitlik, Z. Samra, and M. R. Kramer. 2008. Clinical and radiological features of *Mycobacterium kansasii* infection and *Mycobacterium simiae* infection. *Respir. Med.* **102**:1598–1603.

184. Somoskövi, A., J. Dormandy, A. R. Mayrer, M. Carter, N. Hooper, and M. Salfinger. 2009. "*Mycobacterium canettii*" isolated from a human immunodeficiency virus-positive patient: first case recognized in the United States. *J. Clin. Microbiol.* **47**:255–257.

185. Somoskövi, A., J. E. Hotaling, M. Fitzgerald, D. O'Donnell, L. M. Parsons, and M. Salfinger. 2001. Lessons from a proficiency testing event for acid-fast microscopy. *Chest* **120**:250–257.

186. Somoskövi, A., and P. Magyar. 1999. Comparison of the Mycobacteria Growth Indicator Tube with MB Redox, Löwenstein-Jensen, and Middlebrook 7H11 media for recovery of mycobacteria in clinical specimens. *J. Clin. Microbiol.* **37**:1366–1369.

187. Stephan, C., T. Wolf, U. Goetsch, O. Bellinger, G. Nisius, G. Oremek, Z. Rakus, R. Gottschalk, S. Stark, H. R. Brodt, and S. Staszewski. 2009. Comparing QuantiFERON-tuberculosis Gold, T-SPOT tuberculosis and tuberculin skin test in HIV-infected individuals from a low prevalence tuberculosis country. *AIDS* **22**:2471–2479.

188. Stinear, T. P., T. Seeman, P. F. Harrison, G. A. Jenkin, J. K. Davies, P. D. Johnson, Z. Abdellah, C. Arrowsmith, T. Chillingworth, C. Churcher, K. Clarke, et al. 2008. Insights from the complete genome sequence of *Mycobacterium marinum* on the evolution of *Mycobacterium tuberculosis*. *Genome Res.* **18**:729–741.

189. Supply, P., E. Mazars, S. Lesjean, V. Vincent, B. Gicquel, and C. Locht. 2000. Variable human minisatellite-like regions in the *Mycobacterium tuberculosis* genome. *Mol. Microbiol.* **36**:762–771.

190. Taillard, C., G. Greub, R. Weber, G. E. Pfyffer, T. Bodmer, S. Zimmerli, R. Frei, S. Bassetti, P. Rohner, J. C. Piffaretti, E. Bernasconi, J. Bille, A. Telenti, and G. Prod'hom. 2003. Clinical implications of *Mycobacterium kansasii* species heterogeneity: Swiss national survey. *J. Clin. Microbiol.* **41**:1240–1244.

191. Talati, N. J., U. Seybold, B. Humphrey, A. Aina, J. Tapia, P. Weinfurter, R. Albalak, and H. M. Blumberg. 2009. Poor concordance between interferon-gamma release assays and tuberculin tests in diagnosis of latent tuberculosis infection among HIV-infected individuals. *BMC Infect. Dis.* **9**:15–24.

192. Tavast, E., E. Salo, I. Seppälä, and T. Tuuminen. 2009. IGRA tests perform similarly to TST but cause no adverse reactions: pediatric experience in Finland. *BMC Res. Notes* **2**:9–18.

193. Taylor, L. Q., A. J. Williams, and S. Santiago. 1990. Pulmonary disease caused by *Mycobacterium asiaticum*. *Tubercle* **71**:303–305.

194. **Thorel, M.-F., M. Krichevsky, and V. Levy-Frébault.** 1990. Numerical taxonomy of mycobactin-dependent mycobacteria, emended description of *Mycobacterium avium*, and description of *Mycobacterium avium* subsp. *avium* subsp. nov., *Mycobacterium avium* subsp. *paratuberculosis* subsp. nov., and *Mycobacterium avium* subsp. *silvaticum* subsp. nov. *Int. J. Syst. Bacteriol.* **40:**254–260.

195. **Tortoli, E.** 2003. Impact of genotypic studies in mycobacterial taxonomy: the new mycobacteria of the 1990s. *Clin. Microbiol. Rev.* **16:**319–354.

196. **Tortoli, E., F. Brunello, A. E. Cagni, D. Colombrita, D. Dionisio, L. Grisendi, V. Manfrin, M. Moroni, C. Passerini Tosi, G. Pinsi, C. Scarparo, and M. Tullia Simonetti.** 1998. *Mycobacterium genavense* in AIDS patients, report of 24 cases in Italy and review of the literature. *Eur. J. Epidemiol.* **14:**219–224.

197. **Tortoli, E., R. Mattei, C. Russo, and C. Scarparo.** 2006. *Mycobacterium lentiflavum*, an emerging pathogen? *J. Infect.* **52:**185–187.

198. **Tortoli, E., C. Piersimoni, R. M. Kroppenstedt, J. I. Montoya-Burgos, U. Reischl, A. Giacometti, and S. Emler.** 2001. *Mycobacterium doricum* sp. nov. *Int. J. Syst. Evol. Microbiol.* **51:**2007–2012.

199. **Tortoli, E., L. Rindi, M. J. Garcia, P. Chiaradonna, R. Dei, C. Garzelli, R. M. Kroppenstedt, N. Lari, R. Mattei, A. Mariottini, G. Mazzarelli, et al.** 2004. Proposal to elevate the genetic variant MAC-A, included in the *Mycobacterium avium* complex, to species rank as *Mycobacterium chimaera* sp. nov. *Int. J. Syst. Evol. Microbiol.* **54:**1277–1285.

200. **Tortoli, E., L. Rindi, K. S. Goh, M. L. Katila, A. Mariottini, R. Mattei, G. Mazzarelli, S. Suomalainen, P.Torkko, and N. Rastogi.** 2005. *Mycobacterium florentinum* sp. nov., isolated from humans. *Int. J. Syst. Evol. Microbiol.* **55:**1101–1106.

201. **Tortoli, E., M. Tullia Simonetti, D. Dionisio, and M. Meli.** 1994. Cultural studies on two isolates of *Mycobacterium genavense* from patients with acquired immunodeficiency syndrome. *Diagn. Microbiol. Infect. Dis.* **18:**7–12.

202. **Trifiro, S., A.-M. Bourgault, F. Lebel, and P. René.** 1990. Ghost mycobacteria on Gram stain. *J. Clin. Microbiol.* **28:**146.

203. **Tsai, T. F., C. C. Lai, C. H. Chang, C. H. Hsiao, and P. R. Hsueh.** 2006. Tenosynovitis caused by *Mycobacterium arupense* in a patient with diabetes mellitus. *Clin. Infect. Dis.* **47:**861–863.

204. **Turenne, C. Y., V. J. Cook, T. V. Burdz, R. J. Pauls, L. Thibert, J. N. Wolfe, and A. Kabani.** 2004. *Mycobacterium parascrofulaceum* sp. nov., novel slowly growing, scotochromogenic clinical isolates related to *Mycobacterium simiae*. *Int. J. Syst. Evol. Microbiol.* **54:**1543–1551.

205. **Turenne, C. Y., L. Thibert, K. Williams, T. V. Burdz, V. J. Cook, J. N. Wolfe, D. W. Cockcroft, and A. Kabani.** 2004. *Mycobacterium saskatchewanense* sp. nov., a novel slowly growing scotochromogenic species from human clinical isolates related to *Mycobacterium interjectum* and Accuprobe-positive for *Mycobacterium avium* complex. *Int. J. Syst. Evol. Microbiol.* **54:**659–667.

206. **Turenne, C. Y., R. Wallace, Jr., and M. A. Behr.** 2007. *Mycobacterium avium* in the postgenomic era. *Clin. Microbiol. Rev.* **20:**205–229.

207. **Ucko, M., and A. Colorni.** 2005. *Mycobacterium marinum* infections in fish and humans in Israel. *J. Clin. Microbiol.* **43:**892–895.

208. **van der Werf, T. S., W. T. A. van der Graaf, J. W. Tappero, and K. Asiedu.** 1999. *Mycobacterium ulcerans* infection. *Lancet* **354:**1013–1018.

209. **van Hest, R., A. van der Zanden, M. Boeree, K. Kremer, M. Dessens, P. Westenend, B. Mahara, R. van Uffeklen, R. Schütte, and W. de Lange.** 2004. *Mycobacterium heckeshornense* infection in an immunocompetent patient and identification by 16S rRNA sequence analysis of culture material and a histopathology tissue specimen. *J. Clin. Microbiol.* **42:**4386–4389.

210. **van Ingen, J., S. A. Al-Hajoj, M. Boeree, F. Al-Rabiah, M. Enaimi, R. de Zwaan, E. Tortoli, R. Dekhuijzen, and D. van Soolingen.** 2009. *Mycobacterium riyadhense* sp. nov.,

a non-tuberculous species identified as *Mycobacterium tuberculosis* complex by a commercial line-probe assay. *Int. J. Syst. Evol. Microbiol.* **59:**1049–1053.

211. **van Ingen, J., M. J. Boeree, P. N. Dekhuijzen, and D. van Soolingen.** 2008. Clinical relevance of *Mycobacterium simiae* in pulmonary samples. *Eur. Respir. J.* **31:**106–109.

212. **van Ingen, J., M. J. Boeree, K. Kösters, A. Wieland, E. Tortoli, R. P. Dekhuijzen, and D. van Soolingen.** 2009. Proposal to elevate *Mycobacterium avium* complex ITS sequevar MAC-Q to *Mycobacterium vulneris* sp. nov. *Int. J. Syst. Evol. Microbiol.* **59**(Pt. 9):2277–2282.

213. **van Ingen, J., M. J. Boeree, F. S. Stals, C. C. M. Pitz, J. J. C. M. Rooijmans-Rietjens, A. G. M. van der Zanden, P. N. R. Dekhuijzen, and D. van Soolingen.** 2007. Clinical *Mycobacterium conspicuum* isolation from two immunocompetent patients in The Netherlands. *J. Clin. Microbiol.* **45:**4075–4076.

214. **van Ingen, J., J. A. Lindenboom, N. G. Hartwig, R. E. de Zwaan, E. Tortoli, R. P. Dekhuijzen, M. J. Boeree, and D. van Soolingen.** 2009. *Mycobacterium mantenii* sp. nov., a pathogenic, slowly growing, scotochromogenic mycobacterium. *Int. J. Syst. Evol. Microbiol.* **59:**2782–2787.

215. **van Soolingen, D., T. Hoogenboezem, P. E. W. de Haas, P. W. M. Hermans, M. A. Koedam, K. S. Teppema, P. J. Brennan, G. S. Besra, F. Portaels, J. Top, et al.** 1997. A novel pathogenic taxon of the *Mycobacterium tuberculosis* complex, Canettii: characterization of an exceptional isolate from Africa. *Int. J. Syst. Bacteriol.* **47:**1236–1245.

216. **van Soolingen, D., A. G. M. van der Zanden, P. E. W. de Haas, G. T. Noordhoek, A. Kiers, N. A. Foudraine, F. Portaels, A. H. J. Kolk, K. Kremer, and J. D. A. van Embden.** 1998. Diagnosis of *Mycobacterium microti* infections among humans by using novel genetic markers. *J. Clin. Microbiol.* **36:**1840–1845.

217. **van Zyl-Smit, R. N., M. Pai, K. Peprah, R. Meldau, J. Kieck, J. Jurizu, M. Badri, A. Zumla, L. A. Sechi, E. D. Bateman, and K. Dheda.** 2009. Within-subject variability and boosting of T-cell interferon-γ responses after tuberculin skin testing. *Am. J. Respir. Crit. Care Med.* **180:**49–58.

218. **Viana-Niero, C., C. Gutierrez, C. Sola, I. Filliol, F. Boulahbal, V. Vincent, and N. Rastogi.** 2001. Genetic diversity of *Mycobacterium africanum* clinical isolates based on IS6110-restriction fragment length polymorphism analysis, spoligotyping, and variable number of tandem DNA repeats. *J. Clin. Microbiol.* **39:**57–65.

219. **Villiger, P. M., J. P. Zellweger, and B. Möller.** 2009. Novel screening tools for latent tuberculosis: time to leave an old friend? *Curr. Opin. Rheumatol.* **21:**238–243.

220. **Vuorenmaa, K., I. Ben Salah, V. Barlogis, H. Chambost, and M. Drancourt.** 2009. *Mycobacterium colombiense* and pseudotuberculous lymphadenopathy. *Emerg. Infect. Dis.* **15:**619–629.

221. **Wallace, R.** 1987. Nontuberculous mycobacteria and water: a love affair with increasing clinical importance. *Infect. Dis. Clin. N. Am.* **1:**677–686.

222. **Wallace, R. J., Jr., Y. Zhang, B. A. Brown, D. Dawson, D. T. Murphy, R. Wilson, and D. Griffith.** 1998. Polyclonal *Mycobacterium avium* complex infections in patients with nodular bronchiectasis. *Am. J. Respir. Crit. Care Med.* **158:**1235–1244.

223. **Warren, J. R., M. Bhattacharya, K. N. De Almeida, K. Trakas, and L. R. Peterson.** 2000. A minimum 5.0 ml of sputum improves the sensitivity of acid-fast smear for *Mycobacterium tuberculosis*. *Am. J. Respir. Crit. Care Med.* **161:**1559–1562.

224. **Wayne, L. G., and G. P. Kubica.** 1986. Mycobacteria, p. 1435–1457. In P. H. A. Sneath (ed.), *Bergey's Manual of Systematic Bacteriology*, vol. 2. Williams & Wilkins, Baltimore, MD.

225. **Welch, D., A. Guruswamy, S. Sides, C. Shaw, and M. Gilchrist.** 1993. Timely culture of mycobacteria which utilizes a microcolony method. *J. Clin. Microbiol.* **31:**2178–2184.

226. **Wheeler, P. R., and J. S. Blanchard.** 2005. General metabolism and biochemical pathways of tubercle bacilli, p. 309–339. In S. T. Cole, K. D. Eisenach, D. N. McMurray,

and W. R. Jacobs, Jr. (ed.), *Tuberculosis and the Tubercle Bacillus*. ASM Press, Washington, DC.

227. **White, D. A., T. E. Kiehn, A. Y. Bondoc, and S. A. Massarella.** 1999. Pulmonary nodule due to *Mycobacterium haemophilum* in an immunocompetent host. *Am. J. Respir. Crit. Care Med.* **160:**1366–1368.

228. **Whyte, T., B. Hanahoe, T. Collins, G. Corbett-Feeney, and M. Cormican.** 2000. Evaluation of the BACTEC MGIT 960 and MB/BacT Systems for routine detection of *Mycobacterium tuberculosis. J. Clin. Microbiol.* **38:**3131–3132.

229. **Wolinsky, E.** 1995. Mycobacterial lymphadenitis in children: a prospective study of 105 nontuberculous cases with long-term follow-up. *Clin. Infect. Dis.* **20:**954–963.

230. **Woods, G. L., G. Fish, M. Plaunt, and T. Murphy.** 1997. Clinical evaluation of Difco ESP Culture System II for growth and detection of mycobacteria. *J. Clin. Microbiol.* **35:**121–124.

231. **Woods, G. L., T. A. Long, and F. G. Witebsky.** 1996. Mycobacterial testing in clinical laboratories that participate in the College of American Pathologists Mycobacteriology Surveys. Changes in practices based on responses to 1992, 1993, and 1995 questionnaires. *Arch. Pathol. Lab. Med.* **120:**429–435.

232. **Woods, G. L., E. Pentony, M. J. Boxley, and A. M. Gatson.** 1995. Concentration of sputum by cytocentrifugation for preparation of smears for detection of acid-fast bacilli does not increase sensitivity of the fluorochrome stain. *J. Clin. Microbiol.* **33:**1915–1916.

233. **Woods, G. L., and J. C. Ridderhof.** 1996. Quality assurance in the mycobacteriology laboratory. *Clin. Lab. Med.* **16:**657–675.

234. **World Health Organization.** 1982. Report of the Study Group on chemotherapy of leprosy for control programs. *WHO Tech. Rep. Ser.* no. 847.

235. **World Health Organization.** 2007. *Buruli Ulcer Disease.* WHO Fact Sheet No. 199. World Health Organization, Geneva, Switzerland. http://www.who.int/mediacentre/factsheets/fs199/en/.

236. **World Health Organization.** 2008. Global leprosy situation, beginning of 2008. *Wkly. Epid. Rec.* **33:**293–300. http://www.who.int./wer.

237. **World Health Organization.** 2009. *Global Tuberculosis Control—Epidemiology, Strategy, Financing. WHO Report 2009.* World Health Organization, Geneva, Switzerland. http://www.who/htm/TB/2009.411.

238. **Yajko, D. M., P. S. Nassos, C. A. Sanders, P. C. Gonzalez, A. L. Reingold, C. R. Horsburgh, P. Hopewell, D. P. Chin, and W. K. Hadley.** 1993. Comparison of four decontamination methods for recovery of *Mycobacterium avium* complex from stools. *J. Clin. Microbiol.* **31:**302–306.

239. **Yeboah-Manu, D., T. Bodmer, E. Mensah-Quainoo, S. Owusu, D. Ofori-Adjei, and G. Pluschke.** 2004. Evaluation of decontamination methods and growth media for primary isolation of *Mycobacterium ulcerans* from surgical specimens. *J. Clin. Microbiol.* **42:**5875–5876.

240. **Zellweger, J.-P.** 2008. Latent tuberculosis: which test in which situation? *Swiss Med. Wkly.* **138:**31–37.

241. **Zellweger, J.-P., A. Zellweger, S. Ansermet, B. de Senarclens, and P. Wrighton-Smith.** 2005. Contact tracing using a new T-cell based test: better correlation with tuberculosis exposure than the tuberculin test. *Int. J. Tuberc. Lung Dis.* **9:**1242–1247.

Mycobacterium: Laboratory Characteristics of Slowly Growing Mycobacteria*

ELVIRA RICHTER, BARBARA A. BROWN-ELLIOTT, AND RICHARD J. WALLACE, JR.

29

This chapter represents a transition from previous chapters that detailed phenotypic methods of identification of mycobacteria. Although some phenotypic characterization remains important, it is now well recognized by experts in mycobacterial taxonomy that current accurate identification of organisms of both the *Mycobacterium tuberculosis* complex (MTBC) and the nontuberculous mycobacteria (NTM) requires molecular techniques for definitive identification to species level.

As Tortoli noted in 2003, mycobacterial taxonomy can be divided into two major periods defined by methods used for identification to species level (126). The first period, characterized by utilization of phenotypic studies, lasted from the late 1880s to the end of the 1980s. The second major era, characterized by a shift to genotypic studies, began during the last decade of the 20th century and has continued to the present time.

The MTBC remains the most important group within the genus *Mycobacterium* from a global and clinical perspective. The MTBC currently includes not only the most significant human mycobacterial pathogens, *M. tuberculosis*, *M. bovis*, and *M. bovis* bacillus Calmette-Guérin (BCG), but also less frequently encountered pathogens, *M. caprae*, *M. microti*, *M. africanum*, "*M. canettii*," and *M. pinnipedii*. Further discussion regarding the MTBC can be found in chapter 28 in this *Manual*.

Of the more than 130 currently validated species of NTM, approximately 60 are slowly growing species (Table 1). The most clinically significant and/or most frequently encountered slowly growing NTM species include *Mycobacterium avium*, *M. intracellulare*, *M. kansasii*, *M. marinum*, *M. xenopi*, *M. malmoense*, and *M. ulcerans*. *M. gordonae*, although rarely a pathogen, occurs frequently in human samples, usually as a consequence of contamination from tap water (Table 2). Like the rapidly growing mycobacterial species (see chapter 30 in this *Manual*), the majority of species of the slowly growing NTM have been described since the early 1990s with the advent of molecular technology. Since 2007, 13 new species have been described, including *M. kumamotonense*, *M. seoulense*, *M. senuense*, *M. stomatepiae*, *M. arosiense*, *M. kyorinense*, *M. noviomagense*, *M. paraseoulense*,

M. riyadhense, *M. mantenii*, and four proposed new members of the *Mycobacterium avium* complex (MAC), *M. vulneris*, *M. marseillense*, *M. bouchedurhonense*, and *M. timonense* (6, 61, 67, 77, 78, 84, 95, 109, 138, 139, 141).

EPIDEMIOLOGY AND TRANSMISSION

Unlike *M. tuberculosis*, for which humans are the definitive host, most species of NTM are widely distributed in the environment, and the occurrence of NTM disease is attributed to a combination of host factors, such as age, body weight, the presence of chronic lung diseases (such as cystic fibrosis, bronchiectasis, or chronic obstructive pulmonary disease), alterations of chest structure, and other conditions, along with exposure. Organisms can be found in samples of soil and water, including both natural and treated water sources. For example, *M. kansasii*, *M. xenopi*, and *M. simiae* are almost always recovered from municipal water and rarely, if ever, from other environmental sources.

Furthermore, for NTM there has been no evidence of animal-to-human or human-to-human transmission, unlike with MTBC. Human disease due to NTM is assumed to be acquired from environmental sources either directly by inhaling organisms in aerosols or indirectly by ingesting contaminated food or water, even though the source of infection may not always be detected (39).

Incidence rates of NTM disease are only estimates since, unlike with tuberculosis (TB), all NTM are noncommunicable from human-to-human, and therefore numbers of infections are nonreportable. One publication from 2007 reported that the isolation prevalence of all NTM species (excluding *M. gordonae*) in pulmonary disease in Ontario, Canada, increased from 9.1/100,000 in 1997 to 14.1/100,000 by 2003, with a mean annual increase of 8.4%. Similar increases were noted for individual species. These findings indicate a significant rise in pulmonary disease caused by NTM in Canada (65). Increasing numbers of NTM isolates were also reported for several European countries (66).

The most common infections with NTM currently are pulmonary diseases, but skin and soft tissue, lymphatic, and disseminated infections are also important. The last most often occur in the setting of advanced human immunodeficiency virus (HIV) disease, but non-HIV-infected patients can also be affected. MAC is the most commonly isolated pathogenic slowly growing NTM, but other species of NTM also cause

---

*This chapter contains information presented in chapter 37 by Véronique Vincent and M. Cristina Gutiérrez in the ninth edition of this *Manual*.

TABLE 1 Characteristics of currently recognized species of NTM[h]

Species	Pigmentation	Established pathogenicity	Unique hsp65 gene	Unique 16S rRNA gene	Date of description
M. arosiense	Y	Y	Y	Y	2008
M. arupense	Y	Y	Y	Y	2006
M. asiaticum	Y	Y	Y	Y	1971
M. avium subsp. avium	Y[a]	Y[b]	Y[c]	N	1901
"M. avium subsp. hominissuis"	Y[a]	Y[d]	Y[c]	N	2002
M. avium subsp. paratuberculosis	Y[a]	Y	Y[c]	N	1900
M. bohemicum	Y	Y	U	Y	1998
M. botniense	Y	N	U	Y	2000
M. bouchedurhonense	N	Y	Y	Y	2009
M. branderi	N	Y	U	Y	1995
M. celatum	N	Y	Y	Y	1993
M. chimaera	N	Y	N	N	2004
M. colombiense	N	Y	N	Y	2006
M. conspicuum	Y	Y	U	Y	1996
M. cookii	Y	N	U	Y	1990
M. doricum	Y	Y	U	Y	2001
M. farcinogenes	Y	Q	Y	Y	1973
M. florentinum	N	Y	U	Y	2005
M. gastri	N	N	Y	N	1966
M. genavense	N	Y	U	Y	1993
M. gordonae	Y	N	U	V	1962
M. haemophilum	N	Y	Y	Y	1978
M. heckeshornense	Y	Y	Y	Y	2001
M. heidelbergense	N	Y	Y	Y	1998
M. hiberniae	Y	N	Y	Y	1993
M. interjectum	Y	Y	Y	Y	1993
M. intermedium	Y	Q	Y	Y	1993
M. intracellulare	Y/N	Y	Y	Y	1965
M. kansasii	Y	Y	Y	N	1955
M. kubicae	Y	N	U	Y	2000
M. kumamotonense	U	Q	Y	Y	2006
M. kyorinense	N	Q	Y	Y	2009
M. lacus	N	Q	Y	Y	2002
M. lentiflavum	Y	Y	Y	Y	1996
M. leprae	—[e]	Y	Y	Y	1880
M. lepraemurium	—	Y	Y	Y	1912
M. malmoense	N	Y	Y	Y	1977
M. mantenii	Y	Y	Y	Y	2009
M. marinum	Y	Y	Y	N	1926
M. marseillense	N	Y	Y	Y	2009
M. monteofiorense	N	Y[f]	Y	Y	2003
M. nebraskense	Y	Q	Y	Y	2004
M. nonchromogenicum	N	Q	N	Q	1965
M. noviomagense	N	N	Y	Y	2009
M. palustre	Y	Q	U	Y	2002
M. paraffinicum	Y	U	Y	Y	2009
M. parascrofulaceum	Y	Y	Y	Y	2004
M. paraseoulense	Y	U	Y	N	2010
M. parmense	Y	Y	Y	Y	2004
M. pseudoshottsii	Y	Y[g]	N	N	2005
M. pulveris	N	N	U	Y	1983
M. riyadhense	N	Y	Y	Y	2009
M. saskatchewanense	Y	Y	Y	Y	2004
M. scrofulaceum	Y	Y	Y	Y	1956
M. senuense	N	Q	U	Y	2008
M. seoulense	Y	Q	Y	Y	2007
M. shimoidei	N	Y	Y	Y	1982
M. shottsii	N	Y[g]	U	Y	2003
M. simiae	Y	Y	Y	Y	1965
M. stomatepiae	N	Y[g]	Y	Y	2008
M. szulgai	Y	Y	Y	Y	1972

(Continued on next page)

TABLE 1 *(Continued)*

Species	Pigmentation	Established pathogenicity	Unique *hsp65* gene	Unique 16S rRNA gene	Date of description
M. *terrae*	N	Q	N	Y	1966
M. *timonense*	N	Y	Y	Y	2009
M. *triplex*	N	Y	Y	Y	1997
M. *triviale*	N	N	U	U	1970
M. *tusciae*	Y	Y	U	Y	1999
M. *ulcerans*	N	Y	U	N	1950
M. *vulneris*	Y	Q	Y	Y	2009
M. *xenopi*	N	Y	Y	Y	1959

[a]Most strains (>99%) are nonpigmented.
[b]Birds.
[c]Sequence outside the 441-bp Telenti fragment.
[d]Humans and swine.
[e]—, not grown on artificial media.
[f]Eels.
[g]Fish.
[h]Y, yes; N, no; U, undetermined; Q, questionable.

disease. In the United States, M. *kansasii* infection is the second most frequently recovered pathogenic species (39).

CLINICAL SIGNIFICANCE

Because of the presence of multiple species of NTM in the environment and their opportunistic pathogenic nature, the determination of the clinical significance of the isolation of these species is based upon multiple factors, including clinical setting, host-specific factors, species, the pathogenic potential of the organism, the number of positive cultures, the source of the culture isolate, and quantification of the organisms detected (by smear and culture) (39). For example, although the incidence of a specific NTM such as M. *gordonae* in cultures is high, the pathogenicity of this species is very low, in contrast to that of species such as MAC and M. *kansasii* (7).

Unlike with NTM, the laboratory diagnosis of MTBC is the most important finding in a clinical mycobacteriology laboratory. The finding of this species has vital epidemiologic and public health consequences. Further details on clinical significance of the MTBC may be found in chapter 28 in this *Manual*.

DIRECT EXAMINATION

Microscopy

One of the first, easiest, and least expensive means of detecting the presence of mycobacteria in clinical samples has been microscopic examination. Special acid-fast stains, along with the use of bright field and fluorescence microscopy, are needed for staining of the organisms since the routine Gram stain is not optimal for staining mycobacteria. Further discussion of the specific techniques can be found in chapter 28.

Antigen Detection

Antigen detection is not currently performed for direct detection of mycobacteria in diagnostic laboratories.

Nucleic Acid Detection

Early detection of disease caused by members of the MTBC is essential in controlling transmission of TB. Direct nucleic acid amplification (NAA) techniques for the detection of MTBC bacteria are increasingly being used (26, 28, 31, 63, 85, 86, 87, 88, 93). These tests can provide results in as little as 2 hours, enabling the rapid detection of MTBC from clinical specimens. In addition to "home-brew" in-house polymerase chain reaction (PCR) assays, several commercially available kits which are based on either classical PCR or alternative, isothermal amplification techniques are available (Table 3). Only the Amplified *Mycobacterium tuberculosis* direct test (AMTD) has been approved by the U.S. Food and Drug Administration (FDA) at this time for smear-positive and smear-negative respiratory specimens (16). For nonrespiratory specimens, no FDA-approved test is available.

Many publications have reported on the diagnostic values of the different NAA tests. The most widely used tests in these studies were the AMTD or BD ProbeTec assay (BD Diagnostics, Sparks, MD) (69, 72, 107, 149). Several reviews and meta-analyses have evaluated these publications to estimate the diagnostic accuracy of NAA tests (26, 28, 31, 63, 85, 86, 87, 93).

One main finding among these analyses was the observation of a high degree of variability in accuracy across the studies. Sensitivity values ranged from 36 to 100% (63) or 27 to 100% (93), whereas specificity was more consistent, with values ranging from 54 to 100% (63) or 91 to 100% (93). Subgroup analyses could not explain the high variability found in the study results, even when the same test system was used. An important factor influencing the estimates was the rate of smear-positive samples included in the studies. The specificities and positive-predictive values of the tests were higher and more consistent than the sensitivities, mainly from smear-positive specimens. Thus, a positive NAA test result combined with a high clinical probability provides a rapid diagnosis of TB. In contrast, a patient can be presumed to be infected with an NTM if a negative NAA result with inhibitors excluded was obtained from a smear-positive specimen. As stated above, the sensitivities of the tests are lower, especially for smear-negative specimens. Combined sensitivity values from several studies differed markedly, depending on whether the smears were positive or negative: for AMTD2, the sensitivities were 90 to 100% (smear-positive specimens) and 63.6 to 100% (smear-negative specimens); for ProbeTec,

TABLE 2 Important properties of selected slowly growing NTM species[h]

Species	Optimal growth temp or range (°C)	Colony morphology	Niacin	Nitrate reduction	Features of 16S rRNA gene (GenBank accession no. and/or reference)	Clinical relevance,[a] specimens of first isolation, or important laboratory feature(s)
M. avium subsp. avium, M. avium subsp. paratuberculosis, M. avium subsp. silvaticum	30–37	Smooth (rough)	Neg	Neg	3 subspecies established (124), another subspecies proposed ("M. avium subsp. hominissuis") (74); identical 16S rRNA gene sequences for all subspecies (GQ153272)	Lymphadenitis in children; pulmonary disease in adults[a]; often disseminated infection in HIV patients
M. intracellulare	30–37	Smooth (rough)	Neg	Neg	Several sequence variants known, some elevated to species level (see following rows) (GQ153276)	Pulmonary disease in adults[a], often disseminated infection in HIV-patients
M. chimaera	25–37	Smooth	Neg	Neg	1-bp difference (position 403) from M. intracellulare (AJ548480)	Probably similar to M. intracellulare (131)[b]
M. colombiense	20–37	Rough	Neg	Neg (85%)	7-bp difference from M. intracellulare (AM062764)	HIV patients, blood, sputum (79)[c]
M. arosiense	42	Smooth	ND	Pos	6-bp difference from M. intracellulare (EF054881)	Osteomyelitis in a child (6)[d]
M. vulneris	37	Smooth	Neg	Neg	3-bp difference from M. colombiense (EU834055)	Lymphadenitis in a child and infection after a dog bite (140)[d]
M. bohemicum	37–40	Smooth	Neg	Neg	Unique 16S rRNA gene sequence (81) (U84502)	Lymphadenitis in children (96)
M. celatum	33–42	Smooth	Neg	Neg	3 sequence types are published; type 2 is very different from type 1, type 3 is similar to type 1 (11, 13); unclear taxonomic situation; possesses 2 rRNA operons (97) (L08169, type 1; L08170, type 2; Z46664, type 3)	Pulmonary disease in adults[a]
M. genavense	31–42	Smooth	Neg	Neg	Unique 16S rRNA gene sequence (9) (X60070)	First detection in HIV-patients; single cases also from nonimmunocompromised patients; almost no growth on solid media, scarce growth in liquid media
M. gordonae	30–37	Smooth/rough	Neg	Neg	Several sequence variants of the 16S rRNA gene (54) (AJ581472)	Present in running water systems; usually without clinical relevance
M. haemophilum	25–30	Rough	Neg	Var[f]	Sequence variants (FJ418069[e], EU486080, GU142930); Unique 16S rRNA gene sequence (X88923)	Lymphadenitis in children; skin lesion with immunosuppression; growth usually dependent on the addition of hemin to the medium
M. heidelbergense	30–37	Smooth	Neg	Neg	Unique 16S rRNA gene sequence (X70960)	Lymphadenitis in a child (41)
M. hiberniae	37	Rough	ND	Pos	Unique 16S rRNA gene sequence (1-bp difference from a nonvalidly published species, M. engbaeckii) (AY438069[e])	From environmental specimens; usually without clinical relevance
M. interjectum	31–37	Smooth	Neg	Neg	Unique 16S rRNA gene sequence (X70961)	Lymphadenitis in a child (112)
M. intermedium	31–37	Smooth	Neg	Neg	Unique 16S rRNA gene sequence (X67847)	Isolated from sputum specimens (71)
M. kansasii	35–37	Rough	Neg	Pos	6 subspecies differing in several genes (92, 100); subspecies 1 is prevalent worldwide (49, 119, 151) (AF480601)	Pulmonary disease in adults[a]; rarely associated with lymphadenitis in children

Species	Growth temp (°C)	Colony morphology		AccuProbe	16S rRNA gene sequence	Clinical relevance
M. lentiflavum	22–37	Smooth	Neg	Neg	3 sequence variants (X80769, X80770, X93995)	Most isolates obtained from pulmonary specimens (114)[a]
M. malmoense	30	Smooth	Neg	Neg	Unique 16S rRNA gene sequence yet very similar to that of M. szulgai (GQ153278)	Lymphadenitis in children; pulmonary disease in adults[a]
M. marinum	30	Rough (smooth)	Var[g]	Neg	16S rRNA gene sequence has only a 2-bp difference from that of M. ulcerans (125) (AJ536032)	Swimming pool granuloma
M. scrofulaceum	37	Smooth	Neg	Neg	Unique 16S rRNA sequence (GQ153271)	Pulmonary disease in adults[a]; rarely associated with lymphadenitis in children
M. shimoidei	37	Rough	Neg	Neg	Unique 16S rRNA gene sequence (no correct sequence available)	
M. simiae	37	Smooth	Var	Pos	Unique 16S rRNA gene sequence (GQ153280)	Pulmonary disease in adults[a]
M. szulgai	37	Rough/smooth	Neg	Pos	Unique 16S rRNA gene sequence, yet very similar to that of M. malmoense (AF547969[e])	Pulmonary disease in adults[a]
M. terrae/ M. nonchromogenicum	25–37	Rough/smooth	Neg	Pos/Neg	Group of species with similar genetic and phenotypic characteristics; phylogenetic relationship and position so far uncertain; final species identification difficult, even by sequence analysis (for M. terrae, DQ058407; for M. nonchromogenicum, DQ058406)	Tenosynovitis of the hand; isolates from other sources are usually without clinical relevance
M. ulcerans	30	Rough	Neg	Neg	16S rRNA gene sequence has a 2-bp difference from M. marinum (nucleotides 1248 and 1289) (125) (no correct sequence available)	Extensive skin ulceration in tropical environments
M. xenopi	40-45	Smooth	Neg	Neg	Unique 16S rRNA gene sequence (AJ536033 [at positions 182 and 408 C or T may be present])	Present in hot water systems; often without clinical relevance

[a]Clinical relevance in pulmonary specimens must be proven according to the ATS guidelines.
[b]AccuProbe test is positive for MAC and for M. intracellulare-specific probes but negative for M. avium-specific probe.
[c]AccuProbe test is positive for MAC-specific probe but negative for M. avium- and for M. intracellulare-specific probes.
[d]No data available for AccuProbe tests.
[e]Sequence data exists only for a fragment of the gene.
[f]Different reports with inconsistent data.
[g]The test method differed from the current strip method.
See reference 52a.
[h]Abbreviations: Neg, negative; Pos, positive; ND, not determined; Var, varies.

TABLE 3 Commercially available NAA tests

NAA test	Manufacturer	Method
AMTD[a]	Gen-Probe Inc., San Diego, CA	Transcription-mediated amplification of rRNA
BD ProbeTec ET system	BD Diagnostics, Sparks, MD	Strand displacement amplification of the IS6110 element and 16S rRNA gene of MTBC
COBAS TaqMan *Mycobacterium tuberculosis* test[b]	Roche Diagnostics, Basel, Switzerland	Real-time PCR, amplification of 16S rRNA gene
GenoType Mycobacteria Direct assay	Hain Lifescience, Nehren, Germany	Nucleic acid sequence-based amplification of 23S rRNA of MTBC, M. *avium*, M. *malmoense*, M. *kansasii*, and M. *intracellulare*; line probe assay
artus M. *tuberculosis* PCR kit	Qiagen GmbH, Hilden/Hamburg, Germany	Real-time PCR, amplification of 16S rRNA gene
Loop-mediated isothermal amplification	Eiken Chemical Co. Ltd., Tokyo, Japan	Isothermal amplification, visual observation using UV light
RealArt M. *tuberculosis* TM PCR reagents	Abbott Laboratories, Abbott Park, IL	Real-time PCR using the ABI Prism 7000 system
GeneXpert system	Cepheid, Sunnyvale, CA	Real-time PCR, detection of MTBC and resistance to rifampin; amplification of *rpo*B

[a]Received FDA approval for smear-positive respiratory specimens and smear-negative respiratory specimens from patients suspected of having TB.
[b]Received FDA approval for smear-positive respiratory specimens from patients suspected of having TB.

90 to 100% (smear-positive specimens) and 33.3 to 100% (smear-negative specimens) (93). A negative test result does not rule out MTBC infection.

Quality control for the NAA test performance should include controls for the presence of inhibitors for each specimen to rule out false-negative results. To prevent cross-contamination with amplification products, a strict workflow must be followed, equipment must remain in its respective area, and an adequate cleaning procedure must be performed. The use of closed systems, like real-time analysis, has the advantage that tubes containing amplification products do not need to be reopened, and thus the risk of cross-contamination is reduced.

In general, commercially available tests are preferred over in-house assays because of the standardized protocols and better quality control. A meta-analysis for the use of in-house NAA tests reported a highly heterogeneous estimate of diagnostic accuracy (range of sensitivity, 9.4 to 100%; range of specificity, 5.6 to 100%) (31).

In response to the increasing demand for NAA testing for TB and recognition of the importance of prompt laboratory results in TB diagnosis and control, "Updated Guidelines for the Use of Nucleic Acid Amplification Tests in the Diagnosis of Tuberculosis" have recently been released by the Centers for Disease Control and Prevention (CDC) (16). The new recommendations state that NAA testing should be performed on at least one respiratory specimen from each patient with signs and symptoms of pulmonary TB for whom a diagnosis of TB is being considered but has not yet been established and for whom the test result would alter case management or infection control activities. A detailed testing and interpretation algorithm is proposed. However, culture remains the reference standard for laboratory confirmation of TB and is required for drug susceptibility testing and genotyping.

When NAA tests are being implemented, performance characteristics, such as sensitivity and specificity, need to be established for the laboratory by use of well-known samples. Proficiency should be examined regularly by comparing NAA test results with microbiological and clinical data.

IDENTIFICATION

From a global viewpoint, the rapid detection and identification of M. *tuberculosis* is the most important task of a clinical mycobacteriology laboratory. However, within the last 30 years, the number of currently validated NTM species has increased from approximately 30 to more than 130 species. This development has been paralleled by an increasing incidence of infections due to NTM of mainly slowly growing species. Thus, clinical mycobacteriology laboratories today also encounter the challenge of providing unequivocal identifications of NTM species. The introduction of molecular techniques into the mycobacteriology laboratory has dramatically accelerated the diagnostic process. MTBC bacteria can be detected rapidly in clinical specimens by NAA tests. DNA probes for the confirmation of MTBC and a few NTM species grown on culture media have been available for many years. Historically, species identification has relied, with few exceptions, on the analysis of a series of phenotypic tests for which performance was mostly restricted to specialized laboratories. These tests require a sufficient amount of bacterial cells and several weeks of incubation. As previously discussed, it is now recognized that most of the newer mycobacterial species cannot be reliably identified by biochemical and other phenotypic tests. Several species may exhibit convergent characteristics, and strains of one species may show variability in certain features; such specifics are unknown since most new species have not been studied in detail. The most reliable methods for identification of all mycobacterial species today involve molecular analyses of certain genes. These techniques have the additional advantage that they can be performed from liquid culture media, which in general enable more rapid growth and a more sensitive detection of mycobacteria than solid culture media. Mixed cultures with NTM are not rare, and thus there is a danger of working with cultures in broth only. Thus, all results obtained by molecular methods should be confirmed, even after the reporting of the results, by some important phenotypic characteristics, such as growth rate, colony morphology, and pigmentation (Table 2)

The Clinical and Laboratory Standards Institute (CLSI) recognizes that not all laboratories have unlimited funds or instrumentation to provide state-of-the-art testing in mycobacteriology. Laboratories which have access only to probe technology should probe isolates to rule out MTBC at a minimum and then refer isolates to a reference laboratory for further testing. If no technology is available, it is advisable to refer the isolate to a reference laboratory (18).

Phenotypic Methods

Growth Rate
Growth rate is an obvious property that can be observed with the primary solid culture, at least within some limits (i.e., dependent on appropriate incubation temperature and number of organisms in the primary specimen). The estimation is not reliably applicable for growth in liquid culture medium. To perform a standardized growth test, defined suspensions of mycobacteria are inoculated on solid media and incubated at 30° and 35 to 37°C. Cultures are observed for growth at 5 to 7 days and weekly thereafter. Mycobacteria can thus be classified into the slowly and rapidly growing species. Rapidly growing mycobacteria are able to form visible colonies within 7 days of incubation, whereas slowly growing species require a longer period of time for colony formation.

Temperature
Mycobacterium species differ in the ability to grow at certain temperatures. For determination of the preferred growth temperature, solid culture media are inoculated with defined suspensions of mycobacteria and incubated at various temperatures. For slowly growing species, the minimum set of temperatures for incubation comprises 30 ± 2°C and 35 ± 2°C. Most slowly growing species grow well at 35 to 37°C, although M. *marinum* is an example of a slowly growing pathogen that grows optimally at a lower temperature (30°C) (especially on primary isolation). Additional media incubated at 22 to 25°C and 42°C may be necessary for optimal growth of some species, such as M. *haemophilum* (25°C), M *xenopi* (42°C), and M. *stomatepiae* (22°C). Cultures to determine temperature requirements of known rapidly growing mycobacteria can be read within 1 week, while slowly growing mycobacteria require a longer period of incubation.

Colony Morphology
Colony morphology is a phenotypic property of mycobacteria that can easily be determined. Morphologic characteristics such as size and colony description (flat, raised, etc.) should be noted, but most significant is the smooth or rough growth form of the colonies. M. *tuberculosis* usually grows in rough, nonpigmented colonies on Löwenstein-Jensen slants (Fig. 1) as well as on agar-based media. In contrast, M. *bovis* grows in flat and smooth nonpigmented colonies. The colony morphology may vary when different formulations of solid media are used. Slowly growing NTM species may also exhibit either rough or smooth variants or both types.

Pigmentation and Photoreactivity
Several NTM species may produce pigment, which can range from light yellow, yellow to orange, or even rose. Pigmentation of mycobacteria has been used for primary classification into the nonchromogenic and the chromogenic species (Runyon classification system, named for Ernest Runyon, a pioneer taxonomist in mycobacteriology). Within the pigmented mycobacteria, the photochromogens are nonpigmented in the dark and produce pigmentation only after exposure to light (Fig. 2). This pigment production is an oxygen-dependent reaction. Thus, primary cultures of these

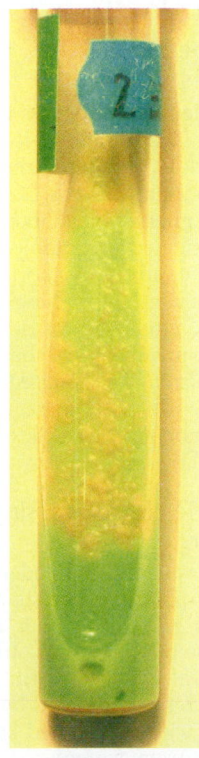

FIGURE 1 M. *tuberculosis* grown on a Löwenstein-Jensen slant for 14 days. Colonies are dry, wrinkled, off-white, and eugenic.

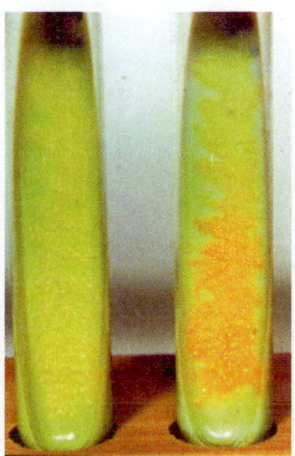

FIGURE 2 M. *marinum* on Löwenstein-Jensen slants after 2 weeks of growth before exposure to light (left) and after exposure to light (photochromogenic) (right).

species may remain nonpigmented even when exposed to light if the caps are tightly closed. Loosening of the caps, done in a biological safety cabinet, may induce the color change. The scotochromogens produce pigment when grown in the dark or when exposed to light (Fig. 3). The color may intensify with the increasing age of the culture. The nonchromogens do not produce pigmentation when grown either in the dark or after exposure to light. The color of nonchromogen colonies may be off-white, buff, or pale yellow and does not intensify when exposed to light (Fig. 4).

No species of the MTBC produce pigment; thus, pigmented mycobacteria per se are NTM.

Niacin Accumulation

Some *Mycobacterium* species cannot use nicotinic acid, although they produce it in their biosynthetic pathways. Consequently, nicotinic acid is excreted into the medium and can be detected. A commercially available paper strip format test is easy to perform and avoids the use of hazardous reagents (BD Diagnostics, Sparks, MD). Better results can be obtained with isoniazid test strips, which are available in the same paper strip format (BD Diagnostics), than with the niacin test strips. The detection of niacin is one of the key phenotypic tests for the identification of *M. tuberculosis*. Within the NTM, *M. simiae* can also be positive in the niacin test. *M. tuberculosis* strain H37 and *M. avium* can be used as positive and negative controls, respectively.

Nitrate Reduction

Several mycobacterial species produce nitrate reductase, which reduces nitrate to nitrite. This ability is assessed by the formation of a diazonium salt, which is finally demonstrated by the production of a red water-soluble dye (18). As for niacin production, a paper strip assay which has proved

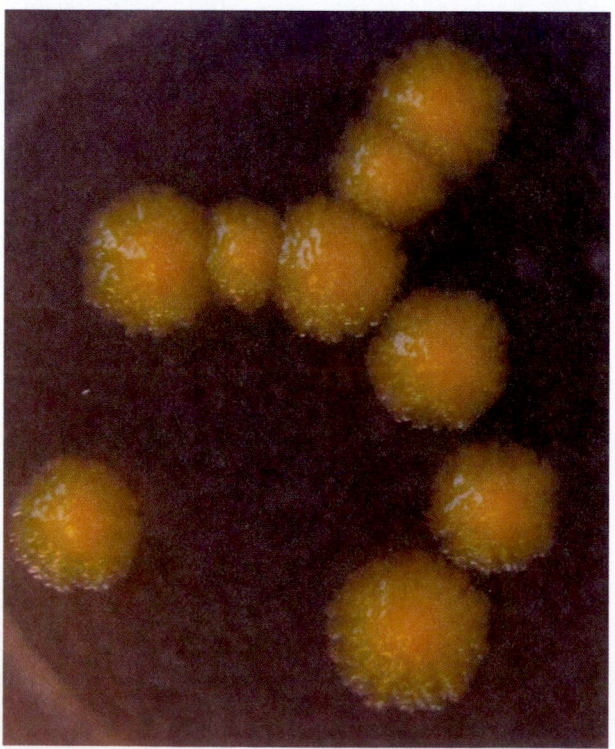

FIGURE 3 *M. gordonae* grown on 7H10 Middlebrook agar for 10 days. Colonies are yellow and smooth (scotochromogenic).

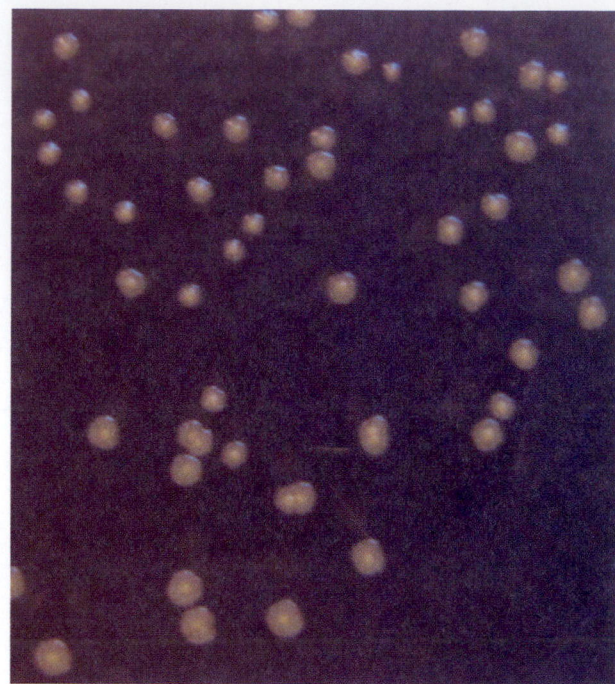

FIGURE 4 *M. celatum* grown on 7H10 Middlebrook agar for 10 days. Colonies are small, colorless, and smooth (nonchromogenic).

to be reliable and efficient is available (BD Diagnostics). The confirmation of the presence of a nitrate reductase is another key phenotypic property for the identification of *M. tuberculosis*. *M. tuberculosis* strain H37 and *M. avium* can be used as positive and negative controls, respectively.

Identification of Species of MTBC Using Phenotypic Markers

If a strain is identified as a member of the MTBC using the AccuProbe test (GenProbe, San Diego, CA) or another molecular method, differentiation of the species *M. tuberculosis*, *M. bovis*, and *M. bovis* BCG can be performed reliably using several phenotypic markers (Table 4). Species identification is considered acceptable if all test results are unambiguous and all controls give correct results.

In case of any deviation in these patterns, molecular techniques should be employed for definite identification. Furthermore, other members of the MTBC, including *M. africanum*, *M. microti*, *M. pinnipedii*, and "*M. canettii*" should always be identified by molecular tests. Sufficient information on phenotypic properties is not available for these rare agents of TB.

Identification of NTM Species Using Phenotypic Markers

As previously emphasized, species identification of NTM is not feasible using phenotypic tests alone. The number of species continues to grow, which highlights the lack of distinctive phenotypic properties. In general, only molecular tests provide a reliable identification. However, as previously stated, all results obtained by molecular methods should be consistent with established key phenotypic characteristics (Table 2). As an example, *M. chelonae* is a rapidly growing species with a preferred temperature of 30 ± 2°C. Incubating media inoculated with *M. chelonae* at higher

TABLE 4 Phenotypic identification of M. *tuberculosis*, M. *bovis*, and M. *bovis* BCG

Species	Niacin	Nitrate reduction	Colony morphology[a]	Susceptibility to:	
				TCH[b]	Pyrazinamide[c]
M. *tuberculosis*	Positive	Positive	Rough	Resistant	Susceptible[f]
M. *bovis*	Negative	Negative	Smooth	Susceptible[e]	Resistant
M. *caprae*	Negative	Negative	Smooth	Susceptible[e]	Susceptible
BCG	Negative[d]	Negative	Rough	Susceptible	Resistant

[a]On Löwenstein-Jensen medium.
[b]TCH, thiophen-2-carboxylic acid hydrazide (tested on solid Löwenstein-Jensen medium).
[c]Preferably tested with the BACTEC 460 or BACTEC MGIT 960 method.
[d]Some strains are weakly positive.
[e]Isoniazid-resistant M. *bovis* strains are also resistant to TCH.
[f]Can be resistant if the strain is already resistant to other first-line drugs.

temperatures may result in delayed growth, which might suggest a slowly growing NTM, rather than a rapid grower.

Mycolic Acid Analysis

The varying composition of the cell wall mycolic acids of different species of mycobacteria has been used for diagnostic purposes for many years (3, 12, 58). Use of high-performance liquid chromatography (HPLC) analysis of the mycolic acid pattern for identification of *Mycobacterium* species can provide identification more rapidly than time-consuming phenotypic tests. Methods for performing HPLC analysis as well as patterns for recognition of mycobacteria are summarized in two manuals available at http://www.cdc.gov/tb/topic/laboratory/default.htm.

For HPLC analysis, mycolic acids are extracted from the cell walls and saponified. The mycolic acids are then derivatized to esters and separated by chromatography. The identification of species is based on the comparison of the test isolate's pattern of peaks with patterns from a library of known reference strains. Reliable databases are an essential prerequisite for exact species identification by this technique. Again, as with molecular testing, results obtained by HPLC analysis should be confirmed by the presence of fundamental specific phenotypic properties, like growth rate, colony morphology, and pigmentation.

HPLC analysis of mycolic acids is not a standard technology for routine laboratories, and equipment costs are high. Once the equipment is available, however, the cost of individual sample testing is relatively inexpensive. It is a rapid alternative to time-consuming phenotypic methods, although not all species can be identified and some isolates can be identified only to a group or complex level. Furthermore, HPLC technology is useful as an additional marker for the recognition of new mycobacterial species and continues to be used in many state and public health laboratories (127, 128). Moreover, MAC and MTBC often can be identified directly from acid-fast bacterium smear-positive samples using the more sensitive fluorescent methodology of HPLC (50).

GENOTYPIC IDENTIFICATION OF MYCOBACTERIAL SPECIES

Complete Genome Sequences

Complete genomic sequences have been determined for a series of mycobacterial species: M. *tuberculosis* strain H37Rv, M. *tuberculosis* strain CDC1551, M. *bovis*, M. *leprae*, "M. *avium* subsp. *hominissuis*" strain 104, M. *avium* subsp. *paratuberculosis* (MAP) strain K-10, M. *marinum*, M. *smegmatis*, and M. *ulcerans*. Detailed information on all genome projects either completed or still in progress can be obtained at http://www.ncbi.nlm.nih.gov/sites/entrez?Db=genomeprj&Cmd=Search&TermToSearch=txid176. The genomic sizes vary markedly among the species, from 3.3 million bp for M. *leprae* (21), with approximately 4.3 million bp for M. *bovis* (35) and 4.4 million bp for M. *tuberculosis* (20), up to 6.6 million bp for M. *marinum* (115) and almost 7 million bp for M. *smegmatis*. Comparative genome analyses of these species repeatedly show that reductive genome evolution has taken place by the process of the adaptation of an environmental bacterium to an intracellular, parasitic lifestyle (38, 116). Genome downsizing, accumulation of pseudogenes, the acquisition of foreign genes that confer fitness advantages, and a high degree of clonality are common characteristics of those mycobacteria that are adapting to a new, stable environment in a host. Complete genome analysis may thus help our understanding of the evolution, host adaptation, and pathobiology of mycobacterial disease and possible targets for antimicrobial chemotherapy. Sequence comparisons may aid the identification of new diagnostic as well as vaccine targets.

Gene Analyses

Partial sequence analysis of selected genes is the most reliable method for identification of mycobacterial species. Sequence variability among species, but homogeneity within species, is the basic prerequisite for this application. For several genes (16S rRNA gene, internal transcribed spacer [ITS], *hsp65*, and *rpoB*), specific regions within the gene which work well for species identification have been identified (1, 32, 53, 55, 56, 70, 88, 94, 105, 147). The most important target for identification of mycobacteria is the 16S rRNA gene. One main advantage of sequence analysis of this gene is the requirement of most journals for simultaneous updating of public databases at the time of publication of a new species. However, quality control and updating of public databases has been a major obstacle in the identification of new species (134). Although the use of public databases for sequence comparisons is widespread among investigators, the lack of quality control and monitoring of these databases, which may include base errors, ambiguous base designations, and incomplete sequences, has contributed to errors in identification. This seems to be particularly problematic for isolates that were identified in the early molecular era, when quality sequences were less available (134).

16S rRNA Gene

For routine identification of mycobacteria, sequence analysis of the complete 16S rRNA gene (approximately 1,500 bp) is not practical and also not necessary. The information content of a sequence stretch of approximately 600 bp located at

TABLE 5 Primers for amplification and sequencing of the mycobacterial 16S rRNA gene

Primer	Sequence	Position[a]	Orientation[b]	Reference
285	5'-GAG AGT TTG ATC CTG GCT CAG	8	F	55
B9	5'-CGT GCT TAA CAC ATG CAA GTC	58	F	98
264	5'-TGC ACA CAG GCC ACA AGG GA	1049	R	55
247	5'-TTT CAC GAA CAA CGC GAC AA	612	R	8

[a]Position in the ribosomal 16S rRNA gene.
[b]F, forward; R, reverse.

the 5' end of the gene is sufficient for identification of most species. This sequence can easily be obtained with one analysis run. Specific primers for amplification and sequencing of the mycobacterial 16S rRNA gene (Table 5) have been described and validated (8, 23, 30, 43, 45, 55, 90, 113, 148).

Primers 264 and 247 target genus-specific sequence regions and can be used for the detection of mycobacteria even in the presence of contaminating bacteria. Furthermore, the 3'-end primers 285 and B9 for the amplification can be used for the sequence reaction. Either of these can be combined with any of the reverse primers. Both forward primers are located upstream of hypervariable regions A and B, which enable the species-specific identification of most mycobacterial species (55). A few species have identical hypervariable regions A and B or a complete 16S rRNA gene sequence. This includes M. marinum, M. ulcerans, M. chelonae, M. abscessus, and M. kansasii (sequence variants I and IV) and M. gastri. For accurate identification of these species, sequence analysis of other genes (e.g., ITS, hsp65, and rpoB) is required. All members of the MTBC have identical 16S rRNA gene sequences and thus cannot be discriminated by this technique, while for some species, minor intraspecies 16S rRNA gene sequence variants which differ in a few base pairs have been observed (M. gordonae, M. kansasii, and M. lentiflavum [54, 100, 114]).

Other Target Genes
Sequencing of several other genes has also been used for identification of mycobacterial species, but the database for these genes is less complete.

23S rRNA Gene
The 23S rRNA gene is also known to contain conserved and variable sequence regions that enable the specific amplification and species identification of mycobacteria (62, 136). Variable regions can also be found in the 5' region. The disadvantage of this target is the length of the gene, approximately 3,100 bp, which is not readily analyzed for most of the Mycobacterium species. Thus, public databases contain few 23S rRNA gene sequence data from mycobacteria.

ITS 1 Gene
Another target is the spacer sequence, which separates the 16S and 23S rRNA genes in the operon and is denominated ITS 1. The sequence of this fragment comprises only 200 to 330 bp and thus can easily be analyzed. Several sets of primers which enable the amplification of the complete fragment and an additional sequence analysis are published (Table 6) (44, 100, 106).

Primers Sp1 and Sp2 allow the genus-specific amplification of the region. Since they target the start site of the ITS, they are not optimal for analysis of the whole sequence. Primers ITS 1 and ITS 2 are located in the 16S and 23S rRNA gene regions, respectively. Using these primers, the entire ITS can be amplified and sequenced. However, they are not genus specific and cannot be used when cultures of mycobacteria are contaminated with other bacteria.

For the ITS 1 sequence, a high variability, which could be used for species identification, has been shown (33, 34, 44, 76, 105, 106). However, for some species, mainly for rapidly growing species but also for some slow growers (M. simiae, M. xenopi) two or more sequence variants have been observed. As with the 16S rRNA gene sequence, M. marinum and M. ulcerans have identical ITS 1 sequences and thus cannot be differentiated by this analysis.

hsp65 Gene
One of the first genetic targets used for the differentiation of mycobacteria is an approximately 440-bp fragment of the hsp65 gene, which codes for the 65-kDa heat shock protein and is also known as the groEL2 gene (94). The amplification of this fragment, followed by a restriction enzyme digestion using the restriction enzymes BstEII and HaeIII and an analysis of the obtained digestion products using agarose gel electrophoresis, provides restriction fragment length polymorphism (RFLP) patterns that are specific for most species (27, 121). An algorithm for the differentiation of the most important species showing the apparent molecular sizes of the fragments has been devised. This PCR-restriction enzyme analysis technique has been used widely, since this is a simple and rapid method with no need for more sophisticated sequencing techniques. However, technical difficulties, such as small size differences between the fragments or the incidence of similar or identical restriction patterns for some species of closely related mycobacteria and, in particular, new species of mycobacteria, are major problems with using this method. With the greater availability and decreasing cost of sequencing, sequence analysis of this hsp65 gene fragment has been increasingly used instead of the PCR-restriction enzyme analysis (70, 104).

TABLE 6 Primers for amplification and sequencing of the mycobacterial ITS 1

Primer	Sequence	Reference
Sp1	5'-ACC TCC TTT CTA AGG AGC ACC	106
Sp2	5'-GAT GCT CGC AAC CAC TAT CCA	106
ITS 1	5'-GAT TGG GAC GAA GTC GTA AC	100
ITS 2	5'-AGC CTC CCA CGT CCT TCA TC	100

TABLE 7 Primers for amplification of a fragment of the *gyrB* gene of MTBC

Primer	Sequence	Position relative to GenBank sequence BX842572
MTUBf	5′-TCG GAC GCG TAT GCG ATA TC	5570–5589
MTUBr	5′-ACA TAC AGT TCG GAC TTG CG	6609–6590

Advantages of sequencing the *hsp65* gene rather than the 16S rRNA gene are especially evident in the identification of closely related species, as the *hsp65* gene is much less conserved than the 16S rRNA gene. *hsp65* gene sequencing allows for differentiation of M. *marinum* from M. *ulcerans*, M. *gastri* from M. *kansasii*, and, with some restrictions, M. *avium* subsp. *avium* from M. *avium* subsp. *hominissuis*.

rpoB Gene

The *rpoB* gene encodes the β subunit of the bacterial RNA polymerase. For M. *tuberculosis*, mutations in a certain region of this gene are known to confer resistance to rifampin. For NTM species, sequence variability that can be used for species identification has been shown (1, 53, 60). Several different sequence fragments of the approximately 3,600-bp gene have been used for amplification and sequence determination. Kim et al. (53) amplified a fragment comprising 306 bp at positions 1362 to 1668 (referred to as region 2/3), whereas Lee et al. (60) targeted a 360-bp sequence at positions 902 to 1261 (referred to as region 1/2) (1). In contrast, Adékambi et al. (1) chose a fragment more distant (region 5). Those authors analyzed an approximately 760-bp fragment at positions 2573 to 3337. In the studies of Kim et al. (53) and Lee et al. (60), type strains of many slowly growing mycobacteria have been included, whereas detailed analyses using region 5 (1) have been performed mainly for rapidly growing mycobacteria. Extensive investigations using clinical isolates of slowly growing mycobacteria are not available for any part of the *rpoB* gene so far. Thus, currently, no final recommendation has been made to determine which fragment is most suitable for the identification of slowly growing mycobacteria.

gyrB Gene

The *gyrB* gene encodes the B subunit of DNA gyrase (topoisomerase II), an enzyme essential for bacterial replication. In 2000, Kasai et al. (52) showed single nucleotide polymorphisms (SNPs) in an approximately 1.2-kbp fragment of the *gyrB* gene which were specific for some species of the MTBC. More-detailed analyses confirmed these results and determined that they could be extended to most members of the MTBC (82).

For M. *microti* and M. *caprae* (previously M. *bovis* subsp. *caprae*), unique characteristic SNPs are known. Identical *gyrB* sequences are shared by M. *tuberculosis* and "M. *canettii*," by M. *africanum* and M. *pinnipedii*, and by M. *bovis* (synonym, M. *bovis* subsp. *bovis*) and BCG. However, "M. *canettii*" is rarely observed outside East Africa and M. *pinnipedii* has so far been exclusively isolated from seals and sea lions, with one exception of infection in a seal trainer (24, 143). Thus, these two species are usually not observed in routine clinical laboratories. In the case of M. *bovis* and BCG, a definite identification is essential for the diagnosis. To finally identify the species, additional techniques, such as estimation of the presence or absence of region of difference 1 (RD1) by PCR analysis, are necessary (120) to differentiate BCG from M. *bovis*. Identification of the characteristic SNPs can be performed by either sequence analysis (Tables 7 and 8) or by restriction enzyme digestion using RsaI, SacII, or TaqI and an additional agarose gel electrophoretic analysis (82).

Use of Sequence Databases for Identification of Mycobacterial Species

For identification of mycobacteria by sequencing analysis, public databases are usually used. Evaluating search results is often difficult for various reasons, including, as previously stated, the lack of quality control of the databases (134). Public databases contain sequences from strains which are not validly published as species, sequences from strains identified as known species but having divergent sequences, and many sequences from uncultured bacteria which are not further characterized. Furthermore, old sequences that are fragmentary or faulty are still included in the public databases (134).

The evaluation of the search result has to be done carefully. For example, in case of an uncommon species, cross-checking of the valid description as a species can easily be performed by using the "List of Prokaryotic Names with Standing in Nomenclature" (http://www.bacterio.cict.fr/m/mycobacterium.html). When obtaining several correct results deriving from different species, it may help to check the database entries if the sequences have been obtained from type strains.

The most important database, the International Nucleotide Sequence Database Collaboration (INSDC), can be used for the analysis of the sequences derived from the different genes as detailed above. There are some curated databases and analysis tools that have been constructed for the analysis of the 16S rRNA gene sequences, such as the commercially available tools SmartGene IDNS

TABLE 8 Position of characteristic SNPs within the *gyrB* gene

Species	Characteristic SNP at position[a]:				
	5671	5752	6307	6406	6446
M. *tuberculosis*/M. *canettii*	GTA **C** GAG	GGT **G** CGG	CGC **T** GTG	TAA **C** GAA	GAC **G** CGA
M. *bovis*/BCG	GTA **C** GAG	GGT **A** CGG	CGC **T** GTG	TAA **T** GAA	GAC **T** CGA
M. *caprae*	GTA **C** GAG	GGT **A** CGG	CGC **G** GTG	TAA **C** GAA	GAC **T** CGA
M. *africanum*/M. *pinnipedii*	GTA **C** GAG	GGT **G** CGG	CGC **T** GTG	TAA **C** GAA	GAC **T** CGA
M. *microti*	GTA **T** GAG	GGT **G** CGG	CGC **T** GTG	TAA **C** GAA	GAC **T** CGA

[a]The SNP is in boldface.

(SmartGene, Lausanne, Switzerland) and MicroSeq microbial identification system (Applied Biosystems, Foster City, CA) or two tools with free access, the Ribosomal Database Project (RDP) (http://rdp.cme.msu.edu/) and the RIDOM-Ribosomal Differentiation of Medical Microorganisms database (http://www3.ridom.de/rdna/). The SmartGene and the RDP packages source their sequences from GenBank, whereas the MicroSeq and RIDOM databases were obtained by sequencing of strains from culture collections and partly from well-known sequevars of certain species (42, 89, 134). The advantage of these databases is the quality control of the entries; thus, most of the difficulties associated with public databases will not be encountered. However, these curated databases lag behind the updates of the INSDC database and may not include sequence variants of species.

Other Molecular Tests

Sequence analysis of target genes for the identification of mycobacteria may not be practical for routine clinical laboratories. Commercially available assays that are based on liquid- or solid-phase hybridization have been shown to be easily implemented into a routine workflow. They are intended for the detection of some of the most important *Mycobacterium* species and can be performed from both solid and liquid media.

AccuProbe Culture Identification Tests

The AccuProbe tests were the first molecular assays for the identification of some important mycobacterial species from positive culture media. They are available for the identification of MTBC, *M. avium*, *M. intracellulare*, MAC, *M. gordonae*, and *M. kansasii*. All tests are FDA approved and commercially available. The recognition is based on the hybridization of specific DNA probes to rRNA of the bacteria. Briefly, by heat treatment and sonication, nucleic acids, including the target 16S rRNA, are released from the mycobacteria. A specific DNA probe hybridizes with the target rRNA. Finally, the DNA-rRNA hybrid molecule can be detected by chemiluminescence. The results are obtained within 2 hours. The tests can be performed from positive solid or liquid media. Using broth culture, an aliquot of approximately 1 to 2 ml of a positive culture is concentrated by centrifugation. The supernatant is discarded and the pellet resuspended in the test reagent. The remaining procedure follows the steps as described in the manufacturer's instructions for performance of the test from solid cultures. The usefulness of these tests has been proven in many studies and by usage in many laboratories worldwide (10, 57, 73, 100, 122, 132). Specificities of the tests are usually reported to be 100%, or sometimes lower (96%), for MAC. Sensitivity values vary with the test used: 100% for *M. gordonae*, 95.2% for MAC, and 97.4 to 100% for *M. kansasii* (10, 57, 100, 132). It has also been shown that MTBC organisms can reliably be identified in the presence of *M. avium* (73). However, there are also some disadvantages of these tests. The probes are limited to a few, although important, mycobacterial species, necessitating the performance of additional tests for mycobacterial identification of species not included on the probe. The need to perform individual tests for each target species renders the tests expensive and, if not performed in parallel, also time-consuming. Furthermore, false-positive results for MAC probes have been reported, but they can be prevented if a higher cutoff value (80,000 relative light units instead of the 30,000 relative light units recommended in the technical insert) is used (19).

Recent studies have shown cross-reactions with the *M. intracellulare* probe and several of the slowly growing mycobacterial species, including *M. arosiense*, *M. chimaera*,

M. nebraskense, and *M. saskatchewanense* (130). Similarly, cross-hybridizations have been documented with the MAC probe and *M. arosiense*, *M. chimaera*, *M. colombiense*, *M. nebraskense*, *M. palustre*, *M. saskatchewanense*, *M. vulneris*, and *M. paraffinicum*. Additional cross-reactivity was seen with the MTBC probe and the less frequently encountered rapidly growing species *M. holsaticum* (130), although this cross-reactivity can be avoided when the selection step of the procedure is performed for 10 min, according to the manufacturer's instructions (99). As with other molecular tests, all results obtained by these tests should be consistent with established phenotypic characteristics of the species.

Line Probe Assays

Alternatively, techniques based on the application of PCR plus reverse hybridization, designed DNA strip assays (line probe assays), have been developed. Briefly, the target sequences are amplified by PCR using biotinylated primers. The amplified PCR products are allowed to hybridize to immobilized, membrane-bound probes covering the species-specific sequence fragment, followed by an enzyme-mediated color reaction. The banding patterns can be analyzed by eye by comparing the patterns on an interpretation chart. The identification of the species relies on specific banding patterns (Fig. 5).

Two tests for the identification of several mycobacterial species are commercially available but are not yet FDA approved. The INNO-LiPA Mycobacteria v2 assay (Innogenetics, Ghent, Belgium) is based on the nucleotide differences in the 16S-23S rRNA gene spacer region and can detect the following *Mycobacterium* species: MTBC, *M. kansasii*, *M. xenopi*, *M. gordonae*, *M. genavense*, *M. simiae*, *M. marinum*, *M. ulcerans*, *M. celatum*, *M. avium*/*M. intracellulare*/*M. scrofulaceum* complex, *M. avium*, *M. intracellulare*, *M. scrofulaceum*, *M. malmoense*, *M. haemophilum*, *M. chelonae* complex, *M. fortuitum* complex, and *M. smegmatis*.

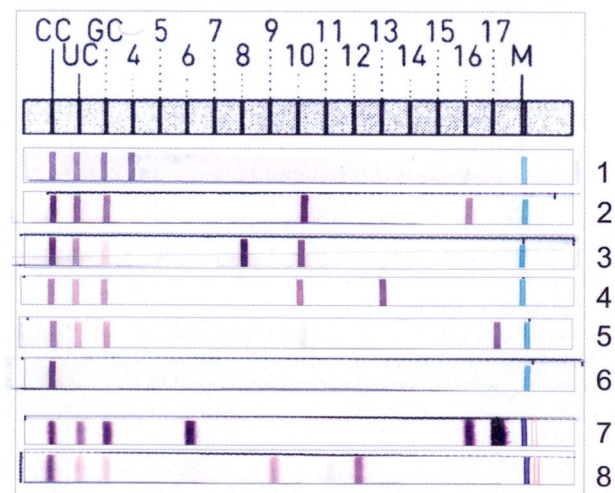

FIGURE 5 Line probe assay (GenoType Mycobacterium CM/AS) for the identification of *Mycobacterium* species. CC, conjugate control; UC, universal control; GC, genus-specific control; 4 to 17, specific bands for identification of the species; M, marker line (flags the upper side of the strip). Lines 1 to 6, CM strips; lines 7 and 8, AS strips. First lane, *M. avium*; second lane, MTBC; third lane, *M. gordonae*; fourth lane, *M. malmoense*; fifth lane, *M. xenopi*; sixth lane, negative control; seventh lane, *M. genavense*; eighth lane, *M. haemophilum*.

The other test is the GenoType Mycobacterium CM/AS test (Hain Lifescience, Nehren, Germany), which is based on the detection of species-specific sequences in the 23S rRNA gene. It is composed of two different strips (strip CM is for common mycobacteria, and strip AS is for additional species) and can identify the following mycobacteria: with strip CM, M. avium, M. abscessus /M. immunogenum, M. chelonae/M. immunogenum, M. fortuitum, M. fortuitum/M. mageritense, M. gordonae, M. intracellulare, M. scrofulaceum/M. paraffinicum/M. parascrofulaceum, M. interjectum, M. kansasii, M. malmoense/M. haemophilum/M. palustre/M. nebraskense, M. marinum/M. ulcerans, MTBC, M. peregrinum/M. alvei/M. septicum, and M. xenopi; and with strip AS, M. simiae, M. mucogenense, M. goodii, M. celatum (types 1 and 3), M. smegmatis, M. genavense/M. triplex, M. lentiflavum, M. heckeshornense, M. szulgai/M. intermedium, M. phlei, M. haemophilum/M. nebraskense, M. kansasii, M. ulcerans, M. gastri, M. asiaticum, and M. shimoidei (two or more species separated by a slash means that they share the same pattern).

Both assays can be conducted from either liquid or solid culture media, and the results are available in approximately 4 to 6 hours. The line probe technique is easy to perform and to incorporate into the workflow of a clinical laboratory. Several studies have evaluated the usefulness of the tests. Concordant results of 89.9 to 98.6% for the GenoType CM and AS assays have been reported (25, 37, 59, 64, 101, 108). Most (up to 96%) of the regularly encountered species already can be identified using the GenoType CM assay alone (101). A limitation of this test is the resolution of patterns that are shared by more than one species, which necessitates additional techniques for further discrimination, e.g., sequencing of additional gene targets or biochemical tests, leading to a delay in obtaining a final result. For the INNO-LiPA assay, 92.2%- to 98.4%-concordant results have been reported (64, 129). The assay can further differentiate M. kansasii and M. chelonae strains into subtypes. The clinical significance of this information so far is unclear, and thus this knowledge is mostly of epidemiological value.

Using line probe assays, more than 90% of the regularly encountered mycobacteria can rapidly be identified. In a few cases, false identification has been reported (101, 129, 130). For the GenoType AS assay, results for M. celatum should be reported only if they are obtained from solid cultures with appropriate growth rates and typical colony morphology.

Recent studies have shown that the GenoType M. intracellulare probe cross-hybridizes with several slowly growing mycobacterial species, including M. arosiense, M. chimaera, M. colombiense, M. mantenii, and M. saskatchewanense. Similarly, the INNO LiPA MAIS assay cross-reacts with M. arosiense, M. heidelbergense, M. mantenii, M. nebraskense, M. parascrofulaceum, and M. paraffinicum (130).

Both assays cannot identify the members of the MTBC to the species level. However, two less frequently encountered species, M. riyadhense and the nonvalidated species "M. simulans," were incorrectly assigned to the MTBC by the GenoType assay in a recent study (130). Importantly, neither line probe system has been reported to misidentify members of the MTBC as NTM (130). All results obtained with these tests should be confirmed by key established phenotypic characteristics, such as growth rate, colony morphology, and pigmentation.

Genotypic Identification of Species of the MTBC

Within the MTBC, the most prevalent species is M. tuberculosis. Identification of M. bovis is of clinical relevance because of the inherent resistance of this species to pyrazinamide, one of the first-line agents for treatment of TB. Moreover, correct identification of M. bovis BCG isolated from the urine of patients treated for bladder cancer is necessary to enable a correct decision for treating or not treating a patient. The identification of the other species is mainly of epidemiological importance and may be an indication of the source of the infection. Although all members of the MTBC are characterized by a high genetic similarity, several sequence polymorphisms which can be used for species identification have been discovered. Several regions of difference that were absent from BCG but present in M. tuberculosis H37Rv were revealed by comparative genomics approaches. The presence or absence of these deletions can be analyzed by PCR assays and additional agarose gel electrophoresis (111). Spoligotyping, a technique applied primarily for strain typing and discussed below, identifies (51) most species within the MTBC. However, with this technique, BCG cannot be discriminated from pathogenic M. bovis strains, as some strains can display identical spoligotype patterns.

A commercially available assay (GenoType MTBC; Hain Lifescience, Nehren, Germany) based on line probe technology enables the identification of species within the MTBC (81, 102, 103, 111). The test can be performed from solid or liquid media, with a total test time of 4 to 6 hours. The assay is based on an MTBC-specific 23S rRNA gene fragment, gyrB DNA sequence polymorphisms, and the RD1 deletion of M. bovis BCG. Specific oligonucleotides targeting these polymorphisms are immobilized on membrane strips. Amplicons derived from a multiplex PCR react with these probes during hybridization. Species can be identified according to the interpretation table provided with the kit. The inclusion of an MTBC-specific 23S rRNA gene fragment confirms the presence of MTBC in order to rule out possible cross-reactivity. Specific patterns can be obtained for M. tuberculosis/"M. canettii," M. africanum/M. pinnipedii, M. microti, M. caprae, M. bovis, and M. bovis BCG. M. tuberculosis and "M. canettii" as well as M. africanum and M. pinnipedii share identical gyrB sequences, and thus they can be identified by specific patterns, but they cannot be differentiated from each other.

The specificity of this test was 100% when strains from culture collections or clinical isolates were compared (102, 103, 111). With strains from culture collections, all species with the exception of an "M. canettii" strain, which was identified as M. tuberculosis, were correctly identified (111). Additionally, 100% of the clinical strains studied were correctly identified (102, 103, 111). No false-positive results were obtained with several NTM strains (111).

Molecular identification of the species of the MTBC may enable a more detailed epidemiological overview. Molecular tests should always be performed if phenotypic characteristics, such as different colony morphologies or negativity in niacin or nitrate reductase tests, are not completely consistent with M. tuberculosis. Furthermore, strains that are monoresistant to pyrazinamide should be analyzed by molecular techniques. These strains can be M. bovis, M. bovis BCG, or, although rare, mono-resistant M. tuberculosis strains. Results obtained by molecular techniques from strains grown in liquid media should be confirmed by selected phenotypic characteristics (i.e., M. tuberculosis should exhibit rough colonies).

TYPING SYSTEMS

Historically, the first strain typing method for M. avium was serotyping based on seroagglutination procedures. Combined use of serotyping and species-specific DNA probes has shown that previously named serovars 1 through 6 and 8 through 11 are M. *avium* and that serovars 7, 12 through 17, 19, 20, and 25 are M. *intracellulare*. Finally, multilocus enzyme electrophoresis has been proven to provide a wider range of polymorphisms than serotyping (150). Serotyping, for both MAC and other mycobacteria, has been replaced by molecular strain typing.

Genotyping of *M. tuberculosis* Strains

The genotyping of M. *tuberculosis* isolates contributes to the knowledge and control of TB by indication of epidemiological links between patients, discrimination between exogenous reinfections and endogenous reactivations, outbreak detection, and the recognition of laboratory cross-contaminations. The CDC has initiated a laboratory program to provide genotyping services for TB control programs to public health laboratories. Further information may be obtained from their website at http://www.cdc.gov/tb/programs/default.htm.

The introduction of the IS*6110*-RFLP technique marked a milestone in determining the molecular epidemiology of M. *tuberculosis* and has been the reference standard for many years. More recently, several alternative PCR-based techniques which are less time-consuming and in part more discriminative than the classical IS*6110*-based technique have been developed.

IS*6110* RFLP Typing

IS*6110* is an insertion sequence that is present in variable numbers (0 to >20 [15]) and has been inserted at various positions in the genomes of MTBC isolates. IS*6110*-based RFLP analysis is performed using an internationally standardized protocol that facilitates comparison of patterns generated by different laboratories (137). High-quality DNA is isolated from mature culture isolates and subjected to restriction enzyme digestion. The DNA fragments are electrophoretically separated, transferred to a membrane, and hybridized with an IS*6110* probe. An internal size standard is also included. The resulting patterns are captured on film. For large-scale comparisons, the patterns should be digitalized by scanning in order for them to be stored in a database. Using computer analysis, the results from separate runs can be compared to detect identical patterns.

The IS*6110* fingerprint patterns are highly discriminatory; only patterns with six or fewer bands provide inadequate discrimination. However, the complete analysis is laborious and time-consuming if the time to obtain sufficient growth on solid media and the multiple technical steps are considered. Furthermore, the analysis of the complex banding patterns requires sophisticated pattern-matching computer software.

Spoligotyping

Spoligotyping (an abbreviation for *spacer oligo*nucleotide *typing*) is a PCR-based technique that targets the variability in the direct repeat (DR) locus of M. *tuberculosis*. The DR region that is present in all MTBC strains consists of multiple DRs of a conserved 36-bp sequence separated by nonrepetitive unique spacer sequences. Of these, 43 spacer sequences identified in the genomes of M. *tuberculosis* and M. *bovis* BCG are used for the spoligotyping assay (51). The spacer segments are amplified by PCR using primers that target the DR sequence. Amplified DNA fragments are hybridized to a membrane with 43 covalently bound oligonucleotides complementary to the 43 spacers.

There are several advantages of spoligotyping compared to IS*6110* RFLP analysis. Since the technique is PCR based, a small amount of DNA is sufficient for analysis. Thus, spoligotyping can be performed from scantily grown solid as well as liquid cultures, enabling a more rapid turnaround time. The technique is less laborious and more rapid than the classical IS*6110* RFLP method. Additionally, the format of the result can easily be transferred into a binary code that can be handled in common computer programs, rendering large-scale comparisons less difficult than the classical method. Unfortunately, spoligotyping is less discriminative than IS*6110* RFLP typing and not sufficient for population-based studies. It can be used for M. *tuberculosis* strains with few IS*6110* copies or M. *bovis* isolates that also have few IS*6110* copies. This technique is very useful for the analysis of assumed laboratory cross-contaminations, as the results can be obtained rapidly.

Spoligotyping also enables the identification of the species of the MTBC by characteristic hybridization patterns of certain spacers. Different genotypes of M. *tuberculosis* which can be identified by specific spoligotype patterns have been described. Most famous is the Beijing genotype, which is frequently encountered in Asia but increasingly distributed worldwide. It can easily be identified by a characteristic spoligotype pattern (144).

MIRU-VNTR Typing

Genotyping may be performed based on the variable numbers of tandem repeats (VNTR) of different classes of genetic elements named mycobacterial interspersed repetitive units (MIRU) (117, 118). This technique is based on the amplification of multiple repeat loci and the subsequent determination of the amplicon size, which depends directly on the number of VNTR copies. Initially, 12 different loci were shown to be suitable for analysis and were considered to possess discriminatory power comparable to that of IS*6110* RFLP analysis (68). This method was adopted in the previously discussed CDC TB genotyping program. Subsequent studies, however, have found the 12-locus assay, even when combined with spoligotyping, to be less discriminatory than the classic RFLP method. The use of a new set of 24 loci for epidemiological studies has been proposed (2, 83, 117). A subset of 15 highly discriminatory loci among the 24 loci provides sufficient discriminatory information for routine epidemiological discrimination.

The amplification of the various loci is usually performed in a multiplex format. The PCR products can be analyzed using an automated DNA sequencer. For small-scale comparisons, analysis of PCR products using classical agarose gel electrophoresis is also possible. The result format is a series of 12, 15, or 24 digits (depending on the MIRU format employed) (Table 9). The number designates the number of repeats at each locus. This format is portable between laboratories and thus simplifies the comparison of large databases. The MIRU-VNTR technique is rapid, with minimal growth required, and is increasingly replacing the IS*6110* RFLP reference standard method.

Genotyping of Slowly Growing NTM

Different approaches have been used for strain comparisons of NTM. Whole-genome analyses have included pulsed-field gel electrophoresis (PFGE) (4, 22, 29, 36, 110), amplified fragment length polymorphism analysis (91), or RFLP typing using specific molecular markers (36, 135). For PFGE and amplified fragment length polymorphism analysis, no genetic information is necessary and the procedures

TABLE 9 MIRU-VNTR patterns of M. *tuberculosis* H37Rv and M. *bovis* BCG (12-locus analysis)

Strain	No. of copies at MIRU locus[a]:											
	2	4	10	16	20	23	24	26	27	31	39	40
M. *tuberculosis* H37Rv	2	3	3	2	2	6	1	3	3	3	2	1
M. *bovis* BCG	2	V[b]	2	3	2	4	2	5	3	3	2	2

[a]According to Supply et al. (118).
[b]V, variable among different BCG strains.

can be performed without further knowledge of the species genome. For RFLP typing, some genetic information, such as the presence of specific IS elements, is a prerequisite.

Pulsed-Field Gel Electrophoresis

The major criterion for molecular strain typing is that the test isolates must all belong to the same species. Thus, definitive identification to the species level is an important prerequisite.

For strain typing of the slowly growing NTM, PFGE has been a useful technique and remains the gold standard for molecular typing. This technique requires an actively growing culture and 3 to 4 weeks for completion. Problems with standardization may result from cell clumping of rough strains. This clumping may also result in different amounts of DNA even from different batches of the same strain, causing problematic uneven (light and overloaded) lanes. Previous studies have detailed the method of PFGE related to clinical and epidemiologic studies of M. *kansasii*, M. *szulgai*, and MAC (40, 46, 92, 145, 146, 151). Recently, PFGE has been applied to study macrolide-susceptible and -resistant isolates and multiple cultures of patients with nodular MAC disease and bronchiectasis (40). Most clinical experts agree that the availability of methods for strain comparison such as PFGE is helpful, if not essential, in making critical decisions about therapy of MAC lung disease (146).

Multilocus Sequence Typing

Another approach for NTM typing is analysis of multiple genes with a high sequence variation, like *hsp65* or ITS. However, available sequences have not provided the level of variability needed for epidemiological analyses. With the progress of whole-genome analysis and the possibility of large-sequence determination, however, this method is likely to prove increasingly useful for multilocus sequencing typing of NTM.

Repetitive-Unit Sequence-Based PCR

Repetitive-unit sequence-based PCR (rep-PCR) has been used for outbreak control of several slowly growing mycobacterial species, including M. *simiae*, M. *gordonae*, M. *terrae*, M. *tuberculosis*, and M. *avium* complex (5, 14, 47). The method is commercially available through bioMérieux DiversiLab System (Durham, NC). The technology is flexible in that it can genotype not only NTM but also other microbial pathogens for epidemiology. Although the technology is proprietary, the company offers a Web-based library of rep-PCR sequences that can be searched for matches with any strain of interest for its users. Moreover, the system has the ability to generate high-resolution DNA fingerprints from small samples in real time, similar to spoligotyping and MIRU typing of M. *tuberculosis*, and has more potential portability than PFGE. The method is semiautomated but does require significant laboratory expenditure.

M. avium

The most extensive investigations for typing of NTM strains have been undertaken for M. *avium*. RFLP analysis based on the insertion sequence IS1245, which is restricted to subspecies of M. *avium*, has been used for genotyping. Standardization of this technique was proposed in 1998 (142), but this technology never became widespread. However, Mijs et al (74) used this method as one tool for distinguishing M. *avium* subsp. *avium* strains obtained from bird specimens from swine- and human-derived strains, for which they proposed the name "M. *avium* subsp. *hominissuis.*" RFLP analysis based on the insertion sequence IS900 can be used for genotyping of MAP.

The availability of the complete genome sequences of the "M. *avium* subsp. *hominisuis*" strain 104 and the MAP strain K-10 allowed the search for divergent regions that can be used for standardization of other techniques for genotyping (135). Based on the genomic sequence data, large-sequence polymorphisms, which were analyzed for their variability among different M. *avium* strains, could be identified. By the use of multilocus sequence typing, many genes that contain multiple sequence variations can now be analyzed in parallel (133). MIRU-VNTRs have also been discovered and to date have been applied mainly to typing of MAP strains (48, 75, 123). Unlike with M. *tuberculosis*, there is currently no widely evaluated and generally accepted protocol for typing of M. *avium* or other NTM species.

ANTIMICROBIAL SUSCEPTIBILITIES

Antimicrobial susceptibility testing (AST) of mycobacteria is crucial for the control of infections caused by many species of mycobacteria. Testing should be performed by experienced laboratories according to the CLSI guidelines (80).

Nontuberculous Slowly Growing Mycobacteria

AST of the NTM requires skill and knowledge of the individual species characteristics. Therefore, the CLSI has advised laboratories that infrequently encounter NTM to refer those isolates to a qualified reference laboratory. Laboratories that elect to perform in-house NTM AST should carefully validate their results and monitor their proficiency regularly, as required by specific accrediting agencies, such as the College of American Pathologists (80).

Generally, broth micro- or macrodilution techniques in serial twofold concentrations are recommended. Testing is most efficiently performed in 96-well microtiter panels. Breakpoints for slowly growing mycobacteria have been proposed for the following antimicrobials: rifampin, rifabutin, amikacin, ethambutol, ciprofloxacin, moxifloxacin, minocycline, doxycycline, clarithromycin, trimethoprim-sulfamethoxazole, and linezolid (80).

The CLSI recommendation specifies testing for slowly growing species, including M. *kansasii*, MAC, and M. *marinum*. Other species of slowly growing NTM have insufficient data to make specific recommendations for testing. Thus, for those species, the CLSI has recommended that testing of these NTM should follow the guidelines for testing rifampin-resistant *M. kansasii*. The CLSI and the statement of the American Thoracic Society and the Infectious Diseases Society of America have recommended that only rifampin and clarithromycin results be reported for *M. kansasii* unless the isolate is rifampin resistant; if so, all of the previously listed antimicrobials should be tested (39, 80).

For isolates of *M. marinum*, experts in mycobacterial susceptibility testing concur that AST is unnecessary in most cases due to the narrow range of MICs for this species. In cases of intolerance to agents typically effective for the treatment of infections due to *M. marinum* (i.e., clarithromycin, rifampin, and ethambutol), antimicrobial testing of the previously listed agents should be performed (80).

Finally, for MAC, because previous studies have shown that no correlation exists between MICs and the clinical response of the patient to agents other than clarithromycin, testing of only clarithromycin is recommended. The exception is for reporting agents such as quinolones (ciprofloxacin or moxifloxacin) and linezolid, for which no correlation studies have been performed to date (80).

Fastidious species which require iron or hemin-containing media for growth, such as *M. haemophilum*, may be tested using an alternative agar disk elution method with commercial antimicrobial disks in molten agar. The CLSI has recommended testing of antimicrobials, including rifampin, clarithromycin, amikacin, ciprofloxacin, trimethoprim-sulfamethoxazole, and doxycycline or minocycline (80).

Specific details and discussion of the AST procedures can be found in chapter 73 of this *Manual*.

Mycobacterium tuberculosis Complex

Currently, methods for testing MTBC are based on the methods of proportion which rely on a clinical definition of drug resistance. Susceptibility testing of MTBC may be performed in agar-based (agar proportion method) or broth-based (commercial) systems. Agar proportion methods may be performed using either commercially prepared or in-house media.

Both the agar proportion and newer liquid detection systems define resistance as growth of >1% of an inoculum of bacterial cells in the presence of a "critical" concentration of the drug. By convention, the critical concentration corresponds to the lowest concentrations of drugs that inhibit 95% of "wild strains" of MTBC that have never been exposed to the antimicrobials without simultaneously inhibiting strains of MTBC from patients who do not respond to treatment and that are considered resistant. The critical concentration is, thus, the standard concentration by which susceptibility and resistance are established.

Generally, the first isolate of MTBC cultures from each patient should be tested, and susceptibility testing should be repeated if the patient fails to respond to therapy or if the cultures remain positive at 3 months. Primary susceptibility testing includes a battery of antimicrobials, including isoniazid at two concentrations (critical and higher concentrations), rifampin, ethambutol, and pyrazinamide. Whenever an isolate is resistant to rifampin or any two of the other primary drugs, a secondary panel including a higher concentration of ethambutol, capreomycin, ethionamide, amikacin, *p*-aminosalicylic acid, rifabutin, streptomycin, and levofloxacin should be tested (80).

Susceptibility testing with MTBC involves direct testing of smear-positive samples (especially from patients known to have or suspected of having MTB). This involves inoculation of drug-containing media with a directly processed sample (i.e., concentrated after decontamination and digestion). Additionally, indirect susceptibility testing may be performed using cultures already growing either in liquid or solid media. This method is usually used on smear-negative samples or if the direct test results are invalid due to contamination, insufficient numbers of colonies in the drug-free quadrants, or insufficient growth after 3 weeks of incubation. Details on both methods of susceptibility testing can be found in chapter 73. Standardized agar proportion methods are not considered rapid methods. Therefore, the addition of a commercial liquid susceptibility system with shorter incubation is strongly recommended for patient testing. It is imperative, however, that any commercial system be validated to produce results that correlate with the standard susceptibility agar proportion methods. As with any other laboratory test, adequate and consistent quality control and proficiency testing should be performed to ensure accurate and consistent results (80).

EVALUATION, INTERPRETATION, AND REPORTING OF RESULTS

Implementation of sensitive and rapid methods for the detection, identification, and susceptibility testing of MTBC and NTM is of paramount importance to the diagnosis and control of TB and NTM disease. The use of the fluorochrome stain for mycobacterial smears, a broth-based culture system, and the use of DNA probes or sequence analysis for identification along with direct susceptibility testing of smear-positive specimens are optimal for the ultimate goal of clinical mycobacteriology in the support of decisions related to the care of patients with mycobacterial infections. As emphasized in this chapter, phenotypic testing of the slowly growing mycobacterial species has limited use and for other mycobacteria (i.e., rapidly growing mycobacteria) should be applied only in conjunction with molecularly based assays. Laboratory work should be organized to prioritize timely and accurate identification and the susceptibility of clinically significant species of mycobacteria.

In order to optimize rapid detection, identification, and AST for the shortest turnaround times, the U.S. Association of Public Health Laboratories has recommended that the Fast Track Referral Model System be implemented. This network system helps to ensure that quality state-of-the-art technology is used, results are reported in a timely manner, and the tracking and fingerprinting of isolates of MTBC occur efficiently for optimal exchange of information between medical centers and the public health sector (18).

Recent CLSI guidelines recommend reports within 24 hours for acid-fast bacterium smears and interim reports if growth is seen on inoculated solid media or when a positive signal is detected on liquid media. A confirmatory report should be issued once growth is evident, and an identification of either NTM or MTBC should be reported. Moreover, reporting should be done as soon as species-level identification is available for NTM and, finally, when susceptibility testing is completed (usually within 7 to 14 days for NTM with broth systems). Additionally, for MTBC, identification from culture results should be reported within an average of 14 days, and a complete culture report with susceptibility results should be reported within an average of 4 to 6 weeks. The use of liquid medium rapid detection systems along with solid medium is critical in order to meet these guidelines (18, 39, 80).

In an effort to develop a more consistent and practical method of reporting identifications performed by molecular techniques, the CLSI (17) has recently published interpretive criteria for the identification of mycobacterial species by DNA target sequencing, including consensus cutoff values for percent identity. The new document states that mycobacteria with 100% 16S rRNA gene identity for genus and species may be definitively reported with both genus and species. However, for those isolates whose identity is 99.0% to 99.9%, the recommendation is to report as "*Mycobacterium* most closely related to the species given." However, if the identity to a recognized species is ≥95 to 98.9%, the results should state that the isolate cannot be definitely identified by 16S rRNA gene sequencing; identification should be given as "most closely related to *Mycobacterium* sp."

Microheterogeneity within an NTM species (i.e., 1 to 5 bases in the 16S rRNA gene are different from the sequence of a known reference strain) has been described for several slowly growing species, including *M. gordonae*, *M. bohemicum*, *M. kansasii*, *M. celatum*, and *M. lentiflavum*. In general, members of the genus *Mycobacterium* are closely related to each other in their 16S rRNA gene sequences and may differ by only a few bases or not at all. In the absence of strong phenotypic differences, definitive NTM identification may be difficult, if not impossible. Turenne et al. advocate that the individual strain ambiguities should be examined carefully using optimum quality sequence databases for comparison, and even then, results may remain inconclusive without resorting to sequencing of alternate targets (134).

As has been discussed previously, 16S rRNA gene sequencing is not useful for separation of some species, including the species within the MTBC. Thus, with MTBC, reporting results of only the 16S rRNA gene sequence should state "*Mycobacterium tuberculosis* complex." When species level identification is necessary, alternate targets, such as *gyrB*, may provide species differentiation, except for MTB and "*M. canetti*."

Among the slowly growing NTM, several species are not identifiable with 16S rRNA gene sequencing alone. For example, *M. kansasii* and *M. gastri* and *M. marinum* and *M. ulcerans* share sequence identity in their 16S rRNA genes, and thus alternate gene targets or determination of photochromogenicity is required to provide species resolution. Alternate gene targets which may help in cases where sequencing of the 16S rRNA gene is not adequate include the ITS 1, *hsp65*, *gyrB*, *rpoB*, *recA*, and *dnaA* genes. Specific numerical cutoff values such as are recommended for the 16S rRNA gene are not yet recommended for these genes.

The more accurate characterization of new species by molecular technology and the enhancement of clinical data with standardized AST results continue to advance our knowledge of the MTBC, NTM, and disease caused by these species. Proper interpretation and reporting of species identification, even by molecular methods, should be checked against fundamentally established phenotypic characteristics, such as growth rate, colony morphology, and pigmentation. Determination of temperature requirements also may be useful for select isolates.

Finally, appropriate AST of clinically significant species is vital to recognize and effectively treat multiple-drug-resistant mycobacterial species, including multidrug-resistant and extensively drug resistant MTBC strains, as well as NTM such as *M. simiae*, MAC, rifampin-resistant *M. kansasii*, and other clinically significant drug-resistant species.

REFERENCES

1. **Adékambi, T., P. Colson, and M. Drancourt.** 2003. *rpoB*-based identification of nonpigmented and late-pigmenting rapidly growing mycobacteria. *J. Clin. Microbiol.* **41:**5699–5708.
2. **Allix-Béguec, C., M. Fauville-Dufaux, and P. Supply.** 2008. Three-year population-based evaluation of standardized mycobacterial interspersed repetitive-unit-variable-number tandem-repeat typing of *Mycobacterium tuberculosis*. *J. Clin. Microbiol.* **46:**1398–1406.
3. **Alshamaony, L., M. Goodfellow, and D. E. Minnikin.** 1976. Free mycolic acids as criteria in the classification of *Nocardia* and the "rhodochrous" complex. *J. Gen. Microbiol.* **92:**188–199.
4. **Alvarez, J., I. G. García, A. Aranaz, J. Bezos, B. Romero, L. de Juan, A. Mateos, E. Gómez-Mampaso, and L. Domínguez.** 2008. Genetic diversity of *Mycobacterium avium* isolates recovered from clinical samples and from the environment: molecular characterization for diagnostic purposes. *J. Clin. Microbiol.* **46:**1246–1251.
5. **Ashworth, M., K. L. Horan, R. Freeman, E. Oren, M. Narita, and G. A. Cangelosi.** 2008. Use of PCR-based *Mycobacterium tuberculosis* genotyping to prioritize tuberculosis outbreak control activities. *J. Clin. Microbiol.* **46:**856–862.
6. **Bang, D., T. Herlin, M. Stegger, A. B. Andersen, P. Torkko, E. Tortoli, and V. O. Thomsen.** 2008. *Mycobacterium arosiense* sp. nov., a slowly growing, scotochromogenic species causing osteomyelitis in an immunocompromised child. *Int. J. Syst. Evol. Microbiol.* **58:**2398–2402.
7. **Behr, M. A., and J. O. Falinkham III.** 2009. Molecular epidemiology of nontuberculous mycobacteria. *Fut. Microbiol.* **4:**1009–1020.
8. **Böddinghaus, B., T. Rogall, T. Flohr, H. Blöcker, and E. C, Böttger.** 1990. Detection and identification of mycobacteria by amplification of rRNA. *J. Clin. Microbiol.* **28:**1751–1759.
9. **Böttger, E. C., B. Hirschel, and M. B. Coyle.** 1993. *Mycobacterium genavense* sp. nov. *Int. J. Syst. Bacteriol.* **43:**841–843.
10. **Bull, T. J., and D. C. Shanson.** 1992. Evaluation of a commercial chemiluminescent gene probe system 'AccuProbe' for the rapid differentiation of mycobacteria, including 'MAIC X,' isolated from blood and other sites, from patients with AIDS. *J. Hosp. Infect.* **21:**143–149.
11. **Bull, T. J., D. C. Shanson, L. C. Archard, M. D. Yates, M. E. Hamid, and D. E. Minnikin.** 1995. A new group (type 3) of *Mycobacterium celatum* isolated from AIDS patients in the London area. *Int. J. Syst. Bacteriol.* **45:**861–862.
12. **Butler, W. R., and L. S. Guthertz.** 2001. Mycolic acid analysis by high-performance liquid chromatography for identification of *Mycobacterium* species. *Clin. Microbiol. Rev.* **14:**704–726.
13. **Butler, W. R., S. P. O'Connor, M. A. Yakrus, R. W. Smithwick, B. B. Plikaytis, C. W. Moss, M. M. Floyd, C. L. Woodley, J. O. Kilburn, F. S. Vadney, and W. M. Gross.** 1993. *Mycobacterium celatum* sp. nov. *Int. J. Syst. Bacteriol.* **43:**539–548. (Author's correction, **43:**868.)
14. **Cangelosi, G. A., R. J. Freeman, K. N. Lewis, D. Livingston-Rosanoff, K. S. Shah, S. J. Milan, and S. V. Goldberg.** 2004. Evaluation of a high-throughput repetitive-sequence-based PCR system for DNA fingerprinting of *Mycobacterium tuberculosis* and *Mycobacterium avium* complex strains. *J. Clin. Microbiol.* **42:**2685–2693.
15. **Cave, M. D., M. Murray, and E. Nardell.** 2005. Molecular epidemiology of *Mycobacterium tuberculosis*, p. 33–46. *In* S. T. Cole, K. D. Eisenach, D. N. McMurray, and W. R. Jacobs, Jr. (ed.), *Tuberculosis and the Tubercle Bacillus.* ASM Press, Washington, DC.
16. **Centers for Disease Control and Prevention.** 2009. Updated guidelines for the use of nucleic acid amplification tests in the diagnosis of tuberculosis. *MMWR Morb. Mortal. Wkly. Rep.* **58:**7–10.

17. **Clinical and Laboratory Standards Institute.** 2008. *Interpretive Criteria for Identification of Bacteria and Fungi by DNA Target Sequencing; Approved Guideline MM18-A.* Clinical and Laboratory Standards Institute, Wayne, PA.

18. **Clinical and Laboratory Standards Institute.** 2008. *Laboratory Detection and Identification of Mycobacteria;* Approved Guideline M48-A. Clinical and Laboratory Standards Institute, Wayne, PA.

19. **Cloud, J. L., K. C. Carroll, S. Cohen, C. M. Anderson, and G. L. Woods.** 2005. Interpretive criteria for use of AccuProbe for identification of *Mycobacterium avium* complex directly from 7H9 broth cultures. *J. Clin. Microbiol.* **43:**347–348.

20. **Cole, S. T., R. Brosch, J. Parkhill, T. Garnier, C. Churcher, D. Harris, S. V. Gordon, K. Eiglmeier, S. Gas, C. E. Barry III, F. Tekaia, K. Badcock, D. Basham, D. Brown, T. Chillingworth, R. Connor, R. Davies, K. Devlin, T. Feltwell, S. Gentles, N. Hamlin, S. Holroyd, T. Hornsby, K. Jagels, A. Krogh, J. McLean, S. Moule, L. Murphy, K. Oliver, J. Osborne, M. A. Quail, M. A. Rajandream, J. Rogers, S. Rutter, K. Seeger, J. Skelton, R. Squares, S. Squares, J. E. Sulston, K. Taylor, S. Whitehead, and B. G. Barrell.** 1998. Deciphering the biology of *Mycobacterium tuberculosis* from the complete genome sequence. *Nature* **393:**537–544. (Erratum, **396:**190.)

21. **Cole, S. T., K. Eiglmeier, J. Parkhill, K. D. James, N. R. Thomson, P. R. Wheeler, N. Honoré, T. Garnier, C. Churcher, D. Harris, K. Mungall, D. Basham, D. Brown, T. Chillingworth, R. Connor, R. M. Davies, K. Devlin, S. Duthoy, T. Feltwell, A. Fraser, N. Hamlin, S. Holroyd, T. Hornsby, K. Jagels, C. Lacroix, J. Maclean, S. Moule, L. Murphy, K. Oliver, M. A. Quail, M. A. Rajandream, K. M. Rutherford, S. Rutter, K. Seeger, S. Simon, M. Simmonds, J. Skelton, R. Squares, S. Squares, K. Stevens, K. Taylor, S. Whitehead, J. R. Woodward, and B. G. Barrell.** 2001. Massive gene decay in the leprosy bacillus. *Nature* **409:**1007–1011.

22. **Conger, N. G., R. J. O'Connell, V. L. Laurel, K. N. Olivier, E. A. Graviss, N. Williams-Bouyer, Y. Zhang, B. A. Brown-Elliott, and R. J. Wallace, Jr.** 2004. *Mycobacterium simae* outbreak associated with a hospital water supply. *Infect. Control. Hosp. Epidemiol.* **25:**1050–1055.

23. **Cook, V. J., C. Y. Turenne, J. Wolfe, R. Pauls, and A. Kabani.** 2003. Conventional methods versus 16S ribosomal DNA sequencing for identification of nontuberculous mycobacteria: cost analysis. *J. Clin. Microbiol.* **41:**1010–1015.

24. **Cousins, D. V., R. Bastida, A. Cataldi, V. Quse, S. Redrobe, S. Dow, P. Duignan, A. Murray, C. Dupont, N. Ahmed, D. M. Collins, W. R. Butler, D. Dawson, D. Rodriguez, J. Loureiro, M. I. Romano, A. Alito, M. Zumarraga, and A. Bernardelli.** 2003. Tuberculosis in seals caused by a novel member of the *Mycobacterium tuberculosis* complex: *Mycobacterium pinnipedii* sp. nov. *Int. J. Syst. Evol. Microbiol.* **53:**1305–1314.

25. **Daley, P., A. Petrich, K. May, K. Luinstra, C. Rutherford, P. Chedore, F. Jamieson, and M. Smieja.** 2008. Comparison of in-house and commercial 16S rRNA sequencing with high-performance liquid chromatography and genotype AS and CM for identification of nontuberculous mycobacteria. *Diagn. Microbiol. Infect. Dis.* **61:**284–293.

26. **Daley, P., S. Thomas, and M. Pai.** 2007. Nucleic acid amplification tests for the diagnosis of tuberculous lymphadenitis: a systematic review. *Int. J. Tuberc. Lung Dis.* **11:**1166–1176.

27. **Devallois, A., K. S. Goh, and N. Rastogi.** 1997. Rapid identification of mycobacteria to species level by PCR-restriction fragment length polymorphism analysis of the *hsp65* gene and proposition of an algorithm to differentiate 34 mycobacterial species. *J. Clin. Microbiol.* **35:**2969–2973.

28. **Dinnes, J., J. Deeks, H. Kunst, A. Gibson, E. Cummins, N. Waugh, F. Drobniewski, and A. Lalvani.** 2007. A systematic review of rapid diagnostic tests for the detection of tuberculosis infection. *Health Technol. Assess.* **11:**1–196.

29. **Doig, C., L. Muckersie, B. Watt, and K. J. Forbes.** 2002. Molecular epidemiology of *Mycobacterium malmoense* infections in Scotland. *J. Clin. Microbiol.* **40:**1103–1105.

30. **El Amin, N. M., H. S. Hanson, B. Pettersson, B. Petrini, and L. V. von Stedingk.** 2000. Identification of nontuberculous mycobacteria: 16S rRNA gene sequence analysis vs. conventional methods. *Scand. J. Infect. Dis.* **32:**47–50.

31. **Flores, L. L., M. Pai, J. M. Colford, Jr., and L. W. Riley.** 2005. In-house nucleic acid amplification tests for the detection of *Mycobacterium tuberculosis* in sputum specimens: meta-analysis and meta-regression. *BMC Microbiol.* **5:**55.

32. **Fox, G. E., E. Stackebrandt, R. B. Hespell, J. Gibson, J. Maniloff, T. A. Dyer, R. S. Wolfe, W. E. Balch, R. S. Tanner, L. J. Magrum, L. B. Zablen, R. Blakemore, R. Gupta, L. Bonen, B. J. Lewis, D. A. Stahl, K. R. Luehrsen, K. N. Chen, and C. R. Woese.** 1980. The phylogeny of prokaryotes. *Science* **209:**457–463.

33. **Frothingham, R., and K. H. Wilson.** 1993. Sequence-based differentiation of strains in the *Mycobacterium avium* complex. *J. Bacteriol.* **175:**2818–2825.

34. **Frothingham, R., and K. H. Wilson.** 1994. Molecular phylogeny of the *Mycobacterium avium* complex demonstrates clinically meaningful divisions. *J. Infect. Dis.* **169:**305–312.

35. **Garnier, T., K. Eiglmeier, J. C. Camus, N. Medina, H. Mansoor, M. Pryor, S. Duthoy, S. Grondin, C. Lacroix, C. Monsempe, S. Simon, B. Harris, R. Atkin, J. Doggett, R. Mayes, L. Keating, P. R. Wheeler, J. Parkhill, B. G. Barrell, S. T. Cole, S. V. Gordon, and R. G. Hewinson.** 2003. The complete genome sequence of *Mycobacterium bovis*. *Proc. Natl. Acad. Sci. USA* **100:**7877–7882.

36. **Garriga, X., P. Cortés, P. Rodríguez, F. March, G. Prats, and P. Coll.** 2000. Comparison of IS1245 restriction fragment length polymorphism and pulsed-field gel electrophoresis for typing clinical isolates of *Mycobacterium avium* subsp. *avium*. *Int. J. Tuberc. Lung Dis.* **4:**463–472.

37. **Gitti, Z., I. Neonakis, G. Fanti, F. Kontos, S. Maraki, and Y. Tselentis.** 2006. Use of the GenoType Mycobacterium CM and AS assays to analyze 76 nontuberculous mycobacterial isolates from Greece. *J. Clin. Microbiol.* **44:**2244–2246.

38. **Gómez-Valero, L., E. P. Rocha, A. Latorre, and F. J. Silva.** 2007. Reconstructing the ancestor of *Mycobacterium leprae*: the dynamics of gene loss and genome reduction. *Genome Res.* **17:**1178–1185.

39. **Griffith, D. E., T. Aksamit, B. A. Brown-Elliott, A. Catanzaro, C. Daley, F. Gordin, S. M. Holland, R. Horsburgh, G. Huitt, M. F. Iademarco, M. Iseman, K. Olivier, S. Ruoss, C. F. von Reyn, R. J. Wallace, Jr., and K. Winthrop; ATS Mycobacterial Diseases Subcommittee, American Thoracic Society; Infectious Disease Society of America.** 2007. An official ATS/IDSA statement: diagnosis, treatment, and prevention of nontuberculous mycobacterial diseases. *Am. J. Respir. Crit. Care Med.* **175:**367–416. (Erratum, **175:**744–745.)

40. **Griffith, D. E., B. A. Brown-Elliott, B. Langsjoen, Y. Zhang, X. Pan, W. Girard, K. Nelson, J. Caccitolo, J. Alvarez, S. Shepherd, R. Wilson, E. A. Graviss, and R. J. Wallace, Jr.** 2006. Clinical and molecular analysis of macrolide resistance in *Mycobacterium avium* complex lung disease. *Am. J. Respir. Crit. Care Med.* **174:**928–934.

41. **Haas, W. H., W. R. Butler, P. Kirschner, B. B. Plikaytis, M. B. Coyle, B. Amthor, A. G. Steigerwalt, D. J. Brenner, M. Salfinger, J. T. Crawford, E. C. Böttger, and H. J. Bremer.** 1997. A new agent of mycobacterial lymphadenitis in children: *Mycobacterium heidelbergense* sp. nov. *J. Clin. Microbiol.* **35:**3203–3209.

42. **Hall, L., K. A. Doerr, S. L. Wohlfiel, and G. D. Roberts.** 2003. Evaluation of the MicroSeq system for identification of mycobacteria by 16S ribosomal DNA sequencing and its integration into a routine clinical mycobacteriology laboratory. *J. Clin. Microbiol.* **41:**1447–1453.

43. **Han, X. Y., A. S. Pham, J. J. Tarrand, P. K. Sood, and R. Luthra.** 2002. Rapid and accurate identification of mycobacteria by sequencing hypervariable regions of the 16S ribosomal RNA gene. *Am. J. Clin. Pathol.* **118:**796–801.

44. **Harmsen, D., S. Dostal, A. Roth, S. Niemann, J. Rothganger, M. Sammeth, J. Albert, M. Frosch, and E. Richter.** 2003. RIDOM: comprehensive and public sequence

database for identification of *Mycobacterium* species. *BMC Infect. Dis.* **3**:26.

45. **Holberg-Petersen, M., M. Steinbakk, K. J. Figenschau, E. Jantzen, J. Eng, and K. K. Melby.** 1999. Identification of clinical isolates of *Mycobacterium* spp. by sequence analysis of the 16S ribosomal RNA gene. Experience from a clinical laboratory. *APMIS* **107**:231–239.

46. **Holmes, G. P., G. B. Bond, R. C. Fader, and S. F. Fulcher.** 2002. A cluster of cases of *Mycobacterium szulgai* keratitis that occurred after laser-assisted in situ keratomileusis. *Clin. Infect. Dis.* **34**:1039–1046.

47. **Horan, K. L., R. Freman, K. Weigel, M. Semret, S. Pfaller, T. C. Covert, D. van Soolingen, S. C. Leão, M. A. Behr, and G. A. Cangelosi.** 2006. Isolation of the genome sequence strain *Mycobacterium avium* 104 from multiple patients over a 17-year period. *J. Clin. Microbiol.* **44**:783–789.

48. **Inagaki, T., K. Nishimori, T. Yagi, K. Ichikawa, M. Moriyama, T. Nakagawa, T. Shibayama, K. Uchiya, T. Nikai, and K. Ogawa.** 2009. Comparison of a variable-number tandem-repeat (VNTR) method for typing *Mycobacterium avium* with mycobacterial interspersed repetitive-unit-VNTR and IS*1245* restriction fragment length polymorphism typing. *J. Clin. Microbiol.* **47**:2156–2164.

49. **Iwamoto, T., and H. Saito.** 2006. Comparative study of two typing methods, *hsp*65 PRA and ITS sequencing, revealed a possible evolutionary link between *Mycobacterium kansasii* type I and II isolates. *FEMS Microbiol. Lett.* **254**:129–133.

50. **Jost, K. C., Jr., D. F. Dunbar, S. S. Barth, V. L. Headley, and L. B. Elliott.** 1995. Identification of *Mycobacterium tuberculosis* and *M. avium* complex directly from smear-positive sputum specimens and BACTEC 12B cultures by high-performance liquid chromatography with fluorescence detection and computer-driven pattern recognition models. *J. Clin. Microbiol.* **33**:1270–1277.

51. **Kamerbeek, J., L. Schouls, A. Kolk, M. van Agterveld, D. van Soolingen, S. Kuijper, A. Bunschoten, H. Molhuizen, R. Shaw, M. Goyal, and J. van Embden.** 1997. Simultaneous detection and strain differentiation of *Mycobacterium tuberculosis* for diagnosis and epidemiology. *J. Clin. Microbiol.* **35**:907–914.

52. **Kasai, H., T. Ezaki, and S. Harayama.** 2000. Differentiation of phylogenetically related slowly growing mycobacteria by their *gyrB* sequences. *J. Clin. Microbiol.* **38**:301–308.

52a. **Kent, P. T., and G. P. Kubica.** 1985. *Public Health Mycobacteriology. A Guide for the Level III Laboratory.* Centers for Disease Control and Prevention, U.S. Department of Health and Human Services, Atlanta, GA.

53. **Kim, B. J., S. H. Lee, M. A. Lyu, S. J. Kim, G. H. Bai, G. T. Chae, E. C. Kim, C. Y. Cha, and Y. H. Kook.** 1999. Identification of mycobacterial species by comparative sequence analysis of the RNA polymerase gene (*rpoB*). *J. Clin. Microbiol.* **37**:1714–1720.

54. **Kirschner, P., and E. C. Böttger.** 1992. Microheterogeneity within rRNA of *Mycobacterium gordonae*. *J. Clin. Microbiol.* **30**:1049–1050.

55. **Kirschner, P., B. Springer, U. Vogel, A. Meier, A. Wrede, M. Kiekenbeck, F. C. Bange, and E. C Böttger.** 1993. Genotypic identification of mycobacteria by nucleic acid sequence determination: report of a 2-year experience in a clinical laboratory. *J. Clin. Microbiol.* **31**:2882–2889.

56. **Lane, D. J., B. Pace, G. J. Olsen, D. A. Stahl, M. L. Sogin, and N. R. Pace.** 1985. Rapid determination of 16S ribosomal RNA sequences for phylogenetic analyses. *Proc. Natl. Acad. Sci. USA* **82**:6955–6959.

57. **Lebrun, L., F. Espinasse, J. D. Poveda, and V. Vincent-Levy-Frebault.** 1992. Evaluation of nonradioactive DNA probes for identification of mycobacteria. *J. Clin. Microbiol.* **30**:2476–2478.

58. **Lechevalier, M. P., A. C. Horan, and H. Lechevalier.** 1971. Lipid composition in the classification of nocardiae and mycobacteria. *J. Bacteriol.* **105**:313–318.

59. **Lee, A. S., P. Jelfs, V. Sintchenko, and G. L. Gilbert.** 2009. Identification of non-tuberculous mycobacteria: utility of the GenoType Mycobacterium CM/AS assay compared with HPLC and 16S rRNA gene sequencing. *J. Med. Microbiol.* **58**:900–904.

60. **Lee, H., H. E. Bang, G. H. Bai, and S. N. Cho.** 2003. Novel polymorphic region of the *rpoB* gene containing *Mycobacterium* species-specific sequences and its use in identification of mycobacteria. *J. Clin. Microbiol.* **41**:2213–2218.

61. **Lee, H. K., S. A. Lee, I. K. Lee, H. K. Yu, Y. G. Park, J. W. Hyun, K. Kim, Y. H. Kook, and B. J. Kim.** 2010. *Mycobacterium paraseoulense* sp. nov., a slowly growing, scotochromogenic species related genetically to *Mycobacterium seoulense*. *Int. J. Syst. Evol. Microbiol.* **60**:439–443.

62. **Liesack, W., S. Sela, H. Bercovier, C. Pitulle, and E. Stackebrandt.** 1991. Complete nucleotide sequence of the *Mycobacterium leprae* 23 S and 5 S rRNA genes plus flanking regions and their potential in designing diagnostic oligonucleotide probes. *FEBS Lett.* **281**:114–118. (Erratum, **286**:238.)

63. **Ling, D. I., L. L. Flores, L. W. Riley, and M. Pai.** 2008. Commercial nucleic-acid amplification tests for diagnosis of pulmonary tuberculosis in respiratory specimens: meta-analysis and meta-regression. *PLoS One* **3**:e1536.

64. **Mäkinen, J., A. Sarkola, M. Marjamäki, M. K. Viljanen, and H. Soini.** 2002. Evaluation of genotype and LiPA MYCOBACTERIA assays for identification of Finnish mycobacterial isolates. *J. Clin. Microbiol.* **40**:3478–3481.

65. **Marras, T. K., P. Chedore, A. M. Ying, and F. Jamieson.** 2007. Isolation prevalence of pulmonary non-tuberculous mycobacteria in Ontario, 1997–2003. *Thorax* **62**:661–666.

66. **Martín-Casabona, N., A. R. Bahrmand, J. Bennedsen, V. O. Thomsen, M. Curcio, M. Fauville-Dufaux, K. Feldman, M. Havelkova, M. L. Katila, K. Köksalan, M. F. Pereira, F. Rodrigues, G. E. Pfyffer, F. Portaels, J. R. Urgell, S. Rüsch-Gerdes, E. Tortoli, V. Vincent, and B. Watt; Spanish Group for Non-Tuberculosis Mycobacteria.** 2004. Non-tuberculous mycobacteria: patterns of isolation. A multi-country retrospective survey. *Int. J. Tuberc. Lung Dis.* **8**:1186–1193.

67. **Masaki, T., K. Ohkusu, H. Hata, N. Fujiwara, H. Iihara, M. Yamada-Noda, P. H. Nhung, M. Hayashi, Y. Asano, Y. Kawamura, and T. Ezaki.** 2006. *Mycobacterium kumamotonense* sp. nov. recovered from clinical specimen and the first isolation report of *Mycobacterium arupense* in Japan: novel slowly growing, nonchromogenic clinical isolates related to *Mycobacterium terrae* complex. *Microbiol. Immunol.* **50**:889–897.

68. **Mazars, E., S. Lesjean, A. L. Banuls, M. Gilbert, V. Vincent, B. Gicquel, M. Tibayrenc, C. Locht, and P. Supply.** 2001. High-resolution minisatellite-based typing as a portable approach to global analysis of *Mycobacterium tuberculosis* molecular epidemiology. *Proc. Natl. Acad. Sci. USA* **98**:1901–1906.

69. **McHugh, T. D., C. F. Pope, C. L. Ling, S. Patel, O. J. Billington, R. D. Gosling, M. C. Lipman, and S. H. Gillespie.** 2004. Prospective evaluation of BDProbeTec strand displacement amplification (SDA) system for diagnosis of tuberculosis in non-respiratory and respiratory samples. *J. Med. Microbiol.* **53**:1215–1219.

70. **McNabb, A., D. Eisler, K. Adie, M. Amos, M. Rodrigues, G. Stephens, W. A. Black, and J. Isaac-Renton.** 2004. Assessment of partial sequencing of the 65-kilodalton heat shock protein gene (*hsp65*) for routine identification of *Mycobacterium* species isolated from clinical sources. *J. Clin. Microbiol.* **42**:3000–3011.

71. **Meier, A., P. Kirschner, K. H. Schröder, J. Wolters, R. M. Kroppenstedt, and E. C. Böttger.** 1993. *Mycobacterium intermedium* sp. nov. *Int. J. Syst. Bacteriol.* **43**:204–209.

72. **Middleton, A. M., P. Cullinan, R. Wilson, J. R. Kerr, and M. V. Chadwick.** 2003. Interpreting the results of the amplified *Mycobacterium tuberculosis* direct test for detection of M. *tuberculosis* rRNA. *J. Clin. Microbiol.* **41**:2741–2743.

73. **Middleton, A. M., M. V. Chadwick, and H. Gaya.** 1997. Detection of *Mycobacterium tuberculosis* in mixed broth cultures using DNA probes. *Clin. Microbiol. Infect.* **3**:668–671.

74. **Mijs, W., P. de Haas, R. Rossau, T. van der Laan, L. Rigouts, F. Portaels, and D. van Soolingen.** 2002. Molecular

evidence to support a proposal to reserve the designation *Mycobacterium avium* subsp. *avium* for bird-type isolates and *M. avium* subsp. *hominissuis* for the human/porcine type of *M. avium. Int. J. Syst. Evol. Microbiol.* **52:**1505–1518.

75. **Möbius, P., G. Luyven, H. Hotzel, and H. Köhler.** 2008. High genetic diversity among *Mycobacterium avium* subsp. *paratuberculosis* strains from German cattle herds shown by combination of IS900 restriction fragment length polymorphism analysis and mycobacterial interspersed repetitive unit-variable-number tandem-repeat typing. *J. Clin. Microbiol.* **46:**972–981.

76. **Mohamed, A. M., D. J. Kuyper, P. C. Iwen, H. H. Ali, D. R. Bastola, and S. H. Hinrichs.** 2005. Computational approach involving use of the internal transcribed spacer 1 region for identification of *Mycobacterium* species. *J. Clin. Microbiol.* **43:**3811–3817.

77. **Mun, H.-S., H.-J. Kim, E.-J. Oh, H. Kim, G.-H. Bai, H.-K. Yu, Y.-G. Park, C.-Y. Cha, Y.-H. Kook, and B.-J. Kim.** 2007. *Mycobacterium seoulense* sp. nov., a slowly growing scotochromogenic species. *Int. J. Syst. Evol. Microbiol.* **57:**594–599.

78. **Mun, H.-S., J.-H. Park, H. Kim, H.-K. Yu, Y.-G. Park, C.-Y. Cha, Y.-H. Kook, and B.-J. Kim.** 2008. *Mycobacterium senuense* sp. nov., a slowly growing, non-chromogenic species closely related to the *Mycobacterium terrae* complex. *Int. J. Syst. Evol. Microbiol.* **58:**641–646.

79. **Murcia, M. I., E. Tortoli, M. C. Menendez, E. Palenque, and M. J. Garcia.** 2006. *Mycobacterium colombiense* sp. nov., a novel member of the *Mycobacterium avium* complex and description of MAC-X as a new ITS genetic variant. *Int. J. Syst. Evol. Microbiol.* **56:**2049–2054.

80. **National Committee for Clinical Laboratory Standards.** 2003. *Susceptibility Testing of Mycobacteria, Nocardiae, and Other Aerobic Actinomycetes; Approved Standard.* Document M24-A. National Committee for Clinical Laboratory Standards, Wayne, PA.

81. **Neonakis, I. K, Z. Gitti, E. Petinaki, S. Maraki, and D. A. Spandidos.** 2007. Evaluation of the GenoType MTBC assay for differentiating 120 clinical *Mycobacterium tuberculosis* complex isolates. *Eur. J. Clin. Microbiol. Infect. Dis.* **26:**151–152.

82. **Niemann, S., D. Harmsen, S. Rüsch-Gerdes, and E. Richter.** 2000. Differentiation of clinical *Mycobacterium tuberculosis* complex isolates by *gyrB* DNA sequence polymorphism analysis. *J. Clin. Microbiol.* **38:**3231–3234.

83. **Oelemann, M. C., R. Diel, V. Vatin, W. Haas, S. Rüsch-Gerdes, C. Locht, S. Niemann, and P. Supply.** 2007. Assessment of an optimized mycobacterial interspersed repetitive-unit-variable-number tandem-repeat typing system combined with spoligotyping for population-based molecular epidemiology studies of tuberculosis. *J. Clin. Microbiol.* **45:**691–697.

84. **Okazaki, M., K. Ohkusu, H. Hata, H. Ohnishi, K. Sugahara, C. Kawamura, N. Fujiwara, S. Matsumoto, Y. Nishiuchi, K. Toyoda, H. Saito, S. Yonetani, Y. Fukugawa, M. Yamamoto, H. Wada, A. Sejimo, A. Ebina, H. Goto, T. Ezaki, and T. Watanabe.** 2009. *Mycobacterium kyorinense* sp. nov., a novel, slow-growing species, related to *Mycobacterium celatum*, isolated from human clinical specimens. *Int. J. Syst. Evol. Microbiol.* **59:**1336–1341.

85. **Pai, M., L. L. Flores, A. Hubbard, L. W. Riley, and J. M. Colford, Jr.** 2004. Nucleic acid amplification tests in the diagnosis of tuberculous pleuritis: a systematic review and meta-analysis. *BMC Infect. Dis.* **4:**6.

86. **Pai, M., L. L. Flores, N. Pai, A. Hubbard, L. W. Riley, and J. M. Colford, Jr.** 2003. Diagnostic accuracy of nucleic acid amplification tests for tuberculous meningitis: a systematic review and meta-analysis. *Lancet Infect. Dis.* **3:**633–643.

87. **Pai, M., S. Kalantri, and K. Dheda.** 2006. New tools and emerging technologies for the diagnosis of tuberculosis. Part II. Active tuberculosis and drug resistance. *Expert Rev. Mol. Diagn.* **6:**423–432.

88. **Park, H., H. Jang, C. Kim, B. Chung, C. L. Chang, S. K. Park, and S. Song.** 2000. Detection and identification of mycobacteria by amplification of the internal transcribed spacer regions with genus- and species-specific PCR primers. *J. Clin. Microbiol.* **38:**4080–4085. (Erratum, **39:**828, 2001.)

89. **Patel, J. B., D. G. Leonard, X. Pan, J. M. Musser, R. E. Berman, and I. Nachamkin.** 2000. Sequence-based identification of *Mycobacterium* species using the MicroSeq 500 16S rDNA bacterial identification system. *J. Clin. Microbiol.* **38:**246–251.

90. **Pauls, R. J., C. Y. Turenne, J. N. Wolfe, and A. Kabani.** 2003. A high proportion of novel mycobacteria species identified by 16S rDNA analysis among slowly growing AccuProbe-negative strains in a clinical setting. *Am. J. Clin. Pathol.* **120:**560–566.

91. **Pfaller, S. L., T. W. Aronson, A. E. Holtzman, and T. C. Covert.** 2007. Amplified fragment length polymorphism analysis of *Mycobacterium avium* complex isolates recovered from southern California. *Med. Microbiol.* **56:**1152–1160.

92. **Picardeau, M., G. Prod'Hom, L. Raskine, M. P. LePennec, and V. Vincent.** 1997. Genotypic characterization of five subspecies of *Mycobacterium kansasii. J. Clin. Microbiol.* **35:**25–32.

93. **Piersimoni, C., and C. Scarparo.** 2003. Relevance of commercial amplification methods for direct detection of *Mycobacterium tuberculosis* complex in clinical samples. *J. Clin. Microbiol.* **41:**5355–5365.

94. **Plikaytis, B. B., B. D. Plikaytis, M. A. Yakrus, W. R. Butler, C. L. Woodley, V. A. Silcox, and T. M. Shinnick.** 1992. Differentiation of slowly growing *Mycobacterium* species, including *Mycobacterium tuberculosis*, by gene amplification and restriction fragment length polymorphism analysis. *J. Clin. Microbiol.* **30:**1815–1822.

95. **Pourahmad, F., F. Cervellione, K. D. Thompson, J. B. Taggart, A. Adams, and R. H. Richards.** 2008. *Mycobacterium stomatepiae* sp. nov., a slowly growing, non-chromogenic species isolated from fish. *Int. J. Syst. Evol. Microbiol.* **58:**2821–2827.

96. **Reischl, U., S. Emler, Z. Horak, J. Kaustova, R. M. Kroppenstedt, N. Lehn, and L. Naumann.** 1998. *Mycobacterium bohemicum* sp. nov., a new slow-growing scotochromogenic mycobacterium. *Int. J. Syst. Bacteriol.* **48:**1349–1355.

97. **Reischl, U., K. Feldmann, L. Naumann, B. J. Gaugler, B. Ninet, B. Hirschel, and S. Emler.** 1998. 16S rRNA sequence diversity in *Mycobacterium celatum* strains caused by presence of two different copies of 16S rRNA gene. *J. Clin. Microbiol.* **36:**1761–1764.

98. **Richter, E., U. Greinert, D. Kirsten, S. Rüsch-Gerdes, C. Schlüter, M. Duchrow, J. Galle, H. Magnussen, M. Schlaak, H. D. Flad, and J. Gerdes.** 1996. Assessment of mycobacterial DNA in cells and tissues of mycobacterial and sarcoid lesions. *Am. J. Respir. Crit. Care Med.* **153:**375–380.

99. **Richter, E., S. Niemann, F. O. Gloeckner, G. E. Pfyffer, and S. Rüsch-Gerdes.** 2002. *Mycobacterium holsaticum* sp. nov. *Int. J. Syst. Evol. Microbiol.* **52:**1991–1996.

100. **Richter, E., S. Niemann, S. Rüsch-Gerdes, and S. Hoffner.** 1999. Identification of *Mycobacterium kansasii* by using a DNA probe (AccuProbe) and molecular techniques. *J. Clin. Microbiol.* **37:**964–970.

101. **Richter, E., S. Rüsch-Gerdes, and D. Hillemann.** 2006. Evaluation of the GenoType Mycobacterium assay for identification of mycobacterial species from cultures. *J. Clin. Microbiol.* **44:**1769–1775.

102. **Richter, E., M. Weizenegger, A. M. Fahr, and S. Rüsch-Gerdes.** 2004. Usefulness of the GenoType MTBC assay for differentiating species of the *Mycobacterium tuberculosis* complex in cultures obtained from clinical specimens. *J. Clin. Microbiol.* **42:**4303–4306.

103. **Richter, E., M. Weizenegger, S. Rüsch-Gerdes, and S. Niemann.** 2003. Evaluation of genotype MTBC assay for differentiation of clinical *Mycobacterium tuberculosis* complex isolates. *J. Clin. Microbiol.* **41:**2672–2675.

104. **Ringuet, H., C. Akoua-Koffi, S. Honore, A. Varnerot, V. Vincent, P. Berche, J. L. Gaillard, and C. Pierre-Audigier.** 1999. *hsp65* sequencing for identification of rapidly growing mycobacteria. *J. Clin. Microbiol.* **37:**852–857.

105. **Roth, A., M. Fischer, M. E. Hamid, S. Michalke, W. Ludwig, and H. Mauch.** 1998. Differentiation of phylogenetically related slowly growing mycobacteria based on

16S-23S rRNA gene internal transcribed spacer sequences. *J. Clin. Microbiol.* **36:**139–147.

106. **Roth, A., U. Reischl, A. Streubel, L. Naumann, R. M. Kroppenstedt, M. Habicht, M. Fischer, and H. Mauch.** 2000. Novel diagnostic algorithm for identification of mycobacteria using genus-specific amplification of the 16S-23S rRNA gene spacer and restriction endonucleases. *J. Clin. Microbiol.* **38:**1094–1104.

107. **Rüsch-Gerdes, S., and E. Richter.** 2004. Clinical evaluation of the semiautomated BD ProbeTec ET system for the detection of *Mycobacterium tuberculosis* in respiratory and nonrespiratory specimens. *Diagn. Microbiol. Infect. Dis.* **48:**265–270.

108. **Russo, C., E. Tortoli, and D. Menichella.** 2006. Evaluation of the new GenoType Mycobacterium assay for identification of mycobacterial species. *J. Clin. Microbiol.* **44:**334–339.

109. **Salah, I. B., C. Cayrou, D. Raoult, and M. Drancourt.** 2009. *Mycobacterium marseillense* sp. nov., *Mycobacterium timonense* sp. nov. and *Mycobacterium bouchedurhonense* sp. nov., members of the *Mycobacterium avium* complex. *Int. J. Syst. Evol. Microbiol.* **59:**2803–2808.

110. **Sevilla, I., L. Li, A. Amonsin, J. M. Garrido, M. V. Geijo, V. Kapur, and R. A. Juste.** 2008. Comparative analysis of *Mycobacterium avium* subsp. *paratuberculosis* isolates from cattle, sheep and goats by short sequence repeat and pulsed-field gel electrophoresis typing. *BMC Microbiol.* **25:**204.

111. **Somoskovi, A., J. Dormandy, J. Rivenburg, M. Pedrosa, M. McBride, and M. Salfinger.** 2008. Direct comparison of the genotype MTBC and genomic deletion assays in terms of ability to distinguish between members of the *Mycobacterium tuberculosis* complex in clinical isolates and in clinical specimens. *J. Clin. Microbiol.* **46:**1854–1857.

112. **Springer, B., P. Kirschner, G. Rost-Meyer, K. H. Schröder, R. M. Kroppenstedt, and E. C. Böttger.** 1993. *Mycobacterium interjectum*, a new species isolated from a patient with chronic lymphadenitis. *J. Clin. Microbiol.* **31:**3083–3089. (Erratum, **32:**1417, 1994.)

113. **Springer, B., L. Stockman, K. Teschner, G. D. Roberts, and E. C. Böttger.** 1996. Two-laboratory collaborative study on identification of mycobacteria: molecular versus phenotypic methods. *J. Clin. Microbiol.* **34:**296–303.

114. **Springer, B., W. K. Wu, T. Bodmer, G. Haase, G. E. Pfyffer, R. M. Kroppenstedt, K. H. Schröder, S. Emler, J. O. Kilburn, P. Kirschner, A. Telenti, M. B. Coyle, and E. C. Böttger.** 1996. Isolation and characterization of a unique group of slowly growing mycobacteria: description of *Mycobacterium lentiflavum* sp. nov. *J. Clin. Microbiol.* **34:**1100–1107.

115. **Stinear, T. P., T. Seemann, P. F. Harrison, G. A. Jenkin, J. K. Davies, P. D. Johnson, Z. Abdellah, C. Arrowsmith, T. Chillingworth, C. Churcher, K. Clarke, A. Cronin, P. Davis, I. Goodhead, N. Holroyd, K. Jagels, A. Lord, S. Moule, K. Mungall, H. Norbertczak, M. A. Quail, E. Rabbinowitsch, D. Walker, B. White, S. Whitehead, P. L. Small, R. Brosch, I. Ramakrishnan, M. A. Fischbach, J. Parkhill, and S. T. Cole.** 2008. Insights from the complete genome sequence of *Mycobacterium marinum* on the evolution of *Mycobacterium tuberculosis*. *Genome Res.* **18:**729–741.

116. **Stinear, T. P., T. Seemann, S. Pidot, W. Frigui, G. Reysset, T. Garnier, G. Meurice, D. Simon, C. Bouchier, L. Ma, M. Tichit, J. L. Porter, J. Ryan, P. D. Johnson, J. K. Davies, G. A. Jenkin, P. L. Small, L. M. Jones, F. Tekaia, F. Laval, M. Daffé, J. Parkhill, and S. T. Cole.** 2007. Reductive evolution and niche adaptation inferred from the genome of *Mycobacterium ulcerans*, the causative agent of Buruli ulcer. *Genome Res.* **17:**192–200.

117. **Supply, P., C. Allix, S. Lesjean, M. Cardoso-Oelemann, S. Rüsch-Gerdes, E. Willery, E. Savine, P. de Haas, H. van Deutekom, S. Roring, P. Bifani, N. Kurepina, B. Kreiswirth, C. Sola, N. Rastogi, V. Vatin, M. C. Gutierrez, M. Fauville, S. Niemann, R. Skuce, K. Kremer, C. Locht, and D. van Soolingen.** 2006. Proposal for standardization of optimized mycobacterial interspersed repetitive unit-variable-number tandem repeat typing of *Mycobacterium tuberculosis*. *J. Clin. Microbiol.* **44:**4498–4510.

118. **Supply, P., E. Mazars, S. Lesjean, V. Vincent, B. Gicquel, and C. Locht.** 2000. Variable human minisatellite-like regions in the *Mycobacterium tuberculosis* genome. *Mol. Microbiol.* **36:**762–771.

119. **Taillard, C., G. Greub, R. Weber, G. E. Pfyffer, T. Bodmer, S. Zimmerli, R. Frei, S. Bassetti, P. Rohner, J. C. Piffaretti, E. Bernasconi, J. Bille, A. Telenti, and G. Prod'hom.** 2003. Clinical implications of *Mycobacterium kansasii* species heterogeneity: Swiss National Survey. *J. Clin. Microbiol.* **41:**1240–1244.

120. **Talbot, E. A., D. L. Williams, and R. Frothingham.** 1997. PCR identification of *Mycobacterium bovis* BCG. *J. Clin. Microbiol.* **35:**566–569.

121. **Telenti, A., F. Marchesi, M. Balz, F. Bally, E. C. Böttger, and T. Bodmer.** 1993. Rapid identification of mycobacteria to the species level by polymerase chain reaction and restriction enzyme analysis. *J. Clin. Microbiol.* **31:**175–178.

122. **Tenover, F. C., J. T. Crawford, R. E. Huebner, L. J. Geiter, C. R. Horsburgh, Jr., and R. C. Good.** 1993. The resurgence of tuberculosis: is your laboratory ready? *J. Clin. Microbiol.* **31:**767–770.

123. **Thibault, V. C., M. Grayon, M. L. Boschiroli, C. Hubbans, P. Overduin, K. Stevenson, M. C. Gutierrez, P. Supply, and F. Biet.** 2007. New variable-number tandem-repeat markers for typing *Mycobacterium avium* subsp. *paratuberculosis* and M. *avium* strains: comparison with IS900 and IS1245 restriction fragment length polymorphism typing. *J. Clin. Microbiol.* **45:**2404–2410.

124. **Thorel, M. F., M. Krichevsky, and V. V. Lévy-Frébault.** 1990. Numerical taxonomy of mycobactin-dependent mycobacteria, emended description of *Mycobacterium avium*, and description of *Mycobacterium avium* subsp. *avium* subsp. nov., *Mycobacterium avium* subsp. *paratuberculosis* subsp. nov., and *Mycobacterium avium* subsp. *silvaticum* subsp. nov. *Int. J. Syst. Bacteriol.* **40:**254–260.

125. **Tønjum, T., D. B. Welty, E. Jantzen, and P. L. Small.** 1998. Differentiation of *Mycobacterium ulcerans*, M. *marinum*, and M. *haemophilum*: mapping of their relationships to M. *tuberculosis* by fatty acid profile analysis, DNA-DNA hybridization, and 16S rRNA gene sequence analysis. *J. Clin. Microbiol.* **36:**918–925.

126. **Tortoli, E.** 2003. Impact of genotypic studies on mycobacterial taxonomy: the new mycobacteria of the 1990s. *Clin. Microbiol. Rev.* **16:**319–354.

127. **Tortoli, E., A. Bartoloni, E. C. Böttger, S. Emler, C. Garzelli, E. Magliano, A. Mantella, N. Rastogi, L. Rindi, C. Scarparo, and P. Urbano.** 2001. Burden of unidentifiable mycobacteria in a reference laboratory. *J. Clin. Microbiol.* **39:**4058–4065.

128. **Tortoli, E., A. Bartoloni, C. Burrini, A. Mantella, and M. T. Simonetti.** 1995. Utility of high-performance liquid chromatography for identification of mycobacterial species rarely encountered in clinical laboratories. *Eur. J. Clin. Microbiol. Infect. Dis.* **14:**240–243.

129. **Tortoli, E., A. Mariottini, and G. Mazzarelli.** 2003. Evaluation of INNO-LiPA MYCOBACTERIA v2: improved reverse hybridization multiple DNA probe assay for mycobacterial identification. *J. Clin. Microbiol.* **41:**4418–4420.

130. **Tortoli, E., M. Pecorari, G. Fabio, M. Messino, and A. Fabio.** 2010. Commercial DNA probes for mycobacteria incorrectly identify a number of less frequently encountered species. *J. Clin. Microbiol.* **48:**307–310.

131. **Tortoli, E., L. Rindi, M. J. Garcia, P. Chiaradonna, R. Dei, C. Garzelli, R. M. Kroppenstedt, N. Lari, R. Mattei, A. Mariottini, G. Mazzarelli, M. I. Murcia, A. Nanetti, P. Piccoli, and C. Scarpaio.** 2004. Proposal to elevate the genetic variant MAC-A, included in the *Mycobacterium avium* complex, to species rank as *Mycobacterium chimaera* sp. nov. *Int. J. Syst. Evol. Microbiol.* **54:**1277–1285.

132. **Tortoli, E., M. T. Simonetti, and F. Lavinia.** 1996. Evaluation of reformulated chemiluminescent DNA probe (AccuProbe) for culture identification of *Mycobacterium kansasii*. *J. Clin. Microbiol.* **34:**2838–2840.

133. Turenne, C. Y., D. M. Collins, D. C. Alexander, and M. A. Behr. 2008. *Mycobacterium avium* subsp. *paratuberculosis* and *M. avium* subsp. *avium* are independently evolved pathogenic clones of a much broader group of *M. avium* organisms. *J. Bacteriol.* **190:**2479–2487.

134. Turenne, C. Y., L. Tschetter, J. Wolfe, and A. Kabani. 2001. Necessity of quality-controlled 16S rRNA gene sequence databases: identifying nontuberculous *Mycobacterium* species. J. Clin. Microbiol. **39:**3637–3648. (Erratum, **40:**2316, 2002.)

135. Turenne, C. Y., R. Wallace, Jr., and M. A. Behr. 2007. *Mycobacterium avium* in the postgenomic era. *Clin. Microbiol. Rev.* **20:**205–229.

136. van der Giessen, J. W., R. M. Haring, and B. A. van der Zeijst. 1994. Comparison of the 23S ribosomal RNA genes and the spacer region between the 16S and 23S rRNA genes of the closely related *Mycobacterium avium* and *Mycobacterium paratuberculosis* and the fast-growing *Mycobacterium phlei*. *Microbiology* **140:**1103–1108.

137. van Embden, J. D., M. D. Cave, J. T. Crawford, J. W. Dale, K. D. Eisenach, B. Giquel, P. Hermans, C. Martin, R. McAdam, T. M. Shinnick, and P. M. Small. 1993. Strain identification of *Mycobacterium tuberculosis* by DNA fingerprinting: recommendations for a standardized methodology. *J. Clin. Microbiol.* **31:**406–409.

138. van Ingen, J., S. A. M. Al-Hajoj, M. Boeree, F. Al-Rabiah, M. Enaimi, R. de Zwaan, E. Tortoli, R. Dekhuijzen, and D. van Soolingen. 2009. *Mycobacterium riyadhense* sp. nov., a non-tuberculous species identified as *Mycobacterium tuberculosis* complex by a commercial line-probe assay. *Int. J. Syst. Evol. Microbiol.* **59:**1049–1053.

139. van Ingen, J., M. J. Boeree, W. C. M. de Lange, P. E. W. de Haas, A. G. M. van der Zanden, W. Mijs, L. Rigouts, R. Dekhuijzen, and D. van Soolingen. 2009. *Mycobacterium noviomagense* sp. nov.; clinical relevance evaluated in 17 patients. *Int. J. Syst. Evol. Microbiol.* **59:**845–849.

140. van Ingen, J., M. J. Boeree, K. Kösters, A. Wieland, E. Tortoli, R. P. Dekhuijzen, and D. van Soolingen. 2009. Proposal to elevate *Mycobacterium avium* complex ITS sequevar MAC-Q to *Mycobacterium vulneris* sp. nov. *Int. J. Syst. Evol. Microbiol.* **59:**2277–2282.

141. van Ingen, J., J. A. Lindeboom, N. G. Hartwig, R. de Zwaan, E. Tortoli, P. N. R. Dekhuijzen, M. J. Boeree, and D. van Soolingen. 2009. *Mycobacterium mantenii* sp. nov., a pathogenic slowly growing, scotochromogenic species. *Int. J. Syst. Evol. Microbiol.* **59:**2782–2787.

142. van Soolingen, D., J. Bauer, V. Ritacco, S. C. Leão, I. Pavlik, V. Vincent, N. Rastogi, A. Gori, T. Bodmer, C. Garzelli, and M. J. Garcia. 1998. IS*1245* restriction fragment length polymorphism typing of *Mycobacterium avium* isolates: proposal for standardization. *J. Clin. Microbiol.* **36:**3051–3054.

143. van Soolingen, D., T. Hoogenboezem, P. E. de Haas, P. W. Hermans, M. A. Koedam, K. S. Teppema, P. J. Brennan, G. S. Besra, F. Portaels, J. Top, L. M. Schouls, and J. D. van Embden. 1997. A novel pathogenic taxon of the *Mycobacterium tuberculosis* complex, Canetti: characterization of an exceptional isolate from Africa. *Int. J. Syst. Bacteriol.* **47:**1236–1245.

144. van Soolingen, D., L. Qian, P. E. de Haas, J. T. Douglas, H. Traore, F. Portaels, H. Z. Qing, D. Enkhsaikan, P. Nymadawa, and J. D. van Embden. 1995. Predominance of a single genotype of *Mycobacterium tuberculosis* in countries of East Asia. *J. Clin. Microbiol.* **33:**3234–3238.

145. Wallace, R. J., Jr., Y. Zhang, B. A. Brown, D. Dawson, D. T. Murphy, R. Wilson, and D. E. Griffith. 1998. Polyclonal *Mycobacterium avium* complex infections in patients with nodular bronchiectasis. *Am. J. Respir. Crit. Care Med.* **158:**1235–1244.

146. Wallace, R. J., Jr., Y. Zhang, B. A. Brown-Elliott, M. A. Yakrus, R. W. Wilson, L. Mann, L. Couch, W. M. Girard, and D. E. Griffith. 2002. Repeat positive cultures in *Mycobacterium intracellulare* lung disease after macrolide therapy represent new infections in patients with nodular bronchiectasis. *J. Infect. Dis.* **186:**266–273.

147. Williams, K. J., C. L. Ling, C. Jenkins, S. H. Gillespie, and T. D. McHugh. 2007. A paradigm for the molecular identification of *Mycobacterium* species in a routine diagnostic laboratory. *J. Med. Microbiol.* **56:**598–602.

148. Woo, P. C., S. K. Lau, J. L. Teng, H. Tse, and K. Y. Yuen. 2008. Then and now: use of 16S rDNA gene sequencing for bacterial identification and discovery of novel bacteria in clinical microbiology laboratories. *Clin. Microbiol. Infect.* **14:**908–934.

149. Woods, G. L., J. S. Bergmann, and N. Williams-Bouyer. 2001. Clinical evaluation of the Gen-Probe amplified *Mycobacterium tuberculosis* direct test for rapid detection of *Mycobacterium tuberculosis* in select nonrespiratory specimens. *J. Clin. Microbiol.* **39:**747–749.

150. Yakrus, M. A., M. W. Reeves, and S. B. Hunter. 1992. Characterization of isolates of *Mycobacterium avium* serotypes 4 and 8 from patients with AIDS by multilocus enzyme electrophoresis. *J. Clin. Microbiol.* **30:**1474–1478.

151. Zhang, Y., L. B. Mann, R. W. Wilson, B. A. Brown-Elliott, V. Vincent, Y. Iinuma, and R. J. Wallace, Jr. 2004. Molecular analysis of *Mycobacterium kansasii* isolates from the United States. *J. Clin. Microbiol.* **42:**119–125.

Mycobacterium: Clinical and Laboratory Characteristics of Rapidly Growing Mycobacteria

BARBARA A. BROWN-ELLIOTT AND RICHARD J. WALLACE, JR.

30

TAXONOMY AND DESCRIPTION OF THE AGENTS

Rapidly growing mycobacteria (RGM) are generally defined as nontuberculous species that grow within 7 days on laboratory media (9). RGM contain long-chain fatty acids known as mycolic acids that can be quantitated using chromatographic techniques, such as high-performance liquid chromatography (HPLC). Before the molecular era, HPLC was used for identification of species of RGM in most major reference laboratories. However, this method has been replaced in most laboratories by more definitive molecular identification methods for more accurate species identification (76).

Currently, there are more than 130 known species of nontuberculous mycobacteria (NTM), of which 70 are species of RGM. More than one-half of RGM species have been described since the early 1990s. Since 2007, 13 new species have been added to the list: M. *aubagnense*, M. *monacense*, M. *phocaicum*, M. *setense*, M. *aromaticivorans*, M. *crocinum*, M. *fluoranthenivorans*, M. *insubricum*, M. *llatzerense*, M. *pallens*, M. *pyrenivorans*, M. *rufum*, and M. *rutilum* (35, 43, 56, 77, 78). The first four species have been associated with human, animal, or fish disease, while the latter nine species have thus far been considered environmental nonpathogens. Additionally, most recently, the species M. *abscessus* has been subdivided into two subspecies. The former species, M. *abscessus*, is now M. *abscessus* subsp. *abscessus*, and two previously described species, M. *massiliense* and M. *bolletii*, were determined to compose another subspecies of M. *abscessus* now known as M. *abscessus* subsp. *bolletii* (39, 43a, 44).

There are currently six major groups or complexes of RGM based on pigmentation and genetic relatedness (Table 1). Nonpigmented pathogen species now are composed of 11 species within the M. *fortuitum* group (43, 87, 90) and the former third biovariant complex (9, 64, 89).

The second group of nonpigmented RGM is the M. *chelonae*/M. *abscessus* group, as listed in Table 1 (1–3, 5, 9, 44). A previously described species, M. *salmoniphilum*, has recently been revived and is also considered to be related to this group. Although this species has been recovered from salmon and trout with disseminated disease, it has not yet been recovered from humans (92).

A third nonpigmented group, the M. *mucogenicum* group, currently includes the three species noted in Table 1 (1, 9, 69).

The fourth group, the M. *smegmatis* group, is currently composed of the two late-pigmenting species, M. *smegmatis* (formerly M. *smegmatis* sensu stricto) and M. *goodii* (7, 9, 89).

The fifth group of RGM includes the early-pigmented species, which traditionally have been difficult to identify by conventional (phenotypic) laboratory methods. The only proven pathogen in this group is M. *neoaurum* (Table 1) and several newly described species, including M. *canariasense*, M. *cosmeticum*, and M. *monacense*. There are a number of previously listed environmental (nonpathogenic) species as well (9, 35, 43, 66, 77, 78).

Current studies based on DNA sequence analysis suggest a sixth group, composed of M. *mageritense* and M. *wolinskyi* (2, 3, 76).

The recent introduction of several new species within the RGM highlights the importance of molecular identification of these organisms to the species level and questions the meaningfulness of the current "group" classification, especially within the M. *fortuitum* group. However, because previous data and publications use this "group" nomenclature, this designation is retained in this chapter for ease of discussion (9).

CLINICAL SIGNIFICANCE

The RGM are opportunistic pathogens that produce disease in a variety of clinical settings. The three major clinically important species of RGM responsible for approximately 80% of disease in humans include M. *fortuitum*, M. *chelonae*, and M. *abscessus* (30). Other potentially pathogenic and clinically significant RGM species have been included in Table 2 (1–5, 7, 9, 28, 43, 52, 56, 63–66, 76–78, 89, 92). RGM are presumed to be common in the environment but have been most often identified in tap water when associated with outbreaks of catheter sepsis in bone marrow transplants, wound infections, and associated pseudo-outbreaks of disease (9). The specific reservoir for M. *abscessus* chronic lung infections has yet to be identified.

Skin and Soft Tissue Infections

The most common infection seen with RGM is a posttraumatic wound infection. Patients are generally healthy, and drug-induced immune suppression results in a minimal increase in risk for this type of infection. The M. *fortuitum*

TABLE 1 Six major groups of RGM

Group or taxon	Species within group or taxon
Mycobacterium fortuitum group	M. fortuitum, M. peregrinum, M. senegalense, M. setense, M. septicum, M. porcinum, M. houstonense, M. boenickei, M. brisbanense, M. neworleansense
M. chelonae/M. abscessus group	M. chelonae, M. immunogenum, M. abscessus subsp. abscessus (formerly M. abscessus), M. abscessus subsp. bolletii (formerly M. massiliense and M. bolletii), M. salmoniphilum
M. mucogenicum group	M. mucogenicum, M. aubagnense, M. phocaicum
M. smegmatis group	M. smegmatis (formerly M. smegmatis sensu stricto), M. goodii
Early-pigmented RGM	M. neoaurum, M. canariasense, M. cosmeticum, M. monacense
M. mageritense/M. wolinskyi group	M. mageritense, M. wolinskyi

group accounts for approximately 60% of cases of localized cutaneous infections, but any of the more than 30 pathogenic RGM species listed in Table 2 can cause disease (9, 21, 48, 64).

Traumatic wound infections, especially open fractures, often involve species within the Mycobacterium fortuitum third biovariant complex (9, 21). More than 75% of the infections reported from a series of 85 isolates of the M. fortuitum third biovariant complex from the United States and the Queensland, Australia, state laboratory were associated with skin, soft tissue, or bone infections (9). The majority of infections occurred 4 to 6 weeks following puncture wounds or open fractures. Metal puncture wounds (48%) and motor vehicle accidents (26%) were the most common antecedent injuries, and approximately 40% of the injury sites involved the foot or leg. Stepping on a nail was the most frequently related scenario. None of the isolates in this series were studied by molecular techniques that would identify them as one of the newly described species within the M. fortuitum third biovariant complex (i.e., M. houstonense, M. boenickei, and M. porcinum).

In a 1989 report (64), approximately 80% of RGM wound isolates related to cardiac surgery were from seven southern coastal states, including Texas, Louisiana, Georgia, Maryland, Alabama, Florida, and South Carolina. A second report published in the same year showed that 92% of 37 identified cases of surgical wound infection following augmentation mammaplasty were also from patients in southern coastal states, with the majority being in Texas, Florida, and North Carolina, suggesting that the disease risk was highest in the southeastern United States (9).

Sporadic cases of localized wound infections following medical or surgical procedures, including needle injections, can occur with M. chelonae but are less common than those with M. fortuitum. The clinical picture of posttraumatic wound infection ranges from localized cellulitis or abscesses to osteomyelitis (9). A 2006 report from a major U.S. clinical referral center of patients from Minnesota, Wisconsin, Iowa, and South Dakota characterized 63 human immunodeficiency virus-negative patients with RGM infections involving M. abscessus or M. chelonae (71%) or the M. fortuitum group (29%). Moreover, patients with M. chelonae or M. abscessus usually had multiple (disseminated) cutaneous lesions, in contrast to those with single (localized) lesions due to M. fortuitum. Most patients with M. fortuitum had

undergone a prior surgical procedure or had experienced a penetrating trauma at the infected site. Patients with M. chelonae or M. abscessus were older and more likely to be on some type of immunosuppressive agent (82). Localized or disseminated infections with M. chelonae most frequently occur in patients receiving long-term corticosteroids and/ or chemotherapy, organ transplant recipients, patients with rheumatoid arthritis or other autoimmune disorders, or patients receiving suppressive therapy (82). Immune suppression in patients with diseases such as AIDS has not been a significant risk factor for development of localized or disseminated M. chelonae infections (9, 82).

Starting in 2000, an outbreak of furunculosis caused by M. fortuitum on the lower extremities was described for 32 otherwise healthy patients who were patrons of a nail salon in California (94). The organism was also cultured from contaminated foot baths and from the inlet suction screens containing hair and other debris, and shaving the legs prior to the footbath and pedicure was an identified risk factor (94, 95). Other species, including M. fortuitum, M. abscessus, and M. mageritense, have subsequently been recovered from cases in California and Georgia (9, 27, 68, 85). Strains from the footbath and from patients were identical by DNA strain typing.

Occasionally, M. wolinskyi, M. mageritense, and members of the M. smegmatis group have been reported from infections following traumatic injury and surgical or medical procedures, such as cardiac surgery, breast reduction surgery, and face-lift plastic surgery. Cellulitis and localized abscess are the most common manifestations (7, 9, 30).

Disseminated Cutaneous Disease

Disseminated cutaneous disease due to members of the M. fortuitum group (including M. fortuitum) is rare even in immunocompromised patients, including those with AIDS (9, 13, 14, 30).

Disseminated cutaneous disease due to M. chelonae is much more common. It typically presents as multiple chronic painful red nodules, usually involving the lower extremities (9, 30). These lesions then drain spontaneously, with the drainage usually being acid fast bacillus smear positive. Almost all patients are immunosuppressed, usually from low-dose corticosteroid therapy. Although the disease is presumably a consequence of hematogenous spread, bacteremia is rarely identified. A portal of entry for the infection is rarely evident (9, 30). In a series of 100 clinical isolates from skin and soft tissue, Brown-Elliott and Wallace reported that 53% were from patients with disseminated cutaneous infections (9).

Disseminated cutaneous disease due to M. abscessus occurs rarely but is serious (9). As with disseminated M. chelonae disease, most cases occur in chronically immunosuppressed patients receiving corticosteroids, and the disease has no apparent portal of entry. Also, as with patients with M. chelonae, patients with disseminated cutaneous infection due to M. abscessus rarely have detectable bacteremia and/or endocarditis but usually present with multiple draining cutaneous nodules, usually in the lower extremities (9, 30).

A rare type of disseminated infection due to RGM in immunocompetent hosts presenting with lymphadenopathy has recently been described (12).

Bone and Joint Infections

RGM may also cause bone and joint infections. Like with bacterial disease, osteomyelitis may follow open bone fractures, puncture wounds, and hematogenous spread from another source. The most common scenario is an open fracture of the femur, often followed by orthopedic surgical procedures. The most frequent pathogen recovered in this setting is a member of the M. fortuitum group, including newly described species, namely, M. houstonense, M. boenickei, and M. setense (9, 20, 43, 64, 75). The two newly described species in the M. smegmatis group, M. goodii and M. wolinskyi, have also been associated with osteomyelitis (7, 9). Bone involvement secondary to a puncture wound is likely the second major cause of osteomyelitis. Infections most commonly involve members of the M. fortuitum group (9). M. fortuitum infections in prosthetic knees and joints have also been reported (20). Vertebral osteomyelitis has also been described (54, 62).

Pulmonary Infections

Chronic lung infections can occur with RGM, most often in nonsmoking older women with bronchiectasis, and are sometimes associated with M. avium complex (MAC) as well. M. abscessus is the causative agent in >80% of cases of pulmonary disease due to RGM (30).

Similarities exist between patients with MAC and those with M. abscessus such that a common pathogenicity or host susceptibility factor may be involved (30). Multiple cultures of M. abscessus from respiratory samples are usually associated with significant pulmonary disease.

Patients with cystic fibrosis (CF) may also become infected with both subspecies of M. abscessus, and this species has been isolated with increasing frequency from the respiratory tracts of patients with CF (9, 18, 19, 36, 51). M. abscessus is the second-most-common species of NTM recovered in CF patients (after MAC) and may be the most-common species associated with clinical disease in this setting (51). Patients with CF also have bronchiectasis in addition to chronic, recurrent airway and parenchymal infections, which may be the primary risk factors for susceptibility to NTM disease (36, 51).

Other RGM, including M. chelonae, members of the M. smegmatis group, and M. fortuitum are less frequently associated with pulmonary disease. M. fortuitum has been reported as a pathogen in half of the cases of chronic aspiration disease secondary to underlying gastroesophageal disorders such as achalasia (9, 30). Pulmonary disease with M. fortuitum in the absence of these disorders is rare. Pulmonary disease with M. chelonae and M. smegmatis has been described for only a few cases, including lipoid pneumonia (9, 30).

Hypersensitivity pneumonitis among metal grinders in industrial plants working with contaminated metalworking fluids has been associated with a newly described species of RGM, M. immunogenum (9, 30, 93). Multiple pseudo-outbreaks associated with this species, resulting from contaminated automated bronchoscope cleaning machines and metalworking fluids, have been reported. This species is able to grow and remain viable in degraded metalworking fluid and is resistant to the routine biocides used for disinfecting the metalworking fluids (9, 93). However, this species has not yet been reported from open-lung biopsy specimens from these patients.

Central Nervous System Disease

Central nervous system disease involving RGM is rare, but morbidity and mortality are high. Most of the reported cases have been associated with M. fortuitum (9, 22, 86).

Corneal Infections (Keratitis)

The number of RGM recovered from ocular infections has been increasing over the last 20 years. A retrospective review of cases of NTM keratitis from 1982 to 1997 at an eye institute in Florida showed that 19 out of 24 cases were due to RGM (24). A recent study which identified 113 ophthalmic isolates by molecular methods showed that the most common RGM were M. chelonae (45%), M. abscessus (42%), and members of the M. fortuitum group (8%) (8).

Since the early 1990s, other descriptions of epidemic and sporadic ocular infections associated with RGM, including after keratoplasty and following laser in situ keratomileusis (LASIK) surgery, have been published (8, 9).

Otitis Media

The most common NTM associated with chronic otitis media is M. abscessus. In a 1988 outbreak of 17 cases of otitis media in two ear, nose, and throat clinics, patients presented with chronic ear drainage, a perforated tympanic membrane, and a prior tympanostomy tube (9). In another series, 20 of 21 cases of sporadic chronic otitis media (some with associated mastoiditis) were due to M. abscessus following ear tube placement. Approximately one-half of the isolates from these cases were aminoglycoside resistant as a result of the patients' long-term use of aminoglycoside ear drops (9).

Health Care-Associated Infections

Previously, health care-associated disease resulting from RGM has been reported most commonly with M. fortuitum, M. chelonae, M. abscessus, and M. mucogenicum, although any species may be involved. Most infections follow contamination with tap water (9, 17, 21, 88). Types of infections include postsurgical wound infections, catheter sepsis, infections following hemodialysis, postinjection abscesses, vaccine-related outbreaks, and otitis media following tympanostomy tube replacement (9, 26, 40). These have been seen as both sporadic cases and localized outbreaks. Recent outbreaks have involved cosmetic procedures such as liposuction, liposculpture, acupuncture, and mesotherapy, a procedure comprised of multiple subcutaneous injections of pharmaceutical or homeopathic medications for cosmetic purposes (6, 25, 26, 40, 47, 48, 83, 84, 97).

Recovery of both subspecies of M. abscessus has been reported from outbreaks of infections associated with laparoscopic surgeries and cosmetic surgeries in Brazil, the Dominican Republic, and Korea (25, 40, 83). These and other recent reports suggest that although few studies have identified these newer subspecies in invasive infections, they have been misclassified in previous studies (67).

TABLE 2 Currently recognized species of RGM[j]

Species	Established clinical significance	Pigmentation	Unique phenotype	Unique hsp65 PRA	Unique (complete) 16S rRNA gene sequence
Common human pathogens					
M. abscessus subsp. abscessus[a]	Yes	No	No	Yes	Yes
M. chelonae	Yes	No	Yes	Yes	Yes
M. fortuitum	Yes	No	Yes	Yes	Yes
Less common human pathogens (>10 clinical isolates or cases)					
M. abscessus subsp. bolletii[b]	Yes	No	No	No	No
M. boenickei	Yes	No	No	Yes	Yes
M. canariasense	Yes	No	No	Yes	Yes
M. cosmeticum	Yes	Yes	Yes	Yes	Yes
M. goodii	Yes	Yes	No	Yes	Yes
M. houstonense	Yes	No	No	No	No[c]
M. immunogenum	Yes	No	No	Yes	Yes
M. mucogenicum	Yes	No	Yes	Yes	Yes
M. neoaurum	Yes	Yes	No	Yes	Yes
M. peregrinum	Yes	No	No	Yes	No[c]
M. porcinum	Yes	No	No	Yes	Yes
M. senegalense	Yes	No	No	Yes	Yes
M. smegmatis	Yes	Yes	No	Yes	Yes
Rare human pathogens (<10 cases or isolates)					
M. aubagnense	Yes	No	No	No	Yes
M. brisbanense	Yes	No	No	Yes	Yes
M. brumae	Yes	No	No	ND	Yes
M. elephantis	Yes	Yes	No	Yes	Yes
"M. lacticola"[d]	Yes	Yes	Unknown	Yes	Yes
M. mageritense	Yes	No	Yes	Yes	Yes
M. monacense	Yes	Yes	No	Yes	Yes
M. moriokaense	Yes	No	No	Yes	Yes
M. neworleansense	Yes	No	No	No	Yes
M. novocastrense	Yes	Yes	No	ND	No
M. phocaicum	Yes	No	No	Yes	No
M. septicum	Yes	No	No	Yes	No[c]
M. setense	Yes	No	Yes	Yes	Yes
M. wolinskyi	Yes	No	No	Yes	Yes
Unproven human pathogens					
M. agri	No	No	No	ND	Yes
M. aichiense	No	No	No	ND	Yes
M. alvei	No	No	No	ND	No
M. aromaticivorans	No	Yes	No	ND	No
M. aurum	No	Yes	No	ND	Yes
M. austroafricanum	No	Yes	No	ND	Yes
M. chitae	No	No	No	ND	Yes
M. chlorophenolicum	No	Yes	No	ND	Yes
M. chubuense	No	Yes	No	ND	Yes
M. confluentis	No	No	No	ND	Yes
M. crocinum	No	Yes	No	ND	No
M. diernhoferi	No	Yes	No	ND	ND
M. duvalii	No	Yes	No	ND	Yes
M. fallax[e]	No	No	No	ND	Yes
M. flavescens	No	Yes	No	ND	Yes
M. fluoranthenivorans	No	No	No	ND	No[f]
M. frederiksbergense	No	Yes	No	ND	No
M. gadium	No	Yes	No	ND	Yes
M. gilvum	No	Yes	No	ND	Yes
M. hassiacum	No	Yes	No[g]	ND	Yes

(Continued on next page)

TABLE 2 (*Continued*)

Species	Established clinical significance	Pigmentation	Unique phenotype	Unique hsp65 PRA	Unique (complete) 16S rRNA gene sequence
M. hodleri[h]	No	Yes	No	ND	No
M. holsaticum	No	Yes	No	Yes	Yes
M. insubricum	No	No	No	Yes	Yes
M. komossense	No	Yes	No	ND	Yes
M. llatzerense	No	No	Yes	ND	Yes
M. madagascariense	No	Yes	No	ND	Yes
M. murale	No	Yes	No	ND	Yes
M. obuense	No	Yes	No	ND	Yes
M. pallens	No	Yes	No	ND	No
M. parafortuitum	No	Yes	No	ND	Yes
M. phlei	No	Yes	No	ND	Yes
M. poriferae	No	Yes	No	ND	ND
M. psychrotolerans	No	Yes	No	ND	Yes
M. pyrenivorans	No	Yes	No	ND	Yes
M. rhodesiae	No	Yes	No	ND	Yes
M. rufum	No	Yes	No	ND	No
M. rutilum	No	Yes	No	ND	No
M. salmoniphilum[i]	Yes	No	No	Yes	Yes
M. sphagni	No	Yes	No	ND	Yes
M. thermoresistibile	No	Yes	No	ND	Yes
M. tokaiense	No	Yes	No	ND	Yes
M. vaccae	No	Yes	No	ND	Yes
M. vanbaalenii	No	Yes	No	ND	Yes

[a]Formerly M. abscessus.
[b]Formerly M. massiliense.
[c]M. houstonense is 100% identical to M. farcinogenes, while M. peregrinum (type I) is 100% identical to M. septicum.
[d]"M. lacticola" is currently a nonvalidated species.
[e]RGM at 30°C/slowly growing at 35°C.
[f]16S rRNA gene sequence is identical to the sequence of the unvalidated species "M. hackensackense."
[g]Grows at 65°C.
[h]Grows on or degrades a variety of organic substrates.
[i]Pathogenic for fish.
[j]ND, no data available.

Central-catheter-associated infections are the most common health care-associated infection due to RGM (9, 55, 63). They are the most common cause of RGM bacteremia, but the disease may also present as local wound drainage as part of an exit site or tunnel infection (9, 55). Other types of catheters can also lead to infections, including peritoneal catheters, ventriculoperitoneal shunts, and shunts for hemodialysis (9). The most common species are M. mucogenicum, M. fortuitum, and M. abscessus. Recently, an outbreak of M. phocaicum and M. mucogenicum was described for five patients with central venous catheters in an oncology unit in a Texas hospital (16). This outbreak represents the first report of clinical isolates of M. phocaicum in a hospital in the United States.

Surgical wound infections due to RGM are a well-recognized clinical entity. In the 1970s and 1980s, these were most commonly associated with augmentation mammaplasty and coronary artery bypass surgery, and multiple disease outbreaks occurred (9, 60). Infections following these types of surgery are now less common, although recently a cluster of 12 cases of postaugmentation mammaplasty surgical-site infection due to M. fortuitum and M. porcinum was reported between 2002 and 2004 in Brazil (60). More often, however, these types of infections have been replaced by infections following other types of cosmetic surgeries, such as liposuction, and other types of prosthetic surgeries, such as knee replacements.

Infections following insertion of prosthetic devices, including prosthetic heart valves, artificial knees and hips, lens implants, and metal rods inserted into the vertebrae to stabilize bones following fractures, have also been described (9, 20). Again, M. fortuitum is the most common pathogen, but any of the pathogenic RGM, including members of the M. smegmatis group, can be associated with this type of infection (9).

In addition to true outbreaks of infection, numerous health care-associated pseudo-outbreaks have been described. Contaminated or malfunctioning bronchoscopes, automated endoscope cleaning machines, and contaminated laboratory reagents and ice have been implicated (9, 31, 33, 42, 88, 91).

RGM are generally resistant to the activities of biocides, such as organomercurials, chlorine, 2% formaldehyde, and alkaline glutaraldehyde, all of which are commonly used disinfectants (9). A report of the contamination of benzalkonium chloride, a widely used antiseptic compound, with M. abscessus and of resulting outbreaks of this species in several patients following steroid injections after skin disinfection emphasizes the limitations of disinfectants against RGM (74).

COLLECTION, TRANSPORT, AND STORAGE OF SPECIMENS

Details of standard methods are included in chapter 28. Transport of species is accomplished by using leak-proof containers and proper safety protocols. Specimens for detection of RGM should be delivered to the laboratory in a timely manner by following appropriate shipping and handling regulations for shipping biological or infectious materials (23).

DIRECT EXAMINATION

Microscopy

The use of mycobacterial smears is a rapid and reasonably sensitive step in the diagnosis of RGM disease. Gram staining of colonies showing faintly staining "ghost-like" beaded gram-positive bacilli is often helpful in establishing a diagnosis of mycobacteriosis. Ziehl-Neelsen or Kinyoun stain may also be useful. However, a smear alone is not sufficient to identify species. A large study found that NTM, including RGM, are likely to be detected by fluorochrome staining of specimens, especially from patients at low risk for AIDS in areas in which lung disease is endemic (23, 98). Further details of the staining procedures are found in chapter 28.

Nucleic Acid Detection

Currently there are no commercial systems available for direct detection of NTM. An indirect test could be an acid-fast bacillus smear-positive sample that is negative by the commercial MTB direct test, but this does not prove the presence of RGM as distinguished from slowly growing NTM.

ISOLATION PROCEDURES

Primary isolation of RGM optimally requires culture at 28 to 30°C rather than 35°C, especially for recovery of M. chelonae and M. immunogenum (9). Direct examination and isolation procedures are detailed in chapter 28.

Recent studies of a murine model suggest that colony morphology, such as a smooth or rough phenotype, may be related to the invasiveness of strains of M. abscessus. The smooth phenotype has been associated with biofilm production and a lack of infectivity; in contrast, strains of the rough phenotype do not form biofilms and invade macrophages (29).

IDENTIFICATION OF RGM

Biochemical Testing

As previously stated, RGM are defined as NTM that grow within 7 days (most species grow within 3 to 4 days) (9). Until the advent of more-modern molecular techniques, traditional laboratory identification of RGM was based primarily upon growth rate, pigmentation, colonial morphology, and a select battery of biochemical tests (9). These standard tests include arylsulfatase production, tolerance to 5% NaCl, nitrate reductase activity, and iron uptake. All members of the M. fortuitum group and M. chelonae/M. abscessus group exhibit a strongly positive arylsulfatase reaction at 3 days. The M. smegmatis group (M. smegmatis and M. goodii) and M. wolinskyi are similar in growth rate but do not exhibit arylsulfatase activity at

3 days (9). Approximately 95% of the isolates of M. smegmatis (sensu stricto) and 80% of M. goodii develop a late (7 to 10 days) yellow-orange pigmentation (5, 9).

The current proposal for clinical laboratories is that biochemical testing of RGM should be replaced with molecular methods. Moreover, biochemical testing should be performed only when a new species is being described as part of a polyphasic identification algorithm.

Supplemental Biochemical Testing: Carbohydrate Utilization

The supplementation of standard biochemical tests with carbohydrate utilization has allowed more complete and accurate laboratory identification of established species and discrimination of some (but not all) new species (9). Identification to the species level and susceptibility testing (see chapter 73) should be performed on isolates of RGM considered to be clinically significant.

However, as previously stated, molecular testing is the only definitive means of identifying RGM species, and laboratories should proceed cautiously when identifying these species by biochemical testing alone.

Antimicrobial Susceptibility Tests for Identification

As discussed above, other adjunctive nonmolecular tests, including antimicrobial susceptibility tests, have also been utilized for the identification of RGM (9). As a screening tool, isolates of the M. fortuitum group and the M. chelonae/M. abscessus group can be differentiated by the use of a polymyxin B disk diffusion method. Generally, isolates of the M. fortuitum group exhibit a partial or clear zone of inhibition (≥10 mm) around the polymyxin disk, whereas isolates of the M. chelonae/M. abscessus group show no zone of inhibition (9). Isolates of the M. fortuitum group are usually susceptible to a broad range of antimicrobials, including amikacin, quinolones, sulfonamides, linezolid, and imipenem. Most of the isolates of this group appear to be intrinsically resistant to the macrolides due to the presence of several related inducible erm genes (9, 49).

Moreover, M. chelonae and M. abscessus also have different antimicrobial susceptibility patterns. One major difference between the two species is resistance to cefoxitin. By agar disk diffusion, M. chelonae shows complete resistance to cefoxitin, with no partial or complete zones of inhibition, in contrast to the partial or complete zones seen with M. abscessus. The MICS of cefoxitin for isolates of M. chelonae are generally ≥256 μg/ml, whereas the modal MIC for isolates of M. abscessus is 32 to 64 μg/ml (9). Furthermore, recent studies have shown that isolates of M. abscessus, but not M. chelonae, have an inducible erm gene similar to the gene in M. fortuitum, which conveys macrolide resistance (49, 50).

The MICs of amikacin for isolates of M. abscessus are lower than those for M. chelonae, and these isolates are resistant to tobramycin, whereas tobramycin is more active than amikacin against M. chelonae. (Amikacin is the preferred aminoglycoside for treatment of M. abscessus, while tobramycin is the preferred agent for M. chelonae.) Additionally, isolates of M. chelonae are more susceptible in vitro to some of the newer antibiotics, including linezolid and moxifloxacin, than are isolates of M. abscessus (5).

With these differences in susceptibility patterns of the rapidly growing species in mind, tentative identification of the most commonly encountered species of RGM is possible and optimal therapeutic regimens can be designed.

However, as with other phenotypic tests, susceptibility testing does not provide definitive species identification. Confirmation of antimicrobial susceptibility patterns in newer species will require testing larger numbers of isolates that have been identified to the species level by molecular techniques.

HPLC Identification

HPLC analysis of mycobacterial cell wall mycolic acid content is routinely used in large reference or state health department laboratories to identify slowly growing isolates of NTM but has been problematic with RGM (9, 10). HPLC can be helpful for placing RGM into groups or complexes but is not specific enough to identify most species with a high degree of accuracy.

Molecular Identification Methods

Nucleic Acid Probes

The INNO LiPA multiplex probe assay (Innogenetics, Ghent, Belgium) is based on the principle of reverse hybridization (79). Although the assay has not received Food and Drug Administration (FDA) clearance, it is being used in some U.S. research laboratories. The assay can identify both rapidly and slowly growing mycobacterial species. Biotinylated DNA obtained by PCR amplification of the 16S–23S internal transcribed spacer region is hybridized with specific oligonucleotide probes immobilized as parallel lines on membrane strips. The main advantage of this system is that a large variety of species may be identified by a single assay without the need to select an appropriate probe. One limitation of the assay is the cross-reactivity that may be detected between species of the M. fortuitum group and several species that are rarely found in clinical samples, such as M. thermoresistibile, M. agri, and M. alvei (9, 79). Additionally, it failed to differentiate isolates of closely related species, such as M. chelonae, from M. abscessus. Since the original studies with the INNO-LiPA assay, however, the system has been improved to include additional probes for the M. fortuitum-M. peregrinum complex and M. smegmatis.

A similar commercial PCR method which targets the 23S rRNA gene, the GenoType Mycobacterium assay (Hain Lifescience, GmbH, Nehren, Germany), provides probes for simultaneous identification of M. chelonae and specific probes for M. peregrinum, M. fortuitum, and M. phlei. These two systems are widely used in Europe for NTM identification (57, 59).

Sequence Analysis for Identification of RGM

Nucleic acid sequence analysis has been performed for the identification of mycobacteria for several years. This identification tool has been useful for the discrimination of most of the newly described species of RGM (32, 41, 52, 81).

16S rRNA Gene Sequence Analysis

Generally, the identification of mycobacteria, including RGM, focuses on two main hypervariable domains known as region A and region B, located on the 5′ end of the 16S rRNA gene. These regions correspond to Escherichia coli positions 129 to 267 and 430 to 500, respectively. Hypervariable region A, especially, contains most of the species-specific sequence variations (so-called "signature sequences") in mycobacterial species, and sequencing of this region allows taxonomic identification of most mycobacteria, including many species of RGM (52, 76).

It is important to note that isolates of two major RGM pathogens, M. chelonae and M. abscessus, require sequencing of sites outside regions A and B, as they are identical in regions A and B but differ at other 16S rRNA gene sites (in the 3′ region), though only at four base pairs (32, 41, 52). To ensure accurate identification, sections of at least 300 bp of quality sequence should be compared between the reference and the query sequences and cover at least one region of the gene where variations are to be expected. Therefore, currently, most clinical laboratories sequence between 450 and 480 bp in order to provide an adequate sequence (53).

In general, members of the genus Mycobacterium are closely related to each other, and closely related species may differ by only a few base pairs or none at all. For example, M. goodii, which is phenotypically difficult to distinguish from M. smegmatis except by susceptibility pattern, has only a four-base difference in its 16S rRNA gene from that of M. smegmatis (5).

A commercial gene sequencing system, the MicroSeq 500 16S rRNA gene bacterial sequencing kit (Applied Biosystems, Foster City, CA), analyzes the first 500-bp sequences and compares the sequences with a commercially prepared database. The use of this commercial system alone cannot differentiate some major species of RGM, such as M. chelonae and M. abscessus, which require sequencing of other regions or other genes for identification (32, 81). This lack of entries makes identification of unknown strains difficult when there is no exact match in the database. For this reason, clinical laboratories have supplemented the commercial database with additional sequences from their own or other libraries, such as RIDOM or GenBank.

A quality-controlled database is indispensable for the evaluation and accurate identification of unknown strains (81). The laboratorian should also recognize that sequence analysis is an important component in a polyphasic approach to the identification of unknown strains. While in some instances, molecule-based identifications without conventional testing may be adequate, more often there are cases in which the broader picture must be reviewed. Some investigators suggest that key phenotypic tests, including colonial morphology, pigmentation, and growth rate analyses, are necessary, especially in the differentiation of closely related species (81).

The lack of consensus for a standard reporting criterion or cutoff value has been a major obstacle in the interpretation of sequence data (53, 81). A reporting criterion such as (i) distinct species, (ii) "related" to a species, or (iii) "most closely related to" a species, depending upon the amount of sequence difference between the unknown isolate and the 16S rRNA gene database entries (40), has been recommended but not validated (52, 81).

A recent Clinical and Laboratory Standards Institute (CLSI) document (53) has recommended guidelines for 16S rRNA gene sequencing in order to identify Mycobacterium sp. in a consistently practical manner. For sequences with 100% sequence probability, a definite genus and species may be assigned. However, for sequence probabilities from 99.0 to 99.9%, the document recommends reporting the isolate as "genus, most closely related to species," and for isolates with a sequence probability of ≥95% to 98.9%, laboratories should consider reporting as "unable to definitively identify by 16S rRNA gene sequencing, most closely related to Mycobacterium sp." (53). We agree that although 100% identity is mandatory for signature sequences, one or a few mismatches at other positions may be acceptable for identification to the species level (53).

Despite the availability of a commercial sequencing method, sequencing remains a complex and often cost-prohibitive procedure for a routine clinical laboratory, which also may not have an adequate volume of isolates to warrant sequencing. Therefore, for these reasons, the general consensus of opinion is that not all laboratories should attempt to incorporate sequencing into their laboratory routine. Moreover, requests for sequencing should instead be sent to a qualified reference laboratory with skill and experience in the method (53, 81).

Sequencing of the *hsp65* Gene

Although the 65-kDa heat shock protein gene (*hsp65*) is highly conserved among species of mycobacteria, it exhibits greater interspecies and intraspecies polymorphism than the 16S rRNA gene sequence (58, 71, 72). This variability can be advantageous to the development of other strategies for the identification of genetically related species of RGM (71, 72). Most sequencing or restriction fragment polymorphism analyses have utilized a 441-bp sequence identified by Telenti et al. (72) and often referred to as the Telenti fragment.

Studies based on DNA sequencing have demonstrated interspecies allelic diversity within RGM. Detailed studies of several RGM species, including *M. peregrinum*, *M. porcinum*, *M. senegalense*, *M. chelonae*, and *M. abscessus*, have shown four to six sequence variants (sequevars) per species that differ by 4 to 6 nucleotides within the 441-bp Telenti fragment (46, 72).

Additionally, unlike the 16S rRNA gene sequencing method, the *hsp65* sequencing method is able to differentiate isolates of *M. abscessus* from *M. chelonae* (they differ by almost 30 bp in their 441-bp *hsp65* sequences, compared to a difference of only 4 bp in their entire 1,500-bp 16S rRNA gene sequences) (46). Unlike with 16S rRNA gene sequencing, with sequencing of the *hsp65* gene, even RGM species with a high degree of 16S rRNA gene similarity, such as *M. fortuitum*, *M. septicum*, *M. peregrinum*, *M. houstonense*, and *M. senegalense*, can be discriminated as distinct species.

As for other sequencing methods, one limitation of sequencing of the *hsp65* gene is that few or no sequences of newer RGM species are available in databases, and detailed sequencing of older species (i.e., multiple strains) has not been done, such that only one sequence per species is generally available. Thus, development of a comprehensive database and in-house validation are essential (46, 76, 81).

rpoB Sequence Analysis

Initial studies using the *rpoB* gene for description of species were based upon analysis of a partial *rpoB* gene sequence, comprising only about 20% of the entire gene length. Other investigators have suggested that species identification of a variety of RGM is possible using a 340- to 360-bp region, but extensive variation may require development of more species-specific probes (1–3, 37, 38, 45).

The utility of *rpoB* has recently been emphasized in a study comparing the phylogenetic relationships of the *rpoB* genes of 19 RGM, including the major pathogens in this group, to several different sequence targets, including 16S rRNA, *hsp65*, *sodA*, and *recA*. All 19 species showed good discrimination with the *rpoB* gene (3, 19).

Not only has the *rpoB* sequence been useful for identification of the established species, but it has also helped to enable the discrimination of species that could not be differentiated by 16S rRNA or the *hsp65* gene sequence

alone. The *rpoB* fragment can be sequenced directly in both directions, allowing identification of most currently recognized species of RGM (2, 3). Newly described species that are usually differentiated by *rpoB* include *M. abscessus* subsp. *bolletii*, *M. phocaicum*, and *M. aubagnense* (1, 2, 5, 39). However, recent studies have shown that multilocus sequencing is necessary to identify *M. abscessus* subsp. *massiliense* (43a, 44, 100).

Sequence Analysis of Other Gene Targets

Other molecular targets for taxonomic identification, including the 32-kDa protein gene, the superoxide dismutase (*sod*) gene, the *dnaJ* gene, the 16S–23S rRNA internal transcribed spacer, the *secA1* gene, and the *recA* gene, have been suggested for mycobacterial identification utilizing either PCR-restriction fragment length polymorphism analysis (PRA) or direct sequencing (3, 14, 15, 99). However, preliminary data suggest that these gene sequences are more varied than the *hsp65* gene sequence and, to date, have been less commonly utilized in laboratory identifications of the species of RGM (3, 100, 101).

Moreover, a major limitation for all sequence-based testing is the lack of sufficient databases (2, 81). Additionally, a multigenic approach for taxonomic evaluation of species has been widely suggested by investigators and has recently been proposed by the ad hoc committee for the reevaluation of the species definition in bacteriology (70).

PCR Restriction Enzyme Analysis (PRA)

PRA of the *hsp65* gene has become a valuable tool used in the identification of RGM. Using the nonsequencing method PRA on the *hsp65* gene (sequevars) of a species to determine minor differences from the *hsp65* genes of other species rarely involves a restriction site, so most species have only one PRA pattern. Currently, the 441-bp Telenti fragment of the *hsp65* gene remains the most useful sequence for PRA identification of RGM, although it has not been evaluated extensively in pigmented RGM and with the newer species and subspecies of RGM, such as *M. phocaicum*, *M. aubagnense*, *M. abscessus* subsp. *bolletii*, and others (9, 71, 72).

The advantages of PRA are that the method of identification does not rely upon growth rate and nutritional requirements, the equipment is relatively inexpensive, and the results for a large number of mycobacterial species can be generated rapidly. The disadvantages are that it requires knowledge of PCR and is a relatively complex procedure that requires extensive in-house validation, since the method is not approved by the FDA. However, as with all sequence-based methods of identification, its utility is limited by the availability of an updated public database. There is no commercial system for *hsp65* PRA. As with all molecular techniques, careful in-house validation with large databases of isolates is essential for laboratories that perform this method.

Algorithms for the identification of mycobacterial species, including RGM, using PRA of the *hsp65* gene have been proposed (23, 71, 72). Figure 1 shows a PRA gel of the RGM most commonly encountered in clinical laboratories.

Pyrosequencing

Pyrosequencing technology (Biotage, Uppsala, Sweden) employs nucleic acid sequencing of a 20- to 30-bp segment of hypervariable region A of the 16S rRNA gene. The

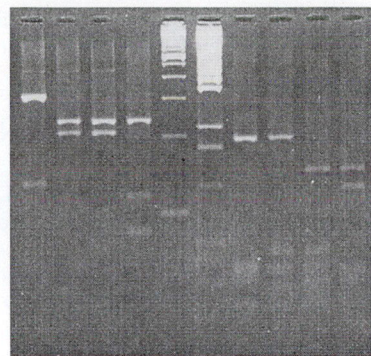

FIGURE 1 PRA patterns of commonly encountered species of RGM. Lanes (left to right): lane 1, M. *chelonae*, BstEII; lane 2, M. *abscessus* subsp. *bolletii*, BstEII; lane 3, M. *abscessus* subsp. *abscessus*, BstEII; lane 4, M. *fortuitum*, BstEII; lane 5, 100-bp ladder; lane 6, pGem ladder; lane 7, M. *chelonae*, HaeIII; lane 8, M. *abscessus* subsp. *bolletii*, HaeIII; lane 9, M. *abscessus* subsp. *abscessus*, HaeIII; lane 10, M. *fortuitum*, HaeIII.

method is based on the detection of pyrophosphate during DNA synthesis. During sequencing, visible light that is proportional to the number of incorporated nucleotides is produced.

The method is not as discriminating as traditional sequencing but is an attractive and less expensive alternative. Another advantage of the pyrosequencing technology is its commercial availability. Like other sequencing methods, however, the major limitation is the quality of the databases for interpretation and comparison of sequences (34). In a recent study of 50 RGM (M. *chelonae*/M. *abscessus* and M. *mucogenicum*), consensus sequences were obtained for 40 isolates, and results were compared to the results of traditional sequencing. Of 10 isolates of M. *fortuitum*, three had a sequence which identically matched M. *fortuitum*/M. *peregrinum*, and the remaining 7 isolates matched M. *fortuitum* (80). To date, this method has provided reliable and rapid identification of a variety of RGM (80).

A real-time PCR with melting curve analysis that consistently detects and differentiates M. *tuberculosis* from NTM has been developed. In a recent study, 20 isolates previously identified as M. *fortuitum* were confirmed as M. *fortuitum*. However, 7 of 24 isolates previously identified as M. *chelonae* or M. *abscessus* were found by pyrosequencing analysis to have been misidentified by traditional methods (65). The application of these methods is currently used only in research or in large reference laboratories after a more extensive evaluation has been done.

TYPING SYSTEMS

Pulsed-Field Gel Electrophoresis

Pulsed-field gel electrophoresis (PFGE) is the most widely used method for molecular strain typing of RGM. Although PFGE has never been standardized for RGM, most investigators concur that small (two- to three-band) differences between isolates indicate that the isolates are closely related; differences of four to six bands indicate that the strains are possibly related, and seven or more differences in bands indicate that the isolates are genetically different

(33, 73, 89, 91). Because unrelated strains of most RGM contain highly diverse PFGE patterns, this technique has been useful in epidemiological investigations. With the addition of thiourea as a recent modification of the original method, it is now possible to obtain reliable results by PFGE of all species of RGM, including isolates previously affected by DNA degradation (102, 103).

Randomly Amplified Polymorphic DNA-PCR

In the randomly amplified polymorphic DNA-PCR (RAPD-PCR) method that uses one arbitrary primer and low-stringency conditions, the primer hybridizes to both strands of template DNA where it is matched or partially matched, resulting in strain-specific heterogeneous DNA products. Zhang and colleagues applied RAPD-PCR or the arbitrarily primed PCR analysis method to compare strains of M. *abscessus* (102). They were able to confirm several previous observations about prior nosocomial RGM outbreaks, including a 1988 epidemic of otitis media due to aminoglycoside-resistant M. *abscessus* in children with prior tympanostomy tubes and an outbreak among cardiac surgery patients (9, 102).

Repetitive-Sequence-Based PCR

Recently, a commercial system, DiversiLab system (Bio-Mérieux, Durham, NC) was developed for strain typing of organisms, including mycobacteria, using repetitive elements interspersed throughout the mycobacterial genome. The system electrophoretically separates repetitive-sequence-based PCR amplicons on microfluidic chips to provide computer-generated readouts. The discriminative power has been reported to equal or exceed that of standard restriction fragment length polymorphism analysis for some species of mycobacteria, with a smaller sample size than that used for standard PFGE and in a much more rapid time frame (11, 101). Limitations of the system include the lack of an extensive established database and the cost of the system.

Enterobacterial Repetitive Intergenic Consensus PCR

Enterobacterial repetitive consensus sequences are repetitive elements distributed along the bacterial chromosome at intergenic regions of polycistronic operons or flanking open reading frames. The method was recently evaluated with isolates of the M. *abscessus*/M. *chelonae* complex and with isolates of M. *fortuitum* (60, 61). Typing of isolates by enterobacterial repetitive intergenic consensus (ERIC) PCR works in mycobacteria as a RAPD-PCR, because the presence of ERIC repeats has never been demonstrated in available *Mycobacterium* genomes and amplification with appropriate ERIC primers can occur in the absence of genuine ERIC sequences (61). In a study of outbreak strains of M. *abscessus* in Brazil, ERIC PCR showed higher discriminatory power than PFGE for typing of strains which had shown smear patterns with PFGE using thiourea (61), although this method was not as discriminatory when isolates of M. *fortuitum* were tested (60, 61).

SEROLOGIC TESTS

Serologic classification of mycobacteria was attempted starting in 1925 with MAC isolates. However, serotyping has not been suitable for routine species identification of mycobacteria, including RGM, and early studies served to emphasize the complexity of the antigenic compositions of mycobacteria, as many antigens are shared by more than one species (96).

ANTIMICROBIAL SUSCEPTIBILITIES

Several different methods have been used for susceptibility testing of RGM for clinical purposes. These methods include agar disk diffusion, broth microdilution, agar disk elution, and the Etest. Each method has proven useful, but none of the methods were well standardized until 2003, with the publication of the CLSI-approved guidelines (98). In the M24-A document, the CLSI recommended broth microdilution as the "gold standard" for susceptibility testing of RGM. Nine antimicrobials, including amikacin, cefoxitin, ciprofloxacin, clarithromycin, doxycycline, linezolid, imipenem, sulfamethoxazole, and tobramycin, have been recommended for testing, and breakpoints have been established for these agents. A proposal to publish CLSI guidelines for additional agents, such as moxifloxacin, minocycline, and trimethoprim-sulfamethoxazole, is under consideration (98).

Briefly, for the broth microdilution method, drug dilutions are prepared using serial twofold dilutions of cation-adjusted Mueller-Hinton broth. Suspensions of organisms are prepared to match a 0.5 McFarland turbidity standard. The suspensions are then diluted to a concentration of approximately 10^6 CFU/ml. From that suspension, 100 μl is delivered into the wells of a 96-well microtiter plate, with a final concentration of approximately 10^4 CFU/well (98). MICs are optimally read after incubation at 30°C for 3 days.

Several specific recommendations about test results have also been made. Tobramycin MICs should be reported only for isolates of M. chelonae. Any RGM isolate for which the amikacin MIC is ≥64 μg/ml should be retested and/or sent to a reference laboratory in order to confirm resistance (although mutational resistance involving the 16S rRNA gene does occur). Imipenem MICs should not be reported for isolates of the M. chelonae/M. abscessus group because the results are not reproducible. Also, if the imipenem MIC for any isolate of the M. fortuitum group is >8 μg/ml, the specimen should be tested again with careful attention paid to inoculum density and with a maximum incubation time of 3 days because of the instability of imipenem over time.

The recent finding of the presence of an erm gene that induces macrolide resistance in isolates of the M. fortuitum group and of M. abscessus but not of M. chelonae has made changes to the manner in which clarithromycin reporting should be done (49, 50). A proposal to the CLSI for an initial 3-day reading of MICs followed by a final reading at 14 days unless the isolate becomes resistant before that time has been made in an attempt to detect isolates that contain the erm gene. The significance of the finding of these genes has not yet been assessed in clinical trials.

Another caveat is that the MICs of sulfamethoxazole and trimethoprim-sulfamethoxazole should be read using 80% inhibition of growth as the susceptibility endpoint, not the 100% inhibition used for the other antimicrobials. Overinoculation of the MIC panels is often most obvious with sulfonamides. An inexperienced laboratorian may interpret an isolate as resistant to sulfonamide when in reality the inoculum was too heavy. Rarely, isolates of the M. fortuitum group are resistant to sulfonamides. If an isolate in this group is found resistant, a repeated test with a lower inoculum is warranted (98).

Further details of antimicrobial susceptibility methods and guidance for patient therapy may be found in chapter 73.

EVALUATION, INTERPRETATION, AND REPORTING OF RESULTS

Dramatic taxonomic changes largely attributed to the advent of molecular testing have occurred over the past 10 to 20 years. Multiple new species have been introduced, and some former subspecies have attained species status. Of the more than 70 valid species of RGM currently described, almost half have been described within the past 10 years.

The recommended methods of identifying species are evolving, with a declining interest in and efficiency of phenotypic testing, including HPLC, and an increasing availability and accuracy of molecular methods. Phenotypic tests have limited utility (e.g., citrate utilization to separate M. chelonae from M. abscessus) and are best applied in conjunction with molecular methods. Currently, molecular methods are preferred and generally are the only way to identify many newer species or subspecies, such as M. goodii, M. abscessus subsp. bolletii, M. wolinskyi, and others. Laboratories in which molecular testing is unavailable should consider referring RGM isolates to a reference laboratory with molecular capabilities.

The major species of RGM (Table 2) have different levels of virulence in different clinical settings and different drug susceptibilities. The diagnostic priorities in terms of disease include bloodstream infection (usually catheter sepsis), disseminated or posttraumatic wound infection, and pulmonary disease (especially in the setting of bronchiectasis). For example, M. mucogenicum is a recognized cause of catheter sepsis, but because of its common presence in tap water, the species is usually considered a contaminant in sputum. The most common RGM isolated from pulmonary specimens and associated with disease is M. abscessus. However, other RGM, such as M. fortuitum, which is rarely considered a pathogen except in the setting of achalasia or lipoid pneumonia, may also be recovered from respiratory samples. The pathogenic potential of RGM is generally related to clinical findings (unexplained fever and dimorphic inflammatory lesions, etc.), the immune status of the patient, the number of positive cultures, the quantity of organisms recovered from smear-positive samples, and the sources of the recovered species. Some established and newly described species have been identified from environmental samples but as yet have not been identified as human or animal pathogens (23). These factors emphasize the need to perform species-level identification and susceptibility testing on clinically significant isolates of RGM.

When species identification of a clinically significant isolate is not available (i.e., susceptibility may be finalized prior to the identification of the species), MICs should be reported for antimicrobials, as recommended by the CLSI. An identification such as "rapidly growing Mycobacterium sp." may be acceptable until identification has been performed. However, the report should include a caveat that tobramycin is validated only for M. chelonae and that imipenem is not validated for the M. chelonae/M. abscessus group (98).

Isolates recovered from a single sample are less likely to be significant than those from multiple samples. Moreover, when MIC results are reported, an interpretation of the isolate (i.e., as "susceptible," "intermediate," or "resistant") should be given for each antimicrobial for which there are recommended breakpoints (98). For agents such as tigecycline, for which no breakpoints have been recommended, an MIC value with a notation that "no CLSI breakpoints have been established for this species" should accompany the report.

Furthermore, for cultures that remain positive for the same species after 6 months of appropriate antimicrobial therapy, confirmation of species identification by molecular methods and repeat antimicrobial susceptibility testing is warranted (98).

Although recent advances in antimicrobial therapies, including those using the new macrolides, fluoroquinolones, oxazolidinones, and tigecycline, have enhanced the therapeutic options and the prognosis for RGM disease, there is still a compelling need for the development of more-efficient, more-effective, and safer oral antimicrobials for treatment. For example, M. abscessus lung disease is still generally considered incurable with the currently available antimicrobials. Susceptibility testing of RGM is necessary in order to select an optimal antimicrobial therapy and to monitor the development of mutational drug resistance which may occur with the prolonged therapy required for RGM disease.

REFERENCES

1. **Adékambi, T., P. Berger, D. Raoult, and M. Drancourt.** 2006. rpoB gene sequence-based characterization of emerging non-tuberculous mycobacteria with descriptions of Mycobacterium bolletii sp. nov., M. phocaicum sp. nov. and Mycobacterium aubagnense sp. nov. Int. J. Syst. Evol. Microbiol. **56:**133–143.

2. **Adékambi, T., P. Colson, and M. Drancourt.** 2003. rpoB-based identification of nonpigmented and late pigmented rapidly growing mycobacteria. J. Clin. Microbiol. **41:**5699–5708.

3. **Adékambi, T., and M. Drancourt.** 2004. Dissection of phylogenetic relationships among 19 rapidly growing Mycobacterium species by 16S rRNA, hsp65, sodA, recA and rpoB gene sequencing. Int. J. Syst. Evol. Microbiol. **54:**2095–2105.

4. **Adékambi, T., D. Raoult, and M. Drancourt.** 2006. Mycobacterium barrassiae sp. nov., a Mycobacterium moriokaense group species associated with chronic pneumonia. J. Clin. Microbiol. **44:**3493–3498.

5. **Adékambi, T., M. Reynaud-Gaubert, G. Greub, M. J. Gevaudan, B. La Scola, D. Raoult, and M. Drancourt.** 2004. Amoebal coculture of "Mycobacterium massiliense" sp. nov. from the sputum of a patient with hemoptoic pneumonia. J. Clin. Microbiol. **42:**5493–5501.

6. **Ara, M., C. S. de Santamaría, P. Zaballos, C. Yus, and M. A. Lezcano.** 2003. Mycobacterium chelonae infection with multiple cutaneous lesions after treatment with acupuncture. Int. J. Dermatol. **42:**642–644.

7. **Brown, B. A., B. Springer, V. A. Steingrube, R. W. Wilson, G. E. Pfyffer, M. J. Garcia, M. C. Menendez, B. Rodriguez-Salgado, K. C. Jost, S. H. Chiu, G. O. Onyi, E. C. Böttger, and R. J. Wallace, Jr.** 1999. Mycobacterium wolinskyi sp. nov. and Mycobacterium goodii sp. nov., two new rapidly growing species related to Mycobacterium smegmatis and associated with human wound infections: a cooperative study from the International Working Group on Mycobacterial Taxonomy. Int. J. Syst. Bacteriol. **49:**1493–1511.

8. **Brown-Elliott, B. A., M. McGlasson, P. Painter, L. Mann, D. Hail, L. Battee, and R. J. Wallace, Jr.** 2009. Comparison of antimicrobials including besifloxacin, ciprofloxacin, gatifloxacin, moxifloxacin, levofloxacin, azithromycin, clarithromycin, amikacin, imipenem, and tobramycin against ophthalmic isolates of nontuberculous mycobacteria, abstr. U-041, p. 583. In Abstr. 109th Gen. Meet. Am. Soc. Microbiol., Philadelphia, PA.

9. **Brown-Elliott, B. A., and R. J. Wallace, Jr.** 2002. Clinical and taxonomic status of pathogenic nonpigmented or late-pigmenting rapidly growing mycobacteria. Clin. Microbiol. Rev. **15:**716–746.

10. **Butler, W. R., and L. S. Guthertz.** 2001. Mycolic acid analysis by high performance liquid chromatography for identification of Mycobacterium species. Clin. Microbiol. Rev. **14:**704–726.

11. **Cangelosi, G. A., R. J. Freeman, K. N. Lewis, D. Livingston-Rosanoff, K. S. Shah, S. J. Milan, and S. V. Goldberg.** 2004. Evaluation of a high-throughput repetitive-sequence-based PCR system for DNA fingerprinting of Mycobacterium tuberculosis and Mycobacterium avium complex strains. J. Clin. Microbiol. **42:**2685–1693.

12. **Chetchotisakd, P., S. Kiertiburanakul, P. Mootsikapun, S. Assanasen, R. Chaiwarith, and S. Anunnatsiri.** 2007. Disseminated nontuberculous mycobacterial infection in patients who are not infected with HIV in Thailand. Clin. Infect. Dis. **45:**421–427.

13. **Chetchotisakd, P., P. Mootsikapun, S. Anunnatsiri, K. Jirarattanapochai, C. Choonhakarn, A. Chaiprasert, P. N. Ubol, L. J. Wheat, and T. E. Davis.** 2000. Disseminated infection due to rapidly growing mycobacteria in immunocompetent hosts presenting with chronic lymphadenopathy: a previously unrecognized clinical entity. Clin. Infect. Dis. **32:**29–34.

14. **Cloud, J. L., K. Hoggan, E. Belousov, S. Cohen, B. A. Brown-Elliott, L. Mann, R. Wilson, W. Aldous, R. J. Wallace, Jr., and G. L. Woods.** 2005. Use of the MGB Eclipse system and SmartCycler PCR for differentiation of Mycobacterium chelonae and M. abscessus. J. Clin. Microbiol. **43:**4205–4207.

15. **Cloud, J. L., H. Neal, R. Rosenberry, C. Y. Turenne, M. Jama, D. R. Hillyard, and K. C. Carroll.** 2002. Identification of Mycobacterium spp. by using a commercial 16S ribosomal DNA sequencing kit and additional sequencing libraries. J. Clin. Microbiol. **40:**400–406.

16. **Cooksey, R. C., M. A. Jhung, M. A. Yakrus, W. R. Butler, T. Adékambi, G. P. Morlock, M. Williams, A. M. Shams, B. J. Jensen, R. E. Morey, N. Charles, S. R. Toney, K. C. Jost, Jr., D. F. Dunbar, V. Bennett, M. Kuan, and A. Srinivasan.** 2008. Multiphasic approach reveals genetic diversity of environmental and patient isolates of Mycobacterium mucogenicum and Mycobacterium phocaicum associated with an outbreak of bacteremias at a Texas hospital. Appl. Environ. Microbiol. **74:**2480–2487.

17. **Covert, T. C., M. R. Rodgers, A. L. Reyes, and G. N. Stelma, Jr.** 1999. Occurrence of nontuberculous mycobacteria in environmental samples. Appl. Environ. Microbiol. **65:**2492–2496.

18. **Cullen, A. R., C. L. Cannon, E. J. Mark, and A. A. Colin.** 2000. Mycobacterium abscessus infection in cystic fibrosis. Am. J. Respir. Crit. Care Med. **161:**641–645.

19. **Devulder, G., M. Pérouse de Montclos, and J. P. Flandrois.** 2005. A multigene approach to phylogenetic analysis using the genus mycobacterium as a model. Int. J. Syst. Evol. Microbiol. **55:**292–302.

20. **Eid, A. J., F. Bergari, I. G. Sia, N. L. Wengenack, D. R. Osmon, and R. R. Razonable.** 2007. Prosthetic joint infection due to rapidly growing mycobacteria: report of 8 cases and review of the literature. Clin. Infect. Dis. **45:**687–694.

21. **Falkinham, J. O., III.** 2003. The changing pattern of nontuberculous mycobacterial disease. Can. J. Infect. Dis. **14:**281–286.

22. **Flor, A., J. A. Capdevila, N. Martin, J. Gavaldà, and A. Pahissa.** 1996. Nontuberculous mycobacterial meningitis: report of two cases and review. Clin. Infect. Dis. **23:**1266–1273.

23. **Forbes, B. A., N. Banaiee, K. G. Beavis, B. A. Brown-Elliott, P. Della Latta, L. B. Elliott, G. S. Hall, B. Hanna, M. D. Perkins, S. H. Siddiqi, R. J. Wallace, Jr., and N. G. Warren.** 2008. Laboratory detection and identification of mycobacteria; approved guideline. Document M48-A. Clinical and Laboratory Standards Institute, Wayne, PA.

24. **Ford, J. G., A. J. W. Huang, S. C. Pfugfelder, E. C. Alfonso, R. K. Forster, and D. Miller.** 1998. Nontuberculous mycobacterial keratitis in south Florida. Ophthalmology **105:**1652–1658.

25. **Furuya, E. Y., A. Paez, A. Srinivasan, R. Cooksey, M. Augenbraun, M. Baron, K. Brudney, P. Della-Latta, C. Estivariz, S. Fischer, M. Flood, P. Kellner, C. Roman, M. Yakrus, D. Weiss, and E. V. Granowitz.** 2008. Outbreak of Mycobacterium abscessus wound infections among "lipotourists" from the United States who underwent abdominoplasty in the Dominican Republic. Clin. Infect. Dis. **46:**1181–1188.

26. Galil, K., L. A. Miller, M. A. Yakrus, R. J. Wallace, Jr., D. G. Mosley, B. England, G. Huitt, M. M. McNeill, and B. A. Perkins. 1999. Abscesses due to *Mycobacterium abscessus* linked to injection of unapproved alternative medication. *Emerg. Infect. Dis.* **5:**681–687.

27. Gira, A. K., H. Reisenauer, L. Hammock, U. Nadiminti, J. T. Macy, A. Reeves, C. Burnett, M. A. Yakrus, S. Toney, B. J. Jensen, H. M. Blumberg, S. W. Caughman, and F. S. Nolte. 2004. Furunculosis due to *Mycobacterium mageritense* associated with footbaths at a nail salon. *J. Clin. Microbiol.* **42:**1813–1817.

28. Gomila, M., A. Ramirez, J. Gascó, and J. Lalucat. 2008. *Mycobacterium llatzerense* sp. nov., a facultatively autotrophic, hydrogen-oxidizing bacterium, isolates from haemodialysis water. *Int. J. Syst. Evol. Microbiol.* **58:**2769–2773.

29. Greendyke, R., and T. F. Byrd. 2008. Differential antibiotics susceptibility of *Mycobacterium abscessus* variants in biofilms and macrophages compared to that of planktonic bacteria. *Antimicrob. Agents Chemother.* **52:**2019–1026.

30. Griffith, D. E., T. Aksamit, B. A. Brown-Elliott, A. Catanzaro, C. Daley, F. Gordin, S. M. Holland, R. Horsburgh, G. Huitt, M. F. Iademarco, M. Iseman, K. Olivier, S. Ruoss, C. F. von Reyn, R. J. Wallace, Jr., and K. Winthrop. 2007. An official ATS/IDSA statement: diagnosis, treatment and prevention of nontuberculous mycobacterial diseases. American Thoracic Society Statement. *Am. J. Respir. Crit. Care Med.* **175:**367–416.

31. Gubler, J. G. H., M. Salfinger, and A. von Graevenitz. 1992. Pseudoepidemic of nontuberculous mycobacteria due to a contaminated bronchoscope cleaning machine: report of an outbreak and review of the literature. *Chest* **101:**1245–1249.

32. Hall, L., K. A. Doerr, S. L. Wohlfiel, and G. D. Roberts. 2003. Evaluation of the MicroSeq system for identification of mycobacteria by 16S ribosomal DNA sequencing and its integration into a routine clinical mycobacteriology laboratory. *J. Clin. Microbiol.* **41:**1447–1453.

33. Hector, J. S. R., Y. Pang, G. H. Mazurek, Y. Zhang, B. A. Brown, and R. J. Wallace, Jr. 1992. Large restriction fragment patterns of genomic *Mycobacterium fortuitum* DNA as strain-specific markers and their use in epidemiologic investigation of four nosocomial outbreaks. *J. Clin. Microbiol.* **30:**1250–1255.

34. Heller, L. C., M. Jones, and R. H. Widen. 2008. Comparison of DNA pyrosequencing with alternative methods for identification of mycobacteria. *J. Clin. Microbiol.* **46:**2092–2094.

35. Hennessee, C. T., J.-S. Seo, A. M. Alvarez, and Q. X. Li. 2009. Polycyclic aromatic hydrocarbon-degrading species isolates from Hawaiian soils: *Mycobacterium crocinum* sp. nov., *Mycobacterium pallens* sp. nov., *Mycobacterium rutilum* sp. nov., *Mycobacterium rufum* sp. nov., and *Mycobacterium aromaticivorans* sp. nov. *Int. J. Syst. Evol. Microbiol.* **59:**378–387.

36. Jönsson, B. E., M. Gilljam, A. Landblad, M. Ridell, A. E. Wold, and C. Welinder-Olsson. 2007. Molecular epidemiology of *Mycobacterium abscessus* with focus on cystic fibrosis. *J. Clin. Microbiol.* **45:**1497–1504.

37. Kim, B. J., S. H. Lee, M. A. Lyu, S. J. Kim, G. H. Bai, G. T. Chae, E. C. Kim, C. Y. Cha, and Y. H. Kook. 1999. Identification of mycobacterial species by comparative sequence analysis of the RNA polymerase gene (*rpoB*). *J. Clin. Microbiol.* **37:**1714–1720.

38. Kim, B.-J., K.-H. Lee, B.-P. Park, S.-J. Kim, G.-H. Bai, S.-J. Kim, and Y.-H. Kook. 2001. Differentiation of mycobacterial species by PCR-restriction analysis of DNA (342 base pairs) of the RNA polymerase gene (*rpoB*). *J. Clin. Microbiol.* **39:**2102–2109.

39. Kim, H.-Y., Y. Kook, Y.-J. Yun, C. G. Park, N. Y. Lee, T. S. Shim, B.-J. Kim, and Y.-H. Kook. 2008. Proportions of *Mycobacterium massiliense* and *Mycobacterium bolletii* in Korean *Mycobacterium chelonae*-*Mycobacterium abscessus* group isolates. *J. Clin. Microbiol.* **46:**3384–3390.

40. Kim, H.-Y., Y.-J. Yun, C. G. Park, D. H. Lee, Y. K. Cho, B. J. Park, S.-I. Joo, E.-C. Kim, Y. J. Hur, B.-J. Kim, and Y. H. Kook. 2007. Outbreak of *Mycobacterium massiliense* infection associated with intramuscular injections. *J. Clin. Microbiol.* **45:**3127–3130.

41. Kirschner, P., B. Springer, U. Vogel, A. Meier, A. Wrede, M. Kiekenbeck, F. C. Bange, and E. C. Böttger. 1993. Genotypic identification of mycobacteria by nucleic acid sequence determination: report of a 2-year experience in a clinical laboratory. *J. Clin. Microbiol.* **31:**2882–2889.

42. Lai, K. K., B. A. Brown, J. A. Westerling, S. A. Fontecchio, Y. Zhang, and R. J. Wallace, Jr. 1998. Long-term laboratory contamination by *Mycobacterium abscessus* resulting in two pseudo-outbreaks: recognition with use of random amplified polymorphic DNA (RAPD) polymerase chain reaction. *Clin. Infect. Dis.* **27:**169–175.

43. Lamy, B., H. Marchandin, K. Hamitouche, and F. Laurent. 2008. *Mycobacterium setense* sp. nov., a *Mycobacterium fortuitum* group organism isolated from a patient with soft tissue infection and osteitis. *J. Syst. Evol. Microbiol.* **58:**486–490.

43a. Leao, S. C., E. Tortoli, J. P. Euzéby, and M. J. Garcia. 19 November 2010. Proposal that the two species *Mycobacterium massiliense* and *Mycobacterium bolletii* be reclassified as *Mycobacterium abscessus* subsp. *bolletii* comb. nov., designation of *Mycobacterium abscessus* subsp. *abscessus* subsp. nov., and emendation of *Mycobacterium abscessus*. *Int. J. Syst. Evol. Microbiol.* [Epub ahead of print.]

44. Leao, S. C., E. Tortoli, C. Viana-Niero, S. Y. M. Ueki, K. V. B. Lima, M. L. Lopes, J. Yubero, M. C. Menendez, and M. J. Garcia. 2009. Characterization of mycobacteria from a major Brazilian outbreak suggests a revision of the taxonomic status of members of the *Mycobacterium chelonae*-*abscessus* group. *J. Clin. Microbiol.* **47:**2691–2698.

45. Lee, H., H.-E. Bang, G.-H. Bai, and S.-N. Cho. 2003. Novel polymorphic region of the *rpoB* gene containing *Mycobacterium* species-specific sequences and its use in identification of mycobacteria. *J. Clin. Microbiol.* **41:**2213–2218.

46. McNabb, A., K. Adie, M. Rodrigues, W. A. Black, and J. Isaac-Renton. 2006. Direct identification of mycobacteria in primary liquid detection media by partial sequencing of the 65-kilodalton heat shock protein gene. *J. Clin. Microbiol.* **44:**60–66.

47. Meyers, H., B. A. Brown-Elliott, D. Moore, J. Curry, C. Truong, Y. Zhang, and R. J. Wallace, Jr. 2002. An outbreak of *Mycobacterium chelonae* following liposuction. *Clin. Infect. Dis.* **34:**1500–1507.

48. Murillo, J., J. Torres, L. Bofill, A. Ríos-Fabra, E. Irausquin, R. Istúriz, M. Guzmán, J. Castro, L. Rubino, and M. Cordido for the Venezuelan Collaborative Infectious and Tropical Diseases Study Group. 2000. Skin and wound infection by rapidly growing mycobacteria. *Arch. Dermatol.* **136:**1347–1352.

49. Nash, K. A., Y. Zhang, B. A. Brown-Elliott, and R. J. Wallace, Jr. 2005. Molecular basis of intrinsic macrolide resistance in clinical isolates of *Mycobacterium fortuitum*. *J. Antimicrob. Chemother.* **55:**170–177.

50. Nash, K. A., B. A. Brown-Elliott, and R. J. Wallace, Jr. 2009. A novel gene, *erm*(41), confers inducible macrolide resistance to clinical isolates of *Mycobacterium abscessus* but is absent from *Mycobacterium chelonae*. *Antimicrob. Agents Chemother.* **53:**1367–1376.

51. Olivier, K. N., D. J. Weber, R. J. Wallace, Jr., A. R. Faiz, J.-H. Lee, Y. Zhang, B. A. Brown-Elliott, A. Handler, R. W. Wilson, M. S. Schechter, L. J. Edwards, S. Chakraborti, and M. R. Knowles, for the Nontuberculous Mycobacteria in Cystic Fibrosis Study Group. 2003. Nontuberculous mycobacteria: I: multicenter prevalence study in cystic fibrosis. *Am. J. Respir. Crit. Care Med.* **167:**828–834.

52. Patel, J. B., D. G. B. Leonard, X. Pan, J. M. Musser, R. E. Berman, and I. Nachamkin. 2000. Sequence-based identification of *Mycobacterium* species using the MicroSeq 500 16S rDNA bacterial identification system. *J. Clin. Microbiol.* **38:**246–251.

53. Petti, C. A., P. P. Bosshard, M. E. Brandt, J. E. Clarridge III, T. V. Feldblyum, P. Foxall, M. R. Furtado, N. Pace, and G. Procop. 2007. Interpretive criteria for microorganism identification by DNA target sequencing: proposed guideline. Document MM18-P. Clinical and Laboratory Standards Institute, Wayne, PA.

54. Pettijean, G., U. Fluckiger, S. Schären, and G. Laifer. 2004. Vertebral osteomyelitis caused by non-tuberculous mycobacteria. *Clin. Microbiol. Infect.* **10**:951–953.

55. Raad, I. I., S. Vartivarian, A. Khan, and G. P. Bodey. 1991. Catheter-related infections caused by the *Mycobacterium fortuitum* complex: 15 cases and review. *Rev. Infect. Dis.* **13**:1120–1125.

56. Reischl, U., H. Melzl, R. M. Kroppenstedt, T. Miethke, L. Naumann, A. Mariottini, G. Mazzarelli, and E. Tortoli. 2006. *Mycobacterium monacense* sp. nov. *Int. J. Syst. Evol. Microbiol.* **56**:2575–2578.

57. Richter, E., S. Rüsch-Gerdes, and D. Hillemann. 2006. Evaluation of the GenoType Mycobacterium assay for identification of mycobacterial species from cultures. *J. Clin. Microbiol.* **44**:1769–1775.

58. Ringuet, H., C. Akoua-Koffi, S. Honore, A. Varnerot, V. Vincent, P. Berche, J. L. Gaillard, and C. Pierre-Audigier. 1999. hsp65 sequencing for identification of rapidly growing mycobacteria. *J. Clin. Microbiol.* **37**:852–857.

59. Russo, C., E. Tortoli, and D. Menichella. 2006. Evaluation of the new GenoType mycobacterium assay for identification of mycobacterial disease. *J. Clin. Microbiol.* **44**:334–339.

60. Sampaio, J. L., E. Chimara, L. Ferrazoli, M. A. da Silva Telles, V. M. Del Guercio, Z. V. Jerico, K. Miyashiro, C. M. Fortaleza, M. C. Padoveze, and S. C. Leao. 2006. Application of four molecular typing methods for analysis of *Mycobacterium fortuitum* group strains causing post-mammaplasty infections. *Clin Microbiol. Infect.* **12**:142–149.

61. Sampaio, J. L., C. Viana-Niero, D. deFreitas, A. O. Hofling-Lima, and S. C. Leao. 2006. Enterobacterial repetitive intergenic consensus PCR is a useful tool for typing *Mycobacterium chelonae* and *Mycobacterium abscessus* isolates. *Diagn. Microbiol. Infect. Dis.* **55**:107–118.

62. Sarria, J. C., N. B. Chutkan, J. E. Figueroa, and A. Hull. 1998. Atypical mycobacterial vertebral osteomyelitis: case report and review. *Clin. Infect. Dis.* **26**:503–505.

63. Schinsky, M. F., M. M. McNeil, A. M. Whitney, A. G. Steigerwalt, B. A. Lasker, M. M. Floyd, G. C. Hogg, D. J. Brenner, and J. M. Brown. 2000. *Mycobacterium septicum* sp. nov. a new rapidly growing species associated with catheter-related bacteraemia. *Int. J. Syst. Evol. Microbiol.* **50**:575–581.

64. Schinsky, M. F., R. E. Morey, A. G. Steigerwalt, M. P. Douglas, R. W. Wilson, M. M. Floyd, W. R. Butler, M. I. Daneshvar, B. A. Brown-Elliott, R. J. Wallace, Jr., M. M. McNeil, D. J. Brenner, and J. M. Brown. 2004. Taxonomic variation in the *Mycobacterium fortuitum* third biovariant complex: description of *Mycobacterium boenickei* sp. nov., *Mycobacterium houstonense* sp. nov., *Mycobacterium neworleansense* sp. nov., and *Mycobacterium brisbanense* sp. nov., and recognition of *Mycobacterium porcinum* from human clinical isolates. *Int. J. Syst. Evol. Microbiol.* **54**:1653–1667.

65. Shrestha, N. B., M. J. Tuohy, G. S. Hall, U. Reischl, S. M. Gordon, and G. W. Procop. 2003. Detection and differentiation of *Mycobacterium tuberculosis* and nontuberculous mycobacterial isolates by real-time PCR. *J. Clin. Microbiol.* **41**:5121–5126.

66. Simmon, K. E., Y. Y. Low, B. A. Brown-Elliott, R. J. Wallace, Jr., and C. A. Petti. 2009. Phylogenetic analysis of *Mycobacterium aurum* and *Mycobacterium neoaurum* with redescription of *M. aurum* culture collection strains. *Int. J. Syst. Evol. Microbiol.* **59**:1371–1375.

67. Simmon, K. E., J. I. Pounder, J. N. Greene, F. Walsh, C. M. Anderson, S. Cohen, C. A. Petti. 2007. Identification of an emerging pathogen, *Mycobacterium massiliense*, by rpoB sequencing of clinical isolates collected in the United States. *J. Clin. Microbiol.* **45**:1978–1980.

68. Sniezek, P. J., B. S. Graham, H. Byers Busch, E. R. Lederman, M. L. Lim, K. Poggemyer, A. Kao, M. Mizrahi, G. Washabaugh, M. Yakrus, and K. L. Winthrop. 2003. Rapidly growing mycobacterial infections after pedicures. *Arch. Dermatol.* **139**:629–634.

69. Springer, B., E. C. Böttger, P. Kirschner, and R. J. Wallace, Jr. 1995. Phylogeny of the *Mycobacterium chelonae*-like organism based on partial sequencing of the 16S rRNA gene and proposal of *Mycobacterium mucogenicum* sp. nov. *Int. J. Syst. Bacteriol.* **45**:262–267.

70. Stackebrandt, E., W. Frederiksen, G. M. Garrity, P. A. D. Grimont, P. Kämpfer, M. C. J. Maiden, X. Nesme, R. Rosselló-Mora, J. Swings, H. G. Trüper, L. Vauterin, A. C. Ward, and W. B. Whitman. 2002. Report of the ad hoc committee for the re-evaluation of the species definition in bacteriology. *Int. J. Syst. Evol. Microbiol.* **52**:1043–1047.

71. Steingrube, V. A., J. L. Gibson, B. A. Brown, Y. Zhang, R. W. Wilson, M. Rajagopalan, and R. J. Wallace, Jr. 1995. PCR amplification and restriction endonuclease analysis of a 65-kilodalton heat shock protein gene sequence for taxonomic separation of rapidly growing mycobacteria. *J. Clin. Microbiol.* **33**:149–153. (Erratum, **33**:1686.)

72. Telenti, A., F. Marchesi, M. Balz, F. Bally, E. C. Böttger, and T. Bodmer. 1993. Rapid identification of mycobacteria to the species level by polymerase chain reaction and restriction enzyme analysis. *J. Clin. Microbiol.* **31**:175–178.

73. Tenover, F. C., R. D. Arbeit, R. V. Goering, P. A. Mickelsen, B. E. Murray, D. H. Persing, and B. Swaminathan. 1995. Interpreting chromosomal DNA restriction patterns produced by pulsed-field gel electrophoresis: criteria for bacterial strain typing. *J. Clin. Microbiol.* **33**:2233–2239.

74. Tiwari, T. S. P., B. Ray, K. C. Jost, Jr., M. K. Rathod, Y. Zhang, B. A. Brown-Elliott, K. Hendricks, and R. J. Wallace, Jr. 2003. Forty years of disinfectant failure: outbreak of postinjection *Mycobacterium abscessus* infection caused by contamination of benzalkonium chloride. *Clin. Infect. Dis.* **36**:954–962.

75. Toro, A., T. Adekambi, F. Cheynet, P.-E. Fournier, and M. Drancourt. 2008. *Mycobacterium setense* infection in humans. *Emerg. Infect. Dis.* **14**:1330–1332. (Letter.)

76. Tortoli, E. 2003. Impact of genotypic studies on mycobacterial taxonomy: the new mycobacteria of the 1990s. *Clin. Microbiol. Rev.* **16**: 319–354.

77. Tortoli, E. 2006. The new mycobacteria: an update. *FEMS Immunol. Med. Microbiol.* **48**:159–178.

78. Tortoli, E., S. Baruzzo, Y. Heijdra, H.-P. Klenk, S. Lauria, A. Mariottini, and J. van Ingen. 2009. *Mycobacterium insubricum* sp. nov. *Int. J. Syst. Evol. Microbiol.* **59**:1518–1523.

79. Tortoli, E., A. Mariottini, and G. Mazzarelli. 2003. Evaluation of INNO-LiPA MYCOBACTERIA v2: improved reverse hybridization multiple DNA probe assay for mycobacterial identification. *J. Clin. Microbiol.* **41**:4418–4420.

80. Tuohy, M. J., G. S. Hall, M. Sholtis, and G. W. Procop. 2005. Pyrosequencing as a tool for the identification of common isolates of *Mycobacterium* sp. *Diagn. Microbiol. Infect. Dis.* **51**:245–250.

81. Turenne, C. Y., L. Tschetter, J. Wolfe, and A. Kabani. 2001. Necessity of quality-controlled 16S rRNA gene sequence databases: identifying nontuberculous *Mycobacterium* species. *J. Clin. Microbiol.* **39**:3637–3648.

82. Uslan, D. Z., T. J. Kowalski, N. L. Wengenack, A. Virk, and J. W. Wilson. 2006. Skin and soft tissue infections due to rapidly growing mycobacteria. *Arch. Dermatol.* **142**:1287–1292.

83. Viana-Niero, C., K. V. B. Lima, M. L. Lopes, M. C. da Silva Rabello, L. R. Marsola, V. C. R. Brilhante, A. M. Durham, and S. C. Leão. 2008. Molecular characterization of *Mycobacterium massiliense* and *Mycobacterium bolletii* in isolates collected from outbreaks of infections after laparoscopic surgeries and cosmetic procedures. *J. Clin. Microbiol.* **46**:850–855.

84. Villaneuva, A., R. V. Calderon, B. A. Vargas, F. Ruiz, S. Aguero, Y. Zhang, B. A. Brown, and R. J. Wallace, Jr. 1997. Report on an outbreak of post-injection abscesses due to *Mycobacterium abscessus*, including management with surgery and clarithromycin therapy and comparison of strains by random amplified polymorphic DNA polymerase chain reaction. *Clin. Infect. Dis.* **24**:1147–1153.

85. **Vugia, D. J., Y. Jang, C. Zizek, J. Ely, K. L. Winthrop, and E. Desmond.** 2005. Mycobacteria in nail salon whirlpool footbaths, California. *Emerg. Infect. Dis.* **11:**616–618.

86. **Wallace, R. J., Jr.** 2004. Infections due to nontuberculous mycobacteria, p. 461–478. *In* W. M. Scheld, R. J. Whitley, and C. M. Marra (ed.), *Infections of the Central Nervous System,* 3rd ed. Lippincott Williams and Wilkins, Philadelphia, PA.

87. **Wallace, R. J., Jr., B. A. Brown, J. Brown, A. G. Steigerwalt, L. Hall, G. Woods, J. Cloud, L. Mann, R. Wilson, C. Crist, K. C. Jost, Jr., D. E. Byrer, J. Tang, J. Cooper, E. Stamenova, B. Campbell, J. Wolfe, and C. Turenne.** 2005. Polyphasic characterization reveals that the human pathogen *Mycobacterium peregrinum* type II belongs to the bovine pathogen species *Mycobacterium senegalense. J. Clin. Microbiol.* **43:**5925–5935.

88. **Wallace, R. J., Jr., B. A. Brown, and D. E. Griffith.** 1998. Nosocomial outbreaks/pseudo-outbreaks caused by nontuberculous mycobacteria. *Annu. Rev. Microbiol.* **2:**453–490.

89. **Wallace, R. J., Jr., B. A. Brown-Elliott, L. Hall, G. Roberts, R. W. Wilson, L. B. Mann, C. J. Crist, S. H. Chiu, R. Dunlap, M. J. Garcia, J. T. Bagwell, and K. C. Jost, Jr.** 2002. Clinical and laboratory features of *Mycobacterium mageritense. J. Clin. Microbiol.* **40:**2930–2935.

90. **Wallace, R. J., Jr., B. A. Brown-Elliott, R. W. Wilson, L. Mann, L. Hall, Y. Zhang, K. C. Jost, Jr., J. M. Brown, A. Kabani, M. F. Schinsky, A. G. Steigerwalt, C. J. Crist, G. D. Roberts, Z. Blacklock, M. Tsukamura, V. Silcox, and C. Turenne.** 2004. Clinical and laboratory features of *Mycobacterium porcinum. J. Clin. Microbiol.* **42:**5689–5697.

91. **Wallace, R. J., Jr., Y. Zhang, B. A. Brown, V. Fraser, G. H. Mazurek, and S. Maloney.** 1993. DNA large restriction fragment patterns of sporadic and epidemic nosocomial strains of *Mycobacterium chelonae* and *Mycobacterium abscessus. J. Clin. Microbiol.* **31:**2697–2701.

92. **Whipps, C. M., W. R. Butler, F. Pourahmad, V. G. Watral, and M. L. Kent.** 2007. Molecular systematics support the revival of *Mycobacterium salmoniphilum* (ex Ross 1960) sp. nov., nom. rev., a species closely related to *Mycobacterium chelonae. Int. J. Syst. Evol. Microbiol.* **57:**2525–2531.

93. **Wilson, R. W., V. A. Steingrube, E. C. Böttger, B. Springer, B. A. Brown-Elliott, V. Vincent, K. C. Jost, Jr., Y. Zhang, M. J. Garcia, S. H. Chiu, G. O. Onyi, H. Rossmoore, D. R. Nash, and R. J. Wallace, Jr.** 2001. *Mycobacterium immunogenum* sp. nov., a novel species related to *Mycobacterium abscessus* and associated with clinical disease, pseudo-outbreaks, and contaminated metalworking fluids: an international cooperative study on mycobacterial taxonomy. *Int. J. Syst. Evol. Microbiol.* **51:**1751–1764.

94. **Winthrop, K. L., M. Abrams, M. Yakrus, I. Swartz, J. Ely, D. Gillies, and D. J. Vugia.** 2002. An outbreak of mycobacterial furunculosis associated with footbaths at a nail salon. *N. Engl. J. Med.* **346:**1366–1371.

95. **Winthrop, K. L., K. Albridge, D. South, P. Albrecht, M. Abrams, M. C. Samuel, W. Leonard, J. Wagner, and D. J. Vugia.** 2004. The clinical management and outcome of nail salon-acquired *Mycobacterium fortuitum* skin infection. *Clin. Infect. Dis.* **38:**38–44.

96. **Wolinsky, E.** 1979. Nontuberculous mycobacteria and associated diseases. *Am. Rev. Respir. Dis.* **119:**107–159.

97. **Woo, P. C. Y., K.-W. Leung, S. S. Y. Wong, K. T. K. Chong, E. Y. L. Cheung, and K.-Y. Yuen.** 2002. Relatively alcohol-resistant mycobacteria are emerging pathogens in patients receiving acupuncture treatment. *J. Clin. Microbiol.* **40:**1219–1224.

98. **Woods, G. L., B. A. Brown-Elliott, E. P. Desmond, G. S. Hall, L. Heifets, G. E. Pfyffer, J. C. Ridderhof, R. J. Wallace, Jr., N. G. Warren, and F. G. Witebsky.** 2003. Susceptibility testing of mycobacteria, nocardiae, and other aerobic actinomycetes; approved standard. Document M24-A. Clinical and Laboratory Standards Institute, Wayne, PA.

99. **Wright, P. W., R. J. Wallace, Jr., N. W. Wright, B. A. Brown, and D. E. Griffith.** 1998. Sensitivity of fluorochrome microscopy for detection of *Mycobacterium tuberculosis* versus nontuberculous mycobacteria. *J. Clin. Microbiol.* **36:**1046–1049.

100. **Zelazny, A. M., L. B. Calhoun, L. Li, Y. R. Shea, and S. H. Fischer.** 2005. Identification of *Mycobacterium* species by *secA1* sequences. *J. Clin. Microbiol.* **43:**1051–1058.

101. **Zelazny, A. M., J. M. Root, Y. R. Shea, R. E. Colombo, I. C. Shamputa, F. Stock, S. McNulty, B. A. Brown-Elliott, R. J. Wallace, Jr., K. N. Olivier, S. M. Holland, and E. P. Sampaio.** 2009. Cohort study of molecular identification and typing of *Mycobacterium abscessus, Mycobacterium massiliense* and *Mycobacterium bolletii. J. Clin. Microbiol.* **47:**1985–1995.

102. **Zhang, Y., M. Rajagopalan, B. A. Brown, and R. J. Wallace, Jr.** 1997. Randomly amplified polymorphic DNA PCR for comparison of *Mycobacterium abscessus* strains from nosocomial outbreaks. *J. Clin. Microbiol.* **35:**3132–3139.

103. **Zhang, Y., M. A. Yakrus, E. A. Graviss, N. Williams-Bouyer, C. Turenne, A. Kabani, and R. J. Wallace, Jr.** 2004. Pulsed-field gel electrophoresis study of *Mycobacterium abscessus* isolates previously affected by DNA degradation. *J. Clin. Microbiol.* **42:**5582–5587.

Approaches to the Identification of Aerobic Gram-Negative Bacteria*

GEORGES WAUTERS AND MARIO VANEECHOUTTE

31

This chapter describes the approach to the identification of gram-negative rods, with emphasis on the greater difficulty in identifying non-glucose-fermenting organisms. In addition to what was presented in the ninth edition of this *Manual*, a scheme is presented to identify these organisms centered around three enzymatic activities, i.e., oxidase, trypsin (benzyl-arginine arylamidase or benzyl-arginine aminopeptidase), and pyrrolidonyl aminopeptidase. These enzymatic reactions are fast and easy to interpret, and they are stable markers in almost all taxa discussed; i.e., there are few species for which these tests yield variable intraspecies results.

Before presenting the identification scheme, several issues of terminology and methodology need to be addressed. First, the use of only the substrate name to designate a biochemical test is imprecise and can lead to confusion. We suggest referring to the specific activity of the biochemical test. For example, we use "gelatin hydrolysis" or "gelatinase" instead of "gelatin" to indicate that this test demonstrates the degradation of and not the production of gelatin.

The term production is used when a specific metabolic product is searched for, as in the case of indole, which is produced as a degradation product of tryptophan. The term hydrolysis is used when it is the disappearance of the substrate (and not the appearance of a degradation product) which is being demonstrated. For instance, tyrosine is present as a granulous deposit in agar and a clearance zone is observed around the colonies or streak when tyrosine is hydrolyzed.

Although all biochemical tests rely on the presence of enzymes, the term enzymatic activity is used for tests when a bacterial suspension is added to a substrate and the enzymatic activity is read without the need for bacterial growth. Enzymatic activity is detected by (i) a chromogenic shift of the substrate, e.g., by the degradation of the colorless *o*-nitrophenyl-β-D-galactopyranoside (ONPG) by β-galactosidase, resulting in liberation of *o*-nitrophenol, a yellow compound); (ii) by the color change of a pH indicator added to the suspension, e.g., phenol red for assessing tributyrate esterase activity; or (iii) by another indicator of enzymatic activity, which causes a color change by interacting with the enzymatic product: e.g., Griess reagents turn red after interacting with nitrite (nitrate reductase activity), Kovács reagents turn red after interacting with indole (indole production), or cinnamaldehyde interacts with free β-naphthylamine (aminopeptidase activity).

This chapter also uses more precise terminology for the terms utilization, oxidation, and glycolysis. "Utilization" is not a precise term to address either assimilation or "usage of any substrate being metabolized," and therefore we avoid using it. "Oxidizer" is often used to describe saccharolytic nonfermenters as opposed to asaccharolytic nonfermenters. However, in strict biochemical terminology, it refers to oxidative phosphorylation as opposed to fermentation as an alternative route after glycolysis. In this chapter we do not use the term oxidation to mean saccharolysis, but we specifically use the term acidification of carbohydrates or saccharolysis. In this respect, we also avoid the use of "glycolysis" for "saccharolysis," because "glycolysis" may be interpreted as referring to the acidification of glucose only or can be understood as the biochemical metabolic cycle preceding fermentation or respiration.

TEST METHODS WITH EMPHASIS ON GRAM-NEGATIVE NONFERMENTERS

Careful attention to testing methods is critical when describing their application for nonfermenters. Slight variations of reagents or incubation conditions can cause numerous misidentifications and have caused erroneous descriptions of new species. Also, although several media and biochemical tests are used for the identification of fermenting *Enterobacteriaceae*, these are not necessarily optimal when testing nonfermenters. Nonfermenters require good aeration because of their strict respiratory metabolism, most often with atmospheric oxygen as the terminal electron acceptor. Growth of most nonfermenters in liquid media is moderate or weak, due to the intrinsically poor aeration of liquid media. Therefore, a small inoculum as used for *Enterobacteriaceae* is not appropriate. Instead, liquid media should be inoculated with a turbid suspension of nonfermenters. Whenever bacterial growth is not required, as is the case for testing enzymatic activity, it is preferable to use a heavy suspension of bacterial cells in an aqueous solution of the substrate, rather than the inoculation of a liquid medium. Further detailed remarks can be found below when describing the different biochemicals used for identification.

---

*This chapter contains information presented in chapter 24 by Paul C. Schreckenberger and David Lindquist in the ninth edition of this *Manual*.

Below we briefly describe some specific tests or modifications used in the identification algorithms of this chapter and of chapter 42, and highlight protocols that should be followed when performing these tests and interpreting the results, with the emphasis on their application for nonfermenters. The descriptions of the other tests discussed in this chapter can be found in chapter 17.

Assimilation or Utilization of Organic Compounds as the Sole Carbon Source for Growth

Different approaches exist to determine the capacities of strains to assimilate, i.e., utilize organic compounds as the sole carbon source for growth. Microbial ID/Characterization (Biolog, Hayward, CA) and API NE and API 32GN (BioMérieux, Marnes-la-Coquette, France) are commercial systems that score growth by assessing the optical density of the minimal broths to which the organic compound has been added. Another method to assess assimilation of an organic compound as the sole carbon source is by observing the alkalinization of a minimal medium to which the sole carbon source and a pH indicator have been added. Therefore, the term alkalinization is frequently used as synonymous to the term assimilation, although "assimilation" may be preferred as a more general term (see below). Simmons' citrate agar base medium is frequently used, with bromothymol blue as the pH indicator (yellow at pH 6.0, green at pH 6.9, and blue at pH 7.6). Citrate, as the sole carbon source, can be replaced by any compound to be tested (12). For most substrates, the medium is also alkalinized as a result of production of hydroxyl radicals and CO_2 by the metabolism of the sole carbon source added. Because CO_2 can escape, the remaining radicals alkalinize the medium. Therefore, it is essential that the tubes be incubated with a loose lid to allow the carbon dioxide to escape. Alkalinization facilitates the interpretation, but as stated above, growth without alkalinization can occur with some substrates and should be interpreted as assimilation positive, as well.

In this chapter, we limit the description of assimilation assays for the identification of nonfermenters to that of acetamide and acetate, used solely as additional characteristics to differentiate between some species. However, as described in chapter 42, *Acinetobacter* identification has been largely based on assimilation tests by supplementing the basal mineral medium of Cruze et al. (5) with a 0.1% (wt/vol) concentration of the carbon source. We refer the reader to that chapter for the basal medium composition, inoculation, and interpretation.

Acid Production from Carbohydrates or Sugars: Saccharolysis

The term "acid production" may refer to acidification of a carbohydrate by fermenters as well as by nonfermenters. Although for diagnostic purposes, while there is no need to differentiate between these modes of acid production (fermentation or oxidation), it is important to distinguish acidification from assimilation. Assimilation is tested on minimal media lacking all carbon sources except the one tested for utilization, whereas more complex media (peptone-rich media), aimed at supporting optimal growth of the organism tested, are used to assess acidification of the single carbohydrate substrate added.

With the exception of the strong acid producers, *Pseudomonas aeruginosa* and *Acinetobacter* spp. and some rare species like those of the genus *Asaia*, acid production by nonfermenters is usually much weaker than acid production by fermenters. Nonfermenters acidify only as a result of the general metabolic activity, which usually leads to weaker

acidification than fermentation, which produces strong acids like lactic acid. Nonfermenters acidify only under well-aerated incubation conditions. Therefore, the conditions to assess this weaker acidification by nonfermenters should be optimized to avoid false-negative results. API kits, like API 20 E (*Enterobacteriaceae*), API 20 NE (non-*Enterobacteriaceae*), and API ID 32 GN (gram negatives), are not suited to detect acidification of carbohydrates by nonfermenters. API 20 NE and API ID 32 GN only score assimilation, which, as already stated above, is sometimes confused with acidification. Two examples are presented to emphasize this point. The results of carbohydrate acidification for *Chryseobacterium caeni* N4^T, obtained by Kämpfer et al. (9), were substantially different from the original description of this species (13). Quan et al. (13) described *C. caeni* as an asaccharolytic species, whereas Kämpfer et al. (9) found the type strain of this species to be one of the most saccharolytic strains among the members of the *Chryseobacterium* genus, rapidly acidifying glucose, maltose, sucrose, trehalose, and L-arabinose. This contradiction may be explained by the fact that Quan et al. (13) used the API 20 E, API 20 NE, and API 32 GN galleries to assess acidification of carbohydrates. Another example comes from the description of *Ralstonia insidiosa* (4), which mentions that no acid is produced from glucose, sucrose, or lactose, as tested with RapID NF Plus (Remel) and API 20 NE (BioMérieux), whereas this species clearly acidifies glucose, L-arabinose, D-xylose, and maltose (14).

Because acid production from carbohydrates by nonfermenting gram-negative rods results in a weaker pH change than that caused by fermentation, the medium and incubation conditions should be optimized to detect the weak acid production. This can be achieved by (i) heavy inoculation; (ii) good aeration; (iii) using media with only small amounts of peptones, because nonfermenters' aerobic metabolism promotes alkalinization and neutralizes the (weak) acidification; and (iv) using media with an appropriate pH indicator.

The oxidation/fermentation medium, with its low peptone content of 0.1%, as originally described by Hugh and Leifson (8) is widely used for this purpose, but acidification of carbohydrates by nonfermenters is better demonstrated on slanted solid media. Ammonium salt agar (ASA) has been recommended (1), but better results can be obtained with low-peptone phenol red (LPPR) agar, as originally described for testing acidification of ethylene glycol (15). The slant is heavily inoculated, and the medium is incubated for up to 7 days. LPPR is more sensitive to acidification of a substrate than ASA, because it is not buffered and because phenol red shifts color to yellow already at pH 6.8, whereas ASA is buffered and the indicator used, i.e., bromocresol purple, only shifts when the pH has dropped to as low as 5.2.

Acid production from the sugar alcohol ethylene glycol, best tested on LPPR agar with 2% ethylene glycol (15), is interesting for the identification of nonfermenters, because it is independent of acid production from sugars. This method is helpful in identifying species, such as *Alcaligenes faecalis*, *Oligella* spp., and *Kerstersia gyiorum*, that acidify ethylene glycol but not sugars. Conversely, species like *Burkholderia* spp. and *Ralstonia pickettii* acidify sugars but not ethylene glycol.

Arginine Dihydrolase

Arginine dihydrolase activity by nonfermenters can best be tested by dense inoculation (McFarland 4 to 5) in Moeller broth with 1% arginine. After inoculation, the broth is overlaid with paraffin oil. Alkalinization, caused by the production of ammonia, is detected by the pH indicators. A positive result is indicated by a purple color, which can be read after 4 h to up to 2 days. These enzymatic reactions can proceed in the absence of oxygen and therefore are not hampered by the presence of paraffin, which is needed to prevent false-positive alkalinization of the broth, due to aerobic metabolic pathways, like the peptone metabolism. This is especially a problem when prolonged incubation is needed, as is the case with some *Haematobacter* strains.

Esculin Hydrolysis

Esculin hydrolysis by nonfermenters is preferably tested on esculin agar without bile, because bile can inhibit some non-fermenters, such as *Moraxella* spp. Broad streak inoculation should be applied. Strains positive for esculin hydrolysis cause a blackening of the agar after overnight incubation.

Flagellum Stains

The detection of flagella is very useful for the identification of some groups of nonfermenters that are otherwise biochemically very similar. Since flagellum staining and microscopy require additional efforts, we limit their use to those species that cannot be differentiated by other methods. There are several types of flagellation. The genera *Achromobacter*, *Alcaligenes*, *Bordetella*, and *Cupriavidus*, including *Cupriavidus gilardii* (originally described as polar [3]), have peritrichous flagella (15). *Ochrobactrum* and *Rhizobium* spp. also exhibit peritrichous flagella, but they frequently have only one or two lateral flagella. *Pseudomonas aeruginosa*, *Pseudomonas stutzeri*, *Pseudomonas alcaligenes*, *Pseudomonas pseudoalcaligenes*, *Pseudomonas oryzihabitans*, the genera *Brevundimonas* and *Shewanella*, *Ralstonia pickettii*, and *Sphingomonas paucimobilis* have polar monotrichous flagellation. In the last two species, the flagella are rarely detected. *Pseudomonas putida*, *Pseudomonas fluorescens*, *Pseudomonas luteola*, the *Burkholderia cepacia* group, and *Stenotrophomonas maltophilia* have polar multitrichous flagella, and the genera *Comamonas*, *Delftia*, and *Herbaspirillum* have bipolar multitrichous tufts.

We have found that flagella are best stained as follows (adapted from Kodaka et al. [10]). Ten volumes of solution A [10 ml of 5% phenol, 2 g of tannic acid, and 10 ml of $KAl(SO_4)_2 \cdot 12 H_2O$ (saturated solution)] are mixed with one volume of solution B (12 g of crystal violet in 100 ml of ethanol, 96%). The mixture is allowed to first stand for 2 to 3 days, without filtration, centrifugation, or shaking. This stain can be used for up to 1 year when stored at room temperature. The stain is carried out by making a less than 0.5 McFarland suspension from fresh colonies on tryptic soy agar (TSA) in a mixture of 30% ethanol and 70% tap water, briefly heating a coverslip (24 by 60 mm) (not a microscopic slide) by holding it in a flame and adding a small drop (5 μl) of the suspension. This drop spreads spontaneously and is allowed to dry. The staining solution is added for 1 to 4 min (longer for longer-stored staining solution), and the coverslip is rinsed with tap water and allowed to dry in an incubator. Pritt glue applicator is applied to the coverslip for better adherence, and the coverslip is then placed onto a slide, with the colored face upwards. It is observed under a ×100 magnification.

Flexirubin Pigment Production

Flexirubin pigment production can be assessed for yellow-pigmented colonies of the *Flavobacteriaceae*. A small mass of bacterial cells is collected with a loop and deposited in a drop of a 20% KOH solution on a slide; a red color indicates the presence of flexirubin pigments (1). *Sphingomonas paucimobilis* produces yellow colonies, but not flexirubin, whereas most *Myroides* strains produce weakly yellow colonies, which are always flexirubin positive.

Gelatin Hydrolysis

Gelatin hydrolysis is best assessed by means of the plate method. Inoculate the plate (nutrient agar plus 0.4% gelatin) with a spot or a streak and incubate until luxuriant growth is obtained. When the isolate is gelatin hydrolysis positive, visual clearing of the agar is usually obvious. If not, add an $HgCl_2$ solution (12 g of $HgCl_2$, 16 ml of HCl [35%], and 80 ml of distilled water [AD]) and observe clearing. The use of $HgCl_2$ solution is generally avoided because of its high toxicity.

Growth at 42°C

Growth at 42°C should be tested by adding 1 drop of a small inoculum (e.g., as for swabbing susceptibility testing plates) in broth tubes incubated in a warm water bath, with a precision of ±0.1°C. Care should be taken that the broth is still completely clear, i.e., not turbid at all, after inoculation. Use of 1.5 to 2 ml of tryptic soy broth (TSB) with a maximal air surface (e.g., in tubes of 16 mm) instead of 5 ml is preferred for better aeration and optimal growth of nonfermenters. The test is read as positive when growth, observed as any presence of turbidity, is present. The use of a positive control tube at 37°C is recommended to exclude that negativity for growth at 42°C is caused by a general loss of viability.

H2S Production or Sulfite Reductase Activity

H_2S production or sulfite reductase activity is best tested on Kligler iron agar (KIA), containing thiosulfate and Fe salt. The H_2S produced from thiosulfate by sulfite reductase will react with the Fe salt to produce FeS, a strong black precipitate which for clinically relevant nonfermenters is only observed for *Shewanella* species. Lead acetate paper, held over the medium to detect evaporating H_2S fumes, is not very useful. This method detects the weak production of H_2S from the amino acids methionine and cysteine. This reaction is widely observed among *Enterobacteriaceae* and is therefore not very discriminative. (Note: when present for nonfermenters, the observed result is usually weak and can yield variable or false-negative results.) Amino acid-derived H_2S production is too weak to be detected on KIA.

Indole Production

Indole production can be detected by different methods. The broth growth method includes inoculation of a broth culture, e.g., heart infusion broth, incubation for 48 h, extraction with xylene, and addition of Ehrlich's reagent (see chapter 17). However, as is the case for the spot indole test (see chapter 17), the broth growth method is not advisable for nonfermenters, because it may lack sensitivity and may be difficult to interpret, yielding a false-negative result for indole production. For example, *Flavobacterium mizutaii*, which is clearly positive for indole production, was described as negative (16), because indole production was assessed using the broth growth method. Similarly, *Elizabethkingia meningoseptica* is mentioned as only 50% indole production positive (7), but using the heavy suspension method, we have never encountered an *E. meningoseptica* isolate that was negative for indole production. In general, most members of the genera *Chryseobacterium*, *Elizabethkingia*, and *Empedobacter* are indole positive, but this reaction is sometimes weak and difficult to demonstrate by conventional broth methods. Therefore, we recommend a simple, rapid, growth-independent method for demonstration of indole production. A heavy suspension (4 to 5 McFarland standard) is prepared in a 0.3% tryptophan solution in AD. After 3 to 4 h of incubation, indole is detected by adding Kovács reagent (for composition, see chapter 17). This method allows detection within a short time of all indole-producing nonfermenting gram-negative rods.

Motility

Motility can be easily determined by microscopic observation of a wet-mount preparation of a young colony from an agar plate. Motility can be studied by inoculation of SIM medium, described in chapter 17. Another culture method, circumventing the need for microscopy, uses inoculation of a large inoculum of a fresh culture in soft agar (0.3% agar), preferably in a small petri dish (5-cm diameter); this provides better aeration than tubes, reducing the potential for false-negative results. For some species, such as *Sphingomonas*, motility can best be demonstrated after incubation of cultures at room temperature, instead of the usual 30 to 35°C for other nonfermenters.

NaCl Requirement

Most commercially available basic media (like TSB) already contain NaCl and should not be used to assess the requirement for NaCl. It is best to use well-aerated tubes with peptone water, i.e., an aqueous solution of 1% tryptone or Casitone, without NaCl in comparison with peptone water to which 1% NaCl was added. Because one is testing the ability of an organism to grow under these conditions, a small inoculum should be used to allow facile detection of turbidity. Also, care should be taken that the inoculum is prepared from a suspension in AD or 1% peptone water without NaCl. The halotolerance of isolates can be studied using peptone water containing increasing concentrations of NaCl, up to 12%.

Nitrite and Nitrate Reductase Activities

Nitrite and nitrate reductase activities can be determined together in nitrate broth (see chapter 17), but for nonfermenters they are best determined by heavy inoculation of separate nitrate and nitrite broths, in which—after incubation—the presence of nitrite is detected by the addition of Griess reagents and, eventually, of zinc dust.

Nitrate can be reduced to nitrite by nitrate reductase, and nitrite can be reduced by nitrite reductase to produce either nitrogen gas (N_2) or ammonium for assimilation into amino compounds. Some species reduce only nitrate, others both nitrate and nitrite, and a few may reduce nitrite without reduction of nitrate.

Nitrate reduction to nitrite by nitrate reductase is best detected in 0.5 or 1 ml of 0.1% KNO_3 broth (for prolonged incubation) or aqueous solution (4 h), using a turbid inoculum (McFarland 4 to 5). The organism is positive for nitrate reductase activity when the addition of Griess reagents (solution A first and then solution B) results in a pink color within 2 min, indicating the presence of nitrite, i.e., the reduction of nitrate to nitrite.

Nitrite reductase activity can be tested by adding a very heavy inoculum (McFarland 8 to 10) to a small volume, e.g., 0.5 or 1 ml, of nitrite broth (0.001% $NaNO_2$ in 1% peptone). The organism is positive for nitrite reductase activity when, after 4 to 24 h of incubation, the addition of Griess' reagents results in a colorless solution, indicating the absence of nitrite, i.e., the reduction of nitrite to N_2 or ammonium.

In summary, certainly for nonfermenters, it may be advisable to use separate nitrate and nitrite broths, eventually with addition of a Durham tube to the nitrite broth—instead of to the nitrate broth, as is usually done—and with addition of zinc dust to the nitrate broth, the latter only for strains where nitrate and nitrite broths both remain colorless after addition of the Griess reagents. Interpretation can be done according to Table 1 in chapter 17.

Pyrrolidonyl Aminopeptidase (Pyrrolidonyl Arylamidase) Activity

Pyrrolidonyl aminopeptidase (pyrrolidonyl arylamidase) activity has been shown to be very helpful in the identification of nonfermenters (2, 11) and is a central characteristic, together with oxidase and trypsin, in the identification scheme proposed here. The test is described in chapter 17.

Starch Hydrolysis

Starch hydrolysis is tested by inoculation onto Mueller-Hinton agar (MHA), which contains starch. Flooding with iodine solution (Lugol) yields a purple-blue color in the presence of starch. Starch hydrolysis is read as a non-purple-stained zone around the streak.

Susceptibility to Colistin

Susceptibility to colistin can be tested on common agars, using 10-μg colistin disks. For diagnostic purposes, any zone of inhibition is interpreted as susceptible.

Susceptibility to Desferrioxamine

Susceptibility to desferrioxamine, an Fe chelator, can be tested on MHA, or on TSA for strains growing poorly on MHA, using paper disks loaded with 250 μg of desferrioxamine or using commercially available Rosco tablets (11). Media should not contain blood, because this provides large amounts of bioavailable Fe, which, in turn, would cause false-positive resistance results. Any inhibition zone is interpreted as susceptible.

Susceptibility to Vancomycin

Susceptibility to vancomycin is tested by disk diffusion, using 30-μg vancomycin disks. Some gram-negative organisms are vancomycin susceptible, and this can be used as a rapid and distinctive identification tool.

Trypsin or Benzyl-Arginine Arylamidase Activity

Trypsin or benzyl-arginine arylamidase activity is very discriminative for nonfermenters, since the strains of almost all taxa exhibit an all-or-nothing positive result, providing a test with high discriminatory value. Therefore, this test can act as a first step in identification. Testing for trypsin activity is described in chapter 17, but it is also easily performed by addition of a trypsin tablet (Rosco) to a dense bacterial suspension in 0.5 ml of AD and can be read within 4 h of incubation, by the addition of cinnamaldehyde [see "Pyrrolidonyl Aminopeptidase (Pyrrolidonyl Arylamidase) Activity)"] (11).

IDENTIFICATION SCHEME AND IDENTIFICATION TABLES

Below, we outline a proposal for rapid and simplified biochemical testing, with emphasis on the identification of gram-negative nonfermenters. Most nonfermenting gram-negative bacteria of clinical relevance have an optimal growth temperature between 30 and 37°C and grow on simple media such as TSA, MHA, and sheep blood agar (SBA). A few species, however, may grow better below 30°C (e.g., *Methylobacterium*), and some *Moraxella* species are more fastidious and require SBA at 37°C for optimal growth.

The scheme below makes it possible in most cases to record within 3 days, starting from KIA, the following characteristics: growth on TSA, MHA, and/or SBA; oxidase; hydrogen sulfide production; fermentation of lactose and glucose; colony pigmentation; motility; susceptibility to colistin, desferrioxamine, and vancomycin; alkaline phosphatase; benzyl-arginine aminopeptidase (trypsin);

pyrrolidonyl aminopeptidase; urease; β-galactosidase; indole production; nitrate reductase; nitrite reductase; lysine decarboxylase; arginine dihydrolase; and acidification of glucose, mannitol, xylose, and ethylene glycol. The reagents used can be prepared once each year and stored at 4°C.

For the sake of manageability, *Advenella incenata* (see chapter 43) and the species of the genus *Pandoraea* (see chapter 41) have not been included in this simplified scheme for aerobically growing gram-negative bacteria. The extreme variability of the phenotypic characteristics within these species and the biochemical inactivity of some *Pandoraea* species would have rendered the scheme proposed here impractical. However, these species are listed below

(see Table 5), and information on their characteristics has been filled out as completely as possible.

Gram-negative bacteria can be identified using the scheme below. It should be mentioned that *Acinetobacter* cells can stain gram variable, whereby sometimes one of two cells in a pair of diplococci is gram negative and the other is gram positive. Also, some phylogenetically gram-positive bacteria may stain gram negative, e.g., *Lactobacillus iners* and *Gardnerella vaginalis* (6). These have not been included in the scheme below. The scheme begins with observation of growth on SBA and takes advantage of observed pigment production.

Table 1 lists the organisms that are very fastidious and grow poorly or not at all on SBA. Species like *Acinetobacter*

TABLE 1 Dichotomous identification algorithm for gram-negative bacteria with poor or no growth on SBA[a]

1a. Growth on SBA p^w → 2
1b. Growth on SBA n → 14
2a. Cells: tiny coccobacilli → 3
2b. Cells: diplococci or coccobacilli → *Neisseria*, except *N. gonorrhoeae* (chapter 32), *Moraxella* (chapter 42)
2c. Cells: rods → 6
2d. Cells: fusiform rods → *Capnocytophaga* (chapter 33)
3a. Urease p → *Brucella* spp. (chapter 44)
3b. Urease n → 4
4a. Oxidase n → *Francisella* (chapter 44)
4b. Oxidase p → 5
5a. Hydrogen sulfide production on KIA p → *Francisella philomiragia* (chapter 44)
5b. Hydrogen sulfide production on KIA n → *Bordetella* spp. (chapter 43)
6a. Colony color pink → *Asaia*, *Azospirillum*, *Methylobacterium*, *Roseomonas* (chapter 42)
6b. Colony color other → 7
7a. Cauliflower-like colonies → *Bartonella* spp. (chapter 46)
7b. Other colonies → 8
8a. Ornithine p, acidification of glucose n → *Eikenella* (chapter 33)
8b. Ornithine n, acidification of glucose p → 9
9a. Acidification of lactose p → 10
9b. Acidification of lactose n → 11
10a. Acidification of sucrose p, xylose n → *Aggregatibacter aphrophilus* (chapter 33)
10b. Acidification of sucrose n, xylose p → *Dysgonomonas* (chapter 33)
11a. Acidification of sucrose p → 12
11b. Acidification of sucrose n → 13
12a. Alkaline phosphatase p → *Suttonella* (chapter 33)
12b. Alkaline phosphatase n → *Cardiobacterium* spp. (chapter 33)
13a. Catalase p → *Aggregatibacter actinomycetemcomitans* (chapter 33)
13b. Catalase n → *Simonsiella* (chapter 33)
14a. Chocolate agar required for growth → 15
14b. Buffered charcoal yeast extract agar required for growth → 18
14c. Brain heart infusion agar with serum required for growth → 19
14d. Regan-Lowe agar or Bordet-Gengou agar required for growth → *Bordetella pertussis* (chapter 43)

15.   Chocolate agar required for growth
15a. Cells: diplococci or coccobacilli → *Neisseria gonorrhoeae* (chapter 32)
15b. Cells: bacilli → 16
16a. Cauliflower-like colonies → *Bartonella*, *Afipia* (chapter 46)
16b. Other colonies → 17
17a. Requirement for hemin (X) and/or adenine dinucleotide (V) p → *Haemophilus* spp. (chapter 34)
17b. Requirement for hemin (X) and/or adenine dinucleotide (V) n → *Francisella* spp. (chapter 44)

18.   Buffered charcoal yeast extract agar required for growth
18a. Cells: long rods → *Legionella* spp. (chapter 45)
18b. Cells: regular rods → *Francisella* spp. (chapter 44)

19.   Brain heart infusion agar with serum required for growth
19a. Cells: pleomorphic, bended filamentous rods → *Streptobacillus* spp. (chapter 33)
19b. Cells: small rods → *Bartonella* spp., *Afipia* spp. (chapter 46)

[a]p, positive; pp, strongly (quickly) positive; (p), delayed positive; p^w, weakly positive; p/(p), positive or delayed positive; p/p^w, positive or weakly positive; n, negative; → [number], go to number indicated further on in the table. Chapter numbers in parentheses indicate the chapters in which the organism(s) is described further in this *Manual*.

TABLE 2 Dichotomous identification algorithm for aerobically growing gram-negative bacteria which form purple or pink colonies on SBA[a]

1a. Colony color purple on SBA → *Chromobacterium* (chapter 33)
1b. Colony color pink on SBA → 2
2a. Fermentation p (butt of KIA yellow) → some *Serratia* species (chapter 37)
2b. Fermentation n (butt of KIA unchanged) → 3
3a. β-Galactosidase p → *Azospirillum* spp. (chapter 42)
3b. β-Galactosidase n → 4
4a. Desferrioxamine S, nitrate reductase p → *Roseomonas* genomospecies 4 (chapter 42)
4b. Desferrioxamine R, nitrate reductase n → 5
5a. Trypsin p → 6
5b. Trypsin n → 7
6a. Urease p → *Methylobacterium* spp. (chapter 42)
6b. Urease n → *Asaia* spp. (chapter 42)
7a. Pyrrolidonyl aminopeptidase p → 8
7b. Pyrrolidonyl aminopeptidase n → 9
8a. Oxidase p[w] → *Roseomonas gilardii* (chapter 42)
8b. Oxidase n → *Roseomonas mucosa* (chapter 42)
9a. Acidification of ethylene glycol p → *Roseomonas cervicalis* (chapter 42)
9b. Acidification of ethylene glycol n → *Roseomonas* genomospecies 5 (chapter 42)

[a]p, positive; pp, strongly (quickly) positive; (p), delayed positive; p[w], weakly positive; p/(p), positive or delayed positive; p/p[w], positive or weakly positive; n, negative; → [number], go to number indicated further on in the table. Chapter numbers in parentheses indicate the chapters in which the organism(s) is described further in this *Manual*.

parvus or most *Moraxella* spp. also grow poorly or slowly, but clearly visible colonies are formed after 48 h at 37°C; these are described elsewhere (see Table 4). The organisms that grow on SBA and that exhibit pink or purple colonies are included in Table 2. For those species that grow well on SBA and do not form pink or purple colonies, proceed following the steps as outlined below.

Day 1
Stab inoculate a KIA tube. Incubate overnight at 30 to 37°C.

Day 2: Interpretation of KIA (differentiation between fermenters and nonfermenters)

Butt and slant yellow: positive for fermentation of both lactose and glucose. Refer to Table 3. Only butt yellow: negative for lactose, positive for glucose fermentation. Refer to Table 3. No yellow color: negative for both lactose and glucose fermentation, i.e., nonfermenters. Proceed with testing outlined for day 3 below.

Day 3: Start of identification of nonfermenters (Table 4)
Inoculate two TSA plates and incubate overnight at 30 to 35°C. Two SBA plates can be used, if more appropriate for more fastidious organisms, but pigmentation is sometimes

(*Text continues on page 549*)

TABLE 3 Dichotomous identification algorithm for aerobically growing gram-negative bacteria fermenting glucose (facultative anaerobes)[a]

1a. Oxidase p → 2
1b. Oxidase n → 6
2a. Growth at 6% NaCl p (halotolerance p) → *Vibrio* spp. (chapter 39)
2b. Growth at 6% NaCl n (halotolerance n) → 3
3a. Motility p → 4
3b. Motility n → 5
4a. Lysine decarboxylase p → *Plesiomonas* spp. (chapter 37), *Aeromonas hydrophila* and *A. veronii* bv. sobria (chapter 37)
4b. Lysine decarboxylase n → other *Aeromonas* spp. (chapter 38)
5a. Fermentation of sucrose p → *Pasteurella* spp., *Actinobacillus* spp. (chapter 33)
5b. Fermentation of sucrose n → *Pasteurella bettyae* (chapter 33)
6a. Growth at 6% NaCl p (halotolerance p) → *Vibrio metschnikovii* (chapter 39)
6b. Growth at 6% NaCl n (halotolerance n) → 7
7a. Growth on MacConkey agar n → *Pasteurella bettyae* (chapter 33)
7b. Growth on MacConkey agar p → 8
8a. Fermentation of lactose, trehalose or xylose p → *Enterobacteriaceae* (chapters 35–37)
8b. Fermentation of lactose, trehalose and xylose n → 9
9a. Phenylalanine deaminase p → *Providencia* spp., *Morganella* spp. (chapter 37)
9b. Phenylalanine deaminase n → 10
10a. Hydrogen sulfide production in KIA p → *Edwardsiella* spp. (chapter 37)
10b. Hydrogen sulfide production in KIA n → *Pasteurella bettyae* (chapter 33)

[a]p, positive; pp, strongly (quickly) positive; (p), delayed positive; p[w], weakly positive; p/(p), positive or delayed positive; p/p[w], positive or weakly positive; n, negative; → [number], go to number indicated further on in the table. Chapter numbers in parentheses indicate the chapters in which the organism(s) is described further in this *Manual*.

TABLE 4 Dichotomous identification algorithm for aerobically growing gram-negative nonfermenters (strict aerobes)[a]

1a. Hydrogen sulfide production in KIA p → 2
1b. Hydrogen sulfide production in KIA n → 3

Hydrogen sulfide production-positive, gram-negative nonfermenters: *Shewanella* (chapter 42)
2a. Requirement for NaCl n, acidification of sucrose p → *Shewanella putrefaciens*
2b. Requirement for NaCl p, acidification of sucrose n → *Shewanella algae*

Hydrogen sulfide production-negative, gram-negative nonfermenters
3a. Green pigment on MHA p (pyoverdin production p[b]) → 4
3b. Green pigment on MHA n (pyoverdin production n) → 10
4a. Growth at 42°C p, assimilation of acetamide p → *P. aeruginosa*, partim pyoverdin p (65%)
4b. Growth at 42°C n, assimilation of acetamide n → 5
5a. Xylose n → 6
5b. Xylose p → 7
6a. Growth at 6% NaCl p (halotolerance p) → *Pseudomonas mosselii*
6b. Growth at 6% NaCl n (halotolerance n) → *Pseudomonas monteilii*
7a. Nitrate reductase p → 8
7b. Nitrate reductase n → 9
8a. Nitrite reductase p → *Pseudomonas veronii* (plus *Pseudomonas fluorescens*, partim pyoverdin p [95%], partim nitrate reductase p [20%], partim nitrite reductase p [5%])
8b. Nitrite reductase n → *Pseudomonas fluorescens*, partim pyoverdin p (95%), partim nitrate reductase p (20%), partim nitrite reductase p (5%)
9a. Gelatinase p → *Pseudomonas fluorescens*, partim pyoverdin p (95%), partim nitrate reductase n (80%)
9b. Gelatinase n → *Pseudomonas putida*, partim pyoverdin p (95%)
10a. Indole p → 11
10b. Indole n → 22

Hydrogen sulfide production-negative, indole production-positive, gram-negative nonfermenters
11a. Trypsin n → *Balneatrix alpica* (chapter 42)
11b. Trypsin p → 12
12a. Pyrrolidonyl aminopeptidase n → *Bergeyella zoohelcum* (chapter 42)
12b. Pyrrolidonyl aminopeptidase p → 13
13a. Acidification of glucose n → *Weeksella virosa* (chapter 42)
13b. Acidification of glucose p → 14
14a. Acidification of mannitol p → 15
14b. Acidification of mannitol n → 16
15a. Urease p → *Elizabethkingia miricola* (chapter 42)
15b. Urease n → *Elizabethkingia meningoseptica* (chapter 42)
16a. Growth at 42°C p → *Chryseobacterium gleum* (chapter 42)
16b. Growth at 42°C n → 17
17a. Urease p → *Wautersiella falsenii* (chapter 42)
17b. Urease n → 18
18a. Esculin hydrolysis p → 19
18b. Esculin hydrolysis n → 21
19a. Acidification of ethylene glycol p → *Chryseobacterium hominis* (chapter 42)
19b. Acidification of ethylene glycol n → 20
20a. Acidification of xylose p, beta-hemolysis on SBA after 3 days n → *Flavobacterium mizutaii* (chapter 42)
20b. Acidification of xylose n, beta-hemolysis on SBA after 3 days p → *Chryseobacterium indologenes* (chapter 42)
21a. Gelatinase pp, growth on MacConkey agar p → *Empedobacter brevis* (chapter 42)
21b. Gelatinase p, growth on MacConkey agar n → *Chryseobacterium anthropi* (chapter 42)

Hydrogen sulfide production-negative, indole production-negative, gram-negative nonfermenters
22a. Oxidase n → 23
22b. Oxidase p → 33

Hydrogen sulfide production-negative, indole production-negative, oxidase negative, gram-negative nonfermenters
23a. Brown pigment on TSA, i.e., tyrosine hydrolase p → 24
23b. Other → 25
24a. Urease p → *Bordetella parapertussis* (chapter 43)
24b. Urease n → *Bordetella holmesii* (chapter 43)
25a. Trypsin p → 26
25b. Trypsin n → 28
26a. Pyrrolidonyl aminopeptidase p → 27
26b. Pyrrolidonyl aminopeptidase n → *Stenotrophomonas maltophilia* (chapter 41)
27a. Arginine dihydrolase p, esculin hydrolysis p → *Pseudomonas luteola* (chapter 40)

(*Continued on next page*)

TABLE 4 Dichotomous identification algorithm for aerobically growing gram-negative nonfermenters (strict aerobes)[a] *(Continued)*

27b. Arginine dihydrolase n, esculin hydrolysis n → *Pseudomonas oryzihabitans* (chapter 40)
28a. Motility n → *Acinetobacter* (chapter 42)
28b. Motility p → 29
29a. Acidification of glucose p → 30
29b. Acidification of glucose n → 31
30a. Alkaline phosphatase p → *Burkholderia cepacia* complex, partim oxidase n (1–4%, up to 14% for *Burkholderia pyrrocinia*) (chapter 41)
30b. Alkaline phosphatase n → *Burkholderia gladioli* (chapter 41)
31a. Gelatinase p → *Bordetella ansorpii* (chapter 43)
31b. Gelatinase n → 32
32a. Desferrioxamine S, growth at 42°C p → *Kerstersia gyiorum* (chapter 43)
32b. Desferrioxamine R, growth at 42°C n → *Bordetella trematum* (chapter 43)

Hydrogen sulfide production-negative, indole production-negative, oxidase-positive, gram-negative nonfermenters
33a. Trypsin p → 34
33b. Trypsin n → 63
34a. Pyrrolidonyl aminopeptidase p → 35
34b. Pyrrolidonyl aminopeptidase n → 49

Hydrogen sulfide production-negative, indole production-negative, oxidase-positive, gram-negative nonfermenters; trypsin positive, pyrrolidonyl aminopeptidase positive
35a. Urease n → 36
35b. Urease p → 40
36a. Vancomycin S → *Sphingomonas* spp., partim pyrrolidonyl aminopeptidase p (25%) (chapter 42)
36b. Vancomycin R → 37
37a. Arginine dihydrolase p → 38
37b. Arginine dihydrolase n → 39
38a. Growth at 42°C p → *Pseudomonas aeruginosa*, partim pyoverdin production n (35%), partim pyrrolidonyl aminopeptidase p (95%) (chapter 40)
38b. Growth at 42°C n → *Pseudomonas fluorescens*, partim pyoverdin production n (5%), partim pyrrolidonyl aminopeptidase p (60%) (chapter 40)
39a. Desferrioxamine S, alkaline phosphatase p/pp, acidification of glucose n, mannitol n and xylose n → *Brevundimonas diminuta*, partim pyrrolidonyl aminopeptidase p (20%) (chapter 41)
39b. Desferrioxamine R, alkaline phosphatase n, acidification of glucose p, mannitol p and xylose p, mucoid colonies → *Inquilinus limosus*, partim urease n (65%) (chapter 42)
40a. Nitrate reductase n → 41
40b. Nitrate reductase p → 45
41a. Desferrioxamine S → *Myroides odoratus* (chapter 42)
41b. Desferrioxamine R → 42
42a. Alkaline phosphatase n, mucoid colonies → *Inquilinus limosus*, partim urease p (35%) (chapter 42)
42b. Alkaline phosphatase p → 43
43a. Nitrite reductase p → *Myroides odoratimimus* (chapter 42)
43b. Nitrite reductase n → 44
44a. Acidification of mannitol p, of ethylene glycol p → *Sphingobacterium spiritivorum* (chapter 42)
44b. Acidification of mannitol n, of ethylene glycol n → *Sphingobacterium multivorum* (chapter 42)
45a. Alkaline phosphatase p, motility n, acidification of ethylene glycol n → *Sphingobacterium thalpophilum* (chapter 42)
45b. Alkaline phosphatase n, motility p, acidification of ethylene glycol p → 46
46a. β-galactosidase (ONPG) p → 47
46b. β-galactosidase (ONPG) n → 48
47a. Tributyrate esterase pp, acidification of raffinose n → *Pannonibacter phragmitetus* (chapter 42)
47b. Tributyrate esterase n/(p), acidification of raffinose p → *Rhizobium radiobacter* (chapter 42)
48a. Colistin S → *Ochrobactrum anthropi* (chapter 42)
48b. Colistin R → *Ochrobactrum intermedium* (chapter 42)

Hydrogen sulfide production-negative, indole production-negative, oxidase-positive, gram-negative nonfermenters; trypsin positive, pyrrolidonyl aminopeptidase negative
49a. Urease p → *Alishewanella fetalis* (chapter 42)
49b. Urease n → 51
50a. Alkaline phosphatase p → 51
50b. Alkaline phosphatase n → 53
51a. Esculin hydrolysis n → *Brevundimonas diminuta*, partim pyrrolidonyl aminopeptidase n (80%) (chapter 41)
51b. Esculin hydrolysis p → 52
52a. Vancomycin S, desferrioxamine R → *Sphingomonas* spp., partim pyrrolidonyl aminopeptidase n (75%) (chapter 42)
52b. Vancomycin R, desferrioxamine S → *Brevundimonas vesicularis* (chapter 41)
53a. Nitrate reductase n → 54

(Continued on next page)

TABLE 4 *(Continued)*

53b. Nitrate reductase p → 56
54a. Desferrioxamine S, arginine dihydrolase n, acidification of glucose n, of xylose n → *Alcaligenes faecalis*, partim trypsin p (30%) (chapter 43)
54b. Desferrioxamine R, arginine dihydrolase p, acidification of glucose p, of xylose p → 55
55a. Gelatinase p → *Pseudomonas fluorescens*, partim pyoverdin n (5%), partim pyrrolidonyl aminopeptidase n (40%), partim nitrate reductase n (80%)
55b. Gelatinase n → *Pseudomonas putida*, partim pyoverdin n (5%) (chapter 40)
56a. Starch hydrolysis p, cauliflower, often yellowish colonies → *Pseudomonas stutzeri* (chapter 40)
56b. Starch hydrolysis n → 57
57a. Nitrite reductase p → 58
57b. Nitrite reductase n → 60
58a. Growth at 42°C p → 59
58b. Growth at 42°C n → *Pseudomonas fluorescens*, partim pyoverdin n (5%), partim pyrrolidonyl aminopeptidase n (40%), partim nitrate reductase p (20%), partim nitrite reductase p (5%) (chapter 40)
59a. Gelatinase n, acidification of mannitol n, often yellowish → *P. mendocina* (chapter 40)
59b. Gelatinase p (80%), acidification of mannitol p (70%) → *P. aeruginosa*, partim pyoverdin n (35%), partim pyrrolidonyl amino-peptidase n (5%), partim nitrite reductase p (95%) (chapter 40)
60a. Acidification of glucose p → 61
60b. Acidification of glucose n → 62
61a. Growth at 42°C p → *P. aeruginosa*: partim pyoverdin n (35%), partim pyrrolidonyl aminopeptidase n (5%), partim nitrite reductase n (5%), or *P. pseudoalcaligenes*, partim acidification of glucose p (10%) (chapter 40)
61b. Growth at 42°C p → *Pseudomonas fluorescens*, partim pyoverdin n (5%), partim pyrrolidonyl aminopeptidase n (40%), partim nitrate reductase p (20%), partim nitrite reductase p (5%) (chapter 40)
62a. Acidification of fructose p^w → *P. pseudoalcaligenes*, partim acidification of glucose n (90%) (chapter 40)
62b. Acidification of fructose n → *P. alcaligenes* (chapter 40)
63a. Pyrrolidonyl aminopeptidase p → 64
63b. Pyrrolidonyl aminopeptidase n → 84

Hydrogen sulfide production-negative, indole production-negative, oxidase-positive, gram-negative nonfermenters; trypsin negative, pyrrolidonyl aminopeptidase positive

64a. Fastidious, small colonies on SBA, plump coccobacilli → *Moraxella atlantae* (chapter 42)
64b. Good growth → 65
65a. Desferrioxamine S → 66
65b. Desferrioxamine R → 67
66a. Urease p/(p), nitrite reductase p, acidification of glucose p, of xylose p, colistin R → *Ralstonia pickettii* (chapter 41)
66b. Urease n, nitrite reductase n, acidification of carbohydrates n, colistin S → *Comamonas terrigena* (chapter 41)
67a. Lysine decarboxylase p → *Burkholderia cenocepacia*, partim pyrrolidonyl aminopeptidase p (few) (chapter 41)
67b. Lysine decarboxylase n → 68
68a. Beta-galactosidase p → *Herbaspirillum* spp. (chapter 41)
68b. Beta-galactosidase n → 69
69a. Motility n → *Bordetella petrii* (chapter 43)
69b. Motility p → 70
70a. Nitrate reductase p → 71
70b. Nitrate reductase n → 78
71a. Urease p/(p), arginine dihydrolase p/(p) → 72
71b. Urease n, arginine dihydrolase n → 73
72a. Gelatinase p → *Acidovorax facilis* (chapter 41)
72b. Gelatinase n → *Acidovorax delafieldii* (chapter 41)
73a. Colistin R → 74
73b. Colistin S → 75
74a. Acidification of mannitol p, of xylose n → *Delftia acidovorans* (chapter 41)
     In addition: assimilation of acetamide p ↔ *Comamonas testosteroni*
74b. Acidification of mannitol n, of xylose p → *Achromobacter xylosoxidans* (chapter 43)
75a. Nitrite reductase p → 76
75b. Nitrite reductase n → 77
76a. Acidification of glucose (p) → *Acidovorax temperans* (chapter 41)
76b. Acidification of glucose n → *Achromobacter denitrificans* (chapter 43)
77a. Alkaline phosphatase p^w → *Cupriavidus gilardii*, partim pyrrolidonyl aminopeptidase p (15%), partim nitrate reductase p (50%)
77b. Alkaline phosphatase n → 78
78a. Flagellation polar or bipolar → *Comamonas testosteroni* (chapter 41)
     In addition: assimilation (alkalinization) of acetamide n ↔ *Delftia acidovorans*
78b. Flagellation peritrichous → *Achromobacter piechaudii* (chapter 43)
79a. Acidification of glucose p, of xylose p → 80
79b. Acidification of glucose n, of xylose n, of mannitol n → 81

(Continued on next page)

TABLE 4 Dichotomous identification algorithm for aerobically growing gram-negative nonfermenters (strict aerobes)[a] *(Continued)*

80a. Acidification of mannitol p → *Ralstonia mannitolilytica* (chapter 43)
80b. Acidification of mannitol n → *Ralstonia insidiosa* (chapter 43)
81a. Urease p → *Cupriavidus pauculus* (chapter 41)
81b. Urease n → 82
82a. Alkaline phosphatase p[w] → *Cupriavidus gilardii*, partim pyrrolidonyl aminopeptidase p (15%), partim nitrate reductase n (50%) (chapter 41)
82b. Alkaline phosphatase n → 83
83a. Acidification of ethylene glycol p → *Bordetella hinzii*
83b. Acidification of ethylene glycol n → *Cupriavidus respiraculi* (chapter 43)

Hydrogen sulfide production-negative, indole production-negative, oxidase-positive, gram-negative nonfermenters; trypsin negative, pyrrolidonyl aminopeptidase negative

84a. Acidification of glucose p → 85
84b. Acidification of glucose n → 92
85a. Colistin R → 86
85b. Colistin S → 90
86a. Acidification of ethylene glycol p → 87
86b. Acidification of ethylene glycol n → 88
87a. Arginine dihydrolase p → *Burkholderia pseudomallei* (chapter 41)
87b. Arginine dihydrolase n → *Psychrobacter immobilis* (chapter 42)
88a. Desferrioxamine S → *Burkholderia multivorans*, partim desferrioxamine S (85%) (chapter 41)
88b. Desferrioxamine R → 89
89a. Sucrose p → *Burkholderia cenocepacia*, partim pyrrolidonyl aminopeptidase n (most), partim sucrose p (90%) (chapter 41)
89b. Sucrose n → *Burkholderia multivorans*, partim desferrioxamine R (15%) (chapter 41), or *Burkholderia cenocepacia*, partim pyrrolidonyl aminopeptidase n (most), partim sucrose n (10%) (chapter 41)
90a. Urease n → *Psychrobacter faecalis* (chapter 42)
90b. Urease p → 91
91a. Nitrate reductase p, arginine dihydrolase n, mucoid, yellowish colonies, O-shaped coccoid cells → *Paracoccus yeei* (chapter 42)
91b. Nitrate reductase n, arginine dihydrolase p → *Haematobacter missouriensis* (chapter 42)
92a. Desferrioxamine S → 93
92b. Desferrioxamine R → 101
93a. Urease p → *Oligella ureolytica* (chapter 42)
93b. Urease n → 94
94a. Motility p → 95
94b. Motility n → 97
95a. Nitrate reductase n, nitrite reductase p → *Alcaligenes faecalis*, partim trypsin n (70%)
95b. Nitrate reductase p, nitrite reductase n → 96
96a. Growth at 42°C p → *Comamonas kerstersii*
96b. Growth at 42°C n → *Comamonas aquatica*
97a. Gelatinase p → *Moraxella lacunata*
97b. Gelatinase n → 98
98a. Acidification of ethylene glycol p → 99
98b. Acidification of ethylene glycol n → 100
99a. Tributyrate esterase p, phenylalanine deaminase n → *Moraxella canis*
99b. Tributyrate esterase n, phenylalanine deaminase p[w] → *Oligella urethralis*
100a. Nitrite reductase p → *Moraxella catarrhalis*
100b. Nitrite reductase n → *Moraxella nonliquefaciens*
101a. Urease p → 102
101b. Urease n → 104
102a. Motility p → *Bordetella bronchiseptica*
102b. Motility n → 103
103a. Arginine dihydrolase p, Tween esterase n → *Haematobacter massiliensis*
103b. Arginine dihydrolase n, Tween esterase p → *Psychrobacter phenylpyruvicus*
104a. Motility p → *Cupriavidus gilardii*, partim pyrrolidonyl aminopeptidase n (85%)
104b. Motility n → 105
105a. Nitrite reductase p → *Psychrobacter pulmonis*
105b. Nitrite reductase n → 106
106a. Acidification of ethylene glycol p → *Moraxella osloensis*
106b. Acidification of ethylene glycol n → *Moraxella lincolnii*

[a]Nonfermenters are usually referred to as strict aerobes, although some nonfermenters, such as all denitrifiers (producing nitrogen gas from nitrite), can grow anaerobically when nitrate and/or nitrite is available as an alternative electron acceptor in oxidative respiration, instead of gaseous oxygen. p, positive; pp, strongly (quickly) positive; (p), delayed positive; p[w], weakly positive; p/(p), positive or delayed positive; p/p[w], positive or weakly positive; n, negative; → [number], go to number indicated further on in the table. Chapter numbers in parentheses indicate the chapters in which the organism(s) is described further in this *Manual*. partim, Latin term used to indicate "the part that is."

[b]*P. monteilii*, *P. mosselii*, and *P. veronii* are 100%, *P. fluorescens* and *P. putida* 95%, and *P. aeruginosa* 65% pyoverdin production p.

more clear on TSA. Inoculation of TSA (or SBA) is used in order to record pigment production, to obtain dense growth on day 4, and to prepare a dense inoculum to carry out rapid enzymatic tests and to inoculate other media, as described below. Two plates are inoculated to keep one for prolonged testing, if necessary. Proceed with day 4.

Day 4: Recording of oxidase and 10 enzymatic tests

A. Perform and record the oxidase test by picking colonies from TSA with a swab to which a drop of oxidase reagent has been added. The test is positive when colonies turn red to purple-blue within 2 min.
B. To perform the following 10 enzymatic tests, use one of the two TSA plates. As previously mentioned and critical to the accuracy of test results, all of these reactions require a heavy inoculum, that is, at least a 4 to 5 McFarland.
   1. Alkaline phosphatase. Prepare inoculum in 0.5 ml of AD containing one alkaline phosphatase tablet (Rosco). Incubate for 4 to 5 h. A yellow color indicates a positive result.
   2. Trypsin, i.e., benzyl-arginine aminopeptidase. Prepare suspension in 0.5 ml of AD containing one trypsin tablet (Rosco). Incubate for 4 to 5 h. Add 1 drop of cinnamaldehyde reagent. An orange to pink color within 5 min indicates a positive result.
   3. Pyrrolidonyl aminopeptidase. Prepare suspension in 0.5 ml of AD containing one pyrrolidonyl aminopeptidase tablet (Rosco). Incubate for 4 to 5 h. Add 1 drop of cinnamaldehyde reagent. An orange to pink color, usually within 5 min, indicates a positive result.
   4. β-Galactosidase. Prepare suspension in 0.5 ml of AD containing one ONPG tablet (Rosco). Incubate for 4 to 5 h. A yellow color indicates a positive result.
   5. Indole production. Prepare suspension in 0.5 ml of 0.3% tryptophan solution. Incubate for 4 to 5 h. Add 8 to 12 drops of Kovács reagent. Indole production is positive when the supernatant turns red.
   6. Urease. Prepare suspension in 1 ml of liquid Christensen urea. Incubate for 4 to 5 h. A pink color indicates a positive result. Record for up to 1 to 2 days, when still negative after 4 to 5 h, and when no final identification has yet been reached.
   7. Nitrate reductase. Prepare a suspension in 1 ml of 0.1% KNO$_3$ broth. Incubate for 4 to 5 h. Take 0.5 ml of the solution and add a drop of Griess A and subsequently 1 drop of Griess B. The test is positive when it immediately turns red, indicating the presence of nitrite. The test may also be positive when colorless, in the case of strong nitrite reductase activity. When the result is not clear, repeat after 24 h with the remaining 0.5 ml of solution.
   8. Nitrite reductase. Prepare a McFarland 6 to 8 suspension in 1 ml of 0.001% NaNO$_2$ broth. Incubate for 4 to 5 h. Take 0.5 ml of the solution and add a drop of Griess A and subsequently add a drop of Griess B. The test is positive when colorless, indicating the absence of nitrite. When the result is not clear, repeat after 24 h with the remaining 0.5 ml of solution.
   9. Lysine decarboxylase. Prepare suspension in 1 ml of Moeller broth plus 1% lysine. Cover with paraffin oil. Incubate for 4 to 5 h. A purple color of the medium indicates a positive result. Record for up to 1 to 2 days.
   10. Arginine dihydrolase. Prepare suspension in 1 ml of Moeller broth plus 1% arginine. Cover with paraffin oil. Incubate for 4 to 5 h. A purple color of the medium indicates a positive result. Record for up to 1 to 2 days, e.g., for some delayed positive strains of *Pseudomonas pseudoalcaligenes* or of *Haematobacter* spp.

Further simplification is possible by preparing a McFarland 4 to 5 suspension in 1.5 ml of AD, dividing this into three aliquots of 0.5 ml to which disks for tests 1 to 3 are added. Also, tests 4 and 5 can be carried out in the same tube, by adding the ONPG disk to the tryptophan solution. In that case, after 4 to 5 h of incubation, first read color for β-galactosidase, before adding Kovács reagent to read the indole production.
C. Testing for susceptibility to colistin, desferrioxamine, and vancomycin. Starting from TSA, prepare a 0.5 McFarland suspension, inoculate one MHA plate to obtain confluent growth, and add colistin (10-μg), desferrioxamine (250-μg), and vancomycin (30-μg) disks. Incubate overnight at 30 to 37°C. → Day 5.A.
D. MHA is preferred for susceptibility testing, because green pigmentation due to pyoverdin (fluorescein production) can be scored more easily on this medium. → Day 5.B.
E. Testing for motility. Starting from TSA, stab inoculate under the surface of soft agar (0.5% TSA), preferably in a small (e.g., 5-ml) petri dish. Incubate overnight at 30°C. → Day 5.C.
F. Testing acidification of carbohydrates. Starting from TSA, inoculate four LPPR tubes, one each with 1% glucose, 1% mannitol, 1% xylose, and 2% ethylene glycol, and incubate for 24 h at 30°C. → Day 5.D.

Day 5: Recording of susceptibility, green colony pigmentation (pyoverdin production), motility, and acidification of carbohydrates

A. Record susceptibility to different antibacterial agents: any clear zone of inhibition is considered as susceptible for diagnostic purposes. A complete lack of a zone of inhibition is interpreted as resistant.
B. Record pyoverdin production as the presence of diffusible green pigment on MHA.
C. Record motility: motility is positive when the culture is spreading from the inoculation zone.
D. Record acidification of glucose, mannitol, xylose, and ethylene glycol. The test is positive when the red color of the medium turns orange to yellow. Extend incubation up to 7 days when necessary.

Prolongation of reading is done when a test is still negative or doubtful and when no final identification (on the basis of the other test results) has yet been reached. When final identification is not reached on the basis of these rapid tests, additional tests should be used (see above, chapter 17, and individual chapters on organism groups). These include flagellum stain, gelatin hydrolysis, esculin hydrolysis, starch hydrolysis, growth on MacConkey agar, acidification of sucrose or of raffinose, tributyrate esterase and Tween 80 esterase, acetamide assimilation (alkalinization), requirement for NaCl, halotolerance, and growth at 42°C. Selection of these tests depends on the group of species that has been suggested already on the basis of the rapid tests and can be deduced from the dichotomous identification algorithm in Table 4 and/or from Table 5.

(Text continues on page 558)

TABLE 5 Overview of biochemical characteristics of the gram-negative nonfermenters[a]

Species	Chapter	Cell morphology	Colony color/pigment/ morphology	Hydrogen sulfide production	Indole production	Oxidase
H₂S production positive						
Shewanella putrefaciens	42	Rods	Often mucoid. Greenish discoloration on SBA.	**p**	n	p
Shewanella algae	42	Rods	Often mucoid. Greenish discoloration on SBA.	**p**	n	p
H₂S production negative, green pigment on MHA						
Pseudomonas aeruginosa, partim pyoverdin p (65%)	40	Rods	**Green diffusible pigment on MHA**	**n**	n	p
Pseudomonas mosselii	40	Rods	**Green diffusible pigment on MHA**	**n**	n	p
Pseudomonas monteilii	40	Rods	**Green diffusible pigment on MHA**	**n**	n	p
Pseudomonas fluorescens, partim pyoverdin p (95%), partim nitrate reductase p (20%)	40	Rods	**Green diffusible pigment on MHA**	**n**	n	p
Pseudomonas veronii	40	Rods	**Green diffusible pigment on MHA**	**n**	n	p
Pseudomonas fluorescens, partim pyoverdin p (95%), partim nitrate reductase n (80%)	40	Rods	**Green diffusible pigment on MHA**	**n**	n	p
Pseudomonas putida, partim pyoverdin p (95%)	40	Rods	**Green diffusible pigment on MHA**	**n**	n	p
H₂S production negative, no green pigment on MHA, indole production positive						
Balneatrix alpica	42	Rods	Yellowish	n	**p**	p
Bergeyella zoohelcum	42	Rods	Mucoid	n	**p**	p
Weeksella virosa	42	Rods	Mucoid	n	**p**	p
Elizabethkingia miricola	42	Rods	Pigment n or pale yellow, flexirubin n	n	**p**	p
Elizabethkingia meningoseptica	42	Rods	Pigment n or pale yellow, flexirubin n	n	**p**	p
Chryseobacterium gleum	42	Rods	Yellow, flexirubin p	n	**p**	p
Wautersiella falsenii	42	Rods	Pigment n or pale yellow, flexirubin n	n	**p**	p
Chryseobacterium hominis	42	Rods	Pigment n or pale yellow, flexirubin n	n	**p**	p
Flavobacterium mizutaii	42	Rods	Pale yellow, flexirubin n	n	**p**	p
Chryseobacterium indologenes	42	Rods	Yellow, flexirubin p (75%)	n	**p**	p
Empedobacter brevis	42	Rods	Pale yellow, flexirubin n	n	**p**	p
Chryseobacterium anthropi	42	Rods	Flexirubin n, often sticky	n	**p**	p
H₂S production negative, no green pigment on MHA, indole production negative, oxidase negative						
Bordetella parapertussis	43	Small cells	**Brown on TSA, i.e., tyrosine hydrolase p**	**n**	**n**	**n**
Bordetella holmesii	43	Small cells	**Brown on TSA, i.e., tyrosine hydrolase p**	**n**	**n**	**n**
Pseudomonas luteola	40	Rods	*Not brown on TSA, yellow*	**n**	**n**	**n**
Pseudomonas oryzihabitans	40	Rods	*Not brown on TSA, yellow*	**n**	**n**	**n**

Trypsin	Pyrrolidonyl aminopeptidase	Susceptibility to desferrioxamine	Urease	Nitrate reductase	Nitrite reductase	Motility	Lysine decarboxylase	Arginine dihydrolase	Alkaline phosphatase	Growth at 42°C	Gelatinase	Acidification of glucose	Acidification of mannitol	Acidification of xylose	Acidification of ethylene glycol	Susceptibility to colistin	Esculin hydrolysis	Starch hydrolysis	β-Galactosidase (ONPG)	Additional characteristics
p	p	R	n	p	n	p	n	n	p	v	p	p^w	n	n	p	S	n	o	o	Requirement for NaCl n
p	p	R	n	p	n	p	n	n	p	v	p	**n**	n	n	p	S	n	o	o	*Requirement for NaCl p*
p	95	R	n	p	95	p	n	p	n	**p**	80	p	70	90	p	S	n	n	n	**Assimilation of acetamide p**
o	o	o	o	n	o	p	n	p	o	n	n	p	75	n	o	o	n	10	o	*Assimilation of acetamide n, growth at 6% NaCl p*
o	o	o	50	n	p	p	n	p	o	n	15	p	n	n	o	o	n	n	o	*Assimilation of acetamide n, growth at 6% NaCl n*
p	n*	R	n	**p**	5	p	n	p	n	n	p	p	55	*p*	38	S	n	n	n	**Assimilation of acetamide n**
o	o	o	25	**p**	*p*	p	n	p	o	n	15	p	o	*p*	o	o	o	o	o	*Assimilation of acetamide n*
p	n*	R	n	**n**	5	p	n	p	n	n	p	**p**	55	*p*	38	S	n	n	n	*Assimilation of acetamide n*
p	n	R	n	**n**	n	p	n	p	n	n	**n**	p	25	*p*	p	S	n	n	n	*Assimilation of acetamide n*
n	n	S	n	p	n	p	n	n	p	p	p	n	n			S	n	p	n	
p	**n**	S	p	n	n	p	n	n	p	p	n	n	n			R	n	n	n	
p	*p*	S	n	n	n	p	n	p	p	**n**	n	n	n			S	n	n	n	
p	*p*	R	p	n	n	p	n	p	p	*p*	*p*	n	n			R	n	n	p	
p	*p*	R	**n**	n	85	p	n	p	50	*p*	*p*	n	p			R	p	n	p	
p	*p*	R	75	75	50	p	n	p	*p*	p	p	n	25	p		R	p	n	p	
p	*p*	S 10	p	n	15	p	n	p	n	p/(p)	*p*	n	n	45		R	55	n	30	
p	*p*	R	**n**	75	75	n	n	p	*p*	n	n	n		p	S 15	p	p	n	
p	*p*	R	**n**	n	75	n	n	p	*p*	n	*p*	n	p		n	R	p	p	n	Beta-hemolysis on SBA after 3 days n
p	*p*	R	n	30	15	n	n	p	n	*p*	*p*	p	n		n	R	p	p	n	*Beta-hemolysis on SBA after 3 days p*
p	*p*	R	**n**	n	n	n	n	p	n	pp	*p*	n	n		n	R	n	60	n	Growth on MCA p
p	*p*	S 80	**n**	n	n	n	n	p	n	*p*	*p*	n	n		n	R	n	v	n	*Growth on MCA n*
n	n	R	**p**	n	n	n	n	n	n	20	n	n	**n**	n	n	S	n	o	n	
o	o	o	**n**	n	o	n	n	n	o	n	n	n	n	n	o	o	n	o	o	
p	p	R	n	95	n	p	n	**p**	30	n	n	p	95	p	p	S	p	n	p	
p	p	R	n	n	n	p	n	**n**	n	n	n	p	p	p	p	S	n	n	n	

(Continued on next page)

Species	Chapter	Cell morphology	Colony color/pigment/morphology	Hydrogen sulfide production	Indole production	Oxidase
Stenotrophomonas maltophilia	41	Rods	**Not brown on TSA**	n	n	n
Acinetobacter	42	Gram variable coccobacilli	**Not brown on TSA**	n	n	n
Burkholderia cepacia complex, partim oxidase n (1–4%, up to 14% for *B. pyrrocinia*)	41	Rods	**Not brown on TSA**	n	n	n
Burkholderia gladioli	41	Rods	**Not brown on TSA**	n	n	n
Bordetella ansorpii	43	Rods	**Not brown on TSA**	n	n	n
Kerstersia gyiorum	43	Rods	**Not brown on TSA, dry, spreading**	n	n	n
Bordetella trematum	43	Rods	**Not brown on TSA**	n	n	n
H₂S production negative, no green pigment on MHA, indole production negative, oxidase positive						
Trypsin positive, pyrrolidonyl aminopeptidase positive						
Sphingomonas spp., partim PYR p (25%)	42	Rods	Yellow, flexirubin n	n	n	*p/p*[w]
Pseudomonas aeruginosa, partim pyoverdin n (35%), partim PYR p (95%)	40	Rods	Pyoverdin n	n	n	*p*
Pseudomonas fluorescens, partim pyoverdin n (5%), partim PYR p (60%)	40	Rods	Pyoverdin n	n	n	*p*
Brevundimonas diminuta, partim PYR p (20%)	41	Rods	Pigment n	n	n	*p*
Inquilinus limosus, partim urease n (65%)	42	Rods	Mucoid	n	n	*p*
Myroides odoratus	42	Rods	Yellow, flexirubin p, spreading	n	n	*p*
Myroides odoratimimus	42	Rods	Yellow, flexirubin p, spreading	n	n	*p*
Sphingobacterium spiritivorum	42	Rods	Yellowish, flexirubin n	n	n	*p*
Sphingobacterium multivorum	42	Rods	Yellowish, flexirubin n	n	n	*p*
Inquilinus limosus, partim urease (p) (35%)	42	Rods	Mucoid	n	n	*p*
Sphingobacterium thalpophilum	42	Rods	Yellowish, flexirubin n	n	n	*p*
Pannonibacter phragmitetus	42	Rods	Creamy	n	n	*p*
Rhizobium radiobacter	42	Rods	Creamy	n	n	*p*
Ochrobactrum anthropi	42	Rods	Creamy or mucoid	n	n	*p*
Ochrobactrum intermedium	42	Rods	Creamy or mucoid	n	n	*p*
Trypsin positive, pyrrolidonyl aminopeptidase negative						
Alishewanella fetalis	42	Rods	Pigment n	n	n	*p*
Sphingomonas spp., partim PYR n (75%)	42	Rods	Yellow, flexirubin n	n	n	*p/p*[w]
Brevundimonas vesicularis	41	Rods	Orange most	n	n	*p*
Brevundimonas diminuta, partim PYR n (80%)	41	Rods	Pigment n	n	n	*p*
Alcaligenes faecalis, partim trypsin p (30%)	42	Rods	Usually dry, often fruity smell	n	n	*p*
Pseudomonas fluorescens, partim pyoverdin n (5%), partim PYR n (40%), partim nitrate reductase n (80%)	40	Rods	Pyoverdin n	n	n	*p*
Pseudomonas putida, partim pyoverdin n (5%)	40	Rods	Pyoverdin n	n	n	*p*
Pseudomonas stutzeri	40	Rods	Cauliflower colonies (rough), often yellowish	n	n	*p*
Pseudomonas mendocina	40	Rods	Often yellowish	n	n	*p*
Pseudomonas aeruginosa, partim pyoverdin n (35%), partim PYR n (5%), partim nitrite reductase p (95%)	40	Rods	Pyoverdin n	n	n	*p*

Trypsin	Pyrrolidonyl aminopeptidase	Susceptibility to desferrioxamine	Urease	Nitrate reductase	Nitrite reductase	Motility	Lysine decarboxylase	Arginine dihydrolase	Alkaline phosphatase	Growth at 42°C	Gelatinase	Acidification of glucose	Acidification of mannitol	Acidification of xylose	Acidification of ethylene glycol	Susceptibility to colistin	Esculin hydrolysis	Starch hydrolysis	β-Galactosidase (ONPG)	Additional characteristics
p	n	R	n	40	n	p	p	n	pp	50	p	(p)	n	35	n	v	40	n	v	
n	n	v	v	v	v	p	v	n	o	v	v	v	n	v	o	o	n	o	v	
n	v	v	v	v	n	p	v	n	p	v	v	p	v	v	n	R	v	o	v	
n	80	R	n	35	n	p	n	n	n	n	70	p	p	p	60	R	10	n	v	
o	o	o	n	n	o	p	o	n	o	o	p	n	n	o	o	S	n	o	o	
n	o	S	n	n	o	p	n	n	n	p	n	n	n	o	p	S	n	o	n	
n	n	R	n	v	n	p	n	n	n	n	n	n	n	o	p	S	n	n	n	
p	p*	R	n	n	n	65	n	n	p	n	n	p	n	85	95	S 5	p	n	p	Vancomycin S
p	p*	R	n	p	95	p	n	p	n	p	80	p	70	90	p	S	n	n	n	*Vancomycin R*
p	p*	R	n	20	5	p	n	p	n	n	p	p	55	p	40	S	n	n	n	*Vancomycin R*
p	p*	S	n	n	n	p	n	n	p/pp	40	70	n	n	n	50	R	n	n	n	*Vancomycin R*
p	p	S R	n*	n	n	65	n	n	n	35	n	p	p	p	n	R	p	o	p	*Vancomycin R*
p	p	S	p	n	p	n	n	n	p	30	p	n	n	n	n	R	n	n	n	
p	p	R	p	n	p	n	n	n	p	30	p	n	n	n	n	R	n	n	n	
p	p	R	p	n	n	n	n	n	p	n	n	p	p	p	p	R	p	n	75	
p	p	R	p	n	n	n	n	n	p	n	n	p	n	p	n	R	p	n	p	
p	p	R	(p)*	n	n	65	n	n	n	35	n	p	p	p	p	R	p	o	p	
p	p	R	p/(p)	p	n	n	n	n	p	p	n	p	n	n	n	R	p	o	p	
p	p	S	p	p	p	p	n	30	n	p	n	p	60	p	p	S	35	n	p	Tributyrate esterase pp, acidification of raffinose n
p	p	S 30	p	p	40	p	n	n	n	30	n	p	p	p	p	S 80	p	o	p	*Tributyrate esterase n/(p), acidification of raffinose p*
p	p	R	p	p	p	p	n	70	n	65	n	p	v	p	p	S	35	o	n	
p	p	R	p	p	p	p	n	70	n	65	n	p	v	p	p	R	35	o	n	
p	n	S	p	p	n	n	n	n	p	p	p	p	n	n	n	S	n	o	n	Vancomycin S
p	n*	S R	n	n	n	65	n	n	p	n	n	p	n	85	95	S 5	p	n	p	*Vancomycin R*
p	n	S	n	n	n	p	n	n	p	20	25	90	n	25	p	R	p	o	p	
p	n*	S	n	n	n	p	n	n	p	40	70	n	n	n	50	R	n	n	n	
p*	n	S	n	n	p	p	n	n	n	20	20	n	n	n	80	R	n	n	n	
p	n*	R	n	n*	5	p	n	p	n	n	p	p	55	p	40	S	n	n	n	
p	n	R	n	n	n	p	n	p	n	n	n	p	25	p	p	S	n	n	n	
p	n	R	n	p	p	p	n	n	n	70	n	p	p	p	p	S	n	p	n	
p	n	R	n	p	p	p	n	p	n	p	n	p	n	p	p	S	n	n	n	
p	n*	R	n	p	p*	p	n	p	n	p	80	p	70	90	p	S	n	n	n	

(Continued on next page)

Species	Chapter	Cell morphology	Colony color/pigment/ morphology	Hydrogen sulfide production	Indole production	Oxidase
Pseudomonas fluorescens, partim pyoverdin n (5%), partim PYR n (40%), partim nitrate reductase p (20%), partim nitrite reductase p (95%)	40	Rods	Pyoverdin n	n	n	p
Pseudomonas aeruginosa, partim pyoverdin n (35%), partim PYR n (5%), partim nitrite reductase n (5%)	40	Rods	Pyoverdin n	n	n	p
Pseudomonas pseudoalcaligenes, partim acidification of glucose p (10%)	40	Rods	Pyoverdin n	n	n	p
Pseudomonas fluorescens, partim pyoverdin n (5%), partim PYR n (40%), partim nitrate reductase p (20%), partim nitrite reductase n (5%)	40	Rods	Pyoverdin n	n	n	p
Pseudomonas pseudoalcaligenes, partim acidification of glucose n (90%)	40	Rods	Pyoverdin n	n	n	p
Pseudomonas alcaligenes	40	Rods	Pyoverdin n	n	n	p
Trypsin negative, pyrrolidonyl aminopeptidase positive						
Moraxella atlantae	42	Plump coccobacilli	**Small**	n	n	p
Ralstonia pickettii	41	Rods	**Pigment n**	n	n	p
Comamonas terrigena	41	Rods	**Pigment n**	n	n	p
Burkholderia cenocepacia, partim PYR p (few)	41	Rods	**Pigment n, often yellowish**	n	n	p/p^w
Herbaspirillum spp.	41	Curved rods	**Pigment n**	n	n	p
Bordetella petrii	43	Small cells	**Pigment n**	n	n	p
Acidovorax facilis	41	Rods	**Pigment n, hemolysis n**	n	n	p
Acidovorax delafieldii	41	Rods	**Pigment n, sometimes yellowish**	n	n	p
Delftia acidovorans	41	Rods	**Pigment n**	n	n	p
Achromobacter xylosoxidans	43	Rods	**Pigment n**	n	n	p
Acidovorax temperans	41	Rods	**Pigment n, sometimes yellowish**	n	n	p
Achromobacter denitrificans	43	Rods	**Pigment n**	n	n	p
Cupriavidus gilardii, partim PYR p (15%), partim nitrate reductase p (50%)	41	Rods	**Pigment n**	n	n	p
Comamonas testosteroni	41	Rods	**Pigment n**	n	n	p
Achromobacter piechaudi	43	Rods	**Pigment n**	n	n	p
Ralstonia mannitolilytica	41	Rods	**Pigment n**	n	n	p
Ralstonia insidiosa	41	Rods	**Pigment n**	n	n	p
Cupriavidus pauculus	41	Rods	**Pigment n**	n	n	p
Cupriavidus gilardii, partim PYR p (15%), partim nitrate reductase n (50%)	41	Rods	**Pigment n**	n	n	p
Bordetella hinzii	43	Small coccobacilli	**Pigment n**	n	n	p
Cupriavidus respiraculi	41	Rods	**Pigment n**	n	n	p
Trypsin negative, pyrrolidonyl aminopeptidase negative						
Burkholderia pseudomallei	41			n	n	p
Psychrobacter immobilis	42	Large coccobacilli	Large, creamy	n	n	p

Trypsin	Pyrrolidonyl aminopeptidase	Susceptibility to desferrioxamine	Urease	Nitrate reductase	Nitrite reductase	Motility	Lysine decarboxylase	Arginine dihydrolase	Alkaline phosphatase	Growth at 42°C	Gelatinase	Acidification of glucose	Acidification of mannitol	Acidification of xylose	Acidification of ethylene glycol	Susceptibility to colistin	Esculin hydrolysis	Starch hydrolysis	β-Galactosidase (ONPG)	Additional characteristics
p	n*	R	n	p*	p*	p	n	p	n	n	p	p	55	p	40	S	n	n	n	
p	n*	R	n	p	n*	p	n	p	n	p	80	p	70	90	p	S	n	n	n	
p	n	S 70	n	p	n	p	n	80	n	p	n	p*	n	70	p	S	n	n	n	
p	n*	R	n	p*	n*	p	n	p	n	n	p	p	55	p	40	S	n	n	n	
p	n	S 70	n	p	n	p	n	80	n	p	n	n*	n	70	p	S	n	n	n	*Fructose p^w*
p	n	R	n	p	n	p	n	v	n	p	n	n	n	n	p	S	n	n	n	*Fructose n*
n	p	S 60	n	n	n	n	n	n	p	v	n	n	n	n	n	S	n	n	n	
n	p	S	p/(p)	p	p	p	n	n	n	v	n	p	n	p	n	R	n	o	n	
n	p	S	n	p	n	p	n	n	n	n	n	p	n	n	n	S	n	o	n	
n	p*	R	n/p	v	n	p	p	n	p/(p)	85	v	p	p	p	n	R	v	o	v	
n	p	R	p	n	n	p	n	n	25	p	n	(p)	p	p	n	S 25	n	o	p	Flagella polar, multitrichous (often bipolar)
n	p	R	n	p	p	n	n	n	o	n	n	n	n	n	n	S	n	o	n	
n	p	R	p	p	n	p	n	n	n	p	p	p	p	p	n	S	n	o	n	
n	p	R	(p)	p	n	p	n	(p)	n	50	n	p	p	(p)	n	S 50	n	o	n	
n	p	R	n	p	n	p	n	n	n	30	n	n	p	n	40	R	n	n	n	Acetamide assimilation p
n	p	R	n	p	60	p	n	n	n	85	n	80	n	p	p	R	n	o	n	
n	p	R	n	p	p	p	n	n	n	p	n	(p)	p^w	n	p(p)	R	n	o	n	
n	p	R	n	p	p	p	n	n	n	25	n	n	n	n	p	S	n	n	n	
n	p*	R	n	p*	n	p	n	p^w	p	n	n	n	n	n	60	S	n	n	n	
n	p	R	n	p	n	p	n	n	n	n	n	n	n	n	20	S	n	n	n	**Flagella polar or bipolar,** acetamide assimilation n
n	p	R	n	p	n	p	n	n	n	60	n	n	n	n	p	S	n	n	n	*Flagella peritrichous*
n	p	R	p	n	n	p	n	n	n	p	n	p	p	p	n	R	n	o	n	Flagellum polar, monotrichous
n	p	R	(p)	n	n	p	n	n	n	p	n	p	n	p	n	R	n	o	n	
n	p	R	p	n	n	p	n	n	n	85	n	n	n	n	n	R	S	n	o	n	
n	p*	R	n	n*	n	p	n	n	p^w	p	n	n	n	n	60	S	S	n	n	n	
n	p	R	n	n	n	p	n	n	n	p	n	n	n	n	p	S	n	n	n	
n	p^w	R	n	n	n	p	n	n	n	n	n	n	n	n	n	S	n	n	n	
n	n	v	n	p	p	p	n	p	p	v	p	p	p	p	p	R	v	o	n	
n	n	R	p	p	n	n	n	n	p	n	p	n	p	p	p	R	R	n	o	n	

(*Continued on next page*)

TABLE 5 Overview of biochemical characteristics of the gram-negative nonfermenters[a] (*Continued*)

Species	Chapter	Cell morphology	Colony color/pigment/morphology	Hydrogen sulfide production	Indole production	Oxidase
Burkholderia multivorans, partim desferrioxamine S (85%)	41	Rods	Pigment n, sometimes yellowish	n	n	**p/p[w]**
Burkholderia cenocepacia, partim PYR n (most), partim sucrose p (90%)	41	Rods	Pigment n, sometimes yellowish	n	n	**p/p[w]**
Burkholderia multivorans, partim desferrioxamine R (15%)	41	Rods	Pigment n, sometimes yellowish	n	n	**p/p[w]**
Burkholderia cenocepacia, partim PYR n (most), partim sucrose n (10%)	41	Rods	Pigment n, sometimes yellowish	n	n	**p/p[w]**
Psychrobacter faecalis	42	Large coccobacilli	Large, creamy	n	n	**p**
Paracoccus yeei	42	Diplococci or coccobacilli, O shaped	Mucoid, yellowish	n	n	**p**
Haematobacter missouriensis	42	Pleomorphic rods or coccobacilli	Variable colony size, mucoid or sticky	n	n	**p**
Oligella ureolytica	42	Small coccobacilli	Small, whitish	n	n	**p**
Alcaligenes faecalis, partim trypsin n (70%)	42	Rods	Usually dry, often fruity smell	n	n	**p**
Comamonas kerstersii	41	Rods	Pigment n	n	n	**p**
Comamonas aquatica	41	Rods	Pigment n	n	n	**p**
Moraxella lacunata	42	Plump rods or coccobacilli	Small	n	n	**p**
Moraxella canis	42	Diplococci	Variable, large; brownish on MHA	n	n	**p**
Oligella urethralis	42	Small coccobacilli	Small, whitish	n	n	**p**
Moraxella catarrhalis	42	Diplococci	White, hockey puck	n	n	**p**
Moraxella nonliquefaciens	42	Plump rods or coccobacilli	Small	n	n	**p**
Bordetella bronchiseptica	43	Small coccobacilli	Pigment n	n	n	**p**
Haematobacter massiliensis	42	Pleomorphic rods or coccobacilli	Variable colony size, mucoid or sticky	n	n	**p**
Psychrobacter phenylpyruvicus	42	Plump rods or coccobacilli	Small	n	n	**p**
Cupriavidus gilardii, partim PYR n (85%)	41	Rods	Pigment n	n	n	**p**
Psychrobacter pulmonis	42	Large coccobacilli	Large, creamy	n	n	**p**
Moraxella osloensis	42	Plump rods or coccobacilli	Small	n	n	**p**
Moraxella lincolnii	42	Plump rods or coccobacilli	Small, weak growth on SBA	n	n	**p**
Species not included in Table 4						
Advenella incenata/Tetrathiobacter kashmirensis (n = 6)	43	Plump rods	Creamy	n	n	p
Pandoraea pulmonicola	41	Rods	Pigment n	n	n	p[w]
Pandoraea apista	41	Rods	Pigment n	n	n	n
Pandoraea norimbergensis/Pandoraea pnomenusa	41	Rods	Pigment n	n	n	n
Pandoraea sp.	41	Rods	Pigment n	n	n	n
Pandoraea sputorum	41	Rods	Pigment n	n	n	n

[a]Characteristics useful for identification according to the dichotomous Table 4 are listed in boldface type; the distinction between groups in each dichotomy is indicated by roman versus italic type. Alphanumeric data are percentages of positive isolates. MCA, MacConkey agar; n, negative; n*, negative, but some isolates of this species are positive for this characteristic, dealt with elsewhere in the table; n/p, most strains negative; o, data not listed; p, positive; pp, strongly positive; p*, positive,

Trypsin	Pyrrolidonyl aminopeptidase	Susceptibility to desferrioxamine	Urease	Nitrate reductase	Nitrite reductase	Motility	Lysine decarboxylase	Arginine dihydrolase	Alkaline phosphatase	Growth at 42°C	Gelatinase	Acidification of glucose	Acidification of mannitol	Acidification of xylose	Acidification of ethylene glycol	Susceptibility to colistin	Esculin hydrolysis	Starch hydrolysis	β-Galactosidase (ONPG)	Additional characteristics
n	n	S*	40	95	n	p	50	n	p/(p)	p	<5	p	p	p	n	R	<5	o	>95	
n	n*	R	40	30	n	p	p	n	p/(p)	85	55	p	p	p	n	R	35	o	>95	Acidification of sucrose p
n	n	R*	40	95	n	p	50	n	p/(p)	p	<5	p	p	p	n	R	<5	o	>95	*Acidification of sucrose n*
n	n*	R	40	30	n	p	p	n	p/(p)	85	55	p	p	p	n	R	35	o	>95	*Acidification of sucrose n*
n	n	R	n	p	p	n	n	n	n	n	n	p	n	p	p	S	n	o	n	
n	n	R	p	p	n	n	n	n	n	35	n	p	45	p	p	S	n	o	n	**Phenylalanine deaminase n**
n	n	R	p	n	n	n	n	p	n	n	n	p	(p)	(p)	p	S	n	o	n	*Phenylalanine deaminase p*
n	n	S	p	p	p	70	n	n	n	20	n	n	n	n	p	S	n	n	n	
n*	n	S	n	n	p	p	n	n	n	20	v	n	n	n	80	S	n	n	n	Phenylalanine deaminase n, flagellation p, peritrichous
n	n	S	n	p	n	p	n	n	n	p	n	n	n	n	n	S	n	n	n	
n	n	S	n	p	n	p	n	n	n	n	n	n	n	n	n	S	n	n	n	
n	n	S	n	p	n	n	n	n	75	n	p	n	n	n	25	S	n	n	n	
n	n	S	n	80	20	n	n	n	n	p	n	n	n	n	p	S	n	n	n	**Tributyrate esterase p, phenylalanine deaminase n**
n	n	S	n	n	p	n	n	n	n	60	n	n	n	n	p	S	n	n	n	*Phenylalanine deaminase p^w*
n	n	S	n	p	p	n	n	n	n	25	n	n	n	n	n	S	n	n	n	
n	n	S	n	p	n	n	n	n	n	15	n	n	n	n	n	S	n	n	n	
n	n	R	p	p	n	p	n	n	n	80	n	n	n	20	n	S	n	n	n	
n	n	R	p	n	n	n	n	p	n	n	n	n	n	n	p	S	n	o	n	Tween esterase n, tributyrate esterase n
n	n	R	p	30	n	n	n	n	n	30	n	n	n	n	60	S	n	n	n	Tween 80 esterase p, tributyrate esterase p
n	n*	R	n	v	n	p	n	n	p^w	p	n	n	n	n	60	S	n	n	n	
n	n	R	n	p	p	n	25	n	n	p	n	n	n	n	p	S	n	n	n	
n	n	R	n	25	n	n	n	n	75	50	n	n	n	n	p	S	n	n	n	
n	n	R	n	n	n	n	n	n	n	n	n	n	n	n	n	S	n	n	n	
n	n	R/S	n/p	n/p	n	p/n	n	n	n/p^w	v	n	p/n	n	p/n	n/p	S	n	o	n	
n	n	R	n	n	n	p	n	n	p	o	o	n	n	n	n	R	n	o	o	
n	p	R	(p)	n	n	p	n	n	n	o	o	(p)^w	n	n	n	S	n	o	o	
n	n	R	(p)	p	n	p	n	n	n	o	o	n	n	n	n	R	n	o	o	
n	n	R	p	n	p	p	n	n	p^w	o	o	(p)^w	n	n	n	R	p	o	o	
n	n	R	p	n	n	p	n	n	n	o	o	n	n	n	n	R	n	o	o	

but some isolates of this species are negative for this characteristic, dealt with elsewhere in the table; p^w, weakly positive; (p), delayed positive; (p)^w, delayed and weakly positive; p/(p), most strains positive, some delayed positive; p/n, most strains positive; p/p^w, most strains positive, some weakly positive; R, resistant; R/S, most strains resistant; S, susceptible; sheep blood agar; S/R: most strains susceptible; S [number], percentage of susceptible strains; v, strain dependent.

REFERENCES

1. **Bernardet, J.-F., Y. Nakagawa, and B. Holmes.** 2002. Proposed minimal standards for describing new taxa of the family *Flavobacteriaceae* and emended description of the family. *Int. J. Syst. Evol. Microbiol.* **52:**1049–1070.

2. **Bombicino, K. A., M. N. Almuzara, A. M. Famiglietti, and V. Vay.** 2007. Evaluation of pyrrolidonyl arylamidase for the identification of nonfermenting Gram-negative rods. *Diagn. Microbiol. Infect. Dis.* **57:**101–103. (Erratum, **57:**473.)

3. **Coenye, T., E. Falsen, M. Vancanneyt, B. Hoste, J. R. W. Govan, K. Kersters, and P. Vandamme.** 1999. Classification of *Alcaligenes faecalis*-like isolates from the environment and human clinical samples as *Ralstonia gilardii* sp. nov. *Int. J. Syst. Bacteriol.* **49:**405–413.

4. **Coenye, T., J. Goris, P. De Vos, P. Vandamme, and J. J. LiPuma.** 2003. Classification of *Ralstonia pickettii*-like isolates from the environment and clinical samples as *Ralstonia insidiosa* sp. nov. *Int. J. Syst. Evol. Microbiol.* **53:**1075–1080.

5. **Cruze, J. A., J. T. Singer, and W. R. Finnerty.** 1979. Conditions for quantitative transformation in *Acinetobacter calcoaceticus. Curr. Microbiol.* **3:**129–132.

6. **De Backer, E., R. Verhelst, H. Verstraelen, M. A. Alqumber, J. P. Burton, J. R. Tagg, M. Temmerman, and M. Vaneechoutte.** 2007. Quantitative determination by real-time PCR of four vaginal *Lactobacillus* species, *Gardnerella vaginalis* and *Atopobium vaginae* indicates an inverse relationship between *L. gasseri* and *L. iners. BMC Microbiol.* **7:**115.

7. **Holmes, B., R. J. Owen, A. G. Steigerwalt, and D. J. Brenner.** 1984. *Flavobacterium gleum*, a new species found in human clinical specimens. *Int. J. Syst. Bacteriol.* **34:**21–25.

8. **Hugh, R., and E. Leifson.** 1953. The taxonomic significance of fermentative versus oxidative metabolism of carbohydrates by various gram negative bacteria. *J. Bacteriol.* **66:**24–26.

9. **Kämpfer, P., M. Vaneechoutte, N. Lodders, T. De Baere, V. Avesani, M. Janssens, H.-J. Busse, and G. Wauters.** 2009. Description of *Chryseobacterium anthropi* sp. nov., to accommodate clinical isolates biochemically similar to *Kaistella koreensis* and *Chryseobacterium haifense*, proposal to reclassify *Kaistella koreensis* as *Chryseobacterium koreense* comb. nov. and emended description of the genus *Chryseobacterium. Int. J. Syst. Evol. Microbiol.* **59:**2421–2428.

10. **Kodaka, H., A. Y. Armfield, G. L. Lombard, and V. R. Dowell, Jr.** 1982. Practical procedure for demonstrating bacterial flagella. *J. Clin. Microbiol.* **16:**948–952.

11. **Laffineur, K., M. Janssens, J. Charlier, V. Avesani, G. Wauters, and M. Delmée.** 2002. Biochemical and susceptibility tests useful for identification of nonfermenting gram-negative rods. *J. Clin. Microbiol.* **40:**1085–1087.

12. **Martin, R., P. S. Riley, D. G. Hollis, R. E. Weaver, and M. I. Krichevsky.** 1981. Characterization of some groups of gram-negative nonfermentative bacteria by the carbon source alkalinization technique. *J. Clin. Microbiol.* **14:**39–47.

13. **Quan, Z.-X., K. K. Kim, M.-K. Kim, L. Jin, and S.-T. Lee.** 2007. *Chryseobacterium caeni* sp. nov., isolated from bioreactor sludge. *Int. J. Syst. Evol. Microbiol.* **57:**141–145.

14. **Vaneechoutte, M., P. Kämpfer, T. De Baere, E. Falsen, and G. Verschraegen.** 2004. *Wautersia* gen. nov., a novel genus accommodating the phylogenetic lineage including *Ralstonia eutropha* and related species, and proposal of *Ralstonia* [*Pseudomonas*] *syzygii* (Roberts *et al.* 1990) comb. nov. *Int. J. Syst. Evol. Microbiol.* **54:**317–327.

15. **Wauters, G., B. Van Bosterhaut, M. Janssens, and J. Verhaegen.** 1998. Identification of *Corynebacterium amycolatum* and other nonlipophilic fermentative corynebacteria of human origin. *J. Clin. Microbiol.* **36:**1430–1432.

16. **Yabuuchi, E., T. Kaneko, I. Yano, C. W. Moss, and N. Miyoshi.** 1983. *Sphingobacterium* gen. nov., *Sphingobacterium spiritivorum* comb. nov., *Sphingobacterium multivorum* com. nov., *Sphingobacterium mizutae* sp. nov., and *Flavobacterium indologenes* sp. nov.: glucose-nonfermenting gram-negative rods in CDC groups IIk-2 and IIb. *Int. J. Syst. Bacteriol.* **33:**580–598.

Neisseria

JOHANNES ELIAS, MATTHIAS FROSCH, AND ULRICH VOGEL

32

TAXONOMY

According to the second edition of *Bergey's Manual of Systematic Bacteriology* the genus *Neisseria* belongs to the family *Neisseriaceae* of the order *Neisseriales* (124), which is placed into the class *Betaproteobacteria*. Since the 1980s, several alterations have been made within the taxonomy and classification of the family *Neisseriaceae* due to knowledge gained from molecular analyses. The exclusion and subsequent reassignment of the genera *Moraxella*, *Acinetobacter*, and *Psychrobacter* to the *Gammaproteobacteria* were first proposed by the use of DNA-rRNA and DNA-DNA hybridization techniques (110) and later confirmed by 16S rRNA gene sequencing (45, 61). Today, the family *Neisseriaceae* is the only family within the order *Neisseriales*, which in addition to the genus *Neisseria* contains *Eikenella*, *Kingella*, and 27 other genera.

DESCRIPTION OF THE GENUS *NEISSERIA*

Most members of the genus *Neisseria* are cocci with a diameter of up to 2 μm, presenting as single bacteria or in pairs. The species *N. elongata*, *N. weaveri*, and the proposed new species *N. bacilliformis* sp. nov. are exceptions and consist of short rods, frequently arranged as diplobacilli or in chains. While *Neisseria* species are gram negative, occasionally a tendency to withstand decolorization is noted. Capsules (*N. meningitidis*) and pili (*N. meningitidis* and *N. gonorrhoeae*) may be present, yet flagella are not formed. *N. meningitidis* is the only species expressing a polysaccharide capsule, of which 12 different serogroups are distinguishable (53). Strains of several species like *N. flavescens*, *N. sicca*, and *N. subflava* may produce a yellowish pigment. *Neisseria* species grow optimally under aerobic conditions and a temperature of 35 to 37°C. Nevertheless, isolation of *N. gonorrhoeae* from body sites with reduced oxygen tensions suggests ability of anaerobic growth, which, given the inability to generate energy from fermentation, was suggested to be due to nitrite respiration (74). Microaerobic growth by denitrification of nitrite via NO has also been shown for *N. meningitidis* (3). While many species are not nutritionally demanding, the human-pathogenic species *N. gonorrhoeae* and *N. meningitidis* are fastidious, showing particular susceptibility to unfavorable environmental factors such as extreme temperatures, desiccation, and alkaline or acidic conditions. All species are oxidase positive and, with the exception of *N. elongata* subsp. *elongata* and *N. elongata* subsp. *nitroreducens*, catalase positive. *Neisseria* species produce acid from carbohydrates by oxidation, not fermentation. Some species, like *N. elongata* and *N. cinerea*, are asaccharolytic. Most members of the genus are able to reduce nitrite. The natural habitat of the members of this genus is the mucous membranes of mammals including humans. The species *N. gonorrhoeae* and *N. meningitidis* are human pathogens. Exotoxins are typically not produced (124). All species classified in the genus *Neisseria* are naturally competent for DNA uptake and display a high frequency of horizontal gene transfer (118). As a consequence, phylogenetic analyses within this genus based on different genes may yield incongruent results (117). Of note, this distortion also applies to 16S rRNA gene sequencing, which has been used to define inter- and intrageneric relationships within the *Neisseriaceae* and *Moraxellaceae* (61). Multiple-locus instead of single-locus approaches might therefore be more suitable for the resolution of species identification within the genus *Neisseria* (10). According to Euzeby's "List of Prokaryotic names with Standing in Nomenclature" (http://www.bacterio.cict.fr/n/neisseria.html), the genus *Neisseria* consists of 25 species.

EPIDEMIOLOGY AND TRANSMISSION

N. gonorrhoeae causes gonorrhea, which is the second most commonly reported notifiable disease in the United States (http://www.cdc.gov/std/stats07/gonorrhea.htm). *N. gonorrhoeae* is always considered pathogenic, and humans are the only hosts of this bacterium. It is mainly transmitted through sexual practices and infects the mucosal surfaces of urethra, cervix, rectum, and pharynx and the eye. The risk of infection is greatly influenced by sexual behavior yet can be reduced, although not eliminated, by the use of condoms (134). Furthermore, the eye can be infected intrapartally during passage of the fetus through the birth canal. The rate of gonorrhea has decreased by 74% from 1975 to 1997 in the United States following the implementation of the gonorrhea control program in the mid-1970s (http://www.cdc.gov/std/stats07/gonorrhea.htm). From 1997 onwards, however, the overall incidence has remained largely unchanged. In 2007, 355,991 cases were reported in the United States, which translates to an overall incidence of 119 cases per 100,000 population. Rates vary considerably among states, with values below 19/100,000 in the Northeast and West to over 250/100,000 in the South. Prior to 1996, disease rates were consistently higher among men, but incidences have been similar or slightly higher among women in recent years. The age groups with the highest burden of disease are adolescents and young adults between 15 and 24 years. In 2007, gonorrhea rates remained highest among African Americans (663 per 100,000), with African American women between 15 and 19 years particularly affected (2,956 per 100,000). Overall rates in the United Kingdom were comparable to those of the United States in 2007 (130 per 100,000), yet a significant downward trend since 2002 has been observed (http://www.hpa.org.uk). While the age distribution is very similar to that of the United States, men have consistently higher rates than women in the United Kingdom. Moreover, Great Britain has observed a threefold increase in the number of individuals diagnosed with gonorrhea among men who have sex with men (MSM).

N. meningitidis also occurs exclusively in humans and plays a dual role of commensal and potential invasive pathogen. On average, the mucosal surfaces of oro- and nasopharynx of 10% of the population is colonized by this bacterium (34). Carriage is strongly age dependent, with adolescents and young adults attaining rates of over 30% in contrast to infants with carriage rates of a few percent (34). As a consequence of repeated episodes of carriage, the percentage of sera with bactericidal activity against pathogenic strain increases with age. Transmission occurs through large droplet secretions from the oropharynx and is favored by repeated or close contact, given the low yield of growth from saliva compared to nasopharyngeal swabs (98). Nevertheless, outbreaks and clusters are rare in developed countries (44). Disease occurs in only a minute proportion of individuals acquiring *N. meningitidis* and follows a typical age distribution with infants and adolescents having the highest incidences. Apart from genetic host polymorphisms (19), individuals with underlying conditions like properdin deficiencies (47), late complement deficiencies (47, 103), and splenic impairment including asplenia (59) are at increased risk for invasive meningococcal disease (IMD). Also, behavioral risk factors, including exposure to smokers (39) and kissing (127), have been described to contribute to acquisition of disease.

IMD is rare in developed countries. In the United States the incidence for the year 2007 was estimated to be 0.34 per 100,000 (26) with serogroups B, C, and Y constituting 91% of all cases. The rate in European countries is rather variable, with the United Kingdom reaching incidences of 2.5/100,000 with an 80% dominance of serogroup B (2007 and 2008) and Germany reporting an incidence of 0.55/100,000 with a 70% proportion of serogroup B in 2008. In contrast, African countries in the so-called meningitis belt regularly report epidemic waves, mainly caused by serogroup A, with rates soaring to over 300 per 100,000 (21). Several predominant clones have successively caused the majority of IMD in Africa (24). A number of vaccines have been developed for the prevention of IMD. In 2005, the Advisory Committee on Immunization Practices recommended vaccination of young adolescents (11 to 12 years of age) with a quadrivalent polysaccharide-protein conjugate vaccine (26) covering serogroups A, C, W135, and Y. Due to high rates of serogroup C disease in the 1990s and early 2000s, several European countries implemented vaccination campaigns with conjugate vaccine against serogroup C, which led to dramatic reduction of disease with this capsule type (126). Until recent times, vaccination against serogroup B had been deemed impossible due to poor immunogenicity of the serogroup B capsule. Nevertheless, outer membrane vesicle vaccines were used to combat local epidemics, e.g., in New Zealand (99). Also, recent advances in the development of vaccines based on outer membrane proteins (55, 104) promise to provide broad coverage against a wide array of disease-causing strains.

CLINICAL SIGNIFICANCE

Members of the genus *Neisseria* have a high affinity to mucosal membranes of mammals and humans. A wide variety of species can be isolated from humans including *N. gonorrhoeae*, *N. cinerea*, *N. elongata*, *N. flavescens*, *N. lactamica*, *N. meningitidis*, *N. mucosa*, *N. polysaccharea*, *N. sicca*, and *N. subflava*. Several species are predominantly recovered from animals, like *N. animalis*, *N. animaloris*, and *N. zoodegmatis* (throat of cats and dogs) (129a), *N. denitrificans* (throat of guinea pigs), *N. dentiae* (dental plaques of domestic cows), *N. macacae* (oropharynges of rhesus monkeys), and *N. weaveri* (oral flora of dogs). Similar to *N. elongata*, the new species *N. bacilliformis* likely colonizes the oral cavity and respiratory tract of humans (58). Most human *Neisseria* species are considered normal inhabitants of the upper respiratory tract, which cause disease in an opportunistic fashion. Rarely, species of animal origin can cause wound infections in humans after bites. *N. meningitidis* mostly appears as a mere commensal of the human oropharynx yet can cause life-threatening, acute disease in previously healthy individuals. *N. gonorrhoeae*, however, is always considered a pathogen, even if obvious signs of disease are absent.

Uncomplicated infection by *N. gonorrhoeae* (gonorrhea) manifests most commonly as acute urethritis in men. The major symptoms are urethral discharge, sometimes associated with dysuria, typically without frequency or urgency. Coinfection of the preputial (Tyson's), urethral (Littré's), and bulbo-urethral (Cowper's) glands is possible. Also, completely asymptomatic infections occur in up to 10% of cases. Most cases of untreated urethritis resolve spontaneously after several weeks. Further localized complications after gonococcal urethritis include acute epididymitis, penile edema, and abscesses of the above-mentioned glands. In women, the endocervix is the primary site of genital infection. Additionally, *N. gonorrhoeae* may infect the urethra, the rectum, the periurethral (Skene's) glands, and the ducts of the greater vestibular (Bartholin's) glands. The squamous epithelium of the vagina is typically not infected in sexually mature women. In contrast to infection in men, asymptomatic infection in women is common (29). Also, if symptoms appear, they often cannot clearly be attributed to infection by *N. gonorrhoeae*, given that concurrent infection by *Chlamydia trachomatis* and *Mycoplasma genitalium* is common. The main complaints include increased vaginal discharge, dysuria, and intermenstrual bleeding. Ascension of the infection may result in pelvic inflammatory disease, which manifests by various combinations of endometritis, salpingitis, tubo-ovarian abscess, and peritonitis. Acute perihepatitis (Fitz-Hugh-Curtis syndrome) can develop following direct extension of *N. gonorrhoeae* from the fallopian tube to the liver capsule and the surrounding peritoneum. While over 80% of rectal infections remain asymptomatic, some patients complain of acute proctitis. Pharyngeal infection is acquired by oral sexual exposure and is mostly asymptomatic (96) yet can also cause overt pharyngitis or tonsillitis (6). While probably less transmissible than rectal or urethral gonorrhea, its silent nature and considerable prevalence among MSM render pharyngeal infection a common reservoir for gonorrhea in sexually active MSM (96). Gonococcal conjunctivitis in adults usually results from autoinoculation, oculogenital, or orogenital exposure. If not treated promptly, corneal ulceration may rapidly develop. Conjunctivitis of the newborn (ophthalmia neonatorum) is transmitted during birth and is favored by premature rupture of the membranes and preterm delivery. Historically a common cause for blindness, it can be prevented by administering a 1% aqueous solution of silver nitrate or an antibiotic ointment (usually containing erythromycin) into the conjunctivae after delivery. Disseminated gonococcal infection (DGI) reflects bacteremic dissemination, possibly generation of immune complexes, and indirect immunological mechanisms. It complicates less than 1% of mucosal infections (63). DGI usually manifests as septic arthritis and a characteristic syndrome of polyarthritis and dermatitis and should be suspected in patients presenting with tenosynovitis, arthritis, and vasculitic skin lesions (69).

IMD commonly presents as meningitis, acute sepsis, or a combination of both. In addition, unusual presentations include transient mild bacteremia, chronic meningococcal sepsis, pneumonia (mainly by serogroup Y), septic arthritis, and endocarditis (23). Symptoms of meningitis vary widely and can include a stiff neck, headache, confusion, and photophobia. Lethality of meningococcal meningitis without sepsis can be as low as 3% (108). Sequelae such as sensorineural hearing loss, developmental delay, and speech defects afflict a substantial part of survivors, yet in a lower proportion than in other forms of acute bacterial meningitis (68). Petechial lesions are telltale signs of meningococcal sepsis, which can coalesce and become ecchymotic. Nevertheless, nonpurpuric maculopapular rashes that can be confused with viral exanthems have also been associated with meningococcemia. Meningococcal septic shock can take a fulminant course with a lethality of 30% (131), and concentrations in plasma can reach up to 10^8 meningococci/ml (18), which in turn lead to massive activation of cytokines and vasoactive anaphylatoxins. Meningococcal shock syndrome is characterized by myocardial depression, vasoplegia, capillary leakage, and disseminated intravascular coagulation (131). Complications of IMD include arthritis, pericarditis, cranial nerve dysfunction, meningococcal pericarditis, and rarely, cerebral or spinal infarction. In addition, adolescent survivors of IMD have been described as suffering from a series of long-term consequences including poorer physical and mental health, quality of life, and educational achievement (13). Bacteremia can also manifest without signs of sepsis in the form of chronic meningococcemia, a condition associated with low-grade relapsing fever, arthritis, and rash (101). Meningococcal pneumonia has been recognized as an infrequent clinical syndrome for more than 100 years (67). Most meningococcal pneumonias are caused by serogroup Y; they are responsible for 45% of IMD in the United States (25) and affect adults disproportionately (138). Preceding viral illness, notably pandemic influenza (49), has been reported to promote its development. *N. meningitidis* is an uncommon cause of acute bacterial conjunctivitis and can also be the etiologic agent of urethritis in men.

The clinical significance of *Neisseria* species other than *N. gonorrhoeae* and *N. meningitidis* is covered under "Evaluation, Interpretation, and Reporting of Results" below.

COLLECTION, TRANSPORT, AND STORAGE OF SPECIMENS

Neisseria gonorrhoeae

The selection of specimens for culture-based diagnosis of gonorrhea depends on the sex of the individual, the level of sexual maturity, and anatomical sites exposed. The anterior portion of the male urethra is sampled by introducing a swab up to 2 cm in a rotatory fashion. Samples from the endocervical canal are obtained by introducing a swab after removal of mucus plugging the cervical orifice. In MSM and women practicing anal intercourse, rectal samples should be taken. Swabs heavily contaminated with feces have to be discarded. In symptomatic patients, direct swabbing of lesions under rectoscopic guidance improves culture yield. A pharyngeal swab should be obtained from individuals who performed fellatio on a person with genital gonorrhea. Vaginal swabs are inadequate for culture-based diagnosis in sexually mature women but can be used in prepubescent females. If the hymen is intact, however, the specimen is collected from the vaginal orifice.

Dacron (polyethylene terephthalate)- or rayon (viscose)-tipped swabs, e.g., Transwab (Medical Wire, Corsham, United Kingdom), Bactiswab (Remel, Lenexa, KS), or Minitip Amies (Copan Innovation, Brescia, Italy), are preferable for culture-based diagnosis of gonorrhea. Calcium alginate swabs should be avoided due to reported toxicity (80). Also, cotton buds and oil-based lubricants can contain unsaturated fatty acids, which inhibit *N. gonorrhoeae*. Although direct plating maximizes the yield of gonococci in culture, this approach is not always practical or possible. Here, Amies-based semisolid transport media can be used to transport swabs to the processing laboratory. There are, however, considerable performance differences of commercial Amies-based transport systems after 24 and 48 hours, which are not uniformly rectifiable by the addition of charcoal (57). Therefore, it is advisable to inoculate swab specimens transported in these media within 6 hours after collection. During the time of transport, media should be kept at room temperature and not refrigerated.

Survival and transport of gonococci for over 24 hours can be achieved by culture medium transport systems, which allow direct plating of specimens in a clinical environment. They usually consist of a solid medium onto which swabs are inoculated directly after collection and a CO_2-generating system within a resealable container. A CO_2-rich atmosphere is generated by tablets containing citric acid and sodium bicarbonate that are activated after contact with water. Commercially available systems include Biocult-GC (Orion Diagnostica, Espoo, Finland) and John E. Martin Biological Environmental Chamber GC-Lect Agar (Becton Dickinson and Company, Franklin Lakes, NJ).

Similar to culture samples, specimens for molecular detection of *N. gonorrhoeae* are best sampled by using rayon- or Dacron-tipped swabs, since calcium alginate was reported to inhibit PCR (38). The inhibitory influence of aluminum shafts is rather contentious, and preliminary testing in conjunction with the employed molecular kit is advisable. Transport and collection systems specifically designed for molecular detection include the Digene Female Swab Specimen Collection Kit (Qiagen Inc., Valencia, CA) and the STD Swab Specimen Collection and Transport Kit (F. Hoffmann-La Roche Ltd., Basel, Switzerland). Some molecular kits can also be used for urine and vaginal swabs (see "Nucleic Acid Amplification Tests" below). For these sample types, recommendations by the producer of the molecular detection kits employed have to be followed.

Neisseria meningitidis

The types of specimens that can be used for the detection of *N. meningitidis* include blood, cerebrospinal fluid (CSF), nasopharyngeal and oropharyngeal swabs, bronchoalveolar lavage fluids, joint aspirates, urethral and endocervical swabs, petechial aspirates, and biopsy specimens. Genital and rectal specimens may be obtained by using the collection and inoculation procedures described above. Pharyngeal swabs used for determination of meningococcal carriage are best taken from the posterior pharyngeal wall through the mouth and plated directly after sampling (109). Alternatively, swabs may be put into Amies-based transport media and plated preferably within 5 hours after collection. Growth of *N. meningitidis* and *N. gonorrhoeae* in commercial blood culture media is adversely affected by the anticoagulant sodium polyanetholesulfonate (107), for which currently no suitable substitute is available. Its inhibitory action is reduced by the addition of gelatin at a concentration of 1 g/liter to most commercially available blood culture media.

Laboratory Safety Issues for Handling of Meningococcal Cultures

Rare cases of fatal meningococcal disease in laboratory staff have been described (114). A risk factor for laboratory-acquired infection is exposure to droplets or aerosols containing *N. meningitidis* (114). Laboratories working with live *N. meningitidis* isolates should comply with biological safety containment level 2 standards, including the use of class II biological safety cabinets whenever infectious splashes or aerosols may be created, e.g., during mobilization of organisms from culture plates, handling of liquid cultures, performing of carbohydrate utilization tests, oxidase testing, and slide agglutination.

DIRECT EXAMINATION

Microscopy

A direct smear for Gram staining should be prepared with a different swab than that used for the collection of specimen for culture. The swab should be rolled softly onto the glass slide to conserve cellular morphology. A presumptive diagnosis of gonococcal urethritis in men is made by visualization of gram-negative diplococci associated with or within polymorphonuclear leukocytes. The sensitivity of microscopy depends on the anatomical site investigated and is highest in urethral slides of men, where it reaches 89% (86). For endocervical and rectal smears of MSM, however, it drops to 51% and 54%, respectively (86). The specificity of microscopic diagnosis for these sites has been reported to be over 90%. Microscopy is not useful for the diagnosis of pharyngeal gonorrhea. Nevertheless, microscopic diagnosis is mandatory from normally sterile material.

A Gram stain of CSF is required for all cases of suspected bacterial meningitis sent to the laboratory. Visualization of gram-negative diplococci is sufficient for the presumptive diagnosis of meningococcal meningitis (Fig. 1). If more than 1 ml of CSF is available, the specimen should be centrifuged at 1,000 × g for 10 minutes and the pellet used for microscopic examination and culture. Cytocentrifugation also increases the sensitivity of microscopic investigation. On Gram-stained smears from CSF, meningococci

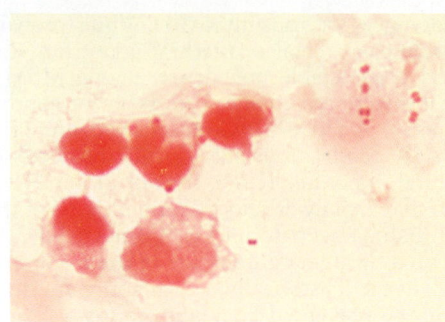

FIGURE 1 Gram stain of cerebrospinal fluid from a patient with meningococcal meningitis.

appear as gram-negative diplococci both inside and outside polymorphonuclear leukocytes, which will typically be abundant in samples from bacterial meningitis. Organisms may tend to resist decolorization.

Antigen Detection

Diagnosis of meningococcal meningitis can be made through the use of commercially available antigen detection kits. These methods are useful, if no or only limited access to microscopes is available. They are of questionable clinical usefulness when compared with Gram stain (102) and should therefore not be used as a substitution for microscopy. Commercially available latex agglutination tests, which consist of latex particles coated with monoclonal antibodies targeting the capsular polysaccharide of common serogroups, include the Pastorex Meningitis kit (Inverness Medical UK Ltd., Stockport, United Kingdom) and Wellcogen N. meningitidis A, C, Y, and W135 (Oxoid Ltd., Basingstoke, United Kingdom). These assays have a reasonable sensitivity and specificity (42) yet are useless for the detection of uncommon serogroups (130). In laboratories handling only a small number of cases the cost for purchase and storage of antigen detection kits outweighs any potential benefits for patient management.

Nucleic Acid Detection

Neisseria gonorrhoeae

Nucleic acid tests permit the rapid and sensitive detection of *N. gonorrhoeae* from clinical samples without the requirement of bacterial viability. They have been in use since the early 1990s and can be categorized in nucleic hybridization assays and nucleic acid amplification tests (NAATs).

Hybridization Assays

The two commercially available hybridization assays include Digene CT/GC Dual ID HC2 (HC2; Qiagen) and Gen-Probe Pace 2 (P2; Gen-Probe Inc., San Diego, CA), which use RNA probes targeting genomic DNA and DNA probes targeting rRNA, respectively. The detection method of the RNA-DNA hybrids in the HC2 assay involves antibody-mediated recognition of the hybrids and subsequent binding of alkaline phosphatase-conjugated antibodies, which act on a chemiluminescent substrate. Signal amplification results from multiple alkaline phosphatase molecules being attached to a conjugated antibody, of which several bind to a single captured hybrid. In the P2 assay the DNA probes are labeled with a chemoluminescent substance, which is quantified after separation of the stable DNA-RNA hybrids from nonhybridized probe. The sensitivity of hybridization tests is probably higher than that of culture (41, 66).

Nucleic Acid Amplification Tests

All main commercial NAATs developed to date use multiplex NAATs, targeting both *N. gonorrhoeae* and *Chlamydia trachomatis* (see chapter 60). Of the first-generation tests, which include Roche Amplicor CT/NG (F. Hoffmann-La Roche Ltd., Basel, Switzerland) and Abbott Ligase Chain Reaction (LCx, Abbott Molecular, Maidenhead, Berkshire, United Kingdom), only Roche Amplicor CT/NG continues to be available. The Amplicor assay uses PCR for amplification of DNA and targets the DNA-cytosine methyltransferase gene. It has shown cross-reactivity with strains of several commensal *Neisseria* species, contributing to low positive predictive values (PPV) on urogenital specimens in several studies (136). The CDC issued guidelines suggesting additional testing for *N. gonorrhoeae* NAATs in cases where the PPV is expected to be lower than 90% (72), which apart from cross-reactivity (i.e., low specificity) can be due to low disease prevalence. With the Amplicor assay, additional testing has been carried out with real-time PCR assays targeting the *porA* pseudogene (135) and the *gyrA* gene (33). A further real-time-based confirmatory test was attempted using gene melt curve analysis with labeled probes hybridizing with variable stretches of the 16S rRNA genes (88), thus enabling distinction of *N. gonorrhoeae* from other *Neisseria* species. Nevertheless, confirmatory tests themselves have differing sensitivities and specificities (88), which can limit their usefulness, as shown for poorly specific assays targeting the *cppB* (cryptic plasmid protein B) gene (20, 88). The Becton Dickinson ProbeTec SDA assay (SDA) (Becton Dickinson) is a second-generation test that uses strand displacement amplification, a technique not requiring thermal cycling, for the multiplication of DNA. It targets a region within the multicopy pilin gene-inverting protein homologue (82). This test was also shown to have a PPV of less than 90% in certain populations (30). Furthermore, cross-reactivity with *N. flavescens*, *N. subflava*, *N. lactamica*, and *N. cinerea* was reported (100). In analogy to Amplicor PCR, *porA* pseudogene and *cppB* were used as a confirmatory test for SDA. The rate of confirmation with *porA*, however, has been reported to be only 74% for anorectal and 30% for oropharyngeal specimens in MSM from Australia (94). Similarly, concordance with *cppB* in urogenital specimens has been only 77% (77), although this figure could represent a shortcoming of the confirmatory assay itself. Additional testing by another NAAT, Aptima Combo 2 and Aptima GC (see below), showed high concordance for cervical and urethral swabs (60) and for male urethral swabs and first-catch urine (31). Aptima Combo 2 (AC2) (Gen-Probe) is a further second-generation test, which uses transcription-mediated amplification for the replication of gonococcal 16S rRNA and a chemiluminescent single-stranded DNA probe for product detection. Aptima GC (AG) represents a confirmatory assay based on the same technology and even uses the same capture probe as AC2 but targets a slightly different region of the rRNA subunit. Evaluations regarding the performance of this assay have largely been favorable. Specificity and sensitivity were shown to be higher than for the Amplicor assay in Australia (83). A study using AC2 with AG as a confirmatory assay demonstrated a PPV of 97% among 60,000 female urine and cervical swabs despite low prevalence (56). Nevertheless, PPV varied between 75% and 100% for urogenital specimens in a multicenter study (31). The specificities of AC2 and those of SDA were very similar and always over 94% in several studies investigating first-void urine (81), vaginal (92), rectal (95, 112), and pharyngeal (5, 112) specimens. Finally, the Abbott RealTime CT/NG (Abbott Molecular) assay is a new real-time PCR test, which like its predecessor, Abbott LCx, targets a region in the *N. gonorrhoeae* opacity (Opa) gene (89). To date, not too many comparative analyses have been published, yet one study analyzing 500 first-void urine specimens (81) reported performance identical to that of AC2. No confirmatory tests have been developed for Abbott RealTime.

In summary, NAATs provide several advantages over culture-based diagnosis yet also have a series of important limitations. The main advantages are their superior sensitivity over culture, evidenced in numerous clinical studies (5, 95, 112, 132), and the less stringent collection and transport conditions. The current list of NAATs with FDA approval includes Amplicor, Abbott RealTime, AC2, and ProbeTec for urine and urethral swab specimens. Some NAATs are licensed for further sample types including self-collected and clinician-collected vaginal swabs (Abbott RealTime and AC2) and endocervical swabs (Amplicor, AC2, and ProbeTec). Importantly, no NAAT is currently cleared for oropharyngeal, rectal, ocular, or pediatric specimens, which to date have to be investigated by culture-based means. Major limitations of NAATs include high cost, carryover contamination, high quality control requirements, and the absence of antibiotic resistance data (136). Furthermore, the assays are susceptible to inhibition by substances present in patient samples, e.g., those commonly found in urine (84), and also to inhibition by competing amplification in the case of coinfection with *C. trachomatis* (136). The complexity of the assay, involving steps such as nucleic acid extraction, amplification, and detection, requires stringent quality control and staff training. Nevertheless, the latest commercial assays such as AC2 and Abbott RealTime can be integrated into fully automated molecular testing systems, such as Tigris-DTS (Gen-Probe, San Diego, CA) and m2000 (Abbott Molecular, Maidenhead, Berkshire, United Kingdom), respectively, thus reducing hands-on processing of samples.

Neisseria meningitidis

Several in-house methods have been developed to enable culture-independent diagnosis of IMD, which are especially useful when previous antibiotic treatment or unfavorable transport conditions lead to a negative culture. The DNA targets used for molecular diagnosis include *ctrA* (52), IS*1106* (16), *siaD* (14, 15) (or *mynA* for serogroup A meningococci), *porA* (111), *porB* (128), *fetA* (123), and housekeeping genes used for multilocus sequence typing (MLST). Specifically, *ctrA* was evaluated as a target in real-time detection of meningococcal DNA (40). Apart from facilitating laboratory confirmation of meningococcal disease, the polysialyltransferase genes (*siaD* or *mynA* in the case of serogroup A) can be used for serogrouping, while *porA*, *porB*, *fetA*, and housekeeping genes allow culture-independent typing (44). False-positive results have been reported for IS*1106*, which should therefore not be used as a single assay for routine screening (16). Moreover, *ctrA* is negative in rare cases of IMD caused by *N. meningitidis* harboring the capsule-null locus (48).

ISOLATION PROCEDURES

Cultivation of *N. gonorrhoeae* requires the use of chocolate agar, which supports the growth of many other commensal bacteria. To isolate *N. gonorrhoeae* from mucosal and other nonsterile body sites, several selective media containing a mixture of inhibitory agents have been developed. All of them contain the antibiotics vancomycin and colistin for the suppression of gram-positive and gram-negative bacteria, respectively. The prototype medium, developed by Thayer and Martin (122), consists of a chocolate agar base, which in addition to the above antibiotics contains nystatin for the inhibition of yeasts. The addition of trimethoprim to the modified Thayer-Martin medium and following formulations prevents swarming of *Proteus* species. The Martin-Lewis medium contains anisomycin instead of nystatin, which has increased activity against *Candida albicans*. Further modifications include the GC-Lect Agar (Becton Dickinson), which provides additional control against *Capnocytophaga* species and against vancomycin-resistant gram-positive contaminants by the addition of lincomycin. Moreover, the reduced vancomycin concentration in GC-Lect Agar enhances the recovery of uncommon vancomycin-sensitive *N. gonorrhoeae*. The media are available in petri-style or John E. Martin Biological Environmental Chamber-style plates. In contrast to above media, the New York City medium is a clear peptone-corn starch agar containing yeast dialysate, citrated horse plasma, and lysed horse erythrocytes. It contains the antibiotics vancomycin, colistin, amphotericin B, and trimethoprim.

Specimens are to be inoculated on warmed or room temperature media. Plates should be incubated at 35 to 37°C with 3 to 7% CO_2 in a moist atmosphere after inoculation. This is accomplished in a commercially available CO_2 incubator equipped with a humidifier. A moist, CO_2-rich atmosphere can also be generated with a candle extinction jar using white, nonscented candles. Cultures should be examined daily for growth and held for a minimum of 72 hours.

For culture-based detection of *N. meningitidis* from primarily sterile materials, such as CSF or joint fluid, specimens should be inoculated onto sheep blood agar and chocolate agar. Specimens from mucosal surfaces (e.g., respiratory material) have to be inoculated additionally on selective media (see above) that exclude growth of most commensal *Neisseria* species. Incubation conditions are identical to those for *N. gonorrhoeae*, at 35 to 37°C under 5% CO_2 tension (109). Nevertheless, in contrast to *N. gonorrhoeae*, *N. meningitidis* tends to grow more readily on solid media and almost invariably grows on blood agar plates. In addition, vancomycin susceptibility, impeding recovery of some gonococcal strains from selective media, has not been described. Media must be examined for suspicious growth at 24, 48, and 72 h. After 72 h a negative culture result can be issued.

IDENTIFICATION

Presumptive Identification

Colonial Morphology

After 48 hours of growth on chocolate agar, colonies of *N. gonorrhoeae* are up to 1 mm in diameter, opaque, grayish white, glistening, and convex. Morphology can vary subject to the presence of pili and opacity proteins. Colonies of *N. gonorrhoeae* expressing pili and opacity proteins are wrinkled and well defined with a clear edge, while nonpiliated colonies have more diffuse edges and are more glistening. Due to rapid pilus phase variation, colonial morphology can appear heterogeneous after primary inoculation.

Colonies of *N. meningitidis* have smooth, entire edges and are about 1 mm in diameter after 18 h of growth on blood agar. They are gray, convex, glistening, and occasionally mucoid. Blood agar beneath the colonies may display a gray-green color.

Microscopic Morphology

A Gram stain must be performed on suspected *N. gonorrhoeae* and *N. meningitidis* colonies to confirm the presence of uniform gram-negative diplococci. Consistent results are obtained with <24-h-old colonies, before autolytic processes appear. Microscopic examination of suspicious colonies growing on selective plates is essential, since gram-negative rods belonging to the genera *Moraxella* (e.g., *M. osloensis*), *Acinetobacter*, and *Kingella* can occasionally grow on them. Nevertheless, the microscopic appearance of gram-negative rods grown on solid media, particularly *Acinetobacter*, can be identical to that of *Neisseria* spp.

Oxidase Test

Performance of the oxidase test is mandatory for colonies suspected to belong to *Neisseria*. Both *N. gonorrhoeae* and *N. meningitidis* give a positive reaction. In the filter paper method, oxidase reagent (1% dimethyl-*p*-phenylene-diamine-dihydrochloride or tetramethyl-*p*-phenylene-diamine-dihydrochloride) is placed on filter paper, onto which a colony is rubbed with a wooden stick (nickel-chrome loops may give a false-positive reaction). A fresh isolate should produce a deep purple color within 10 s. Commercial strips (Microbact Oxidase Strips, Oxoid, United Kingdom) are a useful alternative.

Definitive Identification

Carbohydrate Utilization Assays

Neisseria species produce acid from carbohydrates by oxidation, not fermentation. The only carbohydrate used by *N. gonorrhoeae* is glucose, while *N. meningitidis* additionally catabolizes maltose (Table 1). Rarely, however, *N. gonorrhoeae* (142) and *N. meningitidis* (129) fail to acidify carbohydrate-containing media. Also, several asaccharolytic species including *N. cinerea*, *N. flavescens*, and *N. elongata* never produce acid at all from sugars. The traditional cystine tryptic agar sugar method has been virtually replaced by rapid carbohydrate utilization tests in most routine laboratories. These tests give results within 4 hours and are integrated into commercial kits like ApiNH (bioMerieux, Marcy-l'Etoile, France) and RapID NH (Remel).

Chromogenic Enzyme Substrate Tests

Identification of *N. gonorrhoeae* can be confirmed by direct detection of enzyme activities using chromogenic substrates. The tested enzymes usually include β-galactosidase, γ-glutamyl-aminopeptidase, and proline-iminopeptidase (Pip), which are specific for *N. lactamica*, *N. meningitidis*, and *N. gonorrhoeae*, respectively. The substrates used for the above enzymes, bromo-chloro-indolyl-β-galactoside (or -galactopyranoside), γ-glutamyl-nitroanalide, and proline-methoxynapthylamide, change their colors after a positive reaction to blue, yellow, and red, respectively. The three enzymes can be assayed in a one-tube format in the two commercially available kits, GonoCheck II (EY Laboratories Inc., San Mateo, CA) and Neisseria PET (BioConnections, Wetherby, United Kingdom). In both tests, β-galactosidase and γ-glutamyl-aminopeptidase are assayed first. This requires an incubation step at 37°C for 30 minutes. In a second step, which takes up to 2 minutes, Pip is tested by the addition of the appropriate reagent

TABLE 1 Characteristics of *Neisseria* species of human origin[a]

Species	Morphology	Growth on selective media	Acid production from:					Nitrate reduction	Poly-saccharide from SUC	Reference
			GLU	MAL	LAC	SUC	FRU			
N. bacilliformis	R	0	0	0	0	0	ND	V	ND	58
N. cinerea	C	V	0	0	0	0	0	0	0	
N. elongata	C									124
subsp. *elongata*		0	0	0	0	0	0	0	0	
subsp. *glycolytica*		0	(+)	0	0	0	0	0	0	
subsp. *nitroreducens*		0	0	0	0	0	0	+	0	
N. flavescens	C	0	0	0	0	0	0	0	+	
N. gonorrhoeae	C	+	+	0	0	0	0	0	0	
N. lactamica	C	+	+	+	+	0	0	0	0	
N. meningitidis	C	+	+	+	0	0	0	0	0	
N. mucosa	C	0	+	+	0	+	+	+	+	
N. polysaccharea	C	V	+	+	0	V	0	0	+	
N. sicca	C	0	+	+	0	+	+	0	+	
N. subflava	C									124
bv. *flava*		V	+	+	0	0	+	0	0	
bv. *perflava*		V	+	+	0	+	+	0	+	
bv. *subflava*		V	+	+	0	0	0	0	0	
N. weaveri	R	ND	0	0	0	0	0	0	ND	62

[a]Symbols and abbreviations: 0, negative; +, positive; (+), weakly positive; R, rods; C, cocci; GLU, glucose; MAL, maltose; LAC, lactose; SUC, sucrose; FRU, fructose; V, variable; ND, not determined.

(Neisseria PET) or replacement of the screwcap and subsequent inversion of the tube (GonoCheck II).

A study reported poor sensitivity of these tests in the confirmation of *N. gonorrhoeae* (2). False-negative results were obtained with Pip-negative *N. gonorrhoeae* isolates, which were shown to constitute 4% of all *N. gonorrhoeae* isolates in a recent survey in England and Wales (1). Moreover, *N. meningitidis* may be γ-glutamyl-aminopeptidase negative (142).

Immunologic Methods for Culture Confirmation

All commercially available tests for the culture confirmation of *N. gonorrhoeae* rely on the recognition of gonococcal protein I (with its variants IA and IB) by a pool of monoclonal antibodies. Phadebact Monoclonal GC Test (Bactus AB, Huddinge, Sweden) is a coagglutination assay employing inactivated *Staphylococcus aureus* cells coated with antibodies bound via their Fc portions to staphylococcal protein A. Cross-reactions with M. catarrhalis, N. cinerea, and N. lactamica were reported. Nevertheless, more recent studies found the test to be highly sensitive and specific for culture confirmation of *N. gonorrhoeae* (2, 12). The BD GonoGen II (Becton, Dickinson) is a colorimetric test employing antibodies adsorbed to metal sol particles, which give the reagent its raspberry red color. False-positive reactions with *N. lactamica* and *N. meningitidis* were observed (70). Furthermore, the solubilizing buffer of GonoGen II was described to only insufficiently extract protein I (2), resulting in false-negative reactions for some isolates. However, repeat testing with an extended extraction method led to high specificity and sensitivity of the test (2). The MicroTrak Culture Confirmation Test (Trinity Biotech, Bray, Ireland) uses fluorescein isothiocyanate-labeled antibodies for confirmation of *N. gonorrhoeae*. Positive specimens are identified by apple-green fluorescent diplococci under a fluorescence microscope. Among the immunologic methods, MicroTrak was appraised as the most labor-intensive (2). While earlier evaluations pointed to high specificity yet limited sensitivity (70), false negatives were not observed in a recent study (2).

Multitest Identification Systems

Several kits combine carbohydrate utilization tests and direct enzyme detection assays for rapid confirmation of isolates belonging to *Neisseria*. The Api NH system can be used for the identification of *Neisseria, Haemophilus,* and *Moraxella catarrhalis* and uses 13 miniaturized tests. In total, the test comprises four sugar utilization tests (assessing glucose, fructose, maltose, and sucrose), eight enzyme substrate tests, and an acidimetric penicillinase test. In contrast, the RapID NH (Remel) system contains only two carbohydrate utilization tests (for glucose and sucrose), 10 enzyme substrate tests, and a resazurin reduction test. The Api NH and RapID NH kits are inoculated with dense bacterial suspensions adjusted to McFarland standards of 4 and 3, respectively. Results are obtained after incubation at 37°C for 2 and 4 hours, respectively. The denser bacterial inoculum used in ApiNH might explain the slightly higher sensitivity compared to RapID NH (2). The automated bacterial identification platform Vitek 2 (bioMérieux) can also be used for identification of *Neisseria* species. Its NHI card contains 30 biochemical tests. Valenza and colleagues reported misidentification of *N. gonorrhoeae* as *N. cinerea* in one isolate owing to the lack of glucose utilization (129). In another study, all *N. gonorrhoeae* strains were identified correctly, yet 6% of them received a low-discrimination result (106).

MALDI-TOF MS

Matrix-assisted laser desorption ionization–time-of-flight mass spectrometry (MALDI-TOF MS) has generated a lot of interest as an emerging technique in the identification of bacterial pathogens. A species may be determined within a few minutes from whole cells, cell lysates, or crude bacterial extracts. A recent study analyzing 29, 13, and 15 strains of *N. gonorrhoeae*, *N. meningitidis*, and other *Neisseria* species, respectively, reports that direct bacterial profiles are sufficiently different to allow species identification of pathogenic *Neisseria* organisms (65). Nevertheless, further evaluations on extended strain collections are needed.

Hybridization Test

The Accuprobe culture identification test (Gen-Probe) is a DNA probe assay for *N. gonorrhoeae* isolated from culture. Similar to AC2 and AG, Accuprobe targets gonococcal rRNA. After lysis of bacteria, released rRNA is bound by single-stranded-DNA probes labeled with chemiluminescence. Labeled DNA-RNA hybrids are detected in a luminometer. While the test has not been evaluated of late, a study confirmed high sensitivity and specificity (141).

DNA Sequencing

Interpretive criteria for identification of bacteria and fungi by DNA target sequences have been published by CLSI (36). Harmsen et al. have established a reference database for 16S rRNA sequences including a representative set of *Neisseria* spp. obtained from reference strain collections (http://rdna.ridom.de/). The database in most cases allows the identification to species level of an organism belonging to the genus *Neisseria* (61). Due to the possibility of horizontal gene transfer, however, results obtained from a single locus must be interpreted in light of additional parameters, e.g., growth on selective media, biochemical tests, slide agglutination, and further PCR assays. Differences in 16S rRNA sequences between *N. meningitidis*, *N. cinerea*, *N. gonorrhoeae*, and *N. lactamica* may be as low as 1 to 4% over 700 bp. Other targets such as *gyrB* and *recA* have not been evaluated sufficiently. The pan-*Neisseria* MLST has the capacity to provide sufficient information for accurate species assignment (10).

TYPING SYSTEMS

Neisseria gonorrhoeae

Methods used for typing of *N. gonorrhoeae* include Opa typing, pulsed-field gel electrophoresis, multiantigen sequence typing, and MLST. While both Opa typing and pulsed-field gel electrophoresis are highly discriminatory, they are cumbersome and poorly portable. Multiantigen sequence typing represents a portable, sequence-based typing method of *N. gonorrhoeae* based on the sequencing of coding regions of the highly polymorphic antigens Por and TbpB (β subunit of transferring-binding protein) (91). MLST (85), based on the sequence-based typing of seven household genes, was also highly discriminatory for a sample of 149 *N. gonorrhoeae* isolates (10).

Neisseria meningitidis

N. meningitidis is a highly variable organism, and a vast array of techniques have been developed to describe isolated variants. The simplest method of typing is based on the nature of the polysaccharide capsule. In total, 12 different serogroups can be distinguished, which include A, B, C, H, I, K, L, X, Y, Z, W135, and 29E (53). Serogrouping is usually performed by slide agglutination with a set of commercially available sera (supplied by Remel or Becton Dickinson) (Fig. 2). A further level of differentiation can be achieved

FIGURE 2 Slide agglutination of meningococci with anticapsular sera. Serogroup C strain WUE2120 shows no agglutination with serum against serogroup B (left) but does show a marked reaction with serum against capsular polysaccharide of serogroup C (right). The control for autoagglutination is not shown.

by serotyping and serosubtyping, which designate the serological characterization of the outer membrane proteins PorB and PorA, respectively. Today, DNA sequence-based typing schemes of hypervariable outer membrane proteins have replaced sero(sub)typing. Protocols are available at http://neisseria.org. Sequence-based typing methods have increasingly gained acceptance, and a European consensus recommends serogrouping and MLST in conjunction with the typing of two variable regions of PorA, and the variable region of FetA (50) (Table 2). Protocols for multiple-locus variable-number tandem repeat analysis have also been developed for meningococci (113).

SEROLOGIC TESTS

Serologic tests are used for the determination of protection against invasive meningococcal disease after vaccination or for seroepidemiologic studies. Their use for ascertainment of invasive disease is not helpful, since asymptomatic carriage can also elicit protective (i.e., high) titers. The serum bactericidal assay is a functional assay using an external complement source such as baby rabbit or human complement that determines a bactericidal titer. It is currently regarded as the best surrogate test for vaccine protection across all serogroups (17). In addition to the serum bactericidal assay, serum immunoglobulin G concentrations against serogroups A, C, W135, and Y can be determined with enzyme-linked immunosorbent or bead assays (79).

ANTIMICROBIAL SUSCEPTIBILITIES

Neisseria gonorrhoeae

The Clinical and Laboratory Standards Institute (CLSI) recommends the use of GC agar containing 1% growth supplement for disk diffusion testing of *N. gonorrhoeae* (37). Colony suspensions of isolates have to be adjusted to a 0.5 McFarland standard before inoculation to media. CLSI further recommends agar dilution for the measurement of MICs, yet due to their ease of use, gradient test systems (e.g., Etests) represent an acceptable and frequently used surrogate.

The difficulties in treatment and control of gonorrhea are aggravated by the ability of *N. gonorrhoeae* to mount resistance against a wide range of antibiotics. Although penicillin was the treatment of choice up to the 1970s, the emergence and increase of penicillinase-producing *N. gonorrhoeae* (PPNG) (139) and chromosomally mediated penicillin resistance (Pen^r) led to the abandonment of penicillin as a treatment option. Similarly, plasmid-mediated

TABLE 2 Molecular typing methods for *N. meningitidis*[a]

Target	Method used		Value or use
	Culture isolates	Native samples	
Serogroup	Slide agglutination	PCR (caveat: sequencing required for serogroups W135 and Y [35])	Vaccine preventability
PorA	PCR, DNA sequencing	PCR, DNA sequencing	Routine fine typing (in combination with FetA and serogroup)
FetA	PCR, DNA sequencing	PCR, DNA sequencing	Routine fine typing (in combination with PorA and serogroup)
PorB	PCR, DNA sequencing		Additional typing method
Housekeeping genes: *abcZ, adk, aroE, fumC, gdh, pdhC, pgm* (MLST)	PCR, DNA sequencing	PCR, DNA sequencing	Global epidemiology; species status
penA	PCR, DNA sequencing		Confirmation of reduced penicillin susceptibility
Factor H binding protein	PCR, DNA sequencing		Analysis of possible coverage by new-generation meningococcal vaccines

[a]Abbreviations: PorA, porin A; FetA, ferric enterobactin transport protein A; PorB, porin B; *abcZ*, putative ABC transporter; *adk*, adenylate kinase; *aroE*, shikimate dehydrogenase; *fumC*, fumarate hydratase; *gdh*, glucose-6-phosphate dehydrogenase; *pdhC*, pyruvate dehydrogenase subunit; *pgm*, phosphoglucomutase; *penA*, gene encoding PBP2.

(TRNG) and chromosomally mediated (Tet[r]) resistance against tetracycline resulted in the replacement of this drug by broad-spectrum cephalosporins in the 1980s and later by the fluoroquinolones. Nevertheless, resistance against fluoroquinolones emerged in the 1990s in Southeast Asia (121) and spread widely to many countries, including the United States (51). Since April 2007, quinolones are no longer recommended to treat gonococcal infections in the United States (28). The Gonococcal Isolate Surveillance Project (GISP), which was established in 1986 to monitor trends in antimicrobial resistance in the United States, uses six mutually exclusive categories for the description of chromosomally and plasmid-mediated resistance to penicillin and tetracycline (51): PPNG (β-lactamase positive), TRNG (MIC, ≥16 μg/ml), PPNG-TRNG, Pen[r], Tet[r] (MIC, 2 to 8 μg/ml), and Pen[r] combined with Tet[r] (CMRNG). Quinolone resistance (QRNG) represents an additional nonexclusive category. According to the GISP Annual Report 2007 (27), PPNG, TRNG, and PPNG-TRNG accounted for 0.4%, 5.6%, and 0.5%, respectively, of all sampled strains. Pen[r], Tet[r], and CMRNG increased to 2.2%, 5.1%, and 9.3%, respectively (27). In total, 15% of GISP isolates were resistant to ciprofloxacin in 2007 in the United States (27). In contrast, the rate of QRNG was earlier reported to be 31% in Europe (90) and close to 100% in many Asian settings (137). A total of 27 strains (0.4%) were categorized as azithromycin "nonsusceptible" in GISP isolates in 2007 (37). The CLSI does not define a threshold for resistance of azithromycin and categorizes isolates with MICs of >2 μg/ml as "nonsusceptible." However, the Gonococcal Resistance to Antimicrobials Surveillance Programme (GRASP), which monitors England and Wales, reported 6 "highly" resistant isolates in 2007 with MICs of >256 μg/ml by Etest (32). Nevertheless, in 2008, no highly resistant isolates were collected by GRASP (http://www.hpa.org.uk/GRASP2008). The rise in QRNG and PPNG led to the replacement of quinolones by broad-spectrum cephalosporins as the treatment of choice for gonorrhea. Ceftriaxone is the most active cephalosporin against *N. gonorrhoeae* but has to be given as an intramuscular (i.m.) injection in a preparation containing a local anesthetic.

The most widely recommended oral broad-spectrum cephalosporin is cefixime, yet other oral agents, including ceftibuten, cefozopran, cefdinir, and cefpodoxime, are used as well. Susceptibility testing for cefixime was discontinued in 2007 by GISP, although strains revealing decreased susceptibility with MICs of >0.5 μg/ml were occasionally isolated (27). In addition, treatment failures following therapy with the oral broad-spectrum cephalosporins cefixime and ceftibuten have been reported, but not with the injectable ceftriaxone (121). Alterations in genes including *penA*, encoding penicillin-binding protein 2 (PBP2); *mtrA*, leading to derepression of an efflux pump; *penB1b*, encoding a porin; *ponA*, encoding PBP1; and others have been made responsible for cephalosporin resistance (121). Current treatment guidelines (28) recommend a single dose of ceftriaxone i.m. or cefixime orally for treatment of uncomplicated gonococcal infections of the cervix, urethra, and rectum. Pharyngeal gonorrhea should be treated with ceftriaxone i.m., while a cephalosporin-based intravenous treatment is recommended for the initial treatment of DGI. Fluoroquinolones may be used for treatment only if antimicrobial susceptibility can be documented by culture. Molecular tools for rapid detection of resistance (78, 115) have been developed.

Neisseria meningitidis

According to CLSI, testing is performed by disk diffusion on Mueller-Hinton agar or broth microdilution using cation-adjusted Mueller-Hinton broth (37). Alternatively, gradient test systems (e.g., Etest) are frequently used. In contrast to *N. gonorrhoeae*, *N. meningitidis* is usually penicillin susceptible, and β-lactamase production is rare (133). In many countries penicillin is still regarded as a treatment of choice for IMD. Nevertheless, reduced susceptibility, resulting from modification of PBP2, has been increasingly recorded for several years. Its molecular basis lies in a combination of five amino acid polymorphisms on positions 504, 510, 515, 541, and 566 of the PenA protein's transpeptidase region (119). In a manner analogous to cefixime resistance in *N. gonorrhoeae* (121), *penA* genes of intermediate-resistant strains were found to have a mosaic structure, suggesting multiple events of interspecies horizontal DNA transfer originating from commensal *Neisseria* species (119). Moreover, MICs of cefotaxime were reported to be higher in strains with intermediate resistance to penicillin (4). CLSI defines cefotaxime nonsusceptibility at MICs above 0.12 µg/ml but does not provide a threshold for resistance (37). While cefotaxime nonsusceptibility is rare globally, disquietingly high MICs of up to 8 µg/ml were recently reported from a sample of eight nonsusceptible strains in India (87). Nevertheless, spread to other countries has not taken place and the mechanism of nonsusceptibility remains to be elucidated. Rifampin and ciprofloxacin are used for chemoprophylaxis in close contacts of patients. Rifampin-resistant strains have a MIC of >2 µg/ml and result from point mutations in the RNA polymerase β subunit (*rpoB*) gene (105). Despite this one-step mechanism, the rate of resistance is very low (120). Resistance against ciprofloxacin has recently emerged in the United States (140) and is associated with a point mutation at position 91 of the gene encoding subunit A of DNA gyrase (*gyrA*). While the rate of resistant isolates is low in the United States (140) and Europe, an alarmingly high proportion of 65% was reported from a recent outbreak of IMD in India (97). The CLSI defines ciprofloxacin resistance as a MIC of at least 0.12 µg/ml or a zone diameter of less than 32 mm when using the 5-µg ciprofloxacin disk diffusion method (37). Enríquez and colleagues suggested that a 30-µg nalidixic acid disk is more reliable for screening of ciprofloxacin resistance (46). Azithromycin is used for mucosal eradication of contacts in areas of high rates of ciprofloxacin resistance (140). Due to the lack of resistant strains (73) CLSI only defines nonsusceptibility for strains with a MIC of over 2 µg/ml (37).

EVALUATION, INTERPRETATION, AND REPORTING OF RESULTS

Neisseria gonorrhoeae

Due to the imperfect specificity of many diagnostic methods used for identification of *N. gonorrhoeae*, the PPV of each procedure highly depends on the prevalence of disease. If medicolegal ramifications are likely to result from a positive test, as is the case, for example, in victims of sexual assault, special scrutiny has to be applied to all laboratory procedures involved in the issuing of a positive result.

In cases where probability of a positive test is low, such as in the detection of *N. gonorrhoeae* from pharyngeal samples in a laboratory *not* serving a specialized clinic for genitourinary medicine, special protocols should be in place to ensure confirmation of results. This is especially important for specimens from children and adolescents and the documentation of sexual abuse. Here, suspect *N. gonorrhoeae* should be confirmed by at least two different methods, including (i) multitest identification systems, (ii) immunologic methods, (iii) DNA probe culture confirmation, (iv) sequencing of the 16S rRNA gene, and (v) MALDI-TOF MS. Additionally, strains and DNA need to be conserved.

In settings of high prevalence, such as in laboratories serving genitourinary medicine clinics, tests giving a "yes-no answer" may be preferable over systems identifying the exact species. Here two levels of confidence may be attached to the laboratory report. A presumptive diagnosis of gonorrhea may be issued if one of the following criteria is met: (i) microscopic visualization of typical gram-negative intracellular diplococci on examination of a smear of urethral exudate (male) or endocervical secretions (female), (ii) growth of oxidase-positive bacteria from the male urethra or female

endocervix on selective media with colonial morphology and microscopic appearance (gram-negative diplococci) suggestive of *N. gonorrhoeae*. A definitive diagnosis requires (i) isolation of oxidase-positive gram-negative diplococci from sites of exposure (e.g., urethra, endocervix, throat, and rectum) by culture on selective media; and (ii) confirmation by biochemical or molecular methods. Due to the different performances of available NAATs, the significance of a positive result will differ between settings.

The choice of approach is often determined by workload and prevalence of gonorrhea in the service area of the laboratory. Laboratories that rarely encounter *N. gonorrhoeae* should prefer kits that give a full species identification.

Neisseria meningitidis

N. meningitidis is always considered a pathogen when isolated from usually sterile body fluids such as blood or CSF. Also, when isolated from the urethra, cervix, or the conjunctiva, a pathogenic role is likely. In the above cases, *N. meningitidis* should always be reported and the strain be forwarded to a reference laboratory. As a notable difference from pneumonia and the detection of meningococci from mucosal surfaces, many national guidelines consider meningococcal conjunctivitis to be an indication for chemoprophylaxis of the patient and close contacts, due to high immediate risk of invasive disease (8, 11). Detection of *N. meningitidis* from bronchoalveolar lavage fluid or sputum has to be interpreted in liaison with the clinician. Growth from oropharyngeal or nasopharyngeal specimens usually reflects asymptomatic carriage and may be omitted from laboratory reports, since it can lead to confusion regarding the pathogenic significance. Eradication of the organism in asymptomatic carriers should not be recommended. Similarly, typing of meningococcal carriage isolates should not routinely be performed. Furthermore, obtaining nasopharyngeal swabs to detect meningococci from close contacts of a patient with a case of invasive disease should exclusively be restricted to scientific projects.

Commensal *Neisseria* Species

Neisseria bacilliformis

Like *N. elongata* and *N. weaveri*, *N. bacilliformis* are rods, not cocci. On blood agar, colonies have sizes up to 1 mm after 24 hours and are smooth and glistening (58). The color of colonies ranges from light grey to buff (Fig. 3). Catalase

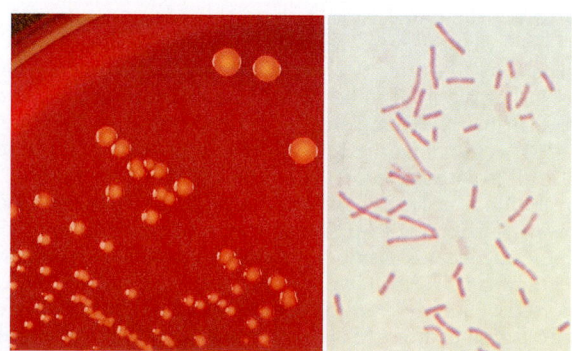

FIGURE 3 Colony morphology (left) and Gram stain (right) of the proposed new species *N. bacilliformis* sp. nov. (58). The strain was isolated from a human periodontal pocket. It was characterized by near-complete sequencing of the 16S rRNA gene. The species is noteworthy due to its rod-like morphology.

reaction and reduction of nitrate are variable, and strains are asaccharolytic (58). Strains are associated with the human respiratory tract and were occasionally recovered as causative agents of endocarditis (58, 93).

Neisseria cinerea

As the species name suggests, colonies of *N. cinerea* have an ash-gray color and are up to 1.5 mm in diameter. Isolates are asaccharolytic; i.e., they do not acidify carbohydrate-containing media. Due to this carbohydrate utilization profile, *N. cinerea* can be confused with glucose-negative *N. gonorrhoeae* (129). Furthermore, growth on selective media is occasionally possible despite colistin sensitivity (76). *N. cinerea* colonizes the oropharynx of over 24% of adults (75). Furthermore, it has been attributed a role in ocular infections in infants (43).

Neisseria elongata

N. elongata forms grayish white, semiopaque colonies, which have a diameter of up to 3 mm after 48 h of incubation. In contrast to the majority of species within *Neisseria*, *N. elongata* cells are short rods of ca. 0.5 μm in diameter. The species consists of three subspecies: *N. elongata* subsp. *elongata*, *N. elongata* subsp. *glycolytica*, and *N. elongata* subsp. *nitroreducens*. As an exception within the genus *Neisseria*, *N. elongata* subsp. *elongata* is catalase negative and does not produce acid from glucose or other carbohydrates. In contrast, subsp. *glycolytica* is catalase positive and weakly acidifies glucose media. Finally, subsp. *nitroreducens* is catalase negative and reduces nitrate. As other *Neisseria* species, *N. elongata* mainly appears as a colonizer of the human oropharynx. Nevertheless, several cases of endocarditis caused by *N. elongata* were published (64).

Neisseria flavescens

N. flavescens produces smooth and opaque yellow colonies. *N. flavescens* does not generate acid from sugars but produces polysaccharide from sucrose, which can be detected by pouring an iodine-containing solution (e.g., Lugol's) over colonies growing on brain heart infusion agar with sucrose. The iodine test is positive if colonies develop a deep-blue color, indicating the presence of a starch-like polysaccharide. *N. flavescens* colonizes the pharynx of humans and only rarely causes disease, such as endocarditis (116).

Neisseria mucosa

N. mucosa typically grows in large, adherent, and mucoid colonies, which are mostly nonpigmented. In carbohydrate utilization tests strains of this species are glucose, maltose, fructose, and sucrose positive. *N. mucosa* is found in the nasopharynx of humans, where it represents an apathogenic commensal. It has been associated with infective endocarditis in rare cases (125), and due to variable susceptibility to penicillin, the choice of antibiotic treatment has to be supported by susceptibility testing.

Neisseria lactamica

N. lactamica is readily confused with *N. meningitidis*, since it is morphologically similar and may grow on selective media. Nevertheless, it acidifies lactose in addition to glucose and maltose and is γ-glutamyl-aminopeptidase negative. *N. lactamica* is a commensal of the upper respiratory tract of infants and children. In contrast to *N. meningitidis*, colonization of the oropharynx with *N. lactamica* begins as soon as 2 weeks after birth (9). It is rarely pathogenic, although exceptional cases of meningitis and septicemia have been described. *N. lactamica* usually displays reduced susceptibility against penicillin.

Neisseria polysaccharea

Strains of *N. polysaccharea* present as small, yellow-grayish, translucent colonies. Like *N. meningitidis*, they acidify glucose and maltose but not fructose or lactose. In addition, they may grow on selective media and are γ-glutamyl-aminopeptidase positive. In contrast to *N. meningitidis*, however, the iodine test is positive, indicating the production of polysaccharide from sucrose (similar to *N. flavescens*). It colonizes the nasopharynx of children and has so far not been associated with disease.

Neisseria sicca

The colonies formed by *N. sicca* are large (≤3 mm), dry, wrinkled, and grayish white, although some strains may produce a yellowish pigment. Its carbohydrate utilization profile is indistinguishable from that of *N. mucosa*, but it does not reduce nitrate. This bacterium is a common oropharyngeal commensal in humans. Nevertheless, it can appear as an opportunistic pathogen. *N. sicca* was recently implicated, for example, as the causative agent of endocarditis (71).

Neisseria subflava

N. subflava appears as smooth, variably transparent colonies with a yellowish pigment. This species contains the previous species *N. subflava*, *N. perflava*, and *N. flava* (124). Strains of *N. subflava* acidify glucose and maltose. In addition, *N. subflava* bv. *subflava* and bv. *flava* produce acid from fructose, while bv. *perflava* acidifies sucrose and produces polysaccharide from sucrose. *N. subflava* is a common commensal of the human oropharynx, yet has occasionally been associated with invasive diseases such as meningitis, endocarditis, and bacteremia (7). Similar to *N. lactamica*, reduced susceptibilities to penicillin and also to cefixime and ciprofloxacin were reported recently (56).

Neisseria weaveri

Colonies of *N. weaveri* are of variable size (1 to 2 mm), smooth, flat, and slightly glistening (124). They have entire edges and are grayish in color. As most species of the genus *Neisseria*, they are strongly catalase and oxidase positive. Like *N. bacilliformis* and *N. elongata*, *N. weaveri* cells are rods, not cocci. *N. weaveri* does not use carbohydrates and does not reduce nitrate (62). Strains are infrequently recovered from human dog bite wounds and oral cavities of dogs (62). While septicemia in an immunosuppressed individual has been described (22), invasive disease is very rare.

REFERENCES

1. **Alexander, S., I. M. C. Martin, K. Fenton, and C. A. Ison.** 2006. The prevalence of proline iminopeptidase negative *Neisseria gonorrhoeae* throughout England and Wales. *Sex. Transm. Infect.* **82:**280–282.
2. **Alexander, S., and C. Ison.** 2005. Evaluation of commercial kits for the identification of *Neisseria gonorrhoeae*. *J. Med. Microbiol.* **54:**827–831.
3. **Anjum, M. F., T. M. Stevanin, R. C. Read, and J. W. B. Moir.** 2002. Nitric oxide metabolism in *Neisseria meningitidis*. *J. Bacteriol.* **184:**2987–2993.
4. **Antignac, A., M. Ducos-Galand, A. Guiyoule, R. Pirès, J. M. Alonso, and M. K. Taha.** 2003. *Neisseria meningitidis* strains isolated from invasive infections in France (1999–2002): phenotypes and antibiotic susceptibility patterns. *Clin. Infect. Dis.* **37:**912–920.

5. Bachmann, L. H., R. E. Johnson, H. Cheng, L. E. Markowitz, J. R. Papp, and E. W. Hook. 2009. Nucleic acid amplification tests for diagnosis of *Neisseria gonorrhoeae* oropharyngeal infections. *J. Clin. Microbiol.* **47:**902–907.

6. Balmelli, C., and H. F. Günthard. 2003. Gonococcal tonsillar infection—a case report and literature review. *Infection* **31:**362–365.

7. Baraldès, M. A., P. Domingo, J. L. Barrio, R. Pericas, M. Gurguí, and G. Vazquez. 2000. Meningitis due to *Neisseria subflava*: case report and review. *Clin. Infect. Dis.* **30:**615–617.

8. Barquet, N., I. Gasser, P. Domingo, F. A. Moraga, A. Macaya, and R. Elcuaz. 1990. Primary meningococcal conjunctivitis: report of 21 patients and review. *Rev. Infect. Dis.* **12:**838–847.

9. Bennett, J. S., D. T. Griffiths, N. D. McCarthy, K. L. Sleeman, K. A. Jolley, D. W. Crook, and M. C. J. Maiden. 2005. Genetic diversity and carriage dynamics of *Neisseria lactamica* in infants. *Infect. Immun.* **73:**2424–2432.

10. Bennett, J. S., K. A. Jolley, P. F. Sparling, N. J. Saunders, C. A. Hart, I. M. Feavers, and M. C. J. Maiden. 2007. Species status of *Neisseria gonorrhoeae*: evolutionary and epidemiological inferences from multilocus sequence typing. *BMC Biol.* **5:**35.

11. Bigham, J. M., M. E. Hutcheon, D. M. Patrick, and A. J. Pollard. 2001. Death from invasive meningococcal disease following close contact with a case of primary meningococcal conjunctivitis—Langley, British Columbia, 1999. *Can. Commun. Dis. Rep.* **27:**13–18.

12. Boehm, D. M., M. Bernhardt, T. A. Kurzynski, D. R. Pennell, and R. F. Schell. 1990. Evaluation of two commercial procedures for rapid identification of *Neisseria gonorrhoeae* using a reference panel of antigenically diverse gonococci. *J. Clin. Microbiol.* **28:**2099–2100.

13. Borg, J., D. Christie, P. G. Coen, R. Booy, and R. M. Viner. 2009. Outcomes of meningococcal disease in adolescence: prospective, matched-cohort study. *Pediatrics* **123:**e502–e509.

14. Borrow, R., H. Claus, U. Chaudhry, M. Guiver, E. B. Kaczmarski, M. Frosch, and A. J. Fox. 1998. siaD PCR ELISA for confirmation and identification of serogroup Y and W135 meningococcal infections. *FEMS Microbiol. Lett.* **159:**209–214.

15. Borrow, R., H. Claus, M. Guiver, L. Smart, D. M. Jones, E. B. Kaczmarski, M. Frosch, and A. J. Fox. 1997. Non-culture diagnosis and serogroup determination of meningococcal B and C infection by a sialyltransferase (siaD) PCR ELISA. *Epidemiol. Infect.* **118:**111–117.

16. Borrow, R., M. Guiver, F. Sadler, E. B. Kaczmarski, and A. J. Fox. 1998. False positive diagnosis of meningococcal infection by the IS1106 PCR ELISA. *FEMS Microbiol. Lett.* **162:**215–218.

17. Borrow, R., P. Balmer, and E. Miller. 2005. Meningococcal surrogates of protection—serum bactericidal antibody activity. *Vaccine* **23:**2222–2227.

18. Brandtzaeg, P., P. Kierulf, P. Gaustad, A. Skulberg, J. N. Bruun, S. Halvorsen, and E. Sørensen. 1989. Plasma endotoxin as a predictor of multiple organ failure and death in systemic meningococcal disease. *J. Infect. Dis.* **159:**195–204.

19. Brouwer, M. C., J. de Gans, S. G. B. Heckenberg, A. H. Zwinderman, T. van der Poll, and D. van de Beek. 2009. Host genetic susceptibility to pneumococcal and meningococcal disease: a systematic review and meta-analysis. *Lancet Infect. Dis.* **9:**31–44.

20. Bruisten, S. M., G. T. Noordhoek, A. J. C. V. D. Brule, B. Duim, C. H. E. Boel, K. El-Faouzi, R. D. Maine, S. Mulder, D. Luijt, and J. Schirm. 2004. Multicenter validation of the cppB gene as a PCR target for detection of *Neisseria gonorrhoeae*. *J. Clin. Microbiol.* **42:**4332–4334.

21. Campagne, G., A. Schuchat, S. Djibo, A. Ousséini, L. Cissé, and J. P. Chippaux. 1999. Epidemiology of bacterial meningitis in Niamey, Niger, 1981–96. *Bull. W. H. O.* **77:**499–508.

22. Carlson, P., S. Kontiainen, P. Anttila, and E. Eerola. 1997. Septicemia caused by *Neisseria weaveri*. *Clin. Infect. Dis.* **24:**739.

23. Cartwright, K., and D. Ala'Aldeen. 1997. *Neisseria meningitidis*: clinical aspects. *J. Infect.* **34:**15–19.

24. Caugant, D. A., and P. Nicolas. 2007. Molecular surveillance of meningococcal meningitis in Africa. *Vaccine* **25:**A8–A11.

25. Centers for Disease Control and Prevention. 2008. *Active Bacterial Core Surveillance (ABCs) Report, Emerging Infections Program Network, Neisseria meningitidis, 2007.* Centers for Disease Control and Prevention, Atlanta, GA.

26. Centers for Disease Control and Prevention. 2005. Prevention and control of meningococcal disease recommendations of the Advisory Committee on Immunization Practices (ACIP). *MMWR Morb. Mortal. Wkly. Rep.* **54**(RR07):1–21.

27. Centers for Disease Control and Prevention. 2009. *Sexually Transmitted Disease Surveillance 2007 Supplement, Gonococcal Isolate Surveillance Project (GISP) Annual Report 2007.* Centers for Disease Control and Prevention, Atlanta, GA.

28. Centers for Disease Control and Prevention. 2007. Update to CDC's sexually transmitted diseases treatment guidelines, 2006: fluoroquinolones no longer recommended for treatment of gonococcal infections. *MMWR Morb. Mortal. Wkly. Rep.* **56:**332–336.

29. Chacko, M. R., C. M. Wiemann, and P. B. Smith. 2004. Chlamydia and gonorrhea screening in asymptomatic young women. *J. Pediatr. Adolesc. Gynecol.* **17:**169–178.

30. Chan, E. L., K. Brandt, K. Olienus, N. Antonishyn, and G. B. Horsman. 2000. Performance characteristics of the Becton Dickinson ProbeTec System for direct detection of *Chlamydia trachomatis* and *Neisseria gonorrhoeae* in male and female urine specimens in comparison with the Roche Cobas System. *Arch. Pathol. Lab. Med.* **124:**1649–1652.

31. Chernesky, M. A., D. H. Martin, E. W. Hook, D. Willis, J. Jordan, S. Wang, J. R. Lane, D. Fuller, and J. Schachter. 2005. Ability of new APTIMA CT and APTIMA GC assays to detect *Chlamydia trachomatis* and *Neisseria gonorrhoeae* in male urine and urethral swabs. *J. Clin. Microbiol.* **43:**127–131.

32. Chisholm, S. A., T. J. Neal, A. B. Alawattegama, H. D. L. Birley, R. A. Howe, and C. A. Ison. 2009. Emergence of high-level azithromycin resistance in *Neisseria gonorrhoeae* in England and Wales. *J. Antimicrob. Chemother.* **64:**353–358.

33. Chui, L., T. Chiu, J. Kakulphimp, and G. J. Tyrrell. 2008. A comparison of three real-time PCR assays for the confirmation of *Neisseria gonorrhoeae* following detection of *N. gonorrhoeae* using Roche COBAS AMPLICOR. *Clin. Microbiol. Infect.* **14:**473–479.

34. Claus, H., M. C. J. Maiden, D. J. Wilson, N. D. McCarthy, K. A. Jolley, R. Urwin, F. Hessler, M. Frosch, and U. Vogel. 2005. Genetic analysis of meningococci carried by children and young adults. *J. Infect. Dis.* **191:**1263–1271.

35. Claus, H., K. Stummeyer, J. Batzilla, M. Mühlenhoff, and U. Vogel. 2009. Amino acid 310 determines the donor substrate specificity of serogroup W-135 and Y capsule polymerases of *Neisseria meningitidis*. *Mol. Microbiol.* **71:**960–971.

36. Clinical and Laboratory Standards Institute. 2008. *Interpretive Criteria for Identification of Bacteria and Fungi by DNA Target Sequencing; Approved Guideline.* Clinical and Laboratory Standards Institute, Wayne, PA.

37. Clinical and Laboratory Standards Institute. 2010. *Performance Standards for Antimicrobial Susceptibility Testing: Twentieth Informational Supplement.* Clinical and Laboratory Standards Institute, Wayne, PA.

38. Cloud, J. L., W. Hymas, and K. C. Carroll. 2002. Impact of nasopharyngeal swab types on detection of *Bordetella pertussis* by PCR and culture. *J. Clin. Microbiol.* **40:**3838–3840.

39. Coen, P. G., J. Tully, J. M. Stuart, D. Ashby, R. M. Viner, and R. Booy. 2006. Is it exposure to cigarette smoke or to smokers which increases the risk of meningococcal disease in teenagers? *Int. J. Epidemiol.* **35:**330–336.

40. Corless, C. E., M. Guiver, R. Borrow, V. Edwards-Jones, A. J. Fox, and E. B. Kaczmarski. 2001. Simultaneous detection of *Neisseria meningitidis*, *Haemophilus influenzae*, and *Streptococcus pneumoniae* in suspected cases of meningitis and septicemia using real-time PCR. *J. Clin. Microbiol.* **39:**1553–1558.

41. **Darwin, L. H., A. P. Cullen, P. M. Arthur, C. D. Long, K. R. Smith, J. L. Girdner, E. W. Hook III, T. C. Quinn, and A. T. Lorincz.** 2002. Comparison of Digene Hybrid Capture 2 and conventional culture for detection of *Chlamydia trachomatis* and *Neisseria gonorrhoeae* in cervical specimens. *J. Clin. Microbiol.* **40:**641–644.

42. **Djibo, S., B. Njanpop Lafourcade, P. Boisier, A. Moussa, G. Kobo, F. Sidikou, A. Hien, G. Bieboure, J. Aguilera, I. Parent du Chatelet, B. D. Gessner, and S. Chanteau.** 2006. Evaluation of the Pastorex meningitis kit for the rapid identification of *Neisseria meningitidis* serogroups A and W135. *Trans. R. Soc. Trop. Med. Hyg.* **100:**573–578.

43. **Dolter, J., J. Wong, and J. M. Janda.** 1998. Association of *Neisseria cinerea* with ocular infections in paediatric patients. *J. Infect.* **36:**49–52.

44. **Elias, J., D. Harmsen, H. Claus, W. Hellenbrand, M. Frosch, and U. Vogel.** 2006. Spatiotemporal analysis of invasive meningococcal disease, Germany. *Emerg. Infect. Dis.* **12:**1689–1695.

45. **Enright, M. C., P. E. Carter, I. A. MacLean, and H. McKenzie.** 1994. Phylogenetic relationships between some members of the genera *Neisseria, Acinetobacter, Moraxella,* and *Kingella* based on partial 16S ribosomal DNA sequence analysis. *Int. J. Syst. Bacteriol.* **44:**387–391.

46. **Enríquez, R., R. Abad, C. Salcedo, and J. A. Vázquez.** 2009. Nalidixic acid disk for laboratory detection of ciprofloxacin resistance in *Neisseria meningitidis. Antimicrob. Agents Chemother.* **53:**796–797.

47. **Fijen, C. A., E. J. Kuijper, M. T. te Bulte, M. R. Daha, and J. Dankert.** 1999. Assessment of complement deficiency in patients with meningococcal disease in The Netherlands. *Clin. Infect. Dis.* **28:**98–105.

48. **Findlow, H., U. Vogel, J. E. Mueller, A. Curry, B. Njanpop-Lafourcade, H. Claus, S. J. Gray, S. Yaro, Y. Traoré, L. Sangaré, P. Nicolas, B. D. Gessner, and R. Borrow.** 2007. Three cases of invasive meningococcal disease caused by a capsule null locus strain circulating among healthy carriers in Burkina Faso. *J. Infect. Dis.* **195:**1071–1077.

49. **Fletcher, W.** 1919. Meningococcus broncho-pneumonia in influenza. *Lancet* **193:**104–105.

50. **Fox, A. J., M. Taha, and U. Vogel.** 2007. Standardized nonculture techniques recommended for European reference laboratories. *FEMS Microbiol. Rev.* **31:**84–88.

51. **Fox, K. K., J. S. Knapp, K. K. Holmes, E. W. Hook, F. N. Judson, S. E. Thompson, J. A. Washington, and W. L. Whittington.** 1997. Antimicrobial resistance in *Neisseria gonorrhoeae* in the United States, 1988–1994: the emergence of decreased susceptibility to the fluoroquinolones. *J. Infect. Dis.* **175:**1396–1403.

52. **Frosch, M., D. Müller, K. Bousset, and A. Müller.** 1992. Conserved outer membrane protein of *Neisseria meningitidis* involved in capsule expression. *Infect. Immun.* **60:**798–803.

53. **Frosch, M., and U. Vogel.** 2006. Structure and genetics of the meningococcal capsule, p. 145–162. *In* M. Frosch and M. Maiden (ed.), *Handbook of Meningococcal Disease.* Wiley-VCH, Weinheim, Germany.

54. **Furuya, R., Y. Onoye, A. Kanayama, T. Saika, T. Iyoda, M. Tatewaki, K. Matsuzaki, I. Kobayashi, and M. Tanaka.** 2007. Antimicrobial resistance in clinical isolates of *Neisseria subflava* from the oral cavities of a Japanese population. *J. Infect. Chemother.* **13:**302–304.

55. **Giuliani, M. M., J. Adu-Bobie, M. Comanducci, B. Aricò, S. Savino, L. Santini, B. Brunelli, S. Bambini, A. Biolchi, B. Capecchi, E. Cartocci, L. Ciucchi, F. Di Marcello, F. Ferlicca, B. Galli, E. Luzzi, V. Masignani, D. Serruto, D. Veggi, M. Contorni, M. Morandi, A. Bartalesi, V. Cinotti, D. Mannucci, F. Titta, E. Ovidi, J. A. Welsch, D. Granoff, R. Rappuoli, and M. Pizza.** 2006. A universal vaccine for serogroup B meningococcus. *Proc. Natl. Acad. Sci. USA* **103:**10834–10839.

56. **Golden, M. R., J. P. Hughes, L. E. Cles, K. Crouse, K. Gudgel, J. Hu, P. D. Swenson, W. E. Stamm, and H. H. Handsfield.** 2004. Positive predictive value of Gen-Probe APTIMA Combo 2 testing for *Neisseria gonorrhoeae* in a population of women with low prevalence of *N. gonorrhoeae* infection. *Clin. Infect. Dis.* **39:**1387–1390.

57. **Graver, M. A., and J. J. Wade.** 2004. Survival of *Neisseria gonorrhoeae* isolates of different auxotypes in six commercial transport systems. *J. Clin. Microbiol.* **42:**4803–4804.

58. **Han, X. Y., T. Hong, and E. Falsen.** 2006. *Neisseria bacilliformis* sp. nov. isolated from human infections. *J. Clin. Microbiol.* **44:**474–479.

59. **Hansen, K., and D. B. Singer.** 2001. Asplenic-hyposplenic overwhelming sepsis: postsplenectomy sepsis revisited. *Pediatr. Dev. Pathol.* **4:**105–121.

60. **Hardwick, R., G. Gopal Rao, and H. Mallinson.** 2009. Confirmation of BD ProbeTec *Neisseria gonorrhoeae* reactive samples by Gen-Probe APTIMA assays and culture. *Sex. Transm. Infect.* **85:**24–26.

61. **Harmsen, D., C. Singer, J. Rothgänger, T. Tønjum, G. S. de Hoog, H. Shah, J. Albert, and M. Frosch.** 2001. Diagnostics of neisseriaceae and moraxellaceae by ribosomal DNA sequencing: ribosomal differentiation of medical microorganisms. *J. Clin. Microbiol.* **39:**936–942.

62. **Holmes, B., M. Costas, S. L. W. On, P. Vandamme, E. Falsen, and K. Kersters.** 1993. *Neisseria weaveri* sp. nov. (formerly CDC Group M-5), from dog bite wounds of humans. *Int. J. Syst. Bacteriol.* **43:**687–693.

63. **Holmes, K. K., G. W. Counts, and H. N. Beaty.** 1971. Disseminated gonococcal infection. *Ann. Intern. Med.* **74:**979–993.

64. **Hsiao, J., M. Lee, J. Chia, W. Ho, J. Chu, and P. Chu.** 2008. *Neisseria elongata* endocarditis complicated by brain embolism and abscess. *J. Med. Microbiol.* **57:**376–381.

65. **Ilina, E. N., A. D. Borovskaya, M. M. Malakhova, V. A. Vereshchagin, A. A. Kubanova, A. N. Kruglov, T. S. Svistunova, A. O. Gazarian, T. Maier, M. Kostrzewa, and V. M. Govorun.** 2009. Direct bacterial profiling by matrix-assisted laser desorption-ionization time-of-flight mass spectrometry for identification of pathogenic *Neisseria. J. Mol. Diagn.* **11:**75–86.

66. **Iwen, P. C., R. A. Walker, K. L. Warren, D. M. Kelly, S. H. Hinrichs, and J. Linder.** 1995. Evaluation of nucleic acid-based test (PACE 2C) for simultaneous detection of *Chlamydia trachomatis* and *Neisseria gonorrhoeae* in endocervical specimens. *J. Clin. Microbiol.* **33:**2587–2591.

67. **Jacobitz, H.** 1907. Der Diplococcus meningitidis cerebrospinalis als Erreger von Erkrankungen der Lunge und Bronchien. *Z. Hyg. Infektionskr.* **56:**175–192.

68. **Jadavji, T., W. D. Biggar, R. Gold, and C. G. Prober.** 1986. Sequelae of acute bacterial meningitis in children treated for seven days. *Pediatrics* **78:**21–25.

69. **Jain, S., H. N. Win, V. Chalam, and L. Yee.** 2007. Disseminated gonococcal infection presenting as vasculitis: a case report. *J. Clin. Pathol.* **60:**90–91.

70. **Janda, W. M., L. M. Wilcoski, K. L. Mandel, P. Ruther, and J. M. Stevens.** 1993. Comparison of monoclonal antibody methods and a ribosomal ribonucleic acid probe test for *Neisseria gonorrhoeae* culture confirmation. *Eur. J. Clin. Microbiol. Infect. Dis.* **12:**177–184.

71. **Jeurissen, A., J. P. Stroy, R. P. Wielenga, and G. I. Andriesse.** 2006. Severe infective endocarditis due to *Neisseria sicca*: case report and review of literature. *Acta Clin. Belg.* **61:**256–258.

72. **Johnson, R. E., W. J. Newhall, J. R. Papp, J. S. Knapp, C. M. Black, T. L. Gift, R. Steece, L. E. Markowitz, O. J. Devine, C. M. Walsh, S. Wang, D. C. Gunter, K. L. Irwin, S. DeLisle, and S. M. Berman.** 2002. Screening tests to detect *Chlamydia trachomatis* and *Neisseria gonorrhoeae* infections—2002. *MMWR Recommend. Rep.* **51:**1–38; quiz CE1–4.

73. **Jorgensen, J. H., S. A. Crawford, L. C. Fulcher, A. Glennen, S. M. Harrington, J. Swenson, R. Lynfield, P. R. Murray, and F. C. Tenover.** 2006. Multilaboratory evaluation of disk diffusion antimicrobial susceptibility testing of *Neisseria meningitidis* isolates. *J. Clin. Microbiol.* **44:**1744–1754.

74. **Knapp, J. S., and V. L. Clark.** 1984. Anaerobic growth of *Neisseria gonorrhoeae* coupled to nitrite reduction. *Infect. Immun.* **46:**176–181.

75. Knapp, J. S., and E. W. Hook. 1988. Prevalence and persistence of *Neisseria cinerea* and other *Neisseria* spp. in adults. *J. Clin. Microbiol.* **26:**896–900.

76. Knapp, J. S., P. A. Totten, M. H. Mulks, and B. H. Minshew. 1984. Characterization of *Neisseria cinerea*, a nonpathogenic species isolated on Martin-Lewis medium selective for pathogenic *Neisseria* spp. *J. Clin. Microbiol.* **19:**63–67.

77. Koenig, M. G., S. L. Kosha, B. L. Doty, and D. G. Heath. 2004. Direct comparison of the BD ProbeTec ET System with in-house LightCycler PCR assays for detection of *Chlamydia trachomatis* and *Neisseria gonorrhoeae* from clinical specimens. *J. Clin. Microbiol.* **42:**5751–5756.

78. Kugelman, G., J. W. Tapsall, N. Goire, M. W. Syrmis, A. Limnios, S. B. Lambert, M. D. Nissen, T. P. Sloots, and D. M. Whiley. 2009. Simple, rapid and inexpensive detection of *Neisseria gonorrhoeae* resistance mechanisms using heat-denatured isolates and SYBR green-based real-time PCR. *Antimicrob. Agents Chemother.* **53:**4211–4216.

79. Lal, G., P. Balmer, H. Joseph, M. Dawson, and R. Borrow. 2004. Development and evaluation of a tetraplex flow cytometric assay for quantitation of serum antibodies to *Neisseria meningitidis* serogroups A, C, Y, and W-135. *Clin. Diagn. Lab. Immunol.* **11:**272–279.

80. Lauer, B. A., and H. B. Masters. 1988. Toxic effect of calcium alginate swabs on *Neisseria gonorrhoeae*. *J. Clin. Microbiol.* **26:**54–56.

81. Levett, P. N., K. Brandt, K. Olenius, C. Brown, K. Montgomery, and G. B. Horsman. 2008. Evaluation of three automated nucleic acid amplification systems for detection of *Chlamydia trachomatis* and *Neisseria gonorrhoeae* in first-void urine specimens. *J. Clin. Microbiol.* **46:**2109–2111.

82. Little, M. C., J. Andrews, R. Moore, S. Bustos, L. Jones, C. Embres, G. Durmowicz, J. Harris, D. Berger, K. Yanson, C. Rostkowski, D. Yursis, J. Price, T. Fort, A. Walters, M. Collis, O. Llorin, J. Wood, F. Failing, C. O'Keefe, B. Scrivens, B. Pope, T. Hansen, K. Marino, and K. Williams. 1999. Strand displacement amplification and homogeneous real-time detection incorporated in a second-generation DNA probe system, BDProbeTecET. *Clin. Chem.* **45:**777–784.

83. Lowe, P., P. O'Loughlin, K. Evans, M. White, P. B. Bartley, and R. Vohra. 2006. Comparison of the Gen-Probe APTIMA Combo 2 assay to the AMPLICOR CT/NG assay for detection of *Chlamydia trachomatis* and *Neisseria gonorrhoeae* in urine samples from Australian men and women. *J. Clin. Microbiol.* **44:**2619–2621.

84. Mahony, J., S. Chong, D. Jang, K. Luinstra, M. Faught, D. Dalby, J. Sellors, and M. Chernesky. 1998. Urine specimens from pregnant and nonpregnant women inhibitory to amplification of *Chlamydia trachomatis* nucleic acid by PCR, ligase chain reaction, and transcription-mediated amplification: identification of urinary substances associated with inhibition and removal of inhibitory activity. *J. Clin. Microbiol.* **36:**3122–3126.

85. Maiden, M. C., J. A. Bygraves, E. Feil, G. Morelli, J. E. Russell, R. Urwin, Q. Zhang, J. Zhou, K. Zurth, D. A. Caugant, I. M. Feavers, M. Achtman, and B. G. Spratt. 1998. Multilocus sequence typing: a portable approach to the identification of clones within populations of pathogenic microorganisms. *Proc. Natl. Acad. Sci. USA* **95:**3140–3145.

86. Manavi, K., H. Young, and D. Clutterbuck. 2003. Sensitivity of microscopy for the rapid diagnosis of gonorrhoea in men and women and the role of gonorrhoea serovars. *Int. J. STD AIDS* **14:**390–394.

87. Manchanda, V., and P. Bhalla. 2006. Emergence of nonceftriaxone-susceptible *Neisseria meningitidis* in India. *J. Clin. Microbiol.* **44:**4290–4291.

88. Mangold, K. A., M. Regner, M. Tajuddin, A. M. Tajuddin, L. Jennings, H. Du, and K. L. Kaul. 2007. *Neisseria* species identification assay for the confirmation of *Neisseria gonorrhoeae*-positive results of the COBAS Amplicor PCR. *J. Clin. Microbiol.* **45:**1403–1409.

89. Marshall, R., M. Chernesky, D. Jang, E. W. Hook, C. P. Cartwright, B. Howell-Adams, S. Ho, J. Welk, J. Lai-Zhang, J. Brashear, B. Diedrich, K. Otis, E. Webb, J. Robinson, and H. Yu. 2007. Characteristics of the m2000 automated sample preparation and multiplex real-time PCR system for detection of *Chlamydia trachomatis* and *Neisseria gonorrhoeae*. *J. Clin. Microbiol.* **45:**747–751.

90. Martin, I. M. C., S. Hoffmann, and C. A. Ison. 2006. European Surveillance of Sexually Transmitted Infections (ESSTI): the first combined antimicrobial susceptibility data for *Neisseria gonorrhoeae* in Western Europe. *J. Antimicrob. Chemother.* **58:**587–593.

91. Martin, I. M. C., C. A. Ison, D. M. Aanensen, K. A. Fenton, and B. G. Spratt. 2004. Rapid sequence-based identification of gonococcal transmission clusters in a large metropolitan area. *J. Infect. Dis.* **189:**1497–1505.

92. Masek, B. J., N. Arora, N. Quinn, B. Aumakhan, J. Holden, A. Hardick, P. Agreda, M. Barnes, and C. A. Gaydos. 2009. Performance of three nucleic acid amplification tests for detection of *Chlamydia trachomatis* and *Neisseria gonorrhoeae* by use of self-collected vaginal swabs obtained via an Internet-based screening program. *J. Clin. Microbiol.* **47:**1663–1667.

93. Masliah-Planchon, J., G. Breton, V. Jarlier, A. Simon, O. Benveniste, S. Herson, and L. Drieux. 2009. Endocarditis due to *Neisseria bacilliformis* in a patient with a bicuspid aortic valve. *J. Clin. Microbiol.* **47:**1973–1975.

94. McNally, L. P., D. J. Templeton, F. Jin, A. E. Grulich, B. Donovan, D. M. Whiley, and P. H. Cunningham. 2008. Low positive predictive value of a nucleic acid amplification test for nongenital *Neisseria gonorrhoeae* infection in homosexual men. *Clin. Infect. Dis.* **47:**e25–e27.

95. Moncada, J., J. Schachter, S. Liska, C. Shayevich, and J. D. Klausner. 2009. Evaluation of self-collected glans and rectal swabs from men who have sex with men for detection of *Chlamydia trachomatis* and *Neisseria gonorrhoeae* by use of nucleic acid amplification tests. *J. Clin. Microbiol.* **47:**1657–1662.

96. Morris, S. R., J. D. Klausner, S. P. Buchbinder, S. L. Wheeler, B. Koblin, T. Coates, M. Chesney, and G. N. Colfax. 2006. Prevalence and incidence of pharyngeal gonorrhea in a longitudinal sample of men who have sex with men: the EXPLORE study. *Clin. Infect. Dis.* **43:**1284–1289.

97. Nair, D., R. Dawar, M. Deb, M. R. Capoor, S. Singal, D. J. Upadhayay, P. Aggarwal, B. DAS, and J. C. Samantaray. 2009. Outbreak of meningococcal disease in and around New Delhi, India, 2005–2006: a report from a tertiary care hospital. *Epidemiol. Infect.* **137:**570–576.

98. Orr, H. J., S. J. Gray, M. Macdonald, and J. M. Stuart. 2003. Saliva and meningococcal transmission. *Emerg. Infect. Dis.* **9:**1314–1315.

99. Oster, P., D. Lennon, J. O'Hallahan, K. Mulholland, S. Reid, and D. Martin. 2005. MeNZB: a safe and highly immunogenic tailor-made vaccine against the New Zealand *Neisseria meningitidis* serogroup B disease epidemic strain. *Vaccine* **23:**2191–2196.

100. Palmer, H. M., H. Mallinson, R. L. Wood, and A. J. Herring. 2003. Evaluation of the specificities of five DNA amplification methods for the detection of *Neisseria gonorrhoeae*. *J. Clin. Microbiol.* **41:**835–837.

101. Parmentier, L., C. Garzoni, C. Antille, L. Kaiser, B. Ninet, and L. Borradori. 2008. Value of a novel *Neisseria meningitidis*–specific polymerase chain reaction assay in skin biopsy specimens as a diagnostic tool in chronic meningococcemia. *Arch. Dermatol.* **144:**770–773.

102. Perkins, M. D., S. Mirrett, and L. B. Reller. 1995. Rapid bacterial antigen detection is not clinically useful. *J. Clin. Microbiol.* **33:**1486–1491.

103. Petersen, B. H., T. J. Lee, R. Snyderman, and G. F. Brooks. 1979. *Neisseria meningitidis* and *Neisseria gonorrhoeae* bacteremia associated with C6, C7, or C8 deficiency. *Ann. Intern. Med.* **90:**917–920.

104. Pillai, S., A. Howell, K. Alexander, B. E. Bentley, H. Jiang, K. Ambrose, D. Zhu, and G. Zlotnick. 2005. Outer membrane protein (OMP) based vaccine for *Neisseria meningitidis* serogroup B. *Vaccine* **23:**2206–2209.

105. Rainbow, J., E. Cebelinski, J. Bartkus, A. Glennen, D. Boxrud, and R. Lynfield. 2005. Rifampin-resistant meningococcal disease. *Emerg. Infect. Dis.* **11:**977–979.

106. **Rennie, R. P., C. Brosnikoff, S. Shokoples, L. B. Reller, S. Mirrett, W. Janda, K. Ristow, and A. Krilcich.** 2008. Multicenter evaluation of the new Vitek 2 Neisseria-Haemophilus identification card. *J. Clin. Microbiol.* **46:**2681–2685.

107. **Rintala, L., and H. M. Pollock.** 1978. Effects of two blood culture anticoagulants on growth of *Neisseria meningitidis. J. Clin. Microbiol.* **7:**332–336.

108. **Robert Koch Institut.** 2008. Invasive Meningokokken-Erkrankungen im Jahr 2007. *Epidemiologisches Bulletin* **32:**331–335.

109. **Roberts, J., B. Greenwood, and J. Stuart.** 2009. Sampling methods to detect carriage of *Neisseria meningitidis*; literature review. *J. Infect.* **58:**103–107.

110. **Rossau, R., E. Vanmechelen, J. De Ley, and H. Van Heuverswijn.** 1989. Specific *Neisseria gonorrhoeae* DNA-probes derived from ribosomal RNA. *J. Gen. Microbiol.* **135:**1735–1745.

111. **Russell, J. E., K. A. Jolley, I. M. Feavers, M. C. J. Maiden, and J. Suker.** 2004. PorA variable regions of *Neisseria meningitidis. Emerg. Infect. Dis.* **10:**674–678.

112. **Schachter, J., J. Moncada, S. Liska, C. Shayevich, and J. D. Klausner.** 2008. Nucleic acid amplification tests in the diagnosis of chlamydial and gonococcal infections of the oropharynx and rectum in men who have sex with men. *Sex. Transm. Dis.* **35:**637–642.

113. **Schouls, L. M., A. van der Ende, M. Damen, and I. van de Pol.** 2006. Multiple-locus variable-number tandem repeat analysis of *Neisseria meningitidis* yields groupings similar to those obtained by multilocus sequence typing. *J. Clin. Microbiol.* **44:**1509–1518.

114. **Sejvar, J. J., D. Johnson, T. Popovic, J. M. Miller, F. Downes, P. Somsel, R. Weyant, D. S. Stephens, B. A. Perkins, and N. E. Rosenstein.** 2005. Assessing the risk of laboratory-acquired meningococcal disease. *J. Clin. Microbiol.* **43:**4811–4814.

115. **Siedner, M. J., M. Pandori, L. Castro, P. Barry, W. L. H. Whittington, S. Liska, and J. D. Klausner.** 2007. Real-time PCR assay for detection of quinolone-resistant *Neisseria gonorrhoeae* in urine samples. *J. Clin. Microbiol.* **45:**1250–1254.

116. **Sinave, C. P., and K. R. Ratzan.** 1987. Infective endocarditis caused by *Neisseria flavescens. Am. J. Med.* **82:**163–164.

117. **Smith, N. H., E. C. Holmes, G. M. Donovan, G. A. Carpenter, and B. G. Spratt.** 1999. Networks and groups within the genus *Neisseria:* analysis of argF, recA, rho, and 16S rRNA sequences from human *Neisseria* species. *Mol. Biol. Evol.* **16:**773–783.

118. **Stein, D. C.** 2006. The Neisseria, p. 602–647. *In* M. Dworkin, S. Falkow, E. Rosenberg, K. H. Schleifer, and E. T. Stackebrandt (ed.), *The Prokaryotes,* 3rd ed. Springer, Berlin, Germany.

119. **Taha, M., J. A. Vázquez, E. Hong, D. E. Bennett, S. Bertrand, S. Bukovski, M. T. Cafferkey, F. Carion, J. J. Christensen, M. Diggle, G. Edwards, R. Enríquez, C. Fazio, M. Frosch, S. Heuberger, S. Hoffmann, K. A. Jolley, M. Kadlubowski, A. Kechrid, K. Kesanopoulos, P. Kriz, L. Lambertsen, I. Levenet, M. Musilek, M. Paragi, A. Saguer, A. Skoczynska, P. Stefanelli, S. Thulin, G. Tzanakaki, M. Unemo, U. Vogel, and M. L. Zarantonelli.** 2007. Target gene sequencing to characterize the penicillin G susceptibility of *Neisseria meningitidis. Antimicrob. Agents Chemother.* **51:**2784–2792.

120. **Taha, M., M. L. Zarantonelli, C. Ruckly, D. Giorgini, and J. Alonso.** 2006. Rifampin-resistant *Neisseria meningitidis. Emerg. Infect. Dis.* **12:**859–860.

121. **Tapsall, J. W.** 2009. *Neisseria gonorrhoeae* and emerging resistance to extended spectrum cephalosporins. *Curr. Opin. Infect. Dis.* **22:**87–91.

122. **Thayer, J. D., and J. E. Martin.** 1964. A selective medium for the cultivation of *N. gonorrhoeae* and *N. meningitidis. Public Health Rep.* **79:**49–57.

123. **Thompson, E. A. L., I. M. Feavers, and M. C. J. Maiden.** 2003. Antigenic diversity of meningococcal enterobactin receptor FetA, a vaccine component. *Microbiology* (Reading) **149:**1849–1858.

124. **Tønjum, T.** 2005. Order IV. Neisseriales, p. 774–862. *In* D. J. Brenner, N. R. Krieg, J. T. Staley, and G. M. Garrity (ed.), *Bergey's Manual of Systematic Bacteriology,* 2nd ed. Springer, Berlin, Germany.

125. **Tronel, H., H. Chaudemanche, N. Pechier, L. Doutrelant, and B. Hoen.** 2001. Endocarditis due to *Neisseria mucosa* after tongue piercing. *Clin. Microbiol. Infect.* **7:**275–276.

126. **Trotter, C. L., and M. E. Ramsay.** 2007. Vaccination against meningococcal disease in Europe: review and recommendations for the use of conjugate vaccines. *FEMS Microbiol. Rev.* **31:**101–107.

127. **Tully, J., R. M. Viner, P. G. Coen, J. M. Stuart, M. Zambon, C. Peckham, C. Booth, N. Klein, E. Kaczmarski, and R. Booy.** 2006. Risk and protective factors for meningococcal disease in adolescents: matched cohort study. *Br. Med. J.* **332:**445–450.

128. **Urwin, R., E. B. Kaczmarski, M. Guiver, A. J. Fox, and M. C. Maiden.** 1998. Amplification of the meningococcal porB gene for non-culture serotype characterization. *Epidemiol. Infect.* **120:**257–262.

129. **Valenza, G., C. Ruoff, U. Vogel, M. Frosch, and M. Abele-Horn.** 2007. Microbiological evaluation of the new VITEK 2 Neisseria-Haemophilus identification card. *J. Clin. Microbiol.* **45:**3493–3497.

129a. **Vandamme, P., B. Holmes, H. Bercovier, and T. Coenye.** 2006. Classification of Centers for Disease Control Group Eugonic Fermenter (EF)-4a and EF-4b as *Neisseria animaloria* sp. nov. and *Neisseria zoodegmatis* sp. nov., respectively. *Int. J. Syst. Evol. Microbiol.* **56:**1801–1805.

130. **van der Ende, A., I. G. Schuurman, C. T. Hopman, C. A. Fijen, and J. Dankert.** 1995. Comparison of commercial diagnostic tests for identification of serogroup antigens of *Neisseria meningitidis. J. Clin. Microbiol.* **33:**3326–3327.

131. **van Deuren, M., P. Brandtzaeg, and J. W. M. van der Meer.** 2000. Update on meningococcal disease with emphasis on pathogenesis and clinical management. *Clin. Microbiol. Rev.* **13:**144–166.

132. **Van Dyck, E., M. Ieven, S. Pattyn, L. Van Damme, and M. Laga.** 2001. Detection of *Chlamydia trachomatis* and *Neisseria gonorrhoeae* by enzyme immunoassay, culture, and three nucleic acid amplification tests. *J. Clin. Microbiol.* **39:**1751–1756.

133. **Vázquez, J. A., A. M. Enriquez, L. De la Fuente, S. Berrón, and M. Baquero.** 1996. Isolation of a strain of beta-lactamase-producing *Neisseria meningitidis* in Spain. *Eur. J. Clin. Microbiol. Infect. Dis.* **15:**181–182.

134. **Warner, L., K. M. Stone, M. Macaluso, J. W. Buehler, and H. D. Austin.** 2006. Condom use and risk of gonorrhea and Chlamydia: a systematic review of design and measurement factors assessed in epidemiologic studies. *Sex. Transm. Dis.* **33:**36–51.

135. **Whiley, D. M., P. J. Buda, J. Bayliss, L. Cover, J. Bates, and T. P. Sloots.** 2004. A new confirmatory *Neisseria gonorrhoeae* real-time PCR assay targeting the porA pseudogene. *Eur. J. Clin. Microbiol. Infect. Dis.* **23:**705–710.

136. **Whiley, D. M., J. W. Tapsall, and T. P. Sloots.** 2006. Nucleic acid amplification testing for *Neisseria gonorrhoeae:* an ongoing challenge. *J. Mol. Diagn.* **8:**3–15.

137. **WHO Western Pacific Region Gonococcal Antimicrobial Surveillance Programme.** 2008. Surveillance of antibiotic resistance in *Neisseria gonorrhoeae* in the WHO Western Pacific Region, 2006. *Commun. Dis. Intell.* **32:**48–51.

138. **Winstead, J. M., D. S. McKinsey, S. Tasker, M. A. De Groote, and L. M. Baddour.** 2000. Meningococcal pneumonia: characterization and review of cases seen over the past 25 years. *Clin. Infect. Dis.* **30:**87–94.

139. **World Health Organization.** 1976. *Neisseria gonorrhoeae* producing beta-lactamase (penicillinase). *Wkly. Epidemiol. Rec.* **51:**385–386.

140. **Wu, H. M., B. H. Harcourt, C. P. Hatcher, S. C. Wei, R. T. Novak, X. Wang, B. A. Juni, A. Glennen, D. J. Boxrud, J. Rainbow, S. Schmink, R. D. Mair, M. J. Theodore, M. A. Sander, T. K. Miller, K. Kruger, A. C. Cohn, T. A. Clark, N. E. Messonnier, L. W. Mayer, and R. Lynfield.** 2009. Emergence of ciprofloxacin-resistant *Neisseria meningitidis* in North America. *N. Engl. J. Med.* **360:**886–892.

141. **Young, H., and A. Moyes.** 1993. Comparative evaluation of AccuProbe culture identification test for *Neisseria gonorrhoeae* and other rapid methods. *J. Clin. Microbiol.* **31:**1996–1999.

142. **Zaia, A., J. M. Griffith, T. R. Hogan, J. W. Tapsall, P. Bainbridge, R. Neill, and D. Tribe.** 2005. Molecular tests can allow confirmation of invasive meningococcal disease when isolates yield atypical maltose, glucose or gamma-glutamyl peptidase test results. *Pathology* **37:**378–379.

Actinobacillus, Capnocytophaga, Eikenella, Kingella, Pasteurella, and Other Fastidious or Rarely Encountered Gram-Negative Rods*

REINHARD ZBINDEN AND ALEXANDER von GRAEVENITZ

33

The bacterial genera covered in this chapter are taxonomically diverse and belong to the families *Cardiobacteriaceae*, *Flavobacteriaceae*, *Fusobacteriaceae*, *Neisseriaceae*, *Pasteurellaceae*, and *Porphyromonadaceae*, but common traits justify their discussion as a group. They are isolated infrequently and constitute part of those gram-negative genera that stand apart from the *Aeromonadaceae*, *Enterobacteriaceae*, *Vibrionaceae*, and *Rickettsiales*. With the exception of *Chromobacterium* and some *Pasteurella* species, for aerobic growth they require supplemented media, on which they often grow slowly (48 h at 35 to 37°C), and fail to grow on enteric media. A 5-to-10% CO_2 atmosphere may be necessary for growth initiation and improves growth on subculture. Some species have varied Gram stain results. With the exception of *Chromobacterium*, they do not possess flagella but may show gliding or twitching motility, resulting in limited spreading of colonies and pitting of the agar surface (68). This chapter discusses only species that can be isolated from humans.

TAXONOMY AND DESCRIPTION OF THE AGENTS

The taxonomy of the family *Pasteurellaceae* has changed in important ways (51, 52, 83). The *Pasteurellaceae* consist of several genera, of which four are known to contain human pathogens: *Actinobacillus*, *Aggregatibacter*, *Haemophilus*, and *Pasteurella*. Minimal standards for the description of genera, species, and subspecies of the *Pasteurellaceae* have been proposed and might create further changes (24). *Aggregatibacter* spp., formerly named *Haemophilus* (106), are included in this chapter. The genus *Haemophilus*, as presently constituted, is described in chapter 34. *Neisseria* spp. with rod forms, and CDC group EF-4a, renamed *Neisseria animaloris* (137), are described in chapter 32 but are included in a differentiation table in this chapter (see Table 4).

Actinobacillus

The genus *Actinobacillus* in the family *Pasteurellaceae* consists of facultatively anaerobic, nonmotile, gram-negative rods and comprises animal (*A. equuli*, *A. lignieresii*, and *A. suis*) and exclusively human (*A. hominis* and *A. suis*) species

but no longer includes *Actinobacillus actinomycetemcomitans* (106). Subspeciation of *A. equuli* could not be upheld by 16S rRNA and *infB* gene sequencing (105). The G+C content of the DNA of *Actinobacillus* spp. is between 40 and 43 mol%.

Aggregatibacter

Earlier, 16S rRNA gene sequencing and DNA-DNA hybridization had placed *Actinobacillus actinomycetemcomitans* closer to the genus *Haemophilus* than to the genus *Actinobacillus* (108), and multilocus sequence analysis of *A. actinomycetemcomitans*, *Haemophilus aphrophilus*, *Haemophilus paraphrophilus*, and *Haemophilus segnis* (106) had suggested a monophyletic group. In addition, DNA-DNA relatedness between *H. aphrophilus* and *H. paraphrophilus* was 77%, and DNA from *H. aphrophilus* was able to transform *H. paraphrophilus* to have an NAD-independent phenotype (106). It was, therefore, proposed to transfer *A. actinomycetemcomitans*, *H. aphrophilus*, *H. paraphrophilus*, and *H. segnis* into a new genus, *Aggregatibacter* in the family *Pasteurellaceae*, with the species *A. aphrophilus* comprising the organisms formerly named *H. aphrophilus* and *H. paraphrophilus*, i.e., including V factor-dependent and -independent isolates (106). The G+C content of the DNA of *Aggregatibacter* spp. is 42 to 44 mol%.

Capnocytophaga

The *Capnocytophaga* genus in the family *Flavobacteriaceae* (51) at present consists of nine species (*C. canimorsus*, *C. cynodegmi*, *C. ochracea*, *C. gingivalis*, *C. sputigena*, *C. haemolytica*, *C. granulosa*, *C. leadbetteri*, and genospecies AHN8471) of facultatively anaerobic, nonmotile, gram-negative rods (43). The G+C content of the DNA of this genus is 34 to 40 mol%.

Cardiobacterium

The *Cardiobacterium* genus in the family *Cardiobacteriaceae* (51) consists of facultatively anaerobic, nonmotile, gram-negative rods, with the species *C. hominis* and *C. valvarum* (61). The G+C content of the DNA of these species is 59 to 60 mol%.

Chromobacterium

The *Chromobacterium* genus in the family *Neisseriaceae* (51) contains several facultatively anaerobic, motile species, of

---

*This chapter contains information presented by Alexander von Graevenitz, Reinhard Zbinden, and Reinier Mutters in chapter 40 of the ninth edition of this *Manual*.

574

which *C. violaceum* is at present the only agent of human disease. Its DNA content is between 65 and 68 mol%. *Chromobacterium haemolyticum*, recently isolated from a sputum culture, is so far represented by one strain only (62) and will not be covered here.

Dysgonomonas

The genus *Dysgonomonas* in the family *Porphyromonadaceae* consists of facultatively anaerobic, nonmotile, gram-negative rods (51). Four species have been described: *D. capnocytophagoides* and *D. gadei* (69), *D. mossii* (91), and "*D. hofstadii*" (90). The G+C content of the DNA of these species is around 38 mol%. The related "DF-3-like" bacteria (30) have not been investigated further.

Eikenella

The genus *Eikenella* in the family *Neisseriaceae* (51) consists of facultatively anaerobic, nonmotile, gram-negative rods. Thus far, only one species, *E. corrodens*, has been recognized, but DNA-DNA hybridization, analysis of the composition of the organism's cellular carbohydrates, and the occurrence of biochemically aberrant (e.g., catalase-positive) isolates suggest that there may be more than one genomospecies (77). The G+C content of the DNA of *Eikenella* is between 56 and 58 mol%.

Kingella

The genus *Kingella* in the family *Neisseriaceae* consists of the facultatively anaerobic, nonmotile species *K. kingae*, *K. denitrificans*, *K. oralis*, and *K. potus* (51). The G+C content of the DNA of these species is between 47 and 58 mol%.

Pasteurella

The taxonomy of the genus *Pasteurella* in the family *Pasteurellaceae* (51) has been in flux for some time (24). *Pasteurella multocida* can be separated into the subspecies *multocida*, *septica*, and *gallicida*; *Pasteurella canis*, *Pasteurella dagmatis*, and *Pasteurella stomatis* are other species isolated from humans. In spite of the genotypical homogeneity of *P. multocida* isolates, phenotypically diverse lineages have been observed, e.g., sucrose-negative variants from infections from bite wounds made by large cats (22). The G+C content of the DNA of *Pasteurella* species is between 38 and 46 mol%. New genera or reclassifications may be necessary for the species discussed below that are preceded by "(*P.*)" or "(*Pasteurella*)" (52, 66).

Simonsiella

The genus *Simonsiella* in the family *Neisseriaceae* (51) consists of several obligately aerobic species which may show gliding motility (85). The only species isolated from humans is *Simonsiella muelleri*. This genus has a G+C content in its DNA of 40 to 50 mol%.

Streptobacillus

The *Streptobacillus* genus in the family *Fusobacteriaceae* (51) consists of one facultatively anaerobic, nonmotile species, *S. moniliformis*, with a G+C content in its DNA of 24 to 26 mol% (40).

Suttonella

The *Suttonella* genus in the family *Cardiobacteriaceae* (51) consists of facultatively anaerobic, nonmotile, gram-negative rods and so far contains only one species, *S. indologenes* (formerly *Kingella indologenes*) (35). The G+C content of its DNA is 49 mol%.

EPIDEMIOLOGY AND TRANSMISSION

Most bacteria in this group are part of the flora of the nasopharynx and/or the oral cavity of animals and/or humans and are parasitic, with the only environmental species being *Chromobacterium*. Transmission from animals occurs by contact (e.g., bites and licking of wounds), from humans to humans by droplets (e.g., directly with *Kingella* spp. or by paraphernalia or human bites with *Eikenella* spp.). They may cause infections anywhere in the human body. Risk factors exist for certain types of septicemia (e.g., liver cirrhosis for *P. multocida*, neutropenia for oxidase-negative *Capnocytophaga* spp., and chronic granulomatous disease for *Chromobacterium violaceum*). Endogenous infections occur as well, e.g., HACEK (*Haemophilus parainfluenzae*, *Aggregatibacter* spp., *Cardiobacterium* spp., *Eikenella corrodens*, and *Kingella* spp.) endocarditis (see "Clinical Significance" below) (16).

Actinobacillus lignieresii (primary habitat in the oral cavities of sheep and cattle), *Actinobacillus equuli* (in the oral cavities of horses and pigs), and *Actinobacillus suis* (in the oral cavities of pigs) can be transmitted to humans by animal contact (21). Exclusively human are *Actinobacillus hominis* and *Actinobacillus ureae*, whose normal habitat is unknown (47, 81).

The habitat of *Aggregatibacter* spp. is the human oral cavity, including dental plaque (81). Infections are endogenous.

The oxidase- and catalase-negative species *Capnocytophaga ochracea*, *Capnocytophaga gingivalis*, *Capnocytophaga sputigena*, *Capnocytophaga haemolytica*, and *Capnocytophaga granulosa*, as well as the recently described *Capnocytophaga leadbetteri* and genospecies AHN8471 (43), are normal but not prominent members of the human oral flora. The first three have been isolated from adults with periodontal disease but also from periodontitis-free adults; the other four have been isolated from supragingival and subgingival plaque in children and adults (43). Infections are endogenous. The oxidase- and catalase-positive species *C. canimorsus* and *C. cynodegmi* reside in the oral cavities of healthy dogs (25% of dogs have *C. canimorsus* as determined by culture and 85 to 100% of dogs have it as determined by PCR) and cats (15%, as determined by culture) (10, 136).

The normal habitat of *Cardiobacterium* spp. is the human oral cavity and nasopharynx but possibly also the gastrointestinal and urogenital tracts (129). Infections are endogenous.

Chromobacterium inhabits soil and water in tropical and subtropical climates between latitudes of 35°N and 35°S (South Africa, Southeast Asia, Australia, southeastern United States and, rarely, South America) (93). The portal of entry is usually the skin, but oral intake has also been reported (125).

Most *Dysgonomonas capnocytophagoides* strains have been isolated from stools of immunocompromised patients, and a few strains have been isolated from other sources (63, 95). The natural habitats of this and the other *Dysgonomonas* spp. are unknown.

The natural habitat of *Eikenella corrodens* is the oral cavities and possibly the gastrointestinal tracts of humans and some mammals, from which it can be transmitted via saliva (bites, syringes) to other individuals (112, 123, 134). Endogenous infections prevail, however.

The natural habitat of *Kingella* spp. is the upper respiratory tract and oral mucosa of humans and possibly other primates. *K. kingae* colonizes the throat but not the nasopharynx of many children aged 6 months to 4 years (142). The natural habitats of *K. denitrificans* and *K. potus* are unknown. *K. oralis* has been isolated from the human mouth (18). Ribotyping and pulsed-field gel electrophoresis have shown that *K. kingae* can be transmitted via respiratory droplets (128), although most infections are endogenous.

Pasteurella spp. are widespread in healthy and diseased wild and domestic animals, including rodents, dogs, and cats, inhabiting the nasopharynx and gingiva (139). Human isolates are transmitted predominantly from animals by contact (bites or licking or scratching of wounds). Of the "related" species, (*Pasteurella*) *aerogenes* occurs primarily in pigs (39), (*Pasteurella*) *caballi* in pigs and equines (23), and (*Pasteurella*) *pneumotropica* in rodents and dogs (44); the natural habitat of (*Pasteurella*) *bettyae* is uncertain.

The natural habitat of *Simonsiella muelleri* is the oral cavities of humans (86).

Streptobacillus moniliformis occurs naturally in the upper respiratory tracts of up to 100% of wild and laboratory rats and other rodents (mice, gerbils, squirrels, ferrets, weasels) and occasionally of dogs and cats preying on rodents. Transmission to humans occurs either from bites of those animals (rat bite fever) or from consumption of contaminated food or water (Haverhill fever) (40).

The natural habitat of *Suttonella indologenes* is not known.

CLINICAL SIGNIFICANCE

Actinobacillus spp.

A. lignieresii causes actinobacillosis, a granulomatous disease in cattle and sheep in which, as with actinomycosis, sulfur granules form in tissues (117). A few human soft tissue infections after a cattle or sheep bite or other contacts have been reported (113). *A. equuli* and *A. suis* have caused a variety of diseases in horses and pigs; human infections are generally due to horse or pig bites or contact (5, 41). Both species have also been isolated, albeit rarely, from the human upper respiratory tract (118, 140). *A. ureae* is most often a commensal in the human respiratory tract, particularly in patients with lower respiratory tract disease (81), but has also been found as an agent of meningitis following trauma or surgery (32) and of other infections in immunocompromised patients (78). *A. hominis* has also been isolated from such patients but has occurred as a commensal as well, albeit rarely (47). Virulence factors belong to the pore-forming protein toxins of the RTX family; RTX toxins have repeats in the structural toxin peptide and exhibit a cytotoxic and often also a hemolytic activity. They are particularly widespread in species of the family *Pasteurellaceae* (46).

Aggregatibacter spp.

A. actinomycetemcomitans is one of the major agents of juvenile and adult periodontitis (104) and may occur together with *Actinomyces* spp. in actinomycotic sulfur granules (76). Furthermore, it may cause HACEK endocarditis (16), soft tissue infections, and other infections (76, 110). HACEK are the causes of approximately 1% of all cases of endocarditis. HACEK endocarditis is characterized by a relatively long interval between first symptoms and diagnosis (range, 2 weeks to 6 months), large vegetations on native or artificial valves of the left side, and frequent embolizations. Prognosis is good with appropriate antibiotic treatment (16).

Virulence factors are an RTX leukotoxin (46), a cytotoxic distending toxin (7), and the adhesin EmaA (132), as well as fimbriae (67).

A. aphrophilus may cause systemic disease, particularly bone and joint infections, spondylodiscitis, and endocarditis (29, 72, 111).

A. segnis, whose frequency may be underestimated due to apparent misdiagnoses, may cause endocarditis and, rarely, other systemic infections (89, 130).

Capnocytophaga spp.

C. ochracea, C. gingivalis, C. sputigena, C. haemolytica, and *C. granulosa* have been reported as agents of septicemia and other endogenous infections (endocarditis, endometritis, osteomyelitis, soft tissue infections, peritonitis, keratitis, noma) (13, 112, 138) in immunocompetent and immunosuppressed (mainly neutropenic) patients. They are able to suppress neutrophilic chemotaxis and lymphocyte proliferation (107). The association with periodontitis remains unclear (43).

Infections with *C. canimorsus* and *C. cynodegmi* are associated mainly with dog or cat bites or contact. Patients infected with *C. canimorsus* most often present with septicemia and have previously been splenectomized or are alcoholics. In fulminant cases with a poor prognosis, disseminated intravascular coagulation, acute renal failure, respiratory distress syndrome, and shock may develop (74). Hemolytic-uremic syndrome and thrombotic thrombocytopenic purpura are other possible sequelae (82, 100). Meningitis (31), eye infections (13), and endocarditis (119) have been reported as well. *C. cynodegmi* has been isolated more rarely, mainly from localized or systemic infections (114). *C. canimorsus* resists phagocytosis by macrophages and killing by complement and leukocytes; macrophages incubated with the bacterium fail to produce several proinflammatory cytokines (124).

Cardiobacterium spp.

Disease caused by both *Cardiobacterium* species is mainly HACEK endocarditis (94); on rare occasions, *C. hominis* has been isolated from other body sites (87, 112). In blood culture-negative cases, the diagnosis has been made by broad-range PCR applied to valve tissue (103).

Chromobacterium violaceum

Localized infections usually arise from contaminated wounds, and septicemia with multiple organ abscesses may follow (93). They are significantly associated with neutrophil dysfunction (glucose-6-phosphate dehydrogenase deficiency, chronic granulomatous disease). Children without these conditions and those with bacteremia show a high fatality rate (125). A number of virulence factors other than endotoxin, i.e., adhesins, invasins, and cytolytic proteins, have been described (15).

Dysgonomonas spp.

Diarrhea was reported to have occurred in 10 of 20 patients with fecal isolates of *C. capnocytophagoides,* whereas routine stool cultures yielded the organism in 1.1 to 2.3% of cultures (95). Bacteremia occurs as well (63); one blood isolate was found to be identical by ribotyping to one in the stool of the same patient (58). One strain of *D. mossii* was isolated from intestinal juice of a patient with pancreatic carcinoma (96). *D. gadei* has been isolated from a human gallbladder (69) and from blood (3), and "*D. hofstadii*" has been isolated from a wound (90).

Eikenella corrodens

E. corrodens is associated with juvenile and adult periodontitis (104) but is also an agent of infections of the upper respiratory tract, pleura and lungs, abdomen, joints, bones, wounds (e.g., from a human bite), and, rarely, other infections, like noma (71, 112, 123, 134). These organisms are often indolent and found mixed with other members of the oropharyngeal biota, particularly staphylococci and streptococci. Risk factors are dental manipulations and intravenous drug abuse. Endocarditis is of the HACEK type if monomicrobial, but polymicrobial non-HACEK cases are known (16). *E. corrodens* can trigger a cascade of events that induce inflammation in periodontal tissue (145).

Kingella spp.

Infections with *K. kingae* show a predilection for bones and joints of previously healthy children under 4 years of age (142). The use of culture and broad-range and *K. kingae*-specific real-time PCR show it to be the most common cause of osteoarthritic infection in this age group (20). Septic arthritis, discitis, and osteomyelitis of the lower extremities as well as occult bacteremia are conspicuous. Stomatitis and/or upper respiratory infections may precede systemic disease, suggesting entry through a damaged mucosa (142). In adults, systemic infections occur in immunocompromised individuals (11) or may present as HACEK endocarditis (16). Virulence factors are an RTX toxin (79) and type IV pili (80).

K. denitrificans has been reported as an agent of endocarditis (99). *K. oralis* has been isolated from patients with periodontitis, but its relationship to the disease is unclear (18). *K. potus* has caused a wound infection following a kinkajou bite (92).

Pasteurella spp.

Human isolates of *P. multocida* are mostly found in wound or soft tissue infections. Less frequent are colonization or infection of the respiratory tract and (by the hematogenous or contiguous route) systemic disease, such as meningitis, dialysis-associated peritonitis, endocarditis, osteomyelitis, and septicemia, with cirrhosis of the liver being a particular risk factor (139). The subspecies most frequently encountered is subsp. *multocida*, which is also more frequent in respiratory infections and bacteremias than subsp. *septica*, which is most often associated with wound infections (36). Infected cat bite wounds contain pasteurellae significantly more often than infected dog bite wounds, reflecting a higher oropharyngeal colonization rate in cats than in dogs (36). In the respiratory tract, colonization may eventually lead to sinusitis or bronchitis as well as pneumonia and empyema, the latter two mostly in patients with prior respiratory disease (101). Virulence factors are capsules (six serotypes, of which A and D account for most human isolates) (36), lipopolysaccharide, an RTX cytotoxin (46), surface adhesins, and iron acquisition proteins (64).

Cases of human infection with *P. canis* (from dogs), *P. dagmatis*, and *P. stomatis* (from dogs or cats) are infrequent (2, 36, 59). In some cases of pasteurellosis, animal contact could not be established. Double infections with two *Pasteurella* spp. have also been observed (70).

Of the "related" species, (*P.) aerogenes* has caused wound infections from pig and hamster bites (39, 45), (*P.) bettyae* has been found in infections of newborns and in infections of the male and female genital tracts (12, 33), and (*P.) caballi* has been isolated from horse bites (42); (*P.) pneumotropica* is a rare agent of systemic infection in humans (44). Reported cases of human infection with *Avibacterium gallinarum*, *Bibersteinia trehalosi*, *Gallibacterium anatis*, and *Mannheimia haemolytica*, all formerly in the genus *Pasteurella*, remain doubtful when stricter identification criteria are employed (60) or require confirmation (52).

Simonsiella spp.

S. muelleri has not been found associated with disease (17, 141).

Streptobacillus moniliformis

Rat bite fever is a systemic illness beginning with fever and chills, followed by migratory, sometimes even suppurative, polyarthritis and a maculopapular rash on the extremities. Rare complications include endocarditis, myo- or pericarditis, pneumonia, septicemia, and abscess formation (37, 40).

Suttonella indologenes

Human isolates of *S. indologenes* have been very rare; they have been isolated from ocular sources (140) and a blood culture in a case of endocarditis (75).

COLLECTION, TRANSPORT, AND STORAGE OF SPECIMENS

Collection of specimens should follow the guidelines described in chapter 16; the low viability of many species makes the use of transport media, e.g., eSwab (Copan Diagnostics Inc., Murrieta, CA), whenever indicated, mandatory. Cultures of most bacteria described in this chapter can be stored at room temperature for 1 to 2 weeks. However, for some other very fastidious bacteria, e.g., *C. canimorsus*, subcultures must be performed frequently. For keeping strains in a culture collection, the isolates should be frozen in a cryoprotective solution, e.g., skim milk, at −70°C.

DIRECT EXAMINATION

Actinobacillus spp. are medium-sized, gram-negative rod-shaped or coccoid bacteria with a tendency to bipolar staining. Their arrangement is single, in pairs, and, rarely, in short chains.

Aggregatibacter spp. are coccoid or rod-shaped gram-negative bacteria, occasionally exhibiting filamentous forms. A PCR for *A. actinomycetemcomitans* has been developed (50).

Capnocytophaga spp. are mainly fusiform, medium-to-long cells with tapered ends (Fig. 1a). PCR has also been devised for their detection (65). *Leptotrichia buccalis* is a long, fusiform, gram-negative rod but with one tapered and one square end (Fig. 1b). Differentiation is supported by biochemical reactions or by analysis of fatty acids (9).

Cardiobacterium spp. are pleomorphic on blood agar. *C. hominis* stains irregularly and appears as straight, gram-negative rods in short chains, pairs, or rosettes, sometimes with bulbous ends; occasionally, filaments are formed. On chocolate agar, this morphology is less distinct than on blood agar. In a few instances, broad-range PCR of valve or emboli have led to the diagnosis (103).

C. violaceum is a medium-sized, gram-negative rod or coccus that is motile by one polar flagellum and one to four lateral flagella. A PCR technique for its detection has been developed (121).

Dysgonomonas spp. are small, gram-negative rods or cocci (Fig. 1c).

E. corrodens is a slender, straight, small, gram-negative rod with rounded ends (Fig. 1d). A PCR has been developed to detect *E. corrodens* in subgingival plaques (50).

Kingella spp. are short, gram-negative rods with square ends that lie together in pairs or clusters (Fig. 1e). They tend to decolorize unevenly on Gram stains. A broad-range PCR has detected *K. kingae*-specific sequences in culture-negative osteoarticular specimens (20).

Pasteurella spp. are small, gram-negative rods or cocci that occur singly, in pairs, or in short chains. Bipolar staining is frequent. "Related" species are more rod-like. A PCR technique for their detection has been developed (73).

Simonsiella spp. are gram-negative, crescent-shaped rods (0.5 to 1.0 μm long) arranged in multicellular filaments (10 to 50 μm by 2 to 8 μm) and segmented into groups of mostly 8 cells, resulting in a caterpillar-like appearance.

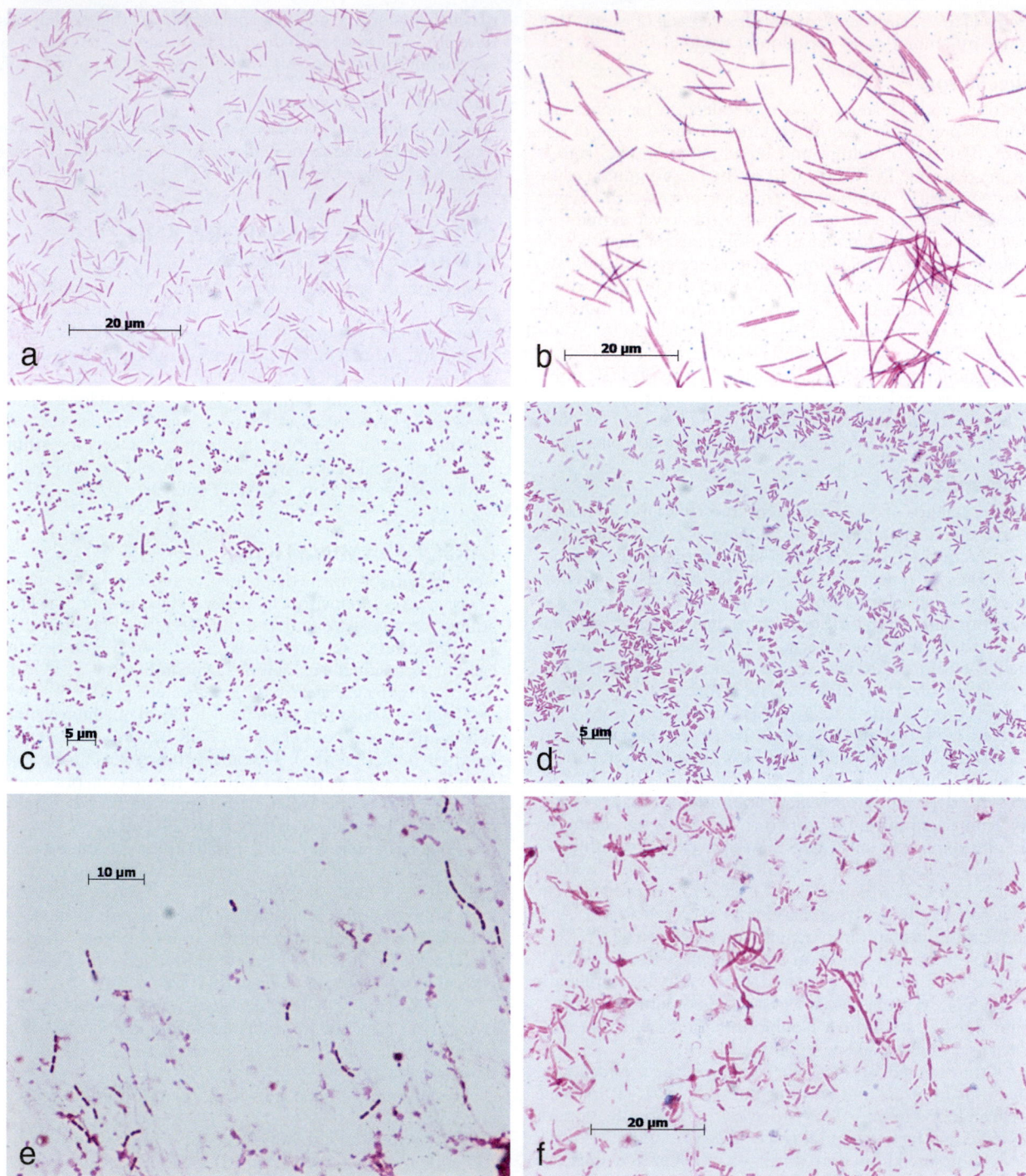

FIGURE 1   (a) *Capnocytophaga ochracea*. Gram stain of a 48-h culture grown on sheep blood agar (Institute of Medical Microbiology, University of Zurich). (b) *Leptotrichia buccalis*. Gram stain of a 48-h culture grown on sheep blood agar (Institute of Medical Microbiology, University of Zurich). (c) *Dysgonomonas capnocytophagoides*. Gram stain of a 48-h culture grown on sheep blood agar (Institute of Medical Microbiology, University of Zurich). (d) *Eikenella corrodens*. Gram stain of a 48-h culture grown on sheep blood agar (Institute of Medical Microbiology, University of Zurich). (e) *Kingella kingae*. Gram stain of a 48-h culture grown in Trypticase soy broth (Institute of Medical Microbiology, University of Zurich). (f) *Streptobacillus moniliformis*. Gram stain of a 48-h culture grown on sheep blood agar (Institute of Medical Microbiology, University of Zurich).

The long axis of each cell is perpendicular to the long axis of the filament. Incomplete decolorization on Gram stains is common.

S. moniliformis is a gram-negative rod with a variable morphology. Depending on age and culture conditions, cells may appear as straight, small to medium-size rods or as 100- to 150-μm-long tangled chains and filaments with bulbar swellings that stain variously with Gram stain (Fig. 1f). In culture-negative cases, broad-range PCR of fluids has been employed (8). A PCR assay which uses primers designed on the basis of 16S rRNA gene sequence data has been described; the PCR product treated with the restriction enzyme BfaI generates three fragments specific for *S. moniliformis* (14).

S. indologenes is a plump, irregularly staining, gram-negative rod; occasionally pairs, chains, or rosettes are formed.

ISOLATION PROCEDURES

For culture of members of this group, the use of blood or chocolate agar and, wherever normal flora and specific bacteria are suspected, of selective media is mandatory. HACEK members do not need more than 5 days of incubation in modern blood culture systems (115).

Actinobacillus spp. require enriched media but not necessarily hemin for growth, and growth is improved by a 5 to 10% CO_2 atmosphere.

Some *A. aphrophilus* (formerly *H. paraphrophilus*) strains and *A. segnis* require V factor; none requires hemin. All of them grow better in a CO_2 atmosphere. Selective media have employed bacitracin and vancomycin (133).

Primary isolation of *Capnocytophaga* spp. requires 5 to 10% CO_2 and enriched media; the composition of the blood agar base influences the ability to grow (38, 146). For detection in mixed cultures, selective media containing bacitracin, polymyxin B, vancomycin, and trimethoprim have been used (26), as have Thayer-Martin and Martin-Lewis agars (116). Inhibition by sodium polyanethol sulfonate in blood culture media has been experimentally verified (122). *C. canimorsus* has most often been isolated from blood. However, it may not be detected by commonly used automated blood culture systems; therefore, clinicians should inform the laboratory about risk factors for *C. canimorsus* infection so that subcultures on enriched media can be performed in a blind manner (146).

Cardiobacterium spp. mostly require 5 to 10% CO_2 and increased humidity for initial growth on blood agar.

C. violaceum grows on routine media, even on most enteric ones, at 30 to 35°C, its optimal temperature.

For *Dysgonomonas* spp., a selective medium containing cefoperazone, vancomycin, and amphotericin B has been used for stool cultures (58).

With a few exceptions, *E. corrodens* strains require hemin for growth unless 5 to 10% CO_2 is present (55). Detection is improved by a selective medium containing clindamycin (126).

Recovery of *K. kingae* from body fluids and pus can be difficult because these specimens seem to be inhibitory. For isolation from mixed cultures, media containing clindamycin or vancomycin as well as Thayer-Martin agar have been recommended (143). The use of various blood culture media has significantly improved the detection rate (142).

In contrast to some *Haemophilus* spp., *Pasteurella* spp. are hemin and CO_2 independent and will, therefore, grow on media without blood. Selective media containing vancomycin, clindamycin, and/or amikacin have been employed (6). "Related" species may even grow on enteric media.

S. muelleri grows well on blood agar but not on enteric agars.

S. moniliformis is best isolated from blood, joint fluid, or abscess material. For culture, media enriched with sheep, horse, or rabbit blood (15% seems to be optimal), serum, or ascitic fluid and a 5 to 10% CO_2 atmosphere at 37°C are required. Sodium polyanethol sulfonate in blood culture media is inhibitory (40).

S. indologenes grows slowly on blood agar (35).

IDENTIFICATION

Phenotypic identification of fastidious gram-negative rods presents several challenges. Triple sugar iron or Kligler's agar may not support the growth of fastidious genera (e.g., *Eikenella*). Media should be rich in peptones (e.g., cystine Trypticase agar); serum (except rabbit serum) should not be used because it may split maltose. The inoculum should be large (cell paste or agar blocks). Unsupplemented media used to check acid formation from carbohydrates may yield false-negative reactions. Gas formation from carbohydrates is scant or absent in most species. Indole may have to be extracted with xylene. Correct identification to the species level often requires multiple substrates that may not be available to routine laboratories (60, 89) and may not even be provided by automated systems (135). In view of the phenotypic closeness of the species, molecular methods (e.g., 16S rRNA gene or *rpoB* gene sequencing) seem optimal for the identification to the species level of *Actinobacillus*, *Aggregatibacter*, *Capnocytophaga,* and *Pasteurella* spp. (44, 52, 83, 89). They have mostly replaced the analysis of cellular fatty acids, which was able to separate only some species from others (140).

Colonies of *Actinobacillus* spp. are approximately 2 mm in diameter after 24 h of growth at 37°C, smooth or rough, viscous, and often adherent to the agar. Smooth colonies are dome shaped and have a bluish hue when viewed by transmitted light. Biochemical reactions are listed in Table 1.

A. actinomycetemcomitans colonies initially show a central dot and a slightly irregular edge and, on further incubation, develop a star-like configuration resembling "crossed cigars" and pit the agar. After several subcultures, this rough morphology may give way to smooth and opaque, nonpitting colonies, reflecting loss of fimbriae. In liquid media, the bacterium forms granules which adhere to the sides and to the bottom of the tube. Colonies of other *Aggregatibacter* spp. are granular or smooth, grayish white to yellowish, and opaque; without CO_2, there is pleomorphism, with small and large colonies. For species identification, a battery of tests (requirements for V- and X-factors, biochemical tests, colonial morphology [Table 1]) is necessary to avoid confusion with *Haemophilus* spp. *Aggregatibacter* spp. have negative reactions for production of indole, ornithine decarboxylase, and urease and are not dependent on X-factor; *Haemophilus* spp. are at least positive for one of those three reactions or cannot synthesize heme components from delta-amino-levulinic acid. Automated systems may present difficulties in identifying to the species level (53, 89, 135).

Colonies of *Capnocytophaga* spp. on blood agar are very small after 24 h at 37°C and reach 2 to 4 mm in diameter after 2 to 4 days; they are convex or flat and often slightly yellow when scraped off agar, show regular or spreading edges, and adhere to the agar surface. Phenotypic

TABLE 1 Biochemical reactions of *Actinobacillus* and *Aggregatibacter* spp.[a]

Reaction	*Actinobacillus lignieresii*	*A. equuli*	*A. suis*	*A. ureae*	*A. hominis*	*Aggregatibacter actinomycetemcomitans*	*A. aphrophilus*	*A. segnis*
Requirement for V-factor	−	−	−	−	−	−	v	+
Beta-hemolysis	−	v	+	−	−	−	−	−
Catalase	v	v	+/+[w]	+	+	+	−	v
Oxidase	+	+	+	+	+	v	v	−
Esculin hydrolysis	−	−	+	−	v	−	−	−
Urease	+	+	+	+	+	−	−	−
ONPG	+	+	v	−	+	−	+	−
Growth on MacConkey agar	v	+	v	−	−	−	v[w]	−
Gas from glucose	−	−	−	−	−	v	+	−
Acid from:								
Lactose	v	+	+	−	+	−	+[D]	−
Sucrose	+	+	+	+	+	−	+	+[w]
D-Xylose	+	+	+	−	+	v	v	−
Maltose	+	+	+	+	+	v	+	+[w]
D-Mannitol	+	+	−	+	+	v	−	−
Trehalose	−	+	+	−	+	−	+[D]	−
D-Melibiose	−	+	+	−	+	−	v	−

[a]Data are from references 21, 47, 113, 118, and 140 and http://www.bacterio.cict.fr.index.html. +, ≥90% of strains positive; −, ≥90% of strains negative; D, delayed reaction; ONPG, *ortho*-nitrophenyl-β-D-galactopyranoside; v, variable; w, weak; /, or. All species are indole negative and reduce nitrate to nitrite.

differentiation of species in the oxidase-negative group may be inconclusive due to the similarity of many biochemical reactions (Table 2) and the lack of suitable substrates even in automated systems (25, 43, 135). This has frequently given rise to identification as "*Capnocytophaga* sp." 16S rRNA gene sequencing is at present the most adequate diagnostic tool (25).

Colonies of *Cardiobacterium* spp. attain a diameter of approximately 1 mm after 48 h at 37°C on blood agar; they are circular, smooth, and opaque, and they may pit the agar. Biochemical tests reactions are recorded in Table 3. Differences between the two species are minimal and concern indole production in some strains, mannitol fermentation, and quantitative composition of cellular fatty acids (61). Some automated systems may misidentify *C. valvarum* (53).

Colonies of *C. violaceum* measure 1 to 2 mm in diameter after 24 h of growth, are round and smooth, have an almond-like smell, and may be beta-hemolytic. Most strains produce a violet pigment called violacein, which is soluble in ethanol but not in water. Identification is easy if this pigment is produced, although the positive oxidase reaction will be detected only by a modified technique (127). Biochemical reactions are listed in Table 3. This species may even grow on most enteric media. Nonpigmented strains may be confused with *Aeromonas* spp. but are lysine, maltose, and mannitol negative. Principal fatty acids do not differentiate between these two genera.

Colonies of *Dysgonomonas* spp. are entire, measure 1 to 2 mm in diameter after 24 h of growth, have a strawberry-like odor, and do not spread or adhere. The species show few biochemical differences (Table 2). Aerobically growing isolates of *Leptotrichia buccalis* may be confused with *Dysgonomonas*; microscopic examination of morphology, different cellular fatty acid profiles,

and determination of the production of lactic acid from glucose in *Leptotrichia* (*Dysgonomonas* produces propionic and succinic acids) are of help if 16S rRNA gene sequencing is not available (9).

Colonies of *Eikenella corrodens* are 1 to 2 mm in diameter after 48 h of growth, show clear centers that are often surrounded by spreading growth, may pit the agar, and assume a slightly yellow hue after several days. In liquid media, granules are produced. Typical isolates fail to form acid from carbohydrates in nonsupplemented media and are ornithine decarboxylase and nitratase positive; lysine decarboxylase activity is variable (Table 3). *E. corrodens* grows poorly or not at all on triple sugar iron or Kligler's agar.

Kingella colonies on blood agar in 5 to 10% CO_2 (which enhances growth) are 1 to 2 mm in diameter after 48 h of growth. One type is smooth with a central papilla, and the other spreads and pits the medium. As the only species, *K. kingae* shows a small but distinct zone of hemolysis on blood agar. Colonies have a short viability and have to be subcultured frequently. Biochemical test results are listed in Table 3. In addition to microscopic and colonial morphology, the tests serve to separate kingellae from rod-shaped members of the genus *Neisseria* (Table 4), with which they may be confused in automated systems (135). Since *K. denitrificans* may grow on Thayer-Martin or Martin-Lewis agar (143), it may be misidentified as *Neisseria gonorrhoeae* unless the catalase reaction, negative for *Kingella*, is performed.

Colonies of *Pasteurella* spp. are 1 to 2 mm in diameter after 24 h of growth at 37°C and are opaque and grayish. Encapsulated strains tend to be mucoid. A slight greening underneath the colonies may be noted. Indole-positive isolates exhibit a mouse-like odor. Biochemical reactions are listed in Table 5. The oxidase test has to be performed on

TABLE 2 Biochemical reactions of *Capnocytophaga* spp., *Dysgonomonas* and related species, and *Streptobacillus*[a]

Reaction	C. ochracea	C. sputigena	C. gingivalis	C. granulosa	C. haemolytica	C. canimorsus	C. cynodegmi	D. capnocytophagoides or D. gadei[b]	D. mossii[b]	"D. hofstadii"	DF-3-like	S. moniliformis
Catalase	−	−	−	−	−	+	+	−	−	−	−	−
Oxidase	−	−	−	−	−	+	+	−	−	−	−	−
Indole	−	−	−	−	−	−	−	−	+	+	+	−
Arginine dihydrolase	−	−	−	ND	ND	+	+	−	−	−	−	+
Nitrate to nitrite	−	v	−	−	+	−	v	−	−	−	−	−
Esculin hydrolysis	+	+	−	−	+	v	+	v	+	+	+	v
Gelatinase	−	v	−	−	−	−	−	−	−	−	v	−
ONPG[c]	+	+	−	+	+	+	+	+	+	+	+	
Acid from:												
Lactose	v	v	−	+	+	+	+	+	+	ND	+	−
Sucrose	+	+	+	+	+	−	+	+	+	ND	−	−
Xylose	−	−	−	−	−	−	−	+	+	ND	−	−
Main cellular fatty acid(s)	iso-15:0, 3-OH-17:0	iso-15:0, 3OH-17:0	iso-15:0, 3-OH-17:0	iso-15:0, 3-OH-17:0	iso-15:0, 3-OH-17:0	iso-15:0, 3-OH-17:0	iso-15:0, 3-OH-17:0	anteiso-15:0, iso-14:0, iso-15:0, iso-3-OH-16:0	anteiso-15:0, iso-15:0, iso-14:0	anteiso-15:0, iso-14:0, iso-3-OH-16:0	anteiso-15:0, iso-15:0, 16:0, 18:2, iso-3-OH-17:0	16:0, 18:1, 18:2, 18:0

[a]Data are from references 9, 30, 69, 90, and 140. +, ≥90% of strains positive; −, ≥90% of strains negative; ND, no data; v, variable. All species are negative for urease and ornithine decarboxylase and form acid from glucose (sometimes only with addition of serum).

[b]The isolates of *D. gadei* were catalase and indole positive and showed a higher percentage of $C_{16:0}$ and a lower percentage of $C_{15:0}$ than *D. capnocytophagoides* (3, 69, 90). *D. mossii* and "*D. hofstadii*" (one strain) differ in a few reactions in the Api Rapid ID32A system (90).

[c]ONPG, *ortho*-nitrophenyl-β-ᴅ-galactopyranoside.

blood agar (57). Nutritionally fastidious, nonmotile strains of *Enterobacteriaceae*, e.g., *Escherichia coli*, may be misidentified as *Pasteurella* unless an oxidase test is performed. In view of the phenotypic closeness of some taxa (22; http://www.bacterio.cict.fr./index.html [last update, 2009]), species identification in automated systems may be unsatisfactory (2, 22, 49, 59). 16S rRNA gene sequencing and *sodA* gene sequencing (52) have provided reliable species identification, the latter with even more discriminatory power.

Colonies of *Simonsiella* spp. are 1 to 2 mm in diameter after 24 h, may show gliding motility, and produce a pale yellow pigment. *S. muelleri* is beta-hemolytic. An optimal medium for recognition is BSTSY agar, which contains bovine serum, glucose, tryptic soy broth, and yeast extract (85). Biochemical tests are listed in Table 3.

S. moniliformis may show eubacterial and L-phase colonies in the same culture. The former are 1 to 3 mm in diameter after 48 to 72 h of growth on blood agar and are round and smooth. L-phase colonies grow better on clear media, yielding the "fried egg" appearance, with irregular outlines and coarse lipid globules. In liquid media, growth occurs mainly in the form of "puff balls" at the bottom of the tube. The organism dies quickly unless subcultured (40). It is biochemically inert; glucose is acidified weakly and in a delayed fashion (Table 2).

Fatty acid analysis can confirm the diagnosis (Table 2), as can 16S rRNA gene sequencing.

Colonies of *S. indologenes* may spread or pit the agar surface of the blood agar. Biochemical tests are listed in Table 3.

TYPING SYSTEMS AND SEROLOGIC TESTS

On the basis of surface polysaccharides, five serotypes of *A. actinomycetemcomitans* can be distinguished, of which a, b, and c are most common (commercial antisera are not available). Serotype b is associated with periodontitis, endocarditis, and penicillin resistance; serotype c is associated with periodontal health and extraoral infections (109).

Typing of *Capnocytophaga* spp. has been done by multilocus enzyme electrophoresis or by restriction fragment length polymorphism analysis (43). Typing of *C. violaceum* has employed *recA* PCR-restriction fragment length polymorphism analysis (120). For *E. corrodens*, typing has been done by arbitrarily primed PCR (48) and by restriction endonuclease analysis (19), which have demonstrated the unstable clonality of *E. corrodens* in the oral cavity. For typing of *Pasteurella* spp., PCR profiling, restriction endonuclease analysis, ribotyping, and pulsed-field gel electrophoresis have been employed (22, 73).

TABLE 3 Biochemical reactions of some rod-shaped species of the *Neisseriaceae* and of the *Cardiobacteriaceae*[a]

Reaction	Chromobacterium violaceum	Eikenella corrodens	Kingella kingae	Kingella denitrificans	Kingella oralis	Kingella potus	Simonsiella muelleri	Cardiobacterium hominis	Cardiobacterium valvarum	Suttonella indologenes
Catalase	+	−	−	−	−	−	−	−	−	v
Oxidase	v	+	+	+	+	+	+	+	+	+
Indole	v	−	−	−	−	−	−	+^{w}	v	+
Arginine dihydrolase	+	−	−	−	−	−	−	−	ND	−
Nitrate to nitrite	+	+	−	+/G	−	−	v	−	−	−
Esculin hydrolysis	−	−	−	−	−	−	−	−	−	−
Ornithine decarboxylase	−	+	−	−	−	−	−	−	ND	−
Growth on MacConkey agar	+	−	−	−	−	−	−	−	−	−
Alkaline phosphatase[b]	+	−	+	−	+	−	+	−	ND	+
Acid from:										
Glucose	+^{c}	−^{d}	+	+	+^{w}	−	+	+	v	+
Sucrose	v	−	−	−	−	−	−	+	v	+
Maltose	−	−	+	−	−	−	+	+	v	+
D-Mannitol	−	−	−	−	−	−	−	+	v	−
Special feature(s)	Violacein v	LD v	Beta-hemolysis			DNase +, yellow pigment	microscopic morphology			
Main cellular fatty acids	18:1ω7c, 16:0, 14:0	16:0, 18:1ω7c, 16:1ω7c	14:0, 16:1ω7c, 16:0	16:0, 14:0, 18:2, 18:1ω9c	ND	16:0, 18:1ω7c, 16:1ω7c	16:1ω7c, 12:0, 14:0	18:1ω7c, 16:0, 14:0	18:1ω7c, 16:0, 14:0	16:0, 18:1ω7c, 16:1ω7c, 14:0

[a]Data are from references 34, 61, 77, 85, 92, and 140. +, ≥90% of strains positive; −, ≥90% of strains negative; G, gas; LD, lysine decarboxylase; ND, no data; v, variable; w, weak. All species are negative for urease and acid production from lactose and D-xylose.
[b]API ZYM system (77).
[c]Some strains form small amounts of gas.
[d]Weakly positive reactions may be observed in O/F media.

Detection of antibodies directed against any of the bacteria discussed in this chapter has been tried on a small scale only and does not seem to offer much value.

ANTIMICROBIAL SUSCEPTIBILITIES

Approved guidelines for broth microdilution susceptibility testing of the HACEK group and for antimicrobial dilution and disk susceptibility testing of *Pasteurella* spp. have recently been published by the CLSI (28) (see chapter 71). Beta-lactamase production among members of the HACEK group is well documented, and beta-lactamase-producing isolates are ampicillin resistant; some isolates may be resistant to ampicillin due to mechanisms other than beta-lactamase production (28).

Susceptibility studies of *Actinobacillus* spp. are extant for a few isolates of the human-pathogenic species that are susceptible to many antimicrobials, including penicillin (47, 78).

Aggregatibacter spp. are susceptible to cephalosporins, tetracyclines, and aminoglycosides (84, 110). Resistance to ampicillin is not uncommon (29, 144), but amoxicillin combined with a beta-lactamase inhibitor has been effective (84).

Capnocytophaga spp. are usually susceptible to broad-spectrum cephalosporins, carbapenems, lincosamides, macrolides, tetracyclines, and fluoroquinolones but are resistant to colistin and aminoglycosides (4). Multidrug-resistant isolates have occasionally been encountered (138).

C. hominis and *C. valvarum* are susceptible to many antimicrobials, including penicillin (61, 84, 94). Beta-lactamase production is rare, and its effect can be neutralized by clavulanic acid (28, 97).

C. violaceum is resistant to many antimicrobials (beta-lactams and colistin) but is mostly susceptible to imipenem, fluoroquinolones, gentamicin, tetracyclines, and co-trimoxazole (1, 93).

D. capnocytophagoides strains are susceptible to tetracyclines, clindamycin, macrolides, and co-trimoxazole, whereas they are resistant to cephalosporins, aminoglycosides, and fluoroquinolones and variably susceptible to other beta-lactam antibiotics and to imipenem (58, 95).

E. corrodens is generally susceptible to penicillin, cephalosporins, carbapenems, doxycycline, azithromycin, and fluoroquinolones but is often resistant to narrow-spectrum cephalosporins, macrolides, and clindamycin (84, 98, 134).

TABLE 4 Differentiation between *Kingella* and rod-shaped *Neisseria* species[a]

Feature	Kingella kingae	Kingella denitrificans	Kingella oralis	Kingella potus	Neisseria elongata subsp. glycolytica	Neisseria elongata subsp. nitroreducens	Neisseria weaveri	Neisseria animaloris (EF-4a)
Catalase	−	−	−	−	+	−	+	+
Nitrate to nitrite	−	+	−	−	−	+	−	+
Nitrate to gas	−	+	−	−	−	−	−	v[c]
Alkaline phosphatase[b]	+	−	+	−	−	−	ND	−
Arginine dihydrolase					−	−	−	v[c]
Glucose acid	+	+	+[w]	−	+[w]	v	−	+[d]
Maltose acid	+	−	−	−	−	−	−	−
Beta-hemolysis	+	−	−	−	−	−	−	−
Main cellular fatty acids	14:0, 16:1ω7c, 16:0	16:0, 14:0, 18:2, 18:1ω9c	ND	16:0, 16:1ω7c, 18:1ω7c	16:0, 16:1ω7c, 18:1ω7c	16:0, 16:1ω7c, 18:1ω7c	16:0, 16:1ω7c, 18:1ω7c	16:0, 16:1ω7c, 18:1ω7c

[a]Data are from references 18, 92, and 140. +, ≥90% of strains positive; −, ≥90% of strains negative; ND, no data available; v, variable; w, weak.
[b]API zym (77).
[c]*Neisseria zoodegmatis* is negative.
[d]*Neisseria zoodegmatis* is positive only in O/F media.

Beta-lactamase-positive strains have been reported, but the enzyme was inhibited by beta-lactamase inhibitors (28, 88).

Kingella spp. are generally susceptible to beta-lactam antibiotics, macrolides, tetracyclines, co-trimoxazole, and quinolones (84, 142). Beta-lactamase-positive isolates have been reported to be susceptible to combinations with beta-lactam inhibitors (99, 131).

Pasteurella spp. are generally susceptible to penicillin, broad-spectrum cephalosporins, tetracyclines, quinolones, and co-trimoxazole but often resistant to oral narrow-spectrum cephalosporins, macrolides, and amikacin; other aminoglycosides are only moderately active (27, 56). Rare penicillin-resistant isolates of *Pasteurella* spp. have been encountered, but their effect can be neutralized by clavulanic acid (28, 102). For isolates of *Pasteurella* spp. from bite wounds, routine testing is usually not necessary; multiple organisms are often present in these specimens. Empirical therapy directed toward these organisms is generally effective for *P. multocida* as well (28). A few beta-lactamase-positive isolates of (*P.*) *bettyae* (12) have also been reported;

they were susceptible to the combination of penicillin and clavulanic acid.

One strain of *S. muelleri* was susceptible to beta-lactam antibiotics, tetracycline, and gentamicin (141).

S. moniliformis is susceptible to penicillin and tetracyclines, the mainstays of treatment, and to cephalosporins, carbapenems, aztreonam, clindamycin, erythromycin, and tetracycline; it shows intermediate susceptibility to aminoglycosides and fluoroquinolones and is resistant to colistin and co-trimoxazole (37, 40).

The susceptibility of *S. indologenes* resembles that of *C. hominis* (75).

EVALUATION, INTERPRETATION, AND REPORTING OF RESULTS

Some bacteria of the group are colonizers of the human or animal oral cavity; therefore, the evaluation of their isolation may be difficult. All should be identified to the species level if isolated as pure cultures from normally sterile body sites.

TABLE 5 Biochemical reactions of human *Pasteurella* and related species[a]

Reaction	P. multocida[b]	P. canis	P. dagmatis	P. stomatis	(P) aerogenes	(P) bettyae	(P) caballi	(P) pneumotropica
Catalase	+	+	+	+	+	−	−	+
Oxidase	+	+	+	+	+	v	+	+
Indole	+	+	+	+	−	+[w]	−	+
Urease	−	−	+	−	+	−	−	+
Ornithine decarboxylase	+	+	−	−	v	−	+	+
Growth on MacConkey agar	−	−	−	−	+	v	−	v
Gas from glucose	−	−	v	−	+	+[w]	+	−
Acid from:								
Lactose	−	−	−	−	v	−	+	−
Sucrose	+	+	+	+	+	−	+	+
D-Xylose	v	−	−	−	v	−	+	+
Maltose	−	−	+	−	+	−	+	+
D-Mannitol	+	−	−	−	−	−	+	−

[a]Data are from references 21 and 140 and http://www.bacterio.cict.fr./index.html. +, ≥90% of strains positive; −, ≥90% of strains negative; v, variable; w, weak. All species reduce nitrate to nitrite and are negative for arginine dihydrolase and esculin hydrolysis.
[b]The three subspecies, *multocida*, *septica*, and *gallicida*, can be separated on the basis of sorbitol and dulcitol fermentation (+/− in subsp. *multocida*, −/− in subsp. *septica*, and −/+ in the mostly avian subsp. *gallicida*); weakly sorbitol-positive strains of subsp. *multocida* can be recognized by a specific PCR profile (54).

Interpretation as infectious agents and results of susceptibility testing should be clearly reported to the physician.

With specimens normally colonized with aerobic and anaerobic bacteria, as well as with specimens from wounds, e.g., bite wounds, the significance of the bacteria discussed in this chapter depends on their predominance and the absence of other potentially pathogenic bacteria. If these conditions are met, identification to the species level is needed for adequate interpretation and reporting as infectious agents and for susceptibility testing. If none of these conditions is present, a repeat culture and close cooperation between the microbiology laboratory and the physician are necessary for interpretation, for identification to the species or genus level, and for susceptibility testing.

REFERENCES

1. **Aldridge, K. E., G. T. Valainis, and C. V. Sanders.** 1988. Comparison of the *in vitro* activity of ciprofloxacin and 24 other antimicrobial agents against clinical strains of *Chromobacterium violaceum*. *Diagn. Microbiol. Infect. Dis.* **10**:31–39.
2. **Allison, K., and J. E. Clarridge.** 2005. Long-term respiratory tract infection with canine-associated *Pasteurella dagmatis* and *Neisseria canis* in a patient with chronic bronchiectasis. *J. Clin. Microbiol.* **43**:4272–4274.
3. **Almuzara, M. N., R. Cittadini, P. J. Ladelfa, L. Olivieri, M. S. Ramirez, C. Zamponi, A. M. R. Famiglietti, and C. A. Vay.** 2009. Bacteremia caused by *Dysgonomonas* spp.: a report of two cases. *Clin. Microbiol. Newsl.* **31**:99–102.
4. **Arlet, G., M. J. Sanson-LePors, I. M. Casin, M. Ortenberg, and Y. Perol.** 1987. In vitro susceptibility of 96 *Capnocytophaga* strains, including a β-lactamase producer, to new β-lactam antibiotics and six quinolones. *Antimicrob. Agents Chemother.* **31**:1283–1284.
5. **Ashhurst-Smith, C., R. Norton, W. Thoreau, and M. M. Peel.** 1998. *Actinobacillus equuli* septicemia: an unusual zoonotic infection. *J. Clin. Microbiol.* **36**:2789–2790.
6. **Avril, J.-L., P.-Y. Donnio, and P. Pouedras.** 1990. Selective medium for *Pasteurella multocida* and its use to detect oropharyngeal carriage in pig breeders. *J. Clin. Microbiol.* **28**:1438–1440.
7. **Belibasakis, G. N., M. Brage, T. Lagergard, and A. Johansson.** 2008. Cytolethal distending toxin upregulates RANKL expression in Jurkat T-cells. *APMIS* **116**:499–506.
8. **Berger, C., M. Altwegg, A. Meyer, and D. Nadal.** 2001. Broad range polymerase chain reaction for diagnosis of rat-bite fever caused by *Streptobacillus moniliformis*. *Pediatr. Infect. Dis. J.* **20**:1181–1182.
9. **Bernard, K., C. Cooper, S. Tessier, and E. P. Ewan.** 1991. Use of chemotaxonomy as an aid to differentiate among *Capnocytophaga* species, CDC group DF-3, and aerotolerant strains of *Leptotrichia buccalis*. *J. Clin. Microbiol.* **29**:2263–2265.
10. **Blanche, P., E. Bloch, and D. Sicard.** 1998. *Capnocytophaga canimorsus* in the oral flora of dogs and cats. *J. Infect.* **36**:134.
11. **Bofinger, J. J., T. Fekete, and R. Samuel.** 2007. Bacterial peritonitis caused by *Kingella kingae*. *J. Clin. Microbiol.* **45**:3118–3120.
12. **Bogaerts, J., J. Verhaegen, W. M. Tello, S. Allen, L. Verbist, E. Van Dyck, and P. Piot.** 1990. Characterization, in vitro susceptibility, and clinical significance of CDC group HB-5 from Rwanda. *J. Clin. Microbiol.* **28**:2196–2199.
13. **Bonatti, H., D. W. Rossboth, D. Nachbaur, M. Fille, C. Aspöck, I. Hend, K. Hourmont, L. White, H. Malnick, and F. J. Allerberger.** 2003. A series of infections due to *Capnocytophaga* spp. in immunosuppressed and immunocompetent patients. *Clin. Microbiol. Infect.* **9**:380–387.
14. **Boot, R., A. Oosterhuis, and H. C. W. Thuis.** 2002. PCR for detection of *Streptobacillus moniliformis*. *Lab. Anim.* **36**:200–208.
15. **Brito, C. F., C. B. Carvalho, F. Santos, R. T. Gazzinelli, S. C. Oliveira, V. Azevedo, and S. M. Teixeira.** 2004. *Chromobacterium violaceum* genome: molecular mechanisms associated with pathogenicity. *Genet. Mol. Res.* **3**:148–161.
16. **Brouqui, P., and D. Raoult.** 2001. Endocarditis due to rare and fastidious bacteria. *Clin. Microbiol. Rev.* **14**:177–207.
17. **Carandina, G., M. Bacchelli, A. Virgili, and R. Strumia.** 1984. *Simonsiella* filaments isolated from erosive lesions of the human oral cavity. *J. Clin. Microbiol.* **19**:931–933.
18. **Chen, C.** 1996. Distribution of a newly described species, *Kingella oralis*, in the human oral cavity. *Oral Microbiol. Immunol.* **11**:425–427.
19. **Chen, C.-K. C., G. J. Sunday, J. J. Zambon, and M. E. Wilson.** 1990. Restriction endonuclease analysis of *Eikenella corrodens*. *J. Clin. Microbiol.* **28**:1265–1270.
20. **Chometon, S., Y. Benito, M. Chaker, S. Boisset, C. Ploton, J. Bérard, F. Vandenesch, and A. M. Freydière.** 2007. Specific real-time polymerase reaction places *Kingella kingae* as the most common cause of osteoarticular infections in young children. *Pediatr. Infect. Dis. J.* **26**:377–381.
21. **Christensen, H., and M. Bisgaard.** 2004. Revised definition of *Actinobacillus sensu stricto* isolated from animals. A review with special emphasis on diagnosis. *Vet. Microbiol.* **99**:13–30.
22. **Christensen, H., M. Bisgaard, O. Angen, W. Frederiksen, and J. E. Olsen.** 2005. Characterization of sucrose-negative *Pasteurella multocida* variants, including isolates from large-cat bite wounds. *J. Clin. Microbiol.* **43**:259–270.
23. **Christensen, H., J. Hommez, J. E. Olsen, and M. Bisgaard.** 2006. (*Pasteurella*) *caballi* infection not limited to horses—a closer look at taxon 42 of Bisgaard. *Lett. Appl. Microbiol.* **43**:424–429.
24. **Christensen, H., P. Kuhnert, H.-J. Busse, W. C. Frederiksen, and M. Bisgaard.** 2007. Proposed minimal standards for the description of genera, species and subspecies of the *Pasteurellaceae*. *Int. J. Syst. Evol. Microbiol.* **57**:166–178.
25. **Ciantar, M., H. N. Newman, M. Wilson, and D. A. Spratt.** 2005. Molecular identification of *Capnocytophaga* spp. via 16S rRNA PCR-restriction fragment length polymorphism analysis. *J. Clin. Microbiol.* **43**:1894–1901.
26. **Ciantar, M., D. A. Spratt, H. N. Newman, and M. Wilson.** 2001. Assessment of five culture media for the growth and isolation of *Capnocytophaga* spp. *Clin. Microbiol. Infect.* **7**:158–160.
27. **Citron, M. D., Y. A. Warren, H. T. Fernandez, M. A. Goldstein, K. L. Tyrell, and E. J. C. Goldstein.** 2005. Broth microdilution and disk diffusion tests for susceptibility testing of *Pasteurella* species isolated from human clinical specimens. *J. Clin. Microbiol.* **43**:2485–2488.
28. **Clinical and Laboratory Standards Institute.** 2006. *Methods for Antimicrobial Dilution and Disk Susceptibility Testing of Infrequently Isolated or Fastidious Bacteria.* Approved guideline M45-A. Clinical and Laboratory Standards Institute, Wayne, PA.
29. **Coll-Vinent, B., X. Suris, A. López-Soto, J. M. Miró, and A. Coca.** 1995. *Haemophilus paraphrophilus* endocarditis: case report and review. *Clin. Infect. Dis.* **20**:1381–1383.
30. **Daneshvar, M. I., D. G. Hollis, and C. W. Moss.** 1991. Chemical characterization of clinical isolates which are similar to CDC group DF-3 bacteria. *J. Clin. Microbiol.* **29**:2351–2353.
31. **De Boer, M. G., P. C. Lambregts, A. P. van Dam, and J. W. van't Wout.** 2007. Meningitis caused by *Capnocytophaga canimorsus*: when to expect the unexpected. *Clin. Neurol. Neurosurg.* **109**:393–398.
32. **De Castro, N., J. Pavie, M. Lagrange-Xélot, D. Bouvry, F. Delisle, A. Parrot, and J. M. Molina.** 2007. Severe *Actinobacillus ureae* meningitis in an immunocompromised patient: report of one case and review of the literature. *Scand. J. Infect. Dis.* **39**:1076–1079.
33. **De Leon, J. P., R. F. Sandfort, and J. D. Wong.** 2000. *Pasteurella bettyae*: report of nine cases and evidence of an emerging neonatal pathogen. *Clin. Microbiol. Newsl.* **22**:190–192.
34. **Dewhirst, F. E., C.-K. C. Chen, B. J. Paster, and J. J. Zambon.** 1993. Phylogeny of species in the family *Neisseriaceae* isolated from human dental plaque and description of *Kingella oralis* sp. nov. *Int. J. Syst. Bacteriol.* **43**:490–499. (Erratum, **44**:376, 1994.)
35. **Dewhirst, F. E., B. J. Paster, S. La Fontaine, and J. I. Rood.** 1990. Transfer of *Kingella indologenes* (Snell and Lapage 1976) to the genus *Suttonella* gen. nov. as *Suttonella indologenes* comb. nov.; transfer of *Bacteroides nodosus* (Beveridge 1941) to the genus *Dichelobacter* gen. nov. as *Dichelobacter nodosus* comb. nov.; and assignment of the genera *Cardiobacterium, Dichelobacter,*

and *Suttonella* to *Cardiobacteriaceae* fam. nov. in the gamma division of *Proteobacteria* on the basis of 16S rRNA sequence comparisons. *Int. J. Syst. Evol. Microbiol.* **40**:426–433.

36. **Donnio, P.-Y., A.-L. Lerestif-Gautier, and J.-L. Avril.** 2004. Characterization of *Pasteurella* spp. strains isolated from human infections. *J. Comp. Pathol.* **130**:137–142.

37. **Dubois, D., F. Robin, D. Bouvier, J. Delmas, R. Bonnet, O. Lesens, and C. Hennequin.** 2008. *Streptobacillus moniliformis* as the causative agent in spondylodiscitis and psoas abscess after rooster scratches. *J. Clin. Microbiol.* **46**:2820–2821.

38. **Dusch, H., R. Zbinden, and A. von Graevenitz.** 1995. Growth differences of *Capnocytophaga canimorsus* strains and some other fastidious organisms on various Columbia-based blood agar media. *Zentralbl. Bakteriol.* **282**:362–366.

39. **Ejlertsen, T., B. Gahrn-Hansen, P. Sogaard, O. Heltberg, and W. Frederiksen.** 1996. *Pasteurella aerogenes* isolated from ulcers or wounds in humans with occupational exposure to pigs: a report of 7 Danish cases. *Scand. J. Infect. Dis.* **28**:567–570.

40. **Elliott, S. P.** 2007. Rat bite fever and *Streptobacillus moniliformis. Clin. Microbiol. Rev.* **20**:13–22.

41. **Escande, F., A. Bailly, S. Bone, and J. Lemozy.** 1996. *Actinobacillus suis* infection after a pig bite. *Lancet* **348**:888.

42. **Escande, F., E. Vallée, and F. Aubart.** 1997. *Pasteurella caballi* infection following a horse bite. *Zentralbl. Bakteriol.* **285**:440–444.

43. **Frandsen, E. V., K. Poulsen, E. Könönen, and M. Kilian.** 2008. Diversity of *Capnocytophaga* species in children and description of *Capnocytophaga leadbetteri* sp. nov. and *Capnocytophaga* genospecies AHN8471. *Int. J. Syst. Evol. Microbiol.* **58**:324–336.

44. **Frebourg, N. B., G. Berthelot, R. Hocq, A. Chibani, and J.-F. Lemeland.** 2002. Septicemia due to *Pasteurella pneumotropica*: 16S rRNA sequencing for diagnosis confirmation. *J. Clin. Microbiol.* **40**:687–689.

45. **Freeman, A. F., X. T. Zheng, J. C. Lane, and S. T. Shulman.** 2004. *Pasteurella aerogenes* hamster bite peritonitis. *Pediatr. Infect. Dis. J.* **23**:368–370.

46. **Frey, J., and P. Kuhnert.** 2002. RTX toxins in *Pasteurellaceae. Int. J. Med. Microbiol.* **292**:149–158.

47. **Friis-Moller, A., J. J. Christensen, V. Fussing, A. Hesselbjerg, J. Christiansen, and B. Bruun.** 2001. Clinical significance and taxonomy of *Actinobacillus hominis. J. Clin. Microbiol.* **39**:930–935.

48. **Fujise, O., W. Chen, S. Rich, and C. Chen.** 2004. Clonal diversity and stability of subgingival *Eikenella corrodens. J. Clin. Microbiol.* **42**:2036–2042.

49. **Funke, G., D. Monnet, C. de Bernardis, A. von Graevenitz, and J. Freney.** 1998. Evaluation of the VITEK 2 system for rapid identification of medically relevant gram-negative rods. *J. Clin. Microbiol.* **36**:1948–1952.

50. **Furcht, C., K. Eschrich, and K. Merte.** 1996. Detection of *Eikenella corrodens* and *Actinobacillus actinomycetemcomitans* by use of the polymerase chain reaction (PCR) in vitro and in subgingival plaque. *J. Clin. Periodontol.* **23**:891–897.

51. **Garrity, G. M., J. A. Bell, and T. G. Lilburn.** 2005. Taxonomic outline of the *Archaea* and *Bacteria*, p. 207–220. In G. M. Garrity et al. (ed.), *Bergey's Manual of Systematic Bacteriology*, 2nd ed., vol. 2. Springer, New York, NY.

52. **Gautier, A.-L., D. Dubois, F. Escande, J.-L. Avril, P. Trieu-Cuot, and O. Gaillot.** 2005. Rapid and accurate identification of human isolates of *Pasteurella* and related species by sequencing the *sodA* gene. *J. Clin. Microbiol.* **43**:2307–2314.

53. **Geissdörfer, W., R. Tandler, C. Schlundt, M. Weyand, W. G. Daniel, and C. Schoerner.** 2007. Fatal bioprosthetic aortic valve endocarditis due to *Cardiobacterium valvarum. J. Clin. Microbiol.* **45**:2324–2326.

54. **Gerardo, S. H., D. M. Citron, M. C. Claros, H. T. Fernandez, and E. J. C. Goldstein.** 2001. *Pasteurella multocida* subsp. *multocida* and *P. multocida* subsp. *septica* differentiation by PCR fingerprinting and α-glucosidase activity. *J. Clin. Microbiol.* **39**:2558–2564.

55. **Goldstein, E. J. C., E. O. Agyare, and R. Silletti.** 1981. Comparative growth of *Eikenella corrodens* on 15 media in three atmospheres of incubation. *J. Clin. Microbiol.* **13**:951–953.

56. **Goldstein, E. J. C., D. M. Citron, and G. A. Richwald.** 1988. Lack of *in vitro* efficacy of oral forms of certain cephalosporins, erythromycin, and oxacillin against *Pasteurella multocida. Antimicrob. Agents Chemother.* **32**:213–215.

57. **Grehn, M., and F. Müller.** 1989. The oxidase reaction of *Pasteurella multocida* strains cultured on Mueller Hinton medium. *J. Microbiol. Methods* **9**:333–336.

58. **Grob, R., R. Zbinden, C. Ruef, M. Hackenthal, I. Diesterweg, M. Altwegg, and A. von Graevenitz.** 1999. Septicemia caused by dysgonic fermenter 3 in a severely immunocompromised patient and isolation of the same microorganism from a stool specimen. *J. Clin. Microbiol.* **37**:1617–1618.

59. **Guillard, T., V. Duval, R. Jobart, L. Brasme, C. David, C. deChamps, M. Begin, and E. Dehoux.** 2009. Dog bite wound infection by *Pasteurella dagmatis* misidentified as *Pasteurella pneumotropica* by automated system Vitek 2. *Diagn. Microbiol. Infect. Dis.* **65**:347–348.

60. **Hamilton-Miller, J. M. T.** 2002. Distinguishing *Pasteurella* spp. from *Haemophilus* spp.: the problem revisited. *Clin. Microbiol. Infect.* **8**:245.

61. **Han, X. Y., and E. Falsen.** 2005. Characterization of oral strains of *Cardiobacterium valvarum* and emended description of the organism. *J. Clin. Microbiol.* **43**:2370–2374.

62. **Han, X. Y., F. S. Han, and J. Segal.** 2008. *Chromobacterium haemolyticum* sp. nov., a strongly haemolytic species. *Int. J. Syst. Evol. Microbiol.* **58**:1398–1403.

63. **Hansen, P. S., T. G. Jensen, and B. Gahrn-Hansen.** 2005. *Dysgonomonas capnocytophagoides* bacteraemia in a neutropenic patient treated for acute myeloid leukemia. *APMIS* **113**:229–231.

64. **Harper, M., J. D. Boyce, and B. Adler.** 2006. *Pasteurella multocida* pathogenesis: 125 years after Pasteur. *FEMS Microbiol Lett.* **265**:1–10.

65. **Hayashi, F., M. Okada, X. Zhong, and K. Miura.** 2001. PCR detection of *Capnocytophaga* species in dental plaque samples from children aged 2 to 12 years. *Microbiol. Immunol.* **45**:17–22.

66. **Hayashimoto, N., A. Takakura, and T. Itoh.** 2005. Genetic diversity on 16 rDNA sequence and phylogenetic tree analysis in *Pasteurella pneumotropica* strains isolated from laboratory animals. *Curr. Microbiol.* **51**:239–243.

67. **Henderson, B., S. P. Nair, J. M. Ward, and M. Wilson.** 2003. Molecular pathogenicity of the oral opportunistic pathogen *Actinobacillus actinomycetemcomitans. Annu. Rev. Microbiol.* **57**:29–55.

68. **Henrichsen, J.** 1983. Twitching motility. *Annu. Rev. Microbiol.* **37**:81–93.

69. **Hofstad, T., I. Olsen, E. R. Eribe, E. Falsen, M. D. Collins, and P. A. Lawson.** 2000. *Dysgonomonas* gen. nov. to accommodate *Dysgonomonas gadei* sp. nov., an organism isolated from a human gall bladder, and *Dysgonomonas capnocytophagoides* (formerly CDC group DF-3). *Int. J. Syst. Evol. Microbiol.* **50**:2189–2195.

70. **Holst, E., J. Rollof, L. Larsson, and J. P. Nielsen.** 1992. Characterization and distribution of *Pasteurella* species recovered from infected humans. *J. Clin. Microbiol.* **30**:2984–2987.

71. **Hombach, M., H. R. Frey, and G. E. Pfyffer.** 2007. Urinary tract infection caused by *Eikenella corrodens. J. Clin. Microbiol.* **45**:675.

72. **Huang, S. T., H. C. Lee, N. Y. Lee, K. H. Liu, and W. C. Ko.** 2005. Clinical characteristics of invasive *Haemophilus aphrophilus* infections. *J. Microbiol. Immunol. Infect.* **38**:271–276.

73. **Hunt, M. L., B. Adler, and K. M. Townsend.** 2000. The molecular biology of *Pasteurella multocida. Vet. Microbiol.* **72**:3–25.

74. **Janda, J. M., M. H. Graves, D. Lindquist, and W. S. Probert.** 2006. Diagnosing *Capnocytophaga canimorsus* infections. *Emerg. Infect. Dis.* **12**:340–342.

75. **Jenny, D. B., P. W. Letendre, and G. Iverson.** 1987. Endocarditis caused by *Kingella indologenes. Rev. Infect. Dis.* **9**:787–789.

76. **Kaplan, A. H., D. J. Weber, E. Z. Oddone, and J. R. Perfect.** 1989. Infection due to *Actinobacillus actinomycetemcomitans*: 15 cases and review. *Rev. Infect. Dis.* **11**:46–63.

77. **Kasten, R., R. Mutters, and W. Mannheim.** 1998. Catalase-positive *Eikenella corrodens* and *Eikenella*-like isolates of human and canine origin. *Zentralbl. Bakteriol.* **288**:319–329.

78. **Kaur, P. P., C. T. Derk, M. Chatterji, and R. J. Dehoratius.** 2004. Septic arthritis caused by *Actinobacillus ureae* in a patient with rheumatoid arthritis receiving anti-tumor necrosis factor-alpha therapy. *J. Rheumatol.* **31:**1663–1666.

79. **Kehl-Fie, T. E., and J. W. St. Geme III.** 2007. Identification and characterization of an RTX toxin in the emerging pathogen *Kingella kingae. J. Bacteriol.* **189:**430–436.

80. **Kehl-Fie, T. E., S. E. Miller, and J. W. St. Geme III.** 2008. *Kingella kingae* expresses type IV pili that mediate adherence to respiratory epithelial and synovial cells. *J. Bacteriol.* **190:**7157–7163.

81. **Kilian, M., and W. Frederiksen.** 1981. Ecology of *Haemophilus, Pasteurella* and *Actinobacillus,* p. 11–38. *In* M. Kilian, W. Frederiksen, and E. L. Biberstein (ed.), *Haemophilus, Pasteurella, and Actinobacillus.* Academic Press, London, United Kingdom.

82. **Kok, R. H., M. J. Wolfhagen, B. M. Mooi, and J. J. Offerman.** 1999. A patient with thrombotic thrombocytopenic purpura caused by *Capnocytophaga canimorsus* septicemia. *Clin. Microbiol. Infect.* **5:**297–298.

83. **Korczak B., H. Christensen, S. Emler, J. Frey, and P. Kuhnert.** 2004. Phylogeny of the family *Pasteurellaceae* based on *rpoB* sequences. *Int. J. Syst. Evol. Microbiol.* **54:**1393–1399.

84. **Kugler, K. C., D. J. Biedenbach, and R. N. Jones.** 1999. Determination of the antimicrobial activity of 29 clinically important compounds tested against fastidious HACEK group organisms. *Diagn. Microbiol. Infect. Dis.* **34:**73–76.

85. **Kuhn, D. A., and D. A. Gregory.** 1978. Emendation of *Simonsiella muelleri* Schmid and description of *Simonsiella steedae* sp. nov., with designations of the respective proposed neotype and holotype strains. *Curr. Microbiol.* **1:**11–14.

86. **Kuhn, D. A., D. A. Gregory, G. E. Buchanan, Jr., M. D. Nyby, and K. R. Daly.** 1978. Isolation, characterization, and numerical taxonomy of *Simonsiella* strains from the oral cavities of cats, dogs, sheep and humans. *Arch. Microbiol.* **118:**235–241.

87. **Kuzucu, C., G. Yetkin, G. Kocak, and V. Nisanoglu.** 2005. An unusual case of pericarditis caused by *Cardiobacterium hominis. J. Infect.* **50:**346–347.

88. **Lacroix, J. M., and C. Walker.** 1991. Characterization of a β-lactamase found in *Eikenella corrodens. Antimicrob. Agents Chemother.* **35:**886–891.

89. **Lau, S. K. P., P. C. Y. Woo, M.-Y. Mok, J. L. L. Teng, V. K. P. Tam, K. K. H. Chan, and K.-Y. Yuen.** 2004. Characterization of *Haemophilus segnis,* an important cause of bacteremia, by 16S rRNA gene sequencing. *J. Clin. Microbiol.* **42:**877–880.

90. **Lawson, P. A., P. Carlson, S. Wernersson, E. R. Moore, and E. Falsen.** 2010. *Dysgonomonas hofstadii* sp. nov., isolated from a human clinical source. *Anaerobe* **16:**161–164.

91. **Lawson, P. A., E. Falsen, E. Inganäs, R. S. Weyant, and M. D. Collins.** 2002. *Dysgonomonas mossii* sp. nov., from human sources. *Syst. Appl. Microbiol.* **25:**194–197.

92. **Lawson, P. A., H. Malnick, M. D. Collins, J. J. Shah, M. A. Chattaway, R. Bendall, and J. W. Hartley.** 2005. Description of *Kingella potus* sp. nov., an organism isolated from a wound caused by an animal bite. *J. Clin. Microbiol.* **43:**3526–3529.

93. **Lee, J., J. S. Kim, C. H. Nahm, J. W. Choi, J. Kim, S. H. Pai, K. H. Moon, K. Lee, and Y. Chong.** 1999. Two cases of *Chromobacterium violaceum* infection after injury in a subtropical region. *J. Clin. Microbiol.* **37:**2068–2070.

94. **Malani, A. N., D. M. Aronoff, S. F. Bradley, and C. A. Kauffmann.** 2006. *Cardiobacterium hominis* endocarditis: two cases and a review of the literature. *Eur. J. Clin. Microbiol. Infect. Dis.* **25:**587–595.

95. **Martinez-Sanchez, L., F. J. Vasallo, F. Garcia-Garrote, L. Alcala, M. Rodriguez-Créixems, and E. Bouza.** 1998. Clinical isolation of a DF-3 microorganism and review of the literature. *Clin. Microbiol. Infect.* **4:**344–346.

96. **Matsumoto, T., Y. Kawakami, K. Oana, T. Honda, K. Yamauchi, Y. Okimura, M. Shiohara, and E. Kasuga.** 2006. First isolation of *Dysgonomonas mossii* from intestinal juice of a patient with pancreatic cancer. *Arch. Med. Res.* **37:**914–916.

97. **Maurissen, W., B. Eyskens, M. Gewillig, and J. Verhaegen.** 2008. Beta-lactamase positive *Cardiobacterium hominis* strain causing endocarditis in a pediatric patient with tetralogy of Fallot. *Clin. Microbiol. Newsl.* **30:**132–133.

98. **Merriam, C. V., D. M. Citron, K. L. Tyrrell, Y. A. Warren, and E. J. C. Goldstein.** 2006. In vitro activity of azithromycin and nine comparator agents against 296 strains of oral anaerobes and 31 strains of *Eikenella corrodens. Int. J. Antimicrob. Agents* **28:**244–248.

99. **Minamoto, G. Y., and E. M. Sordillo.** 1992. *Kingella denitrificans* as a cause of granulomatous disease in a patient with AIDS. *Clin. Infect. Dis.* **15:**1052–1053.

100. **Mulder, A. H., P. G. G. Gerlag, L. H. M. Verhoef, and A. W. L. van den Wall Bake.** 2001. Hemolytic uremic syndrome after *Capnocytophaga canimorsus* (DF-2) septicemia. *Clin. Nephrol.* **55:**167–170.

101. **Muntaner, L., J. M. Suriñach, D. Zuñiga, T. F. De Sevilla, and A. Ferrer.** 2008. Respiratory pasteurellosis: infection or colonization? *Scand. J. Infect. Dis.* **40:**555–560.

102. **Naas, T., F. Benaoudia, L. Lebrun, and P. Nordmann.** 2001. Molecular identification of TEM-1 beta-lactamase in a *Pasteurella multocida* isolate of human origin. *Eur. J. Clin. Microbiol. Infect. Dis.* **20:**210–213.

103. **Nikkari, S., R. Gotoff, P. P. Bourbeau, R. E. Brown, N. R. Kamal, and D. A. Relman.** 2002. Identification of *Cardiobacterium hominis* by broad-range bacterial polymerase chain reaction analysis in a case of culture-negative endocarditis. *Arch. Intern. Med.* **162:**477–479.

104. **Nonnemacher, C., R. Mutters, and L. Flores de Jacoby.** 2001. Microbiological characteristics of subgingival microbiota in adult periodontitis, localized juvenile periodontis and rapidly progressive periodontitis subjects. *Clin. Microbiol. Infect.* **7:**213–217.

105. **Norskov-Lauritsen, N., H. Christensen, H. Okkels, M. Kilian, and B. Bruun.** 2004. Delineation of the genus *Actinobacillus* by comparison of partial *infB* sequences. *Int. J. Syst. Evol. Microbiol.* **54:**635–644.

106. **Norskov-Lauritsen, N., and M. Kilian.** 2006. Reclassification of *Actinobacillus actinomycetemcomitans, Haemophilus aphrophilus, Haemophilus paraphrophilus,* and *Haemophilus segnis* as *Aggregatibacter actinomycetemcomitans* gen. nov., comb. nov., *Aggregatibacter aphrophilus,* com. nov., and *Aggregatibacter segnis* comb. nov., and emended description of *Aggregatibacter aphrophilus* to include V factor-dependent and V factor-independent isolates. *Int. J. Syst. Evol. Microbiol.* **56:**2135–2146.

107. **Ochiai, K., H. Senpuku, and T. Kurita-Ochiai.** 1998. Purification of immunosuppressive factor from *Capnocytophaga ochracea. J. Med. Microbiol.* **47:**1087–1095.

108. **Olsen, J., H. N. Shah, and S. E. Gharbia.** 1999. Taxonomy and biochemical characteristics of *Actinobacillus actinomycetemcomitans* and *Porphyromonas gingivalis. Periodontology* **20:**14–52.

109. **Paju, S., P. Carlson, H. Jousimies-Somer, and S. Asikainen.** 2000. Heterogeneity of *Actinobacillus actinomycetemcomitans* strains in various human infections and relationships between serotype, genotype, and antimicrobial susceptibility. *J. Clin. Microbiol.* **38:**79–84.

110. **Paju, S., P. Carlson, H. Jousimies-Somer, and S. Asikainen.** 2003. *Actinobacillus actinomycetemcomitans* and *Haemophilus aphrophilus* in systemic and nonoral infections in Finland. *APMIS* **111:**653–657.

111. **Pasqualini, L., A. Mencacci, A. M. Scarponi, C. Leli, G. Fabbriciani, L. Callarelli, G. Schillaci, F. Bistoni, and E. Mannarino.** 2008. Cervical spondylodiscitis with spinal epidural abscess caused by *Aggregatibacter aphrophilus. J. Clin. Microbiol.* **57:**652–655.

112. **Paster, B. J., W. A. Falkler, Jr., C. O. Enwonwu, E. O. Idigbe, K. O. Savage, V. A. Levanos, M. A. Tamer, R. L. Ericson, C. N. Lau, and F. E. Dewhirst.** 2002. Prevalent bacterial species and novel phylotypes in advanced noma lesions. *J. Clin. Microbiol.* **40:**2187–2191.

113. **Peel, M. M., K. A. Hornidge, M. Luppino, A. M. Stacpoole, and R. E. Weaver.** 1991. *Actinobacillus* spp. and related bacteria in infected wounds of humans bitten by horses and sheep. *J. Clin. Microbiol.* **29:**2535–2538.

114. **Pers, C., E. Tvedegaard, J. J. Christensen, and J. Bangsborg.** 2007. *Capnocytophaga cynodegmi* peritonitis in a peritoneal dialysis patient. *J. Clin. Microbiol.* **45:**3844–3846.

115. **Petti, C. A., H. S. Bhally, M. P. Weinstein, K. Joho, T. Wakefield, L. B. Reller, and K. C. Carroll.** 2006. Utility of extended blood culture incubation for isolation of *Haemophilus, Actinobacillus, Cardiobacterium, Eikenella,* and *Kingella* organisms: a retrospective evaluation. *J. Clin. Microbiol.* **44:**257–259.

116. **Rummens, J. L., B. Gordts, and H. W. van Landuyt.** 1986. In vitro susceptibility of *Capnocytophaga* species to 29 antimicrobial agents. *Antimicrob. Agents Chemother.* **30:**739–742.

117. **Rycroft, A. N., and L. H. Garside.** 2000. *Actinobacillus* species and their role in animal disease. *Vet. J.* **159:**18–36.

118. **Sakazaki, R., E. Yoshizaki, K. Tamura, and S. Kuramochi.** 1984. Increased frequency of isolation of *Pasteurella* and *Actinobacillus* species and related organisms. *Eur. J. Clin. Microbiol. Infect. Dis.* **3:**244–248.

119. **Sandoe, J. A. T.** 2004. *Capnocytophaga canimorsus* endocarditis. *J. Med. Microbiol.* **53:**245–248.

120. **Scholz, H. C., A. Witte, H. Tomaso, S. Al Dahouk, and H. Neubauer.** 2005. Genotyping of *Chromobacterium violaceum* isolates by *recA* PCR-RFLP analysis. *FEMS Microbiol. Lett.* **244:**347–352.

121. **Scholz, H. C., A. Witte, H. Tomaso, S. Al Dahouk, and H. Neubauer.** 2006. Detection of *Chromobacterium violaceum* by multiplex PCR targeting the *prgI, spaO, invG,* and *sipB* genes. *Syst. Appl. Microbiol.* **29:**45–48.

122. **Shawar, R., J. Sepulveda, and J. E. Clarridge.** 1990. Use of the RapID-ANA system and sodium polyanetholesulfonate disk susceptibility testing in identifying *Haemophilus ducreyi.* *J. Clin. Microbiol.* **28:**108–111.

123. **Sheng, W.-S., P.-R. Hsueh, C.-C. Hung, L.-J. Teng, Y.-C. Chen, and K.-T. Luh.** 2001. Clinical features of patients with invasive *Eikenella corrodens* infections and microbiological characteristics of the causative isolates. *Eur. J. Clin. Microbiol. Infect. Dis.* **20:**231–236.

124. **Shin, H., M. Mally, S. Meyer, C. Fiechter, C. Paroz, U. Zaehringer, and G. R. Cornelis.** 2009. Resistance of *Capnocytophaga canimorsus* to killing by human complement and polymorphonuclear leukocytes. *Infect. Immun.* **77:**2262–2271.

125. **Sirinavin, S., C. Techasaensiri, S. Benjaponpitak, R. Pornkul, and M. Vorachit.** 2005. Invasive *Chromobacterium violaceum* infection in children: case report and review. *Pediatr. Infect. Dis. J.* **24:**559–561.

126. **Slee, A. M., and J. M. Tanzer.** 1978. Selective medium for isolation of *Eikenella corrodens* from periodontal lesions. *J. Clin. Microbiol.* **8:**459–462.

127. **Slesak, G., P. Douangdala, S. Inthalad, J. Silisouk, M. Vongsouvath, A. Sengduangphachanh, C. E. Moore, M. Mayxay, H. Matsuoka, and P. N. Newton.** 2009. Fatal *Chromobacterium violaceum* septicaemia in northern Laos, a modified oxidase test and post-mortem forensic family G6PD analysis. *Ann. Clin. Microbiol. Antimicrob.* **8:**24.

128. **Slonim, A., E. S. Walker, E. Mishori, N. Porat, R. Dagan, and P. Yagupsky.** 1998. Person-to-person transmission of *Kingella kingae* among day care center attendees. *J. Infect. Dis.* **178:**1843–2846.

129. **Slotnick, I. J.** 1968. *Cardiobacterium hominis* in genitourinary specimens. *J. Bacteriol.* **95:**1175.

130. **Somers, C. J., B. C. Millar, J. Xu, D. P. Moore, A. M. Moran, C. Maloney, B. Keogh, P. G. Murphy, and J. E. Moore.** 2003. *Haemophilus segnis:* a rare cause of endocarditis. *Clin. Microbiol. Infect.* **9:**1048–1050.

131. **Sordillo, E. M., M. Rendel, R. Sood, J. Belinfanti, O. Murray, and D. Brook.** 1993. Septicemia due to β-lactamase positive *Kingella kingae.* *Clin. Infect. Dis.* **17:**818–819.

132. **Tang, G., T. Kitten, C. L. Munro, G. C. Wellman, and K. P. Mintz.** 2008. EmaA, a potential virulence determinant of *Aggregatibacter actinomycetemcomitans* in infective endocarditis. *Infect. Immun.* **76:**2316–2324.

133. **Tsuzukibashi, O., K. Takada, M. Saito, C. Kimura, T. Yoshikawa, M. Makimura, and M. Hirasawa.** 2008. A novel selective medium for isolation of *Aggregatibacter (Actinobacillus) actinomycetemcomitans.* *J. Periodont. Res.* **43:**544–548.

134. **Udaka, T., N. Hiraki, T. Shiomori, H. Miyamato, T. Fujimura, T. Inaba, and H. Suzuki.** 2007. *Eikenella corrodens* in head and neck infections. *J. Infect.* **54:**343–348.

135. **Valenza, G., C. Ruoff, U. Vogel, M. Frosch, and M. Abele-Horn.** 2007. Microbiological evaluation of the new VITEK 2 *Neisseria-Haemophilus* identification card. *J. Clin. Microbiol.* **45:**3493–3497.

136. **Van Dam, A. P., A. van Weert, C. Harmanus, K. E. Hovius, E. C. J. Claas, and F. A. G. Reubsaet.** 2009. Molecular characterization of *Capnocytophaga canimorsus* and other canine *Capnocytophaga* spp. and assessment by PCR of their frequencies in dogs. *J. Clin. Microbiol.* **47:**3218–3225.

137. **Vandamme, P., B. Holmes, H. Bercovier, and T. Coenye.** 2006. Classification of Centers for Disease Control group eugonic fermenter (EF)-4a and EF-4b as *Neisseria animaloris* sp. nov. and *Neisseria zoodegmatis* sp. nov., respectively. *Int. J. Syst. Evol. Microbiol.* **56:**1801–1805.

138. **Wang, H.-K., Y.-C. Chen, L.-J. Teng, C.-C. Hung, M.-L. Chen, S.-H. Du, H.-J. Pan, P.-R. Hsueh, and S.-C. Chang.** 2007. Brain abscess associated with multidrug-resistant *Capnocytophaga ochracea* infection. *J. Clin. Microbiol.* **45:**645–647.

139. **Weber, D. J., J. S. Wolfson, M. N. Swartz, and D. C. Hooper.** 1984. *Pasteurella multocida* infections. Report of 34 cases and review of the literature. *Medicine* **63:**133–154.

140. **Weyant, R. S., C. W. Moss, R. E. Weaver, D. G. Hollis, J. G. Jordan, E. C. Cook, and M. I. Daneshvar.** 1996. *Identification of Unusual Pathogenic Gram-Negative Aerobic and Facultatively Anaerobic Bacteria,* 2nd ed. Williams & Wilkins, Baltimore, MD.

141. **Whitehouse, R. L. S., H. Jackson, M. C. Jackson, and M. M. Ramji.** 1987. Isolation of *Simonsiella* sp. from a neonate. *J. Clin. Microbiol.* **25:**522–525.

142. **Yagupsky, P.** 2004. *Kingella kingae:* from medical rarity to an emerging paediatric pathogen. *Lancet Infect. Dis.* **4:**358–367.

143. **Yagupsky, P., M. Merires, J. Bahar, and R. Dagan.** 1995. Evaluation of novel vancomycin-containing medium for primary isolation of *Kingella kingae* from upper respiratory tract specimens. *J. Clin. Microbiol.* **33:**1426–1427.

144. **Yogev, R., D. Shulman, S. T. Shulman, and W. G. Glogowski.** 1986. In vitro activity of antibiotics alone and in combination against *Actinobacillus actinomycetemcomitans.* *Antimicrob. Agents Chemother.* **29:**179–181.

145. **Yumoto, H., M. Yamada, C. Shinohara, H. Nakae, K. Takahashi, H. Azakami, S. Ebisu, and T. Matsuo.** 2007. Soluble products from *Eikenella corrodens* induce cell proliferation and expression of interleukin-8 and adhesion molecules in endothelial cells via mitogen-activated protein kinase pathways. *Oral Microbiol. Immunol.* **22:**36–45.

146. **Zbinden, R.** 1995. *Capnocytophaga canimorsus:* challenge for the clinical microbiologist. *Med. Microbiol. Lett.* **4:**217–223.

Haemophilus

NATHAN A. LEDEBOER AND GARY V. DOERN

34

TAXONOMY AND DESCRIPTION OF THE GENUS

Haemophilus spp. are members of the family *Pasteurellaceae* (51). While the number of *Haemophilus* species described greatly exceeds the number of human pathogens, eight species affecting humans currently included in this genus are *H. influenzae, H. aegyptius, H. ducreyi, H. pittmaniae, H. parainfluenzae, H. haemolyticus, H. parahaemolyticus,* and *H. paraphrohaemolyticus. Aggregatibacter aphrophilus, Aggregatibacter paraphrophilus,* and *Aggregatibacter segnis* were formerly included in the genus *Haemophilus* but have recently been reclassified into the genus *Aggregatibacter* (formerly *Actinobacillus*) based on molecular taxonomy (68). Additionally, *A. aphrophilus* and *A. paraphrophilus* have been combined into the single species *A. aphrophilus* (68). A description of the characteristics and epidemiology of the newly reclassified *A. aphrophilus* species can be found in chapter 33 in this *Manual.* A comprehensive review of the taxonomy of *Haemophilus* species has been provided by Kilian (50) or can be located in reference 45.

In the absence of the recently reclassified species, significant genetic diversity still exists in the *Haemophilus* genus. The genomes of these species range in size from 1.8 Mb for *H. influenzae* to 2.8 Mb for *H. ducreyi* (45). DNA-DNA hybridization studies demonstrate significant heterogeneity between species; studies conducted by Burbach et al. as discussed in reference 45 demonstrate binding ratios between *H. influenzae* and other species to range from 10% (*H. paracuniculus*) to 70% (*H. aegyptius*). *H. influenzae* is most closely related to *H. aegyptius*, with 90% homology, but is most distant from *H. ducreyi*, with only 18% homology. Intraspecies heterogeneity is also significant, ranging from 50 to 100% in *H. influenzae* and *H. parainfluenzae* strains (45).

Members of the *Haemophilus* genus are small, nonmotile, non-spore-forming, non-acid-fast, pleomorphic gram-negative bacilli with fastidious growth requirements. Cells in this genus are coccobacilli or short rods. The cell wall resembles those of other gram-negative bacilli but contains fewer fatty acids than occur in other members of the *Pasteurellaceae* (35, 45, 51); the lipopolysaccharide of *Haemophilus* is structurally different from those of members of the *Enterobacteriaceae* (35, 45, 51). The fatty acid composition of the cell wall includes *n*-tetradecanoate (14:0), 3-hydroxy-tetradecanoate

(3-OH-14:0), *n*-hexadecanoate (16:0), and hexadecanoate (16:1) (48). Fimbriae have been observed on the cell walls of certain species of *H. influenzae* and *H. aegyptius* (45). The genome of *Haemophilus* spp. is characterized by a G+C content of 37 to 45% (45, 51, 83).

Haemophilus spp. are facultatively anaerobic, with requirements for X and/or V factors for growth. X factor is protoporphyrin IX, a metabolic intermediate in the hemin biosynthetic pathway (45). V factor is composed of nicotinamide complexed as NAD or NADP. Both factors are present in erythrocytes ("haemophilus" means "blood loving" in Greek). Requirements for these compounds vary based on the species, with *H. influenzae, H. aegyptius,* and *H. haemolyticus* requiring both X and V factors for growth, whereas others require only a single factor (Table 1). Optimal growth occurs at 35 to 37°C in the presence of 5 to 7% CO_2. All species are CAMP reaction negative and produce alkaline phosphatase (46).

Organisms within the *Haemophilus* genus typically grow on chocolate agar, producing colonies that are usually smooth, with a flat or convex shape. They are nonpigmented (i.e., buff or light tan) or slightly yellow and are 0.5 to 2.0 mm in diameter. Certain *Haemophilus* spp. produce beta-hemolysis when grown on sheep blood agar plates (Table 1). Growth in broth can vary between homogeneous and granular.

Species of *Haemophilus*, other than *H. ducreyi*, typically ferment a wide range of different biochemical substrates. In particular, fermentation of glucose, sucrose, lactose, mannose, and xylose are useful characteristics in the species identification of organisms in this genus. Production of indole, ornithine decarboxylase, urease, catalase, and β-galactosidase plus the ability to produce beta-hemolysis when grown on blood-containing media are other variable properties of *Haemophilus* spp. that aid in the species identification of organisms in this genus (Table 1).

Strains of *H. influenzae* may produce one of six distinct capsular polysaccharides or may be nonencapsulated. Nonencapsulated *H. influenzae* strains are referred to as nontypeable (NTHi) (33) (Fig. 1). The presence of polysaccharide capsular antigen provides the basis for serotype designations, a to f. Capsular serotyping is based on the polysaccharide composition of the capsular structure. Depending on the strain type, the capsule is composed of ribose and fructose

TABLE 1 Differential characteristics of *Haemophilus* species[e]

Haemophilus species	Requirement for:			Fermentation of:					Production of:				Hemolysis
	X factor	V factor	Catalase	Glucose	Sucrose	Lactose	Xylose	Mannose	Indole	Urease	Ornithine decarboxylase	β-Galactosidase	
H. influenzae	+	+	+	+	−	−	+	−	v[a]	v[a]	v[a]	−	−
H. aegyptius	+	+	+	+[b]	−	−	−	−	−	+	−	−	−
H. haemolyticus	+	+	+	+	−	−	−	−	v	+	v[a]	−	+
H. parainfluenzae	−	+	v	+	+	−	v	+	v[a]	v[a]	v[a]	v	−
H. ducreyi	+	−	−	v	−	−	−	−	−	−	−	−	−[c]
H. parahaemolyticus	−	+	v	+	+	−	−	+	−	+	−	v	+
H. pittmaniae	−	+	w	+	+	−	−	+	uk	uk	uk	+	+
H. paraphrohaemolyticus[d]	−	−	+	+	+	−	−	+	−	+	−	v	+

[a] Indole, urease, and ornithine decarboxylase production are the basis for biotyping schemes with *H. influenzae* and *H. parainfluenzae* as depicted in Table 2.
[b] A delayed positive reaction occurs in more than 90% of strains.
[c] Delayed development of hemolysis occurs in 11 to 89% of strains.
[d] Elevated concentrations of CO₂ of ≥10% enhance growth.
[e] +, positive; −, negative; v, variable reaction; w, weak reaction; uk, unknown.

in the furanose ring and Glc, Gal, GlcNAc, or ManANAc in the pyranose ring. The structures of the capsules belonging to each serotype can be found in reference 45. Indole, ornithine decarboxylase, and urease production are the basis for a biotyping scheme with both *H. influenzae* and *H. parainfluenzae* (30) (Table 2).

EPIDEMIOLOGY, PATHOGENESIS, AND TRANSMISSION

Haemophilus influenzae may be found as part of the commensal bacterial flora of the mucosal surfaces of the upper respiratory tracts (URT) of many healthy individuals (65). Asymptomatic colonization of the URT with encapsulated strains of *H. influenzae* type b (Hib) is rare, i.e., 2 to 5% of healthy children in the prevaccine era and significantly fewer (~0.06%) following introduction of the pediatric Hib conjugate antigen vaccine, HIB, in the early 1980s (61). In contrast, NTHi, together with strains of *H. parainfluenzae*, represents a major portion of the cultured bacterial microbiota of the pharynxes and nasopharynxes of >90% of healthy individuals (52, 88). Clones of NTHi present in the URT differ when asymptomatic carriers are compared to those with infection (76, 88). In asymptomatically colonized individuals, the clones vary continuously, with a mean duration of carriage of 1 to 2 months (76). However, during infection, a single clonal group predominates.

The incubation period for *H. influenzae* is poorly understood. The presence of a concomitant or preceding viral infection can potentiate infection. The colonizing bacteria invade the mucosa and enter the bloodstream. The antiphagocytic nature of the Hib capsule and the absence of the anticapsular antibody lead to increasing bacterial proliferation (65). When the bacterial concentration exceeds a critical level, it can disseminate to various sites, including the meninges, subcutaneous tissue, joints, pleura, pericardia, and lungs. The presence of antibody, complement, and phagocytic cells determines the clearance of the bacteremia and can influence dissemination (65).

Host defenses include activation of the alternate and classic complement pathways and antibodies to the polyribosylribitol phosphate (PRP) capsule. Antibody to the Hib capsule plays a primary role in conferring immunity. Newborns have a low risk of infection, likely because of maternal antibodies acquired through colostrum. When these transplacental antibodies to the PRP antigen wane, infants are at high risk of developing invasive *H influenzae* disease, and their immune responses are low even after the disease (65). Therefore, they are at high risk of repeat infections since prior episodes of *H influenzae* do not confer immunity. By the age of 5 years, most children have naturally acquired antibodies. The Hib conjugate vaccine induces protection by inducing antibodies against the PRP capsule.

Colonization of the oral cavity by *H. parainfluenzae* and *H. pittmaniae* superior to the palatal arches is normal. *H. parahaemolyticus* and *H. haemolyticus* colonization in healthy individuals remains rare. Colonization of the cervix with *H. ducreyi* has been documented following sexual intercourse.

CLINICAL SIGNIFICANCE

H. influenzae

Systemic infections caused by *H. influenzae*, such as meningitis, epiglottitis, orbital cellulitis, and bacteremia, are usually caused by capsular type b strains and generally fall

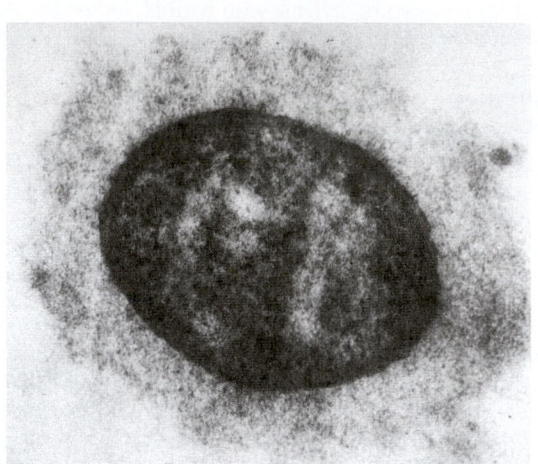
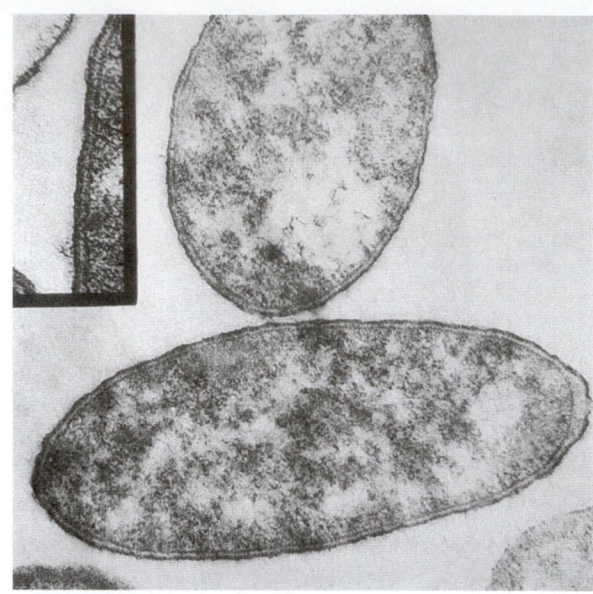

FIGURE 1 Electron micrographs depicting an encapsulated type b strain (left) and a nonencapsulated, nontypeable strain (right) of *Haemophilus influenzae*.

within biotypes I and II of this species (69). Life-threatening *Haemophilus* infections, however, have fortunately become exceedingly uncommon in developed countries since the development and introduction of the pediatric HIB vaccine (14, 79, 91). When infections caused by Hib occur today, it is usually in the setting of an unvaccinated child, although they may also arise in both children and adults as a result of head trauma or cerebrospinal fluid (CSF) leak or following a neurosurgical procedure. Biotype IV strains, at least in the pre-HIB vaccine era, were often found to cause systemic infections in neonates as well as aggressive infections of the genital tract in postpartum women (75, 96).

TABLE 2 Biotypes of *Haemophilus influenzae* and *H. parainfluenzae*

Species	Biotype	Production of:		
		Indole	Ornithine decarboxylase	Urease
H. influenzae	I	+	+	+
	II	+	+	−
	III	−	+	−
	IV	−	+	+
	V	+	−	+
	VI	−	−	+
	VII	+	−	−
	VIII	−	−	−
H. parainfluenzae	I	−	−	+
	II	−	+	+
	III	−	+	−
	IV	+	+	+
	V	−	−	−
	VI	+	−	+
	VII	+	+	−
	VIII	+	−	−

The vast majority of *H. influenzae* infections today are caused by NTHi (33, 88). This organism is an important cause of acute conjunctivitis, acute otitis media, acute maxillary sinusitis, acute bacterial exacerbation of chronic bronchitis, and pneumonia (65). The organism gains access to the site of infection by direct contiguous spread from its reservoir in the URT. Spread via respiratory secretions, usually on the hands of patients, can lead to conjunctival infection. Antecedent viral infections with resultant inflammation of the Eustachian tubes and sinus ostea predispose to infection of the middle ear cavity and maxillary sinuses, respectively, by compromising egress from and ingress to these closed spaces (66). Establishment of infection in the lungs is facilitated by any condition that diminishes mucociliary clearance of organisms from the respiratory tree (65, 67, 86). Examples include smoking, chronic obstructive pulmonary disease, viral infection, recurrent bacterial infection, and physiological alterations, such as those that occur in individuals with cystic fibrosis (65, 67, 86). Persons at risk for systemic NTHi infection include those with functional or anatomic asplenism, sickle cell disease, complement deficiencies, Hodgkin's disease, congenital or acquired hypogammaglobulinemia, and T-cell immunodeficiency states (e.g., human immunodeficiency virus infection). Rarely is NTHi documented to be a cause of bacteremia. This may be due to the relative avirulence of the organism or the inadequacy of conventional blood culture techniques in propagating this fastidious bacterium.

H. ducreyi

Chancroid is a sexually transmitted disease caused by *H. ducreyi* which is usually characterized by the development of a single painful genital ulcer, with associated inguinal lymphadenopathy occurring 2 to 7 days following exposure (23, 26, 60). Keratinocytes are likely the first cell type encountered by *H. ducreyi* upon infection of human skin; thus, the interaction between *H. ducreyi* and keratinocytes is likely important in establishing infection (101). Chancroid occurs most often in developing countries, including much of Asia, Africa, and Latin America. Epidemics of disease are associated with low socioeconomic status, poor hygiene, prostitution, and drug abuse, and commercial sex workers are believed to serve as reservoirs for *H. ducreyi*. Since 1987, reported cases of chancroid declined steadily until 2001. Since then, the number of cases reported has fluctuated from 17 to 55 cases. In 2003, only 54 cases were reported to the CDC, with 24 of these cases from South Carolina. More recently, in 2007, 23 cases of chancroid were reported in the United States, with only eight states (California, Florida, Louisiana, Massachusetts, New York, North Carolina, Texas, and Wisconsin) reporting 1 or more cases. Because of difficulties in establishing an etiologic diagnosis of *H. ducreyi* infection and limited resources in many countries of endemicity, the true incidence of chancroid is unknown.

Other *Haemophilus* spp.

Haemophilus parainfluenzae remains the predominant species colonizing the URT, accounting for fully 75% of the *Haemophilus* biota in the oral cavity and in the pharynx. Interestingly, *H. parainfluenzae* does not routinely colonize the nasal cavity. *H. parainfluenzae* is thought to account for at least some cases of acute otitis media, acute sinusitis, and acute bacterial exacerbation of chronic bronchitis, although its role in these diseases is often inconclusive. Infrequently, it has also been identified as a cause of subacute bacterial endocarditis. As is the case with systemic infections due to NTHi, blood cultures are often negative in patients with *H. parainfluenzae* endocarditis due to the fastidious nature of the pathogen and frequent lysis of the organism, with high concentrations of sodium polyanethol sulfonate (5, 21, 37).

Haemophilus aegyptius, a distinct species of *Haemophilus* that closely resembles biotype III strains of *H. influenzae* and which has been referred to as the Koch-Weeks bacillus, is an important cause of acute purulent conjunctivitis (73). This disease, often called pinkeye, occurs most often in younger children, especially those having extensive contact with other children in closed settings, such as day care centers and grammar school classrooms. It is characterized by the rapid onset of conjunctival inflammation, visual disturbance, and ocular pain and pruritus. It often involves both eyes and is highly transmissible.

Brazilian purpuric fever, a condition that occurs most often in South America, is characterized by rapid onset of high fevers, hypotension, diffuse cutaneous hemorrhaging, and abrupt vascular compromise (4). The causative agent is often mistaken to be *H. aegyptius* but is instead an organism that is classified in biogroup III of *H. influenzae* (4, 8). These strains are characterized by the inability to ferment D-xylose activity, by a particular pattern of their housekeeping genes, by a particular rRNA restriction pattern, and by resistance to serum bactericidal activity, making them unique among other *H. influenzae* biogroups (45).

Other *Haemophilus* species have only rarely been implicated as causes of infection in humans, although lower respiratory tract infection, sinusitis, conjunctivitis, bacteremia, meningitis, wound infections, peritonitis, arthritis, osteomyelitis, and brain abscess have been documented in individual case reports or small case series.

SPECIMEN COLLECTION AND TRANSPORT AND ORGANISM STORAGE

The collection of specimens for the diagnosis of *Haemophilus* infections is predicated on the nature of the infection being evaluated. Details of specimen collection and transport can be found in chapter 16. In patients suspected of having meningitis, blood and CSF cultures should be performed. Middle ear fluid obtained by tympanocentesis is the specimen of choice for patients with otitis media; however, in patients with perforated tympanic membranes and otorrhea, an aseptically collected aspirate of middle ear fluid from the external auditory canal is also satisfactory. In cases of maxillary sinusitis, direct sinus aspirates or middle meatal swab specimens collected under endoscopic guidance should be obtained. Conjunctival swab specimens are required in the evaluation of patients thought to have *Haemophilus* conjunctivitis. In patients suspected of having bronchopulmonary infections due to *Haemophilus* spp., specimens representative of lower respiratory tract secretions should be obtained in such a way as to avoid contamination with oropharyngeal commensal biota. This means that collection of optimal specimens, such as by bronchoalveolar lavage or bronchial washing (less preferable) should be performed to provide optimum specificity when evaluating patients suspected of having *Haemophilus* bronchopulmonary infections. While collection of sputum and tracheal aspirates is less invasive, distinguishing between pathogens and oral biota can be nearly impossible by this means. When bacterial pneumonia is suspected, blood cultures should also be obtained. Importantly, with one exception, nasal, nasopharyngeal, and nasal swab specimens are of no value whatsoever in evaluating patients suspected of having *Haemophilus* infections at any of these respiratory tract sites. The one possible exception is in cystic fibrosis patients experiencing an exacerbation. In this setting, an induced deep-cough specimen collected on a swab inserted into the posterior pharynx may be rewarding (80). Inpatients suspected of having *Haemophilus* infections in normally sterile sites, such as the pleural space, synovium, pericardium, or peritoneum, fluid aspirated aseptically from the site of involvement represents the specimen of choice. Concomitant blood cultures should also be performed.

Finally, specimens for culture of *H. ducreyi* should be collected from the margins of genital lesions with a saline- or broth-moistened swab. The swab should be immediately transported to the laboratory and plated without delay to avoid loss of organism viability. It is imperative that health care providers inform the laboratory of the clinical suspicion of chancroid so that appropriate media for culture of *H. ducreyi* can be employed. If extended transport is required, swab specimens should be plated directly at the time of collection in the patient care area or the specimen swab should be placed in transport medium containing hemin (25). When refrigerated (4°C), the use of Amies transport medium has been demonstrated to maintain the viability of *H. ducreyi* for up to 3 days. Alternatively, specially formulated thioglycolate-hemin-based media containing albumin and glutamine can also be used to preserve organism viability for transport taking longer than 3 days (25, 100). While optimal cultivation of *H. ducreyi* is based on collection of ulcer materials, lymph node aspirates, pus, and aspirates from buboes can also be submitted for culture, albeit with less sensitivity than ulcer material. When cultivating *H. ducreyi* from these specimens, laboratories should consider allowing clinicians to directly plate specimens to maintain optimal recovery. Specimens for *H. ducreyi* nucleic acid amplification techniques should be collected using standard collection techniques for nucleic acid amplification from genital specimens.

Long-term storage of *Haemophilus* spp. is usually accomplished by lyophilization or freezing of isolates at −60°C to −80°C in tryptic soy broth with >10% glycerol or on porous beads (Pro-Lab Diagnostics, Round Rock, TX).

DIRECT EXAMINATION

Microscopy

On Gram stains, *Haemophilus* spp. appear as small pleomorphic gram-negative coccobacilli with coccoid, coccobacillary, rod-shaped, or filamentous forms (Fig. 2). Because of the pleomorphism of *Haemophilus* spp., careful interpretation of the Gram stain smears must be undertaken to avoid confusion with other gram-negative bacteria, such as *Neisseria meningitidis*. Underdecolorization of Gram stains may erroneously suggest the presence of *Streptococcus pneumoniae*, *Listeria monocytogenes*, or *Streptococcus agalactiae*.

Gram stain smears of CSF should be prepared and examined and the results reported within 30 min of receipt of the specimen in the laboratory directly to the health care provider who requested the test. With nonturbid specimens, following centrifugation in a cytocentrifuge at $10,000 \times g$ for 10 min, a concentrated smear is prepared. With visibly turbid specimens, a direct smear should be prepared in addition to the cytospin smear. A Gram stain is performed immediately and examined for the presence of polymorphonuclear leukocytes and bacteria morphologically compatible with *Haemophilus* spp. In rare cases, the CSF Gram stain may reveal many polymorphonuclear leukocytes but no bacteria. When this occurs, prepare another cytospin smear and stain with acridine orange (BD, Sparks, MD, or Remel, Lenexa, KS).

The same approach as that applied to Gram staining should be applied to pleural, peritoneal, synovial, and pericardial fluid specimens. Middle ear fluid specimens and sinus aspirate Gram stains should be prepared directly from the specimen without cytocentrifugation.

Gram stains of lower respiratory tract secretions may be prepared directly from the specimen (e.g., expectorated sputa, endotracheal suction specimens, transbronchial biopsy specimens, bronchial brush biopsy specimens, and thoracotomy specimens) or following cytocentrifugation (e.g., bronchial washes and bronchoalveolar lavage fluid).

Strands of small gram-negative bacilli arranged in a railroad track-like manner on a direct Gram stain are highly

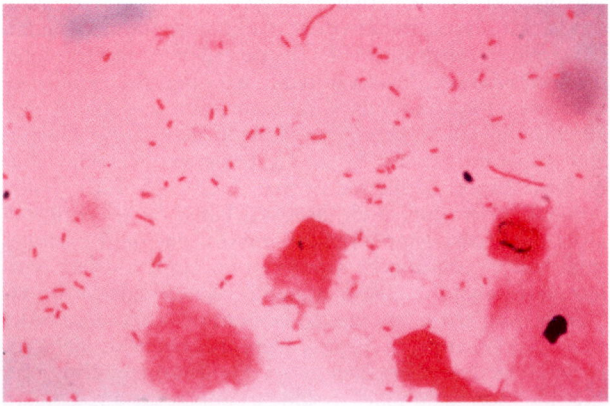

FIGURE 2   Gram stain of *Haemophilus influenzae* present in CSF.

suggestive of *H. ducreyi*. However, Gram staining of genital specimens for *H. ducreyi* is controversial because most genital ulcers contain a mixed bacterial biota, making Gram stain interpretation difficult. Furthermore, the positive yield of a Gram stain for *H. ducreyi* is low in comparison to that of culture or detection with nucleic acid amplification tests.

Antigen Detection

Commercial immunochemical techniques are available for the detection of *S. pneumoniae*, *Streptococcus dysgalactiae*, *H. influenzae*, and *N. meningitidis* directly from CSF and other body fluids. While these techniques provide a rapid identification of the pathogen, they lack sensitivity and specificity compared to Gram staining (59). Thus, the use of *H. influenzae* antigen detection is of limited clinical value, and its use is generally discouraged. However, in certain clinical contexts, such as in resource-constrained regions when the prevalence of disease is high and routine culture is unreliable, antigen-based detection methods may prove useful.

Molecular Techniques

Nucleic acid amplification assays, most notably assays predicated on PCR, have been developed to detect *H. influenzae* directly in various clinical specimens, including CSF, plasma, serum, and whole blood (74, 81). These techniques can be multiplexed to detect other common bacterial causes of specific infectious disease entities, such as meningitis. While publications cite variable detection sensitivities of these techniques, specificity is generally excellent (16, 22, 92).

Studies have demonstrated that the accuracy of clinical diagnosis for chancroid ranges from 33% to 80% (24) and that culture is approximately 75% sensitive (54, 62), making it an ideal candidate for molecular techniques. Molecular strategies have been developed to directly detect *H. ducreyi* from clinical specimens. Primers for these assays have been designed to amplify sequences from either the *H. ducreyi* 16S rRNA gene, the *rrs* (16S)-*rrl* (23S) ribosomal intergenic spacer region, an anonymous fragment of cloned *H. ducreyi* DNA, or the *groEL* gene, which encodes the *H. ducreyi* heat shock protein (54). One strategy includes a chloroform extraction followed by a one-tube nested PCR directed to the 16S rRNA gene, with longer outer primers for annealing at a higher temperature and shorter inner primers labeled with biotin and digoxigenin for binding with streptavidin and colorimetric detection (98). The sensitivity of PCR directly from clinical specimens varies among assays between 83 and 95% compared to culture or clinical diagnosis (54, 98). The adaptations of molecular methods offer superior sensitivity for the diagnosis of chancroid; they are clearly advantageous in areas where the organism is endemic, particularly where testing by culture is difficult or impossible.

The use of molecular methods for the identification of other *Haemophilus* spp. directly from clinical samples has proven difficult. The lack of both sensitivity and specificity has been problematic. In clinical specimens, small numbers of organisms may be present, leading to limitations in detection sensitivity. That is especially the case in patients with *Haemophilus* bacteremia (9). To achieve adequate sensitivity, large volumes of blood or CSF must be processed to achieve adequate sensitivity, creating laborious nucleic acid extraction and concentration processes with little clinical relevance. Further complicating the detection of *Haemophilus* from blood and CSF is the detection of agents following initiation of therapy. While culture frequently becomes negative following administration of the first appropriate dose of antimicrobials, patients can retain bacterial DNA in their blood or CSF for at least 2 weeks following clearance of the organism, leading to false-positive reactions, often making the interpretation of results challenging.

In certain other specimens, particularly specimens from the respiratory tract, commensal strains of *Haemophilus* spp. are often present, rendering positive results inconclusive. Further, the presence of other commensals or use of antimicrobials prior to screening may result in false-positive reactions, thus contributing to a lack of assay specificity. For these reasons, the use of molecular detection techniques is not currently advocated for the detection of *Haemophilus* spp. directly in clinical specimens until clinically significant thresholds for molecular quantification of organisms from respiratory specimens are achieved.

ISOLATION

Media

Optimum recovery of *Haemophilus* spp. in culture requires the use of enriched media that support the growth of these fastidious bacteria. Media must contain at least 10 μg/ml of free X and V factors. High concentrations of both the X and the V factor are found in whole blood, most of it sequestered within erythrocytes. X factor is protoporphyrin IX and can be derived from whole blood or can be added to bacteriological media using crystalline hemin; X factor is readily available in traditional blood agar. V factor is composed of nicotinamide complexed as NAD or NADP and is also readily available in blood. However, nicotinamide is not readily bioavailable because of its intracellular location and the presence of NAD-glycohydrolase enzymes in the blood. For the growth of *Haemophilus* spp. on solid media, crystalline hemin and NAD must be added to a final concentration of 10 μg/ml, or the blood used in the medium must be heated such that the red cells lyse and release free X factor and V factor into the medium. The latter can be accomplished by adding blood to the basal medium as it

cools to 80°C after being autoclaved. This is referred to as "chocolatizing" blood. For optimal growth of *Haemophilus* spp., a concentration of 5% chocolatized sheep blood should be employed (51).

The optimum growth of *Haemophilus* spp., especially of more-fastidious species, such as *H. ducreyi* and *H. aegyptius*, requires, in addition to the X and V factors, supplementation of media with various other growth factors. Two commercially available supplements that supply these growth factor requirements are IsoVitaleX (BD) and Vitox (Remel). These compounds contain glucose, cystine, glutamine, adenine, thiamine, vitamin B_{12}, guanine, iron, and aminobenzoic acid and provide adequate supplementation for the growth of *H. ducreyi* and *H. aegyptius*.

Enriched chocolate agar containing 5% lysed sheep red blood cells and supplemented with 1% IsoVitaleX or 1% Vitox represents one general-purpose medium that is commonly used in clinical laboratories to effectively propagate *Haemophilus* spp. (Fig. 3). Another medium that reliably supports the growth of *Haemophilus* spp. is Levinthal's medium (58). Because it is transparent, Levinthal's medium offers the added benefit of permitting the detection of colony iridescence, a property that is frequently associated with encapsulation (Fig. 4) (12, 72). One recent investigation found that a medium consisting of GC (BD or Remel) agar base, 5% heated sheep red blood cells, and 1% yeast autolysate provided the best growth of all *Haemophilus* spp. other than *H. ducreyi* (77).

A significant challenge in the recovery of *Haemophilus* spp. from respiratory tract specimens is bacterial overgrowth due to the presence of other less fastidious commensal bacteria. Supplementation of media with some combination of bacitracin, vancomycin, and/or clindamycin serves to inhibit overgrowth with commensals, thus permitting the recovery of *Haemophilus* spp. (15). Use of such selective media is particularly relevant to the recovery of *Haemophilus* spp. from respiratory tract specimens from patients with cystic fibrosis, acute exacerbation of chronic bronchitis, conjunctivitis, and epiglottitis (Fig. 5) (28). Several versions of selective *Haemophilus* media are available commercially, including *Haemophilus* isolation agar (Remel) and *Haemophilus* isolation agar with bacitracin (BD). These media contain beef heart infusion agar with casein peptone to supply nutritional requirements, combined with horse blood

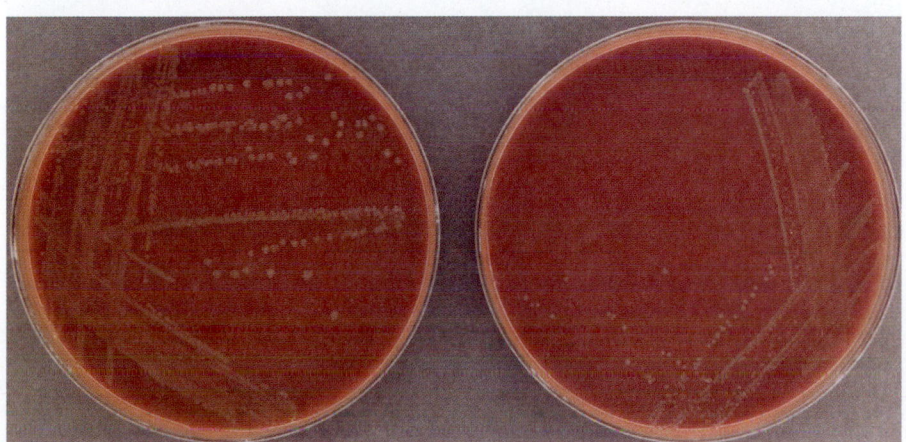

FIGURE 3 Colony morphologies of type b encapsulated (left) and nonencapsulated (right) strains of *Haemophilus influenzae* when propagated on enriched chocolate agar.

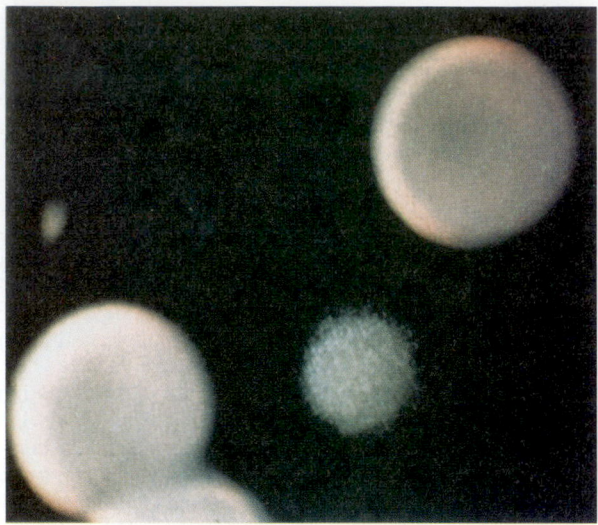

FIGURE 4 Colony morphologies of type b encapsulated (left and right) and nonencapsulated (center) strains of *Haemophilus influenzae* when propagated on Levinthal's agar. Note the conspicuous iridescence apparent with the encapsulated strain.

to supply the X and V factors and to distinguish hemolytic species of *Haemophilus* from those which are not. Bacitracin is added to inhibit normal biotas, including *Neisseria* spp.

The use of selective media is also helpful in recovering *H. ducreyi* from genital tract specimens (100). Selective media may include any of the following: GC agar base with 1% IsoVitaleX, 5% fetal bovine serum, 1% hemoglobin, and 3 μg vancomycin; GC agar base with 5% Fildes enrichment, 5% horse blood, and 3 μg vancomycin; 5% fresh rabbit blood agar with 3 μg vancomycin; or Mueller-Hinton agar with 5% chocolatized horse blood, 1% IsoVitaleX, and 3 μg vancomycin (100). Preferably, two different selective media are employed (100).

Growth of *Haemophilus* spp. may also be achieved on 5% sheep blood agar by use of the microsatellite phenomenon. With the microsatellite test, a single streak line of hemolysin-producing *Staphylococcus* spp. is placed on an agar surface previously inoculated with a specimen suspected of containing *Haemophilus* spp. The hemolysin produced by the *Staphylococcus* species lyses the erythrocytes immediately adjacent to the streak line in the medium, releasing sufficient concentrations of X factor (hemin) and V factor (NAD) into the medium to supply the growth factor requirements of *Haemophilus* spp. *Staphylococcus* also secretes NAD into the medium in proximity to the streak line. Colonies of *Haemophilus* thus appear in a narrow zone adjacent to the staphylococcal streak. This is referred to as "satelliting" growth (Fig. 6). Organisms other than staphylococci can also produce the satellite phenomenon with *Haemophilus*, e.g., enterococci and yeast.

Although not a common cause of bacteremia, special techniques are not necessary for the recovery of *Haemophilus* spp. from blood specimens with modern, continuously monitoring blood culture systems (36, 48). The broth medium used in such systems supports the growth of *Haemophilus* spp. because the blood specimen itself supplies adequate concentrations of both the X and V factors when the erythrocytes present in the specimen lyse as they come into contact with the blood culture broth. However, the common practice of using such systems for the culture of normally sterile body fluids, e.g., synovial, peritoneal, pericardial, and pleural fluid, may be problematic insofar as these specimens may not contain sufficient amounts of blood to supply the necessary levels of the X and V factors to support the growth of *Haemophilus* spp. In situations where *Haemophilus* spp. is strongly suspected in such specimens, blood culture bottles should be supplemented with at least 10 μg of both sterile hemin and NAD/ml prior to inoculation with clinical specimens.

Following inoculation, solid media should be incubated at 35 to 37°C in a moist atmosphere and in the presence of 5 to 7% CO_2. Under these conditions, most *Haemophilus* spp. grow within 24 to 48 h. When specimens for *H. ducreyi* and *H. aegyptius* are cultured, incubation may be necessary for up to 5 days to allow sufficient time for the growth of these fastidious organisms. Further, when technologists attempt to propagate *H. ducreyi*, plates should be incubated at slightly lower temperatures, i.e., 30 to 33°C in 5% CO_2 in a high-moisture environment. Use of lower incubation temperatures will improve the recovery of *H. ducreyi* in comparison to incubation temperatures of 35 to 37°C.

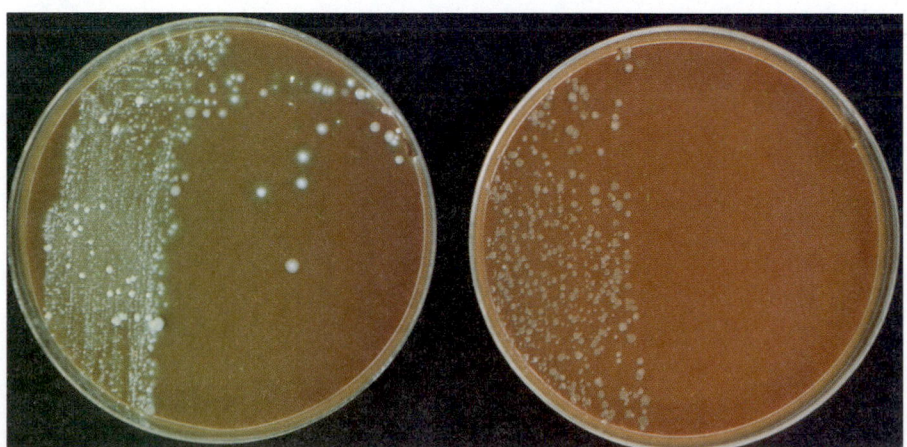

FIGURE 5 Colony growth from an expectorated-sputum specimen containing *Haemophilus influenzae* from a patient with cystic fibrosis propagated on enriched chocolate agar (left) and enriched chocolate agar containing bacitracin, clindamycin, and vancomycin (right).

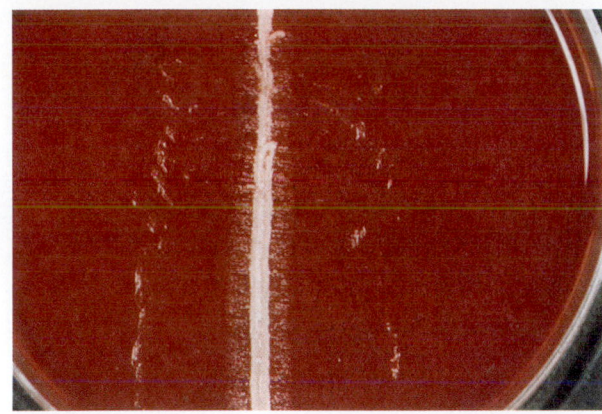

FIGURE 6 Satellite phenomenon observed when *Haemophilus influenzae* is propagated next to a streak of *Staphylococcus aureus* on a 5% sheep blood agar plate.

Colony Appearance

Colonies of *Haemophilus* spp. on suitable solid media, in general, are nonpigmented or slightly yellow and flat to convex, and they have a diameter of 0.5 to 2 mm after 48 h of incubation. Certain species of *Haemophilus* produce beta-hemolysis (Table 1).

Colonies of *H. influenzae* on chocolate agar are smooth, low, convex, grayish, and translucent. Encapsulated strains often have a mucoid appearance, while nonencapsulated strains produce smaller, buff colonies (Fig. 3). Most strains of *H. influenzae* produce indole, emitting a strong amine-like odor. Non-indole-producing strains emit a "mousy" odor. Colonies are 1 to 2 mm in diameter and often grow within 24 h. Colonies grown on clear media, such as Levinthal's agar, demonstrate iridescence under obliquely transmitted light (12, 72). Iridescence is most conspicuous with young colonies and disappears with age. Iridescent colors may include yellow, red, green, or blue. Iridescence is more apparent with capsular type b strains; nonencapsulated strains typically demonstrate a blue-green color (Fig. 4).

Colonies of *H. aegyptius* reach a colony size of only ca. 0.5 mm after 48 h of growth. Colonies are low, convex, and translucent, with a smooth, entire surface. On semisolid media, "comet-like" colonies are produced.

Colonies of *H. parainfluenzae* are typically off-white to yellow and, like *H. influenzae*, 1 to 2 mm in diameter after 24 h of growth. The colony appearance is extremely varied, i.e., flat and smooth, granular with serrated edges, or heaped up and wrinkled. Colonies exhibiting the last morphology may be slid intact across the surface of the agar. The colony morphology of *H. parainfluenzae* may change as the colonies age.

Colonies of *H. haemolyticus* are translucent, smooth, and convex and do not form satellites around *Staphylococcus*. Colonies usually achieve a diameter of 0.5 to 1.5 mm after 24 h, with a clear zone of beta-hemolysis surrounding each colony when the organism is grown on blood agar; *H. haemolyticus* can lose its ability to cause hemolysis following serial subculture on bacteriological media. The growth properties and colony morphology of *H. parahaemolyticus* and *H. paraphrohaemolyticus* are similar to those of *H. haemolyticus*.

H. ducreyi grows poorly, regardless of the medium used, and frequently 3 to 5 days will pass before growth appears. Colonies growing on chocolate agar are small, flat, gray, and smooth. Larger colonies may be interspersed among small colonies but have the same morphology. Growth on blood agar is poor, with a slight beta-hemolysis surrounding the colonies. As with *H. parainfluenzae*, older colonies of *H. ducreyi* are cohesive and can be slid across the agar.

IDENTIFICATION

The identification and differentiation of *Haemophilus* spp. are achieved through determination of X and V factor requirements for growth, performance of the porphyrin test, assessment of hemolysis, determination of carbohydrate fermentation patterns, and production of indole, ornithine decarboxylase, urease, catalase, and β-galactosidase (Table 1). The pattern of X and V growth factor requirements and the porphyrin test provide sufficient information for the presumptive species identification of selected *Haemophilus* spp. Definitive species identification, however, requires assessment of the other phenotypic characteristics listed above (Table 1). Alternatively, sequencing also provides excellent identification of these organisms.

X and V Factor Growth Requirements

X and V factor requirements for the growth of *Haemophilus* spp. may be determined by swab inoculation of a suspension of test organism equivalent in turbidity to a 0.5 McFarland standard across the entire surface of a 100-mm petri dish containing tryptic soy agar. Filter paper disks or strips impregnated with X factor, V factor, and the X and V factors (Remel or BD) are then placed on the agar surface, and the plate is incubated for 20 to 24 h at 35°C in an atmosphere of 5 to 7% CO_2. The pattern of satellite growth around individual disks or strips, in the absence of growth elsewhere on the plate, is used to define the growth factor requirements of the test strain (Fig. 7). Tryptic soy agar is the preferred medium for use when the X and V growth factor requirements for *Haemophilus* spp. are determined, as other media may yield erroneous results (31, 34). Alternatively,

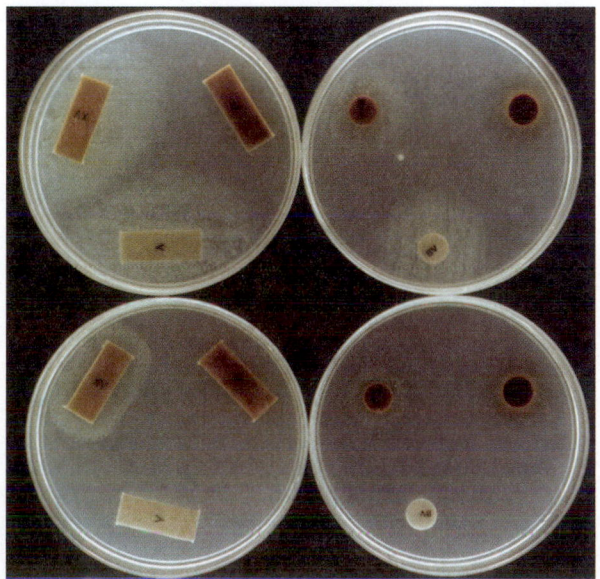

FIGURE 7 Use of X and V factor disks and strips in determining the growth factor requirements of *Haemophilus influenzae* (left disks) and *H. parainfluenzae* (right disks).

tri-plates (Haemophilus ID II; Remel) and quad-plates (Haemophilus ID quad; Remel) can be used to assess X and V growth factor requirements. When performing X and V factor studies, care should be taken to avoid carrying X factor along with the inoculum. This can result in erroneous identification of *H. influenzae* as *H. parainfluenzae*.

All of the X-factor-requiring species of *Haemophilus*, most notably *H. influenzae*, lack the enzymes necessary to convert δ-aminolevulinic acid (ALA) into protoporphyrin, a metabolic intermediate in the biosynthesis of X factor (6). Thus, they require that X factor be supplied exogenously to medium in order to support growth. By taking advantage of this observation, a rapid test, known as the porphyrin or ALA test, can be performed to quickly determine if a test organism requires X factor for growth (49). When positive, the porphyrin test indicates that the test organism is X factor independent; when negative, the porphyrin test indicates that the organism requires X factor. Since the vast majority of X-factor-requiring *Haemophilus* spp. recovered in the clinical laboratory are *H. influenzae*, when the porphyrin test is performed with a clinical isolate and found to be negative, it can be inferred with a high likelihood that the organism is *H. influenzae*.

The porphyrin test is performed using commercially available ALA disks (Remel) or through preparation of liquid porphyrin medium (49). To prepare liquid porphyrin medium, 2 mM ALA and 0.8 mM $MgSO_4$ in 0.1 M phosphate buffer (pH 6.9) are aliquoted in glass tubes with 0.5 ml of porphyrin medium in each tube. Tubes can be stored at 4°C for several months or for years at −20°C. Tubes are inoculated with a loopful of freshly grown bacteria and incubated for 4 h at 35°C in ambient air (51). Following incubation, the tubes are examined for brick-red fluorescence with a device, such as a Wood's lamp, that emits a 360-nm-long-wave UV light (Fig. 8). Tubes with questionable results may be reincubated for up to 24 h. Alternatively, Kovacs' reagent (0.5 ml) can be added to the liquid porphyrin medium, and the tube can be shaken and observed for a red color in the lower water phase (51). A negative-control tube lacking ALA should also be inoculated when the porphyrin test is performed to rule out false-positive reactions due to the presence of indole.

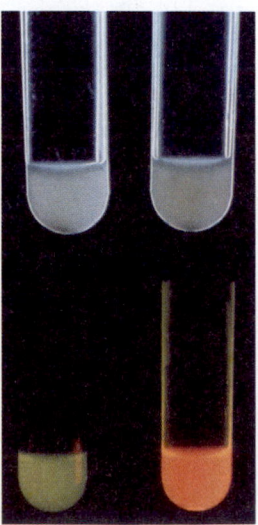

FIGURE 8 Positive (top) and negative (bottom) porphyrin tests.

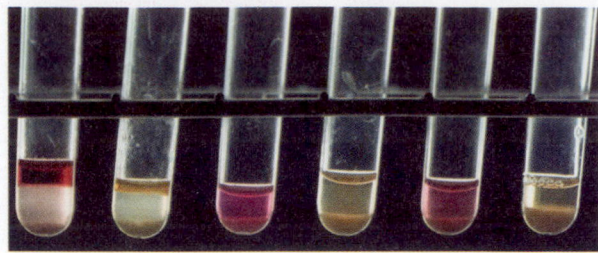

FIGURE 9 Conventional biochemicals depicting positive and negative reactions for indole, urease, and ornithine decarboxylase production (left to right) by *Haemophilus* spp.

The porphyrin test has been shown in several studies to outperform growth-factor-based methods for differentiation of *H. influenzae* from non-*H. influenzae* species (63).

Conventional Biochemical Tests

The list of biochemicals necessary for the differentiation of *Haemophilus* species is provided in Table 1. Carbohydrate fermentation is determined in phenol red broth containing 1% carbohydrate supplemented with 10-μg/ml NAD and hemin. Following heavy inoculation, fermentation tubes are incubated at 35°C without CO_2 for up to 1 week and examined periodically for a red-to-yellow color, indicating a positive reaction. Usually positive reactions become apparent within 24 h; however, *H. aegyptius* and *H. segnis* have been noted to demonstrate weak reactions following a 24-h incubation (7, 51).

Indole production can reliably be determined with most strains of *H. influenzae* and *H. parainfluenzae* using a spot indole test (Remel or BD). However, reliable assessment of indole production by other *Haemophilus* spp. requires use of a solution of 0.1% L-tryptophan in 0.067 M phosphate buffer at pH 6.8. Following inoculation, the suspension is incubated for 4 h at 35°C in ambient air, 0.5 ml of Kovacs' reagent is added to the tube, and the tube is shaken and examined for the appearance of red color in the upper portion of the tube as an indication of a positive reaction (45, 51) (Fig. 9).

Production of ornithine decarboxylase is determined using ornithine decarboxylase medium (see chapter 17) or Moeller's medium. A tube containing either medium is heavily inoculated, incubated for 4 to 24 h at 35°C in ambient air, and examined for a purple coloration as an indication that the organism produces ornithine decarboxylase (45, 51) (Fig. 9). Species of *Haemophilus* positive for ornithine decarboxylase include several biotypes of *H. influenzae* and *H. parainfluenzae*.

As was the case with indole production, in most instances, a spot urease test (Remel or BD) can be used to reliably detect urease production by most strains of *H. influenzae* and *H. parainfluenzae*. Determination of urease production with other species requires the use of urease medium containing 0.1 g KH_2PO_4, 0.1 g K_2HPO_4, 0.5 g NaCl, and 0.5 ml phenol red (1:500) dissolved in 100 ml of distilled water. The pH is adjusted to 7.0 with NaOH, and 10.4 ml of a 20% aqueous solution of urea is added. After inoculation, the tube is incubated for 4 h at 35°C in ambient air and examined for a pink-to-red coloration, indicating a positive reaction (45, 51) (Fig. 9).

Commercial Biochemical Identification Systems

Several commercial identification systems have been developed to identify *Haemophilus* spp. These systems employ a battery of conventional biochemical tests, frequently in a miniaturized form, with results available in shorter time periods than with conventional biochemical tests. The performance characteristics and identification accuracy of these commercial systems are extremely variable (31, 63, 78, 94). The RapID NH system (Remel) contains 11 biochemical reactions in a microwell tray. The reactions used for identification of *Haemophilus* include the production of urease, indole, ornithine decarboxylase, proline, and gamma-glutamyl aminopeptidase, resazurin reduction, glucose and sucrose utilization, nitrate reduction, and phosphate hydrolysis. The kit uses phosphate hydrolysis and nitrate reduction reactions to identify an isolate as belonging to the genus *Haemophilus* and the remaining reactions to identify the isolate to the species level and to determine the biotype of *H. influenzae*. Although various results have been reported with the RapID NH system, when used properly, >95% of clinical isolates of *H. influenzae* should be correctly identified (31).

The BBL Crystal *Neisseria/Haemophilus* ID system (BD) and API NH kit (bioMérieux) provide miniaturized biochemical identification schemes in a microwell tray, with results available in ≤5 h. The Crystal system employs 29 different growth substrates and is predicated on measuring the substrate conversion chromogenically and fluorogenically after 5 h of incubation. The API NH kit consists of 12 dehydrated substrates and a well to detect penicillinase, and it permits the identification of *Haemophilus* spp., *Neisseria* spp., and *Moraxella* spp. The test is performed by inoculating each well with an organism suspension equivalent to a 4 McFarland turbidity standard prepared from 24-h colony growth and incubating the plate for 2 to 2.25 h at 35°C. In addition to testing for penicillinase production, it tests for the following biochemicals: glucose, fructose, maltose, saccharose, ornithine decarboxylase, urease, lipase, alkaline phosphatase, β-galactosidase, proline arylamidase, gamma-glutamyl aminotransferase, and indole (3, 64). Independent research studies evaluating the performances of the Crystal *Neisseria/Haemophilus* and API NH kits compared to accepted gold standards have not been published.

One instrument-based identification system has been developed for the species identification of *Haemophilus* spp., the NH cards for use with the Vitek Legacy and Vitek 2 instruments (bioMérieux). This system is based on colorimetric detection of preformed enzyme complexes using chromogenic substrates. The database supporting these cards encompasses 27 taxa, including *Neisseria*, *Haemophilus*, *Actinobacillus*, *Campylobacter*, *Capnocytophaga*, *Cardiobacterium*, *Eikenella*, *Gardnerella*, *Kingella*, *Moraxella*, *Oligella*, and *Suttonella* species. Studies with the Vitek 2 system using both collections of well-characterized stock strains and clinical isolates have demonstrated identification accuracies of 90 to 95%, with results varying by species (78, 94). In one recent study, >95% of isolates of *H. influenzae*, *H. segnis*, *H. parahaemolyticus*, *H. parainfluenzae*, and *H. actinomycetemcomitans* were correctly identified, while none of the test strains of *H. haemolyticus* were correctly identified (78).

Molecular Identification

Several molecular methods, including 16S rRNA gene sequencing, PCR, and fluorescence in-site hybridization have been described in the literature as being effective tools for the species identification of *Haemophilus* when performed on organisms recovered in culture (17, 71, 74, 99).

Molecular targets for the detection and identification of *Haemophilus* spp. are numerous. Previous studies have described the detection of *H. influenzae* using the cap locus (which includes the capsule *bexA*) (1, 22, 57, 70), the 16S rRNA gene (1, 74, 89, 97), the insertion-like sequence (IS*1016*) (70), the fumarate reductase iron-sulfur gene B (*frdB*) (43), the manganese-dependent superoxide dismutase (*sodA*) (13), and the outer membrane protein P6 gene (*ompP6*) (1, 89, 95). Many of these targets are then combined with PCR (real time or traditional), microarrays, or sequencing to identify the organism. Widely utilized for sequencing, 16S rRNA frequently resolves the identities of strains to the species level; however, identification of *H. influenzae*, *H. aegyptius*, and *H. influenzae* biogroup aegyptius can be problematic due to the high degree of homology in their sequences. In these instances, sequencing of other targets, such as *ropD*, can be considered, or the use of combined sequencing and biochemical studies can be used. Other novel detection methods are also being investigated. One report from Kalogianni et al. (44) describes a simple dipstick test that may identify six pathogens and does not require special instrumentation. Universal primers are used for PCR amplification of the 23S rRNA gene. The amplified product is then labeled with biotin and hybridized to probes specific for the pathogens of interest and applied to the strip. The buffer migrates along the strip by capillary action and binds nanoparticles, producing a characteristic red line. The benefits of these types of technologies are that they can readily be utilized outside large reference laboratories and can be performed in less time than traditional sequencing. However, while microarray, sequencing, and immunoblotting technologies are interesting, a product to detect *Haemophilus* nucleic acid from culture or clinical specimens has yet to be approved by the U.S. Food and Drug Administration (FDA).

Problems in Identification

A significant challenge in the species identification of *H. influenzae*, *H. aegyptius*, and *H. influenzae* biogroup aegyptius is a lack of biochemical diversity and sequence divergence (45, 48, 51). Biochemical profiling and standard 16S rRNA gene sequencing fail to adequately distinguish these organisms (47, 48), necessitating the use of alternate sequencing targets, such as those mentioned in the previous section, or a combination of sequencing and biochemical testing. This is problematic, since *H. aegyptius* lacks the potential to cause Brazilian purpuric fever, while strains of *H. influenzae* biogroup aegyptius cause the disease. Xylose fermentation by most *H. influenzae* isolates combined with the lower growth rate of *H. influenzae* biotype aegyptius and the ability of *H. aegyptius* to agglutinate human erythrocytes may be of some value in distinguishing these organisms (47, 48, 51).

TYPING SYSTEMS

Capsular Serotyping and Biotyping

The capsular antigen of *H. influenzae* is a principal virulence determinant of this organism. Six different capsular antigens have been recognized, each of which is characterized by a distinct carbohydrate chemical composition and given a letter designation from a to f. Prior to the introduction of the pediatric HIB vaccine, capsular type b strains were recovered from human clinical material most often. However, today, at least among populations in which there is widespread use of the HIB vaccine, non-b encapsulated strains occur with nearly equal frequency. For this reason, it may be instructive to know the capsular serotypes of strains of *H. influenzae* recovered from clinical specimens, especially those representative of invasive disease. This may be accomplished using both phenotypic and genotypic methods.

Capsular serotyping of *H. influenzae* is best accomplished by the use of a slide agglutination assay which employs polyclonal antisera, specifically reactive with each of the six capsular antigens (45, 53, 85). It is advisable to perform serotyping as soon as possible after isolation of *H. influenzae*, as the amount of capsular antigen produced may diminish over time, especially with repeated subculture. A thick, homogenous suspension of test organism is prepared in saline, 1 to 2 drops are placed on a glass slide, and then a drop of type-specific antisera is added. The antisera is mixed with the organism suspension, and then the glass slide is rocked gently for ca.1 min before being examined for the presence of clumping, an indication of a positive reaction. The reagents for performing slide agglutination serotyping of *H. influenzae* are commercially available in kit form from Remel and BD.

Alternatively, primary type-specific antibodies can be directly or indirectly detected with fluorescent molecules, and binding of the antibody to the homologous capsular antigen can be determined by fluorescence microscopy (84, 87). While these technologies remain viable, reagents are frequently available on a research-use-only basis.

Whether a slide agglutination test or fluorescent antibodies are used to determine the capsular serotype of an isolate of *H. influenzae*, positive- and negative-control strains should always be processed simultaneously with clinical isolates as a means of validating test results.

As noted above, based on three phenotypic properties, the production of indole, ornithine decarboxylase, and urease, strains of *H. influenzae* and *H. parainfluenzae* can be distinguished into multiple different biotypes (Table 2). Also, as outlined previously, at least with *H. influenzae*, certain biotypes have been found to have specific disease associations. Assessment of indole, ornithine decarboxylase, and urease production with clinical isolates of *H. influenzae* and *H. parainfluenzae* can be accomplished using the conventional methods described above (Fig. 9) or by use of commercially available miniaturized biochemical kit systems (30). In one recent study which compared the API NH strip kit (bioMérieux) with the IDS RapID NH system (Remel) and the NHI card (bioMérieux) as a means for determining the biotypes of a large collection of recent clinical isolates of both *H. influenzae* and *H. parainfluenzae*, the API NH kit yielded the most reliable results, correctly classifying the biotypes of >97% of the strains tested (64).

Typing by Molecular Methods

Molecular methods have the advantage of enhanced specificity due to the use of standardized techniques and a lack of false-positive reactions observed with nonencapsulated strains in slide agglutination tests.

Capsular typing of *H. influenzae* can also be accomplished by use of various molecular methods. Most such assays rely on the amplification of genes in the *cap* locus, the outer membrane protein D gene (*glpQ*), the capsule-producing gene (*bexA*), the 16S rRNA gene, and the insertion-like sequence (55). One algorithm was used for detection of the *cap* genes to determine capsular serotypes a through f, while the capsule-producing gene, *bcxA*, was used to separate strains that produce capsule from those that do not (55). Detection of the *ompP2* (outer membrane lipoprotein P2) gene was used as a control. Using this system,

both a conventional PCR and a real-time PCR assay were found to be more sensitive than a slide agglutination test for serotyping *H. influenzae* (55).

As with the *Enterobacteriaceae*, pulsed-field gel electrophoresis (PFGE) is considered the gold standard for strain typing of *Haemophilus*. The method demonstrates excellent separation of clones but is laborious and time-consuming (2, 10, 82). Other molecular methods for typing have also been applied to *Haemophilus* species. Studies evaluating repetitive-element sequence-based PCR using intergenic dyad sequence (IDS)-specific primers (IDS-PCR) for non-encapsulated *Haemophilus* strains have been developed and demonstrate excellent separation of NTHi strains (10). In one study evaluating the performance of IDS-PCR with 69 NTHi isolates, the assay demonstrated 65 different banding patterns that were epidemiologically classified as fingerprints similar to those obtained by PFGE (10). Other typing technologies applied to *Haemophilus* with a high degree of separation include ribotyping, restriction fragment length polymorphism analysis, multilocus enzyme electrophoresis, randomly amplified polymorphic DNA profile analysis, and multilocus sequence typing (10). While all of these techniques have demonstrated excellent separation, many are laborious and time-consuming (multilocus enzyme electrophoresis, PFGE, and ribotyping), others produce overly complex banding patterns (restriction fragment length polymorphism analyses), and others lack reproducibility (randomly amplified polymorphic DNA profile analysis) (10). Multilocus sequence typing offers the advantage of superior discriminatory power because it combines sequence typing of seven housekeeping genes with results that can readily be compared between laboratories (48).

SEROLOGIC TESTS

Antibody tests have been developed for the detection of *Haemophilus* antibodies; however, they are of little clinical value and are not readily available. Studies evaluating the performances of the enzyme-linked immunosorbent assay (11) and immunofluorescent assays (90) have been conducted; however, because immunity to *Haemophilus* is derived from an eclectic combination of antibodies against the *H. influenzae* capsule and membrane proteins, assays to detect a single class of antibody are of little value. Further complicating the use of *Haemophilus* serologies is the individual variation in antibody level (many adults have undetectable antibody levels), avidity, and persistence (65).

ANTIMICROBIAL SUSCEPTIBILITY TESTING

Resistance Rates

Haemophilus influenzae may produce one of two β-lactamases, TEM-1 and ROB-1. Both enzymes are plasmid associated, extracellular, and produced constitutively in large amounts (39). β-Lactamase-producing strains should be considered resistant to ampicillin and amoxicillin, as these drugs typically have MICs of ≥128 μg/ml against these strains (29). Currently, in the United States, ca. 25% of clinical isolates of NTHi produce β-lactamase (38). Interestingly, this represents a slight decrease in rates, which peaked in the late 1990s (38). One possible explanation for this decrease is the more common use, beginning in the early 1990s, of non-β-lactam antimicrobials, such as the macrolides and fluoroquinolones, in the empirical management of infections such as otitis media, sinusitis, and bronchopulmonary infections, i.e., infections with which NTHi are most often associated. As a consequence of this paradigm shift, β-lactams such as ampicillin and amoxicillin are used less often, with resulting diminished selective pressure on the emergence and persistence of β-lactamase-producing NTHi. β-Lactamase-producing strains of *H. influenzae* remain susceptible to oral and parenteral cephalosporins and carbapenems (29, 32, 38, 40). They are also susceptible to combination agents in which a β-lactamase inhibitor, such as clavulanate, sulbactam, or tazobactam, is combined with a β-lactam agent (29, 32, 38, 40). Examples include amoxicillin-clavulanate, ampicillin-sulbactam, and piperacillin-tazobactam.

Strains of *H. influenzae* that fail to produce β-lactamase but for which the MICs of ampicillin and amoxicillin are elevated have been described (56). These strains, which are often referred to as β-lactamase negative and ampicillin resistant (BLNAR), have altered penicillin binding proteins, which abrogates the binding of drugs such as ampicillin and amoxicillin to their cell wall targets, in turn resulting in elevated MICs (42, 93). The activities of cephalosporins are also diminished with such strains. If one uses an ampicillin or amoxicillin MIC of ≥4 μg/ml to define resistance within *Haemophilus* spp., as is recommended by the Clinical and Laboratory Standards Institute (CLSI) (20), the prevalence of BLNAR strains of *H. influenzae* remains at levels of <1% in the United States (38).

Among other antimicrobials which are relevant to the management of *Haemophilus* infections, with the exception of trimethoprim-sulfamethoxazole (TMP-SMX), resistance rates remain at levels of <1% (29, 38). These antimicrobials include both oral and parenteral cephalosporins, macrolides, fluoroquinolones, and tetracycline. TMP-SMX resistance rates approach 20% (29, 38).

Susceptibility Test Methods

β-Lactamase production by *Haemophilus* spp. can be determined rapidly with either a chromogenic cephalosporin spot test or an acidimetric penicillinase assay, as described in chapter 70 in this *Manual*. Because the β-lactamases of *H. influenzae* are extracellular, constitutive, and produced in large amounts, assuming the test is performed carefully and with adequate positive and negative controls, both methods yield reliable results.

Disk diffusion susceptibility tests can be performed using *Haemophilus* test medium (HTM) agar (41), with incubation of plates for 16 to 18 h at 35°C in 5 to 7% CO_2, as described by the CLSI (19). Zone diameter interpretive criteria have been developed for 39 different antimicrobial agents (20). The details of disk diffusion susceptibility tests are presented in chapter 68.

MICs can be determined with *Haemophilus* spp. by use of broth microdilution (BMD). The CLSI advocates the use of HTM broth (41) when determining MICs by the BMD method (18). Following inoculation, trays are incubated for 20 to 24 h in ambient air at 35°C prior to determination of MICs; MIC interpretive criteria have been developed for 43 different antimicrobial agents (20). The details of BMD MIC tests are presented in chapter 68. In circumstances where HTM is not available or when equivocal results have been obtained with this medium, BMD MICs can be determined with *Haemophilus* spp. using Mueller-Hinton broth supplemented with 3 to 5% sterile lysed horse blood and 10 μg/ml NAD (27). The MIC interpretive criteria for *Haemophilus* promulgated by the CLSI for BMD tests in HTM can also be applied to MICs determined by BMD in medium containing lysed horse blood. Unfortunately,

there exist almost no published data validating the use of the Etest method with *Haemophilus* spp., and therefore, use of this method is not recommended for susceptibility tests with this organism group.

Susceptibility tests with clinical isolates of *H. ducreyi* should not be attempted in routine clinical microbiology laboratories, as standardized susceptibility test methods of proven reliability for this organism have not yet been developed. Similarly, instrument-based susceptibility tests for other *Haemophilus* spp., including *H. influenzae*, have not been proven to be effective and are not recommended for testing this organism group.

Irrespective of the method used for performing susceptibility tests with *Haemophilus* spp., it is essential that adequate quality control is applied using two *H. influenzae* quality control strains, ATCC 49247 and ATCC 49766.

Susceptibility Testing Algorithm

Susceptibility testing with clinical isolates of *Haemophilus* spp. should be applied only to those strains known to be of clinical significance. Further, in the vast majority of instances, only a β-lactamase assay as a means for assessing the activities of ampicillin and amoxicillin need be performed. The prevalence of BLNAR strains of *H. influenzae* and their resistance to other agents that are commonly used to treat the types of infections with which *Haemophilus* spp. are associated are simply too low to justify routine testing. One exception might be resistance to TMP-SMX. This agent, however, is used almost exclusively for oral therapy of community-acquired respiratory tract infections that are invariably managed empirically without performance of laboratory studies aimed at elucidating the specific cause of an individual patient's infection. In other words, in settings where knowledge of the activity profile of TMP-SMX versus *H. influenzae* could be of value, rarely, if ever, is a patient isolate available for testing. In those rare circumstances when the assessment of the activities of agents other than ampicillin or amoxicillin are found to be warranted, either a disk diffusion susceptibility test or a BMD MIC test should be performed.

EVALUATION, INTERPRETATION, AND REPORTING OF RESULTS

The genus *Haemophilus* is a diverse group of organisms which may exist as part of the normal bacterial flora of healthy humans or may be associated with significant disease. As a result, simple recovery of *Haemophilus* from a human clinical sample may not always indicate that the organism is clinically significant. In the following three circumstances, recovery of *Haemophilus* spp. in the laboratory is pathognomonic: (i) isolates from normally sterile sites, including blood cultures, are compatible clinically with illness; (ii) *H. ducreyi* is recovered from genital tract specimens obtained from patients with genital ulcers; and (iii) isolates of *H. aegyptius* from conjunctival specimens are obtained from patients with exudative inflammation of the conjunctiva.

Recovery of *Haemophilus* spp. from specimens that may be contaminated with commensal microbial flora represents a situation in which the clinical significance of the isolate must be questioned. This is often the case, for example, with isolates from respiratory tract sites. In such instances, the quantity of organism recovered, both the absolute quantity and the quantity of the isolate in comparison to quantities of other organisms recovered from the specimen, is of limited value in assessing clinical significance. It may be helpful to try to assess the quality of the specimen, as is possible, for example, with expectorated sputa and endotracheal aspirates. It may also be instructive to compare the results of a given culture with results obtained from previous and subsequent cultures from the same site. Generally speaking, repetitive recovery of the same organism from multiple specimens representative of a specific infectious disease process in an individual patient can be taken as an indication of clinical significance. And finally, it must be recognized that in some cases, it simply is not possible to know with certainty whether a given isolate of *Haemophilus* spp. is clinically significant. In such instances, active dialogue with health care providers is encouraged.

REFERENCES

1. **Abdeldaim, G. M., K. Stralin, L. A. Kirsebom, P. Olcen, J. Blomberg, and B. Herrmann.** 2009. Detection of Haemophilus influenzae in respiratory secretions from pneumonia patients by quantitative real-time polymerase chain reaction. *Diagn. Microbiol. Infect. Dis.* **64:**366–373.

2. **Aparicio, P., F. Roman, and J. Campos.** 1996. Epidemiological characterization of Haemophilus influenzae using molecular markers. *Enferm. Infecc. Microbiol. Clin.* **14:**227–232. (In Spanish.)

3. **Barbe, G., M. Babolat, J. M. Boeufgras, D. Monget, and J. Freney.** 1994. Evaluation of API NH, a new 2-hour system for identification of *Neisseria* and *Haemophilus* species and *Moraxella catarrhalis* in a routine clinical laboratory. *J. Clin. Microbiol.* **32:**187–189.

4. **Barbosa, S. F., S. Hoshino-Shimizu, M. G. Alkmin, and H. Goto.** 2003. Implications of Haemophilus influenzae biogroup aegyptius hemagglutinins in the pathogenesis of Brazilian purpuric fever. *J. Infect. Dis.* **188:**74–80.

5. **Berbari, E. F., F. R. Cockerill III, and J. M. Steckelberg.** 1997. Infective endocarditis due to unusual or fastidious microorganisms. *Mayo Clin. Proc.* **72:**532–542.

6. **Biberstein, E. L., P. D. Mini, and M. G. Gills.** 1963. Action of *Haemophilus* cultures on delta-aminolevulinic acid. *J. Bacteriol.* **86:**814–819.

7. Reference deleted.

8. **Brandileone, M. C., G. W. Ajello, W. F. Bibb, V. S. Vieira, F. O. Sottnek, B. Swaminathan, and the Brazilian Purpuric Fever Study Group.** 1989. Development of diagnostic tests for Haemophilus influenzae biogroup aegyptius, the etiologic agent of Brazilian purpuric fever. *Pediatr. Infect. Dis. J.* **8:**243–245.

9. **Breitkopf, C., D. Hammel, H. H. Scheld, G. Peters, and K. Becker.** 2005. Impact of a molecular approach to improve the microbiological diagnosis of infective heart valve endocarditis. *Circulation* **111:**1415–1421.

10. **Bruant, G., S. Watt, R. Quentin, and A. Rosenau.** 2003. Typing of nonencapsulated *Haemophilus* strains by repetitive-element sequence-based PCR using intergenic dyad sequences. *J. Clin. Microbiol.* **41:**3473–3480.

11. **Burman, L. A., M. Leinonen, and B. Trollfors.** 1994. Use of serology to diagnose pneumonia caused by nonencapsulated Haemophilus influenzae and Moraxella catarrhalis. *J. Infect. Dis.* **170:**220–222.

12. **Catlin, B. W.** 1970. Haemophilus influenzae in cultures of cerebrospinal fluid. Noncapsulated variants typable by immunofluorescence. *Am. J. Dis. Child.* **120:**203–210.

13. **Cattoir, V., O. Lemenand, J. L. Avril, and O. Gaillot.** 2006. The sodA gene as a target for phylogenetic dissection of the genus Haemophilus and accurate identification of human clinical isolates. *Int. J. Med. Microbiol.* **296:**531–540.

14. **Chandran, A., J. P. Watt, and M. Santosham.** 2005. Prevention of Haemophilus influenzae type b disease: past success and future challenges. *Expert Rev. Vaccines* **4:**819–827.

15. **Chapin, K. C., and G. V. Doern.** 1983. Selective media for recovery of *Haemophilus influenzae* from specimens contaminated with upper respiratory tract microbial flora. *J. Clin. Microbiol.* **17:**1163–1165.

16. **Chiba, N., S. Y. Murayama, M. Morozumi, E. Nakayama, T. Okada, S. Iwata, K. Sunakawa, and K. Ubukata.** 2009. Rapid detection of eight causative pathogens for the diagnosis of bacterial meningitis by real-time PCR. *J. Infect. Chemother.* **15:**92–98.

17. **Clarridge, J. E., III.** 2004. Impact of 16S rRNA gene sequence analysis for identification of bacteria on clinical microbiology and infectious diseases. *Clin. Microbiol. Rev.* **17:**840–862.

18. **Clinical and Laboratory Standards Institute.** 2009. *Methods for Dilution Antimicrobial Susceptibility Tests for Bacteria That Grow Aerobically. Approved Standard, Eighth Edition.* Document M07-A8. Clinical and Laboratory Standards Institute, Wayne, PA.

19. **Clinical and Laboratory Standards Institute.** 2009. *Performance Standards for Antimicrobial Disk Susceptibility Tests. Approved Standard, Eighth Edition.* Document M02-A10. Clinical and Laboratory Standards Institute, Wayne, PA.

20. **Clinical and Laboratory Standards Institute.** 2009. *Performance Standards for Antimicrobial Susceptibility Testing; Nineteenth Informational Supplement.* Document M100-S19. Clinical and Laboratory Standards Institute, Wayne, PA.

21. **Cole, R. A., and R. N. Winickoff.** 1979. Hemophilus parainfluenzae endocarditis. *South. Med. J.* **72:**516–518.

22. **Corless, C. E., M. Guiver, R. Borrow, V. Edwards-Jones, A. J. Fox, and E. B. Kaczmarski.** 2001. Simultaneous detection of *Neisseria meningitidis*, *Haemophilus influenzae*, and *Streptococcus pneumoniae* in suspected cases of meningitis and septicemia using real-time PCR. *J. Clin. Microbiol.* **39:**1553–1558.

23. **Czelusta, A., A. Yen-Moore, M. Van der Straten, D. Carrasco, and S. K. Tyring.** 2000. An overview of sexually transmitted diseases. Part III. Sexually transmitted diseases in HIV-infected patients. *J. Am. Acad. Dermatol.* **43:**409–436.

24. **Dangor, Y., R. C. Ballard, F. da L. Exposto, G. Fehler, S. D. Miller, and H. J. Koornhof.** 1990. Accuracy of clinical diagnosis of genital ulcer disease. *Sex. Transm. Dis.* **17:**184–189.

25. **Dangor, Y., F. Radebe, and R. C. Ballard.** 1993. Transport media for Haemophilus ducreyi. *Sex. Transm. Dis.* **20:**5–9.

26. **DiCarlo, R. P., and D. H. Martin.** 1997. The clinical diagnosis of genital ulcer disease in men. *Clin. Infect. Dis.* **25:**292–298.

27. **Doern, G. V.** 1992. In vitro susceptibility testing of *Haemophilus influenzae*: review of new National Committee for Clinical Laboratory Standards recommendations. *J. Clin. Microbiol.* **30:**3035–3038.

28. **Doern, G. V., and B. Brogden-Torres.** 1992. Optimum use of selective plated media in primary processing of respiratory tract specimens from patients with cystic fibrosis. *J. Clin. Microbiol.* **30:**2740–2742.

29. **Doern, G. V., and S. D. Brown.** 2004. Antimicrobial susceptibility among community-acquired respiratory tract pathogens in the USA: data from PROTEKT US 2000–01. *J. Infect.* **48:**56–65.

30. **Doern, G. V., and K. C. Chapin.** 1987. Determination of biotypes of Haemophilus influenzae and Haemophilus parainfluenzae a comparison of methods and a description of a new biotype (VIII) of H. parainfluenzae. *Diagn. Microbiol. Infect. Dis.* **7:**269–272.

31. **Doern, G. V., and K. C. Chapin.** 1984. Laboratory identification of *Haemophilus influenzae*: effects of basal media on the results of the satellitism test and evaluation of the RapID NH system. *J. Clin. Microbiol.* **20:**599–601.

32. **Doern, G. V., J. H. Jorgensen, C. Thornsberry, D. A. Preston, T. Tubert, J. S. Redding, and L. A. Maher.** 1988. National collaborative study of the prevalence of antimicrobial resistance among clinical isolates of Haemophilus influenzae. *Antimicrob. Agents Chemother.* **32:**180–185.

33. **Erwin, A. L., and A. L. Smith.** 2007. Nontypeable Haemophilus influenzae: understanding virulence and commensal behavior. *Trends Microbiol.* **15:**355–362.

34. **Evans, N. M., and D. D. Smith.** 1972. The effect of the medium and source of growth factors on the satellitism test for Haemophilus species. *J. Med. Microbiol.* **5:**509–514.

35. **Flesher, A. R., and R. A. Insel.** 1978. Characterization of lipopolysaccharide of Haemophilus influenzae. *J. Infect. Dis.* **138:**719–730.
36. **Fuller, D. D., T. E. Davis, P. C. Kibsey, L. Rosmus, L. W. Ayers, M. Ott, M. A. Saubolle, and D. L. Sewell.** 1994. Comparison of BACTEC Plus 26 and 27 media with and without fastidious organism supplement with conventional methods for culture of sterile body fluids. *J. Clin. Microbiol.* **32:**1488–1491.
37. **Greene, J. N., R. L. Sandin, L. Villanueva, and J. T. Sinnott.** 1993. Haemophilus parainfluenzae endocarditis in a patient with mitral valve prolapse. *Ann. Clin. Lab. Sci.* **23:**203–206.
38. **Heilmann, K. P., C. L. Rice, A. L. Miller, N. J. Miller, S. E. Beekmann, M. A. Pfaller, S. S. Richter, and G. V. Doern.** 2005. Decreasing prevalence of beta-lactamase production among respiratory tract isolates of *Haemophilus influenzae* in the United States. *Antimicrob. Agents Chemother.* **49:**2561–2564.
39. **Jacobs, M. R., J. Anon, and P. C. Appelbaum.** 2004. Mechanisms of resistance among respiratory tract pathogens. *Clin. Lab. Med.* **24:**419–453.
40. **Jorgensen, J. H., G. V. Doern, L. A. Maher, A. W. Howell, and J. S. Redding.** 1990. Antimicrobial resistance among respiratory isolates of *Haemophilus influenzae, Moraxella catarrhalis*, and *Streptococcus pneumoniae* in the United States. *Antimicrob. Agents Chemother.* **34:**2075–2080.
41. **Jorgensen, J. H., A. W. Howell, and L. A. Maher.** 1990. Antimicrobial susceptibility testing of less commonly isolated *Haemophilus* species using *Haemophilus* test medium. *J. Clin. Microbiol.* **28:**985–988.
42. **Kaczmarek, F. S., T. D. Gootz, F. Dib-Hajj, W. Shang, S. Hallowell, and M. Cronan.** 2004. Genetic and molecular characterization of beta-lactamase-negative ampicillin-resistant *Haemophilus influenzae* with unusually high resistance to ampicillin. *Antimicrob. Agents Chemother.* **48:**1630–1639.
43. **Kais, M., C. Spindler, M. Kalin, A. Ortqvist, and C. G. Giske.** 2006. Quantitative detection of Streptococcus pneumoniae, Haemophilus influenzae, and Moraxella catarrhalis in lower respiratory tract samples by real-time PCR. *Diagn. Microbiol. Infect. Dis.* **55:**169–178.
44. **Kalogianni, D. P., S. Goura, A. J. Aletras, T. K. Christopoulos, M. G. Chanos, M. Christofidou, A. Skoutelis, P. C. Ioannou, and E. Panagiotopoulos.** 2007. Dry reagent dipstick test combined with 23S rRNA PCR for molecular diagnosis of bacterial infection in arthroplasty. *Anal. Biochem.* **361:**169–175.
45. **Kilian, M.** 2005. Genus II. *Haemophilus* Winslow, Broadhurst, Krumwiede, Rogers and Smith 1917,561. *In* G. M. Garrity (ed.), *Bergey's Manual of Systematic Bacteriology*, vol. 2. Springer, New York, NY.
46. **Kilian, M.** 1976. The haemolytic activity of Haemophilus species. *Acta Pathol. Microbiol. Scand. B* **84B:**339–341.
47. **Kilian, M.** 2003. *Haemophilus*, p. 623–635. *In* P. R. Murray, E. J. Baron, J. H. Jorgensen, M. A. Pfaller, and R. H. Yolken (ed.), *Manual of Clinical Microbiology*, 8th ed. ASM Press, Washington, DC.
48. **Kilian, M.** 2007. *Haemophilus*, p. 636–648. *In* P. R. Murray, E. J. Baron, J. H. Jorgensen, M. L. Landry, and M. A. Pfaller (ed.), *Manual of Clinical Microbiology*, 9th ed. ASM Press, Washington, DC.
49. **Kilian, M.** 1974. A rapid method for the differentiation of Haemophilus strains. The porphyrin test. *Acta Pathol. Microbiol Scand. B* **82:**835–842.
50. **Kilian, M.** 1976. A taxonomic study of the genus Haemophilus, with the proposal of a new species. *J. Gen. Microbiol.* **93:**9–62.
51. **Kilian, M., and E. L. Biberstein.** 1984. Genus II. *Haemophilus* Winslow, Broadhurst, Krumwiede, Rogers and Smith 1917, 561, p. 4. *In* D. H. Bergey, N. R. Krieg, and J. G. Holt (ed.), *Bergey's Manual of Systematic Bacteriology*. Williams & Wilkins, Baltimore, MD.
52. **Kuklinska, D., and M. Kilian.** 1984. Relative proportions of Haemophilus species in the throat of healthy children and adults. *Eur. J. Clin. Microbiol.* **3:**249–252.
53. **LaClaire, L. L., M. L. Tondella, D. S. Beall, C. A. Noble, P. L. Raghunathan, N. E. Rosenstein, and T. Popovic.** 2003. Identification of *Haemophilus influenzae* serotypes by standard slide agglutination serotyping and PCR-based capsule typing. *J. Clin. Microbiol.* **41:**393–396.
54. **Lewis, D. A.** 2000. Diagnostic tests for chancroid. *Sex. Transm. Infect.* **76:**137–141.
55. **Maaroufi, Y., J. M. De Bruyne, C. Heymans, and F. Crokaert.** 2007. Real-time PCR for determining capsular serotypes of *Haemophilus influenzae*. *J. Clin. Microbiol.* **45:**2305–2308.
56. **Markowitz, S. M.** 1980. Isolation of an ampicillin-resistant, non-β-lactamase-producing strain of *Haemophilus influenzae*. *Antimicrob. Agents Chemother.* **17:**80–83.
57. **Marty, A., O. Greiner, P. J. Day, S. Gunziger, K. Muhlemann, and D. Nadal.** 2004. Detection of *Haemophilus influenzae* type b by real-time PCR. *J. Clin. Microbiol.* **42:**3813–3815.
58. **McLinn, S. E., J. D. Nelson, and K. C. Haltalin.** 1970. Antimicrobial susceptibility of Hemophilus influenzae. *Pediatrics* **45:**827–838.
59. **Mein, J., and G. Lum.** 1999. CSF bacterial antigen detection tests offer no advantage over Gram's stain in the diagnosis of bacterial meningitis. *Pathology* **31:**67–69.
60. **Mohammed, T. T., and Y. M. Olumide.** 2008. Chancroid and human immunodeficiency virus infection—a review. *Int. J. Dermatol.* **47:**1–8.
61. **Morris, S. K., W. J. Moss, and N. Halsey.** 2008. Haemophilus influenzae type b conjugate vaccine use and effectiveness. *Lancet Infect. Dis.* **8:**435–443.
62. **Morse, S. A., D. L. Trees, Y. Htun, F. Radebe, K. A. Orle, Y. Dangor, C. M. Beck-Sague, S. Schmid, G. Fehler, J. B. Weiss, and R. C. Ballard.** 1997. Comparison of clinical diagnosis and standard laboratory and molecular methods for the diagnosis of genital ulcer disease in Lesotho: association with human immunodeficiency virus infection. *J. Infect. Dis.* **175:**583–589.
63. **Munson, E., M. Pfaller, F. Koontz, and G. Doern.** 2002. Comparison of porphyrin-based, growth factor-based, and biochemical-based testing methods for identification of Haemophilus influenzae. *Eur. J. Clin. Microbiol. Infect. Dis.* **21:**196–203.
64. **Munson, E. L., and G. V. Doern.** 2007. Comparison of three commercial test systems for biotyping *Haemophilus influenzae* and *Haemophilus parainfluenzae*. *J. Clin. Microbiol.* **45:**4051–4053.
65. **Murphy, T. F.** 2005. *Haemophilus* infections, p. 2661–2669. *In* G. L. Mandell, J. E. Bennett, and R. Dolin (ed.), *Principles and Practices of Infectious Diseases*, 6th ed, vol. 2. Elsevier, Philadelphia, PA.
66. **Murphy, T. F., J. M. Bernstein, D. M. Dryja, A. A. Campagnari, and M. A. Apicella.** 1987. Outer membrane protein and lipooligosaccharide analysis of paired nasopharyngeal and middle ear isolates in otitis media due to nontypable Haemophilus influenzae: pathogenetic and epidemiological observations. *J. Infect. Dis.* **156:**723–731.
67. **Murphy, T. F., and S. Sethi.** 2002. Chronic obstructive pulmonary disease: role of bacteria and guide to antibacterial selection in the older patient. *Drugs Aging* **19:**761–775.
68. **Norskov-Lauritsen, N., and M. Kilian.** 2006. Reclassification of *Actinobacillus actinomycetemcomitans, Haemophilus aphrophilus, Haemophilus paraphrophilus* and *Haemophilus segnis* as *Aggregatibacter actinomycetemcomitans* gen. nov., comb. nov., *Aggregatibacter aphrophilus* comb. nov. and *Aggregatibacter segnis* comb. nov., and emended description of *Aggregatibacter aphrophilus* to include V factor-dependent and V factor-independent isolates. *Int. J. Syst. Evol. Microbiol.* **56:**2135–2146.
69. **Oberhofer, T. R., and A. E. Back.** 1979. Biotypes of Haemophilus encountered in clinical laboratories. *J. Clin. Microbiol.* **10:**168–174.
70. **Ohkusu, K., K. A. Nash, and C. B. Inderlied.** 2005. Molecular characterisation of Haemophilus influenzae type a and untypeable strains isolated simultaneously from cerebrospinal fluid and blood: novel use of quantitative real-time PCR based on the cap copy number to determine virulence. *Clin. Microbiol. Infect.* **11:**637–643.

71. **Parsons, L. M., M. Shayegani, A. L. Waring, and L. H. Bopp.** 1989. DNA probes for the identification of *Haemophilus ducreyi. J. Clin. Microbiol.* **27:**1441–1445.

72. **Pittman, M.** 1930. Variation and type-specificity in the bacterial species, *Haemophilus influenzae. J. Exp. Med.* **53:**471–478.

73. **Pittman, M., and D. J. Davis.** 1950. Identification of the Koch-Weeks bacillus (*Hemophilus aegyptius*). *J. Bacteriol.* **59:**413–426.

74. **Poppert, S., A. Essig, B. Stoehr, A. Steingruber, B. Wirths, S. Juretschko, U. Reischl, and N. Wellinghausen.** 2005. Rapid diagnosis of bacterial meningitis by real-time PCR and fluorescence in situ hybridization. *J. Clin. Microbiol.* **43:**3390–3397.

75. **Quentin, R., J. M. Musser, M. Mellouet, P. Y. Sizaret, R. K. Selander, and A. Goudeau.** 1989. Typing of urogenital, maternal, and neonatal isolates of *Haemophilus influenzae* and *Haemophilus parainfluenzae* in correlation with clinical source of isolation and evidence for a genital specificity of *H. influenzae* biotype IV. *J. Clin. Microbiol.* **27:**2286–2294.

76. **Raymond, J., L. Armand-Lefevre, F. Moulin, H. Dabernat, A. Commeau, D. Gendrel, and P. Berche.** 2001. Nasopharyngeal colonization by Haemophilus influenzae in children living in an orphanage. *Pediatr. Infect. Dis. J.* **20:**779–784.

77. **Rennie, R., T. Gordon, Y. Yaschuk, P. Tomlin, P. Kibsey, and W. Albritton.** 1992. Laboratory and clinical evaluations of media for the primary isolation of *Haemophilus* species. *J. Clin. Microbiol.* **30:**1917–1921.

78. **Rennie, R. P., C. Brosnikoff, S. Shokoples, L. B. Reller, S. Mirrett, W. Janda, K. Ristow, and A. Krilcich.** 2008. Multicenter evaluation of the new Vitek 2 *Neisseria-Haemophilus* identification card. *J. Clin. Microbiol.* **46:**2681–2685.

79. **Ribeiro, G. S., J. B. Lima, J. N. Reis, E. L. Gouveia, S. M. Cordeiro, T. S. Lobo, R. M. Pinheiro, C. T. Ribeiro, A. B. Neves, K. Salgado, H. R. Silva, M. G. Reis, and A. I. Ko.** 2007. Haemophilus influenzae meningitis 5 years after introduction of the Haemophilus influenzae type b conjugate vaccine in Brazil. *Vaccine* **25:**4420–4428.

80. **Rosenfeld, M., J. Emerson, F. Accurso, D. Armstrong, R. Castile, K. Grimwood, P. Hiatt, K. McCoy, S. McNamara, B. Ramsey, and J. Wagener.** 1999. Diagnostic accuracy of oropharyngeal cultures in infants and young children with cystic fibrosis. *Pediatr. Pulmonol.* **28:**321–328.

81. **Saha, S. K., G. L. Darmstadt, A. H. Baqui, N. Islam, S. Qazi, M. Islam, S. El Arifeen, M. Santosham, R. E. Black, and D. W. Crook.** 2008. Direct detection of the multidrug resistance genome of Haemophilus influenzae in cerebrospinal fluid of children: implications for treatment of meningitis. *Pediatr. Infect. Dis. J.* **27:**49–53.

82. **Saito, M., A. Umeda, and S. Yoshida.** 1999. Subtyping of *Haemophilus influenzae* strains by pulsed-field gel electrophoresis. *J. Clin. Microbiol.* **37:**2142–2147.

83. **Scott, F. A., C. German, and J. A. Boswick, Jr.** 1981. Hemophilus influenzae cellulitis of the hand. *J. Hand Surg. Am.* **6:**506–509.

84. **Sell, S. H., W. J. Cheatham, B. Young, and K. Welch.** 1963. Hemophilus influenzae in respiratory infections. I. Typing by immunofluorescent techniques. *Am. J. Dis. Child.* **105:**466–469.

85. **Sell, S. H., R. S. Sanders, and W. J. Cheatham.** 1963. Hemophilus influenzae in respiratory infections. II. Specific serological antibodies identified by agglutination and immunofluorescent techniques. *Am. J. Dis. Child.* **105:**470–474.

86. **Sethi, S., and T. F. Murphy.** 2001. Bacterial infection in chronic obstructive pulmonary disease in 2000: a state-of-the-art review. *Clin. Microbiol. Rev.* **14:**336–363.

87. **Slootmans, L., D. A. Vanden Berghe, and P. Piot.** 1985. Typing Haemophilus ducreyi by indirect immunofluorescence assay. *Genitourin. Med.* **61:**123–126.

88. **St. Geme, J. W., III.** 1993. Nontypeable Haemophilus influenzae disease: epidemiology, pathogenesis, and prospects for prevention. *Infect. Agents Dis.* **2:**1–16.

89. **Stralin, K., A. Backman, H. Holmberg, H. Fredlund, and P. Olcen.** 2005. Design of a multiplex PCR for Streptococcus pneumoniae, Haemophilus influenzae, Mycoplasma pneumoniae and Chlamydophila pneumoniae to be used on sputum samples. *APMIS* **113:**99–111.

90. **Stralin, K., H. Holmberg, and P. Olcen.** 2004. Antibody response to the patient's own Haemophilus influenzae isolate can support the aetiology in lower respiratory tract infections. *APMIS* **112:**299–303.

91. **Swingler, G., D. Fransman, and G. Hussey.** 2007. Conjugate vaccines for preventing Haemophilus influenzae type B infections. *Cochrane Database Syst. Rev.* **18:**CD001729.

92. **Tzanakaki, G., M. Tsopanomichalou, K. Kesanopoulos, R. Matzourani, M. Sioumala, A. Tabaki, and J. Kremastinou.** 2005. Simultaneous single-tube PCR assay for the detection of Neisseria meningitidis, Haemophilus influenzae type b and Streptococcus pneumoniae. *Clin. Microbiol. Infect.* **11:**386–390.

93. **Ubukata, K., Y. Shibasaki, K. Yamamoto, N. Chiba, K. Hasegawa, Y. Takeuchi, K. Sunakawa, M. Inoue, and M. Konno.** 2001. Association of amino acid substitutions in penicillin-binding protein 3 with beta-lactam resistance in beta-lactamase-negative ampicillin-resistant *Haemophilus influenzae. Antimicrob. Agents Chemother.* **45:**1693–1699.

94. **Valenza, G., C. Ruoff, U. Vogel, M. Frosch, and M. Abele-Horn.** 2007. Microbiological evaluation of the new VITEK 2 *Neisseria-Haemophilus* identification card. *J. Clin. Microbiol.* **45:**3493–3497.

95. **van Ketel, R. J., B. de Wever, and L. van Alphen.** 1990. Detection of Haemophilus influenzae in cerebrospinal fluids by polymerase chain reaction DNA amplification. *J. Med. Microbiol.* **33:**271–276.

96. **Wallace, R. J., Jr., C. J. Baker, F. J. Quinones, D. G. Hollis, R. E. Weaver, and K. Wiss.** 1983. Nontypable Haemophilus influenzae (biotype 4) as a neonatal, maternal, and genital pathogen. *Rev. Infect. Dis.* **5:**123–136.

97. **Wellinghausen, N., B. Wirths, A. R. Franz, L. Karolyi, R. Marre, and U. Reischl.** 2004. Algorithm for the identification of bacterial pathogens in positive blood cultures by real-time LightCycler polymerase chain reaction (PCR) with sequence-specific probes. *Diagn. Microbiol. Infect. Dis.* **48:**229–241.

98. **West, B., S. M. Wilson, J. Changalucha, S. Patel, P. Mayaud, R. C. Ballard, and D. Mabey.** 1995. Simplified PCR for detection of *Haemophilus ducreyi* and diagnosis of chancroid. *J. Clin. Microbiol.* **33:**787–790.

99. **Woo, P. C., K. H. Ng, S. K. Lau, K. T. Yip, A. M. Fung, K. W. Leung, D. M. Tam, T. L. Que, and K. Y. Yuen.** 2003. Usefulness of the MicroSeq 500 16S ribosomal DNA-based bacterial identification system for identification of clinically significant bacterial isolates with ambiguous biochemical profiles. *J. Clin. Microbiol.* **41:**1996–2001.

100. **York, M. K.** 2004. *Haemophilus ducreyi* cultures, p. 3.9.4.1–3.9.4.5. *In* H. D. Isenberg (ed. in chief), *Clinical Microbiology Procedures Handbook*, 2nd ed., vol. 1. ASM Press, Washington, DC.

101. **Zaretzky, F. R., and T. H. Kawula.** 1999. Examination of early interactions between *Haemophilus ducreyi* and host cells by using cocultured HaCaT keratinocytes and foreskin fibroblasts. *Infect. Immun.* **67:**5352–5360.

Escherichia, *Shigella*, and *Salmonella*

JAMES P. NATARO, CHERYL A. BOPP, PATRICIA I. FIELDS,
JAMES B. KAPER, AND NANCY A. STROCKBINE

35

ESCHERICHIA

Taxonomy

Members of the genus *Escherichia* are classified in the family *Enterobacteriaceae*, which is addressed in chapter 37 of this *Manual* (32, 66, 139, 175). There are six species in this genus: *Escherichia albertii*, *Escherichia blattae*, *Escherichia coli*, *Escherichia fergusonii*, *Escherichia hermannii*, and *Escherichia vulneris*. The G+C content is 48 to 59 mol%, and the type species is *E. coli* (Migula 1895) (39). Average DNA relatedness between the type species and other *Escherichia* species, as assessed by DNA-DNA hybridization, ranges from 38% to 64%. As more genomes become sequenced, refinements to the classification of members of the family *Enterobacteriaceae* will be possible. A recent publication proposes to reclassify *E. blattae* in a newly formed genus as *Shimwellia blattae*, based on sequence analysis of the 16S rRNA gene and four protein coding genes (162). *E. blattae* exhibits about 43% DNA relatedness to *E. coli* by DNA-DNA hybridization.

Members of the genus *Shigella* are phenotypically similar to *Escherichia coli* and, with the exception of *Shigella boydii* serotype 13, would be considered the same species by DNA-DNA hybridization analysis (29) and whole-genome sequence analysis (82). Findings from recent phylogenetic studies with nucleotide sequences of internal fragments from 14 housekeeping genes show that *S. boydii* 13 strains cluster in a neighbor-joining tree with *E. albertii*.

Comparative genomic analysis has provided important insights into the structure and organization of bacterial genomes and the mechanisms by which they evolved. The genomes of more than 20 *E. coli* strains representative of commensal and different pathogenic groups (pathotypes) have been sequenced and compared (2, 26, 46, 60, 146, 167). They range in size from 4,639,221 base pairs for *E. coli* K-12 (26) to 5,945,000 base pairs for a strain of Shiga toxin-producing *E. coli* (STEC) serotype O26:H11 (146). In a comparison of 17 genomes, the number of genes per genome ranged from 4,238 to 5,589, with an average of 2,344 (46.7%) of these being conserved (167). Strains representative of a pathotype contained shared genes as well as unique genes. Enterohemorrhagic *E. coli* (EHEC) strains shared the largest number of genes, with 122 group-specific genes, while uropathogenic *E. coli* (UPEC) strains shared 45 to 56 genes; enteropathogenic *E. coli* (EPEC), enteroaggregative *E. coli* (EAEC), and enterotoxigenic *E. coli* (ETEC) strains each shared 3 to 5 genes; and commensal strains shared 11 genes. The number of strain-specific genes varied widely and was not consistent within a pathotype (167).

Pathogenomic analysis of the numerous plasmids present within representative strains of each of the *E. coli* pathotypes and commensal *E. coli* has revealed considerable diversity and plasticity within these genetic elements (105). In contrast to the overall plasmid diversity, there is limited diversity in the virulence plasmids, which are restricted to a few plasmid backbones, with conservation and linkage of their core components (105). These plasmids contain distinct regions for genetic exchange that appear to evolve via insertion sequence-mediated site-specific recombination. Many such plasmids have also acquired multidrug resistance-encoding islands. In addition to plasmids, bacteriophages play a major role in generating genome diversity by promoting homologous recombination and horizontal gene transfer between bacteria (11, 95). For example, the Sakai strain of *E. coli* O157:H7 contains 18 prophages and 6 prophage-like elements (16% of the total genome), which carry a wide range of virulence genes, including the genes for Shiga toxins 1 and 2 (92, 147). Although many of these prophages carry genetic defects, some are able to be induced and recombine with each other to generate new phages capable of transferring virulence genes to other bacteria (11). The dynamic nature of the Shiga toxin-converting phages has implications for diagnostic testing for STEC. Since STEC strains can lose critical virulence genes, some researchers have proposed that multiple virulence-associated genes, as well as conserved genes, be used to diagnose infections by these bacteria (22, 23). This concept would also apply to other pathotypes of *E. coli*, as most of them carry critical virulence genes on mobile genetic elements.

Description of the Genus

The genus *Escherichia* is composed of motile or nonmotile bacteria that conform to the definitions of the family *Enterobacteriaceae* (66, 175). Species in this genus are gram-negative, oxidase-negative rods that grow well on MacConkey agar (MAC). When these organisms are motile, it is by peritrichous flagella. They can grow aerobically or anaerobically. All ferment D-glucose, and most produce gas from the fermentation of this substrate and other fermentable carbohydrates. Lactose is fermented by most strains of *E. coli*, but its fermentation may be delayed or absent in all or most strains of *E. albertii*, *E. blattae*, *E. fergusonii*, and *E. vulneris*. Typical phenotypic properties are listed in Table 1.

TABLE 1 Biochemical reactions of the six species of *Escherichia* and selected members of the family *Enterobacteriaceae*[a]

Species/biogroup	Indole production	Voges-Proskauer	Motility (35°C)	Yellow pigment	Lysine decarboxylase	Ornithine decarboxylase	Growth in KCN	Acetate utilization	Mucate utilization	D-Glucose, gas	Adonitol, acid	L-Arabinose, acid	D-Arabitol, acid	Cellobiose, acid	Dulcitol, acid	Lactose, acid	Sucrose, acid	D-Mannitol, acid	Raffinose, acid	L-Rhamnose, acid	D-Sorbitol, acid	D-Xylose
Escherichia albertii biogroup 1 (n = 5) (e.g., Albert 19982)	0	0	0	0	100	100	0	20	20	0	0	100	0	0	0	0	0	100	0	0	0	0
Escherichia albertii biogroup 2 (n = 10) (e.g., former *S. boydii* 13)	100	0	0	0	0	100	0	0	0	40	0	100	0	0	0	0	0	100	0	0	100	0
Escherichia blattae	0	0	0	0	100	100	0	0	0	100	0	100	0	0	0	0	0	0	0	100	0	0
Escherichia coli	98	0	95	0	90	65	0	90	50	95	5	99	5	2	60	95	50	98	50	80	94	100
Escherichia coli (inactive biotypes)	80	0	5	0	40	20	1	40	95	5	3	85	5	2	40	25	15	93	15	65	75	95
Escherichia fergusonii	98	0	93	0	95	100	0	96	30	95	98	98	100	96	60	0	0	98	0	92	0	70
Escherichia hermannii	99	0	99	98	6	100	94	78	0	97	0	100	8	97	19	45	45	100	40	97	0	96
Escherichia vulneris	0	0	100	50	85	0	15	30	97	97	0	100	0	100	0	15	8	100	99	93	1	100
Shigella boydii[b]	37	0	0	0	0	0	0	0	78	0	0	94	0	0	12	1	0	99	0	1	59	100
Shigella dysenteriae	40	0	0	0	0	0	0	0	0	0	0	45	0	0	4	0	0	0	0	30	29	27
Shigella flexneri	42	0	0	0	0	0	0	8	0	3	0	60	1	0	2	0	1	91	33	5	30	3
Shigella sonnei	0	0	0	0	0	98	0	0	0	0	0	95	0	5	0	2	1	99	3	77	1	3
Hafnia alvei	0	85	85	0	100	98	95	15	10	98	0	95	0	15	0	5	10	99	2	97	0	1
Hafnia alvei/biogroup 1	0	70	0	0	100	45	0	0	0	0	0	0	0	5	0	0	0	55	0	0	0	98
Salmonella serotype Paratyphi A	0	0	95	0	0	95	0	0	0	99	0	0	0	0	90	0	0	98	1	100	95	0
Salmonella serotype Choleraesuis	0	0	95	0	95	100	0	1	0	95	0	5	1	5	5	0	0	98	1	100	90	98
Yersinia ruckeri	0	10	0	0	50	100	15	0	0	5	0	5	0	0	0	0	0	100	5	0	50	0

[a] Values are percentages of isolates tested with positive test results within 1 or 2 days of incubation at 35 to 37°C. Reactions for isolates that become positive after 2 days are not considered. Data were compiled from findings published by Ewing et al. (68), Wathen-Grady et al. (208, 209), Ansaruzzaman et al. (8), Pryamukhina and Khomenko (163), and Farmer (71) and from unpublished findings from the reference laboratory at the CDC (1972 to 2005).

[b] Excludes strains previously identified as *S. boydii* 13.

Epidemiology and Transmission

E. coli occurs naturally in the lower part of the intestines of humans and warm-blooded animals. In humans, it typically colonizes an infant's gastrointestinal tract within hours of birth and subsequently becomes a prominent facultative anaerobe in the human colonic microbiota, where it exists in a mutually beneficial relationship with its host. *E. coli* generally remains confined to the intestinal lumen; however, in a debilitated or immunosuppressed host or when bacteria are introduced to other tissues following trauma or surgical procedures, even commensal, "nonpathogenic" strains of *E. coli* can cause infection. *E. coli* is typically transmitted through ingestion of contaminated food and water, person-to-person contact, contact with animals, or contact with environments or fomites contaminated with fecal material. Convincing evidence of respiratory transmission has not been reported. Most strains of *E. coli* do not cause disease in healthy persons; however, there are specific pathogenic groups, addressed below, whose members are capable of causing disease in humans and animals. The infectious dose for diarrheagenic *E. coli* varies by strain and pathotype and is estimated to range from 10 to 100 bacteria for *E. coli* O157:H7 to at least 10^8 bacteria for ETEC (72).

Because *E. coli* is ubiquitous in human and animal feces, the presence of this species in water is considered an indicator of fecal contamination. It can be isolated from feces-contaminated foods or water but probably does not occur as a free-living organism in the environment.

E. fergusonii, *E. hermannii*, *E. vulneris*, and *E. albertii* have been isolated from a wide variety of human clinical specimens (stool, urine, sputum, blood, spinal fluid, peritoneal dialysis fluid, and wounds) (13, 33, 70, 100, 119, 157, 179). *E. fergusonii* and *E. albertii* have also been isolated from wild and domestic birds (15, 145). Recently, *E. vulneris* strains with traits common to mammalian pathogens were found actively multiplying within legumes, raising the possibility that plants may represent a niche for transmission of clinically important strains (137). In addition, *E. vulneris* was recovered in combination with other members of the *Enterobacteriaceae* from neonatal enteral feeding tubes, highlighting the potential importance of these devices as risk factors for neonatal infections (99). *E. blattae* occurs naturally in the hindgut of cockroaches and is not known to cause disease in humans.

Clinical Significance

Of the six *Escherichia* species, *E. coli* is the species usually isolated from human specimens and is the one that we know the most about. We know little about the pathogenesis of the other escherichiae; however, it is interesting that strains of *E. albertii*, which have been associated with diarrheal disease in children, contain the locus for enterocyte effacement (LEE) pathogenicity island that is also present in EPEC and EHEC (100, 101, 187).

Extraintestinal *E. coli*

Pathogenic *E. coli* strains are broadly grouped into two categories, namely, extraintestinal pathogenic *E. coli* (ExPEC) and intestinal or diarrheagenic *E. coli*, depending on whether they cause disease outside or within the intestinal tract. Commensal *E. coli* strains, which comprise the majority of the facultative anaerobic intestinal biota in most humans and other mammals, typically do not cause disease but can be opportunistic pathogens when certain conditions exist, such as the presence of a foreign body (e.g., urinary catheter), host compromise (e.g., local anatomical or functional abnormalities, such as urinary or bile tract obstruction or immunocompromise), or

a breach in normally sterile sites causing the introduction of feces or high concentrations of mixed bacteria. ExPEC strains carry a distinct set of virulence genes that enable them to cause disease outside the intestine. This category contains at least two well-recognized pathogenic groups or pathotypes—UPEC and meningitis/sepsis-associated *E. coli* (MNEC)—and a variety of disease-associated strains not yet classified into specific pathotypes.

UPEC

UPEC strains are a major cause of community-acquired urinary tract infections and possess a variety of chromosomally and plasmid-encoded virulence factors that are present in various combinations. Members of this group have a limited number of O antigens (six O groups cause 75% of urinary tract infections) and show combinations of traits, including expression of adhesins (P [Pap], type 1, and other fimbriae), toxins (hemolysin, cytotoxic necrotizing factor, and an autotransported protease [Sat]), or aerobactin, serum resistance, and encapsulation, that are epidemiologically associated with cystitis and acute pyelonephritis in individuals with normal urinary tracts. No single phenotypic profile defining UPEC has emerged. UPEC strains possess large and small pathogenicity islands containing blocks of genes not found in the chromosomes of fecal strains. For a review of the virulence genes and a proposed model of the pathogenesis of UPEC, see the work of Kaper et al. (108) and Johnson and Russo (104).

MNEC

MNEC strains are the most common gram-negative organisms causing neonatal meningitis, which is associated with high morbidity and mortality. The MNEC pathotype is comprised of strains with a limited number of O antigens, and about 80% are positive for the K1 antigen. *E. coli* strains that cause meningitis are spread hematogenously. Levels of bacteremia correlate with the development of meningitis: levels of $>10^3$ CFU/ml of blood are significantly associated with the development of meningitis (59). After entering the blood, these bacteria invade brain microvascular endothelial cells through membrane-bound vacuoles. Within these vacuoles, the organisms control intracellular trafficking to avoid lysosomal fusion and to gain access to the central nervous system without causing apparent damage to the blood-brain barrier. Recent studies have identified several bacterial determinants (IbeA, IbeB, IbeC, AslA, CNF1, FimH, and OmpA) which contribute to the pathogenesis of MNEC in vitro. For reviews, see the work of Kim et al. (113) and Kaper et al. (108).

Diarrheagenic *E. coli*

There are at least five categories of recognized diarrheagenic *E. coli*: STEC, which includes a subset of strains referred to as enterohemorrhagic *E. coli* (EHEC) for their ability to cause bloody diarrhea and hemorrhagic colitis; ETEC; EPEC; EAEC; and enteroinvasive *E. coli* (EIEC) (108, 139). The clinical significance of several other groups of putative diarrheagenic *E. coli*, particularly diffusely adherent *E. coli* (DAEC), is unclear.

STEC

We refer to the STEC category of diarrheagenic *E. coli* according to the toxins that the organisms produce, i.e., as STEC rather than EHEC, because the essential genetic features that define organisms capable of causing hemorrhagic colitis and hemolytic-uremic syndrome (HUS) are not clear. *E. coli* serotypes O157:H7 and O157:nonmotile (O157:NM) (collectively called O157 STEC) produce one

TABLE 2 Frequently encountered serotypes of diarrheagenic *E. coli*[a]

ETEC	EPEC	EIEC	STEC			EAEC
O6:NM	**O55:NM**	O28:NM	O8:H19	O103:H25	O128:H2	O3:H2
O6:H16	**O55:H6**	O29:NM	O22:H8	O104:H7	O128:H45	O15:H18
O8:H9	O55:H7	O112:NM	**O26:NM**	**O104:H21**	**O145:NM**	**O44:H18**
O15:H11	O86:NM	O124:NM	**O26:H11**	**O111:NM**	O146:H21	O51:H11
O20:NM	O86:H34	O124:H7	O28:H25	**O111:H2**	O153:H2	O77:H18
O25:NM	**O111:NM**	**O124:H30**	**O45:H2**	**O111:H8**	O153:H25	O86:H2
O25:H42	**O111:H2**	O136:NM	O55:H7	**O113:H21**	O156:H25	O111ab:H21
O27:NM	O111:H12	**O143:NM**	O69:H11	**O118:H2**	**O157:NM**	O126:H27
O27:H7	O111:H21	O144:NM	O76:H19	O118:H12	**O157:H7**	O141:H49
O27:H20	**O114:NM**	O152:NM	O84:NM	O118:H16	O165:NM	ONT:H21
O49:NM	**O114:H2**	**O164:NM**	O88:H25	O119:NM	O165:H25	ONT:H33
O63:H12	**O119:H6**	O167:NM	O91:NM	O119:H4	O172:NM	
O78:H11	**O125:H21**	**ONT:NM**	O91:H14	O119:H25	O174:H21	
O78:H12	O126:NM		O91:H21	**O121:H19**	O174:H28	
O128:H7	O126:H27		O103:NM	O123:NM	O177:NM	
O148:H28	**O127:NM**		**O103:H2**	O123:H11	O178:H19	
O153:H45	**O127:H6**		O103:H11	O128:NM	O179:H8	
O159:NM	O127:H9					
O159:H4	O127:H21					
O159:H20	**O128:H2**					
O167:H5	O128:H7					
O169:NM	O128:H12					
O169:H41	**O142:H6**					
	O157:H45					

[a]Outbreak-related serotypes are shown in bold. NM, nonmotile; NT, not typeable.

or more Shiga toxins, also called verocytotoxins, and are the most frequently identified diarrheagenic *E. coli* serotypes in North America and Europe. Each year, an estimated 73,000 cases of illness and 60 deaths are caused by O157 STEC in the United States (133).

E. coli O157:H7 and other STEC serotypes cause illness that can present as mild nonbloody diarrhea, severe bloody diarrhea (hemorrhagic colitis), or HUS (reviewed in reference 84). Additional symptoms of *E. coli* O157:H7 infection include abdominal cramps and lack of a high fever. Among patients with O157 STEC diarrhea, 4% or more develop HUS (165), a condition characterized by microangiopathic hemolytic anemia, thrombocytopenia, and acute renal failure. The fatality rate of HUS has declined in recent years due to improvements in case management.

O157 STEC is thought to cause at least 80% of cases of HUS in North America and is recognized as a common cause of bloody diarrhea in developed countries (165). In the United States, the rate of isolation of O157 STEC from fecal specimens is highest in the Northern Tier states, where it may approach the rates for common diarrheal pathogens. Many U.S. clinical laboratories do not routinely culture or otherwise test stools for O157 STEC; as a result, many illnesses are not detected (44, 204). O157 STEC colonizes dairy and beef cattle, and therefore ground beef has caused more O157 STEC outbreaks than any other vehicle of transmission (165, 184). Other known vehicles of transmission include raw milk, sausage, roast beef, unchlorinated municipal water, apple cider, raw vegetables, and sprouts; these vehicles are typically exposed to water contaminated by bovine manure. O157 STEC spreads easily from person to person because the infectious dose is low (<200 CFU); outbreaks associated with person-to-person spread have occurred in schools, long-term care institutions, families, and day care facilities.

More than 150 non-O157 STEC serotypes have been isolated from persons with diarrhea or HUS (http://www .microbionet.com.au/frames/feature/vtec/brief01.html). In some countries, non-O157 STEC strains, particularly *E. coli* serotypes O111:NM and O26:H11, are more commonly isolated than O157 STEC strains, although most outbreaks and cases of HUS are attributed to the latter (serotypes characteristic of diarrheagenic *E. coli* pathotypes are presented in Table 2). In the United States, *E. coli* O157:H7 is the most frequently isolated STEC serotype, but increasingly, non-O157 STEC strains are identified as causes of outbreaks and sporadic illness (36). At the CDC *E. coli* Reference Laboratory, 71% of all non-O157 STEC isolates received between 2003 and 2008 belonged to six serogroups (O26, O103, O111, O121, O45, and O145) (N. A. Strockbine, unpublished data). Because most laboratory methods for the detection of O157 STEC do not detect non-O157 STEC, the numbers of infections with serotypes other than O157:H7 or O157:NM are probably underestimated.

ETEC

ETEC, which produces heat-labile *E. coli* enterotoxin (LT) and/or heat-stable *E. coli* enterotoxin (ST), is an important cause of diarrhea in developing countries, particularly among young children (139). ETEC is also a frequent cause of traveler's diarrhea. From 1975 to 2008, 33 U.S. outbreaks were reported to the Centers for Disease Control and Prevention (CDC) (C. A. Bopp, unpublished data) (54). ETEC is infrequently identified in the United States, but this may be attributable in part to the fact that few laboratories are capable of identifying this pathogen. ETEC strains, particularly those associated with outbreaks, tend to cluster in a few serotypes (Table 2).

The most prominent symptoms of ETEC illness are diarrhea and abdominal cramps, sometimes accompanied by nausea and headache, but usually with little vomiting or fever (54). Although ETEC is usually associated with relatively mild watery diarrhea, illness in some recent ETEC outbreaks has been notable for its prolonged duration (204).

EPEC

In the past, EPEC strains were defined as certain *E. coli* serotypes that were epidemiologically associated with infantile diarrhea but did not produce enterotoxins or Shiga toxins and were not invasive. The traditional EPEC serotypes are listed in Table 2; typically, these serotypes show a distinct pattern of localized adherence to HeLa and HEp-2 cells (203). These serotypes usually also demonstrate actin aggregation in the fluorescent actin stain test, which correlates with the attaching-and-effacing (A/E) lesion in vivo (139). Because of the lack of simple diagnostic methods for detection of EPEC strains, few laboratories attempt to identify these organisms. Full EPEC pathogenicity requires two genetic elements: the EPEC adherence factor (EAF) plasmid, which encodes, most importantly, the bundle-forming pilus, and the chromosomal LEE, which mediates the A/E phenotype. The term "typical EPEC" has been suggested for those organisms harboring both the EAF plasmid and the LEE pathogenicity island (see below). Typical EPEC strains correspond to EPEC strains of the classical serotypes and are important causes of diarrhea in developing countries (62, 139); these organisms were implicated in highly lethal nursery outbreaks in the United States and the United Kingdom before 1970. The infection is currently rare in the industrialized world. More recently, atypical EPEC strains have been implicated as enteric pathogens in the United States, including implication in an outbreak of diarrheal disease (94, 200). These strains possess a functional LEE apparatus but do not carry the EAF plasmid. The full role of these pathogens has yet to be elucidated, but they may be considered potential causes of diarrheal outbreaks when no other pathogens are identified.

Symptoms of severe, prolonged, and nonbloody diarrhea, vomiting, and fever in infants or young toddlers are characteristic of EPEC illness (139). Infection with EPEC has been associated with chronic diarrhea; sequelae may include malabsorption, malnutrition, weight loss, and growth retardation.

EIEC

EIEC strains invade cells of the colon and produce a generally watery, but occasionally bloody, diarrhea by a pathogenic mechanism similar to that of *Shigella*. EIEC is rare in the United States and is less common than ETEC or EPEC in the developing world (139). EIEC strains, like ETEC and EPEC, are associated with a few characteristic serotypes (Table 2). Three large outbreaks of diarrhea caused by EIEC have been reported in the United States (139).

EAEC

EAEC, originally defined by its specific pattern of aggregative adherence to HEp-2 cells in culture, has been associated with diarrhea in a variety of clinical settings, including endemic diarrhea in children of both impoverished and industrialized countries, epidemic diarrhea, diarrhea of travelers to developing countries, and persistent diarrhea among patients with human immunodeficiency virus infection (98). The pathogenicity of EAEC has been confirmed in volunteer studies (138) and by implication of EAEC in diarrhea outbreaks (52). Early studies frequently failed to find an association of EAEC with pediatric diarrhea, but

this association has been strengthened by the use of molecular techniques which discriminate the true pathogens exhibiting the aggregative pattern (53, 174). The term "typical EAEC" describes organisms harboring virulence genes under the control of the global EAEC regulator AggR (174). Typical EAEC may be a common cause of pediatric diarrhea in U.S. infants (53) and should be considered a potential cause of food-borne outbreaks and diarrhea in human immunodeficiency virus-infected patients (98). EAEC diarrhea is accompanied by signs and symptoms of mild inflammation (abdominal pain and fever), but stools usually do not contain blood or fecal leukocytes (98).

Putative Diarrheagenic *E. coli*

Several putative pathotypes have been described. Virulence has not been demonstrated clearly for any of these types by either volunteer studies or outbreak investigations. DAEC strains, which exhibit a characteristic diffuse pattern of adherence to HEp-2 cells, have been implicated as causes of diarrhea in some epidemiologic studies but not others (139), and a prototypical DAEC strain did not elicit diarrhea in adult volunteers (193). In several studies, DAEC infections were significantly associated with watery diarrhea among children of 1 to 5 years of age but were not associated with illness among infants (118). DAEC may occur in industrialized countries (139). A complex signal transduction cascade has been suggested as the mechanism of DAEC pathogenesis (180).

Cytotoxic necrotizing factor (CNF)-producing *E. coli* strains produce a toxin that induces morphological alterations (multinucleation) and death in tissue cultures (38). Two forms have been described: CNF1 and CNF2. CNF1-producing strains were originally detected in infants with enteritis and later in humans with extraintestinal infections (25, 38). Most CNF1-producing strains are also hemolytic, although the toxin is distinct from hemolysin. CNF2-producing strains have been isolated from animals with diarrhea (57, 150, 185). The role of these strains in human diarrheal disease has not been determined definitively (139).

Cytolethal distending toxin-producing *E. coli* strains produce a heat-labile factor that induces cytotonic and cytotoxic changes in Chinese hamster ovary cells similar to those caused by LT (106). This factor does not affect Y-1 cells. The results of one study in Bangladesh suggested that cytolethal distending toxin-producing *E. coli* strains are associated with diarrhea (5, 106), but other studies are needed to establish their status as etiologic agents.

Several diarrheal outbreaks have been linked to *E. coli* strains that do not belong to any of the established pathotypes. Some of these strains carry the gene encoding the enteroaggregative ST-like toxin (EAST1), which is related to the ETEC ST enterotoxin. Further studies are needed to prove the pathogenicity of these strains, but the EAST1 gene can be identified by use of molecular techniques (132).

Collection, Transport, and Storage of Specimens

Information on the collection, transport, and storage of specimens from extraintestinal sites is provided in chapter 16 of this *Manual.* Fecal specimens should be collected in the early stages of any enteric illness (preferably within 4 days of onset), when pathogens are usually present in the stool in the largest numbers and before antimicrobial therapy has been started. Whole stools are usually the specimen of choice, but carefully collected rectal swabs with visible fecal staining may be preferable for diagnosis of *Shigella* (4, 91, 190). Collection of multiple specimens may enhance the recovery rate of *E. coli, Shigella,* and *Salmonella* (65).

Transport of fecal specimens to the laboratory in a timely fashion is critical, particularly for more delicate organisms such as *Shigella* (210). Ideally, fecal specimens should be examined as soon as they are received in the laboratory, but if not processed immediately, they should be either refrigerated or frozen at −70°C. Fecal specimens that will not be examined within 1 to 2 h of collection and all rectal swabs should be placed in cold transport medium and kept at 4°C (80). Transport and storage of fecal specimens at 4°C are very important for *Shigella* as well as *Campylobacter* spp. Manufacturers of commercial transport media, including the acceptable media listed below, commonly state that fecal specimens may be transported and stored at ambient temperature. For *Shigella* and *Campylobacter* spp., this is not advised because there are data showing that transport at ambient temperature may deleteriously affect recovery of these organisms (204, 207).

Many of the commercially available transport media (e.g., Cary-Blair, Stuart's, and Amies transport media) and buffered glycerol saline are satisfactory for *E. coli*, *Salmonella*, and *Shigella*. Although acceptable for the transport of the organisms addressed in this chapter, buffered glycerol saline should not be used for specimens that must also be tested for *Campylobacter* and *Vibrio* (58, 207).

Direct Examination

Microscopy

Gram stains of patient specimens from normally sterile body sites can provide a preliminary indication of which category of bacteria to cultivate from the specimen and if inflammatory cells or blood are present; however, *E. coli* and other *Escherichia* species cannot readily be distinguished from other gram-negative rods by staining or microscopy methods.

Antigen Detection

Several commercial immunoassays are available to diagnose STEC infections by detecting Shiga toxin or the O157 antigen (lipopolysaccharide [LPS]) in fecal specimens (Table 3). These assays are usually more sensitive when performed on enriched specimens than on stool directly. Isolation of STEC from fecal specimens that are positive by one of these rapid diagnostic methods is important for public health purposes. Determination of the subtype of O157 STEC or the serotype of a non-O157 STEC isolate is valuable for outbreak investigations and surveillance purposes (see "Typing Systems" and "Identification" below).

Nucleic Acid Detection

There are no U.S. Food and Drug Administration (FDA)-approved nucleic acid detection methods for the clinical diagnosis of pathogenic *E. coli* or other *Escherichia* infections. Due to the number of inhibitors and amount of competing DNA present in stool specimens, most researchers have found it necessary to perform an enrichment step before testing these specimens by PCR for pathogenic *E. coli*. One group recently reported success for use of an automated DNA extraction system to prepare target DNA (Shiga toxin genes) from unenriched stool specimens for amplification in a home-brew real-time PCR assay (86).

Isolation Procedures

Isolation Procedures for Extraintestinal *E. coli*

Isolation procedures for *E. coli* and other *Escherichia* species from sites outside the intestines are covered in chapter 16 in this *Manual*. Any *E. coli* strain isolated in large numbers (particularly >10^5 CFU/ml of urine) or from normally sterile body sites should be considered a potential pathogen. Although *E. coli* strains with particular virulence in the urinary tract cannot easily be distinguished on differential and selective plating media from organisms of lower virulence, they are commonly hemolytic on sheep blood agar and express one or more of several urinary tract adhesins. Several chromogenic media have been proposed for use in detecting UPEC; these have been compared in published studies (12, 47).

Isolation Procedures for Diarrheagenic *E. coli*

Isolation Procedures for STEC

Guidelines published in 2009 (83) recommend that all stools submitted for testing for routine enteric pathogens (*Salmonella*, *Shigella*, and *Campylobacter*) at clinical diagnostic laboratories and all patients with suspected HUS should be cultured for O157 STEC on selective and differential agar and assayed for non-O157 STEC with a test that detects the Shiga toxins or genes encoding these toxins. The recommendations to isolate O157 STEC and to detect non-O157 STEC were extended to all stools from patients with acute, community-acquired diarrhea because selective testing strategies such as testing only bloody stools or specimens from children, limiting testing to summer months, or basing testing on the presence of indicators such as white blood cells miss many STEC infections. The absence of blood in the stool does not negate the possibility of an STEC-associated diarrheal illness (111, 129). In several studies, most STEC isolates, including both O157 and non-O157 strains, were from patients with apparently nonbloody diarrhea (78, 83, 152, 196, 201). Also, STEC strains are isolated more frequently from children, but almost half of all isolates are obtained from persons of >12 years of age (36, 41, 184, 201), so limiting STEC testing to children would miss many infections. Although infections are more common in summer months, seasonality is not a reliable predictor of STEC infections because infections and outbreaks occur year-round (36, 184, 196). As a sign of STEC, white blood cells are often but not always observed in the stools of patients with STEC infection; thus, determination of white blood cells in stool should not be used as a criterion for STEC specimen selection (87, 184).

Because there is no selective isolation medium for non-O157 STEC strains, testing for the presence of Shiga toxin in fecal specimens is the best approach for detecting these organisms. Commercial enzyme-linked immunoassays (EIAs) are a sensitive means of detecting Shiga toxin (21, 78, 111, 125, 151). Isolation and serotyping of STEC from fecal specimens that are positive by nonculture assays should always be attempted because serotype information is important for public health purposes and may also help in clinical decisions.

Enrichment. Although broth enrichment is widely used for the recovery of O157 STEC from foods, there is little evidence that it enhances isolation from human fecal specimens. However, immunomagnetic separation (IMS), a technique shown to increase the rate of isolation of O157 STEC from food specimens, has been adapted to culture of fecal specimens (109). IMS enhances the detection of O157 STEC from patients with HUS, patients presenting an extended time after the onset of illness, asymptomatic carriers, or specimens that have been stored or transported improperly. IMS beads for O157, O111, and O26 are available commercially (Table 3), or laboratories may produce beads with other O-specific antibodies (153).

Plating media. Because O157 STEC strains ferment lactose, they are impossible to differentiate from other lactose-fermenting

TABLE 3 Partial listing of commercial suppliers of reagents for detection of STEC[a]

Antisera for tube agglutination
    Difco Laboratories (Division of Becton Dickinson and Co., Sparks, MD)
        O157 and H7 antisera
    Statens Serum Institut (Copenhagen, Denmark)
        O157, H7, O26, O103, O111, O145 and other *E. coli* O and H antisera
    Denka Seiken Co., Ltd., Tokyo, Japan
        O157, H7, O26, O103, O111, O145 and other *E. coli* O and H antisera

Latex slide agglutination reagents
    Denka Seiken Co., Ltd., Tokyo, Japan
        O157, O26, and O111 reagents
    Oxoid Inc. (Division of Thermo Fisher Scientific Inc., Waltham, MA)
        O157, O26, O91, O103, O111, and O145 reagents
    ProLab Diagnostics, Inc., Richmond Hill, Ontario, Canada
        O157 and H7 reagents
    Remel, Inc., Lenexa, KS
        O157 and H7 reagents

Immunomagnetic beads
    Dynal Biotech (Division of Invitrogen Corporation, Carlsbad, CA)
        Anti-O157-, anti-O26-, anti-O103-, anti-O111-, and anti-O145-labeled beads
    Denka Seiken Co., Ltd., Tokyo, Japan
        Anti-O157-, anti-O26-, anti-O111-labeled beads

O157 immunoassays
    Meridian Diagnostics Inc., Cincinnati, OH
        For testing stool specimens or enrichment broths for O157 antigen
    Denka Seiken Co., Ltd., Tokyo, Japan
        For testing colony sweeps or individual colonies for O157, O111, or O26 antigen

Shiga toxin immunoassays
    Meridian Diagnostics Inc., Cincinnati, OH
        For testing stool specimens, enrichment broths, colony sweeps, or individual colonies for Shiga toxin
    Remel, Inc., Lenexa, KS
        For testing stool specimens or enrichment broths for Shiga toxin
    Denka Seiken Co., Ltd., Tokyo, Japan
        For testing colony sweeps or individual colonies for Shiga toxin
    Merck KGaA, Darmstadt, Germany
        For testing individual colonies for Shiga Toxin

Chromogenic agars (for visual detection of O157:H7 colonies upon direct inoculation of agar plates)
    Merck KGaA, Darmstadt, Germany
    bioMerieux Inc., Hazelwood, MO
    Biosynth International, Inc., Naperville, IL
    Biolog, Inc., Hayward, CA
    Becton Dickinson and Co., Franklin Lakes, NJ
        Holds license to CHROMagar

[a]This table is not intended to be a comprehensive listing. The FDA has not approved all of these reagents for use with clinical specimens. This table does not include reagents or tests specifically intended for examination of food, water, or environmental specimens. The online version of the *Bacteriological Analytical Manual* lists many tests for food specimens (http://www.fda.gov). Inclusion does not constitute endorsement by the CDC or ASM.

organisms on lactose-containing media. Most O157 STEC strains do not ferment the carbohydrate D-sorbitol overnight, in contrast to the approximately 80% of other *E. coli* strains that ferment sorbitol rapidly. Thus, sorbitol-containing selective media are often used for isolation of O157 STEC. Sorbitol-nonfermenting colonies are suspected (but not definitively known) to be O157:H7 (130). In some areas of central Europe, sorbitol-fermenting O157 STEC strains are commonly isolated from patients with HUS (24); these organisms are very rare in North America (Strockbine, unpublished data).

Specific culture media have been developed to exploit phenotypic and antibiotic resistance traits that are characteristic of STEC strains. Although sorbitol-containing MAC (SMAC) is widely used, cefixime-tellurite-containing SMAC (CT-SMAC) and CHROMAgar O157 have been shown to increase the sensitivity of culture for O157 STEC (49, 213). It has been reported that some O157:NM strains fail to grow on CT-SMAC (109). Several chromogenic agar media are available commercially to assist in rapid identification (Table 3); these media generally perform well for O157:H7 and for some non-O157 STEC strains (19, 127, 144).

Screening procedures for STEC strains. For the isolation of O157 STEC from SMAC, colorless (nonfermenting) colonies are tested with O157 antiserum or latex reagent (186) (Table 3). If the O157 latex reagent is used, it is important to test positive colonies with the latex control reagent to rule out nonspecific reactions. The manufacturers of these kits recommend that strains reacting with both the antigen-specific and control latex reagents be heated and retested. However, in a study that followed this procedure, none of the nonspecifically reacting strains were subsequently identified as O157 STEC (27).

Unlike most other *E. coli* strains, O157 STEC strains do not express beta-glucuronidase; therefore, the MUG reaction (4-methylumbelliferyl-beta-D-glucuronide for detection of beta-glucuronidase activity) is helpful for screening for O157 STEC (177). MUG-positive, urease-positive O157 STEC strains have been isolated in the United States but are still rare 93; Strockbine, unpublished data).

For the recovery of STEC strains from stool specimens which test positive for Shiga toxin, either SMAC or MAC should be inoculated. It is advantageous to use SMAC because O157 STEC can be identified quickly and easily. If sorbitol-nonfermenting colonies are negative with O157 latex, then sorbitol-fermenting colonies (because most non-O157 STEC strains ferment sorbitol) and a representative sample of sorbitol-nonfermenting colonies may be selected for Shiga toxin testing. Latex reagents and antisera (Table 3) for detecting certain non-O157 STEC serotypes are now available and could also be used to test colonies from Shiga toxin-positive specimens or to serogroup Shiga toxin-positive isolates.

Virtually all O157 STEC strains and 60 to 80% of non-O157 STEC strains produce a characteristic *E. coli* hemolysin, referred to as enterohemolysin (Ehly), which is distinct from the alpha-hemolysin produced by other *E. coli* strains (20). Washed sheep blood agar supplemented with calcium (WSBA-Ca) is used as a differential medium for the detection of enterohemolytic activity (20). Ehly-producing colonies can be differentiated from alpha-hemolysin-producing colonies on WSBA-Ca because the latter are visible after 3 to 4 h of incubation. After 3 to 4 h, colonies are marked for the appearance of alpha-hemolysin, and the plates are examined again after 18 to 24 h to detect the enterohemolysin producers.

Incorporation of mitomycin C into WSBA-Ca enhances the appearance of Ehly hemolysis and increases the proportion of non-O157 STEC strains that exhibit this activity (191). Because many non-O157 STEC strains do not demonstrate the enterohemolytic phenotype and because nontoxigenic enterohemolytic strains have been reported, additional screening methods should be used in conjunction with WSBA-Ca medium (176).

Presumptive STEC isolates should be sent to a reference laboratory or a public health laboratory for further characterization.

Isolation Procedures for Other Diarrheagenic *E. coli*

Methods for the isolation of ETEC, EPEC, EIEC, EAEC, and putative diarrheagenic *E. coli* strains are generally available only in reference or research settings. Public health and reference laboratories usually examine specimens for these pathogens only when an outbreak has occurred and specimens are negative for routine bacterial pathogens. ETEC and EAEC should be considered possible etiologic agents of watery diarrhea for which no other pathogen has been identified, especially for travelers (53). EPEC should be considered a possible pathogen in outbreaks of severe nonbloody diarrhea occurring in infants or young toddlers, particularly in nursery or day care settings. EIEC should be considered a possible etiologic agent in outbreaks of nonwatery diarrhea (bloody or nonbloody).

To capture *E. coli* for further testing, fecal specimens should be plated on a differential medium of low selectivity (e.g., MAC). Five to 20 colonies, mostly lactose fermenting but with a representative sample of nonfermenting colonies, should be selected and inoculated onto nonselective agar slants (such as L agar or nutrient agar). These colonies are then sent to a reference laboratory for testing or are screened for virulence-associated characteristics if assays are available. Strains can be kept frozen for long periods in L broth with 15 to 50% glycerol at −80°C. Arrangements for sending *E. coli* isolates from well-characterized outbreaks to the CDC for testing can be made through local and state health departments.

Screening procedures for ETEC, EPEC, EAEC, and EIEC strains. *E. coli* pathotypes other than STEC cannot be distinguished from other *E. coli* strains by phenotypic screening techniques. Many EIEC strains are nonmotile and fail to decarboxylate lysine; however, some EIEC strains are motile or lysine positive. Use of commercial antisera to the classical EPEC somatic (O) and capsular (K) antigens is no longer recommended.

Identification

Phenotypic Identification

With the exception of *E. albertii*, the commercial identification systems do a good job of identifying most *Escherichia* strains. Identification of *E. albertii* with these systems remains problematic because representative strains of this species are not yet included in commercial databases (1). Abbott and colleagues, who extensively characterized five strains of *E. albertii* by conventional phenotypic methods and by commercial identification panels, reported that *E. albertii* is an indole-negative species that ferments D-mannitol but not D-xylose (1). In their study, *E. albertii* strains were identified by commercial systems as *Hafnia alvei*, *Salmonella* or *Salmonella enterica* serotype Choleraesuis, *E. coli* (inactive or serotype O157:H7), or *Yersinia ruckeri*. Although some strains were clearly misidentified, the majority of the strains generated probability scores for the final identification that were unacceptable, or the identification was inconsistent with the source of the specimen (e.g., identification of the fish pathogen *Y. ruckeri* from a human specimen), which should have triggered additional phenotypic tests to establish a more reliable identification. The authors found that the most reliable clue to the possible presence of *E. albertii* was an unacceptable first-choice identification of *H. alvei* for an isolate that is both L-rhamnose and D-xylose negative.

Phenotypic tests that can help discriminate *E. albertii* strains from selected members of the *Enterobacteriaceae* family with similar phenotypic traits are shown in Table 1. Two biogroups of *E. albertii* are listed in Table 1. These correlate with two of the distinct clusters of strains identified in the *E. albertii* lineage by phylogenetic studies (101). Biogroup 1 is comprised of the five strains isolated from Bangladeshi children with diarrhea, while biogroup 2 is comprised of strains formerly identified as *S. boydii* 13. The strains in the two biogroups differ from each other in the abilities to produce indole from tryptophan, decarboxylate lysine, and ferment D-sorbitol. Antigenic relationships between members of the *E. albertii* lineage and other members of the *Enterobacteriaceae* family have been observed (e.g., *S. boydii* 7 and *E. coli* O28). A diagnostic PCR assay using three housekeeping genes was described by Hyma et al. (101) for detection of *E. albertii*; this assay is independent of phenotypic or antigenic traits and should facilitate studies to learn about the diversity within the lineage, the natural habitat of this species, and its role in enteric disease.

Phenotypic identification of presumptive O157 STEC isolates is necessary because other species may cross-react with O157 antiserum or latex reagents, including *Salmonella* O group N (O:30), *Yersinia enterocolitica* serotype O9, *Citrobacter freundii,* and *E. hermannii.* Additional phenotypic tests (cellobiose fermentation and growth in the presence of KCN) may be necessary to differentiate *E. hermannii* from *E. coli,* but because *E. hermannii* is rarely detected in stool specimens, use of these tests is not cost-effective for most laboratories.

Serotyping

The serologic classification of *E. coli* is generally based on the O antigen (somatic) and the H antigen (flagellar) (18). The O and H antigens of *E. coli* are stable and reliable strain characteristics, and although 181 O antigens and 56 H antigens have been described (a few of which are no longer recognized), the actual number of serotype combinations associated with diarrheal disease is limited (Table 2). Determination of the O and H serotypes of *E. coli* strains implicated in diarrheal disease is particularly useful in epidemiologic investigations (Table 2). Even though antisera for the tube agglutination test are available from several manufacturers, most laboratories do not attempt to complete *E. coli* serotyping because it is costly. For well-characterized outbreaks with no identified etiologic agent, arrangements may be made through state health departments to send *E. coli* isolates to the CDC for virulence testing and serotyping.

Serologic Confirmation of O157 STEC

Confirmation of *E. coli* O157:H7 requires identification of the H7 flagellar antigen. H7-specific antisera and latex reagents are commercially available (Table 3), but detection of the H7 flagellar antigen often requires multiple passages (186). Isolates that are nonmotile or negative for the H7 antigen should be tested for the production of Shiga toxins or the presence of Shiga toxin gene sequences.

Approximately 85% of O157 isolates from humans received by the CDC are serotype O157:H7, 12% are nonmotile, and 3% are H types other than H7 (Strockbine, unpublished data). *E. coli* O157:NM strains frequently produce Shiga toxin and are otherwise very similar to O157:H7, but no O157 strain from human illness with an H type other than H7 has been found to produce Shiga toxin (73; Strockbine, unpublished data).

Nucleic Acid-Based Methods

Accurate identification of bacterial isolates is important for directing patient care and management. Compared to traditional phenotypic approaches, which can be influenced by phenotypic variation or subjective interpretation, 16S rRNA gene sequencing is a more objective identification tool and has the potential to reduce laboratory errors. Some clinical laboratories have begun using molecular methods to aid in the identification of organisms that cannot be cultivated due to unusual growth characteristics or antibiotic treatment or cannot be classified by phenotypic methods (76, 134, 155, 166, 181, 213). In one study, results obtained with 16S rRNA gene sequencing and the SmartGene IDNS (Zug, Switzerland) database and software compared favorably to those obtained by conventional phenotypic methods and were better than those obtained with a similar rRNA gene method employing a smaller database for a collection of 300 clinical isolates. The performance differences between the two 16S rRNA gene methods highlight the importance of the size and breadth of the database for successful classification. Difficulties separating *E. coli* from *Shigella* with 16S rRNA gene sequencing should be expected.

These are genetically the same species and have been maintained as separate taxa for medical expediency. The limited findings reported in the studies above and those reported by others (140) show that a small region of the 16S rRNA gene alone will not provide reliable separation of certain medically relevant members of the *Enterobacteriaceae* family (*E. coli/Shigella sonnei* [181] and *Escherichia/Shigella/Hafnia* [134]). The incorporation of virulence genes that define the *Shigella*/EIEC pathotype should help to discriminate it from noninvasive pathotypes or communal *E. coli.* Another approach that has potential to improve microbial identification involves mass spectroscopy. The Ibis T5000 biosensor system (Abbott Molecular, Des Plaines, IL), which is currently used in nonclinical and research settings, uses multiple regions of the 16S and 23S rRNA genes plus several housekeeping genes to discriminate between species within 6 h (63). Validation studies are needed to assess the performance of this technology on clinical specimens.

Virulence Testing

Extraintestinal *E. coli*

Numerous virulence factors have been identified for extraintestinal *E. coli* (108), particularly the K1 antigen, but these are usually identified only in epidemiological studies.

Diarrheagenic *E. coli*

Detection of diarrheagenic pathotypes is typically performed on *E. coli* colonies chosen from selective or nonselective media. If PCR techniques are used, a sweep of confluent growth from a MAC plate may be screened; if the PCR assay is positive, isolated colonies may then be picked and screened individually. Multiplex PCR assays are capable of simultaneously detecting multiple *E. coli* pathotypes (142).

STEC. Two distinct Shiga toxins, Stx1 and Stx2, also referred to as verocytotoxins, have been described. In addition, there are several variant forms of Stx2, including Stx2c, Stx2d, Stx2e, and Stx2f, which in one study were identified more frequently from asymptomatic carriers than from HUS patients (77). All of these toxins are similar to the Shiga toxin expressed by *Shigella dysenteriae* serotype 1, and the Stx1 toxins produced by O157 STEC and other STEC serotypes are virtually identical. STEC may produce either Stx1, Stx2, or both toxins. The production of Stx or the genes encoding Stx can be detected by a variety of biologic, immunologic, or nucleic acid-based assays (139). Protocols for several of these tests (e.g., cell culture, DNA probing, and PCR) are available (149). Stx has also been detected directly in the blood of HUS patients by use of flow cytometry, even in the absence of serologic or microbiologic evidence of STEC infection (198).

STEC strains represent a spectrum of virulence potentials, ranging from the highly virulent O157:H7 serotype that has been responsible for the majority of outbreak cases to apparently avirulent serotypes that have been isolated only from nonhuman sources. The presence of additional virulence factors other than Stx correlates with disease potential. The most important of these virulence factors are the intimin adhesin and the type III secretion system encoded by the LEE pathogenicity island (108). The *eae* gene probe for intimin and the *hlyA* (*ehxA*) gene probe for a plasmid-encoded hemolysin have been the most frequently employed methods to determine virulence potential, but probes for at least 25 different virulence-associated genes have been employed to characterize STEC strains (160). STEC strains have been classified into five "seropathotypes" (A through E) based on the occurrence of serotypes in human disease, in outbreaks, and in severe disease (HUS or hemorrhagic colitis) and on possession of specific virulence genes (110).

ETEC. The ST and LT enterotoxins produced by ETEC may be detected by a variety of biologic, immunologic, and nucleic acid-based assays (139). Two distinct ST variants (STh and STp) have been identified in human strains. Strains that produce ST only or ST in combination with LT have caused most ETEC outbreaks in the United States (54).

Immunoassays for the identification of ST or LT in culture supernatants of ETEC strains are available from at least two commercial sources (Table 3). The ST EIA assay (Denka Seiken Co., Ltd., and Oxoid Ltd.) is a competitive EIA for the detection of ST only (178). A reversed passive latex agglutination assay (VET-RPLA; Oxoid [a similar kit is available from Denka Seiken]) detects both cholera toxin and LT, which are highly related antigenically. The effectiveness of VET-RPLA may be optimized by use of a culture medium designed for LT production, such as Biken's medium, rather than the medium recommended by the manufacturer (214).

EPEC. EPEC, EAEC, and DAEC can be detected by their characteristic patterns of adherence to HEp-2 or HeLa cells in culture (203). These patterns are also observed on formalin- or glutaraldehyde-fixed cells, obviating the need to prepare cells expressly for the assay (135).

EPEC strains are defined on the basis of the A/E histopathology produced on epithelial cells and the lack of Stx (reviewed in references 62 and 108). The A/E phenotype can be detected by tissue culture cell assays or by DNA probe or PCR tests for the *eae* gene, encoding intimin, or the LEE pathogenicity island. The EAF plasmid of typical EPEC (see above) is detected by use of fragment or oligonucleotide probes or PCR primers (139). Atypical EPEC strains possess only the A/E phenotype (LEE pathogenicity island) but do not possess the EAF plasmid.

EAEC. Several simple assays have been described as surrogates for the cell adherence test for identification of EAEC. These include a simple biofilm formation assay on polystyrene (215) and screening for the presence of a pellicle at the surface of broth media (6). EAEC can be identified more definitively by use of a specific DNA probe (the AA or CVD432 probe) (16), which is superior to tissue culture adherence assays for identifying pathogenic strains of EAEC (53). More recent data suggest that the AA probe corresponds to a putative virulence gene called *aatA* (143), which is under the control of a regulator termed AggR. AggR, in turn, controls several other virulence factors (174). Thus, the *aggR* gene (which defines typical EAEC) may represent a superior diagnostic target.

EIEC. EIEC can be identified by various in vivo assays, immunoassays, and nucleic acid-based assays for invasiveness, but no commercial kits or reagents are available. Cell culture invasion assays or DNA-based assays for the *ipaC* or *ipaH* invasion-related factors are, for the most part, practical only in research settings (139). Plasmid DNA electrophoresis may be used to detect the large 120- to 140-MDa plasmid associated with invasiveness, but this plasmid is easily lost when the isolate is subcultured. Because of shared invasiveness-related characteristics, these assays also detect *Shigella* strains.

DAEC. DAEC strains were initially defined on the basis of a diffuse adherence pattern to cultured epithelial cells,

but this phenotype is not specific for enteric strains (180). Various DNA probes and PCR assays have been proposed for DAEC identification, as reviewed previously (139).

Typing Systems

Several methods for subtyping have been used for *E. coli* O157:H7 isolates. In particular, pulsed-field gel electrophoresis (PFGE) methods and multilocus variable-number tandem-repeat analysis methods are useful (102, 139). A national molecular subtyping network, PulseNet, was established in 1996 by the CDC to facilitate subtyping of bacterial food-borne pathogens, including *E. coli* O157:H7, *Shigella,* nontyphoidal *Salmonella* serotypes, and *Listeria monocytogenes* (192). Successful detection of outbreaks by this network of state and local public health laboratories is dependent upon submission of isolates by clinical laboratories for confirmation and subtyping.

Determination of the serotype and the antimicrobial susceptibility pattern is usually adequate for defining outbreak strains of ETEC, EPEC, and EIEC. Plasmid typing or PFGE methods may also be helpful for distinguishing between sporadic isolates and outbreak strains, but neither method has been used widely for these groups of *E. coli.*

Serodiagnostic Tests

At present, serodiagnostic tests for diarrheagenic *E. coli* are valuable only for seroepidemiology surveys and are not useful for the diagnosis of sporadic infections. Assays that measure serum antibody responses to LPS have been used to detect STEC infection in culture-negative HUS patients (139). Enzyme-linked immunosorbent assays have been described to detect saliva antibodies to LPS (124) and serum antibodies to the secreted EspB protein in HUS patients (183).

Antimicrobial Susceptibilities

Extraintestinal *E. coli*

In *E. coli* and other *Enterobacteriaceae,* extended-spectrum β-lactamases (ESBLs) are an important cause of antimicrobial resistance. In the past 20 years, CTX-M β-lactamases and AmpC β-lactamases have emerged. CTX-M-producing *E. coli* strains are often isolated from urinary tract infections, both health care and community acquired, and have also been detected in retail meat samples in the United States (61). AmpC β-lactamases are problematic for clinical laboratories because these enzymes can interfere with β-lactamase ESBL confirmatory tests, resulting in a false report of cephalosporin susceptibility. Carbapenemases are β-lactamases that confer resistance to the carbapenems, and the *Klebsiella pneumoniae* carbapenemase (KPC) is the most frequently encountered enzyme of this class in *E. coli* and other carbapenem-resistant *Enterobacteriaceae.* It is important to detect KPC and other carbapenemases in patients colonized with carbapenem-resistant *Enterobacteriaceae* so that isolation precautions may be instituted to prevent transmission in health care settings (7).

In January 2010, the Clinical and Laboratory Standards Institute (CLSI) published new interpretive criteria for phenotypically assessing the susceptibility of the *Enterobacteriaceae* to the cephalosporins and aztreonam (51). Under the new guidelines, lower breakpoints will be used, thereby eliminating the need to perform routine ESBL tests and to edit the results on reports from susceptible to resistant for cephalosporins, aztreonam, or penicillins. No reduction in breakpoints was proposed for cefepime and cefuroxime (parenteral).

The CLSI suggests that routine antimicrobial susceptibility testing (AST) for *Enterobacteriaceae* include ampicillin, cefazolin (MIC only), gentamicin, and tobramycin testing.

It is noted that *E. coli* and other *Enterobacteriaceae* strains resistant to certain cephalosporins may produce a carbapenemase despite having AST values which fall in the susceptible range. Screening tests such as the modified Hodge test should be performed. Urinary isolates of *E. coli* may be tested against fosfomycin and other drugs used only for urinary tract infections. Current automated susceptibility test systems may not be able to accurately detect ESBLs, AmpCs, and KPCs (75, 173).

Diarrheagenic *E. coli*

STEC

Antimicrobial therapy for O157 STEC diarrhea or HUS is controversial: some publications have suggested that antibiotics increase the risk of HUS (84, 212), while a meta-analysis of published reports found no significantly increased risk (172). There is a lack of evidence to support routine antimicrobial susceptibility testing of STEC strains.

Until recently, *E. coli* O157:H7 isolates were almost uniformly susceptible to antimicrobial agents. However, since the early 1990s, O157 and other STEC strains have demonstrated slowly increasing levels of resistance to certain antibiotics, particularly streptomycin, sulfonamides, and tetracycline (http://www.cdc.gov/narms/).

ETEC, EPEC, EAEC, and EIEC Strains and Other Diarrheagenic *E. coli* Strains

Treatment with an appropriate antibiotic can reduce the severity and duration of symptoms of ETEC infection (139). Antimicrobial resistance, particularly to tetracycline, is common among ETEC strains isolated from outbreaks in the United States (54). Antibiotic treatment may be helpful for diarrhea caused by EPEC (139). Most EPEC strains associated with outbreaks are resistant to multiple antimicrobial agents (62). EAEC strains are commonly resistant to most antibiotics, though these strains are typically susceptible to fluoroquinolones. Clinical studies have demonstrated the effectiveness of ciprofloxacin for travelers with diarrhea caused by EAEC (81). Little information about the efficacy of antimicrobial treatment or the prevalence of resistance is available for EIEC or other putative diarrheagenic *E. coli* strains, but determination of the antimicrobial susceptibility pattern may be helpful in establishing whether the isolates are associated with an outbreak.

Evaluation, Interpretation, and Reporting of Results

Extraintestinal *E. coli*

The final written report should include the final Gram stain result, the final identification as *E. coli*, and the antimicrobial susceptibility test results.

Diarrheagenic *E. coli*

STEC

A presumptive diagnosis of an O157 STEC (isolate positive for O157 antigen) or a non-O157 STEC (isolate positive for Shiga toxin) infection should be reported to the clinician as soon as the laboratory obtains this result. When O157 is not found in a specimen, it is advisable to include a comment on reports stating that non-O157 STEC strains can cause diarrhea and HUS. Cases of STEC infection and HUS should be reported to public health authorities. Presumptive STEC isolates should be confirmed by demonstration of the O157 and H7 antigens or by assay for Shiga toxin and should be identified phenotypically as *E. coli*. STEC isolates should

be forwarded to a local or state public health laboratory for serotyping and/or molecular subtyping.

ETEC, EPEC, EAEC, and EIEC Strains

Generally, the ETEC, EPEC, EAEC, and EIEC classes of diarrheagenic *E. coli* are identified only during outbreak investigations. A laboratory reporting these results, which usually will be a retrospective diagnosis obtained by a reference laboratory, should provide an explanation of the clinical significance of these organisms and may refer the clinician to the reference laboratory for further information. All suspected outbreaks should be reported to public health authorities.

SHIGELLA

Taxonomy

Shigella is classified in the family *Enterobacteriaceae*, which is addressed in chapter 37 of this *Manual* (32, 66). There are four subgroups of *Shigella* that historically have been treated as species, as follows: subgroup A as *S. dysenteriae*, subgroup B as *Shigella flexneri*, subgroup C as *S. boydii*, and subgroup D as *Shigella sonnei*. From a genetic standpoint, the four species of *Shigella*, with the exception of *S. boydii* 13, and *E. coli* represent a single genomospecies (30, 31, 115). Using a genetic definition for species, the four species of *Shigella* would be regarded as serologically defined anaerogenic biotypes of *E. coli*. The current nomenclature for *Shigella* organisms is maintained largely for medical purposes because of the useful association of the genus epithet with the distinctive disease (shigellosis) caused by these organisms. The G+C content of the DNA is 49 to 53 mol%, and the type species for the genus is *S. dysenteriae* (Shiga 1898) (39).

S. boydii 13 strains were first described in 1952 and then added to the *Shigella* scheme in 1958 (69). Early findings from DNA-DNA hybridization showed that these strains represent a new species (30); however, it was not until recently that findings from phylogenetic studies showed that they cluster in a neighbor-joining tree with *E. albertii*, a newly described species of *Escherichia* associated with diarrheal disease in Bangladeshi children (100, 101).

Description of the Genus

The genus *Shigella* is composed of nonmotile bacteria that conform to the definition of the family *Enterobacteriaceae* (66, 188). Species in this genus are gram-negative rods which grow well on MAC. All strains of *Shigella* spp. are nonmotile, do not decarboxylate lysine, do not utilize citrate, malonate, or sodium acetate (with exceptions for *S. flexneri*), and do not grow in KCN or produce H_2S. Compared with *Escherichia*, *Shigella* strains are less active in their use of carbohydrates (Table 4). All ferment D-glucose without the production of gas (a few exceptions produce gas, e.g., certain strains of *S. flexneri* serotype 6 and *S. boydii* serotype 14). *S. sonnei* strains ferment lactose and sucrose on extended incubation, but other species generally do not use these substrates in conventional medium. Salicin, adonitol, and *myo*-inositol are not fermented. There are numerous identical and reciprocal serologic reactions between *Shigella* and *E. coli* (67).

Epidemiology and Transmission

Humans and other large primates are the only natural reservoirs of *Shigella* bacteria. Most transmission is by person-to-person spread, but infection is also caused by ingestion of contaminated food or water. Shigellosis is most common in situations where hygiene is compromised (e.g., child care centers and other institutional settings). In developing populations

TABLE 4 Differentiation of *E. coli* and *Shigella*

Result[a] of test with:	Test					
	Lysine decarboxylase	Motility	Gas from glucose	Acetate utilization	Mucate	Lactose
Shigella	−	−	−	−	−	−
Inactive *E. coli*[b]	d	−	−	d	d	d
E. coli	+	+	+	+	+	+

[a]Abbreviations: +, 90% or more positive within or 2 days; −, no reaction (90% or more) in 7 days; d, different reactions [+, (+), +]. Adapted from Ewing (66).
[b]Nonmotile, anaerogenic biotypes sometimes referred to as Alkalescens-Dispar bioserotypes.

without running water and indoor plumbing, shigellosis can become endemic. Sexual transmission of *Shigella* among men who have sex with men also occurs.

In the United States, an estimated 450,000 cases of shigellosis occur each year, with 70 deaths (133). Up to 20% of all U.S. cases of shigellosis are related to international travel. Most infections in the United States and other developed countries are caused by *S. sonnei*; *S. flexneri* is the second most common subgroup (http://www.cdc.gov/nationalsurveillance/ shigella_surveillance.html). In the developing world, the majority of endemic dysentery cases are caused by *S. flexneri*, with the balance of cases caused by subgroups that vary temporally and geographically (35, 114, 205). Epidemic dysentery is most commonly caused by *S. dysenteriae* 1, whose prevalence rises dramatically during outbreak periods and then falls as the epidemic resolves. Infection with *S. dysenteriae* 1 is associated with high rates of morbidity and mortality in developing countries, particularly when antimicrobial resistance or misdiagnosis delays appropriate treatment. In the United States and other developed countries, *S. sonnei* is endemic and causes large, protracted outbreaks in day care centers (9, 40, 43) and among men who have sex with men (45, 55). The protracted nature of these outbreaks is attributed to a large number of asymptomatically infected individuals in the population and the tendency for secondary spread (88). Most *S. sonnei* strains in the United States have developed resistance to ampicillin and trimethoprim-sulfamethoxazole (55). For most individuals, antibiotic treatment reduces the number of symptomatic days and the length of shedding (123). Resistance to ampicillin and trimethoprim-sulfamethoxazole is common. If resistance to these antibiotics is present, treatment with azithromycin or ciprofloxacin has been effective. To limit the development of resistance, some health care providers treat only the most severe infections.

Clinical Significance

Members of the genus *Shigella* have been recognized since the late 19th century as causative agents of bacillary dysentery. *Shigella* causes bloody diarrhea (dysentery) and nonbloody diarrhea. Shigellosis often begins with watery diarrhea accompanied by fever and abdominal cramps but may progress to classic dysentery with scant stools containing blood, mucus, and pus. Ulcerations, which are restricted to the large intestine and rectum, typically do not penetrate beyond the lamina propria. Bloodstream infections can occur but are rare. Appropriate antimicrobial therapy will decrease the duration, transmission, and severity of symptoms and should be prescribed based on the severity of illness or the need to protect close contacts. Patients in certain occupations (i.e., food handlers, child care providers, and health care workers) and children who attend child care often are required to have a documented negative stool culture following treatment. The infectious dose is low

(1 to 100 organisms), and the incubation period is 1 to 4 days. Shigellae are shed in stool for several days to several weeks after illness, and persons who receive appropriate antimicrobial therapy will be culture negative at 72 h (123). All four subgroups of *Shigella* are capable of causing dysentery, but *S. dysenteriae* serotype 1 has been associated with a particularly severe form of illness thought to be related in part to its production of Shiga toxin. Infection can occasionally be asymptomatic, particularly infection with *S. sonnei* strains. Complications of shigellosis include HUS, which is associated with *S. dysenteriae* 1 infection, and reactive arthritis or Reiter's chronic arthritis syndrome, which is associated with *S. flexneri* infection (3). The identification of *Shigella* species is important for both clinical and epidemiologic purposes.

Collection, Transport, and Storage of Specimens
See "Collection, Transport, and Storage of Specimens" in the *Escherichia* section.

Direct Examination

Microscopy
Shigella cannot readily be distinguished from other gram-negative rods by staining or microscopy methods.

Antigen Detection
Because there is no single somatic antigen common to all *Shigella* strains, antigen detection in clinical specimens is not practical and has not been validated, and no commercial FDA-approved kits are available.

Nucleic Acid Detection
There are no FDA-approved nucleic acid detection methods for clinical diagnosis of *Shigella* infections.

Isolation Procedures

Enrichment and Plating Media
There is no reliable enrichment medium for all *Shigella* isolates, but gram-negative broth and Selenite broth (SEL) are frequently used. For the optimal isolation of *Shigella*, two different selective media should be used: a general purpose plating medium of low selectivity (e.g., MAC) and a more selective agar medium (e.g., xylose-lysine-deoxycholate agar [XLD]). Deoxycholate citrate agar and Hektoen enteric agar (HE) are suitable alternatives to XLD as media with moderate to high selectivities. Salmonella-shigella agar should be used with caution because it inhibits the growth of some strains of *S. dysenteriae* 1.

Screening Procedures
Shigella strains appear as lactose- or xylose-nonfermenting colonies on the isolation media described above. *S. dysenteriae*

1 colonies may be smaller on all of these media, and these strains generally grow best on media with low selectivities (e.g., MAC). *S. dysenteriae* 1 colonies on XLD agar are frequently very tiny, unlike those of other *Shigella* species. *S. sonnei* colonies often appear flattened and spread out on blood agar plates.

Suspect colonies may be screened phenotypically on Kligler iron agar (KIA) or triple sugar iron agar (TSI). *Shigella* species characteristically produce an alkaline slant because strains do not ferment lactose (or sucrose) but do not produce gas or H_2S. A few strains of *S. flexneri* 6 and very few strains of *S. boydii* produce gas in KIA or TSI. Motility and lysine decarboxylase tests are characteristically negative for *Shigella* and can be used to further screen isolates before serologic testing (Table 4). Isolates that react appropriately with the screening tests should then be identified with a complete set of phenotypic tests, with automated systems or self-contained commercial kits being satisfactory, and should be tested with grouping antisera. Confirmation requires both phenotypic and serologic identification, and laboratories that do not perform both types of tests should send *Shigella* isolates to a reference laboratory for confirmation.

Identification

Phenotypic Identification

Because the somatic antigens of most serotypes of *Shigella* are either identical or related to those of *E. coli*, suspicious cultures that are serologically negative should be tested further phenotypically (66). *Shigella* and inactive *E. coli* (anaerogenic or lactose-nonfermenting) strains are frequently difficult to distinguish by routine phenotypic tests. See Table 4 for the phenotypic reactions characteristic of *Shigella* spp. Although *S. dysenteriae* and *S. sonnei* are phenotypically distinct, *S. flexneri* and *S. boydii* are often phenotypically indistinguishable, so serologic grouping is essential.

Serotyping

Serotyping is essential for the identification of *Shigella*. Three of the four subgroups, A (*S. dysenteriae*), B (*S. flexneri*), and C (*S. boydii*), are made up of a number of serotypes. Subgroup A has 15 serotypes; subgroup B has 8 serotypes (with serotypes 1 to 5 subdivided into 11 subserotypes); and subgroup C has 19 serotypes, numbered 1 through 20, with *S. boydii* 13 reclassified as *E. albertii*. Subgroup D (*S. sonnei*) is made up of a single serotype. Subgroups A and C are rare. Several provisional *Shigella* serotypes have also been described, which are held sub judice until findings from the characterization of representative isolates show them to be unique and of sufficient prevalence to merit inclusion in the *Shigella* scheme. Antisera for the identification of provisional serotypes are typically available only at reference laboratories.

Serotyping is typically performed by slide agglutination with polyvalent somatic (O) antigen grouping sera, followed, in some cases, by testing with monovalent antisera for specific serotype identification. Monovalent antiserum to *S. dysenteriae* 1 is required to identify this serotype and is not widely available. Because of the potentially serious nature of illness associated with this serotype, isolates that agglutinate in subgroup A reagent should be sent to a reference laboratory immediately for further serotyping.

Phenotypically typical *Shigella* isolates that agglutinate poorly or that do not agglutinate at all should be suspended in saline and heated in a water bath at 100°C for 15 to 30 min. After cooling, the antigen suspension should be tested in normal saline to determine if it is rough (agglutinates

spontaneously). If the heated and cooled suspension is not rough, it may then be retested for agglutination in antisera.

Typing Systems

A variety of methods have been used to subtype *Shigella*, including colicin typing (particularly for *S. sonnei*), plasmid profiling, restriction fragment length polymorphism analysis, PFGE, and ribotyping (189). For an overview of the epidemiologic use of typing methods, see chapter 8.

Serodiagnostic Tests

Several serodiagnostic assays based on different antigens possessed by *Shigella* have been described (121, 202). These assays are practical only in research settings for seroepidemiology surveys and are not currently used for the diagnosis of infection in individual patients.

Antimicrobial Susceptibilities

Shigella infections are often treated with antimicrobial agents. Because of the widespread antimicrobial resistance among *Shigella* strains, all isolates should undergo susceptibility testing (http://www.cdc.gov/narms/). Because of widespread resistance in the United States, ampicillin and trimethoprim-sulfamethoxazole, two safe drugs that were the most commonly prescribed for treatment of children with *S. sonnei* infections, are no longer options for empiric treatment. Macrolides, in particular azithromycin, are being used to treat these infections, but there are no interpretive criteria for AST for *Shigella*, making it problematic to monitor for development of resistance (9).

Fecal isolates of *Shigella* should be tested against ampicillin, a fluoroquinolone, and trimethoprim-sulfamethoxazole. Strains may produce susceptible AST results for fluoroquinolones, but if they are resistant to nalidixic acid, treatment with a fluoroquinolone may result in a delayed clinical response or treatment failure. *Shigella* should not be reported as susceptible to narrow-spectrum and expanded-spectrum cephalosporins and cephamycins or to aminoglycosides and N1-substituted aminoglycosides because these drugs are not effective clinically.

Reporting of susceptibility results to the clinician is particularly important for *S. dysenteriae* 1 isolates. Infections caused by these strains are often acquired during international travel to areas where most strains are multidrug resistant (197). In many areas of Africa and Asia, *S. dysenteriae* 1 strains are resistant to all locally available antimicrobial agents, including nalidixic acid, but are still susceptible to the fluoroquinolones (35, 171); however, fluoroquinolone-resistant strains have been reported in Asia (114, 194, 195).

Evaluation, Interpretation, and Reporting of Results

A preliminary report of suspected *Shigella* infection may be issued if phenotypic or serologic screening tests are positive. If serotyping results are available, these should also be reported, particularly if the isolate is *S. dysenteriae* 1. All *Shigella* isolates should be tested for antimicrobial susceptibility. Before issuing a final report, isolates should be confirmed by both serologic and phenotypic methods. Isolates, particularly those from individuals with dysentery-like illness, that are phenotypically identified as *Shigella* but that are serologically negative may be new serotypes of *Shigella* and should be sent to a reference laboratory for further characterization. Isolates from sites other than the gastrointestinal tract which resemble *Shigella* should be scrutinized carefully for gas production and other differentiating characteristics because extraintestinal *Shigella* infections are rare. These isolates should be sent to a reference laboratory for confirmation because they are more likely to be anaerogenic *E. coli*, certain strains of which may cross-react with *Shigella* antiserum.

SALMONELLA

Taxonomy

Members of the genus *Salmonella* are classified in the family *Enterobacteriaceae* (32, 66). Species of this genus are motile, gram-negative, facultative rods. Salmonellae are typically defined by their ability to use citrate as a sole carbon source and lysine as a nitrogen source and by the production of H$_2$S on triple sugar agar; exceptions to these traits are used to define specific serotypes (66, 158).

The genus *Salmonella* is composed of two species, *Salmonella enterica* and *Salmonella bongori* (169). *S. enterica* is subdivided into six subspecies: *S. enterica* subsp. *enterica*, often called subspecies I; *S. enterica* subsp. *salamae*, or subspecies II; *S. enterica* subsp. *arizonae*, or subspecies IIIa; *S. enterica* subsp. *diarizonae*, or subspecies IIIb; *S. enterica* subsp. *houtenae*, or subspecies IV; and *S. enterica* subsp. *indica*, or subspecies VI. The type species is *S. enterica* subsp. *enterica*. Subspecies IIIa and IIIb represent organisms originally described in the genus "*Arizona*"; subspecies IIIa contains the monophasic strains, and subspecies IIIb contains the diphasic strains of "*Arizona*" (170). Despite their common history, subspecies IIIa and IIIb are more closely related to some of the other subspecies of *S. enterica* than they are to each other and thus should be considered separate entities (211).

Genome analysis of salmonellae has revealed a high degree of genetic variability. Serotypes within *S. enterica* subspecies I have been shown to differ by as much as 10% in their gene content (i.e., presence or absence of whole genes) (64, 159). Recombination, particularly among strains of *S. enterica* subspecies I, likely contributes to this diversity (116). Whole-genome sequence analysis of many common serotypes, including serotypes with unique virulence properties, such as *S. enterica* serotypes Typhi, Paratyphi A, and Choleraesuis, have been reported and continue to expand our understanding of the pathogenesis and evolutionary history of *Salmonella* (14, 48, 97, 122, 131).

Description of the Genus

Subspecies I strains are commonly isolated from humans and warm-blooded animals. Subspecies II, IIIa, IIIb, IV, and VI strains and *S. bongori* are usually isolated from cold-blooded animals and the environment. Non-subspecies I strains are typically considered rare human pathogens; they make up about 1 to 2% of *Salmonella* isolates reported to the U.S. National *Salmonella* Surveillance System (http://www.cdc .gov/nationalsurveillance/salmonella_surveillance.html). The phenotypic tests useful for identification of *Salmonella* and for subspecies differentiation are given in Table 5.

The nomenclature employed to describe the genus *Salmonella* was problematic for many years due to the use of multiple schemes in the literature and the historical practice of considering different serotypes of *Salmonella* to be different species. The publication of Judicial Opinion 80 in the *International Journal of Systematic and Evolutionary Microbiology* in 2005 (199) hopefully served to clarify nomenclatural issues regarding the genus *Salmonella*, and the conventions set forth in that opinion are used here. *Salmonella* history and nomenclature are reviewed at http://www.bacterio.cict.fr/s/salmonella.html.

Epidemiology and Transmission

Salmonella organisms are isolated most frequently from the intestines of humans and animals. Some serotypes are isolated only from humans (e.g., *Salmonella* serotype Typhi), while others (e.g., *Salmonella* serotype Gallinarum and *Salmonella* serotype IV 48:g,z51:− [formerly serotype Marina]) are strongly associated with certain animal hosts. Members of this genus can be isolated from feces-contaminated foods or water but probably do not occur as free-living organisms in the environment. Historically, *Salmonella* has been considered a pathogen of meat and poultry products but has recently been associated with other food vehicles, such as fresh produce and manufactured products (90).

TABLE 5 Phenotypic reactions useful for differentiating *Salmonella* species and subspecies[a]

Species or subspecies (no. of strains tested)	Dulcitol	Lactose	ONPG	Salicin	Sorbitol	Galacturonate	Malonate	Mucate	Growth in KCN	Gelatin (strip)	L(+)-Tartrate (d-tartrate[j])
S. enterica I (650)	+	−	−	−	+	−	−	+	−	−	+
S. enterica II (146)	+	−	−[f]	−	+	+	+	+	−	+	−
S. enterica IIIa (120)	−	−[c]	−	−	+	−	+	+	−	+	−
S. enterica IIIb (155)	−	−[d]	−	−	+	+	+	−[i]	−	+	−
S. enterica IV (120)	−	−	−	+[h]	+	+	−	−	+	+	−
S. enterica VI (9)	d[b]	d[e]	d[g]	−	−	+	−	+	−	+	−
S. bongori (16)	+	−	+	−	+	+	−	+	+	−	−

[a]Reactions after incubation at 37°C. +, 90% (or more) of stains were positive within 1 or 2 days; (+), positive reaction after 3 or more days; −, no reaction (90% or more) in 7 days; d, different reactions [+, (+), −]; KCN, potassium cyanide; ONPG, o-nitrophenyl-β-D-galactopyranoside. (Adapted from reference 66 with permission of the publisher.)
[b]A total of 67% were positive.
[c]A total of 15% were positive.
[d]A total of 85% were positive.
[e]A total of 22% were positive.
[f]A total of 15% were positive.
[g]A total of 44% were positive.
[h]A total of 60% were positive.
[i]A total of 30% were positive.
[j]Sodium potassium tartrate (66).

Salmonella Serotypes

Salmonella serotyping is a subtyping method based on the immunologic characterization of three surface structures: the O antigen, which is the outermost portion of the LPS layer that covers the bacterial cell; the H antigen, which is the filament portion of the bacterial flagella; and the Vi antigen, which is a capsular polysaccharide present in specific serotypes. Serotyping of *Salmonella* is commonly performed to facilitate public health surveillance of *Salmonella* infections and to aid in the recognition of outbreaks. The serotype of an isolate often correlates with a particular disease syndrome or food vehicle, making serotype data particularly useful in identifying cases and defining outbreaks. For example, *Salmonella* serotype Typhi causes typhoid fever, a more severe disease syndrome than those caZused by most other *Salmonella* serotypes. *Salmonella* serotype Enteritidis is often associated with infections acquired from chicken or egg products (154). Furthermore, *Salmonella* serotyping is performed worldwide and has aided in the recognition of international outbreaks (126). *Salmonella* serotypes Enteritidis and Typhimurium are the two most common serotypes in the United States, making up approximately 35 to 40% of all culture-confirmed infections (http://www.cdc.gov/nationalsurveillance/salmonella_surveillance.html).

Clinical Significance

Strains of *Salmonella* are categorized as typhoidal and nontyphoidal, corresponding to the disease syndrome with which they are associated. Strains of nontyphoidal *Salmonella* usually cause intestinal infections (accompanied by diarrhea, fever, and abdominal cramps) that often last 1 week or longer (96). Less commonly, nontyphoidal *Salmonella* can cause extraintestinal infections (e.g., bacteremia, urinary tract infection, or osteomyelitis), especially in immunocompromised persons. Persons of all ages are affected, but the incidence is highest in infants and young children. *Salmonella* is ubiquitous in animal populations, and human illness is usually linked to foods. Salmonellosis is also transmitted by direct contact with animals, by water, and occasionally by human contact. Each year, an estimated 1.4 million cases of illness and 600 deaths are caused by nontyphoidal salmonellosis in the United States (133).

Typhoid fever, caused by *Salmonella* serotype Typhi, is a serious bloodstream infection common in the developing world. However, it is rare in the United States, where an estimated 800 cases, with fewer than 5 deaths, occur each year; >70% of U.S. cases are related to foreign travel (133). Typhoid fever typically presents with a sustained debilitating high fever and headache. Adults characteristically present without diarrhea. Illness is milder in young children, where it may manifest as nonspecific fever. Humans are the only reservoir for *Salmonella* serotype Typhi, indicating that this serotype is adapted to the human host. Healthy carriers have been noted. Typhoid fever typically has a low infectious dose ($<10^3$ organisms) and a long, highly variable incubation period (1 to 6 weeks). It is transmitted through person-to-person contact or feces-contaminated food and water. Fatal complications of typhoid most commonly occur in the second or third week of illness.

A syndrome similar to typhoid fever is caused by "paratyphoidal" strains of *Salmonella*, i.e., *Salmonella* serotypes Paratyphi A, Paratyphi B, and Paratyphi C. *Salmonella* serotypes Paratyphi A and Paratyphi C are rare in the United States (http://www.cdc.gov/nationalsurveillance/salmonella_surveillance.html). *Salmonella* serotype Paratyphi B is a diverse serotype that is associated with both paratyphoid fever

and gastroenteritis (161). The two pathovars are typically differentiated on the basis of the ability to ferment tartrate; isolates causing paratyphoid fever, the systemic pathovar, are tartrate negative. Isolates associated with gastroenteritis, the enteric pathovar, are typically tartrate positive and are referred to as *Salmonella* serotype Paratyphi B variant L(+)-tartrate + or *Salmonella* serotype Paratyphi B variant Java. The systemic pathovar of *Salmonella* serotype Paratyphi B is considered rare in the United States; however, the tartrate reaction is often not reported, making it impossible to distinguish between the two pathovars (http://www.cdc.gov/nationalsurveillance/salmonella_surveillance.html).

Salmonella serotypes Choleraesuis and Dublin are host adapted to pigs and cattle, respectively, causing serious disease in these two animal species. They rarely cause human infection, but such infections are typically severe, with spread to extraintestinal sites (128, 206). *Salmonella* serotype Dublin has been shown to share virulence traits with *Salmonella* serotype Typhi, which may contribute to its invasiveness in humans (136, 156).

Collection, Transport, and Storage of Specimens

See "Collection, Transport, and Storage of Specimens" in the *Escherichia* section.

Direct Examination

Microscopy

Salmonella cannot be distinguished from other gram-negative rods by microscopy or staining methods. There are no FDA-approved methods for direct examination of clinical specimens for *Salmonella*.

Antigen Detection

A number of commercial rapid diagnostic tests are available for the testing of foods, but to our knowledge, none has been evaluated in the literature for use with fecal specimens, and none are FDA approved for clinical specimens.

Nucleic Acid Detection

There are no FDA-approved methods for nucleic acid detection of *Salmonella* in clinical specimens.

Isolation Procedures

Enrichment

Maximal recovery of *Salmonella* from fecal specimens is obtained by using an enrichment broth, although isolation from acutely ill persons is usually possible by direct plating of specimens. Enrichment broths for *Salmonella* are usually highly selective and inhibit certain serotypes of *Salmonella*, particularly *Salmonella* serotype Typhi. The selective enrichment medium most widely used to isolate *Salmonella* from fecal specimens is SEL. SEL may also be used for the recovery of *Salmonella* serotype Typhi and for *Shigella*, although its value as enrichment for the latter has not been clearly established. Specimens which might contain organisms inhibited by selective enrichment medium should be plated directly or cultured in a nonselective enrichment broth (e.g., gram-negative broth).

Plating Media

Many differential plating media, varying from slightly selective to highly selective, are available for isolation of *Salmonella* from fecal specimens. Media of low selectivity include MAC and eosin-methylene blue. Media of intermediate selectivity include XLD, deoxycholate citrate agar, salmonella-shigella agar, and HE. Highly selective media include bismuth sulfite agar, the preferred medium for the isolation of *Salmonella* serotype Typhi, and brilliant green agar. Bismuth sulfite agar, XLD, and HE all have H$_2$S indicator systems, which are helpful for the detection of lactose-fermenting *Salmonella* strains. Many laboratories use HE or XLD because these media may also be used for the isolation of *Shigella*.

In the developing world, typhoid fever is frequently diagnosed solely on clinical grounds, but isolation of the causative organism is necessary for a definitive diagnosis. *Salmonella* serotype Typhi is isolated more frequently from blood cultures than from fecal specimens. Blood cultures are positive for 80% of typhoid patients during the first week of fever but show decreasing positive results thereafter.

Screening Procedures

A latex agglutination kit has been described for *Salmonella* screening in SEL enrichment broth (Wellcolex Color *Salmonella*; Remel Inc., Lenexa, KS) (28). This kit can also be used to screen individual colonies from primary plates. In using this kit, it should be kept in mind that it identifies only those *Salmonella* isolates belonging to the more common O serogroups and does not differentiate between O groups C$_1$ (O:7) and C$_2$ (O:8).

Suspect colonies may be inoculated onto a screening medium such as KIA or TSI. On KIA or TSI, most *Salmonella* strains produce an alkaline slant, indicating that only glucose is fermented, with gas and H$_2$S. On these media, *Salmonella* serotype Typhi isolates characteristically produce an alkaline slant but do not produce gas, and only a small amount of H$_2$S will be visible at the site of the stab and in the stab line. Lysine iron agar is also a useful screening medium because most *Salmonella* isolates, even those which ferment lactose, decarboxylate lysine and produce H$_2$S. Alternately, isolates may be identified by a battery of phenotypic tests or by slide agglutination with antisera for *Salmonella* O groups. Isolates suspected of being *Salmonella* serotype Typhi should be tested serologically with *Salmonella* Vi and O group D antisera (see below).

If the phenotypic traits for a particular isolate are not characteristic of *Salmonella* but *Salmonella* antigens are found, the cultures should be plated to obtain a pure culture, tested with a complete set of phenotypic tests, or forwarded to a reference laboratory.

Identification

Clinical laboratories may issue a preliminary report of *Salmonella* when an isolate is positive either with *Salmonella* O group antisera or by phenotypic identification methods. An isolate is confirmed as *Salmonella* when the specific O serogroup has been determined and phenotypic identification has been completed.

Phenotypic Identification

Suspect colonies from one of the differential plating media mentioned above can be identified phenotypically as *Salmonella* spp. by use of traditional media in tubes or commercial biochemical systems. Methods for phenotypic identification and specific commercial manual and automated identification systems are covered in chapter 3. The species and subspecies of *Salmonella* can be identified phenotypically, as indicated in Table 5. However, *Salmonella* is a diverse group, and phenotypically atypical strains are not uncommon. Phenotypic identification is commonly combined with serogrouping or serotyping for culture confirmation.

Serogrouping and Serotyping

O serogroup determination is adequate for confirmation of isolates as *Salmonella*. Full serotype determination is useful for public health surveillance but is beyond the scope of most routine clinical laboratories. The methods for serotyping described below are intended primarily for reference laboratories. *Salmonella* isolates are serotyped on the basis of the antigenic properties of their O (somatic) antigens, H (flagellar) antigens, and Vi (capsular) antigens (34, 85). O antigen is a carbohydrate antigen and is the outermost component of LPS. It is a polymer of O subunits; each O subunit is typically composed of four to six sugars, depending on the O antigen. O antigens are designated by numbers and are divided into O serogroups based on antigenic factors associated with the O subunit. Many of the common O groups were originally designated by letter and are still commonly referred to by letter (e.g., *Salmonella* serotype Typhimurium belongs to group O:4 or group B, and *Salmonella* serotype Enteritidis belongs to group O:9 or group D1). Additional O antigenic factors have been identified for specific O groups. They are typically associated with a side sugar that is added to the basic O subunit structure, and they are often variably present or variably expressed within O groups or within serotypes.

H antigen is a protein antigen called flagellin; multiple flagellin subunits make up the flagellar filament. The ends of flagellin are conserved and give the flagellum its characteristic filament structure. The antigenically variable portion of flagellin is the middle region, which is surface exposed. Salmonellae are unique among the enteric bacteria in that they commonly express two different flagellin antigens, although specific serotypes, such as *Salmonella* serotypes Typhi and Enteritidis, possess only one flagellar antigen. The two flagellar antigens are referred to as phase 1 and phase 2 antigens; monophasic and diphasic strains express one and two flagellar antigens, respectively. Individual flagellar antigens can be composed of multiple antigenic factors. For example, the phase 2 flagellar antigen of *Salmonella* serotype Typhimurium is antigen 1,2, which is composed of two antigenic factors, i.e., 1 and 2.

Serotypes are designated according to the conventions of the Kauffmann-White scheme (85). Many of the O and H antigenic types are found in multiple subspecies, and isolates from different subspecies can have the same antigenic profile. Thus, subspecies determination is an integral component of serotype determination for *Salmonella*. The serotypes for all *Salmonella* strains can be designated by antigenic formulae; additionally, serotypes belonging to subspecies I are given a name, which is typically related to the geographical place where the serotype was first isolated. The antigenic formulae of *Salmonella* serotypes are listed in the Kauffmann-White scheme and are expressed as follows: O antigen(s), Vi antigen (when present):phase 1 H antigen(s):phase 2 H antigen(s) (when present). For example, the antigenic formula for *Salmonella* serotype Typhimurium is 4,5,12:i:1,2. Serotype names for subspecies I serotypes are written in roman (not italicized) letters, and the first letter is a capital letter (for example, *Salmonella* serotype Typhimurium). Serotypes belonging to other subspecies are designated by their antigenic formulae following the subspecies name (for example, *S. enterica* subsp. *salamae* serotype 50:z:e,n,x or *Salmonella* serotype II 50:z:e,n,x).

The WHO Collaborating Centre for Reference and Research on *Salmonella*, which is located at the Pasteur Institute in Paris, France, maintains the Kauffmann-White scheme for the designation of *Salmonella* serotypes (85).

Most common serotypes belong to O groups A, B, C1, C2, D1, and E1 (also known as groups O:2, O:4, O:7; O:8; O:9, and O:3,10, respectively). Serotypes belonging to subspecies II (505 serotypes), IIIa (99 serotypes), IIIb (336 serotypes), IV (73 serotypes), and VI (13 serotypes) and to *S. bongori* (22 serotypes) are found primarily in O groups O:11 (F) through O:67 (commonly referred to as the higher O groups).

Determination of O Antigens

O (heat-stable, somatic) antigens are typically identified by first testing the isolate in antisera that detect one or multiple antigenic factors corresponding to the O groups (O grouping antisera). Once the O group is determined, antisera that recognize single antigenic factors are used to confirm the O group and to identify any additional antigenic factors that are associated with that O group (O single-factor antisera) (34). In the clinical laboratory, the approach most commonly used for determining O antigens is to initially test the isolates by slide agglutination in antisera against O groups A to E1 because approximately 95% of *Salmonella* isolates from human specimens belong to one of these O groups. If no agglutination occurs in antisera for these O groups, the isolate is tested in pools containing the remaining *Salmonella* O antisera, for groups O:11 through O:67.

Determination of H Antigens

H (flagellar) antigens are typically determined by tube or slide agglutination tests. Isolates are initially tested with H typing antisera, which recognize individual or multiple antigenic factors, and then with H single-factor antisera, which recognize individual antigenic factors. Typically, the flagellar antigens in a diphasic strain are coordinately regulated so that only one is expressed at a time in a single bacterial cell; however, both phases may be detected in the whole culture, particularly with a fresh clinical isolate. When only one phase is detected (either phase 1 or phase 2), the strain should be inoculated into a semisolid medium to which sterile antiserum to the detected flagellar antigen has been added aseptically. Growth of the strain in this semisolid agar immobilizes cells expressing the detected antigen and allows the movement of bacteria expressing the antigen in the other phase through the semisolid medium. Cells are recovered away from the area of initial inoculation, and the strain is tested in appropriate H typing and single-factor antisera to complete the serotyping. A strain must be actively motile to ensure the good expression of H antigens; sometimes a strain must be passed through one or more tall tubes of semisolid agar to enhance motility before H antigens can be detected.

Detection of the Vi Antigen and Identification of *Salmonella* Serotype Typhi (9,12,[Vi]:d:−)

The Vi antigen, a heat-labile capsular polysaccharide, is useful for the identification of *Salmonella* serotype Typhi. It is also occasionally detected in *Salmonella* serotype Dublin, *Salmonella* serotype Paratyphi C, and some *Citrobacter* strains, so its detection does not constitute definitive evidence of *Salmonella* serotype Typhi. The Vi antigen is identified by slide agglutination with a specific antiserum.

If *Salmonella* serotype Typhi is suspected, the culture is first tested live (unheated) in O group D antiserum (which contains antibodies to O antigens 9 and 12) and Vi antiserum on a slide. The Vi capsular polysaccharide can mask the O antigens, blocking their reactivity with the O grouping antiserum. If only the Vi antiserum is posi-

tive, the bacterial suspension is heated in boiling water for 15 min to remove the capsule, cooled, and tested again in the same antisera. After being heated, *Salmonella* serotype Typhi isolates will be negative in the Vi antiserum but positive in the O group D antiserum. Expression of the Vi antigen by *Salmonella* serotype Typhi is variable but tends to occur more frequently in freshly isolated cultures than in cultures that have been subcultured. If the strain is typical for *Salmonella* serotype Typhi on TSI or KIA (see "Screening Procedures" above), is urease negative, and reacts in O group D or Vi antiserum, a presumptive report is made. The identity of the isolate is typically confirmed by phenotypic testing (Table 5) and determination of the H (flagellar) antigen. However, because *Salmonella* serotype Typhi has a unique phenotypic profile, it can and should be reported based on phenotype alone (i.e., identification of the O and H antigens is not required in order to identify an isolate as *Salmonella* serotype Typhi).

Identification Problems

Several potential problems may prevent accurate serotype determination. The strain may express the Vi capsular antigen, which can block the binding of antibodies against the O antigens. The strain may be rough, i.e., fail to make complete O antigens. Rough strains have a tendency to weakly agglutinate in multiple O grouping antisera. The strain may be mucoid and not agglutinate in any O antisera, or isolates can be nonmotile and not express any flagellar antigens. Among isolates submitted to the National *Salmonella* Reference Laboratory at the CDC, isolates from urine are frequently rough, mucoid, and/or nonmotile. When O antigen and/or H antigen is not detected, a strain is confirmed as a *Salmonella* species by characterization of any antigens that are expressed and by phenotypic testing (Table 5).

Laboratories may overlook *Salmonella* serotype Paratyphi A because they do not screen with O group A antiserum or because its atypical phenotypic profile (H_2S negative, lysine negative, and citrate negative) can be confused with *E. coli*. *Salmonella* serotypes Paratyphi B and Paratyphi B variant L(+)-tartrate + (also known as variant Java) can be confused because they have the same antigenic formula (4,5,12:b:1,2), but they are distinguished phenotypically by their tartrate reactions. Similarly, *Salmonella* serotype Choleraesuis and *Salmonella* serotype Paratyphi C have the same antigenic formula (6,7:c:1,5) but are differentiated phenotypically. *Salmonella* serotype Paratyphi C may express the Vi antigen. *Citrobacter* and *E. coli* strains may possess O, H, or Vi antigens that are related to those of *Salmonella*; biochemical identification may be necessary to confirm that an isolate is *Salmonella* (see Table 5 in this chapter and Table 1 in chapter 31).

Typing Systems

For rarer serotypes, serotype identification may be all that is necessary to identify clusters of temporally related isolates. However, additional subtyping methods are typically required for more common serotypes (e.g., *Salmonella* serotypes Typhimurium, Enteritidis, and Newport). A variety of phenotypic and genotyping methods have been developed for subtyping within serotypes of *Salmonella* (141, 192). PFGE is the current method of choice for the subtyping of most *Salmonella* serotypes, since it is universally applicable and provides good strain discrimination for most serotypes. PulseNet, an international subtyping network that tracks *Salmonella*, is based on PFGE (192). *Salmonella* serotype Enteritidis has limited diversity in PFGE analysis; as a result, phage typing is still necessary to characterize strains, particularly in an outbreak setting (74, 154).

Serodiagnostic Tests

The Widal test, which measures agglutinating antibodies to the O and H antigens of *Salmonella* serotype Typhi, produces false-negative and false-positive reactions and does not provide a definitive diagnosis of individual cases of infection. Two other rapid serodiagnostic tests have proved more useful than the Widal test for the serodiagnosis of typhoid fever (148) (Tubex [IDL Biotech, Sollentuna, Sweden] and TyphiDot [Malaysian Bio-Diagnostics Research Sdn. Bhd., Kuala Lumpur, Malaysia]). These tests are most useful in areas where typhoid fever is endemic and are less useful in the United States, where typhoid fever is rare. Neither of these tests is FDA approved, and TyphiDot is not available in the United States.

Antimicrobial Susceptibilities

Antimicrobial therapy is not recommended for uncomplicated *Salmonella* gastroenteritis, and routine susceptibility testing of fecal isolates is not warranted for treatment purposes. However, determination of antimicrobial resistance patterns is often valuable for surveillance purposes and may be performed periodically to monitor the development and spread of antimicrobial resistance among *Salmonella* isolates.

Salmonella strains may produce susceptible AST results for fluoroquinolones, but if they are resistant to nalidixic acid, treatment with a fluoroquinolone may result in a delayed clinical response or treatment failure. For this reason, nalidixic acid, chloramphenicol, and a broad-spectrum cephalosporin should be tested and reported for extraintestinal isolates of *Salmonella*. *Salmonella* should not be reported as susceptible to narrow-spectrum and expanded-spectrum cephalosporins and cephamycins or to aminoglycosides and N1-substituted aminoglycosides because these drugs are not effective clinically.

In contrast to the case for uncomplicated salmonellosis, treatment with the appropriate antimicrobial agent can be crucial for patients with invasive *Salmonella* and typhoidal infections, and the susceptibilities of these isolates should be reported as soon as possible (117). Testing methods are detailed in chapter 68 in this *Manual*. The untreated case mortality rate for typhoid fever is >10%; when patients with typhoid fever are treated with appropriate antibiotics, the rate should be <1%. However, increasing levels of resistance to one or more antimicrobial agents in *Salmonella* isolates, particularly *Salmonella* serotype Typhi isolates, make selection of an appropriate antibiotic problematic. In particular, reduced susceptibilities to ciprofloxacin among *Salmonella* serotype Typhi isolates and increasing numbers of treatment failures are of concern (107, 164).

Antimicrobial resistance, particularly multiple-drug resistance, has been noted in several nontyphoidal serotypes of *Salmonella*. A strain of *Salmonella* serotype Typhimurium phage type DT104 which was resistant to five antimicrobials (ampicillin, chloramphenicol, streptomycin, sulfonamides, and tetracycline [ACSSuT]) emerged in the late 1990s and is now recognized worldwide. In 2002, 21% of *Salmonella* serotype Typhimurium isolates in the United States had the ACSSuT resistance profile (42). The ACSSuT resistance determinant has been found in *Salmonella* serotype Agona strains (50). The genomic element that carries this ACSSuT determinant has been found to harbor this and other resistance determinants in a variety of serotypes, indicating

that the element may spread horizontally to other serotypes and acquire additional resistance determinants (120).

The emergence of a clone of *Salmonella* serotype Newport which is resistant to at least nine antimicrobials, including expanded-spectrum cephalosporins, was first noted in 2000 in the northeastern United States (89) and has now been found in many regions of the United States (17). In 2002, this strain made up 22% of all *Salmonella* serotype Newport strains in the United States. Similarly resistant strains of *Salmonella* serotype Newport were recently reported in Japan, documenting the potential for worldwide spread of multiply resistant strains (103). Additional information regarding these and other antimicrobial-resistant strains can be found at the CDC's NARMS website (http://www.cdc.gov/narms/).

Evaluation, Interpretation, and Reporting of Results

A preliminary report can be issued as soon as a presumptive identification of *Salmonella* is obtained. In most situations, a presumptive identification is based on phenotypic traits determined by either traditional or commercial systems or by reactivity with *Salmonella* O grouping antisera. A confirmed identification requires both phenotypic identification and O group or serotype determination. Because national surveillance systems depend on the receipt of serotype information for *Salmonella* strains isolated in the United States, laboratories should follow the procedures recommended by their state health departments for submitting *Salmonella* isolates for further characterization, including complete serotyping. The antimicrobial susceptibilities of typhoidal *Salmonella* strains and strains from normally sterile sites should be determined, and the strains should be forwarded to a reference or public health laboratory for complete phenotypic identification and serotyping.

REFERENCES

1. **Abbott, S. L., J. O'Connor, T. Robin, B. L. Zimmer, and J. M. Janda.** 2003. Biochemical properties of a newly described *Escherichia* species, *Escherichia albertii*. *J. Clin. Microbiol.* **41:**4852–4854.
2. **Abu-Ali, G. S., D. W. Lacher, L. M. Wick, W. Qi, and T. S. Whittam.** 2009. Genomic diversity of pathogenic Escherichia coli of the EHEC 2 clonal complex. *BMC Genomics* **10:**296.
3. **Acheson, D. W. K., and G. T. Keusch.** 1995. *Shigella* and enteroinvasive *Escherichia coli*, p. 763–784. *In* M. J. Blaser, P. D. Smith, J. I. Ravdin, H. B. Greenberg, and R. L. Guerrant (ed.), *Infections of the Gastrointestinal Tract*. Raven Press, New York, NY.
4. **Adkins, H. J., and L. T. Santiago.** 1987. Increased recovery of enteric pathogens by use of both stool and rectal swab specimens. *J. Clin. Microbiol.* **25:**158–159.
5. **Albert, M. J., S. M. Faruque, A. S. Faruque, K. A. Bettelheim, P. K. Neogi, N. A. Bhuiyan, and J. B. Kaper.** 1996. Controlled study of cytolethal distending toxin-producing *Escherichia coli* infections in Bangladeshi children. *J. Clin. Microbiol.* **34:**717–719.
6. **Albert, M. J., F. Qadri, A. Haque, and N. A. Bhuiyan.** 1993. Bacterial clump formation at the surface of liquid culture as a rapid test for identification of enteroaggregative *Escherichia coli*. *J. Clin. Microbiol.* **31:**1397–1399.
7. **Anderson, K. F., D. R. Lonsway, J. K. Rasheed, J. Biddle, B. Jensen, L. K. McDougal, R. B. Carey, A. Thompson, S. Stocker, B. Limbago, and J. B. Patel.** 2007. Evaluation of methods to identify the *Klebsiella pneumoniae* carbapenemase in *Enterobacteriaceae*. *J. Clin. Microbiol.* **45:**2723–2725.
8. **Ansaruzzamann, M., A. K. M. G. Kibriya, A. Rahman, P. K. B. Neogi, A. S. G. Faruque, B. Rowe, and M. J. Albert.** 1995. Detection of provisional serovars of *Shigella dysenteriae* and designation as *S. dysenteriae* serotypes 14 and 15. *J. Clin. Microbiol.* **33:**1423–1425.
9. **Arvelo, W., C. J. Hinkle, T. A. Nguyen, T. Weiser, N. Steinmuller, F. Khan, S. Gladbach, M. Parsons, D. Jennings,**

B. P. Zhu, E. Mintz, and A. Bowen. 2009. Transmission risk factors and treatment of pediatric shigellosis during a large daycare center-associated outbreak of multidrug resistant Shigella sonnei: implications for the management of shigellosis outbreaks among children. *Pediatr. Infect. Dis. J.* **28:**976–980.

10. Reference deleted.

11. **Asadulghani, M., Y. Ogura, T. Ooka, T. Itoh, A. Sawaguchi, A. Iguchi, K. Nakayama, and T. Hayashi.** 2009. The defective prophage pool of Escherichia coli O157: prophage-prophage interactions potentiate horizontal transfer of virulence determinants. *PLoS Pathog.* **5:**e1000408.

12. **Aspevall, O., B. Osterman, R. Dittmer, L. Sten, E. Lindback, and U. Forsum.** 2002. Performance of four chromogenic urine culture media after one or two days of incubation compared with reference media. *J. Clin. Microbiol.* **40:**1500–1503.

13. **Awsare, S. V., and M. Lillo.** 1991. A case report of Escherichia vulneris urosepsis. *Rev. Infect. Dis.* **13:**1247–1248.

14. **Baker, S., and G. Dougan.** 2007. The genome of *Salmonella enterica* serovar Typhi. *Clin. Infect. Dis.* **45**(Suppl. 1)**:**S29–S33.

15. **Bangert, R. L., A. C. Ward, E. H. Stauber, B. R. Cho, and P. R. Widders.** 1988. A survey of the aerobic bacteria in the feces of captive raptors. *Avian Dis.* **32:**53–62.

16. **Baudry, B., S. J. Savarino, P. Vial, J. B. Kaper, and M. M. Levine.** 1990. A sensitive and specific DNA probe to identify enteroaggregative *Escherichia coli*, a recently discovered diarrheal pathogen. *J. Infect. Dis.* **161:**1249–1251.

17. **Berge, A. C., J. M. Adaska, and W. M. Sischo.** 2004. Use of antibiotic susceptibility patterns and pulsed-field gel electrophoresis to compare historic and contemporary isolates of multi-drug-resistant *Salmonella enterica* subsp. *enterica* serovar Newport. *Appl. Environ. Microbiol.* **70:**318–323.

18. **Bettelheim, K. A.** 1992. The genus *Escherichia*, p. 2696–2736. *In* A. Balows, H. G. Truper, M. Dworkin, W. Harder, and K.-H. Schleifer (ed.), *The Prokaryotes*, 2nd ed. Springer-Verlag KG, Berlin, Germany.

19. **Bettelheim, K. A.** 2005. Reliability of O157:H7 ID agar (O157 H7 ID-F) for the detection and isolation of verocytotoxigenic strains of *Escherichia coli* belonging to serogroup O157. *J. Appl. Microbiol.* **99:**408–410.

20. **Beutin, L., M. A. Montenegro, I. Orskov, F. Orskov, J. Prada, S. Zimmermann, and R. Stephan.** 1989. Close association of verotoxin (Shiga-like toxin) production with enterohemolysin production in strains of *Escherichia coli*. *J. Clin. Microbiol.* **27:**2559–2564.

21. **Beutin, L., S. Zimmermann, and K. Gleier.** 2002. Evaluation of the VTEC-Screen "Seiken" test for detection of different types of Shiga toxin (verotoxin)-producing *Escherichia coli* (STEC) in human stool samples. *Diagn. Microbiol. Infect. Dis.* **42:**1–8.

22. **Bielaszewska, M., R. Kock, A. W. Friedrich, C. von Eiff, L. B. Zimmerhackl, H. Karch, and A. Mellmann.** 2007. Shiga toxin-mediated hemolytic uremic syndrome: time to change the diagnostic paradigm? *PLoS One* **2:**e1024.

23. **Bielaszewska, M., B. Middendorf, R. Kock, A. W. Friedrich, A. Fruth, H. Karch, M. A. Schmidt, and A. Mellmann.** 2008. Shiga toxin-negative attaching and effacing *Escherichia coli*: distinct clinical associations with bacterial phylogeny and virulence traits and inferred in-host pathogen evolution. *Clin. Infect. Dis.* **47:**208–217.

24. **Bitzan, M., K. Ludwig, M. Klemt, H. Konig, J. Buren, and D. E. Muller-Wiefel.** 1993. The role of *Escherichia coli* O157 infections in the classical (enteropathic) haemolytic uraemic syndrome: results of a Central European, multicentre study. *Epidemiol. Infect.* **110:**183–196.

25. **Blanco, J. E., J. Blanco, M. Blanco, M. P. Alonso, and W. H. Jansen.** 1994. Serotypes of CNF1-producing *Escherichia coli* strains that cause extraintestinal infections in humans. *Eur. J. Epidemiol.* **10:**707–711.

26. **Blattner, F. R., G. Plunkett III, C. A. Bloch, N. T. Perna, V. Burland, M. Riley, J. Collado-Vides, J. D. Glasner, C. K. Rode, G. F. Mayhew, J. Gregor, N. W. Davis, H. A. Kirkpatrick, M. A. Goeden, D. J. Rose, B. Mau, and Y. Shao.** 1997. The complete genome sequence of *Escherichia coli* K-12. *Science* **277:**1453–1462.

27. **Borczyk, A. A., N. Harnett, M. Lombos, and H. Lior.** 1990. False-positive identification of *Escherichia coli* O157 by commercial latex agglutination tests. *Lancet* **336:**946–947.

28. **Bouvet, P. J., and S. Jeanjean.** 1992. Evaluation of two colored latex kits, the Wellcolex Colour Salmonella test and the Wellcolex Colour Shigella test, for serological grouping of *Salmonella* and *Shigella* species. *J. Clin. Microbiol.* **30:**2184–2186.

29. **Brenner, D. J.** 1992. Introduction to the family Enterobacteriaceae, p. 2673–2695. *In* A. Balows, H. G. Truper, M. Dworkin, W. Harder, and K.-H. Schleifer (ed.), *The Prokaryotes*, 2nd ed. Springer-Verlag KG, Berlin, Germany.

30. **Brenner, D. J., G. R. Fanning, G. V. Miklos, and A. G. Steigerwalt.** 1973. Polynucleotide sequence relatedness among *Shigella* species. *Int. J. Syst. Bacteriol.* **23:**1–7.

31. **Brenner, D. J., G. R. Fanning, F. J. Skerman, and S. Falkow.** 1972. Polynucleotide sequence divergence among strains of *Escherichia coli* and closely related organisms. *J. Bacteriol.* **109:**953–965.

32. **Brenner, D. J., and J. J. I. Farmer.** 2005. Order XIII. "Enterobacteriales," p. 587–607. *In* G. M. Garrity, D. J. Brenner, N. R. Krieg, and J. T. Staley (ed.), *Bergey's Manual of Systematic Bacteriology*, 2nd ed., vol. 2. *The* Proteobacteria. *Part B. The* Gammaproteobacteria. Springer Science+Business Media, Inc., New York, NY.

33. **Brenner, D. J., A. C. McWhorter, J. K. Knutson, and A. G. Steigerwalt.** 1982. *Escherichia vulneris*: a new species of *Enterobacteriaceae* associated with human wounds. *J. Clin. Microbiol.* **15:**1133–1140.

34. **Brenner, F. W., and A. C. McWhorter-Murlin.** 1998. *Identification and Serotyping of* Salmonella. Centers for Disease Control and Prevention, Atlanta, GA.

35. **Brooks, J. T., J. B. Ochieng, L. Kumar, G. Okoth, R. L. Shapiro, J. G. Wells, M. Bird, C. Bopp, W. Chege, M. E. Beatty, T. Chiller, J. M. Vulule, E. Mintz, and L. Slutsker.** 2006. Surveillance for bacterial diarrhea and antimicrobial resistance in rural western Kenya, 1997–2003. *Clin. Infect. Dis.* **43:**393–401.

36. **Brooks, J. T., E. G. Sowers, J. G. Wells, K. D. Greene, P. M. Griffin, R. M. Hoekstra, and N. A. Strockbine.** 2005. Non-O157 Shiga toxin-producing *Escherichia coli* infections in the United States, 1983–2002. *J. Infect. Dis.* **192:**1422–1429.

37. Reference deleted.

38. **Caprioli, A., V. Falbo, L. G. Roda, F. M. Ruggeri, and C. Zona.** 1983. Partial purification and characterization of an *Escherichia coli* toxic factor that induces morphological cell alterations. *Infect. Immun.* **39:**1300–1306.

39. **Castellani, A., and A. J. Chalmers.** 1919. *Manual of Tropical Medicine*, 3rd ed. William Wood and Company, New York, NY.

40. **CDC.** 2004. Day care-related outbreaks of rhamnose-negative *Shigella sonnei*—six states, June 2001. *MMWR Morb. Mortal. Wkly. Rep.* **53:**60–63.

41. **CDC.** 2006. *FoodNet Surveillance Report for 2004 (Final Report)*. CDC, Atlanta, GA.

42. **CDC.** 2004. *National Antimicrobial Resistance Monitoring System for Enteric Bacteria (NARMS) 2002 Human Isolates Final Report*. U.S. Department of Health and Human Services, CDC, Atlanta, GA.

43. **CDC.** 2006. Outbreaks of multidrug-resistant *Shigella sonnei* gastroenteritis associated with day care centers—Kansas, Kentucky, and Missouri, 2005. *MMWR Morb. Mortal. Wkly. Rep.* **55:**1068–1071.

44. **CDC.** 2009. Preliminary FoodNet data on the incidence of infection with pathogens transmitted commonly through food—10 states, 2008. *MMWR Morb. Mortal. Wkly. Rep.* **58:**333–337.

45. **CDC.** 2001. *Shigella sonnei* outbreak among men who have sex with men—San Francisco, California, 2000–2001. *MMWR Morb. Mortal. Wkly. Rep.* **50:**922–926.

46. **Chaudhuri, R. R., M. Sebaihia, J. L. Hobman, M. A. Webber, D. L. Leyton, M. D. Goldberg, A. F. Cunningham, A. Scott-Tucker, P. R. Ferguson, C. M. Thomas, G. Frankel, C. M. Tang, E. G. Dudley, I. S. Roberts, D. A. Rasko, M. J. Pallen, J. Parkhill, J. P. Nataro, N. R. Thomson, and I. R. Henderson.** Complete genome sequence and comparative metabolic profiling of the prototypical enteroaggregative *Escherichia coli* strain 042. *PLoS One* **5:**e8801.

47. Chaux, C., M. Crepy, S. Xueref, C. Roure, Y. Gille, and A. M. Freydiere. 2002. Comparison of three chromogenic agar plates for isolation and identification of urinary tract pathogens. *Clin. Microbiol. Infect.* **8:**641–645.

48. Chiu, C. H., P. Tang, C. Chu, S. Hu, Q. Bao, J. Yu, Y. Y. Chou, H. S. Wang, and Y. S. Lee. 2005. The genome sequence of *Salmonella enterica* serovar Choleraesuis, a highly invasive and resistant zoonotic pathogen. *Nucleic Acids Res.* **33:**1690–1698.

49. Church, D. L., D. Emshey, H. Semeniuk, T. Lloyd, and J. D. Pitout. 2007. Evaluation of BBL CHROMagar O157 versus sorbitol-MacConkey medium for routine detection of *Escherichia coli* O157 in a centralized regional clinical microbiology laboratory. *J. Clin. Microbiol.* **45:**3098–3100.

50. Cloeckaert, A., K. Sidi Boumedine, G. Flaujac, H. Imberechts, I. D'Hooghe, and E. Chaslus-Dancla. 2000. Occurrence of a *Salmonella enterica* serovar Typhimurium DT104-like antibiotic resistance gene cluster including the *floR* gene in *S. enterica* serovar Agona. *Antimicrob. Agents Chemother.* **44:**1359–1361.

51. CLSI. 2010. *Performance Standards for Antimicrobial Susceptibility Testing: 20th Information Supplement.* M100-S20, vol. 30, no. 1. Clinical Laboratory Standards Institute, Wayne, PA.

52. Cobeljic, M., B. Miljkovic-Selimovic, D. Paunovic-Todosijevic, Z. Velickovic, Z. Lepsanovic, N. Zec, D. Savic, R. Ilic, S. Konstantinovic, B. Jovanovic, and V. Kostic. 1996. Enteroaggregative *Escherichia coli* associated with an outbreak of diarrhoea in a neonatal nursery ward. *Epidemiol. Infect.* **117:**11–16.

53. Cohen, M. B., J. P. Nataro, D. I. Bernstein, J. Hawkins, N. Roberts, and M. A. Staat. 2005. Prevalence of diarrheagenic *Escherichia coli* in acute childhood enteritis: a prospective controlled study. *J. Pediatr.* **146:**54–61.

54. Dalton, C. B., E. D. Mintz, J. G. Wells, C. A. Bopp, and R. V. Tauxe. 1999. Outbreaks of enterotoxigenic *Escherichia coli* infection in American adults: a clinical and epidemiologic profile. *Epidemiol. Infect.* **123:**9–16.

55. Daskalakis, D. C., and M. J. Blaser. 2007. Another perfect storm: *Shigella*, men who have sex with men, and HIV. *Clin. Infect. Dis.* **44:**335–337.

56. Reference deleted.

57. De Rycke, J., J. F. Guillot, and R. Boivin. 1997. Cytotoxins in nonenterotoxigenic strains of *Escherichia coli* isolated from feces of diarrheic calves. *Vet. Microbiol.* **15:**137–150.

58. DeWitt, W. E., E. J. Gangarosa, I. Huq, and A. Zarifi. 1971. Holding media for the transport of *Vibrio cholerae* from field to laboratory. *Am. J. Trop. Med.* **20:**685–688.

59. Dietzman, D. E., G. W. Fischer, and F. D. Schoenknecht. 1974. Neonatal *Escherichia coli* septicemia—bacterial counts in blood. *J. Pediatr.* **85:**128–130.

60. Dobrindt, U., F. Agerer, K. Michaelis, A. Janka, C. Buchrieser, C. Samuelson, C. Svanborg, G. Gottschalk, H. Karch, and J. Hacker. 2003. Analysis of genome plasticity in pathogenic and commensal *Escherichia coli* isolates by use of DNA arrays. *J. Bacteriol.* **185:**1831–1840.

61. Doi, Y., D. L. Paterson, P. Egea, A. Pascual, L. Lopez-Cerero, M. D. Navarro, J. M. Adams-Haduch, Z. A. Qureshi, H. E. Sidjabat, and J. Rodriguez-Bano. 2010. Extended-spectrum and CMY-type beta-lactamase-producing *Escherichia coli* in clinical samples and retail meat from Pittsburgh, USA and Seville, Spain. *Clin. Microbiol. Infect.* **16:**33–38.

62. Donnenberg, M. S. 2002. Enteropathogenic *Escherichia coli*, p. 595–612. *In* M. J. Blaser, P. D. Smith, J. I. Ravdin, H. B. Greenberg, and R. L. Guerrant (ed.), *Infections of the Gastrointestinal Tract*, 2nd ed. Lippincott Williams & Wilkins, Philadelphia, PA.

63. Ecker, D. J., R. Sampath, C. Massire, L. B. Blyn, T. A. Hall, M. W. Eshoo, and S. A. Hofstadler. 2008. Ibis T5000: a universal biosensor approach for microbiology. *Nat. Rev. Microbiol.* **6:**553–558.

64. Edwards, R. A., G. J. Olsen, and S. R. Maloy. 2002. Comparative genomics of closely related salmonellae. *Trends Microbiol.* **10:**94–99.

65. Ethelberg, S., K. E. Olsen, P. Gerner-Smidt, and K. Molbak. 2007. The significance of the number of submitted samples and patient-related factors for faecal bacterial diagnostics. *Clin. Microbiol. Infect.* **13:**1095–1099.

66. Ewing, W. H. 1986. *Edwards and Ewing's Identification of* Enterobacteriaceae, 4th ed. Elsevier Scientific Publishing Co., Inc., New York, NY.

67. Ewing, W. H. 1986. The genus *Shigella*, p. 135–172. *In Edwards and Ewing's Identification of* Enterobacteriaceae, 4th ed. Elsevier Science Publishing Co., Inc., New York, NY.

68. Ewing, W. H., et al. 1971. *Biochemical Reactions of* Shigella. *Public Health Service Publication 72-8081.* U.S. Department of Health, Education, and Welfare, Atlanta, GA.

69. Ewing, W. H., R. W. Reavis, and B. R. Davis. 1958. Provisional *Shigella* serotypes. *Can. J. Microbiol.* **4:**89–107.

70. Farmer, J. J., III, G. R. Fanning, B. R. Davis, C. M. O'Hara, C. Riddle, F. W. Hickman-Brenner, M. A. Asbury, V. A. Lowery III, and D. J. Brenner. 1985. *Escherichia fergusonii* and *Enterobacter taylorae*, two new species of Enterobacteriaceae isolated from clinical specimens. *J. Clin. Microbiol.* **21:**77–81.

71. Farmer, J. J., III. 2003. *Enterobacteriaceae:* introduction and identification, p. 636–653. *In* P. R. Murray, E. J. Baron, J. H. Jorgensen, M. A. Pfaller, and R. H. Yolken (ed.), *Manual of Clinical Microbiology*, 8th ed, vol. 1. ASM Press, Washington, DC.

72. Feng, P., and S. D. Weagant. 1998. Enumeration of *Escherichia coli* and the coliform bacteria. *In Bacteriological Analytical Manual*, 8th ed. AOAC International, Gaithersburg, MD. (Online.) http://www.fda.gov/Food/ScienceResearch/LaboratoryMethods/BacteriologicalAnalyticalManualBAM/UCM064948.

73. Fields, P. I., K. Blom, H. J. Hughes, L. O. Helsel, P. Feng, and B. Swaminathan. 1997. Molecular characterization of the gene encoding H antigen in *Escherichia coli* and development of a PCR-restriction fragment length polymorphism test for identification of *E. coli* O157:H7 and O157:NM. *J. Clin. Microbiol.* **35:**1066–1070.

74. Fisher, I. S. 2004. Dramatic shift in the epidemiology of *Salmonella enterica* serotype Enteritidis phage types in western Europe, 1998–2003—results from the Enter-net international salmonella database. *Euro. Surveill.* **9:**43–45.

75. Fisher, M. A., P. D. Stamper, K. M. Hujer, Z. Love, A. Croft, S. Cohen, R. A. Bonomo, K. C. Carroll, and C. A. Petti. 2009. Performance of the Phoenix bacterial identification system compared with disc diffusion methods for identifying extended-spectrum beta-lactamase, AmpC and KPC producers. *J. Med. Microbiol.* **58:**774–778.

76. Fontana, C., M. Favaro, M. Pelliccioni, E. S. Pistoia, and C. Favalli. 2005. Use of MicroSeq 500 16S rRNA gene-based sequencing for identification of bacterial isolates that commercial automated systems failed to identify correctly. *J. Clin. Microbiol.* **43:**615–619.

77. Friedrich, A. W., M. Bielaszewska, W. L. Zhang, M. Pulz, T. Kuczius, A. Ammon, and H. Karch. 2002. *Escherichia coli* harboring Shiga toxin 2 gene variants: frequency and association with clinical symptoms. *J. Infect. Dis.* **185:**74–84.

78. Gavin, P. J., L. R. Peterson, A. C. Pasquariello, J. Blackburn, M. G. Hamming, K. J. Kuo, and R. B. Thomson, Jr. 2004. Evaluation of performance and potential clinical impact of ProSpecT Shiga toxin *Escherichia coli* microplate assay for detection of Shiga toxin-producing *E. coli* in stool samples. *J. Clin. Microbiol.* **42:**1652–1656.

79. Reference deleted.

80. Gilligan, P. H., J. M. Janda, M. A. Karmali, and J. M. Miller. 1992. *Cumitech 12A, Laboratory Diagnosis of Bacterial Diarrhea.* ASM Press, Washington, DC.

81. Glandt, M., J. A. Adachi, J. J. Mathewson, Z. D. Jiang, D. DiCesare, D. Ashley, C. D. Ericsson, and H. L. DuPont. 1999. Enteroaggregative *Escherichia coli* as a cause of traveler's diarrhea: clinical response to ciprofloxacin. *Clin. Infect. Dis.* **29:**335–338.

82. Goris, J., K. T. Konstantinidis, J. A. Klappenbach, T. Coenye, P. Vandamme, and J. M. Tiedje. 2007. DNA-DNA hybridization values and their relationship to whole-genome sequence similarities. *Int. J. Syst. Evol. Microbiol.* **57:**81–91.

83. Gould, H. L., C. Bopp, N. Strockbine, R. Atkinson, V. Baselski, B. Body, R. Carey, C. Crandall, S. Hurd, R. Kaplan, M. Neill, S. Shea, P. Somsel, M. Toben-D'Angelo, P. Griffin, and P. Gerner-Smidt. 2009. Recommendations for diagnosis of Shiga toxin-producing *Escherichia coli* infections

by clinical laboratories. *MMWR Morb. Mortal. Wkly. Rep.* **58**(RR-12):1–14.

84. **Griffin, P. M., P. S. Mead, and Sivapalasingam.** 2002. *Escherichia coli* O157:H7 and other enterohemorrhagic *Escherichia coli*, p. 627–642. *In* M. J. Blaser, J. I. Ravdin, H. B. Greenberg, and R. L. Guerrant (ed.), *Infections of the Gastrointestinal Tract*, 2nd ed. Lippincott Williams & Wilkins, New York, NY.

85. **Grimont, P. A. D., and F.-X. Weill.** 2007. *Antigenic Formulae of the* Salmonella *Serovars*, 9th ed. WHO Collaborating Centre for Reference and Research on *Salmonella*, Institut Pasteur, Paris, France.

86. **Grys, T. E., L. M. Sloan, J. E. Rosenblatt, and R. Patel.** 2009. Rapid and sensitive detection of Shiga toxin-producing *Escherichia coli* from nonenriched stool specimens by real-time PCR in comparison to enzyme immunoassay and culture. *J. Clin. Microbiol.* **47**:2008–2012.

87. **Guerrant, R. L., T. J. Van Gilder, T. S. Steiner, N. M. Thielman, L. Slutsker, R. V. Tauxe, T. W. Hennessy, P. M. Griffin, H. DuPont, B. Sack, P. I. Tarr, M. A. Neill, I. Nachamkin, B. Reller, M. T. Osterholm, M. L. Bennish, and L. K. Pickering.** 2001. Practice guidelines for the management of infectious diarrhea. *Clin. Infect. Dis.* **32**:331–350.

88. **Guerrero, L., J. J. Calva, A. L. Morrow, F. R. Velazquez, Y. Lopez-Vidal, H. Ortega, H. Arroyo, T. G. Cleary, and L. K. Pickering.** 1994. Asymptomatic *Shigella* infections in a cohort of Mexican children younger than two years of age. *Pediatr. Infect. Dis. J.* **13**:597–602.

89. **Gupta, A., J. Fontana, C. Crowe, B. Bolstorff, A. Stout, S. Van Duyne, M. P. Hoekstra, J. M. Whichard, T. J. Barrett, and F. J. Angulo.** 2003. Emergence of multidrug-resistant *Salmonella enterica* serotype Newport infections resistant to expanded-spectrum cephalosporins in the United States. *J. Infect. Dis.* **188**:1707–1716.

90. **Hanning, I. B., J. D. Nutt, and S. C. Ricke.** 2009. Salmonellosis outbreaks in the United States due to fresh produce: sources and potential intervention measures. *Foodborne Pathog. Dis.* **6**:635–648.

91. **Hardy, A. V., D. Mackel, D. Frazier, and D. Hamerick.** 1953. The relative efficacy of cultures for *Shigella*. *U. S. Armed Forces Med. J.* **4**:393–394.

92. **Hayashi, T., K. Makino, M. Ohnishi, K. Kurokawa, K. Ishii, K. Yokoyama, C. G. Han, E. Ohtsubo, K. Nakayama, T. Murata, M. Tanaka, T. Tobe, T. Iida, H. Takami, T. Honda, C. Sasakawa, N. Ogasawara, T. Yasunaga, S. Kuhara, T. Shiba, M. Hattori, and H. Shinagawa.** 2001. Complete genome sequence of enterohemorrhagic *Escherichia coli* O157:H7 and genomic comparison with a laboratory strain K-12. *DNA Res.* **8**:11–22.

93. **Hayes, P. S., K. Blom, P. Feng, J. Lewis, N. A. Strockbine, and B. Swaminathan.** 1995. Isolation and characterization of a beta-D-glucuronidase-producing strain of *Escherichia coli* serotype O157:H7 in the United States. *J. Clin. Microbiol.* **33**:3347–3348.

94. **Hedberg, C. W., S. J. Savarino, J. M. Besser, C. J. Paulus, V. M. Thelen, L. J. Myers, D. N. Cameron, T. J. Barrett, J. B. Kaper, and M. T. Osterholm.** 1997. An outbreak of foodborne illness caused by *Escherichia coli* O39:NM, an agent not fitting into the existing scheme for classifying diarrheogenic *E. coli*. *J. Infect. Dis.* **176**:1625–1628.

95. **Herold, S., H. Karch, and H. Schmidt.** 2004. Shiga toxin-encoding bacteriophages—genomes in motion. *Int. J. Med. Microbiol.* **294**:115–121.

96. **Hohmann, E. L.** 2001. Nontyphoidal salmonellosis. *Clin. Infect. Dis.* **32**:263–269.

97. **Holt, K. E., N. R. Thomson, J. Wain, G. C. Langridge, R. Hasan, Z. A. Bhutta, M. A. Quail, H. Norbertczak, D. Walker, M. Simmonds, B. White, N. Bason, K. Mungall, G. Dougan, and J. Parkhill.** 2009. Pseudogene accumulation in the evolutionary histories of *Salmonella enterica* serovars Paratyphi A and Typhi. *BMC Genomics* **10**:36.

98. **Huang, D. B., H. Koo, and H. L. DuPont.** 2004. Enteroaggregative *Escherichia coli*: an emerging pathogen. *Curr. Infect. Dis. Rep.* **6**:83–86.

99. **Hurrell, E., E. Kucerova, M. Loughlin, J. Caubilla-Barron, A. Hilton, R. Armstrong, C. Smith, J. Grant, S. Shoo, and S. Forsythe.** 2009. Neonatal enteral feeding tubes as loci for colonisation by members of the *Enterobacteriaceae*. *BMC Infect. Dis.* **9**:146.

100. **Huys, G., M. Cnockaert, J. M. Janda, and J. Swings.** 2003. *Escherichia albertii* sp. nov., a diarrhoeagenic species isolated from stool specimens of Bangladeshi children. *Int. J. Syst. Evol. Microbiol.* **53**:807–810.

101. **Hyma, K. E., D. W. Lacher, A. M. Nelson, A. C. Bumbaugh, J. M. Janda, N. A. Strockbine, V. B. Young, and T. S. Whittam.** 2005. Evolutionary genetics of a new pathogenic *Escherichia* species: *Escherichia albertii* and related *Shigella boydii* strains. *J. Bacteriol.* **187**:619–628.

102. **Hyytia-Trees, E., S. C. Smole, P. A. Fields, B. Swaminathan, and E. M. Ribot.** 2006. Second generation subtyping: a proposed PulseNet protocol for multiple-locus variable-number tandem repeat analysis of Shiga toxin-producing *Escherichia coli* O157 (STEC O157). *Foodborne Pathog. Dis.* **3**:118–131.

103. **Ishiguro, F., Y. Kyota, M. Mochizuki, T. Fuseda, S. Omoya, H. Izumiya, and H. Watanabe.** 2005. Comparison of multidrug-resistant *Salmonella enterica* serovar Newport isolates from a patient and sewages in Fukui Prefecture. *Kansenshogaku Zasshi* **79**:270–275.

104. **Johnson, J. R., and T. A. Russo.** 2005. Molecular epidemiology of extraintestinal pathogenic (uropathogenic) *Escherichia coli*. *Int. J. Med. Microbiol.* **295**:383–404.

105. **Johnson, T. J., and L. K. Nolan.** 2009. Pathogenomics of the virulence plasmids of *Escherichia coli*. *Microbiol. Mol. Biol. Rev.* **73**:750–774.

106. **Johnson, W. M., and H. Lior.** 1988. A new heat-labile cytolethal distending toxin (CLDT) produced by *Escherichia coli* isolates from clinical material. *Microb. Pathog.* **4**:103–113.

107. **Kadhiravan, T., N. Wig, A. Kapil, S. K. Kabra, K. Renuka, and A. Misra.** 2005. Clinical outcomes in typhoid fever: adverse impact of infection with nalidixic acid-resistant *Salmonella typhi*. *BMC Infect. Dis.* **5**:37.

108. **Kaper, J. B., J. P. Nataro, and H. L. Mobley.** 2004. Pathogenic *Escherichia coli*. *Nat. Rev. Microbiol.* **2**:123–140.

109. **Karch, H., C. Janetzki-Mittmann, S. Aleksic, and M. Datz.** 1996. Isolation of enterohemorrhagic *Escherichia coli* O157 strains from patients with hemolytic-uremic syndrome by using immunomagnetic separation, DNA-based methods, and direct culture. *J. Clin. Microbiol.* **34**:516–519.

110. **Karmali, M. A., M. Mascarenhas, S. Shen, K. Ziebell, S. Johnson, R. Reid-Smith, J. Isaac-Renton, C. Clark, K. Rahn, and J. B. Kaper.** 2003. Association of genomic O island 122 of *Escherichia coli* EDL 933 with verocytotoxin-producing *Escherichia coli* seropathotypes that are linked to epidemic and/or serious disease. *J. Clin. Microbiol.* **41**:4930–4940.

111. **Kehl, K., P. Havens, C. Behnke, and D. Acheson.** 1997. Evaluation of the premier EHEC assay for detection of Shiga toxin-producing *Escherichia coli*. *J. Clin. Microbiol.* **35**:2051–2054.

112. Reference deleted.

113. **Kim, B. Y., J. Kang, and K. S. Kim.** 2005. Invasion processes of pathogenic *Escherichia coli*. *Int. J. Med. Microbiol.* **295**:463–470.

114. **Kuo, C. Y., L. H. Su, J. Perera, C. Carlos, B. H. Tan, G. Kumarasinghe, T. So, P. H. Van, A. Chongthaleong, J. H. Song, and C. H. Chiu.** 2008. Antimicrobial susceptibility of *Shigella* isolates in eight Asian countries, 2001–2004. *J. Microbiol. Immunol. Infect.* **41**:107–111.

115. **Lan, R., M. C. Alles, K. Donohoe, M. B. Martinez, and P. R. Reeves.** 2004. Molecular evolutionary relationships of enteroinvasive *Escherichia coli* and *Shigella* spp. *Infect. Immun.* **72**:5080–5088.

116. **Lan, R., P. R. Reeves, and S. Octavia.** 2009. Population structure, origins and evolution of major *Salmonella enterica* clones. *Infect. Genet. Evol.* **9**:996–1005.

117. **Lee, L. A., N. D. Puhr, E. K. Maloney, N. H. Bean, and R. V. Tauxe.** 1994. Increase in antimicrobial-resistant *Salmonella* infections in the United States, 1989–1990. *J. Infect. Dis.* **170**:128–134.

118. **Levine, M. M., C. Ferreccio, V. Prado, M. Cayazzo, P. Abrego, J. Martinez, L. Maggi, M. M. Baldini, W. Martin, D. Maneval, et al.** 1993. Epidemiologic studies of *Escherichia coli* diarrheal infections in a low socioeconomic level peri-urban community in Santiago, Chile. *Am. J. Epidemiol.* **138:**849–869.

119. **Levine, W. N., and M. J. Goldberg.** 1994. *Escherichia vulneris* osteomyelitis of the tibia caused by a wooden foreign body. *Orthop. Rev.* **23:**262–265.

120. **Levings, R. S., D. Lightfoot, S. R. Partridge, R. M. Hall, and S. P. Djordjevic.** 2005. The genomic island SGI1, containing the multiple antibiotic resistance region of *Salmonella enterica* serovar Typhimurium DT104 or variants of it, is widely distributed in other *S. enterica* serovars. *J. Bacteriol.* **187:**4401–4409.

121. **Lindberg, A. A., P. D. Cam, N. Chan, L. K. Phu, D. D. Trach, G. Lindberg, K. Karlsson, A. Karnell, and E. Ekwall.** 1991. Shigellosis in Vietnam: seroepidemiologic studies with use of lipopolysaccharide antigens in enzyme immunoassays. *Rev. Infect. Dis.* **13**(Suppl. 4):S231–S237.

122. **Liu, W. Q., Y. Feng, Y. Wang, Q. H. Zou, F. Chen, J. T. Guo, Y. H. Peng, Y. Jin, Y. G. Li, S. N. Hu, R. N. Johnston, G. R. Liu, and S. L. Liu.** 2009. Salmonella paratyphi C: genetic divergence from Salmonella choleraesuis and pathogenic convergence with Salmonella typhi. *PLoS One* **4:**e4510.

123. **Lolekha, S., S. Vibulbandhitkit, and P. Poonyarit.** 1991. Response to antimicrobial therapy for shigellosis in Thailand. *Rev. Infect. Dis.* **13:**S342–S346.

124. **Ludwig, K., E. Grabhorn, M. Bitzan, C. Bobrowski, M. J. Kemper, I. Sobottka, R. Laufs, H. Karch, and D. E. Muller-Wiefel.** 2002. Saliva IgM and IgA are a sensitive indicator of the humoral immune response to *Escherichia coli* O157 lipopolysaccharide in children with enteropathic hemolytic uremic syndrome. *Pediatr. Res.* **52:**307–313.

125. **Mackenzie, A. M., P. Lebel, E. Orrbine, P. C. Rowe, L. Hyde, F. Chan, W. Johnson, and P. N. McLaine, and The Synsorb Pk Study Investigators.** 1998. Sensitivities and specificities of Premier *E. coli* O157 and Premier EHEC enzyme immunoassays for diagnosis of infection with verotoxin (Shiga-like toxin)-producing *Escherichia coli*. *J. Clin. Microbiol.* **36:**1608–1611.

126. **Mahon, B. E., A. Ponka, W. N. Hall, K. Komatsu, S. E. Dietrich, A. Siitonen, G. Cage, P. S. Hayes, M. A. Lambert-Fair, N. H. Bean, P. M. Griffin, and L. Slutsker.** 1997. An international outbreak of *Salmonella* infections caused by alfalfa sprouts grown from contaminated seeds. *J. Infect. Dis.* **175:**876–882.

127. **Manafi, M., and B. Kremsmaier.** 2001. Comparative evaluation of different chromogenic/fluorogenic media for detecting *Escherichia coli* O157:H7 in food. *Int. J. Food Microbiol.* **71:**257–262.

128. **Mandal, B. K., and J. Brennand.** 1988. Bacteraemia in salmonellosis: a 15 year retrospective study from a regional infectious diseases unit. *BMJ* **297:**1242–1243.

129. **Manning, S. D., R. T. Madera, W. Schneider, S. E. Dietrich, W. Khalife, W. Brown, T. S. Whittam, P. Somsel, and J. T. Rudrik.** 2007. Surveillance for Shiga toxin-producing *Escherichia coli*, Michigan, 2001–2005. *Emerg. Infect. Dis.* **13:**318–321.

130. **March, S. B., and S. Ratnam.** 1986. Sorbitol-MacConkey medium for detection of *Escherichia coli* O157:H7 associated with hemorrhagic colitis. *J. Clin. Microbiol.* **23:**869–872.

131. **McClelland, M., K. E. Sanderson, J. Spieth, S. W. Clifton, P. Latreille, L. Courtney, S. Porwollik, J. Ali, M. Dante, F. Du, S. Hou, D. Layman, S. Leonard, C. Nguyen, K. Scott, A. Holmes, N. Grewal, E. Mulvaney, E. Ryan, H. Sun, L. Florea, W. Miller, T. Stoneking, M. Nhan, R. Waterston, and R. K. Wilson.** 2001. Complete genome sequence of *Salmonella enterica* serovar Typhimurium LT2. *Nature* **413:**852–856.

132. **McVeigh, A., A. Fasano, D. A. Scott, S. Jelacic, S. L. Moseley, D. C. Robertson, and S. J. Savarino.** 2000. IS*1414*, an *Escherichia coli* insertion sequence with a heat-stable enterotoxin gene embedded in a transposase-like gene. *Infect. Immun.* **68:**5710–5715.

133. **Mead, P. S., L. Slutsker, V. Dietz, L. F. McCaig, J. S. Bresee, C. Shapiro, P. M. Griffin, and R. V. Tauxe.** 1999. Food-related illness and death in the United States. *Emerg. Infect. Dis.* **5:**607–625.

134. **Mignard, S., and J. P. Flandrois.** 2006. 16S rRNA sequencing in routine bacterial identification: a 30-month experiment. *J. Microbiol. Methods* **67:**574–581.

135. **Miqdady, M. S., Z. D. Jiang, J. P. Nataro, and H. L. DuPont.** 2002. Detection of enteroaggregative *Escherichia coli* with formalin-preserved HEp-2 cells. *J. Clin. Microbiol.* **40:**3066–3067.

136. **Morris, C., C. K. Tam, T. S. Wallis, P. W. Jones, and J. Hackett.** 2003. *Salmonella enterica* serovar Dublin strains which are Vi antigen-positive use type IVB pili for bacterial self-association and human intestinal cell entry. *Microb. Pathog.* **35:**279–284.

137. **Muresu, R., G. Maddau, G. Delogu, P. Cappuccinelli, and A. Squartini.** 2010. Bacteria colonizing root nodules of wild legumes exhibit virulence-associated properties of mammalian pathogens. *Antonie Van Leeuwenhoek* **97:**143–153.

138. **Nataro, J. P., Y. Deng, S. Cookson, A. Cravioto, S. J. Savarino, L. D. Guers, M. M. Levine, and C. O. Tacket.** 1995. Heterogeneity of enteroaggregative *Escherichia coli* virulence demonstrated in volunteers. *J. Infect. Dis.* **171:**465–468.

139. **Nataro, J. P., and J. B. Kaper.** 1998. Diarrheagenic *Escherichia coli*. *Clin. Microbiol. Rev.* **11:**142–201.

140. **Naum, M., E. W. Brown, and R. J. Mason-Gamer.** 2008. Is 16S rDNA a reliable phylogenetic marker to characterize relationships below the family level in the *Enterobacteriaceae*? *J. Mol. Evol.* **66:**630–642.

141. **Navarro, F., T. Llovet, M. A. Echeita, P. Coll, A. Aladuena, M. A. Usera, and G. Prats.** 1996. Molecular typing of *Salmonella enterica* serovar Typhi. *J. Clin. Microbiol.* **34:**2831–2834.

142. **Nguyen, T. V., P. Le Van, C. Le Huy, K. N. Gia, and A. Weintraub.** 2005. Detection and characterization of diarrheagenic *Escherichia coli* from young children in Hanoi, Vietnam. *J. Clin. Microbiol.* **43:**755–760.

143. **Nishi, J., J. Sheikh, K. Mizuguchi, B. Luisi, V. Burland, A. Boutin, D. J. Rose, F. R. Blattner, and J. P. Nataro.** 2003. The export of coat protein from enteroaggregative *Escherichia coli* by a specific ATP-binding cassette transporter system. *J. Biol. Chem.* **278:**45680–45689.

144. **Novicki, T. J., J. A. Daly, S. L. Mottice, and K. C. Carroll.** 2000. Comparison of sorbitol MacConkey agar and a two-step method which utilizes enzyme-linked immunosorbent assay toxin testing and a chromogenic agar to detect and isolate enterohemorrhagic *Escherichia coli*. *J. Clin. Microbiol.* **38:**547–551.

145. **Oaks, J. L., T. E. Besser, S. T. Walk, D. M. Gordon, K. B. Beckmen, K. A. Burek, G. J. Haldorson, D. S. Bradway, L. Ouellette, F. R. Rurangirwa, M. A. Davis, G. Dobbin, and T. S. Whittam.** *Escherichia albertii* in wild and domestic birds. *Emerg. Infect. Dis.* **16:**638–646.

146. **Ogura, Y., T. Ooka, Asadulghani, J. Terajima, J. P. Nougayrede, K. Kurokawa, K. Tashiro, T. Tobe, K. Nakayama, S. Kuhara, E. Oswald, H. Watanabe, and T. Hayashi.** 2007. Extensive genomic diversity and selective conservation of virulence-determinants in enterohemorrhagic *Escherichia coli* strains of O157 and non-O157 serotypes. *Genome Biol.* **8:**R138.

147. **Ohnishi, M., K. Kurokawa, and T. Hayashi.** 2001. Diversification of *Escherichia coli* genomes: are bacteriophages the major contributors? *Trends Microbiol.* **9:**481–485.

148. **Olsen, S. J., J. Pruckler, W. Bibb, T. M. Nguyen, M. T. Tran, S. Sivapalasingam, A. Gupta, T. P. Phan, T. C. Nguyen, V. C. Nguyen, D. C. Phung, and E. D. Mintz.** 2004. Evaluation of rapid diagnostic tests for typhoid fever. *J. Clin. Microbiol.* **42:**1885–1889.

149. **Olsvik, O., and N. A. Strockbine.** 1993. PCR detection of heat-stable, heat-labile, and Shiga-like toxin genes in *Escherichia coli*, p. 271–276. *In* D. H. Persing, T. F. Smith, F. C. Tenover, and T. J. White (ed.), *Diagnostic Molecular Microbiology: Principles and Applications*. American Society for Microbiology, Washington, DC.

150. **Oswald, E., J. De Rycke, J. F. Guillot, and R. Boivin.** 1989. Cytotoxic effect of multinucleation in HeLa cell cultures associated with the presence of Vir plasmid in *Escherichia coli* strains. *FEMS Microbiol. Lett.* **49:**95–99.

151. **Park, C. H., H. J. Kim, D. L. Hixon, and A. Bubert.** 2003. Evaluation of the Duopath verotoxin test for detection of

Shiga toxins in cultures of human stools. *J. Clin. Microbiol.* **41:**2650–2653.

152. **Paton, A. W., and J. C. Paton.** 1998. Detection and characterization of Shiga toxigenic *Escherichia coli* by using multiplex PCR assays for *stx₁, stx₂, eaeA,* enterohemorrhagic *E. coli hlyA, rfb*ₒ₁₁₁, and *rfb*ₒ₁₅₇. *J. Clin. Microbiol.* **36:**598–602.

153. **Paton, A. W., R. M. Ratcliff, R. M. Doyle, J. Seymour-Murray, D. Davos, J. A. Lanser, and J. C. Paton.** 1996. Molecular microbiological investigation of an outbreak of hemolytic-uremic syndrome caused by dry fermented sausage contaminated with Shiga-like toxin-producing *Escherichia coli. J. Clin. Microbiol.* **34:**1622–1627.

154. **Patrick, M. E., P. M. Adcock, T. M. Gomez, S. F. Altekruse, B. H. Holland, R. V. Tauxe, and D. L. Swerdlow.** 2004. *Salmonella enteritidis* infections, United States, 1985–1999. *Emerg. Infect. Dis.* **10:**1–7.

155. **Petti, C. A., C. R. Polage, and P. Schreckenberger.** 2005. The role of 16S rRNA gene sequencing in identification of microorganisms misidentified by conventional methods. *J. Clin. Microbiol.* **43:**6123–6125.

156. **Pickard, D., J. Wain, S. Baker, A. Line, S. Chohan, M. Fookes, A. Barron, P. O. Gaora, J. A. Chabalgoity, N. Thanky, C. Scholes, N. Thomson, M. Quail, J. Parkhill, and G. Dougan.** 2003. Composition, acquisition, and distribution of the Vi exopolysaccharide-encoding *Salmonella enterica* pathogenicity island SPI-7. *J. Bacteriol.* **185:**5055–5065.

157. **Pien, F. D., S. Shrum, J. M. Swenson, B. C. Hill, C. Thornsberry, and J. J. Farmer III.** 1985. Colonization of human wounds by *Escherichia vulneris* and *Escherichia hermannii. J. Clin. Microbiol.* **22:**283–285.

158. **Popoff, M. Y., and L. E. Le Minor.** 2005. Genus XXXIII. *Salmonella* Lignieres 1900, 389ᴬᴸ, p. 764–799. *In* G. M. Garrity, D. J. Brenner, N. R. Krieg, and J. T. Staley (ed.), *Bergey's Manual of Systematic Bacteriology,* 2nd ed., vol. 2. *The* Proteobacteria. *Part B. The* Gammaproteobacteria. Springer Science+Business Media, Inc., New York, NY.

159. **Porwollik, S., and M. McClelland.** 2007. Determination of the gene content of *Salmonella* genomes by microarray analysis. *Methods Mol. Biol.* **394:**89–103.

160. **Prager, R., S. Annemuller, and H. Tschape.** 2005. Diversity of virulence patterns among Shiga toxin-producing *Escherichia coli* from human clinical cases—need for more detailed diagnostics. *Int. J. Med. Microbiol.* **295:**29–38.

161. **Prager, R., W. Rabsch, W. Streckel, W. Voigt, E. Tietze, and H. Tschape.** 2003. Molecular properties of *Salmonella enterica* serotype Paratyphi B distinguish between its systemic and its enteric pathovars. *J. Clin. Microbiol.* **41:**4270–4278.

162. **Priest, F. G., and M. Barker.** 2010. Gram-negative bacteria associated with brewery yeasts: reclassification of *Obesumbacterium proteus* biogroup 2 as *Shimwellia pseudoproteus* gen. nov., sp. nov., and transfer of *Escherichia blattae* to *Shimwellia blattae* comb. nov. *Int. J. Syst. Evol. Microbiol.* **60:**828–833.

163. **Pryamukhina, N. S., and N. A. Khomenko.** 1988. Suggestion to supplement *Shigella flexneri* classification scheme with the subserovar *Shigella flexneri* 4c: phenotypic characteristics of strains. *J. Clin. Microbiol.* **26:**1147–1149.

164. **Rahman, M. M., J. A. Haq, M. A. Morshed, and M. A. Rahman.** 2005. *Salmonella enterica* serovar Typhi with decreased susceptibility to ciprofloxacin—an emerging problem in Bangladesh. *Int. J. Antimicrob. Agents* **25:**345–346.

165. **Rangel, J. M., P. H. Sparling, C. Crowe, P. M. Griffin, and D. L. Swerdlow.** 2005. Epidemiology of *Escherichia coli* O157:H7 outbreaks, United States, 1982–2002. *Emerg. Infect. Dis.* **11:**603–609.

166. **Rantakokko-Jalava, K., S. Nikkari, J. Jalava, E. Eerola, M. Skurnik, O. Meurman, O. Ruuskanen, A. Alanen, E. Kotilainen, P. Toivanen, and P. Kotilainen.** 2000. Direct amplification of rRNA genes in diagnosis of bacterial infections. *J. Clin. Microbiol.* **38:**32–39.

167. **Rasko, D. A., M. J. Rosovitz, G. S. Myers, E. F. Mongodin, W. F. Fricke, P. Gajer, J. Crabtree, M. Sebaihia, N. R. Thomson, R. Chaudhuri, I. R. Henderson, V. Sperandio, and J. Ravel.** 2008. The pangenome structure of *Escherichia coli:* comparative genomic analysis of *E. coli* commensal and pathogenic isolates. *J. Bacteriol.* **190:**6881–6893.

168. Reference deleted.

169. **Reeves, M. W., G. M. Evins, A. A. Heiba, B. D. Plikaytis, and J. J. Farmer III.** 1989. Clonal nature of *Salmonella typhi* and its genetic relatedness to other salmonellae as shown by multilocus enzyme electrophoresis, and proposal of *Salmonella bongori* comb. nov. *J. Clin. Microbiol.* **27:**313–320.

170. **Rohde, R.** 1979. Serological integration of all known Arizona species into the Kauffmann-White scheme. *Zentralbl. Bakteriol. Orig. A* **243:**148–176. (In German.)

171. **Sack, R. B., M. Rahman, M. Yunus, and E. H. Khan.** 1997. Antimicrobial resistance in organisms causing diarrheal disease. *Clin. Infect. Dis.* **24**(Suppl. 1):S102–S105.

172. **Safdar, N.** 2002. Risk of hemolytic uremic syndrome after antibiotic treatment of *Escherichia coli* O157:H7 enteritis. *JAMA* **288:**996–1001.

173. **Sanders, C. C., M. Peyret, E. S. Moland, C. Shubert, K. S. Thomson, J.-M. Boeufgras, and W. E. Sanders, Jr.** 2000. Ability of the VITEK 2 advanced expert system to identify beta-lactam phenotypes in isolates of *Enterobacteriaceae* and *Pseudomonas aeruginosa. J. Clin. Microbiol.* **38:**570–574.

174. **Sarantuya, J., J. Nishi, N. Wakimoto, S. Erdene, J. P. Nataro, J. Sheikh, M. Iwashita, K. Manago, K. Tokuda, M. Yoshinaga, K. Miyata, and Y. Kawano.** 2004. Typical enteroaggregative *E. coli* is the most prevalent pathotype among *E. coli* strains causing diarrhea in Mongolian children. *J. Clin. Microbiol.* **42:**133–139.

175. **Scheutz, F., and N. A. Strockbine.** 2005. Genus I. *Escherichia* Castellani and Chalmers 1919, 941Tᴬᴸ, p. 607–624. *In* G. M. Garrity, D. J. Brenner, N. R. Krieg, and J. T. Staley (ed.), *Bergey's Manual of Systematic Bacteriology,* 2nd ed., vol. 2. *The* Proteobacteria. *Part B. The* Gammaproteobacteria. Springer Science+Business Media, Inc., New York, NY.

176. **Schmidt, H., and H. Karch.** 1996. Enterohemolytic phenotypes and genotypes of Shiga toxin-producing *Escherichia coli* O111 strains from patients with diarrhea and hemolytic-uremic syndrome. *J. Clin. Microbiol.* **34:**2364–2367.

177. **Scotland, S. M., T. Cheasty, A. Thomas, and B. Rowe.** 1991. Beta-glucuronidase activity of Vero cytotoxin-producing strains of *Escherichia coli,* including serogroup O157, isolated in the United Kingdom. *Lett. Appl. Microbiol.* **13:**42–44.

178. **Scotland, S. M., G. A. Willshaw, B. Said, H. R. Smith, and B. Rowe.** 1989. Identification of *Escherichia coli* that produces heat-stable enterotoxin STA by a commercially available enzyme-linked immunoassay and comparison of the assay with infant mouse and DNA probe tests. *J. Clin. Microbiol.* **27:**1697–1699.

179. **Senanayake, S. N., A. Jadeer, G. S. Talaulikar, and J. Roy.** 2006. First reported case of dialysis-related peritonitis due to *Escherichia vulneris. J. Clin. Microbiol.* **44:**4283–4284.

180. **Servin, A. L.** 2005. Pathogenesis of Afa/Dr diffusely adhering *Escherichia coli. Clin. Microbiol. Rev.* **18:**264–292.

181. **Simmon, K. E., A. C. Croft, and C. A. Petti.** 2006. Application of SmartGene IDNS software to partial 16S rRNA gene sequences for a diverse group of bacteria in a clinical laboratory. *J. Clin. Microbiol.* **44:**4400–4406.

182. Reference deleted.

183. **Sjogren, A. C., J. B. Kaper, A. Caprioli, and D. Karpman.** 2004. Enzyme-linked immunosorbent assay for detection of Shiga toxin-producing *Escherichia coli* infection by antibodies to *Escherichia coli* secreted protein B in children with hemolytic uremic syndrome. *Eur. J. Clin. Microbiol. Infect. Dis.* **23:**208–211.

184. **Slutsker, L., A. A. Ries, K. D. Greene, J. G. Wells, L. Hutwagner, and P. M. Griffin.** 1997. *Escherichia coli* O157:H7 diarrhea in the United States: clinical and epidemiologic features. *Ann. Intern. Med.* **126:**505–513.

185. **Smith, H. W.** 1974. A search for transmissible pathogenic characters in invasive strains of *Escherichia coli:* the discovery of a plasmid-controlled lethal character closely associated, or identical, with colicine V. *J. Gen. Microbiol.* **83:**95–111.

186. **Sowers, E. G., J. G. Wells, and N. A. Strockbine.** 1996. Evaluation of commercial latex reagents for identification of O157 and H7 antigens of *Escherichia coli. J. Clin. Microbiol.* **34:**1286–1289.

187. **Stock, I., M. Rahman, K. J. Sherwood, and B. Wiedemann.** 2005. Natural antimicrobial susceptibility patterns and biochemical identification of *Escherichia albertii* and *Hafnia alvei* strains. *Diagn. Microbiol. Infect. Dis.* **51:**151–163.

188. **Strockbine, N. A., and A. T. Maurelli.** 2005. Genus XXXV. *Shigella* Castellani and Chalmers 1919, 936[AL], p. 811–823. *In* G. M. Garrity, D. J. Brenner, N. R. Krieg, and J. T. Staley (ed.), *Bergey's Manual of Systematic Bacteriology*, 2nd ed., vol. 2. *The Proteobacteria. Part B. The* Gammaproteobacteria. Springer Science+Business Media, Inc., New York, NY.

189. **Strockbine, N. A., J. Parsonnet, K. Greene, J. A. Kiehlbauch, and I. K. Wachsmuth.** 1991. Molecular epidemiologic techniques in analysis of epidemic and endemic *Shigella dysenteriae* type 1 strains. *J. Infect. Dis.* **163:**406–409.

190. **Stuart, R. D.** 1959. Transport medium for specimens in public health bacteriology. *Public Health Rep.* **74:**431–438.

191. **Sugiyama, K., K. Inoue, and R. Sakazaki.** 2001. Mitomycin-supplemented washed blood agar for the isolation of Shiga toxin-producing *Escherichia coli* other than O157:H7. *Lett. Appl. Microbiol.* **33:**193–195.

192. **Swaminathan, B., T. J. Barrett, S. B. Hunter, R. V. Tauxe, and C. P. T. Force.** 2001. PulseNet: the molecular subtyping network for foodborne bacterial disease surveillance, United States. *Emerg. Infect. Dis.* **7:**382–389.

193. **Tacket, C. O., S. L. Moseley, B. Kay, G. Losonsky, and M. M. Levine.** 1990. Challenge studies in volunteers using *Escherichia coli* strains with diffuse adherence to HEp-2 cells. *J. Infect. Dis.* **162:**550–552.

194. **Talukder, K. A., B. K. Khajanchi, M. A. Islam, D. K. Dutta, Z. Islam, A. Safa, G. Y. Khan, K. Alam, M. A. Hossain, S. Malla, S. K. Niyogi, M. Rahman, H. Watanabe, G. B. Nair, and D. A. Sack.** 2004. Genetic relatedness of ciprofloxacin-resistant *Shigella dysenteriae* type 1 strains isolated in south Asia. *J. Antimicrob. Chemother.* **54:**730–734.

195. **Taneja, N.** 2007. Changing epidemiology of shigellosis and emergence of ciprofloxacin-resistant shigellae in India. *J. Clin. Microbiol.* **45:**678–679.

196. **Tarr, P. I., C. A. Gordon, and W. L. Chandler.** 2005. Shiga toxin-producing *Escherichia coli* and haemolytic uraemic syndrome. *Lancet* **365:**1073–1086.

197. **Tauxe, R. V., N. D. Puhr, J. G. Wells, N. Hargrett-Bean, and P. A. Blake.** 1990. Antimicrobial resistance of *Shigella* isolates in the USA: the importance of international travelers. *J. Infect. Dis.* **162:**1107–1111.

198. **Tazzari, P. L., F. Ricci, D. Carnicelli, A. Caprioli, A. E. Tozzi, G. Rizzoni, R. Conte, and M. Brigotti.** 2004. Flow cytometry detection of Shiga toxins in the blood from children with hemolytic uremic syndrome. *Cytometry B* **61:**40–44.

199. **Tindall, B. J., P. A. Grimont, G. M. Garrity, and J. P. Euzeby.** 2005. Nomenclature and taxonomy of the genus *Salmonella*. *Int. J. Syst. Evol. Microbiol.* **55:**521–524.

200. **Trabulsi, L. R., R. Keller, and T. A. Tardelli Gomes.** 2002. Typical and atypical enteropathogenic *Escherichia coli*. *Emerg. Infect. Dis.* **8:**508–513.

201. **van Duynhoven, Y. T., I. H. Friesema, T. Schuurman, A. Roovers, A. A. van Zwet, L. J. Sabbe, W. K. van der Zwaluw, D. W. Notermans, B. Mulder, E. J. van Hannen, F. G. Heilmann, A. Buiting, R. Jansen, and A. M. Kooistra-Smid.** 2008. Prevalence, characterisation and clinical profiles of Shiga toxin-producing *Escherichia coli* in The Netherlands. *Clin. Microbiol. Infect.* **14:**437–445.

202. **Verbrugh, H. A., D. R. Mekkes, R. P. Verkoyen, and J. E. Landbeer.** 1987. Widal type serology using live antigen for diagnosis of *Shigella flexneri* dysentery. *Eur. J. Clin. Microbiol. Infect. Dis.* **5:**540–542.

203. **Vial, P. A., J. J. Mathewson, H. L. DuPont, L. Guers, and M. M. Levine.** 1990. Comparison of two assay methods for patterns of adherence to HEp-2 cells of *Escherichia coli* from patients with diarrhea. *J. Clin. Microbiol.* **28:**882–885.

204. **Voetsch, A. C., F. J. Angulo, T. Rabatsky-Ehr, S. Shallow, M. Cassidy, S. M. Thomas, E. Swanson, S. M. Zansky, M. A. Hawkins, T. F. Jones, P. J. Shillam, T. J. Van Gilder, J. G. Wells, P. M. Griffin, et al.** 2004. Laboratory practices for stool-specimen culture for bacterial pathogens, including *Escherichia coli* O157:H7, in the FoodNet sites, 1995–2000. *Clin. Infect. Dis.* **38:**S190–S197.

205. **von Seidlein, L., D. R. Kim, M. Ali, H. Lee, X. Wang, V. D. Thiem, G. Canh do, W. Chaicumpa, M. D. Agtini, A. Hossain, Z. A. Bhutta, C. Mason, O. Sethabutr, K. Talukder, G. B. Nair, J. L. Deen, K. Kotloff, and J. Clemens.** 2006. A multicentre study of *Shigella* diarrhoea in six Asian countries: disease burden, clinical manifestations, and microbiology. *PLoS Med.* **3:**e353.

206. **Vugia, D. J., M. Samuel, M. M. Farley, R. Marcus, B. Shiferaw, S. Shallow, K. Smith, F. J. Angulo, et al.** 2004. Invasive *Salmonella* infections in the United States, FoodNet, 1996–1999: incidence, serotype distribution, and outcome. *Clin. Infect. Dis.* **38:**S149–S156.

207. **Wang, W. L., L. B. Reller, B. Smallwood, N. W. Luechtefeld, and M. J. Blaser.** 1983. Evaluation of transport media for *Campylobacter jejuni* in human fecal specimens. *J. Clin. Microbiol.* **18:**803–807.

208. **Wathen-Grady, H. G., L. E. Britt, N. A. Strockbine, and I. K. Wachsmuth.** 1990. Characterization of *Shigella dysenteriae* serotypes 11, 12, and 13. *J. Clin. Microbiol.* **28:**2580–2584.

209. **Wathen-Grady, H. G., B. R. Davis, and G. K. Morris.** 1985. Addition of three new serotypes of *Shigella boydii* to the *Shigella* schema. *J. Clin. Microbiol.* **21:**129–132.

210. **Wells, J. G., and G. K. Morris.** 1981. Evaluation of transport methods for isolating *Shigella* spp. *J. Clin. Microbiol.* **13:**789–790.

211. **Whittam, T. S., and A. C. Bumbaugh.** 2002. Inferences from whole-genome sequences of bacterial pathogens. *Curr. Opin. Genet. Dev.* **12:**719–725.

212. **Wong, C. S., S. Jelacic, R. L. Habeeb, S. L. Watkins, and P. I. Tarr.** 2000. The risk of hemolytic-uremic syndrome after antibiotic treatment of *Escherichia coli* O157:H7 infections. *N. Engl. J. Med.* **342:**1930–1936.

213. **Woo, P. C., P. K. Leung, K. W. Leung, and K. Y. Yuen.** 2000. Identification by 16S ribosomal RNA gene sequencing of an *Enterobacteriaceae* species from a bone marrow transplant recipient. *Mol. Pathol.* **53:**211–215.

214. **Yam, W. C., M. L. Lung, and M. H. Ng.** 1992. Evaluation and optimization of a latex agglutination assay for detection of cholera toxin and *Escherichia coli* heat-labile toxin. *J. Clin. Microbiol.* **30:**2518–2520.

215. **Yamamoto, T., Y. Koyama, M. Matsumoto, E. Sonoda, S. Nakayama, M. Uchimura, W. Paveenkittiporn, K. Tamura, T. Yokota, and P. Echeverria.** 1992. Localized, aggregative, and diffuse adherence to HeLa cells, plastic, and human small intestines by *Escherichia coli* isolated from patients with diarrhea. *J. Infect. Dis.* **166:**1295–1310.

Yersinia*

MARTIN E. SCHRIEFER AND JEANNINE M. PETERSEN

36

The pathogenic *Yersinia* species, *Y. pseudotuberculosis*, *Y. enterocolitica*, and *Y. pestis*, are zoonotic agents that cause disease in humans ranging from mild gastroenteritis to life-threatening plague. Human clinical infections caused by *Y. pseudotuberculosis* and *Y. enterocolitica* most frequently occur after the ingestion of contaminated food or water, whereas the etiologic agent of plague, *Y. pestis*, is naturally vectored to humans by fleas. These species are joined by 11 lesser-known *Yersinia* species which are largely considered environmental species, nonpathogenic to humans (Table 1). Pathogenic *Yersinia* species share a highly conserved virulence plasmid and a chromosomal high pathogenicity island (HPI) and show tropism for lymphoid tissue, where their ability to evade host innate immunity enables extracellular proliferation. Popular awareness of the tens of millions of human deaths caused by the plague bacillus, *Y. pestis*, in each of three pandemics is contrasted by relative ignorance of the current global reach of plague, its firm entrenchment in a number of recent rodent-flea cycles covering much of the western United States and other parts of the world, and its reemergence as a significant human pathogen in parts of eastern Africa and Madagascar. This agent was weaponized by the United States, Japan, and former USSR during and after World War II and remains a high-level biothreat agent. Increased biomedical research, in response to these concerns, has led to a number of recent advances in our understanding of invasiveness and immune system evasion by *Y. pestis* and the closely related *Y. pseudotuberculosis* and *Y. enterocolitica* and exciting new laboratory diagnostic and vaccine development approaches (10, 13, 59, 68).

TAXONOMY AND HISTORY OF THE GENUS

The agent of plague, *Y. pestis* (previously *Bacterium pestis*, *Bacillus pestis*, and *Pasteurella pestis*), was first identified in lymph node aspirates from plague victims in 1894 by Alexander Yersin during his investigation of the leading edge of the third pandemic as it swept quickly from mainland China to Hong Kong and beyond. Further, he demonstrated that laboratory mice and rats inoculated with pure cultures of the gram-negative coccobacillus produced symptoms of plague and death. Four years later, while investigating the advancing epidemic in India, Paul-Louis Simond and Masanori Ogata independently implicated the role of fleas as vectors of disease transmission between rodents and humans. By the early 1900s, plague was introduced along steamship routes to every human-inhabited continent and was responsible for more than 12 million deaths, most of them in India and China (59). Today, plague remains enzootic in parts of Africa, North and South America, and much of Asia.

By 1944, cumulative phenotypic and genotypic peculiarities of *Pasteurella pestis* and *P. pseudotuberculosis* prompted their transfer to the new genus *Yersinia*. Ten years later, *Yersinia* species were included in the family *Enterobacteriaceae*, and in 1964 *Y. enterocolitica* was added to the genus. The diverse group members of *Y. enterocolitica* were further divided into a subgroup initially designated *Y. enterocolitica*-like organisms and later into an additional four species (*Y. intermedia*, *Y. frederiksenii*, *Y. kristensenii*, and *Y. aldovae*) based on sugar fermentation and DNA relatedness. Subsequent species designations include *Y. ruckeri* (serogroup 01, the agent of enteric red mouth disease in rainbow trout), *Y. rohdei*, *Y. mollaretii*, and *Y. bercovieri*. Three additional species have been described since 2005, bringing the total to 14 (www.bacterio.cict.fr/xz/yersinia.html).

Yersinia species have a G+C content of 46 to 50%. By DNA-DNA hybridization, *Yersinia* species are related to other members of the family *Enterobacteriaceae* by 10 to 32%. Intraspecies relatedness is variable, ranging from 55 to 74%, with the notable exception of *Y. pestis* and *Y. pseudotuberculosis*, which demonstrate more than 90% relatedness.

The sequenced and annotated genomes of *Y. pestis* biovar Orientalis and biovar Medievalis were published in 2001 and 2002, respectively (22, 57). Since then the genomes of at least a dozen additional *Y. pestis* strains have been released (13). In 2004, the *Y. pseudotuberculosis* genome was published along with a comparative genomic analysis of *Y. pestis* (16). Completion and analysis of these genomes have solidified a large body of prior genetic evidence suggesting that *Y. pestis* evolved from *Y. pseudotuberculosis* prior to the first plague pandemic (1, 2, 13, 57, 81, 82). Were it not for the profoundly distinct mechanisms of pathogenesis and natural maintenance, taxonomists would likely merge *Y. pseudotuberculosis* and *Y. pestis*. The genome of

---

*This chapter contains information presented in chapter 44 by Audrey Wanger in the ninth edition of this *Manual*.

TABLE 1 Biochemical reactivity of *Yersinia* species[a]

Yersinia species	Motility (25°C)	Ornithine decarboxylase	Urease	VP (25°C)	Citrate (25°C)	Indole	Rhamnose	Sucrose	Cellobiose	Sorbose	Sorbitol	Melibiose	Raffinose	Fucose
Y. pestis	−	−	−	−	−	−	−	−	−	−	−	V	−	ND
Y. pseudotuberculosis	+	−	+	−	−	−	+	−	−	−	−	+	>	−
Y. enterocolitica	+	+	+	+	−	V	−	+	+	+	+	−	−	>
Y. frederiksenii	+	+	+	+	V	+	+	+	+	+	+	−	−	+
Y. kristensenii	V	+	+	−	−	V	−	−	+	+	+	−	−	>
Y. ruckeri	+	+	−	V	+	−	−	+	−	−	−	−	−	ND
Y. mollaretii	+	+	+	+	−	−	−	+	+	+	+	−	−	−
Y. bercovieri	+	+	+	−	−	−	−	+	+	+	+	−	−	+
Y. rohdei	+	V	V	−	−	−	−	+	+	ND	+	V	>	ND
Y. aldovae	+	+	+	+	+	−	+	−	−	ND	+	−	−	>
Y. intermedia	+	+	+	+	+	+	+	+	+	ND	+	+	+	>

Reaction or characteristic[b]

[a]From references 71 and 79.
[b]Incubation is at 35°C except where indicated. VP, Voges-Proskauer; V, variable; ND, not done; −, negative; +, positive.

Y. enterocolitica was published in 2006 (76) and has enabled further understanding of the common and unique genetic lineages and functions of the pathogenic *Yersinia* species.

DESCRIPTION OF THE AGENTS

Yersinia species, as members of the family *Enterobacteriaceae*, are gram-negative, non-spore-forming bacilli that exhibit bipolar staining particularly when seen in primary specimens stained with Giemsa or Wayson's dye. The bacilli are smaller (0.5 to 0.8 μm in diameter and 1 to 3 μm in length) than other members of their family and tend to grow more slowly as well. With the exception of *Y. pestis*, *Yersinia* species are motile at 25°C due to peritrichous or paripolar flagella (Table 1). Interestingly, the pathogenic yersiniae either repress (*Y. pseudotuberculosis* and *Y. enterocolitica*) or, through mutation, have lost the capability to express (*Y. pestis*) the flagellar apparatus; by either mechanism they effectively avoid stimulation of innate immune responses to these potent inducers (52).

Yersinia species are facultative anaerobes that grow at temperatures ranging from 4 to 43°C. Although optimal doubling times are observed between 25 and 28°C, the ability to replicate at 4°C (psychrophile) has important ramifications for blood banking among asymptomatic *Y. enterocolitica*-carrying donors (see "Clinical Significance" below). *Yersinia* species ferment glucose with the production of acid and no gas and are catalase positive and oxidase negative. Most strains grow on MacConkey, blood, and chocolate agars but may be outcompeted by other bacteria in clinical and especially environmental samples (see "Isolation Procedures" below). Yersiniae exhibit poor growth in liquid media and do not form a turbid suspension (79).

The cell walls of *Yersinia* species are very similar to those of other members of the *Enterobacteriaceae* family, and lipopolysaccharide (LPS) is a major component of their outer membrane. The LPS of *Y. pseudotuberculosis* and *Y. enterocolitica* (smooth forms) is complete (lipid A–oligosaccharide core–O antigen polysaccharide), and O-chain variation within these species has enabled serodiscrimination of close to 100 LPS types (6). In contrast, through a genetic defect in the biosynthesis of complete LPS, *Y. pestis* (rough form) lacks the O-specific polysaccharide chain (9, 67).

Several dozen virulence genes, their environment-dependent expression control, and the complex mechanisms of their product action and coordination, which enable immune system evasion and disease progression, have been actively investigated and described. Only a few of the key features will be presented here, and the reader is referred to several excellent reviews for more detailed and comprehensive information (35, 46, 68, 78). Many *Yersinia* virulence genes are conserved across species lines, while others are species specific. Of intrigue, a number of the enteropathogenic *Yersinia* virulence genes have been rendered dysfunctional in the *Y. pestis* lineage, through mutation or insertion sequence interruption, but have been maintained within the species in the absence of apparent function. One of the key features of the pathogenic *Yersinia* species is the ability to scavenge iron from the host by a siderophore called yersiniabactin (Ybt). The *ybt* genes are chromosomally located and clustered on an HPI located in a 102-kb chromosomal region termed the *pgm* (pigmentation) locus. An additional operon within the *pgm* region, and unique to *Y. pestis*, is the *hms* locus. The hemin storage proteins encoded by this locus enable biofilm formation and proventricular blockage required for efficient transmission of *Y. pestis* from vector fleas to mammals (25, 57).

Several other chromosomal virulence genes include *yst*, which encodes a heat-stable toxin unique to the pathogenic members of *Y. enterocolitica*, and *invA*, an epithelial cell adhesin gene common to all three pathogenic *Yersinia* species. In *Y. enterocolitica* and *Y. pseudotuberculosis*, invasin facilitates efficient binding to intestinal mucosal cells and translocation from the lumen to Peyer's patches. An insertion element within the *invA* gene of *Y. pestis* renders it dysfunctional in spite of otherwise >99% nucleic acid identity with the gene of *Y. pseudotuberculosis*.

Although each of the pathogenic *Yersinia* species is associated with different clinical entities, they possess a common and genetically conserved 68- to 75-kb virulence plasmid (termed pCD1 in *Y. pestis* and pYV in *Y. enterocolitica* and *Y. pseudotuberculosis*). This plasmid carries the low calcium response genes, components of the type three secretion system (TTSS), and the associated effectors or *Yersinia* outer membrane proteins (Yops) (65). The TTSS forms a needle structure on the surface of pathogenic *Yersinia* species which interacts with target cells (macrophages, dendritic cells, and granulocytes/neutrophils) and enables injection of six different Yops which effectively interfere with phagocytosis and other innate host cell responses as well as the adaptive inflammatory cascade, ultimately resulting in target cell apoptosis (19). Another virulence plasmid gene product, V antigen, is assembled on the tip of the needle structure and required for injection of Yop effectors (45). Recent experiments also indicate that the anti-inflammatory properties of V antigen enable *Y. pestis*-infected rodent survival while bacterial loads increase to levels beyond 10^8/ml of blood (23). Such levels are required for effective infection of blood-feeding fleas (49).

YadA is an adhesion protein also encoded on the *Yersinia* virulence plasmid. In *Y. enterocolitica* and *Y. pseudotuberculosis,* it too facilitates pathogen binding to M cells of the intestinal mucosa, signal-induced internalization, and subsequent translocation to the Peyer's patches and mesenteric lymph nodes. *Y. pestis*, which does not enter the epithelial cells of mammalian or flea hosts, carries the 70-kb plasmid-encoded *yadA* gene, which is nearly identical to that of *Y. pseudotuberculosis*; but like invasin, *Y. pestis* YadA is dysfunctional, in this case through a base deletion resulting in a frameshift and a truncated product.

Two *Y. pestis* unique plasmids (~110 and 10 kb), acquired after its divergence from *Y. pseudotuberculosis*, carry a variety of genes responsible for several differential attributes of this agent: its ability to utilize a flea vector and its ability to cause acute disease in the infected mammal. The large plasmid encodes the murine toxin (Ymt) and the fraction 1 antigen (F1). Ymt, which is expressed only at temperatures below those of mammalian systems, is a phospholipase whose activity is necessary for pathogen survival within the harsh environment of the flea digestive tract during blood meal digestion (33). In contrast to Ymt, F1 is expressed at temperatures >30°C and during mammalian infection. Upon flea inoculation of *Y. pestis*, some of the bacteria are engulfed and transported to regional lymph nodes by macrophages. Here, during intracellular growth, F1 is expressed and forms a capsule-like structure on the bacterial surface. Subsequent to release of *Y. pestis* from its intracellular location, the antiphagocytic properties of the new F1 surface enable widespread dissemination and replication and result in host sepsis. Plasminogen activator (Pla), one of the small plasmid products, is a surface protease that activates mammalian plasminogen and degrades complement; it has been shown to be essential for dissemination by subcutaneous or intradermal inoculation, experimental proxies for flea-bite transmission, in mouse models of bubonic disease. These are but a few of the *Y. pestis* unique, plasmid-encoded proteins differentially expressed within the temperature and environmental constraints of its arthropod and mammalian hosts which enable pathogen survival, replication, and dissemination (57).

EPIDEMIOLOGY AND TRANSMISSION

Plague is an acute, often fatal disease caused by *Y. pestis*. It exists in natural enzootic cycles between wild rodents and their fleas. The most common mode of transmission to humans is by the bite of infected fleas. Less frequently, infection is the result of handling infected animals, direct contact with infectious body fluids or tissues, or inhaling infectious respiratory droplets or other materials (e.g., laboratory-acquired cases). Epidemics occur occasionally when the disease spreads from wild rodents into populations of rats (genus *Rattus*) that live near human populations. Human risk is greatest when epizootics cause high mortality in these commensal rat populations, thereby forcing fleas to seek alternate hosts, including humans. Although many different species of fleas parasitize rodents and can transmit infection to them, transmission of plague is classically associated with the rat flea (*Xenopsylla cheopis*) (15). *Y. pestis* can survive and multiply in the midgut (stomach) and proventriculus (a valve that connects the esophagus to the midgut) of this flea. Bacterial replication results in blockage of the proventriculus and causes the infected flea to bite multiple hosts in repeated attempts to acquire a blood meal, thereby increasing chances for disease transmission. Interestingly, when the environmental temperature is above 27°C, *Y. pestis* does not produce coagulase and blockage of the proventriculus is unlikely to occur, thus reducing transmission to humans (77).

Approximately 2,500 human cases of plague are identified every year around the world. Although routine reporting of cases to the World Health Organization was discontinued in 2003, between 1989 and 2003, 38,359 human cases with 2,845 deaths were reported from 25 countries. Approximately 80% of these cases were reported from Africa, 15% from Asia, and the remainder from the Americas. Between 1960 and 2006, 447 plague cases (~9 cases/year) were reported in the United States. Although plague occurs among wild animal populations in all of the 17 contiguous states west of the 100th meridian, more than 80% of human cases occur in New Mexico, Arizona, and Colorado, and approximately 10% occur in California (20, 29, 51).

Domestic dogs and cats may serve as carriers of *Y. pestis*-infected fleas into human dwellings. A recent study in New Mexico found that plague victims were significantly more likely than controls to have allowed pets to sleep on their beds (32). Cats are also highly susceptible to plague, acquiring infection by flea bite or ingestion of infected rodents, and develop all of the clinical forms of disease, including pneumonic plague. Infected cats serve as direct sources of human infection via aerosol transmission of organisms, leading to primary pneumonic plague, or by inoculation of organisms through scratches or bites (29). Dogs are most often resistant to clinical infection and develop antibody titers upon exposure.

Hunting in areas where plague is endemic is associated with occasional human infections. Infected animals may not display external or internal signs of disease, and as such, transmission may occur during skinning and handling of animals or ingestion of undercooked meat. Although many animal species are susceptible to plague infection and thus pose a risk factor associated with hunting in areas of endemicity, documented cases of transmission are most frequently associated with rabbits, squirrels, prairie dogs, and bobcats. Direct inoculation into the bloodstream is associated with an increased risk of septicemia and a high fatality rate.

Human-to-human transmission is very rare and occurs only with the pneumonic form of disease; most transmissions are to unprotected/untrained family members and health care providers through close-contact inhalation of particles from infected persons who are coughing copious amounts of bloody sputum. In a number of reports, simple measures such as avoidance of close (<2 meters) contact and/or use of surgical masks and gloves are reported as protective (36, 42). These findings are consistent with limited-distance spread of *Y. pestis*-contaminated respiratory droplets from pneumonic plague patients as opposed to greater dispersal distances of droplet nuclei among other respiratory pathogens, such as *Mycobacterium tuberculosis* from patients with pulmonary tuberculosis. In resource-poor regions, protection of health care providers is often limited to patient contact in well-ventilated wards, minimal time visits, and during such visits, requiring patients to turn their heads away from the provider or examining them from behind (4, 36, 42, 62). In over 60 separate cases of pneumonic plague in the United States since 1924, there have been no human-to-human transmissions (36).

In recorded history there have been three plague pandemics, each originating in different parts of the known world. The earliest pandemic, known as the Justinian plague, spanned the sixth through eighth centuries, began in northeast Africa, and spread through the Middle East and the Mediterranean basin. Methodical and accurate mortality records were not attempted in most affected areas, and competing epidemics such as smallpox have complicated estimates of plague cases and deaths. Nonetheless, it is ventured that from A.D. 541 to 700 there was an overall population loss of 50 to 60% in many locales of affected regions. Historical records of the second pandemic are comparatively numerous and in many cases detailed. Beginning in the Himalaya region of central Asia in the mid 1300s and spreading westward along overland trade routes, it entered Sicily in 1347. The ensuing epidemic, later known as the Black Death, spread quickly by sea to Italy, Greece, and France, and later by land throughout Europe. Between 1347 and 1351, an estimated 17 to 28 million Europeans died of plague. Following epidemics occurred in periodic cycles for over 300 years. Institution of "quarantine," the 40-day isolation of ships and people while waiting to see if symptoms of plague would develop prior to allowing city entrance, originated in Venice in 1377. This and other attempts to slow the spread of plague were futile; the pandemic killed up to one-third of the European population between the 14th and 15th centuries and encompassed the Near and Middle East, Europe, and the British Isles. The cause of plague was still unknown. The third, or modern, plague pandemic originated in southern China in the mid- to late 1800s and spread globally, reintroducing the disease to many regions and establishing new foci in North and South America as well as Madagascar (10, 59, 84).

Four biovars of *Y. pestis*, three of which cause human disease, persist today and are differentiated by their ability to ferment glycerol or arabinose and reduce nitrate (see "Identification" below). Human cases are associated with Antiqua strains found in Asia and Africa, Medievalis strains found in Asia (Near East through the former Soviet Union to China and Mongolia), and Orientalis strains distributed globally. A fourth biovar, Microtus (also known as Pestoides), is pathogenic to the rodent genus *Microtus* (voles), mice, and other small rodents but not to large mammals, including humans (39a, 79a, 83). *Y. pestis* lineage analysis of available strains from the four biovars using multiple-locus variable-number tandem repeat analysis, insertion sequence elements, and single-nucleotide polymorphism genotyping suggest that biovar Microtus is the closest ancestral derivative of *Y. pseudotuberculosis* (2).

Y. enterocolitica is a heterogeneous species with worldwide distribution and both pathogenic (human and animal) as well as nonpathogenic members. Organisms are found in the gastrointestinal tracts of many animal species, most commonly swine, rodents, and dogs. Due to their enhanced growth in cold temperatures, geographic distribution is mostly in subtropical and temperate regions. Food products, particularly raw and undercooked meats, are frequently found to contain these organisms, although the majority of them are nonpathogenic. The genus is divided into six biogroups—1A, 1B, 2, 3, 4, and 5—that are biochemically differentiated (Table 2). Group 1A (which lacks the 68- to 75-kb virulence plasmid) is nonpathogenic, groups 2 through 5 (which lack the chromosomal HPI) are weakly

TABLE 2 Reactions of biotypes of Y. enterocolitica[a] after incubation at 25°C for 48 h

Test	Reaction[b] for biotype:					
	1A	1B	2	3	4	5
Lipase (Tween esterase)	+	+	−	−	−	−
Esculin	+	−	−	−	−	−
Salicin	+	−	−	−	−	−
Indole	+	+	(+)	−	−	−
Xylose	+	+	+	+	−	d
Trehalose	+	+	+	+	+	−
NO₃ → NO₂	+	+	+	+	+	−
DNase	−	−	−	−	+	+
Pyrazinamidase[c]	+	−	−	−	−	−

^{a}Modified from reference 79a with permission of the publisher, S. Karger AG, Basel, Switzerland.
^{b}+, ≥90% of strains are positive; d, 11 to 89% of strains are positive; −, ≥90% of strains are negative; (+), weakly positive reaction.
^{c}According to Kandolo and Wauters (39a).

pathogenic in mice, and group 1B is highly pathogenic and lethal to mice. Group 1B has been frequently isolated in North America, whereas groups 2 through 5 are predominantly isolated in Europe and Japan. Serogroup typing, based on reactivity to O-antigen polysaccharides, has also been developed, and over 70 serotypes are characterized. Many serotypes are geographically focused, and only a few are associated with disease in animals or humans.

Y. pseudotuberculosis is found in the environment (soil and water) and in a diverse group of wild and domesticated animal species. The organism is found worldwide but is most common in northern Europe and Asia, including Japan. The main reservoirs for the organism are rodents, rabbits, and wild birds. Infected animals serve as chronic carriers and sources for infecting water and food, such as meat and dairy products. Like that of *Y. enterocolitica*, the mode of transmission of *Y. pseudotuberculosis* is thought to be largely via ingestion of contaminated food or water.

CLINICAL SIGNIFICANCE

Plague, one of about ten internationally quarantinable diseases, is a severe febrile illness characterized by acute onset, headache, myalgia, malaise, shaking chills, prostration, and gastrointestinal symptoms, and without prompt and appropriate antibiotic treatment, it is often fatal. A formalin-killed whole-cell plague vaccine which demonstrated efficacy for bubonic but not primary pneumonic disease was licensed and available in the United States until 1999. Recent vaccine efforts targeting pneumonic protection have utilized recombinant F1 and V antigens in cocktail or chimeric (rF1V) formulations. Both formulations have demonstrated good protection among immunized mice against pulmonary challenge, and they both appear to be safe, well tolerated, and immunogenic in human trials. Potential licensure by the U.S. FDA will be in accordance with the "animal rule" which requires safety and immunogenicity data from humans along with efficacy in animal models that mimic human disease (68).

There are three major forms of plague: bubonic, septicemic, and pneumonic. Bubonic plague is the most common clinical presentation, accounting for 80 to 90% of cases and characterized by acute development of regional lymphadenopathy. During the bite of an infected flea, up to 10^4 organisms may be inoculated into the skin. Organisms evading neutrophil uptake and other innate surveillance and killing are transported to regional lymph nodes, mainly in macrophages. After a 2- to 8-day incubation period, the patient develops fever and a painful lymph node swelling (bubo). The case fatality rate for untreated bubonic plague cases is 50 to 60%.

Septicemic plague can occur when the organisms inoculated by the infected flea spread to the bloodstream without localizing in regional lymph nodes or when the bacteria are directly introduced into the bloodstream via a cut or wound. This form of the disease is more common in children and is rapidly fatal. Septicemic plague can also occur secondary to bubonic plague that is not adequately treated. In the United States between 1947 and 1977, approximately 10% of plague cases presented with septicemia and approximately 50% of these cases were fatal (30).

Pneumonic plague can be a rare secondary complication of bubonic or septicemic plague or can be the primary infection following direct inhalation of aerosolized organisms from other pneumonic cases (human or animal), infected tissues, or cultured organisms. After an incubation period

of 1 to 6 days, symptoms include high fever and cough with hemoptysis and chest pain (36). Mortality among untreated pneumonic cases is essentially 100%, and even among treated cases mortality often exceeds 50%. Sporadic person-to-person pneumonic outbreaks continue to occur in Madagascar, Uganda, the Democratic Republic of the Congo, and Tibet (4, 62). In 2007, a fatal case of primary pneumonic plague occurred in a Grand Canyon National Park wildlife biologist who had necropsied an infected mountain lion carcass 7 days earlier (80). Between 1925 and 2006, 13 cases of primary and 52 cases of secondary pneumonic plague were described in the United States. Among the primary cases, nine had known exposures: six (67%) were from face-to-face contact with infected pets, and three (33%) were acquired in laboratory settings. Person-to-person transmission of pneumonic plague in the United States has not been reported since 1924.

The most common form of disease due to *Y. enterocolitica* is gastroenteritis associated with consumption of contaminated food or water. It is not unusual to isolate *Y. enterocolitica* from raw meats, including beef, lamb, pork, and chicken. The organism has also been found as a contaminant of cooked, prepackaged deli meat. The majority of strains isolated from human food sources are of the nonpathogenic serotypes. Carriage of the pathogenic serotypes of *Y. enterocolitica* is more common in swine; therefore, consumption of raw or undercooked pork, such as chitterlings, is the main risk factor for gastroenteritis (12, 28, 39). Severity of disease is related to the serotype and can range from self-limited gastroenteritis to terminal ileitis and mesenteric lymphadenitis, often misdiagnosed as appendicitis. Young children most commonly develop gastroenteritis and present with fever, watery diarrhea (occasionally bloody and severe), and abdominal pain following consumption of food contaminated by *Yersinia* species. The heat-stable toxin Yst has been indentified in all enteropathogenic *Y. enterocolitica* strains but is absent in *Y. pseudotuberculosis* (81). Although symptoms typically resolve within approximately 7 days, patients can carry the organism in their gastrointestinal tracts for as long as several months. Organisms can migrate out of the gut via the lymphatics into local lymph nodes. An uncommon complication of gastroenteritis is septicemia. Persons at high risk for septicemia include the elderly and immunocompromised patients, particularly those with underlying metabolic diseases that are associated with iron overload, cancer, liver disease, and steroid therapy.

The production of urease allows *Y. enterocolitica* to survive in the stomach and colonize the small intestine of the human host. Pathogenic strains contain Yops which enable them to resist the normal phagocytic and complement killing process that takes place in Peyer's patches (73). *Y. enterocolitica* is the most common cause of transfusion-related infections due to contaminated red blood cells. Since the organism is able to survive and multiply at refrigeration temperatures, donated blood contaminated with small numbers of organisms from an asymptomatic person can transmit infection to the transfused patient (16, 44). Reactive arthritis is an uncommon sequela of diarrhea due to *Y. enterocolitica*. Patients at increased risk include those who are carriers of the HLA-B27 allele and those with immunologic disorders. Symptoms appear several days to months after the onset of diarrhea and may persist for months. Other less common diseases associated with *Y. enterocolitica* infection include inflammatory bowel disease, most commonly associated with serotype O:3 (63), and autoimmune thyroid disorders, such as Graves' disease and Hashimoto's thyroiditis (15).

Both Y. enterocolitica and Y. pseudotuberculosis have been isolated from patients with Crohn's disease, although a causal relationship has not been proven (34).

Y. pseudotuberculosis usually produces a self-limiting disease, particularly in children and young adults. Rarely, Y. pseudotuberculosis can cause mesenteric lymphadenitis that clinically mimics appendicitis and septicemia and generally occurs in immunocompromised patients (diabetics and those with liver cirrhosis or iron overload) (21). Long-term sequelae of Y. pseudotuberculosis infection include erythema nodosum, Reiter's syndrome, and nephritis. Y. pseudotuberculosis has also recently been implicated in outbreaks of gastroenteritis-pseudoappendicitis associated with consumption of contaminated lettuce and carrots (40, 55).

The lack of classic virulence markers (see "Description of the Agents" above) in the other Yersina species (Table 1) has led to their general classification as nonpathogenic. Nonetheless, several of them (Y. intermedia, Y. frederiksenii, and Y. kristensenii) have been isolated from stool specimens of up to 20% of diarrhea patients for whom etiologic agents were not determined (48). Alternate virulence factors have been suggested for some species, but their proof requires further study. Possible predisposing correlates of infection include corticosteroid, acid suppressant, and antibiotic use and an immunocompromised host status (48, 73).

COLLECTION, TRANSPORT, AND STORAGE OF SPECIMENS

In the United States, Y. pestis is classified as a select agent. To transfer, receive, or possess Y. pestis strains, laboratories must be registered with the Centers for Disease Control and Prevention (CDC). The registration process includes a U.S. Department of Justice investigation of all personnel having access to select agents. Clinical laboratories are exempt from the registration requirement provided that within seven calendar days of identifying one of these agents, they transfer it to a registered entity and/or destroy the agent on site. Laboratories identifying an organism as Y. pestis are required to report this finding immediately to the CDC. Report forms, contact information, laboratory registration information, and pertinent citations of the U.S. Federal Code may be found at www.cdc.gov/od/sap. All routine procedures performed o```n Y. pestis should be done in a facility with a biosafety level of at least 2 (BSL-2), and clinical laboratories should be aware of the sentinel-level clinical microbiology laboratory guidelines as outlined by the American Society for Microbiology (www.asm.org). Processes which increase risk for creating an aerosol, such as liquid culture manipulation, should be performed under BSL-3 conditions. Y. pestis strains lacking either the pgm locus (a 102-kb chromosome region encoding yersiniabactin iron transport, the Hms biofilm, and other systems) or the 60-to-85-kb virulence plasmid (which encodes the TTSS and its effector Yop proteins) are exempt from select agent regulations in the United States and can be handled under BSL-2 conditions. However, pgm mutants are still capable of causing disease; by intravenous injection they are fully virulent, and by peripheral inoculation they require only several log orders increased inocula or iron supplementation for mortality (in mice) comparable to wild-type infections. Strains lacking the virulence plasmid are considered avirulent (25, 38, 58).

Laboratory confirmation of suspected plague diagnosis can be made by detection or growth of Y. pestis. Preferred samples and tissues are dependent on the clinical presentation; lymph node aspirates and blood are recommended in bubonic presentation, blood for septicemic presentation, and respiratory samples and blood for pneumonic presentation. Patients may shed organisms into the blood intermittently, so obtaining multiple sets of blood cultures over a 24-h period increases the sensitivity of detection from this sample source. Blood cultures should be incubated at both 28 and 35°C to increase chances of recovery of the organism (3, 36). Cary-Blair medium and swabs offer an excellent transport medium for preservation of viable organisms if samples cannot be cultured immediately. Other culture sources for pneumonic cases include throat swabs and throat washing specimens; however, due to contamination of these specimens with normal biota (see "Isolation Procedures" below), a broncho-alveolar washing or lavage specimen is preferable (3). Tissue samples from autopsy specimens, lymph node, spleen, liver, and lung can also be utilized for testing. Blood remnants or tissue specimens can also be collected from animals suspected to have died from Y. pestis infection. Convalescent-phase sera can be collected from animals and humans to test for antibody to Y. pestis. Flea triturates can also be tested. Specimens should be sent to the laboratory immediately, and if a delay in transit of more than 2 h is expected, the sample should be transported at 2 to 8°C.

The appropriate specimens for culture of Y. enterocolitica and Y. pseudotuberculosis as well as other Yersinia species are stool, blood, or lymph nodes, depending on the disease form suspected. If food is suspected as the source of an outbreak, the local health department should be involved in the processing of such specimens. Maintain food at 4°C, and transport it as soon as possible. Swabs should be transported to the laboratory at 4°C in Cary-Blair, Amies, or Stuart's medium. Stool specimens can also be placed in transport media and should be maintained at 4°C if transport is expected to take longer than 2 to 4 h. Enrichment broths for recovery of Y. enterocolitica from surface waters have been evaluated, but the ability to recover clinically important strains from this source is uncertain (17).

DIRECT DETECTION

Yersinia species are small (1 to 2 μm by 0.5 μm) gram-negative bacilli that appear either as single cells or as pairs or short chains, particularly when stains are prepared from liquid medium. Direct microscopy of a tissue specimen by using either Wright, Giemsa, Wayson's, or methylene blue stain may be helpful in identification of Y. pestis, since the organisms appear to be safety pin shaped due to bipolar staining (Fig. 1A). Bipolar staining, however, is not a unique feature of Yersinia species and may not always be evident.

A specific staining method for detection of Y. pestis includes the use of a fluorescently labeled antibody (available from CDC) to the capsular F1 antigen. The F1 antigen is expressed at temperatures above 30°C, and fresh cultures, lesions, or tissues (lymph node, liver, spleen, and lung) or their aspirates may be rapidly assessed by this approach (Fig. 1B). Rare Y. pestis strains which lack the caf1 gene have been reported, and Y. pestis should not be ruled out solely on the basis of F1 staining properties. Tissue biopsy specimens fixed in formalin can also be stained with an immunohistochemical stain that is based on a monoclonal antibody to the F1 capsular antigen of Y. pestis. This is a rapid method for diagnosis of plague that does not rely on having fresh tissue or live organisms (80).

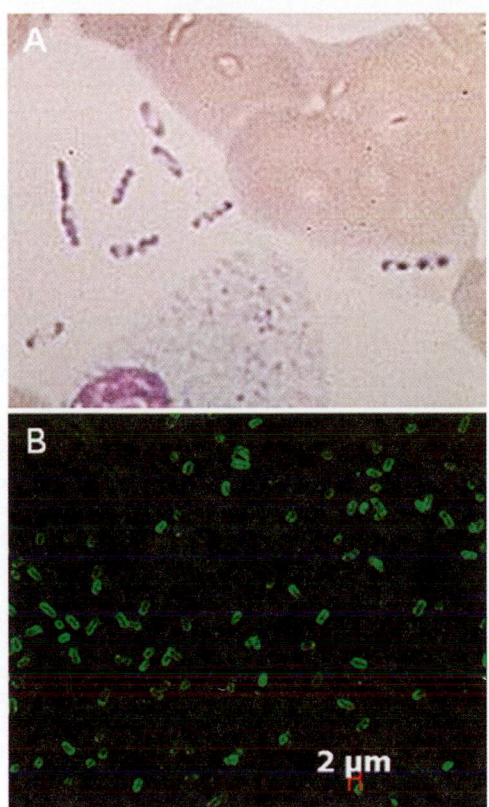

FIGURE 1 (A) Giemsa stain of a blood smear from a patient with *Y. pestis* infection. Note the bipolar-staining "closed safety pin"-shaped cells. (B) Direct fluorescent antibody (F1 conjugate) staining of *Y. pestis*.

A capture enzyme-linked immunosorbent assay for detection of *Y. pestis* F1 antigen in bubo aspirates and serum shows high sensitivity (100% with buboes and 90% with sera; limit of detection, 4 ng/ml) and specificity (approximately 99%) (69). Although this antigen detection approach has been modified to a lateral-flow assay and successfully used under field conditions to diagnose plague infections in humans and animals, this test format is not currently available in the United States (14).

Assays for the direct detection of *Yersinia* nucleic acids in patient specimens have been developed to increase sensitivity. For *Y. pestis*, most assays are directed against the plasminogen activator gene (*pla*) or *caf1* gene, both of which are located on high-copy-number *Y. pestis*-specific plasmids. Following the sequencing of the entire genome of *Y. pestis*, so-called signature genes have been identified on the chromosome of *Y. pestis* that allow for its distinction from *Y. pseudotuberculosis* (57). Recently a multiplex PCR assay for identification of *Y. pestis* and *Y. pseudotuberculosis* was developed based on the *ypo2088* and *pla* genes specific for *Y. pestis* and the *wzz* gene used to identify both *Y. pestis* and *Y. pseudotuberculosis* (50).

PCR has also been used as a sensitive method to detect small numbers of *Y. enterocolitica* in foodstuff (74), as well as in stored red blood cells to prevent transfusion reactions (64). Use of a multiplex PCR assay containing primer sets directed at four different virulence genes to test food samples allows for the distinction between pathogenic and nonpathogenic serotypes and specifically identifies the presence of *Y. enterocolitica* serotype O:3 (74).

ISOLATION PROCEDURES

Yersinia species grow on most routine media, including blood, chocolate, and MacConkey agars incubated at 35°C in ambient air. Eosin-methylene blue, xylose-lysine-deoxycholate agar, and Hektoen enteric agars do not provide any advantage in the isolation of *Y. enterocolitica* and the differentiation of *Yersinia* species from other organisms in the normal stool biota. Due to their ability to ferment sucrose and the fact that *Yersinia* species grow more slowly than most *Enterobacteriaceae*, a selective medium is recommended for specifically culturing *Yersinia* species from nonsterile sites. There are various selective media for the recovery of *Y. enterocolitica*, including cefsulodin-Irgasan-novobiocin (CIN) agar, which inhibits the growth of many other *Enterobacteriaceae*, and salmonella-shigella-deoxycholate calcium chloride agar (27). CIN agar has been found to provide better recovery rates for *Yersinia* than either MacConkey or salmonella-shigella agar incubated at room temperature. Growth of many strains of *Y. pseudotuberculosis* can be inhibited on CIN agar, and therefore MacConkey agar is preferred for isolation (27).

Recovery of *Y. enterocolitica* from food is more difficult than recovery from human clinical specimens, and samples are usually referred to a public health laboratory. Food must be enriched with saline (or a selective broth, such as modified Rappaport broth containing magnesium chloride, malachite green, and carbenicillin [MRB]) at cold temperatures for approximately 21 days (2 to 4 days in MRB) (43).

For isolation of *Y. pestis* from nonsterile sources, MacConkey, CIN, and research formulations (5) are useful, although growth is slower on these than on nonselective agar. As *Y. pestis* also grows at 25°C, incubation of cultures at this lower temperature can aid in isolation from contaminated specimens. Cultures from suspected plague patients should be incubated for 5 days and up to 7 days if the patient has been treated for more than a few days with an appropriate antimicrobial.

Y. pestis colonies are slow growing and are only 1 to 2 mm in diameter after 48 h of incubation, with irregular edges. After 48 to 72 hours, a fried-egg appearance is observed (Fig. 2). No hemolysis is seen on blood agar media. Viewed with a dissecting microscope, the colonies are raised with irregular edges, with a "hammered copper" appearance. Organisms growing in broth appear in clumps along the side of the tube in flocculent or stalactite-like formations if the tube is not shaken. After 24 h of incubation, the clumps settle to the bottom of the tube.

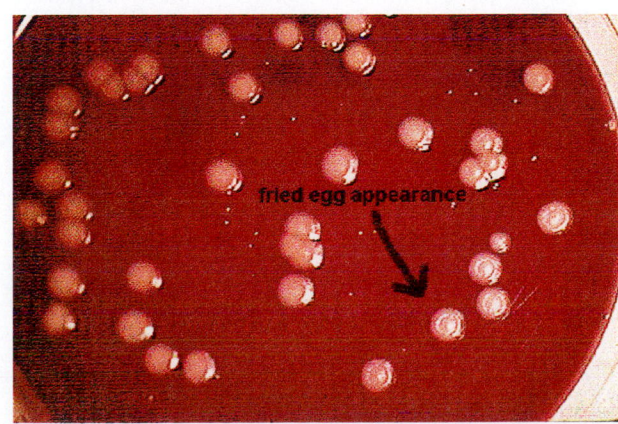

FIGURE 2 Typical fried-egg-shaped colonies of *Y. pestis* on sheep blood agar.

Colonies of *Y. enterocolitica* have a bull's-eye appearance with a red center on CIN agar. Other members of the *Enterobacteriaceae* family which grow on CIN agar, such as *Serratia, Morganella,* and *Citrobacter* species, produce colonies similar in appearance to those of *Yersinia,* but larger. The use of pectin agar has also been described for isolation of *Y. enterocolitica* from stool and for differentiation from other *Enterobacteriaceae.* Although this medium was more sensitive than other currently used selective media and inhibitory to other enterics except *Klebsiella oxytoca* (which demonstrates a similar colony morphology), the medium is currently not commercially available (8).

IDENTIFICATION

Yersinia species are catalase positive and oxidase negative and ferment glucose, as do all other members of the family *Enterobacteriaceae.* *Y. enterocolitica* and *Y. pseudotuberculosis* can be presumptively identified by reactions on triple sugar iron (TSI) and lysine iron agar slants. *Y. enterocolitica* produces a yellow color in the entire TSI tube without gas production, and *Y. pseudotuberculosis* produces an alkaline slant and an acid butt, similar to *Shigella.* Both species are lysine decarboxylase negative and therefore produce a yellow butt in lysine iron agar slants. *Yersinia* species are included in the databases of some automated systems; however, most databases were established with only a few *Yersinia* isolates tested. Automated systems may not adequately identify *Yersinia* species (particularly *Y. pestis*) due in part to their slow growth and biochemical inactivity. In addition, *Y. pestis* has been misidentified by automated systems as *Y. pseudotuberculosis* and as *Shigella, Salmonella,* and *Acinetobacter* species. API 20E was shown to have the highest sensitivity and specificity for the identification of *Y. enterocolitica* and *Y. pseudotuberculosis* (54, 56).

Identification of suspected *Y. pestis* in the clinical laboratory is based on the identification of small gram-negative bacilli which are catalase positive and indole, oxidase, and urease negative as well as characteristic growth on agar, including pinpoint colonies after 24 h on blood and non-lactose-fermenting colonies on MacConkey agar generally after 48 h. See "Sentinel Level Clinical Microbiology Laboratory Guidelines" on the American Society for Microbiology website (www.asm.org) for *Y. pestis*-specific information, pictures, and flowcharts. Following suspected identification of *Y. pestis,* routine clinical laboratories should notify the local public health laboratory and refer the isolate for confirmatory testing. *Y. pseudotuberculosis* and *Y. enterocolitica* can be differentiated from *Y. pestis* by urease activities, which are positive, positive, and negative, respectively. *Y. enterocolitica* can also be differentiated from *Y. pestis* by indole activities, which are positive and negative, respectively. Identification of *Y. enterocolitica* can be made based on typical morphology on CIN agar, reactivity on TSI agar, and urease positivity. Identification of the other *Yersinia* species can be performed by biochemical analysis (Table 1; 53).

Y. enterocolitica has six biogroups which can be differentiated based on reactivity to esculin, indole, D-xylose, trehalose, pyrazinamidase, β-D-glucosidase, and lipase. Although the issue is controversial, biogroup 1A is thought to be nonpathogenic and biotypes 1B and 2 through 5 are pathogenic. Strains belonging to biotype 1A can be differentiated from the others by salicin and pyrazinamidase positivity (Table 2; 37). Serotyping could also help determine the pathogenicity of the isolate, since only a

TABLE 3 Biochemical identification of *Yersinia pestis* biovars

Yersinia pestis biovar	Reaction or characteristic		
	Glycerol	Nitrate	Arabinose
Antiqua	+	+	+
Medievalis	+	−	+
Orientalis	−	+	+
Microtus	+	−	−

small number of the >70 known serotypes are pathogenic; however, antisera are not readily available. Other methods that have been evaluated to determine the pathogenicity of *Y. enterocolitica* are based on the presence of the virulence plasmid and include autoagglutination, calcium-dependent growth at 37°C, and pigmentation on Congo red. Selective media containing Congo red as well as PCR assays have been evaluated for differentiation of virulent from avirulent strains but are currently being used only in research laboratories (75).

Several *Yersinia* species can be differentiated by a number of phenotypic methods, and the four biovars of *Y. pestis* can be separated based on differential reactivity with glycerol, nitrate, and arabinose (Table 3; 47, 83). Recent evidence suggests that biovars based on phenotypic methods do not show a strict correlation to groupings as determined by genotyping methods (1).

TYPING SYSTEMS

Methods used for the evaluation of the relatedness of *Yersinia* species include a number of different phenotypic methods, including serotyping, biotyping, antibiogram analysis, and bacteriophage typing. *Y. enterocolitica* can be divided into six biogroups—1A, 1B, 2, 3, 4, and 5—by using biochemical analysis. These biogroups vary in geographic locations and pathogenic potentials (66). *Y. enterocolitica* also contains more than 70 serotypes, although serotyping is not often performed in routine clinical laboratories, since the antisera are not readily available.

Genotyping methods include pulsed-field gel electrophoresis (PFGE), which has long been considered the gold standard for typing of *Yersinia* species. PFGE was found to be a more useful tool than ribotyping for typing of pathogenic isolates of *Y. enterocolitica* (74) and has been applied to epidemiological tracing of all three pathogenic species. A PFGE method for typing of *Y. pestis* isolates is available through the CDC PulseNet website and has been used in case investigations to identify the source of isolates (81).

SEROLOGIC TESTS

The gold standard for the diagnosis of plague is isolation of the organism; however, serology can play a role, particularly when a culture is not recovered or for retrospective diagnosis or epidemiologic studies in areas where plague is endemic. Most patients with plague seroconvert 1 to 2 weeks following the onset of symptoms. The most commonly used antigen in serologic assays for *Y. pestis* is the capsular F1 antigen. F1 antigen, which is highly immunogenic and stable, is typically present in high concentrations in sera and bubo fluids of plague patients even after several days of appropriate antimicrobial therapy. Serologic diagnosis of plague can be made based only on a fourfold rise in antibody titers between acute and convalescent serum samples. Serologic assay methods include passive hemagglutination, the method recommended by the World Health Organization due to its low cost and ease of performance. The reagents for passive hemagglutination are available only in reference laboratories.

Serology can be used as an adjunct in the diagnosis of disease due to *Y. enterocolitica* or *Y. pseudotuberculosis*. Antibody is detectable within the first week of illness and returns to normal levels 3 to 6 months later. The specificity of serologic assays ranges from 82 to 95% due to cross-reactivity between the two species and also with *Brucella*, *Francisella*, and *Vibrio* species, as well as *Borrelia burgdorferi*, *Chlamydia pneumoniae*, and some *Escherichia coli* serogroups. Another disadvantage of using serology for diagnosis is that antibodies to *Y. enterocolitica* O antigens are often found in healthy subjects due to the frequency of exposure to nonpathogenic serotypes. Most human infections with *Y. enterocolitica* involve serotypes O:3, O:5, 27, O:8, and O:9. Serotype O:3 is the most common cause of gastroenteritis. However, as mentioned above, antisera are available only to public health and research laboratories.

Antibody to outer membrane proteins (Yops) that are present only in virulent strains of *Y. enterocolitica* may be more helpful. In a small study of healthy blood donors, immunoglobulin M (IgM) antibody to Yops was 97% specific for acute infection (72). Testing of blood donors for anti-Yop IgA in New Zealand, which has a high incidence of *Y. enterocolitica* gastroenteritis, showed promise in preventing transfusion-related infections (41). The presence of IgG and IgA antibodies to *Y. enterocolitica* Yops is also used as an aid in the diagnosis of autoimmune disorders that occur postinfection, such as reactive arthritis, erythema nodosum, Graves' disease, and Hashimoto's thyroiditis (15). IgM-, IgA-, and IgG-specific antibody reactivity against Yops in Western immunoblot formats has been correlated with clinical presentation and sequelae (61).

ANTIMICROBIAL SUSCEPTIBILITIES

Pneumonic plague is nearly 100% fatal if not treated within the first 24 h of development of symptoms. The drug of choice for the treatment of plague, pneumonic, septicemic, or bubonic, is streptomycin. However, due to the lack of availability of streptomycin and negative side effects, other agents have been evaluated in vitro and in animal models. The only other antibiotic currently approved for treatment of plague is doxycycline; however, other alternatives would be gentamicin and a fluoroquinolone such as ciprofloxacin or levofloxacin (7, 36). Steward et al. documented the efficacy of fluoroquinolones in a mouse model of systemic and pneumonic plague (70). The treatment of choice for plague meningitis is chloramphenicol. Antibiotic resistance among isolates of *Y. pestis* has only rarely been documented and never in the United States (26). Treatment failure due to antibiotic resistance has never been documented. An isolate of *Y. pestis* from a 1995 plague case in Madagascar was found to be multidrug resistant, with resistance to streptomycin, sulfonamides, tetracycline, and chloramphenicol (31). Routine susceptibility testing of patient isolates in this region of endemicity has failed to identify any further evidence of multidrug resistance during the last 14 years. Antimicrobial susceptibility testing of *Y. pestis* is not usually performed in clinical microbiology laboratories because of safety concerns in working with this organism. The Clinical and Laboratory Standards Institute (www.clsi.org) has published interpretative criteria and quality control limits for broth microdilution of *Y. pestis* using Mueller-Hinton medium (18).

Most cases of *Y. enterocolitica* gastroenteritis do not require treatment; however, treatment is necessary in cases of systemic disease, especially in immunosuppressed patients. Treatment options include trimethoprim-sulfamethoxazole and a fluoroquinolone. *Y. enterocolitica* produces two different β-lactamases, one of which is a class A constitutive enzyme and the other of which is an inducible class C enzyme that is not inhibited by β-lactamase inhibitors. The presence of one or both of these enzymes varies depending on the biogroup (11). Although the β-lactamase confers resistance to penicillin on *Y. enterocolitica*, the organism remains uniformly susceptible to the extended-spectrum cephalosporins (60). Resistance to fluoroquinolones is due to either a mutation in the *gyrA* gene or efflux mechanisms. In a study conducted in Spain, 23% of *Y. enterocolitica* strains isolated from patients with gastroenteritis were nalidixic acid resistant. All resistant isolates had a mutation in *gyrA*, and some were resistant based on an efflux mechanism as well (11). *Y. enterocolitica* strains are susceptible in vitro to aminoglycosides, chloramphenicol, tetracycline, trimethoprim-sulfamethoxazole, and extended-spectrum cephalosporins.

Y. pseudotuberculosis is susceptible to ampicillin, tetracycline, chloramphenicol, cephalosporins, and aminoglycosides. Although infections due to *Y. pseudotuberculosis* are not usually treated, patients with septicemia should be treated with ampicillin, streptomycin, or tetracycline. *Y. aldovae* and *Y. ruckeri* are also susceptible to penicillin. *Y. frederiksenii*, *Y. intermedia*, and *Y. rhodei* produce a β-lactamase similar to that of *Y. enterocolitica*, which is expressed at different levels in different strains (71).

EVALUATION, INTERPRETATION, AND REPORTING OF RESULTS

Y. pestis, *Y. enterocolitica*, and *Y. pseudotuberculosis* are the primary pathogens in the genus *Yersinia*. Isolation of *Y. pestis* from any body site warrants further investigation. Isolation of *Y. enterocolitica* or *Y. pseudotuberculosis* from stool culture is not sufficient for causal evidence of disease, since nonpathogenic serotypes may be normal stool biota. However, no readily available methods except those using routine biochemicals, which are not usually maintained in routine clinical laboratories, are available for differentiation of pathogenic serotypes. Isolation of either species in pure culture from a symptomatic patient with no other diagnosis should be considered suspect. Isolation of either species from blood or other normally sterile sites should also be considered significant.

It has not been shown to be cost-effective to screen all stools for *Y. enterocolitica* by using CIN agar. Isolation rates vary based on geographic locations, with the highest incidence in temperate regions, so the decision to routinely rule out these organisms in stool cultures should be evaluated in individual laboratories after consultation with the infectious disease physicians.

Although the other *Yersinia* species besides *Y. pestis*, *Y. enterocolitica*, and *Y. pseudotuberculosis* are not considered human pathogens, they have been isolated from the gastrointestinal tracts of symptomatic patients with no other diagnosis. It has been recommended that the presence of these *Yersinia* species in pure culture be reported. These organisms may be underrecognized pathogens (24, 48).

Due to the lack of accuracy of commercial systems for the identification of *Y. pestis*, the potential use of *Y. pestis* as a bioweapon, and the seriousness of the disease, all suspected *Y. pestis* isolates should be sent to a local public health laboratory for confirmation.

REFERENCES

1. **Achtman, M., G. Morelli, and P. Zhu.** 2004. Micro-evolution and history of the plague bacillus, *Yersinia pestis. Proc. Natl. Acad. Sci. USA* **101:**17837–17842.

2. **Achtman, M., K. Zurth, G. Morelli, G. Torrea, A. Guiyoule, and E. Carniel.** 1999. *Yersinia pestis,* the cause of plague, is a recently emerged clone of *Yersinia pseudotuberculosis. Proc. Natl. Acad. Sci. USA* **96:**14043–14048.

3. **American Society for Microbiology.** 11 June 2010, posting date. *Sentinel Level Clinical Microbiology Laboratory Guidelines:* Yersinia pestis. American Society for Microbiology, Washington, DC. http://www.asm.org.

4. **Begier, E. M., G. Asiki, Z. Anywaine, B. Yockey, M. E. Schriefer, P. Aleti, A. Ogden-Odoi, J. E. Staples, C. Sexton, S. W. Bearden, and J. L. Kool.** 2006. Pneumonic plague cluster, Uganda, 2004. *Emerg. Infect. Dis.* **12:**460–467.

5. **Ber, R., E. Mamroud, M. Aftalion, A. Tidhar, D. Gur, Y. Flashner, and S. Cohen.** 2003. Development of an improved selective agar medium for isolation of *Yersinia pestis. Appl. Environ. Microbiol.* **69:**5787–5792.

6. **Bogdanovich, T., E. Carniel, H. Fukushima, and M. Skurnik.** 2003. Use of O-antigen gene cluster-specific PCRs for the identification and O-genotyping of *Yersinia pseudotuberculosis* and *Yersinia pestis. J. Clin. Microbiol.* **41:**5103–5112.

7. **Boulanger, L. L., P. Ettestad, J. D. Fogarty, D. T. Dennis, D. Romig, and G. Mertz.** 2004. Gentamicin and tetracyclines for the treatment of human plague: review of 75 cases in New Mexico, 1985–1999. *Clin. Infect. Dis.* **38:**663–669.

8. **Bowen, J. H., and S. D. Kominos.** 1979. Evaluation of a pectin agar medium for isolation of *Yersinia enterocolitica* within 48 hours. *Am. J. Clin. Pathol.* **72:**586–590.

9. **Bruneteau, M., and S. Minka.** 2003. Lipopolysaccharides of bacterial pathogens from the genus Yersinia: a mini-review. *Biochimie* **85:**145–152.

10. **Butler, T.** 2009. Plague into the 21st century. *Clin. Infect. Dis.* **49:**736–742.

11. **Capilla, S., J. Ruiz, P. Goni, J. Castillo, M. C. Rubio, M. T. Jimenez de Anta, R. Gomez-Lus, and J. Vila.** 2004. Characterization of the molecular mechanisms of quinolone resistance in *Yersinia enterocolitica* O:3 clinical isolates. *J. Antimicrob. Chemother.* **53:**1068–1071.

12. **Centers for Disease Control and Prevention.** 2003. *Yersinia enterocolitica* gastroenteritis among infants exposed to chitterlings—Chicago, Illinois, 2002. *Morb. Mortal. Wkly. Rep.* **52:**956–958.

13. **Chain, P. S., E. Carniel, F. W. Larimer, J. Lamerdin, P. O. Stoutland, W. M. Regala, A. M. Georgescu, L. M. Vergez, M. L. Land, V. L. Motin, R. R. Brubaker, J. Fowler, J. Hinnebusch, M. Marceau, C. Medigue, M. Simonet, V. Chenal-Francisque, B. Souza, D. Dacheux, J. M. Elliott, A. Derbise, L. J. Hauser, and E. Garcia.** 2004. Insights into the evolution of *Yersinia pestis* through whole-genome comparison with *Yersinia pseudotuberculosis. Proc. Natl. Acad. Sci. USA* **101:**13826–13831.

14. **Chanteau, S., L. Rahalison, L. Ralafiarisoa, J. Foulon, M. Ratsitorahina, L. Ratsifasoamanana, E. Carniel, and F. Nato.** 2003. Development and testing of a rapid diagnostic test for bubonic and pneumonic plague. *Lancet* **361:**211–216.

15. **Chatzipanagiotou, S., J. N. Legakis, F. Boufidou, V. Petroyianni, and C. Nicolaou.** 2001. Prevalence of Yersinia plasmid-encoded outer protein (Yop) class-specific antibodies in patients with Hashimoto's thyroiditis. *Clin. Microbiol. Infect.* **7:**138–143.

16. **Chen, C. L., J. C. Yu, S. Holme, M. R. Jacobs, R. Yomtovian, and C. P. McDonald.** 2008. Detection of bacteria in stored red cell products using a culture-based bacterial detection system. *Transfusion* **48:**1550–1557.

17. **Cheyne, B. M., M. I. Van Dyke, W. B. Anderson, and P. M. Huck.** 2009. An evaluation of methods for the isolation of Yersinia enterocolitica from surface waters in the Grand River watershed. *J. Water Health* **7:**392–403.

18. **Clinical and Laboratory Standards Institute.** 2009. *Performance Standards Antimicrobial Susceptibility Testing: Nineteenth Informational Supplement.* M100-S19, vol. 29, no. 3. Clinical and Laboratory Standards Institute, Wayne, PA.

19. **Cornelis, G. R.** 2002. Yersinia type III secretion: send in the effectors. *J. Cell Biol.* **158:**401–408.

20. **Craven, R. B., G. O. Maupin, M. L. Beard, T. J. Quan, and A. M. Barnes.** 1993. Reported cases of human plague infections in the United States, 1970–1991. *J. Med. Entomol.* **30:**758–761.

21. **Deacon, A. G., A. Hay, and J. Duncan.** 2003. Septicemia due to *Yersinia pseudotuberculosis:* a case report. *Clin. Microbiol. Infect.* **9:**1118–1119.

22. **Deng, W., V. Burland, G. Plunkett III, A. Boutin, G. F. Mayhew, P. Liss, N. T. Perna, D. J. Rose, B. Mau, S. Zhou, D. C. Schwartz, J. D. Fetherston, L. E. Lindler, R. R. Brubaker, G. V. Plano, S. C. Straley, K. A. McDonough, M. L. Nilles, J. S. Matson, F. R. Blattner, and R. D. Perry.** 2002. Genome sequence of *Yersinia pestis* KIM. *J. Bacteriol.* **184:**4601–4611.

23. **Depaolo, R. W., F. Tang, I. Kim, M. Han, N. Levin, N. Ciletti, A. Lin, D. Anderson, O. Schneewind, and B. Jabri.** 2008. Toll-like receptor 6 drives differentiation of tolerogenic dendritic cells and contributes to LcrV-mediated plague pathogenesis. *Cell Host Microbe* **4:**350–361.

24. **Falcao, J. P., M. Brocchi, J. L. Proenca-Modena, G. O. Acrani, E. F. Correa, and D. P. Falcao.** 2004. Virulence characteristics and epidemiology of Yersinia enterocolitica and Yersiniae other than Y. pseudotuberculosis and Y. pestis isolated from water and sewage. *J. Appl. Microbiol.* **96:**1230–1236.

25. **Fetherston, J. D., and R. D. Perry.** 1994. The pigmentation locus of Yersinia pestis KIM6+ is flanked by an insertion sequence and includes the structural genes for pesticin sensitivity and HMWP2. *Mol. Microbiol.* **13:**697–708.

26. **Frean, J., K. P. Klugman, L. Arntzen, and S. Bukofzer.** 2003. Susceptibility of *Yersinia pestis* to novel and conventional antimicrobial agents. *J. Antimicrob. Chemother.* **52:**294–296.

27. **Fredriksson-Ahomaa, M., and H. Korkeala.** 2003. Low occurrence of pathogenic *Yersinia enterocolitica* in clinical, food, and environmental samples: a methodological problem. *Clin. Microbiol. Rev.* **16:**220–229.

28. **Fredriksson-Ahomaa, M., A. Stolle, and H. Korkeala.** 2006. Molecular epidemiology of Yersinia enterocolitica infections. *FEMS Immunol. Med. Microbiol.* **47:**315–329.

29. **Gage, K. L., D. T. Dennis, K. A. Orloski, P. Ettestad, T. L. Brown, P. J. Reynolds, W. J. Pape, C. L. Fritz, L. G. Carter, and J. D. Stein.** 2000. Cases of cat-associated human plague in the Western US, 1977–1998. *Clin. Infect. Dis.* **30:**893–900.

30. **Gage, K. L., D. T. Dennis, and T. F. Tsai.** 1996. Prevention of plague: recommendations of the Advisory Committee on Immunization Practices (ACIP). *Morb. Mortal. Wkly. Rep.* **45**(RR-14):1–15.

31. **Galimand, M., A. Guiyoule, G. Gerbaud, B. Rasoamanana, S. Chanteau, E. Carniel, and P. Courvalin.** 1997. Multidrug resistance in *Yersinia pestis* mediated by a transferable plasmid. *N. Engl. J. Med.* **337:**677–680.

32. **Gould, L. H., J. Pape, P. Ettestad, K. S. Griffith, and P. S. Mead.** 2008. Dog-associated risk factors for human plague. *Zoonoses Public Health* **55:**448–454.

33. **Hinnebusch, B. J., A. E. Rudolph, P. Cherepanov, J. E. Dixon, T. G. Schwan, and A. Forsberg.** 2002. Role of Yersinia murine toxin in survival of Yersinia pestis in the midgut of the flea vector. *Science* **296:**733–735.

34. **Homewood, R., C. P. Gibbons, D. Richards, A. Lewis, P. D. Duane, and A. P. Griffiths.** 2003. Ileitis due to *Yersinia pseudotuberculosis* in Crohn's disease. *J. Infect.* **47:**328–332.

35. **Huang, X. Z., M. P. Nikolich, and L. E. Lindler.** 2006. Current trends in plague research: from genomics to virulence. *Clin. Med. Res.* **4:**189–199.

36. Inglesby, T. V., D. T. Dennis, D. A. Henderson, J. G. Bartlett, M. S. Ascher, E. Eitzen, A. D. Fine, A. M. Friedlander, J. Hauer, J. F. Koerner, M. Layton, J. McDade, M. T. Osterholm, T. O'Toole, G. Parker, T. M. Perl, P. K. Russell, M. Schoch-Spana, K. Tonat, and the Working Group on Civilian Biodefense. 2000. Plague as a biological weapon: medical and public health management. *JAMA* **283:**2281–2290.

37. Janda, J. M., and S. L. Abbott. 2005. *The Enterobacteria*, 2nd ed. ASM Press, Washington, DC.

38. Jenkins, A. L., P. L. Worsham, and S. L.Welkos. 2009. A strategy to verify the absence of the pgm locus in Yersinia pestis strain candidates for select agent exemption. *J. Microbiol. Methods* **77:**316–319.

39. Jones, T. F. 2003. From pig to pacifier: chitterling-associated yersiniosis outbreak among black infants. *Emerg. Infect. Dis.* **9:**1007–1009.

39a. Kandolo, K., and G. Wauters. 1985. Pyrazinamidase activity in *Yersinia enterocolitica* and related organisms. *J. Clin. Microbiol.* **21:**980–982.

40. Kangas, S., J. Takkinen, M. Hakkinen, U. M. Nakari, T. Johansson, H. Henttonen, L. Virtaluoto, A. Siitonen, J. Ollgren, and M. Kuusi. 2008. Yersinia pseudotuberculosis O:1 traced to raw carrots, Finland. *Emerg. Infect. Dis.* **14:**1959–1961.

41. Kendrick, C. J., B. Baker, A. J. Morris, and P. W. O'Toole. 2001. Identification of *Yersinia*-infected blood donors by anti-Yop IgA immunoassay. *Transfusion* **41:**1365–1372.

42. Kool, J. L. 2005. Risk of person-to-person transmission of pneumonic plague. *Clin. Infect. Dis.* **40:**1166–1172.

43. Laukkanen, R., M. Hakkinen, J. Lunden, M. Fredriksson-Ahomaa, T. Johansson, and H. Korkeala. 2009. Evaluation of isolation methods for pathogenic Yersinia enterocolitica from pig intestinal content. *J. Appl. Microbiol.* **108:**956–964.

44. Leclercq, A., L. Martin, M. L. Vergnes, N. Ounnoughene, J. F. Laran, P. Giraud, and E. Carniel. 2005. Fatal *Yersinia enterocolitica* biotype 4 serovar O:3 sepsis after red blood cell transfusion. *Transfusion* **45:**814–818.

45. Lee, V. T., C. Tam, and O. Schneewind. 2000. LcrV, a substrate for Yersinia enterocolitica type III secretion, is required for toxin targeting into the cytosol of HeLa cells. *J. Biol. Chem.* **275:**36869–36875.

46. Li, B., and R. Yang. 2008. Interaction between *Yersinia pestis* and the host immune system. *Infect. Immun.* **76:**1804–1811.

47. Lindler, L. E. 2009. Typing methods for the plague pathogen, Yersinia pestis. *J. AOAC Int.* **92:**1174–1183.

48. Loftus, C. G., G. C. Harewood, F. R. Cockerill III, and J. A. Murray. 2002. Clinical features of patients with novel *Yersinia* species. *Dig. Dis. Sci.* **47:**2805–2810.

49. Lorange, E. A., B. L. Race, F. Sebbane, and B. J. Hinnebusch. 2005. Poor vector competence of fleas and the evolution of hypervirulence in Yersinia pestis. *J. Infect. Dis.* **191:**1907–1912.

50. Matero, P., T. Pasanen, R. Laukkanen, P. Tissari, E. Tarkka, M. Vaara, and M. Skurnik. 2009. Real-time multiplex PCR assay for detection of Yersinia pestis and Yersinia pseudotuberculosis. *APMIS* **117:**34–44.

51. McNabb, S. J., R. A. Jajosky, P. A. Hall-Baker, D. A. Adams, P. Sharp, C. Worshams, W. J. Anderson, A. J. Javier, G. J. Jones, D. A. Nitschke, A. Rey, and M. S. Wodajo. 2008. Summary of notifiable diseases—United States, 2006. *Morb. Mortal. Wkly. Rep.* **55:**1–92.

52. Minnich, S. A., and H. N. Rohde. 2007. A rationale for repression and/or loss of motility by pathogenic Yersinia in the mammalian host. *Adv. Exp. Med. Biol.* **603:**298–310.

53. Neubauer, H., M. Molitor, L. Rahalison, S. Aleksic, H. Backes, S. Chanteau, and H. Meyer. 2000. A miniaturised semiautomated system for the identification of *Yersinia* species within the genus *Yersinia. Clin. Lab.* **46:**561–567.

54. Neubauer, H., T. Sauer, H. Becker, S. Aleksic, and H. Meyer. 1998. Comparison of systems for identification and differentiation of species within the genus Yersinia. *J. Clin. Microbiol.* **36:**3366–3368.

55. Nuorti, J. P., T. Niskanen, S. Hallanvuo, J. Mikkola, E. Kela, M. Hatakka, M. Fredriksson-Ahomaa, O. Lyytikainen, A. Siitonen, H. Korkeala, and P. Ruutu. 2004. A widespread outbreak of *Yersinia pseudotuberculosis* O:3 infection from iceberg lettuce. *J. Infect. Dis.* **189:**766–774.

56. O'Hara, C. M. 2005. Manual and automated instrumentation for identification of *Enterobacteriaceae* and other aerobic gram-negative bacilli. *Clin. Microbiol. Rev.* **18:**147–162.

57. Parkhill, J., B. W. Wren, N. R. Thomson, R. W. Titball, M. T. Holden, M. B. Prentice, M. Sebaihia, K. D. James, C. Churcher, K. L. Mungall, S. Baker, D. Basham, S. D. Bentley, K. Brooks, A. M. Cerdeno-Tarraga, T. Chillingworth, A. Cronin, R. M. Davies, P. Davis, G. Dougan, T. Feltwell, N. Hamlin, S. Holroyd, K. Jagels, A. V. Karlyshev, S. Leather, S. Moule, P. C. Oyston, M. Quail, K. Rutherford, M. Simmonds, J. Skelton, K. Stevens, S. Whitehead, and B. G. Barrell. 2001. Genome sequence of *Yersinia pestis*, the causative agent of plague. *Nature* **413:**523–527.

58. Perry, R. D., and S. W. Bearden. 2008. Isolation and confirmation of Yersinia pestis mutants exempt from select agent regulations. *Curr. Protoc. Microbiol.* Chapter 5, Unit 5B.2. doi:10.1002/9780471729259.mc05b02s11.

59. Perry, R. D., and J. D. Fetherston. 1997. Yersinia pestis—etiologic agent of plague. *Clin. Microbiol. Rev.* **10:**35–66.

60. Pham, J. N., S. M. Bell, L. Martin, and E. Carniel. 2000. The beta-lactamases and beta-lactam antibiotic susceptibility of *Yersinia enterocolitica. J. Antimicrob. Chemother.* **46:**951–957.

61. Rastawicki, W. 2006. Humoral response to selected antigens of Yersinia enterocolitica and Yersinia pseudotuberculosis in the course of yersiniosis in humans. I. Occurrence of antibodies to Yersinia Yop proteins by Western-blot. *Med. Dosw. Mikrobiol.* **58:**321–328.

62. Ratsitorahina, M., S. Chanteau, L. Rahalison, L. Ratsifasoamanana, and P. Boisier. 2000. Epidemiological and diagnostic aspects of the outbreak of pneumonic plague in Madagascar. *Lancet* **355:**111–113.

63. Saebo, A., E. Vik, O. J. Lange, and L. Matuszkiewicz. 2005. Inflammatory bowel disease associated with *Yersinia enterocolitica* O:3 infection. *Eur. J. Intern. Med.* **16:**176–182.

64. Sen, K. 2000. Rapid identification of *Yersinia enterocolitica* in blood by the 5′ nuclease PCR assay. *J. Clin. Microbiol.* **38:**1953–1958.

65. Shao, F. 2008. Biochemical functions of Yersinia type III effectors. *Curr. Opin. Microbiol.* **11:**21–29.

66. Sharma, S., P. Ramnani, and J. S. Virdi. 2004. Detection and assay of beta-lactamases in clinical and non-clinical strains of *Yersinia enterocolitica* biovar 1A. *J. Antimicrob. Chemother.* **54:**401–405.

67. Skurnik, M., and J. A. Bengoechea. 2003. The biosynthesis and biological role of lipopolysaccharide O-antigens of pathogenic Yersiniae. *Carbohydr. Res.* **338:**2521–2529.

68. Smiley, S. T. 2008. Current challenges in the development of vaccines for pneumonic plague. *Expert Rev. Vaccines* **7:**209–221.

69. Splettstoesser, W. D., L. Rahalison, R. Grunow, H. Neubauer, and S. Chanteau. 2004. Evaluation of a standardized F1 capsular antigen capture ELISA test kit for the rapid diagnosis of plague. *FEMS Immunol. Med. Microbiol.* **41:**149–155.

70. Steward, J., M. S. Lever, P. Russell, R. J. Beedham, A. J. Stagg, R. R. Taylor, and T. J. Brooks. 2004. Efficacy of the latest fluoroquinolones against experimental Yersinia pestis. *Int. J. Antimicrob. Agents* **24:**609–612.

71. Stock, I., and B. Wiedemann. 2003. Natural antimicrobial susceptibilities and biochemical profiles of *Yersinia enterocolitica*-like strains: Y. frederiksenii, Y. intermedia, Y. kristensenii and Y. rohdei. *FEMS Immunol. Med. Microbiol.* **38:**139–152.

72. Strobel, E., J. Heesemann, G. Mayer, J. Peters, S. Muller-Weihrich, and P. Emmerling. 2000. Bacteriological and serological findings in a further case of transfusion-mediated *Yersinia enterocolitica* sepsis. *J. Clin. Microbiol.* **38:**2788–2790.

73. Sulakvelidze, A. 2000. *Yersiniae* other than Y. enterocolitica, Y. pseudotuberculosis, and Y. pestis: the ignored species. *Microbes Infect.* **2:**497–513.

74. Thisted-Lambertz, S., and M.-L. Danielsson-Tham. 2005. Identification and characterization of pathogenic Yersinia enterocolitica isolates by PCR and pulsed-field gel electrophoresis. *Appl. Environ. Microbiol.* **71:**3674–3681.

75. **Thoerner, P., C. I. Bin Kingombe, K. Bogli-Stuber, B. Bissig-Choisat, T. M. Wassenaar, J. Frey, and T. Jemmi.** 2003. PCR detection of virulence genes in *Yersinia entero-colitica* and *Yersinia pseudotuberculosis* and investigation of virulence gene distribution. *Appl. Environ. Microbiol.* **69:**1810–1816.

76. **Thomson, N. R., S. Howard, B. W. Wren, M. T. Holden, L. Crossman, G. L. Challis, C. Churcher, K. Mungall, K. Brooks, T. Chillingworth, T. Feltwell, Z. Abdellah, H. Hauser, K. Jagels, M. Maddison, S. Moule, M. Sanders, S. Whitehead, M. A. Quail, G. Dougan, J. Parkhill, and M. B. Prentice.** 2006. The complete genome sequence and com-parative genome analysis of the high pathogenicity Yersinia enterocolitica strain 8081. *PLoS Genet.* **2:**e206.

77. **Vadyvalkoo, V., C. Jarrett, D. Sturdevant, F. Sebbane, and B. J. Hinnebusch.** 2007. Analysis of Yersinia pestis gene expression in the flea vector. *Adv. Exp. Med. Biol.* **603:**192–200.

78. **Viboud, G. I., and J. B. Bliska.** 2005. *Yersinia* outer proteins: role in modulation of host cell signalling responses and patho-genesis. *Annu. Rev. Microbiol.* **59:**69–89.

79. **Wanger, A.** 1998. *Yersinia,* p. 1051–1063. *In* A. Balows and B. Duerden (ed.), *Topley & Wilson's Microbiology and Microbial Infections,* vol. 2. Arnold, London, United Kingdom.

79a. **Wauters, G., K. Kandolo, and M. Janssens.** 1987. Revised biogrouping scheme of *Yersinia enterocolitica. Contrib. Micro-biol. Immunol.* **9:**14–21.

80. **Wong, D., M. A. Wild, M. A. Walburger, C. L. Higgins, M. Callahan, L. A. Czarnecki, E. W. Lawaczeck, C. E. Levy, J. G. Patterson, R. Sunenshine, P. Adem, C. D. Paddock, S. R. Zaki, J. M. Petersen, M. E. Schriefer, R. J. Eisen, K. L. Gage, K. S. Griffith, I. B. Weber, T. R. Spraker, and P. S. Mead.** 2009. Primary pneumonic plague contracted from a mountain lion carcass. *Clin. Infect. Dis.* **49:**e33–38.

81. **Wren, B. W.** 2003. The yersiniae—a model genus to study the rapid evolution of bacterial pathogens. *Nat. Rev. Micro-biol.* **1:**55–64.

82. **Zhou, D., Y. Han, Y. Song, P. Huang, and R. Yang.** 2004. Comparative and evolutionary genomics of *Yersinia pestis. Microbes Infect.* **6:**1226–1234.

83. **Zhou, D., Z. Tong, Y. Song, Y. Han, D. Pei, X. Pang, J. Zhai, M. Li, B. Cui, Z. Qi, L. Jin, R. Dai, Z. Du, J. Wang, Z. Guo, P. Huang, and R. Yang.** 2004. Genetics of metabolic variations between *Yersinia pestis* biovars and the proposal of a new biovar, microtus. *J. Bacteriol.* **186:**5147–5152.

84. **Zietz, B. P., and H. Dunkelberg.** 2004. The history of the plague and the research on the causative agent Yersinia pes-tis. *Int. J. Hyg. Environ. Health* **207:**165–178.

Klebsiella, Enterobacter, Citrobacter, Serratia, Plesiomonas, and Other Enterobacteriaceae

SHARON L. ABBOTT

37

TAXONOMY

Taxonomically, the *Enterobacteriaceae* remain a challenging group to define on a phylogenetic level, as sequence divergence within the 16S rRNA gene, the most commonly used molecular identification tool, is generally insufficient to accurately discriminate between closely related members of this family (34, 75, 101). Sequencing of other housekeeping genes (i.e., *dnaJ*, *rpoB*, *gyrB*, etc.) often yields different phylogenetic classifications depending on their discriminatory powers. Moreover, 16S rRNA and housekeeping gene sequencing results may not correspond with data generated by the gold standard, DNA-DNA hybridization, or with multilocus enzyme electrophoresis. For instance, *Salmonella bongori* is a distinct species by *dnaJ* sequencing, DNA-DNA hybridization, and multilocus enzyme electrophoresis, while *tuf*, *atpD*, and 23S rRNA sequences place *S. bongori* as a subspecies within *Salmonella enterica* (101). Adoption of a cohesive approach to classification would provide some stability to the taxonomy of this family. Gevers et al. (47) have suggested using multilocus sequence analysis with a set of housekeeping genes selected on the criteria that (i) they are useful for all strains within the taxon being studied, (ii) they present as single copies, and (iii) recombination would not convey a selective advantage. The continuous reclassification of organisms, particularly those with clinical significance, can confuse clinicians, which could have serious consequences for patients.

A number of additions or taxonomic changes within the *Enterobacteriaceae* have occurred in the interval since the ninth edition of this *Manual*; however, only two are of clinical importance. A new species of *Morganella*, *M. psychrotolerans*, has been reported from cold-smoked tuna and has been implicated in an outbreak of histamine (scombroid) poisoning (38). Unlike *Morganella morganii* strains, which produce histamine from the histidine present in seafood at temperatures above normal refrigeration (7 to 10°C), *M. psychrotolerans* produces toxic concentrations of histidine between 0 and 5°C, so even properly refrigerated product could cause disease. The second change of clinical significance is the move of *Enterobacter sakazakii*, a species recognized to be heterogeneous at the DNA level, to a newly created genus, *Cronobacter*, with the subsequent creation of four additional species and an unnamed genomospecies (69). Although not common, *E. sakazakii* is well recognized by infectious disease clinicians as a cause of severe disease (meningitis, necrotizing colitis, and bacteremia) with relatively high mortality rates in neonates. At this time, species of *Cronobacter* cannot be routinely identified in clinical laboratories due to lack of discriminatory biochemical tests. *E. sakazakii* remains an acceptable, validly published name, but PubMed queries indicate that, based on usage, *Cronobacter sakazakii* is gaining acceptance in the literature. The best options available for reporting this organism would be to continue to use *E. sakazakii* or use *Cronobacter sakazakii* complex until such time as the species are readily identifiable by routinely used methodologies. When laboratories adopt taxonomic changes, the older epithet should be included in parentheses following the new name for a minimum of 6 months (11). For infrequently encountered pathogenic organisms, 6 months may be insufficient for physicians to become familiar with the taxonomic change. It is the laboratory's responsibility to ensure that clinicians are aware of the significance of the organism being reported in these cases.

Other genera, including *Pantoea* (*Enterobacter*) *agglomerans* and *Enterobacter cloacae* remain heterogeneous at the DNA level, but because they are not phenotypically separable, genomic groups residing within these species remain unnamed (46, 62). *Hafnia alvei* is composed of two distinct DNA hybridization groups, and studies are in progress to name DNA hybridization group 2 (78).

All the other new species of *Enterobacteriaceae* covered in this chapter that have been added to or transferred between existing genera are included in Tables 1 and 2. The genera listed in the last two columns of Table 2 are not isolated from human clinical specimens or are isolated but may not be significant, and most of these taxa will be unfamiliar to clinical microbiologists. Genera belonging to the *Enterobacteriaceae* that contain one or more species isolated exclusively from insects, plants, fish, marine animals, or birds are not included in the tables or text of this chapter; however, information on them is available elsewhere (72).

DESCRIPTION OF THE GENERA

Members belonging to the family *Enterobacteriaceae* are gram-negative, facultative anaerobic rods or coccobacilli ranging from 0.3 to 1.0 μm wide to 0.6 to 6.0 μm long.

TABLE 1 Nomenclature, isolation source, and significance of selected genera of the family *Enterobacteriaceae*[a]

Current (previous) designation	Clinical data			Environmental data
	Frequency	Source	Significance	
Averyella dalhousiensis	Unk	Wound, blood	2	Unk
Citrobacter				
C. amalonaticus	++	**Feces,** blood, wound, UT, RT	2	Unk, one isolate from an animal
C. braakii	+++	**Feces,** UT, wound	2	Similar to *C. freundii*
C. farmeri	++	**Feces,** UT, blood, wound, RT	2	Unk
C. freundii	++++	All sites, feces most common	1	Water, soil, fish, animals, food
C. koseri (C. diversus)	++	All sites, CSF most common	1	Unk
C. rodentium	−			Pathogenic for mice
C. sedlakii	+	Feces, UT, blood, wound	3	Same as for *C. braakii*
C. werkmanii	+	**Feces,** blood, wound	3	Same as for *C. braakii*
C. youngae	++	**Feces,** UT, blood, wound	3	Same as for *C. braakii*
C. gillenii	+	**Feces,** UT, blood	3	Same as for *C. braakii*
C. murliniae	+	Feces, blood, UT, wound	3	Same as for *C. braakii*
Cronobacter				
C. dublinensis subsp. *dublinensis, lausannensis,* and *lactaridi*	+	Wound, eye, blood	1	Milk powder factory, water
C. malonaticus	+	Blood, wound, RT, ear	1	Same as for *C. sakazakii*
C. muytjensii	+	Bone marrow, blood	1	Same as for *C. sakazakii*
C. sakazakii (Enterobacter)	++	RT, wound, CSF, feces	1	Powdered infant formula
C. turicensis	+	Blood	1	Same as for *C. sakazakii*
Entrobacter				
E. aerogenes	++++	All sites	1	Ubiquitous
E. amnigenus biogroups 1 and 2	−			Plants, water
E. asburiae	++	**UT,** RT, feces, wound, blood	2	Water
E. cancerogenus	++	**Wound,** RT, feces	2	Animals, water
E. cloacae subsp. *cloacae*	++++	All sites	1	Water, soil, sewage, meat
E. cloacae subsp. *dissolvens*	−			Disease corn stalks
E. cowanii	Unk	UT, RT, blood, wound	3	Unk
E. gergoviae	++	RT, UT, blood	2	Water, cosmetics
E. hormaechei subsp. hormaechei	++	RT, wound, blood	1	Unk, one isolate from a frog
E. hormaechei subsp. *oharae* and *steigerwaltii*	++	All sites	1	Plants
E. kobei	+	Blood, RT, UT	2	Food
E. ludwigii	Unk	UT, RT, blood, feces	2	Food
E. nimipressuralis/E. oryzae	−			Diseased elms/wild rice
E. pulveris/E. pyrinus	−			Fruit, milk powder/pear trees
E. radicincitans	−			Phyllosphere of winter wheat
E. turicensis/E. helveticus	−			Fruit powder
Hafnia alvei DNA groups 1 and 2	++	**Feces,** blood, RT	2	Ubiquitous
Klebsiella				
K. granulomatis	++	Genital tract	1	None, restricted to humans
K. pneumoniae subsp. *pneumoniae*	++++	All sites, RT/UT most common	1	Ubiquitous
K. pneumoniae subsp. *ozaenae*	++	**Nasal discharge,** RT, UT, blood	1	None, restricted to humans
K. pneumoniae subsp. *rhinoscleromatis*	++	Nasal discharge	2	None, restricted to humans
K. oxytoca	+++	All sites, common in feces	2	Ubiquitous
K. singaporensis	−			Soil
K. variicola	++	Blood, urine	1	Plants
Morganella				
M. morganii subsp. *morganii* and *sibonii*	++	All sites	1	Unk, mammalian/reptile gastrointestinal tract
M. psychrotolerans	−			Fish, causes scombroid poisoning
Pantoea agglomerans (Enterobacter)	+++	All sites	2	Plants

(Continued on next page)

TABLE 1 *(Continued)*

Current (previous) designation	Clinical data			Environmental data
	Frequency	Source	Significance	
Photorhabdus				
P. asymbiotica subsp. *asymbiotica* and *australis*	++	Wound	2	Unk, possibly insects
P. luminescens/P. temperata	−			Nematodes infecting insects
Plesiomonas shigelloides	+++	**Feces,** blood	1	Aquatic habitats, animals
Proteus				
P. hauseri	+	Unk	Unk	Unk, probably like *P. mirabilis*
P. mirabilis	++++	**UT,** blood, CSF	1	Animals, birds, fish, foods
P. myxofaciens	−			Gypsy moth
P. penneri	++	**UT,** blood, wound, feces, eye	1	Probably like *P. mirabilis*
P. vulgaris	+++	**UT,** wound, stool, RT	1	Probably like *P. mirabilis*
Providencia				
P. alcalifaciens	+++	All sites, UT/feces common	1	Mammals, water
P. burhodogranariea/P. sneebia	−			Both from fruit flies
P. heimbachae/P. rustigianii	+	Feces	3	Penguins/unk
P. rettgeri	+++	All sites, UT most common	1	Same as for *P. alcalifaciens*, insects
P. stuartii	+++	All sites, UT most common	1	Mammals
P. vermicola	−			Nematodes infecting insects
Raoultella				
R. ornithinolytica	+	Wound, UT, blood	2	Food
R. planticola/R. terrigena	Unk	Similar to *K. pneumoniae?*	3	Plants, water
Serratia				
S. entomophila	−			New Zealand grass grub, water
S. ficaria	+	RT, wound	3	Fig wasps, figs, plants
S. fonticola	+	**Wound,** RT	3	Water, birds
S. liquefaciens complex (*S. liquefaciens* sensu stricto, *S. proteamaculans, S. grimesii*)	+++	RT, wound	2	Ubiquitous
S. marcescens subsp. *marcescens*	++++	All sites, RT most common	1	Ubiquitous
S. marcescens subsp. *marcescens* biogroup 1	+	**UT,** RT	2	Unk
S. marcescens subsp. *sakuensis*	−			Wastewater
S. odorifera biogroups 1 and 2	+	RT, wound, feces, blood, UT	2	Plants
S. plymuthica	+	RT	3	Water, plants, small mammals
S. rubidaea	+	RT, wound, blood, UT, feces	2	Water, plants
S. nematodiphila/S. ureilytica	−			Nematodes/water

[a]Abbreviations and symbols: ++++, frequent; +++, occasional; ++, rare; +, very rare; −, not yet isolated from humans; CSF, cerebrospinal fluid; RT, respiratory tract; Unk, unknown; UT, urinary tract; 1, major pathogenic species of humans; 2, proven cause of disease in rare instances; 3, isolated from humans, significance unknown. Bold denotes most common source. Data are from references 2, 3, 14, 16, 18, 36, 43, 46, 50–52, 58, 63–65, 68, 73, 78–80, 83, 85, 87, 92, 95, 99, 104, 106, 107, 111, 112, 121, 127, 131–134, and 149.

Serratia marcescens subsp. *sakuensis* is the only reportedly spore-forming organism in this family (1). Prototrophic strains grow readily on ordinary media. Among these genera, auxotrophic strains from clinical specimens are rare. However, cysteine-requiring urinary isolates of *Klebsiella pneumoniae*, which grow as pinpoint colonies on routine media, do occur. When encountered, these strains require supplementation of biochemical media or commercial identification systems with 0.63 mM cysteine for accurate identification. *K. granulomatis* is culturable only by cell culture techniques.

Of the organisms in Tables 1 and 2 isolated from human specimens, all *Klebsiella, Leminorella, Moellerella, Tatumella,* and *Enterobacter asburiae* strains are nonmotile, although any strain of any genus may be nonmotile and recent data for *E. asburiae* indicate some strains may be motile (64). Some strains of *Serratia plymuthica* may not grow at 37°C, but most other members of the genera discussed in this chapter grow well between 25°C and 37°C. Only *Klebsiella* and *Raoultella* spp. are encapsulated, but strains from all genera may grow as mucoid or rough colonies. Six genera produce pigment. Some strains of *S. marcescens* and most *Serratia rubidaea* and *S. plymuthica* strains produce a red pigment, prodigiosin, which may appear throughout the entire colony or only as a red center or margin. Yellow-pigment-producing organisms include environmental *Enterobacter* species (*E. pulveris* and *E. turicensis* [133, 134]) and most strains of *Cronobacter* (*Enterobacter*) *sakazakii, P. agglomerans, Leclercia adecarboxylata,* and *Photorhabdus asymbiotica.* Yellow pigment may be

TABLE 2 Other members of the family *Enterobacteriaceae*[a]

Human pathogens or opportunists	Primarily environmental strains[b,c]	Nonhuman isolates[c]
Buttiauxella gaviniae (32)	*Budvicia aquatica* (15)	*Buttiauxella* species (32, 100)
Edwardsiella tarda	*Buttiauxella noackiae* (100)	*Erwinia* species (81, 105, 126)
Ewingella americana	*Edwardsiella hoshinae* (53)	*Edwardsiella ictaluri* (57)
Cedecea davisae, C. lapagei, C. neteri,	*Pragia fontium* (5)	*Kluyvera intermedia* (100, 111)
Cedecea genomospecies 3 and 5	*Trabulsiella guamensis* (97)	*Pantoea* species (33, 82)
Kluyvera ascorbata, K. cryocrescens, K. georgiana		
Leclercia adecarboxylata		
Leminorella grimontii, L. richardii,		
Leminorella. genomospecies 3		
Moellerella wisconsensis		
Rahnella aquatilis,		
Rahnella genomospecies 2 and 3 (17)		
Tatumella ptyseos		
Yokenella regensburgei		

[a]References given in parentheses. Genomospecies listed cannot be biochemically separated from other species within their genus and/or only a single strain exists.
[b]Rare human isolates of no, or questionable, significance.
[c]Environmental isolates; fish, marine, animal, or bird isolates; insect isolates or pathogens; plant isolates or phytopathogens.

enhanced by incubation at 25°C; weak pigment producers may only be detected by observing growth placed on a swab or filter paper. *Photorhabdus luminescens* and *P. asymbiotica* cultures are luminescent, giving a visible glow in a darkroom after 5 minutes. *Serratia odorifera*, as indicated by its name, and some *Cedecea* spp. produce a pungent (potato-like) odor due to the production of alkyl-methoxypyrazines (50). Species of *Proteus* and *Providencia* oxidatively deaminate α-amino acids, producing pyruvic acids. L-Phenylalanine deamination yields a green color when ferric chloride is added; however, deamination of *dl*-tryptophan produces the deep reddish brown pigment often seen in media inoculated with these organisms without the addition of ferric chloride (114). *Proteus* species also produce swarmer cells, i.e., elongated forms created when cells fail to septate or divide. These cells, which are profusely covered with flagella, act in concert to produce swarming motility on solid media (12).

Plesiomonas shigelloides organisms are also gram-negative, facultative anaerobes growing as straight rods of sizes similar to those of other *Enterobacteriaceae*. However, unlike other *Enterobacteriaceae*, *P. shigelloides* strains are oxidase positive, do not produce gas from glucose (*Enterobacteriaceae* are variable), and are susceptible to O/129 vibriostatic agent (2,4-diamino-6,7-diisopropylpteridine). Both *P. shigelloides* and enterobacteria grow at similar salt concentrations (0 to 5%) and pH ranges (4.0 to 8.0).

EPIDEMIOLOGY, TRANSMISSION, AND CLINICAL SIGNIFICANCE

The *Enterobacteriaceae* are widely distributed throughout the environment (Tables 1 and 2). Many species of the genera in Table 1 are commonly recognized pathogens, consistently ranking among the top 10 organisms seen in health care-associated infections (42, 61, 94). Between 2002 and 2004, 7 of the 10 most common gram-negative organisms isolated from respiratory tract, urinary tract, and bloodstream infections from intensive care unit patients in the United States were *K. pneumoniae* (15%), *E. cloacae* (9%), *S. marcescens* (6%), *Enterobacter aerogenes* (4%), *Proteus mirabilis* (4%), *Klebsiella oxytoca* (3%), and *Citrobacter freundii* (2%). Between 2006 and 2007, the National Healthcare Safety Network (formerly National Nosoco-

mial Infections Surveillance System) reported *K. pneumoniae, Enterobacter* spp., and *K. oxytoca* among the top 10 most frequently isolated health care-associated infections, making up 6%, 5%, and 2% of the isolates, respectively (61). Notably, *Enterobacter* was reported as the third most common isolate from ventilator-associated pneumonia. European data on infection rates, which are similar to those above, can be found on the following websites: http://ecdc.europa.eu/en/Publications/AER_report.aspx and http://www.hpa.org.uk/web/HPAweb&HPAwebStandard/HPAweb_C/1201767919826. Pediatric patient data collected in 2004 from three continents (North America, Latin America, and Europe) indicated that *Klebsiella* spp., *Enterobacter* spp., *P. mirabilis*, and *Serratia* spp. ranked 4th, 7th, 11th, and 12th, respectively, in the top 15 most frequently isolated organisms (42). Both *Klebsiella* and *Enterobacter* were more prevalent (3rd to 5th versus 10th) in North and Latin America than in Europe. In all geographic areas there was a twofold decrease in prevalence for both *Klebsiella* and *Enterobacter* species in children older than 1 year.

Klebsiella and *Raoultella*

Klebsiella is carried in the nasopharynx and the bowel; however, feces are arguably the most significant source of patient infections (98). Recent data indicate that *K. pneumoniae* bloodstream infection isolation rates are 1.5 times greater during the warmest months of the year (7). These rates most likely reflect increased fecal carriage in humans, which in turn is a reflection of increased organisms in the environment during warm months. This has important implications since colonized patients have a fourfold-increased risk of infection over noncarriers. Similar isolation rate increases were not seen with *Enterobacter* or *Serratia*. *K. pneumoniae*, primarily strains with capsular type K1, have emerged as an important cause of community-acquired pyogenic liver abscess worldwide (19, 91, 117, 146). The majority of patients with *Klebsiella* pyogenic liver abscess are Asian males, 50 to 60 years of age, who present primarily with a right-lobe, solitary, monomicrobial abscess. Studies by Brisse et al. (19) indicate that pyogenic liver abscess-associated K1 isolates belong to a clonal complex designated CC23[K1], whereas K1 strains associated with severe pneumonia isolated from the respiratory tract and bloodstream infections belong to a different complex, CC82^{K1}. *magA* (mucoviscosity-associated gene), which resides within the *cps* (capsular polysaccharide synthesis) operon of all K1 isolates, is not an indicator for primary liver abscess. Conversely, the gene *allS* (an activator of the allantoin regulon) has been detected, to date, only in K1 strains isolated from primary liver abscesses (19, 148). *allS* may confer an advantage in these strains because levels of allantoin, which can serve as a carbon source, are elevated in non-insulin-dependent diabetics (148). Primary liver abscess K1 strains also appear to be separable by conventional biochemical methods (see "Identification" below). Mouse lethality studies show that *Klebsiella* liver abscess isolates that possessed both the hypermucoviscosity phenotype and the *rmpA* (regulator of mucoid phenotype) gene, regardless of the K type, have a 50% lethal dose of $<10^2$ CFU versus $>5 \times 10^7$ CFU for type K1 or K2 urine isolates that were not hypermucoviscous and without *rmpA* or aerobactin genes (148). *Klebsiella rhinoscleromatis* and *Klebsiella ozaenae* are clones of *K. pneumoniae* (not subspecies) that have adapted to cause specific chronic infectious diseases, i.e., rhinoscleroma and atrophic rhinitis (ozena), respectively (19). Neither organism is isolated from the environment or the intestinal tract, and both have lost the ability to utilize substrates involved in plant product degradation pathways; however, isolates from bloodstream, urinary tract, and other infection sites indicate that *K. ozaenae* is more diverse in its ability to cause disease than *K. rhinoscleromatis*. Atrophic rhinitis is restricted to the nose, but rhinoscleroma may spread to the trachea and larynx (73). Both of these tissue-destructive diseases occur more frequently in tropical areas of the world and are spread by person-to-person transmission, although prolonged contact with persons producing airborne nasal secretions is required. A recent retrospective study has updated the epidemiological and clinical features of rhinoscleroma (35). *Klebsiella granulomatis*, also a clone (not species) of *K. pneumoniae*, is the agent of donovanosis or granuloma inguinale, a disease characterized by chronic genital ulcers (19, 56). It also occurs predominantly in tropical countries and is thought to be sexually transmitted, with humans as the only known reservoir. *K. oxytoca* strains carrying a chromosomally encoded heat-labile cytotoxin have been increasingly recognized as a cause of antibiotic-associated hemorrhagic colitis (49, 150). Antibiotic-associated hemorrhagic colitis, associated with the use of β-lactam antibiotics, is self-limiting and resolves spontaneously with the withdrawal of the contributing antibiotic. It differs from *Clostridium difficile* disease in that there is no pseudomembrane formation and *K. oxytoca* antibiotic-associated hemorrhagic colitis stools are bloody. The majority of isolations reported to date for *Klebsiella variicola* are from sterile sites, mainly blood and urine (6, 121). Recent isolates of this organism (three of five from urine), identified by *rpoB* sequencing reported from a Brazilian study, provide increased evidence that this organism is a human pathogen (6). *Raoultella planticola* and *Raoultella terrigena* share pathogenicity characteristics with *K. pneumoniae* and are difficult to distinguish from it biochemically without special tests. In European studies, 3.5% to 19% of clinical strains initially identified as *Klebsiella* were *R. planticola*, while in U.S. and Brazilian surveys of 436 and 122 strains, respectively, only one isolate in each was identified as *R. planticola*, indicating that prevalence of these species may differ geographically (6, 113, 142).

Enterobacter, Pantoea, and Erwinia

Nosocomial *Enterobacter* colonization and infection are frequently associated with contaminated medical devices and instrumentation; however, *Enterobacter* spp. are commonly consumed in foods, so endogenous sources should also be considered (73). *Enterobacter ludwigii* and all *Enterobacter hormaechei* subspecies are isolated from a variety of human sources including blood (63, 65). A nonhuman source for *E. ludwigii* has not been reported, but plants appear to be the natural habitat of *E. hormaechei*. Other environmental organisms including a *Pantoea dispersa*-like organism, *Pantoea ananatis*, and *Erwinia persicina* have been reported from blood or urine (33, 105, 126). *P. agglomerans* is the species of *Pantoea* most commonly isolated from humans. Sporadic infections are associated with penetrating trauma by objects contaminated with soil or vegetation resulting in soft tissue infections, septic arthritis, or osteomyelitis, whereas health care-associated infections and outbreaks often involve contaminated intravenous fluid, parenteral nutrition, or other administered fluids. *P. agglomerans* infections in children, most of whom have severe underlying conditions, are predominantly polymicrobic and therefore of questionable significance even when specimens are from sterile sites (30).

Serratia

Serratia spp. are notorious health care-associated pathogens and colonizers. Transmission is predominately from person to person, but medical apparatuses, intravenous fluids, and other solutions are often implicated as well (73). Indwelling catheters, particularly for urinary tract infections, serve as a primary reservoir for transmission via hospital personnel. In children, the gastrointestinal tract is a common source of infections. Outbreaks transmitted by hand are often insidious, occurring over long periods of time, and may subside and peak a number of times before recognition and infection control efforts can contain them. Pigment production in *S. marcescens* appears to be a marker that the strain is environmental in origin and of low virulence (9). Community-acquired infections are rare except for *S. marcescens* contact lens-induced acute red eye (67). Most of the other species of *Serratia* have also been isolated from humans, in whom they too are usually transients or cause opportunistic infections.

Citrobacter

Citrobacters are primarily inhabitants of the intestinal tract, and their presence in the environment may reflect fecal excretion by humans and animals; the natural habitat of some newer *Citrobacter* species is unknown. The three species most commonly involved in hospital infections are *C. freundii*, *C. koseri*, and *C. braakii*; patients are usually older adults ($\geq$65 years), more often males, and the urinary tract is the most common site of infection (90, 123). One-third to one-half of *Citrobacter* infections, including septicemias, are polymicrobic and are associated with higher mortality rates (18% to 50%) or longer hospital stays (73, 90, 123). Meningitis is almost exclusively associated with *C. koseri* and involves children <2 months of age, with the highest onset rates recorded in neonates with a mean age of 7 days (73). Brain abscesses occur in 75% of infected infants, and neurological defects are common sequelae in surviving infants. The most prominent risk factor is prior colonization; during outbreaks, colonization rates of 27% have been noted versus a normal rate of <1% (93, 143). Person-to-person spread by hospital personnel and, less often, from mother to offspring is the most likely source of infections. Sampling of inanimate or environmental reservoirs in hospitals usually fails to yield *Citrobacter*. Other *Citrobacter* species including *C. gillenii* and *C. murliniae* have been found in human clinical, animal, food, and environmental specimens (16, 18). The role of many *Citrobacter* spp. in human infections is unclear because reports in the literature are insufficient to determine either clinical significance in humans or potential reservoirs for infection. *C. rodentium* causes murine colonic hyperplasia, which is self-limiting in adult mice but causes significant morbidity and mortality in infant mice in mouse colony outbreaks (95).

Proteus, Providencia, and Morganella

Members of *Proteus*, *Providencia*, and *Morganella* genera are widespread in the environment, are normal inhabitants of the gut, and are relatively common in clinical laboratories, especially *P. mirabilis*. In a large six-year population-based survey of *Proteeae*, 85% (4,290 of 5,047) of isolates were community acquired, although providenciae were more likely to be acquired in nursing homes (89). Females (69%) and the elderly (median age, 70) were at highest risk of infection, and the most common specimen sources were urine (86%), soft tissues (7%), blood (3%), miscellaneous fluids (2%), and the respiratory tract (2%). *P. mirabilis*, predominantly from urine, was the most frequently isolated agent (77%). Non-*P. mirabilis* species (primarily *Proteus vulgaris*) were isolated from wounds/soft tissue more often than urine. Of the *Providencia* species, *P. stuartii* was isolated twice as often as other species. *P. mirabilis*, *Proteus penneri*, *Morganella*, and *Providencia alcalifaciens* are seen in diarrheal stools with greater frequency than in normal stools, leading to speculation that they may cause diarrhea. Some strains of *P. alcalifaciens* are invasive in HEp-2 cell assays and elicit diarrhea in the RITARD (reversible intestinal-tie adult rabbit diarrhea) model, while other strains isolated in pure culture or in large numbers from diarrheal stools fail to invade cell lines (4, 76). However, a number of noninvasive *P. alcalifaciens* strains have been shown to be nonadherent to cell lines in vitro, which may provide insight to their inability to invade (86). Yoh et al. (147) used a specialized medium to isolate nine strains of *Providencia rettgeri* from 130 persons with traveler's diarrhea; eight of these strains were invasive in Caco-2 cells, indicating their potential for virulence in humans. Notably, vomiting was present in five *P. rettgeri* cases but was not seen in patients from whom other providenciae were isolated.

Hafnia

Few systematic investigations regarding the ecological distribution of *Hafnia* have been published, although it is a common inhabitant of the gastrointestinal tract of mammals, birds, cold-blooded animals, fish, and insects (74). Isolation from consumables, especially meats, is not uncommon, and presumably its presence indicates prior contact of the item with feces. *Hafnia alvei* has been linked to gastrointestinal disease, although putative virulence characteristics have not been demonstrated (3, 120). However, a toxigenic strain producing a cytopathic effect on Vero cells indistinguishable from Shiga toxin, but not neutralized by anti-Shiga toxin antibody, has been reported (29). Although seen infrequently in extraintestinal disease, such infections occur both in healthy and in immunocompromised patients with monomicrobial infection rates varying from 12 to 75%; the correlation with disease increases when the organism is isolated in pure culture and in high numbers (74). *Hafnia* appears to have a predilection for the biliary tree and may produce abscesses at the site of infection (118).

Plesiomonas shigelloides and Edwardsiella tarda

Plesiomonas is isolated from a wide range of mammals, birds, fish, water-dwelling reptiles, and amphibians, but with the possible exception of cats, there is no evidence it plays a role in diarrheal disease in any of these species (70). Human *P. shigelloides* infections are associated with living in or travel to tropical countries and/or a history of seafood consumption; both acute diarrhea and chronic diarrhea episodes of >2 weeks have been reported (77, 84). Most infections are self-limited with hospitalization required only for severe infections and/or in patients with underlying conditions. *Plesiomonas* typically presents as a secretory (watery) diarrhea, and although it can also manifest as a dysenteric (bloody) diarrhea, the secretory form is seen three times more frequently (144). Possible diarrheal virulence determinants in some isolates include cholera-like, heat-stable, and heat-labile toxins, while other strains have been shown to invade and multiply within human gastrointestinal cells (71, 139). The somatic antigen of *Plesiomonas* may also play a role in pathogenicity, since the gene encoding the most common type, O17, shares almost complete identity with the form 1 (smooth) antigen gene of *Shigella sonnei* (25). Wound infections associated with water contact are not encountered with plesiomonads despite their aquatic reservoir. *Plesiomonas* bacteremia, which is rare and usually polymicrobic, is generally community acquired, and major risk factors include biliary tract disease and advanced age (>75 years) (145). *Edwardsiella tarda* is typically associated with water and animals that inhabit water; it is an infrequent cause of gastroenteritis in humans, with most infections linked to contact with fish or turtles. A low carriage rate in humans, except in tropical areas of the world, and the ability to produce a cell-associated hemolysin and invade HEp-2 cells suggest that *E. tarda* is a diarrheal agent (77). Serious wound infections, including myonecrosis, are reported in immunocompetent individuals with aquatic exposure, but systemic infections usually occur in patients with liver disease or iron overload conditions (129).

Miscellaneous Enterobacteriaceae

Miscellaneous members of *Enterobacteriaceae* that are infrequently encountered in clinical laboratories are primarily opportunistic pathogens in compromised patients or are present as transients or commensals in clinical specimens (73). For some, like *Cedecea* spp., *Leminorella* spp., *Moellerella*, and *Tatumella*, a reservoir has not been determined because they are rarely isolated from nonhuman sources, while *Ewingella*, *Leclercia*, and *Kluyvera* spp. are found in a variety of foods, water, or animals (snails and slugs) and like many enterics appear to be ubiquitous in the environment (40, 54, 55, 59, 60, 66, 73, 137). Other genera isolated from humans have more specific natural habitats such as *Rahnella* (water) or *Yokenella* and *P. asymbiotica* (insects and infections from insect bites) (2, 41, 73, 88). There have been increased reports of clinically significant isolations of *L. adecarboxylata* and *Kluyvera* species, all of which cannot be covered here. *Kluyvera* infections occur in competent and immunosuppressed patients of all age groups (23, 122). The organism is isolated from a broad spectrum of sources including blood, tissue, urine, cerebrospinal fluid, and peritoneal fluid, although urinary tract and bloodstream infections each account for approximately one-third of the infections. When strains are determined to species level, *Kluyvera ascorbata* accounts for more than twice the number of *Kluyvera cryocrescens* infections. Originally considered to be an opportunistic pathogen, *L. adecarboxylata* is quite often isolated from polymicrobial infections in healthy patients without underlying disease (58). This suggests that the coinfecting agent(s) might alter the local tissue environment, allowing growth of *Leclercia*, or that a transfer of genetic factors occurs, enhancing its virulence. The isolation of *Leclercia* in pure culture from previously healthy persons (from a foot abscess and blood and wound caused by a hydrofluoric acid chemical injury) in two recent reports would indicate that at least some strains may be pathogenic (31, 58). *Moellerella wisconsensis*, a rarely reported organism first isolated from stools of diarrheal patients, has been reported from an additional series of five patients with disease ranging from self-limited acute watery diarrhea without mucus to protracted diarrhea, lasting several weeks. No other common diarrheal bacterial pathogens or parasites were present in the stools, and specimens taken after clinical recovery were negative (116).

COLLECTION, TRANSPORT, AND STORAGE OF SPECIMENS

The organisms covered in this chapter are, in general, readily isolated from clinical material, and the principles in chapter 16 of this *Manual* on specimen collection, handling, and processing are applicable. Most of these organisms will survive in culture deeps for approximately a year. Long-term storage methods as recommended in chapter 9 work well for these organisms. *Plesiomonas* cells do not survive for more than 1 to 2 months when held at room temperature and should be maintained at −70°C. In our laboratory, strains of *Tatumella* have failed to survive longer than a year even at −70°C.

ISOLATION PROCEDURES

Few of the clinically relevant strains covered in this chapter present difficulties in isolation from sterile body sites. Isolation from nonsterile body or environmental sites may require specialized media such as CHROMagar Orientation (Becton Dickinson, Sparks, MD) and chromID CPS (bioMerieux, Hazelwood, MO), which perform similarly for the detection of urinary tract pathogens covered in this chapter and can reliably replace MacConkey and blood agars (20, 125). These media prevent swarming of *Proteus* and limit the spread of mucoid colonies, which reduces overgrowth of pathogenic colonies. Additionally, colonies on CHROMagar can be used to inoculate antimicrobial susceptibility tests directly without subculture. CHROMagar media can also be used for specimens from other nonsterile sites; when colony color was combined with indole, lysine, and ornithine decarboxylase tests and serology, 98.7%

(466 of 472) of the above organisms were correctly identified from nonurine samples (109).

Both of the diarrheal pathogens covered in this chapter are easily isolated. *E. tarda* is a lactose-negative, H$_2$S-positive organism, indistinguishable from *Salmonella* on enteric plating media (opaque or opaque with black centers). A positive indole reaction and failure to agglutinate in specific *Salmonella* antisera separate the two organisms. *Plesiomonas* produces non-lactose-, non-sucrose-fermenting colonies on enteric plating media. It does not grow on thiosulfate-citrate-bile salts-sucrose medium, but on cefsulodin-Irgasan-novobiocin medium, opaque colonies without a pink center (mannitol not fermented) are suspicious for plesiomonads. Two other oxidase-positive organisms, *Pseudomonas* and *Aeromonas*, grow on cefsulodin-Irgasan-novobiocin as well, although *Aeromonas* colonies have a pink center with an opaque apron. Inositol fermentation and a positive reaction in Moeller's lysine, arginine, and ornithine tests will differentiate *Plesiomonas* from these agents as well as other organisms.

Other *Enterobacteriaceae* involved in opportunistic infections and that may be isolated from a variety of specimen types generally grow well on commonly used laboratory media (80). Some genera are lactose or sucrose fermenters and give the appearance of normal biota on enteric plating media, while others may produce H$_2$S and appear *Salmonella*-like. *Rahnella*, *Ewingella*, and *Tatumella* may require 48 hours for growth. *Tatumella* also grows poorly on Mueller-Hinton agar, and a broth dilution method may be required for susceptibility testing. *K. granulomatis* does not grow on conventional laboratory media but has been grown in HEp-2 monolayers (22). Detection of Donovan bodies from tissue smears using Giemsa or Wright stains is the method most commonly used to detect this organism. However, these pleomorphic, bipolar staining bodies shaped like a closed safety pin are not always present and are not reliable for diagnosis.

IDENTIFICATION

The biochemical tests most useful for separating members covered in this chapter are given in Tables 3 through 13. A table for the identification of *Plesiomonas* can be found in

TABLE 3 Separation of members of the genus *Citrobacter*[a]

Species	Indole	ODC	Malonate	Acid[b] from:			
				Sucrose	Dulcitol	Melibiose	Adonitol
C. amalonaticus	+	+	−	−	−	−	−
C. braakii	V	+	−	−	V	V	−
C. farmeri	+	+	−	+	−	+	−
C. freundii (sensu stricto)	V	−	−	V	−	+	−
C. koseri	+	+	+	V	V	−	+
C. rodentium	−	+	+	−	−	−	−
C. sedlakii	V	+	+	−	++	−	−
C. werkmanii	−	−	+	−	−	−	−
C. youngae	V	−	−	V	+	−	−
C. gillenii	−	−	+	V	−	V	−
C. murliniae	+	−	−	V	+	V	−

[a]Abbreviations and symbols: ODC, ornithine decarboxylase; +, ≥85%; V, 15 to 84%; −, <15%.
[b]Fermentation reactions in commercial systems should be similar to reactions in conventional fermentation broths (1% carbohydrate in broth with indicator).

TABLE 4 Differentiation of *Pantoea agglomerans* and members of the genus *Enterobacter*[a, b]

Species	LDC	ADH	ODC	VP	Sucrose	Adonitol	D-Sorbitol	L-Rhamnose	α-Methyl-D-glucoside	Esculin	Melibiose	Yellow pigment
					Acid[c] from:							
Human species												
E. aerogenes	+	−	+	+	+	+	+	+	+	+	+	−
P. agglomerans	−	−	−	V	V	−	V	V	−	V	V	V
E. amnigenus biogroup 1	−	−	V	+	+	−	−	+	V	+	+	−
E. asburiae	−	V	+	−	+	−	+	−	+	+	−	−
E. cancerogenus	−	+	+	+	−	−	−	+	−	+	−	−
E. cloacae subsp. cloacae	−	+	+	+	+	V	+	+	V	V	+	−
E. cowanii[d]	−	−	−	+	+	−	+	+	−	+	+	V
E. gergoviae	+	−	+	+	+	−	−	+	−	+	+	−
E. hormaechei subsp. hormaechei	−	V	+	+	+	−	−	+	V	−	−	−
E. kobei	−	+	+	−	+	−	+	+	+	V	+	−
E. sakazakii	−	+	+	+	+	−	−	+	+	+	+	+
Environmental species												
E. amnigenus biogroup 2	−	V	+	+	−	−	+	+	+	+	+	−
E. cloacae subsp. dissolvens	−	+	+	+	+	−	+	+	+	+	+	−
E. nimipressuralis	−	−	+	+	−	−	+	+	+	+	+	−
E. pyrinus[e]	+	−	+	+	+	−	−	+	−	+	+	−
E. radicincitans	−	+	−	+	+	−	+	+	−	+	−	−

[a]See the text for *E. ludwigii* and *E. hormaechei* subsp. *steigerwaltii* and *oharae* identification.
[b]Abbreviations and symbols: LDC, lysine decarboxylase; ADH, arginine dihydrolase; ODC, ornithine decarboxylase; VP, Voges-Proskauer; +, ≥90%; V, 11 to 89%; −, ≤10%.
[c]See Table 3, footnote *b*.
[d]Separated from *P. agglomerans* by a negative malonate reaction and fermentation of D-sorbitol (68).
[e]Separated from *E. gergoviae* by positive reactions in potassium cyanide broth and *myo*-inositol.

chapter 39, which describes vibrios, since these organisms most closely resemble one another biochemically. Correct identification to species level is increasingly important in recognizing strains that are of high risk for carrying extended-spectrum beta-lactamases (ESBLs), cephalosporinases, or carbapenemases.

It should be noted that identification problems arising from the use of commercial systems vary with each genus. The percentage of correct identifications for many commercial systems increases significantly when additional biochemical tests are performed on organisms with "low-probability" identifications. Even when unusual enterobacteria covered in this chapter are included in commercial system databases, the number of strains available to use in challenge studies is very limited; therefore, the ability of these systems to accurately identify these organ-

TABLE 5 Separation of some members of the genera *Klebsiella* and *Raoultella*[a,b]

Species	Indole	ODC	VP	Malonate	ONPG	Growth at: 10°C	Growth at: 44°C	Acid[c] from D-melezitose
R. ornithinolytica	+	+	V	+	+	+	NA	NA
K. oxytoca	+	−	+	+	+	−	+	−
K. ozaenae	−	−	−	−	V	NA	NA	NA
K. pneumoniae[d]	−	−	+	+	+	−	+	−
R. planticola	V	−	+	+	+	+	−	−
R. terrigena	−	−	+	+	+	+	−	+
K. rhinoscleromatis	−	−	−	+	−	NA	NA	NA

[a]*K. singaporensis* biochemicals not available; only a single strain known.
[b]Abbreviations and symbols: ODC, ornithine decarboxylase; VP, Voges-Proskauer; ONPG, *o*-nitrophenyl-β-D-galactopyranoside; NA, not available; +, ≥90%; V, 11 to 89%; −, ≤10%.
[c]See Table 3, footnote *b*.
[d]A negative adonitol reaction may be an indication that the strain is *K. variicola*, but this must be confirmed with gene sequencing (*rpoB*) (6).

TABLE 6 Biochemical characterization of members of the genus *Serratia*[a,b]

Species	LDC	ODC	Mal	Acid[c] from:								Red pigment	Odor
				Arab	L-Rham	D-Xyl	Suc	Adon	D-Sorb	Cello	D-Arabitol		
S. entomophila[d]	−	−	−	−	−	V	+	−	−	−	V	−	−
S. ficaria	−	−	−	+	V	+	+	−	+	+	+	−	V
S. fonticola	+	+	V	+	V	V	V	+	+	−	+	−	−
S. liquefaciens group	+	+	−	+	V	+	+	−	+	−	−	−	−
S. marcescens subsp. marcescens	+	+	−	−	−	−	+	V	+	−	−	V	−
S. marcescens biogroup 1	V	+	−	−	−	−	+	V	+	−	−	NA	−
S. odorifera biogroup 1	+	+	−	+	+	+	+	V	+	+	−	−	+
S. odorifera biogroup 2	+	−	−	+	+	+	−	V	+	+	−	−	+
S. plymuthica[e]	−	−	−	+	−	+	+	−	V	V	−	+	−
S. rubidaea	V	−	+	+	−	+	+	+	−	+	V	+	−

[a]*S. marcescens* subsp. *sakuensis* is reportedly a spore-forming organism; *S. ureilytica* is urea positive; only a single strain is known.
[b]Abbreviations and symbols: LDC, lysine decarboxylase; ODC, ornithine decarboxylase; Mal, malonate; L-Rham, L-rhamnose; D-Xyl, D-xylose; Suc, sucrose; Adon, adonitol; D-Sorb, D-sorbitol; Cello, cellobiose; +, ≥90%; V, 11 to 89%; −, ≤10%; NA, information not available.
[c]See Table 3, footnote *b*.
[d]Growth at 37°C but biochemical characterization optimal at 30°C.
[e]May fail to grow at 37°C.

TABLE 7 Separation of members of the genera *Proteus*, *Providencia*, and *Morganella*[a]

Organism	Indole	H₂S	Urea	ODC	Acid[b] from:				
					Maltose	D-Adonitol	D-Arabitol	Trehalose	myo-Inositol
Proteus									
P. hauseri	+	V	+	−	+	−	−	+	−
P. mirabilis	−	+	+	+	−	−	−	+	−
P. penneri	−	V	+	−	+	−	−	V	−
P. vulgaris[c]	+	V	+	−	+	−	−	−	−
Providencia									
P. alcalifaciens	+	−	−	−	−	+	−	−	−
P. heimbachae	−	−	−	−	V	+	+	−	V
P. rettgeri	+	−	+	−	−	+	+	−	+
P. rustigianii	+	−	−	−	−	−	−	−	−
P. stuartii	+	−	V	−	−	−	−	+	+
Morganella									
M. morganii subsp. morganii	+	−[d]	+	+[e]	−	−	−	−	−
M. morganii subsp. sibonii	V	−[d]	+	+[e]	−	−	−	+	−

[a]Abbreviations and symbols: Ind, indole; H₂S, hydrogen sulfide; ODC, ornithine decarboxylase; +, ≥ 90%; V, 11 to 89%; −, ≤10%.
[b]See Table 3, footnote *b*.
[c]*P. vulgaris* genomospecies 4, 5, and 6 cannot be differentiated phenotypically.
[d]Some members of some biogroups are H₂S positive.
[e]Some members of some biogroups are ornithine decarboxylase negative.

TABLE 8 Separation of *Cedecea* from selected *Enterobacter* and *Cronobacter* species (VP, ADH, and ODC variable or positive)[a]

Organism	Acid[b] from:					
	D-Sorbitol	Raffinose	L-Rhamnose	Melibiose	D-Arabitol	Sucrose
Cedecea davisae	−	−	−	−	−	+
Cedecea lapagei	−	−	−	+	+	−
E. cloacae	+	+	+	+	V	−
Cronobacter sakazakii	−	+	+	+	−	+
E. cancerogenus	−	−	+	−	−	−

[a]Abbreviations and symbols: VP, Voges-Proskauer; ADH, arginine dihydrolase; ODC, ornithine decarboxylase; +, ≥90%; V, 11 to 89%; −, ≤10%.
[b]See Table 3, footnote *b*.

TABLE 9 Differentiation of *Kluyvera* from commonly seen indole-positive, VP-negative organisms[a]

Organism	Citrate	Urea	LDC	KCN
Kluyvera[b]	−	−	+	+
C. koseri	+	V	−	−
Morganella	−	+	−	+
Providencia	V	+	−	+
E. coli	−	−	+	−

[a]Abbreviations and symbols: VP, Voges-Proskauer; LDC, lysine decarboxylase; KCN, potassium cyanide; +, ≥90%; V, 11 to 89%; −, ≤10%. *Leclercia* and *E. tarda* are also indole positive and VP negative and can be found in Tables 10 and 12, respectively.
[b]Includes *K. intermedia* (*K. cochleae* and *Enterobacter intermedius* combined) (111).

isms is really unknown. O'Hara (103) has published a comprehensive review on manual and automated systems for the identification of bacteria in clinical laboratories. It provides the component substrates used and the additional reagents that are needed, if any, as well as quality control, database content, accuracy of identification, important features of each automated identification system, and published evaluations, among other information, for each commercial system. It also emphasizes that the clinical laboratory should not rely solely on the identification provided by commercial systems but rather take into account colony morphology, susceptibility test data, and anatomic site of isolation.

Klebsiella and *Raoultella*

K. pneumoniae CC23[K1] isolates associated with pyogenic liver abscess may be distinguished biochemically from CC82[K1] and type K2 *K. pneumoniae* strains by their utilization of D-ribose, 3-hydroxybutyrate, D-tagatose, and dulcitol as sole carbon sources (19). *K. ozaenae* and *K. rhinoscleromatis* are slow-growing organisms and thus do poorly in commercial systems; however, they can be difficult to separate using conventional biochemicals as well. *R. planticola* and *R. terrigena* require temperature growth and carbon assimilation tests to separate them from *Klebsiella* species. *R. terrigena* can be separated from *R. planticola* by fermentation of β-gentibiose. *K. variicola* is not found in commercial systems, and information from additional isolates has shown that adonitol fermentation is of limited usefulness for its separation from *K. pneumoniae* (6, 121). At this point, sequencing of housekeeping genes (*rpoB* and others) is the only method of correctly identifying this organism. *phoE* and *scrA* (sucrose regulon) genes have been

used to identify and to separate *K. granulomatis* (*phoE* positive and *scrA* negative) from *Klebsiella* species (*phoE* and *scrA* positive) (24).

Enterobacter and *Pantoea*

Because of the genetic heterogeneity in several species, members of the genera *Enterobacter* and *Pantoea* appear to confound commercial systems more often than other genera (73). *E. ludwigii* and *E. hormaechei*, species previously residing within the *E. cloacae* complex, can be separated from *E. cloacae* by growth on 3-0-methyl-D-glucopyranose and putrescine and 3-hydroxybutyrate, respectively (63, 65). By using commercially available tests, the three subspecies of *E. hormaechei* can be separated with adonitol, dulcitol, and D-sorbitol (subsp. *hormaechei* tests negative, positive, and negative, respectively; subsp. *steigerwaltii* tests positive, negative, and positive, respectively; and subsp. *oharae* tests negative, negative, and positive, respectively) (63). *P. agglomerans* is very difficult to identify with either commercial systems or conventional biochemicals (21, 103). Yellow-pigmented and lysine-, arginine,- and ornithine-negative organisms should raise suspicion that the strain is *P. agglomerans*; *Leclercia adecarboxylata* and *P. asymbiotica* also share these characteristics, but they can be separated from *P. agglomerans* by positive indole and negative D-mannitol reactions, respectively. *P. ananatis*, *P. dispersa*, and *E. persicina* most closely resemble *P. agglomerans*, but *P. dispersa* can be separated from *P. agglomerans* by negative reactions for raffinose, salicin, and sucrose and *E. persicina* can be distinguished by negative reactions for maltose and D-xylose, respectively. *P. ananatis* is more difficult to differentiate, and all suspected isolates of this organism, as with other rare Enterobacteriaceae, should be sent to a reference laboratory for confirmation.

Serratia, *Citrobacter*, and *Proteeae*

Serratia spp. are generally easily identified except for the *S. liquefaciens* group; separation of members within this group can be achieved using a combination of API 50 CH (carbohydrate) and API ZYM (enzymatic) (bioMérieux, Hazelwood, MO) strips (50, 73). *Citrobacter* spp. may be included in databases individually or by subgroups (*C. braakii-C. freundii-C. sedlakii*, *C. werkmanii-C. youngae*, or *C. koseri-C. amalonaticus*); however, subgroup identification requires further biochemical testing by standard methodologies, and final species identification is delayed (73). A PYR (L-pyroglutamic acid, Oxoid PYR) disk, which detects pyrrolidonyl peptidase, may be useful for separating biochemically atypical strains of *Citrobacter* (positive)

TABLE 10 Separation of LDC-, ODC-, and ADH-negative unusual *Enterobacteriaceae* found in clinical specimens[a]

Organism	Motility	Gas from glucose	KCN	VP	Acid[b] from: Sucrose	Acid[b] from: L-Arabitol	Acid[b] from: Trehalose
Ewingella	V	−	−	+	−	−	+
Leclercia	+	+	+	−	+	+	+
Moellerella	+	+	V	−	−	+	+
Rahnella	−	+	−	+	+	+	+
Tatumella	−	−	−	−	+	−	+
Photorhabdus asymbiotica[c]	+	−	−	−	−	−	−

[a]Abbreviations and symbols: LDC, lysine decarboxylase; ODC, ornithine decarboxylase; ADH, arginine dihydrolase; KCN, potassium cyanide; VP, Voges-Proskauer; +, ≥90%; V, 11 to 89%; −, ≤10%. *Budvicia* is also LDC, ODC, and ADH negative and can be found in Table 12.
[b]See Table 3, footnote b.
[c]*Photorhabdus* subsp. *australis* can be separated from subsp. *asymbiotica* by fermentation of maltose and glycerol.

Table 11 Separation of *Yokenella* from *Hafnia*[a]

Organism	VP	Malonate	Citrate	Acid[b] from:	
				Melibiose	Glycerol
Yokenella	−	−	+	+	−
Hafnia alvei	+	+	−	−	+
H. alvei biogroup 2	+	−	V	−	+

[a]Abbreviations and symbols: VP, Voges-Proskauer; +, ≥90%; V, 11 to 89%; −, ≤ 10%. Data from reference 78.
[b]See Table 3, footnote *b*.

and *Salmonella* (negative) (13). Gram-negative, oxidase-negative organisms that swarm on blood agar and appear flat with tapered edges on MacConkey agar may be reported as *Proteus*. Spot indole-negative and ampicillin-susceptible strains may be reported as *P. mirabilis*, while spot indole-positive, ampicillin-resistant strains are reported as *P. vulgaris* (10). *P. hauseri*, previously a subgroup of *P. vulgaris*, can be differentiated from *P. vulgaris* by negative salicin/esculin and trehalose reactions (108). *Proteus* organisms that do not fit the above criteria must be fully identified by commercial or conventional biochemical methods (10). *Proteus* species are identified with 95% to 100% accuracy by commercial systems, but *Providencia* identification rates vary from 79% to 100% (108). When *Providencia* spp. are misidentified, they are usually called *Morganella* or *Proteus*. Urea-positive *P. stuartii* may be misidentified as *P. rettgeri*, or the system may require additional tests for identification. Two-hour identification methods misidentify *M. morganii* subsp. *morganii* about 66% of the time.

Other *Enterobacteriaceae*

Averyella dalhousiensis is not in commercial system databases. It may be confused with *K. ascorbata* or misidentified as *S. enterica* in commercial systems. It shares biochemical traits (positive for ONPG [o-nitrophenyl-β-D-galactopyranoside], malonate, potassium cyanide, and fermentation of dulcitol and salicin) with *Salmonella* subspecies 2, 3, and 4. *Ewingella* and *Tatumella* are biochemically inactive, and the latter organism grows poorly in vitro. *Kluyvera* can be identified only to genus level by commercial systems, but species determination requires an ascorbate test and Irgasan susceptibility and/or gas liquid chromatography profiles (73). *P. asymbiotica* is not in most commercial databases.

Molecular Identification

Information on molecular identification techniques is available elsewhere (chapter 4). For laboratories using partial 16S rRNA (~500 bp) sequencing to identify members of the *Enterobacteriaceae*, the Clinical and Laboratory Standards Institute (CLSI) provides extremely useful information, including guidelines with suggested cutoff values for percent identity scores and identification algorithms (27). Specifically, Table 3 of the MM18-A guideline provides information on the usefulness of 16S rRNA for various enteric groups, comments regarding relatedness within groups, alternative DNA targets, and indications for identification to species level and recommendations for resolving species identification. Suggested cutoff values help the laboratory provide clinicians with practical, recognizable identifications of clinically significant organisms and allow the same organisms to be identified with consistency between laboratories. Appropriate cutoff values notwithstanding, accurate organism identification is ultimately dependent upon the availability of a reliable database of known sequences for comparison of the sequences generated for the unknown isolate. Both public and private databases are available, and each offers advantages (128). An evaluation of two commercially available reference sequence libraries, MicroSeq (Applied Biosystems, Foster City, CA) and SmartGene IDNS (SmartGene, Inc., Raleigh, NC), found that the second had a greater diversity of sequences for comparison and provided user-friendly software with enhancements such as the ability to add alternative gene target databases and to store and compare previous clinical sequences (128).

TYPING SYSTEMS

The ability to trace the spread of nosocomial pathogens in outbreaks caused by the *Enterobacteriaceae* has become a major responsibility for the laboratory. Chapters 7 and 8 provide useful information on the molecular epidemiology of enteric outbreaks. Molecular techniques, including plasmid analysis, ribotyping, pulsed-field gel electrophoresis (PFGE), and various PCR methodologies all appear to be satisfactorily discriminatory, with some working better for a specific genus or species than others. PCR techniques, particularly repetitive element-PCR methods for the *Enterobacteriaceae*, have proliferated at an astonishing pace and cannot be covered here more fully. To date, because economic constraints dictate the need for a single method that is applicable for a variety of organisms, PFGE remains the most universally accepted standardized technique for

TABLE 12 Separation of *Enterobacteriaceae* that may be H$_2$S positive[a]

Organism	LDC	ODC	Urea	Acid[b] from L-arabinose	Citrate	KCN	ONPG
Leminorella spp.	−	−	−	+	V[c]	−	−
Edwardsiella tarda	+	+	−	−	−	−	−
Budvicia aquatica[d]	−	−	+	V	−	−	+
Pragia fontium[d]	−	−	−	−	−	−	−
Trabulsiella guamensis[d]	+	+	−	+	V	+	+
Salmonella subgroup 1	+	+	−	+	+	−	−
Citrobacter	−	V	V	+	V	+	+
Proteus	−	V	+	−	V	+	−

[a]Abbreviations and symbols: LDC, lysine decarboxylase; ODC, ornithine decarboxylase; KCN, potassium cyanide; ONPG, o-nitrophenol-β-D-galactopyranoside; +, ≥90%; V, 11 to 89%; −, ≤10%.
[b]See Table 3, footnote *b*.
[c]*L. grimontii* is positive, *L. richardii* is negative.
[d]Found in clinical specimens but of questionable or no significance.

TABLE 13 Resistance mediators of the *Enterobacteriaceae*[a]

Resistance mediators	Ambler class[b]	Resistance to clavulanic acid	Substrates	Enzyme(s)	Location	Organism(s)	Testing procedures
Restricted-spectrum β-lactamases	A	S	Aminopenicillins, carboxypenicillins, narrow-spectrum cephalosporins	TEM 1 and 2, SHV-1	Plasmid or chromosome	*K. pneumoniae*, other genera	Cefpodoxime screen, double disk, MBD, Etest with CTX and CAZ ± clavulanic acid or CPD ± clavulanic acid, chromID agar, automated systems, PCR
Extended-spectrum β-lactamases	A	S	Penicillins, narrow and extended-spectrum cephalosporins, aztreonam	TEM 3, SHV 2 (other types, >130 and 50 types respectively), CTX-M	Plasmid	*Klebsiella* spp. *S. marcescens* *Enterobacter* spp. *Proteus* spp. *C. freundii* *M. morganii*	Same as above, plus induction test with CAZ and FOX
Cephalosporinases	C	R	Extended-spectrum β-lactams, cephamycins, aztreonam	AmpCs (CMY, MOX, FOX, DHA types)	Plasmid Chromosome	*K. pneumoniae* *Enterobacter* spp., *C. freundii*, *S. marcescens*, *Proteus* spp., *M. morganii*	
Carbapenemases	A	S	All β-lactams, aztreonam	KPC type GES SME, IMI, NMC	Plasmid Plasmid Chromosome	*Klebsiella* spp., *Enterobacter* spp., *S. marcescens*, other genera *K. pneumoniae* *Enterobacter* spp., *S. marcescens*	MDB, automated systems, Etest, disk diffusion with ETP, CHROMagar KPC, EDTA disk test, modified Hodge test, MER disk ± boronic acid, PCR
	B	R	All β-lactams	IMP, VIM	Plasmid or chromosome	*K. pneumoniae*, *S. marcescens*, *Enterobacter* spp., *Citrobacter* spp.	Etest (IMI ± EDTA), disk approximation (IMI disk and Tris/EDTA disk), modified Hodge test, PCR

[a]Abbreviations: S, susceptible; R, resistant, BMD, broth microdilution; TEM, from patient's name Temoneira; SHV, sulfhydryl reagent variable; CTX-M, active on cefotaxime, isolated in Munich; CMY, active on cephamycins; MOX, active on moxalactam; FOX, active on cefoxitin; DHA, discovered at Dhahran; KPC, *K. pneumoniae* carbapenemase; GES, Guiana-extended spectrum; SME, *S. marcescens* enzyme; IMI, imipenem-hydrolyzing β-lactamase; NMC, nor metalloenzyme carbapenemase; IMP, active on meropenem; VIM, Verona integron-encoded metallo-β-lactamase. Data are from references 110, 115, 135, 136, 140, and 141.

[b]Class A and C mediators are serine β-lactamases, and class B mediators are metallo-β-lactamases (named for serine or zinc, respectively, present at the active site involved in hydrolysis of the beta-lactam ring).

epidemiological studies. The disadvantage of a long turn-around time (usually 4 days) has been partially overcome by a rapid PFGE protocol that is suitable for most enteric bacteria as well as other common clinical strains (45).

ANTIMICROBIAL SUSCEPTIBILITY

Increasing resistance in members of the *Enterobacteriaceae* (Table 13) has culminated with the emergence of panresistant strains of *K. pneumoniae* for which there are no therapeutic options (37, 110, 135, 136). While *K. pneumoniae* presents the most serious threat, *K. oxytoca*, *S. marcescens*, *Enterobacter* spp., *Proteus* spp., and *Morganella* and *Citrobacter* spp. have all been reported to possess one or more Ambler Class A ESBLs or carbapenemases, Class C cephalosporinase, and/or class B metallo-β-lactamases. Frequently, plasmids encoding these enzymes also carry resistance genes for aminoglycosides, quinolones, and other antimicrobials (37, 102, 140). Although their clinical significance and the need to control intra- and interhospital transmission make detection of these enzymes a priority for the clinical laboratory, they are often unrecognized by routine susceptibility testing because of the difficulty in detecting these enzymes and the lack of standard techniques (110, 135, 136, 140). Both phenotypic and genotypic methods are available for detection of ESBLs, cephalosporinases, and carbapenemases, and while the latter tests are limited to large institutions and research laboratories, they identify specific genes and can detect low-level resistance missed by phenotypic tests. General antimicrobial susceptibility and specialized phenotypic testing procedures are discussed elsewhere in this *Manual* (chapters 67 to 70) and by Patel et al. (110) and Sundin (136).

ESBL-Producing *Enterobacteriaceae*

In addition to screening and confirmatory methods recommended by CLSI (28), a chromogenic agar, chromID ESBL (bioMerieux, Marcy l'Etoile, France), has been developed for detection of ESBLs. Several studies evaluating this medium report chromID ESBL sensitivity equal to or better than that obtained by automated or agar-based methods (39, 48, 119). The specificity for chromID ESBL was similar to that for the comparison methods in two studies (89% and 91%) but was only 11% in the third, causing those authors to recommend that suspected ESBL-producing isolates on this medium be verified with another test (39). The negative predictive value calculated in one study (>99%) indicated that this medium can be used as an effective tool to rule out ESBL-producing strains in clinical samples (119). chromID ESBL uses cefpodoxime as a substrate rather than ceftazidime or cefotaxime, which was noted to increase its sensitivity and was thought to be responsible for the greater recovery of CTX-M type ESBL-producing isolates in one of the studies (48, 119). Strains with hyperproducing AmpC (predominantly *Enterobacter* and *Citrobacter* spp.) and hyperproducing penicillinase (*K. oxytoca*) enzymes produced false positives (strains with correct colony color but ESBL negative on chromID ESBL) in all three studies from both the chromID ESBL agar and the comparison methods (39, 48, 119). In the two studies testing clinical samples, the recovery rate for ESBL-producing strains was 7% and 4%, respectively (48, 119). In addition to chromID ESBL media, Farber et al. (39) tested three Vitek 2 (bioMerieux, Durham, NC) panels and two Phoenix (Becton Dickinson, Sparks, MD) panels with their corresponding expert interpretation software for ESBL detection. Of the two Phoenix

panels, the NMIC/ID-70 panel slightly outperformed the best Vitek 2 panel result (AST-N041) with a sensitivity and specificity of 84% and 75% versus 84% and 50%, respectively. In another study comparing the Phoenix NMIC/ID-108 panel with the MicroScan (Siemens Healthcare Systems, West Sacramento, CA) Neg BP combo panel type 30, both systems did well in detecting ESBL-positive *K. pneumoniae* in clinical strains but MicroScan performed better with various *Enterobacteriaceae* challenge strains (130). When ESBL-producing strains are detected by automated systems, it is generally recommended that they be confirmed using a manual method (39, 130, 135).

Expanded-Spectrum Cephalosporin Resistance

The clinical significance of strains with chromosomal, inducible AmpC enzymes (transient high-level production induced only in the presence of a beta-lactam) is still unclear and the need for treatment controversial. However, the use of a beta-lactam in patients with strains exhibiting permanent AmpC hyperproduction (due to mutations in the regulatory genes that result in more efficient production of the enzyme) can result in treatment failure (135). The fact that AmpC genes are now plasmid mediated in a variety of *Enterobacteriaceae* adds to the need for laboratories to recognize AmpC-positive strains, as they are an even greater risk for transmission within the hospital. Their recognition is also complicated by the fact that reduced susceptibility to cefoxitin, which may be used as a screen for AmpC activity, may reflect a loss of permeability through the outer membranes as well. Incorrect reporting of a strain as AmpC positive may result in the unnecessary use of carbapenems and the concomitant risk of developing resistance to these drugs (136, 138). Nonetheless, intermediate or reduced susceptibility to cefoxitin is still a useful indicator of AmpC presence, signaling the need for further testing (136). Tan et al. (138) evaluated three methods for the detection of AmpC-producing strains of *Escherichia coli*, *Klebsiella*, and *Proteus* spp. This study found that the disk approximation test using imipenem, cefoxitin, and amoxicillin-clavulanic acid as inducing agents against ceftazidime had the least sensitivity (25%) when compared with PCR (94%), agar dilution using cefoxitin ± cloxacillin (90%), or a disk-based test using cefpodoxime or cefoxitin ± cloxacillin or boronic acid (an inhibitor of AmpC and KPC enzymes). In the disk-based inhibitor assay cefoxitin ± cloxacillin, using a zone increase cutoff of ≥4 mm, gave the best overall sensitivity (95%). For the induction test, imipenem performed the best of the agents tested. Overall AmpC activity was detected in 50% (127 of 255) of strains, and AmpC was found to be plasmid-borne in 94% of the 27 strains.

Carbapenem Resistance

Carbapenem resistance genes (which are defined in Table 13) may be plasmid-mediated Class A carbapenemases, most commonly the KPC (*K. pneumoniae* carbapenemase) types, Class A chromosomally encoded SME (*S. marcescens* enzyme), and IMI/NMC (imipenem-hydrolyzing β-lactamase/not metalloenzyme carbapenemase) types; Class B metallo-β-lactamases (MBL), primarily the IMP (active on meropenem) type found in Asia; and Class D OXA (oxacillin-hydrolyzing) carbapenemases (110, 136). Because carbapenem MICs, even when elevated, appear susceptible by CLSI breakpoints, carbapenem-resistant strains are difficult to detect. In testing for carbapenemases, the use of ertapenem as an indicator substrate appears to be more sensitive for the detection of KPCs than imipenem or meropenem (96, 110, 136). McGettigan et al. (96) screened 2,696 *Enterobacteriaceae* by using an ertapenem disk diffusion test or Vitek 2 GN-20 card and obtained equivalent results, detecting 85 ertapenem-intermediate or -resistant strains, of which 63 were KPC-positive *K. pneumoniae*. While all of the *K. pneumoniae* KPC-positive isolates were confirmed by the modified Hodge test and PCR, the four *Enterobacter* spp. isolates were found to be false positives. Anderson et al. (8) found that the broth microdilution test was more sensitive than disk diffusion, Etest, Vitek 2, and MicroScan assays for the detection of carbapenemase resistance regardless of the carbapenem used. Ertapenem was the most sensitive substrate for the disk test, Etest, and automated methods. While sensitive, ertapenem may be less specific than imipenem or meropenem because it detects resistance caused by mechanisms other than carbapenemases (8, 141). Tsakris et al. (141) detected KPC-producing *K. pneumoniae* with 100% sensitivity using disks with imipenem, meropenem, or cefepime alone and with 400 µg of boronic acid, although ertapenem gave false-positive results with five KPC-negative, AmpC-positive isolates. An elevated MIC (≥1 or 2 µg/ml) to meropenem or imipenem in automated assays or a zone of ≤19 mm with an imipenem disk can also be used to screen isolates for KPCs or MBLs (8, 110). Isolates should then be tested by a phenotypic method such as the modified Hodge assay (see chapter 70), which has been found to be 100% sensitive and specific for carbapenemases. Unlike an inhibitor test using a carbapenem or cefepime ± boronic acid, the modified Hodge assay cannot differentiate between KPCs and MBLs, information that is useful for infection control (110, 141). EDTA inhibition assays can also differentiate between KPC and MBL production; Etest markets a double-sided IP/IPI strip with imipenem on one end and imipenem-EDTA on the other end to detect MBLs (110). CHROMagar KPC (CHROMagar, Paris, France) is another product available for the detection of KPC-producing *K. pneumoniae*. When used on rectal swabs, its sensitivity and specificity relative to PCR were 100% and 98%, respectively, compared to 93% and 96% for MacConkey agar with 10-µg carbapenem disks versus PCR (124). Overall, 41 of the 122 (34%) swabs yielded KPC-producing *K. pneumoniae*.

Resistance in Miscellaneous *Enterobacteriaceae*

Strains of *P. mirabilis* are resistant to nitrofurantoin but susceptible to trimethoprim-sulfamethoxazole (SXT), ampicillin, amoxicillin, piperacillin, cephalosporins, aminoglycosides, and imipenem. Although most strains are susceptible to ciprofloxacin, resistance occurs with unrestricted use of the drug (108). *P. penneri* and *P. vulgaris* have a resistance profile similar to that of *Morganella*, although *P. penneri* is more resistant to penicillin than *P. vulgaris*. All three organisms are susceptible to broad-spectrum cephalosporins, cefoxitin, cefepime, aztreonam, aminoglycosides, and imipenem. They are resistant to piperacillin, amoxicillin, ampicillin, cefoperazone, cefuroxime, and cefazolin. *P. rettgeri* and *P. stuartii* are resistant to gentamicin and tobramycin but susceptible to amikacin. Urine isolates are susceptible to broad- and expanded-spectrum cephalosporins, ciprofloxacin, amoxicillin-clavulanic acid, imipenem, and SXT. *Providencia heimbachae*, although infrequently seen in humans, is resistant to tetracycline, most cephalosporins, gentamicin, and amikacin. Human isolates of *E. tarda* are susceptible to cephalosporins, aminoglycosides, imipenem, ciprofloxacin, aztreonam, and antibiotic-β-lactamase inhibitor combination agents (26). Isolates

from fish and fish ponds may be more resistant because of the antibiotics used prophylactically in fish farming. Most strains of *E. tarda* produce β-lactamases, even though they are susceptible to β-lactams. *P. shigelloides* is resistant to ampicillin, carbenicillin, piperacillin, and ticarcillin and is variably resistant to most aminoglycosides and tetracycline (71). Cephalosporins, quinolones, carbapenems, and SXT show good activity against *P. shigelloides*.

Susceptibility results of uncommonly seen species of *Klebsiella*, *Enterobacter*, and *Serratia* are similar to those of conventional species within these genera (44). Susceptibilities for other *Enterobacteriaceae* vary from isolate to isolate, so that no empirical guidelines are available for therapy prior to susceptibility testing of the suspected strain.

EVALUATION, INTREPRETATION, AND REPORTING OF RESULTS

When commercial systems identify species included in this chapter with a high level of accuracy (>90% probability), the identification is probably reliable. However, for organisms isolated from sterile sites that are identified with a probability of <90%, the isolate should be confirmed by conventional or molecular methods or sent to a reference laboratory using these techniques. In the interim, the isolate may be reported to the physician with a presumptive identification. Rare species that are identified with low probabilities should always be sent to a reference laboratory accompanied by a brief history.

An increasing number of patients are infected or colonized with *Enterobacteriaceae* possessing ESBLs and carbapenemases, and they serve as reservoirs for transmission of these enzymes within and between health care institutions. The ability to recognize these strains is critical not only for patient care but also to prevent the emergence of panresistant strains. Reliable, cost-effective methodologies for the detection and reporting of these enzymes that are manageable for all institutions regardless of size and capability are urgently needed. At the very least, all strains of *K. pneumoniae* should be tested for ESBLs, since automated testing methods seem to be reliable with this agent (39). Any strain of *Enterobacteriaceae* that has been shown by susceptibility testing to have an ESBL or AmpC cephalosporinase should be reported as resistant to all penicillins, expanded-spectrum cephalosporins, and aztreonam (136, 140). Data provided by a CDC database of PFGE patterns used to monitor KPC-producing strains isolated in the United States and other areas worldwide indicate that infection control (http://www.cdc.gov/ncidod/dhqp/gl_isolation.html) interventions will be necessary to halt the spread of these organisms (110).

REFERENCES

1. **Ajithkumar, B., V. P. Ajithkumar, R. Iriye, Y. Doi, and T. Sakai.** 2003. Spore-forming *Serratia marcescens* subsp. *sakuensis* subsp. nov. isolated from a domestic wastewater treatment plant. *Int. J. Syst. Evol. Microbiol.* **53:**253–258.
2. **Akhurst, R. J., N. E. Boemare, P. H. Janssen, M. M. Peel, D. A. Alfredson, and C. E. Beard.** 2004. Taxonomy of Australian clinical isolates of the genus *Photorhabdus* and proposal of *Photorhabdus asymbiotica* subsp. *asymbiotica* subsp. nov. and *P. asymbiotica* subsp. *australis* subsp. nov. *Int. J. Syst. Evol. Microbiol.* **54:**1301–1310.
3. **Albert, M. J., K. Alam, M. M. Islam, J. Montanaro, A. S. Rhaman, K. Haider, M. A. Hossain, A. K. Kibriyan, and S. Tzipori.** 1991. *Hafnia alvei*, a probable cause of diarrhea in humans. *Infect. Immun.* **59:**1507–1513.

4. **Albert, M. J., M. Ansaruzzaman, N. A. Bhuiyan, P. K. B. Neogi, and A. S. G. Faruque.** 1995. Characteristics of invasion of HEp-2 cells by *Providencia alcalifaciens*. *J. Med. Microbiol.* **42:**186–190.

5. **Aldova, E., O. Hausner, D. J. Brenner, D. Kocmoud, J. Schindler, B. Potuznikova, and P. Petras.** 1988. *Pragia fontium* gen. nov., sp. nov. of the family *Enterobacteriaceae*, isolated from water. *Int. J. Syst. Bacteriol.* **38:**183–189.

6. **Alves, M. S., R. C. da Silva Dias, A. C. Dias de Castro, L. W. Riley, and B. M. Moreira.** 2006. Identification of clinical isolates of indole-positive and indole-negative *Klebsiella* spp. *J. Clin. Microbiol.* **44:**3640–3646.

7. **Anderson, D. J., H. Richet, L. F. Chen, D. W. Spelman, Y.-J. Hung, A. T. Juang, D. J. Sexton, and D. Raoult.** 2008. Seasonal variation in *Klebsiella pneumoniae* bloodstream infection on 4 continents. *J. Infect. Dis.* **197:**752–756.

8. **Anderson, K. F., D. R. Lonsway, J. K. Rasheed, J. Biddle, B. Jensen, L. K. McDougal, R. B. Carey, A. Thompson, S. Stocker, B. Limbago, and J. B. Patel.** 2007. Evaluation of methods to identify the *Klebsiella pneumoniae* carbapenemase in *Enterobacteriaceae*. *J. Clin. Microbiol.* **45:**2723–2725.

9. **Aucken, H. M., and T. L. Pitt.** 1998. Antibiotic resistance and putative virulence factors of *Serratia marcescens* with respect to O and K serotypes. *J. Med. Microbiol.* **47:**1105–1113.

10. **Baron, E. J.** 2001. Rapid identification of bacteria and yeast: summary of a national committee for clinical laboratory standards proposed guidelines. *Clin. Infect. Dis.* **33:**220–225.

11. **Baron, E. J., and S. D. Allen.** 1993. Should clinical laboratories adopt new taxonomic changes? If so when? *Clin. Infect. Dis.* **16**(Suppl. 4)**:**S449–S450.

12. **Belas, R.** 1992. The swarming phenomenon of *Proteus mirabilis*. *ASM News* **58:**15–21.

13. **Bennett, A. R., S. MacPhee, R. Betts, and D. Post.** 1999. Use of pyrrolidonyl peptidase to distinguish *Citrobacter* from *Salmonella*. *Lett. Appl. Microbiol.* **28:**175–178.

14. **Bhadra, B., P. Roy, and R. Chakraborty.** 2005. *Serratia ureilytica* sp. nov., a novel urea utilizing species. *Int. J. Syst. Evol. Microbiol.* **55:**2155–2158.

15. **Bouvet, O. M. M., P. A. D. Grimont, C. Richard, E. Aldova, O. Hausner, and M. Gabrhelova.** 1985. *Budvicia aquatica* gen. nov.: a hydrogen sulfide-producing member of the *Enterobacteriaceae*. *Int. J. Syst. Bacteriol.* **35:**60–64.

16. **Brenner, D. J., C. M. O'Hara, P. A. D. Grimont, J. M. Janda, E. Falsen, E. Aldova, E. Ageron, J. Schindler, S. L. Abbott, and A. G. Steigerwalt.** 1999. Biochemical identification of *Citrobacter* species defined by DNA hybridization and description of *Citrobacter gillenii* sp. nov. (formerly *Citrobacter* genomospecies 10) and *Citrobacter murliniae* sp. nov. (formerly *Citrobacter* genomospecies 11). *J. Clin. Microbiol.* **37:**2619–2624.

17. **Brenner, D. J., H. E. Muller, A. G. Steigerwalt, A. M. Whitney, C. M. O'Hara, and P. Kampfer.** 1998. Two new *Rahnella* genomospecies that cannot be phenotypically differentiated from *Rahnella aquatilis*. *Int. J. Syst. Bacteriol.* **48:**141–149.

18. **Brenner, D. J., P. A. D. Grimont, A. G. Steigerwalt, G. R. Fanning, E. Ageron, and C. F. Riddle.** 1993. Classification of citrobacteria by DNA hybridization: designation of *Citrobacter farmeri* sp. nov., *Citrobacter youngae* sp. nov., *Citrobacter braakii* sp. nov., *Citrobacter werkmanii* sp. nov., *Citrobacter sedlakii* sp. nov., and three unnamed *Citrobacter* genomospecies. *Int. J. Syst. Bacteriol.* **43:**645–658.

19. **Brisse, S., C. Fevre, V. Passet, S. Issenhuth-Jeanjean, R. Tournebize, L. Diancourt, and P. Grimont.** 2009. Virulent clones of *Klebsiella pneumoniae*: identification and evolutionary scenario based on genomic and phenotypic characterization. *PloS ONE* **4**(3)**:**e4982. http://www.plos.org.

20. **Carricajo, A., S. Boiste, J. Thore, G. Aubert, Y. Gille, and A. M. Freydiere.** 1999. Comparative evaluation of five chromogenic media for detection, enumeration and identification of urinary tract pathogens. *Eur. J. Clin. Microbiol. Infect. Dis.* **18:**796–803.

21. **Carroll, K. C., B. D. Glanz, A. P. Borek, C. Burger, H. S. Bhally, S. Henciak, and D. Flayhart.** 2006. Evaluation of the BD Phoenix Automated Microbiology System for identification and antimicrobial susceptibility testing of *Enterobacteriaceae*. *J. Clin. Microbiol.* **44:**3506–3509.

22. **Carter, J., S. Hutton, K. S. Sriprakash, D. J. Kemp, G. Lum, J. Savage, and F. J. Bowden.** 1997. Culture of the causative organism of donovanosis (*Calymmatobacterium granulomatis*) in HEp-2 cells. *J. Clin. Microbiol.* **35:**2915–2917.

23. **Carter, J. E., and T. N. Evans.** 2005. Clinically significant *Kluyvera* infections. *Am. J. Clin. Pathol.* **123:**334–338.

24. **Carter, J. S., F. J. Bowden, I. Bastain, G. M. Myers, K. S. Sriprakash, and D. J. Kemp.** 1999. Phylogenetic evidence for reclassification of *Calymmatobacterium granulomatis* as *Klebsiella granulomatis* comb. nov. *Int. J. Syst. Bacteriol.* **49:**1695–1700.

25. **Chida, T., N. Okamura, K. Ohtani, Y. Yoshida, E. Arakawa, and H. Watanabe.** 2000. The complete DNA sequence of the O antigen gene region of *Plesiomonas shigelloides* serotype O17 which is identical to *Shigella sonnei* form I antigen. *Microbiol. Immunol.* **44:**161–172.

26. **Clark, R. B., P. D. Lister, and J. M. Janda.** 1991. In vitro susceptibilities of *Edwardsiella tarda* to 22 antibiotics and antibiotic-β-lactamase-inhibitor agents. *Diagn. Microbiol. Infect. Dis.* **14:**173–175.

27. **CLSI.** 2008. *Interpretive Criteria for Identification of Bacteria and Fungi by DNA Target Sequencing; Approved Guidelines.* CLSI Document MM18-A. Clinical and Laboratory Standards Institute, Wayne, PA.

28. **CLSI.** 2009. *Performance Standards for Antimicrobial Susceptibility Testing; Nineteenth Informational Supplement.* CLSI Document M100-S19. Clinical and Laboratory Standards Institute, Wayne, PA.

29. **Crandall, C., S. L. Abbott, Y. Q. Zhao, W. Probert, and J. M. Janda.** 2005. Isolation of toxigenic *Hafnia alvei* from a probable case of hemolytic uremic syndrome. *Infection* **34:**227–229.

30. **Cruz, A. T., A. C. Cazacu, and C. H. Allen.** 2007. *Pantoea agglomerans*, a plant pathogen causing human disease. *J. Clin. Microbiol.* **45:**1989–1992.

31. **Dalamaga, M., M. Pantelaki, K. Marmaniolas, K. Daskalopoulou, and I. Migdalis.** 2009. Isolation of *Leclercia adecarboxylata* from blood and burn wound after a hydrofluoric acid chemical injury. *Burns* **35:**443–445.

32. **De Baere, T., G. Wauters, P. Kampfer, C. Labit, G. Claeys, G. Verschraegen, and M. Vaneechoutte.** 2002. Isolation of *Buttiauxella gaviniae* from a spinal cord patient with urinary bladder pathology. *J. Clin. Microbiol.* **40:**3867–3870.

33. **De Baere, T., R. Verhelst, C. Labit, G. Verschraegen, G. Wauters, G. Claeys, and M. Vaneechoutte.** 2004. Bacteremic infection with *Pantoea ananatis*. *J. Clin. Microbiol.* **42:**4393–4395.

34. **Delmas, J., F. Breysse, G. Devulder, P.-P. Flandrois, and M. Chomarat.** 2006. Rapid identification of *Enterobacteriaceae* by sequencing DNA gyrase subunit B encoding gene. *Diagn. Microbiol. Infect. Dis.* **55:**263–268.

35. **de Pontual, L., P. Ovetchkine, D. Rodriquez, A. Grant, A. Puel, J. Bustamante, S. Plancoulaine, L. Yona, P.-Y. Lienhart, D. Dehesdin, M. Huerre, R. Tournebize, P. Sansonnetti, L. Abel, and L. L. Casanova.** 2008. Rhinoscleroma: a French national retrospective study of epidemiological and clinical features. *Clin. Infect. Dis.* **47:**1396–1402.

36. **Drancourt, M., C. Bollet, A. Carta, and P. Rousselier.** 2001. Phylogenetic analyses of *Klebsiella* species delineate *Klebsiella* and *Raoultella* gen. nov., with description of *Raoultella ornithinolytica* comb. nov. *Int. J. Syst. Evol. Microbiol.* **51:**925–932.

37. **Eleman, A., J. Rahimian, and W. Mandell.** 2009. Infection with panresistant *Klebsiella pneumoniae*: a report of 2 cases and brief review of the literature. *Clin. Infect. Dis.* **49:**271–274.

38. **Emborg, J., P. Dalgaard, and P. Ahrens.** 2006. *Morganella psychrotolerans* sp. nov., a histamine-producing bacterium isolated from various seafoods. *Int. J. Syst. Evol. Microbiol.* **56:**2473–2479.

39. **Farber, J., K.-A. Moder, F. Layer, I. Tammer, W. Konig, and B. Konig.** 2008. Extended-spectrum beta-lactamase detection with different panels for automated susceptibility testing and with a chromogenic medium. *J. Clin. Microbiol.* **46:**3721–3727.

40. **Farmer, J. J., III, G. R. Fanning, G. P. Huntley-Carter, B. Holmes, F. W. Hickman, C. Richard, and D. J. Brenner.** 1981. *Kluyvera,* a new (redefined) genus in the family *Enterobacteriaceae:* identification of *Kluyvera ascorbata* sp. nov. and *Kluyvera cryocrescens* sp. nov. in clinical specimens. *J. Clin. Microbiol.* **13:**919–933.

41. **Farmer, J. J., III, J. H. Jorgeson, P. A. D. Grimont, R. J. Akhurst, G. O. Poinar, E. Ageron, G. V. Pierce, and J. A. Smith.** 1989. *Xenorhabdus luminescens* (DNA hybridization group 5) from human clinical specimens. *J. Clin. Microbiol.* **27:**1594–1600.

42. **Fedler, K. A., D. J. Biedenbach, and R. N. Jones.** 2006. Assessment of pathogen frequency and resistance patterns among pediatric isolates: report from the 2004 SENTRY Antimicrobial Surveillance Program on 3 continents. *Diagn. Microbiol. Infect. Dis.* **56:**427–436.

43. **Fischer-LeSaux, M., V. Viallard, B. Brunel, P. Normand, and N. Boemare.** 1999. Polyphasic classification of the genus *Photorhabdus* and proposal of new taxa: *P. luminescens* subsp. *luminescens* subsp. nov., *P. luminescens* subsp. *akhurstii* subsp. nov., *P. luminescens* subsp. *laumondii* subsp. nov., *P. temperata* sp. nov., and *P. asymbiotica* sp. nov. *Int. J. Syst. Bacteriol.* **49:**1645–1656.

44. **Freney, J., M. O. Husson, F. Gavini, S. Madier, A. Martra, D. Izard, H. Leclerc, and J. Fleurette.** 1988. Susceptibilities to antibiotics and antiseptics of new species of the family *Enterobacteriaceae.* *Antimicrob. Agents Chemother.* **32:**873–876.

45. **Gautom, R. K.** 1997. Rapid pulsed-field gel electrophoresis protocol for typing of *Escherichia coli* O157:H7 and other gram-negative organisms in 1 day. *J. Clin. Microbiol.* **35:**2977–2980.

46. **Gavini, E., J. Mergaert, A. Beji, C. Mielcarek, D. Izard, K. Kersters, and J. De Ley.** 1989. Transfer of *Enterobacter agglomerans* (Beijerinck 1988) Ewing and Fife 1972 to *Pantoea* gen. nov. as *Pantoea agglomerans* comb. nov. and description of *Pantoea dispersa* sp. nov. *Int. J. Syst. Bacteriol.* **39:**337–345.

47. **Gevers, D., F. M. Cohan, J. G. Lawrence, B. G. Spratt, T. Coenye, E. J. Feil, E. Stackebrandt, Y. Van de Peer, P. Vandamne, F. L. Thompson, and J. Swings.** 2005. Re-evaluating prokaryotic species. *Nat. Rev. Microbiol.* **3:**733–739.

48. **Glupczynski, Y., C. Berhin, C. Bauraing, and P. Bogaerts.** 2007. Evaluation of a new selective chromogenic agar medium for detection of extended-spectrum β-lactamase-producing *Enterobacteriaceae.* *J. Clin. Microbiol.* **45:**501–505.

49. **Green, N. M., R. Tran, and J. M. Janda.** 2009. *Klebsiella* and gastrointestinal syndromes with particular emphasis on *Klebsiella oxytoca* antibiotic-associated colitis. *Clin. Microbiol. Newsl.* **31:**111–116.

50. **Grimont, F., and P. A. D. Grimont.** 1981. The genus *Serratia,* p. 2822–2848. *In* M. P. Starr, H. Stolp, H. G. Trüper, and H. G. Schlegel (ed.), *The Prokaryotes: a Handbook on Habitats, Isolation, and Identification of Bacteria.* Springer-Verlag, Berlin, Germany.

51. **Grimont, F., and P. A. D. Grimont.** 1991. The genus *Enterobacter,* p. 2797–2815. *In* A. Balows, H. G. Truper, M. Dworkin, W. Harder, K.-H. Schleifer (ed.), *The Prokaryotes: a Handbook on the Biology of Bacteria: Ecophysiology, Isolation, Identification, Applications,* 2nd ed. Springer-Verlag, Berlin, Germany.

52. **Grimont, F., P. A. D. Grimont, and C. Richard.** 1991. The genus *Klebsiella,* p. 2775–2796. *In* M. P. Starr, H. Stolp, H. G. Trüper, A. Balows, and H. G. Schlegel (ed.), *The Prokaryotes: a Handbook on the Biology of Bacteria: Ecophysiology, Isolation, Identification, Applications.* Springer-Verlag, Berlin, Germany.

53. **Grimont, P. A. D., F. Grimont, C. Richard, and R. Sakazaki.** 1980. *Edwardsiella hoshinae,* a new species of *Enterobacteriaceae.* *Curr. Microbiol.* **4:**347–351.

54. **Grimont, P. A. D., F. Grimont, J. J. Farmer III, and M. A. Asbury.** 1981. *Cedecea davisae* gen. nov., sp. nov., new *Enterobacteriaceae* from clinical specimens. *Int. J. Syst. Bacteriol.* **31:**317–326.

55. **Grimont, P. A. D., J. J. Farmer III, F. Grimont, M. A. Asbury, D. J. Brenner, and C. Deval.** 1983. *Ewingella americana*

56. gen. nov., sp. nov., a new *Enterobacteriaceae* isolated from clinical specimens. *Ann. Microbiol.* (Paris) **134A:**39–52.

56. **Hart, C. A., and S. K. Rao.** 1999. Donovanosis. *J. Med. Microbiol.* **48:**707–709.

57. **Hawke, J. P., A. C. McWhorter, A. G. Steigerwalt, and D. J. Brenner.** 1981. *Edwardsiella ictaluri* sp. nov., the causative agent of enteric septicemia of catfish. *Int. J. Syst. Bacteriol.* **31:**396–400.

58. **Hess, B., A. Burchett, and M. K. Huntington.** 2008. *Leclercia adecarboxylata* in an immunocompetent patient. *J. Med. Microbiol.* **57:**896–898.

59. **Hickman-Brenner, F. W., G. P. Huntley-Carter, Y. Saitoh, A. G. Steigerwalt, J. J. Farmer III, and D. J. Brenner.** 1984. *Moellerella wisconsensis,* a new genus and species of *Enterobacteriaceae* found in human stool specimens. *J. Clin. Microbiol.* **19:**460–463.

60. **Hickman-Brenner, F. W., M. P. Vohra, G. P. Huntley-Carter, G. R. Fanning, V. A. Lowery III, D. J. Brenner, and J. J. Farmer III.** 1985. *Leminorella,* a new genus of *Enterobacteriaceae:* identification of *Leminorella grimontii* sp. nov. and *Leminorella richardii* sp. nov. found in clinical specimens. *J. Clin. Microbiol.* **21:**234–239.

61. **Hidron, A. I., J. R. Edwards, J. Patel, T. C. Horan, D. M. Sievert, D. A. Pollack, S. K. Fridkin for the National Healthcare Safety Network Team and Participating National Healthcare Safety Network Facilities.** 2008. Antimicrobial-resistant pathogens associated with healthcare-associated infections: annual summary of data reported to the National Healthcare Safety Network at the Centers for Disease Control and Prevention, 2006–2007. *Infect. Control Hosp. Epidemiol.* **29:**996–1011.

62. **Hoffmann, H., and A. Roggenkamp.** 2003. Population genetics of the nomenspecies *Enterobacter cloacae.* *Appl. Environ. Microbiol.* **69:**5306–5318.

63. **Hoffmann, H., S. Stindl, W. Ludwig, A. Stumpf, A. Mehlen, D. Monget, D. Pierard, S. Ziesing, J. Heesemann, A. Roggenkamp, and K. H. Schleifer.** 2005. *Enterobacter hormaechei* subsp. *oharae* subsp. nov., *E. hormaechei* subsp. *hormaechei* comb. nov., and *E. hormaechei* subsp. *steigerwaltii* subsp. nov., three new subspecies of clinical importance. *J. Clin. Microbiol.* **43:**3297–3303.

64. **Hoffmann, H., S. Stindl, W. Ludwig, A. Stumpf, A. Mehlen, J. Heesemann, D. Monget, K. H. Schleifer, and A. Roggenkamp.** 2005. Reassignment of *Enterobacter dissolvens* to *Enterobacter cloacae* as *E. cloacae* subspecies *dissolvens* comb. nov. and emended description of *Enterobacter asburiae* and *Enterobacter kobei.* *Syst. Appl. Microbiol.* **28:**196–205.

65. **Hoffmann, H., S. Stindl, A. Stumpf, A. Mehlen, D. Monget, J. Heesemann, K. H. Schleifer, and A. Roggenkamp.** 2005. Description of *Enterobacter ludwigii* sp. nov., a novel *Enterobacter* species of clinical relevance. *Syst. Appl. Microbiol.* **28:**206–212.

66. **Hollis, D. G., F. W. Hickman, G. R. Fanning, J. J. Farmer III, R. E. Weaver, and D. J. Brenner.** 1981. *Tatumella ptyseos* gen. nov., sp. nov., a member of the family *Enterobacteriaceae* found in clinical specimens. *J. Clin. Microbiol.* **14:**79–88.

67. **Hume, E. B. H., M. D. P. Willcox, D. F. Sweeney, and B. A. Holden.** 1996. An examination of the clonal variants of *Serratia marcescens* that infect the eye during contact lens wear. *J. Med. Microbiol.* **45:**127–132.

68. **Inoue, K., K. Sugiyama, Y. Kosako, R. Sakazaki, and S. Yamai.** 2000. *Enterobacter cowanii* sp. nov., a new species of the family *Enterobacteriaceae.* *Curr. Microbiol.* **41:**417–420.

69. **Iversen, C., N. Mullane, B. McCardell, B. D. Tall, A. Lehner, S. Fanning, R. Stephan, and H. Joosten.** 2008. *Cronobacter* gen. nov., a new genus to accommodate the biogroups of *Enterobacter sakazakii,* and proposal of *Cronobacter sakazakii* gen. nov., comb. nov., *Cronobacter malonaticus* sp, nov., *Cronobacter turicensis* sp. nov., *Cronobacter muytjensii* sp. nov., *Cronobacter dublinensis* sp. nov., *Cronobacter* genomospecies 1, and of three subspecies, *Cronobacter dublinensis* subsp. *dublinensis* subsp. nov., *Cronobacter dublinensis* subsp. *lausannensis* subsp. nov., and *Cronobacter dublinensis* subsp. *lactaridi* subsp. nov. *Int J. Syst. Evol. Bacteriol.* **58:**1442–1447.

70. **Jagger, T. D.** 2000. *Plesiomonas shigelloides*—a veterinary perspective. *Infect. Dis. Rev.* **2:**199–210.

71. **Janda, J. M.** 2001. *Aeromonas* and *Plesiomonas*, p. 1237–1270. In M. Sussman (ed.), *Molecular Medical Microbiology*, vol. 2. Academic Press, Ltd., London, United Kingdom.

72. **Janda, J. M.** 2006. New members of the family *Enterobacteriaceae*, p. 5–40. In M. Dworkin, S. Falkow, E. Rosenberg, K.-H. Schleifer, and E. Stackebrandt (ed.), *The Prokaryotes: a Handbook on the Biology of Bacteria*, 3rd ed. Springer-Verlag, New York, NY.

73. **Janda, J. M., and S. L. Abbott.** 2005. *The Enterobacteria*, 2nd ed. ASM Press, Washington, DC.

74. **Janda, J. M., and S. L. Abbott.** 2006. The genus *Hafnia*: from soup to nuts. *Clin. Microbiol. Rev.* **19:**12–18.

75. **Janda, J. M., and S. L. Abbott.** 2007. 16S rRNA gene sequencing for bacterial identification in the diagnostic laboratory: pluses, perils, and pitfalls. *J. Clin. Microbiol.* **45:**2761–2764.

76. **Janda, J. M., S. L. Abbott, D. Woodward, and S. Khashe.** 1998. Invasion of HEp-2 and other eukaryotic cell lines by *Providenciae*: further evidence supporting the role of *Providencia alcalifaciens* in bacterial gastroenteritis. *Curr. Microbiol.* **37:**159–165.

77. **Janda, J. M., S. L. Abbott, and J. G. Morris.** 1995. *Aeromonas, Plesiomonas* and *Edwardsiella*, p. 905–917. In M. J. Blaser, P. D. Smith, J. I. Ravdin, H. B. Greenberg, and R. L. Guerrant (ed.), *Infections of the Gastrointestinal Tract*. Raven Press, Ltd. New York, NY.

78. **Janda, J. M., S. L. Abbott, S. Bystrom, and W. S. Probert.** 2005. Identification of two distinct hybridization groups in the genus *Hafnia* by 16S rRNA gene sequencing and phenotypic methods. *J. Clin. Microbiol.* **43:**3320–3323.

79. **Johnson, A. S., C. Tarr, B. H. Brown, Jr., K. M. Birkhead, and J. J. Farmer III.** 2005. First case of septicemia due to Enteric Group 58 (*Enterobacteriaceae*) and its designation as *Averyella dalhousiensis* gen. nov., sp. nov. based on strains from 20 additional cases. *J. Clin. Microbiol.* **43:**5195–5201.

80. **Juneja, P., and B. P. Lazzaro.** 2009. *Providencia sneebia* sp. nov. and *Providencia burhodogranariea* sp. nov., isolated from wild *Drosophila melanogaster*. *Int. J. Syst. Evol. Microbiol.* **59:**1108–1111.

81. **Kado, C. I.** July 2000. *Erwinia* and related genera. In M. Dworkin, S. Falkow, E. Rosenberg, K.-H. Schleifer, and E. Stackebrandt (ed.), *The Prokaryotes: an Evolving Electronic Resource for the Microbiological Community*, 3rd ed., latest update release 3.2. Springer-Verlag, New York, NY. http://141.150.157.117:8080/prokPUB/index.htm.

82. **Kageyama, B., M. Nakae, S. Yagi, and T. Sonoyama.** 1992. *Pantoea punctata* sp. nov., *Pantoea citrea* sp. nov., and *Pantoea terrea* sp. nov. isolated from fruit and soil samples. *Int. J. Syst. Bacteriol.* **42:**203–210.

83. **Kampfer, P., S. Ruppel, and R. Remus.** 2005. *Enterobacter radicincitans* sp. nov., a plant growth promoting species of the family *Enterobacteriaceae*. *Syst. Appl. Microbiol.* **28:**213–221.

84. **Khan, A. M., A. S. G. Faruque, M. S. Hossain, S. Sattar, G. J. Fuchs, and M. A. Salam.** 2004. *Plesiomonas shigelloides*-associated diarrhoea in Bangladeshi children: a hospital-based surveillance study. *J. Trop. Pediatr.* **50:**354–356.

85. **Kharsany, A. B. M., A. A. Hoosens, P. Kiepela, P. Kirby, and A. W. Sturm.** 1999. Phylogenetic analysis of *Calymmatobacterium granulomatis* based on rRNA gene sequences. *J. Med. Microbiol.* **48:**841–847.

86. **Khashe, S., D. J. Scales, S. L. Abbott, and J. M. Janda.** 2001. Non-invasive *Providencia alcalifaciens* strains fail to attach to HEp-2 cells. *Curr. Microbiol.* **43:**414–417.

87. **Kosako, Y., K. Tamura, R. Sakazaki, and K. Miki.** 1996. *Enterobacter kobei* sp. nov., a new species of the family *Enterobacteriaceae* resembling *Enterobacter cloacae*. *Curr. Microbiol.* **33:**261–265.

88. **Kosako, Y., R. Sakazaki, and E. Yoshizaki.** 1984. *Yokenella regensburgei* gen. nov., sp. nov.: a new genus and species in the family *Enterobacteriaceae*. *Jpn. J. Med. Sci. Biol.* **37:**117–124.

89. **Laupland, K. B., M. D. Parkins, T. Ross, and J. D. D. Pitout.** 2007. Population-based laboratory surveillance for tribe Proteeae isolates in a large Canadian health region. *Clin. Microbiol. Infect.* **13:**683–688.

90. **Lavigne, J.-P., C. Defez, N. Bouziges, A. Mahamat, and A. Sotto.** 2007. Clinical and molecular epidemiology of multidrug-resistant *Citrobacter* spp. infections in a French university hospital. *Eur. J. Clin. Microbiol. Infect Dis.* **26:**439–441.

91. **Lederman, E. R., and N. F. Crum.** 2005. Pyogenic liver abscess with a focus on *Klebsiella pneumoniae* as a primary pathogen: an emerging disease with unique clinical characteristics. *Am. J. Gastroenterol.* **100:**322–331.

92. **Li, X., D. Zhang, F. Chen, J. Ma, Y. Dong, and L. Zhang.** 2004. *Klebsiella singaporensis* sp. nov., a novel isomaltulose-producing bacterium. *Int. J. Syst. Evol. Microbiol.* **54:**2131–2136.

93. **Lin, F.-Y. C., W. F. Devoe, and C. Morrison, J. Libonati, P. Powers, R. J. Gross, B. Rowe, E. Israel, and J. G. Morris.** 1987. Outbreak of neonatal *Citrobacter diversus* meninigitis in a suburban hospital. *Pediatr. Infect. Dis. J.* **6:**50–55.

94. **Lockhart, S. R., M. A. Abramson, S. E. Beekman, G. Gallagher, S. Riedel, D. J. Diekma, J. P. Quinn, and G. V. Doern.** 2007. Antimicrobial resistance among gram-negative bacilli causing infections in intensive care unit patients in the United States between 1993 and 2004. *J. Clin. Microbiol.* **45:**3352–3359.

95. **Luperchio, S. A., J. V. Newman, C. A. Dangler, M. D. Schrenzel, D. J. Brenner, A. G. Steigerwalt, and D. B. Schauer.** 2000. *Citrobacter rodentium*, the causative agent of transmissible murine colonic hyperplasia, exhibits clonality: synonymy of *C. rodentium* and mouse-pathogenic *Escherichia coli*. *J. Clin. Microbiol.* **38:**4343–4350.

96. **McGettigan, S. E., K. Andreacchio, and P. H. Edelstein.** 2009. Specificity of ertapenem susceptibility screening for detection of *Klebsiella pneumoniae* carbapenemases. *J. Clin. Microbiol.* **47:**785–786.

97. **McWhorter, A. C., R. L. Haddock, F. A. Nocon, A. G. Steigerwalt, D. J. Brenner, S. Aleksic, J. Bockmuhl, and J. J. Farmer III.** 1991. *Trabulsiella guamensis*, a new genus and species of the family *Enterobacteriaceae* that resembles *Salmonella* subgroups 4 and 5. *J. Clin. Microbiol.* **29:**1480–1485.

98. **Montgomerie, J. Z.** 1979. Epidemiology of *Klebsiella* and hospital-associated infections. *Rev. Infect. Dis.* **1:**736–753.

99. **Muller, H. E., C. M. O'Hara, G. R. Fanning, F. W. Hickman-Brenner, J. M. Swenson, and D. J. Brenner.** 1986. *Providencia heimbachae*, a new species of *Enterobacteriaceae* isolated from animals. *Int. J. Syst. Bacteriol.* **36:**252–256.

100. **Muller, H. E., D. J. Brenner, G. R. Fanning, P. A. D. Grimont, and P. Kampfer.** 1996. Emended description of *Buttiauxella agrestis* with recognition of six new species of *Buttiauxella* and two new species of *Kluyvera*: *Buttiauxella ferragutiae* sp. nov., *Buttiauxella gaviniae* sp. nov., *Buttiauxella brennerae* sp. nov., *Buttiauxella izardii* sp. nov., *Buttiauxella noackiae* sp. nov., *Buttiauxella warmboldiae* sp. nov., *Kluyvera cochleae* sp. nov., and *Kluyvera georgiana* sp. nov. *Int J. Syst. Bacteriol.* **46:**50–63.

101. **Nhung, P. H., K. Ohsuku, N. Mishima, M. Noda, M. M. Shah, X. Sun, M. Hayashi, and T. Ezaki.** 2007. Phylogeny and species identification of the family *Enterobacteriaceae* based on *dnaJ* sequences. *Diagn. Microbiol. Infect. Dis.* **58:**153–161.

102. **Nordmann, P., G. Cuzon, and T. Naas.** 2009. The real threat of *Klebsiella pneumoniae* carbapenemase-producing bacteria. *Lancet Infect. Dis.* **9:**228–236.

103. **O'Hara, C. M.** 2005. Manual and automated instrumentation for identification of *Enterobacteriaceae* and other aerobic gram-negative bacilli. *Clin. Microbiol. Rev.* **18:**147–162.

104. **O'Hara, C. M., A. G. Steigerwalt, B. C. Hill, J. J. Farmer III, G. R. Fanning, and D. J. Brenner.** 1989. *Enterobacter hormaechei*, a new species of the family *Enterobacteriaceae* formerly known as enteric group 75. *J. Clin. Microbiol.* **27:**2046–2049.

105. O'Hara, C. M., A. G. Steigerwalt, B. C. Hill, J. M. Miller, and D. J. Brenner. 1998. First report of a human isolate of *Erwinia persicinus*. *J. Clin. Microbiol.* **36**:248–250.

106. O'Hara, C. M., A. G. Steigerwalt, D. Green, M. McDowell, B. C. Hill, D. J. Brenner, and J. M. Miller. 1999. Isolation of *Providencia heimbachae* from human feces. *J. Clin. Microbiol.* **37**:3048–3050.

107. O'Hara, C. M., F. W. Brenner, A. G. Steigerwalt, B. C. Hill, B. Holmes, P. A. D. Grimont, P. M. Hawkey, J. L. Penner, J. M. Miller, and D. J. Brenner. 2000. Classification of *Proteus vulgaris* biogroup 3 with recognition of *Proteus hauseri* sp. nov., nom. rev. and unnamed *Proteus* genomospecies 4, 5, and 6. *Int. J. Syst. Evol. Microbiol.* **50**:1869–1875.

108. O'Hara, C. M., F. W. Brenner, and J. M. Miller. 2000. Classification, identification, and clinical significance of *Proteus, Providencia*, and *Morganella*. *Clin. Microbiol. Rev.* **13**:534–546.

109. Ohkusu, K. 2000. Cost-effective and rapid presumptive identification of gram-negative bacilli in routine urine, pus, and stool cultures: evaluation of the use of CHROMagar orientation medium in conjunction with simple biochemical tests. *J. Clin. Microbiol.* **38**:4586–4592.

110. Patel, J. B., J. K. Rasheed, and B. Kitchel. 2009. Carbapenemases in *Enterobacteriaceae*: activity, epidemiology, and laboratory detection. *Clin. Microbiol. Newsl.* **31**:55–62.

111. Pavan, M. E., R. J. Franco, J. M. Rodriguez, P. Gadaleta, S. L. Abbott, J. M. Janda, and J. Zorzopulos. 2005. Phylogenetic relationships of the genus *Kluyvera*: transfer of *Enterobacter intermedius* Izard et al. 1980 to the genus *Kluyvera* as *Kluyvera intermedia* comb. nov. and reclassification of *Kluyvera cochleae* as a later synonym of *K. intermedia*. *Int. J. Syst. Evol. Microbiol.* **55**:437–442.

112. Peng, G., W. Zhang, H. Luo, H. Kie, W. Lai, and Z. Tan. 2009. *Enterobacter oryzae*. sp. nov., a nitrogen-fixing bacterium isolated from the wild rice species *Oryza latifolia*. *Int. J. Syst. Evol. Microbiol.* **59**:1650–1655.

113. Podschun, R., A. Fischer, and U. Ullman. 2000. Expression of putative virulence factors by clinical isolates of *Klebsiella planticola*. *J. Med. Microbiol.* **49**:115–119.

114. Polster, M., and M. Svobodova. 1964. Production of reddish-brown pigment from dl-tryptophan by Enterobacteria of the Proteus-Providencia group. *Experimentia* **20**:637–638.

115. Queenan, A. M., and K. Bush. 2007. Carbapenemases: the versatile β-lactamases. *Clin. Microbiol. Rev.* **20**:440–458.

116. Quevedo, S. M., M. D. Martin, and A. C. Velasco. 2006. *Moellerella wisconsensis*: a hidden enteric pathogen? *Clin. Microbiol. Newsl.* **28**:142–143.

117. Rahimian, J., T. Wilson, V. Oram, and R. S. Holzman. 2004. Pyogenic liver abscess: recent trends in etiology and mortality. *Clin. Infect. Dis.* **39**:1654–1659.

118. Ramos, A., and D. Damaso. 2000. Extraintestinal infection due to *Hafnia alvei*. *Eur. J. Microbiol. Infect. Dis.* **19**:708–710.

119. Reglier-Poupet, H., T. Naas, A. Carrer, A. Cady, J.-M. Adam, N. Fortineau, C. Poyart, and P. Nordmann. 2008. Performance of chromID ESBL, a chromogenic medium for detection of *Enterobacteriaceae* producing extended-spectrum β-lactamases. *J. Med. Microbiol.* **57**:310–315.

120. Ridell, J., A. Siitonen, L. Paulin, L. Mattila, H. Korkeala, and M. J. Albert. 1994. *Hafnia alvei* in stool specimens from patients with diarrhea and healthy controls. *J. Clin. Microbiol.* **32**:2335–2337.

121. Rosenblueth, M., L. Martinez, J. Silva, and E. Martinez-Romero. 2004. *Klebsiella variicola*, a novel species with clinical and plant-associated isolates. *Syst. Appl. Microbiol.* **27**:27–35.

122. Rosso, M., P. Rojas, E. Garcia, J. Marquez, A. Losada, and M. Munoz. 2007. *Kluyvera* meningitis in a newborn. *Pediatr. Infect. Dis. J.* **26**:1070–1071.

123. Samonis, G., D. E. Karageorgopoulos, D. P. Kofteridis, D. K. Matthaiou, V. Sidiropoulou, S. Maraki, and M. E. Falagas. 2009. *Citrobacter* infections in a general hospital: characteristics and outcomes. *Eur. J. Clin. Microbiol. Infect. Dis.* **28**:61–68.

124. Samra, Z., J. Bahar, L. Madar-Shapiro, N. Aziz, S. Israel, and J. Bishara. 2008. Evaluation of CHROMagar KPC for rapid detection of carbapenem-producing *Enterobacteriaceae*. *J. Clin. Microbiol.* **46**:3110–3111.

125. Scarparo, C., P. Piccoli, P. Ricordi, and M. Scagnelli. 2002. Comparative evaluation of two commercial chromogenic media for detection and presumptive identification of urinary tract pathogens. *Eur. J. Clin. Microbiol. Infect. Dis.* **21**:283–289.

126. Schmid, H., C. Weber, J. R. Bogner, and S. Schubert. 2003. Isolation of a *Pantoea dispersa*-like strain from a 71-year-old woman with acute myeloid leukemia and multiple myeloma. *Infection* **31**:66–67.

127. Schonheyder, H. C., K. T. Jensen, and W. Frederiksen. 1994. Taxonomic notes: synonymy of *Enterobacter cancerogenus* (Urosevic 1966) Dickey and Zumoff 1988 and *Enterobacter taylorae* Farmer et al. 1985 and resolution of an ambiguity in the biochemical profile. *Int. J. Syst. Bacteriol.* **44**:586–587.

128. Simmon, K. E., A. C. Croft, and C. A. Petit. 2006. Application of SmartGene IDNS Software to partial 16S rRNA gene sequences for a diverse group of bacteria in a clinical laboratory. *J. Clin. Microbiol.* **44**:4400–4406.

129. Slaven, E. M., F. A. Lopez, S. M. Hart, and C. V. Sanders. 2001. Myonecrosis caused by *Edwardsiella tarda*: a case report and case series of extraintestinal *E. tarda* infections. *Clin. Infect. Dis.* **32**:1430–1433.

130. Snyder, J. W., G. K. Munier, and C. L. Johnson. 2008. Direct comparison of the BD Phoenix System with the MicroScan WalkAway System for identification and antimicrobial susceptibility testing of *Enterobacteriaceae* and nonfermenting gram-negative organisms. *J. Clin. Microbiol.* **46**:2327–2333.

131. Somvanshi, V. S., E. Lang, B. Straubler, C. Sproer, P. Schumann, S. Ganguly, A. K. Saxena, and E. Stackebrandt. 2006. *Providencia vermicola* sp. nov., isolated from infective juveniles of the entomopathogenic nematode *Steinernema thermophilum*. *Int. J. Syst. Evol. Microbiol.* **56**:629–633.

132. Sproer, C., U. Mendrock, J. Swiderski, E. Lang, and E. Stackebrandt. 1999. The phylogenetic position of *Serratia, Buttiauxella* and some other genera of the family *Enterobacteriaceae*. *Int. J. Syst. Bacteriol.* **49**:1433–1438.

133. Stephan, R., S. Van Trappen, I. Cleenwerck, C. Iversen, H. Joosten, P. De Vos, and A. Lehner. 2008. *Enterobacter pulveris* sp. nov., isolated from fruit powder, infant formula and an infant formula production environment. *Int. J. Syst. Evol. Microbiol.* **58**:237–241.

134. Stephan, R., S. Van Trappen, I. Cleenwerck, M. Vancanneyt, P. De Vos, and A. Lehner. 2007. *Enterobacter turicensis* sp. nov. and *Enterobacter helveticus* sp. nov., isolated from fruit powder. *Int. J. Syst. Evol. Microbiol.* **57**: 820–826.

135. Sundin, D. R. 2009. Hidden beta-lactamases in the *Enterobacteriaceae*—dropping the extra disks for detection. Part I. *Clin. Microbiol. Newsl.* **31**:41–44.

136. Sundin, D. R. 2009. Hidden beta-lactamases in the *Enterobacteriaceae*—dropping the extra disks for detection. Part II. *Clin. Microbiol. Newsl.* **31**:47–52.

137. Tamura, K., R. Sakazaki, Y. Kosako, and E. Yoshizaki. 1986. *Leclercia adecarboxylata* gen. nov., comb. nov., formerly known as *Escherichia adecarboxylata*. *Curr. Microbiol.* **13**:179–184.

138. Tan, T. Y., L. S. Y. Ng, J. He, T. H. Koh, and L. Y. Hsu. 2009. Evaluation of screening methods to detect plasmid-mediated AmpC in *Escherichia coli, Klebsiella pneumoniae*, and *Proteus mirabilis*. *J. Clin. Microbiol.* **53**:146–149.

139. Theodoropoulos, T. H. Wong, M. O'Brien, and D. Stenzel. 2001. *Plesiomonas shigelloides* enters polarized human intestinal Caco-2 cells in an in vitro model system. *Infect. Immun.* **69**:2260–2269.

140. Thomson, K. S. 2001. Controversies about extended-spectrum and AmpC beta-lactamases. *Emerg. Infect. Dis.* **7**:333–336.

141. **Tsakris, A., I. Kristo, A. Poulou, K. Themeli-Digalaki, A. Ikonomidis, D. Petropoulou, S. Pournaras, and D. Sofianou.** 2009. Evaluation of boronic acid disk tests for differentiating KPC-possessing *Klebsiella pneumoniae* isolates in the clinical laboratory. *J. Clin. Microbiol.* **47:**362–367.

142. **Westbrook, G. L., C. M. O'Hara, S. B. Roman, and J. M. Miller.** 2000. Incidence and identification of *Klebsiella planticola* in clinical isolates with emphasis on newborns. *J. Clin. Microbiol.* **38:**1495–1497.

143. **Williams, W. W., J. Mariano, M. Spurrier, H. D. Donnell, Jr., R. L. Breckenridge, Jr., R. L. Anderson, I. K. Wachsmuth, C. Thornsberry, D. R. Graham, D. W. Thibeault, and J. R. Allen.** 1984. Nosocomial meningitis due to *Citrobacter diversus* in neonates: new aspects of epidemiology. *J. Infect. Dis.* **150:**229–235.

144. **Wong, T. Y., H. Y. Tsui, M. K. So, J. Y. Lai, C. W. S. Tse, and T. K. Ng.** 2000. *Plesiomonas shigelloides* infection in Hong Kong: retrospective study of 167 laboratory-confirmed cases. *Hong Kong Med. J.* **6:**375–380.

145. **Woo, P. C. Y., S. K. P. Lau, and K.-Y. Yuen.** 2005. Biliary tract disease as a risk factor for *Plesiomonas shigelloides* bacteraemia: a nine-year experience in a Hong Kong hospital and review of the literature. *New Microbiol.* **28:**45–55.

146. **Yang, C.-C., C.-H. Yen, M.-W. Ho, and J.-H. Wang.** 2004. Comparison of pyogenic liver abscess caused by non-*Klebsiella pneumoniae* and *Klebsiella pneumoniae*. *J. Microbiol. Immunol. Infect.* **37:**176–184.

147. **Yoh, M., J. Matsuyama, M. Ohnishi, K. Takagi, H. Miyagi, K. Mori, K.-S. Park, T. Ono, and T. Honda.** 2005. Importance of *Providencia* species as a major cause of travellers' diarrhea. *J. Med. Microbiol.* **54:**1077–1082.

148. **Yu, W.-L., W.-C. Ko, K.-C. Cheng, C.-C. Lee, C.-C. Lai, and Y.-C. Chuang.** 2008. Comparison of prevalence of virulence factors for *Klebsiella pneumoniae* liver abscesses between isolates with capsular K1/K2 and non-K1/K2 serotypes. *Diagn. Microbiol. Infect. Dis.* **62:**1–6.

149. **Zhang, C.-X., S.-Y. Yang, M.-X. Xu, J. Sun, H. Liu, J.-R. Liu, H. Lui, F. Kan, J. Sun, R. Lai, and K.-Y. Zhang.** 2009. *Serratia nematodiphila* sp. nov. associated with the entomopathogenic nematode *Heterorhabditidoides chongmingensis* (Rhabditida: Rhabditidae). *Int. J. Syst. Evol. Microbiol.* **59:**1605–1608.

150. **Zollner-Schwetz, I., C. Hogenauer, M. Joainig, P. Weberhofer, G. Gorkiewicz, T. Valentin, T. A. Hinterleitner, and R. Krause.** 2008. Role of *Klebsiella oxytoca* in antibiotic-associated diarrhea. *Clin. Infect. Dis.* **47:**e74–e78.

Aeromonas*

AMY J. HORNEMAN AND AFSAR ALI

38

TAXONOMY

The genus *Aeromonas* resides within the family *Aeromonadaceae* (16) and the newly proposed order *Aeromonadales*, ord. nov., along with the genera *Oceanimonas* and *Tolumonas* (45). *Aeromonas* is the only one of these three genera that is pathogenic for humans. The use of frequent reclassifications and constant amended or extended descriptions within *Aeromonas* taxonomy can often be initially puzzling to microbiologists not working with these organisms on a daily basis. However, information in this chapter should clarify the identification and significance of those species most often associated with human disease (Table 1). DNA hybridization group numbers, which no longer serve a meaningful purpose, and synonymous species designations for *Aeromonas veronii* bv. sobria (*A. ichthiosmia*) and *A. trota* (*A. enteropelogenes*) (15) are not included, for simplicity. *Aeromonas* group 501, which is made up of *A. schubertii*-like organisms, and *Aeromonas* sp. DNA hybridization group 11 (47), which is made up of *A. eucrenophila*/*A. encheleia*-like organisms, are also not addressed in the table. These groups contain few strains, their taxonomic status has yet to be resolved and is still highly debated, and most importantly, neither group has been shown to be significant in human or animal disease. Newly proposed *Aeromonas* species and subspecies since the publication of the previous edition of this *Manual* include *A. bivalvium* sp. nov., isolated from bivalve mollusks (51); *A. tecta* sp. nov., isolated from both clinical and environmental sources (19); *A. piscicola* sp. nov., isolated from diseased fish (8); and *A. aquariorum* sp. nov., isolated from aquaria of ornamental fish (49). However, there is controversy surrounding the proposal of *A. aquariorum*, since this new species appears to be both phenotypically and genetically identical to *A. hydrophila* subsp. *dhakensis*, proposed in 2002, and isolated from cases of children with diarrhea in Bangladesh (46). Comparative studies between the two laboratories are under way to try to resolve this taxonomic dilemma.

Because of its clinical significance, clinical strains formerly referred to as *A. sobria* are, in fact, *A. veronii* bv. sobria (esculin hydrolysis and ornithine decarboxylase negative and arginine dihydrolase positive) and should be reported as such. Nearly all rapid identification databases, excepting API 20E strips (bioMerieux, Inc., Durham, NC), have converted their *A. sobria* identifications to *A. veronii* bv. sobria. This is especially important because of *A. veronii* bv. sobria's association with more severe, extraintestinal infections, such as septicemia, meningitis following leech therapy, and disseminated intravascular gas production (56, 67). It usually is not necessary to definitively separate members of the *A. hydrophila* complex (*A. hydrophila*, *A. bestiarum*, and *A. salmonicida*) or the *A. caviae* complex (*A. caviae*, *A. media*, and *A. eucrenophila*), especially when they are isolated from feces (see "Evaluation, Interpretation, and Reporting of Results" below).

The type strain *Aeromonas hydrophila* subsp. *hydrophila* ATCC 7966 was the first aeromonad to be completely sequenced, annotated, published, and deposited in GenBank (as CP000462) (66). This was followed just recently by the publication of the complete genome sequence of *Aeromonas salmonicida* subsp. *salmonicida* A449, an agent of furunculosis (a bacterial septicemia of salmonid fish), which was deposited in GenBank as NC 00938. Comparing this aeromonad genome with the *A. hydrophila* ATCC 7966^T genome, which has one chromosome, showed that the A449 *A. salmonicida* genome harbored one chromosome and two large plasmids, carried multiple inversions in the chromosome, and additionally had an approximately 9% difference in gene content compared with the *A. hydrophila* subsp. *hydrophila* ATCC 7966 type strain (60).

DESCRIPTION OF THE GENUS

Members of the genus *Aeromonas* are gram-negative facultative anaerobes that are straight, coccobacillary to bacillary cells with rounded ends, 0.3 to 1.0 μm in diameter and 1.0 to 3.5 μm in length. They can occur singly, in pairs, or, rarely, in short chains. Most species are motile by a single, polar flagellum with a 1.7-μm wavelength, but peritrichous flagella may be formed on solid media in young cultures and lateral flagella occur in some species. Aeromonads are usually oxidase positive and catalase positive and are generally resistant to 150 μg of the vibriostatic agent 2,4-diamino-6,7-diisopropylpteridine (O/129).

---

*This chapter contains information presented in chapter 46 by Amy J. Horneman, Afsar Ali, and Sharon L. Abbott in the ninth edition of this *Manual*.

TABLE 1 Members of the genus *Aeromonas*[a]

Organism	Human isolation (extraintestinal/fecal)	Human pathogen (extraintestinal/fecal)	Frequency in humans	Pathogenic for animals, fish, and reptiles
A. hydrophila complex				
A. hydrophila				
subsp. *hydrophila*	Yes	Yes	Common	Yes
subsp. *dhakensis*[b]	Yes	Yes	Rare	No
subsp. *ranae*	No	No	—	Yes
A. bestiarum	No/yes	—/no	Rare	Yes
A. salmonicida[c]	No/yes	No/no	Rare	
subsp. *salmonicida*				Yes
subsp. *achromogenes*				Yes
subsp. *masoucida*				Yes
subsp. *smithia*				Yes
subsp. *pectinolytica*				No
A. caviae complex				
A. caviae	Yes	Yes	Common	Yes
A. media	No/yes	—/yes	Rare	No
A. eucrenophila	Yes	No/—	Very rare	No
A. veronii complex				
A. veronii bv. sobria	Yes	Yes	Common	Yes
A. veronii bv. veronii	Yes	Yes	Rare	No
A. jandaei	Yes	Yes/unknown	Rare	No
A. trota	Yes	Neither	Rare	No
A. schubertii	Yes/no	Yes/—	Rare	No
A. encheleia	Yes/no	No/—	One case	No
A. allosaccharophila	No/yes	—/no	Very rare	Yes
A. sobria	Neither	—	—	No
A. popoffii	Yes	Yes	Very rare	No
A. culicicola	No	No	—	No
A. simiae	No	No	—	No
A. molluscorum	No	No	—	No
A. bivalvium	No	No	—	No
A. tecta	Yes	No	Rare	No
A. piscicola	No	No	—	Yes

[a]—, not applicable.

[b]May be synonymous with *A. aquariorum*, sp. nov. (49).

[c]There are motile strains of *A. salmonicida* that grow at 37°C and resemble clinical *A. hydrophila* strains that have been isolated from human feces; these can be distinguished using the tests in Table 3.

They are chemoorganotrophic, displaying oxidative and fermentative metabolism of glucose. Acid, and often acid with gas, is produced from many carbohydrates, especially glucose, and nitrate is reduced to nitrite. A variety of exoenzymes such as arylamidases, amylase, DNase, esterases, peptidases, proteases, chitinase, chondroitinase, and hemolysins are produced. The main cellular fatty acids produced are hexadecanoic acid (16:0), hexadecenoic acid (16:1), and octadecenoic acid (18:1). Human (mesophilic) strains grow between 10 and 42°C, but occasional isolates may be more active in some biochemical assays at 22 to 25°C. Psychrophilic strains from fish and the environment (*A. popoffii* and *A. salmonicida*) seldom grow above 37°C and preferentially grow at 22 to 25°C. In brain heart infusion broth at 28°C, growth occurs between pH 4.5 and 9.0 and at salt concentrations between 0 and 4%. The mol% G+C of the DNA is 57 to 63%.

EPIDEMIOLOGY AND TRANSMISSION

Aeromonads are inhabitants of aquatic ecosystems worldwide such as groundwater, reservoirs, and clean or polluted lakes and rivers. *Aeromonas* may also be found in marine environments but only in brackish water or water with a low saline content. Most *Aeromonas* species, particularly those associated with human infections, are found in a wide variety of fresh produce, meat (beef, poultry, and pork), and dairy products (raw milk and ice cream) (32). *A. veronii* bv. sobria is a symbiont in the gut of medicinal leeches, where it may grow as a pure culture (26). Infections in frogs, pigs, cattle, birds, and marine animals have also been reported (32).

Most clinical infections with aeromonads are related to an exposure to some type of aquatic source, whether the clinical specimen is feces or extraintestinal, and, to a lesser extent, to the ingestion of foods. The majority of studies have found a seasonal relationship between the recovery of aeromonads from specimens and the warmer months of the year (37). This is not surprising since the optimal temperature for the growth of mesophilic aeromonads would be that occurring in the warmer months. This would therefore increase the likelihood of recreational human exposure to these bacteria, thereby resulting in an increased risk of colonization and/or infections with these indigenous aquatic microorganisms.

Since *Aeromonas* is not a reportable condition in the United States or in most other countries, the true incidence of *Aeromonas* infections worldwide is not known. Estimates from England/Wales and the United States for septicemia with aeromonads in 2004 revealed an incidence of 1.5 per million population (34). However, any estimates of incidence would most likely be an underestimation, particularly as relates to exposure through drinking water.

CLINICAL SIGNIFICANCE

Aeromonas gastroenteritis ranges from an acute watery diarrhea (most common form) to dysenteric illness to chronic illness. Stools from acute watery diarrhea are loose (take the shape of their container), and erythrocytes and fecal leukocytes are absent. Accompanying symptoms include abdominal pain (60 to 70%), fever and vomiting (20 to 40%), and nausea (40%) (35). Infections are usually self-limiting, but children may require hospitalization due to dehydration. *A. caviae* is the most common species associated with these infections, and *A. caviae* infection can even mimic inflammatory bowel disease in children (74). *A. veronii* bv. sobria strains may be associated with rare cholera-like disease characterized by abdominal pain (60%) and fever and nausea (20%) (32). In dysenteric diarrhea resembling shigellosis, patients suffer from severe abdominal pain and have bloody stools containing mucus and polymorphonuclear leukocytes. About 10 to 15% of patients with either cholera-like or dysenteric diarrhea are coinfected with another enteric pathogen(s).

A comprehensive Bangladesh study found that the presence of loose stools or more severe watery diarrhea was associated with *Aeromonas* strains possessing an *alt* gene (for a heat-labile cytotonic enterotoxin) alone or both *alt* and *ast* (for a heat-stable cytotonic enterotoxin), respectively (6). A large traveler's diarrhea study in Spain found the predominant species to be *A. veronii* bv. veronii and *A. caviae* (75). A third large study in India found seven different species among hospitalized patients with diarrhea, with *A. caviae* predominating, followed by *A. hydrophila* and *A. veronii* bv. sobria, along with the presence of the *alt* and *ast* genes as well as the *act* gene, which encodes a well-established cytotoxic enterotoxin often present in clinical aeromonad isolates (68).

Finally, in a large acute diarrheal outbreak in Brazil that involved 2,170 cases, *Aeromonas* was the species that was recovered in 19.5% of those cases (28). Although most diarrheal cases are generally self-limited, a combination of supportive therapy and antimicrobials are often indicated in the pediatric, geriatric, and immunocompromised populations (35). A 2007 article gives a nice summary of the latest data and theories related to the association of *Aeromonas* with diarrhea (21).

Complications from *Aeromonas* diarrheal disease include hemolytic-uremic syndrome (9, 20) and kidney disease requiring kidney transplantation (23). These more severe infections are usually associated with *A. hydrophila* or *A. veronii* bv. sobria. Also, nonresolvable, intermittent diarrhea can occur months after the initial infection and may persist for months or several years.

Aeromonas can also be isolated from a variety of extraintestinal sites, although blood and wounds are the most common sources. *Aeromonas* septicemia occurs rarely in immunocompetent hosts; most cases are in patients with liver disease and hematological malignancies and can be accompanied by necrotizing fasciitis (40, 41). The species more commonly isolated from septicemia are *A. hydrophila*, *A. veronii* bv. sobria, and *A. jandaei*. Wound infections are usually preceded by traumatic injury that occurs in contact with water, where the predominant species is *A. hydrophila*.

These infections range from uncomplicated cases of cellulitis to myonecrotic infections with a poor prognosis (4, 52). Two such scenarios are the reported outbreaks of wound infections with *A. hydrophila* associated with mud football (73) and wound infections among both the 2004 Asian tsunami survivors (44) and the 2005 Hurricane Katrina survivors in New Orleans, LA (59). Surveys indicate that only 17 to 52% of *Aeromonas* wound infections are monomicrobic (35). Use of medicinal leeches postoperatively to enhance blood flow to surgical sites has resulted in wound infection rates of 20%, primarily with *A. veronii* bv. sobria (26, 65).

Other extraintestinal infections include ocular, respiratory, surgical, and urinary tract infections; meningitis; osteomyelitis; cholecystitis; pneumonia; endocarditis; peritonitis; portal pyemia; and pancreatic abscess (12, 17, 18, 33, 42, 50, 71, 72). A few such examples were the isolation of *A. caviae* from keratitis associated with contact lens wear (58) and isolation of *A. caviae* and *A. popoffii* from separate cases of urinary tract infection (5, 29). The newest disease association with *Aeromonas hydrophila* is spa bath folliculitis, but this is in keeping with the ubiquitous nature of this aquatic microorganism (54).

COLLECTION, TRANSPORT, AND STORAGE OF SPECIMENS

Aeromonads survive well in specimens, and any of the widely used transport media are acceptable for transport (Amies, Cary-Blair, modified Stuart's, and buffered glycerol in saline), with Cary-Blair generally considered to be the best (see chapter 16). Feces are always preferable to rectal swabs for isolation of enteric pathogens, and stools should be collected in the acute phase of disease. Most strains grow equally well at room temperature (20 to 25°C) and incubator temperature (35 to 37°C). Because isolates being kept for long-term storage do not survive well at room or refrigerator temperature in the laboratory for long periods (>1 month), placing aeromonads in media, such as Trypticase soy broth with 30% glycerol, and deep freezing at −80°C is recommended for their long-term storage.

DIRECT EXAMINATION

The direct microscopic examination of wound or skin/superficial specimens or positive blood culture specimens would be somewhat unremarkable, in that the presence of aeromonads would be denoted as straight, gram-negative bacilli with or without the presence of white cells, not unlike the presentation of a similar infection with either enterics or pseudomonads. It is possible to rarely see somewhat elongated bacilli in blood or urine specimens with aeromonads if the patient is undergoing antimicrobial therapy.

Although there have been several DNA probe and real-time PCR methods described for the possible identification of aeromonads from either water, food, or veterinary sources, there are no widely recognized antigen detection and/or nucleic acid detection methods available for detection within clinical specimens.

ISOLATION PROCEDURES

Aeromonads generally grow well on a variety of enteric differential and selective agars, although sucrose- and/or lactose-fermenting strains usually resemble nonpathogens on these media. Blood agar with 20 μg of ampicillin per ml had previously been considered useful for isolating all *Aeromonas* species; however, a substantial percentage (15 to 57%) of *A. caviae* isolates are resistant to ampicillin, and certain species, like *A. trota*, are intrinsically susceptible to ampicillin (10, 38). In fact, a recent environmental sampling study to detect aeromonads showed that when ampicillin is used as a selective agent, a significant portion (17.3%) of the aeromonad population, in at least some environments, could not be isolated using such media (30). Therefore, laboratories should use caution when medium with ampicillin is used in the setup of stool specimens for detecting the presence of all clinically relevant aeromonad species as bacterial enteropathogens.

Modified cefsulodin-Irgasan-novobiocin (CIN) (4 μg of cefsulodin per ml, versus 15 μg/ml in unmodified CIN) is also an excellent isolation medium for aeromonads. On this medium, *Aeromonas* colonies have a pink center with an uneven, clear apron and are indistinguishable from *Yersinia enterocolitica* morphologically. One can incubate CIN at 25°C to enhance the recovery of *Yersinia* and still be able to recover *Aeromonas* within 24 h at this temperature.

Aeromonas agar, available from Lab-M (http://www .lab-m.com), is a relatively new alternative medium to CIN agar that uses D-xylose (which aeromonads do not ferment) as a differential characteristic (7).

Since most clinically relevant species are beta-hemolytic, including an increasing number of *A. caviae* strains, beta-hemolytic colonies on blood agar should be screened with oxidase and a spot indole test. Any colonies positive by both tests should be characterized further, although occasional indole-negative *A. caviae* and nearly all known *A. schubertii* isolates (which are generally associated with severe aquatic wounds) are indole negative (2). Thiosulfate-citrate-bile salts-sucrose medium is usually inhibitory to aeromonads. Enrichment in alkaline peptone water enhances recovery of *Aeromonas* from populations that generally would be expected to shed low numbers of organisms (carriers, convalescent-phase patients, and those with subclinical infections). For patients with acute diarrhea, enrichment is probably unnecessary (61).

IDENTIFICATION

Aeromonas spp. are most easily confused in the laboratory with other oxidase-positive fermenters, i.e., *Vibrio* and *Plesiomonas* spp. *Plesiomonas* is easily differentiated from *Aeromonas* by positive reactions in Moeller's lysine, ornithine, and arginine tests and by fermentation of m-inositol. Vibrios may be more difficult to distinguish from aeromonads (1), which is particularly true for *Vibrio fluvialis* and *A. caviae*,

and in laboratories where the sole means of identification is a rapid miniaturized system (31, 69). Resistance to O/129 vibriostatic agent (150 μg) and the inability to grow in salt concentrations of ≥6% usually indicate the genus *Aeromonas*. *Vibrio cholerae* O139, a cholera toxin-positive, non-salt-requiring, O/129 vibriostatic agent-resistant vibrio, is a major exception to this rule. However, the decarboxylase pattern (positive for lysine and ornithine) and negative reactions for arginine dihydrolase, production of gas from glucose, and fermentation of salicin separate this organism from most aeromonads. Unfortunately, strains of ornithine decarboxylase-positive *A. veronii* bv. veronii will often yield an excellent to very good identification for *V. cholerae* with the rapid identification API-20-E strip (bioMerieux, Inc.), and serotyping and/or additional testing is required to resolve the issue. *A. veronii* bv. veronii would be string test negative, O/129 resistant, and able to produce gas from glucose fermentation; would not require additional salt for growth; and would be inhibited on thiosulfate-citrate-bile salts-sucrose agar. *V. cholerae* strains would have the opposite reactions. Once it has been determined that you have a glucose-fermenting, oxidase-positive, motile gram-negative rod that is resistant to O/129, a small number of biochemical tests can be used for separating *Aeromonas* species into the three major species complexes (Table 2). If warranted, even more discriminatory results for separating members of each complex can be found in bolded text in Table 3 (2), which should replace earlier published tests for species identification (3).

Other Identification Methods

The sequencing of a single housekeeping gene 16S rRNA (48), followed by the development of an extended method using 16S ribosomal DNA (restricted fragment length polymorphism) analysis (22), were both initially promising as methods to identify aeromonads to the species level. However, data on the intragenomic heterogeneity within the 16S rRNA gene in *Aeromonas* strains suggest caution in using this gene for anything beyond genus level identification (53). Therefore, the use of other housekeeping genes as multiple molecular markers, such as *gyraseB* and *rpoD* (70) and *dnaJ* (55), or an even broader approach using multilocus sequence typing with several different genes, seems to be the future avenue for accurate species identification. Extensive studies by Chopra et al. have delineated several DNA probes for the detection of a number of possible virulence-related factors. This was the result of the public release of the *Aeromonas hydrophila* ATCC 7966[T] genome sequence and comparative work with the diarrheal *Aeromonas hydrophila*

TABLE 2 Biochemical identification of *Aeromonas* to complex level

Test	No. of strains identified as belonging to[a]:		
	A. hydrophila complex (A. hydrophila, A. bestiarum, A. salmonicida)	A. caviae complex (A. caviae, A. media, A. eucrenophila)	A. veronii complex (A. veronii HG8,[b] A. jandaei, A. schubertii, A. trota)
Esculin	87 (92, 81, 85)	71 (76, 55, 78)	0
Voges-Proskauer	75 (88, 63, 62)	0	54 (88, 87, 17, 0)
Glucose (gas)	81 (92, 69, 77)	16 (0, 0, 78)	87 (92, 100, 0, 69)
L-Arabinose	93 (84, 100, 100)	96 (100, 100, 78)	4 (12, 0, 0, 0)

[a] The first number is the overall percent positive for each complex for a given trait; the numbers in parentheses are percent positive for each species listed within that complex. Data are derived and modified from Table 5 in reference 2 and reprinted with permission.
[b] Biovar sobria (DNA hybridization group 8); the separation of *A. veronii* bv. veronii (DNA hybridization group 10) from *A. veronii* bv. sobria is achieved with *A. veronii* bv. veronii having positive reactions for ornithine decarboxylase and esculin hydrolysis and a negative reaction for arginine dihydrolase.

TABLE 3 Tests useful in the separation of members within the *Aeromonas* species complexes

Test	A. hydrophila	A. bestiarum	A. salmonicida	A. caviae	A. media	A. eucrenophila	A. veronii[b]	A. jandaei	A. schubertii	A. trota
Utilization of:										
Citrate	+ (92)[c]	V (38)	+ (85)	+ (88)	V (82)	− (0)	V (52)	+ (87)	V (58)	+ (94)
DL-Lactate	V (84)	− (0)	− (0)	+ (96)	V (56)	− (0)	−(0)	− (7)	V (58)	+ (88)
Urocanic acid	V (16)	+ (94)	+ (100)	+ (100)	+ (100)	− (0)	− (0)	− (7)	− (0)	V (75)
Gluconate oxidation	V (64)	− (13)	− (0)	− (0)	− (0)	− (0)	V (60)	V (60)	− (0)	− (0)
Gas from D-glucose	+ (92)	V (69)	V (77)	− (0)	− (0)	V (78)	+ (92)	+ (100)	− (0)	V (69)
PZA	V (24)	V (50)	V (31)	+ (88)	V (18)	+ (100)	ND	ND	ND	ND
Indole	+ (96)	+ (100)	+ (100)	V (84)	+ (100)	+ (89)	+ (100)	+ (100)	V (17)	+ (100)
Voges-Proskauer	+ (92)	V (63)	V (62)	− (0)	− (0)	− (0)	+ (92)	+ (87)	V (17)	− (0)
Lipase (corn oil)	+ (100)	+ (88)	+ (92)	V (76)	V (82)	+ (89)	+ (92)	+ (100)	+ (100)	− (0)
Acid from:										
Cellobiose	− (4)	V (38)	V (69)	+ (100)	+ (100)	V (56)	V (20)	V (20)	− (0)	+ (100)
Lactose	V (64)	− (13)	+ (92)	V (60)	V (64)	− (11)	− (12)	− (0)	− (0)	− (0)
L-Rhamnose	V (24)	V (69)	− (0)	− (0)	− (0)	V (22)	− (0)	− (0)	−(0)	− (0)
D-Sorbitol	− (0)	− (0)	+ (85)	− (4)	− (0)	− (0)	−(0)	− (0)	− (0)	− (0)
Glucose-1-phosphate	ND	ND	ND	− (4)	+ (100)	+ (100)	ND	ND	ND	ND
Glucose-6-phosphate	ND	ND	ND	− (4)	+ (100)	+ (100)	ND	ND	ND	ND
Lactulose	ND	ND	ND	V (68)	V (55)	− (0)	ND	ND	ND	ND
D-Mannose	+ (100)	+ (100)	+ (100)	V (32)	+ (100)	+ (100)	ND	+ (100)	+ (92)	+ (100)
Glycerol	+ (96)	+ (100)	+ (100)	V (68)	V (55)	− (11)	+ (100)	+ (100)	− (0)	+ (94)
D-Mannitol	+ (96)	+(100)	+ (100)	+ (100)	+ (100)	+ (100)	+ (100)	+ (100)	− (0)	V (69)
Sucrose	+ (100)	+ (94)	+ (100)	+ (100)	+ (100)	V (33)	+ (100)	− (0)	− (0)	V (19)
Amp[r]	+ (100)	+ (94)	+ (85)	+ (100)	V (73)	+ (100)	+ (100)	+ (93)	+ (92)	− (6)

[a]Data compiled from Tables 2, 6, 7, and 8 in reference 2 and reprinted with permission. +, ≥85% of the strains positive; −, <15% positive; V, 15 to 85% positive (results at 48 h). Numbers in parentheses indicate percent positive for test at the final day of reading. Gluconate, 2 days; DL-lactate and urocanic acid, 3 days; citrate, 4 days; carbohydrates, indole, and lipase, 7 days; pyrazinamidase (PZA), 2 days; Amp[r], resistance to 10 μg of ampicillin, 1 day; Voges-Proskauer, 3 days. ND, not done.
[b]Biovar sobria (DNA hybridization group 8); the separation of A. *veronii* bv. veronii (DNA hybridization group 10) from A. *veronii* bv. sobria is achieved with A. *veronii* bv. veronii having positive reactions for ornithine decarboxylase and esculin hydrolysis and a negative reaction for arginine dihydrolase.
[c]For each of the three *Aeromonas* species complexes, the discriminatory reactions between the species within each complex are presented in bold type.

TABLE 4 *Aeromonas* species susceptibilities

Susceptibility[a]	Antibiotic agent
Resistant	Ampicillin (except A. *trota* [100% susceptible]), A. *caviae* [35% susceptible][b]
Variable	Ticarcillin or piperacillin (except A. *veronii* bv. veronii [100% resistant], A. *trota* [100% susceptible])
	Cephalothin
	Cefazolin
	Cefoxitin (except A. *veronii* bv. veronii [100% susceptible])
	Cefuroxime
	Ceftriaxone
	Cefotaxime
Susceptible	Ciprofloxacin[c]
	Gentamicin
	Amikacin
	Tobramycin (A. *veronii* bv. veronii [42% resistant])
	Imipenem (A. *jandaei* [65% resistant], A. *veronii* bv. veronii [67% resistant])
	Trimethoprim-sulfamethoxazole

[a]Resistant or susceptible, ≥90% of all isolates resistant or susceptible; variable, 10 to 90% of isolates susceptible (2).
[b]Data for A. *caviae* susceptibility found in references 5 and 38.
[c]Data for resistance to nalidixic acid and pipemidic acid in 26 and 20% of A. *caviae* and A. *hydrophila* strains and 88% of A. *veronii* clinical strains suggest possible future resistance to fluoroquinolones (75).

SSU strain (13). These include, but are not limited to, the discovery of a new hemolysin, the presence of a functional type VI secretion system, a cold shock exoribonuclease R (VacB), and a surface-associated enolase.

SEROLOGIC TESTS

Most serologic assays that have been used to detect antibodies to *Aeromonas* (tube agglutination, immunoblotting, and enzyme-linked immunoassay) have low sensitivity and specificity and are not considered reliable.

ANTIMICROBIAL SUSCEPTIBILITIES

Two of the earliest articles on *Aeromonas* antimicrobial susceptibilities (36, 57) included only strains well characterized to the species level and expanded previously known susceptibility information on aeromonads isolated less frequently from clinical specimens. A general antimicrobial susceptibility profile for *Aeromonas* derived from both of these investigations as well as other studies (32, 39, 76) is given in Table 4. There are CLSI (Clinical and Laboratory Standards Institute) testing guidelines for the major clinical *Aeromonas* species as related to antimicrobial dilution and disk susceptibility testing in document M45-A for infrequently isolated or fastidious bacteria (14).

Ciprofloxacin, commonly used to treat gram-negative infections, was initially reported as active against all species of *Aeromonas*, with little or no resistance reported in studies in the United States and most of Europe (36, 57). However, 2 to 3% of *A. caviae*, *A. hydrophila*, and *A. veronii* bv. sobria strains in Asia have been reported to be ciprofloxacin resistant, as early as 1996 (39). *Aeromonas* species can express three chromosomal β-lactam-induced β-lactamases, including a group 1 molecular class C cephalosporinase, a group 2d molecular class D penicillinase, and a group 3 molecular class B metallo-β-lactamase (carbapenemase) (63). The presence of these β-lactamases in *Aeromonas*, in particular the carbapenemase, may not be detected by conventional susceptibility methods (63). CphA, one of several enzymes responsible for resistance to carbapenems, hydrolyzes nitrocefin poorly or not at all, indicating that the nitrocefin test is not reliable for detecting carbapenemases (27, 63). A case of sepsis due to an extended-spectrum β-lactamase (ESBL)-producing *A. hydrophila* strain in a pediatric patient with diarrhea and pneumonia (62) and a case of *A. hydrophila* necrotizing fasciitis with probable in vivo transfer of a TEM-24 plasmid-borne ESBL gene from *Enterobacter aerogenes* have been reported (24).

A 2009 report on the development of imipenem resistance in an *Aeromonas veronii* bv. sobria clinical isolate recovered from a patient with cholangitis warrants concern among physicians as to the possible emergence of multidrug resistance with this species (64). Much more disturbing are two reports of plasmid-mediated single-resistance and multiresistance determinants among environmental aeromonad isolates (11, 25).

Antimicrobial susceptibility testing of local isolates is necessary for the detection of species-related patterns, because susceptibilities may differ from one geographic area to another. This was very apparent in a study on the in vitro activities of tigecycline, a novel glycylcycline antimicrobial agent, against clinical isolates of *Aeromonas* in Taiwan. It was found that 200 of 201 *Aeromonas* isolates were susceptible to tigecycline, with 1 *A. caviae* isolate having an MIC of 4 μg/ml, and the species-related patterns that varied with geographic areas were confirmed (43).

EVALUATION, INTERPRETATION, AND REPORTING OF RESULTS

Regardless of the site of isolation (intestinal or extraintestinal), aeromonads should be identified either as belonging to the *A. hydrophila* or *A. caviae* complex or as *A. veronii* complex and not "*A. sobria*," which is now *A. veronii* bv. sobria. For routine isolates recovered from uncomplicated cases of gastroenteritis, this level of identification may be sufficient. Although there is strong evidence that some aeromonads are gastrointestinal pathogens, there is no convincing evidence, at present, that all fecal isolates of *Aeromonas* are involved in diarrheal disease. Thus, the significance of the recovery of aeromonads from stool specimens should be interpreted cautiously and must rely on both laboratory information and clinical interpretation. Because of this, the relative quantity of *Aeromonas* organisms recovered on enteric media (few colonies, moderate growth, or predominant organism) should be reported in conjunction with the *Aeromonas* complex or species identification. For complicated cases of diarrhea, e.g., prolonged bloody diarrhea in pediatric patients or chronic gastroenteritis of >1-month duration or in cancer patients with positive fecal cultures (in whom *Aeromonas* tends to disseminate), a definitive species identification is warranted.

For extraintestinal isolates (from blood or wounds), the same general rules should apply to species identification of aeromonads. Although it is clear that both the in vitro and in vivo pathogenic potentials of *Aeromonas* species and strains vary considerably, for the present time, there are no universal markers or indicators available that dictate when isolates should be definitively identified to the species level. Thus, for extraintestinal isolates, identification of aeromonads beyond complexes should be reserved for strains isolated from sterile body sites (blood and cerebrospinal fluid) and serious wound infections (cellulitis and necrotizing fasciitis); for strains exhibiting unusual resistance patterns, associated with nosocomial outbreaks; and for publications describing traditional species associated with new disease processes or newly described species isolated from new anatomic sites.

REFERENCES

1. Abbott, S. L., L. S. Seli, M. Catino, Jr., M. A. Hartley, and J. M. Janda. 1998. Misidentification of unusual *Aeromonas* species as members of the genus *Vibrio*: a continuing problem. *J. Clin. Microbiol.* **36:**1103–1104.
2. Abbott, S. L., W. K. W. Cheung, and J. M. Janda. 2003. The genus *Aeromonas*: biochemical characteristics, atypical reactions, and phenotypic schemes. *J. Clin. Microbiol.* **41:**2348–2357.
3. Abbott, S. L., W. K. W. Cheung, S. Kroske-Bystrom, T. Malekzadeh, and J. M. Janda. 1992. Identification of *Aeromonas* strains to the genospecies level in the clinical laboratory. *J. Clin. Microbiol.* **30:**1262–1266.
4. Adamski, J., M. Koivuranta, and E. Leppanen. 2006. Fatal case of myonecrosis and epticaemia caused by *Aeromonas hydrophila* in Finland. *Scand. J. Infect. Dis.* **38:**1117.
5. Al-Benwan, K., S. Abbott, J. M. Janda, G. Huys, and M. J. Albert. 2007. Cystitis caused by *Aeromonas caviae*. *J. Clin. Microbiol.* **45:**2348–2350.
6. Albert, M. J., M. Ansaruzzaman, K. A. Talukder, A. K. Chopra, I. Kuhn, M. Rahman, A. S. G. Faruque, M. S. Islam, R. B. Sack, and R. Mollby. 2000. Prevalence of enterotoxin genes in *Aeromonas* spp. isolated from children with diarrhea, healthy controls, and the environment. *J. Clin. Microbiol.* **38:**3785–3790.

7. Andelova, A., I. Porazilova, and E. Krejci. 2006. Aeromonas agar is useful selective medium for isolating aeromonads from faecal samples. *J. Med. Microbiol.* **55:**1605–1606.

8. Beaz-Hidalgo, R., A. Alperi, M. J. Figueras, and J. L. Romalde. 30 June 2009. *Aeromonas piscicola* sp. nov., isolated from diseased fish. *Syst. Appl. Microbiol.* **32:**471–479. [Epub ahead of print.]

9. Bogdanovic, R., M. Cobeljic, V. Markovic, V. Nikolic, M. Ognjanovic, L. Sarjanovic, and D. Makic. 1991. Haemolytic-uremic syndrome associated with *Aeromonas hydrophila* enterocolitis. *Pediatr. Nephrol.* **5:**293–295.

10. Carnahan, A. M., and S. W. Joseph. 1993. Systematic assessment of geographically and clinically diverse aeromonads. *Syst. Appl. Microbiol.* **16:**72–84.

11. Cattoir, V., L. Poirel, A. Camille, C.-J. Soussy, and P. Nordmann. 2008. Unexpected occurrence of plasmid-mediated quinolone resistant determinants in environmental *Aeromonas* spp. *Emerg. Infect. Dis.* **14:**231–237.

12. Choi, J., S. Lee, H. Kwon, Y. Kwak, S. Choic, S. Lim, M. Kim, J. Jeong, S. Choi, J. Woo, and Y. Kim. 2008. Clinical significance of spontaneous *Aeromonas* bacterial peritonitis in cirrhotic patients: a matched case-control study. *Clin. Infect. Dis.* **47:**66–72.

13. Chopra, A. K., J. Graf, A. J. Horneman, and J. A. Johnson. 2009. Virulence factor-activity relationships (VFAR) with specific emphasis on *Aeromonas* species (spp.). *J. Water Health* **7**(Suppl. 1):S29–S54.

14. Clinical and Laboratory Standards Institute. 2006. *Methods for Antimicrobial Dilution and Disk Susceptibility Testing of Infrequently Isolated or Fastidious Bacteria; Approved Standard M45-A.* Clinical and Laboratory Standards Institute, Wayne, PA.

15. Collins, M. D., A. J. Martinez-Murcia, and J. Cai. 1993. *Aeromonas enteropelogenes* and *Aeromonas ichthiosmia* are identical to *Aeromonas trota* and *Aeromonas veronii*, respectively, as revealed by small-subunit rRNA sequence analysis. *Int. J. Syst. Bacteriol.* **43:**855–856.

16. Colwell, R. R., M. R. MacDonell, and J. DeLey. 1986. Proposal to recognize the family *Aeromonadaceae* fam. nov. *Int. J. Syst. Bacteriol.* **36:**473–477.

17. Cremonesini, D., and A. Thomson. 2008. Lung colonization with *Aeromonas hydrophila* in cystic fibrosis believed to have come from a tropical fish tank. *J. R. Soc. Med.* **101:**S44–S45.

18. De Gascun, C., L. Rajan, E. O'Neill, P. Downey, and E. Smyth. 2007. Pancreatic abscess due to *Aeromonas hydrophila*. *J. Infect.* **54:**e59–e60.

19. Demarta, A., M. Kupfer, P. Riegel, C. Harf-Monteil, M. Tonolla, R. Peduzzi, A. Monera, M. Jose Saavedra, and A. Martinez-Murcia. 2008. *Aeromonas tecta* sp. nov., isolated from clinical and environmental sources. *Syst. Appl. Microbiol.* **31:**278–286.

20. Figueras, M. J., M. J. Aldea, N. Fernandez, et al. 2007. *Aeromonas* hemolytic uremic syndrome. A case and a review of the literature. *Diagn. Microbiol. Infect. Dis.* **58:**231.

21. Figueras, M. J., A. J. Horneman, A. Martinez-Murcia, and J. Guarro. 2007. Controversial data on the association of *Aeromonas* with diarrhoea in a recent Hong Kong study. *J. Med. Microbiol.* **56:**996–998.

22. Figueras, M. J., L. Soler, M. R. Chacon, J. Guarro, and A. J. Martinez-Murcia. 2000. Extended method for discrimination of *Aeromonas* spp. by 16S rDNA RFLP analysis. *Int. J. Syst. Evol. Microbiol.* **50:**2069–2073.

23. Filler, G., J. H. H. Ehrich, E. Strauch, and L. Beutin. 2000. Acute renal failure in an infant associated with cytotoxic *Aeromonas sobria* isolated from patient's stool and from aquarium water as suspected source of infection. *J. Clin. Microbiol.* **38:**469–470.

24. Fosse, T., C. Giraud-Morin, I. Madinier, F. Mantoux, J. P. Lacour, and J. P. Ortonne. 2004. *Aeromonas hydrophila* with plasmid-borne class A extended-spectrum β-lactamase TEM-24 and three chromosomal class B, C, and D β-lactamases, isolated from a patient with necrotizing fasciitis. *Antimicrob. Agents Chemother.* **48:**2342–2343.

25. Gordon, L., A. Cloeckaert, B. Doublet, S. Schwarz, A. Bouju-Albert, J.-P. Gaiere, H. Le Bris, A. Le Fleche-Mateos, and E. Giraud. 2008. Complete sequence of the *floR*-carrying multiresistance plasmid pAB5S9 from freshwater *Aeromonas bestiarum*. *J. Antimicrob. Chemother.* **62:**65–71.

26. Graf, J. 1999. Symbiosis of *Aeromonas veronii* biovar sobria and *Hirudo medicinalis*, the medicinal leech: a novel model for digestive tract associations. *Infect. Immun.* **67:**1–7.

27. Hayes, M. V., C. J. Thomson, and S. G. B. Amyes. 1996. The "hidden" carbapenemase of *Aeromonas hydrophila*. *J. Antimicrob. Chemother.* **37:**33–44.

28. Hofer, E., C. M. Reis, G. N. Theophilo, et al. 2006. *Aeromonas* associated with an acute diarrhea outbreak in Sao Bento do Una, Pernambuco. *Rev. Soc. Bras. Med. Trop.* **39:**217.

29. Hua, H. T., C. Bollet, S. Tercian, M. Crancourt, and D. Raoult. 2004. *Aeromonas popoffii* urinary tract infection. *J. Clin. Microbiol.* **42:**5427–5428.

30. Huddleston, J., J. Zak, and R. Jeter. 2007. Sampling bias caused by ampicillin in isolation media for *Aeromonas*. *Can. J. Microbiol.* **53:**39–44.

31. Israil, A. M., M. C. Balotescu, I. Alexandru, and G. Dobre. 2003. Discordancies between classical and API 20E microtest biochemical identification of *Vibrio* and *Aeromonas* strains. *Bacteriol. Virusol. Parazitol. Epidemiol.* **48:**141–143. (In Romanian.)

32. Janda, J. M. 2001. *Aeromonas* and *Plesiomonas*, p. 1237–1270. In M. Sussman (ed.), *Molecular Medical Microbiology*, vol. 2. Academic Press, London, United Kingdom.

33. Janda, J. M., and S. L. Abbott. 1998. Evolving concepts regarding the genus *Aeromonas*: an expanding panorama of species, disease presentations, and unanswered questions. *Clin. Infect. Dis.* **27:**332–344.

34. Janda, J. M., and S. L. Abbott. 2010. The genus *Aeromonas*: taxonomy, pathogenicity, and infection. *Clin. Microbiol. Rev.* **23:**35–73.

35. Janda, J. M., S. L. Abbott, and J. G. Morris. 1995. *Aeromonas*, *Plesiomonas* and *Edwardsiella*, p. 905–917. In M. J. Blaser, P. D. Smith, J. I. Ravdin, H. B. Greenberg, and R. L. Guerrant (ed.), *Infections of the Gastrointestinal Tract*. Raven Press, Ltd., New York, NY.

36. Kämpfer, P., C. Christmann, J. Swings, and G. Huys. 1999. In vitro susceptibilities of *Aeromonas* genomic species to 69 antimicrobial agents. *Syst. Appl. Microbiol.* **22:**662–669.

37. Kelly, K. A., E. J. M. Koehler, and L. R. Ashdown. 1993. Spectrum of extraintestinal disease due to *Aeromonas* species in tropical Queensland, Australia. *Clin. Infect. Dis.* **16:**574–579.

38. Kilpatrick, M. E., J. Escamilla, A. L. Bourgeois, H. J. Adkins, and R. C. Rockhill. 1987. Overview of four U.S. Navy overseas research studies on *Aeromonas*. *Experientia* **43:**365–367.

39. Ko, W. C., K. W. Yu, C. Y. Liu, C. T. Huang, H. S. Leu, and Y. C. Chuang. 1996. Increasing antibiotic resistance in clinical isolates of *Aeromonas* strains in Taiwan. *Antimicrob. Agents Chemother.* **40:**1260–1262.

40. Lai, C., L. Ding, and P. Hsueh. 2007. Wound infection and septic shock due to *Aeromonas trota* in a patient with liver cirrhosis. *Clin. Infect. Dis.* **44:**1523.

41. Lee, C., C. Chi, N. Lee, H. Lee, C. Chen, P. Chen, C. Chang, C. Wu, N. Ko, M. Tsai, and W. Ko. 2008. Necrotizing fasciitis in patients with liver cirrhosis: a predominance of monomicrobial gram-negative bacillary infections. *Diagn. Microbiol. Infect. Dis.* **62:**219–225.

42. Li, L., Z. Du, X. Sun, X. Shao, J. Li, L. Zhang, Y. Wang, and Q. Wu. 2008. Severe pneumonia caused by *Aeromonas veronii* biovar sobria: a case report and review of the literature. *Zhonghua Jie He He Hu Xi Za Zhi* **31:**736–739.

43. Liu, C.-Y., Y.-T. Huang, C.-H. Liao, and P.-R. Hsueh. 2008. In vitro activities of tigecycline against clinical isolates of *Aeromonas*, *Vibrio*, and *Salmonella* species in Taiwan. *Antimicrob. Agents Chemother.* **52:**2677–2679.

44. Maegele, M., S. Gregor, E. Steinhausen, B. Bouillon, M. M. Heiss, W. Perbix, F. Wappler, D. Rixen, J. Geisen,

B. Berger-Schreck, and R. Schwarz. 2005. The long-distance tertiary air transfer and care of tsunami victims: injury pattern and microbiological and psychological aspects. *Crit. Care Med.* **33:**1178–1180.

45. **Martin-Carnahan, A., and S. W. Joseph.** 2005. *Aeromonas*, p. 556–578. *In* D. J. Brenner, N. R. Krieg, J. T. Staley, and G. M. Garrity (ed.), *Bergey's Manual of Systematic Bacteriology*, 2nd ed., vol. 2. Springer-Verlag, New York, NY.

46. **Martinez-Murcia, A., A. Monera, A. Alperi, M. Figueras, and M. Saavedra.** 2009. Phylogenetic evidence suggests that strains of *Aeromonas hydrophila* subsp. *dhakensis* belong to the species *Aeromonas aquariorum* sp. nov. *Curr. Microbiol.* **58:**76–80.

47. **Martinez-Murcia, A. J.** 1999. Phylogenetic positions of *Aeromonas encheleia*, *Aeromonas popoffii*, *Aeromonas* DNA hybridization group 11 and *Aeromonas* group 501. *Int. J. Syst. Bacteriol.* **49:**1403–1408.

48. **Martinez-Murcia, A. J., S. Benlloch, and M. D. Collins.** 1992. Phylogenetic interrelationships of members of the genera *Aeromonas* and *Plesiomonas* as determined by 16S ribosomal DNA sequencing: lack of congruence with results of DNA-DNA hybridizations. *Int. J. Syst. Bacteriol.* **42:**412–421.

49. **Martinez-Murcia, A. J., M. Saavedra, V. Mota, T. Maier, E. Stackebrandt, and S. Cousin.** 2008. *Aeromonas aquariorum* sp. nov., isolated from aquaria of ornamental fish. *Int. J. Syst. Evol. Microbiol.* **58:**1169–1175.

50. **Mencacci, A., E. Cenci, R. Mazzolla, S. Farinelli, F. D'Alo, M. Vitali, and F. Bistoni.** 2003. *Aeromonas veronii* biovar veronii septicaemia and acute suppurative cholangitis in a patient with hepatitis B. *J. Med. Microbiol.* **52:**727–730.

51. **Minana-Galbis, D., M. Farfan, M. Fuste, and J. Loren.** 2007. *Aeromonas bivalvium* sp. nov., isolated from bivalve mollusks. *Int. J. Syst. Evol. Microbiol.* **57:**582–587.

52. **Monaghan, S., D. Anjaria, A. Mohr, and D. Livingston.** 2008. Necrotizing fasciitis and sepsis caused by *Aeromonas hydrophila* after crush injury of the lower extremity. *Surg. Infect.* **9:**459–467.

53. **Morandi, A., O. Zhaxybayeva, J. P. Gogarten, and J. Graf.** 2005. Evolutionary and diagnostic implications of intragenomic heterogeneity in the 16S rRNA gene in *Aeromonas* strains. *J. Bacteriol.* **187:**6561–6564.

54. **Mullholland, A., and S. Yong-Gee.** 2008. A possible new cause of spa bath folliculitis: *Aeromonas hydrophila*. *Australas. J. Dermatol.* **49:**39–41.

55. **Nhung, P., H. Hata, K. Ohkusu, M. Noda, M. Shah, K. Goto, and T. Ezaki.** 2007. Use of the novel phylogenetic marker *dnaJ* and DNA-DNA hybridization to clarify interrelationships within the genus *Aeromonas*. *Int. J. Syst. Evol. Microbiol.* **57:**1232–1237.

56. **Ouderkirk, J. P., D. Bekhor, G. S. Turett, and R. Murali.** 2004. *Aeromonas* meningitis complicating medicinal leech therapy. *Clin. Infect. Dis.* **38:**36–37.

57. **Overman, T. L., and J. M. Janda.** 1999. Antimicrobial susceptibility patterns of *Aeromonas jandaei*, *A. schubertii*, *A. trota*, and *A. veronii* biotype veronii. *J. Clin. Microbiol.* **37:**706–708.

58. **Pinna, A., L. A. Sechi, S. Zanetti, D. Usai, and F. Carta.** 2004. *Aeromonas caviae* keratitis associated with contact lens wear. *Ophthalmology* **111:**348–351.

59. **Presley, S., T. Rainwater, G. Austin, S. Platt, J. Zak. G. Cobb, E. Marsland, K. Tian, B. Zhang, T. Anderson, S. Cox, M. Abel, B. Leftwich, J. Huddleston, R. Jeter, and R. Kendall.** 2006. Assessment of pathogens and toxicants in New Orleans, LA following Hurricane Katrina. *Environ. Sci. Technol.* **40:**468–474.

60. **Reith, M., R. Singh, B. Curtis, J. Boyd, A. Bouevitch, J. Kimball, J. Munholland, C. Murphy, D. Sarty, J. Williams, J. Nash, S. Johnson, and L. Brown.** 2008. The genome of *Aeromonas salmonicida* subsp. *salmonicida* A449: insights into the evolution of a fish pathogen. *BMC Genomics* **9:**427–441.

61. **Robinson, J., J. Beaman, L. Wagener, and V. Burke.** 1986. Comparison of direct plating with the use of enrichment culture for isolation of *Aeromonas* spp. from faeces. *J. Med. Microbiol.* **22:**315–317.

62. **Rodriguez, C. N., R. Campos, B. Pastran, I. Jimenez, A. Garcia, P. Meijomil, and A. J. Rodriguez-Morales.** 2005. Sepsis due to extended-spectrum β-lactamase producing *Aeromonas hydrophila* in a pediatric patient with diarrhea and pneumonia. *Clin. Infect. Dis.* **41:**421–422.

63. **Rossolini, G. M., T. Walsh, and G. Amicosante.** 1996. The *Aeromonas* metallo-β-lactamases: genetics, enzymology, and contribution to drug resistance. *Microb. Drug Resist.* **2:**245–251.

64. **Sanchez-Cespedes, J., M. J. Figueras, C. Aspiroz, M. J. Aldea, M. Toledo, A. Alperi, F. Marco, and J. Vila.** 2009. Development of imipenem resistance in an *Aeromonas veronii* biovar sobria clinical isolate recovered from a patient with cholangitis. *J. Med. Microbiol.* **58:**451–455.

65. **Sartor, C., F. Limouzin-Perotti, R. Legre, et al.** 2002. Nosocomial infections with *Aeromonas hydrophila* from leeches. *Clin. Infect. Dis.* **35:**E1.

66. **Seshadri, R., S. W. Joseph, A. K. Chopra, J. Sha, J. Shaw, J. Graf, D. Haft, M. Wu, Q. Ren, M. J. Rosovitz, R. Madupu, L. Tallon, M. Kim, S. Jin, H. Vuong, O. C. Stine, A. Ali, A. J. Horneman, and J. F. Heidelberg.** 2006. Genome sequence of *Aeromonas hydrophila* ATCC 7966ᵀ: jack of all trades. *J. Bacteriol.* **188:**8272–8282.

67. **Shiina, Y., K. Ii, and M. Iwanaga.** 2004. An *Aeromonas veronii* biovar sobria infection with disseminated intravascular gas production. *J. Infect. Chemother.* **10:**37–41.

68. **Sinha, S., T. Shimada, T. Ramamurthy, S. K. Bhattacharya, S. Yamasaki, Y. Takeda, and G. B. Nair.** 2004. Prevalence, serotype distribution, antibiotic susceptibility and genetic profiles of mesophilic *Aeromonas* species isolated from hospitalized diarrhoeal cases in Kolkata, India. *J. Med. Microbiol.* **53:**527–534.

69. **Soler, L., F. Marco, J. Vila, M. R. Chacón, J. Guarro, and M. J. Figueras.** 2003. Evaluation of two miniaturized systems, MicroScan W/A and BBL Crystal E/NF, for identification of clinical isolates of *Aeromonas* spp. *J. Clin. Microbiol.* **41:**5732–5734.

70. **Soler, L., M. A. Yanez, M. R. Chacon, M. G. Aguilera-Arreola, V. Catalan, M. J. Figueras, and A. J. Martinez-Murcia.** 2004. Phylogenetic analysis of the genus *Aeromonas* based on two housekeeping genes. *Int. J. Syst. Evol. Microbiol.* **54:**1511–1519.

71. **Tena, D., C. Aspiroz, M. J. Figueras, A. Gonzalez-Praetorius, M. J. Aldea, A. Alperi, and J. Bisquert.** 2009. Surgical site infection due to *Aeromonas* species: report of nine cases and literature review. *Scand. J. Infect. Dis.* **41:**164–170.

72. **Tulsidas, H., Y. Y. Ong, and K. C. Chan.** 2008. Case report: *Aeromonas hydrophila* bacteraemia and portal pyaemia. *Singapore Med. J.* **49:**346–358.

73. **Vally, H., A. Whittle, S. Cameron, G. K. Dowse, and T. Watson.** 2004. Outbreak of *Aeromonas hydrophila* wound infections associated with mud football. *Clin. Infect. Dis.* **38:**1084–1089.

74. **van der Gaag, E. J., E. Roelofsen, and R. F. Tummers.** 2005. *Aeromonas caviae* infection mimicking inflammatory bowel disease in a child. *Ned. Tijdschr. Geneeskd.* **149:**712–714.

75. **Vila, J., J. Ruiz, F. Gallardo, M. Vargas, L. Soler, M. J. Figueras, and J. Gascon.** 2003. *Aeromonas* spp. and traveler's diarrhea: clinical features and antimicrobial resistance. *Emerg. Infect. Dis.* **9:**552–555.

76. **Vila, J., F. Marco, L. Soler, M. Chacon, and M. J. Figueras.** 2002. *In vitro* antimicrobial susceptibility of clinical isolates of *Aeromonas caviae*, *Aeromonas hydrophila*, and *Aeromonas veronii* biotype sobria. *J. Antimicrob. Chemother.* **49:**701–702.

Vibrio and Related Organisms*

SHARON L. ABBOTT, J. MICHAEL JANDA, AND J. J. FARMER III

39

TAXONOMY

The family *Vibrionaceae* is presently composed of six genera (*Vibrio, Photobacterium, Salinivibrio, Enterovibrio, Grimontia,* and *Aliivibrio*) and over 110 species with standing in bacterial nomenclature (http://www.bacterio.cict.fr/). *Vibrio* is the type genus for the family, and *Vibrio cholerae,* the causative agent of pandemic cholera, is the type species (25). Pathogenic species for humans can be found in three genera, including *Vibrio* (10 species), *Photobacterium,* and *Grimontia* (one species each). Phylogenetic investigations indicate that multiple clades (separate or distinct groups in a phylogenetic sense) exist within this genus, indicating that many *Vibrio* species may eventually be reclassified into different genera. *Photobacterium damselae* is currently the accepted taxon for *Vibrio damsela.* Although definitive DNA relatedness studies are lacking, phylogenetic investigations employing 16S rDNA, *gyrB, rpoA, recA,* and *pyrH* gene sequencing indicate that *P. damselae* clusters within the genus *Photobacterium,* albeit at the extreme periphery to the type species, *P. phosphoreum* (35, 83). *P. damselae* strains also possess defining characters associated with members of the genus *Photobacterium,* including accumulation of poly-β-hydroxybutyrate and the absence of a flagellar sheath (79). Most scientific and medical publications now report infections associated with this taxon as *P. damselae.* When further genetic data become available, the classification of *P. damselae* may need to be reassessed. However, *P. damselae* is clearly not a member of the genus *Vibrio.* One of us (J. J. Farmer III) strongly disagrees with the proposed reclassification of *Vibrio damsela* as *Photobacterium damselae* and will propose (unpublished data) a revised classification in which *Vibrio damsela* will be classified in a new genus rather than in the genus *Photobacterium* (25).

DESCRIPTION OF THE *VIBRIONACEAE*

The *Vibrionaceae* involved in clinical specimens are gram-negative, facultatively anaerobic, straight, curved, or comma-shaped rods, 0.5 to 0.8 μm in width and 1.4 to 2.6 μm in length, that are catalase and oxidase positive (except

Vibrio metschnikovii) (25). Most species are motile by means of sheathed monotrichous or multitrichous polar flagella when grown in liquid media. Strains of some species, such as *V. parahaemolyticus* and *V. alginolyticus,* swarm on solid media by production of numerous lateral flagella (25, 52). All *Vibrionaceae* require Na$^+$ for growth, with the minimal concentration for optimum growth ranging from 0.029 to 4.1% NaCl (25). They also ferment D-glucose but rarely produce gas, reduce nitrate to nitrite (except *Vibrio metschnikovii*), and grow on thiosulfate-citrate-bile salts-sucrose (TCBS) medium. The G+C content of the DNA is 38 to 51 mol% (25). Key properties or characteristics useful in separating clinically significant *Vibrionaceae* from phylogenetically or phenotypically related species are listed in Table 1.

EPIDEMIOLOGY, TRANSMISSION, AND CLINICAL SIGNIFICANCE

The genera covered in this chapter are primarily isolated from marine environments. Vibrios such as *V. cholerae* and *V. mimicus* that require minimal amounts of Na$^+$ for growth can be found in freshwater rivers and lakes as well as estuarine and marine environments. *Vibrionaceae* are commonly isolated from a variety of bivalves and crustaceans, and like other genera found in marine environments, their concentrations peak during the warmer months of the year. In aquatic environments, vibrios can persist in a free-living state or in association with phytoplankton and zooplankton (28, 48, 61, 78). In the environment vibrios may enter a state referred to as viable but nonculturable, in which cells retain basic metabolic processes even though they fail to grow on standard laboratory media (10). Because the viability of these cells is still in question, the term "active but nonculturable" has been proposed (61). Recent studies have shown that in mixed populations of nonculturable and culturable cells of *V. cholerae,* the latter appear to be the main contributors to human infections (61).

The *Vibrionaceae* can be isolated from a wide variety of intestinal and extraintestinal human illnesses. These illnesses include diarrhea, soft tissue disease (cellulitis and necrotizing fasciitis), septicemia, and eye and ear infections (25). In some cases of gastroenteritis and extraintestinal infections it may be difficult to determine if a positive vibrio culture represents true infection or merely colonization because of its widespread occurrence in marine and

---

*This chapter contains information presented in chapter 47 by Sharon L. Abbott, J. Michael Janda, Judith A. Johnson, and J. J. Farmer III in the ninth edition of this *Manual.*

TABLE 1 Properties of the genus *Vibrio* and its relatives: differentiation from other organisms that are phenotypically similar[a]

Test or property	Vibrio	Grimontia	Photobacterium	Aeromonas	Plesiomonas	Enterobacteriaceae
Causes or is associated with intestinal or extraintestinal infections in humans	+	+	+	+	+	+
Oxidase reaction	+	+	+	+	+	−
Enterobacterial common antigen present	−	−	−	−	+	+
Na$^+$ required for, or stimulates, growth	+	+	+	−	−	−
Growth on TCBS agar	+	V[b]	+	−	−	−
Sensitivity to vibriostatic compound O/129[c]	+[d]	+	+	−	+	−
Lipase production	+	−	V	+	−	V
D-Mannitol fermentation	+	−	−	+	−	+

[a]These are general properties of the genera and/or family, but there are exceptions. The properties of *Vibrio* apply to the species that occur in human clinical specimens and may not apply to all nonclinical species. Symbols: +, most strains positive; −, most strains negative.

[b]Strains of *Grimontia hollisae* typically grow poorly or not at all on TCBS agar; those that grow may have a reduced plating efficiency.

[c]O/129, 2,4-diamino-6,7-diisopropylpteridine phosphate (commercially available, 150-μg disks).

[d]Resistance to O/129 has become common in *Vibrio cholerae* strains isolated from India and Bangladesh; *V. cholerae* O139 strains are resistant.

estuarine waters. Ten *Vibrio* species and one species each of *Photobacterium* and *Grimontia* occur in clinical specimens and are listed in Table 2 (25, 56). Extraintestinal *Vibrio* infections are frequently associated with traumatic injuries or inapparent exposure to estuarine or marine waters. Primary septicemia may occur after ingestion of raw seafood (oysters) or as a secondary bacteremia subsequent to a wound infection.

V. cholerae

V. cholerae is the only species that causes endemic, epidemic, and pandemic cholera (20, 68). It is divided into three major subgroups: *V. cholerae* O1, *V. cholerae* O139, and *V. cholerae* non-O1. *Vibrio cholerae* O1 strains may be further subtyped. The three serovars, Inaba, Ogawa, and Hikojima, and the two biotypes, El Tor and classical, can occur in any combination.

V. cholerae O1

In 2007, the WHO reported over 177,000 cases of cholera worldwide, with more than 4,000 deaths (86). In Africa, the current focus of epidemic cholera, case fatality rates approach 5% (54). More than 70,000 infections were reported in Zimbabwe alone between November 2008 and February 2009. The majority of persons ingesting toxigenic *V. cholerae* O1 have asymptomatic infections. Although the ratio of asymptomatic to symptomatic infections is presumed to range from 3 to 100, recent models of infection indicate that the number of asymptomatic infections is much higher and that these undetected infections serve as an ongoing reservoir for cholera in regions of the world where cholera is highly endemic (40). Classic cholera typically results in copious amounts of watery diarrhea passed painlessly, with fluid loss reaching 200 ml/kg of body weight/day. If untreated, the patient becomes prostrate with symptoms of severe dehydration, electrolyte imbalance, painful muscle cramps, watery eyes, loss of skin elasticity, and anuria. Dehydration subsequently leads to hypovolemic shock, acidosis, circulatory collapse, and death, even in previously healthy adults (37). In the United States, occasional cases of classic cholera are seen in travelers returning from regions

of the world where cholera is highly endemic. Traditional therapy consists of fluid replacement by oral rehydration and/or intravenous fluids. The unique ability of *V. cholerae* serogroup O1 to cause this fulminant form of diarrhea is due to the presence of virulence cassette regions and pathogenicity islands on the bacterial chromosome. These regions contain a number of key determinants, including the cholera enterotoxin gene, *ctx*, which is responsible for the large excretion of fluids and electrolytes into the lumen, and a toxin-coregulated pilus gene, *tcpA*, responsible for attachment to the gastrointestinal epithelium (26). Traditional (classical) cholera can be produced by the two biotypes of *V. cholerae* O1, designated classical and El Tor. The first six pandemics were thought to be due to the classical biotype, while the ongoing seventh pandemic, which began in 1961, is caused by the El Tor biotype, which was first isolated in 1905 (68). Recently, genetically evolving hybrid strains of *V. cholerae* O1 have emerged in eastern Africa and Bangladesh (86). These hybrid strains may be more virulent based upon projected case fatality rates. Hybrid strains differ from traditional El Tor or classical isolates in that they carry different combinations of genes from their expected biotype (e.g., El Tor strain with classical *ctxB* on the chromosome) (62). These hybrid strains appear to have evolved via lateral gene transfer and recombination events (81).

V. cholerae O139

In 1992, cholera cases that were attributed to a then new serotype of *V. cholerae*, O139 (synonym: *V. cholerae* O139 Bengal), emerged, particularly in India, Bangladesh, and throughout Asia (3). This serogroup probably resulted from the lateral transfer of a novel somatic antigen and capsule from an unknown bacterium to an El Tor strain (3). O139 and O1 strains carry similar virulence factors, including the *ctx* and *tcpA* genes (56). Clinical diseases due to O1 and O139 *V. cholerae* are also strikingly similar, except that adults are more frequently affected with O139 since previous infection with O1 cholerae is not protective (27). In 2002, O139 reemerged in Bangladesh, causing an estimated 30,000 cases of cholera, primarily in older patients (27). According to the latest WHO report, 41%

TABLE 2 Biochemical test results and other properties of the 12 *Vibrionaceae* species that occur in human clinical specimens[a]

Test[c]	% Positive for[b]:												
	P. shigelloides	*V. cholerae*	*V. mimicus*	*V. metschnikovii*[d]	*V. cincinnatiensis*	*G. hollisae*	*P. damselae*	*V. fluvialis*	*V. furnissii*	*V. alginolyticus*	*V. parahaemolyticus*	*V. vulnificus*[e]	*V. harveyi*
Indole (HIB)	100	99	98	20	8	97	0	13	11	85	98	97	100
VP	0	75	9	96	0	0	95	0	0	95	0	0	50
Moeller's													
Arginine	98	0	0	60	0	0	95	93	100	0	0	0	0
Lysine	99	99	100	35	57	0	50	0	0	99	100	99	100
Ornithine	95	99	99	0	0	100	0	0	0	50	95	55	0
Motility	95	99	98	74	86	0	25	70	89	99	99	99	0
Gelatin	0	90	65	65	0	0	6	85	86	90	95	75	0
hydrolysis (22°C)													
D-Glucose, gas production	0	0	0	0	0	0	10	0	100	0	0	0	
Acid production from:													
L-Arabinose	0	0	1	0	100	97	0	93	100	1	80	0	0
Cellobiose	0	8	0	9	100	0	0	30	11	3	5	99	50
Lactose	80	7	21	50	0	0	0	3	0	0	1	85	0
myo-Inositol	95	0	0	40	100	0	0	0	0	0	0	0	0
Salicin	0	1	0	9	100	0	0	0	0	4	1	95	0
Sucrose	0	100	0	100	100	0	5	100	100	99	1	15	50
ONPG	90	94	90	50	86	0	0	40	35	0	5	75	0
Salt tolerance (growth in nutrient broth with):													
0% NaCl	100	100	100	0	0	0	0	0	0	0	0	0	0
6% NaCl	NA	53	49	78	100	83	95	96	100	100	99	65	100
O/129 susceptibility[f]	100	99	95	90	25	40	90	31	0	19	20	98	100

[a] Abbreviations: HIB, heart infusion broth; VP, Voges-Proskauer; ONPG, o-nitrophenyl-β-D-galactopyranoside; NaCl, sodium chloride; NA, not available.

[b] Percentage of strains positive after 48 h of incubation at 36°C unless otherwise indicated. Most positive reactions occur within 24 h.

[c] 1% NaCl added to all media except salt tolerance tests.

[d] This organism is oxidase negative and does not reduce nitrate to nitrite.

[e] Biogroup 1 strains.

[f] Zone of inhibition present (disk content, 150 μg). Data for *Plesiomonas* are from the Microbial Diseases Laboratory.

of 165 cholera cases reported from China were laboratory confirmed as O139 (86). In contrast, less than 0.5% of >1,400 cholera cases reported by Thailand were O139. To date, no cases of *V. cholerae* O139 infection have been identified in Africa (86).

V. cholerae Non-O1

V. cholerae non-O1 strains (non-O1, non-O139) are the third most commonly isolated vibrios in clinical laboratories in the United States, following *V. parahaemolyticus* and *V. vulnificus*. Unlike O1 strains, non-O1 isolates rarely produce cholera toxin. While the diarrhea produced is watery and severe disease is reported, infections are usually milder than typical cholera. Non-O1 strains of *V. cholerae* that do harbor the cholera toxin gene, such as serogroups O75 and O141, have caused sporadic cases of cholera-like disease in the United States and elsewhere (22, 80). Risk factors for infection appear to be similar to those for other vibrios and include consumption of oysters and other seafoods. Non-O1 vibrios, in contrast to O1 *V. cholerae*, are associated with extraintestinal infections such as septicemia and epidural brain abscess (7, 65). Persons at increased risk of developing non-O1 bacteremia include those with liver disease/cirrhosis or hematologic malignancies (65). The case fatality rate in these patients ranges from 24 to 65% (42, 65). Strains have also been isolated from ears, wounds, the respiratory tract, and urine (57).

V. mimicus

V. mimicus, a nonhalophilic species, is biochemically similar to *V. cholerae* except that it is sucrose negative. Human infections are uncommon, but it is recovered from patients with diarrhea in which it may or may not have a causal role and is usually associated with consumption of uncooked seafood, particularly raw oysters. Rare strains carry the *ctx* gene and can produce cholera-like symptoms. Symptoms generally include abundant watery diarrhea, vomiting, and severe dehydration. Most descriptions of *V. mimicus* gastroenteritis involve individual case reports, but a large-scale foodborne outbreak of gastroenteritis was reported in Thailand in 2004 (16). In that outbreak, over 300 persons were ill, and rectal swabs collected from 24 patients all yielded *V. mimicus*. Presumptive causes of this outbreak included freshwater fish, seafood, and seafood soup. An earlier outbreak was reported from Costa Rica from 1991 to 1993. It involved 33 persons with *V. mimicus*-associated diarrhea, and raw turtle eggs were the implicated vehicle of infection (11).

V. parahaemolyticus

V. parahaemolyticus is the leading cause of bacterial foodborne intestinal infections in Asia and is almost invariably associated with the consumption of raw fish or shellfish (75). In Japan, 50 to 70% of the cases of foodborne diarrhea are due to *V. parahaemolyticus*. In the United States, it is the *Vibrio* species most frequently isolated from clinical specimens and is primarily associated with watery diarrhea. Symptoms of *V. parahaemolyticus*-associated gastroenteritis often include nausea, vomiting, abdominal cramps, low-grade fever, and chills. Fatalities are extremely rare but can occur in cases of severe dehydration. Rehydration is usually the only treatment needed, but antimicrobial therapy may be beneficial in some instances. A recent outbreak of gastroenteritis involving 22 passengers aboard a cruise ship was linked to Alaskan oysters (53). A now widely dispersed clone of *V. parahaemolyticus*, serotype O3:K6, emerged

worldwide in 1997 (59). Strains of this serotype caused an unusually high proportion of *V. parahaemolyticus* foodborne disease outbreaks in Taiwan from 1996 to 1999, which suggests that there is something unusual regarding its ecology, epidemiology, or virulence. This clone, with several of its serovariants, O4:K68, O1:K25, and O4:K12, has continued to spread throughout Asia and to the United States, Canada, Mexico, Russia, France, Italy, Brazil, Chile, Peru, and Mozambique (59). The serologic variants that have arisen since O3:K6 do not appear to have the same capacity to spread or a propensity for causing as severe infections with hospitalization (59).

V. vulnificus

V. vulnificus causes primary septicemia and wound infection and is responsible for more than 90% of deaths due to vibrios in the United States yearly. Primary septicemia has a fatality rate exceeding 50%, even with hospitalization, and occurs predominantly in men over 50 years old (14, 34). Patients usually have predisposing conditions such as liver disease, immunosuppression, increased serum iron, or other chronic diseases (8, 34). CDC data indicate that >95% of patients consumed raw oysters within 7 days of their infection. Patients typically present with a sudden onset of fever and chills, vomiting, diarrhea, and abdominal pain. Secondary skin lesions often appear, progressing to bulla formation and necrosis. Endotoxic shock often occurs and can rapidly lead to death. Both blood cultures and biopsy samples (scrapings) from skin lesions are usually positive. *V. vulnificus* also causes severe wound infections, usually after trauma and exposure to marine animals or the marine environment (34). Wound infections may progress to cellulitis with extensive necrosis (often requiring surgical debridement), myositis, and necrotizing fasciitis that may mimic gas gangrene, and to secondary septicemia. The fatality rate for wound infections ranges from 20 to 30%. Three biogroups have now been defined for *V. vulnificus* (34). Most infections in the United States are due to biogroup 1; biogroup 2 has been principally isolated from diseased eels and also isolated from one human wound infection. *V. vulnificus* biogroup 3 was described in 1999 and has been limited to wound and blood-borne disease in Israeli patients exposed to live tilapia grown in aquaculture.

V. alginolyticus

V. alginolyticus is very common in the marine ecosystem and is the fourth most commonly isolated *Vibrio* species in the United States. It is most frequently isolated from ear and wound infections following seawater exposure. A 2006 European surveillance report detected three cases in which *V. alginolyticus* was isolated (synovial fluid, hand wound, and otitis) in persons who swam in an inlet of the North Sea (70). *V. alginolyticus* has also been isolated from ocular infections and from infrequent cases of monomicrobial or polymicrobial bacteremia, mostly in immunocompromised persons (15, 45). It is occasionally isolated from diarrheal stool, but there is no evidence that it actually causes diarrhea (82).

Photobacterium damselae (V. damsela)

P. damselae is an aggressive marine pathogen causing serious life-threatening illnesses. Fatality rates for *P. damselae* are unknown, but many reports in the literature describe fatal infections, suggesting a fairly high attributable mortality rate (89). Disease syndromes associated with this bacterium include soft tissue infections (cellulitis and necrotizing fasciitis) and bacteremia. Most wound infections develop as indolent processes that progress to more severe disease within a matter of hours, and vibrios are often not suspected as part of the initial diagnosis. Medical intervention, in addition to antibiotics, is often required, including irrigation, fasciotomy, debridement, and sometimes amputation.

Typically, *P. damselae* wound infections occur in fishermen and result from penetrating traumas caused by fish fins, fish hooks, or harpoons (29, 60, 89). More recently, however, other sources of infection have been reported for this organism. These include a case of cellulitis in a healthy teenage surfer who sustained a laceration to his hand from his surfboard, a 30-month-old child with sickle cell anemia who developed bacteremia after handling fish and then scratching an open wound on her buttock, and a urinary tract infection in a pregnant female with increased frequency of urination and dysuria who had sexual intercourse in the Caribbean Sea 1 week prior to infection (2, 6, 41).

V. fluvialis and V. furnissii

V. fluvialis appears to cause sporadic cases of diarrhea worldwide, with severe cases of gastroenteritis sometimes linked to bacteremia or associated with cholera-like symptoms (5, 44). Based upon published reports, there appears to be a small but increasing incidence of extraintestinal *V. fluvialis* infections. These include acute infectious and continuous ambulatory peritoneal dialysis-associated peritonitis, soft tissue infections (cellulitis) associated with cerebritis, and bacteremia (33, 44, 46, 67). For many of these systemic infections, some of which have poor outcomes, vibrios are, again, not initially suspected as a cause. They are eventually associated with seafood consumption or exposure to seawater. *V. furnissii* is rarely isolated from human clinical specimens, but when it is recovered, it is invariably from fecal specimens of patients with diarrhea (23). There is no convincing evidence that it causes diarrhea.

Miscellaneous Vibrios and *Vibrio*-Like Organisms

V. harveyi (*V. carchariae*) is an important pathogen of marine fish and invertebrate species. To date, there are only two confirmed cases of human infection attributed to *V. harveyi*. The first report was of a wound infection resulting from a shark bite (66). The second report involved a 9-year-old boy with anaplastic large cell lymphoma and central-line sepsis who, after completing chemotherapy and autologous stem cell transplantation, developed a febrile episode after swimming in the Mediterranean Sea (85). There is an anecdotal report of two isolates from blood and gallbladder (histories unavailable) that were retrospectively identified by *rpoB* sequencing (77). *Grimontia hollisae* is a halophilic, vibrio-like species primarily associated with moderate to severe cases of diarrhea, sometimes involving hypovolemic shock (31). Most recorded cases of infection involve a history of consumption of seafood, such as oysters. *V. metschnikovii* is frequently isolated from freshwater and brackish and marine waters. It was first reported to cause peritonitis and bacteremia in a patient with an inflamed gallbladder. Subsequently, it has been isolated from additional patients with bacteremia and, rarely, from wound infections; it has also been reported from cases of cholecystitis, diarrhea, and pneumonia (47, 84). *V. cincinnatiensis* was first reported from a patient with bacteremia and meningitis. Subsequent isolates have been from the stool of a person with diarrhea, from aborted bovine fetuses, and from mussels (87).

COLLECTION, TRANSPORT, AND STORAGE OF SPECIMENS

Pertinent clinical history (when known) should accompany specimens to alert the laboratory to include appropriate isolation media for the *Vibrionaceae* in their stool workup; this is especially important in areas where the isolation of vibrios is infrequent (50). Helpful information includes history of travel, consumption of seafood, activity associated with marine or brackish water or wounds associated with such exposure, and hobbies associated with aquaria.

Vibrionaceae, like other enteric organisms, are particularly susceptible to desiccation, so stool specimens that cannot be inoculated onto plating media within 2 to 4 h should be placed in a transport medium. Cary-Blair or any noninhibitory transport medium that does not contain glycerol is acceptable for vibrios; buffered glycerol in saline is unacceptable because some lots of glycerol may be toxic to vibrios. For specimens collected in the field, if necessary, liquid stool may be placed on strips of blotting paper or gauze, then inserted in airtight plastic bags with a few drops of saline to maintain moisture, and then sent to the laboratory. Detailed information on the collection and transport of specimens for vibrio isolation is available elsewhere (12). Special methods for the collection and processing of extraintestinal specimens (blood, wounds, etc.) for vibrio isolation are not required, as vibrios are, as a rule, isolated in pure culture from these sites and the concentration of salt in primary plating media is usually sufficient for their recovery. Upon isolation, however, salt may need to be added to subsequent media to attain growth of salt-requiring vibrios.

Vibrionaceae may die within weeks in vitro, even in moist environments at room temperature, and should be maintained at −70°C as directed in chapter 9.

DIRECT EXAMINATION

Direct microscopic detection of vibrios in stool is not routinely recommended, since it may not be possible to distinguish pathogenic vibrios from other members of the enteric microbiota.

Direct Detection of *V. cholerae* O1 in Stool

Direct detection of *V. cholerae* from stool requires experience to correctly interpret results and is typically done only in laboratories where cholera is common or in field situations where laboratory services are unavailable and rapid diagnosis is required. One of the oldest assays, the microscopic immobilization test, detects loss of motility of *V. cholerae* O1 organisms by the addition of O1 antibody and can be used to detect *V. cholerae* O139 by using O139 antibody. A direct fluorescent-antibody test, Cholera and Bengal SMART, and a membrane antigen rapid test, SMART Cholera O1, are available from New Horizons Diagnostics Corp., Columbia, MD (FDA approval pending), and a *V. cholerae* O1 latex agglutination assay (Denka Seiken, Tokyo, Japan; not FDA approved for human clinical specimens) is commercially available.

Molecular Detection in Clinical Specimens

Publications on molecular methodologies for detection of *V. cholerae*, *V. parahaemolyticus*, and *V. vulnificus* in stool can be found in the literature starting in the 1990s and are too numerous to cover here. Most of the advantages of PCR-based assays over culture methods apply to vibrios and include the ability to freeze stools for epidemiological studies for delayed testing. Also, in areas where vibrios are rarely isolated and laboratory experience or resources are limited, molecular methods may be more reliable and may provide a shorter turnaround time. Inhibitors in stool may affect the analytical sensitivity of an assay of PCR but can be overcome by dilution of the sample. Current PCR assays for *V. cholerae* use a multiplex PCR that includes primers for the *ctx* gene, *rfb* genes (O antigens, O1, and O139, allowing differentiation of serotypes), and *tcpA* genes (specific for the El Tor and classical biotypes, useful for epidemiological purposes) (32, 38). For clinical strains of *V. parahaemolyticus*, the thermostable direct hemolysin, a major virulence determinant, is a common target for detection, but it is not universally present in strains isolated from human infections (9, 72). In reality, other than for surveys, in areas where *V. cholerae* is seldom isolated or in noncoastal areas where *V. parahaemolyticus* is an infrequent pathogen, the use of PCR is impractical and costly by comparison to alkaline peptone water and TCBS medium.

ISOLATION PROCEDURES

Vibrionaceae associated with human disease can be isolated from routine enteric media, but recovery is enhanced when specific media are used. On MacConkey or salmonella-shigella agar, vibrios present as colorless colonies (with the exception of the lactose-fermenting species, *V. vulnificus*). On sucrose-containing media such as Hektoen and xylose-lysine-deoxycholate, sucrose-positive vibrios associated with human disease such as *V. cholerae*, *V. fluvialis*, *V. alginolyticus*, and some strains of *V. vulnificus* cannot be differentiated from normal enteric biotas that ferment sucrose. The addition of a blood agar plate allows colonies to be screened for oxidase, which may improve recovery of vibrios as well as colonies of *Aeromonas* spp. and *Plesiomonas shigelloides*. *G. hollisae* may grow poorly or not at all on any enteric isolation medium, including TCBS; it is probably most reliably isolated from blood agar.

TCBS agar is formulated specifically for the isolation of vibrios (25). Both powdered formulations and prepared plates are readily available from a number of commercial sources. Autoclaving is not required, so powdered media may be kept available in the laboratory and easily prepared by boiling as needed. Inclusion of sucrose allows for preliminary differentiation of *Vibrio* species, with *V. cholerae*, *V. fluvialis*, and *V. alginolyticus* producing yellow colonies while *V. parahaemolyticus*, *V. mimicus*, and most strains of *V. vulnificus* produce green colonies (sucrose not fermented). It should be noted that yellow colonies may convert to green if plates are examined after more than 24 h or are refrigerated after incubation. Oxidase testing is unreliable when performed directly on colonies growing on this medium. Growth from a non-sugar-containing medium such as nutrient agar should be used for oxidase testing.

A chromogenic agar, CHROMagar Vibrio (CHROMagar Microbiology, Paris, France), has been developed primarily for the recovery of *V. parahaemolyticus* from seafood and supports the growth of other vibrios as well (30). *Vibrio* colonies on this medium range in color from milk white to pale blue to violet. Other members of the enteric biota usually do not grow, with the exception of *Proteus mirabilis* and *Providencia rettgeri*, which also produce milk white colonies. Marine agar (BD Biosciences, Sparks, MD), which does not contain any inhibitory or selective ingredients, may be more appropriate for isolation of vibrios from the environment, especially salt-requiring vibrios, because of its high salt content.

It is common for pure cultures of vibrios to produce multiple colony morphologies (as many as five) on any medium, but this phenomenon is most readily noticeable on nonselective media such as blood or heart infusion agars. Variations in morphology include smooth, rough, convex, flat, spreading, and compact in various combinations. Occasionally *V. cholerae* produces rugose (extremely wrinkled) colonies on non-carbohydrate-containing media (4). Like their smooth counterparts, they are fully virulent for humans (90). Rugosity, which is due to production of a unique extracellular polysaccharide, confers biofilm formation and resistance to chlorine, acid pH, and serum killing (4, 90). Although it is believed to enhance survival in aquatic environments, to date it has been demonstrated only in vitro. Classical biotypes of *V. cholerae* also possess the *vps* (vibrio polysaccharide synthesis) gene cluster that encodes this phenotype, but rugose variants have been demonstrated only in El Tor strains (90).

In acute diarrheal disease, stool enrichment is generally not required; however, when enrichment is necessary, alkaline peptone water (1% NaCl, pH 8.5) is the most commonly used enrichment broth for human specimens. It should be incubated at 36°C and subcultured at 18 h. Occasionally, vibrios are recovered only after a shorter incubation (6 h), and for these specimens longer incubation times fail to yield a vibrio, probably due to overgrowth by other organisms (S. Abbott, personal observation).

IDENTIFICATION

Conventional Biochemicals

Biochemical properties that separate members of the *Vibrionaceae* from the *Enterobacteriaceae* (including *Plesiomonas shigelloides*) and the *Aeromonadaceae* are found in Table 1, and biochemical profiles of the 12 species that occur in human clinical specimens are given in Table 2. Generally, species are 0 to 10% positive for the following: H_2S in triple sugar iron, urea (except *V. parahaemolyticus*, 15%), phenylalanine deaminase (except *V. vulnificus* biogroup 1, 35%), malonate, mucate, yellow pigment production, and fermentation of D-adonitol, dulcitol, melibiose (except *V. vulnificus* biogroup 1, 40%), raffinose, L-rhamnose (except *V. furnissii*, 45%), D-sorbitol (except *V. metschnikovii*, 45%), α-methyl-β-D-glucoside, and D-xylose (except for *V. cincinnatiensis*, 57 and 43%, respectively). Variable reactions are seen with methyl red, growth in potassium cyanide broth, D-galactose, glycerol, sodium acetate, DNase at 25°C, and lipase. All species are 99 to 100% positive for growth in 1% NaCl and fermentation of maltose (except *G. hollisae*, 0%) and D-mannose (except *V. cholerae*, 78%, and *V. harveyi*, 50%). Many commercial standard tube tests have sufficient salt to support growth without salt supplementation (0.5 to 1%), but the Microbial Diseases Laboratory, California Department of Public Health, routinely adds 1% salt to all biochemicals (except for the 0% salt broth) for all NaCl-requiring species. Voges-Proskauer, Moeller's decarboxylases and dihydrolase, and nitrate broth may contain no or insufficient NaCl to support growth of some NaCl-requiring strains, and these biochemicals should always have salt added to them (to a final concentration of 1%; for occasional strains, 3%) when these species are tested.

It should be noted that many *V. cholerae* O1 strains from Bangladesh and surrounding areas and all strains of *V. cholerae* O139 are resistant to both 10- and 150-μg disks of the vibriostatic compound O/129 (Remel, Lenexa, KS), a classical test used to distinguish vibrios (Table 1). In areas of the world where cholera is uncommon, complete biochemical testing should be performed and all cultures identified as *V. cholerae* should be sent to public health laboratories for O1 and O139 agglutination and cholera toxin testing. *V. cholerae* O1 isolates should be biotyped to determine whether they are the El Tor or classical biotype. These biotypes can be differentiated by a number of phenotypic tests, including hemolysis of sheep erythrocytes, production of acetylmethylcarbinol (Voges-Proskauer test), and resistance to polymyxin B, all positive for the El Tor biotype. Except for the O serotype and O/129 reaction, *V. cholerae* O139 strains are phenotypically similar to *V. cholerae* O1 El Tor. Strains of *V. cholerae* that fail to agglutinate in either O1 or O139 antiserum are reported as *V. cholerae* non-O1. Serotyping for non-O1 strains is available only in a limited number of reference laboratories and is rarely complete. *V. cholerae* and *V. mimicus* are separated from other species by growth in media lacking NaCl (Difco, BD BioSciences, Nutrient Broth is the only broth that accurately determines NaCl requirement). Strains of *V. parahaemolyticus*, *V. alginolyticus*, and *P. damselae* may be urea positive. Most vibrios isolated from humans produce a buff or tan pigment; however, strains of *V. parahaemolyticus* may produce a dark brown pigment. *G. hollisae* generally grows poorly, especially in Moeller's decarboxylases and dihydrolase broths, even after salt supplementation and produces extremely large zones of inhibition, often necessitating the use of two plates when disk antimicrobial susceptibility testing is performed. *V. metschnikovii* is distinctive because it is an oxidase- and nitrate-negative vibrio. *V. fluvialis* and *V. furnissii* are frequently confused with *Aeromonas caviae*, especially as some strains are weakly halophilic and only moderately susceptible to O/129, and because some strains of *A. caviae* grow on TCBS agar. *V. furnissii* is the only vibrio isolated from humans that is positive for gas production from D-glucose. Rapid, correct identification of *V. vulnificus* strains is critical because of the mortality associated with this organism. Some strains of *V. vulnificus* are sucrose positive, which may add to the confusion in identifying it.

Commercial Systems

There are no recent studies evaluating commercial systems' ability to identify organisms covered in this chapter; however, based on individual case reports, identification of these organisms by commercial systems remains problematic (21, 58, 69). No commercial system includes all 12 clinical species in its database, and some manual systems do not contain any of these species (63, 64). The most recent evaluation indicates that when tested only against those species listed in their databases, the API 20E (bioMerieux Inc., Durham, NC), Crystal E/NF (BD Biosciences), MicroScan Neg ID type 2 and type 3 (Siemens Healthcare Systems, West Sacramento, CA), and Vitek GNI+ and ID-GNB cards (bioMerieux) correctly identified only 63 to 81% of these organisms to the species level (64). Correct identification of the three most commonly isolated species of *Vibrio* from clinical samples varied. For *V. cholerae*, API 20E gave the least (50%) and Crystal the most (97%) accurate identification. For *V. parahaemolyticus*, Rapid Neg ID3 fared the worst (40%) and API 20E and GNI+ the best (97% each), while for *V. vulnificus* biogroup 1 strains, GNI+ (50%) and Crystal E/NF (97%) gave the lowest and highest rates (64). Only Crystal E/NF was able to correctly identify ≥90% of *V. cholerae* or *V. vulnificus* strains, and only API 20E and the two Vitek cards correctly

identified ≥90% of *V. parahaemolyticus* strains. In another study using only *V. vulnificus* biotype 3 strains, MicroScan (98%) and Phoenix (90%) systems did the best in identifying 51 well-characterized isolates to the correct species, while the identification rate on Vitek (13.7%) was much less satisfactory (19). Croci et al. (21) found that for the identification of *V. parahaemolyticus*, API 20NE exhibited greater sensitivity than API 20E (20 versus 16 of 27) but that API 20E was more specific (100% versus 82%). In another study on a mixture of 111 clinical and environmental *V. vulnificus* strains, API 20E, API 20NE, and Biolog (Biolog, Inc., Hayward, CA) correctly identified 60, 0, and 85%, respectively. Of the above products, only Biolog is not FDA approved for use on clinical isolates (69).

Manufacturers' instructions should be checked prior to testing of salt-requiring vibrios to determine if salt supplementation is required. A recent publication indicated that API 20E gave incorrect identifications for clinical isolates of *V. parahaemolyticus* if 2.0% NaCl was used for the diluent, versus 0.85% (51). For clinical isolates of *V. alginolyticus*, either concentration yielded identifications with high probabilities, but for *V. vulnificus*, the 0.85% diluent failed to identify 1 of 2 isolates, whereas the 2.0% NaCl identified both strains with ≥94% probabilities.

Molecular Methods

Molecular identification of vibrios is commonplace in surveys and in research studies. However, it is not commonly employed in clinical laboratories for routine identification because vibrios are relatively rare pathogens in noncoastal areas or regions where cholera is not endemic. Additionally, few, if any, commercial molecular products are FDA approved for human clinical specimens, and insufficient strains are available in most laboratories to validate in-house molecular methods in compliance with Clinical Laboratory Improvement Amendments regulations. The use of 16S rDNA sequencing alone is less than ideal for *Vibrionaceae* identification, as interspecies sequence differences are very small (1 to 6%) and polymorphism has been shown to be fairly common in 16S rRNA genes (55). Tarr et al. (77) developed a multiplex PCR assay, using primers directed at *V. cholerae sodB*, *V. mimicus sodB*, *V. parahaemolyticus flaE*, and *V. vulnificus hsp* genes, that correctly identified 109 isolates and found an additional 4 strains of *V. parahaemolyticus* that either had not been identified to species level (*n* = 3) or had been identified incorrectly as *V. alginolyticus* (*n* = 1). Additionally, *rpoB* gene sequencing was used to identify 12 of 15 isolates not previously identified to species level by biochemical methods. In other studies the *toxR* gene (*V. parahaemolyticus*), *vvhA* (hemolysin, *V. vulnificus*), *vcg* genes (virulence-correlated gene, *V. cholerae*), *wbe* and *wbf* genes (for the O1 and O139 serotypes, respectively), and *tcpA* genes (specific for the El Tor and classical biotypes) have been used for identification (21, 38, 69, 91). Matrix-assisted laser desorption/ionization time-of-flight mass spectrometry promises to be a valuable new tool for identification of closely related bacterial species, with a rapid turnaround time and modest test cost. At this time there are no published studies with vibrios, but future studies should validate the usefulness of this methodology.

V. cholerae and *V. parahaemolyticus* Toxin Detection

In reference laboratories, cholera toxin was traditionally detected by fluid accumulation in animal assays or detection of a cytopathic effect in Y1 adrenal or Chinese hamster ovary cell cultures. A reverse passive latex agglutination assay, VET-RPLA (Denka Seiken), which detects both cholera toxin and the heat-labile toxin of *Escherichia coli*, is commercially available. The majority of human strains of *V. parahaemolyticus* produce a thermostable direct hemolysin encoded by two genes, *tdh* and *tdh2x*. These toxins are rarely produced by environmental strains of *V. parahaemolyticus* but have been detected in *V. cholerae* non-O1, *V. mimicus,* and *G. hollisae* strains. Like cholera toxin, thermostable direct hemolysin can be detected by a commercial latex assay (KAP-RPLA; Denka Seiken), but there are no commercial products that detect the thermostable related hemolysin seen in *V. parahaemolyticus* strains. PCR assays for both hemolysins have been developed but are not commercially available (24).

TYPING SYSTEMS

Serotyping
Serotyping is the most widely utilized conventional procedure. Typing schemes have been described for a number of species, including *V. cholerae*, *V. parahaemolyticus*, and *V. vulnificus*; however, commercial-grade typing sera are available only for *V. cholerae* and *V. parahaemolyticus* (73, 74). *V. cholerae* O1 (polyclonal, Inaba and Ogawa) and O139 antisera are available from BD Biosciences, Denka Seiken, Remel, and New Horizons. *V. parahaemolyticus* antisera (11 O groups and 9 polyvalent and 65 monovalent K groups) are available from Denka Seiken.

Molecular Typing of Vibrios
Because it is well standardized, pulsed-field gel electrophoresis using NotI and SfiI enzymes is probably the "gold standard" for molecular typing of vibrios (36, 80, 90). Ribotyping appears to be less discriminatory (13, 69). Kotetishvili et al. (43) found multilocus sequence typing more discriminatory than pulsed-field gel electrophoresis for *V. cholerae*. Multilocus sequence typing, arbitrarily primed PCR, group-specific PCR of the *toxRS* gene, and PCR for the *orf8* sequence of phage f237 (the last two are species specific) have been used with success for *V. parahaemolyticus*, particularly for serovariants of the O3:K6 clone (9, 59, 72). Likewise, for *V. vulnificus*, repetitive extragenic palindromic PCR is an effective subtyping method (34). Sequencing of genes such as *ctxA*, *ctxB*, *hsp60*, and *recA* has also been used for molecular typing of *Vibrionaceae* (37).

SEROLOGIC TESTS
Reagents for the serodiagnosis of cholera are available only in specialized reference laboratories, but titration of acute- and convalescent-phase sera in agglutination, vibriocidal, or antitoxin tests is extremely reliable (49).

ANTIMICROBIAL SUSCEPTIBILITIES
Generally, for most *V. cholerae* and *V. parahaemolyticus* gastrointestinal infections, treatment by rehydration is recommended over antimicrobial therapy and has the added benefit of reducing the risk of antibiotic resistance. Antimicrobial therapy, however, can reduce the duration of diarrhea, shedding of the organism, and the volume of rehydration fluids needed for recovery, and patients are often treated before culture results are known (80). Clinical and Laboratory Standards Institute (CLSI) document M45-A

includes susceptibility testing guidelines for noncholera vibrios (17). The CLSI interpretive guidelines are limited to ampicillin, tetracyclines, folate pathway inhibitors, and chloramphenicol for *V. cholerae* (18). In vitro susceptibility surveys show *V. cholerae* strains to be susceptible (>90%) to aminoglycosides, azithromycin, fluoroquinolones, extended-spectrum cephalosporins, carbapenems, and monobactams (71, 88). However, a conjugative transposon designated the SXT element and carrying resistance to sulfamethoxazole, trimethoprim, chloramphenicol, and streptomycin emerged first in *V. cholerae* O139 strains in India and is now seen in O1, non-O1, and O139 cholera strains and *V. fluvialis* (1). Ahmed et al. (1) have reported on a *V. fluvialis* isolate with the SXT element and a novel aminoglycoside acetyltransferase gene encoding resistance to gentamicin; resistance to ampicillin, furazolidone, and nalidixic acid was also reported. Multidrug-resistant strains of *V. fluvialis* have also been noted among other strains from India (13). *V. parahaemolyticus* is generally susceptible to most antibiotics used for traveler's diarrhea (72). The fluoroquinolones alone or the synergistic combination of ciprofloxacin and cefotaxime shows excellent in vitro activity against *V. vulnificus* strains (39, 76).

EVALUATION, INTERPRETATION, AND REPORTING OF RESULTS
Isolation of *V. cholerae* O1 or O139 should be reported immediately to the attending physician because of the severe dehydration that cholera can produce. The case should also be phoned to public health authorities and the isolate sent to a public health laboratory for confirmation and toxin testing.

When vibrios are isolated from blood or cerebrospinal fluid (bacteremia and meningitis are associated with high mortality rates) or wound infections which cause extensive tissue damage (*V. vulnificus* and *P. damselae*), the results should also be phoned immediately to the attending physician so that rapid and appropriate antibiotic therapy can be initiated. This is especially true for *V. vulnificus* infections, which have a high mortality rate without rapid, appropriate intervention. The clinical significance of *Vibrio* strains (*V. mimicus*, *V. alginolyticus*, *G. hollisae*, *V. harveyi*, and *V. metschnikovii*) in other specimens, particularly stool, may be more difficult to determine and requires prompt consultation with the attending physician to better understand the clinical context. Most physicians are not familiar with many *Vibrionaceae* species, and a phone consultation would be mutually beneficial to the clinician and laboratory provider. Information helpful to the physician would include the presence or absence of other pathogens and the relative amount of growth (pure or almost pure culture) of the vibrio. *Vibrionaceae* isolates should also be submitted to public health laboratories, as they are monitored under the CDC's International Emerging Infections Program and Vibrio Surveillance System; they may also be needed for confirmation and toxin testing.

Vibrionaceae species that are known to cause diarrhea should be considered clinically significant, particularly if they are present in large numbers and no other potential pathogens are present. Isolation of vibrios from stool in small numbers may only reflect transitory colonization; however, species such as *V. cholerae*, *V. mimicus*, and *V. parahaemolyticus* have documented virulence factors that correlate with their ability to cause intestinal infections. Laboratory tests helpful in determining pathogenic potential are primarily available only in reference laboratories. *Vibrionaceae* isolation from locations such as the ears may represent infection, transient colonization, or merely their presence after exposure to seawater. Again, isolation of *Vibrionaceae* requires prompt consultation with the clinician to better understand the clinical context that can help direct the need for further laboratory investigations.

Finally, readers should also be cautioned that misidentification of *Vibrio* species and their relatives can be a problem in the literature unless investigators used methods that are very sensitive in differentiating all of the species in the family *Vibrionaceae* (25).

REFERENCES

1. **Ahmed, A. M., S. Shinoda, and T. Shimamoto.** 2005. A variant type of *Vibrio cholerae* SXT element in a multi-drug resistant strain of *Vibrio fluvialis. FEMS Microbiol. Lett.* **242:**241–247.

2. **Aigbivbalu, L., and N. Maraqa.** 2009. *Photobacterium damsela* wound infection in a 14-year-old surfer. *South. Med. J.* **102:**425–426.

3. **Albert, M. J., and G. B. Nair.** 2005. *Vibrio cholerae* O139—10 years on. *Rev. Med. Microbiol.* **16:**135–143.

4. **Ali, A., J. G. Morris, and J. A. Johnson.** 2005. Sugars inhibit expression of the rugose phenotype of *Vibrio cholerae. J. Clin. Microbiol.* **43:**1426–1429.

5. **Alton, D. R., M. A. Forgione, Jr., and S. P. Gros.** 2006. Cholera-like presentation in *Vibrio fluvialis* enteritis. *South. Med. J.* **99:**765–767.

6. **Alvarez, J. R., S. Lamba, K. Y. Dyer, and J. J. Apuzzio.** 2006. An unusual case of urinary tract infection in a pregnant woman with *Photobacterium damsela. Infect. Dis. Obstet. Gynecol.* **2006:**80682.

7. **Arnett, M. V., S. L. Fraser, and P. E. McFadden.** 2008. Non-O1 *Vibrio cholerae* epidural brain infection in a 12-year-old boy after a depressed skull fracture. *Pediatr. Infect. Dis. J.* **27:**284–285.

8. **Barton, J. C., and R. C. Ratard.** 2006. *Vibrio vulnificus* bacteremia associated with chronic lymphocytic leukemia, hypogammaglobulinemia, and hepatic cirrhosis: relation to host and exposure factors in 252 *V. vulnificus* infections reported in Louisiana. *Am. J. Med. Sci.* **332:**216–220.

9. **Bhoopong, P., P. Palittapongarnpim, R. Pomwised, A. Kiatkittipong, M. Kamruzzaman, Y. Nakaguchi, M. Nishibuchi, M. Ishibashi, and V. Vuddhakul.** 2007. Variability of properties of *Vibrio parahaemolyticus* strains isolated from individual patients. *J. Clin. Microbiol.* **45:**1544–1550.

10. **Binsztein, N., M. C. Costagliola, M. Pichel, V. Jurquiza, F. C. Ramírez, R. Akselman, M. Vacchino, A. Huq, and R. R. Colwell.** 2004. Viable but nonculturable *Vibrio cholerae* O1 in the aquatic environment. *Appl. Environ. Microbiol.* **70:**7481–7486.

11. **Campos, E., H. Bolaños, M. T. Acuña, G. Díaz, M. C. Matamoros, H. Raventós, L. M. Sanchez, C. Barquero, and Red Nacional de Laboratorios para Colera, Costa Rica.** 1996. *Vibrio mimicus* diarrhea following ingestion of raw turtle eggs. *Appl. Environ. Microbiol.* **62:**1141–1144.

12. **Centers for Disease Control and Prevention.** 1999. *Laboratory Methods for the Diagnosis of Epidemic Dysentery and Cholera.* Centers for Disease Control and Prevention. Atlanta, GA. http://www.cdc.gov/ncidod/dbmd/diseaseinfo/cholera/complete.pdf or http://www.cdc.gov.ncidod/dbmd/diseaseinfo/cholera_lab_manual.htm.

13. **Chakraborty, R., S. Chakraborty, K. De, S. Sinha, A. K. Mukhopadhyay, J. Khanam, T. Ramamurthy, Y. Takeda, S. K. Bhattacharya, and G. B. Nair.** 2005. Cytotoxic and cell vacuolating activity of *Vibrio fluvialis* isolated from paediatric patients with diarrhoea. *J. Med. Microbiol.* **54:**707–716.

14. **Chiang, S.-R., and Y.-C. Chuang.** 2003. *Vibrio vulnificus* infection: clinical manifestations, pathogenesis, and antimicrobial therapy. *J. Microbiol. Immunol.* **36:**81–88.

15. **Chien, J. Y., J. T. Shih, P. R. Hsueh, P. C. Yang, and K. T. Luh.** 2002. *Vibrio alginolyticus* as the cause of pleural empyema

16. **Chitov, T., P. Kirikaew, P. Yungyune, N. Ruengprapan, and K. Sontikum.** 2009. An incidence of large foodborne outbreak associated with *Vibrio mimicus. Eur. J. Clin. Microbiol. Infect. Dis.* **28:**421–424.

17. **Clinical and Laboratory Standards Institute.** 2006. *Methods for Antimicrobial Dilution and Disk Susceptibility Testing of Infrequently Isolated or Fastidious Bacteria; Approved Guideline.* CLSI document M45-A. Clinical and Laboratory Standards Institute, Wayne, PA.

18. **Clinical and Laboratory Standards Institute.** 2009. *Performance Standards for Antimicrobial Susceptibility Testing; Nineteenth Informational Supplement.* CLSI document M100-S19. Clinical and Laboratory Standards Institute, Wayne, PA.

19. **Colodner, R., R. Raz, I. Meir, T. Lazarovich, L. Lerner, J. Kopelowitz, Y. Keness, W. Sakran, S. Ken-Dror, and N. Bisharat.** 2004. Identification of the emerging pathogen *Vibrio vulnificus* biotype 3 by commercially available phenotypic methods. *J. Clin. Microbiol.* **42:**4137–4140.

20. **Colwell, R. R.** 2004. Infectious disease and environment: cholera as a paradigm for waterborne disease. *Int. Microbiol.* **7:**285–289.

21. **Croci, L., E. Suffredini, L. Cozzi, D. Ottaviani, C. Pruzzo, P. Serratore, R. Fischetti, E. Goffredo, G. Loffredo, R. Mioni, and the Vibrio parahaemolyticus Working Group.** 2007. Comparison of different biochemical and molecular methods for the identification of *Vibrio parahaemolyticus. J. Appl. Microbiol.* **102:**229–237.

22. **Crump, J. A., C. A. Bopp, K. D. Greene, K. A. Kubota, R. L. Middendorf, J. G. Wells, and E. D. Mintz.** 2003. Toxigenic *Vibrio cholerae* serogroup O141-associated cholera-like diarrhea and bloodstream infection in the United States. *J. Infect. Dis.* **187:**866–888.

23. **Dalsgaard, A., P. Glerup, L.-L. Hoybe, A.-M. Paarup, R. Meza, M. Bernal, T. Shimada, and D. N. Taylor.** 1997. *Vibrio furnissii* isolated from humans in Peru: a possible human pathogen? *Epidemiol. Infect.* **119:**143–149.

24. **DePaola, A., J. Ulaszek, C. A. Kaysner, B. J. Tenge, J. L. Nordstrom, J. Wells, N. Puhr, and S. M. Gendel.** 2003. Molecular, serological, and virulence characteristics of *Vibrio parahaemolyticus* isolated from environmental, food, and clinical resources in North America and Asia. *Appl. Environ. Microbiol.* **69:**3999–4005.

25. **Farmer, J. J., III, J. M. Janda, F. W. Brenner, D. N. Cameron, and K. M. Birkhead.** 2005. Genus I. *Vibrio* Pacini 1854, 411[AL], p. 494–546. *In* D. Brenner, N. Krieg, J. T. Staley, and G. Garrity (ed.), *Bergey's Manual of Systematic Bacteriology,* vol. 2. *The Proteobacteria, Part B. The Gammaproteobacteria.* Springer, New York, NY.

26. **Faruque, S. H., M. J. Albert, and J. J. Mekalanos.** 1998. Epidemiology, genetics, and ecology of toxigenic *Vibrio cholerae. Microbiol. Mol. Biol. Rev.* **62:**1301–1314.

27. **Faruque, S. M., N. Chowdhury, M. Kamruzzaman, Q. S. Ahmad, A. S. G. Faruque, M. A. Salam, T. Ramamurthy, G. B. Nair, A. Weintraub, and D. A. Sack.** 2003. Reemergence of epidemic *Vibrio cholerae* O139, Bangladesh. *Emerg. Infect. Dis.* **9:**1116–1122.

28. **Feldhusen, F.** 2000. The role of seafood in bacterial foodborne diseases. *Microbes Infect.* **2:**1651–1660.

29. **Goodell, K. H., M. R. Jordan, R. Graham, C. Cassidy, and S. A. Nasraway.** 2004. Rapidly advancing necrotizing fasciitis caused by *Photobacterium (Vibrio) damsela*: a hyperaggressive variant. *Crit. Care Med.* **32:**278–281.

30. **Hara-Kudo, Y., T. Nishina, H. Nakagawa, H. Konuma, J. Hasegawa, and S. Kumagai.** 2001. Improved method for detection of *Vibrio parahaemolyticus* in seafood. *Appl. Environ. Microbiol.* **67:**5819–5823.

31. **Hinestrosa, F., R. G. Madeira, and P. P. Bourbeau.** 2007. Severe gastroenteritis and hypovolemic shock caused by *Grimontia (Vibrio) hollisae* infection. *J. Clin. Microbiol.* **45:**3462–3463.

32. **Hoshino, K., S. Yamasaki, A. K. Mukhopadhyay, S. Chakraborty, A. Basu, S. K. Bhattacharya, G. B. Nair, T. Shimada, and Y. Takeda.** 1998. Development and evaluation of a multiplex PCR assay for rapid detection of toxigenic *Vibrio cholerae* O1 and O139. *FEMS Immunol. Med. Microbiol.* **20:**201–207.

33. **Huang, K.-C., and R. W.-W. Hsu.** 2005. *Vibrio fluvialis* hemorrhagic cellulitis and cerebritis. *Clin. Infect. Dis.* **40:**e75–e77.

34. **Jones, M. K., and J. D. Oliver.** 2009. *Vibrio vulnificus:* disease and pathogenesis. *Infect. Immun.* **77:**1723–1733.

35. **Jung, S.-Y., Y.-T. Jung, T.-K. Oh, and J.-H. Yoon.** 2007. *Photobacterium lutimaris* sp. nov., isolated from a tidal flat sediment in Korea. *Int. J. Syst. Evol. Microbiol.* **57:**332–336.

36. **Kam, K. M., C. K. Y. Leuy, M. B. Parsons, K. L. F. Cooper, G. B. Nair, M. Alam, M. A. Islam, D. T. L. Cheung, Y. W. Chu, T. Ramamurthy, G. P. Pazhani, S. K. Bhattacharya, H. Watanabe, J. Terajima, E. Arakawa, O.-A. Ratchtrachenchai, S. Huttayananont, E. M. Ribot, P. Gerner-Smidt, and B. Swaminathan for the *Vibrio parahaemolyticus* PulseNet Protocol Working Group.** 2008. Evaluation and validation of a PulseNet standardized pulsed-field gel electrophoresis protocol for subtyping *Vibrio parahaemolyticus*. *J. Clin. Microbiol.* **46:**2766–2773.

37. **Kaper, J. B., J. G. Morris, and M. M. Levine.** 1995. Cholera. *Clin. Microbiol. Rev.* **8:**48–86.

38. **Khuntia, H. K., B. B. Pal, and G. P. Chhotray.** 2008. Quadruplex PCR for simultaneous detection of serotype, biotype, toxigenic potential, and central regulating factor of *Vibrio cholerae*. *J. Clin. Microbiol.* **46:**2399–2401.

39. **Kim, D.-M., Y. Lym, S. J. Jang, H. Han, Y. G. Kim, C.-H. Chung, and S. P. Hong.** 2005. In vitro efficacy of the combination of ciprofloxacin and cefotaxime against *Vibrio vulnificus*. *Antimicrob. Agents Chemother.* **49:**3489–3491.

40. **King, A. A., E.-L. Ionides, M. Pascual, and M. J. Bouma.** 2008. Inapparent infections and cholera dynamics. *Nature* **454:**877–880.

41. **Knight-Madden, J. M., M. Barton, N. Gandretti, and A. M. Nicholson.** 2005. *Photobacterium damselae* bacteremia in a child with sickle-cell disease. *Pediatr. Infect. Dis. J.* **24:**654–655.

42. **Ko, W.-C., Y.-C. Chuang, G.-C. Huang, and S.-Y. Hsu.** 1998. Infections due to non-O1 *Vibrio cholerae* in southern Taiwan: predominance in cirrhotic patients. *Clin. Infect. Dis.* **27:**774–780.

43. **Kotetishvili, M., O. C. Stine, Y. Chen, A. Kreger, A. Sulakvelidze, S. Sozhamannan, and J. G. Morris.** 2003. Multilocus sequence typing has better discriminatory ability for typing *Vibrio cholerae* than does pulsed-field gel electrophoresis and provides a measure of phylogenetic relatedness. *J. Clin. Microbiol.* **41:**2191–2196.

44. **Lai, C. H., C. K. Hwang, C. Chin, H. H. Lin, W. W. Wong, and C. Y. Liu.** 2005. Severe watery diarrhea and bacteraemia caused by *Vibrio fluvialis*: a first case report. *J. Infect.* **52:**e95–e98.

45. **Lee, D.-Y., S.-Y. Moon, S.-O. Lee, H.-Y. Yang, H.-J. Lee, and M. S. Lee.** 2008. Septic shock due to *Vibrio alginolyticus* in a cirrhotic patient: the first case in Korea. *Yonsei Med. J.* **49:**329–332.

46. **Lee, J. Y., J. S. Park, S. H. Oh, H. R. Kim, J. N. Lee, and J. H. Shin.** 2008. Acute infectious peritonitis caused by *Vibrio fluvialis*. *Diagn. Microbiol. Infect. Dis.* **62:**216–218.

47. **Linde, H.-J., R. Kobuch, S. Jayasinghe, U. Reischl, N. Lehn, S. Kaulfuss, and L. Beutin.** 2004. *Vibrio metschnikovii*, a rare cause of wound infection. *J. Clin. Microbiol.* **42:**4909–4911.

48. **Lipp, E. K., and J. B. Rose.** 1997. The role of seafood in foodborne diseases in the United States of America. *Rev. Sci. Tech.* **16:**620–640.

49. **Losonsky, G. A., and M. M. Levine.** 1997. Immunologic methods for diagnosis of infections caused by diarrheagenic members of the families *Enterobacteriaceae* and *Vibrionaceae*, p. 484–497. *In* N. R. Rose, E. C. de Macario, J. D. Folds, H. C. Lane, and R. M. Nakamura (ed.), *Manual of Clinical Laboratory Immunology*, 5th ed. ASM Press, Washington, DC.

50. **Marano, N. N., N. A. Daniels, A. N. Easton, A. McShan, B. Ray, J. G. Wells, P. M. Griffin, and F. J. Angulo.** 2000. A survey of stool culturing practices for *Vibrio* species at clinical laboratories in Gulf Coast states. *J. Clin. Microbiol.* **38:**2267–2270.

51. **Martinez-Urtaza, J., A. Lozano-Leon, A. Vina-Feas, J. de Novoa, and O. Garcia-Martin.** 2006. Differences in the API 20E biochemical patterns of clinical and environmental *V. parahaemolyticus* isolates. *FEMS Microbiol. Lett.* **255:**75–81.

52. **McCarter, L. L.** 2001. Polar flagellar motility of the *Vibrionaceae*. *Microbiol. Mol. Biol. Rev.* **65:**445–462.

53. **McLaughlin, J. B., A. DePaola, C. A. Bopp, K. A. Martinek, N. P. Napolilli, C. G. Allison, S. L. Murray, E. C. Thompson, M. M. Bird, and J. P. Middaugh.** 2005. Outbreak of *Vibrio parahaemolyticus* gastroenteritis associated with Alaskan oysters. *N. Engl. J. Med.* **353:**1463–1470.

54. **Mintz, E. D., and R. L. Guerrant.** 2009. A lion in our village—the unconscionable tragedy of cholera in Africa. *N. Engl. J. Med.* **360:**1060–1063.

55. **Moreno, C. O., J. Romero, and R. T. Espejo.** 2002. Polymorphism in repeated 16S rRNA genes is a common property of type strains and environmental isolates of the genus. *Microbiology* **148:**1233–1239.

56. **Morris, J. G., Jr.** 2003. Cholera and other types of vibriosis: a story of human pandemics and oysters on the half shell. *Clin. Infect. Dis.* **37:**272–280.

57. **Morris, J. G., Jr., and G. B. Nair.** 2002. "Non-cholera" *Vibrio* infections, p. 557–571. *In* M. J. Blaser, P. D. Smith, J. I. Ravdin, H. B. Greenberg, and R. L. Guerrant (ed.), *Infections of the Gastrointestinal Tract*, 2nd ed. Lippincott Williams and Wilkins, Philadelphia, PA.

58. **Nagao, M., Y. Shimizu, Y. Kawada, H. Baba, K. Yamada, K. Torii, and M. Ohta.** 2006. Two cases of sucrose-fermenting *Vibrio vulnificus* infection in which 16S rRNA sequencing was useful for diagnosis. *Jpn. J. Infect. Dis.* **59:**108–110.

59. **Nair, G. B., T. Ramamurthy, S. K. Bhattacharya, B. Dutta, Y. Takeda, and D. A. Sack.** 2007. Global dissemination of *Vibrio parahaemolyticus* serotype O3:K6 and its serovariants. *Clin. Microbiol. Rev.* **20:**39–48.

60. **Nakamura, Y., M. Uchihira, M. Ichimiya, K. Morita, and M. Muto.** 2008. Necrotizing fasciitis of the leg due to *Photobacterium damselae*. *J. Dermatol.* **35:**44–45.

61. **Nelson, E. J., J. B. Harris, J. G. Morris, Jr., S. B. Calderwood, and A. Camilli.** 2009. Cholera transmission: the host, pathogen and bacteriophage dynamic. *Nat. Rev. Microbiol.* **7:**693–702.

62. **Nguyen, B. M., J. H. Lee, N. T. Cuong, S. Y. Choi, N. T. Hien, D. D. Anh, H. R. Lee, M. Ansaruzzaman, H. P. Endtz, J. Chun, A. L. Lopez, C. Czerkinsky, J. D. Clemens, and D. W. Kim.** 2009. Cholera outbreaks caused by an altered *Vibrio cholerae* O1 El Tor biotype strain producing classical cholera toxin B in Vietnam in 2007 and 2008. *J. Clin. Microbiol.* **47:**1568–1571.

63. **O'Hara, C. M.** 2005. Manual and automated instrumentation for identification of *Enterobacteriaceae* and other aerobic gram-negative bacilli. *Clin. Microbiol. Rev.* **18:**147–162.

64. **O'Hara, C. M., E. G. Sowers, C. A. Bopp, S. B. Duda, and N. A. Strockbine.** 2003. Accuracy of six commercially available systems for identification of members of the family *Vibrionaceae*. *J. Clin. Microbiol.* **41:**5654–5659.

65. **Patel, N. M., M. Wong, E. Little, A. X. Ramos, K. M. Fox, J. Melvin, A. Moore, and R. Manch.** 2008. *Vibrio cholerae* non-O1 infection in cirrhotics: case report and literature review. *Transpl. Infect. Dis.* **11:**54–56.

66. **Pavia, A. T., J. A. Bryan, K. L. Maher, T. R. Hester, Jr., and J. J. Farmer III.** 1989. *Vibrio carchariae* infection after a shark bite. *Ann. Intern. Med.* **111:**85–86.

67. **Ratnaraja, N., T. Blackmore, J. Byrne, and S. Shi.** 2005. *Vibrio fluvialis* peritonitis in a patient receiving continuous ambulatory peritoneal dialysis. *J. Clin. Microbiol.* **43:**514–515.

68. **Sack, D. A., R. B. Sack, G. B. Nair, and A. K. Siddique.** 2004. Cholera. *Lancet* **363:**223–233.

69. **San Juan, E., B. Fouz, J. D. Oliver, and C. Amaro.** 2009. Evaluation of genotypic and phenotypic methods to distinguish clinical from environmental *Vibrio vulnificus* strains. *Appl. Environ. Microbiol.* **75:**1604–1613.

70. **Schets, F. M., H. H. J. L. van den Berg, A. A. Demeulmeester, E. van Dijk, S. A. Rutjes, H. J. P. van Hooijdonk, and A. M. de Roda Husman.** 2006. *Vibrio alginolyticus* infections in the Netherlands after swimming in the North Sea. *Euro. Surveill.* **11(45):**pii=3077.

71. **Sciortino, C. V., J. A. Johnson, and A. Hamad.** 1996. Vitek system antimicrobial susceptibility testing of O1, O139, and non-O1 *Vibrio cholerae. J. Clin. Microbiol.* **34:**897–900.

72. **Serichantalergs, O., N. A. Bhuiyan, G. B. Nair, O. Chivaratanond, A. Srijan, L. Bodhidatta, S. Anuras, and C. J. Mason.** 2007. The dominance of pandemic serovars of *Vibrio parahaemolyticus* in expatriates and sporadic cases of diarrhoea in Thailand, and new emergent serovar (O3:K6) with pandemic traits. *J. Med. Microbiol.* **56:**608–613.

73. **Shimada, T., E. Arakawa, K. Itoh, T. Okitsu, A. Matushima, Y. Asai, S. Yamai, T. Nakazato, G. B. Nair, M. J. Albert, and Y. Takeda.** 1994. Extended serotyping scheme for *Vibrio cholerae. Curr. Microbiol.* **28:**175–178.

74. **Shimada, T., and R. Sakazaki.** 1984. On the serology of *Vibrio vulnificus. Jpn. J. Med. Sci. Biol.* **37:**241–246.

75. **Su, Y. C., and C. Liu.** 2007. *Vibrio parahaemolyticus:* a concern for seafood safety. *Food Microbiol.* **24:**549–558.

76. **Tang, H.-J., M.-C. Chang, W.-C. Ko, K.-Y. Huang, C.-L. Lee, and Y.-C. Chuang.** 2002. In vitro and in vivo activities of newer fluoroquinolones against *Vibrio vulnificus. Antimicrob. Agents Chemother.* **46:**3580–3584.

77. **Tarr, C. L., J. S. Patel, N. D. Puhr, E. G. Sowers, C. A. Bopp, and N. A. Strockbine.** 2007. Identification of *Vibrio* isolates by multiplex PCR assay and *rpoB* sequence determination. *J. Clin. Microbiol.* **45:**134–140.

78. **Thompson, F. L., T. Iida, and J. Swings.** 2004. Biodiversity of vibrios. *Microbiol. Mol. Biol. Rev.* **68:**403–431.

79. **Thyssen, A., and F. Ollevier.** 2005. Genus II. *Photobacterium* Beijerinck 1889, 401^AL, p. 546–552. *In* D. Brenner, N. Krieg, J. T. Staley, and G. Garrity (ed.), *Bergey's Manual of Systematic Bacteriology*, vol. 2. *The Proteobacteria, Part B. The Gammaproteobacteria.* Springer, New York, NY.

80. **Tobin-D'Angelo, M., A. R. Smith, S. N. Bulens, S. Thomas, M. Hodel, H. Izumiya, E. Arakawa, M. Morita, H. Watanabe, C. Marin, M. B. Parsons, K. Greene, K. Cooper, D. Haydel, C. Bopp, P. Yu, and E. Mintz.** 2008. Severe diarrhea caused by cholera toxin-producing *Vibrio cholerae* serogroup O75 infections acquired in the southeastern United States. *Clin. Infect. Dis.* **47:**1035–1040.

81. **Udden, S. M. N., M. S. H. Zahid, K. Biswas, Q. S. Ahmad, A. Cravioto, G. B. Nair, J. J. Mekalanos, and S. M. Faruque.** 2008. Acquisition of classical CTX prophage from *Vibrio cholerae* O141 by El Tor strains aided by lytic phages and chitin-induced competence. *Proc. Natl. Acad. Sci. USA* **105:**11951–11956.

82. **Uh, Y., J.-S. Park, G.-Y. Hwang, I. H. Jang, K.-J. Yoon, H.-C. Park, and S.-O. Hwang.** 2001. *Vibrio alginolyticus* gastroenteritis: report of two cases. *Clin. Microbiol. Infect.* **7:**104–106.

83. **Urbanczyk, H., J. C. Ast, M. J. Higgins, J. Carson, and P. V. Dunlap.** 2007. Reclassification of *Vibrio fischeri, Vibrio logei, Vibrio salmonicida* and *Vibrio wodanis* as *Aliivibrio fischeri* gen. nov., comb. nov., *Aliivibrio logei* comb. nov., *Aliivibrio salmonicida* comb. nov. and *Aliivibrio wodanis* comb. nov. *Int J. Syst. Evol. Microbiol.* **57:**2823–2829.

84. **Wallet, F., M. Tachon, S. Nseir, R. J. Courcol, and M. Roussel-Delvallez.** 2005. *Vibrio metschnikovii* pneumonia. *Emerg. Infect. Dis.* **11:**1641–1642.

85. **Wilkins, S., M. Millar, S. Hemsworth, G. Johnson, S. Warwick, and B. Pizer.** 2007. *Vibrio harveyi* sepsis in a child with cancer. *Pediatr. Blood Cancer* **50:**891–892.

86. **World Health Organization.** 2008. Cholera, 2007. *Wkly. Epidemiol. Rec.* **83:**269–283.

87. **Wuthe, H.-H., S. Aleksic, and W. Hein.** 1993. Contributions to some phenotypical characteristics of *Vibrio cincinnatiensis.* Studies in one strain of a diarrhoeic human patient and in two isolates from aborted bovine feces. *Zentralbl. Bakteriol.* **279:**458–465.

88. **Yamamoto, T., G. B. Nair, M. J. Albert, C. C. Parodi, and Y. Takeda.** 1995. Survey of in vitro susceptibilities of *Vibrio cholerae* O1 and O139 to antimicrobial agents. *Antimicrob. Agents Chemother.* **39:**241–244.

89. **Yamane, K., J. Asato, N. Kawade, H. Takahashi, B. Kimura, and Y. Arakawa.** 2004. Two cases of fatal necrotizing fasciitis caused by *Photobacterium damselae* in Japan. *J. Clin. Microbiol.* **42:**1370–1372.

90. **Yildiz, F. H., and G. K. Schoolnik.** 1999. *Vibrio cholerae* O1 El Tor: identification of a gene cluster required for the rugose colony type, exopolysaccharide production, chlorine resistance, and biofilm formation. *Proc. Natl. Acad. Sci. USA* **96:**4028–4033.

91. **Zaiderstein, R., C. Sadik, L. Lerner, L. Valinsky, J. Kopelwitz, R. Yishai, V. Agmon, M. Parsons, C. Bopp, and M. Weinberger.** 2008. Clinical characteristics and molecular subtyping of *Vibrio vulnificus* illnesses, Israel. *Emerg. Infect. Dis.* **14:**1875–1882.

Pseudomonas

DEBORAH A. HENRY AND DAVID P. SPEERT

40

TAXONOMY

Pseudomonas is a large and complex genus of gram-negative bacteria of importance, as it includes species with both clinical and environmental implications. Many species are saprophytic or pathogenic for plants. The metabolic versatility of species within this genus allows many to degrade low-molecular-weight organic and aromatic compounds (83). The genus *Pseudomonas* first proposed by Migula in 1894 (113) has undergone many taxonomic revisions as methodologies of species identification continue to improve, and it was comprised of five unrelated groups, as determined by rRNA-DNA hybridization studies in the early 1970s by Palleroni et al. (129). *Pseudomonas* (sensu stricto) is rRNA homology group I (27), in the gamma subclass of the *Proteobacteria* (161). The other rRNA homology groups are II, *Burkholderia* and *Ralstonia*; III, *Comamonas*, *Acidovorax*, *Delftia*, and *Hydrogenophaga*; IV, *Brevundimonas*; and V, *Stenotrophomonas* and *Xanthomonas* (83).

Several of the clinically relevant *Pseudomonas* species demonstrate marked heterogeneity and have been subdivided into biovars or genomovars. Genomovars are genetically distinct groups that warrant species designation but lack phenotypically defining characteristics, and they are determined by DNA-DNA reassociation experiments, 16S rRNA gene sequencing in combination with chemotaxonomic total fatty acid analysis, and total protein pattern analysis (56). Much work in genome sequencing is occurring; 3 strains of *Pseudomonas aeruginosa* and 13 strains from other *Peudomonas* species have been sequenced (http://www.ncbi.nlm.nih .gov/genomes/genlist.cgi?taxid=2&type=0&name= Complete%20Bacteria).

The highest level of genetic diversity of any species known is found in *Pseudomonas stutzeri* (140), as established by multilocus enzyme electrophoresis. *P. stutzeri* has at least nine genomovars, with clinical isolates being found in genomovars 1 and 2. There are no consistent phenotypic differences to justify splitting *P. stutzeri* into unique species (56).

Pseudomonas fluorescens was originally divided into biotypes A, B, C, D, E, F, and G (biotypes A to E are also referred to as biovars I, II, III, IV, and V). Biotype B was reclassified as *Pseudomonas marginalis*. Biotypes D and E (*Pseudomonas chlororaphis* and *Pseudomonas aureofaciens*) have now been combined into the single species *P. chlororaphis*, which is no longer considered a member of the fluorescens group.

Pseudomonas putida consists of biovars A and B. Biovar A should be regarded as the "typical" *P. putida* (35), while biovar B may have a closer affinity with *P. fluorescens*. More biovars of *P. putida* are warranted (35).

Great heterogeneity is found within the species of *P. stutzeri*, *P. fluorescens*, and *P. putida*, and these species are of interest in plant, marine, soil, and biotechnical sciences. They are of limited importance in clinical medicine. As polyphasic taxonomy continues to advance, more changes will doubtlessly arise; the clinical laboratory must keep abreast of such changes, in order to differentiate these isolates from the more clinically important *Pseudomonas* species.

DESCRIPTION OF THE GENUS *PSEUDOMONAS*

Pseudomonas spp. are aerobic non-spore-forming, gram-negative rods which are straight or slightly curved and are 0.5 to 1.0 by 1.5 to 5.0 μm (72). They are usually motile, with one or several polar flagella. They possess a strictly aerobic respiratory metabolism with oxygen as the terminal electron acceptor; in some cases nitrate can be used as an alternative electron acceptor that allows anaerobic growth. Most species of clinical interest are oxidase positive (except *Pseudomonas luteola* and *Pseudomonas oryzihabitans*). *Pseudomonas* spp. are catalase positive and are chemolithotrophs.

EPIDEMIOLOGY AND TRANSMISSION

Autogenous versus Exogenous Infection

Autogenous infection can only occur in those whose colonization resistance has been perturbed: bacteremia secondary to gastrointestinal colonization in neutropenic hosts (170) and pneumonia in individuals who have required endotracheal intubation (ventilator-associated pneumonia) (8, 115). Exogenous infection likely occurs in patients with cystic fibrosis (CF), as their initial infecting isolates usually resemble environmental morphotypes (122), although patient-to-patient spread has occasionally been demonstrated (see below). Most other infections caused by *P. aeruginosa* are probably acquired exogenously, such as in burn wound sepsis, conjunctivitis, otitis externa, and osteochondritis.

Exposure to Inanimate Reservoirs

Although efforts to prevent colonization with *P. aeruginosa* have been made, none has proven uniformly successful. Strict infection control procedures and the practice of compulsory hand hygiene are most effective at preventing patient-to-patient spread, particularly in hospitals.

Special Considerations for Patients with CF

P. aeruginosa is the predominant respiratory tract pathogen in patients with CF (54), but its mode of acquisition is poorly understood (155). Several studies have each demonstrated a common clone in particular groups of patients who have received their care at the same center (5, 18, 79); the most likely explanation for this finding is patient-to-patient spread. Since most patients each tend to carry a unique strain during the course of infection (122, 158), one assumes that the infection was acquired from an environmental source. Indeed, one large study performed in Vancouver, British Columbia, Canada, over more than 20 years failed to demonstrate patient-to-patient spread of *P. aeruginosa* except between siblings who could have acquired it from a common environmental source (158). A recent study has demonstrated that in chronic respiratory infections in CF, sequential isolates of *P. aeruginosa* from 30 patients displayed a high prevalence of DNA mismatch repair system-deficient hypermutable strains on isogenic backgrounds for each patient (42). Infection control policies with CF patients for transmission prevention should be determined by local epidemiological experience (174).

Species other than *P. aeruginosa*

Pseudomonas species other than *P. aeruginosa* are usually acquired from the environment.

CLINICAL SIGNIFICANCE

Normal Host Defenses against *P. aeruginosa*

Individuals with intact host defenses are not at risk for serious infection with *P. aeruginosa*, but those whose circulating neutrophil counts are profoundly depressed (such as patients with cancer receiving chemotherapy) are at risk for invasive infection (156).

Significance of Recovery of *P. aeruginosa* from Clinical Specimens

When *P. aeruginosa* is recovered from a normally sterile body site, such as blood, pleural fluid, or joint space, it usually constitutes a true infection. However, pseudoinfection (36) should be considered when there is a cluster of infections with the same strain of *Pseudomonas*, especially when such infections had not been frequently seen previously, and the patients are neither severely ill nor at enhanced risk of such infection. A search for the source of the cluster should include culture of the antiseptic used for skin preparation for venipuncture or similar procedures.

   P. aeruginosa is able to colonize mucosal surfaces, such as the oropharynx of patients receiving intensive care or the endotracheal tubes of patients receiving mechanical ventilation. Under such circumstances, recovery of *P. aeruginosa* from respiratory tract cultures may not indicate a true infection, and the significance of its presence in the culture should be interpreted with caution.

Infection in Patients with Neutropenia

Not all patients with neutropenia (neutrophil count of less than 0.5×10^9 per liter) are at risk for invasive disease. Patients at greatest risk are adults undergoing cancer che-motherapy or marrow ablation for bone marrow transplantation (9); children with similar conditions are at lesser risk for *P. aeruginosa* bacteremia and are more often infected with gram-positive bacteria.

Infection in Patients with CF

P. aeruginosa is the predominant respiratory tract pathogen in patients with CF, for reasons which remain incompletely explained (54). The organism appears to have a particular tropism for CF epithelial cells and can resist normal respiratory tract host defenses. Once infection is established, it usually persists (48), and the bacteria undergo a transition to the "CF phenotype," consisting of the following: (i) a rough lipopolysaccharide (LPS) (60), in which the O polysaccharide is incompletely expressed, rendering the bacteria susceptible to the bactericidal effect of human serum; (ii) mucoid colonial morphology (95) resulting from the exuberant production of a mucoid exopolysaccharide composed of O-acetylated guluronic and mannuronic acids; (iii) nonmotility (104) in which the bacteria lack normal functional flagellar function; and (iv) hypoexpression of various exotoxins and other exoproducts (12, 185). Some of these changes may be under global regulation, but they can also be expressed individually. Transition of *P. aeruginosa* from nonmucoid to mucoid in the CF lung is usually associated with an accelerated decline in pulmonary function and an adverse prognosis (37), perhaps because of the capacity of the mucoid exopolysaccharide to interfere with normal host phagocytic defenses (54, 157) and to facilitate the formation of biofilms (90). Biofilm formation may also be enhanced by another colonial form, small-colony variants (previously known as dwarf colonies) (48, 64). Furthermore, CF patients receive frequent courses of anti-*Pseudomonas* antimicrobial therapy, often rendering the bacterium with which they are chronically infected resistant to a wide range of antimicrobial agents (61, 86).

Ventilator-Associated and Nosocomial Pneumonia

The normal respiratory tract is well protected against infection by means of mucociliary clearance of inhaled particles and potentially infectious agents. Placement of an endotracheal tube for mechanical ventilation allows upper respiratory tract microbes to gain access to the lower respiratory tract, where infection can be established. Adults receiving mechanical ventilation are at high risk for developing *P. aeruginosa* ventilator-associated pneumonia (17), particularly after or during treatment with broad-spectrum antimicrobial agents. Nosocomial pneumonia most often occurs in neutropenic patients following broad-spectrum antimicrobial therapy (143). Initial empirical therapy, until an etiologic agent is identified, should include a drug effective against *P. aeruginosa*.

Burn Wound Infections

Thermal burns of the skin abrogate an essential component of the body's defense against infection, the physical barrier of the intact dermis (135). The resulting damaged tissue is a rich culture medium and is at great risk for colonization and infection by *P. aeruginosa*; such infections have been one of the leading causes of morbidity and mortality in victims of burns. Topical therapy is designed to prevent *P. aeruginosa* and other pathogens from causing infection. Infections of burn wounds with gram-negative bacteria (in particular *P. aeruginosa*) typically occur about 1 week after the injury. The extent of the burn has a profound influence on risk of infection and prognosis (135). Prevention of bacterial burn wound infection has become so effective over the past decade that it is now very rare, and in many centers fungal infections predominate.

Osteochondritis

P. aeruginosa is the most common cause of osteochondritis of the dorsum of the foot following penetrating wounds (20). The typical scenario involves a child who has stepped on a nail which pierces the foot after passing through the sole of a running shoe. The prevalence of *P. aeruginosa* as the etiological agent in this situation may be due to its propensity to survive in the rubber of old running shoes (38).

Folliculitis and Superficial Infections

Since *P. aeruginosa* is a hydrophilic bacterium and can survive at temperatures as high as 42°C, it has the propensity to cause infection in people who are exposed to heated water for extended periods. Hot tub users are at risk of *P. aeruginosa* folliculitis (55), a condition which is self-limited for healthy hosts and resolves rapidly. People who spend extended periods swimming are at risk of external ear infections ("swimmer's ear"), another self-limiting condition in immunocompetent people which responds readily to therapy with topical antimicrobial agents (7). The cornea is relatively resistant to infection except when its integrity has been broken. Users of contact lenses are at risk of *P. aeruginosa* conjunctivitis, especially if hygiene is poor or lenses are used for extended periods (164).

Other Infections with *P. aeruginosa*

P. aeruginosa can cause meningitis (usually following trauma or surgery) (39), malignant otitis externa in diabetics (144), sepsis and meningitis in newborns (167), endocarditis or osteomyelitis in users of intravenous drugs (148), community-acquired pneumonia (especially in people with underlying lung disease such as bronchiectasis [47]), and urinary tract infections in patients with complex urinary tract abnormalities (118, 142). Each of these presentations is unusual and is superimposed on some abrogation of normal host defenses.

Infections with *Pseudomonas* Species other than *P. aeruginosa*

Healthy individuals are resistant to serious infections by all *Pseudomonas* species, including *P. aeruginosa*. However, immunocompromised hosts are occasionally infected with one of the many non-aeruginosa species, including (but not limited to) *P. fluorescens*, *P. putida*, *P. stutzeri*, *P. oryzihabitans*, *P. luteola*, *P. alcaligenes*, *P. mendocina*, and *P. veronii*. Several of these species have been recovered from the respiratory secretions of patients with CF, but their role in pathogenesis of lung disease has not been determined. Some of these species have the capacity, like *P. aeruginosa*, to grow in hostile environments, such as antiseptic solutions; they can therefore be the cause of pseudobacteremia. Because of their low virulence, infections due to these species are often iatrogenic and are associated with the administration of contaminated solutions, medicines, and blood products or the presence of indwelling catheters (94, 100, 107, 137, 150).

P. fluorescens and *P. putida* have the ability to grow at 4°C, and *P. fluorescens* can be isolated from the skin of a small proportion of blood donors (150), resulting in occasional transfusion-associated septicemia in the recipient. Various *Pseudomonas* species have been implicated in outbreaks of pseudobacteremia (84, 153).

P. stutzeri is an unusual cause of human infection. It can cause bacteremia in immunosuppressed persons (134),

meningitis in human immunodeficiency virus-infected individuals (141), pneumonia in alcoholics (16), and osteomyelitis (139). Iatrogenic infections due to *P. stutzeri* include endophthalmitis following cataract surgery (77) and bacteremia in hemodialysis patients as a result of contaminated dialysis fluid (52). *P. stutzeri* has also been recovered from wounds, the respiratory tract of intubated patients, and the urinary tract, although its pathogenic role in those settings is unclear (119).

P. oryzihabitans is being recognized increasingly as a cause of bacteremia in immunocompromised patients with central venous access devices. Synthetic bath sponges can be a source of bacteremia with this organism in patients with Hickman catheters (107). This organism has also been reported to cause peritonitis in patients undergoing chronic ambulatory peritoneal dialysis, cellulitis, abscesses, wound infections, and meningitis following neurosurgical procedures (94).

P. luteola is a rare cause of infections in humans. There have been case reports of a variety of different infections, including bacteremia, cellulitis, osteomyelitis, peritonitis, endocarditis, and postsurgical meningitis (137, 138).

Other *Pseudomonas* species are found even less frequently in human infection. *P. alcaligenes* has been associated with catheter-related endocarditis in a bone marrow transplant recipient (111). *P. mendocina* has been isolated from two patients with endocarditis (4, 78). *P. veronii* has been reported to be associated with an intestinal inflammatory pseudotumor (19). *P. monteilii* has been recovered from stool, bile, placenta, bronchial aspirates, pleural fluid, and urine, but its clinical significance is uncertain (33, 34). *P. mosselii* has also been isolated from various specimens, but the clinical significance is not known (25).

COLLECTION, TRANSPORT, AND STORAGE OF SPECIMENS

Pseudomonas spp. are able to survive in diverse environments and through a wide temperature range. Some species prefer incubation temperatures lower than 25°C, while *P. aeruginosa* can grow at temperatures up to 42°C. These organisms are easily recovered from clinical specimens using standard collection, transport, and storage techniques as outlined in chapter 16. Samples of *Pseudomonas* spp. can be refrigerated at 2 to 8°C for up to 4 weeks. Organisms can be kept in long-term storage at −80°C using standard laboratory freezing protocols.

DIRECT EXAMINATION

Microscopy

With regard to Gram stain morphology, *Pseudomonas* spp. are motile, gram-negative, non-spore-forming, straight or slightly curved bacilli measuring 0.5 to 0.8 μm by 1.5 to 3.0 μm. The Gram stain morphology cannot easily distinguish *Pseudomonas* spp. from other nonfermenting bacilli, although they are usually thinner than *Enterobacteriaceae*. Among the pseudomonads, there is some variation in Gram stain morphology. Certain strains of *P. putida* can appear elongated. Organisms from older cultures may appear slightly pleomorphic. Flagellar stains reveal one or more polar flagella. *P. aeruginosa* has a single polar flagellum.

Mucoid strains may be distinguished on direct examination by the presence of clusters or long filaments of short gram-negative bacilli surrounded by darker pink-staining material (alginate). It is important to note this on direct examination, as the organisms may grow very slowly or not at all. The presence of these mucoid forms should be documented on clinical reports. Because *Pseudomonas* spp. may be colonizers, their isolation does not always link them to clinical disease. However, their presence intracellularly in polymorphonuclear cells is clinically significant and should be documented and direct further workup.

Nucleic Acid Detection

P. aeruginosa and other *Pseudomonas* species are detected ordinarily by culture techniques; these methods are particularly important for determining antimicrobial susceptibility, as these organisms have a high degree of intrinsic and acquired resistance (61, 98). However, situations exist in which a more rapid method can be instituted, such as for screening environmental niches or for rapidly evaluating the sputum of patients with CF (22, 159, 186). Methods that have been used include PCR amplification of various genomic regions, such as genes for rRNA (76), heat shock protein (22), or exotoxin A (85). Conventional and real-time PCR have both proven to be useful, and the amplification of multiple targets can be particularly valuable in identification of non-aeruginosa *Pseudomonas* species (136). Nucleic acid probes have also been used to detect these bacterial species, the specificity depending upon the unique nature of the genomic region being detected. Probes directed at species-specific 16S rRNA have been most widely used for this purpose (57, 163) and may have a role in the identification of clinically relevant, biochemically inactive *Pseudomonas* species, including certain strains of *P. aeruginosa* (136). PCR amplification of 16S ribosomal DNA (rDNA) followed by restriction fragment length polymorphism (RFLP) analysis has been used to successfully identify and characterize members of the fluorescent pseudomonad group (89). Since RFLP of the 16S rRNA gene does not provide sufficient resolution among genomovars of a species, a more discriminatory test may be used, such as sequencing the internally transcribed 16S-23S rDNA spacer (internal transcribed spacer 1) regions, believed to have more genetic variability among genomovars (56). Recently, peptide nucleic acid fluorescence in situ hybridization (130) has been shown to be highly sensitive and specific for identification of *P. aeruginosa*.

Mechanisms of antimicrobial resistance, such as the identification of extended-spectrum β-lactamases in *P. aeruginosa*, have also been detected using molecular techniques, by real-time PCR detection (180).

ISOLATION PROCEDURES

Pseudomonas species have very simple nutritional requirements and grow well on standard broth and solid laboratory media such as tryptic soy agar with 5% sheep blood, chocolate agar, and MacConkey agar, which are recommended to isolate *Pseudomonas* spp. from clinical specimens. MacConkey agar is also a differential medium helpful in identifying different strains of *Pseudomonas* spp., including mucoid strains of *P. aeruginosa* from CF patients. Multiple selective media containing inhibitors such as acetamide, nitrofurantoin, phenanthroline, 9-chloro-9-[4-(diethyamino)phenyl]-9,10-dihydro-10-phenylacridine hydrochloride (C-390), and cetrimide (15, 66, 82, 87, 91, 109, 169, 171) have been used in the past for the isolation and presumptive identification of *P. aeruginosa* from clinical and environmental samples. Currently, cetrimide and a combination of phenanthroline with C-390 are the most commonly used selective agents. Inhibition of some strains of *P. aeruginosa*

from sputum specimens from CF patients has been reported using a selective agar containing cetrimide (200 mg/liter) and nalidixic acid (15 mg/liter) (40), emphasizing the need to use both selective and nonselective media for recovery of bacteria from these patients. Some of the non-aeruginosa pseudomonads, like *P. fluorescens*, *P. putida*, and *P. oryzihabitans*, may grow better at the lower temperatures of 28 to 30°C. Good growth is usually achieved after 24 to 48 h of incubation. For cultures from CF patients, it is recommended that solid medium plates be held at 35 to 37°C for 5 days.

IDENTIFICATION

Fluorescent Group

Members of the fluorescent pseudomonad group produce pyoverdin, a water-soluble yellow-green or yellow-brown pigment that fluoresces under short-wavelength UV light. Many strains of *P. aeruginosa* can produce the blue pigment pyocyanin. When pyoverdin combines with the blue water-soluble phenazine pigment pyocyanin, the bright green color characteristic of *P. aeruginosa* is created. This organism may also produce other water-soluble pigments such as pyorubrin (red) or pyomelanin (brown-black). Conditions of iron limitation enhance pigment production, as these pigments act as siderophores in iron uptake systems of the bacteria. Non-dye-containing media enhance visualization of pigments.

P. aeruginosa

Most *P. aeruginosa* organisms are easily recognizable on primary isolation media on the basis of characteristic colonial morphology, production of diffusible pigments, and a grape-like odor. Older cultures may exhibit a corn taco-like odor. Colonies are usually flat and spreading and have a serrated edge and a metallic sheen that is often associated with autolysis of the colonies (188). Other morphologies exist, including smooth, mucoid, and dwarf (small-colony variants) (63, 64, 126, 175). Mucoid colonial variants are particularly prevalent in respiratory tract specimens from CF patients (51).

P. aeruginosa is distinct from the rest of the clinically relevant fluorescent pseudomonads in its ability to grow at 42°C. In addition to pigment production, other tests that confirm its identification are positive oxidase and arginine tests and an alkaline over no-change reaction in the triple sugar iron test.

Microbiologists must be aware of certain variations in the phenotypes of *P. aeruginosa*. Isolates lacking oxidase activity have occasionally been reported, but they exhibit the other characteristic features. Prior antibiotic therapy with agents that affect protein synthesis may cause the aberrant phenotype (59, 112). Mucoid isolates of *P. aeruginosa* from CF patients may undergo several phenotypic changes, including slow growth, loss of motility, and loss of pigment production. Small-colony variants may require prolonged incubation, lack motility, be hyperpiliated, adhere to agar surfaces, and show autoaggregative properties in liquid medium (175).

P. fluorescens and P. putida

P. fluorescens and *P. putida* do not possess distinctive colony morphology or odor. Their inability to reduce nitrates to nitrogen gas and their ability to produce acid from xylose distinguish these two species from the other fluorescent pseudomonads. *P. fluorescens* can be differentiated from *P. putida* by its ability to grow at 4°C and to hydrolyze gelatin; *P. putida* can do neither. *P. fluorescens* isolates may require 4 to 7 days of incubation for accurate detection of gelatin hydrolysis. According to the package insert for API 20NE (version 7.0; bioMérieux, Inc., Durham, NC), only 39% of *P. fluorescens* isolates hydrolyze gelatin in 24 to 48 h.

P. veronii, P. monteilii, and *P. mosselii*

P. veronii can reduce nitrates to nitrogen gas but is unable to hydrolyze acetamide. The type strain of *P. veronii* (LMG 17761) is negative for acid from lactose and maltose and does not grow at 36°C (D. A. Henry, unpublished data). *P. monteilii* can be distinguished from the other members of the fluorescent group by its inability to reduce nitrates to nitrites or nitrogen gas, hydrolyze gelatin, or produce acid from xylose. *P. mosselii* can reduce nitrates neither to nitrites nor to nitrogen gas, nor can it produce acid from xylose, but most isolates (92%) can hydrolyze gelatin (Table 1).

Other fluorescent pseudomonads are rarely encountered in clinical specimens. Many of these isolates are negative for arginine dihydrolase activity. Identification as "*Pseudomonas* species, not *aeruginosa*" and susceptibility testing of the isolates, when appropriate, are sufficient in most circumstances. When necessary, these isolates can be referred to reference laboratories.

Nonfluorescent Group

P. stutzeri and *P. mendocina*

Most *P. stutzeri* isolates are easily recognized on primary isolation media by their distinctive dry, wrinkled colony morphology, similar to the morphology of *Burkholderia pseudomallei. P. stutzeri* can be distinguished from the latter species by its lack of arginine dihydrolase activity and inability to produce acid from lactose. *P. stutzeri* colonies can pit or adhere to the agar and are buff to brown. The adherence can make removal of colonies from agar medium difficult. Because of the difficulty in making suspensions of specific turbidity, commercial susceptibility systems may not work well with this organism. Not all isolates of *P. stutzeri* produce wrinkled colonies; such strains can be distinguished from other pseudomonads by their ability to hydrolyze starch, a unique reaction for this species.

P. mendocina colonies are smooth, nonwrinkled, and flat, producing a brownish yellow pigment. Key biochemical characteristics of this species include the ability to reduce nitrates to nitrogen gas, positive arginine dihydrolase activity, and inability to hydrolyze acetamide or starch.

P. alcaligenes and *P. pseudoalcaligenes*

P. alcaligenes and *P. pseudoalcaligenes* have rarely been encountered in clinical samples (111) and do not have a distinctive colony morphology. Compared to other pseudomonads, they are biochemically inert. Characteristics that distinguish them from other biochemically inert gram-negative rods are a positive oxidase reaction, motility due to a polar flagellum, and growth on MacConkey agar. *P. alcaligenes* is distinguished from *P. pseudoalcaligenes* by its inability to oxidize fructose. Although growth at 42°C was thought to be a distinguishing feature between them, further studies now indicate that growth at 41°C (and probably 42°C) is also present in most strains of *P. alcaligenes* (N. Palleroni, personal communication). These organisms are difficult to identify by many commercial systems, and for most clinical situations they can simply be referred to as

"*Pseudomonas* spp., not *aeruginosa.*" If the clinical situation dictates a definitive identification, assistance from reference laboratories should be sought.

P. luteola and *P. oryzihabitans*

P. luteola and *P. oryzihabitans* can be distinguished from other pseudomonads by their negative oxidase reaction and production of an intracellular, nondiffusible yellow pigment. Both organisms typically exhibit rough, wrinkled, adherent colonies or, more rarely, smooth colonies. *P. luteola* can be differentiated from *P. oryzihabitans* on the basis of its ability to hydrolyze o-nitrophenyl-β-D-galactopyranoside and esculin.

Use of Commercial Identification Systems

Commercial identification systems rather than conventional biochemical tests increasingly are used in many laboratories to identify *Pseudomonas* spp. Commercial products can be divided into manual and automated systems (123). The more frequently used manual systems are the API 20NE (bioMérieux), Crystal E/NF (Becton Dickinson), and RapID NF Plus (Innovative Diagnostic Systems). The manual systems usually provide accurate identification of *P. aeruginosa,* including mucoid isolates as well as other *Pseudomonas* species, and are preferred over automated systems for isolates from CF patients.

Automated systems are commonly used in many medium to large clinical laboratories. As *P. aeruginosa* is easily identified by a few conventional biochemical tests, it is often not necessary to use a more expensive commercial system. Several of the automated systems are not very accurate and may require additional testing for non-*P. aeruginosa* species; thus, their labor, cost, and time-saving benefits are lost. Automated systems can identify *P. aeruginosa* from non-CF sources with 90 to 100% accuracy (44, 125), but some systems may require additional tests to achieve these results (124, 168). Most reviews focus on the evaluation of *P. aeruginosa,* with only a few, if any, other *Pseudomonas* species represented in the organisms being tested. When other *Pseudomonas* species were included, the new Vitek 2GN panel performed well (43, 125), while other systems often relied on additional testing to obtain an identification (29, 124, 162, 168). Hence, it is wise to consider carefully the clinical significance, colonial morphology, and other key features before accepting results from automated systems.

Identification of *Pseudomonas* species, especially those isolated from CF patients, is not always optimal with rapid systems. The MicroScan (Dade International, Inc.) system (Negative Combo 15), when incubated for 20 to 24 h according to the manufacturer's method, performed poorly for CF isolates, with only 57% of nonmucoid and 40% of mucoid *P. aeruginosa* isolates correctly identified (147). Extended incubation for 48 h improved accuracy to 86 and 83%, respectively. Misidentified species were most commonly either *Alcaligenes* spp. or *P. fluorescens/P. putida.* For *P. aeruginosa* from non-CF samples, the overall accuracy has been reported as 94% (147). Other automated systems have not been evaluated to date specifically for the identification of CF isolates, so caution in interpreting results is advised. The importance of non-aeruginosa *Pseudomonas* species as the cause of significant infection has not been established in most cases. The need to pursue species identification beyond the ruling out of *P. aeruginosa* will depend on the individual institution's requirements.

TABLE 1 Characteristics of *Pseudomonas* species found in clinical specimens[a]

Test	P. aeruginosa (n = 201)	P. fluorescens (n = 155)	P. putida (n = 16)	P. veronii (n = 8)	P. monteilii (n = 10)	P. mosselii (n =12)	P. stutzeri (n = 28)	P. mendocina (n = 4)	P. pseudoalcaligenes (n = 34)	P. alcaligenes (n = 26)	P. luteola (n = 34)	P. oryzihabitans (n = 36)
Oxidase	99	97	100	100	100	100	100	100	100	96	0	0
Growth												
MacConkey agar	100	100	100	ND[c]	ND	ND	100	100	100	96	100	100
Cetrimide	94	89	81 (6)	ND	90	100	4	75 (25)	56 (18)	15	0	25 (28)
6% NaCl	65	43	100	ND	0	100[e]	80 (16)	100	62 (6)	41	74	62
42°C	100	0	0	0	0	0	69	100	94	V[f]	94	33
Nitrate reduction	98	19	0	100	0	0	100	100	100	54	62	6
Gas from nitrate	93	3	0	100	0	0	100	100	0	0	0	0
Pyoverdin	65	96	93	100	100	100	0	0	0	0	0	0
Arginine dihydrolase	100	97	100	100	100	100	0[d]	100	78	12	100	14
Lysine decarboxylase	0	0	0	ND	0	0	0	0	0	0	0	7
Ornithine decarboxylase	0	0	0	ND	0	0	0	0	0	0	0	3
Hydrolysis												
Urea	48 (9)	21 (31)	31 (44)	25	50	ND	33 (22)	50	3 (6)	0	26 (38)	77
Gelatin (7-day incubation)	82	100	0	13	0	92	0	0	0	0	61	17
Acetamide	100	6 (12)	0	0	0	ND	0	0	ND	ND	ND	ND
Esculin	0	0	0	ND	0	0	0	0	0	0	100	0
Starch	0	0	0	ND	0	8	100	0	0	0	0	0
Acid from[b]:												
Glucose	97	100	100	100	100	100	96 (4)	100	9	0	100	100
Fructose	ND	ND	ND	100	100	100	ND	ND	79 (21)	0	ND	ND
Xylose	90	100	100	100	0	0	93 (7)	75 (25)	18 (12)	0	100	100
Lactose	<1	24	25 (13)	ND	0	17	0	0	0	0	3 (24)	14 (22)
Sucrose	0	48	0	100	0	17	0	0	0	0	12	25
Maltose	<1	2	31	ND	0	75	100	0	0	0	100	97
Mannitol	70	53	25	ND	0	100	89 (4)	0	0	0	76 (18)	100
Simmons citrate	95	93	94 (6)	ND	100	100	82 (14)	100	26 (9)	57 (8)	100	97
No. of flagella	1	>1	>1	>1	ND	1	1	1	1	1	>1	1

[a]Results are given as percentage of positive strains; percentages in parentheses represent strains with delayed reactions. Data are from references 25, 32, 34, and 72.

[b]Oxidative-fermentative basal medium with 1% carbohydrate.

[c]ND, no data.

[d]P. stutzeri-like organisms (formerly CDC group 3b) are arginine dihydrolase positive.

[e]Growth at 3 to 5% NaCl but not at 7% NaCl.

[f]V, variable; many strains can grow at 41°C. See comment in text under identification.

TYPING SYSTEMS

Phenotypic Typing Methods

Historically, typing of *P. aeruginosa* for epidemiological purposes has relied upon phenotypic characteristics of the bacteria. The most widely used method was based upon differences in LPS O polysaccharide (LPS serotyping). This method is good for most clinical isolates but can only differentiate among the 17 different LPS types in the most widely used (Difco) commercial typing set. Antimicrobial susceptibility profiling has been used, but the capacity of *P. aeruginosa* to develop resistance under the pressure of antimicrobial therapy has rendered this method unreliable in conditions of chronic infection such as CF. Each of these methods has its shortcomings, as the phenotypic characteristics of the bacteria are highly plastic. The LPS of CF isolates of *P. aeruginosa* often lack the O polysaccharide, against which most serotyping reagents react. None of these phenotypic methods is reliable in CF, and they have largely been replaced by genotypic methods.

Genotypic Typing Methods

Several genotypic methods have been developed over the past two decades for typing *P. aeruginosa* for epidemiological purposes (155). These are briefly described in the order in which they were developed. Each is useful, even for typing isolates from patients with CF, but they are not available in most clinical diagnostic laboratories.

RFLP

RFLP relies upon the genetic diversity at a specific site within the bacterial genome. Such diversity exists upstream of the gene for exotoxin A (*exoA*) in *P. aeruginosa* (122). In a study of different typing methods, *exoA* RFLP proved superior to all phenotypic methods for typing *P. aeruginosa* (74). This method was also the first to demonstrate convincingly that patients with CF were usually each infected with a unique strain that was usually present durably (without eradication or replacement) for extended periods. Pilin gene RFLP has demonstrated that individual CF patients are durably infected with the same strain despite changes in pilin protein expression (122). The disadvantages of RFLP are its relatively weak discriminatory power (compared to that of newer methods), its cumbersome nature, and its predominant use of radioactive probes.

PFGE

Pulsed-field gel electrophoresis (PFGE) is often considered the "gold standard" for bacterial typing, as it provides a view of the entire genome. The banding pattern is unique to each strain (or clone) and can be used for any bacterial species.

PCR-Based Typing Methods

Several different PCR-based methods have been used for typing *P. aeruginosa*. They are directed at known elements within the genome or against random but relatively frequently encoded sequences. The latter, random amplified polymorphic DNA (RAPD) analysis, has proved quite robust for typing *P. aeruginosa* (105), but it must be run consistently on the same equipment to yield reproducible results. Data from RAPD analysis usually are highly consistent with those from PFGE. PCR-amplified products can be digested with restriction enzymes to yield more discriminatory data (3, 149).

MLST

Multilocus sequence typing (MLST) has only recently been employed for typing *P. aeruginosa*. It is likely to be the most highly discriminatory among the genetic typing tools, but it is extremely time-consuming and expensive to employ. The method entails PCR amplification of specific genes and then sequencing of the gene products. This can be done only in very specialized centers, but it has the power to provide highly reliable data on relatedness among isolates. MLST is particularly useful in typing isolates from patients with CF (176).

SEROLOGIC TESTS

Serologic tests are not recommended for patients with *P. aeruginosa* infections. However, a commercial test system (Mediagnost, Reutlingen, Germany) detecting serum antibodies against three *P. aeruginosa* antigens (alkaline phosphatase, elastase, and exotoxin A) performed favorably for CF patients with negative or intermittent *P. aeruginosa* status, since a rise in antibody titers indicated probable infection (81).

ANTIMICROBIAL SUSCEPTIBILITIES

P. aeruginosa possesses intrinsic resistance to many antibiotic classes and has the ability to develop resistance by mutations in different chromosomal loci or by horizontal acquisition of resistance genes carried on plasmids, transposons, or integrons. The various mechanisms of resistance, substrate specificities, and geographic distributions are discussed below. The frequent acquisition of antimicrobial resistance in *P. aeruginosa* limits the utility of antimicrobial susceptibility patterns as a tool in epidemiological typing.

Mechanisms of Resistance

Intrinsic Resistance

Intrinsic resistance is mediated through multiple mechanisms. *P. aeruginosa* has an inducible chromosomal AmpC β-lactamase that renders it resistant to ampicillin, amoxicillin, amoxicillin-clavulanate, and first- and second-generation cephalosporins, as well as cefotaxime and ceftriaxone (97). Although impermeability was originally thought to be responsible for resistance to other antibiotic classes, efflux pump systems have been identified as a more prevalent intrinsic mechanism of resistance.

Multiple efflux pumps exist in *P. aeruginosa* that can result in expulsion of β-lactams, chloramphenicol, fluoroquinolones, macrolides, novobiocin, sulfonamides, tetracycline, and trimethoprim. Sequencing of the *P. aeruginosa* genome indicates that a high proportion of genes, including regulatory genes, are involved in the efflux of organic compounds, accounting for this organism's ability to adapt to diverse environments and to resist most antimicrobial agents. Efflux systems also export virulence determinants in *P. aeruginosa*, enhancing their toxicity to the host (69).

Acquired Resistance

Various antibiotics overcome the intrinsic resistance of *P. aeruginosa* and are active against this organism. These include extended-spectrum penicillins (piperacillin and ticarcillin), certain third- and fourth-generation cephaloporins (ceftazidime and cefipime), carbapenems (imipenem and meropenem), monobactams (aztreonam), fluoroquinolones (ciprofloxacin and levofloxacin), aminoglycosides (gentamicin, tobramycin, and amikacin), and colistin. Unfortunately, mutational resistance to all the antipseudomonal antibiotics can develop.

Efflux Pumps

Although multidrug efflux pump systems play a significant role in the intrinsic resistance of *P. aeruginosa*, they also are critical to the development of multidrug resistance. MexAB-OprM is expressed constitutively in all strains of *P. aeruginosa*. Upregulation or a mutation in the *mexR* repressor gene (*nalB* mutant) results in efflux pump overproduction and significant increase in the MICs of multiple antibiotics, including quinolones, penicillins, cephalosporins, aztreonam, and meropenem (low-level resistance MIC, 8 to 32 μg/ml), but not imipenem (133).

Impermeability Mutations

Impermeability mutations may result in resistance to carbapenem, aminoglycosides, colistin, and quinolones. They are important in carbapenem resistance and result from the loss of the OprD porin, a protein that forms a narrow transmembrane channel permeable to carbapenems but not β-lactams.

β-Lactamases

The acquisition of β-lactamases (177) is not as common for *P. aeruginosa* as it is for *Enterobacteriaceae* (97). Nevertheless, β-lactamases are being recognized increasingly and are very diverse in this organism. Genes for these enzymes are encoded in plasmids, on transposons or integrons, making their further dissemination likely. They confer resistance predominantly to antipseudomonal penicillins, ceftazidime, cefipime, and aztreonam but not carbapenems. Their activity is inhibited poorly by clavulanic acid or tazobactam.

Carbapenemases

With the exception of GES-2, all carbapenemases in *P. aeruginosa* belong to Ambler class B, commonly referred to as metalloenzymes. Metalloenzymes are not inhibited by clavulanic acid but are susceptible to inhibition by divalent ion chelators such as EDTA. They hydrolyze all β-lactam antibiotics, except aztreonam, and are associated with high-level (MIC > 32 μg/ml) carbapenem resistance. Underreporting of carbapenem resistance may occur, as expression of the carbapenemases varies, resulting in a wide range of MICs (2 to 128 μg/ml) that may go undetected in clinical laboratories that rely only on automated systems.

Genes for these enzymes are plasmid mediated and are located on mobile gene cassettes inserted in variable regions of integrons, resulting in enhanced potential for expression and dissemination. Of concern is the close proximity of these genes to those for aminoglycoside resistance (98).

Carbapenemases are spreading throughout Asia, Europe, and the Americas (24, 50, 88, 93, 131, 145, 172). The plasmid-mediated IMP family of enzymes was first described in Japan (128, 179). The VIM family was first described in Italy (92). Enzymes from both of these carbapenamase families have been found in *Pseudomonas* spp. (75, 120).

Aminoglycoside-Modifying Enzymes

Although impermeability mutations can result in aminoglycoside resistance, especially in CF and intensive care patients, drug inactivation by plasmid-encoded or chromosomally encoded enzymes is the most common mechanism for resistance worldwide to this class of antimicrobials (132). Aminoglycoside-modifying enzymes have been detected

in *P. aeruginosa* for over 30 years; these result in various combinations of resistance to gentamicin, tobramycin, and/or amikacin. *P. aeruginosa* isolates, especially those from Europe and Latin America, increasingly carry multiple modifying enzymes resulting in broad-spectrum aminoglycoside resistance. These enzymes are often encoded on transposons and/or integrons that carry resistance determinants for other classes of antibiotics such as sulfonamides, β-lactams, and chloramphenicol. Multiresistance genes for both aminoglycosides and extended-spectrum β-lactamases and metalloenzymes are of particular concern (132). Aminoglycoside-modifying enzymes can occur together with impermeability mutations (102, 114), resulting in broad-spectrum aminoglycoside resistance. Broad-spectrum aminoglycoside resistance due to a gene (*rmtA*) encoding a 16S rRNA methylase has been described (187).

Other

The discovery of a plasmid-borne quinolone resistance determinant (*qnr*) in gram-negative organisms (110, 178) is of significance for several reasons: (i) it has been transferred by conjugation to multiple organisms, including *P. aeruginosa*; (ii) it is associated with high-level quinolone resistance (up to 250-fold increase in MICs); (iii) it appears to be associated with integrons that carry determinants for resistance to β-lactams and aminoglycosides; and (iv) it expands the spectrum of high-level plasmid-mediated resistance to quinolones.

Antibiotic Tolerance

Biofilm-producing *P. aeruginosa* isolates appear to be protected from killing by antibiotics (166). Although this is widely accepted to indicate antibiotic resistance, a more appropriate term is antibiotic tolerance. Although slower or stationary growth phase has classically been thought to account for relative antibiotic tolerance, many other mechanisms have been proposed. These include quorum sensing (152), decreased diffusion of antibiotics through the matrix polysaccharide alginate (67), synthesis of glucans that specifically bind antibiotics (103), phenotypic variability (30, 41), the presence of persister cells (160), and anaerobic growth of biofilm bacteria, which affects the activity of multiple antibiotics (11, 62).

Multidrug Resistance

Worldwide, despite some geographic variability, antimicrobial resistance, including multidrug (three or more antimicrobial classes) resistance to *P. aeruginosa*, is widespread and increasing (49, 96). In 2003, the European MYSTIC study group reported considerable country-to-country variation in the proportion of multidrug-resistant *P. aeruginosa* isolates within Europe, ranging from 50% to less than 3% (53). The SENTRY Antimicrobial Surveillance Program confirmed geographic variation in Latin America but emphasized the rapid increase in multidrug-resistant strains, with rates approaching 35% (45). From 1993 to 2002, in the United States, the rates of multidrug resistance increased from 4 to 14%, with the highest rates of increase reported for ciprofloxacin, imipenem, tobramycin, and aztreonam (121). Globally, multidrug resistance was found in 10% of *P. aeruginosa* strains analyzed (45).

Antimicrobial Susceptibility Testing

It may be difficult to estimate the true prevalence of antimicrobial resistance in *P. aeruginosa*, as detection of resistance by routine tests agrees poorly with MIC data (2, 68, 73, 99).

Worldwide, susceptibility methods vary in terms of choice of media, inoculum preparation, antimicrobial disc content, breakpoints, and interpretation of those breakpoints. Even when these variables are taken into consideration, susceptibility testing of *P. aeruginosa* remains challenging given the multiple mechanisms of resistance, both intrinsic and acquired, which are frequently expressed concurrently, often at low levels.

In clinical laboratories, susceptibility testing for *Pseudomonas* species may be performed by disc diffusion, agar or broth dilution, Etest (bioMérieux), or automated susceptibility systems using broth microdilution. Disc diffusion tests perform satisfactorily for most clinical isolates of *P. aeruginosa* (23). Limitations to this method include the lack of a quantitative result (MIC) and the potential to miss low-level resistance. Etest has been shown to correlate well with agar dilution for isolates from CF (14, 108) and non-CF (28) patients. Breakpoint interpretation for disc diffusion zones and MICs are standardized, by the Clinical and Laboratory Standards Institute (http://www.clsi.org/) in North America and by the European Committee on Antimicrobial Susceptibility Testing (http://www.eucast.org) in Europe. Due to the differences between these two organizations, susceptibility results should be reported according to an individual institution's operating procedures.

Good correlation with reference methods has been reported for most automated systems (65, 80, 106, 162) when testing *Pseudomonas* isolates from non-CF patients. Results evaluating the performance of various automated systems must be interpreted with caution, as the number of isolates tested is often limited, especially for non-*P. aeruginosa* strains. Whereas most *P. aeruginosa* isolates grow well on agar media, growth of some isolates in broth is variable and may pose difficulties for laboratories that rely solely on automated systems. Alternatively, a liquid medium improves the detection of the efflux resistance phenotype, which may not be detected using solid-medium-based testing (1, 29). This may account for some of the discrepancies reported when comparing different susceptibility testing methods.

Several antibiotics pose specific challenges to susceptibility testing. Carbapenem susceptibility testing results are difficult to interpret due to several factors, including rapid imipenem degradation (173, 183), variable levels of efflux pump expression, and unstable impermeability mutations. Carbapenemase is especially challenging, as it is associated with a wide range of MICs and lacks a simple test for detection. Susceptibility testing of imipenem with and without EDTA (discs or Etest strips) may be used but has been associated with falsely resistant results. Ceftazidime, with or without EDTA, may be a better substrate than imipenem and increases the sensitivity of the test (D. Livermore, presented at the British Society for Antimicrobial Chemotherapy, Standardized Disc Susceptibility Testing Method User Group Meeting, Royal College of Physicians, London, United Kingdom, 25 November 2003). Reproducibility of carbapenem resistance results using various susceptibility test methods is poor, and it is recommended that initial carbapenem resistance be confirmed by a second antimicrobial susceptibility test method (165). Although still restricted to reference laboratories, there are PCR-based methods for detection of carbapenemase production (120, 181).

Colistin is being used more in the treatment of multidrug-resistant *P. aeruginosa*. Disc diffusion testing does not correlate well with MIC results, and underreporting of resistance has been found in 5% of strains (46). Susceptibility testing of colistin should be performed by a MIC method such as agar dilution, Etest, or broth microdilution. Prolonged incubation (for 48 h) is recommended for broth microdilution (70).

Isolates of *P. aeruginosa* from CF patients pose specific difficulties for microbiology laboratories. Isolates from these patients often exhibit mixed morphotypes including mucoid phenotypes, small-colony variants, and bacterial microcolonies in biofilms. Susceptibility testing is complicated by several factors, including lack of correlation between susceptibility results and clinical response (154), different susceptibility patterns within a morphotype (41), lack of reproducibility of susceptibility tests, undercalling resistance, and presence of hypermutable strains (58, 126). Mucoid and nonmucoid phenotypes of *P. aeruginosa* are often coisolated from patients with CF. Mucoid isolates tend to be more susceptible and have lower β-lactamase activity than nonmucoid isolates (21). One explanation may be that these isolates are protected from selective antibiotic pressure. Selective antibiotic pressure, notably from inhalational tobramycin or colistin therapy, gives rise to small-colony variants of *P. aeruginosa* with properties of increased antimicrobial resistance, autoaggregative growth behavior, and enhanced ability to form biofilms (63, 64). In turn, bacterial cells in biofilms adapt into symbiotic bacterial communities in which the mucoid alginate-producing bacterial cells provide physical protection to the biofilm, while the highly antibiotic-resistant nonmucoid cells protect against antibiotic killing (21). Increased ability of biofilm bacteria to acquire resistance phenotypes (26) and selection of hypermutable strains following antimicrobial therapy (58, 126, 127) may further explain the lack of eradication of *P. aeruginosa* from chronically infected CF patients. Since bacteria found in biofilms exhibit MICs 100- to 1,000-fold higher than free-living, planktonic bacteria (71, 117), routine susceptibility testing may underestimate resistance and may contribute to treatment failures. In a study of 597 CF isolates (14), both disc diffusion and Etest were found to be generally acceptable as routine susceptibility testing methods. However, poor correlation was found with disc diffusion testing of mucoid isolates for piperacillin, piperacillin-tazobactam, and meropenem. Underreporting of resistance was more frequent with disc diffusion than with Etest, especially when testing ceftazidime, piperacillin, and piperacillin-tazobactam.

Hypermutable strains may be detected using either disc diffusion or Etest methods by the presence of resistant mutant subpopulations within the inhibition zones of three or more antibiotics (101).

Mucoid isolates pose a specific challenge for automated systems (6, 13, 29). Overestimating susceptibility may occur, as mucoid isolates often demonstrate insufficient growth at 24 h. Automated systems that allow for longer incubation may be preferable. On the other hand, overcalling resistance may result from the presence of large amounts of exopolysaccharide, resulting in turbidity without adequate bacterial growth. These limitations have led many microbiologists who routinely work with mucoid isolates of *P. aeruginosa* to choose alternative methods for susceptibility testing.

Isolating and individually testing all the morphotypes of *P. aeruginosa* is labor-intensive and time-consuming and may not provide clinically relevant susceptibility results. Mixed morphotype testing using phenotypically different colonies directly from sputum cultures, or from subcultures of isolated colonies, has been shown to correlate well with disc diffusion and MIC susceptibility methods (31, 184) and may provide clinically useful susceptibility data with significant time and cost savings. However, the correlation appears to be better for susceptible strains than for resistant strains (116). Direct sputum susceptibility testing using the Etest method has been suggested as an alternative to morphotype testing in assessing the in vivo situation by evaluating bacterial population susceptibility as well as potential interactions with other organisms, including commensal microbes (151; M. Gallagher, presented at the International Cystic Fibrosis Conference, Stockholm, Sweden, 2000).

Other methods have been recommended in an attempt to better predict susceptibility results. Biofilm susceptibility assays have been developed which confirm that biofilm inhibitory concentrations are much higher than conventionally determined MICs for multiple antibiotics (117). Synergy testing using microtiter checkerboard, time-kill test, broth macrodilution breakpoint combination sensitivity test, or Etest methods (10, 151, 182) has been used to assess the activities of antibiotic combinations in vitro in order to predict in vivo synergistic activity. This testing is labor-intensive, time-consuming, and difficult to reproduce, and it remains controversial, as very few clinical data exist demonstrating correlation with prediction of outcomes.

Susceptibility testing of *Pseudomonas* species other than *P. aeruginosa* is rarely indicated, and clinical correlation is required before susceptibility testing is performed. These organisms are generally susceptible to most antipseudomonal antibiotics as well as to trimethoprim-sulfamethoxazole (except most *P. fluorescens/putida* isolates), a property that differentiates them from *P. aeruginosa*. *P. fluorescens*, *P. putida*, and *P. oryzihabitans* may be more resistant to aztreonam and ticarcillin-clavulanate. *P. stutzeri* is usually very susceptible to all antipseudomonal agents (146).

EVALUATION, INTERPRETATION, AND REPORTING OF RESULTS

P. aeruginosa may be associated with colonization or clinically significant infections. Interpretation of the Gram stain often directs the further workup of this organism. The presence of small clusters of gram-negative organisms surrounded by amorphous material is indicative of biofilm formation compatible with a chronic infection. This finding should be reported to physicians, and incubation should be prolonged, as these isolates usually exhibit slower growth characteristics. The presence of these organisms intracellularly in polymorphonuclear cells is a strong indication of true infection rather than colonization. Isolation of *P. aeruginosa* from sterile body sites should always be interpreted as indicative of probable infection. Isolation in mixed culture requires correlation with the direct smear, other organisms isolated, and clinical history. Isolates from sites of chronic infection, such as CF respiratory sites, often exhibit multiple morphotypes that can make identification difficult. Molecular methods increasingly are finding a role in the identification of this organism, especially for epidemiological studies. Susceptibility testing of this organism is difficult, especially for mucoid isolates, due to increasing resistance, lack of reproducibility of results, and lack of clinical correlation. Piperacillin and piperacillin-tazobactam results obtained from automated systems may be unreliable for *Pseudomonas* spp., and in particular for mucoid isolates, and results should be confirmed by disc diffusion or Etest systems. A basic understanding of the multiple mechanisms of resistance, both intrinsic and acquired, is essential to interpret susceptibility testing results and give therapeutic recommendations to physicians. Other *Pseudomonas* species are infrequently isolated in the laboratory and are usually not clinically significant. Clinical correlation and correlation with the Gram stain are essential before further workup is undertaken.

REFERENCES

1. **Aeschlimann, J. R.** 2003. The role of multidrug efflux pumps in the antibiotic resistance of *Pseudomonas aeruginosa* and other gram-negative bacteria. Insights from the Society of Infectious Diseases Pharmacists. *Pharmacotherapy* 23:916–924.
2. **Andrews, J., R. Walker, and A. King.** 2002. Evaluation of media available for testing the susceptibility of *Pseudomonas aeruginosa* by BSAC methodology. *J. Antimicrob. Chemother.* 50:479–486.
3. **Anthony, M., B. Rose, M. B. Pegler, M. Elkins, H. Service, K. Thamotharampillai, J. Watson, M. Robinson, P. Bye, J. Merlino, and C. Harbour.** 2002. Genetic analysis of *Pseudomonas aeruginosa* isolates from the sputa of Australian adult cystic fibrosis patients. *J. Clin. Microbiol.* 40:2772–2778.
4. **Aragone, M. R., D. M. Maurizi, L. O. Clara, J. L. Navarro Estrada, and A. Ascione.** 1992. *Pseudomonas mendocina*, an environmental bacterium isolated from a patient with human infective endocarditis. *J. Clin. Microbiol.* 30:1583–1584.
5. **Armstrong, D. S., G. M. Nixon, R. Carzino, A. Bigham, J. B. Carlin, R. M. Robins-Browne, and K. Grimwood.** 2002. Detection of a widespread clone of *Pseudomonas aeruginosa* in a pediatric cystic fibrosis clinic. *Am. J. Respir. Crit. Care Med.* 166:983–987.
6. **Balke, B., L. Hoy, H. Weissbrodt, and S. Haussler.** 2004. Comparison of the Micronaut Merlin automated broth microtiter system with the standard agar dilution method for antimicrobial susceptibility testing of mucoid and nonmucoid *Pseudomonas aeruginosa* isolates from cystic fibrosis patients. *Eur. J. Clin. Microbiol. Infect. Dis.* 23:765–771.
7. **Beers, S. L., and T. J. Abramo.** 2004. Otitis externa review. *Pediatr. Emerg. Care* 20:250–256.
8. **Bergmans, D. C., M. J. Bonten, E. E. Stobberingh, F. H. van Tiel, S. van der Geest, P. W. de Leeuw, and C. A. Gaillard.** 1998. Colonization with *Pseudomonas aeruginosa* in patients developing ventilator-associated pneumonia. *Infect. Control Hosp. Epidemiol.* 19:853–855.
9. **Bodey, G. P.** 2001. *Pseudomonas aeruginosa* infections in cancer patients: have they gone away? *Curr. Opin. Infect. Dis.* 14:403–407.
10. **Bonapace, C. R., J. A. Bosso, L. V. Friedrich, and R. L. White.** 2002. Comparison of methods of interpretation of checkerboard synergy testing. *Diagn. Microbiol. Infect. Dis.* 44:363–366.
11. **Borriello, G., E. Werner, F. Roe, A. M. Kim, G. D. Ehrlich, and P. S. Stewart.** 2004. Oxygen limitation contributes to antibiotic tolerance of *Pseudomonas aeruginosa* in biofilms. *Antimicrob. Agents Chemother.* 48:2659–2664.
12. **Burke, V., J. O. Robinson, C. J. L. Richardson, and C. S. Bundell.** 1991. Longitudinal studies of virulence factors of *Pseudomonas aeruginosa* in cystic fibrosis. *Pathology* 23:145–148.
13. **Burns, J. L., L. Saiman, S. Whittier, J. Krzewinski, Z. Liu, D. Larone, S. A. Marshall, and R. N. Jones.** 2001. Comparison of two commercial systems (Vitek and MicroScan-WalkAway) for antimicrobial susceptibility testing of *Pseudomonas aeruginosa* isolates from cystic fibrosis patients. *Diagn. Microbiol. Infect. Dis.* 39:257–260.
14. **Burns, J. L., L. Saiman, S. Whittier, D. Larone, J. Krzewinski, Z. Liu, S. A. Marshall, and R. N. Jones.** 2000. Comparison of agar diffusion methodologies for antimicrobial susceptibility testing of *Pseudomonas aeruginosa* isolates from cystic fibrosis patients. *J. Clin. Microbiol.* 38:1818–1822.
15. **Campbell, M. E., S. W. Farmer, and D. P. Speert.** 1988. A new selective medium for *Pseudomonas aeruginosa* with

phenanthroline and 9-chloro-9-[4-(diethylamino)phenyl]-9,10-dihydro-10-phenylacridine (C-390). *J. Clin. Microbiol.* **26:**1910–1912.

16. **Carratala, J., A. Salazar, J. Mascaro, and M. Santin.** 1992. Community-acquired pneumonia due to *Pseudomonas stutzeri. Clin. Infect. Dis.* **14:**792.

17. **Chastre, J., and J. Y. Fagon.** 2002. Ventilator-associated pneumonia. *Am. J. Respir. Crit. Care Med.* **165:**867–903.

18. **Cheng, K., R. L. Smyth, J. R. W. Govan, C. Doherty, C. Winstanley, N. Denning, D. P. Heaf, H. van Saene, and C. A. Hart.** 1996. Spread of β-lactam-resistant *Pseudomonas aeruginosa* in a cystic fibrosis clinic. *Lancet* **348:**639–642.

19. **Cheuk, W., P. C. Woo, K. Y. Yuen, P. H. Yu, and J. K. Chan.** 2000. Intestinal inflammatory pseudotumour with regional lymph node involvement: identification of a new bacterium as the aetiological agent. *J. Pathol.* **192:**289–292.

20. **Chusid, M. J., W. M. Jacobs, and J. R. Sty.** 1979. Pseudomonas arthritis following puncture wounds of the foot. *J. Pediatr.* **94:**429–431.

21. **Ciofu, O., V. Fussing, N. Bagge, C. Koch, and N. Hoiby.** 2001. Characterization of paired mucoid/non-mucoid *Pseudomonas aeruginosa* isolates from Danish cystic fibrosis patients: antibiotic resistance, beta-lactamase activity and RiboPrinting. *J. Antimicrob. Chemother.* **48:**391–396.

22. **Clarke, L., J. E. Moore, B. C. Millar, L. Garske, J. Xu, M. W. Heuzenroeder, M. Crowe, and J. S. Elborn.** 2003. Development of a diagnostic PCR assay that targets a heat-shock protein gene (*groES*) for detection of *Pseudomonas* spp. in cystic fibrosis patients. *J. Med. Microbiol.* **52:**759–763.

23. **Clinical and Laboratory Standards Institute.** 2010. *Performance Standards for Antimicrobial Susceptibility Testing; Twentieth Edition.* Clinical and Laboratory Standards Institute document M100-S20. Clinical and Laboratory Standards Institute, Wayne, PA.

24. **Crespo, M. P., N. Woodford, A. Sinclair, M. E. Kaufmann, J. Turton, J. Glover, J. D. Velez, C. R. Castaneda, M. Recalde, and D. M. Livermore.** 2004. Outbreak of carbapenem-resistant *Pseudomonas aeruginosa* producing VIM-8, a novel metallo-beta-lactamase, in a tertiary care center in Cali, Colombia. *J. Clin. Microbiol.* **42:**5094–5101.

25. **Dabboussi, F., M. Hamze, E. Singer, V. Geoffroy, J. M. Meyer, and D. Izard.** 2002. *Pseudomonas mosselii* sp. nov., a novel species isolated from clinical specimens. *Int. J. Syst. Evol. Microbiol.* **52:**363–376.

26. **Delissalde, F., and C. F. Amabile-Cuevas.** 2004. Comparison of antibiotic susceptibility and plasmid content, between biofilm producing and non-producing clinical isolates of *Pseudomonas aeruginosa. Int. J. Antimicrob. Agents* **24:**405–408.

27. **De Vos, P., and J. De Ley.** 1983. Intra- and intergeneric similarities of *Pseudomonas* and *Xanthomonas* ribosomal ribonucleic acid cistrons. *Int. J. Syst. Bacteriol.* **33:**487–509.

28. **Di Bonaventura, G., E. Ricci, N. Della Loggia, G. Catamo, and R. Piccolomini.** 1998. Evaluation of the E test for antimicrobial susceptibility testing of *Pseudomonas aeruginosa* isolates from patients with long-term bladder catheterization. *J. Clin. Microbiol.* **36:**824–826.

29. **Donay, J. L., D. Mathieu, P. Fernandes, C. Pregermain, P. Bruel, A. Wargnier, I. Casin, F. X. Weill, P. H. Lagrange, and J. L. Herrmann.** 2004. Evaluation of the automated Phoenix system for potential routine use in the clinical microbiology laboratory. *J. Clin. Microbiol.* **42:**1542–1546.

30. **Drenkard, E., and F. M. Ausubel.** 2002. *Pseudomonas* biofilm formation and antibiotic resistance are linked to phenotypic variation. *Nature* **416:**740–743.

31. **Dunne, W. M., Jr., and M. J. Chusid.** 1987. Mixed morphotype susceptibility testing of *Pseudomonas aeruginosa* from patients with cystic fibrosis. *Diagn. Microbiol. Infect. Dis.* **6:**165–170.

32. **Elomari, M., L. Coroler, B. Hoste, M. Gillis, D. Izard, and H. Leclerc.** 1996. DNA relatedness among *Pseudomonas* strains isolated from natural mineral waters and proposal of *Pseudomonas veronii* sp. nov. *Int. J. Syst. Bacteriol.* **46:**1138–1144.

33. **Elomari, M., L. Coroler, D. Izard, and H. Leclerc.** 1995. A numerical taxonomic study of fluorescent *Pseudomonas* strains isolated from natural mineral waters. *J. Appl. Bacteriol.* **78:**71–81.

34. **Elomari, M., L. Coroler, S. Verhille, D. Izard, and H. Leclerc.** 1997. *Pseudomonas monteilii* sp. nov., isolated from clinical specimens. *Int. J. Syst. Bacteriol.* **47:**846–852.

35. **Elomari, M., D. Izard, P. Vincent, L. Coroler, and H. Leclerc.** 1994. Comparison of ribotyping analysis and numerical taxonomy studies of *Pseudomonas putida* biovar A. *Syst. Appl. Microbiol.* **17:**361–369.

36. **Emmerson, A. M.** 2001. Emerging waterborne infections in health-care settings. *Emerg. Infect. Dis.* **7:**272–276.

37. **Farrell, P. M., J. Collins, L. S. Broderick, M. J. Rock, Z. Li, M. R. Kosorok, A. Laxova, W. M. Gershan, and A. S. Brody.** 2009. Association between mucoid *Pseudomonas* infection and bronchiectasis in children with cystic fibrosis. *Radiology* **252:**534–543.

38. **Fisher, M. C., J. F. Goldsmith, and P. H. Gilligan.** 1985. Sneakers as a source of *Pseudomonas aeruginosa* in children with osteomyelitis following puncture wounds. *J. Pediatr.* **106:**607–609.

39. **Fong, I. W., and K. B. Tomkins.** 1985. Review of *Pseudomonas aeruginosa* meningitis with special emphasis on treatment with ceftazidime. *Rev. Infect. Dis.* **7:**604–612.

40. **Fonseca, K., J. MacDougall, and T. L. Pitt.** 1986. Inhibition of *Pseudomonas aeruginosa* from cystic fibrosis by selective media. *J. Clin. Pathol.* **39:**220–222.

41. **Foweraker, J. E., C. R. Laughton, D. F. Brown, and D. Bilton.** 2005. Phenotypic variability of *Pseudomonas aeruginosa* in sputa from patients with acute infective exacerbation of cystic fibrosis and its impact on the validity of antimicrobial susceptibility testing. *J. Antimicrob. Chemother.* **55:**921–927.

42. **Frank, D. N., and N. R. Pace.** 2008. Gastrointestinal microbiology enters the metagenomics era. *Curr. Opin. Gastroenterol.* **24:**4–10.

43. **Funke, G., and P. Funke-Kissling.** 2004. Evaluation of the new VITEK 2 card for identification of clinically relevant gram-negative rods. *J. Clin. Microbiol.* **42:**4067–4071.

44. **Funke, G., and P. Funke-Kissling.** 2004. Use of the BD PHOENIX Automated Microbiology System for direct identification and susceptibility testing of gram-negative rods from positive blood cultures in a three-phase trial. *J. Clin. Microbiol.* **42:**1466–1470.

45. **Gales, A. C., R. N. Jones, J. Turnidge, R. Rennie, and R. Ramphal.** 2001. Characterization of *Pseudomonas aeruginosa* isolates: occurrence rates, antimicrobial susceptibility patterns, and molecular typing in the global SENTRY Antimicrobial Surveillance Program, 1997–1999. *Clin. Infect. Dis.* **32(Suppl. 2):**S146–S155.

46. **Gales, A. C., A. O. Reis, and R. N. Jones.** 2001. Contemporary assessment of antimicrobial susceptibility testing methods for polymyxin B and colistin: review of available interpretative criteria and quality control guidelines. *J. Clin. Microbiol.* **39:**183–190.

47. **Garau, J., and L. Gomez.** 2003. *Pseudomonas aeruginosa* pneumonia. *Curr. Opin. Infect. Dis.* **16:**135–143.

48. **George, A. M., P. M. Jones, and P. G. Middleton.** 2009. Cystic fibrosis infections: treatment strategies and prospects. *FEMS Microbiol. Lett.* **300:**153–164.

49. **Giamarellou, H., and G. Poulakou.** 2009. Multidrug-resistant Gram-negative infections: what are the treatment options? *Drugs* **69:**1879–1901.

50. **Gibb, A. P., C. Tribuddharat, R. A. Moore, T. J. Louie, W. Krulicki, D. M. Livermore, M. F. Palepou, and N. Woodford.** 2002. Nosocomial outbreak of carbapenem-resistant *Pseudomonas aeruginosa* with a new *bla*IMP allele, *bla*IMP-7. *Antimicrob. Agents Chemother.* **46:**255–258.

51. **Gilligan, P. H.** 1991. Microbiology of airway disease in patients with cystic fibrosis. *Clin. Microbiol. Rev.* **4:**35–51.

52. **Goetz, A., V. L. Yu, J. E. Hanchett, and J. D. Rihs.** 1983. *Pseudomonas stutzeri* bacteremia associated with hemodialysis. *Arch. Intern. Med.* **143:**1909–1912.

53. **Goossens, H.** 2003. Susceptibility of multi-drug-resistant *Pseudomonas aeruginosa* in intensive care units: results from the European MYSTIC study group. *Clin. Microbiol. Infect.* **9:**980–983.

54. **Govan, J. R., and V. Deretic.** 1996. Microbial pathogenesis in cystic fibrosis: mucoid *Pseudomonas aeruginosa* and *Burkholderia cepacia*. *Microbiol. Rev.* **60:**539–574.

55. **Gregory, D. W., and W. Schaffner.** 1987. Pseudomonas infections associated with hot tubs and other environments. *Infect. Dis. Clin. N. Am.* **1:**635–648.

56. **Guasp, C., E. R. Moore, J. Lalucat, and A. Bennasar.** 2000. Utility of internally transcribed 16S-23S rDNA spacer regions for the definition of *Pseudomonas stutzeri* genomovars and other *Pseudomonas* species. *Int. J. Syst. Evol. Microbiol.* **50:**1629–1639.

57. **Gunasekera, T. S., M. R. Dorsch, M. B. Slade, and D. A. Veal.** 2003. Specific detection of *Pseudomonas* spp. in milk by fluorescence in situ hybridization using ribosomal RNA directed probes. *J. Appl. Microbiol.* **94:**936–945.

58. **Gustafsson, I., M. Sjolund, E. Torell, M. Johannesson, L. Engstrand, O. Cars, and D. I. Andersson.** 2003. Bacteria with increased mutation frequency and antibiotic resistance are enriched in the commensal flora of patients with high antibiotic usage. *J. Antimicrob. Chemother.* **52:**645–650.

59. **Hampton, K. D., and B. L. Wasilauskas.** 1979. Isolation of oxidase-negative *Pseudomonas aeruginosa* from sputum culture. *J. Clin. Microbiol.* **9:**632–634.

60. **Hancock, R. E., L. M. Mutharia, L. Chan, R. P. Darveau, D. P. Speert, and G. B. Pier.** 1983. *Pseudomonas aeruginosa* isolates from patients with cystic fibrosis: a class of serum-sensitive, nontypable strains deficient in lipopolysaccharide O side chains. *Infect. Immun.* **42:**170–177.

61. **Hancock, R. E., and D. P. Speert.** 2000. Antibiotic resistance in *Pseudomonas aeruginosa*: mechanisms and impact on treatment. *Drug Resist. Updat.* **3:**247–255.

62. **Hassett, D. J., J. Cuppoletti, B. Trapnell, S. V. Lymar, J. J. Rowe, S. S. Yoon, G. M. Hilliard, K. Parvatiyar, M. C. Kamani, D. J. Wozniak, S. H. Hwang, T. R. McDermott, and U. A. Ochsner.** 2002. Anaerobic metabolism and quorum sensing by *Pseudomonas aeruginosa* biofilms in chronically infected cystic fibrosis airways: rethinking antibiotic treatment strategies and drug targets. *Adv. Drug Deliv. Rev.* **54:**1425–1443.

63. **Haussler, S., B. Tummler, H. Weissbrodt, M. Rohde, and I. Steinmetz.** 1999. Small-colony variants of *Pseudomonas aeruginosa* in cystic fibrosis. *Clin. Infect. Dis.* **29:**621–625.

64. **Haussler, S., I. Ziegler, A. Lottel, F. von Gotz, M. Rohde, D. Wehmhohner, S. Saravanamuthu, B. Tummler, and I. Steinmetz.** 2003. Highly adherent small-colony variants of *Pseudomonas aeruginosa* in cystic fibrosis lung infection. *J. Med. Microbiol.* **52:**295–301.

65. **Haussler, S., S. Ziesing, G. Rademacher, L. Hoy, and H. Weissbrodt.** 2003. Evaluation of the Merlin, Micronaut system for automated antimicrobial susceptibility testing of *Pseudomonas aeruginosa* and *Burkholderia* species isolated from cystic fibrosis patients. *Eur. J. Clin. Microbiol. Infect. Dis.* **22:**496–500.

66. **Hedberg, M.** 1969. Acetamide agar medium selective for *Pseudomonas aeruginosa*. *Appl. Microbiol.* **17:**481.

67. **Hentzer, M., G. M. Teitzel, G. J. Balzer, A. Heydorn, S. Molin, M. Givskov, and M. R. Parsek.** 2001. Alginate overproduction affects *Pseudomonas aeruginosa* biofilm structure and function. *J. Bacteriol.* **183:**5395–5401.

68. **Henwood, C. J., D. M. Livermore, D. James, and M. Warner.** 2001. Antimicrobial susceptibility of *Pseudomonas aeruginosa*: results of a UK survey and evaluation of the British Society for Antimicrobial Chemotherapy disc susceptibility test. *J. Antimicrob. Chemother.* **47:**789–799.

69. **Hirakata, Y., R. Srikumar, K. Poole, N. Gotoh, T. Suematsu, S. Kohno, S. Kamihira, R. E. Hancock, and D. P. Speert.** 2002. Multidrug efflux systems play an important role in the invasiveness of *Pseudomonas aeruginosa*. *J. Exp. Med.* **196:**109–118.

70. **Hogardt, M., S. Schmoldt, M. Gotzfried, K. Adler, and J. Heesemann.** 2004. Pitfalls of polymyxin antimicrobial susceptibility testing of *Pseudomonas aeruginosa* isolated from cystic fibrosis patients. *J. Antimicrob. Chemother.* **54:**1057–1061.

71. **Hoiby, N.** 2002. New antimicrobials in the management of cystic fibrosis. *J. Antimicrob. Chemother.* **49:**235–238.

72. **Holt, J., N. R. Kreig, P. H. A. Sneath, J. T. Staley, and S. T. Williams (ed.).** 1994. *Bergey's Manual of Determinative Bacteriology*, 9th ed., p. 93–94. Lippincott Williams & Wilkins, Baltimore, MD.

73. **Ibrahim-Elmagboul, I. B., and D. M. Livermore.** 1997. Sensitivity testing of ciprofloxacin for *Pseudomonas aeruginosa*. *J. Antimicrob. Chemother.* **39:**309–317.

74. **The International *Pseudomonas aeruginosa* Typing Study Group.** 1994. A multicenter comparison of methods for typing strains of *Pseudomonas aeruginosa* predominantly from patients with cystic fibrosis. *J. Infect. Dis.* **169:**134–142.

75. **Jacoby, G. A., and L. S. Munoz-Price.** 2005. The new beta-lactamases. *N. Engl. J. Med.* **352:**380–391.

76. **Jaffe, R. I., J. D. Lane, and C. W. Bates.** 2001. Real-time identification of *Pseudomonas aeruginosa* direct from clinical samples using a rapid extraction method and polymerase chain reaction (PCR). *J. Clin. Lab. Anal.* **15:**131–137.

77. **Jiraskova, N., and P. Rozsival.** 1998. Delayed-onset *Pseudomonas stutzeri* endophthalmitis after uncomplicated cataract surgery. *J. Cataract Refract. Surg.* **24:**866–867.

78. **Johansen, H. K., K. Kjeldsen, and N. Hoiby.** 2001. *Pseudomonas mendocina* as a cause of chronic infective endocarditis in a patient with situs inversus. *Clin. Microbiol. Infect.* **7:**650–652.

79. **Jones, A. M., A. K. Webb, J. R. Govan, C. A. Hart, and M. J. Walshaw.** 2002. *Pseudomonas aeruginosa* cross-infection in cystic fibrosis. *Lancet* **359:**527–528.

80. **Joyanes, P., M. del Carmen Conejo, L. Martinez-Martinez, and E. J. Perea.** 2001. Evaluation of the VITEK 2 system for the identification and susceptibility testing of three species of nonfermenting gram-negative rods frequently isolated from clinical samples. *J. Clin. Microbiol.* **39:**3247–3253.

81. **Kappler, M., A. Kraxner, D. Reinhardt, B. Ganster, M. Griese, and T. Lang.** 2006. Diagnostic and prognostic value of serum antibodies against *Pseudomonas aeruginosa* in cystic fibrosis. *Thorax* **61:**684–688.

82. **Keeven, J. K., and B. T. DeCicco.** 1989. Selective medium for *Pseudomonas aeruginosa* that uses 1,10-phenanthroline as the selective agent. *Appl. Environ. Microbiol.* **55:**3231–3233.

83. **Kersters, K., M. Ludwig, P. Vancanneyt, P. De Vos, M. Gillis, and K.-H. Schleifer.** 1996. Recent changes in the classification of the pseudomonads: an overview. *Syst. Appl. Microbiol.* **19:**465–477.

84. **Keys, T. F., L. J. Melton III, M. D. Maker, and D. M. Ilstrup.** 1983. A suspected hospital outbreak of pseudobacteremia due to *Pseudomonas stutzeri*. *J. Infect. Dis.* **147:**489–493.

85. **Khan, A. A., and C. E. Cerniglia.** 1994. Detection of *Pseudomonas aeruginosa* from clinical and environmental samples by amplification of the exotoxin A gene using PCR. *Appl. Environ. Microbiol.* **60:**3739–3745.

86. **Kirkby, S., K. Novak, and K. McCoy.** 2009. Update on antibiotics for infection control in cystic fibrosis. *Expert Rev. Anti-Infect. Ther.* **7:**967–980.

87. **Krueger, C. L., and W. Sheikh.** 1987. A new selective medium for isolating *Pseudomonas* spp. from water. *Appl. Environ. Microbiol.* **53:**895–897.

88. **Lagatolla, C., E. A. Tonin, C. Monti-Bragadin, L. Dolzani, F. Gombac, C. Bearzi, E. Edalucci, F. Gionechetti, and G. M. Rossolini.** 2004. Endemic carbapenem-resistant *Pseudomonas aeruginosa* with acquired metallo-beta-lactamase determinants in European hospital. *Emerg. Infect. Dis.* **10:**535–538.

89. **Laguerre, G., L. Rigottier-Gois, and P. Lemanceau.** 1994. Fluorescent *Pseudomonas* species categorized by using polymerase chain reaction (PCR)/restriction fragment analysis of 16S rDNA. *Mol. Ecol.* **3:**479–487.

90. **Lam, J., R. Chan, K. Lam, and J. W. Costerton.** 1980. Production of mucoid microcolonies by *Pseudomonas aeruginosa* within infected lungs in cystic fibrosis. *Infect. Immun.* **28:**546–556.

91. **Lambe, D. W., Jr., and P. Stewart.** 1972. Evaluation of Pseudosel agar as an aid in the identification of *Pseudomonas aeruginosa*. *Appl. Microbiol.* **23**:377–381.

92. **Lauretti, L., M. L. Riccio, A. Mazzariol, G. Cornaglia, G. Amicosante, R. Fontana, and G. M. Rossolini.** 1999. Cloning and characterization of bla$_{VIM}$, a new integron-borne metallo-β-lactamase gene from a *Pseudomonas aeruginosa* clinical isolate. *Antimicrob. Agents Chemother.* **43**:1584–1590.

93. **Lee, K., W. G. Lee, Y. Uh, G. Y. Ha, J. Cho, and Y. Chong.** 2003. VIM- and IMP-type metallo-beta-lactamase-producing *Pseudomonas* spp. and *Acinetobacter* spp. in Korean hospitals. *Emerg. Infect. Dis.* **9**:868–871.

94. **Lin, R. D., P. R. Hsueh, J. C. Chang, L. J. Teng, S. C. Chang, S. W. Ho, W. C. Hsieh, and K. T. Luh.** 1997. *Flavimonas oryzihabitans* bacteremia: clinical features and microbiological characteristics of isolates. *Clin. Infect. Dis.* **24**:867–873.

95. **Linker, A., and R. S. Jones.** 1966. A new polysaccharide resembling alginic acid isolated from pseudomonads. *J. Biol. Chem.* **241**:3845–3851.

96. **Lister, P. D., D. J. Wolter, and N. D. Hanson.** 2009. Antibacterial-resistant *Pseudomonas aeruginosa*: clinical impact and complex regulation of chromosomally encoded resistance mechanisms. *Clin. Microbiol. Rev.* **22**:582–610.

97. **Livermore, D. M.** 1995. β-Lactamases in laboratory and clinical resistance. *Clin. Microbiol. Rev.* **8**:557–584.

98. **Livermore, D. M.** 2002. Multiple mechanisms of antimicrobial resistance in *Pseudomonas aeruginosa*: our worst nightmare? *Clin. Infect. Dis.* **34**:634–640.

99. **Livermore, D. M., and H. Y. Chen.** 1999. Quality of antimicrobial susceptibility testing in the UK: a *Pseudomonas aeruginosa* survey revisited. *J. Antimicrob. Chemother.* **43**:517–522.

100. **Lucas, K. G., T. E. Kiehn, K. A. Sobeck, D. Armstrong, and A. E. Brown.** 1994. Sepsis caused by *Flavimonas oryzihabitans*. *Medicine* (Baltimore) **73**:209–214.

101. **Macia, M. D., N. Borrell, J. L. Perez, and A. Oliver.** 2004. Detection and susceptibility testing of hypermutable *Pseudomonas aeruginosa* strains with the Etest and disk diffusion. *Antimicrob. Agents Chemother.* **48**:2665–2672.

102. **MacLeod, D. L., L. E. Nelson, R. M. Shawar, B. B. Lin, L. G. Lockwood, J. E. Dirk, G. H. Miller, J. L. Burns, and R. L. Garber.** 2000. Aminoglycoside-resistance mechanisms for cystic fibrosis *Pseudomonas aeruginosa* isolates are unchanged by long-term, intermittent, inhaled tobramycin treatment. *J. Infect. Dis.* **181**:1180–1184.

103. **Mah, T. F., B. Pitts, B. Pellock, G. C. Walker, P. S. Stewart, and G. A. O'Toole.** 2003. A genetic basis for *Pseudomonas aeruginosa* biofilm antibiotic resistance. *Nature* **426**:306–310.

104. **Mahenthiralingam, E., M. Campbell, and D. P. Speert.** 1994. Nonmotility and phagocytic resistance of *Pseudomonas aeruginosa* isolates from chronically colonized patients with cystic fibrosis. *Infect. Immun.* **62**:596–605.

105. **Mahenthiralingam, E., M. E. Campbell, J. Foster, J. S. Lam, and D. P. Speert.** 1996. Random amplified polymorphic DNA typing of *Pseudomonas aeruginosa* isolates recovered from patients with cystic fibrosis. *J. Clin. Microbiol.* **34**:1129–1135.

106. **Manome, I., M. Ikedo, Y. Saito, K. K. Ishii, and M. Kaku.** 2003. Evaluation of a novel automated chemiluminescent assay system for antimicrobial susceptibility testing. *J. Clin. Microbiol.* **41**:279–284.

107. **Marin, M., D. Garcia de Viedma, P. Martin-Rabadan, M. Rodriguez-Creixems, and E. Bouza.** 2000. Infection of Hickman catheter by *Pseudomonas* (formerly *Flavimonas*) *oryzihabitans* traced to a synthetic bath sponge. *J. Clin. Microbiol.* **38**:4577–4579.

108. **Marley, E. F., C. Mohla, and J. M. Campos.** 1995. Evaluation of E-Test for determination of antimicrobial MICs for *Pseudomonas aeruginosa* isolates from cystic fibrosis patients. *J. Clin. Microbiol.* **33**:3191–3193.

109. **Marold, L. M., R. Freedman, R. E. Chamberlain, and J. J. Miyashiro.** 1981. New selective agent for isolation of *Pseudomonas aeruginosa*. *Appl. Environ. Microbiol.* **41**:977–980.

110. **Martinez-Martinez, L., A. Pascual, and G. A. Jacoby.** 1998. Quinolone resistance from a transferable plasmid. *Lancet* **351**:797–799.

111. **Martino, P., A. Micozzi, M. Venditti, G. Gentile, C. Girmenia, R. Raccah, S. Santilli, N. Alessandri, and F. Mandelli.** 1990. Catheter-related right-sided endocarditis in bone marrow transplant recipients. *Rev. Infect. Dis.* **12**:250–257.

112. **McCleskey, F. K., and E. D. Adams, Jr.** 1980. Isolation of oxidase-negative *Pseudomonas aeruginosa* from urine culture. *J. Clin. Microbiol.* **12**:624–625.

113. **Migula, W.** 1894. Uber ein neues System der Bakterien. *Arb. Bakeriol. Inst. Karlsruhe* **1**:235–238.

114. **Miller, G. H., F. J. Sabatelli, R. S. Hare, Y. Glupczynski, P. Mackey, D. Shlaes, K. Shimizu, K. J. Shaw, and the Aminoglycoside Resistance Study Groups.** 1997. The most frequent aminoglycoside resistance mechanisms—changes with time and geographic area: a reflection of aminoglycoside usage patterns? *Clin. Infect. Dis.* **24**(Suppl. 1): S46–S62.

115. **Morehead, R. S., and S. J. Pinto.** 2000. Ventilator-associated pneumonia. *Arch. Intern. Med.* **160**:1926–1936.

116. **Morlin, G. L., D. L. Hedges, A. L. Smith, and J. L. Burns.** 1994. Accuracy and cost of antibiotic susceptibility testing of mixed morphotypes of *Pseudomonas aeruginosa*. *J. Clin. Microbiol.* **32**:1027–1030.

117. **Moskowitz, S. M., J. M. Foster, J. Emerson, and J. L. Burns.** 2004. Clinically feasible biofilm susceptibility assay for isolates of *Pseudomonas aeruginosa* from patients with cystic fibrosis. *J. Clin. Microbiol.* **42**:1915–1922.

118. **Nakamoto, H., Y. Hashikita, A. Itabashi, T. Kobayashi, and H. Suzuki.** 2004. Changes in the organisms of resistant peritonitis in patients on continuous ambulatory peritoneal dialysis. *Adv. Perit. Dial.* **20**:52–57.

119. **Noble, R. C., and S. B. Overman.** 1994. *Pseudomonas stutzeri* infection. A review of hospital isolates and a review of the literature. *Diagn. Microbiol. Infect. Dis.* **19**:51–56.

120. **Nordmann, P., and L. Poirel.** 2002. Emerging carbapenemases in Gram-negative aerobes. *Clin. Microbiol. Infect.* **8**:321–331.

121. **Obritsch, M. D., D. N. Fish, R. MacLaren, and R. Jung.** 2004. National surveillance of antimicrobial resistance in *Pseudomonas aeruginosa* isolates obtained from intensive care unit patients from 1993 to 2002. *Antimicrob. Agents Chemother.* **48**:4606–4610.

122. **Ogle, J. W., J. M. Janda, D. E. Woods, and M. L. Vasil.** 1987. Characterization and use of a DNA probe as an epidemiological marker for *Pseudomonas aeruginosa*. *J. Infect. Dis.* **155**:119–126.

123. **O'Hara, C. M.** 2005. Manual and automated instrumentation for identification of *Enterobacteriaceae* and other aerobic gram-negative bacilli. *Clin. Microbiol. Rev.* **18**:147–162.

124. **O'Hara, C. M., and J. M. Miller.** 2002. Ability of the MicroScan rapid gram-negative ID type 3 panel to identify nonenteric glucose-fermenting and nonfermenting gram-negative bacilli. *J. Clin. Microbiol.* **40**:3750–3752.

125. **O'Hara, C. M., and J. M. Miller.** 2003. Evaluation of the Vitek 2 ID-GNB assay for identification of members of the family *Enterobacteriaceae* and other nonenteric gram-negative bacilli and comparison with the Vitek GNI+ card. *J. Clin. Microbiol.* **41**:2096–2101.

126. **Oliver, A., R. Canton, P. Campo, F. Baquero, and J. Blazquez.** 2000. High frequency of hypermutable *Pseudomonas aeruginosa* in cystic fibrosis lung infection. *Science* **288**:1251–1254.

127. **Oliver, A., B. R. Levin, C. Juan, F. Baquero, and J. Blazquez.** 2004. Hypermutation and the preexistence of antibiotic-resistant *Pseudomonas aeruginosa* mutants: implications for susceptibility testing and treatment of chronic infections. *Antimicrob. Agents Chemother.* **48**:4226–4233.

128. **Osano, E., Y. Arakawa, R. Wacharotayankun, M. Ohta, T. Horii, H. Ito, F. Yoshimura, and N. Kato.** 1994. Molecular characterization of an enterobacterial metallo β-lactamase found in a clinical isolate of *Serratia marcescens* that shows imipenem resistance. *Antimicrob. Agents Chemother.* **38:**71–78.

129. **Palleroni, N., R. Kunisawa, R. Contopoulou, and M. Doudoroff.** 1973. Nucleic acid homologies in the genus *Pseudomonas. Int. J. Syst. Bacteriol.* **23:**333–339.

130. **Peleg, A. Y., Y. Tilahun, M. J. Fiandaca, E. M. D'Agata, L. Venkataraman, R. C. Moellering, Jr., and G. M. Eliopoulos.** 2009. Utility of peptide nucleic acid fluorescence in situ hybridization for rapid detection of *Acinetobacter* spp. and *Pseudomonas aeruginosa. J. Clin. Microbiol.* **47:**830–832.

131. **Poirel, L., T. Naas, D. Nicolas, L. Collet, S. Bellais, J.-D. Cavallo, and P. Nordmann.** 2000. Characterization of VIM-2, a carbapenem-hydrolyzing metallo-β-lactamase and its plasmid- and integron-borne gene from a *Pseudomonas aeruginosa* clinical isolate in France. *Antimicrob. Agents Chemother.* **44:**891–897.

132. **Poole, K.** 2005. Aminoglycoside resistance in *Pseudomonas aeruginosa. Antimicrob. Agents Chemother.* **49:**479–487.

133. **Poole, K., K. Tetro, Q. Zhao, S. Neshat, D. E. Heinrichs, and N. Bianco.** 1996. Expression of the multidrug resistance operon *mexA-mexB-oprM* in *Pseudomonas aeruginosa: mexR* encodes a regulator of operon expression. *Antimicrob. Agents Chemother.* **40:**2021–2028.

134. **Potvliege, C., J. Jonckheer, C. Lenclud, and W. Hansen.** 1987. *Pseudomonas stutzeri* pneumonia and septicemia in a patient with multiple myeloma. *J. Clin. Microbiol.* **25:**458–459.

135. **Pruitt, B. A., Jr., A. T. McManus, S. H. Kim, and C. W. Goodwin.** 1998. Burn wound infections: current status. *World J. Surg.* **22:**135–145.

136. **Qin, X., J. Emerson, J. Stapp, L. Stapp, P. Abe, and J. L. Burns.** 2003. Use of real-time PCR with multiple targets to identify *Pseudomonas aeruginosa* and other nonfermenting gram-negative bacilli from patients with cystic fibrosis. *J. Clin. Microbiol.* **41:**4312–4317.

137. **Rahav, G., A. Simhon, Y. Mattan, A. E. Moses, and T. Sacks.** 1995. Infections with *Chryseomonas luteola* (CDC group Ve-1) and *Flavimonas oryzihabitans* (CDC group Ve-2). *Medicine* (Baltimore) **74:**83–88.

138. **Rastogi, S., and S. J. Sperber.** 1998. Facial cellulitis and *Pseudomonas luteola* bacteremia in an otherwise healthy patient. *Diagn. Microbiol. Infect. Dis.* **32:**303–305.

139. **Reisler, R. B., and H. Blumberg.** 1999. Community-acquired *Pseudomonas stutzeri* vertebral osteomyelitis in a previously healthy patient: case report and review. *Clin. Infect. Dis.* **29:**667–669.

140. **Rius, N., M. C. Fuste, C. Guasp, J. Lalucat, and J. G. Loren.** 2001. Clonal population structure of *Pseudomonas stutzeri*, a species with exceptional genetic diversity. *J. Bacteriol.* **183:**736–744.

141. **Roig, P., A. Orti, and V. Navarro.** 1996. Meningitis due to *Pseudomonas stutzeri* in a patient infected with human immunodeficiency virus. *Clin. Infect. Dis.* **22:**587–588.

142. **Ronald, A.** 2002. The etiology of urinary tract infection: traditional and emerging pathogens. *Am. J. Med.* **113**(Suppl. 1A):14S–19S.

143. **Rossolini, G. M., and E. Mantengoli.** 2005. Treatment and control of severe infections caused by multiresistant *Pseudomonas aeruginosa. Clin. Microbiol. Infect.* **11**(Suppl. 4):17–32.

144. **Rubin Grandis, J., B. F. Branstetter IV, and V. L. Yu.** 2004. The changing face of malignant (necrotising) external otitis: clinical, radiological, and anatomic correlations. *Lancet Infect. Dis.* **4:**34–39.

145. **Sader, H. S., M. Castanheira, R. E. Mendes, M. Toleman, T. R. Walsh, and R. N. Jones.** 2005. Dissemination and diversity of metallo-beta-lactamases in Latin America: report from the SENTRY Antimicrobial Surveillance Program. *Int. J. Antimicrob. Agents* **25:**57–61.

146. **Sader, H. S., and R. N. Jones.** 2005. Antimicrobial susceptibility of uncommonly isolated non-enteric Gram-negative bacilli. *Int. J. Antimicrob. Agents* **25:**95–109.

147. **Saiman, L., J. L. Burns, D. Larone, Y. Chen, E. Garber, and S. Whittier.** 2003. Evaluation of MicroScan Autoscan for identification of *Pseudomonas aeruginosa* isolates from cystic fibrosis patients. *J. Clin. Microbiol.* **41:**492–494.

148. **Sapico, F. L., and J. Z. Montgomerie.** 1980. Vertebral osteomyelitis in intravenous drug abusers: report of three cases and review of the literature. *Rev. Infect. Dis.* **2:**196–206.

149. **Schutze, G. E., C. H. Gilliam, S. Jin, C. K. Cavenaugh, R. W. Hall, R. W. Bradsher, and R. F. Jacobs.** 2004. Use of DNA fingerprinting in decision making for considering closure of neonatal intensive care units because of *Pseudomonas aeruginosa* bloodstream infections. *Pediatr. Infect. Dis. J.* **23:**110–114.

150. **Scott, J., F. E. Boulton, J. R. Govan, R. S. Miles, D. B. McClelland, and C. V. Prowse.** 1988. A fatal transfusion reaction associated with blood contaminated with *Pseudomonas fluorescens. Vox Sang.* **54:**201–204.

151. **Serisier, D. J., G. Jones, A. Tuck, G. Connett, and M. P. Carroll.** 2003. Clinical application of direct sputum sensitivity testing in a severe infective exacerbation of cystic fibrosis. *Pediatr. Pulmonol.* **35:**463–466.

152. **Shih, P. C., and C. T. Huang.** 2002. Effects of quorum-sensing deficiency on *Pseudomonas aeruginosa* biofilm formation and antibiotic resistance. *J. Antimicrob. Chemother.* **49:**309–314.

153. **Simor, A. E., J. Ricci, A. Lau, R. M. Bannatyne, L. Ford-Jones, G. Verschraegen, G. Claeys, G. Meeus, M. Delanghe, T. F. Keys, L. J. Melton III, M. D. Maker, D. M. Ilstrup, J. J. Farmer III, R. A. Weinstein, C. H. Zierdt, and C. D. Brokopp.** 1985. Pseudobacteremia due to *Pseudomonas fluorescens. Pediatr. Infect. Dis.* **4:**508–512.

154. **Smith, A. L., S. B. Fiel, N. Mayer-Hamblett, B. Ramsey, and J. L. Burns.** 2003. Susceptibility testing of *Pseudomonas aeruginosa* isolates and clinical response to parenteral antibiotic administration: lack of association in cystic fibrosis. *Chest* **123:**1495–1502.

155. **Speert, D. P.** 2002. Molecular epidemiology of *Pseudomonas aeruginosa. Front. Biosci.* **7:**e354–e361.

156. **Speert, D. P.** 1993. *Pseudomonas aeruginosa*-phagocytic cell interaction, p. 163–182. In M. Campa, M. Bendinelli, and H. Friedman (ed.), Pseudomonas aeruginosa *as an Opportunistic Pathogen.* Plenum Press, New York, NY.

157. **Speert, D. P., M. E. Campbell, A. G. Davidson, and L. T. Wong.** 1993. *Pseudomonas aeruginosa* colonization of the gastrointestinal tract in patients with cystic fibrosis. *J. Infect. Dis.* **167:**226–229.

158. **Speert, D. P., M. E. Campbell, D. A. Henry, R. Milner, F. Taha, A. Gravelle, A. G. Davidson, L. T. Wong, and E. Mahenthiralingam.** 2002. Epidemiology of *Pseudomonas aeruginosa* in cystic fibrosis in British Columbia, Canada. *Am. J. Respir. Crit. Care Med.* **166:**988–993.

159. **Spilker, T., T. Coenye, P. Vandamme, and J. J. LiPuma.** 2004. PCR-based assay for differentiation of *Pseudomonas aeruginosa* from other *Pseudomonas* species recovered from cystic fibrosis patients. *J. Clin. Microbiol.* **42:**2074–2079.

160. **Spoering, A. L., and K. Lewis.** 2001. Biofilms and planktonic cells of *Pseudomonas aeruginosa* have similar resistance to killing by antimicrobials. *J. Bacteriol.* **183:**6746–6751.

161. **Stackebrandt, E., R. Murray, and G. Trüper.** 1988. *Proteobacteria* classis nov., a name for the phylogenetic taxon that includes the "purple bacteria and their relatives." *Int. J. Syst. Bacteriol.* **38:**321–325.

162. **Stefaniuk, E., A. Baraniak, M. Gniadkowski, and W. Hryniewicz.** 2003. Evaluation of the BD Phoenix automated identification and susceptibility testing system in clinical microbiology laboratory practice. *Eur. J. Clin. Microbiol. Infect. Dis.* **22:**479–485.

163. **Stender, H., A. Broomer, K. Oliveira, H. Perry-O'Keefe, J. J. Hyldig-Nielsen, A. Sage, B. Young, and J. Coull.** 2000. Rapid detection, identification, and enumeration

of *Pseudomonas aeruginosa* in bottled water using peptide nucleic acid probes. *J. Microbiol. Methods* **42**:245–253.

164. **Stern, G. A.** 1990. Pseudomonas keratitis and contact lens wear: the lens/eye is at fault. *Cornea* **9**(Suppl. 1):S36–S38; discussion, S39–S40.

165. **Steward, C. D., J. M. Mohammed, J. M. Swenson, S. A. Stocker, P. P. Williams, R. P. Gaynes, J. E. McGowan, Jr., and F. C. Tenover.** 2003. Antimicrobial susceptibility testing of carbapenems: multicenter validity testing and accuracy levels of five antimicrobial test methods for detecting resistance in *Enterobacteriaceae* and *Pseudomonas aeruginosa* isolates. *J. Clin. Microbiol.* **41**:351–358.

166. **Stewart, P. S., and J. W. Costerton.** 2001. Antibiotic resistance of bacteria in biofilms. *Lancet* **358**:135–138.

167. **Stoll, B. J., N. Hansen, A. A. Fanaroff, L. L. Wright, W. A. Carlo, R. A. Ehrenkranz, J. A. Lemons, E. F. Donovan, A. R. Stark, J. E. Tyson, W. Oh, C. R. Bauer, S. B. Korones, S. Shankaran, A. R. Laptook, D. K. Stevenson, L. A. Papile, and W. K. Poole.** 2002. Late-onset sepsis in very low birth weight neonates: the experience of the NICHD Neonatal Research Network. *Pediatrics* **110**:285–291.

168. **Sung, L. L., D. I. Yang, C. C. Hung, and H. T. Ho.** 2000. Evaluation of autoSCAN-W/A and the Vitek GNI+ Auto-Microbic system for identification of non-glucose-fermenting gram-negative bacilli. *J. Clin. Microbiol.* **38**:1127–1130.

169. **Szita, G., and G. Biro.** 1990. A synthetic, selective culture medium for *Pseudomonas aeruginosa*. *Acta Vet. Hung.* **38**:187–194.

170. **Tancrede, C. H., and A. O. Andremont.** 1985. Bacterial translocation and gram-negative bacteremia in patients with hematological malignancies. *J. Infect. Dis.* **152**:99–103.

171. **Thom, A. R., M. E. Stephens, W. A. Gillespie, and V. G. Alder.** 1971. Nitrofurantoin media for the isolation of *Pseudomonas aeruginosa*. *J. Appl. Bacteriol.* **34**:611–614.

172. **Tsakris, A., S. Pournaras, N. Woodford, M. F. Palepou, G. S. Babini, J. Douboyas, and D. M. Livermore.** 2000. Outbreak of infections caused by *Pseudomonas aeruginosa* producing VIM-1 carbapenemase in Greece. *J. Clin. Microbiol.* **38**:1290–1292.

173. **Valdezate, S., J. Martinez-Beltran, L. de Rafael, F. Baquero, and R. Canton.** 1996. Beta-lactam stability in frozen microdilution PASCO MIC panels using strains with known resistance mechanisms as biosensors. *Diagn. Microbiol. Infect. Dis.* **26**:53–61.

174. **Vonberg, R. P., and P. Gastmeier.** 2005. Isolation of infectious cystic fibrosis patients: results of a systematic review. *Infect. Control Hosp. Epidemiol.* **26**:401–409.

175. **von Gotz, F., S. Haussler, D. Jordan, S. S. Saravanamuthu, D. Wehmhoner, A. Strussmann, J. Lauber, I. Attree, J. Buer, B. Tummler, and I. Steinmetz.** 2004. Expression analysis of a highly adherent and cytotoxic small colony variant of *Pseudomonas aeruginosa* isolated from a lung of a patient with cystic fibrosis. *J. Bacteriol.* **186**:3837–3847.

176. **Waine, D. J., D. Honeybourne, E. G. Smith, J. L. Whitehouse, and C. G. Dowson.** 2009. Cross-sectional and longitudinal multilocus sequence typing of *Pseudomonas aeruginosa* in cystic fibrosis sputum samples. *J. Clin. Microbiol.* **47**:3444–3448.

177. **Walsh, C., and S. Fanning.** 2008. Antimicrobial resistance in foodborne pathogens—a cause for concern? *Curr. Drug Targets* **9**:808–815.

178. **Wang, M., J. H. Tran, G. A. Jacoby, Y. Zhang, F. Wang, and D. C. Hooper.** 2003. Plasmid-mediated quinolone resistance in clinical isolates of *Escherichia coli* from Shanghai, China. *Antimicrob. Agents Chemother.* **47**:2242–2248.

179. **Watanabe, M., S. Iyobe, M. Inoue, and S. Mitsuhashi.** 1991. Transferable imipenem resistance in *Pseudomonas aeruginosa*. *Antimicrob. Agents Chemother.* **35**:147–151.

180. **Weldhagen, G. F.** 2004. Rapid detection and sequence-specific differentiation of extended-spectrum beta-lactamase GES-2 from *Pseudomonas aeruginosa* by use of a real-time PCR assay. *Antimicrob. Agents Chemother.* **48**:4059–4062.

181. **Weldhagen, G. F., and A. Prinsloo.** 2004. Molecular detection of GES-2 extended spectrum beta-lactamase producing *Pseudomonas aeruginosa* in Pretoria, South Africa. *Int. J. Antimicrob. Agents* **24**:35–38.

182. **White, R. L., D. S. Burgess, M. Manduru, and J. A. Bosso.** 1996. Comparison of three different in vitro methods of detecting synergy: time-kill, checkerboard, and E test. *Antimicrob. Agents Chemother.* **40**:1914–1918.

183. **White, R. L., M. B. Kays, L. V. Friedrich, E. W. Brown, and J. R. Koonce.** 1991. Pseudoresistance of *Pseudomonas aeruginosa* resulting from degradation of imipenem in an automated susceptibility testing system with predried panels. *J. Clin. Microbiol.* **29**:398–400.

184. **Wolter, J. M., G. Kotsiou, and J. G. McCormack.** 1995. Mixed morphotype testing of *Pseudomonas aeruginosa* cultures from cystic fibrosis patients. *J. Med. Microbiol.* **42**:220–224.

185. **Woods, D. E., M. S. Schaffer, H. R. Rabin, G. D. Campbell, and P. A. Sokol.** 1986. Phenotypic comparison of *Pseudomonas aeruginosa* strains isolated from a variety of clinical sites. *J. Clin. Microbiol.* **24**:260–264.

186. **Xu, J., J. E. Moore, P. G. Murphy, B. C. Millar, and J. S. Elborn.** 2004. Early detection of *Pseudomonas aeruginosa*—comparison of conventional versus molecular (PCR) detection directly from adult patients with cystic fibrosis (CF). *Ann. Clin. Microbiol. Antimicrob.* **3**:21.

187. **Yokoyama, K., Y. Doi, K. Yamane, H. Kurokawa, N. Shibata, K. Shibayama, T. Yagi, H. Kato, and Y. Arakawa.** 2003. Acquisition of 16S rRNA methylase gene in *Pseudomonas aeruginosa*. *Lancet* **362**:1888–1893.

188. **Zierdt, C. H.** 1971. Autolytic nature of iridescent lysis in *Pseudomonas aeruginosa*. *Antonie van Leeuwenhoek* **37**:319–337.

Burkholderia, Stenotrophomonas, Ralstonia, Cupriavidus, Pandoraea, Brevundimonas, Comamonas, Delftia, and Acidovorax*

JOHN J. LiPUMA, BART J. CURRIE, SHARON J. PEACOCK, AND PETER A. R. VANDAMME

41

TAXONOMY

In 1973, the taxonomic heterogeneity of the genus *Pseudomonas* was revealed by the work of Palleroni and coworkers, who identified five major species clusters (referred to as rRNA homology groups) among the pseudomonads (187). DNA-rRNA hybridization experiments led to the gradual dissection of the genus during the following decades (144). The name *Pseudomonas* was confined to rRNA homology group I organisms because they comprised the type species, *Pseudomonas aeruginosa* (see chapter 33).

The nomenclatural rearrangements of the genus *Pseudomonas* entailed the creation of several new genera. Some of these encompassed complete rRNA homology groups (e.g., both rRNA homology group IV species were reclassified in the genus *Brevundimonas*), whereas others encompassed only partial groups. rRNA group II pseudomonads belong to the class of the *Gammaproteobacteria* and were reclassified into the genera *Burkholderia* and *Ralstonia* (262, 263). rRNA group II pseudomonads form a remarkable group of primary and opportunistic human, animal, and plant pathogens, as well as environmental species with a considerable potential for biological control, remediation, and plant growth promotion. During the past decade, the interest in several peculiar characteristics of these organisms led to the discovery and description of a multitude of novel species. The genus *Burkholderia* now contains about 60 validly named species, many of which have been isolated from soil and water samples. Some other novel *Burkholderia*-like species were found to represent a distinct phylogenetic lineage with a position intermediate between those of the genera *Burkholderia* and *Ralstonia* and were classified in the novel genus *Pandoraea* (52).

Comparative 16S rRNA gene sequence analysis, further supported by phenotypic differences, indicated that two distinct sublineages existed within the genus *Ralstonia* (229). It was proposed that species of the *Ralstonia eutropha* lineage be classified in a novel genus named *Wautersia*, whereas the name *Ralstonia* was preserved for the lineage comprising *Ralstonia pickettii*, the type species. Shortly thereafter, it became known (225) that *Wautersia eutropha*, the type species

of the genus *Wautersia*, was a junior synonym of *Cupriavidus necator*, the type (and only) species of the genus *Cupriavidus*, an environmental organism which was validly named in 1987, i.e., long before 16S rRNA gene sequence studies were performed routinely (168). To conform to the International Code of Nomenclature of Bacteria (212), the name *Wautersia* had to be replaced by *Cupriavidus* and all species of the genus *Wautersia* became species of the genus *Cupriavidus*.

Several *Burkholderia* species have been isolated from human clinical samples, but only *Burkholderia cepacia* complex, *B. gladioli* (including strains previously classified as *B. cocovenenans* [56]), *B. mallei*, and *B. pseudomallei* are generally recognized as human or animal pathogens. Recent polyphasic taxonomic studies including traditional taxonomic methods, but also multilocus sequence typing (MLST) and whole-genome studies, revealed that *B. cepacia*-like bacteria belong to at least 17 distinct genomic species (genomovars), referred to collectively as the *B. cepacia* complex (66, 228, 230, 231). Ongoing surveys of the diversity of *B. cepacia*-like bacteria recovered from specimens from cystic fibrosis (CF) patients and other specimens revealed the presence of several additional groups in the *B. cepacia* complex that cannot be assigned to one of the established species within this complex by using traditional or molecular identification approaches (200). Further polyphasic taxonomic analyses are needed to determine if these groups represent additional novel species within the *B. cepacia* complex or if they represent new variants of established species. With the exception of *B. ubonensis*, all *B. cepacia* complex species have been recovered from human clinical samples. Within this group, however, *B. multivorans* and *B. cenocepacia* are the most common opportunistic pathogens in CF patients (112, 200).

Apart from the *B. cepacia* complex species, *B. gladioli*, *B. mallei*, and *B. pseudomallei*, the genus *Burkholderia* now comprises an additional 39 validly named species. Most of these organisms are not associated with human disease and are not discussed further here. Species that rarely have been reported as associated with human infections include *B. fungorum*, *B. glumae*, and *B. thailandensis* (21, 57, 240). A complete overview of validly named species can be obtained through Internet sites such as http://www.bacterio.cict.fr/ or http://www.dsmz.de/bactnom/genera1.htm.

There are now five species in the genus *Ralstonia*. The human pathogens include *Ralstonia pickettii*, *R. mannitolilytica* (previously known as *R. pickettii* biovar 3/'thomasii') (85),

*This chapter contains information presented by John J. LiPuma, Bart J. Currie, Gary D. Lum, and Peter A. R. Vandamme in chapter 49 of the ninth edition of this *Manual*.

and *R. insidiosa* (54). *Ralstonia paucula* (previously known as Centers for Disease Control group IVc-2) (226), *Ralstonia gilardii* (53), *R. respiraculi* (68), *R. taiwanensis* (35), and seven additional species, which occur primarily in environmental samples, are now all classified as *Cupriavidus* species (225).

Five distinct species of *Pandoraea*, *Pandoraea apista* (the type species), *P. pulmonicola*, *P. pnomenusa*, *P. sputorum*, and *P. norimbergensis*, and four presently unnamed strains, each representing a distinct additional *Pandoraea* species, have been reported (52, 84). Most of these occur in human clinical specimens.

Organisms in the *Pseudomonas* rRNA homology group III also belong to the *Betaproteobacteria* and are now classified in the family *Comamonadaceae*, which includes the genera *Comamonas*, *Delftia*, and *Acidovorax* (242, 249). The genus *Comamonas* was originally created in 1985 and included a single species, *Comamonas terrigena*. Two years later, *Pseudomonas acidovorans* and *Pseudomonas testosteroni* were reclassified as members of the genus *Comamonas*. *Comamonas acidovorans* was subsequently again reclassified as *Delftia acidovorans* (242). *Comamonas terrigena* encompassed three strain clusters with human clinical isolates (251), which are now known as *C. terrigena*, *Comamonas aquatica*, and *Comamonas kerstersii* (239). Additional novel species have been isolated from environmental samples (265).

Originally, *Acidovorax facilis* was classified as *Hydrogenomonas facilis* based on its ability to oxidize hydrogen. Poly-β-hydroxybutyrate metabolism studies resulted in the transfer of this species to the genus *Pseudomonas*, along with a new species called *Pseudomonas delafieldii*. A new genus, *Acidovorax*, was proposed, which included three species, *A. facilis*, *A. delafieldii*, and *A. temperans*, all members of rRNA homology group III (250). An additional five plant-pathogenic pseudomonads and novel environmental species have now been classified as *Acidovorax* species (100).

The genus *Brevundimonas*, consisting of the species *Brevundimonas diminuta* and *Brevundimonas vesicularis*, was proposed for bacteria originally classified as members of *Pseudomonas* rRNA homology group IV (206) and is a member of the *Alphaproteobacteria*. This genus currently comprises 14 validly named species, most of which are of environmental origin.

Finally, *Pseudomonas maltophilia* represented *Pseudomonas* rRNA homology group V (128). Based on genotypic and phenotypic characteristics, its transfer to the genus *Xanthomonas*, a member of the *Gammaproteobacteria*, was proposed (217). However, many differences were also noted, including number of flagella, nitrate reduction characteristics, fimbriation, and plant pathogenicity. Therefore, the organism was once again reclassified in a novel genus, *Stenotrophomonas* (186). More recently, a novel species, *Stenotrophomonas africana*, was proposed (94). However, Coenye et al. (69) demonstrated that *S. maltophilia* and *S. africana* represented the same species, and nomenclatural priority was given to the former. Seven additional environmental *Stenotrophomonas* species were described recently (124).

DESCRIPTION OF THE AGENTS

Burkholderia, *Ralstonia*, *Cupriavidus*, *Pandoraea*, *Brevundimonas*, *Comamonas*, *Delftia*, and *Acidovorax* spp. are aerobic, non-spore-forming, straight or slightly curved gram-negative rods. They are 1 to 5 μm in length and 0.5 to 1.0 μm in width (126). *Stenotrophomonas* spp. are straight rods and tend to be slightly smaller than members of the other genera (0.7 to 1.8 μm in length and 0.4 to 0.7 μm in width) (126). With the exception of *B. mallei*, these organisms are motile due to the presence of one or more polar flagella (185). These bacteria are catalase positive, and most, with the exception of *Stenotrophomonas* and *B. gladioli*, are either weakly or strongly oxidase positive. All grow on MacConkey agar, except for certain strains of *B. vesicularis*, and appear to be nonfermenters. The majority of species degrade glucose oxidatively, and most degrade nitrate to either nitrite or nitrogen gas. Certain species have distinctive colony morphologies or pigmentation. They are nutritionally quite versatile, with different species being able to utilize a variety of simple and complex carbohydrates, alcohols, and amino acids as carbon sources. Certain species can multiply at 4°C, but most are mesophilic, with optimal growth temperatures between 30 and 37°C (185). For some genera, growth at higher temperatures (i.e., 42°C) can be useful for species identification.

EPIDEMIOLOGY AND TRANSMISSION

Burkholderia, *Ralstonia*, *Cupriavidus*, *Pandoraea*, *Comamonas*, *Delftia*, *Acidovorax*, *Brevundimonas*, and *Stenotrophomonas* spp. are environmental organisms found in water, soil, the rhizosphere, and in and on plants including fruits and vegetables. They have a worldwide distribution. Members of these genera are widely recognized as phytopathogens, and many species were first described in that context. Because of their ability to survive in aqueous environments, these organisms have become particularly problematic as opportunistic nosocomial pathogens in hospitals and health care settings.

The natural distribution of *B. cepacia* complex species is being intensively studied because of interest in their biotechnological properties and their pathogenicity in persons with CF (112, 157). *B. cepacia* complex bacteria often have antifungal, antinematodal, or plant growth-promoting properties, which makes them attractive as biological pesticides and fertilizers (188). Because of their nutritional versatility, *B. cepacia* complex bacteria also have applications for bioremediation of contaminated soils. Unlike *P. aeruginosa*, *B. cepacia* complex bacteria are rarely recovered from environmental sites such as sinks, swimming pools, showers, and salad bars (112, 174). However, some species within the complex, especially *B. ambifaria*, *B. anthina*, and *B. pyrrocinia*, are frequently recovered from soil and environmental water samples (13, 197), provided that appropriate growth conditions are used to inhibit the growth of vast numbers of other environmental bacteria. Of particular note, *B. multivorans*, which is among the most common *B. cepacia* complex species recovered from CF patients, has been relatively infrequently recovered from environmental sources. Studies of a variety of foodstuffs and bottled water have shown that *B. cepacia* complex bacteria have been found in unpasteurized dairy products (18, 173). Due to their intrinsic resistance to antibiotics and disinfectants, *B. cepacia* complex bacteria are also notorious contaminants of pharmaceutical preparations and medical equipment such as nebulizers, which may be sterilized with contaminated anti-infectives (129, 148, 182).

Genotypic and conventional epidemiologic investigations provide compelling evidence for interpatient transmission of common or epidemic *B. cepacia* complex strains among persons with CF (155). One such strain, referred to as the ET12 (for electrophoretic type 12) lineage, is common among CF patients in eastern Canada and the United Kingdom (137, 195). This organism is a *B. cenocepacia* strain that is characterized by the presence of a distinctive cablelike pilus and an associated adhesin that mediates adherence to respiratory epithelium (203). *B. cenocepacia* strain PHDC dominates among infected CF patients in the mid-Atlantic region of the United States and has recently been identified in agricultural soil as well as in CF patients in several European countries (34, 65, 161). *B. cenocepacia* 'Midwest clone' is common among CF patients in the midwestern United States (58).

B. pseudomallei and *B. thailandensis* are found in soil and surface water primarily in tropical and subtropical areas. Both species have been isolated in the rice-growing regions of northeast Thailand, western Cambodia, Laos, and southern and central Vietnam (30, 189, 260). In northern Australia, associations have been made between *B. pseudomallei* and native grasses in undisturbed land and the presence of livestock animals, lower soil pH, and different combinations of soil texture and color in environmentally disturbed sites (140). Recent environmental studies have identified *B. thailandensis*-like organisms from Australia (102).

The known endemic distribution of *B. pseudomallei* is being expanded beyond the traditional regions of endemicity for melioidosis in Southeast Asia and northern Australia, with recent case reports of the disease from the Americas, Madagascar, Mauritius, India, and elsewhere in south Asia, China, and Taiwan. To what extent this reflects a true expansion of endemicity rather than unmasking of the longstanding presence of the bacterium remains unclear (73). What is apparent is that *B. pseudomallei* can occasionally persist in temperate environments after introduction via animals infected with melioidosis (82).

Because of the increasing frequency of nosocomial infections due to *S. maltophilia*, its presence in hospital environments is being more closely examined. Like *P. aeruginosa*, *S. maltophilia* is ubiquitous in aqueous environments and can be readily cultured from water sources in homes and hospitals (91).

Unlike that of certain *B. cepacia* complex strains, evidence for person-to-person transmission of *B. gladioli*, *B. pseudomallei*, *B. mallei*, *S. maltophilia*, and the other species discussed in this chapter is lacking.

CLINICAL SIGNIFICANCE

B. cepacia Complex and B. gladioli

B. cepacia has long been recognized as an occasional opportunistic human pathogen, capable of causing a variety of infections, including bacteremia, urinary tract infection, septic arthritis, peritonitis, and pneumonia in persons with underlying illness (157). Persons with chronic granulomatous disease (CGD) and CF are particularly susceptible to infection (252). *B. cepacia* also has a history as a nosocomial pathogen, causing infections associated with contaminated hospital equipment, medications, and disinfectants including povidone-iodine and benzalkonium chloride (156). Nosocomial outbreaks of respiratory tract infections in patients on mechanical ventilation in intensive care units have been attributed to contamination of nebulizers or nebulized medications such as albuterol (199). Contamination of blood culture systems or disinfectants resulting in pseudo-bacteremia has been described following the isolation of *B. cepacia* from the blood of multiple patients over a short period (72). Early reports of infection in CF described patients with acute pulmonary deterioration and sepsis (referred to as cepacia syndrome) or chronic respiratory tract infections associated with an accelerated decline in lung function

(134, 221). Clinical outcome studies consistently identified *B. cepacia* infection as a significant independent risk factor for morbidity and mortality in CF (71, 153).

The recognition that several closely related species can be distinguished from among organisms previously identified as *B. cepacia* has stimulated interest in the clinical significance of each of these species (154). Approximately 3% of CF patients in the United States are infected with *B. cepacia* complex species, although rates of infection vary from 0 to 20% among CF treatment centers (80). Rates of infection increase with increasing patient age; approximately 5% to 7% of adults with CF are infected (80). Most strains are inherently resistant to currently available antimicrobial agents (see below), and pulmonary infection is generally refractory to therapy. Furthermore, due to the poor postoperative prognosis associated with *B. cepacia* complex, most CF treatment centers consider infection to be an absolute contraindication for lung transplantation, which at present offers the only therapeutic option for successful intermediate-term survival of persons with end-stage pulmonary disease (155). Thus, respiratory tract infection by these species is a cause of great concern to CF patients and their caregivers.

Although 16 of the 17 species of the *B. cepacia* complex have been recovered from persons with CF (the exception is *B. ubonensis*), the distribution of species in this patient population is quite disproportionate. In the United States, *B. multivorans* and *B. cenocepacia* together account for approximately 80% of *B. cepacia* complex infection, with *B. vietnamiensis*, *B. cepacia*, and *B. dolosa* accounting for approximately 7%, 3%, and 3% of infection, respectively (200; J. J. LiPuma, unpublished data). In Canada and some European countries, *B. cenocepacia* alone accounts for as much as 80% of infection (3, 213). Some *B. cepacia* complex species are recovered only rarely. *B. stabilis*, *B. ambifaria*, *B. anthina*, *B. pyrrocinia*, *B. contaminans*, *B. seminalis*, *B. diffusa*, *B. metallidurans*, *B. arboris*, *B. latens*, and *B. lata* each account for less than 1% of *B. cepacia* complex infections among infected CF patients (200; LiPuma, unpublished).

Emerging data suggest that *B. cepacia* complex species also vary with respect to their virulence levels and clinical impacts in CF. Studies involving lung transplant recipients, for example, indicate that rates of postoperative mortality are greater for persons infected preoperatively with *B. cenocepacia* than for patients infected with other *B. cepacia* complex species (4, 8, 93). Carefully conducted multivariate analyses of posttransplant outcomes are less definitive, however (177). Thus, although it is almost certainly true that *B. cenocepacia* is the species most frequently associated with cepacia syndrome, it remains to be shown whether this species, in general, is disproportionately associated with poor outcome; case reports document fatal infection associated with other *B. cepacia* complex species, including *B. multivorans*, *B. stabilis*, and *B. dolosa* (19, 86, 183). Thus, although a positive correlation between species frequency and poor clinical outcome seems likely, firm conclusions regarding the relative virulence of *B. cepacia* complex species must await more definitive study. Evidence also suggests that certain strains are relatively more virulent in human infection. The *B. cenocepacia* ET12 epidemic strain, in particular, appears to be relatively more virulent in CF patients (149). Again, however, further comparative outcome studies are needed before firm conclusions about the relative virulence of specific strains can be drawn.

B. gladioli is most notable as a plant pathogen but is also well recognized to be capable of causing infection in persons with CF or CGD and, occasionally, other immunocompromised patients (114, 202). Anecdotal reports describe acute pulmonary deterioration and recurrent soft tissue abscesses, as well as severe post-lung transplantation infections due to *B. gladioli* in CF patients (16, 138, 145, 177). A more complete appreciation of the epidemiology and clinical significance of *B. gladioli* infection in CF has been confounded by difficulty with accurate identification of this species, which typically is capable of growth on selective media used to isolate *B. cepacia* complex species (49) and is frequently misidentified as a member of the *B. cepacia* complex by commercial test systems (51, 209). Genetic analysis of *Burkholderia* isolates recovered from CF patients indicates that *B. gladioli* is much more commonly involved in infection in this patient population than are most *B. cepacia* complex species, with the exception of *B. multivorans* and *B. cenocepacia*.

B. pseudomallei and *B. mallei*

B. pseudomallei is the causative agent of the human and animal disease melioidosis, which is endemic in Southeast Asia and tropical northern Australia and is being increasingly recognized on the Indian subcontinent and in Central and South America (37, 73). In locations where the disease is endemic, infection is seasonal, with up to 85% of cases occurring during the monsoon wet season. Severe weather events and environmental disturbances have been associated with melioidosis clusters in Australia, and the Asian tsunami of 2004 resulted in cases across the affected region (12, 48). As travel to Southeast Asia and northern Australia has become more frequent, reports of melioidosis in travelers returning to Europe and the United States are becoming more common (81). Melioidosis is an especially important potential travel-related illness for those with CF, and persistent colonization of airways with *B. pseudomallei* can occur in CF despite prolonged therapy, with repeated disease flares and deteriorating lung function (181, 237). Infection with this organism should be considered in the differential diagnosis of any individual with a fever of unknown origin or a tuberculosis-like illness who has a history of travel to a region where *B. pseudomallei* infection is endemic.

B. pseudomallei is acquired from the environment by inoculation through cut or abraded skin, inhalation, or ingestion. Zoonotic disease is described but is exceedingly uncommon, as are person-to-person transmission and laboratory-acquired infection (37). The association of severe weather events with respiratory infection and high mortality rates has been attributed to a shift from percutaneous inoculation to inhalation (78). This idea supports the potential of *B. pseudomallei* as a bioterrorism agent; its isolation from patients who do not give a history of travel to an area where melioidosis is endemic should be immediately reported to local or state public health authorities. For further details, see chapter 12 or http://www.bt.cdc.gov.

The majority of persons exposed to *B. pseudomallei* do not develop clinical infection, with rates of seropositivity in the general population as high as 80% in some locations (141, 256). Latent infection with subsequent reactivation is well recognized, with a recent description of disease onset in the United States, where melioidosis is not endemic, 62 years after presumed infection in Thailand (178). Such cases often achieve notoriety but are rare, and the vast majority of cases of melioidosis are from recent infection, with an incubation period of 1 to 21 days (mean, 9 days). Risk factors for clinical disease following infection with *B. pseudomallei* include diabetes, excessive alcohol consumption, chronic renal disease, and chronic lung disease (79, 152). Twenty to 36%

of cases have no identified risk factor, and mortality in this group is usually low. Disease in children is also uncommon, although parotid abscesses are well recognized as an important manifestation of melioidosis in children in Thailand. Overall rates of mortality from melioidosis vary from 15% in centers where state-of-the-art intensive care therapy is available to over 50% in locations with poor resources (37, 248). Fifty percent of cases present with pneumonia, which can be part of a fatal septicemia or a less severe unilateral infection indistinguishable from other community-acquired pneumonias or a chronic illness mimicking tuberculosis (33). Chronic melioidosis, defined as illness present for over 2 months, occurs in only 10% of cases. Overall, 50% of cases are bacteremic; the presence of >100 CFU/ml of blood and a blood culture showing growth in the first 24 h of incubation are markers for high mortality (222). At the mild end of the clinical spectrum of melioidosis is presentation with a skin ulcer or abscess without systemic illness (103). Other common presentations with or without bacteremia are genitourinary infections, septic arthritis, and osteomyelitis (37, 75, 248). Prostatic abscesses are especially common (75). Abscesses can also occur in spleen, liver, kidneys, and adrenal glands. Parotitis, lymphadenitis, sinusitis, orchitis, myositis (especially psoas abscess), mycotic aneurysms, and pericardial and mediastinal collections have all been described. Lesions can be frankly purulent and may include microabscesses or granulomas or a combination of these features. Clinical meningitis is rare, but melioidosis encephalomyelitis syndrome (74, 75) and brain abscesses have also been reported. The one presentation that has yet to be described is *B. pseudomallei* endocarditis.

B. mallei is the etiologic agent of glanders, a highly communicable disease of livestock, particularly horses, mules, and donkeys. It can be transmitted to humans and is also identified as a potential agent of bioterrorism. Unlike *B. pseudomallei*, *B. mallei* is a host-adapted pathogen that does not persist in the environment outside its host. Glanders has been eradicated from most countries, but enzootic foci persist in the Middle East, Asia, Africa, and South America. The only human case of glanders in the past 50 years in the United States was a recent laboratory-acquired case in a biodefense scientist (27). Like melioidosis, human glanders can be acute or chronic, with the clinical presentation and course depending on the mode of infection, the inoculation dose, and host risk factors. Respiratory inoculation can result in pneumonia with potential for dissemination to internal organs and septicemia. Cutaneous inoculation can result in skin nodules and regional lymphadenitis, also with potential for disseminated disease. Involvement of nodes, both mediastinal and peripheral, is much more common in glanders than in melioidosis, often with suppurative abscesses in untreated cases.

S. maltophilia

S. maltophilia, although typically not pathogenic for healthy persons, is a well-known opportunistic human pathogen. It is among the most common causes of wound infection due to trauma involving agricultural machinery (2). It is also an important nosocomial pathogen associated with substantial morbidity and mortality, particularly in debilitated or immunocompromised patients and patients requiring ventilatory support in intensive care units (5, 99, 119, 176). The incidence of human infection appears to have increased in recent years, and a variety of clinical syndromes have been described, including bacteremia, pneumonia, urinary tract infection, ocular infection, endocarditis, meningitis, soft tissue and wound infection, mastoiditis, epididymitis, cholangitis, osteochondritis, bursitis, and peritonitis (9, 205). Septicemia can be accompanied by ecthyma gangrenosa, a skin lesion more commonly associated with *Pseudomonas aeruginosa* and *Vibrio* spp. (232).

The incidence of *S. maltophilia* respiratory tract infection in persons with CF also appears to be increasing (88, 198, 218); however, the unreliability of historical data limits firm conclusions. Approximately 12% of CF patients included in the CF Foundation's patient registry were culture positive for *S. maltophilia* in 2005 (80). In large multicenter clinical trials, however, *S. maltophilia* was found in a larger proportion of CF patients, being second only to *P. aeruginosa* in frequency of isolation from study subjects (26). Infection or colonization was most frequently transient, with 30% of subjects having at least one sputum culture positive for *S. maltophilia* during the course of 6 months (113). Several case-control studies have drawn conflicting conclusions regarding the role that *S. maltophilia* plays in contributing to pulmonary decline in CF (88, 111).

Ralstonia and *Cupriavidus* spp.

As described above, the taxonomy of the genus *Ralstonia* has been recently revised, with several species being assigned to the genus *Cupriavidus* (225). Among the species in these two genera, *R. pickettii* is best known with respect to human infection. Older reports describe this species as being recovered from a variety of clinical specimens (201) and as causing various infections including bacteremia, meningitis, endocarditis, and osteomyelitis (243). *R. pickettii* also has been identified in pseudobacteremias and nosocomial outbreaks due to contamination of intravenous medications, "sterile" water, saline, chlorhexidine solutions, respiratory therapy solutions, and intravenous catheters (20, 45, 96). This species has also been recovered from the respiratory tract of persons with CF (26). However, *R. pickettii* is easily confused with *Pseudomonas fluorescens* and members of the *B. cepacia* complex based on phenotype (26, 85, 123). Furthermore, several newly recognized *R. pickettii*-like species are also now known to be involved in human infection, particularly in CF (64). Thus, the role of *R. pickettii* as a human pathogen is difficult to assess based on historical data.

R. mannitolilytica (formerly known as *R. pickettii* biovar 3/'thomasii') was recently described as causing nosocomial outbreaks and a case of recurrent meningitis (85). This species accounts for the majority of *Ralstonia* infection in CF patients, being found in more than twice as many CF patients as those infected with *R. pickettii* (64). *R. insidiosa* and *Cupriavidus respiraculi* are recently described species recovered from persons with CF (54, 68). *Cupriavidus gilardii* has been recovered from cerebrospinal fluid (53), and cases of *Cupriavidus pauculus* bacteremia, peritonitis, and tenosynovitis have been reported (226). Both of these species may be found in sputa from patients with CF (64). Although *Cupriavidus metallidurans* and *Cupriavidus basilensis* are not known to cause other human infection, they too have been recovered recently from sputum cultures from patients with CF (64). Despite these observations, the roles of *Ralstonia* and *Cupriavidus* species in human infection, particularly in persons with CF, require further elucidation.

Other Genera

In general, *Brevundimonas, Comamonas, Delftia, Acidovorax,* and *Pandoraea* spp. infrequently cause human infection. Interest in these species focuses primarily on their roles as plant pathogens or in studies of microbial biodiversity and biodegradation.

Brevundimonas spp. are occasionally recovered from clinical specimens (46). *Brevundimonas vesicularis* bacteremia in patients with various underlying illnesses has been reported (104), and the organism has been recognized in cervical specimens because of its ability to produce bright orange colonies on Thayer-Martin agar (184). *Brevundimonas diminuta* has been recovered from blood, urine, and pleural fluid from patients with cancer (117).

Among the *Comamonas* species, *Comamonas testosteroni* has been implicated most often in human infection, with reports describing endocarditis, meningitis, and catheter-associated bacteremia due to this species (7, 70, 150). *D. acidovorans* has similarly been reported to cause infection, being identified in cases of bacteremia, endocarditis, ocular infection, and suppurative otitis (95). *Acidovorax* spp. have been isolated from a variety of clinical sources (250), including blood from a patient with hematological malignancy (261). *Acidovorax* spp., *Comamonas testosteroni,* and *D. acidovorans* have also been recovered from sputa of persons with CF (55; LiPuma, unpublished); however, the roles of these species in contributing to lung disease in CF have not been established.

In addition to causing infection in CF patients (136, 139), *Pandoraea* spp. have been recovered from blood and from patients with chronic obstructive pulmonary disease or CGD (83). Although the roles of these species in contributing to poor outcomes in persons with underlying diseases are unclear, a recent report describes sepsis, multiple organ failure, and death in a patient who underwent lung transplantation due to sarcoidosis (216).

COLLECTION, TRANSPORT, AND STORAGE

The genera described in this chapter include organisms that can survive in a variety of hostile environments and at temperatures found in clinical settings. Therefore, standard collection, transport, and storage techniques as outlined in chapters 9 and 16 are sufficient to ensure the recovery of these organisms from clinical specimens. Recovery of *B. pseudomallei* for the diagnosis of melioidosis is increased by the additional collection of throat and rectal swabs into selective media (see "Culture and Isolation" below) and by collecting larger than standard volumes of cerebrospinal fluid for culture in suspected neurological melioidosis (44).

DIRECT EXAMINATION

Members of the genera discussed here have similar morphologies and, with the exception of *B. pseudomallei,* are not easily distinguished from each other on the basis of Gram staining. *B. pseudomallei* may appear as small gram-negative bacilli with bipolar staining, making the cells resemble safety pins (Fig. 1). This may increase the index of suspicion for the presence of *B. pseudomallei,* but the sensitivity and specificity of this appearance are not high enough to be relied upon for a presumptive clinical diagnosis.

Although PCR-based assays have been described for the identification of *B. cepacia* complex species, *B. pseudomallei, B. gladioli,* several *Ralstonia* and *Cupriavidus* species, *Pandoraea* species, and *S. maltophilia* following culture and isolation (see "Identification" below), the use of PCR for direct detection of these species in clinical specimens remains a research tool (84, 169, 246). Studies of CF sputum samples have indicated that some specimens may be PCR positive but culture negative for certain *B. cepacia* complex species, raising important questions about the natural

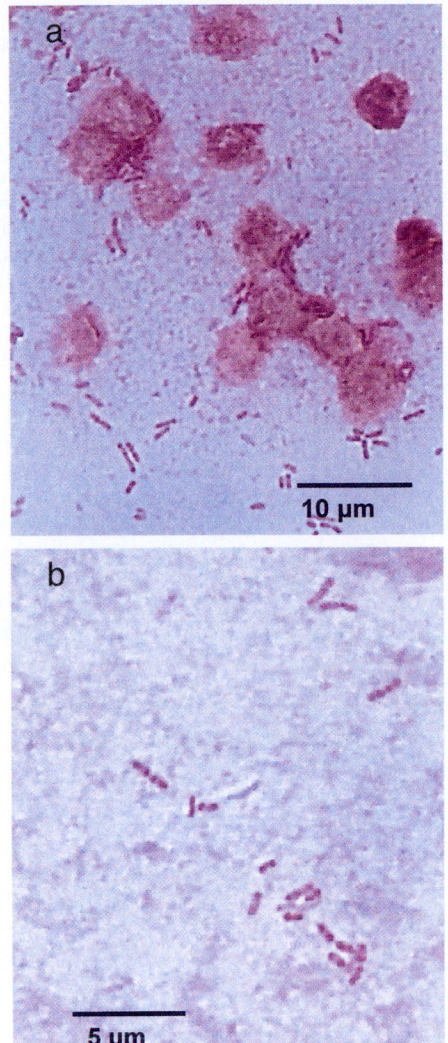

FIGURE 1 (a) Gram stain of *B. pseudomallei* in a blood culture; (b) Gram stain of *B. pseudomallei* from a colony on blood agar.

other urinary tract pathogens including *Klebsiella pneumoniae* and *Escherichia coli* have been reported with EIA but not LA; therefore, EIA results must be interpreted cautiously (92, 211). Antibodies raised against heat-killed whole cells of *B. pseudomallei* have been used to prepare a reagent for DFA staining. When this DFA reagent was used to stain clinical specimens from patients with suspected melioidosis, using a rapid assay that took 10 minutes to prepare and read, it showed a sensitivity of 66% and specificity of 99.5% (258). The reagents described in the literature are largely prepared in-house and are not available commercially.

The evaluation of a conventional PCR assay targeting the 16s rRNA gene for the detection of *B. pseudomallei* in clinical specimens indicated that the assay was sensitive but lacked specificity, resulting in positive predictive values of only 70% (115). Real-time PCR assays targeting *B. pseudomallei* genes encoding 16S rRNA, flagellin (*fliC*), ribosomal protein subunit S21 (*rpsU*), or type III secretion system (TTS) genes have been developed and been shown to have high sensitivities and specificities with pure bacterial cultures (179, 220, 223). Two clinical evaluations of real-time PCR have met with mixed results, with a sensitivity of 91% in one study using an assay targeting a gene in the TSS1 cluster (171) and a considerably lower sensitivity of 61% in a second study that used an assay targeting the 16s rRNA gene (29). Sensitivity of PCR is highest for pus and other body fluids but is low for blood, most likely reflecting a bacterial copy number effect. Loop-mediated isothermal amplification (LAMP) is easy and quick to perform and needs minimal equipment, with amplification being achieved at a fixed temperature in a water bath or heating block. LAMP has been developed and evaluated for the detection of *B. pseudomallei* and diagnosis of melioidosis (28). The assay was sensitive and specific for the laboratory detection of *B. pseudomallei* and had 100% specificity when applied to clinical samples but had a very low diagnostic sensitivity (44%). At present, molecular assays are not sufficiently sensitive to replace conventional culture.

CULTURE AND ISOLATION

The species discussed in this chapter grow well on standard laboratory media such as 5% sheep blood and chocolate agars. Such media can be used to recover the organisms from sterile fluid or tissue where a mixed biota is not anticipated (see chapter 16). All species that have been reported to be recovered from blood, including *B. pseudomallei* (222), grow in broth-based blood culture systems within the standard 5-day incubation period, so that special blood culture techniques such as lysis-centrifugation and extended incubation periods are not required. The use of selective media facilitates the isolation of these organisms from specimens with mixed microbiota. With the exception of *Brevundimonas vesicularis*, MacConkey agar can be used to isolate most species of these genera.

Burkholderia species grow on MacConkey agar (Fig. 2a), but the use of specific selective media with the ability to inhibit *P. aeruginosa* is preferred for the isolation of *B. cepacia* complex and *B. pseudomallei*. Several selective media have been described, and some are commercially available. A multicenter comparison of three media, PC (for *Pseudomonas cepacia*) agar (BD Diagnostics, Franklin Lakes, NJ) (106), OFPBL (for oxidation-fermentation base-polymyxin B-bacitracin-lactose) agar (BD Diagnostics) (241), and BCSA (for *B. cepacia* selective agar; Hardy Diagnostics, Santa Maria, CA) (121), showed that BCSA

history of infection in CF. However, the sensitivities and specificities of such PCR assays for the intended target species are difficult to determine in the absence of reliable "gold standards." The development of assays employing real-time PCR technology may yield reliable approaches to direct detection of these species in clinical specimens in the near future.

Because septicemia with *B. pseudomallei* is frequently fatal and death often occurs in the first few days after presentation to the hospital prior to the availability of culture results, several rapid direct-detection methods have been developed including urinary antigen detection using latex agglutination (LA) and enzyme immunoassay (EIA), and direct fluorescent-antibody (DFA) staining (92, 211, 258). The EIA for the detection of urinary antigen is more sensitive than LA, with an overall sensitivity of 71% for patients with melioidosis compared with an LA sensitivity of 62% (with concentrated urine) or only 17.5% (with unconcentrated urine). The EIA has an even higher sensitivity (84%) for samples from septicemic patients. Cross-reactions with

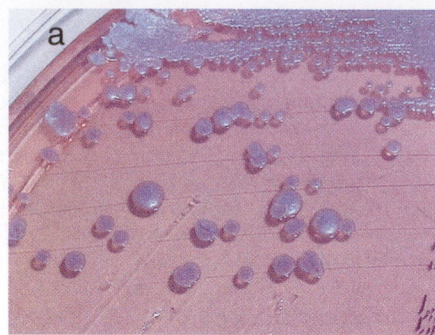

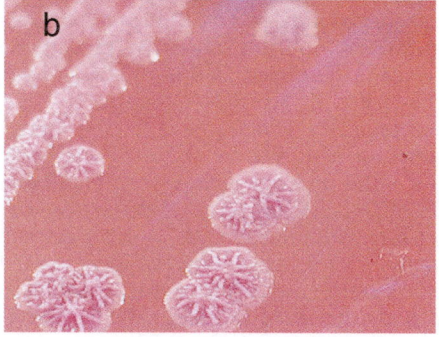

FIGURE 2 (a) *B. pseudomallei* colonies on MacConkey agar; (b) *B. pseudomallei* colonies on blood agar; (c) *B. pseudomallei* colonies on Ashdown medium agar.

was superior, being both more sensitive (more *B. cepacia* isolates were recovered) and more specific (fewer other types of organisms grew) than PC or OFPBL agar (121, 122). The sensitivities of TB-T (for trypan blue-tetracycline) (116), PC-AT (for *Pseudomonas cepacia* azelaic acid) (24), and BCSA (121, 122) were also compared with those of three commercial media, i.e., *B. cepacia* media from MAST Diagnostics (Bootle, Merseyside, United Kingdom), LAB M Ltd. (Bury, United Kingdom), and Oxoid Ltd. (Basingstoke, United Kingdom), through the analysis of 142 clinical and environmental isolates representing all species within the *B. cepacia* complex (235). BCSA and Mast *B. cepacia* medium supported the growth of *B. cepacia* complex isolates most efficiently. The latter two media were also compared in a study to evaluate the sensitivities and specificities for the isolation of *B. cepacia* complex species from sputum specimens from CF patients (253). BCSA was reported as being as sensitive as MAST agar but more selective.

Ashdown medium is effective for the isolation of *B. pseudomallei* (Fig. 2); crystal violet and gentamicin act as selective agents. It has been shown to be superior to MacConkey agar or MacConkey agar supplemented with colistin for the recovery of *B. pseudomallei* from clinical specimens containing mixed bacterial microbiota, such as throat, rectal, and sputum specimens (257). A more recently described selective agar, BPSA (for *B. pseudomallei* selective agar), was reported to improve the recovery of *B. pseudomallei* over that with other media (127); however, this medium is not yet commercially available. BPSA was more inhibitory to *P. aeruginosa* and *B. cepacia* complex species and made recognition of *Burkholderia* species easier due to their distinctive colony morphology. A clinical comparison of BPSA, Ashdown medium, and *Burkholderia cepacia* medium demonstrated equivalent sensitivity for all three media, but the selectivity of BPSA was lower than that for the other two media (191). *Burkholderia cepacia* medium is widely used and represents a good alternative when Ashdown medium is not available. An enrichment broth consisting of Ashdown medium supplemented with 50 mg of colistin is superior to standard enrichment broth such as tryptic soy broth and increases recovery of *B. pseudomallei* from clinical specimens taken from colonized sites compared with plating on Ashdown medium alone (44, 238). Selective broth cultures should be subcultured to Ashdown medium after 48 hours of incubation in air at 37°C, and all inoculated plates should be incubated at 37°C in air and examined daily for 4 days before being discarded, since some colonies become apparent to the naked eye only after extended incubation.

The use of selective media (143) increases the isolation rates of *S. maltophilia* from clinical and environmental samples (89). Denton et al. (89) studied the sensitivity of a selective medium incorporating vancomycin, imipenem, and amphotericin B as selective agents (VIA medium) for isolating *S. maltophilia* from sputum samples collected from children with CF. This study compared the use of VIA medium to an existing in-house method that utilized an imipenem disk placed upon bacitracin-chocolate agar (BC medium) and reported an improved detection using VIA as a selective medium.

IDENTIFICATION

B. cepacia Complex and *B. gladioli*

Accurate identification of *B. cepacia* complex species presents a challenge (170). Commercial bacterial identification systems are not able to reliably distinguish among the species of the *B. cepacia* complex and often fail to differentiate these species from other closely related species such as *B. gladioli* and *Ralstonia, Cupriavidus,* and *Pandoraea* spp. (22, 123, 146, 209). This failure presents a serious problem for CF patients and their caregivers as detailed in "Clinical Significance" above. The identification of *B. cepacia* complex species from CF sputum culture has a dramatic impact on patient management and is a cause of considerable anxiety for patients with CF (155, 156). Consequently, when *Burkholderia, Ralstonia, Cupriavidus,* or *Pandoraea* species are tentatively identified in a patient with CF by using a commercial system, the identity of the isolate should be confirmed by conventional biochemical testing (123) and, if necessary, molecular techniques. To aid clinical microbiologists in the United States, the CF Foundation has established a *B. cepacia* reference laboratory, which uses a combination of phenotypic and genotypic methods (described below) to confirm the identity of suspected *B. cepacia* complex isolates (159). Further information concerning the *B. cepacia* reference laboratory can be found on the CF Foundation website (http://www.cff.org).

TABLE 1 Characteristics of the *B. cepacia* complex, *B. gladioli*, and *Pandoraea* spp.[a]

Test	*B. ambifaria*	*B. anthina*	*B. arboris*	*B. cenocepacia*	*B. cepacia*	*B. contaminans*	*B. diffusa*	*B. dolosa*	*B. lata*	*B. latens*	*B. metallica*	*B. multivorans*	*B. pyrrocinia*	*B. seminalis*	*B. stabilis*	*B. ubonensis*	*B. vietnamiensis*	*B. gladioli*	*Pandoraea* spp.
Oxidase[b]	+	+	+	+	+	V	+	+	V	+	+	+	V	+	+	+	+	V	V
Growth:																			
MacConkey[c]	+	+	+	V	V	+	+	+	+	+	+	+	+	+	+	+	V	+	+
BCSA[b]	+	+	+	+	+	+	+	+	+	+	+	+	+	+	+	+	+	V	V
42°C[c]	V	V	V	V	V	V	V	+	−	+	+	+	V	+	−	V	+	−	V
Yellow pigment[c]	V	−	V	−	V	V	−	−	−	−	V	−	V	V	−	−	−	V	−
Brown pigment[c]	−	−	−	+	−	−	−	−	−	−	−	−	−	−	−	−	−	V	−
Hemolysis[d]	V β	−	V β	−	−	V	−	−	−	−	−	−	V β	−	−	−	V β		
Acid from[e]:																			
Maltose[c]	+	+	+	V	V	V	+	+	+	−	+	+	+	+	+	+	+	−	−
Lactose[b]	+	+	V	+	+	+	+	+	+	−	+	+	+	+	V	+	+	−	−
D-Xylose[c]	+	+	+	+	+	+	+	+	+	−	+	+	+	+	V	+	+	+	−
Sucrose[b]	+	V	V	+	V	+	V	−	V	−	+	V	−	V	V	−	+	−	−
Adonitol[c]	+	V	+	V	V	+	V	+	V	−	+	+	−	V	V	−	+	−	−
Nitrate reduction[c,g]	V	V	V	V	−	V	+	+	V	−	−	+	V	−	−	V	V	V	V
Lysine decarboxylase[b]	+	V	V	+	+	+	+	−	+	+	+	V	+	V	+	−	+	−	−
Ornithine decarboxylase[c]	−	−	+	V	V	−	−	−	−	−	−	V	V	+	−	−	−	−	−
Esculin hydrolase[c,g]	V	−	−	V	V	V	−	−	−	−	+	−	V	−	−	−	−	V	−
Gelatinase[c,g]	+	−	+	V	V	+	V	−	V	V	+	−	V	+	+	+	−	V	−
PNPG or ONPG[b,f]	+	V	+	+	+	+	+	+	V	+	+	+	+	V	−	+	+	+	V

[a] +, >90% of isolates are positive; V, 10 to 90% are positive; −, <10% of isolates are positive.

[b] Number of strains of each species tested: *B. ambifaria*, 51; *B. anthina*, 24; *B. arboris*, 16; *B. cenocepacia*, 928; *B. cepacia*, 181; *B. contaminans*, 54; *B. diffusa*, 16; *B. dolosa*, 57; *B. lata*, 25; *B. latens*, 6; *B. metallica*, 7; *B. multivorans*, 715; *B. pyrrocinia*, 85; *B. seminalis*, 19; *B. stabilis*, 73; *B. ubonensis*, 2; *B. vietnamiensis*, 145; *B. gladioli*, 280; and *Pandoraea* spp., 75. Data from references 123, 227, and 231 and from LiPuma (unpublished) and D. A. Henry (unpublished data).

[c] Number of strains of each species tested: *B. ambifaria*, 18; *B. anthina*, 16; *B. arboris*, 13; *B. cepacia*, 23; *B. cenocepacia*, 139; *B. contaminans*, 7; *B. diffusa*, 6; *B. dolosa*, 12; *B. lata*, 11; *B. latens*, 6; *B. metallica*, 3; *B. multivorans*, 109; *B. pyrrocinia*, 5; *B. seminalis*, 13; *B. stabilis*, 27; *B. ubonensis*, 2; *B. vietnamiensis*, 36; *B. gladioli*, 27; and *Pandoraea* spp., 9. Data from references 123, 227, and 231 and from Henry (unpublished).

[d] Hemolysis of sheep blood; β, beta-hemolysis.

[e] Oxidation test results were recorded after 2 to 7 days of incubation.

[f] PNPG, *p*-nitrophenyl-β-D-glucoside.

[g] Results presented are from the API 20NE test strip.

B. cepacia complex species may require 3 days of incubation before colonies are seen on selective media. On MacConkey or Mueller-Hinton agar, these colonies may be punctate and tenacious, and on blood agar or selective medium such as BCSA, PC agar, or OFPBL agar, the colonies are smooth and slightly raised; occasional isolates are mucoid. On MacConkey agar, colonies of the *B. cepacia* complex frequently become dark pink to red due to oxidation of lactose after extended incubation (4 to 7 days). Most clinical isolates are nonpigmented, but on iron-containing media such as a triple sugar iron slant, many strains produce a bright yellow pigment. *B. cepacia* complex species have a characteristic dirtlike odor.

The species of the *B. cepacia* complex are phenotypically very similar, making their differentiation, even with an extended panel of biochemical tests, rather difficult (Table 1) (123). Further, isolates within these species show considerable phenotypic variability, which is likely due to their unusually large genomes rich in insertion sequences and mobile elements such as plasmids, transposons, and bacteriophages (167). These features can contribute to genetic plasticity and diversity, which, when differentially expressed in isolates, results in variable biochemical phenotypic profiles. Most strains are weakly oxidase positive, although some strains of *B. contaminans*, *B. lata*,

and *B. pyrrocinia* are oxidase negative. *B. multivorans*, *B. stabilis*, and *B. dolosa* rarely oxidize sucrose. *B. stabilis* is ornithine decarboxylase positive, as are most *B. cenocepacia* strains, but is distinctive in that more than two-thirds of strains are *o*-nitrophenyl-β-D-galactopyranoside (ONPG) negative. *B. stabilis*, *B. lata*, and most *B. ambifaria* strains show poor growth at 42°C. *B. dolosa* is usually lysine decarboxylase negative, whereas only approximately one-half of *B. multivorans* strains are negative. Other *B. cepacia* complex species are usually lysine decarboxylase positive. *B. vietnamiensis* and most *B. anthina* strains do not oxidize adonitol. *B. anthina* strains show a distinctive creamy morphology on BCSA, which also turns pink (i.e., alkaline) despite the ability of this species to utilize sucrose (227).

Phenotypic differentiation of *B. cepacia* complex species from *B. gladioli* and *Pandoraea* spp. is also difficult (Table 1). Cellular fatty acid analysis is unable to differentiate *B. cepacia* complex species from *B. gladioli* (215). However, in contrast to *B. cepacia* complex species, most *B. gladioli* strains are oxidase negative, and whereas most *B. cepacia* complex strains oxidize maltose and lactose, *B. gladioli* typically oxidizes neither. *Pandoraea* spp. do not oxidize maltose, lactose, xylose, sucrose, or adonitol, and most are ONPG negative. *B. cepacia* complex species also may be difficult to differentiate from *Ralstonia* and *Cupriavidus* species. However, several of the latter species show a fast and strong oxidase reaction whereas *B. cepacia* complex species produce a slow, weak-positive oxidase test. Further, in contrast to most *B. cepacia* complex species, *Ralstonia* and *Cupriavidus* are lysine decarboxylase negative and most often ONPG negative.

The difficulty in differentiating *B. cepacia* complex species has prompted the development of molecular genetic diagnostic tests capable of identifying these species individually and distinguishing them (as a group) from biochemically similar species. DNA sequence differences in 16S and 23S rRNA genes have been used to develop species-specific PCR assays for the identification of several *B. cepacia* complex species (17, 159, 233), as well as *B. gladioli* (247). *B. multivorans*, *B. vietnamiensis*, and *B. dolosa* can be reliably identified with 16S rRNA-targeted assays, but insufficient sequence variation in rRNA genes exists to enable reliable separation of the remaining *B. cepacia* complex species. Fortunately, species-specific sequence variation does exist in the *recA* gene, and PCR assays targeting this locus enable the reliable identification of the *B. cepacia* complex species most commonly recovered from human specimens (61, 165, 230, 231, 234). Other 16S rRNA- and *recA*-based PCR assays identify all *Burkholderia* spp. (i.e., at the genus level) or all species within the *B. cepacia* complex (i.e., as a group) (159, 165, 190).

Another molecular genetic approach to identifying *B. cepacia* complex species involves restriction fragment length polymorphism (RFLP) analysis of either 16S rRNA or *recA* genes (165, 207). Again, insufficient sequence variation in the 16S rRNA gene limits the use of RFLP analysis of this locus, even when multiple restriction enzymes are used (98, 207, 236). In contrast, *recA* RFLP analysis has proved quite useful in reliably distinguishing all species within the *B. cepacia* complex (165, 190, 230, 231, 234).

Although an MLST scheme for the *B. cepacia* complex was developed primarily as a tool to study the epidemiology and population genetic structure of these species (14), it offers another approach to differentiate species within this group. This scheme was recently modified to allow typing of all species within the genus *Burkholderia* (214). Other genomic approaches, including amplified fragment length polymorphism typing, ribotyping, and whole-cell protein profiling, have been proposed for the differentiation of *B. cepacia* complex species (23, 62, 228). However, these methods are time-consuming and expensive and require an extensive validated database before isolates can be reliably identified. These limitations render them impractical for use in a routine diagnostic laboratory. Cellular fatty acid methyl ester analysis is useful for identification of *Burkholderia* strains at the genus level but is not reliable for identification of individual *B. cepacia* complex species and does not differentiate *B. gladioli* (51, 226).

B. pseudomallei and *B. mallei*

B. pseudomallei colonies on blood agar are typically small, smooth, and creamy in the first 48 hours. On further incubation, this appearance changes to give dry, wrinkled colonies. *B. pseudomallei* on Ashdown agar grows as very small (pinpoint) colonies by 18 h, which are usually purple, flat, dry, and wrinkled ("cornflower head") after 48 hours of incubation (Fig. 2c). The organism is motile, indole negative, oxidase positive, and resistant to colistin and gentamicin, features that aid identification (82). Other typical biochemical reactions are shown in Table 2. *B. pseudomallei* produces a distinctive musty or earthy odor, but sniffing of open plates should never be undertaken on safety grounds (11). *B. thailandensis* may be indistinguishable from *B. pseudomallei* by these simple criteria but can be distinguished based on arabinose assimilation, since *B. thailandensis* can utilize L-arabinose as the sole carbon source but neither *B. pseudomallei* nor *B. mallei* can do so (21, 175, 210). *B. thailandensis*

TABLE 2   Characteristics of *B. mallei*, *B. pseudomallei*, and *B. thailandensis*[a]

Test	*B. mallei*	*B. pseudomallei*	*B. thailandensis*
Oxidase	v	+	+
Growth:			
MacConkey	+	+	+
42°C	−	+	+
Nitrate reduction	+	+	+
Gas from nitrate	−	+	+
Arginine dihydrolase	+	+	+
Lysine decarboxylase	−	−	−
Ornithine decarboxylase	−	−	−
Hydrolysis:			
Urea	v	v	v
Citrate	−	v	v
Gelatin	−	v	v
Esculin	−	v	v
Acid from:			
Glucose	+	+	+
Xylose	v	+	+
Lactose	v	+	+
Sucrose	−	v	v
Maltose	−	+	+
Mannitol	−	+	+
Arabinose	ND	−	+
Motility	0	100%+	100%+
No. of flagella	0	≥2	≥2

[a]Data from references 21 and 244. +, ≥90% positive; −, <10% positive; v, 10% to 90% positive ND, not determined.

is found in clinical samples extremely rarely, and reported cases of human *B. thailandensis* infection in which the bacterial species was fully verified amount to a single patient (108). *B. mallei* is also an extreme rarity in clinical specimens from humans but could be confused with *B. pseudomallei* and *B. thailandensis*. Two differentiating tests in the event that *B. mallei* is suspected or needs to be ruled out are (i) that *B. mallei* is nonmotile and *B. pseudomallei* and *B. thailandensis* are motile and (ii) that *B. mallei* is susceptible to gentamicin (142) while the other two species are inherently resistant. The latter represents a catch for the inexperienced microbiologist, since Ashdown medium normally contains gentamicin and thus fails to support the growth of *B. mallei*. Cellular fatty acid profiles may be useful for differentiating *B. pseudomallei* from other genera, but reports vary on its utility in differentiating *B. thailandensis* and *B. pseudomallei* (130) or other pathogenic *Burkholderia* species including *B. mallei*, *B. cepacia* complex species, and *B. gladioli*.

Multiple evaluations have been performed to determine the accuracy of API 20NE for the identification of *B. pseudomallei*, with the reported percentage of isolates identified correctly ranging from 37% to 99% (6, 82, 87, 108, 131, 132, 162). One possible reason for this interstudy variability is that *B. pseudomallei* is phenotypically distinct in different geographical areas and/or between clinical isolates and those from the environment. A recent study using a large collection (*n* = 800) of *B. pseudomallei* isolates obtained from clinical cases, the environment, and animals from seven Asian countries and northern Australia reported that the API 20NE correctly identified 99% of *B. pseudomallei* isolates (6). This supports the use of API 20NE for the identification of *B. pseudomallei*. API 20NE is unable to identify *B. mallei* or *B. thailandensis* (6). The automated Vitek 1 system provides accurate identification of *B. pseudomallei* (162). Two evaluations of the Vitek 2 colorimetric GN card system have reported an accuracy of around 80% for

B. pseudomallei, the most common incorrect identification being the *Burkholderia cepacia* group (87, 163). The accuracy of Vitek 2 has been reported to be affected by the medium on which *B. pseudomallei* is grown prior to testing, with culture on Columbia horse blood agar being associated with the highest rate of accuracy (163). Because of the difficulty associated with accurate laboratory identification, referral to a reference laboratory is advised when isolation of *B. pseudomallei* or *B. mallei* is suspected. This is especially important with the advent of emerging bioterrorism legislation in many countries (see chapter 12).

B. pseudomallei must be differentiated from *Pseudomonas stutzeri* and *B. cepacia* complex species in clinical specimens. *Pseudomonas stutzeri* appears very similar to *B. pseudomallei* after a few days of incubation, and both *B. pseudomallei* and *B. cepacia* complex species may be isolated from persons with CF (181, 237). Whereas *B. pseudomallei* produces gas from nitrate and is arginine dihydrolase positive, most *B. cepacia* complex isolates are negative for both characteristics. *Pseudomonas stutzeri* is negative for arginine dihydrolase, oxidation-fermentation glucose, and gelatin hydrolysis. Also, *Pseudomonas stutzeri* has only one flagellum, and *B. pseudomallei* has more than one.

Ralstonia and *Cupriavidus* spp.

Although *R. pickettii* was considered to be the *Ralstonia* species most frequently isolated from clinical specimens (201), the recent recognition that several other *Ralstonia* and *Cupriavidus* species can be identified from among *R. pickettii*-like isolates limits previous observations. As is the case with *B. cepacia* complex species, *Ralstonia* and *Cupriavidus* species are phenotypically similar, requiring rather extensive biochemical testing to reliably differentiate them; species level identification with standard biochemical testing is difficult (Table 3). These species may grow slowly on primary isolation media, requiring ≥72 h of incubation before colonies

TABLE 3 Characteristics of *Ralstonia* and *Cupriavidus* spp.[a]

Test	R. pickettii	R. mannitolilytica	R. insidiosa	C. respiraculi	C. gilardii	C. pauculus
Catalase	v	+	+	+	+	+
Oxidase	+	+	+	+	+	+
Growth:						
BCSA	+	+	+	−	−	v
42°C	v	+	ND	ND	+	v
Colistin resistance	+	+	ND	ND	ND	−
Nitrate reduction	+	−	+	v	−	−
Tween 80 hydrolysis	+	+	ND	ND	−	+
Urease	+	+	v	−	−	+
Lysine decarboxylase	−	−	−	−	−	−
ONPG	−	v	v	−	v	ND
Acid from:						
L-Arabinose	+	+	ND	ND	−	−
D-Arabitol	−	+	ND	ND	ND	−
Glucose	+	+	−	−	−	−
Inositol	−	−	ND	ND	ND	−
Lactose	v	+	v	−	−	−
Maltose	v	+	ND	ND	ND	−
Mannitol	−	+	ND	ND	ND	−
Sucrose	−	−	−	−	−	−
Xylose	+	+	ND	ND	−	−
Motility	+	+	ND	ND	+	+
Flagella	1 polar	1 polar	ND	ND	1 polar	Peritrichous

[a]Data from references 53, 54, 85, and 226 and LiPuma, unpublished; +, ≥90% positive; −, <10% positive; v, 10% to 90% positive; ND, not determined.

are visible. They are lysine decarboxylase negative and generally catalase positive, although catalase-negative *R. pickettii* strains have been described (53, 226). Most species show a fast and strong oxidase reaction; however, the intensity of the oxidase reaction varies for *R. mannitolilytica*, *R. pickettii*, and *Cupriavidus gilardii*, with some strains showing a weakly positive reaction (53, 226; LiPuma, unpublished). *R. pickettii*, *R. mannitolilytica*, and *R. insidiosa* grow on BCSA; most *Cupriavidus* strains do not, but growth is strain dependent. These species do not produce acid from sucrose. Most *R. mannitolilytica* strains acidify lactose, whereas most strains from other species do not. *R. insidiosa*, *C. respiraculi*, *Cupriavidus gilardii*, and *Cupriavidus pauculus* are differentiated from *R. pickettii* and *R. mannitolilytica* in failing to acidify glucose. *Cupriavidus* species have a characteristic cellular fatty acid profile different from that of other *Ralstonia* species (53, 85). The main fatty acid components of these species are C16:0, C16:1 w7c, and C18:1 w7c (each accounting for 20 to 30% of the overall fatty acid content); in addition C14:0, C14:0 3OH, and C17:0 cyclo are always present (each accounting for 5 to 10% of the overall fatty acid content) (68, 110).

Molecular genetic tests have proved quite helpful in differentiating these species. A 16S rRNA-directed PCR assay reliably identifies all *Ralstonia* and *Cupriavidus* species (as a group), allowing their differentiation from the phenotypically similar species in the genera *Burkholderia* and *Pandoraea* (64). Species-specific 16S rRNA-based PCR assays have also been developed; these enable the accurate identification of *R. pickettii*, *R. mannitolilytica*, *R. insidiosa*, and *Cupriavidus respiraculi* (64, 67, 68).

Pandoraea spp.

Overall, the biochemical profiles of *Pandoraea* strains are similar to those of *Burkholderia* and *Ralstonia* strains isolated from clinical specimens (Table 1) (52, 83, 123). The lack of saccharolytic activity is indicative of *Pandoraea* but is also seen with some *Ralstonia* species. Definitive identification of putative *Pandoraea* isolates requires molecular confirmation. Coenye et al. (60) described 16S rRNA gene-based PCR assays for the identification of these bacteria. A PCR assay was developed for the identification of *Pandoraea* isolates to the genus level. PCR assays for the identification of *P. apista* and *P. pulmonicola* (as a group), *P. pnomenusa*, *P. sputorum*, and *P. norimbergensis* were also developed. *Pandoraea* strains can be differentiated from *Burkholderia* and *Ralstonia* strains by their specific 16S rRNA gene restriction profile (123, 208) and can be identified at the species level through MspI restriction analysis of the *gyrB* gene (59). A quantitative comparison of the whole-cell fatty acid profiles of the members of these three genera allows the differentiation of *Pandoraea* strains from the others (53, 83). However, with the use of the commercially available microbial identification system database (Microbial ID, Inc., Newark, DE), these organisms are mostly identified with low identification scores as *Burkholderia* or *Ralstonia* species (53, 123) due to a lack of discriminatory fatty acids.

S. maltophilia

Key features for identifying *S. maltophilia* include oxidation of glucose and maltose with a more intense reaction with the latter, positive reactions for DNase and lysine decarboxylase, and a tuft of polar flagella (Table 4) (244). Although most strains were previously believed to be oxidase negative, testing of large numbers of isolates recovered from human specimens and referred to a reference laboratory indicates that as many as 20% may be oxidase positive

(LiPuma, unpublished). This proportion may be higher than expected since strains with an "atypical" phenotype may be preferentially referred for analysis. Detection of extracellular DNase activity by *S. maltophilia* is a key to differentiating this species from most other glucose-oxidizing, gram-negative bacilli. It can be detected on tube-base or plated DNase medium with a methyl green indicator. Care must be taken when interpreting the DNase reaction, since one report documented the misidentification of *S. maltophilia* as *B. cepacia* partially based on false-negative DNase reactions that were finalized with 48 h of incubation rather than 72 h (25). Selected isolates of *Flavobacterium* and *Shewanella* spp. may also be DNase positive. On sheep blood agar, colonies appear rough and lavender-green and have an ammonialike odor. *S. maltophilia* has a characteristic cellular fatty acid profile with large amounts (>30%) of 13-methyl tetradecanoic acid ($C_{15:0\ iso}$) and lesser amounts (>10%) of 12-methyl tetradecanoic acid ($C_{15:0\ anteiso}$) and cis-9-hexadecenoic acid ($C_{16:1}$ cis9) (244). To overcome the problems associated with definitive identification of *S. maltophilia*, Whitby et al. (245) developed a species-specific PCR assay targeting the 23S rRNA gene and reported sensitivity and specificity of 100%. This PCR test was used as a standard to evaluate the identification of *S. maltophilia* using the API 20NE strip and the VITEK 2 ID-GNB card (107). Both systems showed good reliability compared to PCR. A multiplex PCR assay to identify *P. aeruginosa*, *B. cepacia* complex species, and *S. maltophilia* directly in sputum and oropharyngeal specimens from CF patients has been reported, but only a very limited number of *S. maltophilia* isolates were examined (84).

Acidovorax, Brevundimonas, Delftia, and *Comamonas* spp.

Characteristics of *Acidovorax, Brevundimonas, Delftia,* and *Comamonas* are given in Table 4.

Acidovorax species, rarely encountered in clinical and environmental samples, are straight to slightly curved gram-negative bacilli which occur either singly or in short chains. They are oxidase positive and nonpigmented and have a single polar flagellum. Urease activity varies among strains (244, 250).

Brevundimonas diminuta and *Brevundimonas vesicularis*, infrequently encountered in clinical and environmental samples, have growth requirements for specific vitamins, including pantothenate, biotin, and cyanocobalamin. An additional growth requirement for *Brevundimonas diminuta* is cysteine. Most strains of *Brevundimonas diminuta* grow on MacConkey agar, while only approximately 25% of *Brevundimonas vesicularis* strains do so. On primary isolation media, *Brevundimonas diminuta* colonies are chalk white whereas many strains of *Brevundimonas vesicularis* are characterized by an orange intracellular pigment. These organisms are oxidase positive, have a single polar flagellum, and weakly oxidize glucose (*Brevundimonas vesicularis* more so than *Brevundimonas diminuta*), and the vast majority fail to reduce nitrate to nitrite. The most reliable method for differentiating these two species is the test for esculin hydrolysis. Almost all strains of *Brevundimonas vesicularis* (88%) are reported to hydrolyze this substrate, while *Brevundimonas diminuta* strains rarely do (5%) (Table 4) (244).

Comamonas spp. are straight to slightly curved gram-negative bacilli that occur singly or in pairs. The organisms are catalase and oxidase positive and have a single tuft of polar flagella. All human clinical *Comamonas* species reduce nitrate to nitrite. Phenotypic differentiation of *Comamonas*

TABLE 4 Characteristics of *Acidovorax*, *Brevundimonas*, *Delftia*, *Comamonas*, and *Stenotrophomonas* spp. found in clinical specimens[a]

Test	A. delafieldii (n = 2)	A. facilis (n = 2)	A. temperans (n = 2)	B. diminuta (n = 68)	B. vesicularis (n = 94)	D. acidovorans (n = 69)	Comamonas spp. (n = 28)	S. maltophilia (n = 228)
Oxidase	100	100	100	100	98	100	100	20[b]
Growth:								
MacConkey	100	0	100	100	43	100	100	100
Cetrimide	0	0	0	0	0	4	0	2
6.0% NaCl	0	0	0	21	23	6	0	22
42°C	50	0	100	38	19	29	68	48
Nitrate reduction	100	100	100	3	5	99	96	39
Gas from nitrate	0	0	100	0	0	0	0	0
Pigment	Yellow, soluble	None	Yellow, soluble	Brown-tan, soluble	52% yellow-orange, insoluble[e]	26% fluorescent, 44% yellow-tan, soluble	27% yellow-brown, soluble	Brown-tan, soluble
Arginine dihydrolase	100	100	0	0	0	0	0	0
Lysine decarboxylase	0	0	0	0	0	0	0	93
Ornithine decarboxylase	0	0	0	0	0	0	0	0
Indole	0	0	0	0	0	0	0	0
Hemolysis	0	0	0	0	0	0	0	1
Hydrolysis:								
Urea	100	100	50	13	2	0	7	3
Citrate	100	0	0	1	1	94	47	34
Gelatin	0	100	0	68	25	11	0	93
Esculin	0	0	0	5	88	0	0	39
Acid from:								
Glucose[c]	100	100	100	21	87	0	0	85
Xylose	85	100	0	0	27	0	0	35
Lactose	0	0	0	0	0	0	0	60
Sucrose	0	0	0	0	0	0	0	63
Maltose	0	0	0	0	94	0	0	100
Mannitol	50	100	50	0	0	100	0	0
H_2S[d]	100	100	100	34	49	57	0	95
Motility	100	100	100	100	100	100	100	100
No. of flagella	1–2	1–2	1–2	1–2	1–2	>2	>2	>2

[a]Data from reference 244. Values are the percentages of strains positive.
[b]793 isolates tested by using BactiDrop Oxidase (Remel, Dartford, Kent, United Kingdom) (LiPuma, unpublished).
[c]Oxidative-fermentation basal medium with 1% carbohydrate.
[d]Lead acetate paper.
[e]Pigment observed on Thayer-Martin agar.

terrigena from *Comamonas testosteroni* is difficult, and as a result isolates are typically reported as *Comamonas* spp. (Table 4).

D. acidovorans is phenotypically similar to *Comamonas*. Key characteristics of the species include abilities to oxidize fructose and mannitol. One-quarter of the strains produce a fluorescent pigment, while approximately one-half of the strains may produce a soluble yellow to tan one (244, 249).

TYPING SYSTEMS

Several molecular genetic methods are available to assess the relatedness of isolates of these genera during nosocomial or community outbreak investigations. These methods are preferred over phenotypically based systems, which are less discriminatory and reproducible. Analysis of whole-genome macrorestriction profiles with pulsed-field gel electrophoresis (PFGE) has gained acceptance as a preferred genotyping method and has proved useful in numerous studies of *Burkholderia*, *Ralstonia*, and *S. maltophilia* (45, 63, 224). The endonucleases XbaI and SpeI are most frequently used and typically yield a dozen or more DNA fragments for analysis. Care must be taken in interpreting PFGE profiles

of *Burkholderia* species, however. These species have unusually large and dynamic multichromosome genomes that are prone to large-scale alterations in content and arrangement (151). Consequently, epidemiologically irrelevant genomic polymorphisms may arise in the short term and confound outbreak investigations (63). Ribotyping, which relies on polymorphisms in and around rRNA operons, has been used to investigate the epidemiology of *B. cepacia* complex and *B. pseudomallei* (133, 158, 160). Both PFGE and ribotyping are relatively time-consuming and expensive to perform and are therefore not particularly well suited for routine analysis by clinical microbiology laboratories. A variety of PCR-based methods, including randomly amplified polymorphic DNA typing and repetitive-sequence PCR typing, offer attractive alternatives for genotyping *S. maltophilia* and *Burkholderia*, *Ralstonia*, and *Pandoraea* spp. (34, 55, 147, 166, 208). These methods are inexpensive and can provide rapid, reliable results. MLST, which assesses DNA sequence variation at several chromosomal loci, has been developed for numerous species, including the *B. cepacia* complex, *B. pseudomallei*, and *B. mallei* (14, 39, 109). A recent modification of the scheme developed for the *B. cepacia* complex enables MLST analysis of all species within the genus (214). This genotyping strategy provides robust, reproducible, and portable results and is quickly becoming the preferred method for investigating bacterial epidemiology, evolution, and population structure. Both repetitive-sequence PCR using a BOX A1R primer and multilocus variable-number tandem repeat analysis have been developed for *B. pseudomallei* to exclude a clonal outbreak (76, 77). Typing methods have not been reported for *Brevundimonas, Delftia, Comamonas,* or *Acidovorax* spp.

SEROLOGIC TESTS

Of the organisms discussed in this chapter, *B. pseudomallei* is the only one for which serologic tests have been used clinically to diagnose the infection. The indirect hemagglutination assay, although not available commercially, is the most widely used test (10). It is performed by using a prepared antigen from strains of *B. pseudomallei* sensitized to sheep cells and includes unsensitized cells as a control. This assay can be adapted to a microtiter plate test system. The serologic tests currently in use have limited value for the diagnosis of melioidosis in persons who have lived in regions where melioidosis is endemic because the healthy indigenous population is often seropositive (256, 259, 260). Serologic testing is potentially useful for persons who do not normally reside in regions endemic for melioidosis, including returning travellers and laboratory workers following accidental laboratory exposure to *B. pseudomallei* (192). The interpretation of the indirect hemagglutination assay or other serologic assays is complicated by the fact that there are no validated guidelines, and different cutoff points have been used to define seroconversion following exposure and acute infection. Testing should be performed whenever possible on paired samples. Seroconversion with the development of detectable antibodies to *B. pseudomallei* in the second sample is supportive of exposure. A fourfold rise in titer is commonly used to diagnose a range of infectious diseases, but this has not been validated for melioidosis and any reproducible rise between two samples should be viewed as possible evidence of exposure. A single high titer in persons from a nonendemic region with a relevant travel history who presents late after a putative exposure event and for whom paired sera may be less relevant is also suggestive of exposure. Some individuals with culture-proven melioidosis do not have detectable antibodies (41), and so a negative serologic test does not rule out exposure or melioidosis. Given the complexity of this situation, experts in the field should be consulted when serology is used to diagnose melioidosis. Several evaluations of a commercial rapid immunochromatographic test kit (Pan-Bio, Windsor, Queensland, Australia) for the detection of immunoglobulin G and immunoglobulin M antibodies to *B. pseudomallei* have been performed (42, 180, 254), but this test is not currently available.

ANTIMICROBIAL SUSCEPTIBILITIES

Specific susceptibility testing interpretative criteria are not available for all of the species discussed in this chapter. For some species, such as the *B. cepacia* complex and *S. maltophilia*, interpretive criteria for disk diffusion testing are available for only a limited number of antibiotics. In general, MIC broth microdilution tests or Etests are preferred for this group of organisms.

B. cepacia complex species are among the most antimicrobial-resistant bacteria encountered in the clinical laboratory. These species are intrinsically resistant to aminoglycoside and polymyxin antibiotics and are often resistant to β-lactam antibiotics due to inducible chromosomal β-lactamases and altered penicillin-binding proteins (118). Antibiotic efflux pumps may mediate resistance to chloramphenicol, fluoroquinolones, and trimethoprim (196). Clinical strains may be susceptible to only a handful of agents, including trimethoprim-sulfamethoxazole (TMP-SMX), ceftazidime, chloramphenicol, minocycline, imipenem, meropenem, and some fluoroquinolones (1, 125, 194). The glycylcycline antibiotic tigecycline shows highly variable activity in vitro (172). The relatively high MIC observed for some strains and the potential for discoloration of permanent teeth in children younger than 7 years of age limit the use of tigecycline in CF patients. Clinical and Laboratory Standards Institute (CLSI; formerly NCCLS) interpretative criteria for disk diffusion susceptibility testing are available for ceftazidime, meropenem, minocycline, and TMP-SMX (50). MIC broth microdilution tests or Etests are preferred methodologies for susceptibility testing of these species. Because isolates that are initially susceptible may become resistant during the course of therapy, susceptibility testing of repeat isolates may be warranted. Furthermore, strains recovered from patients with CF who have received repeated courses of antibiotic therapy are frequently resistant to all currently available antimicrobial agents (1, 105). Combinations of antimicrobial agents may provide synergistic activity against resistant strains; however, antagonism with combinations is also observed in vitro (1).

B. pseudomallei is intrinsically resistant to penicillins, aminoglycosides, and macrolides. Susceptibility testing should be performed to the antimicrobial agents commonly used to treat melioidosis, which are ceftazidime, imipenem or meropenem, amoxicillin-clavulanate, doxycycline, and trimethoprim-sulfamethoxazole (TMP-SMX). *B. pseudomallei* is usually susceptible to all of these agents with the exception of TMP-SMX, reported rates of resistance for which are in the order of 2% in Australia (135, 193) and 13 to 16% in northeast Thailand (164, 255). Disk diffusion testing of TMP-SMX overestimates resistance and is unreliable (164, 193, 255); acceptable alternatives include Etest, broth microdilution, and agar dilution. Fluoroquinolones are associated with a high rate of therapeutic failure (32) and should not be included in the test panel. Recent studies indicate that tigecycline has good activity against *B. pseudomallei* in vitro and is effective when combined with other agents in an animal model of *B. pseudomallei* infection (97, 219).

Current trends in the management of melioidosis involve an initial 10- to 14-day intensive therapy phase with ceftazidime or meropenem, followed by eradication therapy with TMP-SMX with or without doxycycline for at least 3 months (31, 37, 47, 248). In Australia, TMP-SMX is added to ceftazidime or meropenem during the intensive phase for neurological, prostatic, cutaneous, and bone and joint melioidosis. Amoxicillin-clavulanate is recommended for eradication therapy in pregnancy and is an alternative to TMP-SMX in children (36). In critically ill patients requiring intensive care, meropenem or imipenem may be superior to ceftazidime, and granulocyte colony-stimulating factor is being used in some centers, although a study from Thailand showed no benefit (38, 40, 43, 135). From a molecular genotyping study of cases of recurrent melioidosis, relapse following antimicrobial therapy occurred in 9.7% of patients and a new infection occurred in 3.4% (152).

Because of the potential role of *B. mallei* as a bioterrorism agent, studies have been done recently to determine the activities of a variety of agents against this species. *B. mallei* has a susceptibility profile similar to that of *B. pseudomallei,* except that *B. mallei* is susceptible to aminoglycosides and newer macrolides such as clarithromycin and azithromycin, whereas *B. pseudomallei* is resistant (120, 142). Current recommended treatment and duration of therapy for glanders are the same as those for melioidosis.

Guidelines on the management of accidental laboratory exposure to *B. pseudomallei* and *B. mallei* have been recently published (192).

S. maltophilia is intrinsically resistant to many classes of antibiotics. Resistance can also develop rapidly during infection (101). Resistance to β-lactam agents is mediated by at least two β-lactamases, one of which is zinc dependent and resistant to β-lactamase inhibitors and confers resistance to imipenem. Aminoglycoside and quinolone resistance results from mutations in outer membrane proteins. In a study of isolates recovered from patients with CF, doxycycline was the most active agent in vitro (204). TMP-SMX is usually active and is often used in combination with ticarcillin-clavulanate, minocycline, or piperacillin-tazobactam (204). Other combinations that may be effective include ciprofloxacin paired with ticarcillin-clavulanate, ciprofloxacin and piperacillin-tazobactam, or doxycycline and ticarcillin-clavulanate. Tigecycline is reported to have good activity in vitro (172). CLSI interpretive criteria for disk diffusion susceptibility testing are available for minocycline, levofloxacin, and TMP-SMX (50). However, broth microdilution, Etest, or agar dilution methods are the preferred susceptibility testing methods (9, 264). Many U.S. laboratories comment only on the activity of TMP-SMX but will test additional antibiotics such as minocycline, ceftazidime, ticarcillin-clavulanate, and ciprofloxacin or levofloxacin upon request.

In general, *Comamonas testosteroni* is susceptible to extended- and broad-spectrum cephalosporins, carbapenems, quinolones, and TMP-SMX (15). *D. acidovorans* is frequently resistant to the aminoglycosides.

EVALUATION, INTERPRETATION, AND REPORTING OF RESULTS

The species discussed in this chapter are found in the natural environment and may occasionally contaminate clinical specimens. Nevertheless, they are increasingly recognized as nosocomial and opportunistic pathogens, especially in certain patient populations, such as persons with CF. They are also frequently misidentified by commercial microbial identification systems. Therefore, their recovery in the clinical laboratory must be given careful consideration. In particular, species of the *B. cepacia* complex are not reliably differentiated by phenotypic analyses, and their recovery from persons with CF has serious consequences with respect to patient management and psychosocial well-being (154). Identification of these species should be confirmed by genotypic analyses at a reference laboratory and should promptly be reported to the CF care team. Recovery of *B. pseudomallei* and *B. mallei* in any context should always be considered to reflect clinical disease. Identification of these species should be confirmed by a reference laboratory with experience with these species. Care must be given to ensure that culture handling and shipping comply with current biosafety regulations (see chapters 6 and 12). Identification of these species must be reported to public health officials due to the potential of these species as agents of bioterrorism (see chapter 7). The relevance of the recovery of the other genera described in this chapter, outside the context of CF, is less clear and should be interpreted with caution.

Interpretive criteria for disk diffusion antimicrobial susceptibility testing of most of these species are lacking; MIC broth microdilution and the Etest are therefore the preferred methodologies for susceptibility testing. For multiresistant strains, consideration could be given to testing for synergy with double or triple combinations of antimicrobial agents in reference laboratories (1). It is important to note, however, that neither checkerboard MIC broth microdilution testing nor multiple combination bactericidal antibiotic testing is standardized at present.

REFERENCES

1. **Aaron, S. D., W. Ferris, D. A. Henry, D. P. Speert, and N. E. Macdonald.** 2000. Multiple combination bactericidal antibiotic testing for patients with cystic fibrosis infected with *Burkholderia cepacia. Am. J. Respir. Crit. Care Med.* **161:**1206–1212.
2. **Agger, W. A., T. H. Cogbill, H. Busch, Jr., J. Landercasper, and S. M. Callister.** 1986. Wounds caused by corn-harvesting machines: an unusual source of infection due to Gram-negative bacilli. *Rev. Infect. Dis.* **8:**927–931.
3. **Agodi, A., M. Barchitta, V. Giannino, A. Collura, T. Pensabene, M. L. Garlaschi, C. Pasquarella, F. Luzzaro, F. Sinatra, E. Mahenthiralingam, and S. Stefani.** 2002. *Burkholderia cepacia* complex in cystic fibrosis and non-cystic fibrosis patients: identification of a cluster of epidemic lineages. *J. Hosp. Infect.* **50:**188–195.
4. **Alexander, B. D., E. W. Petzold, L. B. Reller, S. M. Palmer, R. D. Davis, C. W. Woods, and J. J. LiPuma.** 2008. Survival after lung transplantation of cystic fibrosis patients infected with *Burkholderia cepacia* complex. *Am. J. Transplant.* **8:**1025–1030.
5. **Alfieri, N., K. Ramotar, P. Armstrong, M. E. Spornitz, G. Ross, J. Winnick, and D. R. Cook.** 1999. Two consecutive outbreaks of *Stenotrophomonas maltophilia* (*Xanthomonas maltophilia*) in an intensive-care unit defined by restriction fragment-length polymorphism typing. *Infect. Control Hosp. Epidemiol.* **20:**553–556.
6. **Amornchai, P., W. Chierakul, V. Wuthiekanun, Y. Mahakhunkijcharoen, R. Phetsouvanh, B. J. Currie, P. N. Newton, N. van Vinh Chau, S. Wongratanacheewin, N. P. Day, and S. J. Peacock.** 2007. Accuracy of *Burkholderia pseudomallei* identification using the API 20NE system and a latex agglutination test. *J. Clin. Microbiol.* **45:**3774–3776.
7. **Arda, B., S. Aydemir, T. Yamazhan, A. Hassan, A. Tunger, and D. Serter.** 2003. *Comamonas testosteroni* meningitis in a patient with recurrent cholesteatoma. *APMIS* **111:**474–476.
8. **Aris, R. M., J. C. Routh, J. J. LiPuma, D. G. Heath, and P. H. Gilligan.** 2001. Lung transplantation for cystic fibrosis patients with *Burkholderia cepacia* complex. Survival linked to genomovar type. *Am. J. Respir. Crit. Care Med.* **164:**2102–2106.
9. **Arpi, M., M. A. Victor, I. Mortensen, A. Gottschau, and B. Bruun.** 1996. *In vitro* susceptibility of 124 *Xanthomonas maltophilia* (*Stenotrophomonas maltophilia*) isolates: comparison of the agar dilution method with the E-test and two agar diffusion methods. *APMIS* **104:**108–114.
10. **Ashdown, L. R.** 1987. Indirect haemagglutination test for melioidosis. *Med. J. Aust.* **147:**364–365.
11. **Ashdown, L. R.** 1992. Melioidosis and safety in the clinical laboratory. *J. Hosp. Infect.* **21:**301–306.
12. **Athan, E., A. M. Allworth, C. Engler, I. Bastian, and A. C. Cheng.** 2005. Melioidosis in tsunami survivors. *Emerg. Infect. Dis.* **11:**1638–1639.
13. **Balandreau, J., V. Viallard, B. Cournoyer, T. Coenye, S. Laevens, and P. Vandamme.** 2001. *Burkholderia cepacia* genomovar III is a common plant-associated bacterium. *Appl. Environ. Microbiol.* **67:**982–985.
14. **Baldwin, A., E. Mahenthiralingam, K. M. Thickett, D. Honeybourne, M. C. Maiden, J. R. Govan, D. P. Speert, J. J. LiPuma, P. Vandamme, and C. G. Dowson.** 2005. Multilocus sequence typing scheme that provides both species and strain differentiation for the *Burkholderia cepacia* complex. *J. Clin. Microbiol.* **43:**4665–4673.

15. Barbaro, D. J., P. A. Mackowiak, S. S. Barth, and P. M. Southern, Jr. 1987. *Pseudomonas testosteroni* infections: eighteen recent cases and a review of the literature. *Rev. Infect. Dis.* **9:**124–129.

16. Barker, P. M., R. E. Wood, and P. H. Gilligan. 1997. Lung infection with *Burkholderia gladioli* in a child with cystic fibrosis: acute clinical and spirometric deterioration. *Pediatr. Pulmonol.* **23:**123–125.

17. Bauernfeind, A., I. Schneider, R. Jungwirth, and C. Roller. 1999. Discrimination of *Burkholderia multivorans* and *Burkholderia vietnamiensis* from *Burkholderia cepacia* genomovars I, III, and IV by PCR. *J. Clin. Microbiol.* **37:**1335–1339.

18. Berriatua, E., I. Ziluaga, C. Miguel-Virto, P. Uribarren, R. Juste, S. Laevens, P. Vandamme, and J. R. Govan. 2001. Outbreak of subclinical mastitis in a flock of dairy sheep associated with *Burkholderia cepacia* complex infection. *J. Clin. Microbiol.* **39:**990–994.

19. Blackburn, L., K. Brownlee, S. Conway, and M. Denton. 2004. 'Cepacia syndrome' with *Burkholderia multivorans*, 9 years after initial colonization. *J. Cyst. Fibros.* **3:**133–134.

20. Boutros, N., N. Gonullu, A. Casetta, M. Guibert, D. Ingrand, and L. Lebrun. 2002. *Ralstonia pickettii* traced in blood culture bottles. *J. Clin. Microbiol.* **40:**2666–2667.

21. Brett, P. J., D. DeShazer, and D. E. Woods. 1998. *Burkholderia thailandensis* sp. nov., a *Burkholderia pseudomallei*-like species. *Int. J. Syst. Bacteriol.* **48**(Pt. 1):317–320.

22. Brisse, S., S. Stefani, J. Verhoef, A. Van Belkum, P. Vandamme, and W. Goessens. 2002. Comparative evaluation of the BD Phoenix and VITEK 2 automated instruments for identification of isolates of the *Burkholderia cepacia* complex. *J. Clin. Microbiol.* **40:**1743–1748.

23. Brisse, S., C. M. Verduin, D. Milatovic, A. Fluit, J. Verhoef, S. Laevens, P. Vandamme, B. Tummler, H. A. Verbrugh, and A. van Belkum. 2000. Distinguishing species of the *Burkholderia cepacia* complex and *Burkholderia gladioli* by automated ribotyping. *J. Clin. Microbiol.* **38:**1876–1884.

24. Burbage, D. A., M. Sasser, and R. D. Lumsden. 1982. A medium selective for *Pseudomonas cepacia*. *Phytopathology* **72:**706.

25. Burdge, D. R., M. A. Noble, M. E. Campbell, V. L. Krell, and D. P. Speert. 1995. *Xanthomonas maltophilia* misidentified as *Pseudomonas cepacia* in cultures of sputum from patients with cystic fibrosis: a diagnostic pitfall with major clinical implications. *Clin. Infect. Dis.* **20:**445–448.

26. Burns, J. L., J. Emerson, J. R. Stapp, D. L. Yim, J. Krzewinski, L. Louden, B. W. Ramsey, and C. R. Clausen. 1998. Microbiology of sputum from patients at cystic fibrosis centers in the United States. *Clin. Infect. Dis.* **27:**158–163.

27. Centers for Disease Control and Prevention. 2000. Laboratory-acquired human glanders—Maryland, May 2000. *MMWR Morb. Mortal. Wkly. Rep.* **49:**532–535.

28. Chantratita, N., E. Meumann, A. Thanwisai, D. Limmathurotsakul, V. Wuthiekanun, S. Wannapasni, S. Tumapa, N. P. Day, and S. J. Peacock. 2008. Loop-mediated isothermal amplification method targeting the TTS1 gene cluster for detection of *Burkholderia pseudomallei* and diagnosis of melioidosis. *J. Clin. Microbiol.* **46:**568–573.

29. Chantratita, N., V. Wuthiekanun, D. Limmathurotsakul, A. Thanwisai, W. Chantratita, N. P. Day, and S. J. Peacock. 2007. Prospective clinical evaluation of the accuracy of 16S rRNA real-time PCR assay for the diagnosis of melioidosis. *Am. J. Trop. Med. Hyg.* **77:**814–817.

30. Chantratita, N., V. Wuthiekanun, D. Limmathurotsakul, M. Vesaratchavest, A. Thanwisai, P. Amornchai, S. Tumapa, E. J. Feil, N. P. Day, and S. J. Peacock. 2008. Genetic diversity and microevolution of *Burkholderia pseudomallei* in the environment. *PLoS Negl. Trop. Dis.* **2:**e182.

31. Chaowagul, W., W. Chierakul, A. J. Simpson, J. M. Short, K. Stepniewska, B. Maharjan, A. Rajchanuvong, D. Busarawong, D. Limmathurotsakul, A. C. Cheng, V. Wuthiekanun, P. N. Newton, N. J. White, N. P. Day, and S. J. Peacock. 2005. Open-label randomized trial of oral trimethoprim-sulfamethoxazole, doxycycline, and chloramphenicol compared with trimethoprim-sulfamethoxazole and doxycycline for maintenance therapy of melioidosis. *Antimicrob. Agents Chemother.* **49:**4020–4025.

32. Chaowagul, W., Y. Suputtamongkul, M. D. Smith, and N. J. White. 1997. Oral fluoroquinolones for maintenance treatment of melioidosis. *Trans. R. Soc. Trop. Med. Hyg.* **91:**599–601.

33. Chaowagul, W., N. J. White, D. A. Dance, Y. Wattanagoon, P. Naigowit, T. M. Davis, S. Looareesuwan, and N. Pitakwatchara. 1989. Melioidosis: a major cause of community-acquired septicemia in northeastern Thailand. *J. Infect. Dis.* **159:**890–899.

34. Chen, J. S., K. A. Witzmann, T. Spilker, R. J. Fink, and J. J. LiPuma. 2001. Endemicity and inter-city spread of *Burkholderia cepacia* genomovar III in cystic fibrosis. *J. Pediatr.* **139:**643–649.

35. Chen, W. M., S. Laevens, T. M. Lee, T. Coenye, P. De Vos, M. Mergeay, and P. Vandamme. 2001. *Ralstonia taiwanensis* sp. nov., isolated from root nodules of *Mimosa* species and sputum of a cystic fibrosis patient. *Int. J. Syst. Evol. Microbiol.* **51:**1729–1735.

36. Cheng, A. C., W. Chierakul, W. Chaowagul, P. Chetchotisakd, D. Limmathurotsakul, D. A. Dance, S. J. Peacock, and B. J. Currie. 2008. Consensus guidelines for dosing of amoxicillin-clavulanate in melioidosis. *Am. J. Trop. Med. Hyg.* **78:**208–209.

37. Cheng, A. C., and B. J. Currie. 2005. Melioidosis: epidemiology, pathophysiology, and management. *Clin. Microbiol. Rev.* **18:**383–416.

38. Cheng, A. C., D. A. Fisher, N. M. Anstey, D. P. Stephens, S. P. Jacups, and B. J. Currie. 2004. Outcomes of patients with melioidosis treated with meropenem. *Antimicrob. Agents Chemother.* **48:**1763–1765.

39. Cheng, A. C., D. Godoy, M. Mayo, D. Gal, B. G. Spratt, and B. J. Currie. 2004. Isolates of *Burkholderia pseudomallei* from Northern Australia are distinct by multilocus sequence typing, but strain types do not correlate with clinical presentation. *J. Clin. Microbiol.* **42:**5477–5483.

40. Cheng, A. C., D. Limmathurotsakul, W. Chierakul, N. Getchalarat, V. Wuthiekanun, D. P. Stephens, N. P. Day, N. J. White, W. Chaowagul, B. J. Currie, and S. J. Peacock. 2007. A randomized controlled trial of granulocyte colony-stimulating factor for the treatment of severe sepsis due to melioidosis in Thailand. *Clin. Infect. Dis.* **45:**308–314.

41. Cheng, A. C., M. O'Brien, K. Freeman, G. Lum, and B. J. Currie. 2006. Indirect hemagglutination assay in patients with melioidosis in northern Australia. *Am. J. Trop. Med. Hyg.* **74:**330–334.

42. Cheng, A. C., S. J. Peacock, D. Limmathurotsakul, G. Wongsuvan, W. Chierakul, P. Amornchai, N. Getchalarat, W. Chaowagul, N. J. White, N. P. Day, and V. Wuthiekanun. 2006. Prospective evaluation of a rapid immunochromogenic cassette test for the diagnosis of melioidosis in northeast Thailand. *Trans. R. Soc. Trop. Med. Hyg.* **100:**64–67.

43. Cheng, A. C., D. P. Stephens, and B. J. Currie. 2007. Granulocyte-colony stimulating factor (G-CSF) as an adjunct to antibiotics in the treatment of pneumonia in adults. *Cochrane Database Syst. Rev.*, Issue 2, Art. no. CD004400. doi: 10.1002/14651858.CD004400.pub3.ed.

44. Cheng, A. C., V. Wuthiekanun, D. Limmathurosakul, G. Wongsuvan, N. P. Day, and S. J. Peacock. 2006. Role of selective and nonselective media for isolation of *Burkholderia pseudomallei* from throat swabs of patients with melioidosis. *J. Clin. Microbiol.* **44:**2316.

45. Chetoui, H., P. Melin, M. J. Struelens, E. Delhalle, M. M. Nigo, R. De Ryck, and P. De Mol. 1997. Comparison of biotyping, ribotyping, and pulsed-field gel electrophoresis for investigation of a common-source outbreak of *Burkholderia pickettii* bacteremia. *J. Clin. Microbiol.* **35:**1398–1403.

46. Chi, C. Y., C. P. Fung, W. W. Wong, and C. Y. Liu. 2004. *Brevundimonas bacteremia*: two case reports and literature review. *Scand. J. Infect. Dis.* **36:**59–61.

47. Chierakul, W., S. Anunnatsiri, J. M. Short, B. Maharjan, P. Mootsikapun, A. J. Simpson, D. Limmathurotsakul, A. C. Cheng, K. Stepniewska, P. N. Newton, W. Chaowagul, N. J. White, S. J. Peacock, N. P. Day, and P. Chetchotisakd. 2005. Two randomized controlled trials of ceftazidime alone versus ceftazidime in combination with trimethoprim-sulfamethoxazole for the treatment of severe melioidosis. *Clin. Infect. Dis.* **41:**1105–1113.

48. Chierakul, W., W. Winothai, C. Wattanawaitunechai, V. Wuthiekanun, T. Rugtaengan, J. Rattanalertnavee, P. Jitpratoom, W. Chaowagul, P. Singhasivanon, N. J. White, N. P. Day, and S. J. Peacock. 2005. Melioidosis in 6 tsunami survivors in southern Thailand. Clin. Infect. Dis. 41:982–990.

49. Christenson, J. C., D. F. Welch, G. Mukwaya, M. J. Muszynski, R. E. Weaver, and D. J. Brenner. 1989. Recovery of Pseudomonas gladioli from respiratory tract specimens of patients with cystic fibrosis. J. Clin. Microbiol. 27:270–273.

50. Clinical and Laboratory Standards Institute. 2005. Performance Standards for Antimicrobial Susceptibility Testing; Fifteenth Informal Supplement. M100-S15. Clinical and Laboratory Standards Institute, Wayne, PA.

51. Clode, F. E., L. A. Metherell, and T. L. Pitt. 1999. Nosocomial acquisition of Burkholderia gladioli in patients with cystic fibrosis. Am. J. Respir. Crit. Care Med. 160:374–375.

52. Coenye, T., E. Falsen, B. Hoste, M. Ohlen, J. Goris, J. R. Govan, M. Gillis, and P. Vandamme. 2000. Description of Pandoraea gen. nov. with Pandoraea apista sp. nov., Pandoraea pulmonicola sp. nov., Pandoraea pnomenusa sp. nov., Pandoraea sputorum sp. nov. and Pandoraea norimbergensis comb. nov. Int. J. Syst. Evol. Microbiol. 50(Pt. 2):887–899.

53. Coenye, T., E. Falsen, M. Vancanneyt, B. Hoste, J. R. Govan, K. Kersters, and P. Vandamme. 1999. Classification of Alcaligenes faecalis-like isolates from the environment and human clinical samples as Ralstonia gilardii sp. nov. Int. J. Syst. Bacteriol. 49:405–413.

54. Coenye, T., J. Goris, P. De Vos, P. Vandamme, and J. J. LiPuma. 2003. Classification of Ralstonia pickettii-like isolates from the environment and clinical samples as Ralstonia insidiosa sp. nov. Int. J. Syst. Evol. Microbiol. 53:1075–1080.

55. Coenye, T., J. Goris, T. Spilker, P. Vandamme, and J. J. LiPuma. 2002. Characterization of unusual bacteria isolated from respiratory secretions of cystic fibrosis patients and description of Inquilinus limosus gen. nov., sp. nov. J. Clin. Microbiol. 40:2062–2069.

56. Coenye, T., B. Holmes, K. Kersters, J. R. W. Govan, and P. Vandamme. 1999. Burkholderia cocovenenans (van Damme et al. 1960) Gillis et al. 1995 and Burkholderia vandii Urakami et al. 1994 are junior synonyms of Burkholderia gladioli (Severini 1913) Yabuuchi et al. 1993 and Burkholderia plantarii (Azegami et al. 1987) Urakami et al. 1994, respectively. Int. J. Syst. Bacteriol. 49:37–42.

57. Coenye, T., S. Laevens, A. Willems, M. Ohlen, W. Hannant, J. R. W. Govan, M. Gillis, E. Falsen, and P. Vandamme. 2001. Burkholderia fungorum sp. nov. and Burkholderia caledonica sp. nov., two new species isolated from the environment, animals and human clinical samples. Int. J. Syst. Evol. Microbiol. 51:1099–1107.

58. Coenye, T., and J. J. LiPuma. 2002. Population structure analysis of Burkholderia cepacia genomovar III: varying degrees of genetic recombination characterize major clonal complexes. Microbiology 149:77–88.

59. Coenye, T., and J. J. LiPuma. 2002. Use of the gyrB gene for the identification of Pandoraea species. FEMS Microbiol. Lett. 208:15–19.

60. Coenye, T., L. Liu, P. Vandamme, and J. J. LiPuma. 2001. Identification of Pandoraea species by 16S ribosomal DNA-based PCR assays. J. Clin. Microbiol. 39:4452–4455.

61. Coenye, T., E. Mahenthiralingam, D. Henry, J. J. LiPuma, S. Laevens, M. Gillis, D. P. Speert, and P. Vandamme. 2001. Burkholderia ambifaria sp. nov., a novel member of the Burkholderia cepacia complex including biocontrol and cystic fibrosis-related isolates. Int. J. Syst. Evol. Microbiol. 51:1481–1490.

62. Coenye, T., L. M. Schouls, J. R. Govan, K. Kersters, and P. Vandamme. 1999. Identification of Burkholderia species and genomovars from cystic fibrosis patients by AFLP fingerprinting. Int. J. Syst. Bacteriol. 49(Pt 4):1657–1666.

63. Coenye, T., T. Spilker, A. Martin, and J. J. LiPuma. 2002. Comparative assessment of genotyping methods for epidemiologic study of Burkholderia cepacia genomovar III. J. Clin. Microbiol. 40:3300–3307.

64. Coenye, T., T. Spilker, R. Reik, P. Vandamme, and J. J. LiPuma. 2005. Use of PCR analyses to define the distribution of Ralstonia species recovered from patients with cystic fibrosis. J. Clin. Microbiol. 43:3463–3466.

65. Coenye, T., T. Spilker, A. Van Schoor, J. J. LiPuma, and P. Vandamme. 2004. Recovery of Burkholderia cenocepacia strain PHDC from cystic fibrosis patients in Europe. Thorax 59:952–954.

66. Coenye, T., P. Vandamme, J. R. Govan, and J. J. LiPuma. 2001. Taxonomy and identification of the Burkholderia cepacia complex. J. Clin. Microbiol. 39:3427–3436.

67. Coenye, T., P. Vandamme, and J. J. LiPuma. 2002. Infection by Ralstonia species in cystic fibrosis patients: identification of R. pickettii and R. mannitolilytica by polymerase chain reaction. Emerg. Infect. Dis. 8:692–696.

68. Coenye, T., P. Vandamme, and J. J. LiPuma. 2003. Ralstonia respiraculi sp. nov., isolated from the respiratory tract of cystic fibrosis patients. Int. J. Syst. Evol. Microbiol. 53:1339–1342.

69. Coenye, T., E. Vanlaere, E. Falsen, and P. Vandamme. 2004. Stenotrophomonas africana Drancourt et al. 1997 is a later synonym of Stenotrophomonas maltophilia (Hugh 1981) Palleroni and Bradbury 1993. Int. J. Syst. Evol. Microbiol. 54:1235–1237.

70. Cooper, G. R., E. D. Staples, K. A. Iczkowski, and C. J. Clancy. 2005. Comamonas (Pseudomonas) testosteroni endocarditis. Cardiovasc. Pathol. 14:145–149.

71. Corey, M., and V. Farewell. 1996. Determinants of mortality from cystic fibrosis in Canada, 1970–1989. Am. J. Epidemiol. 143:1007–1017.

72. Craven, D. E., B. Moody, M. G. Connolly, N. R. Kollisch, K. D. Stottmeier, and W. R. McCabe. 1981. Pseudobacteremia caused by povidone-iodine solution contaminated with Pseudomonas cepacia. N. Engl. J. Med. 305:621–623.

73. Currie, B. J., D. A. Dance, and A. C. Cheng. 2008. The global distribution of Burkholderia pseudomallei and melioidosis: an update. Trans. R. Soc. Trop. Med. Hyg. 102(Suppl. 1):S1–S4.

74. Currie, B. J., D. A. Fisher, D. M. Howard, and J. N. Burrow. 2000. Neurological melioidosis. Acta Trop. 74:145–151.

75. Currie, B. J., D. A. Fisher, D. M. Howard, J. N. Burrow, D. Lo, S. Selva-Nayagam, N. M. Anstey, S. E. Huffam, P. L. Snelling, P. J. Marks, D. P. Stephens, G. D. Lum, S. P. Jacups, and V. L. Krause. 2000. Endemic melioidosis in tropical northern Australia: a 10-year prospective study and review of the literature. Clin. Infect. Dis. 31:981–986.

76. Currie, B. J., D. Gal, M. Mayo, L. Ward, D. Godoy, B. G. Spratt, and J. J. LiPuma. 2007. Using BOX-PCR to exclude a clonal outbreak of melioidosis, p. 68. BMC Infect. Dis. 7:68.

77. Currie, B. J., A. Haslem, T. Pearson, H. Hornstra, B. Leadem, M. Mayo, D. Gal, L. Ward, D. Godoy, B. G. Spratt, and P. Keim. 2009. Identification of melioidosis outbreak by multilocus variable number tandem repeat analysis. Emerg. Infect. Dis. 15:169–174.

78. Currie, B. J., and S. P. Jacups. 2003. Intensity of rainfall and severity of melioidosis, Australia. Emerg. Infect. Dis. 9:1538–1542.

79. Currie, B. J., S. P. Jacups, A. C. Cheng, D. A. Fisher, N. M. Anstey, S. E. Huffam, and V. L. Krause. 2004. Melioidosis epidemiology and risk factors from a prospective whole-population study in northern Australia. Trop. Med. Int. Health 9:1167–1174.

80. Cystic Fibrosis Foundation. 2008. Patient Registry 2008. Annual Data Report to the Center Directors. Cystic Fibrosis Foundation, Bethesda, MD.

81. Dance, D. A., M. D. Smith, H. M. Aucken, and T. L. Pitt. 1999. Imported melioidosis in England and Wales. Lancet 353:208.

82. Dance, D. A., V. Wuthiekanun, P. Naigowit, and N. J. White. 1989. Identification of Pseudomonas pseudomallei in clinical practice: use of simple screening tests and API 20NE. J. Clin. Pathol. 42:645–648.

83. Daneshvar, M. I., D. G. Hollis, A. G. Steigerwalt, A. M. Whitney, L. Spangler, M. P. Douglas, J. G. Jordan, J. P. MacGregor, B. C. Hill, F. C. Tenover, D. J. Brenner, and R. S. Weyant. 2001. Assignment of CDC weak oxidizer

group 2 (WO-2) to the genus *Pandoraea* and characterization of three new *Pandoraea* genomospecies. *J. Clin. Microbiol.* **39:**1819–1826.

84. **da Silva Filho, L. V. F., A. F. Tateno, L. de F. Velloso, J. E. Levi, S. Fernandes, C. N. O. Bento, J. C. Rodrigues, and S. R. T. S. Ramos.** 2004. Identification of *Pseudomonas aeruginosa*, *Burkholderia cepacia* complex, and *Stenotrophomonas maltophilia* in respiratory samples from cystic fibrosis patients using multiplex PCR. *Pediatr. Pulmonol.* **37:**537–547.

85. **De Baere, T., S. Steyaert, G. Wauters, P. Des Vos, J. Goris, T. Coenye, T. Suyama, G. Verschraegen, and M. Vaneechoutte.** 2001. Classification of *Ralstonia pickettii* biovar 3/'thomasii' strains (Pickett 1994) and of new isolates related to nosocomial recurrent meningitis as *Ralstonia mannitolytica* sp. nov. *Int. J. Syst. Evol. Microbiol.* **51:**547–558.

86. **De Boeck, K., A. Malfroot, L. Van Schil, P. Lebecque, C. Knoop, J. R. Govan, C. Doherty, S. Laevens, and P. Vandamme.** 2004. Epidemiology of *Burkholderia cepacia* complex colonisation in cystic fibrosis patients. *Eur. Respir. J.* **23:**851–856.

87. **Deepak, R. N., B. Crawley, and E. Phang.** 2008. *Burkholderia pseudomallei* identification: a comparison between the API 20NE and VITEK2GN systems. *Trans. R. Soc. Trop. Med. Hyg.* **102**(Suppl. 1):S42–S44.

88. **Demko, C. A., R. C. Stern, and C. F. Doershuk.** 1998. *Stenotrophomonas maltophilia* in cystic fibrosis: incidence and prevalence. *Pediatr. Pulmonol.* **25:**304–308.

89. **Denton, M., M. J. Hall, N. J. Todd, K. G. Kerr, and J. M. Littlewood.** 2000. Improved isolation of *Stenotrophomonas maltophilia* from the sputa of patients with cystic fibrosis using a selective medium. *Clin. Microbiol. Infect.* **6:**397–398.

90. **Denton, M., and K. G. Kerr.** 1998. Microbiological and clinical aspects of infection associated with *Stenotrophomonas maltophilia*. *Clin. Microbiol. Rev.* **11:**57–80.

91. **Denton, M., N. J. Todd, K. G. Kerr, P. M. Hawkey, and J. M. Littlewood.** 1998. Molecular epidemiology of *Stenotrophomonas maltophilia* isolated from clinical specimens from patients with cystic fibrosis and associated environmental samples. *J. Clin. Microbiol.* **36:**1953–1958.

92. **Desakorn, V., M. D. Smith, V. Wuthiekanun, D. A. Dance, H. Aucken, P. Suntharasamai, A. Rajchanuwong, and N. J. White.** 1994. Detection of *Pseudomonas pseudomallei* antigen in urine for the diagnosis of melioidosis. *Am. J. Trop. Med. Hyg.* **51:**627–633.

93. **De Soyza, A., A. McDowell, L. Archer, J. H. Dark, S. J. Elborn, E. Mahenthiralingam, K. Gould, and P. A. Corris.** 2001. *Burkholderia cepacia* complex genomovars and pulmonary transplantation outcomes in patients with cystic fibrosis. *Lancet* **358:**1780–1781.

94. **Drancourt, M., C. Bollet, and D. Raoult.** 1997. *Stenotrophomonas africana* sp. nov., an opportunistic human pathogen in Africa. *Int. J. Syst. Bacteriol.* **47:**160–163.

95. **Ender, P. T., D. P. Dooley, and R. H. Moore.** 1996. Vascular catheter-related *Comamonas acidovorans* bacteremia managed with preservation of the catheter. *Pediatr. Infect. Dis. J.* **15:**918–920.

96. **Fernandez, C., I. Wilhelmi, E. Andradas, C. Gaspar, J. Gomez, J. Romero, J. A. Mariano, O. Corral, M. Rubio, J. Elviro, and J. Fereres.** 1996. Nosocomial outbreak of *Burkholderia pickettii* infection due to a manufactured intravenous product used in three hospitals. *Clin. Infect. Dis.* **22:**1092–1095.

97. **Feterl, M., B. Govan, C. Engler, R. Norton, and N. Ketheesan.** 2006. Activity of tigecycline in the treatment of acute *Burkholderia pseudomallei* infection in a murine model. *Int. J. Antimicrob. Agents* **28:**460–464.

98. **Fiore, A., S. Laevens, A. Bevivino, C. Dalmastri, S. Tabacchioni, P. Vandamme, and L. Chiarini.** 2001. *Burkholderia cepacia* complex: distribution of genomovars among isolates from the maize rhizosphere in Italy. *Environ. Microbiol.* **3:**137–143.

99. **Fujita, J., I. Yamadori, G. Xu, S. Hojo, K. Negayama, H. Miyawaki, Y. Yamaji, and J. Takahara.** 1996. Clinical features of *Stenotrophomonas maltophilia* pneumonia in immunocompromised patients. *Respir. Med.* **90:**35–38.

100. **Gardan, L., D. E. Stead, C. Dauga, and M. Gillis.** 2003. *Acidovorax valerianellae* sp. nov., a novel pathogen of lamb's lettuce [*Valerianella locusta* (L.) Laterr.]. *Int. J. Syst. Evol. Microbiol.* **53:**795–800.

101. **Garrison, M. W., D. E. Anderson, D. M. Campbell, K. C. Carroll, C. L. Malone, J. D. Anderson, R. J. Hollis, and M. A. Pfaller.** 1996. *Stenotrophomonas maltophilia*: emergence of multidrug-resistant strains during therapy and in an in vitro pharmacodynamic chamber model. *Antimicrob. Agents Chemother.* **40:**2859–2864.

102. **Gee, J. E., M. B. Glass, R. T. Novak, D. Gal, M. J. Mayo, A. G. Steigerwalt, P. P. Wilkins, and B. J. Currie.** 2008. Recovery of a *Burkholderia thailandensis*-like isolate from an Australian water source. *BMC Microbiol.* **8:**54.

103. **Gibney, K. B., A. C. Cheng, and B. J. Currie.** 2008. Cutaneous melioidosis in the tropical top end of Australia: a prospective study and review of the literature. *Clin. Infect. Dis.* **47:**603–609.

104. **Gilad, J., A. Borer, N. Peled, K. Riesenberg, S. Tager, A. Appelbaum, and F. Schlaeffer.** 2000. Hospital-acquired *Brevundimonas vesicularis* septicaemia following open-heart surgery: case report and literature review. *Scand. J. Infect. Dis.* **32:**90–91.

105. **Gilligan, P. H.** 1991. Microbiology of airway disease in patients with cystic fibrosis. *Clin. Microbiol. Rev.* **4:**35–51.

106. **Gilligan, P. H., P. A. Gage, L. M. Bradshaw, D. V. Schidlow, and B. T. DeCicco.** 1985. Isolation medium for the recovery of *Pseudomonas cepacia* from respiratory secretions of patients with cystic fibrosis. *J. Clin. Microbiol.* **22:**5–8.

107. **Giordano, A., A. Magni, M. Trancassini, P. Varesi, R. Turner, and C. Mancini.** 2006. Identification of respiratory isolates of *Stenotrophomonas maltophilia* by commercial biochemical systems and species-specific PCR. *J. Microbiol. Methods* **64:**135–138.

108. **Glass, M. B., and T. Popovic.** 2005. Preliminary evaluation of the API 20NE and RapID NF plus systems for rapid identification of *Burkholderia pseudomallei* and *B. mallei*. *J. Clin. Microbiol.* **43:**479–483.

109. **Godoy, D., G. Randle, A. J. Simpson, D. M. Aanensen, T. L. Pitt, R. Kinoshita, and B. G. Spratt.** 2003. Multilocus sequence typing and evolutionary relationships among the causative agents of melioidosis and glanders, *Burkholderia pseudomallei* and *Burkholderia mallei*. *J. Clin. Microbiol.* **41:**2068–2079.

110. **Goris, J., P. De Vos, T. Coenye, B. Hoste, D. Janssens, H. Brim, L. Diels, M. Mergeay, K. Kersters, and P. Vandamme.** 2001. Classification of metal-resistant bacteria from industrial biotopes as *Ralstonia campinensis* sp. nov., *Ralstonia metallidurans* sp. nov. and *Ralstonia basilensis* Steinle et al. 1998 emend. *Int. J. Syst. Evol. Microbiol.* **51:**1773–1782.

111. **Goss, C. H., K. Otto, M. L. Aitken, and G. D. Rubenfeld.** 2002. Detecting *Stenotrophomonas maltophilia* does not reduce survival of patients with cystic fibrosis. *Am. J. Respir. Crit. Care Med.* **166:**356–361.

112. **Govan, J. R., J. E. Hughes, and P. Vandamme.** 1996. *Burkholderia cepacia*: medical, taxonomic and ecological issues. *J. Med. Microbiol.* **45:**395–407.

113. **Graff, G. R., and J. L. Burns.** 2002. Factors affecting the incidence of *Stenotrophomonas maltophilia* isolation in cystic fibrosis. *Chest* **121:**1754–1760.

114. **Graves, M., T. Robin, A. M. Chipman, J. Wong, S. Khashe, and J. M. Janda.** 1997. Four additional cases of *Burkholderia gladioli* infection with microbiological correlates and review. *Clin. Infect. Dis.* **25:**838–842.

115. **Haase, A., M. Brennan, S. Barrett, Y. Wood, S. Huffam, D. O'Brien, and B. Currie.** 1998. Evaluation of PCR for diagnosis of melioidosis. *J. Clin. Microbiol.* **36:**1039–1041.

116. **Hagedorn, C., W. D. Gould, T. R. Bardinelli, and D. R. Gustavson.** 1987. A selective medium for enumeration and recovery of *Pseudomonas cepacia* biotypes from soil. *Appl. Environ. Microbiol.* **53:**2265–2268.

117. **Han, X. Y., and R. A. Andrade.** 2005. *Brevundimonas diminuta* infections and its resistance to fluoroquinolones. *J. Antimicrob. Chemother.* **55:**853–859.

118. **Hancock, R. E.** 1998. Resistance mechanisms in *Pseudomonas aeruginosa* and other nonfermentative Gram-negative bacteria. *Clin. Infect. Dis.* **27**(Suppl. 1):S93–S99.

119. **Hanes, S. D., K. Demirkan, E. Tolley, B. A. Boucher, M. A. Croce, G. C. Wood, and T. C. Fabian.** 2002. Risk factors for late-onset nosocomial pneumonia caused by *Stenotrophomonas maltophilia* in critically ill trauma patients. *Clin. Infect. Dis.* **35**:228–235.

120. **Heine, H. S., M. J. England, D. M. Waag, and W. R. Byrne.** 2001. In vitro antibiotic susceptibilities of *Burkholderia mallei* (causative agent of glanders) determined by broth microdilution and E-test. *Antimicrob. Agents Chemother.* **45**:2119–2121.

121. **Henry, D., M. Campbell, C. McGimpsey, A. Clarke, L. Louden, J. L. Burns, M. H. Roe, P. Vandamme, and D. Speert.** 1999. Comparison of isolation media for recovery of *Burkholderia cepacia* complex from respiratory secretions of patients with cystic fibrosis. *J. Clin. Microbiol.* **37**:1004–1007.

122. **Henry, D. A., M. E. Campbell, J. J. LiPuma, and D. P. Speert.** 1997. Identification of *Burkholderia cepacia* isolates from patients with cystic fibrosis and use of a simple new selective medium. *J. Clin. Microbiol.* **35**:614–619.

123. **Henry, D. A., E. Mahenthiralingam, P. Vandamme, T. Coenye, and D. P. Speert.** 2001. Phenotypic methods for determining genomovar status of the *Burkholderia cepacia* complex. *J. Clin. Microbiol.* **39**:1073–1078.

124. **Heylen, K., B. Vanparys, F. Peirsegaele, L. Lebbe, and P. De Vos.** 2007. *Stenotrophomonas terrae* sp. nov. and *Stenotrophomonas humi* sp. nov., two nitrate-reducing bacteria isolated from soil. *Int. J. Syst. Evol. Microbiol.* **57**:2056–2061.

125. **Hoban, D. J., S. K. Bouchillon, J. L. Johnson, G. G. Zhanel, D. L. Butler, L. A. Miller, J. A. Poupard, et al.** 2001. Comparative in vitro activity of gemifloxacin, ciprofloxacin, levofloxacin and ofloxacin in a North American surveillance study. *Diagn. Microbiol. Infect. Dis.* **40**:51–57.

126. **Holt, J., N. R. Krieg, A. Sneath, T. Staley, and S. T. Williams.** 1994. *Bergey's Manual of Determinative Bacteriology*, 9th ed., vol. 1. The Williams and Wilkins Company, Philadelphia, PA.

127. **Howard, K., and T. J. Inglis.** 2003. Novel selective medium for isolation of *Burkholderia pseudomallei*. *J. Clin. Microbiol.* **41**:3312–3316.

128. **Hugh, R., and E. Ryschenkow.** 1961. *Pseudomonas maltophilia*, an *Alcaligenes*-like species. *J. Gen. Microbiol.* **26**:123–132.

129. **Hutchinson, G. R., S. Parker, J. A. Pryor, F. Duncan-Skingle, P. N. Hoffman, M. E. Hodson, M. E. Kaufmann, and T. L. Pitt.** 1996. Home-use nebulizers: a potential primary source of *Burkholderia cepacia* and other colistin-resistant, gram-negative bacteria in patients with cystic fibrosis. *J. Clin. Microbiol.* **34**:584–587.

130. **Inglis, T. J., M. Aravena-Roman, S. Ching, K. Croft, V. Wuthiekanun, and B. J. Mee.** 2003. Cellular fatty acid profile distinguishes *Burkholderia pseudomallei* from avirulent *Burkholderia thailandensis*. *J. Clin. Microbiol.* **41**:4812–4814.

131. **Inglis, T. J., D. Chiang, G. S. Lee, and L. Chor-Kiang.** 1998. Potential misidentification of *Burkholderia pseudomallei* by API 20NE. *Pathology* **30**:62–64.

132. **Inglis, T. J., A. Merritt, G. Chidlow, M. Aravena-Roman, and G. Harnett.** 2005. Comparison of diagnostic laboratory methods for identification of *Burkholderia pseudomallei*. *J. Clin. Microbiol.* **43**:2201–2206.

133. **Inglis, T. J., L. O'Reilly, N. Foster, A. Clair, and J. Sampson.** 2002. Comparison of rapid, automated ribotyping and DNA macrorestriction analysis of *Burkholderia pseudomallei*. *J. Clin. Microbiol.* **40**:3198–3203.

134. **Isles, A., I. Maclusky, M. Corey, R. Gold, C. Prober, P. Fleming, and H. Levison.** 1984. *Pseudomonas cepacia* infection in cystic fibrosis: an emerging problem. *J. Pediatr.* **104**:206–210.

135. **Jenney, A. W., G. Lum, D. A. Fisher, and B. J. Currie.** 2001. Antibiotic susceptibility of *Burkholderia pseudomallei* from tropical northern Australia and implications for therapy of melioidosis. *Int. J. Antimicrob. Agents* **17**:109–113.

136. **Johnson, L. N., J. Y. Han, S. M. Moskowitz, J. L. Burns, X. Qin, and J. A. Englund.** 2004. *Pandoraea* bacteremia in a cystic fibrosis patient with associated systemic illness. *Pediatr. Infect. Dis. J.* **23**:881–882.

137. **Johnson, W. M., S. D. Tyler, and K. R. Rozee.** 1994. Linkage analysis of geographic and clinical clusters in *Pseudomonas cepacia* infections by multilocus enzyme electrophoresis and ribotyping. *J. Clin. Microbiol.* **32**:924–930.

138. **Jones, A. M., T. N. Stanbridge, B. J. Isalska, M. E. Dodd, and A. K. Webb.** 2001. *Burkholderia gladioli*: recurrent abscesses in a patient with cystic fibrosis. *J. Infect.* **42**:69–71.

139. **Jorgensen, I. M., H. K. Johansen, B. Frederiksen, T. Pressler, A. Hansen, P. Vandamme, N. Hoiby, and C. Koch.** 2003. Epidemic spread of *Pandoraea apista*, a new pathogen causing severe lung disease in cystic fibrosis patients. *Pediatr. Pulmonol.* **36**:439–446.

140. **Kaestli, M., M. Mayo, G. Harrington, L. Ward, F. Watt, J. V. Hill, A. C. Cheng, and B. J. Currie.** 2009. Landscape changes influence the occurrence of the melioidosis bacterium *Burkholderia pseudomallei* in soil in northern Australia. *PLoS Negl. Trop. Dis.* **3**:e364.

141. **Kanaphun, P., N. Thirawattanasuk, Y. Suputtamongkol, P. Naigowit, D. A. Dance, M. D. Smith, and N. J. White.** 1993. Serology and carriage of *Pseudomonas pseudomallei*: a prospective study in 1000 hospitalized children in northeast Thailand. *J. Infect. Dis.* **167**:230–233.

142. **Kenny, D. J., P. Russell, D. Rogers, S. M. Eley, and R. W. Titball.** 1999. In vitro susceptibilities of *Burkholderia mallei* in comparison to those of other pathogenic *Burkholderia* spp. *Antimicrob. Agents Chem.* **43**:2773–2775.

143. **Kerr, K. G., M. Denton, N. Todd, C. M. Corps, P. Kumari, and P. M. Hawkey.** 1996. A new selective differential medium for isolation of *Stenotrophomonas maltophilia*. *Eur. J. Clin. Microbiol. Infect. Dis.* **15**:607–610.

144. **Kersters, K., W. Ludwig, M. Vancanneyt, P. De Vos, M. Gillis, and K. H. Schleifer.** 1996. Recent changes in the classification of the pseudomonads: an overview. *Syst. Appl. Microbiol.* **19**:465–477.

145. **Khan, S. U., S. M. Gordon, P. C. Stillwell, T. J. Kirby, and A. C. Arroliga.** 1996. Empyema and bloodstream infection caused by *Burkholderia gladioli* in a patient with cystic fibrosis after lung transplantation. *Pediatr. Infect. Dis. J.* **15**:637–639.

146. **Kiska, D. L., A. Kerr, M. C. Jones, J. A. Caracciolo, B. Eskridge, M. Jordan, S. Miller, D. Hughes, N. King, and P. H. Gilligan.** 1996. Accuracy of four commercial systems for identification of *Burkholderia cepacia* and other gram-negative nonfermenting bacilli recovered from patients with cystic fibrosis. *J. Clin. Microbiol.* **34**:886–891.

147. **Krzewinski, J. W., C. D. Nguyen, J. M. Foster, and J. L. Burns.** 2001. Use of random amplified polymorphic DNA PCR to examine epidemiology of *Stenotrophomonas maltophilia* and *Achromobacter* (*Alcaligenes*) *xylosoxidans* from patients with cystic fibrosis. *J. Clin. Microbiol.* **39**:3597–3602.

148. **Kutty, P. K., B. Moody, J. S. Gullion, M. Zervos, M. Ajluni, R. Washburn, R. Sanderson, M. A. Kainer, T. A. Powell, C. F. Clarke, R. J. Powell, N. Pascoe, A. Shams, J. J. LiPuma, B. Jensen, J. Noble-Wang, M. J. Arduino, and L. C. McDonald.** 2007. Multistate outbreak of *Burkholderia cenocepacia* colonization and infection associated with the use of intrinsically contaminated alcohol-free mouthwash. *Chest* **132**:1825–1831.

149. **Ledson, M. J., M. J. Gallagher, M. Jackson, C. A. Hart, and M. J. Walshaw.** 2002. Outcome of *Burkholderia cepacia* colonisation in an adult cystic fibrosis centre. *Thorax* **57**:142–145.

150. **Le Moal, G., M. Paccalin, J. P. Breux, F. Roblot, P. Roblot, and B. Becq-Giraudon.** 2001. Central venous catheter-related infection due to *Comamonas testosteroni* in a woman with breast cancer. *Scand. J. Infect. Dis.* **33**:627–628.

151. **Lessie, T. G., W. Hendrickson, B. D. Manning, and R. Devereux.** 1996. Genomic complexity and plasticity of *Burkholderia cepacia*. *FEMS Microbiol. Lett.* **144**:117–128.

152. **Limmathurotsakul, D., W. Chaowagul, W. Chierakul, K. Stepniewska, B. Maharjan, V. Wuthiekanun, N. J. White, N. P. Day, and S. J. Peacock.** 2006. Risk factors for recurrent melioidosis in northeast Thailand. *Clin. Infect. Dis.* **43:**979–986.

153. **Liou, T. G., F. R. Adler, S. C. FitzSimmons, B. C. Cahill, J. R. Hibbs, and B. C. Marshall.** 2001. Predictive 5-year survivorship model of cystic fibrosis. *Am. J. Epidemiol.* **153:**345–352.

154. **LiPuma, J.** 2003. *Burkholderia* and emerging pathogens in cystic fibrosis. *Semin. Respir. Crit. Care Med.* **24:**681–692.

155. **LiPuma, J. J.** 2001. *Burkholderia cepacia* complex: a contraindication to lung transplantation in cystic fibrosis? *Transpl. Infect. Dis.* **3:**149–160.

156. **LiPuma, J. J.** 1998. *Burkholderia cepacia* epidemiology and pathogenesis: implications for infection control. *Curr. Opin. Pulm. Med.* **4:**337–341.

157. **LiPuma, J. J.** 1998. *Burkholderia cepacia.* Management issues and new insights. *Clin. Chest Med.* **19:**473–486.

158. **LiPuma, J. J., S. E. Dasen, D. W. Nielson, R. C. Stern, and T. L. Stull.** 1990. Person-to-person transmission of *Pseudomonas cepacia* between patients with cystic fibrosis. *Lancet* **336:**1094–1096.

159. **LiPuma, J. J., B. J. Dulaney, J. D. McMenamin, P. W. Whitby, T. L. Stull, T. Coenye, and P. Vandamme.** 1999. Development of rRNA-based PCR assays for identification of *Burkholderia cepacia* complex isolates recovered from cystic fibrosis patients. *J. Clin. Microbiol.* **37:**3167–3170.

160. **LiPuma, J. J., J. E. Mortensen, S. E. Dasen, T. D. Edlind, D. V. Schidlow, J. L. Burns, and T. L. Stull.** 1988. Ribotype analysis of *Pseudomonas cepacia* from cystic fibrosis treatment centers. *J. Pediatr.* **113:**859–862.

161. **LiPuma, J. J., T. Spilker, T. Coenye, and C. F. Gonzalez.** 2002. An epidemic *Burkholderia cepacia* complex strain identified in soil. *Lancet* **359:**2002–2003.

162. **Lowe, P., C. Engler, and R. Norton.** 2002. Comparison of automated and nonautomated systems for identification of *Burkholderia pseudomallei. J. Clin. Microbiol.* **40:**4625–4627.

163. **Lowe, P., H. Haswell, and K. Lewis.** 2006. Use of various common isolation media to evaluate the new VITEK 2 colorimetric GN Card for identification of *Burkholderia pseudomallei. J. Clin. Microbiol.* **44:**854–856.

164. **Lumbiganon, P., U. Tattawasatra, P. Chetchotisakd, S. Wongratanacheewin, and B. Thinkhamrop.** 2000. Comparison between the antimicrobial susceptibility of *Burkholderia pseudomallei* to trimethoprim-sulfamethoxazole by standard disk diffusion method and by minimal inhibitory concentration determination. *J. Med. Assoc. Thai.* **83:**856–860.

165. **Mahenthiralingam, E., J. Bischof, S. K. Byrne, C. Radomski, J. E. Davies, Y. Av-Gay, and P. Vandamme.** 2000. DNA-based diagnostic approaches for identification of *Burkholderia cepacia* complex, *Burkholderia vietnamiensis*, *Burkholderia multivorans, Burkholderia stabilis,* and *Burkholderia cepacia* genomovars I and III. *J. Clin. Microbiol.* **38:**3165–3173.

166. **Mahenthiralingam, E., M. E. Campbell, D. A. Henry, and D. P. Speert.** 1996. Epidemiology of *Burkholderia cepacia* infection in patients with cystic fibrosis: analysis by randomly amplified polymorphic DNA fingerprinting. *J. Clin. Microbiol.* **34:**2914–2920.

167. **Mahenthiralingam, E., and P. Drevinek.** 2007. Comparative genomics of *Burkholderia* species, p. 53–79. *In* T. Coenye and P. Vandamme (ed.), *Burkholderia: Molecular Microbiology and Genomics.* Horizon Bioscience, Wymondham, United Kingdom.

168. **Makkar, N. S., and L. E. Casida, Jr.** 1987. *Cupriavidus necator* gen. nov., sp. nov.; a nonobligate bacterial predator of bacteria in soil. *Int. J. Syst. Bacteriol.* **37:**323–326.

169. **McDowell, A., E. Mahenthiralingam, J. E. Moore, K. E. A. Dunbar, A. K. Webb, M. E. Dodd, S. L. Martin, B. C. Millar, C. J. Scott, M. Crowe, and J. S. Elborn.** 2001. PCR-based detection and identification of *Burkholderia cepacia* complex pathogens in sputum from cystic fibrosis patients. *J. Clin. Microbiol.* **39:**4247–4255.

170. **McMenamin, J. D., T. M. Zaccone, T. Coenye, P. Vandamme, and J. J. LiPuma.** 2000. Misidentification of *Burkholderia cepacia* in US cystic fibrosis treatment centers: an analysis of 1,051 recent sputum isolates. *Chest* **117:**1661–1665.

171. **Meumann, E. M., R. T. Novak, D. Gal, M. E. Kaestli, M. Mayo, J. P. Hanson, E. Spencer, M. B. Glass, J. E. Gee, P. P. Wilkins, and B. J. Currie.** 2006. Clinical evaluation of a type III secretion system real-time PCR assay for diagnosing melioidosis. *J. Clin. Microbiol.* **44:**3028–3030.

172. **Milatovic, D., F. J. Schmitz, J. Verhoef, and A. C. Fluit.** 2003. Activities of the glycylcycline tigecycline (GAR-936) against 1,924 recent European clinical bacterial isolates. *Antimicrob. Agents Chemother.* **47:**400–404.

173. **Moore, J. E., B. McIlhatton, A. Shaw, P. G. Murphy, and J. S. Elborn.** 2001. Occurrence of *Burkholderia cepacia* in foods and waters: clinical implications for patients with cystic fibrosis. *J. Food Prot.* **64:**1076–1078.

174. **Moore, J. E., J. Xu, B. C. Millar, M. Crowe, and J. S. Elborn.** 2002. Improved molecular detection of *Burkholderia cepacia* genomovar III and *Burkholderia multivorans* directly from sputum of patients with cystic fibrosis. *J. Microbiol. Methods* **49:**183–191.

175. **Moore, R. A., S. Reckseidler-Zenteno, H. Kim, W. Nierman, Y. Yu, A. Tuanyok, J. Warawa, D. DeShazer, and D. E. Woods.** 2004. Contribution of gene loss to the pathogenic evolution of *Burkholderia pseudomallei* and *Burkholderia mallei. Infect. Immun.* **72:**4172–4187.

176. **Muder, R. R., A. P. Harris, S. Muller, M. Edmond, J. W. Chow, K. Papadakis, M. W. Wagener, G. P. Bodey, and J. M. Steckelberg.** 1996. Bacteremia due to *Stenotrophomonas (Xanthomonas) maltophilia:* a prospective, multicenter study of 91 episodes. *Clin. Infect. Dis.* **22:**508–512.

177. **Murray, S., J. Charbeneau, B. C. Marshall, and J. J. LiPuma.** 2008. Impact of *Burkholderia* infection on lung transplantation in cystic fibrosis. *Am. J. Respir. Crit. Care Med.* **178:**363–371.

178. **Ngauy, V., Y. Lemeshev, L. Sadkowski, and G. Crawford.** 2005. Cutaneous melioidosis in a man who was taken as a prisoner of war by the Japanese during World War II. *J. Clin. Microbiol.* **43:**970–972.

179. **Novak, R. T., M. B. Glass, J. E. Gee, D. Gal, M. J. Mayo, B. J. Currie, and P. P. Wilkins.** 2006. Development and evaluation of a real-time PCR assay targeting the type III secretion system of *Burkholderia pseudomallei. J. Clin. Microbiol.* **44:**85–90.

180. **O'Brien, M., K. Freeman, G. Lum, A. C. Cheng, S. P. Jacups, and B. J. Currie.** 2004. Further evaluation of a rapid diagnostic test for melioidosis in an area of endemicity. *J. Clin. Microbiol.* **42:**2239–2240.

181. **O'Carroll, M. R., T. J. Kidd, C. Coulter, H. V. Smith, B. R. Rose, C. Harbour, and S. C. Bell.** 2003. *Burkholderia pseudomallei:* another emerging pathogen in cystic fibrosis. *Thorax* **58:**1087–1091.

182. **Oie, S., and A. Kamiya.** 1996. Microbial contamination of antiseptics and disinfectants. *Am. J. Infect. Control* **24:**389–395.

183. **Otag, F., G. Ersoz, M. Salcioglu, C. Bal, I. Schneider, and A. Bauernfeind.** 2005. Nosocomial bloodstream infections with *Burkholderia stabilis. J. Hosp. Infect.* **59:**46–52.

184. **Otto, L. A., B. S. Deboo, E. L. Capers, and M. J. Pickett.** 1978. *Pseudomonas vesicularis* from cervical specimens. *J. Clin. Microbiol.* **7:**341–345.

185. **Palleroni, N. J.** 1984. Genus I. *Pseudomonas* Migula 1984 237[AL], p. 141–199. *In* J. Holt and N. R. Krieg (ed.), *Bergey's Manual of Systematic Bacteriology,* vol. 1. The Williams and Wilkins Company, Baltimore, MD.

186. **Palleroni, N. J., and J. F. Bradbury.** 1993. *Stenotrophomonas,* a new bacterial genus for *Xanthomonas maltophilia* (Hugh 1980) Swings et al. 1983. *Int. J. Syst. Bacteriol.* **43:**606–609.

187. **Palleroni, N. J., R. Kunisawa, R. Contopoulou, et al.** 1973. Nucleid acid homologies in the genus *Pseudomonas. Int. J. Syst. Bacteriol.* **23:**333.

188. **Parke, J. L., and D. Gurian-Sherman.** 2001. Diversity of the *Burkholderia cepacia* complex and implications for risk assessment of biological control strains. *Annu. Rev. Phytopathol.* **39:**225–258.

189. **Parry, C. M., V. Wuthiekanun, N. T. Hoa, T. S. Diep, L. T. Thao, P. V. Loc, B. A. Wills, J. Wain, T. T. Hien, N. J. White, and J. J. Farrar.** 1999. Melioidosis in Southern Vietnam: clinical surveillance and environmental sampling. *Clin. Infect. Dis.* **29:**1323–1326.

190. **Payne, G. W., P. Vandamme, S. H. Morgan, J. J. LiPuma, T. Coenye, A. J. Weightman, T. H. Jones, and E. Mahenthiralingam.** 2005. Development of a *recA* gene-based identification approach for the entire *Burkholderia* genus. *Appl. Environ. Microbiol.* **71:**3917–3927.

191. **Peacock, S. J., G. Chieng, A. C. Cheng, D. A. Dance, P. Amornchai, G. Wongsuvan, N. Teerawattanasook, W. Chierakul, N. P. Day, and V. Wuthiekanun.** 2005. Comparison of Ashdown's medium, *Burkholderia cepacia* medium, and *Burkholderia pseudomallei* selective agar for clinical isolation of *Burkholderia pseudomallei. J. Clin. Microbiol.* **43:**5359–5361.

192. **Peacock, S. J., H. P. Schweizer, D. A. Dance, T. L. Smith, J. E. Gee, V. Wuthiekanun, D. DeShazer, I. Steinmetz, P. Tan, and B. J. Currie.** 2008. Management of accidental laboratory exposure to *Burkholderia pseudomallei* and B. *mallei. Emerg. Infect. Dis.* **14:**e2.

193. **Piliouras, P., G. C. Ulett, C. Ashhurst-Smith, R. G. Hirst, and R. E. Norton.** 2002. A comparison of antibiotic susceptibility testing methods for cotrimoxazole with *Burkholderia pseudomallei. Int. J. Antimicrob. Agents* **19:**427–429.

194. **Pitkin, D. H., W. Sheikh, and H. L. Nadler.** 1997. Comparative in vitro activity of meropenem versus other extended-spectrum antimicrobials against randomly chosen and selected resistant clinical isolates tested in 26 North American centers. *Clin. Infect. Dis.* **24**(Suppl. 2):S238–S248.

195. **Pitt, T. L., M. E. Kaufmann, P. S. Patel, L. C. Benge, S. Gaskin, and D. M. Livermore.** 1996. Type characterization and antibiotic susceptibility of *Burkholderia* (*Pseudomonas*) *cepacia* isolates from patients with cystic fibrosis in the United Kingdom and the Republic of Ireland. *J. Med. Microbiol.* **44:**203–210.

196. **Poole, K., and R. Srikumar.** 2001. Multidrug efflux in *Pseudomonas aeruginosa*: components, mechanisms and clinical significance. *Curr. Top. Med. Chem.* **1:**59–71.

197. **Ramette, A., J. J. LiPuma, and J. M. Tiedje.** 2005. Species abundance and diversity of *Burkholderia cepacia* complex in the environment. *Appl. Environ. Microbiol.* **71:**1193–1201.

198. **Razvi, S., L. Quittell, A. Sewall, H. Quinton, B. Marshall, and L. Saiman.** 2009. Respiratory microbiology of patients with cystic fibrosis in the United States, 1995–2005. *Chest* **136:**1554–1560.

199. **Reboli, A. C., R. Koshinski, K. Arias, K. Marks-Austin, D. Stieritz, and T. L. Stull.** 1996. An outbreak of *Burkholderia cepacia* lower respiratory tract infection associated with contaminated albuterol nebulization solution. *Infect. Control Hosp. Epidemiol.* **17:**741–743.

200. **Reik, R., T. Spilker, and J. J. LiPuma.** 2005. Distribution of *Burkholderia cepacia* complex species among isolates recovered from persons with or without cystic fibrosis. *J. Clin. Microbiol.* **43:**2926–2928.

201. **Riley, P. S., and R. E. Weaver.** 1975. Recognition of *Pseudomonas pickettii* in the clinical laboratory: biochemical characterization of 62 strains. *J. Clin. Microbiol.* **1:**61–64.

202. **Ross, J. P., S. M. Holland, V. J. Gill, E. S. DeCarlo, and J. I. Gallin.** 1995. Severe *Burkholderia* (*Pseudomonas*) *gladioli* infection in chronic granulomatous disease: report of two successfully treated cases. *Clin. Infect. Dis.* **21:**1291–1293.

203. **Sajjan, U. S., L. Sun, R. Goldstein, and J. F. Forstner.** 1995. Cable (cbl) type II pili of cystic fibrosis-associated *Burkholderia* (*Pseudomonas*) *cepacia*: nucleotide sequence of the *cblA* major subunit pilin gene and novel morphology of the assembled appendage fibers. *J. Bacteriol.* **177:**1030–1038.

204. **San Gabriel, P., J. Zhou, S. Tabibi, Y. Chen, M. Trauzzi, and L. Saiman.** 2004. Antimicrobial susceptibility and synergy studies of *Stenotrophomonas maltophilia* isolates from patients with cystic fibrosis. *Antimicrob. Agents Chemother.* **48:**168–171.

205. **Sattler, C. A., E. O. Mason, Jr., and S. L. Kaplan.** 2000. Nonrespiratory *Stenotrophomonas maltophilia* infection at a children's hospital. *Clin. Infect. Dis.* **31:**1321–1330.

206. **Segers, P., M. Vancanneyt, B. Pot, U. Torck, B. Hoste, D. Dewettinck, E. Falsen, K. Kersters, and P. De Vos.** 1994. Classification of *Pseudomonas diminuta* Leifson and Hugh 1954 and *Pseudomonas vesicularis* Busing, Doll, and Freytag 1953 in *Brevundimonas* gen. nov. as *Brevundimonas diminuta* comb. nov. and *Brevundimonas vesicularis* comb. nov., respectively. *Int. J. Syst. Bacteriol.* **44:**499–510.

207. **Segonds, C., T. Heulin, N. Marty, and G. Chabanon.** 1999. Differentiation of *Burkholderia* species by PCR-restriction fragment length polymorphism analysis of the 16S rRNA gene and application to cystic fibrosis isolates. *J. Clin. Microbiol.* **37:**2201–2208.

208. **Segonds, C., S. Paute, and G. Chabanon.** 2003. Use of amplified ribosomal DNA restriction analysis for identification of *Ralstonia* and *Pandoraea* species: interest in determination of the respiratory bacterial flora in patients with cystic fibrosis. *J. Clin. Microbiol.* **41:**3415–3418.

209. **Shelly, D. B., T. Spilker, E. J. Gracely, T. Coenye, P. Vandamme, and J. J. LiPuma.** 2000. Utility of commercial systems for identification of *Burkholderia cepacia* complex from cystic fibrosis sputum culture. *J. Clin. Microbiol.* **38:**3112–3115.

210. **Smith, M. D., B. J. Angus, V. Wuthiekanun, and N. J. White.** 1997. Arabinose assimilation defines a nonvirulent biotype of *Burkholderia pseudomallei. Infect. Immun.* **65:**4319–4321.

211. **Smith, M. D., V. Wuthiekanun, A. L. Walsh, N. Teerawattanasook, V. Desakorn, Y. Suputtamongkol, T. L. Pitt, and N. J. White.** 1995. Latex agglutination for rapid detection of *Pseudomonas pseudomallei* antigen in urine of patients with melioidosis. *J. Clin. Pathol.* **48:**174–176.

212. **Sneath, P. H. A.** 1992. *International Code of Nomenclature of Bacteria. 1990 Revision.* American Society for Microbiology, Washington, DC.

213. **Speert, D. P., D. Henry, P. Vandamme, M. Corey, and E. Mahenthiralingam.** 2002. Epidemiology of *Burkholderia cepacia* complex in patients with cystic fibrosis, Canada. *Emerg. Infect. Dis.* **8:**181–187.

214. **Spilker, T., A. Baldwin, A. Bumford, C. G. Dowson, E. Mahenthiralingam, and J. J. LiPuma.** 2009. Expanded multilocus sequence typing for *Burkholderia* species. *J. Clin. Microbiol.* **47:**2607–2610.

215. **Stead, D. E.** 1992. Grouping of plant-pathogenic and some other *Pseudomonas* spp. by using cellular fatty acid profiles. *Int. J. Syst. Evol. Microbiol.* **42:**281–285.

216. **Stryjewski, M. E., J. J. LiPuma, R. H. Messier, Jr., L. B. Reller, and B. D. Alexander.** 2003. Sepsis, multiple organ failure, and death due to *Pandoraea pnomenusa* infection after lung transplantation. *J. Clin. Microbiol.* **41:**2255–2257.

217. **Swings, J., P. De Vos, M. Van den Mooter, and J. De Ley.** 1983. Transfer of *Pseudomonas maltophilia* Hugh 1981 to the genus *Xanthomonas* as *Xanthomonas maltophilia* (Hugh 1981) comb. nov. *Int. J. Syst. Bacteriol.* **33:**409–413.

218. **Talmaciu, I., L. Varlotta, J. Mortensen, and D. V. Schidlow.** 2000. Risk factors for emergence of *Stenotrophomonas maltophilia* in cystic fibrosis. *Pediatr. Pulmonol.* **30:**10–15.

219. **Thamlikitkul, V., and S. Trakulsomboon.** 2006. In vitro activity of tigecycline against *Burkholderia pseudomallei* and *Burkholderia thailandensis. Antimicrob. Agents Chemother.* **50:**1555–1557.

220. **Thibault, F. M., E. Valade, and D. R. Vidal.** 2004. Identification and discrimination of *Burkholderia pseudomallei*, B. *mallei*, and B. *thailandensis* by real-time PCR targeting type III secretion system genes. *J. Clin. Microbiol.* **42:**5871–5874.

221. **Thomassen, M. J., C. A. Demko, J. D. Klinger, and R. C. Stern.** 1985. *Pseudomonas cepacia* colonization among patients with cystic fibrosis. A new opportunist. *Am. Rev. Respir. Dis.* **131:**791–796.

222. **Tiangpitayakorn, C.** 1997. Speed of detection of *Burkholderia pseudomallei* in blood cultures and its correlation with the clinical outcome. *Am. J. Trop. Med. Hyg.* **57:**96–99.

223. Tomaso, H., T. L. Pitt, O. Landt, S. Al Dahouk, H. C. Scholz, E. C. Reisinger, L. D. Sprague, I. Rathmann, and H. Neubauer. 2005. Rapid presumptive identification of *Burkholderia pseudomallei* with real-time PCR assays using fluorescent hybridization probes. *Mol. Cell. Probes* **19:**9–20.

224. Vancouvenberghe, C. 1994. Analysis of epidemic and endemic isolates of *Xanthomonas maltophilia* by contour-clamped homogeneous electric field gel electrophoresis. *Infect. Control Hosp. Epidemiol.* **15:**691–696.

225. Vandamme, P., and T. Coenye. 2004. Taxonomy of the genus *Cupriavidus*: a tale of lost and found. *Int. J. Syst. Evol. Microbiol.* **54:**2285–2289.

226. Vandamme, P., J. Goris, T. Coenye, B. Hoste, D. Janssens, K. Kersters, P. De Vos, and E. Falsen. 1999. Assignment of Centers for Disease Control group IVc-2 to the genus *Ralstonia* as *Ralstonia paucula* sp. nov. *Int. J. Syst. Bacteriol.* **49:**663–669.

227. Vandamme, P., D. Henry, T. Coenye, S. Nzula, M. Vancanneyt, J. J. LiPuma, D. P. Speert, J. R. Govan, and E. Mahenthiralingam. 2002. *Burkholderia anthina* sp. nov. and *Burkholderia pyrrocinia*, two additional *Burkholderia cepacia* complex bacteria, may confound results of new molecular diagnostic tools. *FEMS Immunol. Med. Microbiol.* **33:**143–149.

228. Vandamme, P., B. Holmes, M. Vancanneyt, T. Coenye, B. Hoste, R. Coopman, H. Revets, S. Lauwers, M. Gillis, K. Kersters, and J. R. Govan. 1997. Occurrence of multiple genomovars of *Burkholderia cepacia* in cystic fibrosis patients and proposal of *Burkholderia multivorans* sp. nov. *Int. J. Syst. Bacteriol.* **47:**1188–1200.

229. Vaneechoutte, M., P. Kampfer, T. De Baere, E. Falsen, and G. Verschraegen. 2004. *Wautersia* gen. nov., a novel genus accommodating the phylogenetic lineage including *Ralstonia eutropha* and related species, and proposal of *Ralstonia [Pseudomonas] syzygii* (Roberts et al. 1990) comb. nov. *Int. J. Syst. Evol. Microbiol.* **54:**317–327.

230. Vanlaere, E., A. Baldwin, D. Gevers, D. Henry, E. De Brandt, J. J. LiPuma, E. Mahenthiralingam, D. P. Speert, C. Dowson, and P. Vandamme. 2009. Taxon K, a complex within the *Burkholderia cepacia* complex, comprises at least two novel species, *Burkholderia contaminans* sp. nov. and *Burkholderia lata* sp. nov. *Int. J. Syst. Evol. Microbiol.* **59:**102–111.

231. Vanlaere, E., J. J. LiPuma, A. Baldwin, D. Henry, E. De Brandt, E. Mahenthiralingam, D. Speert, C. Dowson, and P. Vandamme. 2008. *Burkholderia latens* sp. nov., *Burkholderia diffusa* sp. nov., *Burkholderia arboris* sp. nov., *Burkholderia seminalis* sp. nov. and *Burkholderia metallica* sp. nov., novel species within the *Burkholderia cepacia* complex. *Int. J. Syst. Evol. Microbiol.* **58:**1580–1590.

232. Vartivarian, S. E., K. A. Papadakis, J. A. Palacios, J. T. Manning, Jr., and E. J. Anaissie. 1994. Mucocutaneous and soft tissue infections caused by *Xanthomonas maltophilia*. A new spectrum. *Ann. Intern. Med.* **121:**969–973.

233. Vermis, K., T. Coenye, J. J. LiPuma, E. Mahenthiralingam, H. J. Nelis, and P. Vandamme. 2004. Proposal to accommodate *Burkholderia cepacia* genomovar VI as *Burkholderia dolosa* sp. nov. *Int. J. Syst. Evol. Microbiol.* **54:**689–691.

234. Vermis, K., T. Coenye, E. Mahenthiralingam, H. J. Nelis, and P. Vandamme. 2002. Evaluation of species-specific *recA*-based PCR tests for genomovar level identification within the *Burkholderia cepacia* complex. *J. Med. Microbiol.* **51:**937–940.

235. Vermis, K., P. A. Vandamme, and H. J. Nelis. 2003. *Burkholderia cepacia* complex genomovars: utilization of carbon sources, susceptibility to antimicrobial agents and growth on selective media. *J. Appl. Microbiol.* **95:**1191–1199.

236. Vermis, K., C. Vandekerckhove, H. J. Nelis, and P. A. Vandamme. 2002. Evaluation of restriction fragment length polymorphism analysis of 16S rDNA as a tool for genomovar characterisation within the *Burkholderia cepacia* complex. *FEMS Microbiol. Lett.* **214:**1–5.

237. Visca, P., G. Cazzola, A. Petrucca, and C. Braggion. 2001. Travel-associated *Burkholderia pseudomallei* infection (melioidosis) in a patient with cystic fibrosis: a case report. *Clin. Infect. Dis.* **32:**E15–E16.

238. Walsh, A. L., V. Wuthiekanun, M. D. Smith, Y. Suputtamongkol, and N. J. White. 1995. Selective broths for the isolation of *Pseudomonas pseudomallei* from clinical samples. *Trans. R. Soc. Trop. Med. Hyg.* **89:**124.

239. Wauters, G., T. De Baere, A. Willems, E. Falsen, and M. Vaneechoutte. 2003. Description of *Comamonas aquatica* comb. nov. and *Comamonas kerstersii* sp. nov. for two subgroups of *Comamonas terrigena* and emended description of *Comamonas terrigena*. *Int. J. Syst. Evol. Microbiol.* **53:**859–862.

240. Weinberg, J. B., B. D. Alexander, J. M. Majure, L. W. Williams, J. Y. Kim, P. Vandamme, and J. J. LiPuma. 2007. *Burkholderia glumae* infection in an infant with chronic granulomatous disease. *J. Clin. Microbiol.* **45:**662–665.

241. Welch, D. F., M. J. Muszynski, C. H. Pai, M. J. Marcon, M. M. Hribar, P. H. Gilligan, J. M. Matsen, P. A. Ahlin, B. C. Hilman, and S. A. Chartrand. 1987. Selective and differential medium for recovery of *Pseudomonas cepacia* from the respiratory tracts of patients with cystic fibrosis. *J. Clin. Microbiol.* **25:**1730–1734.

242. Wen, A., M. Fegan, C. Hayward, S. Chakraborty, and L. I. Sly. 1999. Phylogenetic relationships among members of the *Comamonadaceae*, and description of *Delftia acidovorans* (den Dooren de Jong 1926 and Tamaoka et al. 1987) gen. nov., comb. nov. *Int. J. Syst. Bacteriol.* **49**(Pt. 2):567–576.

243. Wertheim, W. A., and D. M. Markovitz. 1992. Osteomyelitis and intervertebral discitis caused by *Pseudomonas pickettii*. *J. Clin. Microbiol.* **30:**2506–2508.

244. Weyant, R. S., C. W. Moss, R. E. Weaver, D. G. Hollis, J. G. Jordan, E. C. Cook, and M. I. Daneshvar. 1996. *Identification of Unusual Pathogenic Gram-Negative Aerobic and Facultatively Anaerobic Bacteria*, 2nd ed, vol. 1. The Williams and Wilkins Company, Baltimore, MD.

245. Whitby, P. W., K. B. Carter, J. L. Burns, J. A. Royall, J. J. LiPuma, and T. L. Stull. 2000. Identification and detection of *Stenotrophomonas maltophilia* by rRNA-directed PCR. *J. Clin. Microbiol.* **38:**4305–4309.

246. Whitby, P. W., H. L. Dick, P. W. Campbell III, D. E. Tullis, A. Matlow, and T. L. Stull. 1998. Comparison of culture and PCR for detection of *Burkholderia cepacia* in sputum samples of patients with cystic fibrosis. *J. Clin. Microbiol.* **36:**1642–1645.

247. Whitby, P. W., L. C. Pope, K. B. Carter, J. J. LiPuma, and T. L. Stull. 2000. Species specific PCR as a tool for the identification of *Burkholderia gladioli*. *J. Clin. Microbiol.* **38:**282–285.

248. White, N. J. 2003. Melioidosis. *Lancet* **361:**1715–1722.

249. Willems, A., J. De Ley, M. Gillis, and K. Kersters. 1991. *Comamonadaceae*, a new family encompassing the *Acidovorans* rRNA complex, including *Variovorax paradoxus* gen. nov., comb. nov., for *Alcaligenes paradoxus* (Davis 1969). *Int. J. Syst. Bacteriol.* **41:**445–450.

250. Willems, A., E. Falsen, B. Pot, E. Jantzen, B. Hoste, P. Vandamme, M. Gillis, K. Kersters, and J. De Ley. 1990. *Acidovorax*, a new genus for *Pseudomonas facilis*, *Pseudomonas delafieldii*, E. Falsen (EF) group 13, EF group 16, and several clinical isolates, with the species *Acidovorax facilis* comb. nov., *Acidovorax delafieldii* comb. nov., and *Acidovorax temperans* sp. nov. *Int. J. Syst. Bacteriol.* **40:**384–398.

251. Willems, A., B. Pot, E. Falsen, P. Vandamme, M. Gillis, K. Kersters, and J. De Ley. 1991. Polyphasic taxonomic study of the emended genus *Comamonas*: relationship to *Aquaspirillum aquaticum*, E. Falsen group 10, and other clinical isolates. *Int. J. Syst. Bacteriol.* **41:**427–444.

252. Winkelstein, J. A., M. C. Marino, R. B. Johnston, Jr., J. Boyle, J. Curnutte, J. L. Gallin, H. L. Malech, S. M. Holland, H. Ochs, P. Quie, R. H. Buckley, C. B. Foster, S. J. Chanock, and H. Dickler. 2000. Chronic granulomatous disease. Report on a national registry of 368 patients. *Medicine* (Baltimore) **79:**155–169.

253. Wright, R. M., J. E. Moore, A. Shaw, K. Dunbar, M. Dodd, K. Webb, A. O. Redmond, M. Crowe, P. G. Murphy, S. Peacock, and J. S. Elborn. 2001. Improved cultural detection of *Burkholderia cepacia* from sputum in patients with cystic fibrosis. *J. Clin. Pathol.* **54:**803–805.

254. **Wuthiekanun, V., P. Amornchai, W. Chierakul, A. C. Cheng, N. J. White, S. J. Peacock, and N. P. Day.** 2004. Evaluation of immunoglobulin M (IgM) and IgG rapid cassette test kits for diagnosis of melioidosis in an area of endemicity. *J. Clin. Microbiol.* **42:**3435–3437.

255. **Wuthiekanun, V., A. C. Cheng, W. Chierakul, P. Amornchai, D. Limmathurotsakul, W. Chaowagul, A. J. Simpson, J. M. Short, G. Wongsuvan, B. Maharjan, N. J. White, and S. J. Peacock.** 2005. Trimethoprim/sulfamethoxazole resistance in clinical isolates of *Burkholderia pseudomallei. J. Antimicrob. Chemother.* **55:**1029–1031.

256. **Wuthiekanun, V., W. Chierakul, S. Langa, W. Chaowagul, C. Panpitpat, P. Saipan, T. Thoujaikong, N. P. Day, and S. J. Peacock.** 2006. Development of antibodies to *Burkholderia pseudomallei* during childhood in melioidosis-endemic northeast Thailand. *Am. J. Trop. Med. Hyg.* **74:**1074–1075.

257. **Wuthiekanun, V., D. A. Dance, Y. Wattanagoon, Y. Supputtamongkol, W. Chaowagul, and N. J. White.** 1990. The use of selective media for the isolation of *Pseudomonas pseudomallei* in clinical practice. *J. Med. Microbiol.* **33:**121–126.

258. **Wuthiekanun, V., V. Desakorn, G. Wongsuvan, P. Amornchai, A. C. Cheng, B. Maharjan, D. Limmathurotsakul, W. Chierakul, N. J. White, N. P. Day, and S. J. Peacock.** 2005. Rapid immunofluorescence microscopy for diagnosis of melioidosis. *Clin. Diagn. Lab. Immunol.* **12:**555–556.

259. **Wuthiekanun, V., S. Langa, W. Swaddiwudhipong, W. Jedsadapanpong, Y. Kaengnet, W. Chierakul, N. P. Day, and S. J. Peacock.** 2006. Melioidosis in Myanmar: forgotten but not gone? *Am. J. Trop. Med. Hyg.* **75:**945–946.

260. **Wuthiekanun, V., N. Pheaktra, H. Putchhat, L. Sin, B. Sen, V. Kumar, S. Langla, S. J. Peacock, and N. P. Day.** 2008. *Burkholderia pseudomallei* antibodies in children, Cambodia. *Emerg. Infect. Dis.* **14:**301–303.

261. **Xu, J., J. E. Moore, B. C. Millar, H. D. Alexander, R. McClurg, T. C. Morris, and P. J. Rooney.** 2004. Improved laboratory diagnosis of bacterial and fungal infections in patients with hematological malignancies using PCR and ribosomal RNA sequence analysis. *Leuk. Lymphoma* **45:**1637–1641.

262. **Yabuuchi, E., Y. Kosako, H. Oyaizu, I. Yano, H. Hotta, Y. Hashimoto, T. Ezaki, and M. Arakawa.** 1992. Proposal of *Burkholderia* gen. nov. and transfer of seven species of the genus *Pseudomonas* homology group II to the new genus, with the type species *Burkholderia cepacia* (Palleroni and Holmes 1981) comb. nov. *Microbiol. Immunol.* **36:**1251–1275.

263. **Yabuuchi, E., Y. Kosako, I. Yano, H. Hotta, and Y. Nishiuchi.** 1995. Transfer of two *Burkholderia* and an *Alcaligenes* species to *Ralstonia* gen. nov.: proposal of *Ralstonia pickettii* (Ralston, Palleroni and Doudoroff 1973) comb. nov., *Ralstonia solanacearum* (Smith 1896) comb. nov. and *Ralstonia eutropha* (Davis 1969) comb. nov. *Microbiol. Immunol.* **39:**897–904.

264. **Yao, J. D., M. Louie, L. Louie, J. Goodfellow, and A. E. Simor.** 1995. Comparison of E test and agar dilution for antimicrobial susceptibility testing of *Stenotrophomonas* (*Xanthomonas*) *maltophilia. J. Clin. Microbiol.* **33:**1428–1430.

265. **Young, C. C., J. H. Chou, A. B. Arun, W. S. Yen, S. Y. Sheu, F. T. Shen, W. A. Lai, P. D. Rekha, and W. M. Chen.** 2008. *Comamonas composti* sp. nov., isolated from food waste compost. *Int. J. Syst. Evol. Microbiol.* **58:**251–256.

Acinetobacter, Chryseobacterium, Moraxella, and Other Nonfermentative Gram-Negative Rods*

MARIO VANEECHOUTTE, LENIE DIJKSHOORN, ALEXANDR NEMEC, PETER KÄMPFER, AND GEORGES WAUTERS

42

TAXONOMY

The organisms covered in this chapter belong to a group of taxonomically and phylogenetically diverse, gram-negative nonfermentative rods and coccobacilli. Still, several of the genera dealt with belong to the same family; i.e., *Acinetobacter, Moraxella, Oligella,* and *Psychrobacter* belong to the family *Moraxellaceae (Gammaproteobacteria)* (182), and *Balneatrix, Bergeyella, Chryseobacterium, Elizabethkingia, Empedobacter, Myroides, Sphingobacterium, Wautersiella,* and *Weeksella* belong to the family *Flavobacteriaceae* (Bacteroidetes) (11).

DESCRIPTION OF THE AGENTS

The species dealt with in this chapter all share the common phenotypic features of being catalase positive and failing to acidify the butt of Kligler iron agar (KIA) or triple sugar iron (TSI) agar or of oxidative-fermentative media, indicating their inability to metabolize carbohydrates by the fermentative pathway. These organisms grow significantly better under aerobic than under anaerobic conditions, and many, i.e., those species that can use only oxygen as the final electron acceptor in the respiratory pathway, fail to grow anaerobically at all.

EPIDEMIOLOGY AND TRANSMISSION

Most of the organisms described in this chapter are found in the environment, i.e., soil and water. For methylobacteria, tap water has been implicated as a possible agent of transmission in hospital environments, and methods for monitoring water systems for methylobacteria have been described previously (178). No person-to-person spread has been documented for the species covered in this chapter.

CLINICAL SIGNIFICANCE

Although for almost each of the species in this chapter, as for most other species in other chapters, case reports of, e.g., meningitis and endocarditis can be found, their clinical importance is mostly restricted to that of opportunistic pathogens, except, e.g., for *Elizabethkingia meningoseptica,* *Moraxella lacunata* (eye infections), or *Moraxella catarrhalis* (respiratory tract infections).

The clinical role of *Acinetobacter* species has been reviewed previously (58, 115, 164). These organisms are typical opportunistic pathogens that usually only form a threat to critically ill, hospitalized patients. Hospital-acquired *Acinetobacter* infections comprise ventilator-associated pneumonia, bloodstream infections, urinary tract infections, wound infections, skin and soft tissue infections, and secondary meningitis. *Acinetobacter baumannii* is the species most commonly implicated in hospital-acquired infections. The clinical role of the closely related *Acinetobacter* genomic species 3 and 13TU resembles that of *A. baumannii* (18, 22). For the purpose of this review, we consider *A. baumannii* to comprise these two species as well, unless stated otherwise. *A. baumannii* ventilator-associated pneumonia and bloodstream infections have been documented to be associated with a high degree of mortality and morbidity (41, 188). Particular manifestations of *A. baumannii* are its implication in severely war-wounded soldiers (32, 52), from which stems its popular designation "Iraqibacter," and in victims of natural disasters (161).

The clinical impact of infections with *A. baumannii* is a continuous source of debate (58, 164). Indeed, although severe infections with *A. baumannii* have been documented, colonization is much more frequent than infection, and differentiation between these conditions can be difficult.

Although uncommon, community-acquired infections with *A. baumannii* occur. In particular, community-acquired pneumonia with *A. baumannii* is increasingly reported from tropical areas, like Southeast Asia and tropical Australia (3, 134).

Other *Acinetobacter* species occasionally implicated in nosocomial infections are listed in Table 1. *A. johnsonii, A. lwoffii,* and *A. radioresistens* seem to be natural inhabitants of human skin (186). *A. johnsonii,* which has also been found frequently in feces of nonhospitalized individuals (59), has been implicated in cases of meningitis (189). *A. lwoffii* was a frequent species in clinical specimens during an 8-year study in a university hospital, where it was isolated mainly from blood or intravascular lines (220). *A. ursingii* and *A. junii* have been found to cause bloodstream infections in hospitalized patients (63, 107, 139, 210), while *A. junii* has also been implicated in outbreaks of infection in neonates

*This chapter contains information presented in chapter 50 by Paul C. Schreckenberger, Maryam I. Daneshvar, and Dannie G. Hollis in the ninth edition of this *Manual*.

TABLE 1 Oxidase-negative, indole-negative nonfermenters: the genus *Acinetobacter*[a]

Characteristic	A. calcoaceticus-A. baumannii complex (70)	A. beijerinckii (15)	A. bereziniae (16)	A. guillouiae (17)	A. gyllenbergii (9)	A. haemolyticus (21)	A. junii (21)	A. johnsonii (20)	A. lwoffii (26)	A. parvus (14)	A. radioresistens (22)	A. schindleri (22)	A. ursingii (29)
Growth at:													
44°C	D[b]	−	−	−	−	−	−	−	−	−	D	+	−
41°C	D[c]	−	−	−	−	D	D	−	−	−	D	+	−
37°C	+	+	+[d]	−[d]	+	+	+	−	D	+	+	+	+
Acidification of D-glucose	+	−	D[e]	−	−	D	−	−	D	−	−	−	−
Assimilation of:													
Adipate	+	−	D	+	+	−	−	−	+	−	+	D	+
β-Alanine	+	−	+	+	+	−	−	−	−	−	−	−	−
4-Aminobutyrate	+	+	+	D	D	+	D	D	D	−	+	−	−
L-Arginine	+	−	−	−	+	+	+	D	−	−	+	−	−
L-Aspartate	+	+	+	+	−	D	−	D	−	−	−	−	+
Azelate	+	−	D	+	+	−	D	D	+	−	+	D	+
Citrate (Simmons)	+	+	+	+	+	D	D	+	D	−	−	D	+
Glutarate	+	−	+	+	D	−	−	−	−	−	+	+	+
Histamine	−	−	D	D	−	−	−	−	−	−	−	−	−
L-Histidine	+	+	+	+	+	+	+	−	−	−	−	−	−
DL-Lactate	+	−	+	+	+	−	+	+	+	−	+	+	+
Malonate	D	+	−	D	D	−	−	D	−	−	+	−	−
Phenylacetate	D	−	D	D	+	−	−	−	+	−	+	−	−
Gelatinase	−	D	−	−	+	+	−	−	−	−	−	−	−
Hemolysis of sheep blood	−	+	−	−	+	+	D	−	−	−	−	−	−

[a]Data for the A. calcoaceticus-A. baumannii complex, A. haemolyticus, A. junii, A. johnsonii, A. lwoffii, and A. radioresistens are from Gerner-Smidt et al. (75), except for the results of the assimilation of phenylacetate, L-arginine, and adipate, which were provided by one of us (A. Nemec).
  Data for the other species are from Nemec et al. (149, 150, 154, 155). Numbers between parentheses are the numbers of strains tested. +, positive for 90 to 100% of strains; −, positive for 0 to 10% of strains; D, positive for 11 to 89% of strains.
[b]Typically positive only for A. baumannii and most strains of genomic species 13TU.
[c]Typically negative only for A. calcoaceticus strains.
[d]Growth tested at 38 instead of 37°C.
[e]Positivity, 88%.

(55, 121) and ocular infections (172). A. parvus is regularly isolated from blood cultures (150, 210) but is misidentified by API 20NE as A. lwoffii (M. Vaneechoutte, unpublished data). Many of the infections with these species are related to intravascular catheters or have another iatrogenic origin (9, 63, 194, 238, 248), and their course is generally benign. For various other named or yet-unnamed Acinetobacter species, although recovered from clinical specimens (21, 206), a possible role in infection has not been documented.

Moraxella species are rare agents of infections (conjunctivitis, keratitis, meningitis, septicemia, endocarditis, arthritis, and otolaryngologic infections) (54, 122, 191, 223), but M. catarrhalis has been reported to cause sinusitis and otitis media by contiguous spread of the organisms from a colonizing focus in the respiratory tract (122). However, isolation of M. catarrhalis from the upper respiratory tract (i.e., a throat culture) of children with otitis media or sinusitis does not provide evidence that the isolate is the cause of these infections, because M. catarrhalis is present frequently as a commensal of the upper respiratory tract in children (232). Isolates from sinus aspirates and middle ear specimens obtained by tympanocentesis should be identified and reported. Similarly, little is known about the pathogenesis of lower respiratory tract infection in adults with chronic lung diseases, although a clear pathogenic role may be assigned to this species because M. catarrhalis is not a frequent commensal of the upper respiratory tract in adults (232) and because examination of Gram-stained smears of sputum specimens from patients with exacerbations of bronchitis and pneumonia due to M. catarrhalis usually reveals an abundance of leukocytes, the presence of many gram-negative diplococci as the exclusive or predominant bacterial cell type, and the presence of intracellular gram-negative diplococci. Such specimens may yield M. catarrhalis in virtually pure culture, and the organism should be identified and reported. M. lincolnii is not frequently isolated from clinical samples. M. nonliquefaciens and M. osloensis are the two species most frequently isolated, approximately in equal numbers, from nonrespiratory clinical material, especially blood cultures from patients at risk.

M. *canis* has been isolated from dog bite wounds (111) and from debilitated patients (223). M. *lacunata* has been involved in eye infections (180).

COLLECTION, TRANSPORT, AND STORAGE OF SPECIMENS

Standard methods for collection, transport, and storage of specimens as detailed in chapters 9 and 16 are satisfactory for this group of organisms. The only fastidious species handled in this chapter are *Asaia* species, *Granulibacter bethesdensis*, *Methylobacterium* species, and some *Moraxella* species.

DIRECT EXAMINATION

There are no characteristics available that can help to recognize the species dealt with in this chapter by means of direct microscopic examination of the samples. On Gram stain, organisms appear as gram-negative rods, coccobacilli, or diplococci. Neither direct antigen tests nor molecular genetic tests to use directly on clinical materials have been developed.

ISOLATION PROCEDURES

Initial incubation should be at 35 to 37°C, although some strains, among them many of the pink-pigmented species, grow better at or below 30°C and may be detected only on plates left at room temperature. In such cases, all tests should be carried out at room temperature. In fact, some of the commercial kits, such as the API 20NE, are designed to be incubated at 30°C.

Growth on certain selective primary media, e.g., MacConkey agar, is variable and may be influenced by lot-to-lot variations in the composition of media. Nonfermenters that grow on MacConkey agar generally form colorless colonies, although some form lavender or purple colonies due to uptake of crystal violet contained in the agar medium. Selective media have been described for *Acinetobacter* spp. (8, 113) and for *Moraxella* spp. (231), but their usefulness remains to be assessed.

IDENTIFICATION

This chapter starts with an overview in Fig. 1, which provides a key to the five large groups that can be distinguished among the species described in this chapter. In the previous edition, the simplified scheme for identification of this group of organisms in the clinical laboratory was based on microscopic morphology, oxidase reaction, motility, acidification of carbohydrates, indole production, and the production of pink-pigmented colonies. The identification scheme presented here (Fig. 1) is further simplified and based only on colony color (pink or not) and the presence or absence of oxidase, of benzyl arginine aminopeptidase (trypsin) activity, and of the production of indole.

Figure 1 refers to Tables 1 to 5, which provide further keys to identify the species of these five groups on the basis of biochemical reactions. Results for enzymatic reactions can

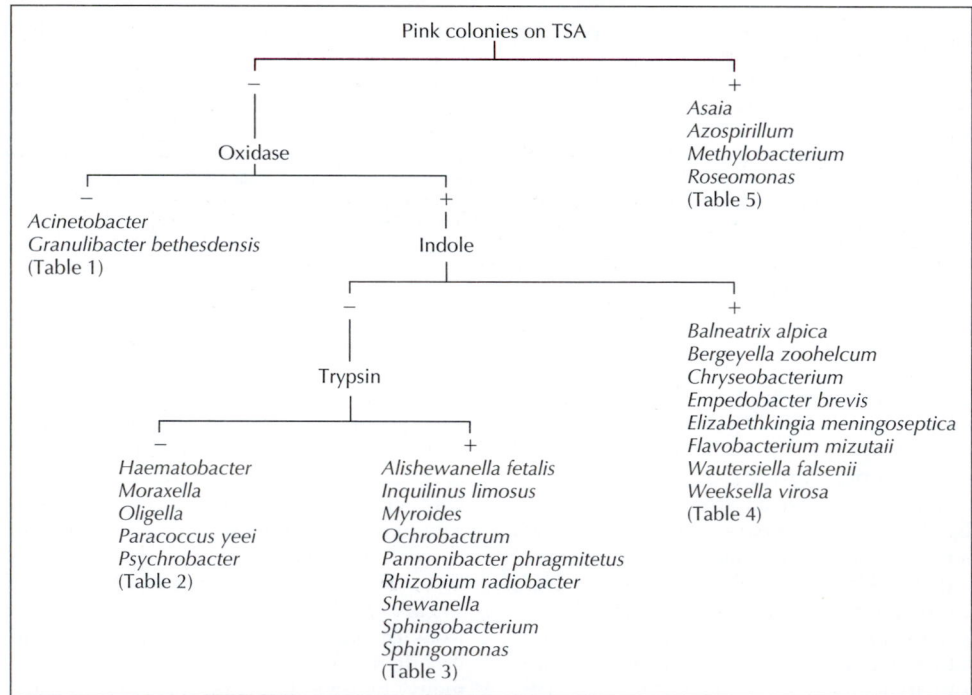

FIGURE 1 Identification of miscellaneous GNF. The organisms covered in this chapter belong to a group of taxonomically diverse, gram-negative nonfermentative rods and coccobacilli. They all share the common phenotypic features of failing to acidify the butt of KIA or TSI agar or of oxidative-fermentative media, indicating their inability to metabolize carbohydrates by the fermentative pathway. These characteristics are shared with those of the species of the emended genus *Pseudomonas* (chapter 40) and those of the species of genera that previously were named as *Pseudomonas* (chapter 41). G. *bethesdensis* grows slowly and poorly on SBA. A. *parvus* forms small colonies as well, but these are already visible after 24 h of incubation.

be read within hours or up to 2 days of incubation, whereas results of carbon source assimilation tests (*Acinetobacter*) and acid production from carbohydrates are read after up to 6 and 7 days, respectively.

For each group of closely related species, we present their taxonomic history (explaining the use of other names in the past and the taxonomic changes introduced since the previous edition), address the clinical importance of the species, and describe the phenotypic data that are useful to differentiate this group from other groups and to differentiate the species within this group (emphasizing the major differences from the previous edition). When relevant, antibiotic susceptibility characteristics and treatment options are discussed immediately; otherwise, they are discussed at the end of each section for the five large groups in this chapter.

The chapter on miscellaneous nonfermentative gram-negative bacteria in this edition of the *Manual* differs from chapter 50 of the previous edition in several aspects. Some of the species described in this chapter in the ninth edition are dealt with in other, more appropriate chapters: *Alcaligenes faecalis* (chapter 43), *Achromobacter denitrificans* and *Achromobacter xylosoxidans* (chapter 43), *Advenella incenata* (chapter 43), *Bordetella* (chapter 43), *Herbaspirillum* (including EF-1 isolates) (chapter 41), *Kerstersia gyiorum* (chapter 43), *Neisseria weaveri* and *N. elongata* (chapter 32), and CDC groups EF-4a and EF-4b (described here as *Neisseria animaloris* and *Neisseria zoodegmatis* [218]) (chapter 32). *Halomonas venusta*, *Laribacter hongkongensis*, and *Massilia timonae* are no longer included.

In addition, we have included only species with validated names and no longer deal with the following groups: *Achromobacter* group F (87); *Agrobacterium* yellow group (247); CDC halophilic nonfermenter group 1 (close to *Halomonas venusta*) (242); CDC groups Ic (247), IIg (85), EO-3 (45), EO-4, EO-5, NO-1 (86), O-1 (close to *Hydrogenophaga pallleronii*) (174), O-2 (close to *Caulobacter vibrioides*), O-3 (47), OFBA-1 (244), *Pseudomonas*-like group 2 (formerly included in the heterogeneous CDC group IVd and close to *Herbaspirillum rubrisubalbicans*), and a group of thermophilic bacteria, some classified as "*Tepidimonas arfidensis*" (128). *Pedobacter* species (199) are also no longer mentioned because they have little or no clinical relevance.

Former unnamed groups have been described as species with validated names in the meantime and are discussed under their appropriate names in this chapter: *Achromobacter* groups B and E have been described as *Pannonibacter phragmitetus* (94), CDC groups IIh and IIc as *Chryseobacterium hominis* (228), part of the CDC group IIe strains as *Chryseobacterium anthropi* (120), and CDC group EO-2 strains as *Paracoccus yeei* (48). Additional new species have been described in the meantime, and those that are included are *Granulibacter bethesdensis* (79) and *Wautersiella falsenii* (119). Although genera like *Acinetobacter* and *Chryseobacterium* comprise many more species than the ones addressed here, we focus on those species that can be isolated from clinical samples.

Classical Biochemical Identification Schemes Presented in This Chapter

For all the species that remain in this chapter, except those of the genus *Acinetobacter*, the biochemical tests listed have been carried out by one of us (G. Wauters), according to standardized protocols, described in detail in chapter 31. This means that for most species the number of strains tested is smaller than the number of strains tested in the previous edition, but that the data listed are not compiled from the literature, whereby different authors may have used different media and protocols. The limited number of tests that have been used to discriminate between the species dealt with in this chapter have been selected because they can be carried out easily and quickly, because they mostly yield uniform results per group or species, and because they are highly discriminatory. For the genus *Acinetobacter*, data based on standardized physiological and nutritional tests were adapted from the literature or were provided by one of the authors (A. Nemec) (see footnotes to Table 1).

Automated, Commercially Available Phenotypic Identification Systems

Traditional diagnostic systems, e.g., those based on oxidation-fermentation media, aerobic low-peptone media, or buffered single substrates, have now been replaced in many laboratories by commercial kits or automated systems like the Vitek 2 (bioMérieux, Marcy L'Etoile, France) and the Phoenix (BD Diagnostic Systems, Sparks, MD). The ability of commercial kits to identify this group of nonfermenters is variable and often results in identification to the genus or group level only, necessitating the use of supplemental biochemical testing for species identification. O'Hara and Miller (160), using the Vitek 2 ID-GNB identification card, reported that of 103 glucose-fermenting and nonfermenting nonenteric strains, 88 (85.4%) were correctly identified at probability levels ranging from excellent to good and that 10 (9.7%) were correctly identified at a low level of discrimination, for a total of 95.1% accuracy within this group. Bosshard et al. (19) compared 16S rRNA gene sequencing for the identification of clinically relevant isolates of nonfermenting gram-negative bacteria (non-*Pseudomonas aeruginosa*) with two commercially available identification systems (API 20NE and Vitek 2 fluorescent card; bioMérieux). By 16S rRNA gene sequence analysis, 92% of the isolates were assigned to species level and 8% to genus level. Using API 20NE, 54% of the isolates were assigned to species level, 7% were assigned to genus level, and 39% of the isolates could not be discriminated at any taxonomic level. The respective numbers for Vitek 2 were 53, 1, and 46%. Fifteen percent and 43% of the isolates corresponded to species not included in the API 20NE and Vitek 2 databases, respectively. Altogether, commercial identification systems can be useful for identification of organisms commonly found in clinical specimens, like *Enterobacteriaceae*. However, for rare organisms the performance of these systems can be poor. This is also illustrated by the performance of API 20NE and Vitek 2 for clinical isolates of *Acinetobacter* (reference 12 and below).

Chemotaxonomic Methods

Identification of nonfermenters by automated cellular fatty acid analysis has also been attempted (237). In view of the difficulties inherent in this approach (162), it is recommended that fatty acid profiles be used only in conjunction with traditional or commercial diagnostic systems. The fatty acid profiles for the most common species of nonfermenting bacteria have been published (247). Unless specifically relevant, we have omitted fatty acid composition data, which were presented in the tables of the previous edition.

A recently developed method of bacterial identification is matrix-assisted laser desorption ionization–time-of-flight mass spectrometry, for which commercial systems, with bacterial mass spectrum databases, have become available recently (Autoflex II mass spectrometer [Bruker Daltonics,

Billerica, MA] and Axima [Shimadzu, Kyoto, Japan]). A recent evaluation showed that 84.1% of 1,660 bacterial isolates analyzed were correctly identified to the species level (190). However, few of the species dealt with in this chapter were included. Another recent application of this technology deals with the *Burkholderia cepacia* complex, indicating its applicability for gram-negative nonfermenters (GNF) (233).

DNA Sequence-Based Methods

Sequence-based methods involving rRNA (16S, 16S-23S spacer, or 23S) and housekeeping genes, such as those encoding RNA polymerase subunit B (*rpoB*), gyrase subunit B (*gyrB*), or the RecA protein (*recA*), have become standard techniques to identify bacteria in general (167) and have contributed to the better delineation of several of these groups and the discovery and description of new species. Because these are generally applicable methods, their application for species of this chapter is not outlined in detail. Other sequence-based methods, based on DNA array hybridization, have been used for some species of these groups (129, 201). DNA sequence-based fingerprinting methods like amplified ribosomal DNA (rDNA) restriction analysis (227, 230), amplified fragment length polymorphism (AFLP) (112), and tDNA PCR (31, 67) have been applied for the identification of species of several groups as well. These fingerprinting approaches are also generally applicable, but they require reference fingerprint libraries and are often poorly exchangeable between different electrophoresis platforms and laboratories.

IDENTIFICATION OF THE FIVE GENOTYPIC GROUPS

Oxidase-Negative GNF

Acinetobacter

The taxonomy of the genus *Acinetobacter* (21, 23, 57, 206, 224) has recently been updated with extended descriptions and formal species names for three species previously designated with provisional designations. These include *A. venetianus* (229) and *A. bereziniae* and *A. guillouiae* (previously designated genospecies 10 and 11, respectively) (21, 154). New species, comprising strains of clinical origin, have been described as well, i.e., *A. beijerinckii* (154), *A. gyllenbergii* (154), *A. parvus* (150), *A. schindleri* (149), and *A. ursingii* (149). Some of the species that were described recently have been shown to be synonymous to already existing species:

A. grimontii (29) was shown to be synonymous to *A. junii* (225), and "*A. septicus*" is synonymous to *A. ursingii* (156). At present, the genus comprises 21 validly named species and 11 species with provisional names. The G+C content of the genus ranges from 38 to 47 mol%. The genomes of seven *Acinetobacter* strains have been sequenced (NCBI, July 2009; http://www.ncbi.nlm.nih.gov/genome?term=acinetobacter).

Members of the genus *Acinetobacter* are widespread in nature and have been cultured from soil, water, sewage, and food and from human and animal specimens. The ecology of most species is unknown. Species of clinical importance are listed in Table 1.

Bacteria belonging to the genus *Acinetobacter* are strictly aerobic, nonfermenting gram-negative coccobacillary microorganisms with a negative oxidase reaction and a positive catalase reaction. Tween 80 esterase activity is frequently present, hemolysis and gelatinase production vary, and nitrate reductase is mostly absent. Motility (hanging drop) is negative, but twitching motility on soft agar occurs occasionally. Individual cell sizes are 0.9 to 1.6 μm in diameter and 1.5 to 2.5 μm in length. In the stationary phase, the organisms are usually coccoid. Cells frequently occur in pairs, resembling *Neisseria* species, but this may be strain or species dependent. In the Gram stain, the organisms can be slightly gram positive. Growth temperature varies, but most species grow between 20 and 35°C. Clinically important species commonly grow well at 37°C or at higher temperatures.

The organisms can form a pellicle on the surface of fluid media. They grow well on complex media, including blood agar, nutrient agar, and MacConkey agar. Colonies are 1 to 2 mm in diameter (sometimes pinpoint), colorless to beige, domed, and smooth to mucoid (Fig. 2). Colonies on MacConkey agar can become pink. Many strains can use a wide variety of carbon sources for growth. Selective enrichment can be obtained in mineral media with acetate as the carbon source and ammonium salt as the nitrogen source with shaking incubation at 30°C (8, 56, 61). General features of *Acinetobacter* species have been reviewed previously (57, 116).

For genus level identification of *Acinetobacter* isolates, the following characters can be used: gram-negative coccobacilli, oxidase negative, aerobic (nonfermenting), and nonmotile. Phenotypic identification of *Acinetobacter* species in the clinical microbiology laboratory by commercial identification systems is problematic (12). This results from the small number of relevant characters tested in these systems and/or from the insufficient quality of reference data in the identification matrices. *A. baumannii* and the closely related species *Acinetobacter* genomic species 3 and 13TU, which are clinically the most important species, and

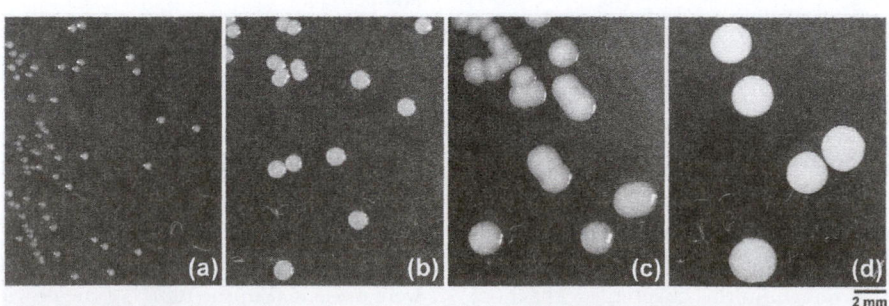

FIGURE 2 Differences in the size of the colonies formed by different *Acinetobacter* species isolated from human clinical specimens. The strains were grown on TSA (Oxoid) at 30°C for 24 h. (a) *A. parvus* NIPH 384^T; (b) *A. ursingii* LUH 3792^T; (c) *A. schindleri* LUH 5832^T; (d) *A. baumannii* ATCC 19606^T.

A. calcoaceticus, an environmental species, together referred to as the *A. calcoaceticus-A. baumannii* complex, are generally not differentiated by these systems. Nonetheless, these systems can be useful for genus level identification and, when supplemented with aerobic acidification of glucose (oxidation-fermentation test), hemolysis, and growth at 44°C, also for presumptive identification of *A. baumannii* (Table 1). We compared Vitek 2 and Phoenix for the ability to identify 76 isolates of 16 clinical *Acinetobacter* species and found that only 19 isolates were correctly identified by Vitek 2 and 5 by Phoenix (M. Vaneechoutte, unpublished data). Phenotypic identification of *Acinetobacter* species can be achieved using physiological, i.e., biochemical and growth temperature, characteristics, and nutritional, i.e., assimilation, characteristics, based on the system of Bouvet and Grimont (22). Table 1 presents a recent update of this system aimed to differentiate all validly named species of clinical importance. Assimilation tests were carried out using the minimal medium of Cruze et al. (44), dispensed into tubes (12-mm inner diameter) in 3-ml volumes inoculated with a small inoculum. Growth on carbon sources was evaluated after 2, 4, 6, and 10 days by means of visual comparison between inoculated tubes containing carbon sources and control tubes containing only inoculated basal medium. Unfortunately, the species of the *A. calcoaceticus-A. baumannii* complex are not clearly distinguished from each other by this approach. In addition, the need for in-house preparation of most of the tests precludes the use of this identification scheme in most diagnostic laboratories.

Therefore, genotypic methods are indispensable for unambiguous identification of *Acinetobacter* species. Well-validated methods are amplified rDNA restriction analysis (60, 227) and whole genomic fingerprinting by AFLP, based on the selective amplification of chromosomal restriction fragments (57, 112). Currently, sequence-based species identification is becoming more and more the standard. Targets for this purpose are the 16S rDNA sequence (224), the *rpoB* gene sequence (81), and the 16S-23S rRNA gene spacer region (34), which has also been used for oligonucleotide array-based identification of species of the *A. calcoaceticus-A. baumannii* complex (129). PCR detection of the *bla*$_{OXA-51-like}$ gene has been shown to be a rapid method for identification of *A. baumannii* isolates (212).

The ecology of most *Acinetobacter* species is still poorly resolved. *A. baumannii* and *Acinetobacter* genomic species 3 and 13TU have been mainly recovered from clinical specimens in hospitals. Human skin carrier rates of *A. baumannii* outside hospitals have been shown to be as low as 0.5 to 3% (10, 186), but higher rates (also for *Acinetobacter* genomic species 3 and 13TU) have been found in tropical areas (40). *A. baumannii* has been isolated from sick animals (15, 226), but an animal or environmental reservoir has not been found. *A. baumannii* is, due to its role as a prominent nosocomial pathogen, the species for which the epidemiology has been studied most intensively. Epidemic strains of this species can survive well in the environment, as they have been found on equipment and on environmental surfaces and materials (219), usually in the vicinity of colonized patients. Multiple sites of the skin and mucosae of patients can be colonized, and colonization may last days to weeks (61, 142).

Genotyping and Epidemiology

A variety of genotyping methods have been described for differentiation between isolates of the same species and study of the epidemiology of acinetobacters, in particular

that of *A. baumannii*. Standardized random amplification PCR-fingerprinting was useful for local typing, but its (interlaboratory) reproducibility was limited (80). Macrorestriction analysis with pulsed-field gel electrophoresis allowed for 95% intra- and 89% interlaboratory reproducibility (187). AFLP fingerprinting also enables genotyping of strains (57, 62, 153), and its robustness makes it suited for setting up a local database for longitudinal studies. Genotyping based on the variable number of tandem repeat loci has allowed for additional subtyping in conjunction with pulsed-field gel electrophoresis analysis (209).

With the introduction of sequence-based methods, it has become possible to set up Internet-based databases to study the global epidemiology of organisms. Three multilocus sequence typing systems, mainly aimed at studying the population biology of *A. baumannii*, have been developed (6, 65; S. Brisse et al., unpublished data [http://www.pasteur.fr/mlst]). Further to typing in the strict sense, specific antibiotic resistance genes like the OXA genes, which confer resistance to carbapenems, are frequently used for additional characterization of *Acinetobacter* isolates (39, 130).

Various methods, often in combination, of genotyping *A. baumannii* isolates from different institutes and countries have identified three major groups of genetically highly related strains, the so-called European clones I to III (151, 221). Many of the strains allocated to these clones are multidrug resistant and have been implicated in outbreaks. Clone I prevailed in the 1980s, but recent studies indicate that subclones of clone II have emerged in the United Kingdom, the Czech Republic, and Portugal (50, 152, 208). Identification of isolates of these clones can be obtained by comparing them to reference sets of the three clones by AFLP analysis (62, 151). Comparative typing of isolates to only one reference strain of each clone may lead to under-identification of the clones, since one reference strain does not cover the intraclonal variation. Multilocus sequence typing with seven genes (http://www.pasteur.fr/mlst) is expected to be the most reliable method for identification of strains of clones I to III (Brisse et al., unpublished). Rapid assignment to the clones by a multiplex PCR targeting the *ompA*, *csuE*, and *bla*$_{OXA-51-like}$ gene sequences is promising (208).

Antimicrobial Susceptibilities

Acinetobacter species are increasingly resistant to multiple antibiotics (108, 134). With the emergence of carbapenem resistance, a last option for treatment of infections with these organisms is disappearing. Multidrug resistance is mainly confined to *A. baumannii*, but strains of the closely related species *Acinetobacter* genomic species 3 can also be multidrug resistant (18, 234). The rates of resistance to different antibiotics can vary among hospitals and regions, depending on the endemic or epidemic presence of multidrug-resistant *A. baumannii*. Resistance mechanisms in *A. baumannii* comprise all currently known mechanisms, including enzymatic breakdown, modification of target sites, active efflux, and decreased influx of antibiotics. The known mechanisms have been reviewed previously (58), and new mechanisms have been discovered since (2, 171).

Recent genomic studies have shed new light on the genetic organization of resistance determinants and their transmission. For example, a resistance island integrated within the ATPase gene has been found in different *A. baumannii* strains for which the genome has been sequenced (1, 71, 109). Among these strains, a variable composition of resistance determinants interspersed with transposons, integrons, and other mobile elements has been identified. Other elements, like insertion sequence elements (211), distributed throughout the genome, are also important for the overall resistance (1).

In vitro determination of antimicrobial susceptibility can be achieved by disk diffusion, agar dilution, or broth microdilution, as recommended by the Clinical and Laboratory Standards Institute (CLSI) (203), or by Etest. The panel of tested antibiotics should cover the spectrum of agents with potential action against *A. baumannii*, including third- or fourth-generation cephalosporins, sulbactam, ureidopenicillins, carbapenems, aminoglycosides, fluoroquinolones, and tetracyclines. Of note, susceptibility to polymyxins, a current last option for treating pandrug-resistant *A. baumannii*, should not be tested by disk diffusion due to poor diffusion of these compounds in agar. Etest and broth microdilution for determination of the MIC for colistin have been compared and showed a good concordance in the MIC range of 0.25 to 1 mg/liter (4). In case of carbapenem resistance, the genes encoding beta-lactamases with carbapenemase activity can be determined by specific PCR (68), to provide better insight into the epidemiology of the resistance.

Granulibacter bethesdensis

Granulibacter bethesdensis (*Acetobacteraceae, Alphaproteobacteria*) (79) is a gram-negative, aerobic, coccobacillary to rod-shaped bacterium, the only species of a new sublineage within the acetic acid bacteria in the family *Acetobacteraceae*. This fastidious organism grows poorly and slowly on sheep blood agar (SBA) at an optimum temperature of 35 to 37°C and an optimum pH of 5.0 to 6.5. It produces a yellow pigment, oxidizes lactate and weakly acetate to carbon dioxide and water, acidifies ethanol, and can use methanol as a sole carbon source, all characteristics that distinguish it from other acetic acid bacteria. The two major fatty acids are C18:1ω7c and C16:0. The DNA base composition is 59.1 mol% G+C. It was first isolated from three patients with chronic granulomatous disease (79) and from an additional patient with chronic granulomatous disease more recently (138).

Oxidase-Positive, Indole-Negative, Trypsin-Negative Nonfermenters

Haematobacter

Three *Haematobacter* species (*Rhodobacteraceae, Alphaproteobacteria*) have been described, i.e., *H. massiliensis* (former *Rhodobacter massiliensis*), *H. missouriensis,* and *Haematobacter* genomospecies 1 (Table 2) (84). These species cannot easily be differentiated phenotypically, and even the 16S rRNA gene sequences are closely related. *Haematobacter* species were described as asaccharolytic, but using low-peptone phenol red agar (see chapter 31), *H. missouriensis* is clearly saccharolytic, producing acid from glucose and xylose and sometimes from mannitol, whereas *H. massiliensis* strains do not acidify carbohydrates. Acid is produced from ethylene glycol by all species. All the species are strongly urease and phenylalanine deaminase positive. Arginine dihydrolase is also positive but sometimes delayed. Asaccharolytic *Haematobacter* strains resemble *Psychrobacter phenylpyruvicus* but can be differentiated by the lack of tributyrine esterase, the lack of growth improvement by Tween 80, and the presence of arginine dihydrolase. Differences from *Psychrobacter faecalis, Psychrobacter pulmonis,*

and related species are the lack of tributyrine and Tween 80 esterase, the lack of nitrate reductase, and a positive arginine dihydrolase test.

Strains received at the CDC have been mainly from patients with septicemia.

Haematobacter strains have low MICs for amoxicillin, fluoroquinolones, aminoglycosides, and carbapenems but variable MICs for cephalosporins, monobactams, and piperacillin.

Moraxella

The genus *Moraxella* comprises approximately 20 species that have been validly named. *M. catarrhalis, M. osloensis, M. nonliquefaciens,* and *M. lincolnii* are part of the normal microbiota of the human respiratory tract. Animal species include *M. bovis,* isolated from healthy cattle and other animals, including horses; *M. boevrei* and *M. caprae* (goats); *M. canis* (dogs, cats, and camels); *M. caviae* (guinea pigs); *M. cuniculi* (rabbits); and *M. ovis* and *M. oblonga* (sheep). The clinical importance of the different species is addressed below.

Both *M. catarrhalis* and *M. canis* grow well on sheep blood agar (SBA) and even on tryptic soy agar (TSA), and their colonies may reach more than 1 mm in diameter after 24 h of incubation. Colonies of *M. catarrhalis* grow well on both blood and chocolate agars, and some strains also grow well on modified Thayer-Martin and other selective media. Colonies are generally gray to white, opaque, and smooth and measure about 1 to 3 mm after 24 h of incubation. Characteristically, the colonies may be nudged intact across the plate with a bacteriological loop like a "hockey puck" and can be removed from the agar entirely, being very consistent. Most *M. canis* colonies resemble those of the *Enterobacteriaceae* (large, smooth colonies) and may produce a brown pigment when grown on starch-containing Mueller-Hinton agar (111). Some strains may also produce very slimy colonies resembling colonies of *Klebsiella pneumoniae* (111). *M. nonliquefaciens* forms smooth, translucent to semiopaque colonies 0.1 to 0.5 mm in diameter after 24 h and 1 mm in diameter after 48 h of growth on SBA plates. Occasionally, these colonies spread and pit the agar. The colonial morphologies of *M. lincolnii* (217), *M. osloensis,* and *Psychrobacter phenylpyruvicus* (formerly *M. phenylpyruvica*) are similar, but pitting is rare. On the other hand, pitting is common with *M. lacunata,* whose colonies are smaller and form dark haloes on chocolate agar. Rod-shaped *Moraxella* species, especially *M. atlantae* and *M. lincolnii,* are more fastidious and display smaller colonies on SBA, less than 1 mm in diameter after 24 h. Colonies of *M. atlantae* are small (usually 0.5 mm in diameter) and show pitting and spreading (24). The growth of *M. atlantae* is stimulated by bile salts, which explains its growth on MacConkey agar. *M. nonliquefaciens* and *M. osloensis* produce colonies that are somewhat larger than those of *M. atlantae* and that are rarely pitting. Colonies of *M. nonliquefaciens* may be mucoid. A selective medium, acetazolamide agar, inhibiting growth of neisseriae when incubated in ambient atmosphere, has been described for *M. catarrhalis* (231).

Moraxella species are coccoid or coccobacillary organisms (plump rods), occurring predominantly in pairs and sometimes in short chains, that tend to resist decolorization in the Gram stain (49). *M. canis* and *M. catarrhalis* are *Neisseria*-like diplococci, and they can easily be distinguished from other moraxellae or other coccoid species by performing a Gram stain on cells cultured in the vicinity of a penicillin disk: cells of *M. canis* and *M. catarrhalis* remain

TABLE 2 Oxidase-positive, indole-negative, trypsin-negative, coccoid nonfermenters[a]

Characteristic	Haematobacter massiliensis (5)	Haematobacter missouriensis (4)	Haematobacter genomospecies 1 (1)	Moraxella atlantae (5)	Moraxella canis (5)	Moraxella catarrhalis (7)	Moraxella lacunata (4)	Moraxella lincolnii (2)	Moraxella nonliquefaciens (15)	Moraxella osloensis (21)	Oligella ureolytica (3)	Oligella urethralis (6)	Paracoccus yeei (11)	Psychrobacter faecalis (10)	Psychrobacter immobilis ATCC 43116[T]	Psychrobacter phenyl pyruvicus (7)[b]	Psychrobacter pulmonis (4)
Motility (flagella)	0	0	0	0	0	0	0	0	0	0	67 (pt)	0	0	0	−	0	0
Growth on MacConkey agar	80	100	100	100	60	0	0	0	0	50	0	50	100	100	+	100	(25)
Alkalinization of acetate	100	100	100	0	100	0	75	0	0	100	100	100	100	100	+	71	100
Susceptibility to desferrioxamine	0	0	0	60	100	100	100	0	100	0	100	100	0	0	−	0	0
Acidification of:																	
Glucose	0	100	0	0	0	0	0	0	0	0	0	0	100	100	+	0	0
Mannitol	0	(50)	(100)	0	0	0	0	0	0	0	0	0	0	(45)	0	−	0
Xylose	0	100	0	0	0	0	0	0	0	0	0	0	100	100	+	0	0
Ethylene glycol	100	100	100	0	100	0	25	0	0	100	100	100	100	100	+	57	0
Gelatinase	0	0	0	0	0	0	100	0	0	0	0	0	0	0	−	0	0
Tween 80 esterase	0	0	0	0	0	0	100	0	0	5	0	0	0	100	+	100	100
Tributyrate esterase	0	0	0	0	100	100	100	0	100	100	0	0	100	100	+	100	100
Alkaline phosphatase	0	0	0	100	0	0	75	0	0	75	0	0	0	0	−	0	0
Phenylalanine deaminase	100	100	100	0	0	0	0	0	0	0	0	0	100[W]	0	10	−	86	0
Pyrrolidonyl aminopeptidase	0	0	0	100	0	0	0	0	0	0	0	0	0	0	−	0	0
Urease	100	100	100	0	0	0	0	0	0	0	100	0	100	0	+	100	0
Nitrate reductase	0	0	0	0	80	100	100	0	100	24	100	0	100	100	+	28	100
Nitrite reductase	0	0	0	0	20	100	0	0	0	0	100	100	0	100	−	0	100
Arginine dihydrolase	100	100	100	0	0	0	0	0	0	0	0	0	0	0	−	0	0

[a]Numbers in parentheses after organism names are numbers of strains tested. Values are percentages; those in parentheses represent delayed positivity. W, weakly positive; pt, peritrichous.
[b]Growth markedly promoted by Tween 80.

spherical diplococci of 0.5 to 1.5 μm in diameter, although of irregular size, whereas coccobacilli show obviously rod-shaped and filamentous cells.

Moraxella species are asaccharolytic and strongly oxidase positive. *M. catarrhalis* and *M. canis* are also strongly catalase positive, and most strains reduce nitrate and nitrite. *M. catarrhalis* and *M. canis* may be easily distinguished from the commensal *Neisseria* species, which are also frequently isolated from respiratory clinical specimens, by the ability of the former to produce DNase and butyrate esterase (tributyrine test). Rapid butyrate esterase tests have been described (198), and the indoxyl-butyrate hydrolysis spot test is commercially available (Remel, Inc., Lenexa, KS). Butyrate esterase is, however, also present in some other *Moraxella* species. *M. canis* acidifies ethylene glycol and alkalinizes acetate, in contrast to *M. catarrhalis*. There are few biochemical differences between *M. catarrhalis* and *M. nonliquefaciens*, which are differentiated from each other mainly on the basis of morphological

characteristics and by nitrite reductase and DNase activity of *M. catarrhalis*.

M. atlantae is the only *Moraxella* species to be pyrrolidonyl aminopeptidase (17) positive. *M. lacunata* is the only proteolytic species with gelatinase activity. Using the plate method (see chapter 31), gelatin hydrolysis occurs usually within 2 to 4 days. A more rapid and almost equally specific test to differentiate *M. lacunata* from other moraxellae is the detection of Tween 80 esterase activity, which is often positive within 2 days, whereas all other species, except for very rare *M. osloensis* strains, remain negative. This species should also be distinguished from *Psychrobacter* species, which are also Tween 80 esterase positive, but *P. phenylpyruvicus* is urease positive and *P. immobilis* and related species exhibit luxuriant growth on plain agar, like TSA, even at 25°C.

M. lincolnii is biochemically quite inactive.

M. osloensis is acetate alkalinization positive, acidifies ethylene glycol, and is resistant to desferrioxamine (250-μg disk).

M. *nonliquefaciens* has opposite properties to those of M. *osloensis* and is, in addition, always nitrate positive.

Antimicrobial Susceptibilities

Most *Moraxella* species are susceptible to penicillin and its derivatives, cephalosporins, tetracyclines, quinolones, and aminoglycosides (70, 197). Production of beta-lactamase has been only rarely reported for *Moraxella* species other than M. *catarrhalis*, of which most isolates produce an inducible, cell-associated beta-lactamase (231). Isolates of M. *catarrhalis* are generally susceptible to amoxicillin-clavulanate, expanded-spectrum and broad-spectrum cephalosporins (i.e., cefuroxime, cefotaxime, ceftriaxone, cefpodoxime, ceftibuten, and the oral agents cefixime and cefaclor), macrolides (e.g., azithromycin, clarithromycin, and erythromycin), tetracyclines, rifampin, and fluoroquinolones.

Oligella urethralis and *O. ureolytica*

The genus *Oligella* comprises two species, *O. ureolytica* (formerly CDC group IVe) and *O. urethralis* (formerly *Moraxella urethralis* and CDC group M-4) (181), which have both been isolated chiefly from the human urinary tract and have been reported to cause urosepsis (173). A case of septic arthritis due to *O. urethralis* has also been reported (144).

Colonies of *O. urethralis* are smaller than those of M. *osloensis* and are opaque to whitish. Colonies of *O. ureolytica* are slow growing on blood agar, appearing as pinpoint colonies after 24 h but large colonies after 3 days of incubation. Colonies are white, opaque, entire, and nonhemolytic.

O. ureolytica and *O. urethralis* are small asaccharolytic coccobacilli that rapidly acidify ethylene glycol and are susceptible to desferrioxamine. Most strains of *O. ureolytica* are motile by peritrichous flagella; all are strongly urease positive (with the urease reaction often turning positive within minutes after inoculation) and reduce nitrate. *Oligella urethralis* strains are nonmotile and urease and nitrate reductase negative, but they reduce nitrite and are weakly phenylalanine deaminase positive. *Bordetella bronchiseptica* and *Cupriavidus pauculus* are also rapidly urease positive but are desferrioxamine resistant.

O. urethralis and M. *osloensis* have biochemical similarities, e.g., accumulation of poly-β-hydroxybutyric acid and failure to hydrolyze urea, but can be differentiated on the basis of nitrite reduction and alkalinization of formate, itaconate, proline, and threonine, all positive for *O. urethralis* (169). Moreover, *O. urethralis* is susceptible to desferrioxamine and tributyrate esterase is negative, in contrast to M. *osloensis*.

O. urethralis is generally susceptible to most antibiotics, including penicillin, while *O. ureolytica* exhibits variable susceptibility patterns (70).

Paracoccus yeei

The genus *Paracoccus* (*Rhodobacteraceae, Alphaproteobacteria*) comprises approximately 25 species, of which only *P. yeei* is of some clinical importance. Daneshvar et al. (48) proposed the name *Paracoccus yeeii*, later changed to *P. yeei*, for the former CDC group EO-2.

Colonies are large and mucoid, with a pale yellow pigmentation. *Paracoccus yeei* organisms are coccoid cells, showing many diplococci and a few very short rods. Microscopically, *P. yeei* is characterized by distinctive O-shaped cells (Fig. 3) upon Gram stain examination due to the presence of vacuolated or peripherally stained cells. The species is saccharolytic and urease positive.

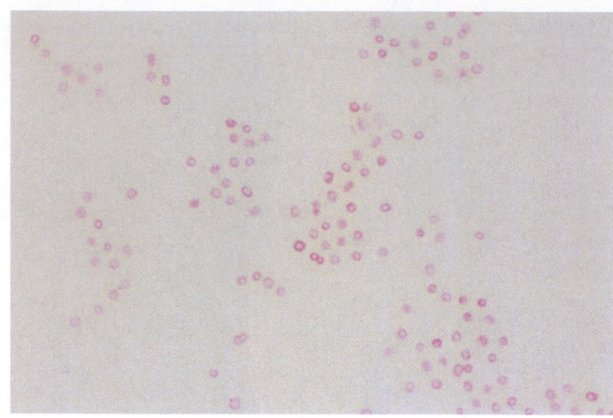

FIGURE 3 Gram stain of *Paracoccus yeei*, showing characteristic doughnut-shaped morphology.

P. yeei has been isolated from various human wound infections (48).

Psychrobacter

The genus *Psychrobacter* (117) comprises more than 30 species, of which only a few are clinically important. Apart from *Psychrobacter phenylpyruvicus*, the *Psychrobacter* strains isolated from clinical material were considered until recently as belonging to the species *Psychrobacter immobilis*. In a recent study, 16 *Psychrobacter* isolates of clinical origin were analyzed. Ten were identified as *P. faecalis*, four were identified as *P. pulmonis*, and two could not be identified but clustered close to *Psychrobacter* when the 16S rRNA gene sequence was determined (G. Wauters, unpublished data). These findings suggest that the majority of the clinical isolates belong to *P. faecalis* and *P. pulmonis*, both first described to occur in animals (pigeons [118] and lambs [235], respectively). *P. immobilis* itself is apparently rarely isolated, if at all, from humans.

P. faecalis and *P. pulmonis* are coccoid gram-negative rods growing on TSA with large, creamy colonies. *P. faecalis* is saccharolytic and acidifies glucose and xylose, while *P. pulmonis* is asaccharolytic. Both species produce acid from ethylene glycol. They are Tween 80 esterase and tributyrate esterase positive. They are nitrate reductase positive and, unlike the type strain of *P. immobilis*, are urease negative and nitrite reductase positive. Colonies may resemble those of *Haematobacter*, but the latter lack nitrate reductase, Tween 80 esterase, and tributyrin esterase and are strongly urease positive, arginine dihydrolase positive, and phenylalanine deaminase positive.

One case of ocular infection (76) and one case of infant meningitis (137) have been reported to be caused by *P. immobilis*, but in light of the data reported here, this might concern infection with one of the other *Psychrobacter* species.

P. phenylpyruvicus, formerly *Moraxella phenylpyruvica* (25), has the morphological and cultural appearance of moraxellae but is urease and phenylalanine deaminase positive. A unique feature of the species is its marked growth improvement by Tween 80. Colonies on TSA with 1% Tween 80 have a size two to three times larger than on SBA. The other *Psychrobacter* species, in contrast to *P. phenylpyruvicus*, grow abundantly on ordinary media such as TSA, and their growth is not promoted by Tween 80. They resemble *Haematobacter* species. *Psychrobacter* species are resistant to penicillin but susceptible to most other antibiotics (76, 137).

Oxidase-Positive, Indole-Negative, Trypsin-Positive Nonfermenters

Alishewanella fetalis

Alishewanella fetalis (*Alteromonadaceae*, *Gammaproteobacteria*) (Table 3) is a gram-negative rod that grows at temperatures between 25 and 42°C, with optimum growth at 37°C. *A. fetalis* can withstand NaCl concentrations of up to 8% but not 10%, which helps differentiate this species from *Shewanella algae*, which can grow in 10% NaCl (240). Also, in contrast to *Shewanella* species, it does not produce H_2S in the butt of TSI and KIA. The type strain tested by us acidifies glucose and does not hydrolyze esculin.

A. *fetalis* has been isolated from a human fetus at autopsy, although its association with clinical infection is unknown (240).

Inquilinus limosus

Inquilinus limosus is a rod-shaped gram-negative bacterium that measures 1.5 to 2 μm in width by 3.5 μm in length; it grows at 35 and 42°C but poorly at 25°C. Colonies are nonpigmented and very mucoid and grow on ordinary media such as TSA. Some strains are motile by one or two polar flagella, but motility is difficult to demonstrate due to the mucoid character of the colonies. In opposition to the original description (42), the species is saccharolytic, acidifying glucose, mannitol, xylose, and other carbohydrates. In contrast, ethylene glycol is not acidified. Beta-galactosidase, pyrrolidonyl aminopeptidase, and trypsin are positive, but alkaline phosphatase is negative. Esculin is hydrolyzed. All strains are positive for catalase, beta-glucosidase, proline aminopeptidase, and pyrrolidonyl aminopeptidase and negative for lysine, arginine, ornithine, denitrification, and indole production (42).

TABLE 3 Oxidase-positive, indole-negative, trypsin-positive nonfermenters[a]

Characteristic	Alishewanella fetalis (1)	Inquilinus limosus (3)	Myroides odoratimimus (20)	Myroides odoratus (4)	Ochrobactrum anthropi (39)/ O. intermedium (3)	Pannonibacter phragmiteus (7)[c]	Rhizobium radiobacter (19)[c]	Shewanella algae (6)[d]	Shewanella putrefaciens (2)[d]	Sphingobacterium multivorum (6)	Sphingobacterium spiritivorum (4)	Sphingobacterium thalpophilum (3)	Sphingomonas spp. (15)
Motility	0	33	0	0	100	100	100	100	100	0	0	0	66
Flagella	0	P, 1	0	0	Pt, L	Pt, L	Pt, L	P, 1	P, 1	0	0	0	P, 1
Growth on MacConkey agar	100	(100)	100	75	100	100	100	100	100	100	(50)	100	0
Acidification of:													
Glucose	100	100	0	0	100	100	100	0	50	100	100	100	87 (13)
Mannitol	0	100	0	0	55	28	100	0	0	0	100	0	0
Xylose	0	100	0	0	100	100	100	0	0	100	100	100	87
Ethylene glycol	0	0	0	0	100	86	100	100	100	0	100	0	93
Urease	100	(33)	100	100	98	100	95	0	0	100	100	(100)	0
Nitrate reductase	100	0	0	0	98	86	89	100	100	0	0	100	7
Nitrite reductase	0	0	100	100	90	100	58	0	0	0	0	0	0
Production of H_2S (on KIA)	0	0	0	0	0	0	0	100	100	0	0	0	0
Esculin hydrolysis	0	100	0	0	12	86	100	0	0	100	100	100	100
Gelatinase	100	0	100	100	0	0	0	100	100	0	0	0	0
Pyrrolidonyl aminopeptidase	0	100	100	100	100	100	100	100	100	100	100	100	27
Alkaline phosphatase	100	0	100	100	0	0	0	100	100	100	100	100	100
Beta-galactosidase (ONPG)[e]	0	100	0	0	0	100	100	0	0	100	75	100	100
Requirement for NaCl	0	0	0	0	0	0	0	100	0	0	0	0	0
Susceptibility to:													
Desferrioxamine	100	0	0	100	0	100	21	0	0	0	0	0	7
Colistin	100	0	0	0	100/0[b]	0	68	66	100	0	0	0	7
Production of flexirubin pigments	0	0	100	100	0	0	0	0	0	0	0	0	0

[a]Numbers in parentheses after organism names are numbers of strains tested. Values are percentages; those in parentheses represent delayed positivity. Pt, peritrichous; P, polar; L, lateral.

[b]*Ochrobactrum anthropi* strains are colistin susceptible, whereas *O. intermedium* strains are colistin resistant (236).

[c]*Pannonibacter* organisms are tributyrate esterase positive within 30 mins. *Rhizobium* organisms are positive only after several hours or remain negative.

[d]Both *Shewanella* species are ornithine decarboxylase positive.

[e]ONPG, o-nitrophenyl-β-D-galactopyranoside.

I. limosus can be distinguished from *Sphingobacterium* spp. by its lack of alkaline phosphatase activity and by its acidification of mannitol. *Sphingobacterium spiritivorum* also produces acid from mannitol but acidifies ethylene glycol, unlike *Inquilinus*. It differs from *Rhizobium radiobacter* and *Pannonibacter phragmitetus* by the absence of acid production from ethylene glycol (also negative in a quarter of the *P. phragmitetus* strains) and by the lack of nitrate reductase activity.

Identifying the species is difficult because it is not contained in the databases of commercial identification kits and its mucoid appearance may lead to confusion with mucoid *P. aeruginosa* strains (170, 246). Isolates can be recovered on colistin-containing *B. cepacia* selective media but are inhibited on *B. cepacia* selective agar, which also contains gentamicin (37).

All isolates are reported to be resistant to penicillins and cephalosporins, kanamycin, tobramycin, colistin, doxycycline, and trimethoprim-sulfamethoxazole and susceptible to imipenem and ciprofloxacin (37, 170, 246).

All strains have been recovered from respiratory secretions of cystic fibrosis patients. The natural habitat of *I. limosus* is unknown to date, and the clinical impact of chronic colonization with *I. limosus* remains unclear. Chiron et al. (37) reported that for one patient, *I. limosus* was the only potential pathogen recovered from the sputum; *Inquilinus* acquisition was followed by a worsening of his lung function.

Myroides odoratimimus and M. odoratus

The genus *Myroides* includes two species, *M. odoratimimus* and *M. odoratus*, formerly *Flavobacterium odoratum* (215), which can be isolated from clinical samples. Cells are thin, middle-sized (0.5 μm in diameter and 1 to 2 μm long) nonmotile rods, but both species display a gliding motility. The spreading colonies develop a typical fruity smell, similar to the odor of *Alcaligenes faecalis*. The yellow pigment, although less pronounced than that of some *Chryseobacterium* species, is of the flexirubin type.

Myroides species grow on most media, including MacConkey agar. Growth occurs at 18 to 37°C but usually not at 42°C. *Myroides* species are asaccharolytic, urease positive, and nitrate reductase negative, but nitrite is reduced. *M. odoratus* can routinely be differentiated by its susceptibility to desferrioxamine, while *M. odoratimimus* is resistant. They also differ by their cellular fatty acid pattern, with *M. odoratimimus* having significant amounts of C13:0i and C15:0 (215).

Organisms identified as *M. odoratus* have been reported mostly from urine but have also been found in wound, sputum, blood, and ear specimens (95). Clinical infection with *Myroides* species is exceedingly rare. However, cases of rapidly progressive necrotizing fasciitis and bacteremia (104) and recurrent cellulitis with bacteremia (5) have been reported. In our experience, based on 24 clinical isolates, *M. odoratimimus* is four to five times more frequently isolated from clinical material than *M. odoratus*.

Most strains are resistant to penicillins, cephalosporins, aminoglycosides, aztreonam, and carbapenems (95).

Ochrobactrum anthropi and O. intermedium

The genus *Ochrobactrum* comprises at present 13 species, of which two are of some clinical importance. *Ochrobactrum anthropi* (93) comprises the so-called urease-positive *Achromobacter* species, formerly designated CDC group Vd (biotypes 1 and 2), and *Achromobacter* groups A, C, and D, described by Holmes et al. (92). Subsequent studies showed

that biogroup C and some strains belonging to biogroup A constitute a homogeneous DNA-DNA hybridization group separate from *O. anthropi*, named *O. intermedium* (236).

Colonies on SBA are small, about 1 mm after overnight incubation, but grow large and creamy after 2 days and appear smooth, circular, and clearly delineated. *Ochrobactrum* species are medium-length gram-negative rods and motile by peritrichous flagella, although most cells have only one or two very long lateral flagella.

Ochrobactrum anthropi and *O. intermedium* have similar phenotypic properties. These species are strongly trypsin and pyrrolidonyl aminopeptidase positive and are saccharolytic, with rapid acidification of glucose and xylose. Acidification of mannitol is irregular and often delayed positive. Ethylene glycol is acidified. Urease is positive. Nitrate is reduced, and the vast majority of the strains also reduce nitrites.

Both *Ochrobactrum* species (*Brucellaceae*, *Alphaproteobacteria*) are closely related to *Brucella* species, with *O. intermedium* occupying a phylogenetic position that is intermediate between *O. anthropi* and *Brucella* (236).

O. anthropi has been isolated from various environmental and human sources, predominantly from patients with catheter-related bacteremias (93, 125, 183) and rarely with other infections (141). One hospital outbreak in transplant patients has been described (69). One case of pyogenic liver infection due to *O. intermedium* has been reported (145), but because of the close phenotypic similarity of *O. anthropi* and *O. intermedium*, it is possible that certain infections thought to be caused by *O. anthropi* were actually caused by *O. intermedium*.

O. anthropi strains are usually resistant to beta-lactams, such as broad-spectrum penicillins, broad-spectrum cephalosporins, aztreonam, and amoxicillin-clavulanate, but are usually susceptible to aminoglycosides, fluoroquinolones, imipenem, tetracycline, and trimethoprim-sulfamethoxazole (13, 125, 183). *O. intermedium* is resistant to colistin, while *O. anthropi* is susceptible.

Pannonibacter phragmitetus

P. phragmitetus, of the family *Rhodobacteraceae* (*Alphaproteobacteria*), has been shown to be identical to the strains formerly designated *Achromobacter* groups B and E (94). The species resembles most strongly *Rhizobium radiobacter*, but saccharolytic activity is somewhat weaker and not as extended; i.e., raffinose is not acidified and mannitol acidification is positive only for the strains belonging to the former *Achromobacter* group B. An easy and reliable differential test is the hydrolysis of tributyrin (diagnostic tablets; Rosco Diagnostica A/S, Taastrup, Denmark), which is positive within 30 min for *P. phragmitetus*, whereas *R. radiobacter* strains are positive only after several hours' to overnight incubation or remain negative. *Ochrobactrum* species do not hydrolyze tributyrin.

Cases of septicemia due to *Achromobacter* group B have been reported (88, 114).

Rhizobium radiobacter

The former genus *Agrobacterium* contained several species of plant pathogens occurring worldwide in soils. Four distinct species of *Agrobacterium* were recognized: *A. radiobacter* (formerly *A. tumefaciens* and CDC group Vd-3), *A. rhizogenes* (subsequently transferred to the genus *Sphingomonas* as *Sphingomona rosa*), *A. vitis*, and *A. rubi* (185). More recently, an emended description of the genus *Rhizobium* (*Rhizobiaceae*, *Alphaproteobacteria*) was proposed to include all species of *Agrobacterium* (252). Following this proposal the new combinations are *Rhizobium radiobacter*, *R. rhizogenes*, *R. rubi*, and *R. vitis* (252). Only *R. radiobacter* is clinically important.

Colonies of *R. radiobacter* are circular, convex, smooth, and nonpigmented to light beige on SBA, with a diameter of 2 mm at 48 h. Colonies may appear wet and become extremely mucoid and pink on MacConkey agar with prolonged incubation. *R. radiobacter* cells measure 0.6 to 1.0 by 1.5 to 3.0 μm and occur singly and in pairs.

R. radiobacter grows optimally at 25 to 28°C but grows at 35°C as well. *R. radiobacter* is phenotypically very similar to the *Ochrobactrum* species, although phylogenetically separate. *R. radiobacter* differs clearly from *Ochrobactrum* species by a positive beta-galactosidase test and by the production of ketolactonate, which is, however, not routinely tested. *R. radiobacter* has a broad saccharolytic activity, including mannitol and raffinose.

R. radiobacter has been most frequently isolated from blood, followed by peritoneal dialysate, urine, and ascitic fluid (64, 105). The majority of cases have occurred in patients with transcutaneous catheters or implanted biomedical prostheses, and effective treatment often requires removal of the device (66). Most strains are susceptible to broad-spectrum cephalosporins, carbapenems, tetracyclines, and gentamicin, but not to tobramycin (64, 241). Testing of individual isolates is recommended for clinically significant cases.

Shewanella algae and S. putrefaciens

The organisms formerly called *Pseudomonas putrefaciens*, *Alteromonas putrefaciens*, *Achromobacter putrefaciens*, and CDC group Ib have been placed in the genus *Shewanella* (140), which comprises over 50 species. *S. putrefaciens* was described with two CDC biotypes. CDC biotype 1 was later described as *S. putrefaciens* sensu stricto, whereas CDC biotype 2 was subsequently assigned to a new species, *S. alga* (158), later corrected to *S. algae*.

Colonies of *Shewanella* species on SBA are convex, circular, smooth, and occasionally mucoid, produce a brown to tan soluble pigment, and cause green discoloration of the medium. Cells are long, short, or filamentous, reminiscent of *Myroides*. Motility is due to a single polar flagellum.

Most strains of both *Shewanella* species produce H_2S in KIA and TSI agar, a unique feature among clinically relevant nonfermenters. Both are also ornithine decarboxylase positive and have strong alkaline phosphatase, strong trypsin, and strong pyrrolidonyl aminopeptidase activities. *S. algae* is halophilic, asaccharolytic, and requires NaCl for growth, with growth occurring already on TSA plus 0.5% NaCl. *S. putrefaciens* does not require NaCl for growth and is saccharolytic, producing acid from maltose and sucrose, and irregularly and weakly from glucose.

Khashe and Janda (126) have reported that *S. algae* is the predominant human clinical isolate (77%), while *S. putrefaciens* represents the majority of nonhuman isolates (89%). Although infrequently isolated in the clinical laboratory, *S. putrefaciens* and *S. algae* have been recovered from a wide variety of clinical specimens and are associated with a broad range of human infections, including skin and soft tissue infections (36), otitis media (99), ocular infection (28), osteomyelitis (20), peritonitis (46), and septicemia (110). The habitat for *S. algae* is saline, whereas *S. putrefaciens* has been isolated mostly from fish, poultry, and meats as well as from freshwater and marine samples.

Shewanella species are generally susceptible to most antimicrobial agents effective against gram-negative rods,

except penicillin and cephalothin (70, 241). The mean MICs of *S. algae* for penicillin, ampicillin, and tetracycline are higher than the corresponding MICs of *S. putrefaciens* (126, 239).

Sphingobacterium

A total of 15 species have been described as belonging to the genus *Sphingobacterium*. Based on 16S rRNA gene sequence data, the indole-producing *Flavobacterium mizutaii* belongs to the genus *Sphingobacterium* (G. Wauters and M. Vaneechoutte, unpublished observation) and should be transferred to the genus *Sphingobacterium* as *Sphingobacterium mizutaii*. As a consequence, the description of the genus *Sphingobacterium* as indole negative will have to be emended.

The species of the genus *Sphingobacterium* encountered in clinical material include *S. multivorum* (formerly *Flavobacterium multivorum* and CDC group IIk-2), *S. spiritivorum* (including the species formerly designated as *Flavobacterium spiritivorum*, *F. yabuuchiae*, and CDC group IIk-3), *S. thalpophilum*, and *Flavobacterium mizutaii* (205, 249).

Colonies are yellowish. *Sphingobacterium* species are middle-sized, nonmotile gram-negative rods. Species of this genus do not produce indole, but *Flavobacterium mizutaii* is indole positive and is therefore dealt with among the indole-positive nonfermenters in Table 4. All species are strongly saccharolytic; i.e., glucose, xylose, and other sugars are acidified. No acid is formed from mannitol, except by *S. spiritivorum*, which is also the only species to produce acid from ethylene glycol. *S. thalpophilum* can be distinguished from other *Sphingobacterium* species by its nitrate reductase and its growth at 42°C.

S. multivorum and *S. spiritivorum* can be distinguished from *Sphingomonas paucimobilis* (formerly CDC group IIk-1) because they are nonmotile, urease positive, and resistant to polymyxin. Many strains of other *Sphingomonas* species are also colistin resistant.

S. multivorum is the most common human species. It has been isolated from various clinical specimens but has only rarely been associated with serious infections (peritonitis and sepsis) (73, 91). Blood and urine have been the most common sources for the isolation of *S. spiritivorum* (90). *F. mizutaii* has been isolated from blood, cerebrospinal fluid (CSF), and wound specimens (247). *S. thalpophilum* has been recovered from wounds, blood, eyes, abscesses, and an abdominal incision (247).

Sphingobacterium species are generally resistant to aminoglycosides and polymyxin B while susceptible in vitro to the quinolones and trimethoprim-sulfamethoxazole. Susceptibility to beta-lactam antibiotics is variable, requiring testing of individual isolates (197).

Sphingomonas Species

On the basis of 16S rRNA gene sequence and the presence of unique sphingoglycolipid and ubiquinone types, the genus *Sphingomonas* (Sphingomoadaceae, Alphaproteobacteria) was created for organisms formerly known as *Pseudomonas paucimobilis* and CDC group IIk-1 (89, 250). Since the original proposal, a total of almost 60 novel species, originating from various environments, have been added to the genus *Sphingomonas*. The former genus *Sphingomonas* can be divided into four phylogenetic groups, each representing a different genus (204), whereby the emended genus *Sphingomonas* contains at least 12 species, of which only *S. paucimobilis* and *S. parapaucimobilis* are thought to be clinically important. However, recent 16S rRNA gene sequencing

TABLE 4 Oxidase-positive, indole-positive nonfermenters[a]

Characteristic	Balneatrix alpica (1)	Bergeyella zoohelcum (6)	Chryseobacterium anthropi (9)	Chryseobacterium gleum (11)	Chryseobacterium hominis (12)	Chryseobacterium indologenes (14)	Elizabethkingia meningoseptica (16)	Empedobacter brevis (7)	Flavobacterium mizutaii (4)	Wautersiella falsenii (45)	Weeksella virosa (10)
Motility	100	0	0	0	0	0	0	0	0	0	0
Beta-hemolysis (after 3 days on SBA)	0	0	0	0	0	100	0	0	0	0	0
Production of flexirubin pigments	0	0	0	100	0	72	0	0	0	0	0
Production of other pigments	PY	−	−/PS	−	−/PY	−	−/PY/PS	PY	PY	−/PY	−
Growth on MacConkey agar	0	0	0	100	0	66	88	100	0	100	0
Growth at 42°C	0	0	0	100	0	0	50	0	0	0	100
Acidification of:											
Glucose	100	0	100	100	100	100	100	100	100	100	0
Mannitol	100	0	0	0	0	0	100	0	0	0	0
Xylose	0	0	0	27	0	0	0	0	100	0	0
L-Arabinose	0	0	0	100	0	0	0	0	75	0	0
Maltose	100	0	100	100	100	100	100	100	100	100	0
Sucrose	0	0	0	0	33	21	0	0	100	0	0
Ethylene glycol	0	0	0	100	100	0	100	0	0	44	0
Esculin hydrolysis	0	0	0	100	100	100	100	0	100	55	0
Gelatinase	0	100	100	100	100	100	100	100	0	55/(45)	100
Urease	0	100	0	73	0	0	0[b]	0	0	100	0
Nitrate reductase	100	0	0	73	75	28	0	0	0	0	0
Nitrite reductase	0	0	0	54	75	14	83	0	75	15	0
Beta-galactosidase (ONPG[c])	0	0	0	0	0	0	100	0	100	31	0
Benzyl-arginine aminopeptidase (trypsin)	0	100	100	100	100	100	100	100	100	100	100
Pyrrolidonyl aminopeptidase	0	0	100	100	100	100	100	100	100	100	100
Susceptibility to:											
Desferrioxamine	100	100	78	0	0	0	0	0	0	12	100
Colistin/polymyxin	100	0	0	0	17	0	0	0	0	0	100

[a]Numbers in parentheses after organism names are numbers of strains tested. Values are percentages; those in parentheses represent delayed positivity. −, none; PY, pale yellow; PS, pale salmon-pink.

[b]*Elizabethkingia miricola* is urease positive (data from reference 127).

[c]ONPG, *o*-nitrophenyl-β-D-galactopyranoside.

of 12 strains of clinical origin (Wauters, unpublished) revealed that several named and unnamed *Sphingomonas* species were present, but no *S. paucimobilis* and only two *S. parapaucimobilis* isolates. Because many phenotypic characteristics are shared by these species, routine laboratories best report them as *Sphingomonas* species.

Sphingomonas colonies are slow growing on blood agar medium, with small colonies appearing after 24 h of incubation. Growth occurs at 37°C but not at 42°C, with optimum growth at 30°C. Almost all strains produce a yellow insoluble pigment, different from flexirubin pigments, as can be established by the KOH test (11). Few strains are nonpigmented or develop a pale yellow color after several days. Older colonies demonstrate a deep yellow (mustard color) pigment.

Sphingomonas species are medium to long motile rods with a single polar flagellum. Motility occurs at 18 to 22°C but not at 37°C. However, few cells are actively motile in broth culture, thus making motility a difficult characteristic to demonstrate.

Oxidase is only weakly positive or even absent. All the strains are saccharolytic, but some acidify glucose only weakly and slowly. Urease is always negative, and nitrate reduction is only very rarely positive. Esculin is hydrolyzed, and beta-galactosidase and alkaline phosphatase are positive. The yellow pigment of some strains may hamper a correct reading of the yellow color shift when nitrophenyl compounds of the latter substrates are used.

Members of this genus are known as decomposers of aromatic compounds and are being developed for use in bioremediation.

Sphingomonas species are widely distributed in the environment, including water, and have been isolated from a variety of clinical specimens, including blood, CSF, peritoneal fluid, urine, wounds, the vagina, and the cervix, as well as from the hospital environment (103, 148, 175). *S. parapaucimobilis* clinical isolates have been obtained from sputum, urine, and the vagina (250).

Most strains are resistant to colistin, but all are susceptible to vancomycin, which is exceptional for gram-negative nonfermenting rods. This is elsewhere only found in *Chryseobacterium* and related genera like *Elizabethkingia* and *Empedobacter*. Most *Sphingomonas* strains are susceptible to tetracycline, chloramphenicol, trimethoprim-sulfamethoxazole, and aminoglycosides. Susceptibility to other antimicrobial agents, including fluoroquinolones, varies (70, 103, 175).

Oxidase-Positive, Indole-Positive Nonfermenters

The natural habitats of most oxidase-positive, indole-positive nonfermenters (Table 4) are soil, plants, and food and water sources, including those in hospitals. Clinically relevant species include *Chryseobacterium* species, *Elizabethkingia meningoseptica*, *Empedobacter brevis*, *Wautersiella falsenii*, *Flavobacterium mizutaii*, *Weeksella virosa*, *Bergeyella zoohelcum*, and *Balneatrix alpica*. All are indole, trypsin, pyrrolidonyl aminopeptidase, and alkaline phosphatase positive, except for *B. zoohelcum*, which is pyrrolidonyl aminopeptidase negative, and *B. alpica*, which is both trypsin and pyrrolidonyl aminopeptidase negative. Table 4 presents an overview of the characteristics useful to differentiate among these species.

Balneatrix alpica

B. alpica was first isolated in 1987 during an outbreak of pneumonia and meningitis among persons who attended a hot (37°C) spring spa in southern France (51). Isolates from eight patients were recovered from blood, CSF, and sputum, and one was recovered from water. This species is only rarely isolated from human clinical specimens.

B. alpica produces colonies that are 2 to 3 mm in diameter, convex, and smooth. The center of the colonies is pale yellow after 2 to 3 days and pale brown after 4 days. *B. alpica* is a straight or curved gram-negative rod. It is the only motile species among the clinically relevant indole-positive nonfermenters. Cells have one or two polar flagella.

The species is strictly aerobic and saccharolytic. Both trypsin and pyrrolidonyl aminopeptidase are negative, unlike with other indole-positive nonfermenters. Growth occurs at 20 to 46°C on ordinary media such as TSA but not on MacConkey agar. It acidifies glucose, mannose, fructose, maltose, sorbitol, mannitol, glycerol, inositol, and xylose. *B. alpica* is nitrate reductase and weakly gelatinase positive. It is similar to *E. meningoseptica* but can be differentiated from this species by its motility and nitrate reductase and by the absence of beta-galactosidase.

B. alpica has been reported to be susceptible to penicillin G and all other beta-lactam antibiotics and to all aminoglycosides, chloramphenicol, tetracycline, erythromycin, sulfonamides, trimethoprim, ofloxacin, and nalidixic acid. It is resistant to clindamycin and vancomycin (30).

Bergeyella zoohelcum

Bergeyella zoohelcum and *Weeksella virosa* are morphologically and biochemically similar organisms with cells measuring 0.6 by 2 to 3 μm, with parallel sides and rounded ends. *B. zoohelcum* colonies are sticky and tan to yellow.

Both species fail to grow on MacConkey agar and are nonsaccharolytic. Both species are susceptible to desferrioxamine and have the unusual feature of being susceptible to penicillin, a feature that allows them to be easily differentiated from the related genera *Chryseobacterium* and *Sphingobacterium*. *B. zoohelcum* can be differentiated from *W. virosa* because it is pyrrolidonyl aminopeptidase negative, strongly urease positive, and resistant to colistin. *B. zoohelcum* comprises formerly CDC group IIj strains (97).

B. zoohelcum is isolated mainly from wounds caused by animal (mostly dog) bites (97, 176). Meningitis or septicemia due to *B. zoohelcum* has occurred in patients either bitten by a dog (146) or with continuous contact with cats (157).

Both *B. zoohelcum* and *W. virosa* are susceptible to most antibiotics. However, at present no specific antibiotic treatment is recommended, and antimicrobial susceptibility testing should be performed on significant clinical isolates.

Chryseobacterium

CDC group IIb comprises the species *Chryseobacterium indologenes*, *C. gleum*, and other strains, which probably represent several unnamed taxa.

Strains included in CDC group IIb are nonmotile rods. Cells of *C. indologenes* are similar to those of *E. meningoseptica*, *C. anthropi*, *C. hominis*, and *F. mizutaii*; i.e., they are thinner in their central than in their peripheral portions and include filamentous forms.

CDC group IIb strains are oxidase and catalase positive, produce flexirubin pigments (11, 168), are moderately saccharolytic, and are esculin and gelatin hydrolysis positive. *C. indologenes* and *C. gleum* can easily be differentiated from each other by four characteristics: *C. indologenes* displays a broad beta-hemolysis area within 3 days of incubation at 37°C on SBA, is always arabinose negative, does not acidify ethylene glycol, and does not grow at 42°C (214). *C. gleum* exhibits pronounced alpha-hemolysis, resembling viridans discoloration; always acidifies ethylene glycol; is arabinose positive or delayed positive; and grows at 42°C.

Beta-hemolysis is absent or very rare in other strains of CDC group IIb and is therefore almost specific for the identification of *C. indologenes*, while the profile of *C. gleum* may be shared by other strains of this group. It should be noted that some *C. indologenes* strains do not produce flexirubin.

Among CDC group IIb species, *C. indologenes* is usually considered most frequently isolated from clinical samples, although it rarely has clinical significance (241). It causes bacteremia in hospitalized patients with severe underlying disease, although the mortality rate is relatively low even among patients who were administered antibiotics without activity against *C. indologenes* (195). Nosocomial infections due to *C. indologenes* have been linked to the use of indwelling devices during hospital stays (7, 102, 159).

Still, the frequency of *C. indologenes* as reported in the literature should be interpreted with caution, because until recently and without molecular biology, *C. indologenes* could almost not be distinguished routinely from other CDC group IIb strains. We have recently examined 21 CDC group IIb strains both phenotypically and by 16S rDNA sequencing and found 9 *C. indologenes* isolates, 5 *C. gleum* isolates, and 7 isolates belonging to unnamed *Chryseobacterium* species.

The production of novel types of metallo-beta-lactamases from *C. indologenes* has been studied in detail (136, 166).

Chryseobacterium anthropi represents part of the strains formerly designated as CDC group IIe (120). Most strains display very sticky colonies, which are nonpigmented but may develop a slightly salmon-pinkish, rarely yellowish color after a few days. In contrast to *C. hominis*, the species is negative for esculin hydrolysis and acidification of ethylene glycol. In addition, many strains are susceptible to desferrioxamine. One case of meningitis caused by CDC group IIe has been reported (245). Most clinical isolates used for the description of the species were from wounds and blood cultures (120).

Chryseobacterium hominis includes the strains formerly included in CDC group IIc and most of the strains of CDC group IIh (228). This species does not produce flexirubin pigments, but some strains exhibit a slightly yellowish pigmentation. Colonies are often mucoid. *C. hominis* can be differentiated from *C. gleum* by the absence of flexirubin pigments and the lack of acid production from arabinose. *C. indologenes* strains lacking flexirubin pigments may resemble *C. hominis*, but the latter is never beta-hemolytic and always acidifies ethylene glycol.

Many strains have been isolated from blood. Others have been isolated from dialysis fluid, pus, the eye, infraorbital drain, and aortic valve, but their clinical significance remains to be assessed (228).

Elizabethkingia meningoseptica and E. miricola

Colonies of *Elizabethkingia meningoseptica*, formerly *Chryseobacterium meningosepticum* (127), are smooth and fairly large, either nonpigmented or producing a pale yellow or slightly salmon-pinkish pigment after 2 or 3 days. Characteristic features are acid production from mannitol and beta-galactosidase activity. Gelatin and esculin hydrolysis are positive. *Elizabethkingia* and *Chryseobacterium* species can be differentiated as well on the basis of 16S rRNA sequence analysis (120, 127).

E. meningoseptica has been reported to be associated with (neonatal) meningitis and nosocomial outbreaks (14, 33, 38, 106, 195, 207), endocarditis (16), cystic fibrosis airway infections (131), retroperitoneal hematoma (133), community-acquired osteomyelitis (132), adult pneumonia and septicemia (14, 135, 192, 241), respiratory colonization and infection following aerosolized polymyxin B treatment (26), and infections reported in dialysis units (135, 165). A clinical case of *E. miricola* was reported only once, in a case of sepsis (77).

Empedobacter brevis

Empedobacter brevis (216) colonies are yellowish pigmented but do not produce flexirubin. *E. brevis* can be differentiated from *C. indologenes*, *C. gleum*, other CDC group IIb strains, and *C. hominis* by its lack of esculin hydrolysis. Growth on MacConkey agar and a stronger gelatinase activity are useful to distinguish it from *C. anthropi*. The species is rarely recovered from clinical material.

Flavobacterium mizutaii

F. mizutaii is saccharolytic, producing acid from a large number of carbohydrates, including xylose, similar to *Sphingobacterium* species, from which it can be distinguished by its indole production and by its failure to grow on MacConkey agar and its usual lack of urease activity (247).

F. mizutaii can be distinguished from *Chryseobacterium* and *Empedobacter* species by its lack of gelatin hydrolysis and of flexirubin production. *F. mizutaii* produces acid from xylose but not from ethylene glycol, allowing differentiation from other indole-positive species. The phenotypic profile of *F. mizutaii* is similar to that of the strains described as *Chryseobacterium* CDC group IIi. Furthermore, 16S rRNA gene sequencing confirms that most CDC group IIi strains actually belong to the species *F. mizutaii*.

F. mizutaii has been described as an indole-negative species (249), but in our hands all strains tested, including the type strain, produce as much indole as the *Chryseobacterium* strains. According to 16S rRNA gene sequencing, this species is closely related to *Sphingobacterium* species, indicating that *F. mizutaii*—formerly *Sphingobacterium mizutae* (98)—should be transferred back to the genus *Sphingobacterium* as *S. mizutaii*. *F. mizutaii* has been isolated from blood, CSF, and wound specimens (247).

Wautersiella falsenii

Wautersiella falsenii is closely related to *E. brevis*, from which it differs by its urease activity. Two genomovars have been described (119): genomovar 1 is always esculin positive and beta-galactosidase negative, whereas 90% of the genomovar 2 strains are esculin negative and 63% are beta-galactosidase positive.

W. falsenii was described as belonging to a separate genus from *Empedobacter*, based on comparison of its 16S rRNA gene sequence with an *E. brevis* EMBL sequence of poor quality. A high-quality sequence of the rRNA gene of the type strain of *E. brevis* indicates that *W. falsenii* probably has to be renamed as *Empedobacter falsenii*.

W. falsenii is much more frequently isolated from clinical samples than *E. brevis* (119). Its clinical significance remains to be assessed.

Weeksella virosa

W. virosa colonies are mucoid and adherent to the agar, reminiscent of the sticky colonies of *B. zoohelcum*. Colonies are not pigmented after 24 h of incubation but may become yellowish, tan to brown, after 2 or 3 days. The cellular morphology of *Weeksella virosa* is dealt with above in the discussion of *Bergeyella zoohelcum*. *W. virosa* can be differentiated from *B. zoohelcum* because it is urease negative and polymyxin B and colistin susceptible, whereas *B. zoohelcum* is rapid urease positive and polymyxin B and colistin resistant. *W. virosa* comprises formerly CDC group IIf strains (96). *W. virosa* is isolated mainly from urine and vaginal samples (96, 177), in contrast to *B. zoohelcum*, which is isolated mostly from animal bites.

The appropriate choice of effective antimicrobial agents for the treatment of chryseobacterial infections is difficult (106). *Chryseobacterium* species and *E. meningoseptica* are inherently resistant to many antimicrobial agents commonly used to treated infections caused by gram-negative bacteria (aminoglycosides, beta-lactam antibiotics, tetracyclines, and chloramphenicol) but are often susceptible to agents generally used for treating infections caused by gram-positive bacteria (rifampin, clindamycin, erythromycin, trimethoprim-sulfamethoxazole, and vancomycin) (70, 197, 241). Although early investigators recommended vancomycin for treating serious infection with *E. meningoseptica* (83), subsequent studies showed greater in vitro activity of minocycline, rifampin, trimethoprim-sulfamethoxazole, and quinolones (14, 72, 197). Among the quinolones, levofloxacin is more active than ciprofloxacin and ofloxacin (197). *C. indologenes* is reported to be uniformly resistant to cephalothin, cefotaxime, ceftriaxone, aztreonam, aminoglycosides, erythromycin, clindamycin, vancomycin, and teicoplanin, while susceptibility to piperacillin, cefoperazone, ceftazidime, imipenem, quinolones, minocycline, and trimethoprim-sulfamethoxazole is variable, requiring testing of individual isolates (133, 197, 243). Several studies reported that administration of quinolone, minocycline, trimethoprim-sulfamethoxazole, or rifampin, and treatment of local infection improve the clinical outcome of patients with *E. meningoseptica* infections. The choice of appropriate antimicrobial therapy is further complicated by the fact that MIC breakpoints for resistance and susceptibility of chryseobacteria have not been established by the CLSI and the results of disk diffusion testing are unreliable in predicting antimicrobial susceptibility of *Chryseobacterium* species (35, 72, 243). The Etest is a possible alternative to the standard agar dilution method for testing cefotaxime, ceftazidime, amikacin, minocycline, ofloxacin, and ciprofloxacin but not piperacillin (101). Definitive therapy for clinically significant isolates should be guided by individual susceptibility patterns determined by an MIC method.

Pink-Pigmented Nonfermenters

It should be noted that colonies of *C. anthropi* and *E. meningoseptica* can be lightly salmon colored on some media after several days of incubation, but this is not to be confused with the clearly pink colonies of the taxa discussed here (Table 5).

Asaia

Asaia is a genus of the family *Acetobacteraceae* (*Alphaproteobacteria*), with some clinically relevant members, such as *A. bogorensis* (251) and *A. siamensis* (123). The natural habitats of *Asaia* species are reported to be the flowers of the orchid tree, plumbago, and fermented glutinous rice, all originating in hot tropical climates, particularly in Indonesia and Thailand.

Growth of *Asaia* species is scant to moderate on SBA. Colonies are pale pink. In opposition to *Methylobacterium*, colonies are not dark under UV light. *Asaia* species are small to middle-sized gram-negative rods, usually motile by one or two polar or lateral flagella. The species are oxidase negative and strongly saccharolytic; i.e., glucose, mannitol, xylose, and L-arabinose are acidified very rapidly, often within 1 h on low-peptone phenol red agar. Acid is also produced from ethylene glycol. Furthermore, *Asaia* species are biochemically rather inert, except for benzyl arginine aminopeptidase (trypsin) activity. *Asaia* species can be distinguished from *Methylobacterium* species by cell morphology, a stronger saccharolytic activity, and acid production from mannitol. *Asaia bogorensis* has been reported as a cause of peritonitis in a patient on automated peritoneal dialysis (196). *Asaia* species have been reported to be resistant to ceftazidime, meropenem, imipenem, trimethoprim, amikacin, vancomycin, aztreonam, penicillin, and ampicillin by disk diffusion (147). The *A. bogorensis* strain reported by Snyder et al. (196) was susceptible to aminoglycosides (amikacin, tobramycin, and gentamicin) and resistant to ceftazidime and meropenem by disk diffusion (196).

Azospirillum

The former *Roseomonas* genomospecies 3 (*Roseomonas fauriae*) and genomospecies 6 have been transferred to the genus *Azospirillum* (*Rhodospirillaceae*, *Alphaproteobacteria*), a genus of nitrogen-fixing plant symbionts that is in a different order of bacteria (43, 82). Some strains of this genus may occasionally be isolated from clinical material (179).

Colonies are pale pink and resemble those of *Roseomonas*. Cells are somewhat more rod shaped than *Roseomonas* and are motile by one or two polar flagella. Oxidase is positive and urea is strongly positive, as in *Roseomonas* species. A positive beta-galactosidase test and esculin hydrolysis allow differentiation of *Azospirillum* from other pink-pigmented species.

Methylobacterium

The genus *Methylobacterium*, of the family *Methylobacteriaceae* (*Alphaproteobacteria*), currently consists of 20 named species plus additional unassigned biovars, recognized on the basis of carbon assimilation type, electrophoretic type, and DNA-DNA homology grouping (74, 78, 213). *Methylobacterium* species are isolated mostly from vegetation but may also occasionally be found in the hospital

TABLE 5 Pink-pigmented nonfermenters[a]

Characteristic	Asaia spp. (2)	Azospirillum spp. (3)	Methylobacterium spp. (4)	Roseomonas cervicalis (2)	Roseomonas gilardii subsp. gilardii and Roseomonas gilardii subsp. rosea (5)	Roseomonas mucosa (8)	Roseomonas genomospecies 4 (1)	Roseomonas genomospecies 5 (3)
Oxidase	0	100	0	100	100[w]	0	100	100[w]
Acidification of:								
Glucose	100	0	(25)	0	(20)	100	(100)	0
Fructose	100	(100)[w]	0	50	60/(40)	100	100	(100)
Mannitol	100	0	0	0	(80)	100	0	0
Xylose	100	100	100	(100)	0	0	0	0
Arabinose	100	100	100	100	100	100	0	0
Ethylene glycol	100	100	100	100	100	100	0	0
Urease	0	100	100	100	100	100	100	100
Nitrate reductase	0	100	0	0	0	0	100	0
Esculin hydrolysis	0	100	0	0	0	0	0	0
Trypsin	100	0	100	0	0	0	0	0
Pyrrolidonyl aminopeptidase	0	100	0	0	100	100	0	0
Beta-galactosidase (ONPG)[b]	0	100	0	0	0	0	0	0
Susceptibility to:								
Colistin	0	0	0	0	40	50	0	33
Desferrioxamine	0	0	0	0	0	0	100	0

[a]Numbers in parentheses after organism names are numbers of strains tested. Values are percentages; those in parentheses represent delayed positivity. w, weak positive reaction.
[b]ONPG, o-nitrophenyl-β-D-galactopyranoside.

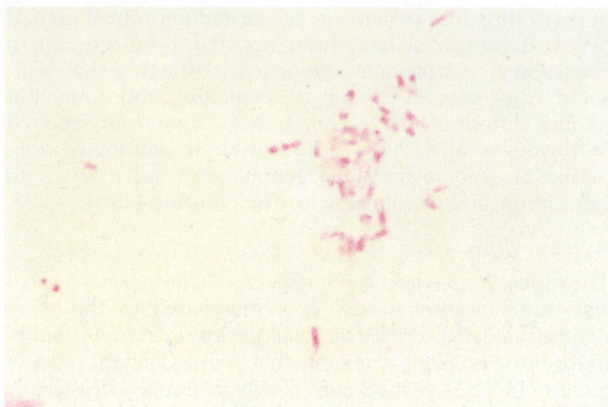

FIGURE 4 Gram stain of *Methylobacterium* showing pleomorphic gram-negative rods with vacuoles.

environment. *Methylobacterium mesophilicum* (formerly *Pseudomonas mesophilica*, *Pseudomonas extorquens*, and *Vibrio extorquens*) and M. *zatmanii* have been the two most commonly reported species isolated from clinical samples.

Colonies of *Methylobacterium* species are small, dry, and coral pink. Under UV light, *Methylobacterium* colonies appear dark due to absorption of UV light (179). Growth is fastidious on ordinary media such as TSA, producing 1-mm-diameter colonies after 4 to 5 days on SBA, modified Thayer-Martin, buffered charcoal-yeast extract, and Middlebrook 7H11 agars, with the best growth occurring on Sabouraud agar and usually no growth on MacConkey agar. Optimum growth occurs between 25 and 30°C. They are able to utilize methanol as a sole source of carbon and energy, although this characteristic may be lost on subculture. Cells are pleomorphic, vacuolated rods that stain poorly and may resist decolorization (Fig. 4). Motility by one polar flagellum is difficult to demonstrate. In the description of the genus (163), methylobacteria were reported to be oxidase positive, but the strains tested by us were all oxidase negative with the dimethyl-paraphenylenediamine reagent. Saccharolytic activity is weaker than in *Asaia* spp., and no acid is produced from mannitol and acid is produced irregularly from glucose. Arabinose, xylose, and ethylene glycol are acidified. Urea and starch are hydrolyzed.

Methylobacterium species have been reported to cause septicemia, continuous ambulatory peritoneal dialysis-related peritonitis, skin ulcers, synovitis, and other infections often in immunocompromised patients, as well as pseudoinfections (100, 124, 184). Tap water has been implicated as a possible agent of transmission in hospital environments, and methods for monitoring water systems for methylobacteria have been described previously (178).

Active drugs include aminoglycosides and trimethoprim-sulfamethoxazole, whereas beta-lactam drugs show variable patterns (27). They are best tested for susceptibility by agar or broth dilution at 30°C for 48 h (27).

Roseomonas

The original description of the genus *Roseomonas* (*Acetobacteraceae*, *Alphaproteobacteria*) included three named species, *R. gilardii* (genomospecies 1), *R. cervicalis* (genomospecies 2), and *R. fauriae* (genomospecies 3), and three unnamed species, *Roseomonas* genomospecies 4, 5, and 6 (179). *Roseomonas* genomospecies 3 and 6 have been transferred to the genus *Azospirillum*.

More recently, Han et al. (82) proposed a new species, *Roseomonas mucosa*, and a new subspecies, *Roseomonas gilardii* subsp. *rosea* (to differentiate from *Roseomonas gilardii* subsp. *gilardii*).

The following *Roseomonas* species can be isolated from clinical samples: *R. gilardii* subsp. *gilardii*, *R. gilardii* subsp. *rosea*, *R. mucosa*, *R. cervicalis*, *Roseomonas* genomospecies 4, and *Roseomonas* genomospecies 5.

Colonies are mucoid and runny (Fig. 5) and grow larger than those of *Asaia* and *Methylobacterium*. Pigmentation varies from pale pink to coral pink. *Roseomonas* cells are nonvacuolated, coccoid, plump rods, mostly in pairs and short chains and usually motile by one or two polar flagella, but motility is often difficult to demonstrate. Genomospecies 5 is nonmotile. Growth occurs at 37°C on ordinary media like SBA, and mostly on MacConkey agar, but the best growth is observed on Sabouraud agar. Oxidase is dependent on the species and often weak. Saccharolytic activity is also species dependent. All *Roseomonas* species strongly hydrolyze urea but not esculin. They are trypsin and beta-galactosidase negative. Phenotypic distinction among the different species is based on oxidase, acid production from carbohydrates, and pyrrolidonyl aminopeptidase and nitrate reductase activities.

R. mucosa acidifies rapidly arabinose, mannitol, and fructose. Glucose is acidified within 1 to 3 days. Oxidase is negative, and pyrrolidonyl aminopeptidase is positive. *R. gilardii* subsp. *gilardii* and *R. gilardii* subsp. *rosea* exhibit a weak oxidase reaction and are pyrrolidonyl aminopeptidase positive. The two subspecies cannot be differentiated by current phenotypic tests. They are less saccharolytic than *R. mucosa* and produce acid from arabinose and fructose but only irregularly and slowly from mannitol and rarely from glucose. *R. cervicalis* is strongly oxidase positive but has no pyrrolidonyl aminopeptidase activity. Only arabinose and fructose are positive within 2 days and xylose within 3 or 4 days. The single strain of genomospecies 4 examined is also oxidase positive and pyrrolidonyl aminopeptidase negative, and its saccharolytic activity is limited to acid production from glucose and fructose. It is the only species displaying nitrate reduction. Genomospecies 5 is weakly oxidase positive and pyrrolidonyl aminopeptidase negative. It is the least saccharolytic species, with only a delayed acid production from fructose. Ethylene glycol is acidified by all species except by genomospecies 4 and 5.

Roseomonas species are uncommon isolates from humans, but they are nevertheless the most frequently isolated pink

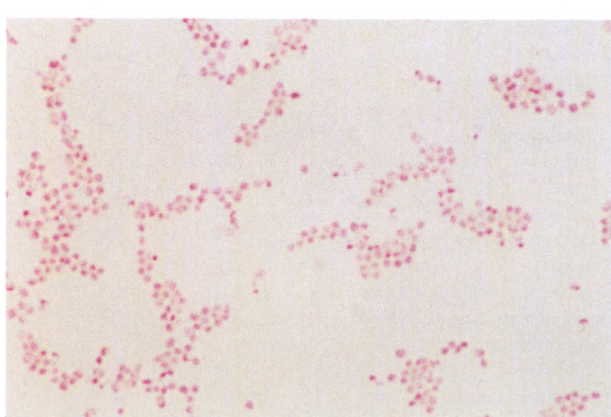

FIGURE 5 *Roseomonas* on Sabouraud dextrose agar showing pink mucoid colonies.

nonfermenters. Clinical isolates have been recovered from blood, wounds, exudates, abscesses, genitourinary sites, continuous ambulatory peritoneal dialysis fluid, and bone (53, 143, 193, 200, 202). A total of 35 cases of opportunistic infections with *Roseomonas* species were reviewed (200). In multiple-case reports, about 60% of the isolates recovered have been from blood, with about 20% from wounds, exudates, and abscesses and about 10% from genitourinary sites (53, 200).

De et al. (53) summarized susceptibility data from three published reports on a combined 80 strains of *Roseomonas*. All strains were susceptible to amikacin (100%); frequently susceptible to imipenem (99%), ciprofloxacin (90%), and ticarcillin (83%); less susceptible to ceftriaxone (38%), trimethoprim-sulfamethoxazole (30%), and ampicillin (13%); and rarely susceptible to ceftazidime (5%). All strains were resistant to cefepime (53). In catheter-related infections, eradication of the organism has proven difficult unless the infected catheter is removed.

ANTIMICROBIAL SUSCEPTIBILITIES

Decisions about performing susceptibility testing are complicated by the fact that the CLSI interpretive guidelines for disk diffusion testing of the nonfermenting gram-negative bacteria are limited to *Pseudomonas* species, *Burkholderia cepacia*, *Stenotrophomonas maltophilia*, and *Acinetobacter* species and therefore, except for *Acinetobacter* species, do not include the organisms covered in this chapter. Furthermore, results obtained with, e.g., *Acinetobacter* species by using disk diffusion do not correlate with results obtained by conventional MIC methods. In general, laboratories should try to avoid performing susceptibility testing on the organisms included in this chapter. When clinical necessity dictates that susceptibility testing be performed, an overnight MIC method, e.g., Etest (bioMérieux) (101), is recommended.

EVALUATION, INTERPRETATION, AND REPORTING OF RESULTS

Although certain nonfermenting bacteria can on occasion be frank pathogens, e.g., *Pseudomonas aeruginosa*, *Burkholderia pseudomallei*, and *Elizabethkingia meningoseptica*, they are generally considered to be of low virulence and often occur in mixed cultures, making it difficult to determine when to work up cultures and when to perform susceptibility studies. *Elizabethkingia meningoseptica* in neonatal meningitis, *Moraxella lacunata* in eye infections, and *M. catarrhalis* in respiratory tract infections should be reported as significant pathogens. Direct Gram stain interpretation of clinical specimens may be of limited importance, because these organisms often occur in mixed infections and because their clinical importance has to be interpreted taking into account the considerations discussed below. Decisions regarding the significance of GNF in a clinical specimen must take into account the clinical condition of the patient and the source of the specimen submitted for culture. In general, the recovery of a GNF in pure culture from a normally sterile site warrants identification and susceptibility testing, whereas predominant growth of a GNF from a nonsterile specimen, such as an endotracheal culture from a patient with no clinical signs or symptoms of pneumonia, would not be worked up further. Because many GNF exhibit multiple-antibiotic resistance, patients who are on antibiotics often become colonized with GNF. GNF species isolated in mixed cultures can usually be reported

by descriptive identification, e.g., "growth of *P. aeruginosa* and two varieties of nonfermenting gram-negative rods not further identified."

REFERENCES

1. **Adams, M. D., K. Goglin, N. Molyneaux, K. M. Hujer, H. Lavender, J. J. Jamison, I. J. MacDonald, K. M. Martin, T. Russo, A. A. Campagnari, A. M. Hujer, R. A. Bonomo, and S. R. Gill.** 2008. Comparative genome sequence analysis of multidrug-resistant *Acinetobacter baumannii*. *J. Bacteriol.* **190:**8053–8064.
2. **Adams, M. D., G. C. Nickel, S. Bajaksouzian, H. Lavender, A. R. Murthy, M. R. Jacobs, and R. A. Bonomo.** 2009. Resistance to colistin in *Acinetobacter baumannii* associated with mutations in the PmrAB two-component system. *Antimicrob. Agents Chemother.* **53:**3628–3634.
3. **Anstey, N. M., B. J. Currie, M. Hassell, D. Palmer, B. Dwyer, and H. Seifert.** 2002. Community-acquired bacteremic *Acinetobacter* pneumonia in tropical Australia is caused by diverse strains of *Acinetobacter baumannii*, with carriage in the throat in at-risk groups. *J. Clin. Microbiol.* **40:**685–686.
4. **Arroyo, L. A., A. Garcia-Curiel, M. E. Pachon-Ibanez, A. C. Llanos, M. Ruiz, J. Pachon, and J. Aznar.** 2005. Reliability of the E-test method for detection of colistin resistance in clinical isolates of *Acinetobacter baumannii*. *J. Clin. Microbiol.* **43:**903–905.
5. **Bachman, K. H., D. L. Sewell, and L. J. Strausbaugh.** 1996. Recurrent cellulitis and bacteremia caused by *Flavobacterium odoratum*. *Clin. Infect. Dis.* **22:**1112–1113.
6. **Bartual, S. G., H. Seifert, C. Hippler, M. A. Luzon, H. Wisplinghoff, and F. Rodriguez-Valera.** 2005. Development of a multilocus sequence typing scheme for characterization of clinical isolates of *Acinetobacter baumannii*. *J. Clin. Microbiol.* **43:**4382–4390.
7. **Bayraktar, M. R., E. Aktas, Y. Ersoy, A. Cicek, and R. Durmaz.** 2007. Postoperative *Chryseobacterium indologenes* bloodstream infection caused by contamination of distillate water. *Infect. Control Hosp. Epidemiol.* **28:**368–369.
8. **Bergogne-Bérézin, E., M. L. Joly-Guillou, and K. J. Towner (ed.).** 1996. Appendix II: selective isolation of *Acinetobacter* spp. by enrichment cultivation, p. 241–242. *In* Acinetobacter: *Microbiology, Epidemiology, Infections, Management.* CRC Press, Boca Raton, FL.
9. **Bergogne-Bérézin, E., and K. J. Towner.** 1996. *Acinetobacter* spp. as nosocomial pathogens: microbiological, clinical, and epidemiological features. *Clin. Microbiol. Rev.* **9:**148–165.
10. **Berlau, J., H. Aucken, H. Malnick, and T. Pitt.** 1999. Distribution of *Acinetobacter* species on skin of healthy humans. *Eur. J. Clin. Microbiol. Infect. Dis.* **18:**179–183.
11. **Bernardet, J.-F., Y. Nakagawa, and B. Holmes.** 2002. Proposed minimal standards for describing new taxa of the family *Flavobacteriaceae* and emended description of the family. *Int. J. Syst. Evol. Microbiol.* **52:**1049–1070.
12. **Bernards, A. T., J. van der Toorn, C. P. A. van Boven, and L. Dijkshoorn.** 1996. Evaluation of the ability of a commercial system to identify *Acinetobacter* genomic species. *Eur. J. Clin. Microbiol. Infect. Dis.* **15:**303–308.
13. **Bizet, C., and J. Bizet.** 1995. Sensibilité comparée de *Ochrobactrum anthropi, Agrobacterium tumefaciens, Alcaligenes faecalis, Alcaligenes denitrificans* subsp. *denitrificans, Alcaligenes denitrificans* subsp. *xylosoxidans* et *Bordetella bronchiseptica* vis-à-vis de 35 antibiotiques dont 17 lactamines. *Pathol. Biol.* **43:**258–263.
14. **Bloch, K. C., R. Nadarajah, and R. Jacobs.** 1997. *Chryseobacterium meningosepticum*: an emerging pathogen among immunocompromised adults. *Medicine* **76:**30–40.
15. **Boerlin, P., S. Eugster, F. Gaschen, R. Straub, and P. Schawalder.** 2001. Transmission of opportunistic pathogens in a veterinary teaching hospital. *Vet. Microbiol.* **82:**347–359.
16. **Bomb, K., A. Arora, and N. Trehan.** 2007. Endocarditis due to *Chryseobacterium meningosepticum*. *Indian J. Med. Microbiol.* **25:**161–162.

17. **Bombicino, K. A., M. N. Almuzara, A. M. Famiglietti, and C. Vay.** 2007. Evaluation of pyrrolidonyl arylamidase for the identification of nonfermenting Gram-negative rods. *Diagn. Microbiol. Infect. Dis.* **57:**101–103. (Erratum, **57:**473.)

18. **Boo, T. W., F. Walsh, and B. Crowley.** 2009. Molecular characterization of carbapenem-resistant *Acinetobacter* species in an Irish university hospital: predominance of *Acinetobacter* genomic species 3. *J. Med. Microbiol.* **58:**209–216.

19. **Bosshard, P. P., R. Zbinden, S. Abels, B. Böddinghaus, M. Altwegg, and E. C. Böttger.** 2006. 16S rRNA gene sequencing versus the API 20 NE system and the VITEK 2 ID-GNB card for identification of nonfermenting gram-negative bacteria in the clinical laboratory. *J. Clin. Microbiol.* **44:**1359–1366.

20. **Botelho-Nevers, E., F. Gouriet, C. Rovery, P. Paris, V. Roux, D. Raoult, and P. Brouqui.** 2005. First case of osteomyelitis due to *Shewanella algae*. *J. Clin. Microbiol.* **43:**5388–5390.

21. **Bouvet, P. J. M., and P. A. D. Grimont.** 1986. Taxonomy of the genus *Acinetobacter* with the recognition of *Acinetobacter baumannii* sp. nov., *Acinetobacter haemolyticus* sp. nov., *Acinetobacter johnsonii* sp. nov., and *Acinetobacter junii* sp. nov. and emended descriptions of *Acinetobacter calcoaceticus* and *Acinetobacter lwoffii*. *Int. J. Syst. Bacteriol.* **36:**228–240.

22. **Bouvet, P. J. M., and P. A. D. Grimont.** 1987. Identification and biotyping of clinical isolates of *Acinetobacter*. *Ann. Inst. Pasteur Microbiol.* **138:**569–578.

23. **Bouvet, P. J. M., and S. Jeanjean.** 1989. Delineation of new proteolytic genomic species in the genus *Acinetobacter*. *Res. Microbiol.* **140:**291–299.

24. **Bovre, K., J. E. Fuglesang, N. Hagen, E. Jantzen, and L. O. Froholm.** 1976. *Moraxella atlantae* sp. nov. and its distinction from *Moraxella phenylpyrouvica*. *Int. J. Syst. Bacteriol.* **26:**511–521.

25. **Bowman, J. P., J. Cavanagh, J. J. Austin, and K. Sanderson.** 1996. Novel *Psychrobacter* species from Antarctic ornithogenic soils. *Int. J. Syst. Bacteriol.* **46:**841–848.

26. **Brown, R. B., D. Phillips, M. J. Barker, R. Pieczarka, M. Sands, and D. Teres.** 1989. Outbreak of nosocomial *Flavobacterium meningosepticum* respiratory infections associated with use of aerosolized polymyxin B. *Am. J. Infect. Control* **17:**121–125.

27. **Brown, W. J., R. L. Sautter, and A. E. Crist, Jr.** 1992. Susceptibility testing of clinical isolates of *Methylobacterium* species. *Antimicrob. Agents Chemother.* **36:**1635–1638.

28. **Butt, A. A., J. Figueroa, and D. H. Martin.** 1997. Ocular infection caused by three unusual marine organisms. *Clin. Infect. Dis.* **24:**740.

29. **Carr, E. L., P. Kämpfer, B. K. Patel, V. Gürtler, and R. J. Seviour.** 2003. Seven novel species of *Acinetobacter* isolated from activated sludge. *Int. J. Syst. Evol. Microbiol.* **53:**953–963.

30. **Casalta, J. P., Y. Peloux, D. Raoult, P. Brunet, and H. Gallais.** 1989. Pneumonia and meningitis caused by a new nonfermentative unknown gram-negative bacterium. *J. Clin. Microbiol.* **27:**1446–1448.

31. **Catry, B., F. Boyen, M. Baele, J. Dewulf, A. de Kruif, M. Vaneechoutte, F. Haesebrouck, and A. Decostere.** 2007. Recovery of *Moraxella ovis* from the bovine respiratory tract and differentiation of *Moraxella* species by tDNA-intergenic spacer PCR. *Vet. Microbiol.* **120:**375–380.

32. **Centers for Disease Control and Prevention.** 2004. *Acinetobacter baumannii* infections among patients at military medical facilities treating injured U.S. service members, 2002–2004. *MMWR Morb. Mortal. Wkly. Rep.* **53:**1063–1066.

33. **Ceyhan, M., I. Yildirim, A. Tekeli, M. Yurdakok, E. Us, B. Altun, T. Kutluk, A. B. Cengiz, V. Gurbuz, C. Barin, A. Bagdat, D. Cetinkaya, D. Gur, and O. Tuncel.** 2008. A *Chryseobacterium meningosepticum* outbreak observed in 3 clusters involving both neonatal and non-neonatal pediatric patients. *Am. J. Infect. Control* **36:**453–457.

34. **Chang, H. C., Y. F. Wei, L. Dijkshoorn, M. Vaneechoutte, C. T. Tang, and T. C. Chang.** 2005. Species-level identification of isolates of the *Acinetobacter calcoaceticus-Acinetobacter baumannii* complex by sequence analysis of the 16S-23S rRNA gene spacer region. *J. Clin. Microbiol.* **43:**1632–1639.

35. **Chang, J.-C., P.-R. Hsueh, J.-J. Wu, S.-W. Ho, W.-C. Hsieh, and K.-T. Luh.** 1997. Antimicrobial susceptibility of flavobacteria as determined by agar dilution and disk diffusion methods. *Antimicrob. Agents Chemother.* **41:**1301–1306.

36. **Chen, Y.-S., Y.-C. Liu, M.-Y. Yen, J.-H. Wang, J.-H. Wang, S.-R. Wann, and D.-L. Cheng.** 1997. Skin and soft-tissue manifestations of *Shewanella putrefaciens* infection. *Clin. Infect. Dis.* **25:**225–229.

37. **Chiron, R., H. Marchandin, F. Counil, E. Jumas-Bilak, A. M. Freydiere, G. Bellon, M. O. Husson, D. Turck, F. Bremont, G. Chabanon, and C. Segonds.** 2005. Clinical and microbiological features of *Inquilinus* sp. isolates from five patients with cystic fibrosis. *J. Clin. Microbiol.* **43:**3938–3943.

38. **Chiu, C.-H., M. Waddingdon, W.-S. Hsieh, D. Greenberg, P. C. Schreckenberger, and A. M. Carnahan.** 2000. Atypical *Chryseobacterium meningosepticum* and meningitis and sepsis in newborns and the immunocompromised, Taiwan. *Emerg. Infect. Dis.* **6:**481–486.

39. **Chu, Y. W., T. K. Cheung, M. Y. Chu, J. Y. Lo, and L. Dijkshoorn.** 2009. OXA-23-type imipenem resistance in *Acinetobacter baumannii* in Hong Kong. *Int. J. Antimicrob. Agents* **34:**285–286.

40. **Chu, Y. W., C. M. Leung, E. T. Houang, K. C. Ng, C. B. Leung, H. Y. Leung, and A. F. Cheng.** 1999. Skin carriage of acinetobacters in Hong Kong. *J. Clin. Microbiol.* **37:**2962–2967.

41. **Cisneros, J. M., M. J. Reyes, J. Pachon, B. Becerril, F. J. Caballero, J. L. Garcia-Garmendia, C. Ortiz, and A. R. Cobacho.** 1996. Bacteremia due to *Acinetobacter baumannii*: epidemiology, clinical findings, and prognostic features. *Clin. Infect. Dis.* **22:**1026–1032.

42. **Coenye, T., J. Goris, T. Spilker, P. Vandamme, and J. J. LiPuma.** 2002. Characterization of unusual bacteria isolated from respiratory secretions of cystic fibrosis patients and description of *Inquilinus limosus* gen. nov., sp. nov. *J. Clin. Microbiol.* **40:**2062–2069.

43. **Cohen, M. F., X. Y. Han, and M. Mazzola.** 2004. Molecular and physiological comparison of *Azospirillum* spp. isolated from *Rhizoctonia solani* mycelia, wheat rhizosphere, and human skin wounds. *Can. J. Microbiol.* **50:**291–297.

44. **Cruze, J. A., J. T. Singer, and W. R. Finnerty.** 1979. Conditions for quantitative transformation in *Acinetobacter calcoaceticus*. *Curr. Microbiol.* **3:**129–132.

45. **Daley, D., S. Neville, and K. Kociuba.** 1997. Peritonitis associated with a CDC group EO-3 organism. *J. Clin. Microbiol.* **35:**3338–3339.

46. **Dan, M., R. Gutman, and A. Biro.** 1992. Peritonitis caused by *Pseudomonas putrefaciens* in patients undergoing continuous ambulatory peritoneal dialysis. *Clin. Infect. Dis.* **14:**359–360.

47. **Daneshvar, M. I., B. Hill, D. G. Hollis, C. W. Moss, J. G. Jordan, J. P. MacGregor, F. Tenover, and R. S. Weyant.** 1998. CDC group O-3: phenotypic characteristics, fatty acid composition, isoprenoid quinone content, and in vitro antimicrobic susceptibilities of an unusual gram-negative bacterium isolated from clinical specimens. *J. Clin. Microbiol.* **36:**1674–1678.

48. **Daneshvar, M. I., D. G. Hollis, R. S. Weyant, A. G. Steigerwalt, A. M. Whitney, M. P. Douglas, J. P. Macgregor, J. G. Jordan, L. W. Mayer, S. M. Rassouli, W. Barchet, C. Munro, L. Shuttleworth, and K. Bernard.** 2003. *Paracoccus yeeii* sp. nov. (formerly CDC group EO-2), a novel bacterial species associated with human infection. *J. Clin. Microbiol.* **41:**1289–1294.

49. **Das, K., S. Shah, and M. H. Levi.** 1997. Misleading Gram stain from a patient with *Moraxella* (*Branhamella*) *catarrhalis* bacteremia. *Clin. Microbiol. Newsl.* **19:**85–88.

50. **Da Silva, G. J., L. Dijkshoorn, T. van der Reijden, B. van Strijen, and A. Duarte.** 2007. Identification of widespread, closely related *Acinetobacter baumannii* isolates in Portugal as a subgroup of European clone II. *Clin. Microbiol. Infect.* **13:**190–195.

51. **Dauga, C., M. Gillis, P. Vandamme, E. Ageron, F. Grimont, K. Kersters, C. de Mahenge, Y. Peloux, and P. A. D. Grimont.** 1993. *Balneatrix alpica* gen. nov., sp. nov., a bacterium associated with pneumonia and meningitis in a spa therapy centre. *Res. Microbiol.* **144:**35–46.

52. **Davis, K. A., K. A. Moran, C. K. McAllister, and P. G. Gray.** 2005. Multidrug-resistant *Acinetobacter* extremity infections in soldiers. *Emerg. Infect. Dis.* **11:**1218–1224.

53. **De, I., K. V. I. Rolston, and X. Y. Han.** 2004. Clinical significance of *Roseomonas* species isolated from catheter and blood samples: analysis of 36 cases in patients with cancer. *Clin. Infect. Dis.* **38:**1579–1584.

54. **De Baere, T., A. Muylaert, E. Everaert, G. Wauters, G. Claeys, G. Verschraegen, and M. Vaneechoutte.** 2002. Bacteremia due to *Moraxella atlantae* in a cancer patient. *J. Clin. Microbiol.* **40:**2693–2695.

55. **de Beaufort, A. J., A. T. Bernards, L. Dijkshoorn, and C. P. van Boven.** 1999. *Acinetobacter junii* causes life-threatening sepsis in preterm infants. *Acta Paediatr.* **88:**772–775.

56. **Dijkshoorn, L., M. F. Michel, and J. E. Degener.** 1987. Cell envelope protein profiles of *Acinetobacter calcoaceticus* strains isolated in hospitals. *J. Med. Microbiol.* **23:**313–319.

57. **Dijkshoorn, L., and A. Nemec.** 2008. The diversity of the genus *Acinetobacter*, p. 1–34. *In* U. Gerischer (ed.), Acinetobacter *Molecular Microbiology.* Caister Academic Press, Norfolk, United Kingdom.

58. **Dijkshoorn, L., A. Nemec, and H. Seifert.** 2007. An increasing threat in hospitals: multidrug-resistant *Acinetobacter baumannii*. *Nat. Rev. Microbiol.* **5:**939–951.

59. **Dijkshoorn, L., E. van Aken, L. Shunburne, T. van der Reijden, A. T. Bernards, A. Nemec, and K. J. Towner.** 2005. Prevalence of *Acinetobacter baumannii* and other *Acinetobacter* spp. in faecal samples from non-hospitalised individuals. *Clin. Microbiol. Infect.* **11:**329–332.

60. **Dijkshoorn, L., B. van Harsselaar, I. Tjernberg, P. J. Bouvet, and M. Vaneechoutte.** 1998. Evaluation of amplified ribosomal DNA restriction analysis for identification of *Acinetobacter* genomic species. *Syst. Appl. Microbiol.* **21:**33–39.

61. **Dijkshoorn, L., W. Van Vianen, J. E. Degener, and M. F. Michel.** 1987. Typing of *Acinetobacter calcoaceticus* strains isolated from hospital patients by cell envelope protein profiles. *Epidemiol. Infect.* **99:**659–667.

62. **Dobrewski, R., E. Savov, A. T. Bernards, M. van den Barselaar, P. Nordmann, P. J. van den Broek, and L. Dijkshoorn.** 2006. Genotypic diversity and antibiotic susceptibility of *Acinetobacter baumannii* isolates in a Bulgarian hospital. *Clin. Microbiol. Infect.* **12:**1135–1137.

63. **Dortet, L., P. Legrand, C. J. Soussy, and V. Cattoir.** 2006. Bacterial identification, clinical significance, and antimicrobial susceptibilities of *Acinetobacter ursingii* and *Acinetobacter schindleri*, two frequently misidentified opportunistic pathogens. *J. Clin. Microbiol.* **44:**4471–4478.

64. **Dunne, W. M., Jr., J. Tillman, and J. C. Murray.** 1993. Recovery of a strain of *Agrobacterium radiobacter* with a mucoid phenotype from an immunocompromised child with bacteremia. *J. Clin. Microbiol.* **31:**2541–2543.

65. **Ecker, J. A., C. Massire, T. A. Hall, R. Ranken, T. T. Pennella, I. C. Agasino, L. B. Blyn, S. A. Hofstadler, T. P. Endy, P. T. Scott, L. Lindler, T. Hamilton, C. Gaddy, K. Snow, M. Pe, J. Fishbain, D. Craft, G. Deye, S. Riddell, E. Milstrey, B. Petruccelli, S. Brisse, V. Harpin, A. Schink, D. J. Ecker, R. Sampath, and M. W. Eshoo.** 2006. Identification of *Acinetobacter* species and genotyping of *Acinetobacter baumannii* by multilocus PCR and mass spectrometry. *J. Clin. Microbiol.* **44:**2921–2932.

66. **Edmond, M. B., S. A. Riddler, C. M. Baxter, B. M. Wicklund, and A. W. Pasculle.** 1993. *Agrobacterium radiobacter*: a recently recognized opportunistic pathogen. *Clin. Infect. Dis.* **16:**388–391.

67. **Ehrenstein, B., A. T. Bernards, L. Dijkshoorn, P. Gerner-Smidt, K. J. Towner, P. J. Bouvet, F. D. Daschner, and H. Grundmann.** 1996. *Acinetobacter* species identification by using tRNA spacer fingerprinting. *J. Clin. Microbiol.* **34:**2414–2420.

68. **Ellington, M. J., J. Kistler, D. M. Livermore, and N. Woodford.** 2007. Multiplex PCR for rapid detection of genes encoding acquired metallo-beta-lactamases. *J. Antimicrob. Chemother.* **59:**321–322.

69. **Ezzedine, H., M. Mourad, C. Van Ossel, C. Logghe, J. P. Squifflet, F. Renault, G. Wauters, J. Gigi, L. Wilmotte, and J. J. Haxha.** 1994. An outbreak of *Ochrobactrum anthropi* bacteraemia in five organ transplant patients. *J. Hosp. Infect.* **27:**35–42.

70. **Fass, R. J., and J. Barnishan.** 1980. In vitro susceptibility of nonfermentative gram-negative bacilli other than *Pseudomonas aeruginosa* to 32 antimicrobial agents. *Rev. Infect. Dis.* **2:**841–853.

71. **Fournier, P. E., D. Vallenet, V. Barbe, S. Audic, H. Ogata, L. Poirel, H. Richet, C. Robert, S. Mangenot, C. Abergel, P. Nordmann, J. Weissenbach, D. Raoult, and J. M. Claverie.** 2006. Comparative genomics of multidrug resistance in *Acinetobacter baumannii*. *PLoS Genet.* **2:**e7.

72. **Fraser, S. L., and J. H. Jorgensen.** 1997. Reappraisal of the antimicrobial susceptibilities of *Chryseobacterium* and *Flavobacterium* species and methods for reliable susceptibility testing. *Antimicrob. Agents Chemother.* **41:**2738–2741.

73. **Freney, J., W. Hansen, C. Ploton, H. Meugnier, S. Madier, N. Bornstein, and J. Fleurette.** 1987. Septicemia caused by *Sphingobacterium multivorum*. *J. Clin. Microbiol.* **25:**1126–1128.

74. **Gallego, V., M. T. Garcia, and A. Ventosa.** 2005. *Methylobacterium isbiliense* sp. nov., isolated from the drinking water system of Sevilla, Spain. *Int. J. Syst. Evol. Microbiol.* **55:**2333–2337.

75. **Gerner-Smidt, P., I. Tjernberg, and J. Ursing.** 1991. Reliability of phenotypic tests for identification of *Acinetobacter* species. *J. Clin. Microbiol.* **29:**277–282.

76. **Gini, G. A.** 1990. Ocular infection caused by *Psychrobacter immobilis* acquired in the hospital. *J. Clin. Microbiol.* **28:**400–401.

77. **Green, O., P. Murray, and J. C. Gea-Banacloche.** 2008. Sepsis caused by *Elizabethkingia miricola* successfully treated with tigecycline and levofloxacin. *Diagn. Microbiol. Infect. Dis.* **62:**430–432.

78. **Green, P. N., I. J. Bousfield, and D. Hood.** 1988. Three new *Methylobacterium* species: *M. rhodesianum* sp. nov., *M. zatmanii* sp. nov., and *M. fujisawaense* sp. nov. *Int. J. Syst. Bacteriol.* **38:**124–127.

79. **Greenberg, D. E., S. F. Porcella, F. Stock, A. Wong, P. S. Conville, P. R. Murray, S. M. Holland, and A. M. Zelazny.** 2006. *Granulibacter bethesdensis* gen. nov., sp. nov., a distinctive pathogenic acetic acid bacterium in the family *Acetobacteraceae*. *Int. J. Syst. Evol. Microbiol.* **56:**2609–2616.

80. **Grundmann, H. J., K. J. Towner, L. Dijkshoorn, P. Gerner-Smidt, M. Maher, H. Seifert, and M. Vaneechoutte.** 1997. Multicenter study using standardized protocols and reagents for evaluation of reproducibility of PCR-based fingerprinting of *Acinetobacter* spp. *J. Clin. Microbiol.* **35:**3071–3077.

81. **Gundi, V. A., L. Dijkshoorn, S. Burignat, D. Raoult, and S. B. La.** 2009. Validation of partial *rpoB* gene sequence analysis for the identification of clinically important and emerging *Acinetobacter* species. *Microbiology* **155:**2333–2341.

82. **Han, X. Y., A. S. Pham, J. J. Tarrand, K. V. Rolston, L. O. Helsel, and P. N. Levett.** 2003. Bacteriologic characterization of 36 strains of *Roseomonas* species and proposal of *Roseomonas mucosa* sp. nov. and *Roseomonas gilardii* subsp. *rosea* subsp. nov. *Am. J. Clin. Pathol.* **120:**256–264.

83. **Hawley, H. B., and D. W. Gump.** 1973. Vancomycin therapy of bacterial meningitis. *Am. J. Dis. Child.* **126:**261–264.

84. **Helsel, L. O., D. G. Hollis, A. G. Steigerwalt, R. E. Morey, J. Jordan, T. Aye, J. Radosevic, D. Jannat-Khah, D. Thiry, D. R. Lonsway, J. B. Patel, M. I. Daneshvar, and P. N. Levett.** 2007. Identification of "*Haematobacter*," a new genus of aerobic gram-negative rods isolated from clinical specimens, and reclassification of *Rhodobacter massiliensis* as "*Haematobacter massiliensis* comb. nov." *J. Clin. Microbiol.* **45:**1238–1243.

85. **Hollis, D. G., M. I. Daneshvar, C. W. Moss, and C. N. Baker.** 1995. Phenotypic characteristics, fatty acid composition, and isoprenoid quinone content of CDC group IIg bacteria. *J. Clin. Microbiol.* **33:**762–764.

86. **Hollis, D. G., C. W. Moss, M. I. Daneshvar, L. Meadows, J. Jordan, and B. Hill.** 1993. Characterization of Centers for Disease Control group NO-1, a fastidious, nonoxidative, gram-negative organism associated with dog and cat bites. *J. Clin. Microbiol.* **31**:746–748.

87. **Holmes, B., M. Costas, A. C. Wood, R. J. Owen, and D. D. Morgan.** 1990. Differentiation of *Achromobacter*-like strains from human blood by DNA restriction endonuclease digest and ribosomal RNA gene probe patterns. *Epidemiol. Infect.* **105**:541–551.

88. **Holmes, B., R. Lewis, and A. Trevett.** 1992. Septicaemia due to *Achromobacter* group B: a report of two cases. *Med. Microbiol. Lett.* **1**:177–184.

89. **Holmes, B., R. J. Owen, A. Evans, H. Malnick, and W. R. Willcox.** 1977. *Pseudomonas paucimobilis*, a new species isolated from human clinical specimens, the hospital environment, and other sources. *Int. J. Syst. Bacteriol.* **27**:133–146.

90. **Holmes, B., R. J. Owen, and D. G. Hollis.** 1982. *Flavobacterium spiritivorum*, a new species isolated from human clinical specimens. *Int. J. Syst. Bacteriol.* **32**:157–165.

91. **Holmes, B., R. J. Owen, and R. E. Weaver.** 1981. *Flavobacterium multivorum*, a new species isolated from human clinical specimens and previously known as group IIK, biotype 2. *Int. J. Syst. Bacteriol.* **31**:21–34.

92. **Holmes, B., C. A. Pinning, and C. A. Dawson.** 1986. A probability matrix for the identification of Gram-negative, aerobic, non-fermentative bacteria that grow on nutrient agar. *J. Gen. Microbiol.* **132**:1827–1842.

93. **Holmes, B., M. Popoff, M. Kiredjian, and K. Kersters.** 1988. *Ochrobactrum anthropi* gen. nov., sp. nov. from human clinical specimens and previously known as group Vd. *Int. J. Syst. Bacteriol.* **38**:406–416.

94. **Holmes, B., P. Segers, T. Coenye, M. Vancanneyt, and P. Vandamme.** 2006. *Pannonibacter phragmitetus*, described from a Hungarian soda lake in 2003, had been recognized several decades earlier from human blood cultures as *Achromobacter* groups B and E. *Int. J. Syst. Evol. Microbiol.* **56**:2945–2948.

95. **Holmes, B., J. J. S. Snell, and S. P. Lapage.** 1979. *Flavobacterium odoratum*: a species resistant to a wide range of antimicrobial agents. *J. Clin. Pathol.* **32**:73–77.

96. **Holmes, B., A. G. Steigerwalt, R. E. Weaver, and D. J. Brenner.** 1986. *Weeksella virosa* gen. nov., sp. nov. (formerly group IIf), found in human clinical specimens. *Syst. Appl. Microbiol.* **8**:185–190.

97. **Holmes, B., A. G. Steigerwalt, R. E. Weaver, and D. J. Brenner.** 1986. *Weeksella zoohelcum* sp. nov. (formerly group IIj), from human clinical specimens. *Syst. Appl. Microbiol.* **8**:191–196.

98. **Holmes, B., R. E. Weaver, A. G. Steigerwalt, and D. J. Brenner.** 1988. A taxonomic study of *Flavobacterium spiritivorum* and *Sphingobacterium mizutae*: proposal of *Flavobacterium yabuuchiae* sp. nov. and *Flavobacterium mizutaii* comb. nov. *Int. J. Syst. Bacteriol.* **38**:348–353.

99. **Holt, H. M., P. Sogaard, and B. Gahrn-Hansen.** 1997. Ear infections with *Shewanella alga*: a bacteriologic, clinical and epidemiologic study of 67 cases. *Clin. Microbiol. Infect.* **3**:329–334.

100. **Hornei, B., E. Luneberg, H. Schmidt-Rotte, M. Maab, K. Weber. F. Heits, M. Frosch, and W. Solbach.** 1999. Systemic infection of an immunocompromised patient with *Methylobacterium zatmanii*. *J. Clin. Microbiol.* **37**:248–250.

101. **Hsueh, P.-R., J.-C. Chang, L.-J. Teng, P.-C. Yang, S.-W. Ho, W.-C. Hsieh, and K.-T. Luh.** 1997. Comparison of Etest and agar dilution method for antimicrobial susceptibility testing of *Flavobacterium* isolates. *J. Clin. Microbiol.* **35**:1021–1023.

102. **Hsueh, P.-R., L.-J. Teng, S.-W. Ho, W.-C. Hsieh, and K.-T. Luh.** 1996. Clinical and microbiological characteristics of *Flavobacterium indologenes* infections associated with indwelling devices. *J. Clin. Microbiol.* **34**:1908–1913.

103. **Hsueh, P.-R., L.-J. Teng, P.-C. Yang, Y.-C. Chen, H.-J. Pan, S.-W. Ho, and K.-T. Luh.** 1998. Nosocomial infections caused by *Sphingomonas paucimobilis*: clinical features and microbiological characteristics. *Clin. Infect. Dis.* **26**:676–681.

104. **Hsueh, P.-R., J.-J. Wu, T.-R. Hsiue, and W.-C. Hsieh.** 1995. Bacteremic necrotizing fasciitis due to *Flavobacterium odoratum*. *Clin. Infect. Dis.* **21**:1337–1338.

105. **Hulse, M., S. Johnson, and P. Ferrieri.** 1993. *Agrobacterium* infections in humans: experience at one hospital and review. *Clin. Infect. Dis.* **16**:112–117.

106. **Hung, P. P., Y. H. Lin, C. F. Lin, M. F. Liu, and Z. Y. Shi.** 2008. *Chryseobacterium meningosepticum* infection: antibiotic susceptibility and risk factors for mortality. *J. Microbiol. Immunol. Infect.* **41**:137–144.

107. **Hung, Y. T., Y. T. Lee, L. J. Huang, T. L. Chen, K. W. Yu, C. P. Fung, W. L. Cho, and C. Y. Liu.** 2009. Clinical characteristics of patients with *Acinetobacter junii* infection. *J. Microbiol. Immunol. Infect.* **42**:47–53.

108. **Huys, G., M. Cnockaert, M. Vaneechoutte, N. Woodford, A. Nemec, L. Dijkshoorn, and J. Swings.** 2005. Distribution of tetracycline resistance genes in genotypically related and unrelated multiresistant *Acinetobacter baumannii* strains from different European hospitals. *Res. Microbiol.* **156**:348–355.

109. **Iacono, M., L. Villa, D. Fortini, R. Bordoni, F. Imperi, R. J. Bonnal, T. Sicheritz-Ponten, B. G. De, P. Visca, A. Cassone, and A. Carattoli.** 2008. Whole-genome pyrosequencing of an epidemic multidrug-resistant *Acinetobacter baumannii* strain belonging to the European clone II group. *Antimicrob. Agents Chemother.* **52**:2616–2625.

110. **Iwata, M., K. Tateda, T. Matsumoto, N. Furuya, S. Mizuiri, and K. Yamaguchi.** 1999. Primary *Shewanella alga* septicemia in a patient on hemodialysis. *J. Clin. Microbiol.* **37**:2104–2105.

111. **Jannes, G., M. Vaneechoutte, M. Lannoo, M. Gillis, M. Vancanneyt, P. Vandamme, G. Verschraegen, H. van Heuverswyn, and R. Rossau.** 1993. Polyphasic taxonomy leading to the proposal of *Moraxella canis* sp. nov. for *Moraxella catarrhalis*-like strains. *Int. J. Syst. Bacteriol.* **43**:438–449.

112. **Janssen, P., K. Maquelin, R. Coopman, I. Tjernberg, P. Bouvet, K. Kersters, and L. Dijkshoorn.** 1997. Discrimination of *Acinetobacter* genomic species by AFLP fingerprinting. *Int. J. Syst. Bacteriol.* **47**:1179–1187.

113. **Jawad, A., P. M. Hawkey, J. Heritage, and A. M. Snelling.** 1994. Description of Leeds Acinetobacter Medium, a new selective and differential medium for isolation of clinically important *Acinetobacter* spp., and comparison with *Herellea* agar and Holton's agar. *J. Clin. Microbiol.* **32**:2353–2358.

114. **Jenks, P. J., and E. J. Shaw.** 1997. Recurrent septicaemia due to "*Achromobacter* group B." *J. Infect.* **34**:143–145.

115. **Joly-Guillou, M. L.** 2005. Clinical impact and pathogenicity of *Acinetobacter*. *Clin. Microbiol. Infect.* **11**:868–873.

116. **Juni, E.** 2005. Genus II. *Acinetobacter* Brisou and Prévot 1954, p. 425–437. *In* G. M. Garrity, D. J. Brenner, N. R. Krieg, and J. T. Staley (ed.), *Bergey's Manual of Systematic Bacteriology*, 2nd ed., vol. 2. Springer-Verlag, New York, NY.

117. **Juni, E., and G. A. Heym.** 1986. *Psychrobacter immobilis* gen. nov., sp. nov.: genospecies composed of gram-negative, aerobic, oxidase-positive coccobacilli. *Int. J. Syst. Bacteriol.* **36**:388–391.

118. **Kämpfer, P., A. Albrecht, S. Buczolitz, and H. J. Busse.** 2002. *Psychrobacter faecalis* sp. nov., a new species from a bioaerosol originating from pigeon faeces. *Syst. Appl. Microbiol.* **25**:31–36.

119. **Kämpfer, P., V. Avesani, M. Janssens, J. Charlier, T. De Baere, and M. Vaneechoutte.** 2006. Description of *Wautersiella falsenii* gen. nov., sp. nov., to accommodate clinical isolates phenotypically resembling members of the genera *Chryseobacterium* and *Empedobacter*. *Int. J. Syst. Evol. Microbiol.* **56**:2323–2329.

120. **Kämpfer, P., M. Vaneechoutte, N. Lodders, T. De Baere, V. Avesani, M. Janssens, H.-J. Busse, and G. Wauters.** 2009. Description of *Chryseobacterium anthropi* sp. nov. to accommodate clinical isolates biochemically similar to *Kaistella koreensis* and *Chryseobacterium haifense*, proposal to reclassify *Kaistella koreensis* as *Chryseobacterium koreense* comb. nov. and emended description of the genus *Chryseobacterium*. *Int. J. Syst. Evol. Microbiol.* **59**:2421–2428.

121. **Kappstein, I., H. Grundmann, T. Hauer, and C. Niemeyer.** 2000. Aerators as a reservoir of *Acinetobacter junii*: an outbreak of bacteraemia in paediatric oncology patients. *J. Hosp. Infect.* **44:**27–30.

122. **Karalus, R., and A. Campagnari.** 2000. *Moraxella catarrhalis*: a review of an important human mucosal pathogen. *Microbes Infect.* **2:**547–559.

123. **Katsura, K., H. Kawasaki, W. Potacharoen, S. Saono, T. Seki, Y. Yamada, T. Uchimura, and K. Komagata.** 2001. *Asaia siamensis* sp. nov., an acetic acid bacterium in the α-Proteobacteria. *Int. J. Syst. Evol. Microbiol.* **51:**559–563.

124. **Kaye, K. M., A. Macone, and P. H. Kazanjian.** 1992. Catheter infection caused by *Methylobacterium* in immunocompromised hosts: report of three cases and review of the literature. *Clin. Infect. Dis.* **14:**1010–1014.

125. **Kern, W. V., M. Oethinger, A. Kaufhold, E. Rozdzinski, and R. Marre.** 1993. *Ochrobactrum anthropi* bacteremia: report of four cases and short review. *Infection* **21:**306–310.

126. **Khashe, S., and J. M. Janda.** 1998. Biochemical and pathogenic properties of *Shewanella alga* and *Shewanella putrefaciens*. *J. Clin. Microbiol.* **36:**783–787.

127. **Kim, K. K., M. K. Kim, J. H. Lim, H. Y. Park, and S.-T. Lee.** 2005. Transfer of *Chryseobacterium meningosepticum* and *Chryseobacterium miricola* to *Elizabethkingia* gen. nov. as *Elizabethkingia meningoseptica* comb. nov. and *Elizabethkingia miricola* comb. nov. *Int. J. Syst. Evol. Microbiol.* **55:**1287–1293.

128. **Ko, K. S., N. Y. Lee, W. S. Oh, J. H. Lee, H. K. Ki, K. R. Peck, and J.-H. Song.** 2005. *Tepidimonas arfidensis* sp. nov., a novel gram-negative and thermophilic bacterium isolated from the bone marrow of a patient with leukemia in Korea. *Microbiol. Immunol.* **49:**785–788.

129. **Ko, W. C., N. Y. Lee, S. C. Su, L. Dijkshoorn, M. Vaneechoutte, L. R. Wang, J. J. Yan, and T. C. Chang.** 2008. Oligonucleotide array-based identification of species in the *Acinetobacter calcoaceticus-A. baumannii* complex in isolates from blood cultures and antimicrobial susceptibility testing of the isolates. *J. Clin. Microbiol.* **46:**2052–2059.

130. **Koh, T. H., L. H. Sng, G. C. Wang, L. Y. Hsu, and Y. Zhao.** 2007. IMP-4 and OXA beta-lactamases in *Acinetobacter baumannii* from Singapore. *J. Antimicrob. Chemother.* **59:**627–632.

131. **Lambiase, A., M. Del Pezzo, V. Raia, A. Sepe, P. Ferri, and F. Rossano.** 2007. *Chryseobacterium* respiratory tract infections in patients with cystic fibrosis. *J. Infect.* **55:**518–523.

132. **Lee, C. H., W. C. Lin, J. H. Chia, L. H. Su, C. C. Chien, A. H. Mao, and J. W. Liu.** 2008. Community-acquired osteomyelitis caused by *Chryseobacterium meningosepticum*: case report and literature review. *Diagn. Microbiol. Infect. Dis.* **60:**89–93.

133. **Lee, S. W., C. A. Tsai, and B. J. Lee.** 2008. *Chryseobacterium meningosepticum* sepsis complicated with retroperitoneal hematoma and pleural effusion in a diabetic patient. *J. Chin. Med. Assoc.* **71:**473–476.

134. **Leung, W. S., C. M. Chu, K. Y. Tsang, F. H. Lo, K. F. Lo, and P. L. Ho.** 2006. Fulminant community-acquired *Acinetobacter baumannii* pneumonia as a distinct clinical syndrome. *Chest* **129:**102–109.

135. **Lin, P. Y., C. Chu, L. H. Su, C. T. Huang, W. Y. Chang, and C. H. Chiu.** 2004. Clinical and microbiological analysis of bloodstream infections caused by *Chryseobacterium meningosepticum* in nonneonatal patients. *J. Clin. Microbiol.* **42:**3353–3355.

136. **Lin, X. H., Y. H. Xu, J. Cheng, T. Li, and Z. X. Wang.** 2008. Heterogeneity of *bla*IND metallo-β-lactamase-producing *Chryseobacterium indologenes* isolates detected in Hefei, China. *Int. J. Antimicrob. Agents* **32:**398–400.

137. **Lloyd-Puryear, M., D. Wallace, T. Baldwin, and D. G. Hollis.** 1991. Meningitis caused by *Psychrobacter immobilis* in an infant. *J. Clin. Microbiol.* **29:**2041–2042.

138. **López, F. C., F. F. de Luna, M. C. Delgado, I. I. de la Rosa, S. Valdezate, J. A. Nieto, and M. Casal.** 2008. *Granulibacter bethesdensis* isolated in a child patient with chronic granulomatous disease. *J. Infect.* **57:**275–277.

139. **Loubinoux, J., L. Mihaila-Amrouche, A. Le Fleche, E. Pigne, G. Huchon, P. A. Grimont, and A. Bouvet.** 2003. Bacteremia caused by *Acinetobacter ursingii*. *J. Clin. Microbiol.* **41:**1337–1338.

140. **MacDonell, M. T., and R. R. Colwell.** 1985. Phylogeny of the *Vibrionaceae*, and recommendation for two new genera, *Listonella* and *Shewanella*. *Syst. Appl. Microbiol.* **6:**171–182.

141. **Mahmood, M. S., A. R. Sarwari, M. A. Khan, Z. Sophie, E. Khan, and S. Sami.** 2000. Infective endocarditis and septic embolization with *Ochrobactrum anthropi*: case report and review of literature. *J. Infect.* **40:**287–290.

142. **Marchaim, D., S. Navon-Venezia, D. Schwartz, J. Tarabeia, I. Fefer, M. J. Schwaber, and Y. Carmeli.** 2007. Surveillance cultures and duration of carriage of multi-drug-resistant *Acinetobacter baumannii*. *J. Clin. Microbiol.* **45:**1551–1555.

143. **Marin, M. E., J. Marco Del Pont, E. Dibar, L. Fernandez Caniggia, G. Greco, Y. Flores, and A. Ascione.** 2001. Catheter-related bacteremia caused by *Roseomonas gilardii* in an immunocompromised patient. *Int. J. Infect. Dis.* **5:**170–171.

144. **Mesnard, R., J. M. Sire, P. Y. Donnio, J. Y. Riou, and J. L. Avril.** 1992. Septic arthritis due to *Oligella urethralis*. *Eur. J. Clin. Microbiol. Infect. Dis.* **11:**195–196.

145. **Moller, L. V. M., J. P. Arends, H. J. M. Harmsen, A. Talens, P. Terpstra, and M. J. H. Slooff.** 1999. *Ochrobactrum intermedium* infection after liver transplantation. *J. Clin. Microbiol.* **37:**241–244.

146. **Montejo, M., K. Aguirrebengoa, J. Ugalde, L. Lopez, J. A. S. Nieto, and J. L. Hernández.** 2001. *Bergeyella zoohelcum* bacteremia after a dog bite. *Clin. Infect. Dis.* **33:**1608–1609.

147. **Moore, J. E., M. McCalmont, J. Xu, B. C. Millar, and N. Heaney.** 2002. *Asaia* sp., an unusual spoilage organism of fruit-flavored bottled water. *Appl. Environ. Microbiol.* **68:**4130–4131.

148. **Morrison, A. J., and J. A. Shulman.** 1986. Community-acquired bloodstream infection caused by *Pseudomonas paucimobilis*: case report and review of literature. *J. Clin. Microbiol.* **24:**853–855.

149. **Nemec, A., T. De Baere, I. Tjernberg, M. Vaneechoutte, T. J. K. van der Reijden, and L. Dijkshoorn.** 2001. *Acinetobacter ursingii* sp. nov. and *Acinetobacter schindleri* sp. nov., isolated from human clinical specimens. *Int. J. Syst. Evol. Microbiol.* **51:**1891–1899.

150. **Nemec, A., L. Dijkshoorn, I. Cleenwerck, T. De Baere, D. Janssens, T. J. K. van der Reijden, P. Jezek, and M. Vaneechoutte.** 2003. *Acinetobacter parvus* sp. nov., a small-colony-forming species isolated from human clinical specimens. *Int. J. Syst. Evol. Microbiol.* **53:**1563–1567.

151. **Nemec, A., L. Dijkshoorn, and T. van der Reijden.** 2004. Long-term predominance of two pan-European clones among multi-resistant *Acinetobacter baumannii* strains in the Czech Republic. *J. Med. Microbiol.* **53:**147–153.

152. **Nemec, A., L. Krizova, M. Maixnerova, L. Diancourt, T. J. van der Reijden, S. Brisse, P. van den Broek, and L. Dijkshoorn.** 2008. Emergence of carbapenem resistance in *Acinetobacter baumannii* in the Czech Republic is associated with the spread of multidrug-resistant strains of European clone II. *J. Antimicrob. Chemother.* **62:**484–489.

153. **Nemec, A., M. Maixnerova, T. J. van der Reijden, P. J. van den Broek, and L. Dijkshoorn.** 2007. Relationship between the AdeABC efflux system gene content, netilmicin susceptibility and multidrug resistance in a genotypically diverse collection of *Acinetobacter baumannii* strains. *J. Antimicrob. Chemother.* **60:**483–489.

154. **Nemec, A., M. Musílek, M. Maixnerová, T. De Baere, T. J. K. van der Reijden, M. Vaneechoutte, and L. Dijkshoorn.** 2009. *Acinetobacter beijerinckii* sp. nov. and *Acinetobacter gyllenbergii* sp. nov., haemolytic organisms isolated from humans. *Int. J. Syst. Evol. Microbiol.* **59:**118–124.

155. **Nemec, A., M. Musílek, O. Šedo, T. De Baere, M. Maixnerová, T. J. K. van der Reijden, Z. Zdráhal, M. Vaneechoutte, and L. Dijkshoorn.** 2010. *Acinetobacter bereziniae* sp. nov. and *Acinetobacter guillouiae* sp. nov., to accommodate *Acinetobacter* genomic species 10 and 11, respectively. *Int. J. Syst. Evol. Microbiol.* **60:**896–903.

156. Nemec, A., M. Musilek, M. Vaneechoutte, E. Falsen, and L. Dijkshoorn. 2008. Lack of evidence for "*Acinetobacter septicus*" as a species different from *Acinetobacter ursingii? J. Clin. Microbiol.* **46:**2826–2827.

157. Noell, F., M. F. Gorce, C. Garde, and C. Bizet. 1989. Isolation of *Weeksella zoohelcum* in septicaemia. *Lancet* **ii:**332.

158. Nozue, H., T. Hayashi, Y. Hashimoto, T. Ezaki, K. Hamasaki, K. Ohwada, and Y. Terawaki. 1992. Isolation and characterization of *Shewanella alga* from human clinical specimens and emendation of the description of *S. alga* Simidu et al., 1990, 335. *Int. J. Syst. Bacteriol.* **42:**628–634.

159. Nulens, E., B. Bussels, A. Bols, B. Gordts, and H. W. Van Landuyt. 2001. Recurrent bacteremia by *Chryseobacterium indologenes* in an oncology patient with a totally implanted intravascular device. *Clin. Microbiol. Infect.* **7:**391–393.

160. O'Hara, C. M., and J. M. Miller. 2003. Evaluation of the Vitek 2 ID-GNB assay for identification of members of the family *Enterobacteriaceae* and other nonenteric gram-negative bacilli and comparison with the Vitek GNI+ card. *J. Clin. Microbiol.* **41:**2096–2101.

161. Oncul, O., O. Keskin, H. V. Acar, Y. Kucukardali, R. Evrenkaya, E. M. Atasoyu, C. Top, S. Nalbant, S. Ozkan, G. Emekdas, S. Cavuslu, M. H. Us, A. Pahsa, and M. Gokben. 2002. Hospital-acquired infections following the 1999 Marmara earthquake. *J. Hosp. Infect.* **51:**47–51.

162. Osterhout, G. J., V. H. Shull, and J. D. Dick. 1991. Identification of clinical isolates of gram-negative nonfermentative bacteria by an automated cellular fatty acid identification system. *J. Clin. Microbiol.* **29:**1822–1830.

163. Patt, T. E., G. C. Cole, and R. S. Hanson. 1976. *Methylobacterium*, a new genus of facultatively methylotrophic bacteria. *Int. J. Syst. Bacteriol.* **26:**226–229.

164. Peleg, A. Y., H. Seifert, and D. L. Paterson. 2008. *Acinetobacter baumannii*: emergence of a successful pathogen. *Clin. Microbiol. Rev.* **21:**538–582.

165. Perera, S., and C. Palasuntheram. 2004. *Chryseobacterium meningosepticum* infections in a dialysis unit. *Ceylon Med J.* **49:**57–60.

166. Perilli, M., B. Caporale, G. Celenza, C. Pellegrini, J. D. Docquier, M. Mezzatesta, G. M. Rossolini, S. Stefani, and G. Amicosante. 2007. Identification and characterization of a new metallo-β-lactamase, IND-5, from a clinical isolate of *Chryseobacterium indologenes*. *Antimicrob. Agents Chemother.* **51:**2988–2990.

167. Petti, C. A., C. R. Polage, and P. Schreckenberger. 2005. Is misidentification of microorganisms by conventional methods a laboratory error? Preventing laboratory errors with 16S rRNA gene sequencing. *J. Clin. Microbiol.* **43:**6123–6125.

168. Pickett, M. J. 1989. Methods for identification of flavobacteria. *J. Clin. Microbiol.* **27:**2309–2315.

169. Pickett, M. J., A. von Graevenitz, G. E. Pfyffer, V. Pünter, and M. Altwegg. 1996. Phenotypic features distinguishing *Oligella urethralis* from *Moraxella osloensis*. *Med. Microbiol. Lett.* **5:**265–270.

170. Pitulle, C., D. M. Citron, B. Bochner, R. Barbers, and M. D. Appleman. 1999. Novel bacterium isolated from a lung transplant patient with cystic fibrosis. *J. Clin. Microbiol.* **37:**3851–3855.

171. Potron, A., L. Poirel, J. Croizé, V. Chanteperdrix, and P. Nordmann. 2009. Genetic and biochemical characterization of the first extended-spectrum CARB-type beta-lactamase, RTG-4, from *Acinetobacter baumannii*. *Antimicrob. Agents Chemother.* **53:**3010–3016.

172. Prashanth, K., M. P. M. Ranga, V. A. Rao, and R. Kanungo. 2000. Corneal perforation due to *Acinetobacter junii*: a case report. *Diagn. Microbiol. Infect. Dis.* **37:**215–217.

173. Pugliese, A., B. Pacris, P. E. Schoch, and B. A. Cunha. 1993. *Oligella urethralis* urosepsis. *Clin. Infect. Dis.* **17:**1069–1070.

174. Purcell, B. K., and D. P. Dooley. 1999. Centers for Disease Control and Prevention group O1 bacterium-associated pneumonia complicated by bronchopulmonary fistula and bacteremia. *Clin. Infect. Dis.* **29:**945–946.

175. Reina, J., A. Bassa, I. Llompart, D. Portela, and N. Borrell. 1991. Infections with *Pseudomonas paucimobilis*: report of four cases and review. *Rev. Infect. Dis.* **13:**1072–1076.

176. Reina, J., and N. Borrell. 1992. Leg abscess caused by *Weeksella zoohelcum* following a dog bite. *Clin. Infect. Dis.* **14:**1162–1163.

177. Reina, J., J. Gil, F. Salva, J. Gomez, and P. Alomar. 1990. Microbiological characteristics of *Weeksella virosa* (formerly CDC group IIf) isolated from the human genitourinary tract. *J. Clin. Microbiol.* **28:**2357–2359.

178. Rice, E. W., D. J. Reasoner, C. H. Johnson, and L. A. DeMaria. 2000. Monitoring for methylobacteria in water systems. *J. Clin. Microbiol.* **38:**4296–4297.

179. Rihs, J. D., D. J. Brenner, R. E. Weaver, A. G. Steigerwalt, D. G. Hollis, and V. L. Yu. 1993. *Roseomonas*, a new genus associated with bacteremia and other human infections. *J. Clin. Microbiol.* **31:**3275–3283.

180. Ringvold, A., E. Vik, and L. S. Bevanger. 1985. *Moraxella lacunata* isolated from epidemic conjunctivitis among teenaged females. *Acta Ophthalmol.* (Copenhagen) **63:**427–431.

181. Rossau, R., K. Kersters, E. Falsen, E. Jantzen, P. Segers, A. Union, L. Nehls, and J. de Ley. 1987. *Oligella*, a new genus including *Oligella urethralis* comb. nov. (formerly *Moraxella urethralis*) and *Oligella ureolytica* sp. nov. (formerly CDC group IVe): relationship to *Taylorella equigenitalis* and related taxa. *Int. J. Syst. Bacteriol.* **37:**198–210.

182. Rossau, R., A. Van Landschoot, M. Gillis, and J. de Ley. 1991. Taxonomy of *Moraxellaceae* fam. nov., a new bacterial family to accommodate the genera *Moraxella*, *Acinetobacter*, and *Psychrobacter* and related organisms. *Int. J. Syst. Bacteriol.* **41:**310–319.

183. Saavedra, J., C. Garrido, D. Folgueira, M. J. Torres, and J. T. Ramos. 1999. *Ochrobactrum anthropi* bacteremia associated with a catheter in an immunocompromised child and review of the pediatric literature. *Pediatr. Infect. Dis. J.* **18:**658–660.

184. Sanders, J. W., J. W. Martin, M. Hooke, and J. Hooke. 2000. *Methylobacterium mesophilicum* infection: case report and literature review of an unusual opportunistic pathogen. *Clin. Infect. Dis.* **30:**936–938.

185. Sawada, H., H. Ieki, H. Oyaizu, and S. Matsumoto. 1993. Proposal for rejection of *Agrobacterium tumefaciens* and revised descriptions for the genus *Agrobacterium* and for *Agrobacterium radiobacter* and *Agrobacterium rhizogenes*. *Int. J. Syst. Bacteriol.* **43:**694–702.

186. Seifert, H., L. Dijkshoorn, P. Gerner-Smidt, N. Pelzer, I. Tjernberg, and M. Vaneechoutte. 1997. Distribution of *Acinetobacter* species on human skin: comparison of phenotypic and genotypic identification methods. *J. Clin. Microbiol.* **35:**2819–2825.

187. Seifert, H., L. Dolzani, R. Bressan, T. van der Reijden, B. van Strijen, D. Stefanik, H. Heersma, and L. Dijkshoorn. 2005. Standardization and interlaboratory reproducibility assessment of pulsed-field gel electrophoresis-generated fingerprints of *Acinetobacter baumannii*. *J. Clin. Microbiol.* **43:**4328–4335.

188. Seifert, H., A. Strate, and G. Pulverer. 1995. Nosocomial bacteremia due to *Acinetobacter baumannii*. Clinical features, epidemiology, and predictors of mortality. *Medicine* (Baltimore) **74:**340–349.

189. Seifert, H., A. Strate, A. Schulze, and G. Pulverer. 1993. Vascular catheter-related bloodstream infection due to *Acinetobacter johnsonii* (formerly *Acinetobacter calcoaceticus* var. *lwoffi*): report of 13 cases. *Clin. Infect. Dis.* **17:**632–636.

190. Seng, P., M. Drancourt, F. Gouriet, B. La Scola, P. E. Fournier, J. M. Rolain, and D. Raoult. 2009. Ongoing revolution in bacteriology: routine identification of bacteria by matrix-assisted laser desorption ionization time-of-flight mass spectrometry. *Clin. Infect. Dis.* **49:**543–551.

191. Shah, S. S., A. Ruth, and S. E. Coffin. 2000. Infection due to *Moraxella osloensis*: case report and review of the literature. *Clin. Infect. Dis.* **30:**179–181.

192. **Sheridan, R. I., C. M. Ryan, M. S. Pasternack, J. M. Weber, and R. G. Tompkins.** 1993. Flavobacterial sepsis in massively burned pediatric patients. *Clin. Infect. Dis.* **17:**185–187.

193. **Shokar, N. K., G. S. Shokar, J. Islam, and A. R. Cass.** 2002. *Roseomonas gilardii* infection: case report and review. *J. Clin. Microbiol.* **40:**4789–4791.

194. **Siegman-Igra, Y., S. Bar-Yosef, A. Gorea, and J. Avram.** 1993. Nosocomial *Acinetobacter* meningitis secondary to invasive procedures: report of 25 cases and review. *Clin. Infect. Dis.* **17:**843–849.

195. **Siegman-Igra, Y., D. Schwartz, G. Soferman, and N. Konforti.** 1987. *Flavobacterium* group IIb bacteremia: report of a case and review of *Flavobacterium* infections. *Med. Microbiol. Immunol.* **176:**103–111.

196. **Snyder, R. W., J. Ruhe, S. Kobrin, A. Wasserstein, C. Doline, I. Nachamkin, and J. H. Lipschutz.** 2004. *Asaia bogorensis* peritonitis identified by 16S ribosomal RNA sequence analysis in a patient receiving peritoneal dialysis. *Am. J. Kidney Dis.* **44:**E15–E17.

197. **Spangler, S. K., M. A. Visalli, M. R. Jacobs, and P. C. Appelbaum.** 1996. Susceptibilities of non-*Pseudomonas aeruginosa* gram-negative nonfermentative rods to ciprofloxacin, ofloxacin, levofloxacin, D-ofloxacin, sparfloxacin, ceftazidime, piperacillin, piperacillin-tazobactam, trimethoprim-sulfamethoxazole, and imipenem. *Antimicrob. Agents Chemother.* **40:**772–775.

198. **Speeleveld, E., J.-M. Fosspre, B. Gordts, and H. W. Landuyt.** 1994. Comparison of three rapid methods, tributyrine, 4-methylumbelliferyl butyrate, and indoxyl acetate, for rapid identification of *Moraxella catarrhalis*. *J. Clin. Microbiol.* **32:**1362–1363.

199. **Steyn, P. L., P. Segers, M. Vancanneyt, P. Sandra, K. Kersters, and J. J. Joubert.** 1998. Classification of heparinolytic bacteria into a new genus, *Pedobacter*, comprising four species: *Pedobacter heparinus* comb. nov., *Pedobacter piscium* comb. nov., *Pedobacter africanus* sp. nov. and *Pedobacter saltans* sp. nov. Proposal of the family *Sphingobacteriaceae* fam. nov. *Int. J. Syst. Bacteriol.* **48:**165–177.

200. **Struthers, M., J. Wong, and J. M. Janda.** 1996. An initial appraisal of the clinical significance of *Roseomonas* species associated with human infections. *Clin. Infect. Dis.* **23:**729–733.

201. **Su, S. C., M. Vaneechoutte, L. Dijkshoorn, Y. F. Wei, Y. L. Chen, and T. C. Chang.** 2009. Identification of nonfermenting Gram-negative bacteria of clinical importance by an oligonucleotide array. *J. Med. Microbiol.* **58:**596–605.

202. **Subudhi, C. P. K., A. Adedeji, M. E. Kaufmann, G. S. Lucas, and J. R. Kerr.** 2001. Fatal *Roseomonas gilardii* bacteremia in a patient with refractory blast crisis of chronic myeloid leukemia. *Clin. Microbiol. Infect.* **7:**573–575.

203. **Swenson, J. M., G. E. Killgore, and F. C. Tenover.** 2004. Antimicrobial susceptibility testing of *Acinetobacter* spp. by NCCLS broth microdilution and disk diffusion methods. *J. Clin. Microbiol.* **42:**5102–5108.

204. **Takeuchi, M., K. Hamana, and A. Hiraishi.** 2001. Proposal of the genus *Sphingomonas sensu stricto* and three new genera, *Sphingobium*, *Novosphingobium* and *Sphingopyxis*, on the basis of phylogenetic and chemotaxonomic analyses. *Int. J. Syst. Evol. Microbiol.* **51:**1405–1417.

205. **Takeuchi, M., and A. Yokota.** 1992. Proposals of *Sphingobacterium faecium* sp. nov., *Sphingobacterium piscium* sp. nov., *Sphingobacterium heparinum* comb. nov., *Sphingobacterium thalpophilum* comb. nov. and two genospecies of the genus *Sphingobacterium*, and synonymy of *Flavobacterium yabuuchiae* and *Sphingobacterium spiritivorum*. *J. Gen. Appl. Microbiol.* **38:**465–482.

206. **Tjernberg, I., and J. Ursing.** 1989. Clinical strains of *Acinetobacter* classified by DNA-DNA hybridization. *APMIS* **97:**595–605.

207. **Tuon, F. F., L. Campos, and D. de Almeida.** 2007. *Chryseobacterium meningosepticum* as a cause of cellulitis and sepsis in an immunocompetent patient. *J. Med. Microbiol.* **56:**1116–1117.

208. **Turton, J. F., S. N. Gabriel, C. Valderrey, M. E. Kaufmann, and T. L. Pitt.** 2007. Use of sequence-based typing and multiplex PCR to identify clonal lineages of outbreak strains of *Acinetobacter baumannii*. *Clin. Microbiol. Infect.* **13:**807–815.

209. **Turton, J. F., J. Matos, M. E. Kaufmann, and T. L. Pitt.** 2009. Variable number tandem repeat loci providing discrimination within widespread genotypes of *Acinetobacter baumannii*. *Eur. J. Clin. Microbiol. Infect. Dis.* **28:**499–507.

210. **Turton, J. F., J. Shah, C. Ozongwu, and R. Pike.** 2010. Incidence of *Acinetobacter* species other than A. *baumannii* among clinical isolates of *Acinetobacter:* evidence for emerging species. *J. Clin. Microbiol.* **48:**1445–1449.

211. **Turton, J. F., M. E. Ward, N. Woodford, M. E. Kaufmann, R. Pike, D. M. Livermore, and T. L. Pitt.** 2006. The role of ISAba1 in expression of OXA carbapenemase genes in *Acinetobacter baumannii*. *FEMS Microbiol. Lett.* **258:**72–77.

212. **Turton, J. F., N. Woodford, J. Glover, S. Yarde, M. E. Kaufmann, and T. L. Pitt.** 2006. Identification of *Acinetobacter baumannii* by detection of the bla$_{OXA-51-like}$ carbapenemase gene intrinsic to this species. *J. Clin. Microbiol.* **44:**2974–2976.

213. **Urakami, T., H. Araki, K.-I. Suzuki, and K. Komagata.** 1993. Further studies of the genus *Methylobacterium* and description of *Methylobacterium aminovorans* sp. nov. *Int. J. Syst. Bacteriol.* **43:**504–513.

214. **Ursing, J., and B. Bruun.** 1991. Genotypic heterogeneity of *Flavobacterium* group IIb and *Flavobacterium breve*, demonstrated by DNA-DNA hybridization. *APMIS* **99:**780–786.

215. **Vancanneyt, M., P. Segers, U. Torck, B. Hoste, J.-F. Bernardet, P. Vandamme, and K. Kersters.** 1996. Reclassification of *Flavobacterium odoratum* (Stutzer 1929) strains to a new genus, *Myroides*, as *Myroides odoratus* comb. nov. and *Myroides odoratimimus* sp. nov. *Int. J. Syst. Bacteriol.* **46:**926–932.

216. **Vandamme, P., J. F. Bernardet, P. Segers, K. Kersters, and B. Holmes.** 1994. New perspectives in the classification of the flavobacteria: description of *Chryseobacterium* gen. nov., *Bergeyella* gen. nov., and *Empedobacter* nom. rev. *Int. J. Syst. Bacteriol.* **44:**827–831.

217. **Vandamme, P., M. Gillis, M. Vancanneyt, B. Hoste, K. Kersters, and E. Falsen.** 1993. *Moraxella lincolnii* sp. nov., isolated from the human respiratory tract, and reevaluation of the taxonomic position of *Moraxella osloensis*. *Int. J. Syst. Bacteriol.* **43:**474–481.

218. **Vandamme, P., B. Holmes, H. Bercovier, and T. Coenye.** 2006. Classification of Centers for Disease Control Group Eugonic Fermenter (EF)-4a and EF-4b as *Neisseria animaloris* sp. nov. and *Neisseria zoodegmatis* sp. nov., respectively. *Int. J. Syst. Evol. Microbiol.* **56:**1801–1805.

219. **van den Broek, P. J., J. Arends, A. T. Bernards, E. De Brauwer, E. M. Mascini, T. J. van der Reijden, L. Spanjaard, E. A. Thewessen, A. van der Zee, J. H. van Zeijl, and L. Dijkshoorn.** 2006. Epidemiology of multiple *Acinetobacter* outbreaks in The Netherlands during the period 1999–2001. *Clin. Microbiol. Infect.* **12:**837–843.

220. **van den Broek, P. J., T. J. K. van der Reijden, E. van Strijen, A. V. Helmig-Schurter, A. T. Bernards, and L. Dijkshoorn.** 2009. Endemic and epidemic *Acinetobacter* species in a university hospital: an 8-year survey. *J. Clin. Microbiol.* **47:**3593–3599.

221. **van Dessel, H., L. Dijkshoorn, T. van der Reijden, N. Bakker, A. Paauw, P. van den Broek, J. Verhoef, and S. Brisse.** 2004. Identification of a new geographically widespread multiresistant *Acinetobacter baumannii* clone from European hospitals. *Res. Microbiol.* **155:**105–112.

222. **van Dessel, H., T. E. Kamp-Hopmans, A. C. Fluit, S. Brisse, A. M. de Smet, L. Dijkshoorn, A. Troelstra, J. Verhoef, and E. M. Mascini.** 2002. Outbreak of a susceptible strain of *Acinetobacter* species 13 (sensu Tjernberg and Ursing) in an adult neurosurgical intensive care unit. *J. Hosp. Infect.* **51:**89–95.

223. **Vaneechoutte, M., G. Claeys, S. Steyaert, T. De Baere, R. Peleman, and G. Verschraegen.** 2000. Isolation of *Moraxella canis* from an ulcerated metastatic lymph node. *J. Clin. Microbiol.* **38:**3870–3871.

224. **Vaneechoutte, M., and T. De Baere.** 2008. Taxonomy of the genus *Acinetobacter*, based on 16S ribosomal RNA gene sequences, p. 35–60. *In* U. Gerischer (ed.), Acinetobacter *Molecular Microbiology.* Caister Academic Press, Norfolk, United Kingdom.

225. **Vaneechoutte, M., T. De Baere, A. Nemec, T. J. K. van der Reijden, and L. Dijkshoorn.** 2008. Reclassification of *Acinetobacter grimontii* Carr et al. 2003 as a later synonym of *Acinetobacter junii* Bouvet and Grimont 1986. *Int. J. Syst. Evol. Microbiol.* **58:**937–940.

226. **Vaneechoutte, M., L. A. Devriese, L. Dijkshoorn, B. Lamote, P. Deprez, G. Verschraegen, and F. Haesebrouck.** 2000. *Acinetobacter baumannii*-infected vascular catheters collected from horses in an equine clinic. *J. Clin. Microbiol.* **38:**4280–4281.

227. **Vaneechoutte, M., L. Dijkshoorn, I. Tjernberg, A. Elaichouni, P. De Vos, G. Claeys, and G. Verschraegen.** 1995. Identification of *Acinetobacter* genomic species by amplified ribosomal DNA restriction analysis. *J. Clin. Microbiol.* **33:**11–15.

228. **Vaneechoutte, M., P. Kämpfer, T. De Baere, V. Avesani, M. Janssens, and G. Wauters.** 2007. *Chryseobacterium hominis* sp. nov., to accommodate clinical isolates biochemically similar to CDC groups II-h and II-c. *Int. J. Syst. Evol. Microbiol.* **57:**2623–2628.

229. **Vaneechoutte, M., A. Nemec, M. Musílek, T. J. K. van der Reijden, M. van den Barselaar, I. Tjernberg, W. Calame, R. Fani, T. De Baere, and L. Dijkshoorn.** 2009. Description of *Acinetobacter venetianus* ex Di Cello et al. 1997 sp. nov. *Int. J. Syst. Evol. Microbiol.* **59:**1376–1381.

230. **Vaneechoutte, M., R. Rossau, P. De Vos, M. Gillis, D. Janssens, N. Paepe, A. De Rouck, T. Fiers, G. Claeys, and K. Kersters.** 1992. Rapid identification of bacteria of the *Comamonadaceae* with amplified ribosomal DNA-restriction analysis (ARDRA). *FEMS Microbiol. Lett.* **93:**227–234.

231. **Vaneechoutte, M., G. Verschraegen, G. Claeys, and A.-M. Van den Abeele.** 1988. A selective medium for *Branhamella catarrhalis*, with acetazolamide as a specific inhibitor of *Neisseria* spp. *J. Clin. Microbiol.* **26:**2544–2548.

232. **Vaneechoutte, M., G. Verschraegen, G. Claeys, B. Weise, and A.-M. Van den Abeele.** 1990. Respiratory tract carrier rates of *Moraxella (Branhamella) catarrhalis* in adults and children and interpretation of the isolation of *M. catarrhalis* from sputum. *J. Clin. Microbiol.* **28:**2674–2680.

233. **Vanlaere, E., K. Sergeant, P. Dawyndt, W. Kallow, M. Erhard, H. Sutton, D. Dare, B. Devreese, B. Samyn, and P. Vandamme.** 2008. Matrix-assisted laser desorption ionisation-time-of of-flight mass spectrometry of intact cells allows rapid identification. *J. Med. Microbiol.* **75:**279–286.

234. **Van Looveren, M., H. Goossens, and the ARPAC Steering Group.** 2004. Antimicrobial resistance of *Acinetobacter* spp. in Europe. *Clin. Microbiol. Infect.* **10:**1106–1107.

235. **Vela, A. I., M. D. Collins, M. V. Latre, A. Mateos, M. A. Moreno, R. Hutson, L. Dominguez, and J. F. Fernandez-Garayzabal.** 2003. *Psychrobacter pulmonis* sp. nov., isolated from the lungs of lambs. *Int. J. Syst. Evol. Microbiol.* **53:**415–419.

236. **Velasco, J., C. Romero, I. Lopez-Goni, J. Leiva, R. Diaz, and I. Moriyon.** 1998. Evaluation of the relatedness of *Brucella* spp. and *Ochrobactrum anthropi* and description of *Ochrobactrum intermedium* sp. nov., a new species with a closer relationship to *Brucella* spp. *Int. J. Syst. Bacteriol.* **48:**759–768.

237. **Veys, A., W. Callewaert, E. Waelkens, and K. van den Abbeele.** 1989. Application of gas-liquid chromatography to the routine identification of nonfermenting gramnegative bacteria in clinical specimens. *J. Clin. Microbiol.* **27:**1538–1542.

238. **Villegas, M. V., and A. I. Hartstein.** 2003. *Acinetobacter* outbreaks, 1977–2000. *Infect. Control Hosp. Epidemiol.* **24:**284–295.

239. **Vogel, B. F., K. Jørgensen, H. Christensen, J. E. Olsen, and L. Gram.** 1997. Differentiation of *Shewanella putrefaciens* and *Shewanella alga* on the basis of whole-cell protein profiles, ribotyping, phenotypic characterization, and 16S rRNA gene sequence analysis. *Appl. Environ. Microbiol.* **63:**2189–2199.

240. **Vogel, B. F., K. Venkateswaran, H. Christensen, E. Falsen, G. Christiansen, and L. Gram.** 2000. Polyphasic taxonomic approach in the description of *Alishewanella fetalis* gen. nov., sp. nov., isolated from a human foetus. *Int. J. Syst. Evol. Microbiol.* **50:**1133–1142.

241. **von Graevenitz, A.** 1985. Ecology, clinical significance, and antimicrobial susceptibility of infrequently encountered glucose-nonfermenting gram-negative rods, p. 181–232. *In* G. L. Gilardi (ed.), *Nonfermentative Gram-Negative Rods: Laboratory Identification and Clinical Aspects.* Marcel Dekker, Inc., New York, NY.

242. **von Graevenitz, A., J. Bowman, C. Del Notaro, and M. Ritzler.** 2000. Human infection with *Halomonas venusta* following fish bite. *J. Clin. Microbiol.* **38:**3123–3124.

243. **von Graevenitz, A., and M. Grehn.** 1977. Susceptibility studies on *Flavobacterium* II-b. *FEMS Microbiol. Lett.* **2:**289–292.

244. **von Graevenitz, A., G. E. Pfyffer, M. J. Pickett, R. E. Weaver, and J. Wüst.** 1993. Isolation of an unclassified nonfermentative gram-negative rod from a patient on continuous ambulatory peritoneal dialysis. *Eur. J. Clin. Microbiol. Infect. Dis.* **12:**568–570.

245. **Watson, K. C., and I. Muscat.** 1983. Meningitis caused by a *Flavobacterium*-like organism (CDC IIe strain). *J. Infect.* **7:**278–279.

246. **Wellinghausen, N., A. Essig, and O. Sommerburg.** 2005. *Inquilinus limosus* in patients with cystic fibrosis, Germany. *Emerg. Infect. Dis.***11:**457–459.

247. **Weyant, R. S., C. W. Moss, R. E. Weaver, D. G. Hollis, J. G. Jordan, E. C. Cook, and M. I. Daneshvar.** 1996. *Identification of Unusual Pathogenic Gram-Negative Aerobic and Facultatively Anaerobic Bacteria,* 2nd ed. The Williams & Wilkins Co., Baltimore, MD.

248. **Wisplinghoff, H., M. B. Edmond, M. A. Pfaller, R. N. Jones, R. P. Wenzel, and H. Seifert.** 2000. Nosocomial bloodstream infections caused by *Acinetobacter* species in United States hospitals: clinical features, molecular epidemiology, and antimicrobial susceptibility. *Clin. Infect. Dis.* **31:**690–697.

249. **Yabuuchi, E., T. Kaneko, I. Yano, C. W. Moss, and N. Miyoshi.** 1983. *Sphingobacterium* gen. nov., *Sphingobacterium spiritivorum* comb. nov., *Sphingobacterium multivorum* com. nov., *Sphingobacterium mizutae* sp. nov., and *Flavobacterium indologenes* sp. nov.: glucose-nonfermenting gram-negative rods in CDC groups IIk-2 and IIb. *Int. J. Syst. Bacteriol.* **33:**580–598.

250. **Yabuuchi, E., I. Yano, H. Oyaizu, Y. Hashimoto, T. Ezaki, and H. Yamamoto.** 1990. Proposals of *Sphingomonas paucimobilis* gen. nov. and comb. nov., *Sphingomonas parapaucimobilis* sp. nov., *Sphingomonas yanoikuyae* sp. nov., *Sphingomonas adhaesiva* sp. nov., *Sphingomonas capsulata* comb. nov., and two genospecies of the genus *Sphingomonas. Microbiol. Immunol.* **34:**99–119.

251. **Yamada, Y., K. Katsura, H. Kawasaki, Y. Widyastuti, S. Saono, T. Seki, T. Uchimura, and K. Komagata.** 2000. *Asaia bogorensis* gen. nov., sp. nov., an unusual acetic acid bacterium in the α-Proteobacteria. *Int. J. Syst. Evol. Microbiol.* **50:**823–829.

252. **Young, J. M., L. D. Kuykendall, E. Martinez-Romero, A. Kerr, and H. Sawada.** 2001. A revision of *Rhizobium* Frank 1889, with an emended description of the genus, and the inclusion of all species of *Agrobacterium* Conn 1942 and *Allorhizobium undicola* de Lajundie et al. 1998 as new combinations: *Rhizobium radiobacter, R. rhizogenes, R. rubi, R. undicola* and *R. vitis. Int. J. Syst. Evol. Microbiol.* **51:**89–103.

Bordetella and Related Genera

CARL-HEINZ WIRSING VON KÖNIG, MARION RIFFELMANN, AND TOM COENYE

43

TAXONOMY

The genera *Bordetella*, *Achromobacter*, *Alcaligenes*, *Kerstersia*, and *Advenella* belong to the family *Alcaligenaceae* (order *Burkholderiales* in the β subclass of the *Proteobacteria*) (22). Other members of this family include *Azohydromonas*, *Brackiella*, *Castellaniella*, *Derxia*, *Oligella*, *Pelistega*, *Pigmentiphaga*, *Pusillimonas*, *Sutterella*, and *Taylorella* (List of Prokaryotic Names with Standing in Nomenclature [http://www.bacterio.cict.fr/]). The genus *Bordetella* contains eight species: *Bordetella avium*, *B. bronchiseptica*, *B. hinzii*, *B. holmesii*, *B. parapertussis*, *B. pertussis* (the type species), *B. petrii*, and *B. trematum* (55, 66, 104, 105, 109, 116). Other putative species, such as "*B. ansorpii*" and other strains similar to *B. trematum* (45, 58), have been described. *B. pertussis*, *B. parapertussis*, and *B. bronchiseptica* could be considered a single species, but chemotaxonomic differences and differences in host range and pathogenesis (66, 76) support their status as separate species. Analysis of their genome sequences revealed that *B. parapertussis* and *B. pertussis* are independent derivatives of a *B. bronchiseptica*-like ancestor (76). The taxonomy of the genus *Achromobacter* is closely intertwined with that of the genus *Alcaligenes*. The genus *Alcaligenes* is now limited to *Alcaligenes aquatilis* and *Alcaligenes faecalis* (the type species) (20, 106), while the genus *Achromobacter* consists of six species: *Achromobacter denitrificans*, *A. insolitus*, *A. piechaudii*, *A. ruhlandii*, *A. spanius*, and *A. xylosoxidans* (the type species) (20, 21, 105, 120). The genus *Kerstersia* was proposed for a set of strains phenotypically resembling *A. faecalis* that were classified as *Kerstersia gyiorum* or as belonging to at least one other (so far unnamed) *Kerstersia* species (20). Similarly, the genus *Advenella* was created to harbor a number of *Alcaligenes*-like strains; these strains belong either to *Advenella incenata* or to one of several additional unnamed genomic species (22) or were previously described as *Tetrathiobacter* species (38).

DESCRIPTION OF THE GENERA

Bordetella

Bordetellae are small (1 to 2 μm), gram-negative, nonsporulating coccoid rods (8). During their adaptation to the human host, *B. pertussis* and *B. parapertussis* underwent a reduction in genome size (4.086 Mbp for *B. pertussis*, 4.774 Mbp for *B. parapertussis*, and 5.338 Mbp for *B. bronchiseptica*). Insertion sequences are found mainly in the genomes of *B. pertussis* (IS481), *B. parapertussis* (IS1001), and *B. holmesii* (IS481) and are found less so in *B. bronchiseptica* (76, 92).

Bordetellae are catalase positive and oxidize amino acids, but no carbohydrates can be fermented. Some species possess peritrichous flagella and are motile. Bordetellae are able to grow in simple synthetic media under aerobic conditions (except for *B. petrii* [see below]). However, *B. pertussis* and *B. parapertussis* are sensitive to toxic substances and metabolites present in many microbiological media and need special transport conditions, special culture media, and prolonged incubation. The other species are less sensitive and can be isolated by routine microbiological procedures.

B. petrii is the most versatile *Bordetella* species, as it can grow aerobically and anaerobically and was initially found as a free-living environmental bacterium. All other bordetellae are found only in warm-blooded animals and humans. *B. avium* is a pathogen for poultry and has only once been isolated from humans (45). *B. bronchiseptica* can cause respiratory infections in many animal species and, infrequently, also in humans. "*B. ansorpii*," *B. hinzii*, *B. holmesii*, *B. petrii*, and *B. trematum* are rarely found in human infections and mainly cause symptomatic diseases in immunocompromised patients. *B. parapertussis* is found in sheep and humans, and *B. pertussis* is thought to be a strictly human pathogen (Table 1).

Bordetellae express many virulence factors that are controlled by a complex virulence expression system operating in response to environmental conditions (BvgAS) (66). In subcultures, these responses were called phases I, II, III, and IV, with phase I being highly pathogenic and phase IV being almost apathogenic. The phases are now called mode X (respiratory tract infection), mode I (intermediate, possibly relevant for transmission), and mode C (starvation). Virulence factors of bordetellae can be classified as adhesins, autotransporters (i.e., filamentous hemagglutinin [FHA], fimbriae [FIM], and pertactin [PRN]), and toxins (i.e., pertussis toxin [PT], adenylate cyclase toxin, and lipopolysaccharide [LPS]) (66). Only *B. pertussis* produces PT, encoded by the *ptx* gene, whereas *B. parapertussis* (and *B. bronchiseptica*) contains the *ptx* gene but normally lacks the promoter (66). PT has ADP-ribosyltransferase activity and

TABLE 1 Members of the genus *Bordetella*

Species	Host	Transmission	Disease
B. pertussis	Humans	Droplets	Pertussis
B. parapertussis	Humans	Droplets	Pertussis-like disease
	Sheep	Unknown	Respiratory disease
B. bronchiseptica	Animals	Droplets (?)	Respiratory disease
	Humans	Droplets (?)	Respiratory disease
			Systemic infection (immunocompromised hosts)
B. hinzii	Poultry	Droplets	Respiratory disease
	Humans	Unknown	Cholangitis, arthritis
B. trematum	Humans	Unknown	Wound infection, otitis
B. holmesii	Humans	Unknown	Systemic infection (immunocompromised hosts)
B. petrii	Environment		
	Humans	Unknown	Osteomyelitis, mastoiditis
"*B. ansorpii*"	Humans	Unknown	Epidermal cyst, systemic infection (immunocompromised hosts)
B. avium	Poultry	Droplets	Respiratory disease
	Humans	Unknown	Respiratory disease

ribosylates G proteins (66). PT induces lymphocytosis and suppresses chemotaxis, oxidative responses, and the overall activity of neutrophils and macrophages. FHA is a large (220-kDa), surface-associated, secreted protein and mediates the adhesion of bordetellae to the ciliated epithelium of the upper respiratory tract. FHA is produced by *B. pertussis*, *B. parapertussis*, and *B. bronchiseptica* (66). FIM types 2 and 3 (FIM2 and FIM3) represent the serotype-specific agglutinogens and are important factors in colonizing the respiratory mucosa. Isolates of *B. pertussis* can display FIM2, FIM3, or both on their surface. Adenylate cyclase toxin is a hemolysin with enzymatic activity (47). *B. pertussis* also produces an LPS without a repetitive O-antigenic chain. PRN is a 68- to 70-kDa surface protein that mediates eukaryotic cell binding in vitro (66). PRN is involved in cell attachment by its Arg-Gly-Asp (RGD) motif and is highly immunogenic (48).

Achromobacter

Achromobacter species are gram-negative, nonsporulating, straight rods of 0.8 to 1.2 by 2.5 to 3.0 μm. They are motile, with peritrichously arranged sheathed flagella; the number of flagella varies from 1 to 20 per cell. They are strictly aerobic and nonfermentative, although strains of some species are able to grow anaerobically with nitrate as an electron acceptor (120). All *Achromobacter* species are oxidase and catalase positive, but none of them exhibits urease, DNase, lysine decarboxylase, ornithine decarboxylase, arginine dihydrolase, or gelatinase activity (21, 120) (Table 2). They grow well on simple media (including nutrient agar), and on nutrient agar, colonies are flat or slightly convex, with smooth margins, and range from white to light brown (21). Under laboratory conditions, growth occurs between 25 and 37°C and in the presence of 0 to 4.5% NaCl (21, 120). *Achromobacter* species contain the Q-8 ubiquinone system (13). The predominant fatty acids are $C_{16:0}$ and $C_{17:0\ cyclo}$ (21). Although detailed information about the natural habitat of these organisms is lacking, soil and water are considered to be primary sources of infection (13, 120).

Alcaligenes, Kerstersia, and Advenella

Following many taxonomic revisions, the genus *Alcaligenes* is now limited to *A. faecalis* (the type species) and *A.*

aquatilis. Within *A. faecalis*, three subspecies (*A. faecalis* subsp. *faecalis*, *A. faecalis* subsp. *parafaecalis*, and *A. faecalis* subsp. *phenolicus*) have been described (84, 90). *A. faecalis* subsp. *parafaecalis* and *A. faecalis* subsp. *phenolicus* are represented by a single environmental isolate each, and *A. aquatilis* strains have been recovered only from lake sediments (106). Some *A. faecalis* strains produce a characteristic fruity odor and/or cause a greenish discoloration of blood agar medium; these strains were previously referred to as "*A. odorans*" (54). *Alcaligenes* species are gram-negative, strictly aerobic rods or coccobacilli that possess oxidase and catalase activity (13). Cells are motile by means of 1 to 12 peritrichous flagella (54). The optimum growth temperature is between 20 and 37°C. They grow well on simple media, and colonies on nutrient agar are generally nonpigmented. The predominant fatty acids in *Alcaligenes* species are $C_{16:0}$ and $C_{17:0\ cyclo}$ (54, 106).

Cells of *Kerstersia* and *Advenella* species are gram-negative, small (1 to 2 μm), rod-shaped or coccoid cells and occur alone, in pairs, or in short chains. Motility is strain dependent. These species grow well on simple media (including nutrient agar). On nutrient agar, colonies are flat or slightly convex, with smooth margins, and range from white to light brown. They are strictly aerobic and nonfermentative. All isolates studied so far are catalase positive, while none of them exhibit β-galactosidase activity (20, 22). *Kerstersia* strains can grow at temperatures between 28 and 42°C; growth also occurs with up to 4.5% NaCl. The predominant fatty acids in *Kerstersia* species are $C_{16:0}$ and $C_{17:0\ cyclo}$ (20). *Advenella* strains can grow at temperatures between 30 and 37°C and at NaCl concentrations between 0 and 3%. The predominant fatty acids in *Advenella* species are $C_{18:1\ w7c}$, $C_{16:0}$, and $C_{16:1\ w7c}$ (22).

EPIDEMIOLOGY AND TRANSMISSION

B. pertussis and B. parapertussis

B. pertussis and *B. parapertussis* cause pertussis, or whooping cough. Infections by *B. parapertussis* tend to take a milder clinical course, with a shorter duration of coughing and less vomiting and whooping (66, 112, 117). *B. pertussis* continues to circulate in populations where high

TABLE 2 Biochemical reactions useful for differentiating *Achromobacter*, *Alcaligenes*, *Kerstersia*, and *Advenella* species[a]

Reaction or characteristic[b]	A. xylosoxidans	A. insolitus	A. spanius	A. denitrificans	A. piechaudii	A. faecalis	K. gyiorum	A. incenata
Oxidase	+	+	+	+	+	+	−	+
Reduction of:								
Nitrate	+	−	−	+	−	−	−	−
Nitrite	+	−	−	+	−	+	−	−
Growth on acetamide	+	+	−	V	V	−	−	−
Assimilation of:								
Glucose	+	−	−	−	−	−	−	V
Xylose	+	−	−	−	−	−	−	V
Mesaconate	+	+	−	V	+	−	−	ND
Aconitate	+	+	−	+	+	V	−	ND
Itaconate	+	+	+	+	+	−	−	ND
Gluconate	+	+	+	−	+	−	V	ND
Caprate	+	+	−	−	−	+	+	−
Phenylacetate	+	+	+	+	+	+	+	−
Citrate	+	+	+	+	−	+	+	+

[a]Data are from references 13, 20, 21, 22, 54, and 120.

[b]Symbols and abbreviations: +, ≥90% of the strains are positive; −, ≤10% of the strains are positive; V, 10 to 89% of the strains are positive; ND, not determined.

vaccination coverage of infants and children is achieved (79, 117), because the protection induced after natural infection and vaccination wanes after several years (79, 107). In vaccinating countries, most cases of pertussis are now observed in neonates, unvaccinated young infants, older schoolchildren, adolescents, and adults (79, 111, 117). A permanent carrier state is not found in pertussis, although in outbreak situations asymptomatic transient carriage of *Bordetella* DNA detected by PCR has been observed in up to ~50% of individuals (66, 113). *B. pertussis* is transmitted by droplets, and in susceptible contacts the transmission rate may be close to 90% (66). In nonprimary cases, transmission rates are probably lower. Transmission of the disease in highly vaccinated populations occurs mainly from adolescents and adults to infants or among older vaccinated children, adolescents, and adults (66, 117). Neonates and young infants are at greatest risk of being infected by their parents, although casual contacts may be important (115). The continuing circulation of *B. pertussis* has prompted many industrialized countries to recommend pertussis vaccination with acellular pertussis vaccines for adolescents and adults, in addition to children, in order to diminish the disease burden in these populations and to reduce morbidity and mortality in newborns and young infants (79).

Other *Bordetella* Species, *Achromobacter*, *Alcaligenes*, *Kerstersia*, and *Advenella*

Data on epidemiology and transmission are limited to *A. xylosoxidans* infections in cystic fibrosis (CF) patients. Persistent infections with this organism can occur, as genotypically identical isolates are recovered from the respiratory tract over prolonged periods (25, 51, 60). There have been several reports of multiple CF patients being colonized or infected by the same *A. xylosoxidans* isolate (60, 80, 103). However, no large-scale outbreaks caused by the same strain and involving multiple treatment centers have been identified, and epidemiological studies revealed that there

are many different *A. xylosoxidans* strains infecting CF patients.

CLINICAL SIGNIFICANCE

B. pertussis and *B. parapertussis*

After an incubation period of 7 to 10 days (range, 4 to 28 days), the primary infection starts, with rhinorrhea, sneezing, and nonspecific coughs (catarrhal phase). The typical clinical symptoms of pertussis are found in primary infections of nonvaccinated children and include coughing spasms, whooping, and vomiting (paroxysmal phase) (77). Cases in neonates and unvaccinated young infants often present with apnea as the only symptom (66, 79). In older schoolchildren, adolescents, and adults, the symptoms can vary widely. Adult pertussis is associated with a long illness, and the persistent cough is often paroxysmal and has a mean duration of approximately 6 weeks. It is frequently accompanied by choking, vomiting, and whooping (117). The CDC clinical case definition for pertussis (http://www.cdc.gov/ncphi/disss/nndss/casedef/pertussis_current.htm) requires 14 days of coughing with paroxysms, whooping, or vomiting. The disease is most dangerous in infants, and most hospitalizations and deaths occur in this age group. Fatal cases of the disease may go undetected in young infants (75, 79).

Pertussis-like symptoms may also be caused by adenovirus, respiratory syncytial virus, human parainfluenza viruses, influenza viruses, *Mycoplasma pneumoniae*, and other agents (79). Coinfections of *B. pertussis* and respiratory syncytial virus are observed frequently in infants (23).

Other *Bordetella* Species

B. bronchiseptica (69, 81), *B. holmesii* (116), and *B. hinzii* (4, 34, 49, 52) can rarely be isolated from respiratory materials from patients with pertussis-like symptoms and other respiratory symptoms. In many cases, patients are systemically or locally immunocompromised, such as human immunodeficiency virus-infected patients or patients suffering from CF (19, 96, 97). As with other gram-negative nonfermentative bacilli, rare cases of bacteremia and septicemia have been described.

B. trematum (24, 104) has been isolated from people working with poultry, and "*B. ansorpii*" (33, 58) is another rare cause of septicemia. *B. petrii* (32, 98), and possibly other environmental bordetellae (110), is rarely found in clinical material, and *B. avium* has so far been isolated from respiratory material from humans only once (45) (Table 1).

Achromobacter

All *Achromobacter* species except *A. ruhlandii* have been recovered from clinical samples or from the hospital environment. *A. xylosoxidans* (previously known as *A. xylosoxidans* subsp. *xylosoxidans*) is an opportunistic human pathogen capable of causing a wide range of infections, such as bacteremia, meningitis, pneumonia, and peritonitis (1, 40). It has also been involved in nosocomial infections attributed to contaminated disinfectants, dialysis fluids, saline solution, and water (70). *A. xylosoxidans* has been reported from CF patients since 1985, and prevalence rates in CF patients vary from 3 to 18% (12, 25, 51, 96). *A. xylosoxidans* infections in CF patients do not seem to have a significant impact on lung function (25, 80, 87). *A. piechaudii* has been isolated from various clinical samples, including pharyngeal swabs, the nose, wounds, blood, and chronic ear discharge (56). There is a single report of recurrent *A. piechaudii* bacteremia associated with an intravenous catheter in an immunocompromised patient (53). *A. denitrificans* (previously known as *A. xylosoxidans* subsp. *denitrificans*) has been recovered from many clinical specimens, such as urine, proctoscopy specimens, prostate secretions, the buccal cavity, pleural fluid, and eye swabs (54), but there are no detailed reports about its clinical significance. *A. insolitus* (in a leg wound and in urine) and *A. spanius* (in blood) have been found in clinical material, but their significance is unclear (21).

Alcaligenes, Kersteria, and Advenella

A. faecalis strains have been isolated from a wide range of clinical samples (54), but the accuracy of the identification (especially in older reports) is difficult to assess. *A. faecalis* was found in cases of bacteremia following surgery or cancer treatment, ocular infections, a pancreatic abscess, infections following bone fractures, urine, and ear discharge (1, 6). There are sporadic reports of the recovery of *A. faecalis* in sputa of CF patients (114). *K. gyiorum* was isolated from human feces, leg wounds, and sputum (20). *A. incenata* has been recovered from human sputum (including sputa from CF patients) and blood, and several unnamed *Advenella* species were isolated from similar sources (22).

COLLECTION, TRANSPORT, AND STORAGE OF SPECIMENS

B. pertussis and B. parapertussis

Sampling for culture and PCR is difficult and markedly influences the sensitivity of these tests. Nasopharyngeal aspirates are adequate samples for infants and young children, and for culture, they are more sensitive than swabs (43). Nasopharyngeal swabs taken by trained personnel from older children, adolescents, and adults provide valid specimens from these age groups. Nasopharyngeal swabs should be taken by gently inserting the swab into the nasopharynx under the inferior nasal choana, and the nose of the patient should be

bent slightly upwards. If possible, two nasopharyngeal swabs should be taken, with one taken from each nostril. Swabs should be small and made of Dacron or rayon. Calcium-alginate swabs and swabs with aluminum shafts should not be used for PCR (86). Flocked nylon swabs, which are more convenient for the patient, may also be used but have not been validated for *B. pertussis* PCR or culture. Samples should be taken before antibiotic treatment is started.

The most sensitive method for culture is direct plating and preincubation at 35 to 37°C for 24 h before transport (73). Transport time is critical, and a transport medium protecting the bacteria from drying is required. Bacteriological transport media such as Casamino Acids or Amies medium with charcoal may be used, but transport time should not exceed 48 h. Half-strength Regan-Lowe (RL) charcoal-blood medium is also used for transport. In contrast to other transport media, RL medium can serve as an enrichment medium for *B. pertussis*. Transport at 4°C increases culture positivity but adds to logistical problems (73). For PCR, swabs can be transported dry at ambient temperature. The use of microbiological transport media such as Amies medium with charcoal does not interfere with PCR (86). Other respiratory samples, such as throat swabs, sputum samples, or throat washes, are less suitable and have not been validated (66, 73).

Other Bordetella Species, Achromobacter, Alcaligenes, Kersteria, and Advenella

For other bordetellae, normal microbiological transport media seem to be suitable for transport. Similarly, *Achromobacter*, *Alcaligenes*, *Kersteria*, and *Advenella* species can survive in a wide range of environments and at various temperatures. Standard collection, transport, and storage techniques are sufficient to ensure recovery of these organisms from clinical specimens, contaminated nosocomial sources, and the environment.

DIRECT DETECTION METHODS

B. pertussis and B. parapertussis

DFA

Direct fluorescent-antibody staining (DFA) requires nasopharyngeal swabs or nasopharyngeal aspirates; it is rapid and simple but lacks sensitivity and specificity (66). Antibodies for DFA are mostly polyclonal or directed against the LPS of *B. pertussis*. DFA is not accepted as proof of infection in notifying countries (73).

PCR

Depending on age, vaccination status, and duration of symptoms of the patients, PCR is between twofold and sixfold more sensitive than culture (35, 86). Block-based and real-time PCR methods seem to have comparable sensitivities (74, 86, 100). Similar to the case for culture, the sensitivity of PCR decreases with the duration of coughing; however, due to its higher sensitivity, it may be a useful tool for diagnosis for up to 4 to 6 weeks of coughing (86). Real-time PCR formats have the advantage of offering a result within several hours. DNA extraction is necessary to limit inhibition of PCR (86). Commercially available extraction kits seem to be comparable and appropriate (86), but no head-to-head comparison has yet been done. These kits are not FDA cleared or CE marked for this purpose. Most laboratories use the IS481 target (copy number, ~200 per cell) (63, 86) for the detection of *B. pertussis* and the IS*1001* target (copy number, ~20 per cell) (41) for the detection of *B. parapertussis*. There has been concern about the specificity of detection of *B. pertussis* due to sequence identity of IS*481* with *B. holmesii* (63, 85). Clinical samples were retested using primer-probe sets specific for *B. holmesii* DNA (3), and *B. holmesii*-specific sequences were not detected in any of the retested samples. These results suggest that IS*481* assays may currently be sufficiently specific for the laboratory diagnosis of *B. pertussis*. However, the periodic appearance of *B. holmesii* in some host populations and a possible carriage of IS*481* by some strains of *B. parapertussis* and *B. bronchiseptica* make it necessary to monitor the specificity of IS*481*-based assays. No specificity problems were reported for the detection of IS*1001* to diagnose *B. parapertussis* infections, although *B. holmesii* shares some sequence identity (86). The PT promoter (*ptxA*-Pr) is another target for *B. pertussis*-specific PCR assays (31, 35, 99), whereas the detection of the PT gene will detect both *B. pertussis* and *B. parapertussis*. Amplification of targets in the FHA gene, the PRN gene, and the porin gene was also used for detection of *B. pertussis* (83). Tests detecting one-copy genes were, however, consistently less sensitive than IS*481*-based PCRs. Detection can be done sequence specifically by use of fluorescence resonance energy transfer hybridization probes, TaqMan probes, and molecular beacons and also by non-sequence-specific formats using Sybr green I (86). For specificity reasons, most laboratories use sequence-specific formats (86). Duplex PCRs for *B. pertussis* (*B. holmesii*) and *B. parapertussis* have been developed. Commercial multiplex PCRs for the detection of various respiratory agents, including bordetellae, are available. External quality control programs have been implemented in European countries (74). In outbreak situations and after household contacts, a positive PCR result may also be found for patients with very few or no symptoms (16, 113).

ISOLATION PROCEDURES

B. pertussis and *B. parapertussis*
Culture is thought to be almost 100% specific, because very rarely have patients been found to harbor *B. pertussis*

without any symptoms (73). Several culture media, such as RL medium (73), Bordet-Gengou (BG) medium (8, 73), and Stainer-Scholte medium, have been used for culture of *B. pertussis* and *B. parapertussis*. RL medium is made with casein digest, beef extract, starch, and charcoal medium supplemented with horse blood. BG medium consists of potato infusion with glycerol and horse blood or sheep blood. Stainer-Scholte medium is a fully synthetic blood-free medium often used in vaccine production (73). Most media are supplemented with cephalexin to suppress concomitant bacteria. RL medium can be stored for 4 to 8 weeks, and BG medium has a shelf life of 5 days. Incubation time should be at least 1 week at 35 to 37°C at ambient atmosphere. The sensitivity of culture depends on the duration of symptoms and the age and vaccination status of the patient, and it varies between ~60% for young unvaccinated infants with symptoms of a few days in duration and <5% for adolescents and adults with more than 3 weeks of coughing (117).

Other *Bordetella* Species and *Achromobacter*
Bordetella spp. other than *B. pertussis* and *B. parapertussis* are encountered in clinical material as gram-negative nonfermentative bacilli in the laboratory. Table 3 gives some information about their growth characteristics and some biochemical reactions that may be used to differentiate them.

Achromobacter species can be isolated from clinical samples by the use of simple media and a selective enteric medium, such as MacConkey agar (54). It has been reported that a minority of *A. xylosoxidans* isolates grow on *Burkholderia cepacia*-selective oxidative-fermentative-polymyxin B-bacitracin-lactose agar or *Pseudomonas cepacia* agar (30% and 20%, respectively) but do not grow on *Burkholderia cepacia*-selective agar (46). Recent data from the U.S. CFF *Burkholderia cepacia* Research Laboratory and Repository (J. J. LiPuma, unpublished data) and a previous study (118) indicate that the majority of *A. xylosoxidans* isolates (~60%) will grow on *Burkholderia cepacia*-selective agar. Results obtained in a small-scale study suggest that particular selective media, such as gram-negative organism-selective agar, may increase the recovery of *A. xylosoxidans* from CF sputa (71).

TABLE 3 Useful characteristics for differentiating *Bordetella* species

Characteristic[a]	B. pertussis	B. parapertussis	B. bronchiseptica	B. avium	"B. ansorpii"	B. hinzii	B. holmesii	B. petrii	B. trematum
Growth on:									
RL medium	3–4 days	2–3 days	1–2 days	ND	ND	ND	ND	ND	ND
Columbia agar	−	V	+	+	+	+	+	+	+
MacConkey agar	−	−	+	+	+	+	V	+	+
Catalase	+	+	+	+	+	+	V	+	+
Oxidase	+	−	+	+	+	+	−	+	−
Motility	−	−	+	−	V	+	−	−	+
Pigment	−	Brown	−	−	−	−	−	Yellow	Yellow
Reduction of:									
Nitrate	−	−	+	−	−	−	−	+	V
Urea	−	+	+	−	−	−	−	−	−
Citrate	−	−	V	V	V	+	−	+	+

[a]Symbols and abbreviations: +, ≥90% of the strains are positive; −0, ≤10% of the strains are positive; V, 10 to 89% of the strains are positive; ND, not determined.

IDENTIFICATION

B. pertussis and *B. parapertussis*

B. pertussis colonies become visible after 3 to 7 days of incubation, and *B. parapertussis* colonies are visible already after 2 to 3 days. On RL medium, colonies are very small, round, and domed and appear silvery (Fig. 1). *B. parapertussis* colonies are larger and less shiny. The minute colonies on BG medium have a small zone of beta-hemolysis. *B. pertussis* is a small, coccoid, gram-negative rod which is catalase and oxidase positive (*B. parapertussis* is oxidase negative). The identities of these two species can best be confirmed by agglutination with specific antibodies. Further biochemical characteristics are given in Table 3. Due to the fastidious growth of *B. pertussis* and *B. parapertussis*, commercial systems for gram-negative rods are not reliable for identifying these species. 16S rRNA gene sequencing (69) and matrix-assisted laser desorption ionization–time-of-flight mass spectrometry (MALDI-TOF) (26) can be applied effectively for identification.

Isolates of *B. pertussis* and, less so, of *B. parapertussis* should not be subcultured because they undergo a phase change as described above. If strains have to be stored, this should be done with primary clinical isolates, and these should be frozen in glycerol at −70°C or in a sucrose-bovine serum albumin medium. Biosafety level 2 is strongly recommended.

Other Bordetellae

Colony morphology is not discriminative, and the bacteria are small coccoid rods that are catalase positive. In most instances, a biochemical system for identification of gram-negative bacilli will be used, such as API-NE, Vitek (bioMérieux), MicroScan (Siemens), Phoenix (Becton Dickinson) (94), and other systems. These systems were validated for nonfermentative rods, among which a few *Bordetella* spp. were also evaluated. Overall, the specificity of these biochemical systems for these bacteria is not very high, and thus an algorithm was recently proposed for the API-NE and Vitek II systems that uses 16S rRNA gene sequencing if the results of the biochemical identification are not reported as "excellent" or "very good" (17). 16S rRNA gene sequencing offers more reliable identification results and is available in many reference laboratories (10, 30, 82, 122). MALDI-TOF offers an alternative to sequencing (26). Apart from *B. bronchiseptica*, isolation of other bordetellae from clinical material is a rare event, and their identification might be confirmed by a reference laboratory.

Achromobacter

Achromobacter species typically show very limited action on carbohydrates (54), which hampers accurate identification at the genus level based on biochemical characteristics. Thus, 16S rRNA gene sequence analysis is recommended (13). Biochemical characteristics that distinguish the various *Achromobacter* species and discern them from *A. faecalis*, *K. gyiorum*, and *A. incenata* are shown in Table 2. Several commercial systems allow the identification of *Achromobacter* species. A comparison indicated that *A. xylosoxidans* was correctly identified in 88%, 71%, 54%, and 21% of cases, using the RapID NF Plus, API Rapid NFT, Vitek, and Remel systems, respectively (57). *A. xylosoxidans* may be misidentified as a member of the *B. cepacia* complex (and the other way around) by some commercial systems (93, 122), and due to its weak biochemical reactivity, prolonged incubation (e.g., for up to 72 h with the API 20 NE system) may be required to obtain a reliable identification. A PCR assay (based on the 16S rRNA gene) was developed for *A. xylosoxidans*, but positive results may also be obtained with strains of other *Achromobacter* species as well as with some *Bordetella* species (62, 97). The use of fluorescent in situ hybridization (FISH) with a probe directed against the 16S rRNA gene has been reported for the identification of *A. xylosoxidans* (114). FISH assays had a high sensitivity and better specificity than the PCR assay (62, 97, 114), although cross-reactivity with *A. ruhlandii* and a *Chryseobacterium* sp. isolate was observed (114). MALDI-TOF and Fourier transform infrared spectroscopy have also been used successfully to identify *A. xylosoxidans* (9, 26).

Alcaligenes, *Kerstersia*, and *Advenella*

For *Alcaligenes*, *Advenella*, and *Kerstersia*, 16S rRNA gene sequence analysis is recommended for accurate identification at the genus level (13). Differential biochemical reactions are listed in Table 2. Members of the genus *Advenella* can be separated from related species by their inability to assimilate phenyl acetate. *Kerstersia* strains are oxidase negative. A distinguishing characteristic of *A. faecalis* isolates is that they reduce nitrite but not nitrate. Molecular techniques have not yet been developed for these organisms, with the exception of a 16S rRNA gene-directed FISH probe for *A. faecalis* (114).

TYPING SYSTEMS

B. pertussis and *B. parapertussis* show only a very small amount of genomic heterogeneity (11). The *ptx* gene and the *prn* genes are polymorphic in the *B. pertussis* genome, and various *ptx* and *prn* types (prn1 to prn8) have been identified (102). The expression of fimbriae undergoes temporal changes, possibly influenced by vaccine coverage (102). Circulating isolates of *B. pertussis* have been typed by various methods, such as pulsed-field gel electrophoresis (PFGE), analysis of variable-number tandem repeats, restriction fragment length polymorphism analysis (102), and others (82). The *prn* types of clinical isolates mostly differ from the *prn* type of the currently used vaccine, but so far no changes in the effectiveness of acellular vaccines have been observed. Studies using PFGE have shown that the overall genomic heterogeneity of clinical isolates decreases (44).

Typing of *A. xylosoxidans* isolates by PFGE of fragments obtained after digestion with XbaI, SpeI, or DraI has been used in several studies (69, 80) and is reported to have a high discriminatory power. Randomly amplified polymorphic DNA PCR (60) and PCR with enter-

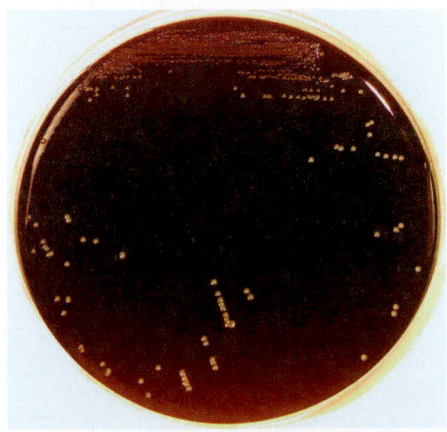

FIGURE 1   Growth of *B. pertussis* on RL medium.

obacterial repetitive intergenic consensus or repetitive extragenic palindromic primers (103) have also been used. The discriminatory power of ribotyping (using the Riboprinter microbial characterization system) was rather low (18). Selective restriction fragment amplification (using EcoRI and MseI) was also successfully applied to *A. xylosoxidans* (103).

SEROLOGIC TESTS

B. pertussis and *B. parapertussis*
Pertussis in older vaccinated children, in adolescents, and in adults is mostly diagnosed by serological tests. The use of enzyme-linked immunosorbent assay (24, 28, 37, 64) to quantify anti-PT antibody levels is a validated and sensitive diagnostic technique and can be performed with paired (acute- and convalescent-phase samples) or single serum samples (73). Paired-sample serology is a standardized method of diagnosis (61), but single-sample serology also provides good sensitivity and specificity to determine cases in older children, adolescents, and adults (5, 15, 27, 121). A WHO reference preparation for human pertussis serology is available (119), and quantitative results of pertussis serology should be reported in international units/milliliter. Immunoglobulin G (IgG) anti-PT antibodies at >100 to 125 IU/ml can be used as an indicator of recent contact with PT-producing bacteria (67, 78, 108). IgG antibodies are those mostly measured, but the roles of other isotypes, such as IgA and IgM, are not clear (66). Serology cannot distinguish between vaccine- and infection-induced immunological responses (symptomatic or asymptomatic infection) (66, 101). Commercial assays are of very variable quality (85a) and are in need of further standardization (101). Pertussis serology may not be used for 1 year after vaccination with acellular vaccines.

ANTIMICROBIAL SUSCEPTIBILITY

B. pertussis and *B. parapertussis*
B. pertussis and *B. parapertussis* are susceptible in vitro to a range of antibiotics, including penicillins, macrolides, ketolides, quinolones, and other antibiotics, including tetracyclines, chloramphenicol, and trimethoprim-sulfamethoxazole, whereas they are resistant to most oral cephalosporins (66, 73). However, in contrast to the case for other bacterial diseases, the exact relationship between the pharmacokinetics and pharmacodynamics of these antibiotics and the in vitro susceptibility of the organism is unknown. Furthermore, the effect on the symptoms of pertussis is not well documented (2, 79).

Methods for antibiotic sensitivity testing of *B. pertussis* and *B. parapertussis* are not standardized. If testing is done, the methods include broth macro- and microdilution methods, agar dilution methods, breakpoint methods, and Etest, whereas the disk diffusion method is mostly not feasible (116). Erythromycin resistance may be evaluated by the disk diffusion method. Erythromycin resistance was documented first in the United States and subsequently in other countries. In retrospect, erythromycin-resistant organisms were found in strain collections from the 1960s, and no data so far suggest that this resistance is spreading (116). Erythromycin resistance is mediated by a mutation in the macrolide binding domain of the 23S rRNA. Routine antibiotic susceptibility testing of *B. pertussis* isolates

is not recommended and should only be done when special clinical or epidemiological circumstances are found (81). Continued surveillance of these isolates, when performed, should also include antimicrobial susceptibility testing.

Other Bordetellae
B. bronchiseptica possesses a β-lactamase (50) and is resistant to many penicillins and cephalosporins and mostly resistant to trimethoprim-sulfamethoxazole (72). A recent study of canine and feline isolates (91) showed that most isolates were sensitive to amoxicillin-clavulanic acid, tetracycline, gentamicin, and a quinolone. *B. avium* was resistant to cefuroxime, trimethoprim-sulfamethoxazole, and tetracycline and sensitive to ampicillin, mezlocillin, and gentamicin (72). A human *B. hinzii* isolate was sensitive to amoxicillin, gentamicin, and meropenem but resistant to cefuroxime, ceftriaxone, and ciprofloxacin (34). A human "*B. ansorpii*" isolate was resistant to aztreonam, cefuroxime, and ceftriaxone and sensitive to amoxicillin, gentamicin, and ciprofloxacin (33). Antimicrobial sensitivity testing of these *Bordetella* isolates should be interpreted in accordance with criteria for other infrequently isolated and fastidious nonfermentative gram-negative rods.

Achromobacter
Methods for antibiotic sensitivity testing of *Achromobacter*, *Alcaligenes*, *Kerstersia*, and *Advenella* species are not standardized. If testing is done, the methods include broth macro- and microdilution, agar dilution methods, breakpoint methods, and Etest.

A. xylosoxidans isolates (39) were sensitive only to imipenem, piperacillin, ticarcillin-clavulanic acid, ceftazidime, and trimethoprim-sulfamethoxazole. Aminoglycosides, expanded-spectrum cephalosporins other than ceftazidime, and quinolones showed no activity. The majority of the strains were resistant to a conventional tobramycin concentration, but 41% of the strains were inhibited by the higher tobramycin concentrations achievable by aerosol delivery of the antibiotic. Similarly, 92% of strains were inhibited by high doses of colistin (100 μg/ml). Little synergistic activity was measured for combinations of antibiotics, and additive activity was noted with chloramphenicol-minocycline, ciprofloxacin-imipenem, and ciprofloxacin-meropenem (89). *A. xylosoxidans* was resistant to azithromycin and clarithromycin, and only modest synergistic and/or additive activities were observed when azithromycin was combined with meropenem or trimethoprim-sulfamethoxazole (88). These data correlate well with many smaller clinical studies and case reports (51, 65, 80, 103). Antimicrobial susceptibility data for other *Achromobacter* species are rare, but *A. spanius* and *A. insolitus* were resistant to most quinolones, macrolides, and cephalosporins tested (22), while a blood isolate of *A. piechaudii* was resistant to ampicillin, cefpodoxime, and gentamicin but susceptible to all other antibiotics tested (53).

Alcaligenes, Kerstersia, and *Advenella*
A. faecalis is more susceptible to antibiotics than *A. xylosoxidans* (95). Most *A. faecalis* strains are resistant to amoxicillin, ticarcillin, aztreonam, kanamycin, gentamicin, and nalidixic acid, while being susceptible to the combination of amoxicillin or ticarcillin with clavulanic acid, to various cephalosporins, and to ciprofloxacin (7). Most *Kerstersia* isolates are susceptible to ciprofloxacin and cefotaxime (20), and antimicrobial susceptibility in *Advenella* spp. has not yet been studied.

EVALUATION, INTERPRETATION, AND REPORTING OF RESULTS

Due to its sensitivity and speed, PCR is the preferred method for the direct detection of *B. pertussis* and *B. parapertussis*. A positive IS*481* PCR from a nasopharyngeal swab or a nasopharyngeal aspirate can be considered to indicate a *B. pertussis* (or *B. holmesii*) infection when the clinical symptoms are in accordance with this result. The specificity may be substantiated by a positive *ptxA*-Pr PCR by reference laboratories. Due to the higher sensitivity of IS*481* PCRs, a few samples may be positive for IS*481* and negative for *ptx*-Pr (35). These results can be reported as *Bordetella* DNA positive (*B. pertussis*, *B. holmesii*, or *B. bronchiseptica*). A positive IS*1001* PCR result from a nasopharyngeal swab or a nasopharyngeal aspirate is indicative of *B. parapertussis* infection, without further tests.

If culture is performed, the isolation of *B. pertussis* and *B. parapertussis* implies an infection, although the sensitivity is sufficiently high only for neonates and unvaccinated infants. Routine antimicrobial sensitivity testing is not necessary.

Serological diagnosis of pertussis is usually based on single-sample serology. Results cannot be interpreted correctly for about 1 year after vaccination with acellular pertussis vaccines. An IgG anti-PT titer of ≥100 to 125 IU/ml is mostly used as an indicator of recent contact. In adolescent and adult populations, an IgG anti-PT titer of <40 IU/ml may be interpreted as not indicative of recent infection. Apart from Massachusetts, serology is not accepted as a confirmation of cases in other U.S. states. Many European countries with statutory notification and laboratory confirmation accept serology as proof of infection.

Similar to the case for other rarely isolated gram-negative nonenteric rods, the clinical relevance of other *Bordetella* spp., *Achromobacter* spp., *Alcaligenes* spp., *Kerstersia* spp., and *Advenella* spp. isolated from clinical material should be discussed on a case-to-case basis between the microbiology laboratory and the clinician. Antimicrobial testing of these species should be performed and can be helpful in guiding therapeutic decisions.

REFERENCES

1. **Aisenberg, G., K. V. Rolston, and A. Safdar.** 2004. Bacteremia caused by *Achromobacter* and *Alcaligenes* species in 46 patients with cancer (1989–2003). *Cancer* **101:**2134–2140.
2. **Altunaiji, S., R. Kukuruzovic, N. Curtis, and J. Massie.** 2007. Antibiotics for whooping cough (pertussis). *Cochrane Database Syst. Rev.* **18:**CD004404.
3. **Antila, M., Q. He, C. de Jong, I. Aarts, H. Verbakel, S. Bruistenm, S. Keller, M. Haanperä, J. Mäkinen, E. Eerola, M. J. Viljanen, J. Mertsola, and A. van der Zee.** 2006. *Bordetella holmesii* DNA is not detected in nasopharyngeal swabs from Finnish and Dutch patients with suspected pertussis. *J. Med. Microbiol.* **55:**1043–1051.
4. **Arvand, M., R. Feldhues, M. Mieth, T. Kraus, and P. Vandamme.** 2004. Chronic cholangitis caused by *Bordetella hinzii* in a liver transplant recipient. *J. Clin. Microbiol.* **42:**2335–2337.
5. **Baughman, A. L., K. M. Bisgard, K. M. Edwards, D. Guris, M. D. Decker, K. Holland, B. D. Meade, and F. Lynn.** 2004. Establishment of diagnostic cutoff points for levels of serum antibodies to pertussis toxin, filamentous hemagglutinin, and fimbriae in adolescents and adults in the United States. *Clin. Diagn. Lab. Immunol.* **11:**1045–1053.
6. **Bizet, J., and C. Bizet.** 1997. Strains of *Alcaligenes faecalis* from clinical material. *J. Infect.* **35:**167–169.
7. **Bizet, C., F. Tekaia, and A. Philippon.** 1993. In-vitro susceptibility of *Alcaligenes faecalis* compared with those of other *Alcaligenes* spp. to antimicrobial agents including seven beta-lactams. *J. Antimicrob. Chemother.* **32:**907–910.
8. **Bordet, J., and U. Gengou.** 1906. Le microbe de la coqueluche. *Ann. Inst. Pasteur* **20:**48–68.
9. **Bosch, A., A. Miñán, C. Vescina, J. Degrossi, B. Gatti, P. Montanaro, M. Messina, M. Franco, C. Vay, J. Schmitt, D. Naumann, and O. Yantorno.** 2008. Fourier transform infrared spectroscopy for rapid identification of nonfermenting gram-negative bacteria isolated from sputum samples from cystic fibrosis patients. *J. Clin. Microbiol.* **46:**2535–2546.
10. **Bosshard, P. P., R. Zbinden, S. Abels, B. Böddinghaus, A. Altwegg, and E. C. Böttger.** 2006. 16S rRNA gene sequencing versus the API 20 NE system and the VITEK 2 ID-GNB card for identification of nonfermenting gram-negative bacteria in the clinical laboratory. *J. Clin. Microbiol.* **44:**1359–1366.
11. **Brinig, M. M., C. A. Cummings, G. N. Sanden, P. Stefanelli, A. Lawrence, and D. A. Relman.** 2006. Significant gene order and expression differences in *Bordetella pertussis* despite limited gene content variation. *J. Bacteriol.* **188:**2375–2382.
12. **Burns, J. L., J. Emerson, J. R. Stapp, D. L. Yim, J. Krzewinski, L. Louden, B. W. Ramsey, and C. R. Clausen.** 1998. Microbiology of sputum from patients at cystic fibrosis centers in the United States. *Clin. Infect. Dis.* **27:**158–163.
13. **Busse, H. J., and A. Stolz.** 2006. *Achromobacter, Alcaligenes* and related genera, p. 675–700. *In* M. Dworkin, S. Falkow, E. Rosenberg, K.-H. Schleifer, and E. Stackebrandt (ed.), *The Prokaryotes*, vol. 5. Springer, Heidelberg, Germany.
14. **Cagney, M., P. B. McIntyre, L. Heron, A. Giammanco, and C. R. MacIntyre.** 2008. The relationship between pertussis symptomatology, incidence and serology in adolescents. *Vaccine* **26:**5547–5553.
15. **Cattaneo, L. A., G. W. Reed, D. H. Haase, M. J. Wills, and K. M. Edwards.** 1996. The seroepidemiology of *Bordetella pertussis* infections: a study in persons ages 1–65 years. *J. Infect. Dis.* **173:**1256–1259.
16. **CDC.** 2007. Outbreaks of respiratory illness mistakenly attributed to pertussis—New Hampshire, Massachusetts, and Tennessee, 2004–2006. *Morb. Mortal Wkly. Rep.* **56:**837–842.
17. **Clarridge, J. E., III.** 2004. Impact of 16S rRNA gene sequence analysis for identification of bacteria on clinical microbiology and infectious diseases. *Clin. Microbiol. Rev.* **17:**840–862.
18. **Clermont, D., C. Harmant, and C. J. Bizet.** 2001. Identification of strains of *Alcaligenes* and *Agrobacterium* by a polyphasic approach. *J. Clin. Microbiol.* **39:**3104–3109.
19. **Coenye, T., J. Goris, T. Spiker, P. Vandamme, and J. J. LiPuma.** 2002. Characterization of unusual bacteria isolated from respiratory secretions of cystic fibrosis patients, and description of *Inquilinus limosus* gen. nov. sp. nov. *J. Clin. Microbiol.* **40:**2062–2069.
20. **Coenye, T., M. Vancanneyt, M. Cnockaert, E. Falsen, J. Swings, and P. Vandamme.** 2003. *Kerstersia gyiorum* gen. nov., sp. nov., a novel *Alcaligenes faecalis*-like organism isolated from human clinical samples, and reclassification of *Alcaligenes denitrificans* Rüger and Tan 1983 as *Achromobacter denitrificans* comb. nov. *Int. J. Syst. Evol. Microbiol.* **53:**1825–1831.
21. **Coenye, T., M. Vancanneyt, E. Falsen, J. Swings, and P. Vandamme.** 2003. *Achromobacter insolitus* sp. nov. and *Achromobacter spanius* sp. nov., from human clinical samples. *Int. J. Syst. Evol. Microbiol.* **53:**1819–1824.
22. **Coenye, T., E. Vanlaere, E. Samyn, E. Falsen, and P. Vandamme.** 2005. *Advenella incenata* gen. nov., sp. nov., a novel member of the *Alcaligenaceae*, isolated from various clinical samples. *Int. J. Syst. Evol. Microbiol.* **55:**251–256.
23. **Cosnes-Lambe, C., J. Raymond, M. Chalumeau, C. Pons-Catalano, F. Moulin, N. de Suremain, H. Reglier-Pupet, P. Lebon, C. Poyart, and E. Grimprel.** 2008. Pertussis and respiratory syncytial virus infections. *Eur. J. Pediatr.* **167:**1017–1019.
24. **Daxboeck, F., E. Goerzer, P. Apfalter, M. Nehr, and R. Krause.** 2004. Isolation of *Bordetella trematum* from a diabetic leg ulcer. *Diabetes Med.* **21:**1247–1248.

25. **De Baets, F., P. Schelstraete, S. Van Daele, F. Haerynck, and M. Vaneechoutte.** 2007. *Achromobacter xylosoxidans* in cystic fibrosis: prevalence and clinical relevance. *J. Cyst. Fibros.* **6:**75–78.

26. **Degand, N., E. Carbonelle, B. Dauphin, J. L. Beretti, M. Le Bourgeois, I. Sermet-Gaudelus, C. Segonds, P. Berche, X. Nassif, and A. Ferroni.** 2008. Matrix-assisted laser desorption ionization–time-of-flight mass spectrometry of nonfermenting gram-negative bacilli isolated from cystic fibrosis patients. *J. Clin. Microbiol.* **46:**3361–3367.

27. **de Melker, H. E., F. G. Versteegh, M. A. Conyn-Van Spaendonck, L. H. Elvers, G. A. Berbers, A. van der Zee, and J. F. Schellekens.** 2000. Specificity and sensitivity of high levels of immunoglobulin G antibodies to pertussis toxin in a single serum sample for diagnosis of infection with *Bordetella pertussis. J. Clin. Microbiol.* **38:**800–806.

28. **Edwards, K. M., B. D. Meade, M. D. Decker, G. F. Reed, M. B. Rennels, M. C. Steinhoff, E. L. Anderson, J. A. Englund, M. A. Pichichichero, M. A. Deloria, and A. Deforest.** 1995. Comparison of 13 acellular pertussis vaccines: overview and serologic response. *Pediatrics* **96:**548–557.

29. **Fenollar, F., V. Roux, A. Stein, M. Drancourt, and D. Raoult.** 2006. Analysis of 525 samples to determine the usefulness of PCR amplification and sequencing of the 16S rRNA gene for diagnosis of bone and joint infections. *J. Clin. Microbiol.* **44:**1018–1028.

30. **Fontana, C., M. Favaro, M. Pellicioni, E. S. Pistoia, and C. Favalli.** 2005. Use of the MicroSeq 500 16S rRNA gene-based sequencing for identification of bacterial isolates that commercial automated systems failed to identify. *J. Clin. Microbiol.* **43:**615–619.

31. **Fry, N. K., O. Tzivra, Y. T. Li, A. McNiff, N. Doshi, P. A. Maple, N. S. Crowcroft, E. Miller, R. C. George, and T. G. Harrison.** 2004. Laboratory diagnosis of pertussis infections: the role of PCR and serology. *J. Med. Microbiol.* **53:**519–525.

32. **Fry, N. K., J. Duncan, H. Malnick, M. Warner, A. J. Smith, M. S. Jackson, and A. Ayoub.** 2005. *Bordetella petrii* clinical isolate. *Emerg. Infect. Dis.* **11:**1131–1133.

33. **Fry, N. K., J. Duncan, H. Malnick, and P. M. Cockcroft.** 2007. The first UK isolate of "*Bordetella ansorpii*" from an immunocompromised patient. *J. Med. Microbiol.* **56:**993–995.

34. **Fry, N. K., J. Duncan, M. T. Edwards, R. E. Tilley, D. Chitvanis, R. Harman, H. Hammerton, and L. Dalton.** 2007. A UK clinical isolate of *Bordetella hinzii* from a patient with myelodysplastic syndrome. *J. Med. Microbiol.* **56:**1700–1703.

35. **Fry, N. K., J. Duncan, K. Wagner, O. Tzivra, N. Doshi, D. J. Litt, N. Crowcroft, E. Miller, R. C. George, and T. G. Harrison.** 2009. Role of PCR in the diagnosis of pertussis infection in infants: 5 years' experience of provision of a same-day real-time PCR service in England and Wales from 2002 to 2007. *J. Med. Microbiol.* **58:**1023–1029.

36. **Gerlach, G., S. Janzen, D. Beier, and R. Gross.** 2004. Functional characterization of the BvgAS two-component system of *Bordetella holmesii. Microbiology* **150:**3715–3729.

37. **Giammanco, A., A. Nardone, R. Pebody, G. Kafatos, N. Andrews, A. Chiarini, S. Taormina, F. de Ory, K. Prossenc, B. Krize, H. Hallander, M. Ljungman, E. Marva, A. Tsakris, D. O'Flanagan, F. Schneider, A. Griskevicius, R. Vranckx, and I. Karacs.** 2008. European Sero-Epidemiology Network 2: standardization of immunoassay results for pertussis requires homogeneity of antigenic preparations. *Vaccine* **26:**4486–4493.

38. **Gibello, A., A. L. Vela, M. Martin, A. Barra-Caracciolo, P. Grenni, and J. F. Fernandez-Garayzabal.** 2009. Reclassification of the members of the genus *Tetrathiobacter* Ghosh et al. 2005 to the genus *Advenella* Coenye et al. 2005. *Int. J. Syst. Evol. Microbiol.* **59:**1914–1918.

39. **Glupczynski, Y., W. Hansen, J. Freney, and E. Yourassowsky.** 1988. In vitro susceptibility of *Alcaligenes denitrificans* subsp. *xylosoxidans* to 24 antimicrobial agents. *Antimicrob. Agents Chemother.* **32:**276–278.

40. **Gómez-Cerezo, J., I. Suárez, J. J. Ríos, P. Peña, M. J. García de Miguel, M. de José, O. Monteagudo, P. Linares, A. Barbado-Cano, and J. J. Vázquez.** 2003. *Achromobacter xylosoxidans* bacteremia: a 10-year analysis of 54 cases. *Eur. J. Clin. Microbiol. Infect. Dis.* **22:**360–363.

41. **Gross, R., C. A. Guzman, M. Sebaiihia, V. A. P. Martins dos Santos, D. H. Pieper, R. Koebnik, M. Lechner, D. Bartels, J. Buhrmeister, J. V. Choudhouri, T. Ebensen, L. Gaigalat, S. Hermann, A. N. Khachane, C. Larisch, S. Link, B. Linke, F. Meyer, S. Mormann, D. Nakunst, C. Rückert, S. Schneiker-Bekel, K. Schulze, F. J. Vorhölter, T. Yevsa, J. T. Engle, W. E. Goldman, A. Pühler, U. B. Göbel, A. Goesmann, H. Blöcker, O. Kaiser, and R. Martinez-Arias.** 2008. The missing link: *Bordetella petrii* is endowed with both the metabolic versatility of environmental bacteria and virulence traits of pathogenic bordetellae. *BMC Genomics* **9:**449.

42. **Haberling, D. L., R. C. Holman, C. D. Paddock, and T. V. Murphy.** 2009. Infant and maternal risk factors for pertussis-related infant mortality in the United States, 1999 to 2004. *Pediatr. Infect. Dis. J.* **28:**194–198.

43. **Hallander, H. O., E. Reizenstein, B. Renemar, G. Rasmuson, L. Mardin, and P. Olin.** 1993. Comparison of nasopharyngeal aspirates with swabs for culture of *Bordetella pertussis. J. Clin. Microbiol.* **31:**50–52.

44. **Hallander, H., A. Advani, M. Riffelmann, C. H. Wirsing von König, V. Caro, N. Guiso, F. R. Mooi, A. Gzyl, M. S. Kaltoft, N. K. Fry, J. Mertsola, and Q. He.** 2007. *Bordetella pertussis* strain circulating in Europe in 1999 to 2004 as determined by pulsed field gel electrophoresis. *J. Clin. Microbiol.* **45:**3257–3261.

45. **Harrington, A. T., J. A. Castellanos, T. M. Ziedalski, J. E. Clarridge III, and B. T. Cookson.** 2009. Isolation of *Bordetella avium* and novel *Bordetella* strain from patients with respiratory disease. *Emerg. Infect. Dis.* **15:**72–74.

46. **Henry, D. A., M. E. Campbell, J. J. LiPuma, and D. P. Speert.** 1997. Identification of *Burkholderia cepacia* isolates from patients with cystic fibrosis and use of a simple new selective medium. *J. Clin. Microbiol.* **35:**614–619.

47. **Hewlett, E. L., G. M. Donato, and M. C. Gray.** 2006. Macrophage cytotoxicity produced by adenylate cyclase toxin from *Bordetella pertussis*: more than just making AMP. *Mol. Microbiol.* **59:**447–459.

48. **Hijnen, M., Q. He, R. Schepp, P. van Gageldonk, J. Mertsola, F. R. Mooi, and G. A. Berbers.** 2008. Antibody responses to defined regions of the *Bordetella pertussis* virulence factor pertactin. *Scand. J. Infect. Dis.* **40:**92–104.

49. **Hristov, A. C., P. G. Auwaerter, M. Romagnoli, and K. C. Caroll.** 2008. *Bordetella hinzii* septicaemia in association with Epstein-Barr virus viremia and an Epstein-Barr virus-associated diffuse large B-cell lymphoma. *Diagn. Microbiol. Infect. Dis.* **61:**484–486.

50. **Kadlec, K., J. Wiegand, C. Kehrenberg, and S. Schwarz.** 2007. Studies on the mechanisms of beta-lactam resistance in *Bordetella bronchiseptica. J. Antimicrob. Chemother.* **59:**396–402.

51. **Kanellopoulou, M., S. Pournaras, H. Iglezos, N. Skarmoutsou, E. Papafrangas, and A. N. Maniatis.** 2004. Persistent colonization of nine cystic fibrosis patients with an *Achromobacter* (*Alcaligenes*) *xylosoxidans* clone. *Eur. J. Clin. Microbiol. Infect. Dis.* **23:**336–339.

52. **Kattar, M. M., J. F. Chavez, A. P. Limaye, S. L. Rassoulian-Barrett, S. L. Yarfitz, L. C. Carlson, Y. Houze, S. Swanzy, B. L. Wood, and B. T. Cookson.** 2000. Application of 16S rRNA sequencing to identify *Bordetella hinzii* as the causative agent of fatal septicaemia. *J. Clin. Microbiol.* **38:**789–794.

53. **Kay, S. E., R. A. Clark, K. L. White, and M. M. Peel.** 2001. Recurrent *Achromobacter piechaudii* bacteremia in a patient with hematological malignancy. *J. Clin. Microbiol.* **39:**808–810.

54. **Kersters, K., and J. De Ley.** 1984. Genus *Alcaligenes* Castellani and Chalmers 1919, 936^(AL), p. 361–373. *In* N. R. Krieg and J. G. Holt (ed.), *Bergey's Manual of Systematic Bacteriology*, vol. 1. Williams & Wilkins Co., Baltimore, MD.

55. Kersters, K., K. H. Hinz, A. Hertle, P. Segers, A. Lievens, O. Siegmann, and J. DeLey. 1984. *Bordetella avium* sp. nov., isolated from the respiratory tracts of turkeys and other birds. *Int. J. Syst. Bacteriol.* **34:**56–70.

56. Kiredjian, M., B. Holmes, K. Kersters, I. Guilvout, and J. De Ley. 1986. *Alcaligenes piechaudii* sp. nov., a new species from human clinical specimens and the environment. *Int. J. Syst. Bacteriol.* **36:**282–287.

57. Kiska, D. L., A. Kerr, M. C. Jones, J. A. Caracciolo, B. Eskridge, M. Jordan, S. Miller, D. Hughes, N. King, and P. H. Gilligan. 1996. Accuracy of four commercial systems for identification of *Burkholderia cepacia* and other gram-negative nonfermenting bacilli recovered from patients with cystic fibrosis. *J. Clin. Microbiol.* **34:**886–891.

58. Ko, K. S., K. R. Pecj, W. S. Oh, N. Y. Lee, J. H. Lee, and J. H. Song. 2005. New species of *Bordetella*, *Bordetella ansorpii* sp. nov., isolated from the purulent exudate of an epidermal cyst. *J. Clin. Microbiol.* **43:**2516–2519.

59. Reference deleted.

60. Krzewinski, J. W., C. D. Nguyen, J. M. Foster, and J. L. Burns. 2001. Use of random amplified polymorphic DNA PCR to examine epidemiology of *Stenotrophomonas maltophilia* and *Achromobacter* (*Alcaligenes*) *xylosoxidans* from patients with cystic fibrosis. *J. Clin. Microbiol.* **39:**3597–3602.

61. Le, T., J. D. Cherry, S. J. Chang, M. D. Knoll, M. L. Lee, S. Barenkamp, D. Bernstein, R. Edelman, K. M. Edwards, D. Greenberg, W. Keitel, J. Treanor, and J. I. Ward. 2004. Immune responses and antibody decay after immunization of adolescents and adults with an acellular pertussis vaccine: the APERT Study. *J. Infect. Dis.* **190:**535–544.

62. Liu, L., T. Coenye, J. L. Burns, P. W. Whitby, T. L. Stull, and J. J. LiPuma. 2002. rDNA-directed PCR for identification of *Alcaligenes* (*Achromobacter*) *xylosoxidans* recovered from cystic fibrosis sputum. *J. Clin. Microbiol.* **40:**1210–1213.

63. Loeffelholz, M. J., C. J. Thompson, K. S. Long, and M. J. R. Gilchrist. 2000. Detection of *Bordetella holmesii* using *Bordetella pertussis* IS481 PCR assay. *J. Clin. Microbiol.* **38:**467.

64. Lynn, F., G. F. Reed, and B. D. Meade. 1996. Collaborative study for the evaluation of enzyme-linked immunosorbent assays used to measure human antibodies to *Bordetella pertussis* antigens. *Clin. Diagn. Lab. Immunol.* **3:**689–700.

65. MacKenzie, F. M., S. V. Smith, K. E. Milne, K. Griffiths, J. Legge, and I. M. Gould. 2004. Antibiograms of resistant gram-negative bacteria from Scottish CF patients. *J. Cyst. Fibros.* **3:**151–157.

66. Mattoo, S., and J. D. Cherry. 2005. Molecular pathogenesis, epidemiology, and clinical manifestations of respiratory infections due to *Bordetella pertussis* and other *Bordetella* subspecies. *Clin. Microbiol. Rev.* **18:**326–382.

67. Mertens, P. L., F. S. Stals, E. W. Steyerberg, and J. H. Richardus. 2007. Sensitivity and specificity of single IgA and IgG antibody concentrations for early diagnosis of pertussis in adults: an evaluation for outbreak management in public health practice. *BMC Infect. Dis.* **7:**53.

68. Moissenet, D., A. Baculard, M. Valcin, V. Marchand, G. Tournier, A. Garbarg-Chenon, and H. Vu-Thien. 1997. Colonization by *Alcaligenes xylosoxidans* in children with cystic fibrosis: a retrospective clinical study conducted by means of molecular epidemiological investigation. *Clin. Infect. Dis.* **24:**274–275.

69. Moissenet, D., E. Bingen, G. Arlet, and H. Vu-Thien. 2005. Use of 16S rRNA gene sequencing for identification of Pseudomonas-like isolates from sputum of patients with cystic fibrosis. *Pathol. Biol.* (Paris) **53:**500–502.

70. Molina-Cabrillana, J., C. Santana-Reyes, A. González-García, A. Bordes-Benítez, and I. Horcajada. 2007. Outbreak of *Achromobacter xylosoxidans* pseudobacteremia in a neonatal care unit related to contaminated chlorhexidine solution. *Eur. J. Clin. Microbiol. Infect. Dis.* **26:**435–437.

71. Moore, J. E., J. Xu, B. C. Millar, J. Courtney, and J. S. Elborn. 2003. Development of a gram-negative selective agar (GNSA) for the detection of gram-negative microflora in sputa in patients with cystic fibrosis. *J. Appl. Microbiol.* **95:**160–166.

72. Mortensen, J. E., A. Brumbach, and T. R. Shrycock. 1989. Antimicrobial susceptibility of *Bordetella avium* and *Bordetella bronchiseptica* isolates. *Antimicrob. Agents Chemother.* **33:**771–772.

73. Müller, F. M., J. E. Hoppe, and C. H. Wirsing von König. 1997. Diagnosis of pertussis: state of the art in 1997. *J. Clin. Microbiol.* **35:**2435–2443.

74. Muyldermans, G., O. Soetens, M. Antoine, S. Bruisten, B. Vincart, K. Doucet, F. Populaire, N. K. Fry, P. Olcen, J. M. Scheftel, J. M. Senterre, A. van der Zee, M. Riffelmann, D. Pierard, and S. Lauwers. 2005. External quality assessment for molecular detection of *Bordetella pertussis* in European laboratories. *J. Clin. Microbiol.* **43:**30–35.

75. Paddock, C. D., G. N. Sanden, J. D. Cherry, A. A. Gal, C. Langston, K. M. Tatti, K. H. Wu, C. S. Goldsmith, P. W. Greer, J. L. Montague, M. T. Eliason, R. C. Holman, J. Guarner, W. J. Shieh, and S. R. Zaki. 2008. Pathology and pathogenesis of fatal *Bordetella pertussis* infections in infants. *Clin. Infect. Dis.* **47:**328–338.

76. Parkhill, J., M. Sebaihia, A. Preston, L. D. Murphy, N. Thomson, D. E. Harris, M. T. Holden, C. M. Churcher, S. D. Bentley, K. L. Mungall, A. M. Cerdeño-Tárraga, L. Temple, K. James, B. Harris, M. A. Quail, M. Achtman, R. Atkin, S. Baker, D. Basham, N. Bason, I. Cherevach, T. Chillingworth, M. Collins, A. Cronin, P. Davis, J. Doggett, T. Feltwell, A. Goble, N. Hamlin, H. Hauser, S. Holroyd, K. Jagels, S. Leather, S. Moule, H. Norberczak, S. O'Neil, D. Ormond, C. Price, E. Rabbinowitsch, S. Rutter, M. Sanders, D. Saunders, K. Seeger, S. Sharp, M. Simmonds, J. Skelton, R. Squares, S. Squares, K. Stevens, L. Unwin, S. Whitehead, B. G. Barrell, and D. J. Maskell. 2003. Comparative analysis of the genome sequences of *Bordetella pertussis*, *Bordetella parapertussis* and *Bordetella bronchiseptica*. *Nat. Genet.* **35:**32–40.

77. Patriarca, P. A., R. J. Biellik, G. Sanden, D. G. Burstyn, P. D. Mitchell, P. R. Silverman, J. P. Davis, and C. R. Manclark. 1998. Sensitivity and specificity of clinical case definitions of pertussis. *Am. J. Public Health* **78:**833–836.

78. Pebody, R. G., N. J. Gay, A. Giammanco, S. Baron, J. Schellekens, A. Tischer, R. M. Olander, N. J. Andrews, W. J. Edmunds, H. Lecoeur, D. Lévy-Bruhl, P. A. Maple, H. de Melker, A. Nardone, M. C. Rota, S. Salmaso, M. A. Conyn-van Spaendonck, S. Swidsinski, and E. Miller. 2005. The seroepidemiology of *Bordetella pertussis* infection in Western Europe. *Epidemiol. Infect.* **133:**159–171.

79. Plotkin, S. (ed.). 2005. The global pertussis initiative. *Pediatr. Infect. Dis. J.* **24:**S5–S98.

80. Raso, T., O. Bianco, B. Grosso, M. Zucca, and D. Savoia. 2008. *Achromobacter xylosoxidans* respiratory tract infections in cystic fibrosis patients. *APMIS* **116:**837–841.

81. Rath, B. A., K. B. Register, J. Wall, D. M. Sokol, and R. B. van Dyke. 2008. Persistent *Bordetella bronchiseptica* pneumonia in an immunocompetent infant and genetic comparison of clinical isolates with kennel cough vaccine strains. *Clin. Infect. Dis.* **46:**905–908.

82. Register, K. B., R. E. Sacco, and G. E. Nordholm. 2003. Comparison of ribotyping and restriction enzyme analysis for inter- and intraspecies discrimination of *Bordetella avium* and *Bordetella hinzii*. *J. Clin. Microbiol.* **41:**1512–1519.

83. Register, K. B., and T. L. Nicholson. 2007. Misidentification of *Bordetella bronchiseptica* as *Bordetella pertussis* using a newly described real-time PCR targeting the pertactin gene. *J. Med. Microbiol.* **56:**1608–1610.

84. Rehfuss, M., and J. Urban. 2005. *Alcaligenes faecalis* subsp. *phenolicus* subsp. nov. a phenol-degrading, denitrifying bacterium isolated from a graywater bioprocessor. *Syst. Appl. Microbiol.* **28:**421–429.

85. Reischl, U., N. Lehn, G. N. Sanden, and M. J. Loeffelholz. 2001. Real-time PCR assay targeting IS481 of *Bordetella pertussis* and molecular basis for detecting *Bordetella holmesii*. *J. Clin. Microbiol.* **39:**1963–1966.

85a. Riffelmann, M., K. Thiel, J. Schmetz, and C. H. Wirsing von Koenig. 2010. Performance of commercial enzyme-linked immunosorbent assays for detection of antibodies to *Bordetella pertussis*. *J. Clin. Microbiol.* **48:**4459–4463.

86. **Riffelmann, M., C. H. Wirsing von König, V. Caro, and N. Guiso.** 2005. Nucleic acid amplification tests for diagnosis of *Bordetella* infections. *J. Clin. Microbiol.* **43:**4925–4929.

87. **Rønne Hansen, C., T. Pressler, N. Høiby, and M. Gormsen.** 2006. Chronic infection with *Achromobacter xylosoxidans* in cystic fibrosis patients; a retrospective case control study. *J. Cyst. Fibros.* **5:**245–251.

88. **Saiman, L., Y. Chen, P. San Gabriel, and C. Knirsch.** 2002. Synergistic activities of macrolide antibiotics against *Pseudomonas aeruginosa, Burkholderia cepacia, Stenotrophomonas maltophilia,* and *Alcaligenes xylosoxidans* isolated from patients with cystic fibrosis. *Antimicrob. Agents Chemother.* **46:**1105–1107.

89. **Saiman, L., Y. Chen, S. Tabibi, P. San Gabriel, J. Zhou, Z. Liu, L. Lai, and S. Whittier.** 2001. Identification and antimicrobial susceptibility of *Alcaligenes xylosoxidans* isolated from patients with cystic fibrosis. *J. Clin. Microbiol.* **39:**3942–3945.

90. **Schroll, G., H. J. Busse, G. Parrer, S. Rölleke, W. Lubitz, and E. B. Denner.** 2001. *Alcaligenes faecalis* subsp. *parafaecalis* subsp. nov., a bacterium accumulating poly-beta-hydroxybutyrate from acetone-butanol bioprocess residues. *Syst. Appl. Microbiol.* **24:**37–43.

91. **Schwarz, S., E. Aleksik, M. Grobbel, A. Lübcke-Becker, C. Werckenthin, L. H. Wieler, and J. Wallmann.** 2007. Antimicrobial susceptibility of *Pasteurella multocida* and *Bordetella bronchiseptica* from dogs and cats as determined in the BfT-GermVet monitoring program 2004–2006. *Berl. Munch. Tierarztl. Woschenschr.* **120:**423–430.

92. **Sebaihia, M., A. Preston, D. J. Maskell, H. Kuzmiak, T. D. Connell, N. D. King, P. E. Orndorff, D. M. Miyamoto, N. R. Thomson, D. Harris, A. Goble, A. Lord, L. Murphy, M. A. Quail, S. Rutter, R. Squares, S. Squares, J. Woodward, J. Parkhill, and L. M. Temple.** 2006. Comparison of the genome sequence of the poultry pathogen *Bordetella avium* with those of *B. bronchiseptica, B. pertussis* and *B. parapertussis* reveals extensive diversity in surface structures associated with host interaction. *J. Bacteriol.* **188:**6002–6015.

93. **Shelly, D. B., T. Spilker, E. J. Gracely, T. Coenye, P. Vandamme, and J. J. LiPuma.** 2000. Utility of commercial systems for identification of *Burkholderia cepacia* complex from cystic fibrosis sputum culture. *J. Clin. Microbiol.* **38:**3112–3115.

94. **Snyder, J. W., G. K. Munier, and C. L. Johnson.** 2008. Direct comparison of the BD Phoenix system with the MicroScan WalkAway system for identification and antimicrobial susceptibility testing of *Enterobacteriaceae* and nonfermenting gram-negative organisms. *J. Clin. Microbiol.* **46:**2327–2333.

95. **Spangler, S. K., M. A. Visalli, M. R. Jacobs, and P. C. Appelbaum.** 1996. Susceptibilities of non-*Pseudomonas aeruginosa* gram-negative nonfermentative rods to ciprofloxacin, ofloxacin, levofloxacin, D-ofloxacin, sparfloxacin, ceftazidime, piperacillin, piperacillin-tazobactam, trimethoprim-sulfamethoxazole, and imipenem. *Antimicrob. Agents Chemother.* **40:**772–775.

96. **Spicuzza, L., C. Sciuto, G. Vitaliti, G. Di Dio, S. Leonardi, and M. La Rosa.** 2009. Emerging pathogens in cystic fibrosis: ten years of follow-up in a cohort of patients. *Eur. J. Clin. Microbiol. Infect. Dis.* **28:**191–195.

97. **Spilker, T., A. A. Liwienski, and J. J. LiPuma.** 2008. Identification of *Bordetella* spp. in respiratory specimens from individuals with cystic fibrosis. *Clin. Microbiol. Infect.* **14:**504–506.

98. **Stark, D., L. A. Riley, J. Harkness, and D. Mariott.** 2007. *Bordetella petrii* from a clinical sample in Australia: isolation and molecular identification. *J. Med. Microbiol.* **56:**435–437.

99. **Tatti, K. M., K. H. Wu, M. L. Tondella, P. K. Cassiday, M. M. Cortese, P. P. Wilkins, and G. N. Sanden.** 2008. Development and evaluation of dual-target real-time polymerase chain reaction assays to detect *Bordetella* spp. *Diagn. Microbiol. Infect. Dis.* **61:**264–272.

100. **Templeton, K. E., S. A. Scheltinga, A. van der Zee, B. M. W. Diederen, A. M. Kruijssen, H. Goossens, E. Kuijper, and E. C. J. Claas.** 2003. Evaluation of real-time PCR for detection of and discrimination between *Bordetella pertussis, Bordetella parapertussis,* and *Bordetella holmesii* for clinical diagnosis. *J. Clin. Microbiol.* **41:**4121–4126.

101. **Tondella, M. L., G. M. Carlone, N. Messonnier, C. P. Quinn, B. D. Meade, D. L. Burns, J. D. Cherry, N. Guiso, E. L. Hewlett, K. M. Edwards, D. Xing, A. Giammanco, C. H. Wirsing von König, L. Han, L. Hueston, J. B. Robbins, M. Powell, C. M. Mink, J. T. Poolman, S. W. Hildreth, F. Lynn, and A. Morris.** 2009. International *Bordetella pertussis* assays standardization and harmonization meeting report. *Vaccine* **27:**803–814.

102. **van Amersfoorth, S. C. M., L. S. Schouls, H. G. J. van der Heide, A. Advani, H. O. Hallander, K. Bondeson, C. H. W. von König, M. Riffelmann, C. Vahrenholz, N. Guiso, V. Caro, E. Njamkepo, Q. He, J. Mertsola, and F. R. Mooi.** 2005. Analysis of *Bordetella pertussis* populations in European countries with different vaccine policies. *J. Clin. Microbiol.* **43:**2837–2843.

103. **Van Daele, S., R. Verhelst, G. Claeys, G. Verschraegen, H. Franckx, L. Van Simaey, C. de Ganck, F. De Baets, and M. Vaneechoutte.** 2005. Shared genotypes of *Achromobacter xylosoxidans* strains isolated from patients at a cystic fibrosis rehabilitation center. *J. Clin. Microbiol.* **43:**2998–3002.

104. **Vandamme, P., J. Hommez, M. Vancanneyt, M. Monsieurs, B. Hoste, B. Cookson, C. H. Wirsing von König, K. Kersters, and P. J. Blackall.** 1995. *Bordetella hinzii* sp. nov., isolated from poultry and humans. *Int. J. Syst. Bacteriol.* **45:**37–45.

105. **Vandamme, P., M. Heyndrickx, M. Vancanneyt, B. Hoste, P. De Vos, E. Falsen, K. Kersters, and K. H. Hinz.** 1996. *Bordetella trematum* sp. nov., isolated from wounds and ear infections in humans, and reassessment of *Alcaligenes denitrificans* Rüger and Tan 1983. *Int. J. Syst. Bacteriol.* **46:**849–858.

106. **Van Trappen, S., T. L. Tan, E. Samyn, and P. Vandamme.** 2005. *Alcaligenes aquatilis* sp. nov., a novel bacterium from sediments of the Weser Estuary, Germany, and a salt marsh on Shem Creek in Charleston Harbor, USA. *Int. J. Syst. Evol. Microbiol.* **55:**2571–2575.

107. **Versteegh, F. G., J. F. Schellekens, A. F. Nagelkerke, and J. J. Roord.** 2002. Laboratory-confirmed reinfection with *Bordetella pertussis. Acta Paediatr.* **91:**95–97.

108. **Versteegh, F. G., P. L. Mertens, H. E. de Melker, J. J. Roord, J. F. Schellekens, and P. F. Teunis.** 2005. Age-specific long-term course of antibodies to pertussis toxin after symptomatic infection with *Bordetella pertussis. Epidemiol. Infect.* **133:**737–748.

109. **Von Witzingerode, F., A. Schattke, R. A. Siddiqui, U. Rösick, U. B. Göbel, and R. Gross.** 2001. *Bordetella petrii* sp. nov., isolated from an anaerobic bioreactor, and emended description of the genus *Bordetella. Int. J. Syst. Evol. Microbiol.* **51:**1257–1265.

110. **Wang, F., S. Grundmann, M. Schmid, U. Dörfler, S. Roherer, J. C. Munch, A. Hartmann, X. Jiang, and R. Schroll.** 2007. Isolation and characterization of 1,2,4-trichlorobenzene mineralizing *Bordetella* sp. and its bioremediation potential in soil. *Chemosphere* **76:**896–902.

111. **Ward, J. I., J. D. Cherry, S. J. Chang, S. Partridge, W. Keitel, K. Edwards, M. Lee, J. Treanor, D. P. Greenberg, S. Barenkamp, D. I. Bernstein, R. Edelman, and the APERT Study Group.** 2006. *Bordetella pertussis* infections in vaccinated and unvaccinated adolescents and adults as assessed in a national prospective randomized acellular pertussis vaccine trial (APERT). *Clin. Infect. Dis.* **43:**151–157.

112. **Watanabe, M., B. Connelly, and A. A. Weiss.** 2006. Characterization of serological responses to pertussis. *Clin. Vaccine Immunol.* **13:**341–348.

113. **Waters, V., F. Jamieson, S. E. Richardson, M. Finkelstein, A. Wormsbecker, and S. A. Halperin.** 2009. Outbreak of atypical pertussis detected by polymerase chain reaction in immunized preschool-aged children. *Pediatr. Infect. Dis. J.* **28:**582–587.

114. **Wellinghausen, N., B. Wirths, and S. Poppert.** 2006. Fluorescence in situ hybridization for rapid identification of *Achromobacter xylosoxidans* and *Alcaligenes faecalis* recovered from cystic fibrosis patients. *J. Clin. Microbiol.* **44:**3415–3417.

115. **Wendelboe, A. M., M. G. Hudgens, C. Poole, and A. van Rie.** 2007. Estimating the role of casual contacts from the community in transmission of *Bordetella pertussis* to young infants. *Emerg. Themes Epidemiol.* **4:**15.

116. **Weyant, R. S., D. G. Hollis, R. E. Weaver, M. F. Amin, A. G. Steigerwalt, S. P. O'Connor, A. M. Whitney, M. I. Daneshvar, C. W. Moss, and D. J. Brenner.** 1995. *Bordetella holmesii* sp. nov., a new gram-negative species associated with septicemia. *J. Clin. Microbiol.* **33:**1–7.

117. **Wirsing von König, C. H., S. Halperin, M. Riffelmann, and N. Guiso.** 2002. Pertussis of adults and infants. *Lancet Infect. Dis.* **2:**744–750.

118. **Wright, R. M., J. E. Moore, A. Shaw, K. Dunbar, M. Dodd, K. Webb, A. O. Redmond, M. Crowe, P. G. Murphy, S. Peacock, and J. S. Elborn.** 2001. Improved cultural detection of *Burkholderia cepacia* from sputum in patients with cystic fibrosis. *J. Clin. Pathol.* **54:**803–805.

119. **Xing, D., C. H. Wirsing von König, P. Newland, M. Riffelmann, B. D. Meade, M. Corbel, and R. Gaines-Das.** 2009. Characterization of proposed reference materials for pertussis antiserum (human) by an international collaborative study. *Clin. Vaccine Immunol.* **16:**303–311.

120. **Yabuuchi, E., Y. Kawamura, Y. Kosako, and T. Ezaki.** 1998. Emendation of the genus *Achromobacter* and *Achromobacter xylosoxidans* (Yabuuchi and Yano) and proposal of *Achromobacter ruhlandii* (Packer and Vishniac) comb. nov., *Achromobacter piechaudii* (Kiredjian et al.) comb. nov., and *Achromobacter xylosoxidans* subsp. *denitrificans* (Rüger and Tan) comb. nov. *Microbiol. Immunol.* **42:**429–438.

121. **Yih, W. K., S. M. Lett, F. N. des Vignes, K. M. Garrison, P. L. Sipe, and C. D. Marchant.** 2000. The increasing incidence of pertussis in Massachusetts adolescents and adults, 1989–1998. *J. Infect. Dis.* **182:**1409–1416.

122. **Zbinden, A., E. C. Bötåtger, P. P. Bosshard, and R. Zbinden.** 2007. Evaluation of the colorimetric VITEK 2 card for identification of gram-negative nonfermentative rods: comparison to 16S rRNA gene sequencing. *J. Clin. Microbiol.* **45:**2270–2273.

Francisella and Brucella*

JEANNINE M. PETERSEN, MARTIN E. SCHRIEFER, AND GEORGE F. ARAJ

44

Francisella and *Brucella*, while not closely related taxonomically, have been traditionally linked in the minds of bacteriologists. Both are zoonotic agents capable of producing severe disease in humans. In the laboratory, they are seen as small gram-negative coccobacilli that grow slowly and are not particularly active biochemically. The two genera also share a reputation for causing laboratory-acquired infections (145, 155). Finally, *Francisella tularensis*, *Brucella melitensis*, *Brucella suis*, and *Brucella abortus* are all considered to be potential bioterrorism agents (152; see also chapter 12 of this *Manual*).

FRANCISELLA

Taxonomy

The family *Francisellaceae*, a member of the gamma subclass of proteobacteria, consists of the single genus *Francisella*. *Francisella tularensis*, *Francisella novicida*, *Francisella philomiragia*, and *Francisella noatunensis* as well as unclassified *Francisella* spp. comprise the genus. Several publications have reviewed the history and descriptions of members of the genus *Francisella* (48, 165, 166).

   F. tularensis is the causative agent of tularemia, a zoonosis affecting a wide range of animals and humans. Three subspecies of *F. tularensis*, *tularensis* (type A), *holarctica* (type B), and *mediasiatica*, displaying >99.8% identity in their 16S rRNA genes, have been described (165). *F. tularensis* subsp. *tularensis* and *F. tularensis* subsp. *holarctica* have been further subdivided into distinct subpopulations using molecular typing methods (117). *F. tularensis* subsp. *tularensis* has been separated into three subclades, termed A1a, A1b, and A2, and within *F. tularensis* subsp. *holarctica*, 10 separate subclades have been identified (117).

   F. novicida and *F. philomiragia*, originally isolated from salty water, are only infrequently associated with human disease (74, 81, 92, 191). *F. novicida* was classifed as a species distinct from *F. tularensis* on the basis of serologic, virulence, and biochemical comparisons (92, 133). Subsequently, similarities between *F. novicida* and *F. tularensis* were identified based on

genome reassociation studies (75% DNA relatedness) and 16S rRNA gene sequences (>99.8% identity) (74, 165). Recent whole-genome comparisons provide evidence that the evolutions of *F. novicida* and *F. tularensis* occurred separately, consistent with *F. novicida* and *F. tularensis* being two separate species (93). Between *F. philomiragia* and *F. tularensis*, genome reassociation studies show 39% average DNA relatedness and >98.3% identity in their 16S rRNA gene sequences (57, 74). *Francisella noatunensis* has been linked only to environmental sources being recovered from a number of saltwater fish species (27, 114, 131). DNA hybridization studies show a mean reassociation value of 68% between *F. noatunensis* and *F. philomiragia*, with the two species displaying 99.3% identity in their 16S rRNA genes (114).

   Several additional *Francisellaceae* members, isolated in culture, including *Wolbachia persica* (165) and *Francisella* spp. recovered from seawater (143), have been described. Additionally, a *Francisella* sp. was isolated from the blood and cerebrospinal fluid (CSF) of two different patients in the United States in 2005 and 2006 (90), while another *Francisella* sp. was isolated from the blood and urine of a patient in Spain (50). Characterization data indicate that these *Francisella* spp. are distinct from *F. tularensis*, *F. novicida*, and *F. philomiragia*.

   Putative *Francisellaceae* family members have also been identified based on shared identities among 16S rRNA gene sequences. These include *Francisella*-like endosymbionts (FLEs) in *Amblyomma maculatum* and multiple *Dermacentor* and *Ornithodoros* tick species (160, 165). DNA from putative *Francisellaceae* family members has also been detected in soil and water samples (22).

Description of the Genus

The genus *Francisella* comprises tiny gram-negative coccobacilli that can be distinguished from similar genera by several features (Table 1). Members of the genus take up Gram's counterstain (safranin) poorly; they are strict aerobes, weakly catalase positive, urease negative, nonmotile, and non-spore-forming, and they react with a limited number of carbohydrates (Table 2). Only a few sugars (glucose, maltose, sucrose, and glycerol) are utilized by most members of the genus. Acid is produced without gas. Unique cellular fatty acids are associated with the genus (Table 1) (74, 165, 192). For most species, in vitro growth is enhanced

---

*This chapter contains information presented in chapter 51 by David Lindquist, May C. Chu, and Will S. Probert in the ninth edition of this *Manual*.

TABLE 1 Presumptive differentiation of *Francisella* and *Brucella* from similar gram-negative genera[a]

Test	*F. tularensis*	*Brucella* spp.	*Bartonella* spp.[b]	*Acinetobacter* spp.	*Psychrobacter phenylpyruvicus*[c]	*Oligella ureolytica*	*Bordetella bronchiseptica*	*Haemophilus* spp.[d]	*Ochrobactrum anthropi*
Oxidase	−	+	−	−	+	+	+	V	+
Urease	−	+	−	−	+	+	+	V	+
Gram stain morphology	Very tiny ccb	Tiny ccb	Thin rod	Broad ccb	Broad ccb	Small to tiny ccb	Thin rod	Small ccb	Medium rod
Specimen source	Ulcer, wound, blood, aspirates	Blood, bone marrow	Blood, bone marrow, lymph node	V	V	Urinary tract	V	Blood, cerebrospinal fluid, other	
X and/or V factor requirement	−	−	−[e]	−	−	−	−	+	−
Cysteine enhancement	+	−	−	−	−	−	−	−	−
Motility	−	−	−	−	−	+[f]	+	−	+
Major CFA[g]	10:0; 14:0; 16:0; 3-OH-16:0; 18:1ω9c; 3-OH-18:0	16:0; 18:1ω7c; 18:0; 19:0cyc[h]	16:0; 17:0; 18:1ω7c	2-OH-12:0; 3-OH-12:0; 16:1ω7c; 16:0; 18:1ω9c	3-OH-12:0; 16:1ω7c; 16:0; 18:2; 18:1ω9c	3-OH-14:0; 16:0; 3-OH-16:0; 18:1ω7c	2-OH-12:0; 3-OH-14:0; 16:1ω7c; 16:0; 17:0cyc	14:0; 3-OH-14:0; 16:1ω7c; 16:0	18:1ω7c; 18:0; 19:0cyc; 2-OH-19:0cyc

[a]+, greater than or equal to 90% positive; −, less than or equal to 10% positive; V, variable (11 to 89% positive); ccb, coccobacilli. Data are from reference 169.
[b]Does not include *Bartonella bacilliformis*, which is the only motile species.
[c]Formerly *Moraxella phenylpyruvica*.
[d]*Haemophilus* spp. requiring X and V factors or V factor only.
[e]While not required, X factor (hemin) enhances growth for many strains.
[f]May be difficult to demonstrate.
[g]The number before the colon indicates the number of carbons; the number after the colon is the number of double bonds, ω indicates the location of the double bond counting from the hydrocarbon end of the carbon chain, OH indicates a hydroxy group at the 2 or 3 position from the carboxyl end, c indicates the *cis* isomer, and cyc indicates a cyclopropane ring structure. Hydroxy acids listed are at least 2% of the total cellular fatty acid (CFA) composition; all others are at least 10%.
[h]*B. canis* lacks 19:0cyc. Cellular fatty acid data for marine mammal strains are not available.

by sulfhydryl supplementation. Cultured members of the genus share >97% identity within their 16S rRNA genes (90, 114, 165).

A few key differences separate species of the *Francisella* genus (Table 2). *F. philomiragia* and *F. novicida* are more biochemically reactive than *F. tularensis*. *F. philomiragia* is oxidase positive by Kovács's modification, whereas *F. novicida* and *F. tularensis* are oxidase negative. *F. novicida* and *F. philomiragia* differ from *F. tularensis* by their ability to grow independently of cysteine supplementation and by their comparatively large cell size. Additionally, levels of virulence in mice differ, with <10 cells of *F. tularensis* being required to kill laboratory mice compared to <100 for *F. novicida* (133). Nucleotide differences within 16S rRNA genes also discriminate *F. tularensis*, *F. novicida*, and *F. philomiragia* (56).

Biochemical, molecular, and virulence differences also differentiate *F. tularensis* subspecies. Glycerol fermentation and citrulline ureidase activity distinguish *F. tularensis* subsp. *tularensis* from *F. tularensis* subsp. *holarctica* (Table 2) (127, 128). PCR-based techniques as well as 16S rRNA gene sequencing can also differentiate *F. tularensis* subsp. *tularensis* from *F. tularensis* subsp. *holarctica* (56, 197). Levels of virulence in rabbits differ, with the 100% lethal dose of *F. tularensis* subsp. *tularensis* being <10 cells when inoculated subcutaneously, compared to 10⁹ cells for *F. tularensis*

subsp. *holarctica* (127). *F. tularensis* subsp. *mediasiatica* differs from both *F. tularensis* subsp. *tularensis* and *F. tularensis* subsp. *holarctica* by its inability to utilize glucose and its moderate pathogenicity in rabbits (128, 165).

Epidemiology and Transmission

Francisellaceae are widely distributed in the natural environment. Some species are obligate pathogens of animals and humans (*F. tularensis*) (Table 3); others are present in the environment (water) and are opportunistic pathogens of humans (*F. novicida* and *F. philomiragia*) (Table 3), while others have been associated only with animals (*F. noatunensis*). *F. tularensis* isolates have been found only within the Northern Hemisphere (Holarctic region), whereas *F. novicida* and *F. noatunensis* have been recovered from both the Northern and Southern Hemispheres (27, 165, 166, 194).

The geographic distribution of *F. tularensis* varies throughout the Northern Hemisphere (128, 165, 166). Infections caused by *F. tularensis* subsp. *tularensis* occur only in North America, whereas *F. tularensis* subsp. *holarctica* has a much wider distribution, causing disease in both the Old and New Worlds. *F. tularensis* subsp. *mediasiatica* has been found only in regions of central Asia. The geographic distributions of *F. tularensis* subsp. *holarctica* and subsp. *tularensis* subclades

TABLE 2 Characteristics of *Francisella* spp.

Characteristic	*F. tularensis* subsp.			*F. novicida*	*F. philomiragia*
	tularensis	*holarctica*	*mediasiatica*		
Gram stain (culture), safranin counterstain	Faintly staining, pleomorphic, single, rarely chained, gram-negative tiny coccobacilli	As for subsp. *tularensis*	As for subsp. *tularensis*	As for subsp. *tularensis*	As for subsp. *tularensis*
Cell size (μm)	0.2–0.7 × 0.2	0.2–0.7 × 0.2	0.2–0.7 × 0.2	0.7 × 1.7	0.7 × 1.7
Growth on standard agar[a]	−	−	−	+	+
CA, 48 h	2- to 4-mm-diam, raised, gray, smooth, moist; butyrous colonies with entire margins; usually no agar discoloration	As for subsp. *tularensis*	As for subsp. *tularensis*	As for subsp. *tularensis* but 5 mm in diam	>5-mm-diam, white, smooth, mucoid, entire colonies; no agar discoloration
Cysteine heart blood agar, 48 h	2–4-mm-diam, raised, smooth, butyrous colonies with entire margins; colonies display green tint and opalescent sheen; green-yellow discoloration of agar	As for subsp. *tularensis*	Not tested	As for subsp. *tularensis* but 5 mm in diam	Colonies are >5 mm in diam, creamy white-gray, mucoid, and smooth, with a purple-tinted opalescent sheen
Requires cystine/cysteine	+	+	+	−	−
Catalase	Weakly +	Weakly +	Weakly +	Weakly +	Weakly +
Oxidase (Kovács)	−	−	−	−	+
Acid from:					
Glucose[b]	+	+	−	+	Weakly +
Maltose	+	+	−	V[c]	+
Sucrose	−	−	+	+	V
Glycerol	+	−	+	+	−
Citrulline ureidase	+	−	+	+	NT[d]
Relative virulence (mice)	High	Intermediate	Low	Low	Low

[a]Standard bacteriological media: blood, Trypticase soy, and brain heart infusion.
[b]Delayed or variable reaction. *F. tularensis* subsp. *mediasiatica* does not ferment glucose (165).
[c]V, variable or slow reaction.
[d]NT, not tested.

also vary. Subclades of *F. tularensis* subsp. *holarctica* within North America are distinct from subclades throughout the rest of the Northern Hemisphere, excepting Scandinavia (188). Within the United States, the geographic distributions of *F. tularensis* subsp. *tularensis* subclades differ. A1a and A1b predominate in the eastern half of the United States, whereas A2 appears restricted to the western United States (91).

F. novicida has been isolated primarily in North America, with occurrences of *F. novicida*-like organisms in Australia and Thailand (94, 194). Of the fewer than 20 known isolates of *F. philomiragia*, most have been from North America, with three single incidences reported from Central and Eastern Europe and Australia (60, 74, 164, 191, 194). *F. noatunensis* has been isolated from Scandinavia, Chile, and Japan (27, 114, 131).

F. tularensis is associated with a wide range of hosts; more than 100 species of wild animals, birds, and arthropods have been found naturally infected (24, 75, 80). Habitats where the Lagomorpha (*Sylvilagus* [rabbits], *Lepus* [hares], and *Oryctolagus* [Old World hares] genera) and the Rodentia (water voles, muskrats, lemmings, voles, and beavers) thrive are believed to be important in maintaining enzootic foci (75, 80). Biting arthropod vectors, primarily tabanid flies (*Chrysops* and *Tabanus*), ticks (*Dermacentor* and *Amblyomma*), and mosquitoes (*Aedes* and *Ochlerotatus* in Sweden and Russia), are implicated in the transmission of tularemia (46, 75, 79, 144). Human infections with *F. tularensis* are acquired usually via inhalation of infective aerosols, ingestion of contaminated water,

handling of sick or dead animals, or ingestion of infected meat or from the bite of an infected arthropod. In contrast to *F. tularensis*, *F. novicida* and *F. philomiragia* do not appear to infect a wide range of hosts. Their primary natural habitat appears to be saltwater. Only a single isolation of *F. philomiragia* from an animal host (muskrat) has been documented (81). Neither *F. novicida* nor *F. philomiragia* has been shown to be transmitted to humans by the bite of an infective arthropod, and arthropods infected with these species have not been identified.

Tularemia has been reported from many countries of the Northern Hemisphere. Foci of endemicity have long been documented in Russia and Kazakhstan, as well as Finland and Sweden (166). Annual cases are usually reported from most countries in Eastern Europe. Cases of tularemia are reported less frequently from Western Europe; however, several outbreaks of tularemia have occurred over the last decade in Spain (5, 108). Other areas reporting outbreaks comprising many hundreds of cases in the last decade include Sweden and Kosovo (139, 150).

In the United States, the incidence of tularemia has steadily declined to 100 to 200 cases each year since the 1940s, when several thousand cases of tularemia were reported annually (31). All states except Hawaii have reported cases. A total of 1,368 human cases from 44 states were reported to the Centers for Disease Control and Prevention (CDC) between 1990 and 2000, with four states, South Dakota, Arkansas, Missouri, and Oklahoma, accounting for

TABLE 3 Epidemiology of *Francisella* spp. affecting humans

Francisella sp.	Infection sources	Geographic distribution (documented cases)	Disease association (humans)
F. tularensis			
subsp. *tularensis* (type A)	Animals (primarily rabbits and cats), ticks, deerflies	North America (United States and Canada)	Tularemia (all forms)
Subclade A2	Animals, ticks, deerflies	Western United States, Alaska	Tularemia (primarily ulceroglandular, glandular)
Subclade A1a	Animals, ticks, deerflies	Eastern United States, California, Utah, Oregon	Tularemia (all forms)
Subclade A1b	Animals, ticks	Eastern United States, California, Idaho, Oregon, Colorado, Alaska	Tularemia (all forms, severe cases)
subsp. *holarctica* (type B)	Animals (primarily rodents), water, ticks, mosquitoes, horseflies	Northern Hemisphere	Tularemia (all forms)
subsp. *mediasiatica*	Animals, ticks	Central Asia	Tularemia
F. novicida	Saltwater	United States, Australia, Thailand	Mild illness (immunocompromised patients)
F. philomiragia	Saltwater	United States, Turkey, Switzerland, Australia	Mild illness (immunocompromised patients)

the majority (56%) of cases (31). Most cases in the United States are sporadic, with patients acquiring tularemia from tick or deerfly bites or from contact with infected animals (e.g., by skinning rabbits) (31, 91). Inhalation of an infective aerosol during landscaping and contact with infected cats are also important modes of transmission (53, 54, 91). The majority of tularemia cases occur in the summer months. Outbreaks of tularemia occur rarely in the United States. An outbreak of pneumonic tularemia associated with landscaping activities occurred on Martha's Vineyard in 2000 (54), and since that time, Martha'a Vineyard has recorded yearly cases (109). The most recent outbreak in the United States occurred in Utah in 2007 and was attributed to deerfly bites (142). Cultures recovered from human cases in the United States from 1996 to 2001 comprise equal proportions of *F. tularensis* subsp. *tularensis* and *F. tularensis* subsp. *holarctica* (174).

Clinical Significance

F. tularensis

Tularemia is caused by *F. tularensis*. The disease has been known historically by a number of synonyms, such as rabbit fever, deerfly fever, market men's disease, the glandular type of tick fever, Ohara's or yato-byo disease, and water rat trappers' disease, attesting to the variety of clinical presentations, the infectious agent's ubiquitous presence in nature, and the means by which humans may acquire the infection.

The clinical spectrum of tularemia depends on the mode of transmission, the virulence of the infecting strain, the immune status of the host, and timely diagnosis and treatment (197). Tularemia can be misdiagnosed since its symptoms are not unique; a sudden onset of chills, fever, headache, and generalized malaise characterize the onset of illness. The differential diagnosis includes a wide range of infectious diseases, such as cat scratch fever, mycobacterial infections, anthrax, brucellosis, legionellosis, and plague (197). The incubation period averages 3 to 5 days.

Patients may present with any one of the clinical forms of tularemia: ulceroglandular, glandular, oculoglandular, oropharyngeal, typhoidal, and pneumonic (197). The most common form is ulceroglandular disease (45 to 80% of the reported cases), where the portal of entry is via an infective arthropod bite or other inoculation through the skin barrier.

Glandular tularemia is similar to ulceroglandular disease but lacks the ulcerated site of infection. Oculoglandular tularemia occurs when the conjunctiva is the initial site of infection, usually as a result of the mechanical transfer of organisms from an infectious source to the eye by the fingers. Oropharyngeal tularemia occurs from ingestion of contaminated water or food and is associated with pharyngeal lymphadenopathy. Pneumonic tularemia occurs by direct inhalation of the organism and is considered the most severe form of the disease. Typhoidal tularemia is the most difficult form to recognize because there is no identified portal of entry and localized signs are absent. If untreated, bacterial dissemination from the primary sites of infection can lead to secondary clinical presentations, such as sepsis and meningitis.

The severity of infection can range from mild and self-limiting to fatal and is largely dependent on the infecting strain. Little to no tularemia-related mortality is reported in Europe and Asia, where only *F. tularensis* subsp. *holarctica* causes tularemia, while mortality in the United States ranges between 2.3% (those diagnosed by culture and serology) and 9% (culture-confirmed cases only) (52, 174). Infections due to *F. tularensis* subsp. *tularensis* are considered to be more severe than infections caused by *F. tularensis* subsp. *holarctica*. Molecular epidemiologic studies have refined this picture and demonstrate that among culture-confirmed cases in the United States, human infections due to the A1b subclade of *F. tularensis* subsp. *tularensis* result in significantly higher mortality (24%) than infections caused by *F. tularensis* subsp. *tularensis* subclades A1a (4%) and A2 (0%) or *F. tularensis* subsp. *holarctica* (7%) (91). Comparisons of levels of virulence in mice corroborate the differences in virulence among *F. tularensis* subsp. *tularensis* clades and also between *F. tularensis* subsp. *tularensis* clades and *F. tularensis* subsp. *holarctica* (118).

F. novicida and *F. philomiragia*

Human infections caused by *F. novicida* and *F. philomiragia* are rare and considered opportunistic infections, infecting primarily patients with underlying immunocompromising conditions. Fewer than 20 cases of *F. philomiragia* infection have been described since the discovery of this species in 1974 (60, 74, 164, 191). All but one case have involved a host with an impaired physical barrier to infection (near drowning) or an impaired immunologic defense system (chronic granulomatous disease or myeloproliferative disease). In most cases, *F. philomiragia* was isolated from normally sterile sites: blood, bone marrow, cerebrospinal fluid, and pericardial fluid. The drowning and water exposure cases were associated with saltwater and brackish water, in contrast to *F. tularensis* infections, which are associated with freshwater sources. Fewer than 10 cases of *F. novicida* or *F. novicida*-like infections have been reported (26, 35, 74, 94, 191, 194). Isolates were recovered from blood, lymph node tissue, and wounds.

Collection, Handling, Storage, and Transport of Specimens

Personnel handling diagnostic cultures of *F. tularensis* are at considerable risk for infection. Due to the extremely low infectious dose for *F. tularensis*, tularemia has been one of the most commonly reported laboratory-associated bacterial infections (132, 145). Even though the use of biological safety cabinets and prophylactic antibiotic therapy (as well as vaccination, where available) provides safeguards for laboratory workers, these precautions have not fully eliminated laboratory exposures or modified practices in the clinical laboratory to minimize risks (155, 162). Manipulation of cultures presents the greatest risk to laboratory workers, due to the high concentration of organisms. Clinical specimens should be handled under biosafety level 2 (BSL-2) conditions with universal precautions, with work being done using BSL-3 practices as soon as a suspect *F. tularensis* is isolated in culture (44). The greatest risk of laboratory-acquired tularemia is by aerosol inhalation while working with cultures. Any work with clinical samples that generates aerosols should be performed using BSL-3 practices. Laboratories may want to consider developing policies that encourage physicians to alert the laboratory if a diagnosis of tularemia is expected.

The choice of specimen for diagnostic testing is generally dependent on the form of clinical illness: ulceroglandular, glandular, oculoglandular, oropharyngeal, pneumonic, or typhoidal tularemia (197). Whole blood is an acceptable specimen for all clinical forms of tularemia, although this sample may be negative, particularly if the disease is in the early stages of progression. Serum for antibody detection is a standard specimen taken for diagnosis of all forms of illness. A first specimen should be collected as early in the course of infection as possible, followed by a second specimen taken in the convalescent period (at least 14 days apart and preferably 3 to 4 weeks after onset of symptoms). Pharyngeal swabs, bronchial/tracheal washes or aspirates, sputum, transthoracic lung aspirates, and pleural fluid are appropriate specimens for pneumonic, typhoidal, or oropharyngeal tularemia. Swabs of visible lesions or affected areas have been used most commonly for ulceroglandular and oculoglandular tularemia. Aspirates from lymph nodes or lesions can be used for diagnosis of ulceroglandular, glandular, and oropharyngeal tularemia. Necropsied materials from animals that are appropriate for testing include samples from visible abscesses as well as samples from lymph node, lung, liver, and spleen tissues and bone marrow.

For specimens to be tested by culture, it is important where possible to decontaminate the surface area prior to specimen collection since contamination of the sample with normal flora could interfere with the interpretation of culture results. To minimize loss in viability, specimens should be delivered to the laboratory within 24 hours and preferably within 2 hours. In general, if transport is >24 hours, specimens should be stored chilled (2 to 8°C)

in an appropriate medium until processed in the laboratory. Freezing of samples, unless in a preservative environment, such as tissue specimens or glycerol-containing solutions, is not recommended because of the lysis of live bacteria upon thawing. Swabs should be placed in Amies agar with charcoal, a commercial transport system designed for anaerobic and aerobic pathogens (Becton, Dickinson and Company, Franklin Lakes, NJ). *F. tularensis* should remain viable for 7 days at ambient room temperature when stored in Amies medium (82). Stuart medium, designed for transporting gonococcal specimens, and saline are inadequate for keeping *F. tularensis* viable during transport (82). For serum samples, separation from blood should take place as soon as possible, preferably within 24 hours. Sera may be stored at 2 to 8°C for up to 10 days. If testing is delayed for a long period, serum samples may be frozen. For PCR, specimens should be collected in guanidine isothiocyanate-containing buffer, which preserves *F. tularensis* DNA for up to 1 month (82). Arthropods may be stored intact in 2% NaCl for culture analysis or in ethanol for molecular testing.

Direct Detection in Specimens

Fresh clinical specimens (ulcer and wound swabs, tissues, and aspirates) where the concentration of organisms might be expected to be high can be directly examined by microscopy by Gram straining, direct fluorescent-antibody (DFA) binding, or immunohistochemistry. Under microscopic examination of Gram-stained specimens, *Francisella* cells (single and pleomorphic) appear tiny and counterstain so faintly with safranin that they can easily be missed. Basic fuchsin counterstains *F. tularensis* better than safranin. Due to the small size of *F. tularensis*, Gram staining of clinical specimens is usually of little diagnostic value. DFA staining using a fluorescein isothiocyanate-labeled hyperimmune rabbit polyclonal antibody directed against whole, killed *F. tularensis* cells can be used to presumptively identify *F. tularensis* subsp. *tularensis* and *F. tularensis* subsp. *holarctica* in clinical specimens (197). This DFA reagent does not react well or at all with *F. novicida* or *F. philomiragia*. Immunohistochemical (IHC) staining using a monoclonal antibody directed against the lipopolysaccharide (LPS) has been used successfully to visualize *F. tularensis* in formalin-fixed tissues (71). Neither the DFA reagent nor the IHC reagent is commercially available. DFA testing of specimens is provided by many reference laboratories in the United States.

Because of the relative rarity of human tularemia, evaluation of molecular diagnostics with clinical specimens has been challenging. PCR-based diagnostic methods have been used most commonly for diagnosis of ulceroglandular tularemia, the most prevalent clinical form. DNA detection by conventional PCR directed at the *tul4* gene (unique to *Francisella* spp.) has been successfully and widely applied for diagnosis of ulceroglandular tularemia (82, 167, 197). The *tul4* PCR assay displays a sensitivity of 75% when applied to wound specimens from patients with ulceroglandular tularemia and was shown to be more sensitive than culture (sensitivity of 62%) (82). More recently, real-time PCR assays using the TaqMan 5′ nuclease assay have been applied to detect *F. tularensis* DNA in a variety of clinical specimens, including ulcer specimens, aspirates, throat swabs, bronchial washes, and pleural fluid (30, 186, 195). These assays target multiple *Francisella* genes (*ISFtu2* element, *iglC*, *tul4*, and *fopA* genes). A limitation of most PCR-based diagnostics for *F. tularensis* is the inability to discriminate *F. tularensis* from *F. novicida*. While this may not be significant for patient management, the correct identification of species has both epidemiologic and public health value. Routine incorporation of real-time PCR into the diagnosis of human tularemia remains in need of further evaluations and standardization.

Detection of *F. tularensis* in ectoparasites is based primarily on PCR methods (65, 203). Of note, FLEs, present in a wide range of tick species, have been shown to cross-react with molecular targets used for the detection of *F. tularensis*, leading to false-positive results (89, 160, 173). If molecular assays are to be used for screening environmental samples for *F. tularensis*, it is important to evaluate the assays for cross-reactivity with other *Francisellaceae* members present in these sample types (22, 143). 16S rRNA gene sequencing can also be helpful for discriminating *F. tularensis* from FLEs or environmental *Francisella* spp. (22, 89).

Isolation Procedures

F. tularensis is slow growing and fastidious, requiring supplementation with sulfhydryl compounds (cysteine, cystine, thiosulfate, and IsoVitaleX) to grow on artificial medium. *F. tularensis* grows on several media common to clinical laboratories, including chocolate agar (CA) (Fig. 1A), buffered charcoal-yeast extract agar (BCYE), and Thayer-Martin agar. It also grows in thioglycolate broth. When supplemented with 1 to 2% IsoVitaleX, general bacteriological media (tryptic soy broth and Mueller-Hinton broth) support the growth of *F. tularensis*. The organisms grow slowly (60-min generation time); good growth, therefore, is obtained by prolonged incubation (48 hours or longer). Suspect cultures should be incubated at 35 to 37°C aerobically and observed daily for up to 14 days; CO_2 does not impede growth. A specialized medium, cysteine heart agar supplemented with 9% chocolatized sheep blood (CHAB), is often used for the growth of *F. tularensis* in reference laboratories (197). *F. tularensis* grows well on CHAB, as this is a high-nutrient medium. Additionally, *F. tularensis* displays distinctive colony morphology on CHAB5 which can aid in identification (Fig. 1). *F. tularensis* does not grow well or at all on general bacteriologic media, such as sheep blood agar. Nutritionally enriched specimens, such as blood or tissue, provide an intrinsic source of sulfhydryl compounds that may initially permit *F. tularensis* growth on general bacteriological media. Upon subculture, the fastidious nature of *F. tularensis* will become evident as the exogenous compounds are depleted, leading to the loss of the bacterium's viability unless the subculture is propagated on cysteine-supplemented medium.

Clinical samples from normally sterile sites can be plated on nonselective agars that support the growth of *F. tularensis*. Care should be taken not to permit laboratory contamination of *F. tularensis* isolates by environmental bacteria such as *Staphylococcus*, as these bacteria rapidly outcompete and inhibit the growth of *F. tularensis* on nonselective media (141). Clinical specimens obtained from nonsterile sites or autopsy and environmental sources should be plated on antibiotic-containing media. Incorporation of an antibiotic supplement (7.5-mg/liter colistin, 2.5-mg/liter amphotericin, 0.5-mg/liter lincomycin, 4.0-mg/liter trimethoprim, and 10-mg/liter ampicillin) into the medium has been demonstrated to prevent other organisms from overwhelming *F. tularensis* (141). Commercially available antibiotic-containing media that support the growth of

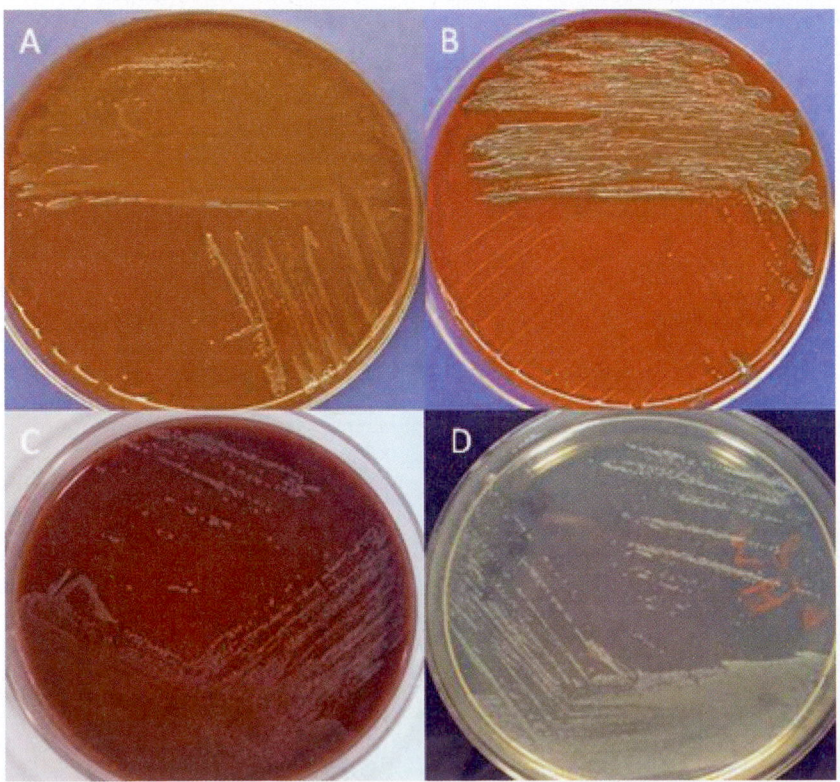

FIGURE 1   *F. tularensis* on CA (A) and CHAB (B) after 48 hours of growth; *B. melitensis* on blood agar (C) and Mueller-Hinton broth (D) after 48 hours of growth.

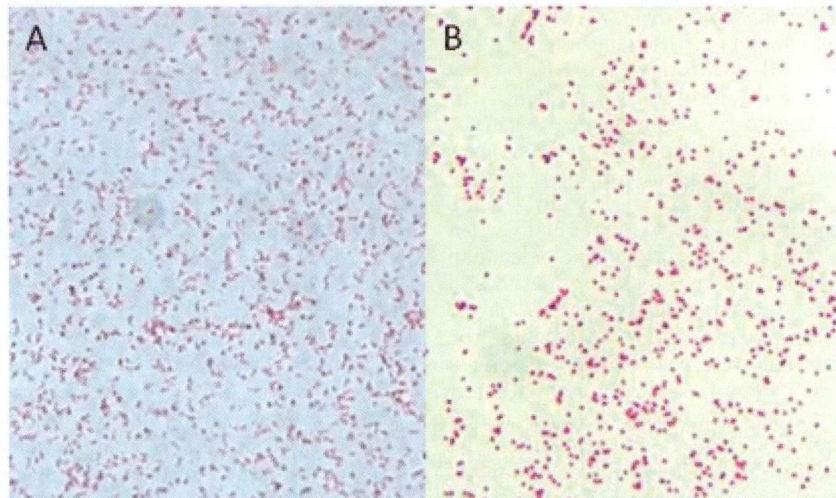

FIGURE 2 Gram stain of *F. tularensis* (A) and *B. melitensis* (B). Magnification, ~×810.

F. tularensis include improved Thayer-Martin agar (Remel, Lenexa, KS), BCYE selective agar containing polymyxin B, anisomycin, and vancomycin (Remel or Becton, Dickinson), and cysteine heart agar containing antibiotics (polymyxin B and penicillin) (Remel).

Specimens for culture should be taken on the basis of clinical presentation and before administration of antibiotics. Fresh clinical material that is likely to contain high concentrations of *F. tularensis* organisms, such as ulcer and wound specimens and lymphoid tissue (liver, spleen, or affected lymph node tissue), is inoculated directly onto an agar plate by using a sample-laden swab or bacteriological loop. Larger inocula are necessary for the recovery of *F. tularensis* from specimens that contain a lower concentration of the organisms, such as aspirates of pharyngeal washes, bronchial wash fluids, pleural fluids, and environmental samples. Whole blood should be directly inoculated into blood culture bottles (197), with subsequent culture of blood culture-positive specimens on agar.

Identification

Because of the rarity as well as the sporadic nature of most tularemia cases, the organism is often not easily identified when it is cultured. The isolation of a very tiny (individual cells may be difficult to discern), poorly counterstaining (by safranin), gram-negative coccobacillus (Fig. 2A) that produces 1- to 2-mm-diameter gray to gray-white colonies on CA after 48 hours (and scant to no growth on blood agar) should raise suspicion for *F. tularensis*. *F. tularensis* is oxidase negative, weakly catalase positive, β-lactamase positive, X and V factor negative, and urease negative. Oxidase, X/V factor, and urease testing can help differentiate *F. tularensis* from other similar gram-negative organisms, including *Brucella* spp., *Haemophilus influenzae*, and *Acinetobacter* spp. (Table 1). If further testing according to the algorithms given in chapter 12 does not rule out *F. tularensis* and the laboratory cannot do further confirmatory tests, the isolate should be sent to a reference laboratory that can confirm (or rule out) its identification as *F. tularensis*. Proper biohazard shipping procedures must be followed (see chapter 12 in this *Manual*). In the United States, all states have at least one reference laboratory that is part of the Laboratory Response Network (LRN). These LRN laboratories are able to confirm the identification of bacterial select agents, including *F. tularensis*. See also http://www.bt.cdc.gov/lrn].

The colonial morphology of *F. tularensis* is most distinctive when it is grown on CHAB. On CHAB, *F. tularensis* exhibits a prominent and unique opalescent sheen due to its production of H$_2$S; this sheen is less prominent in *F. philomiragia* than in *F. tularensis* and is absent in cultures of other gram-negative organisms, such as *Yersinia*, *Brucella*, *Haemophilus*, and *Pasteurella* spp. On CA, BCYE, and Thayer-Martin agar, *F. tularensis* colonies have an entire margin; they are gray, smooth, raised, and moist, with a butyrous consistency. *F. novicida* grows more robustly than *F. tularensis* and is cysteine independent (Table 2). Colonies of *F. philomiragia* on CA are >5 mm in diameter, with an entire margin; they are white, smooth, raised, mucoid, and cysteine independent.

Isolates can be identified as *F. tularensis* using antigen or molecular detection methods, including slide agglutination, DFA staining (Fig. 3), PCR, or sequencing. The slide agglutination test identifies a suspect culture by mixing commercially available (Becton, Dickinson and Company)

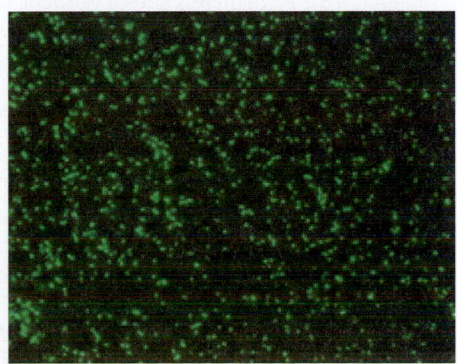

FIGURE 3 DFA staining of a culture of *F. tularensis*. Magnification, ~×490.

polyclonal rabbit anti-*F. tularensis* antibody with suspect cultures; the polyclonal rabbit anti-*F. tularensis* antibody does not react well or at all with *F. novicida* or *F. philomiragia* (197). DFA staining can also be used to identify *F. tularensis* subsp. *tularensis* and *F. tularensis* subsp. *holarctica* isolates (197). Care should be taken to ensure that prepared smears are not too thick, as this can interfere with the performance and interpretation of the test. In general, antigen-based identification methods work optimally when fresh cultures (24 hours) are tested. If a culture older than 24 hours is to be tested by antigen detection methods, a fresh subculture should be prepared. PCR methods targeting *F. tularensis*-specific genes can also be used for the identification of suspect cultures (167, 186). As described earlier in this chapter, it is important to consider that many *F. tularensis* PCR assays cross-react with *F. novicida*. Therefore, it may be important to rule out *F. novicida* as the cause of infection, particularly in areas where tularemia has not been previously reported. 16S rRNA gene sequencing can be useful if the isolate is not easily identified as *F. tularensis* (5, 35). Universal 16S rRNA gene primers or *Francisella*-specific 16S rRNA gene primers can be used (57).

The fatty acid composition is unique to the *Francisella* genus, the species of which are high in saturated even-chain acids ($C_{10:0}$, $C_{14:0}$, $C_{16:0}$) and two long-chain hydroxyl acids (3-OH-$C_{16:0}$, 3-OH-$C_{18:0}$) (78), and can be used to identify the organism as belonging to the *Francisella* genus (74, 165, 192). Commercial biochemical identification systems available in clinical laboratories are not recommended for the diagnosis of *F. tularensis*, as these systems can misidentify *F. tularensis* (197).

Typing Systems

Once an isolate has been identified as a *Francisella* sp., supplemental tests can be used for additional characterization, including typing of species, subspecies, and strain. Oxidase can be used to differentiate *F. philomiragia* from *F. novicida* and *F. tularensis* (Table 2). Glycerol fermentation and citrulline ureidase activity distinguish *F. tularensis* subsp. *tularensis* from *F. tularensis* subsp. *holarctica* (Table 2); conventional assays for these biochemical tests have been described (157). The 96-well automated MicroLog MicroStation system with GN2 microplates (Biolog Inc., Hayward, CA) can also be used to assess the glycerol fermentation of *F. tularensis* (197). Genus, species, and subspecies can be typed by sequence analysis of the 16S rRNA gene (56, 57). PCR methods (both conventional and real-time) can type isolates at the level of genus, species, subspecies (*F. tularensis* subsp. *tularensis* or *F. tularensis* subsp. *holarctica*), and subclades (*F. tularensis* subsp. *tularensis* subclades A1 and A2) (116, 197). Pulsed-field gel electrophoresis can differentiate the three *F. tularensis* subsp. *tularensis* subclades, A1a, A1b, and A2 (91). For discrimination of individual strains, a multilocus variable-number tandem-repeat assay (MLVA) for *F. tularensis*, based on 25 different repeats in the genome (83), has been utilized.

Serologic Tests

Antibodies may be detected as early as 1 week after the onset of symptoms (about 2 weeks after infection). By 2 weeks after onset, antibodies may be detected in 89 to 95.4% of samples. Antibodies can persist for more than 10 years (25, 190). Immunoglobulin M (IgM), IgA, and IgG antibodies may appear simultaneously (178, 187). IgM antibodies can last for many years; thus, their presence does not always indicate early or recent infection (25, 178).

Agglutination testing, either by the tube agglutination (TA) or the microagglutination (MA) method, is a standard serology test for determining the presence of antibodies in tularemia (25, 29, 197). Formalin-killed antigen (prepared from *F. tularensis* subsp. *tularensis* strain Schu S4) is commercially available from Becton, Dickinson. Formalin-killed *F. tularensis* antigen is also prepared within reference laboratories worldwide. In the United States, a single specimen with a TA titer of ≥1:160 or an MA titer of ≥1:128 is considered positive. Formalin-killed *F. tularensis* whole-cell antigen may display low-level cross-reactivity with *Brucella* antibodies (23, 125). No cross-reactivity of *F. novicida* or *F. philomiragia* sera has been observed with *F. tularensis*-killed cells (133). Enzyme-linked immunosorbent assays (ELISAs) have been adopted for use in the parts of Europe where tularemia is endemic (25, 146, 159, 197). The LPS and/or outer membrane fraction remains the primary ELISA antigen used in test applications. Antigenic differences between *F. tularensis* subsp. *tularensis* and subsp. *holarctica* have not been identified for use in serology assays. Thus, serology assays do not distinguish the infecting subspecies. This is of most importance in North America, where both *F. tularensis* subsp. *tularensis* and *F. tularensis* subsp. *holarctica* cause tularemia.

F. tularensis organisms are intracellular bacteria and are capable of eliciting both humoral and cell-mediated immunity (178). The latter response has been known to remain strong 25 years after infection (49). Host T cells retain proliferative responses to unique *F. tularensis* membrane proteins, with concomitant increases in interferon and interleukin-2 levels (49, 175, 176, 178). Tests for measuring the cell-mediated immune response are specialized and are not routinely used for diagnosis of tularemia (47).

Antimicrobial Susceptibilities

F. tularensis infections are treatable with narrow-spectrum antibiotics. All *Francisella* isolates examined to date are β-lactamase positive, so penicillins and cephalosporins are not effective and should not be used to treat tularemia. Antibiotics recommended for treatment and prophylaxis include chloramphenicol, ciprofloxacin, gentamicin, streptomycin, and tetracycline. Antimicrobial susceptibility testing (broth microdilution and Etest) of a large collection of *F. tularensis* isolates worldwide has demonstrated no antimicrobial resistance to drugs used for treating tularemia (77, 177, 181, 182, 184). Some isolates of *F. tularensis* subsp. *holarctica* from Europe and Russia are erythromycin resistant.

Antimicrobial susceptibility testing of *F. tularensis* is not usually performed in clinical microbiology laboratories because of safety concerns in working with this organism and because resistance to antibiotics used for clinical treatment of tularemia has never been reported (179). The Clinical and Laboratory Standards Institute (CLSI) has published interpretative criteria and quality control limits for broth microdilution of *F. tularensis* using Mueller-Hinton medium supplemented with 2% IsoVitaleX (36, 37).

Evaluation, Interpretation, and Reporting of Results

Serology is generally the most common method for laboratory confirmation of *F. tularensis* infection, due largely to the organism being slow growing and fastidious. Nonetheless, culture provides a conclusive diagnosis of infection and whenever possible should be attempted using appropriate biosafety measures. Isolation of a very tiny gram-negative bacterium that shows fastidious growth characteristics and is oxidase negative, weakly catalase positive, urease negative, X/V factor negative, and β-lactamase positive should be strongly suspected as *F. tularensis* and referred to a reference laboratory. Confirmation of *F. tularensis* infections includes (i) identification of a culture as *F. tularensis* and/or (ii) a fourfold difference in titers in acute- and convalescent-phase serum samples, with one of the paired samples having a positive titer. A positive test result for a primary clinical specimen using antigen or molecular detection methods, including DFA staining, IHC staining, or PCR, provides only a presumptive diagnosis of *F. tularensis*. A single positive serum sample is also considered presumptive for tularemia. For all cases presumed to be tularemia, it is necessary to verify that the patients' symptoms are compatible with tularemia and, in the case of a single positive titer, that the patient has not been previously vaccinated.

In the United States, *F. tularensis* is classified as a select agent. To transfer, receive, or possess *F. tularensis*, laboratories must be registered both with the CDC and with the Animal and Plant Health Inspection Service (APHIS) of the U.S. Department of Agriculture. The registration process includes a U.S. Department of Justice investigation of all personnel having access to select agents. Clinical laboratories are exempt from the registration requirement provided that within 7 calendar days of identifying one of these agents, they transfer it to a registered entity and/or destroy the agent on site. Laboratories identifying an organism as *F. tularensis* are required to report this finding immediately to the CDC. Report forms, contact information, laboratory registration information, and pertinent citations of the U.S. Federal Code may be found at http://www.cdc.gov/od/sap.

BRUCELLA

Brucella spp. are common zoonoses among domestic animals and among wildlife, including novel species of marine mammals. *Brucella* spp. also cause infections in humans and can mimic other infectious and noninfectious diseases, posing challenges to physicians in reaching a diagnosis. The remittent/undulant fever of brucellosis was first confused with other diseases, such as malaria and typhoid fever, and was called many synonyms pertaining mainly to the geographic locations where the disease occurred: Mediterranean fever, Malta fever, Gibraltar fever, and Cyprus fever (198). Over the last decade, there has been renewed interest in this organism due to its inclusion in the potential biological weapons lists of most authorities (8, 64, 100, 136, 202; http://www.who.int/csr/resources/publications/Brucellosis.pdf).

Taxonomy and Genome

Brucellaceae is a family of phylogenetically closely related free-living soil organisms composed of *Brucella*, *Ochrobactrum*, and *Mycoplana* spp. The *Brucellaceae* are part of the order *Rhizobiales*, which includes other genera involved in human disease: *Bartonella*, *Afipia*, *Methylobacterium*, and *Roseomonas*. (41, 61).

The taxonomy of *Brucella* spp. remains to be clarified. Studies indicate that terrestrial *Brucella* spp. are homogeneous species harboring >90% interspecies homology by DNA-DNA hybridization studies, identical 16S rRNA gene sequences, and >98% sequence homology by comparative genomics. Because of these findings, a suggestion was made to consider *Brucella* a monospecific genus and the different species as biovars of *Brucella melitensis* (73).

The average size of the genome is 2.37×10^9 Da, with a DNA G+C content of 58 to 59 mol%. Currently, the genus *Brucella* encompasses nine recognized species, six terrestrial and three marine (58, 193). The six terrestrial *Brucella* species are *B. melitensis* (three biovars) (preferred hosts are goats, sheep, and camels), *B. abortus* (seven biovars) (cattle, bison, and buffalo), *B. suis* (five biovars) (swine and a range of wild animals), *B. canis* (dogs), *B. ovis* (rams), and *B. neotomae* (desert and wood rats). The three identified marine species, *B. delphini*, *B. pinnipediae*, and *B. cetaceae*, were recovered from marine mammals (e.g., seals, whales, and dolphins) and were found to differ phenotypically from the six terrestrial species by their patterns of substrate-mediated metabolic activity. *Brucella maris* has been suggested as a name to encompass these marine isolates, but to date this has not been accepted (38). Though preferred or predominant hosts are recognized for *Brucella* spp., cross-infection of other mammalian species, including humans, may occur (41).

Description of the Genus

Brucella spp. are facultative, intracellular, small (0.5- to 1.5-μm), gram-negative coccobacilli that lack capsules, flagellae, endospores, or native plasmids. They are aerobic (some prefer CO_2 for their growth), do not ferment sugars, and are positive in a few oxidative metabolic tests. *Brucella* spp. can grow on a wide range of culture media, and colonies appear after 24 to 48 hours of incubation as mostly smooth colonies, but rough variants can occur (4, 41).

Antigenic Components

Several antigenic determinants of *Brucella*, related mainly to LPS and protein antigens, have been characterized. The LPS is the major antigen that dominates the antibody response. LPS of rough strains is very similar to LPS of smooth strains. Based on their O side chain, smooth strains were reported to be composed of two antigenic epitopes: A (*B. abortus*) and M (*B. melitensis*). The smooth-strain LPS has been reported to be responsible for observed cross-reactions in both the agglutination and complement fixation tests between smooth species of *Brucella* and *Yersinia enterocolitica* O:9, *Escherichia hermannii*, *Escherichia coli* O:157, *Salmonella enterica* serovar O:30, *Stenotrophomonas maltophilia*, and *Vibrio cholerae* O:1. Cross-reaction has been attributed to the similarities of the O-specific side chains of the LPS molecules of these organisms (45).

The characterized protein antigens include outer and inner membrane, cytoplasmic, and periplasmic antigens. Some are recognized by the immune system during infection and are potentially useful in diagnostic tests (41, 66, 120). For example, Omp25 is an outer membrane structural protein that is highly conserved in all brucellae and is associated with both LPS and peptidoglycan. In addition, some proteins, such as ribosomal proteins (e.g., L7/L12) and fusion proteins, demonstrate a protective effect against *Brucella* based on antibody and cell-mediated responses (41, 126). These molecules may be useful in potential vaccines.

Virulence Factors, Pathogenic Mechanisms, and Immune Response

The incubation period is variable but generally is 1 to 4 weeks. The intracellular location and survival of the organism contribute to its virulence and pathogenesis. The exact pathophysiologic aspects of infection remain to be defined (201). Briefly, once the brucellae enter the body by various routes, they are encountered by polymorphonuclear and mononuclear phagocytes, to which lectin facilitates attachment. In the process, several factors are involved in enabling a brucella to enter a host, escape from phagocytic killing by inhibiting the phagosome-lysosome fusion, and evade the immune system, and they aid in its survival and propagation within macrophages and other cells. This is followed up by brucellae being transferred through regional lymph nodes into the circulatory system and subsequently being seeded throughout the body, with tropism for the reticuloendothelial system, resulting in different clinical phases of disease (69). Virulence determinants include urease to avoid stomach stress through oral passage (158) and *Brucella*-containing vacuoles that enable escape from immune system recognition and provide an acidic environment to hamper antibiotic activity. A *Brucella* LPS cell component (containing a poly *N*-formyl perosamine O chain and a CuZn superoxide dismutase) and outer membrane protein 25 (OMP 25) were reported to help the bacteria survive within mononuclear phagocytes (41, 55). Also, the uniqueness of *Brucella* LPS lies in its being a poor inducer of gamma interferon and tumor necrosis factor alpha, both of which are essential for T-helper 1 (Th1)-type-cell-mediated immunity for the elimination of the organism (67). The overall inflammatory process results in a slow degradation of *Brucella* cell wall components by the polymorphonuclear leukocytes and can lead to granuloma formation, which is more often associated with *B. abortus* than *B. melitensis* (69).

Protective immunity, though not long term, is conferred by antibodies to LPS and T-cell-mediated macrophage activation, triggered by protein antigens (41). A study showed a significant increase in the levels of interleukin-12 and gamma interferon in patients with *Brucella* infection compared to levels in controls, indicating that there is induction of Th1-type cytokines during human brucellosis (1). The immune response against *Brucella* involves antigen-specific T-cell activation, CD4+ Th lymphocytes, CD8+ T cells, and humoral responses (67). Lymphocytes are the main stimulant of the immune response. The Th1 response stimulates IgG2a production, which is involved mostly in protection against intracellular pathogens through cell-mediated immunity, and is critical for the clearance of *Brucella* infection. The Th2 response stimulates the production of IgG1 and is mainly responsible for protection against extracellular pathogens through the humoral immune response (67, 201). Recently, a study of *B. abortus* infection in rats showed that the IgG2a response (indicative of a Th1 response) persisted and dominated over the IgG1 response (88). However, the exact nature of the immune response and protective factors involved in this disease are still being investigated, and the pathogenic mechanisms of reinfection remain unknown.

Epidemiology and Transmission

Although *Brucella* can be killed by pasteurization, exposure to UV light, acidity, or many antiseptics and disinfectants, it can survive for long periods under various conditions, e.g., 10 weeks in soil, 11 weeks in aborted fetuses, 17 weeks in bovine stool, around 3 weeks in milk and ice cream, and several months in fresh cheese (41, 202). In terms of the total numbers of infected cases, *B. melitensis* dominates the world arena (especially in the Mediterranean and Arabian Gulf countries). However, *B. abortus* and *B. suis* supersede it in certain geographic locations. *B. canis* has also been reported to cause human diseases, while *B. ovis* and *B. neotomae* have not (41, 100, 137). *Brucella* spp. associated with marine animals have been reported to cause disease in humans (28, 111, 170).

The epidemiologies of human brucellosis differ between areas of endemicity and nonendemicity in terms of age, sex, season, and risk factors. In regions of endemicity, such as the eastern Mediterranean basin, Middle East, the Arabian peninsula, Mexico, Central and South America, the Balkan Peninsula, and the Indian subcontinent, the disease occurs among the general population. In the general population, levels of infection are almost equal among adults and children of both sexes and mostly due to ingestion of unpasteurized goat, sheep, cow, and camel milk or its products (e.g., soft cheese) (59, 100, 137, 163, 202).

In areas where the disease is not endemic, infection is seen predominantly among adult males, acquired occupationally by transmission through direct skin contact (e.g., through cuts and abrasions) with infected animal parts, inhalation of aerosolized infected particles, and accidental inoculation (e.g., sprays or aerosols inoculated into the eye, mouth, and nose). These infections occur mostly among dairy industry professionals, veterinarians, abattoir workers, and clinical and research microbiology staff (16, 200).

Very rare cases transmitted through blood and bone marrow transfusion, suspected sexual intercourse, and banked human sperm have been reported (121, 138, 153, 180, 185). Also, a few cases of neonatal brucellosis have been reported, and the isolation of *Brucella* from human milk may explain it (99, 134).

Laboratory-acquired infection is an important source of transmission. *Brucella* has a very low infectious dose ($\leq 10^2$ organisms), and personnel should adhere to strict safety precautions, especially when handling cultures suspected of containing the organims in clinical, research, and production laboratories (124, 200). Most cases of laboratory-acquired disease result from mishandling and misidentification of the organism (63, 124). The frequent failure of clinical laboratories to correctly identify isolates as *Brucella* species is particularly worrisome from the perspectives of laboratory safety and potential use as a bioweapon. *B. melitensis*, *B. abortus*, and *B. suis* are category B select agents (70, 136).

Clinical Categories of Human Brucellosis

The clinical categories of human brucellosis are based on arbitrary criteria. In 1956, Spink based them on the duration of manifestations (acute, ≤ 2 months; subacute, 2 to 12 months; chronic, ≥ 12 months) (172). Subsequently, others based them primarily on clinical manifestations (e.g., subclinical, localized, chronic, and active, with or without localized disease, including bacteremic and serological classifications) (102, 202). To date, no uniform definition has been adopted.

The incubation period is variable but usually ranges between 1 and 4 weeks. The disease onset is usually insidious, but its presentation encompasses a wide spectrum of nonspecific clinical manifestations, such as fever, sweats, arthralgias, myalgia, fatigue, loss of appetite, weight loss, hepatomegaly, and splenomegaly. Complications can involve many organs and tissues with signs of focal disease. The routine hematology and biochemical profiles are usually within normal limits, with some elevation in erythrocyte sedimentation rate and liver function tests. Thus, to the unaware physician, the diagnosis of brucellosis can be a dilemma and could protract for weeks and, in some complicated cases, for years (59, 100, 106, 156, 202). Increased business and leisure travel to countries where the disease is endemic has led to diagnostic challenges in areas where brucellosis is uncommon, especially when the presentation is unusual (42, 100, 112, 113, 202). Overall, the mortality is very low, but morbidity is high. Previously, brucellosis in childhood was thought to be uncommon, but now it seems to be as prevalent as and presents in a manner similar to that in adults in areas of endemicity (98, 100, 163).

Because of these nonspecific clinical features, human brucellosis was labeled the disease of "mistakes." It can be misdiagnosed and confused with other diseases, such as typhoid fever, rheumatic fever, tuberculosis, malaria, infectious mononucleosis, endocarditis, histoplasmosis, ankylosing spondylitis, pyelitis, cholecystitis, thrombophlebitis, chronic fatigue syndrome, collagen vascular diseases, autoimmune diseases, and tumors (100, 106, 135, 202).

Complications

The most commonly encountered focal complications are osteoarticular (10 to 70%) (mostly joints), genital in both males (6 to 8%) and females (2 to 5%), neurological (3 to 5%), cardiac (1 to 3%), pulmonary (1 to 2%), and renal (< 1%). Mortality is very low (<1%) and is almost exclusively due to cardiac complications (39, 42, 100, 101, 102, 106, 135, 163, 202).

Osteoarticular complications occur mostly as arthritis (10 to 70%) and rarely as osteomyelitis (<1%). The joints most frequently involved are, in descending order, sacroiliac, knee, hip, vertebra, ankle, and multiple other joints. Generally, *Brucella* arthritis can be misdiagnosed as rheumatoid arthritis, rheumatic fever, tuberculosis, and systemic lupus erythematosis.

Neurobrucellosis (3 to 5% of cases) can affect both adults and children with diverse presentations, including fever, headache, meningeal signs, coma, or paresis. Depression and mental fatigue are not uncommon complaints (51, 97, 161). CSF analysis, of both adults and children, is nonspecific and can overlap with other central nervous system diseases, such as mycobacterial, viral, syphilitic or fungal infections, or with noninfectious diseases, such as psychiatric problems, multiple sclerosis, and cancer (51, 97, 161). The yield of *Brucella* culture from CSF is low (5 to 30%). Therefore, the use of *Brucella* serology tests, especially ELISA, on CSF specimens is essential to diagnose neurobrucellosis (9, 161). With appropriate treatment, the prognosis is usually good for acute presentations and varies in the setting of chronic disease.

Genital complications in males (6 to 8% of cases) are mostly orchitis or epididymoorchitis (40, 76, 100). In females, abortion (2 to 5%) has been reported mostly in the first trimester (103). Other rare complications reported for females include cervicitis, salpingitis, tubo-ovarian abscess, and ovarian dermoid cyst (103, 183).

Relapse is considered one of the most important features of brucellosis and its complications (19, 100, 102, 171). Factors associated with relapse include the use of less effective antibiotic therapy, a positive blood culture during the initial presentation, and ≤10 days' duration of symptoms before initiation of treatment.

Collection, Handling, Storage, and Transport of Specimens

Specimens for the laboratory investigation of cases with brucellosis may be sent for culture, serology, and/or molecular testing. Culture can be performed on a wide range of specimen types, including blood (at least two sets), bone marrow, CSF, pleural and synovial fluids, urine, abscess specimens, and tissue specimens. Adequate volumes should be secured prior to initiation of antimicrobial therapy.

Blood (serum) and, when relevant, CSF specimens are used for serologic testing. Molecular testing, though usually for research purposes, can be performed on blood (serum or whole blood, CSF, and bone marrow) specimens.

The guidelines for proper specimen collection, handling, transport, and processing are generally similar to those reported for blood cultures and other specimens submitted for bacterial culture (refer to chapter 16 in this *Manual*). If delay in delivery to the lab is anticipated, specimens can be held in the refrigerator. To avoid/minimize laboratory exposures to the pathogen, specimens from patients suspected of having the disease should be labeled appropriately and referred to a reference laboratory, with the label specifying that the laboratory should rule out brucellosis (44, 196).

Direct Detection

To circumvent the limitations of routine culture and serodiagnostic tests for human brucellosis, in-house-developed conventional PCR and real-time (RT) PCR assays can directly detect *Brucella* from clinical specimens. Several *Brucella*-specific gene targets have been used, including BCS P31 (encodes a 31-kDa cell surface protein) and BP26 (encodes a 26-kDa periplasmic protein), 16S rRNA, and the insertion sequence IS711. The sensitivities of these assays are quite varied, ranging from 50% to 100%. This variation might be related to different DNA extraction methods, detection formats, and different types of specimens (43, 85, 110, 115, 119, 122, 123, 147, 148, 189). The ribosomal 16S-23S ITS region constitutes a suitable target in clinical specimens and formalin-fixed paraffin-embedded archived tissue, as well as for identification of isolates from culture to the species level (85).

Molecular assays constitute a useful adjunct and have promising potential for the diagnosis of human brucellosis in a clinical laboratory setting. Their routine incorporation in the diagnosis of human brucellosis remains in need of further optimization, standardization, and improvement (85, 149).

Culture

Culture is considered the gold standard in the laboratory diagnosis of brucellosis. Conventional methods require long incubation times (6 weeks) and are generally of variable yields, being higher among patients with acute brucellosis (40% to 90%) than in patients in the chronic, focal, and complicated stages (5 to 20%) (10, 41, 100, 199). When positive, culture provides the definitive diagnosis. Bone marrow cultures result in a 15- to 20%-higher yield than peripheral blood cultures. The conventional standard medium for the nonautomated blood culture broth has been the biphasic Ruiz-Castañeda bottle. The growth of the pathogen takes between 7 and 35 days to become positive, and the bottles should be held for 6 weeks, with frequent visual inspection (every 3 days) and terminal subculture before the specimen is discarded as negative (10, 199).

Automated continuously monitored blood culture systems such as Bactec (BD Diagnostics, Sparks, MD) and BacTAlert (bioMérieux, Durham, NC) show higher yields than the conventional culture method and expedite the detection of bacterial growth (majority recovered within 1 week). There is no need to incubate bottles longer than 10 to 14 days (9a; 199). The lysis centrifugation system showed improved and faster yields than conventional methods in those labs that do not have automated blood culture systems (199). However, due to the need for centrifugation and manipulation before direct plating, the system may entail exposure and contamination hazards. Rarely, some patients with brucellosis have a positive blood culture in the absence of positive serology (199, 202).

Recovery of *Brucella* from other clinical material, such as bone marrow, CSF, joint fluid, homogenate of tissues, and bones, in addition to blood specimens, can be achieved by inoculation of specimens into broth media (such as those used for blood cultures) in addition to plated media (blood and CA). The latter medium is incubated at 37°C, preferably under 5 to 10% CO_2, for up to 10 days prior to reporting as negative.

Identification

Clinical microbiology laboratories should report identifications of colonies suspected of being *Brucella* spp. on the basis of a few morphologic, biochemical, and serologic tests. All manipulations of *Brucella* cultures should be done in a biological safety cabinet. In these setups, the colonies are generally recovered directly from inoculated clinical specimens or as a result of subculture from broth media (e.g., biphasic Ruiz-Castañeda medium and blood culture medium showing signs of growth) on blood (Fig. 1C) and CA. Colonies can grow on other media as well (e.g., Mueller-Hinton agar [Fig. 1D] and MacConkey agar [can show variable growth]). Thayer-Martin or Martin-Lewis medium can be used to isolate *Brucella* spp. from contaminated specimens. Generally, colonies are visible after 24 to 48 hours of aerobic incubation or incubation with 5 to 10% CO_2 at 37°C, and there is no need to keep the plates more than 72 to 96 hours before discarding them as negative. The colonies are 1 to 2 mm in diameter, entire, smooth, and glistening. Rough variants can occur with *B. canis* colonies. The presumptive identification of *Brucella* spp. from these colonies entails demonstrating small gram-negative coccobacilli (0.5 to 0.7 μm in diameter and 0.6 to 1.5 μm in length) (Fig. 2B). Biochemical reactions show positive oxidase, catalase, and urease tests, as well as a positive slide agglutination reaction with specific *B. abortus* and/or *B. melitensis* antisera (4, 41). Once these tests are performed and completed, the clinical laboratory may report the organism as presumptively *Brucella* spp. Further characterization and speciation of the pathogen involves extensive testing not routinely performed in most clinical laboratories (4, 95). In the United States, LRN reference laboratories are able to confirm and identify *Brucella* to the species level, and these laboratories can provide guidance and additional pertinent information. See also http://www.bt.cdc.gov/lrn/.

When definitive identification is indicated, conventional and molecular characterizations can be used. Conventional classification/identification to the species level of *Brucella* spp. can be determined from results of certain reactions, such as dye inhibition (thionin, fuchsin, safranin), CO_2 requirement, Tiblisi phage lysis, oxidative metabolic tests (glutamic acid, ornithine, ribose and lysine), and reaction to monospecific sera. *Brucella* is usually subtyped into biovars using multilocus enzyme electrophoresis, pulsed-field gel electrophoresis, randomly amplified polymorphic DNA analysis, enterobacterial repetitive intergenic consensus sequence PCR, repetitive intergenic palindromic sequence PCR, amplified fragment length polymorphism analysis, monolocus (such as *omp2a* and *omp2b*) sequence analysis, or multilocus sequence typing (3, 86, 113, 193).

Typing Systems

One of the most highly discriminatory methodologies for epidemiological subtyping of isolates belonging to monomorphic bacterial species is MLVA (96). In *Brucella*, MLVA schemes with 21 loci (MLVA-21) and MLVA-16, which use a combination of repeat markers distributed across the *Brucella* genome, were able to distinguish isolates of *Brucella* spp. of widespread temporal and geographical origins or of very close origins (3, 86, 193). A *Brucella* MLVA database is hosted at http://mlva.u-psud.f and contains data derived from more than 500 animal and human *Brucella* isolates. Molecular subtyping methods, especially the promising MLVA, may potentially be useful not only for epidemiological trace back purposes or outbreaks but also for distinguishing relapses from reinfection, thereby influencing clinical therapeutic decisions (86).

Serologic Tests

Serologic assays are the most commonly relied upon tests in the laboratory diagnosis of brucellosis. Serological results are optimally interpreted in the context of the evolution of antibody responses after infection with *Brucella* spp. IgM first appears, followed by the appearance of IgG within 10 to 14 days. The general evolution of these and other immunoglobulins depends on response to treatment: in recovery, a gradual and slow decline in titers is observed, while persistent titers alert the clinician to a poor response to treatment due to focal complications, chronic infections, or relapse (18, 62, 140). Persistence, (i.e., detection of antibodies, mostly IgG and some IgM, for a very prolonged time [months and sometime years]) is observed in 15 to 20% of asymptomatic patients who have undergone treatment and cure. The explanation for this remains elusive (100).

Several antigens are used for serologic diagnostic assays, generally obtained from *B. melitensis* and *B. abortus*. Whole-cell preparations are the antigens used in the agglutination and the indirect fluorescent-antibody (IFA) tests, while sonic extracts, purified LPS or protein extracts of *Brucella*, are used mainly in ELISAs (4, 7, 10, 12, 13, 87). Detection of antibodies against infections due to *B. canis* and *B. ovis* require using major outer membrane protein antigens because these strains exist in a rough colony form and do not share cross-reacting antigens with the other *Brucella* spp. (113). Since there is no standardized reference antigen, it is important to note that the source of the antigen, commercial or otherwise, can influence the test results (14).

A wide range of in-house serologic tests and formats have been used for investigating patients with brucellosis (Table 4). These include direct agglutination tests in tubes, e.g., the serum agglutination test (SAT), and on slides, e.g., the rose bengal test, indirect Coombs test, Brucellacapt tests, IFA test, and ELISA for detection of immunoglobulin classes and subclasses (6, 11, 13, 14, 15, 68, 154). Generally, agglutination-based tests cannot differentiate the types of antibodies involved, while the enzyme immunoassay (EIA) and IFA test can. Commercial EIAs detecting *Brucella* IgG and IgM with a high degree of sensitivity and specificity have been available for a number of years (17) and are considered an excellent method for screening sera for *Brucella* antibodies (13, 16).

Brucellacapt (Vircell, Granada, Spain) has been introduced as a rapid (18 to 24 hours) and easy serologic test to carry out. The test is based on immunocapture agglutination methodology that can detect, in a single step, the nonagglutinating IgG and IgA antibodies. The sensitivity and specificity are similar to those of the Coombs test. However, since the latter test is cumbersome because of multiple washing steps, centrifugation, and a long turnaround time (48 hours), Brucellacapt can offer a valuable alternative (129). Immunochromatographic lateral-flow dipstick tests have been advocated for screening/surveillance of patients with brucellosis in areas of endemicity

TABLE 4 Tests commonly used in laboratory diagnosis of brucellosis

Test	General comments
Direct microscopy	Very low sensitivity; not useful routinely; uses differential or immunospecific stains
Culture	If positive, provides definitive diagnosis; variable yield, slow growth; blood culture instruments speed recovery; hazardous
Serology	Most commonly relied upon in diagnosis
Slide agglutination	Simple; rapid (10 min); relatively good in acute cases; high rate of false negatives in complicated and chronic cases; liable to cross-reaction (i.e., false-positive result)
Tube (SAT) or microplate agglutination	Widely used; relatively good in acute cases; high rate of false negatives in complicated and chronic cases; liable to cross-reaction (i.e. false-positive result); takes time to set up and 24 h to read
Indirect Coombs test	Extension of SAT; takes an additional 24 h to read; detects nonagglutinating or incomplete antibodies; good for complicated and chronic cases; misses around 7% of cases compared to ELISA
Brucellacapt	Based on an immunocapture technique to detect, in a single step, the nonagglutinating IgG and IgA antibodies, as well as the agglutinating antibodies. Performance is similar to that of Coombs test, but it is more rapid and easier to carry out.
ELISA	Test of choice for complicated and chronic cases; when other tests are negative, reveals total and individual specific immunoglobulins (IgG, IgM, IgA); rapid (4–6 hours); objective, highly sensitive, and specific.
IFA	Generally like the ELISA, but it is subjective and may fail to detect IgA; rapid (2–3 h)
Molecular/PCR, reverse transcription-PCR	Promising test, theoretically very highly sensitive and specific; additional documentation is needed vs culture and serology prior to making it routine in clinical laboratories

and as outbreak and field tests. They are simple, rapid, and easy to perform and read, with high (>90%) sensitivity and specificity (169).

Antimicrobial Susceptibilities

Routine susceptibility testing of *Brucella* species is not indicated for many reasons. These include the rare development of antibiotic resistance against the tetracyclines, rifampin, and aminoglycosides; the lack of plasmids; concerns for laboratory safety; a poor correlation between high levels of in vitro activity and clinical efficacy for many agents, including β-lactams and quinolones; and a general lack of well-established testing conditions and interpretive standards (37, 202). Recently, the CLSI presented guidelines to determine the MICs of tetracycline and doxycycline against *Brucella* spp., using a Mueller-Hinton broth dilution method (37). The Etest on Mueller-Hinton agar supplemented with sheep blood or horse serum for drug synergy testing has also been described (72, 107, 130).

Anti-*Brucella* Therapy

Appropriate antimicrobial therapy for treatment of human brucellosis reduces morbidity, prevents complications, and minimizes relapses. Several anti-*Brucella* agents have been used (e.g., doxycycline, rifampin, trimethoprim-sulfamethoxazole, streptomycin-gentamicin, some quinolones, and cephalosporins) with various rates of success. Currently, the most effective treatment regimen and optimal duration of treatment remain unclear (20, 59, 84, 98, 168).

Fewer relapses with combined regimens than with monotherapy have been reported. For adults with uncomplicated infection, the WHO recommends oral doxycycline and rifampin for 6 to 8 weeks. Triple regimens using doxycycline, rifampin, and an aminoglycoside for 2 to 3 months are recommended for patients with endocarditis and neurobrucellosis.

Treatment regimens with fluoroquinolones and broad-spectrum cephalosporins have been used. Although these agents have good MICs in vitro against *Brucella* spp., patients treated with these regimens have higher rates of relapses than patients on the standard regimen. The use of fluoroquinolones in combination with rifampin for the treatment of bacteremia and complicated brucellosis has yielded varied results (2, 168).

A recent systematic review and meta-analysis study covering 30 trials and 77 treatment arms showed that among patients with bacteraemia and complicated brucellosis, higher failure and relapse rates and shorter treatment durations (less than 6 weeks) were observed with monotherapy than with multidrug therapy. The preferred treatment should be with dual or triple regimens, including an aminoglycoside (168).

TABLE 5 Interpretation of commonly used serologic tests based on the immunoglobulin type detected and usefulness in the diagnosis of different disease categories/stages of human brucellosis

Test	Type of Ig detected			Usefulness of diagnosis in indicated category			
	IgG	IgM	IgA	Acute	Chronic	Focal	Relapse
Rose bengal/slide	+	+	+	+	−	−	−
Tube (SAT) or microtiter plate agglutination	+	+	+	+	−	−	−
Indirect Coombs	+	−	−	+	+	+	+
Brucellacapt	+	−	+	+	+	+	+
EIA	+	+	+	+	+	+	+

The question about postexposure prophylaxis (doxycycline and rifampin therapy for 3 to 6 weeks) after a high-risk exposure in the lab remains debatable. Guidelines for postexposure management are empirical (32). Upon possible exposure, however, recommendations were made to take a baseline blood sample, monitor for symptoms weekly for 6 months, and perform serological surveillance at 0, 2, 4, 6, and 24 weeks (33).

Prevention

Vaccines have been successful in the control of livestock infections, which can subsequently reduce infections in humans. Most veterinary vaccines focus on live, attenuated *B. abortus* (strain S19) and a more stable rough mutant of *B. abortus* (strain RB51) for cows, *B. melitensis* (strain Rev-1) for sheep and goats, and *B. suis* 2 for swine. However, developed vaccines have had limited efficacy in humans and have been associated with serious medical reactions. Heating of dairy products and related foods has also been effective in preventing disease transmission. The most cost-effective approach to control and prevent brucellosis relies on raising public awareness about the disease and greater cooperation between human and animal health sectors (204).

Evaluation, Interpretation, and Reporting of Results

Interpretation of serologic test results in relation to exposure, diagnosis, and prognosis of the disease necessitates an accurate assessment of the clinical history and current status of patients and understanding the usefulness and pitfalls of the laboratory tests (7, 202). Positive cutoff titers in the *Brucella* agglutination test for diagnosis have generally been considered to be ≥160 in symptomatic patients. However, much lower titers with the SAT have been reported for patients with active disease (100). Moreover, one has to be careful when negative serology is encountered when brucellosis is suspected, since this could be due, for example, to infection with *B. canis*, which can be missed by serologic assays using *B. abortus* or *B. melitensis* antigen. In addition, this could be due to very early disease presentation, and thus repeat testing after 1 to 2 weeks is warranted (18, 85).

In acute brucellosis, elevation in *Brucella*-specific IgG, IgM, IgA, IgE, IgG1, and IgG3 is shown, while in those patients with chronic brucellosis, elevations in IgG, IgA, IgE, IgG1, and IgG4 are usually seen (6, 10, 15, 62). Monitoring the treatment response requires a sequential follow-up for patients with serologic titers. A decline indicates good prognosis, persistently high titers necessitate continuous monitoring, and a resurgence in antibody titers most likely indicates relapse or reinfection. Slide and TA titers fall faster than with the EIA (18, 21, 105, 140). Relapse has also been diagnosed by a detection of a resurgence in *Brucella*-specific IgG and IgA antibodies, not IgM (18, 62, 140). Markers for differentiating active from inactive disease are being sought. For example, anti-*Brucella* cytoplasmic or periplasmic protein antibodies, as determined by ELISA, increased only in patients with active brucellosis and were a better predictor of cure than antilipopolysaccharide antibodies (21, 66, 151). Also, some interleukins show a decrease posttherapy (104).

Though serologic tests are currently of high importance for the investigation of patients with brucellosis, several limitations can be encountered, mainly lack of standardized antigen preparations and assay methodologies, as well as the detection of sustained high antibody titers in some patients, despite treatment and cure (7, 18, 62, 68, 140). False-positive serologic results are rare. However, two cases were recently reported in the United States, a finding which led to initiating not only unnecessary treatment but also a wide range of public health investigations (34).

Based on the above, laboratories should use a combination of two agglutination tests, namely, the SAT and indirect Coombs test, the SAT and Brucellacapt, or ELISAs for IgG and IgM. In doing so, one would be able to detect antibodies in different stages of the disease, since in the acute stage any test can be positive, while in chronic, complicated, or focal disease cases, the SAT can be negative while the Coombs test, Brucellacapt, and ELISA using IgG can be positive (Table 5). Again, one should keep in mind that any serologic test findings need to be interpreted in the context of the patient's clinical history.

REFERENCES

1. **Ahmed, K., K. A. Al-Matrouk, G. Martinez, K. Oishi, V. O. Rotimi, and T. Nagatake.** 1999. Increased serum levels of interferon-gamma and interleukin-12 during human brucellosis. *Am. J. Trop. Med. Hyg.* **61:**425–427.
2. **Akova, M., D. Gür, D. M. Livermore, T. Kocagöz, and H. E. Akalin.** 1999. In vitro activities of antibiotics alone and in combination against *Brucella melitensis* at neutral and acidic pHs. *Antimicrob. Agents Chemother.* **43:**1298–1300.
3. **Al-Dahouk, S., P. Le Flèche, K. Nöckler, I. Jacques, M. Grayon, H. C. Scholz, H. Tomaso, G. Vergnaud, and H. Neubauer.** 2007. Evaluation of *Brucella* MLVA typing for human brucellosis. *J. Microbiol. Methods* **69:**137–145.
4. **Alton, G. G., L. M. Jones, R. D. Angus, and J. M. Verger.** 1988. *Techniques for the Brucellosis Laboratory.* Institut National de la Recherche Agronomique, Paris, France.
5. **Anda, P., J. S. del Pozo, J. M. D. Garcia, R. Escudero, F. J. G. Peña, M. C. L. Velasco, R. E. Sellek, M. R. J. Chillarón, L. P. S. Serrano, and J. F. M. Navarro.** 2001. Waterborne outbreak of tularemia associated with crayfish fishing. *Emerg. Infect. Dis.* **7:**575–582.
6. **Araj, G. F.** 1988. Profiles of brucella specific immunoglobulin G subclass in serum of patients with acute and chronic brucellosis. *Serodiag. Immunother. Infect. Dis.* **2:**401–410.
7. **Araj, G. F.** 1999. Human brucellosis: a classical infectious disease with persistent diagnostic challenges. *Clin. Lab. Sci.* **12:**207–212.
8. **Araj, G. F.** 2000. Human brucellosis revisited: a persistent saga in the Middle East. *BMJ (Middle East)* **7:**6–15.
9. **Araj, G. F., A. R. Lulu, M. A. Saadah, A. M. Mousa, I. L. Strannegard, and R. A. Shakir.** 1986. Rapid diagnosis of central nervous system brucellosis by ELISA. *J. Neuroimmunol.* **12:**73–82.
9a. **Araj, G. F., and M. M. Kattar.** 2003. Rapid diagnosis of human brucellosis using the Bact/Alert continuous culture monitoring system. *Abstr. 103rd Annu. Meet. Am. Soc. Microbiol.,* abstract C-002.
10. **Araj, G. F., A. R. Lulu, M. Y. Mustafa, and M. I. Khateeb.** 1986. Evaluation of ELISA in the diagnosis of acute and chronic brucellosis in human beings. *J. Hyg. Lond.* **97:**457–469.
11. **Araj, G. F., G. M. Brown, M. M. Haj, and N. V. Madhavan.** 1988. Assessment of Brucellosis Card Test in screening patients for brucellosis. *Epidemiol. Infect.* (London) **100:**389–398.
12. **Araj, G. F., A. R. Lulu, M. I. Khateeb, M. A. Saadah, and R. A. Shakir.** 1988. ELISA versus routine tests in the diagnosis of patients with systemic and neurobrucellosis. *Acta Pathlol. Microbiol. Scand.* **96:**171–176.
13. **Araj, G. F., and A. F. Kaufman.** 1989. Determination by enzyme-linked immunosorbent assay of immunoglobulin G (IgG), IgM, and IgA to *Brucella melitensis* major outer membrane proteins and whole-cell heat-killed antigens in sera of patients with brucellosis. *J. Clin. Microbiol.* **27:**1909–1912.
14. **Araj, G. F., R. Dhar, J. L. Lastimoza, and M. Haj.** 1990. Indirect fluorescent-antibody test versus enzyme-linked immunosorbent assay and agglutination tests in the serodiagnosis of patients with brucellosis. *Serodiag. Immunother. Infect. Dis.* **4:**1–8.

15. **Araj, G. F., A. R. Lulu, M. I. Khateeb, and M. M. Haj.** 1990. Specific IgE response in patients with brucellosis. *Epidemiol. Infect.* (London) **105:**571–577.

16. **Araj, G. F., and R. A. Azzam.** 1996. Seroprevalence of brucella antibodies among persons in high-risk occupation in Lebanon. *Epidemiol. Infect.* **117:**281–288.

17. **Araj, G. F., M. Kattar, L. G. Fattouh, O. K. Bajakian, and S. A. Kobeissi.** 2005. Evaluation of the PANBIO *Brucella* immunoglobulin G (IgG) and IgM enzyme-linked immunosorbent assays for diagnosis of human brucellosis. *Clin. Diagn. Lab. Immunol.* **12:**1334–1335.

18. **Ariza, J., T. Pellicer, R. Pallares, Z. Fox, and F. Gudiol.** 1992. Specific antibody profile in human brucellosis. *Clin. Infect. Dis.* **14:**131–140.

19. **Ariza, J., J. Corredoira, R. Pallares, P. F. Viladrich, G. Rufi, M. Pujol, and F. Gudiol.** 1995. Characteristics of and risk factors for relapse of brucellosis in humans. *Clin. Infect. Dis.* **20:**1241–1249.

20. **Ariza, J., M. Bosilkovski, A. Cascio, J. D. Colmenero, M. J. Corbel, M. E. Falagas, Z. A., Memish, M. R. Roushan, E. Rubinstein, N. V. Sipsas, J. Solera, E. J. Young, and G. Pappas.** 2007. Perspectives for the treatment of brucellosis in the 21st century: the Ioannina recommendations. *PLoS Med.* **4:**e317.

21. **Baldi, P.C., S. E. Miguel, C. A. Fossati, and J. C. Wallach.** 1996. Serologic follow-up of human brucellosis by measuring IgG antibodies to LPS and cytoplasmic proteins of *Brucella* species. *Clin. Infect. Dis.* **22:**446–455.

22. **Barns, S. M., C. C. Grow, R. T. Okinaka, P. Keim, and C. R. Kuske.** 2005. Detection of diverse new *Francisella*-like bacteria in environmental samples. *Appl. Environ. Microbiol.* **71:**5494–5500.

23. **Behan, K. A., and G. C. Klein.** 1982. Reduction of *Brucella* species and *Francisella tularensis* cross-reacting agglutinins by dithiothreitol. *J. Clin. Microbiol.* **16:**756–757.

24. **Bell, J. F.** 1980. Tularemia, p. 161–193. In J. H. Steele (ed.), *CRC Handbook Series in Zoonoses.* CRC Press, Boca Raton, FL.

25. **Bevanger, L., J. A. Maeland, and A. I. Kvam.** 1994. Comparative analysis of antibodies to *Francisella tularensis* antigens during the acute phase of tularemia and eight years later. *Clin. Diagn. Lab. Immunol.* **1:**238–240.

26. **Birdsell, D. N., T. Stewart, A. J. Vogler, E. Lawaczeck, A. Diggs, T. L. Sylvester, J. L. Buchhagen, R. K. Auerbach, P. Keim, and D. M. Wagner.** 2009. *Francisella tularensis* subsp. *novicida* isolated from a human in Arizona. *BMC Res. Notes* **2:**223.

27. **Birkbeck, T. H., M. Bordevik, M. K. Frøystad, and A. Baklien.** 2007. Identification of *Francisella* sp. from Atlantic salmon, *Salmo salar* L., in Chile. *J. Fish Dis.* **30:**505–507.

28. **Brew, S. D., L. L. Perrett, J. A. Stack, and A. P. MacMillan.** 1999. Human exposure to *Brucella* recovered from a sea mammal. *Vet. Res.* **24:**483.

29. **Brown, S. L., F. T. McKinney, G. C. Klein, and W. L. Jones.** 1980. Evaluation of a safranin-O-stained antigen microagglutination test for *Francisella tularensis* antibodies. *J. Clin. Microbiol.* **11:**146–148.

30. **Celebi, G., F. Baruönü, F. Ayoğlu, F. Cinar, A. Karadenizli, M. B. Uğur, and S. Gedikoğlu.** 2006. Tularemia, a reemerging disease in northwest Turkey: epidemiological investigation and evaluation of treatment responses. *Jpn. J. Infect. Dis.* **59:**229–234.

31. **Centers for Disease Control and Prevention.** 2002. Tularemia—United States, 1990–2000. *MMWR Morb. Mortal. Wkly. Rep.* **51:**182–184.

32. **Centers for Disease Control and Prevention.** 2008. Update: potential exposures to attenuated vaccine strain *Brucella abortus* RB51 during a laboratory proficiency test—United States and Canada. *MMWR Morb. Mortal. Wkly. Rep.* **57:**36–39.

33. **Centers for Disease Control and Prevention.** 2008. Laboratory-acquired brucellosis—Indiana and Minnesota, 2006. *MMWR Morb. Mortal. Wkly. Rep.* **57:**39–42.

34. **Centers for Disease Control and Prevention.** 2008. Public health consequences of a false-positive laboratory test result for *Brucella*—Florida, Georgia, and Michigan. *MMWR Morb. Mortal. Wkly. Rep.* **57:**603–605.

35. **Clarridge, J. E., III, T. J. Raich, A. Sjöstedt, G. Sandström, R. O. Darouiche, R. M. Shawar, P. R. Georghiou, C. Osting,** and L. Vo. 1996. Characterization of two unusual clinically significant *Francisella* strains. *J. Clin. Microbiol.* **34:**1995–2000.

36. **Clinical and Laboratory Standards Institute.** 2006. Methods for dilution antimicrobial susceptibility tests for bacteria that grow aerobically. Approved standard—seventh edition. CLSI document M7-A7. Clinical and Laboratory Standards Institute, Wayne, PA.

37. **Clinical and Laboratory Standards Institute.** 2009. Performance standards for antimicrobial susceptibility testing; ninteeth informational supplement. M100-S19. Clinical and Laboratory Standards Institute, Wayne, PA.

38. **Cloeckaert, A., J. Verger, M. Grayon, B. Paquet, B. Garin-Bastuji, G. Foster, and J. Godfroid.** 2001. Classification of *Brucella* spp. isolated from marine mammals by DNA polymorphism at the *omp2* locus. *Microbes Infect.* **3:**729–738.

39. **Colmenero, J. D., J. M. Reguera, F. Martos, D. Sanchez-De-Mora, M. Delgado, M. Causse, A. Martin-Farafan, and C. Juarez.** 1996. Complications associated with *Brucella melitensis* infection: a study of 530 cases. *Medicine* (Baltimore) **75:**195–211.

40. **Colmenero, J. D., N. L. Muñoz-Roca, P. Bermudez, A. Plata, A. Villalobos, and J. M. Reguera.** 2007. Clinical findings, diagnostic approach, and outcome of *Brucella melitensis* epididymo-orchitis. *Diagn. Microbiol. Infect. Dis.* **57:**367–372.

41. **Corbel, M. J.** 1997. Brucellosis: an overview. *Emerg. Infect. Dis.* **3:**213–221.

42. **Corbel, M. J., and N. J. Beeching.** 2005. Brucellosis, p. 914–917. In D. L. Kasper, E. Braunwald, A. S. Fauci, S. L. Hauser, D. L. Longo, and J. L. Jameson (ed.), *Harrison's Principles of Internal Medicine,* 16th ed., vol. 1. McGraw-Hill, New York, NY.

43. **DeBeaumont, C., P. A. Falconnet, and M. Maurin.** 2005. Real-time PCR for detection of *Brucella* spp. DNA in serum samples. *Eur. J. Clin. Microbiol. Infect. Dis.* **24:**842–845.

44. **Department of Health and Human Services, Centers for Disease Control and Prevention and National Institutes of Health.** 2007. *Biosafety in Microbiological and Biomedical Laboratories,* 5th ed. Department of Health and Human Services, Centers for Disease Control and Prevention and National Institutes of Health, Washington, DC. http://www.cdc.gov/od/ohs/biosfty/bmbl5/bmbl5toc.htm.

45. **Drancourt, M., P. Brouqui, and D. Raoult.** 1997. *Afipia clevelandensis* antibodies and cross-reactivity with *Brucella* spp. and *Yersinia enterocolitica* O:9. *Clin. Diagn. Lab. Immunol.* **4:**748–752.

46. **Eliasson, H., J. Lindbäck, J. P. Nuorti, M. Arneborn, J. Giesecke, and A. Tegnell.** 2002. The 2000 tularemia outbreak: a case-control study of risk factors in disease-endemic and emergent areas, Sweden. *Emerg. Infect. Dis.* **8:**956–960.

47. **Eliasson, H., P. Olcén, A. Sjöstedt, M. Jurstrand, E. Bäck, and S. Andersson.** 2008. Kinetics of the immune response associated with tularemia: comparison of an enzyme-linked immunosorbent assay, a tube agglutination test, and a novel whole-blood lymphocyte stimulation test. *Clin. Vaccine Immunol.* **15:**1238–1243.

48. **Ellis, J., P. C. Oyston, M. Green, and R. W. Titball.** 2002. Tularemia. *Clin. Microbiol. Rev.* **15:**631–646.

49. **Ericsson, M., G. Sandström, A. Sjöstedt, and A. Tärnvik.** 1994. Persistence of cell-mediated immunity and decline of humoral immunity to the intracellular bacterium *Francisella tularensis. J. Infect. Dis.* **170:**110–114.

50. **Escudero, R., M. Elía, J. A. Sáez-Nieto, V. Menéndez, A. Toledo, G. Royo, M. Rodríguez-Vargas, M. J. Whipp, H. Gil, I. Jado, and P. Anda.** 25 August 2009. A possible novel *Francisella* genomic species isolated from blood and urine of a patient with severe illness. *Clin. Microbiol. Infect.* [Epub ahead of print.] doi:10.1111/j.1469-0691.2009.03029.x.

51. **Estevao, M. H., L. M. Baverosa, L. M. Matos, A. A. Barrosa, and H. C. da Mota.** 1995. Neurobrucellosis in children. *Eur. J. Pediatr.* **154:**120–122.

52. **Evans, M. E., D. W. Gregory, W. Schaffner, and Z. A. McGee.** 1985. Tularemia: a 30-year experience with 88 cases. *Medicine* (Baltimore) **64:**251–269.

53. **Feldman, K. A.,** 2003. Tularemia. *J. Am. Vet. Med. Assoc.* **222:**725–730.

54. Feldman, K. A., R. Enscore, S. Lathrop, B. Matyas, M. McGuill, M. Schriefer, D. Stiles-Enos, D. Dennis, and E. Hayes. 2001. Outbreak of primary pneumonic tularemia on Martha's Vineyard. *N. Engl. J. Med.* **345:**1601–1606.

55. Fernandez-Prada, C. M., E. B. Zelazowska, M. Nikolich, T. L. Hadfield, R. M. Roop, G. L. Robertson, and D. L. Hoover. 2003. Interaction between *Brucella melitensis* and human phagocytes: bacterial surface O-polysaccharide inhibits phagocytosis, bacterial killing, and subsequent host cell apoptosis. *Infect. Immun.* **71:**2110–2119.

56. Forsman, M., G. Sandström, and B. Jaurin. 1990. Identification of *Francisella* species and discrimination of type A and type B strains of *F. tularensis* by 16S rRNA analysis. *Appl. Environ. Microbiol.* **56:**949–955.

57. Forsman, M., G. Sandström, and A. Sjöstedt. 1994. Analysis of 16S ribosomal DNA sequences of *Francisella* strains and utilization for determination of the phylogeny of the genus and for identification of strains by PCR. *Int. J. Syst. Bacteriol.* **44:**38–46.

58. Foster, G., B. S. Osterman, J. Godfroid, I. Jacques, and A. Cloeckaert. 2007. *Brucella ceti* sp. nov., and *Brucella pinnipedialis* sp. nov for *Brucella* strains with cetaceans and seals as their preferred hosts. *Int. J. Syst. Evol. Microbiol.* **57:**2688–2693.

59. Franco, M. P., M. Mulder, R. H. Gilman, and H. L. Smits. 2007. Human brucellosis. *Lancet Infect. Dis.* **7:**775–786.

60. Friis-Møller, A., L. E. Lemming, N. H. Valerius, and B. Bruun. 2004. Problems in identification of *Francisella philomiragia* associated with fatal bacteremia in a patient with chronic granulomatous disease. *J. Clin. Microbiol.* **42:**1840–1842.

61. Garrity, G. M., and J. G. Holt. 2001. Taxonomic outline of the *Archaea* and *Bacteria*, p. 155–166. *In* D. R. Boone and R. C. Castenholz (ed.), *Bergey's Manual of Systematic Bacteriology*, 2nd ed., vol. 1. Springer-Verlag, New York, NY.

62. Gazapo E., J. Gonzalez Lahoz, J. L. Subiza, M. Banquero, J. Jil, and E. G. de la Concha. 1989. Changes in IgM and IgG antibody concentration in brucellosis over time: importance for diagnosis and follow-up. *J. Infect. Dis.* **159:**219–225.

63. Gilligan, P. H., and M. K. York. 2002. *Basic Protocols for Level A Laboratories for the Presumptive Identification of Brucella Species.* American Society for Microbiology, Washington, DC.

64. Godfroid, J., A. Cloeckaert, J. Liautard, S. Kohler, D. Fretin, K. Walravens, B. Garin-Bastuji, and J. Letesson. 2005. From the discovery of the Malta fever's agent to the discovery of a marine mammal reservoir, brucellosis has continuously been a re-emerging zoonosis. *Vet. Res.* **36:**313–326.

65. Goethert, H. K., I. Shani, and S. R. Telford. 2004. Genotypic diversity of *Francisella tularensis* infecting *Dermacentor variabilis* ticks on Martha's Vineyard, Massachusetts. *J. Clin. Microbiol.* **42:**4968–4973.

66. Goldbaum, F. A., J. Leoni, J. C. Wallach, and C. A. Fossati. 1993. Characterization of an 18-kilodalton *Brucella* cytoplasmic protein which appears to be a serological marker of active infection of both human and bovine brucellosis. *J. Clin. Microbiol.* **31:**2141–2145.

67. Golding, B., D. E. Scott, O. Scharf, L. Y. Huang, M. Zaitseva, C. Lapham, N. Eller, and H. Golding. 2001. Immunity and protection against *Brucella abortus*. *Microbes Infect.* **3:**43–48.

68. Gómez, M. C., J. A. Nieto, C. Rosa, P. Geijo, M. A. Escribano, A. Muñoz, and C. López. 2008. Evaluation of seven tests for diagnosis of human brucellosis in an area where the disease is endemic. *Clin. Vaccine Immunol.* **15:**1031–1033.

69. Gorvel, J. P. 2008. *Brucella*: a Mr "Hide" converted into Dr Jekyll. *Microbes Infect.* **10:**1010–1013.

70. Greenfield, R. A., D. A. Drevets, L. J. Machado, G. W. Voskuhl, P. Cornea, and M. S. Bronze. 2002. Bacterial pathogens as biological weapons and agents of bioterrorism. *Am. J. Med. Sci.* **323:**299–315.

71. Guarner, J., P. R. Breer, J. C. Bartlett, M. C. Chu, W. J. Shieh, and S. R. Zaki. 1999. Immunohistochemical detection of *Francisella tularensis* in formalin-fixed paraffin-embedded tissue. *Appl. Immunohistochem. Mol. Morphol.* **7:**122–126.

72. Gür, D., S. Kocagöz, M. Akova, and S. Unal. 1999. Comparison of E test to microdilution for determining in vitro activities of antibiotics against *Brucella melitensis*. *Antimicrob. Agents Chemother.* **43:**2337.

73. Halling, S. M., B. D. Peterson-Burch, B. J. Bricker, R. L. Zuerner, Z. Qing, L. Li, V. Kapur, D. P. Alt, and S. C. Olsen. 2005. Completion of the genome sequence of *Brucella abortus* and comparison to the highly similar genomes of *Brucella melitensis* and *Brucella suis*. *J. Bacteriol.* **187:**2715–2726.

74. Hollis, D. G., R. E. Weaver, A. G. Steigerwalt, J. D. Wenger, C. W. Moss, and D. J. Brenner. 1989. *Francisella philomiragia* comb. nov. (formerly *Yersinia philomiragia*) and *Francisella tularensis* biogroup novicida (formerly *Francisella novicida*) associated with human disease. *J. Clin. Microbiol.* **27:**1601–1608.

75. Hopla, C. E., and A. K. Hopla. 1994. Tularemia, p. 113–126. *In* G. W. Beran and J. H. Steele (ed.), *Handbook of Zoonoses*, 2nd ed. CRC Press, Boca Raton, FL.

76. Ibrahim, A. I. A., R. Awad, S. D. Shetty, M. Saad, and N. E. Bilal. 1988. Genito-urinary complications of brucellosis. *Br. J. Urol.* **61:**294–298.

77. Ikäheimo, I., H. Syrjälä, J. Karhukorpi, R. Schildt, and M. Koskela. 2000. *In vitro* antibiotic susceptibility of *Francisella tularensis* isolated from humans and animals. *J. Antimicrob. Chemother.* **46:**287–290.

78. Jantzen, E., B. P. Berdal, and T. Omland. 1979. Cellular fatty acid composition of *Francisella tularensis*. *J. Clin. Microbiol.* **10:**928–930.

79. Jellison, W. L. 1974. *Tularemia in North America, 1930–1974*, p. 1–276. University of Montana, Missoula, MT.

80. Jellison, W. L., C. R. Owen, J. F. Bell, and G. M. Kohls. 1961. Tularemia and animal populations: ecology and epizootiology. *Wildl. Dis.* **17:**1–15.

81. Jensen, W. I., C. R. Owen, and W. L. Jellison. 1969. *Yersinia philomiragia* sp. n., a new member of the *Pasteurella* group of bacteria, naturally pathogenic for the muskrat (*Ondatra zibethica*). *J. Bacteriol.* **100:**1237–1241.

82. Johansson, A., L. Berglund, U. Eriksson, I. Göransson, R. Wollin, M. Forsman, A. Tärnvik, and A. Sjöstedt. 2000. Comparative analysis of PCR versus culture for diagnosis of ulceroglandular tularemia. *J. Clin. Microbiol.* **38:**22–26.

83. Johansson, A., J. Farlow, P. Larsson, M. Dukerich, E. Chambers, M. Byström, J. Fox, M. Chu, M. Forsman, A. Sjöstedt, and P. Keim. 2004. Worldwide genetic relationships among *Francisella tularensis* isolates determined by multiple-locus variable-number tandem repeat analysis. *J. Bacteriol.* **186:**5808–5818.

84. Joint FAO/WHO Expert Committee on Brucellosis. 1986. Sixth report. World Health Organization Technical Report Series no. 740. World Health Organization, Geneva, Switzerland.

85. Kattar, M. M., P. A. Zallou, G. F. Araj, J. Samaha-Kfoury, H. Shbaklo, S. K. Kanj, S. Khalife, and M. Deeb. 2007. Development and evaluation of real-time polymerase chain reaction assays on whole blood and paraffin-embedded tissues for rapid diagnosis of human brucellosis. *Diagn. Microbiol. Infect. Dis.* **59:**23–32.

86. Kattar, M. M., R. F. Jaafar, G. F. Araj, P. Le Flèche, G. M. Matar, R. Abi Rached, S. Khalife, and G. Vergnaud. 2008. Evaluation of a multilocus variable-number tandem-repeat analysis scheme for typing human *Brucella* isolates in a region of brucellosis endemicity. *J. Clin. Microbiol.* **46:**3935–3940.

87. Kerr, W. R., W. J. McCaughey, J. D. Coghlan, D. J. H. Payn, R. A. Quaife, L. Robertson, and I. D. Farell. 1968. Techniques and interpretation in the serological diagnosis of brucellosis in man. *J. Med. Microbiol.* **1:**181–193.

88. Khatun, M., A. Islam, B. K. Baek, and S. I. Lee. 2009. Characteristics of the immune response during acute brucellosis in Sprague-Dawley rats. *J. Infect. Dev. Ctries.* **3:**392–397.

89. Kugeler, K. J., N. Gurfield, J. G. Creek, K. S. Mahoney, J. L. Versage, and J. M. Petersen. 2005. Discrimination between *Francisella tularensis* and *Francisella*-like endosymbionts when screening ticks by PCR. *Appl. Environ. Microbiol.* **71:**7594–7597.

90. Kugeler, K. J., P. S. Mead, K. L. McGowan, J. M. Burnham, M. D. Hogarty, E. Ruchelli, K. Pollard, B. Husband, C. Conley, T. Rivera, T. Kelesidis, W. M. Lee, W. Mabey, J. M. Winchell, H. L. Stang, J. E. Staples, L. J. Chalcraft, and J. M. Petersen. 2008. Isolation and characterization of a novel *Francisella* sp. from human cerebrospinal fluid and blood. *J. Clin. Microbiol.* **46:**2428–2431.

91. **Kugeler, K. J., P. S. Mead, A. M. Janusz, J. E. Staples, K. A. Kubota, L. G. Chalcraft, and J. M. Petersen.** 2009. Molecular epidemiology of *Francisella tularensis* in the United States. *Clin. Infect. Dis.* **48:**863–870.

92. **Larson, C. L., W. Wicht, and W. L. Jellison.** 1955. A new organism resembling *P. tularensis* isolated from water. *Public Health Rep.* **70:**253–258.

93. **Larsson, P., D. K. Elfsmark, K. Svensson, P. Wikström, M. Forsman, T. Brettin, P. Keim, and A. Johansson.** 2009. Molecular evolutionary consequences of niche restriction in *Francisella tularensis*, a facultative intracellular pathogen. *PLoS Pathog.* **5:**e1000472.

94. **Leelaporn, A., S. Yongyod, S. Limsrivanichakorn, T. Yungyuen, and P. Kiratisin.** 2008. *Francisella novicida* bacteremia, Thailand. *Emerg. Infect. Dis.* **14:**1935–1937.

95. **Lindquist, D., M. C. Chu, and W. S. Probert.** 2007. *Francisella* and *Brucella*, p. 815–834. *In* P. R. Murray, E. J. Baron, J. H. Jorgensen, M. L. Landry, and M. A. Pfaller (ed.), *Manual of Clinical Microbiology*, 9th ed. ASM Press, Washington, DC.

96. **Lista, F., G. Faggioni, S. Valjevac, A. Ciammaruconi, J. Vaissaire, C. Le Doujet, O. Gorgé, R. De Santis, A. Carattoli, A. Ciervo, A. Fasanella, F. Orsini, R. D'Amelio, C. Pourcel, A. Cassone, and G. Vergnaud.** 2006. Genotyping of *Bacillus anthracis* strains based on automated capillary 25-loci multiple locus variable-number tandem repeats analysis. *BMC Microbiol.* **6:**33.

97. **Lubani, M. M., K. Dudin, G. F. Araj, D. S. Manaudhar, and F. Y. Rachid.** 1989. Neurobrucellosis in children. *Pediatr. Infect. Dis. J.* **8:**79–82.

98. **Lubani, M. M., K. I. Dudin, D. C. Sharda, D. S. Manadhar, G. F. Araj, A. H. Hafez, Q. A. Al Saleh, I. Helin, and M. M. Salhi.** 1989. A multicenter therapeutic study of 1100 children with brucellosis. *Pediatr. Infect. Dis. J.* **8:**75–78.

99. **Lubani, M. M., K. I. Dudin, D. C. Sharda, N. M. Abu Sinna, T. Al-Shab, A. A. Al-Refe'ai, S. M. Labani, and A. Nasrallah.** 1998. Neonatal brucellosis. *Eur. J. Pediatr.* **147:**520–522.

100. **Lulu, A. R., G. F. Araj, M. I. Khateeb, M. Y. Mustafa, A. R. Yusuf, and F. F. Fenech.** 1988. Human brucellosis in Kuwait: a prospective study of 400 cases. *Q. J. Med.* **66:**39–54.

101. **Lulu, A. R., and G. F. Araj.** 1991. Pulmonary complications of brucellosis, p. 157–176. *In* O. P. Sharma (ed.), *Lung Disease in the Tropics*. Marcel Dekker Inc., New York, NY.

102. **Madkour, M. M.** 1989. Overview, p. 71–89. *In* M. M. Madkour (ed.), *Brucellosis*. Butterworths, University Press, Cambridge, United Kingdom.

103. **Makhseed, M., A. Harouny, G. F. Araj, M. A. Mousa, and P. Sharma.** 1998. Obstetric and gynecologic implication of brucellosis in Kuwait. *J. Perinatol.* **8:**196–199.

104. **Makis, A. C., E. Galanakis, E. C. Hazmichael, Z. L. Papadopoulou, A. Simopoulou, and K. L. Bourantas.** 2005. Serum levels of soluble interleukin-2 receptor alpha (sIL-2Ralpha) as a predictor of outcome in brucellosis. *J. Infect.* **51:**206–210.

105. **Mantecon, M. A., P. Gutierrez, M. del Pilar Zarzosa, A. I. Duenas, J. Solera, L. Fernández-Lago, N. Vizcaíno, A. Almaraz, M. A. Bratos, A. Rodríguez Torres, and A. Orduña-Domingo.** 2006. Utility of an immunocapture-agglutination test and an enzyme-linked immunosorbent assay test against cytosolic proteins from *Brucella melitensis* B115 in the diagnosis and follow-up of human acute brucellosis. *Diagn. Microbiol. Infect. Dis.* **55:**27–35.

106. **Mantur, B. G., S. K. Amarnath, and R. S. Shinde.** 2007. Review of clinical and laboratory features of human brucellosis. *Ind. J. Med. Microbiol.* **25:**188–202.

107. **Marianelli, C., C. Graziani, C. Santangelo, M. T. Xibilia, A. Imbriani, R. Amato, D. Neri, M. Cuccia, S. Rinnone, V. Di Marco, and F. Ciuchini.** 2007. Molecular epidemiological and antibiotic susceptibility characterization of *Brucella* isolates from humans in Sicily, Italy. *J. Clin. Microbiol.* **45:**2923–2928.

108. **Martín, C. M., T. Gallardo, L. Mateos, E. Vián, M. J. García, J. Ramos, A. C. Berjón, M. del Carmen Viña, M. P. García, J. Yáñez, L. C. González, T. Muñoz, M. Allue, C. Andrés, C. Ruiz, and J. Castrodeza.** 2007. Outbreak of tularaemia in Castilla y León, Spain. *Euro Surveill.* **12:**E071108.1

109. **Matyas, B. T., H. S. Nieder, and S. R. Telford III.** 2007. Pneumonic tularemia on Martha's Vineyard: clinical, epidemiologic, and ecological characteristics. *Ann. N. Y. Acad. Sci.* **1105:**351–377.

110. **Mayefield, J. E., B. J. Bricker, H. Godfrey, R. M. Crosby, D. J. Knight, S. M. Halling, D. Balinsky, and L. B. Tabatabai.** 1988. The cloning, expression and nucleotide sequence of a gene (BCS P31) coding for an immunogenic *B. abortus* protein (31 KDa). *Gene* **63:**1–9.

111. **McDonald, W. L., R. Jamaludin, G. Mackereth, M. Hansen, S. Humphrey, and P. Short.** 2006. Characterization of a *Brucella* sp. strain as a marine-mammal type despite isolation from a patient with spinal osteomyelitis in New Zealand. *J. Clin. Microbiol.* **44:**4363–4370.

112. **Memish, Z. A., and H. H. Balkhy.** 2004. Brucellosis and international travel. *J. Travel Med.* **11:**49–55.

113. **Mercier, E., E. Jumas-Bilak, A. Allardet-Servent, D. O'Callaghan, K. F. Meyer, and E. B. Shaw.** 1996. A comparison of the morphologic, culture and biochemical characteristics of *B. abortus* and *B. melitensis*: studies on the genus *Brucella* nov. gen. I. *J. Infect. Dis.* **27:**173–184.

114. **Mikalsen, J., A. B. Olsen, T. Tengs, and D. J. Colquhoun.** 2007. *Francisella philomiragia* subsp. *noatunensis* subsp. nov., isolated from farmed Atlantic cod (*Gadus morhua* L.). *Int. J. Syst. Evol. Microbiol.* **57:**1960–1965.

115. **Mitka, S., C. Anetakis, E. Souliou, E. Diza, and A. Kansouzidou.** 2007. Evaluation of different PCR assays for the early detection of acute and relapsing human brucellosis in comparison with conventional methods. *J. Clin. Microbiol.* **45:**1211–1218.

116. **Molins, C. R., J. K. Carlson, J. Coombs, and J. M. Petersen.** 2009. Identification of *Francisella tularensis* subsp. *tularensis* A1 and A2 infections by real-time polymerase chain reaction. *Diagn. Microbiol. Infect. Dis.* **64:**6–12.

117. **Molins, C. R., and J. M. Petersen.** 2010. Subpopulations of *F. tularensis* subspecies *tularensis* and *holarctica*: identification and associated epidemiology. *Future Microbiol.* **5:**649–661.

118. **Molins, C. R., M. Delorey, B. M. Yockey, J. W. Young, S. W. Sheldon, S. M. Reese, M. E. Schriefer, and J. M. Petersen.** 2010. Virulence comparison among *Francisella tularensis* subsp. *tularensis* clades in mice. *PLoS One* **5**(4):e10205.

119. **Morata, P., M. I. Quiepo-Ortuno, J. M. Reguera, F. Miralles, J. J. Lopez-Gonzalez, and J. D. Colmenero.** 2001. Diagnostic yield of a PCR assay in focal complications of brucellosis. *J. Clin. Microbiol.* **39:**3743–3746.

120. **Moriyon, I., and I. Lopez-Goni.** 1998. Structure and properties of the outer membranes of *Brucella abortus* and *Brucella melitensis*. *Int. Microbiol.* **1:**19–26.

121. **Naparstek, E., C. S. Block, and S. Slavin.** 1982. Transmission of brucellosis by bone marrow transplantation. *Lancet* **i:**574–575.

122. **Navarro, E., J. C. Segura, M. J. Castaño, and J. Solera.** 2006. Use of real-time quantitative polymerase chain reaction to monitor the evolution of *Brucella melitensis* DNA load during therapy and post-therapy follow-up in patients with brucellosis. *Clin. Infect. Dis.* **42:**1266–1273.

123. **Navarro-Martinez, A., E. Navarro, M. J. Castano, and J. Solera.** 2008. Rapid diagnosis of human brucellosis by quantitative real-time PCR: a case report of brucellar spondylitis. *J. Clin. Microbiol.* **46:**385–387.

124. **Noviello, S., R. Gallo, M. Kelly, R. J. Limberger, K. De Angelis, L. Cain, B. Wallace, and N. Dumas.** 2004. Laboratory-acquired brucellosis. *Emerg. Infect. Dis.* **10:**1848–1850.

125. **Ohara, S., T. Sato, and M. Homma.** 1974. Serological studies on *Francisella tularensis*, *Francisella novicida*, *Yersinia philomiragia*, and *Brucella abortus*. *Int. J. Syst. Bacteriol.* **24:**191–196.

126. **Oliveira, S., and G. A. Splitter.** 1996. Immunization of mice with recombinant L7/L12 ribosomal protein confers protection against *Brucella abortus* infection. *Vaccine* **14:**959–962.

127. **Olsufiev, N. G., O. S. Emelyanova, and T. N. Dunaeva.** 1959. Comparative study of strains of *B. tularense* in the old and new world and their taxonomy. *J. Hyg. Epidemiol. Microbiol. Immunol.* **3:**138–149.

128. **Olsufjev, N. G., and I. S. Meshcheryakova.** 1982. Infraspecific taxonomy of tularemia agent *Francisella tularensis* McCoy et Chapin. *J. Hyg. Epidemiol. Microbiol. Immunol.* **3:**291–299.

129. Orduña, A., A. Almarza, A. Prado, M. P. Gutierrez, A. Garcia-Pascual, A. Duenas, M. Cuervo, R. Abad, B. Hernandez, B. Lorenzo, M. A. Bratos, and A. R. Torres. 2000. Evaluation of an immunocapture-agglutination test (Brucellacapt) for serodiagnosis of human brucellosis. *J. Clin. Microbiol.* **38:**4000–4005.

130. Orhan, G., A. Bayram, Y. Zer, and I. Balci. 2005. Synergy tests by E test and checkerboard methods of antimicrobial combinations against *Brucella melitensis. J. Clin. Microbiol.* **43:**140–143.

131. Ottem, K. F., A. Nylund, E. Karlsbakk, A. Friis-Møller, and T. Kamaishi. 2009. Elevation of *Francisella philomiragia* subsp. *noatunensis* Mikalsen et al. (2007) to *Francisella noatunensis* comb. nov. [syn. *Francisella piscicida* Ottem et al. (2008) syn. nov.] and characterization of *Francisella noatunensis* subsp. *orientalis* subsp. nov., two important fish pathogens. *J. Appl. Microbiol.* **106:**1231–1243.

132. Overholt, E. I., W. D. Tigertt, P. J. Kadull, M. K. Ward, N. D. Charkes, R. M. Rene, T. E. Salzman, and M. Stephens. 1961. An analysis of forty-two cases of laboratory-acquired tularemia. *Am. J. Med.* **30:**785–806.

133. Owen, C. R., E. O. Buker, W. L. Jellison, D. B. Lackman, and J. F. Bell. 1964. Comparative studies of *Francisella tularensis* and *Francisella novicida. J. Bacteriol.* **87:**676–683.

134. Palanduz, A., S. Palanduz, K. Guler, and N. Guler. 2000. Brucellosis in a mother and her young infant: probable transmission by breast milk. *Int. J. Infect. Dis.* **4:**55–56.

135. Pappas, G., N. Akritidis, M. Bosilkovski, and E. Tsianos. 2005. Brucellosis. *New Engl. J. Med.* **35:**2325–2336.

136. Pappas, G., P. Pangopoulou, L. Christou, and N. Akritidis. 2006. Category B potential bioterrorism agents: bacteria, viruses, toxins, and foodborne and waterborne pathogens. *Infect. Dis. Clin. N. Am.* **20:**395–421.

137. Pappas, G., P. Papadimitriou, N. Akritidis, L. Christou, and E. Tsianos. 2006. The new global map of human brucellosis. *Lancet Infect. Dis.* **6:**91–99.

138. Paton, N. I., N. W. Teu, C. F. Vu, and T. P. Teo. 2001. Brucellosis due to blood transfusion. *Clin. Infect. Dis.* **32:**1248.

139. Payne, L., M. Arneborn, A. Tegnell, and J. Giesecke. 2005. Endemic tularemia, Sweden, 2003. *Emerg. Infect. Dis.* **11:**1440–1442.

140. Pellicer, T., J. Ariza, Z. Fox, R. Pallares, and F. Gudiol. 1988. Specific antibodies during relapse of human brucellosis. *J. Infect. Dis.* **157:**918–924.

141. Petersen, J. M., M. E. Schriefer, K. L. Gage, J. A. Montenieri, L. G. Carter, M. Stanley, and M. C. Chu. 2004. Methods for enhanced culture recovery of *Francisella tularensis. Appl. Environ. Microbiol.* **70:**3733–3735.

142. Petersen, J. M., J. K. Carlson, G. Dietrich, R. J. Eisen, J. Coombs, A. M. Janusz, J. Summers, C. B. Beard, and P. S. Mead. 2008. Multiple *Francisella tularensis* subspecies and clades, tularemia outbreak, Utah. *Emerg. Infect. Dis.* **14:**1928–1930.

143. Petersen, J. M., J. Carlson, B. Yockey, S. Pillai, C. Kuske, G. Garbalena, S. Pottumarthy, and L. Chalcraft. 2009. Direct isolation of *Francisella* spp. from environmental samples. **48:**663–667.

144. Petersen, J. M., P. S. Mead, and M. E. Schriefer. 2009. *Francisella tularensis:* an arthropod-borne pathogen. *Vet. Res.* **40:**07.

145. Pike, R. M. 1976. Laboratory-associated infections: summary and analysis of 3921 cases. *Health Lab. Sci.* **13:**105–114.

146. Porsch-Özcürümez, M., N. Kischel, H. Priebe, W. Splettstösser, E. J. Finke, and R. Grunow. 2004. Comparison of enzyme-linked immunosorbent assay, Western blotting, microagglutination, indirect immuno-fluorescence assay, and flow cytometric serological diagnosis of tularemia. *Clin. Diagn. Lab. Immunol.* **11:**1008–1015.

147. Probert, W. S., K. N. Schrader, N. Y. Khuong, S. L. Bystrom, and M. H. Graves. 2004. Real-time multiplex PCR assay for detection of *Brucella* spp., *B. abortus,* and *B. melitensis. J. Clin. Microbiol.* **42:**1290–1293.

148. Quipo-Ortuño, M. I., J. D. Colmenero, M. J. Bravo, M. A. García-Ordoñez, and P. Morata. 2008. Usefulness of a quantitative real-time PCR assay using serum samples to discriminate between inactive, serologically positive and active human brucellosis. *Clin. Microbiol. Infect.* **14:**1128–1134.

149. Quipo-Ortuño, M. I., F. Tena, J. D. Colmenero, and P. Morata. 2008. Comparison of seven commercial DNA extraction kits for the recovery of *Brucella* DNA from spiked human serum samples using real-time PCR. *Eur. J. Clin. Microbiol. Infect. Dis.* **27:**109–114.

150. Reintjes, R., I. Dedushaj, A. Gjini, T. R. Jorgensen, B. Cotter, A. Lieftucht, F. D'Ancona, D. T. Dennis, M. A. Kosoy, G. Mulliqi-Osmani, R. Grunow, A. Kalaveshi, L. Gashi, and I. Humolli. 2002. Tularemia outbreak investigation in Kosovo: case control and environmental studies. *Emerg. Infect. Dis.* **8:**69–73.

151. Rossetti, O. L., A. I. Arese, M. L. Boschiroli, and S. L. Cravero. 1996. Cloning of *B. abortus* gene and characterization of expressed 26-kilodalton periplasmic protein: potential use for diagnosis. *J. Clin. Microbiol.* **34:**165–169.

152. Rotz, L. D., A. S. Kahn, S. R. Lillibridge, S. M. Ostroff, and J. M. Hughes. 2002. Public health assessment of potential biological terrorism agents. *Emerg. Infect. Dis.* **8:**225–230.

153. Ruben, B., J. D. Band, P. Wong, and J. Colvelli. 1991. Person-to-person transmission of *Brucella melitensis. Lancet* **i:**14–15.

154. Ruiz-Mesa, J. D., J. Sánchez-Gonzalez, J. M. Reguera, L. Martin, S. Lopez-Palmero, and J. D. Colmenero. 2005. Rose Bengal test: diagnostic yield and use for the rapid diagnosis of human brucellosis in emergency departments in endemic areas. *Clin. Microbiol. Infect.* **11:**221–225.

155. Rusnak, J. M., M. G. Kortepeter, R. J. Hawley, A. O. Anderson, E. Boudreau, and E. Eitzen. 2004. Risk of occupationally acquired illnesses from biological threat agents in unvaccinated laboratory workers. *Biosecur. Bioterror.* **2:**281–293.

156. Samra, Y., Y. Shaked, M. Hertz, and G. Altman. 1983. Brucellosis: difficulties in diagnosis and a report on 38 cases. *Infection* **11:**310–312.

157. Sandström, G., A. Sjöstedt, M. Forsman, N. V. Pavlovich, and B. N. Mishankin. 1992. Characterization and classification of strains of *Francisella tularensis* isolated in the Central Asian focus of the Soviet Union, and in Japan. *J. Clin. Microbiol.* **30:**172–175.

158. Sangari, F. J., A. Seoane, M. C. Rodriguez, J. Aguero, and M. Garcia Lobo. 2007. Characterization of the urease operon of *Brucella abortus* and assessment of its role in virulence of the bacterium. *Infect. Immun.* **75:**774–780.

159. Schmitt, P., W. Splettstosser, M. Porsch-Özcürümez, E. J. Finke, and R. Grunow. 2005. A novel screening ELISA and a confirmatory Western blot useful for diagnosis and epidemiological studies of tularemia. *Epidemiol. Infect.* **133:**759–766.

160. Scoles, G. A. 2004. Phylogenetic analysis of the *Francisella*-like endosymbionts of *Dermacentor* ticks. *J. Med. Entomol.* **41:**277–286.

161. Shakir, R. A., A. S. N. Al-Din, G. F. Araj, A. R. Lulu, A. R. Mousa, and M. A. Saadah. 1987. Clinical categories of neurobrucellosis: a report on 19 cases. *Brain* **110:**213–223.

162. Shapiro, D. S., and D. R. Schwartz. 2002. Exposure of laboratory workers to *Francisella tularensis* despite a bioterrorism procedure. *J. Clin. Microbiol.* **40:**2278–2281.

163. Sharda, D. C., and M. M. Lubani. 1986. A study of brucellosis in childhood. *Clin. Pediatr.* **25:**492–495.

164. Sicherer, S. H., E. J. Asturias, J. A. Winkelstein, J. D. Dick, and R. E. Willoughby. 1997. *Francisella philomiragia* sepsis in chronic granulomatous disease. *Pediatr. Infect. Dis. J.* **16:**420–422.

165. Sjöstedt, A. 2005. *Francisella*, p. 200–210. *In* D. J. Brenner, N. R. Krieg, J. T. Staley, and G. M. Garrity (ed.), *Bergey's Manual of Systematic Bacteriology*, 2nd ed., vol. 2. *The Proteobacteria.* Springer-Verlag, New York, NY.

166. Sjöstedt, A. 2007. Tularemia: history, epidemiology, pathogen physiology, and clinical manifestations. *Ann. N. Y. Acad. Sci.* **1105:**1–29.

167. Sjöstedt, A., U. Eriksson, L. Berglund, and A. Tärnvik. 1997. Detection of *Francisella tularensis* in ulcers of patients with tularemia by PCR. *J. Clin. Microbiol.* **35:**1045–1048.

168. Skalsky, K., D. Yahav, J. Bishara, S. Pitlik, L. Leibovici, and M. Paul. 2008. Treatment of human brucellosis:

systematic review and meta-analysis of randomised controlled trials. *BMJ* **336:**701–704.

169. **Smits, H. L., T. H. Abdoel, J. Solera, E. Clavijo, and R. Dial.** 2003. Immunochromatographic *Brucella*-specific immunoglobulin M and G lateral flow assays for rapid serodiagnosis of human brucellosis. *Clin. Diagn. Lab. Immunol.* **10:**1141–1146.

170. **Sohn, A. H., W. S. Probert, C. A. Glaser, N. Gupta, A. W. Bollen, J. D. Wong, E. M. Grace, and W. C. McDonald.** 2003. Human neurobrucellosis with intra-cerebral granuloma caused by a marine mammal *Brucella* spp. *Emerg. Infect. Dis.* **9:**485–488.

171. **Solera, J., E. Martinez-Alfaro, A. Espinosa, M. L. Castillejos, P. Geijo, and M. Rodriguez-Zapata.** 1998. Multivariate model for predicting relapse in human brucellosis. *J. Infect.* **36:**85–92.

172. **Spink, W. W.** 1956. *The Nature of Brucellosis.* University of Minnesota Press, Minneapolis.

173. **Sréter-Lancz, Z., Z. Széll, T. Sréter, and K. Márialigeti.** 2008. Detection of a novel *Francisella* in *Dermacentor reticulatus*: a need for careful evaluation of PCR-based identification of *Francisella tularensis* in Eurasian ticks. *Vector Borne Zoonotic Dis.* **9:**123–126.

174. **Staples, J. E., K. A. Kubota, L. G. Chalcraft, P. S. Mead, and J. M. Petersen.** 2006. Epidemiologic and molecular analysis of human tularemia, United States, 1964–2004. *Emerg. Infect. Dis.* **12:**1113–1118.

175. **Surcel, H. M., J. Ilonen, K. Poikonen, and E. Herva.** 1989. *Francisella tularensis*-specific T-cell clones are human leukocyte antigen class II restricted, secrete interleukin-2 and gamma interferon, and induce immunoglobulin production. *Infect. Immun.* **57:**2906–2908.

176. **Surcel, H. M., M. Sarvas, I. M. Helander, and E. Herva.** 1989. Membrane proteins of *Francisella tularensis* LVS differ in ability to induce proliferation of lymphocytes from tularemia-vaccinated individuals. *Microb. Pathog.* **7:**411–419.

177. **Syrjälä, H., R. Schildt, and S. Räisänen.** 1991. *In vitro* susceptibility of *Francisella tularensis* to fluoroquinolones and treatment of tularemia with norfloxacin and ciprofloxacin. *Eur. J. Clin. Microbiol. Infect. Dis.* **10:**68–70.

178. **Tärnvik, A.** 1989. Nature of protective immunity to *Francisella tularensis*. *Rev. Infect. Dis.* **11:**440–451.

179. **Tärnvik, A., and M. C. Chu.** 2007. New approaches to diagnosis and therapy of tularemia. *Ann. N. Y. Acad. Sci.* **1105:**378–404.

180. **Thalhammer, F., G. Eberl, and U. Kopetzki-Kogler.** 1998. Unusual route of transmission for *Brucella abortus*. *Clin. Infect. Dis.* **26:**763–764.

181. **Tomaso, H., S. Al Dahouk, E. Hofer, W. D. Splettstoesser, T. M. Treu, M. P. Dierich, and H. Neubauer.** 2005. Antimicrobial susceptibilities of Austrian *Francisella tularensis holarctica* biovar II strains. *Int. J. Antimicrob. Agents* **26:**279–284.

182. **Urich, S. K., and J. M. Petersen.** 2008. In vitro susceptibility of isolates of *Francisella tularensis* types A and B from North America. *Antimicrob. Agents Chemother.* **52:**2276–2278.

183. **Uwaydah, M., A. Khalil, N. Shamsuddine, F. Matar, and G. F. Araj.** 1998. *Brucella*-ovarian dermoid cyst causing initial treatment failure in a patient with acute brucellosis. *Infection* **26:**131–132.

184. **Valade, E., J. Vaissaire, A. Mérens, E. Hernandez, C. Gros, C. Le Doujet, J. C. Paucod, F. M. Thibault, B. Durand, M. Lapalus, I. Dupuis, A. Caclard, D. R. Vidal, and J. D. Cavallo.** 2008. Susceptibility of 71 French isolates of *Francisella tularensis* subsp. *holarctica* to eight antibiotics and accuracy of the Etest method. *J. Antimicrob. Chemother.* **62:**208–210.

185. **Vanderca, B.** 1990. Isolation of *Brucella melitensis* from human sperm. *Eur. J. Clin. Microbiol. Infect. Dis.* **9:**303–304.

186. **Versage, J. L., D. D. Severin, M. C. Chu, and J. M. Petersen.** 2003. Development of a multitarget real-time TaqMan PCR assay for enhanced detection of *Francisella tularensis* in complex specimens. *J. Clin. Microbiol.* **41:**5492–5499.

187. **Viljanen, M. K., T. Nurmi, and A. Salminen.** 1983. Enzyme-linked immunosorbent assay (ELISA) with bacterial sonicate antigen for IgM, IgA, and IgG antibodies to *Francisella tularensis*: comparison with bacterial agglutination test and ELISA with lipopolysaccharide antigen. *J. Infect. Dis.* **148:**715–720.

188. **Vogler, A. J., D. Birdsell, L. B. Price, J. R. Bowers, S. M. Beckstrom-Sternberg, R. K. Auerbach, J. S. Beckstrom-Sternberg, A. Johansson, A. Clare, J. L. Buchhagen, J. M. Petersen, T. Pearson, J. Vaissaire, M. P. Dempsey, P. Foxall, D. M. Engelthaler, D. M. Wagner, and P. Keim.** 2009. Phylogeography of *Francisella tularensis*: global expansion of a highly fit clone. *J. Bacteriol.* **191:**2474–2484.

189. **Vrioni, G., C. Gartzonika, A. Kostoula, C. Boboyiami, C. Papadopoulou, and S. Levidiotou.** 2004. Application of a polymerase chain reaction enzyme immunoassay in peripheral whole blood and serum specimens for diagnosis of acute human brucellosis. *Eur. J. Clin. Microbiol. Infect. Dis.* **23:**194–199.

190. **Waag, D. M., K. T. McKee, Jr., G. Sandström, L. L. K. Pratt, C. R. Bolt, M. J. England, G. O. Nelson, and J. C. Williams.** 1995. Cell-mediated and humoral immune responses after vaccination of human volunteers with the live vaccine strain of *Francisella tularensis*. *Clin. Diagn. Lab. Immunol.* **2:**143–148.

191. **Wenger, J. D., D. G. Hollis, R. E. Weaver, C. N. Baker, G. R. Brown, D. J. Brenner, and C. V. Broome.** 1989. Infection caused by *Francisella philomiragia* (formerly *Yersinia philomiragia*): a newly recognized human pathogen. *Ann. Intern. Med.* **110:**888–892.

192. **Weyant, R. S., C. W. Moss, R. E. Weaver, D. G. Hollis, J. G. Jordan, E. C. Cook, and M. I. Daneshvar.** 1996. *Identification of Unusual Pathogenic Gram-Negative Aerobic and Facultatively Anaerobic Bacteria,* 2nd ed. The Williams & Wilkins Co., Baltimore, MD.

193. **Whatmore, A. M.** 2009. Current understanding of the genetics diversity of Brucella, an expanding genus of zoonotic pathogens. *Infect. Genet. Evol.* **9:**1168–1184.

194. **Whipp, M. J., J. M. Davis, G. Lum, J. de Boer, Y. Zhou, S. W. Bearden, J. M. Petersen, M. C. Chu, and G. Hogg.** 2003. Characterization of a novicida-like subspecies of *Francisella tularensis* in Australia. *J. Med. Microbiol.* **52:**839–842.

195. **Willke, A., M. Meric, R. Grunow, M. Sayan, E. J. Finke, W. Splettstösser, E. Seibold, S. Erdogan, O. Ergonul, Z. Yumuk, and S. Gedikoglu.** 2009. An outbreak of oropharyngeal tularaemia linked to natural spring water. *J. Med. Microbiol.* **58:**112–116.

196. **World Health Organization.** 2006. *Brucellosis in humans and animals,* p. 36–41. WHO/CDS/EPR/2006.7. World Health Organization, Geneva, Switzerland.

197. **World Health Organization.** 2007. WHO guidelines on tularemia. World Health Organization, Geneva, Switzerland. http://www.cdc.gov/tularemia/resources/whotularemiamanual.pdf.

198. **Wyatt, H. V.** 2000. Sir Themistocles Zammit: his honours and an annotated bibliography of his medical work. *Maltese Med. J.* **12:**27–30.

199. **Yagupsky, P.** 1999. Detection of brucellae in blood cultures. *J. Clin. Microbiol.* **37:**3437–3442.

200. **Yagupsky, P., and E. J. Baron.** 2005. Laboratory exposures to brucellae and implications for bioterrorism. *Emerg. Infect. Dis.* **11:**1180–1185.

201. **Yingst, S., and D. L. Hoover.** 2003. T cell immunity to brucellosis. *Crit. Rev. Microbiol.* **29:**313–331.

202. **Young, E. J.** 2009. Brucella species, p. 2921–2925. *In* G. L. Mandell, J. E. Bennett, and R. Dolin (ed.), *Mandell, Douglas, and Bennett's Principles and Practice of Infectious Diseases,* 7th ed. Elsevier Inc., Philadelphia, PA.

203. **Zhang, F., W. Liu, X. M. Wu, Z. T. Xin, Q. M. Zhao, H. Yang, and W. C. Cao.** 2008. Detection of *Francisella tularensis* in ticks and identification of their genotypes using multiple-locus variable-number tandem repeat analysis. *BMC Microbiol.* **8:**152.

204. **Zinsstag, J., E. Schelling, F. Roth, B. Bonfoh, D. de Savigny, and M. Tanner.** 2007. Human benefits of animal interventions for zoonoses control. *Emerg. Infect. Dis.* **13:**527–531.

*Legionella**

PAUL H. EDELSTEIN

45

TAXONOMY

The *Legionellaceae* are composed of a single genus, *Legionella*, and 52 validly named species (http://www.bacterio.cict .fr/l/legionella.html) (Table 1). *Legionella pneumophila*, *L. micdadei*, *L. longbeachae*, and *L. dumoffii* are the most important from a clinical standpoint, with *L. pneumophila* causing more than 90% of cases of Legionnaires' disease (LD). The *Legionellaceae* are most closely related to the *Coxiellaceae*, and these two families comprise the proposed order "*Legionellales*" within the class *Gammaproteobacteria* and phylum *Proteobacteria* phy. nov. *Coxiella burnetii*, the agent of Q fever, shares many characteristics with *L. pneumophila*, including intracellular parasitism and close homologies of several virulence genes (122). Some investigators proposed the use of *Tatlockia* and *Fluoribacter* as additional genera within the *Legionellaceae* (47), but a subsequent study of 16S rRNA demonstrated that the *Legionellaceae* are monophyletic (44); use of these genus names was never widely accepted and is of historical interest only. A number of *Legionella*-like bacteria have been described to grow only within free-living amoebae, and have been designated LLAP, for *Legionella*-like amoebal pathogen. One of the LLAPs, *Legionella lytica* has been shown to cause human disease. Four have been assigned novel *Legionella* spp.; three of these four have been grown axenically at low temperature (1).

Four different *L. pneumophila* serogroup 1 strains have been completely sequenced: the Philadelphia 1, Lens, Paris, and Corby strains. Analysis of these sequences shows that *L. pneumophila* contains a number of eukaryotic-like genes, some of which have been shown to allow the bacteria to create bacteria-friendly intracellular environments by subverting the normal cellular machinery (11, 12). Analysis of the *L. pneumophila* genome also shows that it is a genetically diverse species and that some virulent strains are disseminated worldwide (11). Genes encoding for the lipopolysaccharide core region and an O side chain predominate in clinical isolates of *L. pneumophila* serogroup 1 and may be the reason why this serogroup predominates as a cause of LD (11).

DESCRIPTION OF THE AGENT

The *Legionellaceae* are a diverse group of mesophilic, motile, asaccharolytic, obligately aerobic, nutritionally fastidious gram-negative rods, sharing common growth dependence for L-cysteine, growth enhancement by iron, and cellular branched-chain fatty acids and ubiquinones that are unusual for gram-negative bacteria (29). *L. pneumophila* is the most extensively studied of the *Legionella* spp., with relatively little known about most of the other *Legionella* spp. Almost all of the *Legionella* spp. have been isolated from aqueous environmental sources, and about a third of the 52 validly named species have been isolated from both humans and the environment. It is assumed that the natural reservoir of all the *Legionellaceae* is our aqueous environment and that humans are an accidental host of the bacterium. Environmental *L. pneumophila* is a facultative intracellular parasite of several different free-living amoebae, such as *Acanthamoeba* and *Naegleria*, existing in microbial consortia in biofilms and free-flowing water.

L. pneumophila grows at a temperature range from 20 to 42°C, with optimal growth occurring at temperatures of 35 to 37°C. Growth on solid media is enhanced by increased humidity. Incubation in 2 to 5% CO_2 can enhance the growth of some *Legionella* spp. Bacterial phenotype, including immunogenicity, cell size, and virulence, can be altered by growth at different temperatures (29).

Amino acids, rather than carbohydrates, are used as energy sources by the *Legionellaceae* growing in vitro; this is true for intracellular bacteria as well, despite the presence of putative carbohydrate utilization genes in the *L. pneumophila* genome (29). Primary isolation of all known *Legionella* spp. requires medium supplementation with L-cysteine, as does successful propagation of all but a few species. Iron supplementation of growth media is required for optimal growth, although many *Legionella* spp. can grow, albeit poorly, in the absence of the mineral. Growth of *L. pneumophila* is enhanced by the addition of α-ketoglutarate (0.1%) to media, via an unknown, nonnutritive, mechanism.

Growth of *L. pneumophila* in artificial media can be inhibited by a number of factors. These include the presence of high (100 mM, or 0.6%) NaCl concentrations, toxic peroxides, products of other bacteria and fungi, and some lipids (29). In addition, optimal growth occurs over a very narrow pH range from 6.7 to 6.9. Solid growth media contain

---

*This chapter contains a figure presented in chapter 52 by Janet E. Stout, John D. Rihs, and Victor L. Yu in the eighth edition of this *Manual*.

TABLE 1 Selected characteristics of *Legionella* spp.[a]

Legionella sp.[b]	Isolated from humans[c]	No. of recognized serogroups	Color under long-wave UV light	Comments
L. adelaidensis	N	1	NC	
L. anisa	Y	1	BW/YG	
L. beliardensis	N	1	YG	
L. birminghamensis	Y	1	YG	
L. bozemanae	Y	2	BW	AN, *Fluoribacter bozemanae*[d]
L. brunensis	N	1	NC	
L. busanensis	N	1	NC	
L. cherrii	N	1	BW	
L. cincinnatiensis	Y	1	YG	
L. drancourtii	N	NK	NK	Amoebic pathogen; no axenic growth
L. drozanskii	N	1	NC	Grows at 30°C but not at 37°C
L. dumoffii	Y	1	BW	AN, *F. dumoffii*[d]
L. erythra	N	2	R	
L. fairfieldensis	N	1	NC	
L. fallonii	N	1	NC	Grows at 30°C but not 37°C
L. feeleii	Y	2	NC	
L. geestiana	N	1	NC	
L. gormanii	Y	1	BW	AN, *F. gormanii*[d]
L. gratiana	N	1	NC	
L. gresiliensis	N	1	YG	
L. hackeliae	Y	2	YG	
L. impletisoli	N	1	NC	
L. israelensis	N	1	NC	
L. jamestowniensis	N	1	YG	
"*L. jeonii*"	N	NK	NK	Amoebic endosymbiont
L. jordanis	Y	1	YG	Partial L-cysteine dependence with serial passage
L. lansingensis	Y	1	NC	
L. londiniensis	N	1	NC	
L. longbeachae	Y	2	YG	
L. lytica	Y	NK	BW	Grows at 30°C but not at 37°C
L. maceachernii	Y	1	YG	AN, *Tatlockia maceachernii*[d]
L. micdadei	Y	1	YG	AN, *T. micdadei*[d]
L. moravica	N	1	NC	
L. nautarum	N	1	NC	
L. oakridgensis	Y	1	YG	Partial L-cysteine dependence with serial passage
L. parisiensis	Y	1	BW	
L. pneumophila	Y	16	YG	Three subspecies recognized
L. quateirensis	N	1	NC	
L. quinlivanii	N	2	YG	
L. rowbothamii	N	1	BW	
L. rubrilucens	N	1	R	
L. sainthelensi	Y	2	YG	
L. santicrucis	N	1	YG	
L. shakespearei	N	1	NC	
L. spiritensis	N	2	YG	Partial L-cysteine dependence with serial passage
L. steigerwaltii	N	1	BW	
L. taurinensis	N	1	R/yg	
L. tucsonensis	Y	1	BW	
L. wadsworthii	Y	1	YG	
L. waltersii	N	1	NC	
L. worsleiensis	N	1	NC	
L. yabuuchiae	N	1	NC	

[a] Abbreviations: Y, yes; N, no; NK, not known; NC, no color; BW, bright blue-white; YG, pale yellow-green; BW/YG, some strains are BW and some YG; R, dark red; R/yg, majority of strains are red, with remainder YG.

[b] All listed species, except "*L. jeonii*," constitute validly published names. Several other species probably exist.

[c] Severely immunosuppressed patients may acquire infections with *Legionella* spp. not previously isolated from humans.

[d] AN, alternative name; while valid, the genus names *Fluoribacter* and *Tatlockia* are not in widespread usage.

activated charcoal to inactivate toxic lipids and peroxides and an organic buffer (MOPS [morpholinepropanesulfonic acid] or ACES [N-(2-acetamido)-2-aminoethanesulfonic acid]) to reduce sodium content and provide the required pH. Preparation of growth media for *Legionella* spp. can be complex and is usually best left to competent commercial sources or to specialized laboratories.

EPIDEMIOLOGY AND TRANSMISSION

LD was first recognized as a distinct entity when epidemic pneumonia with a 15% fatality rate developed during and after a convention of the Pennsylvania American Legion in Philadelphia in July 1976 (30, 41). Joseph McDade and colleagues at the CDC determined that a novel gram-negative bacterium was the cause of the outbreak (83). Neither the disease nor the bacterium was found to be novel, with the first known epidemic of LD having occurred in 1957 (92) and isolation of the bacterium having occurred multiple times from the 1940s on.

Environmental studies found that the bacterium was widespread in natural bodies of water and occasionally in high concentration in warm waters found in plumbing systems, water heaters, warm water spas, and cooling towers. Many different *Legionella* spp. exist in nature within free-living amoebae, and as a result, these otherwise fastidious bacteria can multiply within the amoebae and be protected from biocides (102). *Legionella*-infected amoebae are often found in complex consortia of microorganisms within biofilms. The bacteria are present in very low concentrations in freely flowing cold water and biocide-treated waters but can multiply in warm and, especially, stagnant water. Devices that aerosolize these contaminated waters serve to disseminate the bacteria.

Legionella pneumophila serogroup 1 causes 95 to 98% of community-acquired LD. The Pontiac/MAb 3-1 monoclonal antibody subgroup of *L. pneumophila* serogroup 1 constitutes about 80 to 90% of clinical isolates of this serogroup. Just a few clonal types of *L. pneumophila* serogroup 1, the Pontiac subgroup, are responsible for about 50% of sporadic community-acquired infection (11, 49, 55). Several *L. pneumophila* serogroup 1 strains that predominate as clinical isolates are uncommon in the environment, whereas most *L. pneumophila* strains that are commonly found in the environment are unusual causes of LD (20, 55, 74). Infection caused by *L. pneumophila* serogroup 1 Pontiac subtype is less common in nosocomial LD, especially that involving immunocompromised patients. Up to 60% of nosocomial LD may be caused by other *L. pneumophila* serogroup 1 subtypes, other *L. pneumophila* serogroups, and other *Legionella* species (59, 60).

Infection is acquired by aerosol inhalation of contaminated water, although microaspiration may also be a mechanism of acquiring the disease (30). The majority of community epidemics of LD are from *Legionella*-contaminated cooling towers or other aerosol-generating devices. Contaminated potable water systems, such as water heaters and warm water in pipes can also be a major source of disease, although these sources are not usually the cause of explosive outbreaks of the disease.

Despite the ubiquity of *Legionella* spp. in our environment, LD is an unusual cause of pneumonia. About 0.5 to 5% of adults requiring hospitalization for pneumonia have LD. Passive reporting indicates that the disease incidence is from 4 to 20 cases per million people per year, and a prospective study estimated that the disease incidence is about 80 cases per million people per year, or between 8,000 to 18,000 LD cases annually in the United States (82). This rate may be

an underestimate, as a recent German study found that the annual rate was 180 to 360 cases/million population (117). Underreporting of LD is common in the United States, with only about 2,800 cases reported to the CDC in 2008. Sporadic community-acquired LD is much more common than epidemic-associated disease, in a ratio of about 4:1.

The incubation period of LD is estimated to be between 2 to 14 days, with a median value of about 4 days. A study of a large outbreak extended the incubation period to as long as 19 days, with a median value of 7 days (16).

L. pneumophila causes disease by infecting human mononuclear cells, primarily alveolar macrophages. After the bacterium is inhaled into the lungs, it invades lung macrophages and multiplies in them. Detailed descriptions of pathogenesis can be found elsewhere (2, 30, 46, 67).

CLINICAL SIGNIFICANCE

LD is a type of bacterial pneumonia, caused by *L. pneumophila* and other *Legionella* spp. The pneumonia ranges in severity from mild to fatal, with an average fatality rate of 12% (5). Major risk factors for the disease include immunosuppression of the cellular immune system, cigarette smoking, overnight travel outside the home, use of well water, chronic heart or lung disease, and chronic renal failure. Solid-organ transplant patients are at particularly high risk, as are patients receiving anti-tumor necrosis factor therapy for a variety of autoimmune diseases (30).

LD cannot be readily distinguished from other forms of community-acquired pneumonia by clinical, roentgenographic, or nonspecific laboratory studies (30). Several attempts at developing a clinical scoring system to distinguish LD from other pneumonias have failed.

The severity of pneumonia at presentation, underlying diseases, and promptness of specific antibiotic therapy are important prognostic factors. Promptly treated LD can be cured in 95 to 99% of cases in otherwise healthy persons. Less than half of patients may respond if there is a delay in therapy, immunosuppression, or respiratory failure (30). Untreated disease causes death in about 15% of previously healthy patients and up to 75% of severely immunocompromised ones (30).

Prospective, randomized controlled studies of adequate size have not been performed to determine the optimal therapy for LD, so great reliance is placed on experimental tissue culture and animal model studies, as well as results of nonrandomized studies (23, 30). Erythromycin, clarithromycin, azithromycin, a tetracycline, telithromycin, levofloxacin, ciprofloxacin, and moxifloxacin all appear to have roughly equivalent efficacies for nonimmunocompromised outpatients with mild LD (30). The quinolone antimicrobials, especially levofloxacin, and azithromycin are the drugs of choice for severe disease and for immunocompromised patients (30, 87). Antimicrobial therapy with more than one agent is sometimes used but is of questionable benefit and, in the case of rifampin, may be harmful (52).

Pontiac fever is an acute influenza-like illness that has been associated with exposure to *Legionella* sp.-containing environmental aerosols (40, 51). The etiology and pathogenesis of this disease are unknown, but it appears as if the disease is caused by inhalation of bacterial toxins, such as endotoxin, or perhaps an acute allergic reaction to a bacterium. Since multiple microorganisms, and endotoxin, have been found in aerosols causing Pontiac fever, it is unclear if *Legionella* spp. play any role at all in disease causation. Pontiac fever is self-limited, with no reported deaths, little to no need for hospitalization, and no need for antibiotic therapy.

COLLECTION, TRANSPORT, AND STORAGE OF SPECIMENS

Expectorated sputum and other lower respiratory specimens are the most common sources of *Legionella* spp. Other, less common sources include pleural fluid and blood. Rare sources have included pericardial fluid, kidney, liver, spleen, myocardium, respiratory sinuses, skin and soft tissues, infected wounds, peritoneal fluid, prosthetic heart valves, bone marrow, and intestine. Culture of available sputum, bronchoscopy specimens, lung biopsy specimens, and pleural fluid should be routine for laboratory diagnosis of LD. Lung biopsy specimens have the highest yield but may be negative. Culture of expectorated sputum or other lower respiratory tract secretions, second in yield to lung biopsy, should always be performed for optimal detection of legionella infection. Pleural fluid has low yield but should be cultured if it is available. Routine culture of other specimens for *Legionella* spp. is not indicated unless there is a high clinical suspicion of the disease affecting these sites.

Sputum microscopic scoring criteria cannot be used to determine which sputum specimens should be cultured for legionella bacteria because of limited purulence and scanty secretions in patients with LD. Up to 80% of specimens culture-positive for *Legionella* spp. may be rejected using the criteria of the presence of sputum purulence for processing specimens (39, 66).

Urine for antigen detection should be collected in a sterile container (27). Boric acid preserves the antigen, but use of commercial urine transport systems containing boric acid have not been studied for antigen preservation and freedom from interactions. The urine can be transported to the laboratory at room temperature if no more than a several-hour delay is anticipated. Longer transport times require specimen refrigeration; urine specimens should not be frozen, as this may reduce test sensitivity and specificity.

Blood for serum antibody testing is collected in standard tubes and transported at room temperature (26). Test performance is not adversely affected by storage of the clotted, unseparated blood at room temperature for several days. Long-term storage is at −20°C in aliquots to allow parallel testing without freeze-thawing, which can lower antibody levels.

Legionella spp. are hardy and generally survive for up to a week in clinical specimens. Sputum and other respiratory tract specimens, including lung biopsy specimens, should be collected in sterile containers and transported to the laboratory promptly at room temperature. Transportation and storage should be at 2 to 5°C if more than a several-hour delay is anticipated before the specimen can be plated. Very long term storage is best at −70°C, although this can reduce bacterial concentration to below the level of detection when the starting concentration was low or the specimen was primarily aqueous. Repeated freeze-thawing is harmful to the bacteria. Some tissues, especially spleen, contain growth-preventing substances and must be plated promptly, since even overnight storage at 5°C dramatically reduces culture yield; note that this is not true of lung specimens.

DIRECT EXAMINATION

Microscopy

The morphology of *L. pneumophila* found in lung and sputum specimens is a small coccobacillus to short rod, 3 to 5 μm in length (Fig. 1). This is much different from that observed

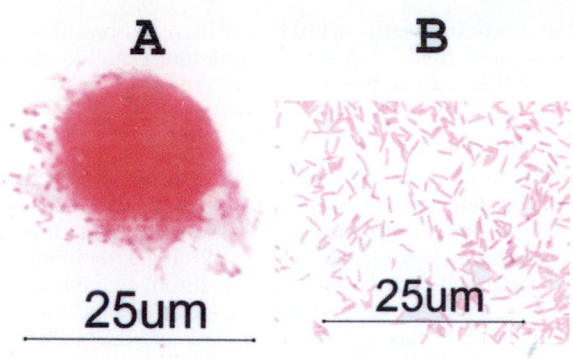

FIGURE 1 Photomicrographs of *L. pneumophila*. (A) Gimenez stain of intracellular bacteria in lung infection. (B) Gram stain using basic fuchsin counterstain of colony taken from BCYEα plate. Note the dramatic size and shape differences between the intracellular and extracellular bacteria.

for the bacterium taken from a culture plate, which is usually a long, filamentous bacillus, 10 to 25 μm in length. *L. pneumophila* is very difficult to detect by Gram staining of sputum or lung biopsy specimens. Use of 0.1% basic fuchsin, rather than safranin, greatly enhances the staining of the bacterium from culture plates, but even with use of this stain, it is very difficult to visualize the bacterium in sputum and tissues. Less than 0.1% of *L. pneumophila* present in lung tissue or sputum can be visualized by Gram stain using basic fuchsin. The small size of intracellular *L. pneumophila*, the form present in human tissues, makes visualization difficult with Gram stain, as does stain uptake by the surrounding proteinaceous material found in sputum and tissue specimens.

Use of the nonspecific Gimenez stain dramatically improves the detection of *L. pneumophila* in sputum and lung tissue by 100- to 1,000-fold over that visualized with Gram stain using basic fuchsin counterstain. In spite of its better performance, this stain is very insensitive for the detection of the bacterium in sputum when compared to immunofluorescent microscopy (34). The Gimenez stain is difficult to prepare, not commercially available, requires filtration before each use, and can be unstable. The stain detects the bacterium in Formalin-fixed, but not embedded, tissues (53).

Enhancement of bacterial staining by silver precipitate stains, such as the Warthin-Starry, and its modifications, and the Dieterle stains (37, 121), was an early approach to the detection of *L. pneumophila* in embedded tissues as well as sputum. These silver stains are useful for detection of the bacterium in embedded tissues but have no present role in the staining of the bacterium in sputum or other nonembedded specimens. Silver stains are not highly sensitive, can produce artifacts, and require expert use and interpretation for optimal sensitivity and specificity.

Some *Legionella* spp., in particular *L. micdadei*, may stain with acid-fast stains, both in fresh specimens and from Formalin-fixed tissues (8, 63). The small coccobacillary morphology of *Legionella* spp. should be a clue that the acid-fast organism is not a mycobacterium.

Immunofluorescent microscopy is the most sensitive and specific microscopic method for the detection of *L. pneumophila* in tissues and sputum (25, 34). Optimal sensitivity and specificity require exacting staining methods and great expertise by the microscopist. Even when well performed, the test sensitivity has been low compared to other diagnostic methods (103). For these reasons, this test is now rarely used for direct examination. Detailed discussions of this test can be found elsewhere (25).

Antigen Detection

LD due to *L. pneumophila* serogroup 1 can often be diagnosed by detection of bacterial antigenuria (27). Several immunoassays are commercially available for this purpose, the most convenient of which is a rapid single test immunochromatographic card assay. Immunochromatographic card assays are made by at least three companies, and two are FDA cleared (Binax, Scarborough, ME, and SA Scientific, San Antonio, TX). Of these, only the Binax NOW assay has been extensively evaluated. Several other assays utilize a microtube-based enzyme immunoassay. Only one non-FDA-cleared kit (Biotest, Dreieich, Germany) is designed to detect non-serogroup 1 *L. pneumophila*, but the kit appears to be no more sensitive than the other available kits (27). The strength of all these assays is their detection of *L. pneumophila* serogroup 1 infections and, in particular, its Pontiac/MAB2/MAB3-1 monoclonal subtype (59–61). The immunochromatographic card assay may be somewhat less sensitive than the microtube-based immunoassays, but its convenience, ease of use, and robustness make up for a slight decrease in sensitivity.

Clinical test performance for all assays is dependent on the pretest probability of *L. pneumophila* serogroup 1 and on the probability of Pontiac monoclonal subtype *L. pneumophila* serogroup 1 infection (59, 61). The assays detect about 60 to 70% of *L. pneumophila* serogroup 1 Pontiac monoclonal subtype epidemic infections and up to 90% of sporadic pneumonia caused by this subtype. The differences in test sensitivity for the same bacterial subtype are probably due to differences in disease severity, the other major factor determining test sensitivity. Patients with severe *L. pneumophila* serogroup 1 LD are the most likely to have positive urine antigen tests, for example, those requiring intensive care nursing and ventilator assistance; test sensitivity in this population is probably in the range of 90 to 95% of those infected with the Pontiac monoclonal subtype. On the other hand, urine testing may detect only 50% of outpatients with mild epidemic disease caused by the same monoclonal subtype, perhaps 40% of hospitalized patients with other *L. pneumophila* serogroup 1 subtypes, and fewer than 5 to 40% of those with infections caused by other serogroups and species (60, 64). The test may be negative during the first day of illness, but those with severe disease are likely to be positive upon presentation to the hospital. Repeat testing 2 to 3 days after the onset of illness may detect a small number of patients who had negative tests initially.

Test sensitivity can be enhanced by concentrating the specimen using ultrafiltration devices such as Amicon concentrators (Millipore, Billerica, MA). In some studies, this has increased test sensitivity by about 30%, without affecting specificity (21, 54). Prolonging incubation time for the Binax NOW assay to 60 minutes also increases sensitivity without decreasing specificity (19, 60). Test sensitivity decreases when specimens are frozen for weeks to months before testing.

The urine antigen assays are very specific, in the range of 99 to 99.9%. False-positive tests can be due to urine rheumatoid-like factors, freeze-thawing of urine, and excessive urinary sediment. All together, these causes of false-positive tests account for no more than a few percent of all positive tests. Regardless, all positive tests should be confirmed after boiling urine clarified by centrifugation.

Molecular Diagnosis of LD

Nucleic acid-based detection of *Legionella* spp. in sputum, urine, and blood samples has been successfully used in reference and research laboratories, with detection of *L. pneumophila* being the most extensively studied. The best results show that molecular diagnosis is a more sensitive method of diagnosis than culture, although some studies showed rough equivalence (86). Test sensitivities have been estimated to be 80 to 100%, 30 to 50%, and 50 to 90% for lower respiratory secretions, serum, and urine analytes, respectively; test specificities are estimated to be >90% (86). Both conventional and real-time assays have been utilized (62, 86). Most laboratories use the macrophage infectivity protein (*mip*) gene target to detect *L. pneumophila*. *Legionella* spp. are most commonly detected using an rRNA target, usually 16S, although 23S is claimed to have advantages (89). Sputum digestion may be important to increase yield (4). Multiplex assays are most commonly used, with no disadvantage over uniplex methods, although one study showed the superiority of a nucleic acid sequence-based amplification uniplex assay over a multiplex format (79, 107). Until recently, only home brew assays were available.

Three commercial assays exist, with only one cleared for marketing by the U.S. FDA (BD ProbeTec ET *Legionella*; BD Diagnostics, Sparks, MD); there are no published evaluations of this product. The other two assays, Chlamylege (Argene, North Massapequa, NY) and Pneumoplex (Prodesse, Waukesha, WI), performed quite well in single published evaluations (48, 70).

The added benefit of nucleic acid amplification-based detection of *Legionella* spp. over that obtained by urine antigen testing appears to be slight, with 11% greater yield than urine testing alone. This is likely because of the predominance of *L. pneumophila* serogroup 1, Pontiac subgroup, in community-acquired disease (18). Performance of nucleic acid testing for the detection of nosocomial LD and LD in immunocompromised patients would probably be significantly higher than urine antigen testing.

Because *Legionella* spp. are commonly found in water, contamination of almost any molecular reagent with *Legionella* spp. nucleic acid is a concern. False-positive PCR tests for *Legionella* spp. have been attributed to contaminated commercially produced "pure" water and nucleic acid extraction columns (35, 104, 114). Since sequencing of false-positive products yielded *Legionella* spp. sequences, contamination cannot be excluded by the ability to sequence the product and assign it to a particular *Legionella* sp. (35). In the case of extraction column contamination, only a few columns of the same lot may be contaminated and not the entire lot. This means that multiple negative controls are required for optimal specificity, including extraction controls as well as no-template controls.

ISOLATION PROCEDURES

Specimen Plating

Optimal yield of *Legionella* spp. from clinical specimens usually requires that specimens be diluted to reduce inhibition by tissue and serum factors as well as antibiotics, that the specimen be pretreated to reduce contaminating microbiota, and that a variety of selective and nonselective media be used (Table 2). Culture of *Legionella* spp. from normally sterile fluids and tissues, such as pleural fluid, aseptically obtained lung tissue, or blood, is often successful without the use of multiple selective media and specimen decontamination.

TABLE 2 Composition and selectivity of media used to grow *Legionella* spp. from clinical and environmental specimens[a]

Medium	Synonym	Selective agents	Main use	Selectivity[b]
BCYEα	CYE	None	Clinical, culture maintenance	None
BMPA	PAC	Cefamandole, polymyxin B, antifungal	Clinical, environmental	Normal respiratory microbiota, 3+; enterics, 3+; yeasts, 3+; molds, 1+; *Legionella* spp., 1+ to 4+
PAV	VAP	Vancomycin, polymyxin B, antifungal	Clinical, environmental	Normal respiratory microbiota, 2+; enterics, 2+; yeasts, 3+; molds, 1+; *Legionella* spp., 1+
MWY	VGP	Vancomycin, polymyxin B, antifungal, glycine	Environmental	Normal respiratory microbiota, 2+; enterics, 2+; yeasts, 3+; molds, 1+; environmental bacteria, 2+; *Legionella* spp., 1+
CCVC		Cephalothin, polymyxin E, vancomycin, cycloheximide	Environmental	Normal respiratory microbiota, 2+; enterics, 3+; yeasts, 2+; molds, 2+; *Legionella* spp., 1+ to 4+
BCYEα-L		None (made without L-cysteine)	Organism identification	*Legionella* spp., 4+ (no growth of *Legionella* spp. on this medium)

[a]Antifungal, either anisomycin or natamycin antifungal compounds; normal respiratory microbiota, normal upper respiratory tract bacteria.
[b]Selectivity scale range 0 to 4+: 0, does not inhibit these organisms; 1+, slight inhibition, allows about 75% growth; 2+, allows about 25 to 50% growth; 3+, allows about 10% growth; 4+, allows less than 1% growth.

Dilution (1:10) in tryptic soy broth increases the culture yield of most specimen types, including sputum and other liquid respiratory tract specimens, lung tissue, lymph nodes and spleen, and probably other organs such as liver and kidney. Sputum and other respiratory specimens should first be examined in a Petri dish for purulent-appearing material, and this material should be selected for culture. Tissues (about 1 g) are ground in a tissue grinder with a small amount (1 ml) of broth, which adequately dilutes most tissues except for spleen; this tissue requires an additional 1:10 dilution for the best recovery of bacteria. Liquid specimens are roughly diluted by adding about 0.1 ml of vortex-mixed liquid specimens to 0.9 ml of the dilution broth. Pleural fluid, joint fluid, and blood subcultured from blood culture bottles do not require dilution before plating; in fact, pleural fluid yield may be enhanced by concentration by centrifugation.

Decontamination is required to reduce contaminating microbiota in most sputum and other respiratory tract secretions. This is done by diluting (1:10) the specimen in a low-pH KCl-HCl buffer (pH 2.2) and incubating it at room temperature (4.0 minutes) before plating the suspension onto culture media. Timing is critical here, with resultant low yield if the timing is off by as little as a minute. The culture medium is sufficiently buffered so that the acidified specimen is neutralized upon being plated. An alternative to specimen acidification is heating at 50°C for 30 minutes. Most aseptically collected tissue specimens do not require decontamination, although occasionally, lung tissues contain multiple contaminating bacteria and fungi. In this case, heat or acid treatment of tissue ground in sterile distilled water may help; sometimes dilutions of the ground tissues are also required for optimal yield, with or without pretreatment.

Inoculation of Plates

Approximately 0.1 ml is inoculated to each plate, with the bulk of the inoculum applied to the first quadrant. Comparative studies are lacking to show whether it is better to streak plates for isolation or to uniformly distribute the inoculum over the entire plate. The plates must be thoroughly dry before being inoculated to aid in absorption of the relatively large volume inoculum and to retard spreading of contaminants throughout the plate.

Culture Media

Buffered charcoal-yeast extract (BCYE) medium supplemented with 0.1% α-ketoglutaric acid (BCYEα), is used for isolation and growth of *Legionella* spp. Use of BCYE without α-ketoglutarate supplementation cannot be recommended for clinical use, as this amino acid greatly enhances growth of the bacterium (32).

BCYEα can be made selective by the addition of antimicrobial agents (Table 2). A variety of different antifungal agents are used in the media. Cycloheximide is a poor choice for media used for clinical specimens, as it fails to inhibit *Candida albicans*. Both anisomycin and natamycin inhibit more yeasts than does cycloheximide. An array of media (Table 2) exists because no one selective medium is best for all purposes. Optimal yield of *Legionella* spp. from clinical specimens requires the use of three different media, one nonselective plate (BCYEα) and two selective media (BMPA [BCYE containing cefamandole, polymyxin B, and eithes anisomycin or natamycin] and PAV [BCYE containing polymyxin B, vancomycin, and either anisomycin or natamycin]). BMPA is an excellent selective medium for the vast majority of *L. pneumophila* strains, but the cefamandole present in the medium inhibits the growth of some other *Legionella* spp. and, rarely, *L. pneumophila* strains. Use of the less-selective medium, PAV, is required for optimal growth of some *Legionella* spp. other than *L. pneumophila*. No selective medium inhibits multiresistant gram-negative bacteria, reducing culture yield in nosocomial disease.

Selective and nonselective media are optimized for the isolation of *L. pneumophila*, and their performance for the isolation of other *Legionella* spp. is not accurately known. One study showed that *L. micdadei* in a guinea pig spleen had enhanced recovery on BCYEα medium prepared with 1% bovine serum albumin; the growth was enhanced because of less growth inhibition by spleen tissue (84). Whether addition of bovine serum albumin to BCYEα medium enhances *L. micdadei* recovery from human lung or sputum is unknown and probably unlikely. A BCYEα-based selective medium containing natamycin, aztreonam, and vancomycin has been reported to be useful for the isolation of *L. longbeachae* from soil (105).

Medium shelf life is around 1 year for nonselective plates and slants. This long shelf life requires thick plates (25-ml pour), complete drying of plates before storage at 2 to 4°C in sealed plastic bags, and protection from light. Selective media lose selectivity after about 3 months of storage time, but depending on the incorporated antibiotic, the media may last considerably longer.

Quality control (QC) testing of media is required before they are put into use. Current CLSI standards are inadequate for proper QC testing of these media. About 1% of commercial media fail laboratory QC testing (personal observations). The CLSI QC testing protocol utilizes a heavy inoculum of medium-adapted *Legionella* sp. strains and a growth/no-growth test. Minor variations in the manufacture of media, such as the addition of excess salt, overlong autoclaving, and degradation of buffers can all seriously affect the ability of the medium to support wild strain growth but not necessarily that of medium-adapted strains. The optimal method for medium QC testing is the inoculation of the test media with several hundred nonartificial medium-passed *L. pneumophila* bacteria (obtained from an infected guinea pig lung) and quantification of the bacterial colonies after 3 to 4 days of incubation (24). In the absence of the availability of lung-passaged *L. pneumophila* bacteria, low-passage clinical strains should be used, taking care to plate only several hundred bacteria per plate. QC testing of selective media for the ability to suppress non-*Legionella* bacteria can be done by inoculation of the plate with relatively antibiotic-susceptible *Escherichia coli* and *Staphylococcus aureus*, such as ATCC 25922 and 25923; the growth should be markedly suppressed.

Medium Incubation

Inoculated media are incubated at 35 to 37°C in humidified air. Regardless of the humidification method, care must be taken to keep the incubators or jars very clean and to regularly sterilize the containers or incubators. A small amount of CO_2 supplementation (2 to 5%) may enhance the growth of some of the more fastidious *Legionella* spp., such as *L. sainthelensi* and *L. oakridgensis*. This low level of CO_2 supplementation will not harm the growth of *L. pneumophila*, but CO_2 levels higher than 5% may inhibit growth. Since the more capnophilic species are very rare human isolates, many laboratories do not use CO_2 incubation of media for *Legionella* spp.

Plate Inspection

Legionella colonies begin to appear on culture plates on day 3 of incubation. It is very unusual for the bacterial colonies to appear on plates after 5 days of incubation. Some very rarely isolated *Legionella* spp. may require up to 14 days of incubation before growth appears; this is an extremely rare event. Regardless, it is reasonable to inspect culture plates on days 1 to 5 and then again at day 14.

The late appearance of *Legionella* spp. on culture plates can be used to great advantage if a careful record is kept of the colonies present on days 1 and 2 postincubation. New colonies appearing after day 2 should be suspected of being *Legionella* spp. Very rarely, *Legionella* spp. may grow from a heavily infected lung (usually from an autopsy of a fatal untreated case) on day 2, so some latitude in growth rate assumptions needs to be applied in the case of autopsy lung cultures. *Legionella* spp. never grow from clinical specimens on day 1 postincubation, a critical point in the distinction of *Pseudomonas aeruginosa* colonies from those of *Legionella* spp., as very early colonies of the latter superficially resemble those of the former.

Proper observation of culture plates requires the use of a dissecting microscope illuminated with direct light aimed at the plate surface at an approximately 30° angle. Failure to use a dissecting microscope or use of improper lighting will result in missed positive cultures, especially when there is mixed bacterial growth on the plates. In addition, very young *Legionella* colonies are very small and difficult to see with the naked eye. Therefore, use of a dissecting microscope can speed up the time to colony detection by as much as a day. *Legionella* growth occurs almost exclusively in the first streak quadrant and sometimes at the edge of the plate.

The size and morphology of *Legionella* colonies change with time. Very young colonies (day 3) are flat, entire, and 0.5 to 1 mm in diameter; when observed with a dissecting microscope and incident visible light, they usually have a speckled blue, blue-green, or red color. Within 6 to 24 h of additional incubation, these colonies become smooth, convex, iridescent, and entire, about 1 to 3 mm in diameter, and look opal-like when observed with a dissecting microscope (Fig. 2). A thick string may form when a loop is inserted in the colony and then removed from the colony. In contrast to several mimics, the edges of the colonies are of the same consistency as the central portion and are not watery and clear. In another 1 to 2 days, the colonies may increase in size up to 5 to 7 mm, become umbonate, sometimes with tuberculated or inhomogeneous texture and develop spready edges; their iridescent nature may be lost at this stage. It is these late-stage colonies that are most difficult to distinguish from

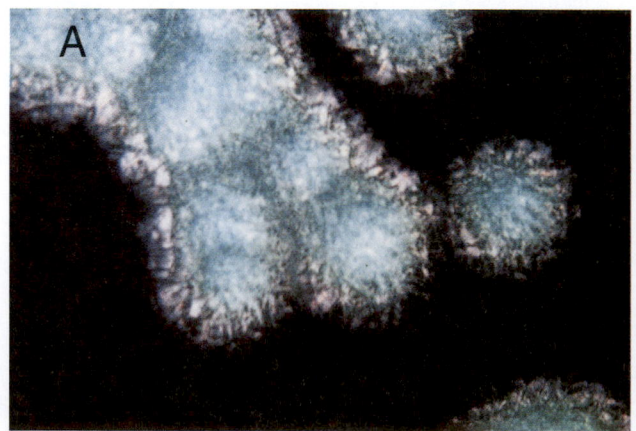
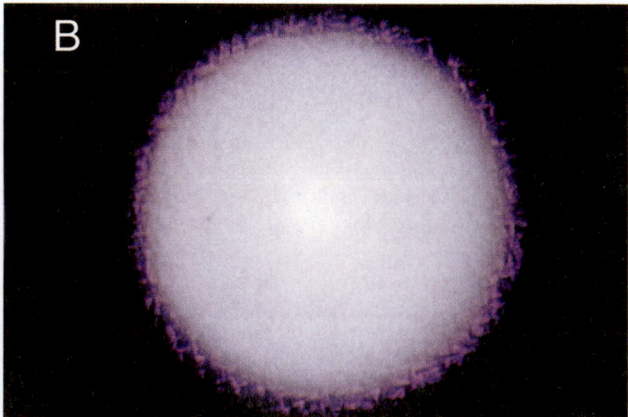

FIGURE 2 Photographs of *L. pneumophila* colonies growing on BCYEα agar. Note the internal speckling and different colors that may be seen, sometimes in the same culture. (Reprinted from Fig. 2A and B, p. 814 of the eighth edition of this *Manual*.)

non-*Legionella* spp., making daily plate observation crucial for accurate detection. Very rarely, some *Legionella* sp. colonies do not change morphology with prolonged incubation.

Biosafety level 2 precautions should be used for the manipulation of *Legionella* sp. cultures. It is safe to inspect culture plates, pick typical colonies, and subculture them on the open bench in a properly ventilated laboratory. Making an organism emulsion on microscope slides for the purposes of Gram staining can also be safely carried out on the open bench. However, vortexing suspensions, sonication, tissue grinding, primary plating, and manipulations that may result in generation of a high concentration aerosol should be performed in a biological safety cabinet. No well-documented cases of laboratory-acquired LD have been reported.

Initial Workup of Suspect Colonies and Look-Alike Bacteria

Colonies suspected of being *Legionella* spp. should first be stained by Gram stain to ascertain that the bacteria are small to sometimes filamentous, gram-negative rods. A small amount of the colony should be emulsified in sterile water or saline on a glass slide. It is important to completely suspend the bacteria in the liquid, as nondispersed clumps may stain as gram-positive rods. It is also crucial to use 0.1% basic fuchsin counterstain because safranin stains these bacteria very poorly. Depending on the colony age and on the strain and species, *Legionella* spp. taken from plates vary in size from short rods, 0.5 by 5 μm, to very long, filamentous bacteria, 1 by 25 μm.

Gram-negative bacteria should then be plated to two different media, BYCEα and either tryptic soy blood (TSB) or BCYEα made without L-cysteine (BCYEα-L), in approximately equal amounts in a small (1-cm²) area; eight or more isolates can be plated to each plate if needed (Fig. 3). Rather large amounts of the picked colony should be inoculated to these media to enable growth after 16 to 18 h of incubation, as the small inocula normally used for other bacteria may otherwise take several days to produce visible colonies on plates. If only a small single colony is available, then it can be emulsified in a small amount (~0.5 ml) of sterile distilled water (not saline) and used for staining, plate inoculation, and seroidentification. *Legionella* spp. should grow in 16 to 36 h on BCYEα medium, but not on TSB agar or BCYEα-L medium; this takes advantage of the L-cysteine growth dependence of *Legionella* spp. Sometimes *Legionella* spp. will grow poorly on TSB or BCYEα-L media, but at most, only about 10% of the amount of growth on BCYEα will occur. Nutrient carryover from the primary isolation plate is the explanation for this light growth; this can be proven by making a subculture of growth on BCYEα-L or TSB on a second plate of the same medium. Rare *Legionella* spp. partially lose growth dependence for L-cysteine on serial passage but even still grow more poorly on BCYEα-L than on BCYEα; these species include *L. spiritensis*, *L. oakridgensis*, and *L. jordanis*, none of which have been reported to cause more than two cases of LD each. TSB performs almost as well as does BCYEα-L for determining L-cysteine dependence for clinical isolates and may be less expensive, depending on the number of isolates tested per plate. If a blood-containing agar medium is used as the screening plate, rather than BCYEα-L, for L-cysteine dependence, great care must be taken that the medium base is not too rich. For example, Brucella blood agar will support *L. pneumophila* growth almost as well as BCYEα medium, and other blood-containing media have been described to do the same (17). The plates are incubated overnight at 35 to 37°C or until there is visible growth on the BCYEα plate. The relative amount of growth on each plate is compared to determine if there is L-cysteine dependence. Most *Legionella* spp. produce a characteristic dank odor when growing in pure growth that is very specific to the trained nose.

Common mimics of *Legionella* spp. colonies on BCYEα plates include *Eikenella corrodens*, *P. aeruginosa*, *Flavobacterium* spp., and some *Bacillus* spp. All of these bacteria grow equally well on BCYEα and BCYEα-L media, but when young, they often grow as speckled colonies on BCYEα plates. *Francisella tularensis* can grow well on BYCEα agar but has no resemblance to *Legionella* spp. colonies. However, *F. tularensis* is the only gram-negative bacterium other than *Legionella* spp. that exhibits L-cysteine growth dependence. The colony morphology of *F. tularensis* is not speckled but rather is opaque and homogeneous. Adding to the confusion is that some serotyping reagents for *Legionella* spp. may cross-react with *F. tularensis*. There is one case report of the misidentification of *F. tularensis* as *L. pneumophila* (118). When tularemia is suspected, more-stringent safety precautions are needed. Of note, some *Bacillus* spp. mimics can stain as gram-negative rods, have unapparent sporulation, and do not grow on TSB (but will grow on BCYEα-L) (109). With prolonged incubation, colonies of both *E. corrodens* and *Flavobacterium* spp. colonies change color and no longer resemble *Legionella* spp.; *E. corrodens* colonies become a light to dark green color and *Flavobacterium* spp. become a bright yellow color. Very young *P. aeruginosa* and *Bacillus* spp. colonies resemble the speckled flat to slightly convex young *Legionella* spp. colonies but, with prolonged incubation, change their morphology, making them easily recognizable as non-*Legionella* sp. colonies. *Bordetella pertussis* colonies may appear late on BCYEα plates, and although this bacterium is not cysteine dependent nor does it possess colony morphology similar to *Legionella* spp., *B. pertussis* has been reported to be misidentified as *Legionella* spp., abetted by serological cross-reactivity (90). Because many different bacteria may cross-react with serological reagents used for typing and identifying *Legionella* spp., it is crucial to become familiar with the morphology and growth characteristics of this genus; relying exclusively on serotyping to identify *Legionella* spp. could result in mistaken identification.

Microbiologists should know that some pathogenic fungi and higher bacteria grow well on BCYEα medium, presenting potential biohazards as well as the opportunity to diagnose unsuspected infections. *Coccidioides* spp. often grow within a day or two on this medium, can rapidly form arthroconidia, and as such, present a biohazard. *Blastomyces dermatitidis* also grows well and converts to the mold phase within a few days. It is likely that other pathogenic fungi grow equally well on this very rich medium. *Nocardia* spp. and rapidly growing mycobacteria often grow quite well on this medium, making BCYEα medium and its selective variants the plating media of choice for the laboratory diagnosis of nocardiosis (69, 116). Bacteremia from *Nocardia* spp. can sometimes be diagnosed by subculture of blood culture bottles to BCYEα.

IDENTIFICATION

Basic Identification

Once L-cysteine dependence has been confirmed, further identification of *Legionella* spp. in a clinical laboratory relies almost exclusively on serotyping the bacteria, using

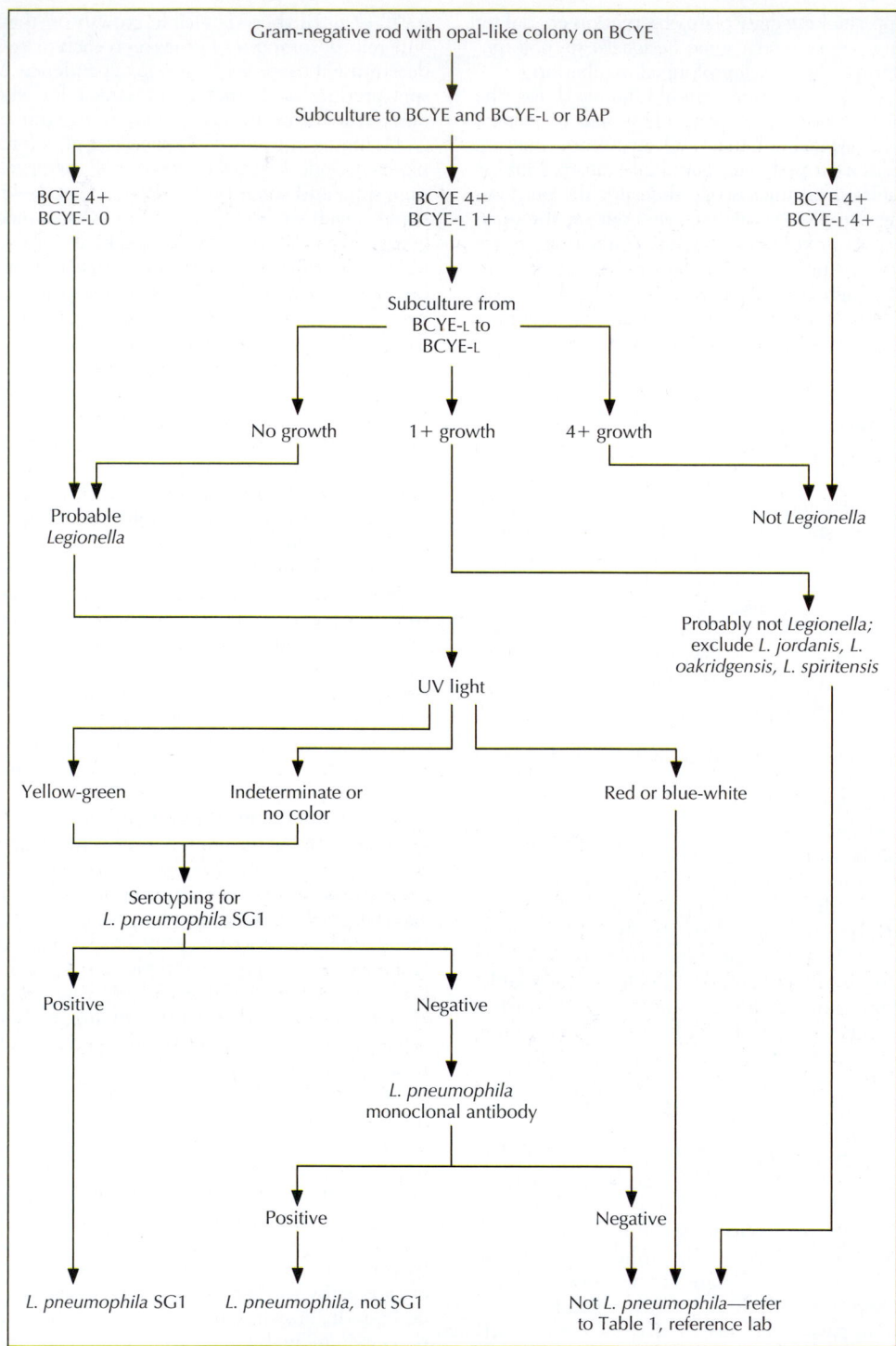

FIGURE 3 Identification flow scheme for basic identification of *Legionella* spp. grown from a BCYEα plate. Abbreviations: BCYE, BCYEα; BCYE-ʟ, BCYEα made without ʟ-cysteine; BAP, tryptic soy blood agar; UV light, colony fluorescence and color when illuminated with long-wave (360 nm) UV light; SG1, serogroup 1. Numbers refer to the amount of growth: 4+, good growth; 1+, poor growth; 0, no growth.

either immunofluorescence or agglutination methods (25, 94). Before identification by serotyping is attempted, the plate should be illuminated with long-wave UV light in a darkroom. Some *Legionella* spp. other than *L. pneumophila* fluoresce a brilliant blue-white color, and some fluoresce a brilliant red. Such bacteria are best identified by a reference laboratory and are not *L. pneumophila*. *L. pneumophila* fluoresces a very pale yellow-green color, usually with diffusion of the fluorescent pigment into the culture medium. This is not specific for this species, and sometimes young cultures are completely nonfluorescent. An excellent and specific FDA-cleared fluorescein isothiocyanate-labeled monoclonal antibody to all serogroups of *L. pneumophila* is available (Monofluo; Bio-Rad). Also, an excellent non-FDA-cleared fluorescein isothiocyanate-labeled *L. pneumophila* serogroup 1 (Philadelphia 1 strain)-specific polyclonal antisera is available (m-TECH, Atlanta, GA [http://www.4m-tech.com/]). Serotyping can also be performed using non-FDA-cleared latex agglutination antisera, available in a variety of formats (Oxoid, Basingstoke, United Kingdom; Denka Seiken, Tokyo, Japan); few data on the performance of these reagents are available.

Since more than 90% of *Legionella* sp. isolates are *L. pneumophila* serogroup 1, a reagent- and time-saving technique is to first test with *L. pneumophila* serogroup 1 antibody; strains negative with this antibody can then be tested with the species-specific monoclonal antibody. Extraordinarily rarely, some *L. pneumophila* serogroup 1 strains do not react with Philadelphia 1 strain antibodies, making it possible that a serogroup 1 strain could be missed with this reagent; additional serogroup 1 antibodies are available (m-TECH). Testing has to be conducted properly for valid results, with the most common errors being false-negative results because of a prozone phenomenon, and false-positive results from contaminated buffers, wash solutions, or cross-contamination from controls (25). Strains that fail to react with *L. pneumophila* antibodies are best identified by reference or public health laboratories that have other typing sera and molecular identification methods in use.

Gram-negative rods isolated from clinical specimens that are morphologically consistent with *Legionella* spp. and are L-cysteine dependent for growth, can be reported as presumptive *Legionella* spp. in the absence of reactivity with typing sera. Gram-negative rods characteristic of *Legionella* spp. that react with *L. pneumophila* monoclonal antibody or *L. pneumophila* serogroup 1 polyclonal antibody can be presumptively identified as *L. pneumophila* or *L. pneumophila* serogroup 1, and the identification can be finalized the next day once L-cysteine growth dependence is confirmed. If the isolate is nonreactive with *L. pneumophila* species-specific antibody or if it is *L. pneumophila* but not serogroup 1, then the isolate should be further typed by a reference laboratory. All clinical isolates should be frozen at −70°C in tryptic soy broth in 10% glycerol and subcultured on a BCYEα slant for possible analysis by public health authorities.

Advanced Identification

Accurate identification of *Legionella* spp. other than *L. pneumophila* and *L. pneumophila* serogroup 1 can be quite difficult because of serologic cross-reactivities between species and serogroups, biochemical inertness, and phenotypic identity of different species. Identification to the species or serogroup level for these bacteria is usually not of major clinical significance but may have significant public health and scientific importance. Infection caused by *Legionella*

spp. other than *L. pneumophila* or *L. longbeachae* almost always occurs in immunocompromised patients, so identification of these other *Legionella* spp. could very rarely be a clue to occult immunosuppression (85). LD caused by *Legionella* spp. other than *L. pneumophila* may respond more poorly to erythromycin therapy (38), but whether knowing the identification of the *Legionella* spp. causing infection would influence patient outcome is debatable, especially since erythromycin is no longer the treatment of choice for severe LD (30). Investigation of LD outbreaks, and sometimes single cases of the disease, requires knowledge of *Legionella* spp. identity and subtype; this identification, if needed, can be performed by a public health or reference laboratory as long as isolates are frozen. The identification techniques used by reference laboratories include serotyping using collections of antisera, biochemical characterization, and sequence-based identification.

Serotyping of *Legionella* spp. is carried out using polyclonal antisera produced by the U.S. CDC, other public health agencies, and commercial laboratories (m-TECH, Denka Seiken, Oxoid, and others). Either immunofluorescence or agglutination reactions are used, with no clear evidence of superiority of one technique over the other (113). Some producers make polyvalent serum pools that react with a large number of species or serogroups, which can be useful to reduce the number of monovalent antisera used. The specificity of the polyvalent antisera has not been studied in great detail, although at least one product reacted with a number of non-*Legionella* spp. (31). This makes it important that monovalent typing be carried out and that the bacteria meet minimal phenotypic criteria for *Legionella* spp. Unfortunately, cross-reactions between different species and serogroups occur even when using monovalent antisera (1, 95, 99, 106, 111, 119). Use of cross-adsorbed polyvalent antisera has been described as a research tool to avoid this problem of cross-reactions, but these reagents are not available outside some research laboratories (6, 110, 112). In addition to intragenus cross-reactions, a large number of cross-reactions of monovalent polyclonal antibodies to non-*Legionella* spp. have been reported, including *P. aeruginosa*, *Flavobacterium* spp., *Bacteroides fragilis*, *Capnocytophaga ochracea*, *B. pertussis*, *Bordetella bronchiseptica*, and possibly *Burkholderia pseudomallei* (7, 14, 15, 33, 50, 68, 71). Antibody to *L. pneumophila* serogroup 1 is quite specific, but otherwise, enough cross-reactions exist to make serological identification only presumptive. Antisera to newer *Legionella* spp. are often unavailable.

Monoclonal typing antibodies reduce the number of cross-reactions with gram-negative bacteria but are only commercially available for the identification of *L. pneumophila* (13, 28, 58, 108). However, great care must be used by experienced microbiologists, as cross-reactions with some non-*Legionella* spp. have been reported with the *L. pneumophila*-specific monoclonal antibody, including *S. aureus*, yeasts, and *Bacillus* spp.

Legionella spp. are relatively inert biochemically and will not be identified using conventional tube or commercial panel biochemical tests. The few biochemical characteristics described for *Legionella* spp. that can be determined in most laboratories, such as oxidase, catalase, and β-lactamase tests, can be nonspecific and, if performed improperly, falsely negative. Use of a research biochemical panel has been described to facilitate the identification of *Legionella* spp. (115).

Determination of cellular fatty acid and isoprenoid quinone composition by gas-liquid chromatography and high-pressure liquid chromatography, respectively, can be successfully used to identify many *Legionella* spp. (75). These techniques require the use of expensive equipment, are highly complex, and have been supplanted by molecular methods. The cellular composition of several newer *Legionella* spp. have not been studied using these techniques, are not in commercial databases, or both, making identification of these newer species by these methods difficult.

The gold standard for the identification of new *Legionella* spp. has been DNA-DNA hybridization analysis (9). This method is tedious, expensive, and labor-intensive and requires special expertise as well as a large collection of reference DNA standards. As such, DNA-DNA hybridization analysis is not used to identify already known species.

Molecular identification of *Legionella* spp. has now replaced other identification techniques in research and specialty laboratories for several reasons. These include the labor cost and time required to serotype a strain, serological cross-reactions, limited availability of antibodies to newer strains, the lack of specific and easy biochemical characterization methods, and the increasing availability of inexpensive DNA sequencing. Molecular identification methods take advantage of the specific 16S rRNA or *mip* gene sequences of the different *Legionella* spp. (44, 78, 97, 101). A *mip* database, procedure instructions, including primer sequences, *mip* sequence alignment software, and other genomic software tools are all available online (http://www.hpa.org.uk/web/HPAweb&HPAwebStandard/HPAweb_C/1195733805138). Sequence analysis of 16S rRNA has been used to identify several new *Legionella* spp. (43, 76, 80, 93). Partial sequencing of 16S rRNA (500 bp) is able to accurately identify all *Legionella* spp. to the genus level and all *L. pneumophila* and about 90% of *Legionella* spp. other than *L. pneumophila* to the species level; incorrect species-level identification is a problem for the more unusual *Legionella* spp. (120). Sequence of the *rpoB* gene has been shown to distinguish between species as well as or better than 16S rRNA or *mip* gene sequencing (72). Intergenic 16S-23S ribosomal spacer PCR analysis has been successful for species identification and does not require DNA sequencing (100). The relative performances of *mip* and 16S rRNA sequencing is not known, but partial 16S rRNA sequencing should not solely be relied upon when an unusual *Legionella* sp. is identified. Limited numbers of reference strains, especially of some unusual species, have been tested by these methods, leaving open the possibility of incorrect classifications. A commercial plate DNA hybridization assay has been reported to correctly identify 23 different *Legionella* spp. (36) and is distributed in Japan (Kobayashi Pharmaceutical, Osaka, Japan).

Molecular methods cannot be used to accurately serogroup *L. pneumophila*, as there are several reports of genotypic discordances for identical serogroups and vice versa (10, 56, 81). Sequencing of the *L. pneumophila dnaJ* gene appeared to be able to distinguish between some, but not all, *L. pneumophila* serogroups (78); different serogroups that had very similar genotypes had been shown by other methods to have discordant genotypes and serogroups. More extensive testing of this method needs to be performed before it is put into routine use.

TYPING SYSTEMS

Typing of *Legionella* spp. is important for public health investigations to help link culture-positive environmental sites with clinical isolates during an epidemic of the disease.

Typing cannot be used by itself to determine the environmental source of an outbreak and must be accompanied by an epidemiologic investigation. Otherwise, incorrect conclusions may be made about epidemic sources (57, 73). This problem is due to clonal distributions of environmental and clinical *Legionella* spp. (3, 65, 77, 96) and to the poor specificity of some typing techniques (22, 96).

Monoclonal antibody typing plays a major role in subtyping *L. pneumophila* serogroup 1 isolates and, when used with molecular methods, can increase typing specificity (42, 45, 96). Used by itself, monoclonal antibody typing may not be specific enough to distinguish between closely related strains.

Sequence-based typing appears to be the most specific and precise molecular subtyping system for both *L. pneumophila* and *L. pneumophila* serogroup 1 (98). A standardized pulsed-field gel electrophoresis method yields reproducible results and is used as a reference typing method by one national laboratory (3).

SEROLOGIC TESTS

LD can be diagnosed by demonstration of an increase in antibodies to killed bacterial cells (26). Indirect immunofluorescent assay is considered the gold standard method. While most patients develop both immunoglobulin G (IgG) and IgM responses, some develop only IgM-only, IgG-only, or IgA-only responses, making it necessary to test for total immunoglobulin response and not just IgG. In addition, IgM antibodies may persist for as long as a year after infection, making IgM presence a poor marker of acute disease (88). About 75% of patients with culture-proven nosocomial *L. pneumophila* serogroup 1 LD develop seroconversion to the bacterium, whereas the test seems to have higher sensitivity in LD epidemics. Seroconversion requires weeks to months after infection, with only about a 50% seroconversion rate after 2 weeks; for optimal test sensitivity, acute-phase serum should be frozen and convalescent-phase sera should be collected at 2, 4, 6, 9, and 12 weeks postinfection. Parallel testing of sera is required for the best specificity. The most specific testing is for seroconversion to *L. pneumophila* serogroup 1 only and the least specific is the use of polyvalent antigen preparations, with approximate test specificities of 99 and 90 to 95%, respectively. Serologic diagnosis is best used for epidemiologic studies because of the retrospective nature of serologic diagnosis and limitations on test specificity and sensitivity.

ANTIMICROBIAL SUSCEPTIBILITIES AND SUSCEPTIBILITY TESTING

The antimicrobial susceptibility of *L. pneumophila* grown in broth or on agar can give results that have no clinical correlate. This is because of the intracellular location of the bacterium in human infection, to which not all antimicrobial agents gain access and retain activity (23). In addition, the complex broth and agar media used to grow *L. pneumophila* inactivate many drugs. There is no indication for performing antimicrobial susceptibility testing against *Legionella* spp. except in a research setting, when correlative studies of intracellular and experimental animal infection models can be performed. The microbiologist must not assume that a particular drug will be effective for the treatment of LD simply because the drug is active against *L. pneumophila* in vitro, nor should there be an assumption that drugs having low MICs against the bacterium in vitro will be more clinically effective than will drugs with higher MICs for the organism. Antimicrobial resistance to drugs used for LD treatment has never been documented to be responsible for clinical treatment failures and has only been demonstrated under laboratory conditions.

Antimicrobial agents that have good intracellular activity against *L. pneumophila* include most macrolide, tetracycline, ketolide, and quinolone antimicrobial agents (23, 30). No β-lactam agent or aminoglycoside has acceptable intracellular activity against the bacterium. It is unknown if the intracellular activity of antimicrobial agents against *L. pneumophila* can be extrapolated to all other *Legionella* spp. and to treatment of infections caused by *Legionella* spp. other than *L. pneumophila*. Some of these other *Legionella* spp. may reside in different subcellular compartments than does *L. pneumophila* and, thus, may respond differently to antimicrobial agents (91). However, macrolide and quinolone antimicrobials appear to be effective for the treatment of LD caused by *L. micdadei*, *L. longbeachae*, *L. bozemanae*, and *L. dumoffii* (85).

EVALUATION, INTERPRETATION, AND REPORTING OF RESULTS

Multiple laboratory methods have to be used for optimal laboratory diagnosis of LD. Culture of *Legionella* bacteria from sputum, lung, or other respiratory sites is the most specific (100%) method for diagnosis of the disease, very sensitive (~80 to 90%) in severe untreated disease, and insensitive (~20%) in those with mild disease. Culture may be the only positive diagnostic test, especially when *Legionella* bacteria other than *L. pneumophila* are causing the infection. In addition, a culture isolate can be used to sort out the source of an epidemic, unlike any of the other diagnostic tests. Because of the technical difficulty of culture diagnosis, its expense, and its low sensitivity for nonsevere disease, several alternative diagnostic methods have been developed. The antigenuria assay is more sensitive than culture for the detection of community-acquired disease, especially epidemic disease. Still, the antigenuria test is only about 60% sensitive in the best of circumstances, performs poorly for detection of nosocomial infection, and detects almost exclusively *L. pneumophila* serogroup 1. Antibody detection complements other laboratory diagnostic methods but is retrospective, as it requires seroconversion for greater test specificity and sensitivity. In addition, antibody results obtained using only polyvalent antigens must be viewed with circumspection. Commercial molecular amplification tests are just being marketed and have yet to be thoroughly evaluated; prior to adoption, more extensive studies are required. The performance of all laboratory diagnostic tests for non-*L. pneumophila* serogroup 1 LD is unknown but presumably is not as good as it is for the diagnosis of *L. pneumophila* serogroup 1 disease.

A major hindrance to the evaluation of all laboratory diagnostic methods is the lack of a good gold standard for diagnosis of LD. Culture diagnosis, while very specific, is known to be imperfect and of limited sensitivity, especially for epidemic LD. Relative performance of the diagnostic tests is often compared to culture diagnosis, which tends to overestimate test sensitivity and underestimate specificity.

Positive cultures for all *Legionella* spp. are virtually diagnostic of LD, providing there are supportive clinical findings such as pneumonia. In contrast, single serum specimens showing elevated antibodies to *Legionella* spp.

or to *L. pneumophila* are often not the result of LD. Only rises in antibody titers to *L. pneumophila* serogroup 1, a test not usually commercially available, are specific enough for diagnosis, but even then, use of appropriate techniques is required for optimal specificity. Detection of *L. pneumophila* serogroup 1 antigenuria is almost as specific as a positive culture once heat-labile factors capable of causing false-positive tests are excluded. Positive test results must be reported promptly to the patient's clinician as well as to infection control and public health authorities.

REFERENCES

1. **Adeleke, A. A., B. S. Fields, R. F. Benson, M. I. Daneshvar, J. M. Pruckler, R. M. Ratcliff, T. G. Harrison, R. S. Weyant, R. J. Birtles, D. Raoult, and M. A. Halablab.** 2001. *Legionella drozanskii* sp. nov., *Legionella rowbothamii* sp. nov. and *Legionella fallonii* sp. nov.: three unusual new *Legionella* species. *Int. J. Syst. Evol. Microbiol.* **51:**1151–1160.
2. **Amer, A. O., and M. S. Swanson.** 2002. A phagosome of one's own: a microbial guide to life in the macrophage. *Curr. Opin. Microbiol.* **5:**56–61.
3. **Aurell, H., J. Etienne, F. Forey, M. Reyrolle, P. Girardo, P. Farge, B. Decludt, C. Campese, F. Vandenesch, and S. Jarraud.** 2003. *Legionella pneumophila* serogroup 1 strain Paris: endemic distribution throughout France. *J. Clin. Microbiol.* **41:**3320–3322.
4. **Bencini, M. A., A. J. van den Brule, E. C. Claas, M. H. Hermans, W. J. Melchers, G. T. Noordhoek, M. M. Salimans, J. Schirm, C. Vink, Z. A. van der, and R. Jansen.** 2007. Multicenter comparison of molecular methods for detection of *Legionella* spp. in sputum samples. *J. Clin. Microbiol.* **45:**3390–3392.
5. **Benin, A. L., R. F. Benson, and R. E. Besser.** 2002. Trends in legionnaires disease, 1980–1998: declining mortality and new patterns of diagnosis. *Clin. Infect. Dis.* **35:**1039–1046.
6. **Benson, R. F., W. L. Thacker, J. A. Lanser, N. Sangster, W. R. Mayberry, and D. J. Brenner.** 1991. *Legionella adelaidensis*, a new species isolated from cooling tower water. *J. Clin. Microbiol.* **29:**1004–1006.
7. **Benson, R. F., W. L. Thacker, B. B. Plikaytis, and H. W. Wilkinson.** 1987. Cross-reactions in *Legionella* antisera with *Bordetella pertussis* strains. *J. Clin. Microbiol.* **25:**594–596.
8. **Bentz, J. S., K. Carroll, J. H. Ward, M. Elstad, and C. J. Marshall.** 2000. Acid-fast-positive *Legionella pneumophila*: a possible pitfall in the cytologic diagnosis of mycobacterial infection in pulmonary specimens. *Diagn. Cytopathol.* **22:**45–48.
9. **Brenner, D. J.** 1987. Classification of the legionellae. *Semin. Respir. Infect.* **2:**190–205.
10. **Brenner, D. J., A. G. Steigerwalt, P. Epple, W. F. Bibb, R. M. McKinney, R. W. Starnes, J. M. Colville, R. K. Selander, P. H. Edelstein, and C. W. Moss.** 1988. *Legionella pneumophila* serogroup Lansing 3 isolated from a patient with fatal pneumonia, and descriptions of *L. pneumophila* subsp. *pneumophila* subsp. nov., *L. pneumophila* subsp. *fraseri* subsp. nov., and *L. pneumophila* subsp. *pascullei* subsp. nov. *J. Clin. Microbiol.* **26:**1695–1703.
11. **Cazalet, C., S. Jarraud, Y. Ghavi-Helm, F. Kunst, P. Glaser, J. Etienne, and C. Buchrieser.** 2008. Multigenome analysis identifies a worldwide distributed epidemic *Legionella pneumophila* clone that emerged within a highly diverse species. *Genome Res.* **18:**431–441.
12. **Cazalet, C., C. Rusniok, H. Bruggemann, N. Zidane, A. Magnier, L. Ma, M. Tichit, S. Jarraud, C. Bouchier, F. Vandenesch, F. Kunst, J. Etienne, P. Glaser, and C. Buchrieser.** 2004. Evidence in the *Legionella pneumophila* genome for exploitation of host cell functions and high genome plasticity. *Nat. Genet.* **36:**1165–1173.
13. **Cercenado, E., P. H. Edelstein, L. H. Gosting, and J. C. Sturge.** 1987. *Legionella micdadei* and *Legionella dumoffii* monoclonal antibodies for laboratory diagnosis of *Legionella* infections. *J. Clin. Microbiol.* **25:**2163–2167.

14. **Chen, S., L. Hicks, M. Yuen, D. Mitchell, and G. L. Gilbert.** 1994. Serological cross-reaction between *Legionella* spp. and *Capnocytophaga ochracea* by using latex agglutination test. *J. Clin. Microbiol.* **32:**3054–3055.

15. **Collins, M. T., F. Espersen, N. Høiby, S. N. Cho, A. Friss-Møller, and J. S. Reif.** 1983. Cross-reactions between *Legionella pneumophila* (serogroup 1) and twenty-eight other bacterial species, including other members of the family *Legionellaceae. Infect. Immun.* **39:**1441–1456.

16. **den Boer, J. W., E. P. Yzerman, J. Schellekens, K. D. Lettinga, H. C. Boshuizen, J. E. Van Steenbergen, A. Bosman, H. S. Van den, H. A. Van Vliet, M. F. Peeters, R. J. van Ketel, P. Speelman, J. L. Kool, and M. A. Conyn-van Spaendonck.** 2002. A large outbreak of Legionnaires' disease at a flower show, the Netherlands, 1999. *Emerg. Infect. Dis.* **8:**37–43.

17. **Dennis, P. J., J. A. Taylor, and G. I. Barrow.** 1981. Phosphate buffered, low sodium chloride blood agar medium for *Legionella pneumophila. Lancet* **ii:**636.

18. **Diederen, B. M., J. A. Kluytmans, C. M. Vandenbroucke-Grauls, and M. F. Peeters.** 2008. Utility of real-time PCR for diagnosis of Legionnaires' disease in routine clinical practice. *J. Clin. Microbiol.* **46:**671–677.

19. **Diederen, B. M., and M. F. Peeters.** 2007. Evaluation of the SAS Legionella Test, a new immunochromatographic assay for the detection of *Legionella pneumophila* serogroup 1 antigen in urine. *Clin. Microbiol. Infect.* **13:**86–88.

20. **Doleans, A., H. Aurell, M. Reyrolle, G. Lina, J. Freney, F. Vandenesch, J. Etienne, and S. Jarraud.** 2004. Clinical and environmental distributions of *Legionella* strains in France are different. *J. Clin. Microbiol.* **42:**458–460.

21. **Domínguez, J. A., J. M. Manterola, R. Blavia, N. Sopena, F. J. Belda, E. Padilla, M. Gimenez, M. Sabria, J. Morera, and V. Ausina.** 1996. Detection of *Legionella pneumophila* serogroup-1 antigen in nonconcentrated urine and urine concentrated by selective ultrafiltration. *J. Clin. Microbiol.* **34:**2334–2336.

22. **Drenning, S. D., J. E. Stout, J. R. Joly, and V. L. Yu.** 2001. Unexpected similarity of pulsed-field gel electrophoresis patterns of unrelated clinical isolates of *Legionella pneumophila,* serogroup 1. *J. Infect. Dis.* **183:**628–632.

23. **Edelstein, P. H.** 1995. Antimicrobial chemotherapy for legionnaires' disease: a review. *Clin. Infect. Dis.* **21:**S265–S276.

24. **Edelstein, P. H.** 1999. The guinea-pig model of Legionnaires' disease, p. 303–314. *In* O. Zak and M. A. Sande (ed.), *Handbook of Animal Models of Infection.* Academic Press, London, United Kingdom.

25. **Edelstein, P. H.** 2004. Detection of *Legionella* antigen by direct immunofluorescence, p. 11.3.1–11.3.7. *In* H. D. Isenberg (ed. in chief), *Clinical Microbiology Procedures Handbook,* 2nd ed. ASM Press, Washington, DC.

26. **Edelstein, P. H.** 2006. Detection of antibodies to *Legionella,* p. 468–476. *In* B. Detrick, R. G. Hamilton, and J. D. Folds (ed.), *Manual of Molecular and Clinical Laboratory Immunology,* 7th ed. ASM Press, Washington, DC.

27. **Edelstein, P. H.** Urinary antigen detection for *Legionella* spp, p. 11.4.1–11.4.7. *In* L. S. Garcia (ed. in chief), *Clinical Microbiology Procedures Handbook,* 3rd ed., vol. 3. ASM Press, Washington, DC.

28. **Edelstein, P. H., K. B. Beer, J. C. Sturge, A. J. Watson, and L. C. Goldstein.** 1985. Clinical utility of a monoclonal direct fluorescent reagent specific for *Legionella pneumophila*: comparative study with other reagents. *J. Clin. Microbiol.* **22:**419–421.

29. **Edelstein, P. H., and N. P. Cianciotto.** 2001. *Legionella* species and Legionnaires' disease. *In* M. Dworkin, S. Falkow, E. Rosenberg, K. H. Schleifer, and E. Stackebrandt (ed.), *The Prokaryotes: an Evolving Electronic Resource for the Microbiological Community.* Springer-Verlag, New York, NY.

30. **Edelstein, P. H., and N. P. Cianciotto.** 2010. *Legionella. In* G. L. Mandell, J. E. Bennett, and R. Dolin (ed.), *Principles and Practice of Infectious Diseases,* 7th ed. Elsevier, Philadelphia, PA.

31. **Edelstein, P. H., and M. A. C. Edelstein.** 1989. Evaluation of the Merifluor-*Legionella* immunofluorescent reagent for identifying and detecting 21 *Legionella* species. *J. Clin. Microbiol.* **27:**2455–2458.

32. **Edelstein, P. H., and S. M. Finegold.** 1979. Use of a semiselective medium to culture *Legionella pneumophila* from contaminated lung specimens. *J. Clin. Microbiol.* **10:**141–143.

33. **Edelstein, P. H., R. M. McKinney, R. D. Meyer, M. A. C. Edelstein, C. J. Krause, and S. M. Finegold.** 1980. Immunologic diagnosis of Legionnaires' disease: cross-reactions with anaerobic and microaerophilic organisms and infections caused by them. *J. Infect. Dis.* **141:**652–655.

34. **Edelstein, P. H., R. D. Meyer, and S. M. Finegold.** 1980. Laboratory diagnosis of Legionnaires' disease. *Am. Rev. Respir. Dis.* **121:**317–327.

35. **Evans, G. E., D. R. Murdoch, T. P. Anderson, H. C. Potter, P. M. George, and S. T. Chambers.** 2003. Contamination of Qiagen DNA extraction kits with Legionella DNA. *J. Clin. Microbiol.* **41:**3452–3453.

36. **Ezaki, T., Y. Hashimoto, H. Yamamoto, M. L. Lucida, S. L. Liu, S. Kusunoki, K. Asano, and E. Yabuuchi.** 1990. Evaluation of the microplate hybridization method for rapid identification of *Legionella* species. *Eur. J. Clin. Microbiol. Infect. Dis.* **9:**213–217.

37. **Faine, S., P. Edelstein, B. D. Kirby, and S. M. Finegold.** 1979. Rapid presumptive bacteriological diagnosis of Legionnaires disease. *J. Clin. Microbiol.* **10:**104–105.

38. **Fang, G.-D., V. L. Yu, and R. M. Vickers.** 1989. Disease due to the *Legionellaceae* (other than *Legionella pneumophila*). Historical, microbiological, clinical, and epidemiological review. *Medicine* (Baltimore) **68:**116–132.

39. **Ferrer, A., P. Bellver, and P. Royo.** 1995. Screening quality of respiratory samples and *Legionella pneumoniae* [sic]. *J. Clin. Microbiol.* **33:**1971.

40. **Fields, B. S., T. Haupt, J. P. Davis, M. J. Arduino, P. H. Miller, and J. C. Butler.** 2001. Pontiac fever due to *Legionella micdadei* from a whirlpool spa: possible role of bacterial endotoxin. *J. Infect. Dis.* **184:**1289–1292.

41. **Fraser, D. W., T. R. Tsai, W. Orenstein, W. E. Parkin, H. J. Beecham, R. G. Sharrar, J. Harris, G. F. Mallison, S. M. Martin, J. E. McDade, C. C. Shepard, and P. S. Brachman.** 1977. Legionnaires' disease: description of an epidemic of pneumonia. *N. Engl. J. Med.* **297:**1189–1197.

42. **Fry, N. K., J. M. Bangsborg, S. Bernander, J. Etienne, B. Forsblom, V. Gaia, P. Hasenberger, D. Lindsay, A. Papoutsi, C. Pelaz, M. Struelens, S. A. Uldum, P. Visca, and T. G. Harrison.** 2000. Assessment of intercentre reproducibility and epidemiological concordance of *Legionella pneumophila* serogroup 1 genotyping by amplified fragment length polymorphism analysis. *Eur. J. Clin. Microbiol. Infect. Dis.* **19:**773–780.

43. **Fry, N. K., T. J. Rowbotham, N. A. Saunders, and T. M. Embley.** 1991. Direct amplification and sequencing of the 16S ribosomal DNA of an intracellular *Legionella* species recovered by amoebal enrichment from the sputum of a patient with pneumonia. *FEMS Microbiol. Lett.* **67:**165–168.

44. **Fry, N. K., S. Warwick, N. A. Saunders, and T. M. Embley.** 1991. The use of 16S ribosomal RNA analyses to investigate the phylogeny of the family *Legionellaceae. J. Gen. Microbiol.* **137:**1215–1222.

45. **Gaia, V., N. K. Fry, B. Afshar, P. C. Luck, H. Meugnier, J. Etienne, R. Peduzzi, and T. G. Harrison.** 2005. Consensus sequence-based scheme for epidemiological typing of clinical and environmental isolates of *Legionella pneumophila. J. Clin. Microbiol.* **43:**2047–2052.

46. **Garduño, R. A., E. Garduño, M. Hiltz, and P. S. Hoffman.** 2002. Intracellular growth of *Legionella pneumophila* gives rise to a differentiated form dissimilar to stationary-phase forms. *Infect. Immun.* **70:**6273–6283.

47. **Garrity, G. M., A. Brown, and R. M. Vickers.** 1980. *Tatlockia* and *Fluoribacter*: two new genera of organisms resembling *Legionella pneumophila. Int. J. Syst. Bacteriol.* **30:**609–614.

48. **Ginevra, C., C. Barranger, A. Ros, O. Mory, J. L. Stephan, F. Freymuth, M. Joannes, B. Pozzetto, and F. Grattard.** 2005. Development and evaluation of Chlamylege, a new commercial test allowing simultaneous detection and identification of *Legionella, Chlamydophila pneumoniae,* and *Mycoplasma pneumoniae* in clinical respiratory specimens by multiplex PCR. *J. Clin. Microbiol.* **43:**3247–3254.

49. **Ginevra, C., F. Forey, C. Campese, M. Reyrolle, D. Che, J. Etienne, and S. Jarraud.** 2008. Lorraine strain of *Legionella pneumophila* serogroup 1, France. *Emerg. Infect. Dis.* **14:**673–675.

50. **Glupczynski, Y., M. Labbe, and E. Yourassowsky.** 1984. Cross-reactivity of environmental bacteria with fluorescent-antibody conjugates for *Legionella pneumophila*. *Eur. J. Clin. Microbiol. Infect. Dis.* **3:**215.

51. **Gotz, H. M., A. Tegnell, J. De, K. A. Broholm, M. Kuusi, I. Kallings, and K. Ekdahl.** 2001. A whirlpool associated outbreak of Pontiac fever at a hotel in Northern Sweden. *Epidemiol. Infect.* **126:**241–247.

52. **Grau, S., J. M. Antonio, E. Ribes, M. Salvado, J. M. Garces, and J. Garau.** 2006. Impact of rifampicin addition to clarithromycin in *Legionella pneumophila* pneumonia. *Int. J. Antimicrob. Agents* **28:**249–252.

53. **Greer, P. W., F. W. Chandler, and M. D. Hicklin.** 1980. Rapid demonstration of *Legionella pneumophila* in unembedded tissue. An adaptation of the Gimenez stain. *Am. J. Clin. Pathol.* **73:**788–790.

54. **Guerrero, C., C. M. Toldos, G. Yagüe, C. Ramírez, T. Rodríguez, and M. Segovia.** 2004. Comparison of diagnostic sensitivities of three assays (Bartels enzyme immunoassay [EIA], Biotest EIA, and Binax NOW immunochromatographic test) for detection of *Legionella pneumophila* serogroup 1 antigen in urine. *J. Clin. Microbiol.* **42:**467–468.

55. **Harrison, T. G., B. Afshar, N. Doshi, N. K. Fry, and J. V. Lee.** 2009. Distribution of *Legionella pneumophila* serogroups, monoclonal antibody subgroups and DNA sequence types in recent clinical and environmental isolates from England and Wales (2000–2008). *Eur. J Clin. Microbiol. Infect. Dis.* **28:**781–791.

56. **Harrison, T. G., N. A. Saunders, A. Haththotuwa, N. Doshi, and A. G. Taylor.** 1992. Further evidence that genotypically closely related strains of *Legionella pneumophila* can express different serogroup specific antigens. *J. Med. Microbiol.* **37:**155–161.

57. **Heath, T. C., C. Roberts, B. Jalaludin, I. Goldthrope, and A. G. Capon.** 1998. Environmental investigation of a legionellosis outbreak in western Sydney: the role of molecular profiling. *Aust. N. Z. J. Public Health* **22:**428–431.

58. **Helbig, J. H., P. C. Luck, and W. Witzleb.** 1994. Serogroup-specific and serogroup-cross-reactive epitopes of *Legionella pneumophila*. *Int. J. Med. Microbiol. Virol. Parasitol. Infect. Dis.* **281:**16–23.

59. **Helbig, J. H., S. A. Uldum, S. Bernander, P. C. Luck, G. Wewalka, B. Abraham, V. Gaia, and T. G. Harrison.** 2003. Clinical utility of urinary antigen detection for diagnosis of community-acquired, travel-associated, and nosocomial legionnaires' disease. *J. Clin. Microbiol.* **41:**838–840.

60. **Helbig, J. H., S. A. Uldum, P. C. Luck, and T. G. Harrison.** 2001. Detection of *Legionella pneumophila* antigen in urine samples by the BinaxNOW immunochromatographic assay and comparison with both Binax Legionella Urinary Enzyme Immunoassay (EIA) and Biotest Legionella Urin Antigen EIA. *J. Med. Microbiol.* **50:**509–516.

61. **Helbig, J. H., S. A. Uldum, P. C. Lück, and T. G. Harrison.** 2002. Detection of *Legionella pneumophila* antigen in urine samples: recognition of serogroups and monoclonal serogroups, p. 204–206. *In* R. Marre, Y. Abu Kwaik, C. Bartlett, N. P. Cianciotto, B. S. Fields, M. Frosch, J. Hacker, and P. C. Lück (ed.), *Legionella*. ASM Press, Washington, DC.

62. **Herpers, B. L., B. M. de Jongh, K. van der Zwaluw, and E. J. van Hannen.** 2003. Real-time PCR assay targets the 23S-5S spacer for direct detection and differentiation of *Legionella* spp. and *Legionella pneumophila*. *J. Clin. Microbiol.* **41:**4815–4816.

63. **Hilton, E., R. A. Freedman, F. Cintron, H. D. Isenberg, and C. Singer.** 1986. Acid-fast bacilli in sputum: a case of *Legionella micdadei* pneumonia. *J. Clin. Microbiol.* **24:**1102–1103.

64. **Horn, J.** 2002. Comparison of non-serogroup 1 detection by Biotest and Binax *Legionella* urinary antigen enzyme immunoassays, p. 207–210. *In* R. Marre, Y. Abu Kwaik, C. Bartlett, N. P. Cianciotto, B. S. Fields, M. Frosch, J. Hacker, and P. C. Lück (ed.), *Legionella*. ASM Press, Washington, DC.

65. **Huang, B., B. A. Heron, B. R. Gray, S. Eglezos, J. R. Bates, and J. Savill.** 2004. A predominant and virulent *Legionella pneumophila* serogroup 1 strain detected in isolates from patients and water in Queensland, Australia, by an amplified fragment length polymorphism protocol and virulence gene-based PCR assays. *J. Clin. Microbiol.* **42:**4164–4168.

66. **Ingram, J. G., and J. F. Plouffe.** 1994. Danger of sputum purulence screens in culture of *Legionella* species. *J. Clin. Microbiol.* **32:**209–210.

67. **Isberg, R. R., T. J. O'Connor, and M. Heidtman.** 2009. The *Legionella pneumophila* replication vacuole: making a cosy niche inside host cells. *Nat. Rev. Microbiol.* **7:**13–24.

68. **Jimenez-Lucho, V., M. Shulman, and J. Johnson.** 1994. *Bordetella bronchiseptica* in an AIDS patient cross-reacts with *Legionella* antisera. *J. Clin. Microbiol.* **32:**3095–3096.

69. **Kerr, E., H. Snell, B. L. Black, M. Storey, and W. D. Colby.** 1992. Isolation of *Nocardia asteroides* from respiratory specimens by using selective buffered charcoal-yeast extract agar. *J. Clin. Microbiol.* **30:**1320–1322.

70. **Khanna, M., J. Fan, K. Pehler-Harrington, C. Waters, P. Douglass, J. Stallock, S. Kehl, and K. J. Henrickson.** 2005. The pneumoplex assays, a multiplex PCR-enzyme hybridization assay that allows simultaneous detection of five organisms, *Mycoplasma pneumoniae, Chlamydia (Chlamydophila) pneumoniae, Legionella pneumophila, Legionella micdadei,* and *Bordetella pertussis,* and its real-time counterpart. *J. Clin. Microbiol.* **43:**565–571.

71. **Klein, G. C.** 1980. Cross-reaction to *Legionella pneumophila* antigen in sera with elevated titers to *Pseudomonas pseudomallei*. *J. Clin. Microbiol.* **11:**27–29.

72. **Ko, K. S., H. K. Lee, M. Y. Park, K. H. Lee, Y. J. Yun, S. Y. Woo, H. Miyamoto, and Y. H. Kook.** 2002. Application of RNA polymerase beta-subunit gene (*rpoB*) sequences for the molecular differentiation of *Legionella* species. *J. Clin. Microbiol.* **40:**2653–2658.

73. **Kool, J. L., U. Buchholz, C. Peterson, E. W. Brown, R. F. Benson, J. M. Pruckler, B. S. Fields, J. Sturgeon, E. Lehnkering, R. Cordova, L. M. Mascola, and J. C. Butler.** 2000. Strengths and limitations of molecular subtyping in a community outbreak of Legionnaires' disease. *Epidemiol. Infect.* **125:**599–608.

74. **Kozak, N. A., R. F. Benson, E. Brown, N. T. Alexander, T. H. Taylor, Jr., B. G. Shelton, and B. S. Fields.** 2009. Distribution of *lag-1* alleles and sequence-based types among *Legionella pneumophila* serogroup 1 clinical and environmental isolates in the United States. *J. Clin. Microbiol.* **47:**2525–2535.

75. **Lambert, M. A., and C. W. Moss.** 1989. Cellular fatty acid compositions and isoprenoid quinone contents of 23 *Legionella* species. *J. Clin. Microbiol.* **27:**465–473.

76. **La Scola, B., R. J. Birtles, G. Greub, T. J. Harrison, R. M. Ratcliff, and D. Raoult.** 2004. *Legionella drancourtii* sp. nov., a strictly intracellular amoebal pathogen. *Int. J. Syst. Evol. Microbiol.* **54:**699–703.

77. **Lawrence, C., M. Reyrolle, S. Dubrou, F. Forey, B. Decludt, C. Goulvestre, P. Matsiota-Bernard, J. Etienne, and C. Nauciel.** 1999. Single clonal origin of a high proportion of *Legionella pneumophila* serogroup 1 isolates from patients and the environment in the area of Paris, France, over a 10-year period. *J. Clin. Microbiol.* **37:**2652–2655.

78. **Liu, H., Y. Li, X. Huang, Y. Kawamura, and T. Ezaki.** 2003. Use of the *dnaJ* gene for the detection and identification of all *Legionella pneumophila* serogroups and description of the primers used to detect 16S rDNA gene sequences of major members of the genus *Legionella*. *Microbiol. Immunol.* **47:**859–869.

79. **Loens, K., T. Beck, D. Ursi, M. Overdijk, P. Sillekens, H. Goossens, and M. Ieven.** 2008. Evaluation of different nucleic acid amplification techniques for the detection of M. *pneumoniae, C. pneumoniae* and *Legionella* spp. in respiratory specimens from patients with community-acquired pneumonia. *J. Microbiol. Methods* **73:**257–262.

80. **LoPresti, F., S. Riffard, H. Meugnier, M. Reyrolle, Y. Lasne, P. A. Grimont, F. Grimont, F. Vandenesch, J. Etienne, J. Fleurette, and J. Freney.** 1999. *Legionella taurinensis* sp. nov., a new species antigenically similar to *Legionella spiritensis*. *Int. J. Syst. Bacteriol.* **49:**397–403.

81. **Luck, P. C., R. J. Birtles, and J. H. Helbig.** 1995. Correlation of MAb subgroups with genotype in closely related *Legionella pneumophila* serogroup 1 strains from a cooling tower. *J. Med. Microbiol.* **43:**50–54.

82. **Marston, B. J., J. F. Plouffe, T. M. File, Jr., B. A. Hackman, S. J. Salstrom, H. B. Lipman, M. S. Kolczak, R. F. Breiman, et al.** 1997. Incidence of community-acquired pneumonia requiring hospitalization. Results of a population-based active surveillance Study in Ohio. *Arch. Intern. Med.* **157:**1709–1718.

83. **McDade, J. E., C. C. Shepard, D. W. Fraser, T. R. Tsai, M. A. Redus, and W. R. Dowdle.** 1977. Legionnaires' disease: isolation of a bacterium and demonstration of its role in other respiratory disease. *N. Engl. J. Med.* **297:**1197–1203.

84. **Morrill, W. E., J. M. Barbaree, B. S. Fields, G. N. Sanden, and W. T. Martin.** 1990. Increased recovery of *Legionella micdadei* and *Legionella bozemanii* on buffered charcoal yeast extract agar supplemented with albumin. *J. Clin. Microbiol.* **28:**616–618.

85. **Muder, R. R., and V. L. Yu.** 2002. Infection due to Legionella species other than *L. pneumophila. Clin. Infect. Dis.* **35:**990–998.

86. **Murdoch, D. R.** 2003. Diagnosis of *Legionella* infection. *Clin. Infect. Dis.* **36:**64–69.

87. **Mykietiuk, A., J. Carratalà, N. Fernández-Sabé, J. Dorca, R. Verdaguer, F. Manresa, and F. Gudiol.** 2005. Clinical outcomes for hospitalized patients with *Legionella* pneumonia in the antigenuria era: the influence of levofloxacin therapy. *Clin. Infect. Dis.* **40:**794–799.

88. **Nagington, J., T. G. Wreghitt, J. O. Tobin, and A. D. Macrae.** 1979. The antibody response in Legionnaires' disease. *J. Hyg. Lond.* **83:**377–381.

89. **Nazarian, E. J., D. J. Bopp, A. Saylors, R. J. Limberger, and K. A. Musser.** 2008. Design and implementation of a protocol for the detection of *Legionella* in clinical and environmental samples. *Diagn. Microbiol. Infect. Dis.* **62:**125–132.

90. **Ng, V., L. Weir, M. K. York, and W. K. Hadley.** 1992. *Bordetella pertussis* versus non-*L. pneumophila Legionella* spp.: a continuing diagnostic challenge. *J. Clin. Microbiol.* **30:**3300–3301.

91. **Ogawa, M., A. Takade, H. Miyamoto, H. Taniguchi, and S. Yoshida.** 2001. Morphological variety of intracellular microcolonies of *Legionella* species in Vero cells. *Microbiol. Immunol.* **45:**557–562.

92. **Osterholm, M. T., T. D. Chin, D. O. Osborne, H. B. Dull, A. G. Dean, D. W. Fraser, P. S. Hayes, and W. N. Hall.** 1983. A 1957 outbreak of Legionnaires' disease associated with a meat packing plant. *Am. J. Epidemiol.* **117:**60–67.

93. **Park, M. Y., K. S. Ko, H. K. Lee, M. S. Park, and Y. H. Kook.** 2003. *Legionella busanensis* sp. nov., isolated from cooling tower water in Korea. *Int. J. Syst. Evol. Microbiol.* **53:**77–80.

94. **Pasculle, A. W., and D. McDevitt.** 2004. *Legionella* cultures, p. 3.11.4.1–3.11.4.14. *In* H. D. Isenberg (ed. in chief), *Clinical Microbiology Procedures Handbook*, 2nd ed. ASM Press, Washington, DC.

95. **Pelaz, C., L. García Albert, and C. M. Bourgon.** 1987. Cross-reactivity among *Legionella* species and serogroups. *Epidemiol. Infect.* **99:**641–646.

96. **Pruckler, J. M., L. A. Mermel, R. F. Benson, C. Giorgio, P. K. Cassiday, R. F. Breiman, C. G. Whitney, and B. S. Fields.** 1995. Comparison of *Legionella pneumophila* isolates by arbitrarily primed PCR and pulsed-field gel electrophoresis: analysis from seven epidemic investigations. *J. Clin. Microbiol.* **33:**2872–2875.

97. **Ratcliff, R. M., J. A. Lanser, P. A. Manning, and M. W. Heuzenroeder.** 1998. Sequence-based classification scheme for the genus *Legionella* targeting the *mip* gene. *J. Clin. Microbiol.* **36:**1560–1567.

98. **Ratzow, S., V. Gaia, J. H. Helbig, N. K. Fry, and P. C. Luck.** 2007. Addition of *neuA*, the gene encoding N-acylneuraminate cytidylyl transferase, increases the discriminatory ability of the consensus sequence-based scheme for typing *Legionella pneumophila* serogroup 1 strains. *J. Clin. Microbiol.* **45:**1965–1968.

99. **Richardson, I. R., and N. F. Lightfoot.** 1992. *Legionella pneumophila* species identification using a commercial latex agglutination kit: a potential cross-reaction problem with serogroup 12. *Med. Lab. Sci.* **49:**144–146.

100. **Riffard, S., F. LoPresti, P. Normand, F. Forey, M. Reyrolle, J. Etienne, and F. Vandenesch.** 1998. Species identification of *Legionella* via intergenic 16S-23S ribosomal spacer PCR analysis. *Int. J. Syst. Bacteriol.* **48:**723–730.

101. **Riffard, S., F. Vandenesch, M. Reyrolle, and J. Etienne.** 1996. Distribution of *mip*-related sequences in 39 species (48 serogroups) of *Legionellaceae. Epidemiol. Infect.* **117:**501–506.

102. **Rowbotham, T. J.** 1986. Current views on the relationships between amoebae, legionellae and man. *Isr. J. Med. Sci.* **22:**678–689.

103. **She, R. C., E. Billetdeaux, A. R. Phansalkar, and C. A. Petti.** 2007. Limited applicability of direct fluorescent-antibody testing for *Bordetella* sp. and *Legionella* sp. specimens for the clinical microbiology laboratory. *J. Clin. Microbiol.* **45:**2212–2214.

104. **Shen, H., S. Rogelj, and T. L. Kieft.** 2006. Sensitive, real-time PCR detects low-levels of contamination by *Legionella pneumophila* in commercial reagents. *Mol. Cell. Probes* **20:**147–153.

105. **Steele, T. W., J. Lanser, and N. Sangster.** 1990. Isolation of *Legionella longbeachae* serogroup 1 from potting mixes. *Appl. Environ. Microbiol.* **56:**49–53.

106. **Tateyama, M.** 1992. Misleading serological identification of *Legionella anisa* as *Legionella bozemanii. Kansenshogaku Zasshi* **66:**149–155.

107. **Templeton, K. E., S. A. Scheltinga, P. Sillekens, J. W. Crielaard, A. P. van Dam, H. Goossens, and E. C. Claas.** 2003. Development and clinical evaluation of an internally controlled, single-tube multiplex real-time PCR assay for detection of *Legionella pneumophila* and other *Legionella* species. *J. Clin. Microbiol.* **41:**4016–4021.

108. **Tenover, F. C., P. H. Edelstein, L. C. Goldstein, J. C. Sturge, and J. J. Plorde.** 1986. Comparison of cross-staining reactions by *Pseudomonas* spp. and fluorescein-labeled polyclonal and monoclonal antibodies directed against *Legionella pneumophila. J. Clin. Microbiol.* **23:**647–649.

109. **Thacker, L., R. M. McKinney, C. W. Moss, H. M. Sommers, M. L. Spivack, and T. F. O'Brien.** 1981. Thermophilic sporeforming bacilli that mimic fastidious growth characteristics and colonial morphology of legionella. *J. Clin. Microbiol.* **13:**794–797.

110. **Thacker, W. L., R. F. Benson, R. B. Schifman, E. Pugh, A. G. Steigerwalt, W. R. Mayberry, D. J. Brenner, and H. W. Wilkinson.** 1989. *Legionella tucsonensis* sp. nov. isolated from a renal transplant recipient. *J. Clin. Microbiol.* **27:**1831–1834.

111. **Thacker, W. L., R. F. Benson, H. W. Wilkinson, N. M. Ampel, E. J. Wing, A. G. Steigerwalt, and D. J. Brenner.** 1986. 11th serogroup of *Legionella pneumophila* isolated from a patient with fatal pneumonia. *J. Clin. Microbiol.* **23:**1146–1147.

112. **Thacker, W. L., J. W. Dyke, R. F. Benson, D. H. Havlichek, Jr., B. Robinson-Dunn, H. Stiefel, W. Schneider, C. W. Moss, W. R. Mayberry, and D. J. Brenner.** 1992. *Legionella lansingensis* sp. nov. isolated from a patient with pneumonia and underlying chronic lymphocytic leukemia. *J. Clin. Microbiol.* **30:**2398–2401.

113. **Thacker, W. L., H. W. Wilkinson, and R. F. Benson.** 1983. Comparison of slide agglutination test and direct immunofluorescence assay for identification of *Legionella* isolates. *J. Clin. Microbiol.* **18:**1113–1118.

114. **van der Zee, A., M. Peeters, C. de Jong, H. Verbakel, J. W. Crielaard, E. C. Claas, and K. E. Templeton.** 2002. Qiagen DNA extraction kits for sample preparation for legionella PCR are not suitable for diagnostic purposes. *J. Clin. Microbiol.* **40:**1126.

115. **Vesey, G., P. J. Dennis, J. V. Lee, and A. A. West.** 1988. Further development of simple tests to differentiate the legionellas. *J. Appl. Bacteriol.* **65:**339–345.

116. **Vickers, R. M., J. D. Rihs, and V. L. Yu.** 1992. Clinical demonstration of isolation of *Nocardia asteroides* on buffered charcoal-yeast extract media. *J. Clin. Microbiol.* **30:**227–228.

117. **von Baum, H., S. Ewig, R. Marre, N. Suttorp, S. Gonschior, T. Welte, and C. Lück.** 2008. Community-acquired *Legionella* pneumonia: new insights from the German competence network for community acquired pneumonia. *Clin. Infect. Dis.* **46:**1356–1364.

118. **Westerman, E. L., and J. McDonald.** 1983. Tularemia pneumonia mimicking legionnaires' disease: isolation of organism on CYE agar and successful treatment with erythromycin. *South. Med. J.* **76:**1169–1170.

119. **Wilkinson, H. W., W. L. Thacker, A. G. Steigerwalt, D. J. Brenner, N. M. Ampel, and E. J. Wing.** 1985. Second serogroup of *Legionella hackeliae* isolated from a patient with pneumonia. *J. Clin. Microbiol.* **22:**488–489.

120. **Wilson, D. A., U. Reischl, G. S. Hall, and G. W. Procop.** 2007. Use of partial 16S rRNA gene sequencing for identification of *Legionella pneumophila* and non-*pneumophila Legionella* spp. *J. Clin. Microbiol.* **45:**257–258.

121. **Winn, W. C., Jr.** 1985. *Legionella* and Legionnaires' disease: a review with emphasis on environmental studies and laboratory diagnosis. *Crit. Rev. Clin. Lab. Sci.* **21:** 323–381.

122. **Zusman, T., G. Yerushalmi, and G. Segal.** 2003. Functional similarities between the *icm/dot* pathogenesis systems of *Coxiella burnetii* and *Legionella pneumophila*. *Infect. Immun.* **71:**3714–3723.

*Bartonella**

RICARDO G. MAGGI, VOLKHARD A. J. KEMPF, BRUNO B. CHOMEL, AND EDWARD B. BREITSCHWERDT

46

TAXONOMY AND DESCRIPTION OF THE GENUS

Bartonella (including some species formerly known as *Rochalimaea*) is a genus of short, facultative intracellular pleomorphic gram-negative coccobacillary or bacillary rods that measure 0.2 to 0.6 μm by 0.5 to 1.0 μm (Fig. 1A and B). Members of this genus can induce acute and persistent intravascular infections in healthy people and animals. *Bartonella* species are members of the alpha-2 subgroup of the class *Alphaproteobacteria*, within the *Rhizobiales* order. There are now more than 22 species or subspecies described, and DNA sequences from numerous other species or strains have been deposited in GenBank. Because of the slow growth of these bacteria on agar plates (dividing time, approximately 24 h), standard biochemical methods for identification have not been useful. *Bartonella* organisms are oxidase and catalase negative and do not produce acid from carbohydrates. On primary culture all members of the genus typically require 15 to 45 days in the presence of 5% CO_2 to form visible colonies on enriched blood-containing media, as these bacteria are highly hemin dependent. The temperatures to achieve optimal growth for various *Bartonella* spp. vary from 25 to 30°C for *Bartonella bacilliformis* to 35 to 37°C for *B. henselae*, *B. koehlerae*, and *B. elizabethae*. On primary isolation, some *Bartonella* species, such as *B. henselae*, *B. clarridgeiae*, *B. vinsonii*, and *B. elizabethae*, form colonies with a white, rough, dry, raised appearance that pit the medium (Fig. 1C). The smooth colony morphology results from phase variation that correlates with the loss of trimeric autotransporter adhesin (TAA) expression. Colonies are hard to extract or transfer to subsequent plates. Other *Bartonella* spp., such as *B. quintana*, have colonies that are usually smaller, gray, translucent, and somewhat gummy or slightly mucoid. A few members of the genus, including *B. bacilliformis*, *B. clarridgeiae*, *B. capreoli*, and *B. schoenbuchensis*, are motile by means of unipolar flagella.

Bartonella bacilliformis, the type species of the genus, is the etiologic agent of Carrion's disease, which is characterized by an acute hemolytic, bacteremic infection called Oroya fever or a chronic vasoproliferative form called verruga peruana, which is characterized by cutaneous nodular vascular eruptions. *Bartonella quintana*, the agent of trench fever, has also been found to be one of the agents of bacillary angiomatosis, a vascular proliferative lesion observed in immunocompromised individuals, mainly with AIDS (76). *B. quintana* has also been associated with endocarditis and bacteremia in homeless people (17). Although the organism is transmitted by the human body louse, *B. quintana* DNA has been amplified from cat fleas and has also been isolated from feral cats and from dogs with endocarditis (8, 16, 44, 70). Bacillary angiomatosis can also be caused by *B. henselae*. Although *B. henselae* has historically been associated with cat scratch disease (CSD), a frequent but self-limiting infection in immunocompetent individuals, more recent findings suggest that this organism may cause persistent bacteremia accompanied by fatigue, arthritis, and neurological or neurocognitive abnormalities (14–16, 93). Similarly, *B. henselae* has been associated with endocarditis in both humans and dogs. A fourth human pathogen, *B. elizabethae*, was isolated in an immunocompetent individual suffering from endocarditis. Since then, *Bartonella vinsonii* subsp. *berkhoffii*, *B. vinsonii* subsp. *arupensis*, *B. koehlerae*, and *B. alsatica* have also been associated with human cases of endocarditis (7) and "*Candidatus* Bartonella washoensis" with a human case of myocarditis. *Bartonella grahamii* has been associated with human cases of neuroretinitis and bilateral retinal artery branch occlusions. *B. vinsonii* subsp. *arupensis* was also isolated from the blood of a rancher with fever and mild neurological symptoms (147). *B. clarridgeiae* is suspected to be a minor agent of CSD, but based on serologic evidence only. Three new proposed *Bartonella* species have been isolated or detected from human cases, including "*B. rochalimae*," "*B. tamiae*," and "*Candidatus* Bartonella melophagi.*"

EPIDEMIOLOGY AND TRANSMISSION

Bartonella species are transmitted by insect vectors such as fleas, sand flies, and body lice and potentially by ticks, biting flies, and wingless flies. In addition, transmission also occurs by animal scratches or possibly bites. Some species are very limited geographically, such as *B. bacilliformis*, found only in the Andes mountain region of South America, in association with the limited distribution of its sand fly vector, *Lutzomyia verrucarum*. Others, such

---

*This chapter contains information presented by David F. Welch and Leonard N. Slater in the eighth edition and by Bruno Chomel and Jean Marc Rolain in the ninth edition of this *Manual*.

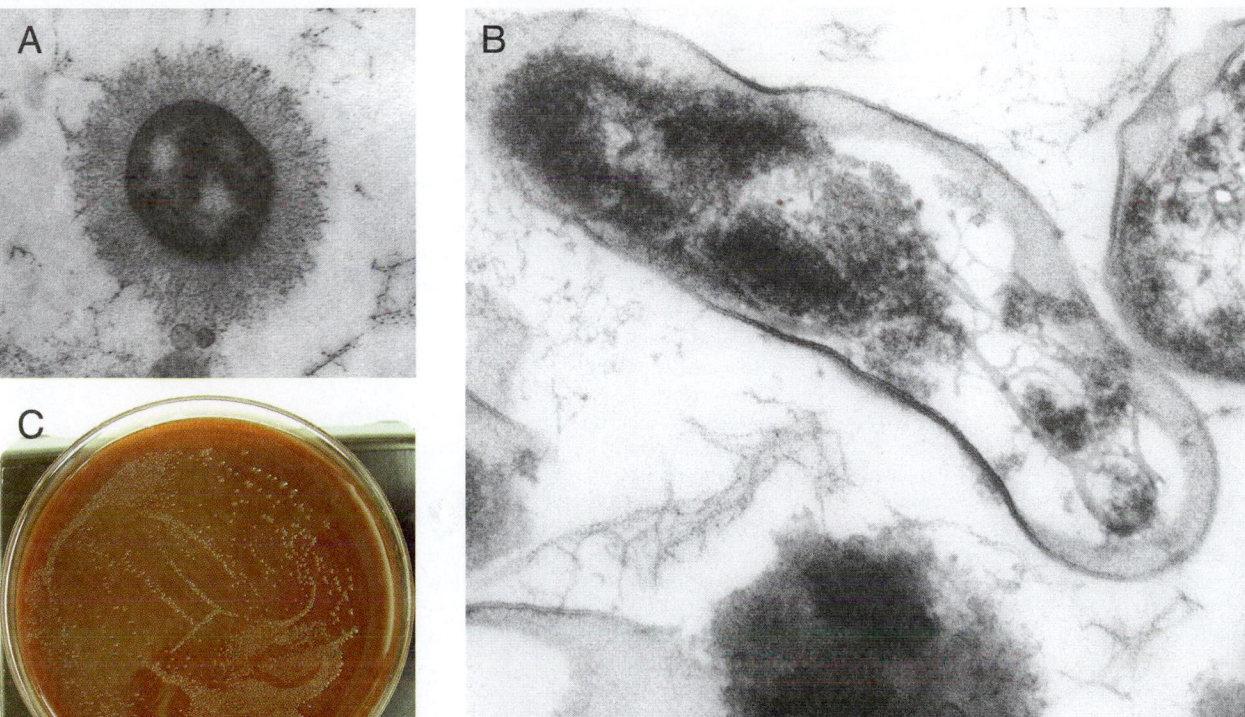

FIGURE 1 (A and B) Electron micrographs of *B. henselae* Marseille (A) and *B. vinsonii* subsp. *berkhoffii* genotype III (B); (C) *B. henselae* strain Houston I isolated on a blood agar plate after 10 days in culture at 36°C and 5% CO_2. Panel A is reprinted from reference 121.

as *B. quintana, B. henselae, B. elizabethae,* and *B. vinsonii* subsp. *berkhoffii,* appear to have a worldwide distribution. *B. quintana* outbreaks are associated with poor sanitation and personal hygiene, particularly in homeless populations worldwide. Infestation by the human body louse, *Pediculus humanus,* results in inoculation of *B. quintana* in arthropod excreta through broken skin (39, 112, 114).

Cats are the main reservoir for *B. henselae, B. clarridgeiae,* and *B. koehlerae.* CSD, caused by *B. henselae* infection, is transmitted from cat to cat mainly by the cat flea, *Ctenocephalides felis* (25); however, cat flea transmission as a cause of human infection has not been confirmed. More likely, human infection results from the inoculation of infective flea feces at the time of the scratch (7). Ticks could be a potential vector for some human *B. henselae* infections (7). Stray cats, cats living outdoors, and young cats are more likely to be bacteremic. The prevalence of *B. henselae* infection is usually highest in warm and humid climates, where cat fleas are abundant. *Bartonella henselae* antibody prevalence in domestic cat populations can range from 14 to 50% (4, 10). Genotype I (Houston) is more common in cats in the Far East (Japan and the Philippines), whereas type II (Marseille) is predominant in Western Europe, North America, and Australia (7). In addition, genotype I seems to have two distinctive variants in the United States: *B. henselae* Houston I and *B. henselae* San Antonio 2, according to sequence differences in the internal transcribed

spacer (ITS) region (15, 43, 44, 56, 92, 94). Coinfection of cats with different *Bartonella* species or genotypes has been reported (53), as well as coinfections in humans or dogs (15, 43, 44). Additionally, *B. quintana, B. koehlerae,* and *B. clarridgeiae* DNA has been detected in cat fleas, suggesting their possible role as vectors for these organisms (123).

Several *Bartonella* species and subspecies, including *B. clarridgeiae, B. quintana, B. elizabethae, B. henselae, B. vinsonii* subsp. *berkhoffii,* "*B. washoensis,*" and "*B. rochalimae*" (58), can infect dogs and humans (Table 1) and may elicit a wide spectrum of disease manifestations, including polyarthritis, cutaneous vasculitis, endocarditis, myocarditis, epistaxis, peliosis hepatis, and granulomatous inflammatory disease. *B. alsatica* (European wild rabbit reservoir) and "*Candidatus* Bartonella melophagi" (sheep reservoir) have been reported in association with endocarditis, lymphadenitis, pericardial effusion and fatigue, joint pain, and tremors (93, 113). Other *Bartonella* species, such as *B. vinsonii* subsp. *vinsonii, B. doshiae, B. taylorii, B. peromysci, B. birtlesii, B. tribocorum, B. talpae, B. bovis, B. chomelii, B. schoenbuchensis,* and *B. capreoli,* have only been isolated from the blood of animals, including wild rodents, squirrels, felids, canids, and ruminants (cattle, deer, and elk). Domestic and wild canids represent the main reservoir of *B. vinsonii* subsp. *berkhoffii,* with high antibody prevalences in dogs from tropical countries (7) and a high prevalence of bacteremia in coyotes (*Canis latrans*) in California (21). Ticks may be

TABLE 1 *Bartonella* species or subspecies presently described, their main reservoirs, their confirmed or possible vectors, and the potential accidental hosts

Bartonella sp.	Nomenclatural status	Main reservoir	Vector or potential vector	Accidental hosts
B. alsatica	Approved	Rabbits (*Oryctolagus cuniculus*)	Fleas? Ticks?	Humans
B. bacilliformis	Approved	Humans; cats? Dogs?	Fleas, sand flies (*Phlebotomus* spp.)	Cats? Dogs?
B. birtlesii	Approved	Wood mice (*Apodemus* spp.)	Fleas?	
B. bovis ("B. weissii")	Approved	Domestic cattle (*Bos taurus*)	Biting flies? Ticks	Cats, humans, dogs
B. capreoli	Approved	Roe deer (*Capreolus capreolus*)	Biting flies? Ticks?	
B. chomelii	Approved	Domestic cattle (*Bos taurus*)	Biting flies? Ticks?	
B. clarridgeiae	Approved	Cats (*Felis catus*)	Fleas; ticks?	Humans, dogs
B. coopersplainsensis	Valid publication	Australian rats	?	?
B. doshiae	Approved	Meadow voles (*Microtus agrestis*), rats (*Rattus* spp.)	Fleas	Humans
B. elizabethae	Approved	Rats (*Rattus norvegicus*)	Fleas	Humans, dogs
B. grahamii	Approved	Voles (*Clethrionomys* spp.), mice (*Apodemus* spp.)	Fleas	Humans
B. henselae	Approved	Cats (*Felis catus*), dogs (*Canis familiaris*)	Fleas; ticks?	Humans, dogs
B. japonica	Valid publication	Field mice (*Apodemus argenteus*)	?	?
B. koehlerae	Approved	Cats (*Felis catus*), gerbils (*Meriones libycus*)?	Fleas	Humans
"Candidatus Bartonella melophagi"	Candidatus	Sheep (*Ovis* spp.)	Keds (*Melophagus ovinus*)	Humans
B. peromysci	Approved	Field mice (*Peromyscus* spp.)	Fleas?	
B. queenslandensis	Valid publication	Australian rats	?	?
B. quintana	Approved	Humans; gerbils (*Meriones libycus*)?	Human body lice, Fleas	Cats, dogs
B. rattaustraliani	Valid publication	Austalian rats	?	?
"B. rattimassiliensis"	Without standing	Rats (*Rattus* spp.)	Fleas?	?
"B. rochlimae"	Without standing	Dogs (*Canis familiaris*)	Sand flies?	Humans
B. schoenbuchensis	Approved	Roe deer (*Capreolus capreolus*)	Deer keds, biting flies; ticks?	Humans
B. silvatica	Valid publication	Japanese field mouse (*Apodemus speciosus*)	?	?
B. talpae	Approved	Moles (*Talpa europaea*)	Fleas?	
"B. tamiae"	Valid publication	Rat (*Rattus* spp.)	Fleas?	Humans
B. taylorii	Approved	Mice (*Apodemus* spp.), gerbils (*Meriones libycus*), voles (*Clethrionomys* spp.)	Fleas	?
B. tribocorum	Approved	Rats (*Rattus* spp.), mice (*Apodemus* spp.)	Fleas?	?
B. vinsonii subsp. arupensis	Approved	White-footed mice (*Peromyscus leucopus*)	Fleas? Ticks?	Humans?
B. vinsonii subsp. berkhoffii	Approved	Coyotes (*C. latrans*), dogs (*Canis familiaris*), foxes (*Urocyon* spp.)	Ticks?	Humans
B. vinsonii subsp. vinsonii	Approved	Meadow voles (*Microtus pennsylvanicus*)	Ear mites (*Trombicula microti*)?	?
"B. volans"	Without standing	Southern flying squirrels (*Glaucomys volans*)	Fleas?	Humans
"Candidatus Bartonella washoensis"	Without standing	California ground squirrels (*Spermophilus beecheyi*), rabbits (*Oryctolagus cuniculus*)	Fleas? Ticks	Humans, dogs

involved in the transmission of *B. vinsonii* subsp. *berkhoffii* to dogs (11). Similarly, *Bartonella* DNA has been identified in questing adult *Ixodes pacificus* ticks from California, including from several *Bartonella* species that are pathogenic for humans (20); *B. henselae* DNA has also been detected in *Ixodes ricinus* ticks collected from humans in Italy (131); and *Bartonella* DNA has been amplified from *Ixodes* ticks from numerous sites throughout the world (5, 35a).

In addition, a wide range of rodent species is reported to be infected with different *Bartonella* species (Table 1). Finally, several *Bartonella* species have been isolated from domestic and wild ruminants (Table 1) among which biting flies could be an important vector for transmission of infection (7).

CLINICAL SIGNIFICANCE

Human Pathogens

Oroya Fever and Verruga Peruana (Carrion's Disease): *B. bacilliformis*

The disease caused by *B. bacilliformis*, especially its chronic form known as verruga peruana, has been recognized since pre-Columbian times in populations of the Andes Mountains. However, the suspected link between the acute form (Oroya fever) and the chronic form was confirmed in 1885 when Daniel Carrion, a medical student, died of Oroya fever after inoculating himself with material from a verruga. The acute form of the disease, usually seen in people who are not natives of the zone of endemicity, is an acute, progressive, severe, and febrile anemia with intravascular hemolysis associated with the presence of *B. bacilliformis* in the erythrocytes. The mortality rate was reported to range from 40 to 90% prior to the antibiotic era. Chronic bacteremia occurs in the general population in regions of endemicity, and evidence for persistent infection has been reported from zones of nonendemicity (19, 80). The second stage of infection occurs weeks to months following the acute infection and is characterized by nodular angioproliferative cutaneous lesions named verruga peruana; mucosal and internal lesions can occur (118, 119). The lesions can persist for several months, but the prognosis for full recovery is good at this stage.

Trench Fever, Bacillary Angiomatosis, Endocarditis, and Prolonged Fever or Bacteremia Caused by *B. quintana*

Trench or quintana fever is a recurrent fever with three to five or more febrile episodes lasting 4 to 5 days each after 15 to 25 days of incubation. Severe headaches and shin pain are common symptoms associated with malaise, anorexia, abdominal pain, restlessness, and insomnia. Mild forms and asymptomatic carriage are also reported (17, 65). Several cases of endocarditis have been associated with *B. quintana* infection (84). In human immunodeficiency virus-infected persons, bacteremia caused by *B. quintana* develops insidiously, involving recurrent fever, headaches, and hepatomegaly. *B. quintana* and *B. henselae* are the two *Bartonella* species involved in the etiology of bacillary angiomatosis. Bacillary angiomatosis, also called epithelioid angiomatosis, is a vasoproliferative disease of the skin characterized by multiple blood-filled, partially endothelial cell-lined cystic structures (135). It is usually characterized by violaceous or colorless papular and nodular skin lesions that clinically suggest Kaposi's sarcoma but histologically

resemble epithelioid hemangiomas. When visceral parenchymal organs are involved, the condition is referred to as bacillary peliosis hepatis, splenic peliosis, or systemic bacillary angiomatosis. Fever, weight loss, malaise, and organomegaly can develop in people with disseminated bacillary angiomatosis. Subcutaneous and lytic bone lesions are also associated with *B. quintana* infection (75).

Zoonotic Bartonellae

CSD

CSD is caused mainly by *B. henselae* (115, 153), whereas *B. clarridgeiae* has been suspected in a few cases, based on serologic evidence (77, 97). There are now strong arguments against *Afipia felis* being one of the etiological agents of CSD (84). In classical CSD, 1 to 3 weeks elapse between the scratch or bite of a cat and the appearance of clinical signs. In 50% of the cases, a small skin lesion, often resembling an insect bite, appears at the inoculation site, usually the hand or forearm. The lesion evolves from a papule to a vesicle and in some instances becomes a partially healed ulcer. These lesions generally resolve within a few days to a few weeks. Lymphadenitis develops approximately 3 weeks after exposure and is generally unilateral. Epitrochlear, axillary, or cervical lymph nodes are most frequently involved. Lymph nodes are usually swollen and painful, and lymphadenopathy persists for several weeks to several months. In 25% of CSD cases, suppuration occurs. The large majority of the cases show signs of systemic infection: fever, chills, malaise, anorexia, and headache. In general, the disease is benign and lymphadenopathy resolves spontaneously without sequelae. Atypical manifestations of CSD occur in 5 to 10% of the cases. The most common of these is Parinaud's oculoglandular syndrome (periauricular lymphadenopathy and palpebral conjunctivitis), but meningitis, encephalitis, osteolytic lesions, and thrombocytopenic purpura may also occur. Encephalopathy is one of the most serious complications of CSD, which usually occurs 2 to 6 weeks after the onset of lymphadenopathy but generally resolves with complete recovery and few or no sequelae. It is estimated that 22,000 human cases of CSD occur yearly in the United States. From 55 to 80% of CSD patients are <20 years old. There is a seasonal pattern, with most cases seen in autumn and winter.

Other clinical presentations associated with *B. henselae* infection are reported to occur in immunocompetent persons, including neuroretinitis or bacteremia accompanied by chronic fatigue syndrome, memory loss, and arthralgia. *Bartonella henselae* is also a frequent cause of prolonged fever and fever of unknown origin in children. Rheumatic manifestations of *Bartonella* infection have been described to occur in children, including cases of myositis, arthritis, and skin nodules. Arthritis is described in a very limited number of cases. Other rheumatic manifestations include erythema nodosum, leukocytoclastic vasculitis, fever of unknown origin with myalgia, osteolytic lesions, and arthralgia (7). Neurological dysfunction and neurocognitive abnormalities are reported for people infected with *B. henselae* (15). Unlike CSD, which appears to be a self-limiting infection in most patients, these cases suggest that *B. henselae* can induce persistent intravascular infections resulting in varied and complex chronic disease manifestations.

Bacillary angiomatosis patients with *B. henselae* infection are epidemiologically linked to cat and flea exposure (75). Fever, weight loss, malaise, and enlargement of affected organs may develop in people with disseminated bacillary angiomatosis. *Bartonella henselae* and *B. quintana* have been implicated in a few cases of human immunodeficiency virus-associated brain lesions, meningoencephalitis and encephalopathy, dementia, and neuropsychological decline (132, 136).

Zoonotic *Bartonella* Species Associated with Endocarditis, Myocarditis, Ocular Lesions, Fever, and Neurological Symptoms

Several zoonotic *Bartonella* spp. have been recognized as causative agents of blood culture-negative endocarditis or myocarditis in humans, including *B. henselae*, *B. koehlerae*, *B. elizabethae*, *B. vinsonii* subsp. *berkhoffii*, *B. vinsonii* subsp. *arupensis* (48), and "*Candidatus* Bartonella washoensis" (7, 30). *Bartonella* spp. account for 3 to 4% of all human cases of endocarditis in France, a percentage similar to that of endocarditis cases caused by *Coxiella burnetii*, the agent of Q fever (60). Some rodent-borne *Bartonella* species are also associated with cases of neuroretinitis (*B. elizabethae* and *B. grahamii*) or fever with bacteremia and neurological symptoms (*B. vinsonii* subsp. *arupensis*) (147).

Other *Bartonella* Species or Subspecies

The clinical impact on animals or humans of many *Bartonella* species is still unknown. Although "*Candidatus* Bartonella melophagi" was isolated from the blood of two women (93) and *B. bovis* DNA was amplified from the heart valves of cows with endocarditis, no other specific pathology has been associated with *Bartonella* species infecting domestic and wild ruminants or for many of the rodent-borne *Bartonella* spp.

Canine and Feline *Bartonella* Species

Several of the 22 species and subspecies known today have been detected in or isolated from pet dogs and cats, thereby highlighting the zoonotic potential of these bacteria for persons with extensive animal contact (26, 28–30, 42, 44, 71, 73, 127, 137, 138). *B. henselae*, *B. clarridgeiae*, *B. koehlerae*, *B. quintana*, *B. bovis*, *B. elizabethae*, and *B. vinsonii* subsp. *berkhoffii* have been recognized as pathogenic for dogs (13, 27), and *B. henselae*, *B. clarridgeiae*, "*Candidatus* Bartonella washoensis," *B. quintana*, *B. rochalimae*, *B. elizabethae*, and *B. vinsonii* subsp. *berkhoffii* also cause feline infections (8, 41, 57, 77, 82, 88, 98). A broad array of manifestations, including endocarditis (22), myocarditis, epistaxis, and lethargy, have been commonly associated with *Bartonella* infection in dogs (9, 12, 13, 78, 79). *Bartonella*-infected cats are more likely to have kidney disease and urinary tract infections, stomatitis, and lymphadenopathy (28). In experimentally infected cats, fever, lymphadenopathy, mild neurological signs, and reproductive disorders have been reported to occur (28). Nevertheless, the clinical spectrum of *Bartonella* infection in dogs and cats may be highly variable, including chronic subclinical infections accompanied by lethargy and weight loss as the only reported abnormalities.

COLLECTION, TRANSPORT, AND STORAGE OF SPECIMENS

Most specimens used for *Bartonella* isolation are either blood or tissue. Approaches typically used for recovery of other pathogens from such sites are suitable. *Bartonella* spp. are difficult to isolate from blood of immunocompetent individuals, as opposed to the relative ease of isolation from blood of immunocompromised patients. Blood samples can be collected either in Isolator blood lysis tubes (Wampole,

Cranbury, NJ), sodium citrate tubes, or plastic EDTA tubes. If storage of specimens prior to culture is necessary, samples should be kept frozen (at least −20°C). It was shown that blood collected from *B. henselae*-infected cats into both EDTA and Isolator blood lysis tubes yielded good recovery and no loss of sensitivity for EDTA tubes kept at −65°C for 26 days (10). Specimens should be collected prior to antimicrobial therapy.

Tissue from enlarged lymph nodes, cutaneous lesions, or various organs can be cultured after homogenization or processed for DNA extraction and PCR. Fresh tissues are preferred for PCR amplification, but paraffin-embedded tissue may be used (23). Fine-needle aspiration has also been successful for detection of *Bartonella* and is less invasive than biopsy (3). *Bartonella* spp. have been successfully cultured from aqueous humor (51, 70).

DIRECT EXAMINATION

Microscopy

With the exception of *B. bacilliformis*, *Bartonella* spp. are not visualized in erythrocytes on stained smears of blood from animal or human patients (84). In rats experimentally infected with *B. birtlesii*, there can be up to eight bacteria per erythrocyte (6a, 29a). Warthin-Starry silver stain is recommended for microscopic detection of *Bartonella* organisms in fixed tissue sections but is not highly specific and is insensitive, even with lymph node biopsy samples from CSD patients. For patients with bacillary angiomatosis, there is usually a larger number of bacilli that are identifiable by Warthin-Starry silver staining.

Antigen Detection

Immunocytochemical labeling is a specific technique but is not widely available (76). Direct immunofluorescence of blood smears allowed rapid diagnosis of *B. quintana* in a patient with acute trench fever (26) and in bacteremic homeless patients (84).

Nucleic Acid Detection

Although PCR and agar plate culture are useful tests to document infection with *Bartonella* species in cats, these traditional techniques are not generally sensitive enough to detect active infection with a *Bartonella* species in human or dog blood samples. Therefore, PCR amplification directly from blood or other diagnostic samples is of limited value for those patients with very-low-level bacteremia. Enrichment culture of the diagnostic sample (blood, cerebrospinal fluid, joint fluid, or effusion) prior to performing PCR (see below) can be used to increase the number of bacteria above the threshold limit of the PCR (10, 14–16, 18, 24, 31, 32, 37, 43, 44, 56, 69, 91, 93, 94, 105, 152; R. Maggi, A. W. Duncan, and E. B. Breitschwerdt, presented at the 20th ASR Meeting and 5th International Conference on Bartonella as Emerging Pathogens, Pacific Grove, CA, 2006).

Advances in PCR methodologies and equipment have facilitated an impressive increase in the sensitivity of molecular detection of *Bartonella* DNA in patient samples. The 16S rRNA gene (*rrs*) was first used by Relman et al. in 1990 for identification of the microbial etiology of bacillary angiomatosis (34, 116). However, this gene does not discriminate among *Bartonella* species (86). The most widely targeted genes are those coding for citrate synthase (*gltA*) (68, 83, 109, 111), a heat shock protein (*groEL*) (154), riboflavin synthase (*ribC*) (2), a cell division protein (*ftsZ*) (155, 156), and a 17-kDa antigen (47). Sequences of *gltA* and *rpoB* (RNA polymerase β-subunit) (117) are congruent with DNA-DNA hybridization for *Bartonella* species identification (86). The ITS region located between the 16S and 23S rRNA genes is a useful diagnostic target for *Bartonella* detection, species identification, and genotyping (14–16, 42, 44, 59, 67, 89, 90). Confirmatory tests (e.g., PCR followed by sequencing or the use of a second target gene PCR assay) must be performed to avoid potential nonspecific amplification and misdiagnosis (89).

ISOLATION PROCEDURES

Blood

Bartonellae can be recovered from the blood of bacteremic patients. In immunocompromised patients, including transplant recipients, the level of bacteremia is often higher than in immunocompetent people (76). Routine cultures of blood from patients with infective endocarditis caused by *Bartonella* spp. are rarely positive. Historically, *Bartonella* species were optimally isolated from blood with the use of the lysis centrifugation system (Isolator) or with EDTA anticoagulant and plating onto fresh chocolate or heart infusion agar containing 5% fresh rabbit blood in the absence of antibiotics. Commercial sheep or horse blood agar plates have also been used. *Bartonella koehlerae* does not grow well on heart infusion agar and requires fresh chocolate agar plates (41). Plates inoculated with blood should be incubated at 35°C for at least 4 weeks in 5% CO_2 and at high humidity. Colonies usually appear after 5 to 15 days (74). Due to prolonged incubation times, other slow-growing pathogens, including *Mycobacterium tuberculosis*, can grow on the plates; therefore, appropriate safety precautions should be taken with all positive cultures. Broth-based or biphasic culture system vials used for blood culture, such as the BACTEC Peds Plus vials (Becton Dickinson, Sparks, MD) can be used for *Bartonella* isolation (54, 99, 143). DNA staining (e.g., acridine orange staining) and blind subculture from negative bottles before discarding them at 7 days may increase the likelihood of identifying *Bartonella* (1). An assay was also developed in which samples of heparinized blood are sedimented and the plasma is collected for inoculation into shell vials (66). Culture is then performed by the centrifugation-shell vial technique using the T24 bladder carcinoma cell line (inaccurately designated ECV304 human endothelial cells) (76).

Preenrichment Culture

In broth, *Bartonella* spp. do not usually produce turbidity or convert enough oxidizable substrate to CO_2; therefore, CO_2 detection-based blood culture systems often fail to indicate growth. Initial efforts to develop an optimized culture media for the isolation of *Bartonella* were aimed at the isolation of these bacteria from sick animals and human patients (22, 51, 84). Novel approaches, such as using an optimized liquid insect cell growth medium as a preenrichment step, have enhanced the detection of *Bartonella* spp. in patient samples (43, 91, 121). One such medium, designated *Bartonella* Alphaproteobacteria growth medium (BAPGM), has enhanced molecular detection and isolation of *Bartonella* species from animal and patient samples and is commercially available from Galaxy Diagnostics (http://www.galaxydx.com). BAPGM supports the growth of at least seven *Bartonella* species and facilitates growth of cocultures combining different *Bartonella* species (43, 91). When used to enhance microbiological documentation of infection, preenrichment culture with BAPGM facilitated the molecular detection and/or isolation of several *Bartonella* species (14–16, 24, 37, 43, 44, 69, 81, 90–94; Maggi et al., presented at the 20th ASR Meeting and 5th International Conference on Bartonella as Emerging Pathogens, Pacific Grove, CA, 2006). Recently, the use of BAPGM has facilitated the isolation of *B. henselae* and *B. vinsonii* subsp. *berkhoffii* from pleural and pericardial effusions from dogs and the documentation of coinfection with *B. henselae* and *B. vinsonii* subsp. *berkhoffii* in blood and joint effusions obtained from a dog with "nonseptic" neutrophilic polyarthritis (23). An optimized BAPGM diagnostic platform could include PCR following preenrichment culture in BAPGM flasks for 7 and 14 days and on colonies if visualized on an agar plate (14, 16, 24, 93). Diagnostic use of the BAPGM platform has also enhanced detection of coinfection with more than one *Bartonella* sp. in dogs (35, 37, 42–44) and in immunocompetent people (14, 16). In addition, BAPGM preenrichment culture has facilitated the isolation of two novel *Bartonella* species, "*Candidatus* Bartonella melophagi" and "*Bartonella tamiae*," from human blood (81, 93).

Tissue

Recovery of *Bartonella* spp. from cutaneous lesions, liver, spleen, or lymph node is possible after homogenization in medium and plating directly onto solid agar. Cocultivation with an endothelial cell line or use of the shell vial method is more laborious but can occasionally yield bacterial growth (76), as with isolation of *Bartonella* from heart valve tissues (84). Although various liquid media have been developed for primary isolation of *B. henselae* from blood, serum, and other tissues (14–16, 22, 24, 35, 37, 43, 44, 56, 69, 81, 91–94, 151; Maggi et al., presented at the 20th ASR Meeting and 5th International Conference on Bartonella as Emerging Pathogens, Pacific Grove, CA, 2006), current evidence best supports the use of an insect cell culture-based medium.

IDENTIFICATION

Colonies of *B. henselae* can be of two morphological types which can be present simultaneously: (i) irregular, raised, whitish, rough (cauliflower-like), and dry or (ii) small, circular, tan, and moist, tending to pit and adhere to the agar (Fig. 1C). *B. quintana* colonies are usually smooth, flat, and shiny and do not pit the agar (76). *B. clarridgeiae* produces small white, raised, indurated, and cohesive colonies which can also appear to spread during primary isolation. Most *Bartonella* spp. usually appear uniformly smooth after repeated subcultures. The bacilli (Fig. 1) are small (2 by 0.5 μm) and stain best with Gimenez stain (76). With Gram staining, *Bartonella* spp. are weakly counterstained with safranin or basic fuchsin. *Bartonella* spp. appear in Gram stains as small, gram-negative, slightly curved rods resembling *Campylobacter*, *Helicobacter*, or *Haemophilus* (148). Colonial morphology in conjunction with slow growth requiring more than 7 days of incubation, and negative catalase and oxidase reactions, is often sufficient for a presumptive identification. DNA sequencing is optimal for confirmation of the genus, species, and strain.

Bartonella bacilliformis, "*Candidatus* Bartonella melophagi," *B. clarridgeiae*, *B. capreoli*, and *B. schoenbuchensis* are the only members of the genus that are motile by means of unipolar flagella. *Bartonella quintana* and *B. henselae* as well as several other *Bartonella* species have a twitching motility on wet mounts associated with the expression of TAAs (e.g., BadA of *B. henselae*; shown in reference 120). These TAAs are responsible for cytoadherence and may mediate specific interactions with extracellular matrix components and endothelial cells (96).

Most species are biochemically inert except for the production of peptidases. None of the various commercially available identification systems contain *Bartonella* spp. in their databases. However, the MicroScan Rapid Anaerobe Panel (Baxter Diagnostics, Deerfield, IL), RapID ANA II, and Rapid ID 32 A have been used for identification. The MicroScan Rapid Anaerobe Panel is reported to provide species identification (code 10077640 for *B. henselae*, code 10073640 for *B. quintana*, and code 10077240 for *B. bacilliformis*) (148). Overall, these identification kits are of limited use for accurate diagnosis of *Bartonella* infections. Measurements of preformed enzymes and standard testing reveal minor differences between species.

Identification of *Bartonella* isolates is largely based on nucleic acid techniques, some of which allow for the species determination, strain determination within a given species, or even genotyping. Methods include Southern blotting, gel and capillary electrophoresis, PCR, DNA hybridization, restriction fragment length polymorphism, and gene sequence analysis (1). As described above, PCR and sequencing of target genes such as *gltA*, *rpoB*, the ITS region, *rrs* (16S rRNA), *groEL*, or *ricC* are the most widely used. Recently, it was demonstrated that mass matrix-assisted laser desorption ionization–time-of-flight mass spectrometry (MALDI-TOF MS) is an accurate and reproducible tool for rapid and inexpensive identification of *Bartonella* species (49a).

TYPING SYSTEMS

Several molecular methods, such as pulsed-field gel electrophoresis, multilocus sequence typing, multispacer typing, and multiple-locus variable-number tandem-repeat analysis (MLVA) (104) can be used to genotype *Bartonella henselae* (and in some cases *B. quintana*) isolates. Also, a genomic fingerprinting technique using infrequent-restriction-site PCR can be used to identify pathogenic *Bartonella* species (55). Diagnostic utility for rapid species or genotype identification is limited when bacterial isolation is not successful. In contrast, even when isolation of the infecting species is not possible, PCR amplification of ITS DNA directly from diagnostic samples and/or from enrichment cultures followed by nucleic acid sequencing is an invaluable tool for primary identification at the species, subspecies, and genotype levels (10, 14–16, 18, 31, 36, 37, 42–44, 89–91, 93, 94; Maggi et al., presented at the 21st Meeting of the American Society for Rickettsiology, Colorado Springs, CO, 2007). *Bartonella vinsonii* subsp. *berkhoffii* can be separated into four distinct genotypes based upon 16S-23S ITS sequences (90).

SEROLOGIC TESTS

Due to difficulties with traditional culture for isolation, serologic testing for *Bartonella* infection, including immunofluorescence antibody assay (IFA), enzyme-linked immunosorbent assay, and Western blotting, has been the cornerstone for clinical diagnosis. Enzyme-linked immunosorbent assay is the simplest to perform and can be easily automated, but it has a low sensitivity (17 to 35%). IFA using commercial antigen slides for *B. henselae* and *B. quintana* has become the most frequently used serologic test worldwide. Human infection with *B. henselae* or *B. quintana* is evaluated by detecting the presence of immunoglobulin M (IgM) and/or IgG antibodies directed against these bacteria. The first serologic test for CSD was an IFA based on *B. henselae* bacilli that were cocultivated with Vero cells to inhibit autoagglutination (115). This test was found to have good sensitivity (84 to 95%) and specificity (94 to 98%) using sera from patients with CSD (33, 115, 153). Titers ranging from 64 to 256 or higher are usually indicative of ongoing infection depending on the differences among laboratory standards; lower titers may indicate an early or late clinical phase of the disease or prior exposure to the bacteria. In cases of endocarditis caused by either *B. henselae* or *B. quintana*, high IgG antibody titers (≥800) are usually detected (50). An IgG antibody titer of ≥800 to either *B. henselae* or *B. quintana* has a positive predictive value of 0.810 for the detection of *Bartonella* infection in the general population and 0.955 for the detection of *Bartonella* infections among patients with endocarditis (50).

Nevertheless, IFA is time-consuming, requires appropriate equipment and expertise, and is subject to interobserver variation due to the difficulty of reading the test (1). For humans, it has been postulated that the sensitivity of different IFAs may range from 14 to 100% depending on the antigen source and cutoff values used by different laboratories (4, 106, 130, 139–142, 144, 145). Antigenic variability among *Bartonella* test strains can result in false-negative serologic results for some patients (38, 45, 49, 52, 139–141, 145, 149). Cross-reactivity can occur among different *Bartonella* species. Antigen adsorption can be used to reduce cross-reactivity and to determine to which antigen the antibodies are truly directed (1). Cross-reactivity for different *Bartonella* species can be present in up to 95% of samples (129). In addition, cross-reactive antibodies to other pathogens, e.g., *Chlamydia pneumoniae*, *Coxiella burnetii*, and spotted-fever group *Rickettsia*, are reported (14, 16, 61, 85, 87, 100, 103, 134, 139, 144, 145). Some studies suggest that genome rearrangement among *B. henselae* strains may play an important role in the establishment of persistent infection and can promote antigenic variation to escape the host immune response (3, 49). In several studies, both *B. henselae* DNA and *B. vinsonii* subsp. *berkhoffii* DNA were repeatedly detected in dogs that were not seroreactive (35, 37, 42, 44). For humans, several reports describe detection and/or isolation of *Bartonella* spp. from seronegative patients (14, 16, 17, 38, 40, 45, 95, 110, 128, 130). The discrepancy between little or no serologic detection of *Bartonella* antibodies and detection of *Bartonella* DNA or bacterial isolation leads one to the conclusion that seronegative infection could be more common in animals and humans than currently recognized.

Dihydrolipoamide succinyltransferase, the TAAs (BadA and Vomps), and other proteins of *B. henselae* and *B. quintana* are immunodominant target proteins potentially useful for diagnostic immunoblotting (6, 46, 146). However, immunoblot-based serologic tests do not show clear immunoreactive profiles, diminishing their utility for routine serologic diagnosis of *Bartonella* infections.

ANTIMICROBIAL SUSCEPTIBILITIES

Antimicrobial susceptibility testing can be performed by agar dilution methods using either blood or chocolate agar or by microdilution techniques using various media supplemented with blood (126). The Etest (AB Biodisk, Solna, Sweden) can also be used to determine antibiotic susceptibility (150). Results of susceptibility testing against *Bartonella* spp. are summarized in Table 2. Evaluation of

TABLE 2 MICs for *Bartonella* spp.[a]

Antibiotic group and drug name	MIC (µg/ml)				
	B. henselae	*B. quintana*	*B. bacilliformis*	*B. vinsonii*	*B. elizabethae*
Aminoglycosides					
Amikacin	2–4	4–8	2–8	4	1
Gentamicin	0.12–0.25	0.12–2	1–2	0.5	0.12
Streptomycin	ND	ND	4	ND	ND
Tobramycin	0.5–1	0.5–4	2–4	2	0.25
Cephalosporins					
Cefotaxime	0.12–0.25	0.12–0.25	0.03–0.12	0.12	0.06
Cefotetan	0.25–0.5	0.12–0.5	2	1	1
Ceftazidime	0.25–0.5	0.25–0.5	0.12–0.25	0.25	0.5
Ceftriaxone	0.12–0.25	0.06–0.25	0.003–0.006	0.06	0.12
Cephalothin	8–16	8–16	4–8	16	8
Macrolides					
Azithromycin	0.006–0.015	0.006–0.03	0.015	0.015	0.006
Clarithromycin	0.006–0.03	0.006–0.03	0.015–0.03	0.03	0.015
Erythromycin	0.06–0.25	0.06–0.12	0.06	0.25	0.12
Roxithromycin	0.015–0.03	0.015–0.06	0.03	0.12	0.06
Telithromycin[a]	0.003	0.006	0.015	ND	ND
Penicillins					
Amoxicillin	0.6–0.12	0.03–0.06	0.03–0.06	0.06	0.03
Oxacillin	1–2	1–4	0.25–0.5	1	4
Penicillin G	0.03–0.06	0.03	0.015–0.03	0.03	0.015
Ticarcillin	0.25	0.06–0.25	0.06–0.12	0.25	0.12
Quinolones					
Ciprofloxacin	0.25–1	0.5–2	0.25–0.5	1	0.5
Pefloxacin	4–8	2–8	1–2	4	2
Sparfloxacin	0.06	0.06–0.12	0.25	0.06	0.06
Tetracyclines					
Doxycycline	0.12	0.06–0.25	0.03–0.06	0.25	0.06
Miscellaneous					
Clindamycin	2–4	4–16	32–64	8	8
Colistin	4–16	4–16	16	8	4
Fosfomycin	16–32	32–64	8–16	16	16
Imipenem	0.5	0.25–1	0.5–1	2	0.25
Rifampin	0.03–0.06	0.06–0.25	0.003	0.12	0.03
TMP-SMX	1/5	0.25/1.25–1/5	0.4/2–0.8/4	1/5	0.5/2.5
Vancomycin	2–8	8–16	4–8	8	8

[a]Determined by the agar dilution technique with Columbia agar supplemented with 5% horse blood. Table adapted from reference 122. Abbreviations: TMP-SMX, trimethoprim-sulfamethoxazole; ND, not done.

susceptibility to antibiotics has been performed either with cell cultures or with axenic media. These methods can also be used for determining the bacteriostatic activity of antibiotics. Determination of antibiotic susceptibility in axenic medium has been carried out both on solid media enriched with 5 to 10% sheep or horse blood and in liquid media (101, 133). It should be noted that the conditions required to grow *Bartonella* during susceptibility testing do not meet standardized criteria established by the Clinical and Laboratory Standards Institute (CLSI). Bacteria of the genus *Bartonella* are susceptible to many antibiotics when grown axenically, including β-lactams, aminoglycosides, chloramphenicol, tetracyclines, macrolide compounds including telithromycin, rifampin, fluoroquinolones, and co-trimoxazole (101, 102, 108, 126).

In vitro antibiotic susceptibilities can also be examined for *Bartonella* species cocultivated with eukaryotic cells. As with agar-based susceptibilities, these studies demonstrate that *Bartonella* spp. are susceptible to many antibiotics in vitro (62). However, all of these antibiotics are bacteriostatic only (63, 64). Only aminoglycosides are bactericidal in vitro when *Bartonella* species are grown either in liquid medium (126), in endothelial cells (107), or in erythrocyte cocultures (125).

Choice and Use of Antibiotics In Vivo

CSD typically does not respond to antibiotic therapy. Most investigators have observed no or minimal benefit with antibiotic treatment, whereas anecdotal reports indicate that ciprofloxacin, rifampin, and co-trimoxazole may be effective (122). Additional efforts are warranted to establish comparative antimicrobial efficacy when treating immunocompetent patients with chronic bacteremia.

EVALUATION, INTERPRETATION, AND REPORTING OF RESULTS

Diagnosis of *Bartonella* infection in humans, especially for typical forms of CSD, is mainly based on serologic data, which is the most cost-effective approach. However, the sensitivity of IFA ranges from 14 to 100%, depending on the antigen, cutoff, and test procedures used (4). For endocarditis, the best approach is serological testing and the performance of nucleic acid amplification methods on cardiac valves. A recent procedure using a single-step serological assay against *Coxiella burnetii* and *Bartonella* species found a sensitivity of 100% and a positive predictive value of 98% for the diagnosis of *Bartonella* infection in blood culture-negative endocarditis (124). New methods of culture in liquid medium are proving diagnostically useful, as direct isolation from blood or tissues is often unsuccessful despite detection of *Bartonella* DNA (10, 14–16, 18, 24, 31, 32, 37, 43, 44, 56, 69, 91, 93, 94, 105, 152; Maggi et al., presented at the 20th ASR Meeting and 5th International Conference on Bartonella as Emerging Pathogens, Pacific Grove, CA, 2006).

REFERENCES

1. **Agan, B. K., and M. J. Dolan.** 2002. Laboratory diagnosis of *Bartonella* infections. *Clin. Lab. Med.* **22:**937–962.
2. **Bereswill, S., S. Hinkelmann, M. Kist, and A. Sander.** 1999. Molecular analysis of riboflavin synthesis genes in *Bartonella henselae* and use of the *ribC* gene for differentiation of *Bartonella* species by PCR. *J. Clin. Microbiol.* **37:**3159–3166.
3. **Berghoff, J., J. Viezens, L. Guptill, M. Fabbi, and M. Arvand.** 2007. *Bartonella henselae* exists as a mosaic of different genetic variants in the infected host. *Microbiology* **153:**2045–2051.
4. **Bergmans, A. M., M. F. Peeters, J. F. Schellekens, M. C. Vos, L. J. Sabbe, J. M. Ossewaarde, H. Verbakel, H. J. Hooft, and L. M. Schouls.** 1997. Pitfalls and fallacies of cat scratch disease serology: evaluation of *Bartonella henselae*-based indirect fluorescence assay and enzyme-linked immunoassay. *J. Clin. Microbiol.* **35:**1931–1937.
5. **Billeter, S. A., M. G. Levy, B. B. Chomel, and E. B. Breitschwerdt.** 2008. Vector transmission of *Bartonella* species with emphasis on the potential for tick transmission. *Med. Vet. Entomol.* **22:**1–15.
6. **Boonjakuakul, J. K., H. L. Gerns, Y. T. Chen, L. D. Hicks, M. F. Minnick, S. E. Dixon, S. C. Hall, and J. E. Koehler.** 2007. Proteomic and immunoblot analyses of *Bartonella quintana* total membrane proteins identify antigens recognized by sera from infected patients. *Infect. Immun.* **75:**2548–2561.
6a. **Boulouis, H. J., F. Barrat, D. Bermond, F. Bernex, D. Thibault, R. Heller, J.-J. Fontaine, Y. Piémont, and B. B. Chomel.** 2001. Kinetics of *Bartonella birtlesii* infection in experimentally infected mice and pathogenic effect on reproductive functions. *Infect. Immun.* **69:**5313–5317.
7. **Boulouis, H. J., C. C. Chang, J. B. Henn, R. W. Kasten, and B. B. Chomel.** 2005. Factors associated with the rapid emergence of zoonotic *Bartonella* infections. *Vet. Res.* **36:**383–410.
8. **Breitschwerdt, E. B.** 2008. Feline bartonellosis and cat scratch disease. *Vet. Immunol. Immunopathol.* **123:**167–171.
9. **Breitschwerdt, E. B., C. E. Atkins, T. T. Brown, D. L. Kordick, and P. S. Snyder.** 1999. *Bartonella vinsonii* subsp. *berkhoffii* and related members of the alpha subdivision of the *Proteobacteria* in dogs with cardiac arrhythmias, endocarditis, or myocarditis. *J. Clin. Microbiol.* **37:**3618–3626.

10. **Breitschwerdt, E. B., B. C. Hegarty, R. Maggi, E. Hawkins, and P. Dyer.** 2005. *Bartonella* species as a potential cause of epistaxis in dogs. *J. Clin. Microbiol.* **43:**2529–2533.
11. **Breitschwerdt, E. B., and D. L. Kordick.** 2000. *Bartonella* infection in animals: carriership, reservoir potential, pathogenicity, and zoonotic potential for human infection. *Clin. Microbiol. Rev.* **13:**428–438.
12. **Breitschwerdt, E. B., and D. L. Kordick.** 1995. Bartonellosis. *J. Am. Vet. Med. Assoc.* **206:**1928–1931.
13. **Breitschwerdt, E. B., D. L. Kordick, D. E. Malarkey, B. Keene, T. L. Hadfield, and K. Wilson.** 1995. Endocarditis in a dog due to infection with a novel *Bartonella* subspecies. *J. Clin. Microbiol.* **33:**154–160.
14. **Breitschwerdt, E. B., R. G. Maggi, A. W. Duncan, W. L. Nicholson, B. C. Hegarty, and C. W. Woods.** 2007. *Bartonella* species in blood of immunocompetent persons with animal and arthropod contact. *Emerg. Infect. Dis.* **13:**938–941.
15. **Breitschwerdt, E. B., R. G. Maggi, W. L. Nicholson, N. A. Cherry, and C. W. Woods.** 2008. *Bartonella* sp. bacteremia in patients with neurological and neurocognitive dysfunction. *J. Clin. Microbiol.* **46:**2856–2861.
16. **Breitschwerdt, E. B., R. G. Maggi, B. Sigmon, and W. L. Nicholson.** 2007. Isolation of *Bartonella quintana* from a woman and a cat following putative bite transmission. *J. Clin. Microbiol.* **45:**270–272.
17. **Brouqui, P., B. Lascola, V. Roux, and D. Raoult.** 1999. Chronic *Bartonella quintana* bacteremia in homeless patients. *N. Engl. J. Med.* **340:**184–189.
18. **Cadenas, M. B., J. Bradley, R. G. Maggi, M. Takara, B. C. Hegarty, and E. B. Breitschwerdt.** 2008. Molecular characterization of *Bartonella vinsonii* subsp. *berkhoffii* genotype III. *J. Clin. Microbiol.* **46:**1858–1860.
19. **Chamberlin, J., L. W. Laughlin, S. Romero, N. Solorzano, S. Gordon, R. G. Andre, P. Pachas, H. Friedman, C. Ponce, and D. Watts.** 2002. Epidemiology of endemic *Bartonella bacilliformis*: a prospective cohort study in a Peruvian mountain valley community. *J. Infect. Dis.* **186:**983–990.
20. **Chang, C. C., B. B. Chomel, R. W. Kasten, V. Romano, and N. Tietze.** 2001. Molecular evidence of *Bartonella* spp. in questing adult *Ixodes pacificus* ticks in California. *J. Clin. Microbiol.* **39:**1221–1226.
21. **Chang, C. C., R. W. Kasten, B. B. Chomel, D. C. Simpson, C. M. Hew, D. L. Kordick, R. Heller, Y. Piemont, and E. B. Breitschwerdt.** 2000. Coyotes (*Canis latrans*) as the reservoir for a human pathogenic *Bartonella* sp.: molecular epidemiology of *Bartonella vinsonii* subsp. *berkhoffii* infection in coyotes from central coastal California. *J. Clin. Microbiol.* **38:**4193–4200.
22. **Chenoweth, M. R., G. A. Somerville, D. C. Krause, K. L. O'Reilly, and F. C. Gherardini.** 2004. Growth characteristics of *Bartonella henselae* in a novel liquid medium: primary isolation, growth-phase-dependent phage induction, and metabolic studies. *Appl. Environ. Microbiol.* **70:**656–663.
23. **Cherry, N. A., P. P. Diniz, R. G. Maggi, J. B. Hummel, E. M. Hardie, E. N. Behrend, E. Rozanski, T. C. Defrancesco, M. B. Cadenas, and E. B. Breitschwerdt.** 2009. Isolation or molecular detection of *Bartonella henselae* and *Bartonella vinsonii* subsp. *berkhoffii* from dogs with idiopathic cavitary effusions. *J. Vet. Intern. Med.* **23:**186–189.
24. **Cherry, N. A., R. G. Maggi, A. L. Cannedy, and E. B. Breitschwerdt.** 2009. PCR detection of *Bartonella bovis* and *Bartonella henselae* in the blood of beef cattle. *Vet. Microbiol.* **135:**308–312.
25. **Chomel, B. B.** 1996. Cat-scratch disease and bacillary angiomatosis. *Rev. Sci. Tech.* **15:**1061–1073.
26. **Chomel, B. B., and H. J. Boulouis.** 2005. Zoonotic diseases caused by bacteria of the genus *Bartonella* genus: new reservoirs? New vectors? *Bull. Acad. Natl. Med.* **189:**465–477; discussion, 477–480. (In French.)
27. **Chomel, B. B., H. J. Boulouis, and E. B. Breitschwerdt.** 2004. Cat scratch disease and other zoonotic *Bartonella* infections. *J. Am. Vet. Med. Assoc.* **224:**1270–1279.
28. **Chomel, B. B., H. J. Boulouis, S. Maruyama, and E. B. Breitschwerdt.** 2006. *Bartonella* spp. in pets and effect on human health. *Emerg. Infect. Dis.* **12:**389–394.

29. Chomel, B. B., R. W. Kasten, J. B. Henn, and S. Molia. 2006. *Bartonella* infection in domestic cats and wild felids. *Ann. N. Y. Acad. Sci.* **1078**:410–415.

29a. Chomel, B. B., R. W. Kasten, J. E. Sykes, H. J. Boulouis, and E. B. Breitschwerdt. 2003. Clinical impact of persistent *Bartonella* bacteremia in humans and animals. *Ann. N. Y. Acad. Sci.* **990**:267–278.

30. Chomel, B. B., R. W. Kasten, C. Williams, A. C. Wey, J. B. Henn, R. Maggi, S. Carrasco, J. Mazet, H. J. Boulouis, R. Maillard, and E. B. Breitschwerdt. 2009. *Bartonella* endocarditis: a pathology shared by animal reservoirs and patients. *Ann. N. Y. Acad. Sci.* **1166**:120–126.

31. Cockwill, K. R., S. M. Taylor, H. M. Philibert, E. B. Breitschwerdt, and R. G. Maggi. 2007. *Bartonella vinsonii* subsp. *berkhoffii* endocarditis in a dog from Saskatchewan. *Can. Vet. J.* **48**:839–844.

32. Cross, J. R., J. H. Rossmeisl, R. G. Maggi, E. B. Breitschwerdt, and R. B. Duncan. 2008. Bartonella-associated meningoradiculoneuritis and dermatitis or panniculitis in 3 dogs. *J. Vet. Intern. Med.* **22**:674–678.

33. Dalton, M. J., L. E. Robinson, J. Cooper, R. L. Regnery, J. G. Olson, and J. E. Childs. 1995. Use of *Bartonella* antigens for serologic diagnosis of cat-scratch disease at a national referral center. *Arch. Intern. Med.* **155**:1670–1676.

34. Dauga, C., I. Miras, and P. A. Grimont. 1996. Identification of *Bartonella henselae* and *B. quintana* 16s rDNA sequences by branch-, genus- and species-specific amplification. *J. Med. Microbiol.* **45**:192–199.

35. De Paiva Diniz, P. P., D. S. Schwartz, H. S. De Morais, and E. B. Breitschwerdt. 2007. Surveillance for zoonotic vector-borne infections using sick dogs from southeastern Brazil. *Vector Borne Zoonotic Dis.* **7**:689–697.

35a. Dietrich, F., T. Schmidgen, R. G. Maggi, D. Ritcher, F.-R. Matuschka, R. Vonthein, E. B. Breitschwerdt, and V. A. Kempf. 2010. Prevalence of *Bartonella henselae* and *Borrelia burgdorferi* sensu lato DNA in *Ixodes ricinus* ticks in Europe. *Appl. Environ. Microbiol.* **76**:1395–1398.

36. Dillon, B., J. Iredell, E. B. Breitschwerdt, and R. G. Maggi. 2005. Potential limitations of the 16S-23S rRNA intergenic region for molecular detection of *Bartonella* species. *J. Clin. Microbiol.* **43**:4921–4922.

37. Diniz, P. P., R. G. Maggi, D. S. Schwartz, M. B. Cadenas, J. M. Bradley, B. Hegarty, and E. B. Breitschwerdt. 2007. Canine bartonellosis: serological and molecular prevalence in Brazil and evidence of co-infection with *Bartonella henselae* and *Bartonella vinsonii* subsp. *berkhoffii*. *Vet. Res.* **38**:697–710.

38. Drancourt, M., R. Birtles, G. Chaumentin, F. Vandenesch, J. Etienne, and D. Raoult. 1996. New serotype of *Bartonella henselae* in endocarditis and cat-scratch disease. *Lancet* **347**:441–443.

39. Drancourt, M., J. L. Mainardi, P. Brouqui, F. Vandenesch, A. Carta, F. Lehnert, J. Etienne, F. Goldstein, J. Acar, and D. Raoult. 1995. *Bartonella (Rochalimaea) quintana* endocarditis in three homeless men. *N. Engl. J. Med.* **332**:419–423.

40. Drancourt, M., V. Moal, P. Brunet, B. Dussol, Y. Berland, and D. Raoult. 1996. *Bartonella (Rochalimaea) quintana* infection in a seronegative hemodialyzed patient. *J. Clin. Microbiol.* **34**:1158–1160.

41. Droz, S., B. Chi, E. Horn, A. G. Steigerwalt, A. M. Whitney, and D. J. Brenner. 1999. *Bartonella koehlerae* sp. nov., isolated from cats. *J. Clin. Microbiol.* **37**:1117–1122.

42. Duncan, A. W., R. G. Maggi, and E. B. Breitschwerdt. 2007. *Bartonella* DNA in dog saliva. *Emerg. Infect. Dis.* **13**:1948–1950.

43. Duncan, A. W., R. G. Maggi, and E. B. Breitschwerdt. 2007. A combined approach for the enhanced detection and isolation of *Bartonella* species in dog blood samples: pre-enrichment liquid culture followed by PCR and subculture onto agar plates. *J. Microbiol. Methods* **69**:273–281.

44. Duncan, A. W., H. S. Marr, A. J. Birkenheuer, R. G. Maggi, L. E. Williams, M. T. Correa, and E. B. Breitschwerdt. 2008. *Bartonella* DNA in the blood and lymph nodes of golden retrievers with lymphoma and in healthy controls. *J. Vet. Intern. Med.* **22**:89–95.

45. Dupon, M., A. M. Savin De Larclause, P. Brouqui, M. Drancourt, D. Raoult, A. De Mascarel, and J. Y. Lacut. 1996. Evaluation of serological response to *Bartonella henselae*, *Bartonella quintana* and *Afipia felis* antigens in 64 patients with suspected cat-scratch disease. *Scand. J. Infect. Dis.* **28**:361–366.

46. Eberhardt, C., S. Engelmann, H. Kusch, D. Albrecht, M. Hecker, I. B. Autenrieth, and V. A. Kempf. 2009. Proteomic analysis of the bacterial pathogen *Bartonella henselae* and identification of immunogenic proteins for serodiagnosis. *Proteomics* **9**:1967–1981.

47. Fenollar, F., and D. Raoult. 2004. Molecular genetic methods for the diagnosis of fastidious microorganisms. *APMIS* **112**:785–807.

48. Fenollar, F., S. Sire, and D. Raoult. 2005. *Bartonella vinsonii* subsp. *arupensis* as an agent of blood culture-negative endocarditis in a human. *J. Clin. Microbiol.* **43**:945–947.

49. Foucault, C., B. La Scola, H. Lindroos, S. G. Andersson, and D. Raoult. 2005. Multispacer typing technique for sequence-based typing of *Bartonella quintana*. *J. Clin. Microbiol.* **43**:41–48.

49a. Fournier, P. E., C. Couderc, S. Buffet, C. Flaudrops, and D. Raoult. 2009. Rapid and cost-effective identification of *Bartonella* species using mass spectrometry. *J. Med. Microbiol.* **58**:1154–1159.

50. Fournier, P. E., J. L. Mainardi, and D. Raoult. 2002. Value of microimmunofluorescence for diagnosis and follow-up of *Bartonella* endocarditis. *Clin. Diagn. Lab. Immunol.* **9**:795–801.

51. Fournier, P. E., J. Robson, Z. Zeaiter, R. McDougall, S. Byrne, and D. Raoult. 2002. Improved culture from lymph nodes of patients with cat scratch disease and genotypic characterization of *Bartonella henselae* isolates in Australia. *J. Clin. Microbiol.* **40**:3620–3624.

52. Goodman, R. A., and E. B. Breitschwerdt. 2005. Clinicopathologic findings in dogs seroreactive to *Bartonella henselae* antigens. *Am. J. Vet. Res.* **66**:2060–2064.

53. Gurfield, A. N., H. J. Boulouis, B. B. Chomel, R. Heller, R. W. Kasten, K. Yamamoto, and Y. Piemont. 1997. Coinfection with *Bartonella clarridgeiae* and *Bartonella henselae* and with different *Bartonella henselae* strains in domestic cats. *J. Clin. Microbiol.* **35**:2120–2123.

54. Guyot, A., A. Bakhai, N. Fry, J. Merritt, H. Malnick, and T. Harrison. 1999. Culture-positive *Bartonella quintana* endocarditis. *Eur. J. Clin. Microbiol. Infect. Dis.* **18**:145–147.

55. Handley, S. A., and R. L. Regnery. 2000. Differentiation of pathogenic *Bartonella* species by infrequent restriction site PCR. *J. Clin. Microbiol.* **38**:3010–3015.

56. Harms, C., R. G. Maggi, E. B. Breitschwerdt, C. L. Clemons-Chevis, M. Solangi, D. S. Rotstein, P. A. Fair, L. J. Hansen, A. A. Hohn, G. N. Lovewell, W. A. McLellan, D. A. Pabst, T. K. Rowles, L. H. Schwacke, F. I. Townsend, and R. S. Wells. 2008. *Bartonella* species detection in captive, stranded and free-ranging cetaceans. *Vet. Res.* **39**:59.

57. Heller, R., M. Artois, V. Xemar, D. De Briel, H. Gehin, B. Jaulhac, H. Monteil, and Y. Piemont. 1997. Prevalence of *Bartonella henselae* and *Bartonella clarridgeiae* in stray cats. *J. Clin. Microbiol.* **35**:1327–1331.

58. Henn, J. B., M. W. Gabriel, R. W. Kasten, R. N. Brown, J. E. Koehler, K. A. MacDonald, M. D. Kittleson, W. P. Thomas, and B. B. Chomel. 2008. Infective endocarditis in a dog and the phylogenic relationship of the associated "*Bartonella rochalimae*" strain with isolates from dogs, gray foxes, and a human. *J. Clin. Microbiol.* **47**:787–790.

59. Houpikian, P., and D. Raoult. 2001. 16S/23S rRNA intergenic spacer regions for phylogenetic analysis, identification, and subtyping of *Bartonella* species. *J. Clin. Microbiol.* **39**:2768–2778.

60. Houpikian, P., and D. Raoult. 2005. Blood culture-negative endocarditis in a reference center: etiologic diagnosis of 348 cases. *Medicine* (Baltimore) **84**:162–173.

61. Houpikian, P., and D. Raoult. 2003. Diagnostic methods. Current best practices and guidelines for identification of difficult-to-culture pathogens in infective endocarditis. *Cardiol. Clin.* **21**:207–217.

62. **Ives, T. J., P. Manzewitsch, R. L. Regnery, J. D. Butts, and M. Kebede.** 1997. In vitro susceptibilities of *Bartonella henselae, B. quintana, B. elizabethae, Rickettsia rickettsii, R. conorii, R. akari,* and *R. prowazekii* to macrolide antibiotics as determined by immunofluorescent-antibody analysis of infected Vero cell monolayers. *Antimicrob. Agents Chemother.* **41:**578–582.

63. **Ives, T. J., E. L. Marston, R. L. Regnery, and J. D. Butts.** 2001. In vitro susceptibilities of *Bartonella* and *Rickettsia* spp. to fluoroquinolone antibiotics as determined by immunofluorescent antibody analysis of infected Vero cell monolayers. *Int. J. Antimicrob. Agents* **18:**217–222.

64. **Ives, T. J., E. L. Marston, R. L. Regnery, J. D. Butts, and T. C. Majerus.** 2000. In vitro susceptibilities of *Rickettsia* and *Bartonella* spp. to 14-hydroxy-clarithromycin as determined by immunofluorescent antibody analysis of infected Vero cell monolayers. *J. Antimicrob. Chemother.* **45:**305–310.

65. **Jackson, L. A., and D. H. Spach.** 1996. Emergence of *Bartonella quintana* infection among homeless persons. *Emerg. Infect. Dis.* **2:**141–144.

66. **Jacomo, V., P. J. Kelly, and D. Raoult.** 2002. Natural history of *Bartonella* infections (an exception to Koch's postulate). *Clin. Diagn. Lab. Immunol.* **9:**8–18.

67. **Jensen, W. A., M. Z. Fall, J. Rooney, D. L. Kordick, and E. B. Breitschwerdt.** 2000. Rapid identification and differentiation of *Bartonella* species using a single-step PCR assay. *J. Clin. Microbiol.* **38:**1717–1722.

68. **Joblet, C., V. Roux, M. Drancourt, J. Gouvernet, and D. Raoult.** 1995. Identification of *Bartonella* (*Rochalimaea*) species among fastidious gram-negative bacteria on the basis of the partial sequence of the citrate-synthase gene. *J. Clin. Microbiol.* **33:**1879–1883.

69. **Jones, S. L., R. Maggi, J. Shuler, A. Alward, and E. B. Breitschwerdt.** 2008. Detection of *Bartonella henselae* in the blood of 2 adult horses. *J. Vet. Intern. Med.* **22:**495–498.

70. **Kelly, P., J. M. Rolain, R. Maggi, S. Sontakke, B. Keene, S. Hunter, H. Lepidi, K. T. Breitschwerdt, and E. B. Breitschwerdt.** 2006. *Bartonella quintana* endocarditis in dogs. *Emerg. Infect. Dis.* **12:**1869–1872.

71. **Keret, D., M. Giladi, Y. Kletter, and S. Wientroub.** 1998. Cat-scratch disease osteomyelitis from a dog scratch. *J. Bone Joint Surg.* **80:**766–767.

72. **Kerkhoff, F. T., A. M. Bergmans, A. van Der Zee, and A. Rothova.** 1999. Demonstration of *Bartonella grahamii* DNA in ocular fluids of a patient with neuroretinitis. *J. Clin. Microbiol.* **37:**4034–4038.

73. **Kerkhoff, F. T., and A. Rothova.** 2000. *Bartonella henselae* associated uveitis and HLA-B27. *Br. J. Ophthalmol.* **84:**1125–1129.

74. **Koehler, J. E., F. D. Quinn, T. G. Berger, P. E. LeBoit, and J. W. Tappero.** 1992. Isolation of *Rochalimaea* species from cutaneous and osseous lesions of bacillary angiomatosis. *N. Engl. J. Med.* **327:**1625–1631.

75. **Koehler, J. E., M. A. Sanchez, C. S. Garrido, M. J. Whitfeld, F. M. Chen, T. G. Berger, M. C. Rodriguez-Barradas, P. E. LeBoit, and J. W. Tappero.** 1997. Molecular epidemiology of bartonella infections in patients with bacillary angiomatosis-peliosis. *N. Engl. J. Med.* **337:**1876–1883.

76. **Koehler, J. E., and J. W. Tappero.** 1993. Bacillary angiomatosis and bacillary peliosis in patients infected with human immunodeficiency virus. *Clin. Infect. Dis.* **17:**612–624.

77. **Kordick, D. L., E. J. Hilyard, T. L. Hadfield, K. H. Wilson, A. G. Steigerwalt, D. J. Brenner, and E. B. Breitschwerdt.** 1997. *Bartonella clarridgeiae,* a newly recognized zoonotic pathogen causing inoculation papules, fever, and lymphadenopathy (cat scratch disease). *J. Clin. Microbiol.* **35:**1813–1818.

78. **Kordick, D. L., B. Swaminathan, C. E. Greene, K. H. Wilson, A. M. Whitney, S. O'Connor, D. G. Hollis, G. M. Matar, A. G. Steigerwalt, G. B. Malcolm, P. S. Hayes, T. L. Hadfield, E. B. Breitschwerdt, and D. J. Brenner.** 1996. *Bartonella vinsonii* subsp. *berkhoffii* subsp. nov., isolated from dogs; *Bartonella vinsonii* subsp. *vinsonii;* and emended description of *Bartonella vinsonii. Int. J. Syst. Bacteriol.* **46:**704–709.

79. **Kordick, S. K., E. B. Breitschwerdt, B. C. Hegarty, K. L. Southwick, C. M. Colitz, S. I. Hancock, J. M. Bradley,** R. Rumbough, J. T. McPherson, and J. N. MacCormack. 1999. Coinfection with multiple tick-borne pathogens in a Walker Hound kennel in North Carolina. *J. Clin. Microbiol.* **37:**2631–2638.

80. **Kosek, M., R. Lavarello, R. H. Gilman, J. Delgado, C. Maguina, M. Verastegui, A. G. Lescano, V. Mallqui, J. C. Kosek, S. Recavarren, and L. Cabrera.** 2000. Natural history of infection with *Bartonella bacilliformis* in a nonendemic population. *J. Infect. Dis.* **182:**865–872.

81. **Kosoy, M., C. Morway, K. W. Sheff, Y. Bai, J. Colborn, L. Chalcraft, S. F. Dowell, L. F. Peruski, S. A. Maloney, H. Baggett, S. Sutthirattana, A. Sidhirat, S. Maruyama, H. Kabeya, B. B. Chomel, R. Kasten, V. Popov, J. Robinson, A. Kruglov, and L. R. Petersen.** 2008. *Bartonella tamiae* sp. nov., a newly recognized pathogen isolated from three human patients from Thailand. *J. Clin. Microbiol.* **46:**772–775.

82. **Lappin, M. R., E. Breitschwerdt, M. Brewer, J. Hawley, B. Hegarty, and S. Radecki.** 2009. Prevalence of *Bartonella* species antibodies and *Bartonella* species DNA in the blood of cats with and without fever. *J. Feline Med. Surg.* **11:**141–148.

83. **Lappin, M. R., D. L. Kordick, and E. B. Breitschwerdt.** 2000. *Bartonella* spp. antibodies and DNA in aqueous humour of cats. *J. Feline Med. Surg.* **2:**61–68.

84. **La Scola, B., and D. Raoult.** 1999. Culture of *Bartonella quintana* and *Bartonella henselae* from human samples: a 5-year experience (1993 to 1998). *J. Clin. Microbiol.* **37:**1899–1905.

85. **La Scola, B., and D. Raoult.** 1996. Serological cross-reactions between *Bartonella quintana, Bartonella henselae,* and *Coxiella burnetii. J. Clin. Microbiol.* **34:**2270–2274.

86. **La Scola, B., Z. Zeaiter, A. Khamis, and D. Raoult.** 2003. Gene-sequence-based criteria for species definition in bacteriology: the *Bartonella* paradigm. *Trends Microbiol.* **11:**318–321.

87. **Liang, Z., and D. Raoult.** 2000. Species-specific monoclonal antibodies for rapid identification of *Bartonella quintana. Clin. Diagn. Lab. Immunol.* **7:**21–24.

88. **Luria, B. J., J. K. Levy, M. R. Lappin, E. B. Breitschwerdt, A. M. Legendre, J. A. Hernandez, S. P. Gorman, and I. T. Lee.** 2004. Prevalence of infectious diseases in feral cats in Northern Florida. *J. Feline Med. Surg.* **6:**287–296.

89. **Maggi, R. G., and E. B. Breitschwerdt.** 2005. Potential limitations of the 16S-23S rRNA intergenic region for molecular detection of *Bartonella* species. *J. Clin. Microbiol.* **43:**1171–1176.

90. **Maggi, R. G., B. Chomel, B. C. Hegarty, J. Henn, and E. B. Breitschwerdt.** 2006. A *Bartonella vinsonii berkhoffii* typing scheme based upon 16S-23S ITS and Pap31 sequences from dog, coyote, gray fox, and human isolates. *Mol. Cell. Probes* **20:**128–134.

91. **Maggi, R. G., A. W. Duncan, and E. B. Breitschwerdt.** 2005. Novel chemically modified liquid medium that will support the growth of seven bartonella species. *J. Clin. Microbiol.* **43:**2651–2655.

92. **Maggi, R. G., C. A. Harms, A. A. Hohn, D. A. Pabst, W. A. McLellan, W. J. Walton, D. S. Rotstein, and E. B. Breitschwerdt.** 2005. *Bartonella henselae* in porpoise blood. *Emerg. Infect. Dis.* **11:**1894–1898.

93. **Maggi, R. G., M. Kosoy, M. Mintzer, and E. B. Breitschwerdt.** 2009. Isolation of Candidatus *Bartonella melophagi* from human blood. *Emerg. Infect. Dis.* **15:**66–68.

94. **Maggi, R. G., S. A. Raverty, S. J. Lester, D. G. Huff, M. Haulena, S. L. Ford, O. Nielsen, J. H. Robinson, and E. B. Breitschwerdt.** 2008. *Bartonella henselae* in captive and hunter-harvested beluga (*Delphinapterus leucas*). *J. Wildl. Dis.* **44:**871–877.

95. **Mainardi, J. L., C. Figliolini, F. W. Goldstein, P. Blanche, M. Baret-Rigoulet, N. Galezowski, P. E. Fournier, and D. Raoult.** 1998. Cat scratch disease due to *Bartonella henselae* serotype Marseille (Swiss cat) in a seronegative patient. *J. Clin. Microbiol.* **36:**2800.

96. **Mandle, T., H. Einsele, M. Schaller, D. Neumann, W. Vogel, I. B. Autenrieth, and V. A. Kempf.** 2005. Infection of human CD34+ progenitor cells with *Bartonella henselae* results in intraerythrocytic presence of *B. henselae. Blood* **106:**1215–1222.

97. **Margileth, A. M., and D. F. Baehren.** 1998. Chest-wall abscess due to cat-scratch disease (CSD) in an adult with antibodies to *Bartonella clarridgeiae*: case report and review of the thoracopulmonary manifestations of CSD. *Clin. Infect. Dis.* **27:**353–357.

98. **Maruyama, S., S. Hiraga, E. Yokoyama, M. Naoi, Y. Tsuruoka, Y. Ogura, K. Tamura, S. Namba, Y. Kameyama, S. Nakamura, and Y. Katsube.** 1998. Seroprevalence of *Bartonella henselae* and *Toxoplasma gondii* infections among pet cats in Kanagawa and Saitama Prefectures. *J. Vet. Med. Sci.* **60:**997–1000.

99. **Mateen, F. J., J. C. Newstead, and K. L. McClean.** 2005. Bacillary angiomatosis in an HIV-positive man with multiple risk factors: a clinical and epidemiological puzzle. *Can. J. Infect. Dis. Med. Microbiol.* **16:**249–252.

100. **Maurin, M., F. Eb, J. Etienne, and D. Raoult.** 1997. Serological cross-reactions between *Bartonella* and *Chlamydia* species: implications for diagnosis. *J. Clin. Microbiol.* **35:**2283–2287.

101. **Maurin, M., S. Gasquet, C. Ducco, and D. Raoult.** 1995. MICs of 28 antibiotic compounds for 14 *Bartonella* (formerly *Rochalimaea*) isolates. *Antimicrob. Agents Chemother.* **39:**2387–2391.

102. **Maurin, M., and D. Raoult.** 1993. Antimicrobial susceptibility of *Rochalimaea quintana, Rochalimaea vinsonii,* and the newly recognized *Rochalimaea henselae. J. Antimicrob. Chemother.* **32:**587–594.

103. **Maurin, M., J. M. Rolain, and D. Raoult.** 2002. Comparison of in-house and commercial slides for detection by immunofluorescence of immunoglobulins G and M against *Bartonella henselae* and *Bartonella quintana. Clin. Diagn. Lab. Immunol.* **9:**1004–1009.

104. **Monteil, M., B. Durand, R. Bouchouicha, E. Petit, B. Chomel, M. Arvand, H. J. Boulouis, and N. Haddad.** 2007. Development of discriminatory multiple-locus variable number tandem repeat analysis for *Bartonella henselae. Microbiology* **153:**1141–1148.

105. **Morales, S. C., E. B. Breitschwerdt, R. J. Washabau, I. Matise, R. G. Maggi, and A. W. Duncan.** 2007. Detection of *Bartonella henselae* DNA in two dogs with pyogranulomatous lymphadenitis. *J. Am. Vet. Med. Assoc.* **230:**681–685.

106. **Murakami, K., M. Tsukahara, H. Tsuneoka, H. Iino, C. Ishida, K. Tsujino, A. Umeda, T. Furuya, S. Kawauchi, and K. Sasaki.** 2002. Cat scratch disease: analysis of 130 seropositive cases. *J. Infect. Chemother.* **8:**349–352.

107. **Musso, D., M. Drancourt, and D. Raoult.** 1995. Lack of bactericidal effect of antibiotics except aminoglycosides on *Bartonella (Rochalimaea) henselae. J. Antimicrob. Chemother.* **36:**101–108.

108. **Myers, W. F., D. M. Grossman, and C. L. Wisseman, Jr.** 1984. Antibiotic susceptibility patterns in *Rochalimaea quintana,* the agent of trench fever. *Antimicrob. Agents Chemother.* **25:**690–693.

109. **Norman, A. F., R. Regnery, P. Jameson, C. Greene, and D. C. Krause.** 1995. Differentiation of *Bartonella*-like isolates at the species level by PCR-restriction fragment length polymorphism in the citrate synthase gene. *J. Clin. Microbiol.* **33:**1797–1803.

110. **Pappalardo, B. L., M. T. Correa, C. C. York, C. Y. Peat, and E. B. Breitschwerdt.** 1997. Epidemiologic evaluation of the risk factors associated with exposure and seroreactivity to *Bartonella vinsonii* in dogs. *Am. J. Vet. Res.* **58:**467–471.

111. **Patel, R., J. O. Newell, G. W. Procop, and D. H. Persing.** 1999. Use of polymerase chain reaction for citrate synthase gene to diagnose *Bartonella quintana* endocarditis. *Am. J. Clin. Pathol.* **112:**36–40.

112. **Raoult, D., C. Foucault, and P. Brouqui.** 2001. Infections in the homeless. *Lancet Infect. Dis.* **1:**77–84.

113. **Raoult, D., F. Roblot, J. M. Rolain, J. M. Besnier, J. Loulergue, F. Bastides, and P. Choutet.** 2006. First isolation of *Bartonella alsatica* from a valve of a patient with endocarditis. *J. Clin. Microbiol.* **44:**278–279.

114. **Raoult, D., and V. Roux.** 1999. The body louse as a vector of reemerging human diseases. *Clin. Infect. Dis.* **29:**888–911.

115. **Regnery, R. L., J. G. Olson, B. A. Perkins, and W. Bibb.** 1992. Serological response to "*Rochalimaea henselae*" antigen in suspected cat-scratch disease. *Lancet* **339:**1443–1445.

116. **Relman, D. A., J. S. Loutit, T. M. Schmidt, S. Falkow, and L. S. Tompkins.** 1990. The agent of bacillary angiomatosis. An approach to the identification of uncultured pathogens. *N. Engl. J. Med.* **323:**1573–1580.

117. **Renesto, P., J. Gouvernet, M. Drancourt, V. Roux, and D. Raoult.** 2001. Use of *rpoB* gene analysis for detection and identification of *Bartonella* species. *J. Clin. Microbiol.* **39:**430–437.

118. **Ricketts, W. E.** 1949. Clinical manifestations of Carrion's disease. *Arch. Intern. Med.* (Chicago) **84:**751–781.

119. **Ricketts, W. E.** 1949. A study of 22 cases of Carrion's disease with intercurrent malaria. *Am. J. Med. Sci.* **218:**525–530.

120. **Riess, T., S. G. Andersson, A. Lupas, M. Schaller, A. Schafer, P. Kyme, J. Martin, J. H. Walzlein, U. Ehehalt, H. Lindroos, M. Schirle, A. Nordheim, I. B. Autenrieth, and V. A. Kempf.** 2004. *Bartonella* adhesin A mediates a proangiogenic host cell response. *J. Exp. Med.* **200:** 1267–1278.

121. **Riess, T., F. Dietrich, K. V. Schmidt, P. O. Kaiser, H. Schwarz, A. Schafer, and V. A. Kempf.** 2008. Analysis of a novel insect cell culture medium-based growth medium for *Bartonella* species. *Appl. Environ. Microbiol.* **74:**5224–5227.

122. **Rolain, J. M., P. Brouqui, J. E. Koehler, C. Maguina, M. J. Dolan, and D. Raoult.** 2004. Recommendations for treatment of human infections caused by *Bartonella* species. *Antimicrob. Agents Chemother.* **48:**1921–1933.

123. **Rolain, J. M., M. Franc, B. Davoust, and D. Raoult.** 2003. Molecular detection of *Bartonella quintana, B. koehlerae, B. henselae, B. clarridgeiae, Rickettsia felis,* and *Wolbachia pipientis* in cat fleas, France. *Emerg. Infect. Dis.* **9:**338–342.

124. **Rolain, J. M., C. Lecam, and D. Raoult.** 2003. Simplified serological diagnosis of endocarditis due to *Coxiella burnetii* and *Bartonella. Clin. Diagn. Lab. Immunol.* **10:**1147–1148.

125. **Rolain, J. M., M. Maurin, M. N. Mallet, D. Parzy, and D. Raoult.** 2003. Culture and antibiotic susceptibility of *Bartonella quintana* in human erythrocytes. *Antimicrob. Agents Chemother.* **47:**614–619.

126. **Rolain, J. M., M. Maurin, and D. Raoult.** 2000. Bactericidal effect of antibiotics on *Bartonella* and *Brucella* spp.: clinical implications. *J. Antimicrob. Chemother.* **46:**811–814.

127. **Rothova, A., F. Kerkhoff, H. J. Hooft, and J. M. Ossewaarde.** 1998. *Bartonella* serology for patients with intraocular inflammatory disease. *Retina* **18:**348–355.

128. **Samson, L., M. Drancourt, J. P. Casalta, and D. Raoult.** 2006. Corpuscular antigenic microarray for the serodiagnosis of blood culture-negative endocarditis. *Ann. N. Y. Acad. Sci.* **1078:**595–596.

129. **Sander, A., R. Berner, and M. Ruess.** 2001. Serodiagnosis of cat scratch disease: response to *Bartonella henselae* in children and a review of diagnostic methods. *Eur. J. Clin. Microbiol. Infect. Dis.* **20:**392–401.

130. **Sander, A., M. Posselt, K. Oberle, and W. Bredt.** 1998. Seroprevalence of antibodies to *Bartonella henselae* in patients with cat scratch disease and in healthy controls: evaluation and comparison of two commercial serological tests. *Clin. Diagn. Lab. Immunol.* **5:**486–490.

131. **Sanogo, Y. O., Z. Zeaiter, G. Caruso, F. Merola, S. Shpynov, P. Brouqui, and D. Raoult.** 2003. *Bartonella henselae* in Ixodes ricinus ticks (Acari: Ixodida) removed from humans, Belluno province, Italy. *Emerg. Infect. Dis.* **9:**329–332.

132. **Schwartzman, W. A., M. Patnaik, F. J. Angulo, B. R. Visscher, E. N. Miller, and J. B. Peter.** 1995. *Bartonella (Rochalimaea)* antibodies, dementia, and cat ownership among men infected with human immunodeficiency virus. *Clin. Infect. Dis.* **21:**954–959.

133. **Sobraques, M., M. Maurin, R. J. Birtles, and D. Raoult.** 1999. In vitro susceptibilities of four *Bartonella bacilliformis* strains to 30 antibiotic compounds. *Antimicrob. Agents Chemother.* **43:**2090–2092.

134. **Solano-Gallego, L., B. Hegarty, Y. Espada, J. Llull, and E. Breitschwerdt.** 2006. Serological and molecular evidence of

exposure to arthropod-borne organisms in cats from north-eastern Spain. *Vet. Microbiol.* **118:**274–277.

135. **Spach, D. H., and J. E. Koehler.** 1998. *Bartonella*-associated infections. *Infect. Dis. Clin. N. Am.* **12:**137–155.

136. **Spach, D. H., L. A. Panther, D. R. Thorning, J. E. Dunn, J. J. Plorde, and R. A. Miller.** 1992. Intracerebral bacillary angiomatosis in a patient infected with human immunodeficiency virus. *Ann. Intern. Med.* **116:**740–742.

137. **Tsukahara, M., H. Iino, C. Ishida, K. Murakami, H. Tsuneoka, and M. Uchida.** 2001. *Bartonella henselae* bacteraemia in patients with cat scratch disease. *Eur. J. Pediatr.* **160:**316.

138. **Tsukahara, M., H. Tsuneoka, H. Iino, K. Ohno, and I. Murano.** 1998. *Bartonella henselae* infection from a dog. *Lancet* **352:**1682.

139. **Tsuneoka, H., R. Fujii, K. Fujisawa, H. Iino, C. Isida, K. Murakami, and M. Tsukahara.** 2000. Clinical evaluation of commercial serological test for *Bartonella* infection. *Kansenshogaku Zasshi* **74:**387–391. (In Japanese.)

140. **Tsuneoka, H., R. Fujii, K. Yamamoto, K. Fujisawa, H. Iino, M. Matsuda, and M. Tsukahara.** 1998. Determination of anti-*Bartonella henselae* antibody by indirect fluorescence antibody test—comparison of two types of antigen: noncocultivated *B. henselae* and cocultivated *B. henselae* with Vero cells. *Kansenshogaku Zasshi* **72:**801–807. (In Japanese.)

141. **Tsuneoka, H., R. Fujii, K. Yamamoto, K. Fujisawa, H. Iino, and M. Tsukahara.** 1999. Prevalence of serum IgG antibody against *Bartonella henselae* in an asymptomatic Japanese population. *Kansenshogaku Zasshi* **73:**90–91. (In Japanese.)

142. **Tsuneoka, H., C. Ishida, and M. Tsukahara.** 2005. Determination of antibody titer to *Bartonella henselae* by indirect fluorescence antibody assay using *B. henselae* from domestic cats as antigen. *Kansenshogaku Zasshi* **79:**826–828. (In Japanese.)

143. **Tsuneoka, H., C. Ishida, A. Umeda, H. Inokuma, and M. Tsukahara.** 2004. Evaluation of isolation media for the detection of *Bartonella henselae*—isolation of *Bartonella henselae* from domestic cats. *Kansenshogaku Zasshi* **78:**574–579. (In Japanese.)

144. **Tsuneoka, H., K. Ouchi, H. Nagaoka, C. Ishida, H. Iino, K. Murakami, K. Tsujino, A. Umeda, and M. Tsukahara.** 2001. Serological cross-reaction among *Bartonella henselae, Chlamydia pneumoniae* and *Coxiella burnetii* by indirect fluorescence antibody method. *Kansenshogaku Zasshi* **75:**406–410. (In Japanese.)

145. **Tsuneoka, H., A. Umeda, M. Tsukahara, and K. Sasaki.** 2004. Evaluation of indirect fluorescence antibody assay for detection of *Bartonella clarridgeiae* and seroprevalence of *B.*

clarridgeiae among patients with suspected cat scratch disease. *J. Clin. Microbiol.* **42:**3346–3349.

146. **Wagner, C. L., T. Riess, D. Linke, C. Eberhardt, A. Schafer, S. Reutter, R. G. Maggi, and V. A. Kempf.** 2008. Use of *Bartonella* adhesin A (BadA) immunoblotting in the serodiagnosis of *Bartonella henselae* infections. *Int. J. Med. Microbiol.* **298:**579–590.

147. **Welch, D. F., K. C. Carroll, E. K. Hofmeister, D. H. Persing, D. A. Robison, A. G. Steigerwalt, and D. J. Brenner.** 1999. Isolation of a new subspecies, *Bartonella vinsonii* subsp. *arupensis,* from a cattle rancher: identity with isolates found in conjunction with *Borrelia burgdorferi* and *Babesia microti* among naturally infected mice. *J. Clin. Microbiol.* **37:**2598–2601.

148. **Welch, D. F., and L. N. Slater.** 2003. *Bartonella* and *Afipia,* p. 824–834. *In* P. R. Murray, E. J. Baron, J. H. Jorgensen, M. A. Pfaller, and R. H. Yolken (ed.), *Manual of Clinical Microbiology,* 8th ed. ASM Press, Washington, DC.

149. **Werner, M., P. E. Fournier, R. Andersson, H. Hogevik, and D. Raoult.** 2003. *Bartonella* and *Coxiella* antibodies in 334 prospectively studied episodes of infective endocarditis in Sweden. *Scand. J. Infect. Dis.* **35:**724–727.

150. **Wolfson, C., J. Branley, and T. Gottlieb.** 1996. The Etest for antimicrobial susceptibility testing of *Bartonella henselae. J. Antimicrob. Chemother.* **38:**963–968.

151. **Wong, M. T., D. C. Thornton, R. C. Kennedy, and M. J. Dolan.** 1995. A chemically defined liquid medium that supports primary isolation of *Rochalimaea (Bartonella) henselae* from blood and tissue specimens. *J. Clin. Microbiol.* **33:**742–744.

152. **Wood, M., R. Maggi, and E. Breitschwerdt.** 2005. The use of pre-enrichment media to enhance detection and isolation of *Bartonella* spp. from dogs. *J. Vet. Intern. Med.* **19:**468.

153. **Zangwill, K. M., D. H. Hamilton, B. A. Perkins, R. L. Regnery, B. D. Plikaytis, J. L. Hadler, M. L. Cartter, and J. D. Wenger.** 1993. Cat scratch disease in Connecticut. Epidemiology, risk factors, and evaluation of a new diagnostic test. *N. Engl. J. Med.* **329:**8–13.

154. **Zeaiter, Z., P. E. Fournier, H. Ogata, and D. Raoult.** 2002. Phylogenetic classification of *Bartonella* species by comparing *groEL* sequences. *Int. J. Syst. Evol. Microbiol.* **52:**165–171.

155. **Zeaiter, Z., P. E. Fournier, and D. Raoult.** 2002. Genomic variation of *Bartonella henselae* strains detected in lymph nodes of patients with cat scratch disease. *J. Clin. Microbiol.* **40:**1023–1030.

156. **Zeaiter, Z., Z. Liang, and D. Raoult.** 2002. Genetic classification and differentiation of *Bartonella* species based on comparison of partial *ftsZ* gene sequences. *J. Clin. Microbiol.* **40:**3641–3647.

Approaches to Identification of Anaerobic Bacteria

ELLEN JO BARON

47

Anaerobic bacteria must be considered etiological agents in a number of clinical syndromes, such as aspiration pneumonia, brain abscess, and intra-abdominal infection, to name a few (19). Infections of prosthetic shoulder joints and corneal implants often involve *Propionibacterium acnes* (27, 39). Thus, complete diagnostic microbiology laboratories must have protocols in place to detect anaerobes, identify them, and determine their antimicrobial susceptibilities. Since the last edition of this *Manual*, *Clostridium difficile* infection has expanded from a largely hospital-acquired syndrome to an international scourge, with highly virulent and drug-resistant strains also causing serious disease in outpatients (6, 17). Lemierre's disease has become more common, and its agent, *Fusobacterium necrophorum*, has been shown to be an important cause of chronic sore throat (1). Many new anaerobic species have been characterized (see the following chapters), and the role of anaerobes in disease has regained respect. Many laboratories have returned to including an anaerobic blood culture bottle in the standard setup, realizing its value (21). This chapter presents an adaptable approach to anaerobic bacteriology based on the resources and capabilities of laboratories.

Specimen choice, collection, transport, and handling are important activities leading to clinically relevant results involving anaerobes. Because of the presence of anaerobes in all mucous membranes of mammals, specimen collection requires extreme caution to avoid contamination by the resident microbiota. Thus, aspirates, curetting specimens from deep wound tissue, and tissue biopsy specimens are recommended (also see chapter 16).

Respiratory tract samples must be collected to avoid oral and nasal secretions. Thus, chronic sinusitis diagnosis requires an aspirate obtained by needle and syringe through the palate or aspirated endoscopically through a protected collector (18). Because transtracheal aspiration is rarely performed today, protected specimen brush samples obtained during endoscopy are the most common acceptable sample for anaerobic culture of lung abscess or other lung infection (4, 11). They must be cultured quantitatively to determine the clinical relevance of isolates. The surgeon should be provided with a freshly boiled tube containing 1 ml chopped-meat broth or anaerobic broth (thioglycolate), into which the brush is dropped after it is cut off the shaft by use of sterile scissors. This protocol requires notifying the laboratory in advance so that the broth can be supplied to the operating attendants. Once received in the laboratory, the broth can be vortexed and a 0.01-ml calibrated loop can be used to inoculate anaerobic and aerobic media. Potential pathogens are usually present in numbers greater than 1,000 CFU/ml (>10 colonies per plate). Physicians often obtain a percutaneous needle aspiration (also called fine-needle aspiration) through intact skin overlying an area of infiltration in the lung, using radiological guidance (7). These samples contain only the tiniest volume of material and must be ground up (if the tissue is solid) and/or diluted in anaerobic broth to stretch the sample for inoculation of all necessary media. This process naturally results in lower recoveries of pathogens present in small numbers. Throat swabs for detection of *F. necrophorum* may be a special case (1).

Because of the relative intolerance of anaerobes to atmospheric oxygen, specimens for anaerobic culture must be transported in containers that exclude air. Some new types of swabs have been shown to maintain the viability of anaerobes during transport (<24 h), but due to the predilection of swabs to pick up contaminating flora and the very small volume that they absorb, they should be reserved for special cases where no other specimen type can be obtained, such as in cases of brain abscess (40). Chapter 16 and the *Wadsworth-KTL Anaerobic Bacteriology Manual* (19) expand on those sites from which anaerobic-bacterial cultures should be performed. Transport devices include small vials with special media and glass beads to break up clumps designed for dental samples (only laboratories with specific expertise should attempt culturing periodontal and other dental infection samples), larger tubes with an anaerobic atmosphere and oxygen-absorbing gel to maintain organism viability, sterile tubes for fluids, citrated or EDTA tubes for serosanguinous fluids in danger of clotting, and plain sterile containers for larger tissue samples (3, 19).

For some anaerobic infections, a Gram stain is a critical step in the diagnosis and allows timely clinical management. Rare urinary tract infections caused by anaerobic bacteria can be detected first by Gram staining (35). Only when urinary tract infections persist and routine aerobic cultures are negative should prolonged incubation in 5% CO_2 or anaerobic-medium inoculation be performed. A sputum Gram stain displaying numerous polymorphonuclear leukocytes (PMNs) or degenerating PMNs, rare or no squamous epithelial cells, and organisms with mixed morphologies, including small gram-positive cocci in chains, fusiform gram-negative rods, and gram-negative coccobacilli, may be the only laboratory test suggesting aspiration pneumonia, as the culture will yield only normal respiratory flora. For serious necrotizing fasciitis, myonecrosis, or clostridial gas gangrene, Gram stains showing rare degenerative PMNs and anaerobic morphotypes (boxcar-shaped gram-positive or variable rods, for example) should be supportive evidence that a patient requires emergent surgery. The special syndrome of bacterial vaginosis, indicated by lack of *Lactobacillus* morphotypes and numerous gram-variable coccobacilli (see chapter 16 for more information) is best diagnosed by Gram staining. In fact, culture is not recommended. Newer studies using molecular methods have shown that many organisms implicated in bacterial vaginosis cannot be recovered in culture (33).

Finally, *Clostridium difficile* infection is best diagnosed by toxigenic culture, with molecular detection of the toxin B gene yielding the next best results (23, 26). Popular enzyme immunoassays for toxins A and B are now known to be not optimal with regard to sensitivity (14, 32). The stool should be inoculated both to selective media and to enrichment broth. Taurocholate-containing agar enhances vegetation of spores and yields the best recovery (5, 17, 25). Stool can be pretreated by heating it at 80°C for 10 min (to select for spores) or, alternatively, by mixing it 1:1 in 95 to 100% ethanol for 1 h (to kill vegetative cells) and then incubated in broth and plated to selective media (19).

Initial anaerobic culture processing should always include Gram staining and, for most specimens, plating to anaerobic blood agar (containing horse or sheep blood, additional hemin, and vitamin K), *Bacteroides* bile esculin agar, and kanamycin-vancomycin agar with laked sheep blood and an anaerobic broth. Commercial media prepared totally without oxygen exposure has been shown to enhance the recovery of some anaerobes (24). If the plates recover organisms, the broth need not be evaluated. However, the broth should be held for up to 14 days in some circumstances, such as for detection of joint infection. As soon as possible after inoculation, media should be placed into an anaerobic atmosphere. Methods such as nitrogen flushing holding jars have been used. Today, smaller incubation containers, such as plastic envelopes, boxes, and shorter jars, and automated gas flushing instruments (Anoxomat [Mart Microbiology, Drachten, The Netherlands]; MAX MICs [Microbiology International, Frederick, MD] are used to shorten the exposure of plated samples to air (toxic oxygen) (10, 13, 37). Use of an anaerobic chamber for all sample manipulations and incubation is the best method to ensure the viability of fastidious anaerobes. If rapid creation of an anaerobic atmosphere is not possible for inoculated plates, it would be better to wait until enough anaerobic samples have been received to fill up one jar and then plate them all at once, closing and gassing the jar as quickly as possible. Jars and boxes should not be opened until after 48 h of incubation to prevent premature death of some slower-growing microbes by exposure to air during their logarithmic growth phase. *Clostridium perfringens*, the agent of gas gangrene, however, grows very quickly and can be identified after overnight incubation. If the clinical situation or initial Gram stain suggests this microbe, it may be prudent to incubate plates individually in plastic anaerobic envelopes (GasPak [Becton Dickinson Microbiology Systems, Cockeysville, MD]; AnaeroPack [Mitsubishi Gas Chemical America, Inc., New York, NY]) so that the plates may be examined early (10).

The initial Gram stain will yield preliminary information about the culture. Clinically important information should be telephoned to the physician or caregiver. For some laboratories, this may be the only anaerobic procedure possible. It is better to interpret Gram stains well and report relevant results quickly than to perform inadequate cultures, which will lead to misleading results. Poor specimen handling or transport, exposure to air, lack of good anaerobic media or atmosphere, early opening of incubation chambers, and other factors will result in the growth of only the hardiest anaerobes, generating incomplete results.

Initial examination of colonies should be performed using a stereomicroscope or at least a strong magnifying glass. Colony morphologies that appear similar when observed at a distance can be differentiated when magnified, and the presence of tiny colonies near larger ones can be discerned. With the pointed end of a broken sterile wooden stick, the tip of a colony should be touched, and then the colony paste should be touched to an anaerobic blood plate, a chocolate agar plate, and a spot on a glass slide. This ensures that the same colony goes onto both plates and the slide. The blood plate should be streaked in quadrants, and special potency disks of 1,000 μg of kanamycin, 5 μg of vancomycin, and 10 μg of colistin can be arranged on the first quadrant. Susceptibility (≥10-mm zone diameter) of the different antibiotics is used to help with further identification (2, 19). The chocolate agar plate is incubated in 5% CO_2 to test a large number of anaerobes in a pie plate format for aerotolerance. Those that grow are not strict anaerobes and can be identified using routine methods. Some organisms can be identified quickly based on colony and Gram stain morphology and a few spot tests; others will require more-extensive methods (19). A new multiparameter anaerobic identification card for the Vitek system (ANC ID card; bioMerieux, Durham, NC) has been favorably reviewed and would be a good choice for those laboratories without molecular-assessment capability (29).

If more-involved methods are necessary, available, and warranted by clinical considerations, prereduced anaerobically sterilized biochemical agents, gas chromatography, and some newer technologies may be employed (19). Analysis of cellular fatty acids has been used to develop extensive databases for anaerobic identification (34, 38). This method, although mostly being replaced by faster modern methods for clinical use, is still valuable for describing new species. Matrix-assisted laser desorption–ionization time of flight (MALDI-TOF) mass spectrometry has been used to identify anaerobes quickly and inexpensively (after initial purchase of the instrument) (20). A commercial MALDI-TOF instrument (MALDI Biotyper; Bruker Daltonics, Billerica, MA) is just beginning to be used in diagnostic laboratories (16). Sequencing of genetic markers, such as portions of the 16S rRNA gene and other useful genetic elements, is the most common method used for anaerobic identification today in clinical laboratories with molecular-assessment capability (22, 29, 31). If the filter "bacteria [ORGN] not uncultured [TITL]" is entered in the BLAST field named "Entry Query," the BLAST database search will not be cluttered with uncultured clones. Modifications such as pyrosequencing are also expected to be useful for anaerobic identifications (12, 28). Chapters 3 and 4 also discuss general principles and the utility of these and other methods. A table listing clinically important pathogens was published in the previous edition of this *Manual* (8). The next chapters of this *Manual* contain up-to-date taxonomic information, including changes from the last edition.

Susceptibilities should be performed for clinically important anaerobes. The Etest can be tailored to the drugs required and can be performed on an individual-organism basis (30). Broth dilution performed in an anaerobic chamber is also acceptable, but interpretation of results may be difficult (9). The Clinical and Laboratory Standards Institute standard method (agar dilution) is not utilized in clinical laboratories, of which only 21% do anaerobic susceptibility testing at all (9, 15, 36). Methods favored in other countries are also available (see http://www.eucast.org, for example).

It is clear that anaerobic bacterial protocols occupy a separate and distinct place in clinical microbiology laboratories. Laboratories must determine the extent of effort that they can devote to anaerobes and then develop their processes to perform only those protocols that they can guarantee will yield reliable, timely, and accurate results. Organisms of importance can always be sent to a reference laboratory for further studies in anaerobic chopped-meat broth or anaerobic transport vials (3).

REFERENCES

1. Amess, J. A., W. O'Neill, C. N. Giollariabhaigh, and J. K. Dytrych. 2007. A six-month audit of the isolation of Fusobacterium necrophorum from patients with sore throat in a district general hospital. *Br. J. Biomed. Sci.* **64**:63–65.
2. Baron, E. J., and D. M. Citron. 1997. Anaerobic identification flowchart using minimal laboratory resources. *Clin. Infect. Dis.* **25**(Suppl. 2):S143–S146.
3. Baron, E. J., C. Strong, M. McTeague, M.-L. Vaisanen, and S. M. Finegold. 1995. Survival of anaerobes in original specimens transported by overnight mail services. *Clin. Infect. Dis.* **20**:S174–S177.
4. Baselski, V. S., M. El-Torky, J. J. Coalson, and J. P. Griffin. 1992. The standardization of criteria for processing and interpreting laboratory specimens in patients with suspected ventilator-associated pneumonia. *Chest* **102**(Suppl.):571S–579S.
5. Bliss, D. Z., S. Johnson, C. R. Clabots, K. Savik, and D. N. Gerding. 1997. Comparison of cycloserine-cefoxitin-fructose agar (CCFA) and taurocholate-CCFA for recovery of Clostridium difficile during surveillance of hospitalized patients. *Diagn. Microbiol. Infect. Dis.* **29**:1–4.
6. Centers for Disease Control and Prevention. 2005. Severe Clostridium difficile-associated disease in populations previously at low risk—four states, 2005. *MMWR Morb. Mortal. Wkly. Rep.* **54**:1201–1205.
7. Chen, C. H., M. L. Kuo, J. F. Shih, T. P. Chang, and R. P. Perng. 1993. Etiologic diagnosis of pulmonary infection by ultrasonically guided percutaneous lung aspiration. *Zhonghua Yi Xue Za Zhi* (Taipei) **51**:333–339.
8. Citron, D. M. 2007. Algorithm for identification of anaerobic bacteria, p. 377–378. *In* P. R. Murray, E. J. Baron, J. H. Jorgensen, M. L. Landy, and M. A. Pfaller (ed.), *Manual of Clinical Microbiology*, 9th ed. ASM Press, Washington, DC.
9. Clinical and Laboratory Standards Institute. 2007. Methods for antimicrobial susceptibility testing of anaerobic bacteria; approved standard—seventh edition. M11-A7. Clinical and Laboratory Standards Institute, Wayne, PA.
10. Doan, N., A. Contreras, J. Flynn, J. Morrison, and J. Slots. 1999. Proficiencies of three anaerobic culture systems for recovering periodontal pathogenic bacteria. *J. Clin. Microbiol.* **37**:171–174.
11. Dore, P., R. Robert, G. Grollier, J. Rouffineau, H. Lanquetot, J. M. Charriere, and J. L. Fauchere. 1996. Incidence of anaerobes in ventilator-associated pneumonia with use of a protected specimen brush. *Am. J. Respir. Crit. Care Med.* **153**:1292–1298.
12. Dowd, S. E., Y. Sun, P. R. Secor, D. D. Rhoads, B. M. Wolcott, G. A. James, and R. D. Wolcott. 2008. Survey of bacterial diversity in chronic wounds using pyrosequencing, DGGE, and full ribosome shotgun sequencing. *BMC Microbiol.* **8**:43.
13. Downes, J., J. I. Mangels, J. Holden, M. J. Ferraro, and E. J. Baron. 1990. Evaluation of two single-plate incubation systems and the anaerobic chamber for the cultivation of anaerobic bacteria. *J. Clin. Microbiol.* **28**:246–248.
14. Eastwood, K., P. Else, A. Charlett, and M. Wilcox. 2009. Comparison of nine commercially available Clostridium difficile toxin detection assays, a real-time PCR assay for C. difficile tcdB, and a glutamate dehydrogenase detection assay to cytotoxin testing and cytotoxigenic culture methods. *J. Clin. Microbiol.* **47**:3211–3217.
15. Goldstein, E. J., D. M. Citron, P. J. Goldman, and R. J. Goldman. 2008. National hospital survey of anaerobic culture and susceptibility methods: III. *Anaerobe* **14**:68–72.
16. Hsieh, S. Y., C. L. Tseng, Y. S. Lee, A. J. Kuo, C. F. Sun, Y. H. Lin, and J. K. Chen. 2008. Highly efficient classification and identification of human pathogenic bacteria by MALDI-TOF MS. *Mol. Cell Proteomics* **7**:448–456.
17. Jarvis, W. R., J. Schlosser, A. A. Jarvis, and R. Y. Chinn. 2009. National point prevalence of Clostridium difficile in US health care facility inpatients, 2008. *Am. J. Infect. Control* **37**:263–270.
18. Joniau, S., S. Vlaminck, L. H. Van, R. Kuhweide, and C. Dick. 2005. Microbiology of sinus puncture versus middle meatal aspiration in acute bacterial maxillary sinusitis. *Am. J. Rhinol.* **19**:135–140.
19. Jousimies-Somer, H., P. Summanen, D. M. Citron, E. J. Baron, H. Wexler, and S. M. Finegold. 2002. *Wadsworth-KTL Anaerobic Bacteriology Manual*. Star Publishing Co., Belmont, CA.
20. Keys, C. J., D. J. Dare, H. Sutton, G. Wells, M. Lunt, T. McKenna, M. McDowall, and H. N. Shah. 2004. Compilation of a MALDI-TOF mass spectral database for the rapid screening and characterisation of bacteria implicated in human infectious diseases. *Infect. Genet. Evol.* **4**:221–242.
21. Lazarovitch, T., S. Freimann, G. Shapira, and H. Blank. 2010. Decrease in anaerobe-related bacteraemias and increase in Bacteroides species isolation rate from 1998 to 2007: a retrospective study. *Anaerobe* **16**:201–205.
22. Levy, P. Y., P. E. Fournier, R. Charrel, D. Metras, G. Habib, and D. Raoult. 2006. Molecular analysis of pericardial fluid: a 7-year experience. *Eur. Heart J.* **27**:1942–1946.
23. Lyras, D., J. R. O'Connor, P. M. Howarth, S. P. Sambol, G. P. Carter, T. Phumoonna, R. Poon, V. Adams, G. Vedantam, S. Johnson, D. N. Gerding, and J. I. Rood. 2009. Toxin B is essential for virulence of Clostridium difficile. *Nature* **458**:1176–1179.
24. Mangels, J. I., and B. P. Douglas. 1989. Comparison of four commercial brucella agar media for growth of anaerobic organisms. *J. Clin. Microbiol.* **27**:2268–2271.
25. Nerandzic, M. M., and C. J. Donskey. 2009. Effective and reduced-cost modified selective medium for isolation of Clostridium difficile. *J. Clin. Microbiol.* **47**:397–400.
26. Peterson, L. R., R. U. Manson, S. M. Paule, D. M. Hacek, A. Robicsek, R. B. Thomson, Jr., and K. L. Kaul. 2007. Detection of toxigenic Clostridium difficile in stool samples by real-time polymerase chain reaction for the diagnosis of C. difficile-associated diarrhea. *Clin. Infect. Dis.* **45**:1152–1160.
27. Piper, K. E., M. J. Jacobson, R. H. Cofield, J. W. Sperling, J. Sanchez-Sotelo, D. R. Osmon, A. McDowell, S. Patrick, J. M. Steckelberg, J. N. Mandrekar, S. M. Fernandez, and R. Patel. 2009. Microbiologic diagnosis of prosthetic shoulder infection by use of implant sonication. *J. Clin. Microbiol.* **47**:1878–1884.
28. Price, L. B., C. M. Liu, J. H. Melendez, Y. M. Frankel, D. Engelthaler, M. Aziz, J. Bowers, R. Rattray, J. Ravel, C. Kingsley, P. S. Keim, G. S. Lazarus, and J. M. Zenilman. 2009. Community analysis of chronic wound bacteria using 16S rRNA gene-based pyrosequencing: impact of diabetes and antibiotics on chronic wound microbiota. *PLoS One* **4**:e6462.

29. **Rennie, R. P., C. Brosnikoff, L. Turnbull, L. B. Reller, S. Mirrett, W. Janda, K. Ristow, and A. Krilcich.** 2008. Multicenter evaluation of the Vitek 2 anaerobe and *Corynebacterium* identification card. *J. Clin. Microbiol.* **46:**2646–2651.

30. **Rosenblatt, J. E., and D. R. Gustafson.** 1995. Evaluation of the Etest for susceptibility testing of anaerobic bacteria. *Diagn. Microbiol. Infect. Dis.* **22:**279–284.

31. **Simmon, K. E., S. Mirrett, L. B. Reller, and C. A. Petti.** 2008. Genotypic diversity of anaerobic isolates from bloodstream infections. *J. Clin. Microbiol.* **46:**1596–1601.

32. **Sloan, L. M., B. J. Duresko, D. R. Gustafson, and J. E. Rosenblatt.** 2008. Comparison of real-time PCR for detection of the *tcdC* gene with four toxin immunoassays and culture in diagnosis of *Clostridium difficile* infection. *J. Clin. Microbiol.* **46:**1996–2001.

33. **Srinivasan, S., and D. N. Fredricks.** 2008. The human vaginal bacterial biota and bacterial vaginosis. *Interdiscip. Perspect. Infect. Dis.* **2008:**750479.

34. **Stoakes, L., T. Kelly, B. Schieven, D. Harley, M. Ramos, R. Lannigan, D. Groves, and Z. Hussain.** 1991. Gas-liquid chromatographic analysis of cellular fatty acids for identification of gram-negative anaerobic bacilli. *J. Clin. Microbiol.* **29:**2636–2638.

35. **Sturm, P. D., E. J. Van, S. Veltman, E. Meuleman, and T. Schulin.** 2006. Urosepsis with *Actinobaculum schaalii* and *Aerococcus urinae*. *J. Clin. Microbiol.* **44:**652–654.

36. **Summanen, P., H. M. Wexler, and S. M. Finegold.** 1992. Antimicrobial susceptibility testing of *Bilophila wadsworthia* by using triphenyltetrazolium chloride to facilitate the endpoint determination. *Antimicrob. Agents Chemother.* **36:**1658–1664.

37. **Summanen, P. H., M. McTeague, M. L. Vaisanen, C. A. Strong, and S. M. Finegold.** 1999. Comparison of recovery of anaerobic bacteria using the Anoxomat, anaerobic chamber, and GasPak jar systems. *Anaerobe* **5:**5–9.

38. **Tuner, K., E. J. Baron, P. Summanen, and S. M. Finegold.** 1992. Cellular fatty acids in *Fusobacterium* species as a tool for identification. *J. Clin. Microbiol.* **30:**3225–3229.

39. **Underdahl, J. P., G. J. Florakis, R. E. Braunstein, D. A. Johnson, P. Cheung, J. Briggs, and D. M. Meisler.** 2000. Propionibacterium acnes as a cause of visually significant corneal ulcers. *Cornea* **19:**451–454.

40. **Van Horn, K. G., C. D. Audette, D. Sebeck, and K. A. Tucker.** 2008. Comparison of the Copan ESwab system with two Amies agar swab transport systems for maintenance of microorganism viability. *J. Clin. Microbiol.* **46:**1655–1658.

Peptostreptococcus, Finegoldia, Anaerococcus, Peptoniphilus, Veillonella, and Other Anaerobic Cocci

YULI SONG AND SYDNEY M. FINEGOLD

48

TAXONOMY

Gram-positive anaerobic cocci comprise a diverse group of organisms. Until recently, most clinical isolates of gram-positive anaerobic cocci were identified as species in the genus *Peptostreptococcus*. *Peptostreptococcus* was described as a genus in 1936 and was considered the anaerobic equivalent of *Streptococcus*. It comprised 16 recognized species, with a G+C range from 27 to 37 mol%, except for *Peptostreptococcus productus* (44 to 45 mol%). In the past decade, molecular techniques such as DNA-DNA hybridization and 16S rRNA gene sequencing have been widely employed in elucidating evolutionary relationships among gram-positive anaerobic coccus species both within and between genera. Most recently, genome sequences of *Finegoldia magna* strain ATCC 29328, *Anaerococcus prevotii* strain DSM 20548, and *Atopobium parvulum* strain DSM 20469 have been published (http://www.ebi.ac.uk/2can/genomes/bacteria.htm).

Polyphasic taxonomic studies have indicated that the gram-positive anaerobic cocci vary markedly in fundamental characteristics, and a number of new genera, including *Anaerococcus*, *Finegoldia*, *Gallicola*, *Parvimonas*, *Peptoniphilus*, and *Murdochiella*, have been proposed (39, 84, 125, 128). Now the genus *Peptostreptococcus* contains only two species, the type species, *P. anaerobius*, and a newly described species, *Peptostreptococcus stomatis* (33). *Peptostreptococcus magnus* and *Peptostreptococcus micros* were placed in two new genera, *Finegoldia* and *Micromonas*, respectively (83). However, the name "*Micromonas*" is illegitimate because of precedence of a microalga *Micromonas*; subsequently, *Parvimonas micra* was proposed as a replacement for "*Micromonas micros*" (125). Ezaki et al. (39) proposed three other genera: *Anaerococcus*, which includes the saccharolytic, butyrate-producing species (*A. hydrogenalis*, *A. lactolyticus*, *A. octavius*, *A. prevotii*, *A. tetradius*, *A. vaginalis*); *Peptoniphilus*, which contains the nonsaccharolytic, butyrate-producing species (*P. asaccharolyticus*, *P. harei*, *P. lacrimalis*, *P. indolicus*, and *P. ivorii*), and *Gallicola*, which contains a single species, *G. barnesae*. Song et al. (119) described two novel species of *Peptoniphilus*, *P. gorbachii* and *P. olsenii*, and one of *Anaerococcus*, *A. murdochii*, isolated from clinical specimens. Most recently, *Murdochiella*, a novel genus which includes a single species (*Murdochiella asaccharolytica*) was proposed. *Peptococcus* is remotely related to other species of gram-positive anaerobic cocci and is rarely cultured from human clinical specimens. *Peptococcus niger* is now the sole remaining representative of this genus.

The taxonomy of other validly published gram-positive anaerobic cocci from human clinical specimens, such as *Streptococcus parvulus*, *Peptostreptococcus productus*, and *Peptostreptococcus saccharolyticus*, has also undergone revision. *Streptococcus parvulus* has been transferred to the genus *Atopobium* as *Atopobium parvulum* (27). *P. productus* was reclassified as *Ruminococcus productus* by Ezaki et al. (38), and a novel genus was recently proposed for this organism, *Blautia* (*Blautia producta*) (68); *Peptostreptococcus saccharolyticus* has been transferred to the genus *Staphylococcus* based on an analysis of nucleic acid relatedness data and cell wall peptidoglycan structure. Table 1 shows the changes in classification of gram-positive anaerobic coccal species from human clinical specimens.

The gram-negative anaerobic cocci are currently classified in five genera of the family *Veillonellaceae*, the genera *Veillonella*, *Acidaminococcus*, *Megasphaera*, *Anaeroglobus*, and *Negativicoccus* (24, 57, 72). The family *Veillonellaceae*, formerly "*Acidaminococcaceae*," is currently classified in the phylum *Firmicutes* (low-G+C-content gram-negative bacteria) and the class *Clostridia* (72).

The family *Veillonellaceae* has been removed from the classification in the latest edition of *Bergey's Manual of Systematic Bacteriology* (45, 72).

The genus *Veillonella* is widely distributed in the oral, genitourinary, respiratory, and intestinal biotas of humans and animals. It is subdivided into 10 species: *Veillonella atypica*, *Veillonella caviae*, *Veillonella criceti*, *Veillonella denticariosi*, *Veillonella dispar*, *Veillonella montpellierensis*, *Veillonella parvula*, *Veillonella ratti*, *Veillonella rodentium*, and *Veillonella rogosae* (56). Of these, only *V. atypica*, *V. denticariosi*, *V. dispar*, *V. parvula*, and *V. rogosae* have been isolated from human oral cavities (2, 4, 23, 62). Four other species, *V. caviae*, *V. criceti*, *V. ratti*, and *V. rodentium*, were found only in animals, except for one *V. ratti* isolate, which was recovered from human semen. Besides *Veillonella* spp., *A. fermentans* and *A. intestini* of the genus *Acidaminococcus*, *M. elsdenii* and *M. micronuciformis* of the genus *Megasphaera*, and *A. geminatus* of the genus *Anaeroglobus* have been isolated from human clinical samples.

DESCRIPTION OF THE GROUP

The organisms included in this chapter are obligately anaerobic, non-spore-forming, sometimes elongated cocci. The genera *Anaerococcus*, *Anaerosphaera*, *Finegoldia*, *Gallicola*, *Parvimonas*, *Peptococcus*, *Peptoniphilus*, and *Peptostreptococcus*,

TABLE 1 Changes in classification of gram-positive anaerobic coccal species from human clinical specimens

Current classification	Previous classification(s)
Peptococcus niger	*Peptococcus niger*
Peptostreptococcus stomatis	*Peptostreptococcus anaerobius*
Peptostreptococcus anaerobius	*Peptostreptococcus anaerobius*
Parvimonas micra	*Peptostreptococcus micros, Micromonas micros*
Peptoniphilus asaccharolyticus	*Peptostreptococcus asaccharolyticus*
Peptoniphilus gorbachii	New species
Peptoniphilus indolicus	*Peptostreptococcus indolicus*
Peptoniphilus harei	*Peptostreptococcus harei*
Peptoniphilus ivorii	*Peptostreptococcus ivorii*
Peptoniphilus lacrimalis	*Peptostreptococcus lacrimalis*
Peptoniphilus olsenii	New species
Anaerococcus murdochii	New species
Anaerococcus prevotii	*Peptostreptococcus prevotii*
Anaerococcus tetradius	*Peptostreptococcus tetradius*
Anaerococcus octavius	*Peptostreptococcus octavius*
Anaerococcus hydrogenalis	*Peptostreptococcus hydrogenalis*
Anaerococcus lactolyticus	*Peptostreptococcus lactolyticus*
Anaerococcus vaginalis	*Peptostreptococcus vaginalis*
Finegoldia magna	*Peptostreptococcus magnus*
Gallicola barnesae	*Peptostreptococcus barnesae*
Slackia heliotrinireducens corrig	*Peptostreptococcus heliotrinreducens*
Atopobium parvulum	*Streptococcus parvulus*
Blautia producta	*Peptostreptococcus productus, Ruminococcus productus*
Blautia coccoides	*Clostridium coccoides*
Blautia wexlerae	New species
Ruminococcus gauvreauii	New species
Staphylococcus saccharolyticus	*Peptostreptococcus saccharolyticus*

as well as the newly described taxon *Murdochiella* (128), are gram-positive, coccobacillary, or, occasionally, coccoid cells. In Gram-stained preparations of pure cultures, cells vary in size from 0.3 mm to 2.0 mm and can be arranged in pairs, short chains, tetrads, small clusters, or irregular masses; most species are present either as chains or as clumps. The ability to utilize carbohydrates varies greatly; some genera are asaccharolytic, but a few are strongly saccharolytic. For most species, the products of protein digestion appear to be the principal energy source. The genus *Staphylococcus* contains two species, *S. saccharolyticus* and *S. aureus* subsp. *anaerobius*, which initially grow under anaerobic conditions and become aerotolerant on subcultures (see chapter 19 in this *Manual*). Strictly anaerobic *Staphylococcus epidermidis* is reported to be occasionally isolated from clinical specimens (105). The genera *Veillonella, Acidaminococcus, Megasphaera, Anaeroglobus,* and *Negativicoccus* (72) are gram-negative cocci. Cells vary in size from 0.3 μm to 2.5 μm. They characteristically occur in pairs, but single cells, masses, or chains may also occur. Carbohydrates are weakly fermented or not fermented. Gas is produced. The metabolic end products are the principal characteristics by which the genera can be differentiated.

EPIDEMIOLOGY AND TRANSMISSION

Gram-positive anaerobic cocci are part of the normal biota of the mouth, upper respiratory and gastrointestinal tracts, female genitourinary system, and skin (82). Gram-positive anaerobic cocci constitute 1 to 15% of the normal oral biota (124); *Parvimonas micra* is usually considered to be the predominant species of gram-positive anaerobic cocci in

the oral biota, and *P. anaerobius* and *F. magna* have been reported to be present. The gastrointestinal tract hosts a wide variety of gram-positive anaerobic cocci, including most recognized species of *Peptostreptococcus*. *B. producta* is one of the most common organisms in the gastrointestinal biota; *F. magna* and *A. prevotii* are also common. *Murdochiella* is also presumably found in the bowel (128). Several other gram-positive anaerobic cocci are found less often. Large numbers of gram-positive anaerobic cocci can be found in the female genitourinary tract. *A. tetradius, A. lactolyticus,* and *A. vaginalis* were first described from vaginal discharges (36, 37, 67); *P. anaerobius, P. asaccharolyticus, P. hydrogenalis, F. magna, Parvimonas micra, A. prevotii,* and *Peptococcus niger* have also been isolated from that site. The skin biota contains gram-positive anaerobic cocci; *F. magna* is the species identified most frequently, followed by *P. asaccharolyticus* (82).

Gram-negative anaerobic cocci form part of the oral, genitourinary, respiratory, and intestinal biota of humans. *Veillonella* species are part of the normal mouth, upper respiratory tract, gastrointestinal tract, and vaginal biotas; *Acidaminococcus* and *Megasphaera* are part of the intestinal biota. *A. geminatus* has also been isolated from the human mouth and gastrointestinal tract (55).

CLINICAL SIGNIFICANCE

Estimation of the clinical significance of anaerobic cocci isolated from clinical specimens is often difficult partly due to their recovery from poorly obtained specimens (failure to exclude normal biota). Anaerobic gram-positive cocci are opportunistic pathogens and comprise approximately one-quarter of all isolates from anaerobic infections (81, 82). They may be present in a great variety of infections involving all areas of the human body, ranging in severity from mild skin abscesses to more serious and life-threatening infections, such as brain abscess, bacteremia, necrotizing pneumonia, and septic abortion. Brain abscess and meningitis are among the more serious infections involving anaerobic cocci (1, 64, 70). In deep-space head and neck infections (13), 9.2% of anaerobic isolates were gram-positive anaerobic cocci (F. magna, P. micra, and P. anaerobius). The incidence of anaerobic cocci in pleuropulmonary infections, such as lung abscess, necrotizing pneumonia, aspiration pneumonia, and empyema, is about 40% (73, 129). Anaerobic cocci are often isolated with other organisms in skin and soft tissue infections, including progressive bacterial synergistic gangrene, necrotizing fasciitis, diabetic foot ulcer, and crepitant cellulitis (10, 82, 86, 123). Other infections in which anaerobic cocci have been recognized as significant pathogens are infections of the female genital tract and intra-abdominal infections (21, 31, 40, 116). In a recent study showing a decrease in anaerobic bacteremia, gram-positive anaerobic cocci increased from 5.4% in an early period to 12% (40). Although most infections involving gram-positive anaerobic cocci are polymicrobial (41), there are many instances of their isolation in pure culture (81, 82); most relate to F. magna, but there are also reports of P. anaerobius, P. asaccharolyticus, P. indolicus, P. micra, A. vaginalis, and P. harei in pure culture.

F. magna is the most pathogenic and one of the most frequently isolated gram-positive anaerobic coccal species found in human clinical specimens. Possible F. magna pathogenicity factors have been identified, including capsule formation (16) and production of various enzymes, such as collagenase, gelatinase (65), and subtilisin-like serine-proteinase (SufA) (59, 60). F. magna was also found to express surface proteins, such as protein L, which is a B-cell superantigen (8), the albumin-binding protein PAB (30), and a protein designated FAF (F. magna adhesion factor) (44); these proteins may play an important role in creating an ecologic niche for F. magna, decreasing antibacterial activity, and suppressing angiogenesis and thus providing an advantage for the survival for this opportunistic pathogen. F. magna has been isolated from a wide variety of infections at various body sites in pure culture. These include cases of endocarditis (43) and meningitis and pneumonia (82, 89), some of which have been fatal. F. magna is most commonly associated with infections of skin and soft tissue, bones, and joints but has also been isolated from cases of septic arthritis (42), prosthetic implant infections (29), breast abscess (34), diabetic foot infections (54), bacterial vaginosis, and upper respiratory tract infections, such as sinusitis and otitis media.

P. anaerobius is involved in polymicrobial infections, including abscess of the brain, ear, jaw, pleural cavity, pelvis, urogenital tract, external genitalia, abdominal regions, and nasal septum (17, 18, 52). The isolation of P. anaerobius from endocarditis specimens has been reported (77). P. anaerobius has been associated with gingivitis (78) and periodontitis (130); it is one of the species found most frequently in the root canals of teeth with periapical abscess and has been isolated from a peritonsillar abscess (26, 103).

P. micra is increasingly recognized as an important oral pathogen (88). It has been shown to produce collagenase, hemolysin, and, occasionally, elastase, all virulence factors (88). Although it is considered a natural commensal of the oral cavity (85, 91), elevated counts of this organism are associated with periodontal destruction (96). It is also commonly isolated from other oral infections, such as endodontic lesions and peritonsillar infections (76). P. micra is not restricted to the oral cavity; it is often isolated in mixed anaerobic infections from different body sites, including brain abscess, otitis media, sinus infection, human bite wounds, pleural empyema, intra-abdominal infection, anorectal abscess, septicemia, gynecological infection, vertebral osteomyelitis, and prosthetic joint infection (82).

Anaerobic gram-negative cocci account for a very small percentage of the anaerobic cocci isolated from human specimens (6). Veillonella sp. strains are frequently isolated from clinical specimens in aerobic-anaerobic polymicrobial cultures. Rarely, Veillonella species have been the only etiologic agents identified in serious infections such as meningitis, osteomyelitis, prosthetic joint infection, pleuropulmonary infection, endocarditis, and bacteremia (5, 19, 20, 69, 71, 73, 113). In most clinical reports of Veillonella infection, the isolates have not been identified to the species level. There have been only four previous reports of confirmed V. parvula discitis or vertebral osteomyelitis (75, 113).

Although the spectrum of infections has remained relatively unchanged since the extensive review by Murdoch in 1998 (82), the prevalence of these organisms as pathogens is clearly increasing.

COLLECTION, TRANSPORTATION, AND STORAGE OF SPECIMENS

Most gram-positive anaerobic cocci isolated from human clinical material are not extremely oxygen sensitive. Specimens suspected of harboring anaerobic cocci should be collected, transported, and stored by methods outlined elsewhere (see chapter 19 in this Manual).

DIRECT EXAMINATION

Microscopy

In clinical samples, direct Gram staining shows that anaerobic cocci vary in size and occur in chains, in pairs, or singly. P. micra cells are less than 0.6 μm in diameter and occur in packets and short chains; other anaerobic cocci, such as A. tetradius, A. prevotii, and F. magnus, have cells greater than 0.6 μm in diameter in pairs and clusters and may resemble staphylococcal cells. The difference in cell size has been used as one characteristic to distinguish between P. micra and F. magna.

Antigen Detection

Serological studies described an indirect fluorescent-antibody test for P. anaerobius, P. micra, and B. producta (28), but they were not taken further.

Nucleic Acid Detection

Molecular diagnostics of infectious diseases, in particular nucleic-acid-based methods, is the fastest-growing field in clinical laboratory diagnostics. These applications are beginning to replace or complement culture-based, biochemical, and immunological assays in microbiology laboratories. Molecular methods, such as nucleic acid probe hybridization and PCR amplification, are not yet standardized or available commercially for the direct demonstration of medically important gram-positive anaerobic cocci from clinical specimens. However, several studies have used molecular techniques to identify and detect anaerobic cocci. DNA probes targeting the 16S rRNA gene have been used to detect *P. anaerobius* and *P. micra*, and PCR assays specific for detection of *F. magna*, *P. anaerobius*, and *P. micra* directly from clinical specimens have been developed (98, 99, 100, 101, 114, 117). More recently, a real-time PCR technique has been applied for quantitative detection of anaerobic cocci. It has been used to detect *P. micra* from prosthetic joint infection, endodontic infections, and periradicular lesions (3, 9, 11, 12, 49, 87, 122). Marrazzo et al. (74) reported using real-time PCR to detect *P. lacrimalis* and *Megasphaera* spp. in vaginal samples. The same approach has also been applied to detect *Veillonella* spp. in human oral and lower intestinal samples, as well as samples from asymptomatic vaginal infections and endodontic infection (7, 95, 102). Several studies reported using a checkerboard DNA-DNA hybridization method to directly detect microbes from oral clinical samples, including *P. micra* (92, 93, 106, 109, 115).

ISOLATION PROCEDURES

Routinely used anaerobic plate media, such as brucella, Columbia, or Schaedler agar base supplemented with 5% sheep blood, vitamin K$_1$, and hemin, support the growth of these microorganisms. However, CDC (Centers for Disease Control and Prevention) agar base (see chapter 17 in this *Manual*) gives better recovery of gram-positive anaerobic cocci than brucella agar or other agars. The usual procedures for anaerobes should be followed (55). Many of these organisms require a high moisture content for optimal growth, so fresh media should be used. Laboratories unable to prepare their own media may wish to consider the use of commercially prepared, prereduced, anaerobically sterilized (PRAS) blood agar (Anaerobe Systems, Morgan Hill, CA). These media have an extended shelf life of up to 6 months and yield results comparable to or better than those obtained with fresh media.

Gram-positive anaerobic cocci are heterogeneous; a single medium is unlikely to support the growth of all representatives and be reasonably selective. Wren (134) showed that nalidixic acid-Tween 80 blood agar gave better isolation than neomycin blood agar, possibly due to the particularly inhibitory nature of neomycin against gram-positive anaerobic cocci, but recommended that a combination of different media be used to maximize recovery rates. Petts et al. (94) reported that oxolinic acid was superior to nalidixic acid for suppression of staphylococci, while permitting the growth of nonsporing anaerobes, including gram-positive anaerobic cocci. Turng et al. (126) described a selective and differential medium for *Parvimonas micra* that contains colistin-nalidixic acid agar (Difco, Detroit, MI), which is a selective base for gram-positive cocci supplemented with glutathione and lead acetate. Strains of *Parvimonas micra* can use the reduced form of glutathione to form hydrogen sulfide, which reacts with lead acetate to form a black precipitate under the colony. Tween 80 supplementation (0.5%) of media may improve the growth of some gram-positive anaerobic cocci.

A recent study (50) tested different media for recovery of *Veillonella* spp. from saliva samples and concluded that a selective medium for *Veillonella* with vancomycin and laked blood gave the greatest recovery of *Veillonella*. This medium can also be used for presumptive identification of *Veillonella*, since the colonies produce a red fluorescence at a wavelength of 365 nm.

IDENTIFICATION

Phenotypic Tests

Some gram-positive anaerobic cocci, particularly strains of *P. asaccharolyticus,* decolorize readily with Gram stain and can be confused with gram-negative anaerobes, such as veillonellae. Gram-positive anaerobic cocci can be distinguished from gram-negative anaerobic cocci by special-potency disks (vancomycin, 5 μg; kanamycin, 1,000 μg; and colistin, 10 μg) (55). Generally, gram-positive anaerobic cocci are sensitive to vancomycin and resistant to colistin, whereas the gram-negative anaerobic cocci are resistant to vancomycin. The cell morphology of older cultures of gram-positive anaerobic cocci can be very irregular, with many coccobacillary and rod-like forms. It is also important to distinguish gram-positive anaerobic cocci from microaerophilic organisms, such as strains of *Streptococcus* species. A simple and reliable test is to apply a 5-μg metronidazole disk to the edge of the inoculum; gram-positive anaerobic cocci show a zone of inhibition of 15 mm or larger, whereas microaerophilic strains show no zones after incubation for 48 h (80).

P. anaerobius is the only gram-positive anaerobic coccus that gives a zone of inhibition of ≥12 mm around a sodium polyanethol sulfonate (SPS) disk. *Parvimonas micra* also exhibits a zone of inhibition with SPS; however, the zone is usually <12 mm in size. Most *P. anaerobius* strains form distinctive colonies on enriched blood agar; they are 1 mm in diameter after 24 h, they are gray with slightly raised off-white centers, and they have a distinctive sweet odor (80). *Parvimonas micra* and *F. magna* can be readily distinguished by a combination of colonial morphology and proteolytic enzyme profiling, supported by Gram-stained cell morphology to assess the cell size. An anaerobic coccus with a milky halo around the colonies on blood agar and small cells (<0.6 μm) can be presumptively identified as *Parvimonas micra* (80, 129). *F. magna* cells are larger than those of most peptostreptococci. Published data (83) also indicate that they can be differentiated by enzymatic tests for proteolytic activity, such as proline arylamidase, phenylalanine arylamidase, and tyrosine arylamidase (see Fig. 1).

P. asaccharolyticus is another gram-positive anaerobic coccal species frequently isolated from human clinical specimens, but strains that were identified phenotypically are genetically diverse. To complicate matters further, the type strain of *P. asaccharolyticus* is highly atypical in its whole-cell composition and some biochemical properties. A recent study of ours (unpublished data) indicated that all strains (a total of 33) that were identified as *P. asaccharolyticus* phenotypically shared only a low sequence similarity (<90%) with the corresponding sequence of the type strain of *P. asaccharolyticus*. They all had almost identical 16S rRNA sequences and shared a high sequence similarity (>99%) with another *P. asaccharolyticus* strain, ATCC 29743. The cellular morphology of this group of bacteria is characteristic: the cell size is more uniform than is observed with most species of gram-positive anaerobic cocci, and cells occur in clumps, retaining Gram's stain poorly and often resembling strains of *Neisseria* species. The colony morphology is also distinctive; after 5 days of incubation on enriched blood agar, colonies are 2 to 3 mm in diameter, glistening, low and convex, and usually whitish to lemon-yellow, and they often have a characteristic musty odor. They produce an enzyme profile very similar to that of strains of *P. harei* (see Fig. 1) (but can be easily differentiated by their clearly different cell and colony morphologies)

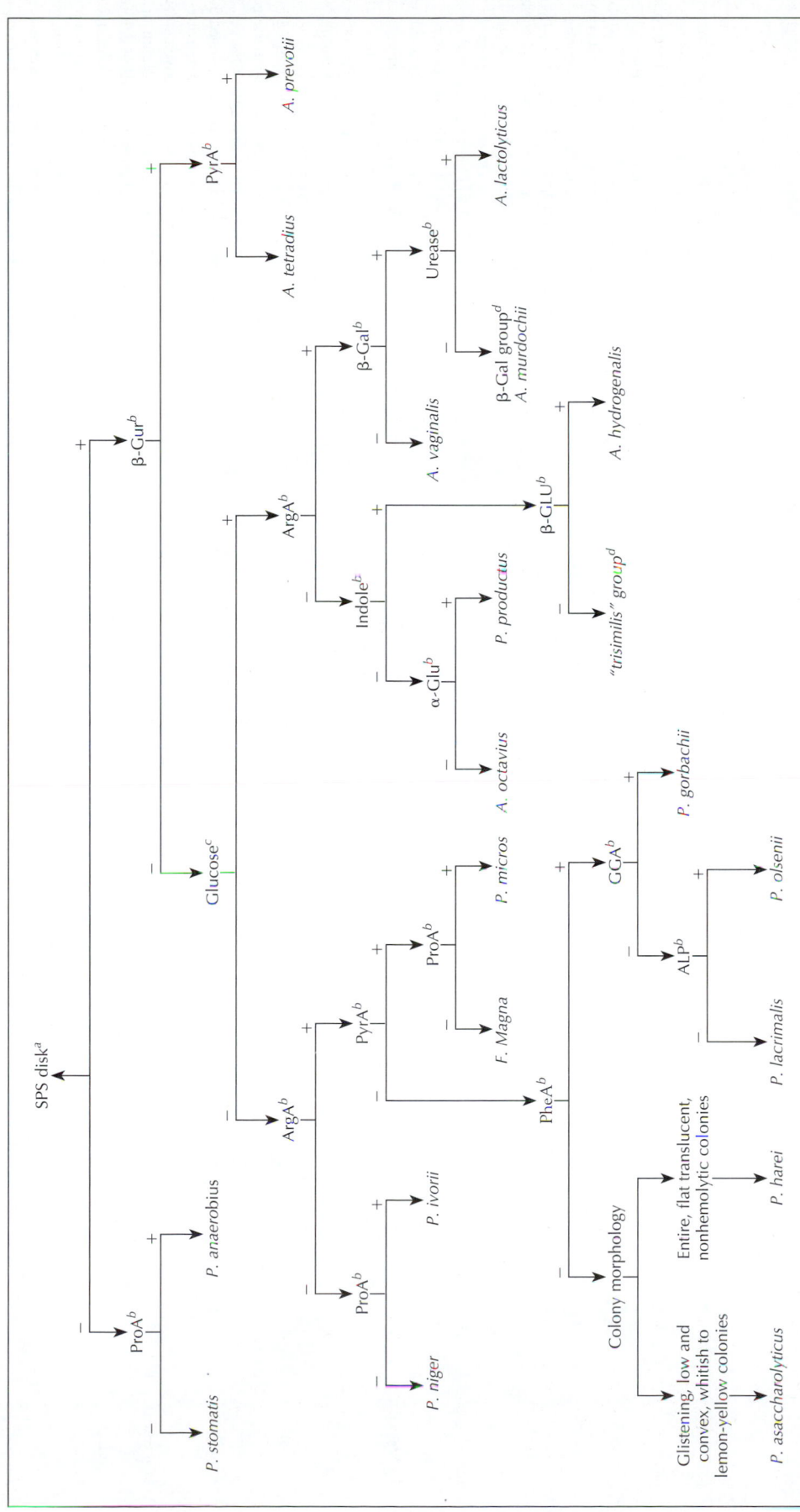

FIGURE 1 Flowchart with key characteristics for identification and differentiation of gram-positive anaerobic cocci. *a*, SPS testing was done using an SPS disk (Anaerobe Systems, Morgan Hill, CA). All gram-positive anaerobic cocci are sensitive to SPS except for *P. anaerobius*, which gives a zone of inhibition of ≥12 mm around an SPS disk. *P. micros* also exhibits a zone of inhibition with SPS; however, the zone is usually <12 mm in size. +, no zone or the zone of inhibition is <12 mm; −, the zone of inhibition is ≥12 mm. *b*, all the enzymatic tests were done by using the Rapid ID 32A system (API bioMérieux, Marcy l'Etoile, France) according to the manufacturer's instructions. β-Gal, β-galactosidase; α-Glu, α-glucosidase; β-Gur, β-glucuronidase; ArgA, arginine arylamidase (AMD); ProA, proline AMD; PheA, phenylalanine AMD; PyrA, pyroglutamyl AMD; GGA, glutamyl glutamic acid AMD; ALP, alkaline phosphatase. *c*, glucose fermentation tests were performed using PRAS peptone-yeast-glucose (PYG) broth (Anaerobe Systems, Morgan Hill, CA). A pH of ≤5.5 in the PYG tubes was interpreted as positive and a pH of ≥5.9 as negative fermentation. *d*, described by D. A. Murdoch and I. J. Mitchelmore (80).

TABLE 2 Differential characteristics of *Peptostreptococcus*, *Peptococcus*, *Peptoniphilus*, *Finegoldia*, and *Anaerococcus*[a]

Species	GLC result(s)	Inhibition by SPS	Indole	Urease	ALP	ADH	Glucose fermentation	α-Gal	β-Gal	α-Glu	β-Gur	ArgA	ProA	PheA	LeuA	PyrA	Gram stain and colony morphology result(s)
P. asaccharolyticus	A, b	−	d	−	−	−	−	−	−	−	−	+	−	−	d	−	Cells are uniform and in clumps; retain Gram's stain poorly; resembling strains of *Neisseria*; glistening, low and convex, usually whitish to lemon-yellow colonies with a musty odor
P. indolicus	A, b	−	+	−	+	−	−	−	−	−	−	+	−	+	+	−	Similar to *P. asaccharolyticus*
P. harei	A, b	−	d	−	−	−	−	−	−	−	−	+	−	−	−/w	−	Cells vary in size and shape; flat, translucent colonies
P. lacrimalis	A, b	−	−	−	−	−	−	−	−	−	−	+	−	+	+	−	Cells are in short chains or clumps; pink-white colonies
P. gorbachii	A, b	−	d	−	−	−	−	−	−	−	−	+	−	+	+	−	Typical cells are ≥0.7 μm; gray, flat or low and convex, circular, entire, opaque
P. olsenii	A, b	−	d	−	+	−	−	−	−	−	−	+	−	+	+	−	Typical cells are ≥0.7 μm; gray, flat or low and convex, circular, entire, opaque with a whiter central peak
"*trisimilis*" group	A, b	−	+	+	d	−	+	−	d	−	−	−	−	−	−	+	Cells are in clumps and tetrads; gray with white centers, entire and circular colonies
A. hydrogenalis	B, a	−	+	d	−/w	−	+	−	−	d	−	−	−	−	−	−	Cells vary in size, arranged in clumps, tetrads, and short chains; gray-white convex colonies, with an unpleasant odor
A. prevotii	B, a	−	−	+	−	−	−	+	−	+	+	+	−	−	−	+	Cells vary in size; arranged in clumps or tetrads; matte-gray, low and convex colonies
A. tetradius	B, a	−	−	+	−	−	+	−	−	+	+	+	−	w	+	w	Cells vary in size; arranged in clumps and tetrads; matte-gray, low and convex colonies
A. lactolyticus	B, a	−	−	+	−	−	+	−	+	−	−	+	−	−	−	−	Cells are in short chains or clumps; pink-white colonies
A. murdochii	B, A	−	−	−	+	+	+	−	+	−	−	+	−	−	+	+	Typical cells are ≥0.7 μm; colonies are gray, flat or low and convex, entire, circular, often matte with a whiter center
A. vaginalis	B, a	−	d	−	−/w	+	+	−	−	−	−	+	−	−	+	−	Cells vary in size; arranged in clumps or tetrads; gray-white, low and convex colonies

808

															Products	Cell and colony morphology
"β-Gal" group	−	−	w	−	+	w/+	−	−/w	−	+	w	d	−	−	B, a	Cells vary in size; arranged in clumps; gray-white, low and convex colonies
A. octavius	−	−	−	−	−	−	−	−	−	+	−	−	+	+	B, a, c	Cells are arranged in clumps; yellowish-white, glistening, circular, raised, entire colonies
P. ivorii	−	−	−	−	−	−	−	−	−	−	−	−	+	+	IV	Cells vary in size; arranged in clumps; yellowish-white, low and convex colonies
P. anaerobius	+	−	−	−	−	−	−	+	−	+	−	−	+	+	A, IC	Cells are highly pleomorphic and in chains; colonies are gray with slightly raised off-white centers and have a distinctive, sweet odor
P. stomatis	+	−	−	−	w	+	−	+	−	w	−	−	−	−	A, IC	Cells are in pairs and have short chains; they are circular, entire, high and convex to pyramidal, opaque, shiny, and cream to off-white, with a narrow gray outer ring (on fastidious anaerobe agar)
F. magna	−	−	−	−	−/w	d	d	−	−	−/w	d	d	+	+	A	Cells are in pairs, tetrads, or clusters; colonies are small, convex, and whitish, while others are flatter and translucent
P. micra	−	−	−	−	−	−	−	−	−	−	+	−	+	+	A	Cells are in pairs, chains, and clusters; colonies are small; typically white, glistening, and domed and often surrounded by a distinctive yellow-brown halo of discolored agar up to 2 mm wide
P. productus	−	+	−	−	+	+	−	+	−	+	−	−	−	−	A	Cells are ovoid and arranged in pairs or chains; glistening gray colonies

[a]Data are mainly from Murdoch (82) and Song et al. (118); Undescribed strains that cluster in whole-cell composition were assessed by pyrolysis mass spectrometry. VFA, volatile fatty acids; A, acetate; B, butyrate; IV, isovalerate; IC, isocaproate; C, n-caproate; SPS, sodium polyanethol sulfonate; ADH, arginine dihydrolase; ALP, alkaline phosphatase; α-Gal, α-galactosidase; β-Gal, β-galactosidase; α-Glu, α-glucosidase; β-Gur, β-glucuronidase; ArgA, arginine arylamidase (AMD); ProA, proline AMD; PheA, phenylalanine AMD; Leu, leucine AMD; PyrA, pyroglutamyl AMD; −, >90% negative; +, >90% positive; w, weakly positive; d, different reactions.

(unpublished data). This group of bacteria can be identified using 16S rRNA gene sequencing. Cells of *P. harei* vary considerably in size (diameter, 0.5 to 1.5 μm) and shape (circular, oval, or elliptical). Colonies of 5-day cultures on enriched blood agar are approximately 1 mm in diameter, entire, flat, and translucent. *P. indolicus* is phenotypically similar to *P. asaccharolyticus* and can be difficult to differentiate but is rarely isolated from human clinical specimens. *P. indolicus* can be tentatively distinguished from *P. asaccharolyticus* by its ability to produce alkaline phosphatase.

A. *prevotii* and A. *tetradius* were reported as common species of gram-positive anaerobic cocci in human clinical material in early surveys. However, nucleic acid studies indicate that they are very heterogeneous. Again, our study based on 16S rRNA gene sequencing indicated that a large percentage of organisms identified as A. *prevotii*/A. *tetradius* are strains of A. *vaginalis*. It is likely that strictly defined strains of A. *prevotii*/A. *tetradius* are only occasionally recovered from most clinical specimens. The activity of pyroglutamic acid arylamidase might be useful for differentiation of A. *prevotii* and A. *tetradius*; however, distinctions cannot be generalized because insufficient numbers of strains of each species have been reliably identified. A. *prevotii* and A. *tetradius* can be distinguished from other recognized species of gram-positive anaerobic cocci by production of α-glucosidase and β-glucuronidase. Strains of other saccharolytic gram-positive anaerobic cocci such as A. *vaginalis* and A. *lactolyticus* can be differentiated by their enzyme profiles (118).

Table 2 summarizes the differential characteristics of gram-positive anaerobic coccal species. Based on published data from our group and others (118), we developed a flow chart for rapid identification of gram-positive anaerobic cocci (Fig. 1). The identification is based on phenotypic tests that can be performed in any diagnostic laboratory. Most of the information presented here relates to the phenotypic characteristics of strains isolated from humans.

Several identification systems, such as the Rapid ID 32A (bioMérieux, Marcy L'Etoile, France) and RapID ANA II (Remel, Inc., Lenexa, KS) systems, are available commercially for the rapid identification of anaerobes. Evaluations of these biochemical kits indicate that they may be of value for characterizing anaerobic cocci; however, these systems are designed to identify as wide a range of anaerobes as possible, and they contain many tests of little relevance for identification of anaerobic cocci. Furthermore, databases accompanying the kits are often incomplete or inaccurate, especially with a number of newly described species. Our most recent evaluation of the Rapid ID 32A kit for identification of gram-positive anaerobic cocci by comparison with 16S rRNA gene sequencing identification showed that the system is good for accurate identification of *Parvimonas micra*, *P. anaerobius*, *F. magna*, and *P. asaccharolyticus* but not other species (unpublished data).

Gram-positive anaerobic cocci are separated into five groups based on fatty acid end products of metabolism as analyzed by gas-liquid chromatography (GLC) (Table 2): (i) an acetate group (containing *F. magna* and *Parvimonas micra*) that produces only acetic acid, (ii) a butyrate-acetate group (containing all of the species in the genus *Anaerococcus*) that produces butyric acid as its major terminal volatile fatty acid (VFA) and acetic acid as a second major acid, (iii) an acetate-butyrate group (containing all of the species in the genus *Peptoniphilus* except *P. ivorii*) that produces acetic acid as its major terminal VFA and butyric acid as the second acid, (iv) a caproate group whose members produce

large quantities of longer-chain VFAs, and (v) an isovaleric acid group (containing *P. ivorii*, the only species of gram-positive anaerobic cocci that produces a major terminal peak of isovaleric acid). The most important species in group iv is *P. anaerobius*, the only species of gram-positive anaerobic cocci to produce a major terminal peak of isocaproic acid. GLC is also useful for identifying the rarely isolated *Peptococcus niger* and *P. octavius*, which produce n-caproic acid.

Veillonella, *Acidaminococcus*, and *Megasphaera* comprise the principal genera of anaerobic gram-negative cocci. The identification of *Veillonella* at the species level remains uncertain and inconvenient owing to the lack of conventional phenotypic and biochemical discriminating tests (62). Moreover, serological groupings (104) are no longer available. Table 3 contains a key for differentiating the genera of anaerobic gram-negative cocci.

Molecular Methods

Direct sequencing of 16S rRNA genes (*rrs*) has proven to be a stable and specific marker for bacterial identification. Two groups have evaluated the utility of 16S rRNA gene sequencing as a means of identifying clinically important gram-positive anaerobic cocci (118, 119, 134). Our studies (118, 119) indicated that problems exist in the public database; for example, among the 13 type strains of gram-positive anaerobic coccal species that we tested, only four "perfectly" matched their corresponding sequences in GenBank, whereas the other nine had lower sequence similarities (<98%). This is due mainly to the poor quality of bacterial sequences deposited in GenBank from early years. Based on the correct 16S rRNA sequences that we deposited in GenBank, a multiplex-PCR scheme was developed for rapid identification of clinically significant gram-positive anaerobic coccal species (120). More recently, Wildeboer-Veloo et al. (132) developed 16S rRNA-based probes for the identification of gram-positive anaerobic cocci isolated from human clinical specimens. However, these assays have not been evaluated for direct bacterial detection from clinical samples.

The MicroSeq 16S rRNA sequencing system could identify only 39% of 23 anaerobic cocci (133). A commercial real-time PCR setup (Septi-Fast; Roche), which is multiplexed for 25 pathogens, does not cover anaerobic cocci at this time (66). There have been favorable reports regarding the Vitek 2 system with an anaerobe identification card but with limited numbers of species and strains of anaerobic cocci (97). Matrix-assisted laser desorption-time of flight mass spectrometry is a promising tool, but the database is limited for gram-positive anaerobic cocci; published studies have involved only a few strains of anaerobic gram-positive cocci and did not detect them well (112).

Beighton et al. (4) reported using *rpoB* gene sequencing for identifying *Veillonella* spp. isolated from tongue samples because 16S rRNA sequence analysis does not reliably differentiate among all members of this genus. Subsequently, a simple two-step PCR procedure was developed for the identification of the recognized oral *Veillonella* species (53).

TYPING SYSTEMS

Molecularly based methods such as PCR amplification of 16S rRNA genes followed by restriction fragment length polymorphism analysis has proved to be useful for gram-positive anaerobic cocci (100) and *Veillonella* species strain typing (110, 111). PCR-amplified rRNA gene spacer polymorphism

TABLE 3 Characteristics of genera of gram-negative cocci[a]

Characteristic	Negativicoccus	Megasphaera	Veillonella	Acidaminococcus	Anaeroglobus
Cell					
Size (μm)	0.4	1.7–2.6	0.3–0.5	0.5–1	0.5–1.1
Growth under microaerophilic conditions	+	−	−	−	−
Nitrate reduction	−	−	+	−	−
Ability to ferment carbohydrates[b]	−	+	−	−	+
Fermentation of lactate	−	+	+	−	−
Decarboxylation of succinate	+	−	+	−	−
Amino acids are the main source of energy	−	−	−	+	−
Gas production	−	+	+	+	−
Metabolic end products	A, P, (L)	A, P, B, V, C	A, P	A, B, (P), (L)	A, P, IB, B, IV

[a]Modified from reference 72. A, acetate; B, butyrate; IB, isobutyrate; V, valerate; IV, isovalerate; C, n-caproate; P, propionate; L, lactate. Parentheses indicate possible production.

[b]Glucose fermentation tests were performed using pre-reduced, anaerobically sterilized PRAS peptone-yeast-glucose broth tubes (Anaerobe Systems, Morgan Hill, CA). The PRAS tubes were inoculated from an actively growing broth culture (without carbohydrate). A pH of ≤5.5 in the PRAS tubes was interpreted as positive, a pH of 5.6 to 5.8 as weakly positive, and a pH of ≥5.9 as negative fermentation.

analysis was also successfully applied in the rapid differentiation of the currently recognized taxa within the group of anaerobic gram-positive cocci (51).

ANTIMICROBIAL SUSCEPTIBILITIES

New information regarding the antimicrobial susceptibilities of gram-positive anaerobic cocci (Table 4) is sparse compared with the information available for other anaerobic species. Many reports fail to give results for specific species, opting instead to combine data for the group. Others have not determined species identification

accurately. Finally, nonstandardized susceptibility testing is sometimes used.

Penicillins are considered to be an effective first-line therapy for gram-positive anaerobic cocci. Most evidence suggests that P. asaccharolyticus, F. magna, and P. micra are usually susceptible to penicillins, although Wren (134) reported 16% and 8% resistance to penicillin among isolates of F. magna and Parvimonas micra, respectively, in their study. Cephalosporins are usually, but not always, effective. Carbapenems are extremely active. Several authorities maintain that almost all gram-positive anaerobic cocci are susceptible to metronidazole, but resistance has frequently been

TABLE 4 Antimicrobial susceptibilities of gram-positive anaerobic cocci[a]

Species (no. of strains)	Range of MICs (mg/ml)[h]								
	Pen (1)	Amp-Sul[i] (8)	Amp-Clav[i] (8)	Pip-Tazo[i] (64)	Cefox (32)	Imi (8)	Clinda (4)	Metro (16)	Cipro (2)
A. lactolyticus (2)	≤0.5	≤0.25	0.25	ND	0.5	0.12	≤0.12	1	ND
A. lactolyticus-I[a] (5)	≤0.5–2[b]	≤0.25–0.5	0.12–0.25	0.5	0.5–2	0.12–0.5	0.25–64[f]	1	0.5–1
A. murdochii (6)	≤0.5–2	≤0.25	ND	ND	0.5–2	0.12–1	≤0.12–4	1–4	ND
A. prevotii (3)	2–16	1–4	2	2	1–4	0.5–1	32–128	1–2	16
A. tetradius (1)	≤0.5	≤0.25	ND	ND	0.5	≤0.062	0.25	2	ND
A. vaginalis (16)	≤0.5	0.12–0.25	0.12–0.25	0.062–0.12	≤0.12–0.25	≤0.062–0.12	0.062–0.5	0.25–4	4 to 8
F. magna (12)	0.12–1	≤ 0.25–0.5	0.12–0.25	ND	0.5–2	0.062–0.5	0.062–2	0.25–2	0.12–2
P. asaccharolyticus (10)	≤0.5	0.12–0.25	0.12–0.25	0.062	≤0.12	≤0.062	≤0.12	0.5–4	ND
P. harei (2)	≤0.5–1	≤0.25	ND	ND	0.25	≤0.062	0.5	2	ND
P. gorbachii (6)	≤0.5–1	≤0.25	ND	ND	≤0.12–0.5	≤0.062	≤0.12–128	0.5–4	ND
P. olsenii (4)	≤0.5	≤0.25	ND	ND	≤0.12	≤0.062	≤0.12–1	0.25–1	ND
P. anaerobius (16)	0.12–32[c]	≤0.25–16[e]	0.12 to 32	ND	0.5 to 32	≤0.062–2	≤0.062–0.5	0.12–8	1
P. stomatis (31)[g]	ND	ND	≤0.016–0.25	ND	≤0.016–1.5	ND	≤0.016–3	≤0.016–0.25	ND
P. micra (15)	0.062–64[d]	0.062–0.5	0.062	0.062	0.5–1	0.062–0.12	0.062–1	0.25–1	1–16

[a]Data were obtained from the Wadsworth Anaerobic Bacteriology Laboratory. Strains were tested by CLSI (formerly NCCLS) agar dilution procedures. Pen, penicillin; Amp-Sul, amoxicillin-sulbactam; Amp-Clav, amoxicillin-clavulanic acid; Pip-Tazo, piperacillin-tazobactam; Cefox, cefoxitin; Imi, imipenem; Clinda, clindamycin; Metro, metronidazole; Cipro, ciprofloxacin; ND, no data.

[b]One of 5 strains showed resistance.

[c]Three of 16 strains showed resistance.

[d]Two of 15 strains showed resistance.

[e]Three of 16 strains showed resistance.

[f]One of 5 strains showed resistance.

[g]Data were obtained from Könönen et al. (63). Strains were tested by the Etest (AB Biodisk).

[h]Numbers in parentheses are applied breakpoints for testing the antimicrobial agents.

[i]Results for this drug combination are given for amoxicillin and piperacillin.

reported. Strains that are microaerophilic (and therefore streptococci) are much more likely to be resistant to metronidazole. Susceptibility to clindamycin varies widely; local geographic variation should be taken into account. A French multicenter study (79) reported 28% clindamycin resistance among *Peptostreptococcus* spp., and an American study by Sanchez et al. (108) noted >10% resistance of *F. magna* to clindamycin. Wren (134) reported 9% of *F. magna* strains to be resistant to clindamycin in London, United Kingdom. Erythromycin and two other macrolides, clarithromycin and azithromycin, have similar efficacies and are probably not active enough to be recommended. Several studies (90, 134) indicated that older quinolones, such as ciprofloxacin, have only moderate activity, but more recently developed agents are extremely active (46, 90, 131). In another recent study, Koeth et al. (61) reported that the rates of susceptibility of *F. magna* to levofloxacin and clindamycin were 72.4% and 84.7%, respectively. It is highly desirable that future investigations present data on different species separately. A recent study by Brazier et al. (15) presented data on different grampositive anaerobic coccal species separately. They found that the highest percentage of overall resistance detected among gram-positive anaerobic cocci was 41.6% resistance to tetracycline, followed by 27.4% resistance to erythromycin. Among gram-positive anaerobic cocci as a group, 7.1% of isolates were resistant to penicillin and clindamycin and 3.5% of isolates were resistant to amoxicillin-clavulanate. There was no resistance among gram-positive anaerobic cocci to piperacillin-tazobactam, chloramphenicol, cefoxitin, imipenem, or metronidazole. A more recent study by the same group found an overall resistance rate of 7% of grampositive anaerobic cocci to penicillin and/or clindamycin (14). Similar results have been reported previously (15), although a higher prevalence of resistance, in particular to clindamycin, has been reported in some studies (61, 79). In another study, one strain of *Ruminococcus gauvreauii* was found to be highly resistant to vancomycin and teicoplanin (>256 µg/ml) (32).

It is worth noting that the resistance rates of *P. stomatis* and *P. anaerobius* are different (63). *P. anaerobius* sensu lato exhibits some resistance to several drugs: amoxicillin, amoxicillin-clavulanate (3 of 30 strains resistant), cefoxitin (2 of 30 strains resistant), and azithromycin and moxifloxacin (1 of 30 strains resistant). There was no resistance found in 31 strains of *P. stomatis*.

Certain newer agents would not be considered primary agents for therapy of infections due to anaerobic cocci, but when they are indicated for another reason in a mixed infection involving anaerobes, it is useful to know about their activity versus anaerobes. Useful references are available regarding the activities against anaerobes of ceftobiprole (35, 47), oritavancin (25), daptomycin (127), dalbavancin (48), and tigecycline (121). A striking example of another use of agents such as these is the report of the successful use of linezolid in a patient with a brain abscess due to a *Peptostreptococcus* sp. after failure of standard treatment (107).

EVALUATION, INTERPRETATION, AND REPORTING OF RESULTS

Because anaerobic bacteriology is time-consuming, several interim reports are desirable. The initial report should give Gram stain results and bacterial and human cell morphologies. The relative quantities of different organisms seen in the smear give a good overall impression of the specimen quality, the nature of the polymicrobial infection, and the relative importance of each organism. In general, bacterial isolates that are predominant and resistant to antimicrobial agents should be given the greatest attention. Bacteria present in pure culture or in large numbers are probably of major importance, as are organisms recovered in multiple cultures and isolated from normally sterile sites. Furthermore, Gram stain results can guide the laboratory in choosing media for optimal recovery of the predicted organisms.

The significance of finding anaerobic gram-positive and gram-negative cocci in clinical specimens depends on the specimen and the likelihood that it was contaminated by the microbiota of the skin or mucous membranes. Hence, interpretation of culture results is dependent on the nature and quality of the specimen submitted to the laboratory.

REFERENCES

1. Al Masalma, M., F. Armougom, W. M. Scheld, H. Dufour, P.-H. Roche, M. Drancurt, and D. Raoult. 2009. The expansion of the microbiological spectrum of brain abscesses with use of multiple 16S ribosomal DNA sequencing. *Clin. Infect. Dis.* **48:**1169–1178.
2. Arif, N., T. Do, R. Byun, E. Sheehy, D. Clark, S. C. Gilbert, and D. Beighton. 2008. *Veillonella rogosae* sp. nov., an anaerobic, Gram-negative coccus isolated from dental plaque. *Int. J. Syst. Evol. Microbiol.* **58:**581–584.
3. Bartz, H., C. Nonnenmacher, C. Bollmann, M. Kuhl, S. Zimmermann, K. Heeg, and R. Mutters. 2005. *Micromonas (Peptostreptococcus) micros:* unusual case of prosthetic joint infection associated with dental procedures. *Int. J. Med. Microbiol.* **294:**465–470.
4. Beighton, D., D. Clark, B. Hanakuka, S. Gilbert, and T. Do. 2008. The predominant cultivable *Veillonella* spp. of the tongue of healthy adults identified using *rpoB* sequencing. *Oral Microbiol. Immunol.* **23:**344–347.
5. Beumont, M. G., J. Duncan, S. D. Mitchell, J. L. Esterhai, Jr., and P. H. Edelstein. 1995. *Veillonella myositis* in an immunocompromised patient. *Clin. Infect. Dis.* **21:**678–679.
6. Bhatti, M. A., and M. O. Frank. 2000. *Veillonella parvula* meningitis: case report and review of *Veillonella* infections. *Clin. Infect. Dis.* **31:**839–840.
7. Biagi, E., B. Vitali, C. Pugliese, M. Candela, G. G. Donders, and P. Brigidi. 2009. Quantitative variations in the vaginal bacterial population associated with asymptomatic infections: a real-time polymerase chain reaction study. *Eur. J. Clin. Microbiol. Infect. Dis.* **28:**281–285.
8. Björck, L. 1988. Protein L: a novel bacterial cell wall protein with affinity for Ig L chains. *J. Immunol.* **140:**1194–1197.
9. Blome, B., A. Braun, V. Sobarzo, and S. Jepsen. 2008. Molecular identification and quantification of bacteria from endodontic infections using real-time polymerase chain reaction. *Oral Microbiol. Immunol.* **23:**384–390.
10. Bourgault, A.-M., J. E. Rosenblatt, and R. H. Fitzgerald. 1980. *Peptococcus magnus:* a significant human pathogen. *Ann. Intern. Med.* **93:**244–248.
11. Boutaga, K., A. J. van Winkelhoff, C. M. Vandenbroucke-Grauls, and P. H. Savelkoul. 2005. Periodontal pathogens: a quantitative comparison of anaerobic culture and real-time PCR. *FEMS Immunol. Med. Microbiol.* **45:**191–199.
12. Boutaga, K., P. H. Savelkoul, E. G. Winkel, and A. J. van Winkelhoff. 2007. Comparison of subgingival bacterial sampling with oral lavage for detection and quantification of periodontal pathogens by real-time polymerase chain reaction. *J. Periodontol.* **78:**79–86.
13. Boyanova, L., R. Kolarov, G. Gergova, E. Deliverska, J. Madjarov, M. Marinov, and I. Mitov. 2006. Anaerobic bacteria in 118 patients with deep-space head and neck infections from the University Hospital of Maxillofacial Surgery, Sofia, Bulgaria. *J. Med. Microbiol.* **55:**1285–1289.
14. Brazier, J., D. Chmelar, L. Dubreuil, G. Feierl, M. Hedberg, S. Kalenic, E. Könönen, B. Lundgren, H. Malamou-Ladas,

E. Nagy, A. Sullivan, and C. E. Nord; ESCMID Study Group on Antimicrobial Resistance in Anaerobic Bacteria. 2008. European surveillance study on antimicrobial susceptibility of Gram-positive anaerobic cocci. *Int. J. Antimicrob. Agents* **31:**316–320.

15. Brazier, J. S., V. Hall, T. E. Morris, M. Gal, and B. I. Duerden. 2003. Antibiotic susceptibilities of Gram-positive anaerobic cocci: results of a sentinel study in England and Wales. *J. Antimicrob. Chemother.* **52:**224–228.

16. Brook, I. 1986. Encapsulated anaerobic bacteria in synergistic infections. *Microbiol. Rev.* **50:**452–457.

17. Brook, I. 1989. Anaerobic bacteria in suppurative genitourinary infections. *J. Urol.* **141:**889–893.

18. Brook, I., and E. H. Frazier. 1990. Aerobic and anaerobic bacteriology of wounds and cutaneous abscesses. *Arch. Surg.* **125:**1445–1451.

19. Brook, I., and E. H. Frazier. 1992. Infections caused by *Veillonella* species. *Infect. Dis. Clin. Pract.* **1:**377–381.

20. Brook, I. 1996. *Veillonella* infections in children. *J. Clin. Microbiol.* **34:**1283–1285.

21. Brook, I. 2004. Intra-abdominal, retroperitoneal, and visceral abscesses in children. *Eur. J. Pediatr. Surg.* **14:**265–273.

22. Buduneli, N., H. Baylas, E. Buduneli, O. Türkoğlu, T. Köse, and G. Dahlen. 2005. Periodontal infections and preterm low birth weight: a case-control study. *J. Clin. Periodontol.* **32:**174–181.

23. Byun, R., J. P. Carlier, N. A. Jacques, H. Marchandin, and N. Hunter. 2007. *Veillonella denticariosi* sp. nov., isolated from human carious dentine. *Int. J. Syst. Evol. Microbiol.* **57:**2844–2848.

24. Carlier, J.-P., H. Marchandin, E. Jumas-Bilak, V. Lorin, C. Henry, C. Carriere, and H. Jean-Pierre. 2002. *Anaeroglobus geminatus* gen. nov., sp. nov., a novel member of the family *Veillonellaceae.* *Int. J. Syst. Evol. Microbiol.* **52:**983–986.

25. Citron, D. M., Y. Y. Kwok, and M. D. Appleman. 2005. In vitro activity of oritavancin (LY333328), vancomycin, clindamycin, and metronidazole against *Clostridium perfringens*, *Propionibacterium acnes*, and anaerobic gram-positive cocci. *Anaerobe* **11:**93–95.

26. Civen, R., M.-L. Väisänen, and S. M. Finegold. 1993. Peritonsillar abscess, retropharyngeal abscess, mediastinitis, and nonclostridial anaerobic myonecrosis: a case report. *Clin. Infect. Dis.* **16**(Suppl. 4):S299–S303.

27. Collins, M. D., and S. Wallbanks. 1992. Comparative sequence analyses of the 16S rRNA genes of *Lactobacillus minutus*, *Lactobacillus rimae* and *Streptococcus parvulus*: proposal for the creation of a new genus, *Atopobium*. *FEMS Microbiol. Lett.* **95:**235–240.

28. Collins, M. L. Z., W. A. Falkler, E. R. Hall, and M. B. Graham. 1989. Serological studies of peptostreptococci using an indirect fluorescent antibody test. *J. Dent. Res.* **68:**1508–1512.

29. Davies, U. M., A. M. Leak, and J. Dave. 1988. Infection of a prosthetic knee joint with *Peptostreptococcus magnus*. *Ann. Rheumat. Dis.* **47:**866–868.

30. de Château, M., and L. Björck. 1994. Protein PAB, a mosaic albumin-binding bacterial protein representing the first contemporary example of module shuffling. *J. Biol. Chem.* **269:**12147–12151.

31. Delaney, M. L., and A. B. Onderdonk. 2001. Nugent score related to vaginal culture in pregnant women. *Obstet. Gynecol.* **98:**79–84.

32. Domingo, M.-C., A. Huletsky, M. Boissinot, K. A. Bernard, F. J. Picard, and M. G. Bergeron. 2008. *Ruminococcus gauvreauii* sp. nov., a glycopeptide-resistant species isolated from a human faecal specimen. *Int. J. Syst. Evol. Microbiol.* **68:**1393–1397.

33. Downes, J., and W. G. Wade. 2006. *Peptostreptococcus stomatis* sp. nov., isolated from the human oral cavity. *Int. J. Syst. Evol. Microbiol.* **56:**751–754.

34. Edmiston, C. E., Jr., A. P. Walker, C. J. Krepel, and C. Gohr. 1990. The nonpuerperal breast infection: aerobic and anaerobic microbial recovery from acute and chronic disease. *J. Infect. Dis.* **162:**695–699.

35. Ednie, L., S. Shapiro, and P. C. Appelbaum. 2007. Antianaerobic activity of ceftobiprole, a new broad-spectrum cephalosporin. *Diagn. Microbiol. Infect. Dis.* **58:**133–136.

36. Egwari, L., V. O. Rotimi, O. O. Abudu, and A. O. Coker. 1995. A study of the anaerobic bacterial flora of the female genital tract in health and disease. *Cent. Afr. J. Med.* **41:**391–397.

37. Ezaki, T., N. Yamamoto, K. Ninomiya. S. Suzuki, and E. Yabuuchi. 1983. Transfer of *Peptococcus indolicus*, *Peptococcus asaccharolyticus*, *Peptococcus prevotii*, and *Peptococcus magnus* to the genus *Peptostreptococcus* and proposal of *Peptostreptococcus tetradius* sp. nov. *Int. J. Syst. Bacteriol.* **33:**683–698.

38. Ezaki, T., N. Li, Y. Hashimoto, H. Miura, and H. Yamamoto. 1994. 16S ribosomal DNA sequences of anaerobic cocci and proposal of *Ruminococcus hansenii* comb. nov. and *Ruminococcus productus* comb. nov. *Int. J. Syst. Bacteriol.* **44:**130–136.

39. Ezaki, T., Y. Kawamura, N. Li, Z. Y. Li, L. Zhao, and S. Shu. 2001. Proposal of the genera *Anaerococcus* gen. nov., *Peptoniphilus* gen. nov. and *Gallicola* gen. nov. for members of the genus *Peptostreptococcus*. *Int. J. Syst. Evol. Microbiol.* **51:**1521–1528.

40. Fenner, L., A. F. Widmer, C. Straub, and R. Frei. 2008. Is the incidence of anaerobic bacteremia decreasing? Analysis of 114,000 blood cultures over a ten-year period. *J. Clin. Microbiol.* **46:**2432–2434.

41. Finegold, S. M. 1995. Anaerobic infections in humans: an overview. *Anaerobe* **1:**3–9.

42. Fitzgerald, R. H., Jr., J. E. Rosenblatt, J. H. Tenney, and A.-M. Bourgault. 1982. Anaerobic septic arthritis. *Clin. Orthop. Rel. Res.* **1982:**141–148.

43. Fournier, P. E., M. V. La, J. P. Casalta, H. Richet, F. Collart, and D. Raoult. 2008. *Finegoldia magna*, an early postoperative cause of infectious endocarditis: report of two cases and review of the literature. *Anaerobe* **14:**310–312.

44. Frick, I. M., C. Karlsson, M. Mörgelin, A. I. Olin, R. Janjusevic, C. Hammarström, E. Holst, M. de Château, and L. Björck. 2008. Identification of a novel protein promoting the colonization and survival of *Finegoldia magna*, a bacterial commensal and opportunistic pathogen. *Mol. Microbiol.* **70:**695–708.

45. Garrity, G. M., and J. G. Holt. 2001. Taxonomic outlines of the Archaea and Bacteria, p. 155–166. *In* D. R. Boone and R. W. Castenholz (ed.), *Bergey's Manual of Systematic Bacteriology*, 2nd ed. Springer, New York, NY.

46. Goldstein, E. J., G. Conrads, D. M. Citron, C. V. Merriam, Y. Warren, and K. Tyrrell. 2002. In vitro activity of gemifloxacin compared to seven other oral antimicrobial agents against aerobic and anaerobic pathogens isolated from antral sinus puncture specimens from patients with sinusitis. *Diagn. Microbiol. Infect. Dis.* **42:**113–118.

47. Goldstein, E. J. C., D. M. Citron, C. V. Merriam, Y. A. Warren, K. L. Tyrrell, and H. T. Fernandez. 2006. In vitro activity of ceftobiprole against aerobic and anaerobic strains isolated from diabetic foot infections. *Antimicrob. Agents Chemother.* **50:**3959–3962.

48. Goldstein, E. J. C., D. M. Citron, Y. A. Warren, K. L. Tyrrell, C. V. Merriam, and H. T. Fernandez. 2006. In vitro activities of dalbavancin and 12 other agents against 329 aerobic and anaerobic gram-positive isolates recovered from diabetic foot infections. *Antimicrob. Agents Chemother.* **50:**2875–2879.

49. Gomes, S. C., C. Nonnenmacher, C. Susin, R. V. Oppermann, R. Mutters, and R. A. Marcantonio. 2008. The effect of a supragingival plaque-control regimen on the subgingival microbiota in smokers and never-smokers: evaluation by real-time polymerase chain reaction. *J. Periodontol.* **79:**2297–2304.

50. Gutierrez de Ferro, M. I., R. E. Ruiz de Valladares, and I. L. Benito de Cardenas. 2005. Recovery of *Veillonella* from saliva. *Rev. Argent. Microbiol.* **37:**22–25.

51. Hill, K. E., C. E. Davies, M. J. Wilson, P. Stephens, M. A. Lewis, V. Hall, J. Brazier, and D. W. Thomas. 2002. Heterogeneity within the gram-positive anaerobic cocci demonstrated by analysis of 16S–23S intergenic ribosomal RNA polymorphisms. *J. Med. Microbiol.* **51:**949–957.

52. **Holdeman-Moore, L. V., J. L. Johnson, and W. E. C. Moore.** 1986. Genus *Peptostreptococcus*, p. 1083–1092. *In* P. H. A. Sneath, N. S. Mair, M. E. Sharpe, and J. G. Holt (ed.), *Bergey's Manual of Systematic Bacteriology*, vol. 2. The Williams & Wilkins Co., Baltimore, MD.

53. **Igarashi, E., A. Kamaguchi, M. Fujita, H. Miyakawa, and F. Nakazawa.** 2009. Identification of oral species of the genus *Veillonella* by polymerase chain reaction. *Oral Microbiol. Immunol.* **24:**310–313.

54. **Johnson, S., F. Lebahn, L. R. Peterson, and D. N. Gerding.** 1995. Use of an anaerobic collection and transport swab device to recover anaerobic bacteria from infected foot ulcers in diabetics. *Clin. Infect. Dis.* **20:**S289–S290.

55. **Jousimies-Somer, H. R., P. Summanen, D. Citron, E. Baron, H. M. Wexler, and S. M. Finegold.** 2002. *Wadsworth-KTL Anaerobic Bacteriology Manual*, 5th ed. Star Publishing, Belmont, CA.

56. **Jumas-Bilak, E., J. P. Carlier, H. Jean-Pierre, C. Teyssier, B. Gay, J. Campos, and H. Marchandin.** 2004. *Veillonella montpellierensis* sp. nov., a novel, anaerobic, Gram-negative coccus isolated from human clinical samples. *Int. J. Syst. Evol. Microbiol.* **54:**1311–1316.

57. **Jumas-Bilak, E., J. P. Carlier, H. Jean-Pierre, F. Mory, C. Teyssier, B. Gay, J. Campos, and H. Marchandin.** 2007. *Acidaminococcus intestini* sp. nov., isolated from human clinical samples. *Int. J. Syst. Evol. Microbiol.* **57:**2314–2319.

58. **Kanno, T., T. Matsuki, M. Oka, H. Utsunomiya, K. Inada, H. Magari, I. Inoue, T. Maekita, K. Ueda, S. Enomoto, M. Iguchi, K. Yanaoka, H. Tamai, S. Akimoto, K. Nomoto, R. Tanaka, and M. Ichinose.** 2009. Gastric acid reduction leads to an alteration in lower intestinal microflora. *Biochem. Biophys. Res. Commun.* **381:**666–670.

59. **Karlsson, C., M.-L. Andersson, M. Collin, A. Schmidtchen, L. Björck, and I.-M. Frick.** 2007. SufA—a novel subtilisin-like serine proteinase of *Finegoldia magna*. *Microbiology* **153:**4208–4218.

60. **Karlsson, C., M. Eliasson, A. I. Olin, M. Morgelin, A. Karlsson, M. Malmsten, A. Egesten, and I. M. Frick.** 2009. SufA of the opportunistic pathogen *Finegoldia magna* modulates actions of the antibacterial chemokine MIG/CXCL9, promoting bacterial survival during epithelial inflammation. *J. Biol. Chem.* **284:**29499–29508.

61. **Koeth, L. M., C. E. Good, P. C. Appelbaum, E. J. Goldstein, A. C. Rodloff, M. Claros, and L. J. Dubreuil.** 2004. Surveillance of susceptibility patterns in 1297 European and US anaerobic and capnophilic isolates to co-amoxiclav and five other antimicrobial agents. *J. Antimicrob. Chemother.* **53:**1039–1044.

62. **Kolenbrander, P. E., and L. V. H. Moore.** 1992. The genus *Veillonella*, p. 2034–2047. *In* A. G. Balows, M. Trüper, W. Dworkin, W. Harder, and K.-H. Schleifer (ed.), *The Prokaryotes*, 2nd ed. Springer, New York, NY.

63. **Könönen, E., A. Bryk, P. Niemi, and A. Kanervo-Nordström.** 2007. Antimicrobial susceptibilities of *Peptostreptococcus anaerobius* and the newly described *Peptostreptococcus stomatis* isolated from various human sources. *Antimicrob. Agents Chemother.* **51:**2205–2207.

64. **Korman, T. M., E. Athan, and D. W. Spelman.** 1997. Anaerobic meningitis due to *Peptostreptococcus* species: case report and review. *Clin. Infect. Dis.* **25:**1462–1464.

65. **Krepel, C. J., C. M. Gohr, A. P. Walker, S. G. Farmer, and C. E. Edmiston.** 1992. Enzymatically active *Peptostreptococcus magnus*: association with site of infection. *J. Clin. Microbiol.* **30:**2330–2334.

66. **Lehmann, L. E., K.-P. Hunfeld, T. Emrich, G. Haberhausen, H. Wissing, A. Hoeft, and F. Stüber.** 2008. A multiplex real-time PCR assay for rapid detection and differentiation of 25 bacterial and fungal pathogens from whole blood samples. *Med. Microbiol. Immunol.* **197:**313–324.

67. **Li, N., Y. Hashimoto, S. Adnan, H. Miura, H. Yamamoto, and T. Ezaki.** 1992. Three new species of the genus *Peptostreptococcus* isolated from humans: *Peptostreptococcus vaginalis* sp. nov., *Peptostreptococcus lacrimalis* sp. nov., and *Peptostreptococcus lactolyticus* sp. nov. *Int. J. Syst. Bacteriol.* **42:**602–605.

68. **Liu, C., S. M. Finegold, Y. Song, and P. A. Lawson.** 2008. Reclassification of *Clostridium coccoides*, *Ruminococcus hansenii*, *Ruminococcus hydrogenotrophicus*, *Ruminococcus luti*, *Ruminococcus productus* and *Ruminococcus schinkii* as *Blautia coccoides* gen. nov., comb. nov., *Blautia hansenii* comb. nov., *Blautia hydrogenotrophica* comb. nov., *Blautia luti* comb. nov., *Blautia producta* comb. nov., *Blautia schinkii* comb. nov. and description of *Blautia wexlerae* sp. nov., isolated from human faeces. *Int. J. Syst. Evol. Microbiol.* **58:**1896–1902.

69. **Liu, J. W., J. J. Wu, L. R. Wang, L. J. Teng, and T. C. Huang.** 1998. Two fatal cases of *Veillonella* bacteraemia. *Eur. J. Clin. Microbiol. Dis.* **17:**62–64.

70. **Maniglia, R. J., T. Roth, and E. A. Blumberg.** 1997. Polymicrobial brain abscess in a patient infected with human immunodeficiency virus. *Clin. Infect. Dis.* **24:**449–451.

71. **Marchandin, H., C. Teyssier, C. Carriere, F. Canovas, H. Daras, and E. Jumas-Bilak.** 2001. Prosthetic joint infection due to *Veillonella dispar*. *Eur. J. Clin. Microbiol. Infect. Dis.* **20:**340–342.

72. **Marchandin, H., C. Teyssier, J. Campos, H. Jean-Pierre, F. Roger, B. Gay, J.-P. Carlier, and E. Jumas-Bilak.** 2010. *Negativicoccus succinovorans* gen. nov., sp. nov., isolated from human clinical samples, emended description of the family *Veillonellaceae* and description of *Negativicutes* classis nov., *Selenomonadales* ord. nov., and *Acidaminococcaceae* fam. nov., in the bacterial phylum *Firmicutes*. *Int. J. Syst. Evol. Microbiol.* **60:**1271–1279

73. **Marina, M., C. A. Strong, R. Civen, E. Molitoris, and S. M. Finegold.** 1993. Bacteriology of anaerobic pleuropulmonary infections: preliminary report. *Clin. Infect. Dis.* **16:**S256–S262.

74. **Marrazzo, J. M., K. K. Thomas, T. L. Fiedler, K. Ringwood, and D. N. Fredricks.** 2008. Relationship of specific vaginal bacteria and bacterial vaginosis treatment failure in women who have sex with women. *Ann. Intern. Med.* **149:**20–28.

75. **Marriott, D., D. Stark, and J. Harkness.** 2007. *Veillonella parvula* discitis and secondary bacteremia: a rare infection complicating endoscopy and colonoscopy? *J. Clin. Microbiol.* **45:**672–674.

76. **Mitchelmore, I. J., A. J. Prior, P. Q. Montgomery, and S. Tabaqchali.** 1995. Microbiological features and pathogenesis of peritonsillar abscesses. *Eur. J. Clin. Microbiol. Infect. Dis.* **14:**870–877.

77. **Montejo, M., G. Ruiz-Irastorza, K. Aguirrebengoa, E. Amutio, J. L. Hernández, and C. Aguirre.** 1995. Prosthetic-valve endocarditis caused by *Peptostreptococcus anaerobius*. *Clin. Infect. Dis.* **20:**1431.

78. **Moore, L. V. H., W. E. C. Moore, and E. P. Cato.** 1987. Bacteriology of human gingivitis. *J. Dent. Res.* **66:**989–995.

79. **Mory, F., A. Lozniewski, S. Bland, A. Sedallian, G. Grollier, F. Girard-Pipau, M. F. Paris, and L. Dubreuil.** 1998. Survey of anaerobic susceptibility patterns: a French multicentre study. *Int. J. Antimicrob. Agents* **10:**229–236.

80. **Murdoch, D. A., and I. J. Mitchelmore.** 1991. The laboratory identification of gram-positive anaerobic cocci. *J. Med. Microbiol.* **34:**295–308.

81. **Murdoch, D. A., I. J. Mitchelmore, and S. Tabaqchali.** 1994. The clinical importance of gram-positive anaerobic cocci isolated at St. Bartholomew's Hospital, London, in 1987. *J. Med. Microbiol.* **41:**36–44.

82. **Murdoch, D. A.** 1998. Gram-positive anaerobic cocci. *Clin. Microbiol. Rev.* **11:**81–120.

83. **Murdoch, D. A., and H. N. Shah.** 1999. Reclassification of *Peptostreptococcus magnus* (Prevot 1933) Holdeman and Moore 1972 as *Finegoldia magna* comb. nov. and *Peptostreptococcus micros* (Prevot 1933) Smith 1957 as *Micromonas micros* comb. nov. *Anaerobe* **5:**555–559.

84. **Murdoch, D. A., H. N. Shah, S. E. Gharbia, and D. Rajendram.** 2000. Proposal to restrict the genus *Peptostreptococcus* (Kluyver & van Niel 1936) to *Peptostreptococcus anaerobius*. *Anaerobe* **6:**257–260.

85. **Natto, S., M. Baljoon, G. Dahlén, and J. Bergström.** 2005. Tobacco smoking and periodontal microflora in a Saudi Arabian population. *J. Clin. Periodontol.* **32:**549–555.

86. Ng, L. S. Y., L. L. Kwang, S. C. S. Yeow, and T. Y. Tan. 2008. Anaerobic culture of diabetic foot infections: organisms and antimicrobial susceptibilities. *Ann. Acad. Med. Singapore* **37**:936–939.

87. Nonnenmacher, C., M. Stelzel, C. Susin, A. M. Sattler, J. R. Schafer, B. Maisch, R. Mutters, and L. Flores-de-Jacoby. 2007. Periodontal microbiota in patients with coronary artery disease measured by real-time polymerase chain reaction: a case-control study. *J. Periodontol.* **78**:1724–1730.

88. Ota-Tsuzuki, C., and M. P. Mayer. 2010. Collagenase production and hemolytic activity related to 16S rRNA variability among *Parvimonas micra* oral isolates. *Anaerobe*, **16**:38–42.

89. Panagou, P., L. Papandreou, and D. Bouros. 1991. Severe anaerobic necrotizing pneumonia complicated by pyopneumothorax and anaerobic monoarthritis due to *Peptostreptococcus magnus*. *Respiration* **58**:223–225.

90. Pankuch, G. A., M. R. Jacobs, and P. C. Appelbaum. 1993. Susceptibilities of 428 gram-positive and -negative anaerobic bacteria to Bay y3118 compared with their susceptibilities to ciprofloxacin, clindamycin, metronidazole, piperacillin, piperacillin-tazobactam, and cefoxitin. *Antimicrob. Agents Chemother.* **37**:1649–1654.

91. Papaioannou, W., S. Gizani, A. D. Haffajee, M. Quirynen, E. Mamai-Homata, and L. Papagiannoulis. 2009. The microbiota on different oral surfaces in healthy children. *Oral Microbiol. Immunol.* **24**:183–189.

92. Paster, B. J., M. K. Russell, T. Alpagot, A. M. Lee, S. K. Bochs, J. L. Galvin, and F. E. Dewhirst. 2002. Bacterial diversity in necrotizing ulcerative periodontitis in HIV-positive subjects. *Ann. Periodontol.* **7**:8–16.

93. Periasamy, S., and P. E. Kolenbrander. 2009. Aggregatibacter actinomycetemcomitans builds mutualistic biofilm communities in saliva with *Fusobacterium nucleatum* and *Veillonella* sp. *Infect. Immun.* **77**:3542–3551.

94. Petts, D. N., W. Champion, and G. Raymond. 1988. Oxolinic acid as a selective agent for the isolation of non-sporing anaerobes from clinical material. *Lett. Appl. Microbiol.* **6**:65–67.

95. Price, R. R., H. B. Viscount, M. C. Stanley, and K. P. Leung. 2007. Targeted profiling of oral bacteria in human saliva and in vitro biofilms with quantitative real-time PCR. *Biofouling* **23**:203–213.

96. Rams, T. E., D. Feik, M. A. Listgarten, and J. Slots. 1992. *Peptostreptococcus micros* in human periodontitis. *Oral Microbiol. Immunol.* **7**:1–6.

97. Rennie, R. P., C. Brosnikoff, L. A. Turnbull, L. B. Reller, S. Mirrett, W. Janda, K. Ristow, and A. Krilcich. 2008. Multicenter evaluation of the Vitek 2 Anaerobe and *Corynebacterium* identification card. *J. Clin. Microbiol.* **46**:2646–2651.

98. Riggio, M. P., A. Lennon, and A. Smith. 2001. Detection of *Peptostreptococcus micros* DNA in clinical samples by PCR. *J. Med. Microbiol.* **50**:249–254.

99. Riggio, M. P., and A. Lennon. 2003. Specific PCR detection of *Peptostreptococcus magnus*. *J. Med. Microbiol.* **52**:309–313.

100. Riggio, M. P., and A. Lennon. 2003. Identification of oral peptostreptococcus isolates by PCR-restriction fragment length polymorphism analysis of 16S rRNA genes. *J. Clin. Microbiol.* **41**:4475–4479.

101. Riggio, M. P., H. Aga, C. A. Murray, M. S. Jackson, A. Lennon, N. Hammersley and J. Bagg. 2007. Identification of bacteria associated with spreading odontogenic infections by16S rRNA gene sequencing. *Oral Surg. Oral Med. Oral Pathol. Oral Radiol. Endod.* **103**:610–617.

102. Rôças, I. N., and J. F. Siqueira, Jr. 2006. Culture-independent detection of *Eikenella corrodens* and *Veillonella parvula* in primary endodontic infections. *J. Endod.* **32**:509–512.

103. Rôças, I. N., and J. F. Siqueira, Jr. 2008. Root canal microbiota of teeth with chronic apical periodontitis. *J. Clin. Microbiol.* **46**:3599–3606.

104. Rogosa, M. 1965. The genus *Veillonella*, IV. Serological groupings, and genus and species emendations. *J. Bacteriol.* **90**:704–709.

105. Rowlinson, M.-C., P. LeBourgeois, K. Ward, Y. L. Song, S. M. Finegold, and D. A. Bruckner. 2006. Isolation of a strictly anaerobic strain of *Staphylococcus epidermidis*. **44**:857–860.

106. Ruviére, D. B., M. R. Leonardo, L. A. da Silva, I. Y. Ito, and P. Nelson-Filho. 2007. Assessment of the microbiota in root canals of human primary teeth by checkerboard DNA-DNA hybridization. *J. Dent. Child.* (Chic.) **74**:118–123.

107. Salin, F., F. Vianello, R. Manara, E. Morelli, A. Cattelan, M. Scarin, and D. Sgarabotto. 2006. Linezolid in the treatment of brain abscess due to Peptostreptococcus. *Scand. J. Infect. Dis.* **38**:203–205.

108. Sanchez, M. L., R. N. Jones, and J. L. Croco. 1992. Use of the Etest to access macrolide-lincosamide resistance patterns among *Peptostreptococcus* species. *Antimicrob. Newsl.* **8**:45–49.

109. Sassone, L., R. Fidel, L. Figueiredo, S. Fidel, M. Faveri, and M. Feres. 2007. Evaluation of the microbiota of primary endodontic infections using checkerboard DNA-DNA hybridization. *Oral Microbiol. Immunol.* **22**:390–397.

110. Sato, T., J. Matsuyama, M. Sato, and E. Hoshino. 1997. Differentiation of *Veillonella atypica*, *Veillonella dispar* and *Veillonella parvula* using restricted fragment-length polymorphism analysis of 16S rDNA amplified by polymerase chain reaction. *Oral Microbiol. Immunol.* **12**:350–353.

111. Sato, T., M. Sato, J. Matsuyama, and E. Hoshino. 1997. PCR-restriction fragment length polymorphism analysis of genes coding for 16S rRNA in *Veillonella* spp. *Int. J. Syst. Bacteriol.* **47**:1268–1270.

112. Seng, P., M. Drancourt, F. Gouriet, B. La Scala, P.-E. Fournier, J. M. Rolain, and D. Raoult. 2009. Ongoing revolution in bacteriology: routine identification of bacteria by matrix-assisted laser desorption ionization time-of-flight mass spectrometry. *Clin. Infect. Dis.* **49**:543–551.

113. Singh, N., and V. L. Yu. 1992. Osteomyelitis due to *Veillonella parvula*: case report and review. *Clin. Infect. Dis.* **14**:361–363.

114. Siqueira, J. F., Jr., I. N. Rôças, A. F. Andrade, and M. de Uzeda. 2003. *Peptostreptococcus micros* in primary endodontic infections as detected by 16S rDNA-based polymerase chain reaction. *J. Endod.* **29**:111–113.

115. Siqueira, J. F., Jr., and I. N. Rôças. 2008. The microbiota of acute apical abscesses. *J. Dent. Res.* **88**:61–65.

116. Smayevsky, J., L. F. Canigia, A. Lanza, and H. Bianchini. 2001. Vaginal microflora associated with bacterial vaginosis in nonpregnant women: reliability of sialidase detection. *Infect. Dis. Obstet. Gynecol.* **9**:17–22.

117. Song, Y., C. Liu, M. McTeague, and S. M. Finegold. 2003. 16S ribosomal DNA sequence-based analysis of clinically significant gram-positive anaerobic cocci. *J. Clin. Microbiol.* **41**:1363–1369.

118. Song, Y., C. Liu, and S. M. Finegold. 2007. Development of a flow chart for identification of gram-positive anaerobic cocci in the clinical laboratory. *J. Clin. Microbiol.* **45**:512–516.

119. Song, Y., C. Liu, and S. M. Finegold. 2007. *Peptoniphilus gorbachii* sp. nov., *Peptoniphilus olsenii* sp. nov., and *Anaerococcus murdochii* sp. nov. isolated from clinical specimens of human origin. *J. Clin. Microbiol.* **45**:1746–1752.

120. Song, Y., C. Liu, M. McTeague, A. Vu, J. Y. Liu, and S. M. Finegold. 2003. Rapid identification of Gram-positive anaerobic coccal species originally classified in the genus *Peptostreptococcus* by multiplex PCR assays using genus- and species-specific primers. *Microbiology* **149**:1719–1727.

121. Sotto, A., N. Bouziges, N. Jordan, J.-L. Richard, and J.-P. Lavigne. 2007. In vitro activity of tigecycline against strains isolated from diabetic foot ulcers. *Pathol. Biologie* **55**:398–406.

122. Subramanian, K., and A. K. Mickel. 2009. Molecular analysis of persistent periradicular lesions and root ends reveals a diverse microbial profile. *J. Endod.* **35**:950–957.

123. Summanen, P. H., D. A. Talan, C. Strong, M. McTeague, R. Bennion, J. E. Thompson, Jr., M.-L. Väisänen, G. Moran, M. Winer, and S. M. Finegold. 1995. Bacteriology

of skin and soft-tissue infections: comparison of infections in intravenous drug users and individuals with no history of intravenous drug use. *Clin. Infect. Dis.* **20**(Suppl. 2): S279–S282.

124. **Sutter, V. L.** 1984. Anaerobes as normal oral flora. *Rev. Infect. Dis.* **6:**S62–S66.

125. **Tindall, B. J., and J. P. Euzéby.** 2002. Proposal of *Parvimonas* gen. nov. and *Quatrionicoccus* gen. nov. as replacements for the illegitimate, prokaryotic, generic names *Micromonas* Murdoch and Shah 2000 and *Quadricoccus* Maszenan et al. 2002, respectively. *Int. J. Syst. Evol. Microbiol.* **56:** 2711–2713.

126. **Turng, B.-F., J. M. Guthmiller, G. E. Minah, and W. A. Falkler, Jr.** 1996. Development and evaluation of a selective and differential medium for the primary isolation of *Peptostreptococcus micros. Oral Microbiol. Immunol.* **5:**356–361.

127. **Tyrrell, K. L., D. M. Citron, Y. A. Warren, H. T. Fernandez, C. V. Merriam, and E. J. C. Goldstein.** 2006. In vitro activities of daptomycin, vancomycin, and penicillin against *Clostridium difficile, C. perfringens, Finegoldia magna,* and *Propionibacterium acnes. Antimicrob. Agents Chemother.* **50:**2728–2731.

128. **Ulger-Toprak, N., C. Liu, P. H. Summanen, and S. M. Finegold.** 2010. *Murdochiella asaccharolytica* gen. nov., sp. nov., a gram-positive, anaerobic coccus isolated from human wound specimens. *Int. J. Syst. Evol. Microbiol.* **60:**1013–1016.

129. **Verma, P.** 2000. Laboratory diagnosis of anaerobic pleuropulmonary infections. *Semin. Respir. Infect.* **15:**114–118.

130. **Wade, W. G., J. Moran, J. R. Morgan, R. Newcombe, and M. Addy.** 1992. The effects of antimicrobial acrylic strips on the subgingival microflora in chronic periodontitis. *J. Clin. Periodontol.* **19:**127–134.

131. **Watt, B., and F. V. Brown.** 1986. Is ciprofloxacin active against clinically important anaerobes? *J. Antimicrob. Chemother.* **17:**605–613.

132. **Wildeboer-Veloo, A. C., H. J. Harmsen, G. W. Welling, and J. E. Degener.** 2007. Development of 16S rRNA-based probes for the identification of Gram-positive anaerobic cocci isolated from human clinical specimens. *Clin. Microbiol. Infect.* **13:**985–992.

133. **Woo, P. C. Y., L. M. W. Chung, J. L. L. Teng, H. Tse, S. S. Y. Pang, V. Y. T. Lau, V. W. K. Wong, K.-L. Kam, S. K. P. Lau, and K.-Y. Yuen.** 2007. In silico analysis of 16S ribosomal RNA gene sequencing-based methods for identification of medically important anaerobic bacteria. *J. Clin. Pathol.* **60:**576–579.

134. **Wren, M. W. D.** 1996. Anaerobic cocci of clinical importance. *Br. J. Biomed. Sci.* **53:**294–301.

Propionibacterium, Lactobacillus, Actinomyces, and Other Non-Spore-Forming Anaerobic Gram-Positive Rods*

WILLIAM G. WADE AND EIJA KÖNÖNEN

49

TAXONOMY AND DESCRIPTION OF THE AGENTS

The anaerobic gram-positive non-spore-forming rods are widely distributed in two gram-positive phyla: *Actinobacteria* and *Firmicutes* (Table 1).

Phylum *Actinobacteria*

The genus *Actinomyces*, and the related clinically relevant genera *Actinobaculum*, *Mobiluncus*, and *Varibaculum*, contain anaerobic and aerotolerant, non-acid-fast, gram-positive organisms with variable morphology, ranging from characteristic branching rods to coccobacilli. The genus *Actinomyces* includes a number of species associated with disease, and the majority of species produce succinic acid from glucose. Recently, a novel *Actinomyces* species, *A. massiliensis*, has been described (146), and the classification of the common oral species *A. naeslundii* has been clarified with the proposal of two new species, *A. johnsonii* and *A. oris* (85). The genus *Actinobaculum* includes *A. massiliense*, *A. schaalii*, and *A. urinale* (71, 76, 112), all of which are associated with urinary tract and other infections, including septicemia and osteomyelitis. The genus *Mobiluncus* contains two species, *M. curtisii* and *M. mulieris*, which are strictly anaerobic, curved bacilli with variable Gram reactions and corkscrew motility. They resemble *Actinomyces* in that succinic acid is the major metabolic end product from glucose. *Varibaculum* (80) is related to *Mobiluncus* on the basis of 16S rRNA gene sequence analysis, as is *Actinomyces neuii*, which is distantly related to *Actinomyces* sensu stricto and would appear to be worthy of proposal as a novel genus (90).

Propionibacterium species are anaerobic and aerotolerant, pleomorphic, gram-positive rods that produce propionic acid from glucose. Five *Propionibacterium* species have been isolated from human clinical infections: *P. acnes*, *P. avidum*, *P. granulosum*, *P. propionicum*, and the recently described *P. acidifaciens* (44). A related species, *Propionimicrobium lymphophilum*, formerly a member of *Propionibacterium*, has also been isolated from clinical material, while *Propioniferax innocua* is a member of the normal skin microbiota.

Members of the genus *Bifidobacterium* and the closely related genera *Alloscardovia* (92), *Parascardovia*, and *Scardovia* (96) are strictly anaerobic or occasionally microaerobic, gram-positive, pleomorphic rods, appearing as uniform to branched or club shaped. Typically, bifidobacteria produce fructose-6-phosphate phosphoketolase as well as acetic and lactic acids as major metabolic end products. Bifidobacteria are aciduric and are nutritionally fastidious. There are currently 32 *Bifidobacterium* species. Of these, 11 species (*B. adolescentis*, *B. angulatum*, *B. bifidum*, *B. breve*, *B. catenulatum*, *B. dentium*, *B. gallicum*, *B. longum*, *B. pseudocatenulatum*, *B. subtile*, and *B. scardovii*) have been isolated from the human gut and oral cavity. *B. longum* now includes the former species *B. infantis* and *B. suis* as subspecies (122, 153).

Numerous taxa have been misassigned to *Lactobacillus* in the past, including the so-called "anaerobic lactobacilli," which are now recognized to constitute two genera, *Atopobium* and *Olsenella*, within the family *Coriobacteriaceae* (37, 41). *Atopobium* species produce lactic acid as the major glucose metabolic end product. *A. minutum* and *A. rimae* were formerly *Lactobacillus* species, and *A. parvulum* and *A. fossor* formerly belonged to the genera *Streptococcus* and *Eubacterium*, respectively (37, 100). The genus *Olsenella* is closely related to *Atopobium* and currently includes two species: *O. uli* (formerly *Lactobacillus uli*) and *O. profusa*, both isolated from the human oral cavity.

The genus *Eggerthella* (191) includes the human pathogens *E. lenta* and *E. sinensis*, while the former *E. hongkongensis* has been moved to the new genus *Paraeggerthella* (200). Other members of the *Coriobacteriaceae* found in human infections include the genera *Collinsella* (101), *Slackia* (191), and *Cryptobacterium* (130), while the genera *Adlercreutzia* and *Gordonibacter* have been isolated recently from feces and the colon, respectively (121, 200).

Phylum *Firmicutes*

Lactobacillus, a large and heterogeneous genus, contains microaerobic, catalase-negative, non-spore-forming, gram-positive rods, which produce lactic acid as their single or major metabolic end product from glucose fermentation. The majority of *Lactobacillus* species are found within the family *Lactobacillaceae* and order *Lactobacillales*. However, *Catenibacterium mitsuokai* (99), isolated from human feces, forms a cluster with *L. vitulinus* and *L. catenaformis*, two misclassified *Lactobacillus* species, within the family *Erysipelotrichaceae* (117).

Organisms assigned to *Eubacterium* are defined by default; they do not produce propionic acid as a major acid product, lactic acid as the sole major acid product, succinic

---

*This chapter contains information presented in chapter 55 by Bernard J. Moncla and Sharon L. Hillier in the eighth edition of this *Manual*.

TABLE 1 Some features of non-spore-forming anaerobic gram-positive genera

Phylum and genus	G+C mol%	Cell characteristics	Aerotolerance[a]	Gram reaction[b]	Major end product(s)[c]	Other features
Actinobacteria						
Actinobaculum	50–57	Straight or slightly curved, branching; singly or in clusters	+/−	(+)	A	Saccharolytic
Actinomyces	55–68	Variable, often branching; singly or in pairs	+/−	+	S, L	Saccharolytic
Adlercreutzia	64–67	Coccobacilli	−	+	None	Asaccharolytic
Alloscardovia	48	Short, irregularly shaped	+	+	ND	Saccharolytic
Atopobium	35–46	Short, elliptical; singly or in pairs or short chains	−/+	+	L	Saccharolytic
Bifidobacterium	57–64	Variable	−/+	+	A, L	Aciduric
Collinsella	60–61	Short; in chains	−	+	A, F, L	Saccharolytic, H_2 production
Cryptobacterium	50–51	Short	−	(+)	None	Asaccharolytic
Eggerthella	62	Coccobacilli or short rods; in pairs or short chains	−	+	(A, L, S)	Asaccharolytic
Gordonibacter	66	Coccobacilli, motile	−	+	ND	Asaccharolytic
Mobiluncus	49–52	Curved with tapered ends; singly or in pairs; motile	−	v	S, L, A	Saccharolytic
Olsenella	63–64	Short, elliptical; singly/in pairs or short chains	−	+	L, A	Saccharolytic
Paraeggerthella	61	Coccobacilli, in chains	−	+	ND	Asaccharolytic
Parascardovia	54–56	Small, slender, variable	−	+	A, L	Saccharolytic
Propionibacterium	59–67	Variable	−/+	+	P	Saccharolytic
Propioniferax	59–63	Variable, in clusters	+	+	P	Saccharolytic
Propionimicrobium	53–54	Variable; often diphtheroid or club-shaped	−	+	P, A, S	Saccharolytic
Scardovia	44–46	Small, coccoid, variable	−	+	A, L	Saccharolytic
Slackia	60–64	Cocci, coccobacilli, or short rods; singly or in clumps	−	(+)	(A)	Asaccharolytic
Varibaculum	52	Short, straight or curved, diphtheroid	−/+	+	L, S	Saccharolytic
Firmicutes						
Anaerofustis	70	Thin rods	−	+	A, B	Saccharolytic
Anaerostipes	46	Thin rods; in short chains	−	(+)	A, B, L	Saccharolytic
Anaerotruncus	54	Thin rods	−	+	A, B	Saccharolytic
Bulleidia	38	Short, straight or slightly curved; singly or in pairs	−	+	A, L	Saccharolytic
"*Catabacter*"	40	Coccobacilli or short rods, motile	−	+	ND	Saccharolytic
Catenibacterium	36–38	Short; in long tangled chains	−	+	A, B, L	Saccharolytic
Dorea	40–46	Short or long; in pairs or chains	−	+	A, F	Saccharolytic, H_2 production
Eubacterium	30–57	Variable	−	v	B, A, L (F)	Saccharolytic
Faecalibacterium	47–57	Pleomorphic rods	−	−	B, F, L	Saccharolytic
Filifactor	34	Short, regular	−	−	B	Asaccharolytic
Flavonifractor	58–62	Straight or slightly curved rods	−	(+)	A, B	Asaccharolytic
Holdemania	38	Short; in pairs or short chains	−	(+)	A, L	Saccharolytic
Lactobacillus	35–53	Short or long, slender; in chains	−/+	+	L	Aciduric
Marvinbryantia	50	Short; in pairs or short chains	−	+	A (S, L)	Formate required
Mogibacterium	41–50	Short; singly or in clumps	−	(+)	PAA	Asaccharolytic
Oribacterium	42	Elongated, ovoid; singly or in pairs; highly motile	−	−	A, L	Saccharolytic
Pseudoramibacter	61	Pleomorphic; in pairs	−	+	A, B, C, F	Saccharolytic
Roseburia	29–42	Thin, pleomorphic rods	−	v	B, L	Saccharolytic, H_2 production
Shuttleworthia	50–51	Short or slightly curved; singly or in pairs or short chains	−	+	B, A (L)	Saccharolytic
Solobacterium	37–39	Short, straight or slightly curved; singly or in pairs	−	+	A, L	Saccharolytic
Turicibacter	37	Irregular, long; in long chains	−	+	L	Saccharolytic

[a] +/− or −/+, variable aerotolerance within the genus; −, the genus contains only strictly anaerobic species.
[b] +, positive; −, negative; v, variable; (+), decolorization in old culture.
[c] A, acetic acid; B, butyric acid; C, caproic acid; F, formic acid; L, lactic acid; P, propionic acid; S, succinic acid; PAA, phenylacetic acid; parentheses, strain variation; ND, not determined.

and lactic acids with small amounts of acetic or formic acids, or acetic and lactic (acetic > lactic) acids, with or without formic acid, as the sole major acid products (125). It has been proposed that *Eubacterium* sensu stricto should be restricted to *E. limosum*, *E. callanderi*, and *E. barkeri* (194). Using this definition, the family *Eubacteriaceae* then includes the genera *Eubacterium* sensu stricto, *Anaerofustis* (with one species, *A. stercorihominis*, isolated from human feces) (56), and *Pseudoramibacter alactolyticus*, a saccharolytic species found in the oral cavity of humans (194). The remaining *Eubacterium* species would therefore require reclassification. Clinically important *Eubacterium* species are widely distributed among the *Firmicutes*. *E. biforme*, *E. cylindroides*, and *E. dolichum* fall within the family *Erysipelotrichaceae* mentioned above, together with the saccharolytic species, *Bulleidia extructa*, isolated from the human mouth (43), and *Holdemania filiformis* (195) and *Solobacterium moorei* (100), isolated from human feces. *Turicibacter sanguinis*, isolated from a blood culture (11), also belongs to this family (117).

Eubacterium brachy, *E. infirmum*, *E. minutum*, *E. nodatum*, *E. saphenum*, and *E. sulci* (formerly *Fusobacterium sulci*), together with *Mogibacterium*, a genus of five species which are difficult to differentiate by phenotypic tests (131, 132), are a group of asaccharolytic taxa isolated from the human mouth. On the basis of 16S rRNA phylogeny and their phenotypic characteristics, novel genera should be created for the majority of these species, with the exception of the pairs of species *E. minutum* and *E. nodatum* and *E. sulci* and *E. infirmum*, which are closely related. Many *Eubacterium* species are closely related to clostridia. Spore formation has long been the primary criterion for assignation of gram-positive anaerobic rods to *Clostridium*, but phylogenetic analysis indicates that the taxonomic importance of this characteristic may have been overemphasized. Numerous phylogenetic clusters contain both sporing and nonsporing representatives. *Eubacterium budayi*, *E. moniliforme*, and *E. nitritogenes* are found in clostridial cluster I described by Collins et al. (36), while *E. siraeum* belongs to a group that includes *Clostridium leptum* and *Anaerotruncus colihominis* (114). *E. tenue* and *E. yurii* belong to cluster XI. *E. tenue* is related to *Clostridium ghonii* and *Clostridium sordellii*; further work is required to determine whether these species constitute a novel genus. Strains of *Eubacterium plautii* and *Clostridium orbiscindens* have been shown to belong to the same taxon and renamed *Flavonifractor plautii* (26). Spore formation is variable among strains of the species; the type and other strains do not produce spores but have sporulation-specific genes. *E. yurii* is related to the genus *Filifactor*, which includes *Filifactor alocis* (formerly *Fusobacterium alocis*) isolated from oral infections in humans (95). *E. contortum*, *E. eligens*, *E. hadrum*, *E. hallii*, *E. ramulus*, *E. rectale*, *E. saburreum*, and *E. ventriosum* belong to the family *Lachnospiraceae*. *E. rectale* and *E. ramulus* are related to *Roseburia intestinalis* (45). This family also includes the recently described formate-requiring species *Marvinbryantia* (formerly *Bryantella*) *formatexigens* (45, 197, 198), isolated from human feces without any disease association so far, and *Oribacterium sinus* (25), a highly motile species isolated from pus of a human sinus. *E. eligens* and *Lachnospira pectinoschiza* are close phylogenetic neighbors and are both motile rods whose growth in broth culture is stimulated by the presence of fermentable carbohydrate. *E. eligens* should therefore be transferred to the genus *Lachnospira*. *Anaerostipes caccae* (163) forms a loose group with *E. hallii*

and *Coprococcus eutactus*, all common species in human feces. "*Catabacter hongkongensis*" is a deep-branching member of the order *Clostridiales*, isolated from blood cultures (109), but as yet not validly published.

EPIDEMIOLOGY AND TRANSMISSION

The majority of the organisms described in this chapter are part of the commensal microbiota associated with the mucocutaneous surfaces of the human and animal digestive tract, being found in the mouth, small and large intestines, urogenital tract, and skin (2, 8, 46, 140, 204). Microbial colonization of an individual occurs in a successive manner during the first weeks and months of life. *Actinomyces* species are among the initial colonizers of the mouth (158), whereas bifidobacteria and lactobacilli play an important role in the development of the healthy gut and its associated immune defenses (20, 164). Where members of this group cause infections, the host itself is the most likely source, although the commensal microbiota of other humans can be responsible, for example, in the case of infections resulting from human bites or clenched fist injuries from striking the face and mouth (17).

CLINICAL SIGNIFICANCE

Non-spore-forming anaerobic gram-positive rods seldom cause infections alone but are typically found in polymicrobial infections associated with mucosal surfaces (Table 2). Many anaerobes involved in infections of the head and neck originate from the oral cavity, and most vaginal and bladder pathogens are of fecal origin. In intra-abdominal infections due to organ perforation, the predominant recoveries reflect the microbiota at the site of the leakage (193). For surgical patients, anaerobes are a significant cause of morbidity and mortality (48). Anaerobic bacteria can occasionally spread to adjacent tissues and even the bloodstream, with serious consequences. For anaerobic bacteremias, the gastrointestinal tract is the most common source, followed by abscesses, gynecologic infections, and wound infections (155). The incidence and range of anaerobic gram-positive bacilli found in blood cultures may be underestimated because many of them are slow growing and have fastidious nutritional requirements. Anaerobic blood culture methods tend to be targeted at *Clostridium* species and *Bacteroides fragilis*, which grow readily and rapidly in commonly used broth media.

Actinomyces and Related Bacteria

Actinomyces and related bacteria are associated with a wide range of infections, normally as part of a polymicrobial consortium (Table 2) (32). Actinomycosis is a chronic, granulomatous infection affecting the cervicofacial, thoracic, and abdominopelvic regions and is caused primarily by *Actinomyces* species, particularly *A. israelii*, *A. gerencseriae*, and *A. graevenitzii*, and *Propionibacterium propionicum* (15, 74). Cervicofacial lesions normally arise as a consequence of untreated dental caries or are associated with dental extractions or trauma. These allow the causative organisms, which are part of the oral commensal biota, to enter the tissues. Although actinomyces are regarded as the primary cause and form the characteristic aggregates of branching bacilli seen macroscopically as sulfur granules, there are always multiple species present, with *Aggregatibacter actinomycetemcomitans* the most typical, together with a variety of oral organisms, including viridans group

TABLE 2 Genera of non-spore-forming anaerobic gram-positive rods detected in human infections

Site or disease association	Genera isolated
Brain and/or central nervous system	*Actinomyces, Eubacterium, Propionibacterium, Pseudoramibacter, Varibaculum*
Eye infections	*Actinomyces, Propionibacterium, Varibaculum*
Mouth	
Abscesses	*Actinomyces, Atopobium, Eubacterium, Filifactor, Mogibacterium, Olsenella, Pseudoramibacter, Slackia, Varibaculum*
Dental caries	*Actinomyces, Bifidobacterium, Lactobacillus, Olsenella, Parascardovia, Propionibacterium, Scardovia*
Endodontic infection	*Actinomyces, Atopobium, Bifidobacterium, Eubacterium, Filifactor, Mogibacterium, Lactobacillus, Olsenella, Propionibacterium, Pseudoramibacter, Slackia*
Periodontal diseases	*Cryptobacterium, Eubacterium, Filifactor, Mogibacterium, Olsenella, Pseudoramibacter, Slackia*
Respiratory tract infections	*Actinomyces, Eubacterium, Lactobacillus, Oribacterium, Propionibacterium*
Abdomen, intestine	
Abscesses	*Actinomyces, Eggerthella, Eubacterium, Lactobacillus*
Appendicitis	*Actinomyces, Eggerthella*
Cholecystitis	*Actinomyces, Lactobacillus*
Peritonitis	*Eggerthella, Lactobacillus*
Genital tract	
Abscesses	*Actinomyces, Atopobium, Eubacterium*
Bacterial vaginosis	*Atopobium, Mobiluncus*
Intrauterine device infections	*Actinomyces, Eubacterium, Varibaculum*
Pelvic inflammatory disease	*Actinomyces, Atopobium, Eubacterium, Lactobacillus*
Preterm labor/delivery	*Mobiluncus*
Urinary tract infections	*Actinobaculum, Actinomyces, Alloscardovia*
Skin and/or soft tissue	
Abscesses	*Actinobaculum, Actinomyces*
Infected atheroma	*Actinomyces*
Acne vulgaris	*Propionibacterium*
Cellulitis	*Actinomyces, Pseudoramibacter*
Necrotizing soft tissue infections	*Actinomyces, Eubacterium, Mogibacterium*
Lymphadenitis	*Propionibacterium, Propionimicrobium*
Bone and joint infections	*Actinobaculum, Actinomyces, Propionibacterium*
Wounds	
Bite wound infections (animal)	*Filifactor, Propionibacterium*
Bite wound infections (human)	*Actinomyces, Collinsella, Eggerthella, Eubacterium, Mogibacterium, Lactobacillus, Propionibacterium*
Postoperative wound infections	*Bifidobacterium, Propionibacterium, Pseudoramibacter*
Diabetic foot infections	*Actinomyces, Propionibacterium*
Cardiovascular sites	
Bacteremia	*Actinobaculum, Actinomyces, Alloscardovia, Atopobium, "Catabacter," Eggerthella, Eubacterium, Lactobacillus, Olsenella, Paraeggerthella, Propionibacterium*
Endocarditis	*Actinomyces, Lactobacillus, Propionibacterium*
Foreign body infections	*Actinomyces, Mogibacterium, Propionibacterium*

streptococci, anaerobic cocci, and gram-negative anaerobic bacilli (143). Thoracic actinomycosis most commonly affects the lungs following aspiration of oral bacteria in saliva, while the majority of pelvic infections are found in women using intrauterine contraceptive devices (177) and abdominal infection normally arises following perforation of the bowel as a result of disease or surgery (192).

Actinomyces make up a significant proportion of the microbiota in dental plaque in healthy individuals but are also associated with a wide range of dental and oral infections, including dental caries, endodontic infections, odontogenic abscesses, and dental implant-associated infections (7, 13, 35, 77, 78, 128, 157). Recently, there has been increasing evidence implicating *Actinomyces* species in infected osteoradionecrosis lesions, based on detection of the organisms within lesions and histological evidence of sulfur granule formation (39, 82). In a study in which anaerobic culture methods were used for sputum of adult cystic fibrosis patients, *Actinomyces* species were frequently isolated (182).

The most frequently isolated *Actinomyces* species from clinical infections are *A. turicensis*, *A. radingae*, and *A. neuii* and are found in a range of soft tissue infections including peri-anal, groin, axillary, breast, and peri-aural abscesses (74). A number of species, especially *A. israelii* and *A. turicensis* but also *A. cardiffensis*, *A. gerencseriae*, *A. naeslundii*, *A. odontolyticus*, *A. urogenitalis*, and a novel, closely related genus and species, *Varibaculum cambriense*, have been isolated from intrauterine device-associated infections in the female genital tract (9, 50, 63, 75, 80). In addition, *A. naeslundii* and *A. israelii* have been isolated from infectious hip prostheses (173, 201). *A. turicensis* and the *Actinobaculum* species *A. massiliense*, *A. schaalii*, and *A. urinale* are particularly associated with genital and urinary tract infections in both females and males (71, 76, 151). Pericarditis cases caused by *A. israelii* and *A. meyeri* have been reported (17). Oral *Actinomyces* species can be detected in the bloodstream following dental procedures (172), while *A. funkei*, *A. massiliensis*, *A. naeslundii*, *A. odontolyticus*, *A. turicensis*, and *Actinobaculum schaalii* and *Actinobaculum urinale* have been demonstrated to cause infections of the blood, particularly in individuals with predisposing conditions (38, 54, 113, 138, 145, 146).

Propionibacterium

Propionibacteria can be found in various systemic or disseminated opportunistic infections (Table 2), such as endocarditis, central nervous system infections, osteomyelitis, osteitis, and arthritis (18, 51, 94), and in about 20% of infected dog and cat bite wounds (179). Because *P. acnes* is a common skin commensal, its isolation from blood is often discounted as contamination of the blood during collection or as clinically insignificant (110, 155). However, *P. acnes* has been shown to be a significant cause of endocarditis, and one third of those cases are complicated by intracardiac abscess formation (171). The pathogenic potential of *P. acnes* should not be underestimated when there are predisposing factors present, such as a foreign body, surgery or trauma, diabetes, or immunosuppression (4, 72, 94, 134, 184, 187). Prosthetic joints are particularly susceptible to *P. acnes* infection (115, 141), and biofilm formation appears to be a specific virulence factor associated with invasive strains (88). *P. acnes* has also been isolated as part of the mixed bacterial community found in the sputum of adult cystic fibrosis patients (182). *P. propionicum* is part of the normal oral microbiota and causes oral and eye infections (14, 27, 167) as well as actinomycosis, in which it displays a spectrum of pathogenicity similar to those of *A. israelii* and *A. gerencseriae* (15). The recently described *P. acidifaciens* is particularly associated with dental caries (44).

Lactobacillus

Despite the reputation of lactobacilli as beneficial organisms, they can be involved in serious infections (Table 2), especially in immunocompromised individuals (16, 19, 24, 53, 133, 154). The *Lactobacillus* species most frequently isolated from various human infections are *L. rhamnosus*, *L. casei*, *L. fermentum*, *L. gasseri*, *L. plantarum*, *L. acidophilus*, and *L. ultunensis* (23, 24, 154). Lactobacilli are particularly associated with advanced dental caries (23, 28, 128), where they are considered a secondary colonizer because of their preference for low-pH habitats, but probably play a role in exacerbating existing lesions (5). The clinical infections most commonly caused by lactobacilli are bacteremia and endocarditis, with an associated relatively high mortality rate (24), with the mouth the primary route of entry to the bloodstream, either as a result of normal chewing and brushing or following dental procedures (24). Detection of lactobacilli, alone or with other microorganisms, in blood cultures of patients with underlying diseases may be clinically significant. *L. rhamnosus* was the most frequent species detected in *Lactobacillus* bacteremia (24, 53, 110, 154). Concern has been expressed that probiotic strains consumed in foodstuffs may cause disease in some individuals. Although such reports are rare (175), there have been reports of sepsis and endocarditis attributed to probiotic *Lactobacillus* strains (106, 203). In some cases, these have been attributed to inappropriate dosages and routes of administration, and it should be remembered that organisms used as probiotics are defined at the strain level and that, although infections may be caused by other strains within the same species, this does not imply that probiotic strains are unsafe. Vancomycin-resistant lactobacilli have been implicated in dialysis-related peritonitis after extended use of glycopeptides (102, 133). In contrast to other *Lactobacillus* species, *L. iners* has been associated with an intermediate state of bacterial vaginosis (190).

Eubacterium and Related Bacteria

The genus *Eubacterium* remains poorly defined, but species belonging to this genus and its relatives in the phylum *Firmicutes* are commonly isolated from oral infections (Table 2), particularly when nutrient-rich media and extended incubation times are used. For example, careful isolation of tiny-colony-forming anaerobes from periodontal pockets in adult patients with advanced periodontitis showed that "*Eubacterium*" species (mainly asaccharolytic) dominated (185), suggesting a role in the etiology of chronic periodontitis. When molecular identification methods were applied to a collection of *Eubacterium*-like strains from oral infections, *Mogibacterium timidum* was one of the most frequently detected species (42). *Mogibacterium vescum*, *Bulleidia extructa*, *Filifactor alocis*, and *Pseudoramibacter alactolyticus* were also found among the isolates from severe (some of them requiring treatment in intensive care units) odontogenic infections. Less frequently isolated were *E. sulci*, *E. saburreum*, and *E. yurii* (42). Many species found in odontogenic infections are also common in endodontic infections (59, 83, 129, 166, 168). *F. alocis*, *E. nodatum*, *E. saphenum*, and *M. timidum* have been associated with periodontal diseases (10, 40, 104, 105, 139), and "*Eubacterium*" species in general with failing dental implants (176). Due to their presence in the oral cavity, various *Eubacterium* and related species are among the anaerobic findings in human bite wound infections (178). *Filifactor villosus*, a species of animal origin, has been isolated from infected cat bite wounds in humans (179). *E. nodatum* has been found in infections of the female genital tract (86). *E. tenue* and *E. callanderi*, an environmental anaerobe, have been detected in clinically significant bacteremia (110, 180).

Eggerthella and Related Bacteria

Species of the genera *Eggerthella* and *Paraeggerthella* are recovered from a wide range of human infections (Table 2). *E. lenta* (formerly *Eubacterium lentum*) is a well-recognized pathogen particularly of intra- and peri-abdominal sites (16, 19, 111, 144). *E. lenta*, *E. sinensis*, and *P. hongkongensis* have been found in blood in association with clinically significant infections of relatively high mortality (110, 111). *Cryptobacterium curtum* and *Slackia exigua* have been associated with chronic periodontitis (10, 104), and the latter has also been associated with endodontic infections (83). An, as yet unnamed, *Eggerthella*-like taxon is associated with bacterial vaginosis (61).

Atopobium

Several species of the genus *Atopobium* are isolated from various infections (Table 2). Although *A. vaginae* is a prominent member of the commensal microbiota of the healthy vagina (148, 202), it has been increasingly reported to be involved in infections of the genital tract, especially bacterial vaginosis (22, 55, 64, 124, 190). *A. minutum* has been isolated from various infections of the lower part of the body, and *A. parvulum* has been isolated from respiratory specimens (136). Although *A. parvulum* and *A. rimae* have been detected in the pockets formed as a result of periodontitis (136, 139), in a comprehensive study of the microbiota of the subgingival region, these species were found to be associated with oral health rather than disease (94). Among *Eubacterium*-like isolates from severe odontogenic infections, *A. rimae* was the most frequently isolated (42).

Olsenella

Olsenella species show disease associations similar to those observed for lactobacilli in the oral cavity and have been found in root caries (142), with *O. profusa* specifically detected in dental caries lesions (128), and *O. uli*, in particular, in endodontic infections (27, 129, 147, 165) and acute dental abscesses (165). Both species can also be found in subgingival sites of periodontitis patients (41, 136). In addition, *O. uli* has been reported as one of the causative organisms in clinically significant bacteremia (110).

Bifidobacterium and Related Bacteria

Culture-independent analyses have shown that although members of the phyla *Bacteroidetes* and *Firmicutes* dominate the gut microbiota numerically, bifidobacteria appear to be functionally of great importance to intestinal health (183). Because of this, they are generally considered to be non-pathogenic but nevertheless are isolated from infections of polymicrobial etiology (Table 2). Dental caries is the most common clinical entity in which *Bifidobacterium*, mainly *B. dentium*, and the related species *Parascardovia denticolens*, *Scardovia inopinata*, and the unnamed *Scardovia* species C1 may have a pathogenic role (1, 7, 28, 119, 120). *B. adolescentis*, *B. dentium*, *B. breve*, and *B. longum* are occasionally isolated from other infections, mainly in immunocompromised individuals (16, 18, 19, 118). Although *B. scardovii* has been isolated from human clinical samples, including blood, urine, and hip (91), its clinical relevance is not known. In addition, a novel species related to *Bifidobacterium*, *Alloscardovia omnicolens*, has been detected in infections at various body sites, including urine and the genitourinary tract, in particular, and the oral cavity, tonsils, lung and aortic abscesses, abdominal wounds, and blood (118).

Mobiluncus

Although the etiology of bacterial vaginosis, the most common infection in the female genital tract, remains unclear, the presence of vibrio-like *Mobiluncus* species in smears of vaginal fluid has been widely used as one of the indicators of bacterial vaginosis (135). Indeed, *Mobiluncus curtisii* is seldom present in the vaginas of healthy women but, instead, is highly associated with bacterial vaginosis and its treatment failure due to persistence of the organism (123, 161). The altered vaginal microbial ecology seen in bacterial vaginosis can be a risk for adverse pregnancy outcome when ascending to the upper genital tract (89). In addition to bacterial vaginosis, *M. curtisii* has been isolated occasionally from endometrial smears and pus specimens of the female genital tract (6) and from blood (70, 152).

COLLECTION, TRANSPORT, AND STORAGE OF SPECIMENS

Many of the organisms described in this chapter are part of the human commensal microbiota and cause disease as opportunistic pathogens. This makes specimen collection difficult because at most sites of infection, the local commensal microbiota is close by. Thus, appropriate and careful specimen collection is critical to avoid contamination of the specimen with the commensal microbiota. Anaerobic transport techniques are also essential for the successful recovery of clinically significant anaerobic bacteria (see chapter 16). Specimens suitable for the isolation of non-spore-forming, gram-positive anaerobic rods present as organisms of etiologic importance include aseptically collected peripheral blood, tissue biopsy specimens, aspirates (e.g., cerebrospinal

fluid, joint fluids, and pus), root canal exudates, and subgingival plaque. Mucosal or cutaneous swabs are not recommended for the reasons mentioned above. Instead of collecting periprosthetic tissue, sonication of the removed implant followed by sonicate fluid culture has proven to be useful for microbiologic diagnosis of prosthetic-joint infection (141, 181). A comprehensive description of different specimen collection and transport methods for anaerobic bacteriology can be found elsewhere (98).

DIRECT EXAMINATION

Direct examination is of unequivocal value in the confirmation of a diagnosis of actinomycosis. The macroscopic presence of "sulfur granules" in pus, which when crushed, Gram stained, and viewed under the microscope reveal a mass of gram-positive branching filaments, is characteristic of this disease. Similarly, in cervical smears of women with an intrauterine contraceptive device, the presence of branching gram-positive organisms suggests an infection with *Actinomyces* (58, 151). Gram stains of vaginal smears have been considered more useful than culture for laboratory confirmation of bacterial vaginosis, and the diagnostic criteria for this common infection have been based on the standardized Nugent scoring system (135). The system relies on Gram stain characteristics of vaginal smears, recognizing individual morphotypes or their combination. Although intercenter reliability for gram-positive cocci was poor, the study documented moderate agreement for large gram-positive rods (lactobacilli), small gram-variable and/ or gram-negative rods (*Gardnerella vaginalis* and *Bacteroides/Prevotella*), and good agreement for curved gram-variable rods (*Mobiluncus*) (135). A simplified assessment of Gram-stained smears, taking lactobacillary and mixed bacterial morphotypes into account, has been proposed (93). It has been noted that the image area observed with microscopes requires standardization, in particular, when interpreting the intermediate state of bacterial vaginosis (108).

In cases in which there is no typical microbiota associated with a particular infection, care should be taken in determining appropriate empiric antimicrobial treatment on the basis of the Gram stain. For example, branching/pleomorphic rods can be tentatively identified as facultatively anaerobic *Actinomyces* or strictly anaerobic *E. nodatum* (86), and the coccoid cells of *Actinomyces radicidentis* are atypical for the genus *Actinomyces* (35), while easily decolorizing species (e.g., *Eubacterium*-like species) can yield a false gram-negative reaction (42). The misinterpretation can lead to antimicrobial coverage targeted against facultative organisms instead of anaerobes and/or gram-negative bacteria.

ISOLATION PROCEDURES

Specimens should be processed without delay using appropriate culture media, including standard anaerobic blood agar enriched with hemin and vitamin K_1 and a variety of selective media based on the expected microbiota at the collection site, or in the case of bite wounds, on the oral microbiota of the attacker (human or animal). Fresh or prereduced culture media, including phenyl ethyl alcohol blood agar and/or colistin nalidixic acid blood agar, can be useful for enhanced recovery rates of gram-positive organisms (29). The growth of many asaccharolytic species on solid media is enhanced by the addition of 0.5% arginine (186). In general, members of the aciduric genera *Bifidobacterium* and *Lactobacillus* can be selectively cultured using agar media with an acidic pH, such as Rogosa or deMan Rogosa Sharpe agar. However, some nutritionally fastidious *Lactobacillus* strains fail to grow on these agar media. Lactobacilli isolated from dental caries were recovered equally well on nonselective blood-containing media and on Rogosa agar, and it was concluded that acidic-pH medium is not required for their detection (128). Notably, *L. iners*, one of the predominant lactobacilli in the vagina, can grow only on blood agar and not on typical solid media used for *Lactobacillus* (52).

Although some members of this group, particularly *Actinomyces* species, are facultative anaerobes and can grow well on aerobically incubated culture media, anaerobic incubation is recommended for optimal recovery. If anaerobic jars are used for incubation, anaerobic growth should not be exposed to oxygen by opening the jar before 48 h of incubation, in order to facilitate the detection of slow-growing, oxygen-sensitive organisms (29). The availability of an anaerobic chamber may enable examination of the culture whenever necessary. For reliable detection of slow-growing organisms, the incubation time should be sufficient; for instance, an extended incubation period may be needed for some clinically relevant *Eubacterium*-like species (42, 130, 131, 180, 185). In heart tissue specimens from endocarditis patients, grinding the tissue can improve the detection of anaerobic bacteria (72, 94). A lytic anaerobic medium can increase the recovery rate of anaerobes and facultative bacteria in automated blood culture systems (149).

IDENTIFICATION

Traditionally, the identification of bacterial isolates in clinical microbiology laboratories is performed by phenotypic tests. For organisms inert in most conventional biochemical tests or with unusual biochemical profiles, as is the case for many *Eubacterium* and related species, or in cases where fastidious organisms require specific nutrients or temperatures, identification strategies based on phenotypic characteristics can be challenging.

Presumptive Identification

The initial differentiation is based on aerotolerance (growth in air or in air plus 5% CO_2), colonial morphology, pigmentation, fluorescence under long-wave UV illumination (365 nm wavelength), and presence of hemolysis. The colonial morphology can provide clues regarding the organism involved; for instance, an easily recognizable "molar tooth" appearance is typical for *A. israelii* but, notably, also for *E. nodatum*, although its colonies are smaller (86). Other rapidly recognizable features are fluorescence and/or pigment production: *E. lenta* shows orange or red fluorescence under UV light (126), and pink/red pigmentation of colonies is typical for *A. odontolyticus*, but some other *Actinomyces* can also produce pigment, especially on rabbit laked blood agar, with *A. graevenitzii* appearing as nearly black, *A. radicidentis* as brown, and *A. urogenitalis* as reddish colonies (81, 159).

Gram stain morphology can contribute to a presumptive identification; it can show whether organisms are gram-positive anaerobic rods, which can be very short (e.g., *C. curtum* and *E. lenta*), long (e.g., many *Lactobacillus* spp.), pleomorphic (e.g., *Bifidobacterium*), branching (e.g., many *Actinomyces* spp.), or curved and motile (e.g., *Mobiluncus* spp.); sometimes a specific cell morphology can be seen, such as "flying birds" (e.g., *P. alactolyticus*). The morphology may vary when cells are grown on different culture media.

The two *Mobiluncus* species can be tentatively separated based on the length of the curved, motile cells: in contrast to the short, gram-variable cells of *M. curtisii*, *M. mulieris* reveals clearly longer cells, which often appear as gram negative (162). Although *Actinomyces* organisms have been traditionally described as branching rods, many new species within the genus are nonbranching, and some have very short or even coccoid cells (35, 188). Staining of cells can vary with different culture conditions. Certain gram-positive anaerobes, e.g., *F. alocis* and *M. mulieris*, routinely stain gram negative, whereas older cultures (>3 days) of *Actinobaculum* and some *Eubacterium* species and species of related genera are gram variable (112, 130, 132). Decolorization of gram-positive organisms may be due to exposure to oxygen or to damage from fixatives and reagents causing a breakdown of the physical integrity of the cell wall; therefore, anaerobic working conditions or, if not available, limited exposure time to oxygen between incubation and staining improves the reliability of the Gram stain for anaerobic bacteria (97). For rapid confirmation of the Gram reaction, a simple test based on dissolution of the gram-negative cell wall and cytoplasmic membrane with a solution of 3% potassium hydroxide ((73) can be used: when suspended in the solution, gram-negative cells display increased viscosity and stringing within 30 s, whereas the absence of stringing, i.e., a negative reaction, suggests that the isolate is gram positive. Routine screening of special-potency antibiotic susceptibility disk patterns is valuable in confirming the accuracy of the Gram stain reaction (98): gram-positive species are generally resistant to colistin (10 μg) and susceptible to vancomycin (5 μg) and often to kanamycin (1 mg). However, the intrinsic resistance of some *Lactobacillus* species/strains, e.g., *L. rhamnosus*, to glycopeptides should be considered (53, 102, 133), in addition to the intrinsic resistance of *Bifidobacterium* to aminoglycosides (127). *Holdemania filiformis* has been reported to be resistant to vancomycin (43).

Additional rapid tests for initial grouping of non-spore-forming gram-positive anaerobes include testing for production of catalase (H_2O_2 at a concentration of 15%) and indole, nitrate reduction, and motility (29). If presumptive identification to the genus level has been made correctly, this may give valuable information to clinicians in deciding the initial treatment. However, differentiating members of the "normal flora" of human skin and mucous membranes from pathogenic non-spore-forming gram-positive rods can be difficult. Identification of nonsporing gram-positive rods to the species level should be performed whenever they are present in pure cultures in clinical specimens or as the predominant organism from normally sterile sites; otherwise, the potential pathogenicity of these less-often suspected species may remain undetected.

Biochemical Testing

For a more advanced phenotypic classification of anaerobic organisms and distinguishing of individual species, sugar fermentation reactions, preferably using prereduced, anaerobically sterilized carbohydrates, and enzyme profiles with individual diagnostic tablets, fluorogenic substrate tests, or preformed enzyme kits must be determined. Insufficient growth or poor reproducibility of reactions can cause difficulties in interpretation of results obtained with biochemical tests; therefore, young cultures and heavy inoculum should be used (159). A well-designed selection of key tests provides a tentative identification of various isolates to the species level prior to confirming their identifications by more definitive methods. Table 3 presents some

TABLE 3 Biochemical characteristics of *Actinomyces* and related bacteria encountered in human infections[a]

Genus and species	Aerotolerance	Pigment[b]	Production of: Catalase	Production of: Urease	Nitrate reduction	Esculin hydrolysis	Production of[e]: α-Glu	Production of[e]: β-NAG	Production of[e]: β-Gal	CAMP test	Fermentation of[f]: Mal	Fermentation of[f]: Man	Fermentation of[f]: Raf	Fermentation of[f]: Suc	Fermentation of[f]: Tre
Actinobaculum															
A. massiliense	+[c]	−	−	−	−	−	+	−	−	−	+	−	+	ND	+
A. schaalii	+	−	−	−	−	−	+	−	−	weak	+	−	−	v	v
A. urinale	(+)[d]	−	−	+	−	−	−	−	−	−	v	−	−	v	−
Actinomyces															
A. cardiffensis	(+)	−	−	−	v	−	+	−	−	−	v	−	v	v	−
A. dentalis	−	−	−	−	−	+	+	−	+	−	+	−	+	+	+
A. europaeus	+	−	−	−	v	v	+	−	+	−	+	−	−	v	v
A. funkei	+	−	−	−	+	−	+	v	v	v	v	−	−	+	−
A. georgiae	+	−	−	−	v	+	+	−	+	−	+	−	v	+	+
A. gerencseriae	+	+	−	−	v	+	+	+	+	−	+	−	v	+	v
A. graevenitzii	+	−	−	−	v	−	v	−	+	−	+	v	−	ND	v
A. hongkongensis	−	−	−	−	−	−	+	−	−	−	ND	ND	+	ND	−
A. israelii	(+)	−	−	−	+	+	+	−	−	−	+	−	+	+	+
A. johnsonii	+	−	v	v	+	−	+	ND	+	ND	ND	ND	ND	ND	v
A. massiliensis	+	−	−	−	+	ND	+	+	+	ND	+	−	−	ND	+
A. meyeri	−	−	−	−	v	−	+	−	−	v	+	−	+	+	−
A. naeslundii	+	−	−	+	+	v	v	+	+	−	+	+	−	+	+
A. nasicola	(+)	−	−	−	−	−	+	−	+	−	−	−	−	−	−
A. neuii															
subsp. anitratus	+	−	+	−	−	−	v	−	+	+	+	+	v	+	
subsp. neuii	+	+	+	−	−	−	+	−	+	+	+	−	v	+	v
A. odontolyticus	+	+	−	−	+	v	+	−	v	+	+	−	−	+	+
A. oricola	+	−	v	−	+	+	+	ND	v	−	−	−	+	ND	+
A. oris	+	+	+	−	v	v	v	−	v	ND	ND	ND	ND	ND	+
A. radicidentis	+	−	+	−	v	+	+	+	−	−	+	+	+	+	+
A. radingae	+	+	−	v	v	+	+	+	v	v	+	−	v	v	v
A. turicensis	+	−	−	−	−	−	+	−	−	−	+	−	v	v	v
A. urogenitalis	+	+	+	v	+	+	v	+	+	−	+	v	−	+	+
A. viscosus	+	−	+	−	+	v	+	−	v	−	+	−	+	+	v
Varibaculum															
V. cambriense	(+)	−	−	−	+	−	+	−	v	−	+	v	−	+	−

[a] Biochemical data from references 62, 71, 75–79, 85, 146, 159, 188, and 199.
[b] *A. graevenitzii* colonies are nonpigmented on brucella agar but almost black on RLB, whereas other pigment-producing *Actinomyces* spp. appear as pinkish/brownish colonies on brucella agar and as darker colonies on RLB.
[c] +, positive; −, negative; v, variable; ND, no data.
[d] (+) better growth in anaerobic conditions.
[e] Abbreviations: α-Glu, α-glucosidase; β-NAG, β-N-acetyl-glucosaminidase; β-gal, β-galactosidase.
[f] Abbreviations: Mal, maltose; Man, mannitol; Raf, raffinose; Suc, sucrose; Tre, trehalose.

TABLE 4 Biochemical characteristics of propionibacteria encountered in human infections[a]

Genus and species	Aerotolerance	Catalase	Indole	Nitrate reduction	Esculin hydrolysis
Propionibacterium					
P. acnes	+	+	+	+	−
P. avidum	+	+	−	−	+
P. granulosum	+	+	−	−	−
P. propionicum	−	−	−	+	−
P. acidifaciens	−	−	−	−	−
Propioniferax					
P. innocua	+	+	−	v	−
Propionimicrobium					
P. lymphophilum	−	v	−	v	ND

[a]Biochemical data compiled from references 42 and 60. Symbols and abbreviations: +, positive; −, negative; v, variable; ND, no data.

biochemical characteristics of *Actinomyces* and related organisms. Since the description of many novel species, such as *A. dentalis*, *A. hongkongensis*, *A. massiliensis*, *A. nasicola*, *A. oricola*, *A. urinale*, and "*Actinobaculum massiliae*," is based on a single strain (71, 76–79, 146, 199), discrepancies in test reactions may appear. In addition, the clarification of the taxonomy of the *A. naeslundii/Actinomyces viscosus* group with the proposal of the new species *A. johnsonii* and *A. oris* (85), while taxonomically valuable and consistent with their ecology, has resulted in a group of species that cannot be differentiated by phenotypic tests alone. Housekeeping gene sequence analysis is required but may be beyond the scope of routine laboratories. Table 4 presents simple enzymatic reactions useful in distinguishing propionibacteria encountered in human infections, and Table 5 shows tests for *Atopobium* and *Olsenella* species. Although the cultivation and identification of *Eubacterium*-like species can be very laborious, not only because of their oxygen sensitivity and slow growth but also due to their nonreactivity in conventional biochemical testing, some simple reactions are helpful for grouping these organisms (Table 6).

In culture-based identification of anaerobic non-spore-forming gram-positive rods, the determination of major volatile fatty acid end products of glucose metabolism, as detected by gas chromatography, is useful for assigning isolates to genus level (Table 1). Typically, *Actinomyces* strains produce succinic and lactic acids as their major metabolic end products, but *A. dentalis* is reported not to produce succinic acid (75). The *Actinomyces*-like *Propionibacterium* species, *P. propionicum*, is easily separated from *Actinomyces*

based on its production of propionic acid (62). For *Lactobacillus* spp., defining characteristics are their ability to grow in acid media and ferment carbohydrates to produce lactic acid as the major end product with or without small amounts of acetate, whereas *Bifidobacterium* spp. produce acetic acid as a major product. A combination of phenotypic tests, specifically the determination of metabolic end products by gas chromatography together with sugar fermentation by prereduced, anaerobically sterilized carbohydrates and enzyme profiles generated by a commercial identification kit (API Rapid ID 32A; bioMérieux, Marcy-l'Etoile, France), have successfully been used to identify oral *Eubacterium*-like isolates to genus and species level (42); for example, the lack of enzyme activity and formation of caproic acid or phenylacetic acid distinguish *P. alactolyticus* or *Mogibacterium* spp., respectively, from other related taxa. However, as already mentioned, phenotypic criteria are particularly unreliable for identification of many *Actinomyces* species (81) and members of the *L. acidophilus* complex and related species (189). In addition, gas chromatographic analysis of cellular fatty acids (98) and examination of protein patterns by polyacrylamide gel electrophoresis have been used taxonomically to distinguish among strains within a species and among organisms within a genus or family.

Preformed enzyme and carbohydrate fermentation profiles can be obtained using commercially available identification test kits, such as the API (bioMérieux), RapID (Remel, Lenexa, KS), and BBL Crystal (Becton Dickinson Diagnostic Systems, Sparks, MD) systems, according to manufacturers' instructions. Although this approach is often

TABLE 5 Enzyme reactions useful in distinguishing species within the genera *Atopobium* and *Olsenella*[a]

Genus and species	Aerotolerance	Production of:		Nitrate reduction	Hydrolysis of:		Acid phosphatase	β-Gal
		Catalase	Indole		Esculin	Arginine		
Atopobium								
A. minutum	−	−	−	−	ND	+	−	−
A. parvulum	−	−	−	−	v	−	+	+
A. rimae	−	−	−	−	v	v	+	−
A. vaginae	(−)[b]	−	−	−	−	+	+	−
Olsenella								
O. profusa	−	−	−	−	+	−	ND	ND
O. uli	−	−	−	−	+	+	ND	ND

[a]Biochemical data compiled from references 35, 39, 40, 135, and 147. Symbols and abbreviations: +, positive; −, negative; v, variable; ND, no data; β-Gal, β-galactosidase.
[b]In the original description, *A. vaginae* is facultatively anaerobic.

TABLE 6 Biochemical characteristics of some human *Eubacterium*-like organisms[a]

Phylum and species	Glucose fermentation	Production of:		Nitrate reduction	Hydrolysis of:	
		Catalase	Indole		Esculin	Arginine
Actinobacteria						
Collinsella aerofaciens	+	−	−	−	v	v
Collinsella intestinalis	+	ND	ND	ND	ND	ND
Collinsella stercoris	+	ND	ND	ND	ND	ND
Cryptobacterium curtum	−	−	−	−	−	+
Eggerthella hongkongensis	−	+	−	−	ND	+
Eggerthella lenta	−	+	−	+	−	+
Eggerthella sinensis	−	+	−	−	ND	+
Slackia exigua	−	−	−	−	−	+
Firmicutes						
Bulleidia extructa	+	−	−	−	−	+
Catenibacterium mitsuokai	+	−	ND	−	−	ND
Eubacterium brachy	−	−	−	−	−	−
Eubacterium limosum	+	−	−	−	+	v
Eubacterium minutum	−	−	−	−	−	−
Eubacterium nodatum	−	−	−	−	−	+
Eubacterium rectale	+	−	−	−	+	−
Eubacterium saburreum	+	−	+	−	+	+
Eubacterium saphenum	−	−	−	−	−	−
Eubacterium sulci	−	−	−	−	−	−
Eubacterium tenue	Weak	−	+	−	−	ND
Eubacterium yurii	Weak	−	+	−	−	−
Filifactor alocis	−	−	−	−	−	+
Flavonifractor plautii	Weak	ND	−	−	−	ND
Holdemania filiformis	+	−	−	−	+	−
Mogibacterium spp.	−	−	−	−	−	−
Pseudoramibacter alactolyticus	+	−	−	−	−	−
Shuttleworthia satelles	+	−	+	−	+	−
Solobacterium moorei	+	−	−	−	+	+

[a]Biochemical data compiled from references 40, 84, 96–98, 110, 129, 130, 193, and 194. Symbols and abbreviations: +, positive reaction; −, negative reaction; v, variable reaction; ND, no data.

hindered by similarities in fermentation profiles of separate species within a genus, kits serve as a widely used adjunct to anaerobe diagnostics in most hospital laboratories (65), since they are easy to use and much faster than conventional anaerobic procedures. The main problem with these kits are their incomplete or inaccurate databases (12, 156). The databases of the API Coryne (bioMérieux) and RapID CB Plus (Remel) tests, designed for coryneform bacteria, currently include some aerotolerant *Actinomyces* and *Propionibacterium* species as well. However, the same test performed by different methodologies may give conflicting results; this is particularly true for the commercial identification kits in which the tests are "poised," to give a definitive positive or negative reaction to aid interpretation. This can have the effect of making the test insufficiently sensitive, giving false negatives compared to conventional tests, or oversensitive, giving rise to false positives (156, 159). Isolates of *A. vaginae* have been misidentified as *Gemella morbillorum* by the API Rapid ID 32A (bioMérieux) and RapID ANA II (Remel) test kits (55, 64). In contrast, a clinically relevant *Bifidobacterium* species, *B. scardovii*, was readily separated from other bifidobacteria by using the Rapid ID 32A kit (bioMérieux) (91). The carbohydrate fermentation test kit API 50 CH (bioMérieux), which is specifically designed for lactobacilli, can be valuable in identification to the genus level but fail at the species level (12). Despite the lack of reliability of species level identifications, commercial test kits can be useful for the detection of positive reactions and

identification of many organisms from clinical sources to the genus level. Clinical microbiologists should be aware of the possibility of erroneous identification and adjust the interpretation of their results accordingly, in conjunction with cellular and colonial morphology and other information available. Indeed, practical, discriminatory, and cost-effective methods are needed for identification of fastidious gram-positive bacteria.

Identification by DNA Sequence Analysis

As discussed above, the use of conventional and biochemical tests for the identification of this group carries a significant risk of misidentification. Far-more-precise identifications can be obtained by 16S rRNA gene sequence analysis (103). DNA can be rapidly and reliably purified from members of this group by using commercially available kits, such as GenElute (Sigma-Aldrich), and the 16S rRNA gene can be amplified using "universal" primers that amplify all members of the domain *Bacteria* (60, 107). Amplicons can be sequenced in-house or submitted to commercial sequencing facilities. The 5′ region of the gene is the most informative for identification purposes; the use of primer 519R for sequencing is recommended (107). Sequences are identified by comparison with those held in the DNA sequence databases, such as GenBank. BLAST interrogation (3) is useful, but care needs to be taken because many sequences in the databases are mislabeled and some pairs or even groups of species have virtually identical 16S rRNA gene sequences. Identification to genus level is ensured, but at species level, some investigation of the phylogenetic status of the genus should be made. This technique, while extremely powerful, should not be regarded as an infallible "black box" method. A major advantage is that methods do not need to be adapted for different groups of organisms; thus, there are no special considerations needed when analyzing gram-positive non-spore-forming anaerobes, except that the DNA extraction method needs to be suitable for lysing the rigid gram-positive cell wall.

A major impetus for the study of as yet uncultured bacteria has been the development of 16S rRNA/PCR amplification/cloning/sequencing methodology (196). The phylum *Firmicutes*, in particular, has been found to harbor a number of lineages without culturable representatives. For example, branches within the families *Eubacteriaceae* and *Lachnospiraceae* have been found in advanced carious lesions, endodontic infections, and subgingival plaque in periodontitis (28, 129, 139). Similarly, the distal esophagus, stomach, and colonic microbiotas include novel branches within the *Clostridiaceae*, *Erysipelotrichaceae*, and *Lachnospiraceae* (8, 140, 174). Culture-independent analysis of the microbiota in bacterial vaginosis identified a novel taxon related to *A. vaginae* (190), and novel taxa belonging to both the *Actinobacteria* and *Firmicutes* were found in a corneal ulcer (160).

SEROLOGIC TESTS

Serological tests are of little diagnostic value for this group of organisms, which are found almost exclusively in polymicrobial infections. Furthermore, infections are frequently opportunistic in nature, with the causative organism being a member of the commensal microbiota, rendering serological tests difficult to interpret.

ANTIMICROBIAL SUSCEPTIBILITIES

In the clinical setting, empirical information is used for the initial diagnosis of infection and choice of antimicrobial therapy, while awaiting culture and susceptibility test results. This is particularly important for this group of organisms because many of them are slow growing, and if they are isolated as part of a mixed infection, it may take some time to obtain pure cultures for testing.

Published data regarding antimicrobial susceptibilities of nonsporing gram-positive anaerobes can be difficult to interpret. Changes in bacterial taxonomy, e.g., among the species of the former *Eubacterium* genus, and more precise classification of tested isolates may result in antimicrobial resistance patterns different from those given in previously published surveys (169). In general, penicillin and other β-lactams are active against gram-positive bacteria together with parenteral carbapenems, such as doripenem, ertapenem, imipenem, and meropenem (21, 49, 66, 68, 87, 116, 127, 169, 170). Metronidazole has been considered a drug of choice for treatment of anaerobic infections; however, the facultative anaerobes among the genera *Propionibacterium*, *Actinobaculum*, *Actinomyces*, *Bifidobacterium*, and *Lactobacillus* are intrinsically resistant, and resistant strains can also be found among the strictly anaerobic genera *Atopobium*, *Eggerthella*, *Eubacterium*, and *Mobiluncus* (6, 30, 55, 87, 116). Failures or relapses are common in the treatment of bacterial vaginosis, but whether metronidazole-resistant *A. vaginae* or *M. curtisii* (6, 55, 64) play a role is not known. Occasional strains among various genera of non-spore-forming gram-positive anaerobic rods show resistance to clindamycin

(21, 30, 47, 69, 84, 137, 169). Although vancomycin and teicoplanin are considered active against most gram-positive bacteria, species-related resistance to glycopeptides is frequent among species of the genus *Lactobacillus*. Less than one-quarter of the isolates from 80 cases of *Lactobacillus* infections were reported as susceptible to vancomycin (24). Notably, the vancomycin-resistant *L. rhamnosus* is the most common *Lactobacillus* species in clinical specimens (53, 154). In contrast to vancomycin and teicoplanin, ramoplanin, a novel glycolipodepsipeptide, showed good activity against lactobacilli (30, 57). A novel glycopeptide, telavancin, has proved to be more active than vancomycin against lactobacilli, except for *L. casei*, and demonstrated very good activity against the tested strains of *Propionibacterium*, *Actinomyces*, *Eggerthella*, and *Eubacterium* (68). Tigecycline, a glycylcycline antimicrobial agent, has been shown to be active against lactobacilli, including *L. casei*, and *Actinomyces* species (67). Oxazolidinones represent a new class of synthetic antimicrobial agents, having relatively good in vitro activities against gram-positive cocci but also against anaerobes, and ranbezolid may have lower MICs than linezolid (21, 49). Also telithromycin, a novel ketolide, and streptogramin antimicrobial agents, such as pristinamycin and quinupristin-dalfopristin, have considerable activities against non-spore-forming gram-positive rods (21, 69, 127). Fluoroquinolones have a broad spectrum of antibacterial activity and good absorption from the gastrointestinal tract. Novel quinolones, such as garenoxacin, gatifloxacin (topical application), and moxifloxacin, exhibit better antianaerobic activity than the older quinolone compounds levofloxacin and ciprofloxacin (21, 47, 84, 116), suggesting their potential in treating mixed organism infections.

The testing of anaerobic isolates for susceptibility to antimicrobials by clinical laboratories remains problematic (see chapter 72). The Clinical and Laboratory Standards Institute defines the agar dilution method as the gold standard but recommends it only for reference laboratories (34). Specific guidance is available for lactobacilli (33). Broth microdilution is recommended for clinical laboratories but is currently limited to fragilis group *Bacteroides*. There are a number of reasons for the current lack of susceptibility testing for this group of organisms. Firstly, anaerobic gram-positive bacilli are frequently isolated from polymicrobial infections from which 10 or more species may be cultivated. The relevance of individual susceptibility testing and its interpretation in this scenario are unclear. Secondly, as has been described in this chapter, there are a large number of species that may be found in clinical material, but each laboratory may encounter them relatively rarely. There are therefore insufficient reference data on the susceptibility profile of each species, but even if appropriate data were available, quality control procedures and strains would be required for each species. A recent survey (65) revealed that the method most commonly used for testing anaerobes was the Etest, which has been found to be useful and reliable (31, 150). Etests should be performed on *Brucella* blood agar and are optimally read after 48 h, to allow sufficient bacterial growth. Some slow-growing species may require longer incubation.

INTERPRETATION AND REPORTING OF RESULTS

Members of this group are commonly found as part of the normal microbiota at mucosal surfaces. The primary considerations then in interpreting laboratory data are the site from which the sample was collected, the method used for collection, and whether the sample was likely to have been contaminated by the commensal biota. Culture plates from samples from mucosal and cutaneous sites should be interpreted with reference to the normal commensal biota expected for that site, and any recent or current antimicrobial therapy. It is important that incubation times are sufficiently long to allow growth of the slow-growing members of this group. Premature reporting of only the fastest growing species can be misleading since growth rates in vivo and in vitro may be very different. Incubation should be continued for at least 7 days before the final report is issued. The commensal microbiota is normally diverse. The finding of a culture from a specimen dominated by a restricted number of organisms is normally suggestive of infection, particularly if suspected clinically, although recent administration of broad-spectrum antimicrobials may also reduce the diversity of the commensal microbiota.

All isolations of members of this group from normally sterile sites, including blood, spinal fluid, internal organs, and body cavities, are significant, and the organism should be identified. Members of the group are generally of low-grade pathogenicity and do not produce classical virulence factors, such as protein toxins. All isolates should be regarded as equally important and reported with sensitivities to antimicrobials appropriate to the clinical diagnosis and the site of the infection. Obtaining pure cultures of all of the organisms present in a polymicrobial infection can be difficult and time consuming but should be attempted. Collation of data regarding the identity and antimicrobial susceptibility profiles of isolates causing confirmed infections will be invaluable in formulating recommendations for empirical treatment, which are lacking at present, and in allowing associations between particular species and diseases to be made.

One specific disease caused by gram-positive nonsporing anaerobes is actinomycosis, typically affecting the cervicofacial region but which can occur at a range of body sites. Pus collected from suspected lesions should be examined macro- and microscopically for the presence of sulfur granules and, if present, should be reported as confirmation of a clinical history consistent with actinomycosis. Culture of *Actinomyces* or related genera alone from a site where the specimen is likely to have been contaminated with the commensal microbiota should be interpreted with caution. This is particularly the case for the head and neck regions since *Actinomyces* is one of the predominant genera among the normal oral microbiota.

REFERENCES

1. **Aas, J. A., A. L. Griffen, S. R. Dardis, A. M. Lee, I. Olsen, F. E. Dewhirst, E. J. Leys, and B. J. Paster.** 2008. Bacteria of dental caries in primary and permanent teeth in children and young adults. *J. Clin. Microbiol.* **46**:1407–1417.
2. **Aas, J. A., B. J. Paster, L. N. Stokes, I. Olsen, and F. E. Dewhirst.** 2005. Defining the normal bacterial flora of the oral cavity. *J. Clin. Microbiol.* **43**:5721–5732.
3. **Altschul, S. F., W. Gish, W. Miller, E. W. Myers, and D. J. Lipman.** 1990. Basic local alignment search tool. *J. Mol. Biol.* **215**:403–410.
4. **Arnell, K., K. Cesarini, A. Lagerqvist-Widh, T. Wester, and J. Sjolin.** 2008. Cerebrospinal fluid shunt infections in children over a 13-year period: anaerobic cultures and comparison of clinical signs of infection with *Propionibacterium acnes* and with other bacteria. *J. Neurosurg. Pediatr.* **1**:366–372.
5. **Badet, C., and N. B. Thebaud.** 2008. Ecology of lactobacilli in the oral cavity: a review of literature. *Open Microbiol. J.* **2**:38–48.
6. **Bahar, H., M. M. Torun, F. Ocer, and B. Kocazeybek.** 2005. *Mobiluncus* species in gynaecological and obstetric infections: antimicrobial resistance and prevalence in a Turkish population. *Int. J. Antimicrob. Agents* **25**:268–271.
7. **Becker, M. R., B. J. Paster, E. J. Leys, M. L. Moeschberger, S. G. Kenyon, J. L. Galvin, S. K. Boches, F. E. Dewhirst, and A. L. Griffen.** 2002. Molecular analysis of bacterial species associated with childhood caries. *J. Clin. Microbiol.* **40**:1001–1009.
8. **Bik, E. M., P. B. Eckburg, S. R. Gill, K. E. Nelson, E. A. Purdom, F. Francois, G. Perez-Perez, M. J. Blaser, and D. A. Relman.** 2006. Molecular analysis of the bacterial microbiota in the human stomach. *Proc. Natl. Acad. Sci. USA* **103**:732–737.
9. **Biyani, D. K., H. Denley, J. Hill, and A. J. Watson.** 2007. IUCD induced abdomino-pelvic actinomycosis presenting as acute large bowel obstruction. *J. Obstet. Gynaecol.* **27**:870–871.
10. **Booth, V., J. Downes, J. Van den Berg, and W. G. Wade.** 2004. Gram-positive anaerobic bacilli in human periodontal disease. *J. Periodontal Res.* **39**:213–220.
11. **Bosshard, P. P., R. Zbinden, and M. Altwegg.** 2002. *Turicibacter sanguinis* gen. nov., sp. nov., a novel anaerobic, gram-positive bacterium. *Int. J. Syst. Evol. Microbiol.* **52**:1263–1266.
12. **Boyd, M. A., M. A. D. Antonio, and S. L. Hillier.** 2005. Comparison of API 50 CH strips to whole-chromosomal DNA probes for identification of *Lactobacillus* species. *J. Clin. Microbiol.* **43**:5309–5311.
13. **Brailsford, S. R., R. B. Tregaskis, H. S. Leftwich, and D. Beighton.** 1999. The predominant *Actinomyces* spp. isolated from infected dentin of active root caries lesions. *J. Dent. Res.* **78**:1525–1534.
14. **Brazier, J. S., and V. Hall.** 1993. *Propionibacterium propionicum* and infections of the lacrimal apparatus. *Clin. Infect. Dis.* **17**:892–893.
15. **Brook, I.** 2008. Actinomycosis: diagnosis and management. *South. Med. J.* **101**:1019–1023.
16. **Brook, I.** 1996. Isolation of non-sporing anaerobic rods from infections in children. *J. Med. Microbiol.* **45**:21–26.
17. **Brook, I.** 2003. Microbiology and management of human and animal bite wound infections. *Prim. Care* **30**:25–39, v.
18. **Brook, I.** 2009. Pericarditis caused by anaerobic bacteria. *Int. J. Antimicrob. Agents* **33**:297–300.
19. **Brook, I., and E. H. Frazier.** 1993. Significant recovery of non-sporulating anaerobic rods from clinical specimens. *Clin. Infect. Dis.* **16**:476–480.
20. **Bruzzese, E., R. B. Canani, G. De Marco, and A. Guarino.** 2004. Microflora in inflammatory bowel diseases: a pediatric perspective. *J. Clin. Gastroenterol.* **38**:S91–S93.
21. **Bryskier, A.** 2001. Anti-anaerobic activity of antibacterial agents. *Expert Opin. Investig. Drugs* **10**:239–267.
22. **Burton, J. P., E. Devillard, P. A. Cadieux, J.-A. Hammond, and G. Reid.** 2004. Detection of *Atopobium vaginae* in postmenopausal women by cultivation-independent methods warrants further investigation. *J. Clin. Microbiol.* **42**:1829–1831.
23. **Byun, R., M. A. Nadkarni, K.-L. Chhour, F. E. Martin, N. A. Jacques, and N. Hunter.** 2004. Quantitative analysis of diverse *Lactobacillus* species present in advanced dental caries. *J. Clin. Microbiol.* **42**:3128–3136.
24. **Cannon, J. P., T. A. Lee, J. T. Bolanos, and L. H. Danziger.** 2005. Pathogenic relevance of *Lactobacillus*: a retrospective review of over 200 cases. *Eur. J. Clin. Microbiol. Infect. Dis.* **24**:31–40.
25. **Carlier, J.-P., G. K'ouas, I. Bonne, A. Lozniewski, and F. Mory.** 2004. *Oribacterium sinus* gen. nov., sp. nov., within the family 'Lachnospiraceae' (phylum Firmicutes). *Int. J. Syst. Evol. Microbiol.* **54**:1611–1615.
26. **Carlier, J. P., M. Bedora-Faure, G. K'Ouas, C. Alauzet, and F. Mory.** 2010. Proposal to unify *Clostridium orbiscindens* Winter et al. 1991 and *Eubacterium plautii* (Seguin 1928) Hofstad and Aasjord 1982 with description of *Flavonifractor plautii* gen. nov., comb. nov. and reassignment of *Bacteroides capillosus* to *Pseudoflavonifractor capillosus* gen. nov., comb. nov. *Int. J. Syst. Evol. Microbiol.* **60**:585–590.

27. Chavez de Paz, L. E., A. Molander, and G. Dahlen. 2004. Gram-positive rods prevailing in teeth with apical periodontitis undergoing root canal treatment. *Int. Endod. J.* **37:**579–587.

28. Chhour, K. L., M. A. Nadkarni, R. Byun, F. E. Martin, N. A. Jacques, and N. Hunter. 2005. Molecular analysis of microbial diversity in advanced caries. *J. Clin. Microbiol.* **43:**843–849.

29. Citron, D. M. 1999. Rapid identification of anaerobes in the clinical laboratory. *Anaerobe* **5:**109–113.

30. Citron, D. M., C. V. Merriam, K. L. Tyrrell, Y. A. Warren, H. Fernandez, and E. J. Goldstein. 2003. In vitro activities of ramoplanin, teicoplanin, vancomycin, linezolid, bacitracin, and four other antimicrobials against intestinal anaerobic bacteria. *Antimicrob. Agents Chemother.* **47:**2334–2338.

31. Citron, D. M., M. I. Ostovari, A. Karlsson, and E. J. Goldstein. 1991. Evaluation of the E test for susceptibility testing of anaerobic bacteria. *J. Clin. Microbiol.* **29:**2197–2203.

32. Clarridge, J. E., III, and Q. Zhang. 2002. Genotypic diversity of clinical *Actinomyces* species: phenotype, source, and disease correlation among genospecies. *J. Clin. Microbiol.* **40:**3442–3448.

33. Clinical and Laboratory Standards Institute. 2006. *Methods for Antimicrobial Dilution and Disk Susceptibility Testing of Infrequently Isolated or Fastidious Bacteria.* Document M45-A. Clinical and Laboratory Standards Institute, Wayne, PA.

34. Clinical and Laboratory Standards Institute. 2007. *Methods for Antimicrobial Susceptibility Testing of Anaerobic Bacteria. Approved Standard,* 7th ed. Clinical and Laboratory Standards Institute, Wayne, PA.

35. Collins, M. D., L. Hoyles, S. Kalfas, G. Sundquist, T. Monsen, N. Nikolaitchouk, and E. Falsen. 2000. Characterization of *Actinomyces* isolates from infected root canals of teeth: description of *Actinomyces radicidentis* sp. nov. *J. Clin. Microbiol.* **38:**3399–3403.

36. Collins, M. D., P. A. Lawson, A. Willems, J. J. Cordoba, J. Fernandez-Garayzabal, P. Garcia, J. Cai, H. Hippe, and J. A. Farrow. 1994. The phylogeny of the genus *Clostridium*: proposal of five new genera and eleven new species combinations. *Int. J. Syst. Bacteriol.* **44:**812–826.

37. Collins, M. D., and S. Wallbanks. 1992. Comparative sequence analyses of the 16S rRNA genes of *Lactobacillus minutus, Lactobacillus rimae* and *Streptococcus parvulus*: proposal for the creation of a new genus *Atopobium. FEMS Microbiol. Lett.* **74:**235–240.

38. Cone, L. A., M. M. Leung, and J. Hirschberg. 2003. *Actinomyces odontolyticus* bacteremia. *Emerg. Infect. Dis.* **9:**1629–1632.

39. Curi, M. M., L. L. Dib, L. P. Kowalski, G. Landman, and C. Mangini. 2000. Opportunistic actinomycosis in osteoradionecrosis of the jaws in patients affected by head and neck cancer: incidence and clinical significance. *Oral Oncol.* **36:**294–299.

40. de Lillo, A., F. P. Ashley, R. M. Palmer, M. A. Munson, L. Kyriacou, A. J. Weightman, and W. G. Wade. 2006. Novel subgingival bacterial phylotypes detected using multiple universal polymerase chain reaction primer sets. *Oral Microbiol. Immunol.* **21:**61–68.

41. Dewhirst, F. E., B. J. Paster, N. Tzellas, B. Coleman, J. Downes, D. A. Spratt, and W. G. Wade. 2001. Characterization of novel human oral isolates and cloned 16S rDNA sequences that fall in the family *Coriobacteriaceae*: description of *Olsenella* gen. nov., reclassification of *Lactobacillus uli* as *Olsenella uli* comb. nov. and description of *Olsenella profusa* sp. nov. *Int. J. Syst. Evol. Microbiol.* **51:**1797–1804.

42. Downes, J., M. A. Munson, D. A. Spratt, E. Kononen, E. Tarkka, H. Jousimies-Somer, and W. G. Wade. 2001. Characterisation of *Eubacterium*-like strains isolated from oral infections. *J. Med. Microbiol.* **50:**947–951.

43. Downes, J., B. Olsvik, S. J. Hiom, D. A. Spratt, S. L. Cheeseman, I. Olsen, A. J. Weightman, and W. G. Wade. 2000. *Bulleidia extructa* gen. nov., sp. nov., isolated from the oral cavity. *Int. J. Syst. Evol. Microbiol.* **50:**979–983.

44. Downes, J., and W. G. Wade. 2009. *Propionibacterium acidifaciens* sp. nov., isolated from the human mouth. *Int. J. Syst. Evol. Microbiol.* **59:**2778–2781.

45. Duncan, S. H., G. L. Hold, A. Barcenilla, C. S. Stewart, and H. J. Flint. 2002. *Roseburia intestinalis* sp. nov., a novel saccharolytic, butyrate-producing bacterium from human faeces. *Int. J. Syst. Evol. Microbiol.* **52:**1615–1620.

46. Eckburg, P. B., E. M. Bik, C. N. Bernstein, E. Purdom, L. Dethlefsen, M. Sargent, S. R. Gill, K. E. Nelson, and D. A. Relman. 2005. Diversity of the human intestinal microbial flora. *Science* **308:**1635–1638.

47. Edmiston, C. E., C. J. Krepel, G. R. Seabrook, L. R. Somberg, A. Nakeeb, R. A. Cambria, and J. B. Towne. 2004. In vitro activities of moxifloxacin against 900 aerobic and anaerobic surgical isolates from patients with intra-abdominal and diabetic foot infections. *Antimicrob. Agents Chemother.* **48:**1012–1016.

48. Edmiston, C. E. J., C. J. Krepel, G. E. Seabrook, and W. G. Jochimsen. 2002. Anaerobic infections in the surgical patient: microbial etiology and therapy. *Clin. Infect. Dis.* **35**(Suppl. 1)**:**S112–S118.

49. Ednie, L. M., A. Rattan, M. R. Jacobs, and P. C. Appelbaum. 2003. Antianaerobe activity of RBX 7644 (ranbezolid), a new oxazolidinone, compared with those of eight other agents. *Antimicrob. Agents Chemother.* **47:**1143–1147.

50. Elsayed, S., A. George, and K. Zhang. 2006. Intrauterine contraceptive device-associated pelvic actinomycosis caused by *Actinomyces urogenitalis. Anaerobe* **12:**67–70.

51. Estoppey, O., G. Rivier, C. H. Blanc, F. Widmer, A. Gallusser, and A. K. So. 1997. *Propionibacterium avidum* sacroiliitis and osteomyelitis. *Rev. Rhum. Engl. Ed.* **64:**54–56.

52. Falsen, E., C. Pascual, B. Sjödén, M. Ohlén, and M. D. Collins. 1999. Phenotypic and phylogenetic characterisation of a novel *Lactobacillus* species from human sources: description of *Lactobacillus iners* sp. nov. *Int. J. Syst. Bacteriol.* **49:**217–221.

53. Felten, A., C. Barreau, C. Bizet, P. H. Lagrange, and A. Philippon. 1999. *Lactobacillus* species identification, H$_2$O$_2$ production, and antibiotic resistance and correlation with human clinical status. *J. Clin. Microbiol.* **37:**729–733.

54. Fendukly, F., and B. Osterman. 2005. Isolation of *Actinobaculum schaalii* and *Actinobaculum urinale* from a patient with chronic renal failure. *J. Clin. Microbiol.* **43:**3567–3569.

55. Ferris, M. J., A. Masztal, K. E. Aldridge, J. D. Fortenberry, P. L. J. Fidel, and D. H. Martin. 2004. Association of *Atopobium vaginae*, a recently described metronidazole resistant anaerobe, with bacterial vaginosis. *BMC Infect. Dis.* **4:**5.

56. Finegold, S. M., P. A. Lawson, M.-L. Vaisanen, D. R. Molitoris, Y. Song, C. Liu, and M. D. Collins. 2004. *Anaerofustis stercorihominis* gen. nov., sp. nov., from human feces. *Anaerobe* **10:**41–45.

57. Finegold, S. M., S. St. John, A. W. Vu, C. M. Li, D. Molitoris, Y. Song, C. M. Liu, and H. M. Wexler. 2004. In vitro activity of ramoplanin and comparator drugs against anaerobic intestinal bacteria from the perspective of potential utility in pathology involving bowel flora. *Anaerobe* **10:**205–211.

58. Fiorino, A. S. 1996. Intrauterine contraceptive device-associated actinomycotic abscess and *Actinomyces* detection on cervical smear. *Obstet. Gynecol.* **87:**142–149.

59. Fouad, A. F., K. Y. Kum, M. L. Clawson, J. Barry, C. Abenoja, Q. Zhu, M. Caimano, and J. D. Radolf. 2003. Molecular characterization of the presence of *Eubacterium* spp and *Streptococcus* spp in endodontic infections. *Oral Microbiol. Immunol.* **18:**249–255.

60. Frank, J. A., C. I. Reich, S. Sharma, J. S. Weisbaum, B. A. Wilson, and G. J. Olsen. 2008. Critical evaluation of two primers commonly used for amplification of bacterial 16S rRNA genes. *Appl. Environ. Microbiol.* **74:**2461–2470.

61. Fredricks, D. N., T. L. Fiedler, K. K. Thomas, B. B. Oakley, and J. M. Marrazzo. 2007. Targeted PCR for detection of vaginal bacteria associated with bacterial vaginosis. *J. Clin. Microbiol.* **45:**3270–3276.

62. Funke, G., A. von Graevenitz, J. E. I. Clarridge, and K. E. Bernard. 1997. Clinical microbiology of coryneform bacteria. *Clin. Microbiol. Rev.* **10:**125–159.

63. Garner, J. P., M. Macdonald, and P. K. Kumar. 2007. Abdominal actinomycosis. *Int. J. Surg.* **5:**441–448.

64. **Geissdörfer, W., C. Böhmer, K. Pelz, C. Schoerner, W. Frobenius, and C. Bogdan.** 2003. Tuboovarian abscess caused by *Atopobium vaginae* following transvaginal oocyte recovery. *J. Clin. Microbiol.* **41:**2788–2790.

65. **Goldstein, E. J., D. M. Citron, P. J. Goldman, and R. J. Goldman.** 2008. National hospital survey of anaerobic culture and susceptibility methods: III. *Anaerobe* **14:**68–72.

66. **Goldstein, E. J., D. M. Citron, C. V. Merriam, Y. Warren, K. L. Tyrrell, and H. Fernandez.** 2003. In vitro activities of telithromycin and 10 oral agents against aerobic and anaerobic pathogens isolated from antral puncture specimens from patients with sinusitis. *Antimicrob. Agents Chemother.* **47:**1963–1967.

67. **Goldstein, E. J., D. M. Citron, C. V. Merriam, Y. A. Warren, K. L. Tyrrell, and H. T. Fernandez.** 2006. Comparative in vitro susceptibilities of 396 unusual anaerobic strains to tigecycline and eight other antimicrobial agents. *Antimicrob. Agents Chemother.* **50:**3507–3513.

68. **Goldstein, E. J., D. M. Citron, C. V. Merriam, Y. Warren, K. L. Tyrrell, and H. T. Fernandez.** 2004. In vitro activities of the new semisynthetic glycopeptide telavancin (TD-6424), vancomycin, daptomycin, linezolid, and four comparator agents against anaerobic gram-positive species and *Corynebacterium* spp. *Antimicrob. Agents Chemother.* **48:**2149–2152.

69. **Goldstein, E. J., D. M. Citron, C. V. Merriam, Y. Warren, K. L. Tyrrell, H. T. Fernandez, and A. Bryskier.** 2005. Comparative in vitro activities of XRP 2868, pristinamycin, quinupristin-dalfopristin, vancomycin, daptomycin, linezolid, clarithromycin, telithromycin, clindamycin, and ampicillin against anaerobic gram-positive species, actinomycetes, and lactobacilli. *Antimicrob. Agents Chemother.* **49:**408–413.

70. **Gomez-Garces, J. L., D. Balas, M. T. Merino, and J. Ignacio Alos.** 1994. *Mobiluncus curtisii* bacteremia following septic abortion. *Clin. Infect. Dis.* **19:**1166–1167.

71. **Greub, G., and D. Raoult.** 2002. "Actinobaculum massiliae," a new species causing chronic urinary tract infection. *J. Clin. Microbiol.* **40:**3938–3941.

72. **Günthard, H., A. Hany, M. Turina, and J. Wüst.** 1994. *Propionibacterium acnes* as a cause of aggressive aortic valve endocarditis and importance of tissue grinding: case report and review. *J. Clin. Microbiol.* **32:**3043–3045.

73. **Halebian, S., B. Harris, S. M. Finegold, and R. D. Rolfe.** 1981. Rapid method that aids in distinguishing gram-positive from gram-negative anaerobic bacteria. *J. Clin. Microbiol.* **13:**444–448.

74. **Hall, V.** 2008. Actinomyces-gathering evidence of human colonization and infection. *Anaerobe* **14:**1–7.

75. **Hall, V., M. D. Collins, R. Hutson, E. Falsen, and B. I. Duerden.** 2002. *Actinomyces cardiffensis* sp. nov. from human clinical sources. *J. Clin. Microbiol.* **40:**3427–3431.

76. **Hall, V., M. D. Collins, R. A. Hutson, E. Falsen, E. Inganas, and B. I. Duerden.** 2003. *Actinobaculum urinale* sp. nov., from human urine. *Int. J. Syst. Evol. Microbiol.* **53:**679–682.

77. **Hall, V., M. D. Collins, R. A. Hutson, E. Inganas, E. Falsen, and B. I. Duerden.** 2003. *Actinomyces oricola* sp. nov., from a human dental abscess. *Int. J. Syst. Evol. Microbiol.* **53:**1515–1518.

78. **Hall, V., M. D. Collins, P. A. Lawson, E. Falsen, and B. I. Duerden.** 2005. *Actinomyces dentalis* sp. nov., from a human dental abscess. *Int. J. Syst. Evol. Microbiol.* **55:**427–431.

79. **Hall, V., M. D. Collins, P. A. Lawson, E. Falsen, and B. I. Duerden.** 2003. *Actinomyces nasicola* sp. nov., isolated from a human nose. *Int. J. Syst. Evol. Microbiol.* **53:**1445–1448.

80. **Hall, V., M. D. Collins, P. A. Lawson, R. A. Hutson, E. Falsen, E. Inganas, and B. I. Duerden.** 2003. Characterization of some *Actinomyces*-like isolates from human clinical sources: description of *Varibaculum cambriensis* gen. nov., sp. nov. *J. Clin. Microbiol.* **41:**640–644.

81. **Hall, V., P. R. Talbot, S. L. Stubbs, and B. I. Duerden.** 2001. Identification of clinical isolates of *Actinomyces* species by amplified 16S ribosomal DNA restriction analysis (ARDRA). *J. Clin. Microbiol.* **39:**3555–3562.

82. **Hansen, T., M. Kunkel, C. J. Kirkpatrick, and A. Weber.** 2006. Actinomyces in infected osteoradionecrosis—underestimated? *Hum. Pathol.* **37:**61–67.

83. **Hashimura, T., M. Sato, and E. Hoshino.** 2001. Detection of *Slackia exigua*, *Mogibacterium timidum* and *Eubacterium saphenum* from pulpal and periradicular samples using the polymerase chain reaction (PCR) method. *Int. Endod. J.* **34:**463–470.

84. **Hecht, D. W., and J. R. Osmolski.** 2003. Activities of garenoxacin (BMS-284756) and other agents against anaerobic clinical isolates. *Antimicrob. Agents Chemother.* **47:**910–916.

85. **Henssge, U., T. Do, D. R. Radford, S. C. Gilbert, D. Clark, and D. Beighton.** 2009. Emended description of *Actinomyces naeslundii* and descriptions of *Actinomyces oris* sp. nov. and *Actinomyces johnsonii* sp. nov., previously identified as *Actinomyces naeslundii* genospecies 1, 2 and WVA 963. *Int. J. Syst. Evol. Microbiol.* **59:**509–516.

86. **Hill, G. B., O. M. Ayers, and A. P. Kohan.** 1987. Characteristics and sites of infection of *Eubacterium nodatum*, *Eubacterium timidum*, *Eubacterium brachy*, and other asaccharolytic eubacteria. *J. Clin. Microbiol.* **25:**1540–1545.

87. **Hoellman, D. B., L. M. Kelly, K. Credito, L. Anthony, L. M. Ednie, M. R. Jacobs, and P. C. Appelbaum.** 2002. In vitro antianaerobic activity of ertapenem (MK-0826) compared to seven other compounds. *Antimicrob. Agents Chemother.* **46:**220–224.

88. **Holmberg, A., R. Lood, M. Morgelin, B. Soderquist, E. Holst, M. Collin, B. Christensson, and M. Rasmussen.** 2009. Biofilm formation by *Propionibacterium acnes* is a characteristic of invasive isolates. *Clin. Microbiol. Infect.* **15:**787–795.

89. **Holst, E., A. R. Goffeng, and B. Andersch.** 1994. Bacterial vaginosis and vaginal microorganisms in idiopathic premature labor and association with pregnancy outcome. *J. Clin. Microbiol.* **32:**176–186.

90. **Hoyles, L., M. D. Collins, E. Falsen, N. Nikolaitchouk, and A. L. McCartney.** 2004. Transfer of members of the genus *Falcivibrio* to the genus *Mobiluncus*, and emended description of the genus *Mobiluncus*. *Syst. Appl. Microbiol.* **27:**72–83.

91. **Hoyles, L., E. Ingana, E. Falsen, M. Drancourt, N. Weiss, A.L. McCartney, and M. D. Collins.** 2002. *Bifidobacterium scardovii* sp. nov., from human sources. *Int. J. Syst. Bacteriol.* **52:**995–999.

92. **Huys, G., M. Vancanneyt, K. D'Haene, E. Falsen, G. Wauters, and P. Vandamme.** 2007. *Alloscardovia omnicolens* gen. nov., sp. nov., from human clinical samples. *Int. J. Syst. Evol. Microbiol.* **57:**1442–1446.

93. **Ison, C. A., and P. E. Hay.** 2002. Validation of a simplified grading of Gram stained vaginal smears for use in genitourinary medicine clinics. *Sex. Transm. Infect.* **78:**413–415.

94. **Jakab, E., R. Zbinden, J. Gubler, C. Ruef, A. von Graevenitz, and M. Krause.** 1996. Severe infections caused by *Propionibacterium acnes*: an underestimated pathogen in late postoperative infections. *Yale J. Biol. Med.* **69:**477–482.

95. **Jalava, J., and E. Eerola.** 1999. Phylogenetic analysis of *Fusobacterium alocis* and *Fusobacterium sulci* based on 16S rRNA gene sequences: proposal of *Filifactor alocis* (Cato, Moore and Moore) comb. nov. and *Eubacterium sulci* (Cato, Moore and Moore) comb. nov. *Int. J. Syst. Bacteriol.* **49:**1375–1379.

96. **Jian, W., and X. Dong.** 2002. Transfer of *Bifidobacterium inopinatum* and *Bifidobacterium denticolens* to *Scardovia inopinata* gen. nov., comb. nov., and *Parascardovia denticolens* gen. nov., comb. nov., respectively. *Int. J. Syst. Evol. Microbiol.* **52:**809–812.

97. **Johnson, M. J., E. Thatcher, and M. E. Cox.** 1995. Techniques for controlling variability in gram staining of obligate anaerobes. *J. Clin. Microbiol.* **33:**755–758.

98. **Jousimies-Somer, H. R., P. Summanen, D. M. Citron, E. J. Baron, H. M. Wexler, and S. M. Finegold.** 2002. *Wadsworth-KTL Anaerobic Bacteriology Manual*, 6th ed. Star Publishing, Belmont, CA.

99. **Kageyama, A., and Y. Benno.** 2000. *Catenibacterium mitsuokai* gen. nov., sp. nov., a gram-positive anaerobic bacterium isolated from human faeces. *Int. J. Syst. Evol. Microbiol.* **50:**1595–1599.

100. **Kageyama, A., and Y. Benno.** 2000. Phylogenic and phenotypic characterization of some *Eubacterium*-like isolates from human feces: description of *Solobacterium moorei* gen. nov., sp. nov. *Microbiol. Immunol.* **44:**223–227.

101. **Kageyama, A., Y. Benno, and T. Nakase.** 1999. Phylogenetic and phenotypic evidence for the transfer of *Eubacterium aerofaciens* to the genus *Collinsella* as *Collinsella aerofaciens* gen. nov., comb. nov. *Int. J. Syst. Bacteriol.* **49:**557–565.

102. **Klein, G., E. Zill, R. Schindler, and J. Louwers.** 1998. Peritonitis associated with vancomycin-resistant *Lactobacillus rhamnosus* in a continuous ambulatory peritoneal dialysis patient: organism identification, antibiotic therapy, and case report. *J. Clin. Microbiol.* **36:**1781–1783.

103. **Kolbert, C. P., and D. H. Persing.** 1999. Ribosomal DNA sequencing as a tool for identification of bacterial pathogens. *Curr. Opin. Microbiol.* **2:**299–305.

104. **Kumar, P. S., A. L. Griffen, J. A. Barton, B. J. Paster, M. L. Moeschberger, and E. J. Leys.** 2003. New bacterial species associated with chronic periodontitis. *J. Dent. Res.* **82:**338–344.

105. **Kumar, P. S., A. L. Griffen, M. L. Moeschberger, and E. J. Leys.** 2005. Identification of candidate periodontal pathogens and beneficial species by quantitative 16S clonal analysis. *J. Clin. Microbiol.* **43:**3944–3955.

106. **Land, M. H., K. Rouster-Stevens, C. R. Woods, M. L. Cannon, J. Cnota, and A. K. Shetty.** 2005. *Lactobacillus* sepsis associated with probiotic therapy. *Pediatrics* **115:**178–181.

107. **Lane, D. J.** 1991. 16S/23S rRNA sequencing, p. 115–175. *In* E. Stackebrandt and M. Goodfellow (ed.), *Nucleic Acid Techniques in Bacterial Systematics.* John Wiley & Sons, Chichester, United Kingdom.

108. **Larsson, P.-G., B. Carlsson, L. Fåhraeus, T. Jakobsson, and U. Forsum.** 2004. Diagnosis of bacterial vaginosis: need for validation of microscopic image area used for scoring bacterial morphotypes. *Sex. Transm. Infect.* **80:**63–67.

109. **Lau, S. K., A. McNabb, G. K. Woo, L. Hoang, A. M. Fung, L. M. Chung, P. C. Woo, and K. Y. Yuen.** 2007. *Catabacter hongkongensis* gen. nov., sp. nov., isolated from blood cultures of patients from Hong Kong and Canada. *J. Clin. Microbiol.* **45:**395–401.

110. **Lau, S. K., P. C. Woo, A. M. Fung, K. M. Chan, G. K. Woo, and K. Y. Yuen.** 2004. Anaerobic, non-sporulating, gram-positive bacilli bacteraemia characterized by 16S rRNA gene sequencing. *J. Med. Microbiol.* **53:**1247–1253.

111. **Lau, S. K., P. C. Woo, G. K. Woo, A. M. Fung, M. K. Wong, K. M. Chan, D. M. Tam, and K. Y. Yuen.** 2004. *Eggerthella hongkongensis* sp. nov. and *Eggerthella sinensis* sp. nov., two novel *Eggerthella* species, account for half of the cases of *Eggerthella* bacteremia. *Diagn. Microbiol. Infect. Dis.* **49:**255–263.

112. **Lawson, P. A., E. Falsen, E. Akervall, P. Vandamme, and M. D. Collins.** 1997. Characterization of some *Actinomyces*-like isolates from human clinical specimens: reclassification of *Actinomyces suis* (Soltys and Spratling) as *Actinobaculum suis* comb. nov. and description of *Actinobaculum schaalii* sp. nov. *Int. J. Syst. Bacteriol.* **47:**899–903.

113. **Lawson, P. A., N. Nikolaitchouk, E. Falsen, K. Westling, and M. D. Collins.** 2001. *Actinomyaces funkei* sp. nov., isolated from human clinical specimens. *Int. J. Syst. Bacteriol.* **51:**853–855.

114. **Lawson, P. A., Y. Song, C. Liu, D. R. Molitoris, M. L. Vaisanen, M. D. Collins, and S. M. Finegold.** 2004. *Anaerotruncus colihominis* gen. nov., sp. nov., from human faeces. *Int. J. Syst. Evol. Microbiol.* **54:**413–417.

115. **Levy, P. Y., F. Fenollar, A. Stein, F. Borrione, E. Cohen, B. Lebail, and D. Raoult.** 2008. *Propionibacterium acnes* postoperative shoulder arthritis: an emerging clinical entity. *Clin. Infect. Dis.* **46:**1884–1886.

116. **Liebetrau, A., A. C. Rodloff, J. Behra-Miellet, and L. Dubreuil.** 2003. In vitro activities of a new des-fluoro(6) quinolone, garenoxacin, against clinical anaerobic bacteria. *Antimicrob. Agents Chemother.* **47:**3667–3671.

117. **Ludwig, W., K.-H. Schleifer, and W. B. Whitman.** 2008. Revised road map to the phylum *Firmicutes*, p. 1–14. *In* P. De Vos, G. Garrity, D. Jones, N. R. Krieg, W. Ludwig, F. A. Rainey, K.-H. Schleifer, and W. B. Whitman (ed.), *Bergey's Manual of Systematic Bacteriology*, vol. 3. Springer-Verlag, New York, NY.

118. **Mahlen, S. D., and J. E. Clarridge III.** 2009. Site and clinical significance of *Alloscardovia omnicolens* and *Bifidobacterium* species isolated in the clinical laboratory. *J. Clin. Microbiol.* **47:**3289–3293.

119. **Mantzourani, M., M. Fenlon, and D. Beighton.** 2009. Association between *Bifidobacteriaceae* and the clinical severity of root caries lesions. *Oral Microbiol. Immunol.* **24:**32–37.

120. **Mantzourani, M., S. C. Gilbert, H. N. Sulong, E. C. Sheehy, S. Tank, M. Fenlon, and D. Beighton.** 2009. The isolation of bifidobacteria from occlusal carious lesions in children and adults. *Caries Res.* **43:**308–313.

121. **Maruo, T., M. Sakamoto, C. Ito, T. Toda, and Y. Benno.** 2008. *Adlercreutzia equolifaciens* gen. nov., sp. nov., an equol-producing bacterium isolated from human faeces, and emended description of the genus *Eggerthella*. *Int. J. Syst. Evol. Microbiol.* **58:**1221–1227.

122. **Mattarelli, P., C. Bonaparte, B. Pot, and B. Biavati.** 2008. Proposal to reclassify the three biotypes of *Bifidobacterium longum* as three subspecies: *Bifidobacterium longum* subsp. *longum* subsp. nov., *Bifidobacterium longum* subsp. *infantis* comb. nov. and *Bifidobacterium longum* subsp. *suis* comb. nov. *Int. J. Syst. Evol. Microbiol.* **58:**767–772.

123. **Meltzer, M. C., R. A. Desmond, and J. R. Schwebke.** 2008. Association of *Mobiluncus curtisii* with recurrence of bacterial vaginosis. *Sex. Transm. Dis.* **35:**611–613.

124. **Menard, J. P., F. Fenollar, M. Henry, F. Bretelle, and D. Raoult.** 2008. Molecular quantification of *Gardnerella vaginalis* and *Atopobium vaginae* loads to predict bacterial vaginosis. *Clin. Infect. Dis.* **47:**33–43.

125. **Moore, W. E. C., and L. V. Holdeman Moore.** 1986. Genus *Eubacterium*, p. 1353–1373. *In* P. H. A. Sneath, N. S. Mair, M. E. Sharpe, and J. G. Holt (ed.), *Bergey's Manual of Systematic Bacteriology*, 1st ed. The Williams and Wilkins Co., Baltimore, MD.

126. **Mosca, A., C. A. Strong, and S. M. Finegold.** 1993. UV red fluorescence of *Eubacterium lentum*. *J. Clin. Microbiol.* **31:**1001–1002.

127. **Moubareck, C., F. Gavini, L. Vaugien, M. J. Butel, and F. Doucet-Populaire.** 2005. Antimicrobial susceptibility of bifidobacteria. *J. Antimicrob. Chemother.* **55:**38–44.

128. **Munson, M. A., A. Banerjee, T. F. Watson, and W. G. Wade.** 2004. Molecular analysis of the microflora associated with dental caries. *J. Clin. Microbiol.* **42:**3023–3029.

129. **Munson, M. A., T. Pitt-Ford, B. Chong, A. J. Weightman, and W. G. Wade.** 2002. Molecular and cultural analysis of the microflora associated with endodontic infections. *J. Dent. Res.* **81:**761–766.

130. **Nakazawa, F., S. E. Poco, T. Ikeda, M. Sato, S. Kalfas, G. Sundqvist, and E. Hoshino.** 1999. *Cryptobacterium curtum* gen. nov., sp. nov., a new genus of gram-positive anaerobic rod isolated from human oral cavities. *Int. J. Syst. Bacteriol.* **49:**1193–1200.

131. **Nakazawa, F., S. E. Poco, M. Sato, T. Ikeda, S. Kalfas, G. Sundqvist, and E. Hoshino.** 2002. Taxonomic characterization of *Mogibacterium diversum* sp. nov. and *Mogibacterium neglectum* sp. nov., isolated from human oral cavities. *Int. J. Syst. Evol. Microbiol.* **52:**115–122.

132. **Nakazawa, F., M. Sato, S. E. Poco, T. Hashimura, T. Ikeda, S. Kalfas, G. Sundqvist, and E. Hoshino.** 2000. Description of *Mogibacterium pumilum* gen. nov., sp. nov. and *Mogibacterium vescum* gen. nov., sp. nov., and reclassification of *Eubacterium timidum* (Holdeman et al. 1980) as *Mogibacterium timidum* gen. nov., comb. nov. *Int. J. Syst. Evol. Microbiol.* **50:**679–688.

133. **Neef, P. A., H. Polenakovik, J. E. Clarridge, M. Saklayen, L. Bogard, and J. M. Bernstein.** 2003. *Lactobacillus paracasei* continuous ambulatory peritoneal dialysis-related peritonitis and review of the literature. *J. Clin. Microbiol.* **41:**2783–2784.

134. **Nisbet, M., S. Briggs, R. Ellis-Pegler, M. Thomas, and D. Holland.** 2007. *Propionibacterium acnes*: an under-appreciated cause of post-neurosurgical infection. *J. Antimicrob. Chemother.* **60:**1097–1103.

135. **Nugent, R. P., M. A. Krohn, and S. L. Hillier.** 1991. Reliability of diagnosing bacterial vaginosis is improved by a standardized method of gram stain interpretation. *J. Clin. Microbiol.* **29:**297–301.

136. **Olsen, I., J. L. Johnson, L. V. Moore, and W. E. Moore.** 1991. *Lactobacillus uli* sp. nov. and *Lactobacillus rimae* sp. nov. from the human gingival crevice and emended descriptions of *Lactobacillus minutus* and *Streptococcus parvulus*. *Int. J. Syst. Bacteriol.* **41:**261–266.

137. **Oprica, C., and C. E. Nord.** 2005. European surveillance study on the antibiotic susceptibility of *Propionibacterium acnes*. *Clin. Microbiol. Infect.* **11:**204–213.

138. **Pajkrt, D., A. M. Simoons-Smit, P. H. Savelkoul, J. van den Hoek, W. W. Hack, and A. M. van Furth.** 2003. Pyelonephritis caused by *Actinobaculum schaalii* in a child with pyeloureteral junction obstruction. *Eur. J. Clin. Microbiol. Infect. Dis.* **22:**438–440.

139. **Paster, B. J., S. K. Boches, J. L. Galvin, R. E. Ericson, C. N. Lau, V. A. Levanos, A. Sahasrabudhe, and F. E. Dewhirst.** 2001. Bacterial diversity in subgingival plaque. *J. Bacteriol.* **183:**3770–3783.

140. **Pei, Z., E. J. Bini, L. Yang, M. Zhou, F. Francois, and M. J. Blaser.** 2004. Bacterial biota in the human distal esophagus. *Proc. Natl. Acad. Sci. USA* **101:**4250–4255.

141. **Piper, K. E., M. J. Jacobson, R. H. Cofield, J. W. Sperling, J. Sanchez-Sotelo, D. R. Osmon, A. McDowell, S. Patrick, J. M. Steckelberg, J. N. Mandrekar, M. Fernandez Sampedro, and R. Patel.** 2009. Microbiologic diagnosis of prosthetic shoulder infection by use of implant sonication. *J. Clin. Microbiol.* **47:**1878–1884.

142. **Preza, D., I. Olsen, J. A. Aas, T. Willumsen, B. Grinde, and B. J. Paster.** 2008. Bacterial profiles of root caries in elderly patients. *J. Clin. Microbiol.* **46:**2015–2021.

143. **Pulverer, G., H. Schutt-Gerowitt, and K. P. Schaal.** 2003. Human cervicofacial actinomycoses: microbiological data for 1997 cases. *Clin. Infect. Dis.* **37:**490–497.

144. **Rautio, M. H., H. Saxen, A. Siitonen, R. Nikku, and H. Jousimies-Somer.** 2000. Bacteriology of histopathologically defined appendicitis in children. *Pediatr. Infect. Dis. J.* **19:**1078–1083.

145. **Reinhard, M., J. Prag, M. Kemp, K. Andresen, B. Klemmensen, N. Højlyng, S. H. Sørensen, and J. J. Christensen.** 2005. Ten cases of *Actinobaculum schaalii* infection: clinical relevance, bacterial identification, and antibiotic susceptibility. *J. Clin. Microbiol.* **43:**5305–5308.

146. **Renvoise, A., D. Raoult, and V. Roux.** 2009. *Actinomyces massiliensis* sp. nov., isolated from a patient blood culture. *Int. J. Syst. Evol. Microbiol.* **59:**540–544.

147. **Rocas, I. N., and J. F. Siqueira.** 2005. Species-directed 16S rRNA gene nested PCR detection of *Olsenella* species in association with endodontic diseases. *Lett. Appl. Microbiol.* **41:**12–16.

148. **Rodriguez Jovita, M., M. D. Collins, B. Sjöden, and E. Falsen.** 1999. Characterization of a novel *Atopobium* isolate from the human vagina: description of *Atopobium vaginae* sp. nov. *Int. J. Syst. Bacteriol.* **49:**1573–1576.

149. **Rohner, P., B. Pepey, and R. Auckenthaler.** 1997. Advantage of combining resin with lytic BACTEC blood culture media. *J. Clin. Microbiol.* **35:**2634–2638.

150. **Rosenblatt, J. E., and D. R. Gustafson.** 1995. Evaluation of the Etest for susceptibility testing of anaerobic bacteria. *Diagn. Microbiol. Infect. Dis.* **22:**279–284.

151. **Sabbe, L. J. M., D. V. D. Merwe, L. Schouls, A. Bergmans, M. Vaneechoutte, and P. Vandamme.** 1999. Clinical spectrum of infections due to the newly described *Actinomyces* species *A. turicensis*, *A. radingae*, and *A. europaeus*. *J. Clin. Microbiol.* **37:**8–13.

152. **Sahuquillo-Arce, J. M., P. Ramirez-Galleymore, J. Garcia, V. Marti, and D. Arizo.** 2008. *Mobiluncus curtisii* bacteremia. *Anaerobe* **14:**123–124.

153. **Sakata, S., M. Kitahara, M. Sakamoto, H. Hayashi, M. Fukuyama, and Y. Benno.** 2002. Unification of *Bifidobacterium infantis* and *Bifidobacterium suis* as *Bifidobacterium longum*. *Int. J. Syst. Evol. Microbiol.* **52:**1945–1951.

154. **Salminen, M. K., H. Rautelin, S. Tynkkynen, T. Poussa, M. Saxelin, V. Valtonen, and A. Järvinen.** 2004. *Lactobacillus* bacteremia, clinical significance, and patient outcome, with special focus on probiotic *L. rhamnosus* GG. *Clin. Infect. Dis.* **38:**62–69.

155. **Salonen, J. H., E. Eerola, and O. Meurman.** 1998. Clinical significance and outcome of anaerobic bacteremia. *Clin. Infect. Dis.* **26:**1413–1417.

156. **Santala, A.-M., N. Sarkonen, V. Hall, P. Carlson, H. Jousimies-Somer, and E. Könönen.** 2004. Evaluation of four commercial test systems for identification of *Actinomyces* and some closely related species. *J. Clin. Microbiol.* **42:**418–420.

157. **Sarkonen, N., E. Könönen, E. Eerola, M. Könönen, H. Jousimies-Somer, and P. Laine.** 2005. Characterization of *Actinomyces* species isolated from failed dental implant fixtures. *Anaerobe* **11:**231–237.

158. **Sarkonen, N., E. Könönen, P. Summanen, A. Kanervo, A. Takala, and H. Jousimies-Somer.** 2000. Oral colonization with *Actinomyces* species in infants by two years of age. *J. Dent. Res.* **79:**864–867.

159. **Sarkonen, N., E. Könönen, P. Summanen, M. Könönen, and H. Jousimies-Somer.** 2001. Phenotypic identification of *Actinomyces* and related species isolated from human sources. *J. Clin. Microbiol.* **39:**3955–3961.

160. **Schabereiter-Gurtner, C., S. Maca, S. Kaminsky, S. Rolleke, W. Lubitz, and T. Barisani-Asenbauer.** 2002. Investigation of an anaerobic microbial community associated with a corneal ulcer by denaturing gradient gel electrophoresis and 16S rDNA sequence analysis. *Diagn. Microbiol. Infect. Dis.* **43:**193–199.

161. **Schwebke, J. R., and L. F. Lawing.** 2001. Prevalence of *Mobiluncus* spp. among women with and without bacterial vaginosis as detected by polymerase chain reaction. *Sex. Transm. Dis.* **28:**195–199.

162. **Schwebke, J. R., S. A. Lukehart, M. C. Roberts, and S. L. Hillier.** 1991. Identification of two new antigenic subgroups within the genus *Mobiluncus*. *J. Clin. Microbiol.* **29:**2204–2208.

163. **Schwiertz, A., G. L. Hold, S. H. Duncan, B. Gruhl, M. D. Collins, P. A. Lawson, H. J. Flint, and M. Blaut.** 2002. *Anaerostipes caccae* gen. nov., sp. nov., a new saccharolytic, acetate-utilising, butyrate-producing bacterium from human faeces. *Syst. Appl. Microbiol.* **25:**46–51.

164. **Servin, A. L.** 2004. Antagonistic activities of lactobacilli and bifidobacteria against microbial pathogens. *FEMS Microbiol. Rev.* **28:**405–440.

165. **Siqueira, J. F., Jr., and I. N. Rocas.** 2009. The microbiota of acute apical abscesses. *J. Dent. Res.* **88:**61–65.

166. **Siqueira, J. F., and I. N. Rocas.** 2003. Detection of *Filifactor alocis* in endodontic infections associated with different forms of periradicular diseases. *Oral Microbiol. Immunol.* **18:**263–265.

167. **Siqueira, J. F., and I. N. Rocas.** 2003. Polymerase chain reaction detection of *Propionibacterium propionicus* and *Actinomyces radicidentis* in primary and persistent endodontic infections. *Oral Surg. Oral Med. Oral Pathol. Oral Radiol. Endod.* **96:**215–222.

168. **Siqueira, J. F., and I. N. Rocas.** 2003. *Pseudoramibacter alactolyticus* in primary endodontic infections. *J. Endod.* **29:**735–738.

169. **Smith, A. J., V. Hall, B. Thakker, and C. G. Gemmell.** 2005. Antimicrobial susceptibility testing of *Actinomyces* species with 12 antimicrobial agents. *J. Antimicrob. Chemother.* **56:**407–409.

170. **Snydman, D. R., N. V. Jacobus, and L. A. McDermott.** 2008. In vitro activities of doripenem, a new broad-spectrum carbapenem, against recently collected clinical anaerobic isolates, with emphasis on the *Bacteroides fragilis* group. *Antimicrob. Agents Chemother.* **52:**4492–4496.

171. **Sohail, M. R., A. L. Gray, L. M. Baddour, I. M. Tleyjeh, and A. Virk.** 2009. Infective endocarditis due to *Propionibacterium* species. *Clin. Microbiol. Infect.* **15:**387–394.

172. **Sonbol, H., D. Spratt, G. J. Roberts, and V. S. Lucas.** 2009. Prevalence, intensity and identity of bacteraemia following conservative dental procedures in children. *Oral Microbiol. Immunol.* **24:**177–182.

173. **Strazzeri, J. C., and S. Anzel.** 1986. Infected total hip arthroplasty due to *Actinomyces israelii* after dental extraction. A case report. *Clin. Orthop.* **210:**128–131.

174. **Suau, A., R. Bonnet, M. Sutren, J. J. Godon, G. R. Gibson, M. D. Collins, and J. Dore.** 1999. Direct analysis of genes encoding 16S rRNA from complex communities reveals many novel molecular species within the human gut. *Appl. Environ. Microbiol.* **65:**4799–4807.

175. **Sullivan, A., and C. E. Nord.** 2006. Probiotic lactobacilli and bacteraemia in Stockholm. *Scand. J. Infect. Dis.* **38:**327–331.

176. **Tabanella, G., H. Nowzari, and J. Slots.** 2009. Clinical and microbiological determinants of ailing dental implants. *Clin. Implant Dent. Relat. Res.* **11:**24–36.

177. **Taga, S.** 2007. Diagnosis and therapy of pelvic actinomycosis. *J. Obstet. Gynaecol. Res.* **33:**882–885.

178. **Talan, D. A., F. M. Abrahamian, G. J. Moran, D. M. Citron, J. O. Tan, and E. J. C. Goldstein.** 2003. Clinical presentation and bacteriologic analysis of infected human bites in patients presenting to emergency departments. *Clin. Infect. Dis.* **37:**1481–1489.

179. **Talan, D. A., D. M. Citron, F. M. Abrahamian, G. J. Moran, and E. J. C. Goldstein.** 1999. Bacteriologic analysis of infected dog and cat bites. *N. Engl. J. Med.* **340:**85–92.

180. **Thiolas, A., C. Bollet, M. Gasmi, M. Drancourt, and D. Raoult.** 2003. *Eubacterium callanderi* bacteremia: report of the first case. *J. Clin. Microbiol.* **41:**2235–2236.

181. **Trampuz, A., K. E. Piper, M. J. Jacobson, A. D. Hanssen, K. K. Unni, D. R. Osmon, J. N. Mandrekar, F. R. Cockerill, J. M. Steckelberg, J. F. Greenleaf, and R. Patel.** 2007. Sonication of removed hip and knee prostheses for diagnosis of infection. *N. Engl. J. Med.* **357:**654–663.

182. **Tunney, M. M., T. R. Field, T. F. Moriarty, S. Patrick, G. Doering, M. S. Muhlebach, M. C. Wolfgang, R. Boucher, D. F. Gilpin, A. McDowell, and J. S. Elborn.** 2008. Detection of anaerobic bacteria in high numbers in sputum from patients with cystic fibrosis. *Am. J. Respir. Crit. Care. Med.* **177:**995–1001.

183. **Turroni, F., A. Ribbera, E. Foroni, D. van Sinderen, and M. Ventura.** 2008. Human gut microbiota and bifidobacteria: from composition to functionality. *Antonie van Leeuwenhoek* **94:**35–50.

184. **Uckay, I., A. Dinh, L. Vauthey, N. Asseray, N. Passuti, M. Rottman, J. Biziragusenyuka, A. Riche, P. Rohner, D. Wendling, S. Mammou, R. Stern, P. Hoffmeyer, and L. Bernard.** 2010. Spondylodiscitis due to *Propionibacterium acnes*: report of twenty-nine cases and a review of the literature. *Clin. Microbiol. Infect.* **16:**353–358.

185. **Uematsu, H., and E. Hoshino.** 1992. Predominant obligate anaerobes in human periodontal pockets. *J. Periodontal Res.* **27:**15–19.

186. **Uematsu, H., N. Sato, M. Z. Hossain, T. Ikeda, and E. Hoshino.** 2003. Degradation of arginine and other amino acids by butyrate-producing asaccharolytic anaerobic gram-positive rods in periodontal pockets. *Arch. Oral Biol.* **48:**423–429.

187. **Vanagt, W. Y., W. J. Daenen, and T. Delhaas.** 2004. *Propionibacterium acnes* endocarditis on an annuloplasty ring in an adolescent boy. *Heart* **90:**e56.

188. **Vandamme, P., E. Falsen, M. Vancanneyt, M. Van Esbroeck, D. Van de Merwe, A. Bergmans, L. Schouls, and L. Sabbe.** 1998. Characterization of *A. turicensis* and *A. radingae* strains from human clinical samples. *Int. J. Syst. Bacteriol.* **48:**503–510.

189. **Vandamme, P., B. Pot, M. Gillis, P. de Vos, K. Kersters, and J. Swings.** 1996. Polyphasic taxonomy, a consensus approach to bacterial systematics. *Microbiol. Rev.* **60:**407–438.

190. **Verhelst, R., H. Verstraelen, G. Claeys, G. Verschraegen, J. Delanghe, L. V. Simaey, C. D. Ganck, M. Temmerman, and M. Vaneechoutte.** 2004. Cloning of 16S rRNA genes amplified from normal and disturbed vaginal microflora suggests a strong association between *Atopobium vaginae*, *Gardnerella vaginalis* and bacterial vaginosis. *BMC Microbiol.* **4:**16.

191. **Wade, W. G., J. Downes, D. Dymock, S. J. Hiom, A. J. Weightman, F. E. Dewhirst, B. J. Paster, N. Tzellas, and B. Coleman.** 1999. The family *Coriobacteriaceae*: reclassification of *Eubacterium exiguum* (Poco et al. 1996) and *Peptostreptococcus heliotrinreducens* (Lanigan 1976) as *Slackia exigua* gen. nov., comb. nov. and *Slackia heliotrinireducens* gen. nov., comb. nov., and *Eubacterium lentum* (Prevot 1938) as *Eggerthella lenta* gen. nov., comb. nov. *Int. J. Syst. Bacteriol.* **49:**595–600.

192. **Wagenlehner, F. M., B. Mohren, K. G. Naber, and H. F. Mannl.** 2003. Abdominal actinomycosis. *Clin. Microbiol. Infect.* **9:**881–885.

193. **Walker, A. P., C. J. Krepel, C. M. Gohr, and C. E. Edmiston.** 1994. Microflora of abdominal sepsis by locus of infection. *J. Clin. Microbiol.* **32:**557–558.

194. **Willems, A., and M. D. Collins.** 1996. Phylogenetic relationships of the genera *Acetobacterium* and *Eubacterium* sensu stricto and reclassification of *Eubacterium alactolyticum* as *Pseudoramibacter alactolyticus* gen. nov., comb. nov. *Int. J. Syst. Bacteriol.* **46:**1083–1087.

195. **Willems, A., W. E. Moore, N. Weiss, and M. D. Collins.** 1997. Phenotypic and phylogenetic characterization of some *Eubacterium*-like isolates containing a novel type B wall murein from human feces: description of *Holdemania filiformis* gen. nov., sp. nov. *Int. J. Syst. Bacteriol.* **47:**1201–1204.

196. **Wilson, M. J., A. J. Weightman, and W. G. Wade.** 1997. Applications of molecular ecology in the characterisation of uncultured microorganisms associated with human disease. *Rev. Med. Microbiol.* **8:**91–101.

197. **Wolin, M. J., T. L. Miller, M. D. Collins, and P. A. Lawson.** 2003. Formate-dependent growth and homoacetogenic fermentation by a bacterium from human feces: description of *Bryantella formatexigens* gen. nov., sp. nov. *Appl. Environ. Microbiol.* **69:**6321–6326.

198. **Wolin, M. J., T. L. Miller, and P. A. Lawson.** 2008. Proposal to replace the illegitimate genus name *Bryantella* Wolin et al. 2004VP with the genus name *Marvinbryantia* gen. nov. and to replace the illegitimate combination *Bryantella formatexigens* Wolin et al. 2004VP with *Marvinbryantia formatexigens* comb. nov. *Int. J. Syst. Evol. Microbiol.* **58:**742–744.

199. **Woo, P. C., A. M. Fung, S. K. Lau, J. L. Teng, B. H. Wong, M. K. Wong, E. Hon, G. W. Tang, and K. Y. Yuen.** 2003. *Actinomyces hongkongensis* sp. nov. a novel *Actinomyces* species isolated from a patient with pelvic actinomycosis. *Syst. Appl. Microbiol.* **26:**518–522.

200. **Wurdemann, D., B. J. Tindall, R. Pukall, H. Lunsdorf, C. Strompl, T. Namuth, H. Nahrstedt, M. Wos-Oxley, S. Ott, S. Schreiber, K. N. Timmis, and A. P. Oxley.** 2009. *Gordonibacter pamelaeae* gen. nov., sp. nov., a new member of the *Coriobacteriaceae* isolated from a patient with Crohn's disease, and reclassification of *Eggerthella hongkongensis* Lau et al. 2006 as *Paraeggerthella hongkongensis* gen. nov., comb. nov. *Int. J. Syst. Evol. Microbiol.* **59:**1405–1415.

201. **Wüst, J., U. Steiger, H. Vuong, and R. Zbinden.** 2000. Infection of a hip prosthesis by *Actinomyces naeslundii*. *J. Clin. Microbiol.* **38:**929–930.

202. **Yamamoto, T., X. Zhou, C. J. Williams, A. Hochwalt, and L. J. Forney.** 2009. Bacterial populations in the vaginas of healthy adolescent women. *J. Pediatr. Adolesc. Gynecol.* **22:**11–18.

203. **Ze-Ze, L., R. Tenreiro, A. Duarte, M. J. Salgado, J. Melo-Cristino, L. Lito, M. M. Carmo, S. Felisberto, and G. Carmo.** 2004. Case of aortic endocarditis caused by *Lactobacillus casei*. *J. Med. Microbiol.* **53:**451–453.

204. **Zhou, X., S. J. Bent, M. G. Schneider, C. C. Davis, M. R. Islam, and L. J. Forney.** 2004. Characterization of vaginal microbial communities in adult healthy women using cultivation-independent methods. *Microbiology* **150:**2565–2573.

Clostridium*

DENNIS L. STEVENS, AMY E. BRYANT, ANJA BERGER,
AND CHRISTOPH von EICHEL-STREIBER

50

TAXONOMY

The genus *Clostridium* comprises obligately anaerobic (or occasionally aerotolerant), gram-positive rods. Currently, >200 clostridial species and subspecies are validly published (http://www.dsmz.de); however, the number of clinically significant clostridia from human infections is limited (Table 1).

Phylogenetically, the genus *Clostridium* is heterogeneous, with many species intermixed with other spore-forming and non-spore-forming genera. Traditionally, the different species have been defined based on morphological, ultrastructural, and physiological features. During the past 2 decades, analyses of 16S rRNA gene sequences indicated that the "clostridia" could be divided into 19 clusters (57). Cluster I forms the basis of the genus *Clostridium* and is analogous to group I proposed by Johnson and Francis over 30 years ago (98). The type species, *Clostridium butyricum*, and most of the clinically relevant *Clostridium* species cluster within rRNA homology group I (reviewed in reference 177). The heterogeneous non-group I clostridia require reclassification; however, 16S rRNA gene sequences may not be adequate alone in distinguishing genera, and it is necessary to find genetic and phenotypic characters that enable rapid discrimination among genera within this group.

Two new species clustering within the *C. coccoides* rRNA group, *C. hathewayi* (179) and *C. bolteae* (173), were described from human feces. Phenotypically, *C. clostridioforme* is a relatively heterogeneous anaerobic species. Sequencing analyses of 16S rRNA genes from 107 strains that were previously identified phenotypically as *C. clostridioforme* in various clinical laboratories revealed that *C. clostridioforme* in fact represents three distinct species: *C. bolteae*, *C. clostridioforme*, and *C. hathewayi* (72). *C. bartlettii* is another new *Clostridium* species described from human feces (174); the clinical significance of this organism remains unknown. "*C. neonatale*" was proposed as a novel species recovered from bacteremia in patients with necrotizing enterocolitis (NEC) (9). *Anaerotruncus colihominis* is a new genus and species within the *C. leptum* rRNA cluster of organisms originally described from human feces (121)

and subsequently found in patients with bacteremia (119). Though it was originally described as a non-spore-forming organism, further studies have revealed that sporulation occurs under some conditions (119) and should therefore be considered in *Clostridium* identification schemes. On the basis of biochemical properties, phylogenetic position, DNA G+C content, and DNA-DNA hybridization, the unification of *Clostridium orbiscindens* and *Eubacterium plautii* into the new genus *Flavonifractor plautii* has been proposed (42).

DESCRIPTION OF THE GENUS

Clostridia belong to the phylum *Firmicutes* and comprise a heterogeneous (paraphyletic) group consisting of at least 12 lineages. Clostridia have a wide range of G+C contents, from 22 to 55 mol%, while the toxigenic species have a much narrower range of G+C contents, 24 to 29 mol% (177). Morphological and phenotypic properties that have traditionally been used to define the genus include (i) the formation of endospores, (ii) anaerobic energy metabolism, (iii) an inability to reduce sulfate to sulfide, and (iv) a gram-positive cell wall structure.

Vegetative cells of *Clostridium* species are pleomorphic, rod shaped, and arranged in pairs or short chains; the cells have rounded or sometimes pointed ends (90). Rods may join to form tight coils or spiral configurations in species such as *C. cocleatum* and *C. spiroforme*. Clostridia stain gram positive in early stages of growth, although some species, such as *C. clostridioforme*, *C. hathewayi*, *C. innocuum*, and *C. ramosum*, may appear gram negative. Several species (e.g., *C. tetani*) appear gram negative by the time that spores have formed. Endospores are often wider than the vegetative organisms, imparting characteristic spindle shapes to clostridia. Most strains are motile by means of peritrichous flagella. Nonmotile species include *C. perfringens*, *C. ramosum*, and *C. innocuum* (90).

Clostridium species are metabolically diverse. As currently designated (57), most species are chemoorganotrophic; some species may be chemoautotrophic and chemolithotrophic. They can be saccharolytic, proteolytic, neither, or both; they do not carry out dissimilatory sulfate reduction. They usually produce mixtures of organic acids and alcohols from carbohydrates, proteins and peptides, or purines and pyrimidines.

---

*This chapter contains information presented by Eric A. Johnson, Paula Summanen, and Sydney M. Finegold in chapter 57 of the ninth edition of this *Manual*.

Most species are obligately anaerobic, although the tolerance to oxygen varies widely; some species (e.g., *C. tertium*) grow but do not sporulate in the presence of air, and a few aerotolerant species, such as *C. carnis*, *C. histolyticum*, and occasional strains of *C. perfringens*, give scant growth on solid media incubated under 5 to 10% CO_2. Aerotolerant clostridia and certain *Bacillus* species may be distinguished by several means: (i) clostridia usually form spores only under anaerobic conditions, (ii) they grow better anaerobically than in air, (iii) they usually do not produce catalase, and (iv) they have straight-chain, saturated, and monounsaturated cellular fatty acid (CFA) compositions, whereas *Bacillus* species have branched-chained CFAs. Although *Clostridium* species are usually catalase and superoxide dismutase negative, trace amounts of these enzyme activities may be detected in some strains, such as *C. perfringens*. In addition, clostridia lack a cytochrome system and are thus oxidase negative. Clostridia often occur in nature and in infections as consortia of mixed species, wherein aerobic and facultative organisms utilize oxygen, provide nutrients or other factors, and create an environment favorable for clostridial growth.

Clostridia produce more kinds of protein toxins than any other bacterial genus, and more than 25 toxins lethal to mice have been identified (reviewed in reference 169). At least 15 species of cluster I *Clostridium* produce protein toxins, and new toxins and virulence proteins have been discovered through traditional isolation techniques and genomic analyses (36, 164). These proteins include neurotoxins, enterotoxins, cytotoxins, collagenases, permeases, necrotizing toxins, lipases, lecithinases, hemolysins, proteinases, hyaluronidases, DNases, ADP-ribosyltransferases, neuraminidases, and some others that are simply known as lethal toxins. Botulinum neurotoxin and tetanus neurotoxin (BoNT and TeNT) are the most potent toxins known, with lethal doses of 0.2 to 10 ng per kg of body weight for various animals, including humans (22). Epsilon toxin is a 33-kDa protein produced by *C. perfringens* types B and D strains, and in animals it causes edema and hemorrhage in the brain, heart, spinal cord, and kidneys. It is among the most lethal of clostridial toxins and is considered a potential bioterrorism agent (22, 167).

Recently, some genomic sequences of pathogenic clostridia have become available (36, 164), which should facilitate a comprehensive approach for understanding virulence factors involved in clostridial pathogenesis.

EPIDEMIOLOGY AND TRANSMISSION

Clostridium species are widespread in nature due to their ability to form resistant endospores. They are commonly found in soil, feces, sewage, and marine sediments. The ecology of *C. perfringens* in soil is greatly influenced by the degree and duration of animal husbandry (reviewed in reference 171), and this has relevance to the incidence of gas gangrene caused by contamination of war wounds with soil. For example, the incidence of clostridial gas gangrene was higher in agricultural lands in Europe than in the Sahara Desert of Africa (171). Similarly, the incidences of tetanus and foodborne botulism are also clearly related to the presence of clostridial spores in soil, water, and many foods (171). Outbreaks of hospital-acquired enteric *C. difficile* infections are often traceable to environmental sources and other typical background factors for nosocomial infection (144). Clostridia are present in large numbers in the indigenous microbiota of the intestinal tracts of humans

and animals, in the female genital tract, and in the oral mucosa as well.

CLINICAL SIGNIFICANCE

Although exogenous clostridial infections or intoxications, such as tetanus, foodborne botulism, and gas gangrene, have been feared for centuries, severe cases of hospital-acquired and community-acquired *C. difficile* colitis have recently emerged. Endogenous clostridia, in association with non-spore-forming anaerobes and facultative or aerobic organisms, also cause severe infections in diabetic patients and in patients in whom the mucosal integrity of the bowel or respiratory system has been compromised. Head and neck infections, brain abscesses, sinusitis, otitis, aspiration pneumonia, lung abscesses, pleural empyemas, cholecystitis, intra-abdominal infections, gynecologic and obstetric infections, soft tissue infections, myonecrosis, and septic arthritis and bone infections all may involve clostridia (82). Common predisposing factors are surgical procedures, trauma, vascular stasis, bowel obstruction, malignancy, immunosuppressive agents, diabetes mellitus, prior aerobic infection, and use of antimicrobial agents with poor activity against clostridia (see the section on *C. difficile* below).

Clostridial Bacteremia

Clostridium species are important causes of bloodstream infections (118, 122, 166). *C. septicum* is isolated only rarely from the feces of healthy individuals but may be found in the appendixes of normal individuals. Over 50% of patients whose blood cultures are positive for this organism have some gastrointestinal anomaly, such as diverticular disease, or an underlying malignancy, such as carcinoma of the colon. Another clinically important association has been observed between *C. septicum* bacteremia and neutropenia of any origin and, more specifically, neutropenic enterocolitis involving the terminal ileum or cecum (112). Patients with diabetes mellitus, severe atherosclerotic cardiovascular disease, or anaerobic myonecrosis (gas gangrene) may also develop *C. septicum* bacteremia (81). The clinical importance of recognizing *C. septicum* bacteremia and starting appropriate treatment immediately cannot be overemphasized. Patients with this condition are usually gravely ill and may have metastatic spread to distant anatomic sites, resulting in spontaneous myonecrosis. Mortality rates are very high. *C. septicum* has also been recovered from cirrhotic patients with bacteremia, as have *C. perfringens*, *C. bifermentans*, and other clostridia (50). Some of these patients have demonstrated septic shock.

Another clostridial species of importance in patients with serious underlying disease, such as malignancy and acute pancreatitis, is *C. tertium*. This organism, as well as *C. septicum* and *C. perfringens*, may be seen among the bacteria in the blood of such patients, with or without neutropenic enterocolitis (124). *C. tertium* may present special problems in terms of both identification and treatment. This organism may appear to be gram negative, and it is aerotolerant and resistant to metronidazole, clindamycin, and cephalosporins. *Clostridium sordellii* and *C. perfringens* have been associated with toxic shock syndrome and abortion (7, 55).

Studies of anaerobic bacteremia by Woo et al. (202) and Simmon et al. (166) identified clostridia based upon sequencing of genes encoding 16S rRNA. *C. perfringens* and *C. tertium* were the two most frequently identified species, causing up to 79% and 5%, respectively, of clostridial bacteremias. The mortality rate of clinically relevant clostridial

TABLE 1 Characteristics of *Clostridium* species of clinical significance[a]

Species	Gelatin hydrolysis	Lecithinase	Lipase	Indole	Esculin hydrolysis	Nitrate	Milk digestion	Fermentation of:		
								Glucose	**Arabinose**	Cellobiose
Saccharolytic, proteolytic										
C. bifermentans[b]	+	+	−	+	+⁻	−	+	+	−	−
C. botulinum[c]										
Types A, B, and F	+	−	+	−	+	−	+	+⁻	−	−
Types B, E and F[d]	+	−	+	−	−	−	−	+	w⁻	−
Types C and D	+	−⁺	+	−⁺	−	−	+	+	−	−
C. cadaveris	+	−	−	+	−	−	+	+	−	−
C. difficile[e]	+	−	−	−	+	−	−	+ʷ	−	v
C. novyi A	+	+	+	−	−	−	−	+	−	−
C. perfringens	+	+	−	−	v	v	+	+	−	−⁺
C. putrificum	+	−	−	−	−⁺	−	+	+ʷ	−	−
C. septicum[f]	+	−	−	−	+	v	+	+	−	+ʷ
C. sordellii[b]	+	+	−	+	−⁺	−	+	+	−	−
C. sporogenes[f]	+	−	+	−	+	−	+	+	−	−ʷ
Saccharolytic, nonproteolytic										
C. baratii	−	+	−	−	+	+⁻	−	+	−	+
C. bolteae[g]	−	−	−	−	−⁺	−	−	+	+	−⁺
C. butyricum	−	−	−	−	+	−	−	+	+⁻	+
C. carnis[h]	−	−	−	−	+	−	−	+	−	w⁺
C. clostridioforme[g]	−	−	−	−	+	−	−	+	+	+
C. glycolicum	−	−	−	−	−⁺	−	−	+	−	−
C. hathewayi[g]	−	−	−	−	+ʷ	−	−	+	V	+
C. indolis	−	−	−	+	+	+⁻	−	+	w⁻	+ʷ
C. innocuum[e]	−	−	−	−	+	−	−	+	−⁺	+
C. paraputrificum	−ʷ	−	−	−	+	−⁺	−	+	−	+
C. ramosum	−	−	−	−	+	−	−	+	−	+
C. sphenoides	−	−	−	+	+	+⁻	−	+	−ʷ	+ʷ
C. symbiosum	−ʷ	−	−	−	−	−	−	+ʷ	V	−
C. tertium[h]	−	−	−	−	+	+⁻	−	+	−	+ʷ
Asaccharolytic										
C. argentinense	+	−	−	−	−	−	+	−	−	−
C. hastiforme	+	−	−	−	−	−⁺	−⁺	−	−	−
C. histolyticum[h]	+	−	−	−	−	−	+	−	−	−
C. limosum	+	+	−	−	−	−	+	−	−	−
C. subterminale	+	−⁺	−	−	−⁺	−	+	−	−	−
C. tetani[f]	+	−	−ʷ	v	−	−	+	−	−	−

[a] +, positive reaction; −, negative reaction; v, variable reaction; w, weakly positive reaction; ST, subterminal; T, terminal. A superscript indicates rare variability. Boldface type indicates key reactions. Capital letters indicate major metabolic products from PYG, lowercase letters indicate minor products, and parentheses indicate a variable reaction for fatty acids as follows: A, acetic; P, propionic; IB, isobutyric; B, butyric; IV, isovaleric; V, valeric; IC, isocaproic; L, lactic; S, succinic; and PA, phenylacetic.

[b] *C. bifermentans* is urease negative, and *C. sordellii* is urease positive. *C. bifermentans* usually forms chalk-white colonies on egg yolk agar.

[c] A toxin neutralization test is required for identification. Send suspected isolates or *C. botulinum*-containing material to the appropriate local or state public health agency.

bacteremia ranged from 29 to 35%, and risk factors for mortality (200) were liver disease and older age. The *C. clostridioforme* group (including *C. clostridioforme*, *C. hathewayi*, and *C. bolteae*) has also caused bacteremia (72, 203).

Enteric Infections

Food Poisoning

C. perfringens is one of the most common bacterial causes of foodborne illness in the United States and Canada (28, 95, 147), and virtually all cases have been due to type A strains (28, 167). In *C. perfringens* type A foodborne disease, the food vehicle is typically improperly cooked meat or a meat product, such as gravy, that has cooled slowly after being cooked or may have been inadequately reheated. Spores surviving the initial cooking germinate, and vegetative cells proliferate during slow cooling or insufficient reheating. Illness results from the ingestion of food containing about 10^8 or more viable vegetative cells, which sporulate in the alkaline environment of the small intestine, producing an enterotoxin (*C. perfringens* enterotoxin [CPE]) in the process. Diarrhea develops within 7

Fructose	**Lactose**	Maltose	Mannitol	Mannose	Melibiose	Ribose	Salicin	**Sucrose**	Xylose	Spore location	Metabolic end products from PYG
$-^{w}$	−	w^{-}	−	$-^{w}$	−	−	−	−	−	ST	A (iv, ic, p, ib, b, l, s)
$-^{w}$	−	$-^{w}$	−	−	−	−	−	−	−	ST	A, B, IV, ib (ic, v, p)
$+^{w}$	−	$+^{-}$	$-^{w}$	$+^{w}$	$-^{w}$	v	−	$+^{w}$	−	ST	B, A (1)
v	−	v	−	v	$-^{w}$	v	−	−	−	T	B, P, A (v, l, s)
v	−	−	−	$-^{w}$	−	−	−	−	−	T	B, A
$+^{w}$	−	−	w^{+}	v	−	$-^{w}$	$-^{w}$	−	$-^{w}$	ST^{T}	B, A, ic, iv, ib (v, l)
$-^{w}$	−	v	−	−	$-^{w}$	v	$-^{w}$	−	−	ST	A, B, P
+	+	+	−	+	v	v	$-^{+}$	+	−	ST	A, B, L (p, s)
$-^{w}$	−	$-^{w}$	−	−	−	−	−	−	−	TST	A, B, ib, iv (p, ic, v, l, s)
+	+	+	−	+	−	v	v	−	−	ST	B, A (p, l)
v	−	w	−	$-^{w}$	−	$-^{w}$	−	−	−	ST	A (IC, p, ib, iv, l)
−	−	$-^{w}$	−	−	−	−	−	−	−	ST	A, B, iv, ib (p, ic, v, l, s)
+	w^{+}	w^{+}	−	+	$-^{w}$	w^{-}	$+^{-}$	+	−	ST	B, A, L (p, s)
+	−	+	−	+	−	−	$-^{+}$	+	+	ST	A (l)
+	+	+	$-^{w}$	+	$+^{w}$	$+^{w}$	$+^{w}$	+	+	ST	B, A (l, s)
v	v	w^{+}	−	w^{+}	−	−	w	w^{+}	−	ST	B, A, L (s)
$+^{w}$	+	+	−	+	v	v	+	$+^{w}$	$+^{w}$	ST	A (l)
$+^{w}$	−	v	−	−	−	−	−	−	$+^{-}$	ST	A, IV, IB (p, l, s)
+	+	+	−	+	+	+	+	+	+	ST	A (l)
w^{+}	w^{+}	w^{+}	$-^{w}$	$-^{w}$	$-^{w}$	$-^{w}$	w^{-}	V	v	T	A
+	$-^{w}$	−	$+^{w}$	+	−	v	$+^{w}$	$+^{w}$	$-^{w}$	T	B, L, a (s)
$+^{w}$	+	+	−	+	−	w^{-}	+	+	−	TST	B, A, L (s)
+	+	+	$+^{-}$	+	$+^{-}$	v	+	+	$-^{w}$	T	A, l (s)
$+^{w}$	w^{+}	$+^{w}$	w^{+}	$+^{w}$	v	$-^{w}$	v	w^{-}	v	ST^{T}	A (l, s)
+	$-^{+}$	−	−	v	−	−	−	−	−	ST	A, B, L
+	+	+	w^{+}	$+^{w}$	$+^{w}$	$+^{w}$	$+^{w}$	+	v	T	A, B, L
−	−	−	−	−	−	−	−	−	−	ST	A, b, ib, iv (l)
−	−	−	−	−	−	−	−	−	−	T	A, B, iv, ib(p, ic)
−	−	−	−	−	−	−	−	−	−	ST	A (l, s)
−	−	−	−	−	−	−	−	−	−	ST	A (l, s)
−	−	−	−	−	−	−	−	−	−	ST	A, B, IV, ib(p, ic, l, s)
−	−	−	−	−	−	−	−	−	−	T	A, B, p (l, s)

[d] Nonproteolytic.

[e] L-Proline aminopeptidase differentiates *C. difficile* and *C. innocuum*. *C. difficile* is positive, and *C. innocuum* is negative.

[f] Swarming.

[g] Cigar shaped. *C. bolteae* is lactose and β-NAG negative, *C. clostridioforme* is lactose positive and β-NAG negative, and *C. hathewayi* is lactose and β-NAG positive.

[h] *C. tertium*, *C. carnis*, and most *C. histolyticum* isolates grow aerobically.

to 30 h of ingestion of such food and is generally mild and self-limiting (167); however, in the very young, the elderly, and the immunocompromised, symptoms are more severe, occasionally resulting in death (29). Enterotoxin-producing *C. perfringens* has been implicated as an etiologic agent of persistent diarrhea in elderly patients in nursing homes and tertiary-care institutions and has been considered to play a role in antibiotic-associated diarrhea (AAD) without pseudomembranous colitis.

C. perfringens strains associated with food poisoning produce the CPE, which generally acts by forming pores in membranes of host cells (167). *C. perfringens* strains isolated from nonfoodborne diseases, such as AAD and sporadic diarrhea, carry *cpe* on a plasmid (41, 73), which may be transmitted to other strains.

Enteritis Necroticans (Pigbel and Darmbrand), Necrotizing Enteritis, and NEC

Enteritis necroticans is caused by alpha-toxin- and beta-toxin-producing strains of *C. perfringens* type C. Beta toxin is located on a plasmid (73) and is responsible mainly for pathogenesis (157, 167, 175). Enteritis necroticans is a life-threatening infection causing ischemic necrosis of the jejunum. In Papua New Guinea during the 1960s, it was found to be the most frequent cause of death in children; it has been associated with pig feasts and occurs both sporadically and in outbreaks. Immunization against the beta toxin decreased the incidence of the disease in New Guinea (120). Enteritis necroticans has also been recognized in the United States, the United Kingdom, Germany, and other developed nations, especially involving adults who are malnourished or who have diabetes, alcoholic liver disease (138, 151), or neutropenia (125). It should be noted that NEC, a disease resembling enteritis necroticans but associated with C. perfringens type A, has been found in North America in previously healthy adults (172).

NEC is a serious gastrointestinal disease affecting low-birth-weight (premature) infants hospitalized in neonatal intensive care units. The etiology and pathogenesis of this disease have remained an enigma for over 4 decades (146). Pathological similarities between NEC and enteritis necroticans include their patterns of bowel necrosis and degrees of inflammation (107). Both diseases may manifest intestinal gas cysts (107). The sources of the gas, which contains hydrogen, methane, and carbon dioxide, are probably the fermentative activities of intestinal bacteria, including clostridia. Epidemiological data support an important role for C. perfringens or other gas-producing microorganisms (e.g., "C. neonatale," certain other clostridia, or Klebsiella spp.) in the pathogenesis of NEC.

Clostridium difficile Infection (CDI)

Prevalence of CDIs
C. difficile, the major cause of antibiotic-associated pseudomembranous colitis, is also the most frequently identified cause of hospital-acquired diarrhea and is responsible for more than 250,000 cases of diarrheal disease per year in the United States, with a cost exceeding $1 billion (114). C. difficile has been isolated from feces of 3 to 5% of the healthy population, 30% of healthy neonates, and 20 to 30% of sedentary patients (185). McFarland et al. (140) reported that 21% of 399 patients with negative cultures on admission to a hospital with a high prevalence of C. difficile-associated disease (CDAD) acquired C. difficile during hospitalization. Of these patients, 63% remained asymptomatic, while 37% developed diarrhea.

Role of the PaLoc in CDI
Only strains that carry the pathogenicity locus (PaLoc) (32) possess the genetic information for the C. difficile enterotoxin, TcdA, and the cytotoxin, TcdB (tcdA and tcdB, respectively). Only strains producing TcdA and/or TcdB cause CDI. A limited number of cases of pseudomembranous colitis are caused by TcdA⁻ TcdB⁺ strains (102, 130, 137, 153) or strains that produce only TcdA (101, 130, 192). Recent results with a hamster model indicate that TcdB may be more important for disease induction than TcdA (131). Strains that carry only the genes for the binary toxin CdtA/B do not cause CDI or pseudomembranous colitis.

TcdA and TcdB, together with toxins from Clostridium sordellii, C. perfringens, and C. novyi (191), belong to the family of large clostridial cytotoxins (LCC). The molecular masses of TcdA and TcdB are 308 kDa and 270 kDa, respectively. Such LCC toxins glycosylate small GTP-binding signal proteins of the Ras family, leading to a breakdown of the cell's cytoskeleton and thus causing apoptosis (104). Both TcdA and TcdB are auto-activated once inside the cell.

However, in contrast to A-B toxins of the diphtheria type, they are single chained.

Two accessory proteins, TcdR and TcdC, of the PaLoc (32) are regulatory elements that control toxin expression (93, 137). Recently, the tcdC gene has gained diagnostic attention since it is shortened in endemic hypervirulent ribotype 027-NAP1 isolates (herein called ribotype 027 isolates) (194). Such strains seem to overproduce toxin but surely lead to more severe causes of CDI (129, 139).

Risk Factors and Course of CDI
Acquisition of C. difficile alone does not induce CDI. Several other risk factors, like age, hospitalization, severe bowel surgery, treatment with proton pump inhibitors plus a change in colonization resistance due to such treatments plus colonization with a TcdA/TcdB-producing C. difficile strain, are necessary for development of CDI.

The spectrum of symptoms ranges from mild self-limiting diarrhea to bloody-slimy diarrhea (called C. difficile-associated diarrhea) to the development of full-scale pseudomembranous colitis (24). The onset of CDI may begin immediately following antibiotic treatment or as long as 4 to 6 weeks after the course of antibiotics has been finished. Antibiotics most commonly associated with CDI are clindamycin, expanded- and broad-spectrum cephalosporins, and fluoroquinolones (189).

Bloody, mucus-filled stools generally indicate greater destruction of the colonic mucosa and hence are associated with more severe disease. Clinical diagnosis may be established by rectoscopy and the identification of pseudomembranes on the colonic mucosa. Severe cases are typically observed among the elderly, in nursing home residents, and in immunocompromised patients (24, 129, 139).

Epidemic Outbreaks
Hypervirulent strains (such as those of ribotype 027) have caused endemic outbreaks in Canada, the United States, Europe, and even worldwide (113, 129, 139). These outbreaks have occurred among younger age groups, in patients with no underlying diseases, and even among outpatients. These cases are associated with megacolon and rupture of the large bowel and are often lethal. There is evidence that use of fluoroquinolones may be an essential trigger in the onset of such endemic outbreaks (176).

Particularly vexing complications of CDIs are relapses after antibiotic treatment caused by the initial causative strain or by reinfection with a second C. difficile strain (99). Published data report relapse rates of 20 to 50%. Even the first relapse should be treated with a vancomycin step therapy (see below). Other forms of treatment, including the use of the probiotic Saccharomyces boulardii (78) and stool transplants, have been suggested, but results are not yet definitive. Eradication of C. difficile from the hospital environment is a worthy objective but a difficult task for infection control practitioners. Commonly used disinfectants are not sporicidal.

Other Etiologies of Antibiotic-Associated Diarrhea
C. difficile is responsible for ≤20% of cases of AAD (23, 198). Enterotoxin-producing C. perfringens type A has been isolated from AAD patients who are negative for C. difficile and who have no other apparent cause of the disease. Coinfection with C. difficile and enterotoxigenic C. perfringens type A has also been reported for AAD patients (1). Though the incidence of C. perfringens-associated AAD has been estimated to be 5 to 20% (15), additional

epidemiological studies are needed to accurately determine the role of this organism in AAD.

Histotoxic Clostridial Skin and Soft Tissue Infections

Histotoxic clostridial species such as *C. perfringens*, *C. histolyticum*, *C. septicum*, *C. novyi*, and *C. sordellii* cause aggressive necrotizing infections of the skin and soft tissues attributable, in part, to the elaboration of bacterial proteases, phospholipases, and cytotoxins (40). Necrotizing clostridial soft tissue infections (gas gangrene) are rapidly progressive and characterized by marked tissue destruction, gas in the tissues, shock, and frequently death (180).

Clostridial Myonecrosis

Traumatic Gas Gangrene due to *C. perfringens*

C. perfringens myonecrosis (gas gangrene) is one of the most fulminant gram-positive infections of humans. Predisposing conditions include crush-type injury, laceration of large- or medium-sized arteries, and open fractures of long bones which are contaminated with soil containing the bacterial spores. Gas gangrene of the abdominal wall and flanks occurs after penetrating injuries, such as knife or gunshot wounds, sufficient to compromise intestinal integrity, with resultant leakage of bowel contents into the soft tissues. In the last few years, cutaneous gas gangrene caused by *C. perfringens*, *C. novyi* type A, and *C. sordellii* have been described in the United States and northern Europe among drug abusers injecting "black-tar heroin" subcutaneously (18, 33, 45, 46, 106).

Clostridial gas gangrene is characterized by the sudden onset of excruciating pain at the infection site (133) and rapid development of a foul-smelling wound containing a thin serosanguinous discharge and gas bubbles. Brawny edema and induration develop and give way to cutaneous blisters containing bluish-to-maroon fluid. Later, such tissue may become liquefied and slough. The margin between healthy and necrotic tissue often advances several inches per hour despite appropriate antibiotic therapy (133), and radical amputation remains the single best life-saving treatment. Shock and organ failure frequently accompany gas gangrene, and when patients become bacteremic, the mortality exceeds 50%.

Diagnosis is not difficult because the infection (i) always begins at the site of significant trauma, (ii) is associated with gas in the tissue, and (iii) is rapidly progressive. A Gram stain of drainage or a tissue biopsy specimen is usually definitive, demonstrating large gram-positive rods and an absence of inflammatory cells. Using experimental models, Bryant and colleagues have recently demonstrated that the severe pain, rapid progression, marked tissue destruction, and absence of neutrophils in *C. perfringens* gas gangrene is caused by alpha-toxin-induced occlusion of blood vessels by platelets and neutrophils (38, 39).

Spontaneous, Nontraumatic Gas Gangrene due to *C. septicum*

The first symptom of spontaneous *C. septicum* gas gangrene may be confusion, followed by the abrupt onset of excruciating pain and rapid progression of tissue destruction, with demonstrable gas in the tissue (100, 133, 171, 181). Swelling increases, and bullae appear filled with clear, cloudy, hemorrhagic, or purplish fluid. The surrounding skin has a purple hue, perhaps reflecting vascular compromise resulting from bacterial toxins diffusing into surrounding tissues (181). The mortality of patients with spontaneous gangrene ranges from 67 to 100%, with the majority of deaths occurring within 24 h of onset. Predisposing host factors include colonic carcinoma, diverticulitis, gastrointestinal surgery, leukemia, lymphoproliferative disorders, cancer chemotherapy, radiation therapy, and, more recently, AIDS (100, 181). Cyclic, congenital, or acquired neutropenia is also strongly associated with an increased incidence of spontaneous gas gangrene due to *C. septicum*, and in such cases, NEC, cecitis, or distal ileitis is commonly found. These gastrointestinal pathologies permit bacterial access to the bloodstream; consequently, the aero-tolerant *C. septicum* can proliferate in normal tissues (171). Patients surviving bacteremia or spontaneous gangrene due to *C. septicum* should have aggressive diagnostic studies to rule out gastrointestinal pathology.

Gynecologic Infections due to *C. sordellii*

Gas gangrene of the uterus, especially that due to *C. sordellii*, has historically occurred as a consequence of illegal or self-induced abortions but in modern times also follows spontaneous abortion, normal vaginal delivery, and cesarean section (reviewed in reference 7). Recently, *C. sordellii* has also been implicated in medically induced abortions (7). Young, previously healthy women with fatal postpartum *C. sordellii* infections present with a unique clinical picture of little or no fever, a lack of a purulent discharge, refractory hypotension, extensive peripheral edema and effusions, hemoconcentration, and a markedly elevated white blood cell count (7). Death in these cases ensues rapidly, and the infection is almost uniformly fatal (7).

Other Clostridial Skin and Soft Tissue Infections

Crepitant cellulitis, also called anaerobic cellulitis, is seen principally in diabetic patients and characteristically involves subcutaneous tissues or retroperitoneal tissues and can progress to fulminant systemic disease; the muscle and fascia are not involved.

Cases of *C. histolyticum* infection with cellulitis, abscess formation, or endocarditis have also been documented in injecting drug users (16). *C. sordellii* was responsible for endophthalmitis after suture removal after a corneal transplant (205). *C. perfringens* endophthalmitis due to penetrating injuries is a fulminant infection (92).

Exotoxins of the Histotoxic Clostridia

Our current understanding of the potent toxins produced by these clostridia is based upon studies done between World Wars I and II, when gas gangrene was a major complication of battlefield injuries. Investigators of this period designated the major lethal toxins of these bacteria with Greek letters, with the letter "α" always used to designate the most potent or most significant lethal factor. A marvelous review of these data can be found in the monograph by Smith (171). Over the ensuing decades, modern technology has provided a greater understanding of the mechanisms of action of some of these factors.

Major Extracellular Toxins of *C. perfringens*

The major *C. perfringens* extracellular toxins implicated in gas gangrene are alpha toxin and theta toxin. Alpha toxin is a lethal lecithinase that has both phospholipase C and sphingomyelinase activities and has been implicated as the major virulence factor based upon the observation that immunization of mice with purified recombinant protein consisting of the C-terminal alpha-toxin domain (amino acids 247 to 370) provided protection against lethal challenge with *C. perfringens* (199). In addition, intravascular activation of platelets by alpha toxin leads to platelet aggregation (38, 184) and formation of occlusive thrombi that completely and irreversibly occlude capillaries, venules, and arterioles (38, 39). Without adequate tissue perfusion, the anaerobic niche is extended and rapid destruction of viable tissue, so characteristic of clostridial gas gangrene, ensues.

Theta toxin from *C. perfringens* (also known as perfringolysin) is a member of the thiol-activated cytolysin family, now termed cholesterol-dependent cytolysins, that includes streptolysin O from group A streptococci, pneumolysin from *Streptococcus pneumoniae*, and several others. Upon contact with cholesterol in the host's cell membranes, theta-toxin monomers oligomerize and insert into the membrane, forming a pore and resulting in cell lysis (161). Theta toxin contributes to the pathogenesis of gas gangrene, likely by its ability to modulate the inflammatory response to infection (37, 182).

Major Extracellular Toxins of *C. septicum*

C. septicum produces four main toxins, alpha toxin (α, lethal, hemolytic, necrotizing activity), beta toxin (β, DNase), gamma toxin (γ, hyaluronidase), and delta toxin (δ, septicolysin, an oxygen-labile hemolysin), as well as a protease and a neuraminidase (171). Unlike the alpha toxin from *C. perfringens*, the *C. septicum* alpha toxin does not possess phospholipase activity. Active immunization against alpha toxin significantly protects against challenge with viable *C. septicum* (17).

Major Extracellular Toxins of *C. sordellii*

Pathogenic strains of *C. sordellii* produce up to seven identified exotoxins. Of these, lethal toxin (LT) and hemorrhagic toxin (HT) are regarded as the major virulence factors. LT and HT are members of the LCC family, all having molecular masses between 250 and 308 kDa. Other members include the *C. difficile* toxins A and B and *C. novyi* alpha toxin. All LCCs possess remarkable amino acid similarity, with identities ranging between 26 and 76%. LT and *C. difficile* toxin B have the highest homology, with amino acid sequences being 76% identical and 90% homologous to one another. All LCCs possess glycosyltransferase activity and modify signaling molecules that control the cell cycle, apoptosis, gene transcription, and the structural functions of actin, such as cell morphology, migration, and polarity. Once modified, these proteins become inoperative. Modification of actin cytoskeletal assembly and organization presumably leads to the massive capillary leakage characteristic of *C. sordellii* infection. The *C. sordellii* neuraminidase has been shown to contribute to the leukemoid reaction, in part, by enhancing the proliferation of granulocyte progenitor cells (6). Other exotoxins include an oxygen-labile hemolysin, DNase, collagenase, and lysolecithinase; however, their roles in pathogenesis have not been extensively investigated.

Botulism

The Organism and Its Toxin

C. botulinum is the cause of the rare but frequently fatal illness known as botulism and which is characterized by sudden flaccid paralysis. Spores of *C. botulinum* are widely distributed in soil and aquatic habitats. *C. botulinum*, along with unique strains of *C. butyricum*, *C. baratii*, and *C. argentinense*, can produce BoNT, the most lethal poison known. The intravenous lethal dose for BoNT has been estimated as 0.1 to 0.5 ng per kg of body weight, and BoNT is among the most potent protein toxins by oral ingestion, with an estimated oral lethal dose of 0.2 to 1 μg per kg (13). There are seven antigenic serotypes of BoNT (A through G) (115), which serve as useful clinical and epidemiological markers (132). Toxin serotypes A, B, and E of *C. botulinum* are the principal causes of botulism in humans (88). Neurotoxigenic strains of *C. butyricum* (70) and *C. baratii* (19, 86, 149) that produce type E and F neurotoxins, respectively, have been implicated mainly in infant botulism. Type E botulinal-toxin-producing *C. butyricum* strains were confirmed by sequencing of the16S rRNA gene (49), leading to the conclusion that neurotoxigenic *C. butyricum* must be regarded as an emergent foodborne pathogen. *C. argentinense*, which produces type G neurotoxin (88), has been isolated from soil in Argentina. Its reported isolation from autopsy materials from five individuals who died suddenly has not been substantiated, and *C. argentinense* has not been clearly implicated in botulism. *C. botulinum* types C and D are associated primarily with botulism in birds and mammals (97, 168). Strains of *C. botulinum* that produce more than one serotype of BoNTs, generally with one serotype being formed in much higher levels, have been isolated from the environment and human and animal botulism cases (88, 96). The BoNTs are coexpressed with nontoxic proteins of toxin gene clusters (31), and evidence suggests that the complexes are much more stable than the labile BoNTs in the gastrointestinal tract. The genes for BoNT complex formation are associated with unstable genetic elements in certain serotypes, enabling toxin gene transfer to nontoxigenic clostridial species that are closely related to *C. botulinum*, such as *C. sporogenes* and *C. subterminale* (64).

There are four naturally occurring types of botulism: (i) classical foodborne botulism, an intoxication caused by the ingestion of preformed botulinal toxin in contaminated food; (ii) wound botulism, which results from elaboration of botulinal toxin in vivo after the growth of *C. botulinum* in an infected wound; (iii) infant botulism, in which botulinal toxin is elaborated in vivo in the gastrointestinal tract of an infant colonized with *C. botulinum*; and (iv) botulism due to intestinal colonization in children and adults (12, 88). Intestinal colonization in adults has been associated with surgery and administration of antibiotics (88). *C. botulinum* has been isolated from patients colonized with *C. difficile* (70), with viral infections (69), or with Crohn's disease (83). Recently, an international outbreak of botulism caused by commercial carrot juice was reported by Sheth et al. (162).

Regardless of the category of botulism, the toxin enters the bloodstream at a peripheral site (e.g., gut, wound, or lung) and is transferred to the neuromuscular junctions of motor neurons, where it binds irreversibly to the presynaptic membranes. The site of action of all serotypes of BoNT is the presynaptic terminal of motor neurons (51, 110, 117, 158). Elucidation of the three-dimensional structures of botulinum and tetanus toxins and their constituent domains has provided considerable insights into their mechanisms of action (116, 117, 158, 186). BoNT penetrates the plasma membrane by receptor-mediated endocytosis, and the light chain of 50 kDa (the catalytic domain) is internalized into the nerve cell through a protein channel (117, 158). Once internalized, BoNT specifically cleaves proteins involved in vesicle trafficking of neurotransmitters to the membrane (158). Exocytosis of acetylcholine is prevented at the nerve terminal to the neuromuscular junction, with consequent blockage of innervation of muscle activity (158). The clinical hallmark of botulism is an acute flaccid paralysis, which begins with bilateral cranial nerve impairment involving muscles of the eyes, face, head, and pharynx and then descends symmetrically to involve muscles of the thorax and extremities. Botulinum toxin, unlike TeNT, probably does not enter the central nervous system (CNS). In naturally occurring foodborne botulism, gastrointestinal symptoms (e.g., abdominal cramps, nausea, vomiting, or diarrhea [more often constipation or obstipation]) may precede the neurologic signs of descending flaccid paralysis. Death results from respiratory failure caused by paralysis of the tongue or muscles of the pharynx, leading to occlusion of the upper airway or from paralysis of the diaphragm and intercostal muscles (13, 51). Generally, the patient's hearing remains normal, consciousness is not lost, and the victim is cognizant of the progression of the disease, which of course can be a terrifying experience.

Wound Botulism in Intravenous Drug Users

An association between botulism and subcutaneous injection of Mexican black-tar heroin into muscle or skin (skin popping) has been reported in the United States and in the United Kingdom (34, 135). A study found 33 clinically diagnosed cases of wound botulism in the United Kingdom and Ireland between 2000 and 2002 (34). The clinical diagnosis was confirmed by laboratory tests in 20 of these cases; 18 cases were caused by type A toxin and 2 by type B toxin. Wound botulism has also occurred after snorting of cocaine (111), cosmetic injection of an unlicensed Botox preparation (52), and a tooth extraction (195).

Infant Botulism

Infant botulism is the most frequently recognized form of botulism in the United States (45% of cases in California) and has been reported in at least 15 other countries (12, 61, 75, 76, 148, 188). The geographic distribution of toxin types in infant botulism cases has paralleled the spore distribution of *C. botulinum* toxin types in soils sampled from different locations (12). Type A has been the most frequent BoNT type in cases of infant botulism in states west of the Mississippi River, whereas type B cases have predominated east of the Mississippi River (12, 170). Three cases have been caused by a strain(s) of *C. botulinum* that produced toxins requiring both type B and F antitoxins for neutralization (88). Type E infant botulism, caused by neurotoxigenic strains of *C. butyricum*, was initially confirmed in two infants from Italy (76), and later in additional patients. Type F infant botulism has been caused by neurotoxigenic *C. baratii* (76).

Most infants that contract botulism are 3 weeks to 6 months old (12), and the only clearly defined risk factors have been exposure to soil, dust, and honey (12, 75). Since *C. botulinum* spores have not been detected in any food or liquid ingested by these infants other than honey (12), it is recommended that honey not be fed to infants less than 1 year of age. Whatever the sources, the ingested spores of *C. botulinum* germinate within the intestinal tract, and the vegetative cells multiply and produce the neurotoxin, which is then absorbed into the bloodstream (12, 88). The first sign of illness is usually constipation, which is often overlooked. Infants develop lethargy and mild weakness, with feeding difficulties, pooled oral secretions, and an altered cry (12). They eventually lose head control and may go on to develop ophthalmoplegia, ptosis, flaccid facial expression, dysphagia, other signs of cranial nerve deficits, generalized muscular weakness, and finally respiratory insufficiency and the inability to swallow. There is likely a spectrum of clinical features in infant botulism, ranging from mild illness not requiring hospitalization to severe botulism requiring intensive care. Human immune globulin that neutralizes BoNT

(BabyBIG; intravenous BIG-IV) has been licensed to the California Department of Public Health Infant Botulism Treatment & Prevention Program [www.infantbotulism.org; 24-h/7-day phone, (510) 231-7600] since 2003 (14, 75). Since 2007, it has been made available to physicians outside the United States on a case-by-case basis. Early treatment has shortened hospital stays and significantly reduced the associated costs of hospitalization (77).

Botulinum Toxin as a Bioterrorism Agent

Inhalational botulism, which results from aerosolization and inhalation of botulinum toxin, has been considered a fifth category of botulism (13, 152, 165). Botulism could also result from covert contamination of foods (13, 196). Inhalational botulism has been demonstrated experimentally in monkeys (13, 152), accidentally in three veterinary personnel in Germany who were exposed to reaerosolized BoNT from rabbits and guinea pigs with aerosolized BoNT on their fur (13), and three researchers who were exposed to an aerosol during BoNT manipulations (91). Terrorists have attempted to use aerosolized botulinum toxin as a bioweapon in Japan but were not successful. Although inhalational botulism is possible, the toxin is unstable in aerosols, and the more likely route of intentional intoxication is by food contamination and oral ingestion.

Tetanus

Tetanus, caused by *C. tetani*, is often associated with puncture wounds that do not appear to be infected. The organism and its spores can be isolated from a variety of sources, including soil and the intestinal contents of numerous animal species. A potent neurotoxin (TeNT), often referred to as tetanospasmin, is elaborated at the site of trauma and rapidly binds to neural tissue, provoking a characteristic paralysis and tonic spasms (26). Tetanus is a totally preventable infection with immunization with tetanus toxoid.

Tetanus is an intoxication analogous to botulism except that it occurs solely through wound infection and production of tetanospasmin (TeNT). TeNT is synthesized as a single, inactive polypeptide chain (150 kDa), which is cleaved by an intrinsic protease to produce an active form, consisting of a heavy chain (100 kDa) and a light chain (50 kDa) linked by a disulfide bond (158). The heavy chain binds to neuronal cells, and the three-dimensional structure of this region has been elucidated (158). The light chain, a zinc endopeptidase, enters the cell cytoplasm and traverses from the nerve terminal to the nerve cell body by retrograde axonal transport (26, 158), eventually reaching neurons in the spinal cord and brain stem, where it affects glycinergic and GABA (γ-amino-*n*-butyric acid)-ergic neurotransmission (26, 158). Inhibitory impulses to CNS neurons are blocked, while uninhibited firing of motor nerve transmission continues, resulting in prolonged muscle spasms of both flexor and extensor muscles that can persist for weeks. The mechanism by which exocytosis of neurotransmitter release is inhibited is analogous to that of BoNT; in fact, TeNT cleaves the vesicle-associated membrane protein (VAMP) at the same peptide bond as BoNT B (117). Unlike with the pathophysiology of botulism, TeNT is retrogradely transported in neurons to the CNS and its site of action (26, 158).

The worldwide incidence of tetanus has been estimated to be as many as 500,000 cases per year (26). Neonatal tetanus is endemic in developing countries due to a lack of vaccine programs for infants or adult women. In developed countries, injection of drugs (i.e., skin popping) has recently become an important risk factor (21, 85).

Additional Clostridial Species of Interest

C. innocuum is associated with bacteremia in immunocompromised hosts and has also been recovered from patients with recurrent CDAD (3). It is often resistant to multiple drugs used to treat anaerobic infections (3). *C. ramosum* was the second-most-common *Clostridium* species (after *C. perfringens*) identified from clinical specimens from children, including those with abscesses, peritonitis, bacteremia, and chronic otitis media (35), and the third-most-common *Clostridium* species in adult cases of bacteremia (122). This species may be resistant to clindamycin and multiple cephalosporins. As noted earlier, *C. tertium* is often isolated from blood cultures from immunocompromised patients and has been reported as a cause of neutropenic enterocolitis and meningitis (56, 109, 124, 183). *C. hathewayi* and *C. bolteae* have been isolated from a variety of human infections (72, 203), including a fatal case of sepsis (128). Phenotypically similar *C. clostridioforme* is one of the clostridia most commonly isolated from human infections and appears to be associated with human infections that are more serious or invasive than infections with *C. hathewayi* or *C. bolteae*.

The emergence of 16S rRNA gene sequencing technology has provided a means of identification of strains that may previously have been misidentified or classified as *Clostridium* without species identification. Examples are from cases of bacteremia caused by *C. hathewayi* (203), *C. intestinale* (66), and *C. symbiosum* (65); fatal sepsis due to *C. fallax* in a previously healthy 16-year-old (89); and abscesses yielding *C. celerecrescens* (80). Microarray analysis of DNA from fecal samples has also been useful in the determination of predominant species in the large bowel (193). It is likely that in this era of molecular identification techniques, a more accurate picture of clostridial infections will emerge.

CLINICAL MICROBIOLOGY OF CLOSTRIDIAL DISEASES

General Methods for Collection, Transport, and Storage of Clinical Specimens

The proper selection, collection, and transport of clinical specimens are extremely important for the laboratory diagnosis of clostridial infections. For recommended collection and transport procedures in general, refer to chapter 16.

Specific Methods for Collection and Direct Examination of Clinical Specimens

In addition to requiring aspirates and tissues, selected clostridial illnesses require special specimens. The methods for collection and direct examination of these specimens are described below.

Suspected Gas Gangrene or Necrotizing Fasciitis

Gas gangrene and necrotizing fasciitis represent extremely urgent situations requiring rapid clinical diagnoses. Multiple tissue specimens should be sampled from the active sites of infection when gas gangrene is suspected, because clostridia are often not distributed uniformly in pathologic lesions. The direct examination of a Gram-stained smear of the wound is of major importance for the early presumptive diagnosis of gas gangrene (10). Characteristic findings in *C. perfringens* infections include the absence of leukocytic infiltration and the presence of clostridia in smears prepared from central areas of the lesion. Special note should be made of Gram-positive rods, with or without spores,

because sporulation in tissue is not common for the two species most frequently encountered in wound and abscess materials, *C. perfringens* and *C. ramosum*. *C. perfringens* usually appears as large, relatively short, fat, gram-positive rods with blunt ends and often in short chains in tissue smears; the cells of *C. ramosum* are more slender and longer (Fig. 1). *C. perfringens* may or may not be encapsulated in smears from wounds; capsules usually are present in smears of endometrial specimens from postabortion *C. perfringens* infections. Spore stains offer no advantage over Gram stains for demonstration of spores, but examination with a phase-contrast or dark-field microscope may be helpful if the spores are close to maturity. If spores are present, shapes (spherical or oval) and positions (terminal, subterminal, or central) in the cells should be noted.

Suspected *C. perfringens* Foodborne Illness

A freshly passed fecal specimen and the suspected food are the preferred specimens for *C. perfringens* culture and toxin assays. These specimens should be placed into sterile containers, stored at 4°C, and shipped on cold packs as soon as possible. For optimal recovery, stool specimens should be processed within 24 h of collection. Swab specimens are inadequate for the toxin assay because the sample volume is insufficient.

Several methods have been described for the detection of CPE in feces, including cell culture assays, enzyme-linked immunosorbent assay (ELISA), and reversed-phase latex agglutination (141, 178). The cell culture assay using Vero cells is not as sensitive or as reproducible as other methods (15, 74). The results of the RPLA kit (PET-RPLA; Oxoid, Hampshire, United Kingdom, and Remel Inc., Lenexa, KS) are reproducible, and the test is reasonably sensitive; however, nonspecific interference by fecal matter has been reported (141). Similarly, the background bacterial DNA in stool has been reported to interfere with PCR amplification of the enterotoxin gene (141). While an in-house ELISA system developed by the Food Safety Microbiology Laboratory of the Central Public Health Laboratory, London, United Kingdom, has been reported to be the most sensitive assay and is considered the gold standard, the TechLab (Blacksburg, Virginia) CPE ELISA system has also provided a specific, reliable, and practical tool for detecting CPE in fecal samples (15, 74).

Suspected Enteritis Necroticans (*C. perfringens* Type C)

If enteritis necroticans is suspected, the appropriate specimens include three blood cultures from three different venipuncture sites, stool (at least 25 g, or 25 ml if liquid), and bowel luminal contents or tissue from the involved bowel (e.g., surgical specimen or autopsy material). Specimens should be transported in tightly sealed, leakproof containers for the following: direct Gram staining, culture, isolation, identification, and typing of *C. perfringens*. PCR assays for genotyping *C. perfringens* are being used in certain research or referral laboratories to aid in diagnosis (175). Accordingly, DNA can be extracted for this purpose from formalin-fixed intestinal tissue or culture and amplified by PCR using primers specific for the *cpa* and *cpb* genes of *C. perfringens* type C.

Suspected CDI

Among the prerequisites for initiating a detailed microbiologic diagnosis of CDI are (i) diarrhea as the lead symptom, (ii) the onset of diarrheal episodes 2 to 3 days after hospitalization without exposure to other obvious inducing microorganisms, (iii) diarrhea for more than 3 days without

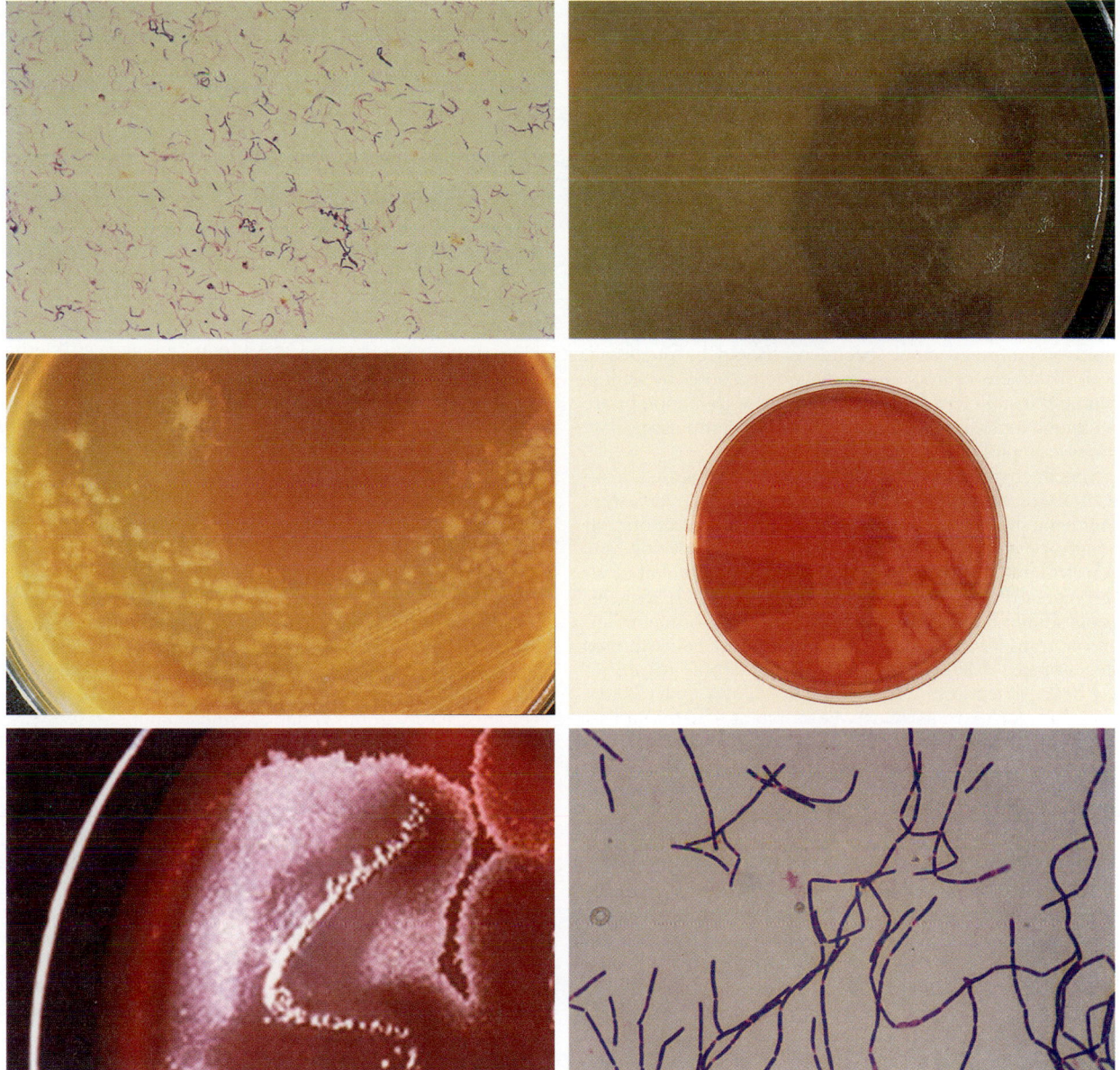

FIGURE 1 (top row, left) Gram stain of C. *ramosum*. Note the thin, Gram stain-variable bacilli with distinct spores. Reprinted with permission from reference 103.
FIGURE 2 (top row, right) Lecithinase reaction on egg yolk agar. Note the opacity of the agar surrounding colonies due to precipitation of complex fats. Reprinted with permission from reference 103.
FIGURE 3 (middle row, left) C. *difficile* on CCFA. Note the yellow, ground-glass appearance of colonies. Reprinted with permission from reference 103.
FIGURE 4 (middle row, right) C. *perfringens* on blood agar showing a double zone of beta-hemolysis. Reprinted with permission from reference 103.
FIGURE 5 (bottom row, left) *Clostridium septicum* on blood agar after 12 h of incubation. Note the spreading colonies. Courtesy of E. J. Baron.
FIGURE 6 (bottom row, right) Gram stain of C. *septicum*. Note the long, filamentous bacilli with rare spores. Courtesy of E. J. Baron.

the causing organism being identified, (iv) a history of antibiotic treatment of the patient, (v) belonging to a risk group (being >65 of age or immunosuppressed or having severe gastrointestinal disease or another severe underlying diseases), and (vi) frequent exposure to C. *difficile*, such as with exposure to nurses or other medical personnel.

Confirming the diagnosis of C. *difficile*-associated enteric disease on the basis of both clinical and laboratory criteria represents the ultimate gold standard. Different algorithms are successfully applied in routine laboratory diagnoses. The different approaches are sometimes governed by the number of stool samples to be processed in a laboratory unit. Generally, laboratory results obtained with immunologic tests must be correlated and interpreted within the context of the patient's clinical presentation. The diagnosis of CDI has gained more attention since the appearance of hypervirulent ribotype 027 strains. However, it needs to be noted that more-severe cases also may arise from strains of other ribotypes.

Submission of Specimens

A single, freshly passed fecal specimen (ideally 10 to 20 ml of watery stool; minimum of 5.0 ml or 5 g) is the preferred specimen for C. difficile culture and toxin assay. To lessen the chance of obtaining positive culture results from patients merely colonized with the organism, only liquid or unformed stool specimens should be processed. Swab specimens of stool are inadequate because the sample volume is insufficient for the toxin assay. Other appropriate specimens include bowel luminal contents and surgical or autopsy samples of the large bowel.

Specimens should be transported in tightly sealed, leak-proof plastic or glass containers. For optimal recovery, stool specimens should be cultured within 2 h of collection. Although spores survive in refrigerated stool for several days, there will probably be a large decrease in the number of viable vegetative cells of C. difficile in refrigerated specimens. Stools should be placed in an anaerobic environment (anaerobic transport vial or bag) if culture must be performed after storage. Adequate recovery of C. difficile organisms may be expected from stools stored at 4°C for up to 2 days. Specimens for toxin assay may be stored at 4°C for up to 3 days or should be frozen at −70°C if performance of the assay is delayed. Freezing at −20°C results in a dramatic loss of cytotoxin activity, so detection limits may no longer be reached.

Cell Culture-Based Methods of Diagnosis of CDI

Cultivation of C. difficile is not necessary for the molecularly based toxin assays described below; however, cultivation is encouraged for subsequent molecular substrain typing and epidemiologic studies. Cytotoxicity testing of cell cultures has long been called the gold standard of C. difficile toxin testing due to its high sensitivity (94 to 100%) and high specificity (99%) (60). However, normally only the activity of the TcdB cytotoxin is monitored, since TcdA needs to be tested on special cells, like HT29 cells (187). Also, the specificity of toxin-induced cytotoxicity is dependent upon neutralization of this effect by a TcdB-specific antitoxin performed in parallel. The need for neutralization of this effect marks a limitation of the test, and not every laboratory should perform neutralization due to time and cost considerations.

Immunologic Methods for Diagnosis of CDI

Commercial tests that are available are listed in Table 2. Currently, the best approach is the detection of TcdA and TcdB by enzyme immunoassay directly from stool specimens; however, immunoassays generally show lower sensitivities and specificities (45 to 95% and 75 to 100%, respectively) than the tissue culture assay (136, 190). The result of toxin testing is the declaration of the sample as being toxin positive or negative without any differentiation of TcdA and TcdB. Immunological toxin detection should be done promptly (within 24 h) following the collection of the sample. Due to the limitations of the specificity and sensitivity of the enzyme immunoassay, the test should be repeated if initial results are negative and if the clinical diagnosis is that of a

CDI. The immunoassays that have been introduced commercially all recognize TcdA effectively but recognize TcdB with a different efficiency. TcdA is the antigen that is more easily detectable, and the tcdA gene is highly conserved. In contrast, TcdB genes differ greatly between strains, and TcdB antibodies are much more difficult to obtain. Single monoclonal antibodies detect only some of the TcdB isoforms.

Testing of TcdA alone is no longer recommended, since some epidemic strains produce only TcdB (198). Difficulties arise especially when C. difficile toxins are detected in strains like ribotype 017 strains, which are TcdA$^-$ and TcdB$^+$, since sensitivity for TcdB is less than for TcdA. Recent work with hamsters has attributed more importance to TcdB (131); in that study, genetically manipulated strains deficient in TcdA production were still lethal, while TcdA-positive strains in which the tcdB gene was interrupted were not (131). Attempts to concentrate on the detection of TcdB (or its gene) alone are problematic since CDI may be caused by strains that produce TcdA only (101, 130, 192).

Lateral-flow quick tests of different formats are being developed as "bedside tests." In the future, with such tests one might even differentiate between both toxins.

Antigen Detection (of GDH) for Diagnosis of CDI

Laboratories with high throughput are increasingly utilizing detection of glutamate dehydrogenase (GDH), the method of choice for screening stool samples for C. difficile. GDH is secreted by C. difficile into the stool and may be detected by commercial enzyme immunoassays. Since GDH is not an enzyme exclusive to C. difficile, its detection is not pathognomonic for CDI and the test does not inform us about the existence of the PaLoc or its toxin profile. Lack of detection of GDH has a high negative predictive value, but false positives occur. Accordingly, it is important to analyze GDH-positive stool samples for TcdA/TcdB, preferably on the same day, to support the diagnosis of CDI. Stools that are GDH positive, while toxin negative, should be routinely cultured, and the strains should be submitted for toxin detection. Strains that remain GDH positive and toxin negative are clearly atoxinogenic and thus apathogenic C. difficile isolates, and this represents a true false-positive GDH test.

DNA-Based Methods for Diagnosis of CDI

Different commercial assays for the detection of the tcdA/tcdB genes have recently become available (e.g., by BD, bioMérieux, and Seegene). A handicap of any genetic analysis is that C. difficile colonization is not necessarily connected to CDI, since healthy carriers exist. It is only when a high quantity of gene product (i.e., toxins) is expressed that CDI results. Thus, if a PCR remains negative, CDI may be excluded to a high degree. The predictive value of a negative PCR is, however, lost if testing is not reliable enough to definitively exclude the presence of genetic variation within the gene of interest. This outcome is also the reason why tests that detect only a single gene of the PaLoc, like tcdB, cannot be recommended for routine use. The known variability of the tcdB gene classifies this gene as a poor candidate for PCR diagnosis.

All tests are performed on DNA extracted from stool specimens by the use of a commercial DNA preparation kit (e.g., those of Qiagen and MN-net). Among the prerequisites of a reliable PCR assay, detection of a C. difficile-specific housekeeping gene (e.g., rrs, encoding the 16S ribosomal subunit, or gluD, encoding the GDH) is

TABLE 2 Commonly used tests for the diagnosis of C. *difficile* disease

Entity detected	Method[a]	Principal advantage(s)	Principal limitation(s)	Available test(s)	Source(s)
Organisms	Culture	Sensitive, specific	Efficiency varies from lab to lab; must add method for toxin detection	CCFA is available from various suppliers; pre-reduced media preferred	Anaerobe Systems, Morgan Hill, CA (www.anaerobesystems.com)
GDH	LA	Rapid, simple	Low sensitivity; does not distinguish between toxigenic and nontoxigenic C. *difficile* strains	C. *difficile* test kit	Thermo Fisher Scientific-Remel Products, Lenexa, KS (www.remel.com)
	EIA	Rapid, simple; higher sensitivity than LA	Does not distinguish between toxigenic and nontoxigenic C. *difficile* strains	ImmunoCard C. *difficile* C. *diff* Chek	Meridian Bioscience, Cincinnati, OH (www.meridianbioscience.com) TechLab, Inc., Blacksburg, VA (www.techlab.com)
GDH + toxin A	EIA	Rapid, simple; higher sensitivity than LA	Cannot distinguish between toxin B-positive and -negative strains	Triage C. *difficile* panel	Biosite Diagnostics Inc., San Diego, CA (www.biosite.com)
Toxin A	LA	Rapid, simple	Low sensitivity	Culturette CDT kit	Becton Dickinson (BD), Sparks, MD (www.bd.com)
	EIA	Rapid, simple	Sensitivity and specificity vary considerably; does not detect A⁻/B⁺ isolates	C. *difficile* toxin A	Thermo Fisher Scientific-Remel/Oxoid
	ICA	Rapid, simple	Less sensitive than EIA	ColorPAC toxin A test kit Clearview C. *difficile* toxin A	bioMérieux, Marcy-l'Etoile, France (www.biomerieux-diagnostics.com) Inverness Medical Professional Diagnostics, Princeton, NJ (www.invernessmedicalpd.com)
Toxin B	CTA	Sensitive, specific	Requires 24–48 h to complete; toxin B can be inactivated, resulting in false-negative results	C. *difficile* Tox-B test	TechLab, Inc.
Toxins A and B	EIA	Rapid, simple, detects A⁻/B⁺ isolates	Sensitivity and specificity vary considerably	Premier toxins A and B ProSpecT C. *difficile* toxin A/B microplate C. *difficile* Tox A/B II ImmunoCard toxins A and B Xpert C. *difficile* toxin A/B Tox A/B Quik Chek	Meridian Bioscience Thermo Fisher Scientific-Remel Products TechLab, Inc. Meridian Bioscience Thermo Fisher Scientific-Remel Products Inverness Medical Professional Diagnostics
	Automated		Requires automated system	VIDAS C. *difficile* A & B	bioMérieux (www.biomerieux-diagnostics.com)
GDH + toxins A and B	EIA	Rapid, simple	Detects and differentiates between toxigenic and nontoxigenic strains	C. diff Quik Chek Complete	TechLab, Inc.

[a]CTA, cell culture-based cytotoxicity assay; LA, latex agglutination; EIA, enzyme immunoassay; ICA, immunochromatographic assay.

necessary to be sure that C. *difficile* is in the sample at all. In samples positive for the housekeeping gene but negative for genes of the PaLoc, a nontoxinogenic C. *difficile* isolate is highly probable. Since it was reported that such strains may protect against colonization with toxigenic strains (68), this may even argue against a cause of CDI. Thus, PCR-based approaches that detect only a single gene should be considered unreliable for CDI diagnosis because of the adverse consequences that a negative test result would have on treatment decisions.

Approaches that simultaneously detect a variety of species-specific genes and virulence factors (e.g., *tcdA* and *tcdB* genes, *cdtA* and *cdtB* genes, and *tcdC* [Cepheid]) should be developed and evaluated for their usefulness in routine diagnosis. Such assays would be of a high predictive value since, for example, infection with a hypervirulent 027 strain could be diagnosed. A potential dilemma that must be considered is that hypervirulence is not solely associated with ribotype 027, and so a singular focus on this ribotype may be misleading.

Suspected Neutropenic Enterocolitis Involving *C. septicum*

The specimens of choice for suspected neutropenic enterocolitis involving *C. septicum* are (i) three blood cultures collected from three different venipuncture sites, (ii) stool (at least 25 g, or 25 ml if liquid), and (iii) luminal contents or tissue from the involved ileocecal area collected at surgery or autopsy and transported in tightly sealed leakproof containers. In addition, a biopsy sample of muscle (or an aspirate of fluid from the involved area, taken with a needle and syringe) should be collected if the patient is also suspected of having myonecrosis or another form of progressive infection.

Suspected *C. botulinum* or *C. tetani* Infection or Intoxication

Most hospital laboratories are not properly equipped to process specimens from patients suspected of having botulism. Before collecting any specimens, the medical care providers who suspect a diagnosis of botulism in a patient should immediately call their state health department's emergency 24-h telephone number or the CDC in Atlanta, GA [(770) 488-7100, 24-h/7-day emergency service] so that appropriate action can be taken to establish the diagnosis, initiate treatment, and investigate the case. Acceptable specimens include feces, enema fluid, gastric aspirates or vomitus, tissue or exudates, and postmortem specimens. These specimens should be placed into sterile unbreakable containers. Serum specimens (preferably >10 ml) should be collected as soon as possible after the onset of symptoms. Clinical swabs should be collected in an anaerobic transport medium; environmental swabs (from which spores may be isolated) may be sent in plastic containers without any medium. Food specimens should be left in their original containers, if possible, or placed in sterile unbreakable containers. All specimens should be stored at 4°C and shipped on cold packs as soon as possible. Further information can be found at the CDC botulism website (http://www .bt.cdc.gov/agent/botulism). Laboratories should have all of the pertinent information and contact numbers handy. During investigations of possible bioterrorism, sera, gastric aspirates, feces, and environmental or nasal swabs could be useful for detecting aerosolized botulinum toxin that may have been inhaled (10, 204). All specimens should be refrigerated until they can be transported to the laboratory for testing.

Certain clostridial toxins, particularly BoNT, TeNT, and iota toxin, are extremely toxic molecules and are considered very potent poisons. The CDC recommends biosafety level 3 primary containment and personnel precautions for facilities producing BoNTs for study. Ideally, personnel who work in laboratories should be immunized with a pentavalent (A to E) toxoid; however, the vaccine is no longer available from the CDC. A biosafety manual should be posted in the laboratory and should contain the proper emergency phone numbers and procedures for emergency response. Regulations governing personnel safety for research with select agents are outlined in the *Code of Federal Regulations* (67a) and the manual *Biosafety in Microbiological and Biomedical Laboratories* (46a).

Direct Toxin Detection

Bioassays for BoNT and TeNT are currently the most important laboratory tests for the diagnosis of botulism and tetanus (44, 63, 88). The definitive diagnosis of botulism is the detection of BoNT (not the organism) (88). Currently, the only reliable assay for BoNT is the mouse bioassay, together with neutralization of mouse toxicity with type-specific antitoxins (88, 197). Detection of neurotoxins is usually performed on fecal specimens, blood (serum), suspect foods in cases of foodborne botulism, and culture fluid following enrichment by growth of the organism (44, 88). ELISAs, cell culture systems (87), and biosensor platforms (62, 160) have also been used to detect BoNT (63, 160). Real-time PCR assays for detection of *C. botulinum* BoNT gene fragments specific to BoNT A, B, and E have been developed as alternatives to the mouse bioassay; this approach was found to demonstrate a sensitivity and specificity similar to those of conventional approaches (5, 59). Potential problems with PCR detection are strains that have the gene but do not produce toxin. Thus, the bioassay remains the study of choice.

ISOLATION PROCEDURES

Isolation and Appearance on Plated Media

A summary of useful procedures for culture and isolation of clostridia is provided below. Clostridia usually produce good growth on commercially available CDC anaerobe blood agar and phenylethyl alcohol blood agar (PEA) after 1 to 2 days of incubation. Brucella agar with 5% sheep blood, Columbia agar, or brain-heart infusion agar supplemented with yeast extract, vitamin K, and hemin may also be used as the non-selective blood agar medium. Colony characteristics vary on different media. A few species, such as *C. perfringens*, form colonies after overnight incubation or in as little as 6 h. When clostridia are suspected in wound or abscess specimens (e.g., gas gangrene), egg yolk agar (modified McClung-Toabe formula [see chapter 17]) should also be inoculated.

After incubation, the blood agar and PEA cultures should be examined under a dissecting microscope, with attention being paid to the hemolysis pattern, colony structure, and evidence of swarming or motile colonies. Egg yolk agar should be examined for evidence of lecithinase (Fig. 2) or lipase production. Lecithinase activity is indicated by the development of an insoluble, opaque, whitish precipitate within the agar. An iridescent sheen or oil-on-water appearance (pearly layer) indicates lipase activity. Proteolysis, the third reaction that can be seen on egg yolk agar, is indicated by a zone of translucent clearing in the medium around the colonies. The same reactions can be visualized on the hemin-supplemented egg yolk agar formulation recommended by Jousimies-Somer et al. (103) or on Lombard-Dowell egg yolk agar (201), in addition to on the modified McClung-Toabe egg yolk agar formulation.

Isolation of additional strains in the presence of swarming *Proteus* species or *C. septicum* may require short incubation times (18 to 24 h), subculture onto PEA, or use of anaerobe blood agar with 4% agar ("stiff blood agar"). When isolated colonies can be picked, they should be subcultured to chopped-meat medium and incubated overnight for the inoculation of differential media. Prereduced, anaerobically sterilized (PRAS) peptone-yeast-glucose media may be inoculated for detection of metabolic products by gas-liquid chromatography (GLC) if the laboratory has that capability.

Spore Selection Techniques

Heat or ethanol treatment procedures can aid in detecting spores (103, 108). Ethanol may be more effective than heat if the specimen contains relatively heat-sensitive clostridia (e.g., *C. botulinum* type E and some strains of *C. perfringens* involved in foodborne outbreaks). Heat treatment may be more effective than alcohol if homogenization is incomplete and the specimen contains particulate matter that is not penetrated adequately by the alcohol. For any spore selection technique, an untreated control subculture should be prepared.

For alcohol treatment, an equal volume of absolute (or 95%) ethanol is added to a 1-ml sample of a fecal suspension or homogenate of a wound or exudate in a sterile screw-cap tube. The specimen is gently mixed at room temperature (22 to 25°C for 1 h). An Ames aliquot mixer (Miles Laboratories, Inc., Elkhart, IN) is a convenient way to provide continuous mixing. The treated material is used to inoculate chopped-meat–glucose or thioglycolate medium, anaerobe blood agar, or egg yolk agar. The culture is incubated and inspected for growth.

For heat treatment, a tube of chopped-meat–glucose or thioglycolate medium (5 ml) is preheated in an 80°C water bath for 5 min, and 1 ml of sample suspension is added. The culture is incubated for 10 min at 80°C, and the tube is removed and cooled in cold water. The treated sample suspension is subcultured into an unheated tube of chopped-meat–glucose or thioglycolate medium, anaerobe blood agar, or egg yolk agar. The cultures are incubated anaerobically and examined for growth.

Isolation of *C. difficile*

Since *C. difficile* can be isolated from stool in asymptomatic patients, culture alone is not sufficient to diagnose CDI and may misdiagnose AAD caused by other agents unless stool samples are also assayed for the presence of *C. difficile* toxins. However, the recent emergence of the epidemic, hypervirulent ribotype 027 strain has reinforced the need for cultivation of *C. difficile* for subsequent typing, molecular studies, and determination of antimicrobial susceptibility.

Currently, routine cultivation is done at 35 to 37°C on cycloserine-cefoxitin-fructose (CCF) agar (see chapter 17) with or without blood. With prereduced medium, strains grow better. Best results are achieved in CCF broth supplemented with pure taurocholate; however, 7 days of culture is recommended. Growth depends on strict anaerobic conditions. Typically, the culturing time ranges from 3 to 7 days. Alcohol shock is a potential alternative to improve *C. difficile* isolation (103, 108). Following incubation, plates should be examined using a dissecting microscope. Colonies of *C. difficile* are yellowish to white, circular to irregular, and flat, with a rhizoid or erose edge and a ground-glass appearance (Fig. 3). The colonies have a distinctive odor like *para*-cresol (or horse manure). In addition, *C. difficile* colonies on CCFA (cycloserine-cefoxitin-fructose agar) fluoresce chartreuse under UV light (103).

Gram staining of *C. difficile* reveals rods that are gram positive to gram variable, thin, with parallel sides, and 0.5 μm wide by 3- to 5-μm long. Isolation may be difficult due to the presence of both vegetative and spore-forming bacteria. Presumptive identification of *C. difficile* can be made by demonstrating typical colonies, Gram stain morphology, and characteristic odor. Biochemical differentiation is easiest with detection of proline-aminopeptidase. Definitive identification depends on demonstration of the unique pattern of short-chain fatty acid metabolic products by GLC, by biochemical characterization of isolates, or by 16S rRNA gene sequencing (11, 25, 79, 90) (Table 1).

IDENTIFICATION

Preliminary Identification

Identification of *Clostridia* in specimens from sites of infection due to mixed organisms can be time-consuming and expensive. Use of selective and differential media for initial processing can provide rapid and relevant information to the clinician. When isolated from normally sterile sites and sites of serious infection, bacteria should always be completely identified. Some of the organisms that warrant identification include *C. septicum* (associated with gastrointestinal malignancy), *C. ramosum*, *C. innocuum*, and *C. clostridioforme* (which are frequently resistant to antibiotics), and *C. perfringens* (53).

Clostridia are typically gram-positive rods by microscopic morphology. Some clostridia appear to be gram negative, especially *C. ramosum*, *C. innocuum*, and the *C. clostridioforme* group, but the special-potency antibiotic disk pattern (see below) verifies the presence of gram-positive organisms. Second, it may be difficult to detect spores, so an ethanol treatment, heat spore treatment, or malachite green stain may be necessary, and phase-contrast or dark-field microscopy may be helpful. Third, the colonial morphology of pure cultures may be variable, so the culture may appear to be mixed. Subcultures of single, well-isolated colonies yield the same variable morphologies. Examination of colonies by stereomicroscopy is helpful for noting colonial characteristics. Fourth, the aerotolerant clostridia may be confused with *Bacillus* or *Lactobacillus* spp. *Clostridium* species sporulate anaerobically only, grow much better anaerobically (larger colonies), and are almost always catalase negative. *Bacillus* spp. sporulate aerobically only, usually grow better aerobically, and are usually catalase positive. Aerobically grown *C. tertium* has colonial and cellular morphologies similar to those of *Lactobacillus* spp. Certain clostridia can be identified with relative ease by Gram staining, colony morphology determination, a positive indole reaction, hemolysis on blood agar, and the tests described below (Table 3).

Special-Potency Disks

The isolate should be subcultured on blood agar with special-potency disks containing vancomycin (5 μg), kanamycin (1 mg), or colistin (10 μg) and incubated anaerobically for 48 to 72 h at 35 to 37°C. Clostridia are colistin and kanamycin resistant and vancomycin susceptible (Table 3), except for occasional *C. innocuum* isolates, which may be only moderately susceptible to vancomycin (8).

Lecithinase and Lipase

The isolate should be subcultured on egg yolk agar and incubated anaerobically for 48 to 72 h at 35 to 37°C. Lecithinase activity is demonstrated by a white, opaque, diffuse zone around the colonies that extends into the medium (Fig. 2). Lipase activity is indicated by an iridescent sheen on the surface of bacterial growth and on the agar surface around the colonies.

Spore Test

Media for the demonstration of spores include chopped-meat agar or broth and thioglycolate medium. The culture should be incubated anaerobically at 5 to 7°C below the optimum temperature (30°C) for the growth and sporulation of clostridia, except with *C. perfringens* (should be induced at 37°C). Actively growing cultures

TABLE 3 Rapid identification of some lecithinase-positive and/or swarming *Clostridium* spp. of clinical significance[a]

Species	Lecithinase	Lipase	Indole	Swarming	Urease	Spore location	Other characteristic(s)
C. bifermentans	+	−	+	−	−	ST	Chalk-white colonies on EYA
C. novyi A	+	+	−	+	−	ST	Robust beta-hemolysis
C. perfringens	+	−	−	−	−	ST	Double zone of beta-hemolysis, reverse CAMP test positive
C. sordellii	+	−	+	−	+	ST	Large, gram-positive bacilli
C. septicum	−	−	−	+	−	ST	Rare spores; spreading, adherent colonies
C. sporogenes	−	+	−	+	−[+]	ST	Abundant oval spores
C. tetani	−	−[w]	v	+	−	T	Drumstick shaped

[a]EYA, egg yolk agar. For other abbreviations and symbols, see Table 1, footnote *a*.

may stand at room temperature for several days to 1 week, and ethanol or heat spore treatments can be performed as described above.

Definitive Identification of *Clostridium* Species

The traditional method for the phenotypic characterization and identification of clostridia is the use of PRAS media for the determination of fermentation profiles and other characteristics, combined with GLC analysis of metabolic end products (58, 150). However, only a few laboratories have PRAS media or GLC available. Table 1 lists characteristics that are useful for definitive identification of clinically relevant clostridia. The key reactions (bold in Table 1) require minimal PRAS medium and can be used in conjunction with commercial identification kits or individual preformed-enzyme tests, such as Wee Tabs (Key Scientific, Round Rock, TX) or Rosco diagnostic tablets (Rosco, Taastrup, Denmark). Gelatin and esculin hydrolysis, carbohydrate fermentation reactions, and metabolic end product analysis are based on results obtained with PRAS media (Anaerobe Systems, Morgan Hill, CA).

PRAS Biochemical Inoculation

Actively growing broth cultures (without carbohydrate) or cell pastes suspended in broth medium (e.g., peptone-yeast or thioglycolate) may be used to inoculate PRAS media. Cultures are incubated for 48 to 72 h at 35 to 37°C, but overnight incubation is sufficient for many clostridia.

Gelatin Hydrolysis

A PRAS gelatin tube with an actively growing culture is refrigerated along with an uninoculated tube for at least 1 h. The tubes are removed to room temperature, inverted immediately, and observed for liquefaction every 5 min. In a positive reaction, the gelatin is hydrolyzed and thus fails to solidify, dropping to the top of the inverted tube immediately. In a negative reaction, the medium fails to liquefy when it reaches room temperature (>30 min). A weakly positive reaction yields liquid medium at the time that it reaches room temperature (<30 min).

Esculin Hydrolysis

Five drops of 1% ferric ammonium citrate are added to a tube of actively growing bacteria in a PRAS esculin tube, and the tube is observed for a color change and fluorescence under UV (366-nm) light. In a positive reaction, a black or dark-brown color develops, and there is no fluorescence

under UV light. In a negative reaction, no color develops, and the tube fluoresces white-blue under UV light. Since many clostridia produce hydrogen sulfide (H_2S), which also reacts with the reagent to form a black complex, all tubes that darken after the addition of reagent should be confirmed under UV light.

Carbohydrate Fermentation

The pH of actively growing organisms (>2+ turbidity) should be measured in a PRAS carbohydrate tube. A positive reaction ("acid") yields a pH below 5.5, and a negative reaction results in a pH exceeding 5.9. "Weak acid" is indicated by a pH of 5.6 to 5.8. Details of GLC procedures used for the analyses of metabolic end products listed in Table 1 are outlined elsewhere (103).

Commercial kits, based on the detection of preformed enzymes with chromogenic or fluorogenic substrates, have been marketed for the rapid identification of anaerobes. These panels include RapID ANA II (Remel), Api 20A and RapID 32A (bioMérieux, Durham, NC), Vitek ANI card and Vitek 2ANC card (bioMérieux), and the BBL Crystal anaerobe identification system (BD, Franklin Lakes, NJ). The overall performances of these panels vary, and the panels are not always satisfactory as the sole identification method for clostridia (8, 43, 127, 134, 142, 154, 159). In general, Gram stain reaction, cellular morphologies, colonial characteristics, and aerotolerance of isolates (characteristics noted above and in Tables 1 and 3) should be determined in conjunction with the use of commercial microsystems. Supplementation of tests in these kits with individual tablets (e.g., Wee tabs or Rosco tablets) can be helpful. Other useful supplemental tests for clostridia include the tests outlined above, such as lipase and lecithinase production, the reduction of nitrate, gelatin and esculin hydrolysis, carbohydrate fermentation, and metabolic end product analysis using GLC.

Clostridial biochemical activity is quite variable, being saccharolytic/proteolytic and saccharolytic/nonproteolytic to asaccharolytic. The identification of asaccharolytic species are most sophisticated. Liquid chromatography-mass spectroscopy (67) and molecular biological methods such as 16S rRNA gene sequencing (166, 202) can be useful in these cases. 16S rRNA gene sequencing is becoming more popular, though interpretation of results must be done by those with special training. Other promising methods for the identification of *Clostridium* species are fluorescent in situ hybridization (FISH) (27, 163) and matrix-assisted laser desorption–time of flight mass spectrometry (84).

Characteristics of Commonly Encountered Clostridia

Key characteristics that aid in the presumptive identification of the most common species are listed below. See also Tables 1 and 3.

C. *bifermentans*: colonies chalk-white on egg yolk agar, irregular, scalloped edge; many free spores, often in chains; urease negative; indole and lecithinase positive. C. *sordellii* is similar but is usually urease positive.

C. *bolteae*: colonies usually have a slightly irregular edge; greening of agar around colonies; gram negative; tapered ends; spores are rare; lactose negative and β-N-acetylglucosaminidase (β-NAG) negative.

C. *butyricum*: very large, irregular colonies with mottled-to-mosaic internal structure; subterminal spores; ferments many carbohydrates.

C. *cadaveris*: white-gray, entire or slightly irregular, raised to slightly convex; oval terminal spores; spot indole positive.

C. *clostridioforme*: same as for C. *bolteae* but lactose positive and β-NAG negative.

C. *difficile*: colonies creamy yellow to gray-white (Fig. 3); irregular, coarse, mottled-to-mosaic internal structure; matte or dull surface; horse stable odor (*para*-cresol); subterminal and free spores or spores infrequent; gelatin hydrolysis can be slow; mannitol and proline positive; colonies fluoresce chartreuse on selective CCFA.

C. *glycolicum*: colonies are gray-white with an entire or scalloped edge and convex; subterminal and free spores.

C. *hathewayi*: same as for C. *bolteae* but lactose and β-NAG positive.

C. *innocuum*: gray-white-to-brilliant-greenish colonies, coarsely mottled-to-mosaic internal structure, entire edge usually; terminal spores may be difficult to find; nonmotile; mannitol positive; lactose, maltose, and proline negative.

C. *novyi* type A: lecithinase and lipase positive, may swarm, strong beta-hemolysis.

C. *perfringens*: double zone of beta-hemolysis around colonies (Fig. 4), boxcar-shaped rods, spores rare, lecithinase positive (Fig. 2).

C. *ramosum*: colonies resemble *Bacteroides fragilis* but usually have a slightly irregular edge; Gram stain variable, palisading, slender rods; small round or oval terminal spores (Fig. 1); nonmotile; mannitol positive.

C. *septicum*: swarms (Fig. 5); large, filamentous bacilli (Fig. 6); subterminal spores often in "lemon" forms; DNase positive and sucrose negative.

C. *sporogenes*: Medusa-head colonies, possible swarming, colonies adhere firmly to agar; subterminal and many free spores; lipase positive.

C. *symbiosum*: rods with tapered ends, football shaped, may form chains, often has spores.

C. *tertium*: aerotolerant, terminal spores when anaerobically incubated.

C. *tetani*: may form a thin film of growth over entire agar plate, especially on moist media; drumstick spores.

Toxin tests are necessary for the identification of a few species. C. *sporogenes* cannot be differentiated with certainty from the proteolytic group I strains of C. *botulinum* unless toxin tests are used. A few strains of C. *botulinum* produce lecithinase as well as lipase and are difficult to distinguish from C. *novyi* type A except by toxin tests. As a supplement to the methods described, the various types of C. *botulinum* and other clostridia can be presumptively identified on the basis of differences in their CFA profiles (11, 79, 90) and by typing methods such as pulsed-field gel electrophoresis (PFGE) or other molecular analyses. Finegold et al. (72) described a multiplex PCR procedure for rapid distinction of the three species of the C. *clostridioforme* group.

TYPING SYSTEMS

In the event of severe cases of disease and lethal outcomes for patients, typing of strains is recommended. Physicians should be aware of their local C. *difficile* situation and should be sure that hypervirulent strains are not present. Monitoring of the local situation gives a hint about the local standard of hygiene, the education of nurses (and other colleagues), and the risks for patients. It is obvious from investigations of C. *difficile* strains that every region may have its particular pattern of strains, with ribotypes differing between different countries in Europe but also between different regions of a single state (20).

To resolve endemic-disease situations, to monitor the spread of infection, and to assess the genetic relatedness of the associated strains, the successful cultivation of C. *difficile* is required. Starting with the pure culture, several approaches have been used for such analyses, including restriction endonuclease analysis, PFGE, PCR-ribotyping, multilocus sequence typing, and others (105). For example, the recent hypervirulent isolates have been typed as 027 by ribotyping, designated toxinotype III by typing the toxin A and B genes of the PaLoc, and designated NAP1/2 by restriction fragment length polymorphism analysis (North American PFGE type 1/2) (139). Recently, Bouvet and Popoff used triple-locus sequence analysis of the toxin regulatory genes *tcdC*, *tcdR*, and *cdtR* to assess the evolutionary relatedness of strains isolated from humans and food animals (30). The variety of methods used for this analysis already indicates the difficulties in setting a standard procedure that may be used routinely and worldwide.

PCR-ribotyping could become such a reference method; however, type strains are not easy enough to receive and are available only from a very few places. Therefore, only a limited number of labs have enough standard strains available to qualify the ribotypes of the strains that are posted. Normally the isolated strains should be sent to such labs; the use of Amies transport medium is an appropriate means for doing so. PCR-ribotyping is done with two specific primers that amplify the spacer region in between the 16S and the 23S ribosomal RNAs. The spacer region is known for its heterogenous nature, as opposed to the highly conserved rRNA genes themselves. C. *difficile* contains 10 rRNA copies, and variations in the spacer regions are seen between different strains but also between different rRNA copies of a single strain.

Multilocus sequence typing has been successfully used as a reproducible and discriminating system for strain typing of *Clostridium botulinum* type A using clinical and food isolates (94), C. *perfringens* isolates from necrotic enteritis outbreaks in broiler chicken populations (47), and C. *septicum* isolates recovered from poultry flocks experiencing episodes of gangrenous dermatitis (145). Leclair et al. described a modified PFGE protocol to be the most useful method for typing epidemiologically related C. *botulinum* type E strains, in comparison with randomly amplified polymorphic DNA analysis and automated ribotyping using clinical and food isolates associated with four botulism outbreaks (123). Furthermore, analysis of the variable numbers of tandem repeats (VNTRs) within the genome, called multiple-locus VNTR analysis, has been described for *C. perfringens* (48, 156). Epidemiologically related isolates previously typed by PFGE were also examined by multiple-locus VNTR analysis, and the congruency of the two methods was found to be very high. Macdonald et al. described VNTR regions in *Clostridium botulinum* strains, providing a rapid and highly discriminatory tool to distinguish among *C. botulinum* BoNT/A1 strains for investigations of botulism outbreaks (132).

SEROLOGIC TESTS

Serologic procedures are not practical for secure strain identification from colonies. Furthermore, no standardized tests are available for the detection of antibodies against *Clostridium* species in clinical specimens to confirm diagnoses of clostridial infections. To evaluate the vaccination status, determination of immunoglobulin G antibodies against tetanus toxin may be useful, but in cases of an unclear immunization status, preventable vaccination should be done.

ANTIMICROBIAL SUSCEPTIBILITIES

Antimicrobial susceptibility studies with strains of a number of clostridial species are summarized in Table 4. Now that more laboratories are identifying anaerobes by 16S rRNA gene sequencing, more-accurate species identification will be available and more-reliable susceptibility data can be generated. Drugs lacking antimicrobial activities against various clostridia include trimethoprim-sulfamethoxazole, ampicillin, and clindamycin. No resistance of clostridia to ampicillin-sulbactam or piperacillin-tazobactam has been noted, and antimicrobial resistance is uncommon among clostridia with respect to imipenem, metronidazole, and vancomycin. Five species (all with small numbers of strains) and *C. perfringens* show little or no resistance to the antimicrobial agents under consideration (Table 4). Organisms with some resistance to three drugs include *C. ramosum*, *C. innocuum*, and *C. clostridioforme*.

Multiple studies have described resistance to various antibiotics among clostridia. Resistance to penicillin is especially common in *C. ramosum*, *C. clostridioforme*, and *C. butyricum*; these species produce β-lactamases that are induced by β-lactam antibiotics. *C. tertium* has resistance features unusual among clostridia, including resistance to β-lactam antibiotics, metronidazole, and clindamycin. When treating *C. difficile* infections with metronidazole, a considerable time lag in the onset of its antibiotic activity has to be considered due to its prodrug nature (25). Resistance to clindamycin has been documented for strains of *C. perfringens* (as noted above), *C. ramosum*, *C. difficile*, *C. tertium*, *C. subterminale*, *C. butyricum*, *C. sporogenes*, and *C. innocuum* (201).

Chloramphenicol, piperacillin, metronidazole, imipenem, and combinations of β-lactams with β-lactam inhibitors (e.g., ampicillin-sulbactam) were active against most clostridia (201) and this has not changed significantly over the last 10 years (155). In a recent study of Finegold et al., ampicillin-sulbactam and nitazoxanide had the best activities in comparison with neomycin, rifaximin, teicoplanin, and vancomycin (71). The clostridia are variably resistant to cephalosporins and tetracyclines, and they are usually resistant to the aminoglycosides. Many clostridia other than *C. perfringens* (particularly *C. ramosum*, *C. clostridioforme*, and *C. innocuum*) are resistant to cefoxitin, cefotaxime, ceftazidime, ceftizoxime, cefoperazone, and other broad-spectrum β-lactams (8, 201). Most strains of *C. innocuum* were only moderately susceptible to vancomycin (8, 71, 143).

Earlier quinolones, such as ciprofloxacin, levofloxacin, and lomefloxacin, have demonstrated low or intermediate activities against anaerobes, but more recently introduced quinolones, like moxifloxacin, gatifloxacin, and garenoxacin, have good activities in vitro against most anaerobes, including clostridia (2, 126). A high frequency of moxifloxacin resistance has been described among *C. difficile* isolates (4), and quinolone resistance is a problem among pathogens.

EVALUATION, INTERPRETATION, AND REPORTING OF RESULTS

The isolation of a *Clostridium* species from a clinical specimen, even a blood culture, may or may not be significant clinically, and culture results should be interpreted in relation to the patient's clinical findings. Clostridia of the patient's own intestinal microbiota may be present on the skin and may contaminate blood samples or other specimens. Bacteremia may be transient or clinically insignificant. In addition, most clostridia currently encountered in wounds, exudates, blood, and other normally sterile body fluids are opportunistic and may not cause serious or progressive disease unless conditions are suitable in the host. As discussed earlier in this chapter, one exception to this generalization is *C. septicum*, which is rarely encountered in blood cultures except from patients who have an underlying malignancy or neutropenic sepsis. *C. septicum* sepsis is an infectious disease emergency that requires prompt and clear communication between the laboratory and the clinician in order to institute early surgical measures and treatment with antimicrobial agents to improve outcomes. *C. tertium*, *C. perfringens*, and other clostridia, to a lesser extent, may be involved in serious infections that require emergency measures. The best approach for preventing tragic consequences that may be avoidable is good communication between microbiologists and clinicians.

The accurate and timely reporting of preliminary results (e.g., findings from direct microscopic examinations of clinical specimens), as well as early culture results (after 24 and 48 h of incubation), can be extremely valuable to the physician. For smaller laboratories without anaerobic chambers, incubation of the appropriate media in anaerobic jars provides acceptable recovery for most clinically significant anaerobes, assuming that optimal collection and transport of specimens are performed. The colony characteristics and microscopic features of some clostridia (e.g., *C. perfringens*, *C. sordellii*, and *C. sporogenes*) may be distinctive, so preliminary or presumptive reports may be released before aerotolerance studies are completed. Accurate, definitive identification is needed to better define the role of clostridia in disease, to aid the clinician in selecting optimal treatment, and for public health purposes (e.g., hospital-acquired *C. difficile* disease).

Potentially life-threatening diseases due to *Clostridium* species or their toxins, such as botulism, tetanus, or severe cases of *C. difficile* infection, should be carefully examined by the physician and the microbiologist together to ensure optimal sample collection and transport, immediate processing,

TABLE 4 Activities of various drugs against *Clostridium* spp. (Wadsworth agar dilution procedure)[a]

Antimicrobial agent	CLSI MIC breakpoint (μg/ml) Susceptible	Intermediate	% Susceptible[b] C. bifermentans	C. bolteae	C. butyricum	C. cadaveris	C. clostridioforme	C. difficile	C. disporicum	C. glycolicum	C. hathewayi	C. innocuum	C. paraputrificum	C. perfringens	C. ramosum	C. septicum	C. sordellii	C. sporogenes	C. subterminale	C. tertium
Ampicillin[c]	0.5	1	100	67	86	100[d]	67	26	100	100	ND[e]	100	94	100	100	100[d]	100	100	100	100
Amoxicillin-clavulanate	4/2	8/4	100	66	100	ND	75	100	100	100	100	100	100	100	100	ND	100	100	100[d]	100[d]
Piperacillin-tazobactam	32/4	64/4	100[d]	ND	ND	ND	ND	100	ND	ND	ND	100	ND	100	100	ND	100	100[d]	ND	ND
Ticarcillin	32	64	ND	ND	ND	ND	ND	100	ND	ND	ND	ND	ND	100	100	ND	100	100[d]	ND	ND
Clindamycin	2	4	100	100	100	100[d]	90	56	100	92	93	83	87	100	82	100[d]	94	8	85	100[d]
Vancomycin	8	16	100	91	100	100[d]	100	100	100	100	100	98	100	100	100	100[d]	100	100	100	100
Imipenem	4	8	100[d]	100[d]	100[d]	100[d]	ND	94	ND	ND	ND	100	100[d]	100	100	ND	100	100	ND	ND
Linezolid	2	4	100	100	85	ND	86	91	100	100	100	94	75	100	12	ND	100	100	83	100[d]
Metronidazole	8	16	100	100	100	100	100	100	100	100	100	98	100	97	98	100[d]	95	100	100	100
Trimethoprim-sulfamethoxazole	32	64	0	67	50	0[d]	100	26	78	0		3	31	4	57	100[d]	0	0[d]	0	14

[a]Clinical and Laboratory Standards Institute (CLSI) approved method M11-A6 (54) data from the Wadsworth Anaerobic Bacteriology Laboratory.
[b]According to the CLSI-approved breakpoints (M11-A6) (54), the intermediate category is susceptible.
[c]Strains producing β-lactamase should be considered resistant.
[d]Five or fewer strains were tested.
[e]ND, no data.

and initiation of specific therapy. Furthermore, health care institutions require accurate and rapid diagnosis for early detection of possible outbreaks and to implement effective control measures.

REFERENCES

1. **Abrahao, C., R. J. Carman, H. Hahn, and O. Liesenfeld.** 2001. Similar frequency of detection of *Clostridium perfringens* enterotoxin and *Clostridium difficile* toxins in patients with antibiotic-associated diarrhea. *Eur. J. Clin. Microbiol. Infect. Dis.* **20:**676–677.
2. **Ackermann, G., R. Schaumann, B. Pless, M. C. Claros, E. J. Goldstein, and A. C. Rodloff.** 2000. Comparative activity of moxifloxacin in vitro against obligately anaerobic bacteria. *Eur. J. Clin. Microbiol. Infect. Dis.* **19:**228–232.
3. **Ackermann, G., Y. J. Tang, S. S. Jang, J. Silva, A. C. Rodloff, and S. H. Cohen.** 2001. Isolation of *Clostridium innocuum* from cases of recurrent diarrhea in patients with prior *Clostridium difficile* associated diarrhea. *Diagn. Microbiol. Infect. Dis.* **40:**103–106.
4. **Ackermann, G., Y. J. Tang, R. Kueper, P. Heisig, A. C. Rodloff, J. Silva, Jr., and S. H. Cohen.** 2001. Resistance to moxifloxacin in toxigenic *Clostridium difficile* isolates is associated with mutations in *gyrA*. *Antimicrob. Agents Chemother.* **45:**2348–2353.
5. **Akbulut, D., K. A. Grant, and J. McLauchlin.** 2005. Improvement in laboratory diagnosis of wound botulism and tetanus among injecting illicit-drug users by use of real-time PCR assays for neurotoxin gene fragments. *J. Clin. Microbiol.* **43:**4342–4348.
6. **Aldape, M. J., A. E. Bryant, Y. Ma, and D. L. Stevens.** 2007. The leukemoid reaction in *Clostridium sordellii* infection: neuraminidase induction of promyelocytic cell proliferation. *J. Infect. Dis.* **195:**1838–1845.
7. **Aldape, M. J., A. E. Bryant, and D. L. Stevens.** 2006. *Clostridium sordellii* infection: epidemiology, clinical findings, and current perspectives on diagnosis and treatment. *Clin. Infect. Dis.* **43:**1436–1446.
8. **Alexander, C. J., D. M. Citron, J. S. Brazier, and E. J. Goldstein.** 1995. Identification and antimicrobial resistance patterns of clinical isolates of *Clostridium clostridioforme*, *Clostridium innocuum*, and *Clostridium ramosum* compared with those of clinical isolates of *Clostridium perfringens*. *J. Clin. Microbiol.* **33:**3209–3215.
9. **Alfa, M. J., D. Robson, M. Davi, K. Bernard, C. P. Van, and G. K. Harding.** 2002. An outbreak of necrotizing enterocolitis associated with a novel clostridium species in a neonatal intensive care unit. *Clin. Infect. Dis.* **35:**S101–S105.
10. **Allen, S. D., C. L. Emery, and J. A. Siders.** 2002. Anaerobic bacteriology, p. 50–81. *In* A. L. Truant (ed.), *Manual of Commercial Methods in Clinical Microbiology.* ASM Press, Washington, DC.
11. **Allen, S. D., J. A. Siders, M. J. Riddell, J. A. Fill, and W. S. Wegener.** 1995. Cellular fatty acid analysis in the differentiation of *Clostridium* in the clinical microbiology laboratory. *Clin. Infect. Dis.* **20**(Suppl. 2):S198–S201.
12. **Arnon, S. S.** 2004. Infant botulism, p. 1758–1766. *In* R. D. Feigen, J. D. Cherry, G. Demmler, and S. Kaplan (ed.), *Textbook of Pediatric Infectious Diseases.* W. B. Saunders, Philadelphia, PA.
13. **Arnon, S. S., R. Schechter, T. V. Inglesby, D. A. Henderson, J. G. Bartlett, M. S. Ascher, E. Eitzen, A. D. Fine, J. Hauer, M. Layton, S. Lillibridge, M. T. Osterholm, T. O'Toole, G. Parker, T. M. Perl, P. K. Russell, D. L. Swerdlow, and K. Tonat.** 2001. Botulinum toxin as a biological weapon: medical and public health management. *JAMA* **285:**1059–1070.
14. **Arnon, S. S., R. Schechter, S. E. Maslanka, N. P. Jewell, and C. L. Hatheway.** 2006. Human botulism immune globulin for the treatment of infant botulism. *N. Engl. J. Med.* **354:**462–471.
15. **Asha, N. J., D. Tompkins, and M. H. Wilcox.** 2006. Comparative analysis of prevalence, risk factors, and molecular epidemiology of antibiotic-associated diarrhea due to *Clostridium difficile*, *Clostridium perfringens*, and *Staphylococcus aureus*. *J. Clin. Microbiol.* **44:**2785–2791.
16. **Assadian, O., A. Assadian, C. Senekowitsch, A. Makristathis, and G. Hagmuller.** 2004. Gas gangrene due to *Clostridium perfringens* in two injecting drug users in Vienna, Austria. *Wien. Klin. Wochenschr.* **116:**264–267.
17. **Ballard, J., A. Bryant, D. Stevens, and R. K. Tweten.** 1992. Purification and characterization of the lethal toxin (alpha-toxin) of *Clostridium septicum*. *Infect. Immun.* **60:**784–790.
18. **Bangsberg, D. R., J. I. Rosen, T. Aragon, A. Campbell, L. Weir, and F. Perdreau-Remington.** 2002. Clostridial myonecrosis cluster among injection drug users: a molecular epidemiology investigation. *Arch. Intern. Med.* **162:**517–522.
19. **Barash, J. R., T. W. Tang, and S. S. Arnon.** 2005. First case of infant botulism caused by *Clostridium baratii* type F in California. *J. Clin. Microbiol.* **43:**4280–4282.
20. **Barbut, F., P. Mastrantonio, M. Delmee, J. Brazier, E. Kuijper, and I. Poxton.** 2007. Prospective study of *Clostridium difficile* infections in Europe with phenotypic and genotypic characterisation of the isolates. *Clin. Microbiol. Infect.* **13:**1048–1057.
21. **Barsam, A., M. Kerins, and P. Jaye.** 2005. Tetanus and intravenous drug use. *Eur. J. Clin. Microbiol. Infect. Dis.* **24:**497–498.
22. **Barth, H., K. Aktories, M. R. Popoff, and B. G. Stiles.** 2004. Binary bacterial toxins: biochemistry, biology, and applications of common *Clostridium* and *Bacillus* proteins. *Microbiol. Mol. Biol. Rev.* **68:**373–402.
23. **Bartlett, J. G.** 2002. Clinical practice. Antibiotic-associated diarrhea. *N. Engl. J. Med.* **346:**334–339.
24. **Bartlett, J. G., and D. N. Gerding.** 2008. Clinical recognition and diagnosis of *Clostridium difficile* infection. *Clin. Infect. Dis.* **46**(Suppl. 1):S12–S18.
25. **Belmares, J., D. N. Gerding, J. P. Parada, S. Miskevics, F. Weaver, and S. Johnson.** 2007. Outcome of metronidazole therapy for *Clostridium difficile* disease and correlation with a scoring system. *J. Infect.* **55:**495–501.
26. **Bleck, T. P.** 1991. Tetanus: pathophysiology, management, and prophylaxis. *Dis. Mon.* **37:**545–603.
27. **Bloedt, K., M. Riecker, S. Poppert, and N. Wellinghausen.** 2009. Evaluation of new selective culture media and a rapid fluorescence in situ hybridization assay for identification of *Clostridium difficile* from stool samples. *J. Med. Microbiol.* **58:**874–877.
28. **Borriello, S. P., F. E. Barclay, A. R. Welch, M. F. Stringer, G. N. Watson, R. K. Williams, D. V. Seal, and K. Sullens.** 1985. Epidemiology of diarrhoea caused by enterotoxigenic *Clostridium perfringens*. *J. Med. Microbiol.* **20:**363–372.
29. **Bos, J., L. Smithee, B. McClane, R. F. Distefano, F. Uzal, J. G. Songer, S. Mallonee, and J. M. Crutcher.** 2005. Fatal necrotizing colitis following a foodborne outbreak of enterotoxigenic *Clostridium perfringens* type A infection. *Clin. Infect. Dis.* **40:**e78–e83.
30. **Bouvet, P. J., and M. R. Popoff.** 2008. Genetic relatedness of *Clostridium difficile* isolates from various origins determined by triple-locus sequence analysis based on toxin regulatory genes *tcdC*, *tcdR*, and *cdtR*. *J. Clin. Microbiol.* **46:**3703–3713.
31. **Bradshaw, M., S. S. Dineen, N. D. Maks, and E. A. Johnson.** 2004. Regulation of neurotoxin complex expression in *Clostridium botulinum* strains 62A, Hall A-hyper, and NCTC 2916. *Anaerobe* **10:**321–333.
32. **Braun, V., T. Hundsberger, P. Leukel, M. Sauerborn, and C. von Eichel-Streiber.** 1996. Definition of the single integration site of the pathogenicity locus in *Clostridium difficile*. *Gene* **181:**29–38.
33. **Brazier, J. S., M. Gal, V. Hall, and T. Morris.** 2004. Outbreak of *Clostridium histolyticum* infections in injecting drug users in England and Scotland. *Euro Surveill.* **9:**15–16.
34. **Brett, M. M., G. Hallas, and O. Mpamugo.** 2004. Wound botulism in the UK and Ireland. *J. Med. Microbiol.* **53:**555–561.
35. **Brook, I.** 1995. Clostridial infection in children. *J. Med. Microbiol.* **42:**78–82.

36. **Bruggemann, H., and G. Gottschalk.** 2004. Insights in metabolism and toxin production from the complete genome sequence of *Clostridium tetani. Anaerobe* **10**:53–68.

37. **Bryant, A. E., R. Bergstrom, G. A. Zimmerman, J. L. Salyer, H. R. Hill, R. K. Tweten, H. Sato, and D. L. Stevens.** 1993. *Clostridium perfringens* invasiveness is enhanced by effects of theta toxin upon PMNL structure and function: the roles of leukocytotoxicity and expression of CD11/CD18 adherence glycoprotein. *FEMS Immunol. Med. Microbiol.* **7**:321–336.

38. **Bryant, A. E., R. Y. Z. Chen, Y. Nagata, Y. Wang, C. H. Lee, S. Finegold, P. H. Guth, and D. L. Stevens.** 2000. Clostridial gas gangrene I: cellular and molecular mechanisms of microvascular dysfunction induced by exotoxins of *C. perfringens. J. Infect. Dis.* **182**:799–807.

39. **Bryant, A. E., R. Y. Z. Chen, Y. Nagata, Y. Wang, C. H. Lee, S. Finegold, P. H. Guth, and D. L. Stevens.** 2000. Clostridial gas gangrene II: phospholipase C-induced activation of platelet gpIIb/IIIa mediates vascular occlusion and myonecrosis in *C. perfringens* gas gangrene. *J. Infect. Dis.* **182**:808–815.

40. **Bryant, A. E., and D. L. Stevens.** 1997. The pathogenesis of gas gangrene, p. 185–196. *In* J. I. Rood, R. Titball, B. McClane, and G. Songer (ed.), *The Clostridia: Molecular Biology and Pathogenesis.* Academic Press Limited, San Diego, CA.

41. **Brynestad, S., M. R. Sarker, B. A. McClane, P. E. Granum, and J. I. Rood.** 2001. Enterotoxin plasmid from *Clostridium perfringens* is conjugative. *Infect. Immun.* **69**:3483–3487.

42. **Carlier, J. P., M. Bedora-Faure, G. K'ouas, C. Alauzet, and F. Mory.** 2009. Proposal to unify *Clostridium orbiscindens* Winter et al. 1991 and *Eubacterium plautii* (Seguin 1928) Hofstad and Aasjord 1982 with description of *Flavonifractor plautii* gen. nov., comb. nov. and reassignment of *Bacteroides capillosus* to *Pseudoflavonifractor capillosus* gen. nov., comb. nov. *Int. J. Syst. Evol. Microbiol.* **60**:585–590.

43. **Cavallaro, J. J., L. S. Wiggs, and J. M. Miller.** 1997. Evaluation of the BBL Crystal Anaerobe identification system. *J. Clin. Microbiol.* **35**:3186–3191.

44. **Centers for Disease Control and Prevention.** 1998. *Botulism in the United States 1899–1996. Handbook for Epidemiologists, Clinicians, and Laboratory Workers.* U.S. Department of Health and Human Services, Public Health Service, Centers for Disease Control and Prevention, Atlanta, GA.

45. **Centers for Disease Control and Prevention.** 2000. Update: *Clostridium novyi* and unexplained illness among injecting-drug users—Scotland, Ireland, and England, April–June 2000. *MMWR Morb. Mortal. Wkly. Rep.* **49**:543–545.

46. **Centers for Disease Control and Prevention.** 2001. Soft tissue infections among injection drug users—San Francisco, California, 1996–2000. *MMWR Morb. Mortal. Wkly. Rep.* **50**:381–384.

46a. **Centers for Disease Control and Prevention.** 2009. *Biosafety in Microbiological and Biomedical Laboratories,* 5th ed. Centers for Disease Control and Prevention, Atlanta, GA. http://www.cdc.gov/biosafety/publications/bmbl5/index.htm.

47. **Chalmers, G., H. L. Bruce, D. B. Hunter, V. R. Parreira, R. R. Kulkarni, Y. F. Jiang, J. F. Prescott, and P. Boerlin.** 2008. Multilocus sequence typing analysis of *Clostridium perfringens* isolates from necrotic enteritis outbreaks in broiler chicken populations. *J. Clin. Microbiol.* **46**:3957–3964.

48. **Chalmers, G., S. W. Martin, J. F. Prescott, and P. Boerlin.** 2008. Typing of *Clostridium perfringens* by multiple-locus variable number of tandem repeats analysis. *Vet. Microbiol.* **128**:126–135.

49. **Chaudhry, R., B. Dhawan, D. Kumar, R. Bhatia, J. C. Gandhi, R. K. Patel, and B. C. Purohit.** 1998. Outbreak of suspected *Clostridium butyricum* botulism in India. *Emerg. Infect. Dis.* **4**:506–507.

50. **Chen, Y. M., H. C. Lee, C. M. Chang, Y. C. Chuang, and W. C. Ko.** 2001. Clostridium bacteremia: emphasis on the poor prognosis in cirrhotic patients. *J. Microbiol. Immunol. Infect.* **34**:113–118.

51. **Cherington, M.** 2004. Botulism: update and review. *Semin. Neurol.* **24**:155–163.

52. **Chertow, D. S., E. T. Tan, S. E. Maslanka, J. Schulte, E. A. Bresnitz, R. S. Weisman, J. Bernstein, S. M. Marcus, S. Kumar, J. Malecki, J. Sobel, and C. R. Braden.** 2006. Botulism in 4 adults following cosmetic injections with an unlicensed, highly concentrated botulinum preparation. *JAMA* **296**:2476–2479.

53. **Citron, D. M., and P. C. Appelbaum.** 1993. How far should a clinical laboratory go in identifying anaerobic isolates, and who should pay? *Clin. Infect. Dis.* **16**(Suppl. 4):S435–S438.

54. **Clinical and Laboratory Standards Institute.** 2004. *Methods for Antimicrobial Susceptibility Testing of Anaerobic Bacteria.* Approved method M11-A6. Clinical and Laboratory Standards Institute, Wayne, PA.

55. **Cohen, A. L., J. Bhatnagar, S. Reagan, S. B. Zane, M. A. D'Angeli, M. Fischer, G. Killgore, T. S. Kwan-Gett, D. B. Blossom, W. J. Shieh, J. Guarner, J. Jernigan, J. S. Duchin, S. R. Zaki, and L. C. McDonald.** 2007. Toxic shock associated with *Clostridium sordellii* and *Clostridium perfringens* after medical and spontaneous abortion. *Obstet. Gynecol.* **110**:1027–1033.

56. **Coleman, N., G. Speirs, J. Khan, V. Broadbent, D. G. Wight, and R. E. Warren.** 1993. Neutropenic enterocolitis associated with *Clostridium tertium. J. Clin. Pathol.* **46**:180–183.

57. **Collins, M. D., P. A. Lawson, A. Willems, J. J. Cordoba, J. Fernandez-Garayzabal, P. Garcia, J. Cai, H. Hippe, and J. A. Farrow.** 1994. The phylogeny of the genus *Clostridium*: proposal of five new genera and eleven new species combinations. *Int. J. Syst. Bacteriol.* **44**:812–826.

58. **Cresci, A., C. Orpianesi, R. F. La, F. Pannelli, G. Saltalamacchia, G. Scaloni, F. Trotta, and V. Mastrandrea.** 1988. Characterization of some *Clostridium* species by gas-liquid chromatography using numerical analysis. *Microbiologica* **11**:179–199.

59. **De Medici, D., F. Anniballi, G. M. Wyatt, M. Lindstrom, U. Messelhausser, C. F. Aldus, E. Delibato, H. Korkeala, M. W. Peck, and L. Fenicia.** 2009. Multiplex PCR to detect botulinum neurotoxin-producing clostridia in clinical, food, and environmental samples. *Appl. Environ. Microbiol.* **75**:6457–6461.

60. **Doern, G. V., R. T. Coughlin, and L. Wu.** 1992. Laboratory diagnosis of *Clostridium difficile*-associated gastrointestinal disease: comparison of a monoclonal antibody enzyme immunoassay for toxins A and B with a monoclonal antibody enzyme immunoassay for toxin A only and two cytotoxicity assays. *J. Clin. Microbiol.* **30**:2042–2046.

61. **Domingo, R. M., J. S. Haller, and M. Gruenthal.** 2008. Infant botulism: two recent cases and literature review. *J. Child Neurol.* **23**:1336–1346.

62. **Dong, M., W. H. Tepp, E. A. Johnson, and E. R. Chapman.** 2004. Using fluorescent sensors to detect botulinum neurotoxin activity in vitro and in living cells. *Proc. Natl. Acad. Sci. USA* **101**:14701–14706.

63. **Downes, F. P., and K. Ito.** 2001. *Compendium of Methods for the Microbiological Examination of Foods.* American Public Health Association, Washington, DC.

64. **Eklund, M. W., F. T. Poysky, and W. H. Habig.** 1989. Bacteriophages and plasmids in *Clostridium botulinum* and *Clostridium tetani* and their relationship to production of toxins, p. 25–51. *In* L. L. Simpson (ed.), *Botulinum Toxin and Tetanus Toxin.* Academic Press, San Diego, CA.

65. **Elsayed, S., and K. Zhang.** 2004. Bacteremia caused by *Clostridium symbiosum. J. Clin. Microbiol.* **42**:4390–4392.

66. **Elsayed, S., and K. Zhang.** 2005. Bacteremia caused by *Clostridium intestinale. J. Clin. Microbiol.* **43**:2018–2020.

67. **Everley, R. A., T. M. Mott, D. M. Toney, and T. R. Croley.** 2009. Characterization of *Clostridium* species utilizing liquid chromatography/mass spectrometry of intact proteins. *J. Microbiol. Methods* **77**:152–158.

67a. **Federal Register.** Title 29, Code of Federal Regulations, part 1910, subpart I. Personal Protective Equipment.

68. **Fedorko, D. P., H. D. Engler, E. M. O'Shaughnessy, E. C. Williams, C. J. Reichelderfer, and W. I. Smith, Jr.** 1999. Evaluation of two rapid assays for detection of *Clostridium difficile* toxin A in stool specimens. *J. Clin. Microbiol.* **37**:3044–3047.

69. **Fenicia, L., F. Anniballi, S. Pulitano, O. Genovese, G. Polidori, and P. Aureli.** 2004. A severe case of infant botulism caused by *Clostridium botulinum* type A with concomitant intestinal viral infections. *Eur. J. Pediatr.* **163:**501–502.

70. **Fenicia, L., D. L. Da, F. Anniballi, G. Franciosa, S. Zanconato, and P. Aureli.** 2002. A case of infant botulism due to neurotoxigenic *Clostridium butyricum* type E associated with *Clostridium difficile* colitis. *Eur. J. Clin. Microbiol. Infect. Dis.* **21:**736–738.

71. **Finegold, S. M., D. Molitoris, and M. L. Vaisanen.** 2009. Study of the in vitro activities of rifaximin and comparator agents against 536 anaerobic intestinal bacteria from the perspective of potential utility in pathology involving bowel flora. *Antimicrob. Agents Chemother.* **53:**281–286.

72. **Finegold, S. M., Y. Song, C. Liu, D. W. Hecht, P. Summanen, E. Kononen, and S. D. Allen.** 2005. *Clostridium clostridioforme:* a mixture of three clinically important species. *Eur. J. Clin. Microbiol. Infect. Dis.* **24:**319–324.

73. **Fisher, D. J., K. Miyamoto, B. Harrison, S. Akimoto, M. R. Sarker, and B. A. McClane.** 2005. Association of beta2 toxin production with *Clostridium perfringens* type A human gastrointestinal disease isolates carrying a plasmid enterotoxin gene. *Mol. Microbiol.* **56:**747–762.

74. **Forward, L. J., D. S. Tompkins, and M. M. Brett.** 2003. Detection of *Clostridium difficile* cytotoxin and *Clostridium perfringens* enterotoxin in cases of diarrhoea in the community. *J. Med. Microbiol.* **52:**753–757.

75. **Fox, C. K., C. A. Keet, and J. B. Strober.** 2005. Recent advances in infant botulism. *Pediatr. Neurol.* **32:**149–154.

76. **Franciosa, G., P. Aureli, and R. Schechter.** 2003. *Clostridium botulinum*, p. 61–89. *In* M. D. Bier and J. W. Miliotis (ed.), *International Handbook of Foodborne Pathogens.* Marcel Dekker, Inc., New York, NY.

77. **Francisco, A. M., and S. S. Arnon.** 2007. Clinical mimics of infant botulism. *Pediatrics* **119:**826–828.

78. **Gerding, D. N., C. A. Muto, and R. C. Owens, Jr.** 2008. Treatment of *Clostridium difficile* infection. *Clin. Infect. Dis.* **46**(Suppl. 1):S32–S42.

79. **Ghanem, F. M., A. C. Ridpath, W. E. Moore, and L. V. Moore.** 1991. Identification of *Clostridium botulinum*, *Clostridium argentinense*, and related organisms by cellular fatty acid analysis. *J. Clin. Microbiol.* **29:**1114–1124.

80. **Glazunova, O. O., D. Raoult, and V. Roux.** 2005. First identification of *Clostridium celerecrescens* in liquid drained from an abscess. *J. Clin. Microbiol.* **43:**3007–3008.

81. **Goon, P. K., M. O'Brien, and O. G. Titley.** 2005. Spontaneous *Clostridium septicum* septic arthritis of the shoulder and gas gangrene. A case report. *J. Bone Joint Surg. Am.* **87:**874–877.

82. **Gorbach, S. L.** 1998. Gas gangrene and other clostridial skin and soft tissue infections, p. 915–922. *In* S. L. Gorbach, J. G. Bartlett, and N. R. Blacklow (ed.), *Infectious Diseases*, 2nd ed. W. B. Saunders, Philadelphia, PA.

83. **Griffin, P. M., C. L. Hatheway, R. B. Rosenbaum, and R. Sokolow.** 1997. Endogenous antibody production to botulinum toxin in an adult with intestinal colonization botulism and underlying Crohn's disease. *J. Infect. Dis.* **175:**633–637.

84. **Grosse-Herrenthey, A., T. Maier, F. Gessler, R. Schaumann, H. Bohnel, M. Kostrzewa, and M. Kruger.** 2008. Challenging the problem of clostridial identification with matrix-assisted laser desorption and ionization–time-of-flight mass spectrometry (MALDI-TOF MS). *Anaerobe* **14:**242–249.

85. **Hahne, S. J., J. M. White, N. S. Crowcroft, M. M. Brett, R. C. George, N. J. Beeching, K. Roy, and D. Goldberg.** 2006. Tetanus in injecting drug users, United Kingdom. *Emerg. Infect. Dis.* **12:**709–710.

86. **Hall, J. D., L. M. McCroskey, B. J. Pincomb, and C. L. Hatheway.** 1985. Isolation of an organism resembling *Clostridium baratii* which produces type F botulinal toxin from an infant with botulism. *J. Clin. Microbiol.* **21:**654–655.

87. **Hall, Y. H., J. A. Chaddock, H. J. Moulsdale, E. R. Kirby, F. C. Alexander, J. D. Marks, and K. A. Foster.** 2004. Novel application of an in vitro technique to the detection and quantification of botulinum neurotoxin antibodies. *J. Immunol. Methods* **288:**55–60.

88. **Hatheway, C. I.** 2009. Botulism, p. 111–133. *In* A. Balows, W. J. Hausler, M. Ohashi, and A. Turano (ed.), *Laboratory Diagnosis of Infectious Diseases.* Pringer, New York, NY.

89. **Hausmann, R., F. Albert, W. Geissdorfer, and P. Betz.** 2004. *Clostridium fallax* associated with sudden death in a 16-year-old boy. *J. Med. Microbiol.* **53:**581–583.

90. **Holdeman, L. V., E. P. Cato, and W. E. C. Moore.** 1977. *Anaerobe Laboratory Manual.* Virginia Polytechnic Institute and State University, Blacksburg.

91. **Holzer, E.** 1962. Botulism caused by inhalation. *Med. Klin.* **57:**1735–1738. (In German.)

92. **Hsu, H. Y., S. F. Lee, M. E. Hartstein, and G. J. Harocopos.** 2008. *Clostridium perfringens* keratitis leading to blinding panophthalmitis. *Cornea* **27:**1200–1203.

93. **Hundsberger, T., V. Braun, M. Weidmann, P. Leukel, M. Sauerborn, and C. von Eichel-Streiber.** 1997. Transcription analysis of the genes *tcdA-E* of the pathogenicity locus of *Clostridium difficile*. *Eur. J. Biochem.* **244:**735–742.

94. **Jacobson, M. J., G. Lin, T. S. Whittam, and E. A. Johnson.** 2008. Phylogenetic analysis of *Clostridium botulinum* type A by multi-locus sequence typing. *Microbiology* **154:**2408–2415.

95. **Johansson, A., A. Aspan, E. Bagge, V. Baverud, B. E. Engstrom, and K. E. Johansson.** 2006. Genetic diversity of *Clostridium perfringens* type A isolates from animals, food poisoning outbreaks and sludge. *BMC Microbiol.* **6:**47.

96. **Johnson, E. A., and M. Bradshaw.** 2001. *Clostridium botulinum* and its neurotoxins: a metabolic and cellular perspective. *Toxicon* **39:**1703–1722.

97. **Johnson, E. A., and M. C. Goodnough.** 1998. Botulism, p. 723–741. *In* L. Collier, B. W. Mahy, and A. Balows (ed.), *Topley and Wilson's Microbiology and Microbial Infections*, 9th ed. Arnold Publishing, London, United Kingdom.

98. **Johnson, J. L., and B. S. Francis.** 1975. Taxonomy of the Clostridia: ribosomal ribonucleic acid homologies among the species. *J. Gen. Microbiol.* **88:**229–244.

99. **Johnson, S.** 2009. Recurrent *Clostridium difficile* infection: a review of risk factors, treatments, and outcomes. *J. Infect.* **58:**403–410.

100. **Johnson, S., M. R. Driks, R. K. Tweten, J. Ballard, D. L. Stevens, D. J. Anderson, and E. N. Janoff.** 1994. Clinical courses of seven survivors of *Clostridium septicum* infection and their immunologic responses to α toxin. *Clin. Infect. Dis.* **19:**761–764.

101. **Johnson, S., and D. N. Gerding.** 1998. *Clostridium difficile*-associated diarrhea. *Clin. Infect. Dis.* **26:**1027–1034.

102. **Johnson, S., S. A. Kent, K. J. O'Leary, M. M. Merrigan, S. P. Sambol, L. R. Peterson, and D. N. Gerding.** 2001. Fatal pseudomembranous colitis associated with a variant *Clostridium difficile* strain not detected by toxin A immunoassay. *Ann. Intern. Med.* **135:**434–438.

103. **Jousimies-Somer, H. R., P. Summanen, D. M. Citron, E. J. Baron, H. M. Wexler, and S. M. Finegold.** 2002. *Anaerobic Bacteriology Manual.* Star Publishing Company, Belmont, CA.

104. **Just, I., J. Selzer, M. Wilm, C. von Eichel-Streiber, M. Mann, and K. Aktories.** 1995. Glucosylation of Rho proteins by *Clostridium difficile* toxin B. *Nature* **375:**500–503.

105. **Killgore, G., A. Thompson, S. Johnson, J. Brazier, E. Kuijper, J. Pepin, E. H. Frost, P. Savelkoul, B. Nicholson, R. J. van den Berg, H. Kato, S. P. Sambol, W. Zukowski, C. Woods, B. Limbago, D. N. Gerding, and L. C. McDonald.** 2008. Comparison of seven techniques for typing international epidemic strains of *Clostridium difficile*: restriction endonuclease analysis, pulsed-field gel electrophoresis, PCR-ribotyping, multilocus sequence typing, multilocus variable-number tandem-repeat analysis, amplified fragment length polymorphism, and surface layer protein A gene sequence typing. *J. Clin. Microbiol.* **46:**431–437.

106. **Kimura, A. C., J. I. Higa, R. M. Levin, G. Simpson, Y. Vargas, and D. J. Vugia.** 2004. Outbreak of necrotizing fasciitis due to *Clostridium sordellii* among black-tar heroin users. *Clin. Infect. Dis.* **38:**e87–e91.

107. **Kliegman, R. M., and A. A. Fanaroff.** 1984. Necrotizing enterocolitis. *N. Engl. J. Med.* **310:**1093–1103.

108. **Koransky, J. R., S. D. Allen, and V. R. Dowell, Jr.** 1978. Use of ethanol for selective isolation of spore-forming microorganisms. *Appl. Environ. Microbiol.* **35:**762–765.

109. **Kourtis, A. P., R. Weiner, K. Belson, and F. O. Richards, Jr.** 1997. *Clostridium tertium* meningitis as the presenting sign of a meningocele in a twelve-year-old child. *Pediatr. Infect. Dis. J.* **16:**527–529.

110. **Koussoulakos, S.** 2009. Botulinum neurotoxin: the ugly duckling. *Eur. Neurol.* **61:**331–342.

111. **Kudrow, D. B., D. A. Henry, D. A. Haake, G. Marshall, and G. E. Mathisen.** 1988. Botulism associated with *Clostridium botulinum* sinusitis after intranasal cocaine abuse. *Ann. Intern. Med.* **109:**984–985.

112. **Kudsk, K. A.** 1992. Occult gastrointestinal malignancies producing metastatic *Clostridium septicum* infections in diabetic patients. *Surgery* **112:**765–770.

113. **Kuijper, E. J., B. Coignard, J. S. Brazier, C. Suetens, D. Drudy, C. Wiuff, H. Pituch, P. Reichert, F. Schneider, A. F. Widmer, K. E. Olsen, F. Allerberger, D. W. Notermans, F. Barbut, M. Delmee, M. Wilcox, A. Pearson, B. C. Patel, D. J. Brown, R. Frei, T. Akerlund, I. R. Poxton, and P. Tull.** 2007. Update of *Clostridium difficile*-associated disease due to PCR ribotype 027 in Europe. *Euro Surveill.* **12:**E1–E2.

114. **Kyne, L., M. B. Hamel, R. Polavaram, and C. P. Kelly.** 2002. Health care costs and mortality associated with nosocomial diarrhea due to *Clostridium difficile*. *Clin. Infect. Dis.* **34:**346–353.

115. **Lacy, D. B., and R. C. Stevens.** 1999. Sequence homology and structural analysis of the clostridial neurotoxins. *J. Mol. Biol.* **291:**1091–1104.

116. **Lacy, D. B., W. Tepp, A. C. Cohen, B. R. DasGupta, and R. C. Stevens.** 1998. Crystal structure of botulinum neurotoxin type A and implications for toxicity. *Nat. Struct. Biol.* **5:**898–902.

117. **Lalli, G., S. Bohnert, K. Deinhardt, C. Verastegui, and G. Schiavo.** 2003. The journey of tetanus and botulinum neurotoxins in neurons. *Trends Microbiol.* **11:**431–437.

118. **Lassmann, B., D. R. Gustafson, C. M. Wood, and J. E. Rosenblatt.** 2007. Reemergence of anaerobic bacteremia. *Clin. Infect. Dis.* **44:**895–900.

119. **Lau, S. K., P. C. Woo, G. K. Woo, A. M. Fung, A. H. Ngan, Y. Song, C. Liu, P. Summanen, S. M. Finegold, and K. Yuen.** 2006. Bacteraemia caused by *Anaerotruncus colihominis* and emended description of the species. *J. Clin. Pathol.* **59:**748–752.

120. **Lawrence, G. W., D. Lehmann, G. Anian, C. A. Coakley, G. Saleu, M. J. Barker, and M. W. Davis.** 1990. Impact of active immunisation against enteritis necroticans in Papua New Guinea. *Lancet* **336:**1165–1167.

121. **Lawson, P. A., Y. Song, C. Liu, D. R. Molitoris, M. L. Vaisanen, M. D. Collins, and S. M. Finegold.** 2004. *Anaerotruncus colihominis* gen. nov., sp. nov., from human faeces. *Int. J. Syst. Evol. Microbiol.* **54:**413–417.

122. **Leal, J., D. B. Gregson, T. Ross, D. L. Church, and K. B. Laupland.** 2008. Epidemiology of Clostridium species bacteremia in Calgary, Canada, 2000–2006. *J. Infect.* **57:**198–203.

123. **Leclair, D., F. Pagotto, J. M. Farber, B. Cadieux, and J. W. Austin.** 2006. Comparison of DNA fingerprinting methods for use in investigation of type E botulism outbreaks in the Canadian Arctic. *J. Clin. Microbiol.* **44:**1635–1644.

124. **Leegaard, T. M., P. Sandven, and P. Gaustad.** 2005. *Clostridium tertium*: 3 case reports. *Scand. J. Infect. Dis.* **37:**230–232.

125. **Li, D. Y., A. O. Scheimann, J. G. Songer, R. E. Person, M. Horwitz, L. Resar, and K. B. Schwarz.** 2004. Enteritis necroticans with recurrent enterocutaneous fistulae caused by *Clostridium perfringens* in a child with cyclic neutropenia. *J. Pediatr. Gastroenterol. Nutr.* **38:**213–215.

126. **Liebetrau, A., A. C. Rodloff, J. Behra-Miellet, and L. Dubreuil.** 2003. In vitro activities of a new des-fluoro(6) quinolone, garenoxacin, against clinical anaerobic bacteria. *Antimicrob. Agents Chemother.* **47:**3667–3671.

127. **Lindstrom, M. K., H. M. Jankola, S. Hielm, E. K. Hyytia, and H. J. Korkeala.** 1999. Identification of *Clostridium botulinum* with API 20 A, Rapid ID 32 A and RapID ANA II. *FEMS Immunol. Med. Microbiol.* **24:**267–274.

128. **Linscott, A. J., R. B. Flamholtz, D. Shukla, Y. Song, C. Liu, and S. M. Finegold.** 2005. Fatal septicemia due to *Clostridium hathewayi* and *Campylobacter hominis*. *Anaerobe* **11:**97–98.

129. **Loo, V. G., L. Poirier, M. A. Miller, M. Oughton, M. D. Libman, S. Michaud, A. M. Bourgault, T. Nguyen, C. Frenette, M. Kelly, A. Vibien, P. Brassard, S. Fenn, K. Dewar, T. J. Hudson, R. Horn, P. Rene, Y. Monczak, and A. Dascal.** 2005. A predominantly clonal multi-institutional outbreak of *Clostridium difficile*-associated diarrhea with high morbidity and mortality. *N. Engl. J. Med.* **353:**2442–2449.

130. **Lyerly, D. M., L. M. Neville, D. T. Evans, J. Fill, S. Allen, W. Greene, R. Sautter, P. Hnatuck, D. J. Torpey, and R. Schwalbe.** 1998. Multicenter evaluation of the *Clostridium difficile* TOX A/B TEST. *J. Clin. Microbiol.* **36:**184–190.

131. **Lyras, D., J. R. O'Connor, P. M. Howarth, S. P. Sambol, G. P. Carter, T. Phumoonna, R. Poon, V. Adams, G. Vedantam, S. Johnson, D. N. Gerding, and J. I. Rood.** 2009. Toxin B is essential for virulence of *Clostridium difficile*. *Nature* **458:**1176–1179.

132. **Macdonald, T. E., C. H. Helma, L. O. Ticknor, P. J. Jackson, R. T. Okinaka, L. A. Smith, T. J. Smith, and K. K. Hill.** 2008. Differentiation of *Clostridium botulinum* serotype A strains by multiple-locus variable-number tandem-repeat analysis. *Appl. Environ. Microbiol.* **74:**875–882.

133. **MacLennan, J. D.** 1962. The histotoxic clostridial infections of man. *Bacteriol. Rev.* **26:**177–276.

134. **Marler, L. M., J. A. Siders, L. C. Wolters, Y. Pettigrew, B. L. Skitt, and S. D. Allen.** 1991. Evaluation of the new RapID-ANA II system for the identification of clinical anaerobic isolates. *J. Clin. Microbiol.* **29:**874–878.

135. **Maselli, R. A., W. Ellis, R. N. Mandler, F. Sheikh, G. Senton, S. Knox, H. Salari-Namin, M. Agius, R. L. Wollmann, and D. P. Richman.** 1997. Cluster of wound botulism in California: clinical, electrophysiologic, and pathologic study. *Muscle Nerve* **20:**1284–1295.

136. **Massey, V., D. B. Gregson, A. H. Chagla, M. Storey, M. A. John, and Z. Hussain.** 2003. Clinical usefulness of components of the Triage immunoassay, enzyme immunoassay for toxins A and B, and cytotoxin B tissue culture assay for the diagnosis of *Clostridium difficile* diarrhea. *Am. J. Clin. Pathol.* **119:**45–49.

137. **Matamouros, S., P. England, and B. Dupuy.** 2007. *Clostridium difficile* toxin expression is inhibited by the novel regulator TcdC. *Mol. Microbiol.* **64:**1274–1288.

138. **Matsuda, T., Y. Okada, E. Inagi, Y. Tanabe, Y. Shimizu, K. Nagashima, J. Sakurai, M. Nagahama, and S. Tanaka.** 2007. Enteritis necroticans 'pigbel' in a Japanese diabetic adult. *Pathol. Int.* **57:**622–626.

139. **McDonald, L. C., G. E. Killgore, A. Thompson, R. C. Owens, Jr., S. V. Kazakova, S. P. Sambol, S. Johnson, and D. N. Gerding.** 2005. An epidemic, toxin gene-variant strain of *Clostridium difficile*. *N. Engl. J. Med.* **353:**2433–2441.

140. **McFarland, L. V., M. E. Mulligan, R. Y. Kwok, and W. E. Stamm.** 1989. Nosocomial acquisition of *Clostridium difficile* infection. *N. Engl. J. Med.* **320:**204–210.

141. **Modi, N., and M. H. Wilcox.** 2001. Evidence for antibiotic induced *Clostridium perfringens* diarrhoea. *J. Clin. Pathol.* **54:**748–751.

142. **Mory, F., C. Alauzet, C. Matuszewski, P. Riegel, and A. Lozniewski.** 2009. Evaluation of the new Vitek 2 ANC card for identification of medically relevant anaerobic bacteria. *J. Clin. Microbiol.* **47:**1923–1926.

143. **Mory, F., A. Lozniewski, V. David, J. P. Carlier, L. Dubreuil, and R. Leclercq.** 1998. Low-level vancomycin resistance in *Clostridium innocuum*. *J. Clin. Microbiol.* **36:**1767–1768.

144. **Mulligan, M. E., L. R. Peterson, R. Y. Kwok, C. R. Clabots, and D. N. Gerding.** 1988. Immunoblots and plasmid fingerprints compared with serotyping and polyacrylamide gel

electrophoresis for typing *Clostridium difficile. J. Clin. Microbiol.* **26**:41–46.

145. **Neumann, A. P., and T. G. Rehberger.** 2009. MLST analysis reveals a highly conserved core genome among poultry isolates of *Clostridium septicum. Anaerobe* **15**:99–106.

146. **Obladen, M.** 2009. Necrotizing enterocolitis—150 years of fruitless search for the cause. *Neonatology* **96**:203–210.

147. **Olsen, S. J., L. C. MacKinnon, J. S. Goulding, N. H. Bean, and L. Slutsker.** 2000. Surveillance for foodborne-disease outbreaks—United States, 1993–1997. *MMWR Surveill. Summ.* **49**:1–62.

148. **Paerregaard, A., O. Angen, M. Lisby, K. Molbak, M. E. Clausen, and J. J. Christensen.** 2008. Denmark: botulism in an infant or infant botulism? *Euro Surveill.* **13**:pii=19072.

149. **Paisley, J. W., B. A. Lauer, and S. S. Arnon.** 1995. A second case of infant botulism type F caused by *Clostridium baratii. Pediatr. Infect. Dis. J.* **14**:912–914.

150. **Pepersack, F., M. Labbe, C. Nonhoff, and E. Schoutens.** 1983. Use of gas-liquid chromatography as a screening test for toxigenic *Clostridium difficile* in diarrhoeal stools. *J. Clin. Pathol.* **36**:1233–1236.

151. **Petrillo, T. M., C. M. Beck-Sague, J. G. Songer, C. Abramowsky, J. D. Fortenberry, L. Meacham, A. G. Dean, H. Lee, D. M. Bueschel, and S. R. Nesheim.** 2000. Enteritis necroticans (pigbel) in a diabetic child. *N. Engl. J. Med.* **342**:1250–1253.

152. **Pitt, M. L., and R. D. LeClaire.** 2005. Pathogenesis by aerosol, p. 65–78. *In* L. E. Lindler, F. J. Lebeda, and G. W. Korch (ed.), *Biological Weapons Defense. Infectious Diseases and Counterbioterrorism.* Humana Press, Inc., Totowa, NJ.

153. **Reineke, J., S. Tenzer, M. Rupnik, A. Koschinski, O. Hasselmayer, A. Schrattenholz, H. Schild, and C. von Eichel-Streiber.** 2007. Autocatalytic cleavage of *Clostridium difficile* toxin B. *Nature* **446**:415–419.

154. **Rennie, R. P., C. Brosnikoff, L. Turnbull, L. B. Reller, S. Mirrett, W. Janda, K. Ristow, and A. Krilcich.** 2008. Multicenter evaluation of the Vitek 2 anaerobe and Corynebacterium identification card. *J. Clin. Microbiol.* **46**:2646–2651.

155. **Roberts, S. A., K. P. Shore, S. D. Paviour, D. Holland, and A. J. Morris.** 2006. Antimicrobial susceptibility of anaerobic bacteria in New Zealand: 1999–2003. *J. Antimicrob. Chemother.* **57**:992–998.

156. **Sawires, Y. S., and J. G. Songer.** 2005. Multiple-locus variable-number tandem repeat analysis for strain typing of *Clostridium perfringens. Anaerobe* **11**:262–272.

157. **Sayeed, S., F. A. Uzal, D. J. Fisher, J. Saputo, J. E. Vidal, Y. Chen, P. Gupta, J. I. Rood, and B. A. McClane.** 2008. Beta toxin is essential for the intestinal virulence of *Clostridium perfringens* type C disease isolate CN3685 in a rabbit ileal loop model. *Mol. Microbiol.* **67**:15–30.

158. **Schiavo, G., M. Matteoli, and C. Montecucco.** 2000. Neurotoxins affecting neuroexocytosis. *Physiol. Rev.* **80**:717–766.

159. **Schreckenberger, P. C., D. M. Celig, and W. M. Janda.** 1988. Clinical evaluation of the Vitek ANI card for identification of anaerobic bacteria. *J. Clin. Microbiol.* **26**:225–230.

160. **Sharma, S. K., and R. C. Whiting.** 2005. Methods for detection of *Clostridium botulinum* toxin in foods. *J. Food Prot.* **68**:1256–1263.

161. **Shepard, L. A., A. P. Heuck, B. D. Hamman, J. Rossjohn, M. W. Parker, K. R. Ryan, A. E. Johnson, and R. K. Tweten.** 1998. Identification of a membrane-spanning domain of the thiol-activated pore-forming toxin *Clostridium perfringens* perfringolysin O: an alpha-helical to beta-sheet transition identified by fluorescence spectroscopy. *Biochemistry* **37**:14563–14574.

162. **Sheth, A. N., P. Wiersma, D. Atrubin, V. Dubey, D. Zink, G. Skinner, F. Doerr, P. Juliao, G. Gonzalez, C. Burnett, C. Drenzek, C. Shuler, J. Austin, A. Ellis, S. Maslanka, and J. Sobel.** 2008. International outbreak of severe botulism with prolonged toxemia caused by commercial carrot juice. *Clin. Infect. Dis.* **47**:1245–1251.

163. **Shimizu, S., M. Ootsubo, Y. Kubosawa, I. Fuchizawa, Y. Kawai, and K. Yamazaki.** 2009. Fluorescent in situ hybridization in combination with filter cultivation (FISHFC) method for specific detection and enumeration of viable *Clostridium perfringens. Food Microbiol.* **26**:425–431.

164. **Shimizu, T., K. Ohtani, H. Hirakawa, K. Ohshima, A. Yamashita, T. Shiba, N. Ogasawara, M. Hattori, S. Kuhara, and H. Hayashi.** 2002. Complete genome sequence of *Clostridium perfringens*, an anaerobic flesh-eater. *Proc. Natl. Acad. Sci. USA* **99**:996–1001.

165. **Shukla, H. D., and S. K. Sharma.** 2005. *Clostridium botulinum*: a bug with beauty and weapon. *Crit. Rev. Microbiol.* **31**:11–18.

166. **Simmon, K. E., S. Mirrett, L. B. Reller, and C. A. Petti.** 2008. Genotypic diversity of anaerobic isolates from bloodstream infections. *J. Clin. Microbiol.* **46**:1596–1601.

167. **Smedley, J. G., III, D. J. Fisher, S. Sayeed, G. Chakrabarti, and B. A. McClane.** 2004. The enteric toxins of *Clostridium perfringens. Rev. Physiol. Biochem. Pharmacol.* **152**:183–204.

168. **Smith, G. R.** 1987. Botulism in water birds and its relation to comparative medicine, p. 73–86. *In* M. W. Elklund and V. R. Dowell, Jr. (ed.), *Avian Botulism.* Charles C Thomas, Springfield, IL.

169. **Smith, L. D. S.** 1975. Clostridium, p. 109–114. *In* L. D. S. Smith (ed.), *The Pathogenic Anaerobic Bacteria.* Charles C Thomas, Springfield, IL.

170. **Smith, L. D. S., and H. Sugiyama.** 1988. *Botulism. The Organism, Its Toxins, the Diseases.* Charles C Thomas, Springfield, IL.

171. **Smith, L. D. S., and B. L. Williams.** 1984. *The Pathogenic Anaerobic Bacteria.* Charles C Thomas, Springfield, IL.

172. **Sobel, J., C. G. Mixter, P. Kolhe, A. Gupta, J. Guarner, S. Zaki, N. A. Hoffman, J. G. Songer, M. Fremont-Smith, M. Fischer, G. Killgore, P. H. Britz, and C. MacDonald.** 2005. Necrotizing enterocolitis associated with *Clostridium perfringens* type A in previously healthy north american adults. *J. Am. Coll. Surg.* **201**:48–56.

173. **Song, Y., C. Liu, D. R. Molitoris, T. J. Tomzynski, P. A. Lawson, M. D. Collins, and S. M. Finegold.** 2003. *Clostridium bolteae* sp. nov., isolated from human sources. *Syst. Appl. Microbiol.* **26**:84–89.

174. **Song, Y. L., C. X. Liu, M. McTeague, P. Summanen, and S. M. Finegold.** 2004. *Clostridium bartlettii* sp. nov., isolated from human faeces. *Anaerobe* **10**:179–184.

175. **Songer, J. G.** 1997. Molecular and immunological methods for the diagnosis of clostridial diseases, p. 491–503. *In* J. I. Rood, B. A. McClane, J. G. Songer, and R. W. Titball (ed.), *The Clostridia: Molecular Biology and Pathogenesis.* Academic Press, New York, NY.

176. **Spigaglia, P., F. Barbanti, P. Mastrantonio, J. S. Brazier, F. Barbut, M. Delmee, E. Kuijper, and I. R. Poxton.** 2008. Fluoroquinolone resistance in *Clostridium difficile* isolates from a prospective study of *C. difficile* infections in Europe. *J. Med. Microbiol.* **57**:784–789.

177. **Stackebrandt, E., and F. A. Rainey.** 1997. Phylogenic relationships, p. 3–19. *In* J. I. Rood, B. A. McClane, J. G. Songer, and R. W. Titball (ed.), *The Clostridia: Molecular Biology and Pathogenesis*, 1st ed. Academic Press, New York, NY.

178. **Statius van Eps, R. G., and G. M. LaMuraglia.** 1997. Photodynamic therapy inhibits transforming growth factor beta activity associated with vascular smooth muscle cell injury. *J. Vasc. Surg.* **25**:1044–1052.

179. **Steer, T., M. D. Collins, G. R. Gibson, H. Hippe, and P. A. Lawson.** 2001. *Clostridium hathewayi* sp. nov., from human faeces. *Syst. Appl. Microbiol.* **24**:353–357.

180. **Stevens, D. L., A. L. Bisno, H. F. Chambers, E. D. Everett, P. Dellinger, E. J. Goldstein, S. L. Gorbach, J. V. Hirschmann, E. L. Kaplan, J. G. Montoya, and J. C. Wade.** 2005. Practice guidelines for the diagnosis and management of skin and soft-tissue infections. *Clin. Infect. Dis.* **41**:1373–1406.

181. **Stevens, D. L., D. M. Musher, D. A. Watson, H. Eddy, R. J. Hamill, F. Gyorkey, H. Rosen, and J. Mader.** 1990. Spontaneous, nontraumatic gangrene due to *Clostridium septicum. Rev. Infect. Dis.* **12**:286–296.

182. **Stevens, D. L., R. K. Tweten, M. M. Awad, J. I. Rood, and A. E. Bryant.** 1997. Clostridial gas gangrene: evidence that alpha and theta toxins differentially modulate the

immune response and induce acute tissue necrosis. *J. Infect. Dis.* **176:**189–195.

183. **Steyaert, S., R. Peleman, M. Vaneechoutte, B. T. De, G. Claeys, and G. Verschraegen.** 1999. Septicemia in neutropenic patients infected with *Clostridium tertium* resistant to cefepime and other expanded-spectrum cephalosporins. *J. Clin. Microbiol.* **37:**3778–3779.

184. **Sugahara, T., T. Takahashi, Yamaya S, and A. Ohsaka.** 1976. In vitro aggregation of platelets induced by alpha toxin (phospholipase C) of *Clostridium perfringens. Jpn. J. Med. Sci. Biol.* **29:**255–263.

185. **Sunenshine, R. H., and L. C. McDonald.** 2006. *Clostridium difficile*-associated disease: new challenges from an established pathogen. *Cleve. Clin. J. Med.* **73:**187–197.

186. **Swaminathan, S., and S. Eswaramoorthy.** 2000. Structural analysis of the catalytic and binding sites of *Clostridium botulinum* neurotoxin B. *Nat. Struct. Biol.* **7:**693–699.

187. **Torres, J., M. Camorlinga-Ponce, and O. Munoz.** 1992. Sensitivity in culture of epithelial cells from rhesus monkey kidney and human colon carcinoma to toxins A and B from *Clostridium difficile. Toxicon* **30:**419–426.

188. **Underwood, K., S. Rubin, T. Deakers, and C. Newth.** 2007. Infant botulism: a 30-year experience spanning the introduction of botulism immune globulin intravenous in the intensive care unit at Childrens Hospital Los Angeles. *Pediatrics* **120:**e1380–e1385.

189. **Valiquette, L., B. Cossette, M. P. Garant, H. Diab, and J. Pepin.** 2007. Impact of a reduction in the use of high-risk antibiotics on the course of an epidemic of *Clostridium difficile*-associated disease caused by the hypervirulent NAP1/027 strain. *Clin. Infect. Dis.* **45**(Suppl. 2):S112–S121.

190. **Vanpoucke, H., B. T. De, G. Claeys, M. Vaneechoutte, and G. Verschraegen.** 2001. Evaluation of six commercial assays for the rapid detection of *Clostridium difficile* toxin and/or antigen in stool specimens. *Clin. Microbiol. Infect.* **7:**55–64.

191. **von Eichel-Streiber, C., P. Boquet, M. Sauerborn, and M. Thelestam.** 1996. Large clostridial cytotoxins—a family of glycosyltransferases modifying small GTP-binding proteins. *Trends Microbiol.* **4:**375–382.

192. **Voth, D. E., and J. D. Ballard.** 2005. *Clostridium difficile* toxins: mechanism of action and role in disease. *Clin. Microbiol. Rev.* **18:**247–263.

193. **Wang, R. F., M. L. Beggs, B. D. Erickson, and C. E. Cerniglia.** 2004. DNA microarray analysis of predominant human intestinal bacteria in fecal samples. *Mol. Cell. Probes* **18:**223–234.

194. **Warny, M., J. Pepin, A. Fang, G. Killgore, A. Thompson, J. Brazier, E. Frost, and L. C. McDonald.** 2005. Toxin production by an emerging strain of *Clostridium difficile* associated with outbreaks of severe disease in North America and Europe. *Lancet* **366:**1079–1084.

195. **Weber, J. T., H. C. Goodpasture, H. Alexander, S. B. Werner, C. L. Hatheway, and R. V. Tauxe.** 1993. Wound botulism in a patient with a tooth abscess: case report and review. *Clin. Infect. Dis.* **16:**635–639.

196. **Wein, L. M., and Y. Liu.** 2005. Analyzing a bioterror attack on the food supply: the case of botulinum toxin in milk. *Proc. Natl. Acad. Sci. USA* **102:**9984–9989.

197. **Wheeler, C., G. Inami, J. Mohle-Boetani, and D. Vugia.** 2009. Sensitivity of mouse bioassay in clinical wound botulism. *Clin. Infect. Dis.* **48:**1669–1673.

198. **Wilkins, T. D., and D. M. Lyerly.** 2003. *Clostridium difficile* testing: after 20 years, still challenging. *J. Clin. Microbiol.* **41:**531–534.

199. **Williamson, E. D., and R. W. Titball.** 1993. A genetically engineered vaccine against alpha-toxin of *Clostridium perfringens* protects against experimental gas gangrene. *Vaccine* **11:**1253–1258.

200. **Wilson, J. R., and A. P. Limaye.** 2004. Risk factors for mortality in patients with anaerobic bacteremia. *Eur. J. Clin. Microbiol. Infect. Dis.* **23:**310–316.

201. **Winn, W. C., S. D. Allen, W. M. Janda, E. W. Koneman, G. Procop, P. C. Schrechenberger, and G. Woods.** 2005. *Koneman's Color Atlas and Textbook of Diagnostic Microbiology.* Lippincott Williams & Wilkins, Philadelphia, PA.

202. **Woo, P. C., S. K. Lau, J. L. Teng, H. Tse, and K. Y. Yuen.** 2008. Then and now: use of 16S rDNA gene sequencing for bacterial identification and discovery of novel bacteria in clinical microbiology laboratories. *Clin. Microbiol. Infect.* **14:**908–934.

203. **Woo, P. C., S. K. Lau, G. K. Woo, A. M. Fung, V. P. Yiu, and K. Y. Yuen.** 2004. Bacteremia due to *Clostridium hathewayi* in a patient with acute appendicitis. *J. Clin. Microbiol.* **42:**5947–5949.

204. **Woodruff, B. A., P. M. Griffin, L. M. McCroskey, J. F. Smart, R. B. Wainwright, R. G. Bryant, L. C. Hutwagner, and C. L. Hatheway.** 1992. Clinical and laboratory comparison of botulism from toxin types A, B, and E in the United States, 1975–1988. *J. Infect. Dis.* **166:**1281–1286.

205. **Zink, J. M., R. Singh-Parikshak, A. Sugar, and M. W. Johnson.** 2004. *Clostridium sordellii* endophthalmitis after suture removal from a corneal transplant. *Cornea* **23:**522–523.

Bacteroides, Porphyromonas, Prevotella, Fusobacterium, and Other Anaerobic Gram-Negative Rods

EIJA KÖNÖNEN, WILLIAM G. WADE, AND DIANE M. CITRON

51

TAXONOMY AND DESCRIPTION OF THE GROUP

Most of the obligately anaerobic, gram-negative, non-spore-forming rods of clinical relevance belong to the phylum *Bacteroidetes*, including the families *Bacteroidaceae*, *Porphyromonadaceae*, *Prevotellaceae*, and *Rikenellaceae*, and to the phylum *Fusobacteria*, including the family *Fusobacteriaceae*. In addition, clinically important taxa representing anaerobic, gram-negative, non-spore-forming rods exist in some other phyla, such as *Firmicutes* and *Proteobacteria* and the recently described *Synergistetes*. There have been a considerable number of recent changes in the taxonomy of the taxa that are covered in this chapter; some new genera have been named, and a plethora of novel species have been described in the past few years. The changes made since the ninth edition of this *Manual* are listed in Table 1.

Within the family *Bacteroidaceae*, the genus *Bacteroides* consists of saccharolytic, bile-resistant, and nonpigmented species, mainly isolated from the gut (178). Currently, the genus is limited to species within the *Bacteroides fragilis* group, which includes more than 20 species (212). Of these, especially *B. fragilis*, *B. thetaiotaomicron*, and *B. ovatus* are highly relevant in human infections. Since 2006, few taxonomic changes have occurred within the genus; some novel species have been described, and some former *Bacteroides* species have been moved to other genera. Novel species of the *B. fragilis* group (Table 1) have been isolated from feces of healthy subjects (8–10, 28, 76, 96, 161, 210). *B. distasonis*, *B. goldsteinii*, and *B. merdae* now reside in a novel genus, *Parabacteroides* (167), and *B. splanchinus* is now in another novel genus, *Odoribacter* (74). *B. capillosus*, which is both phenotypically and genotypically distinct from the genus *Bacteroides*, has been assigned to a novel genus, *Pseudoflavonifractor*, as *P. capillosus* (26). This represents a distinct lineage in clostridial cluster IV of the phylum *Firmicutes*. The genus *Bacteroides* still contains organisms for which the taxonomic position remains uncertain; for example, further studies are needed for *B. ureolyticus*, which is an asaccharolytic, formate- and fumarate-requiring species, i.e., phenotypically close to *Campylobacter gracilis* (205). A novel genus, distantly related to the genus *Bacteroides*, contains one species isolated from a human brain abscess, *Phocaeicola abscessus*, which is asaccharolytic and motile (4).

The genus *Alistipes*, which belongs to the family *Rikenellaceae*, currently includes five species, *A. finegoldii*, *A. indistinctus*, *A. onderdonkii*, *A. putredinis*, and *A. shahii* (136, 157, 191), which are anaerobic, nonmotile, and, except for coccoid-shaped *A. indistinctus* cells, straight or slightly curved rods. The type species of the genus, *A. putredinis* (formerly *Bacteroides putredinis*), is asaccharolytic, nonpigmented, and bile sensitive. *A. indistinctus* is also nonpigmented and bile sensitive but it is saccharolytic, whereas the other *Alistipes* species are saccharolytic, pigmented, and bile resistant.

The family *Porphyromonadaceae* includes five genera with species detected in humans: *Barnesiella*, *Odoribacter*, *Parabacteroides*, *Porphyromonas*, and *Tannerella*. Of these genera, *Porphyromonas* is clinically most relevant. There are currently 17 validly published *Porphyromonas* species, and many of them are of animal origin. *P. asaccharolytica*, *P. bennonis*, *P. catoniae*, *P. endodontalis*, *P. gingivalis*, *P. somerae*, and *P. uenonis* are rather frequently detected in humans (56, 101, 102, 177, 195, 196). Most species are asaccharolytic and, except for *P. catoniae*, pigmented, and they are generally considered pathogens. The genus *Parabacteroides*, consisting of *P. distasonis*, *P. goldsteinii*, *P. gordonii*, *P. johnsonii*, and *P. merdae* (167, 168, 171), is phylogenetically closely related to the genera *Tannerella* (166) and *Barnesiella* (169). *Parabacteroides* organisms are saccharolytic and resistant to 20% bile. The genus *Tannerella* contains only one species, *T. forsythia* (formerly *T. forsythensis*) (166), which is an important oral pathogen, and the genus *Barnesiella* contains one human species, *B. intestinihominis*, isolated from feces (129). Both of these species are anaerobic, nonpigmented, nonmotile, pleomorphic rods. The new genus *Odoribacter* includes two human-derived species; *O. splanchnicus* (formerly *Bacteroides*) is saccharolytic and bile resistant, while the newly described *O. laneus* (136) is asaccharolytic and susceptible to 20% bile.

The family *Prevotellaceae* includes saccharolytic or moderately saccharolytic short rods that produce acetic and succinic acids as their major end products of fermentation (179). This family has been confronted by a tremendously increasing number of species in the past few years. Most novel *Prevotella* species (Table 1) have been isolated from the oral cavity (43–45, 47, 172) but also from feces (75) and other sites of the body, where they have been associated with various clinical conditions (2, 42, 60, 109, 170). Two

TABLE 1 Recently classified or reclassified genera and species (from 2006 onwards) within non-spore-forming anaerobic gram-negative rods isolated from humans

Phylum and genus	Species	Previous nomenclature	Reference(s)
Bacteroidetes			
Alistipes	*A. indistinctus*	New species	136
	A. onderdonkii	New species	191
	A. shahii	New species	191
Bacteroides	*B. cellulosilyticus*	New species	161
	B. clarus	New species	210
	B. coprophilus	New species	76
	B. dorei	New species	10
	B. faecis	New species	96
	B. finegoldii	New species	9
	B. fluxus	New species	210
	B. intestinalis	New species	8
	B. oleiciplenus	New species	210
	B. xylanisolvens	New species	28
Barnesiella (new genus)	*B. intestinihominis*	New species	129, 169
Odoribacter (new genus)	*O. laneus*	New species	136
	O. splanchnicus	*Bacteroides splanchnicus*	74
Parabacteroides (new genus)	*P. distasonis*	*Bacteroides distasonis*	167
	P. goldsteinii	*Bacteroides goldsteinii*	167
	P. gordonii	New species	171
	P. johnsonii	New species	168
	P. merdae	*Bacteroides merdae*	167
Paraprevotella (new genus)	*P. clara*	New species	130
	P. xylaniphila	New species	130
Phocaeicola (new genus)	*P. abscessus*	New species	4
Porphyromonas	*P. bennonis*	New species	196
Prevotella	*P. amnii*	New species	109
	P. aurantiaca	New species	172
	P. bergensis	New species	42
	P. copri	New species	75
	P. histicola	New species	44
	P. maculosa	New species	43
	P. micans	New species	45
	P. nanceiensis	New species	2
	P. pleuritidis	New species	170
	P. saccharolytica	New species	47
	P. stercorea	New species	75
	P. timonensis	New species	60
Synergistetes (new phylum)			92
Jonquetella (new genus)	*J. anthropi*	New species	91
Pyramidobacter (new genus)	*P. piscolens*	New species	46
Firmicutes			
Dialister	*D. succinatiphilus*	New species	129
Megamonas	*M. funiformis*	New species	173
Proteobacteria			
Sutterella	*S. parvirubra*	New species	173
Parasutterella (new genus)	*P. excrementihominis*	New species	135

species, *P. heparinolytica* and *P. zoogleoformans*, are only loosely connected to other *Prevotella* species and, instead, they cluster phylogenetically with *Bacteroides* species (146), while *P. tannerae*, together with some as-yet-uncultivable taxa, appears to represent a novel genus, related to but distinct from *Prevotella*. Recently, a novel genus, *Paraprevotella*, consisting of two new species (Table 1) from human feces, was described (130).

In the family *Fusobacteriaceae* of the phylum *Fusobacteria*, the genera of clinical interest are *Fusobacterium*, *Leptotrichia*,

and *Sneathia*. These organisms are nonmotile, pleomorphic rods, mainly isolated from the oral cavity. In a study using sequencing of the 16S-23S rRNA gene internal transcribed spacer regions of *Fusobacterium* species (35), three phylogenetic clusters were formed: the first cluster included *F. mortiferum*, *F. varium*, and *F. ulcerans*; the second cluster contained *F. nucleatum* subspecies, *F. naviforme* (note that there are considerable inconsistencies in the phenotypic and genotypic characteristics between *F. naviforme* strains obtained by different laboratories; the strain used

TABLE 2 Characteristics of genera representing gram-negative anaerobic rods isolated from clinical specimens[a]

Characteristic	Bacteroides[b]	Alistipes[c]	Odoribacter[d]	Porphyromonas[e]	Parabacteroides	Tannerella	Prevotella
Growth in microaerobic atmosphere	−	−	−	−	−	−	−
Cell morphology	Short	Short	Pleomorphic	v	Short	Pleomorphic	Coccobacillary
Motility	−	−	−	−	−	−	−
Pigment production[h]	−	v	−	+	−	−	v
Growth in 20% bile	+	v	v	−	+	−	−
Susceptibility to[i]:							
Vancomycin (5 μg)	R	R	R	S	R	R	R
Kanamycin (1,000 μg)	R	R	R	R	R	S	v
Colistin (10 μg)	R	R	R	R	R	S	v
Catalase production	−	v	v	v	v	v	−
Indole production	v	v	+	v	−	−	v
Nitrate reduction	−	−	−	−	−	−	−
Carbohydrate fermentation	+	+	v	v	+	−	+
Major metabolic end product(s)[j]	A, S	S	A, P, S	A, B, P	A, S	A, B, IV, P, PA	A, S
Type species	B. fragilis	A. putredinis	O. splanchnicus	P. asaccharolytica	P. distasonis	T. forsythia	P. melaninogenica

[a]Symbols: +, positive; −, negative; v, variable reaction.
[b]Bacteroides sensu stricto.
[c]A. putredinis is asaccharolytic.
[d]Susceptibility pattern of O. laneus not reported.
[e]P. catoniae is nonpigmented, is resistant to vancomycin, and does not produce butyric acid. P. bennonis produces succinic acid but neither butyric nor propionic acids.

in this study by Conrads et al. [35] fits with the original description of the species), *F. simiae*, and *F. periodonticum*; the third cluster included *F. necrophorum* subspecies and *F. gonidiaformans*. *F. russii* and *F. perfoetens* formed separate branches. The somewhat fuzzy phylogeny of fusobacteria and wide heterogeneity of *F. nucleatum*, in particular, have been recently explained by potential horizontal gene transfer that occurred in the close interaction of oral bacteria within dental biofilms (123). The genus *Leptotrichia* consists of nonmotile, highly saccharolytic, long rods that typically produce lactic acid. Currently, there are six validly described *Leptotrichia* species: *L. buccalis*, *L. goodfellowii*, *L. hofstadii*, *L. shahii*, *L. trevisanii*, and *L. wadei* (50, 51), while a former species, *L. sanguinegens*, isolated from blood, was moved to a novel genus, *Sneathia* (34). "*L. amnionii*" (180) is not validly published and, in fact, phylogenetically clusters closer to *Sneathia sanguinegens* than to other *Leptotrichia* species (50).

Recently, a novel phylum named *Synergistetes* was proposed by Jumas-Bilak et al. (92). So far, only two cultivable genera, including obligately anaerobic, nonmotile, gram-negative species, *Jonquetella anthropi* (91) and *Pyramidobacter piscolens* (46), have been isolated from humans. However, fluorescent in situ hybridization analysis has revealed that the oral cavity harbors a diverse population of unculturable *Synergistetes*, which are large curved bacilli (206).

In the gram-positive phylum *Firmicutes*, the family *Veillonellaceae* includes some clinically important genera, which have traditional gram-negative cell walls. The genus *Dialister* includes five species of human origin: *D. invisus* (41) and *D. pneumosintes* (formerly *Bacteroides pneumosintes*) isolated from the oral cavity, *D. micraerophilus* and *D. propionicifaciens* (90) from clinical specimens, and a novel species, *D. succinatiphilus*, from feces (129). These anaero-

bic or microaerobic, gram-negative coccobacilli are asaccharolytic and largely unreactive in biochemical tests (90). The two human species of the genus *Megamonas*, *M. hypermegale* and the novel *M. funiformis* (173), are anaerobic, gram-negative, very large rods. In the genus *Selenomonas*, *S. sputigena*, *S. artemidis*, *S. dianae*, *S. flueggei*, *S. infelix*, and *S. noxia*, and also the closely related *Centipeda periodontii*, have been isolated from the human oral cavity (126). They are anaerobic, gram-negative, curved motile rods.

Various families in the phylum *Proteobacteria* include genera and species with clinical importance in humans. The genera *Sutterella* and *Parasutterella* in the family *Alcaligenaceae* consist of asaccharolytic, bile-resistant, gram-negative short rods, of which *S. wadsworthensis* and the novel *S. parvirubra* (173) and *P. excrementihominis* (135) have been isolated from human specimens. The family *Desulfovibrionaceae* contains two genera of clinical interest, *Bilophila* and *Desulfovibrio*. *Bilophila wadsworthia* is an anaerobic, asaccharolytic, bile-resistant, gram-negative rod and is a significant pathogen in humans (11). Of the more than 30 *Desulfovibrio* species, some infrequently cause a variety of human infections (64). In the family *Desulfomicrobiaceae*, the genus *Desulfomicrobium* includes one human species, *D. orale*, which is associated with periodontal diseases (106). The genus *Anaerobiospirillum* of the family *Succinivibrionaceae* includes two species, *A. succiniciproducens* and *A. thomasii*, isolated from feces of humans, cats, and dogs (121). *Anaerobiospirillum*, *Desulfovibrio*, and *Desulfomicrobium* organisms are strictly anaerobic, gram-negative, motile, spiral-shaped bacteria that reduce sulfate.

Complete genome sequences are available for the following members of this group: *Bacteroides thetaiotaomicron* strain VPI-5482 (accession no. NC_004663) (215); *Bacteroides fragilis* NCTC 9343 (NC_003228) (27); *B. fragilis* YCH46 (NC_006347) (105); *Bacteroides vulgatus*

Fusobacterium	Leptotrichia[f]	Dialister	Selenomonas	Sutterella	Bilophila	Desulfovibrio[g]	Anaerobiospirillum
—	—	v	—	v	—	—	—
v	v	Coccoid	Curved	Straight	Straight	Curved	Spiral, long
—	—	—	+	—	—	+	+
—	—	—	—	—	—	+	—
v	—	—	—	v	+	v	v
R	R	R	R	R	R	R	R
S	S	S	S	S	S	S	S
S	S	v	v	S	S	R	v
—	v	—	—	—	+	v	—
v	—	—	—	—	—	—	—
—	—	—	+	v	+	v	—
v	+	—	+	—	—	—	+
B	L	A, P	A, P	S	A	A	A, S
F. nucleatum	L. buccalis	D. pneumosintes	S. sputigena	S. wadsworthensis	B. wadsworthia	D. desulfuricans	A. succiniproducens

[f]Some strains can grow in a microaerobic atmosphere in subsequent cultures.

[g]D. piger is nonmotile.

[h]Pigmentation on blood agar varies from tan to black. In some cases, it may take up to 2 weeks. Rabbit laked blood agar enhances pigment production.

[i]Special-potency antimicrobial identification disks. Symbols: R, resistant; S, susceptible; v, variable reaction. A zone size of ≥10 mm in diameter is considered susceptible.

[j]Symbols: A, acetic acid; B, butyric acid; IV, isovaleric acid; P, propionic acid; PA, phenylacetic acid; S, succinic acid.

ATCC 8482 (NC_009614) (216); *Parabacteroides distasonis* ATCC 8503 (NC_009615) (216); *Porphyromonas gingivalis* W83 (NC_002950) (140); *Porphyromonas gingivalis* ATCC 33277 (NC_010729) (138); *Desulfovibrio desulfuricans* G20 (NC_007519) (unpublished); *D. desulfuricans* 27774 (NC_011883) (unpublished); *Desulfovibrio magneticus* RS-1 (NC_012796) (139); *Desulfovibrio salexigens* DSM 2638 (NC_012881) (unpublished); *Desulfovibrio vulgaris* DP4 (NC_008751) (207); *D. vulgaris* "Hildenborough" (NC_002937) (79); *D. vulgaris* "Miyazaki" (NC_011769) (unpublished); *Fusobacterium nucleatum* ATCC 25586 (NC_003454) (93); *Leptotrichia buccalis* C-1013-b (NC_013192) (83). Interestingly, the genome sequence for *F. nucleatum* revealed that although this species has a gram-negative cell wall, including an outer membrane, a significant proportion of genes were related to homologues from gram-positive species in the phylum *Firmicutes*, suggesting that *Fusobacterium* has a gram-positive evolutionary history (93).

Current methods used for taxonomic studies are mainly based on nucleic acid analyses, in particular, sequencing of the 16S rRNA gene and comparison of these sequences, in order to reveal the phylogenetic relatedness of taxa. This approach does not necessarily correlate with phenotypic characteristics, such as cell and colony morphologies, atmospheric growth requirements, and various biochemical test results, which are still widely used in clinical microbiology laboratories. However, appropriate atmospheric requirements should be determined for all isolates, because the true anaerobes can be differentiated from facultatively anaerobic bacteria by their inability to grow in the presence of oxygen and by their susceptibility to metronidazole (89). Table 2 presents differential characteristics of clinically relevant genera within the gram-negative anaerobic rods.

EPIDEMIOLOGY AND TRANSMISSION

Gram-negative anaerobic rods inhabit the mucosal surfaces of the oral cavity and gastrointestinal tract of animals and humans. In fact, some of these organisms, such as *Fusobacterium* and *Prevotella*, are ubiquitous members of the mouth from the early months of life (102) and, when teeth erupt, are an integral part of dental biofilms (99). Recently, *Prevotella* has been shown among the dominant genera in other habitats, such as the esophagus and stomach (13, 149), which have previously been considered to have a very limited microbial diversity. In the gut, *Bacteroides* becomes part of the microbiota in early infancy, although as a result of cesarean section, the colonization of the *B. fragilis* group organisms can be delayed and the levels are greatly reduced (150). Two bacterial phyla, *Firmicutes* and *Bacteroidetes*, dominate in the gut, and changes in their relative proportion seem to have an impact on host physiology, with the proportion of *Bacteroidetes* being decreased in obese people (113, 212). In the female genital tract, when the vaginal hydrogen peroxide-producing lactobacilli decrease in numbers, *Prevotella* species increase and become an important part of the microbiota with other commensal vaginosis-associated microorganisms (186).

CLINICAL SIGNIFICANCE

Anaerobes, originating mainly from the indigenous microbiota, are detected typically in polymicrobial infections associated with mucosal surfaces close to the site where they reside. Most infections are acquired when the integrity of the colonized mucosa or lumen is breached by trauma, underlying disease, or during surgery. Exceptions to this endogenous acquisition include clenched-fist wounds and animal and human bite wounds. Gram-negative anaerobes,

TABLE 3 Common genera of anaerobic gram-negative rods detected in human infections

Site of isolation	Genera isolated
Brain and/or central nervous system	*Bacteroides, Dialister, Fusobacterium, Porphyromonas*
Mouth	
Abscesses	*Dialister, Fusobacterium, Prevotella, Porphyromonas*
Endodontic infection	*Centipeda, Dialister, Fusobacterium, Porphyromonas, Prevotella, Tannerella*
Periodontal diseases	*Desulfomicrobium, Dialister, Fusobacterium, Porphyromonas, Prevotella, Selenomonas, Tannerella*
Peri-implant diseases	*Fusobacterium, Porphyromonas, Prevotella, Tannerella*
Spreading odontogenic infection	*Fusobacterium, Prevotella*
Ear, nose, and throat	*Fusobacterium, Prevotella*
Lower respiratory tract	*Bacteroides, Dialister, Fusobacterium, Porphyromonas, Prevotella, Selenomonas*
Abdomen or intestine	
Abscesses	*Alistipes, Bacteroides, Bilophila, Fusobacterium, Parabacteroides, Porphyromonas, Sutterella*
Appendicitis	*Alistipes, Bacteroides, Bilophila, Fusobacterium, Parabacteroides, Porphyromonas, Sutterella*
Peritonitis	*Alistipes, Bacteroides, Desulfovibrio, Parabacteroides, Porphyromonas, Sutterella*
Diarrhea	*Anaerobiospirillum, Bacteroides*
Urogenital tract	
Abscesses	*Bacteroides, Prevotella*
Bacterial vaginosis	*Leptotrichia, Porphyromonas, Prevotella, Sneathia, Tannerella*
Intra-amniotic infection	*Dialister, Fusobacterium, Leptotrichia, Porphyromonas, Sneathia*
Preterm delivery	*Fusobacterium, Leptotrichia, Sneathia*
Urinary tract infection	*Bacteroides, Dialister, Leptotrichia, Prevotella*
Skin and/or soft tissue	
Abscesses	*Bacteroides, Dialister, Fusobacterium, Jonquetella, Porphyromonas, Prevotella*
Ulcer or chronic wound	*Bacteroides, Dialister, Porphyromonas, Prevotella*
Bite wound infection (animal)	*Bacteroides, Fusobacterium, Porphyromonas, Prevotella*
Bite wound infection (human)	*Dialister, Fusobacterium, Prevotella*
Bones and joints	
Arthritis	*Bacteroides, Porphyromonas, Tannerella*
Osteomyelitis	*Bacteroides, Fusobacterium, Porphyromonas*
Cardiovascular sites	
Bacteremia	*Alistipes, Anaerobiospirillum, Bacteroides, Bilophila, Desulfovibrio, Dialister, Fusobacterium, Leptotrichia, Parabacteroides, Porphyromonas, Prevotella, Sneathia*
Endocarditis	*Bacteroides, Fusobacterium, Leptotrichia*
Pericarditis	*Bacteroides, Fusobacterium*

such as *B. fragilis*, are involved in a variety of infections associated with considerable morbidity and mortality (212). Table 3 summarizes the infectious sites where gram-negative anaerobic organisms have been frequently isolated from clinical specimens. Anaerobic bacteria can occasionally spread to adjacent tissues and the bloodstream with serious consequences. Localized dentoalveolar infections can result in life-threatening spread of oral anaerobes along tissue spaces of the head and neck up to the mediastinum (55). In cases when gram-negative anaerobes gain entrance to the bloodstream and trigger a systemic inflammatory response, this may result in sepsis or infective endocarditis with a fatal outcome. The gastrointestinal tract and the oropharynx are the most common sources for anaerobic bacteremias, with gastrointestinal surgery and underlying malignancies being the major predisposing factors (17, 108). In the oral cavity, inflamed periodontal tissues offer an open portal for a myriad of oral anaerobes to the circulation via the daily practices of oral hygiene and chewing food (7, 116). This calls attention to the importance of prevention of oral infections, especially in patients at increased risk for infective endocarditis.

Bacteroides and Related Genera

Among the anaerobes in clinical specimens, members of the bile-resistant *B. fragilis* group are the most commonly encountered and are more virulent and resistant to antimicrobial agents than most other anaerobes. Although other intestinal *Bacteroides* species outnumber *B. fragilis* 10- to 100-fold, *B. fragilis* proved to be the most frequent *Bacteroides* found in specimens from blood, ulcers, abscesses, bronchial secretion, bone, intra-abdominal infections, inflamed appendix, and the head (212). In the Wadsworth Anaerobe Collection database, consisting of more than 3,000 clinical specimens, *B. thetaiotaomicron* and *B. ovatus*, as well as *B. capillosus* (currently known as a *Pseudoflavonifractor* species), in descending order, were also detected in these specimens, but less frequently. Another U.S. study that included over 5,000 isolates of the *B. fragilis* group from clinical specimens confirmed this: *B. fragilis* was most common (52%), followed by *B. thetaiotaomicron* (19%) and *B. ovatus* (10%) (185). In children, *B. fragilis* is the main anaerobic organism recovered from intra-abdominal infections (114, 212); for instance, it is isolated from nearly all tissue specimens of acute appendicitis (156). Around 10 to 20% of the *B. fragilis* strains are able to produce enterotoxin; these strains have been associated with diarrhea and, in addition, their proportion seems to be higher than that of nontoxigenic strains among blood culture isolates (175). The *B. fragilis* group organisms (here also including *Parabacteroides distasonis*) and other *Bacteroides* species are the most frequently isolated pathogens from bloodstream infections with involvement of anaerobes (17, 108, 181, 212). Recently, the first recoveries of two novel *Bacteroides* species, *B. dorei* and *B. finegoldii*, were reported from blood (181). *Bacteroides* involvement in infective endocarditis, where *B. fragilis* of gastrointestinal origin is the most frequent finding, tends to be more serious than that of other anaerobes, sometimes with a fatal outcome (14, 23). The *B. fragilis* group has been recovered from pericarditis samples (24) and, often as a single isolate, from septic arthritis as well as from osteomyelitis samples (22). Although spondylodiscitis caused by anaerobes is not common, the involvement of *B. fragilis* needs to be taken into account in cases with potential bacteremia of intestinal origin (48). By hematogeneous spread, the *B. fragilis* group and other *Bacteroides* organisms can reach the brain, causing abscesses (111, 154, 194). In addition, members of this group are among the predominant isolates from burn wound infections, with potential involvement in sepsis in this context (133). *Bacteroides* species can be involved in part in polymicrobial necrotizing soft tissue infections (212), and the *B. fragilis* group is, after gram-positive anaerobic cocci, one of the most common anaerobic findings in infected moderate to severe diabetic foot wounds (32, 141). In cat and dog bite infections, *B. tectus* was the most common *Bacteroides* isolate (197).

Pigmented, bile-resistant *Alistipes* species, *A. finegoldii*, *A. onderdonkii*, and *A. shahii*, have been strongly connected to appendicitis, both in children and in adults (156, 191). In addition, *A. finegoldii* has been isolated from blood, *A. shahii* from intra-abdominal fluid, and *A. onderdonkii* from intra-abdominal abscesses and urine (54, 181, 191).

Porphyromonas and Related Genera

Pathogenic potential varies between different *Porphyromonas* species. Of the three oral *Porphyromonas* species, *P. endodontalis* and *P. gingivalis* are known significant pathogens. The detection rate of *P. gingivalis*, one of the major periodontal pathogens, increases with age (80, 103). In addition to periodontitis, it has been frequently detected in oral specimens from necrotizing ulcerative gingivitis, infected root canals, peri-implant lesions, and acute apical abscesses (62, 67, 155, 183). Besides the oral cavity, it has been detected in clinical specimens from various body sites, e.g., intra-abdominal sites (122), vaginal samples in women with bacterial vaginosis (151), amniotic fluid (112), synovial specimens of rheumatoid arthritis and psoriatic arthritis patients (124) and, together with some other periodontal organisms, in occluded arteries of lower extremities of Buerger's disease patients (84). *P. endodontalis* is one of the dominant organisms in infected root canals and in acute dental abscesses (67, 164, 183) but may also be involved in chronic periodontitis (104). *P. uenonis*, which is phenotypically similar to *P. endodontalis* and *P. asaccharolytica*, has been detected in polymicrobial infections below the waistline: appendicitis, peritonitis, pilonidal abscess, an infected sacral decubitus ulcer, and bacterial vaginosis (56, 57). *P. asaccharolytica*

and *P. somerae* were among the anaerobic isolates from moderate to severe diabetic foot infections (32). At the VA Wadsworth Medical Center laboratory, the 58 *P. somerae* isolates originated from a variety of specimens, including lower extremity skin and soft tissue or bone, in particular, and inguinal or sacral area abscess, intra-abdominal abscess, transtracheal aspirate, axillary abscess, mastoiditis, blood culture, brain tissue, and infected scalp (presented in order of their frequency) (195). A novel *Porphyromonas* species, *P. bennonis*, has been detected in human wound infections and abscesses, especially in patients with chronic skin and soft tissue lesions in the perirectal, buttock, and groin regions (196). Although *P. catoniae* inhabits the oral cavity without any disease association described to date, it has been isolated from an abdominal abscess (101). *P. gingivalis* and *Porphyromonas* species of animal origin, e.g., *P. cangingivalis*, *P. canoris*, *P. cansulci*, and *P. macacae*, have been encountered in humans with animal bite infections (197).

Parabacteroides species are common inhabitants of the human gut, and *P. distasonis* is one of the anaerobes of clinical importance in specimens from intra-abdominal infections and inflamed appendixes, where *P. goldsteinii* and *P. merdae* can also be found (189, 212). In addition, *P. distasonis*, *P. merdae*, and a novel species, *P. gordonii*, have been isolated from human blood (85, 171, 181, 212).

Tannerella forsythia is considered one of the major periodontal pathogens (80, 200). In addition, it is one of the predominant organisms in root canal infections (164) and has been found in infected sites around dental implants (155). This oral bacterium has been recovered from vaginal samples in women with bacterial vaginosis (151) as well as from synovial specimens of rheumatoid arthritis and psoriatic arthritis patients (124).

Prevotella and Related Genera

Prevotella species are among the dominating microorganisms of the oral cavity, where they, despite their commensalism, can be involved in nearly all types of oral infections. Interestingly, *P. melaninogenica*, which is a common anaerobic organism in saliva (100, 102), is also one of the most prevalent anaerobes, together with *F. nucleatum*, *P. intermedia*, and *P. buccae*, in infected human bite lesions (198). Although the cariogenic microbiota mainly consists of gram-positive species, some proteolytic gram-negative taxa, including *P. denticola* and *P. tannerae*, can be frequently encountered in advanced carious lesions (29). *P. intermedia* (sensu stricto) is strongly linked to periodontitis (103, 148), and *P. intermedia* and/or the phenotypically identical *P. nigrescens* has been detected in samples from pregnancy gingivitis, necrotizing ulcerative gingivitis, pericoronitis, peri-implantitis, root canal infections, and dentoalveolar abscesses (62, 67, 69, 122, 155, 183, 184). Also, *P. baroniae*, a recently described *Prevotella* species, proved to be common in root canal infections and acute dental abscess aspirates (164, 183). In noma (cancrum oris) lesions, *P. intermedia* (sensu lato) is considered a key organism (49). In spreading odontogenic infections, members of the genus *Prevotella* seem to play an important role, with *P. buccae* and *P. oris* the most prominent findings in this context (55, 159). Recently, a new concept of the polymicrobial bacteriology of cystic fibrosis has been presented and, indeed, not only aerobic *Pseudomonas aeruginosa* and *Staphylococcus aureus* but also some anaerobes, especially *Prevotella*, such as *P. melaninogenica*, *P. denticola*, *P. oris*, and *P. salivae*, have been detected as one of the persistently dominating organisms in the sputum of these patients (16). Also, *Prevotella* taxa were recovered from bronchoalveolar lavage fluid of ventilator-associated pneumonia (6). Furthermore, various *Prevotella* species are found in extraoral infections and abscesses in a wide range of body sites, for instance, *P. amnii*, *P. bivia*, *P. corporis*, *P. disiens*, *P. intermedia*, and *P. nigrescens* in the female genital tract (21, 109, 148, 151); *P. buccalis* in urine (40); *P. bergensis*, *P. bivia*, and *P. melaninogenica* in infectious lesions of the skin and soft tissues, including diabetic foot lesions (32, 42); *P. intermedia* and *P. nigrescens* in intra-abdominal and soft tissue abscesses (122); *P. intermedia* (sensu lato) and *P. melaninogenica* in peritonsillar and retropharyngeal abscesses (21); *P. timonensis* in breast abscesses (60); *P. intermedia* in synovial fluid of arthritis patients (124); and *P. intermedia* and *P. nigrescens* (with some other periodontal bacteria) in occluded arteries of lower extremities of Buerger's disease patients (84). Several *Prevotella* species, such as *P. bivia*, *P. buccae*, *P. denticola*, *P. disiens*, and *P. nigrescens*, have been among anaerobic findings in bloodstream infections (122, 181). *P. heparinolytica* is a relatively common anaerobic isolate from animal bite wounds (197).

Fusobacterium and Related Genera

Clinically, the most important *Fusobacterium* species are *F. nucleatum* and *F. necrophorum* (19, 20, 31, 160). *F. nucleatum* is an oral species which has been divided into several subspecies with variable pathogenic potentials (19). It is a key organism in maturation of pathogenic biofilms in periodontal pockets (187) and considered an important pathogen in peri-implantitis, root canal infections, dentoalveolar abscesses, and spreading odontogenic infections (155, 159, 164, 183). It is also an important etiologic agent in extraoral infections and abscesses at a wide range of body sites, being detected from blood, brain, chest, heart, lung, liver, appendix, joint, abdomen, genitourinary tract, and fetal membranes as well as infected human bite lesions (14, 22, 24, 31, 39, 71, 73, 82, 111, 156, 181, 198). In a tertiary care hospital where all episodes of documented brain abscess cases between 1991 and 2000 were reviewed, in 40% of cerebral puncture specimens, only anaerobes were found; of these, *F. nucleatum* proved to be the most frequently isolated organism, found in one of three of the patients diagnosed (111). The presence of a novel adhesin, *Fusobacterium* adhesin A, seems to allow separation of oral fusobacteria, *F. nucleatum*, *F. periodonticum*, and *F. simiae*, from nonoral fusobacteria, including *F. gonidiaformans*, *F. mortiferum*, *F. naviforme*, *F. russii*, and *F. ulcerans* (72). Because the adhesin was present in *F. nucleatum* isolated from intrauterine infections but absent among the vaginal species *F. gonidiaformans* and *F. naviforme*, it was hypothesized that intrauterine *F. nucleatum* originates from the oral cavity rather than the vaginal tract. Of the two *F. necrophorum* subspecies, *F. necrophorum* subsp. *funduliforme* (biovar B) is a human pathogen (20, 160). *F. necrophorum* is best known for its connection to Lemierre's syndrome (necrobacillosis), which can be considered an invasive *F. necrophorum* disease, often with pleuropulmonar involvement (20, 70, 160). It is notable that invasive disease with *F. necrophorum* may be on the increase (20). In Denmark, the overall mortality of Lemierre's syndrome, originating mainly from oropharyngeal sites, was reported to be 9% in adolescents, and that of disseminated *F. necrophorum* infections, originating from lower parts of the body, was 26% in elderly with predisposing diseases (70). In the latter type of cases, underlying cancers should be considered. Interestingly, *F. necrophorum* can be found in adolescents as the causative agent in approximately 10% of cases of tonsillitis

(persistent sore throat) not caused by group A streptococci (5, 20, 160). In a Danish retrospective study of 847 patients with peritonsillar abscesses from 2001 to 2006, *F. necrophorum* was detected in 23% of the pus aspirate or swab specimens, most of them growing as a pure culture (97). Recently, Riordan (160), in his extensive review on *F. necrophorum*, presented a wide variety of infections caused by this organism: in the head and neck, infections included tonsillitis, peritonsillar abscess, deep neck space infection, mediastinitis, otogenic infection, mastoiditis, sinusitis, and odontogenic infection; as intracranial complications, infections included sinus thrombosis, cerebral abscess, and meningitis; systemic manifestations included bacteremia, septicemia, pleuropulmonary infections, bone and joint infections, soft tissue infections, intra-abdominal sepsis, endocarditis, and pericarditis. Other *Fusobacterium* taxa, such as *F. necrogenes*, *F. ulcerans*, and the *F. mortiferum-F. varium* group, have been only occasionally isolated from human clinical specimens (31, 32, 110, 115). *F. nucleatum*, an *F. nucleatum*-like species of animal origin, *F. canifelinum*, and *F. russii* are of importance in cat and dog bite wounds (36, 197).

Commensal *Leptotrichia* species have been implicated in anaerobic bacteremias in immunocompromised patients with lesions of the oral mucosa but are also occasionally considered etiologic agents of bacteremia and infective endocarditis in immunocompetent individuals (17, 25, 51, 201, 203). *L. buccalis*, *L. goodfellowii*, *L. trevisanii*, and *L. wadei* are the main *Leptotrichia* findings in blood specimens. In addition, *L. wadei* was reported as a causative organism of a severe pneumonia in an immunocompetent subject (95). In the female genital tract, some infectious cases, including intrauterine fetal demise and septic abortion, have been reported in connection with *L. amnionii* (18, 48, 167). However, *L. amnionii* was recently isolated from a knee joint specimen of a male patient (68), i.e., the case was unrelated to either the female genital tract or delivery. Based on the high number of *L. amnionii* bacteria in urine samples from renal transplant recipients, it may be considered one of the etiologic agents of urinary tract infections (38). In addition to *L. amnionii*, *Sneathia* (formerly *Leptotrichia*) *sanguinegens*, which was originally isolated from blood (32), has been reported from various infectious conditions of the female genital tract, such as preterm labor, peripartum bacteremia, and pyosalpinx, and in amniotic fluid in association with various clinical syndromes (36, 37, 48). *Leptotrichia* and *Sneathia* are among the taxa of which concentrations have been suggested for use as potential markers of bacterial vaginosis and its treatment response (58). Moreover, these taxa are considered clinically relevant intra-amniotic pathogens (37, 70) and, in fact, it has been suggested that the role of *L. amnionii* and *S. sanguinegens* in preterm labor is currently underestimated.

Other Gram-Negative Anaerobic Rods

In the novel phylum *Synergistetes*, there are two cultivable species representing two genera, i.e., *Jonquetella anthropi* and *Pyramidobacter piscolens*, which both have been isolated from human clinical specimens. The *J. anthropi* isolates came from breast abscess, pelvic abscess, sebaceous cyst, wound, and peritoneal fluid specimens (91), while *P. piscolens* isolates were from odontogenic abscesses and the periodontal pocket and gingival crevice (46).

Two *Dialister* species, *D. pneumosintes* and *D. invisus*, are inhabitants of the oral cavity, where they have been implicated as pathogens in endodontal and periodontal infections as well as acute dental abscesses (37, 41, 147, 163, 183). In addition, they have been recovered from infectious specimens from sites such as blood, brain abscesses, bronchoalveolar lavage fluids from patients with ventilator-associated pneumonia or cystic fibrosis, urine, and human bite wounds (6, 7, 16, 40, 128, 165, 198). A considerable portion of *D. pneumosintes* isolates originate from various cutaneous or soft tissue infections (128). It may be that a patient's poor dental hygiene is a predisposing factor in certain nonoral cases, e.g., bacteremia and brain abscess (6, 165). *D. micraerophilus*, which is not a strict anaerobe, and *D. propionicifaciens* have been isolated from a variety of clinical specimens, mainly below the waistline (90, 128).

Selenomonas species and *Centipeda periodontii* are motile organisms recovered from the oral cavity, where they are components of dental biofilms (98, 102). *S. sputigena* has been found in specimens from necrotizing ulcerative gingivitis, generalized aggressive periodontitis, and acute dental abscesses (52, 62, 183), *S. noxia* has been reported in chronic and aggressive periodontitis lesions (52, 199), and *C. periodontii* has been isolated from endodontic infections (182). Furthermore, there have been a few reports on the involvement of *Selenomonas* in nonoral infections, including cystic fibrosis and bacteremia (15, 16, 88).

S. wadsworthensis, a microaerobic organism phenotypically but not phylogenetically close to fastidious *Campylobacter* species, has been isolated from a variety of infections, such as appendicitis, peritonitis, and rectal or perirectal abscesses (125, 211).

B. wadsworthia is a significant human pathogen in polymicrobial intra-abdominal infections, especially in appendicitis, at an increasing frequency with deteriorating disease status (11). In gangrenous appendixes of children, *B. wadsworthia* is even more common than in those of adults (156). Moreover, *B. wadsworthia* has been isolated from abscesses at various body sites as well as from blood (11, 204).

Some *Anaerobiospirillum* and *Desulfovibrio* organisms reside in the gastrointestinal tract of humans but can also be infrequently encountered in clinical specimens; typical cases are bacteremia and abdominal infections in immunocompromised patients (64, 88, 120, 152). Of the two *Anaerobiospirillum* species, *A. succiniciproducens* has been connected to bacteremia and diarrheal illness, whereas *A. thomasii* is considered a potential cause of diarrhea but not of bacteremia (121). In the case of diarrhea, the possibility of zoonotic transmission exists (120). The main *Desulfovibrio* species isolated from human infections include *D. desulfuricans*, *D. fairfieldensis*, *D. piger*, and *D. vulgaris* (64, 88, 118, 153, 209). *D. desulfuricans* is common also in the environment, whereas *D. fairfieldensis* and *D. piger* have been detected only in humans so far. *D. fairfieldensis*, which may have a higher pathogenic potential than the other species, has been isolated from blood, in particular, but also from various intra-abdominal sites, urine, and periodontal pockets (153). In addition to *D. fairfieldensis*, an oral *Desulfomicrobium* species, *D. orale*, has been connected to periodontitis (106).

COLLECTION, TRANSPORT, AND STORAGE OF SPECIMENS

General guidelines for collection, transport, and storage of specimens are discussed in chapters 9 and 16 of this *Manual*. Specimens suitable for the isolation of anaerobes include aseptically obtained blood, tissue biopsies, aspirates (e.g., cerebrospinal fluid, joint fluids, and pus), root canal exudates, and subgingival plaque. Appropriate respiratory tract specimens include bronchoscopic protected bronchoalveolar lavage fluid, and expectorated sputum samples may be collected from patients with cystic fibrosis (202). Also, wound and ulcer specimens should preferably be taken by tissue biopsy, wound curettage, or aspiration. For example, for diabetic foot ulcers, the lesion is cleaned and carefully debrided, and tissue samples are collected from the base or progressive edge, where bacteria actively multiply (32). Infected tissue, obtained by excision or biopsy, is always preferable to pus as a clinical specimen. However, when pus is collected, it is best aspirated into a syringe through a needle and injected into an anaerobic transport vial containing an oxidation-reduction indicator (e.g., products from Anaerobe Systems, Morgan Hill, CA, and Becton Dickinson, Sparks, MD). It is notable that syringes used for aspiration should not be used as transporters because of the potential danger of needle stick injuries or accidental expulsion and because oxygen diffuses through plastic syringes (89). Mucosal or cutaneous swabs are not recommended. In cases where bacteremia is suspected, a 20-ml volume of blood (at least two separate samples) is recommended for cultures. Anaerobic culture is important, especially in patients with complex underlying diseases and when the source of bacteremia is unknown (85, 108). Also, blood collected from patients with abdominal or gynecological processes, peritoneal abscess, dirty wound, decubitus ulcers, osteomyelitis, or spreading oropharyngeal disease should be examined for anaerobes.

Specimens must be transported to the laboratory under anaerobic conditions without delay for further processing. An optimal transport system is one that is able to maintain the viability of anaerobic organisms without allowing the overgrowth of aerobic bacteria. However, if clinical specimens contain fastidious organisms, the transport to the clinical laboratory should occur within 24 h (30). Tissue samples are best transported in specific anaerobic transport vials or in loosely capped containers sealed in gas-impermeable bags in which an anaerobic atmosphere has been generated. For small tissue and biopsy specimens and for subgingival and root canal samples, a semisolid anaerobic transport medium (e.g., those of Anaerobe Systems and Becton Dickinson), in which the specimen can be submerged, can be used.

Further guidance for the collection of specimens from different body sites and by various methods as well as transport systems and anaerobic techniques can be found in more detail elsewhere (89).

For long-term storage, 2- to 3-day-old cultures can be transferred into vials containing sterilized 20% skim milk and kept frozen at −70°C.

DIRECT EXAMINATION

The gross appearance, fluorescence under long-wave UV light, and odor of the specimen can give the laboratory valuable clues to the presence of anaerobes. A fetid or putrid odor due to volatile short-chain fatty acids and amines is always associated with the presence of anaerobes in the sample. Black necrotic tissue and/or red fluorescence of the sample may be indicative of the presence of pigmented gram-negative rods (89).

The Gram stain is still the fastest, simplest, and most likely to yield significant information and should be prepared from all specimens accepted for anaerobic culture. Many gram-negative anaerobic rods, e.g., different species within the genus *Fusobacterium*, have unique cell morphology. For instance, a Gram-stained smear with highly pleomorphic gram-negative rods in blood culture from a septic patient following a sore throat may indicate invasive *F. necrophorum* infection (20). The morphotypes and relative quantities of the bacteria and host inflammatory cells present in the preparation should be reported. Gram stain using the Nugent criteria for interpretation of vaginal discharge is still considered the best method for diagnosis of bacterial vaginosis (107).

Molecular Detection

Molecular methods are increasingly used for direct detection of bacteria from clinical specimens. As yet, they are not widely used for routine diagnostics but are mainly used in specialized oral and other research microbiology laboratories.

For the detection of fastidious organisms and potential pathogens, sequencing of the 16S rRNA gene has been successfully used not only for bacterial identification in typical polymicrobial lesions, such as periodontitis, endodontic infections, and spreading odontogenic infections (104, 147, 159, 183, 206), but also in infections where the involvement of anaerobic bacteria has not been traditionally taken into account, e.g., cystic fibrosis (16). It is notable that a culture-based approach can underestimate the presence of etiologic but fastidious or uncultivable organisms in clinical specimens. For example, *Prevotella* species are highly prevalent in the lungs of cystic fibrosis patients (16, 202), but routine culture of sputum does not include anaerobes and potential anaerobic pathogens are not reported. Furthermore, in women with preterm labor whose amniotic fluid tested positive by culture or PCR, seven species, including *S. sanguinegens* and *L. amnionii*, were detected by PCR only (39). In addition, in a study of urinary tract specimens from renal transplant recipients (40), the 16S rRNA PCR method detected a wide range of bacteria, including gram-negative anaerobes, such as *B. vulgatus*, *D. invisus*, *F. nucleatum*, *L. amnionii*, *P. buccalis*, and *P. ruminicola*, in culture-negative samples.

A checkerboard DNA-DNA hybridization method, in which a set of DNA samples are hybridized against large numbers of DNA probes on a single support membrane, was first developed to investigate the presence of DNA of target organisms (up to 40 species at a time) in dental plaque (187). Recently, it has been used for other clinical specimens, such as serum and synovial fluid of patients with active arthritis (124) and vaginal samples for detecting selected target microbes in bacterial vaginosis (151).

ISOLATION PROCEDURES

Except for blood and joint fluid cultures, the use of liquid medium as the only anaerobic culture technique is not acceptable (89). The use of solid nonselective medium together with selective medium increases the yield and saves time in terms of recognition and isolation of colonies. The selective media are chosen based on the expected microbiota at the collection site, or in the case of bite wounds, on the oral microbiota of the biter (human or animal). Freshly prepared or prereduced and anaerobically sterilized medium should be used (89). Different basal media differ in their abilities to support the growth of anaerobes; brucella base and fastidious anaerobe agar (Lab M, Bury, United Kingdom) may be the best basal media for isolation of gram-negative anaerobic rods. In particular, fastidious anaerobe

agar enhances the growth of fusobacteria (20). In academic centers performing large-scale anaerobic bacteriology, it would be ideal to use two different basal media to maximize isolation efficiency.

Culture methods are found in chapter 17. The minimum medium setup for isolating gram-negative anaerobic rods includes (i) a nonselective, enriched, brucella base sheep blood agar plate supplemented with vitamin K$_1$ and hemin (BA); (ii) a kanamycin-vancomycin laked sheep blood agar plate for the selection of *Bacteroides* and *Prevotella* species; and (iii) a *Bacteroides* bile-esculin (BBE) agar plate for specimens from areas below the diaphragm for the selection and presumptive identification of the *B. fragilis* group and *Bilophila* species. BBE and kanamycin-vancomycin laked sheep blood are also available as biplates. A phenylethyl alcohol sheep blood agar plate used to prevent overgrowth by aerobic gram-negative rods and swarming of some clostridia is indicated for purulent specimens and in the case of mixed infections. Use of a metronidazole disk on nonselective agar is useful for the detection of gram-negative obligate anaerobes; however, it may mask the presence of infrequently encountered metronidazole-resistant organisms.

After inoculation, the anaerobic plates are immediately incubated at 36 to 37°C in an anaerobic environment, such as an anaerobic bag, jar, or chamber. Alternatively, setup and incubation may all be done in an anaerobic chamber. Plates should not be exposed to air during the first 48 h, to avoid loss of the more oxygen-sensitive species. The availability of an anaerobic chamber enables the examination of the culture whenever necessary. An incubation period of 48 h will reveal the presence of rapidly growing strains, such as *Bacteroides* or clostridia, but reincubation for 5 to 7 days for primary plates is recommended, since some species, such as *Bilophila*, *Desulfovibrio*, and *Porphyromonas*, may not be detected with shorter incubation times and require at least 4 to 5 days for growth (11, 64, 89).

Increased awareness of the importance of anaerobic organisms as a cause of systemic infections may contribute to the increase of their isolation and detection in blood samples in clinical microbiology laboratories (78). To reliably detect anaerobic organisms, the LYTIC 10 Anaerobic/F Bactec medium (Becton Dickinson) has been shown to be a rapid and reliable method, improving the detection of low levels of anaerobic bacteria, such as *Prevotella* and *Fusobacterium*, in the sample (7).

IDENTIFICATION

After anaerobic incubation, the relative quantities of distinct colony types are recorded. Plates should be examined with a dissecting microscope to facilitate detection. Even after incubation for 7 days, certain species, such as *Desulfovibrio* and *Dialister*, grow as transparent colonies that are pinpoint in size and are easily overlooked in mixed cultures (64, 90, 118, 153). The isolates should then be subcultured onto BA and, at this point, a rabbit laked blood agar plate for the rapid demonstration of pigment production and an egg yolk agar plate for the demonstration of lipase, lecithinase, and proteolytic activities may also be inoculated. The primary plates are reincubated along with the purity and test plates.

Presumptive Identification

Colony morphology of an isolate in pure culture can be useful for presumptive identification. For example, *F. nucleatum* can appear on the plate as speckled, iridescent, or bread crumb-like colonies, while *B. wadsworthensis* has typical black-centered colonies on BBE (89). Colony morphology, together with the capability of erythrocyte agglutination, is among the features that can be used to separate the two *F. necrophorum* subspecies by using phenotypic tests (87). The agglutination procedure, using human and chicken erythrocytes, is performed by a glass slide method, where agglutination is observed by mixing a drop of bacterial suspension and a drop of erythrocyte suspension on a microscope slide. *F. necrophorum* subsp. *funduliforme* (agglutination-negative) colonies are pulvinate, creamy, and glistening with entire margins, whereas *F. necrophorum* subsp. *necrophorum* (agglutination-positive) colonies are convex or umbonate, waxy, and dull with erose margins. Also, observation of hemolysis may be of diagnostic value; for instance, both *F. necrophorum* subspecies exhibit beta-hemolysis when grown on horse blood agar (87). Hemolytic properties on human blood may aid in separation of different *Leptotrichia* species (50). Production of pigment is another visible characteristic valuable in presumptive identification; the pigmented gram-negative anaerobic rods are composed of saccharolytic and asaccharolytic species of the genera *Prevotella* and *Porphyromonas* and three pigment-producing *Alistipes* species, *A. finegoldii*, *A. onderdonkii*, and *A. shahii*. In this context, it is notable that the statement "after 4 days incubation on laked rabbit blood agar, colonies appear black" in the original description of *A. onderdonkii* and *A. shahii* (191) is incorrect. Instead, the grade of pigmenting is light or moderately brown on rabbit laked blood agar, and pigment also appears on BA after extended incubation. The pigmented *Prevotella* and *Porphyromonas* species vary greatly in the degree and rapidity of pigment production (2 to 21 days), which ranges from buff to tan to black, depending primarily on the type of blood and the composition of the base medium used in the agar (89). Fluorescence under long-wavelength UV light can be helpful in presumptive identification; pigmented *Prevotella* and *Porphyromonas* colonies typically fluoresce red, *F. nucleatum* and *F. necrophorum* fluoresce yellow-green, and *Desulfovibrio* and *Bilophila* species, when tested with a drop of NaOH on a swab of cell paste, fluoresce red due to the presence of desulfoviridin pigment (87, 89, 209).

Microscopic determination of the morphology of Gram-stained bacterial cells can aid presumptive identification of the organisms present. Among fusiforms, *F. nucleatum* usually exhibits long, spindle-shaped cells with tapered ends, while *F. necrophorum* and *F. mortiferum* have highly pleomorphic cells, with or without swollen areas and large round bodies (20, 87, 89). *Leptotrichia* cells, which often stain gram-positive in fresh cultures, have been usually considered long rods; however, this description fits only with *L. buccalis*, *L. hofstadii*, *L. shahii*, and *L. trevisanii* (50, 201). *Dialister* species are small coccobacilli, making their separation from gram-negative cocci difficult (90). *Desulfovibrio piger* typically stains bipolar (209). Wet slide preparation for microscopic examination reveals the motility of gram-negative anaerobes: *Selenomonas* displays a characteristic tumbling motility, often moving laterally across the field; *Anaerobiospirillum* cells are spiral with corkscrew-like motility; *Desulfovibrio* species, except for *D. piger*, appear as curved rods with rapid, progressive motility (64, 117, 121).

The *B. fragilis* group, in particular, and most *Bacteroides* species are typically bile resistant (89, 212). Pigment-producing *Alistipes* can be readily distinguished from pigmented *Porphyromonas* and *Prevotella* species by the resistance to 20% bile (191). Among fusobacteria, *F. mortiferum*, *F. varium*, and some strains of *F. necrophorum* grow

in the presence of bile, whereas *F. nucleatum* does not. The profile of susceptibility to special-potency antimicrobial disks (a zone size of ≥10 mm is considered susceptible), containing vancomycin (5 μg), kanamycin (1,000 μg), and colistin (10 μg), is useful in presumptive identification of many gram-negative anaerobic taxa (Table 2). Gram-negative anaerobic rods are typically resistant to vancomycin, with pigmented *Porphyromonas* species the only exception. Susceptibility to both kanamycin and colistin is characteristic of *Fusobacterium* and *Leptotrichia* species and *S. wadsworthensis*. To differentiate members of the genera *Dialister* and *Veillonella*, special potency disks can be helpful; *Dialister* species are resistant to colistin, whereas *Veillonella* species are usually susceptible, except for *V. montpellierensis* and *V. ratti* (90). Among motile gram-negative organisms, *Anaerobiospirillum* is usually susceptible to colistin, unlike most *Desulfovibrio* and *Selenomonas* isolates.

In addition to the characteristics listed above, there are some simple tests that are within the scope of most clinical laboratories. For example, a bile-resistant organism with typical darkening of the center of colonies on BBE can be easily recognized as *B. wadsworthia* by its strong catalase reaction with 10 to 15% H_2O_2 (11), and by combining positive indole and lipase reactions, a *Fusobacterium*-like organism can be tentatively identified as *F. necrophorum* (20). An indole- and lipase-positive short rod that forms black-pigmented colonies and fluoresces red can be identified as *P. intermedia/P. nigrescens*, while *P. pallens* resembles these indole-positive species but has lighter pigment and is lipase negative. *Bilophila* and *Sutterella* typically reduce nitrate. A characteristic smell may guide the identification; a foul smell produced by butyric acid and other metabolic products is typical for *Fusobacterium* species (89), while a strong sulfur smell is typical for the presence of *Desulfovibrio* species (64, 209).

Biochemical Testing

In culture-based biochemical testing, the main techniques for classification of anaerobic organisms and distinction of individual species include sugar fermentation reactions, using prereduced, anaerobically sterilized carbohydrates or commercial test kits, and the determination of enzyme profiles with individual diagnostic tablets or preformed enzyme kits. In addition, the determination of major volatile fatty acid end products of glucose metabolism, as detected by gas liquid chromatography (GLC), is a useful adjunct to biochemical and physiological tests (89), but together with analysis of the long-chain fatty acids found in bacterial cell walls it is beyond the scope of most clinical laboratories.

Commercially available test kits, such as the API 20A, API ZYM, and Rapid ID 32A (bioMeriéux, Marcy-l'Etoile, France), RapID ANA II (Remel, Lenexa, KS), BBL crystal identification (Becton Dickinson), and AN microplates (Biolog Inc., Hayward, CA) systems, are used for testing preformed enzyme and carbohydrate fermentation profiles in clinical microbiology laboratories (66). Diagnostic tablets (e.g., from Rosco, Taastrup, Denmark, and Key Scientific, Stamford, TX) are also useful for determining individual enzyme reactions of anaerobic isolates. A heavy inoculum from 2- to 3-day-old cultures should be used for testing to obtain optimal reactions. When using different test systems, variation of test results is expected due to differences in the substrate specificities. These rapid, easy-to-use systems are best suited for fast-growing and biochemically reactive anaerobes, such as the *B. fragilis* group organisms, but even then it may not be possible to reliably identify the isolate to the species level. The Vitek 2ANC card (bioMeriéux) is a new automated system for rapid identification of anaerobic bacteria from clinical specimens (132, 158). According to the results of a clinical trial performed in three large tertiary care centers (158), the Vitek 2 ANC card (bioMeriéux) proved to be acceptable for routine use in laboratories; however, the system incorrectly identified a considerable number of clinically relevant species, such as *F. necrophorum*, *P. intermedia*, and *P. melaninogenica*, and did not include clinical isolates that were not in the system's rather limited database. However, skillful reading of the Gram stain preparation considerably improves the percentage of correct identifications (132).

The most commonly encountered bile-resistant organisms in clinical specimens belong to the *B. fragilis* group organisms. They grow as gray, circular, convex, and entire colonies on BA and, in addition, grow well on BBE where they (except for *B. vulgatus*) blacken the agar by hydrolyzing esculin. Based on their resistance to special-potency antibiotic disks (vancomycin, kanamycin, and colistin) and a few rapid tests, such as the catalase, indole, esculin, and α-fucosidase tests, they can be initially reported as *B. fragilis* group or organisms most closely related to this group (89). The genus *Parabacteroides* now includes the former *B. distasonis* and *B. merdae* (167), and *B. slanchnicus* has been moved to the genus *Odoribacter* (74). In addition, some newly described, clinically relevant species include *B. massiliensis*, *B. nordii*, *B. salyersiae*, *P. goldsteinii*, and *P. gordonii* (53, 171, 188, 189). All *Parabacteroides* species are negative for indole and α-fucosidase, distinguishing them from the *B. fragilis* group organisms. *P. goldsteinii* is phylogenetically and phenotypically very similar to *P. merdae*; however, *P. goldsteinii* is positive for α-glucosidase and β-glucosidase (Rosco), whereas *P. merdae* is not (189). Furthermore, the positive β-glucuronidase reaction of *P. goldsteinii* and *P. merdae* separates them from *P. distasonis*. Unlike other *Parabacteroides* species, *P. gordonii* does not hydrolyze esculin and does not ferment trehalose (171). Most of the *B. fragilis* group and related organisms are highly fermentative. Table 4 presents the key characteristics for distinguishing the *B. fragilis* group organisms, including *Parabacteroides* species and *O. splanchnicus*.

TABLE 4 Identification scheme for the *B. fragilis* group, *Parabacteroides*, and *Odoribacter* organisms isolated from humans[a]

Species	Production of:			Fermentation of:							
	Indole	Catalase	α-Fuc[b]	Arabinose	Cellobiose	Rhamnose	Salicin	Sucrose	Trehalose	Xylan	Xylose
B. caccae	−	−	+	+	v	v	v	+	+	−	+
B. cellulosilyticus	ND	−	w	w	w	ND	w	+	−	w	+
B. clarus[c]	+	−	−	−	+	+	w	+	w	ND	+
B. coprocola	−	−	+	−	+	+	+	+	−	ND	+
B. coprophilus	−	ND	+	−	w	−	−	+	ND	ND	−
B. dorei	−	ND	+	+	−	+	−	+	−	ND	+
B. eggerthii	+	−	−	+	v	v	−	−	−	+	+
B. faecis	+	−	+	+	+	+	−	+	−	ND	+
B. finegoldii	−	ND	−	+	+	+	+	+	−	ND	+
B. fluxus[c]	+	−	+	+	+	+	+	+	+	ND	+
B. fragilis	−	+	+	−	v	−	−	+	−	−	+
B. intestinalis	+	ND	+	+	+	+	−	+	−	ND	+
B. massiliensis	−	−	+	−	−	−	−	+	−	ND	
B. nordii	+	−	−	−	+	+	−	+	−	−	+
B. oleiciplenus[c]	+	+	−	+	+	+	+	+	+	ND	+
B. ovatus	+	+	+	+	+	+	+	+	+	+	+
B. plebeius	−	−	+	+	+	+	−	+	−	ND	+
B. salyersiae	+	−	−	+	+	+	−	+	−	−	+
B. stercoris	+	v	v	+	−	+	+	+	+	+	+
B. thetaiotaomicron	+	+	+	+	v	+	−	+	+	−	+
B. uniformis	+	−	+	+	+	−	+	+	−	−	+
B. vulgatus	−	−	+	+	−	+	−	+	−	v	+
B. xylanisolvens	−	−	+	+	+	+	+	+	+	+	+
O. laneus[c]	+	−	+	−	−	−	−	−	−	−	−
O. splanchnicus	+	v	+	+	−	−	−	−	−	−	−
P. distasonis	−	+	−	−	+	v	+	+	+	−	+
P. goldsteinii	−	v	−	−	+	+	−	+	+	−	+
P. gordonii	−	v	−	+	−	−	−	+	−	ND	+
P. johnsonii	−	+	−	+	−	+	−	+	+	ND	+
P. merdae	−	−	−	−	v	v	v	+	+	−	+

[a]Data were compiled from references 8 to 10, 28, 76, 89, 96, 136, 161, 168, 171, 188 to 190, and 210. Symbols: +, positive; −, negative; v, variable; w, weak reaction; ND, no data.
[b]α-Fuc, α-fucosidase.
[c]Results are based on testing of a single strain.

A. putredinis (formerly *Bacteroides putredinis*), the type species of the genus *Alistipes*, is nonpigmented, asaccharolytic, bile sensitive, and positive for indole and catalase (157). In contrast, most *Alistipes* species can be separated from *Bacteroides* and *A. putredinis* by their pigment production, although demonstration of this trait may require prolonged incubation. *A. finegoldii*, *A. onderdonkii*, and *A. shahii* strains grow well on solid media, where colonies appear beta-hemolytic, but not in liquid media, with or without supplements (191). They are variably saccharolytic due to their poor growth in liquid media and are bile resistant and catalase negative. Two enzyme reactions may be able to separate pigmented *Alistipes* species: *A. finegoldii* is positive for α-fucosidase but negative for β-glucosidase, whereas *A. onderdonkii* is negative and *A. shahii* is positive for both enzymes (191).

Tannerella forsythia is a fastidious oral pathogen, and human strains require exogenous *N*-acetylmuramic acid for growth in pure cultures (166, 200). Key characteristics of *T. forsythia* are its sensitivity to bile and positive trypsin and esculin reactions. Notably, animal strains from bite wound infections are positive for catalase and indole (81).

Porphyromonas species, except for *P. catoniae*, produce pigment. The identification of the closely related and phenotypically similar *P. asaccharolytica*, *P. endodontalis*, and *P. uenonis* is difficult due to their slow pigment production and inactivity in biochemical testing. Testing with prereduced, anaerobically sterilized carbohydrates is not helpful in distinguishing these species, but glyoxylic acid and glycerol in the AN microplate system (Biolog Inc.) enable their separation: *P. asaccharolytica* is positive for glyoxylic acid and *P. uenonis* is positive for glycerol (56). *P. asaccharolytica* is also positive for α-fucosidase, while the other two species are negative. In addition, the differences in the degrees of pigmentation may be helpful, with *P. uenonis* being the most and *P. endodontalis* the least pigmenting (56). Positive indole, *N*-acetyl-β-glucosaminidase, and trypsin reactions comprise a typical pattern for *P. gingivalis* (89). Unlike most *Porphyromonas* species, *P. bennonis*, *P. somerae*, and *P. catoniae* are indole negative, and the two latter species

also weakly saccharolytic (101, 195, 196), which may lead to their misidentification as *Prevotella* species in clinical laboratories. However, the sensitivity to vancomycin and satellite-like growth pattern (i.e., larger colonies surrounded by smaller colonies), together with negative indole and α-fucosidase but positive *N*-acetyl-β-glucosaminidase reactions, identify the isolate as *P. somerae* (195). Also, *P. catoniae* isolates grow as satellite-like colonies but are nonpigmented, resistant to vancomycin but susceptible to sodium polyanethol sulfonate in the special-potency antimicrobial disk test, and produce major amounts of propionic acid as shown by GLC (101). *P. bennonis* is a slow-growing organism with very slight pigmentation after extended incubation of at least 10 days and has a variable susceptibility to vancomycin (196). Unlike other *Porphyromonas* species, it produces major amounts of acetic and succinic acids in GLC, and some strains are catalase positive (196). Most *Porphyromonas* species of animal origin have been differentiated from the human strains by a positive catalase reaction (89). Table 5 presents the key reactions for distinguishing *Porphyromonas* species.

A small number of *Prevotella* species produce indole: *P. intermedia*, *P nigrescens*, *P. pallens*, *P. micans*, and "*P. massiliensis*" (12, 45, 89). Except for *P. massiliensis*, these species are pigment producers, as are *P. corporis*, *P. denticola*, *P. loescheii*, *P. melaninogenica*, *P. shahii*, *P. tannerae*, and *P. histicola* (44, 89). Some strains of *P. histicola* have a bull's-eye appearance due to pigmentation of the colony center (44). Noteworthy is that pigment production, as well as its degree, on BA may take up to 14 days and vary from tan to brown to black depending on the species. Detection of lipase on egg yolk agar may be useful: *P. intermedia* and *P. nigrescens* and many *P. loescheii* strains are positive. Notably, the separation of *P. intermedia* from *P. nigrescens* is not possible by phenotypic methods. Besides the production of pigment and indole, *Prevotella* organisms are characterized by their capability of fermenting a variety of sugars. *P. massiliensis* is an exception, being very unreactive; however, the description of the species is based on one strain (12). *Prevotella* organisms produce acetic and succinic acids as

TABLE 5 Some phenotypic characteristics of *Porphyromonas* species of human or animal origin[a]

| Species | Production of[b]: | | | | | | | Sugar fermentation |
	Pigment	Indole	Catalase	α-Fuc	β-NAG	Trypsin	Chymotrypsin	
P. asaccharolytica	+	+	−	+	−	−	−	−
P. bennonis	w	−	v	−	+	−	+	−
P. catoniae	−	−	−	+	+	v	+	w
P. endodontalis	+	+	−	−	−	−	−	−
P. gingivalis	+	+	−	−	+	+	+	−
P. somerae	+	−	−	−	+	−	+	w
P. uenonis	+	+	−	−	−	−	−	−
P. cangingivalis	+	+	+	−	−	−	−	−
P. canoris	+	+	+	−	+	−	−	−
P. cansulci	+	+	+	−	−	−	−	−
P. circumdentaria	+	+	+	−	−	−	−	−
P. crevioricanis	+	+	+	−	−	−	−	−
P. gingivicanis	+	+	+	−	−	−	−	−
P. gulae	+	+	+	−	+	+	+	−
P. levii	+	−	−	−	+	−	+	w
P. macacae	+	+	−	−	+	+	+	w

[a]Data were compiled from references 56, 89, 195, and 196. Symbols: +, positive; −, negative; v, variable; w, weak reaction.
[b]α-Fuc, α-fucosidase; β-NAG, *N*-acetyl-β-glucosaminidase.

TABLE 6 Biochemical identification scheme for *Prevotella* species[a]

Species	Production of[b]:					Hydrolysis of[c]:		Fermentation of:						
	Pigment	Ind	Lip	α-Fuc	β-NAG	Gel	Esc	Arabinose	Cellobiose	Lactose	Salicin	Sucrose	Mannose	Raffinose
P. amnii	−	−	−	−	+	−	+	ND	−	+	−	−	ND	ND
P. baroniae	−	−	−	+	+	w	+	−	+	+	+	+	+	+
P. bergensis	−	−	−	−	v	−	+	+	+	+	+	−	+	−
P. bivia	−	−	−	+	+	+	−	−	−	+	−	−	+	−
P. buccae	−	−	−	−	−	+	+	+	+	+	+	+	+	+
P. buccalis	−	−	−	+	+	−	+	+	+	+	−	+	+	+
P. copri	−	−	−	−	−	−	+	+	+	+	+	+	−	+
P. corporis	+	−	−	−	−	+	−	−	−	−	−	−	+	−
P. dentalis	−	−	−	−	+	−	−	+	+	+	−	w	+	+
P. denticola	v	−	−	+	+	+	+	−	−	+	−	+	+	+
P. disiens	−	−	−	−	−	+	−	−	−	−	−	−	−	−
P. enoeca	−	−	−	+	+	+	v	−	−	+	−	−	v	−
P. heparinolytica	−	+	−	+	+	−	+	+	+	+	+	+	+	−
P. histicola	v	−	−	+	+	+	−	−	−	+	−	+	+	+
P. intermedia	+	+	+	+	−	+	−	−	−	−	−	+	v	v
P. loescheii	+	−	v	+	+	+	−	−	+	+	−	+	+	+
P. maculosa	−	−	−	−	+	−	+	+	+	+	+	+	+	+
P. marshii	−	−	−	−	−	+	−	−	−	−	−	−	v	−
P. melaninogenica	+	−	−	+	+	+	v	−	−	+	−	+	+	+
P. micans	+	+	−	+	+	+	−	−	+	+	+	+	+	+
P. multiformis	−	−	−	v	+	+	−	−	+	+	−	+	+	+
P. multisaccharivorax	−	−	−	+	+	+	+	v	+	+	v	+	+	+
P. nanceiensis	−	−	−	+	+	−	+	−	v	+	−	+	+	+
P. nigrescens	+	+	+	+	−	+	−	−	−	−	−	+	+	+
P. oralis	−	−	−	+	+	v	+	−	+	+	+	+	+	+
P. oris	−	−	−	+	+	v	+	+	+	+	+	+	+	+
P. oulorum	−	−	−	+	+	−	−	−	−	+	−	−	+	+
P. pallens	+	+	−	−	+	−	+	−	−	−	−	+	−	+
P. pleuritidis[d]	−	−	−	+	+	+	−	−	−	−	−	+	−	−
P. saccharolytica	−	−	ND	−	+	w	+	+	+	+	+	+	+	+
P. salivae	−	−	−	w	+	−	+	+	+	+	+	+	+	+
P. shahii	+	−	−	w	+	+	−	−	−	+	−	+	+	+
P. stercorea	−	−	−	+	+	−	−	−	−	+	−	−	+	+
P. tannerae	v	−	−	+	+	+	−	−	−	v	−	v	v	v
P. timonensis[d]	−	−	−	+	+	+	−	−	−	+	−	−	−	−
P. veroralis	−	−	−	+	+	v	+	−	+	+	−	+	+	+
P. zoogleoformans	−	v	−	+	+	v	+	v	+	+	v	+	v	v

[a]Data were compiled from references 2, 12, 42 to 45, 47, 60, 75, 89, 109, and 170. Symbols: +, positive; −, negative; v, variable; w, weak reaction; ND, no data.
[b]Ind, indole; Lip, lipase; α-Fuc, α-fucosidase; β-NAG, *N*-acetyl-β-glucosaminidase.
[c]Gel, gelatin; Esc, esculin.
[d]Results shown are based on testing of a single strain.

their major metabolic end products of glucose fermentation in GLC; however, *P. marshii*, unusually, also produces propionic acid. Due to the high and still increasing number of *Prevotella* species, which have been described based on 16S rRNA gene sequencing, their precise identification by biochemical tests alone is challenging. Table 6 lists enzyme and sugar fermentation reactions that could be of value in their identification.

Fusobacteria can be presumptively identified by a limited number of simple laboratory tests, including cell morphology with Gram stain, growth in 20% bile, and indole production, but their definitive identification to the species level may require additional biochemical testing (Table 7). *F. nucleatum*, appearing as white, speckled, or bread crumb-like colonies, is known for its wide heterogeneity.

It includes five subspecies, *F. nucleatum* subsp. *animalis*, *F. nucleatum* subsp. *fusiforme*, *F. nucleatum* subsp. *nucleatum*, *F. nucleatum* subsp. *polymorphum*, and *F. nucleatum* subsp. *vincentii*, but phenotypic tests are not able to identify the organism to the subspecies level. Also, *F. periodonticum* is indistinguishable from *F. nucleatum* by phenotypic methods. In the case of the increasingly clinically important *F. necrophorum*, there are two subspecies, *F. necrophorum* subsp. *funduliforme*, isolated from human infections, and *F. necrophorum* subsp. *necrophorum* from animal infections (20, 87, 160). Both subspecies are indole and lipase positive, but colony morphology and few phenotypic tests, including erythrocyte agglutination, are able to distinguish them (87). A *Fusobacterium* egg yolk agar test has been described for selective isolation of fusobacteria and rapidly differentiating

TABLE 7 Some phenotypic characteristics of *Fusobacterium* species[a]

Species	Cell morphology	Growth in 20% bile	Production of:		Conversion to propionate from:	
			Indole	Lipase	Lactate	Threonine
F. gonidiaformans	Gonidial	−	+	−	−	+
F. mortiferum	Pleomorphic with large, round bodies	+	−	−	−	+
F. naviforme	Boat shape	−	+	−	−	−
F. necrophorum subsp. *funduliforme*	Coccoid/pleomorphic, curling, tangling	v	+	+	+	+
F. necrophorum subsp. *necrophorum*	Pleomorphic (entire)	v	+	+	+	+
F. nucleatum	Slender, long	−	+	−	−	+
F. periodonticum	Slender, long	−	+	−	−	+
F. russii	Large with rounded ends	−	−	−	−	−
F. varium	Large with rounded ends	+	v	v	−	+
F. ulcerans	Large with rounded ends	+	−	−	−	+

[a]Data were compiled from references 31, 87, and 89. Symbols: +, positive; −, negative; v, variable reaction.

F. necrophorum (127). An indole-negative pleomorphic organism that grows on BBE may be presumptively identified as *F. mortiferum* (89). *F. ulcerans* closely resembles indole-negative *F. varium* strains but reduces nitrate. All fusobacteria produce major amounts of butyric acid as their metabolic end product (Table 2) and, in addition, *F. naviforme*, *F. russii*, and *F. varium* produce lactic acid, as detected in GLC (89).

Although *Leptotrichia* species are anaerobic on first isolation, in subcultures some strains can grow aerobically in the presence of CO_2 (51). These organisms have been known as large fusiforms, but their cell morphology varies between the species: *L. buccalis*, *L. hofstadii*, *L. shahii*, and *L. trevisanii* are long rods, and *L. goodfellowii* and *L. wadei* are relatively short rods, while *L. amnionii* appears as pleomorphic coccobacilli and fusiforms and *S. sanguinegens* appears as pleomorphic rods with some filaments (34, 50, 180, 201). Fresh cells may stain gram positive (51). Lactate production as the major end product of glucose fermentation is characteristic for *Leptotrichia* and *Sneathia* (Table 2). *S. sanguinegens* and *L. amnionii* are extremely fastidious, and thus very little is known about their biochemical characteristics (34, 38, 180); however, positive reactions by Rapid ID 32A (bioMeriéux) have been reported for β-glucuronidase, alkaline phosphatase, arginine arylaminidase activity, and raffinose fermentation (34, 38). Table 8 presents some characteristics helpful in their biochemical identification.

Within the newly described phylum *Synergistetes* (92), *Jonquetella anthropi* (91) and *Pyramidobacter piscolens* (46) are the two human-derived species that have been cultured so far. They are asaccharolytic rods with acetic acid as their major metabolic end product of glucose fermentation. *J. anthropi* is susceptible to bile and forms pinpoint colonies on blood agar, while the colonies of *P. piscolens* are somewhat bigger and highly convex to pyramidal. Both species are unreactive to most biochemical tests; however, two reactions in the Rapid ID 32 A system (bioMeriéux) are able to separate these species, as *J. anthropi* is positive for glycine arylamidase and leucyl glycine arylamidase and *P. piscolens* is highly positive for glycine arylamidase (46, 91).

Dialister species are coccobacilli that form tiny colonies on blood agar. They are asaccharolytic and grow poorly in liquid media; lack of reactivity in conventional biochemical tests hampers their identification. They are often confused with *Veillonella* because of their tiny cell size. There are a few

enzymes in the Rapid ID 32 A kit (bioMeriéux) that may be useful in distinguishing three *Dialister* species: *D. pneumosintes* is positive for glycine arylamidase, *D. micraerophilus* for alanine, phenylalanine, serine, and tyrosine arylamidases and arginine dihydrolase, and *D. succinatiphilus* for alkaline phosphatase (90, 129). However, *D. invisus* and *D. propionifaciens* are negative for all tests in this kit. The latter species produces propionate, which can be detected by GLC (90). Molecular methods, such as 16S rRNA gene sequencing, are often needed for the accurate detection of *Dialister* species in clinical specimens (90, 165).

B. wadsworthensis isolates are asaccharolytic, bile resistant, and strongly positive for catalase, and most strains are urease positive (11). This species also produces hydrogen sulfide, and its growth is stimulated by bile (ox gall) and pyruvate. This pattern, together with its typical colony characteristics on BBE, may result in its reliable identification.

Two human *Sutterella* species, *S. wadsworthensis* and *S. parvirubra*, and the novel *Parasutterella excrementihominis* are asaccharolytic and very unreactive organisms, of which only *S. wadsworthensis* has been isolated from infections so far. *P. excrementihominis* and *S. parvirubra* are strictly anaerobic, have coccoid cells, and are negative for nitrate reduction (135, 173), while *S. wadsworthensis* is a straight rod that is able to grow under microaerobic conditions and to reduce nitrate (211).

Of the motile gram-negative anaerobic genera isolated from human specimens, *Selenomonas* and *Anaerobiospirillum* are saccharolytic, while *Phocaeicola* and *Desulfovibrio* are asaccharolytic. Unlike the others, *Desulfovibrio* species are positive for desulfoviridin, which can be detected by adding 2 N NaOH to cell paste on a swab and observing for red fluorescence under UV light (64, 209). *Desulfomicrobium orale* is a straight rod and is negative for desulfoviridin but, typically, both *D. orale* and *Desulfovibrio* species reduce sulfate (106). *P. abscessus* is a slow-growing coccobacillus with a lophotrichous flagellar arrangement (4). Flagellae of *Selenomonas* are arranged on the concave side of the cell, while those of *Centipeda* are around the cell (126). *Anaerobiospirillum* species have a corkscrew shape and a jerky motility. *A. succiniciproducens* is sensitive to colistin, and it ferments glucose, maltose, lactose, and sucrose. *A. thomasii* can be differentiated from *A. succiniciproducens* by carbohydrate fermentations and by α-glucosidase and β-galactosidase activities, the former being negative and the latter positive for both reactions (121).

TABLE 8 Some phenotypic characteristics of *Leptotrichia* species and *Sneathia sanguinegens*[a]

Species	Beta-hemolysis	Production of[b]:						
		Catalase	α-Gal	β-Gal	α-Glu	β-Glu	β-NAG	PAL
L. amnionii	ND	−	−	−	−	−	−	+
L. buccalis	−	−	+	−	+	+	−	+
L. goodfellowii	+	+	−	+	−	+	+	+
L. hofstadii	+	+	−	−	+	+	−	+
L. shahii	−	+	−	−	+	−	−	−
L. trevisanii	ND	+	−	−	+	+	+	+
L. wadei	+	+	−	−	+	+	−	−
S. sanguinegens	ND	−	−	−	−	−	−	+

[a]Data were compiled from references 34, 50, 180, and 201. Symbols: +, positive reaction; −, negative reaction; ND, no data.
[b]α-Gal, α-galactosidase; β-Gal, β-galactosidase; α-Glu, α-glucosidase; β-Glu, β-glucosidase; β-NAG, N-acetyl-β-glucosaminidase; PAL, alkaline phosphatase.

Desulfovibrio species are curved rods with a rapid, progressive motility (except for the nonmotile *D. piger*) and are resistant to colistin and to 20% bile (except for the bile-sensitive *D. desulfuricans*) (209). A rather simple test scheme, including catalase, indole, nitrate, and urease, is able to separate the four *Desulfovibrio* species isolated from human clinical specimens: *D. desulfuricans* is positive for nitrate and urease, *D. fairfieldensis* is positive for catalase and nitrate, and *D. vulgaris* is positive for indole, while *D. piger* is negative for all these reactions (209). Table 9 presents an identification scheme for motile gram-negative anaerobic genera.

Advanced Techniques for Identification

Whole-cell bacterial identification by matrix-assisted laser desorption ionization–time-of-flight mass spectrometry has proven to be a promising method for the identification of gram-negative anaerobic bacteria (137, 192). Peptides and small proteins, which are assumed to be characteristic for each bacterial species, can be measured from whole cells, cell lysates, or crude bacterial extracts. The method is cost-effective, accurate, and rapid (176), making it a potential alternative for traditional identification. However, accurate identification depends on the unknown organism being present in the database. There are numerous unnamed species among the anaerobic gram-negative bacilli which can confound this type of analytical approach.

Another method which can reliably detect as-yet-un-named taxa as well as identify known species is 16S rRNA gene sequence analysis (33). For clinical purposes, a 500-bp sequence from the 5′ end of the gene is able to identify most, but not all, members of this group to species level. This method is being increasingly used for identification of anaerobic bacteria, because sequencing of the gene is faster and more accurate than biochemical testing and, notably, independent of the growth characteristics (181, 190). Recently, sequencing of the *rpoB* gene has also proven its potential for bacterial identification (1). For instance, *rpoB* gene analysis has been successfully used for distinguishing two closely related *Fusobacterium* species, *F. nucleatum* and *F. periodonticum*, and for oral isolates versus those isolated from intestinal biopsies (193). However, sequencing, as a routine method, may not be feasible for many clinical laboratories. The development of algorithms to screen for those isolates that can be adequately identified by conventional methods and to refer difficult-to-identify isolates for 16S rRNA gene sequencing has been proposed (33, 181). Also, commercial 16S rRNA gene sequence-based identification

kits, containing reagents for DNA extraction and amplification, are available (MicroSeq; Applied Biosystems, Foster City, CA). However, they require instruments, including a thermal cycler and automated gene sequencer, and software for interpretation, and the data needed to assess their value in identifying gram-negative anaerobes are not available.

Although sequencing of the 16S rRNA gene is a useful method for identification of fastidious anaerobic organisms, providing a much faster turnaround time than conventional methods, molecular analysis alone should not replace culturing in the clinical setting. Phenotypic characteristics, obtained by culture and biochemical testing, assist in correlating the sequence-based data, which can be sometimes difficult to interpret, for example, due to incomplete sequences stored in the database. More importantly, culture is necessary for antibiotic susceptibility testing of isolates from clinical specimens.

Unculturable Anaerobic Gram-Negative Rods

In many chronic infections, if not in all, several as-yet-uncultivated phylotypes representing gram-negative anaerobic phyla can be detected. These include two deep branches of the phylum *Bacteroidetes* found in the human mouth and gut (104, 134) and a similar group within the newly described phylum *Synergistetes* (92), for which no cultivable representatives are available (206). In the female genital tract, several *Prevotella*-like phylotypes have been strongly associated with bacterial vaginosis (143). Currently, chronic venous leg ulcers are considered polymicrobial infections in which unknown bacteroidales are among the most ubiquitous organisms (213).

SEROLOGIC TESTS

Because infections caused by gram-negative anaerobic taxa are polymicrobial and opportunistic in nature, serological procedures are not practical for their identification from colonies. Furthermore, no standardized tests that would be useful for these bacteria are available for the detection of antibodies or antigens.

ANTIMICROBIAL SUSCEPTIBILITIES

Trends of increasing resistance among gram-negative anaerobes to antimicrobial agents have been observed (77). Although susceptibility to antibiotics can vary considerably among species within the same genus, most clinical

TABLE 9 Biochemical identification of motile gram-negative anaerobic rods[a]

Genus and species	Nitrate reduction	Esculin hydrolysis	Production of[b]:									Fermentation of[c]:					
			Cat	Ind	Urea	α-Glu	α-Gal	β-Gal	α-Fuc	β-NAG	Glu	Man	Sor	Tre	Raf	Suc
Anaerobiospirillum																
A. *succiniproducens*	−	−	−	−	−	+	−	+	−	+	+	ND	−	−	+	+
A. *thomasii*	−	−	−	−	−	−	−	−	−	+	+	ND	−	−	−	−
Selenomonas																
S. *artemidis*	v	−	−	−	−	v	−	−	−	−	+	+	v	−	−	+
S. *dianae*	+	−	−	−	−	−	−	−	−	−	+	+	−	+	v	+
S. *flueggei*	+	−	−	−	−	+	v	−	−	−	+	+	+	−	v	+
S. *infelix*	+	+	−	−	−	v	v	−	−	−	+	+	v	−	+	+
S. *noxia*	−	−	−	−	−	−	−	−	−	−	w	−	−	−	−	−
S. *sputigena*	v	−	−	−	−	w	+	v	−	−	+	−	−	−	+	+
Desulfovibrio																
D. *desulfuricans*	+	ND	−	−	+	ND	ND	ND	ND	ND	"−"	"−"	"−"	"−"	"−"	"−"
D. *fairfieldensis*	+	ND	+	−	−	ND	ND	ND	ND	ND	"−"	"−"	"−"	"−"	"−"	"−"
D. *piger*[d]	−	ND	−	−	−	ND	ND	ND	ND	ND	"−"	"−"	"−"	"−"	"−"	"−"
D. *vulgaris*	−	ND	−	+	−	ND	ND	ND	ND	ND	"−"	"−"	"−"	"−"	"−"	"−"
Phocaeicola																
P. *abscessus*	−	−	−	−	ND	w	+	+	+	+	"−"	"−"	"−"	"−"	"−"	"−"

[a]Data were compiled from references 4, 119, 121, 126, and 209. Symbols: +, positive; −, negative; v, variable; w, weak reaction; ND, no data.

[b]Cat, catalase; Ind, indole; α-Glu, α-glucosidase; α-Gal, α-galactosidase; β-Gal, β-galactosidase; α-Fuc, α-fucosidase; β-NAG, N-acetyl-β-glucosaminidase.

[c]Glu, glucose; Man, mannose; Sor, sorbitol; Tre, trehalose; Raf, raffinose; Suc, sucrose. "−" for *Desulfovibrio* and *Phocaeicola* species indicates that the species is asaccharolytic.

[d]Nonmotile.

laboratories neither perform the accurate species-level identification of the isolated organism nor test the susceptibilities of anaerobic isolates (66). Without knowledge of the local susceptibility patterns, the choice of proper antimicrobial therapy can be hampered and make the treatment outcomes of anaerobic infections less predictable. According to recent surveys conducted in the United States, Europe, Kuwait, Taiwan, and New Zealand, members of the B. fragilis group are among the most resistant anaerobes to various antimicrobial agents; this situation is independent of the geographical location (61, 86, 115, 144, 162, 185, 214). Some variation, however, exists in resistance rates between countries and areas. In a large U.S. survey, including 10 geographically diverse medical centers, yearly changes in the B. fragilis group susceptibility patterns to ertapenem, imipenem, meropenem, ampicillin-sulbactam, piperacillin-tazobactam, cefoxitin, clindamycin, moxifloxacin, tigecycline, chloramphenicol, and metronidazole were followed from 1997 to 2004 (185). Among the >5,000 isolates tested, the most resistant organism proved to be a *Parabacteroides* species, *P. distasonis*. Its resistance rate (17%) to ampicillin-sulbactam nearly doubled during the follow-up period, compared to an average resistance rate of 2% for all the other species combined, during the later years. Moreover, one of three of the tested *P. distasonis* strains proved to be resistant to cefoxitin. Of the B. fragilis group organisms, B. fragilis was the most susceptible (<2% of the tested strains resistant) to carbapenems and β-lactam–β-lactamase inhibitor combinations (185). In another large survey, conducted at the National Taiwan University Hospital, the proportion of susceptible isolates

of *Bacteroides*, *Prevotella*, and/or *Fusobacterium* species to many antimicrobials, especially cefmetazole, clindamycin, and the combination ampicillin-sulbactam, decreased during the period from 2000 to 2007 (115). Noteworthy was the presence of intermediate or resistant strains to carbapenems among the tested B. fragilis, Fusobacterium, and Prevotella isolates from blood; one B. fragilis isolate was even resistant to all four carbapenems tested (115). Indeed, blood isolates seem to be less susceptible than those from intra-abdominal, obstetric, or other infections (3). Newer fluoroquinolones have been considered to have good antianaerobic effects, but this situation may be worsening among gram-negative anaerobes (63, 145). *Pseudoflavonifractor capillosus* (formerly a non-fragilis group *Bacteroides*) has shown to be prevalent and to exhibit high resistance rates to moxifloxacin in Greece (145), with the caveat that the isolates examined in the study were not identified using sequence-based methods. In general, carbapenems, some β-lactam–β-lactamase inhibitor combinations, chloramphenicol, and metronidazole are the most useful antianaerobic agents, whereas most cephalosporins, clindamycin, and most fluoroquinolones are currently considered less active for use against gram-negative anaerobic bacteria in severe infections (3, 61, 77, 86, 115, 144, 185, 212). In addition, the relatively new antimicrobial drugs tigecycline and linezolid have demonstrated good antianaerobic effects against gram-negative anaerobes; however, some resistant *Bacteroides* and *Prevotella* strains have been reported (65, 185, 214). A few cases of multidrug-resistant B. fragilis isolated from blood and drainage fluid after gastric surgery have been reported (94, 208), with the strains being resistant to antianaerobic

TABLE 10 Antimicrobial activities of antimicrobial agents against common gram-negative anaerobes[a]

Antimicrobial agent(s)	Resistance rate (%) of tested strains			
	Bacteroides	Porphyromonas	Prevotella	Fusobacterium
Penicillin	96–100	26	61–95	4–15
Amoxicillin-clavulanate	4–33	0	0–8	0–7
Piperacillin-tazobactam	0–7	0	0	0
Cefoxitin	0–18	ND	0–1	0
Doripenem	0–7	ND	0	0
Ertapenem	<1–5	ND	0	0
Imipenem	0–4	0	6	0–4
Meropenem	0–5	0	0–3	0–8
Tigecycline	4–8	ND	0	0
Moxifloxacin	7–35	ND	16–38	0–13
Clindamycin	6–59	0	4–32	0–8
Metronidazole	0–2	0	0–8	0
Chloramphenicol	0–4	ND	0	4

[a]Data were compiled from references 61, 86, 115, 145, 162, and 185. ND, no data.

agents, such as carbapenems, β-lactam–β-lactamase inhibitors, clindamycin, and/or metronidazole. Interestingly, one of these cases was successfully treated with linezolid (208). Despite the extensive use of metronidazole against anaerobes, acquired resistance has been considered rare (<5%). However, prolonged exposure of *nim* gene-carrying *Bacteroides* species to metronidazole can select for therapeutic resistance (59). A considerable number of *Dialister* strains, isolated from a variety of clinical specimens, showed decreased susceptibility to metronidazole but without harboring *nim* genes (128). Also, rare strains of *Prevotella* species may appear highly resistant to metronidazole, resulting in poor treatment outcome (131).

Although the agar dilution method is recommended as the method of choice for susceptibility testing of anaerobic species, many studies have shown that the Etest (bioMeriéux) provides reliable results on susceptibilities of anaerobic isolates from clinical specimens (59, 61, 86, 214). The Etest is simple to perform and readily available when needed, offering a useful method for susceptibility testing in clinical microbiology laboratories. It has been observed that some slow-growing metronidazole-resistant clones can be overlooked when using the standard incubation time of 48 h; therefore, it has been recommended that laboratories reexamine the Etest plates after 72 h to look for small colonies within the metronidazole inhibition zone (59, 131). Susceptibility testing methods for anaerobic bacteria are described further in chapter 72.

Table 10 summarizes the current antimicrobial activity rates of the clinically most relevant gram-negative anaerobic taxa.

EVALUATION, INTERPRETATION, AND REPORTING OF RESULTS

Knowledge about the resident microbiota and awareness of the role of anaerobic bacteria in disease permit the clinician to anticipate the likely infecting species at different body sites. Training for anaerobic techniques, in general, and introduction of more advanced methods for the detection and precise identification of anaerobic organisms are urgently needed in clinical microbiology laboratories, considering the current reports of increasing frequencies of anaerobic

bacteremia and septicemia (108), increasing numbers of patients with *F. necrophorum*-associated invasive diseases (20), and also the increasing resistance rates of anaerobes to various antimicrobials (77, 86, 115, 185, 212, 214). In cases of inaccurate microbiology and inappropriate choices of antimicrobial agents in treating an infection, mortality rates and other treatment failures increase significantly (142, 174). Collecting of clinical specimens should avoid the mucosal microbiota, and proper transport medium and times should be used for keeping the anaerobes alive. Factors such as foul-smelling discharge, proximity of infection to mucosal surfaces, abscess formation, and necrotic tissue indicate the presence of anaerobes in the specimen. A definitive identification of an anaerobic isolate should be obtained for all isolates from normally sterile body sites, including blood, spinal fluid, and organs or body cavities; when the patient is gravely ill and not responding to treatment; and when prolonged treatment is necessary. It would be desirable for reference laboratories to periodically provide information on local susceptibility patterns of anaerobic species within the clinically important taxa. However, not only an accurate antimicrobial therapy but also proper surgery, such as the drainage of abscesses and excision of necrotic tissue, are important in resolving anaerobic infections. It is notable that chronic infectious lesions, in particular, include consortia of bacteria organized in biofilms.

The most important, and often difficult, task in the reporting of results of the isolation of gram-negative anaerobes is determination of whether the organism is involved in the infectious process or is merely a bystander originating from the patient's commensal microbiota. All isolations from normally sterile sites should be regarded as significant. A secondary challenge is that these organisms are often found in polymicrobial infections, with a number of different species present and often as a biofilm. Obtaining pure cultures for susceptibility testing can therefore be time-consuming, and the resulting susceptibility profiles may be conflicting, making the recommendation of appropriate antimicrobial therapy difficult. Fortunately, such infections typically respond well to empirical treatment, as partial disruption of the bacterial consortium responsible is sufficient to allow the body's defenses to deal with the infection.

REFERENCES

1. **Adékambi, T., M. Drancourt, and D. Raoult.** 2009. The *rpoB* gene as a tool for clinical microbiologists. *Trends Microbiol.* **17:**37–45.

2. **Alauzet, C., F. Mory, J. P. Carlier, H. Marchandin, E. Jumas-Bilak, and A. Lozniewski.** 2007. *Prevotella nanceiensis* sp. nov., isolated from human clinical samples. *Int. J. Syst. Evol. Microbiol.* **57:**2216–2220.

3. **Aldridge, K. E., D. Ashcraft, K. Cambre, C. L. Pierson, S. G. Jenkins, and J. E. Rosenblatt.** 2001. Multicenter survey of the changing in vitro antimicrobial susceptibilities of clinical isolates of *Bacteroides fragilis* group, *Prevotella*, *Fusobacterium*, *Porphyromonas*, and *Peptostreptococcus* species. *Antimicrob. Agents Chemother.* **45:**1238–1243.

4. **Al Masalma, M., D. Raoult, and V. Roux.** 2009. *Phocaeicola abscessus* gen. nov., sp. nov., an anaerobic bacterium isolated from human brain abscess sample. *Int. J. Syst. Evol. Microbiol.* **59:**2232–2237.

5. **Amess, J. A., W. O'Neill, C. N. Giollariabhaigh, and J. K. Dytrych.** 2007. A six-month audit of the isolation of *Fusobacterium necrophorum* from patients with sore throat in a district general hospital. *Br. J. Biomed. Sci.* **64:**63–65.

6. **Bahrani-Mougeot, F. K., B. J. Paster, S. Coleman, S. Barbuto, M. T. Brennan, J. Noll, T. Kennedy, P. C. Fox, and P. B. Lockhart.** 2007. Molecular analysis of oral and respiratory bacterial species associated with ventilator-associated pneumonia. *J. Clin. Microbiol.* **45:**1588–1593.

7. **Bahrani-Mougeot, F. K., B. J. Paster, S. Coleman, J. Ashar, S. Barbuto, and P. B. Lockhart.** 2008. Diverse and novel oral bacterial species in blood following dental procedures. *J. Clin. Microbiol.* **46:**2129–2132.

8. **Bakir, M. A., M. Kitahara, M. Sakamoto, M. Matsumoto, and Y. Benno.** 2006. *Bacteroides intestinalis* sp. nov., isolated from human faeces. *Int. J. Syst. Evol. Microbiol.* **56:**151–154.

9. **Bakir, M. A., M. Kitahara, M. Sakamoto, M. Matsumoto, and Y. Benno.** 2006. *Bacteroides finegoldii* sp. nov., isolated from human faeces. *Int. J. Syst. Evol. Microbiol.* **56:**931–935.

10. **Bakir, M. A., M. Sakamoto, M. Kitahara, M. Matsumoto, and Y. Benno.** 2006. *Bacteroides dorei* sp. nov., isolated from human faeces. *Int. J. Syst. Evol. Microbiol.* **56:**1639–1643.

11. **Baron, E. J.** 1997. *Bilophila wadsworthia*: a unique gram-negative anaerobic rod. *Anaerobe* **3:**83–86.

12. **Berger, P., T. Adékambi, M. N. Mallet, and M. Drancourt.** 2005. *Prevotella massiliensis* sp. nov. isolated from human blood. *Res. Microbiol.* **156:**967–973.

13. **Bik, E. M., P. B. Eckburg, S. R. Gill, K. E. Nelson, E. A. Purdom, F. Francois, G. Perez-Perez, M. J. Blaser, and D. A. Relman.** 2006. Molecular analysis of the bacterial microbiota in the human stomach. *Proc. Natl. Acad. Sci. USA* **103:**732–737.

14. **Bisharat, N., L. Goldstein, R. Raz, and M. Elias.** 2001. Gram-negative anaerobic endocarditis: two case reports and review of the literature. *Eur. J. Clin. Microbiol. Infect. Dis.* **20:**651–654.

15. **Bisiaux-Salauze, B., C. Perez, M. Sebald, and J. C. Petit.** 1990. Bacteremias caused by *Selenomonas artemidis* and *Selenomonas infelix*. *J. Clin. Microbiol.* **28:**140–142.

16. **Bittar, F., H. Richet, J. C. Dubus, M. Reynaud-Gaubert, N. Stremler, J. Sarles, D. Raoult, and J. M. Rolain.** 2008. Molecular detection of multiple emerging pathogens in sputa from cystic fibrosis patients. *PLoS One* **3:**e2908.

17. **Blairon, L., Y. De Gheldre, B. Delaere, A. Sonet, A. Bosly, and Y. Glupczynski.** 2006. A 62-month retrospective epidemiological survey of anaerobic bacteraemia in a university hospital. *Clin. Microbiol. Infect.* **12:**527–532.

18. **Boennelycke, M., J. J. Christensen, M. Arpi, and S. Krause.** 2007. *Leptotrichia amnionii* found in septic abortion in Denmark. *Scand. J. Infect. Dis.* **39:**382–383.

19. **Bolstad, A. I., H. B. Jensen, and V. Bakken.** 1996. Taxonomy, biology, and periodontal aspects of *Fusobacterium nucleatum*. *Clin. Microbiol. Rev.* **9:**55–71.

20. **Brazier, J. S.** 2006. Human infections with *Fusobacterium necrophorum*. *Anaerobe* **12:**165–172.

21. **Brook, I.** 2002. Microbiology of polymicrobial abscesses and implications for therapy. *J. Antimicrob. Chemother.* **50:**805–810.

22. **Brook, I.** 2008. Microbiology and management of joint and bone infections due to anaerobic bacteria. *J. Orthop. Sci.* **13:**160–169.

23. **Brook, I.** 2008. Infective endocarditis caused by anaerobic bacteria. *Arch. Cardiovasc. Dis.* **101:**665–676.

24. **Brook, I.** 2009. Pericarditis caused by anaerobic bacteria. *Int. J. Antimicrob. Agents* **33:**297–300.

25. **Caram, L. B., J. P. Linefsky, K. M. Read, D. R. Murdoch, T. Lalani, C. W. Woods, L. B. Reller, S. S. Kanj, M. M. Premru, S. Ryan, M. Al-Hegelan, P. Y. Donnio, C. Orezzi, M. G. Paiva, C. Tribouilloy, R. Watkin, O. Harris, D. P. Eisen, G. R. Corey, C. H. Cabell, C. A. Petti, et al.** 2008. *Leptotrichia* endocarditis: report of two cases from the International Collaboration on Endocarditis (ICE) database and review of previous cases. *Eur. J. Clin. Microbiol. Infect. Dis.* **27:**139–143.

26. **Carlier, J. P., M. Bedora-Faure, G. K'ouas, C. Alauzet, and F. Mory.** 2009. Proposal to unify *Clostridium orbiscindens* Winter et al. 1991 and *Eubacterium plautii* (Seguin 1928) Hofstad and Aasjord 1982, with description of *Flavonifractor plautii* gen. nov., comb. nov. and reassignment of *Bacteroides capillosus* to *Pseudoflavonifractor capillosus* gen. nov., comb. nov. *Int. J. Syst. Evol. Microbiol.* **60:**585–590.

27. **Cerdeno-Tarraga, A. M., S. Patrick, L. C. Crossman, G. Blakely, V. Abratt, N. Lennard, I. Poxton, B. Duerden, B. Harris, M. A. Quail, A. Barron, L. Clark, C. Corton, J. Doggett, M. T. Holden, N. Larke, A. Line, A. Lord, H. Norbertczak, D. Ormond, C. Price, E. Rabbinowitsch, J. Woodward, B. Barrell, and J. Parkhill.** 2005. Extensive DNA inversions in the *B. fragilis* genome control variable gene expression. *Science* **307:**1463–1465.

28. **Chassard, C., E. Delmas, P. A. Lawson, and A. Bernalier-Donadille.** 2008. *Bacteroides xylanisolvens* sp. nov., a xylan-degrading bacterium isolated from human faeces. *Int. J. Syst. Evol. Microbiol.* **58:**1008–1013.

29. **Chhour, K. L., M. A. Nadkarni, R. Byun, F. E. Martin, N. A. Jacques, and N. Hunter.** 2005. Molecular analysis of microbial diversity in advanced caries. *J. Clin. Microbiol.* **43:**843–849.

30. **Citron, D. M., Y. A. Warren, M. K. Hudspeth, and E. J. Goldstein.** 2000. Survival of aerobic and anaerobic bacteria in purulent clinical specimens maintained in the Copan Venturi Transystem and Becton Dickinson Port-a-Cul transport systems. *J. Clin. Microbiol.* **38:**892–894.

31. **Citron, D. M.** 2002. Update on the taxonomy and clinical aspects of the genus *Fusobacterium*. *Clin. Infect. Dis.* **35**(Suppl. 1)**:**S22–S27.

32. **Citron, D. M., E. J. Goldstein, C. V. Merriam, B. A. Lipsky, and M. A. Abramson.** 2007. Bacteriology of moderate-to-severe diabetic foot infections and in vitro activity of antimicrobial agents. *J. Clin. Microbiol.* **45:**2819–2828.

33. **Clarridge, J. E., III.** 2004. Impact of 16S rRNA gene sequence analysis for identification of bacteria on clinical microbiology and infectious diseases. *Clin. Microbiol. Rev.* **17:**840–862.

34. **Collins, M. D., L. Hoyles, E. Tornqvist, R. von Essen, and E. Falsen.** 2001. Characterization of some strains from human clinical sources which resemble "*Leptotrichia sanguinegens*": description of *Sneathia sanguinegens* sp. nov., gen. nov. *Syst. Appl. Microbiol.* **24:**358–361.

35. **Conrads, G., M. C. Claros, D. M. Citron, K. L. Tyrrell, V. Merriam, and E. J. Goldstein.** 2002. 16S-23S rDNA internal transcribed spacer sequences for analysis of the phylogenetic relationships among species of the genus *Fusobacterium*. *Int. J. Syst. Evol. Microbiol.* **52:**493–499.

36. **Conrads, G., D. M. Citron, R. Mutters, S. Jang, and E. J. Goldstein.** 2004. *Fusobacterium canifelinum* sp. nov., from the oral cavity of cats and dogs. *Syst. Appl. Microbiol.* **27:**407–413.

37. **Contreras, A., N. Doan, C. Chen, T. Rusitanonta, M. J. Flynn, and J. Slots.** 2000. Importance of *Dialister pneumosintes* in human periodontitis. *Oral Microbiol. Immunol.* **15:**269–272.

38. **De Martino, S. J., I. Mahoudeau, J. P. Brettes, Y. Piemont, H. Monteil, and B. Jaulhac.** 2004. Peripartum bacteremias due to *Leptotrichia amnionii* and *Sneathia sanguinegens*, rare causes of fever during and after delivery. *J. Clin. Microbiol.* **42:**5940–5943.

39. **DiGiulio, D. B., R. Romero, H. P. Amogan, J. P. Kusanovic, E. M. Bik, F. Gotsch, C. J. Kim, O. Erez, S. Edwin, and D. A. Relman.** 2008. Microbial prevalence, diversity and abundance in amniotic fluid during preterm labor: a molecular and culture-based investigation. *PLoS One* **3:**e3056.

40. **Domann, E., G. Hong, C. Imirzalioglu, S. Turschner, J. Kühle, C. Watzel, T. Hain, H. Hossain, and T. Chakraborty.** 2003. Culture-independent identification of pathogenic bacteria and polymicrobial infections in the genitourinary tract of renal transplant recipients. *J. Clin. Microbiol.* **41:**5500–5510.

41. **Downes, J., M. Munson, and W. G. Wade.** 2003. *Dialister invisus* sp. nov., isolated from the human oral cavity. *Int. J. Syst. Evol. Microbiol.* **53:**1937–1940.

42. **Downes, J., I. C. Sutcliffe, T. Hofstad, and W. G. Wade.** 2006. *Prevotella bergensis* sp. nov., isolated from human infections. *Int. J. Syst. Evol. Microbiol.* **56:**609–612.

43. **Downes, J., I. C. Sutcliffe, V. Booth, and W. G. Wade.** 2007. *Prevotella maculosa* sp. nov., isolated from the human oral cavity. *Int. J. Syst. Evol. Microbiol.* **57:**2936–2939.

44. **Downes, J., S. J. Hooper, M. J. Wilson, and W. G. Wade.** 2008. *Prevotella histicola* sp. nov., isolated from the human oral cavity. *Int. J. Syst. Evol. Microbiol.* **58:**1788–1791.

45. **Downes, J., M. Liu, E. Kononen, and W. G. Wade.** 2009. *Prevotella micans* sp. nov., isolated from the human oral cavity. *Int. J. Syst. Evol. Microbiol.* **59:**771–774.

46. **Downes, J., S. R. Vartoukian, F. E. Dewhirst, J. Izard, T. Chen, W. H. Yu, I. C. Sutcliffe, and W. G. Wade.** 2009. *Pyramidobacter piscolens* gen. nov., sp. nov., a member of the phylum "Synergistetes" isolated from the human oral cavity. *Int. J. Syst. Evol. Microbiol.* **59:**972–980.

47. **Downes, J., A. C. Tanner, F. E. Dewhirst, and W. G. Wade.** 2010. *Prevotella saccharolytica* sp. nov., isolated from the human oral cavity. *Int. J. Syst. Evol. Microbiol.* **60:** 2458–2461.

48. **Elgouhari, H., M. Othman, and W. H. Gerstein.** 2007. *Bacteroides fragilis* vertebral osteomyelitis: case report and a review of the literature. *South. Med. J.* **100:**506–511.

49. **Enwonwu, C. O., W. A. Falkler, and E. O. Idigbe.** 2000. Oro-facial gangrene (noma/cancrum oris): pathogenetic mechanisms. *Crit. Rev. Oral Biol. Med.* **11:**159–171.

50. **Eribe, E. R., B. J. Paster, D. A. Caugant, F. E. Dewhirst, V. K. Stromberg, G. H. Lacy, and I. Olsen.** 2004. Genetic diversity of *Leptotrichia* and description of *Leptotrichia goodfellowii* sp. nov., *Leptotrichia hofstadii* sp. nov., *Leptotrichia shahii* sp. nov. and *Leptotrichia wadei* sp. nov. *Int. J. Syst. Evol. Microbiol.* **54:**583–592.

51. **Eribe, E. R., and I. Olsen.** 2008. *Leptotrichia* species in human infections. *Anaerobe* **14:**131–137.

52. **Faveri, M., M. P. Mayer, M. Feres, L. C. de Figueiredo, F. E. Dewhirst, and B. J. Paster.** 2008. Microbiological diversity of generalized aggressive periodontitis by 16S rRNA clonal analysis. *Oral Microbiol. Immunol.* **23:**112–118.

53. **Fenner, L., V. Roux, M. N. Mallet, and D. Raoult.** 2005. *Bacteroides massiliensis* sp. nov., isolated from blood culture of a newborn. *Int. J. Syst. Evol. Microbiol.* **55:**1335–1337.

54. **Fenner, L., V. Roux, P. Ananian, and D. Raoult.** 2007. *Alistipes finegoldii* in blood cultures from colon cancer patients. *Emerg. Infect. Dis.* **13:**1260–1262.

55. **Fihman, V., L. Raskine, F. Petitpas, J. Mateo, R. Kania, J. Gravisse, M. Resche-Rigon, I. Farhat, B. Berçot, D. Payen, M. J. Sanson-Le Pors, P. Herman, and A. Mebazaa.** 2008. Cervical necrotizing fasciitis: 8-years' experience of microbiology. *Eur. J. Clin. Microbiol. Infect. Dis.* **27:**691–695.

56. **Finegold, S. M., M. L. Vaisanen, M. Rautio, E. Eerola, P. Summanen, D. Molitoris, Y. Song, C. Liu, and H. Jousimies-Somer.** 2004. *Porphyromonas uenonis* sp. nov., a pathogen for humans distinct from *P. asaccharolytica* and *P. endodontalis.* *J. Clin. Microbiol.* **42:**5298–5301.

57. **Fredricks, D. N., T. L. Fiedler, and J. M. Marrazzo.** 2005. Molecular identification of bacteria associated with bacterial vaginosis. *N. Engl. J. Med.* **353:**1899–1911.

58. **Fredricks, D. N., T. L. Fiedler, K. K. Thomas, C. M. Mitchell, and J. M. Marrazzo.** 2009. Changes in vaginal bacterial concentrations with intravaginal metronidazole therapy for bacterial vaginosis as assessed by quantitative PCR. *J. Clin. Microbiol.* **47:**721–726.

59. **Gal, M., and J. S. Brazier.** 2004. Metronidazole resistance in *Bacteroides* spp. carrying *nim* genes and the selection of slow-growing metronidazole-resistant mutants. *J. Antimicrob. Chemother.* **54:**109–116.

60. **Glazunova, O. O., T. Launay, D. Raoult, and V. Roux.** 2007. *Prevotella timonensis* sp. nov., isolated from a human breast abscess. *Int. J. Syst. Evol. Microbiol.* **57:**883–886.

61. **Glupczynski, Y., C. Berhin, and H. Nizet.** 2009. Antimicrobial susceptibility of anaerobic bacteria in Belgium as determined by E-test methodology. *Eur. J. Clin. Microbiol. Infect. Dis.* **28:**261–267.

62. **Gmür, R., C. Wyss, Y. Xue, T. Thurnheer, and B. Guggenheim.** 2004. Gingival crevice microbiota from Chinese patients with gingivitis or necrotizing ulcerative gingivitis. *Eur. J. Oral Sci.* **112:**33–41.

63. **Golan, Y., L. A. McDermott, N. V. Jacobus, E. J. Goldstein, S. Finegold, L. J. Harrell, D. W. Hecht, S. G. Jenkins, C. Pierson, R. Venezia, J. Rihs, P. Iannini, S. L. Gorbach, and D. R. Snydman.** 2003. Emergence of fluoroquinolone resistance among *Bacteroides* species. *J. Antimicrob. Chemother.* **52:** 208–213.

64. **Goldstein, E. J. C., D. M. Citron, V. A. Peraino, and S. A. Cross.** 2003. *Desulfovibrio desulfuricans* bacteremia and review of human *Desulfovibrio* infections. *J. Clin. Microbiol.* **41:**2752–2754.

65. **Goldstein, E. J. C., D. M. Citron, C. V. Merriam, Y. A. Warren, K. L. Tyrrell, and H. T. Fernandez.** 2006. Comparative in vitro susceptibilities of 396 unusual anaerobic strains to tigecycline and eight other antimicrobial agents. *Antimicrob. Agents Chemother.* **50:**3507–3513.

66. **Goldstein, E. J., D. M. Citron, P. J. Goldman, and R. J. Goldman.** 2008. National hospital survey of anaerobic culture and susceptibility methods: III. *Anaerobe* **14:**68–72.

67. **Gomes, B. P., R. C. Jacinto, E. T. Pinheiro, E. L. Sousa, A. A. Zaia, C. C. Ferraz, and F. J. Souza-Filho.** 2005. *Porphyromonas gingivalis, Porphyromonas endodontalis, Prevotella intermedia* and *Prevotella nigrescens* in endodontic lesions detected by culture and by PCR. *Oral Microbiol. Immunol.* **20:**211–215.

68. **Goto, M., S. Hitomi, and T. Ishii.** 2007. Bacterial arthritis caused by *Leptotrichia amnionii.* *J. Clin. Microbiol.* **45:**2082–2083.

69. **Gürsoy, M., G. Haraldsson, M. Hyvönen, T. Sorsa, R. Pajukanta, and E. Könönen.** 2009. Does the frequency of *Prevotella intermedia* increase during pregnancy? *Oral Microbiol. Immunol.* **24:**299–303.

70. **Hagelskjaer Kristensen, L., and J. Prag.** 2008. Lemierre's syndrome and other disseminated *Fusobacterium necrophorum* infections in Denmark: a prospective epidemiological and clinical survey. *Eur. J. Clin. Microbiol. Infect. Dis.* **27:**779–789.

71. **Han, X. Y., J. S. Weinberg, S. S. Prabhu, S. J. Hassenbusch, G. N. Fuller, J. J. Tarrand, and D. P. Kontoyiannis.** 2003. Fusobacterial brain abscess: a review of five cases and an analysis of possible pathogenesis. *J. Neurosurg.* **99:**693–700.

72. **Han, Y. W., A. Ikegami, C. Rajanna, H. I. Kawsar, Y. Zhou, M. Li, H. T. Sojar, R. J. Genco, H. K. Kuramitsu, and C. X. Deng.** 2005. Identification and characterization of a novel adhesin unique to oral fusobacteria. *J. Bacteriol.* **187:**5330–5340.

73. **Han, Y. W., T. Shen, P. Chung, I. A. Buhimschi, and C. S. Buhimschi.** 2009. Uncultivated bacteria as etiologic agents of intra-amniotic inflammation leading to preterm birth. *J. Clin. Microbiol.* **47:**38–47.

74. **Hardham, J. M., K. W. King, K. Dreier, J. Wong, C. Strietzel, R. R. Eversole, C. Sfintescu, and R. T. Evans.** 2008. Transfer of *Bacteroides splanchnicus* to *Odoribacter* gen. nov. as *Odoribacter splanchnicus* comb. nov., and description of *Odoribacter denticanis* sp. nov., isolated from the crevicular spaces of canine periodontitis patients. *Int. J. Syst. Evol. Microbiol.* **58:**103–109.

75. **Hayashi, H., K. Shibata, M. Sakamoto, S. Tomita, and Y. Benno.** 2007. *Prevotella copri* sp. nov. and *Prevotella stercorea* sp. nov., isolated from human faeces. *Int. J. Syst. Evol. Microbiol.* **57:**941–946.

76. Hayashi, H., K. Shibata, M. A. Bakir, M. Sakamoto, S. Tomita, and Y. Benno. 2007. *Bacteroides coprophilus* sp. nov., isolated from human faeces. *Int. J. Syst. Evol. Microbiol.* **57:**1323–1326.

77. Hecht, D. W. 2004. Prevalence of antibiotic resistance in anaerobic bacteria: worrisome developments. *Clin. Infect. Dis.* **39:**92–97.

78. Hecht, D. W. 2007. Routine anaerobic blood cultures: back where we started? *Clin. Infect. Dis.* **44:**901–903.

79. Heidelberg, J. F., R. Seshadri, S. A. Haveman, C. L. Hemme, I. T. Paulsen, J. F. Kolonay, J. A. Eisen, N. Ward, B. Methe, L. M. Brinkac, S. C. Daugherty, R. T. Deboy, R. J. Dodson, A. S. Durkin, R. Madupu, W. C. Nelson, S. A. Sullivan, D. Fouts, D. H. Haft, J. Selengut, J. D. Peterson, T. M. Davidsen, N. Zafar, L. Zhou, D. Radune, G. Dimitrov, M. Hance, K. Tran, H. Khouri, J. Gill, T. R. Utterback, T. V. Feldblyum, J. D. Wall, G. Voordouw, and C. M. Fraser. 2004. The genome sequence of the anaerobic, sulfate-reducing bacterium *Desulfovibrio vulgaris* Hildenborough. *Nat. Biotechnol.* **22:**554–559.

80. Holt, S. C., and J. L. Ebersole. 2005. *Porphyromonas gingivalis*, *Treponema denticola*, and *Tannerella forsythia*: the "red complex," a prototype polybacterial pathogenic consortium in periodontitis. *Periodontol. 2000* **38:**72–122.

81. Hudspeth, M. K., S. Hunt Gerardo, M. F. Maiden, D. M. Citron, and E. J. C. Goldstein. 1999. Characterization of *Bacteroides forsythus* strains from cat and dog bite wounds in humans and comparison with monkey and human oral strains. *J. Clin. Microbiol.* **37:**2003–2006.

82. Huggan, P. J., and D. R. Murdoch. 2008. Fusobacterial infections: clinical spectrum and incidence of invasive disease. *J. Infect.* **57:**283–289.

83. Ivanova, N., S. Gronow, A. Lapidus, A. Copeland, T. G. Del Rio, M. Nolan, S. Lucas, F. Chen, H. Tice, J.-F. Cheng, E. Saunders, D. Bruce, L. Goodwin, T. Brettin, J. C. Detter, C. Han, S. Pitluck, N. Mikhailova, A. Pati, K. Mavrommatis, A. Chen, K. Palaniappan, M. Land, L. Hauser, Y.-J. Chang, C. D. Jeffries, P. Chain, C. Rohde, M. Goker, J. Bristow, J. A. Eisen, V. Markowitz, P. Hugenholtz, N. C. Kyrpides, and H.-P. Klenk. 2009. Complete genome sequence of *Leptotrichia buccalis* type strain (C-1013-bT). *Stand. Genom. Sci.* **1:**126–132.

84. Iwai, T., Y. Inoue, M. Umeda, Y. Huang, N. Kurihara, M. Koike, and I. Ishikawa. 2005. Oral bacteria in the occluded arteries of patients with Buerger disease. *J. Vasc. Surg.* **42:**107–115.

85. Iwata, K., and M. Takahashi. 2008. Is anaerobic blood culture necessary? If so, who needs it? *Am. J. Med. Sci.* **336:**58–63.

86. Jamal, W., M. Shahin, and V. O. Rotimi. 2010. Surveillance and trends of antimicrobial resistance among clinical isolates of anaerobes in Kuwait hospitals from 2002 to 2007. *Anaerobe* **16:**1–5.

87. Jensen, A., L. Hagelskjaer Kristensen, H. Nielsen, and J. Prag. 2008. Minimum requirements for a rapid and reliable routine identification and antibiogram of *Fusobacterium necrophorum*. *Eur. J. Clin. Microbiol. Infect. Dis.* **27:**557–563.

88. Johnson, C. C., and S. M. Finegold. 1987. Uncommonly encountered, motile, anaerobic gram-negative bacilli associated with infection. *Rev. Infect. Dis.* **9:**1150–1162.

89. Jousimies-Somer, H., P. Summanen, D. M. Citron, E. J. Baron, H. M. Wexler, and S. M. Finegold. 2002. *Wadsworth-KTL Anaerobic Bacteriology Manual*, 6th ed. Star Publishing, Belmont, CA.

90. Jumas-Bilak, E., H. Jean-Pierre, J. P. Carlier, C. Teyssier, K. Bernard, B. Gay, J. Campos, F. Morio, and H. Marchandin. 2005. *Dialister micraerophilus* sp. nov. and *Dialister propionicifaciens* sp. nov., isolated from human clinical samples. *Int. J. Syst. Evol. Microbiol.* **55:**2471–2478.

91. Jumas-Bilak, E., J. P. Carlier, H. Jean-Pierre, D. Citron, K. Bernard, A. Damay, B. Gay, C. Teyssier, J. Campos, and H. Marchandin. 2007. *Jonquetella anthropi* gen. nov., sp. nov., the first member of the candidate phylum 'Synergistetes' isolated from man. *Int. J. Syst. Evol. Microbiol.* **57:**2743–2748.

92. Jumas-Bilak, E., L. Roudière, and H. Marchandin. 2009. Description of 'Synergistetes' phyl. nov. and emended description of the phylum 'Deferribacteres' and of the family Syntrophomonadaceae, phylum 'Firmicutes.' *Int. J. Syst. Evol. Microbiol.* **59:**1028–1035.

93. Kapatral, V., I. Anderson, N. Ivanova, G. Reznik, T. Los, A. Lykidis, A. Bhattacharyya, A. Bartman, W. Gardner, G. Grechkin, L. Zhu, O. Vasieva, L. Chu, Y. Kogan, O. Chaga, E. Goltsman, A. Bernal, N. Larsen, M. D'Souza, T. Walunas, G. Pusch, R. Haselkorn, M. Fonstein, N. Kyrpides, and R. Overbeek. 2002. Genome sequence and analysis of the oral bacterium *Fusobacterium nucleatum* strain ATCC 25586. *J. Bacteriol.* **184:**2005–2018.

94. Katsandri, A., J. Papaparaskevas, A. Pantazatou, G. L. Petrikkos, G. Thomopoulos, D. P. Houhoula, and A. Avlamis. 2006. Two cases of infections due to multidrug-resistant *Bacteroides fragilis* group strains. *J. Clin. Microbiol.* **44:**3465–3467.

95. Kawanami, T., K. Fukuda, T. Yatera, T. Kido, C. Yoshii, H. Taniguchi, and M. Kido. 2009. Severe pneumonia with *Leptotrichia* sp. detected predominantly in bronchoalveolar lavage fluid by use of 16S rRNA gene sequencing analysis. *J. Clin. Microbiol.* **47:**496–498.

96. Kim, M. S., S. W. Roh, and J. W. Bae. 2010. *Bacteroides faecis* sp. nov., isolated from human faeces. *Int. J. Syst. Evol. Microbiol.* **60:**2572–2576.

97. Klug, T. E., M. Rusan, K. Fuursted, and T. Ovesen. 2009. *Fusobacterium necrophorum*: most prevalent pathogen in peritonsillar abscess in Denmark. *Clin. Infect. Dis.* **49:**1467–1472.

98. Kolenbrander, P. E., R. N. Andersen, and L. V. Moore. 1989. Coaggregation of *Fusobacterium nucleatum*, *Selenomonas flueggei*, *Selenomonas infelix*, *Selenomonas noxia*, and *Selenomonas sputigena* with strains from 11 genera of oral bacteria. *Infect. Immun.* **57:**3194–3203.

99. Kolenbrander, P. E. 2000. Oral microbial communities: biofilms, interactions, and genetic systems. *Annu. Rev. Microbiol.* **54:**413–437.

100. Könönen, E., H. Jousimies-Somer, and S. Asikainen. 1994. The most frequently isolated gram-negative anaerobes in saliva and subgingival samples taken from young women. *Oral Microbiol. Immunol.* **9:**126–128.

101. Könönen, E., M.-L. Väisänen, S. M. Finegold, R. Heine, and H. Jousimies-Somer. 1996. Cellular fatty acid analysis and enzyme profiles of *Porphyromonas catoniae*, a frequent colonizer of the oral cavity in children. *Anaerobe* **2:**329–335.

102. Könönen, E. 2000. Development of oral bacterial flora in young children. *Ann. Med.* **32:**107–112.

103. Könönen, E., S. Paju, P. J. Pussinen, M. Hyvönen, P. Di Tella, L. Suominen-Taipale, and M. Knuuttila. 2007. Population-based study of salivary carriage of periodontal pathogens in adults. *J. Clin. Microbiol.* **45:**2446–2451.

104. Kumar, P. S., A. L. Griffen, J. A. Barton, B. J. Paster, M. L. Moeschberger, and E. J. Leys. 2003. New bacterial species associated with chronic periodontitis. *J. Dent. Res.* **82:**338–344.

105. Kuwahara, T., A. Yamashita, H. Hirakawa, H. Nakayama, H. Toh, N. Okada, S. Kuhara, M. Hattori, T. Hayashi, and Y. Ohnishi. 2004. Genomic analysis of *Bacteroides fragilis* reveals extensive DNA inversions regulating cell surface adaptation. *Proc. Natl. Acad. Sci. USA* **101:**14919–14924.

106. Langendijk, P.S., E. M. Kulik, H. Sandmeier, J. Meyer, and J. S. van der Hoeven. 2001. Isolation of *Desulfomicrobium orale* sp. nov. and *Desulfovibrio* strain NY682, oral sulfate-reducing bacteria involved in human periodontal disease. *Int. J. Syst. Evol. Microbiol.* **51:**1035–1044.

107. Larsson, P.-G., B. Carlsson, L. Fåhraeus, T. Jakobsson, and U. Forsum. 2004. Diagnosis of bacterial vaginosis: need for validation of microscopic image area used for scoring bacterial morphotypes. *Sex. Transm. Infect.* **80:**63–67.

108. Lassmann, B., D. R. Gustafson, C. M. Wood, and J. E. Rosenblatt. 2007. Reemergence of anaerobic bacteremia. *Clin. Infect. Dis.* **44:**895–900.

109. Lawson, P. A., E. Moore, and E. Falsen. 2008. *Prevotella amnii* sp. nov., isolated from human amniotic fluid. *Int. J. Syst. Evol. Microbiol.* **58:**89–92.

110. Legaria, M. C., G. Lumelsky, V. Rodriguez, and S. Rosetti. 2005. Clindamycin-resistant *Fusobacterium varium* bacteremia and decubitus ulcer infection. *J. Clin. Microbiol.* **43:**4293–4295.

111. Le Moal, G., C. Landron, G. Grollier, B., Bataille, F. Roblot, P. Nassans, and B. Becq-Giraudon. 2003. Characteristics of brain abscess with isolation of anaerobic bacteria. *Scand. J. Infect. Dis.* **35:**318–321.

112. León, R., N. Silva, A. Ovalle, A. Chaparro, A. Ahumada, M. Gajardo, M. Martinez, and J. Gamonal. 2007. Detection of *Porphyromonas gingivalis* in the amniotic fluid in pregnant women with a diagnosis of threatened premature labor. *J. Periodontol.* **78:**1249–1255.

113. Ley, R. E., P. J. Turnbaugh, S. Klein, and J. I. Gordon. 2006. Microbial ecology: human gut microbes associated with obesity. *Nature* **444:**1022–1023.

114. Lin, W. J., W. T. Lo, C. C. Chu, M. L. Chu, and C. C. Wang. 2006. Bacteriology and antibiotic susceptibility of community-acquired intra-abdominal infection in children. *J. Microbiol. Immunol. Infect.* **39:**249–254.

115. Liu, C. Y., Y. T. Huang, C. H. Liao, L. C. Yen, H. Y. Lin, and P. R. Hsueh. 2008. Increasing trends in antimicrobial resistance among clinically important anaerobes and *Bacteroides fragilis* isolates causing nosocomial infections: emerging resistance to carbapenems. *Antimicrob. Agents Chemother.* **52:**3161–3168.

116. Lockhart, P. B., M. T. Brennan, H. C. Sasser, P. C. Fox, B. J. Paster, and F. K. Bahrani-Mougeot. 2008. Bacteremia associated with toothbrushing and dental extraction. *Circulation* **117:**3118–3125.

117. Loubinoux, J., F. M. Valente, I. A. Pereira, A. Costa, P. A. Grimont, and A. E. Le Faou. 2002. Reclassification of the only species of the genus *Desulfomonas*, *Desulfomonas pigra*, as *Desulfovibrio piger* comb. nov. *Int. J. Syst. Evol. Microbiol.* **52:**1305–1308.

118. Loubinoux, J., B. Jaulhac, Y. Piemont, H. Monteil, and A. E. Le Faou. 2003. Isolation of sulfate-reducing bacteria from human thoracoabdominal pus. *J. Clin. Microbiol.* **41:**1304–1306.

119. Maiden, M. F., A. Tanner, and W. E. Moore. 1992. Identification of *Selenomonas* species by whole-genomic DNA probes, sodium dodecyl sulfate-polyacrylamide gel electrophoresis, biochemical tests and cellular fatty acid analysis. *Oral Microbiol. Immunol.* **7:**7–13.

120. Malnick, H., K. Williams, J. Phil-Ebosie, and A. S. Levy. 1990. Description of a medium for isolating *Anaerobiospirillum* spp., a possible cause of zoonotic disease, from diarrheal feces and blood of humans and use of the medium in a survey of human, canine, and feline feces. *J. Clin. Microbiol.* **28:**1380–1384.

121. Malnick, H. 1997. *Anaerobiospirillum thomasii* sp. nov., an anaerobic spiral bacterium isolated from the feces of cats and dogs and from diarrheal feces of humans, and emendation of the genus *Anaerobiospirillum*. *Int. J. Syst. Evol. Microbiol.* **47:**381–384.

122. Mättö, J., S. Asikainen, M. L. Väisänen, M. Rautio, M. Saarela, P. Summanen, S. Finegold, and H. Jousimies-Somer. 1997. Role of *Porphyromonas gingivalis*, *Prevotella intermedia*, and *Prevotella nigrescens* in extraoral and some odontogenic infections. *Clin. Infect. Dis.* **25**(Suppl. 2):S194–S198.

123. Mira, A., R. Pushker, B. A. Legault, D. Moreira, and F. Rodríguez-Valera. 2004. Evolutionary relationships of *Fusobacterium nucleatum* based on phylogenetic analysis and comparative genomics. *BMC Evol. Biol.* **4:**50.

124. Moen, K., J. G. Brun, M. Valen, L. Skartveit, E. K. Eribe, I. Olsen, and R. Jonsson. 2006. Synovial inflammation in active rheumatoid arthritis and psoriatic arthritis facilitates trapping of a variety of oral bacterial DNAs. *Clin. Exp. Rheumatol.* **24:**656–663.

125. Molitoris, E., H. M. Wexler, and S. M. Finegold. 1997. Sources and antimicrobial susceptibilities of *Campylobacter gracilis* and *Sutterella wadsworthensis*. *Clin. Infect. Dis.* **25**(Suppl. 2):S264–S265.

126. Moore, L. V. H., J. L. Johnson, and W. E. C. Moore. 1987. *Selenomonas noxia* sp. nov., *Selenomonas flueggei* sp. nov., *Selenomonas infelix* sp. nov., *Selenomonas dianae* sp. nov., and *Selenomonas artemidis* sp. nov., from the human gingival crevice. *Int. J. Syst. Evol. Microbiol.* **37:**271–280.

127. Morgenstein, A. A., D. M. Citron, and S. M. Finegold. 1981. New medium selective for *Fusobacterium* species and differential for *Fusobacterium necrophorum*. *J. Clin. Microbiol.* **13:**666–669.

128. Morio, F., H. Jean-Pierre, L. Dubreuil, E. Jumas-Bilak, L. Calvet, G. Mercier, R. Devine, and H. Marchandin. 2007. Antimicrobial susceptibilities and clinical sources of *Dialister* species. *Antimicrob. Agents Chemother.* **51:**4498–4501.

129. Morotomi, M., F. Nagai, H. Sakon, and R. Tanaka. 2008. *Dialister succinatiphilus* sp. nov. and *Barnesiella intestinihominis* sp. nov., isolated from human faeces. *Int. J. Syst. Evol. Microbiol.* **58:**2716–2720.

130. Morotomi, M., F. Nagai, H. Sakon, and R. Tanaka. 2009. *Paraprevotella clara* gen. nov., sp. nov., and *Paraprevotella xylaniphila* sp. nov., members of the family 'Prevotellaceae' isolated from human faeces. *Int. J. Syst. Evol. Microbiol.* **59:**1895–1900.

131. Mory, F., J. P. Carlier, C. Alauzet, M. Thouvenin, H. Schuhmacher, and A. Lozniewski. 2005. Bacteremia caused by a metronidazole-resistant *Prevotella* sp. strain. *J. Clin. Microbiol.* **43:**5380–5383.

132. Mory, F., C. Alauzet, C. Matuszeswski, P. Riegel, and A. Lozniewski. 2009. Evaluation of the new Vitek 2 ANC card for identification of medically relevant anaerobic bacteria. *J. Clin. Microbiol.* **47:**1923–1926.

133. Mousa, H. A. 1997. Aerobic, anaerobic and fungal burn wound infections. *J. Hosp. Infect.* **37:**317–323.

134. Munson, M. A., T. Pitt-Ford, B. Chong, A. Weightman, and W. G. Wade. 2002. Molecular and cultural analysis of the microflora associated with endodontic infections. *J. Dent. Res.* **81:**761–766.

135. Nagai, F., M. Morotomi, H. Sakon, and R. Tanaka. 2009. *Parasutterella excrementihominis* gen. nov., sp. nov., a novel member of the family *Alcaligenaceae*, isolated from human faeces. *Int. J. Syst. Evol. Microbiol.* **59:**1793–1797.

136. Nagai, F., M. Morotomi, Y. Watanabe, H. Sakon, and R. Tanaka. 2010. *Alistipes indistinctus* sp. nov. and *Odoribacter laneus* sp. nov., common members of the human intestinal microbiota isolated from faeces. *Int. J. Syst. Evol. Microbiol.* **60:**1296–1302.

137. Nagy, E., T. Maier, E. Urban, G. Terhes, and M. Kostrzewa, on behalf of the ESCMID Study Group on Antimicrobial Resistance in Anaerobic Bacteria. 2009. Species identification of clinical isolates of *Bacteroides* by matrix-assisted laser-desorption/ionization time-of-flight mass spectrometry. *Clin. Microbiol. Infect.* **15:**796–802.

138. Naito, M., H. Hirakawa, A. Yamashita, N. Ohara, M. Shoji, H. Yukitake, K. Nakayama, H. Toh, F. Yoshimura, S. Kuhara, M. Hattori, T. Hayashi, and K. Nakayama. 2008. Determination of the genome sequence of *Porphyromonas gingivalis* strain ATCC 33277 and genomic comparison with strain W83 revealed extensive genome rearrangements in *P. gingivalis*. *DNA Res.* **15:**215–225.

139. Nakazawa, H., A. Arakaki, S. Narita-Yamada, I. Yashiro, K. Jinno, N. Aoki, A. Tsuruyama, Y. Okamura, S. Tanikawa, N. Fujita, H. Takeyama, and T. Matsunaga. 2009. Whole genome sequence of *Desulfovibrio magneticus* strain RS-1 revealed common gene clusters in magnetotactic bacteria. *Genome Res.* **19:**1801–1808.

140. Nelson, K. E., R. D. Fleischmann, R. T. DeBoy, I. T. Paulsen, D. E. Fouts, J. A. Eisen, S. C. Daugherty, R. J. Dodson, A. S. Durkin, M. Gwinn, D. H. Haft, J. F. Kolonay, W. C. Nelson, T. Mason, L. Tallon, J. Gray, D. Granger, H. Tettelin, H. Dong, J. L. Galvin, M. J. Duncan, F. E. Dewhirst, and C. M. Fraser. 2003. Complete genome sequence of the oral pathogenic bacterium *Porphyromonas gingivalis* strain W83. *J. Bacteriol.* **185:**5591–5601.

141. Ng, L. S., L. L. Kwang, S. C. Yeow, and T. Y. Tan. 2008. Anaerobic culture of diabetic foot infections: organisms and antimicrobial susceptibilities. *Ann. Acad. Med. Singapore* **37:**936–939.

142. Nguyen, M. H., V. L. Yu, A. J. Morris, L. McDermott, M. W. Wagener, L. Harrell, and D. R. Snydman. 2000.

Antimicrobial resistance and clinical outcome of *Bacteroides* bacteraemia: findings of a multicenter prospective observational trial. *Clin. Infect. Dis.* **30**:870–876.

143. **Oakley, B. B., T. L. Fiedler, J. M. Marrazzo, and D. N. Fredricks.** 2008. Diversity of human vaginal bacterial communities and associations with clinically defined bacterial vaginosis. *Appl. Environ. Microbiol.* **74**:4898–4909.

144. **Papaparaskevas, J., A. Pantazatou, A. Katsandri, N. J. Legakis, A. Avlamis, et al.** 2005. Multicentre survey of the in-vitro activity of seven antimicrobial agents, including ertapenem, against recently isolated gram-negative anaerobic bacteria in Greece. *Clin. Microbiol. Infect.* **11**:820–824.

145. **Papaparaskevas, J., A. Pantazatou, A. Katsandri, D. P. Houhoula, N. J. Legakis, A. Tsakris, and A. Avlamis.** 2008. Moxifloxacin resistance is prevalent among *Bacteroides* and *Prevotella* species in Greece. *J. Antimicrob. Chemother.* **62**:137–141.

146. **Paster, B. J., F. E. Dewhirst, I. Olsen, and G. J. Fraser.** 1994. Phylogeny of *Bacteroides*, *Prevotella*, and *Porphyromonas* spp. and related bacteria. *J. Bacteriol.* **176**:725–732.

147. **Paster, B. J., S. K. Boches, J. L. Galvin, R. E. Ericson, C. N. Lau, V. A. Levanos, A. Sahasrabudhe, and F. E. Dewhirst.** 2001. Bacterial diversity in human subgingival plaque. *J. Bacteriol.* **183**:3770–3783.

148. **Pearce, M. A., D. A. Devine, R. A. Dixon, and T. J. van Steenbergen.** 2000. Genetic heterogeneity in *Prevotella intermedia*, *Prevotella nigrescens*, *Prevotella corporis* and related species isolated from oral and nonoral sites. *Oral Microbiol. Immunol.* **15**:89–95.

149. **Pei, Z., E. J. Bini, L. Yang, M. Zhou, F. Francois, and M. J. Blaser.** 2004. Bacterial biota in the human distal esophagus. *Proc. Natl. Acad. Sci. USA* **101**:4250–4255.

150. **Penders, J., C. Thijs, C. Vink, F. F. Stelma, B. Snijders, I. Kummeling, P. A. van den Brandt, and E. E. Stobberingh.** 2006. Factors influencing the composition of the intestinal microbiota in early infancy. *Pediatrics* **118**:511–521.

151. **Persson, R., J. Hitti, R. Verhelst, M. Vaneechoutte, R. Persson, R. Hirschi, M. Weibel, M. Rothen, M. Temmerman, K. Paul, and D. Eschenbach.** 2009. The vaginal microflora in relation to gingivitis. *BMC Infect. Dis.* **9**:6.

152. **Pienaar, C., A. J. Kruger, E. C. Venter, and J. D. Pitout.** 2003. *Anaerobiospirillum succiniciproducens* bacteraemia. *J. Clin. Pathol.* **56**:316–318.

153. **Pimentel, J. D., and R. C. Chan.** 2007. *Desulfovibrio fairfieldensis* bacteremia associated with choledocholithiasis and endoscopic retrograde cholangiopancreatography. *J. Clin. Microbiol.* **45**:2747–2750.

154. **Prasad, K. N., A. M. Mishra, D. Gupta, N. Husain, M. Husain, and R. K. Gupta.** 2006. Analysis of microbial etiology and mortality in patients with brain abscess. *J. Infect.* **53**:221–227.

155. **Pye, A. D., D. E. Lockhart, M. P. Dawson, C. A. Murray, and A. J. Smith.** 2009. A review of dental implants and infection. *J. Hosp. Infect.* **72**:104–110.

156. **Rautio, M., H. Saxén, A. Siitonen, R. Nikku, and H. Jousimies-Somer.** 2000. Bacteriology of histopathologically defined appendicitis in children. *Pediatr. Infect. Dis. J.* **19**:1078–1083.

157. **Rautio, M., E. Eerola, M. L. Väisänen-Tunkelrott, D. Molitoris, P. Lawson, M. D. Collins, and H. Jousimies-Somer.** 2003. Reclassification of *Bacteroides putredinis* (Weinberg et al., 1937) in a new genus *Alistipes* gen. nov., as *Alistipes putredinis* comb. nov., and description of *Alistipes finegoldii* sp. nov., from human sources. *Syst. Appl. Microbiol.* **26**:182–188.

158. **Rennie, R. P., C. Brosnikoff, L. Turnbull, L. B. Reller, S. Mirrett, W. Janda, K. Ristow, and A. Krilcich.** 2008. Multicenter evaluation of the Vitek 2 anaerobe and *Corynebacterium* identification card. *J. Clin. Microbiol.* **46**:2646–2651.

159. **Riggio, M. P., H. Aga, C. A. Murray, M. S. Jackson, A. Lennon, N. Hammersley, and J. Bagg.** 2007. Identification of bacteria associated with spreading odontogenic infections by 16S rRNA gene sequencing. *Oral Surg. Oral Med. Oral Pathol. Oral Radiol. Endod.* **103**:610–617.

160. **Riordan, T.** 2007. Human infection with *Fusobacterium necrophorum* (necrobacillosis), with a focus on Lemierre's syndrome. *Clin. Microbiol. Rev.* **20**:622–659.

161. **Robert, C., C. Chassard, P. A. Lawson, and A. Bernalier-Donadille.** 2007. *Bacteroides cellulosilyticus* sp. nov., a cellulolytic bacterium from the human gut microbial community. *Int. J. Syst. Evol. Microbiol.* **57**:1516–1520.

162. **Roberts, S. A., K. P. Shore, S. D. Paviour, D. Holland, and A. J. Morris.** 2006. Antimicrobial susceptibility of anaerobic bacteria in New Zealand: 1999–2003. *J. Antimicrob. Chemother.* **57**:992–998.

163. **Rôças, I. N., and J. F. Siqueira, Jr.** 2006. Characterization of *Dialister* species in infected root canals. *J. Endod.* **32**:1057–1061.

164. **Rôças, I. N., and J. F. Siqueira, Jr.** 2008. Root canal microbiota of teeth with chronic apical periodontitis. *J. Clin. Microbiol.* **46**:3599–3606.

165. **Rousée, J. M., D. Bermond, Y. Piémont, C. Tournoud, R. Heller, P. Kehrli, M. L. Harlay, H. Monteil, and B. Jaulhac.** 2002. *Dialister pneumosintes* associated with human brain abscesses. *J. Clin. Microbiol.* **40**:3871–3873.

166. **Sakamoto, M., M. Suzuki, M. Umeda, I. Ishikawa, and Y. Benno.** 2002. Reclassification of *Bacteroides forsythus* (Tanner et al. 1986) as *Tannerella forsythensis* corrig., gen. nov., comb. nov. *Int. J. Syst. Evol. Microbiol.* **52**:841–849.

167. **Sakamoto, M., and Y. Benno.** 2006. Reclassification of *Bacteroides distasonis*, *Bacteroides goldsteinii* and *Bacteroides merdae* as *Parabacteroides distasonis* gen. nov., comb. nov., *Parabacteroides goldsteinii* comb. nov. and *Parabacteroides merdae* comb. nov. *Int. J. Syst. Evol. Microbiol.* **56**:1599–1605.

168. **Sakamoto, M., M. Kitahara, and Y. Benno.** 2007. *Parabacteroides johnsonii* sp. nov., isolated from human faeces. *Int. J. Syst. Evol. Microbiol.* **57**:293–296.

169. **Sakamoto, M., P. T. Lan, and Y. Benno.** 2007. *Barnesiella viscericola* gen. nov., sp. nov., a novel member of the family *Porphyromonadaceae* isolated from chicken caecum. *Int. J. Syst. Evol. Microbiol.* **57**:342–346.

170. **Sakamoto, M., K. Ohkusu, T. Masaki, H. Kako, T. Ezaki, and Y. Benno.** 2007. *Prevotella pleuritidis* sp. nov., isolated from pleural fluid. *Int. J. Syst. Evol. Microbiol.* **57**:1725–1728.

171. **Sakamoto, M., N. Suzuki, N. Matsunaga, K. Koshihara, M. Seki, H. Komiya, and Y. Benno.** 2009. *Parabacteroides gordonii* sp. nov., isolated from human blood cultures. *Int. J. Syst. Evol. Microbiol.* **59**:2843–2847.

172. **Sakamoto, M., N. Suzuki, and M. Okamoto.** 2010. *Prevotella aurantiaca* sp. nov., isolated from the human oral cavity. *Int. J. Syst. Evol. Microbiol.* **60**:500–503.

173. **Sakon, H., F. Nagai, M. Morotomi, and R. Tanaka.** 2008. *Sutterella parvirubra* sp. nov. and *Megamonas funiformis* sp. nov., isolated from human faeces. *Int. J. Syst. Evol. Microbiol.* **58**:970–975.

174. **Salonen, J. H., E. Eerola, and O. Meurman.** 1998. Clinical significance and outcome of anaerobic bacteremia. *Clin. Infect. Dis.* **26**:1413–1417.

175. **Sears, C. L.** 2009. Enterotoxigenic *Bacteroides fragilis*: a rogue among symbiotes. *Clin. Microbiol. Rev.* **22**:349–369.

176. **Seng, P., M. Drancourt, F. Gouriet, B. La Scola, P. E. Fournier, J. M. Rolain, and D. Raoult.** 2009. Ongoing revolution in bacteriology: routine identification of bacteria by matrix-assisted laser desorption ionization time-of-flight mass spectrometry. *Clin. Infect. Dis.* **49**:543–551.

177. **Shah, H. N., and M. D. Collins.** 1988. Proposal for reclassification of *Bacteroides asaccharolyticus*, *Bacteroides gingivalis*, and *Bacteroides endodontalis* in a new genus, *Porphyromonas*. *Int. J. Syst. Evol. Microbiol.* **38**:128–131.

178. **Shah, H. N., and M. D. Collins.** 1989. Proposal to restrict the genus *Bacteroides* (Castellani and Chalmers) to *Bacteroides fragilis* and closely related species. *Int. J. Syst. Evol. Microbiol.* **39**:85–87.

179. **Shah, H. N., and D. M. Collins.** 1990. *Prevotella*, a new genus to include *Bacteroides melaninogenicus* and related species formerly classified in the genus *Bacteroides*. *Int. J. Syst. Evol. Microbiol.* **40**:205–208.

180. **Shukla, S. K., P. R. Meier, P. D. Mitchell, D. N. Frank, and K. D. Reed.** 2002. *Leptotrichia amnionii* sp. nov., a novel bacterium isolated from the amniotic fluid of a woman after intrauterine fetal demise. *J. Clin. Microbiol.* **40**:3346–3349.

181. Simmon, K. E., S. Mirrett, L. B. Reller, and C. A. Petti. 2008. Genotypic diversity of anaerobic isolates from bloodstream infections. *J. Clin. Microbiol.* **46:**1596–1601.

182. Siqueira, J. F., Jr., and I. N. Rôças. 2004. Nested PCR detection of *Centipeda periodontii* in primary endodontic infections. *J. Endod.* **30:**135–137.

183. Siqueira, J. F., Jr., and I. N. Rôças. 2009. The microbiota of acute apical abscesses. *J. Dent. Res.* **88:**61–65.

184. Sixou, J. L., C. Magaud, A. Jolivet-Gougeon, M. Cormier, and M. Bonnaure-Mallet. 2003. Evaluation of the mandibular third molar pericoronitis flora and its susceptibility to different antibiotics prescribed in France. *J. Clin. Microbiol.* **41:**5794–5797.

185. Snydman, D. R., N. V. Jacobus, L. A. McDermott, R. Ruthazer, Y. Golan, E. J. Goldstein, S. M. Finegold, L. J. Harrell, D. W. Hecht, S. G. Jenkins, C. Pierson, R. Venezia, V. Yu, J. Rihs, and S. L. Gorbach. 2007. National survey on the susceptibility of *Bacteroides fragilis* group: report and analysis of trends in the United States from 1997 to 2004. *Antimicrob. Agents Chemother.* **51:**1649–1655.

186. Sobel, J. D. 2000. Bacterial vaginosis. *Annu. Rev. Med.* **51:**349–356.

187. Socransky, S. S., A. D. Haffajee, M. A. Cugini, C. Smith, and R. L. Kent, Jr. 1998. Microbial complexes in subgingival plaque. *J. Clin. Periodontol.* **25:**134–144.

188. Song, Y. L., C. X. Liu, M. McTeague, and S. M. Finegold. 2004. "*Bacteroides nordii*" sp. nov. and "*Bacteroides salyersae*" sp. nov. isolated from clinical specimens of human intestinal origin. *J. Clin. Microbiol.* **42:**5565–5570.

189. Song, Y., C. Liu, J. Lee, M. Bolanos, M. L. Vaisanen, and S. M. Finegold. 2005. "*Bacteroides goldsteinii*" sp. nov. isolated from clinical specimens of human intestinal origin. *J. Clin. Microbiol.* **43:**4522–4527.

190. Song, Y., C. Liu, M. Bolanos, J. Lee, M. McTeague, and S. M. Finegold. 2005. Evaluation of 16S rRNA sequencing and reevaluation of a short biochemical scheme for identification of clinically significant *Bacteroides* species. *J. Clin. Microbiol.* **43:**1531–1537.

191. Song, Y., E. Könönen, M. Rautio, C. Liu, A. Bryk, E. Eerola, and S. M. Finegold. 2006. *Alistipes onderdonkii* sp. nov. and *Alistipes shahii* sp. nov., of human origin. *Int. J. Syst. Evol. Microbiol.* **56:**1985–1990.

192. Stîngu, C. S., A. C. Rodloff, H. Jentsch, R. Schaumann, and K. Eschrich. 2008. Rapid identification of oral anaerobic bacteria cultivated from subgingival biofilm by MALDI-TOF-MS. *Oral Microbiol. Immunol.* **23:**372–376.

193. Strauss, J., A. White, C. Ambrose, J. McDonald, and E. Allen-Vercoe. 2008. Phenotypic and genotypic analyses of clinical *Fusobacterium nucleatum* and *Fusobacterium periodonticum* isolates from the human gut. *Anaerobe* **14:**301–309.

194. Su, T. M., C. M. Lan, Y. D. Tsai, T. C. Lee, C. H. Lu, and W. N. Chang. 2008. Multiloculated pyogenic brain abscess: experience in 25 patients. *Neurosurgery* **62**(Suppl. 2):556–561.

195. Summanen, P. H., B. Durmaz, M. L. Väisänen, C. Liu, D. Molitoris, E. Eerola, I. M. Helander, and S. M. Finegold. 2005. *Porphyromonas somerae* sp. nov., a pathogen isolated from humans and distinct from *Porphyromonas levii*. *J. Clin. Microbiol.* **43:**4455–4459.

196. Summanen, P. H., P. A. Lawson, and S. M. Finegold. 2009. *Porphyromonas bennonis* sp. nov., isolated from human clinical specimens. *Int. J. Syst. Evol. Microbiol.* **59:**1727–1732.

197. Talan, D. A., D. M. Citron, F. M. Abrahamian, G. J. Moran, E. J. Goldstein, et al. 1999. Bacteriologic analysis of infected dog and cat bites. *N. Engl. J. Med.* **340:**85–92.

198. Talan, D. A., F. M. Abrahamian, G. J. Moran, D. M. Citron, J. O. Tan, E. J. Goldstein, et al. 2003. Clinical presentation and bacteriologic analysis of infected human bites in patients presenting to emergency departments. *Clin. Infect. Dis.* **37:**1481–1489.

199. Tanner, A., M. F. Maiden, P. J. Macuch, L. L. Murray, and R. L. Kent, Jr. 1998. Microbiota of health, gingivitis, and initial periodontitis. *J. Clin. Periodontol.* **25:**85–98.

200. Tanner, A. C., and J. Izard. 2006. *Tannerella forsythia*, a periodontal pathogen entering the genomic era. *Periodontology 2000* **42:**88–113.

201. Tee, W., P. Midolo, P. H. Janssen, T. Kerr, and M. L. Dyall-Smith. 2001. Bacteremia due to *Leptotrichia trevisanii* sp. nov. *Eur. J. Clin. Microbiol. Infect. Dis.* **20:**765–769.

202. Tunney, M. M., T. R. Field, T. F. Moriarty, S. Patrick, G. Doering, M. S. Muhlebach, M. C. Wolfgang, R. Boucher, D. F. Gilpin, A. McDowell, and J. S. Elborn. 2008. Detection of anaerobic bacteria in high numbers in sputum from patients with cystic fibrosis. *Am. J. Respir. Crit. Care Med.* **177:**995–1001.

203. Ulstrup, A. K., and S. H. Hartzen. 2006. *Leptotrichia buccalis*: a rare cause of bacteraemia in non-neutropenic patients. *Scand. J. Infect. Dis.* **38:**712–716.

204. Urbán, E., A. Hortobágyi, K. Szentpáli, and E. Nagy. 2004. Two intriguing *Bilophila wadsworthia* cases from Hungary. *J. Med. Microbiol.* **53:**1167–1169.

205. Vandamme, P., M. I. Daneshvar, F. E. Dewhirst, B. J. Paster, K. Kersters, H. Goossens, and C. W. Moss. 1995. Chemotaxonomic analyses of *Bacteroides gracilis* and *Bacteroides ureolyticus* and reclassification of *B. gracilis* as *Campylobacter gracilis* comb. nov. *Int. J. Syst. Evol. Microbiol.* **45:**145–152.

206. Vartoukian, S. R., R. M. Palmer, and W. G. Wade. 2009. Diversity and morphology of members of the phylum "*Synergistetes*" in periodontal health and disease. *Appl. Environ. Microbiol.* **75:**3777–3786.

207. Walker, C. B., S. Stolyar, D. Chivian, N. Pinel, J. A. Gabster, P. S. Dehal, Z. He, Z. K. Yang, H. C. Yen, J. Zhou, J. D. Wall, T. C. Hazen, A. P. Arkin, and D. A. Stahl. 2009. Contribution of mobile genetic elements to *Desulfovibrio vulgaris* genome plasticity. *Environ. Microbiol.* **11:**2244–2252.

208. Wareham, D. W., M. Wilks, D. Ahmed, J. S. Brazier, and M. Millar. 2005. Anaerobic sepsis due to multidrug-resistant *Bacteroides fragilis*: microbiological cure and clinical response with linezolid therapy. *Clin. Infect. Dis.* **40:**e67–e68.

209. Warren, Y. A., D. M. Citron, C. V. Merriam, and E. J. Goldstein. 2005. Biochemical differentiation and comparison of *Desulfovibrio* species and other phenotypically similar genera. *J. Clin. Microbiol.* **43:**4041–4045.

210. Watanabe, Y., F. Nagai, M. Morotomi, H. Sakon, and R. Tanaka. 2010. *Bacteroides clarus* sp. nov., *Bacteroides fluxus* sp. nov. and *Bacteroides oleiciplenus* sp. nov., isolated from human faeces. *Int. J. Syst. Evol. Microbiol.* **60:**1864–1869.

211. Wexler, H. M., D. Reeves, P. H. Summanen, E. Molitoris, M. McTeague, J. Duncan, K. H. Wilson, and S. M. Finegold. 1996. *Sutterella wadsworthensis* gen. nov., sp. nov., bile-resistant microaerophilic *Campylobacter gracilis*-like clinical isolates. *Int. J. Syst. Evol. Microbiol.* **46:**252–258.

212. Wexler, H. M. 2007. *Bacteroides*: the good, the bad, and the nitty-gritty. *Clin. Microbiol. Rev.* **20:**593–621.

213. Wolcott, R. D., V. Gontcharova, Y. Sun, and S. E. Dowd. 2009. Evaluation of the bacterial diversity among and within individual venous leg ulcers using bacterial tag-encoded FLX and titanium amplicon pyrosequencing and metagenomic approaches. *BMC Microbiol.* **9:**226.

214. Wybo, I., D. Piérard, I. Verschraegen, M. Reynders, K. Vandoorslaer, G. Claeys, M. Delmée, Y. Glupczynski, B. Gordts, M. Ieven, P. Melin, M. Struelens, J. Verhaegen, and S. Lauwers. 2007. Third Belgian multicentre survey of antibiotic susceptibility of anaerobic bacteria. *J. Antimicrob. Chemother.* **59:**132–139.

215. Xu, J., M. K. Bjursell, J. Himrod, S. Deng, L. K. Carmichael, H. C. Chiang, L. V. Hooper, and J. I. Gordon. 2003. A genomic view of the human-*Bacteroides thetaiotaomicron* symbiosis. *Science* **299:**2074–2076.

216. Xu, J., M. A. Mahowald, R. E. Ley, C. A. Lozupone, M. Hamady, E. C. Martens, B. Henrissat, P. M. Coutinho, P. Minx, P. Latreille, H. Cordum, A. Van Brunt, K. Kim, R. S. Fulton, L. A. Fulton, S. W. Clifton, R. K. Wilson, R. D. Knight, and J. I. Gordon. 2007. Evolution of symbiotic bacteria in the distal human intestine. *PLoS Biol.* **5:**e156.

Algorithms for Identification of Curved and Spiral-Shaped Gram-Negative Rods

IRVING NACHAMKIN

52

Curved and spiral-shaped bacteria have a common microscopic morphology but represent diverse bacterial pathogens. These organisms are curved, helical, or spiral-shaped gram-negative rods. Specific detection of these organisms may require a combination of tests, including microscopy, histologic staining of tissue, biochemical tests, antigen tests, serologic tests, bacteriologic culture, and molecular approaches.

Most bacteria in this group of organisms are isolated from patients with gastrointestinal tract-related infections. *Campylobacter jejuni* subsp. *jejuni* is the most frequently isolated curved gram-negative rod associated with diarrheal illness, but under proper culture conditions, other *Campylobacter* spp., *Helicobacter* spp., *Arcobacter* spp., and *Vibrio* species may be detected in routine stool cultures (Fig. 1). *Helicobacter cinaedi* and *Helicobacter fennelliae* are two important *Helicobacter* species isolated from fecal specimens (see chapter 54). *Helicobacter pylori* is the most common curved gram-negative

rod isolated from gastric tissue, but other *Helicobacter* species have also been reported in this site.

Other less commonly isolated curved gram-negative rods include the anaerobes *Desulfovibrio* spp., *Sutterella wadsworthensis*, *Wolinella succinogenes*, and *Anaerobiospirillum succiniciproducens*, which may be isolated from blood, abscess material, or other clinical samples (Table 1). Several oxidase-positive nonfermenters, including *Herbaspirillum* species (see chapter 41), may also have a curved appearance.

The spirochetes *Borrelia* spp. and *Leptospira* spp. cause systemic infections and are infrequently isolated in clinical laboratories, usually only with specialized media. These bacteria are strictly aerobic and have optimal growth temperatures at 28 to 30°C (*Leptospira* spp.) and 30 to 33°C (*Borrelia* spp.). *Treponema* spp. of clinical importance are diagnosed based on clinical and epidemiologic findings, as well as microscopic, serologic, and molecular test procedures.

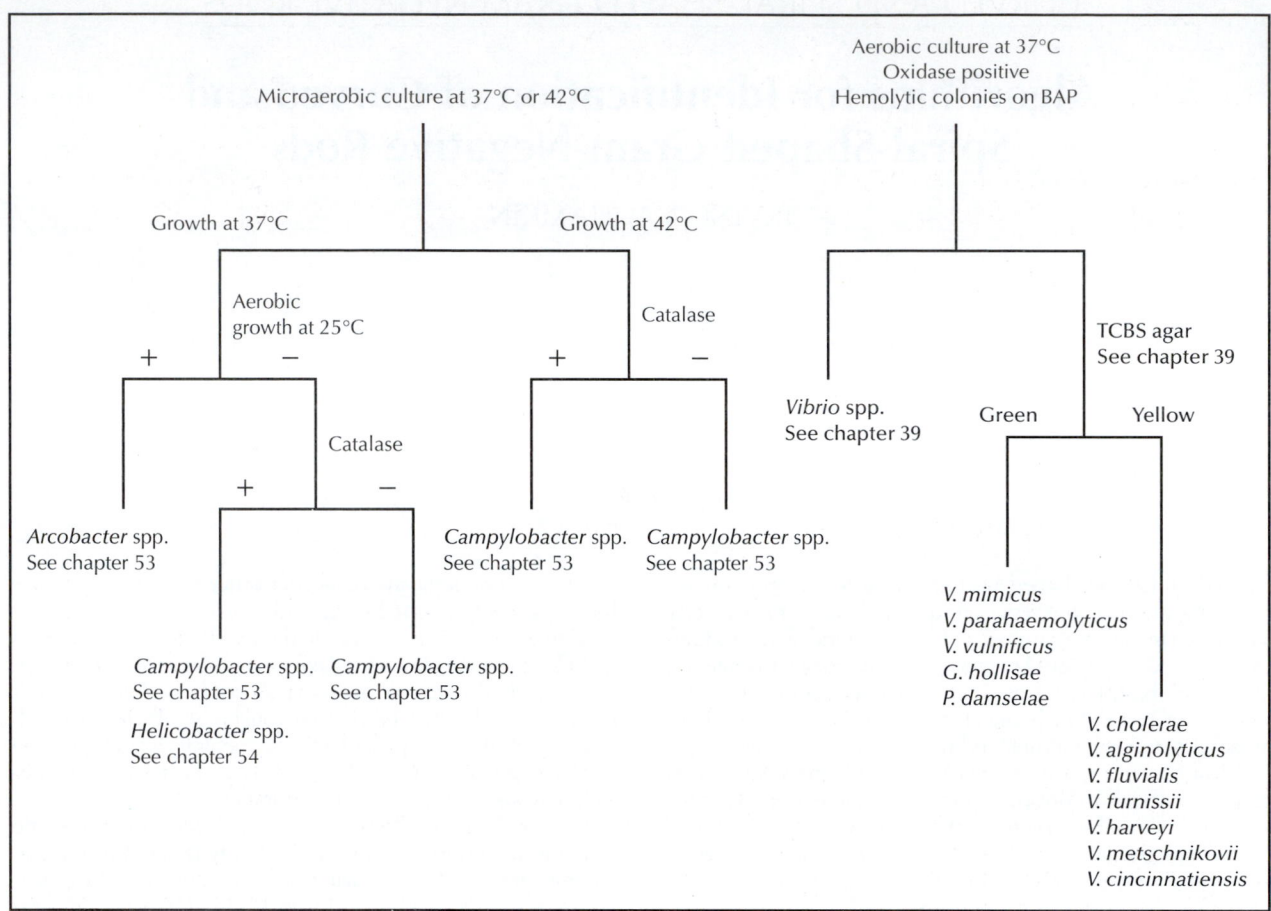

FIGURE 1 Algorithm for identification of curved gram-negative bacilli from fecal samples. Abbreviations: BAP, sheep blood agar plate; TCBS, thiosulfate-citrate-bile salts-sucrose agar.

TABLE 1 Curved gram-negative bacilli that may be encountered in clinical specimens[a]

Clinical entity	Specimen type(s)	Curved gram-negative organisms encountered	Species[b]	Microscopic appearance in specimen	Culture conditions and media	Chapter
Gastroenteritis	Stool, intestinal biopsy	Arcobacter	A. butzleri A. cryaerophilus A. skirrowii	Slightly curved, curved, S-shaped, or helical	Microaerobic, may grow aerobically or anaerobically, nonhemolytic, grows on nonselective blood agar (with filtration method), may grow on Campy-CVA	53
		Brachyspira	B. aalborgi B. pilosicoli	Spirochete	Anaerobic, prolonged incubation (1–2 wk) on anaerobic media, selective media may be required	57
		Campylobacter	C. jejuni subsp. jejuni C. jejuni subsp. doylei C. coli C. upsaliensis C. fetus subsp. fetus C. lari C. curvus C. concisus C. insulaenigrae C. rectus C. hominis C. lanienae C. hyointestinalis C. peloridis C. sputorum	Curved, spiral, gull-wing-shaped, S-shaped GNR	Microaerobic, 37 or 42°C, increased H_2 required for some non-C. jejuni/C. coli species, requires selective media, such as Campy-CVA, and charcoal-based media, such as CCDA; filtration method for less common species and H_2-requiring species	57
		Helicobacter		Curved, spiral, gull-wing-shaped, S-shaped GNR	Microaerobic, 37°C, increased H_2 required for intestinal species, nonselective blood agar for H. pylori, selective supplements (Skirrow's, Dent's) may be needed for contaminated gastric samples	54
		Gastric	H. pylori H. bizzozeronii H. suis			
		Intestinal	H. bilis H. canis H. canadensis H. cinaedi H. fennelliae H. pullorum			
		Vibrio	V. cholerae V. parahaemolyticus V. fluvialis V. alginolyticus V. cincinnatiensis V. furnissii V. metschnikovii V. mimicus Grimontia hollisae (formerly V. hollisae) Photobacterium damselae (formerly V. damselae)	Comma-shaped or straight rods, larger than Campylobacter spp.	Aerobic conditions, 37°C, grows on routine laboratory media, blood agar, MacConkey agar; use selective medium for primary isolation from stool samples, such as TCBS	39
Bacteremia	Blood	Borrelia	Lyme group B. afzelii B. burgdorferi B. garinii Relapsing fever group B. recurrentis B. hermsii	Not seen in routine BC bottles	Difficult to isolate, special media required for isolation; BSK, MKP	56

(Continued on next page)

TABLE 1 Curved gram-negative bacilli that may be encountered in clinical specimens *(Continued)*

Clinical entity	Specimen type(s)	Curved gram-negative organisms encountered	Species[b]	Microscopic appearance in specimen	Culture conditions and media	Chapter
		Campylobacter	*C. jejuni* subsp. *jejuni* *C. fetus* subsp. *fetus* *C. upsaliensis* *C. lari* *C. concisus*	Curved, spiral, gull-wing-shaped, S-shaped GNR	Microaerobic, incubate subcultures at 37°C, increased H$_2$ required for some non-C. jejuni/C. coli strains	53
		Herbaspirillum	*Herbaspirillum* species 3	Curved or helical GNR	Growth properties not described	41
		Helicobacter	*H. cinaedi* *H. fennelliae*	Curved, spiral, gull-wing-shaped, S-shaped GNR	Microaerobic, incubate subcultures at 37°C, increased H$_2$ required	54
		Leptospira	*L. biflexa* *L. interrogans*	Not seen in routine BC bottles	Aerobic growth, 28–30°C, specialized media required for isolation, such as EMJH, PLM-5	55
		Vibrio	*V. vulnificus* *V. metschnikovii* *V. cincinnatiensis* *Photobacterium damselae* (formerly *V. damselae*)	Comma-shaped or straight rods	Aerobic growth, 37°C, grows on routine blood agar, MacConkey agar	39
Tissue infection, oral	Tissue biopsy, abscess fluid	*Campylobacter*	*C. concisus* *C. curvus* *C. rectus* *C. gracilis* *C. showae* *C. ureolyticus*	Curved, spiral, gull-wing-shaped, S-shaped GNR	Microaerobic, incubate cultures at 37°C, increased H$_2$ required for oral species, use nonselective blood agar or CCDA with filtration method	53
Tissue infection, skin, wound, other	Skin biopsy, lesion fluid	*Borrelia*	Lyme group	Histologic stains required	Difficult to isolate, special media required for isolation; BSK, MKP	56
		Treponema	*T. pallidum* (syphilis) "*T. carateum*" (pinta) "*T. pallidum* subsp. *pertenue*" (yaws) "*T. pallidum* subsp. *endemicum*" (endemic)	Spirochetes (silver staining, dark-field microscopy, DFA)	Has not been isolated in vitro	57
		Vibrio	*V. vulnificus* *V. alginolyticus* *V. harveyi* *Photobacterium damselae* (formerly *V. damselae*)	Comma-shaped or straight rods, larger than *Campylobacter* spp.	Aerobic, grows on routine laboratory media, blood agar, MacConkey agar	39
		Anaerobes	*Desulfovibrio* spp. *Sutterella wadsworthensis* *Wolinella succinogenes* *Anaerobiospirillum succiniciproducens*	Curved rods	Growth under anaerobic conditions, use anaerobe media	51
		Herbaspirillum	*Herbaspirillum* species 3	Curved or helical GNR	Growth properties not described	41
Urine		*Leptospira*	*L. biflexa* *L. interrogans*	Spirochete with curved ends (observed by dark-field microscopy)	Aerobic growth, 28–30°C, specialized media required for isolation, such as EMJH, PLM-5	55

[a]BC, blood culture; GNR, gram-negative rod; DFA, direct fluorescent antibody assay; Campy CVA, Campy-cefoperazone, vancomycin, amphotericin; CCDA, charcoal-cefoperazone-deoxycholate agar; TCBS, thiosulfate-citrate-bile salts-sucrose agar; BSK, Barbour-Stoenner-Kelly medium; MKP, modified Kelley's medium; EMJH, Ellinghausen-McCullough-Johnson-Harris medium; PLM-5, prepared leptospira medium.

[b]Not all species listed in this category have been shown to cause human diseases; they are listed if they have been isolated from human clinical specimens.

Campylobacter and *Arcobacter*

COLLETTE FITZGERALD AND IRVING NACHAMKIN

53

TAXONOMY

Three closely related genera, *Campylobacter*, *Arcobacter*, and *Sulfurospirillum*, are included in the family *Campylobacteraceae* (99, 126). The family *Campylobacteraceae* includes 22 species within the genus *Campylobacter*, 7 species in the genus *Arcobacter*, and 6 species in the genus *Sulfurospirillum*. Since the completion of the first genome sequence of *Campylobacter jejuni* subsp. *jejuni* (103), additional complete genome sequences of *C. jejuni*, *C. coli*, *C. lari*, and *C. upsaliensis* have been published (42, 54, 107) with genome sizes varying from 1.59 to 1.85 Mb. Two reviews on comparative genomics of *Campylobacter* have been published (18, 80). Since the last edition of this *Manual*, several new species and subspecies of *Campylobacter* have been proposed including *C. canadensis* (61), isolated from whooping cranes at the Calgary Zoo; *C. avium* from poultry (113), *C. peloridis* (26) isolated from human feces, dialysis fluid, and shellfish; two subspecies of *C. lari* (26); and *C. cuniculorum* from rabbits (140); as well as two *Arcobacter* species, *Arcobacter mytili* (23), isolated from mussels and *A. thereius*, from pigs and ducks (55). *Bacteroides ureolyticus* was reclassified as *Campylobacter ureolyticus* (129). A detailed review on the taxonomy of *Campylobacteraceae* was recently published (25).

DESCRIPTION OF THE AGENTS

Campylobacter spp. are curved, S-shaped, or spiral rods that are 0.2 to 0.9 μm wide and 0.5 to 5 μm long. Occasional species such as *C. hominis* form straight rods. *Campylobacter* species are gram-negative, non-spore-forming rods that may form spherical or coccoid bodies in old cultures or cultures exposed to air for prolonged periods. Organisms are usually motile by means of a single polar unsheathed flagellum at one or both ends, but some may lack flagella. Species are generally microaerobic with a respiratory type of metabolism; however, some strains grow aerobically or anaerobically. An atmosphere containing increased hydrogen is required by some species for microaerobic growth (128).

Arcobacter spp. are gram-negative, slightly curved, curved, S-shaped, or helical non-spore-forming rods that are 0.2 to 0.9 μm wide and 1 to 3 μm long. Organisms are motile with a single polar unsheathed flagellum. *Arcobacter* spp. grow microaerobically at 15, 25, and 30°C but have variable growth at 37 and 42°C. Organisms are microaerobic and do not require increased hydrogen for growth. *Arcobacter* spp. may grow aerobically at 30°C and anaerobically at 35 to 37°C. Most strains are nonhemolytic. *A. skirrowii* may be alpha-hemolytic (130). *A. halophilus* is an obligate halophile and grows poorly on media containing less than 2% NaCl (31).

Originally classified as free-living *Campylobacter* species, *Sulfurospirillum* spp. are slender, curved gram-negative rods, 0.1 to 0.5 μm wide and 1 to 3 μm long. All of the species are sulfur reducers and exhibit variable metabolic activity. *S. deleyianum* is the type species of the genus. These species have no known pathogenicity for humans or animals, are environmental organisms isolated from water sediments, and are not further discussed in this chapter (126).

EPIDEMIOLOGY AND TRANSMISSION

Campylobacter species are primarily zoonotic, with a variety of animals implicated as reservoirs for human infection (Table 1). In addition to food animals such as poultry, cattle, sheep, and pigs, *Campylobacter* species may be present in domestic pets. Humans appear to be the only recognized reservoirs for the periodontal-disease-related species *C. concisus*, *C. rectus*, *C. curvus*, and *C. showae*.

Campylobacter infections are common both in the developed and developing worlds. The reported incidence of culture-confirmed infections varies considerably from country to country, and as culturing practices and reporting requirements can vary, direct comparison of the reported incidences can be complex. In the United States, where reporting practices vary from state to state, the foodborne diseases active surveillance program FoodNet (www.cdc.gov/foodnet) provides uniform reporting from a panel of sentinel sites, giving an accurate incidence of diagnosed infections. Since FoodNet surveillance began in 1996, the incidence of culture-confirmed *Campylobacter* infections in FoodNet sites has been found to have declined 30% when 2006 data are compared to the 1996–1998 baseline (2). Most of the decline occurred from 1996 to 1999; there was a more moderate decrease between 1999 and 2006. In 2008, the incidence of laboratory-confirmed *Campylobacter* infections in FoodNet was 12.68 per 100,000 persons, ranging from 30.23 in California to 6.66 per 100,000 in Maryland (17); this estimated incidence of infections caused by *Campylobacter* did not change significantly compared with the incidence

TABLE 1 Reservoirs for and diseases associated with *Campylobacter* and *Arcobacter* species[a]

Species	Humans	Cattle	Sheep	Pigs	Wild birds	Poultry	Pets	Rodents	Types of infections[b]
C. avium						X			NR
C. canadensis					X				NR
C. cuniculorum							X[c]		
C. jejuni subsp. *jejuni*	X	X			X	X	X		GI, B
C. jejuni subsp. *doylei*	X								GI, B
C. coli				X	X	X			GI, B
C. fetus subsp. *fetus*		X	X						B, GI
C. upsaliensis						X	X		GI, B
C. lari					X		X		GI, B
C. hyointestinalis		X		X		X	X	X	GI
C. helveticus							X		NR
C. sputorum	X[d]	X[e,f]	X[f]						GI[d]
C. concisus	X								D
C. curvus	X								D
C. rectus	X								D, GI
C. showae	X								D
C. gracilis	X								D
C. mucosalis				X					NR
A. butzleri		X		X		X			GI, B, T
A. cibarius						X			NR
A. cryaerophilus		X	X	X		X			GI
A. thereius				X		X			NR
A. skirrowii		X	X	X		X			GI

[a]The information on this table is from references 70, 88, 117, and 127.
[b]GI, gastrointestinal; B, bloodstream infection; D, dental/oral; T, soft tissue; NR, not reported to be associated with human infections.
[c]rabbits.
[d]Biovar sputorum.
[e]Biovar paraureolyticus.
[f]Biovar faecalis.

for the preceding 3 years (2005 to 2007). However, *C. jejuni* subsp. *jejuni* (referred to as *C. jejuni*) continues to be the most common enteric pathogen isolated from patients reported from some states in FoodNet with 1.4 million cases estimated in the United States annually (115). Because of underdiagnosis and underreporting, the actual incidence in any country is substantially greater than the reported incidence. For example, in the United States, it was estimated that the true incidence was 35-fold higher than reported incidence, or 515/100,000 in 1999 (115). In Europe, campylobacter infection is quite common, with an incidence rate of approximately 50/100,000 population (96).

The epidemiology of campylobacteriosis in the United States does not appear to have changed over the last 20 years (96). *Campylobacter* infections are usually sporadic; the incidence starts to rise in March with a peak in the summer months and declines in early fall (96). Infection usually follows ingestion of improperly handled or cooked food, primarily poultry products. Case-control studies both in the United States and Europe continue to find eating poultry to be a significant risk factor for developing campylobacteriosis (96). Outbreaks usually occur in the spring and fall months, and in recent years, most outbreaks have been associated with food (poultry or unpasteurized dairy products) or water. Approximately one-half of the outbreaks in the United States from 1998 to 2004 were associated with dairy products or water; the remaining outbreaks were mostly foodborne, and 44% were attributed to poultry (96). The number of foodborne *Campylobacter* outbreaks in the United States appears to be increasing; from 1998 to 2002 there were 64 foodborne *Campylobacter*

outbreaks causing 1,628 illnesses, compared to 92 outbreaks and 1,431 illnesses during 2003 to 2007. (http://www.cdc.gov/foodborneoutbreaks/outbreak_data.htm). Outbreaks in other developed countries are also associated with food, water, or dairy contamination (96). The incidence of *Campylobacter* infection in developing countries such as Mexico and Thailand is much higher than in the United States. In developing countries, *Campylobacter* is frequently isolated from individuals who may or may not have diarrheal disease. Most symptomatic infections occur in infancy and early childhood, and incidence decreases with age. Travelers to developing countries are at risk for developing *Campylobacter* infection, with isolation rates from 0 to 39% reported in different studies. The incidence of infection follows a bimodal age distribution with the highest incidence in infants and young children followed by a second peak in young adults 20 to 40 years old (115). Secondary transmission of *Campylobacter* from ill persons to other individuals is rare, even though the infectious dose for developing illness is not particularly high (96).

CLINICAL SIGNIFICANCE

C. jejuni and *C. coli*

C. jejuni and *C. coli* have been recognized since the early 1970s as agents of gastrointestinal infection. *C. jejuni* is one of the most common causes of bacterial enteritis in the United States. *C. jejuni* and *C. coli* continue to be the most common *Campylobacter* species associated with diarrheal illness and produce clinically indistinguishable infections. Most laboratories do not routinely distinguish between these organisms. In patients with gastroenteritis caused by *C. jejuni*/*C. coli*, patients' symptoms range from none to severe, including fever, abdominal cramping, and diarrhea (with or without blood/fecal white cells) that lasts several days to more than 1 week (10). The usual incubation period is about 3 days with a general range of 1 to 7 days. Symptomatic infections are usually self-limited, but relapses may occur in 5 to 10% of untreated patients (10). *Campylobacter* infection may mimic acute appendicitis and result in unnecessary surgery. Extraintestinal infections have been reported following *Campylobacter* enteritis and include bacteremia, hepatitis, cholecystitis, pancreatitis, abortion and neonatal sepsis, nephritis, prostatitis, urinary tract infection, peritonitis, myocarditis, and focal infections including meningitis, septic arthritis, and abscess formation (10). Bacteremia has been reported to occur at a rate of 1.5 per 1,000 intestinal infections with the highest rate in the elderly (118). Persistent diarrheal illness and bacteremia may occur in immunocompromised hosts, such as patients with human immunodeficiency virus infection, and may be difficult to treat (10). Deaths attributable to *C. jejuni* infection are uncommon (10). The health burden of campylobacteriosis appears to be substantial and may be underrecognized (84).

C. jejuni is the most often recognized infection preceding the development of Guillain-Barré syndrome (GBS), an acute paralytic disease of the peripheral nervous system (89). Certain heat-stable (HS) serotypes appear to be overrepresented in some GBS cases, such as HS:19 and HS:41; however, other more common serotypes are frequently reported (89). The pathogenesis of *Campylobacter*-induced GBS involves host immune responses to gangliosidelike epitopes present in the core region of the lipooligosaccharide (44), which in the susceptible host mediate damage to the peripheral nerves, where ganglioside targets are highly enriched (138).

Reactive arthritis sometimes follows *Campylobacter* infection, with the onset of pain and joint swelling averaging 2 weeks, with an average range lasting from a few weeks to nearly a year. Reiter's syndrome may also occur in some patients (10). The literature is mixed on the role of HLA B27 as a risk factor for reactive arthritis (10).

The pathogenesis of *Campylobacter* enteric infection is still not well understood. The infective dose of *Campylobacter* is not well defined, but as few as 500 organisms may be capable of causing illness (10). The signs and symptoms of infection suggest an invasive mechanism of disease. A variety of determinants may be important in the virulence of *C. jejuni* infection, including adherence to the intestinal mucosa, bacterial effects on the cell, and inflammatory responses by the host (68). *Campylobacter* does not produce a classic, choleralike enterotoxin (137).

Campylobacter Species Other than *C. jejuni* and *C. coli*

Campylobacter species other than *C. jejuni* and *C. coli* are increasingly isolated from human infections by improved culture methods that are more optimal for the non-*C. jejuni* and non-*C. coli* species.

C. fetus subsp. fetus is primarily associated with bacteremia and extraintestinal infections during pregnancy or in the compromised host (11). Although gastroenteritis does occur with this species, the incidence is probably underestimated because the organism may not grow well at 42°C and is usually susceptible to cephalothin (cefalotin), an antimicrobial agent used in some common selective media for

stool culture (132). *C. fetus* subsp. *fetus* produces a surface protein microcapsule composed of a high-molecular-weight surface layer protein that is essential for virulence (11). *C. fetus* subsp. *venerealis* causes bovine venereal campylobacteriosis and is a cause of bovine infertility but is rarely the cause of human infection (11).

C. upsaliensis is a thermotolerant species that causes diarrhea and bacteremia in humans and is also associated with canine and feline gastroenteritis (69). Over a 10-year period, *C. upsaliensis* was the most common non-*C. jejuni*/ coli species isolated from stool samples submitted to the laboratory for culture (133). *C. upsaliensis* is susceptible to many antimicrobial agents present in *C. jejuni* selective media and thus is usually not isolated on routine primary isolation media; it can be recovered using the filtration technique described below.

C. lari is a nalidixic acid-resistant, thermophilic species first isolated from gulls of the genus *Larus* and from other avian species, dogs, cats, and chickens. *C. lari* has been infrequently reported from humans with bacteremia and gastrointestinal and urinary tract infections (69). Recent phylogenetic studies have described two subspecies, *C. lari* subsp. *concheus* and *C. lari* subsp. *lari* (26).

Other *Campylobacter* species have been isolated from clinical specimens of patients with a variety of diseases, but their pathogenic role has not been determined (69). *C. jejuni* subsp. *doylei* is a nitrate-negative subspecies of *C. jejuni* rarely recovered from patients with upper gastrointestinal tract infections and gastroenteritis (69). *C. hyointestinalis* has been occasionally associated with proctitis and diarrhea in human infection. *C. concisus* is associated primarily with periodontal disease but has also been isolated from patients with bacteremia, foot ulcer, and upper and lower gastrointestinal tract infections (69). Although *C. concisus* has been isolated from many patients with diarrheal illness, it can also be isolated from the feces of healthy individuals, and there is no convincing evidence to date that it causes diarrhea (35). *C. sputorum* has been associated with lung, axillary, scrotal, and groin abscesses (70). *C. sputorum* bv. paraureolyticus, formerly referred to as catalase-negative urease-positive campylobacter, has been isolated from patients with diarrhea, but the significance of this finding is unknown (101). *C. mucosalis* was reported to have been isolated from two children with enteritis, but subsequent testing showed that the isolates were actually *C. concisus* (100). *C. helveticus* (119) has been recovered from domestic cats and dogs and has not been reported from human sources. *C. rectus* is primarily isolated from patients with active periodontal infections but has also been isolated from a patient with pulmonary infection (69, 111) and breast abscess (49). There is some suggestion that *C. curvus* may be an etiologic agent in diarrheal illness (1), but it was rarely isolated from stool samples in another large study (35). *C. curvus* is also isolated from patients with periodontal infections and in patients with a liver abscess and pneumonia (49). *C. showae* has been isolated from the human gingival crevice (36). *C. gracilis* has been isolated from patients with appendicitis/peritonitis, bacteremia, soft-tissue abscesses, and pulmonary infections (85). *C. hominis* has been isolated from fecal samples of healthy individuals and may be a commensal of the oral cavity (71). *C. lanienae* was isolated from two asymptomatic abattoir workers, but its clinical significance is unknown (73). *C. canadensis* (61) has been isolated from whooping cranes at the Calgary Zoo and *C. peloridis* (26) from human feces, dialysis fluid, and shellfish. *C. cuniculorum* was isolated from the cecum of rabbits but not reported from humans (140). *C. avium* is a hippurate hydrolase-positive species that was isolated from broiler chickens and turkeys but has not been reported from human samples (113). A review on the clinical significance of non-*C. jejuni*/*C. coli* species was published previously (69).

Arcobacter

Arcobacter spp. are aerotolerant, *Campylobacter*-like organisms frequently isolated from bovine and porcine products of abortion and feces of animals with enteritis (39). Two of the seven *Arcobacter* species have been associated with human infection. *A. butzleri* has been isolated from patients with bacteremia, endocarditis, peritonitis, and diarrhea (70, 132). *A. cryaerophilus* has been previously characterized into two DNA related groups, 1A and 1B (65). *A. cryaerophilus* group 1B has been isolated from patients with bacteremia and diarrhea (70, 132) and also from healthy individuals (57), suggesting a commensal role for this species. Group 1A has been isolated from animal sources (65). *Arcobacter butzleri* was reported to be the fourth most common *Campylobacter*-like organism isolated from patients with diarrhea by Vandenberg et al. (132) and was also one of the most common non *C. jejuni*/*coli* species isolated over a 10-year period from over 73,000 stool samples (133). Thus, *A. butzleri* may be underrecognized if appropriate culture conditions are not used. In a survey of 2,855 *Campylobacter*-like isolates submitted for characterization from laboratories in France, *A. butzleri* was identified in 1%, primarily from fecal samples of patients with a diarrheal illness (109). *A. skirrowii* was reported to be isolated from a human stool culture in a patient with chronic diarrhea, but the role of this species in human disease is unknown (139). *A. nitrofigilis*, a nitrogen-fixing bacterium found on the roots of a small marsh plant in Nova Scotia, is not associated with human disease (39). *Arcobacter cibarius* has been isolated only from poultry carcasses; the medical significance of this species is unknown (56). *Arcobacter halophilus* requires increased salt for growth in culture; however, the medical significance of this species is unknown (31). *Arcobacter thereius* has been isolated from liver and kidney of spontaneous porcine abortions and from the cloacae of ducks but has not been reported from human samples (55). *Arcobacter mytili* was recently isolated from shellfish from northeastern Spain and has not been reported from human samples (23).

COLLECTION, TRANSPORT, AND STORAGE OF SPECIMENS

Fecal Samples

Fecal specimens are preferred for isolating *Campylobacter* species from patients with gastrointestinal infections; however, rectal swabs are acceptable for culture. For hospitalized patients, the "3-day" rule (rejection of specimens collected >72 h after admission) should be used as a criterion for acceptability of routine culture requests (48, 53). For routine purposes, a single stool sample has high sensitivity for common enteric pathogens, but two samples may be desirable, depending upon clinical circumstances such as a >2-h delay in transport of the first sample that could affect recovery (39). A transport medium should be used when a delay of more than 2 h is anticipated and for transporting rectal swabs. Several types of transport media are useful for *Campylobacter* including alkaline peptone water with thioglycolate and cystine, modified Stuart medium, and Cary-Blair medium (39). Transport media such as commercial Stuart medium and buffered glycerol saline do not appear to perform well. Modified Cary-Blair medium containing reduced agar (1.6 g/liter) appears to be the most suitable single transport medium for *Campylobacter* as well as other enteric pathogens. Specimens received in Cary-Blair medium should be stored at 4°C if processing is not performed immediately. Use of Cary-Blair medium supplemented with laked sheep blood may be useful for prolonged storage of stool samples and recovery of *C. jejuni* (136).

Blood

Campylobacter species, primarily *C. fetus*, *C. jejuni*, and *C. upsaliensis*, have been isolated from blood; however, in only a few studies have optimal conditions for isolating *Campylobacter* from blood culture systems been evaluated. Both the Bactec system (BD, Sparks, MD) (aerobic bottles) and Septi-Chek system (BD, Sparks, MD) appear to support the growth of the common *Campylobacter* species (39). The BacT/Alert system (bioMérieux, Inc.) also supports the growth of *Campylobacter fetus* (22). Other systems such as anaerobic broth or lysis centrifugation may not be as sensitive (39).

DIRECT EXAMINATION

Microscopy

Clinical microbiologists do not normally consider performing Gram stain analysis of stool samples for diagnosis of bacterial gastroenteritis; however, this is a rapid and sensitive method for presumptive diagnosis of *Campylobacter* enteritis. *Campylobacter* spp. are not easily visualized with the safranin counterstain commonly used in the Gram stain procedure and are somewhat thinner than other enteric gram-negative bacteria; carbol-fuchsin or 0.1% aqueous basic fuchsin should be used as the counterstain for smears of stools or pure cultures (39). Because of their characteristic morphology, *Campylobacter* spp. may be detected by direct Gram stain examination of stools obtained from patients with acute enteritis, with sensitivity ranging from 66% to 94% and specificity above 95%. Phase-contrast and dark-field microscopy have also been used to directly detect motile campylobacters in fresh stool samples; however, the sensitivity of these approaches has not been studied widely, and in our opinion these methods require significant microscopic expertise (39).

Fecal white cells may be present during *Campylobacter* infection and have been reported in 25% to 80% of culture-proven cases (53). There is no known correlation between the number of cells present and infection. While the likelihood of infection with *Campylobacter* or other enteroinvasive pathogens may be higher in the qualitative presence of fecal leukocytes, the absence of fecal leukocytes does not rule out the diagnosis. Thus, routine examination of stool samples for fecal leukocytes is not recommended as a test for predicting bacterial infection or for selective culturing for *Campylobacter* or other stool pathogens (39, 48).

Antigen Detection

Several commercially available antigen detection systems for *Campylobacter* in stool samples are now currently available; the ProSpecT *Campylobacter* assay (Alexon-Trend, Inc., distributed through Remel), the Premier Campy *Campylobacter* assay (Meridian Biosciences), and the ImmunoCard Stat!

Campy assay (Meridian Biosciences). When compared with culture, the ProSpecT immunoassay has been shown to vary in sensitivity from 80 to 96% and has a specificity of >97% (28, 52, 124). This enzyme immunoassay (EIA) was found to cross-react with *C. upsaliensis* (28). Antigen may be detected in stored stool samples at 4°C for several days (32). The Premier Campylobacter assay is a microtiter plate-based EIA, while the Immuno*Card* STAT! Campy assay is a one-step lateral flow immunoassay; both are reported to be specific for the detection of *Campylobacter jejuni* and *C. coli*, but there are limited available data on their performance characteristics. Other EIAs available outside the United States have variable performance (123). Given that a *Campylobacter* infection is a low-incidence disease, the specificity values described to date for the *Campylobacter* antigen detection assays mentioned above suggest that these tests can lead to poor positive predictive values.

Nucleic Acid Detection Techniques

Amplification techniques have been used directly to detect *Campylobacter* in stool samples (105, 116). Molecular approaches to detecting *Campylobacter* directly may improve the time to detection, identification to the species level, and identification of the less common *Campylobacter* species often missed by conventional culture. A commercially available molecular test for detection of *Campylobacter* spp. in fecal samples is not currently available. This approach is also more expensive than culture and does not provide an isolate for further characterization.

ISOLATION PROCEDURES

Most *Campylobacter* species require a microaerobic atmosphere containing approximately 5% O_2, 10% CO_2, and 85% N_2 for optimal recovery. Several manufacturers produce microaerobic gas generator packs that are suitable for routine use. A trigas incubator or evacuation and replacement of an anaerobic jar with the approximate gas mixture may also be used for routine cultures (39). The anoxomat (Mart Microbiology, distributed through Spiral BioTech) is a convenient automated system for the evacuation and gas replacement of jars used for generating different atmospheric conditions, including microaerobic conditions (13). The concentration of oxygen generated in candle jars is suboptimal for the isolation of *Campylobacter* and should not be used for routine laboratory isolation procedures (39).

Some species of *Campylobacter*, such as *C. sputorum*, *C. concisus*, *C. mucosalis*, *C. curvus*, *C. rectus*, and *C. hyointestinalis*, require increased hydrogen for primary isolation and growth. These species will usually not be recovered under the conventional microaerobic conditions, since the amount of hydrogen generated in properly used commercial gas-packs is <2%. A gas mixture of 10% CO_2, 6% H_2, and the balance N_2 used in an evacuation-replacement jar is sufficient for isolating hydrogen-requiring species. A study by Vandenberg and colleagues reemphasized the requirement of increased hydrogen for isolating certain *Campylobacter* spp. (132).

A number of selective media have been recommended for isolating *C. jejuni* and *C. coli*. These include two blood-free media, charcoal cefoperazone deoxycholate agar (CCDA) and charcoal-based selective medium (CSM); and two blood-containing media, Campy-CVA (cefoperazone, vancomycin, amphotericin) medium and Skirrow medium (39). Although CVA medium is commonly used in the United States for isolating *Campylobacter* from clinical stool specimens, there are limited data available to assess the ability of CVA to recover *Campylobacter* species from stool specimens, when compared to other *Campylobacter*-selective media; additional evaluation studies are warranted. Charcoal-based media containing cefoperazone, amphotericin, and teicoplanin (CAT media) are selective media for the primary isolation of *C. upsaliensis* (7). Two studies, however, did not isolate *C. upsaliensis* from any stool samples by use of this medium (35, 52). *C. upsaliensis* may occasionally be recovered on some other selective media. *C. upsaliensis* isolates can also be recovered by using the filtration method, and some strains may grow better in a hydrogen-enriched atmosphere (46, 70).

To achieve the highest yield of *Campylobacter* from stool samples, a combination of media that includes either CCDA or CSM appears to be the optimal method (33) and may increase the recovery of *Campylobacter* by as much as 10 to 15% over the use of a single medium. If only a single medium is used, we suggest using Campy-CVA, CCDA, or CSM. In a comparative study, CCDA medium was found to be the most sensitive for detecting *C. jejuni* and *C. coli* compared with Skirrow's medium, CAT agar, and filtration technique (35).

If *Campylobacter* infection is suspected at the time blood specimens are drawn, broth media should be subcultured after 24 to 48 h to a nonselective blood agar medium and plates incubated under microaerobic conditions at 37°C, preferably with increased hydrogen. This allows for the isolation of thermophilic and nonthermophilic species. While commonly used blood culture systems should support the growth of *Campylobacter* and give appropriate signals if positive, it may be prudent to perform a blind subculture. Similarly, blood drawn in Isolator (Wampole Laboratories, Cranbury, NJ) tubes for bacterial culture should include a nonselective blood agar plate incubated under microaerobic conditions at 37°C if *Campylobacter* infection is suspected. If a curved, gram-negative rod is observed upon Gram stain examination of a positive blood culture bottle, an aliquot should be cultured on a nonselective blood agar plate and incubated under microaerobic conditions at 37°C. An alternative staining method such as acridine orange may also be useful for detecting campylobacters in blood culture bottles if the Gram stain is negative.

Optimal conditions for recovery of *Arcobacter* from clinical specimens have not been determined. *Arcobacter* spp. were first isolated on semisolid media designed to isolate *Leptospira* spp. (39). *Arcobacter* species are aerotolerant and have been recovered on certain selective media such as Campy-CVA (5) incubated under microaerobic conditions at 37°C and on nonselective media used in the filtration method (132). Selective media for isolation of *Arcobacter* spp. from human stool samples were evaluated by Houf and Stephan (57). Both selective plates and enrichment broth containing selective supplements with 5-fluorouracil, amphotericin B, cefoperazone, novobiocin, and trimethoprim showed good recovery of *Arcobacter* sp. (57). Several other media have been reported to recover *Arcobacter* species but have not been studied in clinical settings (5, 24, 130).

Enrichment Cultures

Enrichment broths formulated to enhance the recovery of *Campylobacter* from stool include Preston enrichment, Campy-thio, and *Campylobacter* enrichment broth (39). Enrichment cultures may be beneficial in instances where low numbers of organisms may be expected due to delayed transport to the laboratory or after the acute stage of disease when the concentration of organisms may be low, such as in the investigation of GBS following acute *Campylobacter* infection (87). The clinical advantage and cost-effectiveness of using enrichment cultures as part of the routine stool culture setup have not been studied adequately.

Filtration

Filtration techniques designed to isolate *C. jejuni* and *C. coli* as well as other *Campylobacter* species (35, 39, 132) and *Arcobacter* spp. (65, 132, 133) that are susceptible to antibiotics present in most selective media should be used to complement direct culture to selective plating media. As only stool samples containing ~10^5 CFU/ml of *Campylobacter* will be detected with filtration, it should not be used as a replacement for direct culture, because the filtration method is not as sensitive as primary culture with selective media (46).

The method is based on the principle that campylobacters can pass through membrane filters (0.45-μm to 0.65-μm pore size) with relative ease (because organisms are thin and highly motile) while other elements of the stool microbiota are retained during the short processing time. Cellulose acetate membrane filters with a 0.65-μm pore size are recommended for routine use and available from a number of suppliers (39). Filtration is performed by placing a sterile 0.65-μm-pore-size cellulose acetate filter onto the surface of an agar medium such as antibiotic-free CCDA, CSM, or blood-containing medium. Ten to 15 drops of fecal suspension are placed on the filter, and the plate is incubated at 37°C for 45 to 60 min. The filter is then removed, and the plate incubated at 37°C under microaerobic conditions, preferably with an atmosphere containing increased hydrogen (for the hydrogen-requiring species).

Species within the genus *Campylobacter* and *Arcobacter* have different optimal temperatures for growth. The choice of incubation temperature for routine stool cultures is critical in determining the spectrum of species that will be isolated. By convention, most laboratories use 42°C as the primary incubation temperature for *Campylobacter*. This temperature allows growth of *C. jejuni* and *C. coli* on selective media while inhibiting other fecal microbiota. *C. upsaliensis* also grows well at 42°C but usually is not recovered on selective media. *C. fetus* exhibits variable growth at this temperature and may not be recovered. *Arcobacter* species will generally not be recovered at 42°C.

In contrast, most *Campylobacter* and *Arcobacter* species grow well at 37°C. Selective media, such as Skirrow medium, were devised for use at 42°C and have poor selective properties at 37°C, whereas CCDA and CSM show good selective properties at 37°C (33). Plates should be incubated a minimum of 72 h before being reported as negative. It has been reported that incubation of CCDA medium for 5 to 6 days increased the yield of *C. jejuni* and *C. coli* compared with 2 days of incubation (35).

Because of the expense of including several types of media and the filtration method in the initial workup for *Campylobacter*, a practical approach is to use a single medium for isolation of thermophilic *Campylobacter* spp. in the workup of acute bacterial gastroenteritis, such as Campy-CVA, CCDA, or CSM incubated at 42°C. If the primary culture workup is unrevealing and for patients with persistent diarrhea, cultures for non-*C. jejuni*/*C. coli* species may be appropriate. Additional stool samples should be plated on multiple selective media (e.g., CCDA or CVA),

processed by the filtration method as well, and incubated at 37°C under microaerobic conditions with increased hydrogen.

IDENTIFICATION

The identification of *Campylobacter* species is made difficult because of their complex and rapidly evolving taxonomy, fastidious growth requirements, and biochemical inertness (Table 2). These problems have resulted in a proliferation of phenotypic and genotypic methods for identifying members of this group (39).

Campylobacter spp. and *Arcobacter* spp.

Depending on the growth medium used, *Campylobacter* colonies may have different appearances. In general, *Campylobacter* spp. produce gray, flat, irregular, and spreading colonies. Spreading along the streak line is commonly seen, particularly on freshly prepared media. As the moisture content decreases, colonies may form round, convex, and glistening colonies with little spreading observed. Thus, proper storage of media to ensure moisture content is important for optimal isolation and recognition of *Campylobacter* spp. Hemolysis on blood agar is not observed. *Arcobacter* colonies are morphologically similar to those of *Campylobacter* (126, 130).

The Gram stain appearance of *Arcobacter* may differ from that of typical *Campylobacter*. *A. butzleri* is only slightly curved, while *A. cryaerophilus* tends to be much more helical in appearance than *Campylobacter*. Commercial systems for identification of *Campylobacter* species were not found to be more accurate than conventional tests (60). Unfortunately, *Campylobacter* species are difficult to differentiate from *Arcobacter* species based on phenotypic tests. However, an aerotolerant species (i.e., exhibiting growth under aerobic conditions) that grows on MacConkey agar under microaerobic conditions could be presumptively identified as *Arcobacter*. The failure to grow on MacConkey, however, does not rule out *Arcobacter* species.

C. jejuni and *C. coli*

For initial analysis, a Gram stain examination of the colony should be performed along with an oxidase test. Oxidase-positive colonies exhibiting a characteristic Gram stain appearance (e.g., gram-negative, curved to S-shaped rods) isolated from selective media incubated at 42°C under microaerobic conditions can be reliably reported as *Campylobacter* spp. The most common species, *C. jejuni*, is relatively easy to identify phenotypically; hydrolysis of sodium hippurate is the major test for distinguishing *C. jejuni* (and also *C. jejuni* subsp. *doylei*) from other *Campylobacter* species. Strains isolated on selective media that grow at 42°C, are oxidase positive, show characteristic microscopic morphology, and are positive for hippurate hydrolysis should be reported as *C. jejuni*, and for routine clinical purposes no other tests need to be performed (Fig. 1). Methods for this test are described elsewhere (74). Occasional strains of *C. jejuni* are hippurate negative, making them more difficult to identify. Gas-liquid chromatography for detecting benzoic acid (liberated from hydrolysis of sodium hippurate) is the most sensitive assay for hippurate hydrolysis and can be used for more definitive determination. Molecular detection of the *hipO* (hippuricase) gene or other *C. jejuni*-specific markers (Table 3) by PCR may be useful for identifying phenotypically negative isolates (50) and weakly positive isolates (15) and to clarify false-positive results for non-*C. jejuni* species (27, 29). A comparison of different PCR targets

TABLE 2 Useful phenotypic properties of *Campylobacter* and *Arcobacter* species[a]

Organism	Catalase	H$_2$ required	Urease	H$_2$S (TSI)	Hippurate hydrolysis	Indoxyl acetate hydrolysis	Aryl sulfatase	Selenite reduction	Growth in 1% glycine	Growth at 25°C	Aerobic growth
Commonly encountered species of known or presumed clinical importance											
C. jejuni subsp. jejuni	+	V	–	–	+	+	V	V	+	–	–
C. jejuni subsp. doylei	V	–	–	–	V	+	–	–	+	–	–
C. coli	+	–	–	V	–	+	–	+	+	+	–
C. fetus subsp. fetus	+	–	–	–	–	–	–	V	+	+	–
C. lari subsp. lari/ concheus[b]	+	–	V	–	–	–	–	V	+	–	–
C. upsaliensis	–	–	–	–	+	+	–	+	+	–	–
Infrequently encountered species											
C. avium	V	V	–	–	+	+	ND	–	–	–	–
C. canadensis	V	V	V	V	–	+	ND	ND	V	–	–
C. concisus	–	+	–	V	–	–	+	V	V	–	–
C. cuniculorum	+	–	–	–	–	+	ND	–	–	–	–
C. curvus	V	+	–	V	V	V	+	V	V	+	–
C. fetus subsp. venerealis	V	–	–	–	–	–	–	–	V	ND	–
C. gracilis	V	ND	–	–	–	V	ND	–	+	–	–
C. helveticus	–	+[c]	–	–	–	+	ND	–	V	–	–
C. hominis	–	V	ND	+	–	–	ND	+	+	v	–
C. hyointestinalis subsp. hyointestinalis	+	V	–	+[d]	–	–	–	+	+	–	–
C. hyointestinalis subsp. lawsonii	+	V	+	–	–	–	–	+	V	–	–
C. insulaenigrae	+	–	–	–	–	–	ND	ND	+	–	–
C. lanienae	+	+	–	+	–	–	ND	+	v	–	–
C. mucosalis	+	ND	–	ND	–	+	–	V	V	–	ND
C. peloridis	V	+	ND	–	–	V	ND	ND	+	ND	ND
C. rectus	V	+	–	+	–	+	+	–	+	–	–
C. showae	+	+	–	+	–	–	+	V	V	–	–
C. sputorum[d] bv. sputorum	+	–	–	+	–	–	+	V	+	–	–
C. sputorum bv. faecalis	–	+	–	+	–	–	+	V	+	–	–
C. sputorum bv. paraureolyticus	V	+	–	–	–	–	+	–	+	–	–
C. ureolyticus	V	+[c]	+	–	–	+	ND	–	+	–	–
A. cibarius	V	–	+	–	+	+	ND	–	–	+	V
A. cryaerophilus	V	–	–	–	+	+	–	ND	V	+	+
A. butzleri	+	–	–	–	+	+	–	–	+	V	+
A. mytili	+	–	–	–	+	ND	ND	ND	ND	+	+
A. nitrofigilis	+	–	+	–	+	+	–	ND	–	ND	ND
A. skirrowii	+	+	–	–	+	+	–	ND	V	+	+
A. thereius	+	–	–	–	+	+	–	ND	+	+	+

[a] Adapted from references 23, 26, 39, 55, 56, 61, 113, 129, and 140. +, positive reaction; –, negative reaction; V, variable reaction; ND, not determined; TSI, triple sugar iron.
[b] C. lari subsp. concheus can be differentiated from C. lari subsp. lari by lack of growth on media containing 0.05% safranin (26).
[c] Anaerobic growth only.
[d] Strains of C. sputorum and C. hyointestinalis subsp. lawsonii normally produce large amounts of H$_2$S in TSI agar (71).

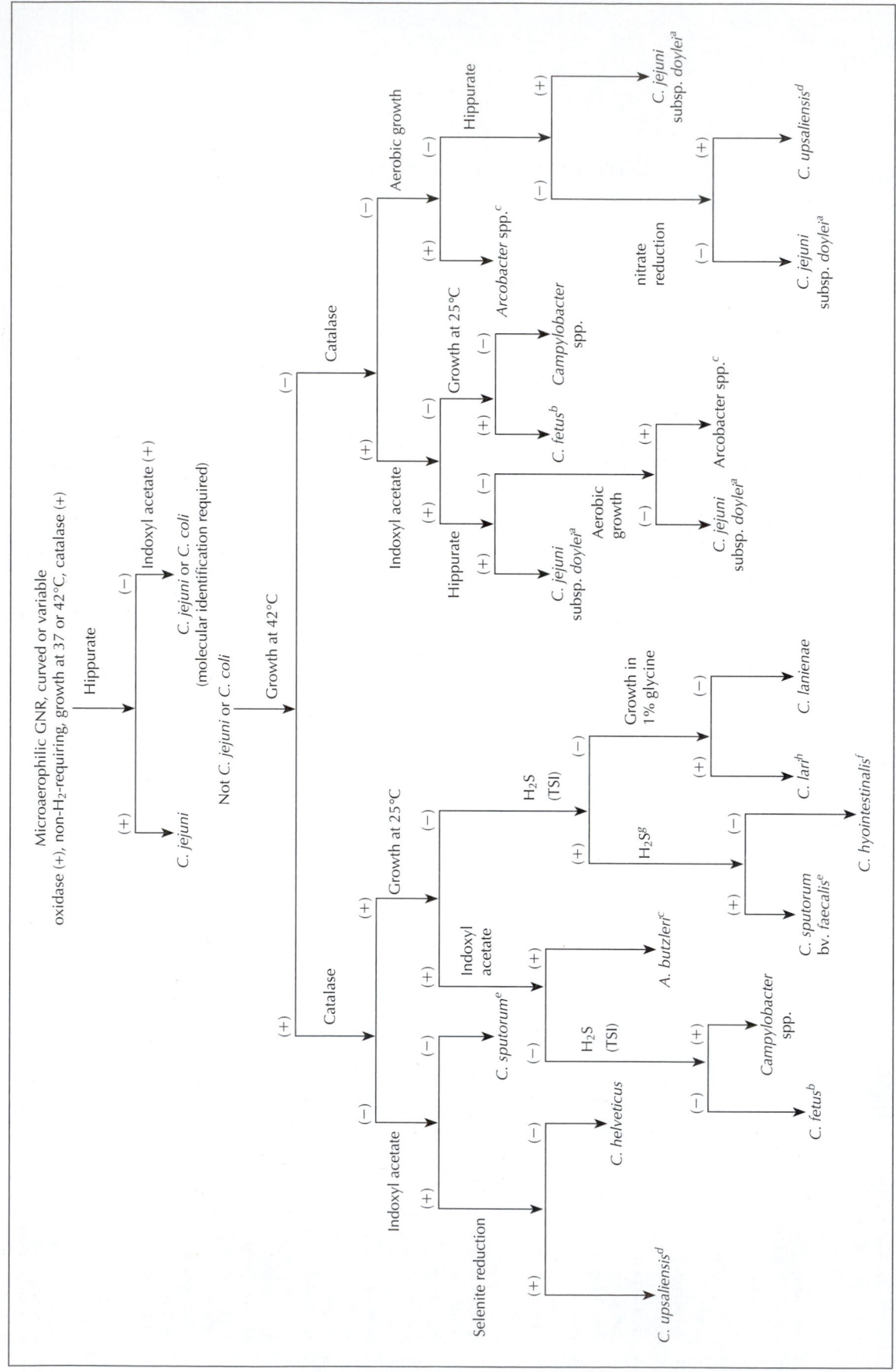

FIGURE 1 Practical algorithm for identifying *Campylobacter* and *Arcobacter* spp. that do not require increased hydrogen for primary isolation in the clinical laboratory. GNR, gram-negative rods; TSI, triple sugar iron agar. [a]*C. jejuni* subsp. *doylei* is variable for catalase and hippurate tests. [b]Strains of *C. fetus* subsp. *fetus* can be variable for growth at 42°C. [c]*A. butzleri* is variable for growth at 42°C and in the catalase test. *A. cryaerophilus* is variable for growth at 42°C. [d]*C. upsaliensis* is variable for the catalase test. [e]Results for the catalase test are biovar dependent; *C. sputorum* bv. faecalis is catalase positive. Some strains of *C. sputorum* may grow better in an increased hydrogen environment. [f]*C. hyointestinalis* grows under microaerophilic conditions, but some strains require additional hydrogen. [g]Rapid H₂S test. [h]Urease-positive *C. lari* strains are referred to as the urease-positive thermophilic campylobacter group.

TABLE 3   Differentiation of *Campylobacter jejuni* and *C. coli* by PCR

Assay	Target gene	Primers (5′–3′)[a]	Reference
C. jejuni specific	*hip*O (hippuricase)	HIP400F: GAA GAG GGT TTG GGT GGT G HIP1134R: AGC TAG CTT CGC ATA ATA ACT TG	72
C. coli specific	*asp* (putative aspartokinase)	CC18F: GGT ATG ATT TCT ACA AAG CGA G CC519R: ATA AAA GAC TAT CGT CGC GTG	72
C. jejuni/C. coli multiplex	Unknown	JUN3: CAT CTT CCC TAG TCA AGC CT JUN4: AAG ATA TGG CTC TAG CAA GAC COL1: AGG CAA GGG AGC CTT TAA TC COL2: TAT CCC TAT CTA CAA ATT CGC	131
C. jejuni/C. coli multiplex	*ceu-oxr* [iron(III)-ABC transporter/putative oxidoreductase]	(cc) CeuE-F: ATG AAA AAA TAT TTA GTT TTT GCA (cc) CeuE-R: ATT TTA TTA TTT GTA GCA GCG (cj) Oxr-F: CAA ATA AAG TTA GAG GTA GAA TGT (cj) Oxr-R: GGA TAA GCA CTA GCT AGC TGA T	92

[a]Abbreviations: cc, *C. coli*; cj, *C. jejuni*.

to differentiate *C. jejuni* from *C. coli* has been published (31, 112). Evaluations of these *C. jejuni*-specific PCR tests have shown no one test to be entirely specific or sensitive; therefore, the use of more than one target for molecular identification of *C. jejuni* is recommended. In addition, false negatives or nonspecifically amplified product(s) have been noted for some of the *C. jejuni*-specific assays; therefore, a second PCR, targeting another *C. jejuni*-specific gene, may be necessary in some instances. The use of heated lysates rather than purified DNA may not always be a suitable reaction template for these PCR assays (83, 97).

With the exception of hippuricase activity, which *C. coli* is lacking, *C. coli* and *C. jejuni* are similar biochemically (Table 2). Therefore, molecular methods are needed to accurately identify *C. coli* and differentiate it from hippurate-negative *C. jejuni*; most have proved both accurate and sensitive (97). If molecular testing is not available, strains isolated on selective media that grow at 42°C, are oxidase positive, show characteristic microscopic morphology, and are hippurate negative and indoxyl acetate positive should be reported as hippurate-negative *C. jejuni/C. coli* (Fig. 1). Susceptibility (inhibition) or resistance of *Campylobacter* spp. to nalidixic acid and cephalothin were historically used as an aid for species identification. However, with the increasing prevalence of fluoroquinolone resistance in these species, the use of these disk identification assays can no longer be relied upon.

For species other than *C. jejuni*, phenotypic characterization is more problematic. An algorithm for identification of the thermophilic *Campylobacter* spp. is shown in Fig. 1. The most useful tests for initial identification include growth at 25°C, 37°C, and 42°C, catalase production, hippurate hydrolysis (74), indoxyl acetate hydrolysis (75), and production of H$_2$S (8).

Additional tests can be performed to aid in the identification of *Campylobacter* spp.(Fig. 1). To obtain consistent and reproducible results, a standardized suspension and inoculum should be used for performing phenotypic tests. For growth temperature and oxygen tolerance studies, a suspension of the organism in heart infusion broth or tryptic soy broth with turbidity at a McFarland standard of 1 should be used. A fiber-tipped swab dipped in the broth suspension should be used to make a single streak across the plate (Mueller-Hinton agar with 5% sheep blood is a suitable medium), and the plates should be incubated at the desired temperature and/or atmospheric conditions (8, 86).

Several commercial systems have been developed as an aid to identifying *Campylobacter* spp. to the genus level. Two immunologic reagents are currently available in the United States for culture identification: Campy-JCL (Scimedx Corp., Denville, NJ) and Dryspot Campylobacter Test Kit (Remel). Campy-JCL was previously evaluated and does not differentiate between *C. jejuni* and *C. coli* (90). The Dryspot Campylobacter latex test is reported by the manufacturer to identify but not differentiate *C. jejuni*, *C. coli*, *C. lari*, and *C. upsaliensis* and to yield variable results for *C. fetus* subsp. *fetus* (Oxoid USA, www.oxoid.com). A DNA probe (Accuprobe; Gen-Probe Inc., San Diego, CA) directed against *Campylobacter* rRNA sequences identifies *Campylobacter* to the genus level and detects *C. jejuni* subsp. *jejuni*, *C. jejuni* subsp. *doylei*, *C. coli*, and *C. lari* (108, 122). However, the probe also hybridized with 2 of 17 *C. hyointestinalis* strains (108). Thus, these methods may be useful for confirming *Campylobacter* to the genus level if other tests are not conclusive. However, they cannot be used to rule out *Campylobacter*, and the cross-reactivity of these tests with closely related taxa and/or more newly described species needs to be determined.

Because many species of *Campylobacter* and *Arcobacter* are difficult to identify by phenotypic testing alone, tests for detection of species-specific sequences via PCR have been developed. The 16S rRNA gene and 23S rRNA gene are widely used for genus- and species-specific tests; PCR assays based on these targets have been described for 12 different *Campylobacter* species (98) and three *Arcobacter* species (14, 58). Broad-range molecular identification schemes involving restriction fragment analysis of PCR-amplified regions of the 16S or 23S rRNA genes have also been described for identification of *Campylobacter* and *Arcobacter* species (16, 37, 38).

Many other gene targets have been used in species-specific PCR assays, including *gyrA* (79, 134), *glyA* (4), *ceuE* gene (45), *asp* (72), *lpxA* (67), and a GTPase gene (134). Subspecies identification by PCR within *C. fetus* (59, 125) and *C. jejuni* (81) has also been described. While the use of such PCR tests combines the advantages of being quick and easy to perform with low cost and high-throughput capability, amenable to automation, it is important to validate PCR tests to fully determine their specificity and sensitivity before use. More recently, species-specific microarrays have been described for identification of several *Campylobacter* species, including *C. jejuni*, *C. coli*, *C. lari*, and *C. upsaliensis*

(64, 110, 135). While these methods are promising tools for both identification and further genetic characterization of *Campylobacter* spp., the cost and limited availability of the technology in the clinical laboratory make this approach not currently practical for routine application in the clinical setting.

Comparison of 16S rRNA gene sequences is also a useful tool for differentiation of *Campylobacter* spp. from closely related taxa, such as *Arcobacter* and *Helicobacter*. However, it is important to note that species level identification based on 16S is much more difficult, particularly for the common species of *Campylobacter*. At or above 97% identity, some groups of closely related species such as *C. jejuni*, *C. coli*, and *C. lari*; *C. upsaliensis* and *C. helveticus*; and *C. fetus*, *C. hyointestinalis*, and *C. lanienae* cannot be confidently distinguished from each other based on 16S rRNA gene sequences (98). Conversely, intraspecies 16S rRNA gene diversity is seen in other species, such as *C. hyointestinalis* (51). A commercial 16S rRNA gene microbial identification system, MicroSEQ (Applied Biosystems), is available to identify and classify unidentified bacteria, including *Campylobacter* and *Arcobacter* species, by comparing either full- or partial-length (500-bp)16S rRNA gene sequences to a validated microbial 16S rRNA gene sequence library. However, partial gene sequencing using the MicroSEQ 500 system is not recommended for accurate identification of some of the commonly encountered *Campylobacter* species, as sequencing of the first 500 bp of the gene only examines two of the four variable regions within the 16S rRNA gene of *Campylobacter* species (47); this can lead to misidentification of the groups of closely related *Campylobacter* species described above.

TYPING SYSTEMS

Typing systems for *Campylobacter* epidemiologic studies vary in complexity and ability to discriminate between strains. Common phenotypic methods that have been applied include biotyping, phage typing, and serotyping (94, 104). The heat-labile serotyping scheme, originally described by Lior, can detect over 100 serotypes of *C. jejuni*, *C. coli*, and *C. lari* (104). Uncharacterized bacterial surface antigens and, in some serotypes, flagellar antigens are the serodeterminants for this serotyping system (3). The heat-stable Penner (HS) serotyping scheme detects 60 types of *C. jejuni* and *C. coli* (104). Initially thought to detect lipopolysaccharide antigenic determinants, the HS system has been shown to detect a *Campylobacter* capsular polysaccharide (62). Serotyping (HS) is performed in only a few reference laboratories worldwide because of the time and expense needed to maintain quality antisera. A serotyping reagent kit is also commercially available (Denka Seiken USA Inc., Campbell, CA).

The limitations of phenotypic subtyping methods and the rapid growth of molecular biology techniques in the 1990s led to the development of a range of molecular subtyping methods such as restriction endonuclease analysis, ribotyping, PCR-based techniques, pulsed-field gel electrophoresis of macrorestricted chromosomal DNA (PFGE), and amplified fragment length polymorphism (94, 104). The development of a rapid 1-day standardized PFGE protocol (112), which is used by participants of the PulseNet national surveillance network for foodborne pathogens (www.cdc.gov/pulsenet), has facilitated the use of this approach for outbreak investigations of campylobacteriosis (95). However, interpretation of data can be difficult since genomic rearrangements can lead to changes in PFGE

profiles (40). Advances in DNA sequencing technology have provided a means to investigate strain variation at the nucleotide level and have led to the emergence of DNA-sequencing-based subtyping systems such as multilocus sequence typing (MLST) (30). MLST is useful for studies of the population structure and molecular epidemiology of *C. jejuni* (30), although commonly circulating sequence types can make recognition of outbreaks caused by these strains problematic (19, 114). In addition, the generation of *Campylobacter* whole-genome sequences has led the way for the development of a new technique, genomotyping based on microarray technology (66). At present, no method alone is adequate for all applications, and a combination of methods such as serotyping and molecular methods should be used for reliable determination of strain relatedness and for studying the epidemiology of *Campylobacter* infections (94). A more detailed discussion of molecular typing methods and their application for use in epidemiological studies of *Campylobacter* species has been recently published elsewhere (102).

An MLST system for *Arcobacter* spp. was recently reported (82). Using a set of 374 isolates comprising different species, from different sources and geographic locations, no association of MLST type and location or source was observed.

SEROLOGIC TESTS

Serum immunoglobulin G (IgG), IgM, and IgA levels rise in response to infection, but serum and fecal IgA levels appear during the first few weeks of infection and then fall rapidly (9, 121). Serum antibody assays vary in both sensitivity and specificity for detecting *Campylobacter* infection, and test performance appears to be population dependent. Campylobacter antibody assays have been used to study patients with GBS and reactive arthritis (6). Patients with *Campylobacter* infection may give false-positive *Legionella* antibody test results (12). Serologic testing appears to be useful for epidemiologic investigations and is not recommended for routine diagnosis (120).

ANTIMICROBIAL SUSCEPTIBILITIES

C. jejuni and *C. coli* have variable susceptibility to a variety of antimicrobial agents, including macrolides, fluoroquinolones, aminoglycosides, chloramphenicol, nitrofurantoin, and tetracycline (www.cdc.gov/NARMS). Azithromycin and erythromycin are drugs of choice for treating *C. jejuni* gastrointestinal infections, and for susceptible organisms, ciprofloxacin or norfloxacin may also be used. Early therapy of susceptible *Campylobacter* infection with erythromycin or ciprofloxacin is effective in eliminating the organism from stool and may also reduce the duration of symptoms associated with infection (10).

C. jejuni is generally susceptible to erythromycin, with resistance rates of less than 10% (10, 34, 43). Rates of erythromycin resistance in *C. coli* are generally higher than in *C. jejuni* and vary considerably, with up to 25 to 50% of strains showing resistance in some studies (10, 43). Although ciprofloxacin has been effective in treating *Campylobacter* infections, emergence of ciprofloxacin resistance during therapy has been reported (106). Several in vitro studies show significant rates of resistance to fluoroquinolones (34, 63, 91). Resistance to fluoroquinolones has ranged from <5% in Australia to approximately 80% reported in Thailand (10, 41). In 2006, approximately 20%

of *Campylobacter* strains reported through the National Antimicrobial Resistance Monitoring System at CDC were fluoroquinolone resistant (http://www.cdc.gov/NARMS/). Individuals with fluoroquinolone-resistant C. *jejuni* have been shown to have a longer duration of diarrhea, and thus, routine testing of isolates may be indicated (10, 93). C. *jejuni* and C. *coli* are resistant to β-lactam antibiotics, generally penicillins and narrow-spectrum cephalosporins, but imipenem has good anticampylobacter activity.

Parenteral therapy is used to treat systemic C. *fetus* infections; drugs used include ampicillin, aminoglycosides, imipenem, and chloramphenicol, depending upon the type of infection. C. *lari* is resistant to nalidixic acid but may be susceptible to fluoroquinolones, and resistance to macrolides is generally low (41). C. *upsaliensis* is generally susceptible to a variety of antimicrobial agents and shows low rates of resistance to macrolides and fluoroquinolones (41). *Arcobacter butzleri* and A. *cryaerophilus* have variable resistance to macrolides and fluoroquinolones (41).

Agar dilution is the method recognized by the Clinical Laboratory Standards Institute (CLSI) for testing *Campylobacter* spp.; quality control ranges for several antimicrobial agents have been published (21, 76). A broth microdilution method with published quality control ranges for several antimicrobial agents and a disk diffusion method are also approved by CLSI (20, 77). Studies testing *Campylobacter* with the Etest have been published (78).

EVALUATION, INTERPRETATION, AND REPORTING OF RESULTS

Campylobacter species, including the common thermophilic species C. *jejuni* and C. *coli*, should be sought in all diarrheic stools submitted to the laboratory for routine culture. Except for epidemiological purposes, cultures of formed stools should not be performed. Isolation of *Campylobacter* from a patient with acute diarrhea is usually significant, since the carrier rate in developed countries is quite low; however, in developing countries, isolation might be more difficult to interpret, especially in the presence of other enteric pathogens. In acute infection, there are usually a high number of organisms in the stool, but the quantity of organisms is not related to the severity of infection or indicative of a carrier state. Gram stain analysis of fecal samples to look for organisms with typical *Campylobacter* morphology is a highly sensitive and specific test that is currently underutilized; it should be performed for rapid preliminary diagnosis of *Campylobacter* infection. Other species, such as C. *fetus* subsp. *fetus* and C. *upsaliensis*, may be important causes of diarrhea and are not isolated on routine selective media. Special methods including alternative incubation techniques are required as described in this chapter and should be performed by special request. Oxidase-positive, curved, gram-negative rods that are hippurate hydrolysis positive should be reported as C. *jejuni* without further workup. The importance of identifying other species depends upon the clinical circumstance, but identification tests should always be performed with isolates from blood or other sterile sites, since this could influence antimicrobial therapy decisions. Given that fluoroquinolone resistance is present in a significant proportion of C. *jejuni* isolates, fluoroquinolone susceptibility testing is suggested for patients that are receiving or being considered for therapy of gastroenteritis. Susceptibility testing should be performed with all isolates from sterile clinical sites.

Use of trade names is for identification only and does not imply endorsement by the Public Health Service or by the U.S. Department of Health and Human Services.

REFERENCES

1. **Abbott, S. L., M. Waddington, D. Lindquist, J. Ware, W. Cheung, J. Ely, and J. M. Janda.** 2005. Description of *Campylobacter curvus* and C. *curvus*-like strains associated with sporadic episodes of bloody gastroenteritis and Brainerd's diarrhea. *J. Clin. Microbiol.* **43:**585–588.

2. **Ailes, E., L. Demma, S. Hurd, J. Hatch, T. F. Jones, D. Vugia, A. Cronquist, M. Tobin-D'Angelo, K. Larson, E. Laine, K. Edge, S. Zansky, and E. Scallan.** 2008. Continued decline in the incidence of *Campylobacter* infections, FoodNet 1996–2006. *Foodborne Pathog. Dis.* **5:**329–337.

3. **Alm, R. A., P. Guerry, M. E. Power, H. Lior, and T. J. Trust.** 1991. Analysis of the role of flagella in the heat-labile Lior serotyping scheme of thermophilic campylobacters by mutant allele exchange. *J. Clin. Microbiol.* **29:**2438–2445.

4. **Al Rashid, S. T., I. Dakuna, H. Louie, D. Ng, P. Vandamme, W. Johnson, and V. L. Chan.** 2000. Identification of *Campylobacter jejuni*, C. *coli*, C. *lari*, C. *upsaliensis*, *Arcobacter butzleri*, and A. *butzleri*-like species based on the glyA gene. *J. Clin. Microbiol.* **38:**1488–1494.

5. **Anderson, K. F., J. A. Kiehlbauch, D. C. Anderson, H. M. McClure, and I. K. Wachsmuth.** 1993. *Arcobacter* (*Campylobacter*) *butzleri*-associated diarrheal illness in a nonhuman primate. *Infect. Immun.* **61:**2220–2223.

6. **Ang, C. W., K. A. Krogfelt, P. Herbrink, J. Keijser, W. van Pelt, T. Dalby, M. Kuiif, B. C. Jacobs, M. P. Bergman, P. Schiellerup, and C. E. Visser.** 2007. Validation of an ELISA for the diagnosis of recent *Campylobacter* infections in Guillain-Barré and reactive arthritis patients. *Clin. Microbiol. Infect.* **13:**915–922.

7. **Aspinall, S. T., D. R. Wareing, P. G. Hayward, and D. N. Hutchinson.** 1996. A comparison of a new selective medium (CAT) with membrane filtration for the isolation of thermophilic campylobacters including *Campylobacter upsaliensis*. *J. Appl. Bacteriol.* **80:**645–650.

8. **Barrett, T. J., C. M. Patton, and G. K. Morris.** 1988. Differentiation of *Campylobacter* species using phenotypic characterization. *Lab. Med.* **19:**96–102.

9. **Black, R. E., D. Perlman, M. L. Clements, M. M. Levine, and M. J. Blaser.** 1992. Human volunteer studies with *Campylobacter jejuni*, p. 207–215. *In* I. Nachamkin, M. J. Blaser, and L. S. Tompkins (ed.), Campylobacter jejuni: *Current Status and Future Trends.* American Society for Microbiology, Washington, DC.

10. **Blaser, M. J., and J. Engberg.** 2008. Clinical aspects of *Campylobacter jejuni* and *Campylobacter coli* infections, p. 99–121. *In* I. Nachamkin, C. M. Szymanski, and M. J. Blaser (ed.), *Campylobacter*, 3rd ed. ASM Press, Washington, DC.

11. **Blaser, M. J., D. G. Newell, S. A. Thompson, and E. L. Zechner.** 2008. Pathogenesis of *Campylobacter fetus*, p. 401–428. *In* I. Nachamkin, C. M. Szymanski, and M. J. Blaser (ed.), *Campylobacter*, 3rd ed. ASM Press, Washington, DC.

12. **Boswell, T. C. J., and G. Kudesia.** 1992. Serological cross-reactions between *Legionella pneumophila* and *Campylobacter* in the indirect fluorescent antibody test. *Epidemiol. Infect.* **109:**291–295.

13. **Brazier, J. S., and S. A. Smith.** 1989. Evaluation of the anoxomat: new technique for anaerobic and microaerophilic clinical bacteriology. *J. Clin. Pathol.* **42:**640–644.

14. **Brightwell, G., E. Mowat, R. Clemens, J. Boerema, D. J. Pulford, and S. L. W. On.** 2007. Development of a multiplex and real time PCR assay for the specific detection of *Arcobacter butzleri* and *Arcobacter cryaerophilus*. *J. Microbiol. Methods* **68:**318–325.

15. **Burnett, T. A., A. Hornitzky, P. Kuhnert, and S. P. Djordjevic.** 2002. Speciating *Campylobacter jejuni* and *Campylobacter coli* isolates from poultry and humans using six PCR-based assays. *FEMS Microbiol. Lett.* **216:**201–209.

16. **Cardarelli-Leite, P., K. Blom, C. M. Patton, M. A. Nich-olson, A. G. Steigerwalt, S. B. Hunter, D. J. Brenner, T. J. Barrett, and B. Swaminathan.** 1996. Rapid identification of *Campylobacter* species by restriction fragment length poly-morphism analysis of a PCR amplified fragment of the gene coding for 16S rRNA. *J. Clin. Microbiol.* **34:**62–67.

17. **Centers for Disease Control and Prevention.** 2009. Prelimi-nary FoodNet data on the incidence of infection with patho-gens transmitted commonly through food—10 states. *MMWR Morb. Mortal. Wkly. Rep.* **58:**333–337.

18. **Champion, O. L., S. Al-Jaberi, R. A. Stabler, and B. W. Wren.** 2008. Comparative genomics of *Campylobacter jejuni*, p. 63–71. *In* I. Nachamkin, C. Szymanski, and M. J. Blaser (ed.), *Campylobacter*, 3rd ed. ASM Press, Washington, DC.

19. **Clark, C. G., L. Bryden, W. R. Cuff, P. L. Johnson, F. Jamieson, B. Ciebin, and G. Wang.** 2005. Use of the Ox-ford multilocus sequence typing protocol and sequencing of the flagellin short variable region to characterize isolates from a large outbreak of waterborne *Campylobacter* sp. strains in Walkerton, Ontario, Canada. *J. Clin. Microbiol.* **43:**2080–2091.

20. **Clinical and Laboratory Standards Institute.** 2006. *Methods for Antimicrobial Dilution and Disk Susceptibility Testing of Infrequently Isolated or Fastidious Bacteria.* Approved guide-line M45-A. Clinical and Laboratory Standards Institute, Wayne, PA.

21. **Clinical and Laboratory Standards Institute.** 2005. *Per-formance Standards for Antimicrobial Susceptibility Testing: Fifteenth Informational Supplement.* M100-S15. Clinical and Laboratory Standards Institute, Wayne, PA.

22. **Cochennec, F., L. Gazaigne, P. Lesprit, P. Desgranges, E. Allaire, and J. Becquemin.** 2008. Aortoiliac aneurysms infected by *Campylobacter fetus*. *J. Vasc. Surg.* **48:**815–820.

23. **Collado, L., I. Cleenwerck, S. Van Trappen, P. De Vos, and M. J. Figueras.** 2009. *Arcobacter mytili* sp. nov., an in-doxyl acetate-hydrolysis-negative bacterium isolated from mussels. *Int. J. Syst. Evol. Microbiol.* **59:**1391–1396.

24. **de Boer, E., J. J. H. C. Tilburg, D. L. Woodward, H. Lior, and W. M. Johnson.** 1996. A selective medium for the isolation of *Arcobacter* from meats. *Lett. Appl. Microbiol.* **23:**64–66.

25. **Debruyne, L., D. Gevers, and P. Vandamme.** 2008. Taxon-omy of the family *Campylobacteraceae*, p. 3–25. *In* I. Nacham-kin, C. M. Szymanski, and M. J. Blaser (ed.), *Campylobacter*, 3rd ed. ASM Press, Washington, DC.

26. **Debruyne, L., S. L. W. On, E. De Brandt, and P. Van-damme.** 2009. Novel *Campylobacter lari*-like bacteria from humans and molluscs: description of *Campylobacter peloridis* sp. nov., *Campylobacter lari* subsp. *concheus* subsp. nov. and *Campylobacter lari* subsp. *lari* subsp. nov. *Int. J. Syst. Evol. Microbiol.* **59:**1126–1132.

27. **Debruyne, L., E. Samyn, E. DeBrandt, O. Vandenberg, M. Heyndrickx, and P. Vandamme.** 2008. Comparative performance of different PCR assays for the identification of *Campylobacter jejuni* and *Campylobacter coli*. *Res. Microbiol.* **159:**88–93.

28. **Dediste, A., O. Vandenberg, L. Vlaes, A. Ebraert, N. Douat, P. Bahwere, and J.-P. Butzler.** 2003. Evaluation of the ProSpecT microplate assay for detection of *Campylobacter*: a routine laboratory perspective. *Clin. Microbiol. Infect.* **9:**1085–1090.

29. **Denis, M., C. Soumet, K. Rivoal, G. Ermel, D. Blivet, G. Salvat, and P. Colin.** 1999. Development of a m-PCR assay for simultaneous identification of *Campylobacter jejuni* and *C. coli*. *Lett. Appl. Microbiol.* **29:**406–410.

30. **Dingle, K. E., F. M. Colles, D. R. A. Wareing, R. Ure, A. J. Fox, F. E. Bolton, H. J. Bootsma, R. J. L. Willems, R. Ur-win, and M. C. J. Maiden.** 2001. Multilocus sequence typing system for *Campylobacter jejuni*. *J. Clin. Microbiol.* **39:**14–23.

31. **Donachie, S. P., J. P. Bowman, S. L. W. On, and M. Alam.** 2005. *Arcobacter halophilus* sp. nov., the first obligate halophile in the genus *Arcobacter*. *Int. J. Syst. Evol. Microbiol.* **55:**1271–1277.

32. **Endtz, H. P., C. W. Ang, N. Van Den Braak, A. Lui-jendijk, B. C. Jacobs, P. de Man, J. M. van Duin, A. van Belkum, and H. A. Verbrugh.** 2000. Evaluation of a new commercial immunoassay for rapid detection of *Campylobacter jejuni* in stool samples. *Eur. J. Clin. Microbiol. Infect. Dis.* **19:**794–797.

33. **Endtz, H. P., G. J. Ruijs, A. H. Zwinderman, T. van der Reijden, M. Biever, and R. P. Mouton.** 1991. Comparison of six media, including a semisolid agar, for the isolation of various *Campylobacter* species from stool specimens. *J. Clin. Microbiol.* **29:**1007–1010.

34. **Engberg, J., F. M. Aarestrup, D. E. Taylor, P. Gerner-Smidt, and I. Nachamkin.** 2001. Quinolone and macrolide resistance in *Campylobacter jejuni* and *C. coli*: resistance mechanisms and trends in human isolates. *Emerg. Infect. Dis.* **7:**24–34.

35. **Engberg, J., S. L. W. On, C. S. Harrington, and P. Gerner-Smidt.** 2000. Prevalence of *Campylobacter*, *Arcobacter*, *Helico-bacter*, and *Sutterella* spp. in human fecal samples as estimated by a reevaluation of isolation methods for *Campylobacter*. *J. Clin. Microbiol.* **38:**286–291.

36. **Etoh, Y., F. E. Dewhirst, B. J. Paster, A. Yamamoto, and N. Goto.** 1993. *Campylobacter showae* sp. nov., isolated from the human oral cavity. *Int. J. Syst. Bacteriol.* **43:**631–639.

37. **Fermer, C., and E. O. Engvall.** 1999. Specific PCR identifica-tion and differentiation of the thermophilic campylobacters, *Campylobacter jejuni*, *C. coli*, *C. lari*, and *C. upsaliensis*. *J. Clin. Microbiol.* **37:**3370–3373.

38. **Figueras, M. J., L. Collado, and J. Guarro.** 2008. A new 16S rDNA RFLP method for the discrimination of the accepted species of *Arcobacter*. *Diagn. Microbiol. Infect. Dis.* **62:**11–15.

39. **Fitzgerald, C., and I. Nachamkin.** 2007. *Campylobacter* and *Arcobacter*, p. 933–946. *In* P. R. Murray, E. J. Baron, J. H. Jorgensen, M. L. Landry, and M. A. Pfaller (ed.), *Manual of Clinical Microbiology*, 9th ed. ASM Press, Washington DC.

40. **Fitzgerald, C., A. Sails, and B. Swaminathan.** 2005. Genetic techniques: molecular subtyping methods, p. 271–293. *In* T. McMeekin (ed.), *Detecting Pathogens in Food*. Woodhouse Publishing, Cambridge, United Kingdom.

41. **Fitzgerald, C., J. Whichard, and I. Nachamkin.** 2008. Diagno-sis and antimicrobial susceptibility of *Campylobacter* species, p. 227–243. *In* I. Nachamkin, C. M. Szymanski, and M. J. Blaser (ed.), *Campylobacter*, 3rd ed. ASM Press, Washington, DC.

42. **Fouts, D. E., E. F. Mongodin, R. E. Mandrell, W. G. Miller, D. A. Rasko, J. Ravel, L. M. Brinkac, R. T. DeBoy, C. T. Parker, S. C. Daugherty, R. J. Dodson, A. S. Durkin, R. Madupu, S. A. Sullivan, J. U. Shetty, M. A. Ayodeji, A. Shvartsveyn, M. C. Schatz, J. H. Badger, C. M. Fraser, and K. E. Nelson.** 2005. Major structural differences and novel potential virulence mechanisms from the genomes of multiple *Campylobacter* species. *PLoS Biol.* **3:**72–85.

43. **Gibreel, A., and D. E. Taylor.** 2006. Macrolide resistance in *Campylobacter jejuni* and *Campylobacter coli*. *J. Antimicrob. Chemother.* **58:**243–255.

44. **Gilbert, M., P. C. R. Godschalk, C. T. Parker, H. P. Endtz, and W. W. Wakarchuk.** 2005. Genetic basis for the variation in the lipooligosaccharide outer core of *Campylobacter jejuni* and possible association of glycotransferase genes with post-infectious neuropathies, p. 219–248. *In* J. M. Ketley and M. E. Konkel (ed.), *Campylobacter: Molecular and Cellular Biology*. Horizon Bioscience, Norfolk, United Kingdom.

45. **Gonzalez, I., K. A. Grant, P. T. Richardson, S. F. Park, and M. D. Collins.** 1997. Specific identification of the enteropathogens *Campylobacter jejuni* and *Campylobacter coli* by using a PCR test based on the *ceuE* gene encoding a putative virulence determinant. *J. Clin. Microbiol.* **35:**759–763.

46. **Goossens, H., L. Vlaes, M. De Boeck, B. Pot, K. Kersters, J. Levy, P. de Mol, J. P. Butzler, and P. Vandamme.** 1990. Is "*Campylobacter upsaliensis*" an unrecognised cause of human diarrhoea? *Lancet* **335:**584–586.

47. **Gorkiewicz, G., G. Feierl, C. Schober, F. Dieber, J. Kofer, R. Zechner, and E. L. Zechner.** 2003. Species-specific identi-fication of campylobacters by partial 16S rRNA gene sequenc-ing. *J. Clin. Microbiol.* **41:**2537–2546.

48. **Guerrant, R. L., T. Van Gilder, T. S. Steiner, N. M. Thielman, L. Slutsker, R. V. Tauxe, T. Hennessy, P. M. Griffin, H. L. DuPont, R. B. Sack, P. I. Tarr, M. Neill, I. Nachamkin, L. B. Reller, M. T. Osterholm, M. L. Bennish, and L. K. Pickering.** 2001. Practice guidelines for managing infectious diarrhea. *Clin. Infect. Dis.* **32:**331–351.

49. **Han, X. Y., J. J. Tarrand, and D. C. Rice.** 2005. Oral *Campylobacter* species involved in extraoral abscess: a report of three cases. *J. Clin. Microbiol.* **43:**2513–2515.

50. **Hani, E., and V. L. Chan.** 1995. Expression and characterization of *Campylobacter jejuni* benzoylglycine amidohydrolase (hippuricase) gene in *Escherichia coli*. *J. Bacteriol.* **177:**2396–2402.

51. **Harrington, C. S., and S. L. W. On.** 1999. Extensive 16S rRNA gene sequence diversity in *Campylobacter hyointestinalis* strains: taxonomic and applied implications. *Int. J. Syst. Bacteriol.* **49:**1171–1175.

52. **Hindiyeh, M., S. Jense, S. Hohmann, H. Benett, C. Edwards, W. Aldeen, A. Croft, J. Daly, S. Mottice, and K. C. Carroll.** 2000. Rapid detection of *Campylobacter jejuni* in stool specimens by an enzyme immunoassay and surveillance for *Campylobacter upsaliensis* in the greater Salt Lake City area. *J. Clin. Microbiol.* **38:**3076–3079.

53. **Hines, J., and I. Nachamkin.** 1996. Effective use of the clinical microbiology laboratory for diagnosing diarrheal diseases. *Clin. Infect. Dis.* **23:**1292–1301.

54. **Hofreuter, D., J. Tsai, R. O. Watson, V. Novik, B. Altman, M. Benitez, C. Clark, C. Perbost, T. Jarvic, L. Du, and J. E. Galan.** 2006. Unique features of a highly pathogenic *Campylobacter jejuni* strain. *Infect. Immun.* **74:**4694–4707.

55. **Houf, K., S. L. W. On, T. Coenye, L. Debruyne, S. De Smet, and P. Vandamme.** 2009. *Arcobacter thereius* sp. nov. isolated from pigs and ducks. *Int. J. Syst. Evol. Microbiol.* **59:**2599–2604.

56. **Houf, K., S. L. W. On, T. Coenye, J. Mast, J. Van Hoof, and P. Vandamme.** 2005. *Arcobacter cibarius* sp. nov., isolated from broiler carcasses. *Int. J. Syst. Evol. Microbiol.* **55:**713–717.

57. **Houf, K., and R. Stephan.** 2007. Isolation and characterization of the emerging foodborne pathogen *Arcobacter* from human stool. *J. Microbiol. Methods* **68:**408–413.

58. **Houf, K., A. Tutenel, L. De Zutter, J. Van Hoof, and P. Vandamme.** 2000. Development of a multiplex PCR assay for the simultaneous detection and identification of *Arcobacter butzleri*, *Arcobacter cryaerophilus*, and *Arcobacter skirrowii*. *FEMS Microbiol. Lett.* **193:**89–94.

59. **Hum, S., K. Quinn, J. Brunner, and S. L. On.** 1997. Evaluation of a PCR assay for identification and differentiation of *Campylobacter fetus* subspecies. *Aust. Vet. J.* **75:**827–831.

60. **Huysmans, M. B., J. D. Turnidge, and J. H. Williams.** 1995. Evaluation of API Campy in comparison with conventional methods for identification of thermophilic campylobacters. *J. Clin. Microbiol.* **33:**3345–3346.

61. **Inglis, G. D., B. M. Hoar, D. P. Whiteside, and D. W. Morck.** 2007. *Campylobacter canadensis* sp. nov., from captive whooping cranes in Canada. *Int. J. Syst. Evol. Microbiol.* **57:**2636–2644.

62. **Karlyshev, A. V., D. Linton, N. A. Gregson, A. J. Lastovica, and B. W. Wren.** 2000. Genetic and biochemical evidence of a *Campylobacter jejuni* capsular polysaccharide that accounts for Penner serotype specificity. *Mol. Microbiol.* **35:**529–541.

63. **Kassenborg, H. D., K. E. Smith, D. J. Vugia, T. Rabatsky-Ehr, M. R. Bates, M. A. Carter, N. B. Dumas, M. P. Cassidy, N. Marano, R. V. Tauxe, and F. J. Angulo.** 2004. Fluoroquinolone-resistant *Campylobacter* infections: eating poultry outside of the home and foreign travel are risk factors. *Clin. Infect. Dis.* **38**(Suppl. 3)**:**279–284.

64. **Keramas, G., D. D. Bang, M. Lund, M. Madsen, S. E. Rasmussen, H. Bunkenborg, P. Telleman, and C. B. Christensen.** 2003. Development of a sensitive DNA microarray suitable for rapid detection of *Campylobacter* spp. *Mol. Cell. Probes* **17:**187–196.

65. **Kiehlbauch, J. A., D. J. Brenner, M. A. Nicholson, C. N. Baker, C. M. Patton, A. G. Steigerwalt, and I. K. Wachsmuth.** 1991. *Campylobacter butzleri* sp. nov. isolated from humans and animals with diarrheal illness. *J. Clin. Microbiol.* **29:**376–385.

66. **Klena, J. D., and M. E. Konkel.** 2005. Methods for epidemiologic analysis of *Campylobacter jejuni*, p. 165–179. *In* J. M. Ketley and M. E. Konkel (ed.), Campylobacter: *Molecular and Cellular Biology*. Horizon Bioscience, Norfolk, United Kingdom.

67. **Klena, J. D., C. T. Parker, K. Knibb, J. C. Ibbitt, P. M. Devane, S. T. Horn, W. G. Miller, and M. E. Konkel.** 2004. Differentiation of *Campylobacter coli*, *Campylobacter jejuni*, *Campylobacter lari*, and *Campylobacter upsaliensis* by a multiplex PCR developed from the nucleotide sequence of the lipid A gene *lpxA*. *J. Clin. Microbiol.* **42:**5549–5557.

68. **Larson, C. L., J. E. Christensen, S. A. Pacheco, S. A. Minnich, and M. E. Konkel.** 2008. *Campylobacter jejuni* secretes proteins via the flagellar type II secretion system that contribute to host cell invasion and gastroenteritis, p. 315–332. *In* I. Nachamkin, C. M. Szymanski, and M. J. Blaser (ed.), *Campylobacter*, 3rd ed. ASM Press, Washington, DC.

69. **Lastovica, A. J., and B. M. Allos.** 2008. Clinical significance of *Campylobacter* and related species other than *Campylobacter jejuni* and *Campylobacter coli*, p. 123–149. *In* I. Nachamkin, C. M. Szymanski, and M. J. Blaser (ed.), *Campylobacter*, 3rd ed. ASM Press, Washington, DC.

70. **Lastovica, A. J., and M. B. Skirrow.** 2000. Clinical significance of *Campylobacter* and related species other than *Campylobacter jejuni*, p. 89–121. *In* I. Nachamkin and M. J. Blaser (ed.), *Campylobacter*. ASM Press, Washington, DC.

71. **Lawson, A. J., S. L. W. On, J. M. J. Logan, and J. Stanley.** 2001. *Campylobacter hominis* sp. nov., from the human gastrointestinal tract. *Int. J. Syst. Evol. Microbiol.* **51:**651–660.

72. **Linton, D., A. J. Lawson, R. J. Owen, and J. Stanley.** 1997. PCR detection, identification to species level, and fingerprinting of *Campylobacter jejuni* and *Campylobacter coli* direct from diarrheic samples. *J. Clin. Microbiol.* **35:**2568–2572.

73. **Logan, J. M. J., A. Burnens, D. Linton, A. J. Lawson, and J. Stanley.** 2000. *Campylobacter lanienae* sp. nov., a new species isolated from workers in an abattoir. *Int. J. Syst. Evol. Microbiol.* **50:**865–872.

74. **MacFaddin, J. F.** 2000. Hippurate hydrolysis test, p. 188–204. *In* J. F. MacFaddin (ed.), *Biochemical Tests for Identification of Medical Bacteria*. Lippincott Williams & Wilkins, Philadelphia, PA.

75. **MacFaddin, J. F.** 2000. Indoxyl substrate hydrolysis tests, p. 233–238. *In* J. F. MacFaddin (ed.), *Biochemical Tests for Identification of Medical Bacteria*. Lippincott Williams & Wilkins, Philadelphia, PA.

76. **McDermott, P. F., S. M. Bodeis, F. M. Aarestrup, S. Brown, M. Traczewski, P. l. Fedorka-Cray, M. Wallace, I. A. Critchley, C. Thornsberry, S. Graff, R. Flamm, J. Beyer, D. Shortridge, L. J. Piddock, V. Ricci, M. M. Johnson, R. N. Jones, B. Reller, S. Mirrett, J. Aldrobi, R. Rennie, C. Brosnikoff, L. Turnbull, G. Stein, S. Schooley, R. A. Hanson, and R. D. Walker.** 2005. Development of a standardized susceptibility test for *Campylobacter* with quality-control ranges for ciprofloxacin, doxycycline, erythromycin, gentamicin and meropenem. *Microb. Drug Resist.* **10:**124–131.

77. **McDermott, P. F., S. M. Bodeis-Jones, T. R. Fritsche, R. D. Walker, and the Campylobacter Susceptibility Testing Group.** 2005. Broth microdilution susceptibility testing of *Campylobacter jejuni* and the determination of quality control ranges for fourteen antimicrobial agents. *J. Clin. Microbiol.* **43:**6136–6138.

78. **McGill, K., L. Kelley, R. H. Madden, L. Moran, C. Carroll, A. O'Leary, J. E. Moore, E. McNamara, M. O'Mahony, S. Fanning, and P. Whyte.** 2009. Comparison of disc diffusion and epsilometer (E-test) testing techniques to determine antimicrobial susceptibility of *Campylobacter* isolates of food and human clinical origin. *J. Microbiol. Methods* **79:**238–241.

79. **Menard, A., F. Dachet, V. Prouzet-Mauleon, M. Oleastro, and F. Megraud.** 2005. Development of a real-time fluorescence resonance energy transfer PCR to identify the main pathogenic *Campylobacter* spp. *Clin. Microbiol. Infect.* **11:**281–287.

80. **Miller, W. G.** 2008. Comparative genomics of *Campylobacter* species other than *Campylobacter jejuni*, p. 73–95. *In* I. Nachamkin, C. Szymanski, and M. J. Blaser (ed.), *Campylobacter*, 3rd ed. ASM Press, Washington, DC.

81. **Miller, W. G., C. T. Parker, S. Heath, and A. J. Lastovica.** 2007. Identification of genomic differences between *Campylobacter jejuni* subsp. *jejuni* and *C. jejuni* subsp. *doylei* at the nap locus leads to the development of a *C. jejuni* subspeciation multiplex PCR method. *BMC Microbiol.* **7:**11.

82. **Miller, W. G., I. V. Wesley, S. L. W. On, K. Houf, F. Megraud, G. Wang, E. Yee, A. Srijan, and C. J. Mason.** 2009. First multi-locus sequence typing scheme for *Arcobacter* spp. *BMC Microbiol.* **9:**196.

83. **Mohran, Z. S., R. R. Arthur, B. A. Oyofo, L. F. Peruski, M. O. Wasfy, T. F. Ismail, and J. R. Murphy.** 1998. Differentiation of *Campylobacter* isolates on the basis of sensitivity to boiling in water as measured by PCR-detectable DNA. *Appl. Environ. Microbiol.* **64:**363–365.

84. **Molbak, K., and A. H. Havelaar.** 2008. Burden of illness of campylobacteriosis and sequelae, p. 151–162. *In* I. Nachamkin, C. M. Szymanski, and M. J. Blaser (ed.), *Campylobacter*, 3rd ed. ASM Press, Washington, DC.

85. **Molitoris, E., H. M. Wexler, and S. M. Finegold.** 1997. Sources and antimicrobial susceptibilies of *Campylobacter gracilis* and *Sutterella wadsworthensis*. *Clin. Infect. Dis.* **25S:**S264–S265.

86. **Morris, G. K., and C. M. Patton.** 1985. *Campylobacter*, p. 302–308. *In* E. Lennette, A. Balows, W. J. Hausler, Jr., and H. J. Shadomy (ed.), *Manual of Clinical Microbiology*. American Society for Microbiology, Washington, DC.

87. **Nachamkin, I.** 1997. Microbiologic approaches for studying *Campylobacter* in patients with Guillain-Barré syndrome. *J. Infect. Dis.* **176**(Suppl. 2)**:**S106–S114.

88. **Nachamkin, I.** 2001. *Campylobacter jejuni*, p. 179–192. *In* M. P. Doyle, L. R. Beuchat, and T. J. Montville (ed.), *Food Microbiology: Fundamentals and Frontiers*, 2nd ed. ASM Press, Washington, DC.

89. **Nachamkin, I., B. M. Allos, and T. W. Ho.** 1998. *Campylobacter* and Guillain-Barré Syndrome. *Clin. Microbiol. Rev.* **11:**555–567.

90. **Nachamkin, I., and S. Barbagallo.** 1990. Culture confirmation of *Campylobacter* spp. by latex agglutination. *J. Clin. Microbiol.* **28:**817–818.

91. **Nachamkin, I., B. S. Ung, and M. Li.** 2002. Increasing fluoroquinolone resistance in *Campylobacter jejuni*, Pennsylvania, USA, 1982–2001. *Emerg. Infect. Dis.* **8:**1501–1503.

92. **Nayak, R., T. M. Stewart, and M. S. Nawaz.** 2005. PCR identification of *Campylobacter coli* and *Campylobacter jejuni* by partial sequencing of virulence genes. *Mol. Cell. Probes* **19:**187–193.

93. **Nelson, J. M., K. E. Smith, D. J. Vugia, T. Rabatsky-Ehr, S. D. Segler, H. D. Kassenborg, S. M. Zansky, K. Joyce, N. Marano, R. M. Koekstra, and F. J. Angulo.** 2004. Prolonged diarrhea due to ciprofloxacin-resistant *Campylobacter* infection. *J. Infect. Dis.* **190:**1150–1157.

94. **Newell, D. G., J. A. Frost, B. Duim, J. A. Wagenaar, R. H. Madden, J. van der Plas, and S. L. W. On.** 2000. New developments in the subtyping of *Campylobacter* species, p. 27–44. *In* I. Nachamkin and M. J. Blaser (ed.), *Campylobacter*. ASM Press, Washington, DC.

95. **Olsen, S. J., G. R. Hansen, L. Bartlett, C. Fitzgerald, A. Sonder, R. Manjrekar, T. Riggs, J. Kim, R. Flahart, G. Pezzino, and D. L. Swerdlow.** 2001. An outbreak of *Campylobacter jejuni* infections associated with food handler contamination: the use of pulsed-field gel electrophoresis. *J. Infect. Dis.* **183:**164–167.

96. **Olson, C. K., S. Ethelberg, W. van Pelt, and R. V. Tauxe.** 2008. Epidemiology of *Campylobacter jejuni* infections in industrialized nations, p. 163–189. *In* I. Nachamkin, C. M. Szymanski, and M. J. Blaser (ed.), *Campylobacter*, 3rd ed. ASM Press, Washington, DC.

97. **On, S. L., and P. J. Jordan.** 2003. Evaluation of 11 PCR assays for species-level identification of *Campylobacter jejuni* and *Campylobacter coli*. *J. Clin. Microbiol.* **41:**330–336.

98. **On, S. L. W.** 2005. Taxonomy, phylogeny and methods for the identification of *Campylobacter* species, p. 13–42. *In* J. M. K. Konkel (ed.), Campylobacter: *Molecular and Cellular Biology*. Horizon Biosciences, Norwich, United Kingdom.

99. **On, S. L. W.** 2001. Taxonomy of *Campylobacter*, *Arcobacter*, *Helicobacter* and related bacteria: current status, future prospects and immediate concerns. *J. Appl. Microbiol.* **90:**1S–15S.

100. **On, S. L. W.** 1994. Confirmation of human *Campylobacer concisus* isolates misidentified as *Campylobacter mucosalis* and suggestions for improved differentiation between the two species. *J. Clin. Microbiol.* **32:**2305–2306.

101. **On, S. L. W., H. I. Atabay, J. E. L. Corry, C. S. Harrington, and P. Vandamme.** 1998. Emended description of *Campylobacter sputorum* and revision of its infrasubspecific (biovar) divisions, including *C. sputorum* biovar paraureolyticus, a urease-producing variant from cattle and humans. *Int. J. Syst. Bacteriol.* **48:**195–206.

102. **On, S. L. W., N. McCarthy, W. G. Miller, and B. J. Gilpin.** 2008. Molecular epidemiology of *Campylobacter* species, p. 191–211. *In* I. Nachamkin, C. M. Szymanski, and M. J. Blaser (ed.), *Campylobacter*, 3rd ed. ASM Press, Washington, DC.

103. **Parkhill, J., B. W. Wren, K. Mungall, J. M. Ketley, C. Churcher, D. Basham, T. Chillingworth, R. M. Davies, T. Feltwell, S. Holroyd, K. Jagels, A. V. Karlyshev, S. Moule, M. J. Pallen, C. W. Penn, M. A. Quail, M. A. Rajandream, K. M. Rutherford, A. H. M. van Vliet, S. Whitehead, and B. G. Barrell.** 2000. The genome sequence of the foodborne pathogen *Campylobacter jejuni* reveals hypervariable sequences. *Nature* **403:**665–668.

104. **Patton, C. M., and I. K. Wachsmuth.** 1992. Typing schemes: are current methods useful?, p. 110–128. *In* I. Nachamkin, M. J. Blaser, and L. S. Tompkins (ed.), Campylobacter jejuni: *Current Status and Future Trends*. American Society for Microbiology, Washington, DC.

105. **Persson, S., and K. E. Olsen.** 2005. Multiplex PCR for identification of *Campylobacter coli* and *Campylobacter jejuni* from pure cultures and directly on stool samples. *J. Med. Microbiol.* **54:**1043–1047.

106. **Petruccelli, B. P., G. S. Murphy, J. L. Sanchez, S. Walz, R. DeFraites, J. Gelnett, R. L. Haberberger, P. Echeverria, and D. N. Taylor.** 1992. Treatment of traveler's diarrhea with ciprofloxacin and loperamide. *J. Infect. Dis.* **165:**557–560.

107. **Poly, F., T. Read, D. R. Tribble, S. Baqar, M. Lorenzo, and P. Guerry.** 2007. Genome sequence of a clinical isolate of *Campylobacter jejuni* from Thailand. *Infect. Immun.* **75:**3425–3433.

108. **Popovic-Uroic, T., C. M. Patton, I. K. Wachsmuth, and P. Roeder.** 1991. Evaluation of an oligonucleotide probe for identification of *Campylobacter* species. *Lab. Med.* **22:**533–539.

109. **Prouzet-Mauleon, V., L. Labadi, N. Bouges, A. Menard, and F. Megraud.** 2006. *Arcobacter butzleri*: underestimated enteropathogen. *Emerg. Infect. Dis.* **12:**307–309.

110. **Quinones, B., C. T. Parker, J. M. Janda, Jr., W. G. Miller, and R. E. Mandrell.** 2007. Detection and genotyping of *Arcobacter* and *Campylobacter* isolates from retail chicken samples by use of DNA oligonucleotide arrays. *Appl. Environ. Microbiol.* **73:**3645–3655.

111. **Rams, T. E., D. Feik, and J. Slots.** 1993. *Campylobacter rectus* in human periodontitis. *Oral Microbiol. Immun.* **8:**230–235.

112. **Ribot, E. M., C. Fitzgerald, K. Kubota, B. Swaminathan, and T. J. Barrett.** 2001. Rapid pulsed-field gel electrophoresis protocol for subtyping *Campylobacter jejuni*. *J. Clin. Microbiol.* **39:**1889–1894.

113. **Rossi, M., L. Debruyne, R. G. Zanoni, G. Manfreda, J. Revez, and P. Vandamme.** 2009. *Campylobacter avium* sp. nov., a hippurate-positive species isolated from poultry. *Int. J. Syst. Evol. Microbiol.* **59:**2364–2369.

114. **Sails, A. D., B. Swaminathan, and P. I. Fields.** 2003. Utility of multilocus sequence typing as an epidemiological tool for investigation of outbreaks of gastroenteritis caused by *Campylobacter jejuni*. *J. Clin. Microbiol.* **41:**4733–4739.

115. **Samuel, M. C., D. J. Vugia, S. Shallow, R. Marcus, S. Segler, T. McGivern, H. Kassenborg, K. Reilly, M. Kennedy, F. Angulo, and R. V. Tauxe.** 2004. Epidemiology of sporadic *Campylobacter* infection in the United States and declining trend in incidence, FoodNet 1996–1999. *Clin. Infect. Dis.* **38**(Suppl. 3):165–174.

116. **Schuurman, T., R. F. de Boer, E. van Zanten, K. R. van Slochteren, H. R. Scheper, B. G. Dijk-Alberts, A. V. M. Moller, and A. M. D. Kooistra-Smid.** 2007. Feasibility of a molecular screening method for detection of *Salmonella enterica* and *Campylobacter jejuni* in a routine community-based clinical microbiology laboratory. *J. Clin. Microbiol.* **45**:3692–3700.

117. **Skirrow, M. B.** 1994. Diseases due to *Campylobacter, Helicobacter* and related bacteria. *J. Comp. Pathol.* **111**:113–149.

118. **Skirrow, M. B., D. M. Jones, E. Sutcliffe, and J. Benjamin.** 1993. *Campylobacter* bacteremia in England and Wales, 1981–1991. *Epidemiol. Infect.* **110**:567–573.

119. **Stanley, J., A. P. Burnens, D. Linton, S. L. W. On, M. Costas, and R. J. Owen.** 1992. *Campylobacter helveticus* sp. nov., a new thermophilic species from domestic animals: characterization, and cloning of a species-specific DNA probe. *J. Gen. Microbiol.* **138**:2293–2303.

120. **Taylor, B. V., J. Williamson, J. Luck, D. Coleman, D. Jones, and A. McGregor.** 2004. Sensitivity and specificity of serology in determining recent acute *Campylobacter* infection. *Int. Med. J.* **34**:250–258.

121. **Taylor, D. N., D. M. Perlman, P. D. Echeverria, U. Lexomboon, and M. J. Blaser.** 1993. *Campylobacter* immunity and quantitative excretion rates in Thai children. *J. Infect. Dis.* **168**:754–758.

122. **Tenover, F. C., L. Carlson, S. Barbagallo, and I. Nachamkin.** 1990. DNA probe culture confirmation assay for identification of thermophilic *Campylobacter* species. *J. Clin. Microbiol.* **28**:1284–1287.

123. **Tissari, P., and H. Rautelin.** 2007. Evaluation of an enzyme immunoassay-based stool antigen test to detect *Campylobacter jejuni* and *Campylobacter coli*. *Diagn. Microbiol. Infect. Dis.* **58**:171–175.

124. **Tolcin, R., M. M. LaSalvia, B. A. Kirkley, E. A. Vetter, F. Cockerill, and G. W. Procop.** 2000. Evaluation of the Alexon-Trend ProSpecT *Campylobacter* Microplate Assay. *J. Clin. Microbiol.* **38**:3853–3855.

125. **van Bergen, M. A., G. Simons, van der Graaf-van Bloois, J. P. van Putten, J. Rombout, I. Wesley, and J. A. Wagenaar.** 2005. Amplified fragment length polymorphism based identification of genetic markers and novel PCR assay for differentiation of *Campylobacter fetus* subspecies. *J. Med. Microbiol.* **54**:1217–1224.

126. **Vandamme, P.** 2000. Taxonomy of the Family Campylobacteraceae, p. 3–26. *In* I. Nachamkin and M. J. Blaser (ed.), *Campylobacter*. ASM Press, Washington, DC.

127. **Vandamme, P., M. I. Daneshvar, F. E. Dewhirst, B. J. Paster, K. Kersters, H. Goossens, and C. W. Moss.** 1995. Chemotaxonomic analyses of *Bacteroides gracilis* and *Bacteroides ureolyticus* and reclassification of *B. gracilis* as *Campylobacter gracilis* comb. nov. *Int. J. Syst. Bacteriol.* **45**:145–152.

128. **Vandamme, P., and J. De Ley.** 1991. Proposal for a new family, *Campylobacteraceae*. *Int. J. Syst. Bacteriol.* **41**:451–455.

129. **Vandamme, P., L. Debruyne, E. De Brandt, and E. Falsen.** 2010. Reclassification of *Bacteroides ureolyticus* as *Campylobacter ureolyticus* comb. nov. *Int. J. Syst. Evol. Microbiol.* **60**:2016–2022.

130. **Vandamme, P., M. Vancanneyt, B. Pot, L. Mels, B. Hoste, D. Dewettinck, L. Vlaes, C. Van den Borre, R. Higgins, J. Hommez, K. Kersters, J.-P. Butzler, and H. Goossens.** 1992. Polyphasic taxonomic study of the emended genus *Arcobacter* with *Arcobacter butzleri* comb. nov. and *Arcobacter skirrowii* sp. nov., an aerotolerant bacterium isolated from veterinary specimens. *Int. J. Syst. Bacteriol.* **42**:344–356.

131. **Vandamme, P., L. J. VanDoorn, S. T. Alrashid, W. G. V. Quint, J. VanderPlas, V. L. Chan, and S. L. W. On.** 1997. *Campylobacter hyoilei* Alderton et al. 1995 and *Campylobacter coli* Veron and Chatelain 1973 are subjective synonyms. *Int. J. Syst. Bacteriol.* **47**:1055–1060.

132. **Vandenberg, O., A. Dediste, K. Houf, S. Ibekwem, H. Souayah, S. Cadranel, N. Douat, G. Zissis, J.-P. Butzler, and P. Vandamme.** 2004. *Arcobacter* species in humans. *Emerg. Infect. Dis.* **10**:1863–1867.

133. **Vandenberg, O., K. Houf, N. Douat, L. Vlaes, P. Retore, J. P. Butzler, and A. Dediste.** 2006. Antimicrobial susceptibility of clinical isolates of non-jejuni/coli campylobacters and arcobacters from Belgium. *J. Antimicrob. Chemother.* **57**:908–913.

134. **van Doorn, L. J., A. V. Van Haperen, A. Burnens, M. Huysmans, P. Vandamme, B. A. J. Giesendorf, M. J. Blaser, and W. G. V. Quint.** 1999. Rapid identification of thermotolerant *Campylobacter jejuni, Campylobacter coli, Campylobacter lari*, and *Campylobacter upsaliensis* from various geographic regions by a GTPase-based PCR-reverse hybridization assay. *J. Clin. Microbiol.* **37**:1790–1796.

135. **Volokhov, D., V. Chizhikov, K. Chumakov, and A. Rasooly.** 2003. Microarray-based identification of thermophilic *Campylobacter jejuni, C. coli, C. lari*, and *C. upsaliensis*. *J. Clin. Microbiol.* **41**:4071–4080.

136. **Wasfy, M., B. Oyofo, A. Elgindy, and A. Churilla.** 1995. Comparison of preservation media for storage of stool samples. *J. Clin. Microbiol.* **33**:2176–2178.

137. **Wassenaar, T. M.** 1997. Toxin production by *Campylobacter* spp. *Clin. Microbiol. Rev.* **10**:466–476.

138. **Willison, H. J.** 2005. The immunobiology of Guillain-Barre syndromes. *J. Peripher. Nerv. Syst.* **10**:94–112.

139. **Wybo, I., J. Breynaert, S. Lauwers, F. Lindenburg, and K. Houf.** 2004. Isolation of *Arcobacter skirrowii* from a patient with chronic diarrhea. *J. Clin. Microbiol.* **42**:1851–1852.

140. **Zanoni, R. G., L. Debruyne, M. Rossi, J. Revez, and P. Vandamme.** 2009. *Campylobacter cuniculorum* sp. nov. from rabbits. *Int. J. Syst. Evol. Microbiol.* **59**:1666–1671.

Helicobacter*

ANDREW J. LAWSON

54

TAXONOMY

The genus *Helicobacter* is classified in the family "*Helicobacteraceae*" of the class *Epsilonproteobacteria*, formerly known as the epsilon subclass of the *Proteobacteria*, with *Helicobacter pylori* as the type species (101). The other genus in the family is *Wolinella*, with the type species *Wolinella succinogenes*, and both genera are phenotypically similar to the genus *Campylobacter*. *Helicobacter* is a genus of expanding diversity. Since the genus name was formally proposed in 1989 (48) with two species (*H. pylori* and *Helicobacter mustelae*) and revised in 1991 to include *Helicobacter cinaedi* and *Helicobacter fennelliae* (132), it has grown to comprise some 32 species, including two species with *Candidatus* status (Table 1). Species of *Helicobacter* have genomic G+C base contents ranging from 30 (*H. acinonychis*) to 48 (*H. canis*) mol%, which is similar to the G+C content range of *Campylobacter* species. In addition, there are a number of unique *Helicobacter* 16S rRNA gene sequences listed in GenBank that represent sound taxa that have not yet met the criteria for official recognition but could be the basis of future new species. All species described in this chapter except "*Helicobacter winghamensis*" have formally validated names by international rules of nomenclature (101).

The intense interest in gastric spiral bacteria, observed for more than 100 years in animals and humans but rarely cultured, was triggered in 1982 by the discovery of *Campylobacter pyloridis* (later renamed *Helicobacter pylori*) which was cultured from stomach biopsy specimens from human patients with gastritis (138). Phylogenetic analyses based on 16S rRNA gene sequences indicate distinct groups of species within the genus; these fall broadly into groups of gastric (stomach) and enterohepatic (intestine, liver, or biliary tract) origins and include a subgroup of enterohepatic species lacking the characteristic sheathed flagella (Fig. 1). Phylogenetic analyses reliant on 16S rRNA gene sequences alone have sensitivity limitations in investigations of closely related helicobacters, which have a high degree of natural transformation and genetic plasticity. Additional phylogenetically informative genes, such as those encoding 23S rRNA and heat shock protein 60,

have been used to construct phylogenies of taxa closely related by 16S rRNA gene sequences and to resolve any discordancies (5, 29, 96).

The classification of non-*H. pylori* gastric helicobacters has proved particularly problematic because they are difficult to culture and closely related by 16S rRNA gene sequence analysis (Fig. 1). Large gastric spiral bacteria originally referred to as "*Gastrospirillum hominis*" were subsequently designated "*Helicobacter heilmannii*" and shown by 16S rRNA gene sequences to comprise two genospecies referred to as "*H. heilmannii*" 1 and "*H. heilmannii*" 2 (121). Further developments have provided clarification that *Helicobacter suis*, recently cultured and formally recognized and named (5), includes samples identified as "*Candidatus* Helicobacter suis" and "*H. heilmannii*" 1 and some clones of "*Gastrospirillum hominis*." "*H. heilmannii*" 2 taxonomy is more complex, as it encompasses samples identified as "*Candidatus* H. heilmannii" 2 (noncultivable) and closely related cultured species (*Helicobacter bizzozeronii*, *Helicobacter salomonis*, and *Helicobacter felis*), typically found in dogs and cats (52). For convenience, "*H. heilmannii*" and allied species of gastric origin are collectively referred to in this chapter as "*H. heilmannii*"-like organisms (HHLO), as the accuracy of identifications is uncertain in earlier clinical reports. In addition, the classification is not fully resolved for organisms with spindle-shaped cells surrounded by periplasmic fibrils and bipolar tufts of sheathed flagella originally referred to as "*Flexispira rappini*" (121). Phylogenetic analysis identified 10 different taxa, of which several grouped with named species of *Helicobacter* (30). Flexispira taxa 2, 3, and 8 are now considered to constitute a single species, *Helicobacter bilis* (55), while taxa 1, 4, and 5 are assigned to *Helicobacter trogontum* (54).

Further insights into the taxonomy of the genus are now possible with the availability of complete genome sequences for five strains of *H. pylori* (86), and for strains of *Helicobacter acinonychis*, *Helicobacter canadensis*, and *Helicobacter hepaticus*. Comparative genomics should enable deeper levels of taxonomic analysis as further *Helicobacter* genomes become available.

DESCRIPTION OF THE AGENTS

Members of the genus *Helicobacter* typically are curved, helical or spiral, or fusiform rod-shaped bacteria with or

---

*This chapter contains information presented by James G. Fox and Francis Megraud in chapter 60 of the ninth edition of this *Manual*.

TABLE 1 *Helicobacter* species, hosts, and disease spectrum

Helicobacter species	Primary hosts	Primary site(s)	Diseases in humans
Gastric			
H. acinonychis	Large felines (cheetahs)	Stomach	Not reported
H. baculiformis	Cats	Stomach	Not reported
H. bizzozeronii	Dogs, cats	Stomach	Gastritis, ulcer
Candidatus "H. bovis"	Cattle	Stomach	Gastritis
H. cetorum	Dolphins, whales	Stomach	Not reported
H. cynogastricus	Dogs	Stomach	Not reported
H. felis	Cats, dogs	Stomach	Gastritis, ulcer
Candidatus "H. heilmannii"	Humans	Stomach	Gastritis, ulcer
H. pylori	Humans	Stomach	Gastritis, ulcer, MALT lymphoma, gastric cancer
H. salomonis	Dogs	Stomach	Gastritis, ulcer
H. suis	Pigs	Stomach	Gastritis, ulcer
Enterohepatic			
H. anseris	Geese	Intestine	Not reported
H. aurati	Rodents (hamsters)	Intestine	Not reported
H. bilis	Rodents, dogs	Intestine, liver	Sepsis
H. brantae	Geese	Intestine	Not reported
H. canis	Dogs	Intestine	Not reported
H. cholecystus	Rodents (hamster)	Liver	Not reported
H. cinaedi	Rodents, dogs, primates	Intestine	Colitis, sepsis, cellulitis
H. equorum	Horses	Intestine	Not reported
H. fennelliae	Dogs	Intestine	Colitis, sepsis
H. hepaticus	Rodents	Intestine, liver	Not reported
H. marmotae	Rodents (woodchucks), cats	Intestine, liver	Not reported
H. mastomyrinus	Rodents (*Mastomys*)	Intestine, liver	Not reported
H. muridarum	Rodents	Intestine	Not reported
H. mustelae	Ferrets, minks	Stomach	Not reported
H. pametensis	Birds (terns), pigs	Intestine	Not reported
H. trogontum	Rodents	Intestine	Not reported
H. typhlonius	Rodents	Intestine	Not reported
Unsheathed			
H. canadensis	Chickens, Geese	Intestine	Gastroenteritis
H. ganmani	Rodents (mice)	Intestine	Liver disease?
H. mesocricetorum	Rodents (hamsters)	Intestine	Not reported
H. pullorum	Chickens	Intestine	Gastroenteritis
H. rodentium	Rodents	Intestine	Not reported
"*H. winghamensis*"	Rodents	Intestine	Gastroenteritis

without periplasmic fibers. The cells have sizes ranging from 0.3 to 0.60 μm in width and 1 to 10 μm in length. Cells may become spheroid or form coccoid bodies if they are cultured for a prolonged period or if growth conditions are not optimal. Such forms typically cannot be subcultured. Helicobacters are all gram negative, cytochrome oxidase producing, and non-spore-forming. Cells are motile and possess either single or multiple flagella. There is considerable diversity among species in flagellum morphology. Flagella are typically sheathed; for example, *H. pylori* has multiple (four to eight per cell) monopolar sheathed flagella with terminal knobs (Table 2). In contrast, *Helicobacter pullorum*, *H. canadensis*, and five other species with unsheathed flagella form a distinct phylogenetic group within the genus (Fig. 1). Gastric helicobacters found in animals, with the exception of *Helicobacter baculiformis*, have distinctive, tightly spiraled morphologies and can exhibit tufts of up to 20 multiple flagella per cell. The optimum temperature for growth is 37°C. Helicobacters are organotrophs, possess a respiratory type of metabolism, and are microaerobic. The optimal atmosphere for growth varies, as some species, such as *Helicobacter ganmani*, a rodent enteric organism (115), grow best in an anaerobic cabinet, although strict anaerobiosis can be lethal. Successful cultivation of helicobacters typically requires a humid atmosphere maintained at 37°C with reduced levels of oxygen (5 to 10%) and increased levels of carbon dioxide (5 to 12%). *Helicobacter* species grow poorly, if at all, in routine aerobic atmospheres. Key biochemical characteristics, such as urease hydrolysis, nitrate reduction, indoxyl acetate hydrolysis, and alkaline phosphatase activity, vary among species of *Helicobacter* and so are utilized in species identification (Table 2). However, there is no single common feature which reliably distinguishes all species of *Helicobacter* from those of *Campylobacter*. All helicobacters lack the carbohydrate utilization pathways typically exploited in conventional laboratory biochemical tests. Genomic analysis of *H. pylori* shows that it does not appear capable of using complex carbohydrates as energy sources,

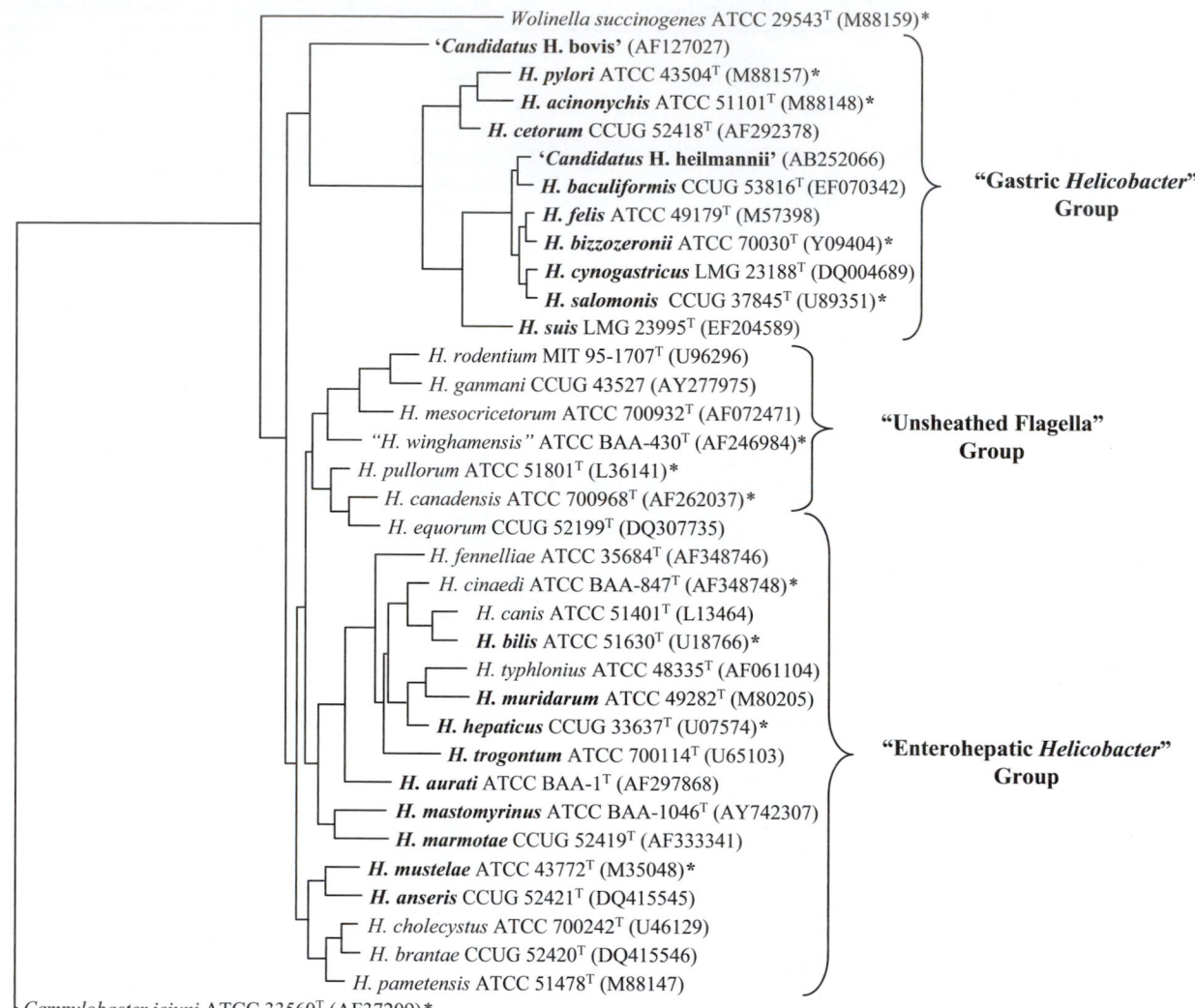

FIGURE 1 Phylogenetic tree of the genus *Helicobacter* based on 16S rRNA gene sequence similarity constructed using the neighbor-joining method. The bar represents percentage sequence divergence. Species marked in boldface type are urease positive; those in lightface are urease negative. * indicates species for which a genome sequence either is available or currently is being determined. Strain collection catalogue and 16S rRNA gene sequence reference numbers (in parentheses) are given where available.

and comparisons with the *Campylobacter jejuni* genome indicate significant differences in energy metabolism and chemotaxis systems (1).

EPIDEMIOLOGY AND TRANSMISSION

Helicobacter species are isolated from the gastrointestinal and hepatobiliary tracts of a variety of mammalian hosts that include humans, dogs, cats, cattle, sheep, swine, rodents, nonhuman primates, cheetahs, ferrets, rabbits, dolphins, whales, and horses, as well as chickens and wild birds (Table 1).

H. pylori

H. pylori, with its characteristic strong urealytic ability, is the gastric helicobacter of humans and is found almost exclusively in the human stomach, which provides the reservoir of infection. Exceptions are isolates from primates previously named *Helicobacter nemestrinae*, which is now considered a synonym of *H. pylori*. There is no evidence of animal-to-human transmission. The organism colonizes the cardia, corpus, and antrum of the stomach and may also be found in areas of gastric metaplasia of the proximal duodenum. Sero-epidemiology shows a widespread distribution, with estimates that close to half the human global population is colonized, with clinical disease being the exception rather than the rule (85). In North America and in Europe, up to 15% of children and up to 60% of adults are infected, although there is evidence that prevalence rates are declining in developed societies with improvements in sanitation and living standard (8, 127). The prevalence of *H. pylori* infection differs markedly between developing

TABLE 2 Key characteristics for identification of *Helicobacter* species[a]

Helicobacter species	Catalase	Urease	Nitrate	Indoxyl acetate hydrolysis	Alkaline phosphatase	γ-Glutamyl transpeptidase	Growth		Resistance to:		Mol% G+C	Flagellum type[b] (no.)	Flagellum sheath
							At 42°C	With 1% glycine	Nal	Ceph			
Gastric													
H. acinonychis	+	+	−	−	+	+	−	−	R	S	30	B (2–5)	+
H. baculiformis	+	+	+	−	+	+	−	−	I	R	ND	B (11)	+
H. bizzozeronii	+	+	+	+	+	+	+	−	R	S	ND	B (10–20)	+
"Candidatus H. bovis"	ND	+	ND	ND	ND	ND	ND	ND	ND	ND	ND	M/B (1–4)	?
H. cetorum	+	+	−	−	−	+	+	−	I	S	ND	B (2)	+
H. cynogastricus	+	+	+	−	+	+	−	−	ND	ND	ND	B (6–12)	+
H. felis	+	+	+	−	+	+	−	−	R	S	42	B (14–20)	+
"Candidatus H. heilmannii"	ND	+	ND	ND	ND	ND	ND	ND	ND	ND	ND	B (10–20)	+
H. pylori	+	+	−	−	+	+	−	−	R	S	35–37	B (4–8)	+
H. salomonis	+	+	+	+	+	+	−	−	R	S	ND	B (10–23)	+
H. suis	+	+	−	−	+	+	−	−	ND	ND	ND	B (4–10)	+
Enterohepatic													
H. anseris	−	+	−	+	−	−	+	W	S	R	ND	B (2)	+
H. aurati	−	+	−	+	+	+	+	+	S	R	ND	B (7–10)	+
H. bilis	+	+	+	+	−	+	+	+	R	R	ND	B (3–14)	+
H. brantae	−	+	−	+	−	−	+	W	S	R	ND	B (2)	+
H. canis	−	+	−	−	+	+	+	+	S	I	48	B (2)	+
H. cholecystus	+	+	+	−	+	−	−	+	I	R	ND	M (1)	+
H. cinaedi	+	+	+	−	+	−	−	+	S	I	37–38	B (1–2)	+
H. equorum	+	+	+	−	−	−	−	+	R	R	ND	M (1)	+
H. fennelliae	+	+	−	−	+	−	−	+	S	S	35	M/B (1–2)	+
H. hepaticus	+	+	+	−	+	−	−	+	R	R	35	B (2)	+
H. marmotae	+	+	+	−	+	−	−	+	R	R	ND	B (2)	+
H. mastomyrinus	+	+	−	−	+	−	+	+	R	R	ND	B (2)	+
H. muridarum	+	+	+	−	+	+	−	+	R	R	34	B (10–14)	+
H. mustelae	+	+	+	+	+	+	+	+	S	S	36	P (4–8)	+
H. pametensis	+	+	+	+	+	−	+	ND	S	S	38	B (2)	+
H. trogontum	+	+	+	+	+	+	−	+	R	R	ND	B (4–7)	+
H. typhlonius	+	+	−	−	+	−	+	+	S	R	ND	B (2)	+
Unsheathed													
H. canadensis	+	−	W	+	−	−	+	+	R	R	33	B (2)	−
H. ganmani	−	−	+	−	−	ND	+	+	R	S	ND	B (2)	−
H. mesocricetorum	+	−	+	ND	+	−	+	+	S	R	ND	B (2)	−
H. pullorum	+	−	+	−	−	ND	+	−	R	S	34–35	M (1)	−
H. rodentium	+	−	+	−	−	−	+	+	R	R	ND	B (2)	−
"H. winghamensis"	−	−	+	+	+	ND	+	+	R	R	ND	B (2)	−

[a] Test results from Baele et al. (5) and Fox and Megraud (39) and formal species descriptions. +, positive; −, negative; W, weakly positive; ND, not determined; Nal, nalidixic acid; Ceph, cephalexin; R, resistant; S, susceptible.
[b] B, bipolar; M, monopolar; P, peritrichous.

903

and developed countries (124). In developing countries, infection occurs early in life; most children are infected by the age of 10, and prevalence remains high (up to 90%) for all adult age groups. In contrast, in developed countries, a progressive increase in prevalence is observed, from a low percentage of infection in children to 40 to 50% infection rates in the older age groups. This is not the consequence of a progressive acquisition of the infection but rather the result of a cohort effect (124). Reported incidences of culture confirm that infections vary considerably from country to country depending on local treatment guidelines and culturing practices.

The modes and routes of transmission of *H. pylori* from person to person remain to be definitely proven. There is epidemiological evidence for both oral-oral and fecal-oral transmission, with the latter being more likely in developing countries, where sanitation and contaminated water supplies may pose a greater risk (8). The role of contaminated public water supplies has never been convincingly proven because of the rarity of culture-positive water samples (139). There is no evidence that viable cells of *H. pylori* can survive the disinfection levels in properly maintained main supplies, although survival may be possible as a viable nonculturable form (94). Biofilms within water distribution systems have been suggested as possible sites of passive accumulation (9).The rationale for oral-oral transmission relies on the presence of *H. pylori* in regurgitated gastric juice, thus allowing *H. pylori* to temporarily colonize the oral cavity. Another possibility is via vomitus, in which *H. pylori* can remain viable for hours (108). Person-to-person transmission appears to be most frequent in intrafamilial settings during childhood, particularly between mothers and siblings, as well as among siblings and between other household contacts (106). Family groups provide the best opportunity to study person-to-person transmission, but interpretation of evidence is complex. Patterns of frequent horizontal spread deduced from DNA sequence types were found both within families and between unrelated individuals in rural South Africa, which may be a situation representative of high-prevalence areas in large parts of the developing world (119). In urban families, in contrast, clonal transmission of *H. pylori* was more frequent between first-degree relatives.

"H. heilmannii"-Like Organisms

Human infections with HHLO are generally considered uncommon, with prevalence rates detected by histological observation ranging from <0.3% in developed countries to about 6% in other regions (102). A higher rate of 2% was indicated for some United Kingdom patients by a direct biopsy PCR assay designed to detect multiple HHLO species (16). Now that individual HHLO taxa are better defined, retrospective reassessment using species-specific assays of past cases attributed to "*H. heilmannii*" provide evidence of infection with one or more species of zoonotic origin, notably *H. salomonis*, *H. felis*, "*H. suis*," and "*Candidatus* Helicobacter bovis" (26, 52, 134). These findings indicate cats, dogs, and swine as possible sources of infection, but modes of transmission are unknown.

Enterohepatic Helicobacters

Enterohepatic helicobacters inhabit the intestinal and hepatobiliary tracts of various mammal and bird hosts, and several species, such as *H. bilis*, *H. canadensis*, *H. canis*, *H. cinaedi*, *H. fennelliae*, *H. pullorum*, and "*H. winghamensis*," infect humans with clinical symptoms (Table 1). Little is known

about prevalence and routes of transmission of these species, but the implications are that they are transmitted to humans from animals (102). *H. pullorum* is a recognized zoonotic risk, as it has been identified in carcasses of broiler chickens and laying hens (144) and on uncooked retail chicken (47).

CLINICAL SIGNIFICANCE

H. pylori

Warren and Marshall (138) first proposed the association of *H. pylori* with peptic ulcer disease, and since then it has become established as the most clinically important species of *Helicobacter*. It is recognized as the main cause of peptic ulcer disease and a major risk factor for gastric cancer (124). *H. pylori* infection is also an independent risk factor for the development of atrophic gastritis, gastric ulcer disease, gastric adenocarcinomas, and gastric mucosa-associated lymphoid tissue (MALT) lymphomas (124). Individuals infected with *H. pylori* may develop acute gastritis (abdominal pain, nausea, and vomiting) within 2 weeks following infection. The species establishes a chronic infection in the majority of infected people, represented by chronic gastritis. Prominent mucosal inflammation is often evident in the antrum (antrum-predominant gastritis), predisposing to hyperacidity and duodenal ulcer disease. Many patients infected with *H. pylori* have recurrent abdominal symptoms (nonulcer dyspepsia) without ulcer disease, and there appears to be a clinical benefit in eradicating *H. pylori* in these patients (92). Duodenitis often occurs with *H. pylori* infection, and duodenal ulcers develop in as many as 16% of infected individuals (39). Gastric MALT lymphoma, a rare stomach cancer, is caused by *H. pylori* infection and is the only cancer which can possibly be cured by antibiotics (141). Eradication of *H. pylori* is also recommended in cases of unexplained iron deficiency anemia and chronic idiopathic thrombocytopenic purpura (82). The clinical significance of *H. pylori* infection remains speculative in a number of other chronic conditions, notably ischemic heart disease, inflammatory bowel disease, and liver and biliary tract diseases (27, 68, 97).

"H. heilmannii"-Like Organisms

HHLO infection has been associated with mild-to-moderate gastritis, peptic ulcer disease, and gastric MALT lymphomas in adults, although it has not unequivocally been established as a causative agent (52, 95). HHLO infection is a rare finding in children (114). The etiology of HHLO infections is unclear because they are uncommon and organisms are unculturable in a routine clinical laboratory.

Enterohepatic Helicobacters

Isolated cases of infections in adults and children with enterohepatic helicobacters have been reported over the past 20 years, but their clinical significance is often not clearly established. Isolates are mainly from blood and, to a lesser extent, from fecal samples (36, 102). The bacteremia-associated helicobacters, although rare, are the most clinically significant, as they occur more frequently in patients with underlying conditions. It is presumed that these helicobacters are able to invade the bloodstream via colonization of the human lower gastrointestinal tract, possibly from mucosal cells damaged by combined chemo- and radiotherapy.

H. cinaedi was initially described in homosexual men with proctitis (129). Infections may present in various clinical manifestations (proctocolitis, gastroenteritis, neonatal meningitis, localized pain and rash, and bacteremia), particularly in individuals with underlying immunosuppressive conditions, such as AIDS, malignant diseases, and chronic alcoholism (98, 102, 131). *H. fennelliae* was also first described from rectal swabs of homosexual men with symptoms of proctitis (129) and has subsequently been implicated as a cause of human gastroenteritis and bacteremia, particularly in immunocompromised individuals (102). *H. pullorum* has been associated with several cases of human gastroenteritis (11, 122, 123). Furthermore, DNA of this species was detected by PCR in the hepatobiliary tracts of patients with chronic cholecystitis (38) as well as in intestinal biopsy specimens of Crohn's disease patients (68). The clinical significance of the latter findings is unclear.

Other species of *Helicobacter* isolated occasionally from infected humans but of unclear clinical significance include *H. canadensis* (37) and "*H. winghamensis*" (90) from cases of gastroenteritis, *H. canis* from cases of bacteremia and multifocal cellulitis (74, 111), and *H. bilis* from cases of bacteremia (36, 102). The presence of *H. bilis* in human gallbladder tissue (38) and of *H. ganmani* in the liver tissue of children with chronic liver disease (128) was indicated by PCR assays, but clinical relevance was not established. Unspecified *Helicobacter* DNA has been detected in liver specimens from patients with various diseases, including hepatocellular carcinoma and cholangiocarcinoma (4, 23, 99, 116).

COLLECTION, TRANSPORT, AND STORAGE OF SPECIMENS

Gastric Biopsy Specimens

Gastric biopsy specimens for the direct diagnosis of *H. pylori* are routinely obtained from the antrum and corpus by esophagogastroduodenoscopy. While sterile normal saline may be sufficient for short-term (up to approximately 2 h) transport of gastric biopsy specimens, a transport medium should be used if available to maintain the viability of the organisms for culture. *H. pylori* is sensitive to desiccation and to ambient atmosphere and temperature. A semisolid transport medium may be used (e.g., Portagerm pylori [bioMerieux Inc., Durham, NC]) or an in-house transport medium that comprises brain heart infusion broth (3.5%), yeast extract (2.5%), sterile horse serum (5%), and *Helicobacter pylori* selective supplement (Dent's; 10-μg/ml vancomycin, 5-μg/ml trimethoprim, 5-μg/ml cefsulodin, and 5-μg/ml amphotericin B [Oxoid Ltd., Basingstoke, United Kingdom]). Alternative media include Stuart's transport medium or Brucella broth with 20% glycerol. If culture of *H. pylori* is not possible within 24 h, it is recommended that biopsy specimens be stored overnight at 4°C in a transport medium and then transported at ambient temperature. For longer-term storage, biopsy specimens should be frozen at −70°C in a 10%-glycerol-containing medium.

Fecal Specimens

H. pylori and other gastric helicobacters cannot ordinarily be isolated from human fecal specimens, so samples are not recommended for routine culture. Fecal samples are used for *H. pylori* stool antigen testing and either should be tested immediately or should be stored immediately at −20°C. Repeated thawing and freezing of samples should be avoided. As enterohepatic helicobacters can cause enteric disease, fecal specimens may be required for culture. However, campylobacters are more likely to be tested for in the first

instance, and relevant protocols for their collection, transport, and storage also can be used for enterohepatic species of *Helicobacter* (as for *Campylobacter* [see chapter 53]).

Blood Specimens

Blood specimens are required for serological diagnosis of an *H. pylori* infection and may be collected, transported, and stored by standard protocols. Also, as the enterohepatic helicobacters may translocate across the intestinal barrier and cause invasive infections, peripheral venous blood from suspected cases may be required for microbiological testing. Blood may be collected in commercially available aerobic and anaerobic blood culture bottles and transported and stored according to the protocols used for campylobacters, which are more likely be tested for in the first instance (for *Campylobacter*, see chapter 53).

Other Clinical Specimens

Laboratory tests requiring the collection of other types of specimen have been developed to assist in the diagnosis of *H. pylori* infection and may be undertaken under some circumstances (89).

Gastric Juice

Gastric juice, obtained from the patient either by aspiration after the introduction of a nasogastric tube or by the so-called string test, has been used as a possible source of *H. pylori* for culture and PCR (39). Gastric juice does not offer a satisfactory alternative to a biopsy specimen as a routine specimen because of problems caused in culture by overgrowth of nasopharyngeal microbiota unless preventive steps such as acid pretreatment are taken (140). Specimens, if used, should be transported at 4°C and processed without delay.

Urine

Fresh urine samples required for serological tests should be collected and transported by standard protocols. Urine samples cannot be frozen because any resultant protein precipitation may interfere with the tests (39).

Saliva

Saliva samples required for serological tests can be collected easily by having the patient spit into a tube. An alternative that may be preferable is use of a special swab device rubbed over the gums that is designed to obtain gingival transudate enriched in immunoglobulin G (IgG) (39, 81). Specimens should then be transported by routine protocols.

DIRECT EXAMINATION

Microscopic Examination of Gastric Biopsy Specimens

Histopathological examination of gastric biopsy specimen sections preserved in a fixative (10% formaldehyde) and embedded in paraffin is widely used for diagnosis of *H. pylori* infection. Standard hematoxylin and eosin tissue staining is not sufficient to detect *H. pylori* (110), whereas the Warthin-Starry stain allows excellent visualization of bacteria if performed by trained histology personnel. Although the specificity is usually adequate, the presence of bacteria with atypical morphologies may result in misinterpretations. Under optimal conditions, histological diagnosis has a sensitivity and specificity of 95% (39). Immunohistological staining with specific *H. pylori* antibodies can improve specificity. Histological methods and interpretation of histological findings are outside the scope of this chapter, but from the microbiology laboratory perspective, microscopic examinations of a smear prepared directly from a biopsy specimen or from imprint cytology provide rapid bacteriological test results for observation of cells of *H. pylori* (39, 89). Staining can be performed using Gram stain, rapid Giemsa stain, or the fluorescent acridine orange stain. The less common gastric HHLO can also be Giemsa stained and, when observed microscopically, can be distinguished from *H. pylori* by their distinct tightly spiral morphology (59).

Microscopic Examination of Stool and Other Pathological Specimens

Direct Gram stain analysis of stool smears and other clinical samples is not routinely performed for the detection of *H. pylori* or other helicobacters. Direct identification of helicobacters in positive blood cultures may require special stains, particularly if tests are performed by personnel unaccustomed to looking for such organisms. Thin, gull-shaped bacteria such as *H. cinaedi* can be difficult to observe by Gram staining and require acridine orange staining, darkfield microscopy, or Giemsa staining (62). A modified Gram stain with carbol (0.5%) or basic fuchsin (0.1%) as the counterstain is also recommended for detection (39).

Urease Testing of Gastric Biopsy Specimens for *H. pylori*

H. pylori produces large amounts of extracellular urease, which can rapidly be detected following introduction of gastric biopsy tissue into a urea-containing medium. Urease catalyzes the hydrolysis of urea into ammonia and carbonate. The net effect of ammonia production is to increase local pH. Detection of urease activity forms the basis of several simple, inexpensive, and easy-to-perform tests that are usually performed in an endoscopy unit by clinicians (39, 89). Biopsy specimens are placed either in an agar gel or on a paper strip containing a pH indicator. If organisms are present in sufficient numbers, a color change will occur as a result of urea breakdown and ammonia production. Commercial rapid urease tests that include agar gel-based tests (e.g., CLOtest [Kimberly-Clark, Neenah, WI]) and paper-based strip tests (e.g., PyloriTek [BARD, Murray Hill, NJ]) have been critically evaluated, and specificities are usually excellent (89, 143). Detection sensitivity also is high but is dependent on the *H. pylori* density in mucosal biopsy specimens and the number of biopsy specimens sampled. Agar gel-based tests have their optimal sensitivity after 24 h of incubation, whereas strip tests are optimal within an hour, making them truly rapid tests (39). Urease broth media commonly available in microbiology laboratories, such as modified Christensen medium and urea-indole medium, can be used but are not optimized to have sensitivities equivalent to those of commercially available kits.

Urea Breath Test

Another important clinically performed test, based on the ability of *H. pylori* to produce urease and developed specifically for detection of an active infection, is the urea breath test (UBT). The UBT test has the advantage of being noninvasive, as urea, labeled with either a carbon radioactive isotope (^{14}C) or a nonradioactive natural isotope (^{13}C), is ingested by the patient. The labeled CO_2 is absorbed by the blood and exhaled in expired air. The testing methodology and factors influencing the result, standardization, and application in different clinical

settings have been comprehensively reviewed (39, 89). The use of the UBT has high diagnostic accuracy (>95%) (82) and, where available, is consistently recommended for the diagnosis of *H. pylori* infections in adults in both pre- and posttreatment settings (82, 89). A recent prospective multicenter study indicated that the ^{13}C UBT was also simple and accurate for diagnosis of *H. pylori* infections in children (32).

H. pylori Fecal Antigen Detection

Stool antigen tests using an enzyme-linked immunosorbent assay (ELISA) provide another valuable aid in the diagnosis of an active *H. pylori* infection. The test is easy to perform and has the advantage of being noninvasive. Since becoming commercially available, kits consisting of a polyclonal antibody fixed on microwells (e.g., Premier Platinum HpSA [Meridian Bioscience Inc., Cincinnati, OH]) have been extensively evaluated on samples from adults and children (41) and have proved to be an excellent diagnostic tool. A systematic review of published data up to 2004 confirmed the value of such kits for primary pretreatment as well as for follow-up posttreatment diagnosis (41). The test was further developed by using specific monoclonal antibodies (89), and reviews and meta-analysis based on evaluations of kits (e.g., IDEIA HpStAR [Oxoid Ltd., United Kingdom] and Premier Platinum HpSA PLUS [Meridian, Bioscience Inc., Cincinnati, OH]) indicated improved sensitivity compared to those of polyclonal tests (6, 42, 89). For example, high sensitivity (94%) and specificity (100%) were reported for tests on pretreatment adult stools in England (18), and the performance of tests was reported to be excellent for young children in Finland (67). If the UBT is not available, the laboratory-based stool antigen test is recommended for confirmation of eradication at least 4 weeks after treatment (82). The presence of some false positives has been noted in the use of stool antigen tests for posteradication diagnosis, possibly attributable to the presence of antigen in stools from degraded coccoid forms (6). Some stool samples that were transiently positive by ELISA also have been reported for children and were thought to have transient infections with *H. pylori* or *Helicobacter* spp. (53). Monoclonal antibodies are used also in immunoenzymatic rapid point-of-care tests for diagnosis of *H. pylori* infection (e.g., the ImmunoCard STAT! HpSA [Meridian Bioscience Inc., Cincinnati, OH] and *RAPID* Hp StAR [Oxoid Ltd., Basingstoke, United Kingdom]), and their performance in the clinical/near-patient setting has been critically evaluated (6, 18, 24, 89).

Nucleic Acid Detection

Detection of *H. pylori* in Gastric Biopsy Specimens

Nucleic acid assays based on PCR amplification and on fluorescence in situ hybridization with species-specific probes provide useful approaches for the detection of *H. pylori* in gastric biopsy specimens, as they are significantly faster than culture. The commonest targets for amplification are 16S rRNA, *ureA*, *glmM* (formerly named *ureC*), *vacA*, and *cagA* genes (125), and in addition 23S rRNA genes have been targeted for both detection and antibiotic susceptibility testing (21, 118). There is currently no "gold standard" method for use in the clinical laboratory setting for PCR of gastric biopsy specimens, and so it is advised that PCR-based assays should not be the sole basis of determining the *H. pylori* status of a patient (125). Nevertheless, PCR assays can provide added value in investigating culture-negative gastric biopsy specimens, particularly those from cases for which other clinical tests indicate an *H. pylori* infection (21). A systematic study of primers for *H. pylori* detection found that the four best-performing assays each attained a detection limit of <100 CFU/ml from gastric tissue (125). However, no assay had 100% specificity or sensitivity, and all produced false positives. Two of the best all-around assays based on the HP64-f/HP64-r primers for the *ureA* gene and HP1/HP2 primers for the 16S rRNA genes had sensitivities and specificities of >90% with gastric biopsy specimens.

Detection of *H. pylori* in Feces

The PCR assays developed for biopsy specimen testing, in particular those using primers targeting the 16S rRNA and *ureA* genes, have been applied to stools to detect *H. pylori* with various success rates (89), and their value for routine laboratory use is questionable. Feces is a complex material containing a number of PCR inhibitors (93), and complex DNA purification methods are needed to either eliminate or reduce the levels of such compounds (61). The performance of the assays is restricted by the low numbers of *H. pylori* cells in feces and by degradation of DNA during transit through the intestinal tract. Another test uses a biprobe 23S rRNA gene real-time PCR assay (118), and a modified version (ClariRes assay [Ingenetix, Vienna, Austria]), as well as clarithromycin susceptibility testing of stool specimens of symptomatic children (77), has been applied to detection (for further details, see "Antimicrobial Susceptibility" below).

Detection of HHLO in Gastric Biopsy Specimens

Specialist assays have been developed for direct PCR detection of species of HHLO in gastric biopsy specimens (134), and simultaneous testing for both *H. pylori* and HHLO can be performed using a multiplex PCR assay (16). Fluorescence in situ hybridization tests with species-specific probes can also be applied to detect HHLO in human gastric biopsy specimens (130).

Detection of Other Helicobacters in Clinical Samples

With the exception of an unvalidated 16S rRNA gene PCR assay for detection of *H. pullorum* in human fecal extracts (11), there are no assays suitable for fecal detection of enterohepatic *Helicobacter* species of clinical relevance. Genus-level PCR-based assays targeting mainly 16S rRNA genes have been developed and used for direct detection of other helicobacters in a variety of clinical samples that include dental plaque and saliva (49, 126), intestinal tissue biopsy specimens (68), and liver biopsy specimens and associated tissues (bile and gallbladder) (4, 116). These assays are generally undertaken for specific epidemiological and disease association investigations and so are unlikely to be used in the routine laboratory. Results of such PCR-based assays performed in the absence of other evidence therefore should be interpreted with caution (125).

ISOLATION PROCEDURES

Isolation of *H. pylori*

H. pylori is readily isolated by culture from gastric biopsy specimens. Tissue should be streaked over the culture medium with a minimum of delay or first homogenized to facilitate a higher yield of bacteria. Agar-based media such as brain heart infusion agar, brucella agar, Wilkins Chalgren agar, and Trypticase soy agar, can be used for primary

culture. In our experience, Columbia agar base supplemented with 10% defibrinated horse blood gives excellent results. A selective medium (e.g., *Helicobacter pylori* selective medium [Oxoid Ltd., Basingstoke, United Kingdom]) containing Dent's antibiotic supplement (see "Collection, Transport, and Storage of Specimens" above) also gives adequate isolation results. Plates should be incubated at 35 to 37°C in a humid microaerobic atmosphere (4% O_2, 5% CO_2, 5% H_2, and 86% N_2) achieved using either a gas jar and gas-generating system or an incubator (e.g., the MACS VA500 microaerophilic workstation [Microbiology International, Frederick, MD]). The exact gas mixes used vary between laboratories, but the presence of 5% H_2 in the atmosphere enhances growth. Culture plates should be observed daily for the appearance of small, smooth, circular colonies, which should appear after 48 h of incubation. Plates must be incubated for 10 days before a negative result is given. Colonies should be subcultured on nonselective medium for further investigation. Isolates may be stored at −80°C in cryovials (e.g., the Microbank bacterial preservation system [PRO-LAB Diagnostics, Austin, TX]).

Isolation of Other Helicobacters

There are no recommended culture methods available currently for use in routine clinical laboratories for isolation of "*H. heilmannii*" and HHLO from human gastric biopsy specimens. The first and only reported successful isolation of "*H. heilmannii*" from a human, achieved after 7 days with a nonselective medium (7% lysed horse blood) in a 5% O_2 and 10% CO_2 atmosphere (2), was subsequently identified as *Helicobacter bizzozeronii* (57). A novel isolation method using high acidity and modified gaseous conditions has now been developed for isolation of *H. suis* from pig gastric tissue but has not yet been evaluated on human gastric biopsy specimens (5).

Enterohepatic helicobacters such as *H. bilis*, *H. canadensis*, *H. canis*, *H. cinaedi*, *H. fennelliae*, *H. pullorum*, and "*H. winghamensis*" are isolated typically during investigation for campylobacters in feces from humans with gastroenteritis. These organisms grow at 37°C but not uniformly at 42°C, the temperature most often used for isolation of *C. jejuni*. Fresh stool specimens should be examined using a selective medium or the nonselective membrane filter method (70) with incubation for a minimum of 7 days at 37°C in a microaerobic atmosphere (36, 133). Strains of some species may require 5 to 10% H_2 for optimum growth, and recovery may be hindered if they are susceptible to antibiotics present in the selective isolation medium.

Some enterohepatic helicobacters, such as *H. cinaedi*, *H. canis*, and *H. fennelliae*, are isolated occasionally from blood of patients with suspected bacteremia using commercial blood culture systems (e.g., the Bactec system [BD, Sparks, MD]). Isolates are usually detected in aerobic blood culture bottles only and may be problematic to recover as they are difficult to see microscopically and will probably grow poorly on subculture if plates are not incubated for an extended period (minimum of 6 days) in a microaerobic atmosphere. The isolation of *Helicobacter* species from other sterile body fluids is rare, but a notable example is the isolation of *H. cinaedi* from joint fluid using a nonselective blood medium (56, 133).

IDENTIFICATION

Identification of *Helicobacter* species is based on a limited range of morphological, physiological, and biochemical characteristics (Table 2). Helicobacters have various colony phenotypes on blood agar, ranging from the discrete, gray, and translucent colonies of *H. pylori* to swarming phenotypes of some gastric helicobacters (e.g., *H. felis*). Most isolates are motile and should be routinely tested for oxidase, catalase, and urease activities according to recommended procedures (28).

H. pylori and Other Gastric Helicobacters

In stained gastric biopsy samples, *H. pylori* cells usually have a curved or helical morphology. However, on subculture, this "classical" morphology is often lost, and in Gram-stained preparations, cells may appear curved, U shaped, or even as straight rods. HHLO cells are larger in size and have a more pronounced helical morphology in histological examinations of gastric biopsy specimens (59). *Helicobacter* cells may appear faint on conventional Gram staining and require prolonged counterstaining with carbol fuchsin (0.5%) for enhanced visualization. Urease-negative organisms may be present occasionally in gastric biopsy specimens, as *H. cinaedi*, although not cultured, has been identified by DNA analysis (109). It is important therefore to perform other key biochemical tests, such as indoxyl acetate hydrolysis and hippurate hydrolysis, to identify isolates of any unexpected species.

Enterohepatic Helicobacters

Enterohepatic helicobacters may appear as a swarming thin film (e.g., *H. cinaedi* and *H. fennelliae*) or as discrete single colonies (e.g., *H. canadensis* and *H. pullorum*). By light microscopy, they morphologically resemble other gram-negative spiral or curved bacteria. The enterohepatic species possess several distinguishing characteristics (Table 2), and biochemical and tolerance tests should be carried out according to the recommended procedures (28). Species lacking urease activity isolated from humans, such as *H. canadensis*, *H. canis*, *H. cinaedi*, *H. fennelliae*, and *H. pullorum*, superficially resemble enteric campylobacters, and definitive identification may not be possible from phenotype alone. Useful distinguishing tests are growth at 42°C, as both *H. cinaedi* and *H. fennelliae* are negative, and indoxyl acetate hydrolysis, for which *C. jejuni* and *Campylobacter coli* are positive and *H. pullorum* is negative. A PCR assay is described for identification of *H. pullorum* (122), but the assay does not distinguish *H. pullorum* from *H. canadensis*, which characteristically hydrolyzes indoxyl acetate and is resistant to nalidixic acid (37). *H. canis* is unlike most other helicobacters in being both catalase negative and urease negative, features that may cause confusion with "*H. winghamensis*" and *H. bilis*. Growth at 42°C and the nitrate reduction and indoxyl acetate hydrolysis tests may be useful to distinguish *H. canis* from other catalase-negative campylobacters. It is important to be aware that fecal specimens occasionally can be cocolonized with multiple *Helicobacter* and *Campylobacter* species, so making a complete diagnostic evaluation is challenging (70). *Helicobacter* genus-specific PCR assays may be useful (76), and sequencing of 16S rRNA genes may be required for a definitive identification.

TYPING SYSTEMS

Typing of *H. pylori*

Typing isolates of *H. pylori* has no role in direct patient management (82). Even so, typing data may be useful in monitoring the effects of therapy and to establish whether a persistent infection is due to eradication failure or reinfection, in investigating associations between strain type and disease severity, in epidemiological investigations of routes and modes of transmission, and in investigating the ancestry of strains worldwide that might be relevant in vaccine development. There is no generally agreed-upon system for typing isolates of *H. pylori*, although many different methods have been applied and evaluated (104). While a somatic antigen serotyping scheme was proposed (91), genotypic methods are the most widely used means of characterizing individual isolates of *H. pylori*. A key feature of *H. pylori* is its high genetic diversity, with almost every isolate having a unique genotype arising from within-genome diversification and reassortment by natural homologous recombination (119). This diversification is thought to aid *H. pylori* in persistence during chronic infection and in adapting to new gastric environments.

The highly polymorphic vacuolating cytotoxin (*vacA*) gene provides the basis of a widely adopted PCR-based genotyping scheme with recommended primers (3). The *vacA* allelic type is determined by the presence or absence of short, conserved nucleotide inserts within the signal and middle regions (107). Common *vacA* allelic types identified worldwide are s1/m1 (vacuolating), s1/m2 (selectively vacuolating), and s2/m2 (nonvacuolating). The signal region alleles can be further divided into s1a, s1b, and s1c subfamilies, and likewise the midregion is subdivided into m2a and m2b subfamilies (104). Genotyping can be performed either by using individual PCR assays or multiplex PCR assays (14) or by using the reverse hybridization line probe assay (104). Molecular fingerprinting methods applied to *H. pylori* include electrophoretic protein profiling, ribotyping, restriction fragment length polymorphism (RFLP) analysis, pulsed-field gel electrophoresis (PFGE), amplified fragment length polymorphism analysis, and plasmid profiling (104). These methods have limited discriminatory power and have been superseded by PCR-RFLP analysis because of its relative technical simplicity and versatility. The technique has been applied widely in genotyping *H. pylori*, using in particular urease (*ureA*) and flagellin (*flaA*) gene polymorphisms, and also as a primary typing technique to differentiate among *H. pylori* in gastric biopsy specimens without the need for culture (75). Furthermore, analysis of stool samples based on two species-specific biprobe real-time PCR assays targeting the *glmM* and *recA* genes offers potential as a noninvasive genotyping method for *H. pylori* (113). Direct nucleotide sequencing is now a feasible approach to typing *H. pylori*, with the availability of high-throughput sequencing technology. Sequence data are readily comparable by access to publically available curated databases of sequences of loci for individual species (79) that include *H. pylori* (http://pubmlst.org/perl/mlstdbnet/mlstdbnet.pl?file=pub-hp_profiles.xml). This database contains 1,933 unique sequence types (November 2009) based on seven loci and provides an invaluable reference resource for typing.

Typing of Other Helicobacters

The need to type species of *Helicobacter* other than *H. pylori* is unlikely, and the genotyping schemes described are of questionable value for routine use. These include amplified fragment length polymorphism analysis and PFGE of *H. pullorum* (12, 40), plasmid profiling and ribotyping of *H. cinaedi* and *H. fennelliae* (62), and PFGE and random amplified polymorphism DNA analysis of *H. cinaedi* (66).

SEROLOGIC TESTS

Detection of *H. pylori* Antibody in Blood

H. pylori infection induces a specific systemic immune response to multiple antigens, with only 2% of patients failing to seroconvert (89). The immune response typically shows a transient rise in specific IgM antibodies followed by a rise in IgG and IgA antibodies that persists during infection. Serology is widely used in primary screening for *H. pylori* infection, as it is a simple, noninvasive test. A number of in-house and commercial kits have been developed over the past 20 years for antibody detection, with the essential laboratory technique being the standard ELISA. The performance and diagnostic utility of laboratory ELISA kits (e.g., Cobas Core enzyme immunoassay [Roche, Mannheim, Germany]) and rapid near-patient immunochromatographic tests (e.g., FlexSure HP [Beckman Coulter Inc., Brea, CA]) have been critically evaluated in several reviews and meta-analyses (69, 73, 89, 120). Serology (ELISA) kits that measure IgG antibodies are recommended based on overall performance as an accurate means of diagnosing infection (69). The relevance of IgA in testing is more controversial (69, 120). Some investigators have observed IgA to be equal to IgG in performance, but a recent evaluation concluded that IgA alone yielded poorer overall sensitivity and specificity, although it performed better in samples from children than those from adults (120). IgM has been found to have little diagnostic value, with an unacceptably low sensitivity (120). The Maastricht III Consensus Report recommended serological test kits with high accuracy (>90%) in validated settings (82).

Serology is not recommended for posteradication follow-up when tests detecting an active infection are preferable (82, 89). Antibody titers decrease very slowly after eradication, so a singe serum sample does not differentiate past and ongoing infections. Some 30% of patients have elevated IgG antibodies even after 5 years of successful eradication therapy (135). False-positives therefore could result in some patients being inappropriately treated for presumed *H. pylori* infection, particularly in low-prevalence populations (87). Serology is useful in epidemiological studies of *H. pylori* infections, but such analyses likewise need to take into account that some asymptomatic individuals without an active infection may test positive.

Immunoblot analysis may also be used for the diagnosis of *H. pylori* infections, and the commercial Helico Blot 2.1 test (Genelabs Diagnostics, Singapore) has been evaluated in studies of adults and children (73, 136). The test may not be commonly performed in a routine clinical laboratory setting, but its high sensitivity and high specificity (96%) in patients <50 years old indicate that it could be used as a confirmatory test in some situations (136). It may have applications also in detecting a past infection, especially by monitoring the persistence of antibodies to CagA, a product of the *cagA* gene within the *cag* pathogenicity island (136). While it is recognized that CagA protein and also VacA protein, a cytotoxin produced in various amounts, are important *H. pylori* pathogenicity factors, they are of little relevance in the management of infections (82).

Detection of *H. pylori* Antibodies in Urine

Specific *H. pylori* IgG antibodies are present in urine at low concentrations. A review of 18 published studies over the period 1998 to 2004 using kits that included commercial ELISAs and rapid immunoenzymatic tests, listed sensitivities and specificities ranging from 82 to 100% and from 68 to 100%, respectively (89). While the accuracy is not affected by the pH or the presence of bacteriuria, it may be influenced by a large amount of total IgG. Detection of *H.pylori* antibody in urine is attractive because it is noninvasive and it could be useful for epidemiological studies (82).

Detection of *H. pylori* Antibodies in Saliva

Salivary antibodies are secreted during the immune response to *H. pylori* infections (78). Several commercial kits and in-house ELISAs been developed to detect *H. pylori*-specific IgG in saliva, and a review of 15 published studies between 1994 and 2002 listed sensitivities and specificities ranging from 64 to 94% and from 58 to 95%, respectively (89). The detection of *H. pylori* antibody in saliva can be helpful for epidemiological studies (82).

Detection of Other *Helicobacter* Antibodies in Clinical Samples

Serology has no application in the routine diagnosis of human infections with gastric HHLO and enterohepatic helicobacters, as there are no validated IgG or IgA assays currently available. Sustained immunoglobulin responses to multiple antigens of *H. cinaedi* and *H. fennelliae* have been documented (35), and there is recent evidence that a 30-kDa putative membrane protein, identified as a major antigen of *H. cinaedi*, could be useful for immunological and serological testing for clinical diagnosis and epidemiology (58).

ANTIMICROBIAL SUSCEPTIBILITY

H. pylori Antibiotic Therapy and Relevance of Resistance

The first-choice standard triple therapy to eradicate *H. pylori* comprises a proton pump inhibitor, clarithromycin, and either amoxicillin or metronidazole (82). Therapy should ideally be based on pretreatment antibiotic susceptibility testing, although this is not always practical (50). The main cause of failure to eradicate *H. pylori* with the standard antimicrobial regimen is clarithromycin resistance (89). Prevalence rates are 10 to 15% in the United States (31, 103) and about 10% in Europe, with distinct regional variations (20, 65, 89). The clinical impact of resistance is marked, with an eradication rate for the standard therapy decreased by 70% (from 88 to 18%) (89). The key risk factor for clarithromycin resistance is previous consumption of macrolides, and prevalence of resistance after failure of treatment is extremely high, with rates of resistance to clarithromycin of up to 63% (19, 65). Monitoring local clarithromycin prevalence rates is important, as the recommended threshold at which clarithromycin should not be used or susceptibility testing should be performed is 15 to 20% (82).

Resistance to metronidazole, a key component of the triple-therapy regimen, is also widespread and is estimated to decrease treatment success rates by 25% (89). Resistance rates are 20 to 40% in the United States, with similar levels in Europe (typically 27%) (89). In some other countries, resistance rates may be as high as 60 to 90%. In vitro resistance to metronidazole may not accurately reflect in vivo resistance (34), and for that reason, routine susceptibility testing is not recommended in Maastricht III guidelines (82). Nevertheless, laboratory testing is important for surveillance of resistance, as a threshold of resistance in the population of 40% provides a guide in deciding choice of treatment (82).

Resistance of *H. pylori* to other antibiotics used in therapy, such as amoxicillin and tetracycline (an antibiotic used in second-choice treatment), is rarely found ($< 1\%$) in the United States and Europe (89), although higher rates to both antibiotics have been reported in some Asian populations (64). Two other classes of antibiotics have emerged as third-choice (rescue therapy) in the treatment of *H. pylori* infection: a fluoroquinolone, levofloxacin, and a rifamycin, rifabutin. Increasing consumption of fluoroquinolones may lead to higher prevalence of resistance in *H. pylori*, as rates of resistance to levofloxacin are currently about 9% in the United States (10) and even higher in some other countries, such as Italy, where resistance rates are up to 22% (7, 22). Resistance to rifabutin is virtually absent in *H. pylori* (22, 44), although its use in eradication therapy has been limited. The efficacy of furazolidone has also been evaluated (117), but no data are available on resistance rates.

Phenotypic Susceptibility Testing of *H. pylori* Cultures

Gastric biopsy isolates of *H. pylori* should be tested against the antibiotics commonly used in eradication therapy, in particular, clarithromycin, as resistance in vitro is clinically relevant. Phenotypic methods of susceptibility testing, such as broth microdilution, disk diffusion, the Etest, and agar dilution, can be applied to *H. pylori*. The Clinical and Laboratory Standards Institute (CLSI; formerly NC-CLS) and a workgroup of the European Helicobacter Study Group have made a similar recommendation of an agar dilution method and breakpoint for testing susceptibility to clarithromycin (25, 45, 89). In this method, Mueller-Hinton agar base with 5% aged sheep blood is incubated for 72 h at 35°C, with an MIC breakpoint for resistance of 1 µg/ml. The Etest (bioMerieux Inc., Durham, NC) may also be used to determine MIC (20), and its results correlate well with broth dilution results. The disc diffusion method is cost-effective for routine testing, and an inhibitory zone of less than 17 mm around a clarithromycin disk indicates a resistant strain (51).

Metronidazole in vitro susceptibility testing is intrinsically less reliable in terms of inter- and intralaboratory reproducibility and is more difficult to standardize, as results appear to be highly dependent on atmospheric conditions (89). Elevated MICs (>8 µg/ml) have been correlated with treatment failures, and 8 µg/ml is the threshold commonly used to define metronidazole resistance (89). The Etest is also used to determine metronidazole MICs for resistant isolates, but comparisons with broth dilution results may not correlate fully (89). The agar diffusion method with disks can be used for testing susceptibility to other antibiotics less commonly used in eradication, such as tetracycline, ciprofloxacin, and rifabutin. For instance, isolates were recorded as resistant if the growth inhibition zone for tetracycline was <30 mm (10-µg disk) (21) and if any inhibition zone was observed for ciprofloxacin (1-µg disk) and rifampin (5-µg disk) (22). The present tentative agar dilution MIC interpretive criteria for resistance to these antibiotics are >1 µg/ml for tetracycline, >0.5 µg/ml for levofloxacin, and >1 µg/ml for rifabutin (22, 44, 89). For resistant isolates, the MICs can be determined using the Etest.

Genotypic Susceptibility Testing of *H. pylori* Cultures and in Biopsy Specimens

Resistance to clarithromycin in *H. pylori* is attributed to point mutations at sites (A2142G and A2143G) in the peptidyltransferase region of domain V of the 23S rRNA gene which inhibit macrolide binding (137). Several methods involving gene amplification, rapid sequencing by pyrosequencing, or fluorescent in situ hybridization have been developed for the rapid detection of mutations associated with clarithromycin resistance (89, 105). PCR-RFLP analysis was initially used on isolates to detect relevant mutations, but real-time PCR now provides a simpler and more rapid approach. Adaptations allow detection with excellent sensitivity of both *H. pylori* and its resistance to clarithromycin directly from gastric biopsy specimens (13, 21, 100, 118). Real-time PCR assays also are available to ascertain resistance to tetracycline by rapid detection of 16S rRNA gene point mutations (72) and to ciprofloxacin/levofloxacin by rapid detection of point mutations in the quinolone resistance-determining region of the *gyrA* gene (43). Likewise, a real-time PCR test has been developed to ascertain resistance to rifabutin by rapid detection of point mutations in the *rpoB* gene (142). In contrast, development of a DNA-based assay to detect *H. pylori* resistance to metronidazole has proved more problematic, as the mechanisms of in vitro resistance have yet to be fully elucidated. Multiple null mutations in the NADPH nitroreductase gene (*rdxA*) and in the NAD(P)H flavin oxidoreductase gene (*frxA*) may contribute to the induction of resistance, but neither provides consistent markers for in vitro resistance testing (15, 17). The metronidazole resistance phenotype may involve more-complex metabolic changes than inactivation of the *rdxA* and *frxA* genes, as there is evidence of a role for oxygen and the intracellular redox status (60). Detection of RdxA protein by immunoblotting is possible but needs further development (71).

Genotypic Susceptibility Testing of *H. pylori* in Feces

A biprobe 23S rRNA gene real-time PCR assay has been developed for direct clarithromycin susceptibility testing of *H. pylori* in stool specimens (118), and an evaluation of a modified version, the *Helicobacter pylori* ClariRes assay (Ingenetix, Vienna, Austria), reported that it was at least as sensitive and more specific than the stool antigen test (112). However, another evaluation of the assay on stool specimens from symptomatic children reported a sensitivity of only 63% (77), and the resultant discussion highlighted the importance of appropriate laboratory practice, especially in handling of the stool sample, to ensure accurate performance of the assay (80).

Susceptibility Testing of Gastric HHLO

Optimal treatment remains to be established for HHLO, although there is evidence that eradication by antimicrobial therapy, such as that used in conventional *H. pylori* eradication, results in the resolution of gastritis and peptic ulcer disease (46, 59) as well as "*H. heilmannii*"-associated, primary, low-grade MALT lymphoma (95). Although susceptibilities in vitro were described for multiple isolates (from one patient) of an HHLO subsequently identified as *H. bizzozeronii* (2, 57), usually there are no cultures of HHLO available for testing. Consequently, there is no information for HHLO on their frequency of resistance to clarithromycin and other antibiotics. To ascertain possible treatment options for HHLO, triple therapy was shown to significantly reduce burden in experimentally infected mouse stomachs (83). However, no PCR assays, such as those used to determine *H. pylori* clarithromycin and tetracycline resistance in gastric biopsy tissue, have been developed for direct testing of resistance in HHLO.

Susceptibility Testing of Enterohepatic Helicobacters

No recommended guidelines are available for treatment of a diagnosed infection with the enterohepatic helicobacters *H. cinaedi*, *H. canis*, *H. fennelliae*, and *H. pullorum* and intestinal flexispira-like helicobacters. Various antibiotic agents alone or in combination have been successfully used in treating such infections, but there is insufficient information to determine resistance rates for individual species. For the more commonly reported *H. cinaedi*, effective therapy for infection may require prolonged courses for at least 2 to 3 weeks of multiple antibiotics, such as erythromycin, ciprofloxacin, gentamicin, levofloxacin, tetracycline, and beta-lactams (63, 84, 102). Susceptibility testing of *H. cinaedi* appears to be meaningful, as resistance in vitro has been correlated with treatment failures (63). However, there are no guidelines for antimicrobial susceptibility testing with interpretive criteria currently recommended for enterohepatic helicobacters. As a guide, it may be noted that in testing *H. cinaedi* from a recurrent-bacteremia case, the approach used was interpretation of susceptibility for clarithromycin based on the CLSI guidelines for *H. pylori* and on published reports for metronidazole and amoxicillin but that for other antibiotics, interpretation was based on CLSI guidelines for gram-negative bacilli (131).

EVALUATION, INTERPRETATION, AND REPORTING OF RESULTS

The principal noninvasive tests for diagnosis of an *H. pylori* infection before treatment are the UBT, enzyme immunoassay-based stool antigen tests, and high-accuracy ELISA-based IgG serology. According to the clinical setting, endoscopic investigation may be indicated, and then rapid urease testing, histology, and culture of gastric biopsy specimens can be used. To assess *H. pylori* status for posttreatment follow-up, the UBT and stool antigen tests are the recommended noninvasive tests, but not IgG serology, as serum antibody concentrations fall slowly after eradication. In addition to test performance, other factors, such as cost-effectiveness and patient attitudes, need to be considered in test selection (33, 88). To perform antimicrobial susceptibility testing, bacteriological culture of *H. pylori* from gastric biopsy specimens is recommended, especially in cases of repeated treatment failure. Successful culture may be reported if the organism is microaerobic, has a gram-negative morphology, and is oxidase, catalase, and urease positive. If culture is not positive after 10 days of incubation, it can be reported as negative, but if clinical tests indicate an *H. pylori* infection, it may be informative to perform a species-specific PCR assay directly on the gastric biopsy specimen. Because of the potential unreliability of PCR assays, resulting in false positives, such tests should not be used as the sole basis for diagnosis. Testing for clarithromycin susceptibility should be performed using either the CLSI reference method or a substantially equivalent method. Direct PCR testing of cultures or biopsy specimens provides a rapid alternative to phenotypic testing to detect the presence of discrete mutations conferring macrolide resistance. Eradication therapies are also likely to include other agents, such as amoxicillin, metronidazole, and tetracycline and in problem cases possibly rifabutin, levofloxacin, and furazolidone, depending on local clinical practice. Interpretive criteria for these antimicrobials, where available, may be "tentative" but should be used in the absence of recommended guidelines.

Gastric infection with non-*pylori Helicobacter* species is less common and should be diagnosed from bacterial morphology in gastric biopsy specimens. In the microbiology laboratory, they may be detected by an HHLO-specific PCR assay. Because of the lack of rapid diagnostic methods for the enterohepatic species, these must be cultured for a definitive identification. Enteric species such as *H. canadensis* and *H. pullorum* may occasionally be isolated by techniques employed for the isolation of *Campylobacter* species, particularly if nonselective media and incubation at 37°C are employed. As *Campylobacter* isolates are typically only cursorily identified routinely, enteric *Helicobacter* species are likely to be missed. Although they may have a limited role in human gastroenteritis, their significance remains unclear. Other species, such as *H. cinaedi*, *H. canis*, and *H. fennelliae*, may be rarely encountered from blood culture and other sites of infection. They are unlikely to grow well aerobically but may be apparent after prolonged incubation in an atmosphere containing additional CO_2 or on plates incubated "anaerobically" (conditions of strict anaerobiosis will not support growth). As these enterohepatic helicobacters are typically urease negative and can be confused with campylobacters, accurate identification is often difficult, and a reference laboratory should be consulted. The clinical significance of isolates may be unclear and should be assessed on a case-by-case basis. Determination of antibiotic susceptibilities should be performed if needed to guide antibiotic therapy decisions.

I thank Robert Owen for his substantial contribution to the preparation of this chapter.

Use of trade names of, or details about, specific products does not imply endorsement of those products or their manufacturers by the author or the Health Protection Agency.

REFERENCES

1. **Alm, R. A., and B. Noonan.** 2001. The genome, p. 295–311. *In* H. L. T. Mobley, G. L. Mendz, and S. L. Hazell (ed.), Helicobacter pylori: *Physiology and Genetics.* ASM Press, Washington, DC.
2. **Andersen, L. P., K. Boye, J. Blom, S. Holck, A. Norgaard, and L. Elsborg.** 1999. Characterization of a culturable "*Gastrospirillum hominis*" (Helicobacter heilmannii) strain isolated from human gastric mucosa. *J. Clin. Microbiol.* **37:**1069–1076.
3. **Atherton, J. C., T. L. Cover, R. J. Twells, M. R. Morales, C. J. Hawkey, and M. J. Blaser.** 1999. Simple and accurate PCR-based system for typing vacuolating cytotoxin alleles of *Helicobacter pylori. J. Clin. Microbiol.* **37:**2979–2982.
4. **Avenaud, P., A. Marais, L. Monteiro, B. Le Bail, P. Bioulac Sage, C. Balabaud, and F. Megraud.** 2000. Detection of *Helicobacter* species in the liver of patients with and without primary liver carcinoma. *Cancer* **89:**1431–1439.
5. **Baele, M., A. Decostere, P. Vandamme, L. Ceelen, A. Hellemans, J. Mast, K. Chiers, R. Ducatelle, and F. Haesebrouck.** 2008. Isolation and characterization of Helicobacter suis sp. nov from pig stomachs. *Int. J. Syst. Evol. Microbiol.* **58:**1350–1358.
6. **Blanco, S., M. Forne, A. Lacoma, C. Prat, M. A. Cuesta, I. Latorre, J. M. Viver, G. Fernandez, S. Molinos, and J. Dominguez.** 2008. Comparison of stool antigen immunoassay methods for detecting Helicobacter pylori infection before and after eradication treatment. *Diagn. Microbiol. Infect. Dis.* **61:**150–155.
7. **Branca, G., T. Spanu, G. Cammarota, A. M. Schito, A. Gasbarrini, G. B. Gasbarrini, and G. Fadda.** 2004. High levels of dual resistance to clarithromycin and metronidazole and in vitro activity of levofloxacin against Helicobacter pylori isolates from patients after failure of therapy. *Int. J. Antimicrob. Agents* **24:**433–438.

8. **Bruce, M. G., and H. I. Maaroos.** 2008. Epidemiology of *Helicobacter pylori* infections. *Helicobacter* **13**(Suppl. 1):1–6.

9. **Bunn, J. E., W. G. MacKay, J. E. Thomas, D. C. Reid, and L. T. Weaver.** 2002. Detection of *Helicobacter pylori* DNA in drinking water biofilms: implications for transmission in early life. *Lett. Appl. Microbiol.* **34**:450–454.

10. **Carothers, J. J., M. G. Bruce, T. W. Hennessy, M. Bensler, J. M. Morris, A. L. Reasonover, D. A. Hurlburt, A. J. Parkinson, J. M. Coleman, and B. J. McMahon.** 2007. The relationship between previous fluoroquinolone use and levofloxacin resistance in *Helicobacter pylori* infection. *Clin. Infect. Dis.* **44**:e5–e8.

11. **Ceelen, L., A. Decostere, G. Verschraegen, R. Ducatelle, and F. Haesebrouck.** 2005. Prevalence of *Helicobacter pullorum* among patients with gastrointestinal disease and clinically healthy persons. *J. Clin. Microbiol.* **43**:2984–2986.

12. **Ceelen, L. M., A. Decostere, K. Van den Bulck, S. L. On, M. Baele, R. Ducatelle, and F. Haesebrouck.** 2006. *Helicobacter pullorum* in chickens, Belgium. *Emerg. Infect. Dis.* **12**:263–267.

13. **Chisholm, S. A., R. J. Owen, E. L. Teare, and S. Saverymuttu.** 2001. PCR-based diagnosis of *Helicobacter pylori* infection and real-time determination of clarithromycin resistance directly from human gastric biopsy samples. *J. Clin. Microbiol.* **39**:1217–1220.

14. **Chisholm, S. A., E. L. Teare, B. Patel, and R. J. Owen.** 2002. Determination of *Helicobacter pylori* vacA allelic types by single-step multiplex PCR. *Lett. Appl. Microbiol.* **35**:42–46.

15. **Chisholm, S. A., and R. J. Owen.** 2003. Mutations in *Helicobacter pylori* rdxA gene sequences may not contribute to metronidazole resistance. *J. Antimicrob. Chemother.* **51**:995–999.

16. **Chisholm, S. A., and R. J. Owen.** 2003. Development and application of a novel screening PCR assay for direct detection of "*Helicobacter heilmannii*"-like organisms in human gastric biopsies in southeast England. *Diagn. Microbiol. Infect. Dis.* **46**:1–7.

17. **Chisholm, S. A., and R. J. Owen.** 2004. Frameshift mutations in frxA occur frequently and do not provide a reliable marker for metronidazole resistance in UK isolates of *Helicobacter pylori*. *J. Med. Microbiol.* **53**:135–140.

18. **Chisholm, S. A., C. L. Watson, E. L. Teare, S. Saverymuttu, and R. J. Owen.** 2004. Non-invasive diagnosis of *Helicobacter pylori* infection in adult dyspeptic patients by stool antigen detection: does the rapid immunochromatography test provide a reliable alternative to conventional ELISA kits? *J. Med. Microbiol.* **53**:623–627.

19. **Chisholm, S. A., and R. J. Owen.** 2006. From Nobel to no cure: a case for monitoring antibiotic resistance in the gastric pathogen *Helicobacter pylori*. *Expert. Rev. Anti Infect. Ther.* **4**:349–351.

20. **Chisholm, S. A., E. L. Teare, K. Davies, and R. J. Owen.** 2007. Surveillance of primary antibiotic resistance of *Helicobacter pylori* at centres in England and Wales over a six-year period (2000–2005). *Euro Surveill.* **12**:E3–E4.

21. **Chisholm, S. A., and R. J. Owen.** 2008. Application of polymerase chain reaction-based assays for rapid identification and antibiotic resistance screening of *Helicobacter pylori* in gastric biopsies. *Diagn. Microbiol. Infect. Dis.* **61**:67–71.

22. **Chisholm, S. A., and R. J. Owen.** 2009. Frequency and molecular characteristics of ciprofloxacin- and rifampicin-resistant *Helicobacter pylori* from gastric infections in the United Kingdom. *J. Med. Microbiol.* **58**:1322–1328.

23. **Cindoruk, M., M. Y. Cirak, S. Unal, T. Karakan, G. Erkan, D. Engin, S. Dumlu, and S. Turet.** 2008. Identification of *Helicobacter* species by 16S rDNA PCR and sequence analysis in human liver samples from patients with various etiologies of benign liver diseases. *Eur. J. Gastroenterol. Hepatol.* **20**:33–36.

24. **Cirak, M. Y., Y. Akyon, and F. Megraud.** 2007. Diagnosis of *Helicobacter pylori*. *Helicobacter* **12**(Suppl. 1):4–9.

25. **Clinical and Laboratory Standards Institute.** 2006. Methods for antimicrobial dilution and disk susceptibility testing of infrequently isolated or fastidious bacteria, vol. 26 (no. 19). Approved guideline M45-A. Clinical and Laboratory Standards Institute, Wayne, PA.

26. **De Groote, D., L. J. Van Doorn, B. K. Van den, P. Vandamme, M. Vieth, M. Stolte, J. C. Debongnie, A. Burette, F. Haesebrouck, and R. Ducatelle.** 2005. Detection of non-pylori *Helicobacter* species in "*Helicobacter heilmannii*"-infected humans. *Helicobacter* **10**:398–406.

27. **de Martel, C., M. Plummer, J. Parsonnet, L. J. Van Doorn, and S. Franceschi.** 2009. *Helicobacter* species in cancers of the gallbladder and extrahepatic biliary tract. *Br. J. Cancer* **100**:194–199.

28. **Dewhirst, F. E., J. G. Fox, and S. L. On.** 2000. Recommended minimal standards for describing new species of the genus *Helicobacter*. *Int. J. Syst. Evol. Microbiol.* **50**:2231–2237.

29. **Dewhirst, F. E., Z. Shen, L. Stokes, M. Scimeca, and J. G. Fox.** 2005. Discordant 16S rRNA and 23S rRNA phylogenies for the genus *Helicobacter*: implications for phylogenetic inference and systematics. *J. Bacteriol.* **187**:6106–6118.

30. **Dewhirst, F. E., J. G. Fox, E. N. Mendes, B. J. Paster, C. E. Gates, C. A. Kirkbride, and K. A. Eaton.** 2000. '*Flexispira rappini*' strains represent at least 10 *Helicobacter* taxa. *Int. J. Syst. Evol. Microbiol.* **50**:1781–1787.

31. **Duck, W. M., J. Sobel, J. M. Pruckler, Q. Song, D. Swerdlow, C. Friedman, A. Sulka, B. Swaminathan, T. Taylor, M. Hoekstra, P. Griffin, D. Smoot, R. Peek, D. C. Metz, P. B. Bloom, S. Goldschmidt, J. Parsonnet, G. Triadafilopoulos, G. I. Perez-Perez, N. Vakil, P. Ernst, S. Czinn, D. Dunne, and B. D. Gold.** 2004. Antimicrobial resistance incidence and risk factors among *Helicobacter pylori*-infected persons, United States. *Emerg. Infect. Dis.* **10**:1088–1094.

32. **Elitsur, Y., V. Tolia, M. A. Gilger, J. Reeves-Garcia, E. Schmidt-Sommerfeld, A. R. Opekun, H. El Zimaity, D. Y. Graham, and K. Enmei.** 2009. Urea breath test in children: the United States prospective, multicenter study. *Helicobacter* **14**:134–140.

33. **Elwyn, G., M. Taubert, S. Davies, G. Brown, M. Allison and C. Phillips.** 2007. Which test is best for *Helicobacter pylori*? A cost-effectiveness model using decision analysis. *Br. J. Gen. Pract.* **57**:401–403.

34. **Fischbach, L., and E. L. Evans.** 2007. Meta-analysis: the effect of antibiotic resistance status on the efficacy of triple and quadruple first-line therapies for *Helicobacter pylori*. *Aliment. Pharmacol. Ther.* **26**:343–357.

35. **Flores, B. M., C. L. Fennell, and W. E. Stamm.** 1989. Characterization of *Campylobacter cinaedi* and *C. fennelliae* antigens and analysis of the human immune response. *J. Infect. Dis.* **159**:635–640.

36. **Fox, J. G.** 2002. The non-*H. pylori* helicobacters: their expanding role in gastrointestinal and systemic diseases. *Gut* **50**:273–283.

37. **Fox, J. G., C. C. Chien, F. E. Dewhirst, B. J. Paster, Z. Shen, P. L. Melito, D. L. Woodward, and F. G. Rodgers.** 2000. *Helicobacter canadensis* sp. nov. isolated from humans with diarrhea as an example of an emerging pathogen. *J. Clin. Microbiol.* **38**:2546–2549.

38. **Fox, J. G., F. E. Dewhirst, Z. Shen, Y. Feng, N. S. Taylor, B. J. Paster, R. L. Ericson, C. N. Lau, P. Correa, J. C. Araya, and I. Roa.** 1998. Hepatic *Helicobacter* species identified in bile and gallbladder tissue from Chileans with chronic cholecystitis. *Gastroenterology* **114**:755–763.

39. **Fox, J. G., and F. Megraud.** 2007. *Helicobacter*, p. 947–963. In P. R. Murray, E. J. Baron, J. H. Jorgensen, M. L. Landry, and M. A. Pfaller (ed.), *Manual of Clinical Microbiology*, 9th ed. ASM Press, Washington, DC.

40. **Gibson, J. R., M. A. Ferrus, D. Woodward, J. Xerry, and R. J. Owen.** 1999. Genetic diversity in *Helicobacter pullorum* from human and poultry sources identified by an amplified fragment length polymorphism technique and pulsed-field gel electrophoresis. *J. Appl. Microbiol.* **87**:602–610.

41. **Gisbert, J. P., and J. M. Pajares.** 2004. Stool antigen test for the diagnosis of *Helicobacter pylori* infection: a systematic review. *Helicobacter* **9**:347–368.

42. **Gisbert, J. P., M. F. de la Morena, and V. Abraira.** 2006. Accuracy of monoclonal stool antigen test for the diagnosis of *H. pylori* infection: a systematic review and meta-analysis. *Am. J. Gastroenterol.* **101**:1921–1930.

43. **Glocker, E., and M. Kist.** 2004. Rapid detection of point mutations in the *gyrA* gene of *Helicobacter pylori* conferring resistance to ciprofloxacin by a fluorescence resonance energy transfer-based real-time PCR approach. *J. Clin. Microbiol.* **42:**2241–2246.

44. **Glocker, E., C. Bogdan, and M. Kist.** 2007. Characterization of rifampicin-resistant clinical *Helicobacter pylori* isolates from Germany. *J. Antimicrob. Chemother.* **59:**874–879.

45. **Glupczynski, Y., N. Broutet, A. Cantagrel, L. P. Andersen, T. Alarcon, M. Lopez-Brea, and F. Megraud.** 2002. Comparison of the E test and agar dilution method for antimicrobial susceptibility testing of *Helicobacter pylori. Eur. J. Clin. Microbiol. Infect. Dis.* **21:**549–552.

46. **Goddard, A. F., R. P. Logan, J. C. Atherton, D. Jenkins, and R. C. Spiller.** 1997. Healing of duodenal ulcer after eradication of *Helicobacter heilmannii. Lancet* **349:**1815–1816.

47. **González, A., P. Piqueres, Y. Moreno, I. Cañigral, R. J. Owen, J. Hernández, and M. A. Ferrús.** 2008. A novel real-time PCR assay for the detection of *Helicobacter pullorum*-like organisms in chicken products. *Int. Microbiol.* **11:**203–208.

48. **Goodwin, C., T. Armstrong, T. Chilvers, M. Peters, M. J. Collins, L. Sly, W. McConnell, and W. Harper.** 1989. Transfer of *Campylobacter pylori* and *Campylobacter mustelae* to *Helicobacter* gen. nov. as *Helicobacter pylori* comb. nov. and *Helicobacter mustelae* comb. nov., respectively. *Int. J. Syst. Bacteriol.* **39:**397–405.

49. **Goosen, C., J. Theron, M. Ntsala, F. F. Maree, A. Olckers, S. J. Botha, A. J. Lastovica, and S. W. van der Merwe.** 2002. Evaluation of a novel heminested PCR assay based on the phosphoglucosamine mutase gene for detection of *Helicobacter pylori* in saliva and dental plaque. *J. Clin. Microbiol.* **40:**205–209.

50. **Graham, D. Y., and A. Shiotani.** 2008. New concepts of resistance in the treatment of *Helicobacter pylori* infections. *Nat. Clin. Pract. Gastroenterol. Hepatol.* **5:**321–331.

51. **Grignon, B., J. Tankovic, F. Megraud, Y. Glupczynski, M. O. Husson, M. C. Conroy, J. P. Emond, J. Loulergue, J. Raymond, and J. L. Fauchere.** 2002. Validation of diffusion methods for macrolide susceptibility testing of *Helicobacter pylori. Microb. Drug Resist.* **8:**61–66.

52. **Haesebrouck, F., F. Pasmans, B. Flahou, K. Chiers, M. Baele, T. Meyns, A. Decostere, and R. Ducatelle.** 2009. Gastric *helicobacters* in domestic animals and nonhuman primates and their significance for human health. *Clin. Microbiol. Rev.* **22:**202–223.

53. **Haggerty, T. D., S. Perry, L. Sanchez, G. Perez-Perez, and J. Parsonnet.** 2005. Significance of transiently positive enzyme-linked immunosorbent assay results in detection of *Helicobacter pylori* in stool samples from children. *J. Clin. Microbiol.* **43:**2220–2223.

54. **Hanninen, M. L., M. Utriainen, I. Happonen, and F. E. Dewhirst.** 2003. *Helicobacter* sp. flexispira 16S rDNA taxa 1, 4, and 5 and Finnish porcine *Helicobacter* isolates are members of the species *Helicobacter trogontum* (taxon 6). *Int. J. Syst. Evol. Microbiol.* **53:**425–433.

55. **Hanninen, M. L., R. I. Karenlampi, J. M. Koort, T. Mikkonen, and K. J. Bjorkroth.** 2005. Extension of the species *Helicobacter bilis* to include the reference strains of *Helicobacter* sp. flexispira taxa 2, 3 and 8 and Finnish canine and feline flexispira strains. *Int. J. Syst. Evol. Microbiol.* **55:**891–898.

56. **Husmann, M., C. Gries, P. Jehnichen, T. Woelfel, G. Gerken, W. Ludwig, and S. Bhakdi.** 1994. *Helicobacter* sp. strain Mainz isolated from an AIDS patient with septic arthritis: case report and nonradioactive analysis of 16S rRNA sequence. *J. Clin. Microbiol.* **32:**3037–3039.

57. **Jalava, K., S. L. On, C. S. Harrington, L. P. Andersen, M. L. Hanninen and P. Vandamme.** 2001. A cultured strain of 'Helicobacter heilmannii,' a human gastric pathogen identified as *H. bizzozeronii*: evidence for zoonotic potential of *Helicobacter. Emerg. Infect. Dis.* **7:**1036–1038.

58. **Iwashita, H., S. Fujii, Y. Kawamura, T. Okamoto, T. Sawa, T. Masaki, A. Nishizono, S. Higashi, T. Kitamura, F. Tamura, Y. Sasaki, and T. Akaike.** 2008. Identification of the major antigenic protein of *Helicobacter cinaedi* and its immunogenicity in humans with *H. cinaedi* infections. *Clin. Vac. Immunol.* **15:**513–521.

59. **Jothimani, D. K., U. Zanetto, R. J. Owen, A. J. Lawson, and P. G. Wilson.** 2009. A rare case of gastric erosions. *Gut* **58:**1669.

60. **Kaakoush, N. O., C. Asencio, F. Megraud, and G. L. Mendz.** 2009. A redox basis for metronidazole resistance in *Helicobacter pylori. Antimicrob. Agents Chemother.* **53:**1884–1891.

61. **Kabir, S.** 2004. Detection of *Helicobacter pylori* DNA in feces and saliva by polymerase chain reaction: a review. *Helicobacter* **9:**115–123.

62. **Kiehlbauch, J. A., D. J. Brenner, D. N. Cameron, A. G. Steigerwalt, J. M. Makowski, C. N. Baker, C. M. Patton, and I. K. Wachsmuth.** 1995. Genotypic and phenotypic characterization of *Helicobacter cinaedi* and *Helicobacter fennelliae* strains isolated from humans and animals. *J. Clin. Microbiol.* **33:**2940–2947.

63. **Kiehlbauch, J. A., R. V. Tauxe, C. N. Baker, and I. K. Wachsmuth.** 1994. *Helicobacter cinaedi*-associated bacteremia and cellulitis in immunocompromised patients. *Ann. Intern. Med.* **121:**90–93.

64. **Kim, J. M., J. S. Kim, N. Kim, S. G. Kim, H. C. Jung, and I. S. Song.** 2006. Comparison of primary and secondary antimicrobial minimum inhibitory concentrations for *Helicobacter pylori* isolated from Korean patients. *Int. J. Antimicrob. Agents* **28:**6–13.

65. **Kist, M.** 2007. *Helicobacter pylori*: primary antimicrobial resistance and first-line treatment strategies. *Euro Surveill.* **12:**E1–E2.

66. **Kitamura, T., Y. Kawamura, K. Ohkusu, T. Masaki, H. Iwashita, T. Sawa, S. Fujii, T. Okamoto, and T. Akaike.** 2007. *Helicobacter cinaedi* cellulitis and bacteremia in immunocompetent hosts after orthopedic surgery. *J. Clin. Microbiol.* **45:**31–38.

67. **Kolho, K. L., T. Klemola, A. Koivusalo, and H. Rautelin.** 2006. Stool antigen tests for the detection of *Helicobacter pylori* in children. *Diagn. Microbiol. Infect. Dis.* **55:**269–273.

68. **Laharie, D., C. Asencio, J. Asselineau, P. Bulois, A. Bourreille, J. Moreau, P. Bonjean, D. Lamarque, A. Pariente, J. C. Soule, A. Charachon, B. Coffin, P. Perez, F. Megraud, and F. Zerbib.** 2009. Association between enterohepatic *Helicobacter* species and Crohn's disease: a prospective cross-sectional study. *Aliment. Pharmacol. Ther.* **30:**283–293.

69. **Laheij, R. J., H. Straatman, J. B. Jansen, and A. L. Verbeek.** 1998. Evaluation of commercially available *Helicobacter pylori* serology kits: a review. *J. Clin. Microbiol.* **36:**2803–2809.

70. **Lastovica, A. J., and E. le Roux.** 2000. Efficient isolation of campylobacteria from stools. *J. Clin. Microbiol.* **38:**2798–2799.

71. **Latham, S. R., R. J. Owen, N. C. Elviss, A. Labigne, and P. J. Jenks.** 2001. Differentiation of metronidazole-sensitive and -resistant clinical isolates of *Helicobacter pylori* by immunoblotting with antisera to the RdxA protein. *J. Clin. Microbiol.* **39:**3052–3055.

72. **Lawson, A. J., N. C. Elviss, and R. J. Owen.** 2005. Real-time PCR detection and frequency of 16S rDNA mutations associated with resistance and reduced susceptibility to tetracycline in *Helicobacter pylori* from England and Wales. *J. Antimicrob. Chemother.* **56:**282–286.

73. **Leal, Y. A., L. F. Flores, L. B. Garcia-Cortes, R. Cedillo-Rivera, and J. Tores.** 2008. Antibody-based detection tests for the diagnosis of *Helicobacter pylori* infection in children: a meta-analysis. *PLoS ONE* **3:**e3751. doi:10.1371/journal.pone.0003751.

74. **Leemann, C., E. Gambillara, G. Prod'hom, K. Jaton, R. Panizzon, J. Bille, P. Francioli, G. Greub, E. Laffitte, and P. E. Tarr.** 2006. First case of bacteraemia and multifocal cellulitis due to *Helicobacter canis* in an immunocompetent patient. *J. Clin. Microbiol.* **44:**4598–4600.

75. **Li, C., T. Ha, D. S. Chi, D. A. Ferguson, Jr., C. Jiang, J. J. Laffan, and E. Thomas.** 1997. Differentiation of *Helicobacter pylori* strains directly from gastric biopsy specimens by PCR-based restriction fragment length polymorphism analysis without culture. *J. Clin. Microbiol.* **35:**3021–3025.

76. **Logan, J. M. J., A. Burnens, D. Linton, A. Lawson, and J. Stanley.** 2000. *Campylobacter lanienae* sp. nov., a new species isolated from workers in an abattoir. *Int. J. Syst. Evol. Microbiol.* **50:**865–872.

77. Lottspeich, C., A. Schwarzer, K. Panthel, S. Koletzko, and H. Russmann. 2007. Evaluation of the novel *Helicobacter pylori* ClariRes real-time PCR assay for detection and clarithromycin susceptibility testing of *H. pylori* in stool specimens from symptomatic children. *J. Clin. Microbiol.* **45:**1718–1722.

78. Luzza, F., M. Maletta, M. Imeneo, A. Marcheggiano, C. Iannoni, L. Biancone, and F. Pallone. 1995. Salivary-specific immunoglobulin G in the diagnosis of *Helicobacter pylori* infection in dyspeptic patients. *Am. J. Gastroenterol.* **90:**1820–1823.

79. Maiden, M. C. 2006. Multilocus sequence typing of bacteria. *Annu. Rev. Microbiol.* **60:**561–588.

80. Makristathis, A., A. M. Hirschl, H. Russmann, and S. Koletzko. 2007. Detection and clarithromycin susceptibility testing of *Helicobacter pylori* in stool specimens by real-time PCR: how to get accurate test results. *J. Clin. Microbiol.* **45:**2756–2757.

81. Malaty, H. M., N. D. Logan, D. Y. Graham, J. E. Ramchatesingh, and S. G. Reddy. 2000. *Helicobacter pylori* infection in asymptomatic children: comparison of diagnostic tests. *Helicobacter* **5:**155–159.

82. Malfertheiner, P., F. Megraud, C. O'Morain, F. Bazzoli, E. El Omar, D. Graham, R. Hunt, T. Rokkas, N. Vakil, and E. J. Kuipers. 2007. Current concepts in the management of *Helicobacter pylori* infection: the Maastricht III Consensus Report. *Gut* **56:**772–781.

83. Matsui, H., C. Aikawa, Y. Sekiya, S. Takahashi, S. Y. Murayama, and M. Nakamura. 2008. Evaluation of antibiotic therapy for eradication of "*Candidatus* Helicobacter heilmannii.*" Antimicrob. Agents Chemother.* **52:**2988–2989.

84. Matsumoto, T., M. Kawakubo, M. Shiohara, T. Kumagai, E. Hidaka, K. Yamauchi, K. Oana, K. Matsuzawa, H. Ota, and Y. Kawakami. 2009. Phylogeny of a novel "*Helicobacter heilmannii*" organism from a Japanese patient with chronic gastritis based on DNA sequence analysis of 16S rRNA and urease genes. *J. Microbiol.* **47:**201–207.

85. Mbulaiteye, S. M., M. Hisada, and E. M. El Omar. 2009. *Helicobacter pylori* associated global gastric cancer burden. *Front. Biosci.* **14:**1490–1504.

86. McClain, M. S., C. L. Shaffer, D. A. Israel, R. M. Peek, Jr., and T. L. Cover. 2009. Genome sequence analysis of *Helicobacter pylori* strains associated with gastric ulceration and gastric cancer. *BMC Genomics* **10:**3. doi.:10.1186/1471-2164-10-3.

87. McNulty, C., L. Teare, R. Owen, D. Tompkins, P. Hawtin, and K. McColl. 2005. Test and treat for dyspepsia—but which test? *BMJ* **330:**105–106.

88. McNulty, C. A. M., and J. W. Whiting. 2007. Patients' attitudes to *Helicobacter pylori* breath and stool antigen tests compared to blood serology. *J. Infect.* **55:**19–22.

89. Mégraud, F., and P. Lehours. 2007. *Helicobacter pylori* detection and antimicrobial susceptibility testing. *Clin. Microbiol. Rev.* **20:**280–322.

90. Melito, P. L., C. Munro, P. R. Chipman, D. L. Woodward, T. F. Booth, and F. G. Rodgers. 2001. *Helicobacter winghamensis* sp. nov., a novel *Helicobacter* sp. isolated from patients with gastroenteritis. *J. Clin. Microbiol.* **39:**2412–2417.

91. Mills, S. D., L. A. Kurjanczyk, and J. L. Penner. 1992. Antigenicity of *Helicobacter pylori* lipopolysaccharides. *J. Clin. Microbiol.* **30:**3175–3180.

92. Moayyedi, P., J. Deeks, N. J. Talley, B. Delaney, and D. Forman. 2003. An update of the Cochrane systematic review of *Helicobacter pylori* eradication therapy in nonulcer dyspepsia: resolving the discrepancy between systematic reviews. *Am. J. Gastroenterol.* **98:**2621–2626.

93. Monteiro, L., N. Gras, R. Vidal, J. Cabrita, and F. Megraud. 2001. Detection of *Helicobacter pylori* DNA in human feces by PCR: DNA stability and removal of inhibitors. *J. Microbiol. Methods* **45:**89–94.

94. Moreno, Y., P. Piqueres, J. L. Alonso, A. Jimenez, A. Gonzalez, and M. A. Ferrus. 2007. Survival and viability of *Helicobacter pylori* after inoculation into chlorinated drinking water. *Water Res.* **41:**3490–3496.

95. Morgner, A., N. Lehn, L. P. Andersen, C. Thiede, M. Bennedsen, K. Trebesius, B. Neubauer, A. Neubauer, M. Stolte, and E. Bayerdörffer. 2000. *Helicobacter heilmannii*-associated primary gastric low-grade MALT lymphoma: complete remission after curing the infection. *Gastroenterology* **118:**821–828.

96. Moyaert, H., A. Decostere, P. Vandamme, L. Debruyne, J. Mast, M. Baele, L. Ceelen, R. Ducatelle, and F. Haesebrouck. 2007. *Helicobacter equorum* sp. nov., a urease-negative *Helicobacter* species isolated from horse faeces. *Int. J. Syst. Evol. Microbiol.* **57:**213–218.

97. Moyaert, H., F. Franceschi, D. Roccarina, R. Ducatelle, F. Haesebrouck, and A. Gasbarrini. 2008. Extragastric manifestations of *Helicobacter pylori* infection: other helicobacters. *Helicobacter* **13**(Suppl. 1):47–57.

98. Murakami, H., M. Goto, E. Ono, E. Sawabe, M. Iwata, K. Okuzumi, K. Yamaguchi, and T. Takahashi. 2003. Isolation of *Helicobacter cinaedi* from blood of an immunocompromised patient in Japan. *J. Infect. Chemother.* **9:**344–347.

99. Nilsson, H. O., R. Mulchandani, K. G. Tranberg, U. Stenram, and T. Wadstrom. 2001. *Helicobacter* species identified in liver from patients with cholangiocarcinoma and hepatocellular carcinoma. *Gastroenterology* **120:**323–324.

100. Oleastro, M., A. Menard, A. Santos, H. Lamouliatte, L. Monteiro, P. Barthelemy, and F. Megraud. 2003. Real-time PCR assay for rapid and accurate detection of point mutations conferring resistance to clarithromycin in *Helicobacter pylori*. *J. Clin. Microbiol.* **41:**397–402.

101. On, S. L. W., A. Lee, J. L. O'Rourke, F. E. Dewhirst, B. J. Paster, J. G. Fox, and P. Vandamme. 2005. Genus I. *Helicobacter*, p. 1169–1189. *In* D. J. Brenner, N. R. Krieg, J. T. Staley, and G. Garrity (ed.), *Bergey's Manual of Systematic Bacteriology*, 2nd ed. Springer, New York, NY.

102. O'Rourke, J. L., M. Grehan, and A. Lee. 2001. Non-pylori *Helicobacter* species in humans. *Gut* **49:**601–606.

103. Osato, M. S., R. Reddy, S. G. Reddy, R. L. Penland, H. M. Malaty, and D. Y. Graham. 2001. Pattern of primary resistance of *Helicobacter pylori* to metronidazole or clarithromycin in the United States. *Arch. Intern. Med.* **161:**1217–1220.

104. Owen, R. J., D. E. Taylor, G. Wang, and L.-J. van Doorn. 2001. Heterogeneity and subtyping, p. 363–378. *In* H. L. T. Mobley, G. L. Mendz, and S. L. Hazell (ed.), Helicobacter pylori: *Physiology and Genetics*. ASM Press, Washington, DC.

105. Owen, R. J. 2002. Molecular testing for antibiotic resistance in *Helicobacter pylori*. *Gut* **50:**285–289.

106. Owen, R. J., and J. Xerry. 2003. Tracing clonality of *Helicobacter pylori* infecting family members from analysis of DNA sequences of three housekeeping genes (*ureI, atpA* and *ahpC*), deduced amino acid sequences, and pathogenicity-associated markers (*cagA* and *vacA*). *J. Med. Microbiol.* **52:**515–524.

107. Owen, R. J., and J. Xerry. 2007. Geographical conservation of short inserts in the signal and middle regions of the *Helicobacter pylori* vacuolating cytotoxin gene. *Microbiology* **153:**1176–1186.

108. Parsonnet, J., H. Shmuely, and T. Haggerty. 1999. Fecal and oral shedding of *Helicobacter pylori* from healthy infected adults. *JAMA* **282:**2240–2245.

109. Pena, J. A., K. McNeil, J. G. Fox, and J. Versalovic. 2002. Molecular evidence of *Helicobacter cinaedi* organisms in human gastric biopsy specimens. *J. Clin. Microbiol.* **40:**1511–1513.

110. Powers, C. N. 1998. Diagnosis of infectious diseases: a cytopathologist's perspective. *Clin. Microbiol. Rev.* **11:**341–365.

111. Prag, J., J. Blom, and K. A. Krogfelt. 2007. *Helicobacter canis* bacteraemia in a 7-month-old child. *FEMS Immunol. Med. Microbiol.* **50:**264–267.

112. Puz, S., Z. Kovach, A. M. Hirschl, M. Hafner, A. Innerhofer, M. Rotter, and A. Makristathis. 2006. Evaluation of the novel *Helicobacter pylori* ClariRes real-time PCR assay for detection and clarithromycin susceptibility testing of *H. pylori* in stool specimens and gastric biopsies; comparison with the stool antigen test. *Helicobacter* **11:**396.

113. Puz, S., A. Innerhofer, M. Ramharter, M. Haefner, A. M. Hirschl, Z. Kovach, M. Rotter, and A. Makristathis. 2008. A novel noninvasive genotyping method of *Helicobacter pylori* using stool specimens. *Gastroenterology* **135**:1543–1551.

114. Qualia, C. M., P. J. Katzman, M. R. Brown, and K. Kooros. 2007. A report of two children with *Helicobacter heilmannii* gastritis and review of the literature. *Pediatr. Dev. Pathol.* **10**:391–394.

115. Robertson, B. R., J. L. O'Rourke, P. Vandamme, S. L. On, and A. Lee. 2001. *Helicobacter ganmani* sp. nov., a urease-negative anaerobe isolated from the intestines of laboratory mice. *Int. J. Syst. Evol. Microbiol.* **51**:1881–1889.

116. Rocha, M., P. Avenaud, A. Menard, B. Le Bail, C. Balabaud, P. Bioulac-Sage, D. M. de Magalhaes Queiroz, and F. Megraud. 2005. Association of *Helicobacter* species with hepatitis C cirrhosis with or without hepatocellular carcinoma. *Gut* **54**:396–401.

117. Sanches, B., L. Coelho, L. Moretzsohn, and G. Vieira, Jr. 2008. Failure of *Helicobacter pylori* treatment after regimes containing clarithromycin: new practical therapeutic options. *Helicobacter* **13**:572–576.

118. Schabereiter-Gurtner, C., A. M. Hirschl, B. Dragosics, P. Hufnagl, S. Puz, Z. Kovach, M. Rotter, and A. Makristathis. 2004. Novel real-time PCR assay for detection of *Helicobacter pylori* infection and simultaneous clarithromycin susceptibility testing of stool and biopsy specimens. *J. Clin. Microbiol.* **42**:4512–4518.

119. Schwarz, S., G. Morelli, B. Kusecek, A. Manica, F. Balloux, R. J. Owen, D. Y. Graham, S. van der Merwe, M. Achtman, and S. Suerbaum. 2008. Horizontal versus familial transmission of *Helicobacter pylori*. *PLoS Pathog.* **4**:e1000180.

120. She, R. C., A. R. Wilson, and C. M. Litwin. 2009. Evaluation of *Helicobacter pylori* immunoglobulin G (IgG), IgA, and IgM serologic testing compared to stool antigen testing. *Clin. Vac. Immunol.* **16**:1253–1255.

121. Solnick, J. V., and D. B. Schauer. 2001. Emergence of diverse *Helicobacter* species in the pathogenesis of gastric and enterohepatic diseases. *Clin. Microbiol. Rev.* **14**:59–97.

122. Stanley, J., D. Linton, A. P. Burnens, F. E. Dewhirst, S. L. On, A. Porter, R. J. Owen, and M. Costas. 1994. *Helicobacter pullorum* sp. nov.—genotype and phenotype of a new species isolated from poultry and from human patients with gastroenteritis. *Microbiology* **140**:3441–3449.

123. Steinbrueckner, B., G. Haerter, K. Pelz, S. Weiner, J. A. Rump, W. Deissler, S. Bereswill, and M. Kist. 1997. Isolation of *Helicobacter pullorum* from patients with enteritis. *Scand. J. Infect. Dis.* **29**:315–318.

124. Suerbaum, S., and P. Michetti. 2002. *Helicobacter pylori* infection. *N. Engl. J. Med.* **347**:1175–1186.

125. Sugimoto, M., J. Y. Wu, S. Abudayyeh, J. Hoffman, H. Brahem, K. Al Khatib, Y. Yamaoka, and D. Y. Graham. 2009. Unreliability of results of PCR detection of *Helicobacter pylori* in clinical or environmental samples. *J. Clin. Microbiol.* **47**:738–742.

126. Suzuki, N., M. Yoneda, T. Naito, T. Iwamoto, Y. Masuo, K. Yamada, K. Hisama, I. Okada, and T. Hirofuji. 2008. Detection of *Helicobacter pylori* DNA in the saliva of patients complaining of halitosis. *J. Med. Microbiol.* **57**:1553–1559.

127. Tan, H. J., and K. L. Goh. 2008. Changing epidemiology of *Helicobacter pylori* in Asia. *J. Dig. Dis.* **9**:186–189.

128. Tolia, V., H. O. Nilsson, A. Boyer, A. Wuerth, W. A. Al Soud, R. Rabah, and T. Wadstrom. 2004. Detection of *Helicobacter ganmani*-like 16S rDNA in pediatric liver tissue. *Helicobacter* **9**:460–468.

129. Totten, P. A., C. L. Fennell, F. C. Tenover, J. M. Wezenberg, P. L. Perine, W. E. Stamm, and K. K. Holmes. 1985. *Campylobacter cinaedi* (sp. nov.) and *Campylobacter fennelliae* (sp. nov.): two new *Campylobacter* species associated with enteric disease in homosexual men. *J. Infect. Dis.* **151**:131–139.

130. Trebesius, K., K. Adler, M. Vieth, M. Stolte, and R. Haas. 2001. Specific detection and prevalence of *Helicobacter heilmannii*-like organisms in the human gastric mucosa by fluorescent in situ hybridization and partial 16S ribosomal DNA sequencing. *J. Clin. Microbiol.* **39**:1510–1516.

131. Uçkay, I., J. Garbino, P. Y. Dietrich, B. Ninet, P. Rohner, and V. Jacomo. 2006. Recurrent bacteraemia with *Helicobacter cinaedi*: case report and review of the literature. *BMC Infect. Dis.* **23**:86.

132. Vandamme, P., E. Falsen, R. Rossau, B. Hoste, P. Segers, R. Tytgat, and J. De Ley. 1991. Revision of *Campylobacter*, *Helicobacter*, and *Wolinella* taxonomy: emendation of generic descriptions and proposal of *Arcobacter* gen. nov. *Int. J. Syst. Bacteriol.* **41**:88–103.

133. Vandamme, P., C. S. Harrington, K. Jalava, and S. L. On. 2000. Misidentifying helicobacters: the *Helicobacter cinaedi* example. *J. Clin. Microbiol.* **38**:2261–2266.

134. Van den Bulck, K., A. Decostere, M. Baele, A. Driessen, J. C. Debongnie, A. Burette, M. Stolte, R. Ducatelle, and F. Haesebrouck. 2005. Identification of non-*Helicobacter pylori* spiral organisms in gastric samples from humans, dogs, and cats. *J. Clin. Microbiol.* **43**:2256–2260.

135. Veijola, L., A. Oksanen, A. Linnala, P. Sipponen, and H. Rautelin. 2007. Persisting chronic gastritis and elevated *Helicobacter pylori* antibodies after successful eradication therapy. *Helicobacter* **12**:605–608.

136. Veijola, L., A. Oksanen, P. Sipponen, and H. Rautelin. 2008. Evaluation of a commercial immunoblot, Helicoblot 2.1, for diagnosis of *Helicobacter pylori* infection. *Clin. Vaccine Immunol.* **15**:1705–1710.

137. Versalovic, J., D. Shortridge, K. Kibler, M. V. Griffy, J. Beyer, R. K. Flamm, S. K. Tanaka, D. Y. Graham, and M. F. Go. 1996. Mutations in 23S rRNA are associated with clarithromycin resistance in *Helicobacter pylori*. *Antimicrob. Agents Chemother.* **40**:477–480.

138. Warren, J. R., and B. J. Marshall. 1983. Unidentified curved bacilli on gastric epithelium in active chronic gastritis. *Lancet* **i**:1273–1275.

139. Watson, C. L., R. J. Owen, B. Said, S. Lai, J. V. Lee, S. Surman-Lee, and G. Nichols. 2004. Detection of *Helicobacter pylori* by PCR but not culture in water and biofilm samples from drinking water distribution systems in England. *J. Appl. Microbiol.* **97**:690–698.

140. Williams, M. P., J. C. Sercombe, A. J. Lawson, E. Slater, R. J. Owen, and R. E. Pounder. 1999. The effect of omeprazole dosing on the isolation of *Helicobacter pylori* from gastric aspirates. *Aliment. Pharmacol. Ther.* **13**:1161–1169.

141. Wundisch, T., C. Thiede, A. Morgner, A. Dempfle, A. Gunther, H. Liu, H. Ye, M. Q. Du, T. D. Kim, E. Bayerdorffer, M. Stolte, and A. Neubauer. 2005. Long-term follow-up of gastric MALT lymphoma after *Helicobacter pylori* eradication. *J. Clin. Oncol.* **23**:8018–8024.

142. Wueppenhorst, N., H. P. Stueger, M. Kist, and E. Glocker. 2009. Identification and molecular characterization of triple- and quadruple-resistant *Helicobacter pylori* clinical isolates in Germany. *J. Antimicrob. Chemother.* **63**:648–653.

143. Yousfi, M. M., H. M. El-Zimaity, R. A. Cole, R. M. Genta, and D. Y. Graham. 1997. Comparison of agar gel (CLOtest) or reagent strip (PyloriTek) rapid urease tests for detection of *Helicobacter pylori* infection. *Am. J. Gastroenterol.* **92**:997–999.

144. Zanoni, R. G., M. Rossi, D. Giacomucci, V. Sanguinetti, and G. Manfreda. 2007. Occurrence and antibiotic susceptibility of *Helicobacter pullorum* from broiler chickens and commercial laying hens in Italy. *Int. J. Food Microbiol.* **116**:168–173.

Leptospira

PAUL N. LEVETT

55

TAXONOMY

Serologic Classification

The genus *Leptospira* is comprised of spiral-shaped bacteria with hooked ends (29). This genus, along with the genera *Leptonema* and *Turneriella*, makes up the family *Leptospiraceae* within the order *Spirochaetales* and class *Spirochaetes* of the proposed phylum *Spirochaetes* (24). The genus was formerly divided into two species: *Leptospira interrogans*, comprising all pathogenic strains, and *L. biflexa*, containing the saprophytic strains isolated from the environment (29). *L. biflexa* and *L. interrogans* were differentiated by a number of biochemical tests (29).

Leptospires are divided into serovars defined by agglutination after cross-absorption with homologous antigen (15, 29, 31). Serovars are considered distinct if more than 10% of the homologous titer remains in at least one of the two antisera on repeated testing (65). Over 60 serovars of *L. biflexa* sensu lato and more than 200 serovars of *L. interrogans* sensu lato are recognized. Serovars that are antigenically related have traditionally been grouped into serogroups (31). Serogroups have no taxonomic standing, but the concept has proved useful for epidemiological understanding, particularly when interpreting the serological results from the microscopic agglutination test (MAT). The serogroups of *L. interrogans* sensu lato and some common serovars are shown in Table 1.

Genotypic Classification

The phenotypic classification of leptospires was replaced by a genotypic one, in which 20 genomospecies include all serovars of *Leptospira* (35, 43, 59, 60, 81). Table 2 lists all validly named species of *Leptospira*. DNA hybridization studies have also confirmed the taxonomic status of the monospecific genera *Leptonema* (6) and *Turneriella* (40). The genetically defined species of *Leptospira* do not correspond to the previous two species (*L. interrogans* sensu lato and *L. biflexa* sensu lato), and both pathogenic and nonpathogenic serovars occur within some species (36). Neither serogroup nor serovar reliably predicts the true species of *Leptospira*. Moreover, genetic heterogeneity resulting from horizontal transfer of genes coding for cell surface antigens occurs within serovars (6, 21), resulting in strains of some serovars being classified in multiple species (Table 3). In addition, the phenotypic characteristics formerly used to differentiate

L. interrogans sensu lato from *L. biflexa* sensu lato do not differentiate the genetically defined species (6, 81). Both *L. interrogans* and *L. biflexa* are retained as specific names in the genomic classification, and in this chapter, specific names refer to the genetically defined species, including *L. interrogans* sensu stricto and *L. biflexa* sensu stricto.

The molecular classification of leptospires requires the identification of both species and serovar of each isolate. Identification of *Leptospira* species is readily accomplished by *rrs* (16S rRNA gene) sequencing, and sequences are available in GenBank (48). Phylogenetic analysis of *rrs* sequences demonstrates three clades of leptospires, representing pathogens, saprophytes, and a group of species of uncertain pathogenicity (Fig. 1). However, sequences within the saprophyte clade differ by only a few base pairs. Other housekeeping gene sequences, such as *rpoB* (33) and *gyrB* (61), may provide better discrimination between species. Serovar identification is discussed below.

DESCRIPTION OF THE FAMILY

Leptospires are tightly coiled spirochetes, usually 0.1 μm by 6 to 20 μm. The helical conformation is right-handed, while the amplitude is approximately 0.1 to 0.15 μm and the wavelength approximately 0.5 μm (19). The cells have pointed ends, either or both of which are usually bent into a distinctive hook (Fig. 2). Two axial filaments (periplasmic flagella), with polar insertions, are located in the periplasmic space. Leptospires exhibit two distinct forms of movement, either translational (rapid back-and-forth movements) or rotational (spinning rapidly about the long axis of the cell) (26). Morphologically, all leptospires are indistinguishable.

Leptospires are obligate aerobes with an optimum growth temperature of 28 to 30°C. The optimum pH for growth is 7.2 to 7.6. They produce both catalase and oxidase. They grow in simple media enriched with vitamins (vitamins B2 and B12 are growth factors), long-chain fatty acids, and ammonium salts (29).

EPIDEMIOLOGY AND TRANSMISSION

Leptospires are ubiquitous, either free-living in water or associated with renal infection of animals (32). Leptospirosis is presumed to be the most widespread zoonosis in the

TABLE 1 Serogroups and selected serovars of *Leptospira interrogans* sensu lato

Serogroup	Serovars
Icterohaemorrhagiae	Copenhageni
	Icterohaemorrhagiae
	Lai
Hebdomadis	Hebdomadis
	Jules
Autumnalis	Autumnalis
	Bim
	Fortbragg
Pyrogenes	Pyrogenes
Bataviae	Bataviae
Grippotyphosa	Canalzonae
	Grippotyphosa
Canicola	Canicola
Australis	Australis
	Bratislava
Pomona	Pomona
Javanica	Arenal
	Javanica
Sejroe	Sejroe
	Hardjo
Panama	Mangus
	Panama
Cynopteri	Cynopteri
Djasiman	Djasiman
Sarmin	Sarmin
Mini	Mini
	Georgia
Tarassovi	Tarassovi
Ballum	Arborea
	Ballum
Celledoni	Celledoni
Louisiana	Lanka
	Louisiana
Ranarum	Ranarum
Manhao	Manhao
Shermani	Shermani
Hurstbridge	Hurstbridge

TABLE 2 Genospecies of *Leptospira*

L. alexanderi[a]
L. biflexa[b]
L. borgpetersenii[a]
L. broomii[c]
L. fainei[c]
L. inadai[c]
L. interrogans[a]
L. kirschneri[a]
L. kmetyi[a]
L. licerasiae[c]
L. meyeri[a]
L. noguchii[a]
L. santarosai[a]
L. weilii[a]
L. wolbachii[b]
L. wolffii[c]

[a]These species comprise the clade of pathogenic *Leptospira* species.
[b]Currently only nonpathogenic strains of these species are known.
[c]These species comprise the clade of *Leptospira* species intermediate between the pathogenic and nonpathogenic clades (Fig. 1).

world (79). The source of infection in humans is usually either direct or indirect contact with the urine of an infected animal. The incidence is very much higher in warm-climate countries than in temperate regions, due mainly to longer survival of leptospires in the environment in warm, humid conditions. Leptospirosis is seasonal. Peak incidence occurs in summer or fall in temperate regions, where temperature is the limiting factor in survival of leptospires, and during rainy seasons in warm-climate regions where rapid desiccation would otherwise prevent survival.

Animals, including humans, can be categorized as maintenance hosts or accidental (incidental) hosts. A maintenance host is defined as a species in which infection is endemic, usually transferred from animal to animal by direct contact. Infection is usually acquired at an early age, and the prevalence of chronic excretion in the urine increases with the age of the animal. Other animals (such as humans) may become infected by indirect contact with the maintenance host. Animals may be maintenance hosts of some serovars but incidental hosts of others, infection with which may cause severe or fatal disease. The most important maintenance hosts are small mammals, which

may transfer infection to domestic farm animals, dogs, and humans. Different rodent species may be reservoirs of distinct serovars, but rats are generally maintenance hosts for serovars of the serogroup Icterohaemorrhagiae serovars, and mice for serogroup Ballum serovars. Domestic animals are also maintenance hosts; dairy cattle may harbor serovars Hardjo and Pomona, pigs Pomona, Tarassovi, or Bratislava, and dogs Canicola. Distinct variations in maintenance hosts and the serovars they carry occur throughout the world, and these associations may change over time.

Knowledge of the prevalent serovars and their maintenance hosts is essential in understanding the epidemiology of the disease. For example, canine leptospirosis is increasing in the northeastern region of North America. Very few cases have been diagnosed by culture, but serology suggests that they are caused largely by serovar Grippotyphosa (7, 76). Epidemiological evidence implicates raccoons and possibly skunks as the reservoir. Cases are clustered particularly in newly suburbanized areas (76). This change in epidemiology has led to the inclusion of serovars Grippotyphosa and Pomona in canine vaccines.

Human infections may be acquired through occupational, recreational, or avocational exposures. Occupation

TABLE 3 Leptospiral serovars found in multiple species[a]

Serovar	Species
Bataviae	*L. interrogans, L. santarosai*
Bulgarica	*L. interrogans, L. kirschneri*
Grippotyphosa	*L. kirschneri, L. interrogans*
Hardjo	*L. borgpetersenii, L. interrogans, L. meyeri*
Icterohaemorrhagiae	*L. interrogans, L. inadai*
Kremastos	*L. interrogans, L. santarosai*
Mwogolo	*L. kirschneri, L. interrogans*
Paidjan	*L. kirschneri, L. interrogans*
Pomona	*L. interrogans, L. noguchii*
Pyrogenes	*L. interrogans, L. santarosai*
Szwajizak	*L. interrogans, L. santarosai*
Valbuzzi	*L. interrogans, L. kirschneri*

[a]Based on data reported by Brenner et al. (6) and by Feresu et al. (21).

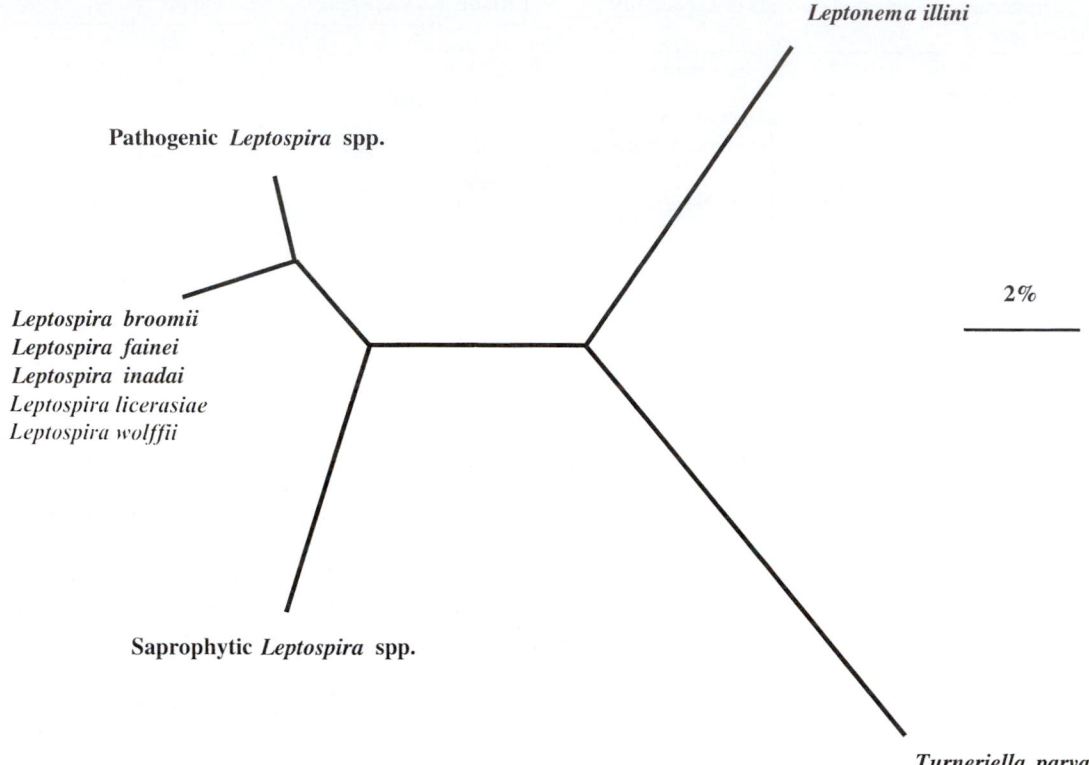

FIGURE 1 Phylogenetic relationships based on *rrs* (16S rRNA gene) sequences between the genera of the *Leptospiraceae*. The scale bar represents a 2% difference in sequence.

remains a significant risk factor for humans. Direct contact with infected animals accounts for most infections in farmers, veterinarians, abattoir workers, rodent control workers, and those in other occupations which require contact with animals, while indirect contact is important for sewer workers, miners, soldiers, septic tank cleaners, fish farmers, rice field workers, and sugar cane cutters. Livestock farming is a major occupational risk factor throughout the world. The highest risk is associated with dairy farming, in particular with milking of dairy cattle, and is associated with serovar Hardjo. There is a significant risk associated with recreational exposures occurring in water sports (47). The increasing popularity of adventure sports and ecotourism has led to an increase in leptospirosis in travelers (34).

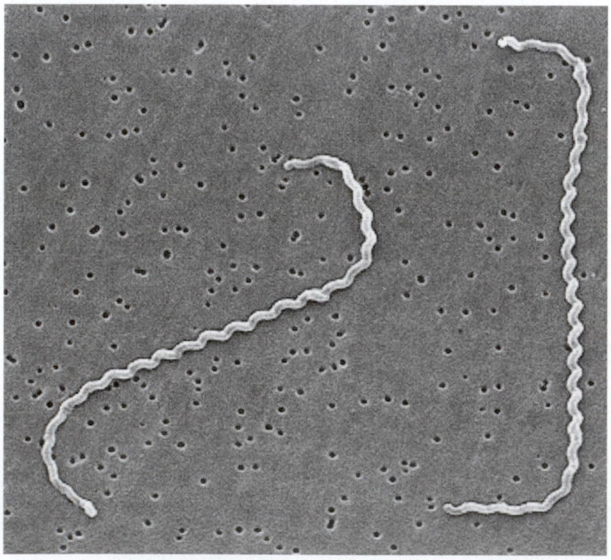

CLINICAL SIGNIFICANCE

The usual portal of entry is through abrasions or cuts in the skin, or via the conjunctiva. The great majority of infections are either subclinical or of very mild severity, and patients generally do not seek or are not brought to medical attention. The clinical presentation of leptospirosis is biphasic, with a septicemic phase lasting about a week, followed by the immune phase, characterized by antibody production and excretion of leptospires in the urine. Most of the complications of leptospirosis are associated with localization of leptospires within the tissues during the immune phase, and thus occur during the second week of the illness.

The overwhelming majority of the recognized cases present with a febrile illness of sudden onset, the symptoms of which include chills, headache, myalgia, abdominal pain, and conjunctival suffusion. Aseptic meningitis may be found in ≤25% of all leptospirosis cases. Between 5 and 10% of all patients with leptospirosis have the icteric form of the disease (Weil's disease), in which the clinical course is often very rapidly progressive. In addition to jaundice, patients with icteric leptospirosis may develop acute renal failure, pulmonary

FIGURE 2 Scanning electron micrograph of leptospiral cells bound to a 0.2-μm-pore-size filter. Magnification, approximately ×3,500. Source: Public Health Image Library.

hemorrhage, and cardiac arrhythmias. Severe cases often present late in the course of the disease, and this contributes to the high mortality rate, which ranges between 5 and 15%.

COLLECTION, TRANSPORT, AND STORAGE OF SPECIMENS

Leptospires can be isolated from blood, cerebrospinal fluid (CSF), and peritoneal dialysate fluids during the first 10 days of illness. Specimens should be collected before antibiotic therapy is initiated and while the patient is febrile. Under optimal conditions, 1 or 2 drops of venous blood are inoculated directly into culture medium at the bedside. Survival of leptospires in commercial blood culture media for several days has been reported (52). There are no transport media available, but blood can be collected and shipped at ambient temperature in tubes containing heparin, oxalate, or citrate (19). Citrate- or EDTA-containing tubes are optimal for PCR detection, whereas tubes containing heparin, sodium polyanethol sulfonate, or saponin are inhibitory to PCRs (41, 64).

Urine can be cultured after the first week of illness. Specimens should be collected aseptically into sterile containers without preservatives and must be processed within a short time of collection; the best results are obtained when the delay is less than 1 h. If culture is not possible, urine specimens intended for PCR testing may be stabilized using one of several commercial products for this purpose, allowing for transport over long distances (41).

DIRECT EXAMINATION

Microscopy

Leptospires may be visualized in clinical material by dark-field microscopy ($\times$100 and $\times$400 magnification) or by immunofluorescence or light microscopy after appropriate staining. Dark-field microscopic examination of body fluids such as blood, urine, CSF, or dialysate fluid is insensitive and lacks specificity (75). Approximately 10^4 leptospires/ml are necessary for one cell per field to be visible by dark-field microscopy (72). Direct dark-field microscopy of blood is also subject to misinterpretation of fibrin or protein threads, which may demonstrate Brownian motion (19, 72). Leptospires in tissues were first visualized by silver staining (66), and the Warthin-Starry stain is widely used for histologic examination. More recently, immunohistochemical methods have been applied (73, 82). Immunohistochemical staining can be performed at the Centers for Disease Control and Prevention (CDC), Atlanta, GA (contact Sherif Zaki [szaki@cdc.gov]).

Antigen Detection

Antigen detection is generally regarded as insensitive. There are no commercial antigen detection assays.

Nucleic Acid Techniques

Several primer pairs for detection of leptospire nucleic acids by conventional PCR have been described (36). Two methods subjected to extensive clinical evaluation (9, 45) were found to be more sensitive than culture, and leptospiral DNA has been amplified from serum, urine, aqueous humor, CSF, and tissues obtained at autopsy (8, 45). Both studies showed that the sensitivity of PCR was comparable to that of serologic diagnosis by testing acute- and convalescent-phase sera using the MAT, while offering more rapid diagnosis, during the acute illness (9, 45).

Real-time PCR assays have been developed, targeting either *rrs* or pathogen-specific sequences (20, 41, 46, 51, 58, 67). These assays have yet to be evaluated in large clinical studies, but they appear to be comparable in sensitivity with culture (58). Real-time PCR assays have been applied to quantify the burden of infecting organisms in human cases and animal models (23, 42, 57). A limitation of PCR-based diagnosis of leptospirosis is the inability of most PCR assays to identify the infecting serovar. While this is not significant for individual patient management, the identity of the serovar has both epidemiological and public health value.

ISOLATION PROCEDURES

Leptospiremia occurs during the first stage of the disease, beginning before the onset of symptoms, and has usually finished by the end of the first week of the acute illness (44). Therefore, blood cultures should be taken as soon as possible after the patient's presentation. One or two drops of blood (approximately 50 µl) are inoculated into 10-ml semisolid oleic acid-albumin medium (18, 30), such as Ellinghausen-McCullough-Johnson-Harris (EMJH) medium or Fletcher's medium (Difco EMJH or Difco Fletcher's medium; BD Diagnostic Systems, Sparks, MD), containing 0.1% agar and 200 µg of 5-fluorouracil/ml, at the patient's bedside. Blood is allowed to drop onto the surface of the medium; mixing is not necessary. Care should be taken to avoid overinoculation of the medium, as blood contains inhibitors of leptospiral growth. For the greatest recovery rate, multiple cultures should be performed, but this is rarely possible. Survival of leptospires in commercial blood culture media for up to a week has been reported (25, 52). Since the organism does not grow in conventional media, positive signals in automated systems are most unlikely. However, if a diagnosis of leptospirosis is suspected after the collection of conventional blood cultures, it is possible to detect leptospires using PCR assays.

Other samples that can be cultured during the first week of illness include CSF and peritoneal dialysate. Urine cultures can yield growth from the beginning of the second week of symptomatic illness. Survival of leptospires in voided human urine is limited, so urine should be processed immediately, by neutralization of pH with sodium bicarbonate followed by centrifugation. After centrifugation in 15-ml tubes for 30 min at 1,500 $\times$ g, the sediment is resuspended in 1 ml of phosphate-buffered saline and 1 or 2 drops are inoculated into semisolid EMJH medium containing 5-fluorouracil as described above.

Cultures in EMJH medium are incubated in sealed bottles at 28 to 30°C and examined weekly by dark-field microscopy for up to 13 weeks before being discarded. Growth often develops in a discrete band, several millimeters below the surface of the medium, known as a Dinger's ring. Cultures that show growth of other bacteria may be passed through a 0.2- or 0.45-µm-pore-size filter before subculture into fresh medium.

IDENTIFICATION

Isolated leptospires are identified either by serologic methods or, more recently, by molecular techniques. Traditional methods relied on cross-agglutinin absorption (15). The number of laboratories that can perform these identification methods is very small. The use of panels of monoclonal antibodies allows laboratories which can perform the MAT to identify isolates of frequently encountered serovars with relative rapidity (69). Monoclonal antibodies are available from the WHO/OIE Leptospirosis Reference Laboratory at the Royal Tropical Institute, Amsterdam, The Netherlands.

The molecularly based taxonomy of *Leptospira* necessitates the identification of isolates to both the species and serovar levels. Species identification is most practically done by sequence analysis (11), using *rrs* (16s rRNA) (48), *gyrB* (61), *rpoB* (33), or *secY* (74).

TYPING PROCEDURES

Because of the difficulties associated with serologic identification of leptospiral isolates, there has been great interest in molecular methods for identification and subtyping (11). Methods employed have included digestion of chromosomal DNA by restriction endonucleases, restriction fragment length polymorphisms, ribotyping, pulsed-field gel electrophoresis, and a number of PCR-based approaches (11). The most widely applicable molecular method for identification of serovars is pulsed-field gel electrophoresis, because this technique is widely used for infection control studies and for public health typing of enteric pathogens (22, 28). This approach has been standardized, using the PulseNet model, in which standardized profiles can be exchanged electronically (22).

More recently, the availability of the full genome sequences of several *Leptospira* strains has led to the development of sequence-based methods, such as amplified fragment length polymorphism and variable-number tandem-repeat methods. Several studies have applied multilocus sequence typing to understand the epidemiology of leptospirosis (2, 70). The application of these powerful tools will lead to greater understanding of leptospiral epidemiology at a population level (11, 37).

SEROLOGIC TESTS

Most cases of leptospirosis are diagnosed by serology. Antibodies are detectable in the blood approximately 5 to 7 days after the onset of symptoms. The definitive serologic investigation in leptospirosis remains the MAT, in which patients' sera are reacted with live or killed antigen suspensions of leptospiral serovars. After incubation, the serum-antigen mixtures are examined microscopically for agglutination and the titers are determined. The MAT is a complex test to control, perform, and interpret (71), the use of which is limited to regional or national reference laboratories. Protocols for performing the MAT have been described in detail elsewhere (3, 19). An international proficiency testing scheme under the auspices of the International Leptospirosis Society has stimulated improvement in the performance of the MAT by participating laboratories (12). The range of antigens used should include serovars representative of all serogroups (19, 71). The wide range of antigens is used in order to detect infections with uncommon, or previously undetected, serovars. The test is read by dark-field microscopy. The endpoint is the highest dilution of serum in which 50% agglutination occurs and is determined by the presence of approximately 50% free, unagglutinated leptospires, by comparison with the control suspension (19). Considerable effort is required to reduce the subjective effect of observer variation, even within laboratories.

Interpretation of the MAT is complicated by the high degree of cross-reaction that occurs between different serogroups, especially in acute-phase samples. Paradoxical reactions, in which the highest titers are detected to a serogroup unrelated to the infecting one, are also common (36). The broad cross-reactivity in the acute phase, followed by relative serogroup specificity in convalescent-phase samples, results from the detection in the MAT of both immunoglobulin M (IgM) and IgG antibodies and the presence of several common antigens among leptospires (1).

Paired sera are required to confirm a diagnosis with certainty. A fourfold or greater rise in titer between paired sera confirms the diagnosis, regardless of the interval between samples. The interval between first and second samples depends very much on the delay between onset of symptoms and presentation of the patient. If symptoms typical of leptospirosis are present, an interval of 3 to 5 days may be adequate to detect rising titers. However, if the patient presents earlier in the course of the disease, or if the date of onset is not known precisely, then an interval of 10 to 14 days between samples is more appropriate. Less often, seroconversion does not occur with such rapidity, and a longer interval between samples (or repeated sampling) is necessary. MAT serology is insensitive, particularly in early acute-phase specimens (5, 14). Moreover, patients with fulminant leptospirosis may die before seroconversion occurs (14, 55).

A presumptive diagnosis can be made by detection of a single elevated titer in association with an acute febrile illness. The magnitude of such a titer is dependent upon the background level of exposure in the population, and hence the seroprevalence. In the current CDC case definition, a titer of ≥200 in a patient with a clinically compatible illness is used to indicate a probable case (10).

Titers following acute infection may be extremely high (≥25,600) and may take months, or even years, to fall to low levels (13, 56). Thus, in a high-incidence population, a low cutoff titer for presumptive diagnosis is inappropriate and will generate many false-positive diagnoses. In areas where leptospirosis is endemic, a single titer of ≥800 in symptomatic patients is generally indicative of leptospirosis, but titers as high as ≥1,600 have been recommended (3). Rarely, seroconversion may be delayed for many weeks after recovery, and longer serologic follow-up will be necessary to confirm the diagnosis.

Formalized antigens have been used in the MAT in order to overcome some of the difficulties associated with the use of live antigens. Titers obtained with these antigens are somewhat lower, and more cross-reactions are detected (19). These antigens are not available commercially but may be obtained from WHO Collaborating Centres.

The MAT is the most appropriate test to employ in epidemiological serosurveys, since it can be applied to sera from any animal species, and because the range of antigens utilized can be expanded or decreased as required. It is usual to use a titer of ≥100 as evidence of past exposure (71). Contrary to a widely held belief, the MAT is a serogroup-specific assay. However, conclusions about infecting serovars cannot be drawn without isolates; at best, the MAT data can give a general impression of which serogroups are present within a population (38).

Because of the complexity of the MAT, rapid screening tests for leptospiral antibodies in acute infection have been developed. Traditional methods based upon agglutination have largely been superceded by IgM detection assays. IgM antibodies become detectable during the first week of illness, allowing the diagnosis to be confirmed and treatment to be initiated while it is likely to be most effective. IgM detection has repeatedly been shown to be more sensitive than the MAT when the first specimen is taken early in the acute phase of the illness (14, 77). IgM dipstick assays have been shown to be as sensitive as microtiter plate IgM enzyme-linked immunosorbent assay (4, 27, 39). Other rapid assays include a latex agglutination assay (63) and a lateral-flow assay (62).

ANTIMICROBIAL SUSCEPTIBILITIES

Leptospires are susceptible to many antimicrobial agents, including β-lactams, macrolides, tetracyclines, fluoroquinolones, and streptomycin. Problems in the determination of susceptibility include the long incubation time required (17), the use of media containing serum (50, 80), and the difficulty in quantifying growth accurately. These constraints limited the development of rapid, standardized methods for susceptibility testing. However, broth microdilution methods have been described recently (49) which have facilitated the testing of larger numbers of isolates against a wide range of antimicrobial agents (54). Such studies are expected to lead to the identification of potential new agents for inclusion in clinical trials.

Penicillin and doxycycline are both effective for treatment of leptospirosis and remain the drugs of choice (16); clinical studies have shown that broad-spectrum cephalosporins may be equally effective (53, 68). Prophylaxis with doxycycline is effective at preventing disease but not seroconversion (16).

EVALUATION, INTERPRETATION, AND REPORTING OF RESULTS

A diagnosis of leptospirosis can be made by isolation of the organism or by amplification of leptospiral DNA from blood, urine, or other specimens, by demonstration of leptospires in tissues by immunohistochemical staining, or by detection of a fourfold or greater rise in titers between acute- and convalescent-phase serum samples tested by the same methodology at the same time. In populations and/or regions where leptospirosis is not endemic, MAT titers of ≥200 in a single specimen obtained after the onset of symptoms are suggestive but not diagnostic of acute or recent leptospirosis. A titer of ≥800 in the presence of compatible symptoms is strong evidence of recent or current leptospirosis. Delayed seroconversions are common. Assays that detect IgM antibodies give presumptive evidence of recent exposure to leptospirosis but require confirmation by another method, since IgM titers are persistent (13). Negative test results in the presence of compatible symptoms do not rule out the diagnosis of leptospirosis, and further samples should be examined. The isolation of leptospires, the demonstration of leptospiral DNA by molecular methods, or the detection of leptospires in tissues by immunohistochemistry confirms the diagnosis and differentiates between current infection and past exposure, which may not be clearly differentiated by serology.

Despite recent advances in molecular detection and characterization of leptospires and in the development of rapid serologic tests, there are still relatively few laboratories throughout the world with the appropriate capabilities

for *Leptospira* diagnostics. Additional information regarding leptospirosis and diagnostic centers of expertise (78) is available for downloading from the International Leptospirosis Society website (http://www.med.monash.edu.au/microbiology/staff/adler/ils.html).

REFERENCES

1. **Adler, B., and S. Faine.** 1978. The antibodies involved in the human immune response to leptospiral infection. *J. Med. Microbiol.* **11:**387–400.
2. **Ahmed, N., S. M. Devi, L. Valverde Mde, P. Vijayachari, R. S. Machang'u, W. A. Ellis, and R. A. Hartskeerl.** 2006. Multilocus sequence typing method for identification and genotypic classification of pathogenic *Leptospira* species. *Ann. Clin. Microbiol. Antimicrob.* **5:**28.
3. **Alexander, A. D.** 1986. Serological diagnosis of leptospirosis, p. 435–439. *In* N. R. Rose, H. Friedman, and J. L. Fahey (ed.), *Manual of Clinical Laboratory Immunology*, 3rd ed. American Society for Microbiology, Washington, DC.
4. **Bajani, M. D., D. A. Ashford, S. L. Bragg, C. W. Woods, T. Aye, R. A. Spiegel, B. D. Plikaytis, B. A. Perkins, M. Phelan, P. N. Levett, and R. S. Weyant.** 2003. Evaluation of four commercially available rapid serologic tests for diagnosis of leptospirosis. *J. Clin. Microbiol.* **41:**803–809.
5. **Brandão, A. P., E. D. Camargo, E. D. da Silva, M. V. Silva, and R. V. Abrão.** 1998. Macroscopic agglutination test for rapid diagnosis of human leptospirosis. *J. Clin. Microbiol.* **36:**3138–3142.
6. **Brenner, D. J., A. F. Kaufmann, K. R. Sulzer, A. G. Steigerwalt, F. C. Rogers, and R. S. Weyant.** 1999. Further determination of DNA relatedness between serogroups and serovars in the family *Leptospiraceae* with a proposal for *Leptospira alexanderi* sp. nov. and four new *Leptospira* genomospecies. *Int. J. Syst. Bacteriol.* **49:**839–858.
7. **Brown, C. A., A. W. Roberts, M. A. Miller, D. A. David, S. A. Brown, C. A. Bolin, J. Jarecki-Black, C. E. Greene, and D. Miller-Liebl.** 1996. *Leptospira interrogans* serovar *grippotyphosa* infection in dogs. *J. Am. Vet. Med. Assoc.* **209:**1265–1267.
8. **Brown, P. D., D. G. Carrington, H. van de Kemp, C. N. Edwards, S. R. Jones, P. R. Prussia, S. Garriques, W. J. Terpstra, and P. N. Levett.** 2003. Direct detection of leptospiral material in human postmortem samples. *Res. Microbiol.* **154:**581–586.
9. **Brown, P. D., C. Gravekamp, D. G. Carrington, H. Van de Kemp, R. A. Hartskeerl, C. N. Edwards, C. O. R. Everard, W. J. Terpstra, and P. N. Levett.** 1995. Evaluation of the polymerase chain reaction for early diagnosis of leptospirosis. *J. Med. Microbiol.* **43:**110–114.
10. **Centers for Disease Control and Prevention.** 1997. Case definitions for infectious conditions under public health surveillance. *MMWR Morb. Mortal. Wkly. Rep.* **46**(RR-10):49.
11. **Cerqueira, G. M., and M. Picardeau.** 2009. A century of *Leptospira* strain typing. *Infect. Genet. Evol.* **9:**760–768.
12. **Chappel, R. J., M. G. Goris, M. F. Palmer, and R. A. Hartskeerl.** 2004. Impact of proficiency testing on results of the microscopic agglutination test for diagnosis of leptospirosis. *J. Clin. Microbiol.* **42:**5484–5488.
13. **Cumberland, P., C. O. R. Everard, J. G. Wheeler, and P. N. Levett.** 2001. Persistence of anti-leptospiral IgM, IgG and agglutinating antibodies in patients presenting with acute febrile illness in Barbados 1979–1989. *Eur. J. Epidemiol.* **17:**601–608.
14. **Cumberland, P. C., C. O. R. Everard, and P. N. Levett.** 1999. Assessment of the efficacy of the IgM enzyme-linked immunosorbent assay (ELISA) and microscopic agglutination test (MAT) in the diagnosis of acute leptospirosis. *Am. J. Trop. Med. Hyg.* **61:**731–734.
15. **Dikken, H., and E. Kmety.** 1978. Serological typing methods of leptospires. *Methods Microbiol.* **11:**259–307.
16. **Edwards, C. N., and P. N. Levett.** 2004. Prevention and treatment of leptospirosis. *Expert Rev. Anti-Infect. Ther.* **2:**293–298.

17. **Ellinghausen, H. C.** 1983. Growth, cultural characteristics, and antibacterial sensitivity of *Leptospira interrogans* serovar *hardjo. Cornell Vet.* **73:**225–239.

18. **Ellinghausen, H. C., and W. G. McCullough.** 1965. Nutrition of *Leptospira pomona* and growth of 13 other serotypes: fractionation of oleic albumin complex and a medium of bovine albumin and polysorbate 80. *Am. J. Vet. Res.* **26:**45–51.

19. **Faine, S., B. Adler, C. Bolin, and P. Perolat.** 1999. Leptospira *and Leptospirosis*, 2nd ed. MedSci, Melbourne, Australia.

20. **Fearnley, C., P. R. Wakeley, J. Gallego-Beltran, C. Dalley, S. Williamson, C. Gaudie, and M. J. Woodward.** 2008. The development of a real-time PCR to detect pathogenic *Leptospira* species in kidney tissue. *Res. Vet. Sci.* **85:**8–16.

21. **Feresu, S. B., C. A. Bolin, H. van de Kemp, and H. Korver.** 1999. Identification of a serogroup Bataviae *Leptospira* strain isolated from an ox in Zimbabwe. *Zentralbl. Bakteriol.* **289:**19–29.

22. **Galloway, R. L., and P. N. Levett.** 2010. Application and validation of PFGE for serovas identification of *Leptospira* clinical isolates. *PLoS Neglected Trop. Dis.* **4:**e824.

23. **Ganoza, C. A., M. A. Matthias, D. Collins-Richards, K. C. Brouwer, C. B. Cunningham, E. R. Segura, R. H. Gilman, E. Gotuzzo, and J. M. Vinetz.** 2006. Determining risk for severe leptospirosis by molecular analysis of environmental surface waters for pathogenic *Leptospira. PLoS Med.* **3:**1329–1340.

24. **Garrity, G. M., and J. G. Holt.** 2001. The road map to the Manual, p. 119–166. *In* D. R. Boone, R. W. Castenholtz, and G. M. Garrity (ed.), *Bergey's Manual of Systematic Bacteriology*, 2nd ed., vol. 1. Springer-Verlag, New York, NY.

25. **Gelman, S. S., A. V. Gundlapalli, D. Hale, A. Croft, M. Hindiyeh, and K. C. Carroll.** 2002. Spotting the spirochete: rapid diagnosis of leptospirosis in two returned travelers. *J. Travel Med.* **9:**165–167.

26. **Goldstein, S. F., and N. W. Charon.** 1988. Motility of the spirochete *Leptospira. Cell Motil. Cytoskeleton* **9:**101–110.

27. **Gussenhoven, G. C., M. A. W. G. van der Hoorn, M. G. A. Goris, W. J. Terpstra, R. A. Hartskeerl, B. W. Mol, C. W. van Ingen, and H. L. Smits.** 1997. LEPTO dipstick, a dipstick assay for detection of *Leptospira*-specific immunoglobulin M antibodies in human sera. *J. Clin. Microbiol.* **35:**92–97.

28. **Herrmann, J. L., E. Bellenger, P. Perolat, G. Baranton, and I. Saint Girons.** 1992. Pulsed-field gel electrophoresis of NotI digests of leptospiral DNA: a new rapid method of serovar identification. *J. Clin. Microbiol.* **30:**1696–1702.

29. **Johnson, R. C., and S. Faine.** 1984. *Leptospira*, p. 62–67. *In* N. R. Krieg and J. G. Holt (ed.), *Bergey's Manual of Systematic Bacteriology*, vol. 1. Williams & Wilkins, Baltimore, MD.

30. **Johnson, R. C., and V. G. Harris.** 1967. Differentiation of pathogenic and saprophytic leptospires. 1. Growth at low temperatures. *J. Bacteriol.* **94:**27–31.

31. **Kmety, E., and H. Dikken.** 1993. Classification of the species *Leptospira interrogans* and history of its serovars. University Press Groningen, Groningen, The Netherlands.

32. **Ko, A. I., C. Goarant, and M. Picardeau.** 2009. Leptospira: the dawn of the molecular genetics era for an emerging zoonotic pathogen. *Nat. Rev. Microbiol.* **7:**736–747.

33. **La Scola, B., L. T. M. Bui, G. Baranton, A. Khamis, and D. Raoult.** 2006. Partial *rpoB* gene sequencing for identification of *Leptospira* species. *FEMS Microbiol. Lett.* **263:**142–147.

34. **Lau, C., L. Smythe, and P. Weinstein.** 2010. Leptospirosis: an emerging disease in travellers. *Travel Med. Infect. Dis.* **8:**33–39.

35. **Levett, P. N.** 2007. *Leptospira*, p. 963–970. *In* P. R. Murray, E. J. Baron, J. H. Jorgensen, M. L. Landry, and M. A. Pfaller (ed.), *Manual of Clinical Microbiology*, 9th ed. ASM Press, Washington, DC.

36. **Levett, P. N.** 2001. Leptospirosis. *Clin. Microbiol. Rev.* **14:**296–326.

37. **Levett, P. N.** 2007. Sequence-based typing of *Leptospira*: epidemiology in the genomic era. *PLoS Neglected Trop. Dis.* **1:**e120.

38. **Levett, P. N.** 2003. Usefulness of serologic analysis as a predictor of the infecting serovar in patients with severe leptospirosis. *Clin. Infect. Dis.* **36:**447–452.

39. **Levett, P. N., S. L. Branch, C. U. Whittington, C. N. Edwards, and H. Paxton.** 2001. Two methods for rapid serological diagnosis of acute leptospirosis. *Clin. Diagn. Lab. Immunol.* **8:**349–351.

40. **Levett, P. N., R. E. Morey, R. Galloway, A. G. Steigerwalt, and W. A. Ellis.** 2005. Reclassification of *Leptospira parva* Hovind-Hougen et al. 1982 as *Turneriella parva* gen. nov., comb. nov. *Int. J. Syst. Evol. Microbiol.* **55:**1497–1499.

41. **Levett, P. N., R. E. Morey, R. L. Galloway, D. E. Turner, A. G. Steigerwalt, and L. W. Mayer.** 2005. Detection of pathogenic leptospires by real-time quantitative PCR. *J. Med. Microbiol.* **54:**45–49.

42. **Lourdault, K., F. Aviat, and M. Picardeau.** 2009. Use of quantitative real-time PCR for studying the dissemination of *Leptospira interrogans* in the guinea pig infection model of leptospirosis. *J. Med. Microbiol.* **58:**648–655.

43. **Matthias, M. A., J. N. Ricaldi, M. Cespedes, M. M. Diaz, R. L. Galloway, M. Saito, A. G. Steigerwalt, K. P. Patra, C. V. Ore, E. Gotuzzo, R. H. Gilman, P. N. Levett, and J. M. Vinetz.** 2008. Human leptospirosis caused by a new, antigenically unique *Leptospira* associated with a *Rattus* species reservoir in the Peruvian Amazon. *PLoS Neglected Trop. Dis.* **2:**e213.

44. **McCrumb, F. R., J. L. Stockard, C. R. Robinson, L. H. Turner, D. G. Levis, C. W. Maisey, M. F. Kelleher, C. A. Gleiser, and J. E. Smadel.** 1957. Leptospirosis in Malaya. I. Sporadic cases among military and civilian personnel. *Am. J. Trop. Med. Hyg.* **6:**238–256.

45. **Merien, F., G. Baranton, and P. Pérolat.** 1995. Comparison of polymerase chain reaction with microagglutination test and culture for diagnosis of leptospirosis. *J. Infect. Dis.* **172:**281–285.

46. **Merien, F., D. Portnoi, P. Bourhy, F. Charavay, A. Berlioz-Arthaud, and G. Baranton.** 2005. A rapid and quantitative method for the detection of *Leptospira* species in human leptospirosis. *FEMS Microbiol. Lett.* **249:**139–147.

47. **Monahan, A. M., I. S. Miller, and J. E. Nally.** 2009. Leptospirosis: risks during recreational activities. *J. Appl. Microbiol.* **107:**707–716.

48. **Morey, R. E., R. L. Galloway, S. L. Bragg, A. G. Steigerwalt, L. W. Mayer, and P. N. Levett.** 2006. Species-specific identification of *Leptospiraceae* by 16S rRNA gene sequencing. *J. Clin. Microbiol.* **44:**3510–3516.

49. **Murray, C. K., and D. R. Hospenthal.** 2004. Broth microdilution susceptibility testing for *Leptospira* spp. *Antimicrob. Agents Chemother.* **48:**1548–1552.

50. **Oie, S., K. Hironaga, A. Koshiro, H. Konishi, and Z. Yoshii.** 1983. In vitro susceptibilities of five *Leptospira* strains to 16 antimicrobial agents. *Antimicrob. Agents Chemother.* **24:**905–908.

51. **Palaniappan, R. U., Y. F. Chang, C. F. Chang, M. J. Pan, C. W. Yang, P. Harpending, S. P. McDonough, E. Dubovi, T. Divers, J. Qu, and B. Roe.** 2005. Evaluation of *lig*-based conventional and real time PCR for the detection of pathogenic leptospires. *Mol. Cell. Probes* **19:**111–117.

52. **Palmer, M. F., and W. J. Zochowski.** 2000. Survival of leptospires in commercial blood culture systems revisited. *J. Clin. Pathol.* **53:**713–714.

53. **Panaphut, T., S. Domrongkitchaiporn, A. Vibhagool, B. Thinkamrop, and W. Susaengrat.** 2003. Ceftriaxone compared with sodium penicillin G for treatment of severe leptospirosis. *Clin. Infect. Dis.* **36:**1507–1513.

54. **Ressner, R. A., M. E. Griffith, M. L. Beckius, G. Pimentel, R. S. Miller, K. Mende, S. L. Fraser, R. L. Galloway, D. R. Hospenthal, and C. K. Murray.** 2008. Antimicrobial susceptibilities of geographically diverse clinical human isolates of *Leptospira. Antimicrob. Agents Chemother.* **52:**2750–2754.

55. **Ribeiro, M. A., C. S. N. Assis, and E. C. Romero.** 1994. Serodiagnosis of human leptospirosis employing immunodominant antigen. *Serodiagn. Immunother. Infect. Dis.* **6:**140–144.

56. **Romero, E. C., C. R. Caly, and P. H. Yasuda.** 1998. The persistence of leptospiral agglutinins titers in human sera diagnosed by the microscopic agglutination test. *Rev. Inst. Med. Trop. São Paulo* **40:**183–184.

57. **Segura, E. R., C. A. Ganoza, K. Campos, J. N. Ricaldi, S. Torres, H. Silva, M. J. Cespedes, M. A. Matthias, M. A. Swancutt,**

R. Lopez Linan, E. Gotuzzo, H. Guerra, R. H. Gilman, and J. M. Vinetz. 2005. Clinical spectrum of pulmonary involvement in leptospirosis in a region of endemicity, with quantification of leptospiral burden. *Clin. Infect. Dis.* **40:**343–351.

58. Slack, A., M. Symonds, M. Dohnt, C. Harris, D. Brookes, and L. Smythe. 2007. Evaluation of a modified Taqman assay detecting pathogenic *Leptospira* spp. against culture and *Leptospira*-specific IgM enzyme-linked immunosorbent assay in a clinical environment. *Diagn. Microbiol. Infect. Dis.* **57:**361–366.

59. Slack, A. T., T. Kalambaheti, M. L. Symonds, M. F. Dohnt, R. L. Galloway, A. G. Steigerwalt, W. Chaicumpa, G. Bunyaraksyotin, S. Craig, B. J. Harrower, and L. D. Smythe. 2008. *Leptospira wolffii* sp. nov., isolated from a human with suspected leptospirosis in Thailand. *Int. J. Syst. Evol. Microbiol.* **58:**2305–2308.

60. Slack, A. T., S. Khairani-Bejo, M. L. Symonds, M. F. Dohnt, R. L. Galloway, A. G. Steigerwalt, A. R. Bahaman, S. Craig, B. J. Harrower, and L. D. Smythe. 2009. *Leptospira kmetyi* sp. nov., isolated from an environmental source in Malaysia. *Int. J. Syst. Evol. Microbiol.* **59:**705–708.

61. Slack, A. T., M. L. Symonds, M. F. Dohnt, and L. D. Smythe. 2006. Identification of pathogenic *Leptospira* species by conventional or real-time PCR and sequencing of the DNA gyrase subunit B encoding gene. *BMC Microbiol.* **6:**95.

62. Smits, H. L., C. K. Eapen, S. Sugathan, M. Kuriakose, M. H. Gasem, C. Yersin, D. Sasaki, B. Pujianto, M. Vestering, T. H. Abdoel, and G. C. Gussenhoven. 2001. Lateral-flow assay for rapid serodiagnosis of human leptospirosis. *Clin. Diagn. Lab. Immunol.* **8:**166–169.

63. Smits, H. L., M. A. van Der Hoorn, M. G. Goris, G. C. Gussenhoven, C. Yersin, D. M. Sasaki, W. J. Terpstra, and R. A. Hartskeerl. 2000. Simple latex agglutination assay for rapid serodiagnosis of human leptospirosis. *J. Clin. Microbiol.* **38:**1272–1275.

64. Smythe, L. D., I. L. Smith, G. A. Smith, M. F. Dohnt, M. L. Symonds, L. J. Barnett, and D. B. McKay. 2002. A quantitative PCR (TaqMan) assay for pathogenic *Leptospira* spp. *BMC Infect. Dis.* **2:**13.

65. Stallman, N. D. 1987. International Committee on Systematic Bacteriology Subcommittee on the Taxonomy of *Leptospira*. Minutes of the meeting, 5 and 6 September 1986, Manchester, England. *Int. J. Syst. Bacteriol.* **37:**472–473.

66. Stimson, A. M. 1907. Note on an organism found in yellow-fever tissue. *Public Health Rep.* **22:**541.

67. Stoddard, R. A., J. E. Gee, P. P. Wilkins, K. McCaustland, and A. R. Hoffmaster. 2009. Detection of pathogenic *Leptospira* spp. through TaqMan polymerase chain reaction targeting the LipL32 gene. *Diagn. Microbiol. Infect. Dis.* **64:**247–255.

68. Suputtamongkol, Y., K. Niwattayakul, C. Suttinont, K. Losuwanaluk, R. Limpaiboon, W. Chierakul, V. Wuthiekanun, S. Triengrim, M. Chenchittikul, and N. J. White. 2004. An open, randomized, controlled trial of penicillin, doxycycline, and cefotaxime for patients with severe leptospirosis. *Clin. Infect. Dis.* **39:**1417–1424.

69. Terpstra, W. J. 1992. Typing leptospira from the perspective of a reference laboratory. *Acta Leidensia* **60:**79–87.

70. Thaipadungpanit, J., V. Wuthiekanun, W. Chierakul, L. D. Smythe, W. Petkanchanapong, R. Limpaiboon, A. Apiwatanaporn, A. T. Slack, Y. Suputtamongkol, N. J. White, E. J. Feil, N. P. Day, and S. J. Peacock. 2007. A dominant clone of *Leptospira interrogans* associated with an outbreak of human leptospirosis in Thailand. *PLoS Neglected Trop. Dis.* **1:**e56.

71. Turner, L. H. 1968. Leptospirosis II. Serology. *Trans. R. Soc. Trop. Med. Hyg.* **62:**880–889.

72. Turner, L. H. 1970. Leptospirosis III. Maintenance, isolation and demonstration of leptospires. *Trans. R. Soc. Trop. Med. Hyg.* **64:**623–646.

73. Uip, D. E., V. Amato Neto, and M. S. Duarte. 1992. Diagnóstico precoce da leptospirose por demonstração de antígenos através de exame imuno-histoquímino em músculo da panturrilha. *Rev. Inst. Med. Trop. São Paulo* **34:**375–381.

74. Victoria, B., A. Ahmed, R. L. Zuerner, N. Ahmed, D. M. Bulach, J. Quinteiro, and R. A. Hartskeerl. 2008. Conservation of the *S10-spc-α* locus within otherwise highly plastic genomes provides phylogenetic insight into the genus *Leptospira*. *PLoS One* **3:**e2752.

75. Vijayachari, P., A. P. Sugunan, T. Umapathi, and S. C. Sehgal. 2001. Evaluation of darkground microscopy as a rapid diagnostic procedure in leptospirosis. *Indian J. Med. Res.* **114:**54–58.

76. Ward, M. P., L. F. Guptill, A. Prahl, and C. C. Wu. 2004. Serovar-specific prevalence and risk factors for leptospirosis among dogs: 90 cases (1997–2002). *J. Am. Vet. Med. Assoc.* **224:**1958–1963.

77. Winslow, W. E., D. J. Merry, M. L. Pirc, and P. L. Devine. 1997. Evaluation of a commercial enzyme-linked immunosorbent assay for detection of immunoglobulin M antibody in diagnosis of human leptospiral infection. *J. Clin. Microbiol.* **35:**1938–1942.

78. World Health Organization. 2003. *Human Leptopirosis: Guidance for Diagnosis, Surveillance and Control.* World Health Organization, Geneva, Switzerland.

79. World Health Organization. 1999. Leptospirosis worldwide, 1999. *Wkly. Epidemiol. Rec.* **74:**237–242.

80. Wylie, J. A. H., and E. Vincent. 1947. The sensitivity of organisms of the genus *Leptospira* to penicillin and streptomycin. *J. Pathol. Bacteriol.* **59:**247–254.

81. Yasuda, P. H., A. G. Steigerwalt, K. R. Sulzer, A. F. Kaufmann, F. Rogers, and D. J. Brenner. 1987. Deoxyribonucleic acid relatedness between serogroups and serovars in the family *Leptospiraceae* with proposals for seven new *Leptospira* species. *Int. J. Syst. Bacteriol.* **37:**407–415.

82. Zaki, S. R., W.-J. Shieh, and The Epidemic Working Group. 1996. Leptospirosis associated with outbreak of acute febrile illness and pulmonary haemorrhage, Nicaragua, 1995. *Lancet* **347:**535.

*Borrelia**

MARTIN E. SCHRIEFER

56

Borreliosis, in the form of louse-borne relapsing fever (LBRF), has been known to man for thousands of years and has been the cause of massive epidemics as recently as the early 1900s (41). This human-specific disease is caused by *Borrelia recurrentis* and is vectored by the human-specific body louse, *Pediculus humanus humanus*. Although improved personal hygiene and use of antibiotics and dichlorodiphenyltrichloroethane (DDT) in the 20th century resulted in global case and morbidity declines, LBRF continues to severely impact impoverished and displaced populations in parts of east Africa (30). In contrast, tick-borne borrelioses, both tick-borne relapsing fever (TBRF) and Lyme borreliosis (LB), are caused by over a dozen *Borrelia* species (Table 1) and were first described about 100 years ago (1, 24, 36). With the exception of *Borrelia duttoni*, all tick-borne borrelioses are zoonotic diseases and humans are a dead-end host.

In the first half of the 20th century, borrelia research literature focused largely on TBRF, with particular interest in multiphasic antigen variation of the spirochete and the associated clinical relapses and immune response of the infected host (14). TBRF is vectored by soft-bodied ticks of the genus *Ornithodoros* (Table 1; Fig. 1). Although TBRF only occurs sporadically and in focal areas throughout most of the world, it is one of the most common bacterial infections in parts of northwest Africa and a leading cause of prenatal and child mortality in central Tanzania (30, 120).

LB, first known as erythema chronicum migrans, was reported in the late 19th century medical literature from Europe. Numerous reports described its association with hard-bodied tick bites of the genus *Ixodes* (Fig. 1), its responsiveness to penicillin, and its likely spirochetal etiology (1, 56). Despite these latter proven correct deductions, the disease garnered little notoriety and, outside Europe, was largely unknown until the late 1900s. In 1969, a North American case of erythema migrans (EM) in a patient from Wisconsin was described and successfully treated with penicillin (110). However, active investigation of the etiology and natural biology of the disease was not initiated until the mid-1970s. In 1975, a group of parents in Lyme, Connecticut, expressed concerns to the state health department

about a seeming epidemic of inflammatory arthritis among local children. Ensuing epidemiological and clinical investigations linked antecedent tick bites with EM and subsequent arthritis among children and adults in this and other regions in the United States (116). The causative agent of LB, or Lyme disease as it is known in North America, *Borrelia burgdorferi*, and transmission by its vector tick, *Ixodes scapularis*, were described a few years later (23). Since that time, LB has become and remains the most prevalent vector-borne disease in North America, with approximately 20,000 cases reported per year in the United States (10). Although LB is a nonreportable disease in many countries and underreported in others, estimates of annual LB incidence range from 85,000 to well over 100,000 (58).

TAXONOMY

Borrelia belongs to the order *Spirochaetales*, which encompasses the families *Spirochaetaceae* and *Leptospiraceae*. Within the *Spirochaetaceae*, two genera, *Borrelia* and *Treponema*, cause human disease. Borreliae are agents of LBRF and both tick-borne LB and relapsing fever. The type species of the genus *Borrelia* is *Borrelia anserina*, which causes borreliosis in birds. Based on *rrs* (16S rRNA gene) sequence analyses, spirochetes form a distinct entity (division D) within the eubacterial kingdom. They are neither gram positive nor gram negative. In case of the spirochetes, morphological criteria and DNA data produce concordant phylogenies, a rare trait in other bacterial groups.

DESCRIPTION OF THE GENUS

Common Characteristics

Borreliae (Fig. 2 and 3) are similar in length (8 to 30 μm) but wider (0.2 to 0.5 μm) than the two other human-pathogenic spirochetes, the treponemes and the leptospires (14). They are highly motile organisms, with corkscrew and oscillating motility enabling movement through highly viscous mediums such as connective tissue. In contrast to the exoflagella of other bacteria, the flagella of spirochetes are endoflagella. The endoflagella (7 to 20 per terminus) are localized beneath the outer membrane and insert subterminally at one end or the other of the protoplasmic cylinder. The protoplasmic cylinder consists of a peptidoglycan layer

---

*This chapter contains information presented in chapter 62 by Bettina Wilske, Barbara J. B. Johnson, and Martin E. Schriefer in the ninth edition of this *Manual*.

TABLE 1 Characteristics of arthropod-borne borreliae[a]

Borrelia sp.	Arthropod vector(s)	Animal reservoir	Geographic distribution	Disease
Relapsing fever borreliae				
B. recurrentis	Pediculus humanus humanus	Humans	East Africa	LBRF (epidemic)
B. duttonii	O. moubata	Humans	Central, eastern, and southern Africa	TBRF (endemic)
B. hispanica	O. erraticus	Rodents	Mediterranean region	Hispano-African TBRF
B. crocidurae	O. sonrai, O. erraticus	Rodents	Morocco, Libya, Egypt, Turkey, Senegal	North African TBRF
B. merionesi				
B. microti				
B. dipodilli				
B. persica	O. tholozani	Rodents	Western China, India, Kashmir, central Asia, Iraq, Iran, Egypt	Asiatic-African TBRF
B. caucasica	O. verrucosus	Rodents	Caucasus to Iraq	Caucasian TBRF
B. hermsii	O. hermsi	Rodents	Western North America	American TBRF
B. turicatae	O. turicata	Rodents	Southwestern United States	American TBRF
B. parkeri	O. parkeri	Rodents	Western United States	American TBRF
B. mazzottii	O. talajé	Rodents	Southern United States, Mexico, Central and South America	American TBRF
B. venezuelensis	O. rudis (O. venezuelensis)	Rodents	Central and South America	American TBRF
B. burgdorferi sensu lato				
B. burgdorferi	I. scapularis	Rodents	Eastern and north-central United States	LB
	I. pacificus	Rodents	Western United States	LB
	I. ricinus	Rodents	Europe	LB
B. garinii	I. ricinus, I. persulcatus	Rodents	Europe, Asia	LB
	I. uriae	Birds	Europe, Asia	?
B. afzelii	I. ricinus, I. persulcatus	Rodents	Europe, Asia	LB
B. spielmanii	I. ricinus	Rodents	Europe	LB (few cases)
B. japonica	I. ovatus	Rodents	Japan	?
B. andersonii	I. dentatus	Rabbits	United States	?
B. bissettii	I. scapularis, I. pacificus	Rodents	United States	?
B. tanukii	I. tanukii, I. ovatus	Rodents	Japan	?
B. turdi	I. turdus	?	Japan	?
B. sinica	I. ovatus		China	?
B. valaisiana	I. ricinus	Birds	Europe, Asia	LB (one case)
B. lusitaniae	I. ricinus	Reptiles (birds?)	Europe, North Africa	LB (few cases)
B. californiensis	?	Rodents	Western United States	?
B. carolinensis	I. minor	Rodents	Southeastern United States	?
Other borreliae				
B. lonestari	Amblyomma americanum	?	United States	?
B. miyamotoi	I. persulcatus	Rodents	Japan	?
B. theileri	Rhipicephalus, Boophilus spp.	Cattle, horses, sheep	South Africa, Australia, North America, Europe	Bovine borreliosis
B. coriaceae	O. coriaceus	Deer?	Western United States	Epizootic bovine abortion?
B. anserina	Argas spp.	Fowl	Worldwide	Avian borreliosis

[a] Modified from reference 132.

and an inner membrane which encloses the internal components of the cell (14). If cultivable, borreliae grow slowly under microaerophilic (13) or anaerobic (96) conditions. They require *N*-acetylglucosamine and long-chain saturated and unsaturated fatty acids and produce lactic acid through glucose fermentation (65).

Species Diversity

The causative agent of LB, *B. burgdorferi*, was first described by Burgdorfer et al. in the early 1980s (23). Studies published since 1992 have divided *B. burgdorferi* sensu lato into 3 prevalent, human-pathogenic species—*B. burgdorferi* sensu stricto, *B. afzelii*, and *B. garinii* (12)—and 11 other species, some of which have been linked to human cases (Table 1) (122). In North America, *B. burgdorferi* sensu stricto is the only human-pathogenic species, whereas all three species have been isolated from humans in Europe. From central to eastern Asia, *B. garinii* and *B. afzelii* are the agents of almost all human cases of LB.

There is a high prevalence of *B. afzelii* among human skin isolates from Europe, whereas isolates from cerebrospinal fluid (CSF) in Europe are most often *B. garinii*

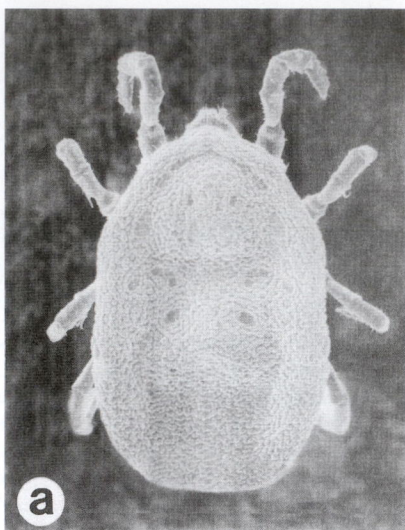
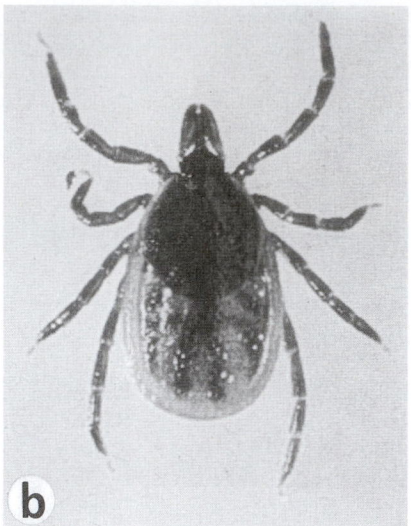

FIGURE 1 Two genera of ticks are vectors for relapsing fever and LB: *Ornithodoros* (a) and *Ixodes* (b).

(Table 2) (39, 104). All three genospecies cause Lyme arthritis in Europe (Table 2) (38, 44, 119).

A few studies have reported the detection of other *Borrelia* species (*B. valaisiana*, *B. spielmanii*, and *B. lusitaniae*) in patient samples in Europe (28, 100, 101, 121). Similarly, *B. lonestari*, a species carried by a hard tick but genetically more closely related to the relapsing fever spirochetes vectored by soft ticks, has been reported from the southeastern United States. This spirochete has been implicated in at least one case of EM, although a prospective investigation of skin biopsy and serum samples from 30 Missouri patients who presented with EM-like rashes failed to detect genetic evidence of *B. lonestari* or *B. burgdorferi* (138).

In North America, *B. turicatae*, *B. parkeri*, and *B. hermsii* have been isolated from *Ornithodoros parkeri*, *Ornithodoros turicatae*, and *Ornithodoros hermsi* ticks, respectively, but they may be a single species because their DNA-DNA similarity is greater than 70%. The species status of other cultivable borreliae, such as *B. anserina*, *B. crocidurae*, *B. recurrentis*, and *B. coriaceae*, has been supported by greater DNA-DNA dissimilarity findings (31, 65).

The Genome

The genomes of the borreliae are unusual among prokaryotes in having a small linear chromosome of approximately 1,000 kb and both linear and circular plasmids. Also atypical of most bacteria, borreliae have a low G+C content, approximately 30 mol%. The complete nucleotide sequence of the chromosome and 21 plasmids (9 circular and 12 linear) has been published for the type strain, *B. burgdorferi* B31 (43). A total of 59% of the chromosomal open reading frames (ORFs) have homologs in other bacterial species; in contrast, homologs have been identified for

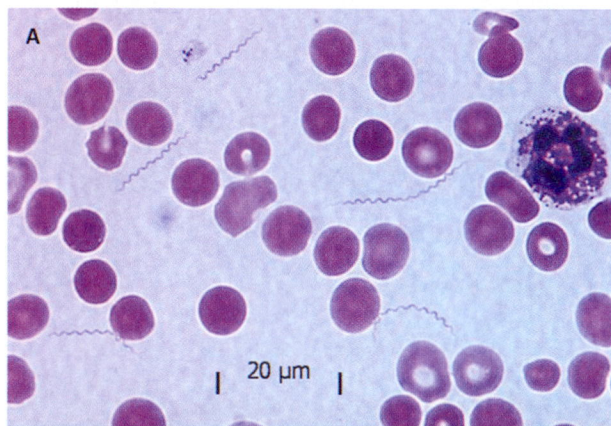

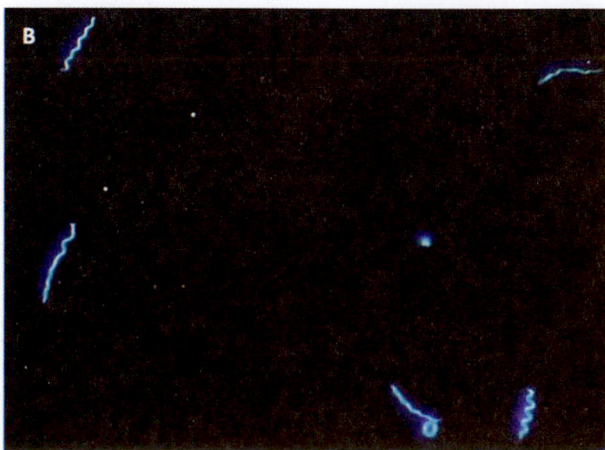

FIGURE 3 *Borrelia* spirochetes. (A) *B. hermsii* in a thin smear of patient blood (bright-field microscopy, Giemsa stain); (B) *B. burgdorferi* culture (dark-field microscopy).

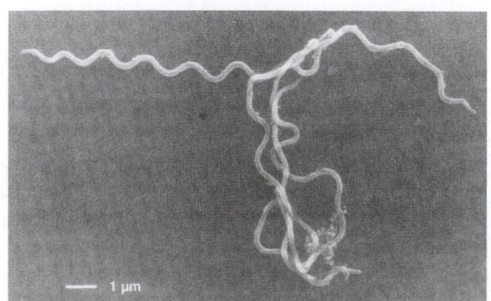

FIGURE 2 Scanning electron micrograph of *B. burgdorferi* (provided by Gerhard Wanner, Munich, Germany).

TABLE 2 Distribution of species of *B. burgdorferi* sensu lato in European isolates from CSF, skin, and synovial fluid specimens[a]

Species	% Distribution in specimens from[b]:		
	CSF (n = 78)	Skin (n = 560)	Synovial fluid (n = 20)
B. burgdorferi sensu stricto	12	1	33
B. afzelii	17	88	29
B. garinii	71	10	38

[a]Data from references 38, 104, and 119.

[b]*B. burgdorferi* sensu lato species identifications from CSF and skin are based on culture; species identification from synovial fluid samples is based on *ospA* PCR results. Culture isolates from synovial fluid are too few to estimate *Borrelia* species distribution.

only one-third of the plasmid ORFs. The genome encodes a basic set of proteins for DNA replication, transcription, and energy metabolism but, interestingly, lacks most cellular biosynthetic pathways. Of some surprise is the tremendous number (>150) of genes that encode putative lipoproteins, suggesting an essential role for these molecules in the life cycle of the spirochete. Genome analysis of another Lyme disease spirochete, *B. garinii* (strain PBi), revealed that most of the chromosome is conserved (>90% DNA and amino acid level identity) in the two species. Furthermore, two co-linear plasmids (lp54 and cp26) seem to belong to the basic genome inventory of the *Borrelia* species that causes Lyme disease. However, the authors did not find counterparts of the *B. burgdorferi* plasmids lp36 and lp38 or their respective gene repertoires in the *B. garinii* genome (45). The large linear plasmid lp54 encodes two major outer surface proteins, OspA and OspB, which are tandemly arrayed in one operon (17). OspC, another major outer surface protein, is encoded on a circular plasmid (cp26), and sequence analysis of *ospC* from different strains suggests that gene exchange might play a role in the diversity and immune evasion of Lyme disease borreliae (62).

Whole-genome microarray analysis revealed that a total of 215 ORFs, 136 of which are plasmid borne, were differentially expressed at 23 and 35°C. These findings highlight the potential importance of plasmid-borne genes in the adaptation of *B. burgdorferi* sensu lato to mammal hosts and tick vectors (84). The linear plasmids of *B. hermsii* and *B. turicatae* contain genes encoding outer membrane lipoproteins, called variable major proteins (Vmp). These genes are silent except when they are translocated to an expression site immediately adjacent to one of the linear plasmid telomeres. Antigenic variation of Vmp-like proteins due to recombination of *vls* (Vmp-like small) gene sequence cassettes has also been described for *B. burgdorferi*. These *vls* genes have highly variable regions as well as highly conserved sequences which encode immunogenic epitopes important for serodiagnosis (78, 139).

EPIDEMIOLOGY AND TRANSMISSION

The ecological components that maintain *Borrelia* species in nature are quite diverse and are spread throughout the world (Table 1).

Relapsing Fever Borreliae

Most relapsing fever borreliae have rodents as reservoirs and are transmitted by soft-bodied ticks of the genus *Ornithodoros* (Fig. 1). One exception, *B. recurrentis*, the agent of LBRF, has only humans as reservoirs and is transmitted only by the human-specific body louse, *Pediculus humanus humanus*. It has been commonly accepted that *B. duttoni*, a prevalent agent of TBRF in east Africa, also had humans as reservoirs, although recent studies challenge this understanding. Endemic cycles of TBRF between rodents and *Ornithodoros* ticks are recognized globally (Table 1). Human infections occur in western Canada and the United States (reportable in 11 western states), portions of Mexico, Central and South America, the Mediterranean, Central Asia, and much of Africa. *Ornithodoros* ticks are rapid (10 to 30 minutes) and typically nocturnal feeders; human victims most often do not recall tick bites. Although LBRF had a global distribution only 100 years ago, recent outbreaks have been limited to parts of east Africa. LBRF is not communicable between its human hosts, but rapid transfer of the infected louse between persons by direct contact and shared clothing and bedding enables efficient disease dissemination among crowded populations, particularly when personal hygiene is compromised.

B. burgdorferi Sensu Lato

The Lyme disease borreliae of *B. burgdorferi* sensu lato are transmitted by hard-bodied ticks (genus *Ixodes*) (Fig. 1). Globally, LB is limited to temperate regions of the northern hemisphere (Table 1). The prevalence of vector-competent ticks and their infection-permissive vertebrate hosts largely defines human risk and case numbers. For example, in the United States during the 15-year period from 1992 to 2006, 93% of the total cases (n = 248,074) reported to the CDC by health departments were from 10 (Connecticut, Delaware, Massachusetts, Maryland, Minnesota, New Jersey, New York, Pennsylvania, Rhode Island, and Wisconsin) of 50 states, and these case incidences were mirrored by *B. burgdorferi* sensu stricto infection rates among *I. scapularis* ticks and reservoir vertebrates (10).

Ixodes species feed on three different hosts depending on the developmental stage of the tick. The larvae and nymphs feed primarily on small rodents, whereas adult ticks feed on a variety of mammals (deer, raccoons, domestic and wild carnivores, larger domestic animals, and birds). The feeding period of *Ixodes* ticks is rather long (several days to over a week) and contributes to their geographic dispersal along with the movement of the host. Birds, particularly migratory seabirds, can transport the ticks (*Ixodes uriae*) over very long distances and thus distribute borreliae (especially *B. garinii*) worldwide (44).

There appears to be an association between *B. afzelii* and small rodents and *B. garinii* and birds, likely due to different serum sensitivities of the borreliae (59) mediated by complement regulator-acquiring surface proteins (73). In unfed ticks, *B. burgdorferi* sensu lato lives in the midgut. During the blood meal, transcriptional changes are induced in the borreliae and precede their migration to the salivary glands (108). Migration of spirochetes from the feeding *I. scapularis* midgut to the skin of the animal host takes >36 h (32). For *Ixodes ricinus*, however, spirochete migration has been observed with ticks feeding for as few as 17 h (67).

CLINICAL SIGNIFICANCE

Relapsing Fever

Relapsing fever is an infectious disease with an acute onset of clinical signs and symptoms including high fever, shaking chills, severe headache, nausea, myalgias, and severe malaise. Initial physical findings often are conjunctival effusion, petechiae, and diffuse abdominal tenderness. Fever attacks of 3 to 7 days are interspersed with afebrile periods of days to weeks. Detailed descriptions and reviews have been published elsewhere for LBRF (98) and TBRF (8, 37).

LBRF is, in general, more severe than TBRF. An exception to this rule is *B. duttoni* TBRF in east Africa. TBRF studies in Tanzania and the Democratic Republic of the Congo have documented severe morbidity among pregnant women, the young, and the elderly; pregnancy loss rates of 47% have been reported in some areas of endemicity (30). In TBRF, up to 13 febrile attacks have been documented, and a rash is more often reported than in LBRF (28% versus 8%). Splenomegaly, hepatomegaly, and jaundice are observed in 77%, 66%, and 36% of LBRF cases, respectively, whereas these signs are reported in only 41%, 17%, and 7% of TBRF cases. In LBRF, 34% of the patients have respiratory symptoms and 30% have central nervous system (CNS) involvement; in patients with TBRF, these figures are 16% and 9%, respectively (66). Complications leading to death (mortality rate of up to 40% in LBRF) are acute heart and hepatic failure and cerebral hemorrhage. Disease severity increases with compromising conditions common to many areas of endemicity.

The initial treatment of relapsing fever cases with appropriate antibiotics may elicit the Jarisch-Herxheimer reaction (JHR) (37). This reaction, associated with the rapid clearance of spirochetes from circulation and an overwhelming release of cytokines, typically occurs within 1 to 4 hours of antibiotic treatment. Signs include hypotension, tachycardia, chills, rigors, diaphoresis, and sudden elevation of body temperature. Death caused by JHR associated with LBRF has been reported. While generally not as severe, JHR associated with TBRF in the United States is reported in approximately 50% of cases. Therefore, patients with either LBRF or TBRF should be monitored closely upon initial treatment.

Acute respiratory distress syndrome (ARDS) may occur more frequently in TBRF than previously recognized. In 2004 and 2005, three cases of posttreatment ARDS in patients with severe TBRF were reported from California, Washington, and Nevada. A retrospective investigation of 111 TBRF cases reported from these states during the preceding 10 years revealed two additional ARDS cases, both occurring after 2001. Continued surveillance is needed to determine whether the risk of ARDS in TBRF is increasing. If so, possible correlates might include changed medical practices, use of newer antimicrobials, or the emergence of more-virulent TBRF strains (27).

Lyme Borreliosis

LB can be defined by early localized, early disseminated, and late-stage manifestations similar to the three stages of syphilis (115). The natural course of untreated *B. burgdorferi* infections varies considerably, and clinical manifestations can occur alone or in various combinations (112, 115). In the majority of cases, the infection is self-limiting, but in some cases, *B. burgdorferi* will disseminate to other skin sites, the nervous system, the joints, the heart, or occasionally, to other organs.

EM at the site of the infectious tick bite is the most common manifestation of early (stage I) LB and occurs in 60 to 90% of patients. The center of the expanding annular lesion often fades to produce a bull's-eye appearance. However, the extension, color intensity, and duration of EM vary considerably. In Europe, the skin lesion often develops more slowly and persists longer; hence, the initial description of chronicum migrans (1). One or more general symptoms, such as fatigue, arthralgia, myalgias, and headache accompany a majority of primary EM cases (118, 134).

In some patients, hematogenous dissemination of spirochetes to other organs and tissues occurs within days to weeks of infection (stage II). Patients often feel quite ill and can present with fatigue, headache, fever, malaise, arthralgia, and myalgia. Multiple (secondary) erythemata are common in the United States but uncommon in Europe. Neurologic structures, including the meninges, brain, spinal cord, peripheral nerves, and nerve roots, are also potential sites of early disseminated infection. In the United States, 15 to 20% of untreated patients develop neurologic signs, most commonly facial nerve palsy (unilateral or bilateral), meningitis, and radiculoneuropathy. CSF findings in cases of Lyme meningitis almost always include a mononuclear pleocytosis (10 to 1,000 cells/μl) and elevated protein concentration. Meningitis, or even facial palsy without meningismus, is more common among children than adults. Severe encephalitis is occasionally observed in stage II. Bannwarth's syndrome is the most common neurologic manifestation of early, disseminated LB in Europe. The syndrome is characterized initially by intense, migratory or focal, radicular pain, particularly at night, and by cranial nerve palsy. Paresis of the extremities and the trunk are less frequent. Further clinical manifestations of stage II may include Lyme carditis, most often with atrioventricular conduction blocks, and ophthalmic involvement. Borrelial lymphocytoma, a reddish to livid swelling of the skin that typically occurs in locations such as the earlobe, nipple, or scrotum, is manifested among some patients in Europe (112, 115).

Lyme arthritis and acrodermatitis chronica atrophicans (ACA), occurring months to years after the initial infection, are the most common manifestations of late (stage III) disease. Lyme arthritis can be monoarticular or oligoarticular, typically affecting the knee, and usually takes an intermittent course. Patients with ACA initially develop an infiltrative stage, followed by alterations characteristic of the atrophic stage: creased skin with livid discolorations and plastic protrusion of vessels. ACA is observed almost exclusively in Europe, a finding highly correlated with *B. afzelii* infections. Chronic neuroborreliosis is a very rare manifestation of late (stage III) disease. Paraparesis and tetraparesis are the most common symptoms. Examination of the CSF reveals a marked elevation of protein concentration with a low to moderate increase of cells in the CSF. The detection of intrathecally produced specific antibodies is currently regarded as the best marker of neuroborreliosis (49, 112, 115).

Early manifestations of LB are observed most frequently in the spring, summer, and autumn, coinciding with tick activity. Late manifestations do not show a seasonal pattern.

COLLECTION, TRANSPORT, AND STORAGE OF SPECIMENS

General Remarks for Collection and Transport

For culture, collection and preparation of specimens under sterile conditions are of utmost importance. Body fluids should be transported without any additives, and biopsy specimens should be placed in a small quantity of sterile saline or suitable culture medium (see "Isolation Procedures" below). Samples should reach the laboratory as quickly as possible (within 2 to 4 h). Before specimens are collected and transported, the laboratory should be contacted so that details of methodology can be agreed upon. If postal transport is unavoidable, overnight delivery is recommended. Specimens for laboratory confirmation of LB are presented in Table 3.

Blood and Serum

For relapsing fever, blood is the specimen of choice. During febrile attacks, borreliae may be easily detected by dark-field or bright-field microscopy of a wet mount blood sample or a stained blood smear, respectively (see "Microscopy" below) (Fig. 3). During early febrile periods, the spirochetemia may reach 10^6 to 10^8 cells per ml (65). Blood from acutely ill patients is also the best source for culture confirmation (31). However, the spirochetemia diminishes with each successive relapse, and visualization or culture isolation of borreliae is often unsuccessful during afebrile periods. In contrast to relapsing fever, spirochetemia in LB patients is below the level of microscopic detection, with estimates of 0.1 spirochetes/ml of whole blood. The rate of culture recovery from EM patient's blood has generally been 5% or less (4). However, in a series of experiments, it was demonstrated that *B. burgdorferi* culture recovery from untreated adult patients with EM was better from plasma than from serum or from an identical volume of whole blood. Approximately 50% of large-volume plasma cultures from EM patients have yielded *B. burgdorferi* (135). Serum is suitable for indirect (antibody) evidence of *Borrelia* exposure. Specific antibody detection tests are the most widely utilized tests for laboratory confirmation of LB (see "Serologic Tests" below). Serodiagnosis of relapsing fever is performed only in a few specialized laboratories.

Cerebrospinal Fluid

Patients with suspected Lyme neuroborreliosis (LNB) may have evidence of immunoglobulin synthesis against *B. burgdorferi* antigens in the CSF, elevated CSF inflammatory cells (usually lymphocytes, monocytes, or plasma cells), and elevated protein. CSF along with serum drawn at the same time should be obtained for laboratory demonstration of *Borrelia*-specific, intrathecal (CSF/serum antibody index) antibody production (see "Serologic Tests" below). For culture or PCR, detection rates are only about 20% (76). Positive PCR results with CSF also seem to correlate inversely with the duration of neurologic disease. Among neuroborreliosis patients, 7 of 14 (50%) with a disease duration of less than 2 weeks had a positive PCR result compared with only 2 of 16 (13%) patients in whom the illness duration was greater than 2 weeks ($P = 0.045$) (76).

Synovial Fluid or Synovial Biopsy Specimens

Investigation of synovial fluid or a synovial biopsy specimen by PCR can be useful in special circumstances where Lyme arthritis is suspected or the efficacy of antibiotic treatment is questioned (see "Nucleic Acid Detection Techniques" below) (4, 82). Culture is usually negative, with few exceptions. Due to the high protein permeability of the synovium, synovial fluid and serum display roughly equivalent antibody titers. Thus, it is sufficient to monitor antibody in serum.

Skin Biopsy Specimens

Skin biopsy samples are the best sources for isolation of *B. burgdorferi*; spirochetes can be isolated in most untreated cases of EM and acrodermatitis (Table 4). In cases of EM, culture success is highest (up to 86%) with biopsy samples taken close to (4 mm inside) the expanding border of the lesion (16), although this is primarily a technique for research, not for routine diagnosis. There are indications that the number of spirochetes in the skin is rather low or unevenly distributed, since an increase in the sensitivity is observed if more than one biopsy sample is investigated (140). Without treatment, *B. burgdorferi* sensu lato can persist for long periods in the skin, as shown by isolation from a 10-year-old acrodermatitis lesion (7). Biopsy samples (taken after thorough disinfection of the skin) should be sent in a

TABLE 3 Specimen types used for the diagnosis of LB

Clinical manifestation	Specimens for:	
	Direct pathogen detection (culture, PCR)	Antibody detection
Stage I (early/localized; days through weeks after tick bite)		
EM	Skin biopsy	Serum
Stage II (early/disseminated; weeks through months after tick bite)		
Multiple erythemata	Skin biopsy	Serum
Borrelial lymphocytoma	Skin biopsy	Serum
Lyme carditis	Endomyocardial biopsy	Serum
Neuroborreliosis	CSF	Paired serum/CSF[a]
Stage III (late/persistent; months through years after tick bite)		
Arthritis	Synovial fluid, synovial biopsy	Serum
ACA	Skin biopsy	Serum
Chronic neuroborreliosis	CSF	Paired serum/CSF[a]

[a] From the same day for AI determination.

TABLE 4 Sensitivity of methods for pathogen detection (PCR and culture) in LB

Specimen	Sensitivity
Skin (EM, acrodermatitis)	50–70% with culture or PCR
CSF (neuroborreliosis, stage II)	10–30% with culture or PCR[a]
Synovial fluid[b] (Lyme arthritis)	50–70% with PCR (culture is rarely positive)
Blood (EM)	15–40% with PCR or culture

[a] Up to 50% in patients with disease duration of less than 2 weeks compared with only 13% in patients for whom the illness duration was greater than 2 weeks.
[b] Higher sensitivity of direct pathogen detection from synovial biopsy specimen.

small amount of sterile saline or Barbour-Stoenner-Kelly (BSK) medium (with or without rifampin) as soon as possible to a microbiology laboratory capable of culturing *B. burgdorferi*.

Other Materials

Ticks are often tested for borreliae as part of epidemiological studies to assess risk to human populations in a given geographic area. Although specialized laboratories offer diagnostic services for individual ticks, detection of spirochetes within ticks by PCR or other methods has not been shown to provide clinically useful information.

DIRECT EXAMINATION

Microscopy

Direct microscopic visualization of borreliae in clinical samples is applicable only to cases of relapsing fever. During acute phases, spirochetemia often reaches 10^6 to 10^8 borreliae/ml, and motile spirochetes can be visualized by dark-field microscopy from wet preparations made from a drop of blood. This simple confirmatory test is often overlooked because of the increasingly common use of automated differential blood counts. Spirochetes can be visualized by stained (e.g., Giemsa) thin or thick films (Fig. 3). Detection of low-level spirochetemias may be assisted by a microhematocrit concentration technique. The hematocrit capillary is filled 75% with anticoagulated (e.g., EDTA or citrate treated) blood and centrifuged for 2 min. The buffy coat is then examined directly under the microscope at ×400 to ×1,000 (132). Failure to observe spirochetes does not rule out disease, and culture isolation (see "Isolation Procedures" below) can be considered.

Antigen Detection

Enzyme-linked immunosorbent assay and immunoblotting have been used for the detection of borrelial antigen in body fluids, including CSF and urine (29, 60). However, a commercial assay for antigen in urine was shown to lack reproducibility, and its use is not recommended (72).

Nucleic Acid Detection Techniques

Nucleic acid amplification techniques (NAAT) may serve as an adjunct to clinical diagnosis but should be restricted to experienced and specialized laboratories (102, 133). A variety of chromosomal and plasmid targets for NAAT have been developed (for reviews, see references 4, 35, 47, and 105). For PCR, an analytical sensitivity of approximately 10 to 20 borreliae per test sample has been demonstrated. Test sensitivities for both NAAT and culture are greater with

tissue specimens than with body fluids, except for synovial fluid, with which NAAT is superior. Sensitivities of 96% (82) and 86% (19) were reported for NAAT with synovial fluid from American patients with Lyme arthritis. European authors found NAAT sensitivities ranging between 50 and 70% (38, 44, 97, 119). Patients with Lyme arthritis are nearly always seropositive, so PCR of synovial samples is not used as a primary diagnostic technique. A positive PCR result after antibiotic therapy is of uncertain significance, since the presence of *B. burgdorferi* DNA does not necessarily mean that spirochetes are viable (19).

With skin biopsy and CSF specimens, NAAT demonstrated diagnostic sensitivities of approximately 60% and 20%, respectively (20, 39, 76). A prospective study of PCR and culture detection of *B. burgdorferi* in EM biopsy samples from Slovenian patients showed comparable sensitivities (36% culture positive in modified Kelly Preac-Mursic medium, 24% culture positive in BSK II medium, and 25% PCR positive) (91). PCR targeting *ospA*, a plasmid-borne gene, is more sensitive than flagellin PCR, which uses a chromosomal target (88, 140). Borreliae can shed blebs containing plasmids, leading to greater abundance of plasmid than chromosomal genes.

PCR amplification of *B. burgdorferi* sequences from urine has been described (99, 105) but is not recommended. Although *Borrelia*-specific DNA was demonstrated in over 70% of skin biopsy samples from patients with florid EM, parallel testing of urine samples was uniformly negative (20).

ISOLATION PROCEDURES

Many Lyme and relapsing fever borreliae are successfully cultured in artificial media. However, for diagnostic purposes, culturing is a slow, time-consuming method characterized by low sensitivity, especially from body fluids of patients with LB (Table 4). For these reasons, culture attempts are most often limited to research applications and performed by reference laboratories (e.g., the National Reference Center for Borreliae in Germany and the Centers for Disease Control and Prevention [CDC] in the United States).

Several media (modified Kelly medium, e.g., BSK II, BSK-H, or modified Kelly Preac-Mursic) (13, 92, 96) are capable of supporting growth of borreliae. It is important to verify the quality of each lot of medium by growing a reference strain from a small inoculum (<10 cells). Optimum growth (the generation time of *B. burgdorferi* is about 7 to 20 h) in these media is obtained at 30 to 33°C under microaerophilic conditions. Positive cultures from EM and synovial biopsy or fluid samples (blood and CSF) may be obtained in as few as 4 days, but most isolates require several weeks of incubation and negative cultures should be monitored by dark-field microscopy (Fig. 3) for at least 6 weeks.

IDENTIFICATION

Molecular Techniques

Relapsing fever borreliae have been typed on the basis of DNA-DNA reassociation analysis and flagellin gene analysis (31, 65). *B. burgdorferi* has an arrangement of its rRNA genes (a single *rrs* and tandemly repeated *rrl* and *rrf* genes) which distinguishes it from the relapsing fever borreliae (which have single copies of each) (109). Sequencing of 5S-23S intergenic spacers and a number of genes, pulsed-field gel electrophoresis of large restriction fragments, PCR, and restriction fragment length polymorphism analysis of multiple targets have all been utilized for species differentiation (15, 39, 77, 93, 122, 129, 130). However, in most cases, diagnosis and effective management of individual patients are independent of species determinations beyond the Lyme disease and relapsing fever groupings.

Immunological Techniques

Serotyping methods to identify *Borrelia* species and strains within a species have been described (125, 126). However, as with molecular techniques, diagnosis and effective management of individual patients have yet to utilize characterizations beyond the Lyme disease and relapsing fever groupings.

SEROLOGIC TESTS

Borrelia Antigens and Human Humoral Immune Response

B. burgdorferi possesses at least 30 immunogenic proteins which include the outer surface proteins A to F, a number of tissue binding proteins, and components of the flagellar apparatus. Proper detection and interpretation of the humoral response against *B. burgdorferi* must consider several variables. All LB genospecies (or strains within a genospecies) do not produce qualitatively or quantitatively identical sets of antigens. In serologic assays that utilize whole-cell culture extracts as the source of reactive antigens, these variables may result in different sizes of a given antigen (e.g., OspC, 21 to 25 kDa), quantitative antigen differences, or even their absence. This is particularly problematic in Europe and Asia, where multiple genospecies are present. Thus, it is imperative, even in North America, that diagnostic laboratories and manufacturers of serologic assays verify that all diagnostic antigens are present in relevant amounts. In the case of Western immunoblots, diagnostic antigens must also be discernable from each other. For many diagnostic proteins, sequence heterogeneity, even between strains in a given genospecies, may result in amino acid variations and reduced detection of an antibody response from a patient with a heterologous infection. Again, OspC serves as an example: with 21 major OspC types recognized among North American and European isolates (111), patient reactivity in an assay with one selected OspC type may not be sufficiently cross-reactive to enable its detection (61, 137). In addition to genospecies and strain-dependent protein profiles as well as antigenic heterogeneity, many antigens are variably expressed in response to environmental cues both in culture and during infection. OspC and VlsE serve as examples; while both of these potent immunogens are expressed during early infection, they are variably produced in culture, often in very low amounts. Thus, their presence in diagnostic assays must be verified. Similarly, while OspA expression is turned off in early infection (55) and is therefore an insensitive marker of this stage of disease, it is an abundant protein in most cultures. During progression to later stage II and III disease, particularly in North America, expression of OspA is often triggered and patient antibody to this antigen is strongly correlated with arthritic involvement (70).

Among *B. burgdorferi* immunogenic proteins, some have both heterogeneous and conserved antigen epitopes. Despite the overall antigenic heterogeneity of OspC, its C-terminal 10 amino acids harbor a highly conserved and immunodominant epitope (pepC10) which has been used

successfully in peptide based serodiagnostic enzyme immunoassays (EIAs) (81). Finally, at least one protein of great and recent diagnostic interest is capable of switching antigen epitopes during infection. The VlsE (variable major-protein-like sequence expressed) of *B. burgdorferi* is a surface lipoprotein that is expressed early in infection. It contains both variable and invariable regions, and extensive antigenic switching within the variable regions likely contributes to immune evasion (11, 83, 139). Nonetheless, and of some surprise, studies in the late 1990s found that LB patients developed strong antibody responses to VlsE, particularly to the sixth invariant region of the protein (78), and that this region was highly conserved among the three major LB genospecies. These findings served as the basis of EIAs in which synthetic peptides representing the sixth invariant (or conserved) region, C6, were developed. Accumulating published studies over the last 10 years have shown that VlsE and C6-based assays have high sensitivities in most stages of LB and suggest that they may serve as future, single-tier assays for serodiagnosis (4, 9, 46, 78, 106, 117).

The earliest immunoglobulin M (IgM) responses to all *B. burgdorferi* infections are directed against OspC (21 to 25 kDa), the flagellar antigens, p41 (FlaB) and p37 (FlaA), and p35 (BBK32, fibronectin binding protein) and are typically detectable within the first few weeks. Detectable IgM against BmpA (39 kDa) is in part strain dependent and most often appears after the response to OspC, FlaB, and FlaA (2, 4, 34, 40). Although the level of IgM antibody to most spirochetal antigens peaks within the first weeks, it often persists at detectable levels for many months.

The IgG response increases and broadens slowly over the first weeks of disease. Among the reactive antigens to which there is an early IgG response are OspC, p35 (BBK32), p37 (FlaA), VlsE, and p41 (FlaB) (2, 5, 74, 78, 86). During early disseminated (stage II) disease, IgG levels increase, and reactivity against Osp17 (DbpA, decorin binding protein A), p39 (BmpA), and p58 often appears (53). The late-stage immune response (stage III) is characterized by IgG antibodies to a wide variety of antigens (34, 53). Approximately 80% of the sera from European patients with late disease (arthritis and ACA) react with p14, Osp17 (DbpA), p21 (not OspC), p30 (not OspA), p39, p43, p58, and p83/100 (homolog of p93) of *B. afzelii* strain PKo (53). Similarly, among North American patients with chronic neurologic abnormalities or arthritis, close to 100% react with 5 or more of the diagnostic antigens p18, p23 (OspC), p28, p30, p39 (BmpA), p41 (FlaB), p45, p58, p66, and p93 (4, 34, 117).

Notable differences in late-stage disease antibody responses between European and North American patients include those to OspC and OspA. While IgG antibodies against OspC are detected in only 20% of European patients with late-stage disease (53), the frequency of IgG reactivity to OspC in American patients with late-stage disease is 48% (34). Similarly, while only 5 to 7% of European patients with late-stage disease are reactive to OspA (53, 127) over 40% of American patients with late-stage disease are reactive to this antigen (5, 34).

Two-Step Approach in Serodiagnosis

For serodiagnosis of LB, a two-step approach is recommended by the Association of State and Territorial Public Health Laboratory Directors (ASTPHLD) and the CDC (25, 63). All serum specimens submitted for Lyme disease testing should be evaluated in a two-step process, in which the first step is a sensitive serologic test, such as an EIA or immunofluorescence assay (IFA). Specimens found to be negative should not be tested further. All specimens found to be positive or equivocal by a sensitive first-tier test should be further tested by a standardized immunoblot procedure (25). This procedure is also recommended in the MiQ LB standard published by the German expert group on the diagnosis of LB of the German Society for Hygiene and Microbiology (DGHM) (Fig. 4) (133). The concept of a two-step approach, which aims at increasing the predictive value of a positive result with each step, requires that the tests be performed in succession (64, 133). Omitting the first step, a quantitative assay, and proceeding directly with qualitative immunoblots reduces the specificity of the procedure.

Immunofluorescence Assay

For the IFA, borreliae fixed on glass slides are used as the antigen. IFA for serodiagnosis of relapsing fever, however, is challenging, since expression of the major membrane proteins is variable. The specificity of IFA serodiagnosis for Lyme disease may be improved by adsorption of sera with *Treponema phagedenis* sonicate (IFA-ABS) (133). For the IgM test, pretreatment of the sera with anti-IgG immune serum is recommended to avoid false-positive test results due to rheumatoid factor as well as false-negative results due

to high IgG antibody levels. As in all antibody detection assays, it is important to verify expression of OspC within the antigen source cultures. Although IFA is relatively easy to perform, it is not easy to standardize, and evaluation of test results requires expertise not always available in the routine laboratory. In general, antibody titers of ≥64 and ≥256 are regarded as positive on the IFA-ABS and unadsorbed IFA, respectively. Sera from patients with syphilis are often positive in the unadsorbed assay and are rarely positive on the IFA-ABS (133).

Enzyme Immunoassay

Different modifications of the EIA have been used for the diagnosis of LB. In the indirect EIA, antigen is used to coat the plates, followed by incubation with patient serum, enzyme-labeled anti-IgM or anti-IgG, and the EIA substrate. Capture IgM-EIA (μ-capture EIA) has been specially designed to avoid false-positive reactivity due to rheumatoid factor (52). Rheumatoid factor false-positive reactivity can also be overcome by pretreatment of the sera with anti-IgG (127). EIA has the advantage of objective measurement, quantification, and high throughput. Many different antigen preparations have been used, including whole-cell sonicates (103), isolated flagella (50), detergent extracts (127), recombinant protein antigens (68, 75, 127), and synthetic peptides (78). Use of crude antigen preparations,

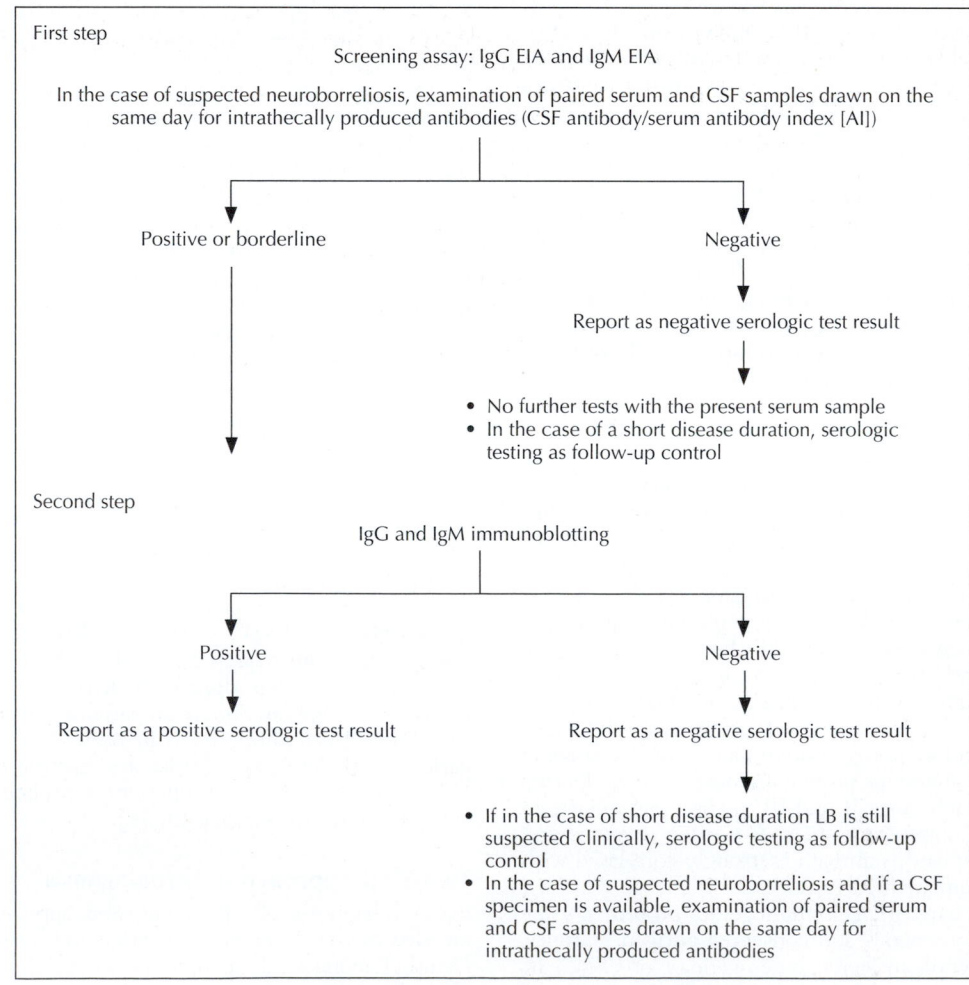

FIGURE 4 Two-step approach for serodiagnosis.

such as whole-cell sonicates, often results in unacceptable specificity. Improved tests which utilize enriched, specific, or recombinant protein antigens are now widely used. Tests using an octyl β-D-glucopyranoside detergent extract and Reiter treponeme absorbent, isolated flagella, recombinant VlsE, or the C6 peptide of VlsE are commercially available (Dade-Behring, Marburg, Germany; Dakopatts, Copenhagen, Denmark; Diasorin, Turin, Italy; and Immunetics, Boston, MA). Since VlsE is not present in relevant amounts in cultivated borreliae, recombinant VlsE has been added to whole-cell extracts to increase sensitivity in some products (Dade-Behring).

Immunoblotting

The Western immunoblot is regarded as a supplementary (United States) or confirmatory (Europe) assay. This implies that it should be employed only when a screening assay is reactive (positive or indeterminate, sometimes called equivocal). Western immunoblotting enables assessment of the humoral immune response to protein antigens as separated by sodium dodecyl sulfate-polyacrylamide gel electrophoresis (SDS-PAGE). Antigen preparations for Western immunoblotting include whole-cell lysates or recombinant protein antigen mixtures that are resolved (largely by molecular weight) by SDS-PAGE and then transferred to blot membranes. Patient antibody against dozens of borrelial antigens can be discerned by the experienced diagnostic laboratorian. However, the procedure is considered technically complex. An alternative test format is the line immunoblot, whereby recombinant or native borrelia antigens, which have been resolved or purified by means other than SDS-PAGE, are directly striped on membranes for immunoprobing. This approach enables discrete spacing or placement of individual antigens in quantified deliveries on the membrane and avoids the overlap of comigrating antigens that often complicate reading on Western immunoblots. With either method, Western immunoblot or line immunoblot, it is imperative that antigen identification and cutoff (minimal band intensity) controls are employed in each diagnostic run. These calibration controls may include antibody preparations provided with commercial kits, monoclonal antibodies (MAbs) available from commercial and other sources (e.g., CDC), or calibrated patient samples.

Numerous immunoblot tests which use antigens of various strains or genospecies of *B. burgdorferi* sensu lato are commercially available. The ASTPHLD and the CDC, as well as the DGHM, have published recommendations for interpretation of the *Borrelia* immunoblot (25, 133). In the United States, immunoblot interpretation rules have been recommended which refer to detection of antibody against whole-cell antigens of specific *B. burgdorferi* sensu stricto strains (34, 40). The IgM immunoblot is interpreted as positive if ≥2 bands of the following proteins are reactive: p23 (OspC), p39 (BmpA), and p41 (FlaB). The IgG blot is interpreted as positive if ≥5 bands of the following proteins are reactive: p18, p23 (OspC), p28, p30, p39 (BmpA), p41 (FlaB), p45, p58, p66, and p93. If the immunoblot is used within the first 4 weeks of disease onset (early, stage I or II), both IgM and IgG immunoblots should be performed. Due to specificity concerns of the IgM immunoblotting criteria potentially yielding false-positive findings in persons with a low pretest likelihood of infection, initial recommendations limited application of the IgM Western blot to the first 4 weeks of infection. Beyond this time point,

a more-specific IgG-reactive Western blot is expected. Recent studies, however, indicate that some patients do not develop a robust IgG response during the first 4 weeks of infection (117).

Interpretation of the antibody response among European patients is complicated by the risk of infection with different *Borrelia* species. In addition, immunoblot studies have shown that the immune response to European infections, compared with North American infections, is restricted to a narrower spectrum of *Borrelia* proteins (33). Interpretive rules defined in a species- and strain-specific manner have been determined (53, 62) and independently corroborated (59). *B. afzelii* strain PKo is preferred to PBi (*B. garinii*) and PKa2 (*B. burgdorferi* sensu stricto) strains because it permits a two-band criterion for the IgG test: at least two bands positive for p14, p17 (DbpA), p21, OspC, p30, p39 (BmpA), p43, p58, and p83/100 (Fig. 5) (133). According to the general Deutsches Institut für Normung (DIN) recommendations on the immunoblot (DIN 58967, part 40), at least a two-band criterion should be required for the positive interpretation of the IgG immunoblot. In IgM immunoblots, a detectable immune response is restricted to only a few bands. Therefore, the IgM blot is regarded as positive if there is strong reactivity to OspC (133). Specific DIN recommendations for the *Borrelia* immunoblot (DIN 58969, part 44) have been published which include new antigens (i.e., VlsE) and the line immunoblot as a new technique.

Recombinant immunoblots with Osp17 (DbpA), OspC, p39 (BmpA), truncated p41 (FlaB), p58, and p83/100

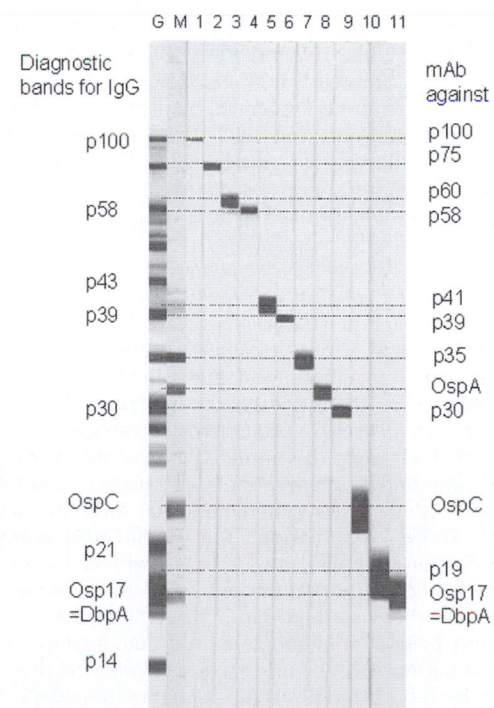

FIGURE 5 Whole-cell immunoblot for identification of diagnostic bands with MAbs. The antigen used is *B. afzelii* strain PKo. Lanes: G, IgG blot from a patient with late disease; M, IgM blot from a patient with early disease; 1 to 11, different MAbs against the respective reactive proteins. (Modified from reference 53.)

have demonstrated sensitivity comparable to that of the whole-cell immunoblot, except for patients with isolated EM (128). The recombinant immunoblot was substantially improved by the addition of several homologs of VlsE and DbpA, which increased the sensitivity of antibody detection in early disease (46, 106). Recombinant blots containing DbpA, OspC, p39 (BmpA), truncated p41 (FlaB), VlsE, and p83/100 are commercially available (Mikrogen, Munich, Germany). Using the line blot technique, sensitivity among early neuroborreliosis patients was significantly increased compared to the conventional sonicate immunoblot (92% versus 69%, respectively) (46). Listings of FDA, 510K-approved seroassays for commercial distribution can be found at http://www.accessdata.fda.gov/scripts/cdrh/cfdocs/cfPMN/pmn.cfm by entering "LSR" in the product code field.

Detection of Intrathecally Produced (CSF) Antibodies

Approximately 15% of untreated LB patients will develop neurologic manifestations. LNB has been divided into early disseminated and late stages. Both the CNS and peripheral nervous system, as well as blood vessels and meningeal coverings, may be involved in either stage. Laboratory testing should only be used to confirm the diagnosis, and the presence of B. burgdorferi-specific antibody in CSF or serum may be indicative of past or present infection. The pattern of nervous system involvement is largely stage dependent and may affect the correlation between clinical spectrum and serologic test utility. Thus, careful evaluation of a thorough clinical history and presentation are critical to the selection of appropriate diagnostic tests and proper interpretation of their findings (49, 54, 85, 94).

In patients in whom the CNS is involved, there should be evidence of CNS inflammation. Rarely, this may be localized to the brain or spinal cord, but in most cases, it involves the CSF and is evidenced by pleocytosis, elevated protein concentrations, and in cases of protracted infection, anti-borrelia-specific immunoglobulin synthesis. In contrast, for peripheral nervous system-limited disease, the CSF findings may be normal, as it is in most patients who have toxic-metabolic encephalopathy (49).

Although <10% of LNB cases are culture confirmed, subtle differences in clinical presentation between European and North American LNB are linked to causative genospecies. North American cases are limited to B. burgdorferi sensu stricto, while most European culture-positive LNB cases are B. afzelii and much smaller percentages of cases are B. garinii and B. burgdorferi sensu stricto.

The triad of early disseminated LNB, also known as meningoradiculoneuropathy, includes aseptic meningitis, cranial neuropathy, and radiculoneuritis; these may occur singularly or in combination. The single most common presentation of early disseminated LNB in North America is meningitis. Examination of the CSF shows mononuclear pleocytosis and elevated protein. CSF-specific anti-B. burgdorferi (IgA or IgG) immunoglobulin is demonstrated in 80 to 90% of patients. Standard two-tier serology in these patients is also most often positive. Cranial neuropathy occurs both in North America and Europe in about 10% of early disseminated LNB cases. Most frequently, this involves the facial nerve and is manifested by unilateral or bilateral facial palsy. Only about 50% of these cases will demonstrate CSF pleocytosis. European early disseminated LNB often presents as Bannwarth's syndrome and is highly associated with B. garinii infection. This radiculoneuropathy

also occurs in up to 5% of untreated North American LB patients. Most patients with Lyme radiculoneuritis are reactive in two-tier serologic testing, and CSF findings include pleocytosis and B. burgdorferi-specific antibody (49, 54, 85, 94, 113).

Late neurological manifestations usually develop months to years after initial infection. Encephalopathy is more common in North America, while encephalomyelitis is more frequent in Europe. For cases of late encephalopathy, serum immunoreactivity is nearly universal, while CSF pleocytosis, elevated protein, and B. burgdorferi-specific antibody are found in only 5%, 20 to 45%, and ~50% of cases, respectively. Most cases of chronic encephalomyelitis are reported from Europe, although North American cases have been described. In these cases, CSF pleocytosis and marked B. burgdorferi-specific antibody are almost universal.

Although there are no well-accepted criteria for seroconfirmation of neuroborreliosis in the United States, detection of intrathecal Borrelia-specific immune response is a valuable tool and is widely utilized in Europe (18). Methods taking into account potential dysfunction of the blood-CSF barrier, a common finding in neuroborreliosis, are required for accurate assessment of intrathecal antibody production. Long-used procedures for detection of specific intrathecal antibody production in the diagnosis of neurosyphilis have been modified for the diagnosis of neuroborreliosis (51, 114, 131). The most frequently used method is the determination of the CSF/serum antibody index (specific antibody index [AI]). CSF and serum must be obtained at the same time. By calculating the AI, CSF and serum are compared with regard to the portion of pathogen-specific IgG antibodies in the total IgG content. An AI of ≥2.0 is considered significantly elevated (79, 133). Lower indices (e.g., ≥1.3) are also considered significant by some investigators. False-positive AI results are likely with neurosyphilis patients when tested with whole-cell or flagellum sonicates in EIA. Here, EIAs with T. phagedenis adsorption (Dade-Behring) or recombinant antigens not cross-reacting with Treponema pallidum can be helpful for differential diagnosis. Other suitable methods for determination of intrathecal antibody production are the μ- or γ-capture EIA (Dakopatts) (51) and the IgG-matched immunoblot (131). The latter allows comparison of the antibody spectrum (against various Borrelia proteins) in serum and in CSF and thus permits conclusions as to the specificity of the intrathecal antibody response.

Vaccination: Past, Future, and Impact on Serology

The recombinant OspA vaccine (LYMErix), was withdrawn from the United States market in 2002. However, persistent titers among previous vaccinees may still be encountered and complicate interpretation of whole-cell-based serologic tests (3). Use of recently available commercial recombinant immunoblots will avoid false test results among OspA vaccinees.

Controversial Methods

A variety of diagnostic approaches have been developed as alternatives or adjuncts to the more widely practiced methods described above. T-lymphocyte proliferation assays have been used in various scientific studies to investigate the human T-cell response to Borrelia antigens (71). However, T-lymphocyte proliferation assays cannot be recommended as diagnostic tests due to their cumbersome nature and concerns about their specificity and standardization (26, 57, 124, 141). Antigen detection tests also are not recommended, as discussed above.

Detection of *B. burgdorferi*-specific antibodies in immune complexes has been proposed to be superior for serodiagnosis of acute Lyme disease (107) and as a marker of active infection (22). Recent work demonstrates that test results for antibodies precipitated from serum as immune complexes are highly correlated with enzyme-linked immunosorbent assay results obtained using unprocessed serum and are not more likely to reflect active infection than standard serology (80). Transformation of *B. burgdorferi* into spheroplasts (L-forms) in vitro in response to deprivation of serum or culture in CSF has been observed (6, 21). When visualized under a microscope, spheroplasts sometimes appear to be enclosed in a sac, so they have also been called "cysts." If apparently pure L-forms are injected into mice, they are infectious (48). The clinical and diagnostic significance of L-forms has not been demonstrated but warrants further study. There are commercial tests offered that purport to specifically detect cell wall-deficient or "cystic" forms of *B. burgdorferi* by IFA (123a) and culture (90), but they have not been validated with appropriate controls and are not recommended.

ANTIMICROBIAL SUSCEPTIBILITIES

The antimicrobial susceptibility of *Borrelia* species has been studied intensively in vitro (65, 95). Standard methods for the determination of the minimal bactericidal concentration have not been established. However, there is general agreement on the in vitro susceptibility of borreliae to antimicrobials, as follows. *B. burgdorferi* sensu lato is susceptible to macrolides, tetracyclines, semisynthetic penicillins, and the expanded- and broad-spectrum cephalosporins; moderately susceptible to penicillin G and chloramphenicol; and resistant to trimethoprim, sulfamethoxazole, rifampin, the aminoglycosides, and the quinolones (65). No significant differences between the Lyme disease borreliae and relapsing fever borreliae (*B. hermsii* and *B. turicatae*) were found with regard to penicillin G, amoxicillin, ceftriaxone, erythromycin, azithromycin, doxycycline, or tetracycline (65). There is no indication for routine antimicrobial susceptibility testing in either Lyme disease or relapsing fever.

Recommendations for Antibiotic Therapy

All clinical manifestations of *B. burgdorferi* infection should be treated with antibiotics. The antibiotic, dosage, duration, and route of application depend on the clinical picture and stage of the disease (123, 136). In cases of solitary EM, oral treatment with doxycycline, amoxicillin, or cefuroxime axetil is recommended. In acrodermatitis, the same antibiotics and daily doses as in EM are recommended. In arthritis, oral treatment with doxycycline may be tried first, but in cases of poor therapeutic response, patients should be treated intravenously with cephalosporins or penicillin G. Intravenous cephalosporins or penicillin G is also recommended for stage III neuroborreliosis.

EVALUATION, INTERPRETATION, AND REPORTING OF RESULTS

General Aspects

Clinical criteria (case history and clinical findings) are decisive factors in the diagnosis and ordering of microbiological laboratory testing. The predictive value of laboratory tests is directly related to the pretest probability. It should be kept in mind that the lower the probability based on the clinical diagnosis, the lower the predictive value of a positive test result. For example, a negative serologic result has a high

negative predictive value for Lyme arthritis, since nearly all cases are seropositive. Whether or not a positive test corresponds with the patient's presentation is a question that can only be answered by the clinician, e.g., by means of clinical case definitions applied to the various manifestations of LB. Therefore, the laboratory report should not contain any therapy recommendations.

Serologic Report

The serologic report should contain the following points:

1. Recording of individual test results. Results of the first assay, generally an EIA, are reported as positive, indeterminate, or negative. The immunoblot results are reported as positive or negative. In the case of a positive result, the reactive diagnostic bands may be reported (135). Caution against overinterpretation of minimally reactive blots must be emphasized (e.g., IgG reactivity against p41 is expected in approximately 50% of healthy adults in the United States and Europe and is excluded from the European scoring criteria).

2. Assessment of the final result of the two-step approach regarding its immunodiagnostic significance (e.g., whether specific antibodies have been detected or not).

3. Assessment of serologic findings as to the stage of the immune response, as far as test results allow pertinent statements to this effect (see below).

4. Recommendations for further reasonable diagnostic methods (PCR or culture) or for serologic follow-up, if indicated.

Patterns of Serologic Results in Various Stages of LB

Antibody tests performed in the early stage of LB, particularly in cases lacking evidence of spirochetal dissemination, may show a negative or an indeterminate result (Table 5), often due to insufficient time for the full evolution of the immune response. In some cases, seroconversion does not occur until after initiation of treatment. Serologic testing of patients with EM alone is not recommended because of the low predictive value of a negative result and the highly characteristic appearance of most rashes. In the presence of a suggestive clinical presentation and inadequate response to therapy, serologic testing is warranted up to 6 weeks after onset of disease. During the first 4 weeks of a positive clinical correlation, detection of IgM is consistent with an active infection. A robust IgG response is expected thereafter. Usually, only a few bands (IgM and/or IgG) are detected by immunoblotting during the first weeks of early disease. In late disease, a positive test for IgG antibodies is mandatory for seroconfirmation and the IgM test is not useful for establishing the diagnosis; the absence of IgG rules out the diagnosis of late Lyme disease even in the presence of IgM. False-positive IgM results due to a polyclonal B-cell activation immune response in the

TABLE 5 Sensitivity of antibody detection methods in the diagnosis of Lyme disease

Stage	Sensitivity (%)	Remarks
I	20–50	Predominance of IgM
II	70–90	Presence of IgM and IgG; in cases of long disease duration, predominance of IgG
III	Nearly 100[a]	Usually only IgG

[a]Negative only for patients with a very short duration of symptoms.

context of herpesvirus infections or autoimmune diseases and rheumatoid disorders also need to be considered. In many cases, the origin of such IgM responses remains unclear. Both IgM and IgG may persist for many months, and their presence may be compatible with past, asymptomatic, spontaneously resolved, or treated and clinically cured infections. Such patterns are often found among members of high-risk groups with frequent tick exposure (for example, forest workers) who do not show any clinical manifestations.

In cases of CNS neuroborreliosis, detection of pathogen-specific, intrathecal antibodies provides critical laboratory evidence of past or present infection. Anti-borrelia antibodies (IgM, IgG, and IgA) in the absence of CSF pleocytosis suggests previous infection, and since specific antibody and positive AI may be detectable years after treatment and cure, repeat testing is not appropriate for monitoring therapy success.

Influence of Antimicrobial Therapy on Serodiagnosis

Clinicians are often tempted to order repeated posttreatment serologies in an effort to correlate cure and decreasing antibody titers. However, IgG antibodies against *B. burgdorferi* (especially those against whole-cell antigens) persist for a long time even after successful therapy. Significant titer changes can only be expected several months after the end of therapy; in cases of late manifestations, even years may elapse. Moreover, a decrease in antibody titer does not rule out persistence of the pathogen. Since there is practically no indication for follow-up serologic tests, therapeutic success should be based on clinical criteria. A fourfold decline in titer of antibody to VlsE peptide C6 was shown to be an indicator of successful therapy for early Lyme disease (89), but this was not demonstrated for late disease (87) or posttreatment Lyme disease syndrome (42).

Sources of Error in Serodiagnosis

False results, both negative and positive, can occur from the test itself or the nature of the immune response. Seronegative results within the first days of disease are the norm. In Europe, differences between the test antigen and the species causing infection can also contribute to seronegative findings. Deficiencies in diagnostic antigen expression among cultivated borreliae will compromise the sensitivity of tests (important diagnostic antigens such as OspC and DbpA are often not expressed in cultivated borreliae, and VlsE is poorly expressed in vitro). The high background reactivity of many first-generation whole-cell-based assays often results in lower specificity and, therefore, frequent false-positive results. Cross-reactivity with treponemes can be largely avoided by use of Reiter treponeme adsorbent, although syphilis serology should be performed in cases where treponeme exposure cannot be ruled out. Second- and third-generation assays with improved sensitivity and specificity are preferable to the first-generation tests. Nonetheless, critical assessment of pretest risk factors, clinical history, and presentation will provide the best guidance for laboratory test use and minimize false test outcomes of current and future diagnostic tests.

REFERENCES

1. **Afzelius, A.** 1921. Erythema chronicum migrans. *Acta. Dermato-Venereol.* **2:**120–125.
2. **Aguero-Rosenfeld, M. E., J. Nowakowski, S. Bittker, D. Cooper, R. B. Nadelman, and G. P. Wormser.** 1996. Evolution of the serologic response to *Borrelia burgdorferi* in treated patients with culture-confirmed erythema migrans. *J. Clin. Microbiol.* **34:**1–9.
3. **Aguero-Rosenfeld, M. E., J. Roberge, C. A. Carbonaro, J. Nowakowski, R. B. Nadelman, and G. P. Wormser.** 1999. Effects of OspA vaccination on Lyme disease serologic testing. *J. Clin. Microbiol.* **37:**3718–3721.
4. **Aguero-Rosenfeld, M. E., G. Wang, I. Schwartz, and G. P. Wormser.** 2005. Diagnosis of Lyme borreliosis. *Clin. Microbiol. Rev.* **18:**484–509.
5. **Akin, E., G. L. McHugh, R. A. Flavell, E. Fikrig, and A. C. Steere.** 1999. The immunoglobulin (IgG) antibody response to OspA and OspB correlates with severe and prolonged Lyme arthritis and the IgG response to P35 correlates with mild and brief arthritis. *Infect. Immun.* **67:**173–181.
6. **Alban, P. S., P. W. Johnson, and D. R. Nelson.** 2000. Serum-starvation-induced changes in protein synthesis and morphology of *Borrelia burgdorferi*. *Microbiology* **146:**119–127.
7. **Asbrink, E., and A. Hovmark.** 1988. Early and late cutaneous manifestations in Ixodes-borne borreliosis (erythema migrans borreliosis, Lyme borreliosis). *Ann. N. Y. Acad. Sci.* **539:**4–15.
8. **Assous, M. V., and A. Wilamowski.** 2009. Relapsing fever in Eurasia—forgotten, but certainly not gone! *Clin. Microbiol. Infect.* **15:**407–414.
9. **Bacon, R. M., B. J. Biggerstaff, M. E. Schriefer, R. D. Gilmore, Jr., M. T. Philipp, A. C. Steere, G. P. Wormser, A. R. Marques, and B. J. Johnson.** 2003. Serodiagnosis of Lyme disease by kinetic enzyme-linked immunosorbent assay using recombinant VlsE1 or peptide antigens of *Borrelia burgdorferi* compared with 2-tiered testing using whole-cell lysates. *J. Infect. Dis.* **187:**1187–1199.
10. **Bacon, R. M., K. J. Kugeler, and P. S. Mead.** 2008. Surveillance for Lyme disease—United States, 1992–2006. *MMWR Surveill. Summ.* **57:**1–9.
11. **Bankhead, T., and G. Chaconas.** 2007. The role of VlsE antigenic variation in the Lyme disease spirochete: persistence through a mechanism that differs from other pathogens. *Mol. Microbiol.* **65:**1547–1558.
12. **Baranton, G., D. Postic, G. Saint, I. P. Boerlin, J. C. Piffaretti, M. Assous, and P. A. Grimont.** 1992. Delineation of *Borrelia burgdorferi* sensu stricto, *Borrelia garinii* sp. nov., and group VS461 associated with Lyme borreliosis. *Int. J. Syst. Bacteriol.* **42:**378–383.
13. **Barbour, A. G.** 1984. Isolation and cultivation of Lyme disease spirochetes. *Yale J. Biol. Med.* **57:**521–525.
14. **Barbour, A. G., and S. F. Hayes.** 1986. Biology of *Borrelia* species. *Microbiol. Rev.* **50:**381–400.
15. **Belfaiza, J., D. Postic, E. Bellenger, G. Baranton, and I. S. Girons.** 1993. Genomic fingerprinting of *Borrelia burgdorferi* sensu lato by pulsed-field gel electrophoresis. *J. Clin. Microbiol.* **31:**2873–2877.
16. **Berger, B. W., R. C. Johnson, C. Kodner, and L. Coleman.** 1992. Cultivation of *Borrelia burgdorferi* from erythema migrans lesions and perilesional skin. *J. Clin. Microbiol.* **30:**359–361.
17. **Bergstrom, S., V. G. Bundoc, and A. G. Barbour.** 1989. Molecular analysis of linear plasmid-encoded major surface proteins, OspA and OspB, of the Lyme disease spirochaete *Borrelia burgdorferi*. *Mol. Microbiol.* **3:**479–486.
18. **Blanc, F., B. Jaulhac, M. Fleury, J. de Seze, S. J. de Martino, V. Remy, G. Blaison, Y. Hansmann, D. Christmann, and C. Tranchant.** 2007. Relevance of the antibody index to diagnose Lyme neuroborreliosis among seropositive patients. *Neurology* **69:**953–958.
19. **Bradley, J. F., R. C. Johnson, and J. L. Goodman.** 1994. The persistence of spirochetal nucleic acids in active Lyme arthritis. *Ann. Intern. Med.* **120:**487–489.
20. **Brettschneider, S., H. Bruckbauer, N. Klugbauer, and H. Hofmann.** 1998. Diagnostic value of PCR for detection of *Borrelia burgdorferi* in skin biopsy and urine samples from patients with skin borreliosis. *J. Clin. Microbiol.* **36:**2658–2665.
21. **Brorson, O., and S. H. Brorson.** 1998. In vitro conversion of *Borrelia burgdorferi* to cystic forms in spinal fluid, and transformation to mobile spirochetes by incubation in BSKH medium. *Infection* **26:**144–150.

22. **Brunner, M., and L. H. Sigal.** 2001. Use of serum immune complexes in a new test that accurately confirms early Lyme disease and active infection with *Borrelia burgdorferi. J. Clin. Microbiol.* **39:**3213–3221.

23. **Burgdorfer, W., A. G. Barbour, S. F. Hayes, J. L. Benach, E. Grunwaldt, and J. P. Davis.** 1982. Lyme disease—a tick-borne spirochetosis? *Science* **216:**1317–1319.

24. **Carlisle, R. J.** 1906. Two cases of relapsing fever with notes on the occurrence of the disease throughout the world at the present day. *J. Infect. Dis.* **3:**233–265.

25. **Centers for Disease Control and Prevention.** 1995. Recommendations for test performance and interpretation from the Second National Conference on Serologic Diagnosis of Lyme Disease. *Morb. Mortal. Wkly. Rep.* **44:**590.

26. **Centers for Disease Control and Prevention.** 2005. Caution regarding testing for Lyme disease. *Morb. Mortal. Wkly. Rep.* **54:**125.

27. **Centers for Disease Control and Prevention.** 2007. Acute respiratory distress syndrome in persons with tick-borne relapsing fever—three states, 2004–2005. *Morb. Mortal. Wkly. Rep.* **56:**1073–1076.

28. **Collares-Pereira, M., S. Couceiro, I. Franca, K. Kurtenbach, S. M. Schafer, L. Vitorino, L. Goncalves, S. Baptista, M. L. Vieira, and C. Cunha.** 2004. First isolation of *Borrelia lusitaniae* from a human patient. *J. Clin. Microbiol.* **42:**1316–1318.

29. **Coyle, P. K., S. E. Schutzer, A. L. Belman, L. B. Krupp, and Z. Dheng.** 1992. Cerebrospinal fluid immunologic parameters in neurologic Lyme disease, p. 31–44. *In* S. E. Schutzer (ed.), *Lyme Disease: Molecular and Immunologic Approaches.* Cold Spring Harbor Laboratory Press, Cold Spring Harbor, N.Y.

30. **Cutler, S. J., A. Abdissa, and J. F. Trape.** 2009. New concepts for the old challenge of African relapsing fever borreliosis. *Clin. Microbiol. Infect.* **15:**400–406.

31. **Cutler, S. J., J. Moss, M. Fukunaga, D. J. Wright, D. Fekade, and D. Warrell.** 1997. *Borrelia recurrentis* characterization and comparison with relapsing-fever, Lyme-associated, and other *Borrelia* spp. *Int. J. Syst. Bacteriol.* **47:**958–968.

32. **de Silva, A. M., and E. Fikrig.** 1995. Growth and migration of *Borrelia burgdorferi* in *Ixodes* ticks during blood feeding. *Am. J. Trop. Med. Hyg.* **53:**397–404.

33. **Dressler, F., R. Ackermann, and A. C. Steere.** 1994. Antibody responses to the three genomic groups of *Borrelia burgdorferi* in European Lyme borreliosis. *J. Infect. Dis.* **169:**313–318.

34. **Dressler, F., J. A. Whalen, B. N. Reinhardt, and A. C. Steere.** 1993. Western blotting in the serodiagnosis of Lyme disease. *J. Infect. Dis.* **167:**392–400.

35. **Dumler, J. S.** 2001. Molecular diagnosis of Lyme disease: review and meta-analysis. *Mol. Diagn.* **6:**1–11.

36. **Dutton, J. E., and J. L. Todd.** 1905. The nature of tick fever in the eastern part of the Congo Free State, with notes on the distribution and bionomics of the ticks. *Br. Med. J.* **2:**1259–1260.

37. **Dworkin, M. S., T. G. Schwan, D. E. Anderson, Jr., and S. M. Borchardt.** 2008. Tick-borne relapsing fever. *Infect. Dis. Clin. N. Am.* **22:**449–468, viii.

38. **Eiffert, H., A. Karsten, R. Thomssen, and H. J. Christen.** 1998. Characterization of *Borrelia burgdorferi* strains in Lyme arthritis. *Scand. J. Infect. Dis.* **30:**265–268.

39. **Eiffert, H., A. Ohlenbusch, H. J. Christen, R. Thomssen, A. Spielman, and F. R. Matuschka.** 1995. Nondifferentiation between Lyme disease spirochetes from vector ticks and human cerebrospinal fluid. *J. Infect. Dis.* **171:**476–479.

40. **Engstrom, S. M., E. Shoop, and R. C. Johnson.** 1995. Immunoblot interpretation criteria for serodiagnosis of early Lyme disease. *J. Clin. Microbiol.* **33:**419–427.

41. **Felsenfeld, O.** 1965. *Borrelia; Strains, Vectors, Human and Animal Borreliosis.* Warren H. Green, Inc., St. Louis, MO.

42. **Fleming, R. V., A. R. Marques, M. S. Klempner, C. H. Schmid, L. G. Dally, D. S. Martin, and M. T. Philipp.** 2004. Pre-treatment and post-treatment assessment of the C(6) test in patients with persistent symptoms and a history of Lyme borreliosis. *Eur. J. Clin. Microbiol. Infect. Dis.* **23:**615–618.

43. **Fraser, C. M., S. Casjens, W. M. Huang, G. G. Sutton, R. Clayton, R. Lathigra, O. White, K. A. Ketchum, R. Dodson, E. K. Hickey, M. Gwinn, B. Dougherty, J. F. Tomb, R. D. Fleischmann, D. Richardson, J. Peterson, A. R. Kerlavage, J. Quackenbush, S. Salzberg, M. Hanson, R. van Vugt, N. Palmer, M. D. Adams, J. Gocayne, J. Weidman, T. Utterback, L. Watthey, L. McDonald, P. Artiach, C. Bowman, S. Garland, C. Fuji, M.D. Cotton, K. Horst, K. Roberts, B. Hatch, H. O. Smith, and J. C. Venter.** 1997. Genomic sequence of a Lyme disease spirochaete, *Borrelia burgdorferi. Nature* **390:**580–586.

44. **Gern, L.** 2009. Life cycle of Borrelia burgdorferi sensu lato and transmission to humans. *Curr. Probl. Dermatol.* **37:**18–30.

45. **Glöckner, G., R. Lehmann, A. Romualdi, S. Pradella, U. Schulte-Spechtel, M. Schilhabel, B. Wilske, J. Suhnel, and M. Platzer.** 2004. Comparative analysis of the *Borrelia garinii* genome. *Nucleic Acids Res.* **32:**6038–6046.

46. **Goettner, G., U. Schulte-Spechtel, R. Hillermann, G. Liegl, B. Wilske, and V. Fingerle.** 2005. Improvement of Lyme borreliosis serodiagnosis by a newly developed recombinant IgG and IgM line immunoblot and addition of VlsE and DbpA homologues. *J. Clin. Microbiol.* **43:**3602–3609.

47. **Goodman, J. L., J. F. Bradley, A. E. Ross, P. Goellner, A. Lagus, B. Vitale, B. W. Berger, S. Luger, and R. C. Johnson.** 1995. Bloodstream invasion in early Lyme disease: results from a prospective, controlled, blinded study using the polymerase chain reaction. *Am. J. Med.* **99:**6–12.

48. **Gruntar, I., T. Malovrh, R. Murgia, and M. Cinco.** 2001. Conversion of *Borrelia garinii* cystic forms to motile spirochetes in vivo. *APMIS* **109:**383–388.

49. **Halperin, J. J.** 2008. Nervous system Lyme disease. *Infect. Dis. Clin. N. Am.* **22:**261–274, vi.

50. **Hansen, K., P. Hindersson, and N. S. Pedersen.** 1988. Measurement of antibodies to the *Borrelia burgdorferi* flagellum improves serodiagnosis in Lyme disease. *J. Clin. Microbiol.* **26:**338–346.

51. **Hansen, K., and A. M. Lebech.** 1991. Lyme neuroborreliosis: a new sensitive diagnostic assay for intrathecal synthesis of *Borrelia burgdorferi*—specific immunoglobulin G, A, and M. *Ann. Neurol.* **30:**197–205.

52. **Hansen, K., K. Pii, and A. M. Lebech.** 1991. Improved immunoglobulin M serodiagnosis in Lyme borreliosis by using a μ-capture enzyme-linked immunosorbent assay with biotinylated *Borrelia burgdorferi* flagella. *J. Clin. Microbiol.* **29:**166–173.

53. **Hauser, U., G. Lehnert, R. Lobentanzer, and B. Wilske.** 1997. Interpretation criteria for standardized Western blots for three European species of *Borrelia burgdorferi* sensu lato. *J. Clin. Microbiol.* **35:**1433–1444.

54. **Hildenbrand, P., D. E. Craven, R. Jones, and P. Nemeskal.** 2009. Lyme neuroborreliosis: manifestations of a rapidly emerging zoonosis. *AJNR Am. J. Neuroradiol.* **30:**1079–1087.

55. **Hodzic, E., S. Feng, K. J. Freet, D. L. Borjesson, and S. W. Barthold.** 2002. Borrelia burgdorferi population kinetics and selected gene expression at the host-vector interface. *Infect. Immun.* **70:**3382–3388.

56. **Hollstrom, E.** 1951 Successful treatment of erythema migrans Afzelius. *Acta. Derm. Venereol.* **31:**235–243.

57. **Horowitz, H. W., C. S. Pavia, S. Bittker, G. Forseter, D. Cooper, R. B. Nadelman, D. Byrne, R. C. Johnson, and G. P. Wormser.** 1994. Sustained cellular immune responses to *Borrelia burgdorferi*: lack of correlation with clinical presentation and serology. *Clin. Diagn. Lab. Immunol.* **1:**373–378.

58. **Hubalek, Z.** 2009. Epidemiology of lyme borreliosis. *Curr. Probl. Dermatol.* **37:**31–50.

59. **Humair, P., and L. Gern.** 2000. The wild hidden face of Lyme borreliosis in Europe. *Microbes Infect.* **2:**915–922.

60. **Hyde, F. W., R. C. Johnson, T. J. White, and C. E. Shelburne.** 1989. Detection of antigens in urine of mice and humans infected with *Borrelia burgdorferi*, etiologic agent of Lyme disease. *J. Clin. Microbiol.* **27:**58–61.

61. **Ivanova, L., I. Christova, V. Neves, M. Aroso, L. Meirelles, D. Brisson, and M. Gomes-Solecki.** 2009. Comprehensive seroprofiling of sixteen B. burgdorferi OspC: implications for Lyme disease diagnostics design. *Clin. Immunol.* **132:**393–400.

62. Jauris-Heipke, S., G. Liegl, V. Preac-Mursic, D. Rössler, E. Schwab, E. Soutschek, G. Will, and B. Wilske. 1995. Molecular analysis of genes encoding outer surface protein C (OspC) of *Borrelia burgdorferi* sensu lato: relationship to *ospA* genotype and evidence of lateral gene exchange of *ospC*. *J. Clin. Microbiol.* **33**:1860–1866.

63. Johnson, B. J. 2006. Lyme disease: serologic assays for antibodies to *Borrelia burgdorferi*, p. 493–500. *In* B. Detrick, R. G. Hamilton, and J. D. Folds (ed.), *Manual of Molecular and Clinical Laboratory Immunology*, 7th ed. ASM Press, Washington, DC.

64. Johnson, B. J., K. E. Robbins, R. E. Bailey, B. L. Cao, S. L. Sviat, R. B. Craven, L. W. Mayer, and D. T. Dennis. 1996. Serodiagnosis of Lyme disease: accuracy of a two-step approach using a flagella-based ELISA and immunoblotting. *J. Infect. Dis.* **174**:346–353.

65. Johnson, R. C. 1998. *Borrelia*, p. 1277–1286. *In* L. H. Collier and W. W. Topley (ed.), *Topley & Wilson's Microbiology and Microbial Infections*. Arnold, London, Great Britain.

66. Johnson, W. D., Jr. 1995. *Borrelia* species (relapsing fever), p. 2141–2143. *In* G. L. Mandell, J. E. Bennett, and R. Dolin (ed.), *Mandell, Douglas and Bennett's Principles and Practice of Infectious Diseases*, 4th ed. Churchill Livingstone, New York, NY.

67. Kahl, O., C. Janetzki-Mittmann, J. S. Gray, R. Jonas, J. Stein, and R. de Boer. 1998. Risk of infection with *Borrelia burgdorferi* sensu lato for a host in relation to the duration of nymphal Ixodes ricinus feeding and the method of tick removal. *Zentbl. Bakteriol.* **287**:41–52.

68. Kaiser, R., and S. Rauer. 1999. Advantage of recombinant borrelial proteins for serodiagnosis of neuroborreliosis. *J. Med. Microbiol.* **48**:5–10.

69. Kaiser, R., and S. Rauer. 1999. Serodiagnosis of neuroborreliosis: comparison of reliability of three confirmatory assays. *Infection* **27**:177–182.

70. Kalish, R. A., J. M. Leong, and A. C. Steere. 1993. Association of treatment-resistant chronic Lyme arthritis with HLA-DR4 and antibody reactivity to OspA and OspB of Borrelia burgdorferi. *Infect. Immun.* **61**:2774–2779.

71. Kalish, R. S., J. A. Wood, W. Golde, R. Bernard, L. E. Davis, R. C. Grimson, P. K. Coyle, and B. J. Luft. 2003. Human T lymphocyte response to *Borrelia burgdorferi* infection: no correlation between human leukocyte function antigen type 1 peptide response and clinical status. *J. Infect. Dis.* **187**:102–108.

72. Klempner, M. S., C. H. Schmid, L. Hu, A. C. Steere, G. Johnson, B. McCloud, R. Noring, and A. Weinstein. 2001. Intralaboratory reliability of serologic and urine testing for Lyme disease. *Am. J. Med.* **110**:217–219.

73. Kraiczy, P., J. Hellwage, C. Skerka, H. Becker, M. Kirschfink, M. M. Simon, V. Brade, P. F. Zipfel, and R. Wallich. 2004. Complement resistance of *Borrelia burgdorferi* correlates with the expression of BbCRASP-1, a novel linear plasmid-encoded surface protein that interacts with human factor H and FHL-1 and is unrelated to Erp proteins. *J. Biol. Chem.* **279**:2421–2429.

74. Lahdenne, P., J. Panelius, H. Saxen, T. Heikkila, H. Sillanpaa, M. Peltomaa, M. Arnez, H. I. Huppertz, and I. J. Seppala. 2003. Improved serodiagnosis of erythema migrans using novel recombinant borrelial BBK32 antigens. *J. Med. Microbiol.* **52**:563–567.

75. Lawrenz, M. B., J. M. Hardham, R. T. Owens, J. Nowakowski, A. C. Steere, G. P. Wormser, and S. J. Norris. 1999. Human antibody responses to VlsE antigenic variation protein of *Borrelia burgdorferi*. *J. Clin. Microbiol.* **37**:3997–4004.

76. Lebech, A. M., K. Hansen, F. Brandrup, O. Clemmensen, and L. Halkier-Sorensen. 2000. Diagnostic value of PCR for detection of *Borrelia burgdorferi* DNA in clinical specimens from patients with erythema migrans and Lyme neuroborreliosis. *Mol. Diagn.* **5**:139–150.

77. Le Fleche, A., D. Postic, K. Girardet, O. Peter, and G. Baranton. 1997. Characterization of *Borrelia lusitaniae* sp. nov. by 16S ribosomal DNA sequence analysis. *Int. J. Syst. Bacteriol.* **47**:921–925.

78. Liang, F. T., E. Aberer, M. Cinco, L. Gern, C. M. Hu, Y. N. Lobet, M. Ruscio, P. E. Voet, Jr., V. E. Weynants, and M. T. Philipp. 2000. Antigenic conservation of an immunodominant invariable region of the VlsE lipoprotein among European pathogenic genospecies of *Borrelia burgdorferi* SL. *J. Infect. Dis.* **182**:1455–1462.

79. Luft, B. J., C. R. Steinman, H. C. Neimark, B. Muralidhar, T. Rush, M. F. Finkel, M. Kunkel, and R. J. Dattwyler. 1992. Invasion of the central nervous system by *Borrelia burgdorferi* in acute disseminated infection. *JAMA* **267**:1364–1367.

80. Marques, A. R., R. L. Hornung, L. Dally, and M. T. Philipp. 2005. Detection of immune complexes is not independent of detection of antibodies in Lyme disease patients and does not confirm active infection with *Borrelia burgdorferi*. *Clin. Diagn. Lab. Immunol.* **12**:1036–1040.

81. Mathiesen, M. J., M. Christiansen, K. Hansen, A. Holm, E. Asbrink, and M. Theisen. 1998. Peptide-based OspC enzyme-linked immunosorbent assay for serodiagnosis of Lyme borreliosis. *J. Clin. Microbiol.* **36**:3474–3479.

82. Nocton, J. J., F. Dressler, B. J. Rutledge, P. N. Rys, D. H. Persing, and A. C. Steere. 1994. Detection of *Borrelia burgdorferi* DNA by polymerase chain reaction in synovial fluid from patients with Lyme arthritis. *N. Engl. J. Med.* **330**:229–234.

83. Norris, S. J. 2006. Antigenic variation with a twist–the Borrelia story. *Mol. Microbiol.* **60**:1319–1322.

84. Ojaimi, C., C. Brooks, S. Casjens, P. Rosa, A. Elias, A. Barbour, A. Jasinskas, J. Benach, L. Katona, J. Radolf, M. Caimano, J. Skare, K. Swingle, D. Akins, and I. Schwartz. 2003. Profiling of temperature-induced changes in *Borrelia burgdorferi* gene expression by using whole genome arrays. *Infect. Immun.* **71**:1689–1705.

85. Pachner, A. R., and I. Steiner. 2007. Lyme neuroborreliosis: infection, immunity, and inflammation. *Lancet Neurol.* **6**:544–552.

86. Panelius, J., P. Lahdenne, H. Saxen, S. A. Carlsson, T. Heikkila, M. Peltomaa, A. Lauhio, and I. Seppala. 2003. Diagnosis of Lyme neuroborreliosis with antibodies to recombinant proteins DbpA, BBK32, and OspC, and VlsE IR6 peptide. *J. Neurol.* **250**:1318–1327.

87. Peltomaa, M., G. McHugh, and A. C. Steere. 2003. Persistence of the antibody response to the VlsE sixth invariant region (IR6) peptide of *Borrelia burgdorferi* after successful antibiotic treatment of Lyme disease. *J. Infect. Dis.* **187**:1178–1186.

88. Persing, D. H., B. J. Rutledge, P. N. Rys, D. S. Podzorski, P. D. Mitchell, K. D. Reed, B. Liu, E. Fikrig, and S. E. Malawista. 1994. Target imbalance: disparity of *Borrelia burgdorferi* genetic material in synovial fluid from Lyme arthritis patients. *J. Infect. Dis.* **169**:668–672.

89. Philipp, M. T., A. R. Marques, P. T. Fawcett, L. G. Dally, and D. S. Martin. 2003. C6 test as an indicator of therapy outcome for patients with localized or disseminated Lyme borreliosis. *J. Clin. Microbiol.* **41**:4955–4960.

90. Phillips, S. E., L. H. Mattman, D. Hulinska, and H. Moayad. 1998. A proposal for the reliable culture of *Borrelia burgdorferi* from patients with chronic Lyme disease, even from those previously aggressively treated. *Infection* **26**:364–367.

91. Picken, M. M., R. N. Picken, D. Han, Y. Cheng, E. Ruzic-Sabljic, J. Cimperman, V. Maraspin, S. Lotric-Furlan, and F. Strle. 1997. A two year prospective study to compare culture and polymerase chain reaction amplification for the detection and diagnosis of Lyme borreliosis. *Mol. Pathol.* **50**:186–193.

92. Pollack, R. J., S. R. Telford III, and A. Spielman. 1993. Standardization of medium for culturing Lyme disease spirochetes. *J. Clin. Microbiol.* **31**:1251–1255.

93. Postic, D., M. V. Assous, P. A. Grimont, and G. Baranton. 1994. Diversity of *Borrelia burgdorferi* sensu lato evidenced by restriction fragment length polymorphism of rrf (5S)-rrl (23S) intergenic spacer amplicons. *Int. J. Syst. Bacteriol.* **44**:743–752.

94. Prasad, A., and D. Sankar. 1999. Overdiagnosis and overtreatment of Lyme neuroborreliosis are preventable. *Postgrad. Med. J.* **75**:650–656.

95. **Preac-Mursic, V.** 1993. Antibiotic susceptibility of *Borrelia burgdorferi*, in vitro and in vivo, p. 301–311. *In* K. Weber and W. Burgdorfer (ed.), *Aspects of Lyme Borreliosis*. Springer Verlag, Berlin, Germany.

96. **Preac-Mursic, V., B. Wilske, and S. Reinhardt.** 1991. Culture of *Borrelia burgdorferi* on six solid media. *Eur. J. Clin. Microbiol. Infect. Dis.* **10:**1076–1079.

97. **Priem, S., M. G. Rittig, T. Kamradt, G. R. Burmester, and A. Krause.** 1997. An optimized PCR leads to rapid and highly sensitive detection of *Borrelia burgdorferi* in patients with Lyme borreliosis. *J. Clin. Microbiol.* **35:**685–690.

98. **Ramos, J. M., E. Malmierca, F. Reyes, W. Wolde, A. Galata, A. Tesfamariam, and M. Gorgolas.** 2004. Characteristics of louse-borne relapsing fever in Ethiopian children and adults. *Ann. Trop. Med. Parasitol.* **98:**191–196.

99. **Rauter, C., M. Mueller, I. Diterich, S. Zeller, D. Hassler, T. Meergans, and T. Hartung.** 2005. Critical evaluation of urine-based PCR assay for diagnosis of Lyme borreliosis. *Clin. Diagn. Lab. Immunol.* **12:**910–917.

100. **Richter, D., D. Postic, N. Sertour, I. Livey, F.-R. Matuschka, and G. Baranton.** 2006. Delineation of *Borrelia burgdorferi* sensu lato species by multilocus sequence analysis and confirmation of the delineation of *B. spielmanii* sp. nov. *Int. J. Syst. Evol. Microbiol.* **56:**873–881.

101. **Rijpkema, S. G., D. J. Tazelaar, M. J. Molkenboer, G. T. Noordhoek, G. Plantinga, L. M. Schouls, and J. F. Schellekens.** 1997. Detection of *Borrelia afzelii, Borrelia burgdorferi* sensu stricto, *Borrelia garinii* and group VS116 by PCR in skin biopsies of patients with erythema migrans and acrodermatitis chronica atrophicans. *Clin. Microbiol. Infect.* **3:**109–116.

102. **Roth, A., H. Mauch, and U. B. Göbel.** 1997. MIQ 1, nucleic acid amplification techniques. *In* H. Mauch and (ed.), *Qualitätsstandards in der Mikrobiologisch-Infektiologischen Diagnostik.* Gustav Fischer Verlag, Stuttgart, Germany. (In German.)

103. **Russell, H., J. S. Sampson, G. P. Schmid, H. W. Wilkinson, and B. Plikaytis.** 1984. Enzyme-linked immunosorbent assay and indirect immunofluorescence assay for Lyme disease. *J. Infect. Dis.* **149:**465–470.

104. **Ruzic-Sabljic, E., V. Maraspin, S. Lotric-Furlan, T. Jurca, M. Logar, A. Pikelj-Pecnik, and F. Strle.** 2002. Characterization of *Borrelia burgdorferi* sensu lato strains isolated from human material in Slovenia. *Wien. Klin. Wochenschr.* **114:**544–550.

105. **Schmidt, B. L.** 1997. PCR in laboratory diagnosis of human *Borrelia burgdorferi* infections. *Clin. Microbiol. Rev.* **10:**185–201.

106. **Schulte-Spechtel, U., G. Lehnert, G. Liegl, V. Fingerle, C. Heimerl, B. J. Johnson, and B. Wilske.** 2003. Significant improvement of the recombinant *Borrelia*-specific immunoglobulin G immunoblot test by addition of VlsE and a DbpA homologue derived from *Borrelia garinii* for diagnosis of early neuroborreliosis. *J. Clin. Microbiol.* **41:**1299–1303.

107. **Schutzer, S. E., P. K. Coyle, P. Reid, and B. Holland.** 1999. *Borrelia burgdorferi*-specific immune complexes in acute Lyme disease. *JAMA* **282:**1942–1946.

108. **Schwan, T. G.** 2003. Temporal regulation of outer surface proteins of the Lyme-disease spirochaete Borrelia burgdorferi. *Biochem. Soc. Trans.* **31:**108–112.

109. **Schwartz, J. J., A. Gazumyan, and I. Schwartz.** 1992. rRNA gene organization in the Lyme disease spirochete, *Borrelia burgdorferi. J. Bacteriol.* **174:**3757–3765.

110. **Scrimenti, R. J.** 1970. Erythema chronicum migrans. *Arch. Dermatol.* **102:**104–105.

111. **Seinost, G., D. E. Dykhuizen, R. J. Dattwyler, W. T. Golde, J. J. Dunn, I. N. Wang, G. P. Wormser, M. E. Schriefer, and B. J. Luft.** 1999. Four clones of Borrelia burgdorferi sensu stricto cause invasive infection in humans. *Infect. Immun.* **67:**3518–3524.

112. **Stanek, G., and F. Strle.** 2003. Lyme borreliosis. *Lancet* **362:**1639–1647.

113. **Steere, A. C.** 2006. Lyme borreliosis in 2005, 30 years after initial observations in Lyme Connecticut. *Wien. Klin. Wochenschr.* **118:**625–633.

114. **Steere, A. C., V. P. Berardi, K. E. Weeks, E. L. Logigian, and R. Ackermann.** 1990. Evaluation of the intrathecal antibody response to *Borrelia burgdorferi* as a diagnostic test for Lyme neuroborreliosis. *J. Infect. Dis.* **161:**1203–1209.

115. **Steere, A. C., J. Coburn, and L. Glickstein.** 2004. The emergence of Lyme disease. *J. Clin. Investig.* **113:**1093–1101.

116. **Steere, A. C., S. E. Malawista, D. R. Snydman, R. E. Shope, W. A. Andiman, M. R. Ross, and F. M. Steele.** 1977. Lyme arthritis: an epidemic of oligoarticular arthritis in children and adults in three Connecticut communities. *Arthritis Rheum.* **20:**7–17.

117. **Steere, A. C., G. McHugh, N. Damle, and V. K. Sikand.** 2008. Prospective study of serologic tests for Lyme disease. *Clin. Infect. Dis.* **47:**188–195.

118. **Strle, F., R. B. Nadelman, J. Cimperman, J. Nowakowski, R. N. Picken, I. Schwartz, V. Maraspin, M. E. Aguero-Rosenfeld, S. Varde, S. Lotric-Furlan, and G. P. Wormser.** 1999. Comparison of culture-confirmed erythema migrans caused by *Borrelia burgdorferi* sensu stricto in New York State and by *Borrelia afzelii* in Slovenia. *Ann. Intern. Med.* **130:**32–36.

119. **Vasiliu, V., P. Herzer, D. Rössler, G. Lehnert, and B. Wilske.** 1998. Heterogeneity of *Borrelia burgdorferi* sensu lato demonstrated by an *ospA*-type-specific PCR in synovial fluid from patients with Lyme arthritis. *Med. Microbiol. Immunol.* **187:**97–102.

120. **Vial, L., G. Diatta, A. Tall, H. Bael, H. Bouganali, P. Durand, C. Sokhna, C. Rogier, F. Renaud, and J. F. Trape.** 2006. Incidence of tick-borne relapsing fever in west Africa: longitudinal study. *Lancet* **368:**37–43.

121. **Wang, G., A. P. van Dam, and J. Dankert.** 1999. Phenotypic and genetic characterization of a novel *Borrelia burgdorferi* sensu lato isolate from a patient with lyme borreliosis. *J. Clin. Microbiol.* **37:**3025–3028.

122. **Wang, G., A. P. van Dam, I. Schwartz, and J. Dankert.** 1999. Molecular typing of *Borrelia burgdorferi* sensu lato: taxonomic, epidemiological, and clinical implications. *Clin. Microbiol. Rev.* **12:**633–653.

123. **Weber, K., and H. W. Pfister.** 1994. Clinical management of Lyme borreliosis. *Lancet* **343:**1017–1020.

123a. **Whitaker, J. A., E. G. Fort, and D. M. Hamilton.** January 2005. U.S. patent 6,838,247.

124. **Wilske, B.** 2005. Epidemiology and diagnosis of Lyme borreliosis. *Ann. Med.* **37:**568–579.

125. **Wilske, B., U. Busch, H. Eiffert, V. Fingerle, H. W. Pfister, D. Rössler, and V. Preac-Mursic.** 1996. Diversity of OspA and OspC among cerebrospinal fluid isolates of *Borrelia burgdorferi* sensu lato from patients with neuroborreliosis in Germany. *Med. Microbiol. Immunol.* **184:**195–201.

126. **Wilske, B., U. Busch, V. Fingerle, S. Jauris-Heipke, V. Preac Mursic, D. Rössler, and G. Will.** 1996. Immunological and molecular variability of OspA and OspC. Implications for *Borrelia* vaccine development. *Infection* **24:**208–212.

127. **Wilske, B., V. Fingerle, P. Herzer, A. Hofmann, G. Lehnert, H. Peters, H. W. Pfister, V. Preac-Mursic, E. Soutschek, and K. Weber.** 1993. Recombinant immunoblot in the serodiagnosis of Lyme borreliosis. Comparison with indirect immunofluorescence and enzyme-linked immunosorbent assay. *Med. Microbiol. Immunol.* **182:**255–270.

128. **Wilske, B., C. Habermann, V. Fingerle, B. Hillenbrand, S. Jauris-Heipke, G. Lehnert, I. Pradel, D. Rössler, and U. Schulte-Spechtel.** 1999. An improved recombinant IgG immunoblot for serodiagnosis of Lyme borreliosis. *Med. Microbiol. Immunol.* **188:**139–144.

129. **Wilske, B., S. Jauris-Heipke, R. Lobentanzer, I. Pradel, V. Preac-Mursic, D. Rössler, E. Soutschek, and R. C. Johnson.** 1995. Phenotypic analysis of outer surface protein C (OspC) of *Borrelia burgdorferi* sensu lato by monoclonal antibodies: relationship to genospecies and OspA serotype. *J. Clin. Microbiol.* **33:**103–109.

130. **Wilske, B., V. Preac-Mursic, U. B. Göbel, B. Graf, S. Jauris, E. Soutschek, E. Schwab, and G. Zumstein.** 1993. An OspA serotyping system for *Borrelia burgdorferi* based on

reactivity with monoclonal antibodies and OspA sequence analysis. *J. Clin. Microbiol.* **31:**340–350.

131. **Wilske, B., G. Schierz, V. Preac-Mursic, K. von Busch, R. Kuhbeck, H. W. Pfister, and K. Einhäupl.** 1986. Intrathecal production of specific antibodies against *Borrelia burgdorferi* in patients with lymphocytic meningoradiculitis (Bannwarth's syndrome). *J. Infect. Dis.* **153:**304–314.

132. **Wilske, B., B. J. B. Johnson and M. E. Schriefer.** 2007. *Borrelia*, p. 971–986. *In* P.R. Murray, E. J. Baron, J. H. Jorgensen, M. L. Landry, and M. A. Pfaller (ed.), *Manual of Clinical Microbiology*, 9th ed. ASM Press, Washington, DC.

133. **Wilske, B., L. Zöller, V. Brade, H. Eiffert, U. B. Göbel, G. Stanek, and H. W. Pfister.** 2000. MIQ 12, Lyme-Borreliose, p. 1–59. *In* H. Mauch and R. Lütticken (ed.), *Qualitätsstandards in der Mikrobiologisch-Infektiologischen Diagnostik*. Urban & Fischer Verlag, Munich, Germany.

134. **Wormser, G. P.** 2006. Early Lyme disease. *N. Engl. J. Med.* **354:**2794–2801.

135. **Wormser, G. P., S. Bittker, D. Cooper, J. Nowakowski, R. B. Nadelman, and C. Pavia.** 2000. Comparison of the yields of blood cultures using serum or plasma from patients with early Lyme disease. *J. Clin. Microbiol.* **38:**1648–1650.

136. **Wormser, G. P., R. J. Dattwyler, E. D. Shapiro, J. J. Halperin, A. C. Steere, M. S. Klempner, P. J. Krause, J. S. Bakken, F. Strle, G. Stanek, L. Bockenstedt, D. Fish, J. S. Dumler, and R. B. Nadelman.** 2006. The clinical assessment, treatment, and prevention of Lyme disease, human granulocytic anaplasmosis, and babesiosis: clinical practice guidelines by the Infectious Diseases Society of America. *Clin. Infect. Dis.* **43:**1089–1134.

137. **Wormser, G. P., D. Liveris, K. Hanincova, D. Brisson, S. Ludin, V. J. Stracuzzi, M. E. Embers, M. T. Philipp, A. Levin, M. Aguero-Rosenfeld, and I. Schwartz.** 2008. Effect of Borrelia burgdorferi genotype on the sensitivity of C6 and 2-tier testing in North American patients with culture-confirmed Lyme disease. *Clin. Infect. Dis.* **47:**910–914.

138. **Wormser, G. P., E. Masters, D. Liveris, J. Nowakowski, R. B. Nadelman, D. Holmgren, S. Bittker, D. Cooper, G. Wang, and I. Schwartz.** 2005. Microbiologic evaluation of patients from Missouri with erythema migrans. *Clin. Infect. Dis.* **40:**423–428.

139. **Zhang, J. R., J. M. Hardham, A. G. Barbour, and S. J. Norris.** 1997. Antigenic variation in Lyme disease borreliae by promiscuous recombination of VMP-like sequence cassettes. *Cell* **89:**275–285.

140. **Zore, A., E. Ruzic-Sabljic, V. Maraspin, J. Cimperman, S. Lotric-Furlan, A. Pikelj, T. Jurca, M. Logar, and F. Strle.** 2002. Sensitivity of culture and polymerase chain reaction for the etiologic diagnosis of erythema migrans. *Wien. Klin. Wochenschr.* **114:**606–609.

141. **Zoschke, D. C., A. A. Skemp, and D. L. Defosse.** 1991. Lymphoproliferative responses to *Borrelia burgdorferi* in Lyme disease. *Ann. Intern. Med.* **114:**285–289.

Treponema and *Brachyspira*, Human Host-Associated Spirochetes

JUSTIN D. RADOLF, ALLAN PILLAY, AND DAVID L. COX

57

TAXONOMY

The recognition of spirochetes as human host-associated organisms is believed to date from nearly 400 years ago, when Van Leeuwenhoek described spiral, nimble "animalcules" in human oral plaque (61). Determination of taxonomic relationships among spirochetes has been complicated by their fastidious nature and the refractoriness of many to cultivation. Numerous phenotypic traits have been examined in attempts to establish taxonomic hierarchies (113). Paster et al. (119) demonstrated using 16S rRNA sequences that spirochetes can be grouped into a phylum of five clusters, *Treponema*, *Spirochaeta*, *Borrelia*, *Serpula* (now *Brachyspira*), and *Leptospira*. The relatedness among members of clusters varied considerably. Interspecies similarities among borrelia were >97%, suggesting recent evolutionary divergence. In contrast, the approximate 10% sequence differences among treponemes pointed toward divergence over a much greater evolutionary time frame.

Many investigators formerly believed that cultivatable treponemes were closely related, nonpathogenic forms of *Treponema pallidum* (32, 129, 157). Miao and Fieldsteel (96, 97) dispelled this idea by demonstrating that *T. pallidum* DNA shared less than 5% homology with DNAs of cultivatable treponemes but was indistinguishable from that of a *Treponema pertenue* (yaws) strain. Consistent with rRNA data (119), they were unable to detect cross-hybridization between DNAs from many cultivatable treponemes. Their work led to the reclassification of the agents of venereal syphilis, endemic syphilis, and yaws as *T. pallidum* subsp. *pallidum*, *T. pallidum* subsp. *endemicum*, and *T. pallidum* subsp. *pertenue*, respectively, while *Treponema carateum*, the cause of the skin disease pinta, retained its status as a distinct species primarily because no isolates were available for study (142). While *Treponema denticola* has long been considered the prototype oral treponeme, it represents only a small fraction of the resident treponemes in patients with gingivitis and periodontitis (118). In 1997, all *Serpulina* species were reclassified as *Brachyspira* (112). Two *Brachyspira* species, *B. aalborgi* and *B. pilosicoli*, have been identified as causes of human intestinal spirochetosis (HIS) (14, 98).

DESCRIPTION OF THE AGENTS

Treponema pallidum Subspecies

The four members of the genus *Treponema* that cause venereal syphilis, endemic syphilis, yaws, and pinta are morphologically identical (65) and, despite advances in molecular differentiation, are distinguished primarily by differences in geographic distribution, epidemiology, clinical manifestations, and host range in experimental animals (Table 1) (95, 136). Only *T. pallidum* subsp. *pallidum* is transmitted routinely by sexual contact and vertically from a pregnant woman to her fetus (95, 127). It also is the only subspecies that regularly breaches the blood-brain barrier (127). The type strain of *T. pallidum* subsp. *pallidum* (Nichols) was isolated in 1912 from the cerebrospinal fluid of an individual with secondary syphilis (108) and has been propagated since by intratesticular inoculation of rabbits (87). No strain or subspecies of *T. pallidum* can be cultivated continuously in vitro, although limited replication has been achieved by cocultivation with mammalian cells (29). Rabbits are the animals of choice for studying syphilitic infection and can be used to recover strains from clinical specimens by rabbit infectivity testing (RIT) (87).

T. pallidum is approximately 0.2 μm in diameter, has tapering ends, and ranges in length from 6 to 20 μm (Fig. 1). Cells typically consist of 6 to 14 waves, with a wavelength of 1.1 μm and an amplitude of ~0.3 μm (Fig. 1). Because of their small diameter, pathogenic treponemes cannot be visualized by bright-field microscopy, nor do they take up Gram stain; they are best visualized by dark-field (DF) or phase-contrast microscopy. *T. pallidum* grows slowly (doubling time of 30 to 33 h in rabbits) and poorly tolerates desiccation, elevated temperatures, and high oxygen tensions (111). Once considered an anaerobe, it was reclassified as a microaerophile based on the finding that it replicates best in vitro in ambient oxygen concentrations of 3 to 5% (30). *T. pallidum* relies entirely upon glycolysis for energy production and is unable to synthesize fatty acids, nucleotides, enzyme cofactors, and most amino acids (43). The molecular architecture and cell envelope composition differ markedly from gram-negative bacteria (17). In addition to lacking lipopolysaccharide (43), the outer membrane contains an extraordinarily low density of integral

TABLE 1 Characteristics and major clinical features of the treponematoses

Venereal syphilis (*Treponema pallidum* subsp. *pallidum*)
World distribution
Transmitted predominantly sexually, also congenitally, and rarely, by transfusion
Stages/manifestations
  Primary (local): 10–90 days postinoculation (avg, 21 days)
    Single or multiple ulcers (chancres) on skin or mucous membranes
    Regional lymphadenopathy
  Secondary (disseminated): 6 wk–6 mo postinfection (also seen with early latent relapses)
    Diffuse lesions, most typically skin, but also visceral
    Other mucocutaneous lesions: condyloma lata, alopecia
    Generalized lymphadenopathy
    Occasionally constitutional symptoms
    CNS involvement common (usually asymptomatic invasion by *T. pallidum*) but also
      symptomatic (usually "aseptic" meningitis)
  Latent (early latency, ≤1 yr duration; late latency, >1 yr duration)
    Reactive serologic tests for syphilis without manifestations
    Relapses are common during early latency and are infectious
    Late latency is noninfectious, chronic, "asymptomatic" (may just be clinically inapparent)
  Tertiary
    Gummatous (skin, bones, or viscera)
    Cardiovascular (classically involving proximal thoracic aorta)
    Neurosyphilis (classically paresis, tabes dorsalis)
  Congenital
    Early (perinatal): ranges from asymptomatic to disseminated to fulminant
    Late: interstitial keratitis, bone and tooth deformities, deafness, neurosyphilis

Yaws (*Treponema pallidum* subsp. *pertenue*)
Tropical areas (sub-Saharan Africa), South America, Caribbean
Transmitted by nonvenereal person-to-person contact
Infection usually occurs in childhood
Typically does not involve CNS or cause congenital infection
Stages/manifestations
  Early: 10–90 days postinoculation (avg, 21 days)
    Primary lesion (mother yaw): papular, nontender, often pruritic, crusted, or ulcerated
    Disseminated lesions (frambesia)
    Malaise, fever, lymphadenopathy
    Osteitis, periostitis
  Latent: positive serologic tests but without other signs of infection
  Late: 10% of untreated individuals
    Destructive lesions of bone and cartilage
    Hyperkeratotic skin lesions

Endemic syphilis (*Treponema pallidum* subsp. *endemicum*)
Saharan Africa, Middle East
Transmitted by nonvenereal person-to-person contact, utensils
Infection of children or adults, rarely congenital infection
Stages/manifestations
  Early
    Primary: mucosal or cutaneous lesions, often undetected
    Secondary: disseminated oropharyngeal, cutaneous lesions
    Generalized lymphadenopathy
    Periostitis
  Latent: positive serologic tests, no other signs of infection
  Late: destructive skin, bone, and cartilage lesions

Pinta (*Treponema carateum*)
Semiarid warm areas of Central and South America
Transmitted by nonvenereal person-to-person contact, usually children or adolescents
Restricted to skin
Stages/manifestations
  Early
    Primary lesion: hyperkeratotic, pigmented papule or plaque
    Disseminated skin lesions
    Regional lymphadenopathy
  Late: pigmentary changes in skin (hyper- and hypopigmentation)

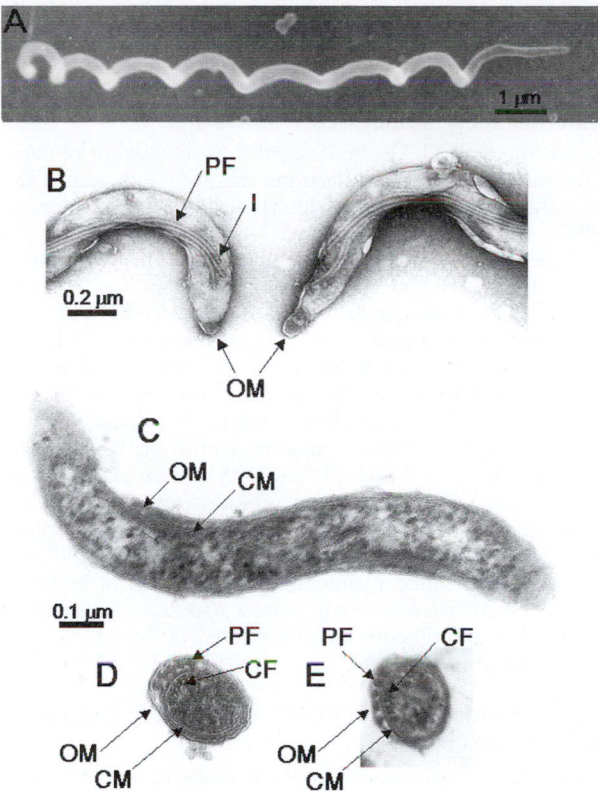

FIGURE 1 Morphology of *T. pallidum*. (A) Scanning electron micrograph showing spiral shape. (B) Negatively stained view of the tips of two organisms. Note the insertion points (I) of periplasmic flagella (PF) near the ends. (C to E) Electron micrographs of ultrathin sections, showing the outer membrane (OM), the cytoplasmic membrane (CM), periplasmic flagella (PF), and the location of the cytoplasmic filaments (CF). Reprinted from reference 109 with permission of Kluwer.

membrane proteins (17). Many of the bacterium's dominant immunogens are lipid-modified periplasmic proteins involved in transport of nutrients across the cytoplasmic membrane (17).

Host-Associated Spirochetes

Treponemes

Oral treponemes are anaerobic, spiral-shaped organisms ranging from 0.15 to 0.30 μm in diameter and from 5 to 16 μm in length (80). They can be differentiated based on genotypic characteristics and biochemical parameters, such as growth requirements, carbohydrate fermentation, and enzymatic activities (142). *T. denticola* has been identified in specimens from healthy patients and in individuals with periodontal disease (104). *T. phagedenis*, *T. refringens*, and *T. minutum* inhabit the smegma found beneath the prepuce and in other epithelial folds of the genital region. *T. phagedenis* and *T. refringens* are 0.20 to 0.25 μm in diameter, whereas *T. minutum* tends to be smaller in diameter (0.15 to 0.20 μm) (80). *T. denticola* binds to host cells and extracellular matrix components and also coaggregates with other bacteria (*Porphyromonas gingivalis* and *Fusobacterium nucleatum*) in periodontal pockets (34). Although less invasive than *T. pallidum*, *T. denticola* forms abscesses and demonstrates a limited degree of hematogenous dissemination in a SCID mouse model (42).

Brachyspira

B. aalborgi was first isolated in 1982 (66) but remains poorly characterized (150). The type strain is comma-shaped or helical, 2 to 6 μm long and approximately 0.2 μm in width, with tapered ends and 4 flagella at each end (66). Isolation requires weeks of incubation under anaerobic conditions (37). *B. aalborgi* has not been isolated from animals. *B. pilosicoli* colonizes the large intestine of a number of animal species, causes intestinal spirochetosis in pigs, and is thought to have greater human pathogenic potential (11, 98). Compared to *B. aalborgi*, isolates of *B. pilosicoli* are longer (4 to 12 μm), more coiled, and have more-pointed ends (153). On blood agar plates, *B. pilosicoli* isolates display 2 morphologically distinct weakly β-hemolytic colony types (149). Intestinal spirochetes can be found in all regions of the colon but increase in number from cecum to rectum (75). They reside in the brush border surrounded by microvilli with their proximal tips embedded in invaginations of the host cell membrane (Fig. 2). Because of high density and orientation perpendicular to the mucosal surface, they form a characteristic basophilic fringe often described as a "false brush border" in histologic samples stained with hematoxylin and eosin (H&E) (Fig. 2, top) (75). Though generally noninvasive and minimally inflammatory, they have been observed within colonic epithelial cells, subepithelial cells, and Schwann cells (117) as well as causing crypt abscesses, ulceration, and necrosis (76). Spirochetemia has been reported in a small number of critically ill patients with multiple-organ failure (151).

EPIDEMIOLOGY AND TRANSMISSION

Venereal Syphilis

The incidence of syphilis in the United States fell precipitously in the late 1940s following the introduction of penicillin (107). After a nadir in the 1950s, syphilis rates began to rise with peaks occurring every 10 years. Grassly et al. (49) contended that the oscillating nature of syphilis epidemics can be explained by waxing and waning immunity in at-risk populations. Fenton et al. (39) argued forcefully against this thesis, maintaining that epidemiologic determinants are the major drivers of syphilis transmission in developed countries. After steady declines throughout most of the 1990s to historically low levels, and despite the launching of the National Plan to Eliminate Syphilis in the United States in 1999, rates have increased annually since 2001 (21). These trends, mirrored throughout Western Europe (154), reflect the resurgence of risky sexual behaviors among men who have sex with men (MSM) (56) and also increases in syphilis among women (21). Hispanics and African Americans, particularly those in the southeastern United States, continue to be disproportionately affected; a recent serosurvey found the seroprevalence among all adults aged 18 to 49 years to be 0.71% but 4.3% among non-Hispanic blacks (48, 121). In 1999, the World Health Organization (WHO) estimated that 12 million persons acquire syphilis each year (63). The majority of cases occur in underdeveloped countries, particularly sub-Saharan Africa and South Asia. Eastern Europe and Russia reported dramatic increases in the incidence of syphilis with the fall of Communism (78). Alarming increases in syphilis rates in China, attributed to the enormous societal and economic changes in that country during the past two decades, also have been noted (26).

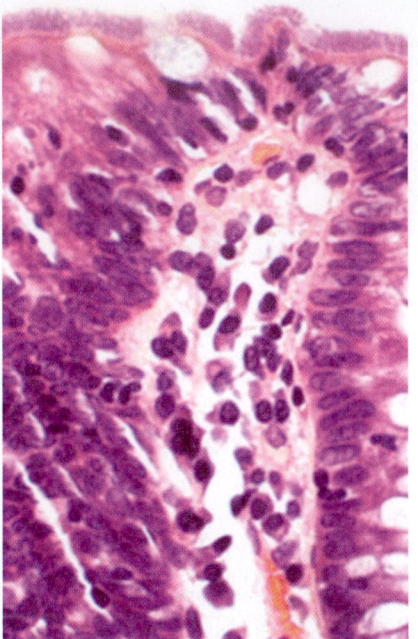

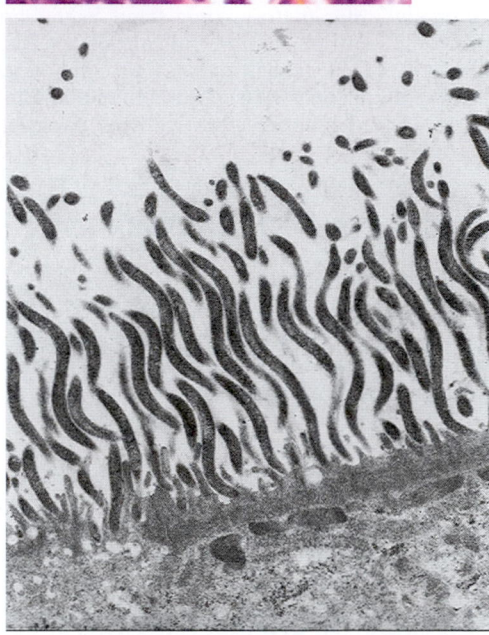

FIGURE 2 Human intestinal spirochetosis. (Top) H&E staining of a colonic biopsy sample showing a false brush border covering the luminal surface of the colon as observed by light microscopy. Reproduced from reference 36 with permission from Blackwell Publishing Asia Pty Ltd. (Bottom) TEM showing *Brachyspira aalborgi* attached end-on to the colonic mucosa, forming a false brush border. Magnification, ×11,000. Reproduced from reference 77 with permission from the American Society for Microbiology.

Transmission of syphilis occurs after contact with primary- and secondary-stage lesions (Table 1 and Fig. 3). Estimates of the risk of sexual transmission vary greatly, from 10 to 80%, with the 30% transmission rate reported by Schroeter et al. (138) a commonly quoted figure. Vertical transmission of syphilis has been recognized for several

centuries (139). Neonates also can become infected from exposure to lesional exudate or infected maternal blood within the birth canal (139).

Endemic Treponematoses

According to WHO estimates, prior to the advent of penicillin, as many as 200 million persons were exposed to the endemic treponematoses during their lifetimes. In the early 1950s, the WHO and United Nations Children's Fund launched an extremely successful program that decreased the global prevalence of endemic treponematoses by more than 95% over an approximately 10-year period (95). Unfortunately, the failure of local health services has led to their comeback in many areas where they were formerly endemic (95). In contrast to yaws and pinta, which occur in moist tropical regions, endemic syphilis is a disease of hot, dry countries; major foci of endemic syphilis still exist in the Sahelian region of Africa (Table 1) (95). Pinta is now confined to native populations in remote Central and South America (Table 1) (95). The agents of yaws and pinta are transmitted by contact with lesions during childhood or early adolescence (Table 1). Transmission of endemic syphilis occurs via nonsexual contact with infectious lesions on the skin and mucous membranes or via shared drinking and eating utensils (95).

Oral Treponemes: Gingivitis, Periodontal Disease, and Atherosclerosis

The epidemiologic importance of *T. denticola* and other oral treponemes arises from their occurrence as components of the polymicrobial consortium that causes gingivitis (62). Gingivitis is ubiquitous globally in children and adults and is associated with poor oral hygiene; comprehensive oral hygiene programs are effective in preventing or reducing gingival inflammation (4). Chronic periodontitis is most common in adults and seniors and is more common with cigarette smoking, obesity, diabetes, and alcohol consumption (3). The National Survey of Employed Adults and Seniors and the Third National Health and Nutrition Examination Survey found periodontal disease in 24% of employed adults and more than 60% of seniors (3, 24). Accumulating evidence links periodontal disease with coronary artery disease and ischemic stroke (6, 55), although risk varies considerably among studies (105, 120).

Intestinal Spirochetosis

The frequency of spirochetal colonization of the intestinal tract has declined dramatically in developed countries during the 20th century but remains high in the developing world (75). *B. aalborgi*, lacking animal reservoirs, is probably transmitted via the fecal-oral route (11). Infection with *B. pilosicoli* likely occurs by ingestion of water contaminated by feces of birds, animals, or infected humans (11). In developed countries, HIS prevalence is greatest in MSM with or without human immunodeficiency virus (HIV) infection, with oral-anal contact being the presumed mode of transmission (35, 149).

CLINICAL SIGNIFICANCE

Venereal Syphilis

Figure 3 illustrates the natural history of untreated syphilis, emphasizing the relationship among the stages of the disease, the presence of infectious treponemes, and reactivity in serologic tests (see below), while Table 2 describes the

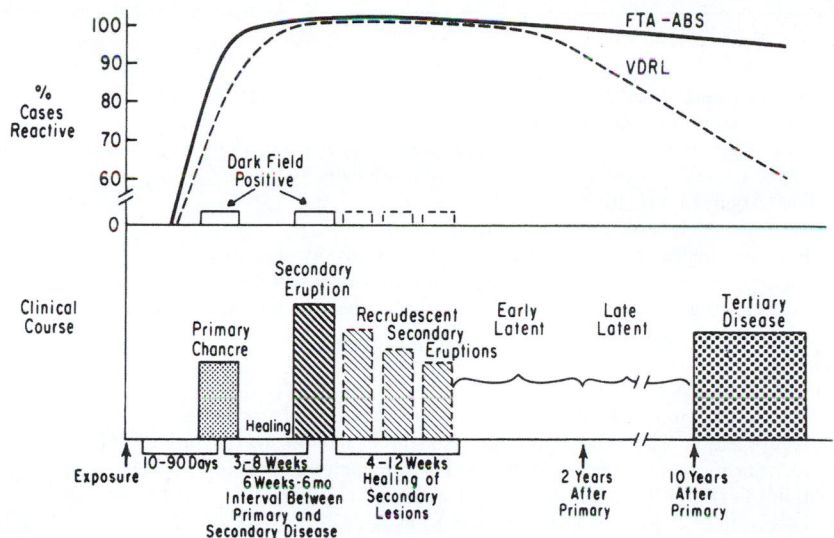

FIGURE 3 The course of untreated syphilis. The presence of treponemes in mucocutaneous lesions and serologic responses (top) are juxtaposed with disease stage and manifestations (bottom). Reprinted with permission from reference 50.

criteria required for staging syphilitic infection. Although the clinical consequences of syphilitic infection may be delayed for months to years, venereal syphilis typically commences with the appearance of one or more mucocutaneous lesions days to weeks following inoculation (85). Primary syphilis occurs when spirochetes replicating at the site of inoculation induce a local inflammatory response, giving rise to one or more chancres, the defining lesion(s) of primary syphilis. The clinical consequences of spirochete dissemination, collectively referred to as secondary syphilis, become manifest 4 to 10 weeks after the chancre. Because chancres often are not visible in females, women tend to present with secondary disease; a similar trend has been noted in MSM (160). Although mucocutaneous lesions are the most common presentation, secondary syphilis can affect any organ (85). Mucocutaneous lesions of secondary syphilis usually resolve in 3 to 12 weeks, leading to the asymptomatic stage referred to as latency. The Oslo Study of Untreated Syphilis showed that 25% of patients experience secondary relapses, mostly within the first year but as late as 5 years (85). All forms of tertiary syphilis have decreased markedly in incidence in the postantibiotic era; there are no reliable figures on the relative frequency of late complications.

A statistical association between HIV infection and syphilis became evident in the AIDS epidemic (72). Although initially thought to reflect similar risk factors, complex epidemiologic and biologic relationships have been identified (72). Chancres facilitate HIV transmission by increasing susceptibility or infectiousness (44). A multicenter prospective study sponsored by the Centers for Disease Control and Prevention found that HIV infection had only a minimal effect on early syphilis (133).

Early congenital syphilis is analogous to secondary syphilis and can involve almost any fetal organ, with liver, kidneys, bone, pancreas, spleen, lungs, heart, and brain the most frequently afflicted (115, 139). Two years of age is used to demarcate early from late congenital syphilis, which corresponds to tertiary syphilis in the adult. The best known stigmata of late congenital syphilis are Hutchinson's teeth,

interstitial keratitis, saddle nose deformity, frontal bossing, and saber shins (139).

Endemic Treponematoses

Clinical features of the endemic treponematoses are summarized in Table 1. Primary yaws (frambesia) consists of a papule at the site of inoculation that enlarges to a hyperkeratotic papilloma ("mother yaw") before forming a shallow ulcer that can persist for months to years. Highly infectious secondary lesions appear weeks to months later, frequently accompanied by painful periostitis (95). After a several-year period of infectious relapses, patients enter an asymptomatic late latent period; approximately 10% of untreated patients progress to tertiary disease, generally consisting of solitary destructive lesions of bone or mucocutaneous surfaces. Endemic syphilis usually begins as a generalized infection in the absence of an obvious primary lesion and is characterized by ulcerative lesions of the oropharyngeal mucosa (mucous patches), angular stomatitis and split papules at the corners of the mouth, intertrigial condylomata (similar to those of venereal syphilis), painful periostitis, and rashes (95). Tertiary gummas, most commonly on the skin, in the nasopharynx, and in bone, may result in severe disfigurement. Pinta is unique in being limited to skin (95). The initial lesions of primary pinta, small papules, appear after an incubation period of 1 week to 4 months. Secondary lesions (pintids) usually appear 2 to 6 months later. Tertiary lesions consist of well-defined hyperchromic, hypochromic, achromic, or dyschromic patches of skin.

Intestinal Spirochetosis

In 1967, Harland and Lee (53) coined the term intestinal spirochetosis to describe a noninflammatory condition of the large bowel in which spirochetes attached end-on to the colonic epithelium in a dense, palisade-like arrangement, forming a basophilic "false brush border" that was easily overlooked on casual inspection (Fig. 2, top). Although they identified spirochetes in 9 of 100 consecutive biopsy specimens examined, they were unable to relate these findings to symptomatology. The

TABLE 2 Criteria for diagnosis of syphilis

Early syphilis
  Primary
    Confirmed (requires 1 *and* 2 or 3)
      1. One or more chancres (ulcers)
      2. Identification of *T. pallidum* in lesion exudate by microscopy (DF or DFA-TP)
      3. Detection of *T. pallidum* DNA in lesion exudate by PCR
    Probable (requires 1 *and* either 2, 3, or 4)
      1. One or more lesions compatible with chancres
      2. Reactive nontreponemal test without a previous history of syphilis
      3. Reactive treponemal test without a previous history of syphilis
      4. For persons with a history of syphilis, a 4-fold increase in nontreponemal test titer in comparison with previous result
  Secondary
    Confirmed (requires 1 *and* either 2, 3, or 4)
      1. Skin or mucous membrane lesions consistent with secondary syphilis
      2. Identification of *T. pallidum* in lesion exudates by microscopy (DF or DFA-TP)
      3. Identification of treponemes in skin biopsy specimen by silver, immunofluorescence (DFAT-TP), or immunohistochemical staining
      4. Detection of *T. pallidum* DNA in tissue by PCR
    Probable (requires 1 *and* either 2 or 3)
      1. Skin or mucous membrane lesions consistent with secondary syphilis
        a. Macular, papular, follicular, papulosquamous, or pustular rash
        b. Condylomata lata (anogenital region or mouth)
        c. Mucous patches (oropharynx or cervix)
      2. In persons with no prior history, reactive nontreponemal test titer of ≥4 and a reactive confirmatory treponemal test
      3. For persons with a prior history of syphilis, a 4-fold increase in the most recent nontreponemal test titer compared with previous test results
  Early latent
    Probable (requires 1 *and* either 2 or 3)
      1. Absence of signs and symptoms of syphilis
      2. Reactive nontreponemal and treponemal tests without a prior history of syphilis
      3. For persons with a prior history of syphilis, a 4-fold increase in the most recent nontreponemal test titer compared with previous test results (obtained ≤1 yr ago)
  Late latent or latent of unknown duration
    Probable (requires 1 *and* either 2 or 3)
      1. Absence of signs and symptoms
      2. No past diagnosis of syphilis and reactive nontreponemal and treponemal test results; if a reactive treponemal screening test is followed by a nonreactive nontreponemal test, a second, different treponemal test is also reactive
      3. A history of syphilis therapy and a current nontreponemal test titer demonstrating 4-fold or greater increase from the last nontreponemal test titer (obtained >1 yr ago)

Late syphilis
  Benign (gummatous) and cardiovascular
    Confirmed (requires 1 *and* 2 or 3)
      1. Clinically compatible case
      2. Identification of treponemes in tissue sections (usually skin biopsy) by silver, immunofluorescence (DFAT-TP), or immunohistochemical staining
      3. Detection of *T. pallidum* DNA in tissue by PCR
    Probable (requires 1, 2, *and* 3)
      1. Clinically compatible case
      2. A reactive serum treponemal test
      3. No known history of treatment for syphilis
  Neurosyphilis
    Confirmed (requires 1, 2, *and* either 3, 4, or 5)
      1. Clinical signs consistent with neurosyphilis
      2. A reactive serum treponemal test
      3. A reactive VDRL in CSF
      4. Detection of *T. pallidum* DNA in CSF by PCR
      5. Identification of treponemes in nervous tissue by silver, immunofluorescence (DFAT-TP), or immunohistochemical staining

(*Continued on next page*)

TABLE 2 *(Continued)*

Probable (requires 1, 2, *and* 3)
  1. Clinical signs consistent with neurosyphilis
  2. A reactive serum treponemal test
  3. Elevated CSF protein or leukocyte count in the absence of other known causes

Congenital syphilis (neonatal)
  Confirmed (requires 1 *and* 2 or 3)
    1. Clinically compatible case
    2. Demonstration of *T. pallidum* by microscopic examination of specimens from lesions, amniotic fluid (antenatal), placenta, umbilical cord, nasal discharge, or autopsy material
    3. Detection of *T. pallidum* DNA in lesions, tissue, blood, and/or CSF by PCR
  Probable (requires 1, 2, *and* 3)
    1. Infant born to a mother who had untreated or inadequately treated syphilis at delivery, regardless of findings in the infant
    2. An infant with a reactive treponemal test result
    3. One of the following additional criteria
      a. Clinical signs or symptoms of congenital syphilis on physical examination
      b. Abnormal CSF finding without other cause
      c. Reactive VDRL in CSF
      d. Reactive IgM antibody test specific for syphilis
Syphilitic stillbirth
  1. A fetal death that occurs after a 20-wk gestation or in which the fetus weighs <500 g
  2. Mother had untreated or inadequately treated syphilis at delivery

confusion and controversy over the clinical significance of HIS have not abated over the years despite extensive phylogenetic and biochemical characterization of intestinal spirochetes (see above) and advances in methodologies for their isolation and/or detection (see below).

COLLECTION, TRANSPORT, AND STORAGE OF SPECIMENS

Treponema pallidum: Syphilis

Because *T. pallidum* cannot be cultivated on artificial medium, the diagnosis of syphilis has to rely on the direct detection of the organism in clinical specimens in conjunction with serologic tests. Due to the complex nature of syphilitic infection, there is no ideal test for the direct detection of *T. pallidum*; test selection is dependent upon clinical presentation and type of specimen obtained (Table 3). *T. pallidum* can be detected in lesion exudate by DF microscopy, direct fluorescent antibody test for *T. pallidum* (DFA-TP), or PCR, while in some circumstances, touch preparations or tissue impressions can also be used for DFA-TP. Cerebral spinal fluid (CSF) is used primarily for VDRL testing, but it also can be examined by PCR. Tissue biopsies are rarely performed on genital ulcers but are used for diagnosing nongenital manifestations of secondary and

TABLE 3 Laboratory tests used for direct detection of *T. pallidum* in clinical samples obtained during the various stages of syphilis

Stage of disease	Test(s) used for specimen type						
	Lesion exudate	Lymph node aspirate	Tissue biopsy	Blood/plasma/serum	Cerebrospinal fluid	Amniotic fluid	Placenta or cord
Primary	DF[a], DFA-TP[b], PCR	DF, DFA-TP, PCR	—	—	—	—	—
Secondary	DF[a], DFA-TP, PCR	DF, DFA-TP, PCR	Silver stain, IHC, DFAT-TP[b], PCR	PCR	PCR[d]	—	—
Neurosyphilis	—[c]	—	Silver stain, IHC, DFAT-TP[b], PCR	—	PCR	—	—
Tertiary (not neurosyphilis)	—	—	Silver stain, IHC, DFAT-TP, PCR	—	PCR	—	—
Fetal/congenital[e]	DF, DFA-TP, PCR	—	Silver stain, IHC, DFAT-TP, PCR	PCR	PCR	DF, DFA-TP, PCR	Silver stain, IHC, DFAT-TP, PCR

[a]Applicable to all except oral lesions.
[b]There is no commercial kit for this test, but FITC-conjugated polyclonal or monoclonal antibody can be purchased commercially.
[c]—, not applicable.
[d]CDC recommends against routine lumbar puncture, but it needs to be done for neurologic symptoms.
[e]Nasal discharge or autopsy material can also be examined for *T. pallidum*.

tertiary disease. PCR can be performed on either fixed or unfixed tissue, although unfixed tissue is recommended. Other specimens, such as lymph node aspirate and amniotic fluid, although rarely obtained, can be examined by DF microscopy, DFA-TP, and PCR, while placenta or cord tissue can be examined by silver staining, immunohistochemistry (IHC), direct fluorescent antibody tissue test for *T. pallidum* (DFAT-TP), and PCR.

Serum is the specimen of choice for conventional treponemal and nontreponemal serodiagnostic tests, but whole blood and plasma also can be used in some assays. When screening for congenital syphilis, the CDC recommends testing of the mother's serum rather than cord blood. Infant's serum is the specimen of choice for immunoglobulin M (IgM)-specific tests, since cord blood specimens can be contaminated by maternal blood. Plasma can be used for the rapid plasma reagin (RPR) and toluidine red unheated serum test (TRUST) assays but not for the VDRL test because heat inactivation of plasma enhances fibrin formation, leading to false-positive results. Also, plasma should be tested within 24 hours to avoid false-positive test results. Whole blood, serum, or plasma can be used for rapid point-of-care (RPOC) treponemal tests although they are designed for use with whole blood. Whole blood for PCR testing should be collected in tubes containing EDTA as an anticoagulant.

The order of sample collection from genital ulcers or moist lesions depends on the tests to be performed. Samples should be collected first for DF microscopy followed by DFA-TP and PCR. Ideally, the specimen for both DF microscopy and DFA-TP should be free of red blood cells, other microorganisms, and tissue debris. A detailed procedure for collecting a specimen for DF examination has been described by Wheeler et al. (156). Briefly, the site is gently cleansed and abraded with sterile gauze moistened with physiological saline until serous fluid appears; the specimen is collected directly onto a clean glass slide and a coverslip is applied. A specimen for DFA-TP is collected in the same manner but left to air dry for 15 minutes. To collect a specimen for PCR, a sterile dacron- or cotton-tipped swab should be rolled firmly along the base of the ulcer or lesion. The swab then should be suspended in a cryotube containing 1 to 2 ml of nucleic acid transport medium such as Genelock (Sierra Molecular Corporation, Sonora, CA) or universal transport medium (Copan Diagnostics, Murrieta, CA). Tissue or fine-needle aspirates (e.g., lymph nodes) for silver staining, IHC, or DFAT-TP should be fixed in 10% buffered formalin at room temperature immediately and sent to the laboratory for paraffin embedding and sectioning. To test products of conception for congenital syphilis, a 3- to 4-cm section of umbilical cord that hasn't been cleansed with soap or antimicrobial-containing solution should be obtained distal from the placenta. The specimen should be taken soon after delivery and fixed in formalin or refrigerated if not being processed immediately.

Lesion exudates air dried on slides for DFA-TP staining can be sent to the laboratory at ambient temperature or on dry ice if slides were frozen after collection (80). Samples collected in Genelock or universal transport medium for PCR can be shipped at room temperature or with cool packs overnight. Serum and plasma should be shipped with cool packs. Transportation of whole blood for serologic testing can be done at ambient temperature if testing is done on-site; otherwise, samples should be stored at 4°C and transported overnight with cool packs. Previously frozen plasma or serum must be shipped on dry ice. CSF for serology can be transported at ambient temperature overnight

or on cold packs if also being used for PCR testing. Tissue samples for silver staining, IHC, and DFAT-TP can be shipped in formalin at ambient temperature for paraffin embedding. Whole blood for serology can be stored at 4°C for 48 to 72 h. Serum, plasma, and CSF for serology should be stored at 4°C if testing will be delayed by more than 4 h and at −20°C or lower if testing will be done more than 5 days from collection. Slides containing air-dried lesion exudates and touch preparations for DFA-TP staining can be stored in a slide container at 4 to 29°C for up to 2 weeks; otherwise, specimens should be fixed with acetone and stored at −20°C until testing. Samples of unfixed tissue, ulcer exudate, mucosal or skin lesions, CSF, and amniotic fluid should be stored at −70°C if PCR testing cannot be performed immediately. Formalin-fixed samples should be stored at room temperature prior to embedding and sectioning or DNA extraction.

T. denticola and Other Oral Treponemes

Specimen collection for detection, isolation, or identification of *T. denticola* and other commensal treponemes is not normally performed in the routine clinical management of gingivitis or periodontitis; however, detailed methods and information for propagating these organisms for research purposes are available (38).

Brachyspira: Intestinal Spirochetosis

Fecal samples should be collected in sterile containers and transported at ambient temperature to the laboratory or overnight on ice if culture or DF microscopy will be performed off-site. Rectal swabs (148) can be collected and transported in Stuart's medium (Becton Dickinson, Sparks, MD). Fecal samples and swabs should be processed for culture within 24 h of collection (16, 148). Fresh colonic or rectal biopsy samples should be used for culture, while samples for histological examination should be processed as described for *T. pallidum*. Biopsy samples placed in physiological saline have been successfully used to culture *B. aalborgi* (16). Fecal samples or rectal swabs can be used for isolation of strains (10) or examination by DF microscopy (135). Cultured spirochetes from solid- or broth-based media can be observed by phase-contrast microscopy (10). Biopsy specimens obtained from the colon or rectum can serve as material for culture, PCR, or histological examination by light microscopy or transmission electron microscopy (TEM) (77, 99, 135).

DIRECT DETECTION

T. pallidum

DF Microscopy

Touch preparations of primary, secondary, and early congenital syphilis lesions should be examined by DF microscopy, but other specimens (e.g., lymph node aspirates and amniotic fluid) may contain enough spirochetes for DF microscopy examination (Table 3). The test must be performed within 20 min, since it relies on the observation of motile treponemes. The DF microscopy procedure has been described in detail by Wheeler et al. (156). A step-by-step instructional video can be obtained without charge from David Cox, Laboratory Reference and Research Branch, Division of STD Prevention, CDC [(404) 639-3446; dlc6@cdc.gov]. *T. pallidum* cannot be distinguished from the other human pathogenic treponemes using DF microscopy. DF microscopy should not be performed on oral lesions, since *T. pallidum* cannot be distinguished easily from commensal oral spirochetes.

DFA-TP

Touch preparations of lesion exudates (64) or tissue impressions (23) can serve as samples for DFA-TP, which utilizes either a fluorescein isothiocyanate (FITC)-conjugated polyclonal or monoclonal antibody for staining. There is no FDA-approved DFA-TP test in the United States, although labeled polyclonal antibodies can be obtained commercially (Meridian Life Sciences, Saco, ME; ViroStat, Portland, ME). Results with polyclonal antibodies should be interpreted with caution, since they are not specific for pathogenic treponemes.

Silver Staining, DFAT-TP, IHC

Silver staining (either Warthin-Starry or Steiner) is used for visualizing treponemes in paraffin-embedded samples. DFAT-TP is a modification of the DFA-TP test that enables immunofluorescent labeling of treponemes in tissue samples (68). For DFAT-TP, tissue sections are deparaffinized and pretreated prior to immunostaining to enhance epitope accessibility (22). Unabsorbed polyclonal antibodies for IHC are available commercially (Biocare Medical, Concord, CA; ViroStat, Portland, ME).

PCR

PCR is not used routinely for syphilis testing, and a commercial test is not available. However, since 1991, numerous studies have been published using PCR for *T. pallidum* detection based on several gene targets. Of these, the *polA* (tp0105) (92) and *tpn47* (tp0574) (116) are most commonly used. Although PCR can be performed on many sample types, the test is most useful for genital ulcers and exudative lesions, which can be sampled noninvasively and typically contain large numbers of treponemes.

Genomic DNA for PCR testing is usually extracted from 200 µl of nucleic acid transport medium containing a genital ulcer swab sample using a commercial kit (e.g., QIAamp DNA mini kit; Qiagen Inc., Valencia, CA). Laboratories with real-time PCR capability can use the TaqMan-based multiplex PCR assay developed in the Laboratory Reference and Research Branch, Division of STD Prevention at the CDC for testing genital ulcer disease (GUD) samples. This assay simultaneously detects *T. pallidum*, *Haemophilus ducreyi*, and herpes simplex viruses 1 and 2 (HSV-1 and -2), the major causative agents of GUD. Gene targets, primers, and probes for the assay are shown in Table 4. Laboratories that lack real-time PCR capability can use the conventional multiplex PCR assay for detection of *T. pallidum*, *H. ducreyi*, and HSV described by Mackay et al. (Table 5) (88). If testing for *H. ducreyi* will not be performed, PCR products from the multiplex reaction can be analyzed by agarose gel electrophoresis. Otherwise, an enzyme-linked amplicon hybridization assay (88) can be used because the amplicons for *H. ducreyi* and HSV cannot be distinguished on agarose gels. A TaqMan-based real-time PCR targeting the *polA* gene can be used when the primary diagnostic objective is to determine if a specimen contains just *T. pallidum* (22). The primers consist of TP-1 (5'-CAGGATCCGGCATATGTCC-3') and TP-2 (5'-AAGTGTGAGCGTCTCATCATTCC-3') and a probe, TP-3 (5'-CTGTCATGCACCAGCTTCGACGTCTT-3'), which is labeled with 6-carboxyfluorescein (FAM) at the 5' end and black hole quencher 1 (BHQ1) at the 3' end. Laboratories unable to perform real-time PCR can use a conventional assay targeting the *polA* gene of *T. pallidum* with primers F1 (5'-TGCGCGTGTGCGAATGGTGT-GGTC-3') and R1 (5'-CACAGTGCTCAAAAACGC-CTGCACG-3') using PCR conditions described by Liu et al. (84).

Brachyspira

Fresh stool specimens or rectal swabs can be examined by DF microscopy for the presence of spirochetes (135). Colonic and rectal biopsy specimens can be examined by using periodic acid-Schiff (PAS), H&E, or silver staining: spirochetes appear as a "fuzzy coat" on the brush border of the epithelium (Fig. 2, top) (16, 146). Using TEM,

TABLE 4 Oligonucleotide primers and probes used for real-time multiplex PCR for GUD

Organism or control	Gene target	Sequence of primer/probe (5'–3')	Nucleotide position	Concn[a] (nM)
HSV-1 and -2	*gD*[b]	CCCCGCTGGAACTACTATGACA	472–493	200
		GCATCAGGAACCCCAGGTTA	535–516	300
		FAM[f]-TTTAGCGCCGTCAGCGAGG-BHQ[g]	496–514	200
H. ducreyi	*hhdA*[c]	AATCGTTAACTGCGGGATTAGG	5153–5174	200
		CAATAGACACATTATCGCCCTTTAAA	5245–5220	300
		JOE[f]-ATGGCCATGGTAGTGAGGTAAATCAGGCTGT-BHQ	5180–5210	200
T. pallidum	*tpn47*[d]	CAACACGGTCCGCTACGACTA	864–884	300
		TGCCATAACTCGCCATCAGA	931–912	300
		ROX[f]-ACGGTGATGACGCGAGCTACACCA-BHQ	887–910	200
Human	RNase P[e]	CCAAGTGTGAGGGCTGAAAAG	826–846	80
		TGTTGTGGCTGATGAACTATAAAAGG	905–880	80
		CY5[f]-CCCCAGTCTCTGTCAGCACTCCCTTC-BHQ	851–876	80

[a]Indicates final concentration of primer or probe in multiplex reaction.
[b]Glycoprotein D gene.
[c]Hemolysin A gene.
[d]47-kDa immunogen gene.
[e]Human ribonuclease P gene target is used as an internal control.
[f]Fluorescent dyes.
[g]Black hole quencher.

TABLE 5 Oligonucleotide primers and probes used for conventional multiplex PCR for GUD[a]

Organism or control	Oligonucleotide	Sequence (5'–3')	Gene target	Amplicon length (bp)
HSV-1 and -2	HSV01.16	GCCGTAAAACGGGGACATGTACACAAAGT	gB[b]	432
	HSV02.16	TTCAAGGCCACCATGTACTACAAAGACGT		
	HSV1_P01.16	GCGTTGGCCGGTTTCAGCTCC		
	HSV2_P02.16	GACCTTCGCCGGCTTGAGCTC		
H. ducreyi	HD01.1	CAAGTCGAACGGTAGCACGAAG	16S rRNA	439
	HD02.1	TTCTGTGACTAACGTCAATCAATTTTG		
	HD_P02.1	CCGAAGGTCCCACCCTTTAATCCGA		
T. pallidum	TPAL01.3	CAGAGCCATCAGCCCTTTTCA	tpn47[c]	260
	TPAL02.3	GAAGTTTGTCCCAGTTGCGGTT		
	TPAL_P01.3	CGGGCTCTCCATGCTGCTTACCTTA		
Endogenous retrovirus 3[d]	ERV01.1	CATGGGAAGCAAGGGAACTAATG	env[e]	136
	ERV02.1	CCCCAGCGAGCAATACAGAATT		
	ERV_P01.3	TCTTCCCTCGAACCTGCACCATCAAGTCA		

[a]Adapted from reference 88.
[b]Glycoprotein B gene.
[c]47-kDa immunogen gene.
[d]Used as an internal control.
[e]Envelope gene.

the organisms appear to attach end-on to the host cell membrane (Fig. 2, bottom) (15, 77). IHC also has been performed with polyclonal antibodies to *T. pallidum*, *Mycobacterium bovis*, and an uncharacterized intestinal spirochete (77, 146). Detection of *B. pilosicoli* and *B. aalborgi* DNA can be achieved with the PCR assays described in Table 6 (99, 100).

ISOLATION PROCEDURES

T. pallidum

RIT is the only means available for isolating *T. pallidum* from clinical specimens and, because of its extraordinary sensitivity (1 to 2 organisms), has long been considered the gold standard for treponeme detection. The RIT method has been described in detail by Lukehart and Marra (87).

Brachyspira

Fecal samples, rectal swabs, or colon or rectum biopsy specimens can be cultured using brain heart infusion agar

(10, 77) or Trypticase soy agar medium (77) with 10% bovine blood, 400 μg/ml of spectinomycin, and 5 μg/ml of polymyxin incubated anaerobically at 37°C. Specimens should be streaked onto agar plates within 1 h of collection (77). Colonies of *B. aalborgi* appear light gray and weakly beta-hemolytic with a diameter of 1.2 mm on brain heart infusion agar medium after 21 days of incubation (10). *B. pilosicoli* and *B. aalborgi* appear as a thin film or as discrete, pinpoint colonies on Trypticase soy agar medium after 5 to 14 days (10). *B. aalborgi* cultures usually require a longer incubation period. *B. aalborgi* has been successfully subcultured on brain heart infusion agar (10) and propagated in Trypticase soy broth containing 10% fetal calf serum (16). *B. pilosicoli* is less fastidious than *B. aalborgi* and can be subcultured on media used for its isolation.

IDENTIFICATION

Brachyspira

B. pilosicoli and *B. aalborgi* strains can be characterized using API-ZYM (bioMérieux, Inc., Durham, NC) and using

TABLE 6 Primers and thermocycling conditions for *B. aalborgi*- and *B. pilosicoli*-specific PCR[a]

Organism	Primer sequence (name) (5'–3')	Predicted product size (bp)	Thermocycling conditions
B. aalborgi 16S rRNA	TAC CGC ATA TAC TCT TGA C (F, Ba 16S) CCT ACA ATA TCC AAG AAC C (R, Ba 16S)	471	94°C for 4.5 min; 33 cycles of 94°C for 30 s, 46°C for 30 s, 72°C for 30 s
B. aalborgi nox	GGT TGA CTC AAG CAC TAC (F, Ba nox) AAA CCG TAT TTT GTT CCA GG (R, Ba nox)	334	94°C for 4.5 min; 30 cycles of 94°C for 30 s, 46°C for 30 s, 72°C for 30 s
B. pilosicoli 16S rRNA	AGA GGA AAG TTT TTT CGC TTC (Acoli 1) CCCCTACAATATCCAAGACT	439	94°C for 4.5 min; 33 cycles of 94°C for 30 s, 51°C for 30 s, 72°C for 30 s
B. pilosicoli nox	GTA ACT CCT CCT ATT GAG (F, Sp nox) GCA CCA TTA GGT AAA GTC (R, Sp nox)	465	94°C for 4.5 min; 30 cycles of 94°C for 30 s, 45°C for 30 s, 72°C for 30 s

[a]Adapted from references 99 and 100.

biochemical tests such as indole production and hippurate hydrolysis (16, 77, 151). A strong hippurate reaction and weak α-galactosidase activity is often used to identify *B. pilosicoli*, while *B. aalborgi* is negative for α-galactosidase activity and gives a weak hippurate reaction (77).

TYPING SYSTEMS

T. pallidum

Identification of variable regions within the *T. pallidum* genome has made possible the development of a molecular typing system for *T. pallidum* (123). Typing is based on PCR amplification and restriction fragment length polymorphism (RFLP) analysis of 3 members of the *tpr* gene family (*tprE* [*tp0313*], *tprG* [*tp0317*], and *tprJ* [*tp0621*]) (Fig. 4, top) and amplification of a variable number of 60-bp tandem repeats within *arp* (*tp0433*) (Fig. 4, bottom). To type *T. pallidum* strains, an approximately 1.8-kb region of *tprE*, *G*, and *J* is simultaneously amplified using a nested PCR and primer pairs B1, 5'-ACTGGCTCTGCCACACTTGA-3', and A2, 5'-CTACCAGGAGAGGGTGACGC-3', and IP6, 5'-CAGGTTTTGCCGTTAAGC-3', and IP7, 5'-AATCAAGGGAGAATACCGTC-3', followed by restriction digestion with MseI and RFLP analysis (124). The 60-bp repeat region of *arp* is amplified with PCR primers 1A (5'-CAAGTCAGGACGGACTGTCCCTTGC-3') and 2A (5'-GGTATCACCTGGGGATGCGCACG-3'); an improved method has recently been developed (73). Strain typing is performed primarily on specimens from genital ulcers and mucosal lesions, but other specimens also have been typed (102, 145). The major strain types identified are 14*a*, 14*d*, and 14*f* (124, 145). Only a few specimens from epidemiologically linked cases have been typed (41).

Brachyspira

B. pilosicoli strains can be characterized by pulsed-field gel electrophoresis (PFGE) and multilocus enzyme electrophoresis, but the PFGE method appears more discriminatory. Studies using PFGE show that *B. pilosicoli* strains belong to a genetically diverse group (11, 152). There are no reports on typing of *B. aalborgi* strains.

SEROLOGIC TESTS

General Principles

Syphilis elicits two different types of antibody responses, traditionally designated "nontreponemal" and "treponemal" (Fig. 3) (80). Nontreponemal tests, which detect antibodies directed against lipoidal antigens, were the first to be developed and are still used for screening and evaluation of disease activity following therapy (Table 7). Nontreponemal tests have 2 inherent problems: they lack sensitivity in primary and late syphilis (Fig. 3) and they lack specificity because reactive antibodies can be elicited in diseases and conditions unrelated to syphilis, giving rise to biological false positives (BFPs) (128). Conventional treponemal tests, beginning with fluorescent treponemal antibody absorption (FTA-ABS), were developed using *T. pallidum* or *T. pallidum* lysates to address the lack of specificity of the nontreponemal tests (80). The need for high throughput and decreased costs prompted development of automated enzyme immunoassays (EIAs), most that now use recombinant antigens (Tables 8 to 11). The challenge of syphilis diagnosis in developing countries necessitated the development of RPOC dual tests which simultaneously provide both qualitative nontreponemal and treponemal test results from finger stick blood.

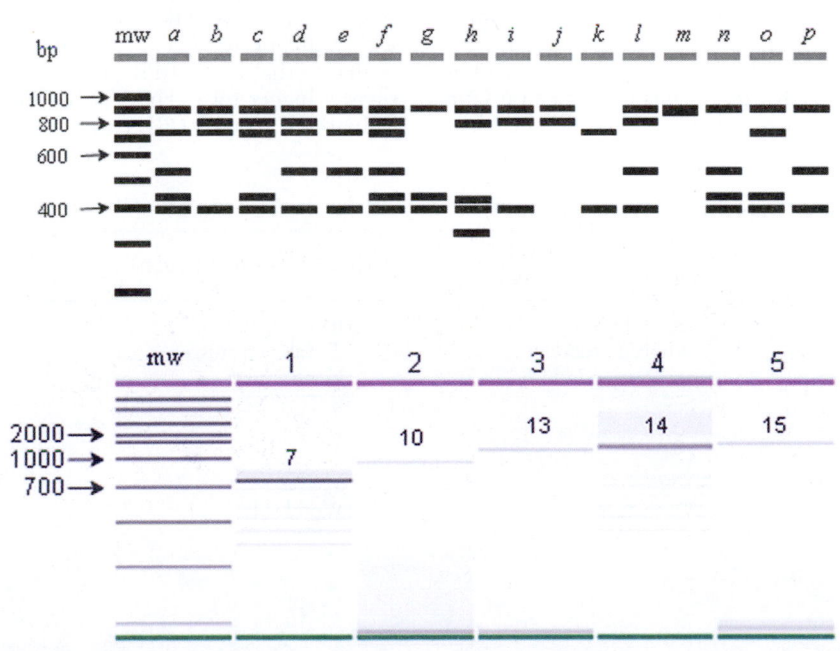

FIGURE 4 PCR-based molecular typing of *T. pallidum* "street strains." (Top) Schematic representation of all *tpr* gene MseI RFLP patterns identified to date. (Bottom) Schematic showing different *arp* repeat sizes obtained by PCR. The size of each repeat is indicated above the amplicon. mw, molecular weight.

TABLE 7 Nontreponemal tests for syphilis serodiagnosis

Parameter	VDRL	USR	RPR	TRUST	ChemBio DPP[a]	SPAN Spirolipin[a]	ViraMed
Method	Flocculation	Flocculation	Flocculation	Flocculation	Lateral immuno-chromatography	Flowthrough	Pseudo-WB
Specimen[b]	S, C	S	S, P	S, P	S, P, B	S, P, B	S
Sample vol (μl)[c]	50–100	50–100	50–100	50–100	5	100	20
Time to complete (min)[c]	15	15	15	15	20	15	90
FDA approved	Yes	Yes	Yes	Yes	No	No	No
Sensitivity (%)					91.1	96.5	84
Primary	67–78	80	60–86	70–85			
Secondary	96–100	100	100	100			
Tertiary	85–95	95	98	98			
Specificity (%)	96–99	98–99	93–99	98–99	98.6	97.7	91.0
Reference(s)	31, 80, 89, 159	80, 81	31, 80, 81, 125	80, 81	CDC, unpublished data	Package insert; CDC, unpublished data	Package insert

[a]Point-of-care test; FDA license in progress; trials in North and South America and Europe.
[b]S, serum; C, CSF; P, plasma; B, blood.
[c]For technical details, see *Manual of Tests for Syphilis* (http://www.cdc.gov/std/syphilis/manual-1998/).

Nontreponemal Tests

Table 7 presents the salient features of the commercially available nontreponemal tests along with the corresponding information for the nontreponemal components of three dual tests, Vira Med ViraBlot (Planegg, Germany), Span SpiroLipin (Surat, India), and ChemBio DPP Screen and Confirm (Medford, NY), that are not FDA approved. Detailed protocols for performing the RPR, VDRL, unheated serum reagin (USR), and TRUST assays can be found in *A Manual of Tests for Syphilis* published by the American Public Health Association (http://www.apha.org) (81); an online version can be accessed at http://www.cdc.gov/std/syphilis/manual-1998/.

The VDRL test is a quantitative flocculation reaction between a cardiolipin-based antigen and serum performed on special glass slides (81). The results are read microscopically at ×100; the highest titer causing flocculation is the endpoint. The VDRL test also is performed on CSF to identify and manage cases of neurosyphilis. The USR

microflocculation test uses a modified VDRL antigen containing choline chloride, which eliminates the need for heating of the serum sample (81), and is read microscopically like the VDRL. The USR test is rarely used, since the RPR test is essentially equivalent but does not require a microscope for determination of results. The RPR card test, performed on serum or plasma, contains finely divided charcoal particles as a visualizing agent (81). In the RPR card test, serial dilutions of serum or plasma (heated or unheated) are prepared on a plastic-coated card after which the RPR antigen is added. The presence of antibodies causes flocculation, while suspensions without antibodies remain uniformly gray. The TRUST is a macroflocculation assay, very similar to the RPR, in which the charcoal is replaced with toluidine red (81). The sensitivity of the TRUST is similar to that of the RPR (Table 7), while its specificity is slightly higher (80). The VDRL-CSF is performed identically to the serum VDRL except that the VDRL antigen is

TABLE 8 Conventional treponemal tests for syphilis

Characteristic	FTA-ABS (indirect immunofluorescence)	MHA-TP (agglutination)	TP-PA (agglutination)
Detects	IgG + IgM	IgG + IgM	IgG + IgM
Captures antibody with	Whole *T. pallidum*	*T. pallidum* antigen	*T. pallidum* lysate
Conjugate	anti-human Ig-FITC	None	None
Specimen[a]	S, C[b]	S	S
Sample vol (μl)	50	100	100
Time to complete (h)	1.5	2	2
Available/FDA approved	Yes/yes	Yes/yes	Yes/yes
Usage	Worldwide	Worldwide	Worldwide
Sensitivity (%)			
Primary	82–90	57–88	85–97.5
Secondary	100	96–100	100
Latent	96	96–97	100
Tertiary	100	98–100	96.2–100
Specificity (%)	94.5–97	99	100
Reference(s)	1, 80	25, 91	19, 31, 125

[a]S, serum; C, CSF
[b]Some authorities use FTA-ABS on CSF as a means of ruling out neurosyphilis (see the text).

TABLE 9 Treponemal EIAs for syphilis[a]

Characteristic	Captia IgM	TrepCheck IgM	Captia IgG	TrepCheck IgG	Murex ICE	TrepSure	Bioelisa 3.0	Enzywell	Syphilis EIA II	Pathozyme syphilis	Trepanostika	Enzygost
Type	Direct	Direct	Indirect	Indirect	Capture & direct	Indirect	Indirect	Indirect	Indirect	Competitive	Competitive	Competitive
Detects	IgM	IgM	IgG	IgG	IgG + IgM	IgG + IgM	IgG + IgM	IgG + IgM	IgG + IgM	IgG + IgM	IgG + IgM	IgG + IgM
Captures antibody with	Rabbit anti-human IgM	Rabbit anti-human IgM	Whole T. pallidum	r T. pallidum; 15, 17, 44, 47-kDa forms	r T. pallidum + anti-human IgG/IgM	r T. pallidum: 15, 17, 44, 47-kDa forms	r T. pallidum; 15, 17, 44, 47-kDa forms	r T. pallidum Ag	r T. pallidum; 15, 17, 47-kDa forms	T. pallidum Ag	r T. pallidum	T. pallidum Ag
Conjugate	T. pallidum Ag-HRP	r T. pallidum Ag-HRP[c]	Anti-human IgG-HRP	Anti-human IgG-HRP	r T. pallidum-HRP	r T. pallidum Ag-HRP	r T. pallidum; (15, 17, 47-kDa forms)- HRP	r T. pallidum Ag-HRP	r T. pallidum; (15, 17, 47-kDa forms)- HRP	Anti-T. pallidum Ab-HRP	r T. pallidum Ag-HRP	Anti-T. pallidum Ab-HRP
Specimen	S	S	S	S	S	S	S, P	S, P	S, P	S, P	S, P	S
Sample vol (µl)	5	10	10	100	50	100	50	30	50	25	30	30
Time to complete (h)	3	3	3	3	2.83	2	2	1.33	1.5	2.5	1.5	2.66
FDA approved	Yes	Yes	Yes	Yes	No	Yes	No	Yes	No	No	No	No
Usage area	Worldwide	Worldwide	Worldwide	Worldwide	Europe, United Kingdom	North America	Europe, United Kingdom	Europe, United Kingdom	Europe, United Kingdom	Europe, United Kingdom	Europe, United Kingdom	Europe, United Kingdom
Sensitivity (%)												
Primary	89.9–94.1		83–95		75–98.2		98.2	98.2	99.1	97.4	99.1	98.2
Primary, MHATP negative[b]	86.5		23		75.0		67.3			69	76.9	69.2
Secondary	65–100		76.5		100		100	100	100	100	100	100
Latent	19–75		97–100		100		100	100	100	100	100	100
Tertiary	100											
Sensitivity, stages not determined (%)		97.4		99.5		98.90						
Specificity (%)	100	100.0	99–100	100.0	99	99.9	100	100	100	98.5–100	100	100
Reference(s)	82, 94	Package insert	27, 82	Package insert	1, 27	Package insert; CDC, unpublished data	1, 27	1, 27	27	1, 27	1, 27	1, 27, 90

[a]S, serum; P, plasma: r, recombinant antigen; Ag, antigen; Ab, antibody, HRP, horseradish peroxidase.
[b]See reference 137.
[c]Different conjugates required.

953

TABLE 10 Treponemal immunoblots and rapid tests for syphilis

Characteristic	Immunoblotting			Rapid tests (immunochromatographic strips)				
	MarDx	ViraMed	Inno-LIA	Determine	Espline	Bioline	SPAN Spirolipin	ChemBio DPP
Manufacturer	Trinity Biotech, Wicklow, Ireland	ViraMed Biotech, Planegg, Germany	Innogenetics NV, Ghent, Belgium	Abbott Laboratories, Abbott Park, IL	Fujirebio, Inc., Tokyo, Japan	Standard Diagnostics, Inc, Yongin-Si, South Korea	Span Diagnostics Ltd., Surat, India	ChemBio Diagnostic Systems, Inc, Medford, NY
Type				Lateral flow	Lateral flow	Lateral flow	Flowthrough	Lateral flow
Detects	IgG or IgM	IgG/IgM	IgG + IgM	IgG + IgM	IgG + IgM	IgG + IgM	IgG + IgM	IgG + IgM
Captures antibody with	Whole T. pallidum	r T. pallidum; 15, 17, 44, 47 kDa[a]	r T. pallidum; 15, 17, 43, 47 kDa	r T. pallidum; 47 kDa	r T. pallidum; 15, 17, 47 kDa	r T. pallidum; 15, 17, 47 kDa	r T. pallidum; 48 kDa	r T. pallidum; 17 kDa, cardiolipin
Conjugate	Anti-human Ig-AlkP[c]	Anti-human Ig-AlkP	Anti-human Ig-AlkP	Anti-human IgG-gold	Anti-human IgG-gold	Anti-human IgG-gold	Anti-human IgG-gold	Anti-human IgG-gold
Specimen[b]	S	S	S	S, P, B	S, P	S, P, B	S, P, B	S, P, B
Sample vol (µl)	20	20	10	50	25	10-20	100	5
Time to complete	2 h	1.5 h	4-6 h	5-20 min	15 min	5-20 min	2-5 min	20 min
Available/FDA approved	Yes/no	Yes/no	Yes/no	Yes/yes	Yes/no	Yes/no	Yes/no	Yes/in progress
Usage area	Europe	Europe	Europe, Canada	United States	Worldwide	Worldwide	Worldwide, not United States	United States
Sensitivity (%)								
Primary			94.0					
Secondary			100					
Latent								
Tertiary			100					
Sensitivity, stages not determined (%)		100/97		91.8-100	97.7	95.5-98.9	97.3	97.0
Specificity (%)		100/97	99.3	98.5-98.9	93.4	94.9-98.2	99.1	95.5
Reference(s)	Insert, 51	Insert	33, 51, 89	59, 83, 147	59, 147	59, 83	Package insert; CDC, unpublished data	Package insert; CDC, unpublished data

[a] Recombinant antigen.
[b] S, serum; C, CSF; P, plasma; B, blood.
[c] AlkP, alkaline phosphatase.

TABLE 11 Treponemal light-based tests for syphilis

Characteristic	BioPlex IgG	Architect	AtheNA	Liaison
Manufacturer	Bio-Rad Laboratories, Hercules, CA	Abbott Laboratories, Abbott Park, IL	Zeus Scientific, Branchburg, NJ	Diasorin S.p.A, Vercelli, Italy
Type	Bead capture	Bead capture	Bead capture	Bead capture
Detects	IgG + IgM	IgG + IgM	IgG	IgG + IgM
Captures antibody with	r *T. pallidum*; 15, 17, 47 kDa[a]	r *T. pallidum*; 15, 17, 47 kDa	r *T. pallidum*; 17 kDa	r *T. pallidum*; 17 kDa
Conjugate	Anti-human phycoerythrin	Anti-human Ig-acridinium	Anti-human phycoerythrin	Isoluminol-antigen conjugate
Specimen[b]	S	S/P	S	S
Sample vol (μl)	5	30/150	10	70
Time to complete (min)	45	30	75	40
Available / FDA Approved	Yes/yes	Yes/yes	No/in development	Yes/yes
Usage area	Europe, United States	Europe, United Kingdom	In development	Europe, United States
Sensitivity (%)				
Primary	91.40	97.5		100.0
Secondary	89.3	100		100.0
Latent	100			
Tertiary	86.4	100		98.7
Sensitivity, stages not determined (%)			94.3	
Specificity (%)	98.10	98.4	98.1	99.1
References	Package insert; CDC, unpublished data	Package insert, 90, 159	Package insert; CDC, unpublished data	Package insert; CDC, unpublished data; 91

[a]Recombinant antigen.
[b]S, serum; P, plasma.

diluted 1:1 with 10% saline (79). RPR testing of CSF is not recommended.

Treponemal Tests

The salient features of the commercially available treponemal tests, as well as some that are still developmental are summarized in Tables 8 to 11. Detailed protocols for the FTA-ABS, microhemagglutination assay for antibodies to *T. pallidum* (MHA-TP), and *T. pallidum* particle agglutination (TP-PA) tests can be found in *A Manual of Tests for Syphilis* (81).

FTA-ABS Test

In the FTA-ABS test (Table 8), a serum sample, adsorbed with an extract of *T. phagedenis* Reiter (Sorbent) to remove cross-reactive antibodies, is reacted with treponemes fixed to glass slides; FITC-conjugated anti-human immunoglobulin is used to visualize antibody-labeled organisms. The FTA-ABS test cannot distinguish between IgG or IgM antibodies. The serum is subjectively scored based upon the fluorescence intensity. Standardized controls which produce negative, weak, and strong fluorescence readings must be included in each assay. The test can be performed with unheated CSF for diagnosis of neurosyphilis (see below). Because of the subjectivity involved in reading samples and the need for expensive microscopy equipment, the FTA-ABS is used much less frequently than in the past.

MHA-TP and TP-PA Tests

The MHA-TP test (Table 8) is a passive hemagglutination assay of formalinized, tanned erythrocytes sensitized with *T. pallidum* antigen that can be used to test preabsorbed patient sera; it has been supplanted by the TP-PA. The TP-PA test (Fujirebio, Inc., Tokyo, Japan) is a modification of the MHA-TP test that uses gelatin particles sensitized with

T. pallidum antigens to reduce the number of nonspecific interactions (125). With both tests, agglutination indicates the presence of IgG and/or IgM antitreponemal antibodies.

EIAs

With the exception of the Captia IgG (Trinity Biotech Plc; Bio-Rad Laboratories, Hercules, CA), all of the EIAs (Table 9) currently being used for syphilis diagnosis employ recombinant antigens and detect IgG, IgM, or both. The 15-, 17-, 44.5-, and 47-kDa antigens are the most frequently utilized because they induce strong, persistent antibody responses (52) and are thought to be expressed only by pathogenic treponemes (110). Although EIAs using recombinant antigens might be expected to perform better than assays using *T. pallidum* lysates (67), this has not been borne out (137). EIAs utilize one of three basic formats or combinations: (i) direct or "sandwich," (ii) indirect, and (iii) competitive. The direct format uses antibody immobilized on the plastic matrix to capture serum antibodies. Examples are the Captia IgM, TrepCheck IgM (Phoenix Bio-Tech Corporation, Mississauga, Ontario, Canada), and Murex ICE (Murex Biotech Ltd., Dartford, United Kingdom) which use recombinant antigen enzyme conjugates to detect serum antibodies captured by the immobilized antibodies. In contrast, the indirect format uses immobilized antigens to capture reactive serum antibodies. Reactive antibodies are then detected in one of two ways: either with anti-antibody enzyme conjugates or with recombinant antigen enzyme conjugates. The Captia IgG, TrepCheck IgG, and Murex ICE detect reactive antibodies using anti-antibody conjugates, while the Trep-Sure (Phoenix Bio-Tech Corporation, Mississauga, Ontario, Canada), Bioelisa 3.0 (Biokit, Barcelona, Spain), Enzwell (Diesse, Siena, Italy), and Syphilis EIA II (Newmarket Laboratories Ltd., Newmarket, United Kingdom) use antigen conjugates for detection. One disadvantage of indirect

EIAs using anti-antibody conjugates can be high background signals which give rise to false-positive results. In the direct and indirect formats, an increasing signal indicates a more-reactive serum. The competitive format (Pathozyme Syphilis [Omega Diagnostics, Alloa, United Kingdom], Biomerieux Trepanostika [Organon, Turnhout, Belgium], and Behring Enzygost [Behring, Marburg, Germany]) uses immobilized antigen to capture specific IgG and IgM antibodies from patient sera, which then block binding of an antibody conjugate of identical specificity. With this format, optical density is inversely related to the amount of antibody bound.

Immunoblot (WB) Tests

Immunoblotting techniques (Table 10) add specificity because they identify specific treponemal proteins recognized by serum antibodies; they also can separately detect IgG or IgM antibodies. Three Western blot (WB) tests are available: MarDx (Trinity Biotech, Wicklow, Ireland), INNO-LIA (Innogenetics NV, Ghent, Belgium), and ViraBlot (ViraMed Biotech, Planegg, Germany). The MarDx test, which uses whole *T. pallidum* lysate, is used to define serum reactivity when screening and confirmatory treponemal tests are discrepant (51). A positive test requires reactivity with 2 of the 3 major antigens (15, 17, and 47 kDa).

The INNO-LIA and ViraBlot tests are pseudo-WBs that employ four recombinant antigens (15, 17, 44, and 47 kDa) applied onto a nitrocellulose membrane (33, 51, 89). For the INNO-LIA, a positive test requires reactivity with 3 of the 4 major antigens; if only 1 or 2 lines react, the result is considered indeterminate. In addition to the same 4 recombinant antigens as the INNO-LIA, the ViraBlot strip (IgG or IgM) has 5 stripes with increasing quantities of VDRL antigen, which allows for semiquantitative nontreponemal results. A negative nontreponemal test has a combined score of 0 (i.e., 0 of 5 stripes reactive), a weak reaction has a combined score of 1 or 2, a medium reaction has a combined score of 3 to 6, and a strong reaction has a combined score of 6 to 10. A weak reaction is equivalent to RPR titers between 1 and 8, a medium reaction is equivalent to RPR titers between 8 to 32, and a strong reaction is equivalent to RPR titers of >32. A positive treponemal reaction requires reactivity with 2 or more of the recombinant antigens.

RPOC and Other Rapid Tests

Dual rapid tests that can use finger stick blood for nontreponemal and treponemal tests are RPOC tests (Table 10) and are distinguished from rapid tests that require serum and provide only treponemal test results. Rapid tests come in 2 formats: lateral flow and flowthrough cassette. The ChemBio Screen and Confirm (ChemBio Diagnostic Systems, Inc., Medford, NY) is a lateral-flow RPOC test that requires only 5 μl of whole blood or serum and can be read visually or with a digital card reader for quantitative results. The Span Spirolipin (Span Diagnostics Ltd., Surat, India) is a flowthrough RPOC test in which control, nontreponemal, and 17-kDa antigens are located, respectively, at the 12, 4, and 8 o'clock positions. Both RPOCs have undergone testing at the CDC and currently are being evaluated under field conditions (18a, 18b).

Light-Based Bead-Capture Technology

The final group of serologic tests which use bead-capture technology consists of two platforms: Luminex and chemiluminescence. Performed in 96-well microtiter plates, this format enables high throughput. The Luminex assay differs from EIAs in two ways: (i) the capture antibody is attached to a suspension of polystyrene beads instead of the wells, and

(ii) the polystyrene beads are dyed with fluorophores of differing intensities that confer on each bead a unique fingerprint, enabling multiplex antibody detection. After the sandwich immunoassay, the bead suspension is analyzed using a dual laser flow cytometry detection system. Currently, there are three Luminex-based assays, all treponemal tests: the Abbott Architect (Abbott Laboratories, Abbott Park, IL), the Bio-Rad BioPlex (Bio-Rad Laboratories, Hercules, CA), and the Zeus Athena (Zeus Scientific, Branchburg, NJ). The first two are FDA-approved and currently in use; only the Abbott Architect has been evaluated in a published independent study (90, 159). The DiaSorin Liaison (DiaSorin S.p.A., Vercelli, Italy) is a chemiluminescence-based assay which captures reactive patient antibodies on magnetic beads. Unbound antibodies are removed by wash cycles, and an isoluminol-antigen conjugate is used to bind to reactive antibodies. Positive sera are detected by the addition of chemical reagents which produce a flash-chemiluminescent signal (91).

ANTIMICROBIAL SUSCEPTIBILITIES

T. pallidum

Routine antimicrobial susceptibility testing of *T. pallidum* is not practical due to the lack of a suitable in vitro cultivation system. *T. pallidum* strains are highly susceptible to penicillin G, which has been used successfully for the treatment of syphilis over the past 65 years (158). Ceftriaxone is highly active against *T. pallidum* in vitro and is unquestionably effective in the treatment of early syphilis when a sufficient number of doses is given (158). Because efficacy data for ceftriaxone are limited, its use as an alternative therapy for syphilis is recommended only when better-established regimens are contraindicated (158). Tetracycline has long been the second-line drug recommended for treatment of syphilis in patients allergic to penicillin; doxycycline, which has a much longer half-life, is equivalent to tetracycline (47, 158). Erythromycin treatment failures were recognized many years ago and, in one case from which an isolate was obtained, was shown to be due to infection with an erythromycin-resistant strain (144). Enthusiasm for azithromycin, which can be administered orally in a single 2-g dose, has been tempered by the discovery of geographically widespread macrolide-resistant strains of *T. pallidum* associated with an A2058G mutation in both copies of the bacterium's 23S rRNA genes (86). In vitro studies indicate that quinolone compounds have low antimicrobial activity against *T. pallidum* (111).

Brachyspira

The in vitro antimicrobial susceptibilities of *B. pilosicoli* isolates from a number of geographic locations have been tested using an agar dilution method (10). Isolates were found to be susceptible to amoxicillin-clavulanic acid, ceftriaxone, chloramphenicol, meropenem, tetracycline, and metronidazole. Metronidazole remains the drug of choice for treating *B. pilosicoli* infections; resistance has not been reported (8).

EVALUATION, INTERPRETATION, AND REPORTING OF RESULTS

Direct Detection of *T. pallidum*

DF Microscopy and DFA-TP

Identification of a single motile *T. pallidum* by DF microscopy is sufficient for diagnosis. The predictive value of DF microscopy has been difficult to discern (54), with one study (156) claiming a 97% positivity rate in patients with clinically diagnosed primary syphilis (80% for patients positive on their first clinic visit). The development of PCR has provided a much needed standard for assessing the sensitivity and specificity of DF microscopy. In two independent studies in which conventional multiplex PCR was used to evaluate the etiology of genital ulcers (116, 130), the sensitivity and specificity of DF microscopy ranged from 39 to 81% and 82 to 100%, respectively. DF microscopy has fallen into disfavor because it requires a specialized microscope and highly trained laboratory personnel. However, the continued need for DF microscopy proficiency is underscored by studies demonstrating that substantial percentages of DF microscopy-positive primary syphilis patients lack detectable antibodies (Fig. 3) (80). Although DFA-TP is at least as sensitive as DF microscopy and more specific (80), it has never gained wide acceptance and is unlikely to see increased usage in the PCR era.

Visualization of *T. pallidum* in Tissues

Silver impregnation is the traditional method for *T. pallidum* detection in formalin-fixed tissues (155) and should be performed when routine histopathologic findings suggest syphilis. When performed by a credible laboratory and accompanied by reactive serologic tests, visualization of spirochetes by silver staining can be considered definitive evidence for syphilis (Table 2). Of note, rare cases of seronegative secondary syphilis in HIV-infected patients are described in which silver staining was instrumental in establishing a diagnosis (60, 74). Silver staining has three principal drawbacks. First, it is prone to staining artifacts. Second, its sensitivity is limited but not well determined. The Dieterle stain is said to be more sensitive than the Warthin-Starry stain (9). Third, it is not *T. pallidum* specific (e.g., *Borrelia burgdorferi* might be mistaken for *T. pallidum*). Recently, impressive results have been obtained using commercially available polyclonal anti-*T. pallidum* antibodies and avidin-biotin immunoperoxidase staining in paraffin-embedded skin biopsy specimens from secondary syphilis patients (13, 126).

PCR Detection of *T. pallidum*

PCR enhances detection of *T. pallidum* in genital ulcer exudates. An additional advantage of PCR for diagnosis of GUD is that multiplex analysis for other causes of GUD, most importantly HSV-1 and HSV-2 (see above), is possible. CSF has also been examined extensively by PCR. In a multicenter study, PCR in conjunction with RIT confirmed the long-held view that neuroinvasion by *T. pallidum* occurs at high frequency in early syphilis patients without neurologic symptoms (133). Unfortunately, very little is known about the utility of CSF PCR for diagnosing symptomatic neurosyphilis. A study from South Africa found that 56% of 50 patients with suspected neurosyphilis had positive CSF PCRs (102), but these findings need corroboration. Cumulative evidence suggests that PCR is also useful for detection of treponemes in fresh and processed tissues. Comparative analysis of paraffin-embedded secondary syphilis skin biopsy specimens revealed that PCR is equivalent to IHC staining and is easier to perform (9). Studies using conventional and real-time PCR indicate that analysis of blood has diagnostic utility, although results have varied (46, 92, 145). Nevertheless, PCR assays of blood should be used sparingly in suspected cases of acquired syphilis pending a consensus on the specific clinical scenarios in which it complements conventional diagnostic methods.

Serologic Tests

Serologic tests supplement the direct detection methods for diagnosis of primary and open lesions of secondary syphilis, essential for confirming a diagnosis in suspected tertiary disease, and are the only means for diagnosing latent infection when patients are asymptomatic (Table 2 and Fig. 3). Many problems in syphilis management stem from the fact that antibody responses are poor surrogate markers for syphilitic infection. Moreover, available assays measure two distinctly different kinds of antibody reactivities with different kinetics during untreated and treated infection (Fig. 3). None of the currently available serologic tests can distinguish venereal syphilis from the endemic treponematoses (Table 1).

Nontreponemal Tests

Nontreponemal antibody tests are reported as the highest dilution giving a fully reactive result. A fourfold change in titer is required for a clinically significant difference between two nontreponemal test results using the same assay. Titers for the same serum can differ by two- to fourfold when tested using microscopic versus macroscopic nontreponemal tests, underscoring the importance of using the same method for serial serologic tests, preferably in the same laboratory. Sera with extremely high nontreponemal test titers can give weak, atypical, or even negative "rough" reactions at low dilutions when antibody excess prevents agglutination. This prozone phenomenon occurs in 1 to 2% of patients with secondary syphilis (71). Most laboratories circumvent this problem by routinely determining the titers of all samples to at least 16 dilutions.

Traditional algorithms utilize nontreponemal tests as the primary screening tests for suspected syphilis. Nontreponemal tests must be interpreted according to the suspected stage of syphilis as well as the population being tested. Reactive results should be confirmed using a treponemal test, since the proportion of false-positive tests increases with decreasing prevalence of syphilis. Approximately 30% of those with early primary syphilis have nonreactive nontreponemal test results on the initial visit (Fig. 3 and Table 7), underscoring the importance of direct detection methods for genital ulcers and the use of treponemal tests for diagnosis. In secondary syphilis, nearly all patients have nontreponemal test endpoint titers of >8. Approximately one-third of patients with tertiary disease have nonreactive nontreponemal tests (85).

Conditions other than treponemal infection can elicit antilipoidal antibodies that cause BFP reactions, defined as reactivity in a nontreponemal test with a negative treponemal test result. Review articles cite a number of conditions and diseases that cause BFPs (106); in our opinion, many of these lack strong scientific evidence. It is important to emphasize that BFPs are not necessarily indicative of any disease state. A study of 19,067 Jamaicans revealed that 0.59% of the general population were BFP by the VDRL test (143), and in some populations, the frequency may be as high as 1% (106). BFP reactions can be classified into two groups. Acute BFP reactions, which last less than 6 months, are associated with transient diseases or conditions such as malaria (70), brucellosis (18), mononucleosis (90, 131), viral hepatitis (58), lymphogranuloma venereum (141), viral pneumonias (5), tuberculosis (131), and chancroid (141). More recently, smallpox vaccination was confirmed to cause an increased frequency of BFP reactions (103). Causes of chronic BFP reactions, which last more than 6 months, include autoimmune diseases, particularly systemic lupus erythematosus (28), HIV infection (7, 58), intravenous drug use (58), and leprosy (45). Aging (132) and pregnancy (90, 132) also have been cited as causes of BFP reactions, but it is likely that these studies did not identify the true causes of the false-positive tests. For example, in a Swedish study of 5,170 pregnancies, 9 pregnant women with BFPs and

13 matched negative controls were examined for autoimmune antibodies to ascertain the nature of their reactions (57). Eight of the 9 BFPs were positive for reasons other than pregnancy, including antinuclear antibodies, lupus anticoagulant antibodies, anti-DNA and antimitochondrial antibodies, and several other factors. In the matched control group, the rate of these conditions was not significantly different. Another study (106) reported that the rate of true BFPs was about 14 per 10,000 pregnancies. These findings indicate that the frequency of pregnancy as a contributing factor of BFP reactions may be far less than previously believed.

A drop in nontreponemal test titer is the only means for monitoring therapeutic response once disease manifestations resolve. It was once believed that nontreponemal tests revert to nonreactive in the majority of treated patients with primary and secondary syphilis (40). However, a substantial percentage of patients do not serorevert during the monitoring period (12). In a longitudinal study of syphilis patients following therapy, Romanowski and coworkers (134) confirmed that the serologic response to therapy is slow and often incomplete. This study, as well as anecdotal experience, brought about a substantial loosening in the accepted criteria for an adequate therapeutic response, currently defined as a fourfold decrease in nontreponemal titer by 1 year (158). It is important to note, however, that 15% of patients treated for early syphilis do not achieve a twofold titer decline (133). The clinical relevance of persistent nontreponemal test reactivity is uncertain and a matter of debate.

Treponemal Tests

Conventional treponemal tests (i.e., FTA-ABS and TP-PA) and the vast majority of commercially available treponemal EIAs measure both IgG and IgM without distinguishing the class responsible for reactivity. This property accounts for the primary strength of treponemal tests, namely, their high level of sensitivity for syphilitic infection of all stages, and also their cardinal weakness, the inability to distinguish active from inactive disease. The greatest value of the treponemal tests is in distinguishing between true- and false-positive nontreponemal test results. In contrast to nontreponemal tests, treponemal tests are performed at a fixed titer or serum dilution and titers are not normally determined.

FTA-ABS reactivity is graded on a scale of 1 to 4+; 1+ reactivity, which is highly observer dependent, is considered equivocal evidence for syphilis, while 2+ reactivity also has a significant probability of being due to naturally occurring cross-reacting antibodies (101). Another type of false positivity, beaded fluorescence due to anti-DNA antibodies, is observed in sera from patients with systemic lupus erythematosus and other autoimmune diseases (140). Authorities now question the long-held belief that the FTA-ABS should be considered the gold standard treponemal test (2). In head-to-head comparisons, the TP-PA has been shown to be as sensitive and specific for all stages of syphilis as any treponemal test currently on the market, including EIAs using recombinant antigens (27, 89, 94).

Two head-to-head comparisons of a large number of EIAs provide some guidance on their use (27, 137). All of the commercially available EIAs have high specificities (at or near 100% in tested panels) and, not surprisingly, nearly 100% sensitivities in diagnosing secondary syphilis. Schmidt et al. (137) evaluated nine EIAs using highly selected sera from patients with primary syphilis, all with nonreactive MHA-TP tests. Higher sensitivity correlated with (i) the volume and dilution of serum used, (ii) assay format (i.e., capture and competitive tests showed higher sensitivities than

sandwich-based assays), and (iii) detection of IgM as well as IgG antibodies. The higher sensitivity for primary syphilis of assays that include IgM detection is presumed to be due to the earlier appearance of IgM versus IgG antitreponemal antibodies. IgM-specific assays are not currently recommended by the CDC for diagnosis of acquired syphilis (158).

The availability of high-throughput EIAs has resulted in a dramatic shift in serologic screening for syphilis. In recent years, numerous laboratories have switched from the traditional (i.e., nontreponemal test followed by treponemal test confirmation) to a reverse algorithm in which screening is performed with a treponemal test, usually an EIA, followed by a nontreponemal test when the former is reactive (20). While the two algorithms should be comparable for identifying individuals likely to have active disease, the new testing sequence also identifies seropositive individuals who would have been missed with nontreponemal test screening but for whom no means exists to ascertain their true infection status. Some could have either very early or longstanding latent syphilis and require therapy, while others have treated infection or are uninfected with cross-reactive antibodies. A careful clinical history is important, since previously treated individuals require no further management and a sexual history can identify at-risk individuals for whom a reactive test has a higher probability of being a true positive (114). For persons without a history of treatment, a TP-PA test should be performed (20). A reactive second test confirms syphilis while leaving unresolved the issue of disease activity. If the second treponemal test is nonreactive, the clinician could decide that no further evaluation or treatment is indicated or that treatment is indicated for individuals at high risk.

Neurosyphilis

CSF abnormalities are common in early syphilis patients without neurologic symptoms, and a high proportion of such individuals have treponemes in their central nervous system (CNS) yet do not require enhanced therapy (133). For these reasons, routine lumbar puncture is not recommended in early syphilis (158). Some groups argue that this recommendation should not apply to HIV-infected patients with serum RPR titers of ≥32 or CD4 counts below 350 (93). The diagnosis of neurosyphilis is based on a combination of clinical and laboratory test criteria (Table 2). CSF examination should include the VDRL-CSF slide test and total protein and leukocyte counts. The VDRL-CSF test is considered to have high specificity but low sensitivity for neurosyphilis (85). A nonreactive VDRL-CSF test result, therefore, does not rule out neurosyphilis. The FTA-ABS CSF test has high sensitivity but low specificity for neurosyphilis because reactivity may be due to the passive transfer of IgG antitreponemal antibodies across the blood-brain barrier rather than intrathecal production of antibodies (69). A negative FTA-ABS CSF test, however, is strong evidence against neurosyphilis (69).

Syphilis and HIV

There is a clear consensus that serologic tests for syphilis perform well for persons coinfected with HIV and can be relied upon for accurate diagnosis in such individuals (158). However, some caveats to this statement exist. First, HIV-infected individuals can have a higher incidence of false-positive nontreponemal tests (7, 58). Second, nontreponemal test titers in HIV-infected individuals tend to be higher than those in patients without HIV infection, and they decline more slowly or not at all following recommended therapy (133). Third, there are a small number of documented cases in which HIV-infected patients with secondary syphilis had nonreactive syphilis serologies (60, 74).

Congenital Syphilis

In 1990 and 1996, the CDC issued revised criteria for congenital syphilis surveillance (139, 161) (Table 2). A confirmed diagnosis requires demonstration of *T. pallidum* in neonatal tissues, lesion exudates, and/or secretions or in the products of conception (i.e., placenta or umbilical cord) using a direct detection method. Congenital syphilis is diagnosed presumptively in a symptomatic or asymptomatic infant whose mother had untreated or inadequately treated syphilis at delivery *or* in an infant with a reactive treponemal test and any one of the following: (i) clinical (i.e., physical exam or laboratory) evidence of congenital syphilis; (ii) a reactive VDRL-CSF test; and (iii) elevated CSF cell count or protein (without other cause). These extremely broad criteria were formulated to ensure treatment of virtually all at-risk infants. Serologic testing is the mainstay for diagnosis of congenital syphilis but is even more problematic than in adults because infant sera are contaminated by the transplacental passage of maternal IgG. It is generally accepted that a nontreponemal test titer in the infant fourfold greater than that of the mother constitutes serologic evidence for congenital infection Unfortunately, infant nontreponemal test titers usually do not exceed those in maternal sera (139). Currently, no commercially available IgM test for congenital syphilis is recommended by CDC.

This work was supported in part by grant R01 AI26756 from NI-AID/NIH to J.D.R.

REFERENCES

1. **Aktas, G., H. Young, A. Moyes, and S. Badur.** 2005. Evaluation of the serodia *Treponema pallidum* particle agglutination, the Murex Syphilis ICE and the Enzywell TP tests for serodiagnosis of syphilis. *Int. J. STD AIDS* **16:**294–298.
2. **Aktas, G., H. Young, A. Moyes, and S. Badur.** 2007. Evaluation of the fluorescent treponemal antibody absorption test for detection of antibodies (immunoglobulins G and M) to *Treponema pallidum* in serologic diagnosis of syphilis. *Int. J. STD AIDS* **18:**255–260.
3. **Albandar, J. M.** 2005. Epidemiology and risk factors of periodontal diseases. *Dent. Clin. North Am.* **49:**517–532.
4. **Albandar, J. M., Y. A. Buischi, M. P. Mayer, and P. Axelsson.** 1994. Long-term effect of two preventive programs on the incidence of plaque and gingivitis in adolescents. *J. Periodontol.* **65:**605–610.
5. **Allison, A., and A. Dick.** 1954. False-positive serological reactions in virus pneumonia. *Lancet* **267:**364–365.
6. **Arbes, S. J., Jr., G. D. Slade, and J. D. Beck.** 1999. Association between extent of periodontal attachment loss and self-reported history of heart attack: an analysis of NHANES III data. *J. Dent. Res.* **78:**1777–1782.
7. **Augenbraun, M. H., J. A. DeHovitz, J. Feldman, L. Clarke, S. Landesman, and H. M. Minkoff.** 1994. Biological false-positive syphilis test results for women infected with human immunodeficiency virus. *Clin. Infect. Dis.* **19:**1040–1044.
8. **Bait-Merabet, L., A. Thille, P. Legrand, C. Brun-Buisson, and V. Cattoir.** 2008. *Brachyspira pilosicoli* bloodstream infections: case report and review of the literature. *Ann. Clin. Microbiol. Antimicrob.* **7:**19.
9. **Behrhof, W., E. Springer, W. Brauninger, C. J. Kirkpatrick, and A. Weber.** 2008. PCR testing for *Treponema pallidum* in paraffin-embedded skin biopsy specimens: test design and impact on the diagnosis of syphilis. *J. Clin. Pathol.* **61:**390–395.
10. **Brooke, C. J., T. V. Riley, and D. J. Hampson.** 2003. Evaluation of selective media for the isolation of *Brachyspira aalborgi* from human faeces. *J. Med. Microbiol.* **52:**509–513.
11. **Brooke, C. J., T. V. Riley, and D. J. Hampson.** 2006. Comparison of prevalence and risk factors for faecal carriage of the intestinal spirochaetes *Brachyspira aalborgi* and *Brachyspira pilosicoli* in four Australian populations. *Epidemiol. Infect.* **134:**627–634.
12. **Brown, S. T., A. Zaidi, S. A. Larsen, and G. H. Reynolds.** 1985. Serological response to syphilis treatment. A new analysis of old data. *JAMA* **253:**1296–1299.
13. **Buffet, M., P. A. Grange, P. Gerhardt, A. Carlotti, V. Calvez, A. Bianchi, and N. Dupin.** 2007. Diagnosing *Treponema pallidum* in secondary syphilis by PCR and immunohistochemistry. *J. Investig. Dermatol.* **127:**2345–2350.
14. **Calderaro, A., S. Bommezzadri, C. Gorrini, G. Piccolo, S. Peruzzi, V. Villanacci, C. Zambelli, G. Dettori, and C. Chezzi.** 2007. Infective colitis associated with human intestinal spirochetosis. *J. Gastroenterol. Hepatol.* **22:**1772–1779.
15. **Calderaro, A., C. Gorrini, S. Peruzzi, G. Piccolo, G. Dettori, and C. Chezzi.** 2007. Occurrence of human intestinal spirochetosis in comparison with infections by other enteropathogenic agents in an area of the Northern Italy. *Diagn. Microbiol. Infect. Dis.* **59:**157–163.
16. **Calderaro, A., V. Villanacci, M. Conter, P. Ragni, G. Piccolo, C. Zuelli, S. Bommezzadri, R. Guegan, C. Zambelli, F. Perandin, M. C. Arcangeletti, M. C. Medici, N. Manca, G. Dettori, and C. Chezzi.** 2003. Rapid detection and identification of *Brachyspira aalborgi* from rectal biopsies and faeces of a patient. *Res. Microbiol.* **154:**145–153.
17. **Cameron, C. E.** 2006. The *T. pallidum* outer membrane and outer membrane proteins, p. 237–266. *In* J. D. Radolf and S. A. Lukehart (ed.), *Pathogenic Treponema: Molecular and Cellular Biology.* Caister Academic Press, Norwich, United Kingdom.
18. **Casao, M. A., J. Leiva, R. Diaz, and C. Gamazo.** 1998. Anti-phosphatidylcholine antibodies in patients with brucellosis. *J. Med. Microbiol.* **47:**49–54.
18a. **Castro, A., J. Esfandiari, S. Kumar, M. Ashton, S. Kikkert, M. Park, and R. Ballard.** 2010. Novel point-of-care test for simultaneous detection of nontreponemal and treponemal antibodies in patients with syphilis. *J. Clin. Microbiol.* **48:**4615–4619.
18b. **Castro, A., H. Mody, S. Parab, M. Patel, S. Kikkert, M. Park, and R. Ballard.** 2010. An immunofiltration device for the simultaneous detection of non-treponemal and treponemal antibodies in patients with syphilis. *Sex. Transm. Infect.* **86:**532–536.
19. **Castro, R. R., E. S. Prieto, I. Santo, J. Azevedo, and F. L. Exposto.** 2001. Evaluation of the passive particle agglutination test in the serodiagnosis and follow-up of syphilis. *Am. J. Clin. Pathol.* **116:**581–585.
20. **Centers for Disease Control and Prevention.** 2008. Syphilis testing algorithms using treponemal tests for initial screening—four laboratories, New York City, 2005–2006. *MMWR Morb. Mortal. Wkly. Rep.* **57:**872–875.
21. **Centers for Disease Control and Prevention.** 2009. *Sexually Transmitted Disease Surveillance 2007 Supplement: Syphilis Surveillance Report.* Centers for Disease Control and Prevention, U.S. Department of Health and Human Services, Atlanta, GA.
22. **Chen, C. Y., K. H. Chi, R. W. George, D. L. Cox, A. Srivastava, S. M. Rui, F. Carneiro, G. Y. Lauwers, and R. C. Ballard.** 2006. Diagnosis of gastric syphilis by direct immunofluorescence staining and real-time PCR testing. *J. Clin. Microbiol.* **44:**3452–3456.
23. **Choi, Y. J., and L. Reiner.** 1979. Syphilitic lymphadenitis: immunofluorescent identification of spirochetes from imprints. *Am. J. Surg. Pathol.* **3:**553–555.
24. **Cobb, C. M., K. B. Williams, and M. M. Gerkovitch.** 2009. Is the prevalence of periodontitis in the USA in decline? *Periodontol. 2000* **50:**13–24.
25. **Coffey, E. M., L. L. Bradford, L. S. Naritomi, and R. M. Wood.** 1972. Evaluation of the qualitative and automated quantitative microhemagglutination assay for antibodies to *Treponema pallidum*. *Appl. Microbiol.* **24:**26–30.
26. **Cohen, M. S., S. Hawkes, and D. Mabey.** 2006. Syphilis returns to china ... With a vengeance. *Sex. Transm. Dis.* **33:**724–725.

27. Cole, M. J., K. R. Perry, and J. V. Parry. 2007. Comparative evaluation of 15 serological assays for the detection of syphilis infection. *Eur. J. Clin. Microbiol. Infect. Dis.* **26:**705–713.

28. Costello, P. B., G. L. Powell, and F. A. Green. 1990. The structural requirements for anti-cardiolipin antibody binding in sera from patients with syphilis and SLE. *Clin. Immunol. Immunopathol.* **56:**393–400.

29. Cox, D. L. 1994. Culture of *Treponema pallidum. Methods Enzymol.* **236:**390–405.

30. Cox, D. L., B. Riley, P. Chang, S. Sayahtaheri, S. Tassell, and J. Hevelone. 1990. Effects of molecular oxygen, oxidation-reduction potential, and antioxidants upon in vitro replication of *Treponema pallidum* subsp. *pallidum. Appl. Environ. Microbiol.* **56:**3063–3072.

31. Creegan, L., H. M. Bauer, M. C. Samuel, J. Klausner, S. Liska, and G. Bolan. 2007. An evaluation of the relative sensitivities of the venereal disease research laboratory test and the *Treponema pallidum* particle agglutination test among patients diagnosed with primary syphilis. *Sex. Transm. Dis.* **34:**1016–1018.

32. DeLamater, E. D., M. Haanes, R. H. Wiggall, and D. M. Pillsbury. 1951. Studies on the life cycle of spirochetes. VIII. Summary and comparison of observations on various organisms. *J. Investig. Dermatol.* **16:**231–256.

33. Ebel, A., L. Vanneste, M. Cardinaels, E. Sablon, I. Samson, B. K. De, F. Hulstaert, and M. Zrein. 2000. Validation of the INNO-LIA syphilis kit as a confirmatory assay for *Treponema pallidum* antibodies. *J. Clin. Microbiol.* **38:**215–219.

34. Ellen, R. P. 2006. Virulence determinants of oral treponemes, p. 357–386. *In* J. D. Radolf and S. A. Lukehart (ed.), *Pathogenic Treponema: Molecular and Cellular Biology.* Caister Academic Press, Norwich, United Kingdom.

35. Ena, J., A. Simon-Aylon, and F. Pasquau. 2009. Intestinal spirochetosis as a cause of chronic diarrhoea in patients with HIV infection: case report and review of the literature. *Int. J. STD AIDS* **20:**803–805.

36. Esteve, M., A. Salas, F. Fernandez-Banares, J. Lloreta, M. Marine, C. I. Gonzalez, M. Forne, J. Casalots, R. Santaolalla, J. C. Espinos, M. A. Munshi, D. J. Hampson, and J. M. Viver. 2006. Intestinal spirochetosis and chronic watery diarrhea: clinical and histological response to treatment and long-term follow up. *J. Gastroenterol. Hepatol.* **21:**1326–1333.

37. Fellstrom, C., T. Rasback, K. E. Johansson, T. Olofsson, and A. Aspan. 2008. Identification and genetic fingerprinting of *Brachyspira* species. *J. Microbiol. Methods* **72:**133–140.

38. Fenno, J. C. 2005. Laboratory maintenance of *Treponema denticola. Curr. Protoc. Microbiol.* **12:**12B.1.

39. Fenton, K. A., R. Breban, R. Vardavas, J. T. Okano, T. Martin, S. Aral, and S. Blower. 2008. Infectious syphilis in high-income settings in the 21st century. *Lancet Infect. Dis.* **8:**244–253.

40. Fiumara, N. J. 1986. Treatment of primary and secondary syphilis: serologic response. *J. Am. Acad. Dermatol.* **14:**487–491.

41. Florindo, C., V. Reigado, J. P. Gomes, J. Azevedo, I. Santo, and M. J. Borrego. 2008. Molecular typing of *Treponema pallidum* clinical strains from Lisbon, Portugal. *J. Clin. Microbiol.* **46:**3802–3803.

42. Foschi, F., J. Izard, H. Sasaki, V. Sambri, C. Prati, R. Muller, and P. Stashenko. 2006. *Treponema denticola* in disseminating endodontic infections. *J. Dent. Res.* **85:**761–765.

43. Fraser, C. M., S. J. Norris, G. M. Weinstock, O. White, G. G. Sutton, R. Dodson, M. Gwinn, E. K. Hickey, R. Clayton, K. A. Ketchum, E. Sodergren, J. M. Hardham, M. P. McLeod, S. Salzberg, J. Peterson, H. Khalak, D. Richardson, J. K. Howell, M. Chidambaram, T. Utterback, L. McDonald, P. Artiach, C. Bowman, M. D. Cotton, and J. C. Venter. 1998. Complete genome sequence of *Treponema pallidum*, the syphilis spirochete. *Science* **281:**375–388.

44. Galvin, S. R., and M. S. Cohen. 2004. The role of sexually transmitted diseases in HIV transmission. *Nat. Rev. Microbiol.* **2:**33–42.

45. Garner, M. F., J. L. Backhouse, G. Daskalopoulos, and J. L. Walsh. 1973. The Treponema pallidum haemagglutination (TPHA) test in biological false positive and leprosy sera. *J. Clin. Pathol.* **26:**258–260.

46. Gayet-Ageron, A., B. Ninet, L. Toutous-Trellu, S. Lautenschlager, H. Furrer, V. Piguet, J. Schrenzel, and B. Hirschel. 2009. Assessment of a real-time PCR test to diagnose syphilis from diverse biological samples. *Sex. Transm. Infect.* **85:**264–269.

47. Ghanem, K. G., E. J. Erbelding, W. W. Cheng, and A. M. Rompalo. 2006. Doxycycline compared with benzathine penicillin for the treatment of early syphilis. *Clin. Infect. Dis.* **42:**e45–e49.

48. Gottlieb, S. L., V. Pope, M. R. Sternberg, G. M. McQuillan, J. F. Beltrami, S. M. Berman, and L. E. Markowitz. 2008. Prevalence of syphilis seroreactivity in the United States: data from the National Health and Nutrition Examination Surveys (NHANES) 2001–2004. *Sex. Transm. Dis.* **35:**507–511.

49. Grassly, N. C., C. Fraser, and G. P. Garnett. 2005. Host immunity and synchronized epidemics of syphilis across the United States. *Nature* **433:**417–421.

50. Gutman, L. T. 1992. The spirochetes, p. 657–675. *In* W. K. Joklik, H. P. Willett, D. B. Amos, and C. M. Wilfert (ed.), *Zinsser Microbiology*, 20th ed. Appleton & Lange, Norwalk, CT.

51. Hagedorn, H. J., A. Kraminer-Hagedorn, K. De Bosschere, F. Hulstaert, H. Pottel, and M. Zrein. 2002. Evaluation of INNO-LIA syphilis assay as a confirmatory test for syphilis. *J. Clin. Microbiol.* **40:**973–978.

52. Hanff, P. A., T. E. Fehniger, J. N. Miller, and M. A. Lovett. 1982. Humoral immune response in human syphilis to polypeptides of *Treponema pallidum. J. Immunol.* **129:**1287–1291.

53. Harland, W. A., and F. D. Lee. 1967. Intestinal spirochaetosis. *Br. Med. J.* **3:**718–719.

54. Hart, G. 1986. Syphilis tests in diagnosing and therapeutic decision making. *Ann. Intern. Med.* **104:**368–376.

55. Haynes, W. G., and C. Stanford. 2003. Periodontal disease and atherosclerosis: from dental to arterial plaque. *Arterioscler. Thromb. Vasc. Biol.* **23:**1309–1311.

56. Heffelfinger, J. D., E. B. Swint, S. M. Berman, and H. S. Weinstock. 2007. Trends in primary and secondary syphilis among men who have sex with men in the United States. *Am. J. Public Health* **97:**1076–1083.

57. Henriksen, R., P. E. Sogaard, L. Grennert, B. U. Hansen, R. Manthorpe, and I. M. Nilsson. 1989. Autoimmune antibodies and pregnancy outcome in women with false-positive syphilis test results. A retrospective controlled investigation of women from 5170 deliveries. *Acta Obstet. Gynecol. Scand.* **68:**537–540.

58. Hernandez-Aguado, I., F. Bolumar, R. Moreno, F. J. Pardo, N. Torres, J. Belda, A. Espacio, et al. 1998. False-positive tests for syphilis associated with human immunodeficiency virus and hepatitis B virus infection among intravenous drug abusers. *Eur. J. Clin. Microbiol. Infect. Dis.* **17:**784–787.

59. Herring, A. J., R. C. Ballard, V. Pope, R. A. Adegbola, J. Changalucha, D. W. Fitzgerald, E. W. Hook III, A. Kubanova, S. Mananwatte, J. W. Pape, A. W. Sturm, B. West, Y. P. Yin, and R. W. Peeling. 2006. A multi-centre evaluation of nine rapid, point-of-care syphilis tests using archived sera. *Sex. Transm. Infect.* **82**(Suppl. 5)**:**v7–v12.

60. Hicks, C. B., P. M. Benson, G. P. Lupton, and E. C. Tramont. 1987. Seronegative secondary syphilis in a patient infected with the human immunodeficiency virus (HIV) with Kaposi sarcoma. A diagnostic dilemma. *Ann. Intern. Med.* **107:**492–495.

61. Holt, S. C. 1978. Anatomy and chemistry of spirochetes. *Microbiol. Rev.* **42:**114–160.

62. Holt, S. C., and J. L. Ebersole. 2006. The oral spirochetes: their ecology and role in the pathogenesis of periodontal disease, p. 323–356. *In* J. D. Radolf and S. A. Lukehart (ed.), *Pathogenic Treponema: Molecular and Cellular Biology.* Caister Academic Press, Norwich, United Kingdom.

63. Hook, E. W., III, and R. W. Peeling. 2004. Syphilis control-a continuing challenge. *N. Engl. J. Med.* **351:**121–124.

64. Hook, E. W., III, R. E. Roddy, S. A. Lukehart, J. Hom, K. K. Holmes, and M. R. Tam. 1985. Detection of *Treponema pallidum* in lesion exudate with a pathogen-specific monoclonal antibody. *J. Clin. Microbiol.* **22:**241–244.

65. **Hovind-Hougen, K.** 1983. Morphology, p. 3–28. *In* R. F. Schell and D. M. Musher (ed.), *Pathogenesis and Immunology of Treponemal Infection.* Marcel Dekker, New York, NY.

66. **Hovind-Hougen, K., A. Birch Andersen, R. Henrik Nielsen, M. Orholm, J. O. Pedersen, P. S. Teglbjaerg, and E. H. Thaysen.** 1982. Intestinal spirochetosis: morphological characterization and cultivation of the spirochete *Brachyspira aalborgi* gen. nov., sp. nov. *J. Clin. Microbiol.* **16:**1127–1136.

67. **Isaacs, R. D., and J. D. Radolf.** 1989. Molecular approaches to improved syphilis serodiagnosis. *Serodiagn. Immunother. Infect. Dis.* **3:**299–306.

68. **Ito, F., E. F. Hunter, R. W. George, V. Pope, and S. A. Larsen.** 1992. Specific immunofluorescent staining of pathogenic treponemes with a monoclonal antibody. *J. Clin. Microbiol.* **30:**831–838.

69. **Jaffe, H. W., S. A. Larsen, M. Peters, D. F. Jove, B. Lopez, and A. L. Schroeter.** 1978. Tests for treponemal antibody in CSF. *Arch. Intern. Med.* **138:**252–255.

70. **Jaffe, H. W., and D. M. Musher.** 1992. Management of the reactive syphilis serology, p. 935–939. *In* K. K. Holmes, P.-A. Mårdh, P. F. Sparling, P. J. Wiesner, W. Cates, Jr., S. M. Lemon, and W. E. Stamm (ed.), *Sexually Transmitted Diseases,* 2nd ed. McGraw-Hill, New York, NY.

71. **Jurado, R. L., J. Campbell, and P. D. Martin.** 1993. Prozone phenomenon in secondary syphilis. Has its time arrived? *Arch. Intern. Med.* **153:**2496–2498.

72. **Karp, G., F. Schlaeffer, A. Jotkowitz, and K. Riesenberg.** 2009. Syphilis and HIV co-infection. *Eur. J. Intern. Med.* **20:**9–13.

73. **Katz, K. A., A. Pillay, K. Ahrens, R. P. Kohn, K. Hermanstyne, K. T. Bernstein, R. C. Ballard, and J. D. Klausner.** 2010. Molecular epidemiology of syphilis—San Francisco, 2004–2007. *Sex. Transm. Dis.* **37:**660–663.

74. **Kingston, A. A., J. Vujevich, M. Shapiro, C. M. Hivnor, D. M. Jukic, J. M. Junkins-Hopkins, D. M. Jih, J. R. Kostman, and W. D. James.** 2005. Seronegative secondary syphilis in 2 patients coinfected with human immunodeficiency virus. *Arch. Dermatol.* **141:**431–433.

75. **Korner, M., and J. O. Gebbers.** 2003. Clinical significance of human intestinal spirochetosis—a morphologic approach. *Infection* **31:**341–349.

76. **Kostman, J. R., M. Patel, E. Catalano, J. Camacho, J. Hoffpauir, and M. J. DiNubile.** 1995. Invasive colitis and hepatitis due to previously uncharacterized spirochetes in patients with advanced human immunodeficiency virus infection. *Clin. Infect. Dis.* **21:**1159–1165.

77. **Kraaz, W., B. Pettersson, U. Thunberg, L. Engstrand, and C. Fellstrom.** 2000. *Brachyspira aalborgi* infection diagnosed by culture and 16S ribosomal DNA sequencing using human colonic biopsy specimens. *J. Clin. Microbiol.* **38:**3555–3560.

78. **Kuklova, I., M. Kojanova, H. Zakoucka, R. Pankova, P. Velcevsky, Z. Rozehnalova, and J. Hercogova.** 2008. Dermatovenereology in the post-communist era: syphilis in Prague during 1999 to 2005. *Dermatol. Clin.* **26:**231–237.

79. **Larsen, S. A., and E. A. Hambie.** 1985. Cerebrospinal fluid serologic test for syphilis: treponemal and nontreponemal tests, p. 157–162. *In* R. Morisset and E. Kurstak (ed.), *Advances in Sexually Transmitted Diseases.* VNW Science Press, Ultrecht, The Netherlands.

80. **Larsen, S. A., B. M. Steiner, and A. H. Rudolph.** 1995. Laboratory diagnosis and interpretation of tests for syphilis. *Clin. Microbiol. Rev.* **8:**1–21.

81. **Larsen, S. A., V. Pope, R. E. Johnson, and E. J. Kennedy, Jr.** 1998. *A Manual of Tests for Syphilis.* American Public Health Association, Washington, DC.

82. **Lefevre, J. C., M. A. Bertrand, and R. Bauriaud.** 1990. Evaluation of the Captia enzyme immunoassays for detection of immunoglobulins G and M to *Treponema pallidum* in syphilis. *J. Clin. Microbiol.* **28:**1704–1707.

83. **Li, J., H. Y. Zheng, L. N. Wang, Y. X. Liu, X. F. Wang, and X. R. Liu.** 2009. Clinical evaluation of four recombinant *Treponema pallidum* antigen-based rapid diagnostic tests for syphilis. *J. Eur. Acad. Dermatol. Venereol.* **23:**648–650.

84. **Liu, H., B. Rodes, C. Y. Chen, and B. Steiner.** 2001. New tests for syphilis: rational design of a PCR method for detection of *Treponema pallidum* in clinical specimens using unique regions of the DNA polymerase I gene. *J. Clin. Microbiol.* **39:**1941–1946.

85. **Lukehart, S. A.** 2008. Syphilis, p. 1038–1046. *In* A. S. Fauci, E. Braunwald, D. L. Kasper, S. J. Hauser, D. L. Longo, and J. L. Jameson (ed.), *Harrison's Principles of Internal Medicine,* 17th ed. McGraw Hill, New York, NY.

86. **Lukehart, S. A., C. Godornes, B. J. Molini, P. Sonnett, S. Hopkins, F. Mulcahy, J. Engelman, S. J. Mitchell, A. M. Rompalo, C. M. Marra, and J. D. Klausner.** 2004. Macrolide resistance in *Treponema pallidum* in the United States and Ireland. *N. Engl. J. Med.* **351:**154–158.

87. **Lukehart, S. A., and C. M. Marra.** 2007. Isolation and laboratory maintenance of *Treponema pallidum. Curr. Protoc. Microbiol.* **12:**12A.1.

88. **Mackay, I. M., G. Harnett, N. Jeoffreys, I. Bastian, K. S. Sriprakash, D. Siebert, and T. P. Sloots.** 2006. Detection and discrimination of herpes simplex viruses, *Haemophilus ducreyi, Treponema pallidum,* and *Calymmatobacterium* (*Klebsiella*) *granulomatis* from genital ulcers. *Clin. Infect. Dis.* **42:**1431–1438.

89. **Manavi, K., H. Young, and A. McMillan.** 2006. The sensitivity of syphilis assays in detecting different stages of early syphilis. *Int. J. STD AIDS* **17:**768–771.

90. **Marangoni, A., A. Moroni, S. Accardo, and R. Cevenini.** 2009. Laboratory diagnosis of syphilis with automated immunoassays. *J. Clin. Lab. Anal.* **23:**1–6.

91. **Marangoni, A., V. Sambri, S. Accardo, F. Cavrini, A. D'Antuono, A. Moroni, E. Storni, and R. Cevenini.** 2005. Evaluation of LIAISON *Treponema* Screen, a novel recombinant antigen-based chemiluminescence immunoassay for laboratory diagnosis of syphilis. *Clin. Diagn. Lab. Immunol.* **12:**1231–1234.

92. **Marfin, A. A., H. Liu, M. Y. Sutton, B. Steiner, A. Pillay, and L. E. Markowitz.** 2001. Amplification of the DNA polymerase I gene of *Treponema pallidum* from whole blood of persons with syphilis. *Diagn. Microbiol. Infect. Dis.* **40:**163–166.

93. **Marra, C. M., C. L. Maxwell, S. L. Smith, S. A. Lukehart, A. M. Rompalo, M. Eaton, B. P. Stoner, M. Augenbraun, D. E. Barker, J. J. Corbett, M. Zajackowski, C. Raines, J. Nerad, R. Kee, and S. H. Barnett.** 2004. Cerebrospinal fluid abnormalities in patients with syphilis: association with clinical and laboratory features. *J. Infect. Dis.* **189:**369–376.

94. **McMillan, A., and H. Young.** 2008. Qualitative and quantitative aspects of the serological diagnosis of early syphilis. *Int. J. STD AIDS* **19:**620–624.

95. **Meheus, A., and F. J. Ndowa.** 2008. Endemic treponematoses, p. 685–688. *In* K. K. Holmes, P. F. Sparling, W. E. Stamm, P. Piot, J. N. Wasserheit, L. Corey, M. S. Cohen, and D. H. Watts (ed.), *Sexually Transmitted Diseases,* 4th ed. McGraw Hill, New York, NY.

96. **Miao, R., and A. H. Fieldsteel.** 1978. Genetics of *Treponema*: relationship between *Treponema pallidum* and five cultivable treponemes. *J. Bacteriol.* **133:**101–107.

97. **Miao, R. M., and A. H. Fieldsteel.** 1980. Genetic relationship between *Treponema pallidum* and *Treponema pertenue,* two noncultivable human pathogens. *J. Bacteriol.* **141:**427–429.

98. **Mikosza, A. S., and D. J. Hampson.** 2001. Human intestinal spirochetosis: *Brachyspira aalborgi* and/or *Brachyspira pilosicoli? Anim. Health Res. Rev.* **2:**101–110.

99. **Mikosza, A. S., T. La, C. J. Brooke, C. F. Lindboe, P. B. Ward, R. G. Heine, J. G. Guccion, W. B. de Boer, and D. J. Hampson.** 1999. PCR amplification from fixed tissue indicates frequent involvement of *Brachyspira aalborgi* in human intestinal spirochetosis. *J. Clin. Microbiol.* **37:**2093–2098.

100. **Mikosza, A. S., T. La, K. R. Margawani, C. J. Brooke, and D. J. Hampson.** 2001. PCR detection of *Brachyspira aalborgi* and *Brachyspira pilosicoli* in human faeces. *FEMS Microbiol. Lett.* **197:**167–170.

101. **Miller, J. N.** 1975. Value and limitations of nontreponemal and treponemal tests in the laboratory diagnosis of syphilis. *Clin. Obstet. Gynecol.* **18:**191–203.

102. **Molepo, J., A. Pillay, B. Weber, S. A. Morse, and A. A. Hoosen.** 2007. Molecular typing of *Treponema pallidum* strains from patients with neurosyphilis in Pretoria, South Africa. *Sex. Transm. Infect.* **83:**189–192.

103. **Monath, T. P., and S. E. Frey.** 2009. Possible autoimmune reactions following smallpox vaccination: the biologic false positive test for syphilis. *Vaccine* **27:**1645–1650.

104. **Moter, A., B. Riep, V. Haban, K. Heuner, G. Siebert, M. Berning, C. Wyss, B. Ehmke, T. F. Flemmig, and U. B. Gobel.** 2006. Molecular epidemiology of oral treponemes in patients with periodontitis and in periodontitis-resistant subjects. *J. Clin. Microbiol.* **44:**3078–3085.

105. **Mustapha, I. Z., S. Debrey, M. Oladubu, and R. Ugarte.** 2007. Markers of systemic bacterial exposure in periodontal disease and cardiovascular disease risk: a systematic review and meta-analysis. *J. Periodontol.* **78:**2289–2302.

106. **Nandwani, R., and D. T. Evans.** 1995. Are you sure it's syphilis? A review of false positive serology. *Int. J. STD AIDS* **6:**241–248.

107. **Nell, E. E.** 1954. Comparative sensitivity of treponemes of syphilis, yaws, and bejel to penicillin in vitro, with observations on factors affecting its treponemicidal action. *Am. J. Syph.* **38:**92–106.

108. **Nichols, H. J. and H. H. Hough.** 1913. Demonstration of *Spirochaeta pallida* in the cerebrospinal fluid. From a patient with nervous relapse following the use of salvarsan. *JAMA* **40:**108–110.

109. **Norris, S. J.** 1988. Syphilis, p. 1–31. *In* D. J. M. Wright (ed.), *Immunology of Sexually Transmitted Diseases.* Kluwer Academic Publishers, Boston, MA.

110. **Norris, S. J., et al.** 1993. Polypeptides of *Treponema pallidum*: progress toward understanding their structural, functional, and immunologic roles. *Microbiol. Rev.* **57:**750–779.

111. **Norris, S. J., D. L. Cox, and G. M. Weinstock.** 2001. Biology of *Treponema pallidum*: correlation of functional activities with genome sequence data. *J. Mol. Microbiol. Biotechnol.* **3:**37–62.

112. **Ochiai, S., Y. Adachi, and K. Mori.** 1997. Unification of the genera *Serpulina* and *Brachyspira*, and proposals of *Brachyspira hyodysenteriae* comb. nov., *Brachyspira innocens* comb. nov. and *Brachyspira pilosicoli* comb. nov. *Microbiol. Immunol.* **41:**445–452.

113. **Olsen, I., B. J. Paster, and F. E. Dewhirst.** 2000. Taxonomy of spirochetes. *Anaerobe* **6:**39–47.

114. **Ooi, C., P. Robertson, and B. Donovan.** 2002. Investigation of isolated positive syphilis enzyme immunoassay (ICE Murex) results. *Int. J. STD AIDS* **13:**761–764.

115. **Oppenheimer, E. H., and J. B. Hardy.** 1971. Congenital syphilis in the newborn infant: clinical and pathological observations in recent cases. *Johns Hopkins Med. J.* **129:**63–82.

116. **Orle, K. A., C. A. Gates, D. H. Martin, B. A. Body, and J. B. Weiss.** 1996. Simultaneous detection of *Haemophilus ducreyi*, *Treponema pallidum*, and herpes simplex virus types 1 and 2 from genital ulcers. *J. Clin. Microbiol.* **34:**49–4.

117. **Padmanabhan, V., J. Dahlstrom, L. Maxwell, G. Kaye, A. Clarke, and P. J. Barratt.** 1996. Invasive intestinal spirochetosis: a report of three cases. *Pathology* **28:**283–286.

118. **Paster, B. J., S. K. Boches, J. L. Galvin, R. E. Ericson, C. N. Lau, V. A. Levanos, A. Sahasrabudhe, and F. E. Dewhirst.** 2001. Bacterial diversity in human subgingival plaque. *J. Bacteriol.* **183:**3770–3783.

119. **Paster, B. J., F. E. Dewhirst, W. G. Weisburg, L. A. Tordoff, G. J. Fraser, R. B. Hespell, T. B. Stanton, L. Zablen, L. Mandelco, and C. R. Woese.** 1991. Phylogenetic analysis of the spirochetes. *J. Bacteriol.* **173:**6101–6109.

120. **Persson, G. R., and R. E. Persson.** 2008. Cardiovascular disease and periodontitis: an update on the associations and risk. *J. Clin. Periodontol.* **35:**362–379.

121. **Peterman, T. A., J. D. Heffelfinger, E. B. Swint, and S. L. Groseclose.** 2005. The changing epidemiology of syphilis. *Sex. Transm. Dis.* **32:**S4–S10.

122. Reference deleted.

123. **Pillay, A., H. Liu, C. Y. Chen, B. Holloway, A. W. Sturm, B. Steiner, and S. A. Morse.** 1998. Molecular subtyping of *Treponema pallidum* subspecies *pallidum*. *Sex. Transm. Dis.* **25:**408–414.

124. **Pillay, A., H. Liu, S. Ebrahim, C. Y. Chen, W. Lai, G. Fehler, R. C. Ballard, B. Steiner, A. W. Sturm, and S. A. Morse.** 2002. Molecular typing of *Treponema pallidum* in South Africa: cross-sectional studies. *J. Clin. Microbiol.* **40:**256–258.

125. **Pope, V., M. B. Fears, W. E. Morrill, A. Castro, and S. E. Kikkert.** 2000. Comparison of the Serodia *Treponema pallidum* particle agglutination, Captia Syphilis-G, and SpiroTek Reagin II tests with standard test techniques for diagnosis of syphilis. *J. Clin. Microbiol.* **38:**2543–2545.

126. **Quatresooz, P., and G. E. Pierard.** 2009. Perivascular cuff and spread of *Treponema pallidum*. *Dermatology* **219:**259–262.

127. **Radolf, J. D., K. R. O. Hazlett, and S. A. Lukehart.** 2006. Pathogenesis of syphilis, p. 197–236. *In* J. D. Radolf and S. A. Lukehart (ed.), *Pathogenic Treponema: Molecular and Cellular Biology.* Caister Academic Press, Norwich, United Kingdom.

128. **Ratnam, S.** 2005. The laboratory diagnosis of syphilis. *Can. J. Infect. Dis. Med. Microbiol.* **16:**45–51.

129. **Reiter, H.** 1960. An account of the so-called Reiter treponeme (history, isolation, cultivation, specificity, and utilization). *Br. J. Vener. Dis.* **36:**18–20.

130. **Risbud, A., K. Chan-Tack, D. Gadkari, R. R. Gangakhedkar, M. E. Shepherd, R. Bollinger, S. Mehendale, C. Gaydos, A. Divekar, A. Rompalo, and T. C. Quinn.** 1999. The etiology of genital ulcer disease by multiplex polymerase chain reaction and relationship to HIV infection among patients attending sexually transmitted disease clinics in Pune, India. *Sex. Transm. Dis.* **26:**55–62.

131. **Rodriguez, I., E. L. Alvarez, C. Fernandez, and A. Miranda.** 2002. Comparison of a recombinant-antigen enzyme immunoassay with *Treponema pallidum* hemagglutination test for serological confirmation of syphilis. *Mem. Inst. Oswaldo Cruz* **97:**347–349.

132. Reference deleted.

133. **Rolfs, R. T., M. R. Joesoef, E. F. Hendershot, A. M. Rompalo, M. H. Augenbraun, M. Chiu, G. Bolan, S. C. Johnson, P. French, E. Steen, J. D. Radolf, S. Larsen, et al.** 1997. A randomized trial of enhanced therapy for early syphilis in patients with and without human immunodeficiency virus infection. *N. Engl. J. Med.* **337:**307–314.

134. **Romanowski, B., R. Sutherland, G. Fick, D. Mooney, and E. J. Love.** 1991. Serologic response to treatment of infectious syphilis. *Ann. Intern. Med.* **114:**1005–1009.

135. **Ruane, P. J., M. M. Nakata, J. F. Reinhardt, and W. L. George.** 1989. Spirochete-like organisms in the human gastrointestinal tract. *Rev. Infect. Dis.* **11:**184–196.

136. **Schell, R. F.** 1983. Rabbit and hamster models of treponemal infection, p. 121–135. *In* R. F. Schell and D. M. Musher (ed.), *Pathogenesis and Immunology of Treponemal Infection.* Marcel Dekker, Inc., New York, NY.

137. **Schmidt, B. L., M. Edjlalipour, and A. Luger.** 2000. Comparative evaluation of nine different enzyme-linked immunosorbent assays for determination of antibodies against *Treponema pallidum* in patients with primary syphilis. *J. Clin. Microbiol.* **38:**1279–1282.

138. **Schroeter, A. L., R. H. Turner, J. B. Lucas, and W. J. Brown.** 1971. Therapy for incubating syphilis. Effectiveness of gonorrhea treatment. *JAMA* **218:**711–713.

139. **Shafii, T., J. D. Radolf, P. J. Sanchez, K. F. Schulz, and F. K. Murphy.** 2008. Congenital syphilis, p. 1577–1612. *In* K. K. Holmes, P. F. Sparling, W. E. Stamm, P. Piot, J. N. Wasserheit, L. Corey, M. S. Cohen, and D. H. Watts (ed.), *Sexually Transmitted Diseases*, 4th ed. McGraw Hill, New York, NY.

140. **Shore, R. N., and J. A. Faricelli.** 1977. Borderline and reactive FTA-ABS. Results in lupus erythematosus. *Arch. Dermatol.* **113:**37–41.

141. **Sischy, A., F. da L'Exposto, Y. Dangor, H. G. Fehler, F. Radebe, D. D. Walkden, S. D. Miller, and R. C. Ballard.** 1991. Syphilis serology in patients with primary syphilis and non-treponemal sexually transmitted diseases in southern Africa. *Genitourin. Med.* **67:**129–132.

142. **Smibert, R. M.** 1984. Genus III: *Treponema,* p. 49–57. *In* N. R. Krieg and J. G. Holt (ed.), *Bergey's Manual of Systematic Bacteriology.* Williams & Wilkins Co., Baltimore, MD.

143. **Smikle, M. F., O. James, and P. Prabhakar.** 1990. Prevalence of reactive serological tests for syphilis in the Jamaican population. *West Indian Med. J.* **39:**170–173.

144. **Stamm, L. V., and H. L. Bergen.** 2000. A point mutation associated with bacterial macrolide resistance is present in both 23S rRNA genes of an erythromycin-resistant *Treponema pallidum* clinical isolate. *Antimicrob. Agents Chemother.* **44:**806–807.

145. **Sutton, M. Y., H. Liu, B. Steiner, A. Pillay, T. Mickey, L. Finelli, S. Morse, L. E. Markowitz, and M. E. St. Louis.** 2001. Molecular subtyping of *Treponema pallidum* in an Arizona county with increasing syphilis morbidity: use of specimens from ulcers and blood. *J. Infect. Dis.* **183:**1601–1606.

146. **Tanahashi, J., T. Daa, A. Gamachi, K. Kashima, Y. Kondoh, N. Yada, and S. Yokoyama.** 2008. Human intestinal spirochetosis in Japan; its incidence, clinicopathologic features, and genotypic identification. *Mod. Pathol.* **21:**76–84.

147. **Tinajeros, F., D. Grossman, K. Richmond, M. Steele, S. G. Garcia, L. Zegarra, and R. Revollo.** 2006. Diagnostic accuracy of a point-of-care syphilis test when used among pregnant women in Bolivia. *Sex. Transm. Infect.* **82**(Suppl. 5):v17–v21.

148. **Tompkins, D. S., S. J. Foulkes, P. G. Godwin, and A. P. West.** 1986. Isolation and characterisation of intestinal spirochaetes. *J. Clin. Pathol.* **39:**535–541.

149. **Trivett-Moore, N. L., G. L. Gilbert, C. L. Law, D. J. Trott, and D. J. Hampson.** 1998. Isolation of *Serpulina pilosicoli* from rectal biopsy specimens showing evidence of intestinal spirochetosis. *J. Clin. Microbiol.* **36:**261–265.

150. **Trott, D. J., and D. J. Hampson.** 1998. Evaluation of day-old specific pathogen-free chicks as an experimental model for pathogenicity testing of intestinal spirochaete species. *J. Comp. Pathol.* **118:**365–381.

151. **Trott, D. J., N. S. Jensen, G. Saint, I, S. L. Oxberry, T. B. Stanton, D. Lindquist, and D. J. Hampson.** 1997. Identification and characterization of *Serpulina pilosicoli* isolates recovered from the blood of critically ill patients. *J. Clin. Microbiol.* **35:**482–485.

152. **Trott, D. J., A. S. Mikosza, B. G. Combs, S. L. Oxberry, and D. J. Hampson.** 1998. Population genetic analysis of *Serpulina pilosicoli* and its molecular epidemiology in villages in the eastern Highlands of Papua New Guinea. *Int. J. Syst. Bacteriol.* **48**(Pt. 3):659–668.

153. **Trott, D. J., T. B. Stanton, N. S. Jensen, and D. J. Hampson.** 1996. Phenotypic characteristics of *Serpulina pilosicoli* the agent of intestinal spirochaetosis. *FEMS Microbiol. Lett.* **142:**209–214.

154. **Velicko, I., M. Arneborn, and A. Blaxhult.** 2008. Syphilis epidemiology in Sweden: re-emergence since 2000 primarily due to spread among men who have sex with men. *Euro Surveill.* **13:**pii=19063. http://www.eurosurveillance.org/ViewArticle .aspx?ArticleId=19063.

155. **Warthin, A. S., and A. C. Starry.** 1920. A more rapid and improved method of demonstrating spirochetes in tissues. *Am. J. Syph. Gonorrhea Vener. Dis.* **4:**97–103.

156. **Wheeler, H. L., S. Agarwal, and B. T. Goh.** 2004. Dark ground microscopy and treponemal serological tests in the diagnosis of early syphilis. *Sex. Transm. Infect.* **80:**411–414.

157. **Willcox, R. R., and T. Guthe.** 1966. *Treponema pallidum.* A bibliographical review of the morphology, culture and survival of *T. pallidum* and associated organisms. *Bull. W. H. O.* **35:**1–169.

158. **Workowski, K. A.** 2010. Sexually transmitted diseases treatment guidelines. *MMWR Recommend. Rep.* **59:**1–110.

159. **Young, H., J. Pryde, L. Duncan, and J. Dave.** 2009. The Architect Syphilis assay for antibodies to *Treponema pallidum:* an automated screening assay with high sensitivity in primary syphilis. *Sex. Transm. Infect.* **85:**19–23.

160. **Zellan, J., and M. Augenbraun.** 2004. Syphilis in the HIV-infected patient: an update on epidemiology, diagnosis, and management. *Curr. HIV/AIDS Rep.* **1:**142–147.

161. **Zenker, P.** 1991. New case definition for congenital syphilis reporting. *Sex. Transm. Dis.* **18:**44–45.

General Approaches to Identification of *Mycoplasma, Ureaplasma,* and Obligate Intracellular Bacteria

J. STEPHEN DUMLER

58

The bacteria discussed in chapters 59 to 64 differ from bacteria described in other parts of this *Manual* by several characteristics, including lack of efficient characterization with the Gram stain method and, except for *Mycoplasma* and *Ureaplasma* species and to a limited degree for *Tropheryma whipplei,* the requirement for intracellular growth. Thus, the most frequently used tests in clinical microbiology laboratories, the Gram stain and culture on artificial media, are unable to detect these organisms if present in clinical samples. Diagnosis of infections caused by these bacteria has traditionally been accomplished by Romanowsky staining (Giemsa and Wright stains) of clinical samples, by detection of antibody responses to infection using a variety of serological tests, or by histopathologic analysis of biopsy samples. Molecular diagnostic tools and better culture methods have significantly improved the ability to detect these agents and to diagnose the diseases that they cause. For some of these infections, molecular tools are standard practice. The following tables summarize the epidemiology of these infections (Table 1) and the diagnostic tests most often used for the detection of the causative bacteria (Table 2).

TABLE 1 Epidemiology and clinical diseases associated with *Anaplasma*, *Chlamydia*, *Coxiella*, *Ehrlichia*, *Mycoplasma*, *Orientia*, *Rickettsia*, *Tropheryma*, and *Ureaplasma* infections

Organism	Disease	Reservoir(s)	Vector and mode of transmission
Anaplasma phagocytophilum	Human granulocytotropic anaplasmosis (HGA); fever, headache, myalgia, systemic involvement except for central nervous system	White-footed mouse, other small mammals, ruminants, deer	*Ixodes scapularis* (deer or black-legged tick), *I. pacificus* (western black-legged tick), *I. ricinus* (rabbit tick), *I. persulcatus* tick bites
Chlamydia trachomatis	Endemic trachoma, inclusion keratoconjunctivitis, urethritis, epididymitis, endometritis, salpingitis, perihepatitis, pneumonia, lymphogranuloma venereum	Humans	Sexual contact, hand-eye contact, insect fomites, infected birth canal
Chlamydia pneumoniae	Pneumonia, bronchitis, sinusitis, pharyngitis	Humans	Inhalation of infected aerosols
Chlamydia psittaci	Psittacosis (pneumonia), systemic infections	Birds, domestic animals	Direct contact with or inhalation of infected aerosols
Coxiella burnetii	Acute Q fever (self-limited febrile illness ± pneumonia, hepatitis); chronic Q fever (endocarditis, endovascular infections)	Cattle, sheep, goats, cats, rabbits, dogs, ticks	Inhalation of infected aerosols; ingestion of nonpasteurized dairy products
Ehrlichia chaffeensis	Human monocytotropic ehrlichiosis (HME): fever, headache, myalgia, systemic involvement including central nervous system	White-tailed deer, dogs and other canids, raccoons	*Amblyomma americanum* (Lone Star tick) and potentially *Dermacentor variabilis* (American dog tick) tick bites
Ehrlichia ewingii	"Ewingii" ehrlichiosis: fever, headache, myalgia, predominantly in immunocompromised individuals	Dogs and other canids	*Amblyomma americanum* (Lone Star tick) tick bites
Mycoplasma genitalium	Urethritis, cervicitis, endometritis, conjunctivitis	Humans	Sexual contact, vertical transmission in utero or intrapartum
Mycoplasma hominis	Acute pyelonephritis, bacterial vaginosis, pelvic inflammatory disease, postabortion bacteremia	Humans	Sexual contact, vertical transmission in utero or intrapartum
Mycoplasma pneumoniae	Tracheobronchitis, pneumonia, pharyngitis, extrapulmonary complications (meningoencephalitis, arthritis, etc.)	Humans	Contact with infectious aerosols or fomites
Orientia tsutsugamushi	Scrub typhus	Chiggers (larval mites)	*Leptotrombidium* spp. (chigger) bites
Rickettsia africae	African tick-bite fever	Not established	*Amblyomma* spp. tick bites
Rickettsia akari	Rickettsialpox	Mice and other small mammals	*Allodermanyssus sanguineus* (mouse mite) bites
Rickettsia conorii	Boutonneuse fever or Mediterranean spotted fever	Small mammals and ticks	*Rhipicephalus sanguineus* (Brown dog) tick bites
Rickettsia felis	Flea-borne spotted fever	Fleas, opossums, cats, dogs	*Ctenocephalides felis* (cat fleas); contamination of infected flea feces into flea bite
Rickettsia honei	Flinders Island spotted fever	Not established (reptiles?)	*Aponomma hydrosauri* (reptile tick)
Rickettsia prowazekii	Louse-borne typhus	Humans, lice, flying squirrels	*Pediculus humanus* subsp. *corporis* (body louse); contamination of infected louse feces into louse bite
Rickettsia rickettsii	Rocky Mountain spotted fever	Ticks, small and medium-size mammals	*Dermacentor variabilis* (American dog tick), *Dermacentor andersoni* (wood tick), *Rhipicephalus sanguineus* (North and Central America), *Amblyomma cajennense* (Central and South America) tick bites
Rickettsia slovaca	Tick-borne lymphadenopathy	Not determined	*Dermacentor marginatus* ticks (Europe)
Rickettsia typhi	Murine typhus	Rats and other rodents, opossums	*Xenopsylla cheopis* (Rat fleas) and *Ctenocephalides felis* (Cat fleas); contamination of flea bite wound with infected flea feces
Tropheryma whipplei	Weight loss, diarrhea, malabsorption, arthropathy, lymphadenopathy, culture-negative endocarditis, encephalitis	Humans	Environmental contacts (sewage, human stool, saliva); genetic predispositions
Ureaplasma urealyticum	Urethritis, epididymo-orchitis, urinary calculi, abortion, chorioamnionitis	Humans	Sexual contact, in utero or peripartum vertical transmission

TABLE 2 Diagnostic tests for *Anaplasma*, *Chlamydia*, *Coxiella*, *Ehrlichia*, *Mycoplasma*, *Orientia*, *Rickettsia*, *Tropheryma*, and *Ureaplasma*

Organism	Diagnostic test[a]
Anaplasma phagocytophilum	**Microscopy:** Giemsa or Wright stain of peripheral blood or buffy coat smears is positive in approximately 60% of infected persons. **Antigen tests:** None commercially available; immunohistochemistry offered at CDC. **Molecular tests:** EDTA-anticoagulated blood collected during the pretreatment acute phase of illness is used for PCR amplification. Species- and genus-specific tests are described. Current test of choice for diagnosis during active infection. **Culture:** EDTA-anticoagulated peripheral blood is inoculated onto HL-60, THP1, or other myelocytic cell lines. Positive cultures may be obtained between 3 and 30 days from many samples if inoculated within 24 h and if obtained before antimicrobial therapy. Lack of timely results precludes frequent use. **Serologic tests:** IFA is the most frequently used test. In a patient with typical clinical features of human granulocytotropic anaplasmosis, a fourfold or greater rise in IgG titer confirms infection, and a single peak IgG titer of ≥80 provides supportive evidence. IgG test sensitivity is between 90 and 100%; specificity is approximately 95%. IgM testing is not recommended.
Chlamydia trachomatis	**Microscopy:** Organisms can be detected by DFA test or Giemsa stain. DFA is more sensitive, but neither test should be used alone. **Antigen tests:** Commercial EIAs for *C. trachomatis* vary in sensitivity but may cross-react with other bacterial LPSs and are not suitable alone for screening. EIA using blocking antibodies may increase specificity to 99.5%. Point-of-care tests are only 62–72% sensitive compared to culture and less sensitive than molecular tests. **Molecular tests:** Commercial NAATs (PCR, transcription-mediated amplification, strand displacement amplification) are available and are tests of choice for confirmation of *C. trachomatis* infections. **Culture:** Recovered in many different cell cultures including McCoy and HeLa cells. Test sensitivity is dependent on the quality of the submitted specimen. **Serologic tests:** MIF test is most sensitive and specific (test of choice) for neonatal pneumonia but is not recommended for other *C. trachomatis* infections. Fourfold or greater rises in titers are significant, but rising titers may not be observed with chronic, repeated, or systemic infections. A single IgM titer of ≥32 supports a diagnosis of neonatal pneumonia.
Chlamydia pneumoniae	**Microscopy:** Organisms may be detected by Giemsa stain or DFA test directed against LPS, but both tests are relatively insensitive. **Antigen tests:** Available EIAs directed against LPS detect all *Chlamydiaceae* but are licensed only for *C. trachomatis*. **Molecular tests:** None commercially available. **Culture:** Recovered best if inoculated onto HL cells or Hep-2 cells. **Serologic tests:** MIF test is the test of choice. Diagnosis confirmed by fourfold or greater rise in titer or single samples with IgM titer of ≥16 and/or IgG titer of ≥512.
Chlamydia psittacii	**Microscopy:** Organisms may be detected by Giemsa stain or DFA test directed against LPS, but both tests are relatively insensitive. **Antigen tests:** Available EIAs directed against LPS detect all *Chlamydiaceae* but are licensed only for *C. trachomatis*. **Molecular tests:** None commercially available. **Culture:** Recovered in many different cell cultures including McCoy and HeLa cells. **Serologic tests:** MIF test is most sensitive and specific (test of choice).
Coxiella burnetii	**Microscopy:** DFA or immunohistochemistry may be performed, but these tests are not widely available. **Antigen tests:** None commercially available. **Molecular tests:** PCR available through reference laboratories; more sensitive than serology during first few weeks; whole blood or leukocyte fractions are preferred, and serum is less useful. Cardiac valve tissue more sensitive than blood for chronic Q fever endocarditis. **Culture:** Requires BSL3 facility and practices; U.S. category B select agent. Animal (mouse) inoculation is most sensitive. May be cultivated in a variety of cell lines, especially HEL, Vero, RK13, THP1, or A549 cells in flasks or shell vials. **Serologic tests:** Most frequently used diagnostic test. Acute Q fever is confirmed by a fourfold or greater rise in titer to phase II antigens or by a single IgM titer of ≥50 and IgG of titer ≥200. Chronic Q fever is confirmed in a single serum with a ≥800 IgG titer to phase I antigen. A decreasing antibody titer suggests successful therapy. The IFA test that detects both phase I and II IgG and IgM is recommended. IgM phase II antigen enzyme-linked immunosorbent assay is commercially available but is for acute Q fever diagnosis only.
Ehrlichia chaffeensis	**Microscopy:** Giemsa or Wright staining of peripheral blood or buffy coat smears is positive in up to 29% of infected persons. **Antigen tests:** None commercially available; immunohistochemistry offered at CDC. **Molecular tests:** EDTA-anticoagulated blood collected during the pretreatment acute phase of illness is used for PCR amplification. Species- and genus-specific tests are described. Current test of choice for diagnosis during active infection. Sensitivity ranges from 56 to100%. **Culture:** EDTA-anticoagulated peripheral blood or CSF is inoculated onto DH82, THP1, HEL-22, Vero, HL-60, or other cell lines. Positive cultures may be obtained between 5 and >30 days from most samples if inoculated within 12 hours and if obtained before antimicrobial therapy. Lack of timely results precludes frequent use. **Serologic tests:** IFA is the most frequently used test. In a patient with typical clinical features of human monocytic ehrlichiosis, a fourfold or greater rise in IgG titer confirms infection, and a single peak IgG titer of ≥64 provides supportive evidence. IgG test sensitivity is believed to be high; specificity is approximately 95%. IgM testing is not recommended.

(Continued on next page)

TABLE 2 (*Continued*)

Organism	Diagnostic test[a]
Ehrlichia ewingii	**Microscopy:** Giemsa or Wright stain of peripheral blood or buffy coat smears occasionally reveals bacterial clusters (morulae) in neutrophils of infected persons. **Antigen tests:** None available. **Molecular tests:** EDTA-anticoagulated blood collected during the pretreatment acute phase of illness is used for PCR amplification. Species- and genus-specific tests are available in some reference and public health laboratories. Current test of choice for diagnosis during active infection. Sensitivity is not currently known but is suspected to be high. **Culture:** No method of in vitro culture has been developed. **Serologic tests:** No specific antibody test is available. Antibody tests are based largely on cross-reactivity with *E. chaffeensis* and alone are not diagnostic.
Mycoplasma genitalium	**Microscopy:** May be detected in genital fluids by use of DNA fluorochrome stains (Hoechst 33258 or acridine orange), but these are not specific. **Antigen tests:** Not recommended for diagnostic purposes. **Molecular tests:** PCR amplification may be the only practical means for detection of the pathogen. Commercial kits are not currently available in the United States. **Culture:** Organisms are isolated from a variety of genital fluids. Growth conditions are not well established but can require 6 weeks or more. Widely considered insensitive for diagnosis confirmation. **Serologic tests:** MIF and Western immunoblot methods have been described, although none are commercially available.
Mycoplasma hominis	**Microscopy:** May be detected in body fluids by use of DNA fluorochrome stains (Hoechst 33258 or acridine orange), but these are not specific. **Antigen tests:** None commercially available. **Molecular tests:** PCR tests have been developed but because of rapid growth are less useful than culture. **Culture:** Organisms are isolated from a variety of clinical samples. Dacron or polyester swabs are preferred; wood shafted cotton swabs should be avoided. Mycoplasmas are extremely labile, and appropriate transport medium should be used. Can be recovered on SP4 broth and agar supplemented with arginine (best overall), on Shepard's 10B broth, or on A8 agar. Growth occurs within 2 to 4 days. **Serologic tests:** Not recommended for routine use.
Mycoplasma pneumoniae	**Microscopy:** May be detected in body fluids by using DNA fluorochrome stains (Hoechst 33258 or acridine orange), but these are not specific. **Antigen tests:** Not recommended for diagnostic purposes. **Molecular tests:** PCR amplification is the test of choice and is highly sensitive, but clinical studies have yielded variable results when compared with culture and serology. Commercial kits are not currently available in the United States. **Culture:** Organisms are isolated from a variety of clinical samples. Dacron or polyester swabs are preferred; wood-shafted cotton swabs should be avoided. Mycoplasmas are extremely labile, and appropriate transport medium should be used. Can be recovered on SP4 glucose broth or agar. Growth occurs after 21 days or longer. Blind subculture may improve yield. Widely considered insensitive for diagnosis confirmation. **Serologic tests:** EIAs are more sensitive and specific than CF and IFA; detection of seroconversion by demonstration of a fourfold increase in antibody titer is preferred, but detection of IgM antibodies in single sera may be useful. The cold agglutinin test is not recommended for diagnosis of *M. pneumoniae* infection.
Orientia tsutsugamushi	**Microscopy:** DFA or immunohistochemistry on skin or other tissues may be performed, but tests are not widely available. **Antigen tests:** Not available. **Molecular tests:** PCR amplification performed on EDTA-anticoagulated blood, buffy coat leukocytes, plasma, or tissue samples obtained during acute phase of illness; available only through reference laboratories. **Culture:** Isolation is performed by intraperitoneal inoculation of mice. Performed only in reference and research laboratories. **Serologic tests:** With the IFA test in a region of endemicity, a titer of ≥400 is 98% specific and 48% sensitive. Lower cutoffs are used for populations in which the infection is not endemic. Indirect immunoperoxidase is also sensitive and specific with diagnostic cutoffs of ≥128 for IgG and ≥32 for IgM. Dot EIA kits are available and have lower sensitivity and specificity than IFA. Weil-Felix (*Proteus*) febrile agglutinins test is insensitive and nonspecific.
Rickettsia africae and *Rickettsia conorii*	**Microscopy:** DFA or immunohistochemistry on skin biopsy specimen of rash or eschar is sensitive and specific for spotted fever group rickettsiae. Antibodies are not commercially available. **Antigen tests:** Not available. **Molecular tests:** PCR amplification performed on EDTA-anticoagulated blood, buffy coat leukocytes, plasma, skin biopsy specimens, or tissue samples obtained during acute phase of illness; available only through reference laboratories. **Culture:** Heparin-anticoagulated plasma or buffy coat cells, or triturated skin biopsy specimens are inoculated into shell vials seeded with cell lines such as Vero, L-929, HEL, or MRC5. Infected cells are detected by immunofluorescence or PCR after 48 to 72 h; sensitivity is up to 59%. **Serologic tests:** IFA is sensitive using *R. africae*, *R. conorii*, or other spotted fever group rickettsial antigens (e.g., *R. rickettsii*) but is low during the acute phase of illness. A fourfold increase in titer is generally considered most specific, but single titers of ≥128 for IgG and ≥32 for IgM are considered diagnostically significant. A Dot EIA test that is modestly less sensitive and specific is available for *R. conorii*.

(*Continued on next page*)

TABLE 2 Diagnostic tests for *Anaplasma, Chlamydia, Coxiella, Ehrlichia, Mycoplasma, Orientia, Rickettsia, Tropheryma,* and *Ureaplasma (Continued)*

Organism	Diagnostic test[a]
Rickettsia akari	**Microscopy:** DFA or immunohistochemistry on skin biopsy specimen of rash or eschar is sensitive and specific for spotted fever group rickettsiae. Antibodies are not commercially available. **Antigen tests:** Not available. **Molecular tests:** PCR amplification performed on skin biopsy specimen of eschars obtained during acute phase of illness; available only through reference laboratories. **Culture:** Heparin-anticoagulated blood plasma or buffy coat cells are inoculated into shell vials seeded with cell lines such as Vero, L-929, HEL, or MRC-5. Infected cells are detected by Giemsa, Gimenez, or fluorescent antibody staining after 48 to 72 h. Sensitivity is not known. **Serologic tests:** IFA is sensitive using either *R. akari* or other spotted fever group rickettsial antigens (e.g., *R. rickettsii*) but is low during the acute phase of illness. A fourfold increase in titer is generally considered most specific, but single titers of ≥128 for IgG and ≥32 for IgM are considered diagnostically significant. *R. akari*-specific testing can be obtained in reference or public health laboratories.
Rickettsia felis	**Microscopy:** Not available. **Antigen tests:** Not available. **Molecular tests:** PCR amplification performed on EDTA-anticoagulated blood, buffy coat leukocytes, plasma, or tissue samples obtained during acute phase of illness; available only through reference laboratories. **Culture:** Not available except through research laboratories **Serologic tests:** IFA is sensitive using either *R. felis* or other spotted fever or typhus group rickettsial antigens but is low during the acute phase of illness. A fourfold increase in titer is generally considered most specific; diagnostic titers have not been established. *R. felis*-specific testing can be obtained in reference or public health laboratories.
Rickettsia prowazekii	**Microscopy:** Not available. **Antigen tests:** Not available. **Molecular tests:** PCR amplification performed on EDTA-anticoagulated blood, buffy coat leukocytes, plasma, or tissue samples obtained during acute phase of illness; available only through reference laboratories. **Culture:** Heparin-anticoagulated blood plasma or buffy coat cells are inoculated into shell vials seeded with cell lines such as Vero, L-929, HEL, or MRC-5. Infected cells are detected by Giemsa, Gimenez, or fluorescent antibody staining after 48 to 72 h. Sensitivity is not known. **Serologic tests:** IFA is sensitive using either *R. prowazekii* or *R. typhi* as antigen. A fourfold increase in titer is generally considered most specific, but single titers of ≥128 for IgG and ≥ 32 for IgM are considered diagnostically significant.
Rickettsia rickettsii	**Microscopy:** DFA or immunohistochemistry on skin biopsy specimen of rash is 70% sensitive and 100% specific. Antibodies are not commercially available. **Antigen tests:** Not available. **Molecular tests:** PCR amplification performed on EDTA-anticoagulated blood, buffy coat leukocytes, plasma, or tissue samples obtained during acute phase of illness; available only through reference laboratories. **Culture:** Heparin-anticoagulated blood plasma or buffy coat cells are inoculated into shell vials seeded with cell lines such as Vero, L-929, HEL, or MRC-5. Infected cells are detected by Giemsa, Gimenez, or fluorescent antibody staining after 48 to 72 h. Sensitivity is not known. **Serologic tests:** IFA is sensitive using *R. rickettsii* or other spotted fever group rickettsial antigens (for example), but is low during the acute phase of illness. A fourfold increase in titer is generally considered most specific, but single titers of ≥128 for IgG and ≥32 for IgM are considered diagnostically significant.
Rickettsia typhi	**Microscopy:** DFA or immunohistochemistry on skin biopsy specimen of rash is sensitive and specific. Antibodies are not commercially available. **Antigen tests:** Not available. **Molecular tests:** PCR amplification performed on EDTA-anticoagulated blood, buffy coat leukocytes, plasma, or tissue samples obtained during acute phase of illness; available only through reference laboratories. **Culture:** Heparin-anticoagulated blood plasma or buffy coat cells are inoculated into shell vials seeded with cell lines such as Vero, L-929, HEL, or MRC-5. Infected cells are detected by Giemsa, Gimenez, or fluorescent antibody staining after 48 to 72 h. Sensitivity is not known. **Serologic tests:** IFA is sensitive using either *R. prowazekii* or *R. typhi* as antigen. A fourfold increase in titer is generally considered most specific, but single titers of ≥128 for IgG and ≥32 for IgM are considered diagnostically significant. A Dot EIA that is modestly less sensitive and specific is available for *R. typhi*.
Tropheryma whipplei	**Microscopy:** Tissue biopsy with periodic acid-Schiff stain or immunohistochemistry; electron microscopy. **Antigen tests:** None available. **Molecular tests:** PCR tests are currently the preferred method for specific diagnosis; performed on fresh, frozen, or paraffin-embedded small intestinal biopsy specimens, cardiac valve tissues, lymph nodes, liver, synovium, CNS samples. Available through reference laboratories. **Culture:** Blood, small intestine tissue, cardiac valves, CSF, aqueous humor, and synovial fluid can be inoculated onto HEL or MRC5 cell lines. Sensitivity of culture is not known, and at least 30 days are required before detection. **Serologic tests:** Not currently useful.

(Continued on next page)

TABLE 2 *(Continued)*

Organism	Diagnostic test[a]
Ureaplasma urealyticum	**Microscopy:** May be detected in body fluids using DNA fluorochrome stains (Hoechst 33258 or acridine orange), but these are not specific. **Antigen tests:** None commercially available. **Molecular tests:** PCR tests have been developed but are less useful than culture. **Culture:** Organisms are isolated from a variety of clinical samples. Dacron or polyester swabs are preferred; wood-shafted cotton swabs should be avoided. Ureaplasmas are extremely labile, and appropriate transport medium should be used. Can be recovered on Shepard's 10B urea broth and A8 urea agar. Growth occurs within 2 to 4 days. **Serologic tests:** Not recommended for routine use.

[a]Abbreviations: CF, complement fixation; CNS, central nervous system; CSF, cerebrospinal fluid; DFA, direct fluorescent antibody; EIA, enzyme immunoassay; IFA, indirect fluorescent antibody; Ig, immunoglobulin; MIF, microimmunofluorescence; NAAT, nucleic acid amplification tests; LPS, lipopolysaccharide.

Mycoplasma and *Ureaplasma*

KEN B. WAITES AND DAVID TAYLOR-ROBINSON

59

TAXONOMY

Bacteria commonly referred to as mycoplasmas ("fungus form") are included within the class *Mollicutes* ("soft skin"), which comprises 4 orders, 5 families, 8 genera, and more than 200 known species, as shown in Table 1. Table 2 lists 16 species isolated from humans on multiple occasions. This list excludes species of animal origin that are generally considered transient colonizers and that are detected occasionally in humans. Mollicutes are believed to have evolved from clostridium-like gram-positive cells by gene deletion. The availability of species-specific PCR technology is ameliorating difficulties of both culture and identification for fastidious mollicutes. Therefore, additional species are likely to be discovered.

DESCRIPTION OF *MOLLICUTES*

Mollicutes are smaller than conventional bacteria in cellular dimensions as well as genome size, making them the smallest free-living organisms known. Mycoplasmas associated with humans range from coccoid cells of about 0.2 to 0.3 µm in diameter, as in *Ureaplasma* spp. and *Mycoplasma hominis* (112), to tapered rods 1 to 2 µm in length and 0.1 to 0.2 µm in width, as in the case of *Mycoplasma pneumoniae* (152). Mollicutes are contained by a trilayered cell membrane and do not possess a cell wall. The permanent lack of a cell wall barrier makes the mollicutes unique among prokaryotes and differentiates them from bacterial L forms for which the lack of the cell wall is but a temporary reflection of environmental conditions. Lack of a cell wall also renders the mollicutes insensitive to the activity of beta-lactam antimicrobials, prevents them from staining by the Gram reaction, and is largely responsible for their pleomorphic form. The extremely small genome (<600 kb in the case of *Mycoplasma genitalium*) and limited biosynthetic capabilities explain the parasitic or saprophytic existence of these organisms, their sensitivity to environmental conditions, and their fastidious growth requirements which can complicate cultural detection. Mollicutes require enriched growth medium supplemented with nucleic acid precursors. Except for acholeplasmas, asteroleplasmas, and mesoplasmas, mollicutes require sterols in growth media, supplied by the addition of serum. Growth rates in culture medium vary among individual species, with generation times of approximately 1 hour for *Ureaplasma* spp., 6 hours for M. *pneumoniae*, and 16 hours for M. *genitalium* (68).

Typical mycoplasmal colonies vary from 15 to 300 µm in diameter. Colonies of some species, such as M. *hominis*, often exhibit a "fried egg" appearance owing to the contrast between deeper growth in the center of the colony, with more shallow growth at the periphery (Fig. 1). Other species, such as M. *pneumoniae*, produce spherical colonies (Fig. 2). Whereas colonies of mycoplasmal species may be observed with the naked eye, those produced by ureaplasmas are typically 15 to 60 µm in diameter and require low-power microscopic magnification for visualization (Fig. 3).

Mycoplasmas of human origin can be classified according to whether they ferment glucose, utilize arginine, or hydrolyze urea (Table 2). Except for hydrolysis of urea, which is unique for ureaplasmas, these biochemical features are not sufficient for species distinction. Anaeroplasmas and asteroleplasmas, which occur in ruminants, are strictly anaerobic, while most other mollicutes are facultative anaerobes.

Attachment of M. *pneumoniae* to host cells in the respiratory tract of humans is a prerequisite for colonization and infection. Cytadherence, mediated by the P1 adhesin and other accessory proteins, described in detail in recent reviews (139, 147), is followed by induction of chronic inflammation and cytotoxicity mediated by hydrogen peroxide, which also acts as a hemolysin. M. *pneumoniae* stimulates B and T lymphocytes and induces formation of autoantibodies which react with a variety of host tissues and the I antigen on erythrocytes, which is responsible for production of cold agglutinins (147). Recently, an ADP-ribosylating toxin with significant sequence homology to the pertussis toxin S1 subunit, now known as the community-acquired respiratory distress syndrome toxin that causes vacuolation and ciliostasis in cultured host cells, was described in M. *pneumoniae* (74). M. *genitalium* also possesses a terminal structure, the MgPa adhesin, which facilitates its attachment to epithelial cells (60). Factors involved with *Ureaplasma* and M. *hominis* attachment have not been characterized to the same extent as for M. *pneumoniae*, and these mycoplasmas do not have prominent attachment organelles. Henrich et al. (58) demonstrated the presence of the variable adherence-associated antigen that is believed to be a major adhesin of M. *hominis* and could also assist in evasion of host immune responses through antigenic variation. Ureaplasmas also attach to a variety of cell types, mediated by adhesin proteins expressed on the surface of the bacterial cell. The multiple-banded

TABLE 1 Classification and some distinguishing features of mollicutes

Classification of the class *Mollicutes*	Distinguishing features			
	Sterol required	Genome size (kbp)	G+C content of DNA (mol%)	Other
Order I: *Mycoplasmatales*				Human/animal hosts
Family I: *Mycoplasmataceae*				
Genus I: *Mycoplasma* (130 species)[a]	Yes	580–1,350	23–40	
Genus II: *Ureaplasma* (7 species)[b]	Yes	730–1,170	25–32	Hydrolyze urea
Order II: *Entomoplasmatales*				Plant/insect hosts
Family I: *Entomoplasmataceae*				Nonhelical structure
Genus I: *Entomoplasma* (6 species)	Yes	870–900	27–34	
Genus II: *Mesoplasma* (11 species)	No	825–930	26–32	
Family II: *Spiroplasmataceae*				Helical structure
Genus I: *Spiroplasma* (34 species)	Yes/No	780–2,200	24–31	
Order III: *Acholeplasmatales*[c]				Animal/plant hosts
Family I: *Acholeplasmataceae*				
Genus I: *Acholeplasma* (15 species)	No	1,500–1,650	26–36	
Order IV: *Anaeroplasmatales*				Animal hosts
Family I: *Anaeroplasmataceae*				Obligate anaerobes
Genus I: *Anaeroplasma* (4 species)	Yes	1,500–1,600	29–33	
Genus II: *Asteroleplasma* (1 species)	No	1,500	40	
"*Candidatus* Phytoplasma"[c] (26 species)	Unknown	530–1,350	23–29	Noncultivable

[a]The total number includes subspecies. The genus *Mycoplasma* also includes four species not validly published and nine "*Candidatus*" species of cell wall-less uncultivated parasitic bacteria, eight of which attach to the surface of erythrocytes and may also occur free in the plasma, plus one pneumotrophic "*Candidatus*" species. Some were previously classified in the genera *Haemobartonella* and *Eperythrozoon*. Their G+C contents and sterol requirements are unknown.
[b]*U. urealyticum* and *U. parvum*, formerly considered biovars of *U. urealyticum*, are now classified as two separate species and are the only ureaplasmas of human origin.
[c]Phytoplasmas are "*Candidatus*" species of uncultivable mollicutes of plants and insects genetically related to the *Acholeplasmatales*.

(MB) antigen contains serotype-specific and cross-reactive epitopes and is a prominent antigen recognized during human ureaplasmal infections (146). Ureaplasmas also produce immunoglobulin A (IgA) protease and release ammonia through urealytic activity (146).

EPIDEMIOLOGY AND TRANSMISSION

Mollicutes are common in practically all mammalian species as well as many other vertebrates in which they have been sought. Although most mollicutes have species-specific host-organism associations, some mycoplasmas and acholeplasmas

TABLE 2 Primary sites of colonization, metabolism, and pathogenicity of mollicutes of human origin[a]

Species	Primary site of colonization		Metabolism of:		Pathogenicity
	Respiratory tract	Genitourinary tract	Glucose	Arginine	
M. *salivarium*	+	−	−	+	−
M. *orale*	+	−	−	+	−
M. *buccale*	+	−	−	+	−
M. *faucium*	+	−	−	+	−
M. *lipophilum*	+	−	−	+	−
M. *amphoriforme*[b]	?+	−	+	−	?
M. *pneumoniae*	+	−	+	−	+
M. *hominis*	+	+	−	+	+
M. *genitalium*[c]	?+	+	+	−	+
M. *fermentans*	+	+	+	+	+
M. *primatum*	−	+	−	+	−
M. *spermatophilum*	−	+	−	+	−
M. *pirum*	?	?	+	+	−
M. *penetrans*	−	+	+	+	?
Ureaplasma spp.[d]	+	+	−	−	+
Acholeplasma laidlawii	+	−	+	−	−

[a]Symbols: +, positive for trait; −, negative for trait; ?, unknown.
[b]All isolates reported to date have been from the lower respiratory tract, but no other sites have been sampled.
[c]The organism has been found in the oropharynx, but it seems unlikely that this is a common or primary location.
[d]These species metabolize urea.

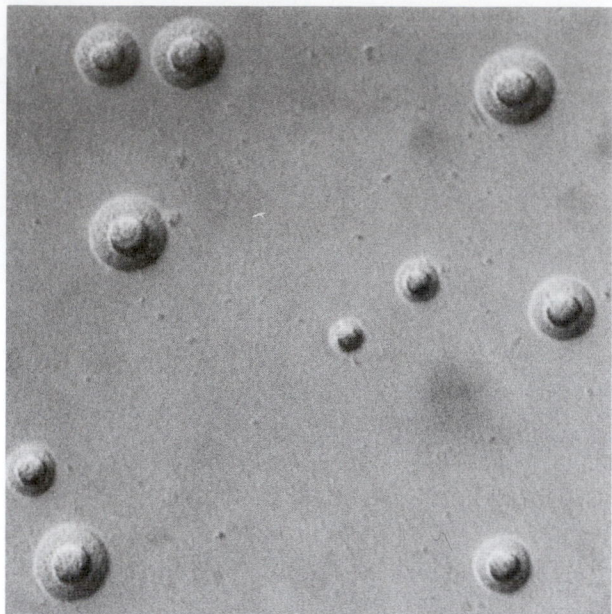

FIGURE 1 Fried-egg-type colonies of *Mycoplasma hominis* of up to 110 µm in diameter growing on A8 agar. Magnification, ×132.

of animal origin occur in a wide variety of different hosts. Mollicutes in the genera *Spiroplasma*, *Mesoplasma*, *Entomoplasma*, and *Acholeplasma* can be isolated from insects and plants.

In humans, mycoplasmas and ureaplasmas are associated with the mucosa, residing predominantly in the respiratory or urogenital tract, rarely penetrating the submucosa, except in cases of immunosuppression or instrumentation, when they may invade the bloodstream and disseminate to various organs and tissues. Many *Mycoplasma* spp. exist as commensals in the oropharynx (Table 2) and are associated with invasive disease only in very rare circumstances. Oral commensal mycoplasmas may occasionally spread to the lower respiratory tract but should not cause diagnostic confusion with *M. pneumoniae* if appropriate means of organism identification are employed. *Mycoplasma fermentans* has been detected in various body sites, including the urogenital tract, throat, lower respiratory tract, and other body locations, including joints (146), but

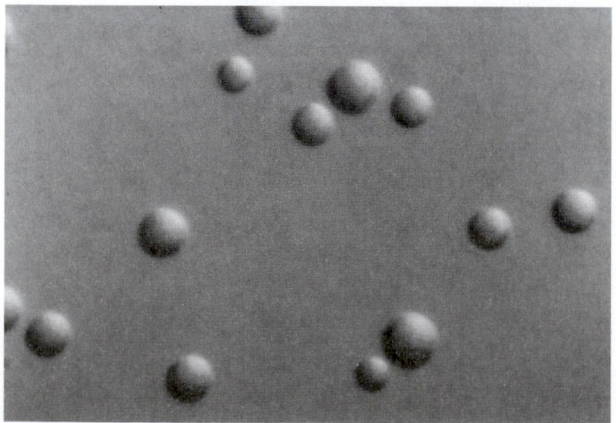

FIGURE 2 Spherical colonies of *Mycoplasma pneumoniae* of up to 100 µm in diameter growing on SP4 agar. Magnification, ×126.

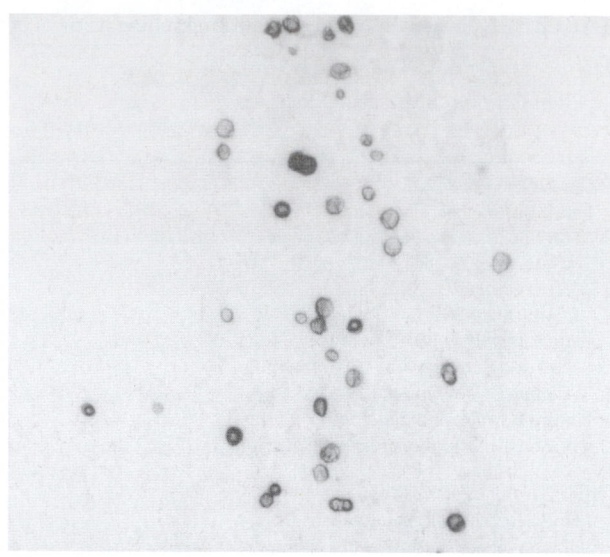

FIGURE 3 Granular, brown, urease-positive colonies of *Ureaplasma* species, 15 to 60 µm in diameter, from a vaginal specimen growing on A8 agar. Magnification, ×100.

its primary site of colonization and true disease potential are incompletely understood. The frequent occurrence of pathogenic species such as *M. hominis* and ureaplasmas in the lower urogenital tract in healthy men and women has complicated understanding of their disease-producing capabilities. *Mycoplasma primatum* and *Mycoplasma spermatophilum* have been detected in the urogenital tract but have not been associated with disease. PCR assays have demonstrated the frequent occurrence of *M. genitalium* in the urogenital tract in men with urethritis and in the lower and upper genital tract sites in women and of *Mycoplasma penetrans* in the urine of homosexual males with human immunodeficiency virus (64, 84). Although mycoplasmas are generally considered extracellular organisms, intracellular localization is now appreciated for *M. fermentans*, *M. penetrans*, *M. genitalium*, and *M. pneumoniae* (11, 33, 139, 147). Intracellular localization may be responsible for protecting the organisms from antibodies and antibiotics as well as contributing to disease chronicity and difficulty in cultivation in some cases. Variation in surface antigens of *M. hominis* and *Ureaplasma* spp. may be related to persistence of these organisms at invasive sites. In humans, mycoplasmas and ureaplasmas may be transmitted by direct contact between hosts, i.e., venereally through genital-genital or oral-genital contact, vertically from mother to offspring either at birth or in utero, by respiratory aerosols or fomites in the case of *M. pneumoniae*, or even by nosocomial acquisition through transplanted tissues.

CLINICAL SIGNIFICANCE

Respiratory Infections

M. pneumoniae causes approximately 20% of all community-acquired pneumonias in the general population and up to 50% of pneumonias in certain confined groups (139, 147). Although *M. pneumoniae* has long been associated with pneumonias in school-aged children, adolescents, and young adults, in recent years this organism was also shown to occur endemically and occasionally epidemically in older persons, as well as in children under 5 years of age (147).

The most typical clinical syndrome is tracheobronchitis, often accompanied by upper respiratory tract manifestations, such as acute pharyngitis. Pneumonia develops in about one-third of persons who are infected. The incubation period is generally 2 to 3 weeks, and spread throughout households is common. The organism can persist in the respiratory tract for several months after initial infection and sometimes for years in hypogammaglobulinemic patients, possibly because it attaches strongly to and invades epithelial cells. Disease tends not to be seasonal, subclinical infections are common, and the disease is ordinarily mild. However, severe infections requiring hospitalization and even death are known to occur (147).

Extrapulmonary complications of M. pneumoniae infections may include meningoencephalitis, ascending paralysis, transverse myelitis, Bell's palsy, possibly some cases of involuntary movements, pericarditis, hemolytic anemia, arthritis, nephritis, and mucocutaneous lesions (123, 139, 147). An autoimmune response is thought to play a role in some extrapulmonary complications. However, M. pneumoniae has been isolated directly from cerebrospinal, pericardial, and synovial fluids as well as other extrapulmonary sites, and additional evidence of direct invasion by this organism has been documented by the use of the PCR assay (123). Clinical manifestations are not sufficiently unique to allow differentiation from infections caused by other common bacteria, particularly Chlamydophila pneumoniae. Data from animal models as well as clinical studies suggest a role for M. pneumoniae and C. pneumoniae as etiologic or exacerbating factors in bronchial asthma (94, 138), and additional clinical studies linked these microorganisms to stable as well as exacerbating disease (56, 72).

M. fermentans has been recovered from the throats of children with pneumonia, some of whom had no other etiologic agent identified, but the frequency of its occurrence in healthy children is not known (128). It has been detected in adults with an acute influenza-like illness (86) and in bronchoalveolar lavage specimens, peripheral blood lymphocytes, and bone marrow from patients with AIDS and respiratory disease (3, 4). Respiratory infection with M. fermentans is not necessarily linked with immunodeficiency, but it may also behave as an opportunistic pathogen.

Very little is known about Mycoplasma amphoriforme beyond what has been described in the initial reports of its detection in the lower respiratory tract by culture and/or PCR in a series of patients with antibody deficiency and chronic bronchitis or bronchiectasis (151). Its biochemical reactivity, colonial appearance, growth characteristics, and gliding motility (57) are similar to these features of M. pneumoniae, but it is distinct genetically. Repeated isolations over time and clinical improvement after antimicrobial therapy which resulted in the elimination of the mycoplasma suggest a possible pathogenic role, but more work must be done to determine the extent of disease that may be due to this organism.

Genitourinary Infections

Following puberty, Ureaplasma spp. and M. hominis can be isolated from the lower genital tract in many healthy sexually active adults, but there is evidence that these organisms play etiologic roles in some genital tract diseases. Results of human and animal inoculation studies and observations of immunocompromised persons are supportive of ureaplasmas being a cause of nonchlamydial, nongonococcal urethritis (NGU) in men, with further evidence supplied by therapeutic and serologic studies (128). Since identification of two distinct biovars of Ureaplasma urealyticum, now considered separate species, biovar 2 (U. urealyticum) has been

implicated in NGU, whereas biovar 1 (Ureaplasma parvum) has not been implicated in this manner according to some investigators (38), although doubt about this species specificity in association with NGU has been raised by others (19). Evidence that M. hominis causes NGU is lacking. M. genitalium has been detected by PCR technology significantly more often in urethral specimens from men with acute NGU than from those without urethritis and is now considered to be one of the causes of the disease (63, 64, 127). M. genitalium-positive men have been found to have symptomatic urethritis significantly more often than those infected with Chlamydia trachomatis (53). Antibody responses have been detected in some men with acute disease, and this mycoplasma has also produced urethritis in nonhuman primates (127). M. genitalium also could be a rare cause of conjunctivitis associated with urethritis (16). M. fermentans, M. penetrans, and Mycoplasma pirum were not detected in the urethras of men with urethritis by PCR assays, suggesting that these organisms are unlikely to have a pathogenic role in this condition (36). In women, there is no evidence that M. hominis is a cause of the urethral syndrome, but ureaplasmas may be involved (121).

M. hominis and Ureaplasma spp. have not been detected by culture of prostatic biopsy samples from patients with chronic abacterial prostatitis (39), and M. genitalium has been found rarely by using a PCR assay (80). In contrast, ureaplasmas have been recovered in an epididymal aspirate from a patient suffering with nonchlamydial, nongonococcal acute epididymo-orchitis accompanied by a specific antibody response (62) and may be an infrequent cause of this disease. Ureaplasma spp. produce urease and induce crystallization of struvite and calcium phosphates in urine in vitro and calculi in animal models (55, 137). They have been found in urinary calculi of patients with infection-type stones more frequently than those with metabolic-type stones (55). M. hominis has been isolated from the upper urinary tract only in patients with symptoms of acute pyelonephritis, often with an antibody response, and may cause about 5% of cases of this disease (133). Obstruction or instrumentation of the urinary tract may be predisposing factors. Ureaplasmas have not been associated in the same way.

Mollicutes do not cause vaginitis but are among various microorganisms that proliferate in patients with bacterial vaginosis (BV). Some studies suggest that M. hominis may contribute independently to BV, but evidence is lacking for an independent association of ureaplasmas with BV (146). BV may lead to pelvic inflammatory disease, and M. hominis has been isolated from the endometrium and fallopian tubes of about 10% of women with salpingitis accompanied by a specific antibody response (137). Serological evidence suggests that M. hominis could be an independent factor in tubal factor infertility (7). Ureaplasma spp. have been isolated directly from affected fallopian tubes but not alone. This latter observation, together with the negative results of serologic tests, animal models, and fallopian tube organ cultures (128), does not support a causal relationship for ureaplasmas in pelvic inflammatory disease. M. genitalium, however, may play a role, as indicated by its significant association with cervicitis (52) and endometritis (30). In addition, there is serologic evidence that M. genitalium causes some cases of tubal infertility (28). That ureaplasmas might cause infertility still remains speculative (126).

Ureaplasmas have been isolated from the internal organs of spontaneously aborted fetuses and from stillborn and premature infants more often than from induced abortions or normal full-term infants (146). The results from some serologic and therapeutic studies have also supported a role for these organisms in fetal morbidity (25). BV is a possible confounding factor which must be considered in the association between ureaplasmas in the chorioamnion and low birth weight. Ureaplasmas at this site are directly associated with inflammation (51) and may invade the amniotic sac early in pregnancy in the presence of intact fetal membranes, causing persistent infection and adverse pregnancy outcome (23, 129).

The notion that *M. hominis* causes fever in some women after abortion, or after normal delivery, is based on its isolation from the blood of about 10% of such women but not from afebrile women who had abortions or from healthy pregnant women (127). In addition, antibody responses have been detected in about half of febrile aborting women but in few of those who remain afebrile (127). Similar observations have been made for the isolation of *Ureaplasma* spp. which may be responsible for some cases of postpartum endometritis (26). The ability of *U. parvum* and *M. hominis* to upregulate amniotic fluid leukocytes, proinflammatory cytokines, prostaglandins, metalloproteinases and uterine activity to induce chorioamnionitis, a systemic fetal inflammatory response, and contribute to preterm labor and fetal lung injury is supported by experimental studies in rhesus monkeys (100). There are conflicting opinions about the importance of *U. urealyticum* as opposed to *U. parvum* in premature delivery, a situation that needs to be resolved (146). There is no evidence that *M. genitalium* is a cause of preterm labor or abortion (87, 101).

Neonatal Infections

Colonization of infants by genital mycoplasmas may occur by ascension from the lower genital tract of the mother at the time of delivery or in utero earlier in gestation and may be transient and without sequelae. The rate of vertical transmission may be 18 to 55% among infants born to colonized mothers (146). *Ureaplasma* spp. and *M. hominis* may be isolated from neonates born to mothers with intact membranes and delivered by cesarean section (146). Congenital pneumonia, bacteremia, progression to chronic lung disease of prematurity with the development of inflammatory cytokines in tracheal aspirates, and even death have occurred in very-low-birth-weight infants due to ureaplasmal infection of the lower respiratory tract (118, 146). A meta-analysis of the literature accumulated since the 1980s supports the association of ureaplasmal infection with development of chronic lung disease, but so far there has been no evidence of a reduction in the incidence of chronic lung disease or death when preterm infants have been treated with erythromycin (118). Both *M. hominis* and *Ureaplasma* spp. have been isolated from maternal and umbilical cord blood as well as the blood of neonates. Both species can also invade the cerebrospinal fluid of neonates (146). Either mild, subclinical meningitis without sequelae or neurological damage with permanent handicaps may ensue. Colonization of healthy full-term infants declines after 3 months of age, and fewer than 10% of older children and sexually inexperienced adults are colonized with genital mycoplasmas (146). Vertical transmission of *M. genitalium* from mother to neonate has been reported (88), but its significance in neonates is unknown.

Routine screening of neonates for genital mycoplasmas is not clinically justified based on the available evidence that many healthy neonates may be colonized without consequence. However, if there is clinical, radiological, or laboratory evidence of pneumonia, meningitis, or overall instability, particularly in preterm neonates in whom there are no obvious alternative etiologies, infection with *M. hominis* or *Ureaplasma* spp. should be considered.

Systemic Infections and Immunosuppressed Hosts

Extrapulmonary and extragenital mycoplasmal infections probably occur more often than currently recognized. *M. hominis* is alone among pathogenic mycoplasmas of human origin which may occasionally be detected in routine bacteriologic cultures, so there have been many instances of accidental discovery when mycoplasmas were not specifically sought. The number of published case reports implicating *Mycoplasma* and *Ureaplasma* species in a variety of systemic infections involving persons with and without impaired host defenses has increased in recent years as a result of a more widespread utilization of universal PCR primers when infection is suspected and no conventional microbes are detected by culture. Mollicutes can cause invasive disease of the joints as a result of dissemination from the genital or respiratory tracts in immunosuppressed persons, especially individuals with hypogammaglobulinemia (137). *M. hominis* bacteremia has been demonstrated after renal transplantation (114), trauma, and genitourinary manipulations and also in brain abscesses, osteomyelitis lesions (95), and wound infections (128). Numerous mycoplasmal species, including *M. fermentans, U. urealyticum,* and *Mycoplasma salivarium,* have been detected by culture and/or PCR in synovial fluid of persons with various arthritides, although the precise contribution of these organisms to these disease conditions is still uncertain (71, 116, 117). The significance of *M. fermentans* and other mycoplasmas in persons with AIDS and as possible agents of Gulf War syndrome has received a great deal of attention. However, there is no credible evidence supporting an association or causal role in either condition (136).

COLLECTION, TRANSPORT, AND STORAGE OF SPECIMENS

Specimen Type and Collection

Body fluids appropriate for mycoplasmal culture or detection by noncultural methods include blood, synovial fluid, amniotic fluid, cerebrospinal fluid, urine, prostatic secretions, semen, wound aspirates, sputum, pleural fluid, bronchoalveolar lavage fluid, or other tracheobronchial secretions, depending on the clinical condition and organisms of interest. Swabs from the nasopharynx, throat, cervix/vagina, wounds, and urethra are also acceptable. Tissue from biopsy or autopsy, including placenta, endometrium, bone chips, and urinary calculi can also be used. When swabs are used, care must be taken to sample the desired site vigorously to obtain as many cells as possible, since mycoplasmas are cell associated. Urine specimens may sometimes prove more sensitive than urethral swabs for detection of fastidious mycoplasmas such as *M. genitalium* by PCR (65). If determination of the localization of mycoplasmas in the genitourinary tract is desired, urine specimens can be obtained at various stages during urination or after prostatic massage. Care should be taken to avoid collection of specimens that are contaminated by lubricants or antiseptics commonly used in gynecologic practice. Dacron or polyester swabs with aluminum or plastic shafts are preferred. Wooden shaft cotton swabs should be avoided because of potential inhibitory effects. Swabs should always be removed from specimens before transportation to the laboratory.

Successful isolation of mycoplasmas from blood can be achieved by inoculating blood, free of anticoagulant, into liquid mycoplasmal growth media at the bedside in a 1:5 to 1:10 ratio, using as much blood as possible (at least 10 ml is desirable for adults). Mycoplasmas are inhibited by sodium polyanethol sulfonate, the anticoagulant used in most commercial blood culture media, but the inhibitory effect can be overcome by addition of gelatin (1% [wt/vol]) (108). Use of commercial blood culture media with or without automated blood culture instruments is not recommended for detection of mycoplasmas. None of the newer continuously monitored automated blood culture systems will flag bottles containing M. *hominis*, even when additional metabolic substrate and gelatin are added. The organism may survive in these media for several days, however (141).

Transport and Storage

Mycoplasmas are extremely sensitive to adverse environmental conditions, particularly drying and heat. Specimens should be inoculated at bedside whenever possible, using appropriate transport and/or culture media. Specific mycoplasma media such as SP4 or Shepard's 10B broth or 2 SP (10% heat-inactivated fetal calf serum with 0.2 M sucrose in 0.02 M phosphate buffer, pH 7.2) are acceptable transport media. Other media available commercially for transport and storage of specimens are Stuart's medium, Trypticase soy broth with 0.5% bovine serum albumin, and Mycotrans (Irvine Scientific, Irvine, CA). A3B broth (Remel, Inc.) is available as a transport medium, whereas Remel arginine broth, 10B, and SP4 transport broths also serve as growth media. Liquid specimens do not require special transport media if cultures can be inoculated within 1 hour, provided the specimens are protected from evaporation. Tissues can be placed in a sterile container which can be tightly closed and delivered to the laboratory immediately. Otherwise, tissue specimens should be placed in transport media if delay in culture inoculation is anticipated. Specimens should be refrigerated if immediate transportation to the laboratory is not possible. If specimens must be shipped and/or if the storage time is likely to exceed 24 h prior to processing, the specimen in transport medium should be frozen at −80°C to prevent loss of viability and to minimize bacterial overgrowth. Mollicutes can be stored for long periods in appropriate growth or transport media at −80°C or in liquid nitrogen. Frozen specimens can be shipped with dry ice to a reference laboratory if necessary. Storage at −20°C is deleterious to detection, even by non-culture methods. When frozen specimens are to be examined, they should be thawed rapidly in a water bath at 37°C.

DIRECT EXAMINATION

Microscopy

Lack of a cell wall precludes visualization of mycoplasmas by Gram staining, but this procedure may prove useful to exclude contaminating bacteria. A DNA fluorochrome stain such as Hoechst 33258 (ICN Biomedicals, Costa Mesa, CA) or acridine orange stain may be useful to assist in organism visualization when applied to body fluids such as amniotic fluid after cytocentrifugation, but it is not specific for mycoplasmas.

Antigen Detection

Rapid methods for antigenic detection of M. *pneumoniae* were developed in the 1980s, but these techniques were hampered by low sensitivity and cross-reactivity with other commensal mycoplasmas. This approach for rapid diagnosis has now been abandoned in favor of nucleic acid amplification methods.

Nucleic Acid Detection Techniques

PCR systems have been developed for all of the clinically important *Mycoplasma* and *Ureaplasma* species that infect humans. The advantages they have over culture and serology include the ability to complete the procedure in 1 day, utilizing a single specimen containing organisms that do not have to be viable, as well as the ability to detect nucleic acid in preserved tissues.

Some examples of gene targets used in PCR assays include 16S rRNA (65, 73, 90, 104, 117, 157); other repetitive sequences such as the insertion-like elements of M. *fermentans* and repMp1 of M. *pneumoniae* (47, 150); the P1 adhesin (34, 69, 110), ATPase operon (15), and *tuf* genes of M. *pneumoniae* (89); *gap* in M. *hominis* (8); and the MgPa adhesin (34, 70) and *gyrA* genes (18) of M. *genitalium*. Urease genes (17, 157) and the MB antigen gene (78, 107) have been used as targets in *Ureaplasma* spp. Real-time PCR assays have been described for M. *pneumoniae* (93), M. *genitalium* (66, 73, 120), M. *hominis* (8), and *Ureaplasma* spp. (92). Advantages of real-time PCR assays include more rapid turnaround time, less handling of PCR product, and improved diagnostic sensitivity. For slowly growing organisms, such as M. *pneumoniae*, and especially for extremely fastidious species for which optimum cultivation techniques are not established, such as M. *genitalium* and M. *fermentans*, the use of PCR assays may be the only practical means of detecting their presence in clinical specimens. The sensitivity of PCR is very high, theoretically corresponding to a single organism when purified DNA is used.

Comparison of the PCR technique with culture and/or serology, in the case of M. *pneumoniae*, has yielded varied results that are not always in agreement. Positive PCR results in culture-negative persons without evidence of respiratory disease suggest inadequate assay specificity, persistence of the organism after infection, or its existence in asymptomatic carriers. Positive PCR results in serologically negative persons may be due to an inadequate immune response or from the collection of specimens before specific antibody synthesis could occur. Negative PCR results in culture or serologically proven infections raises the possibility of inhibitors or other technical problems with the assay. Use of a second PCR assay with a different gene target may help interpret results and resolve such discrepancies. This is particularly important in the setting of a positive PCR assay when culture and/or serology is negative. If mycoplasmacidal antibiotics have been administered, PCR results may be negative even though serology is positive. There is some evidence suggesting that PCR inhibition may occur more commonly with nasopharyngeal specimens than throat swabs being assayed for M. *pneumoniae* (42, 111). Commercial reagents available for purification of nucleic acid can be helpful in overcoming PCR inhibition.

Multiplex PCR assays have been developed to detect M. *pneumoniae* and other respiratory pathogens (110). Assays to detect M. *genitalium* and other urogenital pathogens (91) have also been described. A PCR-microtiter plate hybridization assay (158) and a microwell-plate-based PCR assay have been developed for large-scale screening for M. *genitalium* (48). Strong associations between serology and PCR for M. *genitalium* have been described (149), but the analytical sensitivity of a single PCR assay for M. *genitalium* was questioned by Baseman et al. (10), who reported that 61% of culture-positive women tested negative by PCR, despite apparently good quality control parameters for their assay. Assuming culture positivity was not due to cross-contamination, this highlights the fact that reduced sensitivity of a single PCR assay may be related to quality of the specimen or presence of inhibitors.

PCR technology is less valuable for routine diagnostic purposes in the case of the more rapidly growing and relatively easily cultivable organisms, such as M. hominis and Ureaplasma spp., but this method can be valuable in clinical studies of ureaplasmal infections. The newest PCR-based techniques permit identification and differentiation of U. urealyticum versus U. parvum (75, 78, 79, 92, 107). PCR is also a very good tool for identification of an unknown mycoplasma previously obtained by culture.

PCR is now the diagnostic method of choice for detection of M. pneumoniae infection in laboratories that can develop their own assays, but no complete PCR diagnostic kits are sold commercially for diagnostic use in the United States. However, several complete PCR assays are sold commercially in various European countries. Recent comparisons to in-house techniques were generally favorable (46, 134).

ISOLATION PROCEDURES

Biosafety Considerations
M. pneumoniae, M. hominis, and ureaplasmas are considered category 2 pathogens. Work with these microorganisms and other mycoplasmas of human origin can be safely undertaken on the laboratory bench and/or in a class 2 safety cabinet.

Growth Media and Inoculation
Growth of mycoplasmas pathogenic for humans requires the presence of serum, growth factors such as yeast extract, and a metabolic substrate. No single formulation is ideal for all species due to different properties, optimum pH, and substrate requirements. SP4 broth and agar (pH 7.5) are the best media overall and can be used for both M. pneumoniae and M. hominis, provided arginine is added for the latter. Shepard's 10B broth (pH 6.0) can be used for M. hominis and Ureaplasma spp., with A8 as the corresponding solid medium. Penicillin G should be added to minimize bacterial overgrowth. The addition of a pH indicator, such as phenol red, is important for detection because mycoplasmas usually do not produce turbidity in broth culture owing to their small cell size. Media formulations are provided elsewhere (140).

For self-prepared media, quality control is crucial for each of the main components. These controls must consist of the quantitative growth of a mycoplasma strain(s) in two media that differ only in the component to be tested. New lots or batches of broth are satisfactory if the numbers of organisms that grow are within one 10-fold dilution of the reference batch. Agar plates should ideally support growth of at least 90% of the colonies that are supported by the reference media. The sterility of commercially purchased media components, such as horse serum, must be confirmed prior to their use. Quality control test organisms should include type strains and low-passage clinical isolates of the species of interest. When testing ureaplasmas, it is recommended to include at least one serovar representative from each of the two species. Testing inhibitory properties of media against growth of various other organisms likely present in specimens from nonsterile sites may also be worthwhile to prevent loss of mycoplasmas due to overgrowth of contaminating organisms.

Specimens should always be mixed well before inoculating media, fluids should be centrifuged (600 × g for 15 min), and the pellet should be inoculated. Urine can be filtered through a 0.45-μm-pore-size filter if bacterial contamination is suspected. Furthermore, it is wise to mince, not grind, tissues in broth prior to dilution. Serial dilution of specimens in broth to at least 10^{-3}, with subculture of each dilution onto agar, is an extremely important step in the cultivation process, since it will help overcome possible interference by antibiotics, antibodies, and other inhibitors, including bacteria that may be present in clinical specimens. Omission of this critical dilution step can be one reason why some laboratories have difficulty in recovering organisms. Dilution also helps to overcome the problem of rapid decline in culture viability, which is particularly common with ureaplasmas, and it also provides information about the number of organisms present.

Incubation Conditions and Subcultures
Broths should be incubated at 37°C under atmospheric conditions. Agar plates yield the best growth if they are incubated in an atmosphere of room air supplemented with 5 to 10% CO_2 or in an anaerobic environment of 95% N_2 plus 5% CO_2. The relatively rapid growth rates of M. hominis and Ureaplasma spp. make identification of most positive cultures possible within 2 to 4 days, whereas M. pneumoniae may require up to 3 weeks or longer. All broths that change color should be subcultured into a fresh tube of the corresponding broth (0.1 ml into 0.9 ml) and onto agar (0.02 ml). Subcultures of Ureaplasma spp. must be performed soon after the color change occurs because the culture can lose viability within a few hours. Subculture also increases the diagnostic yield, since some strains may not grow sufficiently from the original specimen inoculated initially onto solid media. Blind subculture periodically during incubation may improve the yield of M. pneumoniae, since a color change may not always be evident, even if growth occurs, but culture is still relatively insensitive for detection of this mycoplasma. Cultures should be incubated for at least 7 days before being designated negative for genital mycoplasmas and 4 weeks for M. pneumoniae. The growth rate of M. fermentans is similar to that of M. pneumoniae. However, for M. fermentans, M. genitalium, and mycoplasmas of human origin other than M. pneumoniae, M. hominis, or Ureaplasma spp., cultivation conditions are not well established.

Development of Colonies
Broth cultures for Ureaplasma spp. should be examined for color change resulting from hydrolysis of urea twice daily for up to 7 days because of the steep death phase of this organism in culture. This is less critical for Mycoplasma spp., for which once daily inspection of broth cultures is sufficient. Agar plates should be examined, using a stereomicroscope at a magnification of ×20 to 60, daily for Ureaplasma spp., at 1- to 3-day intervals for M. hominis, and every 3 to 5 days for M. pneumoniae and other slower-growing species. Ureaplasma colonies (Fig. 3) can be identified on A8 agar by urease production in the presence of $CaCl_2$ indicator contained in the medium. The larger M. hominis colonies are urease negative and often have the typical fried-egg appearance (Fig. 1). Other species, such as M. pneumoniae and M. genitalium, will produce much smaller spherical colonies which may or may not demonstrate the fried-egg appearance (Fig. 2). Methylene blue stain applied directly to the agar plate to turn the colonies blue is sometimes useful if there is uncertainty about whether or not mycoplasmal colonies are present. M. hominis is the only pathogenic mycoplasma of humans cultivable on bacteriological media such as chocolate agar or blood agar. However, the pinpoint translucent colonies are easily overlooked, and routine bacterial cultures may be discarded sooner than the time needed for M. hominis colonies to develop, which may be 4 days or more in some cases. Occurrence of suspicious colonies warrants subculture to appropriate mycoplasma media.

Commercial Media and Culture Kits

A variety of kits for detection, quantitation, identification, and antimicrobial susceptibility testing of *Ureaplasma* spp. and *M. hominis* from urogenital specimens are available in Europe. Some of these products, such as Mycoscreen Plus and Mycofast US (Wescor Inc., Logan, UT), are now being sold commercially in the United States along with older products such as Mycoscreen GU, Mycotrim GU agar, and the Mycotrim GU triphasic flask system (Irvine Scientific). A comparable system, Mycotrim RS, has been adapted for detection of *M. pneumoniae* in respiratory specimens. Remel, Inc., has developed several formulations of transport and growth media, including 10B broth, A7 agar, A8 agar, SP4 broth, and SP4 agar.

Some kits and other commercial products and media have been evaluated by independent investigators (1, 20, 27, 29, 106, 119, 154). Commercial products and kits may be of particular value if the need to detect mycoplasmas arises infrequently in laboratories which do not specialize in mycoplasma detection, but users should be aware of the potential limitations of existing products. If commercially prepared media are to be utilized, it is advisable that laboratories perform internal quality control tests.

IDENTIFICATION

Even though the numerous large-colony mycoplasmal species which may be isolated from humans cannot be identified based on colonial morphology or a particular biochemical profile, the body site of origin and rate of growth, in conjunction with biochemical features and colonial appearance, give some clues. Utilization of glucose by a mycoplasma in SP4 broth will produce an acidic shift (red to yellow), whereas utilization of arginine will produce a red to deeper red color change in this broth in the presence of the phenol red pH indicator. Urea or arginine hydrolysis in 10B broth causes an alkaline shift of orange to deep red. Thus, a slow-growing glycolytic organism from the respiratory tract that produces spherical colonies on SP4 agar after approximately 5 to 20 days of incubation is likely to be *M. pneumoniae*. An alkaline color change which occurs after overnight incubation without turbidity in 10B broth containing urea is almost certainly due to *Ureaplasma* spp., whereas a urogenital specimen that produces an alkaline reaction within 24 to 72 hours in broth supplemented with arginine is likely to contain *M. hominis*. Examination of colonial morphology is sufficient to identify *Ureaplasma* spp., and it is important to keep in mind that these organisms often coexist with *M. hominis* in urogenital specimens.

To identify a large-colony mycoplasma completely to species level, a number of different techniques are available, but PCR is now considered the best overall choice for species identification, since it is much simpler to perform than other methods and it does not require immunological reagents that are not readily available. The PCR assay is also less subjective to interpret than some of the older methods such as epi-immunofluorescence.

TYPING SYSTEMS

Several methods for typing mollicutes are described and used to study the epidemiology of *M. pneumoniae* and the differential pathogenicity for the two genomic clusters and 14 serotypes of *Ureaplasma* spp. Techniques used initially to serotype ureaplasmas from clinical specimens include monoclonal and polyclonal antibodies (49, 159), immunofluorescence (98), immunoperoxidase (109), and agar growth inhibition (130). Results of earlier studies have been varied and inconsistent due to the inefficient and imprecise methods available, occurrence of multiple cross-reactions, and the fact that many persons may harbor more than one serotype in their urogenital tract in the presence or absence of disease. Development of monoclonal antibodies enabled identification of MB antigens responsible for ureaplasma serotype specificity on the cell surface (159). PCR-based assays have enabled more accurate characterization of the two genomic clusters of *Ureaplasma* spp. that led to their designation as two separate species. Pulsed-field gel electrophoresis has been applied to *Ureaplasma* spp. to determine the size of the genome (99, 113), and this technique can distinguish among the majority of the 14 *Ureaplasma* serotypes and detect differences within serotypes (97).

Restriction fragment length polymorphism, multiple-locus variable-number tandem-repeat analysis, Western blotting, two-dimensional gel electrophoresis, nucleic acid sequence-based amplification, and other types of PCR assays have been used to characterize *M. pneumoniae* clinical isolates (31, 35, 41, 45, 61, 102, 115). Most evaluations have determined that there are two major genomic groups or subtypes distinguishable by analysis of the P1 adhesin gene, ORF6 gene, P65 gene, and typical DNA restriction fragment pattern. Typing of human mycoplasmas or ureaplasmas for diagnostic or epidemiological purposes is not recommended at the present time, and the methods are unavailable except in specialized research or reference laboratories.

SEROLOGIC TESTS

M. pneumoniae Respiratory Disease

Historically, serology has been the most common laboratory means for diagnosis of *M. pneumoniae* respiratory tract infections. Although culture and PCR are also used to detect the presence of *M. pneumoniae* in respiratory specimens, persistence of the organism for variable lengths of time following acute infection makes it difficult in some cases to assess the significance of a positive culture or PCR assay without additional confirmatory tests such as seroconversion.

M. pneumoniae has both lipid and protein antigens which elicit antibody responses that can be detected after about 1 week of illness, peaking at 3 to 6 weeks, followed by a gradual decline, allowing several different types of serologic assays based on different antigens and technologies. Serology is a very useful epidemiologic tool in circumstances where the likelihood of mycoplasmal disease is high, but it is less suited for assessment of individual patients in a timely manner. Its main disadvantage is the need for both acute- and convalescent-phase paired sera collected 2 to 3 weeks apart that are tested simultaneously for IgM and IgG to confirm seroconversion. This is especially important in adults over 40 years of age who may not mount an IgM response, presumably because of reinfection (132, 147). Moreover, IgM antibodies can sometimes persist for several weeks to months, making it risky to base diagnosis of acute infection on a single assay for IgM even in children (132, 147). Antibody production may also be delayed in some infections, or even absent if the patient is immunosuppressed. False-negative tests for IgM can also occur if serum is collected too soon after the onset of illness. Since *M. pneumoniae* is a mucosal pathogen, IgA is typically produced early in the course of infection. Measurement of serum IgA has been suggested as an alternative approach for diagnosis of acute infection because of its rapid rise and decline, but very few commercial assays include reagents for its detection (139).

Complement fixation (CF) was the primary method for serological testing for M. pneumoniae in the past. Although CF measures mainly the early IgM response, the test does not differentiate among antibody classes. Cross-reactions with other organisms, most notably M. genitalium (82), are well recognized, and false-positive results due to cross-reactive autoantibodies induced by acute inflammation from other unrelated causes may occur. In most clinical laboratories, CF has been replaced by alternative techniques. Table 3 provides examples of various assays used to detect M. pneumoniae infection. More detailed descriptions of individual assay kits are available in other reference texts (148).

Immunofluorescent antibody (IFA) assays, direct and indirect hemagglutination using IgM capture, and other particle agglutination antibody assays (PAs) have been developed to detect antibody to M. pneumoniae (5, 50, 81). IFA assays consist of M. pneumoniae antigen affixed to microscope slides and measures IgM and IgG separately. This assay is technically simple to perform but subjective in interpretation, it requires a fluorescent microscope, and the presence of M. pneumoniae-specific IgG may interfere with IgM results (5). Qualitative and semiquantitative PAs using either latex beads or gelatin that detect IgM and IgG simultaneously can be technically easy to perform. However, PAs do not offer any significant advantages over enzyme immunoassays (EIAs) and are not available commercially in the United States.

EIAs have become the most widely used methods for detection of M. pneumoniae antibody in the United States. All are classified as having either moderate or high complexity according to the Clinical Laboratory Improvement Amendment. They may be qualitative or quantitative and may or may not require specialized equipment. EIAs are more sensitive than CF and can be performed with very small volumes of serum. A membrane-based EIA specific for IgM, the ImmunoCard (Meridian Diagnostics, Cincinnati, OH), was developed for rapid detection of acute M. pneumoniae infection using a single serum specimen. However, a recent study found this EIA had a sensitivity of only 31.8% when a single serum was analyzed from seropositive children with pneumonia, increasing to 88% when paired sera were analyzed (103). The Remel EIA (Remel, Inc.) is another rapid point-of-care qualitative assay that detects both IgM and IgG simultaneously in an easy-to-read format without the need for instrumentation. This test has shown good

TABLE 3 Examples of test kits sold in the United States for detection of serum antibodies to M. pneumoniae[a]

Product name	Manufacturer	Antibody(ies) measured	Assay format and description	No. of tests/kit	Specimen throughput	Assay time	
						Start to finish	Hands on
M. pneumoniae antibody (MP) test system	Zeus Scientific, Inc., Branchburg, NJ	IgM and IgG separately	Indirect immunofluorescence assay available as a slurry of M. pneumoniae antigenic substrate or a Crown Titer of M. pneumoniae colonies affixed to microscope slides	100	Each slide contains 10 wells	2.5 h	30 min
ETI-MP IgM or IgG	Savyon Diagnostics, Ltd., Ashdod, Israel	IgM and IgG separately	EIA using a 96-well microtiter plate coated with a membrane preparation containing M. pneumoniae P1 protein	192	Strips of 8 wells	2.5 h	15–20 min
ImmunoCard	Meridian Diagnostics, Cincinnati, OH	IgM only	Qualitative, membrane-based, EIA in a single-sample-card format consisting of a test port containing M. pneumoniae antigen and a control port containing immobilized human IgM	30	1 specimen per card	12 min	10 min
M. pneumoniae IgG/IgM antibody test system	Remel, Inc., Lenexa, KS	IgM and IgG simultaneously	Qualitative, membrane-based, enzyme immunobinding assay consisting of a single sample test containing inactivated M. pneumoniae cytadhesin protein	10 or 40	1 specimen per card	10 min	2–3 min
Mycoplasma IgG and IgM ELISA test system	Zeus Scientific, Inc.	IgM and IgG separately	Qualitative EIA in multiwell breakaway strips containing partially purified inactivated M. pneumoniae	96	Strips of 8 wells	50 min	5–10 min
GenBio Immuno-WELL M. pneumoniae IgM or IgG	Alexon-Trend, Inc., Ramsey, MN	IgM and IgG separately	EIA using a 96-well microtiter plate coated with purified glycolipid M. pneumoniae antigen (strain FH, ATCC 15531)	96	Strips of 8 wells	IgG, 2.35 h; IgM, 2.75 h	15–20 min

[a]This table does not include all commercially available test kits for serological diagnosis of M. pneumoniae infections sold in the United States. It provides descriptions of tests representing various formats and is limited to those products which have been evaluated in independent studies.

sensitivity and specificity when compared to other EIAs, IFA assays, and CF. Several comparison studies have been performed, evaluating each of the EIA kits listed in Table 3 and various others (5, 6, 9, 13, 50, 81, 122, 131). A comprehensive evaluation of 12 commercial EIAs and PAs using PCR as a reference standard found that most assays had problems with sensitivity and specificity. This evaluation indicated limitations for their use in the diagnosis of acute infections, reaffirmed the necessity of testing both IgM and IgG in paired sera from adults, and suggested the PCR assay may be a better diagnostic approach (13). Another study (32) reported sera from a substantial proportion of healthy blood donors have measurable antibody against M. *pneumoniae*, suggesting cross-reactivity of the antigens used in some of the commercial EIAs and the likelihood their use results in overdiagnosis of mycoplasmal infections. A combination of IgM or IgA serology and PCR can be a logical diagnostic approach if only a single specimen is available, but it may be less useful in adults who do not mount an IgM response and would add considerable cost to laboratory testing (139). Cold agglutinins, detected by agglutination of type O Rh-negative erythrocytes at 4°C, occur in association with M. *pneumoniae* infection in about 50% of cases (24). Titers of 64 to 128 or a fourfold or greater rise in titer suggest a recent M. *pneumoniae* infection, but the test is nonspecific and is not recommended for diagnostic use.

Infections Due to Genital Mycoplasmas

Serological tests for M. *hominis* and *Ureaplasma* spp. using metabolism inhibition, microimmunofluorescence, and EIA have been described previously (21, 22, 85, 125, 130). A microimmunofluorescence assay for M. *genitalium* has also been developed (54) and was shown to detect antibody responses in men with NGU (124) and women with salpingitis (96). A sensitive and specific serological assay for M. *genitalium* using lipid-associated membrane proteins as antigens has been used in combination with Western immunoblots to assess the immunoreactivity of women who were regarded as culture positive for M. *genitalium* (10). No serological tests for genital mycoplasmas have been standardized and made commercially available for diagnostic use in the United States. Therefore, they cannot be recommended for routine diagnostic purposes.

ANTIBIOTIC SUSCEPTIBILITIES

Methods Used for Testing

Several methods of susceptibility testing used for conventional bacteria have been employed for testing mycoplasmas. Agar dilution has been used as a reference method (77). It has the advantages of a relatively stable endpoint over time, the inoculum size does not have a great effect, and it allows detection of mixed cultures readily. However, this technique is not practical for testing small numbers of strains or occasional isolates which may be encountered in diagnostic laboratories. Agar disk diffusion is not useful for testing mycoplasmas, since there has been no correlation between inhibitory zones and MICs, and the relatively slow growth of some of these organisms further limits this technology. Microbroth dilution to determine MICs is the most practical and widely used method. It is economical and allows several antimicrobials to be tested in the same microtiter plate, but it has numerous disadvantages in that preparation of antimicrobial dilutions is labor-intensive and the endpoint tends to shift over time (140). Limited comparisons of agar dilution

versus microbroth dilution indicated that the two methods provided similar results for various antimicrobials tested against *Ureaplasma* spp. and M. *hominis* (59, 76, 145).

Studies using the Etest (bioMérieux, Durham, NC) agar gradient diffusion technique for detection of tetracycline resistance in M. *hominis* yielded results comparable to microbroth dilution (143). Additional comparative studies have also validated this method for determination of susceptibilities of M. *hominis* to fluoroquinolones (142) and susceptibilities of ureaplasmas to various antimicrobials (43).The Etest has the advantages of simplicity of agar-based testing, has an endpoint which does not shift over time, does not have a large inoculum effect, and can easily be adapted for testing single isolates.

There have been no universally accepted standards for pH, media, incubation conditions, or duration of incubation for performing mycoplasmal or ureaplasmal susceptibility tests. No MIC breakpoints specific for these organisms are endorsed by any regulatory agency. Lack of specific guidelines for susceptibility testing methods, quality control reference strains, MIC ranges, and interpretation of results has led to diverse and often inconsistent susceptibility profiles. The Human Mycoplasma Susceptibility Testing Subcommittee of the Clinical and Laboratory Standards Institute (CLSI) has submitted recommendations for standard methods for agar- and broth-based susceptibility testing of human mycoplasmas and ureaplasmas. A forthcoming CLSI guideline will also designate quality control reference strains, expected MIC ranges, and proposed MIC interpretive breakpoints for selected drugs.

MIC assays must include control strains for validation purposes. M. *pneumoniae* strain M129 ATCC 29342, M. *hominis* strain PG21ATCC 23114, and U. *urealyticum* (serovar 9) ATCC 33175 have been shown to provide reproducible MICs for several antimicrobials by multiple laboratories participating in studies to collect data for the proposed CLSI guideline. An inoculum of 10^4 to 10^5 CFU/ml has been recommended as the optimum inoculum for broth-based testing (140, 144). Nonstandardized conditions at low pH (6.0) can affect MICs, especially for macrolides, but such conditions are required for growth of *Ureaplasma* spp. Step-by-step procedures for performance of in vitro susceptibility tests for mycoplasmas and ureaplasmas of human origin have been published previously (144). These procedures have been modified somewhat in the forthcoming CLSI guideline.

Commercial 10B and SP4 broths (Remel, Inc.) perform in an acceptable manner for determining broth dilution antimicrobial susceptibilities of *Ureaplasma* spp. and M. *pneumoniae*, respectively. A modified nonproprietary Hayflick's broth has been recommended for testing M. *hominis* by the Mycoplasma Susceptibility Testing Subcommittee of the CLSI. Agar-based tests can utilize A8, SP4, and modified Hayflick's media for these same organisms, respectively.

Tetracycline-resistant M. *hominis* and *Ureaplasma* spp. can easily be distinguished by broth- or agar-based methods, since the resistant strains generally have MICs of ≥2 μg/ml. Commercial MIC test kits are available in some countries. Details on these products are provided in reference texts (148).

Susceptibility Profiles and Treatment

A comparison of MICs for several antimicrobial agents is shown in Table 4. Mollicutes are innately resistant to all beta-lactams, sulfonamides, trimethoprim, and rifampin. Resistance to macrolides and lincosamides is variable according to species, with M. *hominis* being resistant to erythromycin and other 14- and 15-membered macrolides but susceptible to clindamycin. For *Ureaplasma* spp., the reverse is true. Newer

TABLE 4 Ranges of MIC of various antimicrobials for M. pneumoniae, M. hominis, M. fermentans, M. genitalium, and Ureaplasma spp.[a]

Antimicrobial	MIC (μg/ml) for:				
	M. pneumoniae	M. hominis	M. genitalium	M. fermentans	Ureaplasma spp.
Tetracycline	0.063–0.25	0.2–2[c]	≤0.01–0.05	0.1–1	0.05–2[b]
Doxycycline	0.02–0.5	0.1–2[c]	≤0.01–0.3	0.05–1	0.02–1[b]
Tigecycline	0.06–0.25	0.125–0.5	ND	ND	1–16
Erythromycin	≤0.004–0.06[b]	32–>1,000	≤0.01	0.5–64	0.02–8[d]
Roxithromycin	≤0.01	>16	0.01	32–64	0.1–2
Dirithromycin	<0.015–0.5	>64	<0.015–0.125	≥64	0.25–4
Clarithromycin	≤0.004–0.125[b]	16–>256	≤0.01	1–64	≤0.004–2
Azithromycin	≤.004–0.01[b]	4–64	≤0.01	≤0.003–0.05	0.5–4[d]
Josamycin	≤0.01–0.03	0.05–2	0.01–0.03	0.1–0.5	0.03–4
Clindamycin	≤0.008–2	≤0.008–2	0.2–1	0.01–0.25	0.2–64
Lincomycin	4–8	0.2–1	1–8	ND	8–256
Pristinamycin	0.02–0.05	0.1–0.5	≤0.01–0.02	ND	0.1–1
Spiramycin	<0.015–0.25	32–>64	0.125–1	2–4	4–32
Telithromycin	<0.008–0.06[b]	2–32	<0.015	0.06–0.25	<0.015–0.25
Cethromycin	<0.001–0.016	<0.008–0.031	ND	<0.008	<0.008–0.031
Chloramphenicol	2	2–25	ND	0.5–10	0.4–8
Gentamicin	4	2–16	ND	0.25–>500	0.1–13
Ciprofloxacin	0.5–2	0.1–4	2	0.02–>64	0.1–16
Ofloxacin	0.05–2	0.1–4	1–2	0.02–0.25	0.2–4
Levofloxacin	0.5–1	0.1–2	0.5–1	0.05–1	0.2–2
Sparfloxacin	≤0.008–0.5	<0.008–0.1	0.05–0.1	≤0.01–0.05	0.003–1
Gatifloxacin	0.031–1	0.016–0.25	0.125	<0.008–0.25	0.125–2
Moxifloxacin	0.06–0.125	0.06–0.125	0.03–0.06	≤0.015–0.06	0.125–1
Garenoxacin	<0.008–0.125	<0.008–0.063	0.06–0.125	<0.008–0.015	0.016–1
Gemifloxacin	0.05–0.125	0.0025–0.01	0.05–0.125	0.001–0.01	0.03–0.5
Rifampin	>8	>1,000	ND	25–>50	>1,000
Quinupristin/dalfopristin	0.008–0.06	0.03–8	0.05	0.1–0.5	0.03–0.5
Linezolid	32–128	1–8	4–128	0.063–4	>64

[a]Data were compiled from multiple published studies in which different methodologies, and often different antimicrobial concentrations, were used. Elevated MICs (≥8 μg/ml) for the occasionally encountered fluoroquinolone-resistant M. hominis and Ureaplasma spp. have not been included in the MIC ranges. ND, no data available.
[b]Macrolide-susceptible strains only. MICs for M. pneumoniae isolates containing mutations in domain V of rRNA usually exceed 32 μg/ml.
[c]Tetracycline-susceptible strains only. MICs for isolates containing tet(M) are generally 2–>64 μg/ml.
[d]Macrolide-susceptible strains only. MICs for Ureaplasma spp. containing mutations in rRNA usually exceed 32 μg/ml.

macrolides and ketolides have shown in vitro activity comparable to that of erythromycin for M. pneumoniae.

M. pneumoniae has historically been predictably susceptible to fluoroquinolones, tetracyclines, and macrolides, so susceptibility testing has not been recommended except for the in vitro evaluation of new and previously untested agents. However, recent studies from Japan, China, France, and the United States found that high-level macrolide resistance in M. pneumoniae due to mutations in domain V on the 23S rRNA gene is increasing in patients with acute respiratory infections (83, 105, 153, 155, 156). This resistance is greatest in China, where the percentage of resistant organisms has exceeded 80% (83, 156). Molecular-based methods to detect mutations in rRNA directly in clinical specimens by PCR enables monitoring resistance trends without having to isolate M. pneumoniae in culture and can provide rapid diagnostic information (105, 153, 155). Tetracycline resistance has been well documented in both M. hominis and Ureaplasma spp. since the mid-1980s, mediated by the tet(M) determinant which codes for a protein that binds to the ribosomes, protecting them from the actions of these drugs. The extent to which tetracycline resistance occurs in M. hominis and Ureaplasma spp. varies geographically and according to prior antimicrobial exposure in different populations but may approach 40 to 50% (146). High-level macrolide-resistant U. parvum in which there was a deletion of 2 amino acids in the L4 ribosomal protein was recently

reported from the United Kingdom, but such resistance is believed to be rare (14). We have recently encountered occasional Ureaplasma isolates in the United States with high-level macrolide resistance that have mutations in the 23S rRNA gene. Men with M. genitalium NGU and women with cervicitis respond better to azithromycin than tetracycline, possibly because of the lower MICs, but there has also been documentation of clinically significant macrolide-resistant M. genitalium due to rRNA gene mutations (67).

Fluoroquinolones such as levofloxacin and moxifloxacin are usually active against all human mycoplasmal and ureaplasmal species. Occasional fluoroquinolone-resistant strains of M. hominis, Ureaplasma spp., and M. genitalium with mutations in the DNA gyrase and/or topoisomerase IV genes have been reported (12, 37, 44). Other agents such as streptogramins, aminoglycosides, and chloramphenicol may show in vitro inhibitory activity, but these agents are rarely used to treat infections caused by these organisms. Oxazolidinones are inactive in vitro against mycoplasmas.

Extragenital infections, often in immunocompromised hosts, may be caused by multidrug-resistant mycoplasmas and ureaplasmas, making guidance of chemotherapy by in vitro susceptibility tests important in this clinical setting. Eradication of infection under these circumstances can be extremely difficult, requiring prolonged therapy, even when the organisms are susceptible to the expected agents. This difficulty highlights the facts that mollicutes are inhibited but not killed by most commonly used bacteriostatic antimicrobial agents in concentrations achievable in vivo and that a functioning immune system plays an integral part in their eradication. Treatment of mycoplasmal and ureaplasmal infections has been described in detail elsewhere (138).

EVALUATION, INTERPRETATION, AND REPORTING OF RESULTS

Tests offered through diagnostic microbiology laboratories should focus on the species known to cause human disease and for which cultivation techniques are best defined. Unusual organisms, or those for which cultivation conditions are not established, may be detectable by PCR technology offered through specialized research or reference laboratories. Such organisms should be sought only after consultation with clinicians and personnel from the reference laboratory. Except for *Ureaplasma* spp., which can be identified by urease production and distinct colonial morphology, and until species identification can be confirmed, a preliminary report of "large-colony *Mycoplasma* species" is appropriate. In many instances, as in culturing specimens from the lower genital tract, this may be sufficient. Isolates from normally sterile sites and/or from immunosuppressed persons should be identified to species level by PCR if possible.

M. pneumoniae

Detection of M. *pneumoniae* in culture is time-consuming, not overly sensitive, and rarely performed. However, isolation of the organism from respiratory tract specimens is clinically significant in most instances and should be correlated with the presence of clinical respiratory disease, since a small proportion of asymptomatic carriers can exist. Detection by PCR is becoming more widely available, but a positive result must still be correlated with clinical events. A fourfold rise in antibody titer between acute- and convalescent-phase sera is considered diagnostic of acute infection. In children, adolescents, and young adults, a single positive IgM result using appropriate immunoglobulin class-specific reagents can be considered diagnostic of acute infection in most, but not necessarily all, cases because of the possibility of prolonged IgM elevation that sometimes occurs. Mild respiratory infections due to M. *pneumoniae* may not merit a costly and time-consuming microbiological work-up, since empiric treatment will be effective in most instances. However, the emergence of clinically significant macrolide resistance may influence choices of empiric antimicrobial agents.

M. hominis

M. *hominis* can be detected in culture within a few days. It may occasionally be discovered in routine bacteriologic media from appropriate clinical material, but this should not be relied upon. Its isolation in any quantity from normally sterile body fluids or tissues is significantly associated with disease, but quantitation of organisms may be of value in other circumstances. When mycoplasmas are detected in nonsterile sites, such as the female lower genital tract in numbers exceeding 10^5 organisms, they are likely to be associated with BV.

Ureaplasma Species

Isolation of *Ureaplasma* spp. in any quantity from normally sterile body fluids or tissues is significantly associated with disease. Fewer than 10^4 organisms in the male urethra are unlikely to be significant. Distinguishing between the 2 *Ureaplasma* spp. by PCR may become more important in view of possible differences in pathogenicity in some circumstances such as NGU. The presence of *Ureaplasma* spp.

in the lower respiratory tract of neonates with respiratory distress may be clinically significant, but there are no definitive guidelines for antibiotic treatment (2, 38, 40).

M. genitalium

Growing evidence for the role of M. *genitalium* as a urogenital pathogen has generated interest in the development of diagnostic methods for its detection, though no molecular biology-based assays for direct detection or serology test kits are sold commercially thus far. Even though cultivation techniques for M. *genitalium* have been described previously (10, 68, 135), relatively few clinical isolates have actually been attained since the initial description of this mycoplasma in the early 1980s. The slow growth, requiring 6 weeks or longer, makes culture impractical. The potential importance of this organism in sexually transmitted urogenital infections underscores the need for improved and standardized methods for its detection. At present, noncommercial, nonstandardized PCR-based assays are all that are available. When M. *genitalium* is detected in clinical specimens from the urogenital tract, such as the male urethra or female cervix, in persons with clinical evidence of urethritis or cervicitis, it should be considered medically significant.

REFERENCES

1. **Abele-Horn, M., C. Blendinger, C. Becher, P. Emmerling, and G. Ruckdeschel.** 1996. Evaluation of commercial kits for quantitative identification and tests on antibiotic susceptibility of genital mycoplasmas. *Zentralbl. Bakteriol.* **284:**540–549.
2. **Abele-Horn, M., C. Wolff, P. Dressel, F. Pfaff, and A. Zimmermann.** 1997. Association of *Ureaplasma urealyticum* biovars with clinical outcome for neonates, obstetric patients, and gynecological patients with pelvic inflammatory disease. *J. Clin. Microbiol.* **35:**1199–2202.
3. **Ainsworth, J. G., J. Clarke, R. Goldin, and D. Taylor-Robinson.** 2000. Disseminated *Mycoplasma fermentans* in AIDS patients: several case reports. *Int. J. STD AIDS* **11:**751–755.
4. **Ainsworth, J. G., J. Clarke, M. Lipman, D. Mitchell, and D. Taylor-Robinson.** 2000. Detection of *Mycoplasma fermentans* in broncho-alveolar lavage fluid specimens from AIDS patients with lower respiratory tract infection. *HIV Med.* **1:**219–223.
5. **Alexander, T. S., L. D. Gray, J. A. Kraft, D. S. Leland, M. T. Nikaido, and D. H. Willis.** 1996. Performance of Meridian ImmunoCard Mycoplasma test in a multicenter clinical trial. *J. Clin. Microbiol.* **34:**1180–1183.
6. **Aubert, G., B. Pozzetto, O. G. Gaudin, J. Hafid, A. D. Mbida, and A. Ros.** 1992. Evaluation of five commercial tests: complement fixation, microparticle agglutination, indirect immunofluorescence, enzyme-linked immunosorbent assay and latex agglutination, in comparison to immunoblotting for *Mycoplasma pneumoniae* serology. *Ann. Biol. Clin.* (Paris) **50:**593–597.
7. **Baczynska, A., H. Friis Svenstrup, J. Fedder, S. Birkelund, and G. Christiansen.** 2005. The use of enzyme-linked immunosorbent assay for detection of *Mycoplasma hominis* antibodies in infertile women serum samples. *Hum. Reprod.* **20:**1277–1285.
8. **Baczynska, A., H. F. Svenstrup, J. Fedder, S. Birkelund, and G. Christiansen.** 2004. Development of real-time PCR for detection of *Mycoplasma hominis.* *BMC Microbiol.* **4:**35.
9. **Barker, C. E., M. Sillis, and T. G. Wreghitt.** 1990. Evaluation of Serodia Myco II particle agglutination test for detecting *Mycoplasma pneumoniae* antibody: comparison with mu-capture ELISA and indirect immunofluorescence. *J. Clin. Pathol.* **43:**163–165.
10. **Baseman, J. B., M. Cagle, J. E. Korte, C. Herrera, W. G. Rasmussen, J. G. Baseman, R. Shain, and J. M. Piper.** 2004. Diagnostic assessment of *Mycoplasma genitalium* in culture-positive women. *J. Clin. Microbiol.* **42:**203–211.
11. **Baseman, J. B., and J. G. Tully.** 1997. Mycoplasmas: sophisticated, reemerging, and burdened by their notoriety. *Emerg. Infect. Dis.* **3:**21–32.
12. **Bebear, C. M., H. Renaudin, A. Charron, M. Clerc, S. Pereyre, and C. Bebear.** 2003. DNA gyrase and topoisomerase

IV mutations in clinical isolates of *Ureaplasma* spp. and *Mycoplasma hominis* resistant to fluoroquinolones. *Antimicrob. Agents Chemother.* **47**:3323–3325.

13. **Beersma, M. F., K. Dirven, A. P. van Dam, K. E. Templeton, E. C. Claas, and H. Goossens.** 2005. Evaluation of 12 commercial tests and the complement fixation test for *Mycoplasma pneumoniae*-specific immunoglobulin G (IgG) and IgM antibodies, with PCR used as the "gold standard." *J. Clin. Microbiol.* **43**:2277–2285.

14. **Beeton, M. L., V. J. Chalker, N. C. Maxwell, S. Kotecha, and O. B. Spiller.** 2009. Concurrent titration and determination of antibiotic resistance in *Ureaplasma* species with identification of novel point mutations in genes associated with resistance. *Antimicrob. Agents Chemother.* **53**:2020–2027.

15. **Bernet, C., M. Garret, B. de Barbeyrac, C. Bebear, and J. Bonnet.** 1989. Detection of *Mycoplasma pneumoniae* by using the polymerase chain reaction. *J. Clin. Microbiol.* **27**:2492–2496.

16. **Bjornelius, E., J. S. Jensen, and P. Lidbrink.** 2004. Conjunctivitis associated with *Mycoplasma genitalium* infection. *Clin. Infect. Dis.* **39**:e67–e69.

17. **Blanchard, A., J. Hentschel, L. Duffy, K. Baldus, and G. H. Cassell.** 1993. Detection of *Ureaplasma urealyticum* by polymerase chain reaction in the urogenital tract of adults, in amniotic fluid, and in the respiratory tract of newborns. *Clin. Infect. Dis.* **17**(Suppl. 1):S148–S153.

18. **Blaylock, M. W., O. Musatovova, J. G. Baseman, and J. B. Baseman.** 2004. Determination of infectious load of *Mycoplasma genitalium* in clinical samples of human vaginal cells. *J. Clin. Microbiol.* **42**:746–752.

19. **Bradshaw, C. S., S. N. Tabrizi, T. R. Read, S. M. Garland, C. A. Hopkins, L. M. Moss, and C. K. Fairley.** 2006. Etiologies of nongonococcal urethritis: bacteria, viruses, and the association with orogenital exposure. *J. Infect. Dis.* **193**:336–345.

20. **Broitman, N. L., C. M. Floyd, C. A. Johnson, L. M. de la Maza, and E. M. Peterson.** 1992. Comparison of commercially available media for detection and isolation of *Ureaplasma urealyticum* and *Mycoplasma hominis*. *J. Clin. Microbiol.* **30**:1335–1337.

21. **Brown, M. B., G. H. Cassell, W. M. McCormack, and J. K. Davis.** 1987. Measurement of antibody to *Mycoplasma hominis* by an enzyme-linked immunoassay and detection of class-specific antibody responses in women with postpartum fever. *Am. J. Obstet. Gynecol.* **156**:701–708.

22. **Brown, M. B., G. H. Cassell, D. Taylor-Robinson, and M. C. Shepard.** 1983. Measurement of antibody to *Ureaplasma urealyticum* by an enzyme-linked immunosorbent assay and detection of antibody responses in patients with nongonococcal urethritis. *J. Clin. Microbiol.* **17**:288–295.

23. **Cassell, G. H., R. O. Davis, K. B. Waites, M. B. Brown, P. A. Marriott, S. Stagno, and J. K. Davis.** 1983. Isolation of *Mycoplasma hominis* and *Ureaplasma urealyticum* from amniotic fluid at 16–20 weeks of gestation: potential effect on outcome of pregnancy. *Sex. Transm. Dis.* **10**:294–302.

24. **Cassell, G. H., G. Gambill, and L. B. Duffy.** 1996. ELISA in respiratory infections of humans, p. 123–136. *In* J. G. Tully and S. Razin (ed.), *Molecular and Diagnostic Procedures in Diagnostic Mycoplasmology*. Academic Press, New York, NY.

25. **Cassell, G. H., K. B. Waites, and D. T. Crouse.** 2001. Mycoplasmal infections, p. 733–767. *In* J. S. Remington and J. O. Klein (ed.), *Infectious Diseases of the Fetus and Newborn Infant*, 5th ed. W.B. Saunders Co., Inc., Philadelphia, PA.

26. **Chaim, W., S. Horowitz, J. B. David, F. Ingel, B. Evinson, and M. Mazor.** 2003. *Ureaplasma urealyticum* in the development of postpartum endometritis. *Eur. J. Obstet. Gynecol. Reprod. Biol.* **109**:145–148.

27. **Cheah, F. C., T. P. Anderson, B. A. Darlow, and D. R. Murdoch.** 2005. Comparison of the Mycoplasma Duo test with PCR for detection of *Ureaplasma* species in endotracheal aspirates from premature infants. *J. Clin. Microbiol.* **43**:509–510.

28. **Clausen, H. F., J. Fedder, M. Drasbek, P. K. Nielsen, B. Toft, H. J. Ingerslev, S. Birkelund, and G. Christiansen.** 2001. Serological investigation of *Mycoplasma genitalium* in infertile women. *Hum. Reprod.* **16**:1866–1874.

29. **Clegg, A., M. Passey, M. Yoannes, and A. Michael.** 1997. High rates of genital mycoplasma infection in the highlands of Papua New Guinea determined both by culture and by a commercial detection kit. *J. Clin. Microbiol.* **35**:197–200.

30. **Cohen, C. R., L. E. Manhart, E. A. Bukusi, S. Astete, R. C. Brunham, K. K. Holmes, S. K. Sinei, J. J. Bwayo, and P. A. Totten.** 2002. Association between *Mycoplasma genitalium* and acute endometritis. *Lancet* **359**:765–766.

31. **Cousin-Allery, A., A. Charron, B. de Barbeyrac, G. Fremy, J. Skov Jensen, H. Renaudin, and C. Bebear.** 2000. Molecular typing of *Mycoplasma pneumoniae* strains by PCR-based methods and pulsed-field gel electrophoresis. Application to French and Danish isolates. *Epidemiol. Infect.* **124**:103–111.

32. **Csango, P. A., J. E. Pedersen, and R. D. Hess.** 2004. Comparison of four *Mycoplasma pneumoniae* IgM-, IgG- and IgA-specific enzyme immunoassays in blood donors and patients. *Clin. Microbiol. Infect.* **10**:1094–1098.

33. **Dallo, S. F., and J. B. Baseman.** 2000. Intracellular DNA replication and long-term survival of pathogenic mycoplasmas. *Microb. Pathog.* **29**:301–309.

34. **de Barbeyrac, B., C. Bernet-Poggi, F. Febrer, H. Renaudin, M. Dupon, and C. Bebear.** 1993. Detection of *Mycoplasma pneumoniae* and *Mycoplasma genitalium* in clinical samples by polymerase chain reaction. *Clin. Infect. Dis.* **17**(Suppl. 1):S83–S89.

35. **Degrange, S., C. Cazanave, A. Charron, H. Renaudin, C. Bebear, and C. M. Bebear.** 2009. Development of multiple-locus variable-number tandem-repeat analysis for molecular typing of *Mycoplasma pneumoniae*. *J. Clin. Microbiol.* **47**:914–923.

36. **Deguchi, T., C. B. Gilroy, and D. Taylor-Robinson.** 1996. Failure to detect *Mycoplasma fermentans*, *Mycoplasma penetrans*, or *Mycoplasma pirum* in the urethra of patients with acute nongonococcal urethritis. *Eur. J. Clin. Microbiol. Infect. Dis.* **15**:169–171.

37. **Deguchi, T., S. Maeda, M. Tamaki, T. Yoshida, H. Ishiko, M. Ito, S. Yokoi, Y. Takahashi, and S. Ishihara.** 2001. Analysis of the gyrA and parC genes of *Mycoplasma genitalium* detected in first-pass urine of men with non-gonococcal urethritis before and after fluoroquinolone treatment. *J. Antimicrob. Chemother.* **48**:742–744.

38. **Deguchi, T., T. Yoshida, T. Miyazawa, M. Yasuda, M. Tamaki, H. Ishiko, and S. Maeda.** 2004. Association of *Ureaplasma urealyticum* (biovar 2) with nongonococcal urethritis. *Sex. Transm. Dis.* **31**:192–195.

39. **Doble, A., B. J. Thomas, P. M. Furr, M. M. Walker, J. R. W. Harris, R. O. Witherow, and D. Taylor-Robinson.** 1989. A search for infectious agents in chronic abacterial prostatitis using ultrasound guided biopsy. *Br. J. Urol.* **64**:297–301.

40. **Domingues, D., L. T. Tavira, A. Duarte, A. Sanca, E. Prieto, and F. Exposto.** 2002. *Ureaplasma urealyticum* biovar determination in women attending a family planning clinic in Guine-Bissau, using polymerase chain reaction of the multiple-banded antigen gene. *J. Clin. Lab. Anal.* **16**:71–75.

41. **Dorigo-Zetsma, J. W., J. Dankert, and S. A. Zaat.** 2000. Genotyping of *Mycoplasma pneumoniae* clinical isolates reveals eight P1 subtypes within two genomic groups. *J. Clin. Microbiol.* **38**:965–970.

42. **Dorigo-Zetsma, J. W., R. P. Verkooyen, H. P. van Helden, H. van der Nat, and J. M. van den Bosch.** 2001. Molecular detection of *Mycoplasma pneumoniae* in adults with community-acquired pneumonia requiring hospitalization. *J. Clin. Microbiol.* **39**:1184–1186.

43. **Dosa, E., E. Nagy, W. Falk, I. Szoke, and U. Ballies.** 1999. Evaluation of the Etest for susceptibility testing of *Mycoplasma hominis* and *Ureaplasma urealyticum*. *J. Antimicrob. Chemother.* **43**:575–578.

44. **Duffy, L., J. Glass, G. Hall, R. Avery, R. Rackley, S. Peterson, and K. Waites.** 2006. Fluoroquinolone resistance in *Ureaplasma parvum* in the United States. *J. Clin. Microbiol.* **44**:1590–1591.

45. **Dumke, R., I. Catrein, E. Pirkil, R. Herrmann, and E. Jacobs.** 2003. Subtyping of *Mycoplasma pneumoniae* isolates based on extended genome sequencing and on expression profiles. *Int. J. Med. Microbiol.* **292**:513–525.

46. **Dumke, R., and E. Jacobs.** 2009. Comparison of commercial and in-house real-time PCR assays used for detection of *Mycoplasma pneumoniae*. *J. Clin. Microbiol.* **47**:441–444.

47. **Dumke, R., N. Schurwanz, M. Lenz, M. Schuppler, C. Luck, and E. Jacobs.** 2007. Sensitive detection of *Mycoplasma pneumoniae* in human respiratory tract samples by optimized real-time PCR approach. *J. Clin. Microbiol.* **45:**2726–2730.

48. **Dutro, S. M., J. K. Hebb, C. A. Garin, J. P. Hughes, G. E. Kenny, and P. A. Totten.** 2003. Development and performance of a microwell-plate-based polymerase chain reaction assay for *Mycoplasma genitalium. Sex. Transm. Dis.* **30:**756–763.

49. **Echahidi, F., G. Muyldermans, S. Lauwers, and A. Naessens.** 2000. Development of monoclonal antibodies against *Ureaplasma urealyticum* serotypes and their use for serotyping clinical isolates. *Clin. Diagn. Lab. Immunol.* **7:**563–567.

50. **Echevarria, J. M., P. Leon, P. Balfagon, J. A. Lopez, and M. V. Fernandez.** 1990. Diagnosis of *Mycoplasma pneumoniae* infection by microparticle agglutination and antibody-capture enzyme-immunoassay. *Eur. J. Clin. Microbiol. Infect. Dis.* **9:**217–220.

51. **Eschenbach, D. A.** 1993. *Ureaplasma urealyticum* and premature birth. *Clin. Infect. Dis.* **17**(Suppl. 1):S100–S106.

52. **Falk, L., H. Fredlund, and J. S. Jensen.** 2005. Signs and symptoms of urethritis and cervicitis among women with or without *Mycoplasma genitalium* or *Chlamydia trachomatis* infection. *Sex. Transm. Infect.* **81:**73–78.

53. **Falk, L., H. Fredlund, and J. S. Jensen.** 2004. Symptomatic urethritis is more prevalent in men infected with *Mycoplasma genitalium* than with *Chlamydia trachomatis. Sex. Transm. Infect.* **80:**289–293.

54. **Furr, P. M., and D. Taylor-Robinson.** 1984. Microimmunofluorescence technique for detection of antibody to *Mycoplasma genitalium. J. Clin. Pathol.* **37:**1072–1074.

55. **Grenabo, L., H. Hedelin, and S. Pettersson.** 1988. Urinary infection stones caused by *Ureaplasma urealyticum*: a review. *Scand. J. Infect. Dis. Suppl.* **53:**46–49.

56. **Hahn, D. L.** 2009. Macrolide therapy in asthma: limited treatment, long-term improvement. *Eur. Respir. J.* **33:**1239.

57. **Hatchel, J. M., R. S. Balish, M. L. Duley, and M. F. Balish.** 2006. Ultrastructure and gliding motility of *Mycoplasma amphoriforme*, a possible human respiratory pathogen. *Microbiology* **152:**2181–2189.

58. **Henrich, B., R. C. Feldmann, and U. Hadding.** 1993. Cytoadhesins of *Mycoplasma hominis. Infect. Immun.* **61:**2945–2951.

59. **Hilliard, N. J., L. B. Duffy, D. M. Crabb, and K. B. Waites.** 2005. In vitro comparison of agar and microbroth dilution methods for determination of MICs for *Mycoplasma hominis. J. Microbiol. Methods* **60:**285–288.

60. **Hu, P. C., U. Schaper, A. M. Collier, W. A. Clyde, Jr., M. Horikawa, Y. S. Huang, and M. F. Barile.** 1987. A *Mycoplasma genitalium* protein resembling the *Mycoplasma pneumoniae* attachment protein. *Infect. Immun.* **55:**1126–1131.

61. **Jacobs, E., A. Pilatschek, B. Gerstenecker, K. Oberle, and W. Bredt.** 1990. Immunodominant epitopes of the adhesin of *Mycoplasma pneumoniae. J. Clin. Microbiol.* **28:**1194–1197.

62. **Jalil, N., A. Doble, C. Gilchrist, and D. Taylor-Robinson.** 1988. Infection of the epididymis by *Ureaplasma urealyticum. Genitourin. Med.* **64:**367–368.

63. **Jensen, J. S.** 1994. *Mycoplasma genitalium*: a cause of nongonococcal urethritis? *Genitourin. Med.* **70:**363.

64. **Jensen, J. S.** 2004. *Mycoplasma genitalium*: the aetiological agent of urethritis and other sexually transmitted diseases. *J. Eur. Acad. Dermatol. Venereol.* **18:**1–11.

65. **Jensen, J. S., E. Bjornelius, B. Dohn, and P. Lidbrink.** 2004. Comparison of first void urine and urogenital swab specimens for detection of *Mycoplasma genitalium* and *Chlamydia trachomatis* by polymerase chain reaction in patients attending a sexually transmitted disease clinic. *Sex. Transm. Dis.* **31:**499–507.

66. **Jensen, J. S., E. Bjornelius, B. Dohn, and P. Lidbrink.** 2004. Use of TaqMan 5;pr nuclease real-time PCR for quantitative detection of *Mycoplasma genitalium* DNA in males with and without urethritis who were attendees at a sexually transmitted disease clinic. *J. Clin. Microbiol.* **42:**683–692.

67. **Jensen, J. S., C. S. Bradshaw, S. N. Tabrizi, C. K. Fairley, and R. Hamasuna.** 2008. Azithromycin treatment failure in *Mycoplasma genitalium*-positive patients with nongonococcal urethritis is associated with induced macrolide resistance. *Clin. Infect. Dis.* **47:**1546–1553.

68. **Jensen, J. S., H. T. Hansen, and K. Lind.** 1996. Isolation of *Mycoplasma genitalium* strains from the male urethra. *J. Clin. Microbiol.* **34:**286–291.

69. **Jensen, J. S., J. Sondergard-Andersen, S. A. Uldum, and K. Lind.** 1989. Detection of *Mycoplasma pneumoniae* in simulated clinical samples by polymerase chain reaction. *APMIS* **97:**1046–1048.

70. **Jensen, J. S., S. A. Uldum, J. Sondergard-Andersen, J. Vuust, and K. Lind.** 1991. Polymerase chain reaction for detection of *Mycoplasma genitalium* in clinical samples. *J. Clin. Microbiol.* **29:**46–50.

71. **Johnson, S., D. Sidebottom, F. Bruckner, and D. Collins.** 2000. Identification of *Mycoplasma fermentans* in synovial fluid samples from arthritis patients with inflammatory disease. *J. Clin. Microbiol.* **38:**90–93.

72. **Johnston, S. L., F. Blasi, P. N. Black, R. J. Martin, D. J. Farrell, and R. B. Nieman.** 2006. The effect of telithromycin in acute exacerbations of asthma. *N. Engl. J. Med.* **354:**1589–1600.

73. **Jurstrand, M., J. S. Jensen, H. Fredlund, L. Falk, and P. Molling.** 2005. Detection of *Mycoplasma genitalium* in urogenital specimens by real-time PCR and by conventional PCR assay. *J. Med. Microbiol.* **54:**23–29.

74. **Kannan, T. R., D. Provenzano, J. R. Wright, and J. B. Baseman.** 2005. Identification and characterization of human surfactant protein A binding protein of *Mycoplasma pneumoniae. Infect. Immun.* **73:**2828–2834.

75. **Katz, B., P. Patel, L. Duffy, R. L. Schelonka, R. A. Dimmitt, and K. B. Waites.** 2005. Characterization of ureaplasmas isolated from preterm infants with and without bronchopulmonary dysplasia. *J. Clin. Microbiol.* **43:**4852–4854.

76. **Kenny, G. E., and F. D. Cartwright.** 1993. Effect of pH, inoculum size, and incubation time on the susceptibility of *Ureaplasma urealyticum* to erythromycin in vitro. *Clin. Infect. Dis.* **17**(Suppl. 1):S215–S218.

77. **Kenny, G. E., F. D. Cartwright, and M. C. Roberts.** 1986. Agar dilution method for determination of antibiotic susceptibility of *Ureaplasma urealyticum. Pediatr. Infect. Dis. J.* **5:**S332–S334.

78. **Knox, C. L., and P. Timms.** 1998. Comparison of PCR, nested PCR, and random amplified polymorphic DNA PCR for detection and typing of *Ureaplasma urealyticum* in specimens from pregnant women. *J. Clin. Microbiol.* **36:**3032–3039.

79. **Kong, F., Z. Ma, G. James, S. Gordon, and G. L. Gilbert.** 2000. Molecular genotyping of human *Ureaplasma* species based on multiple-banded antigen (MBA) gene sequences. *Int. J. Syst. Evol. Microbiol.* **50**(Pt. 5):1921–1929.

80. **Krieger, J. N., D. E. Riley, M. C. Roberts, and R. E. Berger.** 1996. Prokaryotic DNA sequences in patients with chronic idiopathic prostatitis. *J. Clin. Microbiol.* **34:**3120–3128.

81. **Lieberman, D., S. Horowitz, O. Horovitz, F. Schlaeffer, and A. Porath.** 1995. Microparticle agglutination versus antibody-capture enzyme immunoassay for diagnosis of community-acquired *Mycoplasma pneumoniae* pneumonia. *Eur. J. Clin. Microbiol. Infect. Dis.* **14:**577–1584.

82. **Lind, K.** 1982. Serological cross-reactions between "*Mycoplasma genitalium*" and M. *pneumoniae. Lancet* **ii:**1158–1159.

83. **Liu, Y., X. Ye, H. Zhang, X. Xu, W. Li, D. Zhu, and M. Wang.** 2009. Antimicrobial susceptibility of *Mycoplasma pneumoniae* isolates and molecular analysis of macrolide-resistant strains from Shanghai, China. *Antimicrob. Agents Chemother.* **53:**2160–2162.

84. **Lo, S. C., M. M. Hayes, R. Y. Wang, P. F. Pierce, H. Kotani, and J. W. Shih.** 1991. Newly discovered mycoplasma isolated from patients infected with HIV. *Lancet* **338:**1415–1418.

85. **Lo, S. C., R. Y. Wang, T. Grandinetti, N. Zou, C. L. Haley, M. M. Hayes, D. J. Wear, and J. W. Shih.** 2003. *Mycoplasma hominis* lipid-associated membrane protein antigens for effective detection of M. *hominis*-specific antibodies in humans. *Clin. Infect. Dis.* **36:**1246–1253.

86. **Lo, S. C., D. J. Wear, S. L. Green, P. G. Jones, and J. F. Legier.** 1993. Adult respiratory distress syndrome with or without systemic disease associated with infections due to *Mycoplasma fermentans. Clin. Infect. Dis.* **17**(Suppl. 1):S259–S263.

87. Lu, G. C., J. R. Schwebke, L. B. Duffy, G. H. Cassell, J. C. Hauth, W. W. Andrews, and R. L. Goldenberg. 2001. Midtrimester vaginal *Mycoplasma genitalium* in women with subsequent spontaneous preterm birth. *Am. J. Obstet. Gynecol.* **185:**163–165.

88. Luki, N., P. Lebel, M. Boucher, B. Doray, J. Turgeon, and R. Brousseau. 1998. Comparison of polymerase chain reaction assay with culture for detection of genital mycoplasmas in perinatal infections. *Eur. J. Clin. Microbiol. Infect. Dis.* **17:**255–263.

89. Luneberg, E., J. S. Jensen, and M. Frosch. 1993. Detection of *Mycoplasma pneumoniae* by polymerase chain reaction and nonradioactive hybridization in microtiter plates. *J. Clin. Microbiol.* **31:**1088–1094.

90. Maeda, S., T. Deguchi, H. Ishiko, T. Matsumoto, S. Naito, H. Kumon, T. Tsukamoto, S. Onodera, and S. Kamidono. 2004. Detection of *Mycoplasma genitalium*, *Mycoplasma hominis*, *Ureaplasma parvum* (biovar 1) and *Ureaplasma urealyticum* (biovar 2) in patients with non-gonococcal urethritis using polymerase chain reaction-microtiter plate hybridization. *Int. J. Urol.* **11:**750–754.

91. Mahony, J. B., D. Jang, S. Chong, K. Luinstra, J. Sellors, M. Tyndall, and M. Chernesky. 1997. Detection of *Chlamydia trachomatis*, *Neisseria gonorrhoeae*, *Ureaplasma urealyticum*, and *Mycoplasma genitalium* in first-void urine specimens by multiplex polymerase chain reaction. *Mol. Diagn.* **2:**161–168.

92. Mallard, K., K. Schopfer, and T. Bodmer. 2005. Development of real-time PCR for the differential detection and quantification of *Ureaplasma urealyticum* and *Ureaplasma parvum*. *J. Microbiol. Methods* **60:**13–19.

93. Maltezou, H. C., B. La-Scola, H. Astra, I. Constantopoulou, V. Vlahou, D. A. Kafetzis, A. G. Constantopoulos, and D. Raoult. 2004. *Mycoplasma pneumoniae* and *Legionella pneumophila* in community-acquired lower respiratory tract infections among hospitalized children: diagnosis by real time PCR. *Scand. J. Infect. Dis.* **36:**639–642.

94. Martin, R. J., M. Kraft, H. W. Chu, E. A. Berns, and G. H. Cassell. 2001. A link between chronic asthma and chronic infection. *J. Allergy. Clin. Immunol.* **107:**595–601.

95. Meyer, R. D., and W. Clough. 1993. Extragenital *Mycoplasma hominis* infections in adults: emphasis on immunosuppression. *Clin. Infect. Dis.* **17**(Suppl. 1):S243–S249.

96. Moller, B. R., D. Taylor-Robinson, and P. M. Furr. 1984. Serological evidence implicating *Mycoplasma genitalium* in pelvic inflammatory disease. *Lancet* **i:**1102–1103.

97. Moser, S. A., C. A. Mayfield, L. B. Duffy, and K. B. Waites. 2006. Genotypic characterization of *Ureaplasma* species by pulsed field gel electrophoresis. *J. Microbiol. Methods* **67:**606–610.

98. Naessens, A., W. Foulon, J. Breynaert, and S. Lauwers. 1988. Serotypes of *Ureaplasma urealyticum* isolated from normal pregnant women and patients with pregnancy complications. *J. Clin. Microbiol.* **26:**319–322.

99. Neimark, H. C., and C. S. Lange. 1990. Pulse-field electrophoresis indicates full-length mycoplasma chromosomes range widely in size. *Nucleic Acids Res.* **18:**5443–5448.

100. Novy, M. J., L. Duffy, M. K. Axthelm, D. W. Sadowsky, S. S. Witkin, M. G. Gravett, G. H. Cassell, and K. B. Waites. 2009. *Ureaplasma* parvum or *Mycoplasma hominis* as sole pathogens cause chorioamnionitis, preterm delivery, and fetal pneumonia in rhesus macaques. *Reprod. Sci.* **16:**56–70.

101. Oakeshott, P., P. Hay, D. Taylor-Robinson, S. Hay, B. Dohn, S. Kerry, and J. S. Jensen. 2004. Prevalence of *Mycoplasma genitalium* in early pregnancy and relationship between its presence and pregnancy outcome. *Br. J. Obstet. Gynecol.* **111:**1464–1467.

102. Ovyn, C., D. van Strijp, M. Ieven, D. Ursi, B. van Gemen, and H. Goossens. 1996. Typing of *Mycoplasma pneumoniae* by nucleic acid sequence-based amplification, NASBA. *Mol. Cell. Probes* **10:**319–324.

103. Ozaki, T., N. Nishimura, J. Ahn, N. Watanabe, T. Muto, A. Saito, N. Koyama, K. Nakane, and K. Funahashi. 2007. Utility of a rapid diagnosis kit for *Mycoplasma pneumoniae* pneumonia in children, and the antimicrobial susceptibility of the isolates. *J. Infect. Chemother.* **13:**204–207.

104. Perni, S. C., S. Vardhana, I. Korneeva, S. L. Tuttle, L. R. Paraskevas, S. T. Chasen, R. B. Kalish, and S. S. Witkin. 2004. *Mycoplasma hominis* and *Ureaplasma urealyticum* in midtrimester amniotic fluid: association with amniotic fluid cytokine levels and pregnancy outcome. *Am. J. Obstet. Gynecol.* **191:**1382–1386.

105. Peuchant, O., A. Menard, H. Renaudin, M. Morozumi, K. Ubukata, C. M. Bebear, and S. Pereyre. 2009. Increased macrolide resistance of *Mycoplasma pneumoniae* in France directly detected in clinical specimens by real-time PCR and melting curve analysis. *J. Antimicrob. Chemother.* **64:**52–58.

106. Phillips, L. E., K. H. Goodrich, R. M. Turner, and S. Faro. 1986. Isolation of *Mycoplasma* species and *Ureaplasma urealyticum* from obstetrical and gynecological patients by using commercially available medium formulations. *J. Clin. Microbiol.* **37:**377–379.

107. Pitcher, D., M. Sillis, and J. A. Robertson. 2001. Simple method for determining biovar and serovar types of *Ureaplasma urealyticum* clinical isolates using PCR-single-strand conformation polymorphism analysis. *J. Clin. Microbiol.* **39:**1840–1844.

108. Pratt, B. C. 1991. Recovery of *Mycoplasma hominis* from blood culture media. *Med. Lab. Sci.* **48:**350.

109. Quinn, P. A., L. U. Arshoff, and H. C. Li. 1981. Serotyping of *Ureaplasma urealyticum* by immunoperoxidase assay. *J. Clin. Microbiol.* **13:**670–676.

110. Ramirez, J. A., S. Ahkee, A. Tolentino, R. D. Miller, and J. T. Summersgill. 1996. Diagnosis of *Legionella pneumophila*, *Mycoplasma pneumoniae*, or *Chlamydia pneumoniae* lower respiratory infection using the polymerase chain reaction on a single throat swab specimen. *Diagn. Microbiol. Infect. Dis.* **24:**7–14.

111. Reznikov, M., T. K. Blackmore, J. J. Finlay-Jones, and D. L. Gordon. 1995. Comparison of nasopharyngeal aspirates and throat swab specimens in a polymerase chain reaction-based test for *Mycoplasma pneumoniae*. *Eur. J. Clin. Microbiol. Infect. Dis.* **14:**58–61.

112. Robertson, J. A., M. Alfa, and E. S. Boatman. 1983. Morphology of the cells and colonies of *Mycoplasma hominis*. *Sex. Transm. Dis.* **10:**232–239.

113. Robertson, J. A., L. E. Pyle, G. W. Stemke, and L. R. Finch. 1990. Human ureaplasmas show diverse genome sizes by pulsed-field electrophoresis. *Nucleic Acids Res.* **18:**1451–1455.

114. Rohner, P., I. Schnyder, B. Ninet, J. Schrenzel, D. Lew, T. Ramla, J. Garbino, and V. Jacomo. 2004. Severe *Mycoplasma hominis* infections in two renal transplant patients. *Eur. J. Clin. Microbiol. Infect. Dis.* **23:**203–204.

115. Sasaki, T., T. Kenri, N. Okazaki, M. Iseki, R. Yamashita, M. Shintani, Y. Sasaki, and M. Yayoshi. 1996. Epidemiological study of *Mycoplasma pneumoniae* infections in Japan based on PCR-restriction fragment length polymorphism of the P1 cytadhesin gene. *J. Clin. Microbiol.* **34:**447–449.

116. Schaeverbeke, T., C. B. Gilroy, C. Bebear, J. Dehais, and D. Taylor-Robinson. 1996. *Mycoplasma fermentans*, but not *M. penetrans*, detected by PCR assays in synovium from patients with rheumatoid arthritis and other rheumatic disorders. *J. Clin. Pathol.* **49:**824–828.

117. Schaeverbeke, T., H. Renaudin, M. Clerc, L. Lequen, J. P. Vernhes, B. De Barbeyrac, B. Bannwarth, C. Bebear, and J. Dehais. 1997. Systematic detection of mycoplasmas by culture and polymerase chain reaction (PCR) procedures in 209 synovial fluid samples. *Br. J. Rheumatol.* **36:**310–314.

118. Schelonka, R. L., B. Katz, K. B. Waites, and D. K. Benjamin, Jr. 2005. Critical appraisal of the role of *Ureaplasma* in the development of bronchopulmonary dysplasia with metaanalytic techniques. *Pediatr. Infect. Dis J.* **24:**1033–1039.

119. Sillis, M. 1993. Genital mycoplasmas revisited—an evaluation of a new culture medium. *Br. J. Biomed. Sci.* **50:**89–91.

120. Simms, I., K. Eastick, H. Mallinson, K. Thomas, R. Gokhale, P. Hay, A. Herring, and P. A. Rogers. 2003. Associations between *Mycoplasma genitalium*, *Chlamydia trachomatis* and pelvic inflammatory disease. *J. Clin. Pathol.* **56:**616–618.

121. Stamm, W. E., K. Running, J. Hale, and K. K. Holmes. 1983. Etiologic role of *Mycoplasma hominis* and *Ureaplasma urealyticum* in women with the acute urethral syndrome. *Sex. Transm. Dis.* **10:**318–322.

122. **Talkington, D. F., S. Shott, M. T. Fallon, S. B. Schwartz, and W. L. Thacker.** 2004. Analysis of eight commercial enzyme immunoassay tests for detection of antibodies to *Mycoplasma pneumoniae* in human serum. *Clin. Diagn. Lab. Immunol.* **11:**862–867.

123. **Talkington, D. F., K. B. Waites, S. B. Schwartz, and R. E. Besser.** 2001. Emerging from obscurity: understanding pulmonary and extrapulmonary syndromes, pathogenesis, and epidemiology of human *Mycoplasma pneumoniae* infections, p. 57–84. *In* W. M. Scheld, W. A. Craig, and J. M. Hughes (ed.), *Emerging Infections 5.* ASM Press, Washington, DC.

124. **Taylor-Robinson, D.** 1989. Genital mycoplasma infections. *Clin. Lab. Med.* **9:**501–523.

125. **Taylor-Robinson, D.** 1983. Metabolism inhibition test, p. 411–417. *In* J. G. Tully and S. Razin (ed.), *Methods in Mycoplasmology,* vol. 1. Academic Press, New York, NY.

126. **Taylor-Robinson, D.** 1986. Evaluation of the role of *Ureaplasma urealyticum* in infertility. *Pediatr. Infect. Dis. J.* **5:**S262–S265.

127. **Taylor-Robinson, D.** 2002. *Mycoplasma genitalium*—an update. *Int. J. STD AIDS* **13:**145–151.

128. **Taylor-Robinson, D.** 1996. Infections due to species of *Mycoplasma* and *Ureaplasma:* an update. *Clin. Infect. Dis.* **23:**671–682.

129. **Taylor-Robinson, D.** 2007. The role of mycoplasmas in pregnancy outcome. *Best Pract. Res. Clin. Obstet. Gynaecol.* **21:**425–438.

130. **Taylor-Robinson, D., and C. W. Csonka.** 1981. Laboratory and clinical aspects of mycoplasmal infections of the human genitourinary tract, p. 151–186. *In* J. W. Harris (ed.), *Recent Advances in Sexually Transmitted Diseases,* vol. 2. Churchill Livingstone, Ltd., Edinburgh, United Kingdom.

131. **Thacker, W. L., and D. F. Talkington.** 2000. Analysis of complement fixation and commercial enzyme immunoassays for detection of antibodies to *Mycoplasma pneumoniae* in human serum. *Clin. Diagn. Lab. Immunol.* **7:**778–780.

132. **Thacker, W. L., and D. F. Talkington.** 1995. Comparison of two rapid commercial tests with complement fixation for serologic diagnosis of *Mycoplasma pneumoniae* infections. *J. Clin. Microbiol.* **33:**1212–1214.

133. **Thomsen, A. C.** 1978. Mycoplasmas in human pyelonephritis: demonstration of antibodies in serum and urine. *J. Clin. Microbiol.* **8:**197–202.

134. **Touati, A., A. Benard, A. Ben Hassen, C. M. Bebear, and S. Pereyre.** 2009. Evaluation of five commercial real-time PCR assays for the detection of *Mycoplasma pneumoniae* in respiratory tract specimens. *J. Clin. Microbiol.* **47:**2269–2271.

135. **Tully, J. G., D. Taylor-Robinson, D. L. Rose, R. M. Cole, and J. M. Bove.** 1983. *Mycoplasma genitalium,* a new species from the human urogenital tract. *Int. J. Syst. Bacteriol.* **33:**387–396.

136. **Uno, M., T. Deguchi, H. Komeda, M. Hayasaki, M. Iida, M. Nagatani, and Y. Kawada.** 1997. *Mycoplasma genitalium* in the cervices of Japanese women. *Sex. Transm. Dis.* **24:**284–286.

137. **Waites, K., and D. Talkington.** 2005. New developments in human diseases due to mycoplasmas, p. 289–354. *In* A. Blanchard and G. Browning (ed.), *Mycoplasmas: Pathogenesis, Molecular Biology, and Emerging Strategies for Control.* Horizon Scientific Press, Norwich, United Kingdom.

138. **Waites, K. B.** 2008. Mycoplasma, p. 1145–1156. *In* D. Schlossberg (ed.), *Clinical Infectious Disease.* Cambridge University Press, Cambridge, United Kingdom.

139. **Waites, K. B., M. F. Balish, and T. P. Atkinson.** 2008. New insights into the pathogenesis and detection of *Mycoplasma pneumoniae* infections. *Future Microbiol.* **3:**635–648.

140. **Waites, K. B., C. M. Bebear, J. A. Robertson, D. F. Talkington, and G. E. Kenny (ed.).** 2001. *Cumitech 34, Laboratory Diagnosis of Mycoplasmal Infections,* ASM Press, Washington, DC.

141. **Waites, K. B., and K. C. Canupp.** 2001. Evaluation of BacT/ALERT system for detection of *Mycoplasma hominis* in simulated blood cultures. *J. Clin. Microbiol.* **39:**4328–4331.

142. **Waites, K. B., K. C. Canupp, and G. E. Kenny.** 1999. In vitro susceptibilities of *Mycoplasma hominis* to six fluoroquinolones as determined by E test. *Antimicrob. Agents Chemother.* **43:**2571–2573.

143. **Waites, K. B., D. M. Crabb, L. B. Duffy, and G. H. Cassell.** 1997. Evaluation of the Etest for detection of tetracycline resistance in *Mycoplasma hominis. Diagn. Microbiol. Infect. Dis.* **27:**117–122.

144. **Waites, K. B., L. B. Duffy, S. Schwartz, and D. F. Talkington.** 2004. *Mycoplasma* and *Ureaplasma,* p. 3.15.1–3.15.17. *In* H. Isenberg (ed.), *Clinical Microbiology Procedures Handbook,* 2nd ed. ASM Press, Washington, DC.

145. **Waites, K. B., T. A. Figarola, T. Schmid, D. M. Crabb, L. B. Duffy, and J. W. Simecka.** 1991. Comparison of agar versus broth dilution techniques for determining antibiotic susceptibilities of *Ureaplasma urealyticum. Diagn. Microbiol. Infect. Dis.* **14:**265–271.

146. **Waites, K. B., B. Katz, and R. L. Schelonka.** 2005. Mycoplasmas and ureaplasmas as neonatal pathogens. *Clin. Microbiol. Rev.* **18:**757–789.

147. **Waites, K. B., and D. F. Talkington.** 2004. *Mycoplasma pneumoniae* and its role as a human pathogen. *Clin. Microbiol. Rev.* **17:**697–728.

148. **Waites, K. B., D. F. Talkington, and C. M. Bebear.** 2002. Mycoplasmas, p. 201–224. *In* A. L. Truant (ed.), *Manual of Commercial Methods in Clinical Microbiology.* ASM Press, Washington, DC.

149. **Wang, R. Y., T. Grandinetti, J. W. Shih, S. H. Weiss, C. L. Haley, M. M. Hayes, and S. C. Lo.** 1997. *Mycoplasma genitalium* infection and host antibody immune response in patients infected by HIV, patients attending STD clinics and in healthy blood donors. *FEMS Immunol. Med. Microbiol.* **19:**237–245.

150. **Wang, R. Y., W. S. Hu, M. S. Dawson, J. W. Shih, and S. C. Lo.** 1992. Selective detection of *Mycoplasma fermentans* by polymerase chain reaction and by using a nucleotide sequence within the insertion sequence-like element. *J. Clin. Microbiol.* **30:**245–248.

151. **Webster, D., H. Windsor, C. Ling, D. Windsor, and D. Pitcher.** 2003. Chronic bronchitis in immunocompromised patients: association with a novel *Mycoplasma* species. *Eur. J. Clin. Microbiol. Infect. Dis.* **22:**530–534.

152. **Wilson, M. H., and A. M. Collier.** 1976. Ultrastructural study of *Mycoplasma pneumoniae* in organ culture. *J. Bacteriol.* **125:**332–339.

153. **Wolff, B. J., W. L. Thacker, S. B. Schwartz, and J. M. Winchell.** 2008. Detection of macrolide resistance in *Mycoplasma pneumoniae* by real-time PCR and high-resolution melt analysis. *Antimicrob. Agents Chemother.* **52:**3542–3549.

154. **Wood, J. C., R. M. Lu, E. M. Peterson, and L. M. de la Maza.** 1985. Evaluation of Mycotrim-GU for isolation of *Mycoplasma* species and *Ureaplasma urealyticum. J. Clin. Microbiol.* **22:**789–792.

155. **Xiao, L., T. P. Atkinson, J. Hagood, C. Makris, L. B. Duffy, and K. B. Waites.** 2009. Emerging macrolide resistance in *Mycoplasma pneumoniae* in children: detection and characterization of resistant isolates. *Pediatr. Infect. Dis.* **28:**693–698.

156. **Xin, D., Z. Mi, X. Han, L. Qin, J. Li, T. Wei, X. Chen, S. Ma, A. Hou, G. Li, and D. Shi.** 2009. Molecular mechanisms of macrolide resistance in clinical isolates of *Mycoplasma pneumoniae* from China. *Antimicrob. Agents Chemother.* **53:**2158–2159.

157. **Yoon, B. H., R. Romero, J. H. Lim, S. S. Shim, J. S. Hong, J. Y. Shim, and J. K. Jun.** 2003. The clinical significance of detecting *Ureaplasma urealyticum* by the polymerase chain reaction in the amniotic fluid of patients with preterm labor. *Am. J. Obstet. Gynecol.* **189:**919–924.

158. **Yoshida, T., S. Maeda, T. Deguchi, T. Miyazawa, and H. Ishiko.** 2003. Rapid detection of *Mycoplasma genitalium, Mycoplasma hominis, Ureaplasma parvum,* and *Ureaplasma urealyticum* organisms in genitourinary samples by PCR-microtiter plate hybridization assay. *J. Clin. Microbiol.* **41:**1850–1855.

159. **Zheng, X., L. J. Teng, H. L. Watson, J. I. Glass, A. Blanchard, and G. H. Cassell.** 1995. Small repeating units within the *Ureaplasma urealyticum* MB antigen gene encode serovar specificity and are associated with antigen size variation. *Infect. Immun.* **63:**891–898.

Chlamydiaceae*

CHARLOTTE GAYDOS AND ANDREAS ESSIG

60

TAXONOMY AND NOMENCLATURE

Chlamydia spp. are nonmotile, obligate intracellular prokaryotic pathogens characterized by a unique biphasic developmental cycle bearing two chlamydial forms that differ essentially in terms of morphology and function. According to the *Approved List of Bacterial Names*, published in 1980, the *Chlamydiaceae* contained one genus with just two species, *Chlamydia trachomatis* and *Chlamydia psittaci*, which were separated by their capability to accumulate glycogen in inclusions (Fig. 1A) and their susceptibility to sulfadiazine. In the 1990s, the application of DNA-based classification methods contributed to the recognition of the emerging human pathogen *Chlamydia pneumoniae* (31) and of *Chlamydia pecorum* (21), a pathogen of ruminants, as new species of the *Chlamydiaceae*. Phylogenetic analyses of the 16S and 23S rRNA genes were the rationale for the proposal of an emended description of the order *Chlamydiales* and a revised taxonomy of the family *Chlamydiaceae* in 1999 (19). According to this proposal, members of the order *Chlamydiales* are obligately intracellular bacteria that have the unique chlamydia-like developmental cycle and more than 80% sequence identity with chlamydial 16S rRNA genes and/or 23S rRNA genes. The emended order now includes four families: *Chlamydiaceae*, *Parachlamydiaceae*, *Simkaniaceae* (46), and *Waddliaceae* (83).

Early divergence of *C. trachomatis*-like strains in the *Chlamydiaceae* was postulated on the basis of sequence data from the ribosomal genes and supported by other data, such as genome size, glycogen production, and *ompA* sequence analysis. This led to the proposal to divide the family *Chlamydiaceae* into two genera, *Chlamydia* and *Chlamydophila* (19). As a consequence, *Chlamydia pneumoniae*, *Chlamydia psittaci*, and *Chlamydia pecorum* were proposed to be placed into the new genus *Chlamydophila*. However, the newly proposed nomenclature was controversial. The division into two genera was especially objected to by experts in the field who argued that the new genus designations ignore the unique, highly conserved biology shared by these organisms that was recognized when they were in a single genus (90). Although the new taxonomy was validly

published, the scientific chlamydia community has consistently rejected use of the term *Chlamydophila*, and its use has declined (96).

DESCRIPTION OF THE *CHLAMYDIACEAE*

The *Chlamydiaceae* contain the known human pathogens *C. trachomatis*, *C. pneumoniae*, and *C. psittaci* as well as organisms such as *C. abortus* and *C. felis* that have been associated only rarely with human infections. Members of the *Chlamydiaceae* show less than 10% overall 16S rRNA gene diversity and less than 10% overall 23S rRNA gene diversity. The genome sizes of the *Chlamydiaceae* range from 1.0 to 1.24 Mbp, with a G+C content of about 40%.

The cell wall harbors a common lipopolysaccharide (LPS) that differs from the LPS of other bacteria in its relatively low endotoxic activity. Accounting for about 60% of the protein mass, the 40-kDa chlamydial major outer membrane protein (MOMP) encoded by the *ompA* gene, is an important structural component of the organisms' outer membrane. The variable domains (VD1 through VD4) lead to multiple *C. trachomatis* serovars associated with different clinical manifestations of oculogenital infections. In contrast, *C. pneumoniae* isolates possess a strikingly high MOMP homology, and serovars of *C. pneumoniae* have not been described.

Members of the *Chlamydiaceae* share a unique biphasic developmental cycle leading to important consequences in laboratory diagnosis, clinical course, and antibiotic therapy. The elementary body (EB) of chlamydiae infects eukaryotic host cells and can survive for only a limited period of time outside the host cell. Once inside the host cell, EBs differentiate to metabolically active reticulate bodies (RB) that multiply by binary fission (Fig. 1D) within vacuoles that are continuously growing and that develop into large intracytoplasmic inclusions (Fig. 1C). Reticulate bodies reorganize back to EBs at the end of the chlamydial developmental cycle (Fig. 1D). After 48 to 72 h, hundreds of EBs are released from the host cell using two mutually exclusive pathways to perpetuate the infectious cycle (41). Genomic transcriptional analysis of the chlamydial developmental cycle revealed a small subset of genes that control the differentiation stages of the cycle and have evolutionary origins in eukaryotic lineages (2).

---

*This chapter contains material presented in chapter 63 by James B. Mahony, Brian K. Coombes, and Max A. Chernesky in the eighth edition of this *Manual*.

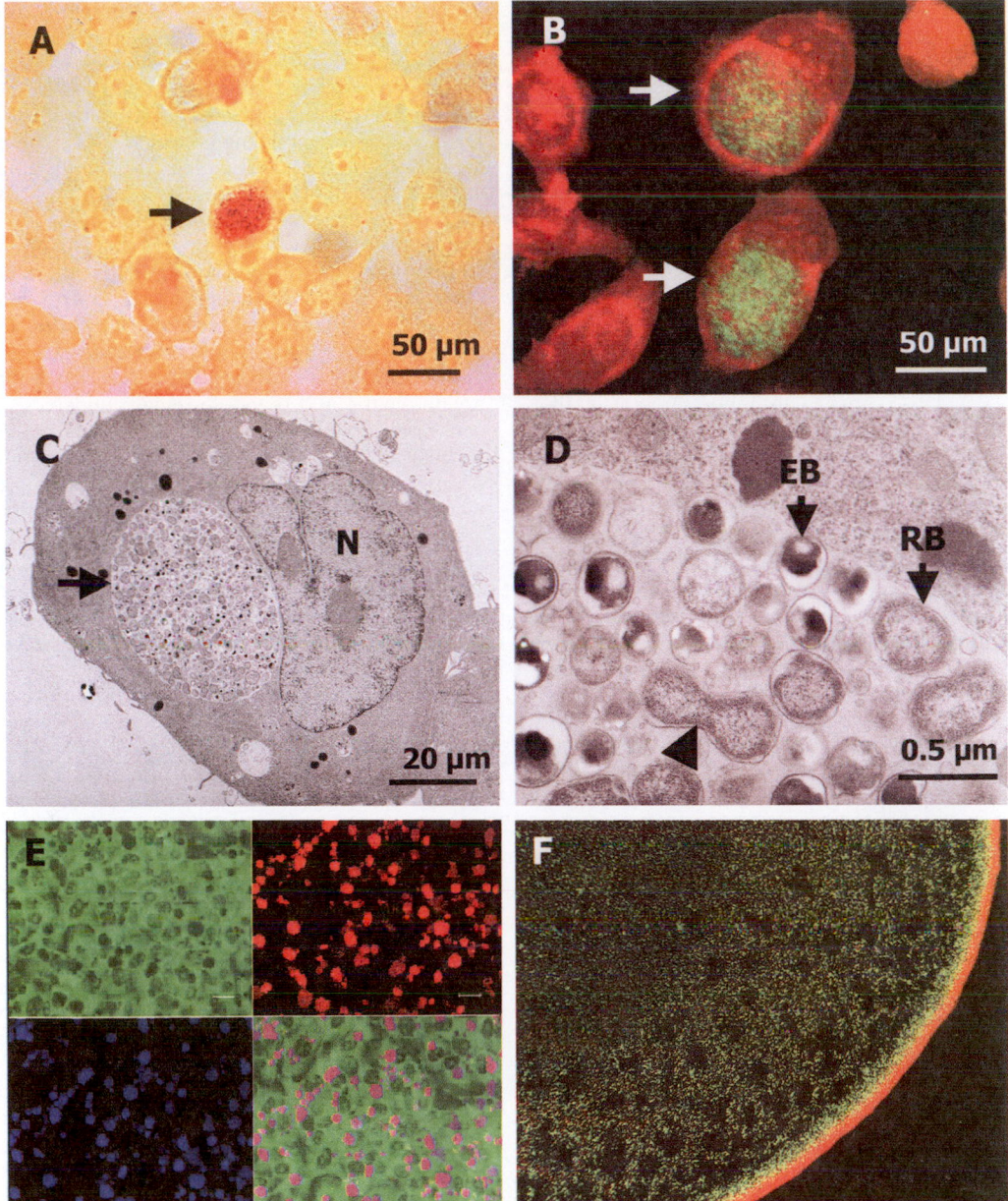

FIGURE 1 Identification of *C. trachomatis* by staining intracytoplasmic inclusions with iodine (A) and an FITC-conjugated monoclonal antibody directed at the MOMP (B). Transmission electron microscopy of a *C. pneumoniae*-infected cell shows an intracytoplasmic inclusion impressing the cell nucleus (C) and filled with EBs and RBs (D) at 60 h postinfection; the arrowhead shows a dividing RB. Identification of culture-grown *C. pneumoniae* by fluorescence in situ hybridization using rRNA targeted oligonucleotide probes (E). Simultaneous use of a Cy5-labeled probe that targets a chlamydial 16S rRNA sequence common to all members of the *Chlamydiaceae* (blue) and a Cy3-labeled probe specific for *C. pneumoniae* (red). Due to the overlap of colors, *C. pneumoniae* appears purple in the composite image; host cells are counterstained by a 5(6)-carboxyfluorescein-*N*-hydroxysuccinimide ester (FLUOS)-labeled eukaryotic probe (green). IgG-MIF image (magnification, ×400) showing bright homogeneous fluorescence of *C. pneumoniae* EBs at a serum dilution of 1:512 (F). (Photographs courtesy of Sonja Maier, Sven Poppert, and Ulrike Simnacher, Department of Medical Microbiology and Hygiene, University of Ulm; and Matthias Horn, Division of Microbial Ecology, University of Vienna.)

Evidence is accumulating that factors including gamma interferon, antibiotics, and nutrient deprivation may drive chlamydiae into a state of persistence. Persistent chlamydial forms are morphologically characterized by aberrant enlarged RBs located within small intracellular inclusions that are arrested in a viable but noninfectious state. It was proposed that persistence is an alternative life cycle used by chlamydiae to avoid the host immune response. As a consequence, chronic infections have been attributed to chlamydial persistence (14). However, the clinical significance of chlamydial persistence is still a matter of debate because diagnostic tools to detect persistence in the human host are lacking.

The chlamydiae can elicit the induction of apoptosis under some circumstances and actively inhibit apoptosis under others (9). This points to an important strategy that chlamydiae have evolved to promote their survival through the modulation of programmed cell death pathways in infected host cells.

Sequence information is now available for C. trachomatis, including lymphogranuloma venereum (LGV) isolates (95, 101), C. pneumoniae (47), C. caviae (78), C. abortus (102), and a Chlamydia-like endosymbiont of Acanthamoeba (39), and is in progress for C. muridarum. Genome analysis of this environmental chlamydial strain showed that about 700 million years ago the last common ancestor of pathogenic and symbiotic chlamydiae was already adapted to intracellular survival in early eukaryotes and contained many virulence factors found in modern pathogenic chlamydiae, including a type III secretion system (39). Comparison of the C. pneumoniae genome with the C. trachomatis genome has provided an understanding of the common biological processes required for infection and survival in mammalian cells. Prominent comparative findings include expansion of a novel family of 21 sequence-variant outer membrane proteins, conservation of a type III secretion virulence system, three serine/threonine protein kinases and a pair of paralogous phospholipase D-like proteins, additional purine and biotin biosynthetic capability, a homologue for aromatic amino acid (tryptophan) hydroxylase, and the loss of tryptophan biosynthesis genes (47).

CLINICAL SIGNIFICANCE, EPIDEMIOLOGY, AND TRANSMISSION

C. trachomatis

Based on the antigenic reactivity of the MOMP, C. trachomatis is currently divided into 18 serovars. Serovars A, B, Ba, and C can be isolated from patients with clinical trachoma in areas of endemicity in poor countries in Africa, the Middle East, Asia, and South America. Acute manifestations of trachoma include primarily a follicular kerato-conjunctivitis, while late-stage manifestations include tarsoconjunctival scarring with trichiasis, entropium, and subsequent loss of vision (93). According to estimates of the World Health Organization (WHO), approximately 1.3 million people in the world suffer from preventable blindness due to trachoma. Trachoma is transmitted under poor hygienic conditions between members of the same family or between families with shared facilities via discharges from the eyes of infected patients. Flies feeding from the mucopurulent eye discharges of infected and weakened humans may carry the organisms on their legs from one person to another across relatively long distances. A WHO global initiative aims to eliminate blinding trachoma by 2020.

The C. trachomatis serovars D through K, including the serovars Da and Ia and the genovariant Ja, are associated with genital tract disease and are among the most common sexually transmitted bacterial organisms in industrialized countries. According to surveillance data of the Centers for Disease Control and Prevention (CDC), these organisms are responsible for an estimated 2 to 3 million new cases every year in the United States, with 1,108,374 cases reported in 2007 in the United States. They typically cause nongonococcal urethritis in men and cervicitis in women. Infection of the urethra and the lower genital tract may cause dysuria, whitish or clear urethral or mucopurulent vaginal discharge, and postcoital bleeding. Urethritis and the rarer manifestations proctitis and conjunctivitis are observed with both men and women. The majority of infections are asymptomatic and therefore remain undetected (73). This can result in ascending infections, such as epididymitis in men and endometritis, salpingitis, pelvic inflammatory disease, and perihepatitis (Fitz-Hugh-Curtis syndrome) in women. Manifestations of upper genital infection in women are irregular uterine bleeding, pelvic discomfort, or chronic abdominal pain. Salpingitis may lead to tubal scarring and severe reproductive complications, such as tubal-factor infertility and ectopic pregnancy. Tubal-factor infertility attributable to C. trachomatis is the most frequent form of infection-induced infertility. C. trachomatis-infected pregnant women may transmit the organisms during delivery to the infants, who are therefore at risk to develop neonatal conjunctivitis and/or pneumonia (81, 82).

Sequelae of C. trachomatis infection in both men and women can involve HLA-B27-associated reactive arthritis, presenting most frequently as an acute asymmetric oligoarthritis with or without enthesopathic and extra-musculoskeletal symptoms (117). The young age of sexually active people is strongly associated with infection, with the highest prevalence in those 25 years or less (11). Additionally, sex workers, persons with a new sex partner, or persons who have had several sex partners are at increased risk of infection. In addition, high prevalence rates were found among incarcerated females entering juvenile and adult correctional facilities (43). Screening women who are at risk for C. trachomatis infection can prevent serious complications such as pelvic inflammatory disease (73). Consequently, female screening programs have been established in some European countries and the United States to identify and treat infections of asymptomatic individuals and their partners. Screening asymptomatic men has been discussed, and guidance for screening men was issued by the CDC in 2007 (http://www.cdc.gov/std/chlamydia/ChlamydiaScreening-males.pdf). However, the USPSTF concluded that the current evidence is insufficient to assess the balance of benefits and harms of screening for chlamydial infection for men (http://www.ahrq.gov/clinic/uspstf07/chlamydia/chlamydiars.htm#clinical).

The C. trachomatis serovars L1, L2, L2a, and L3 cause LGV, a systemic sexually transmitted disease that is endemic in parts of Africa, Asia, South America, and the Caribbean but rare in industrialized countries. However, ongoing reports about outbreaks with the newly identified variant L2b in Europe, Australia, and the United States show that health care providers should be vigilant for LGV especially among men who have sex with men (30, 70, 94, 114). The primary lesion, a small, painless papule that tends to ulcerate at the site of inoculation, often escapes attention. Proctitis is more common in people who practice receptive anal intercourse, and elevated white blood cell counts in anorectal smear specimens may predict LGV in these patients (105). Ulcer formation favors transmission of human immunodeficiency virus and other sexually transmitted and blood-borne diseases. The cardinal feature of LGV is the presence of painful inguinal and/or femoral lymphadenopathy. Complications of LGV include development of coalescing fluctuant lymph nodes (buboes) that result in discharging sinuses and fistula formation. If untreated, fibrosis can lead to lymphatic obstruction causing elephantiasis of the genitalia.

C. pneumoniae

C. pneumoniae causes infections of the upper and lower respiratory tract, such as sinusitis, pharyngitis, bronchitis, and pneumonia (51). C. pneumoniae was identified as the causative agent in 10 to 15% of cases of community-acquired pneumonia in adults (54) as well as in children (77) . However, data from studies yielding prevalence rates under 1% for C. pneumoniae pose the question of whether its role in community-acquired pneumonia is overestimated (97, 113). Severe and life-threatening C. pneumoniae infections have been described for patients with acute leukemia and treatment-induced neutropenia (35). Chronic infection with C. pneumoniae was reported among patients with chronic obstructive pulmonary disease and could also play a role in the natural history of asthma, including exacerbations. The clinical symptoms of C. pneumoniae infection are nonspecific and do not differ significantly from those caused by respiratory viruses and Mycoplasma pneumoniae. Persistent cough seems not to be strongly associated with C. pneumoniae (108). Primary infection occurs mainly in school-age children, while reinfection has been observed with adults. Seroprevalence rates from 40 to 70% show that C. pneumoniae is a widely spread organism in industrialized as well as developing countries.

The role of C. pneumoniae in the etiology of atherosclerosis, a chronic inflammatory disease of the artery vessel wall (80), has been discussed since 1988 when Saikku and coworkers presented serological evidence of an association of C. pneumoniae with coronary heart disease and acute myocardial infarction (85). In subsequent studies, the organisms were identified in atherosclerotic lesions of patients by culture, PCR, immunohistochemistry, and transmission electron microscopy; however, the discrepancies of study results (112), including those of animal studies and the failure of large-scale treatment studies (32), have raised skepticism about the organism's causative role in atherosclerosis (42). In addition, a heterogeneous spectrum of extrapulmonary diseases have been linked to C. pneumoniae, including multiple sclerosis, Alzheimer's disease, and chronic fatigue syndrome; however, a causal relationship between these diseases and C. pneumoniae infection has not been substantiated.

C. psittaci

Psittacine birds and a wide range of other avian species can act as natural reservoirs for C. psittaci. In the C. psittaci taxon (19), only the avian chlamydial strains previously designated Chlamydia psittaci are retained. Others have been placed into several animal-associated species, such as C. abortus, C. muridarum, C. suis, C. felis, and C. caviae. All birds are susceptible; however, pet birds (parrots, parakeets, macaws, and cockatiels) and poultry (turkeys and ducks) are the most frequently involved in C. psittaci transmission to humans. Exposure is greatest for poultry breeders and the processing workers, as well as in households with pet birds.

Infectious forms of the organisms are shed from symptomatic and from apparently healthy birds and may remain viable for several months. C. psittaci can be readily transmitted to humans either by direct contact with infected birds or following inhalation of aerosols from nasal discharges and from infectious fecal or feather dust. Transmission from person to person has been suggested but has never been proven. Symptomatic C. psittaci infection in humans may present as a severe chronic pneumonia (18), although mild illness and asymptomatic infections in persons exposed to infected birds have also been observed (66). Typical symptoms include fever, chills, muscular aches and pains, severe headache, hepato- and/or splenomegaly, and gastrointestinal symptoms. Cardiac complications may involve endocarditis and myocarditis. Fatal cases were common in the preantibiotic era. Due to quarantine of imported birds and improved veterinary-hygienic measures, outbreaks and sporadic cases of psittacosis are rarely observed nowadays. Since 1996, fewer than 50 confirmed cases have been reported in the United States each year.

C. abortus

Chlamydiae associated with ruminant abortion and formerly contained within the Chlamydia psittaci taxon were transferred to a new species: C. abortus (107). C. abortus has been acknowledged as a cause of abortion and fetal loss in sheep and has also been detected broadly in calves. There are a number of reports of pregnant women who have had spontaneous abortions following exposure to animals infected with C. abortus (76, 109). The incidence of this animal-acquired infection is not known, but sheep and goats during the birthing season represent a potential risk to pregnant women. Obstetricians should consider this diagnosis along with early antibiotic treatment and cesarean section delivery in the context of the patient's case history.

Environmental Chlamydiae

The host range of chlamydiae was further broadened with the discovery of Chlamydia-related endosymbionts in free-living amoebae. The so-called environmental chlamydiae that have been placed in the family Parachlamydiaceae share the chlamydial developmental cycle and represent an evolutionary early-diverging sister of the pathogenic chlamydiae (39). Environmental chlamydiae were discussed as potential emerging pathogens (33); however, clinical evidence for their importance in human infection is still pending. Simkania negevensis, currently the only member of the Simkaniaceae, is a recently discovered Chlamydia-like intracellular agent which has been associated with respiratory infections in infants (46). The natural host of Simkania is not known; however, the organisms were successfully grown in various cell lines as well as in free-living amoebae and were identified in drinking water and in reclaimed wastewater.

COLLECTION, TRANSPORT, AND STORAGE

General Comments

Since chlamydiae are obligate intracellular pathogens, the objective of specimen collection should usually be to include the host cells that harbor the organisms. Outside their host, chlamydiae survive only briefly, and efforts must be undertaken to maintain the organisms' viability for successful culture. Commercial diagnostic nonculture assays do not require the presence of viable chlamydiae in the specimen; nevertheless, the instructions of the manufacturer given in the package insert should be followed for appropriate collection, transport, and storage of specimens. This includes the use of swabs and transport media specified by the manufacturer.

For successful culture of chlamydiae, the time between collection and processing of the specimens in the laboratory should be minimized while keeping specimens cold (4 to 8°C). Specimens should be forwarded to the laboratory within 24 h in a special chlamydial transport medium, such as 2-sucrose phosphate or sucrose phosphate glutamate supplemented with fetal bovine serum (5 to 10%), gentamicin (10 μg/ml), vancomycin (25 to 100 μg/ml), and amphotericin B (2 μg/ml) or nystatin (25 U/ml). Tetracyclines, macrolides, and penicillins cannot be used in the transport media since they have activity against chlamydiae. If specimens cannot be processed within 24 h, storage at −70°C in transport media is acceptable. Specimens for culture should not be stored at −20°C or in frost-free freezers. Swab specimens should be collected on swabs with a Dacron tip and an aluminum or plastic shaft. Swab tips made of calcium alginate and swabs with wooden shafts may inhibit the growth of chlamydiae. It is recommended to check new lots of swabs that are used to collect specimens for culture of chlamydiae for possible inhibition of chlamydial growth (16).

C. trachomatis

The type and anatomical site of specimen collection for laboratory diagnosis of C. trachomatis infection depend on both the clinical picture and the laboratory test selection, as comprehensively reviewed elsewhere (4, 23, 44, 56, 93). Table 1 gives an overview about ranges of sensitivity and specificity for common diagnostic tests for C. trachomatis in urogenital specimens. Noninvasively collected specimens such as first-void urine (FVU; first 10 to 30 ml of urine) and vaginal swab specimens are excellent for diagnosis of C. trachomatis genital tract infection by nucleic acid amplification techniques (NAATs). Sensitivity and specificity of NAATs for C. trachomatis on noninvasively collected specimens are similar to those obtained on samples collected directly from the cervix or urethra (25, 88). Patients and clinicians may prefer self-sampling to the standard collection methods (40). FVU specimens should be obtained at least 2 h after the last micturition. Ambient-temperature storage of fresh unprocessed urine should not exceed 24 h to avoid denaturation of chlamydial DNA. Subsequent processing of the urine specimens for NAAT varies depending on the manufacturer's instructions. Neither urine nor vaginal specimens are recommended for testing by culture and nonamplification assays, such as enzyme immunoassay (EIA), direct fluorescence assay (DFA), and nucleic acid hybridization (NAH), because of their relatively very low sensitivity with these assays (44).

Traditional sites for specimen collection in C. trachomatis genital tract infection involve the endocervix in females and the urethra in males. Newly recommended specimen additions include vaginal samples for women and urine for men, but only when highly sensitive nucleic acid amplification tests are used (23, 86). Proficient specimen collection including speculum examination in females is required to obtain appropriate samples that contain sufficient columnar or squamocolumnar cells. Purulent discharges have to be cleaned before a swab is inserted 1 to 2 cm into the cervical os past the squamocolumnar junction, rotated more than two times, and removed without touching the vaginal mucosa (4). Urethral specimens from males are collected by placing a dry swab 3 or 4 cm into the urethra and rotating prior to removal. Urination prior to specimen collection may reduce test sensitivity by washing out infected columnar cells. Since culture and older less-sensitive tests are falling into disuse, the preferred samples recommended for screening asymptomatic women are vaginal swabs, which can be self-collected for some assays. Self-obtained vaginal swabs are gaining in practical use and have been recommended as highly accurate and acceptable samples by the NIH and CDC (38). It was shown that for women, self-collected vaginal swabs had a clearly higher mean chlamydial load than did first-void urine specimens (115).

Table 1 Ranges of sensitivity and specificity for diagnostic tests for C. trachomatis in urogenital specimens [a]

Diagnostic method	Sensitivity (%)	Specificity (%)
Tissue culture	70–85	100
DFA	80–85	>99
EIA	53–76	95
Direct hybridization	65–83	99
PCR		
Cervical swabs	89.7	99.4
Female urine	89.2	99.0
Male urine	90.3	98.4
Strand displacement amplification		
Cervical swabs	92.8	98.1
Female urine	80.5	98.4
Male urine	94.5	91.4
Male urethral swabs	94.6	94.2
Transcription-mediated amplification		
Cervical swabs	94.2	97.6
Vaginal swabs	96.6–96.7	97.6–97.1
Female urine	94.7	98.9
Male urine	97.0	99.1
Male urethral	95.2	98.2

[a] Sensitivities and specificities are adapted from clinical trial data and are published in package inserts.

In women with salpingitis, samples may be collected by needle aspiration of the involved fallopian tube. Endometrial specimens have also yielded chlamydiae. Further appropriate sites include the conjunctiva in chlamydial eye infection (trachoma, inclusion conjunctivitis, and newborn conjunctivitis) and the nasopharynx and deeper respiratory tract of infants in newborn pneumonia. For men who have sex with men, screening of rectal and pharyngeal specimens is recommended since some reports support the utility of commercial NAATs as a screening test for this population (49, 89). In cases of suspected LGV, ulcer swabs, aspirates of bubo fluid, and rectal or urethral swabs should be collected in transport medium. Buboes of LGV may contain only small amounts of thin milky fluid, and it may be necessary to inject 2 to 5 ml of sterile saline to obtain any fluid by aspiration (56).

C. pneumoniae

The optimal sites for specimen collection in C. *pneumoniae* infection are poorly defined. Respiratory specimens from which the organisms were cultured include sputum, bronchoalveolar lavage fluid, nasopharyngeal aspirates, throat washings, and throat swabs (tonsil area). Swab specimens should be collected using a Dacron tip and a plastic shaft (16) and placed immediately in transport medium. Specimens need to be kept at 4 to 8°C in chlamydial transport medium, since the organisms are inactivated rapidly at room temperature. Rapid freezing or freezing and thawing of specimens should be avoided (51). Liquid specimens are collected in transport medium at a specimen-to-medium ratio of 1:2 (16). Testing of vascular tissue specimens and blood samples, except for research studies, is of questionable value.

C. psittaci

C. *psittaci* strains seem to be the most stable organisms among the pathogenic chlamydiae. Nevertheless, specimens should be collected in chlamydial transport medium. Appropriate specimens include sputum, bronchoalveolar lavage fluid, pleural fluid, blood, and tissue biopsy specimens from various anatomical sites. Culture is no longer recommended because of the potential for laboratory acquired infections. There are only single commercial nonculture tests for C. *psittaci* (7) available; however, a panel of research nucleic acid amplification assays has been published (28, 57, 64).

DIRECT EXAMINATION

Nucleic Acid Amplification Techniques

C. trachomatis

Due to their high sensitivity and specificity, NAATs are the tests of choice for diagnosis of genital C. *trachomatis* infections in routine clinical laboratories. NAATs can be used to detect C. *trachomatis* without a pelvic examination or intraurethral swab specimen by testing self- or clinician-collected vaginal swabs or urine, respectively (13, 86). This facilitates the establishment of screening programs in asymptomatic individuals and may enhance the compliance for testing asymptomatic contact persons of infected individuals. NAATs on urine, with confirmation, were shown to be adequate for use as a new forensic standard for diagnosis of C. *trachomatis* and *Neisseria gonorrhoeae* in children suspected of being sexual abused (5). Increasing experience

is available for the use of NAATs in conjunctival, oropharyngeal, and rectal samples (49, 89) and in LGV (12, 98). Thus far, no commercial company has an FDA-cleared test for these alternative sample types, but it is possible for laboratories to use these samples for testing by NAATs if they perform a verification study to indicate their performance. If such verification is performed, CLIA compliance can be demonstrated (http://www.aphl.org/aphlprograms/infectious/std/Pages/stdtestingguidelines.aspx). Commercial NAATs seem to work in newborn conjunctivitis (82), but no one has an FDA claim. For research studies of trachoma patients, NAATs have been recommended as the "gold standard" and are now being used by many research laboratories. However, the commercial assays presently available may be too expensive and too complex for use in some national trachoma programs (93). In many evaluations, NAATs detected 20 to 30% more positive specimens than could be detected by earlier technologies.

Licensed NAATs for detection of C. *trachomatis* include (in the order of their introduction) the PCR-based Roche Amplicor (Roche Diagnostics, Basel, Switzerland), the Aptima transcription-mediated amplification assay (Gen-Probe, Inc., San Diego, CA) and the BD ProbeTec strand displacement amplification (SDA) assay (Becton Dickinson and Company, Diagnostic Systems, Franklin Lakes, NJ). The former, frequently used Abbott LCx ligase chain reaction was withdrawn from the commercial market by the manufacturer in 2003. Licensed assays working on fully automated platforms for use in high-volume laboratories include the Cobas TaqMan, Abbott m2000, BD ProbeTec (Viper), and Aptima (Tigris) (53, 61).

Both the PCR and SDA assay amplify nucleotide sequences of the 7.5-kbp cryptic plasmid of C. *trachomatis*, which is present in an average copy number of about four plasmids per chromosome in EBs and up to seven plasmids per chromosome in replicating RBs (74). C. *trachomatis* strains that do not harbor the cryptic plasmid have been isolated sporadically from urethral specimens. A new variant of C. *trachomatis* with clinical and epidemiological relevance was recently discovered in Sweden. Due to a 377-bp deletion in the target sequence for nucleic acid amplification, this strain has initially escaped detection by some of the licensed NAATs (37, 65), but manufacturers affected by this discovery moved quickly to modify their primers to enable this variant's detection. The transcription-mediated amplification-based assays target specific sequences of the 23S rRNA, which is also present in multiple copies. Each of the three commercially available NAAT systems offers the option for combination testing of C. *trachomatis* and *Neisseria gonorrhoeae* in the same specimen. The transcription-mediated amplification platform is also offered as individual assays for chlamydia infection or gonorrhea.

Considering the multiplicity of target sites for the amplification procedures being used, NAATs should be able to produce a positive signal from less than one EB; however, the actual sensitivity with clinical specimens is lower because of sampling variability and inefficient nucleic acid isolation. Since inhibitor problems of NAATs can be reduced by dilution of specimens, heating, freeze-thaw cycles, or overnight storage at 4°C, the use of internal inhibitor controls of the amplification assays (as supplied by the manufacturers of PCR and SDA) is helpful for identification of clinical specimens containing inhibitory factors (59). Extraction of nucleic acids by target capture and magnetic bead procedures by second-generation NAATs has almost completely eliminated the presence of inhibitors in processed clinical samples. All these NAAT assays are highly specific for chlamydiae if problems with cross-contamination, labeling errors, and mistakes in specimen collection can be avoided (Table 1). Confirmatory testing of positive specimens was recommended by the CDC if a low positive predictive value was expected (<90%) or if a false-positive result would have serious psychosocial or legal consequences (44). However, supplemental testing is no longer recommended for chlamydia (http://www.aphl.org/aphlprograms/infectious/std/Pages/stdtestingguidelines.aspx) or for diagnosis of C. trachomatis and Neisseria gonorrhoeae in children suspected of having been sexually abused (5, 87).

In settings where resources are limited, including developing countries, the concept of pooling to detect C. trachomatis by NAATs has proved to be a simple, accurate, and cost-effective procedure compared to individual testing (45, 55). Specimen pools may consist of aliquots from 4 to 10 processed specimens (FVU or genital swab) combined into one amplification tube. Subsequent testing of individual samples is required only if the pooled sample gives a positive result. Following this strategy, considerable savings of reagent costs can be obtained, especially in low-prevalence populations.

C. pneumoniae

A vast number of PCR-based protocols using different formats and target genes have been developed in research laboratories for detection of C. pneumoniae in both respiratory and nonrespiratory samples (50). However, the lack of a reliable gold standard for C. pneumoniae infection has made it difficult to evaluate the published protocols thoroughly. Broad application of NAATs for diagnosis of C. pneumoniae infection has been hampered because many PCR protocols are not reliable or robust enough to provide reproducible results in routine clinical laboratories. Even in specialized laboratories, there seems to be a substantial interlaboratory variation in the performance of C. pneumoniae NAATs, and the need for quality control and standardization of these assays has been recognized (16, 50). Subsequently, specific recommendations for standardizing C. pneumoniae PCR assays were made, and it was suggested that the performance of newly developed PCR protocols be compared with that of at least one of four recommended assays that target the PSTI fragment (10), the ompA gene (104), or the 16S rRNA gene (24, 57). However, all of these assays must be considered research tools (16), because commercial FDA-cleared assays are currently not available. Real-time PCR technology provides promising results that warrant further evaluation of this approach for detection of C. pneumoniae infection (1, 79, 103). A recent review again stated that standardization and validation, particularly of PCR assays, are urgently needed because the true role of the organism in respiratory infections as well as in extrapulmonary diseases cannot be ascertained at the moment (50).

C. psittaci

NAATs could be helpful for detection of avian C. psittaci strains from clinical samples since culture of these organisms is dangerous and requires biosafety level 3 (BSL-3) facilities and is not recommended. Some PCR-based assays have been developed for diagnosis of human ornithosis (7, 18, 57, 63, 104), and a commercially available DNA microarray assay for detection and species identification of human and zoonotic chlamydiae has been introduced (7). Due to the rarity of the disease, the performance characteristics of these assays have been poorly evaluated in clinical specimens.

Nucleic Acid Hybridization

Two NAH tests are commercially available for detection of C. trachomatis. The Gen-Probe PACE 2 test (Gen-Probe, Inc.) hybridizes to a species-specific sequence of chlamydial 16S rRNA that is present in a high copy number in replicating chlamydiae. Available data suggest that it is about as sensitive as the better antigen detection and cell culture methods and is relatively specific. However, it was shown that commercial NAATs improved the detection of infections in women by 17 to 38% compared to PACE 2 (6). The second NAH test, the Digene Hybrid Capture II, is a nucleic acid probe-signal amplification assay (Digene Corp., Gaithersburg, MD) that uses RNA hybridization probes for DNA sequences encoding both genomic and cryptic plasmid sequences of C. trachomatis. This assay was shown to reach the sensitivity of a commercial NAAT when cervical specimens were investigated (106). NAHs are considered highly robust test methods for detection of C. trachomatis. NAH tests have been recommended for endocervical swabs or urethral swabs from men when a NAAT is not available or not economical. As is the case with other non-NAATs, NAH tests have not been recommended for use in noninvasive-collection specimens, such as urine and vaginal swabs (44). Both NAH systems also offer a test format that enables detection of C. trachomatis and N. gonorrhoeae in a single specimen. However, their use is rapidly being replaced by NAAT assays, which is now the test platform of choice for chlamydia tests.

Antigen Detection Assays

DFA

The presence of typical intracytoplasmic inclusions in columnar epithelial cells of the conjunctiva, urethra, or cervix of infected patients can be demonstrated when air-dried smears are fixed on a slide with absolute methanol and stained with Giemsa stain. Cytological testing was particularly useful in diagnosing acute inclusion conjunctivitis of the newborn, but the more sensitive immunofluorescence procedures have largely replaced this method. DFAs use fluorescein isothiocyanate (FITC)-conjugated monoclonal antibodies directed at a C. trachomatis-specific epitope of the MOMP (Chlamydia Cel [Cellabs, Brookvale, Australia] or Pathfinder [Bio-Rad Laboratories, Redmond, WA]). DFAs are based on detecting EBs in smears, although staining of inclusions can also succeed if intact infected host cells are collected. Checking for the presence of columnar cells allows assessment of the adequacy of the sample. The procedure offers rapid diagnosis, taking only 30 min to perform, making DFAs useful, especially for laboratories that test only a limited number of specimens. However, this method requires an experienced microscopist who can distinguish between fluorescing chlamydial particles and nonspecific fluorescence. The DFA has approximately 75 to 85% sensitivity and 98 to 99% specificity compared with culture and a lower sensitivity than NAATs (8, 69). DFAs can be another alternative for testing endocervical swabs from females or urethral swabs from males when a NAAT is not available or not economical. In addition, DFAs have been recommended for use with conjunctival specimens and for testing of individuals with possible rectal and pharyngeal exposure to C. trachomatis, if a C. trachomatis MOMP-specific antibody is used (44). Non-trachomatis chlamydial conjunctivitis should be considered if the DFA reveals the presence of chlamydial LPS but not C. trachomatis-specific MOMP.

EIA

EIAs for the detection of *C. trachomatis* use either monoclonal or polyclonal antibodies to detect chlamydial LPS, which is more soluble than MOMP. Although they can theoretically detect all chlamydiae, EIAs have not been well evaluated for the diagnosis of infections with *C. pneumoniae* or *C. psittaci*. The performance characteristics of EIAs for laboratory diagnosis of *C. trachomatis* have been reviewed comprehensively elsewhere (4). Using cultures as reference standards, the sensitivities of EIAs applied to endocervical swabs were in a range from 62 to 72% (69). EIAs are never recommended for testing of noninvasively collected specimens, such as urine and vaginal swabs. EIAs are now considered substandard and are not recommended for use as a diagnostic platform by the CDC.

Rapid or point-of-care (POC) tests designed for office- or clinic-based settings have been developed and provide test results in less than 30 min for *C. trachomatis* infection in women. Similar to EIAs, they also use antibodies against chlamydial LPS, with the potential to yield false-positive results due to cross-reaction with other gram-negative bacteria. Current POC tests are not recommended in laboratory settings because sensitivity and specificity are lower, quality controls are less rigorous, and costs are higher than for tests designed for laboratory use (44). Although some POC assays are FDA cleared, they were compared to culture as the gold standard and now that the new gold standard is NAATs, the package inserts often overstate sensitivities. When compared to PCR, the Clearview POC demonstrated a sensitivity of 32.8% for vaginal swabs and 49.7% for cervical swabs (116). New POC assays are being developed and appear promising but are not yet FDA cleared (58).

ISOLATION PROCEDURES

Biosafety Considerations

C. pneumoniae and *C. trachomatis* are BSL-2 organisms, whereas *C. psittaci* is a BSL-3 organism. Transmission of the organisms from patient specimens or infected cell cultures can occur through aerosols, splashes onto the mucous membranes of the eyes, and hand-to-face actions. In recent years, fewer laboratory-acquired infections have been reported, probably due to the common usage of class II biosafety cabinets in laboratories that work with *Chlamydia*-infected cell cultures. Use of a class II biosafety cabinet protects laboratory staff from exposure to aerosols as well as specimens and cell cultures from contamination. Additional means of preventing laboratory-acquired infection include the use of gloves, alcohol-based hand disinfectants, safety centrifuge caps, and face protection, if appropriate. Laboratory infections with *C. trachomatis* usually manifest as follicular conjunctivitis. The LGV strains are more invasive, and severe cases of laboratory-associated pneumonia and lymphadenitis are reported. *C. psittaci* must be considered a potentially dangerous organism, requiring appropriate BSL-3 facilities. Laboratory-acquired *C. pneumoniae* infections might be underestimated since the mild clinical course may not prompt infected laboratory workers to seek medical attention.

Specimen Processing

Ocular and Genital Tract Specimens

For culture of chlamydiae from ocular and genital tract sites, only swabs that are rapidly forwarded to the laboratory in a special chlamydial transport medium are acceptable (see above). Specimens to be assayed by commercial EIA, DFA, NAH, or NAAT should be processed as directed by the manufacturer.

Bubo Pus

To prepare bubo pus, the aspirate fluid of fluctuant lymph nodes is ground and then suspended in nutrient broth or cell culture medium to at least 20% by weight. Even when the pus is not viscous, dilution is advisable. The material should be tested for bacterial contaminants and inoculated onto monolayer cultures of McCoy or HeLa 229 cells.

Blood

Blood samples from clotted blood tubes have been used in the past for diagnosis of *C. psittaci* endocarditis. The blood clot was ground, and cell culture medium was added to make a 10% solution. However culture is no longer recommended for *C. psittaci* due to the possibility of laboratory acquired infections, so this method is reserved for specialized research laboratories

Sputum, Throat Washings, and Other Secretions from the Respiratory Tract

Sputum and other respiratory samples are suspended in antibiotic-containing transport medium or cell culture medium at a ratio of specimen to medium of 1:2 to 1:10, depending on specimen consistency. Specimens are homogenized by adding sterile glass beads to the sample and vigorously vortexing for 1 to 2 min in a tightly stoppered container. Extracts should be centrifuged for 20 to 30 min at $100 \times g$ to remove coarse material before the supernatant fluid is inoculated onto cell monolayers. Serial dilutions may be required if the inoculum is toxic to cells.

Fecal Samples

Human rectal swabs for *C. trachomatis* and avian material for *C. psittaci* are suspended in chlamydial transport medium or antibiotic-containing cell culture medium. The suspension is shaken thoroughly and centrifuged at $300 \times g$ for 10 min, and the supernatant is removed. It may be further diluted (1:2 and 1:20) with medium before being inoculated into cell culture. Rectal swabs for a commercial NAAT are processed in accordance with the corresponding protocol of the manufacturer.

Tissue Samples

Frozen tissue is thawed in a refrigerator at 4°C. The specimen is weighed, minced with sterile scissors or a scalpel, and ground with a mortar and pestle or homogenizer. A volume of cell culture medium required to make a 10 to 20% suspension is added, and the suspension is thoroughly mixed. For tissue specimens, serial dilutions (1:10 to 1:100) are often required for inoculation to prevent toxicity.

Isolation

Cell culture was considered the gold standard for diagnosis of genital *C. trachomatis* infection because its sensitivity and specificity were thought to be close to 100%. Problems associated with cell culture isolation of chlamydiae, including technical complexity and long turnaround time, and stringent requirements related to collection, transport, and storage of specimens have driven the development of commercially available nonculture methods that have found widespread application in many routine laboratories. With the advent of antigen detection methods, it became clear that the sensitivity of culture was substantially lower than previously thought, probably due mostly to the presence of nonviable chlamydiae that died during transport and processing. Culture for detection of chlamydiae in clinical specimens is now performed generally only in specialized laboratories (4). Culture is recommended in treatment failures (when a viable isolate is needed for susceptibility testing) and in cases related to possible sexual assault for medicolegal reasons (44), although NAATs on urine have been shown to be adequate for children suspected of being sexually abused (5).

Historically, chlamydiae were cultivated in the yolk sac of embryonated eggs. The yolk sac method (for details, see reference 91) is still used for preparing antigens for the microimmunofluorescence (MIF) test. The ability to propagate chlamydiae in the laboratory has greatly increased the understanding of diagnosis and pathogenesis of chlamydial infections (92). For isolation of chlamydiae from clinical specimens, appropriately collected and transported samples are inoculated onto preformed cell monolayers. A number of susceptible permanent cell lines, including McCoy, HeLa 229, HEp-2, HL, BGMK, Vero, and L cells, have been used. Clinical samples are centrifuged onto monolayers to enhance infection. Strains of *C. psittaci* and LGV biovars are capable of serial growth in cell culture without centrifugation. Cultures are incubated for 48 to 72 h in the presence of the host cell protein synthesis inhibitor cycloheximide. McCoy and HeLa 229 cells are most commonly used for *C. trachomatis*. HL and HEp-2 cells seem to be more sensitive for recovery of the fastidious *C. pneumoniae* from clinical specimens. Visualization of cell culture-grown chlamydiae is achieved by the immunostaining of inoculated cell monolayers for intracytoplasmic inclusions. A positive culture shows one or more typical intracellular inclusions (Fig. 1B).

Cell culture methods can vary among laboratories. Host cells are plated either onto 12-mm glass coverslips contained in 15-mm-diameter (1 dram [1 dram = 3.697 ml]) disposable glass vials (shell vial method) or in 6-, 12-, or 24-well tissue culture plates. The cells are seeded in concentrations of 1×10^5 to 2×10^5 cells/ml to give a healthy and confluent monolayer after 24 to 48 h of incubation. For optimal results, cell monolayers should be inoculated with patient specimens within 24 h after reaching confluency. Clinical specimens are thoroughly vortexed with glass beads in tightly closed screw-cap vials to facilitate release of chlamydiae before inoculation. The cell culture medium of the cell monolayers to be inoculated is discarded and replaced by a volume of 0.2 to 2 ml of the vortexed specimen. The inoculated specimen is centrifuged onto the cell monolayers at 900 to 3,000 × *g* for 1 h at 22 to 35°C. Cells are incubated at 35°C for 1 to 2 h to allow uptake of chlamydiae before the medium is replaced with chlamydial isolation medium consisting of the cell culture medium supplemented with fetal calf serum (10%), L-glutamine (2 mM), cycloheximide (1 to 2 μg/ml), gentamicin (10 μg/ml), vancomycin (25 μg/ml), and amphotericin B (2 μg/ml). Cultures are incubated at 35°C in 5% CO_2 for 48 to 72 h. Then, one coverslip per specimen is removed for immunostaining of inoculated monolayers. Both cell detritus and toxic effects of the inoculum may make it difficult to read slides. Dilution of cell-rich material (bubo pus, sputum, tissue samples, and rectal swabs) and blind performance of subpassages can be helpful for microscopic interpretation of slides.

If a blind subpassage or passage of positive material is to be performed, the corresponding cell monolayers of duplicate wells are scraped and disrupted by vortexing with glass beads. Cell debris of harvested material is removed by low-speed centrifugation (300 × *g*) for 10 min, and the supernatant is passed onto preformed cell monolayers as described above. For *C. pneumoniae*, most laboratories agree that at least two passages are needed to maximize the recovery of the organisms from respiratory specimens. Modifications of the standard procedure, including use of serum-free culture medium, pretreatment of cell monolayers with polyethylene glycol or diethylaminoethyl-dextran, and extension of culture times, have not been sufficiently tested to warrant their routine recommendation (16). Laboratories processing large numbers of specimens may use flat-bottom 48- or 96-well microtiter plates onto which cells are plated directly. Processing and incubation are as described above, but microscopy is modified because cells are stained directly in the well, requiring use of inverted microscopes and long working objectives.

Continuous quality control is important for maintaining a sensitive and specific culture system. Because of its technical complexity, there are multiple opportunities to modify factors in the culture system that may impact the isolation efficiency (92, 93). Therefore, positive controls with a known number of inclusion-forming units should be run routinely to check the sensitivity of the culture system. Negative controls with uninfected human cells may help to evaluate episodes of cross-contamination as a result of handling positive patient specimens or positive controls. Routine testing of cell culture systems for *Mycoplasma* contamination has been recommended because *Mycoplasma* contamination may impair the growth of chlamydiae and may decrease the sensitivity of the culture system (16).

IDENTIFICATION

The basic procedure for detection of isolated chlamydiae involves demonstration of intracytoplasmic inclusions by fluorescent-antibody staining that provides both morphological and immunological identification of chlamydiae. Screening of cultures can be performed with a commercially available FITC-conjugated monoclonal anti-LPS antibody (Pathfinder; Bio-Rad), which recognizes all chlamydiae known to cause infections in humans. Confirmation of positive genital cultures can be done by the use of a *C. trachomatis* MOMP-specific monoclonal antibody (Fig. 1B). For respiratory cultures, a *C. pneumoniae*-specific monoclonal antibody may additionally be appropriate. Monoclonal antibodies specific for *C. psittaci* are not commercially available. Using DFA procedures, inclusions of *C. trachomatis*-infected cells are visible at 24 h postinfection. Less expensive but also less sensitive methods that were commonly used before the advent of monoclonal antibodies include Giemsa staining (which needs an experienced and well-trained microscopist for interpretation) and iodine staining for identification of glycogen-containing inclusions that are produced by *C. trachomatis* but not by *C. psittaci* or *C. pneumoniae* (Fig. 1A).

Identification of replicating chlamydiae can also be done by fluorescence in situ hybridization using fluorescently labeled oligonucleotide probes complementary to order-, genus-, and species-specific target sites on the chlamydial 16S rRNA molecules (75). The risk of false-positive signals caused by nonspecific binding of the fluorescent dyes to nontarget organisms or structures of the host cells can be minimized by the simultaneous application of multiple probes with hierarchical specificity labeled with different dyes, leading to a characteristic hybridization pattern (Fig. 1E)

TYPING SYSTEMS

Serotyping and genotyping procedures are important tools for epidemiological studies. They are of clinical use if medicolegal issues are involved or if LGV is suspected. The most convenient method for serotyping *C. trachomatis* isolates appears to be the microwell typing system (100), in which inclusions in microtiter plates are stained with pools of monoclonal antibodies (available at Washington Research Foundation, Seattle, WA) that recognize serovar- and subspecies-specific epitopes of the MOMP. Genotyping of *C. trachomatis* isolates usually involves either restriction fragment length polymorphism analysis of the MOMP-encoding *ompA* gene or sequence analysis of the VDs in the *ompA* gene. These variable regions include the peptides responsible for species, serovar, and serogroup specificities. PCR amplification and sequencing of *ompA* using extracted DNA from patient specimens, such as urine or genital samples, allows direct genotyping from *C. trachomatis*-positive individuals without isolation of the organisms. In addition, new high-resolution genotyping methods applying a multilocus variable number tandem repeat assay or multilocus sequence typing have been introduced (71). *ompA*-based procedures (27), including real-time PCR with high-resolution melt analysis (64) and DNA microarray technology (84) are used to identify all known and additional new genotypes of avian *C. psittaci* strains. Different serotypes or genotypes of *C. pneumoniae* have not been described.

SEROLOGIC TESTS

Serologic testing may be helpful in the diagnosis of human ornithosis, LGV, neonatal pneumonia caused by *C. trachomatis*, and respiratory *C. pneumoniae* infections. Serological testing for diagnosis of uncomplicated genital infections of the urethra and the lower genital tract as well as for *C. trachomatis* screening in asymptomatic individuals is not recommended (44). *C. trachomatis* antibody testing has been proposed as the first screening test for tubal factor subfertility (15). Antibodies to *C. trachomatis* were independently associated with reduced rates of pregnancy and elevated rates of recurrent pelvic inflammatory disease (68).

Since a reference standard has not been defined, the diagnostic value of some serological assays for detection of chronic or persistent chlamydial infections is difficult to estimate. General problems of chlamydial serodiagnosis arise from the difficulty in obtaining paired serum samples, the high seroprevalence of *C. pneumoniae* in adult populations, and the lack of standardized species-specific test methods. The most commonly used serological assay formats include the complement fixation (CF) test, the MIF test, and the EIA to detect immunoglobulin M (IgM), IgA, IgG, or total classes of antibodies, with either family, species, or serotype specificity. Some of these assays have been commercialized and are being used by clinical laboratories, although their performance characteristics have been evaluated only in a limited number of studies.

CF Test

The CF test is based on antibody reactivity to the chlamydial LPS antigen common to all members of the *Chlamydiaceae*. The CF test may be useful in diagnosing LGV in patients who present compatible clinical symptoms. A titer of ≥256 strongly supports the clinical diagnosis, while a titer of <32 rules it out except in the very early stages of the disease (56). In addition, the CF test is useful for diagnosis of psittacosis; however, in the absence of a typical

patient history (exposure to birds), *C. pneumoniae* infection might be considered for patients with positive test results. However, due to its potential for cross-reactivity and its low sensitivity for reinfection, CF is not recommended for serodiagnosis of *C. pneumoniae* infections (16). The CF test also lacks sensitivity for the diagnosis of trachoma, inclusion conjunctivitis, and uncomplicated genital infections caused by *C. trachomatis*. The CF test is widely becoming unavailable in many laboratories, which may limit its usefulness in the near future.

MIF Test

The MIF test developed by Wang and Grayston in the early 1970s is still considered the method of choice for serodiagnosis of chlamydial infections. With this procedure, species- and serovar-specific antibody responses in human chlamydial infection can be detected. The MIF test allows quantitative detection of IgM and IgG antibodies that may be helpful in distinguishing recent from past infections.

The MIF test is the diagnostic test of choice for *C. trachomatis* pneumonitis in infants because elevated levels of IgM antibodies are regularly associated with disease (4). A single IgM titer of ≥32 may support the diagnosis of neonatal pneumonia caused by *C. trachomatis*. IgG antibodies are less useful because infants may present with typical symptoms when they still have a high level of maternal IgG. In LGV-infected individuals, a MIF IgG titer of ≥128 strongly supports the clinical diagnosis, although invasive genital infection with *C. trachomatis* serovars D through K, such as pelvic inflammatory disease, salpingitis, or epididymitis, can also give rise to high serum titers of antichlamydial antibody (56). The MIF test may be useful in the diagnosis of psittacosis and is the serological testing method of choice for diagnosis of acute *C. pneumoniae* infection. Criteria for acute infection of *C. pneumoniae* generally include paired sera demonstrating at least a fourfold rise in titer and single serum samples with IgM titers of ≥16 and/or IgG titers of ≥512. However, single IgG titers of ≥512 should be interpreted with caution because elevated IgG titers may persist for several years in the absence of clinically apparent disease (16). IgG titers in the range of 16 to 256 are suggestive of past infection. The usefulness of IgA as a diagnostic marker in acute or chronic *C. pneumoniae* infections has not been substantiated (50).

The MIF assay is performed using purified formalinized EBs of representative strains or serovars of *C. trachomatis*, *C. psittaci*, and *C. pneumoniae* that are dotted in a specific pattern onto glass slides. MIF antigens are commercially available from the Washington Research Foundation. Serial dilutions of patient sera are placed over the fixed antigen dots and incubated, and bound antibody is detected with fluorescein-conjugated anti-IgG or anti-IgM antibody (Fig. 1F). A more detailed description of the MIF procedure has been summarized elsewhere (110). In addition, recommendations for standardizing the MIF assay in terms of antigen preparation, testing, interpretation of results, and quality assurance should be followed (16).

The MIF assay format is technically demanding, time-consuming, and less useful for higher volume testing. In addition, subjective reading of titers may contribute to intra- and interlaboratory variation in MIF assay results (72). For these reasons, well-trained and experienced laboratory staff are required. A few standardized kits based on the MIF format have been developed and marketed (Focus Diagnostics, Cypress, CA; Labsystems Oy, Helsinki, Finland; and Savyon Diagnostics Ltd., Ashdod, Israel). Initial studies suggest that their performance characteristics are similar and seem to correspond well to those of the classical MIF method (3). However, at the time of this writing, none of these assays are cleared by the FDA for use in the United States for the diagnosis of *C. pneumoniae* or *C. trachomatis* infection.

Enzyme Immunoassay

To overcome the problems associated with MIF testing, EIAs have been developed that offer a more automated workflow and objective end points for serodiagnosis of chlamydial infections. EIAs based on synthetic peptides from the VD4 of the *C. trachomatis* MOMP have been marketed for detection of *C. trachomatis*-specific IgG and IgA antibodies (CT-EIA [Labsystems], SeroCT [Savyon Diagnostics], and CT pELISA [Medac, Wedel, Germany]). These assays performed as well as the MIF assay in a few studies (67); however, little is known regarding how long specific antibodies may persist in individuals with resolved infections. For this reason they cannot reliably differentiate current and past infections. They are not useful in *C. trachomatis* infections of the lower genital tract for which adequate specimens for direct detection of the organisms can be noninvasively obtained. Further studies are needed to clarify if *C. trachomatis* species-specific antibody tests based on recombinant antigens are convenient tools for the diagnosis of upper-genital tract infections (20).

The major antigenic determinants of *C. pneumoniae* that are broadly immunodominant among infected individuals are elusive. Commercial assays designed for specific diagnosis of *C. pneumoniae* infection are based on either whole elementary bodies (Savyon Diagnostics) or (to obtain more specificity) on LPS-extracted EB preparations (Labsystems and Medac). Most kits have been compared only to MIF (36), but none has been evaluated adequately with sera from culture- or PCR-positive patients. Thus, their diagnostic value for acute *C. pneumoniae* infections remains to be determined (16).

ANTIMICROBIAL SUSCEPTIBILITIES AND TREATMENT

Evaluation of antimicrobial resistance and potential clinical treatment failure in chlamydial infection is hampered by the lack of standardized antimicrobial susceptibility tests and the fact that in vitro resistance does not correlate with the patient's clinical outcome (99). For these reasons, antimicrobial susceptibility testing of *Chlamydia* organisms has little clinical utility and is currently performed only in some research laboratories. Antimicrobial susceptibility testing of chlamydiae requires growing the organisms in epithelial cells cultured in medium containing increasing concentrations of antibiotics. Cells are stained with an FITC-labeled anti-chlamydial antibody, and the lowest concentration of antibiotic that inhibits inclusion formation after 48 h of incubation is reported as the MIC (99, 111). The minimum chlamydicidal concentration has been defined as the lowest concentration of antibiotic producing no viable bacterial progeny as determined after passage from antimicrobial-containing medium to antimicrobial-free medium. However, variation of antimicrobial susceptibility results is common because they depend on many factors, including the cell type used, the inoculum size, and the time between infection and the addition of an antimicrobial.

Tetracyclines, macrolides, fluoroquinolones, and rifampin are commonly used for antibiotic treatment of chlamydial infections. A single 1-gram dose of azithromycin has been shown to be as effective for the treatment of uncomplicated genital *C. trachomatis* infections in adults as a standard 7-day course of doxycycline (29, 52). Alternative regimens include a 7-day course of erythromycin, ofloxacin, or levofloxacin. More data and clinical experience are available to support the efficacy and safety of azithromycin in pregnant women (29). Cotreatment or testing for chlamydiae should be considered among gonorrhea-infected patients because of the frequency of coinfection. Systemic treatment with erythromycin has been recommended for ophthalmia neonatorum as well as for infant pneumonia caused by *C. trachomatis*. In the treatment of adult inclusion conjunctivitis, a single azithromycin dose was as effective as a standard 10-day treatment with doxycycline (48). Doxycycline for 21 days is the antibiotic treatment of choice for both bubonic and anogenital LGV (62). Doxycycline, azithromycin, erythromycin, levofloxacin, and newer macrolides, such as clarithromycin and roxithromycin, have been recommended for treatment of *C. pneumoniae* infection; however, evidence from clinical trials supporting their use is limited.

Chlamydial resistance to recommended antimicrobial agents appears to be rare and confined to only a few clinical isolates of *C. trachomatis* and has not yet been reported for *C. pneumoniae* or *C. psittaci* infections. Nevertheless, concern has been raised about resistance because recurrent or persistent chlamydial infections were observed with women adequately treated for *C. trachomatis* infection and in a few cases of *C. pneumoniae* infections (34).

In vitro, chlamydial resistance to fluoroquinolones, macrolides, tetracyclines, and rifampin can be induced with large numbers of organisms cultured in the presence of antimicrobials. In an animal model, persistence of *C. pneumoniae* after antimicrobial therapy has been demonstrated (60). The emergence of *Chlamydia suis* strains isolated from livestock and displaying a chromosomally stable *tet*(C) resistance gene raises concern about the issue of antibiotic use in animal feeds (17).

INTERPRETATION AND REPORTING OF RESULTS

Licensed commercially available NAATs enable the reliable detection of uncomplicated genital *C. trachomatis* infection, even from noninvasively obtained specimens such as first void urine and (self-collected) vaginal swabs. These specimens are also recommended for screening asymptomatic individuals. Reporting of test results for chlamydiae should include the type of test used and a clinical interpretation if possible. Sexual partners of infected patients should be notified, examined, and treated for *C. trachomatis*. Patients and their partners should be instructed to abstain from sexual intercourse until therapy is completed. Due to the presence of nonviable bacteria, nonculture tests for *C. trachomatis*, especially NAATs, may remain positive when performed ≤3 weeks after completion of therapy (22). The use of EIAs, DFAs, and NAH-based assays are increasingly discouraged due to their relatively low sensitivity compared to those of NAATs. In cases of repeated treatment failure, isolation should be attempted and specimens should be forwarded to a specialized reference laboratory.

NAATs could also be helpful for diagnosis of *C. pneumoniae* and *C. psittaci* infections. However, commercial FDA-cleared assays are currently not available. Therefore, respiratory specimens of patients with clinical suspicion of ornithosis or *C. pneumoniae* infection should be directed to a specialized laboratory.

Interpretation of serological results is particularly challenging with chlamydial infections. Serological testing may be helpful for diagnosis of human ornithosis, LGV, neonatal pneumonia, and respiratory *C. pneumoniae* infections. A reliable serologic marker for chronic or persistent chlamydial infection is not available. Especially in *C. pneumoniae*, there is poor agreement between the presence of chlamydial antibody and direct markers of current infection, such as culture or PCR (26). Single-point serology for diagnosis of *C. pneumoniae* infection is discouraged, except when specific IgM antibodies are positive. Paired sera should be tested in the same assay on the same day, and seroconversion or a fourfold rise or fall in titer is diagnostic for a recent infection. Obviously, there is a general lack of reliable and standardized assays for laboratory diagnosis of *C. pneumoniae*, and this basically hampers the current understanding of the organism's true prevalence and role in respiratory infections as well as in extrapulmonary diseases.

REFERENCES

1. **Apfalter, P., W. Barousch, M. Nehr, A. Makristathis, B. Willinger, M. Rotter, and A. M. Hirschl.** 2003. Comparison of a new quantitative ompA-based real-time PCR TaqMan assay for detection of *Chlamydia pneumoniae* DNA in respiratory specimens with four conventional PCR assays. *J. Clin. Microbiol.* **41:**592–600.

2. **Belland, R. J., G. Zhong, D. D. Crane, D. Hogan, D. Sturdevant, J. Sharma, W. L. Beatty, and H. D. Caldwell.** 2003. Genomic transcriptional profiling of the developmental cycle of Chlamydia trachomatis. *Proc. Natl. Acad. Sci. USA* **100:**8478–8483.

3. **Bennedsen, M., L. Berthelsen, and I. Lind.** 2002. Performance of three microimmunofluorescence assays for detection of *Chlamydia pneumoniae* immunoglobulin M, G, and A antibodies. *Clin. Diagn. Lab. Immunol.* **9:**833–839.

4. **Black, C. M.** 1997. Current methods of laboratory diagnosis of *Chlamydia trachomatis* infections. *Clin. Microbiol. Rev.* **10:**160–184.

5. **Black, C. M., E. M. Driebe, L. A. Howard, N. N. Fajman, M. K. Sawyer, R. G. Girardet, R. L. Sautter, E. Greenwald, C. M. Beck-Sague, E. R. Unger, J. U. Igietseme, and M. R. Hammerschlag.** 2009. Multicenter study of nucleic acid amplification tests for detection of Chlamydia trachomatis and Neisseria gonorrhoeae in children being evaluated for sexual abuse. *Pediatr. Infect. Dis. J.* **28:**608–613.

6. **Black, C. M., J. Marrazzo, R. E. Johnson, E. W. Hook III, R. B. Jones, T. A. Green, J. Schachter, W. E. Stamm, G. Bolan, M. E. St. Louis, and D. H. Martin.** 2002. Head-to-head multicenter comparison of DNA probe and nucleic acid amplification tests for *Chlamydia trachomatis* infection in women performed with an improved reference standard. *J. Clin. Microbiol.* **40:**3757–3763.

7. **Borel, N., E. Kempf, H. Hotzel, E. Schubert, P. Torgerson, P. Slickers, R. Ehricht, T. Tasara, A. Pospischil, and K. Sachse.** 2008. Direct identification of chlamydiae from clinical samples using a DNA microarray assay: a validation study. *Mol. Cell. Probes* **22:**55–64.

8. **Boyadzhyan, B., T. Yashina, J. H. Yatabe, M. Patnaik, and C. S. Hill.** 2004. Comparison of the APTIMA CT and GC assays with the APTIMA combo 2 assay, the Abbott LCx assay, and direct fluorescent-antibody and culture assays for detection of *Chlamydia trachomatis* and *Neisseria gonorrhoeae*. *J. Clin. Microbiol.* **42:**3089–3093.

9. **Byrne, G. I., and D. M. Ojcius.** 2004. Chlamydia and apoptosis: life and death decisions of an intracellular pathogen. *Nat. Rev. Microbiol.* **2:**802–808.

10. **Campbell, L. A., M. M. Perez, D. J. Hamilton, C. C. Kuo, and J. T. Grayston.** 1992. Detection of *Chlamydia pneumoniae* by polymerase chain reaction. *J. Clin. Microbiol.* **30:**434–439.

11. **Centers for Disease Control and Prevention.** 2009. Sexually transmitted disease surveillance, 2007. CDC, U.S. Department of Health and Human Services, Atlanta, GA. http://www.cdc.gov/std/stats07/toc.htm.

12. **Chen, C. Y., K. H. Chi, S. Alexander, C. A. Ison, and R. C. Ballard.** 2008. A real-time quadriplex PCR assay for the diagnosis of rectal lymphogranuloma venereum and non-lymphogranuloma venereum Chlamydia trachomatis infections. *Sex. Transm. Infect.* **84:**273–276.

13. **Chernesky, M. A., D. H. Martin, E. W. Hook, D. Willis, J. Jordan, S. Wang, J. R. Lane, D. Fuller, and J. Schachter.** 2005. Ability of new APTIMA CT and APTIMA GC assays to detect *Chlamydia trachomatis* and *Neisseria gonorrhoeae* in male urine and urethral swabs. *J. Clin. Microbiol.* **43:**127–131.

14. **Dean, D., R. J. Suchland, and W. E. Stamm.** 2000. Evidence for long-term cervical persistence of Chlamydia trachomatis by omp1 genotyping. *J. Infect. Dis.* **182:**909–916.

15. **den Hartog, J. E., C. M. Lardenoije, J. L. Severens, J. A. Land, J. L. Evers, and A. G. Kessels.** 2008. Screening strategies for tubal factor subfertility. *Hum. Reprod.* **23:**1840–1848.

16. **Dowell, S. F., R. W. Peeling, J. Boman, G. M. Carlone, B. S. Fields, J. Guarner, M. R. Hammerschlag, L. A. Jackson, C. C. Kuo, M. Maass, T. O. Messmer, D. F. Talkington, M. L. Tondella, and S. R. Zaki.** 2001. Standardizing Chlamydia pneumoniae assays: recommendations from the Centers for Disease Control and Prevention (USA) and the Laboratory Centre for Disease Control (Canada). *Clin. Infect. Dis.* **33:**492–503.

17. **Dugan, J., D. D. Rockey, L. Jones, and A. A. Andersen.** 2004. Tetracycline resistance in Chlamydia suis mediated by genomic islands inserted into the chlamydial inv-like gene. *Antimicrob. Agents Chemother.* **48:**3989–3995.

18. **Essig, A., P. Zucs, M. Susa, G. Wasenauer, U. Mamat, M. Hetzel, U. Vogel, S. Wieshammer, H. Brade, and R. Marre.** 1995. Diagnosis of ornithosis by cell culture and polymerase chain reaction in a patient with chronic pneumonia. *Clin. Infect. Dis.* **21:**1495–1497.

19. **Everett, K. D., R. M. Bush, and A. A. Andersen.** 1999. Emended description of the order *Chlamydiales*, proposal of *Parachlamydiaceae* fam. nov. and *Simkaniaceae* fam. nov., each containing one monotypic genus, revised taxonomy of the family *Chlamydiaceae*, including a new genus and five new species, and standards for the identification of organisms. *Int. J. Syst. Bacteriol.* **49:**415–440.

20. **Forsbach-Birk, V., U. Simnacher, K. I. Pfrepper, E. Soutschek, A. O. Kiselev, M. F. Lampe, T. Meyer, E. Straube, and A. Essig.** 2010. Identification and evaluation of a combination of chlamydial antigens to support the diagnosis of severe and invasive Chlamydia trachomatis infections. *Clin. Microbiol. Infect.* **16:**1237–1244.

21. **Fukushi, H., and K. Hirai.** 1992. Proposal of *Chlamydia pecorum* sp. nov. for *Chlamydia* strains derived from ruminants. *Int. J. Syst. Bacteriol.* **42:**306–308.

22. **Gaydos, C. A., K. A. Crotchfelt, M. R. Howell, S. Kralian, P. Hauptman, and T. C. Quinn.** 1998. Molecular amplification assays to detect chlamydial infections in urine specimens from high school female students and to monitor the persistence of chlamydial DNA after therapy. *J. Infect. Dis.* **177:**417–424.

23. **Gaydos, C. A., D. V. Ferrero, and J. Papp.** 2008. Laboratory aspects of screening men for Chlamydia trachomatis in the new millennium. *Sex. Transm. Dis.* **35:**S45–S50.

24. **Gaydos, C. A., T. C. Quinn, and J. J. Eiden.** 1992. Identification of *Chlamydia pneumoniae* by DNA amplification of the 16S rRNA gene. *J. Clin. Microbiol.* **30:**796–800.

25. **Gaydos, C. A., T. C. Quinn, D. Willis, A. Weissfeld, E. W. Hook, D. H. Martin, D. V. Ferrero, and J. Schachter.** 2003. Performance of the APTIMA Combo 2 assay for detection of *Chlamydia trachomatis* and *Neisseria gonorrhoeae* in female urine and endocervical swab specimens. *J. Clin. Microbiol.* **41:**304–309.

26. **Gaydos, C. A., P. M. Roblin, M. R. Hammerschlag, C. L. Hyman, J. J. Eiden, J. Schachter, and T. C. Quinn.** 1994. Diagnostic utility of PCR-enzyme immunoassay, culture, and serology for detection of *Chlamydia pneumoniae* in symptomatic and asymptomatic patients. *J. Clin. Microbiol.* **32:**903–905.

27. **Geens, T., A. Desplanques, M. Van Loock, B. M. Bonner, E. F. Kaleta, S. Magnino, A. A. Andersen, K. D. Everett, and D. Vanrompay.** 2005. Sequencing of the *Chlamydophila psittaci ompA* gene reveals a new genotype, E/B, and the need for a rapid discriminatory genotyping method. *J. Clin. Microbiol.* **43:**2456–2461.

28. **Geens, T., A. Dewitte, N. Boon, and D. Vanrompay.** 2005. Development of a Chlamydophila psittaci species-specific and genotype-specific real-time PCR. *Vet. Res.* **36:**787–797.

29. **Geisler, W. M.** 2007. Management of uncomplicated Chlamydia trachomatis infections in adolescents and adults: evidence reviewed for the 2006 Centers for Disease Control and Prevention sexually transmitted diseases treatment guidelines. *Clin. Infect. Dis.* **44**(Suppl. 3)**:**S77–S83.

30. **Gomes, J. P., A. Nunes, C. Florindo, M. A. Ferreira, I. Santo, J. Azevedo, and M. J. Borrego.** 2009. Lymphogranuloma venereum in Portugal: unusual events and new variants during 2007. *Sex. Transm. Dis.* **36:**88–91.

31. **Grayston, J. T., L. A. Campbell, C. C. Kuo, C. H. Mordhorst, P. Saikku, D. H. Thom, and S. P. Wang.** 1990. A new respiratory tract pathogen: Chlamydia pneumoniae strain TWAR. *J. Infect. Dis.* **161:**618–625.

32. **Grayston, J. T., R. A. Kronmal, L. A. Jackson, A. F. Parisi, J. B. Muhlestein, J. D. Cohen, W. J. Rogers, J. R. Crouse, S. L. Borrowdale, E. Schron, and C. Knirsch.** 2005. Azithromycin for the secondary prevention of coronary events. *N. Engl. J. Med.* **352:**1637–1645.

33. **Greub, G.** 2009. Parachlamydia acanthamoebae, an emerging agent of pneumonia. *Clin. Microbiol. Infect.* **15:**18–28.

34. **Hammerschlag, M. R., K. Chirgwin, P. M. Roblin, M. Gelling, W. Dumornay, L. Mandel, P. Smith, and J. Schachter.** 1992. Persistent infection with Chlamydia pneumoniae following acute respiratory illness. *Clin. Infect. Dis.* **14:**178–182.

35. **Heinemann, M., W. V. Kern, D. Bunjes, R. Marre, and A. Essig.** 2000. Severe Chlamydia pneumoniae infection in patients with neutropenia: case reports and literature review. *Clin. Infect. Dis.* **31:**181–184.

36. **Hermann, C., K. Gueinzius, A. Oehme, S. Von Aulock, E. Straube, and T. Hartung.** 2004. Comparison of quantitative and semiquantitative enzyme-linked immunosorbent assays for immunoglobulin G against *Chlamydophila pneumoniae* to a microimmunofluorescence test for use with patients with respiratory tract infections. *J. Clin. Microbiol.* **42:**2476–2479.

37. **Herrmann, B., A. Torner, N. Low, M. Klint, A. Nilsson, I. Velicko, T. Soderblom, and A. Blaxhult.** 2008. Emergence and spread of Chlamydia trachomatis variant, Sweden. *Emerg. Infect. Dis.* **14:**1462–1465.

38. **Hobbs, M. M., P. B. Van Der, P. Totten, C. A. Gaydos, A. Wald, T. Warren, R. L. Winer, R. L. Cook, C. D. Deal, M. E. Rogers, J. Schachter, K. K. Holmes, and D. H. Martin.** 2008. From the NIH: proceedings of a workshop on the importance of self-obtained vaginal specimens for detection of sexually transmitted infections. *Sex. Transm. Dis.* **35:**8–13.

39. **Horn, M., A. Collingro, S. Schmitz-Esser, C. L. Beier, U. Purkhold, B. Fartmann, P. Brandt, G. J. Nyakatura, M. Droege, D. Frishman, T. Rattei, H. W. Mewes, and M. Wagner.** 2004. Illuminating the evolutionary history of chlamydiae. *Science* **304:**728–730.

40. **Hsieh, Y. H., M. R. Howell, J. C. Gaydos, K. T. McKee, Jr., T. C. Quinn, and C. A. Gaydos.** 2003. Preference among female Army recruits for use of self-administrated vaginal swabs or urine to screen for Chlamydia trachomatis genital infections. *Sex. Transm. Dis.* **30:**769–773.

41. **Hybiske, K., and R. S. Stephens.** 2007. Mechanisms of host cell exit by the intracellular bacterium Chlamydia. *Proc. Natl. Acad. Sci. USA* **104:**11430–11435.

42. **Ieven, M. M., and V. Y. Hoymans.** 2005. Involvement of *Chlamydia pneumoniae* in atherosclerosis: more evidence for lack of evidence. *J. Clin. Microbiol.* **43:**19–24.

43. **Joesoef, M. R., H. S. Weinstock, C. K. Kent, J. M. Chow, M. R. Boudov, F. M. Parvez, T. Cox, T. Lincoln, J. L. Miller, and M. Sternberg.** 2009. Sex and age correlates of Chlamydia prevalence in adolescents and adults entering correctional facilities, 2005: implications for screening policy. *Sex. Transm. Dis.* **36:**S67–S71.

44. **Johnson, R. E., W. J. Newhall, J. R. Papp, J. S. Knapp, C. M. Black, T. L. Gift, R. Steece, L. E. Markowitz, O. J. Devine, C. M. Walsh, S. Wang, D. C. Gunter, K. L. Irwin, S. DeLisle, and S. M. Berman.** 2002. Screening tests to detect Chlamydia trachomatis and Neisseria gonorrhoeae infections—2002. *MMWR Recommend. Rep.* **51:**1–38.

45. **Kacena, K. A., S. B. Quinn, M. R. Howell, G. E. Madico, T. C. Quinn, and C. A. Gaydos.** 1998. Pooling urine samples for ligase chain reaction screening for genital *Chlamydia trachomatis* infection in asymptomatic women. *J. Clin. Microbiol.* **36:**481–485.

46. **Kahane, S., K. D. Everett, N. Kimmel, and M. G. Friedman.** 1999. *Simkania negevensis* strain ZT: growth, antigenic and genome characteristics. *Int. J. Syst. Bacteriol.* **49:**815–820.

47. **Kalman, S., W. Mitchell, R. Marathe, C. Lammel, J. Fan, R. W. Hyman, L. Olinger, J. Grimwood, R. W. Davis, and R. S. Stephens.** 1999. Comparative genomes of Chlamydia pneumoniae and C. trachomatis. *Nat. Genet.* **21:**385–389.

48. **Katusic, D., I. Petricek, Z. Mandic, I. Petric, J. Salopek-Rabatic, V. Kruzic, K. Oreskovic, J. Sikic, and G. Petricek.** 2003. Azithromycin vs doxycycline in the treatment of inclusion conjunctivitis. *Am. J. Ophthalmol.* **135:**447–451.

49. **Kent, C. K., J. K. Chaw, W. Wong, S. Liska, S. Gibson, G. Hubbard, and J. D. Klausner.** 2005. Prevalence of rectal, urethral, and pharyngeal chlamydia and gonorrhea detected in 2 clinical settings among men who have sex with men: San Francisco, California, 2003. *Clin. Infect. Dis.* **41:**67–74.

50. **Kumar, S. and M. R. Hammerschlag.** 2007. Acute respiratory infection due to Chlamydia pneumoniae: current status of diagnostic methods. *Clin. Infect. Dis.* **44:**568–576.

51. **Kuo, C. C., L. A. Jackson, L. A. Campbell, and J. T. Grayston.** 1995. *Chlamydia pneumoniae* (TWAR). *Clin. Microbiol. Rev.* **8:**451–461.

52. **Lau, C. Y., and A. K. Qureshi.** 2002. Azithromycin versus doxycycline for genital chlamydial infections: a meta-analysis of randomized clinical trials. *Sex. Transm. Dis.* **29:**497–502.

53. **Levett, P. N., K. Brandt, K. Olenius, C. Brown, K. Montgomery, and G. B. Horsman.** 2008. Evaluation of three automated nucleic acid amplification systems for detection of Chlamydia trachomatis and Neisseria gonorrhoeae in first-void urine specimens. *J. Clin. Microbiol.* **46:**2109–2111.

54. **Lim, W. S., J. T. Macfarlane, T. C. Boswell, T. G. Harrison, D. Rose, M. Leinonen, and P. Saikku.** 2001. Study of community acquired pneumonia aetiology (SCAPA) in adults admitted to hospital: implications for management guidelines. *Thorax* **56:**296–301.

55. **Lindan, C., M. Mathur, S. Kumta, H. Jerajani, A. Gogate, J. Schachter, and J. Moncada.** 2005. Utility of pooled urine specimens for detection of *Chlamydia trachomatis* and *Neisseria gonorrhoeae* in men attending public sexually transmitted infection clinics in Mumbai, India, by PCR. *J. Clin. Microbiol.* **43:**1674–1677.

56. **Mabey, D., and R. W. Peeling.** 2002. Lymphogranuloma venereum. *Sex. Transm. Infect.* **78:**90–92.

57. **Madico, G., T. C. Quinn, J. Boman, and C. A. Gaydos.** 2000. Touchdown enzyme time release-PCR for detection and identification of *Chlamydia trachomatis, C. pneumoniae*, and *C. psittaci* using the 16S and 16S-23S spacer rRNA genes. *J. Clin. Microbiol.* **38:**1085–1093.

58. **Mahilum-Tapay, L., V. Laitila, J. J. Wawrzyniak, H. H. Lee, S. Alexander, C. Ison, A. Swain, P. Barber, I. Ushiro-Lumb, and B. T. Goh.** 2007. New point of care Chlamydia Rapid Test—bridging the gap between diagnosis and treatment: performance evaluation study. *BMJ* **335:**1190–1194.

59. Mahony, J., S. Chong, D. Jang, K. Luinstra, M. Faught, D. Dalby, J. Sellors, and M. Chernesky. 1998. Urine specimens from pregnant and nonpregnant women inhibitory to amplification of *Chlamydia trachomatis* nucleic acid by PCR, ligase chain reaction, and transcription-mediated amplification: identification of urinary substances associated with inhibition and removal of inhibitory activity. *J. Clin. Microbiol.* **36:**3122–3126.

60. Malinverni, R., C. C. Kuo, L. A. Campbell, and J. T. Grayston. 1995. Reactivation of Chlamydia pneumoniae lung infection in mice by cortisone. *J. Infect. Dis.* **172:**593–594.

61. Marshall, R., M. Chernesky, D. Jang, E. W. Hook, C. P. Cartwright, B. Howell-Adams, S. Ho, J. Welk, J. Lai-Zhang, J. Brashear, B. Diedrich, K. Otis, E. Webb, J. Robinson, and H. Yu. 2007. Characteristics of the m2000 automated sample preparation and multiplex real-time PCR system for detection of Chlamydia trachomatis and Neisseria gonorrhoeae. *J. Clin. Microbiol.* **45:**747–751.

62. McLean, C. A., B. P. Stoner, and K. A. Workowski. 2007. Treatment of lymphogranuloma venereum. *Clin. Infect. Dis.* **44**(Suppl. 3)**:**S147–S152.

63. Messmer, T. O., S. K. Skelton, J. F. Moroney, H. Daugharty, and B. S. Fields. 1997. Application of a nested, multiplex PCR to psittacosis outbreaks. *J. Clin. Microbiol.* **35:**2043–2046. (Erratum, **36:**1821, 1998.)

64. Mitchell, S. L., B. J. Wolff, W. L. Thacker, P. G. Ciembor, C. R. Gregory, K. D. Everett, B. W. Ritchie, and J. M. Winchell. 2009. Genotyping of Chlamydophila psittaci by real-time PCR and high-resolution melt analysis. *J. Clin. Microbiol.* **47:**175–181.

65. Moller, J. K., L. N. Pedersen, and K. Persson. 2008. Comparison of Gen-probe transcription-mediated amplification, Abbott PCR, and Roche PCR assays for detection of wild-type and mutant plasmid strains of *Chlamydia trachomatis* in Sweden. *J. Clin. Microbiol.* **46:**3892–3895.

66. Moroney, J. F., R. Guevara, C. Iverson, F. M. Chen, S. K. Skelton, T. O. Messmer, B. Plikaytis, P. O. Williams, P. Blake, and J. C. Butler. 1998. Detection of chlamydiosis in a shipment of pet birds, leading to recognition of an outbreak of clinically mild psittacosis in humans. *Clin. Infect. Dis.* **26:**1425–1429.

67. Morre, S. A., C. Munk, K. Persson, S. Kruger-Kjaer, R. van Dijk, C. J. Meijer, and A. J. van Den Brule. 2002. Comparison of three commercially available peptide-based immunoglobulin G (IgG) and IgA assays to microimmunofluorescence assay for detection of Chlamydia trachomatis antibodies. *J. Clin. Microbiol.* **40:**584–587.

68. Ness, R. B., D. E. Soper, H. E. Richter, H. Randall, J. F. Peipert, D. B. Nelson, D. Schubeck, S. G. McNeeley, W. Trout, D. C. Bass, K. Hutchison, K. Kip, and R. C. Brunham. 2008. Chlamydia antibodies, chlamydia heat shock protein, and adverse sequelae after pelvic inflammatory disease: the PID Evaluation and Clinical Health (PEACH) Study. *Sex. Transm. Dis.* **35:**129–135.

69. Newhall, W. J., R. E. Johnson, S. DeLisle, D. Fine, A. Hadgu, B. Matsuda, D. Osmond, J. Campbell, and W. E. Stamm. 1999. Head-to-head evaluation of five chlamydia tests relative to a quality-assured culture standard. *J. Clin. Microbiol.* **37:**681–685.

70. Nieuwenhuis, R. F., J. M. Ossewaarde, H. M. Gotz, J. Dees, H. B. Thio, M. G. Thomeer, J. C. den Hollander, M. H. Neumann, and W. I. van der Meijden. 2004. Resurgence of lymphogranuloma venereum in Western Europe: an outbreak of Chlamydia trachomatis serovar l2 proctitis in The Netherlands among men who have sex with men. *Clin. Infect. Dis.* **39:**996–1003.

71. Pedersen, L. N., B. Herrmann, and J. K. Moller. 2009. Typing Chlamydia trachomatis: from egg yolk to nanotechnology. *FEMS Immunol. Med. Microbiol.* **55:**120–130.

72. Peeling, R. W., S. P. Wang, J. T. Grayston, F. Blasi, J. Boman, A. Clad, H. Freidank, C. A. Gaydos, J. Gnarpe, T. Hagiwara, R. B. Jones, J. Orfila, K. Persson, M. Puolakkainen, P. Saikku, and J. Schachter. 2000. Chlamydia

pneumoniae serology: interlaboratory variation in microimmunofluorescence assay results. *J. Infect. Dis.* **181**(Suppl. 3)**:**S426–S429.

73. Peipert, J. F. 2003. Clinical practice. Genital chlamydial infections. *N. Engl. J. Med.* **349:**2424–2430.

74. Pickett, M. A., J. S. Everson, P. J. Pead, and I. N. Clarke. 2005. The plasmids of Chlamydia trachomatis and Chlamydophila pneumoniae (N16): accurate determination of copy number and the paradoxical effect of plasmid-curing agents. *Microbiology* **151:**893–903.

75. Poppert, S., A. Essig, R. Marre, M. Wagner, and M. Horn. 2002. Detection and differentiation of chlamydiae by fluorescence in situ hybridization. *Appl. Environ. Microbiol.* **68:**4081–4089.

76. Pospischil, A., R. Thoma, M. Hilbe, P. Grest, and J. O. Gebbers. 2002. Abortion in woman caused by caprine Chlamydophila abortus (Chlamydia psittaci serovar 1). *Swiss Med. Wkly.* **132:**64–66.

77. Principi, N., S. Esposito, F. Blasi, and L. Allegra. 2001. Role of Mycoplasma pneumoniae and Chlamydia pneumoniae in children with community-acquired lower respiratory tract infections. *Clin. Infect. Dis.* **32:**1281–1289.

78. Read, T. D., G. S. Myers, R. C. Brunham, W. C. Nelson, I. T. Paulsen, J. Heidelberg, E. Holtzapple, H. Khouri, N. B. Federova, H. A. Carty, L. A. Umayam, D. H. Haft, J. Peterson, M. J. Beanan, O. White, S. L. Salzberg, R. C. Hsia, G. McClarty, R. G. Rank, P. M. Bavoil, and C. M. Fraser. 2003. Genome sequence of Chlamydophila caviae (Chlamydia psittaci GPIC): examining the role of niche-specific genes in the evolution of the Chlamydiaceae. *Nucleic Acids Res.* **31:**2134–2147.

79. Reischl, U., N. Lehn, U. Simnacher, R. Marre, and A. Essig. 2003. Rapid and standardized detection of Chlamydia pneumoniae using LightCycler real-time fluorescence PCR. *Eur. J. Clin. Microbiol. Infect. Dis.* **22:**54–57.

80. Ross, R. 1999. Atherosclerosis—an inflammatory disease. *N. Engl. J. Med.* **340:**115–126.

81. Rours, I. G., M. M. Hammerschlag, G. G. Van Doornum, W. W. Hop, R. R. de Groot, D. H. Willemse, H. H. Verbrugh, and R. R. Verkooyen. 2009. Chlamydia trachomatis respiratory infection in Dutch infants. *Arch. Dis. Child.* **94:**705–707.

82. Rours, I. G., M. R. Hammerschlag, A. Ott, T. J. De Faber, H. A. Verbrugh, R. de Groot, and R. P. Verkooyen. 2008. Chlamydia trachomatis as a cause of neonatal conjunctivitis in Dutch infants. *Pediatrics* **121:**e321–e326.

83. Rurangirwa, F. R., P. M. Dilbeck, T. B. Crawford, T. C. McGuire, and T. F. McElwain. 1999. Analysis of the 16S rRNA gene of micro-organism WSU 86-1044 from an aborted bovine foetus reveals that it is a member of the order *Chlamydiales*: proposal of *Waddliaceae* fam. nov., *Waddlia chondrophila* gen. nov., sp. nov. *Int. J. Syst. Bacteriol.* **49:**577–581.

84. Sachse, K., K. Laroucau, F. Vorimore, S. Magnino, J. Feige, W. Muller, S. Kube, H. Hotzel, E. Schubert, P. Slickers, and R. Ehricht. 2009. DNA microarray-based genotyping of Chlamydophila psittaci strains from culture and clinical samples. *Vet. Microbiol.* **135:**22–30.

85. Saikku, P., M. Leinonen, K. Mattila, M. R. Ekman, M. S. Nieminen, P. H. Makela, J. K. Huttunen, and V. Valtonen. 1988. Serological evidence of an association of a novel Chlamydia, TWAR, with chronic coronary heart disease and acute myocardial infarction. Lancet ii:983–986.

86. Schachter, J., M. A. Chernesky, D. E. Willis, P. M. Fine, D. H. Martin, D. Fuller, J. A. Jordan, W. Janda, and E. W. Hook III. 2005. Vaginal swabs are the specimens of choice when screening for Chlamydia trachomatis and Neisseria gonorrhoeae: results from a multicenter evaluation of the APTIMA assays for both infections. *Sex. Transm. Dis.* **32:**725–728.

87. Schachter, J., J. M. Chow, H. Howard, G. Bolan, and J. Moncada. 2006. Detection of *Chlamydia trachomatis* by nucleic acid amplification testing: our evaluation suggests that CDC-recommended approaches for confirmatory testing are ill-advised. *J. Clin. Microbiol.* **44:**2512–2517.

88. **Schachter, J., W. M. McCormack, M. A. Chernesky, D. H. Martin, P. B. Van Der, P. A. Rice, E. W. Hook III, W. E. Stamm, T. C. Quinn, and J. M. Chow.** 2003. Vaginal swabs are appropriate specimens for diagnosis of genital tract infection with Chlamydia trachomatis. *J. Clin. Microbiol.* **41:**3784–3789.

89. **Schachter, J., J. Moncada, S. Liska, C. Shayevich, and J. D. Klausner.** 2008. Nucleic acid amplification tests in the diagnosis of chlamydial and gonococcal infections of the oropharynx and rectum in men who have sex with men. *Sex. Transm. Dis.* **35:**637–642.

90. **Schachter, J., R. S. Stephens, P. Timms, C. Kuo, P. M. Bavoil, S. Birkelund, J. Boman, H. Caldwell, L. A. Campbell, M. Chernesky, G. Christiansen, I. N. Clarke, C. Gaydos, J. T. Grayston, T. Hackstadt, R. Hsia, B. Kaltenboeck, M. Leinonnen, D. Ojcius, G. McClarty, J. Orfila, R. Peeling, M. Puolakkainen, T. C. Quinn, R. G. Rank, J. Raulston, G. L. Ridgeway, P. Saikku, W. E. Stamm, D. T. Taylor-Robinson, S. P. Wang, and P. B. Wyrick.** 2001. Radical changes to chlamydial taxonomy are not necessary just yet. *Int. J. Syst. Evol. Microbiol.* **51:**249.

91. **Schachter, J., and W. E. Stamm.** 1999. *Chlamydia*, p. 795–806. *In* P. R. Murray, E. J. Baron, J. H. Jorgensen, M. A. Pfaller, and R. H. Yolken (ed.), *Manual of Clinical Microbiology*, 7th ed. ASM Press, Washington, DC.

92. **Scidmore, M. A.** 2005. Cultivation and laboratory maintenance of Chlamydia trachomatis. *Curr. Protoc. Microbiol.* **Chapter 11:**Unit 11A1.

93. **Solomon, A. W., R. W. Peeling, A. Foster, and D. C. Mabey.** 2004. Diagnosis and assessment of trachoma. *Clin. Microbiol. Rev.* **17:**982–1011.

94. **Stark, D., S. van Hal, R. Hillman, J. Harkness, and D. Marriott.** 2007. Lymphogranuloma venereum in Australia: anorectal *Chlamydia trachomatis* serovar L2b in men who have sex with men. *J. Clin. Microbiol.* **45:**1029–1031.

95. **Stephens, R. S., S. Kalman, C. Lammel, J. Fan, R. Marathe, L. Aravind, W. Mitchell, L. Olinger, R. L. Tatusov, Q. Zhao, E. V. Koonin, and R. W. Davis.** 1998. Genome sequence of an obligate intracellular pathogen of humans: Chlamydia trachomatis. *Science* **282:**754–759.

96. **Stephens, R. S., G. Myers, M. Eppinger, and P. M. Bavoil.** 2009. Divergence without difference: phylogenetics and taxonomy of Chlamydia resolved. *FEMS Immunol. Med. Microbiol.* **55:**115–119.

97. **Stralin, K., E. Tornqvist, M. S. Kaltoft, P. Olcen, and H. Holmberg.** 2006. Etiologic diagnosis of adult bacterial pneumonia by culture and PCR applied to respiratory tract samples. *J. Clin. Microbiol.* **44:**643–645.

98. **Sturm, P. D., P. Moodley, K. Govender, L. Bohlken, T. Vanmali, and A. W. Sturm.** 2005. Molecular diagnosis of lymphogranuloma venereum in patients with genital ulcer disease. *J. Clin. Microbiol.* **43:**2973–2975.

99. **Suchland, R. J., W. M. Geisler, and W. E. Stamm.** 2003. Methodologies and cell lines used for antimicrobial susceptibility testing of *Chlamydia* spp. *Antimicrob. Agents Chemother.* **47:**636–642.

100. **Suchland, R. J., and W. E. Stamm.** 1991. Simplified microtiter cell culture method for rapid immunotyping of *Chlamydia trachomatis. J. Clin. Microbiol.* **29:**1333–1338.

101. **Thomson, N. R., M. T. Holden, C. Carder, N. Lennard, S. J. Lockey, P. Marsh, P. Skipp, C. D. O'Connor, I. Goodhead, H. Norbertzcak, B. Harris, D. Ormond, R. Rance, M. A. Quail, J. Parkhill, R. S. Stephens, and I. N. Clarke.** 2008. Chlamydia trachomatis: genome sequence analysis of lymphogranuloma venereum isolates. *Genome Res.* **18:**161–171.

102. **Thomson, N. R., C. Yeats, K. Bell, M. T. Holden, S. D. Bentley, M. Livingstone, A. M. Cerdeno-Tarraga, B. Harris, J. Doggett, D. Ormond, K. Mungall, K. Clarke, T. Feltwell, Z. Hance, M. Sanders, M. A. Quail, C. Price, B. G. Barrell, J. Parkhill, and D. Longbottom.** 2005. The

Chlamydophila abortus genome sequence reveals an array of variable proteins that contribute to interspecies variation. *Genome Res.* **15:**629–640.

103. **Tondella, M. L., D. F. Talkington, B. P. Holloway, S. F. Dowell, K. Cowley, M. Soriano-Gabarro, M. S. Elkind, and B. S. Fields.** 2002. Development and evaluation of real-time PCR-based fluorescence assays for detection of *Chlamydia pneumoniae. J. Clin. Microbiol.* **40:**575–583.

104. **Tong, C. Y., and M. Sillis.** 1993. Detection of Chlamydia pneumoniae and Chlamydia psittaci in sputum samples by PCR. *J. Clin. Pathol.* **46:**313–317.

105. **Van der Bij, A. K., J. Spaargaren, S. A. Morre, H. S. Fennema, A. Mindel, R. A. Coutinho, and H. J. de Vries.** 2006. Diagnostic and clinical implications of anorectal lymphogranuloma venereum in men who have sex with men: a retrospective case-control study. *Clin. Infect. Dis.* **42:**186–194.

106. **Van Der Pol, B., J. A. Williams, N. J. Smith, B. E. Batteiger, A. P. Cullen, H. Erdman, T. Edens, K. Davis, H. Salim-Hammad, V. W. Chou, L. Scearce, J. Blutman, and W. J. Payne.** 2002. Evaluation of the Digene Hybrid Capture II Assay with the Rapid Capture System for detection of *Chlamydia trachomatis* and *Neisseria gonorrhoeae. J. Clin. Microbiol.* **40:**3558–3564.

107. **Van Loock, M., D. Vanrompay, B. Herrmann, S. J. Vander, G. Volckaert, B. M. Goddeeris, and K. D. Everett.** 2003. Missing links in the divergence of *Chlamydophila abortus* from *Chlamydophila psittaci. Int. J. Syst. Evol. Microbiol.* **53:**761–770.

108. **Wadowsky, R. M., E. A. Castilla, S. Laus, A. Kozy, R. W. Atchison, L. A. Kingsley, J. I. Ward, and D. P. Greenberg.** 2002. Evaluation of *Chlamydia pneumoniae* and *Mycoplasma pneumoniae* as etiologic agents of persistent cough in adolescents and adults. *J. Clin. Microbiol.* **40:**637–640.

109. **Walder, G., H. Hotzel, C. Brezinka, W. Gritsch, R. Tauber, R. Wurzner, and F. Ploner.** 2005. An unusual cause of sepsis during pregnancy: recognizing infection with Chlamydophila abortus. *Obstet. Gynecol.* **106:**1215–1217.

110. **Wang, S.** 2000. The microimmunofluorescence test for Chlamydia pneumoniae infection: technique and interpretation. *J. Infect. Dis.* **181**(Suppl. 3):S421–S425.

111. **Wang, S. A., J. R. Papp, W. E. Stamm, R. W. Peeling, D. H. Martin, and K. K. Holmes.** 2005. Evaluation of antimicrobial resistance and treatment failures for Chlamydia trachomatis: a meeting report. *J. Infect. Dis.* **191:**917–923.

112. **Weiss, S. M., P. M. Roblin, C. A. Gaydos, P. Cummings, D. L. Patton, N. Schulhoff, J. Shani, R. Frankel, K. Penney, T. C. Quinn, M. R. Hammerschlag, and J. Schachter.** 1996. Failure to detect Chlamydia pneumoniae in coronary atheromas of patients undergoing atherectomy. *J. Infect. Dis.* **173:**957–962.

113. **Wellinghausen, N., E. Straube, H. Freidank, H. von Baum, R. Marre, and A. Essig.** 2006. Low prevalence of Chlamydia pneumoniae in adults with community-acquired pneumonia. *Int. J. Med. Microbiol.* **296:**485–491.

114. **White, J. A.** 2009. Manifestations and management of lymphogranuloma venereum. *Curr. Opin. Infect. Dis.* **22:**57–66.

115. **Wiggins, R., S. Graf, N. Low, and P. J. Horner.** 2009. Real-time quantitative PCR to determine chlamydial load in men and women in a community setting. *J. Clin. Microbiol.* **47:**1824–1829.

116. **Yin, Y. P., R. W. Peeling, X. S. Chen, K. L. Gong, H. Zhou, W. M. Gu, H. P. Zheng, Z. S. Wang, G. Yong, W. L. Cao, M. Q. Shi, W. H. Wei, X. Q. Dai, X. Gao, Q. Chen, and D. Mabey.** 2006. Clinic-based evaluation of Clearview Chlamydia MF for detection of Chlamydia trachomatis in vaginal and cervical specimens from women at high risk in China. *Sex. Transm. Infect.* **82**(Suppl. 5):v33–v37.

117. **Zeidler, H., J. Kuipers, and L. Kohler.** 2004. Chlamydia-induced arthritis. *Curr. Opin. Rheumatol.* **16:**380–392.

Rickettsia and *Orientia*

DAVID H. WALKER AND DONALD H. BOUYER

61

TAXONOMY

The family *Rickettsiaceae* comprises two genera of small, obligately intracellular bacteria that reside free within the host cell's cytosol, namely, *Rickettsia* and *Orientia*. Although the number and diversity of pathogenic strains in these genera are similar, the practices of species designation differ remarkably. The second edition of *Bergey's Manual of Systematic Bacteriology* lists 20 validated names of *Rickettsia* species, and others have been proposed (115). Strains of *Orientia tsutsugamushi*, the single species of the genus, have 0.8% divergence of the *rrs* (16S rRNA) gene. Similarly, other obligately intracellular bacteria have 0.5% *rrs* divergence within a species (e.g., *Ehrlichia chaffeensis*, *Coxiella burnetii*, and *Chlamydia trachomatis*). A proposal of criteria for the limits of divergence of *Rickettsia* species based upon the unacceptable criterion of historical designations would allow different species to be as closely related as 0.2% divergence for *rrs*, 0.8% for citrate synthetase (*gltA*), 1.2% for outer membrane protein A (*ompA*), 0.8% for outer membrane protein B (*ompB*), and 0.7% for the cytoplasmic antigen encoded by *sca4* (21, 24). There are no common or universal concepts that can be utilized to delineate prokaryotic species as there are with eukaryotes. However, among prokaryotes 1% divergence of the *rrs* gene is considered as a natural separation between species. Thus, the genus *Rickettsia* has a disproportionate number of designated species relative to the genetic divergence of the bacteria.

The genus is divided by the phylogenetic clustering of species into the typhus group (TG) and spotted fever group (SFG), defined originally by their distinctive lipopolysaccharide antigens, and the transitional and other basal groups that are widely distributed in arthropods (111). The TG consists of only two members, *Rickettsia prowazekii* and *R. typhi*, whereas the SFG contains bacteria that are generally recognized as human pathogens (*R. rickettsii*, *R. conorii*, *R. africae*, *R. sibirica*, *R. japonica*, *R. honei*, *R. parkeri*, *R. massiliae*, *R. monacensis*, *R. slovaca*, *R. aeschlimannii*, and *R. helvetica*) as well as others that have been identified only in arthropods (6, 32, 64, 76, 78, 111, 115). The transitional group, a clade between the TG and SFG, contains the pathogens *R. akari*, *R. australis*, and *R. felis* (26). Most *Rickettsia* species of undetermined pathogenicity, including *R. montanensis*, *R. bellii*, *R. peacockii*, and *R. rhipicephali*, are much more prevalent in U.S. ticks than is pathogenic *R. rickettsii*. SFG isolates from Israel and the Astrakhan region

of Russia, which have wider geographic distributions, are genetic variants of *R. conorii*. There are reports of SFG rickettsioses in southern Asia for which the agents have not been determined (75, 85).

Orientia tsutsugamushi diverges from *Rickettsia* by approximately 10% in the *rrs* gene and differs greatly in its cell wall structure, containing completely unrelated proteins and lacking lipopolysaccharide (Table 1). Phylogeny based upon *groEL*, a member of the molecular chaperone family, reveals similar genetic diversity for the unispecies genus *Orientia* as for SFG *Rickettsia*, for which it may be that too many species have been named (Fig. 1) (50, 99). *O. tsutsugamushi*, originally classified serologically, has subsequently been analyzed genetically (40). In each geographic area there are several genetic variants. Phylogeny reveals nine clusters that are not identical with serotypes. The genotypes do not have strong evidence of geographic differentiation (40). Genetic variants of *O. tsutsugamushi* appear to correspond to particular arthropod hosts in which divergence most likely occurred.

DESCRIPTION OF THE GENERA

Species of *Rickettsia* are small (0.3 to 0.5 μm by 1 to 2 μm), obligately intracellular bacteria of the *Alphaproteobacteria* with a gram-negative cell wall structure that contains lipopolysaccharide, peptidoglycan, a major 135-kDa S-layer protein (OmpB), a 17-kDa lipoprotein, and, for SFG rickettsiae, a surface-exposed protein (OmpA) containing different numbers of nearly identical tandem repeat units (27, 98). *Rickettsia* organisms have small (1.1 to 1.5 Mb), A+T-rich genomes resulting from reductive evolution with a high proportion (19 to 24%) of noncoding sequence. Among SFG and TG rickettsiae the genomes have remarkable synteny (57). The lack of genes for enzymes for sugar metabolism, lipid biosynthesis, nucleotide synthesis, and amino acid synthesis and the presence of genes encoding enzymes for the complete tricarboxylic acid cycle and several copies of ATP/ADP translocase suggest both independent synthesis of ATP and acquisition of host ATP and rickettsial utilization of host sources for nutrition and building blocks. Rickettsiae adhere to the host cell receptor Ku70 by OmpB (and also by OmpA to an unknown receptor for SFG rickettsiae), trigger signaling pathways leading to recruitment and activation of induced phagocytosis, and

TABLE 1 Characteristics of *Rickettsia* and *Orientia*
tsutsugamushi[a]

Organism(s)	LPS	OmpA	OmpB	17-kDa lipo-protein	56-kDa protein
SFG	S	+	+	+	0
T group	T	0	+	+	0
R. canadensis	T	+	+	+	0
R. bellii	B	0	+	+	0
O. tsutsugamushi	0	0	0	0	+

[a]LPS, lipopolysaccharide; S, SFG LPS present; T, TG LPS present; B,
R. bellii-type LPS present. Symbols: +, present; 0, absent.

escape from the phagosome by membranolytic activities
of rickettsial phospholipase D and TlyC (54, 55, 112). O.
tsutsugamushi (0.3 to 0.5 μm by 0.8 to 1.5 μm) has a 2.1-Mb
genome with high proportions of genes encoding mobile
genetic elements, identical repeats, and fragmented genes
and a low coding capacity (13). The organisms have a major
surface protein of 54 to 58 kDa as well as 110-, 80-, 47-,
42-, 35-, 28-, and 25-kDa surface proteins but lack muramic
acid, glucosamine, 2-keto-3-deoctulonic acid, and hydroxy
fatty acids, suggesting the absence of lipopolysaccharide and
peptidoglycan. *Orientia* has a more plastic gram-negative
cell wall with a thicker outer leaflet and thinner inner leaflet of the outer envelope than those of *Rickettsia*.

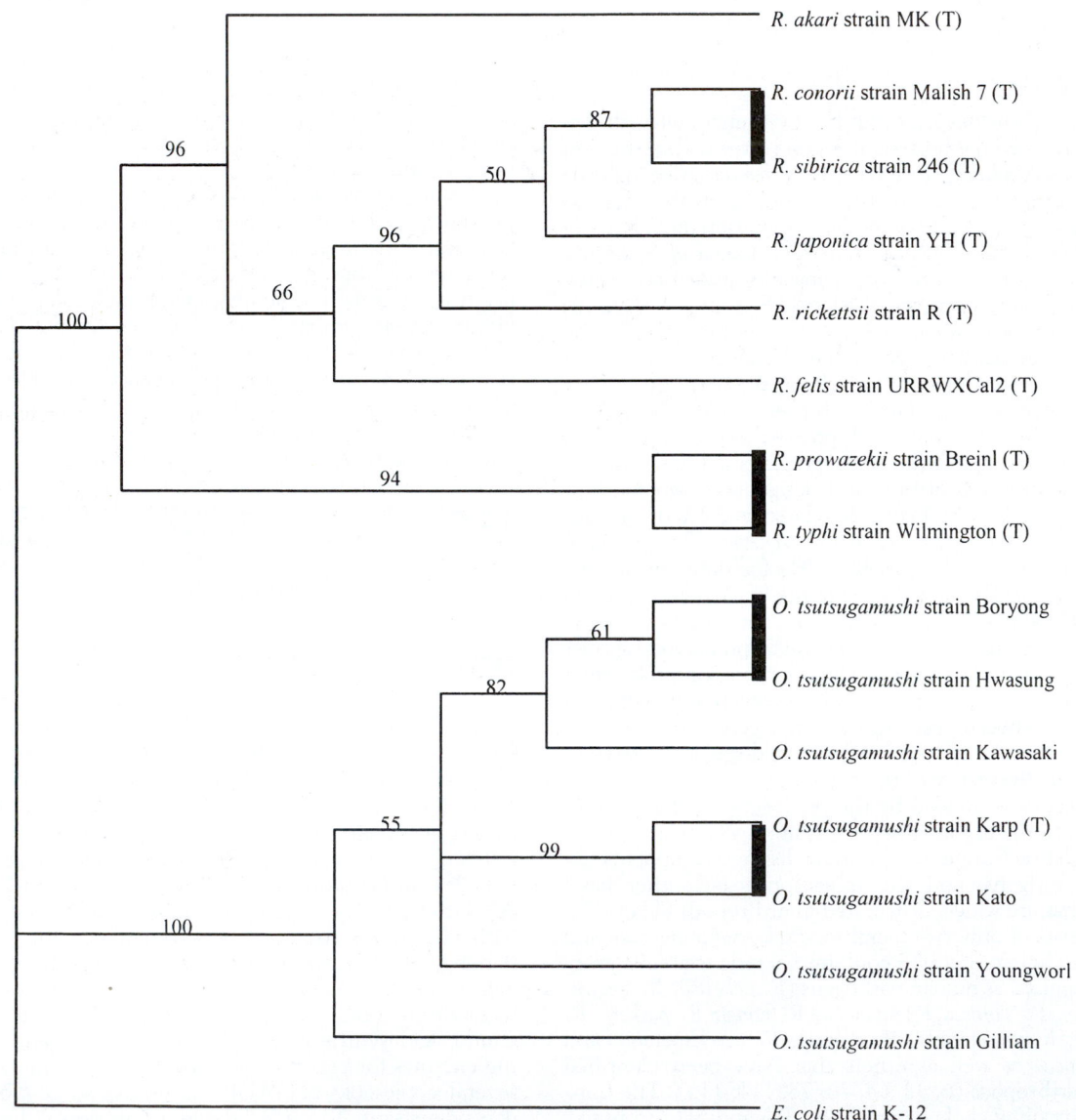

FIGURE 1 Phylogeny of *Rickettsia* and *Orientia* as determined by unweighted maximum-parsimony
analyses of *groEL* gene sequences prepared by PAUP 4.0 software with *Escherichia coli* as the outgroup.
Numerical values on the branches represent the quantity of genetic divergence from the nearest node.
(T) indicates type strain.

EPIDEMIOLOGY AND TRANSMISSION

Rickettsia spp. reside in an arthropod host (tick, mite, louse, flea, or other insect) for at least a part of their life cycle, during which they are maintained by transovarian transmission and/or cycles involving horizontal transmission to vertebrate hosts (7, 17, 31, 46, 56, 69, 70, 92) (Table 2). *Orientia* resides free in the cytosol and is maintained in nature by transovarian transmission in trombiculid mites, which transmit the infection to humans during feeding at the larval stage (Table 2).

CLINICAL SIGNIFICANCE

In addition to Rocky Mountain spotted fever (RMSF), rickettsialpox, murine typhus, flying squirrel-associated *R. prowazekii* infection, flea-borne spotted fever, and *R. parkeri* infection, which are indigenous to the United States, the potential for imported cases is significant for African tick bite fever, boutonneuse fever, murine typhus, and scrub typhus (Table 2) (10, 18, 38, 39, 71, 77, 86, 103, 109). Other rickettsioses, either because of their geographic distribution and the infrequency of travelers' exposure to them or because of their incidence, are unlikely to be imported. RMSF, louse-borne typhus, and scrub typhus are life-threatening illnesses even for young, previously healthy persons. Murine typhus and boutonneuse fever can have a fatal outcome in patients who are elderly or have underlying diseases or other risk factors. A recent study of 140 patients infected with *R. conorii* who were admitted to Portuguese hospitals indicated that alcoholism and infection with the Israeli strain are risk factors for a fatal outcome. Fatal cases more frequently have acute renal failure, hyperbilirubinemia, obtundation, tachypnea, petechial rash, gastrointestinal symptoms, and coagulopathy (16).

An average of 7 days after tick bite inoculation of rickettsiae, patients with RMSF develop fever, severe headache, malaise, and myalgia, frequently accompanied by nausea, vomiting, and abdominal pain and sometimes cough (38). A rash typically appears only after 3 to 5 days of illness. Rickettsiae infect endothelial cells, frequently leading to increased vascular permeability and focal hemorrhages. In severe cases, noncardiogenic pulmonary edema and rickettsial encephalitis with coma and seizures are grave conditions that often presage death (30, 102).

Rickettsia parkeri causes a milder illness with tick inoculation site eschar, fever, headache, myalgia, usually a maculopapular or vesiculopapular rash, less frequently tender regional lymphadenitis, and no reported deaths (66). Rickettsialpox has been recognized mainly as a nonfatal urban disease with disseminated vesicular rash and an eschar at the location of rickettsial inoculation by the feeding mite (39). The complete spectrum of clinical manifestations of *R. felis* infections has yet to be determined. This disease suffers from diagnostic neglect despite its widening recognized geographic distribution and the prevalence of cat flea exposure (86, 96, 116, 119, 120).

Murine typhus causes a rash in only slightly more than one-half of patients, cough and chest radiographic infiltrates suggesting pneumonia in many patients, and in some patients severe illness with seizures, coma, and renal and respiratory failure necessitating intensive care unit admission in 10% of hospitalized cases (18).

Travelers who have returned from Africa and develop fever, one or more eschars, and, in some cases, regional lymphadenopathy and a maculopapular or vesicular rash are very likely infected with *R. africae* (77).

Rickettsia prowazekii, *R. rickettsii*, *R. typhi*, and *R. conorii* are bioterror threats via aerosol exposure to organisms that are infectious at a low dose (100).

Scrub typhus caused by *O. tsutsugamushi* occurs in the geographic area that is bordered by Japan, Korea, and Russia on the north, Australia and Indonesia on the south, Pakistan and Afghanistan on the west, and the Philippines and Micronesia on the east (90). Clinical signs and symptoms of the disease include fever, headache, maculopapular rash, eschar, interstitial pneumonia, temporary deafness, lymphadenopathy, and central nervous system involvement (11, 74, 88, 90, 106). Without treatment, mortality can reach up to 30% (11, 51, 95, 106).

COLLECTION, TRANSPORT, AND STORAGE OF SPECIMENS

Blood should be collected as early as possible in the course of illness. For the isolation of rickettsiae, blood should be obtained in a sterile heparin-containing vial prior to the administration of antimicrobial agents that are active against rickettsiae (38, 48). For isolation and immunocytologic diagnosis, blood may be stored temporarily at 4°C and should be processed as promptly as possible. If inoculation of cell culture or animals must be delayed for more than 24 h, plasma, buffy coat, whole blood, or biopsied tissue should be frozen rapidly and stored at −70°C or in liquid nitrogen. EDTA- or sodium citrate-anticoagulated blood collected in the acute state has been used effectively for the diagnosis of boutonneuse fever, murine typhus, epidemic typhus, Japanese spotted fever, scrub typhus, and, with lower sensitivity, RMSF and African tick bite fever by PCR (23, 77, 84, 86, 91, 118). PCR provides a higher diagnostic yield when applied to biopsy specimens of rickettsia-infected lesions, particularly eschars (5, 16, 44, 61, 65). If whole blood, plasma, buffy coat, or tissue cannot be processed for PCR within several days, it should be stored at −20°C or lower. Serum has a lower sensitivity for PCR but is often diagnostic in fatal cases (52, 62).

For serologic diagnosis, blood is collected as early in the course of disease as possible, a second sample is collected after 1 or 2 weeks, and if a fourfold rise in antibodies has not occurred, a third sample is collected 3 or 4 weeks after onset. The serum may be stored for several days at 4°C but should be stored frozen at −20°C or lower for longer periods to avoid degradation of the antibodies. However, blood samples collected by finger stick on appropriate blotting paper in remote areas and sent by ordinary mail can be used for serologic diagnosis (20, 72). Even after transport at ambient temperature, this collection method yields a serologic sensitivity similar to that of testing of fresh serum for indirect immunofluorescence assay (IFA) diagnosis of scrub typhus (72).

A 3-mm-diameter punch biopsy specimen of a skin lesion, preferably a maculopapule containing a petechia or the margin of an eschar, should be collected as soon as possible (59, 101). Although treatment should not be delayed, it is best to perform the biopsy prior to the completion of 24 h of treatment with a tetracycline or chloramphenicol. For immunohistologic detection of rickettsiae, the specimen can be snap-frozen for frozen sectioning or fixed in formaldehyde for the preparation of paraffin-embedded sections (27, 38, 39, 59, 101–105). The former approach yields an answer more rapidly, but freezing artifacts distort the architecture of the tissue, and fixed tissue is more convenient for shipping to a reference laboratory. Aseptically

TABLE 2 Etiology, epidemiology, and ecology of rickettsial diseases

Organism(s)	Disease	Geographic distribution	Typical mode of transmission to humans	Natural cycle
SFG				
R. rickettsii	RMSF	Western hemisphere	Tick bite	Transovarian in ticks and vertebrate-tick cycles
R. conorii	Boutonneuse fever	Southern Europe, Africa, Middle East	Tick bite	Transovarian in ticks and likely vertebrate-tick cycles
R. africae	African tick bite fever	Sub-Saharan Africa, Caribbean	Tick bite	Transovarian in ticks
R. parkeri	Maculatum disease	North and South America	Tick bite	Transovarian in ticks
R. sibirica	North Asian tick typhus; Lymphangitis-associated rickettsiosis	Asia, Europe, Africa	Tick bite	Transovarian in ticks
R. japonica	Japanese spotted fever	Japan, Korea	Tick bite	Ticks
R. heilongjiangensis	Far Eastern tick-borne rickettsiosis	Russia	Tick bite	Ticks
R. honei	Flinders Island spotted fever	Australia, Thailand	Tick bite	Transovarian in ticks
R. slovaca	Tick-borne lymphadenopathy	Eurasia	Tick bite	Unknown
R. massiliae, R. monacensis, R. aeschlimannii, R. helvetica	Few case reports of unnamed diseases	Varied	Presumed tick bite	Ticks
TG				
R. prowazekii	Primary louse-borne typhus	Worldwide	Infected louse feces rubbed into broken skin or mucous membranes or inhaled as an aerosol	Human-louse cycle; flying squirrel-flea and/or louse cycle
R. prowazekii	Brill-Zinsser disease	Worldwide	Recrudescence years after primary attack of louse-borne typhus	
R. typhi	Murine typhus	Worldwide	Infected flea feces rubbed into broken skin or mucous membranes or inhaled as an aerosol	Rat-flea cycle; opossum-flea cycle
Transitional group				
R. akari	Rickettsialpox	United States, Ukraine, Croatia, Korea, Turkey, Mexico	Mite bite	Transovarian in mites and mite-mouse cycles
R. australis	Queensland tick typhus	Australia	Tick bite	Ticks
R. felis	Flea-borne spotted fever	North and South America, Europe, Africa	Not known	Transovarian in cat fleas
Scrub typhus group				
O. tsutsugamushi	Scrub typhus	Japan, eastern Asia, northern Australia, west and southwest Pacific and Indian Oceans	Chigger bite	Transovarian in mites

collected autopsy tissues, e.g., spleen and lung, are useful for rickettsial isolation, ideally inoculated fresh, or held for 24 h at 4°C or stored frozen at −70°C for longer periods if the specimen must be shipped to a public health or reference laboratory. Autopsy tissues can also be examined for rickettsiae by immunohistochemistry or PCR.

Body lice (*Pediculus humanus corporis*) removed from the clothing of patients with suspected epidemic typhus can be examined for the presence of rickettsiae. Body lice acquire rickettsiae and remain infected for life, thus providing a useful specimen for PCR diagnosis even after a prolonged period of shipping at ambient temperature and humidity, which do not ensure survival of the lice (82).

DIRECT DETECTION

General Considerations

Molecular and immunohistochemical diagnostic tests, the most useful methods for establishing a diagnosis during the acute stage of illness (when therapeutic decisions are critical), are available at this time, to the best of our knowledge, in only a few reference laboratories, including ours. Individual cases for immunohistochemistry may be referred to the following laboratories after contacting the directors for consultation: David H. Walker, Department of Pathology, University of Texas Medical Branch, 301 University Blvd., Keiller Building, Room 1.116, Galveston, TX 77555-0609 [telephone, (409) 772-3989; fax, (409) 772-1850; e-mail, dwalker@utmb.edu]; J. Stephen Dumler, Division of Medical Microbiology, Department of Pathology, The Johns Hopkins Medical Institutions, Meyer B1-193, 600 North Wolfe St., Baltimore, MD 21287 [telephone, (410) 955-8654; fax, (410) 287-3665; e-mail, sdumler@jhmi.edu]; Sherif Zaki, Infectious Disease Pathology Branch, National Center for Emerging and Zoonotic Infectious Diseases, Centers for Disease Control and Prevention, 1600 Clifton Rd., Mail Stop G-32, Atlanta, GA 30333 [telephone, (404) 639-3133; e-mail, sxz1@cdc.gov]; and Robert Massung, Rickettsial Zoonosis Branch, Centers for Disease Control and Prevention, 1600 Clifton Rd., Mail Stop G-13, Atlanta, GA 30333 [telephone, (404) 639-1082; e-mail, rmassung@cdc.gov].

Immunologic Detection

The diagnoses of RMSF, *R. parkeri* infection, boutonneuse fever, African tick bite fever, murine typhus, louse-borne typhus, and rickettsialpox have been established by immunohistochemical detection of rickettsiae in formalin-fixed, paraffin-embedded sections of biopsy specimens of rash and eschar lesions (30, 38, 61, 101, 103, 105) (Fig. 2, left). Monoclonal antibodies that are specific for lipopolysaccharides of either SFG or TG rickettsiae have been used to detect rickettsiae by immunohistochemical staining (Fig. 2, right). There is no antibody commercially available (103, 104). The sensitivity and specificity of immunohistochemical detection of *R. rickettsii* in cutaneous biopsy specimens are 70 and 100%, respectively (38, 101). Eschar biopsies yield sensitive specimens for the diagnosis of SFG rickettsioses that manifest that lesion and should be considered for diagnostic evaluation for patients suspected to have rickettsialpox, *R. parkeri* infection, boutonneuse fever, or African tick bite fever. Because histologic processing results in heat denaturation of species-specific antigens, immunohistochemistry only distinguishes *Rickettsia* at the SFG or TG level.

Immunocytochemical detection of *R. conorii* in circulating endothelial cells has been accomplished by capture of the endothelial cells from blood samples using magnetic beads coated with a monoclonal antibody to a human

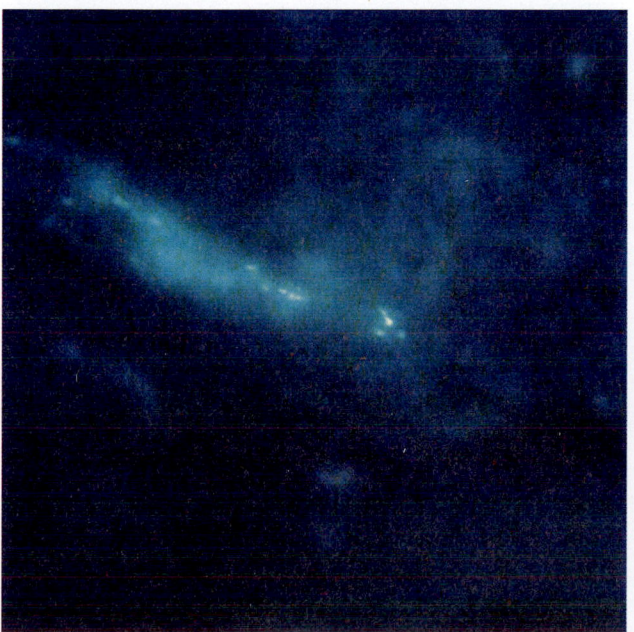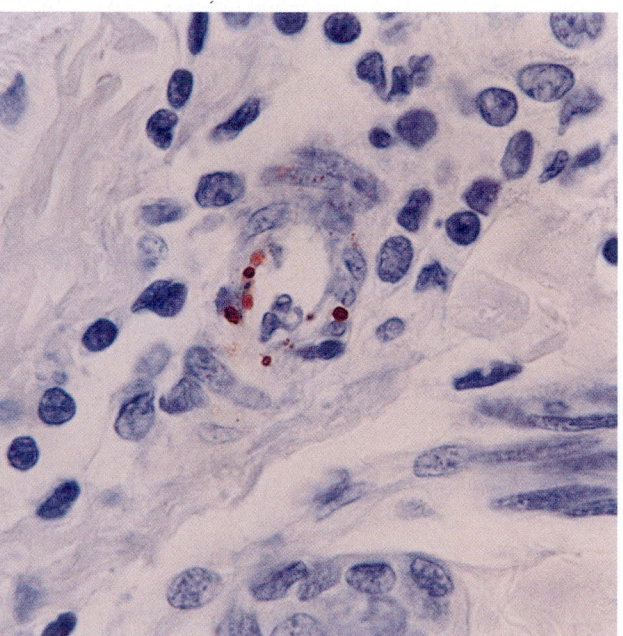

FIGURE 2 (Left) Direct immunofluorescence staining of skin biopsy specimens with anti-SFG *Rickettsia* antibodies facilitates rapid diagnosis. Rickettsiae are present in the vessel wall. (Right) Demonstration of rickettsial organisms in the microvasculature of the dermis in a patient with a history of RMSF. Rickettsiae are seen in the vessel wall. An immunoperoxidase stain, using monoclonal antibodies directed against SFG lipopolysaccharide, was used. Skin biopsy magnification, ×800.

endothelial cell surface antigen followed by immunofluorescent staining of the intracellular rickettsiae (48). This method has a sensitivity of 50% and a specificity of 94%. Rickettsiae are detected in 56% of untreated patients and in 29% of patients receiving antirickettsial treatment. *O. tsutsugamushi* has been identified using immunohistochemistry in human endothelial cells, macrophages, and cardiac myocytes (60). The technique of in situ hybridization has been developed but has not been reported for the detection of rickettsiae in clinical samples.

Molecular Detection

PCR has been applied to the amplification of the DNA of *R. rickettsii, R. parkeri, R. conorii, R. japonica, R. typhi, R. prowazekii, R. africae, R. sibirica, R. felis, R. akari, R. slovaca,* and *O. tsutsugamushi,* usually from peripheral blood, buffy coat, or plasma but occasionally from fresh, frozen, or paraffin-embedded tissue or arthropod vectors from patients (14, 23, 53, 65, 77, 82, 84, 86, 87, 89, 97). Nested PCR applied to skin biopsy specimens, particularly of eschars prior to treatment, has a sensitivity of 78% (22). For all pathogenic *Rickettsia* spp., the 17-kDa lipoprotein gene is a target, employing the primers CAT-TACTTGGTTCTCAATTCGGT and GTTTTATTAGTG-GTTACGTAACC, which amplify a 231-bp DNA fragment (86). The *gltA, rrs, groEL, ompA,* and *ompB* genes have also been amplified diagnostically, with the *Rickettsia* being identified through either restriction fragment length polymorphism analysis using AluI and XbaI or sequencing of the PCR product. The availability of rickettsial genome sequences offers the possible design of an enormous number of primer sets. The approach of using primer sets on a single occasion to reduce the chances of amplicon contamination and false-positive results seems impractical. With batch processing, the delay in laboratory results reduces the clinical value (22). The single use of primers requires that their utility and sensitivity be unknown. The potential for amplicon contamination originating from a positive patient sample remains even if there is no positive control. Recent advances in technology, such as real-time PCR, allow for increased sensitivity in the detection of rickettsiae (43, 47, 63, 67, 68, 73, 93, 97, 114). The advantage of real-time PCR is detection of rickettsial organisms during the early or acute phase of disease before the generation of antibody. The targets for primer design have ranged from housekeeping genes (*gltA*) to antigen genes (*ompA* and *ompB*). The sensitivities for detection vary among primer sets. For example, real-time assays utilizing primer set RR.190.547F (CCTGCCGATAATTAT-ACAGGTTTA) and RR.190.701R (GTTCCGTTAATG-GCAGCAT), which generates a product of 154 bp, can detect five copies of rickettsial DNA. The primer set CS-5 and CS-6 detects 1 copy of *R. rickettsii* DNA and 10 copies of *R. bellii* DNA. Perhaps the best potential demonstration of real-time PCR as a diagnostic assay was observed in a recent study that compared real-time PCR evaluation with serology (114). In this study, primer set PanRick_2_for (5'-ATAGGACAACCGTTTATTT-3') and PanRick_2_rev (5'-CAAACATCATATGCAGAAA-3') and a probe, PanRick_3_taq (5'-FAM-CCTGATAATTCGTTA-GATTTTACCG-TMR-3'), targeting a 70-bp region of the rickettsial *gltA* gene, were utilized for diagnosis of a febrile returned traveler who also presented with a macular rash and an eschar on his leg. DNA was extracted from a small biopsied sample of the eschar and the leukocyte layer of the EDTA-treated blood samples collected from the patient and analyzed by real-time PCR. The assay was able to detect 1,476 copies of PCR target per ml (1.4 copies per μl) from the initial patient sample. The acute-phase serum of the patient had a positive IFA titer for SFG immunoglobulin M (IgM) antibodies of 64 and no IgG antibodies. Intracellular bacterial growth was observed in Gimenez-stained Vero cells on day 5 after inoculation. An IgG seroconversion was detected using convalescent-phase sera obtained 4 weeks later. This rapid (total processing time is 3 to 4 h) molecular approach is currently being evaluated further for its effectiveness as a rapid diagnostic tool (114).

For *O. tsutsugamushi,* the 56-kDa protein gene is the usual target of diagnostic PCR. The nested 56-kDa gene PCR assay is useful for the diagnosis of *O. tsutsugamushi* infections during the acute phase of the disease (84). PCR amplification of DNA from blood samples, using primers p34 (TCAAGCTT-ATTGCTAGTGCAATGTCTGC) and p55 (AGGGAT-CCCTGCTGCTGTGCTTGCTGCG), which generate a 1,003-bp product, followed by nested PCR with primers p10 (GATCAAGCTTCCTCAGCCTACTATAATGCC) and p11 (CTAGGGATCCCGACAGATGCACTATT-AGGC), yields a 483-bp product. This assay detects 10 prototype strains of *O. tsutsugamushi* and does not amplify *R. typhi* or *R. honei.* Real-time PCR assays utilizing the *Orientia htrA* gene have been applied to diagnosis with clinical samples (35, 89), and the most sensitive levels of detection (two copies per μl of buffy coat extracted DNA) have been observed when using the *groEL* gene as a target for analysis of blood collected from 61 Thai patients at the time of clinic admission (67). In this assay, a set of primers (forward primer, 5'-TTGCAACRAATCGTGAAAAG-3', and reverse primer, 5'-TCTCCGTCTACATCATCAGCA-3') were used to amplify a 459-bp fragment of the gene. This method shows promise as a diagnostic tool for the acute stage of scrub typhus. The development of a loop-mediated isothermal PCR targeting *groEL* of *O. tsutsugamushi* offers the possibility of a simple method that can be used in locations lacking costly infrastructure (68).

ISOLATION PROCEDURES

Due to their high infectivity at a low dose, rickettsial isolation is performed in biosafety level 3 laboratories. Cumbersome historic methods, such as inoculation of adult male guinea pigs, mice, or the yolk sac of embryonated chicken eggs, have been supplanted by cell culture methods, except for isolation of *O. tsutsugamushi,* which is often achieved by intraperitoneal inoculation of mice (38, 48). Vero, L-929, HEL, and MRC5 cells have been used in antibiotic-free media to isolate rickettsiae. The best results are achieved with heparin-anticoagulated plasma, buffy coat, or skin lesion biopsy specimens collected prior to administration of antirickettsial therapy.

Samples containing 0.5 ml of triturated clinical material mixed with 0.5 ml of tissue culture medium are inoculated as promptly as possible onto 3.7-ml shell vials with 12-mm-diameter round coverslips having a confluent layer of cells and centrifuged at 700 × g for 1 h at room temperature to enhance attachment and entry of rickettsiae into host cells (3, 48). After removal of the inoculum, the shell vials are washed with phosphate-buffered saline and incubated with minimal essential medium containing 10% fetal calf serum in an atmosphere containing 5% CO_2 at 34°C. At 48 and 72 h, a coverslip is examined by Giemsa or Gimenez stain or by immunofluorescence with antibodies against SFG and TG rickettsiae. Detection of four or more organisms is interpreted as a positive result. This method has yielded a diagnosis in 59% of samples from patients with boutonneuse fever who had neither been treated nor developed antibodies to *R. conorii* prior to collection of the sample (48). Rickettsiae were detected at 48 h of growth in 82% of the positive samples. Universal precautions should be exercised, and work should be performed in a laminar-flow biosafety hood with use of gloves, mask, and gown. Although the quantity of rickettsiae in the cell culture is relatively low, care to avoid aerosol, internal, or contact exposure should be taken as for mycobacteria, fungi, and viruses.

IDENTIFICATION OF *RICKETTSIA* AND *ORIENTIA* ISOLATES

Rickettsiae isolated in cell culture can be identified by indirect immunofluorescence with group-, species-, and strain-specific monoclonal antibodies. Rickettsial isolates are frequently identified by molecular methods such as PCR amplification of genes that are genus specific (17-kDa protein, citrate synthase [*gltA*], or *ompB*) or SFG specific (*ompA*) (80). Determination of DNA sequences identifies unique isolates. *O. tsutsugamushi*, being more distantly related to *Rickettsia* spp., lacks the above-mentioned cell wall genes but can be identified by PCR of the gene encoding the major immunodominant 56-kDa surface protein, *groEL*, or *rrs* (44, 68).

Identifying the species of rickettsial isolates by microimmunofluorescence serotyping requires intravenous inoculation of mice with rickettsiae on days 0 and 7 and collection of sera on day 10. The high-titer antibodies react with conformational species-specific epitopes of OmpA and OmpB. Antibodies against group-specific lipopolysaccharide develop later in the murine immune response to high doses of *Rickettsia*. This rather cumbersome and expensive method requires propagation of large quantities of the isolate and of the prototype strains for immunofluorescence titration as well as for development of the typing sera. Genetic analysis is currently favored for identification of isolates. An isolate that is known to be a *Rickettsia* should be identified in a biosafety level 3 laboratory, and isolates of *R. rickettsii* and *R. prowazekii* must be handled as required by U.S. federal regulations for select agents.

SEROLOGIC TESTS

For most clinical microbiology laboratories, assays for antibodies to rickettsiae are the only tests performed. This situation is unfortunate for the patient with a life-threatening, acutely incapacitating rickettsial disease because these assays are useful principally for serologic confirmation of the diagnosis in convalescence and usually do not provide information that is helpful in making critical therapeutic decisions during the acute stage of illness. Patients who die of rickettsioses usually have received many antibiotics, none of which have antirickettsial activity owing in part to the lack of laboratory data providing clinical guidance for a rickettsial diagnosis. The earlier a diagnosis is established, the shorter the course of rickettsial illness after an appropriate antirickettsial antibiotic is administered.

Serologic assays for the diagnosis of rickettsial infections focus on the "gold standard," the IFA. Other approaches include indirect immunoperoxidase assay, latex agglutination, enzyme immunoassay (EIA), *Proteus vulgaris* OX-19 and OX-2 and *Proteus mirabilis* OX-K agglutination, line blot, Western immunoblotting, and rapid lateral flow assays (8, 12, 15, 18, 19, 28, 33, 36–39, 41, 42, 77, 101, 110, 113).

Only some of these assays are available as commercial kits or in reference laboratories, and not for all rickettsial diseases. Other serologic tests, such as indirect hemagglutination, microagglutination, and complement fixation, are no longer in general use.

The IFA contains all the rickettsial heat-labile protein antigens and group-shared lipopolysaccharide antigen and thus provides group-reactive serology. IFA reagents are available commercially for SFG and TG rickettsiae from Scimedx Corp., Denville, NJ; Focus Technologies, Cypress, CA; and Fuller Laboratories, Fullerton CA; they are also available for *O. tsutsugamushi* from Scimedx Corp. In cases of RMSF, IFA detects antibodies at a titer of ≥64, usually in the second week of illness. Effective antirickettsial treatment of RMSF must be initiated by day 5 of illness to avoid a potentially fatal outcome. For boutonneuse fever, an IFA titer of ≥40 occurs in 46% of patients between days 5 and 9 of illness, in 90% of patients between 20 and 29 days, and in 100% of patients thereafter. In murine typhus, diagnostic IFA titers are present in 50% of cases by the end of the first week of illness and in nearly all cases by 15 days after onset (18). In areas where particular rickettsial diseases are endemic, a higher diagnostic cutoff titer is required. For example, for the IFA diagnosis of scrub typhus in patients residing in zones of endemicity, an IFA titer of antibody to *O. tsutsugamushi* of ≥400 is 96% specific and 48% sensitive, with sensitivity rising from 29% in the first week to 56% in the second week (4). Lowering the diagnostic cutoff titer to 100 raises the sensitivity only to 84% and reduces the specificity to 78%. These considerations are not as important when testing patients who have visited regions of endemicity for only a short period. Each laboratory performing the test should establish its own cutoff titers for the patient population, the microscope and reagents used, and the laboratorian's judgment of the minimal positive signal. Meta-analysis of IFA serology for the diagnosis of scrub typhus led to recommendations that diagnosis be based on a fourfold or greater rise in titer and that diagnosis not be based on a single antibody titer unless previous studies had determined the seroprevalence in the local population justifying the cutoff titer (4).

Indirect immunoperoxidase assays for scrub typhus, murine typhus, boutonneuse fever, and presumably other rickettsioses yield results similar to those of IFA when the IgG diagnostic titer is set at 128 and that of IgM is set at 32 (42). Advantages include the use of a light microscope rather than a fluorescence microscope and the production of a permanent slide result. Latex agglutination test reagents are available commercially from Scimedx Corp., only for *R. rickettsii* in the United States. Latex beads coated with an extracted rickettsial protein-carbohydrate complex containing rickettsial lipopolysaccharide are agglutinated mainly by IgM antibodies, with reports of a sensitivity of 71 to 94% and a specificity of 96 to 99% (28). A diagnostic titer of 128 is often detected early in the second week of illness.

EIAs have been developed in various formats, including antigens coating microtiter wells or immobilized on nitrocellulose or other sheets for use in the commercial reference laboratory setting. Dot EIA kits are commercially available in the United States from Scimedx Corp. for detecting antibodies against *R. rickettsii*, *R. conorii*, *R. typhi*, and *O. tsutsugamushi* (41, 110). No peer-reviewed publications have described evaluation of the use of the dot EIA for the diagnosis of RMSF. Compared with an IFA titer of ≥64 for the diagnosis of murine typhus, the dot EIA showed a sensitivity of 88% and specificity of 91% (41). The dot EIA for diagnosis of scrub typhus had sensitivities and specificities of only 80 and 77%, respectively, compared with an IFA cutoff titer of 64, and 89 and 66%, respectively, at an IFA cutoff titer of 128 (110). These SFG rickettsia and *R. typhi* kits detect cross-reactive antibodies, as demonstrated in an outbreak of African tick bite fever by clinical and epidemiological data. The dot EIA of *R. conorii* antigen provided early diagnostic evidence of an SFG rickettsiosis. Subsequent analysis revealed poor specificity with a high rate of false-positive results. These assays are diagnostic tools that do not require expensive, specialized equipment, but they suffer from apparent low specificity. Standard EIAs for detecting IgG or IgM antibodies against SFG rickettsiae or *O. tsutsugamushi* are also available from Panbio Diagnostics internationally but are not currently available for purchase in the United States. The utilization of these tests for paired sera from populations with clinical (fever, headache, or rash) and epidemiological (vector exposure) features consistent with rickettsiosis would most likely yield useful information. A multitest dot EIA for scrub typhus, murine typhus, and leptospirosis was not useful in Thailand, where nearly all patients had antibodies to more than one agent and others had antibodies to an agent that was not the cause of the illness (108). The diagnosis of scrub typhus by detection of antibodies in clinical samples in an IgM capture enzyme-linked immunosorbent assay can be utilized for single serum samples from early-stage infections (33). The performance values of this assay are a sensitivity of 96.3% and a specificity of 99%. A comparison of serologic methods for scrub typhus revealed that an EIA containing recombinant p56 of Karp, Kato, and Gilliam strains was most sensitive (100%) and that rapid lateral-flow assay of antibodies against recombinant Karp p56 had a sensitivity of 86% (33). The latter, which is especially useful in situations with limited laboratory facilities and a low number of specimens, is available from Panbio Ltd., Brisbane, Australia.

The assays that were historically most widely used for the diagnosis of rickettsial diseases are agglutination of the OX-19 and OX-2 strains of *Proteus vulgaris* for TG and SFG rickettsioses and the OX-K strain of *Proteus mirabilis* for *O. tsutsugamushi* infections. These assays have poor sensitivity and specificity (37, 101). They should be replaced by more accurate serologic methods such as IFA or EIA. However, there are situations in developing countries where the choice is between the *Proteus* agglutination tests and none at all for the detection of important public health problems such as outbreaks of louse-borne typhus (1). In fact, the evidence leading to the discovery of Japanese spotted fever and Flinders Island spotted fever included *Proteus* agglutinating antibodies.

Shared antigens of OmpA, OmpB, and group-specific lipopolysaccharide impede establishment of a species-specific diagnosis by serologic methods. The criterion of a fourfold or greater difference in IFA titers between the two suspected agents distinguished infections by *R. prowazekii* and *R. typhi* in only 34% of cases and infections by *R. africae* from those by *R. conorii* in only 26% (49, 77). Western immunoblotting detection of antibodies against OmpA or OmpB of only one *Rickettsia* species has also been proposed as a criterion for species-specific diagnosis. However, it was effective in distinguishing *R. prowazekii* and *R. typhi* infections or *R. africae* and *R. conorii* infections in only one-half of the cases (34, 49, 77). Cumbersome, expensive cross-absorption of sera prior to IFA or Western immunoblotting is more effective in establishing a species-specific diagnosis. However, interpretation of these results requires careful

evaluation of the performance of valid controls, the quality and quantity of each antigen preparation, and the potential for the occurrence of infection by an untested, even as-yet-discovered, agent. In the past, knowledge of the geographic origin of the case sufficed to designate the specific diagnosis. However, the increasing number and geographic overlap of rickettsioses challenge the old assumptions. The report of the reactivity of sera from patients with flea-borne spotted fever but not patients with RMSF, rickettsialpox, or murine typhus with a recombinant fragment of *R. felis* OmpA suggests that species-specific peptide antigens may be identified and incorporated into assays that identify the disease more precisely (117).

ANTIMICROBIAL SUSCEPTIBILITY TESTING

Data supporting the use of doxycycline or another tetracycline antibiotic as the drug of choice for the treatment of infections caused by *Rickettsia* spp. and *O. tsutsugamushi* and the use of chloramphenicol as an alternative drug have been derived principally by empirical experience, retrospective case studies, and a few prospective studies (2, 9, 25, 29, 45, 58, 79, 81, 83, 94). In addition to historic studies of the activity of antimicrobial agents against these obligately intracellular bacteria in infected animals and embryonated eggs, studies of the effects of antimicrobial agents in cell culture have supported the consideration of alternative drugs such as fluoroquinolones, josamycin, azithromycin, and clarithromycin. Indeed, several fluoroquinolones, josamycin, and azithromycin have been used successfully for the treatment of boutonneuse fever under certain circumstances but cannot be recommended for more pathogenic rickettsioses (2, 9, 58, 79). Mediterranean spotted fever has also been treated effectively in clinical trials with fluoroquinolones such as ciprofloxacin and macrolides such as azithromycin or clarithromycin. A retrospective study of patients with murine typhus demonstrated that ciprofloxacin is an effective drug. Except for cases of scrub typhus in Thailand which have not responded to doxycycline or chloramphenicol but for which azithromycin has been reported to be effective, there is little concern regarding rickettsial development of antimicrobial resistance (45, 94, 107). During pregnancy, chloramphenicol has been used to treat RMSF and josamycin for boutonneuse fever. Antimicrobial susceptibility studies of rickettsiae are not routinely performed clinical laboratory tests.

INTERPRETATION AND REPORTING OF RESULTS

When reporting the results of an assay for antibodies in a single serum sample, the laboratorian seldom knows the duration of illness and whether the serum sample is from the acute or the convalescent phase of the disease. For sera that are nonreactive by dot EIA, by IFA at a dilution of 1:64, by indirect immunoperoxidase assay at a dilution of 1:128, by latex agglutination at a dilution of 1:64, or by Weil-Felix *Proteus* agglutination at a titer of 1:160, the laboratory report should state that no antibodies were detected at the particular cutoff dilution, which may differ among some laboratories and some patient populations, that negative results are expected in the acute stage of rickettsial illness, and that a second sample should be submitted to evaluate the possibility of seroconversion if no alternative diagnosis has been established. If paired acute- and convalescent-phase sera separated by an appropriate interval are available, they should be tested simultaneously. It is wise to test for all the rickettsial and ehrlichial agents to which the patient is likely to have been exposed in the United States. SFG rickettsiae, *Ehrlichia chaffeensis*, *Anaplasma phagocytophilum*, and *R. typhi* are the likely agents unless travel to an area where scrub typhus is endemic has occurred. If the paired sera are negative, the report should state that the results do not support the diagnosis of rickettsial infection but that occasionally antibody synthesis is delayed, particularly in cases with early antirickettsial therapy. If a single serum sample contains an IFA antibody titer of ≥64, an IgM IFA titer of ≥32, an indirect immunoperoxidase antibody titer of ≥128, a latex agglutination titer of ≥64, or a Weil-Felix titer of ≥320, the laboratory report should state that antibodies reactive with the particular rickettsial antigen were detected at the measured titer, that the result provides supportive evidence for the diagnosis of the rickettsial disease, and that a convalescent-phase sample should be submitted to assess the possibility of a diagnostic rise in titer. If paired sera measured simultaneously show a fourfold or greater rise in titer, the interpretation is stated that the results strongly support the rickettsial diagnosis indicated by the tested antigen. If a significant titer was detected in the acute-phase sample, but no rise or only a single doubling dilution rise was measured, it should be stated that an additional later sample should be tested to evaluate a fourfold rise or fall in titer. The concept that recrudescent typhus could be distinguished from primary louse-borne typhus by the absence of IgM antibodies to *R. prowazekii* and of *Proteus* OX-19 agglutinating antibodies has been challenged (19). The manufacturers of the dot EIA have recommended the interpretation that strongly reactive samples (three or four dots) may indicate the presence of a specific antibody response and that weakly reactive samples (one or two dots) are infrequent but possible in normal populations. Retesting 2 to 3 weeks later would establish the diagnosis if three or four dots develop in the convalescent-phase serology and should always be performed.

Isolation of a rickettsia from blood or tissue may be interpreted as indicating an etiologic role. The level of identification of the isolate should be stated, whether identified only as to a group containing particular organisms or to the species level.

Immunohistologic and immunocytologic diagnostic interpretation states the method, reactivity of the method (e.g., antibody reactive with SFG rickettsiae), and location of the antigen (e.g., in vascular endothelium and frequently adjacent vascular smooth muscle for *R. rickettsii*). Detection of three or more rickettsiae in vascular endothelium in biopsy specimens or four or more rickettsiae in captured circulating endothelial cells is diagnostic of rickettsial infection.

Interpretation of PCR results should state the target gene, the organisms that would be detected, and the presence or absence of a DNA product. If a specific oligonucleotide probe or DNA sequencing confirmed the specificity of the identification, this result should be stated. For negative immunohistologic, immunocytologic, and PCR results, it should always be stated that the failure to detect the agent does not exclude the diagnosis, along with data regarding the sensitivity and specificity of the assay in the particular laboratory and the effects of antirickettsial treatment on the sensitivity.

Special efforts should be made to establish the diagnosis of fatal cases, including rickettsial isolation, immunohistology, PCR, and serology on samples collected at necropsy.

REFERENCES

1. **Animut, A., Y Mekonnen, D. Shimelis, and E. Ephraim.** 2009. Febrile illnesses of different etiology among outpatients in four health centers in northwestern Ethiopia. *Jpn. J. Infect. Dis.* **62:**104–110.

2. **Bella, F., B. Font, S. Uriz, T. Munoz, E. Espejo, J. Traveria, J. A. Serrano, and F. Segura.** 1990. Randomized trial of doxycycline versus josamycin for Mediterranean spotted fever. *Antimicrob. Agents Chemother.* **34:**937–938.

3. **Birg, M. L., B. La Scola, V. Roux, P. Brouqui, and D. Raoult.** 1999. Isolation of *Rickettsia prowazekii* from blood by shell vial cell culture. *J. Clin. Microbiol.* **37:**3722–3724.

4. **Blacksell, S. D., N. J. Bryant, D. H. Paris, J. A. Doust, Y. Sakoda, and N. P. J. Day.** 2007. Scrub typhus serologic testing with the indirect immunofluorescence method as a diagnostic gold standard: a lack of consensus leads to lots of confusion. *Clin. Infect. Dis.* **44:**391–401.

5. **Boudebouch, N., M. Sarih, C. Socolovschi, T. Fatihi, A. Chakib, H. Amarouch, M. Hassar, J.-M. Rolain, P. Parola, and D. Raoult.** 2008. Spotted fever group rickettsioses documented in Morocco. *Clin. Microbiol. Infect.* **15:**257–258.

6. **Bouyer, D. H., J. Stenos, P. Crocquet-Valdes, C. G. Moron, V. L. Popov, J. E. Zavala-Velazquez, L. D. Foil, D. R. Stothard, A. F. Azad, and D. H. Walker.** 2001. *Rickettsia felis:* molecular characterization of a new member of the spotted fever group. *Int. J. Syst. Evol. Microbiol.* **51:**339–347.

7. **Brouqui, P., P. Parola, P. E. Fournier, and D. Raoult.** 2007. Spotted fever rickettsioses in southern and eastern Europe. *FEMS Immunol. Med. Microbiol.* **49:**2–12.

8. **Brown, G. W., A. Shirai, C. Rogers, and M. G. Groves.** 1983. Diagnostic criteria for scrub typhus: probability values for immunofluorescent antibody and *Proteus* OXK agglutinin titers. *Am. J. Trop. Med. Hyg.* **32:**1101–1107.

9. **Cascio, A., C. Colomba, D. Di Rosa, L. Salsa, L. di Martino, and L. Titone.** 2001. Efficacy and safety of clarithromycin as treatment for Mediterranean spotted fever in children: a randomized controlled trial. *Clin. Infect. Dis.* **33:**409–411.

10. **Chapman, A. S., in collaboration with the Tickborne Rickettsial Diseases Working Group.** 2006. Diagnosis and management of tickborne rickettsial diseases: Rocky Mountain spotted fever, ehrlichioses, and anaplasmosis—United States. *MMWR Recommend. Rep.* **55**(RR-4):1–27.

11. **Charoensak, A., O. Charwalparit, C. Suttinont, K. Niwattayakul, K. Losuwanaluk, S. Silpasakor, and Y. Suputtamongkol.** 2006. Scrub typhus: chest radiographic and clinical findings in 130 Thai patients. *J. Med. Assoc. Thai.* **89:**600–606.

12. **Ching, W. M., D. Rowland, Z. Zhang, A. L. Bourgeois, D. Kelly, G. A. Dasch, and P. L. Devine.** 2001. Early diagnosis of scrub typhus with a rapid flow assay using recombinant major outer membrane protein antigen (r56) of *Orientia tsutsugamushi*. *Clin. Diagn. Lab. Immunol.* **8:**409–414.

13. **Cho, N.-H., H.-R. Kim, J.-H. Lee, S.-Y. K. J. Kim, S. Cha, S.-Y. Kim, A. C. Darby, H.-H. Fuxelius, J. Yin, J. H. Kim, H. Kim, S. J. Lee, Y.-S. Koh, W.-J. Jang, K.-H. Park, S. G. E. Andersson, M.-S. Choi, and K.-S. Kim.** 2007. The *Orientia tsutsugamushi* genome reveals massive proliferation of conjugative type IV secretion system and host-cell interaction genes. *Proc. Natl. Acad. Sci. USA* **104:**7981–7986.

14. **Choi, Y.-J., W.-J. Jang, J.-H. Kim, J.-S. Ryu, S.-H. Lee, K.-H. Park, H.-S. Paik, Y.-S. Koh, M.-S. Choi, and I.-S. Kim.** 2005. Spotted fever group and typhus group rickettsioses in humans, South Korea. *Emerg. Infect. Dis.* **11:**237–244.

15. **Coleman, R. E., V. Sangkasuwan, N. Suwanabun, C. Eamsila, S. Mungviriya, P. Devine, A. L. Richards, D. Rowland, W.-M. Ching, J. Sattabongkot, and K. Lerdthusnee.** 2002. Comparative evaluation of selected diagnostic assays for the detection of IgG and IgM antibody to *Orientia tsutsugamushi* in Thailand. *Am. J. Trop. Med. Hyg.* **67:**497–503.

16. **de Sousa, R., A. Franca, S. D. Nobrega, A. Belo, M. Amaro, T. Abreu, J. Pocas, P. Proenca, J. Vaz, J. Torgal, F. Bacellar, N. Ismail, and D. H. Walker.** 2008. Host- and microbe-related risk factors for and pathophysiology of fatal

Rickettsia conorii infection in Portuguese patients. *J. Infect. Dis.* **198:**576–585.

17. Dobler, G., and R. Wolfel. 2009. Typhus and other rickettsioses. *Dtsch. Arztebl. Int.* **106:**348–354.

18. Dumler, J., J. P. Taylor, and D. H. Walker. 1991. Clinical and laboratory features of murine typhus in south Texas, 1980 through 1987. *JAMA* **266:**1365–1370.

19. Eremeeva, M. E., N. M. Balayeva, and D. Raoult. 1994. Serological response of patients suffering from primary and recrudescent typhus: comparison of complement fixation reaction, Weil-Felix test, microimmunofluorescence, and immunoblotting. *Clin. Diagn. Lab. Immunol.* **1:**318–324.

20. Fenollar, F., and D. Raoult. 1999. Diagnosis of rickettsial diseases using samples dried on blotting paper. *Clin. Diagn. Lab. Immunol.* **6:**483–488.

21. Fournier, P. E., J. S. Dumler, G. Greub, J. Zhang, Y. Wu, and D. Raoult. 2003. Gene sequence-based criteria for identification of new *Rickettsia* isolates and description of *Rickettsia heilongjiangensis* sp. nov. *J. Clin. Microbiol.* **41:**5456–5465.

22. Fournier, P. E., and D. Raoult. 2004. Suicide PCR on skin biopsy specimens for diagnosis of rickettsioses. *J. Clin. Microbiol.* **42:**3428–3434.

23. Furuya, Y., T. Katayama, Y. Yoshida, and I. Kaiho. 1995. Specific amplification of *Rickettsia japonica* DNA from clinical specimens by PCR. *J. Clin. Microbiol.* **33:**487–489.

24. Gevers, D., F. M. Cohan, J. G. Lawrence, B. G. Spratt, T. Coenye, E. J. Feil, E. Stackebrandt, Y. Van de Peer, P. Vandamme, F. L. Thompson, and J. Swings. 2005. Re-evaluating prokaryotic species. *Nat. Rev. Microbiol.* **3:**733–739.

25. Gikas, A., S. Doukakis, J. Pediaditis, S. Kastanakis, A. Psaroulaki, and Y. Tselentis. 2002. Murine typhus in Greece: epidemiological, clinical, and therapeutic data from 83 cases. *Trans. R. Soc. Trop. Med. Hyg.* **96:**250–253.

26. Gillespie, J. J., K. Williams, M. Shukla, E. E. Snyder, E. K. Norkberg, S. M. Ceraul, C. Dharmanolla, D. Rainery, J. Soneja, J. M. Shallom, N. Dongre Vishnubhat, R. Wattam, A. Purkayastha, M. Czar, O. Crasta, J. C. Setubal, A. F. Azad, and B. S. Sobral. 2008. *Rickettsia* phylogenomics: unwinding the intricacies of obligate intracellular life. *PLoS One* **3:**e2018.

27. Gilmore, R. D., Jr. 1993. Comparison of the *rompA* gene repeat regions of *Rickettsiae* reveals species-specific arrangements of individual repeating units. *Gene* **125:**97–102.

28. Hechemy, K. E., R. L. Anacker, R. N. Philip, K. T. Kleeman, J. N. MacCormack, S. J. Sasowski, and E. E. Michaelson. 1980. Detection of Rocky Mountain spotted fever antibodies by a latex agglutination test. *J. Clin. Microbiol.* **12:**144–150.

29. Holman, R. C., C. D. Paddock, A. T. Curns, J. W. Krebs, J. H. McQuiston, and J. E. Childs. 2001. Analysis of risk factors for fatal Rocky Mountain spotted fever: evidence for superiority of tetracyclines for therapy. *J. Infect. Dis.* **184:**1437–1444.

30. Horney, L. F., and D. H. Walker. 1988. Meningoencephalitis as a major manifestation of Rocky Mountain spotted fever. *South. Med. J.* **81:**915–918.

31. Horta, M. C., J. Moraes-Filho, R. A. Casagrande, T. B. Saito, S. C. Rosa, M. Ogrzewalska, E. R. Matushima, and M. B. Labruna. 2009. Experimental infection of opossums *Didelphis aurita* by *Rickettsia rickettsii* and evaluation of the transmission of the infection to ticks *Amblyomma cajennense*. *Vector Borne Zoonotic Dis.* **9:**109–118.

32. Jado, I., J. A. Oteo, M. Aldamiz, H. Gil, R. Escudero, V. Ibarra, J. Portu, A. Portillo, M. J. Lezaun, C. Garcia-Amil, I. Rodríguez-Moreno, and P. Anda. 2007. *Rickettsia monacensis* and human disease, Spain. *Emerg. Infect. Dis.* **13:**1405–1407.

33. Jang, W. J., M. S. Huh, K. H. Park, M. S. Choi, and I. S. Kim. 2003. Evaluation of an immunoglobulin M capture enzyme-linked immunosorbent assay for diagnosis of *Orientia tsutsugamushi* infection. *Clin. Diagn. Lab. Immunol.* **10:**394–398.

34. Jensenius, M., P. E. Fournier, S. Vene, S. H. Ringertz, B. Myrvang, and D. Raoult. 2004. Comparison of immunofluo-

rescence, Western blotting, and cross-adsorption assays for diagnosis of African tick bite fever. *Clin. Diagn. Lab. Immunol.* **11:**786–788.

35. Jiang, J., T. C. Chan, J. J. Temenak, G. A. Dasch, W. M. Ching, and A. L. Richards. 2004. Development of a quantitative real-time polymerase chain reaction assay specific for *Orientia tsutsugamushi*. *Am. J. Trop. Med. Hyg.* **70:**351–356.

36. Jiang, J., K. J. Marienau, L. A. May, H. J. Beecham III, R. Wilkinson, W.-M. Ching, and A. L. Richards. 2003. Laboratory diagnosis of two scrub typhus outbreaks at Camp Fuji, Japan in 2000 and 2001 by enzyme-linked immunosorbent assay, rapid flow assay, and Western blot assay using outer membrane 56-kD recombinant proteins. *Am. J. Trop. Med. Hyg.* **69:**60–66.

37. Kaplan, J. E., and L. B. Schonberger. 1986. The sensitivity of various serologic tests in the diagnosis of Rocky Mountain spotted fever. *Am. J. Trop. Med. Hyg.* **35:**840–844.

38. Kaplowitz, L. G., J. V. Lange, J. J. Fischer, and D. H. Walker. 1983. Correlation of rickettsial titers, circulating endotoxin, and clinical features in Rocky Mountain spotted fever. *Arch. Intern. Med.* **143:**1149–1151.

39. Kass, E. M., W. K. Szaniawski, H. Levy, J. Leach, K. Srinivasan, and C. Rives. 1994. Rickettsialpox in a New York City hospital, 1980 to 1989. *N. Engl. J. Med.* **331:**1612–1617.

40. Kelly, D. J., P. A. Fuerst, W-M. Ching, and A. L. Richards. 2009. Scrub typhus: the geographic distribution of phenotypic and genotypic variants of *Orientia tsutsugamushi*. *Clin. Infect. Dis.* **48:**S203–S230.

41. Kelly, D. J., C. T. Chan, H. Paxton, K. Thompson, R. Howard, and G. A. Dasch. 1995. Comparative evaluation of a commercial enzyme immunoassay for the detection of human antibody to *Rickettsia typhi*. *Clin. Diagn. Lab. Immunol.* **2:**356–360.

42. Kelly, D. J., P. W. Wong, E. Gan, and G. E. Lewis, Jr. 1988. Comparative evaluation of the indirect immunoperoxidase test for the serodiagnosis of rickettsial disease. *Am. J. Trop. Med. Hyg.* **38:**400–406.

43. Kidd, L., R. Maggi, P. P. V. P. Diniz, B. Hegarty, M. Tucker, and E. Breitschwerdt. 2008. Evaluation of conventional and real-time PCR assays for detection and differentiation of spotted fever group *Rickettsia* in dog blood. *Vet. Microbiol.* **129:**294–303.

44. Kim, D.-M., H. L. Kim, C. Y. Park, T. Y. Yang, J. H. Lee, J. T. Yang, S.-K. Shim, and S.-H. Lee. 2006. Clinical usefulness of eschar polymerase chain reaction for the diagnosis of scrub typhus: a prospective study. *Clin. Infect. Dis.* **43:**1296–1300.

45. Kim, Y.-S., H.-J. Yun, S. K. Shim, S. H. Koo, S. Y. Kim, and S. Kim. 2004. A comparative trial of a single dose of azithromycin versus doxycycline for the treatment of mild scrub typhus. *Clin. Infect. Dis.* **39:**1329–1335.

46. Labruna, M. B., M. Ogrzewalska, T. F. Martins, A. Pinter, and M. C. Horta. 2008. Comparative susceptibility of larval stages of *Amblyomma aureolatum*, *Amblyomma cajennense*, and *Rhipicephalus sanguineus* to infection by *Rickettsia rickettsii*. *J. Med. Microbiol.* **45:**1156–1159.

47. Labruna, M. B., T. Whitworth, M. C. Horta, D. H. Bouyer, J. W. McBride, A. Pinter, V. Popov, S. M. Gennari, and D. H. Walker. 2004. *Rickettsia* species infecting *Amblyomma cooperi* ticks from an area in the state of São Paulo, Brazil, where Brazilian spotted fever is endemic. *J. Clin. Microbiol.* **42:**90–98.

48. La Scola, B., and D. Raoult. 1996. Diagnosis of Mediterranean spotted fever by cultivation of *Rickettsia conorii* from blood and skin samples using the centrifugation-shell vial technique and by detection of *R. conorii* in circulating endothelial cells: a 6-year follow-up. *J. Clin. Microbiol.* **34:**2722–2727.

49. La Scola, B., L. Rydkina, J. B. Ndihokubwayo, S. Vene, and D. Raoult. 2000. Serological differentiation of murine typhus and epidemic typhus using cross-adsorption and Western blotting. *Clin. Diagn. Lab. Immunol.* **7:**612–616.

50. Lee, J.-H., H.-S. Park, W.-J. Jang, S.-E. Koh, J.-M. Kim, S.-K. Shim, M.-Y. Park, Y.-W. Kim, B.-J. Kim, Y.-H. Kook,

K.-H. Park, and S.-H. Lee. 2003. Differentiation of rickett-siae by *groEL* gene analysis. *J. Clin. Microbiol.* **41:**2952–2960.

51. **Lee, N., M. Ip, B. Wong, G. Lui, W. T. Y. Tsang, J. Y. Lai, K. W. Choi, R. Lam, T. K. Ng, J. Ho, Y. Y. Chan, C. S. Cockram, and S. T. Lai.** 2008. Risk factors associated with life-threatening rickettsial infections. *Am. J. Trop. Med. Hyg.* **78:**973–978.

52. **Leitner, M., S. Yitzhaki, S. Rzotkiewicz, and A. Keysary.** 2002. Polymerase chain reaction-based diagnosis of Mediter-ranean spotted fever in serum and tissue samples. *Am. J. Trop. Med. Hyg.* **67:**166–169.

53. **Liu, Y.-X., W.-C. Cao, Y. Gao, J.-L. Zhang, Z.-Q. Yang, Z.-T. Zhao, and J. E. Foley.** 2006. *Orientia tsutsugamushi* in eschars from scrub typhus patients. *Emerg. Infect. Dis.* **12:**1109–1112.

54. **Martinez, J. J., S. Seveau, E. Veiga, S. Matsuyama, and P. Cossart.** 2005. Ku70, a component of DNA-dependent pro-tein kinase, is a mammalian receptor for *Rickettsia conorii.* *Cell* **123:**1013–1023.

55. **Martinez, J. J., and P. Cossart.** 2004. Early signaling events involved in the entry of *Rickettsia conorii* into mammalian cells. *J. Cell Sci.* **117:**5097–5106.

56. **McDade, J. E., C. C. Shepard, M. A. Redus, V. F. Newhouse, and J. D. Smith.** 1980. Evidence of *Rickettsia prowazekii* infections in the United States. *Am. J. Trop. Med. Hyg.* **29:**277–284.

57. **McLeod, M. P., X. Qin, S. E. Karpathy, J. Gioia, S. K. Highlander, G. E. Fox, T. Z. McNeill, J. Jiang, D. Muzny, L. S. Jacob, A. C. Hawes, E. Sodergren, R. Gill, J. Hume, M. Morgan, G. Fan, A. A. Amin, R. A. Gibbs, C. Hong, X-Y. Yu, D. H. Walker, and G. M. Weinstock.** 2004. Com-plete genome sequence of *Rickettsia typhi* and comparison with sequences of other rickettsiae. *J. Bacteriol.* **186:**5842–5855.

58. **Meloni, G., and T. Meloni.** 1996. Azithromycin vs. doxycy-cline for Mediterranean spotted fever. *Pediatr. Infect. Dis. J.* **15:**1042–1044.

59. **Montenegro, M. R., S. Mansueto, B. C. Hegarty, and D. H. Walker.** 1983. The histology of "taches noires" of bouton-neuse fever and demonstration of *Rickettsia conorii* in them by immunofluorescence. *Virchows Arch.* **400:**309–317.

60. **Moron, C. L., H.-M. Feng, D. J. Wear, and D. H. Walker.** 2000. Identification of the target cells of *Orientia tsutsugamushi* in human cases of scrub typhus. *Mod. Pathol.* **14:**752–759.

61. **Mouffok, N., P. Parola, H. Lepidi, and D. Raoult.** 2009. Mediterranean spotted fever in Algeria—new trends. *Int. J. Infect. Dis.* **13:**227–235.

62. **Nascimento, E. M. M., S. Colombo, T. K. Nagasse-Sugahara, R. N. Angerami, M. R. Resende, L. J. da Silva, G. Katz, and F. C. P. dos Santos.** 2009. Evaluation of PCR-based assay in human serum samples for diagnosis of fatal cases of spotted fever group rickettsiosis. *Clin. Microbiol. Infect.* **15:**232–234.

63. **Ndip, L. M., E. B. Fokam, D. H. Bouyer, R. N. Ndip, V. P. Titanji, D. H. Walker, and J. W. McBride.** 2004. Detec-tion of *Rickettsia africae* in patients and ticks along the coastal region of Cameroon. *Am. J. Trop. Med. Hyg.* **71:**363–366.

64. **Nilsson, K.** 2009. Septicaemia with *Rickettsia helvetica* in a pa-tient with acute febrile illness, rash and myasthenia. *J. Infect.* **58:**79–82.

65. **Ono, A., K. Nakamura, S. Higuchi, Y. Miwa, K. Naka-mura, T. Tsunoda, H. Kuwabara, Y. Furuya, K. Dobashi, and M. Mori.** 2002. Successful diagnosis using scab for PCR specimen in tsutsugamushi disease. *Intern. Med.* **41:**408–411.

66. **Paddock, C. D., R. W. Finley, C. S. Wright, H. N. Robin-son, B. J. Schrodt, C. C. Lane, O. Ekenna, M. A. Blass, C. L. Tamminga, C. A. Ohl, S. L. F. McLellan, J. Goddard, R. C. Holman, J. J. Openshaw, J. W. Sumner, S. R. Zaki, and M. E. Ermeeva.** 2008. *Rickettsia parkeri* rickettsiosis and its clinical distinction from Rocky Mountain spotted fever. *Clin. Infect. Dis.* **47:**1188–1196.

67. **Paris, D. H., N. Aukkanit, K. Jenjaroen, S. D. Blacksell, and N. P. J. Day.** 2009. A highly sensitive quantitative real-time PCR assay based on the *groEL* gene of contemporary Thai strains of *Orientia tsutsugamushi. Clin. Microbiol. Infect.* **15:**488–495.

68. **Paris, D. H., S. D. Blacksell, P. N. Newton, and N. P. J. Day.** 2008. Simple, rapid and sensitive detection of *Orientia tsutsugamushi* by loop-isothermal DNA amplification. *Trans. R. Soc. Trop. Med. Hyg.* **102:**1239–1246.

69. **Parola, P., R. S. Miller, P. McDaniel, S. R. Telford III, J.-M. Rolain, C. Wongsrichanalai, and D. Raoult.** 2003. Emerging rickettsioses of the Thai-Myanmar border. *Emerg. Infect. Dis.* **9:**592–595.

70. **Parola, P., C. D. Paddock, and D. Raoult.** 2005. Tick-borne rickettsioses around the world: emerging diseases challenging old concepts. *Clin. Microbiol. Rev.* **18:**719–756.

71. **Parola, P., D. Vogelaers, C. Roure, F. Janbon, and D. Raoult.** 1998. Murine typhus in travelers returning from In-donesia. *Emerg. Infect. Dis.* **4:**677–680.

72. **Phetsouvanh, R., S. D. Blacksell, K. Jenjaroen, N. P. J. Day, and P. N. Newton.** 2009. Comparison of indirect im-munofluorescence assays for diagnosis of scrub typhus and murine typhus using venous blood and finger prick filter paper blood spots. *Am. J. Trop. Med. Hyg.* **80:**837–840.

73. **Prakash, J. A. J., M. E. Reller, N. Barat, and J. S. Dumler.** 2009. Assessment of a quantitative multiplex 5′ nuclease real-time PCR for spotted fever and typhus group rickettsioses and *Orientia tsutsugamushi. Clin. Microbiol. Infect.* **15:**292–293.

74. **Premaratna, R., T. G. A. N. Chandrasena, A. S. Dassayake, A. D. Loftis, G. A. Dasch, and H. D. de Silva.** 2006. Acute hearing loss due to scrub typhus: a forgotten complication of a reemerging disease. *Clin. Infect. Dis.* **42:**e6–e8.

75. **Premaratna, R., A. D. Loftis, T. G. A. N. Chandrasena, G. A. Dasch, and J. J. de Silva.** 2008. Rickettsial infections and their clinical presentations in the western province of Sri Lanka: a hospital-based study. *Int. J. Infect. Dis.* **12:**198–202.

76. **Pretorius, A.-M., and R. J. Birtles.** 2002. *Rickettsia aeschli-mannii:* a new pathogenic spotted fever group rickettsia, South Africa. *Emerg. Infect. Dis.* **8:**874.

77. **Raoult, D., P.-E. Fournier, F. Fenollar, M. Jensenius, T. Prioe, J. J. De Pina, G. Caruso, N. Jones, H. Laferl, J. E. Rosenblatt, and T. J. Marrie.** 2001. *Rickettsia africae,* a tick-borne pathogen in travelers to sub-Saharan Africa. *N. Engl. J. Med.* **344:**1501–1510.

78. **Raoult, D., A. Lakos, F. Fenollar, J. Beytout, P. Brouqui, and P.-E. Fournier.** 2002. Spotless rickettsiosis caused by *Rickettsia slovaca* and associated with *Dermacentor* ticks. *Clin. Infect. Dis.* **34:**1331–1336.

79. **Raoult, D., and M. Maurin.** 2002. *Rickettsia* species, p. 913–921. *In* V. L. Yu, R. Webber, and D. Raoult (ed.), *Antimi-crobial Therapy and Vaccines,* 2nd ed. Apple Trees Production, LLC, New York, NY.

80. **Regnery, R. L., C. L. Spruill, and B. D. Plikaytis.** 1991. Genotypic identification of rickettsiae and estimation of in-traspecies sequence divergence for portions of two rickettsial genes. *J. Bacteriol.* **173:**1576–1589.

81. **Rolain, J. M., L. Stuhl, M. Maurin, and D. Raoult.** 2002. Evaluation of antibiotic susceptibilities of three rickettsial species including *Rickettsia felis* by a quantitative PCR DNA assay. *Antimicrob. Agents Chemother.* **46:**2747–2751.

82. **Roux, V., and D. Raoult.** 1999. Body lice as tools for diagno-sis and surveillance of reemerging diseases. *J. Clin. Microbiol.* **37:**596–599.

83. **Ruiz-Beltrán, R., and J. I. Herrero-Herrero.** 1992. Evalu-ation of ciprofloxacin and doxycycline in the treatment of Mediterranean spotted fever. *Eur. J. Clin. Microbiol. Infect. Dis.* **11:**427–431.

84. **Saisongkorh, W., M. Chenchittikul, and K. Silpapojakul.** 2004. Evaluation of nested PCR for the diagnosis of scrub typhus among patients with acute pyrexia of unknown origin. *Trans. R. Soc. Trop. Med. Hyg.* **98:**360–366.

85. **Sangkasuwan, V., T. Chatyingmongkol, S. Sukwit, C. Eamsila, T. Chuenchitra, W. Rodkvamtook, J. Jiang, A. L. Richards, K. Lerdthusnee, and J. W. Jones.** 2007. Description of the first reported human case of spotted fever group rickettsi-osis in urban Bangkok. *Am. J. Trop. Med. Hyg.* **77:**891–892.

86. **Schriefer, M. E., J. B. Sacci, Jr., J. S. Dumler, M. G. Bul-len, and A. F. Azad.** 1994. Identification of a novel rickettsial

infection in a patient diagnosed with murine typhus. *J. Clin. Microbiol.* **32:**949–954.

87. **Shpynov, S., P. E. Fournier, N. Rudakov, I. Arsen'eva, M. Granitov, I. Tarasevich, and D. Raoult.** 2009. Tick-borne rickettsiosis in the Altay region of Russia. *Clin. Microbiol. Infect.* **15:**313–314.

88. **Silpapojakul, K.** 1997. Scrub typhus in the Western Pacific region. *Ann. Acad. Med. Singapore* **26:**794–800.

89. **Singhsilarak, T., W. Leowattana, S. Looareesuwan, V. Wongchotigul, J. Jiang, A. L. Richards, and G. Watt.** 2005. Short report: detection of *Orientia tsutsugamushi* in clinical samples by quantitative real-time polymerase chain reaction. *Am. J. Trop. Med. Hyg.* **72:**640–641.

90. **Sirisanthana, V., T. Puthanakit, and T. Sirisanthana.** 2003. Epidemiologic, clinical and laboratory features of scrub typhus in thirty Thai children. *Pediatr. Infect. Dis.* **22:**341–345.

91. **Sonthayanon, P., W. Chierakul, K. Wuthiekanun, K. Phimda, S. Pukrittayakamee, N. P. Day, and S. J. Peacock.** 2009. Association of high *Orientia tsutsugamushi* DNA loads with disease of greater severity in adults with scrub typhus. *J. Clin. Microbiol.* **47:**430–434.

92. **Souza, C. E., J. Moraes-Filho, M. Ogrzewalska, F. C. Uchoa, M. C. Horta, S. S. L. Souza, R. C. M. Borba, and M. B. Labruna.** 2009. Experimental infection of capybaras *Hydrochoerus hydrochaeris* by *Rickettsia rickettsii* and evaluation of the transmission of the infection to ticks *Amblyomma cajennense*. *Vet. Parasitol.* **161:**116–121.

93. **Stenos, J., S. R. Graves, and N. B. Unsworth.** 2005. A highly sensitive and specific real-time PCR assay for the detection of spotted fever and typhus group rickettsiae. *Am. J. Trop. Med. Hyg.* **73:**1083–1085.

94. **Strickman, D., T. Sheer, K. Salata, J. Hershey, G. Dasch, D. Kelly, and R. Kuschner.** 1995. In vitro effectiveness of azithromycin against doxycycline-resistant and -susceptible strains of *Rickettsia tsutsugamushi*, etiologic agent of scrub typhus. *Antmicrob. Agents Chemother.* **39:**2406–2410.

95. **Suputtamongkol, Y., C. Suttinont, K. Niwatayakul, S. Hoontrakul, R. Limpaiboon, W. Chierakul, K. Losuwanaluk, and W. Saisongkork.** 2009. Epidemiology and clinical aspects of rickettsioses in Thailand. *Ann. N. Y. Acad. Sci.* **1166:**172–179.

96. **Tsai, K.-H., H. Y. Lu, J. J. Tsai, S. K. Yu, J. H. Huang, and P. Y. Shu.** 2008. Human case of *Rickettsia felis* infection, Taiwan. *Emerg. Infect. Dis.* **14:**1970–1972.

97. **Valbuena, G., W. Bradford, and D. H. Walker.** 2003. Expression analysis of the T-cell-targeting chemokines CXCL9 and CXCL10 in mice and humans with endothelial infections caused by rickettsiae of the spotted fever group. *Am. J. Pathol.* **163:**1357–1369.

98. **Vishwanath, S.** 1991. Antigenic relationships among the rickettsiae of the spotted fever and typhus groups. *FEMS Microbiol. Lett.* **81:**341–344.

99. **Vitorino, L., S.-M. Chen, F. Bacellar, and L. Ze-Ze.** 2007. Rickettsiae phylogeny: a multigenic approach. *Microbiology* **153:**160–168.

100. **Walker, D. H.** 2003. Principles of the malicious use of infectious agents to create terror: reasons for concern for organisms of the genus *Rickettsia*. *Ann. N. Y. Acad. Sci.* **990:**739–742.

101. **Walker, D. H., M. S. Burday, and J. D. Folds.** 1980. Laboratory diagnosis of Rocky Mountain spotted fever. *South. Med. J.* **73:**1443–1447.

102. **Walker, D. H., C. G. Crawford, and B. G. Cain.** 1980. Rickettsial infection of pulmonary microcirculation: the basis for interstitial pneumonitis in Rocky Mountain spotted fever. *Hum. Pathol.* **11:**263–272.

103. **Walker, D. H., H-M. Feng, S. Ladner, A. N. Billings, S. R. Zaki, D. J. Wear, and B. Hightower.** 1997. Immunohistochemical diagnosis of typhus rickettsioses using an anti-lipopolysaccharide monoclonal antibody. *Mod. Pathol.* **10:**1038–1042.

104. **Walker, D. H., S. D. Hudnall, W. K. Szaniawski, and H.-M. Feng.** 1999. Monoclonal antibody-based immunohistochemical diagnosis of rickettsialpox: the macrophage is the principal target. *Mod. Pathol.* **12:**529–533.

105. **Walker, D. H., F. M. Parks, T. G. Betz, J. P. Taylor, and J. W. Muehlberger.** 1989. Histopathology and immunohistologic demonstration of the distribution of *Rickettsia typhi* in fatal murine typhus. *Am. J. Clin. Pathol.* **91:**720–724.

106. **Wang, C.-C., S.-F. Liu, J.-W. Liu, Y.-H. Chung, M.-C. Su, and M.-C. Lin.** 2007. Acute respiratory distress syndrome in scrub typhus. *Am. J. Trop. Med. Hyg.* **76:**1148–1152.

107. **Watt, G., C. Chouriyagune, R. Ruangweerayud, P. Watcharapichat, D. Phulsuksombati, K. Jongsakul, P. Teja-Isavadharm, D. Bhodhidatta, K. D. Corcoran, G. A. Dasch, and D. Strickman.** 1996. Scrub typhus infections poorly responsive to antibiotics in northern Thailand. *Lancet* **348:**86–89.

108. **Watt, G., K. Jongsakul, R. Ruangvirayuth, P. Kantipong, and K. Silpapojakul.** 2005. Short report: prospective evaluation of a multi-test strip for the diagnoses of scrub and murine typhus, leptospirosis, dengue fever, and *Salmonella typhi* infection. *Am. J. Trop. Med. Hyg.* **72:**10–12.

109. **Watt, G., and D. Strickman.** 1994. Life-threatening scrub typhus in a traveler returning from Thailand. *Clin. Infect. Dis.* **18:**624–626.

110. **Weddle, J. R., T.-C. Chan, K. Thompson, H. Paxton, D. J. Kelly, G. Dasch, and D. Strickman.** 1995. Effectiveness of a dot-blot immunoassay of anti-*Rickettsia tsutsugamushi* antibodies for serologic analysis of scrub typhus. *Am. J. Trop. Med. Hyg.* **53:**43–46.

111. **Weinert, L. A., J. H. Werren, A. Aebi, G. N. Stone, and F. M. Jiggins.** 2009. Evolution and diversity of *Rickettsia* bacteria. *BMC Biol.* **7:**6. http://www.biomedcentral.com/1741-7007/7/6.

112. **Whitworth, T., V. L. Popov, X. J. Yu, D. H. Walker, and D. H. Bouyer.** 2005. Expression of *Rickettsia prowazekii pld* or *tlyC* gene in *Salmonella enterica* serovar Typhimurium mediates phagosomal escape. *Infect. Immun.* **73:**6668–6673.

113. **Wilkinson, R., D. Rowland, and W. M. Ching.** 2003. Development of an improved rapid lateral flow assay for the detection of *Orientia tsutsugamushi*-specific IgG/IgM antibodies. *Ann. N. Y. Acad. Sci.* **990:**386–390.

114. **Wolfel, R., S. Essbauer, and G. Gobler.** 2008. Concepts of modern rickettsial diagnosis. *Int. J. Med. Microbiol.* **298:**368–374.

115. **Yu, X. J., and D. H. Walker.** 2005. Family I. Rickettsiaceae, p. 96–116. *In* G. M. Garrity et al. (ed.), *Bergey's Manual of Systematic Bacteriology*, 2nd ed., vol. 2. Williams & Wilkins, Baltimore, MD.

116. **Zavala-Castro, J., J. Zavala-Velazquez, D. H. Walker, J. Perez-Osorio, and G. Peniche-Lara.** 2009. Severe human infection with *Rickettsia felis* associated with hepatitis in Yucatan, Mexico. *Int. J. Med. Microbiol.* **299:**529–533.

117. **Zavala-Castro, J., E. K. R. Dzul-Rosado, J. J. A. Leon, D. H. Walker, and J. E. Zavala-Velazquez.** 2008. Short report: *Rickettsia felis* outer membrane protein A: a potential tool for diagnosis of patients with flea-borne spotted fever. *Am. J. Trop. Med. Hyg.* **79:**903–906.

118. **Zavala-Castro, J. E., K. R. Dzul-Rosado, J. J. A. Leon, D. H. Walker, and J. E. Zavala-Velazquez.** 2008. An increase in human cases of spotted fever rickettsiosis in Yucatan, Mexico, involving children. *Am. J. Trop. Med. Hyg.* **79:**907–910.

119. **Zavala-Velazquez, J. E., J. A. Ruiz-Sosa, R. A. Sanchez-Elias, G. Becerra-Carmona, and D. H. Walker.** 2000. *Rickettsia felis* rickettsiosis in Yucatan. *Lancet* **356:**1079–1080.

120. **Znazen, A., J.-M. Rolain, N. Hammami, A. Hammami, M. B. Jemaa, and D. Raoult.** 2006. *Rickettsia felis* infection, Tunisia. *Emerg. Infect. Dis.* **12:**138–140.

Ehrlichia, Anaplasma, and Related Intracellular Bacteria*

MEGAN E. RELLER AND J. STEPHEN DUMLER

62

TAXONOMY

Members of the genus *Ehrlichia* and *Anaplasma* are now recognized to be important human pathogens. They are obligate intracellular bacteria currently placed in the *Proteobacteria* phylum (*Alphaproteobacteria*), order *Rickettsiales*, and family *Anaplasmataceae*. Although most closely related to the genera *Rickettsia* and *Orientia*, organisms classically considered ehrlichiae are divided into four major clades. Taxonomic classification (Fig. 1) is largely based upon sequence analysis of *rrs* (16S rRNA genes) and *groESL* (heat shock operon) (47, 72), but also that of citrate synthase (*gltA*), the β subunit of RNA polymerase (*rpoB*), FtsZ protein (*ftsZ*), and other rRNA genes (71–73, 80, 89, 130). Serologic cross-reactions, similarities among major immunodominant surface proteins, and the cellular tropisms of these bacteria further support the phylogenetic approach (43, 74). All members of the former tribes *Ehrlichieae* and *Wolbachieae* are now included in the family *Anaplasmataceae* instead of the family *Rickettsiaceae*. Table 1 delineates current, proposed, and former names of selected *Ehrlichia* and *Anaplasma* species that are known human and veterinary pathogens. All tick-borne *Anaplasmataceae* are grouped within two closely related genera, *Ehrlichia* and *Anaplasma*. *A. phagocytophilum*, within the genus *Anaplasma*, now includes *Ehrlichia phagocytophila*, *Ehrlichia equi*, and the human granulocytic ehrlichiosis (HGE) agent. Minor sequence differences in *rrs* exist between these organisms, which could reflect biological and ecological differences (33, 91, 127). Genetic variants of *A. phagocytophilum* have been reported in ticks and mammals in the northeastern United States and Europe, including some that probably do not cause disease in humans (91, 127).

Although *Ehrlichia* species infect predominantly leukocytes of humans and other mammals, individual *Anaplasma* species infect bone marrow-derived cells of each lineage in different animal hosts. *Neorickettsia* species infect predominantly mononuclear phagocytes and occasionally enterocytes in mammalian hosts (98). Recently, a new bacterium that is equally distant from the *Ehrlichia* and *Anaplasma* genera and present in *Ixodes* spp. ticks has been proposed as a member of a new genus, "*Candidatus* Neoehrlichia mikurensis" (26, 76, 78, 120). The genus *Aegyptianella* is currently listed as *incertae sedis*, most closely related to *Anaplasma* (115). *Wolbachia* spp. are "endosymbionts" of insects, helminths, and crustaceans that are transmitted only by transovarial and transstadial (between stages of development) passage (133).

DESCRIPTION OF THE GENERA

Ehrlichia and *Anaplasma* spp. are gram-negative obligate intracellular bacteria that reside and propagate within membrane-lined vacuoles found in the cytoplasm of bone marrow-derived cells, such as granulocytes, monocytes, erythrocytes, and platelets. *E. ruminantium* and several other species also infect endothelial cells (51, 135). These intracytoplasmic clusters of bacteria resemble elementary bodies of *Chlamydia* as small dense core forms (0.2 to 0.4 μm); larger forms (0.8 to 1.5 μm) resemble reticulate bodies (110). Both are capable of binary fission. At least in some species, specific ligands associated with cell adhesion are differentially expressed on the infective dense form but not on the metabolically active reticulate form. After a few days, the elementary bodies dividing in the phagosome form an inclusion, also called a morula, that can be seen microscopically. *Neorickettsia sennetsu* grows as bacterial cells that can maintain individual vacuolar membranes when they undergo binary fission. Cell lysis leads to the release of bacteria that can infect other competent cells (22). Unlike *Rickettsia*, *Ehrlichia* and *Anaplasma* do not have a thickened outer membrane leaflet. The outer membrane appears more ruffled in *A. phagocytophilum* than in *N. sennetsu* or *Ehrlichia chaffeensis* (111). By transmission electron microscopy, *Ehrlichia* and *Anaplasma* spp. have a very limited region that corresponds to the peptidoglycan layer, and genes necessary for its synthesis are not present within the genomes of *Ehrlichia*, *Anaplasma*, or *Neorickettsia* spp. (21, 53, 58). The full genome sequences of 15 *Anaplasmataceae* members are established and range in length from 860 kb in *N. sennetsu* and 1,176 kb in *Ehrlichia chaffeensis* to 1,471 kb in *A. phagocytophilum*. Genome sequencing has identified a low G+C content common to endosymbionts (except for *Anaplasma marginale*) and a large proportion of noncoding sequences. Many of the genes required for glycolysis are absent (53). Carbon sources are proline and glutamine. In contrast to

---

*This chapter contains information presented by Juan P. Olano and Maria E. Aguero-Rosenfeld in chapter 67 of the ninth edition of this *Manual*. Table 1 and Fig. 1 are modified and Fig. 2 is reprinted from that chapter.

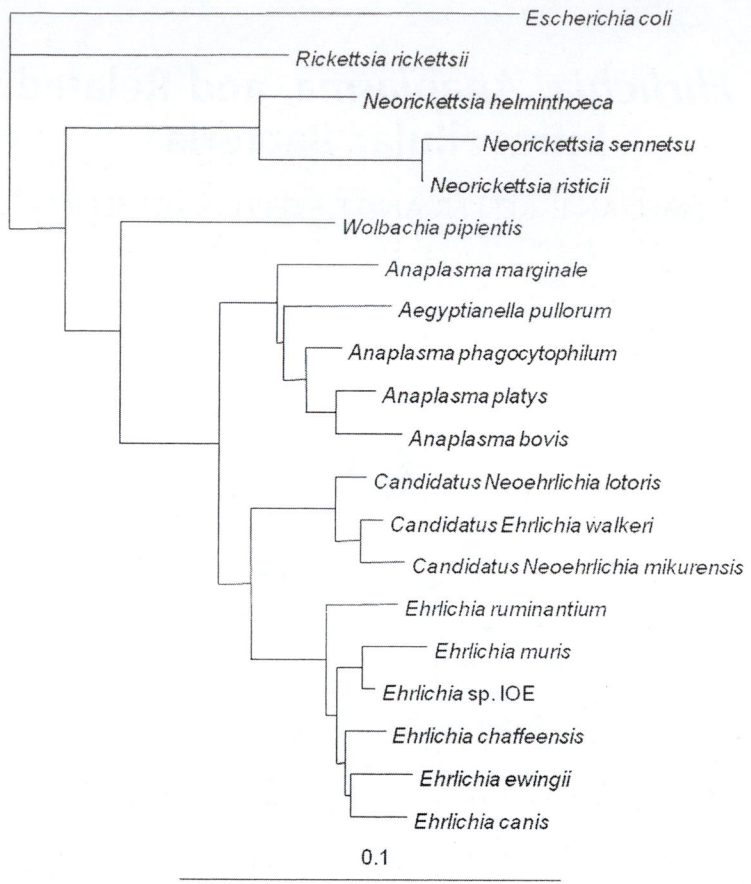

FIGURE 1 Neighbor-joining phylogenetic tree inferred from 16S rRNA gene sequences of selected *Ehrlichia*, "*Candidatus* Neoehrlichia," *Anaplasma*, *Neorickettsia*, and *Wolbachia* spp. *Escherichia coli* and *Rickettsia rickettsii* are used as outgroups. The bar represents the estimated number of substitutions per site.

Rickettsiaceae, all enzymes necessary for the Krebs cycle and for metabolism of purine and pyrimidine are present. ATP synthesis is possible, since these organisms possess the ATP synthase complex and other enzymes required for aerobic respiration. However, unlike *Rickettsia*, ATP/ADP translocases are absent. Genes for type IV secretion systems most likely contribute to virulence and are present as they are in other *Alphaproteobacteria* (99). In contrast to the reductive evolution seen in other intracellular bacteria, these organisms have many pseudogenes, which document gene duplication events (21, 53). The active duplication of tandemly repeated sequences likely results in new genes, antigenic variation, immune evasion, and thereby enhanced survival.

Anaplasma marginale infects ruminants, and *Aegyptianella* spp. infect birds, amphibians, and reptiles. These organisms also reside in small membrane-bound inclusions (19, 115) and are not known to cause human disease.

EPIDEMIOLOGY AND TRANSMISSION

Ehrlichia and *Anaplasma* spp. are zoonotic agents transmitted to animals and humans by ticks. *Neorickettsia sennetsu* rarely causes human disease and is likely acquired by ingestion of fish infested with *Neorickettsia*-infected flukes (98). *Wolbachia* spp. are symbionts of a broad range of arthropods, helminths, and crustaceans (131). Thus, most species can infect vertebrates and invertebrates (Table 1). Transovarial transmission of these organisms in ticks does not occur, but transstadial, interstadial, and intrastadial transmission do. *Ehrlichia* spp. are acquired when the immature tick (larva or nymph) feeds on an infected animal and are transmitted when the next stage (nymph or adult) feeds on another mammalian host. Ticks and mammals, the latter with high-grade and/or persistent bacteremia, may serve as reservoirs (83). In contrast, humans are only inadvertently infected and represent an end-stage host. Therefore, maintenance of tick-borne ehrlichiae in nature depends upon the presence of appropriate tick vectors and mammalian hosts in the local environment (6, 84, 114, 132).

Recognized natural reservoirs for *E. chaffeensis* include deer (*Odocoileus virginianus* and *Blastocerus dichotomus)*, domestic dogs, and perhaps other animals that host *Amblyomma* ticks (41, 82). Less important reservoirs include opossums, raccoons, voles, coyotes, and goats (101). White-tailed deer (*Odocoileus virginianus*) also are a reservoir of *Ehrlichia ewingii* and of another ehrlichial agent closely related to *Anaplasma platys*, the white-tailed deer agent, which has not yet been associated with human disease (8). The major reservoirs for *A. phagocytophilum* are incompletely investigated. However, small mammals are frequent hosts of the immature stages of *Ixodes scapularis* or *Ixodes ricinus* (132, 138). These include the white-footed mouse (*Peromyscus leucopus*) in the eastern United States,

TABLE 1 Selected features of *Ehrlichia, Anaplasma, Neorickettsia,* and *Aegyptianella* species of human and veterinary interest

Organism name	Former or other name(s)	Vector(s)	Disease[a]	Hosts developing disease	Infected cells	Reservoir host(s)
Anaplasma						
Anaplasma phagocytophilum	*E. equi, E. phagocytophila,* HGE agent	*Ixodes persulcatus* group	EGE Tick-borne fever HGA	Horses Ruminants Humans, dogs	Granulocytes	Deer, sheep White-footed mice
Anaplasma marginale, A. centrale, A. ovis		Several tick species	Ruminant anaplasmosis	Cattle, sheep, goats	Erythrocytes	Ruminants; wild cervids?
Anaplasma platys	*Ehrlichia platys*	*Rhipicephalus sanguineus?, Amblyomma* spp.?	Canine cyclic thrombocytopenia	Dogs	Platelets	Ruminants?
Anaplasma bovis	*Ehrlichia bovis*	*Rhipicephalus appendiculatus, Amblyomma variegatum*	Bovine ehrlichiosis	Cattle	Mononuclear leukocytes	Ruminants, rabbits?
Ehrlichia						
Ehrlichia chaffeensis		*Amblyomma americanum, Dermacentor variabilis*	HME	Humans, dogs	Mononuclear leukocytes	White-tailed deer, domestic dogs; others?
Ehrlichia ewingii		*Amblyomma americanum*	CGE Ewingii ehrlichiosis	Dogs Humans	Granulocytes	Canids
Ehrlichia canis		*Rhipicephalus sanguineus*	CME	Dogs Humans?	Mononuclear leukocytes	Canids
Ehrlichia ruminantium	*Cowdria ruminantium*	*Amblyomma* species	Cowdriosis (heartwater)	Domestic and wild ruminants	Granulocytes, endothelial cells	Ruminants
Ehrlichia muris		*Haemaphysalis flava*	Not named	Laboratory mice	Mononuclear leukocytes	Not known
Ehrlichia species	*Ixodes ovatus Ehrlichia* (IOE)	*Ixodes ovatus*	Not named	Laboratory and wild mice and rodents	Mononuclear leukocytes, Kupffer cells, endothelial cells	Not known
Neorickettsia						
Neorickettsia sennetsu	*Ehrlichia sennetsu*	Unknown; possibly acquired by ingestion	Sennetsu fever	Humans	Mononuclear leukocytes	Fluke-infested fish?
Neorickettsia risticii	*Ehrlichia risticii*	Ingestion of fluke-infested insects	Potomac horse fever	Horses	Mononuclear leukocytes	*Juga* sp. flukes
Neorickettsia helminthoeca		Ingestion of fluke-infested salmonid fish	Salmon poisoning disease	Dogs, bears	Mononuclear leukocytes	Fluke-infested fish
Genus and species incertae sedis						
Aegyptianella spp.		*Amblyomma* spp.	Aegyptianellosis	Birds, amphibians, reptiles	Erythrocytes	Not known
Neoehrlichia mikurensis	*Ehrlichia walkeri*	*Ixodes ricinus, Ixodes ovatus, Ixodes persulcatus*	No disease	Rodents	Endothelial cells	Rodents
Neoehrlichia lotoris		*Ixodes* spp.?	No disease	Not known	Not known	Raccoons

[a]EGE, equine granulocytic ehrlichiosis; CGE, canine granulocytic ehrlichiosis; CME, canine monocytic ehrlichiosis.

chipmunks (*Tamias striatus*), voles (*Clethrionomys gapperi*), and wild mice (*Apodemus* spp.). Although white-tailed deer can be persistently infected by *A. phagocytophilum*, the *A. phagocytophilum* strains (AP variant 1) that naturally infect deer are not infectious for small mammals, have not been identified in humans, and may represent nonpathogenic variants (90, 96). Persistent or prolonged infection in animal reservoir hosts is essential for maintenance of zoonoses. Mice infected with *A. phagocytophilum* can remain infected for months, which contributes to transmission to different stages of developing *I. scapularis* ticks (124). In Europe, red deer, sheep, cattle, and goats are persistently infected and serve as reservoirs of *A. phagocytophilum*. The reservoir for *N. sennetsu* is not known; however, epidemiological data suggest that consumption of raw fish is a risk factor for sennetsu fever (98). Other species of *Neorickettsia* have complex transmission processes involving trematodes. *N. risticii*, the agent of Potomac horse fever, is transmitted to horses by accidental ingestion of insects carrying *N. risticii*-infected cercariae (85). Similarly, *N. helminthoeca* infects dogs through ingestion of trematode-infested fish.

CLINICAL SIGNIFICANCE

Human Diseases

HME

The causative agent of human monocytic ehrlichiosis (HME) is *E. chaffeensis*, a monocytotropic ehrlichia that was first identified as a human pathogen in a patient with a severe febrile illness after tick bites in 1986 (86). More than 5,490 cases of HME were reported to CDC through 2009; however, data from active surveillance efforts suggest that HME occurs much more frequently than is reported (44, 50). The seroprevalence of *E. chaffeensis* ranges from 1.3% to 12.5% in the regions of Arkansas and Tennessee in which it is endemic. In contrast, active surveillance in Tennessee and Missouri identified 330 to 414 cases/100,000 population (44, 50). Most cases are identified in the south-central and southeastern United States, but increasingly infections are identified in the middle Atlantic states. Prospective evaluation of heavily exposed cohorts shows that approximately 75% of seroconversions are subclinical (57). Recent reports from Latin America, Africa, Europe, and Asia indicate that *E. chaffeensis*, or closely related microorganisms, are also found there (23, 59, 95, 106, 117, 139). Using PCR to amplify ehrlichial *rrs*, *E. chaffeensis* nucleotide sequences have been found in various tick species from different regions of China (29).

The median incubation period for HME is 9 days. The median age is 44 years, and 66% of patients are males (42, 101). Patients often present with high fever (96%), headache (72%), malaise (77%), myalgia (68%), and no localizing physical findings (50). Gastrointestinal (nausea, vomiting, and diarrhea), respiratory (cough), and osteoarticular (joint pain) symptoms are present in less than 50% of patients. Central nervous system involvement (stiff neck, confusion, and meningitis), have been described (125). Petechial, macular, and maculopapular rashes occur with varied distribution and onset (100, 101). Rashes are more frequent in children (67% of cases) (121). Abnormal laboratory parameters occur in at least 86% of patients and include thrombocytopenia (70 to 90%), leukopenia (60%) with lymphopenia and/or neutropenia, and increased serum aspartate transaminases (50%). Severe complications

include meningoencephalitis and a toxic shock-like syndrome with multiorgan failure, including adult respiratory distress syndrome. Fulminant infections are more common in patients immunocompromised by HIV, high-dose corticosteroids, and medications related to organ transplantation (56, 88, 102–104, 119, 126). The case fatality rate is 2 to 3%. Male sex, advanced age, and an immunocompromised status are independent risk factors for death (42).

HGA

The causative agent of human granulocytic anaplasmosis (HGA) is *Anaplasma phagocytophilum*. HGA was first identified in 1990 in a patient from Wisconsin who reported tick bites. Neither *E. chaffeensis* nor its tick vector was known to exist in that area (12, 33). Although tick bite is likely the most frequent route of transmission, there are others (30, 67, 148). Perinatal transmission has been reported (67), as has transmission by accidental inoculation of infected blood and blood transfusion (30, 148).

HGA, like HME, is not a reportable illness in all states; thus, the true incidence and prevalence of the infection are unknown. However, passive surveillance in northwestern Wisconsin and Connecticut reveals yearly incidence rates of 24 to 58 cases per 100,000 population (44). As of 2009, more than 6,200 cases had been reported nationwide, with the highest annual incidence rates in the Northeast and upper Midwest. Infected patients have been identified in other states, as well as in several European and Asian countries (9, 18, 38, 106, 109, 113, 148). Most infections are likely subclinical, since between 0.6% and 14.9% of the population in Connecticut and northwestern Wisconsin, respectively, are seropositive (14, 69). The tick vectors for HME and HGA coexist in the middle Atlantic and southern New England states, and in the southern Midwest. Thus, both diseases can occur in these areas (32, 38, 42). Furthermore, human ehrlichioses, including HME, HGA, and *E. ewingii* infections, are clinically indistinguishable.

HGA has a median incubation period of 5 to 11 days after the bite of an *Ixodes* sp. tick. The median age is 43 to 60 years (1, 3, 16), and the male/female ratio is 2:1 (11). Patients most often present with high fever (91%), myalgias (77%), headache (77%), and malaise (94%). Gastrointestinal, respiratory, musculoskeletal, and central nervous system involvement occurs in fewer patients. Rash is observed in 6% of patients, all attributable to erythema migrans with concurrent Lyme disease (13). Leukopenia with lymphopenia, thrombocytopenia, and increased serum aspartate transaminase activities are common early in the disease and may normalize before antimicrobial treatment. Lymphocytosis with atypical lymphocytes can occur after the first week of infection (11, 68). Severe complications of HGA include a septic shock-like illness with multiorgan failure, adult respiratory distress syndrome, and opportunistic infections (16, 63, 68, 81, 136). Meningitis has not been documented. At least 6 deaths have been reported, 3 of which had opportunistic infections including *Candida* esophagitis, *Cryptococcus* pneumonia, invasive pulmonary aspergillosis, and herpes esophagitis (16, 63, 81, 136).

Ehrlichia ewingii Ehrlichiosis

E. ewingii was recognized to cause human infection when its DNA was found in the blood of patients with an HME-like disease in Missouri (28). As with *E. chaffeensis*, the main vector is the lone star tick (*Amblyomma americanum*); therefore, the distribution of the disease is similar to that of HME. Evidence of *E. ewingii* in *Dermacentor variabilis* ticks has also been documented (140, 145). White-tailed deer are also reservoirs, and recent epidemiological studies suggest that dogs may be as well (8, 145). Ewingii ehrlichiosis seems to affect mostly immunosuppressed patients, including those with HIV, but is clinically milder than coinfection with HIV and *E. chaffeensis* (28, 102). In dogs, *E. ewingii* is responsible for canine granulocytotropic ehrlichiosis.

Sennetsu Ehrlichiosis (Neorickettsiosis)
Named after the Japanese term for glandular fever, *Neorickettsia sennetsu* was first isolated from patients with suspected infectious mononucleosis in 1953 (94). It is rarely identified now. Patients develop a self-limited febrile illness with chills, headache, malaise, sore throat, anorexia, and generalized lymphadenopathy. Cases were identified in Japan and possibly Malaysia, although at least one new case was recently recognized in Laos (98). Laboratory findings include early leukopenia and atypical lymphocytes in the peripheral blood during early convalescence. No fatalities or severe complications have been reported.

Other Human Ehrlichioses
In 1996, *Ehrlichia canis* was isolated from the blood of an asymptomatic man from Venezuela. Since then, six additional symptomatic patients were identified as infected by an *E. canis* strain that differs from canine strains by a single nucleotide polymorphism in *rrs* (107, 108).

While *Wolbachia* spp. are not known to be directly pathogenic for humans or animals, emerging evidence indicates a potential role for the intracellular bacterial components ("symbionts") of such helminths as *Brugia malayi*, *Onchocerca volvulus*, and *Wuchereria bancrofti* as potentiators of the inflammatory reactions associated with parasitic infections (65, 133).

COLLECTION, TRANSPORT, AND STORAGE OF SPECIMENS
Currently, there are three methods for diagnosis of active infection with HME or HGA: (i) PCR amplification of nucleic acids from *Ehrlichia* or *Anaplasma* species; (ii) detection of morulae in the cytoplasm of infected leukocytes by nonspecific Romanowsky stains (e.g., Giemsa or Wright) or by specific immunocytologic or immunohistologic stains, using *E. chaffeensis* or *A. phagocytophilum* antibodies; and (iii) culture of *Ehrlichia* or *Anaplasma* from blood or cerebrospinal fluid (CSF). In contrast, testing of single serum samples (acute or convalescent phase) is rarely useful. However, concurrent testing of paired sera (obtained during acute illness and in convalescence, 2 to 4 weeks later) does provide definitive retrospective diagnosis.

EDTA-anticoagulated blood is a useful specimen for most tests (PCR, smears, and culture) and should be obtained during the active phase of illness (1, 60, 100). Peripheral blood buffy coat smears or cytocentrifuged preparations of CSF cells should also be obtained at the acute phase and should be prepared within hours of obtaining the samples, since leukocytes degenerate rapidly. Once prepared, air-dried blood smears and cytocentrifuged CSF preparations are stable at room temperature for months or years.

Whole blood is the preferred sample for PCR since it contains infected leukocytes; serum should not be used. Samples for PCR should be tested promptly or frozen at −80°C.

The preferred specimen for culture of *Ehrlichia* and *Anaplasma* is peripheral blood. Samples should be obtained by sterile venipuncture or lumbar puncture and processed as soon as possible. The culture conditions for *Ehrlichia* and *Anaplasma* species are still being optimized. Culture is currently performed only in a few public health and research laboratories. Samples for culture should be maintained at approximately 4°C during shipping but not frozen. *A. phagocytophilum* is easier to culture than *E. chaffeensis*, including from EDTA-anticoagulated blood stored for up to 18 days at 4°C (75). *Ehrlichia*- and *Anaplasma*-infected cells can be stored frozen within infected host cells at −80°C for months. Storage of infected cells is best accomplished when more than 50 to 90% of the host cells are infected and is achieved by suspension of at least 10^6 cells per ml in tissue culture medium that contains 10% dimethyl sulfoxide and at least 30% fetal bovine serum.

LABORATORY CONFIRMATION OF *EHRLICHIA CHAFFEENSIS*

Direct Examination

Microscopy by Romanowsky Staining of Peripheral Blood
Patients with suspected HME should have Romanowsky-stained (Giemsa or Wright stain) peripheral blood or buffy coat leukocytes examined for the presence of ehrlichial morulae. However, the sensitivity is low (≤29%) compared to culture (125). *E. chaffeensis* is detected predominantly in monocytes and is more frequently detected in severe infection. When present, morulae are small (1 to 3 μm in diameter) round-to-oval clusters of bacteria that appear as basophilic to amphophilic stippling within cytoplasmic vacuoles with Romanowsky stains (Fig. 2C). Detection of morulae is accomplished more frequently in immunocompromised patients. Since the percentage of cells infected ranges from 0.2% to 10%, up to 500 cells should be examined.

Antigen Detection by Immunohistology
Immunohistochemistry may identify *E. chaffeensis* in bone marrow, liver, and spleen. However, the sensitivity of detecting active infection with examination of bone marrow is only 40% (49). A monoclonal antibody can specifically detect *E. chaffeensis* in human tissues (146), but most studies use polyclonal antibodies that react with other *Ehrlichia* species. Commercial assays are not currently available.

Nucleic Acid Detection Techniques
The most widely used method is PCR amplification of DNA from *E. chaffeensis* in clinical samples using the HE1/HE3 primer set (7, 55, 125). This primer pair amplifies a 389-bp fragment of *rrs* (16S rRNA gene). The product may be detected by simple nucleic acid staining (e.g., ethidium bromide) after agarose gel electrophoresis, by Southern hybridization of the amplified products using an internal probe, or by real-time PCR with either 5′-nuclease or molecular beacon probes that increase analytical sensitivity (37). A clinical evaluation of *E. chaffeensis* PCR using the HE1/HE3 system showed a sensitivity of 79 to 100% compared with serology; however, nucleic acids from *E. chaffeensis* were frequently detected in patients who never developed antibodies (7, 125). Similar sensitivity was shown with a nested PCR that employs broad-range "*Ehrlichia* genus" primers in an initial step followed by PCR with the HE1/HE3 primer pair (77). A nested-PCR assay with broad-range *rrs* primers (8F and

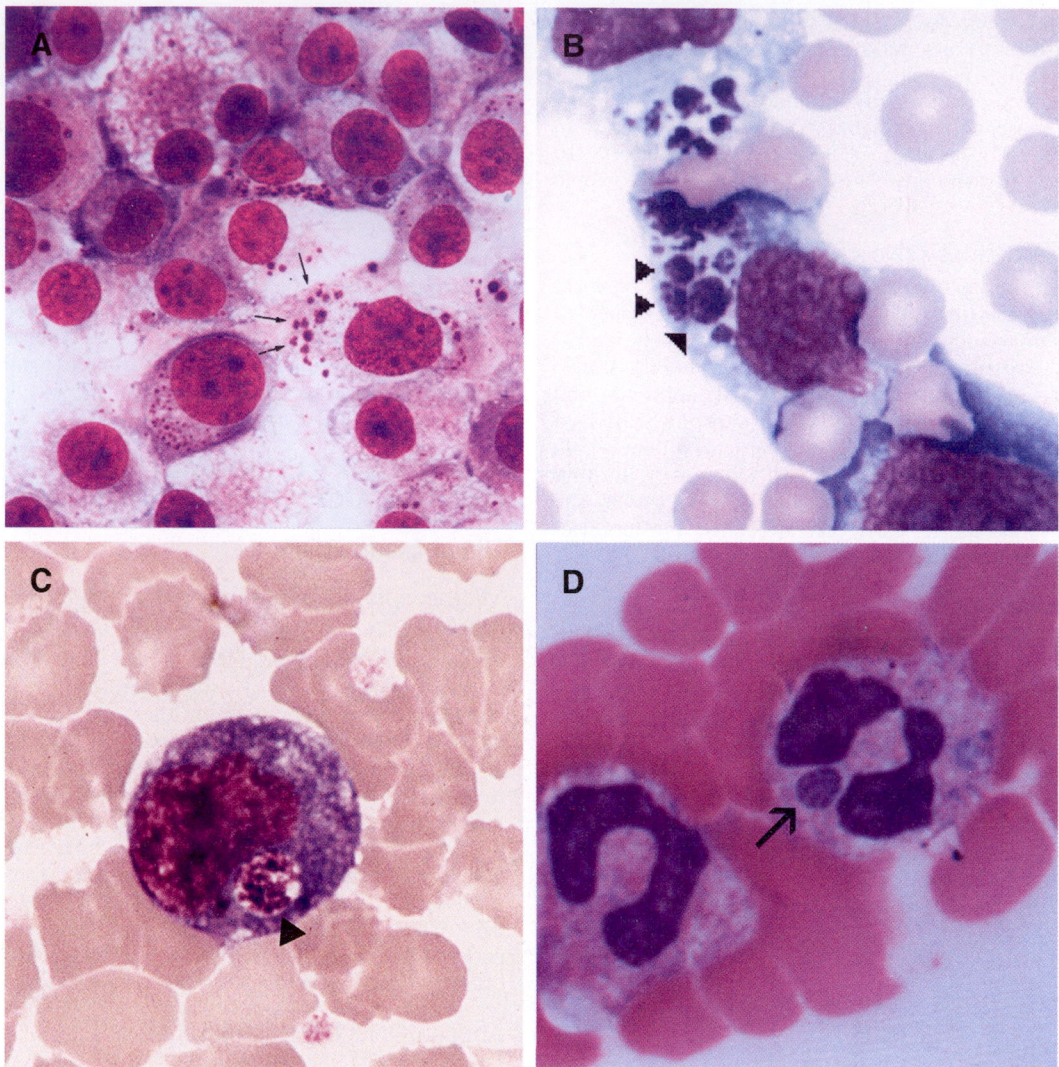

FIGURE 2 (A) *E. chaffeensis* cultured in the canine histiocyte cell line DH82. Note the presence of basophilic, stippled, intracytoplasmic inclusions approximately 2 to 3 μm in diameter (arrows). The smaller intracytoplasmic granules may also be ehrlichial morulae. Romanowsky (Leukostat) stain; original magnification, ×1,000. (B) *A. phagocytophilum* cultured in the human promyelocytic cell line HL-60 from the blood of an infected patient. Note the presence of multiple basophilic, stippled, intracytoplasmic inclusions (arrowheads) in an HL-60 cell. Wright stain; original magnification, ×1,000. (C and D) *E. chaffeensis* (C) and *A. phagocytophilum* (D) in peripheral blood leukocytes. Note that an *E. chaffeensis* morula (arrowhead) is present in a monocyte (C) and that an *A. phagocytophilum* morula (arrow) is present in a neutrophil (D). Wright stain; original magnification, ×1,000.

1448R) followed by a second (nested) reaction with primers 15F and 208R on whole blood yielded results similar to those obtained with culture (125). Other targets for PCR that have not been fully evaluated for clinical sensitivity or specificity include the *groESL* operon, the outer-surface variable-length PCR target protein gene present in *E. chaffeensis* (102, 125, 129), the 120-kDa antigen gene that encodes an immunodominant antigen with tandemly repeated subunits that vary among *E. chaffeensis* isolates, the quinolinate synthase A gene, *nadA*, the disulfide bond formation protein gene (*dsb*), and the p28 multigene family (43, 102, 134, 147). In a prospective study, the overall sensitivity and specificity of PCR were 56% and 100%, respectively, using the 16S rRNA subunit, *nadA*, and 120-kDa protein genes (100). However, in this study

several samples had high titers of antiehrlichial antibodies by immunofluorescence assay (IFA), suggesting that the pathogen may have already been cleared (few circulating ehrlichiae). When sensitivity was calculated using seroconversion as the gold standard, it increased to 84%. Posttest probabilities for a positive and negative PCR result were 96% and 11.1%, respectively. Posttest probabilities depend critically on prevalence (100).

Real-time multicolor PCR and real-time multiplex reverse transcriptase PCR assays have been developed recently with extremely high analytical sensitivity and specificity comparable to that of nested PCR (43, 123). Advantages include improved specificity (lower risk of contamination), increased speed, lower cost, and the detection of multiple ehrlichial pathogens simultaneously.

Isolation Procedures

Ehrlichia chaffeensis has been isolated from peripheral blood of a limited number of patients with HME, and an *E. canis*-like organism was isolated only once from an asymptomatic human (40, 48, 104, 108, 125). The most frequently used cell for primary isolation is the canine histiocytic cell line DH82; however, *E. chaffeensis* has been successfully cultivated in other cells including the human macrophage-like THP-1 cells, the fibroblast-like HEL-22 cells, Vero cells, and HL-60 cells (human promyelocytic cell line differentiated to monocytic pathway), among others (64). Isolation may be successful even when infected leukocytes are not observed on peripheral blood examination (125). Isolation usually involves direct inoculation of leukocyte fractions or whole blood into flasks with confluent layers of adherent cells or into flasks that contain approximately 2×10^5 to 1×10^6 nonadherent cells per ml of tissue culture medium. Macrophage-like cells that are highly phagocytic may be adversely affected by the presence of erythrocytes; thus, it is recommended that either (i) leukocytes be fractionated from erythrocytes by density gradient centrifugation (e.g., Ficoll-Paque); or (ii) leukocytes be harvested after erythrocyte lysis (hypotonic lysis, NH_4Cl lysis, etc.); or (iii) cell confluency be reestablished after cultivation with erythrocyte-containing samples by addition of uninfected host cells. Since *E. chaffeensis* may be present in few peripheral blood leukocytes, it is advisable to inoculate cultures with as many peripheral blood leukocytes as possible (which may be difficult with leukopenia). Use of 2 to 3 ml of EDTA-anticoagulated blood diluted in 2 volumes of sterile Hanks' balanced salt solution followed by Histopaque (Sigma, St. Louis, MO) gradient separation of leukocytes has been effective (125).

The blood mononuclear cells are resuspended in a 2-ml volume of tissue culture medium supplemented with 5% fetal bovine serum and allowed to interact with adherent host cells in a 25-cm^2 flask for 3 h, usually enhanced by incubation with rocking at 37°C in 5% CO_2. The inoculum is removed if significant erythrocyte contamination is present, and the monolayer is replenished with 5 ml of fresh tissue culture medium. Since *Ehrlichia* species are bacteria, antibiotics in the medium must be avoided. The generation time of *E. chaffeensis* is approximately 19 h (22), and thus, cultures must be maintained to allow a slow logarithmic or stable growth phase to avoid the host cells outgrowing the ehrlichiae.

Identification

The presence of infected cells is determined by sampling the medium (DH82 cells and THP-1 cells) or by lightly scraping part of the monolayer. Aliquots of the culture are cytocentrifuged and then stained with Romanowsky or immunofluorescent stains, and cells are examined for the presence of intracytoplasmic morulae or *Ehrlichia chaffeensis* antigen (Fig. 2A). Culture may require one month or more but has been achieved in as short a time as a few days (40, 48, 125). Confirmation of the infectious agent is currently best achieved by PCR amplification using species-specific primers (5).

Serologic Tests

The gold standard for the diagnosis of HME is demonstration of a fourfold rise in immunoglobulin G (IgG) titer or seroconversion by examination of paired (acute- and convalescent-phase) sera. Thus, diagnosis is at best retrospective. The most frequently used serologic method is the indirect IFA. Other methods have included enzyme immunoassays (enzyme-linked immunosorbent assay [ELISA]) and protein (Western) immunoblotting. Ehrlichial antigens may be difficult to prepare and are available mostly through public health and research laboratories, although commercial production and distribution are now available. Commercial sources of IFA serodiagnostic kits include Focus Technologies (Cypress, CA), Scimedx Corp. (Denville, NJ), and PanBio Diagnostics (no longer available in the United States).

Currently, there is little standardization for any method of ehrlichial serology, and cutoff titers are dependent upon validation in individual laboratories that perform these assays. The algorithm for serologic testing by IFA includes an initial screen at a dilution of 1:64 or 1:80 for IgG antibodies to *E. chaffeensis*. Reactive samples are then titrated to the end point.

Ehrlichia chaffeensis IFA

E. chaffeensis IgG is detected by IFA using *E. chaffeensis* Arkansas strain-infected DH82 canine macrophage-like cells. Reactive sera are serially diluted starting at a dilution of 1:64. The presence of antibodies is detected after incubation with fluorescein isothiocyanate-conjugated anti-human IgG. The test is positive if classic intracytoplasmic morulae are seen. It is important to identify the appropriate proportion of infected cells as determined by a positive control serum and the appropriate morphology for each antigen preparation to preclude false-positive interpretations. Prescreening for autoantibodies or routine removal of rheumatoid factors will lessen the risk of misinterpretation due to antibodies reactive with cellular components including nuclear or cytoplasmic antigens that could have the morphologic appearance of morulae. A fourfold increase in IgG antibody titer or seroconversion confirms the diagnosis of acute HME. A single specific IgG titer of ≥64, like identification of morulae in monocytes or macrophages for *E. chaffeensis* by microscopy, is suggestive. Antibody titers may be detected in a small proportion of subjects without HME owing to the presence of antigens that are highly conserved among bacterial species (39, 141). Acute-phase sera should be obtained at the time of presentation with acute illness, and convalescent-phase sera are best obtained 3 to 6 weeks later (39).

The sensitivity and specificity of IFA for the diagnosis of infection with *E. chaffeensis* are not known but are assumed to be high because of documented correlation between new or rising antibody titers against *E. chaffeensis* and characteristic clinical findings (57). In the early phase of infection, IFA testing is not sensitive compared to PCR (36). A systematic evaluation of the usefulness of IgM testing has not been conducted, but a preliminary evaluation based on nine culture-confirmed cases suggests that it might be slightly more sensitive than IgG for the diagnosis of HME during the acute phase (36). Previously, the serologically cross-reactive *E. canis* was used as a surrogate antigen; however, this serodiagnostic assay has a lower sensitivity than that obtained using *E. chaffeensis*, and its use should be discouraged (7). The role of immunoblots in diagnosis is not well established; however, many patients with *E. chaffeensis* infection can be differentiated from patients with HGA by the demonstration of antibodies reactive with one or more of the 22-, 28-, 29-, 46-, 54-, or 120-kDa antigens of *E. chaffeensis* (24, 34). Alternative methods based on recombinant proteins show promise but are not commercially available (147). Antibodies to *E. chaffeensis* have also been detected in patients diagnosed with Rocky Mountain spotted fever, Q fever, brucellosis, Lyme disease, and Epstein-Barr virus infections, suggesting that false-positive reactions do occur (39, 141). Antigenic diversity among *E. chaffeensis* isolates is well described (35) but may not affect the detection of polyclonal antibody responses generated with human infection. Several reports characterized patients with suspected HME who lacked antibody responses, even long after onset of symptoms (55, 118, 125). However, in the few cases in which *E. chaffeensis* infection was proven by isolation of the agent, patients who survived developed clear convalescent serologic reactions by IFA (35, 40, 48, 102, 125). Hypothetical reasons for false-negative results include infection by antigenically diverse strains (unproven) and abrogation of antibody response by early therapy (125).

LABORATORY CONFIRMATION OF *ANAPLASMA PHAGOCYTOPHILUM*

Direct Examination

Microscopy by Romanowsky Staining of Peripheral Blood

Examination of Romanowsky-stained (Giemsa or Wright stain) peripheral blood or buffy coat leukocytes for the presence of morulae is highly valuable in the diagnosis of HGA. Usually, 800 to 1,000 granulocytes are examined under magnification of ×500 to ×1,000 for the presence of morulae (1, 3, 16). Since most patients presenting with positive smears have <1% of infected granulocytes and usually have leukopenia, buffy coat preparations yield more than peripheral smears. Infection rates as high as 40% of granulocytes have been described (12). As for HME, the presence of detectable infected granulocytes in peripheral blood correlates modestly with severity of infection (3, 11, 12). The sensitivity of the buffy coat smear examination in the acute phase of HGA is approximately 60% (11). When present, ehrlichial morulae are small (1 to 3 μm in diameter) round-to-oval clusters of bacteria that stain basophilic to amphophilic with Romanowsky stains (Fig. 2D). These clusters are present in the cytoplasm of neutrophils or eosinophils and have a stippled appearance owing to individual bacteria within the vacuole.

Immunohistology for Antigen Detection

Immunohistologic methods may also be used to identify *A. phagocytophilum* within human tissues, including bone marrow, liver, and spleen (81).

Nucleic Acid Detection Techniques

Multiple PCR assays for detection of *A. phagocytophilum* nucleic acids have been published (54, 62, 92, 123, 128). Most utilize regions of *rrs* (16S rRNA gene) that are relatively specific as targets for amplification. The most frequently applied and evaluated method employs the primer set ge9f and ge10r, which amplifies a 919-bp fragment, most often used as a single-stage reaction, with or without a hybridization probe to enhance sensitivity (33, 54). A popular alternative is the use of nested PCR with an outer set of primers that anneal to and amplify eubacterial 16S rRNA genes, followed by a nested internal PCR with *A. phagocytophilum*-specific primers (92, 125). Amplification of the *groESL* region using a nested PCR has also been useful to detect ehrlichial DNA in blood during the acute phase. Primers HS1 and HS6 are used in the primary reaction followed by primers HS43 and HS45. The size of the amplified product distinguishes *E. chaffeensis* from *A. phagocytophilum*, 528 bp versus 480 bp, respectively (128). The analytical sensitivity and specificity of

several published primer sets were evaluated by using DNA extracted from serial dilutions of *A. phagocytophilum*-infected HL-60 cells (92). Specificity was evaluated using DNA extracted from cultures of *E. chaffeensis*, *Rickettsia rickettsii*, and *Bartonella henselae*. The primer sets with the greatest sensitivity and specificity were those used in a nested reaction to amplify *rrs*, i.e., ge3a-ge10 and ge9-ge2, and those amplifying *msp2* gene, i.e., msp2-3f-msp2-3r (92). Both PCR assays detected as few as 0.25 infected HL-60 cell per μl of blood. Additional recent methods employ real-time PCR and the 5′ nuclease (TaqMan) approach and target the >100-copy *msp2* gene family, which provides increased sensitivity to as low as 1 infected cell per μl of blood (122). A multiplex assay to detect *Ehrlichia* and *Anaplasma* spp. by real-time reverse transcriptase PCR was developed and evaluated in peripheral blood of dogs suspected of ehrlichiosis (123). The assay has a sensitivity of 100 *rrs* transcripts, which corresponds to about 1 infected cell in a test sample, can detect single or multiple infections, and has the potential for automation.

Isolation Procedures

A. phagocytophilum has been successfully cultivated more often from human patients than has *E. chaffeensis*, *E. canis*, or *N. sennetsu*, probably owing to the quantity of organisms present in the peripheral blood of infected patients (1). HGA is described in Europe and Asia, and several successes at isolating the organism have been reported. At least one human isolate of *A. phagocytophilum* from outside the United States (Slovenia) has been verified (61). Isolation is best achieved in the human promyelocytic cell line HL-60 (60) and has been accomplished even when morulae are not observed in peripheral blood smears. The optimal conditions for recovery of these bacteria have not been conclusively determined. Because erythrocytes do not adversely affect HL-60 cells, direct inoculation of EDTA-anticoagulated blood is effective. Fractionation of blood into buffy coat or granulocyte fractions by density gradient centrifugation is also effective (116). Approximately 100 to 500 μl of EDTA-anticoagulated blood, containing 10^2 to 10^4 infected granulocytes, is inoculated into 100-fold more uninfected HL-60 cells that are in the exponential growth phase. Cultures are subsequently maintained at a concentration between 2×10^5 and 1×10^6 cells per ml of tissue culture medium.

Identification

Cultures are examined every 2 to 3 days by Romanowsky staining of cytocentrifuged preparations of 20 to 50 μl of culture suspensions. *Anaplasma* morulae appear as small aggregates of basophilic bacteria in the cytoplasm of the HL-60 cells (Fig. 2B). Since HL-60 cells can contain a variety of cytoplasmic granules, immunocytochemistry or immunofluorescence is very helpful for the inexperienced laboratorian. Unfortunately, immunohistological reagents are currently not commercially available. Cultures usually require between 5 and 10 days before morulae are clearly identified; but infected cells may be detected as early as 3 days postinoculation. Time to detection of organisms in culture correlates with the number of bacteria present in blood at the time of culture (75). Definitive identification is achieved by PCR amplification using species-specific primers (33, 60) or by sequence analysis of PCR-amplified *rrs* (33). The exact length of incubation before cultures are considered negative is not determined, but they should be kept for at least 14 days, maintaining the cell density adjusted to about 2×10^5/ml.

Serologic Tests

Anaplasma phagocytophilum IFA

Although testing can be performed using *A. phagocytophilum* antigens prepared from infected circulating leukocytes of horses, the preferred method for testing human sera is the use of a human isolate propagated in the HL-60 promyelocyte cell line (4, 38, 60, 70, 112, 137). It is now well demonstrated that antigenic diversity exists among isolates of *A. phagocytophilum,* but such diversity has not been shown to affect detection in clinical specimens (10, 137). Interpretation of immunofluorescent patterns is similar to that for *E. chaffeensis* and requires an experienced microscopist. Commercial sources of IFA serodiagnostic kits include Focus Technologies (Cypress, CA), Scimedx Corp. (Denville, NJ), and PanBio Diagnostics (no longer available in the United States).

Sera should be screened at a single dilution (1:64 or 1:80), and the presence of antibodies is determined after incubation with fluorescein isothiocyanate-conjugated anti-human IgG. If specimens test reactive, they are serially diluted to determine the end point titer. A serologic confirmation diagnosis is achieved when a fourfold rise in titer is demonstrated in convalescence with a minimum IgG titer of 80 or when a single antibody titer of ≥80 is demonstrated in a patient with typical clinical features of HGA (3, 15, 16). Approximately 25 to 45% of infected patients have antibodies at the time of presentation (3, 4, 15, 16); however, up to 11 to 14% of the population possess antibodies in some regions of high endemicity, rendering a single serologic test less useful (2, 14). The typical response during acute infection is a rapid rise (within 2 weeks of onset) in antibody levels reaching high titers (≥640) within the first month (4, 15). In treated patients whose diagnosis was confirmed by culture, antibody titers declined gradually over the several months, and about one-half of these patients had antibodies detectable by IFA 1 year after infection. However, many patients have antibodies detectable for months to years after the initial infection (15).

The sensitivity and specificity of the HGA serologic tests are both believed to be high because of good correlation between typical clinical cases and serologic reactions to *A. phagocytophilum* group antigens (3, 4, 15). Seroconversion was documented in 21 of 23 patients (91.3%) with culture-confirmed HGA from whom a convalescent-phase sample was available (4). In an inter- and intralaboratory evaluation, paired serology had a median sensitivity of 95% for the detection of acute HGA in a group of 28 patients diagnosed by culture, PCR, or the presence of morulae in blood smears (137). IgM testing appears to be a useful tool for identification of recent infection, but neither the sensitivity nor the specificity is as high as testing paired sera for IgG (137). Although ELISA and immunoblots have been described (45, 70, 112), they are not routinely used methods for the serodiagnosis of HGA. Patients with HGA have serologic reactions to *E. chaffeensis* in up to 15% of cases but often show higher titers with antigens of the homologous infecting agent (3, 137). Thus, when ehrlichiosis is clinically suspected, screening for antibodies against *E. chaffeensis* and *A. phagocytophilum* is recommended (31). Immunoblots may be used to differentiate among *A. phagocytophilum* and *E. chaffeensis* infections by demonstration of a major *A. phagocytophilum* antigen of approximately 44 kDa in sera of HGA patients (45, 70, 141).

False-positive reactions can be observed in patients infected with other rickettsiae, Q fever, and Epstein-Barr virus. Many patients with HGA develop antibodies that react with *Borrelia burgdorferi* by ELISA and demonstrate diagnostic IgG or IgM immunoblots (144). Most of these likely represent false positives for *B. burgdorferi,* although some patients have been confirmed by culture to have concurrent infection with *A. phagocytophilum* and *B. burgdorferi* (97, 141). Another explanation is previous exposure to another tick-borne agent (sequential tick bites). Indeed, antibodies to multiple agents are common in individuals living in areas of high endemicity (14, 87). Autoantibodies to platelets and other leukocyte components also can cause false-positive IFA tests (142).

Technologies that use commercially prepared recombinant *A. phagocytophilum* msp2 proteins or peptides in devices that enable rapid detection have been employed for serologic diagnosis in veterinary laboratories, but these antigens have not been evaluated for diagnosis of human infections (17).

ANTIMICROBIAL SUSCEPTIBILITIES

Routine antimicrobial susceptibility testing of *Ehrlichia* or *Anaplasma* species isolates is unnecessary. These bacteria are maintained enzootically by transmission among ticks and feral mammalian reservoir hosts (5, 82, 105, 132, 138). The level of exposure of such vertebrate and invertebrate hosts to antimicrobial selection factors is very low, and thus, antimicrobial pressure that results in resistance is very unlikely. Most patients with either HME or HGA defervesce within 48 hours of therapy with doxycycline, the drug of choice (13, 57). Tetracyclines are uniformly bactericidal for *Ehrlichia* and *Anaplasma* species, whereas the MICs of chloramphenicol cannot be safely achieved in humans with HME or HGA (20, 25, 66, 77, 93). In contrast, many antibiotics prescribed for undifferentiated fever, such as penicillins, cephalosporins, aminoglycosides, and macrolides, do not inhibit the growth of ehrlichiae in vitro. The rifamycins (rifampin and rifabutin) can achieve effective inhibition or killing of *Ehrlichia* and *Anaplasma* species in vitro, and the fluoroquinolones (ofloxacin and levofloxacin) have very low MICs for human isolates of *A. phagocytophilum* (66, 93). However, at least one report documents recrudescence of infection with *A. phagocytophilum* after levofloxacin was discontinued; the patient ultimately responded appropriately to doxycycline treatment (143). Rifampin has been successfully used to treat HGA during pregnancy and could be a useful alternative for patients who cannot receive tetracyclines (27, 79). In vitro susceptibility testing by real-time PCR found that *E. chaffeensis* was susceptible to doxycycline and rifampin and was partially susceptible to the fluoroquinolones. Resistance to macrolides, co-trimoxazole, and beta-lactam compounds was confirmed (20).

Whereas persistent infections with *Ehrlichia* and *Anaplasma* species may occur in naturally and experimentally infected animals even after treatment with tetracycline, persistence of ehrlichiae in humans is rarely documented and is not believed to have any clinical importance (46, 52, 118). Therapy is usually highly effective at eliminating ehrlichiae from the blood of infected humans.

EVALUATION, INTERPRETATION, AND REPORTING OF RESULTS

Identification of infections with *Ehrlichia* and *Anaplasma* species requires clinical suspicion followed by laboratory confirmation. Since rapid specific diagnosis is infrequently possible, empiric therapy should be initiated when the diagnosis is suspected, since delays may lead to increased morbidity and perhaps mortality. Collection of diagnostic samples should ideally occur before therapy is initiated, and patients should be encouraged to return for clinical and serologic follow-up 2 to 4 weeks later.

The presence of intracytoplasmic inclusions within a leukocyte in peripheral blood is helpful, but they can be difficult to distinguish from overlying platelets, Döhle bodies, toxic granulation, nuclear fragments, Auer rods, other bacteria, yeast, inorganic materials, or normal granules. If the typical morphology of an *Ehrlichia* or *Anaplasma* spp. morula is observed, an assessment as to the hematopoietic lineage and the percentage of cells that contain morulae should be made and reported.

A positive PCR result should be reported as such, indicating the presence of *E. chaffeensis* or *A. phagocytophilum* DNA, and it should be made clear that a positive PCR is not equivalent to the culture of ehrlichiae from blood. Laboratories that use a broad-range PCR to identify *Ehrlichia* or *Anaplasma* spp. DNA in blood may also detect *E. ewingii* infection that may mimic either HME or HGA (28).

IFA serologic results should be reported as the titer of antibodies determined to be reactive with *E. chaffeensis* or *A. phagocytophilum*, including the positive cutoff values determined in the laboratory. The gold standard for the diagnosis of *E. chaffeensis* or *A. phagocytophilum* infection by serology is a fourfold increase in IgG titer or documentation of seroconversion. An interpretation should indicate whether the titers are considered "significant" or "positive" based on a fourfold increase or fourfold decrease or only as a single high serum IgG titer. The use of IgM titers is not advocated to establish a diagnosis, since it is not as sensitive as IgG alone. It should be remembered that infections with *E. ewingii* yield serologic patterns considered diagnostic for *E. chaffeensis*. Although not routinely available, immunoblot analyses could provide information about antibodies that react with specific antigens considered unique or diagnostic of infection with a single species of *Ehrlichia* or *Anaplasma*.

Human ehrlichioses became nationally notifiable in 1999, but not all states report these diseases. For the purpose of surveillance, the Council of State and Territorial Epidemiologists and the CDC developed a case definition that was amended in 2008 to include HME, HGA, *E. ewingii* infection, and ehrlichiosis/anaplasmosis—undetermined (http://www.cdc.gov/ncphi/disss/nndss/casedef/ehrlichiosis_2008.htm). According to this definition, a case presenting with fever, headache, myalgia, anemia, leukopenia, thrombocytopenia, or any hepatic transaminase elevation as described above could be classified as confirmed based on specific laboratory findings. A confirmed HME or HGA case is supported by (i) a fourfold change in IgG antibody titer to *E. chaffeensis* or *A. phagocytophilum* antigen, respectively, by IFA in paired serum samples; or (ii) positive PCR and confirmation of *E. chaffeensis* or *A. phagocytophilum* DNA, respectively; or (iii) immunostaining of *E. chaffeensis* or *A. phagocytophilum* antigen, respectively, in a biopsy or autopsy sample; or (iv) culture of *E. chaffeensis* or *A. phagocytophilum*, respectively, from a clinical sample. Supportive laboratory evidence is provided by an IFA IgG titer of ≥64 to *E. chaffeensis* or *A. phagocytophilum* antigen or by identification of morulae in monocytes (HME) or neutrophils (HGA). The diagnosis of *E. ewingii* infection can only be established by nucleic acid amplification methods since specific antigens and serologic methods are not available. The statement "ehrlichiosis or anaplasmosis 'undetermined'" is used when serological tests cannot distinguish between *E. chaffeensis* and *A. phagocytophilum* as agents of infection.

REFERENCES

1. **Aguero-Rosenfeld, M. E.** 2002. Diagnosis of human granulocytic ehrlichiosis: state of the art. *Vector Borne Zoonotic Dis.* **2:**233–239.
2. **Aguero-Rosenfeld, M. E., L. Donnarumma, L. Zentmaier, J. Jacob, M. Frey, R. Noto, C. A. Carbonaro, and G. P. Wormser.** 2002. Seroprevalence of antibodies that react with *Anaplasma phagocytophila*, the agent of human granulocytic ehrlichiosis, in different populations in Westchester County, New York. *J. Clin. Microbiol.* **40:**2612–2615.
3. **Aguero-Rosenfeld, M. E., H. W. Horowitz, G. P. Wormser, D. F. McKenna, J. Nowakowski, J. Munoz, and J. S. Dumler.** 1996. Human granulocytic ehrlichiosis: a case series from a medical center in New York State. *Ann. Intern. Med.* **125:**904–908.
4. **Aguero-Rosenfeld, M. E., F. Kalantarpour, M. Baluch, H. W. Horowitz, D. F. McKenna, J. T. Raffalli, T. Hsieh, J. Wu, J. S. Dumler, and G. P. Wormser.** 2000. Serology of culture-confirmed cases of human granulocytic ehrlichiosis. *J. Clin. Microbiol.* **38:**635–638.
5. **Anderson, B. E., J. E. Dawson, D. C. Jones, and K. H. Wilson.** 1991. *Ehrlichia chaffeensis*, a new species associated with human ehrlichiosis. *J. Clin. Microbiol.* **29:**2838–2842.
6. **Anderson, B. E., K. G. Sims, J. G. Olson, J. E. Childs, J. F. Piesman, C. M. Happ, G. O. Maupin, and B. J. Johnson.** 1993. *Amblyomma americanum*: a potential vector of human ehrlichiosis. *Am. J. Trop. Med. Hyg.* **49:**239–244.
7. **Anderson, B. E., J. W. Sumner, J. E. Dawson, T. Tzianabos, C. R. Greene, J. G. Olson, D. B. Fishbein, M. Olsen-Rasmussen, B. P. Holloway, E. H. George, and A. F. Azad.** 1992. Detection of the etiologic agent of human ehrlichiosis by polymerase chain reaction. *J. Clin. Microbiol.* **30:**775–780.
8. **Arens, M. Q., A. M. Liddell, G. Buening, M. Gaudreault-Keener, J. W. Sumner, J. A. Comer, R. S. Buller, and G. A. Storch.** 2003. Detection of *Ehrlichia* spp. in the blood of wild white-tailed deer in Missouri by PCR assay and serologic analysis. *J. Clin. Microbiol.* **41:**1263–1265.
9. **Arnez, M., M. Petrovec, S. Lotric-Furlan, T. A. Zupanc, and F. Strle.** 2001. First European pediatric case of human granulocytic ehrlichiosis. *J. Clin. Microbiol.* **39:**4591–4592.
10. **Asanovich, K. M., J. S. Bakken, J. E. Madigan, M. Aguero-Rosenfeld, G. P. Wormser, and J. S. Dumler.** 1997. Antigenic diversity of granulocytic *Ehrlichia* isolates from humans in Wisconsin and New York and a horse in California. *J. Infect. Dis.* **176:**1029–1034.
11. **Bakken, J. S., M. E. Aguero-Rosenfeld, R. L. Tilden, G. P. Wormser, H. W. Horowitz, J. T. Raffalli, M. Baluch, D. Riddell, J. J. Walls, and J. S. Dumler.** 2001. Serial measurements of hematologic counts during the active phase of human granulocytic ehrlichiosis. *Clin. Infect. Dis.* **32:**862–870.
12. **Bakken, J. S., J. S. Dumler, S. M. Chen, M. R. Eckman, L. L. Van Etta, and D. H. Walker.** 1994. Human granulocytic ehrlichiosis in the upper Midwest United States. A new species emerging? *JAMA* **272:**212–218.
13. **Bakken, J. S., and S. Dumler.** 2008. Human granulocytic anaplasmosis. *Infect. Dis. Clin. N. Am.* **22:**433–448, viii.
14. **Bakken, J. S., P. Goellner, M. Van Etten, D. Z. Boyle, O. L. Swonger, S. Mattson, J. Krueth, R. L. Tilden, K. Asanovich, J. Walls, and J. S. Dumler.** 1998. Seroprevalence of human granulocytic ehrlichiosis among permanent residents of northwestern Wisconsin. *Clin. Infect. Dis.* **27:**1491–1496.
15. **Bakken, J. S., I. Haller, D. Riddell, J. J. Walls, and J. S. Dumler.** 2002. The serological response of patients infected with the agent of human granulocytic ehrlichiosis. *Clin. Infect. Dis.* **34:**22–27.
16. **Bakken, J. S., J. Krueth, C. Wilson-Nordskog, R. L. Tilden, K. Asanovich, and J. S. Dumler.** 1996. Clinical and laboratory characteristics of human granulocytic ehrlichiosis. *JAMA* **275:**199–205.
17. **Beall, M. J., R. Chandrashekar, M. D. Eberts, K. E. Cyr, P. P. Diniz, C. Mainville, B. C. Hegarty, J. M. Crawford, and E. B. Breitschwerdt.** 2008. Serological and molecular prevalence of *Borrelia burgdorferi*, *Anaplasma phagocytophilum*, and *Ehrlichia* species in dogs from Minnesota. *Vector Borne Zoonotic Dis.* **8:**455–464.

18. **Blanco, J. R., and J. A. Oteo.** 2002. Human granulocytic ehrlichiosis in Europe. *Clin. Microbiol. Infect.* **8:**763–772.

19. **Blouin, E. F., and K. M. Kocan.** 1998. Morphology and development of *Anaplasma marginale* (Rickettsiales: Anaplasmataceae) in cultured *Ixodes scapularis* (Acari: Ixodidae) cells. *J. Med. Entomol.* **35:**788–797.

20. **Branger, S., J. M. Rolain, and D. Raoult.** 2004. Evaluation of antibiotic susceptibilities of *Ehrlichia canis, Ehrlichia chaffeensis,* and *Anaplasma phagocytophilum* by real-time PCR. *Antimicrob. Agents Chemother.* **48:**4822–4828.

21. **Brayton, K. A., L. S. Kappmeyer, D. R. Herndon, M. J. Dark, D. L. Tibbals, G. H. Palmer, T. C. McGuire, and D. P. Knowles, Jr.** 2005. Complete genome sequencing of *Anaplasma marginale* reveals that the surface is skewed to two superfamilies of outer membrane proteins. *Proc. Natl. Acad. Sci. USA* **102:**844–849.

22. **Brouqui, P., M. L. Birg, and D. Raoult.** 1994. Cytopathic effect, plaque formation, and lysis of *Ehrlichia chaffeensis* grown on continuous cell lines. *Infect. Immun.* **62:**405–411.

23. **Brouqui, P., C. Le Cam, P. J. Kelly, R. Laurens, A. Tounkara, S. Sawadogo, M. Velo, L. Gondao, B. Faugere, J. Delmont, A. Bourgeade, and D. Raoult.** 1994. Serologic evidence for human ehrlichiosis in Africa. *Eur. J. Epidemiol.* **10:**695–698.

24. **Brouqui, P., C. Lecam, J. Olson, and D. Raoult.** 1994. Serologic diagnosis of human monocytic ehrlichiosis by immunoblot analysis. *Clin. Diagn. Lab. Immunol.* **1:**645–649.

25. **Brouqui, P., and D. Raoult.** 1992. In vitro antibiotic susceptibility of the newly recognized agent of ehrlichiosis in humans, *Ehrlichia chaffeensis. Antimicrob. Agents Chemother.* **36:**2799–2803.

26. **Brouqui, P., Y. O. Sanogo, G. Caruso, F. Merola, and D. Raoult.** 2003. Candidatus *Ehrlichia walkerii:* a new *Ehrlichia* detected in *Ixodes ricinus* tick collected from asymptomatic humans in Northern Italy. *Ann. N. Y. Acad. Sci.* **990:**134–140.

27. **Buitrago, M. I., J. W. Ijdo, P. Rinaudo, H. Simon, J. Copel, J. Gadbaw, R. Heimer, E. Fikrig, and F. J. Bia.** 1998. Human granulocytic ehrlichiosis during pregnancy treated successfully with rifampin. *Clin. Infect. Dis.* **27:**213–215.

28. **Buller, R. S., M. Arens, S. P. Hmiel, C. D. Paddock, J. W. Sumner, Y. Rikihsa, A. Unver, M. Gaudreault-Keener, F. A. Manian, A. M. Liddell, N. Schmulewitz, and G. A. Storch.** 1999. *Ehrlichia ewingii,* a newly recognized agent of human ehrlichiosis. *N. Engl. J. Med.* **341:**148–155.

29. **Cao, W. C., Y. M. Gao, P. H. Zhang, X. T. Zhang, Q. H. Dai, J. S. Dumler, L. Q. Fang, and H. Yang.** 2000. Identification of *Ehrlichia chaffeensis* by nested PCR in ticks from Southern China. *J. Clin. Microbiol.* **38:**2778–2780.

30. **Centers for Disease Control and Prevention.** 2008. *Anaplasma phagocytophilum* transmitted through blood transfusion—Minnesota, 2007. *MMWR Morb. Mortal. Wkly. Rep.* **57:**1145–1148.

31. **Centers for Disease Control and Prevention.** 2009. Anaplasmosis and ehrlichiosis—Maine, 2008. *MMWR Morb. Mortal. Wkly. Rep.* **58:**1033–1036.

32. **Chapman, A. S., J. S. Bakken, S. M. Folk, C. D. Paddock, K. C. Bloch, A. Krusell, D. J. Sexton, S. C. Buckingham, G. S. Marshall, G. A. Storch, G. A. Dasch, J. H. McQuiston, D. L. Swerdlow, S. J. Dumler, W. L. Nicholson, D. H. Walker, M. E. Eremeeva, and C. A. Ohl.** 2006. Diagnosis and management of tickborne rickettsial diseases: Rocky Mountain spotted fever, ehrlichioses, and anaplasmosis—United States: a practical guide for physicians and other health-care and public health professionals. *MMWR Recommend. Rep.* **55:**1–27.

33. **Chen, S. M., J. S. Dumler, J. S. Bakken, and D. H. Walker.** 1994. Identification of a granulocytotropic *Ehrlichia* species as the etiologic agent of human disease. *J. Clin. Microbiol.* **32:**589–595.

34. **Chen, S. M., J. S. Dumler, H. M. Feng, and D. H. Walker.** 1994. Identification of the antigenic constituents of *Ehrlichia chaffeensis. Am. J. Trop. Med. Hyg.* **50:**52–58.

35. **Chen, S. M., X. J. Yu, V. L. Popov, E. L. Westerman, F. G. Hamilton, and D. H. Walker.** 1997. Genetic and antigenic diversity of *Ehrlichia chaffeensis:* comparative analysis of a novel human strain from Oklahoma and previously isolated strains. *J. Infect. Dis.* **175:**856–863.

36. **Childs, J. E., J. W. Sumner, W. L. Nicholson, R. F. Massung, S. M. Standaert, and C. D. Paddock.** 1999. Outcome of diagnostic tests using samples from patients with culture-proven human monocytic ehrlichiosis: implications for surveillance. *J. Clin. Microbiol.* **37:**2997–3000.

37. **Chu, F. K.** 1998. Rapid and sensitive PCR-based detection and differentiation of aetiologic agents of human granulocytotropic and monocytotropic ehrlichiosis. *Mol. Cell. Probes* **12:**93–99.

38. **Comer, J. A., W. L. Nicholson, J. G. Olson, and J. E. Childs.** 1999. Serologic testing for human granulocytic ehrlichiosis at a national referral center. *J. Clin. Microbiol.* **37:**558–564.

39. **Dawson, J., D. Fishbein, T. Eng, M. Redus, and N. Greene.** 1990. Diagnosis of human ehrlichiosis with the indirect fluorescent antibody test: kinetics and specificity. *Ann. N. Y. Acad. Sci.* **590:**308.

40. **Dawson, J. E., B. E. Anderson, D. B. Fishbein, J. L. Sanchez, C. S. Goldsmith, K. H. Wilson, and C. W. Duntley.** 1991. Isolation and characterization of an *Ehrlichia* sp. from a patient diagnosed with human ehrlichiosis. *J. Clin. Microbiol.* **29:**2741–2745.

41. **Dawson, J. E., and S. A. Ewing.** 1992. Susceptibility of dogs to infection with *Ehrlichia chaffeensis,* causative agent of human ehrlichiosis. *Am. J. Vet. Res.* **53:**1322–1327.

42. **Demma, L. J., R. C. Holman, J. H. McQuiston, J. W. Krebs, and D. L. Swerdlow.** 2005. Epidemiology of human ehrlichiosis and anaplasmosis in the United States, 2001–2002. *Am. J. Trop. Med. Hyg.* **73:**400–409.

43. **Doyle, C. K., M. B. Labruna, E. B. Breitschwerdt, Y. W. Tang, R. E. Corstvet, B. C. Hegarty, K. C. Bloch, P. Li, D. H. Walker, and J. W. McBride.** 2005. Detection of medically important *Ehrlichia* by quantitative multicolor TaqMan real-time polymerase chain reaction of the dsb gene. *J. Mol. Diagn.* **7:**504–510.

44. **Dumler, J. S.** 2005. Anaplasma and ehrlichia infection. *Ann. N. Y. Acad. Sci.* **1063:**361–373.

45. **Dumler, J. S., K. M. Asanovich, J. S. Bakken, P. Richter, R. Kimsey, and J. E. Madigan.** 1995. Serologic cross-reactions among *Ehrlichia equi, Ehrlichia phagocytophila,* and human granulocytic *Ehrlichia. J. Clin. Microbiol.* **33:**1098–1103.

46. **Dumler, J. S., and J. S. Bakken.** 1996. Human granulocytic ehrlichiosis in Wisconsin and Minnesota: a frequent infection with the potential for persistence. *J. Infect. Dis.* **173:**1027–1030.

47. **Dumler, J. S., A. F. Barbet, C. P. Bekker, G. A. Dasch, G. H. Palmer, S. C. Ray, Y. Rikihisa, and F. R. Rurangirwa.** 2001. Reorganization of genera in the families *Rickettsiaceae* and *Anaplasmataceae* in the order *Rickettsiales:* unification of some species of *Ehrlichia* with *Anaplasma, Cowdria* with *Ehrlichia* and *Ehrlichia* with *Neorickettsia,* descriptions of six new species combinations and designation of *Ehrlichia equi* and 'HGE agent' as subjective synonyms of *Ehrlichia phagocytophila. Int. J. Syst. Evol. Microbiol.* **51:**2145–2165.

48. **Dumler, J. S., S. M. Chen, K. Asanovich, E. Trigiani, V. L. Popov, and D. H. Walker.** 1995. Isolation and characterization of a new strain of *Ehrlichia chaffeensis* from a patient with nearly fatal monocytic ehrlichiosis. *J. Clin. Microbiol.* **33:**1704–1711.

49. **Dumler, J. S., J. E. Dawson, and D. H. Walker.** 1993. Human ehrlichiosis: hematopathology and immunohistologic detection of *Ehrlichia chaffeensis. Hum. Pathol.* **24:**391–396.

50. **Dumler, J. S., J. E. Madigan, N. Pusterla, and J. S. Bakken.** 2007. Ehrlichioses in humans: epidemiology, clinical presentation, diagnosis, and treatment. *Clin. Infect. Dis.* **45**(Suppl. 1):S45–S51.

51. **Dumler, J. S., Y. Rikihisa, and G. A. Dasch.** 2005. Genus I. *Anaplasma,* p. 117–125. *In* G. M. Garrity, D. J. Brenner, N. R. Krieg, and J. T. Staley (ed.), *Bergey's Manual of Systematic Bacteriology,* 2nd ed., vol. 2. *The Proteobacteria, Part C. The Alpha-, Beta-, Delta-, and Epsilon-Proteobacteria.* Springer, East Lansing, MI.

52. **Dumler, J. S., W. L. Sutker, and D. H. Walker.** 1993. Persistent infection with *Ehrlichia chaffeensis. Clin. Infect. Dis.* **17:**903–905.

53. Dunning Hotopp, J. C., M. Lin, R. Madupu, J. Crabtree, S. V. Angiuoli, J. Eisen, R. Seshadri, Q. Ren, M. Wu, T. R. Utterback, S. Smith, M. Lewis, H. Khouri, C. Zhang, H. Niu, Q. Lin, N. Ohashi, N. Zhi, W. Nelson, L. M. Brinkac, R. J. Dodson, M. J. Rosovitz, J. Sundaram, S. C. Daugherty, T. Davidsen, A. S. Durkin, M. Gwinn, D. H. Haft, J. D. Selengut, S. A. Sullivan, N. Zafar, L. Zhou, F. Benahmed, H. Forberger, R. Halpin, S. Mulligan, J. Robinson, O. White, Y. Rikihisa, and H. Tettelin. 2006. Comparative genomics of emerging human ehrlichiosis agents. PLoS Genet. 2:e21.

54. Edelman, D. C., and J. S. Dumler. 1996. Evaluation of an improved PCR diagnostic assay for human granulocytic ehrlichiosis. Mol. Diagn. 1:41–49.

55. Everett, E. D., K. A. Evans, R. B. Henry, and G. McDonald. 1994. Human ehrlichiosis in adults after tick exposure. Diagnosis using polymerase chain reaction. Ann. Intern. Med. 120:730–735.

56. Fichtenbaum, C. J., L. R. Peterson, and G. J. Weil. 1993. Ehrlichiosis presenting as a life-threatening illness with features of the toxic shock syndrome. Am. J. Med. 95:351–357.

57. Fishbein, D. B., J. E. Dawson, and L. E. Robinson. 1994. Human ehrlichiosis in the United States, 1985 to 1990. Ann. Intern. Med. 120:736–743.

58. Frutos, R., A. Viari, C. Ferraz, A. Morgat, S. Eychenie, Y. Kandassamy, I. Chantal, A. Bensaid, E. Coissac, N. Vachiery, J. Demaille, and D. Martinez. 2006. Comparative genomic analysis of three strains of Ehrlichia ruminantium reveals an active process of genome size plasticity. J. Bacteriol. 188:2533–2542.

59. Gongora-Biachi, R. A., J. Zavala-Velazquez, C. J. Castro-Sansores, and P. Gonzalez-Martinez. 1999. First case of human ehrlichiosis in Mexico. Emerg. Infect. Dis. 5:481.

60. Goodman, J. L., C. Nelson, B. Vitale, J. E. Madigan, J. S. Dumler, T. J. Kurtti, and U. G. Munderloh. 1996. Direct cultivation of the causative agent of human granulocytic ehrlichiosis. N. Engl. J. Med. 334:209–215.

61. Grzeszczuk, A., A. Milstone, K. S. Choi, N. Barat, J. C. Garcia-Garcia, M. Petrovec, and J. S. Dumler. 2009. Differential impairment of neutrophil function by strains of Anaplasma phagocytophilum. Clin. Microbiol. Infect. 15:19–20.

62. Halasz, C. L., G. W. Niedt, C. P. Kurtz, D. G. Scorpio, J. S. Bakken, and J. S. Dumler. 2005. A case of Sweet syndrome associated with human granulocytic anaplasmosis. Arch. Dermatol. 141:887–889.

63. Hardalo, C. J., V. Quagliarello, and J. S. Dumler. 1995. Human granulocytic ehrlichiosis in Connecticut: report of a fatal case. Clin. Infect. Dis. 21:910–914.

64. Heimer, R., D. Tisdale, and J. E. Dawson. 1998. A single tissue culture system for the propagation of the agents of the human ehrlichioses. Am. J. Trop. Med. Hyg. 58:812–815.

65. Hoerauf, A. 2008. Filariasis: new drugs and new opportunities for lymphatic filariasis and onchocerciasis. Curr. Opin. Infect. Dis. 21:673–681.

66. Horowitz, H. W., T. C. Hsieh, M. E. Aguero-Rosenfeld, F. Kalantarpour, I. Chowdhury, G. P. Wormser, and J. M. Wu. 2001. Antimicrobial susceptibility of Ehrlichia phagocytophila. Antimicrob. Agents Chemother. 45:786–788.

67. Horowitz, H. W., E. Kilchevsky, S. Haber, M. Aguero-Rosenfeld, R. Kranwinkel, E. K. James, S. J. Wong, F. Chu, D. Liveris, and I. Schwartz. 1998. Perinatal transmission of the agent of human granulocytic ehrlichiosis. N. Engl. J. Med. 339:375–378.

68. Hossain, D., M. E. Aguero-Rosenfeld, H. W. Horowitz, J. M. Wu, T. C. Hsieh, N. Sachdeva, S. J. Peterson, J. S. Dumler, and G. P. Wormser. 1999. Clinical and laboratory evolution of a culture-confirmed case of human granulocytic ehrlichiosis. Conn. Med. 63:265–270.

69. IJdo, J. W., J. I. Meek, M. L. Cartter, L. A. Magnarelli, C. Wu, S. W. Tenuta, E. Fikrig, and R. W. Ryder. 2000. The emergence of another tickborne infection in the 12-town area around Lyme, Connecticut: human granulocytic ehrlichiosis. J. Infect. Dis. 181:1388–1393.

70. IJdo, J. W., Y. Zhang, E. Hodzic, L. A. Magnarelli, M. L. Wilson, S. R. Telford III, S. W. Barthold, and E. Fikrig. 1997. The early humoral response in human granulocytic ehrlichiosis. J. Infect. Dis. 176:687–692.

71. Inokuma, H., P. Brouqui, M. Drancourt, and D. Raoult. 2001. Citrate synthase gene sequence: a new tool for phylogenetic analysis and identification of Ehrlichia. J. Clin. Microbiol. 39:3031–3039.

72. Inokuma, H., K. Fujii, M. Okuda, T. Onishi, J. P. Beaufils, D. Raoult, and P. Brouqui. 2002. Determination of the nucleotide sequences of heat shock operon groESL and the citrate synthase gene (gltA) of Anaplasma (Ehrlichia) platys for phylogenetic and diagnostic studies. Clin. Diagn. Lab. Immunol. 9:1132–1136.

73. Inokuma, H., Y. Terada, T. Kamio, D. Raoult, and P. Brouqui. 2001. Analysis of the 16S rRNA gene sequence of Anaplasma centrale and its phylogenetic relatedness to other ehrlichiae. Clin. Diagn. Lab. Immunol. 8:241–244.

74. Jongejan, F., L. A. Wassink, M. J. Thielemans, N. M. Perie, and G. Uilenberg. 1989. Serotypes in Cowdria ruminantium and their relationship with Ehrlichia phagocytophila determined by immunofluorescence. Vet. Microbiol. 21:31–40.

75. Kalantarpour, F., I. Chowdhury, G. P. Wormser, and M. E. Aguero-Rosenfeld. 2000. Survival of the human granulocytic ehrlichiosis agent under refrigeration conditions. J. Clin. Microbiol. 38:2398–2399.

76. Kawahara, M., Y. Rikihisa, E. Isogai, M. Takahashi, H. Misumi, C. Suto, S. Shibata, C. Zhang, and M. Tsuji. 2004. Ultrastructure and phylogenetic analysis of 'Candidatus Neoehrlichia mikurensis' in the family Anaplasmataceae, isolated from wild rats and found in Ixodes ovatus ticks. Int. J. Syst. Evol. Microbiol. 54:1837–1843.

77. Klein, M. B., C. M. Nelson, and J. L. Goodman. 1997. Antibiotic susceptibility of the newly cultivated agent of human granulocytic ehrlichiosis: promising activity of quinolones and rifamycins. Antimicrob. Agents Chemother. 41:76–79.

78. Koutaro, M., A. S. Santos, J. S. Dumler, and P. Brouqui. 2005. Distribution of 'Ehrlichia walkeri' in Ixodes ricinus (Acari: Ixodidae) from the northern part of Italy. J. Med. Entomol. 42:82–85.

79. Krause, P. J., C. L. Corrow, and J. S. Bakken. 2003. Successful treatment of human granulocytic ehrlichiosis in children using rifampin. Pediatrics 112:e252–e253.

80. Lee, K. N., I. Padmalayam, B. Baumstark, S. L. Baker, and R. F. Massung. 2003. Characterization of the ftsZ gene from Ehrlichia chaffeensis, Anaplasma phagocytophilum, and Rickettsia rickettsii, and use as a differential PCR target. DNA Cell Biol. 22:179–186.

81. Lepidi, H., J. E. Bunnell, M. E. Martin, J. E. Madigan, S. Stuen, and J. S. Dumler. 2000. Comparative pathology, and immunohistology associated with clinical illness after Ehrlichia phagocytophila-group infections. Am. J. Trop. Med. Hyg. 62:29–37.

82. Lockhart, J. M., W. R. Davidson, D. E. Stallknecht, J. E. Dawson, and E. W. Howerth. 1997. Isolation of Ehrlichia chaffeensis from wild white-tailed deer (Odocoileus virginianus) confirms their role as natural reservoir hosts. J. Clin. Microbiol. 35:1681–1686.

83. Long, S. W., X. Zhang, J. Zhang, R. P. Ruble, P. Teel, and X. J. Yu. 2003. Evaluation of transovarial transmission and transmissibility of Ehrlichia chaffeensis (Rickettsiales: Anaplasmataceae) in Amblyomma americanum (Acari: Ixodidae). J. Med. Entomol. 40:1000–1004.

84. Macleod, J. R., and W. S. Gordon. 1933. Studies in tickborne fever of sheep. I. Transmission by the tick, Ixodes ricinus, with a description of the disease produced. Parasitology 25:273–285.

85. Madigan, J. E., N. Pusterla, E. Johnson, J. S. Chae, J. B. Pusterla, E. Derock, and S. P. Lawler. 2000. Transmission of Ehrlichia risticii, the agent of Potomac horse fever, using naturally infected aquatic insects and helminth vectors: preliminary report. Equine Vet. J. 32:275–279.

86. Maeda, K., N. Markowitz, R. C. Hawley, M. Ristic, D. Cox, and J. E. McDade. 1987. Human infection with Ehrlichia canis, a leukocytic rickettsia. N. Engl. J. Med. 316:853–856.

87. **Magnarelli, L. A., J. S. Dumler, J. F. Anderson, R. C. Johnson, and E. Fikrig.** 1995. Coexistence of antibodies to tick-borne pathogens of babesiosis, ehrlichiosis, and Lyme borreliosis in human sera. *J. Clin. Microbiol.* **33:**3054–3057.

88. **Marty, A. M., J. S. Dumler, G. Imes, H. P. Brusman, L. L. Smrkovski, and D. M. Frisman.** 1995. Ehrlichiosis mimicking thrombotic thrombocytopenic purpura. Case report and pathological correlation. *Hum. Pathol.* **26:**920–925.

89. **Massung, R. F., K. Lee, M. Mauel, and A. Gusa.** 2002. Characterization of the rRNA genes of *Ehrlichia chaffeensis* and *Anaplasma phagocytophila. DNA Cell Biol.* **21:**587–596.

90. **Massung, R. F., T. N. Mather, and M. L. Levin.** 2006. Reservoir competency of goats for the Ap-variant 1 strain of *Anaplasma phagocytophilum. Infect. Immun.* **74:**1373–1375.

91. **Massung, R. F., M. J. Mauel, J. H. Owens, N. Allan, J. W. Courtney, K. C. Stafford III, and T. N. Mather.** 2002. Genetic variants of *Ehrlichia phagocytophila,* Rhode Island and Connecticut. *Emerg. Infect. Dis.* **8:**467–472.

92. **Massung, R. F., and K. G. Slater.** 2003. Comparison of PCR assays for detection of the agent of human granulocytic ehrlichiosis, *Anaplasma phagocytophilum. J. Clin. Microbiol.* **41:**717–722.

93. **Maurin, M., J. S. Bakken, and J. S. Dumler.** 2003. Antibiotic susceptibilities of *Anaplasma (Ehrlichia) phagocytophilum* strains from various geographic areas in the United States. *Antimicrob. Agents Chemother.* **47:**413–415.

94. **Misao, T., and Y. Kobayashi.** 1955. Studies on infectious mononucleosis (glandular fever). I. Isolation of etiologic agent from blood, bone marrow, and lymph node of a patient with infectious mononucleosis by using mice. *Kyushu J. Med. Sci.* **6:**145–152.

95. **Morais, J. D., J. E. Dawson, C. Greene, A. R. Filipe, L. C. Galhardas, and F. Bacellar.** 1991. First European case of ehrlichiosis. *Lancet* **338:**633–634.

96. **Morissette, E., R. F. Massung, J. E. Foley, A. R. Alleman, P. Foley, and A. F. Barbet.** 2009. Diversity of *Anaplasma phagocytophilum* strains, USA. *Emerg. Infect. Dis.* **15:**928–931.

97. **Nadelman, R. B., H. W. Horowitz, T. C. Hsieh, J. M. Wu, M. E. Aguero-Rosenfeld, I. Schwartz, J. Nowakowski, S. Varde, and G. P. Wormser.** 1997. Simultaneous human granulocytic ehrlichiosis and Lyme borreliosis. *N. Engl. J. Med.* **337:**27–30.

98. **Newton, P. N., J. M. Rolain, B. Rasachak, M. Mayxay, K. Vathanatham, P. Seng, R. Phetsouvanh, T. Thammavong, J. Zahidi, Y. Suputtamongkol, B. Syhavong, and D. Raoult.** 2009. Sennetsu neorickettsiosis: a probable fish-borne cause of fever rediscovered in Laos. *Am. J. Trop. Med. Hyg.* **81:**190–194.

99. **Ohashi, N., N. Zhi, Q. Lin, and Y. Rikihisa.** 2002. Characterization and transcriptional analysis of gene clusters for a type IV secretion machinery in human granulocytic and monocytic ehrlichiosis agents. *Infect. Immun.* **70:**2128–2138.

101. **Paddock, C. D., and J. E. Childs.** 2003. *Ehrlichia chaffeensis:* a prototypical emerging pathogen. *Clin. Microbiol. Rev.* **16:**37–64.

102. **Paddock, C. D., S. M. Folk, G. M. Shore, L. J. Machado, M. M. Huycke, L. N. Slater, A. M. Liddell, R. S. Buller, G. A. Storch, T. P. Monson, D. Rimland, J. W. Sumner, J. Singleton, K. C. Bloch, Y. W. Tang, S. M. Standaert, and J. E. Childs.** 2001. Infections with *Ehrlichia chaffeensis* and *Ehrlichia ewingii* in persons coinfected with human immunodeficiency virus. *Clin. Infect. Dis.* **33:**1586–1594.

103. **Paddock, C. D., D. P. Suchard, K. L. Grumbach, W. K. Hadley, R. L. Kerschmann, N. W. Abbey, J. E. Dawson, B. E. Anderson, K. G. Sims, J. S. Dumler, and B. Herndier.** 1993. Brief report: fatal seronegative ehrlichiosis in a patient with HIV infection. *N. Engl. J. Med.* **329:**1164–1167.

104. **Paddock, C. D., J. W. Sumner, G. M. Shore, D. C. Bartley, R. C. Elie, J. G. McQuade, C. R. Martin, C. S. Goldsmith, and J. E. Childs.** 1997. Isolation and characterization of *Ehrlichia chaffeensis* strains from patients with fatal ehrlichiosis. *J. Clin. Microbiol.* **35:**2496–2502.

105. **Pancholi, P., C. P. Kolbert, P. D. Mitchell, K. D. Reed, Jr., J. S. Dumler, J. S. Bakken, S. R. Telford III, and D. H. Persing.** 1995. *Ixodes dammini* as a potential vector of human granulocytic ehrlichiosis. *J. Infect. Dis.* **172:**1007–1012.

106. **Park, J. H., E. J. Heo, K. S. Choi, J. S. Dumler, and J. S. Chae.** 2003. Detection of antibodies to *Anaplasma phagocytophilum* and *Ehrlichia chaffeensis* antigens in sera of Korean patients by Western immunoblotting and indirect immunofluorescence assays. *Clin. Diagn. Lab. Immunol.* **10:**1059–1064.

107. **Perez, M., M. Bodor, C. Zhang, Q. Xiong, and Y. Rikihisa.** 2006. Human infection with *Ehrlichia canis* accompanied by clinical signs in Venezuela. *Ann. N. Y. Acad. Sci.* **1078:**110–117.

108. **Perez, M., Y. Rikihisa, and B. Wen.** 1996. *Ehrlichia canis*-like agent isolated from a man in Venezuela: antigenic and genetic characterization. *J. Clin. Microbiol.* **34:**2133–2139.

109. **Petrovec, M., S. Lotric Furlan, T. A. Zupanc, F. Strle, P. Brouqui, V. Roux, and J. S. Dumler.** 1997. Human disease in Europe caused by a granulocytic *Ehrlichia* species. *J. Clin. Microbiol.* **35:**1556–1559.

110. **Popov, V. L., S. M. Chen, H. M. Feng, and D. H. Walker.** 1995. Ultrastructural variation of cultured *Ehrlichia chaffeensis. J. Med. Microbiol.* **43:**411–421.

111. **Popov, V. L., V. C. Han, S. M. Chen, J. S. Dumler, H. M. Feng, T. G. Andreadis, R. B. Tesh, and D. H. Walker.** 1998. Ultrastructural differentiation of the genogroups in the genus *Ehrlichia. J. Med. Microbiol.* **47:**235–251.

112. **Ravyn, M. D., J. L. Goodman, C. B. Kodner, D. K. Westad, L. A. Coleman, S. M. Engstrom, C. M. Nelson, and R. C. Johnson.** 1998. Immunodiagnosis of human granulocytic ehrlichiosis by using culture-derived human isolates. *J. Clin. Microbiol.* **36:**1480–1488.

113. **Remy, V., Y. Hansmann, S. De Martino, D. Christmann, and P. Brouqui.** 2003. Human anaplasmosis presenting as atypical pneumonitis in France. *Clin. Infect. Dis.* **37:**846–848.

114. **Richter, P. J., Jr., R. B. Kimsey, J. E. Madigan, J. E. Barlough, J. S. Dumler, and D. L. Brooks.** 1996. *Ixodes pacificus (Acari: Ixodidae)* as a vector of *Ehrlichia equi (Rickettsiales: Ehrlichieae). J. Med. Entomol.* **33:**1–5.

115. **Rikihisa, Y.** 2006. New findings on members of the family Anaplasmataceae of veterinary importance. *Ann. N. Y. Acad. Sci.* **1078:**438–445.

116. **Rikihisa, Y., N. Zhi, G. P. Wormser, B. Wen, H. W. Horowitz, and K. E. Hechemy.** 1997. Ultrastructural and antigenic characterization of a granulocytic ehrlichiosis agent directly isolated and stably cultivated from a patient in New York state. *J. Infect. Dis.* **175:**210–213.

117. **Ripoll, C. M., C. E. Remondegui, G. Ordonez, R. Arazamendi, H. Fusaro, M. J. Hyman, C. D. Paddock, S. R. Zaki, J. G. Olson, and C. A. Santos-Buch.** 1999. Evidence of rickettsial spotted fever and ehrlichial infections in a subtropical territory of Jujuy, Argentina. *Am. J. Trop. Med. Hyg.* **61:**350–354.

118. **Roland, W. E., G. McDonald, C. W. Caldwell, and E. D. Everett.** 1995. Ehrlichiosis—a cause of prolonged fever. *Clin. Infect. Dis.* **20:**821–825.

110. **Safdar, N., R. B. Love, and D. G. Maki.** 2002. Severe *Ehrlichia chaffeensis* infection in a lung transplant recipient: a review of ehrlichiosis in the immunocompromised patient. *Emerg. Infect. Dis.* **8:**320–323.

120. **Sanogo, Y. O., P. Parola, S. Shpynov, J. L. Camicas, P. Brouqui, G. Caruso, and D. Raoult.** 2003. Genetic diversity of bacterial agents detected in ticks removed from asymptomatic patients in northeastern Italy. *Ann. N. Y. Acad. Sci.* **990:**182–190.

121. **Schutze, G. E., S. C. Buckingham, G. S. Marshall, C. R. Woods, M. A. Jackson, L. E. Patterson, and R. F. Jacobs.** 2007. Human monocytic ehrlichiosis in children. *Pediatr. Infect. Dis. J.* **26:**475–479.

122. **Scorpio, D. G., M. Akkoyunlu, E. Fikrig, and J. S. Dumler.** 2004. CXCR2 blockade influences *Anaplasma phagocytophilum* propagation but not histopathology in the mouse model of human granulocytic anaplasmosis. *Clin. Diagn. Lab. Immunol.* **11:**963–968.

123. Sirigireddy, K. R., and R. R. Ganta. 2005. Multiplex detection of *Ehrlichia* and *Anaplasma* species pathogens in peripheral blood by real-time reverse transcriptase-polymerase chain reaction. *J. Mol. Diagn.* **7:**308–316.

124. Stafford, K. C., III, R. F. Massung, L. A. Magnarelli, J. W. Ijdo, and J. F. Anderson. 1999. Infection with agents of human granulocytic ehrlichiosis, Lyme disease, and babesiosis in wild white-footed mice (*Peromyscus leucopus*) in Connecticut. *J. Clin. Microbiol.* **37:**2887–2892.

125. Standaert, S. M., T. Yu, M. A. Scott, J. E. Childs, C. D. Paddock, W. L. Nicholson, J. Singleton, Jr., and M. J. Blaser. 2000. Primary isolation of *Ehrlichia chaffeensis* from patients with febrile illnesses: clinical and molecular characteristics. *J. Infect. Dis.* **181:**1082–1088.

126. Stone, J. H., K. Dierberg, G. Aram, and J. S. Dumler. 2004. Human monocytic ehrlichiosis. *JAMA* **292:**2263–2270.

127. Stuen, S., I. Van De Pol, K. Bergstrom, and L. M. Schouls. 2002. Identification of *Anaplasma phagocytophila* (formerly *Ehrlichia phagocytophila*) variants in blood from sheep in Norway. *J. Clin. Microbiol.* **40:**3192–3197.

128. Sumner, J. W., W. L. Nicholson, and R. F. Massung. 1997. PCR amplification and comparison of nucleotide sequences from the *groESL* heat shock operon of *Ehrlichia* species. *J. Clin. Microbiol.* **35:**2087–2092.

129. Sumner, J. W., K. G. Sims, D. C. Jones, and B. E. Anderson. 1993. *Ehrlichia chaffeensis* expresses an immunoreactive protein homologous to the *Escherichia coli* GroEL protein. *Infect. Immun.* **61:**3536–3539.

130. Taillardat-Bisch, A. V., D. Raoult, and M. Drancourt. 2003. RNA polymerase beta-subunit-based phylogeny of *Ehrlichia* spp., *Anaplasma* spp., *Neorickettsia* spp. and *Wolbachia pipientis*. *Int. J. Syst. Evol. Microbiol.* **53:**455–458.

131. Taylor, M. J. 2002. *Wolbachia* endosymbiotic bacteria of filarial nematodes. A new insight into disease pathogenesis and control. *Arch. Med. Res.* **33:**422–424.

132. Telford, S. R., III, J. E. Dawson, P. Katavolos, C. K. Warner, C. P. Kolbert, and D. H. Persing. 1996. Perpetuation of the agent of human granulocytic ehrlichiosis in a deer tick-rodent cycle. *Proc. Natl. Acad. Sci. USA* **93:**6209–6214.

133. Turner, J. D., R. S. Langley, K. L. Johnston, K. Gentil, L. Ford, B. Wu, M. Graham, F. Sharpley, B. Slatko, E. Pearlman, and M. J. Taylor. 2009. *Wolbachia* lipoprotein stimulates innate and adaptive immunity through Toll-like receptors 2 and 6 to induce disease manifestations of filariasis. *J. Biol. Chem.* **284:**22364–22378.

134. Wagner, E. R., W. G. Bremer, Y. Rikihisa, S. A. Ewing, G. R. Needham, A. Unver, X. Wang, and R. W. Stich. 2004. Development of a p28-based PCR assay for *Ehrlichia chaffeensis*. *Mol. Cell. Probes* **18:**111–116.

135. Walker, D. H., and J. S. Dumler. 1996. Emergence of the ehrlichioses as human health problems. *Emerg. Infect. Dis.* **2:**18–29.

136. Walker, D. H., and J. S. Dumler. 1997. Human monocytic and granulocytic ehrlichioses. Discovery and diagnosis of emerging tick-borne infections and the critical role of the pathologist. *Arch. Pathol. Lab. Med.* **121:**785–791.

137. Walls, J. J., M. Aguero-Rosenfeld, J. S. Bakken, J. L. Goodman, D. Hossain, R. C. Johnson, and J. S. Dumler. 1999. Inter- and intralaboratory comparison of *Ehrlichia equi* and human granulocytic ehrlichiosis (HGE) agent strains for serodiagnosis of HGE by the immunofluorescent-antibody test. *J. Clin. Microbiol.* **37:**2968–2973.

138. Walls, J. J., B. Greig, D. F. Neitzel, and J. S. Dumler. 1997. Natural infection of small mammal species in Minnesota with the agent of human granulocytic ehrlichiosis. *J. Clin. Microbiol.* **35:**853–855.

139. Wen, B., W. Cao, and H. Pan. 2003. Ehrlichiae and ehrlichial diseases in China. *Ann. N. Y. Acad. Sci.* **990:**45–53.

140. Wolf, L., T. McPherson, B. Harrison, B. Engber, A. Anderson, and P. Whitt. 2000. Prevalence of *Ehrlichia ewingii* in *Amblyomma americanum* in North Carolina. *J. Clin. Microbiol.* **38:**2795.

141. Wong, S. J., G. S. Brady, and J. S. Dumler. 1997. Serological responses to *Ehrlichia equi*, *Ehrlichia chaffeensis*, and *Borrelia burgdorferi* in patients from New York State. *J. Clin. Microbiol.* **35:**2198–2205.

142. Wong, S. J., and J. A. Thomas. 1998. Cytoplasmic, nuclear, and platelet autoantibodies in human granulocytic ehrlichiosis patients. *J. Clin. Microbiol.* **36:**1959–1963.

143. Wormser, G. P., A. Filozov, S. R. Telford III, S. Utpat, R. S. Kamer, D. Liveris, G. Wang, L. Zentmaier, I. Schwartz, and M. E. Aguero-Rosenfeld. 2006. Dissociation between inhibition and killing by levofloxacin in human granulocytic anaplasmosis. *Vector Borne Zoonotic Dis.* **6:**388–394.

144. Wormser, G. P., H. W. Horowitz, J. Nowakowski, D. McKenna, J. S. Dumler, S. Varde, I. Schwartz, C. Carbonaro, and M. Aguero-Rosenfeld. 1997. Positive Lyme disease serology in patients with clinical and laboratory evidence of human granulocytic ehrlichiosis. *Am. J. Clin. Pathol.* **107:**142–147.

145. Yabsley, M. J., A. S. Varela, C. M. Tate, V. G. Dugan, D. E. Stallknecht, S. E. Little, and W. R. Davidson. 2002. *Ehrlichia ewingii* infection in white-tailed deer (*Odocoileus virginianus*). *Emerg. Infect. Dis.* **8:**668–671.

146. Yu, X., P. Brouqui, J. S. Dumler, and D. Raoult. 1993. Detection of *Ehrlichia chaffeensis* in human tissue by using a species-specific monoclonal antibody. *J. Clin. Microbiol.* **31:**3284–3288.

147. Yu, X. J., P. Crocquet-Valdes, L. C. Cullman, and D. H. Walker. 1996. The recombinant 120-kilodalton protein of *Ehrlichia chaffeensis*, a potential diagnostic tool. *J. Clin. Microbiol.* **34:**2853–2855.

148. Zhang, L., Y. Liu, D. Ni, Q. Li, Y. Yu, X. J. Yu, K. Wan, D. Li, G. Liang, X. Jiang, H. Jing, J. Run, M. Luan, X. Fu, J. Zhang, W. Yang, Y. Wang, J. S. Dumler, Z. Feng, J. Ren, and J. Xu. 2008. Nosocomial transmission of human granulocytic anaplasmosis in China. *JAMA* **300:**2263–2270.

Coxiella*

STEPHEN R. GRAVES AND ROBERT F. MASSUNG

63

TAXONOMY

Coxiella burnetii is a small gram-negative rod that grows within a parasitophorous vacuole located in the cytoplasm of a host eucaryotic cell (invertebrate or vertebrate animal). It is a member of the γ subgroup of the *Proteobacteria* microbial phylum. The closest related bacterium is in the genus *Legionella*. *Bergey's Manual of Systematic Microbiology* (2005) classifies it under the order *Legionellales*, family *Coxiellaceae* (7). The only other member of the genus *Coxiella* is the proposed "*C. cheraxi*" bacterium, a pathogen of the Australian freshwater crayfish *Cherax quadricarinatus* (14).

DESCRIPTION OF THE AGENT

C. burnetii consists of different morphological forms, depending on the stage of its life cycle. Large-cell variants (LCV; 0.4 to 1.5 μm by 0.2 to 0.5 μm) are metabolically active and divide by binary fission inside the parasitophorous vacuole of the host eukaryotic cell. Small-cell variants (SCV; 0.5 μm by 0.2 μm) are electron dense and form when conditions are no longer conducive to active growth (13) (Fig. 1). SCV are filterable (0.22 μm), and this quiescent form of the cell differentially expresses certain proteins compared to LCV (26, 64, 66, 79). SCV are functionally spores, although chemically different from the gram-positive bacterial spore, as it lacks diaminopimelic acid. They act as the survival and transmissible form of the bacterium when it is extracellular and in the environment. SCV can survive in animal-contaminated environments (e.g., soil, hay, etc.) for many years, probably decades. However, they are not as heat stable as normal bacterial spores and can be inactivated at 63°C for 40 minutes (56). The cell wall, while gram-negative, stains poorly by Gram stain and better by Gimenez stain.

The complete genome sequences of Nine Mile and other strains of *C. burnetii* have demonstrated a circular genome with approximately 2 million base pairs, including many insertion sequences, and a single plasmid is found in most strains (65). The presence of many pseudogenes implies a process of ongoing gene degradation presumably associated with an evolutionarily recent adaptation to an intracellular

lifestyle. Unlike the *Rickettsiaceae*, *C. burnetii* does not transport ATP across its cell membrane and has almost full biosynthetic capabilities. It is metabolically active in the extracellular phase, utilizes glucose and glutamate at low pH, and has recently been grown in cell-free medium (48). Using microarray and whole-genome sequence analysis, variability in open reading frames and transposon-mediated genomic plasticity have been demonstrated (4).

The virulent form of *C. burnetii* is referred to as "phase I" because it is first isolated from humans with Q fever, infected vertebrate animals (especially cattle, sheep, and goats), and ticks. When these isolates are grown in the laboratory in tissue culture or embryonated eggs, the population of bacteria gradually change to a second form ("phase II") and become avirulent. This population change can involve loss of genetic material (29), such that the microbe cannot synthesize a full-length polysaccharide, lacking a terminal sugar chain as part of its cell wall lipopolysaccharide (LPS) (78). However, in some strains, loss of virulence does not seem to involve genomic changes (15), presumably due to changes in the expression of genes coding for virulence determinants. The in vitro change from virulent phase I to avirulent phase II is analogous to the "smooth"-to-"rough" transition that occurs in bacteria of the *Enterobacteriaceae* group. In phase I cells, the terminal glycan chain of the LPS contains three unique sugars, L-virenose, dihydrohydroxystreptose, and galactosaminuronyl-α-(1,6)- glucosamine, that are not present in phase II LPS (1). Phase I LPS appears to be a key virulence determinant of *C. burnetii*.

EPIDEMIOLOGY AND TRANSMISSION

Coxiella burnetii is associated with vertebrate animals, especially cattle, sheep, and goats. At parturition, when large concentrations of *C. burnetii* are present in the placenta, fetus, and associated membranes and fluids, the microbe readily contaminates the animal's environment. It can remain viable in soil, hay, etc., for many years (possibly decades), presumably in its "spore-like" form (63, 85). Milk from infected cows and other lactating animals may contain *C. burnetii* (30), which is destroyed by the temperature reached during pasteurization (39). Goats are a significant source of infection (19).

A number of other vertebrate animals can be hosts for *C. burnetii*, especially native animals, for example, native

---

*This chapter contains material presented by Philippe Brouqui, Thomas Marrie, and Didier Raoult in chapter 68 of the ninth edition of this *Manual*.

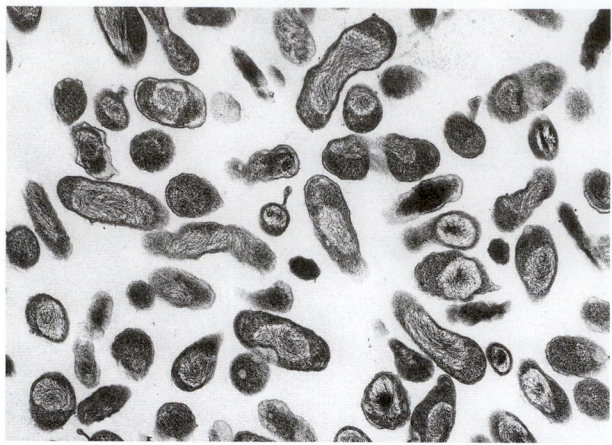

FIGURE 1 Electron micrograph of purified *C. burnetii* showing both LCV and SVC forms. (Courtesy of Rocky Mountain Laboratories, NIAID, NIH.)

rats, wombats, bandicoots, and kangaroos in Australia. Infections have been described for pets, including cats and dogs, with human outbreaks in North America linked to parturition by these animals (8, 32, 53). Birds are also hosts (70), and various other domestic and wildlife species have been reported as potential host species, including mice, horses, rabbits, and buffalo (43).

Numerous tick species either harbor or transmit *C. burnetii* and may be important for maintenance of the agent in veterinary populations, but tick transmission is not considered a major route of transmission to humans. Although there are a few reports of probable human infection by tick bite, the great bulk of human infections are by aerosol transmission from an infected animal focus, such as a herd of parturient goats. Infection in animals appears to be almost always asymptomatic, with recrudescence only during parturition usually followed by recovery of the maternal animal. Australian studies showed the importance of the bandicoot (*Isoodon macrourus)* (a marsupial) and its tick *Haemaphysalis humerosa* (17) and the kangaroo and its tick *Amblyomma triguttatum* (54) in sylvatic cycles of *C. burnetii* in Australia.

Derrick described Q fever in a large number of Australian patients, including some probably infected by tick bite, although most were infected by inhalation of dust associated with cattle (16). Now, Q fever is thought to be endemic in every country except New Zealand (28). In the United States, 22% of veterinarians are seropositive compared to approximately 3% of the population overall (2, 86). Travelers and military personnel can also be infected (12, 25). Transmission by aerosol and wind is well recognized (73). Nosocomial transmission, presumably by coughing with aerosol production, has rarely been reported (49), as has infection of surgical and obstetric staff during a Caesarean section on an infected patient (60). Sexual transmission has also been noted, as presumably *C. burnetii* was present in semen, from a chronic focus in the prostate gland or testis (45).

The epidemiology of human Q fever is a combination of the worldwide ubiquitous distribution of *C. burnetii;* the extremely low infectious dose required for human infection (probably between 1 and 10 viable *C. burnetii* cells) (72); the environmental conditions favoring transmission, such

as high concentrations of infected animals, high pregnancy rates, appropriate environmental conditions (transmission is greater under dry conditions), and the strength and direction of prevailing winds (73); and the inherent variability in human susceptibility to *C. burnetii*. While some people are exposed and become sick, others are exposed and seroconvert asymptomatically or have only mild symptoms, not sufficient to seek medical assistance. The proportion of persons that become ill after natural exposure may be as low as 50% (18, 76).

CLINICAL SIGNIFICANCE

Q fever can present in many forms: (i) as an acute undifferentiated febrile illness, (ii) as a chronic infection (usually involving the cardiovascular system), or (iii) as a postinfectious chronic fatigue syndrome (only recently recognized). Q fever can be latent and recrudesce during periods of relative immunosuppression, such as late pregnancy, causing fetal infection. Infection can also result in asymptomatic seroconversion and complete clearance of the microbe, with the patient being unaware of infection or being only mildly ill.

Other features of Q fever include a higher incidence of symptomatic disease in men than women and a higher incidence in middle-age men than those of other age groups. Although it is claimed that occupational and exposure differences explain the gender differences, it is probably not the complete picture. For example, female hormones appear to be protective in mice (59).

Pathogenesis

Because *C. burnetii* is an intracellular pathogen, growing in a membrane-bound vacuole in the cytoplasm of a host cell, its survival in the host animal (or patient) depends on its ability to survive and grow intracellularly in the host cell (82). This in turn depends on its ability to keep the host cell alive, and this requires microbe-directed immunomodulation of the host (84). Normally a host cell would deal with an invasion by an intracellular microbe by activating the host-cell self-destructing apoptotic process. Indeed, this is what happens in phase II (avirulent) *C. burnetii* infection. The microbe is rapidly internalized (involving receptor αVβ3 integrin and complement receptor 3) (10), and it grows until the host's cell-mediated immune response (involving gamma interferon and other molecules) induces apoptosis and the infected host cell is destroyed, along with the microbe. Certain Toll-like receptors are involved in the initial microbe-host cell interaction (88).

However, in the case of phase I (virulent) *C. burnetii*, a different sequence of events occurs, leading to the survival and growth of the microbe (36, 81). The type 1 LPS fails to activate dendritic cells (67), and the initial contact between the host cell membrane and the bacterium bypasses complement receptor 3 (44). This leads to a different sequence of intracellular events. Genes of a type IV secretion system (similar to the Dot/Icm system of *Legionella pneumophila*) are expressed, leading to secretion of bacterial proteins into the cytoplasm of the host cell (89). These proteins divert the normal intracellular autophagy pathway, which results in the formation of a parasitophorous vacuole. It gradually enlarges by incorporating recycled endoplasmic reticulum membrane into its own vesicular membrane, allowing the phase I *C. burnetii* to grow. The inhibition of apoptosis is mediated by host kinases (80), which allow the microbe to survive by preserving the infected host cell. The metabolically active *C. burnetii* LCV continues to grow in the absence of any effective host immune response despite the presence of circulating antibodies and cell-mediated immunity mediated by T lymphocytes. Eventually the conditions inside the parasitophorous vacuole become unsuitable for ongoing logarithmic bacterial growth, presumably due to nutrient depletion, and *C. burnetii* converts to the SCV, the nonreplicating survival form. Even then, the host cell may not be destroyed, leading to a state of chronicity or latent infection. Host responses keep the microbe in check, but should immunosuppression develop, such as during pregnancy, the bacterium starts growing again, causing a Q fever relapse. This is well recognized during the third trimester of pregnancy. In patients with chronic Q fever, there is impaired maturation of phagolysosomes, permitting ongoing survival of *C. burnetii* (23).

Acute Q Fever

Q fever is a difficult disease to diagnose, as there are no pathognomic symptoms or signs that give health care providers a clue to the etiology. Many doctors rarely consider Q fever in the differential diagnosis of an acute febrile illness unless a link with animal contact is established from the patient's history. In fact, many patients without any significant animal contact or tick bite develop Q fever, due to its dispersal by wind (73). Living downwind of a herd of parturient animals, an animal-holding yard, or an abattoir is a risk for Q fever. Presenting features include fever, headache, myalgia, elevated liver transaminases, and interstitial pneumonia. It is claimed that the disease may differ in its presentation in different countries, especially with respect to pneumonia.

The great diversity in acute symptoms is probably due to (i) differences in strains of *C. burnetii*; (ii) differences in human immune response genes and how they process and eliminate *C. burnetii* (27); (iii) route of infection (patients infected by the respiratory route [the most common route] are likely to develop pneumonia, and patients infected by other routes [e.g. tick bite, oral, sexually transmitted, and needle stick accident] can manifest the illness differently); and (iv) infecting dose, since the dose of *C. burnetii* (phase I) needed to infect a person is between 1 and 10 bacteria. An increased dose leads to a reduced incubation period (72). Infecting dose is likely to influence the symptoms and clinical course of the illness. Those with higher infecting doses are more likely to have severe symptoms. Reviews of Q fever from Australia (16, 55, 68) and elsewhere (41, 43, 57) show the diversity of symptoms in this disease.

Occasionally, acute Q fever can be fulminant (46). However, most patients survive acute Q fever and defervesce in about 10 to 14 days, at which time they develop either sterilizing or nonsterilizing immunity. It is the latter patients who can go on to develop chronic Q fever.

Chronic Q Fever

As a result of the early dissemination of *C. burnetii*, many organ systems are exposed and can become chronically infected. The cardiovascular system is particularly susceptible. Most cases of chronic Q fever involve endocarditis (5), including infection of congenitally abnormal (e.g., bicuspid) or previously damaged aortic and mitral valves, aneurysms, and vascular grafts. Pericarditis, myocarditis, and splenic rupture have been reported. Other systems that are often involved in chronic Q fever include the gastrointestinal tract, with chronic granulomatous hepatitis (Fig. 2), acalculous cholecystitis, and diarrhea; central nervous system, characterized by meningitis and meningoencephalitis; and

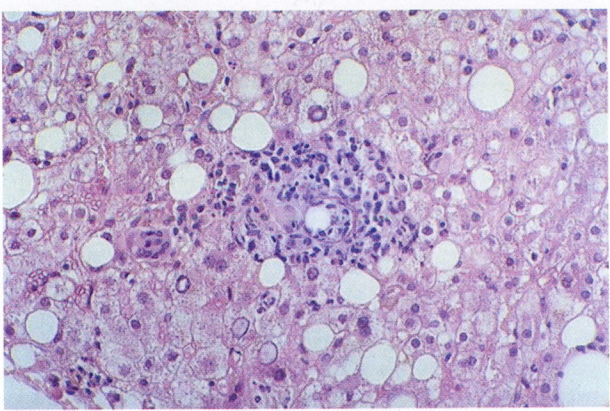

FIGURE 2 Hematoxylin and eosin stain of liver biopsy in a patient with acute Q fever. A doughnut ring granuloma is shown. Original magnification, ×400. (Courtesy of H. Lepidi, Marseille, France.)

bones and tendons, with infections. Rare features include lymphadenopathy, migratory thrombophlebitis, rash, and prostatitis. Many of these pathogenic features appear to involve autoimmunity, and the presence of autoantibodies is a feature of chronic Q fever (9, 87).

Pregnancy and Q Fever

Q fever in pregnancy is an underrecognized problem rarely mentioned as a cause of congenital infection, yet it is clearly a problem in many countries where Q fever is significant. As pregnancy develops, latent, viable *C. burnetii* starts growing in the placenta and the fetus, leading to infection and fetal death (71). While not recognized as one of the classical "TORCH" agents of congenital infection, it should be included under "O" (for "other").

Q Fever in Children

Children appear to be less susceptible to symptomatic Q fever than adults, as do young mice compared to older mice (34). Nevertheless, infections, mainly febrile or influenza like, have been reported (37, 47, 75).

Post-Q Fever Fatigue Syndrome

While a postinfectious fatigue syndrome, lasting weeks to months after an infectious disease is well recognized, post-Q fever fatigue syndrome is not yet universally acknowledged. First described in 1996 (3, 40) in the United Kingdom and Australia, post-Q fever fatigue syndrome is defined as fatigue persisting more than 12 months after the onset of acute Q fever.

COLLECTION, TRANSPORT, AND STORAGE OF SPECIMENS

Specimens for the diagnosis of Q fever in humans include blood and tissue, the latter most commonly from heart valves following valve replacement surgery. The sample collected will depend on the diagnostic test(s) available. Whole blood may be used for isolation and nucleic acid detection methods, and serum or plasma for serologic methods. Tissue samples are most commonly used for isolation, PCR, and immunohistochemistry (IHC). Whole blood may be collected in sodium citrate or EDTA tubes. Samples to be used for isolation should be collected aseptically and shipped promptly, while maintaining refrigeration. If storage of specimens prior to culture is necessary, samples should be kept frozen before and during shipment (at least −20°C; −80°C is preferable). Blood or tissue samples to be tested by PCR or IHC should be frozen (−20°C) prior to and during shipment, although tissues fixed by the diagnostic laboratory for IHC may be shipped at room temperature.

For the diagnosis of a suspected acute infection by molecular methods or isolation, whole blood should be collected during the acute phase, preferably prior to antibiotic therapy. For serologic diagnosis of an acute infection, a serum sample should be collected during the acute phase and a second sample at 3 or 4 weeks after onset. While the same specimens may be used for the diagnosis of chronic infection as for acute infection, the timing of collection is not as critical. Blood and tissue samples may be persistently positive by culture and/or PCR in chronic infections, and serum antibody levels are typically elevated (phase I and phase II immunoglobulin G [IgG] titers of >1,000) and sustained relative to acute infections, which have generally lower peak titers that decrease postinfection.

C. burnetii can be isolated from blood or tissue samples, but since it is an obligate intracellular bacterium, this must be done in cell culture or embryonated chicken eggs or by animal inoculation. Isolation must currently be performed in specialized high-containment biosafety level 3 (BSL-3) facilities, as the agent is highly infectious and classified as a select agent and a CDC category B bioterrorism agent (86a). If an isolate is propagated by a diagnostic laboratory, U.S. federal regulations require that it be transported to a registered select agent laboratory or destroyed, within 7 days (National Select Agent Registry, Centers for Disease Control and Prevention; http://www.selectagents.gov/cdForm.html). Diagnostic samples can be evaluated by PCR and serologic methods in BSL-2 facilities with the use of appropriate personal protective equipment.

DIRECT EXAMINATION

Microscopy and Antigen Detection

IHC is an excellent method for the detection of C. burnetii antigens in tissue samples (Fig. 3), particularly cardiac valve tissues that are colonized during chronic Q fever. Organisms in heart valve tissues have also been demonstrated by direct immunofluorescent methods or visualized by electron microscopy (Fig. 1). However, these methods are rarely used for the diagnosis of acute Q fever, as the appropriate tissue samples are not often collected and will vary among patients and because other methods (PCR and serology) that are simpler to perform on blood samples are available.

Nucleic Acid Detection

PCR can be a useful diagnostic tool for acute and chronic Q fever infections (62). It is important that the sample is collected during the early period of an acute infection while the patient is bacteremic (optimally within 4 weeks of onset of symptoms). A recent study showed that PCR can be more sensitive than serology during the first 2 weeks after the onset of symptoms and provide an earlier diagnosis than with serology alone (22). Whole blood is most commonly used for the analysis of acute infections, although enrichment of the white cell fraction (buffy coat) may increase sensitivity. Serum may be used if whole blood is not available, although it is less likely to be positive due to the lack

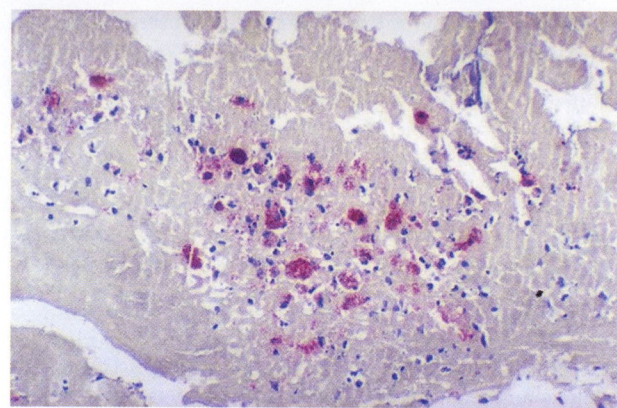

FIGURE 3 Alkaline phosphatase IHC on the heart valve from a patient with chronic Q fever endocarditis. C. burnetii microorganisms are stained pink within mononuclear cells. Original magnification, ×400.

of infected cells. For chronic Q fever with endocarditis, the valve tissue is typically positive, while blood may be positive or negative. It has been reported that PCR is generally positive in chronically infected patients with phase I IgG antibody titers between 1:800 and 1:6,400, but PCR is often negative in those with higher titers. A number of PCR assays are described that amplify the multicopy IS1111 insertion sequence (31, 50), and these generally provide increased sensitivity compared to assays that amplify single-copy genes (com1, 16S, 23S, etc.). However, the potential for false positives with PCR makes it imperative that these results be interpreted relative to other diagnostic assays, such as serology and other clinical data.

ISOLATION PROCEDURES

Isolation of C. burnetii from human blood or tissue must be performed in a BSL-3 containment facility due to the low infectious dose of the agent and potential for generating aerosols. Isolation can be accomplished in tissue culture cells or embryonated chicken eggs or by inoculation into animals such as mice or guinea pigs; the last requires BSL-3 containment facilities. Any infected tissue sample can be used for isolation, and PCR assays are quite useful for screening tissue samples prior to isolation to determine those potentially containing organisms. The organism can be stable in tissue samples for months before isolation attempts. Animal inoculation is the most sensitive method for isolation. A mouse can be injected intraperitoneally with up to 0.5 ml of inoculum, and the spleen harvested at 10 to 14 days postinjection. The spleen is homogenized and injected into another mouse, inoculated onto uninfected tissue culture cells, or used to infect embryonated eggs for further propagation. Isolation by animal inoculation is particularly useful for tissue or environmental samples that could be contaminated with organisms other than C. burnetii, as the animal serves to amplify Coxiella while killing other agents. Aseptically collected tissues that likely contain only C. burnetii can be inoculated directly onto tissue culture cells or embryonated chicken eggs. A shell vial method that works well is described for isolation in human embryonic lung fibroblast tissue culture cells (61) and can be used with many commonly available cell lines (e.g., Vero, RK13, THP1, and A549)

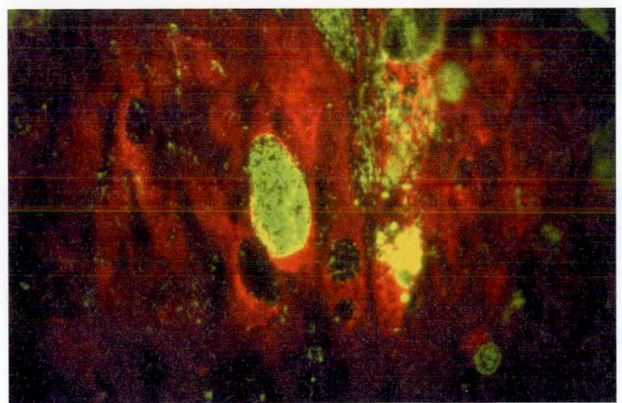

FIGURE 4 Identification of *C. burnetii* in shell vial culture at day 6 by the use of specific monoclonal antibody-based direct fluorescent-antibody test. Original magnification, ×1,000.

susceptible to infection by *C. burnetii*. Egg inoculations work particularly well for propagating large amounts of *C. burnetii* for antigen preparation.

IDENTIFICATION

Only reference laboratories are likely to isolate *C. burnetii* in pure culture and be required to confirm its identification by classical means. In recent years, identification is more often accomplished by amplifying and sequencing key genes (e.g. *com1* and IS*1111a*). A routine diagnostic laboratory that inadvertently isolates *C. burnetii* in tissue culture could identify it by direct fluorescent-antibody assay (Fig. 4), although specific antisera are not commercially available.

TYPING SYSTEMS

Typing systems, based on genetic differences between isolates, are not standardized and are still undergoing development. While no typing scheme is universally accepted, it is clear that there is considerable strain/isolate variability within the species *C. burnetii*.

SEROLOGIC TESTS

The detection of antibodies to *C. burnetii* is the most commonly used and effective method for the diagnosis of Q fever. The primary serologic assays in use today are the indirect immunofluorescent antibody (IFA) assay, the complement fixation (CF) test, and the enzyme-linked immunosorbent assay (ELISA), with the IFA assay being the gold standard and most commonly used method. CF methods generally lack sensitivity and are used less commonly today, while ELISAs are growing in use and availability. The diagnosis of infection by any serologic assay may be complicated by the facts that *C. burnetii* has a worldwide distribution in nature and many humans have been exposed and may be seropositive. All serologic methods make use of *C. burnetii* antigen grown in either tissue culture cells or embryonated chicken eggs. Serologic methods also take advantage of the antigenic differences between naturally occurring virulent phase I *C. burnetii* and attenuated phase II isolates (69). Phase I strains contain intact LPS antigens, while phase II strains lack complete LPS antigens. The antibodies produced during natural human infection respond in a unique time sequence to the phase I and phase II forms, with the acute response directed primarily to phase II antigens while the response in chronic infections is a mixture of phase I and phase II antibodies.

IFA Test

IFA tests detect IgG, IgM, and IgA antibodies for both phase I and phase II antigens and allow for the detection of, and discrimination between, acute and chronic infection (51). The IFA test has excellent specificity and sensitivity for the diagnosis of Q fever if the appropriate samples are available. The diagnosis of acute Q fever is dependent on seroconversion, defined as a fourfold increase in the IgG titer for phase II between acute and convalescent samples. Alternately, a single serum sample with a phase II IgG titer of ≥200 and a phase II IgM titer of ≥50 has been used to diagnose acute Q fever (74). Chronic infections typically present with phase I IgG titers of >800 (43). However, the choice of cutoff titer for acute or chronic disease should be determined in each laboratory, as methods for antigen preparations, assays, and interpretation can vary. Ideally, reference laboratories should provide controls with known positive and negative samples that could be used for in-laboratory assay validation and cutoff determination. FDA-approved, commercial *C. burnetii* IFA tests are available for the diagnosis of acute Q fever (IgG and IgM assays for phase II antigens) and provide the best source for laboratories not equipped to prepare their own antigens (Focus Diagnostics, Cypress, CA). The diagnosis of chronic Q fever is best performed at reference laboratories that have BSL-3 facilities for the propagation and storage of phase I organisms since *C. burnetii* is classified as a U.S. category B bioterrorism agent.

ELISA

ELISAs are reported to be as sensitive and specific as IFA tests (33, 52, 77, 83). FDA-approved, commercial ELISAs that detect IgG or IgM antibodies to phase II antigens are available (Inverness, Brisbane, Australia) and are useful for detection of IgM antibodies (20), although not currently marketed in the United States. A number of reference laboratories and research institutions have also developed in-house ELISAs. In general, ELISAs are qualitative and have not been evaluated as thoroughly as IFA tests. Commercial and in-house ELISAs can be automated to require minimal interpretation and are particularly useful for the detection of IgG antibodies to phase II antigens when employed in seroprevalence studies. However, their lack of standardization and quantification make them less than ideal for the diagnosis of acute Q fever, and the lack of phase I antigens in commercial assays limits their use for the diagnosis of chronic Q fever.

CF Test

Whereas CF is still commonly used as a diagnostic assay for veterinary testing, the assay is rarely used for human diagnostics due to advances in IFA and ELISA methods and the demonstration that the CF test has lower sensitivity, is more time consuming, and detects seroconversion at a later date than the other assays (21). False negatives with the CF assay have also been described for chronic infections with high titers due to a prozone effect.

ANTIMICROBIAL SUSCEPTIBILITIES, TREATMENT, AND PREVENTION

In vitro antimicrobial susceptibility testing is not routinely performed. *C. burnetii* is an intracellular pathogen, and correlations between in vitro MICs of antibiotics in an infected tissue culture system and antibiotic activity in infected patients are uncertain.

The recommended treatment for acute Q fever is doxycycline, although strains with partial doxycycline resistance have been reported. Erythromycin and azithromycin are not recommended, as many strains are resistant (MIC of >8 μg/ml) (35, 58). Neither ciprofloxacin nor chloramphenicol are recommended, as they do not inhibit in vitro growth (6, 61). Rifampin (rifampicin) may be used, although it is not recommended in the United States. Treatment in pregnancy with co-trimoxazole is recommended, as adverse outcomes are well recognized (11).

Chronic Q fever, especially Q fever endocarditis, requires long-term antibiotics and often valve replacement. Doxycycline and hydroxychloroquine are recommended for a minimum of 1 year and possibly longer. Hydroxychloroquine increases the pH of the phagolysosome from 4.8 to 5.7 and renders doxycycline bactericidal rather than bacteriostatic (42).

A human Q fever vaccine (QVAX) is commercially available only in Australia (24, 38).

EVALUATION, INTERPRETATION, AND REPORTING OF RESULTS

Serological and nucleic acid amplification (PCR) reports for a patient evaluated for Q fever can be difficult to understand. Interpretation should always be provided and should include (i) the significance of the antibody titer, particularly the difference between antibodies to phase I and phase II C. burnetii and the different antibody classes detected (IgM, IgG, and IgA); (ii) whether the serologic result supports recent Q fever (phase II IgM high), past Q fever (phase II IgG high), or chronic Q fever (phase I IgG and IgA high); (iii) if there is only one serum sample available for testing, the importance of receiving a second serum sample to detect a fourfold increase in antibody titer (for example, a raised phase II IgM only in one serum sample may represent very early acute Q fever or a false-positive result); (iv) in locales where vaccination occurs or where the post-Q fever fatigue syndrome is considered, a comment that no antibody pattern can currently define either condition should be provided; and (v) an indication that detection of C. burnetii DNA in blood usually indicates acute, very early Q fever, often before seroconversion. Tissue specimens (e.g., heart valve, liver, and bone marrow) are most often positive in chronic Q fever, although peripheral blood leukocytes from such patients can be positive or negative.

REFERENCES

1. Amano, K.-I., J. C. Williams, S. R. Missler, and V. N. Reinhold. 1987. Structure and biological relationships of Coxiella burnetii lipopolysaccharides. J. Biol. Chem. 262:4740–4747.
2. Anderson, A. D., D. Kruszon-Moran, A. D. Loftis, G. McQuillan, W. L. Nicholson, R. A. Priestley, A. J. Candee, N. E. Patterson, and R. F. Massung. 2009. Seroprevalence of Q fever in the United States, 2003–2004. Am. J. Trop. Med. Hyg. 81:691–694.
3. Ayres, J. G., E. G. Smith, and N. Flint. 1996. Protracted fatigue and debility after acute Q fever. Lancet 347:978–979.
4. Beare, P. A., N. Unsworth, M. Andoh, D. E. Voth, A. Omsland, S. D. Gilk, K. P. Williams, B. W. Sobral, J. J. Kupko III, S. F. Porcella, J. E. Samuel, and R. A. Heinzen. 2009. Comparative genomics reveal extensive transposon-mediated genomic plasticity and diversity among potential effector proteins within the genus Coxiella. Infect. Immun. 77:642–656.
5. Botelho-Nevers, E., P. E. Fournier, H. Richet, F. Fenollar, H. Lepidi, C. Foucault, A. Branchereau, P. Piquet, M. Maurin, and D. Raoult 2007. Coxiella burnetii infection of aortic aneurysms or vascular grafts: report of 30 new cases and evaluation of outcome. Eur. J. Clin. Microbiol. Infect. Dis. 26:635–640.
6. Brennan, R. E., and J. E. Samuel. 2003. Evaluation of Coxiella burnetii antibiotic susceptibilities by real-time PCR assay. J. Clin. Microbiol. 41:1869–1874.
7. Brenner, D., N. R. Krieg, and J. T. Staley. 2005. Bergey's Manual of Systematic Bacteriology, 2nd ed., vol. 2. The Proteobacteria. Part B, the Gammaproteobacteria, 210–241. Springer, New York, NY.
8. Buhariwalla, F., B. Cann, and T. J. Marrie. 1996. A dog-related outbreak of Q fever. Clin. Infect. Dis. 23:753–755.
9. Camacho, M. T., I. Outschoorn, A. Tellez, and J. Sequi. 2005. Autoantibody profiles in the sera of patients with Q fever: characterization of antigens by immunofluorescence, immunoblot and sequence analysis. J. Autoimmun. Dis. 2:10.
10. Capo, C., A. Moynault Y. Collette, D. Olive, E. J. Brown, D. Raoult, and J.-L. Mege. 2003. Coxiella burnetii avoids macrophage phagocytosis by interfering with the spatial distribution of complement receptor 3. J. Immunol. 170:4217–4225.
11. Carcopino, X., D. Raoult, F. Bretelle, L. Boubli, and A. Stein. 2007. Managing Q fever during pregnancy: the benefits of long-term cotrimoxazole therapy. Clin. Infect. Dis. 45:548–555.
12. Cohen, N. J., M. Papernik, J. Singleton, J. Segreti, and M. E. Eremeeva. 2007. Q fever in an American tourist returning from Australia. Travel Med. Infect. Dis. 5(3):194–195.
13. Coleman, S. A., E. R. Fischer, D. Howe, D. J. Mead, and R. A. Heinzen. 2004. Temporal analysis of Coxiella burnetii morphological differentiation. J. Bacteriol. 186:7344–7352.
14. Cooper, A., R. Layton, L. Owens, N. Ketheesan, and B. Govan. 2007. Evidence for classification of a crayfish pathogen as a member of the genus Coxiella. Lett. Appl. Microbiol. 45:558–563.
15. Denison, A., R. F. Massung, and H. A Thompson. 2007. Analysis of the O-antigen biosynthesis regions of phase II isolates of Coxiella burnetii. FEMS Microbiol. Lett. 267:102–107.
16. Derrick, E. H. 1973. The course of infection with Coxiella burnetii. Med. J. Aust. 1:1051–1057.
17. Derrick, E. H., and D. J. W. Smith. 1940. Studies in the epidemiology of Q fever. 2. The isolation of three strains of Rickettsia burnetii from the bandicoot Isoodon torosus. Aust. J. Exp. Biol. Med. Sci. 18:99–102.
18. Dupuis, G., J. Petite, O. Peter, and M. Vouilloz. 1987. An important outbreak of human Q fever in a Swiss alpine valley. Int. J. Epidemiol. 16:282–287.
19. Enserick, M. 2010. Questions abound in Q fever explosion in the Netherlands. Science 327:266–267.
20. Field, P. R., J. L. Mitchell, A. Santiago, D. J. Dickeson, S. W. Chan, D. W. Ho, A. M. Murphy, A. J. Cuzzubbo, and P. L. Devine. 2000. Comparison of a commercial enzyme-linked immunosorbent assay with immunofluorescence and complement fixation tests for detection of Coxiella burnetii (Q fever) immunoglobulin M. J. Clin. Microbiol. 38:1645–1647.
21. Field, P. R., J. G. Hunt, and A. M. Murphy. 1983. Detection and persistence of specific IgM antibody to Coxiella burnetii by enzyme-linked immunosorbent assay: a comparison with immunofluorescence and complement fixation tests. J. Infect. Dis. 148:477–487.
22. Fournier, P. E., and D. Raoult. 2003. Comparison of PCR and serology assays for early diagnosis of acute Q fever. J. Clin. Microbiol. 41:5094–5098.
23. Ghigo, E., A. Honstettre, C. Capo, J. P. GorVel, D. Raoult, and J.-L. Mege. 2004. Link between impaired maturation of phagosomes and defective Coxiella burnetii killing in patients with chronic Q fever. J. Infect. Dis. 190:1767–1772.
24. Gidding, H. F., C. Wallace, G. L. Lawrence, and P. B McIntyre. 2009. Australia's natural Q fever vaccination program. Vaccine 27:2037–2041.

25. **Hartzell, J. D., S. W. Peng, R. N. Wood-Morris, D. M. Sarmiento, J. F. Collen, P. M. Robben, and K. A. Moran.** 2007. Atypical Q fever in U.S. soldiers. *Emerg. Infect. Dis.* **13:**1247–1249.

26. **Heinzen, R. A., and T. Hackstadt.** 1996. A developmental stage-specific histone H1 homolog of *Coxiella burnetii*. *J. Bacteriol.* **178:**5049–5052.

27. **Helbig, K. J., R. J. Harris, J. Ayres, H. Dunckley, A. Lloyd, J. Robson, and B. P. Marmion.** 2005. Immune response genes in the post Q fever fatigue syndrome, Q fever endocarditis and uncomplicated acute primary Q fever. *QJM* **98:**565–574.

28. **Hilbink, F., M. Penrose, E. Kovacova, and J. Kozar.** 1993. Q fever is absent from New Zealand. *Int. J. Epidemiol.* **22:**945–949.

29. **Hoover, T. A., D. W. Culp, M. H. Vodkin, J. C. Williams, and H. A. Thompson.** 2002. Chromosomal DNA deletions explain phenotypic characteristics of two antigenic variants, phase II and RSA 514 (crazy) of the *Coxiella burnetii* Nine Mile strain. *Infect. Immun.* **70:**6726–6733.

30. **Kim, S. G., E. H. Kim, C. J. Lafferty, and E. Dubovi.** 2005. *Coxiella burnetii* in bulk tank milk samples, United States. *Emerg. Infect. Dis.* **11:**619–621.

31. **Klee, S. R., J. Tyczka, H. Ellerbrok, T. Franz, S. Linke, G. Baljer, and B. Appel.** 2006. Highly sensitive real-time PCR for specific detection and quantification of *Coxiella burnetii*. *BMC Microbiol.* **6:**2.

32. **Kosatsky, T.** 1984. Household outbreak of Q-fever pneumonia related to a parturient cat. *Lancet* **ii:**1447–1449.

33. **Kovácová, E., J. Gallo, S. Schramek, J. Kazár, and R. Brezina.** 1987. *Coxiella burnetii* antigens for detection of Q fever antibodies by ELISA in human sera. *Acta Virol.* **31:**254–259.

34. **Leone, M., Y. Bechah, S. Meghari, H. Lepidi, C. Capo, D. Raoult, and J.-L. Mege.** 2007. *Coxiella burnetii* infection in C57BL/6 mice aged 1 or 14 months. *FEMS Immunol. Med. Microbiol.* **50:**396–400.

35. **Lever, M. S., K. R. Bewley, B. Dowsett, and G. Lloyd.** 2004. In vitro susceptibility of *Coxiella burnetii* to azithromycin, doxycycline, ciprofloxacin and a range of newer fluoroquinolones. *Int. J. Antimicrob. Agents* **24:**194–196.

36. **Luhrmann, A., and C. R. Roy.** 2007. *Coxiella burnetii* inhibits activation of host cell apoptosis through a mechanism that involves preventing cytochrome *c* release from mitochondria. *Infect. Immun.* **75:**5282–5289.

37. **Maltezou, H. C., and D. Raoult.** 2002. Q fever in children. *Lancet Infect. Dis.* **2:**686–689.

38. **Marmion, B. P.** 2007. Q fever: the long journey to control by vaccination. *Med. J. Aust.* **186:**164–165.

39. **Marmion, B. P., F. O. MacCallum, A. Rowlands, and C. C. Thiel.** 1951. The effect of pasteurization on milk containing *Rickettsia burnetii*. *Mon. Bull. Minist. Health Public Health Lab. Serv.* **10:**119–128.

40. **Marmion, B. P., M. Shannon, I. Maddocks, P. Storm, and I. Penttila.** 1996. Protracted debility and fatigue after Q fever. *Lancet* **347:**977–978.

41. **Marrie, T. J., N. Campbell, S. A. McNeil, D. Webster, and T. F. Hatchette.** 2008. Q fever update, maritime Canada. *Emerg. Infect. Dis.* **14:**67–69.

42. **Maurin, M., A. M. Benoliel, P. Bongrand, and D. Raoult.** 1992. Phagolysosomal alkalinization and the bacteriocidal effect of antibiotics: the *Coxiella burnetii* paradigm. *J. Infect. Dis.* **166:**1097–1102.

43. **Maurin, M., and D. Raoult.** 1999. Q fever. *Clin. Microbiol. Rev.* **12:**518–553.

44. **Mege, J. L., M. Maurin, C. Capo, and D. Raoult.** 1997. *Coxiella burnetii*: the 'query' bacterium. A model of immune subversion by a strictly intracellular microorganism. *FEMS Microbiol. Rev.* **19:**209–217.

45. **Milazzo, A., R. Hall, P. A. Storm, R. J. Harris, W. Winslow, and B. P Marmion.** 2001. Sexually transmitted Q fever. *Clin. Infect. Dis.* **33:**399–402.

46. **Munckhof, W. J., N. Runnegar, T. J. Gray, C. Taylor, C. Palmer, and A. Holley.** 2007. Two rare severe and fulminant presentations of Q fever in patients with minimal risk factors for this disease. *Int. Med. J.* **37:**775–778.

47. **Nagaoka H., M. Akiyama, M. Sugieda, T. Nishio, S. Akahane, H. Hattori, T. Ho, H. Fukushi, and K. Harai.** 1996. Isolation of *Coxiella burnetii* from children with influenza-like symptoms in Japan. *Microbiol. Immunol.* **40:**147–151.

48. **Omsland, A., D. C. Cockrell, D. Howe, E. R. Fischer, K. Virtaneva, D. E. Sturdevant, S. F. Porcella, and R. A. Heinzen.** 2009. Host cell-free growth of the Q fever bacterium *Coxiella burnetii*. *Proc. Natl. Acad. Sci. USA* **106:**4430–4434.

49. **Osorio, S., C. Sarria, P. Gonzalez-Ruano, E. C. Casal, and A. Garcia.** 2003. Nosocomial transmission of Q fever. *J. Hosp. Infect.* **54:**162–168.

50. **Panning, M., J. Kilwinski, S. Greiner-Fischer, M. Peters, S. Kramme, D. Frangoulidis, H. Meyer, K. Henning, and C. Drosten.** 2008. High throughput detection of Coxiella burnetii by real-time PCR with internal control system and automated DNA preparation. *BMC Microbiol.* **8:**77.

51. **Peacock, M. G., R. N. Philip, J. C. Williams, and R. S. Faulkner.** 1983. Serological evaluation of Q fever in humans: enhanced phase I titers of immunoglobulins G and A are diagnostic for Q fever endocarditis. *Infect. Immun.* **41:**1089–1098.

52. **Péter, O., G. Dupuis, D. Bee, R. Lüthy, J. Nicolet, and W. Burgdorfer.** 1988. Enzyme-linked immunosorbent assay for diagnosis of chronic Q fever. *J. Clin. Microbiol.* **26:**1978–1982.

53. **Pinsky, R. L., D. B. Fishbein, C. R. Greene, and K. F. Gensheimer.** 1991. An outbreak of cat-associated Q fever in the United States. *J. Infect. Dis.* **164:**202–204.

54. **Pope, J. H., W. Scott, and R Dwyer.** 1960. *Coxiella burnetii* in kangaroos and kangaroo ticks in western Queensland. *Aust. J. Exp. Biol.* **38:**17–28.

55. **Powell, O.** 1960. Q fever: clinical features in 72 cases. *Aust. Ann. Med.* **9:**214–223.

56. **Ransom, S. E., and R. J. Huebner.** 1951. Studies on the resistance of *Coxiella burnetii* to physical and chemical agents. *Am. J. Hyg.* **53:**110–119.

57. **Raoult, D.** 2000. Q fever 1985–1998. Clinical and epidemiologic features of 1,383 infections. *Medicine* **79:**109–123.

58. **Raoult, D.** 2003. Use of macrolides for Q fever. *Antimicrob. Agents Chemother.* **47:**446.

59. **Raoult, D., T. Marrie, and J. Mege.** 2005. Natural history and pathophysiology of Q fever. *Lancet Infect. Dis.* **5:**219–226.

60. **Raoult, D., and A. Stein.** 1994. Q fever during pregnancy—a risk for women, fetuses and obstetricians. *N. Engl. J. Med.* **330:**371.

61. **Raoult, D., H. Torres, and M. Drancourt.** 1991. Shell-vial assay: evaluation of a new technique for determining antibiotic susceptibility, tested in 13 isolates of *Coxiella burnetii*. *Antimicrob. Agents Chemother.* **35:**2070–2077.

62. **Rolain, J. M., and D. Raoult.** 2005. Molecular detection of *Coxiella burnetii* in blood and sera during Q fever. *QJM* **98:**615–617.

63. **Rustscheff, S., L. Norlander, A. Macellaro, A. Sjostedt, S. Vene, and M. Carlsson.** 2000. A case of Q fever acquired in Sweden and isolation of the probable etiological agent, *Coxiella burnetii*, from an indigenous source. *Scand. J. Infect. Dis.* **32:**605–607.

64. **Seshadri, R., L. R. Hendrix, and J. E. Samuel.** 1999. Differential expression of translational elements by life cycle variants of *Coxiella burnetii*. *Infect. Immun.* **67:**6026–6033.

65. **Seshadri, R., I. Paulsen, and J. A. Eisen, T. D. Read, K. E. Nelson, W. C. Nelson, N. L. Ward, H. Tettelin, T. M. Davidsen, M. J. Beanan, R. T. Deboy, S. C. Daugherty, L. M. Brinkac, R. Madupu, R. J. Dodson, H. M. Khouri, K. H. Lee, H. A. Carty, D. Scanlan, R. A. Heinzen, H. A. Thompson, J. E. Samuel, C. M. Fraser, and J. F. Heidelberg.** 2003. Complete genome sequence of the Q fever pathogen *Coxiella burnetii*. *Proc. Natl. Acad. Sci. USA* **100:**5455–5460.

66. **Seshadri, R., and J. E. Samuel.** 2001. Characterization of a stress-induced alternative sigma factor, RpoS, of *Coxiella burnetii* and its expression during the development cycle. *Infect. Immun.* **69:**4874–4883.

67. **Shannon, J. G., D. Howe, and R. A. Heinzen.** 2005. Virulent *Coxiella burnetii* does not activate human dendritic cells: role of lipopolysaccharide as a shielding molecule. *Proc. Natl. Acad. Sci. USA* **102:**8722–8727.

68. **Spellman, D. W.** 1982. Q fever: a study of 111 consecutive cases. *Med. J. Aust.* **1:**547–553.

69. **Stoker, M. G., and P. Fiset.** 1956. Phase variation of the Nine Mile and other strains of *Rickettsia burneti. Can. J. Microbiol.* **2:**310–321.

70. **Syrucek, L., and K. Raska.** 1956. Q fever in domestic and wild birds. *Bull. W. H. O.* **15:**329–337.

71. **Syrucek, L., O. Sobelavsky, and I. Gutvirth.** 1958. Isolation of *Coxiella burnetii* from human placentas. *J. Hyg. Epidemiol. Microbiol. Immunol.* **11:**29–35.

72. **Tigertt, W. D., A. S. Benenson, and R. E. Shope.** 1956. Studies on Q fever in man. *Trans. Assoc. Am. Physicians* **69:** 98–104.

73. **Tissot-Dupont, H., M.-A. Amadei, M. Nezri, and D. Raoult.** 2004. Wind in November, Q fever in December. *Emerg. Infect. Dis.* **10:**1264–1269.

74. **Tissot-Dupont, H., X. Thirion, and D. Raoult.** 1994. Q fever serology: cutoff determination for microimmunofluorescence. *Clin. Diagn. Lab. Immunol.* **1:**189–196.

75. **To, H., N. Kako, G. Q. Zhang, H. Otsuka, M. Ogawa, O. Ochiai, S. A. V. Nguyen, T. Yamaguchi, H. Fukushi, N. Nagaoka, M. Akiyama, K. Amano, and K. Hirai.** 1996. Q fever pneumonia in children in Japan. *J. Clin. Microbiol.* **34:**647–651.

76. **Tonge, J. I., and J. M. Kennedy.** 1963. An outbreak of Q fever in an abattoir near Brisbane. *Med. J. Aust.* **50:**340–343.

77. **Uhaa, I. J., D. B. Fishbein, J. G. Olson, C. C. Rives, D. M. Waag, and J. C. Williams.** 1994. Evaluation of specificity of indirect enzyme-linked immunosorbent assay for diagnosis of human Q fever. *J. Clin. Microbiol.* **32:**1560–1565.

78. **Vadovic, P., K. Slaba, M. Fodorova, L. Skultety, and R. Toman.** 2005. Stuctural and functional characterization of the glycan antigens involved in immunobiology of Q fever. *Ann. N. Y. Acad. Sci.* **1063:**149–153.

79. **Varghees, S., K. Kiss, G. Frans, O. Braha, and J. E. Samuel.** 2002. Cloning and porin activity of the major outer membrane protein P1 from *Coxiella burnetii. Infect. Immun.* **70:**6741–6750.

80. **Voth, D. E., and R. A. Heinzen.** 2009. Sustained activation of Akt and Erk1/2 is required for *Coxiella burnetii* antiapoptotic activity. *Infect. Immun.* **77:**205–213.

81. **Voth, D. E., D. Howe, and R. A. Heinzen.** 2007. *Coxiella burnetii* inhibits apoptosis in human THP-1 cells and monkey primary alveolar macrophages. *Infect. Immun.* **75:**4263–4271.

82. **Voth, D. E., and R. A. Heinzen.** 2007. Lounging in a lysosome: the intracellular life of *Coxiella burnetii. Cell. Microbiol.* **9:**829–840.

83. **Waag, D., J. Chulay, T. Marrie, M. England, and J. Williams.** 1995. Validation of an enzyme immunoassay for serodiagnosis of acute Q fever. *Eur. J. Clin. Microbiol. Infect. Dis.* **14:**421–427.

84. **Wagg, D. M., and J. C. Williams.** 1988. Immune modulation by *Coxiella burnetii*: characterization of a phase I immunosuppressive complex differentially expressed among strains. *Immunopharmacol. Immunotoxicol.* **10:**231–260.

85. **Welsh, H. H., E. H. Lennette, F. R. Abinanti, J. F. Winn, and W. Kaplan.** 1959. Q fever studies. XXI. The recovery of *Coxiella burnetii* from the soil and surface water of premises harboring infected sheep. *Am. J. Hyg.* **70:**14–20.

86. **Whitney, E. A., R. F. Massung, A. J. Candee, E. C. Ailes, L. M. Myers, N. E. Patterson, and R. L. Berkelman.** 2009. Seroepidemiologic and occupational risk survey for *Coxiella burnetii* antibodies among US veterinarians. *Clin. Infect. Dis.* **48:**550–557.

86a. **Wilson, D. E., and L. C. Chosewood (ed.).** 2007. *Biosafety in microbiological and biomedical laboratories,* 5th ed. U.S. Department of Health and Human Services, Centers for Disease Control and Prevention, and National Institutes of Health. Washington, DC. http://www.cdc.gov/OD/ohs/biosfty/bmbl5/bmbl5toc.htm.

87. **Wong, R. C. W., R. Wilson, R. Silcock, L. M. Kratzing, and D. Looke.** 2001. Unusual combination of positive IgG autoantibodies in acute Q fever. *Int. Med. J.* **31:**432–435.

88. **Zamboni, D. S., M. A. Campos, A. C. T. Torrecilhas, K. Kiss, J. E. Samuel, D. T. Golenbock, F. N. Lauw, C. R. Roy, I. C. Almeida, and R. T. Gazzinelli.** 2004. Stimulation of Toll-like receptor 2 by *Coxiella burnetii* is required for macrophage production of pro-inflammatory cytokines and resistance to infection. *J. Biol. Chem.* **279:**54405–54415.

89. **Zamboni, D. S., S. McGrath, M. Rabinovitch, and C. R. Roy.** 2003. *Coxiella burnetii* expresses type IV secretion system proteins that function similarly to components of the *Legionella pneumophila* Dot/Icm system. *Mol. Microbiol.* **49:**965–976.

Tropheryma

THOMAS MARTH

64

Tropheryma whipplei, a rod-shaped, environmental actinomycete with a distinct genome and typical periodic acid-Schiff (PAS) stain reaction, is the causative bacterium of Whipple's disease (WD). The genus name *Tropheryma* is derived from the Greek words *trophe* (nourishment) and *eryma* (barrier).

TAXONOMY

In 1991 and 1992, fragments of the 16S rRNA gene from tissues of WD patients were sequenced. These sequences indicated that the causative agent of WD was in a new genus that belongs to the subdivision of gram-positive bacteria with high GC content, the actinomycetes, and is a member of the phylum *Actinobacteria* (25, 30). The name *Tropheryma whipplei* was assigned after its culture and deposition (14, 23). The organism is closely related to several actinobacteria, nocardioforms, and cellulomonads, including *Dermatophilus congolensis*, *Arthrobacter globiformis*, *Cellulomonas hominis*, the human pathogen *Rothia dentocariosa*, and *Rhodococcus* spp.; *T. whipplei* is distantly related to *Streptomyces* spp. and *Mycobacterium* spp. The organism is now placed in an intermediate position between cellulomonads and a group of actinomycetes with a group B peptidoglycan.

DESCRIPTION OF THE AGENT

Genomes of two different *T. whipplei* strains have been sequenced (2, 24). Both are very similar (>99% identity) and contain approximately 925 kbp with 800 protein-coding genes and have a GC content of 47%. The bacterium possesses a unique circular chromosome and is the only known reduced-genome species (<1 Mb) within the *Actinobacteria*. The genome is deficient in genes that encode energy metabolism and amino acid synthesis (e.g., no thioredoxin), suggesting a host-dependent life style. Alignment of genome sequences reveals a large chromosomal inversion and the presence of a common repeat, highly conserved at the nucleotide level. This results in the expression of different subsets of cell surface proteins and represents a potential mechanism for evasion of the host immune response (2, 24).

EPIDEMIOLOGY AND TRANSMISSION

The bacterium, like some of its phylogenetic relatives, is present in the environment. PCR studies have shown the presence of *T. whipplei* in sewage plants and in human stools and saliva (29). It has been speculated that *T. whipplei* is acquired via the oral route and may infect people through drinking water.

While *T. whipplei* is genetically heterogeneous, as shown by sequencing of the 16S–23S rRNA gene interspacer and of the 23S rRNA gene, genomic variants are neither associated with the geographic residence of patients nor with the agent's organotropism (16).

Genetic host factors are probably disease determinants, as WD occurs very rarely (approximate yearly incidence, 0.5 to 1 per million), usually late in life (mean age at diagnosis, about 50 years), and is eight times more common in men than in women. Recently, an HLA association with DRB1*13 and DQB1*06 but not B27 was observed in a large European cohort (20). In addition, recent findings described subtle and persistent immune disturbances that caused impaired phagocytosis and intracellular degradation of *T. whipplei* (18). These immunological deficits include decreased gamma interferon and increased interleukin-4 (IL-4) expression by T cells and an impaired monocyte and macrophage function, with decreased IL-12 and increased IL-16 expression by macrophages (4, 18, 21, 22). Apparently, the mucosal immune response is not sufficient to kill ingested bacteria in patients with WD.

CLINICAL SIGNIFICANCE

WD may occur in the following clinical categories and courses (28): (i) classical WD, which presents with weight loss, diarrhea, and arthropathy in 75% of patients by the time of diagnosis; (ii) isolated infection of cardiac valves without classical WD; (iii) asymptomatic carriers of *T. whipplei*. In these cases it is still unclear whether the asymptomatic carriers are only passing the agent through their stool.

Although WD has traditionally been regarded as a gastrointestinal disease, arthropathy often precedes the diagnosis by a mean of 8 years in two-thirds of patients (5, 19, 28).

Weight loss is the major sign by the time of diagnosis and is present in two-thirds of patients at more than 4 years before diagnosis. Watery diarrhea resulting from small intestine involvement is episodic and accompanied by colicky abdominal pain. Steatorrhea occurs rarely, and 20 to 30% of patients have evidence of occult blood in stool. These symptoms with concomitant anorexia can lead to malabsorption syndrome. In about half of WD patients systemic symptoms occur. Intermittent low-grade fever, night sweats, and peripheral and intra-abdominal lymphadenopathy are frequent features. *T. whipplei* infection also results quite often in cardiac, lung, and central nervous system (CNS) signs and symptoms, which can occur even in the absence of gastrointestinal manifestations (5, 19, 28).

COLLECTION, TRANSPORT, AND STORAGE OF SPECIMENS

The most frequent diagnostic samples are small bowel biopsy specimens. Endoscopic biopsies, at least four to six, from the distal duodenum and/or the jejunum, even in the absence of intestinal symptoms, should also be obtained systematically in suspected WD, because involvement could be patchy (19). The samples should be fixed in 10% formalin for histopathologic examination, PAS staining, and immunohistochemistry. Samples from other affected or potentially affected organs, such as other gastrointestinal specimens, lymph nodes, heart valves, liver, synovia, and in rare cases, CNS samples, can be processed in a similar fashion. To confirm the diagnosis of WD, a PCR should be performed from diagnostic samples. In this instance, and if culture is to be performed, fresh samples (solid or liquid, e.g., saliva, synovial fluid, or ascites fluid; each at least 2 to 3 ml) should be frozen at −80°C and transported on dry ice (8, 23). It is important to note that cerebrospinal fluid (CSF) should be analyzed in every confirmed WD patient, as 50% of patients carry *T. whipplei* in the CNS even without neurologic or psychiatric symptoms (12). In suspected WD endocarditis, the excised cardiac valve should be tested by PAS staining and additionally by PCR or immunohistochemistry (7, 19, 28). For monitoring of treatment success in terms of bacterial eradication with long-term therapy, saliva and stools for PCR and blood for PCR and immunohistochemistry may be sampled (sampling amounts are specified above) and tested after 6 and 12 months of treatment. However, these test results should be interpreted with caution, and in concert with the clinic and the PAS stain, as there may be a high number of false test results (19).

DIRECT EXAMINATION

Microscopy

PAS Staining

The diagnosis of WD is highly suspected if typical PAS-positive staining is present in histopathologic sections (Fig. 1). Light microscopic examination of duodenal or jejunal biopsy specimens in WD typically reveals infiltration of the lamina propria by large macrophages containing granular foamy PAS-positive inclusions that are diastase resistant. These are also silver stain positive and often gram positive, representing remnants of ingested bacteria (5). The PAS positivity, also found in many other organ samples, is believed to be a reaction with bacterial cell wall

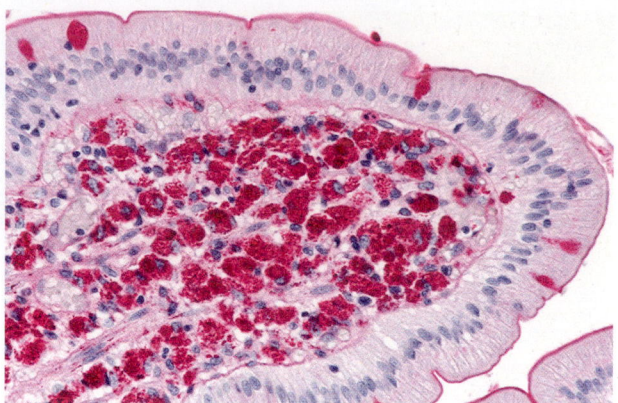

FIGURE 1 PAS stain of a duodenal biopsy specimen in a patient with WD. Large numbers of purple-stained macrophages in the lamina propria can be seen. Magnification, ×31.

capsular mucopolysaccharides. However, there are several pitfalls in the histopathologic diagnosis of WD. Involvement of the gastrointestinal tract or lymphatic tissue can be accompanied by noncaseating, epithelioid cells (sarcoid-like granulomas) which are PAS negative (5, 19, 28). Infection with *Rhodococcus equi* or nontuberculous mycobacteria in patients with AIDS (1) or infection with fungi, *Histoplasma* spp., or other organisms may appear histologically similar to WD. Some of these organisms may be ruled out by using Ziehl-Neelsen stain. Biopsy specimens taken from the colon or the rectum, sites that are only infrequently involved, can be misleading due to other conditions that are accompanied by PAS-positive cells (e.g., melanosis coli or histiocytosis) (7, 19, 28).

Electron Microscopy

The characteristic, rod-shaped (0.25 μm by 1.5 to 2.5 μm) organism can be observed by electron microscopy in various stages of degradation within cells and in the extracellular space (5) (Fig. 2). The organism uniformly possesses a trilaminar plasma membrane and a surrounding homogeneous cell wall of 20-nm thickness with two inner layers

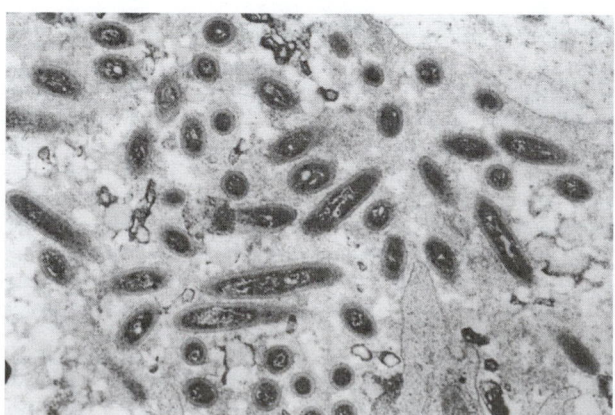

FIGURE 2 Electron microscopic appearance of *T. whipplei*. Magnification, ×23,100.

and an outer trilaminar membrane-like structure usually seen in gram-negative bacteria. Other characteristics, including the central location of tubules and vesicles, are typical of gram-positive organisms. Electron microscopy may be used in rare instances if the diagnosis is not achieved by other means (5).

Antigen Detection

Immunohistochemistry

As polyclonal antibodies have become available after the culture of *T. whipplei* (23), immunohistochemical staining of various tissues (gastrointestinal samples, lymph nodes, and heart valves), fluids (such as CSF or synovial fluid), and blood cells (monocytes) has been reported (15, 23, 28). The technique was used on fixed samples from the original case reported by G. H. Whipple in 1907 (6). By using immunohistochemistry, *T. whipplei* can be directly visualized, and this method provides a sensitive and specific addition to the PAS staining method.

Nucleic Acid Detection

PCR

After sampling and adequate storage of a variety of tissues and fluids, PCR is preceded by DNA extraction, for which different protocols have been used, including DNA binding columns, phenol-chloroform-ethanol purification, Chelex suspension, and chaotropic lysis. For optimal PCR results, the use of fresh tissues (or samples frozen at −80°C until analysis) is recommended; paraffin-embedded tissues can be used as well (8, 14, 23, 25). PCR amplification of a bacterial gene (e.g., targeting the 16S or the 16S–23S intergenic region) has been reliably successful for diagnosis of *T. whipplei* infection (8, 10). Real-time PCR provides a higher sensitivity and can be used for quantitation (8, 27). However, in view of a potentially high rate of false-positive results due to contamination, PCR assays should (i) include adequate positive and negative controls (e.g., water and DNA extracted from control tissues) or (ii) when in doubt be redone using a different DNA sample, and the PCR assay results should (iii) be confirmed by sequencing or hybridization and (iv) be interpreted in concert with other test results (PAS staining and immunohistochemistry).

ISOLATION AND IDENTIFICATION

T. whipplei has only recently been cultured in human fibroblasts based on specific cell culture techniques (using, for example, HEL and MRC5 cell lines) (3, 23). Because *T. whipplei* lacks some amino acid biosynthetic pathways as predicted by genome analysis, a specially supplemented medium has been generated which allows the organism to grow axenically (24, 26). Raoult et al. have thus obtained a larger number of isolates from cardiac valves, duodenal biopsy samples, blood, and synovial fluid in serial cultures (10, 16, 17, 26). Culture from sterile fluids is easier, as contaminated specimens require the use of antimicrobials. The primary detection of *T. whipplei* can require several weeks due to its very long doubling time (up to 18 days) (9, 23, 26).

The identification procedure was initially and extensively described by Raoult et al. (23, 26). During culture,

medium is changed every 15 days, for up to 180 days or longer. To detect bacterial growth, supernatant is examined with each medium change by centrifugation followed by (i) immunofluorescence staining using *T. whipplei* polyclonal rabbit antibodies and (ii) PCR (with positive results confirmed by sequencing or hybridization) (9, 14, 23, 26).

SEROLOGIC TESTS

Serologic assays for WD have been described (23), but assays still need to be developed with higher specificity and should be tested more broadly.

ANTIMICROBIAL SUSCEPTIBILITIES AND TREATMENT

Due to the difficulties in culturing the organism and the organism's long doubling time, routine susceptibility testing for *T. whipplei* currently is not, and never may be, available. A cell culture approach with three bacterial strains suggested that doxycycline, macrolides, aminoglycosides, penicillin, rifampin, teicoplanin, chloramphenicol, and sulfamethoxazole may be active, with MICs ranging from 0.25 to 2 µg/ml, while cephalosporins and aztreonam may not be active (3, 23). However, in axenic medium, all of the aforementioned antimicrobials exhibit MICs ranging from 0.06 to 1 µg/ml (26). Trimethoprim may not be effective in vitro, based on predictions from genomic analysis (24). In another in vitro assay, a combination of doxycycline and hydroxychloroquine was described as bactericidal, perhaps as a result of the alkalinized milieu generated by these antimicrobials and the observation that *T. whipplei* resides and grows in acidic vacuoles (10, 13).

Untreated WD is chronic, progressive, and fatal. Prior to 1980, many patients were treated with penicillin, streptomycin, or tetracycline. However, these treatments were associated with a high frequency (up to one in three cases) of organ relapses and sometimes isolated CNS relapses, resulting in a poor prognosis (5, 19). Since then, trimethoprim-sulfamethoxazole (160 and 800 mg, respectively, orally twice daily), which has a lower relapse rate (5 to 15%), administered for a duration of 1 to 2 years has been recommended (11, 12, 19).

Oral therapy should be preceded by a 2-week course of parenteral therapy with either ceftriaxone (2 g daily) or, with equally good results, meropenem (1 g three times daily) (12). The use of parenteral therapy was recently clarified in a randomized controlled trial (the SIMW study) with 40 WD patients; this study also demonstrated a very high clinical remission rate if antimicrobial therapy was closely monitored (12). Another alternative parenteral regimen, e.g., in cases of allergies, combines streptomycin (1 g daily) and penicillin G (1 million units four times daily) for 2 to 4 weeks. The combination of doxycycline (200 mg daily) plus hydrochloroquine (200 mg three times daily) for 1 year was used successfully in four patients (10).

In response to treatment, diarrhea and fever resolve within 1 week and other symptoms improve in many cases after a few weeks. Follow-up duodenal biopsy samples and CSF samples should each be obtained after 6 and 12 months of treatment. If no PAS-positive material is present or if *T. whipplei* is not identified by molecular or immunohistochemistry testing, antibiotic treatment can be stopped

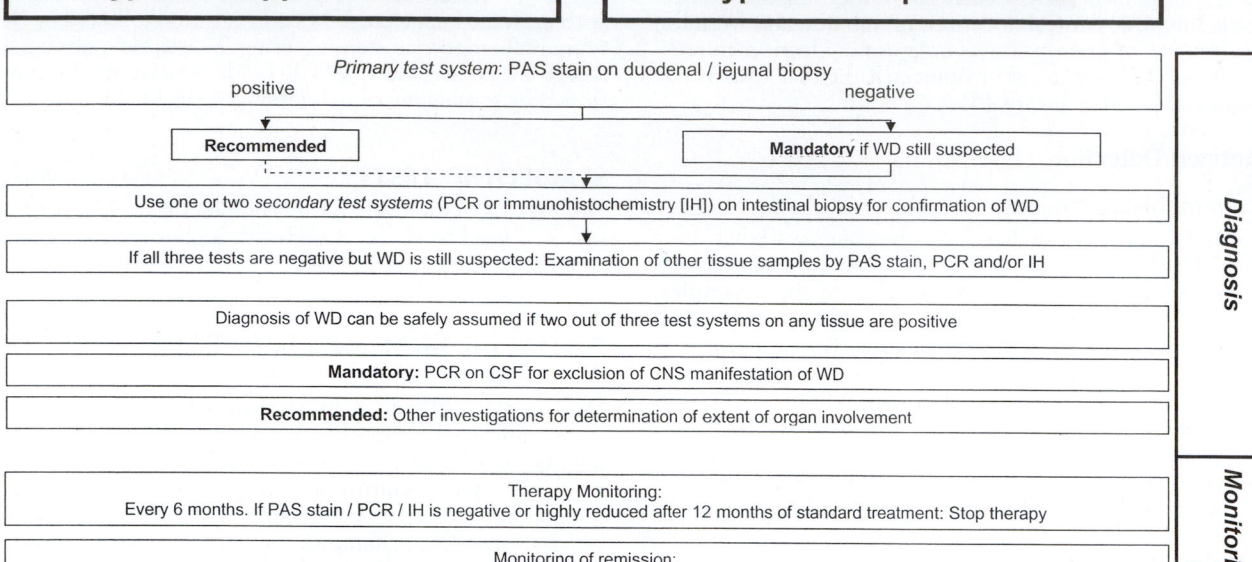

FIGURE 3 Algorithm for WD diagnosis and monitoring.

(Fig. 3). In some patients, PAS-positive cells persist for a long time, and a few patients have an antibiotic-refractory disease (5, 19).

EVALUATION, INTERPRETATION, AND REPORTING OF RESULTS

As results from single diagnostic tests may be misleading or false positive, adequate control tests have to be performed. More importantly, in view of the protean course of WD and its often difficult diagnosis, the histopathologic, molecular, and laboratory findings—in diagnostic and monitoring situations—have to be interpreted in the context of the clinical features of the patient, i.e., a positive PCR or immunohistochemistry test without clinical correlation should not result in the initiation of treatment. The advantages

and disadvantages of the different diagnostic tests are delineated in Table 1. Real-time PCR has advantages in terms of sensitivity and quantitation; usually, sequencing of the DNA should be performed. The use of fresh tissues (highest diagnostic yields are from duodenum, jejunum, and CSF) is preferable, and analysis of blood, saliva, or stool may be problematic. In cases of doubt, or in cases of severe CNS disease, endocarditis, complicated or rare organ manifestation, or lack of treatment response after 2 weeks, specialists should be consulted and an individualized treatment regimen is recommended. Also, when a severe or CNS relapse occurs, an expert opinion should be obtained. In case of negative results (e.g., negative PCR results which could be due to antecedent antimicrobial therapy), other test systems may be applied. An algorithm for a diagnostic approach is given in Fig. 3.

TABLE 1 Diagnostic tools for the diagnosis of WD

Technique	Sample(s)	Advantage(s)	Disadvantage(s)	Diagnostic value
PAS stain	Small bowel, organ tissues, body fluids	Widely available, simple, reproducible	Not pathognomonic, as believed in the past	Very high; usually first diagnostic test; diagnostic if additional technique detects *T. whipplei*
PCR	Small bowel, organ tissues, body fluids, stool, saliva, (blood)	High sensitivity	Specificity varies, not widely available	High; diagnostic if additional technique detects *T. whipplei*
Immunodetection	Small bowel, organ tissues, body fluids, stool, saliva, blood	High sensitivity and specificity, reproducible on same tissue	Not widely available	High; diagnostic if additional technique detects *T. whipplei*
Electron microscopy	Small bowel, organ tissues, body fluids	High sensitivity and specificity	Not widely available, laborious	Very high
Serology	Serum	Simple procedure	Experimental technique	Currently not clear

REFERENCES

1. **Autran, B., I. Gorin, M. Leibowitch, L. Laroche, J. P. Escande, J. Hewitt, and C. Marche.** 1983. AIDS in a Haitian woman with cardiac Kaposi's sarcoma and Whipple's disease. *Lancet* i:767–768.

2. **Bentley, S. D., M. Maiwald, L. D. Murphy, M. J. Pallen, C. A. Yeats, L. G. Dover, H. T. Nobertczak, G. S. Besra, M. A. Quail, D. E. Harris, A. von Herbay, A. Goble, S. Rutter, R. Squares, S. Squares, B. G. Barrell, J. Parkhill, and D. A. Relman.** 2003. Sequencing and analysis of the genome of the Whipple's disease bacterium *Tropheryma whipplei*. *Lancet* **361:**637–644.

3. **Boulos, A., J. M. Rolain, and D. Raoult.** 2004. Antibiotic susceptibility of *Tropheryma whipplei* in MRC5 cells. *Antimicrob. Agents Chemother.* **48:**747–752.

4. **Desnues, B., H. Lepidi, D. Raoult, and J. L. Mege.** 2005. Whipple disease: intestinal infiltrating cells exhibit a transcriptional pattern of M2/alternatively activated macrophages. *J. Infect. Dis.* **9:**1642–1646.

5. **Dobbins, W. O., III.** 1987. *Whipple's Disease.* Charles C Thomas, Springfield, IL.

6. **Dumler, J. S., B. L. Baisden, J. H. Yardley, and D. Raoult.** 2003. Immunodetection of *Tropheryma whipplei* in intestinal tissues from Dr. Whipple's 1907 patient. *N. Engl. J. Med.* **348:**1411–1412.

7. **Fenollar, F., H. Lepidi, and D. Raoult.** 2001. Whipple's endocarditis: review of the literature and comparisons with Q fever, *Bartonella* infection, and blood culture-positive endocarditis. *Clin. Infect. Dis.* **33:**1309–1316.

8. **Fenollar, F., P. E. Fournier, D. Raoult, R. Girolami, H. Lepidi, and C. Poyart.** 2002. Quantitative detection of *Tropheryma whipplei* DNA by real-time PCR. *J. Clin. Microbiol.* **40:**1119–1120.

9. **Fenollar, F., M. L. Birg, V. Gauduchon, and D. Raoult.** 2003. Culture of *Tropheryma whipplei* from human samples: a 3-year experience (1999 to 2002). *J. Clin. Microbiol.* **41:** 3816–3822.

10. **Fenollar, F., X. Puechal, and D. Raoult.** 2007. Whipple's disease. *N. Engl. J. Med.* **356:**55–66.

11. **Feurle, G. E., and T. Marth.** 1994. An evaluation of antimicrobial treatment for Whipple's disease: tetracycline versus trimethoprim-sulfomethoxazole. *Dig. Dis. Sci.* **39:**1642–1648.

12. **Feurle, G. E., N. S. Junga, and T. Marth.** 2010. Efficacy of ceftriaxone or meropenem as initial therapies in Whipple's disease. *Gastroenterology* **138:**478–486.

13. **Ghigo, E., C. Capo, M. Aurouze, J. Gorvel, D. Raoult, and J. Mege.** 2002. Survival of *Tropheryma whipplei*, the agent of Whipple's disease, requires phagosome acidification. *Infect. Immun.* **70:**1501–1506.

14. **La Scola, B., F. Fenollar, P. Fournier, M. Altwegg, M. Mallet, and D. Raoult.** 2001. Description of *Tropheryma whipplei* gen. nov., sp. nov., the Whipple's disease bacillus. *Int. J. Syst. Evol. Microbiol.* **51:**1471–1479.

15. **Lepidi, H., N. Costedoat, J. C. Piette, J. R. Harlé, and D. Raoult.** 2002. Immunohistological detection of *Tropheryma whipplei* (Whipple bacillus) in lymph nodes. *Am. J. Med.* **113:**334–336.

16. **Li, W., F. Fenollar, J. M. Rolain, P. E. Fournier, G. E. Feurle, C. Müller, V. Moos, T. Marth, M. Altwegg, R. C. Calligaris-Maibach, T. Schneider, F. Biagi, B. La Scola, and D. Raoult.** 2008. Genotyping reveals a wide heterogeneity of *Tropheryma whipplei*. *Microbiology* **154:**521–527.

17. **Maiwald, M., A. von Herbay, D. N. Fredricks, C. C. Ouverney, J. C. Kosek, and D. A. Relman.** 2003. Cultivation of *Tropheryma whipplei* from cerebrospinal fluid. *J. Infect. Dis.* **188:**801–808.

18. **Marth, T., N. Kleen, A. Stallmach, S. Ring, S. Aziz, C. Schmidt, W. Strober, M. Zeitz, and T. Schneider.** 2002. Dysregulated peripheral and mucosal Th1/Th2 response in Whipple's disease. *Gastroenterology* **123:**1468–1477.

19. **Marth, T., and D. Raoult.** 2003. Whipple's disease. *Lancet* **361:**239–246.

20. **Martinetti, M., F. Biagi, C. Badulli, G. E. Feurle, C. Müller, V. Moos, T. Schneider, T. Marth, A. Marchese, L. Trotta, S. Sachetto, A. Pasi, A. De Silvestri, L. Salvaneschi, and G. R. Corazza.** 2009. The HLA alleles DRB1*13 and DQB1*06 are associated to Whipple's disease. *Gastroenterology* **136:**2289–2294.

21. **Moos, V., D. Kunkel, T. Marth, G. E. Feurle, B. La Scola, R. Ignatius, M. Zeitz, and T. Schneider.** 2006. Reduced peripheral and mucosal T. *whipplei*-specific Th1 response in patients with Whipple's disease. *J. Immunol.* **177:**2015–2022.

22. **Moos, V., C. Schmidt, A. Geelhaar, D. Kunkel, K. Allers, K. Schinnerling, C. Loddenkemper, F. Fenollar, A. Moter, D. Raoult, R. Ignatius, and T. Schneider.** 2010. Impaired immune functions of monocytes and macrophages in Whipple's disease. *Gastroenterology* **138:**210–220.

23. **Raoult, D., M. L. Birg, B. La Scola, P. E. Fournier, M. Enea, H. Lepidi, V. Roux, J. C. Piette, F. Vandenesch, D. Vital Durand, and T. J. Marrie.** 2000. Cultivation of the bacillus of Whipple's disease. *N. Engl. J. Med.* **342:**620–625.

24. **Raoult, D., H. Ogata, S. Audic, C. Robert, K. Suhre, and M. Drancourt.** 2003. *Tropheryma whipplei* Twist: a human pathogenic Actinobacteria with a reduced genome. *Genome Res.* **13:**1800–1809.

25. **Relman, D. A., T. M. Schmidt, R. P. Mac Dermot, and S. Falkow.** 1992. Identification of the uncultured bacillus of Whipple's disease. *N. Engl. J. Med.* **327:**293–301.

26. **Renesto, P., N. Crapoulet, H. Ogata, B. La Scola, G. Vestris, J. M. Claverie, and D. Raoult.** 2003. Genome-based design of a cell-free culture medium for *Tropheryma whipplei*. *Lancet* **362:**447–449.

27. **Rolain, J. M., F. Fenollar, and D. Raoult.** 2007 False positive PCR detection of *Tropheryma whipplei* in the saliva of healthy people. *BMC Microbiol.* **7:**48–55.

28. **Schneider, T., V. Moos, C. Loddenkemper, T. Marth, F. Fenollar, and D. Raoult.** 2008. Whipple's disease: new aspects of pathogenesis and treatment. *Lancet Infect. Dis.* **8:**179–190.

29. **Schöniger-Hekele, M., D. Petermann, B. Weber, and C. Muller.** 2007. *Tropheryma whipplei* in the environment: survey of sewage plant influxes and sewage plant workers. *Appl. Environ. Microbiol.* **73:**2033–2035.

30. **Wilson, K. H., R. Blichington, R. Frontingham, and J. A. P. Wilson.** 1991. Phylogeny of the Whipple's disease associated bacterium. *Lancet* **338:**474–475.

section III

ANTIBACTERIAL AGENTS AND SUSCEPTIBILITY TEST METHODS

VOLUME EDITOR: JAMES H. JORGENSEN
SECTION EDITOR: JEAN B. PATEL

Antibacterial Agents

JOSEPH D. C. YAO AND ROBERT C. MOELLERING, JR.

65

Antimicrobial chemotherapy has played a vital role in the treatment of human infectious diseases since the discovery of penicillin in the 1920s. Hundreds of antimicrobial agents have been developed or synthesized to date, and a broad number and variety of agents are currently available for clinical use. However, the sheer numbers and continuing development of agents make it difficult for clinicians to keep up with progress in the field. Similarly, this variety presents significant challenges for the clinical microbiologist who must decide which agents are appropriate for inclusion in routine and specialized susceptibility testing.

This chapter provides an overview of the antibacterial agents currently marketed in the United States, with major emphasis on their mechanisms of action, spectra of activity, important pharmacologic parameters, and toxicities. Antibiotics that have fallen into disuse or remained investigational are mentioned only briefly.

PENICILLINS

The penicillins (Table 1) are a group of natural and semisynthetic antibiotics containing the chemical nucleus 6-aminopenicillanic acid, which consists of a β-lactam ring fused to a thiazolidine ring (Fig. 1a). The naturally occurring compounds are produced by a number of *Penicillium* spp. The penicillins differ from one another in the substitution at position 6, where changes in the side chain may modify the pharmacokinetic and antibacterial properties of the drug.

Mechanism of Action

The major antibacterial action of penicillins is derived from their ability to inhibit a number of bacterial enzymes, namely penicillin-binding proteins (PBPs), that are essential for peptidoglycan synthesis (367). This ability to inhibit bacterial cell wall enzymes such as the transpeptidases usually confers on the penicillins bactericidal activity against gram-positive bacteria. The bactericidal activity of the penicillins is often related to their ability to trigger membrane-associated autolytic enzymes that destroy the cell wall. Other minor mechanisms of action include inhibition of bacterial endopeptidase and glycosidase, enzymes involved in bacterial cell growth. There is also recent evidence suggesting that penicillins may inhibit RNA synthesis in some bacteria, causing death without cell lysis, but the significance of these observations remains to be determined (222).

Pharmacology

Oral absorption differs markedly among the penicillins. As a natural congener of penicillin G, penicillin V resists gastric acid inactivation and is better absorbed from the gastrointestinal tract than is penicillin G. Amoxicillin is a semisynthetic analog of ampicillin and has greater gastrointestinal absorption than ampicillin (95% versus 40% absorption). Bacampicillin is an ampicillin ester that is absorbed considerably better from the gastrointestinal tract than is ampicillin or amoxicillin. This ester is inactive until naturally occurring esterases in the intestinal mucosa and serum hydrolyze them to release the parent compound, ampicillin, into the serum. The isoxazolyl penicillins, such as oxacillin, cloxacillin, and dicloxacillin, as well as nafcillin are acid stable and are also absorbed from the gastrointestinal tract, in contradistinction to certain other antistaphylococcal penicillins, such as methicillin, which are not acid resistant and cannot be given via the oral route.

Repository forms of penicillin G, available in procaine or benzathine, delay absorption from an intramuscular depot. Procaine penicillin G provides detectable levels for 12 to 24 h, suitable for treatment of uncomplicated pneumococcal pneumonia and gonorrhea due to fully susceptible organisms. Benzathine penicillin G achieves very low levels in blood for prolonged periods (3 to 4 weeks) and is useful for the therapy of syphilis and for prophylaxis of streptococcal pharyngitis and rheumatic fever.

Penicillins are well distributed to many body compartments, including lung, liver, kidney, muscle, bone, and placenta. Penetration into the eye, brain, cerebrospinal fluid (CSF), and prostate is poor in the absence of inflammation. These drugs are metabolized to a small degree and are rapidly excreted, essentially unchanged, via the kidney. With average half-lives of 0.5 to 1.5 h, they are usually administered every 4 to 6 h to maintain effective blood levels. The renal tubular excretion of penicillins can be blocked by probenecid, thus prolonging their half-lives in serum.

Dosage reduction of most penicillins is necessary only in severe renal insufficiency (creatinine clearance of ≤10 ml/min). Dosages of all penicillins except nafcillin and the isoxazolyl penicillins are adjusted for hemodialysis. Peritoneal dialysis requires dosage reduction of carbenicillin and ticarcillin.

1043

TABLE 1 Penicillins

Natural
    Benzylpenicillin (penicillin G)
    Phenoxymethyl penicillin (penicillin V)

Semisynthetic
    Penicillinase resistant
        Cloxacillin
        Dicloxacillin
        Methicillin
        Nafcillin
        Oxacillin
    Extended spectrum
        Aminopenicillins
            Amoxicillin
            Ampicillin
            Bacampicillin
            Pivampicillin
        Carboxypenicillins
            Carbenicillin
            Ticarcillin
        Ureidopenicillins
            Azlocillin
            Mezlocillin
            Piperacillin

Penicillin + β-lactamase inhibitor combinations
    Ampicillin-sulbactam (Unasyn)
    Ticarcillin-clavulanate (Timentin)
    Amoxicillin-clavulanate (Augmentin)
    Piperacillin-tazobactam (Zosyn)

Spectrum of Activity

The penicillins have antibacterial activity against most gram-positive and many gram-negative and anaerobic organisms. Penicillin G is very effective against penicillin-susceptible *Staphylococcus aureus*, *Streptococcus pneumoniae*, *Streptococcus pyogenes*, viridans group streptococci, *Streptococcus bovis*, *Neisseria gonorrhoeae*, *Neisseria meningitidis*, *Pasteurella multocida*, anaerobic cocci, *Clostridium* spp., *Fusobacterium* spp., *Prevotella* spp., and *Porphyromonas* spp. However, the occurrence of penicillin-resistant pneumococci has increased worldwide (166, 306, 307). Penicillin G is the drug of choice for treatment of syphilis and *Actinomyces* infections. Penicillin V has a spectrum of activity similar to that of penicillin G, except that it is less active against *N. gonorrhoeae*. Both drugs are drugs of choice for the treatment of streptococcal tonsillopharyngitis and for the primary and secondary prevention of rheumatic fever (121). Penicillinase-resistant penicillins, of which methicillin is the prototype, are primarily effective against penicillinase-producing staphylococci. The agents are at least 25 times more active than other penicillins against penicillinase-positive staphylococci. Although they are also active against *S. pneumoniae* and *S. pyogenes*, their MICs for these organisms are higher than those of penicillin G. They are not active against enterococci, members of the family *Enterobacteriaceae*, *Pseudomonas* spp., or members of the *Bacillus fragilis* group.

Ampicillin and amoxicillin have spectra of activity similar to that of penicillin G, but they are more active against enterococci and *Listeria monocytogenes*. These are the drugs of choice for prevention of infective endocarditis in patients with high-risk cardiac conditions undergoing

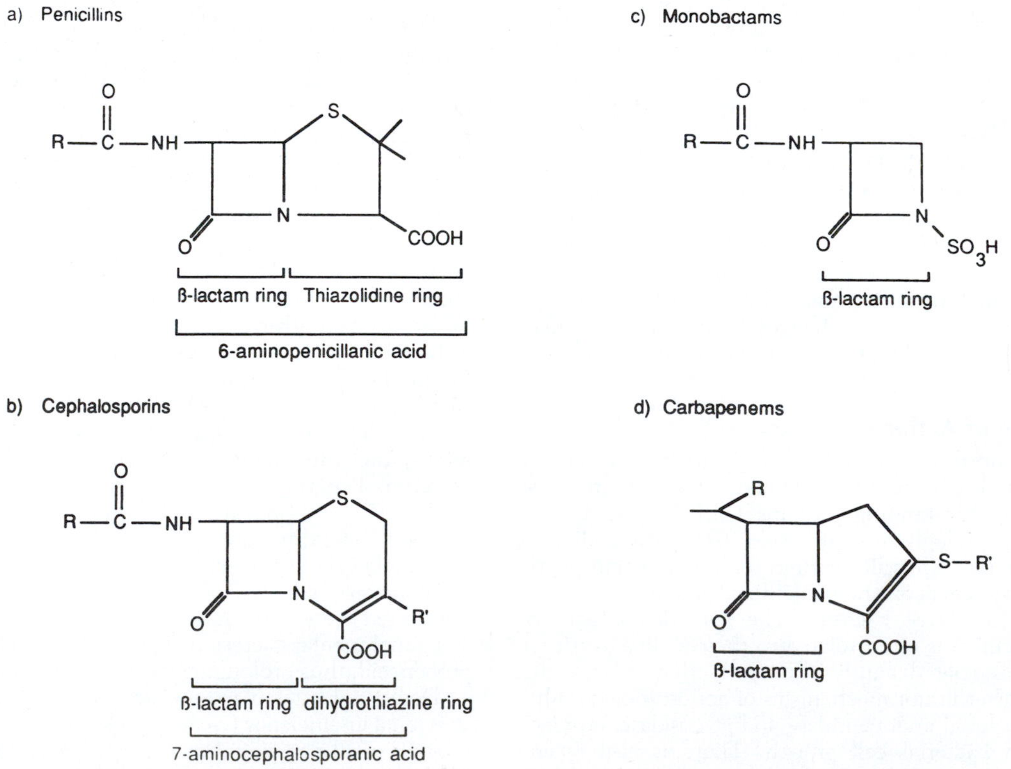

a) Penicillins

b) Cephalosporins

c) Monobactams

d) Carbapenems

FIGURE 1 Chemical structures of β-lactam antibiotics.

invasive dental, respiratory tract, gastrointestinal, and genitourinary procedures (376). Although they are also more active against *Haemophilus influenzae* and *Haemophilus parainfluenzae*, up to 25% of *H. influenzae* isolates are resistant, usually because of β-lactamase production. *Salmonella* and *Shigella* spp., including *Salmonella enterica* serovar Typhi, and many strains of *Escherichia coli* and *Proteus mirabilis* are susceptible to these agents. Ampicillin is more effective against shigellae, whereas amoxicillin is more effective against salmonellae. Both of these agents are degraded by β-lactamase and are inactive against many *Enterobacteriaceae* and *Pseudomonas* spp.

The carboxypenicillins and ureidopenicillins have increased activity against gram-negative bacteria that are resistant to ampicillin. Although these drugs are susceptible to staphylococcal penicillinase, they are more stable against hydrolysis by the β-lactamases of *Enterobacteriaceae* and *Pseudomonas aeruginosa*. Carbenicillin and ticarcillin are relatively active against streptococci as well as against *Haemophilus* spp., *Neisseria* spp., and a variety of anaerobes. They inhibit *Enterobacteriaceae* but are inactive against *Klebsiella* spp. Although carboxypenicillins are not particularly active against the enterococci, they may act synergistically with aminoglycosides against these organisms.

The ureidopenicillins have greater in vitro activity against streptococci and enterococci than do the carboxypenicillins, and they inhibit more than 75% of *Klebsiella* spp. (81). They have excellent activity against many *Enterobacteriaceae* and anaerobic bacteria, including members of the *B. fragilis* group. On a weight basis, their activities in decreasing order of potency against *P. aeruginosa* are as follows: piperacillin, azlocillin > mezlocillin, ticarcillin > carbenicillin (64). These agents also act synergistically with aminoglycosides against *P. aeruginosa*.

Adverse Effects

Common reactions to penicillins include allergic skin rashes, diarrhea, and drug fever. Severe anaphylactic reactions, which can be fatal, may occur in previously sensitized patients rechallenged with penicillins, but fortunately, such reactions are quite rare. At high doses (usually $>30 \times 10^6$ U/day), penicillin G can cause myoclonic twitching and seizures due to central nervous system toxicity. All of the penicillins may cause interstitial nephritis on an allergic basis, but methicillin is more likely than the other penicillins to cause this complication. Hepatitis has been associated with prolonged use of oxacillin. High-dose carbenicillin can result in sodium overload and hypokalemia. Neutropenia may occur with any of the penicillins. Thrombocytopenia and Coombs-positive hemolytic anemia are rare complications of penicillin therapy. Bleeding tendencies due to interference with platelet function can occur with the use of carboxypenicillins and ureidopenicillins (96). Although pseudomembranous colitis has been associated with all the penicillins, it occurs more frequently with ampicillin (27).

CEPHALOSPORINS

Cephalosporins are derivatives of the fermentation products of *Cephalosporium acremonium* (also designated *Acremonium chrysogenum*). They contain a 7-aminocephalosporanic acid nucleus, which consists of a β-lactam ring fused to a dihydrothiazine ring (Fig. 1b). Various substitutions at positions 3 and 7 alter their antibacterial activities and pharmacokinetic properties. Addition of a methoxy group at position 7 of the β-lactam

ring results in a new group of compounds called cephamycins, which are highly resistant to a variety of β-lactamases.

Mechanism of Action

Similar to the penicillins, cephalosporins act by binding to PBPs of susceptible organisms, thereby interfering with synthesis of peptidoglycan of the bacterial cell wall. In addition, these β-lactam agents may produce bactericidal effects by triggering autolytic enzymes in the cell envelope (367). Of note are the unique chemical structure-activity relationships for ceftaroline and ceftobiprole, which contain a thiazole moiety and a vinylpyrrolidinone moiety, respectively, at position 3 of the cephem ring. These chemical side chains promote binding of the drugs to PBP 2a, thereby conferring anti-methicillin-resistant *S. aureus* (MRSA) bactericidal activity (355, 392).

Pharmacology

Most cephalosporins require parenteral administration, but quite a few are available in oral form. Cephalexin, cephradine, cefadroxil, cefaclor, cefuroxime axetil, cefprozil, loracarbef, cefdinir, cefditoren pivoxil, cefixime, cefpodoxime proxetil, and ceftibuten are given orally with good gastrointestinal absorption (60 to 90% of oral dose). Cefuroxime axetil is an acetoxyethyl ester of cefuroxime, and it is de-esterified at the intestinal mucosa and absorbed into the bloodstream as cefuroxime. Cefditoren pivoxil and cefpodoxime proxetil are prodrugs that are absorbed and hydrolyzed by esterases in vivo to release the active drugs cefditoren and cefpodoxime, respectively. Relatively high concentrations of these agents are attained across the placenta and in synovial, pleural, pericardial, and peritoneal fluids. Levels in bile are usually high, especially with cefoperazone, which is excreted mainly in the bile. Ceftizoxime, cefotaxime, ceftriaxone, cefoperazone, moxalactam, and cefepime penetrate well into the CSF and are useful for the treatment of meningitis. Cefuroxime penetrates inflamed meninges, but levels in CSF are inadequate in providing bactericidal activity against susceptible bacteria.

Cephalothin, cephapirin, and cefotaxime are converted to the desacetyl forms before excretion. All cephalosporins except cefoperazone are excreted primarily by the kidney, and for these drugs, dosage adjustments are necessary in patients with renal insufficiency (creatinine clearance of <50 ml/min). Like that of the penicillins, the renal excretion of cephalosporins, except for ceftriaxone, is impeded by probenecid. In general, these agents are removed by hemodialysis but not by peritoneal dialysis. Of the cephalosporins, cefonicid and ceftriaxone have the longest elimination half-lives, at 4.5 and 8 hours, respectively, permitting once- or twice-daily drug administration in the treatment of serious infections.

Ceftaroline fosamil and ceftobiprole medocaril are developed as water-soluble prodrugs of ceftaroline and ceftobiprole, respectively, and they undergo rapid conversion (<1 h) to the respective active drugs after intravenous administration. With a half-life of 2.5 h, infusion of 500 mg and 1 g of ceftaroline results in maximum concentrations of 16 and 30 μg/ml in serum, respectively (334). Following infusion of ceftobiprole medocaril at 500 mg and 1 g, maximum concentrations achieved in serum are 35 and 72 μg/ml, respectively (355). With a half-life of 3 to 4 h, the drug undergoes minimal hepatic metabolism and is primarily eliminated in the urine. Dosage adjustment is necessary for both drugs in patients with renal insufficiency.

Spectrum of Activity

Cephalosporins are classified by a well-accepted but somewhat arbitrary scheme of grouping by generations based on general features of their antibacterial activity (Table 2). The first-generation (narrow-spectrum) drugs, exemplified by cephalothin and cefazolin, have good gram-positive activity and relatively modest gram-negative activity. They are active against penicillin-susceptible and -resistant *S. aureus* as well as *S. pneumoniae*, *S. pyogenes*, and other aerobic and anaerobic streptococci. Methicillin-resistant staphylococci and enterococci are resistant. Some *Enterobacteriaceae*, including many strains of *E. coli*, *Klebsiella* spp., and *Proteus mirabilis*, are susceptible. *Pseudomonas* spp., including *P. aeruginosa*, many *Proteus* spp., and *Serratia* and *Enterobacter* spp. are resistant. These agents are active against penicillin-susceptible anaerobes except members of the *B. fragilis* group. They have only modest activity against *H. influenzae*.

The second-generation (expanded-spectrum) cephalosporins are stable against certain β-lactamases found in gram-negative bacteria and, as a result, have increased activity against gram-negative organisms. The agents are more active than narrow-spectrum drugs against *E. coli*, *Klebsiella* spp., and *Proteus* spp. Their activity also extends to cover some *Enterobacter* and *Serratia* strains, and they have good activity against *Haemophilus* spp., *Neisseria* spp., and many anaerobes. Cefaclor, cefuroxime, cefamandole,

TABLE 2 Cephalosporins

Narrow spectrum (first generation)
  Cefadroxil
  Cefazolin
  Cephalexin
  Cephaloridine
  Cephalothin
  Cephapirin
  Cephradine

Expanded spectrum (second generation)
  Cefaclor
  Cefamandole
  Cefmetazole
  Cefonicid
  Ceforanide
  Cefotetan
  Cefoxitin
  Cefuroxime
  Cefprozil
  Loracarbef

Broad spectrum (third generation)
  Cefdinir
  Cefditoren
  Cefixime
  Cefoperazone
  Cefotaxime
  Cefpodoxime
  Ceftazidime
  Ceftibuten
  Ceftizoxime
  Ceftriaxone

Extended spectrum (fourth generation)
  Cefepime
  Cefpirome[a]
  Ceftaroline
  Ceftobiprole[a]

[a]Not licensed for clinical use in the United States.

cefonicid, and cefprozil are active against ampicillin-resistant *H. influenzae* and *Moraxella catarrhalis* (34, 345). However, cefamandole exhibits a significant inoculum effect and is not suitable for treating life-threatening infections due to *H. influenzae*. Ceforanide and cefonicid have spectra of antibacterial activities similar to that of cefamandole, but they are less active than cefamandole against gram-positive cocci. Loracarbef belongs to a new class of cephalosporin derivatives known as carbacephems, in which the sulfur atom of the dihydrothiazine ring is replaced by a methylene group to form a tetrahydropyridine ring (65). Since this structural modification of the cephalosporin nucleus is minor, loracarbef is considered to be a cephalosporin. Its spectrum of antibacterial activity is very similar to those of cefaclor, cefuroxime, and cefprozil. None of the expanded-spectrum agents is active against *Pseudomonas* spp.

Cefoxitin, cefotetan, and cefmetazole belong to a unique group of expanded-spectrum cephalosporins that have marked activity against anaerobes, including members of the *B. fragilis* group (168, 372). Cefotetan is two to four times less active than cefoxitin and cefmetazole against gram-positive cocci, but it is more potent than these two drugs against susceptible *Enterobacteriaceae*. The three drugs are equally active against *H. influenzae*, *M. catarrhalis*, and *N. gonorrhoeae*, including penicillin-resistant strains. While these drugs are comparable in their activities against the *B. fragilis* group, cefoxitin is the most active against *Prevotella* spp., *Porphyromonas* spp., and gram-positive anaerobic cocci. Cefotetan and cefmetazole have the advantage of more prolonged half-lives in serum.

Third-generation (broad-spectrum) cephalosporins are generally less active than the narrow-spectrum agents against gram-positive cocci, but they are much more active against the *Enterobacteriaceae* and *P. aeruginosa*. Their potent broad spectra of gram-negative activity are due to their stability to β-lactamases and their ability to pass through the outer cell envelopes of gram-negative bacilli (95, 251). There are two subgroups among these agents: those with potent activity against *P. aeruginosa* (ceftazidime and cefoperazone) and those without such activity (ceftizoxime, cefotaxime, and ceftriaxone).

Cefotaxime inhibits more than 90% of strains of *Enterobacteriaceae*, including those resistant to aminoglycosides. The MIC$_{90}$s for *E. coli*, *Proteus* spp., and *Klebsiella* spp. are <0.5 μg/ml. Its activity against strains of *S. marcescens*, *Enterobacter cloacae*, and *Acinetobacter* spp. is variable, and it is inactive against *P. aeruginosa*. It has moderate activity against anaerobes but is inferior to cefoxitin and cefotetan against most of these isolates.

Ceftizoxime and ceftriaxone have spectra of activity similar to that of cefotaxime with a few exceptions. Ceftriaxone is the most active agent against penicillinase-positive or -negative strains of *N. gonorrhoeae*, and it is effective as single-dose therapy for infections caused by these organisms (51). However, *N. gonorrhoeae* strains with reduced susceptibility to these drugs have emerged (198). Because of its long half-life in serum (the longest of the currently available cephalosporins), ceftriaxone is used frequently in outpatient antibiotic therapy of serious infections, including Lyme disease (228).

Cefoperazone is less active than cefotaxime against many *Enterobacteriaceae* and gram-positive cocci. However, it has activity against *P. aeruginosa*, with an MIC$_{50}$ of ≤16 μg/ml. Its activity against anaerobes is similar to that of cefotaxime (169). Ceftazidime has potent activity against *P. aeruginosa*, with an MIC$_{90}$ of <8 μg/ml (251). It is more active than the ureidopenicillins against these strains. This agent has activity similar to that of cefotaxime against the Enterobacteriaceae but is not as active against gram-positive cocci. It has little activity against gram-negative anaerobes.

Cefdinir (62), cefditoren (34, 165, 170), cefixime (23), cefpodoxime (108, 305), and ceftibuten (169, 378) are extended-spectrum oral cephalosporins that are more stable than the narrow- and expanded-spectrum oral cephalosporins against gram-negative bacterial β-lactamases. Compared with the earlier cephalosporins, the newer drugs are equally active against streptococci (MIC$_{90}$s, ≤0.06 μg/ml) but less active against methicillin-susceptible staphylococci (MIC$_{90}$s of 2 μg/ml). With potent activities similar to that of ceftizoxime against many Enterobacteriaceae, H. influenzae, M. catarrhalis, and N. gonorrhoeae (including β-lactamase-producing strains), they are inactive against Pseudomonas, Enterobacter, Serratia, and Morganella spp. and anaerobes. None of the currently available cephalosporins is clinically useful against enterococci.

Cefepime is a so-called fourth-generation (extended-spectrum) cephalosporin approved for clinical use in the United States. Together with cefpirome (not licensed for clinical use in the United States), they have the unique features of reduced affinity for and increased stability to the Bush class I β-lactamases. Therefore, these agents are active against stably derepressed class I β-lactamase mutants of Enterobacteriaceae and P. aeruginosa. In addition, cefepime and cefpirome penetrate well through gram-negative bacterial outer membrane, due to a quaternary nitrogen substitution that makes them zwitterions (net neutral charge). They are more active in vitro than cefotaxime and ceftriaxone against some Enterobacteriaceae (MIC$_{90}$s of ≤0.1 μg/ml) (116). Cefepime has activity comparable to that of ceftazidime against P. aeruginosa with MIC$_{90}$s of ≤4 μg/ml, and it is active against some ceftazidime-resistant strains (282). Against staphylococci (MIC$_{90}$s of ≤2 μg/ml) and streptococci (MIC$_{90}$s of ≤0.12 μg/ml), the activities of this group of drugs are comparable to those of the narrow-spectrum cephalosporins (116). However, they are not active clinically against enterococci or anaerobes.

Ceftaroline and ceftobiprole are active against all staphylococci, including methicillin-susceptible S. aureus (MSSA), MRSA, heterogeneous vancomycin-intermediate S. aureus (hVISA), VISA, and vancomycin-resistant S. aureus (VRSA) at MIC$_{90}$s of ≤1 μg/ml, and against multidrug-resistant pneumococci at MIC$_{90}$s of 0.5 μg/ml (46, 223, 241, 316, 334). Viridans group streptococci and beta-hemolytic streptococci are inhibited at MIC$_{90}$s of ≤1 μg/ml. While ceftaroline has minimal activity against enterococci, ceftobiprole exhibits good activity against both vancomycin-susceptible and -resistant enterococci, with MIC$_{90}$s of 1 and 4 μg/ml, respectively (9). The gram-negative activity of ceftaroline is limited mainly to gram-negative respiratory tract pathogens, including β-lactamase-producing H. influenzae and M. catarrhalis (MIC$_{90}$s of 0.125 and 0.25 μg/ml, respectively), and N. gonorrhoeae (MIC$_{90}$ of 0.25 μg/ml) as well as Enterobacteriaceae that do not contain extended-spectrum β-lactamases (ESBLs). It is weakly active against P. aeruginosa, Acinetobacter, and gram-negative bacilli with inducible AmpC β-lactamases. Ceftobiprole is somewhat more active than ceftriaxone and ceftazidime against P. aeruginosa and Enterobacteriaceae with derepressed AmpC β-lactamases (MIC$_{90}$s of 8 to 16 μg/ml), but it is inactive against ESBL-producing Enterobacteriaceae

and multidrug-resistant Acinetobacter baumannii isolates. Both drugs display variable activity against anaerobes, with good activity against Clostridium spp. (except C. difficile), Fusobacterium, Lactobacillus, Peptostreptococcus, Porphyromonas, Propionibacterium acnes, and Veillonella, but are inactive against B. fragilis, B. fragilis group, and Prevotella (58).

Adverse Effects

Cephalosporins are generally very well tolerated. The most common side effects are diarrhea and hypersensitivity reactions such as rash, drug fever, and serum sickness. Cross-reactions with these drugs occur in only 3% to 7% of penicillin-allergic patients (177). Other infrequent side effects include pseudomembranous colitis, elevated serum creatinine and transaminase levels, leukopenia, thrombocytopenia, and Coombs-positive hemolytic anemia. These abnormalities are usually mild and reversible. Prolonged use of ceftriaxone has been associated with formation of gallbladder sludge, which usually resolves after the drug is discontinued (313), and rarely cholecystitis.

Disulfiram-like reactions have been described in patients receiving cefamandole, cefotetan, and cefoperazone. This reaction is attributed to the N-methylthiotetrazole side chains of these antibiotics, which are similar to the chemical structure of disulfiram. Hypoprothrombinemia and bleeding tendencies have been observed with these cephalosporins. Causes of the coagulopathy included (i) alteration to healthy gut biota by the antibiotics, thus inhibiting the synthesis of vitamin K and its precursors; and (ii) the N-methylthiotetrazole side chain, which inhibits the vitamin K-dependent carboxylase enzyme responsible for converting clotting factors II, VII, IX, and X to their active forms and also prevents regeneration of active vitamin K from its inactive form (310).

OTHER β-LACTAM ANTIBIOTICS

■ Monobactams

Aztreonam is the only monobactam antibiotic currently in clinical use. The monobactams are β-lactams with various side chains affixed to a monocyclic nucleus (Fig. 1c).

Mechanism of Action

Aztreonam binds primarily to PBP 3 of gram-negative aerobes, including P. aeruginosa, thereby disrupting bacterial cell wall synthesis. It is not hydrolyzed by most commonly occurring plasmid- and chromosomally mediated β-lactamases, and it does not induce the production of these enzymes (45).

Pharmacology

Given intravenously, aztreonam is widely distributed to body tissues and fluids. Average drug concentrations in serum exceed the MIC$_{90}$s of most Enterobacteriaceae by four to eight times for 8 h and are inhibitory to P. aeruginosa for 4 h. It crosses inflamed meninges in sufficient amount to be potentially therapeutic for meningitis caused by susceptible organisms. Its half-life in serum is about 1.7 h, and it is excreted mainly unchanged by the kidney. Dosage modification is necessary for patients with renal failure. The drug is removed by both hemodialysis and peritoneal dialysis.

Spectrum of Activity

The antibacterial activity of aztreonam is limited to aerobic gram-negative bacilli, inhibiting most Enterobacteriaceae,

Neisseria spp., and *Haemophilus* spp. with MIC$_{90}$s of ≤0.5 μg/ml (25, 342). It has significant activity against *Enterobacter* spp., and *Serratia marcescens*, with most strains being inhibited at ≤16 μg/ml. However, many *Acinetobacter* spp., *Burkholderia cepacia*, and *S. maltophilia* are resistant. It shows in vitro synergism when combined with aminoglycosides against 30 to 60% of aztreonam-susceptible organisms, including *P. aeruginosa* and aminoglycoside-resistant gram-negative bacilli (44). Bacterial tolerance and inoculum effect are generally not seen with this agent. Aztreonam is not active against gram-positive bacteria or anaerobes.

Adverse Effects

Aztreonam is generally a safe agent, with a toxicity profile similar to those of other β-lactam drugs. Nausea, diarrhea, skin rash, eosinophilia, mild elevation of serum transaminase levels, and transiently elevated serum creatinine level have occurred. It has minimal cross-reactivity with other β-lactams and can be used safely in patients allergic to penicillins or cephalosporins (311). Hematologic abnormalities have not been reported.

■ Carbapenems

Carbapenems are a unique class of β-lactam agents with the widest spectrum of antibacterial activity of the currently available antibiotics. Structurally, they differ from other β-lactams in having a hydroxyethyl side chain in *trans* configuration at position 6 and lacking a sulfur or oxygen atom in the bicyclic nucleus (Fig. 1d). The unique stereochemistry of the hydroxyethyl side chain confers stability against β-lactamases. Doripenem, ertapenem, imipenem, and meropenem are the carbapenems currently available for clinical use (258). Other members of this class currently undergoing preclinical evaluation or clinical trials include biapenem, faropenem, and panipenem (123, 124, 271).

Mechanism of Action

Carbapenems bind to PBP 1 and PBP 2 of gram-negative and gram-positive bacteria, causing cell elongation and lysis (328). They are stable toward most plasmid- or chromosomally mediated β-lactamases except those produced by *Stenotrophomonas maltophilia* and some strains of *B. fragilis* (249). Bacterial resistance arises from production of carbapenemases, such as *Klebsiella pneumoniae* carbapenemases, serine carbapenemases (MSE, NMC-A, IMI, and GES), and metallo-β-lactamases (IMI and VIM), capable of hydrolyzing the carbapenem nucleus and from alteration of the porin channels in the bacterial cell wall, thereby reducing the permeability of the drugs.

Pharmacology

After intravenous administration, the carbapenems distribute widely in the body but undergo no significant biliary excretion. Imipenem is metabolized and inactivated in the kidneys by a dehydropeptidase-I (DHP-I) enzyme found in the brush border of proximal renal tubular cells. To achieve adequate concentrations in serum and urine, a DHP inhibitor, cilastatin, was developed; it is combined with imipenem in a 1:1 dosage ratio for clinical use. Cilastatin has no antibacterial activity, nor does it alter the activity of imipenem. It has a renal protective effect by preventing excessive accumulation of potentially toxic imipenem metabolites in the renal tubular cells. Meropenem, ertapenem, faropenem, and biapenem contain a β-methyl group substitution at position C-1 of the bicyclic nucleus, resulting in increased stability to inactivation by human renal DHP-I. These agents do not require concomitant administration of a DHP-I inhibitor.

The pharmacokinetics of doripenem, imipenem, and meropenem are very similar, with elimination half-lives in serum of about 1 h. Peak concentrations of the drugs in serum are about 25 to 35 μg/ml and 55 to 70 μg/ml following 0.5-g and 1-g doses, respectively. These drugs penetrate inflamed meninges well, with drug levels of 0.5 to 6 μg/ml in the CSF (67, 258). Ertapenem is highly (>95%) bound to human plasma proteins, with poor penetration into the CSF. Its relatively long plasma half-life of 4 h allows for once-daily dosing frequency. Peak serum concentration of 155 μg/ml is reached following a single intravenous dose of 1 g of ertapenem (257). Dosage adjustment of these carbapenem drugs is necessary for creatinine clearance of ≤30 ml/min. These agents, including cilastatin, are effectively removed by hemodialysis.

Spectrum of Activity

In general, all the carbapenems have similar antibacterial potencies with minor differences. They have excellent in vitro activity against aerobic gram-positive species: staphylococci (penicillin-susceptible and -resistant isolates); viridans group streptococci; group A, B, C, and G streptococci; *Bacillus* spp.; and *L. monocytogenes*. Doripenem and imipenem are two to four times more active than meropenem and ertapenem against streptococci and methicillin-susceptible staphylococci (MIC$_{90}$s of ≤0.5 μg/ml), but methicillin-resistant staphylococci are usually resistant to all carbapenems. Although the MICs of carbapenems for penicillin-resistant pneumococci are elevated (MIC$_{90}$s of 0.25 to 2 μg/ml), many strains remain susceptible to these drugs, with doripenem and imipenem being most potent (16, 175, 280). Ertapenem has poor activity against *Enterococcus faecalis*, but these isolates are inhibited by other carbapenems at ≤4 μg/ml. However, *Enterococcus faecium* is usually resistant to all carbapenems.

More than 90% of *Enterobacteriaceae*, including those resistant to other β-lactams and aminoglycosides, are susceptible to carbapenems, with the following decreasing order of activity: doripenem, ertapenem, meropenem > biapenem > faropenem, imipenem (172, 275). These agents are highly active against clinical isolates of ESBL-producing *K. pneumoniae* and *E. coli* with MIC$_{90}$s of 0.015 to 0.125 μg/ml (171, 172). Most *Enterobacter* spp., *Citrobacter* spp., and *Serratia* spp. are inhibited by ≤2 μg/ml. Although ertapenem is inactive against *Acinetobacter* and *Pseudomonas*, it is 5- to 10-fold more active than other carbapenems against fastidious gram-negative bacteria such as *Haemophilus*, *Moraxella*, *Neisseria*, and *Pasteurella*. Most strains of *P. aeruginosa* are inhibited by other carbapenems at 4 to 8 μg/ml, with meropenem as the most potent agent, including against imipenem-resistant strains (172, 244). While they inhibit *B. cepacia* and *Pseudomonas stutzeri*, carbapenems are inactive against *S. maltophilia* (77). Emergence of resistant *Pseudomonas* spp. has been observed during therapy with carbapenems. Imipenem may show in vitro antagonism with broad-spectrum cephalosporins or extended-spectrum penicillins as a result of its ability to induce class I β-lactamase production (249).

Carbapenems are the most potent β-lactams against anaerobes, with activities comparable to those of clindamycin and metronidazole. The MIC$_{90}$s for anaerobic gram-positive cocci, *Clostridium*, the *B. fragilis* group, *Fusobacterium*, *Porphyromonas*, and *Prevotella* are ≤4 μg/ml (323, 324, 371).

This class of drugs is also active in vitro against *Actinomyces, Nocardia,* and atypical mycobacteria (86, 130).

Adverse Effects

The side effects of carbapenems are similar to those of other β-lactam antibiotics. Nausea, vomiting, and diarrhea occur in up to 5% of patients, usually associated with parenteral administration of ertapenem and imipenem. Pseudomembranous colitis can occur with carbapenems. Allergic reactions such as drug fever, skin rashes, and urticaria are seen in about 3% of patients. Cross-reactivity with other β-lactam agents is possible but has not been fully studied. Seizures of unclear etiology have occurred in up to 5% of patients receiving imipenem, particularly in the elderly age group and in patients with renal insufficiency or underlying neurologic disorders, while other carbapenems have low seizure-inducing potential (<1%) (391). Reversible elevation of serum transaminases, leukopenia, and thrombocytopenia have been described for carbapenems, but coagulopathy has not been reported.

β-LACTAMASE INHIBITORS

Clavulanic Acid

Clavulanic acid is a naturally occurring weak antimicrobial agent found initially in cultures of *Streptomyces clavuligerus* (253). It inhibits β-lactamases from staphylococci and many gram-negative bacteria. This agent acts primarily as a "suicide inhibitor" by forming an irreversible acyl enzyme complex with the β-lactamase, leading to loss of activity of the enzyme.

Clavulanic acid acts synergistically with various penicillins and cephalosporins against β-lactamase-producing staphylococci, klebsiellae, *H. influenzae*, *M. catarrhalis*, *N. gonorrhoeae*, *E. coli*, *Proteus* spp., the *B. fragilis* group, *Prevotella* spp., and *Porphyromonas* spp. (20, 105). Plasmid-mediated TEM β-lactamases present in ceftazidime-resistant strains of *K. pneumoniae* and *E. coli* are inactivated by this drug (161). However, the inducible β-lactamases (chromosomal class I) of *Enterobacter, Citrobacter, Proteus, Acinetobacter, Serratia,* and *Pseudomonas* spp. are not inhibited by clavulanic acid (181). The combination of clavulanic acid with ampicillin, amoxicillin, or ticarcillin is active in vitro against *Mycobacterium tuberculosis*, which is known to produce β-lactamases (69, 383).

In the United States, clavulanic acid is available for clinical use in combination with oral amoxicillin at dosage ratios of 1:2, 1:4, 1:7, and 1:16 and in a 1:15 or 1:30 parenteral combination with ticarcillin. Intravenous combinations of clavulanic acid and amoxicillin at ratios of 1:5 and 1:10 are also used outside North America. The pharmacologic parameters of amoxicillin and ticarcillin are not significantly altered when either drug is combined with clavulanic acid. Amoxicillin-clavulanate is moderately well absorbed from the gastrointestinal tract, with a half-life in serum of about 1 h for each component. One-third of a dose is metabolized, while the remainder is excreted unchanged in the urine. The drug is widely distributed to various body tissues and fluids, but it penetrates uninflamed meninges very poorly.

Adverse reactions are similar to those reported for amoxicillin or ticarcillin used alone. Nausea, vomiting, abdominal cramps, and diarrhea occur in 5 to 10% of patients taking amoxicillin-clavulanate. The incidence of allergic skin reactions is similar to that of ampicillin alone.

Sulbactam

Sulbactam is a semisynthetic 6-desaminopenicillin sulfone with weak antibacterial activity (10). It functions as an effective inhibitor of certain plasmid- and chromosomally mediated β-lactamases of *S. aureus,* many *Enterobacteriaceae, H. influenzae, M. catarrhalis, Neisseria* spp., *Legionella* spp., the *B. fragilis* group, *Prevotella* spp., *Porphyromonas* spp., and *Mycobacterium* spp. (236). Sulbactam alone is active against *N. gonorrhoeae, N. meningitidis,* some *Acinetobacter* spp., and *B. cepacia* (162, 238). It acts synergistically with penicillins and cephalosporins against organisms that are otherwise resistant to the β-lactam drugs because of the production of β-lactamases. A combination of sulbactam (8 μg/ml) and ampicillin (16 μg/ml) inhibits most strains of staphylococci, *Klebsiella* spp., *E. coli, H. influenzae, M. catarrhalis, Neisseria* spp., the *B. fragilis* group, *Prevotella* spp., and *Porphyromonas* spp. that are ampicillin resistant (288, 373). Like clavulanic acid, sulbactam does not inhibit the β-lactamases of *Enterobacter, Citrobacter, Providencia,* indole-positive *Proteus, Pseudomonas* spp., or *S. maltophilia.*

For clinical use, sulbactam is combined with ampicillin as a parenteral preparation in a 1:2 ratio. The pharmacologic properties of the drugs are not affected by each other in this combination. Ampicillin-sulbactam penetrates well into body tissues and fluids, including peritoneal and blister fluids. It enters the CSF in the presence of inflamed meninges. Like ampicillin, sulbactam has a half-life in serum of 1 h, and 85% of the drug is excreted unchanged via the kidneys. Since clearances of both sulbactam and ampicillin are affected similarly in patients with impaired renal function, dosage adjustments are similar for the two drugs.

The most common side effects of the ampicillin-sulbactam combination have been nausea, diarrhea, and skin rash. Transient eosinophilia and transaminasemia have been reported. Adverse reactions attributed to ampicillin may also occur with the use of ampicillin-sulbactam.

Tazobactam

Tazobactam is a penicillanic acid sulfone derivative structurally related to sulbactam. Like clavulanic acid and sulbactam, tazobactam acts as a suicidal β-lactamase inhibitor and binds to bacterial PBP 1 or PBP 2 (238). Despite having very poor intrinsic antibacterial activity by itself, it is comparable to clavulanate and sulbactam in lowering the MICs up to 20-fold for many organisms when combined with various β-lactams against β-lactamase-producing organisms. Tazobactam actively inhibits the β-lactamases of staphylococci, *H. influenzae, N. gonorrhoeae, E. coli,* the *B. fragilis* group, *Prevotella* spp., and *Porphyromonas* spp. (6, 139, 186). It also has activity against the class I β-lactamases of *Acinetobacter, Citrobacter, Proteus, Providencia,* and *Morganella* spp., but it remains inactive against those of *Enterobacter* spp., *Pseudomonas* spp., *S. maltophilia,* and some *Klebsiella* spp. (181, 186, 238). Of the penicillin-β-lactamase inhibitor combinations, piperacillin-tazobactam is the one most active (two- to eightfold-lower MICs) against β-lactamase-producing aerobic and anaerobic gram-negative bacilli (88, 186).

Available as a 1:8 ratio dosage combination with piperacillin, tazobactam is administered parenterally. The two drugs do not affect each other's metabolism or pharmacokinetics. High concentrations of both agents are achieved in the intestinal mucosa, lung, and skin, with relatively poor distribution to muscle, fat, prostate, and CSF (in the absence of inflamed meninges). With a half-life in serum of about 1 h, elimination of tazobactam is mainly via the renal route and is not affected by hepatic failure (327). Major adverse effects of the piperacillin-tazobactam combination are similar to those of piperacillin alone, such as diarrhea, skin rash, and allergic reactions. Mild elevation in serum transaminase levels may be encountered in about 10% of patients.

NXL104

NXL104 is a novel non-β-lactam inhibitor of class A and C β-lactamases through the formation of stable covalent carbamoyl linkages (28, 79). It is currently undergoing preclinical and clinical studies in combination with ceftazidime and ceftaroline for the treatment of nosocomial gram-negative infections. When tested at a concentration of 4 μg/ml in combination with ceftazidime and cefotaxime against *Enterobacteriaceae*, this drug potentiated the activity of the cephalosporins 4- to 8,000-fold with MICs of ≤1.0 μg/ml for all organisms, including those producing AmpC β-lactamases, ESBLs of TEM, SHV, or CTX-M types, and *K. pneumoniae* carbapenemases (202). Although it effectively restores the activity of imipenem against isolates producing class A carbapenemases, NXL104 does not potentiate the activity of ceftazidime and cefotaxime against *Enterobacteriaceae* containing IMP or VIM metallo-β-lactamases.

AMINOGLYCOSIDES AND AMINOCYCLITOLS

Since the first aminoglycoside (aminoglycosidic aminocyclitol), streptomycin, was introduced in 1944, this class of antibiotic has played a vital role in the treatment of serious gram-negative infections. Among the unique features of the aminoglycosides are the bactericidal activity against aerobic gram-negative bacilli (including *Pseudomonas* spp.), activity against *M. tuberculosis*, and a relatively low incidence of bacterial resistance. The currently available aminoglycosides are derived from *Micromonospora* spp. (gentamicin, netilmicin, and sisomicin) or from *Streptomyces* spp. (kanamycin, neomycin, paromomycin, streptomycin, and tobramycin). The difference in origin of these compounds accounts for the differences of their suffixes, "micin" versus "mycin." Streptomycin, neomycin, kanamycin, tobramycin, and gentamicin are naturally occurring aminoglycosides, whereas amikacin and netilmicin are semisynthetic derivatives of kanamycin and sisomicin, respectively. Structurally, each of these aminoglycosides contains two or more amino sugars linked by glycosidic bonds to an aminocyclitol ring nucleus.

Spectinomycin is an aminocyclitol antibiotic isolated from *Streptomyces spectabilis*. Although it contains an aminocyclitol nucleus, it is not strictly an aminoglycoside because it does not contain an amino sugar or a glycosidic bond.

Mechanism of Action

Aminoglycosides are bactericidal agents that inhibit bacterial protein synthesis by binding irreversibly to the bacterial 30S ribosomal subunit. The aminoglycoside-bound bacterial ribosomes then become unavailable for translation of mRNA during protein synthesis, thereby leading to cell death (75). The aminoglycosides also cause misreading of the genetic code, with resultant production of nonsense proteins. To reach the intracellular ribosomal binding targets, an aerobic energy-dependent process is necessary to enable successful penetration of the bacterial inner cell membrane

by the aminoglycosides. Bacterial uptake of these agents is facilitated by inhibitors of bacterial cell wall synthesis such as β-lactams and vancomycin. This interaction forms the basis of antibacterial synergism between aminoglycosides and β-lactam antibiotics. There are three known mechanisms of bacterial resistance to aminoglycosides: (i) decreased intracellular accumulation of the antibiotic by altering the outer membrane permeability, decreasing inner membrane transport, or active efflux; (ii) modification of the target site by mutation in the ribosomal proteins or 16S RNA or posttranscriptional methylation of 16S RNA (117); and (iii) enzymatic modification of the drug (the most common resistance mechanism) (318).

Spectinomycin acts similarly to the aminoglycosides by binding to the 30S ribosomal subunits and inhibiting protein synthesis. However, it does not cause misreading of the mRNA and is not bactericidal.

Pharmacology

All aminoglycosides have similar pharmacologic properties. Gastrointestinal absorption of these agents is unpredictable and always low. Because of its severe toxicity with systemic administration, neomycin is available only for oral and topical use. After intravenous administration, aminoglycosides are freely distributed in the extracellular space but penetrate poorly into the CSF, vitreous fluid of the eye, biliary tract, prostate, and tracheobronchial secretions, even in the presence of inflammation.

In adults with normal renal function, the aminoglycosides have half-lives in serum of about 2 to 3 h. They are primarily excreted, essentially unchanged, via the kidneys. There is considerable variation in the elimination of aminoglycosides among individuals, especially in patients with impaired renal function. Monitoring of serum aminoglycoside levels in these patients is essential for providing adequate therapy and reducing toxicity. With their features of concentration-dependent killing and prolonged postantibiotic effect, aminoglycosides may be administered once daily to achieve maximum bactericidal activity at high concentrations in serum without increased risk of toxicities (29). In renal failure, the drugs accumulate and dosage reductions are necessary. Aminoglycosides are substantially removed by hemodialysis and to a lesser extent by peritoneal dialysis.

Spectrum of Activity

Aminoglycoside antibiotics are active primarily against aerobic gram-negative bacilli and *S. aureus*. As a group, they are particularly potent against the *Enterobacteriaceae*, *P. aeruginosa*, and *Acinetobacter* spp. Certain differences in antimicrobial spectra among the various aminoglycosides do exist. Kanamycin is limited in its spectrum because of the common resistance of *P. aeruginosa* and frequent occurrence of plasmid-mediated inactivating enzymes among other gram-negative bacilli (75). It is now used occasionally as a "second-line" drug in combination with other antibiotics for the therapy of mycobacterial infections (361). Similarly, widespread resistance among *Enterobacteriaceae* has limited the usefulness of streptomycin. As a single agent, streptomycin is used in the therapy of infections due to *Francisella tularensis* (tularemia) and *Yersinia pestis* (plague) (219). It is often used in conjunction with tetracycline for the treatment of brucellosis. It has the greatest in vitro activity of the aminoglycosides against *M. tuberculosis*. It may also be used in combination with penicillin or vancomycin for the treatment of infective endocarditis due to viridans group streptococci or enterococci, provided that the organisms do not possess high-level ribosomal or enzymatic resistance to streptomycin (14, 377).

Although gentamicin and tobramycin have very similar antibacterial activity profiles, gentamicin is more active in vitro against *Serratia* spp., whereas tobramycin is more active against *P. aeruginosa* (252). However, these minor differences have not been correlated with greater efficacy of one agent over the other. For the most part, gentamicin and tobramycin are susceptible to inactivation by the same modifying enzymes produced by resistant bacteria, except that in contrast to gentamicin, tobramycin can be inactivated by 6-acetyltransferase and 4'-adenyltransferase and has variable susceptibility to 3-acetyltransferase. Netilmicin and amikacin are resistant to many of these aminoglycoside-modifying enzymes and therefore are active against most *Enterobacteriaceae* that are resistant to gentamicin and tobramycin (243). Netilmicin is intrinsically less active than gentamicin or tobramycin against *P. aeruginosa*, and most gentamicin-resistant *Serratia, Proteus, Providencia,* and *Pseudomonas* isolates are also usually resistant to netilmicin (114). Amikacin is often used as the aminoglycoside of choice when gentamicin and tobramycin resistances are prevalent. In addition, amikacin is active against many *Mycobacterium* spp. (361). Aminoglycosides are only moderately active against *Haemophilus* and *Neisseria* spp. Of the agents active against *Bartonella* spp., aminoglycosides are the only drugs consistently bactericidal toward this group of organisms (219).

Although active against staphylococci, aminoglycosides are not recommended as single agents for the treatment of staphylococcal infections. Gentamicin is often combined with a penicillin or vancomycin for synergy in the treatment of serious infections due to staphylococci, enterococci, or viridans group streptococci (14, 366, 377). The aminoglycosides are not active against anaerobes.

Paromomycin is an aminoglycoside notable for its amebicidal and antihelminthic effects, and it is used clinically for the treatment of intestinal amebiasis and tapeworm infections (229). It has modest antibacterial activity against gram-positive cocci and *Enterobacteriaceae*, but *P. aeruginosa* isolates are generally resistant (74).

Spectinomycin is used primarily for uncomplicated anogenital infections due to *N. gonorrhoeae* in patients with penicillin or cephalosporin allergy and contraindications to fluoroquinolone therapy (51). It is effective against β-lactamase-producing and fluoroquinolone-resistant strains, and gonococci are rarely resistant to this drug (98). However, spectinomycin is ineffective for pharyngeal gonococcal infections, syphilis, or chlamydial infections.

Adverse Effects

Considerable intrinsic toxicity, mainly in the form of nephrotoxicity and auditory or vestibular toxicity, is characteristic of all of the aminoglycosides. The nephrotoxic potential varies among the aminoglycosides, with neomycin being the most toxic and streptomycin the least. This effect is usually reversible when the drug is discontinued. The presence of hypotension, prolonged duration of therapy, preexisting renal insufficiency, and possibly excessive trough serum aminoglycoside concentrations increase the risk of nephrotoxicity.

All aminoglycosides are capable of causing damage to the eighth cranial nerve in humans. Vestibular toxicity is more frequently associated with streptomycin, gentamicin, and tobramycin, whereas auditory toxicity is more typical of kanamycin and amikacin. This frequently irreversible side effect may occur even after discontinuation of the drug and is cumulative with repeated courses of the agent. The ototoxicity is a result of selective destruction of the hair cells in the cochlea. Clinically detectable auditory and vestibular dysfunction has been reported to occur in 3 to 5% of patients receiving gentamicin, tobramycin, or amikacin who underwent audiometric testing (97).

Neuromuscular paralysis, which is usually reversible, can occur after rapid intravenous infusion of aminoglycosides. This phenomenon occurs particularly in the setting of myasthenia gravis or concurrent use of succinylcholine during anesthesia. Other minor adverse reactions include local pain and allergic skin rashes. Serious adverse reactions have not been reported for spectinomycin.

QUINOLONES

Quinolones belong to a group of potent antibiotics biochemically related to nalidixic acid, which was developed initially as a urinary antiseptic. Nalidixic acid and its early analogs, oxolinic acid and cinoxacin, have limited clinical applications as a result of the widespread emergence of bacterial resistance. Newer quinolones have been synthesized by modifying the original two-ring quinolone (or naphthyridone) nucleus with different side chain substitutions (18). These new agents, also known as fluoroquinolones, each contain a fluorine atom attached to the nucleus at position 6. Quinolones that are currently available for clinical use in the United States are listed in Table 3. Grepafloxacin, temafloxacin, and trovafloxacin have been withdrawn from clinical use due to toxicities, while sparfloxacin and lomefloxacin are no longer available for use in the United States. Garenoxacin and sitafloxacin are currently undergoing clinical investigation in the United States. Several closely related fluoroquinolones (e.g., sarafloxacin) are approved for agricultural and veterinary use in the United States and elsewhere.

TABLE 3 Quinolones

Narrow spectrum (first generation)
  Cinoxacin[a]
  Nalidixic acid
  Oxolinic acid[a]

Broad spectrum (second generation)
  Ciprofloxacin
  Enoxacin
  Fleroxacin[b]
  Levofloxacin
  Norfloxacin
  Ofloxacin
  Pefloxacin[b]
  Rufloxacin[b]

Expanded spectrum (third generation)
  Tosufloxacin[b]

Extended spectrum (fourth generation)
  Besifloxacin
  Garenoxacin[b]
  Gatifloxacin
  Gemifloxacin
  Moxifloxacin
  Sitafloxacin[b]

[a]Discontinued for clinical use in the United States.
[b]Not licensed for clinical use in the United States.

Mechanism of Action

The primary bacterial target of the quinolones is DNA gyrase, a type II DNA topoisomerase enzyme essential for DNA replication, recombination, and repair (143). Newer fluoroquinolones also inhibit DNA topoisomerase IV. DNA gyrase A subunit is the main target of quinolones in gram-negative bacteria, whereas topoisomerase IV is the primary target in gram-positive bacteria. Inhibition of these bacterial enzyme targets causes relaxation or decatenation of the supercoiled DNA, leading to termination of chromosomal replication and interference with cell division and gene expression. By inhibiting bacterial DNA synthesis, these agents are bactericidal. However, the antibacterial activity of quinolones is reduced in the presence of low pH, urine, and divalent cations (Mg^{2+} and Ca^{2+}).

Bacterial resistance to quinolones may occur by several mechanisms: (i) single-step chromosomal mutations in the structural genes (*gyrA*, *gyrB*, *parC*, and *parE*) encoding the DNA gyrase and topoisomerase IV; (ii) mutations in the regulatory genes governing bacterial outer membrane permeability to the drug; (iii) expression or overexpression of energy-dependent multidrug efflux pump AcrAB; (iv) acquisition of plasmid-mediated resistance genes (*qnrA*, *qnrB*, and *qnrS*) encoding proteins that prevent the binding of quinolones to bacterial DNA gyrase and topoisomerase IV; and (v) acquisition of a plasmid containing the resistance gene *aac(6)-Ib-cr*, which encodes a variant aminoglycoside acetyltransferase capable of modifying quinolones (selective only for ciprofloxacin and norfloxacin) and reducing their activity. The last two mechanisms confer low-level resistance to quinolones (239, 339).

Pharmacology

Fluoroquinolones are generally well absorbed from the gastrointestinal tract, with the exception of norfloxacin. The oral bioavailability varies from 60% to 95% for the various fluoroquinolones (336). After oral administration, serum concentrations peak in 1 to 2 h. The presence of food does not significantly alter the absorption of these drugs. However, coadministration with iron- or zinc-containing multivitamins or with antacids containing aluminum, magnesium, or calcium substantially reduces the gastrointestinal absorption and subsequent peak concentrations of quinolones in serum. The degree of serum protein binding is generally low, ranging from 8% for ofloxacin to 60% for rufloxacin. The prolonged elimination half-lives of fluoroquinolones allow for twice- or once-daily dosing (133, 349). Ciprofloxacin, ofloxacin, levofloxacin, gatifloxacin, and moxifloxacin are also available for intravenous use, while besifloxacin, ciprofloxacin, gatifloxacin, levofloxacin, moxifloxacin, and ofloxacin are available commercially as ophthalmic preparations.

Quinolones have good penetration into lung, kidney, muscle, bone, intestinal wall, and extravascular body fluids. Concentrations in prostate are about two times those in the serum, and concentrations of 25 to 100 times those above peak serum concentrations are achieved in the urine. In the presence of meningeal inflammation, only ofloxacin, levofloxacin, gatifloxacin, and moxifloxacin achieve concentrations of >1 μg/ml in the CSF (221). Quinolones penetrate well into phagocytes, such that concentrations within neutrophils and macrophages are as high as 14 times those of serum concentrations (352). This feature accounts for their excellent in vivo activity against such intracellular pathogens as *Brucella*, *Listeria*, *Salmonella*, and *Mycobacterium* spp.

Pefloxacin is metabolized mainly by the liver to form glucuronide conjugates, and it is converted into norfloxacin in vivo. Ofloxacin exhibits little or no in vivo metabolism, and it is excreted mainly (90%) via the kidney. The other quinolones are cleared by both hepatic and renal routes in varying proportions, with elimination primarily via the kidneys. This renal elimination is blocked by probenecid. Small amounts of these drugs are also excreted in the bile.

Hepatic insufficiency prolongs the elimination half-lives of pefloxacin, whereas the clearance of other fluoroquinolones is significantly diminished in the presence of renal failure. All of these drugs are only partially removed by hemodialysis (<15%) and are minimally affected by peritoneal dialysis because of their marked extravascular penetration, as reflected in their very large volumes of distribution.

Spectrum of Activity

Quinolones may be categorized into groups with similar spectra of antibacterial activity (Table 3), analogous to the classification of cephalosporins (18). The narrow-spectrum quinolones are inactive against gram-positive cocci, and their clinical utility is limited by widespread prevalence and rapid emergence of bacterial resistance. Broad-spectrum (second-generation) fluoroquinolones are active against both gram-positive and gram-negative bacteria (5). Increased activity against gram-positive cocci and favorable pharmacodynamic properties (high ratios of area-under-the-curve from 0 to 24 h to MIC) are major features of the newer fluoroquinolones (third and fourth generations), with potencies two- to eightfold greater than those of broad-spectrum agents (5, 70). MIC$_{90}$s for MSSA, MRSA, and coagulase-negative staphylococci are in the range of 0.03 to 1 μg/ml, while methicillin-resistant staphylococci are becoming increasingly resistant to these agents. Although potency against enterococci is lower, gatifloxacin is two- to fourfold (MIC$_{90}$s of 0.25 to 0.5 μg/ml) and gemifloxacin and moxifloxacin are four- to eightfold (MIC$_{90}$s of 0.03 to 0.25 μg/ml) more active than levofloxacin against multidrug-resistant *S. pneumoniae*.

In contrast to earlier drugs of this class, many of the expanded- and extended-spectrum quinolones possess potent activity against anaerobes, including members of the *B. fragilis* group and *C. difficile* (337). The relative activities of these newer drugs against all anaerobes in decreasing order of potency are as follows: sitafloxacin > garenoxacin > gatifloxacin > moxifloxacin, tosufloxacin. The more active of these agents inhibit the *B. fragilis* group, *Prevotella*, *Porphyromonas*, *Fusobacterium*, *Clostridium*, and anaerobic gram-positive cocci at concentrations of 0.06 to 2 μg/ml. However, increasing fluoroquinolone resistance has emerged among *Bacteroides* spp. since the introduction of the newer drugs (33, 125, 324).

The fluoroquinolones possess excellent activity in vivo against *Enterobacteriaceae*, *P. aeruginosa*, *Citrobacter*, *Serratia*, and *Acinetobacter* spp., *H. influenzae*, and gram-negative cocci such as *N. gonorrhoeae*, *N. meningitidis*, and *M. catarrhalis* (5). Enteropathogenic gram-negative bacilli such as *Salmonella*, *Shigella*, *Yersinia enterocolitica*, *Vibrio* spp., *Aeromonas* spp., *Plesiomonas* spp., *Campylobacter jejuni*, enteroinvasive and enterotoxigenic *E. coli* are all susceptible to the quinolones (87). Clinical studies have shown these drugs to be effective in the prophylaxis and treatment of infectious diarrheas. However, reduced susceptibility and resistance to quinolones have emerged in clinical isolates of *Salmonella*, *Shigella*, and *Campylobacter* spp. (89). *Legionella* spp. are susceptible to these agents, with MICs of most fluoroquinolones of 0.12 to 1.0 μg/ml for these organisms (5). Fluoroquinolones are the first class of oral antibiotics with outstanding potency against *P. aeruginosa*. Ciprofloxacin is the most active among these drugs against *P. aeruginosa*, with MIC$_{90}$s of 0.5 to 1 μg/ml. However, *Burkholderia* spp. and *S. maltophilia* are variably resistant to quinolones (356).

The fluoroquinolones, especially ciprofloxacin, levofloxacin, and ofloxacin, are active in vitro against *Mycobacterium* species *M. tuberculosis*, *M. fortuitum* group, *M. chelonae*, *M. kansasii*, and *M. xenopi* (76, 346, 389). Their activity against *Mycobacterium avium* complex is fair to poor. They also exhibit activity against *Chlamydia trachomatis*, *Chlamydophila pneumoniae*, and *Mycoplasma hominis*, with MIC$_{90}$s of 0.1 to 1 μg/ml, but are less potent against *Ureaplasma urealyticum* (87, 178). Ciprofloxacin and pefloxacin have been shown to inhibit *Rickettsia conorii*, *Rickettsia rickettsii*, and *Coxiella burnetii* (285, 286, 388). The broad-spectrum fluoroquinolones also possess potent activity against *Bartonella* spp. (218) and *Brucella melitensis* (90). Although quinolones possess in vitro activity against *Plasmodium falciparum* at achievable serum concentrations, they are relatively ineffective when used clinically for the treatment of malaria. *Nocardia* spp. are relatively resistant to the quinolones (32).

No significant inoculum effect has been observed among the bacteria susceptible to quinolones. Combinations of quinolones with β-lactam drugs or aminoglycosides are usually indifferent or additive in their effects against gram-negative and gram-positive bacteria and mycobacteria (380). However, bactericidal activities of quinolones can be antagonized by rifampin or chloramphenicol.

Adverse Effects

Gastrointestinal symptoms, occurring in up to 10% of patients as nausea, vomiting, abdominal discomfort, and diarrhea, are the most common side effects (19, 200, 329). However, *C. difficile* colitis occurs infrequently with the use of quinolones. Headaches, fatigue, insomnia, dizziness, agitation, and rarely, seizures, can occur. These adverse neurologic effects are usually associated with high dosages in elderly patients or concurrent use of nonsteroidal anti-inflammatory drugs.

Allergic reactions are uncommon and often manifest as rash, urticaria, and generalized pruritus. Dose-related photosensitivity occurs most frequently with fleroxacin and lomefloxacin. Rare laboratory abnormalities occurring during fluoroquinolone therapy include elevations in serum transaminases, eosinophilia, leukopenia, and thrombocytopenia. Gatifloxacin can cause hypoglycemia and hyperglycemia, and its use is contraindicated in diabetic patients.

Enoxacin and, to a lesser extent, ciprofloxacin and pefloxacin increase the levels of theophylline and caffeine in serum as a result of decreased hepatic clearance (19, 277). Other reported drug interactions include augmentation of the anticoagulant effects of warfarin by ciprofloxacin, norfloxacin, and ofloxacin and an increase in serum cyclosporin levels with ciprofloxacin (277).

Although irreversible cartilage erosions and skeletal abnormalities were observed in studies of quinolone toxicity in animals (19), such effects have not yet been documented unequivocally in humans. However, use of quinolones is generally contraindicated in children and in pregnant or nursing mothers. Tendinitis and tendon rupture, mainly involving the Achilles tendon, can occur with incidence up to 0.5% in the general population and increased risk in patients >60 years old or on corticosteroid therapy (227).

MACROLIDES

Macrolides have been in use since the early 1950s, with erythromycin as the prototypical antibiotic of this class for over 30 years (365). Their chemical structures consist of a macrocyclic lactone ring attached to two sugar moieties, desosamine and cladinose. They differ from each other in the size (14 to 16 atoms) and substitution pattern of the lactone ring. Erythromycin is a naturally occurring 14-membered macrolide derived from *Streptomyces erythreus*, and other natural analogs include oleandomycin, spiramycin, and josamycin. Clarithromycin and dirithromycin are 14-membered-ring semisynthetic macrolides, while azithromycin is a 15-membered-ring derivative, also known as an azalide, with a nitrogen atom incorporated in its lactone ring. These new macrolides offer significant advantages over erythromycin because of expanded antimicrobial spectra, improved pharmacokinetic parameters, and less frequent adverse effects and drug interactions. Roxithromycin, flurithromycin, and rokitamycin are new macrolides available for clinical use currently in Europe, Asia, and South America (179).

Mechanism of Action

Macrolides are generally bacteriostatic agents that inhibit bacterial RNA-dependent protein synthesis. They may be bactericidal at high drug concentrations and against a low inoculum of bacteria. They bind reversibly to the 23S rRNA of the 50S ribosomal subunits of susceptible organisms, thereby blocking the translocation reaction of polypeptide chain elongation (353). The presence of *erm*(B) gene-encoded rRNA methyltransferases that modify the bacterial 23S rRNA target-binding site is the primary mechanism of macrolide resistance and confers macrolide-lincosamide-streptogramin B (MLS$_B$) coresistance (84). Expression of *erm* may be constitutive or inducible. If inducible, the bacterial strains appear to be resistant to erythromycin (an inducer) but susceptible to clindamycin. However, treatment with clindamycin may lead to selection of resistant mutants and therapeutic failure (323). Other uncommon mechanisms of resistance to macrolides include production of macrolide-inactivating enzymes (esterases, phosphorylases, and glycosidases), *mef*- and *msr*-encoded active efflux of drug, *mtrR* promoter gene mutation-induced overproduction of an *mtrCDE*-encoded efflux pump, and mutations in 23S rRNA (109, 215).

Pharmacology

Erythromycin is available in various topical, parenteral (lactobionate and gluceptate), and oral (base stearate, ethylsuccinate, and estolate) preparations. While clarithromycin and dirithromycin are available only in oral forms, azithromycin is formulated for oral and intravenous administration. When administered orally, erythromycin base is rapidly inactivated by gastric acid, whereas the newer macrolides are stable against acid degradation. Intestinal absorption of erythromycin (except for the estolate form) and azithromycin is reduced up to 50% in the presence of food. Peak levels in serum of 2 to 3, 1 to 2, 0.2 to 0.6, and 0.4 µg/ml are reached at 3 h after oral doses of erythromycin (500 mg), clarithromycin (250 mg), dirithromycin (500 mg), and azithromycin (500 mg), respectively. Much higher concentrations of erythromycin are achieved with intravenous infusion. Tissue distributions of macrolides are excellent, with concentrations in various tissues 10- to 100-fold higher than that in serum (375). The high concentrations reached rapidly within neutrophils and macrophages account for their potent activity against intracellular pathogens (315). They penetrate poorly into the brain and CSF, but they do cross the placenta and are excreted in breast milk.

Erythromycin, clarithromycin, and dirithromycin are metabolized by the liver and primarily excreted in the bile. Azithromycin is excreted largely unchanged in the bile. Clarithromycin exhibits first-pass metabolism, producing a microbiologically active 14-hydroxy derivative that is two to four times more potent than the parent drug against some organisms. Following gastrointestinal absorption, dirithromycin is rapidly converted by nonenzymatic hydrolysis to erythromycyclamine, an active derivative with microbiologic activity similar to that of its parent compound. Erythromycin, clarithromycin, 14-hydroxy clarithromycin, azithromycin, and dirithromycin have terminal half-lives in serum of 1.5, 5, 8.5, 41, and 44 h, respectively. Because of its exceptionally high tissue penetration, azithromycin has a half-life in tissue of 2 to 4 days (315). Dosage adjustment of clarithromycin is necessary with moderate to severe renal failure (creatinine clearance of <30 ml/min). Except for clarithromycin, macrolides are removed minimally by hemodialysis or peritoneal dialysis.

Spectrum of Activity

Macrolides are relatively broad-spectrum antibiotics, with activity against gram-positive and some gram-negative bacteria, mycoplasmas, chlamydiae, treponemes, and rickettsiae (315, 375). Erythromycin shows good activity against staphylococci and streptococci, including S. pneumonia, but the emergence of resistance among these isolates (especially group A streptococci) is a problem in certain parts of the world (55, 166, 306, 307). Erythromycin and dirithromycin exhibit similar in vitro antibacterial activities (30). Clarithromycin is two- to fourfold more active than the other macrolides, and azithromycin is less active than erythromycin against most staphylococci and streptococci (24). These drugs are bactericidal against susceptible strains of streptococci but bacteriostatic toward staphylococci and enterococci. Erythromycin-resistant strains display cross-resistance to these drugs, and methicillin-resistant staphylococci and many enterococci are resistant to all macrolides. These drugs are also active against Corynebacterium spp., L. monocytogenes, and Actinomyces israelii (24).

The antibacterial activity of macrolides against gram-negative bacilli is influenced by pH, with increasing potency (lower MICs) as the pH rises to 8.5. H. influenzae and M. catarrhalis are more susceptible to azithromycin (MIC$_{90}$ of 0.5 µg/ml) than to other macrolides (8- to 16-fold-higher MIC$_{90}$s) (203, 273). However, additive (and possibly synergistic) activity between clarithromycin and its 14-hydroxy metabolite reduces the MIC of clarithromycin for H. influenzae two- to fourfold (250). Clarithromycin is the most active drug in this class against C. pneumoniae (MIC$_{90}$ of 0.25 µg/ml) and Legionella isolates (MIC$_{90}$ of 0.25 µg/ml) (24).

All four macrolides are equally potent against Bordetella pertussis and M. pneumoniae, and erythromycin has long been established as the drug of choice for the therapy of infections due to these pathogens and Legionella spp. Macrolides are active against Campylobacter spp., Helicobacter pylori, P. multocida, N. meningitidis, and B. burgdorferi (24, 273). Unlike other macrolides, azithromycin is also active in vitro against E. coli, Shigella spp., Salmonella spp., and Y. enterocolitica (203, 250).

Macrolide antibiotics are effective in vitro against many pathogens that cause sexually transmitted diseases. N. gonorrhoeae, Haemophilus ducreyi, C. trachomatis, and U. urealyticum are all susceptible, but only azithromycin is active against Mycoplasma hominis (24, 203). Erythromycin may be used for the treatment of gonorrhea and syphilis in patients who cannot tolerate penicillin G (51), but data on the new macrolides for these indications are limited. Azithromycin is effective as an alternative to tetracyclines for the treatment of genital chlamydial infections (331). As a group, macrolides are among the most potent agents inhibitory toward Bartonella spp. (218).

The macrolides have good activity against anaerobic bacteria such as the B. fragilis group, Fusobacterium spp., Prevotella spp., Porphyromonas spp., P. acnes, and anaerobic gram-positive cocci, with MIC$_{90}$s of 1 to 4 µg/ml (24). Except for dirithromycin, they are active against most Clostridium spp., especially C. perfringens, with most strains inhibited at ≤1 µg/ml. For this reason, erythromycin is commonly used preoperatively with or without neomycin as oral bowel preparations.

Atypical mycobacteria are more susceptible than M. tuberculosis to macrolide antibiotics (203). The MIC$_{90}$s of clarithromycin and azithromycin for Mycobacterium avium complex are in the range of 2 to 4 µg/ml, allowing additive or synergistic killing activity of these organisms within infected macrophages when these drugs are combined with other antimycobacterial drugs (24). Erythromycin is used occasionally to treat infections due to Mycobacterium scrofulaceum, Mycobacterium kansasii, and Mycobacterium chelonae (361) and in combination with ampicillin against Nocardia asteroides (104).

Spiramycin and the new macrolides offer comparable in vitro activity against Toxoplasma gondii, and they are effective in the treatment of toxoplasmosis (229).

Adverse Effects

The incidence of serious side effects related to the use of erythromycin is relatively low. Gastrointestinal irritation, such as abdominal cramps, nausea, vomiting, and diarrhea, is common with oral administration and can occur when the drug is given intravenously. These side effects occur less frequently with dirithromycin, clarithromycin, and azithromycin. Thrombophlebitis is associated with intravenous infusion, but it can be avoided by dilution of the dose in a large volume of fluid and by a slow infusion rate. Hypersensitivity reactions may include skin rash, fever, and eosinophilia. Cholestatic hepatitis occurring in adults has frequently been associated with the estolate form but has also been reported with other forms of erythromycin (340) and azithromycin (13). For this reason, erythromycin estolate is no longer recommended for use in adults.

Reversible hearing loss may occur with use of large doses and very high serum concentrations of erythromycin (≥4 g/day), usually in elderly patients with renal insufficiency (43). Ototoxicity has also been reported with high doses of clarithromycin and azithromycin used to treat *M. avium* complex infections. Pseudomembranous colitis and superinfection of the gastrointestinal tract or vagina with *Candida* spp. or gram-negative bacilli occur rarely. Concurrent erythromycin therapy increases the levels of theophylline, cyclosporine, and digoxin in serum by interfering with their hepatic metabolism (357). It also increases the anticoagulant effect of warfarin. To date, no clinically significant interactions have been observed between these drugs and dirithromycin, clarithromycin, or azithromycin. However, cardiac arrhythmias have occurred during concurrent use of terfenadine with erythromycin or clarithromycin.

KETOLIDES

Ketolides are semisynthetic derivatives of erythromycin A, having a ketone group instead of an L-cladinose moiety at the 3 position on the erythronolide A ring. This modification of the chemical structure results in increased stability in acid media, noninducibility of MLS$_B$ resistance, and enhanced activity against gram-positive cocci. The ketolides currently under clinical development also have a substituted carbamate link between carbon atoms 11 and 12 in the macrolide nucleus. This modification enables them to retain activity against bacteria whose ribosomes have been methylated at position A2058 as a result of acquired methylase genes (1). Telithromycin is the first and only ketolide currently approved for clinical use in the United States. Another ketolide, cethromycin, is currently undergoing clinical studies (141, 284).

Mechanism of Action

Like the macrolide antibiotics, ketolides inhibit the translation function in susceptible organisms at the level of the 50S ribosomal subunit. Specifically, ketolides interact with the bacterial 23S rRNA at domains II and V of the peptidyltransferase site (142). These drugs are also able to inhibit the formation of the 30S ribosomal unit. Although ketolides do not induce MLS$_B$ resistance, staphylococci with constitutively expressed MLS$_B$ resistance encoded by *erm* genes are resistant to telithromycin. Although these drugs do not appear to be affected by efflux, mutations in 23S rRNA and ribosomal proteins L4 and L22 (147) or *ermB* gene mutation-induced rRNA methylation (381) can lead to in vitro resistance to ketolides. This class of drugs has a low potential to select for resistance or induce cross-resistance among other MLS$_B$ antimicrobials.

Pharmacology

Telithromycin is administered orally as a once-daily dose of 800 mg, with rapid gastrointestinal absorption yielding a mean peak concentration in plasma of 2 μg/ml in 1 to 2 h and steady state in 2 days. A mean trough concentration in plasma of 0.07 μg/ml is attained at 24 h after dosing (248). The oral bioavailability of 57% is unaffected by food ingestion. With about 70% of the drug protein bound, telithromycin exhibits biphasic elimination from plasma with initial and terminal half-lives of 2 to 3 h and 9 to 10 h, respectively. The drug penetrates well into bronchopulmonary, tonsillar, and sinus tissues and into middle ear fluid, and it is accumulated by polymorphonuclear neutrophils with an intracellular-to-plasma concentration ratio of >500 at 24 h. Hepatic metabolism with elimination via feces (~80%) is the main route of excretion, and <15% of the administered dose is eliminated in the urine. Dosage adjustments are not necessary in patients with renal or hepatic impairment.

Spectrum of Activity

Ketolides possess a good spectrum of potent activity against respiratory pathogens as well as intracellular bacteria, and telithromycin is designed specifically for the treatment of community-acquired respiratory tract infections. It is more active than macrolides against *S. pneumoniae* isolates, irrespective of penicillin susceptibility, with MIC$_{90}$ of ≤1 μg/ml for telithromycin, and 90% of penicillin-resistant strains are inhibited at 0.25 μg/ml (93, 100, 173, 208). Almost all macrolide-resistant strains of pneumococci are inhibited at ≤0.5 μg/ml, regardless of the underlying mechanism of macrolide resistance (166, 306, 307). Telithromycin is more active than erythromycin and clarithromycin and as potent as azithromycin against *H. influenzae* (MIC$_{90}$s of 2 to 4 μg/ml) and *M. catarrhalis* (MIC$_{90}$s of 0.06 to 0.125 μg/ml). The activity of telithromycin is unaffected by β-lactamase production in these strains, but the MICs are increased twofold in the presence of 5% CO_2. Significant postantibiotic effect may be observed for up to 9 h with this drug against the major respiratory pathogens (80).

Telithromycin is also active against staphylococci, with MIC$_{90}$s of 0.125 to 0.25 μg/ml for *S. aureus* and coagulase-negative staphylococci, regardless of the susceptibility to oxacillin. However, isolates harboring the constitutive MLS$_B$ mechanism of resistance are resistant to ketolides. Enterococci without underlying resistance to macrolides and clindamycin are susceptible to telithromycin, with MIC$_{90}$s of 0.125 μg/ml for *E. faecalis* and *E. faecium*. Higher MIC$_{90}$s (4 to 8 μg/ml) are observed with erythromycin- or clindamycin-resistant enterococci (317). Telithromycin displays good in vitro activity against betahemolytic streptococci and viridans group streptococci, regardless of their susceptibility to penicillin G, with all isolates inhibited at ≤0.5 μg/ml. While streptococcal isolates with the *mefA* gene-mediated drug efflux mechanism of resistance to erythromycin remain susceptible to telithromycin, MICs are higher (2 to 16 μg/ml) among the strains with inducible or constitutive *erm* gene-mediated resistance to erythromycin. Other gram-positive cocci, such as *Pediococcus, Leuconostoc, Stomatococcus,* and *Rhodococcus equi*, are susceptible to telithromycin, with MIC$_{90}$s of 0.03 to 0.25 μg/ml.

This drug is also very active against gram-positive bacilli, inhibiting *Corynebacterium* (including *C. diphtheriae* and *C. jeikeium*), *Listeria, Lactobacillus, Actinomyces,* and *Erysipelothrix* at concentrations of ≤0.125 μg/ml (317). Telithromycin is inhibitory (MIC$_{90}$s of 0.125 to 0.5 μg/ml) to *Peptostreptococcus* spp., *Prevotella* spp., *Porphyromonas* spp., *Bilophila* spp. and *Clostridium perfringens*, but it is not active against other *Clostridium* spp., *Fusobacterium*, and the *B. fragilis* group (374). This drug has poor activity against other gram-negative bacilli, including the Enterobacteriaceae, *Acinetobacter* spp., *P. aeruginosa*, and *Borrelia burgdorferi* (159).

Intracellular pathogens, such as *Legionella, Mycoplasma, Chlamydia*, and *Chlamydophila*, are highly susceptible to telithromycin, with MIC$_{90}$s of 0.004 to 0.25 μg/ml (100). *Rickettsia* spp., *Bartonella* spp., *C. burnetii*, and *F. tularensis* are also susceptible to this agent. Telithromycin is comparable to the macrolides in its activity against mycobacteria, with MIC$_{90}$ of 4 μg/ml for *M. chelonae* and *M. avium* complex, and it is not active against M. *tuberculosis,* M. *bovis,* and other atypical mycobacteria (102).

Adverse Effects

Telithromycin is well tolerated by all patient populations, with gastrointestinal adverse effects as the most frequent adverse effects, such as diarrhea (15%), nausea (9%), vomiting, and dizziness (17). Occurrence of C. *difficile*-associated diarrhea has not been reported in clinical trial studies. While elevation of serum transaminase levels is found in <10% of patients, rare cases of severe hepatotoxicity can occur (60). Since ketolides are substrates and inhibitors of the hepatic cytochrome P450 CYP3A4 isoenzyme pathway, their potential to lengthen the QT interval is augmented by concomitant administration of other CYP3A4 inhibitors, such as the triazole antifungal agents (31).

TETRACYCLINES AND GLYCYLCYCLINES

Tetracyclines are broad-spectrum bacteriostatic antibiotics with the hydronaphthacene nucleus, which contains four fused rings. The congeners form three groups based on their duration of action. Chlortetracycline, oxytetracycline, and tetracycline are short-acting, demeclocycline and methacycline are intermediate-acting, and doxycycline and minocycline are long-acting drugs. Glycylcyclines are a group of semisynthetic tetracycline derivatives containing a glycylamido substitution at position 9, and tigecycline (a 9-*t*-butylglycylamido derivative of minocycline) is the first in this class of drugs available for clinical use (337).

Mechanism of Action

Tetracyclines and glycylcyclines act against susceptible microorganisms by inhibiting protein synthesis. They enter bacteria by an energy-dependent process and bind reversibly to the 30S ribosomal subunits, preventing the attachment of aminoacyl-tRNA to the ribosomal acceptor A-site in the RNA-ribosome complex (56, 260). Resistance to tetracyclines occurs among clinical isolates as a result of active efflux of the drug from of the cell, an altered ribosomal target site that prevents binding of the drug (ribosomal protection), or production of modifying enzymes that inactivate the drug. With stearic hindrance from the bulky side group at position 9, glycylcyclines are unaffected by bacterial ribosomal protection proteins and evade the efflux pumps present in tetracycline-resistant strains. These drugs also have higher binding affinity for the bacterial ribosomes than tetracyclines (260). Reduced susceptibility to tigecycline has been found in clinical strains of *Enterobacteriaceae,* A. *baumannii,* P. *aeruginosa,* and S. *aureus* possessing chromosomally encoded multicomponent efflux pumps (220, 268, 299), and in some *Bacteroides* spp. with the *tet*(X) gene-mediated monooxygenase enzyme that degrades tetracyclines (237).

Pharmacology

Tetracyclines are incompletely absorbed from the gastrointestinal tract, but their absorption is improved in the fasting state. Ingestion of food, especially dairy products, and other substances such as antacids and iron preparations impairs the absorption of these drugs. Less interference with absorption by foods occurs with doxycycline and minocycline. These long-acting tetracyclines are more readily absorbed, and therefore, lower doses are required. Peak concentrations in serum of 3 to 5 μg/ml are reached in 2 h after standard oral dosages. Intravenous preparations are available, and peak concentrations in serum of 10 to 20 μg/ml are reached in 1 h after intravenous administration (2). Tetracyclines are usually bacteriostatic at these clinically achievable concentrations in serum.

Tissue penetration of these drugs is excellent, but CSF levels are low even in the presence of meningeal inflammation. Tetracyclines cross the placenta and are incorporated into fetal bone and teeth. They are excreted in high concentrations in human milk. Therefore, tetracyclines are not advised for pregnant or lactating women. Minocycline, the most lipophilic tetracycline at physiologic pH, reaches relatively high concentrations in saliva and tears, making it an ideal antibiotic to eradicate the meningococcal carrier state (152).

Tetracyclines are metabolized by the liver and concentrated in the bile. Biliary concentrations of tetracyclines are three to five times higher than concurrent levels in plasma, with significant drug accumulation in the blood of patients with hepatic insufficiency or biliary obstruction. These drugs are excreted primarily in the urine except for doxycycline, which is excreted primarily (90%) as an inactive conjugate via the biliary tract in the feces. Renal failure prolongs the half-lives of the tetracyclines except doxycycline. Therefore, doxycycline is considered the tetracycline of choice for extrarenal infections in the presence of renal failure.

Tigecycline is administered as an intravenous formulation because of limited oral bioavailability. After multiple doses of 50 mg infused every 12 h, peak serum concentration is reached at ~0.8 μg/ml (213, 226). Despite having plasma protein binding of 80%, the drug has a rapid and wide distribution into tissues, including bone. Penetration into CSF with or without meningitis is marginal, with drug level of 0.025 μg/ml in CSF at 12 h after infusion of a single 100-mg dose (290). It is eliminated primarily by the liver via glucuronidation and biliary excretion of unchanged drug, and the mean elimination half-life is 36 h. With <30% of the drug excreted unchanged in the urine, dosage adjustment is not required for renal insufficiency, hemodialysis, or mild to moderate hepatic dysfunction.

Spectrum of Activity

All tetracyclines have similar antimicrobial spectra, with activity against many gram-positive and gram-negative bacteria, mycoplasmas, chlamydiae, rickettsiae, and some protozoa. Many gram-positive aerobic cocci, including S. *aureus,* S. *pyogenes,* and S. *pneumoniae,* are susceptible at concentrations achievable in the serum. However, tetracycline-resistant strains of S. *pneumoniae* are common (166, 306, 307). Although many E. *coli* isolates are susceptible to tetracyclines, pseudomonads and many *Enterobacteriaceae* are resistant. Most strains of *Shigella* and *Salmonella* spp. are resistant to these agents. Tetracyclines are used mainly for the treatment of acute, uncomplicated urinary tract infections due to E. *coli* (155) and as effective prophylactic therapy for traveler's diarrhea caused by enterotoxigenic E. *coli* (110). With activity against *Burkholderia pseudomallei,* *Brucella* spp., *Vibrio* spp., and *Mycobacterium marinum* (362), they have been used successfully in the treatment of infections due to these bacteria. Their efficacy in the therapy of cholera is diminishing owing to the emergence of resistant *Vibrio cholerae* isolates (303). Minocycline is active against *Nocardia* spp.

(78). Many anaerobic bacteria, including members of the *B. fragilis* group and *Actinomyces* spp., are susceptible to tetracyclines (263).

These drugs are useful in the treatment of urethritis and acute pelvic inflammatory diseases caused by *N. gonorrhoeae*, *C. trachomatis*, *U. urealyticum*, and *M. hominis*. Resistance to tetracyclines is prevalent among *N. gonorrhoeae* strains (98). The drugs are effective for the treatment of other chlamydial infections (psittacosis, lymphogranuloma venereum, and trachoma) (51). Other infections responsive to tetracyclines include granuloma inguinale, chancroid, relapsing fever, and tularemia. Tetracyclines are the drug of choice for treating rickettsial infections (Rocky Mountain spotted fever, endemic and scrub typhus, and Q fever). Many pathogenic spirochetes, including *Treponema pallidum* and *B. burgdorferi*, are susceptible (51, 228). Protozoans such as *Plasmodium falciparum* and *Entamoeba histolytica* are also inhibited by these drugs (229, 262).

Due to its potent and wide-spectrum antimicrobial activity against gram-positive, gram-negative, and anaerobic organisms, tigecycline is useful for treatment of complicated skin and skin structure infections, intra-abdominal infections, and nosocomial infections due to multidrug-resistant pathogens except *P. aeruginosa* (176, 337). All staphylococci, including methicillin-resistant and vancomycin-intermediate strains, are inhibited at ≤ 1 μg/ml. Vancomycin-susceptible and -resistant enterococci typically show MIC_{90}s of 0.25 to 0.5 μg/ml, and *E. faecium* and *E. faecalis* are inhibited equally well by this drug. However, tigecycline exhibits no bactericidal activity (minimum bactericidal concentration at which 90% of the isolates are inhibited [MBC_{90}] >32 μg/ml) against staphylococci and enterococci in time-kill studies. Viridans group streptococci, beta-hemolytic streptococci, and multidrug-resistant pneumococci are highly susceptible, with MIC_{90}s ranging from ≤ 0.25 to 0.5 μg/ml. The drug is also very active against the *Enterobacteriaceae* and nonfermentative gram-negative bacilli, including strains producing ESBLs, with MIC_{90}s of ≤ 2 μg/ml. It inhibits multidrug-resistant *A. baumannii* and *S. maltophilia* with MIC_{90}s of 2 μg/ml (149, 160). Among fastidious respiratory tract pathogens, MIC_{90}s are 0.5 μg/ml and 1 μg/ml for *H. influenzae* and *M. catarrhalis*, respectively. *Proteus*, *Morganella*, *Providencia*, and *P. aeruginosa* are generally resistant (MIC_{90}s of >16 μg/ml). Tigecycline also exhibits some activity against most *B. fragilis* group isolates (MIC_{90} of 8 μg/ml), peptostreptococci (MIC_{90} of 4 μg/ml), *Clostridium* spp. (MIC_{90} of 0.5 μg/ml), *Prevotella* spp., *Propionibacterium*, and *Fusobacterium* (127, 324).

Compared to tetracyclines, tigecycline exhibits more potent activity against *M. pneumoniae*, *M. hominis*, *C. pneumoniae*, and *C. trachomatis*, with MIC_{90}s in the range of 0.125 to 0.5 μg/ml. It is less active toward *U. urealyticum* and *Legionella* spp., with MIC_{90}s of 8 μg/ml. Rapidly growing mycobacteria, including *M. abscessus*, *M. chelonae*, and the *M. fortuitum* group, are 4- to 11-fold more susceptible ((MIC_{90}s of ≤ 0.25 μg/ml) to this drug than to tetracyclines (358). However, slowly growing nontuberculous mycobacteria, such as *M. kansasii*, *M. marinum*, and *M. xenopi*, are less susceptible to tigecycline than to minocycline.

Susceptibility testing with tigecycline should be done using freshly prepared media or media containing a biocatalytic oxygen-reducing reagent (e.g., Oxyrase), because the drug is prone to oxidative degradation. Testing using aged broth media (prepared >12 h prior to inoculation) yielded MIC results that were generally 1 to 2 dilutions higher than those obtained using fresh media (40, 156). Commercial media high in Mn^{2+} content (>2.5 ppm) have been reported to increase MICs of tigecycline in susceptibility testing (101).

Adverse Effects

Tetracyclines have irritative effects on the upper gastrointestinal tract, producing esophageal ulcerations, nausea, vomiting, and epigastric distress. Alterations in the enteric biota occur with the use of tetracyclines, often resulting in diarrhea, and pseudomembranous colitis can develop with prolonged use. Hypersensitivity reactions are unusual, generally manifesting themselves as urticaria, fixed drug eruptions, morbilliform rashes, and anaphylaxis. Cross-reactivity among tetracyclines is the rule. Photosensitivity reactions consist of an erythematous rash on areas exposed to sunlight and can occur with all analogs, especially demeclocycline (113).

Minocycline has been known to cause vertigo, and benign intracranial hypertension (pseudotumor cerebri) has been described with many of the analogs (363). Tetracycline can aggravate preexisting renal failure by inhibiting protein synthesis, increasing the azotemia from amino acid metabolism. Tetracyclines cause depression of bone growth, permanent discoloration of the teeth, and enamel hypoplasia when given during tooth and skeletal development (137). Therefore, these drugs are usually avoided in childhood (<8 years of age) and during pregnancy.

Tigecycline is generally well tolerated, with nausea, vomiting, headache, and diarrhea reported as the most common side effects. Due to similar adverse effects as tetracyclines on bone and tooth development, use of this drug is contraindicated in pregnancy, nursing mothers, and those <18 years of age. It may also show cross-hypersensitivity to tetracyclines (390).

LINCOSAMIDES

The lincosamide antibiotics include lincomycin, which was initially isolated from *Streptomyces lincolnensis*, and clindamycin, which is a chemical modification of lincomycin. The chemical structure of each drug consists of an amino acid linked to an amino sugar. Compared with lincomycin, clindamycin has increased antibacterial activity and improved absorption after oral administration (224). Both drugs are available for parenteral and oral use, but lincomycin is rarely used now in the United States.

Mechanism of Action

Lincosamides bind to the 50S ribosomal subunits of susceptible bacteria and prevent elongation of peptide chains by interfering with peptidyl transfer, thereby suppressing protein synthesis. The ribosomal binding sites are the same as, or closely related to, those that bind macrolides, streptogramins, and chloramphenicol (191). Lincosamides can be bactericidal or bacteriostatic, depending on the drug concentration, bacterial species, and inoculum of bacteria.

Pharmacology

About 90% of an oral clindamycin dose is absorbed from the gastrointestinal tract, with no interference from the ingestion of food. A single oral dose of 150 mg yields a peak concentration in serum of 2 to 3 μg/ml in 1 h. Peak levels in serum of 10 to 12 μg/ml are obtained at 1 h after a 600-mg intravenous dose. Therapeutic serum drug levels are maintained for 6 to 9 h after these dosages (193).

Clindamycin distributes well into bone, lungs, pleural fluid, and bile, but it penetrates poorly into CSF, even with meningitis. It readily crosses the placenta and enters fetal tissues. Clindamycin is actively concentrated in neutrophils and macrophages.

The normal half-life of clindamycin is 2.4 h. Most of the drug is metabolized by the liver and excreted in an inactive form in the urine. Its half-life is prolonged by severe liver dysfunction, necessitating dosage reduction in patients with severe liver disease. Although the serum drug levels are increased in patients with severe renal failure, dose modification is not essential. The drug is not removed significantly by hemodialysis or peritoneal dialysis.

Spectrum of Activity

Lincosamides have a broad spectrum of activity against the aerobic gram-positive cocci and anaerobes. Clindamycin is more potent than lincomycin against methicillin-susceptible *Staphylococcus* spp., *S. pneumoniae*, and group A and viridans group streptococci (193, 224). The MIC$_{90}$s are in the range of 0.01 to 0.1 µg/ml for these strains. However, resistance to clindamycin has emerged in clinical isolates of these bacteria that are also resistant to erythromycin (55, 166, 306, 307). The prevalence of clindamycin-resistant *S. aureus* may be 15 to 20% in some institutions. Enterococci are uniformly resistant to the lincosamides. All of the *Enterobacteriaceae* are resistant to lincosamides.

Clindamycin is one of the most active antibiotics available against anaerobes, including members of the *B. fragilis* group and *C. perfringens*, with MIC$_{90}$s of ≤2 µg/ml (26, 193). However, clindamycin resistance (which appears to be increasing) is found in 10 to 15% of the *B. fragilis* group, 15 to 20% of *Prevotella* spp. and *Porphyromonas* spp., 10 to 20% of clostridial species, 10% of peptococci, and most *Fusobacterium varium* strains (4, 325). Clindamycin has been used successfully as single-agent therapy for actinomycosis (291), babesiosis (229, 379), and malaria (194). It is also effective in combination with pyrimethamine for toxoplasma encephalitis (71) and in combination with primaquine for *Pneumocystis jirovecii* pneumonia (347).

Adverse Effects

Clindamycin-associated diarrhea occurs in up to 20% of patients, and use of this drug has been associated with pseudomembranous colitis caused by toxin-producing *C. difficile* (27). This complication is not dose related and may occur after oral or parenteral therapy. Prompt cessation of the antibiotic in conjunction with oral vancomycin, metronidazole, or bacitracin therapy is effective in reversing this complication.

Other uncommon side effects include skin rashes, fever, and reversible elevation of serum transaminases. Clindamycin can block neuromuscular transmission and may potentiate the action of neuromuscular blocking agents during anesthesia.

GLYCOPEPTIDES AND LIPOPEPTIDES

Vancomycin, a bactericidal antibiotic obtained from *Streptomyces orientalis*, is the only glycopeptide marketed for clinical use in the United States. Initially introduced for its efficacy against penicillin-resistant staphylococci, it has become most useful against methicillin-resistant staphylococci and in patients allergic to penicillins or cephalosporins. Teicoplanin (formerly teichomycin A), a new complex glycopeptide chemically related to vancomycin (326), is currently available for clinical use in most countries of the world except the United States. Dalbavancin, oritavancin, and telavancin are semisynthetic lipoglycopeptides (glycopeptide derivatives with hydrophobic substituents), with the last having been recently approved for clinical use in the United States (12, 15, 197, 261). Daptomycin is a unique, naturally occurring cyclic lipopeptide antibiotic found among the fermentation by-products of *Streptomyces roseosporus* and has potent activity against gram-positive bacteria. Ramoplanin is an investigational semisynthetic lipoglycodepsipeptide with a spectrum of activity similar to those of the glycopeptides (94), but systemic toxicity limits its clinical trials to oral administration and topical application only.

Mechanism of Action

Glycopeptides inhibit peptidoglycan synthesis in the bacterial cell wall by complexing with the D-alanyl–D-alanine portion of the cell wall precursor. Resistance to vancomycin and teicoplanin can occur by one of two mechanisms: (i) presence of a complex series of bacterial cytoplasmic enzymes present in vancomycin-resistant enterococci synthesizing abnormal peptidoglycan precursors terminating in D-alanyl–D-lactate residues (instead of D-alanyl–D-alanine), thereby markedly lowering the binding affinity with the glycopeptides; or (ii) increased accumulation of peptidoglycan precursors (murein monomers) resulting in a thickened cell wall with "trapping" of drug molecules, thereby preventing further diffusion of the drug into the inner part of cell wall layers of VISA (66).

Daptomycin binds irreversibly to the cytoplasmic membrane of susceptible bacteria via a calcium ion-dependent insertion of the hydrophobic tail of the molecule and causes generalized disruption of membrane permeability (150). The end effect is cell death without cell lysis, providing potent bactericidal activity of this drug. It is unable to penetrate the outer membrane of gram-negative bacteria. Reduced susceptibility and resistance to daptomycin have occurred in enterococci (206, 302) and *S. aureus* (144, 321), possibly due to the physical barrier of a thickened bacterial cell wall similar to those found in VISA, alteration of the charge of the outer cell envelope (68), or cumulative point mutations in genes encoding various bacterial enzymes (112).

Ramoplanin acts by binding to lipid II intermediate present in the cell membrane of gram-positive bacteria and inhibiting bacterial transglycosylase (PBP 1b), an enzyme essential for peptidoglycan synthesis. With this unique mechanism of action, this drug is bactericidal against vancomycin-resistant strains of enterococci and staphylococci.

Oritavancin and telavancin have a dual mechanism of action: (i) inhibition of the transglycosylation process of peptidoglycan cell wall synthesis by forming a complex with the D-alanyl–D-alanine residues and (ii) depolarization of the bacterial cell membrane. The depolarization effect on membrane potential depends both on the presence of lipid II and on an interaction between telavancin and D-alanyl–D-alanine residues, affecting diverse *S. aureus* strains including those with decreased susceptibility to vancomycin and daptomycin (210).

Pharmacology

Vancomycin and teicoplanin can be administered orally or parenterally. After oral administration, the drugs are poorly absorbed, and high concentrations in stools are achieved, accounting for their efficacy in treating pseudomembranous colitis (99). Desirable peak and trough levels in serum of

20 to 50 μg/ml and 5 to 15 μg/ml, respectively, are obtained after a 1-g intravenous dose of vancomycin every 12 h in healthy subjects (301). Similar drug concentrations in serum are reached with intravenous teicoplanin, which has the advantage of longer serum half-life and can be administered once daily. Therapeutic levels of both drugs are achieved in synovial, ascitic, pericardial, and pleural fluids, with variable penetration into the CSF only in the presence of inflamed meninges (3, 235).

Vancomycin and teicoplanin have half-lives in serum of 6 and 45 h, respectively, in patients with healthy renal function, and they are eliminated from the body by glomerular filtration. In severe renal insufficiency, their excretion is prolonged to about 9 days, and they are not removed by hemodialysis or peritoneal dialysis.

Intravenous infusion of daptomycin at a dosage of 6 mg/kg results in peak and trough concentrations of 82 and 6 μg/ml, respectively, in serum. About 90% of the drug is bound to plasma proteins, with limited metabolism. Despite its wide distribution into various body sites and tissues, daptomycin shows poor penetration into the CSF and alveolar space, where it is bound by surfactant, precluding its use for the treatment of meningitis and pneumonia (335). Its elimination half-life is 9 h, and 80% of the drug is excreted via the kidney with two-thirds as intact drug (305). The dosing interval is increased to every 48 h when creatinine clearance is ≤30 ml/min.

Without systemic absorption or intestinal degradation of the drug, ramoplanin administered orally at doses of 200 mg or 400 mg twice daily reaches high concentrations in the stool, with mean minimum drug levels of ~460 μg/g and ~760 μg/g in the feces, respectively. This feature enables the drug to be developed for clinical trials in treatment of C. difficile-associated diarrhea and gastrointestinal decolonization to prevent nosocomial bacteremia due to vancomycin-resistant enterococci.

Telavancin is ~95% protein bound in human plasma with good penetration into tissues and a prolonged half-life of 7 to 9 h, and it exhibits time-dependent bactericidal activity in vivo (145). The drug is eliminated from the body via urinary excretion with 75% of the drug unchanged. Hemodialysis removes ~6% of telavancin, and dosage reduction is necessary in renal insufficiency with creatinine clearance of <50 ml/min (309).

Spectrum of Activity

Glycopeptides and lipopeptides are active mainly against aerobic and anaerobic gram-positive organisms, including methicillin-susceptible and -resistant staphylococci, streptococci, enterococci, Corynebacterium spp., Bacillus spp., L. monocytogenes, Clostridium spp., and Actinomyces spp. The MICs of vancomycin against S. aureus, Staphylococcus epidermidis, streptococci, and enterococci are typically in the range of 0.25 to 2 μg/ml (167). The bactericidal activity varies, with MBCs 20-fold higher than MICs for viridans group streptococci. These agents are essentially bacteriostatic against enterococci and staphylococci. Teicoplanin (132, 135, 209), ramoplanin (63), and daptomycin (22, 378) are two- to fourfold more active than vancomycin against these gram-positive cocci. Resistance to vancomycin has emerged among clinical isolates of enterococci (53) and staphylococci (146). Cross-resistance with teicoplanin is variable in these strains, but most are susceptible to daptomycin and ramoplanin (164) with MICs of ≤2 μg/ml. Other naturally vancomycin-resistant gram-positive organisms, such as Leuconostoc,

Lactobacillus, and Pediococcus spp., are susceptible to ramoplanin (63, 164, 298).

Vancomycin is useful in the prevention and treatment of endocarditis due to gram-positive bacteria in patients who are allergic to penicillin (14, 377). It is the drug of choice for treating C. jeikeum infections (120) and is useful for Flavobacterium meningosepticum meningitis (138) and antibiotic-associated C. difficile colitis (27).

The glycopeptides and lipopeptides are not active against gram-negative organisms or mycobacteria. They show no cross-resistance with other unrelated antibiotics. They act synergistically with aminoglycosides or rifampin against staphylococci, streptococci, and enterococci (240, 348, 366), and they are bactericidal with aminoglycosides against Listeria spp.

Daptomycin exhibits concentration-dependent bactericidal activity in vitro against most gram-positive bacteria in their growing and stationary phases (300). The MIC_{90}s for multidrug-resistant isolates of staphylococci (including VISA), pneumococci, and streptococci are ≤1 μg/ml (304, 385). Vancomycin-susceptible and -resistant enterococci are inhibited equally at MIC_{90} of ≤4 μg/ml. The drug is active (MIC_{90}s of ≤2 μg/ml) against Listeria, Corynebacterium spp., Propionibacterium, C. difficile, C. perfringens, and peptostreptococci (128, 350). While Leuconostoc, Pediococcus, and Lactobacillus are susceptible, other Clostridium spp., Actinomyces, and Eubacterium showed MIC_{90}s in the range of 4 to 16 μg/ml. Since optimal in vitro activity of daptomycin depends on the calcium ion concentration in the growth medium, media used for susceptibility testing with this drug should contain the recommended calcium concentration of 50 μg/ml. Current Etest strips of daptomycin used in the drug gradient diffusion method are manufactured with added calcium. Inconsistent results have been observed with the disk diffusion method, and the agar dilution method has not been validated for testing this drug.

With antimicrobial spectra of activity similar to those of glycopeptides, lipoglycopeptides are more active than vancomycin and teicoplanin against a broad range of gram-positive bacteria (8, 15, 35, 185, 281). MIC_{90}s for MSSA, MRSA, and coagulase-negative staphylococci range from 0.06 μg/ml for dalbavancin to 1 μg/ml for oritavancin. Although the MICs are higher than those of glycopeptide-susceptible strains, VISA, hVISA, and VRSA isolates are susceptible to these drugs, with MICs ranging from 0.5 to 4 μg/ml (279, 309). Lipoglycopeptides retain activity against staphylococci that exhibit reduced susceptibility to daptomycin and linezolid. Vancomycin-susceptible enterococci are inhibited by dalbavancin, oritavancin, and telavancin in the range of 0.06 to 1 μg/ml, with MICs twofold higher for E. faecalis than E. faecium. Vancomycin-resistant enterococci of the VanA and VanB phenotypes are usually resistant, with MIC_{90}s of 4 to >64 μg/ml to dalbavancin and telavancin but not oritavancin (8, 392). These drugs are most active against streptococci, including multidrug-resistant pneumococci, with MIC_{90} ranging from 0.015 to 0.125 μg/ml (255). Telavancin also exhibits potent activity against Actinomyces spp., C. difficile, C. perfringens, Corynebacterium spp. (including C. jeikeium), Lactobacillus spp., and P. acnes, with MIC_{90}s ranging from 0.06 to 1 μg/ml (129).

Adverse Effects

The most frequent side effects of vancomycin are fever, chills, and phlebitis at the site of infusion. Rapid or bolus infusion of vancomycin causes tingling and flushing of the face, neck and thorax, known as the red man syndrome, as a result of histamine release by basophils and mast cells (278). This phenomenon is not due to allergic hypersensitivity, and it may also occur with telavancin. Allergic maculo-papular or diffuse erythematous rashes can occur in up to 5% of patients. Reversible leukopenia or eosinophilia can rarely develop with glycopeptide use.

High-frequency hearing loss due to ototoxicity has been reported in patients receiving high daily doses of vanco-mycin, especially among those who were >50 years of age (106). Vancomycin-induced nephrotoxicity is rare, but this risk increases with use of large doses of the drug at >4 g per day (204) and during combination therapy with vancomy-cin and aminoglycosides.

Teicoplanin is generally well tolerated and does not pro-duce the red man syndrome or nephrotoxicity. It does cause irritation at the site of intravenous infusion, and ototoxicity has been reported (73).

Common adverse reactions of daptomycin include diar-rhea, rash, dizziness, and dyspnea. Elevated serum creatinine phosphokinase levels, myalgias, and myopathy can occur but are reversible (7, 48), and they are significantly reduced with lower dosages and once-daily dosing frequency. Taste disturbance, nausea, vomiting, and foamy urine are the most common adverse reactions (<10%) to telavancin, and reversible renal dysfunction occurred in 3% of patients receiving this drug (195). Use of telavancin is contraindi-cated in pregnant women.

STREPTOGRAMINS

Streptogramins are natural cyclic peptides produced by *Streptomyces* spp. They are a unique class of antibiot-ics in which each member is a combination of at least two structurally unrelated components, groups A and B streptogramins, acting synergistically against susceptible bacteria (267). Group A streptogramins are polyunsatu-rated macrolactones consisting of lactam and lactone linkages with an oxazole ring, and the main compounds in this group are pristinamycin II_A and pristinamycin II_B. Group B streptogramins are cyclic hexadepsipeptides, with pristinamycin I_A and pristinamycin I_C as the principal compounds. Quinupristin-dalfopristin is the first injectable streptogramin antibiotic combination developed for clini-cal use in the United States. It is a 30:70 mixture of the semisynthetic streptogramins quinupristin and dalfopristin, which are water-soluble derivatives of pristinamycin I_A and pristinamycin II_A, respectively.

Mechanism of Action

The streptogramins exert synergistic bactericidal effect on susceptible organisms by inhibiting bacterial protein synthesis. They enter bacterial cells via passive diffu-sion and then bind specifically and irreversibly to the 50S subunits of the 70S bacterial ribosomes. Binding of group A streptogramins to the ribosome induces a conformational change in the ribosome that increases its affinity for group B compounds. Group A streptogramins prevent peptide bond formation during the chain elon-gation step, while group B components cause release of the incomplete peptide chains from the 50S ribosomal subunit (353).

Acquired bacterial resistance to the streptogramins, which may be chromosomal or plasmid mediated, is mainly due to modification of the drug target by methylation of the bacterial 23S rRNA, resulting in resistance to all mac-rolides, lincosamides, and group B streptogramins (MLS_B resistance phenotype) but not to group A streptogramins. Mutations in the L22 ribosomal protein gene (*rpIV*), active efflux of groups A and B streptogramins, and drug inacti-vation by streptogramin A acetylase and streptogramin B hydrolase have been described.

Pharmacokinetics

Quinupristin-dalfopristin is administered intravenously with distribution into most tissues. Both components are highly protein bound (70 to 90%) and rapidly cleared from plasma via biliary excretion by hepatic conjugation processes (207). Less than 20% of the administered drug combina-tion is excreted in the urine. Following intravenous doses of 7.5 mg/kg of body weight, peak concentrations in serum of quinupristin and dalfopristin reach 2.7 and 7.2 μg/ml, re-spectively, with elimination half-lives of 1 and 0.75 h. The two components penetrate and accumulate in macrophages, and the ratio of peak in vitro cellular-to-extracellular con-centrations is 50:35. The drug combination does not cross noninflamed blood-brain barrier or placenta to any signifi-cant degree. Dosage adjustment is needed for patients with renal insufficiency (creatinine clearance, <30 ml/min), and the drug combination is removed in modest amounts by dialysis.

Spectrum of Activity

Streptogramins are active mainly against gram-positive bac-teria, with modest activities against selected gram-negative and anaerobic pathogens. Quinupristin-dalfopristin has potent bactericidal activity against MSSA, MRSA, coagu-lase-negative staphylococci, and streptococci, with MIC_{90}s of ≤1 μg/ml and MBCs within two- to fourfold of the MICs (38, 103). Staphylococci and streptococci, including *S. pneumoniae*, that are resistant to β-lactam drugs, mac-rolides, and fluoroquinolones usually remain susceptible to quinupristin-dalfopristin, but staphylococci with MLS_B resistance due to methylation of the 23S rRNA-binding site are inhibited but not killed by quinupristin-dalfopristin (38). While most *E. faecium* (MIC_{90}s of ≤4 μg/ml) strains are susceptible, *E. faecalis* is intrinsically resistant (MIC_{90}s of ≥32 μg/ml) to the drug combination because of active efflux of dalfopristin. Although it is not bactericidal against enterococci, quinupristin-dalfopristin inhibits vancomycin-resistant *E. faecium* (VanA or VanB phenotype), including multidrug-resistant strains, at MIC_{90}s of ≤2 μg/ml (207). This drug combination offers a therapeutic option for serious multidrug-resistant gram-positive bacterial infec-tions (187, 199, 234, 266). *N. meningitidis*, *N. gonorrhoeae*, *M. pneumoniae*, *C. pneumoniae*, and *L. pneumophila* are all highly susceptible to the drug (MIC_{90}s of ≤2 μg/ml). Quinupristin-dalfopristin is also active against *M. catarrhalis* and *H. influenzae*, with MIC_{90}s of ≤4 μg/ml. Enterobac-teriaceae and other nonfermenting gram-negative bacilli are resistant.

Among the anaerobes, *C. perfringens* and *C. difficile* are the most susceptible (MIC_{90}s of 0.25 μg/ml). Quinupristin-dalfopristin is active against the *B. fragilis* group (MIC_{90} of 4 μg/ml) as well as other anaerobic bacteria including *Prevotella*, *Porphyromonas*, *Fusobacterium*, *P. acnes*, *Lactoba-cillus*, and peptostreptococci, with MIC_{90}s of 2 to 4 μg/ml.

Adverse Effects

Phlebitis at the site of intravenous infusion is the major local adverse reaction, and the incidence and severity are dose and concentration related (207, 296). The most common systemic side effects that may lead to discontinuation of therapy are arthralgias and myalgia, both of which are reversible on discontinuation of the combination (234, 283). Elevated levels of serum transaminases and cutaneous reactions such as itching, burning, and erythema of the face, neck, or upper body have been also reported.

OXAZOLIDINONES

Oxazolidinones are a unique group of synthetic antibiotics originally discovered in the 1970s (216). Linezolid is currently the only oxazolidinone available for clinical use (233), while other analogs are undergoing preclinical development (72, 134, 151).

Mechanism of Action

Oxazolidinones inhibit bacterial protein synthesis by preventing the formation of a functional initiation complex consisting of $tRNA^{fMet}$, mRNA, initiation factors, and the ribosome (341). Linezolid binds to the domain V region of 23S rRNA in the 50S ribosomal subunit, thereby distorting the binding site for $tRNA^{fMet}$ and inhibiting formation of a functional 70S initiation complex, thus preventing initiation of mRNA translation. In this regard, this class of antibiotics is unique, without cross-resistance with other antibiotics that also inhibit ribosomal protein synthesis. Resistance to linezolid has occurred in clinical isolates of MRSA, vancomycin-resistant enterococci, and pneumococci, as a result of point mutations in domain V of the 23S rRNA gene (37, 230) or L4 ribosomal protein (382). Oxazolidinones are generally inactive against gram-negative bacteria because of endogenous efflux pumps present in these organisms (341).

Pharmacology

Linezolid is available in oral and parenteral forms. Rapid and extensive absorption occurs after oral administration (>95% bioavailability), reaching maximum serum concentrations of 15 to 20 µg/ml within 2 h after an oral dose of 600 mg (330). The drug is metabolized primarily in the liver, and the elimination half-life is about 5 h. With 30% of the drug being protein bound, it is well distributed in all body tissues, including the CSF (245). The drug is eliminated via the kidneys, with 30% being excreted unchanged in the urine. No dose adjustment is necessary in patients with renal insufficiency or mild to moderate hepatic impairment, while 20% of a dose is removed by hemodialysis (212).

Spectrum of Activity

As a group, oxazolidinones have varying activity against most gram-positive bacteria and mycobacteria. Linezolid has excellent activity against staphylococci (including methicillin-resistant strains), streptococci, and multidrug-resistant enterococci, with MIC_{90}s ranging from 1 to 4 µg/ml (61, 201, 393). The MIC_{90}s are in the range of 0.5 to 2 µg/ml for pneumococci. Although the antibacterial effect of linezolid is generally bacteriostatic, the drug is bactericidal against most strains of staphylococci and pneumococci. Other bacteria that are inhibited by linezolid include *Actinomyces* spp., *B. cereus*, *Corynebacterium* spp., *Leuconostoc*, *Pediococcus*, *R. equi*, *L. monocytogenes*, *Clostridium* spp., and gram-positive anaerobic cocci (128). Both slowly and rapidly growing *Mycobacterium* spp. and *Nocardia* spp. are also susceptible to linezolid, with MIC_{90}s of ≤8 µg/ml (42,

359). Linezolid is an important therapeutic option for skin and soft tissue infections (369), respiratory tract infections (294), and infections due to methicillin-resistant staphylococci (90, 320, 338) and vancomycin-resistant enterococci (92, 272, 276).

Adverse Effects

The most common drug-related adverse events (≤5% incidence) are diarrhea, headache, and nausea (111, 295). Prolonged use of linezolid (usually >28-day duration) has led to rare optic neuropathy (192), peripheral neuropathy (41), and myelosuppression, including anemia, leukopenia, thrombocytopenia, and pancytopenia, which are reversible upon discontinuation of therapy (11, 122). As a mild nonselective inhibitor of monoamine oxidase, linezolid can interact with adrenergic or serotonergic drugs, and rare cases of serotonin syndrome have occurred with concomitant use of selective serotonin reuptake inhibitor drugs (189).

SULFONAMIDES AND TRIMETHOPRIM (TMP)

Sulfonamides were the first effective systemic antimicrobial agents used in the United States during the 1930s. They are derived from sulfanilamide, which shares chemical similarities with *para*-aminobenzoic acid, a factor essential for bacterial folic acid synthesis. Various substitutions at the sulfonyl radical attached to the benzene ring nucleus enhance the antibacterial activity and also determine the pharmacologic properties of the drug.

TMP is a pyrimidine analog that inhibits the enzyme dihydrofolate reductase, interfering with folic acid metabolism, subsequent pyrimidine synthesis, and one-carbon fragment metabolism in the bacteria. Since TMP and sulfonamides block the bacterial folic acid metabolic pathway at different sites, they potentiate the antibacterial activity of one another and act synergistically against a wide variety of organisms. Such a combination, TMP-sulfamethoxazole (TMP-SMX), also called co-trimoxazole, was introduced clinically in 1968 and has proven to be very effective in the treatment of many infections (293, 308). Iclaprim is a new-generation diaminopyrimidine that potently and selectively inhibits bacterial dihydrofolate reductase. It has undergone phase III trials as single-agent therapy for gram-positive coccal infections, but it has not been approved for clinical use in the United States or Europe (183, 269, 304).

Mechanism of Action

Sulfonamides competitively inhibit bacterial modification of *para*-aminobenzoic acid into dihydrofolate, whereas TMP inhibits bacterial dihydrofolate reductase. This sequential inhibition of folate metabolism ultimately prevents the synthesis of bacterial DNA (148). Since mammalian cells do not synthesize folic acid, human purine synthesis is not affected significantly by sulfonamides or TMP. The antibacterial effect of these agents may be reduced in patients receiving high doses of folinic acid.

Pharmacology

Sulfonamides are usually administered in the oral and topical forms; the intravenous preparations (sulfadiazine and sulfisoxazole) are rarely used. The sulfonamides vary in their durations of action. Thus, sulfamethizole and sulfisoxazole are short-acting, sulfadiazine and SMX are intermediate-acting, and sulfadoxine is a long-acting compound. Mafenide acetate (Sulfamylon cream) and silver sulfadiazine are applied topically in burn patients and have significant percutaneous absorption. Sulfacetamide is available as an ophthalmic preparation, and various combinations of other sulfonamides are available orally (triple sulfa, or trisulfapyrimidine) or as vaginal creams or suppositories.

The orally administered sulfonamides are absorbed rapidly and completely from the gastrointestinal tract. They are metabolized in the liver by acetylation and glucuronidation and are excreted by the kidney as free drug and inactive metabolites. Sulfonamides compete for bilirubin-binding sites on plasma albumin and increase levels of unconjugated bilirubin in blood. For this reason they should not be given to neonates, in whom increased serum bilirubin levels may cause kernicterus.

Sulfonamides are well distributed throughout the body, with levels in the cerebrospinal, synovial, pleural, and peritoneal fluids being about 80% of the concentrations in serum. They readily cross the placenta and enter the fetal circulation. Sulfonamides may be used in renal failure, but the drugs may accumulate during prolonged therapy as a result of reduced renal excretion.

TMP is available only for oral use and is absorbed almost completely from the gastrointestinal tract. After the usual 100-mg dose, peak levels in serum reach 1 μg/ml in 1 to 4 h. This drug distributes widely in body tissues, including the kidney, lung, and prostate, and in body fluids (264). Concentrations in CSF are about 40% of levels in serum. Its half-life in serum is about 10 h in healthy subjects and is prolonged in those with renal insufficiency. Up to 80% of a dose is excreted unchanged in the urine by tubular secretion; the remaining fraction is excreted as inactive metabolites by the kidney or in the bile.

A fixed combination of TMP-SMX in a dose ratio of 1:5 is available for oral and intravenous use. An intravenous dose of 160 mg of TMP with 800 mg of SMX produces average peak levels in serum of 3.4 and 47.3 μg/ml, respectively, in 1 h. Similar peak levels are reached at 2 to 4 h after the same dose is taken orally. Widely distributed in the body, both drugs reach therapeutic levels in the CSF (40% of levels in serum). Excretion is primarily by the kidney; dosage reduction is necessary in patients with creatinine clearances of ≤30 ml/min. Both TMP and SMX are removed by hemodialysis and partially by peritoneal dialysis.

Spectrum of Activity

Sulfonamides are inhibitory to a variety of gram-positive and gram-negative bacteria, actinomycetes, chlamydiae, toxoplasmas, and plasmodia. Their in vitro antimicrobial activities are irregular, being strongly influenced by inoculum size and composition of the test media. Susceptibility testing end points are often difficult to determine because of the presence of hazy growth within zones of inhibition in disk diffusion tests and because of the phenomenon of "trailing" in dilution tests. Sulfadiazine and sulfisoxazole are effective for rheumatic fever prophylaxis, but they are not useful in treating established group A beta-hemolytic streptococcal pharyngitis. These drugs may be used for prophylaxis of close contacts of patients with meningitis due to sulfonamide-susceptible N. meningitidis. Sulfisoxazole can be used to treat chlamydial urethritis, and sulfacetamide ophthalmic solution is effective for trachoma and inclusion conjunctivitis.

Sulfadiazine in combination with pyrimethamine has been used successfully to treat toxoplasmosis, and sulfadox-ine combined with pyrimethamine (Fansidar) is effective in the prophylaxis and therapy of P. falciparum malaria (226, 229). Sulfonamides are active against N. asteroides (78), and they show moderate activity against M. kansasii, M. fortuitum group, M. marinum, and M. scrofulaceum (289). Other uses of sulfonamides include therapy of meliodosis, dermatitis herpetiformis, lymphogranuloma venereum, and chancroid.

Among the gram-negative bacilli, E. coli strains were initially susceptible to the sulfonamides, especially at levels achievable in the urine. Therefore, these drugs have been used primarily in the treatment of first-episode acute urinary tract infections due to E. coli. However, increasing bacterial resistance has limited their efficacy in recent years. S. marcescens, P. aeruginosa, enterococci, and anaerobes are usually resistant to the sulfonamides.

TMP is active in vitro against many gram-positive cocci and most gram-negative bacilli. P. aeruginosa, most anaerobes, M. pneumoniae, and mycobacteria are resistant. The MIC varies considerably with the test media used. Like the sulfonamides, TMP is used primarily in the therapy of uncomplicated and recurrent urinary tract infections due to susceptible organisms (155). However, resistance to TMP is prevalent among Enterobacteriaceae.

Combinations of TMP with other agents, such as rifampin, polymyxins, and aminoglycosides, have demonstrated in vitro synergistic antibacterial activity against various gram-negative bacilli. TMP combined with dapsone is effective in the treatment of P. jirovecii pneumonia in immunocompromised patients.

Many gram-positive cocci, including staphylococci and streptococci, and most gram-negative bacilli except P. aeruginosa are susceptible to TMP-SMX (47). However, 10% to 50% of strains of S. pneumoniae are resistant in many parts of the world (180). The drug combination has variable bactericidal effects on enterococci in vitro, depending on the test media used for susceptibility testing (247). Unlike many bacteria that can utilize only thymidine for growth, enterococci can use thymidine, thymine, exogenous folinic acid, dihydrofolate, and tetrahydrofolate, resulting in higher MICs (25- to 50-fold increase) on media containing these compounds (242). This fact also explains the ineffectiveness of TMP-SMX against enterococci in vivo.

With excellent activity against M. catarrhalis and H. influenzae, including β-lactamase-producing strains, TMP-SMX is useful for the therapy of acute otitis media, sinusitis, acute bronchitis, and pneumonia. It has shown excellent results in the prophylaxis and therapy of acute and chronic urinary tract infections (155, 332). It is an effective alternative therapy for uncomplicated urogenital gonorrhea, including cases caused by penicillinase-producing N. gonorrhoeae (51). It can be used also for the treatment of chancroid, but resistance to TMP-SMX in H. ducreyi is increasing. The drug combination is also useful in treating infections due to salmonellae, shigellae, enteropathogenic E. coli, and Y. enterocolitica (246). It has been used successfully for prophylaxis and treatment of traveler's diarrhea (83), but resistance to TMP-SMX in Shigella spp. and E. coli now severely limits its usefulness in many parts of the world.

Other microorganisms susceptible to TMP-SMX include Brucella spp., B. pseudomallei, B. cepacia, S. maltophilia, M. kansasii, M. marinum, and M. scrofulaceum. M. tuberculosis and M. chelonae are generally resistant. It is a valuable antibiotic for the treatment of N. asteroides infections

(360), *B. cepacia* and *S. maltophilia* bacteremia, *L. monocytogenes* meningitis, gastroenteritis due to *Isospora belli* and *Cyclospora* spp. (229), and Whipple's disease. In immunocompromised hosts (e.g., those with leukemia or AIDS or organ transplant recipients), TMP-SMX is effective for the prophylaxis and treatment of *P. jirovecii* pneumonia (52).

Adverse Effects

Sulfonamides are known to cause nausea, vomiting, headache, and fever. Hypersensitivity reactions can occur as rashes, vasculitis, erythema nodosum, erythema multiforme, and Stevens-Johnson syndrome (49). Very high doses of less-water-soluble sulfonamides such as sulfadiazine may result in crystalluria, with renal tubular deposits of sulfonamide crystals. Bone marrow toxicity with anemia, leukopenia, or thrombocytopenia can occur. Sulfonamides should be avoided in patients with glucose-6-phosphate dehydrogenase deficiency because of associated hemolytic anemia. Sulfonamides also potentiate the effects of warfarin, phenytoin, and oral hypoglycemic agents.

In general, TMP is well tolerated. With prolonged use, megaloblastic anemia, neutropenia, and thrombocytopenia can develop, especially in folate-deficient patients. Adverse reactions to TMP-SMX due to either the TMP or, more commonly, the SMX component can occur. Mild gastrointestinal symptoms and allergic skin rashes occur in about 3% of patients (190). Megaloblastic bone marrow changes with leukopenia, thrombocytopenia, or granulocytopenia may develop, usually in patients with preexisting folate deficiency. Nephrotoxicity usually occurs in patients with underlying renal dysfunction. Patients with AIDS have a much higher frequency (as much as 70%) of adverse reactions (131).

POLYMYXINS

Polymyxins are a group of cationic cyclic polypeptides originally derived from *Bacillus polymyxa*. They consist of five different compounds (polymyxins A to E) and have limited spectra of antimicrobial activity and significant toxicity (188). Only polymyxins B and E (colistin) are used clinically in humans.

Mechanism of Action

Acting like detergents or surfactants, members of this group of antibiotics interact with the phospholipids of the bacterial cell membrane, thereby increasing cell permeability and disrupting osmotic integrity. This process results in leakage of intracellular constituents, leading to cell death. The bactericidal action is reduced in the presence of calcium, which interferes with the attachment of drugs to the cell membrane. With almost complete cross-resistance existing between polymyxin B and colistin, gram-negative bacteria can become resistant by alterations of the outer cell membrane from reduction in lipopolysaccharides, reduced levels of specific outer membrane proteins, reduced cell envelope Mg^{2+} and Ca^{2+} contents, and lipid alterations. In addition, the presence of a polymyxin B efflux pump system and colistinase, which inactivates colistin, has been reported (91).

Pharmacology

Polymyxins are usually administered parenterally, orally, or topically. They are not significantly absorbed when given orally or topically, and intramuscular injections can be painful. Peak concentrations in serum of 5 μg/ml are obtained with a total daily dose of intravenous polymyxin B at 2.5 mg (or 25,000 U)/kg (196). Polymyxin E is available commercially as colistin sulfate and colistimethate sodium (a sulfomethyl derivative of colistin), with the former given orally for local antibacterial effect in the gut and the latter used for intravenous or intramuscular injections. The half-life of polymyxin B in serum is about 6 to 7 h, and that of colistin is 2 to 4 h. They do not penetrate well into pleural fluid, synovial fluid, or CSF even in the presence of inflammation (217). Excretion is mostly via the kidneys by glomerular filtration. Levels in serum and toxicity are increased in states of renal insufficiency. These drugs are not removed by hemodialysis, but small amounts can be removed by peritoneal dialysis.

Polymyxin is often used topically as 0.1% polymyxin in combination with bacitracin or neomycin for treatment of skin, mucous membrane, eye, and ear infections. It is poorly absorbed from these surfaces. When the drug is used for irrigation of serous or wound cavities, systemic absorption can be significant enough to produce toxicity.

Spectrum of Activity

Polymyxins are active only against gram-negative bacilli, especially *Pseudomonas* spp. The MIC$_{90}$s for *Pseudomonas* spp., including *P. aeruginosa*, are <8 μg/ml. *Proteus*, *Providencia*, *Serratia*, and *Neisseria* isolates are usually resistant (188). Emergence of resistance during therapy is rare, and there is no cross-resistance with other antibiotics. Polymyxins B and E have identical antimicrobial spectra and show complete cross-resistance to one another.

The combination of polymyxins with TMP-SMX may be synergistic in the treatment of serious infection due to multiply resistant *Serratia* spp., *P. aeruginosa*, *B. cepacia*, and *S. maltophilia* (77, 292). The polymyxins are usually reserved for serious, life-threatening *Pseudomonas* or gram-negative bacillary infections caused by organisms resistant to all other antibiotics (91). Aerosolized polymyxins have been used successfully to treat respiratory tract colonization and nosocomial pneumonia due to multidrug-resistant gram-negative bacilli or *P. aeruginosa* in patients with or without cystic fibrosis or bronchiectasis (196, 232).

Adverse Effects

Neurotoxicity and nephrotoxicity are the two major side effects of polymyxins (196). Paresthesia with flushing, dizziness, vertigo, ataxia, slurred speech, drowsiness, or mental confusion occurs when levels in serum exceed 1 to 2 μg/ml (91). Polymyxins also have a curare-like effect that can block neuromuscular transmission. Dose-related renal dysfunction occurs in about 20% of patients receiving appropriate therapeutic dosages. Allergic reactions such as fever and skin rashes are rare, but urticaria and shock after rapid intravenous infusion have occurred.

CHLORAMPHENICOL

Chloramphenicol is a unique antibiotic originally derived from *Streptomyces venezuelae*. It contains a nitrobenzene ring. It is a highly effective broad-spectrum antimicrobial agent with specific indications for use in seriously ill patients. Thiamphenicol is an analog of chloramphenicol with a similar spectrum of antimicrobial activity (254). Only chloramphenicol is available for clinical use in the United States.

Mechanism of Action

The drug is a bacteriostatic agent that inhibits protein synthesis by binding reversibly to the peptidyltransferase component of the 50S ribosomal subunit and preventing the transpeptidation process of peptide chain elongation. At therapeutic concentrations achievable in the serum, it can be bactericidal against common meningeal pathogens such as *S. pneumoniae*, *N. meningitidis*, and *H. influenzae* (211, 254). Bacterial resistance occurs with plasmid-mediated, *cat* gene-encoded production of chloramphenicol acetyltransferase enzyme, which inactivates the drug (319).

Pharmacology

Chloramphenicol is available for topical, oral, or parenteral use. It is not absorbed in any significant amount when applied topically, but it is rapidly and completely absorbed from the gastrointestinal tract. After an oral or intravenous dose of 1 g, peak concentrations in serum at 2 h can reach 10 to 15 μg/ml. It diffuses well into many tissues and body fluids, including CSF, where levels are generally 30 to 50% of concentrations in serum even without meningeal inflammation (322). The antibiotic readily crosses the placental barrier and is present in human milk.

Chloramphenicol is metabolized and inactivated by glucuronidation in the liver, with a half-life of 4 h in adults. The active drug (5 to 10%) and its inactive metabolites are excreted by the kidneys. Careful monitoring of serum chloramphenicol levels, maintaining peak concentrations in serum in the therapeutic range of 10 to 20 μg/ml, is useful for ensuring therapeutic efficacy and reduced toxicity. Patients with hepatic failure have high levels of active drug in serum owing to prolonged half-life. Dosage modification is not necessary in the presence of renal insufficiency, since the metabolites are not as toxic as the active drug. Levels in serum are not affected by hemodialysis or peritoneal dialysis.

Spectrum of Activity

Chloramphenicol is very active against many gram-positive and gram-negative bacteria, chlamydiae, mycoplasmas, and rickettsiae. MIC$_{90}$s for most gram-positive aerobic and anaerobic cocci are ≤12.5 μg/ml (254). However, the drug is usually inactive against MRSA and methicillin-resistant *S. epidermidis* and is variably active against enterococci. *N. meningitidis*, *H. influenzae* (ampicillin-resistant and -susceptible strains), and *Enterobacteriaceae* are susceptible. Its activity against *Serratia* and *Enterobacter* isolates is variable, and *Pseudomonas* spp. are usually resistant. Salmonellae, including *Salmonella enterica* serovar Typhi, are also susceptible, but resistant isolates are being encountered with increasing frequency (54).

Chloramphenicol has excellent activity against anaerobic bacteria, including members of the *B. fragilis* group. Almost all of these isolates are inhibited at concentrations of ≤10 μg/ml (4, 325). It is also active against *Rickettsia* spp. and *Coxiella burnetii*.

Adverse Effects

Bone marrow toxicity is the major complication of chloramphenicol use. This side effect may occur as either dose-related bone marrow suppression or idiosyncratic aplastic anemia. Reversible bone marrow depression with anemia, leukopenia, and thrombocytopenia occurs as a result of a direct pharmacologic effect of the drug on hematopoiesis. High doses (>4 g/day), prolonged therapy, and excessively high levels in serum (>20 μg/ml) predispose patients to develop this type of complication. The second form of bone marrow toxicity is a rare but usually fatal complication that manifests as aplastic anemia. This response is not dose related, and the precise mechanism is unknown. It can occur weeks to months after the use of chloramphenicol, and it can develop after the use of oral, intravenous, or topical preparations.

Gray baby syndrome, characterized by vomiting, abdominal distention, cyanosis, hypothermia, and circulatory collapse, may occur in premature infants and neonates. This toxicity results from the immature hepatic function of neonates, which impairs hepatic inactivation of the drug. Reversible optic neuritis causing decreased visual acuity has been reported in patients receiving prolonged therapy. Chloramphenicol can occasionally cause hypersensitivity reactions, including skin rashes, drug fevers, and anaphylaxis. It potentiates the action of warfarin, phenytoin, and oral hypoglycemic agents by competitive inhibition of hepatic microsomal enzymes.

METRONIDAZOLE

Metronidazole is a 5-nitroimidazole derivative that was first introduced in 1959 for the treatment of *Trichomonas vaginalis* infections. It now has an important therapeutic role in the treatment of infections due to anaerobic bacteria and certain protozoan parasites. Tinidazole, a second-generation 5-nitroimidazole compound, is approved in the United States for treatment of trichomoniasis, giardiasis, and amebiasis.

Mechanism of Action

Metronidazole owes its bactericidal activity to the nitro group of its chemical structure. After the drug gains entry into the cells of susceptible organisms, the nitro group is reduced by a nitroreductase enzyme in the cytoplasm, generating certain short-lived, highly cytotoxic intermediate compounds or free radicals that disrupt host DNA (85). Resistance to nitroimidazoles may be due to decreased uptake of the drug or inducible production of 5-nitroimidazole reductase enzyme that can scavenge the free-radical intermediates (205).

Pharmacology

Metronidazole can be administered via the topical, oral, or intravenous route. It is absorbed rapidly and almost completely when given orally. Peak levels in serum of 6 μg/ml are obtained 1 h after an oral dose of 250 mg. Intravenous doses of 7.5 mg/kg result in peak concentrations in serum of 20 to 25 μg/ml. The drug has a half-life in serum of 8 h. Therapeutic levels are achieved in all body tissues and fluids, including abscess cavities and CSF, even without meningeal inflammation. The drug crosses the placenta and is secreted in breast milk. It is metabolized mainly in the liver, and 60 to 80% is excreted in the kidney. With impaired hepatic function, plasma clearance of metronidazole is delayed and dosage adjustments are necessary. The pharmacokinetics are minimally affected by renal insufficiency. Metronidazole and its metabolites are removed completely by dialysis.

Spectrum of Activity

Metronidazole exhibits potent activity against almost all anaerobic bacteria, including the *B. fragilis* group, *Fusobacterium*, and *Clostridium* (26). It is the only antimicrobial agent with consistent bactericidal activity against members of the *B. fragilis* group. However, the susceptibility of gram-positive anaerobic cocci is somewhat variable, with MIC$_{90}$s of 16 μg/ml for these organisms. Most strains of the genera *Actinomyces, Arachnia,* and *Propionibacterium* are resistant. Frequencies of metronidazole-resistant *B. fragilis* group isolates (MICs of >16 μg/ml) in the range of 2% to 5% have been reported from various institutions (4, 325). Tinidazole is somewhat more potent than metronidazole in its antianaerobe activities (57). Nitroimidazoles have no activity against aerobic bacteria, including the *Enterobacteriaceae.*

The drug is effective in the treatment of antibiotic-associated colitis caused by *C. difficile* (27), with efficacy equivalent to that of oral vancomycin for this indication (344). It is also useful in combination with an aminoglycoside for treating polymicrobial soft tissue infections and mixed aerobic-anaerobic intra-abdominal and pelvic infections.

Metronidazole and tinidazole are active against the protozoa *Trichomonas vaginalis, Giardia lamblia,* and *Entamoeba histolytica.* It is the drug of choice for the treatment of trichomoniasis, giardiasis, and intestinal and invasive amebiasis, including amebic liver abscess (118, 229).

Adverse Effects

Metronidazole is generally well tolerated, and adverse side effects are uncommon. It can cause mild gastrointestinal symptoms such as nausea, abdominal cramps, and diarrhea. An unpleasant, metallic taste may be experienced with oral therapy. Metronidazole can potentiate the effect of warfarin and prolong the prothrombin time.

Although metronidazole is carcinogenic in mice and rats, there is no evidence for carcinogenicity in humans. However, use of this agent in pregnancy, especially during the first trimester, and in nursing mothers should be avoided.

RIFAMYCINS

Rifamycins are a group of macrocyclic compounds produced by the mold *Streptomyces mediterranei.* Rifampin, also known as rifampicin and a semisynthetic antibiotic derived from rifamycin B, was the first of this class of drugs introduced for clinical use in 1968 as an effective antituberculous drug. A closely related compound, rifabutin, a derivative of rifamycin S, is another potent antimycobacterial agent, especially against *M. avium* complex (259). Rifaximin, a derivative of rifampin, possesses an additional pyridoimidazole ring and is a nonabsorbed oral drug used for therapy of uncomplicated traveler's diarrhea.

Mechanism of Action

Rifamycins exert their bactericidal effects by forming a stable complex with bacterial DNA-dependent RNA polymerase, preventing the chain initiation process of DNA transcription (368). Mammalian RNA synthesis is not affected, because the mammalian enzyme is much less sensitive to the drug. Rifampin-resistant isolates possess an altered RNA polymerase enzyme that arises easily from single-step mutations during monotherapy with rifampin.

Pharmacology

Rifampin is well absorbed after oral administration, reaching peak concentrations in serum of 5 to 10 μg/ml in 2 to 4 h following a 600-mg dose. A parenteral preparation is also available. Rifampin is deacetylated in the liver to an active metabolite and excreted in the bile, and it undergoes enterohepatic circulation. The normal half-life in serum varies from 1.5 to 5 h. The drug distributes well to almost all body tissues and fluids, reaching concentrations equal to or exceeding that in the serum. Levels in the CSF are highest in the presence of inflamed meninges. Rifampin is able to enter phagocytes and kill living intracellular organisms (214), and it crosses the placenta. About 30 to 40% of the drug is excreted in the urine, and it does not accumulate in patients with impaired renal function. Hemodialysis and peritoneal dialysis do not eliminate the drug. Dosage adjustments are necessary for patients with severe hepatic dysfunction.

Due to an additional pyridoimidazole ring in its chemical structure, rifaximin is largely unabsorbed after oral administration, with >99% of the drug present in the stool, and <1% of an oral dose is detectable in plasma of both healthy volunteers and persons with damaged intestinal mucosa (157). Average fecal concentrations of the drug reach 8,000 μg/g on the third day of therapy at an oral dose of 400 mg twice daily (163).

Spectrum of Activity

In addition to its well-known antimycobacterial effects (59), rifampin has a wide spectrum of antimicrobial activity. It is bactericidal against gram-positive cocci such as staphylococci (including methicillin-resistant strains), streptococci, and anaerobic cocci, with MICs in the range of 0.01 to 0.5 μg/ml. It remains an important adjunct in the combination therapy of serious and chronic staphylococcal infections (36, 107, 270). However, it is bacteriostatic against enterococci, with usual MICs of <16 μg/ml (240).

N. gonorrhoeae, N. meningitidis, and *H. influenzae,* including β-lactamase-producing strains, are susceptible to rifampin, which is used frequently in the prophylaxis of meningococcal and *H. influenzae* type b meningitis (140). MICs for *Enterobacteriaceae* are ≤12 μg/ml, while MICs for *S. marcescens* and *P. aeruginosa* are higher (240). Besides fluoroquinolones, rifampin is one of the most active agents against *L. pneumophila* and other *Legionella* spp., with MICs of ≤0.03 μg/ml. Because of its ability to enter phagocytes, rifampin inhibits the intracellular growth of *Brucella* spp. and *C. burnetii* (286), and it is used frequently in the combination therapy of infections due to these organisms. Although *Chlamydia* spp. are very susceptible to rifampin in vitro, resistance emerges rapidly when rifampin is used alone.

Rifaximin has broad-spectrum inhibitory activity against enteric bacterial pathogens, including enterotoxigenic and enteroaggregative strains of *E. coli, Aeromonas, Shigella,* and *Salmonella,* with MIC$_{90}$s ranging from 4 to 16 μg/ml (157, 297). Although it is less active against *C. jejuni* (MIC$_{90}$ of 512 μg/ml), *Y. enterocolitica* (MIC$_{90}$ of 128 μg/ml), *C. difficile* (MIC$_{90}$ of 128 μg/ml), and *H. pylori* (MIC$_{50}$ of 4 μg/ml), concentrations of rifaximin achieved in the intestinal lumen are >10-fold higher than the MICs of the drug for these pathogens. This drug has been used successfully to treat and prevent uncomplicated traveler's diarrhea (184).

Adverse Effects

Rifampin has many side effects, including gastrointestinal discomfort and hypersensitivity reactions, such as drug fever, skin rashes, and eosinophilia. It produces a harmless, orange-red coloration of saliva, tears, urine, and sweat. In up to 20% of patients, an influenza-like syndrome with fever, chills, arthralgias, and myalgias may develop after several months of intermittent therapy (136). This immunologic reaction may be associated with hemolytic anemia, thrombocytopenia, and renal failure. Rifampin-induced hepatitis occurs in <1% of patients and is more frequent during concurrent isoniazid therapy for tuberculosis. As a result of its ability to induce human hepatic cytochrome P450 enzyme, rifampin has clinically significant interactions with many drugs, such as antagonizing the effect of oral contraceptives and diminishing the anticoagulant activity of warfarin.

Headache, nausea, abdominal pain, and fatigue are the most frequent side effects reported for rifaximin. Rare hypersensitivity reactions, including allergic dermatitis, rash, angioneurotic edema, urticaria, and pruritus, can occur with rifaximin, which is contraindicated in those who are allergic to rifampin (157). However, unlike rifampin, rifaximin does not cause clinically relevant interactions with drugs, because of lack of systemic absorption of this drug.

NITROFURANTOIN

Nitrofurantoin belongs to a class of compounds consisting of a primary nitro group joined to a heterocyclic ring. Its role in human therapeutics is limited to treatment of urinary tract infections (155).

Mechanism of Action

Nitrofurantoin exerts its antibacterial effects via multiple mechanisms. At high concentrations, nitrofurantoin is converted by bacterial nitroreductases to highly reactive electrophilic intermediates that bind nonspecifically to bacterial ribosomal proteins and rRNA, causing complete cessation of synthesis of bacterial DNA, RNA, and proteins (225). It inhibits the inducible synthesis of essential bacterial enzymes (β-galactosidase and galactokinase) at concentrations near the MICs of susceptible organisms and disrupts bacterial metabolism, in the absence of reductive activation of the drug (225). Despite nearly 60 years of clinical use, development of bacterial resistance has not been a significant problem for this drug.

Pharmacology

The drug is available in microcrystalline (Furadantin) and macrocrystalline (Macrodantin) forms. It is administered orally and is well absorbed from the gastrointestinal tract. Very low levels of the drug are achieved in serum and most body tissues after usual oral doses. With a half-life in serum of about 20 min, two-thirds of the drug is rapidly metabolized and inactivated in various tissues. The remaining one-third is excreted unchanged into the urine. An average dose of nitrofurantoin yields a concentration in urine of 50 to 250 μg/ml in patients with healthy renal function. In alkaline urine, more of the drug is dissociated into the ionized form, with lowered antibacterial activity. Nitrofurantoin accumulates in the sera of patients with creatinine clearances of <60 ml/min. The drug is removed by hemodialysis. The risk of systemic toxicity increases in the presence of severe uremia. It is contraindicated in patients with significant renal impairment and hepatic failure.

Spectrum of Activity

Nitrofurantoin has a broad spectrum of antibacterial activity against gram-positive and gram-negative bacteria, particularly the common urinary tract pathogens. It is active against gram-positive cocci, such as *S. aureus*, *S. epidermidis*, *Staphylococcus saprophyticus*, and *E. faecalis*, with MICs in the range of 4 to 25 μg/ml (153). *S. pneumoniae*, *S. pyogenes*, and *Corynebacterium* spp. are also susceptible, but they rarely cause urinary tract infections. Over 90% of *E. coli* and many coliform bacteria are susceptible to nitrofurantoin at MICs of <32 μg/ml. However, only one-third of *Enterobacter* and *Klebsiella* isolates are susceptible. *Pseudomonas* and most *Proteus* spp. are resistant. Susceptible organisms rarely become resistant to this drug during therapy.

Adverse Effects

Gastrointestinal irritation with anorexia, nausea, and vomiting is the most common side effect. Diarrhea and abdominal cramps may occur. Hypersensitivity reactions, such as drug fever, chills, arthralgia, skin rashes, and a lupus-like syndrome, have been observed (154). Pulmonary reactions are the most common serious side effects associated with nitrofurantoin use. Acute pneumonitis with fever, cough, dyspnea, eosinophilia, and pulmonary infiltrates present on chest radiographs can occur after a few days of therapy (154). This immunologically mediated reaction is more common in elderly patients and is rapidly reversible after cessation of therapy. Chronic pulmonary reactions with interstitial pneumonitis leading to irreversible pulmonary fibrosis can occur in patients on continuous therapy for 6 months or more (231).

Peripheral polyneuropathy is a serious side effect that occurs more often in patients with renal failure. Hemolytic anemia, megaloblastic anemia, and bone marrow suppression with leukopenia can occur. Rare hepatotoxic reactions, such as cholestatic jaundice and chronic active hepatitis, have been reported (314).

FOSFOMYCIN

Fosfomycin, first isolated from cultures of *Streptomyces* spp. in 1969, is a phosphonic acid derivative originally named phosphonomycin (333). In the United States, it is used as single-dose therapy for uncomplicated urinary tract infections due to susceptible organisms (155).

Mechanism of Action

Fosfomycin is bactericidal by inhibiting UDP-*N*-acetyl-glucosamine enolpyruvyl transferase (MurA), a bacterial cytoplasmic enzyme that catalyzes the formation of uridine diphosphate-*N*-acetylmuramic acid during the initial step of peptidoglycan synthesis (174). There is little cross-resistance between fosfomycin and other antibacterial agents, most likely because it differs from other agents in its chemical structure and site of action. Resistance to fosfomycin can occur by three mechanisms: (i) mutations of the structural or regulatory genes for the bacterial proteins (GlpT and UhpT) that transport the drug into the cell, (ii) plasmid-mediated production of a drug-inactivating enzyme (FosA), and (iii) overproduction of the target enzyme MurA (256, 343).

Pharmacology

Originally formulated as sodium and calcium salts for oral and intravenous use, fosfomycin is available in the United

States as an oral, water-soluble tromethamine salt. Following oral administration, it is rapidly absorbed and converted to the free acid fosfomycin. With markedly improved oral bioavailability (35 to 40%), fosfomycin has a mean elimination half-life of 5.5 h, and it is primarily excreted unchanged in the urine (265). Following a single oral dose of 3 g, peak serum concentrations (range, 22 to 32 μg/ml) are achieved in 2 h after administration, with peak urinary concentrations (1,000 to 4,400 μg/ml) occurring within 4 h and remaining high (>128 μg/ml) for 24 to 48 h, sufficient to inhibit most urinary tract pathogens. Peak urinary concentrations are reached later and lowered when the drug is administered with food or antiperistaltic agents. In patients with renal impairment (creatinine clearance, <30 ml/min), peak serum concentrations of fosfomycin are increased, with decreased urinary elimination and reduced urinary concentrations of the drug.

While not bound to plasma protein, it is widely distributed in various body fluids and tissues, including kidneys, prostate, and seminal vesicles, from which it is cleared slowly. Although it crosses the placental barrier, the drug can be used safely during pregnancy if clearly needed.

Spectrum of Activity

Fosfomycin has a broad spectrum of antibacterial activity against most gram-positive and gram-negative bacteria isolated from patients with lower urinary tract infections. *E. coli, Serratia, Klebsiella, Citrobacter, Enterobacter* spp., *S. aureus*, and enterococci are generally inhibited by fosfomycin at concentrations of <64 μg/ml (21, 265). Fosfomycin is bactericidal at concentrations that are similar to the MIC values, at ≤2-fold differences. It is more active than TMP and nalidixic acid, while similar to norfloxacin and cotrimoxazole, in its activity against these organisms (21). At a breakpoint concentration of ≤128 μg/ml, 60%, 20%, and 80% of isolates of *Pseudomonas* spp., *Morganella morganii*, and *S. saprophyticus*, respectively, are susceptible to fosfomycin (274). In multiple-dose use, bacterial resistance to fosfomycin emerges rapidly, and it can be chromosomal or, more rarely, plasmid mediated. However, cross-resistance with other antimicrobials has been uncommon (287).

The in vitro activity of fosfomycin is affected by test medium and conditions (265, 274). Fosfomycin has much greater in vitro activity, and closer correlation with in vivo activity, when the test medium is supplemented with glucose-6-phosphate at 25 μg/ml, which is recommended for susceptibility testing with the agar and broth dilution methods. The disk diffusion testing method utilizes disks containing 200 μg of fosfomycin tromethamine and 50 or 100 μg of glucose-6-phosphate.

Adverse Effects

Mild, self-limiting gastrointestinal disturbances, mainly diarrhea, are the most frequent side effects (3% to 5%). Other minor adverse events include headaches, dizziness, rash, and vaginitis.

METHENAMINE

Methenamine is a tertiary amine with properties of a monoacidic base; it is used as a urinary antiseptic. To be activated, it is combined chemically with a poorly metabolized acid and administered as the mandelate (Mandelamine) or hippurate (Hiprex or Urex) salt.

Mechanism of Action

Methenamine has no antibacterial action by itself, but it is converted at acid pH to ammonia and formaldehyde, which provides the antiseptic action. This hydrolytic process occurs in the urine, and an effective bacteriostatic concentration of formaldehyde is reached at a urine pH of <5.5. Since the serum is at physiologic pH, formaldehyde is not released while methenamine circulates in the body.

Pharmacology

The agent is well absorbed from the gastrointestinal tract and is rapidly excreted in the urine. The elimination half-life of methenamine is about 4 h. At a urinary pH of 5.0, about 20% of methenamine excreted in the urine is hydrolyzed to formaldehyde and ammonia. Bactericidal levels (>20 mg/ml) of formaldehyde are generated in the bladder urine at 2 h after oral administration and may be maintained for at least 6 h or until the patient voids (182). The mandelate and hippurate moieties are also rapidly excreted in the urine in active, unchanged forms by glomerular filtration and tubular secretion. The agent is contraindicated in patients with hepatic insufficiency because of the ammonia produced.

Spectrum of Activity

With the liberation of enough formaldehyde into the urine, methenamine is essentially active against all gram-positive and gram-negative bacteria and also against fungi (182). However, it is not effective for treating urinary tract infections due to urea-splitting organisms such as *Proteus* and *Morganella*, which can convert urea to ammonium hydroxide, thereby preventing the hydrolysis of methenamine to formaldehyde. Combination with acetohydroxamic acid, a urease inhibitor, has been suggested for treating these infections by *Proteus* and *Morganella*. Since bacteria and fungi do not become resistant to formaldehyde, emergence of resistance to methenamine is not a problem.

Methenamine is not useful for acute urinary tract infections. It has been used successfully as prophylactic therapy for recurrent bacteriuria, particularly those caused by highly resistant gram-negative bacilli or yeasts. It is also effective as prolonged suppressive therapy for chronic bacteriuria in the absence of structural abnormalities of the urinary tract.

Adverse Effects

Methenamine and its acid salts are generally well tolerated. Some patients may develop nausea, vomiting, abdominal cramps, and diarrhea. High doses or prolonged administration of the drug can cause urinary tract irritation by the free formaldehyde, resulting in urinary frequency, dysuria, albuminuria, and hematuria. Skin rashes may also occur. To avoid precipitation of urate crystals in the urine, methenamine salts should not be used in patients with gout or hyperuricemia.

BACITRACIN

Originally isolated from *Bacillus licheniformis* (formerly *B. subtilis*), bacitracin is a peptide antibiotic consisting of peptide-linked amino acids. Although it was introduced initially for the systemic treatment of severe staphylococcal infections, it is now mainly restricted to topical use because of its systemic toxicity.

Bacitracin inhibits dephosphorylation of a lipid pyrophosphate, a step essential for bacterial cell wall synthesis. It also disrupts the bacterial cytoplastic membrane. Bacitracin is often used in various topical preparations, such as creams, ointments, antibiotic sprays and powders, and solutions for wound irrigation or bladder instillation. When used as a topical antibiotic, no significant amount of bacitracin is absorbed systemically. Large doses used to irrigate serous cavities may be associated with systemic toxicity.

This drug is active mainly against gram-positive bacteria, especially staphylococci and group A beta-hemolytic streptococci. However, group C and G streptococci are less susceptible, while group B streptococci are resistant (104). *Neisseria* spp. are also susceptible, but gram-negative bacilli are resistant. Bacitracin is often combined with neomycin, polymyxin B, or both in topical preparations to provide broad-spectrum antibacterial coverage. Orally administered bacitracin is effective in treating antibiotic-associated C. *difficile* colitis (82).

Systemic administration of bacitracin results in significant nephrotoxicity. Side effects are rare when the drug is given orally or applied topically. The drug is nonirritating to skin or mucous membranes. Allergic skin sensitization is rare. ■

MUPIROCIN

Mupirocin, formerly pseudomonic acid A, is a topical antibacterial agent derived from the fermentation products of *Pseudomonas fluorescens* (115). It contains a unique 9-hydroxynonanoic acid moiety in its chemical structure, and it inhibits isoleucyl-tRNA synthetase, resulting in cessation of bacterial protein synthesis (158). Low-level resistance (MICs of 4 to 256 µg/ml) results from an altered synthetase enzyme due to mutations in the bacterial chromosomal *ileS* gene, whereas high-level, transferable resistance (MIC of ≥512 µg/ml) is mediated by the *mupA* gene that encodes an entirely different synthetase.

Originally developed for the topical treatment of superficial soft tissue infections, particularly those due to staphylococci, mupirocin is available as a 2% ointment or cream in the United States. After topical application, <1% of the drug is absorbed systemically, with no detectable levels in the urine or feces. Penetration into deeper dermal layers of the skin is increased with traumatized skin or use of occlusive dressings. The drug is highly protein bound (95%), and its activity is lowered in the presence of serum. It is most active at moderately acid pH, with no inoculum effect (364). Mupirocin is slowly metabolized in the skin to the inactive monic acid.

It has excellent in vitro activity, primarily against the gram-positive cocci. S. *aureus*, including MRSA, and coagulase-negative staphylococci are uniformly very susceptible, with MIC90s of <0.5 µg/ml (50). Emergence of resistant strains of staphylococci can occur with widespread use of mupirocin (39, 40, 351). Most streptococci (including S. *pneumoniae*, beta-hemolytic streptococci of groups A, B, C, and G, and viridans group streptococci) are inhibited by concentrations of ≤1 µg/ml. Resistant bacteria include enterococci, *Corynebacterium* spp., *Erysipelothrix* spp., *P. acnes*, gram-positive anaerobes, and most gram-negative bacteria. However, H. *influenzae*, N. *gonorrhoeae*, N. *meningitidis*, M. *catarrhalis*, B. *pertussis*, and *P. multocida* are quite susceptible, with MICs in the range of 0.02 to 0.025 µg/ml. There is no cross-resistance between mupirocin and other major groups of antibiotics. Clinically, mupirocin is efficacious in the therapy of superficial skin infections, such as impetigo, folliculitis, and burn wound infections that are caused by staphylococci or streptococci (126). Although this drug has been used successfully to eradicate nasal carriage of S. *aureus*, including methicillin-resistant strains (354), it may not prevent nosocomial S. *aureus* infections (370).

No systemic toxic effects have been reported with mupirocin. Local irritation, such as burning, stinging, itch, and rash, which may be due to the polyethylene glycol base in the vehicle ointment, may occur.

RETAPAMULIN

Retapamulin belongs to a new class of antibiotics called pleuromutilins, which are derived from a fermentation product of *Pleurotus mutilus* (an edible mushroom). This class of agents selectively inhibits the elongation phase of bacterial protein synthesis by preventing normal formation of active 50S ribosomal subunits and interfering with peptide bond formation (386). Low-level resistance to retapamulin has been induced in vitro with stepwise mutations in the *rplC* gene that encodes the bacterial ribosomal protein L3 (119), but the frequency of such resistance is very low and high-level mutational resistance is unlikely to occur. However, a recently described plasmid-mediated gene (*cfr*) encodes an enzyme that methylates the ribosomal binding site for pleuromutilins and leads to cross-resistance to lincosamides, oxazolidinones, chloramphenicol, and streptogramin B (229).

Retapamulin is active against S. *aureus*, S. *pyogenes*, S. *agalactiae*, and viridans group streptococci at very low concentrations (MIC90s of 0.03 to 0.5 µg/ml), including MRSA and isolates resistant to β-lactams, macrolides, quinolones, and mupirocin, without target-specific cross-resistance to other antibacterial agents (312, 387). More than one-half of the strains of MRSA and S. *aureus* highly resistant to mupirocin and fusidic acid remain susceptible to this drug (384). It is also active against S. *pneumoniae*, H. *influenzae*, M. *catarrhalis*, and most anaerobes, including P. *acnes*. Retapamulin is licensed in the United States as a 1% ointment for the topical treatment of impetigo caused by MSSA and S. *pyogenes*.

No systemic toxic effects have occurred with the topical use of retapamulin. Irritation, itching, pain, rash, and contact dermatitis at the application site were reported in <2% of patients in clinical studies of this drug.

APPENDIX
Approximate Concentrations of Antibacterial Agents in Serum

The concentrations of antimicrobial agents listed in the table below are approximations taken from various reports and publications. Several factors can influence the level of antimicrobial agent in individual patients, including inherent differences in the patients themselves, their physical condition, the dosages, and the routes of administration. The values can also be influenced by the assay methods used to obtain them. Therefore, these concentrations should be used only as approximate values, and clinicians should use their knowledge of the patient and the drugs, the recommendations from U.S. Food and Drug Administration-approved package inserts, or other reputable sources in planning their therapeutic regimens.

Approximate antibacterial concentrations in serum

Antimicrobial agent	Serum half-life (h)	Unit dose	Avg peak level in serum (μg/ml) [a]		
			p.o.	i.m.	i.v.[b]
Amikacin	2–2.5	7.5 mg/kg		15–20	20–40
Amoxicillin	1	500 mg	6–8		
Amoxicillin/clavulanate	1.3/1.0	250/125 mg	3.3 (amox)		
			1.5 (clav)		
		500/125 mg	6.5 (amox)		
			1.8 (clav)		
		875/125 mg	11.6 (amox)		
			2.2 (clav)		
		1,000/62.5 mg	17 (amox)		
			2.1 (clav)		
Ampicillin	1.1	500 mg	2.5–5	8–10	
		1 g			40
Ampicillin/sulbactam	1.1/1.0	3 g			120 (amp)
					60 (sulb)
		1.5 g			18 (amp)
					13 (sulb)
Azithromycin	48	500 mg	0.4		3.5
Azlocillin	1	2 g			130
Aztreonam	1.7	1 g		45	90–160
Bacampicillin	1.1	800 mg	13		
Carbenicillin	1.1	1 g		20–30	150
Carbenicillin indanyl sodium	1.1	764 mg	10		
Cefaclor	0.6	500 mg	16		
Cefadroxil	1.5	500 mg	10		
Cefamandole	0.5–1	1 g		20–36	90–140
Cefazolin	1.8	1 g		65	185
Cefepime	2	1 g		30	82
Cefdinir	1.7	300 mg	1.6		
Cefditoren	1.6	200 mg	3.1		
		400 mg	4.4		
Cefixime	3–4	400 mg	3.5		
Cefmetazole	1.5	1 g			70
Cefonicid	4	1 g		98	220
Cefoperazone	2	1 g		65–75	153
Ceforanide	3	1 g		70	125
Cefotaxime	1	1 g		20	40–45
Cefotetan	3–4.5	1 g		50–80	160
Cefoxitin	1	1 g		20–25	55–110
Cefpirome	2	1 g		45	85
Cefpodoxime	2.5	200 mg	2.3		
Cefprozil	1.5	500 mg	10.5		
Ceftazidime	2	1 g		40	70
Cethromycin[c]	5	150 mg	0.2		
		300 mg	0.5		
Ceftibuten	2.5	400 mg	15		
Ceftizoxime	1.5	1 g		39	80–90
Ceftobiprole[c]	3–4	500 mg			44
		750 mg			60
Ceftriaxone	6–9	500 mg		40–45	
		1 g			150
Cefuroxime	1.5	750 mg		27	50
Cefuroxime axetil	1.5	500 mg	9		
Cephalexin	0.9	500 mg	18		
Cephalothin	0.6	1 g			30–60
Cephapirin	0.6	1 g			40–70
Cephradine	0.8	500 mg	16		
Cefpirome[c]	2	1 g			80
		2 g			180
Ceftaroline[c]	2.6	600 mg		8.5	21

(Continued on next page)

Approximate antibacterial concentrations in serum (*Continued*)

Antimicrobial agent	Serum half-life (h)	Unit dose	Avg peak level in serum (μg/ml)[a]		
			p.o.	i.m.	i.v.[b]
Chloramphenicol	4	1 g	10–18		10–15
Chlortetracycline	6–9	500 mg	2–4	12	
Cinoxacin	1–1.5	500 mg	15		
Ciprofloxacin	5–6	400 mg			4.5
		500 mg	3.0		
		500 mg XR[d]	1.6		
		750 mg	4.0		
		1,000 mg XR[d]	3.1		
Clarithromycin	5–7	250 mg	1–2		
		500 mg	3–4		
		1,000 mg XL[d]	2–3		
Clinafloxacin	5.2	200 mg	1.5		
Clindamycin	2.5	300 mg	3	6	
		600 mg			10–12
Cloxacillin	0.5	500 mg	10		
Colistimethate sodium	2	150 mg		5–6	
Dalbavancin[c]	149–198	1 g			285
Daptomycin	9	4 mg/kg			70
		6 mg/kg			82
Demeclocycline	12	300 mg	1–2		
Dicloxacillin	0.5–0.7	500 mg	15		
Dirithromycin	40	500 mg	0.5		
Doxycycline	18–22	100 mg	2.5		4
Enoxacin	4–6	400 mg	3–5		
Ertapenem	4	1 g		70	155
Erythromycin	1.5	500 mg	2–3		
		1 g			10
Fleroxacin	12	400 mg	5		7–8
Fosfomycin	5.7	3 g	25		
		50 mg/kg			275
Fusidic acid	13–19	500 mg	25–30		50
Gatifloxacin	7	400 mg	4		4.5
Gemifloxacin	7–8	320 mg	1.8		
Gentamicin	2–3	1.5 mg/kg	4–6		4–8
Iclaprim[c]	2.3–3.6	60 mg			1.2
		160 mg	0.5		
Imipenem	1	500 mg			25–35
Kanamycin	2.2–3	7.5 mg/kg		20–25	
Levofloxacin	6–8	500 mg	5.5		6.5
		750 mg	8.5		12
Lincomycin	5	500 mg	3.5		
		600 mg		10	16–21
Linezolid	5	400 mg	11		
		600 mg	13		13
Loracarbef	1	400 mg	14		
Meropenem	1	500 mg			25–35
Methicillin	0.5	1 g	15		60
Metronidazole	8	500 mg	12		20–25
Mezlocillin	1	1 g			15
		3 g			260
Minocycline	14–16	100 mg	1		
Moxifloxacin	12	400 mg	4.5		4.5
Nafcillin	0.5	500 mg			5–8
		1 g			20–40
Nalidixic acid	1.5	1 g	20–50		
Netilmicin	2.5	2 mg/kg		5–7	6–8
Nitrofurantoin	0.3	100 mg	<2		
Norfloxacin	3.3	400 mg	1.5		
Ofloxacin	5	400 mg	4		

(*Continued on next page*)

Approximate antibacterial concentrations in serum (*Continued*)

Antimicrobial agent	Serum half-life (h)	Unit dose	Avg peak level in serum (μg/ml)[a]		
			p.o.	i.m.	i.v.[b]
Oritavancin[c]	136–274	0.5 mg/kg			6.5
		200 mg			25–35
Ornidazole	13	500 mg	10		20
Oxacillin	0.5	500 mg	4–6	14–16	
		1 g			40
Oxytetracycline	9	500 mg	1–2		
Pefloxacin[c]	10	400 mg	3		5.5
Penicillin G	0.5	500 mg	1.5–2.5		
Aqueous		1×10^6 U		8–10	10
Benzathine		1.2×10^6 U		0.1–0.15	
Procaine		1.2×10^6 U		3	
Penicillin V	0.5	500 mg	3–5		
Piperacillin	1.1	2 g			36
		4 g			240
Piperacillin-tazobactam	1.1/1.0	3.375 g			242 (pip)
					24 (tazo)
		4.5 g			298 (pip)
					34 (tazo)
Pivampicillin	0.5–1	350 mg	2		
Polymyxin B	6–7	2.5 mg/kg			5
Quinupristin-dalfopristin	1/0.75	7.5 mg/kg			3 (Q)
					7.5 (D)
Rifampin	2–5	600 mg	7–9		10
Spectinomycin	1–2	2 g		100	
Spiramycin	3.8	2 g	3		
Streptomycin	2–3	1 g		25–50	
Sulfadiazine	17	2 g	100–150		
Sulfadoxine	150–200	1 g	50–75		
Sulfamethizole	4–7	2 g	60		
Sulfamethoxazole	10–12	1 g	40		
Sulfisoxazole	5–7	2 g	170		
Teicoplanin[c]	45	200 mg		7	
		400 mg			20–40
Telavancin	6–8	7.5 mg/kg			88
		10 mg/kg			108
Telithromycin	9–10	800 mg	2		
Tetracycline	8	500 mg	4		8
Ticarcillin	1.2	1 g		20–30	
		3 g			190
Ticarcillin–clavulanate	1.2/1.0	3.1 g			330 (ticar)
					8 (clav)
Tigecycline	36	50 mg			0.8
Tinidazole	12–14	2 g	48		
Tobramycin	2–2.8	1.5 mg/kg		4–6	4–8
Trimethoprim	10–12	100 mg	1		
TMP–SMX		160/800 mg	3 (TMP)		9 (TMP)
			46 (SMX)		106 (SMX)
Vancomycin	6	500 mg			20–40

[a]p.o., oral; i.m., intramuscular; i.v., intravenous; amox, amoxicillin; clav, clavulanate; amp, ampicillin; sulb, sulbactam.
[b]At 30 min following intravenous infusion.
[c]Not licensed for clinical use in the United States.
[d]XR or XL, extended-release formulation.

REFERENCES

1. **Ackermann, G., and A. C. Rodloff.** 2003. Drugs of the 21st century: telithromycin (HMV 3647)—the first ketolide. *J. Antimicrob. Chemother.* **51:**497–511.

2. **Agwuh, K. N., and A. MacGowan.** 2006. Pharmacokinetics and pharmacodynamics of the tetracyclines including glycylcyclines. *J. Antimicrob. Chemother.* **58:**256–265.

3. **Albanese, J., M. Leone, B. Bruguerolle, M. L. Ayem, B. Lacarelle, and C. Martin.** 2000. Cerebrospinal fluid penetration and pharmacokinetics of vancomycin administered by continuous infusion to mechanically ventilated patients in an intensive care unit. *Antimicrob. Agents Chemother.* **44:**1356–1358.

4. **Aldridge, K. E., D. Ashcraft, K. Cambre, C. L. Pierson, S. G. Jenkins, and J. E. Rosenblatt.** 2001. Multicenter survey of the changing in vitro antimicrobial susceptibilities of clinical isolates of *Bacteroides fragilis* group, *Prevotella*, *Fusobacterium*, *Porphyromonas*, and *Peptostreptococcus* species. *Antimicrob. Agents Chemother.* **45:**1238–1243.

5. **Anderson, V. R., and C. M. Perry.** 2008. Levofloxacin: a review of its use as a high-dose, short-course treatment for bacterial infection. *Drugs* **68:**535–565.

6. **Appelbaum, P. C., M. R. Jacobs, S. K. Spangler, and S. Yamabe.** 1986. Comparative activity of beta-lactamase inhibitors YTR 830, clavulanate, and sulbactam combined with beta-lactams against beta-lactamase-producing anaerobes. *Antimicrob. Agents Chemother.* **30:**789–791.

7. **Arbeit, R. D., D. Maki, F. P. Tally, E. Campanaro, B. I. Eisenstein, and the Daptomycin Investigators, 98-01 and 99-01.** 2004. The safety and efficacy of daptomycin for the treatment of complicated skin and skin-structure infections. *Clin. Infect. Dis.* **38:**1673–1681.

8. **Arhin, F. F., D. C. Draghi, C. M. Pillar, T. R. Parr, Jr., G. Moeck, and D. F. Sahm.** 2009. Comparative in vitro activity profile of oritavancin against recent gram-positive clinical isolates. *Antimicrob. Agents Chemother.* **53:**4762–4771.

9. **Arias, C. A., K. V. Singh, D. Panesso, and B. E. Murray.** 2007. Time-kill and synergism studies of ceftobiprole against *Enterococcus faecalis*, including beta-lactamase-producing and vancomycin-resistant isolates. *Antimicrob. Agents Chemother.* **51:**2043–2047.

10. **Aswapokee, N., and H. C. Neu.** 1978. A sulfone beta-lactam compound which acts as a beta-lactamase inhibitor. *J. Antibiot.* (Tokyo) **31:**1238–1244.

11. **Attassi, K., E. Hershberger, R. Alam, and M. J. Zervos.** 2002. Thrombocytopenia associated with linezolid therapy. *Clin. Infect. Dis.* **34:**695–698.

12. **Attwood, R. J., and K. L. LaPlante.** 2007. Telavancin: a novel lipoglycopeptide antimicrobial agent. *Am. J. Health Syst. Pharm.* **64:**2335–2348.

13. **Baciewicz, A. M., A. Al-Nimir, and P. Whelan.** 2005. Azithromycin-induced hepatotoxicity. *Am. J. Med.* **118:**1438–1439.

14. **Baddour, L. M., W. R. Wilson, A. S. Bayer, V. G. Fowler, Jr., A. F. Bolger, M. E. Levison, P. Ferrieri, M. A. Gerber, L. Y. Tani, M. H. Gewitz, D. C. Tong, J. M. Steckelberg, R. S. Baltimore, S. T. Shulman, J. C. Burns, D. A. Falace, J. W. Newburger, T. J. Pallasch, M. Takahashi, and K. A. Taubert.** 2005. Infective endocarditis: diagnosis, antimicrobial therapy, and management of complications. *Circulation* **111:**394–434.

15. **Bailey, J., and K. M. Summers.** 2008. Dalbavancin: a new lipoglycopeptide antibiotic. *Am. J. Health Syst. Pharm.* **65:**599–610.

16. **Baldwin, C. M., K. A. Lyseng-Williamson, and S. J. Keam.** 2008. Meropenem: a review of its use in the treatment of serious bacterial infections. *Drugs* **68:**803–838.

17. **Balfour, J. A., and D. P. Figgitt.** 2001. Telithromycin. *Drugs* **61:**815–829.

18. **Ball, P.** 2000. Quinolone generations: natural history or natural selection? *J. Antimicrob. Chemother.* **46**(Suppl. 1):17–24.

19. **Ball, P., L. Mandell, Y. Niki, and G. Tillotson.** 1999. Comparative tolerability of the newer fluoroquinolone antibacterials. *Drug Saf.* **21:**407–421.

20. **Bansal, M. B., S. K. Chuah, and H. Thadepalli.** 1985. In vitro activity and in vivo evaluation of ticarcillin plus clavulanic acid against aerobic and anaerobic bacteria. *Am. J. Med.* **79:**33–38.

21. **Barry, A. L., and S. D. Brown.** 1995. Antibacterial spectrum of fosfomycin trometamol. *J. Antimicrob. Chemother.* **35:**228–230.

22. **Barry, A. L., P. C. Fuchs, and S. D. Brown.** 2001. In vitro activities of daptomycin against 2,789 clinical isolates from 11 North American medical centers. *Antimicrob. Agents Chemother.* **45:**1919–1922.

23. **Barry, A. L., and R. N. Jones.** 1987. Cefixime: spectrum of antibacterial activity against 16,016 clinical isolates. *Pediatr. Infect. Dis. J.* **6:**954–957.

24. **Barry, A. L., R. N. Jones, and C. Thornsberry.** 1988. In vitro activities of azithromycin (CP 62,993), clarithromycin (A-56268; TE-031), erythromycin, roxithromycin, and clindamycin. *Antimicrob. Agents Chemother.* **32:**752–754.

25. **Barry, A. L., C. Thornsberry, R. N. Jones, and T. L. Gavan.** 1985. Aztreonam: antibacterial activity, beta-lactamase stability, and interpretive standards and quality control guidelines for disk-diffusion susceptibility tests. *Rev. Infect. Dis.* **7**(Suppl. 4):S594–S604.

26. **Bartlett, J. G.** 1982. Anti-anaerobic antibacterial agents. *Lancet* **ii:**478–481.

27. **Bartlett, J. G.** 1992. Antibiotic-associated diarrhea. *Clin. Infect. Dis.* **15:**573–581.

28. **Bassetti, M., E. Righi, and C. Viscoli.** 2008. Novel beta-lactam antibiotics and inhibitor combinations. *Expert Opin. Investig. Drugs* **17:**285–296.

29. **Bates, R. D., and M. C. Nahata.** 1994. Once-daily administration of aminoglycosides. *Ann. Pharmacother.* **28:**757–766.

30. **Bauernfeind, A.** 1993. In-vitro activity of dirithromycin in comparison with other new and established macrolides. *J. Antimicrob. Chemother.* **31**(Suppl. C):39–49.

31. **Bearden, D. T., M. M. Neuhauser, and K. W. Garey.** 2001. Telithromycin: an oral ketolide for respiratory infections. *Pharmacotherapy* **21:**1204–1222.

32. **Berkey, P., D. Moore, and K. Rolston.** 1988. In vitro susceptibilities of *Nocardia* species to newer antimicrobial agents. *Antimicrob. Agents Chemother.* **32:**1078–1079.

33. **Betriu, C., I. Rodriguez-Avial, M. Gomez, E. Culebras, and J. J. Picazo.** 2005. Changing patterns of fluoroquinolone resistance among *Bacteroides fragilis* group organisms over a 6-year period (1997–2002). *Diagn. Microbiol. Infect. Dis.* **53:**221–223.

34. **Biedenbach, D. J., R. N. Jones, and T. R. Fritsche.** 2008. Antimicrobial activity of cefditoren tested against contemporary (2004–2006) isolates of Haemophilus influenzae and Moraxella catarrhalis responsible for community-acquired respiratory tract infections in the United States. *Diagn. Microbiol. Infect. Dis.* **61:**240–244.

35. **Billeter, M., M. J. Zervos, A. Y. Chen, J. R. Dalovisio, and C. Kurukularatne.** 2008. Dalbavancin: a novel once-weekly lipoglycopeptide antibiotic. *Clin. Infect. Dis.* **46:**577–583.

36. **Bliziotis, I. A., F. Ntziora, K. R. Lawrence, and M. E. Falagas.** 2007. Rifampin as adjuvant treatment of gram-positive bacterial infections: a systematic review of comparative clinical trials. *Eur. J. Clin. Microbiol. Infect. Dis.* **26:**849–856.

37. **Bonora, M. G., M. Solbiati, E. Stepan, A. Zorzi, A. Luzzani, M. R. Catania, and R. Fontana.** 2006. Emergence of linezolid resistance in the vancomycin-resistant *Enterococcus faecium* multilocus sequence typing C1 epidemic lineage. *J. Clin. Microbiol.* **44:**1153–1155.

38. **Bouanchaud, D. H.** 1997. In-vitro and in-vivo antibacterial activity of quinupristin/dalfopristin. *J. Antimicrob. Chemother.* **39**(Suppl. A):15–21.

39. **Boyce, J. M.** 1996. Preventing staphylococcal infections by eradicating nasal carriage of *Staphylococcus aureus*: proceeding with caution. *Infect. Control. Hosp. Epidemiol.* **17:**775–779.

40. **Bradley, S. F., M. A. Ramsey, T. M. Morton, and C. A. Kauffman.** 1995. Mupirocin resistance: clinical and molecular epidemiology. *Infect. Control Hosp. Epidemiol.* **16:**354–358.

41. **Bressler, A. M., S. M. Zimmer, J. L. Gilmore, and J. Somani.** 2004. Peripheral neuropathy associated with prolonged use of linezolid. *Lancet Infect. Dis.* **4:**528–531.

42. **Brown-Elliott, B. A., C. J. Crist, L. B. Mann, R. W. Wilson, and R. J. Wallace, Jr.** 2003. In vitro activity of linezolid against slowly growing nontuberculous mycobacteria. *Antimicrob. Agents Chemother.* **47:**1736–1738.

43. **Brummett, R. E., and K. E. Fox.** 1989. Vancomycin- and erythromycin-induced hearing loss in humans. *Antimicrob. Agents Chemother.* **33:**791–796.

44. **Buesing, M. A., and J. H. Jorgensen.** 1984. In vitro activity of aztreonam in combination with newer beta-lactams and amikacin against multiply resistant gram-negative bacilli. *Antimicrob. Agents Chemother.* **25:**283–285.

45. **Bush, K., J. S. Freudenberger, and R. B. Sykes.** 1982. Interaction of azthreonam and related monobactams with beta-lactamases from gram-negative bacteria. *Antimicrob. Agents Chemother.* **22:**414–420.

46. **Bush, K., M. Heep, M. J. Macielag, and G. J. Noel.** 2007. Anti-MRSA beta-lactams in development, with a focus on ceftobiprole: the first anti-MRSA beta-lactam to demonstrate clinical efficacy. *Expert Opin. Investig. Drugs* **16:**419–429.

47. **Bushby, S. R.** 1973. Trimethoprim-sulfamethoxazole: in vitro microbiological aspects. *J. Infect. Dis.* **128**(Suppl.)**:**S442–S462.

48. **Carpenter, C. F., and H. F. Chambers.** 2004. Daptomycin: another novel agent for treating infections due to drug-resistant gram-positive pathogens. *Clin. Infect. Dis.* **38:**994–1000.

49. **Carroll, O. M., P. A. Bryan, and R. J. Robinson.** 1966. Stevens-Johnson syndrome associated with long-acting sulfonamides. *JAMA* **195:**691–693.

50. **Casewell, M. W., and R. L. Hill.** 1985. In-vitro activity of mupirocin (pseudomonic acid) against clinical isolates of *Staphylococcus aureus. J. Antimicrob. Chemother.* **15:**523–531.

51. **Centers for Disease Control and Prevention.** 2010. Sexually transmitted diseases treatment guidelines, 2010. *MMWR Morb. Mortal. Wkly. Rep.* **59**(RR-12)**:**1–110.

52. **Centers for Disease Control and Prevention.** 2009. Guidelines for the prevention and treatment of opportunistic infections among HIV-exposed and HIV-infected children. *MMWR Morb. Mortal. Wkly. Rep.* **58**(RR-11)**:**1–166.

53. **Cetinkaya, Y., P. Falk, and C. G. Mayhall.** 2000. Vancomycin-resistant enterococci. *Clin. Microbiol. Rev.* **13:**686–707.

54. **Cherubin, C. E.** 1981. Antibiotic resistance of *Salmonella* in Europe and the United States. *Rev. Infect. Dis.* **3:**1105–1126.

55. **Cherubin, C. E., and D. B. Azabache.** 1992. While nearly no one was watching: the rise of erythromycin and clindamycin resistance in *Streptococcus pneumoniae* and *Streptococcus pyogenes. Antimicrobic Newsl.* **8:**37–44.

56. **Chopra, I., and M. Roberts.** 2001. Tetracycline antibiotics: mode of action, applications, molecular biology, and epidemiology of bacterial resistance. *Microbiol. Mol. Biol. Rev.* **65:**232–260.

57. **Citron, D. M., K. L. Tyrrell, H. Fernandez, C. V. Merriam, and E. J. C. Goldstein.** 2005. In vitro activities of tinidazole and metronidazole against *Clostridium difficile, Prevotella bivia* and *Bacteroides fragilis. Anaerobe* **11:**315–317.

58. **Citron, D. M., K. L. Tyrrell, C. V. Merriam, and E. J. Goldstein.** 2010. In vitro activity of ceftaroline against 623 diverse strains of anaerobic bacteria. *Antimicrob. Agents Chemother.* **54:**1627–1632.

59. **Clark, J., and A. Wallace.** 1967. The susceptibility of mycobacteria to rifamide and rifampicin. *Tubercle* **48:**144–148.

60. **Clay, K. D., J. S. Hanson, S. D. Pope, R. W. Rissmiller, P. P. Purdum, and P. M. Banks.** 2006. Severe hepatotoxicity of telithromycin: three case reports and literature review. *Ann. Intern. Med.* **144:**E1–E6.

61. **Clemett, D., and A. Markham.** 2000. Linezolid. *Drugs* **59:**815–827.

62. **Cohen, M. A., E. T. Joannides, G. E. Roland, M. A. Meservey, M. D. Huband, M. A. Shapiro, J. C. Sesnie, and C. L. Heifetz.** 1994. In vitro evaluation of cefdinir (FK482), a new oral cephalosporin with enhanced antistaphylococcal activity and beta-lactamase stability. *Diagn. Microbiol. Infect. Dis.* **18:**31–39.

63. **Collins, L. A., G. M. Eliopoulos, C. B. Wennersten, M. J. Ferraro, and R. C. Moellering, Jr.** 1993. In vitro activity of ramoplanin against vancomycin-resistant gram-positive organisms. *Antimicrob. Agents Chemother.* **37:**1364–1366.

64. **Coppens, L., and J. Klastersky.** 1979. Comparative study of anti-pseudomonas activity of azlocillin, mezlocillin, and ticarcillin. *Antimicrob. Agents Chemother.* **15:**396–399.

65. **Copper, R. D.** 1992. The carbacephems: a new beta-lactam antibiotic class. *Am. J. Med.* **92**(Suppl. 6A)**:**2S–6S.

66. **Courvalin, P.** 2006. Vancomycin resistance in gram-positive cocci. *Clin. Infect. Dis.* **42**(Suppl. 1)**:**S25–S34.

67. **Craig, W. A.** 1997. The pharmacology of meropenem, a new carbapenem antibiotic. *Clin. Infect. Dis.* **24**(Suppl. 2)**:**S266–S275.

68. **Cui, L., E. Tominaga, H.-M. Neoh, and K. Hiramatsu.** 2006. Correlation between reduced daptomycin susceptibility and vancomycin resistance in vancomycin-intermediate *Staphylococcus aureus. Antimicrob. Agents Chemother.* **50:**1079–1082.

69. **Cynamon, M. H., and G. S. Palmer.** 1983. In vitro activity of amoxicillin in combination with clavulanic acid against *Mycobacterium tuberculosis. Antimicrob. Agents Chemother.* **24:**429–431.

70. **Dalhoff, A., and F. J. Schmitz.** 2003. In vitro antibacterial activity and pharmacodynamics of new quinolones. *Eur. J. Clin. Microbiol. Infect. Dis.* **22:**203–221.

71. **Dannemann, B., J. A. McCutchan, D. Israelski, D. Antoniskis, C. Leport, B. Luft, J. Nussbaum, N. Clumeck, P. Morlat, J. Chiu, J. L. Vilde, P. Haseltine, J. Leedom, J. Remington, M. Orellana, D. Feigal, A. Bartok, et al.** 1992. Treatment of toxoplasmic encephalitis in patients with AIDS: a randomized trial comparing pyrimethamine plus clindamycin to pyrimethamine plus sulfadiazine. *Ann. Intern. Med.* **116:**33–43.

72. **Das, B., A. V. Rajarao, S. Rudra, A. Yadav, A. Ray, M. Pandya, A. Rattan, and A. Mehta.** 2009. Synthesis and biological activity of novel oxazolidinones. *Bioorg. Med. Chem. Lett.* **19:**6424–6428.

73. **Davey, P. G., and A. H. Williams.** 1991. A review of the safety profile of teicoplanin. *J. Antimicrob. Chemother.* **27**(Suppl. B)**:**69–73.

74. **Davidson, R. N., M. den Boer, and K. Ritmeijer.** 2009. Paromomycin. *Trans. R. Soc. Trop. Med. Hyg.* **103:**653–660.

75. **Davies, J. E.** 1983. Resistance to aminoglycosides: mechanisms and frequency. *Rev. Infect. Dis.* **5**(Suppl. 2)**:**S261–S267.

76. **Davies, S., P. D. Sparham, and R. C. Spencer.** 1987. Comparative in-vitro activity of five fluoroquinolones against mycobacteria. *J. Antimicrob. Chemother.* **19:**605–609.

77. **Denton, M., and K. G. Kerr.** 1998. Microbiological and clinical aspects of infection associated with *Stenotrophomonas maltophilia. Clin. Microbiol. Rev.* **11:**57–80.

78. **Dewsnup, D. H., and D. N. Wright.** 1984. In vitro susceptibility of *Nocardia asteroides* to 25 antimicrobial agents. *Antimicrob. Agents Chemother.* **25:**165–167.

79. **Drawz, S. M., and R. A. Bonomo.** 2010. Three decades of beta-lactamase inhibitors. *Clin. Microbiol. Rev.* **23:**160–201.

80. **Drusano, G.** 2001. Pharmacodynamic and pharmacokinetic considerations in antimicrobial selection: focus on telithromycin. *Clin. Microbiol. Infect.* **7**(Suppl. 3)**:**24–29.

81. **Drusano, G. L., S. C. Schimpff, and W. L. Hewitt.** 1984. The acylampicillins: mezlocillin, piperacillin, and azlocillin. *Rev. Infect. Dis.* **6:**13–32.

82. **Dudley, M. N., J. C. McLaughlin, G. Carrington, J. Frick, C. H. Nightingale, and R. Quintiliani.** 1986. Oral bacitracin vs vancomycin therapy for *Clostridium difficile*-induced diarrhea: a randomized double-blind trial. *Arch. Intern. Med.* **146:**1101–1104.

83. **DuPont, H. L.** 2005. Travelers' diarrhea: antimicrobial therapy and chemoprevention. *Nat. Clin. Pract. Gastroenterol. Hepatol.* **2:**191–198.

84. **Eady, E. A., J. I. Ross, and J. H. Cove.** 1990. Multiple mechanisms of erythromycin resistance. *J. Antimicrob. Chemother.* **26:**461–465.

85. **Edwards, D. I.** 1993. Nitroimidazole drugs—action and resistance mechanisms. I. Mechanisms of action. *J. Antimicrob. Chemother.* **31:**9–20.

86. **Edwards, J. R.** 1995. Meropenem: a microbiological overview. *J. Antimicrob. Chemother.* **36**(Suppl. A):1–17.

87. **Eliopoulos, G. M., and C. T. Eliopoulos.** 1993. Activity in vitro of the quinolones, p. 161–193. *In* D. C. Hooper and J. S. Wolfson (ed.), *Quinolone Antimicrobial Agents,* 2nd ed. American Society for Microbiology, Washington, DC.

88. **Eliopoulos, G. M., K. Klimm, M. J. Ferraro, G. A. Jacoby, and R. C. Moellering, Jr.** 1989. Comparative in vitro activity of piperacillin combined with the beta-lactamase inhibitor tazobactam (YTR 830). *Diagn. Microbiol. Infect. Dis.* **12:**481–488.

89. **Engberg, J., F. M. Aarestrup, D. E. Taylor, P. Gerner-Smidt, and I. Nachamkin.** 2001. Quinolone and macrolide resistance in *Campylobacter jejuni* and *C. coli*: resistance mechanisms and trends in human isolates. *Emerg. Infect. Dis.* **7:**24–34.

90. **Falagas, M. E., and I. A. Bliziotis.** 2006. Quinolones for treatment of human brucellosis: critical review of the evidence from microbiological and clinical studies. *Antimicrob. Agents Chemother.* **50:**22–33.

91. **Falagas, M. E., and S. K. Kasiakou.** 2005. Colistin: the revival of polymyxins for the management of multidrug-resistant gram-negative bacterial infections. *Clin. Infect. Dis.* **40:**1333–1341.

92. **Falagas, M. E., I. I. Siempos, and K. Z. Vardakas.** 2008. Linezolid versus glycopeptide or beta-lactam for treatment of gram-positive bacterial infections: meta-analysis of randomised controlled trials. *Lancet Infect. Dis.* **8:**53–66.

93. **Farrell, D. J., and D. Felmingham.** 2004. Activities of telithromycin against 13,874 *Streptococcus pneumoniae* isolated collected between 1999 and 2003. *Antimicrob. Agents Chemother.* **48:**1882–1884.

94. **Farver, D. K., D. D. Hedge, and S. C. Lee.** 2005. Ramoplanin: a lipoglycodepsipeptide antibiotic. *Ann. Pharmacother.* **39:**863–868.

95. **Fass, R. J.** 1983. Comparative in vitro activities of third-generation cephalosporins. *Arch. Intern. Med.* **143:**1743–1745.

96. **Fass, R. J., E. A. Copelan, J. T. Brandt, M. L. Moeschberger, and J. J. Ashton.** 1987. Platelet-mediated bleeding caused by broad-spectrum penicillins. *J. Infect. Dis.* **155:**1242–1248.

97. **Fee, W. E., Jr.** 1980. Aminoglycoside ototoxicity in the human. *Laryngoscope* **90**(Suppl. 24):1–19.

98. **Fekete, T.** 1993. Antimicrobial susceptibility testing of *Neisseria gonorrhoeae* and implications for epidemiology and therapy. *Clin. Microbiol. Rev.* **6:**22–33.

99. **Fekety, R., J. Silva, B. Buggy, and H. G. Deery.** 1984. Treatment of antibiotic-associated colitis with vancomycin. *J. Antimicrob. Chemother.* **14**(Suppl. D):97–102.

100. **Felmingham, D.** 2001. Microbiological profile of telithromycin, the first ketolide antimicrobial. *Clin. Microbiol. Infect.* **7**(Suppl. 3):2–10.

101. **Fernandez-Mazarrasa, C., O. Mazarrasa, J. Calvo, A. del Arco, and L. Martinez-Martinez.** 2009. High concentrations of manganese in Mueller-Hinton agar increase MICs of tigecycline determined by Etest. *J. Clin. Microbiol.* **47:**827–829.

102. **Fernandez-Roblas, R., J. Esteban, F. Cabria, J. C. Lopez, M. S. Jimenez, and F. Soriano.** 2000. In vitro susceptibilities of rapidly growing mycobacteria to telithromycin (HMR 3647) and seven other antimicrobials. *Antimicrob. Agents Chemother.* **44:**181–182.

103. **Finch, R. G.** 1996. Antibacterial activity of quinupristin/dalfopristin: rationale for clinical use. *Drugs* **51**(Suppl. 1):31–37.

104. **Finland, M., C. Garner, C. Wilcox, and L. D. Sabath.** 1976. Susceptibility of beta-hemolytic streptococci to 65 antibacterial agents. *Antimicrob. Agents Chemother.* **9:**11–19.

105. **Finlay, J., L. Miller, and J. A. Poupard.** 2003. A review of the antimicrobial activity of clavulanate. *J. Antimicrob. Chemother.* **52:**18–23.

106. **Forouzesh, A., P. A. Moise, and G. Sakoulas.** 2009. Vancomycin ototoxicity: a reevaluation in an era of increasing doses. *Antimicrob. Agents Chemother.* **53:**483–486.

107. **Forrest, G. N., and K. Tamura.** 2010. Rifampin combination therapy for nonmycobacterial infections. *Clin. Microbiol. Rev.* **23:**14–34.

108. **Frampton, J. E., R. N. Brogden, H. D. Langtry, and M. M. Buckley.** 1992. Cefpodoxime proxetil: a review of its antibacterial activity, pharmacokinetic properties and therapeutic potential. *Drugs* **44:**889–917.

109. **Franceschi, F., Z. Kanyo, E. C. Sherer, and J. Sutcliffe.** 2004. Macrolide resistance from the ribosome perspective. *Curr. Drug Targets Infect. Disord.* **4:**177–191.

110. **Freeman, L. D., D. R. Hooper, D. F. Lathen, D. P. Nelson, W. O. Harrison, and D. S. Anderson.** 1983. Brief prophylaxis with doxycycline for the prevention of traveler's diarrhea. *Gastroenterology* **84:**276–280.

111. **French, G.** 2003. Safety and tolerability of linezolid. *J. Antimicrob. Chemother.* **51**(Suppl. S2):ii45–ii53.

112. **Friedman, L., J. D. Alder, and J. A. Silverman.** 2006. Genetic changes that correlate with reduced susceptibility to daptomycin in *Staphylococcus aureus*. *Antimicrob. Agents Chemother.* **50:**2137–2145.

113. **Frost, P., G. D. Weinstein, and E. C. Gomez.** 1972. Phototoxic potential of minocycline and doxycycline. *Arch. Dermatol.* **105:**681–683.

114. **Fu, K. P., and H. C. Neu.** 1976. In vitro study of netilmicin compared with other aminoglycosides. *Antimicrob. Agents Chemother.* **10:**526–534.

115. **Fuller, A. T., G. Mellows, M. Woolford, G. T. Banks, K. D. Barrow, and E. B. Chain.** 1971. Pseudomonic acid: an antibiotic produced by *Pseudomonas fluorescens*. *Nature* **234:**416–417.

116. **Fung-Tomc, J. C.** 1997. Fourth-generation cephalosporins. *Clin. Microbiol. Newsl.* **19:**129–136.

117. **Galimand, M., P. Courvalin, and T. Lambert.** 2003. Plasmid-mediated high-level resistance to aminoglycosides in *Enterobacteriaceae* due to 16S rRNA methylation. *Antimicrob. Agents Chemother.* **47:**2565–2571.

118. **Gardner, T. B., and D. R. Hill.** 2001. Treatment of giardiasis. *Clin. Microbiol. Rev.* **14:**114–128.

119. **Gentry, D. R., S. F. Rittenhouse, L. McCloskey, and D. J. Holmes.** 2007. Stepwise exposure of *Staphylococcus aureus* to pleuromutilins is associated with stepwise acquisition of mutations in *rplC* and minimally affects susceptibility to retapamulin. *Antimicrob. Agents Chemother.* **51:**2048–2052.

120. **Geraci, J. E., and W. R. Wilson.** 1981. Vancomycin therapy for infective endocarditis. *Rev. Infect. Dis.* **3**(Suppl.): S250–S258.

121. **Gerber, M. A., R. S. Baltimore, C. B. Eaton, M. Gewitz, A. H. Rowley, S. T. Shulman, and K. A. Taubert.** 2009. Prevention of rheumatic fever and diagnosis and treatment of acute streptococcal pharyngitis. *Circulation* **119:**1541–1551.

122. **Gerson, S. L., S. L. Kaplan, J. B. Bruss, V. Le, F. M. Arellano, B. Hafkin, and D. J. Kuter.** 2002. Hematologic effects of linezolid: summary of clinical experience. *Antimicrob. Agents Chemother.* **46:**2723–2726.

123. **Gettig, J. P., C. W. Crank, and A. H. Philbrick.** 2008. Faropenem medoxomil. *Ann. Pharmacother.* **42:**80–90.

124. **Goa, K. L., and S. Noble.** 2003. Panipenem/betamipron. *Drugs* **63:**913–925; discussion 926.

125. **Golan, Y., L. A. McDermott, N. V. Jacobus, E. J. C. Goldstein, S. Finegold, L. J. Harrell, D. W. Hecht, S. G. Jenkins, C. Pierson, R. Venezia, J. Rihs, P. Iannini, S. L. Gorbach, and D. R. Snydman.** 2003. Emergence of fluoroquinolones resistance among *Bacteroides* species. *J. Antimicrob. Chemother.* **52:**208–213.

126. **Goldfarb, J., D. Crenshaw, J. O'Horo, E. Lemon, and J. L. Blumer.** 1988. Randomized clinical trial of topical mupirocin versus oral erythromycin for impetigo. *Antimicrob. Agents Chemother.* **32:**1780–1783.

127. **Goldstein, E. J., D. M. Citron, C. V. Merriam, Y. A. Warren, K. L. Tyrrell, and H. T. Fernandez.** 2006. Comparative in vitro susceptibilities of 396 unusual anaerobic strains to tigecycline and eight other antimicrobial agents. *Antimicrob. Agents Chemother.* **50:**3507–3513.

128. **Goldstein, E. J., D. M. Citron, C. V. Merriam, Y. A. Warren, K. L. Tyrrell, and H. T. Fernandez.** 2003. In vitro activities of daptomycin, vancomycin, quinupristin-dalfopristin, linezolid, and five other antimicrobials against 307 gram-positive anaerobic and 31 *Corynebacterium* clinical isolates. *Antimicrob. Agents Chemother.* **47:**337–341.

129. **Goldstein, E. J., D. M. Citron, K. L. Tyrrell, and Y. A. Warren.** 2004. Bactericidal activity of telavancin, vancomycin and metronidazole against Clostridium difficile. *Anaerobe* **48:**2149–2152.

130. **Goldstein, E. J., D. M. Citron, C. Vreni Merriam, Y. Warren, and K. L. Tyrrell.** 2000. Comparative in vitro activities of ertapenem (MK-0826) against 1,001 anaerobes isolated from human intra-abdominal infections. *Antimicrob. Agents Chemother.* **44:**2389–2394.

131. **Gordin, F. M., G. L. Simon, C. B. Wofsy, and J. Mills.** 1984. Adverse reactions to trimethoprim-sulfamethoxazole in patients with the acquired immunodeficiency syndrome. *Ann. Intern. Med.* **100:**495–499.

132. **Gorzynski, E. A., D. Amsterdam, T. R. Beam, Jr., and C. Rotstein.** 1989. Comparative in vitro activities of teicoplanin, vancomycin, oxacillin, and other antimicrobial agents against bacteremic isolates of gram-positive cocci. *Antimicrob. Agents Chemother.* **33:**2019–2022.

133. **Grasela, D. M.** 2000. Clinical pharmacology of gatifloxacin, a new fluoroquinolone. *Clin. Infect. Dis.* **31**(Suppl. 2):S51–S58.

134. **Gravestock, M. B.** 2005. Recent developments in the discovery of novel oxazolidinone antibacterials. *Curr. Opin. Drug Discov. Dev.* **8:**469–477.

135. **Greenwood, D.** 1988. Microbiological properties of teicoplanin. *J. Antimicrob. Chemother.* **21**(Suppl. A):1–13.

136. **Grosset, J., and S. Leventis.** 1983. Adverse effects of rifampin. *Rev. Infect. Dis.* **5**(Suppl. 3):S440–S450.

137. **Grossman, E. R., A. Walchek, and H. Freedman.** 1971. Tetracyclines and permanent teeth: the relation between dose and tooth color. *Pediatrics* **47:**567–570.

138. **Gump, D. W.** 1981. Vancomycin for treatment of bacterial meningitis. *Rev. Infect. Dis.* **3**(Suppl.):S289–S292.

139. **Gutmann, L., M. D. Kitzis, S. Yamabe, and J. F. Acar.** 1986. Comparative evaluation of a new beta-lactamase inhibitor, YTR 830, combined with different beta-lactam antibiotics against bacteria harboring known beta-lactamases. *Antimicrob. Agents Chemother.* **29:**955–957.

140. **Guttler, R. B., G. W. Counts, C. K. Avent, and H. N. Beaty.** 1971. Effect of rifampin and minocycline on meningococcal carrier rates. *J. Infect. Dis.* **124:**199–205.

141. **Hammerschlag, M. R., and R. Sharma.** 2008. Use of cethromycin, a new ketolide, for treatment of community-acquired respiratory infections. *Expert Opin. Investig. Drugs* **17:**387–400.

142. **Hansen, L. H., P. Mauvais, and S. Douthwaite.** 1999. The macrolide-ketolide antibiotic binding site is formed by structures in domains II and V of 23S ribosomal RNA. *Mol. Microbiol.* **31:**623–631.

143. **Hawkey, P. M.** 2003. Mechanisms of quinolone action and microbial response. *J. Antimicrob. Chemother.* **51**(Suppl. 1):29–35.

144. **Hayden, M. K., K. Rezai, R. A. Hayes, K. Lolans, J. P. Quinn, and R. A. Weinstein.** 2005. Development of daptomycin resistance in vivo in methicillin-resistant *Staphylococcus aureus*. *J. Clin. Microbiol.* **43:**5285–5287.

145. **Hegde, S. S., N. Reyes, T. Wiens, N. Vanasse, R. Skinner, J. McCullough, K. Kaniga, J. Pace, R. Thomas, J. P. Shaw, G. Obedencio, and J. K. Judice.** 2004. Pharmacodynamics of telavancin (TD-6424), a novel bactericidal agent, against gram-positive bacteria. *Antimicrob. Agents Chemother.* **48:**3043–3050.

146. **Hiramatsu, K.** 2001. Vancomycin-resistant *Staphylococcus aureus*: a new model of antibiotic resistance. *Lancet Infect. Dis.* **1:**147–155.

147. **Hisanaga, T., D. J. Hoban, and G. G. Zhanel.** 2005. Mechanisms of resistance to telithromycin in *Streptococcus pneumoniae*. *J. Antimicrob. Chemother.* **56:**447–450.

148. **Hitchings, G. H.** 1973. Mechanism of action of trimethoprim-sulfamethoxazole. *J. Infect. Dis.* **128**(Suppl.):433–436.

149. **Hoban, D. J., S. K. Bouchillon, and M. J. Dowzicky.** 2007. Antimicrobial susceptibility of extended-spectrum beta-lactamase producers and multidrug-resistant *Acinetobacter baumannii* throughout the United States and comparative in vitro activity of tigecycline, a new glycylcycline antimicrobial. *Diagn. Microbiol. Infect. Dis.* **57:**423–428.

150. **Hobbs, J. K., K. Miller, A. J. O'Neill, and I. Chopra.** 2008. Consequences of daptomycin-mediated membrane damage in Staphylococcus aureus. *J. Antimicrob. Chemother.* **62:**1003–1008.

151. **Hoellman, D. B., G. Lin, L. M. Ednie, A. Rattan, M. R. Jacobs, and P. C. Appelbaum.** 2003. Antipneumococcal and antistaphylococcal activities of ranbezolid (RBX 7644), a new oxazolidinone, compared to those of other agents. *Antimicrob. Agents Chemother.* **47:**1148–1150.

152. **Hoeprich, P. D., and D. M. Warshauer.** 1974. Entry of four tetracyclines into saliva and tears. *Antimicrob. Agents Chemother.* **5:**330–336.

153. **Hof, H., O. Zak, E. Schweizer, and A. Denzler.** 1984. Antibacterial activities of nitrothiazole derivatives. *J. Antimicrob. Chemother.* **14:**31–39.

154. **Holmberg, L., G. Boman, L. E. Bottiger, B. Eriksson, R. Spross, and A. Wessling.** 1980. Adverse reactions to nitrofurantoin: analysis of 921 reports. *Am. J. Med.* **69:**733–738.

155. **Hooton, T. M., and W. E. Stamm.** 1997. Diagnosis and treatment of uncomplicated urinary tract infection. *Infect. Dis. Clin. N. Am.* **11:**551–581.

156. **Hope, R., M. Warner, S. Mushtaq, M. E. Ward, T. Parsons, and D. M. Livermore.** 2005. Effect of medium type, age and aeration on the MICs of tigecycline and classical tetracyclines. *J. Antimicrob. Chemother.* **56:**1042–1046.

157. **Huang, D. B., and H. L. DuPont.** 2005. Rifaximin: a novel antimicrobial for enteric infections. *J. Infect. Dis.* **50:**97–106.

158. **Hughes, J., and G. Mellows.** 1978. Inhibition of isoleucyl-transfer ribonucleic acid synthetase in *Escherichia coli* by pseudomonic acid. *Biochem. J.* **176:**305–318.

159. **Hunfeld, K.-P., T. A. Wichelhaus, R. Rodel, G. Acker, V. Brade, and P. Kraiczy.** 2004. Comparison of in vitro activities of ketolides, macrolides, and an azalide against the spirochete *Borrelia burgdorferi*. *Antimicrob. Agents Chemother.* **48:**344–347.

160. **Insa, R., E. Cercenado, M. J. Goyanes, A. Morente, and E. Bouza.** 2007. In vitro activity of tigecycline against clinical isolates of *Acinetobacter baumannii* and *Stenotrophomonas maltophilia*. *J. Antimicrob. Chemother.* **59:**583–585.

161. **Jacoby, G. A., and L. S. Munoz-Price.** 2005. The new beta-lactamases. *N. Engl. J. Med.* **352:**380–391.

162. **Jacoby, G. A., and L. Sutton.** 1989. *Pseudomonas cepacia* susceptibility to sulbactam. *Antimicrob. Agents Chemother.* **33:**583–584.

163. **Jiang, Z. D., S. Ke, E. Palazzini, L. Riopel, and H. Dupont.** 2000. In vitro activity and fecal concentration of rifaximin after oral administration. *Antimicrob. Agents Chemother.* **44:**2205–2206.

164. **Johnson, A. P., A. H. Uttley, N. Woodford, and R. C. George.** 1990. Resistance to vancomycin and teicoplanin: an emerging clinical problem. *Clin. Microbiol. Rev.* **3:**280–291.

165. **Johnson, D. M., D. J. Biedenbach, M. L. Beach, M. A. Pfaller, and R. N. Jones.** 2000. Antimicrobial activity and in vitro susceptibility test development for cefditoren against *Haemophilus influenzae, Moraxella catarrhalis,* and *Streptococcus* species. *Diagn. Microbiol. Infect. Dis.* **37:**99–105.

166. **Johnson, D. M., M. G. Stilwell, T. R. Fritsche, and R. N. Jones.** 2006. Emergence of multidrug-resistant *Streptococcus pneumoniae*: report from the SENTRY Antimicrobial Surveillance Program (1999–2003). *Diagn. Microbiol. Infect. Dis.* **56:**69–74.

167. **Jones, R. N.** 2006. Microbiological features of vancomycin in the 21st century: minimum inhibitory concentration creep, bactericidal/static activity, and applied breakpoints to predict clinical outcomes or detect resistant strains. *Clin. Infect. Dis.* **42**(Suppl. 1):S13–S24.

168. **Jones, R. N.** 1989. Review of the in-vitro spectrum and characteristics of cefmetazole (CS-1170). *J. Antimicrob. Chemother.* **23**(Suppl. D):1–12.

169. **Jones, R. N., and A. L. Barry.** 1983. Cefoperazone: a review of its antimicrobial spectrum, beta-lactamase stability, enzyme inhibition, and other in vitro characteristics. *Rev. Infect. Dis.* **5**(Suppl. 1):S108–S126.

170. **Jones, R. N., D. J. Biedenbach, and D. M. Johnson.** 2000. Cefditoren activity against nearly 1,000 non-fastidious bacterial isolates and the development of in vitro susceptibility test methods. *Diagn. Microbiol. Infect. Dis.* **37**:143–146.

171. **Jones, R. N., H. K. Huynh, and D. J. Biedenbach.** 2004. Activities of doripenem (S-4661) against drug-resistant clinical pathogens. *Antimicrob. Agents Chemother.* **48**:3136–3140.

172. **Jones, R. N., J. T. Kirby, and P. R. Rhomberg.** 2008. Comparative activity of meropenem in US medical centers (2007): initiating the 2nd decade of MYSTIC program surveillance. *Diagn. Microbiol. Infect. Dis.* **61**:203–213.

173. **Jorgensen, J. H., S. A. Crawford, M. L. McElmeel, and C. G. Whitney.** 2004. Activities of cethromycin and telithromycin against recent North American isolates of *Streptococcus pneumoniae. Antimicrob. Agents Chemother.* **48**:605–607.

174. **Kahan, F. M., J. S. Kahan, P. J. Cassidy, and H. Kropp.** 1974. The mechanism of action of fosfomycin (phosphonomycin). *Ann. N. Y. Acad. Sci.* **235**:364–386.

175. **Keam, S. J.** 2008. Doripenem: a review of its use in the treatment of bacterial infections. *Drugs* **68**:2021–2057.

176. **Kelesidis, T., D. E. Karageorgopoulos, I. Kelesidis, and M. E. Falagas.** 2008. Tigecycline for the treatment of multidrug-resistant *Enterobacteriaceae*: a systematic review of the evidence from microbiological and clinical studies. *J. Antimicrob. Chemother.* **62**:895–904.

177. **Kelkar, P. S., and J. T. Li.** 2001. Cephalosporin allergy. *N. Engl. J. Med.* **345**:804–809.

178. **Kenny, G. E., T. M. Hooton, M. C. Roberts, F. D. Cartwright, and J. Hoyt.** 1989. Susceptibilities of genital mycoplasmas to the newer quinolones as determined by the agar dilution method. *Antimicrob. Agents Chemother.* **33**:103–107.

179. **Kirst, H. A., and G. D. Sides.** 1989. New directions for macrolide antibiotics: structural modifications and in vitro activity. *Antimicrob. Agents Chemother.* **33**:1413–1418.

180. **Klugman, K. P.** 1990. Pneumococcal resistance to antibiotics. *Clin. Microbiol. Rev.* **3**:171–196.

181. **Knapp, C. C., J. Sierra-Madero, and J. A. Washington.** 1989. Activity of ticarcillin/clavulanate and piperacillin/tazobactam (YTR 830; CL-298,741) against clinical isolates and against mutants derepressed for class I beta-lactamase. *Diagn. Microbiol. Infect. Dis.* **12**:511–515.

182. **Knight, V., J. W. Draper, E. A. Brady, and C. A. Attmore.** 1952. Methenamine mandelate: antimicrobial activity, absorption and excretion. *Antibiot. Chemother.* **2**:615–635.

183. **Kohlhoff, S. A., and R. Sharma.** 2007. Iclaprim. *Expert Opin. Investig. Drugs* **16**:1441–1448.

184. **Koo, H. L., H. L. Dupont, and D. B. Huang.** 2009. The role of rifaximin in the treatment and chemoprophylaxis of travelers' diarrhea. *Ther. Clin. Risk Manag.* **5**:841–848.

185. **Kosowska-Shick, K., C. Clark, K. Pankuch, P. McGhee, B. Dewasse, L. Beachel, and P. C. Appelbaum.** 2009. Activity of telavancin against staphylococci and enterococci determined by MIC and resistance selection studies. *Antimicrob. Agents Chemother.* **53**:4217–4224.

186. **Kuck, N. A., N. V. Jacobus, P. J. Petersen, W. J. Weiss, and R. T. Testa.** 1989. Comparative in vitro and in vivo activities of piperacillin combined with the beta-lactamase inhibitors tazobactam, clavulanic acid, and sulbactam. *Antimicrob. Agents Chemother.* **33**:1964–1969.

187. **Lamb, H. M., D. P. Figgitt, and D. Faulds.** 1999. Quinupristin/dalfopristin: a review of its use in the management of serious gram-positive infections. *Drugs* **58**:1061–1097.

188. **Landman, D., C. Georgescu, D. A. Martin, and J. Quale.** 2008. Polymyxins revisited. *Clin. Microbiol. Rev.* **21**:449–465.

189. **Lawrence, K. R., M. Adra, and P. K. Gillman.** 2006. Serotonin toxicity associated with the use of linezolid: a review of postmarketing data. *Clin. Infect. Dis.* **42**:1578–1583.

190. **Lawson, D. H., and B. J. Paice.** 1982. Adverse reactions to trimethoprim-sulfamethoxazole. *Rev. Infect. Dis.* **4**:429–433.

191. **Leclercq, R.** 2002. Mechanisms of resistance to macrolides and lincosamides: nature of the resistance elements and their clinical implications. *Clin. Infect. Dis.* **34**:482–492.

192. **Lee, E., S. Burger, J. Shah, C. Melton, M. Mullen, F. Warren, and R. Press.** 2003. Linezolid-associated toxic optic neuropathy: a report of 2 cases. *Clin. Infect. Dis.* **37**:1389–1391.

193. **Leigh, D. A.** 1981. Antibacterial activity and pharmacokinetics of clindamycin. *J. Antimicrob. Chemother.* **7**(Suppl. A):3–9.

194. **Lell, B., and P. G. Kremsner.** 2002. Clindamycin as an antimalarial drug: review of clinical trials. *Antimicrob. Agents Chemother.* **46**:2315–2320.

195. **Leonard, S. N., C. M. Cheung, and M. J. Rybak.** 2008. Activities of ceftobiprole, linezolid, vancomycin, and daptomycin against community-associated and hospital-associated methicillin-resistant *Staphylococcus aureus. Antimicrob. Agents Chemother.* **52**:2974–2976.

196. **Li, J., R. L. Nation, J. D. Turnidge, R. W. Milne, K. Coulthard, C. R. Rayner, and D. L. Paterson.** 2006. Colistin: the re-emerging antibiotic for multidrug-resistant Gram-negative bacterial infections. *Lancet Infect. Dis.* **6**:589–601.

197. **Lin, S. W., P. L. Carver, and D. D. DePestel.** 2006. Dalbavancin: a new option for the treatment of gram-positive infections. *Ann. Pharmacother.* **40**:449–460.

198. **Lindberg, R., H. Fredlund, R. Nicholas, and M. Unemo.** 2007. *Neisseria gonorrhoeae* isolates with reduced susceptibility to cefixime and ceftriaxone: association with genetic polymorphisms in *penA, mtrR, porB1b*, and *ponA. Antimicrob. Agents Chemother.* **51**:2117–2122.

199. **Linden, P. K., R. C. Moellering, Jr., C. A. Wood, S. J. Rehm, J. Flaherty, F. Bompart, and G. H. Talbot.** 2001. Treatment of vancomycin-resistant *Enterococcus faecium* infections with quinupristin/dalfopristin. *Clin. Infect. Dis.* **33**:1816–1823.

200. **Lipsky, B. A., and C. A. Baker.** 1999. Fluoroquinolone toxicity profiles: a review focusing on newer agents. *Clin. Infect. Dis.* **28**:352–364.

201. **Livermore, D. M.** 2003. Linezolid in vitro: mechanism and antibacterial spectrum. *J. Antimicrob. Chemother.* **51**(Suppl. 2):ii9–ii16.

202. **Livermore, D. M., S. Mushtaq, M. Warner, C. Miossec, and N. Woodford.** 2008. NXL104 combinations versus *Enterobacteriaceae* with CTX-M extended-spectrum beta-lactamases and carbapenemases. *J. Antimicrob. Chemother.* **62**:1053–1056.

203. **Lode, H., K. Borner, P. Koeppe, and T. Schaberg.** 1996. Azithromycin: review of key chemical, pharmacokinetic and microbiological features. *J. Antimicrob. Chemother.* **37**(Suppl. C):1–8.

204. **Lodise, T. P., B. Lomaestro, J. Graves, and G. L. Drusano.** 2008. Larger vancomycin doses (at least four grams per day) are associated with an increased incidence of nephrotoxicity. *Antimicrob. Agents Chemother.* **52**:1330–1336.

205. **Lofmark, S., H. Fang, M. Hedberg, and C. Edlund.** 2005. Inducible metronidazole resistance and *nim* genes in clinical *Bacteroides fragilis* group isolates. *Antimicrob. Agents Chemother.* **49**:1253–1256.

206. **Long, J. K., T. K. Choueiri, G. S. Hall, R. K. Avery, and M. A. Sekeres.** 2005. Daptomycin-resistant *Enterococcus faecium* in a patient with acute myeloid leukemia. *Mayo Clin. Proc.* **80**:1215–1216.

207. **Low, D. E.** 1995. Quinupristin/dalfopristin: spectrum of activity, pharmacokinetics, and initial clinical experience. *Microb. Drug Resist.* **1:**223–234.

208. **Low, D. E., S. Brown, and D. Felmingham.** 2004. Clinical and bacteriological efficacy of the ketolide telithromycin against isolates of key respiratory pathogens: a pooled analysis of phase III studies. *Clin. Microbiol. Infect.* **10:**27–36.

209. **Low, D. E., A. McGeer, and R. Poon.** 1989. Activities of daptomycin and teicoplanin against *Staphylococcus haemolyticus* and *Staphylococcus epidermidis*, including evaluation of susceptibility testing recommendations. *Antimicrob. Agents Chemother.* **33:**585–588.

210. **Lunde, C. S., S. R. Hartouni, J. W. Janc, M. Mammen, P. P. Humphrey, and B. M. Benton.** 2009. Telavancin disrupts the functional integrity of the bacterial membrane through targeted interaction with the cell wall precursor lipid II. *Antimicrob. Agents Chemother.* **53:**3375–3383.

211. **Lutsar, I., G. H. McCracken, Jr., and I. R. Friedland.** 1998. Antibiotic pharmacodynamics in cerebrospinal fluid. *Clin. Infect. Dis.* **27:**1117–1127.

212. **MacGowan, A. P.** 2003. Pharmacokinetic and pharmacodynamic profile of linezolid in healthy volunteers and patients with gram-positive infections. *J. Antimicrob. Chemother.* **51**(Suppl. S2)**:**ii17–ii25.

213. **MacGowan, A. P.** 2008. Tigecycline pharmacokinetic/pharmacodynamic update. *J. Antimicrob. Chemother.* **62**(Suppl. 1)**:**i11–i16.

214. **Mandell, G. L.** 1983. The antimicrobial activity of rifampin: emphasis on the relation to phagocytes. *Rev. Infect. Dis.* **5**(Suppl. 3)**:**S463–S467.

215. **Maravic, G.** 2004. Macrolide resistance based on the *erm*-mediated rRNA methylation. *Curr. Drug Targets Infect. Disord.* **4:**193–202.

216. **Marchese, A., and G. C. Schito.** 2001. The oxazolidinones as a new family of antimicrobial agent. *Clin. Microbiol. Infect.* **7**(Suppl. 4)**:**66–74.

217. **Markantonis, S. L., N. Markou, M. Fousteri, N. Sakellaridis, S. Karatzas, I. Alamanos, E. Dimopoulou, and G. Baltopoulos.** 2009. Penetration of colistin into cerebrospinal fluid. *Antimicrob. Agents Chemother.* **53:**4907–4910.

218. **Maurin, M., S. Gasquet, C. Ducco, and D. Raoult.** 1995. MICs of 28 antibiotic compounds for 14 *Bartonella* (formerly *Rochalimaea*) isolates. *Antimicrob. Agents Chemother.* **39:**2387–2391.

219. **Maurin, M., and D. Raoult.** 2001. Use of aminoglycosides in treatment of infections due to intracellular bacteria. *Antimicrob. Agents Chemother.* **45:**2977–2986.

220. **McAleese, F., P. Petersen, A. Ruzin, P. M. Dunman, E. Murphy, S. J. Projan, and P. A. Bradford.** 2005. A novel MATE family efflux pump contributes to the reduced susceptibility of laboratory-derived *Staphylococcus aureus* mutants to tigecycline. *Antimicrob. Agents Chemother.* **49:**1865–1871.

221. **McCracken, G. H., Jr.** 2000. Pharmacodynamics of gatifloxacin in experimental models of pneumococcal meningitis. *Clin. Infect. Dis.* **31**(Suppl. 2)**:**S45–S50.

222. **McDowell, T. D., and K. E. Reed.** 1989. Mechanism of penicillin killing in the absence of bacterial lysis. *Antimicrob. Agents Chemother.* **33:**1680–1685.

223. **McGee, L., D. Biek, Y. Ge, M. Klugman, M. du Plessis, A. M. Smith, B. Beall, C. G. Whitney, and K. P. Klugman.** 2009. In vitro evaluation of the antimicrobial activity of ceftaroline against cephalosporin-resistant isolates of *Streptococcus pneumoniae*. *Antimicrob. Agents Chemother.* **53:**552–556.

224. **McGehee, R. F., Jr., C. B. Smith, C. Wilcox, and M. Finland.** 1968. Comparative studies of antibacterial activity in vitro and absorption and excretion of lincomycin and clinimycin. *Am. J. Med. Sci.* **256:**279–292.

225. **McOsker, C. C., and P. M. Fitzpatrick.** 1994. Nitrofurantoin: mechanism of action and implications for resistance development in common uropathogens. *J. Antimicrob. Chemother.* **33**(Suppl. A)**:**23–30.

226. **Meagher, A. K., P. G. Ambrose, T. H. Grasela, and E. J. Ellis-Grosse.** 2005. The pharmacokinetic and pharmacodynamic profile of tigecycline. *Clin. Infect. Dis.* **41**(Suppl. 5)**:**S333–S340.

227. **Medical Letter on Drugs and Therapeutics.** 2008. Fluoroquinolones and tendon injuries. *Med. Lett. Drugs Ther.* **50:**93.

228. **Medical Letter on Drugs and Therapeutics.** 2007. Treatment of Lyme disease. *Med. Lett. Drugs Ther.* **49:**49–51.

229. **Medical Letter on Drugs and Therapeutics.** 2007. Drugs for parasitic infections. *Treat. Guidel. Med. Lett.* **5**(Suppl.)**:**e1–e15.

230. **Meka, V. G., and H. S. Gold.** 2004. Antimicrobial resistance to linezolid. *Clin. Infect. Dis.* **39:**1010–1015.

231. **Mendez, J. L., H. F. Nadrous, T. E. Hartman, and J. H. Ryu.** 2005. Chronic nitrofurantoin-induced lung disease. *Mayo Clin. Proc.* **80:**1298–1302.

232. **Michalopoulos, A., and E. Papadakis.** 2010. Inhaled anti-infective agents: emphasis on colistin. *Infection* **38:**81–88.

233. **Moellering, R. C.** 2003. Linezolid: the first oxazolidinone antimicrobial. *Ann. Intern. Med.* **138:**135–142.

234. **Moellering, R. C., P. K. Linden, J. Reinhardt, E. A. Blumberg, F. Bompart, and G. H. Talbot for the Synercid Emergency Use Group.** 1999. The efficacy and safety of quinupristin/dalfopristin for the treatment of infections caused by vancomycin-resistant *Enterococcus faecium*. *J. Antimicrob. Chemother.* **44:**251–261.

235. **Moellering, R. C., Jr.** 1984. Pharmacokinetics of vancomycin. *J. Antimicrob. Chemother.* **14**(Suppl. D)**:**43–52.

236. **Monk, J. P., and D. M. Campoli-Richards.** 1987. Ofloxacin: a review of its antibacterial activity, pharmacokinetic properties and therapeutic use. *Drugs* **33:**346–391.

237. **Moore, I. F., D. W. Hughes, and G. D. Wright.** 2005. Tigecycline is modified by the flavin-dependent monooxygenase TetX. *Biochemistry* **44:**11829–11835.

238. **Moosdeen, F., J. D. Williams, and S. Yamabe.** 1988. Antibacterial characteristics of YTR 830, a sulfone beta-lactamase inhibitor, compared with those of clavulanic acid and sulbactam. *Antimicrob. Agents Chemother.* **32:**925–927.

239. **Morgan-Linnell, S. K., L. Becnel Boyd, D. Steffen, and L. Zechiedrich.** 2009. Mechanisms accounting for fluoroquinolone resistance in *Escherichia coli* clinical isolates. *Antimicrob. Agents Chemother.* **53:**235–241.

240. **Morris, A. B., R. B. Brown, and M. Sands.** 1993. Use of rifampin in nonstaphylococcal, nonmycobacterial disease. *Antimicrob. Agents Chemother.* **37:**1–7.

241. **Morrissey, I., Y. Ge, and R. Janes.** 2009. Activity of the new cephalosporin ceftaroline against bacteraemia isolates from patients with community-acquired pneumonia. *Int. J. Antimicrob. Agents* **33:**515–519.

242. **Murray, B. E.** 1990. The life and times of the *Enterococcus*. *Clin. Microbiol. Rev.* **3:**46–65.

243. **Muscato, J. J., D. W. Wilbur, J. J. Stout, and R. A. Fahrlender.** 1991. An evaluation of the susceptibility patterns of gram-negative organisms isolated in cancer centres with aminoglycoside usage. *J. Antimicrob. Chemother.* **27**(Suppl. C)**:**1–7.

244. **Mushtaq, S., Y. Ge, and D. M. Livermore.** 2004. Doripenem versus *Pseudomonas aeruginosa* in vitro: activity against characterized isolates, mutants, and transconjugants and resistance selection potential. *Antimicrob. Agents Chemother.* **48:**3086–3092.

245. **Myrianthefs, P., S. L. Markantonis, K. Vlachos, M. Anagnostaki, E. Boutzouka, D. Panidis, and G. Baltopoulos.** 2006. Serum and cerebrospinal fluid concentrations of linezolid in neurosurgical patients. *Antimicrob. Agents Chemother.* **50:**3971–3976.

246. **Nadelman, R. B., S. W. Luger, E. Frank, M. Wisniewski, J. J. Collins, and G. P. Wormser.** 1992. Comparison of cefuroxime axetil and doxycycline in the treatment of early Lyme disease. *Ann. Intern. Med.* **117:**273–280.

247. **Najjar, A., and B. E. Murray.** 1987. Failure to demonstrate a consistent in vitro bactericidal effect of trimethoprim-sulfamethoxazole against enterococci. *Antimicrob. Agents Chemother.* **31:**808–810.

248. **Namour, F., D. H. Wessels, M. H. Pascual, D. Reynolds, E. Sultan, and B. Lenfant.** 2001. Pharmacokinetics of the

new ketolide telithromycin (HMR 3647) administered in ascending single and multiple doses. *Antimicrob. Agents Chemother.* **45**:170–175.

249. Neu, H. C. 1985. Carbapenems: special properties contributing to their activity. *Am. J. Med.* **78**(Suppl. 6A):33–40.

250. Neu, H. C. 1991. The development of macrolides: clarithromycin in perspective. *J. Antimicrob. Chemother.* **27**(Suppl. A):1–9.

251. Neu, H. C. 1982. The new beta-lactamase-stable cephalosporins. *Ann. Intern. Med.* **97**:408–419.

252. Neu, H. C. 1976. Tobramycin: an overview. *J. Infect. Dis.* **134**(Suppl.):S3–S19.

253. Neu, H. C., and K. P. Fu. 1978. Clavulanic acid, a novel inhibitor of beta-lactamases. *Antimicrob. Agents Chemother.* **14**:650–655.

254. Neu, H. C., and K. P. Fu. 1980. In vitro activity of chloramphenicol and thiamphenicol analogs. *Antimicrob. Agents Chemother.* **18**:311–316.

255. Nicolau, D. P., H. K. Sun, E. Seltzer, M. Buckwalter, and J. A. Dowell. 2007. Pharmacokinetics of dalbavancin in plasma and skin blister fluid. *J. Antimicrob. Chemother.* **60**:681–684.

256. Nilsson, A. I., O. G. Berg, O. Aspevall, G. Kahlmeter, and D. I. Andersson. 2003. Biological costs and mechanisms of fosfomycin resistance in *Escherichia coli. Antimicrob. Agents Chemother.* **47**:2850–2858.

257. Nix, D. E., A. K. Majumdar, and M. J. DiNubile. 2004. Pharmacokinetics and pharmacodynamics of ertapenem: an overview for clinicians. *J. Antimicrob. Chemother.* **53**(Suppl. 2):ii23–ii28.

258. Norrby, S. F., K. L. Faulkner, and P. A. Newell. 1997. Differentiating meropenem and imipenem/cilastatin. *Infect. Dis. Clin. Pract.* **6**:291–303.

259. O'Brien, R. J., M. A. Lyle, and D. E. Snider, Jr. 1987. Rifabutin (ansamycin LM 427): a new rifamycin-S derivative for the treatment of mycobacterial diseases. *Rev. Infect. Dis.* **9**:519–530.

260. Olson, M. W., A. Ruzin, E. Feyfant, T. S. Rush III, J. O'Connell, and P. A. Bradford. 2006. Functional, biophysical, and structural bases for antibacterial activity of tigecycline. *Antimicrob. Agents Chemother.* **50**:2156–2166.

261. Pace, J. L., and G. Yang. 2006. Glycopeptides: update on an old successful antibiotic class. *Biochem. Pharmacol.* **71**:968–980.

262. Pang, L. W., N. Limsomwong, E. F. Boudreau, and P. Singharaj. 1987. Doxycycline prophylaxis for falciparum malaria. *Lancet* **i**:1161–1164.

263. Pankuch, G. A., T. A. Davies, M. R. Jacobs, and P. C. Appelbaum. 2002. Antipneumococcal activity of ertapenem (MK-0826) compared to those of other agents. *Antimicrob. Agents Chemother.* **46**:42–46.

264. Patel, R. B., and P. G. Welling. 1980. Clinical pharmacokinetics of co-trimoxazole (trimethoprim-sulphamethoxazole). *Clin. Pharmacokinet.* **5**:405–423.

265. Patel, S. S., J. A. Balfour, and H. M. Bryson. 1997. Fosfomycin tromethamine: a review of its antibacterial activity, pharmacokinetic properties and therapeutic efficacy as a single-dose oral treatment for acute uncomplicated lower urinary tract infections. *Drugs* **53**:637–656.

266. Pechere, J. C. 1999. Current and future management of infections due to methicillin-resistant staphylococci infections: the role of quinupristin/dalfopristin. *J. Antimicrob. Chemother.* **44**(Suppl. A):11–18.

267. Pechere, J. C. 1996. Streptogramins: a unique class of antibiotics. *Drugs* **51**(Suppl. 1):13–19.

268. Peleg, A. Y., J. Adams, and D. L. Paterson. 2007. Tigecycline efflux as a mechanism for nonsusceptibility in *Acinetobacter baumannii. Antimicrob. Agents Chemother.* **51**:2065–2069.

269. Peppard, W. J., and C. D. Schuenke. 2008. Iclaprim, a diaminopyrimidine dihydrofolate reductase inhibitor for the potential treatment of antibiotic-resistant staphylococcal infections. *Curr. Opin. Investig. Drugs* **9**:210–225.

270. Perlroth, J., M. Kuo, J. Tan, A. S. Bayer, and L. G. Miller. 2008. Adjunctive use of rifampin for the treatment of *Staphylococcus aureus* infections: a systematic review of the literature. *Arch. Intern. Med.* **168**:805–819.

271. Perry, C. M., and T. Ibbotson. 2002. Biapenem. *Drugs* **62**:2221–2234.

272. Perry, C. M., and B. Jarvis. 2001. Linezolid: a review of its use in the management of serious gram-positive infections. *Drugs* **61**:525–551.

273. Peters, D. H., H. A. Friedel, and D. McTavish. 1992. Azithromycin: a review of its antimicrobial activity, pharmacokinetic properties and clinical efficacy. *Drugs* **44**:750–799.

274. Pfaller, M. A., A. L. Barry, and P. C. Fuchs. 1993. Evaluation of disk susceptibility testing of fosfomycin tromethamine. *Diagn. Microbiol. Infect. Dis.* **17**:67–70.

275. Pillar, C. M., M. K. Torres, N. P. Brown, D. Shah, and D. F. Sahm. 2008. In vitro activity of doripenem, a carbapenem for the treatment of challenging infections caused by gram-negative bacteria, against recent clinical isolates from the United States. *Antimicrob. Agents Chemother.* **52**:4388–4399.

276. Plouffe, J. F. 2000. Emerging therapies for serious gram-positive bacterial infections: a focus on linezolid. *Clin. Infect. Dis.* **31**(Suppl. 4):S144–S149.

277. Polk, R. E. 1989. Drug-drug interactions with ciprofloxacin and other fluoroquinolones. *Am. J. Med.* **87**(Suppl. 5A):76S–81S.

278. Polk, R. E., D. P. Healy, L. B. Schwartz, D. T. Rock, M. L. Garson, and K. Roller. 1988. Vancomycin and the red-man syndrome: pharmacodynamics of histamine release. *J. Infect. Dis.* **157**:502–507.

279. Pope, S. D., and A. M. Roecker. 2006. Dalbavancin: a novel lipoglycopeptide antibacterial. *Pharmacotherapy* **26**:908–918.

280. Poulakou, G., and H. Giamarellou. 2008. Doripenem: an expected arrival in the treatment of infections caused by multidrug-resistant Gram-negative pathogens. *Expert Opin. Investig. Drugs* **17**:749–771.

281. Poulakou, G., and H. Giamarellou. 2008. Oritavancin: a new promising agent in the treatment of infections due to gram-positive pathogens. *Expert Opin. Investig. Drugs* **17**:225–243.

282. Qadri, S. M., B. A. Cunha, Y. Ueno, F. Abumustafa, H. Imambaccus, D. D. Tullo, and P. Domenico. 1995. Activity of cefepime against nosocomial blood culture isolates. *J. Antimicrob. Chemother.* **36**:531–536.

283. Raad, I., R. Hachem, H. Hanna, E. Girgawy, K. Rolston, E. Whimbey, R. Husni, and G. Bodey. 2001. Treatment of vancomycin-resistant enterococcal infections in the immunocompromised host: quinupristin-dalfopristin in combination with minocycline. *Antimicrob. Agents Chemother.* **45**:3202–3204.

284. Rafie, S., C. MacDougall, and C. James. 2010. Cethromycin: a promising new ketolide antibiotic for respiratory infections. *Pharmacotherapy* **30**:290–303.

285. Raoult, D., P. Roussellier, V. Galicher, R. Perez, and J. Tamalet. 1986. In vitro susceptibility of *Rickettsia conorii* to ciprofloxacin as determined by suppressing lethality in chicken embryos and by plaque assay. *Antimicrob. Agents Chemother.* **29**:424–425.

286. Raoult, D., H. Torres, and M. Drancourt. 1991. Shell-vial assay: evaluation of a new technique for determining antibiotic susceptibility, tested in 13 isolates of *Coxiella burnetii. Antimicrob. Agents Chemother.* **35**:2070–2077.

287. Reeves, D. S. 1994. Fosfomycin trometamol. *J. Antimicrob. Chemother.* **34**:853–858.

288. Retsema, J. A., A. R. English, A. Girard, J. E. Lynch, M. Anderson, L. Brennan, C. Cimochowski, J. Faiella, W. Norcia, and P. Sawyer. 1986. Sulbactam/ampicillin: in vitro spectrum, potency, and activity in models of acute infection. *Rev. Infect. Dis.* **8**(Suppl. 5):S528–S534.

289. Rodloff, A. C. 1982. In-vitro susceptibility test of non-tuberculous mycobacteria to sulphamethoxazole, trimethoprim, and combinations of both. *J. Antimicrob. Chemother.* **9**:195–199.

290. Rodvold, K. A., M. H. Gotfried, M. Cwik, J. M. Korth-Bradley, G. Dukart, and E. J. Ellis-Grosse. 2006. Serum, tissue and body fluid concentrations of tigecycline after a single 100 mg dose. J. Antimicrob. Chemother. 58:1221–1229.

291. Rose, H. D., and M. W. Rytel. 1972. Actinomycosis treated with clindamycin. JAMA 221:1052.

292. Rosenblatt, J. E., and P. R. Stewart. 1974. Combined activity of sulfamethoxazole, trimethoprim, and polymyxin B against gram-negative bacilli. Antimicrob. Agents Chemother. 6:84–92.

293. Rubin, R. H., and M. N. Swartz. 1980. Trimethoprim-sulfamethoxazole. N. Engl. J. Med. 303:426–432.

294. Rubinstein, E., S. Cammarata, T. Oliphant, and R. Wunderink. 2001. Linezolid (PNU-100766) versus vancomycin in the treatment of hospitalized patients with nosocomial pneumonia: a randomized, double-blind, multicenter study. Clin. Infect. Dis. 32:402–412.

295. Rubinstein, E., R. Isturiz, H. C. Standiford, L. G. Smith, T. H. Oliphant, S. Cammarata, B. Hafkin, V. Le, and J. Remington. 2003. Worldwide assessment of linezolid's clinical safety and tolerability: comparator-controlled phase III studies. Antimicrob. Agents Chemother. 47:1824–1831.

296. Rubinstein, E., P. Prokocimer, and G. H. Talbot. 1999. Safety and tolerability of quinupristin/dalfopristin: administration guidelines. J. Antimicrob. Chemother. 44(Suppl. A): 37–46.

297. Ruiz, J., L. Mensa, C. O'Callaghan, M. J. Pons, A. Gonzalez, J. Vila, and J. Gascon. 2007. In vitro antimicrobial activity of rifaximin against enteropathogens causing traveler's diarrhea. Diagn. Microbiol. Infect. Dis. 59:473–475.

298. Ruoff, K. L., D. R. Kuritzkes, J. S. Wolfson, and M. J. Ferraro. 1988. Vancomycin-resistant gram-positive bacteria isolated from human sources. J. Clin. Microbiol. 26:2064–2068.

299. Ruzin, A., M. A. Visalli, D. Keeney, and P. A. Bradford. 2005. Influence of transcriptional activator RamA on expression of multidrug efflux pump AcrAB and tigecycline susceptibility in Klebsiella pneumoniae. Antimicrob. Agents Chemother. 49:1017–1022.

300. Rybak, M. J. 2006. The efficacy and safety of daptomycin: first in a new class of antibiotics for gram-positive bacteria. Clin. Microbiol. Infect. 12(Suppl. 1):24–32.

301. Rybak, M. J. 2006. The pharmacokinetic and pharmacodynamic properties of vancomycin. Clin. Infect. Dis. 42(Suppl. 1):S35–S39.

302. Sabol, K., J. E. Patterson, J. S. Lewis, A. Owens, J. Cadena, and J. H. Jorgensen. 2005. Emergence of daptomycin resistance in Enterococcus faecium during daptomycin therapy. Antimicrob. Agents Chemother. 49:1664–1665.

303. Sack, D. A., R. B. Sack, G. B. Nair, and A. K. Siddique. 2004. Cholera. Lancet 363:223–233.

304. Sader, H. S., and R. N. Jones. 2009. Antimicrobial susceptibility of gram-positive bacteria isolated from US medical centers: results of the Daptomycin Surveillance Program (2007–2008). Diagn. Microbiol. Infect. Dis. 65:158–162.

305. Safdar, N., D. Andes, and W. A. Craig. 2004. In vivo pharmacodynamic activity of daptomycin. Antimicrob. Agents Chemother. 48:63–68.

306. Sahm, D. F., N. P. Brown, D. C. Draghi, A. T. Evangelista, Y. C. Yee, and C. Thornsberry. 2008. Tracking resistance among bacterial respiratory tract pathogens: summary of findings of the TRUST Surveillance Initiative, 2001–2005. Postgrad. Med. 120:8–15.

307. Sahm, D. F., N. P. Brown, C. Thornsberry, and M. E. Jones. 2008. Antimicrobial susceptibility profiles among common respiratory tract pathogens: a GLOBAL perspective. Postgrad. Med. 120:16–24.

308. Salter, A. J. 1982. Trimethoprim-sulfamethoxazole: an assessment of more than 12 years of use. Rev. Infect. Dis. 4:196–236.

309. Saravolatz, L. D., G. E. Stein, and L. B. Johnson. 2009. Telavancin: a novel lipoglycopeptide. Clin. Infect. Dis. 49:1908–1914.

310. Sattler, F. R., M. R. Weitekamp, and J. O. Ballard. 1986. Potential for bleeding with the new beta-lactam antibiotics. Ann. Intern. Med. 105:924–931.

311. Saxon, A., A. Hassner, E. A. Swabb, B. Wheeler, and N. F. Adkinson, Jr. 1984. Lack of cross-reactivity between aztreonam, a monobactam antibiotic, and penicillin in penicillin-allergic subjects. J. Infect. Dis. 149:16–22.

312. Scangarella-Oman, N. E., R. M. Shawar, S. Bouchillon, and D. Hoban. 2009. Microbiological profile of a new topical antibacterial: retapamulin ointment 1%. Expert Rev. Anti-Infect. Ther. 7:269–279.

313. Schaad, U. B., J. Wedgwood-Krucko, and H. Tschaeppeler. 1988. Reversible ceftriaxone-associated biliary pseudolithiasis in children. Lancet ii:1411–1413.

314. Schattner, A., J. Von der Walde, N. Kozak, N. Sokolovskaya, and H. Knobler. 1999. Nitrofurantoin-induced immune-mediated lung and liver disease. Am. J. Med. Sci. 317:336–340.

315. Schentag, J. J., and C. H. Ballow. 1991. Tissue-directed pharmacokinetics. Am. J. Med. 91(Suppl. 3A):5S–11S.

316. Schirmer, P. L., and S. C. Deresinski. 2009. Ceftobiprole: a new cephalosporin for the treatment of skin and skin structure infections. Expert Rev. Anti-Infect. Ther. 7:777–791.

317. Schulin, T., C. B. Wennersten, R. C. Moellering, Jr., and G. M. Eliopoulos. 1998. In-vitro activity of the new ketolide antibiotic HMR 3647 against gram-positive bacteria. J. Antimicrob. Chemother. 42:297–301.

318. Shaw, K. J., P. N. Rather, R. S. Hare, and G. H. Miller. 1993. Molecular genetics of aminoglycoside resistance genes and familial relationships of the aminoglycoside-modifying enzymes. Microbiol. Rev. 57:138–163.

319. Shaw, W. V. 1984. Bacterial resistance to chloramphenicol. Br. Med. Bull. 40:36–41.

320. Shorr, A. F., M. J. Kunkel, and M. Kollef. 2005. Linezolid versus vancomycin in Staphylococcus aureus bacteremia: pooled analysis of randomized studies. J. Antimicrob. Chemother. 56:923–929.

321. Skiest, D. J. 2006. Treatment failure resulting from resistance of Staphylococcus aureus to daptomycin. J. Clin. Microbiol. 44:655–656.

322. Smith, A. L., and A. Weber. 1983. Pharmacology of chloramphenicol. Pediatr. Clin. N. Am. 30:209–236.

323. Snydman, D. R., N. V. Jacobus, and L. A. McDermott. 2008. In vitro activities of doripenem, a new broad-spectrum carbapenem, against recently collected clinical anaerobic isolates, with emphasis on the Bacteroides fragilis group. Antimicrob. Agents Chemother. 52:4492–4496.

324. Snydman, D. R., N. V. Jacobus, L. A. McDermott, Y. Golan, D. W. Hecht, E. J. Goldstein, L. Harrell, S. Jenkins, D. Newton, C. Pierson, J. D. Rihs, V. L. Yu, R. Venezia, S. M. Finegold, J. E. Rosenblatt, and S. L. Gorbach. 2010. Lessons learned from the anaerobe survey: historical perspective and review of the most recent data (2005–2007). Clin. Infect. Dis. 50(Suppl. 1):S26–S33.

325. Snydman, D. R., N. V. Jacobus, L. A. McDermott, R. Ruthazer, Y. Golan, E. J. Goldstein, S. M. Finegold, L. J. Harrell, D. W. Hecht, S. G. Jenkins, C. Pierson, R. Venezia, V. Yu, J. Rihs, and S. L. Gorbach. 2007. National survey on the susceptibility of Bacteroides fragilis group: report and analysis of trends in the United States from 1997 to 2004. Antimicrob. Agents Chemother. 51:1649–1655.

326. Somma, S., L. Gastaldo, and A. Corti. 1984. Teicoplanin, a new antibiotic from Actinoplanes teichomyceticus nov. sp. Antimicrob. Agents Chemother. 26:917–923.

327. Sorgel, F., and M. Kinzig. 1993. The chemistry, pharmacokinetics and tissue distribution of piperacillin/tazobactam. J. Antimicrob. Chemother. 31(Suppl. A):39–60.

328. Spratt, B. G., V. Jobanputra, and W. Zimmermann. 1977. Binding of thienamycin and clavulanic acid to the penicillin-binding proteins of Escherichia coli K-12. Antimicrob. Agents Chemother. 12:406–409.

329. Stahlmann, R., and H. Lode. 1999. Toxicity of quinolones. Drugs 58(Suppl. 2):37–42.

330. **Stalker, D. J., G. L. Jungbluth, N. K. Hopkins, and D. H. Batts.** 2003. Pharmacokinetics and tolerance of single- and multiple-dose oral or intravenous linezolid, an oxazolidinone antibiotic, in healthy volunteers. *J. Antimicrob. Chemother.* **51:**1239–1246.

331. **Stamm, W. E.** 1991. Azithromycin in the treatment of uncomplicated genital chlamydial infections. *Am. J. Med.* **91**(Suppl. 3A):19S–22S.

332. **Stapleton, A., and W. E. Stamm.** 1997. Prevention of urinary tract infection. *Infect. Dis. Clin. N. Am.* **11:**719–733.

333. **Stapley, E. O., D. Hendlin, J. M. Mata, M. Jackson, H. Wallick, S. Hernandez, S. Mochales, S. A. Currie, and R. M. Miller.** 1969. Phosphonomycin: discovery and in vitro biological characterization. *Antimicrob. Agents Chemother.* **9:**284–290.

334. **Steed, M. E., and M. J. Rybak.** 2010. Ceftaroline: a new cephalosporin with activity against resistant gram-positive pathogens. *Pharmacotherapy* **30:**375–389.

335. **Steenbergen, J. N., J. Alder, G. M. Thorne, and F. P. Tally.** 2005. Daptomycin: a lipopeptide antibiotic for the treatment of serious gram-positive infections. *J. Antimicrob. Chemother.* **55:**283–288.

336. **Stein, G. E.** 1996. Pharmacokinetics and pharmacodynamics of newer fluoroquinolones. *Clin. Infect. Dis.* **23**(Suppl. 1): S19–S24.

337. **Stein, G. E., and W. A. Craig.** 2006. Tigecycline: a critical analysis. *Clin. Infect. Dis.* **43:**518–524.

338. **Stevens, D. L., D. Herr, H. Lampiris, J. L. Hunt, D. H. Batts, and B. Hafkin.** 2002. Linezolid versus vancomycin for the treatment of methicillin-resistant *Staphylococcus aureus* infections. *Clin. Infect. Dis.* **34:**1481–1490.

339. **Strahilevitz, J., G. A. Jacoby, D. C. Hooper, and A. Robicsek.** 2009. Plasmid-mediated quinolone resistance: a multifaceted threat. *Clin. Microbiol. Rev.* **22:**664–689.

340. **Sullivan, D., M. E. Csuka, and B. Blanchard.** 1980. Erythromycin ethylsuccinate hepatotoxicity. *JAMA* **243**–1074.

341. **Swaney, S. M., H. Aoki, M. C. Ganoza, and D. L. Shinabarger.** 1998. The oxazolidinone linezolid inhibits initiation of protein synthesis in bacteria. *Antimicrob. Agents Chemother.* **42:**3251–3255.

342. **Sykes, R. B., and D. P. Bonner.** 1985. Aztreonam: the first monobactam. *Am. J. Med.* **78**(Suppl. 2A):2–10.

343. **Takahata, S., T. Ida, T. Hiraishi, S. Sakakibara, K. Maebashi, S. Terada, T. Muratani, T. Matsumoto, C. Nakahama, and K. Tomono.** 2010. Molecular mechanisms of fosfomycin resistance in clinical isolates of *Escherichia coli.* *Int. J. Antimicrob. Agents* **35:**333–337.

344. **Teasley, D. G., D. N. Gerding, M. M. Olson, L. R. Peterson, R. L. Gebhard, M. J. Schwartz, and J. T. Lee, Jr.** 1983. Prospective randomised trial of metronidazole versus vancomycin for *Clostridium-difficile*-associated diarrhoea and colitis. *Lancet* **ii:**1043–1046.

345. **Thornsberry, C.** 1992. Review of the in vitro antibacterial activity of cefprozil, a new oral cephalosporin. *Clin. Infect. Dis.* **14**(Suppl. 2):S189–S194.

346. **Todd, P. A., and D. Faulds.** 1991. Ofloxacin: a reappraisal of its antimicrobial activity, pharmacology and therapeutic use. *Drugs* **42:**825–876.

347. **Toma, E., S. Fournier, M. Dumont, P. Bolduc, and H. Deschamps.** 1993. Clindamycin/primaquine versus trimethoprim-sulfamethoxazole as primary therapy for *Pneumocystis carinii* pneumonia in AIDS: a randomized, double-blind pilot trial. *Clin. Infect. Dis.* **17:**178–184.

348. **Tuazon, C. U., and H. Miller.** 1984. Comparative in vitro activities of teichomycin and vancomycin alone and in combination with rifampin and aminoglycosides against staphylococci and enterococci. *Antimicrob. Agents Chemother.* **25:**411–412.

349. **Turnidge, J.** 1999. Pharmacokinetics and pharmacodynamics of fluoroquinolones. *Drugs* **58**(Suppl. 2):29–36.

350. **Tyrrell, K. L., D. M. Citron, Y. A. Warren, H. T. Fernandez, C. V. Merriam, and E. J. Goldstein.** 2006. In vitro activities of daptomycin, vancomycin, and penicillin against *Clostridium difficile, C. perfringens, Finegoldia magna,* and *Propionibacterium acnes. Antimicrob. Agents Chemother.* **50:**2728–2731.

351. **Upton, A., S. Lang, and H. Heffernan.** 2003. Mupirocin and *Staphylococcus aureus*: a recent paradigm of emerging antibiotic resistance. *J. Antimicrob. Chemother.* **51:**613–617.

352. **Van der Auwera, P., T. Matsumoto, and M. Husson.** 1988. Intraphagocytic penetration of antibiotics. *J. Antimicrob. Chemother.* **22:**185–192.

353. **Vannuffel, P., and C. Cocito.** 1996. Mechanism of action of streptogramins and macrolides. *Drugs* **51**(Suppl. 1):20–30.

354. **van Rijen, M. M., M. Bonten, R. P. Wenzel, and J. A. Kluytmans.** 2008. Intranasal mupirocin for reduction of *Staphylococcus aureus* infections in surgical patients with nasal carriage: a systematic review. *J. Antimicrob. Chemother.* **61:**254–261.

355. **Vidaillac, C., and M. J. Rybak.** 2009. Ceftobiprole: first cephalosporin with activity against methicillin-resistant *Staphylococcus aureus. Pharmacotherapy* **29:**511–525.

356. **Visalli, M. A., S. Bajaksouzian, M. R. Jacobs, and P. C. Appelbaum.** 1997. Comparative activity of trovafloxacin, alone and in combination with other agents, against gram-negative nonfermentative rods. *Antimicrob. Agents Chemother.* **41:**1475–1481.

357. **von Rosensteil, N. A., and D. Adam.** 1995. Macrolide antibacterials: drug interactions of clinical significance. *Drug Saf.* **13:**105–122.

358. **Wallace, R. J., Jr., B. A. Brown-Elliott, C. J. Crist, L. Mann, and R. W. Wilson.** 2002. Comparison of the in vitro activity of the glyclycline tigecycline (formerly GAR-936) with those of tetracycline, minocycline, and doxycycline against isolates of nontuberculous mycobacteria. *Antimicrob. Agents Chemother.* **46:**3164–3167.

359. **Wallace, R. J., Jr., B. A. Brown-Elliott, S. C. Ward, C. J. Crist, L. B. Mann, and R. W. Wilson.** 2001. Activities of linezolid against rapidly growing mycobacteria. *Antimicrob. Agents Chemother.* **45:**764–767.

360. **Wallace, R. J., Jr., E. J. Septimus, T. W. Williams, Jr., R. H. Conklin, T. K. Satterwhite, M. B. Bushby, and D. C. Hollowell.** 1982. Use of trimethoprim-sulfamethoxazole for treatment of infections due to *Nocardia. Rev. Infect. Dis.* **4:**315–325.

361. **Wallace, R. J., Jr., J. M. Swenson, V. A. Silcox, and M. G. Bullen.** 1985. Treatment of nonpulmonary infections due to *Mycobacterium fortuitum* and *Mycobacterium chelonei* on the basis of in vitro susceptibilities. *J. Infect. Dis.* **152:**500–514.

362. **Wallace, R. J., Jr., and K. Wiss.** 1981. Susceptibility of *Mycobacterium marinum* to tetracyclines and aminoglycosides. *Antimicrob. Agents Chemother.* **20:**610–612.

363. **Walters, B. N., and S. S. Gubbay.** 1981. Tetracycline and benign intracranial hypertension: report of five cases. *Br. Med. J.* **282:**19–20.

364. **Ward, A., and D. M. Campoli-Richards.** 1986. Mupirocin: a review of its antibacterial activity, pharmacokinetic properties and therapeutic use. *Drugs* **32:**425–444.

365. **Washington, J. A., II, and W. R. Wilson.** 1985. Erythromycin: a microbial and clinical perspective after 30 years of clinical use. *Mayo Clin. Proc.* **60:**189–203.

366. **Watanakunakorn, C., and J. C. Tisone.** 1982. Synergism between vancomycin and gentamicin or tobramycin for methicillin-susceptible and methicillin-resistant *Staphylococcus aureus* strains. *Antimicrob. Agents Chemother.* **22:**903–905.

367. **Waxman, D. J., and J. L. Strominger.** 1983. Penicillin-binding proteins and the mechanism of action of beta-lactam antibiotics. *Annu. Rev. Biochem.* **52:**825–869.

368. **Wehrli, W.** 1983. Rifampin: mechanisms of action and resistance. *Rev. Infect. Dis.* **5**(Suppl. 3):S407–S411.

369. **Weigelt, J., K. Itani, D. Stevens, W. Lau, M. Dryden, and C. Knirsch for the Linezolid CCSTI Study Group.** 2005. Linezolid versus vancomycin in treatment of complicated skin and soft tissue infections. *Antimicrob. Agents Chemother.* **49:**2260–2266.

370. **Wertheim, H. F., M. C. Vos, A. Ott, A. Voss, J. A. Kluytmans, C. M. Vandenbroucke-Grauls, M. H. Meester,**

P. H. van Keulen, and H. A. Verbrugh. 2004. Mupirocin prophylaxis against nosocomial *Staphylococcus aureus* infections in nonsurgical patients: a randomized study. *Ann. Intern. Med.* **140:**419–425.

371. Wexler, H. M., A. E. Engel, D. Glass, and C. Li. 2005. In vitro activities of doripenem and comparator agents against 364 anaerobic clinical isolates. *Antimicrob. Agents Chemother.* **49:**4413–4417.

372. Wexler, H. M., and S. M. Finegold. 1988. In vitro activity of cefotetan compared with that of other antimicrobial agents against anaerobic bacteria. *Antimicrob. Agents Chemother.* **32:**601–604.

373. Wexler, H. M., B. Harris, W. T. Carter, and S. M. Finegold. 1985. In vitro efficacy of sulbactam combined with ampicillin against anaerobic bacteria. *Antimicrob. Agents Chemother.* **27:**876–878.

374. Wexler, H. M., E. Molitoris, D. Molitoris, and S. M. Finegold. 2001. In vitro activity of telithromycin (HMR 3647) against 502 strains of anaerobic bacteria. *J. Antimicrob. Chemother.* **47:**467–469.

375. Williams, J. D., and A. M. Sefton. 1993. Comparison of macrolide antibiotics. *J. Antimicrob. Chemother.* **31**(Suppl. C):11–26.

376. Wilson, W., K. A. Taubert, M. Gewitz, P. B. Lockhart, L. M. Baddour, M. Levison, A. Bolger, C. H. Cabell, M. Takahashi, R. S. Baltimore, J. W. Newburger, B. L. Strom, L. Y. Tani, M. Gerber, R. O. Bonow, T. Pallasch, S. T. Shulman, A. H. Rowley, J. C. Burns, P. Ferrieri, T. Gardner, D. Goff, and D. T. Durack. 2007. Prevention of infective endocarditis: guidelines from the American Heart Association. *Circulation* **116:**1736–1754.

377. Wilson, W. R., A. W. Karchmer, A. S. Dajani, K. A. Taubert, A. Bayer, D. Kaye, A. L. Bisno, P. Ferrieri, S. T. Shulman, and D. T. Durack. 1995. Antibiotic treatment of adults with infective endocarditis due to streptococci, enterococci, staphylococci, and HACEK microorganisms. *JAMA* **274:**1706–1713.

378. Wise, R., J. M. Andrews, and J. P. Ashby. 2001. Activity of daptomycin against gram-positive pathogens: a comparison with other agents and the determination of a tentative breakpoint. *J. Antimicrob. Chemother.* **48:**563–567.

379. Wittner, M., K. S. Rowin, H. B. Tanowitz, J. F. Hobbs, S. Saltzman, B. Wenz, R. Hirsch, E. Chisholm, and G. R. Healy. 1982. Successful chemotherapy of transfusion babesiosis. *Ann. Intern. Med.* **96:**601–604.

380. Wolfson, J. S., and D. C. Hooper. 1989. Fluoroquinolone antimicrobial agents. *Clin. Microbiol. Rev.* **2:**378–424.

381. Wolter, N., A. M. Smith, D. J. Farrell, J. B. Northwood, S. Douthwaite, and K. P. Klugman. 2008. Telithromycin resistance in *Streptococcus pneumoniae* is conferred by a deletion in the leader sequence of *erm*(B) that increases rRNA methylation. *Antimicrob. Agents Chemother.* **52:**435–440.

382. Wolter, N., A. M. Smith, D. J. Farrell, W. Schaffner, M. Moore, C. G. Whitney, J. H. Jorgensen, and K. P. Klugman. 2005. Novel mechanism of resistance to oxazolidinones, macrolides, and chloramphenicol in ribosomal protein L4 of the pneumococcus. *Antimicrob. Agents Chemother.* **49:**3554–3557.

383. Wong, C. S., G. S. Palmer, and M. H. Cynamon. 1988. In-vitro susceptibility of *Mycobacterium tuberculosis*, *Mycobacterium bovis* and *Mycobacterium kansasii* to amoxycillin and ticarcillin in combination with clavulanic acid. *J. Antimicrob. Chemother.* **22:**863–866.

384. Woodford, N., M. Afzal-Shah, M. Warner, and D. M. Livermore. 2008. In vitro activity of retapamulin against *Staphylococcus aureus* isolates resistant to fusidic acid and mupirocin. *J. Antimicrob. Chemother.* **62:**766–768.

385. Wootton, M., A. P. MacGowan, and T. R. Walsh. 2006. Comparative bactericidal activities of daptomycin and vancomycin against glycopeptide-intermediate *Staphylococcus aureus* (GISA) and heterogeneous GISA isolates. *Antimicrob. Agents Chemother.* **50:**4195–4197.

386. Yan, K., L. Madden, A. E. Choudhry, C. S. Voigt, R. A. Copeland, and R. R. Gontarek. 2006. Biochemical characterization of the interactions of the novel pleuromutilin derivative retapamulin with bacterial ribosomes. *Antimicrob. Agents Chemother.* **50:**3875–3881.

387. Yang, L. P., and S. J. Keam. 2008. Retapamulin: a review of its use in the management of impetigo and other uncomplicated superficial skin infections. *Drugs* **68:**855–873.

388. Yeaman, M. R., L. A. Mitscher, and O. G. Baca. 1987. In vitro susceptibility of *Coxiella burnetii* to antibiotics, including several quinolones. *Antimicrob. Agents Chemother.* **31:**1079–1084.

389. Young, L. S., O. G. Berlin, and C. B. Inderlied. 1987. Activity of ciprofloxacin and other fluorinated quinolones against mycobacteria. *Am. J. Med.* **82**(Suppl. 4A):23S–26S.

390. Zhanel, G. G., K. Homenuik, K. Nichol, A. Noreddin, L. Vercaigne, J. Embil, A. Gin, J. A. Karlowsky, and D. J. Hoban. 2004. The glycylcyclines: a comparative review with the tetracyclines. *Drugs* **64:**63–88.

391. Zhanel, G. G., G. Sniezek, F. Schweizer, S. Zelenitsky, P. R. Lagace-Wiens, E. Rubinstein, A. S. Gin, D. J. Hoban, and J. A. Karlowsky. 2009. Ceftaroline: a novel broad-spectrum cephalosporin with activity against meticillin-resistant *Staphylococcus aureus*. *Drugs* **69:**809–831.

392. Zhanel, G. G., S. Trapp, A. S. Gin, M. DeCorby, P. R. Lagace-Wiens, E. Rubinstein, D. J. Hoban, and J. A. Karlowsky. 2008. Dalbavancin and telavancin: novel lipoglycopeptides for the treatment of gram-positive infections. *Expert Rev. Anti-Infect. Ther.* **6:**67–81.

393. Zurenko, G. E., B. H. Yagi, R. D. Schaadt, J. W. Allison, J. O. Kilburn, S. E. Glickman, D. K. Hutchinson, M. R. Barbachyn, and S. J. Brickner. 1996. In vitro activities of U-100592 and U-100766, novel oxazolidinone antibacterial agents. *Antimicrob. Agents Chemother.* **40:**839–845.

Mechanisms of Resistance to Antibacterial Agents

LOUIS B. RICE AND ROBERT A. BONOMO

66

GENERAL CONCEPTS, INOCULUM EFFECTS, AND TOLERANCE

When the growing problem of antimicrobial resistance in bacteria is considered, it is worth remembering that resistance is not a new phenomenon, nor is it unexpected in an environment in which potent antimicrobial agents are used. The diversity of the microbial world and the relatively specific activities of our antimicrobial agents virtually ensure widespread resistance among bacteria. In many cases, this resistance is recognized when an antibiotic is first tested for development. For example, it is not considered a problem or threat that *Escherichia coli* is resistant to vancomycin. We simply understand that *E. coli* is not among vancomycin's spectrum of activity, and we avoid using vancomycin when *E. coli* infection is known or highly suspected (i.e., it has natural or primary resistance to vancomycin). Conversely, the increasing resistance of *E. coli* to ciprofloxacin represents an important problem, since we frequently use the fluoroquinolone class of antimicrobial agents to treat infections in which *E. coli* is likely to be involved. So when we speak of the problem of resistance, we must recognize that most problems result from expression of resistance by bacteria that are intrinsically susceptible to the antibiotic in question (i.e., acquired resistance).

It is also important to recognize that resistance as a clinical entity is essentially a relative phenomenon, in many ways a problem only indirectly related to the microbiological techniques often used to detect it. For example, it is possible to incorporate enough ticarcillin into an agar plate to inhibit an ampicillin-resistant *Enterococcus faecium* (in many cases this requires about 10,000 μg/ml). So in one sense, ampicillin-resistant *E. faecium* is susceptible to high concentrations of ticarcillin. However, such concentrations cannot be achieved at the site of infection, so ampicillin-resistant *E. faecium* is not considered susceptible to ticarcillin. It is the responsibility of the Clinical and Laboratory Standards Institute (CLSI; formerly National Committee for Clinical Laboratory Standards), the Food and Drug Administration, and other standard-setting bodies in different countries to make determinations on susceptible, intermediate, and resistant breakpoints for new antimicrobial agents, considering factors of in vitro susceptibility, pharmacokinetics, and pharmacodynamics. These issues become very important in treating meningitis, in which

relatively minor increases in the *Streptococcus pneumoniae* MIC for penicillin can foil treatment, but in many cases are less relevant in the treatment of simple urinary tract infections, given the tendency of many antibiotics to concentrate in the urine.

The relativity of resistance is no better exemplified than by considerations of susceptibility in bacterial strains that exhibit significant inoculum effects, such as those resistant by virtue of producing β-lactamase. β-Lactamase-mediated resistance results from a chemical interaction in which the β-lactamase molecule binds to the β-lactam antibiotic in a manner that ultimately results in the hydrolysis of the critical β-lactam ring structure (Fig. 1). The rapidity and efficiency with which binding and hydrolysis proceed are dependent upon the affinity with which the β-lactamase molecule binds the antibiotic and the efficiency of the subsequent hydrolysis. High affinity and rapid hydrolysis mean that the cell wall synthesis machinery (penicillin-binding proteins [PBPs]) can be defended with relatively few β-lactamase molecules compared to the number of β-lactam molecules likely to be present in the vicinity of the PBPs. Low affinity and slow hydrolysis mean that more β-lactamase molecules are necessary for effective resistance, but also that resistance can be more easily overcome by adding more antibiotic molecules. Increasing the inoculum of organisms in a solution with a fixed concentration of β-lactam antibiotic has the effect of increasing the number of β-lactamase molecules and can in some instances result in clinically important levels of resistance. A *Klebsiella pneumoniae* strain that produces extended-spectrum β-lactamase (ESBL) TEM-26, for example, may exhibit a standard inoculum (ca. 10^5 CFU/ml) MIC for cefotaxime of 1 μg/ml. However, when the inoculum is increased to 10^7 CFU/ml, the MIC increases to >256 μg/ml (240).

A second, more amorphous and difficult-to-evaluate concept in considering antimicrobial resistance is that of tolerance, or resistance to killing at antimicrobial concentrations sufficient to inhibit further growth. Tolerance is an unimportant concept for the treatment of most infections, since for therapeutic success it is usually sufficient to inhibit further growth of bacteria (bacteriostatic activity), allowing the patient's immune defenses to kill the growth-inhibited organisms and clean up the debris. In some instances, however, antimicrobial killing of the bacteria (bactericidal

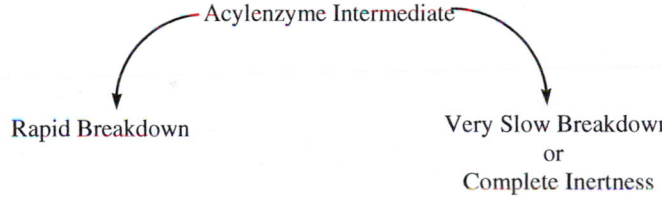

FIGURE 1 Serine β-lactamases and their reactions with β-lactam carbonyl donors. Modified from reference 101.

activity) is required to yield a high percentage of treatment success. Instances where bactericidal activity is preferred include endocarditis, meningitis, and osteomyelitis, in which the immune system has limited access to the infection site. They also include circumstances in which the immune system is severely compromised, such as in patients undergoing high-dose chemotherapy for hematologic malignancies. In these instances, antibiotics that are primarily bacteriostatic, such as the tetracyclines or the macrolides, are considered poor choices for therapy, whereas β-lactam antibiotics, which are primarily bactericidal, are preferred. Some bacteria are naturally tolerant to β-lactam antibiotics. Bactericidal activity against the enterococcus, for example, requires two agents, one active against cell wall synthesis and an aminoglycoside (179). Recognition of this bactericidal synergism raised cure rates for enterococcal endocarditis from about 40 to 70% or greater (235). Unfortunately, expression of aminoglycoside-modifying enzymes (AMEs) negates the synergism and appears to decrease the cure rates for enterococcal endocarditis. Although some level of tolerance to β-lactam antibiotics can be demonstrated for

several different bacterial species, the impact on the treatment of clinical infections appears to be less dramatic than with the enterococcus.

Emergence and Spread of Antibiotic Resistance

The emergence of antimicrobial resistance phenotypes is inevitably linked to the clinical (or other) use of the antimicrobial agent against which resistance is directed. One reason for this association is trivial—we do not generally test for resistance to antibiotics that are not in clinical use. The second reason is that nature abhors a vacuum, so when an effective antibiotic eliminates a susceptible biota, resistant varieties soon fill the niche. Once a resistance phenotype has emerged within a previously susceptible species, the rapidity and efficiency with which it spreads are affected by a host of different factors, including the degree of resistance expressed, the ability of the organism to tolerate the resistance mechanism, linkage to other genes, site of primary colonization, and others. The rapidity and completeness of resistance gene spread are often unpredictable. For example, the staphylococcal β-lactamase gene

TABLE 1 Common associations of resistance mechanisms

Antibiotic class	Resistance type	Resistance mechanism	Common example
Aminoglycosides	Decreased uptake	Changes in outer membrane permeability	*P. aeruginosa*
	Enzymatic modification (AMEs)	Phosphotransferase	Wide range of enteric gram-negative bacteria
		Adenyltransferase	Wide range of enteric gram-negative bacteria
		Acetyltransferase	Wide range of enteric gram-negative bacteria
		Bifunctional enzyme	*aac(6′)-aph(2″)* in *S. aureus*, *E. faecium*, and *E. faecalis*
β-Lactams	Altered PBP(s)	PBP 2a (additional PBP)	*mecA* in *S. aureus* and coagulase-negative staphylococci
		PBP 2x, PBP 2b, PBP 1a (acquired from other streptococci by transformation	*S. pneumoniae*
		PBP 5 (point mutation)	*E. faecium*
	Enzymatic degradation (β-lactamases)	Ambler class A	TEM-1 in *E. coli*, *H. influenzae*, and *N. gonorrhoeae*
			SHV-1 in *K. pneumoniae*
			K-1 (OXY-1) in *K. oxytoca*
			ESβLs (TEM-3+, SHV-2+, and CTX-M types) in *K. pneumoniae* and *E. coli*
			BRO-1 in *Moraxella catarrhalis*
			PC1 in *S. aureus*
			PSE-1 in *P. aeruginosa*
			KPC β-lactamases
		Ambler class B	L-1 in *S. maltophilia*
			Ccr-A in *B. fragilis*
		Ambler class C	AmpC in *E. cloacae*, *C. freundii*, and similar enzymes in *S. marcescens*, *M. morganii*, *P. stuartii*, and *Providencia rettgeri*
		Ambler class D	OXA-1 in *E. coli*
Chloramphenicol	Enzymatic degradation Efflux	CATs	CAT in *S. pneumoniae*
		Membrane transporters	*cmlA* and *flo*-encoded efflux in *E. coli* and *Salmonella* spp.
Glycopeptides	Altered target	Altered peptidoglycan cross-link target (D-Ala–D-Ala to D-Ala–D-Lac or D-Ala–D-Ser) encoded by complex gene cluster	VanA gene cluster in *E. faecium*, *E. faecalis*, and *S. aureus*; VanB gene cluster in *E. faecium* and *E. faecalis*
	Target overproduction	Excess peptidoglycan	Glycopeptide intermediate strains of *S. aureus* and *Staphylococcus haemolyticus*
Oxazolidinones	Altered target	Mutation leading to reduced binding to active site	G2576U mutation in rRNA in *E. faecium* and *S. aureus*
MLS$_B$	Altered target	Ribosomal active-site methylation with reduced binding	*erm*-encoded methylases in *S. aureus*, *S. pneumoniae*, and *S. pyogenes*
Macrolides	Efflux	Mef efflux pump	*mef*-encoded efflux in *S. pneumoniae* and *S. pyogenes*
Streptogramin A	Enzymatic degradation	Acetyltransferases	*vat[A]*, *vat[B]*, and *vat[C]*, encoded enzymes in *S. aureus*
			vat[D] and *vat[E]* encoded enzymes in *E. faecium*
Quinolones	Altered target	Mutation leading to reduced binding to active site(s) (quinolone-resistance determining region)	Mutations in *gyrA* in enteric gram-negative bacteria and *S. aureus*
			Mutations in *gyrA* and *parC* in *S. pneumoniae*
	Efflux	New membrane transporters	NorA in *S. aureus*
	Protection from DNA binding	Acquired protection protein	*qnr* gene and variants
	Enzymatic modification	Mutated aminoglycoside acetyltransferase	*aac6′-Ib* variant in *E. coli*
Rifampin	Altered target	Mutations leading to reduced binding to RNA polymerase	Mutations in *rpoB* in *S. aureus* and *M. tuberculosis*

(Continued on next page)

TABLE 1 (*Continued*)

Antibiotic class	Resistance type	Resistance mechanism	Common example
Tetracyclines	Efflux	New membrane transporters	*tet* genes encoding efflux proteins in gram-positive bacteria (mainly group 2) and gram-negative bacteria (mainly group 1)
	Altered target	Production of proteins that bind to the ribosome and alter the conformation of the active site (ribosomal protection proteins)	*tet*(M) in a variety of gram-positive bacteria
Sulfonamides	Altered target	Mutation or recombination of genes encoding DHPS	Found in a wide range of species, e.g., *E. coli*, *S. aureus*, and *S. pneumoniae*
		Acquisition of new low-affinity DHPS genes	*sulI* and *sulII* in enteric gram-negative bacteria
Trimethoprim	Altered target	Mutations in gene encoding DHFR	*S. aureus*, *S. pneumoniae*, and *H. influenzae*
		Acquisition of new low-affinity DHFR genes	*dhfrI* and *dhfrII* encoded, found in a wide range of species
	Overproduction of target	Promoter mutation leading to overproduction of DHFR	*E. coli*

(conferring resistance to penicillin) was first described shortly after the introduction of penicillin into clinical use and is now almost universally present within staphylococci in the hospital and the community. It was not until the early 1980s that this gene was described to occur in *Enterococcus*, and it has never spread widely in this genus. The reverse appears to be true with the vancomycin resistance genes, which are found widely in *E. faecium* but remain exceedingly rare in *Staphylococcus aureus*.

An important cause of the spread of antimicrobial resistance is the failure to adhere to appropriate infection control techniques, both within and outside the hospital. It is well established that strains of methicillin-resistant *S. aureus* (MRSA) within individual hospitals, and even within entire cities, are often clonally related, as determined by genetic techniques such as pulsed-field gel electrophoresis, multilocus sequence typing, and staphylococcal protein A typing (241). The spread of these problematic pathogens has been attributed to transmission from patient to patient, presumably by transiently or persistently colonized health care workers (262). The primary site of *S. aureus* colonization is the anterior nares. Colonization of the nares facilitates aerosol transmission of the resistant bacteria, particularly during periods of viral upper respiratory infection in the colonized worker. It also facilitates direct transmission, given the frequent contact between hands and nose in many people and the frequently poor hand washing practices of health care workers. The clinical consequences of patient colonization can be significant. Studies have shown a correlation between patient colonization with MRSA and subsequent infection during periods of high risk, such as the postoperative period (210).

Although antibiotic resistance is predominantly a nosocomial problem, resistant bacteria are also spread in the community setting. Sites in which resistant bacteria have been known to spread include day care centers and nursing homes (2, 310). Penicillin-resistant pneumococci have been found to colonize as many as 25% of a day care center's population. Transmission probably reaches its peak in the winter months, when viral upper respiratory infections are prevalent. The prevalence of viral upper respiratory infections works in two ways to increase transmission: (i) it probably increases the inoculum of resistant organisms being spread by those already colonized (see above references

for *S. aureus* colonization), and (ii) it makes those who are not colonized more likely to become colonized because of the increased likelihood that they will receive antimicrobial therapy. Nursing homes are predisposed to resistance for a variety of reasons, including the debilitated state of much of their population, frequent movement back and forth to tertiary care hospitals, and frequent use of antimicrobial agents in an effort to ward off infections that necessitate hospital admissions.

A final important source of the emergence and spread of antibiotic-resistant bacteria is nonhuman niches in which antibiotics are used. It is now well established that antimicrobial use in food animals is associated with both resistance in bacterial species that contaminate food and infect humans, primarily *Salmonella* and *Campylobacter*, and the transfer of resistance determinants to their human counterparts, such as *Enterococcus* (80). Compelling evidence also exists that high rates of ciprofloxacin resistance in *E. coli* can be associated with the use of fluoroquinolones in poultry (75). Finally, the European outbreak of vancomycin-resistant enterococci with the *vanA* determinant in the 1990s was almost certainly fueled by the use of avoparcin (a glycopeptide antibiotic) as a growth promoter in food animals (302). Data are also emerging that the use of antibiotics to promote growth of animals is often expensive and unnecessary, which has prompted many stakeholders in this issue to outline specific instances in which such antimicrobial use will be permitted.

Genetic Bases of Resistance

Acquired antimicrobial resistance results from biochemical processes that are encoded by bacterial genes. A general list of mechanisms of resistance is presented in Table 1. In order to understand the biochemical processes, it is useful to first discuss the genetic underpinnings of resistance and its evolution. Antimicrobial resistance arises by (i) mutation of cellular genes, (ii) acquisition of exogenous resistance genes, or (iii) mutation of acquired genes.

Mutation of Cellular Genes

All antibiotics have targets, which are often (but not always) proteins with important functional responsibilities for cell growth or maintenance. Cellular genes encode these proteins. Interactions between antibiotics and target proteins are often quite specific, and changing a single amino acid, frequently as a result of a single base change in the gene, can sometimes alter these interactions. Perhaps the most familiar example of this mechanism is resistance to rifampin. Rifampin targets the cellular RNA polymerase (encoded by *rpoB*), and a single point mutation in this gene may confer complete resistance. These mutations occur in most bacterial species at a relatively high frequency (ca. 10^{-8}/CFU). Incubating enough cells with inhibitory concentrations of rifampin eliminates susceptible cells and allows the resistant mutants to proliferate. The rifampin in the medium does not actually cause resistance but, rather, selects mutants that occur naturally but which have no selective advantage for survival in the absence of rifampin in the environment. Other examples of mutational resistance include resistance to streptomycin by ribosomal mutation (74), resistance to fluoroquinolones through mutations of cellular topoisomerases (167), and resistance to linezolid by mutations in the rRNA (224), among others.

Resistance mutations may also be found in genes that regulate cellular processes. Perhaps the most completely studied example of regulatory mutation resulting in resistance is the derepression of the chromosomal β-lactamase of *Enterobacter* spp. (127). Mutations in a cellular amidase gene (designated *ampD*) result in buildup of a cell wall breakdown product that has the effect of dramatically increasing expression of a chromosomal β-lactamase gene (*ampC*). Other examples of regulatory changes include the downregulation of expression of the porin OMPD2 in *Pseudomonas aeruginosa* associated with resistance to imipenem (157), or the insertion of an insertion sequence (IS) element upstream of a chromosomal carbapenemase conferring imipenem resistance on *Bacteroides fragilis* (214).

Whether mutational resistance is likely to persist depends in some measure on whether the resistance mutation is tolerable to the cell. For example, although decreased expression of OMPD2 appears to be readily achievable for *P. aeruginosa*, the fact that these resistant strains have not spread widely in the nearly 20 years of carbapenem use probably reflects the fact that this porin has functions that are beneficial to the bacterium, favoring reexpression of the porin once the imipenem threat has been dissipated. Similarly, intermediate levels of susceptibility to vancomycin in *S. aureus* have thus far been attributed to marked changes in the composition of the cell wall (265). These changes are unlikely to be favored in an environment free of vancomycin, since *S. aureus* likely "decided" a long time ago the optimal size and composition of its cell wall. The deleterious effects of acquiring resistance are often referred to as fitness cost.

Disadvantageous resistance mutations do not always disappear. Although initial point mutations in the *rpoB* gene that confer rifampin resistance on *Salmonella enterica* serotype Typhimurium appear to decrease the fitness of the organism for survival in vivo, persistence in a live host is frequently associated with compensatory mutations that at least partially restore fitness to the strain while retaining the resistance (rather than mutating back to susceptibility) (24). Similarly, transfer of mutated *pbp5* into *E. faecium* strains is often associated with decreases in the expression of ampicillin resistance, but growth on increased concentrations of ampicillin easily yields colonies that grow well at higher concentrations (237). Similar findings have been reported for *S. aureus* strains transformed with the *mecA* gene, encoding methicillin resistance (181). In summary, while mutational resistance often confers a fitness cost, subsequent adaptations may make expression of resistance less costly.

Acquisition of Resistance Genes

If resistance is not achievable through mutation, resistance determinants can be acquired. Most antimicrobial agents are natural products or derivatives of natural products. Therefore, resistance genes for most antibiotics must exist in the microbial world, either in the species that produce the antibiotic or within species that live in the same ecological niche as the antibiotic producers (62). The challenge for susceptible human pathogens is to find and acquire these resistance determinants. To assist in this acquisition, bacteria have evolved a range of mechanisms that promote gene exchange. Perhaps the simplest of these techniques is natural transformation, referring to the ability of some bacterial species to absorb naked DNA molecules from the environment under the appropriate circumstances (108). Once taken up by the susceptible bacterium, these foreign pieces of DNA enter the bacterial chromosome by recombining across regions of sufficient homology. In some cases, functional genes result from this recombination. If the acquired gene encodes a protein that is less susceptible to inhibition than the native protein, a reduction in susceptibility may result. Perhaps the best-studied example of the formation of these "mosaic" genes to confer resistance is penicillin and cephalosporin resistance in *Streptococcus pneumoniae* (108). A variety of mosaic *pbp* genes have been described to occur in resistant strains, with the level and degree of resistance determined by the number and nature of gene recombinations. Mosaic topoisomerase genes have also been described to occur in fluoroquinolone-resistant transformable bacteria (63).

Most bacteria are incapable of natural transformation and so have developed other mechanisms for acquiring useful genetic determinants. A commonly employed mechanism for genetic exchange is the transfer of conjugative plasmids. These extrachromosomal replicative DNA forms may bear a variety of important genes. Some plasmids are relatively narrow in their host range, while others transfer into and replicate within several different species. Transfer frequencies can be very high, as in the F factor of *E. coli* (virtual complete transfer in 1 h) or the pheromone-responsive plasmids found in *E. faecalis* (ca. 10^{-1} transconjugant/recipient CFU in 24 h), or more modest, as observed with the broad-host-range enterococcal plasmids such as pAMβ1 (10^{-7} to 10^{-6} transconjugant/recipient CFU in 24 h) (35). Having entered into a new genus on broad-host-range plasmids, resistance determinants can readily transfer onto more frequently transferable plasmids to increase their movement through the new genus. In the first case of true vancomycin-resistant *S. aureus* described in the literature, it appears that vancomycin resistance transposon Tn*1546* entered into *S. aureus* from *Enterococcus faecalis* on a broad-host-range plasmid and then transposed to a conjugative plasmid native to the staphylococcus (89, 304). Plasmids may also integrate into the chromosome of the recipient strains, potentially increasing the stability of the genetic information they carry.

Bacteria also take advantage of bacterial viruses (bacteriophages) for genetic exchange. These discreet packages deliver to uninfected cells a quantity of DNA approximating the size of their genome (in most cases roughly 40 kb). Designed to incorporate their own genome into the manufactured phage head, they sometimes incorporate bits of chromosomal DNA adjacent to the phage integration site (specialized transduction) and other times incorporate an appropriate-size plasmid or chromosomal DNA segment unrelated to the integrated phage genome (generalized transduction). Since the staphylococcal β-lactamase gene is frequently identified on nonconjugative plasmids of approximately 35 to 40 kb, and since bacteriophages have been well described for staphylococci for decades, it has been speculated that the high prevalence of β-lactamase production in staphylococci has resulted from bacteriophage-mediated transfer of these plasmids. Bacteriophages have also been implicated in the transfer of virulence determinants (82).

Nonreplicative mobile elements known as transposons have also been implicated in the transfer of resistance genes (232). Transposons encode their own ability to transfer between replicons (autonomously replicating DNA segments). In some cases, the transposons themselves encode conjugation functions, which allow them to transfer from bacterial chromosome to bacterial chromosome. The best characterized of these conjugative transposons is Tn916, an 18-kb element originally described for E. faecalis but which has a very broad host range (233). Tn916 encodes resistance to tetracycline and minocycline through the tet(M) resistance gene. Many different Tn916-like transposons have now been described for enterococci and other organisms, and some of them, such as Tn1545 from S. pneumoniae, possess additional resistance genes (conferring resistance to erythromycin and kanamycin) (233). Some investigators have suggested that the conjugation events associated with Tn916-like transposons are akin to cell fusion events, in which portions of the genome distinct from that adjacent to the inserted transposon can exchange via homologous recombination (284). Transposons with structural similarity to Tn916 have been implicated in the transfer of vancomycin resistance between E. faecium strains (40).

Transposons lacking conjugative functions may also transfer between strains. The most common mechanism by which this transfer is presumed to occur is either transient or more permanent integration into transferable plasmids. Among the more common classes of nonconjugative transposons are the Tn3 family elements (including Tn917, conferring erythromycin resistance, and Tn1546, conferring VanA-type vancomycin resistance) (14, 257) and the composite elements formed by mobile IS elements flanking resistance genes (including Tn4001, conferring high-level gentamicin resistance on many gram-positive species) (94).

In recent years the importance of "common regions" has been increasingly recognized (282). These regions, which are often found near the 3′ conserved regions of integrons, have been implicated in the movement of a range of different antimicrobial resistance determinants. These regions represent an atypical type of IS element (IS91-like). They lack typical inverted repeats and transpose by a rolling-circle mechanism that allows them to transpose adjacent DNA without a flanking second copy of the element.

The precise origin of resistance genes is often difficult to discern, but in some cases it is at least possible to determine that acquired resistance determinants originated in other genera. The VanB-type vancomycin resistance gene in enterococci, for example, has a G+C content of nearly 50% (78). The enterococcal genome, in contrast, has a G+C content of approximately 35 to 38%. These differences virtually confirm the origin of the vanB determinant in a genus other than Enterococcus. The likely origin appears to be streptomycetes, probably species that manufacture glycopeptide antibiotics, with entry into the enterococcus facilitated by the incorporation of these resistance operons into transposons.

It is worth noting at this point that any concept of the bacterial genome as a fixed entity is untenable. Comparisons of E. coli genomes reveal striking differences between enteropathogenic and uropathogenic strains, with the different regions constituting pathogenicity islands that confer specific virulence traits that give the strains their clinical profiles (111, 306). Data emanating from a comparative study of 36 S. aureus genomes indicate that 22% of the genome is dispensable, with many of these variable regions constituting presumed pathogenicity islands and regions of antimicrobial resistance (88). Finally, it is estimated that 25% of the genome of E. faecalis strain V583 was acquired from outside the genus (208).

Mutation of Acquired Genes

As bacteria have responded to the challenge of antimicrobial agents, so have we responded to the challenge of antibiotic resistance. Our typical response to the appearance of antimicrobial resistance has been a concerted effort to develop novel antimicrobial agents that are active against resistant strains. The emergence of β-lactamase-mediated resistance to antibiotics is an instructive example of this interplay. Ampicillin was developed as the first penicillin with clinically significant activity against gram-negative rods, primarily E. coli. Within a few years of the clinical introduction of ampicillin, strains of E. coli were described that were resistant to this antibiotic by virtue of production of a plasmid-mediated β-lactamase designated TEM (named after the patient from whom the resistant strain was isolated). S. aureus expressed a similar β-lactamase, prompting a concerted effort on the part of the pharmaceutical industry to develop β-lactam antibiotics resistant to hydrolysis. Among the more successful compounds that were developed were methicillin (with activity against β-lactamase-producing S. aureus), the cephalosporins and carbapenems (with widespread activity against many β-lactamase-producing species), and the β-lactamase inhibitors, which restored the activity of β-lactams susceptible to hydrolysis.

The most successful and widely developed class of β-lactamase-resistant β-lactam antibiotics is the cephalosporins. So many of these agents have been developed for clinical use that they are frequently lumped into "generations" to facilitate remembering their spectra of activity. The third-generation, or extended-spectrum, cephalosporins cefotaxime, ceftizoxime, ceftriaxone, and ceftazidime are particularly potent antibiotics that are resistant to hydrolysis by the original TEM enzyme. Unfortunately, increasing clinical use of these agents, particularly ceftazidime, was associated with the emergence of resistant gram-negative rods, particularly K. pneumoniae (131). Molecular analysis of these resistant strains revealed that the resistance was mediated by β-lactamase and that many of these β-lactamases were derived from the native TEM enzyme through one or more point mutations in the bla_{TEM} gene.

Biochemical Mechanisms of Resistance

Modification of the Antibiotic

Many antibiotic-modifying enzymes have been described, including the β-lactamases, the AMEs, and chloramphenicol acetyltransferases (CATs). Although these enzymes are in many cases acquired, some are intrinsic to certain genera. For example, chromosomal β-lactamases are intrinsic to almost all gram-negative rods. Expression of these enzymes is often only at a very low level, conferring resistance to only very susceptible β-lactams, as with *K. pneumoniae* resistance to ampicillin through expression of the chromosomal SHV-1 enzyme (236), or to no β-lactams at all, as with wild-type *E. coli* strains. In some bacterial genera (notably *Enterobacter* and *Pseudomonas*), chromosomal β-lactamases are under regulatory control, with derangements in these regulatory mechanisms resulting in high-level, broad-spectrum β-lactam resistance (128). In some instances AMEs are intrinsic to bacterial species as well, as with the chromosomal acetyltransferases of *Providencia stuartii* and *Serratia marcescens* (231, 258).

Modifying enzymes in general confer high levels of resistance to the antibiotics against which they have activity. Expression of the TEM-1 β-lactamase by *E. coli*, for example, can increase the ampicillin MIC from 8 μg/ml to >10,000 μg/ml. Similarly, expression of the bifunctional aminoglycoside resistance enzyme in *E. faecalis* raises the gentamicin MIC from 32 to 64 μg/ml to >2,000 μg/ml. As effective as these mechanisms are, however, some antibiotics appear to be immune to inactivating enzymes. Vancomycin has been in clinical use since 1958, yet there are still no examples of vancomycin-modifying enzymes in bacteria.

Modification of the Target Molecule

Since antibiotic interaction with target molecules is generally quite specific, minor alterations of the target molecule can have important effects on antibiotic binding. Numerous examples exist of antibiotic target modification as a mechanism of resistance, including the many erythromycin ribosomal methylases that confer resistance to the macrolide-lincosamide-streptogramin B (MLS$_B$) class of antibiotics (305). Modifications of PBPs can affect the affinities of these molecules for β-lactam antibiotics, as noted above for *S. pneumoniae*, and especially for ampicillin-resistant *E. faecium* through mutations in PBP 5 (108, 237). Modifications of PBPs seem to be a favored mechanism of β-lactam resistance in gram-positive bacteria, whereas β-lactamase production is favored in gram-negative rods. Although the reason for this difference is unknown, it is interesting that β-lactamases produced by gram-positive bacteria diffuse into the external medium once produced, whereas those produced by gram-negative rods are kept within the periplasmic space by the outer membrane. The ability to concentrate β-lactamases enhances their efficacy and may help explain the preference for this mechanism among gram-negative rods.

Other important examples of target modifications include the altered cell wall precursors that confer resistance to glycopeptide antibiotics, mutated DNA gyrase and topoisomerase IV conferring resistance to fluoroquinolone antimicrobial agents, ribosomal protection mechanisms conferring resistance to tetracyclines, and RNA polymerase mutations conferring resistance to rifampin. The degree of resistance conferred by target modifications is variable and may be dependent upon the ability of the mutated target to perform its normal function. Mutations in PBPs of *S. pneumoniae*, for example, confer a relatively low level of resistance (although one that is significant in the treatment of meningitis) (108), whereas VanA-type vancomycin resistance confers a very high level of resistance to vancomycin in enterococci (15).

Restricted Access to the Target

It is axiomatic that an antibiotic must reach its target in order to be effective. Therefore, for targets for which barriers must be crossed by the antibiotic, strengthening these barriers can be a highly effective mechanism of resistance. All gram-negative bacteria have an outer membrane that must be traversed before the cytoplasmic membrane can be reached. Reductions in the quantities of known or presumed porins (channels for movement of materials across the outer membrane) have been documented as important contributors to resistance to imipenem in *P. aeruginosa*, cefepime in *Enterobacter cloacae,* and cefoxitin or ceftazidime in *K. pneumoniae* (151, 157, 168). In most instances, this restricted entry must be in combination with production of an at least moderately active β-lactamase to confer high-level resistance. Barriers to entry can also exist in the cytoplasmic membrane. Movement of aminoglycosides across the cytoplasmic membrane is an oxygen-dependent process, so these antibiotics are inactive in anaerobic environments (and hence against strictly anaerobic species) (149).

Efflux Pumps

Among the most active areas of research in antimicrobial resistance is the identification and characterization of pumps that extrude one or more antibiotic classes from the bacterial cell. Several classes of pumps have been described for gram-positive and/or gram-negative bacteria. They may be quite selective, or they may have a broad substrate specificity. The majority of these pumps are located in the cytoplasmic membrane and use proton motive force to drive drug efflux. The major families of efflux transporters are (i) the major facilitator superfamily (MFS), which includes QacA and NorA/Bmr of gram-positive bacteria and EmrB of *E. coli*; (ii) the small multidrug resistance family, including Smr of *S. aureus* and EmrE of *E. coli*; and (iii) the resistance-nodulation-cell division (RND) family, including AcrAB-TolC of *E. coli* and MexAB-OprM of *P. aeruginosa*. The structure of the AcrAB-TolC RND-type efflux pump is shown in Fig. 2. Deciphering the crystal structure of this pump was a major achievement (182). Among other things, it revealed that there was a periplasmic opening in the pump that could allow passage of molecules, explaining the previously confusing observation that RND pumps included β-lactam antibiotics (which do not enter the cytoplasm) among their substrates. In some instances, combinations of different types of pumps can result in higher levels of resistance than are achieved by the activity of a single pump alone (150).

Attribution of resistance to a specific mechanism may be difficult when more than one mechanism is involved. For example, resistance to imipenem in *P. aeruginosa* is contributed to by reduced access (through downregulation of OMPD2) and production of AmpC β-lactamase (157). Neither mechanism alone is sufficient to yield clinically significant levels of resistance, yet both are required for high levels of resistance to result.

RESISTANCE MECHANISMS FOR DIFFERENT ANTIMICROBIAL CLASSES

Aminoglycoside Resistance

In explaining resistance to aminoglycosides (amikacin, gentamicin, kanamycin, neomycin, netilmicin, paromomycin, streptomycin, and tobramycin), we first explain how aminoglycosides reach their target in bacterial cells and then review their mechanism of action. The clinical indications for aminoglycoside therapy are also summarized.

The aminoglycosides contain an aminocyclitol ring (streptidine or 2-deoxystreptamine) and two or more amino sugars linked by glycosidic bonds. They are hydrophilic antibiotics whose antimicrobial activity is concentration dependent. They are particularly active against aerobic, gram-negative

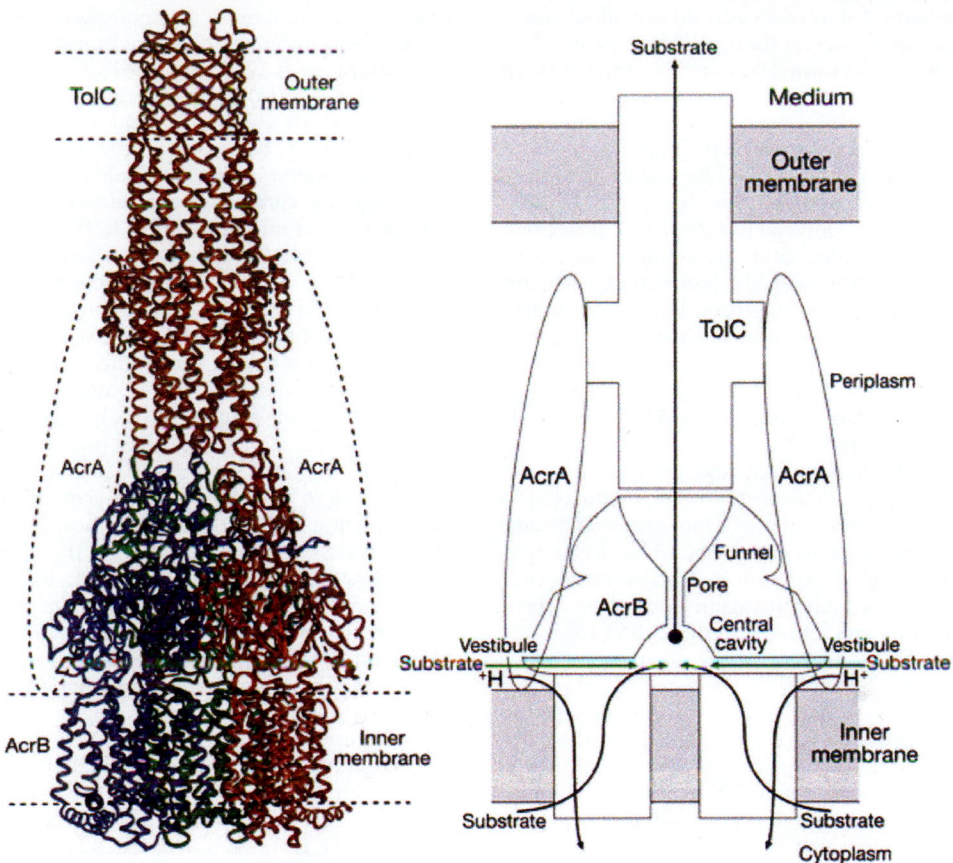

FIGURE 2 Representation of the crystal structure of the AcrAB-TolC three-component RND multidrug efflux pump. On the left are the three components of the pumps as they link the cytoplasmic (inner) membrane to the outer membrane. The periplasmic linker protein (AcrA) is shown only in outline to allow visualization of the linkage between AcrB and TolC. On the right, an outline of the pump shown at the left is presented, detailing the functional regions of the pump. Reprinted with permission from reference 182.

rods. As a class, these agents have other highly desirable qualities: they are rapidly bactericidal, demonstrate a postantibiotic effect, and exhibit predictable pharmacodynamics.

Mechanism of Action of Aminoglycosides

Aminoglycosides have unique effects on protein translation in prokaryotes. These effects may explain why aminogolycosides are bactericidal, whereas most other antibiotics that target the ribosome (chloramphenicol, macrolides, and tetracyclines) are bacteriostatic.

First, aminoglycosides penetrate bacteria by three main steps. The positively charged aminoglycoside binds to the negatively charged bacterial cell. Next, in an energy-dependent process driven by the membrane-bound electron transport system present only in aerobic bacteria, a small fraction of the aminoglycosides that are attached to the bacterium are taken into the cell.

Once inside the cell, the principal target of aminoglycoside action is the 30S subunit of the ribosome. The molecular details of aminoglycoside binding to the ribosome are unique. Gentamicin attaches to the highly conserved tRNA acceptor A site of the *E. coli* 16S rRNA (176). This binding prevents the elongation of the growing peptide chain by causing misreading or premature termination of peptide synthesis. By interfering with translation of mRNA,

protein production is altered, aberrant proteins are synthesized and inserted in the cell membrane, cell permeability is increased, more aminoglycosides are taken up into the cell, and cell death ensues.

Mistranslated proteins may also affect the bacterial cell. Paromomycin increases the error rate of protein translation by allowing the incorporation of the wrong tRNAs (the missense substitution rate of amino acids at specified positions in proteins is 1 in 3,000). Spectinomycin, a non-aminoglycoside aminocyclitol, inhibits translocation of the peptidyl-tRNA from the A site to the P site. Streptomycin also makes the ribosome error prone by allowing the binding of different tRNAs (43).

Resistance to aminoglycosides can occur by four mechanisms: (i) loss of cell permeability (decreased uptake), (ii) alterations in the ribosome that prevent binding, (iii) expulsion by efflux pumps, and (iv) enzymatic inactivation by AMEs.

Resistance due to Decreased Uptake and Altered Electrical Potential, Divalent Cations, and Efflux

It is well known that bacterial respiration generates an electrical potential across the membrane. Hence, anaerobes and facultative anaerobes (e.g., enterococci or certain small-colony variants of staphylococci) do not allow movement of aminoglycosides across their cell membranes. This intrinsic resistance confers low-level cross-resistance to all aminoglycosides.

Studies of *P. aeruginosa* and *E. coli* indicate that movement across the outer membrane may be due to a self-promoted uptake mechanism. The cationic aminoglycosides displace divalent cations (e.g., Mg^{2+}) that cross-bridge adjacent lipopolysaccharide (LPS) molecules, thereby permeabilizing the outer membrane and allowing entry of aminoglycosides (136). Consistent with this model, divalent cations have long been known to antagonize the activity of aminoglycosides against gram-negative bacteria (38).

Recent data indicate that *P. aeruginosa* possesses an inducible RND-type pump (MexXY-OprM) that extrudes aminoglycosides (132, 164). In *E. coli*, aminoglycosides are captured from both periplasm and cytoplasm by the AcrD multidrug efflux transporter (3). Evaluating a multidrug-resistant (MDR) strain of *Acinetobacter baumannii* BM4454 that was resistant to aminoglycosides, Magnet et al. found an RND-type efflux pump in *A. baumannii* (162) and showed that it was under stringent control by a two-component regulatory and sensor system, *adeRS* (165).

Modification of the Ribosome

Bacterial cells have multiple copies of the rRNA genes. Mutations that affect aminoglycoside binding to the ribosome include alterations in ribosomal proteins, 16S rRNA, and enzymatic methylation of the rRNA. Ribosomal mutations have been demonstrated to confer resistance to spectinomycin and streptomycin (294) and, more recently, to other aminoglycosides as well (171). The newly identified 16S rRNA methylases (RmtA, RmtB, and ArmA) in gram-negative rods have been noted as emerging problems (316). The first such novel enzyme was found in *K. pneumoniae* BM4536 and designated *armA* (aminoglycoside resistance methylase A) (95, 96).

AMEs

As in the case with β-lactamases (see below), aminoglycoside inactivation by AMEs is the most important mechanism in terms of frequency and level of resistance (17). AMEs are believed to originate from *Actinomycetes* that synthesize these antibiotics (*Streptomyces* and *Micromonospora* spp.). It is also possible that AMEs originated from enzymes involved in normal cellular respiration (housekeeping functions)

(230). These enzymes are phosphotransferases (APHs), nucleotidyltransferases or adenyltransferases (ANTs), and acetyltransferases (AACs). AMEs covalently modify specific amino or hydroxyl groups, resulting in aminoglycosides that bind poorly (higher K_m and less affinity) to the ribosome. AMEs can be passed from one bacterium to another by mobile genetic elements. These resistance determinants are frequently carried on specialized transposable genetic elements called integrons (259, 309).

Sites of AME modification of aminoglycosides are delineated by a standard numbering system. The streptidine or 2-deoxystreptamine nucleus forms the center for the numbering scheme (from 2-deoxystreptamine derive all aminoglycosides except streptomycin and spectinomycin). The first sugar moiety at the 4 position has positions numbered with a single prime (1′ to 6′); the second sugar moiety at the 6 position gets positions numbered with a double prime (1″ to 6″). Hence, AAC(6′) acetylates an amino group at the 6′ position (via an acetyltransferase) on the amino sugar attached to the 4 position (Fig. 3). Each AME class consists of numerous enzymes that can modify different OH or NH_2 groups. These are divided into subclasses. In each subclass, there are different enzyme types that are designated by a roman numeral, e.g., AAC(3)-I. Isoenzymes are also described and are designated by a lowercase letter a or b, etc. These isoenzymes are functionally identical and confer identical resistance phenotypes.

Currently, there are seven major phosphotransferases [APH(3′), APH(2″), APH(3″), APH(6), APH(9), APH(4), and APH(7″)], four nucleotidyltransferases [ANT(6), ANT(3″), ANT(4′), and ANT(2″)], and four acetyltransferases [AAC(2′), AAC(6), AAC(1), and AAC(3)]. A bifunctional AME also exists able to acetylate and phosphorylate [AAC(6′)-APH(2″)]. This enzyme is found in *Staphylococcus*, *Streptococcus*, and *Enterococcus* and is responsible for high-level resistance to aminoglycosides (81). The gene *aac(6′)-aph(2″)*, which encodes the synthesis of this enzyme, is present in Tn*4001*-like transposons which are inserted in both plasmids and the chromosomes of aminoglycoside-resistant isolates. Most aminoglycoside-resistant health care-associated MRSA strains express this enzyme.

Resistance to β-Lactam Antibiotics

PBP-Mediated Resistance

β-Lactam antibiotics (penicillins, cephalosporins, monobactams, and carbapenems) are the safest and mostly widely

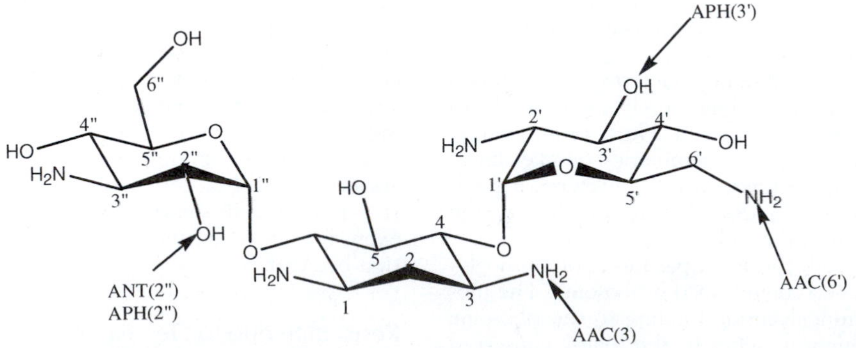

FIGURE 3 Sites of modification on kanamycin B by various AMEs. The arrows point to the sites of modification by the specific enzymes, namely, acetyltransferases, phosphotransferases, and nucleotidyltransferases. Reprinted with permission from reference 145.

used class of antibiotics ever developed. They act by inhibiting the PBPs, the transpeptidases that manufacture peptidoglycan. The specific functions of different PBPs have been identified for some bacteria, but the precise ways in which they interact with each other and with cell wall precursors remain largely a mystery. Some are clearly essential for cell viability (generally the high-molecular-weight transpeptidases and their partner transglycosylases), while others appear to be dispensable, with no apparent deleterious effects on cellular structure or function resulting from their absence (most commonly the low-molecular-weight carboxypeptidases). It has long been suspected that some PBPs are redundant and can perform the functions of others. For example, *E. faecium* strains in which all of the PBPs except low-affinity PBP 5 are saturated grow normally, implying that PBP 5 can perform all of the penicillin-inhibitable functions required for cell wall synthesis (311). On the other hand, *E. faecium* strains in which *pbp5* has been deleted grow normally as well, implying that the other PBPs can provide all of these functions (237).

PBPs are all members of a larger family of serine peptidases that includes most of the β-lactamases. PBPs and β-lactamases interact with β-lactam molecules (themselves structural analogues of the peptidyl-D-alanyl–D-alanine termini of peptidoglycan precursors) by catalytically disrupting the β-lactam bond, resulting in a serine ester-linked acyl enzyme derivative (Fig. 1). In the case of β-lactamases, a water molecule then hydrolyzes the ester linkage of the acyl enzyme intermediate, releasing the irreversibly damaged penicilloyl (or cephalosporyl) moiety and regenerating the active enzyme. PBP–β-lactam acyl enzyme derivatives are in general less accommodating to nucleophilic attack by the water molecule, resulting in a persistence of the covalent bond and inactivation of the PBP. The stability of this interaction allows identification of these proteins by binding to radiolabeled penicillin and is the genesis of their designation as PBPs. Because β-lactamases have no definable function in the cell other than to interact with β-lactam molecules, their affinity for the β-lactam and the rapidity with which the reaction proceeds determine their effectiveness, and hence the level of resistance. Conversely, since PBPs have a very important alternative function (manufacture of cell wall), the affinity of the interaction between PBPs and the β-lactam is a measure of distraction from their primary functions and thereby often defines the level of susceptibility of the strain.

Inhibition of PBPs interrupts cell wall synthesis, which by itself should inhibit cell growth rather than kill the cell. However, the interaction of β-lactam molecules with PBPs triggers the activity of cell wall-degrading molecules known as autolysins, which rupture the cell, leading to cell death (283). The extent to which these autolytic enzymes are activated correlates in most cases with the killing activity of a β-lactam against a particular bacterial strain.

Some bacterial species are intrinsically resistant to some β-lactam antibiotics by virtue of decreased PBP affinity. For example, enterococci are resistant to clinically achievable levels of cephalosporin antibiotics because of the presence of low-affinity PBP 5. Similar low affinity is demonstrated for the semisynthetic antistaphylococcal penicillins nafcillin and oxacillin, as well as for the antipseudomonal penicillins carbenicillin and ticarcillin. Enterococcal PBP 5 is bound with a diminished affinity by ampicillin and the ureidopenicillins mezlocillin and piperacillin, resulting in MICs that are higher than for streptococci, but within the concentration range achievable in human serum.

PBP-mediated resistance for normally susceptible bacteria takes several forms, including (i) overproduction of a PBP, (ii) acquisition of a foreign PBP with low affinity, (iii) recombination of a susceptible PBP with more resistant varieties, and (iv) point mutations within PBPs that lower affinity for the β-lactam antibiotic. PBP-mediated resistance is predominantly found in gram-positive bacteria. However, there are examples of gram-negative bacteria with PBP-mediated resistance, and we point these out as they come up.

PBP Overexpression

Increased expression of a PBP as a mechanism of conferring resistance is relatively uncommon. Clear examples of settings in which increased quantities of a PBP are associated with resistance include the increased levels of methicillin resistance found in *S. aureus* strains overexpressing PBP 4 (115) and increased levels of penicillin resistance in *Enterococcus hirae* and *E. faecium* strains that overexpress PBP 5 (90, 237). The existence of this mechanism serves as a reminder that, like with β-lactamases, susceptibility or resistance depends on the number of β-lactam molecules relative to the number of targets. Increasing the number of target molecules can, under the correct circumstances, result in resistance. Conversely, imipenem's effectiveness against *E. coli* has been partially attributed to the fact that its primary target is PBP 2, which is present in roughly 200 copies, in contrast to PBP 3, estimated at 2,000 copies. In any case, overproduction of PBPs is a rare mechanism of resistance to β-lactam antibiotics.

Acquisition of Foreign PBPs

Acquisition of a foreign PBP as a mechanism of resistance is best exemplified by the expression of methicillin resistance in *S. aureus* strains by virtue of the expression of PBP 2a, a low-affinity PBP not native to *S. aureus* (47). PBP 2a is classified as a class B PBP, meaning that it has a function C-terminal transpeptidase domain but an N-terminal domain whose function has yet to be determined. This contrasts with class A PBPs, which have N termini with glycosyltransferase activities and C termini with transpeptidase activities. As a result, the transglycosylase domain of *S. aureus* PBP 2 is required for expression of β-lactam resistance by PBP 2a (213). The cooperation of specific class A PBPs with low-affinity class B PBPs has also been shown for *E. faecalis* and, more recently, for *E. faecium* (9, 239).

The origin of the *mecA* gene (which encodes PBP 2a) is unknown. A *mecA* homologue has been identified in *Staphylococcus sciuri*, a primitive staphylococcal species associated with rodents and primitive mammals (56). The deduced amino acid sequences of the two enzymes exhibited 88% similarity across the entire protein and 91% identity within the transpeptidase domain. *S. sciuri* strains are not methicillin resistant, however, which may owe to the lack of an effective promoter upstream of the gene. *S. sciuri mecA* homologues in which the promoter has spontaneously mutated express higher levels of methicillin resistance both in *S. sciuri* and when cloned on a high-copy-number vector in *S. aureus* (315). Expression of methicillin resistance in *S. aureus* is commonly under regulatory control, either by the product of the upstream *mecI* gene or in *trans* by the homologous *blaI* gene, which regulates expression of β-lactamase (the promoter regions of *mecA* and the *blaZ* β-lactamase genes are similar) (106). The *mecI/blaI* repressors are, in turn, controlled by the *mecR1/blaR1* sensors/transducers, although the precise mechanism of this interaction is incompletely understood. The efficiency of induction varies with the mechanism (*blaR1-blaI*-mediated induction is faster), leading to complications in detecting the methicillin resistance phenotype. In fact, only a small minority of a resistant population may express high levels of resistance. Several techniques are used in the laboratory to "bring out" the resistance (prolonged incubation, increased salt in the media, and cefoxitin susceptibility testing), and more recently, techniques have been developed to bypass phenotypic expression in favor of directly identifying the *mecA* gene or directly detecting PBP 2a.

Expression of PBP 2a-mediated resistance to β-lactams in *S. aureus* is also influenced by the expression of other genetic loci called the *fem* (factors essential for methicillin resistance) or *aux* (auxiliary) genes (47). The *fem* and *aux* genes were first identified by transposon mutagenesis of MRSA looking for insertions that would reduce the expression of resistance. Many *fem* and *aux* factors have now been identified, and all are involved in the formation of the staphylococcal cell wall (47). These data indicate that minor perturbations of the normal processes prevent PBP 2a from functioning, suggesting that it is a very particular enzyme. However, when cloned into a heterologous (*E. faecalis*) background, PBP 2a was found to be capable of synthesizing peptidoglycan polymers using precursors distinctly different from those found in *S. aureus* (8).

The *mecA* gene is located within a larger (ca. 21- to 67-kb) region of the chromosome known as the staphylococcal chromosomal cassette (SCC*mec*) region (126). SCC*mec* is a mobile element, with mobility conferred by the presence of the *ccrA/B* or *ccrC* gene. The basic elements of SCC*mec* are the *mecR1/mecI/pbp2a* region and *ccrA*. In recent community-acquired *S. aureus* isolates, little else is included in the SCC*mec* complexes (types IV to VII) (65). Hence, the SCC*mec* region in these isolates is relatively small (20 to 30 kb), and the isolates themselves tend to be resistant to only β-lactams. As of this writing, seven (and possibly eight) different *mec* regions (SCC*mec* I to VII) have been described (65, 320). Nosocomial isolates have larger SCC*mec* regions, owing to the accumulation over time of integrated plasmids or transposons that contribute to the multiresistance of these isolates (126). Although the SCC*mec* element has never been shown to be transferable in vitro, compelling data have emerged from the study of clinical isolates that the type IV SCC*mec* element has been recently acquired (83). Transfer of the *mec* region between staphylococcal strains has never been conclusively documented. The spread of MRSA within institutions is therefore largely due to the transmission of resistant organisms from patient to patient, probably on the hands of transiently colonized health care workers (262). Single strains have spread through entire hospitals and even cities (241). *mecA* stabilities differ among different *S. aureus* clones (138), suggesting one potential explanation for the limited lineages within which the resistance determinant has been found.

Resistance Mutations by Recombination with Foreign DNA

Resistance through recombination between native, susceptible PBPs and those of less susceptible species is largely restricted to species that are capable of natural transformation, or taking up naked DNA from the environment. Prominent among these species are *S. pneumoniae*, viridans group streptococci, *Neisseria gonorrhoeae*, and *Neisseria meningitidis* (108). *S. pneumoniae* contains six PBPs (1a,

1b, 2a, 2b, 2x, and 3), all of which are subject to recombination with foreign PBPs taken up by transformation. In most cases, resistant *pbp* genes demonstrate mosaic patterns (individual segments of foreign *pbp* genes integrated with the native *pbp* gene) with the foreign DNA in the less penicillin-susceptible viridans group streptococci (108). In fact, genetic exchange appears common between these closely related species, with mosaic patterns demonstrable even in PBPs from susceptible *Streptococcus mitis* strains (7). Penicillin resistance in *S. pneumoniae* can be established by alterations in PBPs 2x, 2b, and 1a, whereas only alterations in PBPs 2x and 1a are required for cephalosporin resistance (19). Penicillin resistance has been described to occur in *S. pneumoniae* for some time, with cephalosporin resistance emerging more recently, most commonly in strains already resistant to penicillin. However, strains resistant to cephalosporins but susceptible to penicillin have also been reported (268). High-level resistance (≥2 μg/ml) usually implies modification of more than one PBP, sometimes with several mosaic regions in each one (19).

As with PBP 2a-mediated resistance to methicillin in *S. aureus*, expression of penicillin and cephalosporin resistance in *S. pneumoniae* is dependent on the proper functioning of auxiliary genes. The *fib* locus of *S. pneumoniae* (*fibA* and *fibB*) is analogous to *femA* and *femB* in *S. aureus*. It is involved in formation of interpeptide bridges, and inactivation of the *fib* locus is associated with reduction of cross-linked muropeptides and loss of penicillin resistance even in the presence of low-affinity mosaic PBPs (301). The *murM/murN* operon encodes enzymes involved in the biosynthesis of branched structured cell wall muropeptides commonly found in penicillin-resistant pneumococci (85). Inactivation of *murM/murN* results in loss of branched-chain muropeptides as well as loss of penicillin resistance.

Among gram-negative species, *Neisseria* organisms are well known to be naturally transformable. It is therefore not entirely surprising that strains of both *Neisseria gonorrhoeae* and *Neisseria meningitidis* have been described in which mosaic PBP genes are associated with decreased susceptibility to penicillin (108). Similar to the *S. pneumoniae* picture, the resistant portions of the PBP genes have been acquired from closely related commensal *Neisseria* species that are more resistant to penicillin (272). While penicillin resistance in *N. meningitidis* remains, thankfully, extremely rare, both β-lactamase-mediated resistance and PBP-mediated resistance to β-lactams in *N. gonorrhoeae* are quite common.

Point Mutations

The final mechanism of PBP-mediated β-lactam resistance results from point mutations within the *pbp* genes that result in lower affinity for the β-lactam in question. This form of mutational resistance is seen most commonly in PBP 5 of *E. faecium* strains, raising penicillin MICs from 4 to 16 μg/ml to as high as >1,000 μg/ml. High-level penicillin-resistant strains now represent the majority of clinical *E. faecium* isolates in the United States (249). These mutations further reduce the affinity for cephalosporins and other β-lactams with lower affinity for the nonmutated version, leading to an increase in resistance that may have implications for the likelihood that antibiotic use will promote colonization with MDR *E. faecium* (68). Most of the mutations occur in the vicinity of one or more of several conserved boxes important for β-lactam binding (247). A systematic study of several common mutations of PBP 5 has revealed that resistance increases with increasing number of mutations, with some loci conferring higher levels of resistance than others (234).

In rare instances, point mutations of the *S. aureus pbp2* gene have been associated with methicillin resistance, but the importance of this mechanism pales in comparison to that of expression of PBP 2a (107). Among gram-negative species, point mutations of the *ftsI* gene of *Haemophilus influenzae* (encoding the transpeptidase domain of PBP 3a and/or PBP 3b) have been associated with non-β-lactamase-mediated resistance to ampicillin and cephalosporins in this species (291). Although mutations have also been noted within PBP 4 in this species, it is not clear that these have a significant impact on β-lactam susceptibility.

β-Lactamase-Mediated Resistance

Classification of β-Lactamases

Two major schemes are currently used to classify β-lactamases: the Ambler classification system and the Bush-Jacoby classification system (35a). The Ambler classification separates β-lactamases into four distinct classes (A to D) based on similarities in amino acid sequence. Classes A, C, and D are serine β-lactamases, whereas class B enzymes are metallo-β-lactamases that require one or two zinc atoms for activity (see above). The Bush-Jacoby classification system (formerly referred to as Bush-Medeiros-Jacoby scheme [7, 36, 37]) classifies β-lactamases according to functional similarities (substrate and inhibitor profiles). There are four categories (groups) and multiple subgroups in the updated Bush-Jacoby system (groups 1, 2 [2a, 2b, 2br, 2d, 2be, 2c, and 2f], etc.) (36). A comparison of the two classification systems is summarized in Table 2. In the discussions that ensue, we refer to both classification systems.

At the time of this writing, more than 890 β-lactamases are reported (K. Bush, personal communication). The largest increases in numbers occurred in the class A and class D families. To illustrate, there are currently more than 165 TEM β-lactamases, more than 75 ESBLs of the TEM family, 36 inhibitor-resistant TEMs (IRTs), 9 complex mutants of TEM (CMTs), 126 SHVs, more than 160 OXA enzymes, and 91 CTX-M ESBLs. The number of class C β-lactamases has also increased to 44, and the numbers of IMP and VIM metallo-β-lactamases have increased to 25 and 23, respectively (these families are discussed below). Most worrisome is the number of β-lactamases that are able to hydrolyze carbapenems. As these carbapenemases (e.g., *Klebsiella pneumoniae* carbapenemase [KPC]) are being recovered from clinical isolates, the threat to our "last line" therapy is ever increasing. Presently, there are nine variants of KPC β-lactamases. The reader is referred to the following website for updates: http://www.lahey.org/studies.

β-Lactamase Mechanism

β-Lactamases are members of a superfamily of active-site serine proteases or D,D-peptidases (170). The mechanism of hydrolysis of β-lactams by β-lactamases is best studied for TEM-1. TEM-1 β-lactamase disrupts the amide bond of a β-lactam in a two-step reaction. First, the negatively charged carboxylate group of the β-lactam antibiotic is attracted to the active site by the enzyme's positively charged residues. There, the β-lactam is properly positioned, making key hydrogen bonding interactions with the enzyme (142). The residues in the active site that facilitate this attraction in the serine β-lactamases are often called the oxyanion hole or electrophilic center. Next, the β-lactam is acylated (Fig. 1). A conserved serine, Ser70, in the active site of TEM-1 serves as the reactive nucleophile in this acylation reaction. Recent ultrahigh-resolution x-ray crystallography studies of TEM-1 (0.85 Å) indicate that Glu166, acting through the catalytic water, activates Ser70 for nucleophilic attack of the β-lactam ring. Then, a strategically positioned water molecule is activated by a general base (e.g., again Glu166 and the same water molecule). This water molecule deacylates the β-lactam and regenerates the active β-lactamase. This symmetric mechanism is also supported by the ultrahigh-resolution structure (0.90 Å) of another common class A β-lactamase, SHV-2, found in *K. pneumoniae* (196). There is general consensus on the mechanics of deacylation by the class A TEM-1 β-lactamase (attention to Glu166), but the details of acylation still remain contentious. Debate centers on which residue in the active site (Lys73 or Glu166) deprotonates the reactive Ser70 or whether either pathway is in competition with the other (174).

β-Lactamase Processing

Generally speaking, β-lactamases are secreted into the periplasmic space in gram-negative bacteria or into the surrounding medium by gram-positive organisms.

TABLE 2 β-Lactamase classification

Bush-Jacoby system classification	Major subgroup	Ambler system classification	Main attributes
Group 1 cephalosporinases		C (cephalosporinases)	Usually chromosomal; resistance to all β-lactams except carbapenems; not inhibited by clavulanate
Group 2 penicillinases (clavulanic acid susceptible)	2a	A (serine β-lactamases)	Staphylococcal penicillinases
	2b	A	Broad spectrum: TEM-1, TEM-2, and SHV-1
	2be	A	Extended spectrum: TEM and SHV variants, predominantly
	2br	A	IRTs
	2c	A	Carbenicillin hydrolyzing
	2e	A	Cephalosporinases inhibited by clavulanate
	2f	A	Carbapenemases inhibited by clavulanate
	2d	D (oxacillin hydrolyzing)	Oxacillin-hydrolyzing (OXA)
Group 3 metallo-β-lactamase	3a	B (metalloenzymes)	Zinc-dependent carbapenemases
	3b	B	
	3c	B	
Group 4		Not classified	Miscellaneous enzymes, most not yet sequenced

Membrane-associated enzymes have been rarely reported (*Bacillus licheniformis*, *Bacillus cereus*, and *Bacteroides vulgatus*). β-Lactamases are synthesized as precursor proteins. As in other bacteria, the export of proteins into the periplasmic space is mediated by an amino-terminal signal peptide. After transport, the signal peptide of the β-lactamase is cleaved by a processing enzyme, signal peptidase I.

Genetic Environment of β-Lactamases

β-Lactamases can be chromosome-, plasmid-, or transposon-encoded enzymes that are produced in a constitutive or inducible manner. An increasing number of β-lactamases have been found that are encoded on integrons.

Integrons are genetic elements of variable length that contain a 5′ conserved integrase gene (*int*), mobile antibiotic resistance genes (called cassettes), and an integration site for the gene cassette, *attI* (att, attachment). To date, five distinct integron classes have been found to be associated with cassettes that contain antibiotic resistance genes. Three main classes of integrons (classes 1 to 3) have been described for gram-negative bacteria. Integrons capture antibiotic resistance gene cassettes by using a site-specific recombination mechanism. In the class 1 integrons, the 3′ conserved segment includes three open reading frames, *qacEΔ1*, a deletion derivative of the antiseptic resistance gene *qacE*, and *sul1*, a sulfonamide resistance gene. As integrons carry multiple resistance determinants and can be readily mobilized, their impact on antibiotic resistance is significant. In the words of Hall and Collis, "integrons thus act both as natural cloning systems and as expression vectors" (109). The capture and spread of antibiotic resistance determinants by integrons underlie the rapid evolution of multiple antibiotic resistance among diverse gram-negative clinical isolates (244). As reviewed by Stokes and Hall (273a), integrons were originally found on mobile elements from pathogenic bacteria and were found to be a major reservoir of antibiotic resistance genes. Analysis of their gene content suggests that integrons are phylogenetically diverse and have been with bacteria for a long time. Interestingly, integrons have been found in approximately 9% of sequenced bacterial genomes. It is maintained that the integron/gene cassette system has a function in evolution rather than just conferring resistance to antibiotics. Consequently, integrons may be the agents of change that drive bacterial evolution and adaptation. It should be noted that gene cassettes are mobile and can also exist in free circular form. However, these cassettes do not include all functions required for their mobility. Cassettes are formally part of the integron only when they are integrated at the integron receptor site. The genes within the cassette do not have promoters.

Integrons are an important source for the spread of *bla* genes. Integrons containing β-lactamases have been found in *A. baumannii*, *P. aeruginosa*, and other species of gram-negative bacteria encompassing Ambler class A, B, and D β-lactamases (307). The β-lactamase enzymes/families found on integrons are VEB-1, VEB-2, GES-1, GES-2, IBI-1, IBI-1, CTX-M-2, CTX-M-9, PSE-1, and numerous OXA β-lactamases (189, 216, 217). OXA and metallo-β-lactamases that confer resistance to carbapenems (IMP-1 to IMP-4, IMP-6 to IMP-8, IMP-12, VIM-1, VIM-2, and GIM-1) are also included in integron-encoded β-lactamases (45, 307).

Class A β-Lactamases (Bush Group 2b Penicillinases)

Class A β-lactamases possess four important structural motifs that create a complex hydrogen-bonding network to fix the β-lactam in the substrate-binding pocket. Residues Ser70-Xaa-Xaa-Lys73, Ser130-Asp131-Asn132 (SDN loop), and Lys/Arg234-Thr/Ser235-Gly236 define the conserved residues critical for β-lactam binding and hydrolysis (142). The Ω loop (amino acids Arg164 to Asn179) is unique in class A β-lactamases. A highly conserved Glu166 that functions as a general base (electron donor) in the catalytic process is located in the Ω loop (see above). The salt bridge formed between Arg164 and Asn179 define the limits, or "neck," of the Ω loop.

The two commonly encountered class A β-lactamases found in *Enterobacteriaceae* are designated TEM-1 and SHV-1. TEM-1 and SHV-1 β-lactamases are primarily penicillinases with diminished activity against cephalosporin substrates. These two families of β-lactamases have received considerable attention over the past three decades since they are the progenitors of the ESBLs and IRT β-lactamases, now common in many hospitals.

Bush group 2be. ESBLs are generally class A β-lactamases that have "expanded" or changed their substrate profile as a result of amino acid substitutions. Normally, extended-spectrum cephalosporins are very poor substrates for hydrolysis by Bush group 2be enzymes (high K_m and low k_{cat}). Extended-spectrum cephalosporins are extremely potent β-lactams. Mutations at critical amino acids expand the spectrum of these enzymes and allow the hydrolysis of extended-spectrum cephalosporins (211). In most cases, ESBL mutations render the enzymes more susceptible to inhibition by mechanism-based inactivators (clavulanic acid, sulbactam, and tazobactam). Until recently, an explanation for this increased susceptibility was not apparent. Studying reactions using Raman spectroscopy and stopped-flow kinetics, it is now maintained that increased amounts of certain key intermediates of SHV-2 and SHV-5 are formed (i.e., the enamine intermediate). As a result, the K_i values of the mechanism-based inhibitors are reduced (increased susceptibility to inhibitors) up to 50-fold in SHV-2 and SHV-5. The impact of enteric gram-negative rods possessing ESBLs on the choice of empirical and definitive antimicrobial therapy has been substantial (143, 158, 203, 205, 206).

Among the TEM family enzymes, five amino acid residues appear to be most important for conferring the ESBL phenotype: Gly238 and Ala237 (located on the b3 β-pleated sheet), Arg164 and Asp179 (located on the neck of the Ω loop), and Asp104 (located directly across from G238 and A237 at the opening of the active-site cavity) (142, 228). Of note, the substitution of Gly to Ser, Ala, or Asp at Ambler position (ABL) 238 is a common mutation in both TEM and SHV ESBLs (http://www.lahey.org/studies/webt.html).

Non-TEM, non-SHV ESBLs. Among the non-TEM, non-SHV ESBLs, the CTX-M β-lactamases are the most prevalent. They can be divided into distinct clusters (see http://www.lahey.org/studies/webt.html). Unlike most (but not all) TEM- and SHV-derived ESBLs, CTX-M β-lactamases hydrolyze cefotaxime and ceftriaxone better than they do ceftazidime. Current data show that CTX-M enzymes are more readily inhibited by tazobactam than they are by clavulanic acid. The first CTX-M-type β-lactamase (MEN-1) was described nearly a decade ago. There are now nearly 60 members of this family.

CTX-M β-lactamases are commonly found in *K. pneumoniae*, *E. coli*, typhoidal and nontyphoidal *Salmonella*, *Shigella* spp., *Citrobacter freundii*, *Enterobacter* spp., and *Serratia marcescens* (141, 146, 204). The chromosome-encoded β-lactamase of *Kluyvera ascorbata* is a probable progenitor for some plasmid-encoded CTX-M enzymes (141). Other CTX-M β-lactamases may derive from *Kluyvera georgiana* (199). A recent comprehensive review delineates the lineage of many CTX-M enzymes resulting from *Kluyvera* spp. (27). Of note, different genetic elements may be involved in the mobilization of *bla*CTX-M genes.

Many other clinically important non-TEM, non-SHV ESBLs have been described (K1, GES-1, PER-1, PER-2, VEB-1, BES-1, IBI-1, IBI-2, and OXA-type) (30, 31, 219).

Structural biology of ESBLs. Important insights have emerged from the study of a number of atomic structures of class A ESBLs. The common theme that emerges is that the active site is selectively remodeled and expanded to accommodate the bulky R1 side chain of extended-spectrum cephalosporin. Although the details of this modification are different for many of the ESBLs, the remodeling comes at a price. Many of these ESBLs are not as catalytically efficient (e.g., redcuced k_{cat}/K_m) as are the wild-type progenitors against certain substrates. With the expanded substrate spectrum, one uniformly observes decreases in penicillin MICs and in k_{cat}/K_m ratios. In addition, these enzymes are less stable to proteolysis and heat. The structures of Toho-1, TEM-52, TEM-64, the Gly238Ala ESBL in TEM, SHV-2, and K1 β-lactamases all reveal insights into why expanded-spectrum cephalosporins fit in the active site (49, 124, 125, 196, 200, 263, 287, 300).

Serine carbapenemases of Bush group 2f or class A type. In the past, β-lactamases able to hydrolyze carbapenems were rare. It is regrettable that this is no longer the case. Representatives of these carbapenemases are Sme-1, Sme-2, NMC-A, IMI-1, GES-2, and KPC-2 (217, 317). Usually, class A carbapenemases hydrolyze imipenem but are not resistant to clavulanic acid inhibition (the exception may be KPC enzymes). *bla*NMC-A and *bla*IMI-1 are chromosomally located genes in *Enterobacter cloacae* and are induced by cefoxitin and imipenem (194, 229). *bla*NMC-A is regulated by a LysR-type regulatory protein (186). It is felt that *bla*IMI-1 is also regulated in the same manner (229). *bla*Sme-1 is a chromosomally located gene encoding serine carbapenemase of class A in *E. cloacae* and *Serratia marcescens*.

A notable increase in bacteria expressing class A carbapenemases has occurred in the United States. Numerous studies are revealing that KPC β-lactamases are becoming endemic in East Coast cities. First found in *K. pneumoniae*, these β-lactamases have been detected in *Salmonella enterica* serotype Cubana, *Klebsiella oxytoca*, and *Enterobacter* sp. strain MS 412 (121, 177, 317, 318), among others. *bla*KPC-2 is located on a nonconjugative plasmid (317). In *Salmonella* and *K. oxytoca*, *bla*KPC-2 was isolated from conjugative plasmids (177, 318). The plasmid bearing *bla*KPC-3 from New York was also transferable by conjugation (314). Currently, *bla*KPC has been localized to two genetic elements, Tn*4401* and the KQ element (186, 238). *K. pneumoniae* organisms bearing KPCs are now found in North and South America, the Caribbean, Europe, Israel, and Asia. These isolates are highly resistant to penicillins, cephalosporins, and commercially available β-lactam–β-lactamase inhibitor combinations and show reduced susceptibility to carbapenems.

Detection of KPC β-lactamases may be a problem for clinical laboratories because of the positive ESBL confirmation tests (clavulanate-potentiated activities of ceftriaxone, ceftazidime, cefepime, and aztreonam). To improve detection of KPC-expressing *K. pneumoniae*, care in inoculum preparation for broth-based susceptibility methods must be taken. Investigators in this area have found that resistant isolates were readily detected by agar-based methods but not by broth methods (33). Bratu et al. first found that using ertapenem or meropenem improves detection (33).

We stress that the clinical detection systems (i.e., automated systems like Vitek 1 and 2, Phoenix, and MicroScan) that are currently used by most hospital laboratories may not be completely accurate for detection of KPC in all strains of *K. pneumoniae*. Thus, the true prevalence of KPC-producing isolates may be underappreciated, and therapeutic decisions based upon susceptibility testing can be adversely affected. We now generally recognize that screening with ertapenem increases the sensitivity for detecting KPCs by Etest, disk diffusion, and automated methods, while testing with meropenem and imipenem increases specificity. Currently, the major phenotypic test that is used is the modified Hodge test (MHT). In this test, a lawn of susceptible *E. coli* (e.g., strain ATCC 25922), a carbapenem disk (ertapenem or meropenem), and a streak of the suspected KPC producer are placed upon an agar plate and incubated overnight. Growth up to the disk is checked the next day and, if present, suggests carbapenemase production. Unfortunately, there may be false positivities. Chromogenic agar tests are also now employed in selected circumstances, but clinical experience is limited. Chromogenic agar for KPC detection (CHROMagar KPC) demonstrated a sensitivity and specificity of 100 and 98.4% compared with PCR for *bla*KPC for detection of KPC-producing *Enterobacteriaceae* directly from rectal swab specimens. The rectal swabs were obtained from 122 unique patients (41 KPC-producing *K. pneumoniae* isolates were detected). The study had certain limitations (the sample size was small, and the study was performed at one institution and involved predominantly a single clone of carbapenem-resistant *K. pneumoniae*). In practical terms, the strains turn red when *E. coli* producing a carbapenemase is detected and metallic blue when *K. pneumoniae* produces a carbapenemase. Currently, there are two different tests available: the CHROMagar KPC and the CHROM ID ESBL (42, 250). The latter CHROM method can detect producers of IMP-, VIM-, and KPC-type carbapenemases with high levels of resistance to cephalosporins and to carbapenems.

Boronic acid disks have also been used to detect KPC producers. In this assay, the boronic acid disks (e.g., 3-aminophenylboronic acid) when combined with a carbapenem have a senstivity and specificity that approaches 100% (67, 288). These assays can be performed more readily than others and can add to the current need to define the mechanism of resistance and detect KPCs. In our experience, PCR still remains the "gold standard" and is readily performed in many reference laboratories throughout the United States.

So far, the crystal structure of only KPC-2 has been determined. KPC-2 has an overall structure similar to that of other class A enzymes, and, interestingly, this β-lactamase has only 50% protein sequence conservation compared to CTX-M-1, 39% to SHV-1, and 35% to TEM-1 (140). The KPC-2 β-lactamase possesses a large and shallow active site, allowing it to accommodate "bulkier" β-lactams. As a result of these structural changes, KPC-2 is regarded as a versatile β-lactamase (226). Microbiologists and clinicians observed that many *bla*KPC-2-containing strains are resistant to β-lactam–β-lactamase inhibitor combinations. At present, β-lactam therapeutic options do seem to work against these highly resistant strains.

Among these serine carbapenemases exists a notable curiosity. bla_{GES-2} is a plasmid-borne β-lactamase gene found in *P. aeruginosa* (221). bla_{GES-2} is a point mutation mutant of bla_{GES-1}, which encodes a clavulanic acid-inhibited ESBL (a non-TEM, non-SHV ESBL). It is curious that GES-1 is an ESBL and that a single point mutation (Gly → Asp at position 170 in the Ω loop) can add an imipenemase activity to GES-2 (93). The OXA carbapenemases are discussed below.

Inhibitor-resistant class A β-lactamase: Bush group 2br. Amino acid mutations within TEM and SHV that confer resistance to inhibition by β-lactamase inhibitors have also been characterized at the following amino acid positions: Met69, Ser130, Arg244, Arg275, and Asn276 (28, 64, 79, 223, 254, 276, 281, 293, 296). Most inhibitor-resistant β-lactamases are variants of the TEM-1 enzyme, with only two descriptions of clinical isolates expressing SHV β-lactamases that are resistant to inhibitors at the time of this writing (SHV-10 and SHV-49) (70, 223). It is possible that the frequency of inhibitor-resistant β-lactamases in TEM and SHV family enzymes is underestimated, since many laboratories in the United States do not identify these strains routinely (139). Cephalosporins or high-dose piperacillin-tazobactam may be effective for the treatment of *E. coli* expressing some inhibitor-resistant β-lactamases.

Mutants of TEM β-lactamases are being recovered that maintain the ESBL phenotype but also demonstrate inhibitor resistance. These are referred to as CMTs. There are now four CMTs (84, 190, 218, 266). It is still unknown how these enzymes will affect empirical treatment. At this time, clinical microbiology laboratories do not have the resources to detect these complex phenotypes.

Class B β-Lactamases (Bush Group 3 Enzymes)
In contrast to the serine-dependent β-lactamases (classes A, C, and D), class B β-lactamases are metalloenzymes. These enzymes contain an αββα motif with a central β sandwich and two α helices on each side. Consequently, class B β-lactamases require zinc or another heavy metal for catalysis, and their activities are inhibited by chelating agents (EDTA). This zinc atom is held in place by three histidines and a water molecule. Some metallo-β-lactamases contain a second Zn binding site. These two sites function separately, with the primary Zn binding site assisted by the secondary site. A coordinated water molecule also plays a critical role in catalysis (299).

With few exceptions (see below), class B β-lactamases confer resistance to a wide range of β-lactam compounds, including cephamycins and carbapenems. The class B β-lactamases are resistant to inactivation by clavulanate, sulbactam, and tazobactam. Aztreonam, a monobactam, may act as an inhibitor, but there are metallo-β-lactamases that hydrolyze aztreonam. Of note, isolates expressing VIM-2 can be susceptible to aztreonam (215).

Class B β-lactamases can be grouped into three different subclasses (B1, B2, and B3) depending on their requirements for zinc. B1 enzymes (IMP-1, VIM-2, and CcrA) are fully active with one or two zinc ions, B3 enzymes (e.g., L1) require two zinc ions, and B2 enzymes (e.g., CphA) are inhibited by the addition of a second zinc ion. Amino acid positions can be assigned according to a specific numbering system, designated BBL, that is based upon structural alignment (97). Although the genes encoding metallo-β-lactamases show very little primary structure sequence identity (17 to 37%), the three-dimensional structures of the known metallo-β-lactamases appear to be similar (39, 54, 271, 292).

Because of the metal ion, the catalytic pathway of metallo-β-lactamases does not involve an acyl enzyme intermediate as it does in classes A and C. The catalytic pathway in class B also incorporates a hydrolytic water molecule (the "bridging" water molecule) that possesses enhanced nucleophilicity due to the proximity to the metal ion. The zinc ions coordinate two water molecules. The addition of the hydroxide to the carbonyl carbon of the β-lactam leads to the formation of a transient, noncovalent reaction intermediate. The mechanistic details of this pathway have been recently summarized by Crowder et al. (58) and are beyond the scope of this chapter.

The majority of metallo-β-lactamases are chromosomally encoded, and their expression may be constitutive or inducible. The metallo-β-lactamases of *B. cereus, Stenotrophomonas maltophilia, Aeromonas hydrophila,* and *Aeromonas jandaei* are inducible. In *A. jandaei,* regulation of the metallo-β-lactamase appears to involve two-component signal transduction systems (5).

The metallo-β-lactamases of the VIM and IMP types are now established as important threats to our antimicrobial armamentarium. These metallo-β-lactamases are broad-spectrum enzymes and are active against most β-lactams, including carbapenems, and have been found in various gram-negative clinical isolates mostly in the Far East and the Mediterranean regions. bla_{VIM} is an integron-borne metallo-β-lactamase that is usually found in *P. aeruginosa* isolates. Unfortunately, the VIM metallo-β-lactamase has spread to other enteric bacilli (*E. coli, Enterobacter aerogenes, E. cloacae,* and *Klebsiella* spp.). bla_{VIM-2} has now spread to more than 20 countries (243). The majority of metallo-β-lactamases are mobilized on integrons, transposons, and mobile common regions (299). A curious finding is the coisolation of VIM-1 with KPC-2 in Greece (102). Similarly, IMP metallo-β-lactamases are very widespread. IMP metallo-β-lactamases have been found as part of integrons in the following bacteria: *P. aeruginosa, Pseudomonas putida, Serratia marcescens, Pseudomonas stutzeri, Acinetobacter baumannii, Pseudomonas fluorescens, K. pneumoniae, K. oxytoca, E. aerogenes, Achromobacter xylosoxidans,* and *Escherichia coli* (299). In an unusual parallel to what has been found with VIM and KPC-2 (see above), IMP-1 has also been discovered in combination with OXA carbapenemases (275).

Recently, a novel class B enzyme that has raised significant concern has been described. NDM-1 (New Delhi metallo-β-lactamase) is a class B β-lactamase encoded by a very mobile genetic element, and the pattern of spread is providing to be more complex and apparently more unpredictable than that of the gene encoding KPC. Moreover, the number of patients possessing bacteria containing bla_{NDM-1} is growing. The gene has moved from India and Pakistan to the United Kingdom, the United States, Kenya, Japan, Canada, Belgium, The Netherlands, Taiwan, Oman, and Australia. bla_{NDM-1} has been found on plasmids of different sizes and has been located near a pathogenicity island. The resistance determinants flanking this *bla* gene seem to be numerous, including chromosomal β-lactamases (bla_{CMY} and bla_{DHA}) and chloramphenicol and aminoglycoside resistance genes. The global impact of this gene and its spread must be carefully monitored.

As stated above, the atomic structures of a number of class B β-lactamases have been solved (39, 54, 97, 98). The structures are being used to design novel inhibitors of class B β-lactamases.

Class C β-Lactamases

Ambler class C (Bush-Jacoby-Medeiros group 1) chromosomal β-lactamases are produced to a greater or lesser degree by almost all gram-negative bacteria (*Salmonella*, *Klebsiella*, *Proteus mirabilis*, *Proteus vulgaris*, and *Stenotrophomonas maltophilia* being the major exceptions) (129). Chromosomally encoded (and inducible) enzymes are particularly important in clinical isolates of *C. freundii*, *E. aerogenes*, *E. cloacae*, *Morganella morganii*, *P. aeruginosa*, and *S. marcescens*. Although class C β-lactamases hydrolyze cephalosporins (including extended-spectrum cephalosporins) more effectively than they do penicillins, it should be kept in mind that these enzymes have a great efficiency for hydrolysis of penicillins (the K_m is very low). Most class C enzymes are resistant to inhibition by clavulanate, sulbactam, and tazobactam (in the case of tazobactam, the resistance to inhibition is generally less).

Class C β-lactamases have larger active-site cavities than do class A enzymes, which may allow them to bind the bulky extended-spectrum cephalosporins (oxyimino-β-lactams) (57, 159). It is claimed that this conformational expansion and flexibility facilitate hydrolysis of oxyimino-β-lactams by making the acyl enzyme intermediate more open to attack by water (57, 159, 175).

The important structural elements described for class A enzymes are also present in class C β-lactamases. The active-site serine (Ser64) is located near the N terminus of a long helix and is followed on the next helix turn by a lysine (Ser64-Xaa-Xaa-Lys67). The second element contains a Tyr-Xaa-Asn (Tyr150) or Ser-Xaa-Asn pattern corresponding to the Ser130-Asp131-Asn132 loop of class A β-lactamases. The opposite side of the active site is marked by Lys315/Arg/His-Thr/Ser-Gly corresponding to the KTG motif of class A enzymes.

Class C cephalosporinases acylate β-lactams in the same manner as class A enzymes do. In many ways the reaction mechanism of class C β-lactamases remains enigmatic (51, 100). First, the catalytic Ser64 attacks the β-lactam carbonyl carbon and the acyl enzyme forms. The approach of the activated water molecule is different between AmpC and class A enzymes (class C from the β-face). This implies that the deacylation mechanism is distinct. Unlike with class A enzymes, the ring amine of the acyl enzyme of class C facilitates deacylation. This "substrate-assisted catalysis" generally distinguishes class C from class A (although there are reports of substrate-assisted catalysis occurring in class A TEM as well) (34). Examining the catalytic mechanism, a "Glu166 equivalent" in class C β-lactamases is not readily apparent; this role may be filled by the tyrosine (Tyr150) in the Tyr-Xaa-Asn motif. The current thinking is that the conserved residue, Tyr150, acts as a general base in the acylation mechanism by increasing the nucleophilicity of Ser64. However, Tyr150 may stay protonated during the reaction and is thus not able to serve as an anionic base during hydrolysis. The proton on Tyr150 helps stabilize the water's developing negative charge. However, mutagenesis studies do not rule out a role for Lys67 in the coordinate base mechanism as well (50).

The first class C β-lactamase structure determined was for the AmpC cephalosporinase of *C. freundii*, determined by Oefner et al. (197). The structures of P99 β-lactamase of *E. cloacae*, AmpC β-lactamase from *E. coli*, and *E. cloacae* GC1 and *E. cloacae* 908R β-lactamases have ensued (57, 160) (http://www.rcsb.org). The GC1 β-lactamase of *E. cloacae* has improved hydrolytic activity for oxyimino-β-lactam antibiotics because of a tripeptide insertion in

the Ω loop (a tandem repeat Ala211-Val212-Arg213). In a strict sense, this is a class C ESBL. As a result of this addition, the width of the opening of the active-site binding cavity is larger and the substrate spectrum has expanded (57). As stated in the paragraph above, a number of other structures of the *E. coli* class C β-lactamase have been solved in an attempt to decipher the mechanism of catalysis. In the clinically important class C enzyme-producing gram-negative rods, β-lactamase production is normally repressed. The details of the repression have been mostly elucidated for *Enterobacter* spp. (127). Repression and activation are closely linked to the processes of cell wall synthesis and breakdown. The molecule that serves as both the repressor and the activator of *ampC* transcription is AmpR, a transcriptional regulator of the LysR family. AmpR is present as a repressor by virtue of its interaction with UDP-MurNAc pentapeptide, a peptidoglycan precursor molecule. In this form AmpR is incapable of activating *ampC* and in fact serves as a repressor of *ampR* expression. In the setting of high concentrations of cell wall breakdown product anhydro-MurNAc tripeptide (or anhydro-MurNAc pentapeptide), however, UDP-MurNAc pentapeptide is displaced from its site in AmpR, resulting in the conversion of AmpR to an activator of *ampC* transcription.

Increases in *ampC* expression may result from the action of β-lactam antibiotics, certain of which cause the release of significant quantities of anhydro-MurNAc tripeptide and/or pentapeptide from the peptidoglycan. This anhydro-UDP-MurNAc tripeptide enters the cell through a channel (AmpG) and overwhelms the recycling ability of the cytosolic amidase (AmpD) specific for recycling of muropeptides. Under these circumstances (induction), β-lactamase is produced only as long as the antibiotic is present in the medium.

Constitutive high-level production of AmpC β-lactamase most commonly results from a mutation in the *ampD* gene, reducing the quantity of (or eliminating) AmpD from the cytoplasm. Under these circumstances, a constant high level of anhydro-MurNAc tripeptide is present in the cytoplasm, and AmpR serves as a constitutive activator of *ampC* transcription. Constitutive production can also result from deletion of *ampR*, but in this circumstance β-lactamase production is generally at a low level.

The widespread dissemination of *ampC*-type β-lactamase genes on transferable plasmids is a continuing challenge. These plasmid-encoded AmpC cephalosporinases are separated into four general groups. Group 1 plasmid-encoded AmpC cephalosporinases consist of those which originated from the chromosomal AmpC of *C. freundii* (BIL-1, CMY-2, LAT-1, and LAT-2). Members of group 2 are related to the chromosomal cephalosporinase of *E. cloacae* (MIR-1 and ACT-1), group 3 β-lactamases belong to the AmpC of *P. aeruginosa* (CMY-1, FOX-1, and MOX-1), and group 4 enzymes belong to the CMY-1 β-lactamase (CMY-1 cluster). Plasmid-mediated class C β-lactamases have been described to occur in many gram-negative organisms from all parts of the world. Host strains harboring these enzymes include *K. pneumoniae*, *E. aerogenes*, *Salmonella enterica* serotype Senftenberg, *E. coli*, *Proteus mirabilis*, *M. morganii*, and *K. oxytoca*. The loss of porin proteins in clinical isolates with plasmid-encoded AmpC enzymes may result in resistance to carbapenems (32, 273).

Class D β-Lactamases

The OXA-type (oxacillin-hydrolyzing) β-lactamases have been most commonly described for *Enterobacteriaceae*,

Acinetobacter spp., and *P. aeruginosa* (187). In terms of their genetic background in these gram-negative organisms, many class D β-lactamase genes are associated with class 1 integrons or with ISs (220). OXA enzymes confer resistance to a wide variety of penicillins. They are only weakly inhibited by clavulanic acid. There are some interesting exceptions to this rule in that OXA-2 and OXA-32 are inhibited by tazobactam but not sulbactam or clavulanate. In an unusual manner, OXA β-lactamases are inhibited by sodium chloride (50 to 75 mM NaCl). Mutagenesis studies suggest that susceptibility to inhibition by NaCl is related to the presence of a Tyr residue at position 144. Overall, the amino acid identities between class D and class A or class C β-lactamases are less than 20%. Their frequent location on mobile genetic elements (plasmids or integrons) facilitates spread (188, 216, 297).

Several OXA β-lactamases (OXA-11 and OXA-14 to OXA-20) are associated with an ESBL phenotype. These OXA types have been found exclusively in *P. aeruginosa*. A comparison of the crystal structure of the OXA-10 β-lactamase with those of the class C enzyme from *E. cloacae* P99 and of the class A TEM-1 enzyme from *E. coli* shows that the class D and class A enzymes share an common fold (α helices and β-pleated sheets), although the distribution of secondary structure elements is different. A remarkable feature is the nearly perfect symmetry of all atoms that constitute the catalytic machinery for acylation (Ser67, Lys70, Ser115, and Lys205 in OXA-10 and Ser70, Lys73, Ser130, and Lys234 in TEM-1). There seems to be an extension of the substrate-binding site (tripeptide strand) in OXA-10. The role of the peptide extension is not known. The "oxyanion hole" is provided by the main-chain nitrogen atoms of Ser67 and Phe208. In class D, the same residue (Lys70) is involved in acylation and deacylation (172, 201).

OXA enzymes are assuming greater importance due to the ability of members of this class to hydrolyze carbapenems. The first description of a serine carbapenemase in *A. baumannii* was ARI-1 (OXA-23) in 1985 (207). Although OXA carbapenemases hydrolyze imipenem inefficiently, their presence in an organism with an active efflux pump or a porin mutation may confer clinically significant levels of resistance (117). It is notable that *A. baumannii* isolates possess a chromosomally encoded oxacillinase, OXA-69, that confers very-low-level imipenem resistance. This gene is ubiquitous in *A. baumannii* and is referred to as a housekeeping gene (116).

Our understanding of the hydrolytic mechanism of class D β-lactamases is based on the careful study of OXA-10, -13, and -1. OXA β-lactamases are unique because of the direct role of carboxylation of the active-site Lys70. The carbamic acid on Lys70 can ionize to yield a carbamate that hydrogen bonds with the nucleophilic Ser67 residue. In this manner, the carboxylated Lys70 may serve as the general base by activating both Ser67 for acylation and the hydrolytic water for deacylation.

More relevant to the issue of carbapenem resistance are the crystal structures of OXA-24/40 and OXA-48. OXA-24/40 is one of the most widespread carbapenemases found in *A. baumannii* (29). This enzyme was originally part of a clinical epidemic in Spain that involved a 10-month-long outbreak affecting 29 patients, 23 of them hospitalized in five intensive care units. The work by Santillana et al. showed that OXA-24/40 has a hydrophobic barrier formed by Tyr112 and Met223 side chains, which define a tunnel-like entrance to the active site (253). OXA-48 was initially isolated from *K. pneumoniae*. Docquier et al. (66) found that OXA-48 is similar to OXA-10 in structure and not like OXA-24/40. Molecular dynamics simulation showed that meropenem may position itself between Leu158 and Thr213, with the C-6 ethoxy group approaching Val120. In this manner, H_2O gets near Lys73 and can attack C=O at the amide bond.

Resistance to Chloramphenicol

Acetyltransferases

Chloramphenicol is a broad-spectrum antimicrobial agent whose use has waned in recent years due to well-characterized hematologic toxicity and a wealth of less toxic therapeutic options. The most common mechanism of resistance to chloramphenicol is the elaboration of CATs. A large number of CAT genes have been reported, and these determinants generally confer extremely high levels of resistance on the organisms expressing them. Substantial structural similarities exist among the different CAT variants, although their nucleotide sequences may be quite divergent (184). Relationships among the different CATs have been described in detail in a review by Schwarz and colleagues (256). Chloramphenicol contains two hydroxyl groups that are acetylated in a reaction catalyzed by CAT in which acetyl coenzyme A serves as the acyl donor. Initial acetylation occurs at the C-3 hydroxyl group to yield 3-acetoxy-chloramphenicol (260). Following nonenzymatic rearrangement to 1-acetoxy-chloramphenicol and reacetylation, the 1,3-diacetoxy-chloramphenicol product is formed. Neither the mono- nor the di-acetoxy derivatives are able to bind to the 50S ribosomal subunit and inhibit prokaryotic peptidyltransferase (260).

CATs are generally divided into two types: type A (classical) CATs and type B (xenobiotic) CATs (256). For *S. aureus*, five structurally similar type A CATs (A, B, C, D, and that encoded by the prototypic plasmid pC194) have been described (87). The *cat* genes encoding these enzymes are commonly located on small, multicopy plasmids, and expression is inducible by a translational attenuation mechanism (256). *E. faecalis* and *S. pneumoniae* also express inducible CAT genes that are similar to the type D gene of *S. aureus*. Two *cat* genes encoding constitutive CAT expression have been described to occur in *Clostridium perfringens*. *catP* is generally found within transposon Tn*4451*, whereas *catQ* (nearly identical to *catD* of *Clostridium difficile*) is chromosomal (256).

Three types of type A CATs (I, II, and III) have been identified in gram-negative bacteria. The widely prevalent type I enzymes are distinguished by their ability to bind and inhibit (without acetylation) the activity of fusidic acid. These enzymes are frequently found to be associated with transposon Tn9 or related elements. Type II CATs are notable for their sensitivity to inhibition by thiol-reactive agents and by their association with *H. influenzae* (183). Most knowledge of the structural features of the type A CAT enzymes comes from the study of the type III enzyme, for which the tertiary structure is known at high resolution (184). The structural determinants of binding for each substrate are also known for this enzyme.

Type B (xenobiotic) acetyltransferases (184) are structurally unrelated to classic CATs, and those that have been demonstrated to acetylate chloramphenicol confer only low levels of chloramphenicol resistance even when present in high copy number. Their natural substrate is likely something other than chloramphenicol, explaining their limited ability to acetylate this antibiotic. First described to occur in *Agrobacterium tumefaciens*, they have now been identified in a wide range of species (256). Included among this class of agents are the virginiamycin acetyltransferases found in *S. aureus* and *E. faecium* (see section on macrolides below). In fact, although they are members of this class, the *vat* genes do not confer resistance to chloramphenicol, nor have they been demonstrated to be able to acetylate chloramphenicol in vitro (184). They are, however, quite adept at acetylating streptogramins. The crystal structures of two trimeric type B CATs have been determined (20, 225).

Decreased Accumulation of Chloramphenicol

It is now well recognized that chloramphenicol serves as a substrate for many of the MDR efflux pumps that exist in gram-positive and gram-negative bacteria, including those found in *E. coli*, *P. aeruginosa*, *Bacillus subtilis*, and *S. aureus* (191). In addition, there are efflux systems that are specific for chloramphenicol. The first chloramphenicol-specific efflux gene that was described was *cmlA* within the In4 integron of Tn1696 (23). *cmlA* encodes an efflux mechanism that uses chloramphenicol but not florfenicol (a chloramphenicol derivative licensed for use in animals in 1996 in the United States for the treatment of bovine respiratory pathogens) as a substrate. Gram-negative bacteria also express efflux genes specific for both chloramphenicol and florfenicol (flo_{Pp} and flo_{St}). These resistance genes are being reported with increasing frequency for animal-derived *E. coli* and *Salmonella* isolates (26, 308). In fact, the chloramphenicol resistance expressed by MDR *Salmonella enterica* serovar Typhimurium DT104 is most commonly encoded by flo_{St} (26), emphasizing again the potential negative impact of using similar antimicrobial agents in humans and animals. Very recently, chloramphenicol resistance in *Acinetobacter baumannii* has been attributed to the activity of an MFS-type pump designated CraA (242).

Resistance to Daptomycin

Daptomycin is a cyclic lipopeptide antibiotic with activity exclusively against gram-positive bacteria. It has bactericidal activity against most strains and acts by a cooperative interaction in the presence of physiological concentrations of calcium that result in the formation of pores in the cytoplasmic membranes of target bacterial cells. The end result is leakage of ions from the cell and cell death. Resistance to daptomycin has been found in both enterococci and staphylococci. Resistance to daptomycin is very rare in surveys, but in the clinical setting resistance may arise associated with prolonged therapy. The precise mechanisms of resistance have not been defined, but overexpression of genes associated with increasing the positive charge of the cytoplasmic membrane has been implicated, although actual changes in membrane charge have been difficult to demonstrate (178). Exposure to daptomycin strongly induces the autoregulatory hVISA-associated (see below) VraRS two-component regulatory system in *S. aureus* (185) and a similar system in *Bacillus subtilis* (105). Perhaps as a result of these common pathways, hVISA strains frequently express reduced susceptibility to daptomycin (59) and strains expressing reduced susceptibility to daptomycin exhibit the hVISA (see below) phenotype (37). Unfortunately, *S. aureus* strains with reduced susceptibility have been isolated with some frequency during prolonged treatment of deep-seated infections (91).

Resistance to Glycopeptides

Glycopeptide antibiotics (vancomycin and teicoplanin) inhibit cell wall synthesis by binding to the pentapeptide peptidoglycan precursor molecule as it exits the cytoplasmic membrane. This binding prevents the cross-linking (transpeptidation) of peptidoglycan precursors necessary for the formation of normal, stable cell walls. The large size of the glycopeptide molecules also appears to inhibit the other major peptidoglycan linkage reaction (transglycosylation) by steric hindrance. The specific moiety bound by vancomycin is the terminal D-alanyl–D-alanine of the pentapeptide. The vast majority of bacteria that have been studied have peptidoglycan precursors that are pentapeptides terminating in D-Ala–D-Ala, and therefore are theoretically susceptible to vancomycin. However, the large size of vancomycin exceeds the exclusion limits of the porins in the outer membranes of gram-negative bacteria, so vancomycin cannot access the target in these species. Hence, vancomycin is active only against bacteria lacking outer membranes, which are predominantly gram positive.

Acquired resistance to vancomycin in gram-positive bacteria comes in three varieties largely defined by the species within which they have been described: (i) altered precursor formation in enterococci, (ii) mutational cell wall changes in staphylococci, and (iii) tolerance in pneumococci. The importance of the first type of resistance is characterized by both its prevalence and the importance of the species as a cause of infection, whereas the other two are defined more by the importance of the species than by their prevalence.

To date, six varieties of enterococcal glycopeptide resistance have been described (VanA through VanE and VanG). Of these, the most clinically important are VanA and VanB (15). VanA and VanB are encoded by similar operons in which three genes (*vanH*, *vanA*, and *vanX* or *vanH*$_B$, *vanB*, and *vanX*$_B$) are required for expression of resistance (15). Two other genes (*vanY* and *vanZ* or *vanY*$_B$ and *vanW*) serve to amplify resistance but are not required for its expression (11, 12), and two more genes (*vanS* and *vanR* or *vanS*$_B$ and *vanR*$_B$) regulate the transcription of the three essential genes (13, 77). The ultimate purpose of these genes is to alter the structure of the pentapeptide precursor from terminating in D-alanyl–D-alanine to D-alanine–D-lactate, in so doing reducing the binding affinity of vancomycin to its target roughly 1,000-fold. The sequence of reactions resulting in this structure is outlined in reference 122. Since the terminal amino acid is cleaved off of the pentapeptide in the transpeptidation reaction, the final composition of the cell wall is indistinguishable from that of strains lacking the resistance determinant. Apparently the enterococcal PBPs, which facilitate transpeptidation, have no trouble processing the altered precursors.

VanA enterococci are phenotypically resistant to vancomycin and teicoplanin, whereas VanB strains are resistant to vancomycin but appear to be susceptible to teicoplanin. This susceptibility results from the fact that teicoplanin does not induce expression of resistance (77). Once the VanB operon is expressed, however, resistance to teicoplanin results. Consequently, teicoplanin has been disappointing as a therapy for infections caused by VanB enterococci, since mutations in the VanB regulatory apparatus resulting in either inducibility by teicoplanin or constitutive expression occur readily during therapy (16, 112, 135).

Both VanA and VanB operons are carried by transposons. VanA is found exclusively within transposon Tn1546, a 10.4-kb Tn3 family element that is presumed to disseminate among enterococci by integrating into conjugative plasmids (14). The genes of the VanA operon are found to be highly conserved in their sequence when different strains are compared, but the restriction maps of the operons and of Tn1546 often differ markedly among clinical strains (61). These differences result from insertions of a variety of IS elements with or without subsequent deletions of parts of the mobile element and have been used by some investigators to establish lineages of strains within defined clinical settings. The VanB operon is most commonly encoded on highly similar transposons designated Tn5382 or Tn1549 (40, 99). These transposons exhibit significant homology to prototype enterococcal conjugative transposon Tn916. In contrast to the vanA gene, three allelic variants of vanB (vanB1, vanB2, and vanB3) have been described. The vanB2 gene is associated with Tn5382 (60).

The overwhelming majority of clinical vancomycin-resistant enterococcal strains are E. faecium, a predilection that remains unexplained (249). The vast majority of vancomycin-resistant E. faecium strains that cause clinical infection are also resistant to ampicillin, owing to the expansion of a group of hospital-adapted clones (referred to as clonal complex 17) that have emerged around the world. Clonal complex 17 strains are found worldwide and are characterized by their resistance to ampicillin and by the fact that they frequently harbor putative virulence determinants such as esp_{Efm} and hyl_{Efm} (147, 148).

Despite in vitro transfer of the VanA determinant to S. aureus (193), and at least 11 instances in which VanA-expressing S. aureus have been described for clinical samples (209), vancomycin-resistant S. aureus remains exceedingly rare. In all cases resistance has been conferred by the VanA operon, and in one well-characterized case transfer appears to have been facilitated by the presence of Tn1546 on a broad-host-range plasmid in E. faecalis, with transposition of Tn1546 to a staphylococcal plasmid once entry into the staphylococcus occurred (89, 304).

The VanC operon is intrinsic to the cell wall synthesis machinery of the minor enterococcal species Enterococcus casseliflavus (including the biotype formerly classified as E. flavescens) and Enterococcus gallinarum (71, 298). The peptidoglycan precursor in VanC strains terminates in D-alanine–D-serine, reducing vancomycin affinity about sevenfold and resulting in low levels of resistance. Precursors terminate in D-alanine–D-serine strains of E. faecalis with VanE (86), whereas VanD E. faecium terminates in D-alanine–D-lactate. The failure to observe dissemination of VanD may be explained in part by the fact that the VanX equivalent enzyme in E. faecium BM4339 appears to be ineffective in an enterococcal background. Resistance was expressed in BM4339 because that strain lacked a functional cellular ligase (ddl) gene, eliminating the need for VanX activity to express resistance (44).

Mutational resistance to glycopeptides in S. aureus commonly takes the form of reduced susceptibility, rather than frank resistance. These strains, alternately called hVISA (hetero-vancomycin-intermediate S. aureus) or hGISA (hetero-glycopeptide-intermediate S. aureus), express vancomycin MICs in the 4- to 8-μg/ml range (156). However, within these cultures are smaller populations of cells that express higher levels of resistance. The resistance phenotype is characterized by thickened cell wall, which may decrease glycopeptide susceptibility by providing an excess of false targets for glycopeptide binding. In many, but not all, cases, conversion to the hVISA phenotype is associated with the vraRS two-component regulatory circuit, which responds to cell wall damage in S. aureus and regulates more than 40 genes, some of which are associated with the biosynthesis of peptidoglycan (21). Interestingly, recent

work suggests that the hVISA phenotype can be selected by exposure to β-lactam antibiotics as well as by exposure to glycopeptides (137). Animal studies suggest that the level of resistance expressed by hVISA strains reduces the effectiveness of vancomycin therapy (53).

Glycopeptide resistance has also been reported for coagulase-negative species of staphylococci. In contrast to S. aureus, resistance in Staphylococcus haemolyticus has been associated with changes in the composition of the cross-links of the peptidoglycan (22). The mechanism by which this would lead to vancomycin resistance is incompletely understood.

Vancomycin is, in general, a less bactericidal antibiotic than are the β-lactams. Evidence for the importance of this observation can be found in several species. The bacteremia associated with S. aureus endocarditis, for example, takes roughly twice as much time to clear with vancomycin treatment than with treatment by β-lactam oxacillin (154). Recent clinical data also suggest that vancomycin treatment was associated with higher rates of failure and relapse than was nafcillin treatment for bacteremia due to methicillin-susceptible S. aureus (48). Vancomycin efficacy appears to be particularly poor against some strains of MRSA. In a recent clinical trial, vancomycin successfully treated left-sided endocarditis in only 2 of 9 cases, a success rate that was similar to that of daptomycin (2 of 10) (91). Reports of vancomycin tolerance in Streptococcus pneumoniae first appeared in 1990 (289). S. pneumoniae is the most common cause of bacterial meningitis in most patient populations, and bactericidal therapy is optimal for treatment of this condition. At least one case of presumed recrudescence of meningitis after treatment of a case of vancomycin-tolerant pneumococcal meningitis has been reported (114). Tolerance appears to involve mutations within an operon (vex123) encoding an ABC transporter, but the mechanism by which this occurs remains undefined (104). Further work will be required before we understand the true importance of pneumococcal tolerance for the treatment of clinical infections.

Resistance to Linezolid

The oxazolidinone antibiotic linezolid inhibits bacterial protein synthesis by interacting with the N-formylmethionyl-tRNA–ribosome–mRNA ternary complex commonly referred to as the initiation complex (264). Linezolid exerts excellent bacteriostatic activity against a wide range of gram-positive pathogens, including methicillin-resistant staphylococci and MDR enterococci. Clinical use of this agent has been associated with the emergence of resistant strains, most commonly after prolonged therapy of difficult-to-eradicate bacteria. Resistance has now been described for both enterococci and staphylococci, but overall rates several years after clinical introduction of this agent remain very low (134). Resistance is most often associated with a G2576U (Escherichia coli numbering scheme) point mutation in the 23S rRNA, although mutations at other positions may also contribute to resistance (224). Resistance to linezolid, macrolides, and chloramphenicol has been attributed to a 6-bp deletion in the gene encoding riboprotein L4 in S. pneumoniae (313). Since the 23S subunit genes exist in multiple copies in different bacteria (four in E. faecalis and S. pneumoniae, six in E. faecium, and five or six in S. aureus), more than one copy of the genes must be mutated to confer resistance, with strains having a higher percentage of mutated 23S genes expressing greater levels of resistance (166). Gene conversion, or recombination between mutated genes and wild-type genes, can rapidly increase the levels of resistance once the first gene muta-tion has occurred (161). In this fashion, persistent selective pressure exerted by linezolid can lead to rapid development of high-level (MIC > 128 μg/ml) resistance.

Plasmid-mediated resistance to linezolid through the ex-pression of the *cfr* rRNA methylase gene has been reported for staphylococci (10), but the prevalence of this type of linezolid resistance remains very low (134).

Resistance to Macrolides

Erythromycin (the first macrolide) was initially isolated from *Streptomyces erythraeus,* a soil organism found in the Philippines. There are currently four macrolides in com-mon use: erythromycin, clarithromycin, azithromycin, and roxithromycin. Macrolides inhibit protein synthesis in susceptible organisms by binding reversibly to the peptidyl-tRNA binding region of the 50S ribosomal subunit, inhib-iting translocation of a newly synthesized peptidyl-tRNA molecule from the acceptor site on the ribosome to the peptidyl (or donor site). Erythromycin does not bind to mammalian ribosomes. Most gram-negative organisms are resistant to erythromycin because entry of erythromycin into the cell is restricted.

Resistance to macrolides occurs by several mechanisms. Among the more important of these mechanisms is methy-lation of the ribosome, preventing erythromycin binding (305). This methylation is most commonly accomplished by different *erm* (erythromycin ribosomal methylase) genes. Methylated ribosomes confer resistance to macrolides, the re-lated lincosamides (clindamycin and lincomycin), and strep-togramins B (MLS$_B$ resistance). Many *erm* genes have been described—*erm*(A) and the related *erm*(TR), plus *erm*(B) and the related *erm*(AM)—and resistance is frequently in-ducible by macrolides but not by clindamycin (iMLS$_B$). In some strains, *erm*-type resistance is expressed constitutively (cMLS$_B$), resulting in resistance to clindamycin as well.

The second major mechanism of resistance to macrolides is expression of efflux pumps encoded by *mef* genes (Mef in gram-positive bacteria and Acr-AB-TolC in *H. influenzae* and *E. coli*) (321). The efflux pumps confer resistance to the macrolides but not to clindamycin, hence the phenotypic description of this resistance as "M" type. *mef* genes have been studied most extensively for *Streptococcus pneumoniae* [*mef*(E)] and *Streptococcus pyogenes* [*mef*(A)], but similar genes have been described for a variety of gram-positive genera. The prevalences of *mef*-mediated resistance versus that mediated by MLS$_B$-type mechanisms in *S. pneumoniae* vary in different parts of the world. Minor mechanisms of resistance to macrolides include esterases that hydrolyze the antibiotics and point mutations within the 50S rRNA gene.

Resistance to Ketolides

Ketolides belong to a new class of semisynthetic 14-membered-ring macrolides, which differ from erythromycin by having a 3-keto group instead of the neutral sugar L-cladinose. Ketolides bind to an additional site on the bac-terial ribosome, increasing their binding affinity relative to that of other macrolides (69). Telithromycin, a ketolide, is uniformly and highly active against pneumococci (regardless of their susceptibility or resistance to erythromycin and/or penicillin), erythromycin-susceptible *S. pyogenes* and eryth-romycin-resistant *S. pyogenes* strains of the M phenotype or iMLS$_B$ or cMLS$_B$ phenotype [in which resistance is mediated by a methylase encoded by the *erm*(TR) gene] (18). Ketolides are less active against erythromycin-resistant *S. pyogenes* strains with the cMLS$_B$ phenotype or the iMLS$_A$ subtype (in

which resistance is mediated by a methylase encoded by the *ermB* gene), these strains ranging in phenotype from the up-per limits of susceptibility to resistant. Methicillin-resistant staphylococci, which commonly express a cMLS$_B$ phenotype, are not susceptible to telithromycin (18).

Resistance to Quinupristin-Dalfopristin

Quinupristin-dalfopristin is a mixture of semisynthetic strep-togramins A and B licensed in Europe and the United States. A related streptogramin A and B combination, virginiamy-cin, has been used for years as a growth promoter in animal feed. Resistance to these mixtures can result from resistance to streptogramin A alone and was first described for staphy-lococci conferred by genes encoding streptogramin A acetyl-transferases [*vat*(A), *vat*(B), and *vat*(C)] or ATP-binding efflux genes [*vga*(A) and *vga*(B)]. Quinupristin-dalfopristin's excellent activities against *E. faecium* and MRSA make it an alternative for the treatment of MDR *E. faecium* and health care-associated MRSA infections, especially since the com-bination retains in vitro activity against streptogramin B-resistant strains. Two acetyltransferase-encoding resistance genes have now been described that confer resistance to quinupristin-dalfopristin in *E. faecium*: *vat*(D) [previously *sat*(A)] and *vat*(E) [previously *sat*(G)]. In most cases, these resistance genes are found along with an *erm* gene (270), suggesting that resistance to both streptogramins A and B may be necessary to confer clinically significant levels of resistance to quinupristin-dalfopristin in *E. faecium*. These resistance genes are frequently present on transferable plas-mids. Although quinupristin-dalfopristin remains active against the majority of human *E. faecium* strains, the use of virginiamycin in animal feeds has been associated with high percentages of resistance in isolates derived from animals (113). In many cases, the known mechanisms of resistance to quinupristin-dalfopristin are not present in these isolates (113), indicating that there is still much to be learned about resistance to quinupristin-dalfopristin in *E. faecium*.

Resistance to Metronidazole

Metronidazole is a member of the nitroimidazole family of bactericidal antimicrobials. The 5-nitroimidazole molecule is a prodrug whose activation depends upon reduction of the ni-tro group in the absence of oxygen. An exception to this rule occurs in *Helicobacter pylori,* with which the RdxA protein re-duces metronidazole in a microaerophilic environment (295). The nitro group of metronidazole accepts a single electron from electron transport proteins (ferredoxins) in bacteria, yielding a toxic radical anion. Metronidazole's activity appears to result in DNA damage and cell death (73). Resistance to metronidazole is rare. Decreased uptake and/or a reduced rate of reduction is believed to be responsible for metronidazole resistance in some cases (72). Five *Bacteroides* genes, *nimA* to *nimE*, have been implicated in resistance to 5-nitroimidazole antibiotics. Analysis of the NimA susceptible and resistant *Bacteroides* strains and recent crystal structure analysis suggest that the enzyme utilizes pyruvate for a two-electron reaction resulting in an amine that prevents the formation of the toxic anion radical (41, 152). Expression of *nim* genes varies depending on the positioning of a variety of IS elements that supply active promoters (269). Recent data indicate that the enzyme thioredoxin reductase is responsible for reduction of metronidazole in *Trichomonas vaginalis* (153).

Resistance to Nitrofurantoin

The antibiotics nitrofurazone and nitrofurantoin are used in the treatment of genitourinary infections and as topical antibacterial agents. Nitrofurazone is primarily used as a topical antiseptic (103). Nitrofurantoin, 1-[(5-nitrofurfurylidene)amino]hydantoin, is a synthetic antibacterial agent used primarily in the treatment of urinary tract infections. The mechanism of action of nitrofurazone and nitrofurantoin has not been fully elucidated. Investigators have reported that the ability of nitrofurantoin to kill bacteria correlates with the presence of bacterial nitroreductases which convert nitrofurantoin to highly reactive electrophilic intermediates (173). These intermediates are believed to attack bacterial ribosomal proteins nonspecifically, causing complete inhibition of protein synthesis. In *E. coli*, nitroreductases are type 1 oxygen-insensitive enzymes, encoded by the *nfnA* (*nfsA*) and *nfnB* (*nfsB*) genes. Strains of bacteria that are resistant to nitrofurantoin have been shown to possess diminished nitroreductase activity (227), which may seriously compromise their fitness (252). Resistance to nitrofurantoin from reduced nitroreductase activity seems to be present in other genera as well.

Resistance to Polymyxin B and Polymyxin E (Colistin)

Clinical and scientific interest in the cationic polypeptides is increasing. Although they were first used in the early 1960s, colistin (polymyxin E) and polymyxin B are now often used as first-line therapy of infections caused by MDR gram-negative bacterial infections. The polymyxins are polycationic peptide antibiotics isolated from *Bacillus polymyxa* (133). They exert their bactericidal activity by binding to the cell membrane of gram-negative bacteria and disrupting its permeability, resulting in leakage of intracellular components. They also disrupt bacterial biofilm formation. In mechanistic terms, polymyxin binds to phosphorylated head groups of lipid A. Hence, by disrupting cell membranes, these agents become rapidly bactericidal against certain gram-negative bacteria (278, 290).

Not all gram-negative bacteria are susceptible to polymyxins. Organisms that are resistant to polymyxins have cell walls that prevent access of the drug to the cell membrane. In general, polymyxins are bactericidal against *P. aeruginosa*, *Acinetobacter* spp., some *Proteus mirabilis* strains, and some strains of *Serratia marcescens*. *Proteus* spp., *Providencia* spp., *Neisseria* spp., and gram-positive bacteria are resistant to polymyxins (278, 290).

Polymyxin-resistant mutants and bacteria exhibit a modified LPS. In *E. coli*, *Salmonella* serovar Typhimurium, and many other pathogenic gram-negative bacteria, modification of the phosphate groups of lipid A confers resistance to polymyxin and cationic antimicrobial peptides. LPS modifications that include alteration of the fatty acid content of lipid A, phosphoethanolamine addition to the core and lipid A head groups, and 4-amino-4-deoxy-L-arabinose addition to the core and lipid A regions have been well studied (290). Recent evidence also implicates the presence of the MtrC-MtrD-MtrE efflux pump and lipid A modification as well as the type IV pilin secretion system to modulate levels of polymyxin resistance in *Neisseria meningitidis* (290) and the PmrAB two-component system in resistance to colistin in *Acinetobacter baumannii* (1).

Resistance to Quinolones

The fluoroquinolones are among the most widely used antimicrobial agents in both the hospital and community settings. Quinolone antibiotics all act by directly inhibiting DNA synthesis. Their targets include two type 2 topoisomerases: DNA gyrase and topoisomerase IV. These two enzymes are structurally related in that both exist as tetramers composed of two different subunits (GyrA and GyrB of DNA gyrase and ParC and ParE of topoisomerase IV). DNA gyrase acts to maintain negative supercoiling of DNA, whereas topoisomerase IV separates interlocked daughter DNA strands formed during replication, facilitating segregation into daughter cells. Fluoroquinolones bind to the topoisomerase-DNA complexes and disrupt various cellular processes involving DNA (replication fork, transcription of RNA, and DNA helicase) (118, 261, 312). The end result is cellular death by unclear mechanisms.

The affinities of fluoroquinolones for the two targets vary, explaining to some degree the differing potencies of the various agents against different bacterial species. The enzyme for which a particular fluoroquinolone exerts the greatest affinity is referred to as the primary target (6, 25, 202). In general, the primary target of fluoroquinolones in gram-negative bacteria is DNA gyrase, whereas in gram-positive bacteria it is topoisomerase IV.

Alterations in Target Enzymes

The most common mechanism of clinically significant levels of fluoroquinolone resistance is through alterations of the topoisomerase enzymes. These alterations are created by spontaneous mutations that occur within the respective genes. In GyrA and ParC, resistance-associated mutations are often localized to a region in the amino terminus of the enzyme containing the active-site tyrosine that is covalently linked to the broken DNA strand. This 130-bp region of *gyrA* has been referred to as the quinolone resistance-determining region. X-ray crystallographic studies of a fragment of the GyrA enzyme suggest that these mutations are clustered in three dimensions, lending support to the hypothesis that the region constitutes a part of the quinolone binding site (180). Particularly frequent sites for resistance-associated mutations are serine 83 and aspartate 87 of GyrA and serine 79 and aspartate 83 of ParC (212).

Experimental data suggest that point mutations occur singly in roughly 1 in 10^6 to 10^9 cells. The level of resistance conferred by a single point mutation in the primary target enzyme depends upon the reduction of enzyme affinity created by the mutation, as well as the affinity of the fluoroquinolone for the secondary target. In this scenario, it is expected that fluoroquinolones exhibiting strong affinity for both target enzymes would be less likely to be associated with the emergence of resistant strains, since the retained activity against the secondary target would be enough to inhibit the bacterium even in the presence of a primary target mutation. Fluoroquinolone-species combinations for which single mutations result in significantly higher MICs (such as ciprofloxacin and *S. aureus* or *P. aeruginosa*) would be expected to readily select out (and have readily selected out [55]) resistant mutants in the clinical setting.

Most highly resistant strains exhibit more than one mutation in both the GyrA and ParC enzymes, a phenomenon that can be reproduced in the laboratory by serial passage of strains on progressively higher concentrations of fluoroquinolones. It is noteworthy in this context that fluoroquinolone resistance conferred by enzyme mutations is essentially class resistance. In other words, the activity of all fluoroquinolones is affected by mutations that result in resistance. Therefore, while single point mutations that confer resistance to one fluoroquinolone may not result in MICs conferring clinical resistance to another, the MICs of the second fluoroquinolone will inevitably be increased. In the setting of such preexisting mutations, the second fluoro-quinolone could then select for an additional mutation that would result in clinically significant levels of resistance. This reasoning has led to the recommendation that the most potent and broadly active fluoroquinolone always be used first, to prevent the emergence of resistance. The wisdom of this recommendation remains to be tested.

Mutations in GyrB and ParE are far less common than in their companion subunits and tend to cluster in the mid-portion of the subunit (120). A clear understanding of the impact these mutations have on enzyme structure or function awaits detailed crystallographic studies of enzyme-fluoroquinolone complexes.

Resistance Due to Decreased Intracellular Accumulation

Fluoroquinolones penetrate the outer membrane of gram-negative bacteria through porins, so the absence of specific porins can affect the level of susceptibility. However, their ability to diffuse through outer and cytoplasmic membranes is sufficient to retain activity against strains solely lacking porins (192). More important in reducing intracellular accumulation of fluoroquinolones is the expression of MDR pumps (212). The intrinsic efflux pump complexes in gram-negative bacteria extend from the cytoplasmic membrane through the outer membrane, whereas gram-positive pumps need only traverse the cytoplasmic membrane. These pumps move compounds across the bacterial membranes by proton motive force and are presumed to represent systems by which bacteria rid themselves of toxic materials. Resistance results when expression of pumps is increased due to mutations within their regulatory genes (322). By themselves, pumps generally confer only a low level of resistance to fluoroquinolones. However, their expression may amplify the level of resistance conferred by point mutations within the topoisomerase genes. By so doing, they may increase the risk that use of a given fluoroquinolone will select for resistant mutants through single point mutations. In recent years, a plasmid-mediated efflux pump (QepA) has been recognized among strains of *Enterobacteriaceae* (46). This pump extrudes the hydrophilic fluoroquinolones (ciprofloxacin, enrofloxacin, and norfloxacin).

The major type of plasmid-mediated fluoroquinolone resistance present in gram-negative bacteria is conferred by the Qnr proteins (130, 195), which protect DNA from quinolone binding (285, 286). In general, only low levels of resistance are conferred by this mechanism, but as with other accessory mechanisms, the presence of Qnr can facilitate the clinical emergence of strains resistant by virtue of point mutations in the topoisomerase genes. Five variants of Qnr have now been described (A, B, C, D, and S). There are several alleles within the A, B, and S variants (http://www.lahey.org/qnrStudies/). The prevalence of this mechanism is increasing, which may be partly explained by the frequent presence of *qnr* within complex *sulI*-type integrons (195) often associated with insertion elements (282).

Plasmid-mediated fluoroquinolone resistance can also be conferred by the AAC(6′)-Ib-cr protein, which is a mutant of the AAC(6′)-Ib AME (46). This confers low levels of resistance to ciprofloxacin and norfloxacin.

Resistance to Rifampin

Rifampin is particularly active against gram-positive bacteria and mycobacteria. It acts by inhibiting bacterial DNA-dependent RNA polymerase. Point mutations in the chromosomal *rpoB* gene confer resistance to rifampin (303).

The frequency with which these point mutations occur precludes using rifampin as a single agent for the treatment of bacterial infections.

Resistance to Tetracyclines

The tetracyclines are a group of bacteriostatic antibiotics that act by inhibiting attachment of aminoacyl-tRNA to the ribosome acceptor site, thereby preventing elongation of the peptide chains of nascent proteins (255). In order to gain access to the bacterial ribosome, tetracyclines need to enter the cell. In *E. coli* and presumably other gram-negative bacteria, they enter the periplasmic space through outer membrane porins OmpC and OmpF, probably chelated to magnesium ions (255). Once in the periplasmic space, the weakly lipophilic tetracycline molecule dissociates from the magnesium ion and crosses into the cell by diffusing though the lipid bilayer in an energy-dependent process. Once inside the cell, tetracycline-ion complexes bind to the ribosome at a single, high-affinity binding site on the 30S subunit, blocking access of the aminoacyl-tRNA to the ribosome acceptor site. Although of high affinity, binding of tetracycline to the ribosome is reversible (52).

Tetracyclines are broad-spectrum and effective anti-microbial agents. Unfortunately, widespread use of tetra-cyclines to treat clinical infections and for promotion of growth in livestock has been associated with the emergence and dissemination of a variety of resistance determinants. As a consequence, the number of infections for which tet-racyclines are recommended as first-line therapy has been limited for many years (248). The vast majority of tetracy-cline resistance determinants fall into one of two classes: (i) efflux or (ii) ribosomal protection. The designations of the different resistance determinants and their classes can be found in detail in an excellent review of tetracy-clines by Chopra and Roberts (52). Initial designations of tetracycline resistance determinants used the prefix *tet* or *otr* with letters (A, for example) designating the different determinants. Since the number of resistance determinants now exceeds the number of letters in the alphabet, a system using numbers has been devised (155).

Tetracycline efflux proteins are all membrane associated and members of the MFS proteins. They expel tetracycline from the cell by exchanging a proton for a tetracycline-cation complex. In general, the efflux proteins confer resistance to tetracyclines but tend to spare minocycline (52). The single exception to this rule is the Tet(B) protein of gram-negative organisms, which confers resistance to both tetracycline and minocycline. The efflux proteins have been divided into six groups based on amino acid identity. Group 1 consists of Tet efflux proteins that are found primarily in gram-negative species [with the exception of Tet(Z)], whereas group 2 [consisting only of Tet(K) and Tet(L)] is found primarily in gram-positive species. Groups 3 through 6 are small groups consisting of one or two efflux proteins each.

Ribosome protection proteins comprise the other major mechanism of tetracycline resistance. These proteins exhibit homology to elongation factors EF-Tu and EF-G and exhibit ribosome-dependent GTPase activity (251). They act by binding to the ribosome, thereby changing its conformation and inhibiting binding of tetracycline. Tet(M) and Tet(O) are the best characterized of these proteins. Ribosome protection genes are widespread in bacteria, in many cases as a result of their incorporation into broad-host-range conjugative transposons.

Both efflux proteins and ribosomal protection proteins are regulated in ways that their expression is increased in the presence of tetracyclines. The efflux proteins of gram-negative organisms are regulated by repressors that are divergently transcribed relative to the efflux proteins (119). Binding of the repressors to tetracycline changes the conformation of the repressor so that it can no longer bind to the operator region, resulting in increased transcription of both the efflux protein and the repressor genes. The gram-positive efflux genes are not associated with specific protein repressors; sequence analysis suggests that these determinants may be regulated by mechanisms similar to translational attenuation, but study of this area has been limited (274). Transcription of ribosomal protection genes is augmented by growth in the presence of tetracycline.

Intrinsic mechanisms of tetracycline resistance exist in many, if not all, gram-negative bacteria. Among the best characterized of these systems is the *mar* (multiple antibiotic resistance) operon (4). This locus consists of a repressor (MarR) that represses transcription of *marA*, which encodes a transcriptional activator of a variety of genes. Overexpression of MarA results in decreased expression of OmpF, a porin through which tetracycline enters the periplasmic space, and increased expression of multidrug efflux pump AcrAB, a member of the RND family of efflux proteins, which includes tetracyclines among its substrates. Several similar pump systems have been described for *P. aeruginosa* and other gram-negative bacteria (222). As our knowledge of the genomes of different bacterial species becomes more complete, we will no doubt discover several other pump systems that affect levels of susceptibility to tetracyclines and other antibiotics.

The remarkable diversity of species within which tetracycline resistance determinants are found owes much to the inclusion of these resistance genes within broad-host-range transferable genetic elements. These include transferable plasmids in gram-negative species, where *tet* genes may be found included within integrons, and conjugative transposons. Among the best studied of the conjugative transposons is the Tn*916* family, originally described for *E. faecalis* (233). The complete sequence of Tn*916* has been determined and is remarkable for its dearth of restriction enzyme digestion sites [except in the region of the *tet*(M) gene, which appears to be a late arrival to the element] (198). This lack of restriction sites likely facilitates its entry into a variety of different bacterial species. Transfer of Tn*916*-like elements from enterococci into many other species has been demonstrated in vitro and in animal models, and the remnants of Tn*916*-like sequences in *N. gonorrhoeae* are impressive testimony to its ability to travel widely (233). Transfer of Tn*916*-like elements, which is increased after exposure to tetracycline, has also been suggested to facilitate transfer of unlinked genes, further amplifying the risks of overexposure to tetracycline in the environment.

Resistance to Tigecycline

The recent licensing of the glycylcycline tigecycline offers a broad-spectrum antimicrobial alternative for treating infections due to resistant pathogens, including MRSA and ESBL-producing *K. pneumoniae*. Tigecycline's broad spectrum of antimicrobial activity is due to its resistance to the common efflux or ribosomal protection mechanisms that confer resistance to older tetracyclines. Some bacterial species, notably *P. aeruginosa* and *Proteus* spp., are intrinsically resistant to tigecycline because they express RND-type efflux pumps that effectively extrude the antibiotic (245). Resistance to

tigecycline in other gram-negative species has also been reported, generally resulting from activation of normally repressed AcrAB-type RND efflux pumps (246). The ultimate importance of these pump activations for clinical resistance to tigecycline awaits more extensive clinical use.

Resistance to Trimethoprim-Sulfamethoxazole

Biosynthesis of several amino acids and purines depends upon the availability of tetrahydrofolate. With few exceptions, bacteria are unable to absorb preformed folic acid, and hence rely upon their ability to synthesize it. Sulfamethoxazole and trimethoprim are inhibitors of two enzymes (dihydropteroic acid synthase [DHPS] and dihydrofolate reductase [DHFR]) that act sequentially in the manufacture of tetrahydrofolate. It is thought that the two inhibitors act synergistically to inhibit folate synthesis, although the mechanism for possible synergism (since sequential blockage of a fully inhibited pathway should not augment resistance) is not clear.

Intrinsic Resistance

Trimethoprim-sulfamethoxazole is a remarkably broad-spectrum antimicrobial agent. Intrinsic resistance is relatively rare and may occur by decreased access to the target enzymes (*P. aeruginosa*) (279) or low-affinity DHFR enzymes (*Neisseria* spp., *Clostridium* spp., *Brucella* spp., *Bacteroides* spp., *Moraxella catarrhalis*, and *Nocardia* spp.) (280) or by the ability to absorb exogenous folate (*Enterococcus* spp. and *Lactobacillus* spp.) (319) or thymine (*Enterococcus* spp.) (110). The decreased access to the target enzyme in *P. aeruginosa* appears to be due to both a permeability barrier and active efflux from the cell (144, 169). The percentage contribution of each of these mechanisms to resistance remains unclear.

Acquired Resistance to Trimethoprim

Mutational resistance to trimethoprim has been described for several species and involves promoter mutations leading to overproduction of DHFR (in *E. coli*), point mutations within the *dhfr* gene leading to resistance (in *S. aureus* and *S. pneumoniae*), or both mechanisms (in *H. influenzae*) (123). More common is the acquisition of low-affinity *dhfr* genes, of which approximately 20 have been described (123). Expression of the *dhfrI* and variants of *dhfrII* genes, which are most commonly found on plasmids in gram-negative bacteria, increases resistance to levels greatly exceeding clinically achievable concentrations.

Acquired Resistance to Sulfonamides

Point mutations or small insertions of DNA segments within chromosomal *dhps* genes conferring resistance to sulfonamides have been reported for many different species (76, 123). More extensive changes within *dhps* genes resulting in resistance have been reported for *N. meningitidis* and *S. pyogenes*. In these instances, the extensive changes have suggested acquisition of at least some parts of the *dhps* genes from other species via transformation and recombination (267, 277). Plasmid-mediated, transferable resistance to sulfonamides has been reported for gram-negative bacteria (123). In contrast to the diversity in *dhfr* genes, only two acquired low-affinity *dhps* genes (*sulI* and *sulII*) have been described. Genes conferring resistance to sulfonamides are frequently incorporated into MDR integrons, which are themselves frequently integrated into transferable plasmids. The transferability of these resistance plasmids and the frequent association with other resistance genes explain in part the widespread nature and persistence of resistance to this antimicrobial combination. One trimethoprim-sulfamethoxazole-resistant *E. coli* strain was reported to have spread widely in the United States, causing urinary tract infections in young women in at least two states (163), although more recent data suggest that this widespread prevalence may owe more to parallel emergence of related strains than to direct spread of an outbreak isolate (92).

REFERENCES

1. **Adams, M. D., G. C. Nickel, S. Bajaksouzian, H. Lavender, A. R. Murthy, M. R. Jacobs, and R. A. Bonomo.** 2009. Resistance to colistin in *Acinetobacter baumannii* associated with mutations in the PmrAB two-component system. *Antimicrob. Agents Chemother.* **53:**3628–3634.

2. **Adcock, P. M., P. Pastor, F. Medley, J. E. Patterson, and T. V. Murphy.** 1998. Methicillin-resistant *Staphylococcus aureus* in two child care centers. *J. Infect. Dis.* **178:**577–580.

3. **Aires, J. R., and H. Nikaido.** 2005. Aminoglycosides are captured from both periplasm and cytoplasm by the AcrD multidrug efflux transporter of *Escherichia coli. J. Bacteriol.* **187:**1923–1929.

4. **Alekshun, M. N., and S. B. Levy.** 1997. Regulation of chromosomally mediated multiple antibiotic resistance: the *mar* regulon. *Antimicrob. Agents Chemother.* **41:**2067–2075.

5. **Alksne, L. E., and B. A. Rasmussen.** 1997. Expression of the AsbA1, OXA-12, and AsbM1 β-lactamases in *Aeromonas jandaei* AER 14 is coordinated by a two-component regulon. *J. Bacteriol.* **179:**2006–2013.

6. **Alovero, F. L., X. S. Pan, J. E. Morris, R. H. Manzo, and L. M. Fisher.** 2000. Engineering the specificity of antibacterial fluoroquinolones: benzenesulfonamide modifications at C-7 of ciprofloxacin change its primary target in *Streptococcus pneumoniae* from topoisomerase IV to gyrase. *Antimicrob. Agents Chemother.* **44:**320–325.

7. **Amoroso, A., D. Demares, M. Mollerach, G. Gutkind, and J. Coyette.** 2001. All detectable high-molecular-mass penicillin-binding proteins are modified in a high-level β-lactam-resistant clinical isolate of *Streptococcus mitis. Antimicrob. Agents Chemother.* **45:**2075–2081.

8. **Arbeloa, A., J. E. Hugonnet, A. C. Sentilhes, N. Josseaume, L. Dubost, C. Monsempes, D. Blanot, J. P. Brouard, and M. Arthur.** 2004. Synthesis of mosaic peptidoglycan cross-bridges by hybrid peptidoglycan assembly pathways in gram-positive bacteria. *J. Biol. Chem.* **279:**41546–41556.

9. **Arbeloa, A., H. Segal, J. E. Hugonnet, N. Josseaume, L. Dubost, J. P. Brouard, L. Gutmann, D. Mengin-Lecreulx, and M. Arthur.** 2004. Role of class A penicillin-binding proteins in PBP5-mediated β-lactam resistance in *Enterococcus faecalis. J. Bacteriol.* **186:**1221–1228.

10. **Arias, C. A., M. Vallejo, J. Reyes, D. Panesso, J. Moreno, E. Castaneda, M. V. Villegas, B. E. Murray, and J. P. Quinn.** 2008. Clinical and microbiological aspects of linezolid resistance mediated by the *cfr* gene encoding a 23S rRNA methyltransferase. *J. Clin. Microbiol.* **46:**892–896.

11. **Arthur, M., F. Depardieu, H. Snaith, P. Reynolds, and P. Courvalin.** 1995. The *vanZ* gene of Tn*1546* from *Enterococcus faecium* BM4147 confers resistance to teicoplanin. *Gene* **154:**87–92.

12. **Arthur, M., C. Molinas, and P. Courvalin.** 1992. Sequence of the *vanY* gene required for production of a vancomycin-inducible D,D-carboxypeptidase in *Enterococcus faecium* BM4147. *Gene* **120:**111–114.

13. **Arthur, M., C. Molinas, and P. Courvalin.** 1992. The VanS-VanR two-component regulatory system controls synthesis of depsipeptide peptidoglycan precursors in *Enterococcus faecium* 4147. *J. Bacteriol.* **174:**2582–2591.

14. **Arthur, M., C. Molinas, F. Depardieu, and P. Courvalin.** 1993. Characterization of Tn*1546*, a Tn*3*-related transposon conferring glycopeptide resistance by synthesis of depsipeptide peptidoglycan precursors in *Enterococcus faecium* BM4147. *J. Bacteriol.* **175:**117–127.

15. **Arthur, M., P. Reynolds, and P. Courvalin.** 1996. Glycopeptide resistance in enterococci. *Trends Microbiol.* **4:**401–407.

16. **Aslangul, E., M. Baptista, B. Fantin, F. Depardieu, M. Arthur, P. Courvalin, and C. Carbon.** 1997. Selection of glycopeptide-resistant mutants of VanB-type *Enterococcus faecalis* BM4281 in vitro and in experimental endocarditis. *J. Infect. Dis.* **175:**598–605.

17. **Azucena, E., and S. Mobashery.** 2001. Aminoglycoside-modifying enzymes: mechanisms of catalytic processes and inhibition. *Drug Resist. Updates* **4:**106–117.

18. **Balfour, J. A., and D. P. Figgitt.** 2001. Telithromycin. *Drugs* **61:**815–829.

19. **Barcus, V. A., K. Ghanekar, M. Yeo, T. J. Coffey, and C. G. Dowson.** 1995. Genetics of high level penicillin resistance in clinical isolates of *Streptococcus pneumoniae.* FEMS *Microbiol. Lett.* **126:**299–303.

20. **Beaman, T. W., M. Sugantino, and S. L. Roderick.** 1998. Structure of the hexapeptide xenobiotic acetyltransferase from *Pseudomonas aeruginosa. Biochemistry* (Moscow) **37:**6689–6696.

21. **Belcheva, A., and D. Golemi-Kotra.** 2008. A close-up view of the VraSR two-component system. A mediator of *Staphylococcus aureus* response to cell wall damage. *J. Biol. Chem.* **283:**12354–12364.

22. **Billot-Klein, D., L. Gutmann, D. Bryant, D. Bell, J. van Heijenoort, J. Grewal, and D. M. Shlaes.** 1996. Peptidoglycan synthesis and structure in *Staphylococcus haemolyticus* expressing increasing levels of resistance to glycopeptide antibiotics. *J. Bacteriol.* **178:**4696–4703.

23. **Bissonnette, L., S. Champetier, J. P. Buisson, and P. H. Roy.** 1991. Characterization of the nonenzymatic chloramphenicol resistance (*cmlA*) gene of the In4 integron of Tn*1696*: similarity of the product to transmembrane transport proteins. *J. Bacteriol.* **173:**4493–4502.

24. **Bjorkman, J., I. Nagaev, O. G. Berg, D. Hughes, and D. I. Andersson.** 2000. Effects of environment on compensatory mutations to ameliorate costs of antibiotic resistance. *Science* **287:**1479–1482.

25. **Blanche, F., B. Cameron, F. X. Bernard, L. Maton, B. Manse, L. Ferrero, N. Ratet, C. Lecoq, A. Goniot, D. Bisch, and J. Crouzet.** 1996. Differential behaviors of *Staphylococcus aureus* and *Escherichia coli* type II DNA topoisomerases. *Antimicrob. Agents Chemother.* **40:**2714–2720.

26. **Bolton, L. F., L. C. Kelley, M. D. Lee, P. J. Fedorka-Cray, and J. J. Maurer.** 1999. Detection of multidrug-resistant *Salmonella enterica* serotype Typhimurium DT104 based on a gene which confers cross-resistance to florfenicol and chloramphenicol. *J. Clin. Microbiol.* **37:**1348–1351.

27. **Bonnet, R.** 2004. Growing group of extended-spectrum β-lactamases: the CTX-M enzymes. *Antimicrob. Agents Chemother.* **48:**1–14.

28. **Bonomo, R. A., C. G. Dawes, J. R. Knox, and D. M. Shlaes.** 1995. β-Lactamase mutations far from the active site influence inhibitor binding. *Biochim. Biophys. Acta* **1247:**121–125.

29. **Bou, G., A. Oliver, and J. Martinez-Beltran.** 2000. OXA-24, a novel class D β-lactamase with carbapenemase activity in an *Acinetobacter baumannii* clinical strain. *Antimicrob. Agents Chemother.* **44:**1556–1561.

30. **Bradford, P. A.** 2001. Extended-spectrum β-lactamases in the 21st century: characterization, epidemiology, and detection of this important resistance threat. *Clin. Microbiol. Rev.* **14:**933–951.

31. **Bradford, P. A.** 2001. What's new in beta-lactamases? *Curr. Infect. Dis. Rep.* **3:**13–19.

32. **Bradford, P. A., C. Urban, N. Mariano, S. J. Projan, J. J. Rahal, and K. Bush.** 1997. Imipenem resistance in *Klebsiella pneumoniae* is associated with the combination of ACT-1, a plasmid-mediated AmpC β-lactamase, and the loss of an outer membrane protein. *Antimicrob. Agents Chemother.* **41:**563–569.

33. **Bratu, S., M. Mooty, S. Nichani, D. Landman, C. Gullans, B. Pettinato, U. Karumudi, P. Tolaney, and J. Quale.**

2005. Emergence of KPC-possessing *Klebsiella pneumoniae* in Brooklyn, New York: epidemiology and recommendations for detection. *Antimicrob. Agents Chemother.* **49:**3018–3020.

34. **Brown, N. G., S. Shanker, B. V. Venkataram Prasad, and T. Palzkill.** 2009. Structural and biochemical evidence that a TEM-1 β-lactamase N170G active site mutant acts via substrate-assisted catalysis. *J. Biol. Chem.* **284:**33703–33712.

35. **Bruand, C., L. Chatelier, S. D. Ehrlich, and L. Janniere.** 1993. A fourth class of theta-replicating plasmids: the pAMβ1 family from Gram-positive bacteria. *Proc. Natl. Acad. Sci. USA* **90:**11668–11672.

35a. **Bush, K., and G. A. Jacoby.** 2010. Updated functional classification of β-lactamases. *Antimicrob. Agents Chemother.* **54:**969–976.

36. **Bush, K., G. A. Jacoby, and A. A. Medeiros.** 1995. A functional classification scheme for β-lactamases and its correlation with molecular structure. *Antimicrob. Agents Chemother.* **39:**1211–1233.

37. **Camargo, I. L., H. M. Neoh, L. Cui, and K. Hiramatsu.** 2008. Serial daptomycin selection generates daptomycin-nonsusceptible *Staphylococcus aureus* strains with a heterogeneous vancomycin-intermediate phenotype. *Antimicrob. Agents Chemother.* **52:**4289–4299.

38. **Campbell, B. D., and R. J. Kadner.** 1980. Relation of aerobiosis and ionic strength to the uptake of dihydrostreptomycin in *Escherichia coli. Biochim. Biophys. Acta* **593:**1–10.

39. **Carfi, A., S. Pares, E. Duee, M. Galleni, C. Duez, J. M. Frere, and O. Dideberg.** 1995. The 3-D structure of a zinc metallo-β-lactamase from *Bacillus cereus* reveals a new type of protein fold. *EMBO J.* **14:**4914–4921.

40. **Carias, L. L., S. D. Rudin, C. J. Donskey, and L. B. Rice.** 1998. Genetic linkage and cotransfer of a novel, *vanB*-containing transposon (Tn*5382*) and a low-affinity penicillin-binding protein 5 gene in a clinical vancomycin-resistant *Enterococcus faecium* isolate. *J. Bacteriol.* **180:**4426–4434.

41. **Carlier, J. P., N. Sellier, M. N. Rager, and G. Reysset.** 1997. Metabolism of a 5-nitroimidazole in susceptible and resistant isogenic strains of *Bacteroides fragilis. Antimicrob. Agents Chemother.* **41:**1495–1499.

42. **Carrër, A., N. Fortineau, and P. Nordmann.** 2010. Use of ChromID extended-spectrum β-lactamase medium for detecting carbapenemase-producing *Enterobacteriaceae. J. Clin. Microbiol.* **48:**1913–1914.

43. **Carter, A. P., W. M. Clemons, D. E. Brodersen, R. J. Morgan-Warren, B. T. Wimberly, and V. Ramakrishnan.** 2000. Functional insights from the structure of the 30S ribosomal subunit and its interactions with antibiotics. *Nature* **407:**340–348.

44. **Casadewall, B., P. E. Reynolds, and P. Courvalin.** 2001. Regulation of expression of the *vanD* glycopeptide resistance gene cluster from *Enterococcus faecium* BM4339. *J. Bacteriol.* **183:**3436–3446.

45. **Castanheira, M., M. A. Toleman, R. N. Jones, F. J. Schmidt, and T. R. Walsh.** 2004. Molecular characterization of a β-lactamase gene, *bla*GIM-1, encoding a new subclass of metallo-beta-lactamase. *Antimicrob. Agents Chemother.* **48:**4654–4661.

46. **Cattoir, V., and P. Nordmann.** 2009. Plasmid-mediated quinolone resistance in gram-negative bacterial species: an update. *Curr. Med. Chem.* **16:**1028–1046.

47. **Chambers, H. F.** 1997. Methicillin resistance in staphylococci: molecular and biochemical basis and clinical implications. *Clin. Microbiol. Rev.* **10:**781–791.

48. **Chang, F. Y., J. E. Peacock, Jr., D. M. Musher, P. Triplett, B. B. MacDonald, J. M. Mylotte, A. O'Donnell, M. M. Wagener, and V. L. Yu.** 2003. *Staphylococcus aureus* bacteremia: recurrence and the impact of antibiotic treatment in a prospective multicenter study. *Medicine* (Baltimore) **82:**333–339.

49. **Chen, Y., J. Delmas, J. Sirot, B. Shoichet, and R. Bonnet.** 2005. Atomic resolution structures of CTX-M beta-lactamases: extended spectrum activities from increased mobility and decreased stability. *J. Mol. Biol.* **348:**349–362.

50. **Chen, Y., A. McReynolds, and B. K. Shoichet.** 2009. Reexamining the role of Lys67 in class C beta-lactamase catalysis. *Protein Sci.* **18:**662–669.

51. **Chen, Y., G. Minasov, T. A. Roth, F. Prati, and B. K. Shoichet.** 2006. The deacylation mechanism of AmpC beta-lactamase at ultrahigh resolution. *J. Am. Chem. Soc.* **128:**2970–2976.

52. **Chopra, I., and M. Roberts.** 2001. Tetracycline antibiotics: mode of action, applications, molecular biology, and epidemiology of bacterial resistance. *Microbiol. Mol. Biol. Rev.* **65:**232–260.

53. **Climo, M. W., R. L. Patron, and G. L. Archer.** 1999. Combinations of vancomycin and β-lactams are synergistic against staphylococci with reduced susceptibilities to vancomycin. *Antimicrob. Agents Chemother.* **43:**1747–1753.

54. **Concha, N. O., C. A. Janson, P. Rowling, S. Pearson, C. A. Cheever, B. P. Clarke, C. Lewis, M. Galleni, J. M. Frere, D. J. Payne, J. H. Bateson, and S. S. Abdel-Meguid.** 2000. Crystal structure of the IMP-1 metallo β-lactamase from *Pseudomonas aeruginosa* and its complex with a mercaptocarboxylate inhibitor: binding determinants of a potent, broad-spectrum inhibitor. *Biochemistry* (Moscow) **39:**4288–4298.

55. **Coronado, V. G., J. R. Edwards, D. H. Culver, and R. P. Gaynes.** 1995. Ciprofloxacin resistance among nosocomial *Pseudomonas aeruginosa* and *Staphylococcus aureus* in the United States. National Nosocomial Infections Surveillance (NNIS) System. *Infect. Control Hosp. Epidemiol.* **16:**71–75.

56. **Couto, I., H. de Lencastre, E. Severina, W. Kloos, J. A. Webster, R. J. Hubner, I. S. Sanches, and A. Tomasz.** 1996. Ubiquitous presence of a *mecA* homologue in natural isolates of *Staphylococcus sciuri. Microb. Drug Resist.* **2:**377–391.

57. **Crichlow, G. V., A. P. Kuzin, M. Nukaga, K. Mayama, T. Sawai, and J. R. Knox.** 1999. Structure of the extended-spectrum class C beta-lactamase of *Enterobacter cloacae* GC1, a natural mutant with a tandem tripeptide insertion. *Biochemistry* (Moscow) **38:**10256–10261.

58. **Crowder, M. W., J. Spencer, and A. J. Vila.** 2006. Metallo-beta-lactamases: novel weaponry for antibiotic resistance in bacteria. *Acc. Chem. Res.* **39:**721–728.

59. **Cui, L., A. Iwamoto, J. Q. Lian, H. M. Neoh, T. Maruyama, Y. Horikawa, and K. Hiramatsu.** 2006. Novel mechanism of antibiotic resistance originating in vancomycin-intermediate *Staphylococcus aureus. Antimicrob. Agents Chemother.* **50:**428–438.

60. **Dahl, K. H., E. W. Lundblad, T. P. Rokenes, O. Olsvik, and A. Sundsfjord.** 2000. Genetic linkage of the *vanB2* gene cluster to Tn*5382* in vancomycin-resistant enterococci and characterization of two novel insertion sequences. *Microbiology* **146:**1469–1479.

61. **Darini, A. L., M. F. Palepou, and N. Woodford.** 2000. Effects of the movement of insertion sequences on the structure of VanA glycopeptide resistance elements in *Enterococcus faecium. Antimicrob. Agents Chemother.* **44:**1362–1364.

62. **D'Costa, V. M., K. M. McGrann, D. W. Hughes, and G. D. Wright.** 2006. Sampling the antibiotic resistome. *Science* **311:**374–377.

63. **de la Campa, A. G., L. Balsalobre, C. Ardanuy, A. Fenoll, E. Perez-Trallero, and J. Linares.** 2004. Fluoroquinolone resistance in penicillin-resistant *Streptococcus pneumoniae* clones, Spain. *Emerg. Infect. Dis.* **10:**1751–1759.

64. **Delaire, M., R. Labia, J. P. Samama, and J. M. Masson.** 1992. Site-directed mutagenesis at the active site of *Escherichia coli* TEM-1 beta-lactamase. Suicide inhibitor-resistant mutants reveal the role of arginine 244 and methionine 69 in catalysis. *J. Biol. Chem.* **267:**20600–20606.

65. **Deurenberg, R. H., and E. E. Stobberingh.** 2008. The evolution of *Staphylococcus aureus. Infect. Genet. Evol.* **8:**747–763.

66. **Docquier, J. D., V. Calderone, F. De Luca, M. Benvenuti, F. Giuliani, L. Bellucci, A. Tafi, P. Nordmann, M. Botta, G. M. Rossolini, and S. Mangani.** 2009. Crystal structure of the OXA-48 beta-lactamase reveals mechanistic diversity among class D carbapenemases. *Chem. Biol.* **16:**540–547.

67. **Doi, Y., B. A. Potoski, J. M. Adams-Haduch, H. E. Sidjabat, A. W. Pasculle, and D. L. Paterson.** 2008. Simple disk-based method for detection of *Klebsiella pneumoniae* carbapenemase-type β-lactamase by use of a boronic acid compound. *J. Clin. Microbiol.* **46:**4083–4086.

68. **Donskey, C. J., J. A. Hanrahan, R. A. Hutton, and L. B. Rice.** 2000. Effect of parenteral antibiotic administration on establishment of colonization with vancomycin-resistant *Enterococcus faecium* in the mouse gastrointestinal tract. *J. Infect. Dis.* **181:**1830–1833.

69. **Douthwaite, S., L. H. Hansen, and P. Mauvais.** 2000. Macrolide-ketolide inhibition of MLS-resistant ribosomes is improved by alternative drug interaction with domain II of 23S rRNA. *Mol. Microbiol.* **36:**183–193.

70. **Dubois, V., L. Poirel, C. Arpin, L. Coulange, C. Bebear, P. Nordmann, and C. Quentin.** 2004. SHV-49, a novel inhibitor-resistant β-lactamase in a clinical isolate of *Klebsiella pneumoniae. Antimicrob. Agents Chemother.* **48:**4466–4469.

71. **Dutka-Malen, S., B. Blaimont, G. Wauters, and P. Courvalin.** 1994. Emergence of high-level resistance to glycopeptides in *Enterococcus gallinarum* and *Enterococcus casseliflavus. Antimicrob. Agents Chemother.* **38:**1675–1677.

72. **Edwards, D. I.** 1993. Nitroimidazole drugs—action and resistance mechanisms. I. Mechanisms of action. *J. Antimicrob. Chemother.* **31:**9–20.

73. **Edwards, D. I.** 1993. Nitroimidazole drugs—action and resistance mechanisms. II. Mechanisms of resistance. *J. Antimicrob. Chemother.* **31:**201–210.

74. **Eliopoulos, G. M., B. F. Farber, B. E. Murray, C. Wennersten, and R. Moellering, Jr.** 1984. Ribosomal resistance of clinical enterococcal isolates to streptomycin. *Antimicrob. Agents Chemother.* **25:**398–399.

75. **Ena, J., M. M. Lopez-Perezagua, C. Martinez-Peinado, M. A. Cia-Barrio, and I. Ruiz-Lopez.** 1998. Emergence of ciprofloxacin resistance in *Escherichia coli* isolates after widespread use of fluoroquinolones. *Diagn. Microbiol. Infect. Dis.* **30:**103–107.

76. **Enne, V. I., A. King, D. M. Livermore, and L. M. Hall.** 2002. Sulfonamide resistance in *Haemophilus influenzae* mediated by acquisition of *sul2* or a short insertion in chromosomal *folP. Antimicrob. Agents Chemother.* **46:**1934–1939.

77. **Evers, S., and P. Courvalin.** 1996. Regulation of VanB-type vancomycin resistance gene expression by the VanS$_B$-VanR$_B$ two-component regulatory system in *Enterococcus faecalis* V583. *J. Bacteriol.* **178:**1302–1309.

78. **Evers, S., D. F. Sahm, and P. Courvalin.** 1993. The *vanB* gene of vancomycin-resistant *Enterococcus faecalis* V583 is structurally-related to genes encoding D-ala:D-ala ligases and glycopeptide-resistance proteins VanA and VanC. *Gene* **124:**143–144.

79. **Farzaneh, S., E. B. Chaibi, J. Peduzzi, M. Barthelemy, R. Labia, J. Blazquez, and F. Baquero.** 1996. Implication of Ile-69 and Thr-182 residues in kinetic characteristics of IRT-3 (TEM-32) β-lactamase. *Antimicrob. Agents Chemother.* **40:**2434–2436.

80. **Ferber, D.** 2000. Antibiotic resistance. Superbugs on the hoof? *Science* **288:**792–794.

81. **Ferretti, J. J., K. S. Gilmore, and P. Courvalin.** 1986. Nucleotide sequence of the gene specifying the bifunctional 6′-aminoglycoside acetyltransferase-2″ aminoglycoside phosphotransferase enzyme in *Streptococcus faecalis* and identification and cloning of the gene regions specifying the two activities. *J. Bacteriol.* **167:**631–638.

82. **Ferretti, J. J., W. M. McShan, D. Ajdic, D. J. Savic, G. Savic, K. Lyon, C. Primeaux, S. Sezate, A. N. Suvorov, S. Kenton, H. S. Lai, S. P. Lin, Y. Qian, H. G. Jia, F. Z. Najar, Q. Ren, H. Zhu, L. Song, J. White, X. Yuan, S. W. Clifton, B. A. Roe, and R. McLaughlin.** 2001. Complete genome sequence of an M1 strain of *Streptococcus pyogenes. Proc. Natl. Acad. Sci. USA* **98:**4658–4663.

83. **Fey, P. D., B. Said-Salim, M. E. Rupp, S. H. Hinrichs, D. J. Boxrud, C. C. Davis, B. N. Kreiswirth, and P. M. Schlievert.** 2003. Comparative molecular analysis of community- or hospital-acquired methicillin-resistant *Staphylococcus aureus. Antimicrob. Agents Chemother.* **47:**196–203.

84. **Fiett, J., A. Palucha, B. Miaczynska, M. Stankiewicz, H. Przondo-Mordarska, W. Hryniewicz, and M. Gniadkowski.** 2000. A novel complex mutant β-lactamase, TEM-68, identified in a *Klebsiella pneumoniae* isolate from an outbreak of extended-spectrum β-lactamase-producing klebsiellae. *Antimicrob. Agents Chemother.* **44:**1499–1505.

85. **Filipe, S. R., and A. Tomasz.** 2000. Inhibition of the expression of penicillin resistance in *Streptococcus pneumoniae* by inactivation of cell wall muropeptide branching genes. *Proc. Natl. Acad. Sci. USA* **97:**4891–4896.

86. **Fines, M., B. Perichon, P. Reynolds, D. F. Sahm, and P. Courvalin.** 1999. VanE, a new type of acquired glycopeptide resistance in *Enterococcus faecalis* BM4405. *Antimicrob. Agents Chemother.* **43:**2161–2164.

87. **Fitton, J. E., and W. V. Shaw.** 1979. Comparison of chloramphenicol acetyltransferase variants in staphylococci. Purification, inhibitor studies and N-terminal sequences. *Biochem. J.* **177:**575–582.

88. **Fitzgerald, J. R., D. E. Sturdevant, S. M. Mackie, S. R. Gill, and J. M. Musser.** 2001. Evolutionary genomics of *Staphylococcus aureus:* insights into the origin of methicillin-resistant strains and the toxic shock syndrome epidemic. *Proc. Natl. Acad. Sci. USA* **98:**8821–8826.

89. **Flannagan, S. E., J. W. Chow, S. M. Donabedian, W. J. Brown, M. B. Perri, M. J. Zervos, Y. Ozawa, and D. B. Clewell.** 2003. Plasmid content of a vancomycin-resistant *Enterococcus faecalis* isolate from a patient also colonized by *Staphylococcus aureus* with a VanA phenotype. *Antimicrob. Agents Chemother.* **47:**3954–3959.

90. **Fontana, R., M. Aldegheri, M. Ligozzi, H. Lopez, A. Sucari, and G. Satta.** 1994. Overproduction of a low-affinity penicillin-binding protein and high-level ampicillin resistance in *Enterococcus faecium. Antimicrob. Agents Chemother.* **38:**1980–1983.

91. **Fowler, V. G., Jr., H. W. Boucher, G. R. Corey, E. Abrutyn, A. W. Karchmer, M. E. Rupp, D. P. Levine, H. F. Chambers, F. P. Tally, G. A. Vigliani, C. H. Cabell, A. S. Link, I. DeMeyer, S. G. Filler, M. Zervos, P. Cook, J. Parsonnet, J. M. Bernstein, C. S. Price, G. N. Forrest, G. Fatkenheuer, M. Gareca, S. J. Rehm, H. R. Brodt, A. Tice, and S. E. Cosgrove.** 2006. Daptomycin versus standard therapy for bacteremia and endocarditis caused by *Staphylococcus aureus. N. Engl. J. Med.* **355:**653–665.

92. **France, A. M., K. M. Kugeler, A. Freeman, C. A. Zalewski, M. Blahna, L. Zhang, C. F. Marrs, and B. Foxman.** 2005. Clonal groups and the spread of resistance to trimethoprim-sulfamethoxazole in uropathogenic *Escherichia coli. Clin. Infect. Dis.* **40:**1101–1107.

93. **Frase, H., Q. Shi, S. A. Testero, S. Mobashery, and S. B. Vakulenko.** 2009. Mechanistic basis for the emergence of catalytic competence against carbapenem antibiotics by the GES family of beta-lactamases. *J. Biol. Chem.* **284:**29509–29513.

94. **Galas, D. J., and M. Chandler.** 1989. Bacterial insertion sequences, p. 109–162. *In* D. E. Berg and M. M. Howe (ed.), *Mobile DNA.* American Society for Microbiology, Washington, DC.

95. **Galimand, M., P. Courvalin, and T. Lambert.** 2003. Plasmid-mediated high-level resistance to aminoglycosides in *Enterobacteriaceae* due to 16S rRNA methylation. *Antimicrob. Agents Chemother.* **47:**2565–2571.

96. **Galimand, M., S. Sabtcheva, P. Courvalin, and T. Lambert.** 2005. Worldwide disseminated *armA* aminoglycoside resistance methylase gene is borne by composite transposon Tn*1548. Antimicrob. Agents Chemother.* **49:**2949–2953.

97. **Galleni, M., J. Lamotte-Brasseur, G. M. Rossolini, J. Spencer, O. Dideberg, and J. M. Frere.** 2001. Standard numbering scheme for class B β-lactamases. *Antimicrob. Agents Chemother.* **45:**660–663.

98. **Garau, G., C. Bebrone, C. Anne, M. Galleni, J. M. Frere, and O. Dideberg.** 2005. A metallo-beta-lactamase enzyme in action: crystal structures of the monozinc carbapenemase CphA and its complex with biapenem. *J. Mol. Biol.* **345:**785–795.

99. **Garnier, F., S. Taourit, P. Glaser, P. Courvalin, and M. Galimand.** 2000. Characterization of transposon Tn*1549,* conferring VanB-type resistance in *Enterococcus* spp. *Microbiology* **146:**1481–1489.

100. **Gherman, B. F., S. D. Goldberg, V. W. Cornish, and R. A. Friesner.** 2004. Mixed quantum mechanical/molecular mechanical (QM/MM) study of the deacylation reaction in

a penicillin binding protein (PBP) versus in a class C beta-lactamase. *J. Am. Chem. Soc.* **126:**7652–7664.

101. **Ghuysen, J. M.** 1991. Serine β-lactamases and penicillin-binding proteins. *Annu. Rev. Microbiol.* **45:**37–67.

102. **Giakkoupi, P., O. Pappa, M. Polemis, A. C. Vatopoulos, V. Miriagou, A. Zioga, C. C. Papagiannitsis, and L. S. Tzouvelekis.** 2009. Emerging *Klebsiella pneumoniae* isolates coproducing KPC-2 and VIM-1 carbapenemases. *Antimicrob. Agents Chemother.* **53:**4048–4050.

103. **Guay, D. R.** 2001. An update on the role of nitrofurans in the management of urinary tract infections. *Drugs* **61:**353–364.

104. **Haas, W., J. Sublett, D. Kaushal, and E. I. Tuomanen.** 2004. Revising the role of the pneumococcal *vex-vncRS* locus in vancomycin tolerance. *J. Bacteriol.* **186:**8463–8471.

105. **Hachmann, A. B., E. R. Angert, and J. D. Helmann.** 2009. Genetic analysis of factors affecting susceptibility of *Bacillus subtilis* to daptomycin. *Antimicrob. Agents Chemother.* **53:**1598–1609.

106. **Hackbarth, C. J., and H. F. Chambers.** 1993. *blaI* and *blaR1* regulate β-lactamase and PBP 2a production in methicillin-resistant *Staphylococcus aureus*. *Antimicrob. Agents Chemother.* **37:**1144–1149.

107. **Hackbarth, C. J., T. Kocagoz, S. Kocagoz, and H. F. Chambers.** 1995. Point mutations in *Staphylococcus aureus* PBP 2 gene affect penicillin-binding kinetics and are associated with resistance. *Antimicrob. Agents Chemother.* **39:**103–106.

108. **Hakenbeck, R., and J. Coyette.** 1998. Resistant penicillin-binding proteins. *Cell. Mol. Life Sci.* **54:**332–340.

109. **Hall, R. M., and C. M. Collis.** 1995. Mobile gene cassettes and integrons: capture and spread of genes by site-specific recombination. *Mol. Microbiol.* **15:**593–600.

110. **Hamilton-Miller, J. M.** 1988. Reversal of activity of trimethoprim against gram-positive cocci by thymidine, thymine and 'folates.' *J. Antimicrob. Chemother.* **22:**35–39.

111. **Hayashi, T., K. Makino, M. Ohnishi, K. Kurokawa, K. Ishii, K. Yokoyama, C. G. Han, E. Ohtsubo, K. Nakayama, T. Murata, M. Tanaka, T. Tobe, T. Iida, H. Takami, T. Honda, C. Sasakawa, N. Ogasawara, T. Yasunaga, S. Kuhara, T. Shiba, M. Hattori, and H. Shinagawa.** 2001. Complete genome sequence of enterohemorrhagic *Escherichia coli* O157:H7 and genomic comparison with a laboratory strain K-12. *DNA Res.* **8:**11–22.

112. **Hayden, M. K., G. M. Trenholm, J. E. Schultz, and D. F. Sahm.** 1993. In vivo development of teicoplanin resistance in a VanB *Enterococcus faecium* isolate. *J. Infect. Dis.* **167:**1224–1227.

113. **Hayes, J. R., D. D. Wagner, L. L. English, L. E. Carr, and S. W. Joseph.** 2005. Distribution of streptogramin resistance determinants among *Enterococcus faecium* from a poultry production environment of the USA. *J. Antimicrob. Chemother.* **55:**123–126.

114. **Henriques Normark, B., R. Novak, A. Ortqvist, G. Kallenius, E. Tuomanen, and S. Normark.** 2001. Clinical isolates of *Streptococcus pneumoniae* that exhibit tolerance of vancomycin. *Clin. Infect. Dis.* **32:**552–558.

115. **Henze, U. U., and B. Berger-Bachi.** 1995. *Staphylococcus aureus* penicillin-binding protein 4 and intrinsic β-lactam resistance. *Antimicrob. Agents Chemother.* **39:**2415–2422.

116. **Heritier, C., L. Poirel, P. E. Fournier, J. M. Claverie, D. Raoult, and P. Nordmann.** 2005. Characterization of the naturally occurring oxacillinase of *Acinetobacter baumannii*. *Antimicrob. Agents Chemother.* **49:**4174–4179.

117. **Heritier, C., L. Poirel, T. Lambert, and P. Nordmann.** 2005. Contribution of acquired carbapenem-hydrolyzing oxacillinases to carbapenem resistance in *Acinetobacter baumannii*. *Antimicrob. Agents Chemother.* **49:**3198–3202.

118. **Hiasa, H., D. O. Yousef, and K. J. Marians.** 1996. DNA strand cleavage is required for replication fork arrest by a frozen topoisomerase-quinolone-DNA ternary complex. *J. Biol. Chem.* **271:**26424–26429.

119. **Hillen, W., and C. Berens.** 1994. Mechanisms underlying expression of Tn*10* encoded tetracycline resistance. *Annu. Rev. Microbiol.* **48:**345–369.

120. **Hooper, D. C.** 2001. Emerging mechanisms of fluoroquinolone resistance. *Emerg. Infect. Dis.* **7:**337–341.

121. **Hossain, A., M. J. Ferraro, R. M. Pino, R. B. Dew III, E. S. Moland, T. J. Lockhart, K. S. Thomson, R. V. Goering, and N. D. Hanson.** 2004. Plasmid-mediated carbapenem-hydrolyzing enzyme KPC-2 in an *Enterobacter* sp. *Antimicrob. Agents Chemother.* **48:**4438–4440.

122. **Hughes, D.** 2003. Exploiting genomics, genetics and chemistry to combat antibiotic resistance. *Nat. Rev. Genet.* **4:**432–441.

123. **Huovinen, P.** 2001. Resistance to trimethoprim-sulfamethoxazole. *Clin. Infect. Dis.* **32:**1608–1614.

124. **Ibuka, A., A. Taguchi, M. Ishiguro, S. Fushinobu, Y. Ishii, S. Kamitori, K. Okuyama, K. Yamaguchi, M. Konno, and H. Matsuzawa.** 1999. Crystal structure of the E166A mutant of extended-spectrum β-lactamase Toho-1 at 1.8 Å resolution. *J. Mol. Biol.* **285:**2079–2087.

125. **Ibuka, A. S., Y. Ishii, M. Galleni, M. Ishiguro, K. Yamaguchi, J. M. Frere, H. Matsuzawa, and H. Sakai.** 2003. Crystal structure of extended-spectrum beta-lactamase Toho-1: insights into the molecular mechanism for catalytic reaction and substrate specificity expansion. *Biochemistry* (Moscow) **42:**10634–10643.

126. **Ito, T., Y. Katayama, K. Asada, N. Mori, K. Tsutsumimoto, C. Tiensasitorn, and K. Hiramatsu.** 2001. Structural comparison of three types of staphylococcal cassette chromosome *mec* integrated in the chromosome in methicillin-resistant *Staphylococcus aureus*. *Antimicrob. Agents Chemother.* **45:**1323–1336.

127. **Jacobs, C., J.-M. Frere, and S. Normark.** 1997. Cytosolic intermediates for cell wall biosynthesis and degradation control inducible β-lactam resistance in gram-negative bacteria. *Cell* **88:**823–832.

128. **Jacobs, C., B. Joris, M. Jamin, K. Klarsov, J. Van Beeumen, D. Mengin-Lecreuix, J. van Heijenoort, J. T. Park, S. Normark, and J.-M. Frère.** 1995. AmpD, essential for both β-lactamase regulation and cell wall recycling, is a novel cytosolic *N*-acetylmuramyl-L-alanine amidase. *Mol. Microbiol.* **15:**553–559.

129. **Jacoby, G. A.** 2009. AmpC β-lactamases. *Clin. Microbiol. Rev.* **22:**161–182.

130. **Jacoby, G. A.** 2005. Mechanisms of resistance to quinolones. *Clin. Infect. Dis.* **41**(Suppl. 2)**:**S120–S126.

131. **Jacoby, G. A., and A. A. Medeiros.** 1991. More extended-spectrum β-lactamases. *Antimicrob. Agents Chemother.* **35:**1697–1704.

132. **Jeannot, K., M. L. Sobel, F. El Garch, K. Poole, and P. Plesiat.** 2005. Induction of the MexXY efflux pump in *Pseudomonas aeruginosa* is dependent on drug-ribosome interaction. *J. Bacteriol.* **187:**5341–5346.

133. **Jones, R. N., T. R. Anderegg, and J. M. Swenson.** 2005. Quality control guidelines for testing gram-negative control strains with polymyxin B and colistin (polymyxin E) by standardized methods. *J. Clin. Microbiol.* **43:**925–927.

134. **Jones, R. N., J. E. Ross, M. Castanheira, and R. E. Mendes.** 2008. United States resistance surveillance results for linezolid (LEADER Program for 2007). *Diagn. Microbiol. Infect. Dis.* **62:**416–426.

135. **Kaatz, G. W., S. M. Seo, N. J. Dorman, and S. A. Lerner.** 1990. Emergence of teicoplanin resistance during therapy of *Staphylococcus aureus* endocarditis. *J. Infect. Dis.* **162:**103–108.

136. **Kadurugamuwa, J. L., J. S. Lam, and T. J. Beveridge.** 1993. Interaction of gentamicin with the A band and B band lipopolysaccharides of *Pseudomonas aeruginosa* and its possible lethal effect. *Antimicrob. Agents Chemother.* **37:**715–721.

137. **Katayama, Y., H. Murakami-Kuroda, L. Cui, and K. Hiramatsu.** 2009. Selection of heterogeneous vancomycin-intermediate *Staphylococcus aureus* by imipenem. *Antimicrob. Agents Chemother.* **53:**3190–3196.

138. Katayama, Y., D. A. Robinson, M. C. Enright, and H. F. Chambers. 2005. Genetic background affects stability of *mecA* in *Staphylococcus aureus*. *J. Clin. Microbiol.* **43**:2380–2383.

139. Kaye, K. S., H. S. Gold, M. J. Schwaber, L. Venkataraman, Y. Qi, P. C. De Girolami, M. H. Samore, G. Anderson, J. K. Rasheed, and F. C. Tenover. 2004. Variety of β-lactamases produced by amoxicillin-clavulanate-resistant *Escherichia coli* isolated in the northeastern United States. *Antimicrob. Agents Chemother.* **48**:1520–1525.

140. Ke, W., C. R. Bethel, J. M. Thomson, R. A. Bonomo, and F. van den Akker. 2007. Crystal structure of KPC-2: insights into carbapenemase activity in class A beta-lactamases. *Biochemistry* (Moscow) **46**:5732–5740.

141. Kim, J., Y. M. Lim, Y. S. Jeong, and S. Y. Seol. 2005. Occurrence of CTX-M-3, CTX-M-15, CTX-M-14, and CTX-M-9 extended-spectrum β-lactamases in *Enterobacteriaceae* clinical isolates in Korea. *Antimicrob. Agents Chemother.* **49**:1572–1575.

142. Knox, J. R. 1995. Extended-spectrum and inhibitor-resistant TEM-type β-lactamases: mutations, specificity, and three-dimensional structure. *Antimicrob. Agents Chemother.* **39**:2593–2601.

143. Ko, W. C., D. L. Paterson, A. J. Sagnimeni, D. S. Hansen, A. Von Gottberg, S. Mohapatra, J. M. Casellas, H. Goossens, L. Mulazimoglu, G. Trenholme, K. P. Klugman, J. G. McCormack, and V. L. Yu. 2002. Community-acquired *Klebsiella pneumoniae* bacteremia: global differences in clinical patterns. *Emerg. Infect. Dis.* **8**:160–166.

144. Kohler, T., M. Kok, M. Michea-Hamzehpour, P. Plesiat, N. Gotoh, T. Nishino, L. K. Curty, and J. C. Pechere. 1996. Multidrug efflux in intrinsic resistance to trimethoprim and sulfamethoxazole in *Pseudomonas aeruginosa*. *Antimicrob. Agents Chemother.* **40**:2288–2290.

145. Kotra, L. P., J. Haddad, and S. Mobashery. 2000. Aminoglycosides: perspectives on mechanisms of action and resistance and strategies to counter resistance. *Antimicrob. Agents Chemother.* **44**:3249–3256.

146. Lartigue, M. F., L. Poirel, J. W. Decousser, and P. Nordmann. 2005. Multidrug-resistant *Shigella sonnei* and *Salmonella enterica* serotype Typhimurium isolates producing CTX-M beta-lactamases as causes of community-acquired infection in France. *Clin. Infect. Dis.* **40**:1069–1070.

147. Leavis, H., J. Top, N. Shankar, K. Borgen, M. Bonten, J. van Embden, and R. J. Willems. 2004. A novel putative enterococcal pathogenicity island linked to the *esp* virulence gene of *Enterococcus faecium* and associated with epidemicity. *J. Bacteriol.* **186**:672–682.

148. Leavis, H. L., R. J. Willems, W. J. van Wamel, F. H. Schuren, M. P. Caspers, and M. J. Bonten. 2007. Insertion sequence-driven diversification creates a globally dispersed emerging multiresistant subspecies of *E. faecium*. *PLoS Pathog.* **3**:e7.

149. Leclerq, R., S. Dutka-Malen, A. Brisson-Noel, C. Molinas, E. Derlot, M. Arthur, J. Duval, and P. Courvalin. 1992. Resistance of enterococci to aminoglycosides and glycopeptides. *Clin. Infect. Dis.* **15**:495–501.

150. Lee, A., W. Mao, M. S. Warren, A. Mistry, K. Hoshino, R. Okumura, H. Ishida, and O. Lomovskaya. 2000. Interplay between efflux pumps may provide either additive or multiplicative effects on drug resistance. *J. Bacteriol.* **182**:3142–3150.

151. Lee, E. H., M. H. Nicolas, M. D. Kitzis, G. Pialoux, E. Collatz, and L. Gutmann. 1991. Association of two resistance mechanisms in a clinical isolate of *Enterobacter cloacae* with high-level resistance to imipenem. *Antimicrob. Agents Chemother.* **35**:1093–1098.

152. Leiros, H. K., S. Kozielski-Stuhrmann, U. Kapp, L. Terradot, G. A. Leonard, and S. M. McSweeney. 2004. Structural basis of 5-nitroimidazole antibiotic resistance: the crystal structure of NimA from *Deinococcus radiodurans*. *J. Biol. Chem.* **279**:55840–55849.

153. Leitsch, D., D. Kolarich, M. Binder, J. Stadlmann, F. Altmann, and M. Duchene. 2009. *Trichomonas vaginalis*: metronidazole and other nitroimidazole drugs are reduced by the flavin enzyme thioredoxin reductase and disrupt the cellular redox system. Implications for nitroimidazole toxicity and resistance. *Mol. Microbiol.* **72**:518–536.

154. Levine, D. P., B. S. Fromm, and B. R. Reddy. 1991. Slow response to vancomycin or vancomycin plus rifampin in methicillin-resistant *Staphylococcus aureus* endocarditis. *Ann. Intern. Med.* **115**:674–680.

155. Levy, S. B., L. M. McMurry, T. M. Barbosa, V. Burdett, P. Courvalin, W. Hillen, M. C. Roberts, J. I. Rood, and D. E. Taylor. 1999. Nomenclature for new tetracycline resistance determinants. *Antimicrob. Agents Chemother.* **43**:1523–1524.

156. Linares, J. 2001. The VISA/GISA problem: therapeutic implications. *Clin. Microbiol. Infect.* **7**:8–15.

157. Livermore, D. M. 1992. Interplay of impermeability and chromosomal β-lactamase activity in imipenem-resistant *Pseudomonas aeruginosa*. *Antimicrob. Agents Chemother.* **36**:2046–2048.

158. Livermore, D. M., D. F. Brown, J. P. Quinn, Y. Carmeli, D. L. Paterson, and V. L. Yu. 2004. Should third-generation cephalosporins be avoided against AmpC-inducible Enterobacteriaceae? *Clin. Microbiol. Infect.* **10**:84–85.

159. Lobkovsky, E., E. M. Billings, P. C. Moews, J. Rahil, R. F. Pratt, and J. R. Knox. 1994. Crystallographic structure of a phosphonate derivative of the *Enterobacter cloacae* P99 cephalosporinase: mechanistic interpretation of a beta-lactamase transition-state analog. *Biochemistry* (Moscow) **33**:6762–6772.

160. Lobkovsky, E., P. C. Moews, H. Liu, H. Zhao, J. M. Frere, and J. R. Knox. 1993. Evolution of an enzyme activity: crystallographic structure at 2-Å resolution of cephalosporinase from the *ampC* gene of *Enterobacter cloacae* P99 and comparison with a class A penicillinase. *Proc. Natl. Acad. Sci. USA* **90**:11257–11261.

161. Lobritz, M., R. Hutton-Thomas, S. Marshall, and L. B. Rice. 2003. Recombination proficiency influences frequency and locus of mutational resistance to linezolid in *Enterococcus faecalis*. *Antimicrob. Agents Chemother.* **47**:3318–3320.

162. Magnet, S., P. Courvalin, and T. Lambert. 2001. Resistance-nodulation-cell division-type efflux pump involved in aminoglycoside resistance in *Acinetobacter baumannii* strain BM4454. *Antimicrob. Agents Chemother.* **45**:3375–3380.

163. Manges, A. R., J. R. Johnson, B. Foxman, T. T. O'Bryan, K. E. Fullerton, and L. W. Riley. 2001. Widespread distribution of urinary tract infections caused by a multidrug-resistant *Escherichia coli* clonal group. *N. Engl. J. Med.* **345**:1007–1013.

164. Mao, W., M. S. Warren, A. Lee, A. Mistry, and O. Lomovskaya. 2001. MexXY-OprM efflux pump is required for antagonism of aminoglycosides by divalent cations in *Pseudomonas aeruginosa*. *Antimicrob. Agents Chemother.* **45**:2001–2007.

165. Marchand, I., L. Damier-Piolle, P. Courvalin, and T. Lambert. 2004. Expression of the RND-type efflux pump AdeABC in *Acinetobacter baumannii* is regulated by the AdeRS two-component system. *Antimicrob. Agents Chemother.* **48**:3298–3304.

166. Marshall, S. H., C. J. Donskey, R. Hutton-Thomas, R. A. Salata, and L. B. Rice. 2002. Gene dosage and linezolid resistance in *Enterococcus faecium* and *Enterococcus faecalis*. *Antimicrob. Agents Chemother.* **46**:3334–3336.

167. Martinez, J. L., A. Alonso, J. M. Gomez-Gomez, and F. Baquero. 1998. Quinolone resistance by mutations in chromosomal gyrase genes. Just the tip of the iceberg? *J. Antimicrob. Chemother.* **42**:683–688.

168. Martinez-Martinez, L., S. Hernandez-Alles, S. Alberti, J. M. Tomas, V. J. Benedi, and G. A. Jacoby. 1996. In vivo selection of porin-deficient mutants of *Klebsiella pneumoniae* with increased resistance to cefoxitin and expanded-spectrum cephalosporins. *Antimicrob. Agents Chemother.* **40**:342–348.

169. Maseda, H., H. Yoneyama, and T. Nakae. 2000. Assignment of the substrate-selective subunits of the MexEF-OprN multidrug efflux pump of *Pseudomonas aeruginosa*. *Antimicrob. Agents Chemother.* **44**:658–664.

170. **Matagne, A., J. Lamotte-Brasseur, and J. M. Frere.** 1998. Catalytic properties of class A beta-lactamases: efficiency and diversity. *Biochem. J.* **330:**581–598.

171. **Maus, C. E., B. B. Plikaytis, and T. M. Shinnick.** 2005. Molecular analysis of cross-resistance to capreomycin, kanamycin, amikacin, and viomycin in *Mycobacterium tuberculosis. Antimicrob. Agents Chemother.* **49:**3192–3197.

172. **Maveyraud, L., D. Golemi, L. P. Kotra, S. Tranier, S. Vakulenko, S. Mobashery, and J. P. Samama.** 2000. Insights into class D beta-lactamases are revealed by the crystal structure of the OXA10 enzyme from *Pseudomonas aeruginosa. Structure Fold Des.* **8:**1289–1298.

173. **McOsker, C. C., and P. M. Fitzpatrick.** 1994. Nitrofurantoin: mechanism of action and implications for resistance development in common uropathogens. *J. Antimicrob. Chemother.* **33**(Suppl. A):23–30.

174. **Meroueh, S. O., J. F. Fisher, H. B. Schlegel, and S. Mobashery.** 2005. Ab initio QM/MM study of class A beta-lactamase acylation: dual participation of Glu166 and Lys73 in a concerted base promotion of Ser70. *J. Am. Chem. Soc.* **127:**15397–15407.

175. **Minasov, G., X. Wang, and B. K. Shoichet.** 2002. An ultrahigh resolution structure of TEM-1 beta-lactamase suggests a role for Glu166 as the general base in acylation. *J. Am. Chem. Soc.* **124:**5333–5340.

176. **Mingeot-Leclercq, M. P., Y. Glupczynski, and P. M. Tulkens.** 1999. Aminoglycosides: activity and resistance. *Antimicrob. Agents Chemother.* **43:**727–737.

177. **Miriagou, V., L. S. Tzouvelekis, S. Rossiter, E. Tzelepi, F. J. Angulo, and J. M. Whichard.** 2003. Imipenem resistance in a *Salmonella* clinical strain due to plasmid-mediated class A carbapenemase KPC-2. *Antimicrob. Agents Chemother.* **47:**1297–1300.

178. **Mishra, N. N., S. J. Yang, A. Sawa, A. Rubio, C. C. Nast, M. R. Yeaman, and A. S. Bayer.** 2009. Analysis of cell membrane characteristics of in vitro-selected daptomycin-resistant strains of methicillin-resistant *Staphylococcus aureus. Antimicrob. Agents Chemother.* **53:**2312–2318.

179. **Moellering, R. C., and A. N. Weinberg.** 1971. Studies on antibiotic synergism against enterococci. II. Effect of various antibiotics on the uptake of 14C-labelled streptomycin by enterococci. *J. Clin. Investig.* **50:**2580–2584.

180. **Morais Cabral, J. H., A. P. Jackson, C. V. Smith, N. Shikotra, A. Maxwell, and R. C. Liddington.** 1997. Crystal structure of the breakage-reunion domain of DNA gyrase. *Nature* **388:**903–906.

181. **Murakami, K., and A. Tomasz.** 1989. Involvement of multiple genetic determinants in high-level methicillin resistance in *Staphylococcus aureus. J. Bacteriol.* **171:**874–879.

182. **Murakami, S., R. Nakashima, E. Yamashita, and A. Yamaguchi.** 2002. Crystal structure of bacterial multidrug efflux transporter AcrB. *Nature* **419:**587–593.

183. **Murray, I. A., J. V. Martinez-Suarez, T. J. Close, and W. V. Shaw.** 1990. Nucleotide sequences of genes encoding the type II chloramphenicol acetyltransferases of *Escherichia coli* and *Haemophilus influenzae,* which are sensitive to inhibition by thiol-reactive reagents. *Biochem. J.* **272:**505–510.

184. **Murray, I. A., and W. V. Shaw.** 1997. O-Acetyltransferases for chloramphenicol and other natural products. *Antimicrob. Agents Chemother.* **41:**1–6.

185. **Muthaiyan, A., J. A. Silverman, R. K. Jayaswal, and B. J. Wilkinson.** 2008. Transcriptional profiling reveals that daptomycin induces the *Staphylococcus aureus* cell wall stress stimulon and genes responsive to membrane depolarization. *Antimicrob. Agents Chemother.* **52:**980–990.

186. **Naas, T., and P. Nordmann.** 1994. Analysis of a carbapenem-hydrolyzing class A beta-lactamase from *Enterobacter cloacae* and of its LysR-type regulatory protein. *Proc. Natl. Acad. Sci. USA* **91:**7693–7697.

187. **Naas, T., and P. Nordmann.** 1999. OXA-type beta-lactamases. *Curr. Pharm. Des.* **5:**865–879.

188. **Navia, M. M., J. Ruiz, and J. Vila.** 2002. Characterization of an integron carrying a new class D beta-lactamase (OXA-37) in *Acinetobacter baumannii. Microb. Drug Resist.* **8:**261–265.

189. **Navia, M. M., J. Ruiz, and J. Vila.** 2004. Molecular characterization of the integrons in Shigella strains isolated from patients with traveler's diarrhea. *Diagn. Microbiol. Infect. Dis.* **48:**175–179.

190. **Neuwirth, C., S. Madec, E. Siebor, A. Pechinot, J. M. Duez, M. Pruneaux, M. Fouchereau-Peron, A. Kazmierczak, and R. Labia.** 2001. TEM-89 β-lactamase produced by a *Proteus mirabilis* clinical isolate: new complex mutant (CMT 3) with mutations in both TEM-59 (IRT-17) and TEM-3. *Antimicrob. Agents Chemother.* **45:**3591–3594.

191. **Nikaido, H.** 1998. Multiple antibiotic resistance and efflux. *Curr. Opin. Microbiol.* **1:**516–523.

192. **Nikaido, H., and D. G. Thanassi.** 1993. Penetration of lipophilic agents with multiple protonation sites into bacterial cells: tetracyclines and fluoroquinolones as examples. *Antimicrob. Agents Chemother.* **37:**1393–1399.

193. **Noble, W. C., Z. Virani, and R. G. A. Gee.** 1992. Cotransfer of vancomycin and other resistance genes from *Enterococcus faecalis* NCTC 12201 to *Staphylococcus aureus. FEMS Microbiol. Lett.* **93:**195–198.

194. **Nordmann, P., S. Mariotte, T. Naas, R. Labia, and M. H. Nicolas.** 1993. Biochemical properties of a carbapenem-hydrolyzing β-lactamase from *Enterobacter cloacae* and cloning of the gene into *Escherichia coli. Antimicrob. Agents Chemother.* **37:**939–946.

195. **Nordmann, P., and L. Poirel.** 2005. Emergence of plasmid-mediated resistance to quinolones in *Enterobacteriaceae. J. Antimicrob. Chemother.* **56:**463–469.

196. **Nukaga, M., K. Mayama, A. M. Hujer, R. A. Bonomo, and J. R. Knox.** 2003. Ultrahigh resolution structure of a class A beta-lactamase: on the mechanism and specificity of the extended-spectrum SHV-2 enzyme. *J. Mol. Biol.* **328:**289–301.

197. **Oefner, C., A. D'Arcy, J. J. Daly, K. Gubernator, R. L. Charnas, I. Heinze, C. Hubschwerlen, and F. K. Winkler.** 1990. Refined crystal structure of beta-lactamase from *Citrobacter freundii* indicates a mechanism for beta-lactam hydrolysis. *Nature* **343:**284–288.

198. **Oggioni, M. R., C. G. Dowson, J. M. Smith, R. Provvedi, and G. Pozzi.** 1996. The tetracycline resistance gene *tet*(M) exhibits mosaic structure. *Plasmid* **35:**156–163.

199. **Olson, A. B., M. Silverman, D. A. Boyd, A. McGeer, B. M. Willey, V. Pong-Porter, N. Daneman, and M. R. Mulvey.** 2005. Identification of a progenitor of the CTX-M-9 group of extended-spectrum β-lactamases from *Kluyvera georgiana* isolated in Guyana. *Antimicrob. Agents Chemother.* **49:**2112–2115.

200. **Orencia, M. C., J. S. Yoon, J. E. Ness, W. P. Stemmer, and R. C. Stevens.** 2001. Predicting the emergence of antibiotic resistance by directed evolution and structural analysis. *Nat. Struct. Biol.* **8:**238–242.

201. **Paetzel, M., F. Danel, L. de Castro, S. C. Mosimann, M. G. Page, and N. C. Strynadka.** 2000. Crystal structure of the class D beta-lactamase OXA-10. *Nat. Struct. Biol.* **7:**918–925.

202. **Pan, X. S., and L. M. Fisher.** 1999. *Streptococcus pneumoniae* DNA gyrase and topoisomerase IV: overexpression, purification, and differential inhibition by fluoroquinolones. *Antimicrob. Agents Chemother.* **43:**1129–1136.

203. **Paterson, D. L.** 2001. Extended-spectrum beta-lactamases: the European experience. *Curr. Opin. Infect. Dis.* **14:**697–701.

204. **Paterson, D. L., K. M. Hujer, A. M. Hujer, B. Yeiser, M. D. Bonomo, L. B. Rice, and R. A. Bonomo.** 2003. Extended-spectrum β-lactamases in *Klebsiella pneumoniae* bloodstream isolates from seven countries: dominance and widespread prevalence of SHV- and CTX-M-type β-lactamases. *Antimicrob. Agents Chemother.* **47:**3554–3560.

205. **Paterson, D. L., W. C. Ko, A. Von Gottberg, S. Mohapatra, J. M. Casellas, H. Goossens, L. Mulazimoglu, G. Trenholme, K. P. Klugman, R. A. Bonomo, L. B. Rice, M. M. Wagener, J. G. McCormack, and V. L. Yu.** 2004. Antibiotic therapy for *Klebsiella pneumoniae* bacteremia: implications of production of extended-spectrum beta-lactamases. *Clin. Infect. Dis.* **39:**31–37.

206. Paterson, D. L., W. C. Ko, A. Von Gottberg, S. Mohapatra, J. M. Casellas, H. Goossens, L. Mulazimoglu, G. Trenholme, K. P. Klugman, R. A. Bonomo, L. B. Rice, M. M. Wagener, J. G. McCormack, and V. L. Yu. 2004. International prospective study of *Klebsiella pneumoniae* bacteremia: implications of extended-spectrum beta-lactamase production in nosocomial infections. *Ann. Intern. Med.* **140:**26–32.

207. Paton, R., R. S. Miles, J. Hood, and S. G. B. Amyes. 1993. ARI-1: beta-lactamase-mediated imipenem resistance in *Acinetobacter baumannii*. *Int. J. Antimicrob. Agents* **2:**81–88.

208. Paulsen, I. T., L. Banerjei, G. S. Myers, K. E. Nelson, R. Seshadri, T. D. Read, D. E. Fouts, J. A. Eisen, S. R. Gill, J. F. Heidelberg, H. Tettelin, R. J. Dodson, L. Umayam, L. Brinkac, M. Beanan, S. Daugherty, R. T. DeBoy, S. Durkin, J. Kolonay, R. Madupu, W. Nelson, J. Vamathevan, B. Tran, J. Upton, T. Hansen, J. Shetty, H. Khouri, T. Utterback, D. Radune, K. A. Ketchum, B. A. Dougherty, and C. M. Fraser. 2003. Role of mobile DNA in the evolution of vancomycin-resistant *Enterococcus faecalis*. *Science* **299:**2071–2074.

209. Périchon, B., and P. Courvalin. 2009. VanA-type vancomycin-resistant *Staphylococcus aureus*. *Antimicrob. Agents Chemother.* **53:**4580–4587.

210. Perl, T. M., J. J. Cullen, R. P. Wenzel, M. B. Zimmerman, M. A. Pfaller, D. Sheppard, J. Twombley, P. P. French, and L. A. Herwaldt. 2002. Intranasal mupirocin to prevent postoperative *Staphylococcus aureus* infections. *N. Engl. J. Med.* **346:**1871–1877.

211. Philippon, A., R. Labia, and G. A. Jacoby. 1989. Extended-spectrum β-lactamases. *Antimicrob. Agents Chemother.* **33:**1131–1136.

212. Piddock, L. J. V. 1999. Mechanisms of fluoroquinolone resistance: an update 1994–1998. *Drugs* **58:**11–18.

213. Pinho, M. G., H. de Lencastre, and A. Tomasz. 2001. An acquired and a native penicillin-binding protein cooperate in building the cell wall of drug-resistant staphylococci. *Proc. Natl. Acad. Sci. USA* **98:**10886–10891.

214. Podglajen, I., J. Breuil, A. Rohaut, C. Monsempes, and E. Collatz. 2001. Multiple mobile promoter regions for the rare carbapenem resistance gene of *Bacteroides fragilis*. *J. Bacteriol.* **183:**3531–3535.

215. Poirel, L., L. Collet, and P. Nordmann. 2000. Carbapenem-hydrolyzing metallo-beta-lactamase from a nosocomial isolate of *Pseudomonas aeruginosa* in France. *Emerg. Infect. Dis.* **6:**84–85.

216. Poirel, L., P. Gerome, C. De Champs, J. Stephanazzi, T. Naas, and P. Nordmann. 2002. Integron-located *oxa-32* gene cassette encoding an extended-spectrum variant of OXA-2 β-lactamase from *Pseudomonas aeruginosa*. *Antimicrob. Agents Chemother.* **46:**566–569.

217. Poirel, L., D. Girlich, T. Naas, and P. Nordmann. 2001. OXA-28, an extended-spectrum variant of OXA-10 β-lactamase from *Pseudomonas aeruginosa* and its plasmid- and integron-located gene. *Antimicrob. Agents Chemother.* **45:**447–453.

218. Poirel, L., H. Mammeri, and P. Nordmann. 2004. TEM-121, a novel complex mutant of TEM-type β-lactamase from *Enterobacter aerogenes*. *Antimicrob. Agents Chemother.* **48:**4528–4531.

219. Poirel, L., T. Naas, M. Guibert, E. B. Chaibi, R. Labia, and P. Nordmann. 1999. Molecular and biochemical characterization of VEB-1, a novel class A extended-spectrum β-lactamase encoded by an *Escherichia coli* integron gene. *Antimicrob. Agents Chemother.* **43:**573–581.

220. Poirel, L., T. Naas, and P. Nordmann. 2010. Diversity, epidemiology, and genetics of class D β-lactamases. *Antimicrob. Agents Chemother.* **54:**24–38.

221. Poirel, L., G. F. Weldhagen, T. Naas, C. De Champs, M. G. Dove, and P. Nordmann. 2001. GES-2, a class A β-lactamase from *Pseudomonas aeruginosa* with increased hydrolysis of imipenem. *Antimicrob. Agents Chemother.* **45:**2598–2603.

222. Poole, K., K. Krebes, C. McNally, and S. Neshat. 1993. Multiple antibiotic resistance in *Pseudomonas aeruginosa*: evidence for involvement of an efflux operon. *J. Bacteriol.* **175:**7363–7372.

223. Prinarakis, E. E., V. Miriagou, E. Tzelepi, M. Gazouli, and L. S. Tzouvelekis. 1997. Emergence of an inhibitor-resistant beta-lactamase (SHV-10) derived from an SHV-5 variant. *Antimicrob. Agents Chemother.* **41:**838–840.

224. Prystowsky, J., F. Siddiqui, J. Chosay, D. L. Shinabarger, J. Millichap, L. R. Peterson, and G. A. Noskin. 2001. Resistance to linezolid: characterization of mutations in rRNA and comparison of their occurrences in vancomycin-resistant enterococci. *Antimicrob. Agents Chemother.* **45:**2154–2156.

225. Qiu, W., R. Shi, M. L. Lu, M. Zhou, P. H. Roy, J. Lapointe, and S. X. Lin. 2004. Crystal structure of chloramphenicol acetyltransferase B2 encoded by the multiresistance transposon Tn*2424*. *Proteins* **57:**858–861.

226. Queenan, A. M., and K. Bush. 2007. Carbapenemases: the versatile β-lactamases. *Clin. Microbiol. Rev.* **20:**440–458.

227. Race, P. R., A. L. Lovering, R. M. Green, A. Ossor, S. A. White, P. F. Searle, C. J. Wrighton, and E. I. Hyde. 2005. Structural and mechanistic studies of *Escherichia coli* nitroreductase with the antibiotic nitrofurazone. Reversed binding orientations in different redox states of the enzyme. *J. Biol. Chem.* **280:**13256–13264.

228. Raquet, X., J. Lamotte-Brasseur, E. Fonze, S. Goussard, P. Courvalin, and J. M. Frere. 1994. TEM beta-lactamase mutants hydrolysing third-generation cephalosporins. A kinetic and molecular modelling analysis. *J. Mol. Biol.* **244:**625–639.

229. Rasmussen, B. A., K. Bush, D. Keeney, Y. Yang, R. Hare, C. O'Gara, and A. A. Medeiros. 1996. Characterization of IMI-1 β-lactamase, a class A carbapenem-hydrolyzing enzyme from *Enterobacter cloacae*. *Antimicrob. Agents Chemother.* **40:**2080–2086.

230. Rather, P. N. 1998. Origins of aminoglycoside modifying enzymes. *Drug Resist. Updates* **1:**285–291.

231. Rather, P. N., E. Orosz, K. J. Shaw, R. Hare, and G. Miller. 1993. Characterization and transcriptional regulation of the 2'-N-acetyltransferase gene from *Providencia stuartii*. *J. Bacteriol.* **175:**6492–6498.

232. Rice, L. B. 2000. Bacterial monopolists: the bundling and dissemination of antimicrobial resistance genes in gram-positive bacteria. *Clin. Infect. Dis.* **31:**762–769.

233. Rice, L. B. 1998. Tn*916* family conjugative transposons and dissemination of antimicrobial resistance determinants. *Antimicrob. Agents Chemother.* **42:**1871–1877.

234. Rice, L. B., S. Bellais, L. L. Carias, R. Hutton-Thomas, R. A. Bonomo, P. Caspers, M. G. Page, and L. Gutmann. 2004. Impact of specific *pbp5* mutations on expression of β-lactam resistance in *Enterococcus faecium*. *Antimicrob. Agents Chemother.* **48:**3028–3032.

235. Rice, L. B., S. B. Calderwood, G. M. Eliopoulos, B. F. Farber, and A. W. Karchmer. 1991. Enterococcal endocarditis: a comparison of native and prosthetic valve disease. *Rev. Infect. Dis.* **13:**1–7.

236. Rice, L. B., L. L. Carias, A. M. Hujer, M. Bonafede, R. Hutton, C. Hoyen, and R. A. Bonomo. 2000. High-level expression of chromosomally encoded SHV-1 β-lactamase and an outer membrane protein change confer resistance to ceftazidime and piperacillin-tazobactam in a clinical isolate of *Klebsiella pneumoniae*. *Antimicrob. Agents Chemother.* **44:**362–367.

237. Rice, L. B., L. L. Carias, R. Hutton-Thomas, F. Sifaoui, L. Gutmann, and S. D. Rudin. 2001. Penicillin-binding protein 5 and expression of ampicillin resistance in *Enterococcus faecium*. *Antimicrob. Agents Chemother.* **45:**1480–1486.

238. Rice, L. B., L. L. Carias, R. A. Hutton, S. D. Rudin, A. Endimiani, and R. A. Bonomo. 2008. The KQ element, a complex genetic region conferring transferable resistance to carbapenems, aminoglycosides, and fluoroquinolones in *Klebsiella pneumoniae*. *Antimicrob. Agents Chemother.* **52:**3427–3429.

239. Rice, L. B., L. L. Carias, S. Rudin, R. Hutton, S. Marshall, M. Hassan, N. Josseaume, L. Dubost, A. Marie, and M. Arthur. 2009. Role of class A penicillin-binding proteins in the expression of β-lactam resistance in *Enterococcus faecium*. *J. Bacteriol.* **191:**3649–3656.

240. Rice, L. B., J. D. C. Yao, K. Klimm, G. M. Eliopoulos, and R. C. Moellering, Jr. 1991. Efficacy of different β-lactams against an extended-spectrum β-lactamase-producing *Klebsiella pneumoniae* strain in the rat intra-abdominal abscess model. *Antimicrob. Agents Chemother.* **35:**1243–1244.

241. Roberts, R. B., A. de Lancastre, W. Eisner, E. P. Severina, B. Shopsin, B. N. Kreiswirth, A. Tomasz, and the MRSA Collaborative Study Group. 1998. Molecular epidemiology of methicillin-resistant *Staphylococcus aureus* in 12 New York hospitals. *J. Infect. Dis.* **178:**164–171.

242. Roca, I., S. Marti, P. Espinal, P. Martínez, I. Gibert, and J. Vila. 2009. CraA, a major facilitator superfamily efflux pump associated with chloramphenicol resistance in *Acinetobacter baumannii*. *Antimicrob. Agents Chemother.* **53:**4013–4014.

243. Rodriguez-Martinez, J. M., P. Nordmann, N. Fortineau, and L. Poirel. 2010. VIM-19, a metallo-β-lactamase with increased carbapenemase activity from *Escherichia coli* and *Klebsiella pneumoniae*. *Antimicrob. Agents Chemother.* **54:**471–476.

244. Rowe-Magnus, D. A., A. M. Guerout, and D. Mazel. 2002. Bacterial resistance evolution by recruitment of super-integron gene cassettes. *Mol. Microbiol.* **43:**1657–1669.

245. Ruzin, A., D. Keeney, and P. A. Bradford. 2005. AcrAB efflux pump plays a role in decreased susceptibility to tigecycline in *Morganella morganii*. *Antimicrob. Agents Chemother.* **49:**791–793.

246. Ruzin, A., M. A. Visalli, D. Keeney, and P. A. Bradford. 2005. Influence of transcriptional activator RamA on expression of multidrug efflux pump AcrAB and tigecycline susceptibility in *Klebsiella pneumoniae*. *Antimicrob. Agents Chemother.* **49:**1017–1022.

247. Rybkine, T., J.-L. Mainardi, W. Sougakoff, E. Collatz, and L. Gutmann. 1998. Penicillin-binding protein 5 sequence alterations in clinical isolates of *Enterococcus faecium* with different levels of β-lactam resistance. *J. Infect. Dis.* **178:**159–163.

248. Sabath, L. D. 1969. Drug resistance of bacteria. *N. Engl. J. Med.* **280:**91–94.

249. Sahm, D. F., M. K. Marsilio, and G. Piazza. 1999. Antimicrobial resistance in key bloodstream bacterial isolates: electronic surveillance with The Surveillance Network Database—USA. *Clin. Infect. Dis.* **29:**259–263.

250. Samra, Z., J. Bahar, L. Madar-Shapiro, N. Aziz, S. Israel, and J. Bishara. 2008. Evaluation of CHROMagar KPC for rapid detection of carbapenem-resistant *Enterobacteriaceae*. *J. Clin. Microbiol.* **46:**3110–3111.

251. Sanchez-Pescador, R., J. T. Brown, M. Roberts, and M. S. Urdea. 1988. Homology of the TetM with translational elongation factors: implications for potential modes of tetM conferred tetracycline resistance. *Nucleic Acids Res.* **16:**1218.

252. Sandegren, L., A. Lindqvist, G. Kahlmeter, and D. I. Andersson. 2008. Nitrofurantoin resistance mechanism and fitness cost in *Escherichia coli*. *J. Antimicrob. Chemother.* **62:**495–503.

253. Santillana, E., A. Beceiro, G. Bou, and A. Romero. 2007. Crystal structure of the carbapenemase OXA-24 reveals insights into the mechanism of carbapenem hydrolysis. *Proc. Natl. Acad. Sci. USA* **104:**5354–5359.

254. Saves, I., O. Burlet-Schiltz, P. Swaren, F. Lefevre, J. M. Masson, J. C. Prome, and J. P. Samama. 1995. The asparagine to aspartic acid substitution at position 276 of TEM-35 and TEM-36 is involved in the beta-lactamase resistance to clavulanic acid. *J. Biol. Chem.* **270:**18240–18245.

255. Schnappinger, D., and W. Hillen. 1996. Tetracyclines: antibiotic action, uptake, and resistance mechanisms. *Arch. Microbiol.* **165:**359–369.

256. Schwarz, S., C. Kehrenberg, B. Doublet, and A. Cloeckaert. 2004. Molecular basis of bacterial resistance to chloramphenicol and florfenicol. *FEMS Microbiol. Rev.* **28:**519–542.

257. Shaw, J. H., and D. B. Clewell. 1985. Complete nucleotide sequence of macrolide-lincosamide-streptogramin B resistance transposon Tn917 in *Streptococcus faecalis*. *J. Bacteriol.* **164:**782–796.

258. Shaw, K. J., P. Rather, F. Sabatelli, P. Mann, H. Munayyer, R. Mierzwa, G. Petrikkos, R. S. Hare, G. H. Miller, P. Bennett, and P. Downey. 1992. Characterization of the chromosomal *aac(6′)-Ic* gene from *Serratia marcescens*. *Antimicrob. Agents Chemother.* **36:**1447–1455.

259. Shaw, K. J., P. N. Rather, R. S. Hare, and G. H. Miller. 1993. Molecular genetics of aminoglycoside resistance genes and familial relationships of the aminoglycoside-modifying enzymes. *Microbiol. Rev.* **57:**138–163.

260. Shaw, W. V. 1983. Chloramphenicol acetyltransferase: enzymology and molecular biology. *CRC Crit. Rev. Biochem.* **14:**1–46.

261. Shea, M. E., and H. Hiasa. 1999. Interactions between DNA helicases and frozen topoisomerase IV-quinolone-DNA ternary complexes. *J. Biol. Chem.* **274:**22747–22754.

262. Sherertz, R. J., D. R. Reagan, K. D. Hampton, K. L. Robertson, S. A. Streed, H. M. Hoen, R. Thomas, and J. M. Gwaltney, Jr. 1996. A cloud adult: the *Staphylococcus aureus*-virus interaction revisited. *Ann. Intern. Med.* **124:**539–547.

263. Shimamura, T., A. Ibuka, S. Fushinobu, T. Wakagi, M. Ishiguro, Y. Ishii, and H. Matsuzawa. 2002. Acyl-intermediate structures of the extended-spectrum class A beta-lactamase, Toho-1, in complex with cefotaxime, cephalothin, and benzylpenicillin. *J. Biol. Chem.* **277:**46601–46608.

264. Shinabarger, D. L., K. R. Marotti, R. W. Murray, A. H. Lin, E. P. Melchior, S. M. Swaney, D. S. Dunyak, W. F. Demyan, and J. M. Buysse. 1997. Mechanism of action of oxazolidinones: effects of linezolid and eperezolid on translation reactions. *Antimicrob. Agents Chemother.* **41:**2132–2136.

265. Sieradzki, K., R. B. Roberts, S. W. Haber, and A. Tomasz. 1999. The development of vancomycin resistance in a patient with methicillin-resistant *Staphylococcus aureus* infection. *N. Engl. J. Med.* **340:**517–523.

266. Sirot, D., C. Recule, E. B. Chaibi, L. Bret, J. Croize, C. Chanal-Claris, R. Labia, and J. Sirot. 1997. A complex mutant of TEM-1 β-lactamase with mutations encountered in both IRT-4 and extended-spectrum TEM-15, produced by an *Escherichia coli* clinical isolate. *Antimicrob. Agents Chemother.* **41:**1322–1325.

267. Skold, O. 2000. Sulfonamide resistance: mechanisms and trends. *Drug Resist. Updates* **3:**155–160.

268. Smith, A. M., R. F. Botha, H. J. Koornhof, and K. P. Klugman. 2001. Emergence of a pneumococcal clone with cephalosporin resistance and penicillin susceptibility. *Antimicrob. Agents Chemother.* **45:**2648–2650.

269. Soki, J., M. Gal, J. S. Brazier, V. O. Rotimi, E. Urban, E. Nagy, and B. I. Duerden. 2005. Molecular investigation of genetic elements contributing to metronidazole resistance in *Bacteroides* strains. *J. Antimicrob. Chemother.* **57:**212–220.

270. Soltani, M., D. Beighton, J. Philpott-Howard, and N. Woodford. 2000. Mechanisms of resistance to quinupristin-dalfopristin among isolates of *Enterococcus faecium* from animals, raw meat, and hospital patients in Western Europe. *Antimicrob. Agents Chemother.* **44:**433–436.

271. Spencer, J., A. R. Clarke, and T. R. Walsh. 2001. Novel mechanism of hydrolysis of therapeutic beta-lactams by *Stenotrophomonas maltophilia* L1 metallo-beta-lactamase. *J. Biol. Chem.* **276:**33638–33644.

272. Spratt, B. G., Q.-Y. Zhang, D. M. Jones, A. Hutchison, J. A. Brannigan, and C. G. Dowson. 1989. Recruitment of a penicillin-binding protein gene from *Neisseria flavescens* during the emergence of penicillin resistance in *Neisseria meningitidis*. *Proc. Natl. Acad. Sci. USA* **86:**8988–8992.

273. Stapleton, P. D., K. P. Shannon, and G. L. French. 1999. Carbapenem resistance in *Escherichia coli* associated with plasmid-determined CMY-4 β-lactamase production and loss of an outer membrane protein. *Antimicrob. Agents Chemother.* **43:**1206–1210.

273a. Stokes, H. W., and R. M. Hall. 1989. A novel family of potentially mobile DNA elements encoding site-specific gene integration function integrons. *Mol. Microbiol.* **3:**1669–1683.

274. Su, Y. A., P. He, and D. B. Clewell. 1992. Characterization of the *tetM* determinant of Tn916: evidence for regulation by transcriptional attenuation. *Antimicrob. Agents Chemother.* **36:**769–778.

275. Sung, J. Y., K. C. Kwon, J. W. Park, Y. S. Kim, J. M. Kim, K. S. Shin, J. W. Kim, C. S. Ko, S. Y. Shin, J. H. Song, and S. H. Koo. 2008. Dissemination of IMP-1 and OXA type beta-lactamase in carbapenem-resistant *Acinetobacter baumannii*. *Korean J. Lab. Med.* **28**:16–23.

276. Swaren, P., D. Golemi, S. Cabantous, A. Bulychev, L. Maveyraud, S. Mobashery, and J. P. Samama. 1999. X-ray structure of the Asn276Asp variant of the *Escherichia coli* TEM-1 beta-lactamase: direct observation of electrostatic modulation in resistance to inactivation by clavulanic acid. *Biochemistry* (Moscow) **38**:9570–9576.

277. Swedberg, G., S. Ringertz, and O. Skold. 1998. Sulfonamide resistance in *Streptococcus pyogenes* is associated with differences in the amino acid sequence of its chromosomal dihydropteroate synthase. *Antimicrob. Agents Chemother.* **42**:1062–1067.

278. Tam, V. H., A. N. Schilling, G. Vo, S. Kabbara, A. L. Kwa, N. P. Wiederhold, and R. E. Lewis. 2005. Pharmacodynamics of polymyxin B against *Pseudomonas aeruginosa*. *Antimicrob. Agents Chemother.* **49**:3624–3630.

279. Then, R. L. 1982. Mechanisms of resistance to trimethoprim, the sulfonamides, and trimethoprim-sulfamethoxazole. *Rev. Infect. Dis.* **4**:261–269.

280. Then, R. L., and P. Angehrn. 1979. Low trimethoprim susceptibility of anaerobic bacteria due to insensitive dihydrofolate reductases. *Antimicrob. Agents Chemother.* **15**:1–6.

281. Thomson, C. J., and S. G. Amyes. 1992. TRC-1: emergence of a clavulanic acid-resistant TEM beta-lactamase in a clinical strain. *FEMS Microbiol. Lett.* **70**:113–117.

282. Toleman, M. A., P. M. Bennett, and T. R. Walsh. 2006. ISCR elements: novel gene-capturing systems of the 21st century? *Microbiol. Mol. Biol. Rev.* **70**:296–316.

283. Tomasz, A. 1983. Murein hydrolases: enzymes in search of a physiologic function, p. 155–172. *In* R. Hackenbeck, J. Holtje, and H. Labischinski (ed.), *The Target of Penicillin*. Walter de Gruyter, Berlin, Germany.

284. Torres, O. R., R. Z. Korman, S. A. Zahler, and G. M. Dunny. 1991. The conjugative transposon Tn925: enhancement of conjugal transfer by tetracycline in *Enterococcus faecalis* and mobilization of chromosomal genes in both *Bacillus subtilis* and *E. faecalis*. *Mol. Gen. Genet.* **225**:395–400.

285. Tran, J. H., and G. A. Jacoby. 2002. Mechanism of plasmid-mediated quinolone resistance. *Proc. Natl. Acad. Sci. USA* **99**:5638–5642.

286. Tran, J. H., G. A. Jacoby, and D. C. Hooper. 2005. Interaction of the plasmid-encoded quinolone resistance protein Qnr with *Escherichia coli* DNA gyrase. *Antimicrob. Agents Chemother.* **49**:118–125.

287. Tranier, S., A. T. Bouthors, L. Maveyraud, V. Guillet, W. Sougakoff, and J. P. Samama. 2000. The high resolution crystal structure for class A beta-lactamase PER-1 reveals the bases for its increase in breadth of activity. *J. Biol. Chem.* **275**:28075–28082.

288. Tsakris, A., I. Kristo, A. Poulou, K. Themeli-Digalaki, A. Ikonomidis, D. Petropoulou, S. Pournaras, and D. Sofianou. 2009. Evaluation of boronic acid disk tests for differentiating KPC-possessing *Klebsiella pneumoniae* isolates in the clinical laboratory. *J. Clin. Microbiol.* **47**:362–367.

289. Tuomanen, E., and A. Tomasz. 1990. Mechanism of phenotypic tolerance of nongrowing pneumococci to beta-lactam antibiotics. *Scand. J. Infect. Dis. Suppl.* **74**: 102–112.

290. Tzeng, Y. L., K. D. Ambrose, S. Zughaier, X. Zhou, Y. K. Miller, W. M. Shafer, and D. S. Stephens. 2005. Cationic antimicrobial peptide resistance in *Neisseria meningitidis*. *J. Bacteriol.* **187**:5387–5396.

291. Ubukata, K., Y. Shibasaki, K. Yamamoto, N. Chiba, K. Hasegawa, Y. Takeuchi, K. Sunakawa, M. Inoue, and M. Konno. 2001. Association of amino acid substitutions in penicillin-binding protein 3 with β-lactam resistance in β-lactamase-negative ampicillin-resistant *Haemophilus influenzae*. *Antimicrob. Agents Chemother.* **45**:1693–1699.

292. Ullah, J. H., T. R. Walsh, I. A. Taylor, D. C. Emery, C. S. Verma, S. J. Gamblin, and J. Spencer. 1998. The crystal structure of the L1 metallo-β-lactamase from *Stenotrophomonas maltophilia* at 1.7 Å resolution. *J. Mol. Biol.* **284**:125–136.

293. Vakulenko, S. B., B. Geryk, L. P. Kotra, S. Mobashery, and S. A. Lerner. 1998. Selection and characterization of β-lactam–β-lactamase inactivator-resistant mutants following PCR mutagenesis of the TEM-1 β-lactamase gene. *Antimicrob. Agents Chemother.* **42**:1542–1548.

294. Vakulenko, S. B., and S. Mobashery. 2003. Versatility of aminoglycosides and prospects for their future. *Clin. Microbiol. Rev.* **16**:430–450.

295. van der Wouden, E. J., J. C. Thijs, J. G. Kusters, A. A. van Zwet, and J. H. Kleibeuker. 2001. Mechanism and clinical significance of metronidazole resistance in *Helicobacter pylori*. *Scand. J. Gastroenterol. Suppl.* **2001**:10–14.

296. Vedel, G., A. Bellaouaj, L. Gilly, R. Labia, A. Phillipon, P. Nevot, and G. Paul. 1992. Clinical isolates of *Escherichia coli* producing TRI β-lactamases: novel TEM enzymes conferring resistance to β-lactamase inhibitors. *J. Antimicrob. Chemother.* **30**:449–462.

297. Vila, J., M. Navia, J. Ruiz, and C. Casals. 1997. Cloning and nucleotide sequence analysis of a gene encoding an OXA-derived β-lactamase in *Acinetobacter baumannii*. *Antimicrob. Agents Chemother.* **41**:2757–2759.

298. Vincent, S., P. Minkler, B. Bincziewski, L. Etter, and D. M. Shlaes. 1992. Vancomycin resistance in *Enterococcus gallinarum*. *Antimicrob. Agents Chemother.* **36**:1392–1399.

299. Walsh, T. R., M. A. Toleman, L. Poirel, and P. Nordmann. 2005. Metallo-β-lactamases: the quiet before the storm? *Clin. Microbiol. Rev.* **18**:306–325.

300. Wang, X., G. Minasov, and B. K. Shoichet. 2002. Evolution of an antibiotic resistance enzyme constrained by stability and activity trade-offs. *J. Mol. Biol.* **320**:85–95.

301. Weber, B., K. Ehlert, A. Diehl, P. Reichmann, H. Labischinski, and R. Hakenbeck. 2000. The *fib* locus in *Streptococcus pneumoniae* is required for peptidoglycan cross-linking and PBP-mediated beta-lactam resistance. *FEMS Microbiol. Lett.* **188**:81–85.

302. Wegener, H. C., F. M. Aarestrup, L. B. Jensen, A. M. Hammerum, and F. Bager. 1999. Use of antimicrobial growth promoters in food animals and *Enterococcus faecium* resistance to therapeutic antimicrobial drugs in Europe. *Emerg. Infect. Dis.* **5**:329–335.

303. Wehrli, W. 1983. Rifampin: mechanisms of action and resistance. *Rev. Infect. Dis.* **5**(Suppl. 3):S407–S411.

304. Weigel, L. M., D. B. Clewell, S. R. Gill, N. C. Clark, L. K. McDougal, S. E. Flannagan, J. F. Kolonay, J. Shetty, G. E. Killgore, and F. C. Tenover. 2003. Genetic analysis of a high-level vancomycin-resistant isolate of *Staphylococcus aureus*. *Science* **302**:1569–1571.

305. Weisblum, B. 1995. Erythromycin resistance by ribosome modification. *Antimicrob. Agents Chemother.* **39**:577–585.

306. Welch, R. A., V. Burland, G. Plunkett III, P. Redford, P. Roesch, D. Rasko, E. L. Buckles, S. R. Liou, A. Boutin, J. Hackett, D. Stroud, G. F. Mayhew, D. J. Rose, S. Zhou, D. C. Schwartz, N. T. Perna, H. L. Mobley, M. S. Donnenberg, and F. R. Blattner. 2002. Extensive mosaic structure revealed by the complete genome sequence of uropathogenic *Escherichia coli*. *Proc. Natl. Acad. Sci. USA* **99**:17020–17024.

307. Weldhagen, G. F. 2004. Integrons and beta-lactamases—a novel perspective on resistance. *Int. J. Antimicrob. Agents* **23**:556–562.

308. White, D. G., C. Hudson, J. J. Maurer, S. Ayers, S. Zhao, M. D. Lee, L. Bolton, T. Foley, and J. Sherwood. 2000. Characterization of chloramphenicol and florfenicol resistance in *Escherichia coli* associated with bovine diarrhea. *J. Clin. Microbiol.* **38**:4593–4598.

309. White, P. A., C. J. McIver, and W. D. Rawlinson. 2001. Integrons and gene cassettes in the Enterobacteriaceae. *Antimicrob. Agents Chemother.* **45**:2658–2661.

310. Wiener, J., J. P. Quinn, P. A. Bradford, R. V. Goering, C. Nathan, K. Bush, and R. A. Weinstein. 1999. Multiple antibiotic-resistant *Klebsiella* and *Escherichia coli* in nursing homes. *JAMA* **281**:517–523.

311. **Williamson, R., C. LaBouguenec, L. Gutmann, and T. Horaud.** 1985. One or two low affinity penicillin-binding proteins may be responsible for the range of susceptibility of *Enterococcus faecium* to penicillin. *J. Gen. Microbiol.* **131:**1933–1940.

312. **Willmott, C. J., S. E. Critchlow, I. C. Eperon, and A. Maxwell.** 1994. The complex of DNA gyrase and quinolone drugs with DNA forms a barrier to transcription by RNA polymerase. *J. Mol. Biol.* **242:**351–363.

313. **Wolter, N., A. M. Smith, D. J. Farrell, W. Schaffner, M. Moore, C. G. Whitney, J. H. Jorgensen, and K. P. Klugman.** 2005. Novel mechanism of resistance to oxazolidinones, macrolides, and chloramphenicol in ribosomal protein L4 of the pneumococcus. *Antimicrob. Agents Chemother.* **49:**3554–3557.

314. **Woodford, N., P. M. Tierno, Jr., K. Young, L. Tysall, M. F. Palepou, E. Ward, R. E. Painter, D. F. Suber, D. Shungu, L. L. Silver, K. Inglima, J. Kornblum, and D. M. Livermore.** 2004. Outbreak of *Klebsiella pneumoniae* producing a new carbapenem-hydrolyzing class A beta-lactamase, KPC-3, in a New York medical center. *Antimicrob. Agents Chemother.* **48:**4793–4799.

315. **Wu, S. W., H. de Lencastre, and A. Tomasz.** 2001. Recruitment of the *mecA* gene homologue of *Staphylococcus sciuri* into a resistance determinant and expression of the resistant phenotype in *Staphylococcus aureus.* *J. Bacteriol.* **183:**2417–2424.

316. **Yamane, K., J. Wachino, Y. Doi, H. Kurokawa, and Y. Arakawa.** 2005. Global spread of multiple aminoglycoside resistance genes. *Emerg. Infect. Dis.* **11:**951–953.

317. **Yigit, H., A. M. Queenan, G. J. Anderson, A. Domenech-Sanchez, J. W. Biddle, C. D. Steward, S. Alberti, K. Bush, and F. C. Tenover.** 2001. Novel carbapenem-hydrolyzing β-lactamase, KPC-1, from a carbapenem-resistant strain of *Klebsiella pneumoniae. Antimicrob. Agents Chemother.* **45:**1151–1161.

318. **Yigit, H., A. M. Queenan, J. K. Rasheed, J. W. Biddle, A. Domenech-Sanchez, S. Alberti, K. Bush, and F. C. Tenover.** 2003. Carbapenem-resistant strain of *Klebsiella oxytoca* harboring carbapenem-hydrolyzing β-lactamase KPC-2. *Antimicrob. Agents Chemother.* **47:**3881–3889.

319. **Zervos, M. J., and D. R. Schaberg.** 1985. Reversal of in vitro susceptibility of enterococci to trimethoprim-sulfamethoxazole by folinic acid. *Antimicrob. Agents Chemother.* **28:**446–448.

320. **Zhang, K., J. A. McClure, S. Elsayed, and J. M. Conly.** 2009. Novel staphylococcal cassette chromosome *mec* type, tentatively designated type VIII, harboring class A *mec* and type 4 *ccr* gene complexes in a Canadian epidemic strain of methicillin-resistant *Staphylococcus aureus. Antimicrob. Agents Chemother.* **53:**531–540.

321. **Zhong, P., and V. D. Shortridge.** 2000. The role of efflux in macrolide resistance. *Drug Resist. Updates* **3:**325–329.

322. **Ziha-Zarifi, I., C. Llanes, T. Kohler, J. C. Pechere, and P. Plesiat.** 1999. In vivo emergence of multidrug-resistant mutants of *Pseudomonas aeruginosa* overexpressing the active efflux system MexA-MexB-OprM. *Antimicrob. Agents Chemother.* **43:**287–291.

Susceptibility Test Methods: General Considerations

JOHN D. TURNIDGE, MARY JANE FERRARO, AND JAMES H. JORGENSEN

67

Determination of the antimicrobial susceptibilities of significant bacterial isolates is one of the principal functions of the clinical microbiology laboratory. From the physician's pragmatic point of view, the results of susceptibility tests are often considered important or more important than the identification of the pathogen involved. This is particularly true in an era of increasing antimicrobial resistance in which treatment options are at times limited to newer, more costly antibacterial agents. As a result, the laboratory must give high priority not only to producing technically accurate data but also to reporting those data to physicians in an easily interpretable manner.

The main objective of susceptibility testing is to predict the outcome of treatment with the antimicrobial agents tested. Results are generally reported as categories of susceptibility. The implication of the result category "susceptible" is that there is a high probability that the patient will respond to treatment with the appropriate dosage regimen for that antimicrobial agent. The result "resistant" implies that treatment with the antimicrobial agent is likely to fail. One group has coined the term "90–60 rule"; that is, for many infections we can expect treatment success about 90% of the time when the organism tests as "susceptible" to that treatment, and success may still occur in around 60% of cases when the organism tests as "resistant" to the agent used (41). The apparent 60% response rate to ineffective antimicrobials is said to reflect the natural response to many bacterial infections in an immunologically normal host (36).

Most test methods also include an "intermediate" category of susceptibility, which can have several meanings. With agents that can be safely administered at higher doses (e.g., penicillins and cephalosporins), this category may imply that higher doses may be required to ensure efficacy or that the agent may prove efficacious if it is normally concentrated in an infected body fluid, e.g., urine. Conversely, for body compartments where drug penetration is restricted even in the presence of inflammation (e.g., cerebrospinal fluid), it suggests that extreme caution should be taken in the use of the agent. It may also represent a buffer zone that prevents truly resistant strains from being incorrectly categorized as susceptible, and vice versa.

A further aim of susceptibility testing is to guide the clinician in the selection of the most appropriate agent for a particular clinical problem. In most clinical settings, susceptibility test results are usually obtained 24 to 48 h or more after the patient has been given empirical treatment. The test results may confirm the susceptibility of the organism to the drug initially prescribed or may indicate resistance, in which case alternative therapy will likely be required. The report describing the susceptibility testing results should provide the clinician with alternative agents to which the organism is susceptible. These alternatives also may be useful if the patient subsequently develops an adverse reaction to the initial antimicrobial agent. There is a growing emphasis from professional societies and managed care organizations to use susceptibility test results to direct therapy toward the most narrow spectrum, least expensive agent to which the pathogen should respond. This is particularly true for hospitalized patients, in whom the rate of antimicrobial resistance tends to be higher, and it is easier to make therapeutic changes for inpatients than for outpatients. This makes the accuracy of susceptibility testing even more critical for effective patient care.

The clinical microbiology laboratory should perform susceptibility testing only for pathogens for which well-standardized methods are available and for pathogens whose resistance is known or suspected to be a clinical problem; susceptibility testing should not be performed on normal biota or colonizing organisms. Currently, routine susceptibility testing methods are best standardized for the common aerobic and facultative bacteria and systemic antibacterial agents. For some uncommon or highly fastidious bacteria and for most topical antibacterial agents, simple routine test methods have not been standardized. Taking into account this limitation, the Clinical and Laboratory Standards Institute (CLSI; formerly the NCCLS) has released recommendations on how some of these bacteria may be tested and the results interpreted (11). With some pathogens (e.g., *Mycobacterium tuberculosis* and invasive fungi), routine testing is important for patient management, but testing is best performed by specialized laboratories in which test volumes are sufficient to maintain technical proficiency and where unusual or inaccurate results are likely to be recognized. Susceptibility testing methods for certain other pathogens (e.g., mycoplasmas, chlamydiae, legionellae, spirochetes, viruses, protozoa, and helminths) may not be well established at present and/or are limited to a few specialty laboratories. A number of choices exist in antibacterial susceptibility testing with respect to methodology and selection of agents for routine testing.

SELECTING AN ANTIMICROBIAL SUSCEPTIBILITY TESTING METHOD

Clinical microbiology laboratories can choose from among several conventional or novel methods of routine antibacterial susceptibility testing. These include the broth microdilution, disk diffusion, antimicrobial gradient, and automated-instrument methods. In recent years, there has been a trend toward the use of commercial broth microdilution and automated-instrument methods instead of the disk diffusion procedure. However, there remains ongoing interest in the disk diffusion test because of its inherent flexibility in drug selection, its ability to respond quickly to changes in interpretive breakpoints or when new agents are introduced, and its low cost. The availability of numerous antibacterial agents and the diversity of antimicrobial agent formularies of different institutions have made it difficult for manufacturers of commercial test systems to provide standard test panels that fit everyone's needs. Thus, the inherent flexibility in drug selection that is provided by the disk diffusion test is an undeniable asset of the method. The test is also one of the most established and best proven of all susceptibility tests and continues to be updated and refined through frequent (usually annual) CLSI publications (13, 14). Instrumentation is now available for reading and interpreting zone diameters as well as for storing this information and may reduce interobserver reading errors (31–33).

Advantages of the microdilution and agar gradient diffusion methods include the generation of a quantitative result (i.e., an MIC) rather than a category result and the ability to test accurately some anaerobic or fastidious species that may not be tested by the disk diffusion method (7, 9, 11, 24, 27); ancillary benefits are computer systems that accompany many of the microdilution and automated systems (24). Indeed, computerized data management systems are very important in laboratories that may have limited or inflexible laboratory information systems. However, an MIC method should not be chosen on the basis that MICs are routinely more useful to physicians. There is no clear evidence that MICs are more relevant than susceptibility category results to the selection of appropriate antibacterial therapy for most infections (17).

A laboratory may choose to perform rapid, automated antibacterial susceptibility testing in order to generate results faster than manual methods can generate them. The provision of susceptibility results 1 day sooner than that provided by conventional methods seems a logical advance in patient care. Three studies have demonstrated both the clinical and economic benefits derived from the use of rapid susceptibility testing and reporting (2, 21, 30), while a further study has not shown such a benefit (4). However, rapid susceptibility testing results may not have substantial impact unless the laboratory uses more aggressive means of communication to make physicians aware of the results (51). A previously cited shortcoming of rapid susceptibility testing methods was the failure to detect some inducible or subtle resistance mechanisms (23, 29, 49, 50). However, the instruments most notorious for such problems are no longer marketed, and the manufacturers of the remaining instruments have made substantial efforts to correct earlier problems (34, 40, 44, 54) or to extend testing to include fastidious organisms (26). It is important to emphasize that accuracy should not be sacrificed in an effort to generate a rapid susceptibility testing result.

SELECTING ANTIBACTERIAL AGENTS FOR ROUTINE TESTING

The laboratory has the responsibility to test antimicrobial agents and report on those that are most appropriate for the organism isolated, the site of infection, and the clinical practice setting in which the laboratory functions. The battery of antimicrobial agents routinely tested and reported on by the laboratory will depend on the characteristics of the patients under care in the institution and the likelihood of encountering highly resistant organisms (25). A laboratory serving a tertiary-care medical center, which specializes in the care of immunosuppressed patients, may need to test routinely agents that are broader in spectrum than those tested by a laboratory that supports a primary-care outpatient practice in which antibiotic-resistant organisms are less commonly encountered (46).

When a laboratory's routine susceptibility testing batteries are determined, several principles should be followed. First, the antimicrobial agents that are included in the institution's formulary and that physicians prescribe on a daily basis should be tested. Second, the species tested strongly influences the choice of antimicrobial agents for testing. The CLSI publishes tables that list the antimicrobial agents appropriate for testing against various groups of aerobic and fastidious bacteria (14). The guidelines indicate the drugs that are most appropriate for testing against each organism group and for treatment based upon the specimen source (e.g., cerebrospinal fluid, blood, urine, or feces). The lists also include a few agents that may be tested as surrogates for other agents because of the greater ability of a particular agent to detect resistance to closely related drugs (e.g., the use of the cefoxitin disk test to predict overall β-lactam resistance in staphylococci) (14). This initial list of agents must be tailored to an individual institution's specific needs through discussions with infectious disease physicians, pharmacists, and committees concerned with infection control and the institutional formulary (25).

A third important step in defining routine testing batteries is ascertaining the availability of specific antimicrobial agents for testing by the laboratory's routine testing methodology. Certain methods (e.g., the disk diffusion, gradient diffusion, and in-house-prepared broth and agar dilution methods) allow the greatest flexibility in the selection of test batteries. In contrast, some commercial systems may have less flexibility or may experience delays in adding the latest antimicrobial agents approved for clinical use. However, practicality limits the maximum number of drugs that can be tested simultaneously with an isolate by any susceptibility testing method. For example, a maximum of 12 disks can be placed on a 150-mm-diameter Mueller-Hinton agar plate, and a similar number can ordinarily be accommodated in a microdilution panel if full concentration ranges of each agent are to be included for routine determination of MICs. Some commercial test panels attempt to resolve this problem by testing a larger array of antimicrobial agents, although in a very limited concentration range (perhaps 2 to 4 dilutions for each agent).

ESTABLISHING SUSCEPTIBILITY BREAKPOINTS

There is general agreement that the MIC is the most basic laboratory measurement of the activity of an antimicrobial agent against an organism. It is defined as the lowest concentration that will inhibit the growth of a test organism over a defined interval related to the organism's growth rate, most commonly 18 to 24 h. The MIC is the fundamental measurement that forms the basis of most susceptibility testing methods and against which the levels of drug achieved in human body fluids may be compared to determine breakpoints for defining susceptibility.

The conventional technique for measuring the MIC involves exposing the test organism to a series of twofold dilutions of the antimicrobial agent in a suitable culture system, e.g., broth or agar for bacteria. The twofold-dilution scheme was originally used because of the convenience of preparing dilutions from a single starting concentration in broth and agar dilution methods. Subsequently, this system proved to be meaningful because an antibiotic's MICs for a single bacterial species in the absence of resistance mechanisms have a statistically normal distribution when plotted on a logarithmic scale. This provides investigators with the opportunity to examine the distributions of MICs for bacterial populations and distinguish strains for which the MICS are abnormally high (potentially resistant strains) from those for which MICs are normal (susceptible strains) (28; http://www.srga.org/eucastwt/WT_EUCAST.htm).

MIC measurements are influenced in vitro by a number of factors, including the composition of the medium, the size of the inoculum, the duration of incubation, and the presence of resistant subpopulations of the organism. The in vitro test conditions also do not encompass other factors that can have an influence on in vivo antimicrobial activity. These include sub-MIC effects, postantibiotic effects, protein binding, effects on organism virulence or toxin production, variations in redox potential at sites of infection, and the pharmacokinetic changes resulting from different drug levels in blood and at the site of infection over time. Nevertheless, if determined under standardized conditions, MIC measurements provide a fixed reference point for the setting of pharmacodynamic breakpoints with the power to predict efficacy in vivo. Pharmacological breakpoints can be applied directly to routine dilution testing methods that generate MICs, such as broth microdilution, agar dilution, gradient methods, and some automated instruments. They also provide reference values for deriving breakpoints for disk diffusion methods.

Breakpoints (or interpretative criteria) are the values that determine the categories susceptible, intermediate, and resistant. The approach to setting breakpoints varies by organization or regulatory body. Depending on the approach taken, up to four sources of data can be examined in establishing breakpoints (52).

MIC Distributions

Examination of MIC distributions can indicate the range of MICs of a population of strains that lack any known mechanisms of resistance to a particular drug (wild-type population). These distributions may aid in the recognition of new resistance mechanisms by highlighting strains for which the MICs fall outside the normal distribution. However, distributions of MICs have limited direct application since they vary between species, and for some strains for which the MICs are outside the normal range, the MICs may be below clinically derived breakpoints. Such strains may or may not respond to treatment. Knowledge of the presence of specific resistance mechanisms that inactivate compounds of a particular drug class assists in deriving microbiological breakpoints often called epidemiological cutoff values.

Pharmacokinetics and Pharmacodynamics

Pharmacokinetics examines the absorption, distribution, accumulation, and elimination (metabolism and excretion) of a drug in the body over time. These parameters are usually determined using healthy volunteers. A drug's MICs can be compared with the concentration of the drug achievable in blood or other body fluids (e.g., cerebrospinal fluid). In the past, breakpoints were chosen generally such that the MICs for susceptible pathogens would be exceeded by the drug level for most or all of the dosing interval. Newer data that are now considered when establishing breakpoints include pharmacodynamic calculations. Pharmacodynamics is the study of the time course of drug action against the microorganism. For antimicrobial agents, the desired action is pathogen eradication. In vitro pharmacodynamic studies have revealed that agents fall into three classes: those with principally time-dependent antimicrobial action and no or short postantibiotic effects, those with time-dependent action and long postantibiotic effects, and those with prominent concentration-dependent action (17). For drugs with time-dependent action and no or short postantibiotic effects, the critical determinant of bacterial killing in vivo is the percentage of time in a dosing interval that the drug concentration is above the MIC. For the other two classes, the important determinant is the ratio of the area under the concentration-time curve to the MIC and/or the ratio of the peak concentration to the MIC. For β-lactams, short-acting macrolides, and clindamycin, the relevant measure is the percentage of time that the drug concentration is above the MIC, and the ratio of the area under the concentration-time curve or of the peak concentration to the MIC is the relevant parameter for aminoglycosides, long-acting macrolides, tetracyclines, glycopeptides, and fluoroquinolones (18). These values can be used to calculate the maximum MICs or breakpoints that allow the achievement of optimum efficacy with standard drug dosing schedules.

Clinical and Bacteriological Response Rates

During clinical trials, the clinical and/or bacteriologic eradication response rates of organisms for which the MICs of new antimicrobial agents have been determined give an indication of the relevance of breakpoints selected by using the MIC distributions and the pharmacokinetic/pharmacodynamic properties of the drug. Response rates of at least 80% may be expected for organisms classified as susceptible, although the rates can be lower depending on the site and type of infection. While in some countries breakpoints are determined primarily from clinical and bacteriological response rates, the CLSI evaluates clinical and bacteriological response rates in conjunction with population distributions, pharmacokinetics, and pharmacodynamics in establishing the breakpoints in an attempt to provide the best correlation between in vitro test results and clinical outcome (8).

Inhibition Zone Diameter Distributions for Disk Diffusion Methods

Once the MIC breakpoints are selected, disk diffusion breakpoints can be chosen by plotting the inhibition zone diameters against the MICs derived from the testing of a large number of strains of various species. A statistical approach that uses the linear regression formula may be used to calculate the appropriate zone diameter intercepts for the predetermined MIC breakpoints. An alternative, pragmatic approach to deriving disk diffusion breakpoints is the use of the error rate-bounded method, in which the zone diameter criteria are selected on the basis of the minimization of the disk interpretive errors, especially the very major errors (5, 38) (Fig. 1). Newer statistical techniques are being studied to improve the correlation with MICs (16). The newest CLSI approach focuses on the rate of interpretive errors near the proposed breakpoint versus rates of errors with MICs more than a single $\log_2$ dilution from the MIC breakpoints (8). The concept is that errors that occur with isolates for which MICs are very close to the

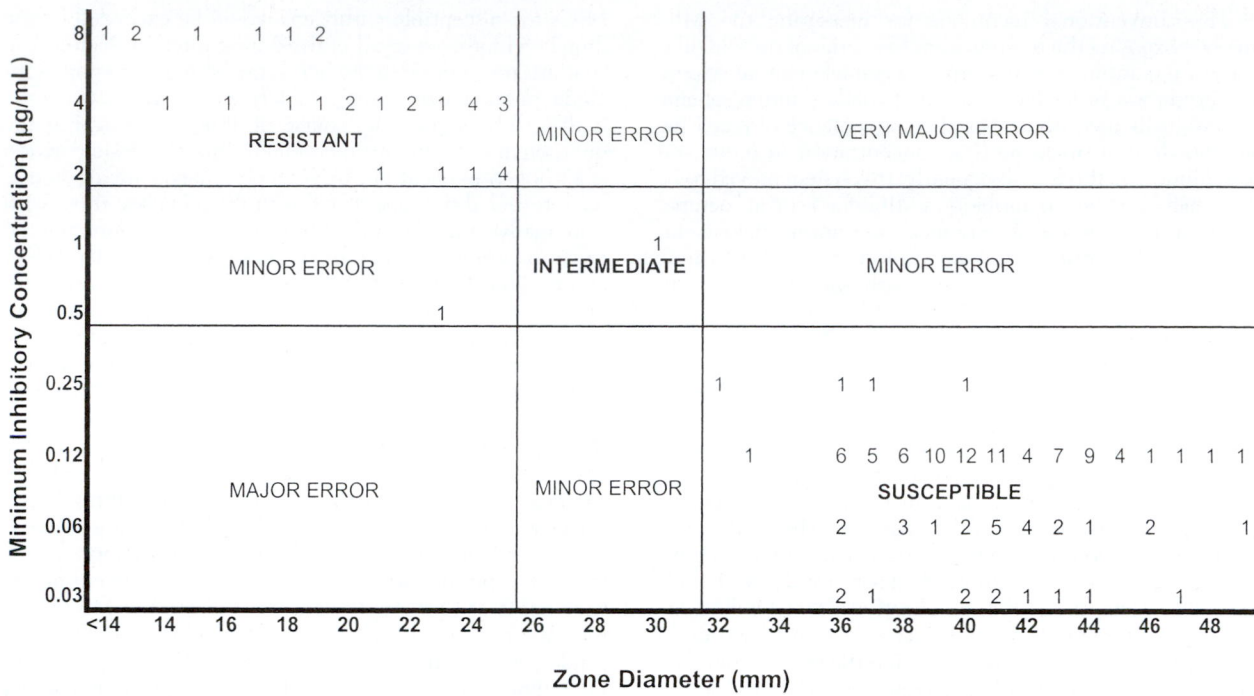

FIGURE 1 Comparison of zone diameters with MICs of a hypothetical antimicrobial agent.

MIC breakpoints are less of a concern than errors with more highly resistant or susceptible strains.

Breakpoints derived by professional groups or regulatory bodies in various countries are often quite similar. For instance, there is a small number of breakpoint discrepancies between the CLSI and the U.S. Food and Drug Administration, which are under review by both groups. However, there can be notable differences in the breakpoints used in different countries or regions for the same agents. The reasons for the differences may be that certain countries use different dosages or administration intervals for some drugs. In addition, some countries are more conservative in assessing the susceptibility to antimicrobial agents and place greater emphasis on the detection of emerging resistance, noted primarily by examination of microorganism population distributions. Technical factors such as the inoculum density, atmosphere of incubation, and test medium can also affect MICs and zone diameters, thereby justifying different interpretive criteria in some countries. These technical differences are summarized in chapter 68 of this *Manual*. Two non-U.S. methods minimize or avoid the use of an intermediate category of susceptibility, based on the rationale that such results are of little value to clinicians (3, 36). The lack of a buffer between susceptible and resistant categories can result in higher rates of incorrect categorization. It may be safer for a laboratory to employ a method that uses an intermediate category or, if not, to report intermediate results as resistant.

Information on a range of international susceptibility testing methods and/or breakpoints can be downloaded or purchased from the following websites:

- the CLSI website at http://www.clsi.org;
- the European Committee on Antimicrobial Susceptibility Testing website at http://www.eucast.org (EUCAST now sets or harmonizes breakpoints for all its member countries);
- the British Society for Antimicrobial Chemotherapy website at http://www.bsac.org.uk;
- the Deutsches Institut für Normung website at http://www.beuth.de/;
- the Swedish Reference Group for Antibiotics website at http://www.srga.org;
- a website featuring the Danish commercial disk diffusion method at http://www.rosco.dk;
- a website featuring the Australian Calibrated Dichotomous Sensitivity disk diffusion method at http://www.med.unsw.edu.au/pathology-cds/.

MOLECULAR DETECTION OF RESISTANCE

As highlighted in chapter 74, there is now a range of molecular techniques for the detection of many resistance genes. While none are currently recommended for routine testing, some have found a place in larger laboratories, where detection of certain important resistance genes can be implemented in cost-effective manner. Examples include the detection of *mecA* in *Staphylococcus* species, especially *S. aureus*, and detection of the *vanA* and *vanB* genes in *Enterococcus* species. In addition, molecular techniques are becoming available for the rapid detection of methicillin-resistant *S. aureus* from positive blood culture bottles. These molecular tests have been increasingly valuable for infection control purposes (48). Molecular methods are also valuable for confirming unusual resistances and for determining which mechanism of resistance is present when this has epidemiological significance. For example, there is currently great interest in the emergence and spread of plasmid-mediated varieties of carbapenem resistance (53), quinolone resistance (45), and resistance to aminoglycosides attributable to ribosomal methylases (6) in enteric gram-negative bacteria.

SELECTED USE OF CONFIRMATORY AND SUPPLEMENTARY TESTS

Besides performing routine susceptibility testing, laboratories will encounter isolates or tests results that are unexpected, i.e., for which there is no testing guidance available or which are considered to be of major epidemiological importance. The CLSI provides some guidance on what resistances might be considered unexpected (either uncommon or never reported [14]). Recommendations of how to proceed vary, but if results are not attributable to simple laboratory errors and are reproducible, then testing by an alternative method and, if necessary, referral to a reference laboratory is warranted. For some key resistances, e.g., carbapenem resistance in *Enterobacteriaceae*, the most effective confirmatory method is resistance gene detection, as described in chapter 74. In other circumstances, one of the special phenotypic tests described in chapter 70 will suffice.

Inducible resistance is considered to be clinically important for a small number of antimicrobial-bacterial combinations. At present, only methods for detecting inducible resistance to clindamycin in *Staphylococcus* and *Streptococcus* species have been sufficiently evaluated and standardized to be recommended for routine laboratory use (12, 13).

For some clinical conditions, e.g., bacterial meningitis caused by *Streptococcus pneumoniae*, susceptibility test interpretation and clinician guidance can be enhanced by performing MIC measurements if these data were not generated by the laboratory's routine method. Customized or locally prepared microtiter trays or, alternatively, a commercial gradient diffusion method may be used (39).

REPORTING OF RESULTS

The reporting of results is the crucial final step in susceptibility testing. There are no universally agreed upon practices for generating reports, but the following elements should be considered. Categorical reporting, in which the tests results are susceptible, intermediate, or resistant, is standard practice and widely understood by clinicians. When available, MIC data may be reported but should appear only along with a categorical interpretation. Susceptibility test reports should be formatted in such a way that the results are unambiguous in either printed or electronic form, especially if more than one organism is being reported. Most importantly, so-called cascade reporting is recommended to reduce the chance of the clinician choosing a broader-spectrum antimicrobial agent inappropriately (19). Cascade reporting involves the withholding of results for broader-spectrum antimicrobials from the report when the isolate tested is susceptible to narrower-spectrum agents, e.g., withholding a vancomycin result when an isolate of *Staphylococcus aureus* tests as susceptible to oxacillin or cefoxitin. Such reporting is considered to be an essential part of hospital antimicrobial stewardship programs (20), as is the production of annual reports that summarize overall susceptibility and resistance patterns (antibiograms) (10).

FUTURE DIRECTIONS AND NEEDS IN ANTIMICROBIAL SUSCEPTIBILITY TESTING

Antimicrobial resistance is becoming widespread among a variety of clinically significant bacterial species (47, 55). Therefore, microbiology laboratories play a key role in the patient management process by providing accurate data on which physicians can base therapy decisions. Susceptibility testing results, however, are also used by investigators in surveillance studies and by infection control practitioners to detect and control the spread of antibiotic-resistant organisms (10, 43). Surveillance can be performed at laboratories at the local, regional, national, and international level through direct interchange of data from laboratory information systems to centralized databases (42). Thus, the accuracy of stored results becomes almost as important as the accuracy of test performance and interpretation.

To meet these challenges and responsibilities, clinical microbiologists must continuously assess and update their susceptibility testing strategies. The first priority is to use accurate and reliable methods, whether they are conventional or perhaps newer molecular methods. Then, careful monitoring of test performance with well-characterized control strains that challenge the capabilities of the testing methods becomes essential. Today, laboratories must use a variety of testing methods, each tailored specifically to a particular species or group of organisms. It is not likely that a single method, whether conventional or commercial, will be optimal for all antimicrobial agents, organisms, and resistance mechanisms. This will require increased education and training for clinical microbiologists in the future. Some assistance may be sought from the computer-based "expert" systems that allow a rapid and accurate view of antimicrobial susceptibility profiles and recognition of potentially aberrant results or novel resistance mechanisms (15, 44). Rapid progress is also being made on molecular methods that are starting to have practical application in routine clinical laboratories (1, 35, 37; see also chapter 74).

More-effective means of conveying critical antimicrobial susceptibility testing information to clinicians in a time frame that allows efficient and effective management of patients and in a format that is unambiguous to clinicians in various practice specialties are still needed. Clinical microbiologists should become more proactive in the reporting of antimicrobial susceptibility results and in cross-linking that information to other databases (e.g., those for pharmacy prescriptions) to ensure that patients receive the most efficacious cost-effective therapy.

REFERENCES

1. **Allaouchiche, B., H. Jaumain, G. Zambardi, D. Chassard, and J. Freney.** 1999. Clinical impact of rapid oxacillin susceptibility testing using a PCR assay in *Staphylococcus aureus* bacteraemia. *J. Infect.* **39**:198–204.
2. **Barenfanger, J., C. Drake, and G. Kacich.** 1999. Clinical and financial benefits of rapid identification and antimicrobial susceptibility testing. *J. Clin. Microbiol.* **37**:1415–1418.
3. **Bell, S. M.** 1988. Additions and modifications to the range of antibiotics tested by the CDS method of antibiotic sensitivity testing. *Pathology* **20**:303–304.
4. **Bruins, M., H. Oord, P. Bloembergen, M. Wolfhagen, A. Casparie, J. Degener, and G. Ruijs.** 2005. Lack of effect of shorter turnaround time of microbiological procedures on clinical outcomes: a randomised controlled trial among hospitalised patients in the Netherlands. *Eur. J. Clin. Microbiol. Infect. Dis.* **24**:305–313.
5. **Brunden, M. N., G. E. Zurenko, and B. Kapik.** 1992. Modification of the error-rate bounded classification scheme for use with two MIC break points. *Diagn. Microbiol. Infect. Dis.* **15**:135–140.
6. **Cantón, R.** 2009. Antibiotic resistance genes from the environment: a perspective through newly identified antibiotic resistance mechanisms in the clinical setting. *Clin. Microbiol. Infect.* **15**(Suppl. 1):20–25.
7. **Citron, D. M., M. I. Ostoravi, A. Karlsson, and E. J. C. Goldstein.** 1991. Evaluation of the E test for susceptibility testing of anaerobic bacteria. *J. Clin. Microbiol.* **29**:2197–2203.
8. **Clinical and Laboratory Standards Institute.** 2008. Development of *in vitro* susceptibility testing criteria and quality

control parameters. Approved guideline M23-A3. Clinical and Laboratory Standards Institute, Wayne, PA.

9. **Clinical and Laboratory Standards Institute.** 2007. Methods for antimicrobial susceptibility testing of anaerobic bacteria. Approved standard M11-A7. Clinical and Laboratory Standards Institute, Wayne, PA.

10. **Clinical and Laboratory Standards Institute.** 2009. Analysis and presentation of cumulative antimicrobial susceptibility test data. Approved guideline M39-A3. Clinical and Laboratory Standards Institute, Wayne, PA.

11. **Clinical and Laboratory Standards Institute.** 2010. Methods for antimicrobial dilution and disk susceptibility testing of infrequently-isolated or fastidious bacteria. Approved guideline M45-A2. Clinical and Laboratory Standards Institute, Wayne, PA.

12. **Clinical and Laboratory Standards Institute.** 2009. Methods for dilution antimicrobial susceptibility tests for bacteria that grow aerobically. Approved standard M7-A8. Clinical and Laboratory Standards Institute, Wayne, PA.

13. **Clinical and Laboratory Standards Institute.** 2009. Performance standards for antimicrobial disk susceptibility tests. Approved standard M2-A10. Clinical and Laboratory Standards Institute, Wayne, PA.

14. **Clinical and Laboratory Standards Institute.** 2010. Performance standards for antimicrobial susceptibility testing. Supplement M100-S20. Clinical and Laboratory Standards Institute, Wayne, PA.

15. **Courvalin, P.** 1992. Interpretive reading of antimicrobial susceptibility tests. *ASM News* **58:**368–375.

16. **Craig, B. A.** 2000. Modeling approach to diameter breakpoint determination. *Diagn. Microbiol. Infect. Dis.* **36:**193–202.

17. **Craig, W. A.** 2002. Pharmacodynamics of antimicrobials: general concepts and applications, p. 1–22. *In* C. H. Nightingale, T. Murakawa, and P. G. Ambrose (ed.), *Antimicrobial Pharmacodynamics in Theory and Clinical Practice.* Marcel Dekker, New York, NY.

18. **Craig, W. A.** 1998. Pharmacokinetic/pharmacodynamic parameters: rationale for antibacterial dosing of mice and men. *Clin. Infect. Dis.* **26:**1–10.

19. **Cunney, R. J., and E. G. Smyth.** 2000. The impact of laboratory reporting practices on antibiotic utilisation. *Int. J. Antimicrob. Agents* **14:**13–19.

20. **Dellit, T. H., R. C. Owens, J. E. McGowan, Jr., D. N. Gerding, R. A. Weinstein, J. P. Burke, W. C. Huskins, D. L. Paterson, N. O. Fishman, C. F. Carpenter, P. J. Brennan, M. Billeter, and T. M. Hooton.** 2007. Infectious Diseases Society of America and the Society for Healthcare Epidemiology of America guidelines for developing an institutional program to enhance antimicrobial stewardship. *Clin. Infect. Dis.* **44:**159–177.

21. **Doern, G. V., R. Vautour, M. Gaudet, and B. Levy.** 1994. Clinical impact of rapid in vitro antimicrobial susceptibility testing and bacterial identification. *J. Clin. Microbiol.* **32:**1757–1762.

22. **International Organization for Standardization.** 2006. *Susceptibility Testing of Infectious Agents and Evaluation of Performance of Antimicrobial Susceptibility Devices. Part 1. Reference Method for Testing the In Vitro Activity of Antimicrobial Agents against Bacteria Involved in Infectious Diseases.* ISO/DIS 20776-1. International Organization for Standardization, Geneva, Switzerland.

23. **Jett, B., L. Free, and D. F. Sahm.** 1996. Factors influencing the Vitek gram-positive susceptibility system's detection of *vanB*-encoded vancomycin resistance among enterococci. *J. Clin. Microbiol.* **34:**701–706.

24. **Jorgensen, J. H.** 1993. Selection criteria for an antimicrobial susceptibility testing system. *J. Clin. Microbiol.* **31:**2841–2844.

25. **Jorgensen, J. H.** 1993. Selection of antimicrobial agents for routine testing in a clinical microbiology laboratory. *Diagn. Microbiol. Infect. Dis.* **16:**245–249.

26. **Jorgensen, J. H.** 2000. Rapid automated antimicrobial susceptibility testing of *Streptococcus pneumoniae* by use of the bioMerieux VITEK 2. *J. Clin. Microbiol.* **38:**2814–2818.

27. **Jorgensen, J. H., M. J. Ferraro, M. L. McElmeel, J. Spargo, J. M. Swenson, and F. C. Tenover.** 1994. Detection of penicillin and extended-spectrum cephalosporin resistance among *Streptococcus pneumoniae* clinical isolates by use of the E test. *J. Clin. Microbiol.* **32:**159–163.

28. **Kahlmeter, G., D. F. J. Brown, F. W. Goldstein, A. P. MacGowan, J. W. Mouton, A. Österland, A. Rodloff, M. Steinbakk, P. Urbanskova, and A. Vatopoulos.** 2003. European harmonization of MIC breakpoints for antimicrobial susceptibility testing of bacteria. *J. Antimicrob. Chemother.* **52:**145–148.

29. **Katsanis, G. P., J. Spargo, M. J. Ferraro, L. Sutton, and G. A. Jacoby.** 1994. Detection of *Klebsiella pneumoniae* and *Escherichia coli* strains producing extended-spectrum β-lactamases. *J. Clin. Microbiol.* **32:**691–696.

30. **Kerremans, J. J., P. Verboom, T. Stijnen, L. Hakkart-van Roijen, W. Goessens, H. A. Verbrugh, and M. C. Vos.** 2008. Rapid identification and antimicrobial susceptibility testing reduce antibiotic use and accelerate pathogen-directed antibiotic use. *J. Antimicrob. Chemother.* **61:**428–435.

31. **Kolbert, M., F. Chegani, and P. M. Shah.** 2004. Evaluation of the OSIRIS video reader as an automated measurement system for the agar disk diffusion technique. *Clin. Microbiol. Infect.* **10:**416–420.

32. **Korgenski, E. K., and J. A. Daly.** 1998. Evaluation of the BIOMIC video reader system for determining interpretive categories of isolates on the basis of disk diffusion susceptibility results. *J. Clin. Microbiol.* **36:**302–304.

33. **Lestari, E. S., J. A. Severin, P. M. Filius, K. Kuntaman, D. Offra Duerink, U. Hadi, H. Wahjono, H. A. Verbrugh, and Antimicrobial Resistance in Indonesia: Prevalence and Prevention (AMRIN).** 2008. Comparison of the accuracy of disk diffusion diameters obtained by manual zone measurements to that by automated zone measurements to determine antimicrobial susceptibility. *J. Microbiol. Methods* **75:**177–181.

34. **Ling, T. K. W., P. C. Tam, Z. K. Liu, and A. F. B. Cheng.** 2001. Evaluation of VITEK 2 rapid identification and susceptibility testing system against gram-negative clinical isolates. *J. Clin. Microbiol.* **39:**2964–2966.

35. **Louie, L., S. O. Matsumura, E. Choi, M. Louie, and A. E. Simor.** 2000. Evaluation of three rapid methods for detection of methicillin resistance in *Staphylococcus aureus*. *J. Clin. Microbiol.* **38:**2170–2173.

36. **MacGowan, A. P., and R. Wise.** 2001. Establishing MIC breakpoints and the interpretation of in vitro susceptibility tests. *J. Antimicrob. Chemother* **48**(Suppl. S1):17–28.

37. **Martineau, F., F. J. Picard, L. Grenier, P. H. Roy, M. Ouellette, and M. G. Bergeron.** 2000. Multiplex PCR assays for the detection of clinically relevant antibiotic resistance genes in staphylococci isolated from patients infected after cardiac surgery. The ESPRIT trial. *J. Antimicrob. Chemother.* **46:**527–534.

38. **Metzler, D. M., and R. M. DeHaan.** 1974. Susceptibility tests of anaerobic bacteria: statistical and clinical considerations. *J. Infect. Dis.* **130:**588–594.

39. **Mittman, S. A., R. C. Huard, P. Della-Latta, and S. Whittier.** 2009. Comparison of BD phoenix to Vitek 2, MicroScan MICroSTREP, and Etest for antimicrobial susceptibility testing of *Streptococcus pneumoniae*. *J. Clin. Microbiol.* **47:**3557–3561.

40. **Nadler, H. L., C. Dolan, L. Mele, and S. R. Kurtz.** 1985. Accuracy and reproducibility of the AutoMicrobic System Gram-Negative General Susceptibility-Plus Card for testing selected challenge organisms. *J. Clin. Microbiol.* **22:**355–360.

41. **Rex, J. H., and M. A. Pfaller.** 2002. Has antifungal susceptibility testing come of age? *Clin. Infect. Dis.* **35:**982–989.

42. **Sahm, D. F., J. A. Karlowsky, L. J. Kelly, I. A. Critchley, M. E. Jones, C. Thornsberry, Y. Mauriz, and J. Kahn.** 2001. Need for annual surveillance of antimicrobial resistance in *Streptococcus pneumoniae* in the United States: 2-year longitudinal analysis. *Antimicrob. Agents Chemother.* **45:**1037–1042.

43. **Sahm, D. F., and F. C. Tenover.** 1997. Surveillance for the emergence and dissemination of antimicrobial resistance in bacteria. *Infect. Dis. Clin. N. Am.* **11:**767–785.

44. **Sanders, C. C., M. Peyret, E. S. Moland, S. J. Cavalieri, C. Shubert, K. S. Thomson, J.-M. Boeufgras, and W. E. Sanders, Jr.** 2001. Potential impact of the VITEK 2 System and the Advanced Expert System on the clinical laboratory of a university-based hospital. *J. Clin. Microbiol.* **39:**2379–2385.

45. **Strahilevitz, J., G. A. Jacoby, D. C. Hooper, and A. Robicsek.** 2009. Plasmid-mediated quinolone resistance: a multifaceted threat. *Clin. Microbiol. Rev.* **22:**664–689.

46. **Tan, T. Y., C. McNulty, A. Charlett, N. Nessa, C. Kelly, and T. Beswick.** 2003. Laboratory antibiotic susceptibility reporting and antibiotic prescribing in general practice. *J. Antimicrob. Chemother.* **51:**379–384.

47. **Tenover, F. C.** 2001. Development and spread of bacterial resistance to antimicrobial agents. An overview. *Clin. Infect. Dis.* **15**(Suppl.):S108–S115.

48. **Tenover, F. C.** 2007. Rapid detection and identification of bacterial pathogens using novel molecular technologies: infection control and beyond. *Clin. Infect. Dis.* **44:**418–423.

49. **Tenover, F. C., J. M. Swenson, C. O'Hara, and S. A. Stocker.** 1995. Ability of commercial and reference antimicrobial susceptibility testing methods to detect vancomycin resistance in enterococci. *J. Clin. Microbiol.* **33:**1524–1527.

50. **Tenover, F. C., J. Tokars, J. Swenson, S. Paul, K. Splitalny, and W. Jarvis.** 1993. Ability of clinical laboratories to detect antimicrobial-resistant enterococci. *J. Clin. Microbiol.* **31:**1695–1699.

51. **Trenholme, G. M., R. L. Kaplan, P. H. Karahusis, T. Stine, J. Fuhrer, W. Landau, and S. Levin.** 1989. Clinical impact of rapid identification and susceptibility testing of bacterial blood culture isolates. *J. Clin. Microbiol.* **27:**1342–1345.

52. **Turnidge, J. D., and D. L. Paterson.** 2007. Setting and revising antibacterial susceptibility breakpoints. *Clin. Microbiol. Rev.* **20:**391–408.

53. **Walsh, T. R.** 2008. Clinically significant carbapenemases: an update. *Curr. Opin. Infect. Dis.* **21:**367–371.

54. **Washington, J. A., C. C. Knapp, and C. C. Sanders.** 1988. Accuracy of microdilution and the AutoMicrobic System in detection of β-lactam resistance in gram-negative bacterial mutants with derepressed β-lactamase. *Rev. Infect. Dis.* **10:**824–829.

55. **Williams, R. M.** 2001. Globalization of antimicrobial resistance: epidemiological challenges. *Clin. Infect. Dis.* **15**(Suppl.):S116–S117.

Susceptibility Test Methods: Dilution and Disk Diffusion Methods

JEAN B. PATEL, FRED C. TENOVER, JOHN D. TURNIDGE,
AND JAMES H. JORGENSEN

68

There are a number of methods for antimicrobial suscepti-bility testing of bacteria, and they are categorized into dilu-tion methods that generate MIC results and disk diffusion methods that generate zone diameter results. Susceptibility testing methods can also be categorized as generic reference methods, which are described by standards-setting organiza-tions (e.g., the Clinical and Laboratory Standards Institute [CLSI], European Union Committee on Antimicrobial Susceptibility Testing [EUCAST], and British Society for Antimicrobial Chemotherapy [BSAC]), and commer-cial methods, which are mostly automated systems (e.g., MicroScan [Siemens Healthcare Diagnostics, Deerfield, IL], Vitek [bioMérieux, Durham, NC], Phoenix [BD, Sparks, MD], or Sensititre [Trek Diagnostics Systems, Cleveland, OH]) or gradient diffusion methods (e.g., Etest [bio-Mérieux] or M.I.C.Evaluators [Oxoid, Cambridge, United Kingdom]). Generic reference methods are those in which the reagents for testing can be obtained from multiple sources and prepared in a laboratory without the need for sophisticated manufacturing processes. The CLSI reference methods are broth macrodilution, broth microdilution, agar dilution, and disk diffusion (20, 21).

The choice of methods to be used in individual laborato-ries is based on factors such as relative ease of performance, cost, flexibility in selection of drugs for testing, availability of automated or semiautomated devices to facilitate testing, and perceived accuracy of the methodology (50). Refer-ence dilution methods are typically used by pharmaceutical companies to establish MIC data for new antimicrobial agents, by research laboratories and device manufacturers as a standard to which new susceptibility testing methods are evaluated, and by reference laboratories for confirming unusual susceptibility test results. Although it has become increasingly uncommon, some clinical microbiology labora-tories use reference dilution methods for routine diagnostic testing. More frequently, clinical microbiology laboratories use automated systems or a combination of MIC and disk diffusion methods for routine susceptibility testing.

Interpretive categories for antimicrobial agent test re-sults (i.e., susceptible, intermediate, and resistant) are established for disk diffusion methods based on MIC data so that interpretive errors between methods are minimized (18). Briefly, interpretive categories, or breakpoints, are first established for MIC results generated by either the broth or agar reference method. These breakpoints are based upon the normal MIC distributions for a bacterial species, phar-macokinetic/pharmacodynamic modeling data, and data from clinical outcome studies. Subsequently, disk diffusion breakpoints are set by comparing disk diffusion data to MIC data and choosing breakpoints so that interpretive er-rors between methods are within acceptable limits (a more detailed description is provided later in this chapter). Inter-pretive categories for MIC methods and disk diffusion are established after both intralaboratory and interlaboratory reproducibilities are verified for these methods. Since inter-pretive criteria for disk diffusion data are set so that there is optimal correlation with MIC results, in most cases, one method of susceptibility testing is not superior to the other. However, there are specific examples of when one method may be preferred. Daptomycin, polymyxin B, and colistin are antimicrobial agents that do not diffuse well in agar, so in most cases disk diffusion is not an accurate method for these agents and MIC methods are recommended (38, 47). MIC tests are also recommended for testing of susceptibil-ity of staphylococci to vancomycin because vancomycin susceptibility testing by disk diffusion is not an accurate method for distinguishing vancomycin-intermediate from vancomycin-susceptible staphylococci (70). Also, MIC testing is necessary for accurate category assignment of *Streptococcus pneumoniae* isolates that produce zones of inhibition of ≤ 19 mm around a 1-μg oxacillin disk (51). For some bacteria, there are limited or no disk diffusion data available from well-controlled studies; thus, establish-ing interpretive criteria is not feasible (e.g., *Pseudomonas* spp. other than *Pseudomonas aeruginosa*, *Bacillus* spp., and *Corynebacterium* spp.). An example of a disk diffusion test being preferred to MIC testing is the cefoxitin disk test that predicts *mecA* carriage by coagulase-negative staphylococci. The disk test is more accurate than cefoxitin MIC testing for detecting *mecA*-mediated resistance in these species. The MIC testing produced inaccurate results in part be-cause some lots of Mueller-Hinton broth did not adequately support growth of all coagulase-negative staphylococcus isolates tested (71).

For MIC testing, the CLSI recommends reporting the MIC along with the interpretive category, but for disk diffusion testing, only the interpretive category should be reported. In most instances, the actual MIC does not affect patient management, except for cases of endocarditis, osteomyelitis, and meningitis, when MICs close to the nonsusceptible breakpoint can significantly influence the choice of antimicrobial agents. However, most clinicians typically use only the interpretive category to make their treatment decisions. MIC results also can be informative for epidemiological purposes for multiply resistant isolates. For epidemiological purposes, emerging resistance mechanisms may be identified among those isolates for which the antimicrobial agent MIC is above the normal MIC distribution for isolates of the same species. A valuable source of normal MIC distributions for various bacterium-antimicrobial agent combinations is the EUCAST website (http://www.escmid.org/research_projects/eu_cast/). Isolates for which MICs are greater than the normal distribution that still test as susceptible to the antimicrobial agent may possess a resistance mechanism, such that a successful therapeutic outcome with the agent cannot be predicted. There are several instances where information about elevated but susceptible MICs is useful. For example, isolates of *Enterobacteriaceae* that show elevated fluoroquinolone MICs but that are still in the susceptible category may possess a first-step fluoroquinolone mutation or possibly a plasmid-mediated fluoroquinolone resistance mechanism that may either reduce the effectiveness of the drug, as with *Salmonella enterica* serovar Typhi infections, or allow the organism to survive long enough to develop high-level resistance (56). This information would be particularly useful in an outbreak setting in which fluoroquinolones were being considered for treatment or prophylaxis. Similarly, an elevated but susceptible-range cephalosporin MIC in an isolate of *Enterobacteriaceae* may indicate production of an extended-spectrum β-lactamase (ESBL). When using the revised CLSI cephalosporin breakpoints for *Enterobacteriaceae*, tests for ESBL detection are no longer required, but ESBL production is useful information for epidemiological and infection control purposes. When treating an infection caused by a multiresistant isolate, which may be susceptible only to a single indicated agent, clinicians may consider using agents that give intermediate or even resistant results at an alternative dose, a different route of administration to optimize drug concentrations at the site of infection, or combinations

of agents to try to effect a cure. An MIC result combined with agent-specific pharmacokinetic/pharmacodynamic data may be used to guide this decision.

The selection of antibacterial agents for testing is complicated by the large number of agents available today and the diversity of institutional formularies. Some of these compounds, however, exhibit similar, if not identical, activities in vitro, so in some cases, one compound can be tested as a surrogate to represent one or more closely related compounds. Such extrapolations are listed in Table 1. Use of drug surrogates (also referred to as class representatives) can substantially reduce the number of agents required for testing and in some cases provide necessary flexibility in adapting commercial test systems for routine use in a variety of institutions. For instance, the susceptibility of *Staphylococcus* spp. to oxacillin (or cefoxitin) can be extrapolated to apply to all currently available penicillinase-stable penicillins, most cephalosporins (with the exception of the cephalosporins against methicillin-resistant *Staphylococcus aureus* [MRSA], e.g., ceftaroline and ceftobiprole), and essentially all carbapenems. Thus, it is unnecessary to test any of the agents in these chemical classes (20). Other extrapolations are possible, especially if there is demonstrated susceptibility to a less potent member of the chemical class of antimicrobial agent.

It is important that microbiologists work with the representatives of the hospital's pharmacy and formulary committees to ensure that the antibacterial agents being tested in the laboratory reflect those in the institution's current formulary (49). Doing so can contribute to the hospital's efforts to improve antimicrobial stewardship (31). Guidelines for the selection of antibacterial agents to be tested routinely are published annually by the CLSI (22) and are summarized in Table 2. While this listing is sometimes regarded rigidly as the standard for selecting the agents that must be tested, it is a list of agents that should be considered for routine testing only; many variables go into the decision as to which agents should be tested in any particular setting (48). The CLSI also cautions that the decision about testing and reporting of some agents selectively should be made by the clinical microbiologist in conjunction with the infectious disease practitioners, the pharmacy, and/or the infection control committees (20, 22).

TABLE 1 Antibacterial susceptibility results that may be extrapolated from other test results

Test drug (result)	Organism(s)	Drug(s) for which result can be extrapolated
Penicillin G	*Staphylococcus* spp., *Neisseria gonorrhoeae*	Phenoxymethylpenicillin, phenethicillin, ampicillin, amoxicillin, bacampicillin, cyclacillin, hetacillin, carbenicillin, mezlocillin, azlocillin, ticarcillin, piperacillin
Ampicillin	All	Amoxicillin, bacampicillin, cyclacillin, hetacillin
Ampicillin	*Enterococcus* spp.	Penicillin
Oxacillin	*Staphylococcus* spp.	All penicillins, including antistaphylococcal penicillins; all cephalosporins (except cephalosporins with anti-MRSA activity); all β-lactamase inhibitor combinations; all carbapenems; loracarbef
Cephalothin	*Enterobacteriaceae*	Cefadroxil, cefpodoxime, cephalexin, loracarbef; not other cephalosporins
Erythromycin	Gram-positive cocci	Azithromycin, clarithromycin, dirithromycin, roxithromyxin
Tetracycline	All (except *Staphylococcus*, *Enterococcus*, and *Acinetobacter* spp.)	Doxycycline, minocycline, chlortetracycline, demeclocycline and oxytetracycline, methacycline
Sulfisoxazole	All	All sulfonamides

TABLE 2 Antimicrobial agents recommended for routine dilution and disk diffusion susceptibility testing[a]

Antimicrobial agent	Group[b] recommended for testing with:							
	Enterobacteriaceae	P. aeruginosa	Other non-Enterobacteriaceae[c,d]	Acinetobacter spp.[d]	Burkholderia cepacia[d]	Stenotrophomonas maltophilia[d]	Staphylococci[d]	Enterococci[d]
Penicillins								
Penicillin G							A	A[e,f]
Ampicillin	A							A[e,f]
Oxacillin[g] or methicillin							A	
Ticarcillin		B						
Piperacillin	B	A	A[*]	B				
Ampicillin-sulbactam	B			A				
Amoxicillin-clavulanic acid	B							
Piperacillin-tazobactam	B	B	B[*]	B	B[*]			
Ticarcillin-clavulanic acid	B		B[*]	B	B[*]	B[*]		
Cephalosporins								
Cephalothin	U[h]							
Cefazolin	A							
Cefuroxime	B							
Cefoxitin	B						A[i]	
Cefotetan	B							
Cefotaxime	B		C[*]	B				
Ceftriaxone	B		C[*]	B				
Ceftazidime	C	A	A[*]	A	B	B[*]		
Cefepime	B	B	B[*]	B				
Carbapenems								
Ertapenem	B							
Imipenem	B	B	B[*]	A				
Meropenem	B	B	B[*]	A	B			
Other β-lactams								
Aztreonam	C	B	B[*]					
Aminoglycosides								
Gentamicin	A	A	A[*]	A			C	C[j]
Netilmicin				A				
Tobramycin	A	A	A[*]	A				
Amikacin	B	B	B[*]	B				
Streptomycin								C[j]
Macrolides								
Azithromycin							A	
Clarithromycin							A	
Erythromycin							A	

Quinolones								
Ciprofloxacin	B	B	B*	A			C	U
Levofloxacin	B	B	B*	A	B*	B	C	U
Lomefloxacin	U	U	U*				U	
Moxifloxacin							C	
Norfloxacin	U	U	U*				U	U
Ofloxacin	U	U	U*				C	
Miscellaneous								
Chloramphenicol	C		C*		B*	B*	C	
Clindamycin							A	
Daptomycin							B*	B*
Doxycycline				B			B	
Linezolid							B	B
Minocycline				B	B	B		
Nitrofurantoin	U						U	U
Quinupristin-dalfopristin							C	B
Rifampin							B	
Sulfisoxazole	U		U*				U	
Tetracycline	C		U*[k]	B			B[k]	U
Telithromycin							B	
Trimethoprim-sulfamethoxazole	B		B*	B	A	A	A	
Trimethoprim	U						U	
Vancomycin							B	B[f]

[a]Modified from CLSI document M100-S20 (22) with permission. Current standards and supplements to them may be obtained from the CLSI, 940 West Valley Rd., Suite 1400, Wayne, PA 19087-1898.

[b]Group A comprises primary drugs to be tested and reported, group B comprises those to be tested as primary drugs but reported selectively, group C comprises supplemental drugs to be reported selectively, and group U comprises drugs to be tested with urinary isolates only.

[c]Non-*Enterobacteriaceae* include *Pseudomonas* spp. and other nonfastidious, non-glucose-fermenting gram-negative bacilli but exclude *P. aeruginosa*, *Acinetobacter* spp., *Burkholderia cepacia*, *Burkholderia mallei*, *Burkholderia pseudomallei*, and *Stenotrophomonas maltophilia*, since there are separate listings of suggested drugs to test and report for them.

[d]Those agents marked with an asterisk should be tested only by using an MIC method and not by using disk diffusion.

[e]Results of tests with penicillin apply to other penicillins (e.g., ampicillin, amoxicillin, carboxypenicillins, and ureidopenicillins) against β-lactamase-negative enterococci.

[f]Combination therapy consisting of penicillin, ampicillin, or vancomycin and an aminoglycoside is recommended for serious infections.

[g]Staphylococci resistant to the penicillinase-resistant penicillins should also be considered resistant to penicillins, β-lactam–β-lactamase-inactivating combinations, cephalosporins (except cephalosporins with anti-MRSA activity), and carbapenems.

[h]Cephalothin test results should only be used to represent oral agents, i.e., cefadroxil, cefpodoxime, cephalexin, and loracarbef. Older data which suggest that cephalothin results could predict susceptibility to some other cephalosporins may still be correct, but there are no recent data to confirm this.

[i]Cefoxitin is used as a surrogate for oxacillin for staphylococci.

[j]For use of aminoglycosides to screen enterococci for synergy resistance, see the sections "Breakpoint Susceptibility Tests" and "Resistance Screens."

[k]Doxycycline or minocycline may be tested on a supplemental basis because of their greater activities against some nonfermentative gram-negative bacilli and staphylococci.

DILUTION METHODS

Broth and agar dilution susceptibility testing methods are used to determine the minimal concentration, usually in micrograms per milliliter, of an antimicrobial agent required to inhibit or kill a microorganism. Antimicrobial agents are usually tested at $\log_2$ (twofold) serial dilutions, and the lowest concentration that inhibits visible growth of an organism is designated the MIC. The concentration range used may vary with the drug, the organism being tested, and the site of infection. Ranges should encompass the concentrations defining the interpretive categories (i.e., susceptible, intermediate, and resistant) and also the ranges that include the expected MICs for quality control reference strains. Other dilution methods include those that test a single concentration or a selected few concentrations of antimicrobial agents (i.e., breakpoint susceptibility tests and single-drug-concentration screens; see below).

Dilution methods offer flexibility in the sense that the standard medium used to test frequently encountered organisms (e.g., staphylococci, enterococci, *Pseudomonas aeruginosa*, and members of the family *Enterobacteriaceae*) may be supplemented or even replaced with another medium to allow accurate testing of certain fastidious bacterial species that may not be reliably tested by disk diffusion. Dilution methods are also readily adaptable to automated test systems.

DILUTION TESTING: AGAR METHOD

Dilution of Antimicrobial Agents

The solvents and diluents needed to prepare stock solutions of most commonly used antimicrobial agents are listed in the CLSI document on dilution testing (20).

Preparation, Supplementation, and Storage of Media

Mueller-Hinton agar is the recommended medium for testing most commonly encountered aerobic and facultatively anaerobic bacteria (20). The dehydrated agar base is commercially available and should be prepared as described by the manufacturer. Before sterilization, the molten agar is usually distributed into screw-cap tubes in exact aliquots sufficient to dilute the desired antimicrobial concentrations 10-fold. Tubes of agar, one for each drug concentration to be tested, are sterilized by autoclaving at 121°C for 15 min, and the agar is allowed to equilibrate to 48 to 50°C in a preheated water bath. Once the agar has equilibrated, the appropriate volume of antimicrobial agent is added, the tube contents are mixed by gentle inversion and poured into 100-mm-diameter round or square sterile plastic petri plates set on a level surface, and the agar is allowed to solidify. For growth controls, agar plates without antimicrobial agents are also prepared. All plates should be filled to a depth of 3 to 4 mm (20 to 25 ml of agar per round plate and 30 ml per square plate), and the pH of each batch should be checked to confirm the acceptable pH range of 7.2 to 7.4 (20).

After sterilization and temperature equilibration of the molten agar, any necessary supplements are aseptically added to the Mueller-Hinton agar at the time of addition of the drug solutions. For testing of streptococci, supplementation with 5% defibrinated sheep or horse blood is recommended (20). However, sheep blood supplementation may antagonize the activities of sulfonamide and trimethoprim with some organisms (8). The presence of blood also affects results with novobiocin and nafcillin as well as the in vitro activities of cephalosporins against enterococci (12, 67); therefore, blood

supplementation should not be used unless necessary for bacterial growth (see chapter 75 for acceptable methods for testing of fastidious bacterial species). Performance standards for Mueller-Hinton agar have been defined sufficiently such that calcium and magnesium supplementation is unnecessary (23). The agar should be supplemented with 2% NaCl for testing of oxacillin against staphylococci (42).

Once prepared, plates should be sealed in plastic bags and stored at 4 to 8°C. In general, they should be used within 5 days of preparation or as long as the MICs for control strains that are tested routinely are within the acceptable ranges. However, certain agents are sufficiently labile that plates may not be stored prior to use, e.g., carbapenems, cefaclor, and clavulanic acid. Before inoculation, plates that have been stored under refrigeration should be allowed to equilibrate to room temperature and the agar surface should be dry.

Inoculation Procedures

Variations in inoculum size may substantially affect MICs; therefore, careful inoculum standardization is required to obtain accurate results. The recommended final inoculum for agar dilution is 10^4 CFU per spot (20). This may be achieved in either of two ways. Four or five colonies are picked from overnight growth cultures on agar-based medium and inoculated into 4 to 5 ml of suitable broth that will support good growth (usually tryptic soy broth). Broths are incubated at 35°C until visibly turbid, and then the suspension is diluted until it matches the turbidity of a 0.5 McFarland, barium sulfate (BaSO$_4$), or latex particle turbidity standard (ca. 10^8 CFU/ml). The 0.5 McFarland standard may be purchased or the barium sulfate standard may be prepared as described in the CLSI document (20). The accuracy of the standard should be verified by using a spectrophotometer with a 1-cm light path; for the 0.5 McFarland standard, the absorbance at 625 nm should be 0.08 to 0.13 (20). An alternative inoculum standardization method, one that is preferred by many microbiologists, utilizes direct suspension of colonies from overnight growth cultures on a nonselective agar medium in saline or broth to a turbidity that matches the 0.5 McFarland standard. This approach eliminates the time needed for growing the inoculum in broth (20). In either case, normal saline or sterile broth is used to make a 1:10 dilution of the suspension to obtain an adjusted concentration of 10^7 CFU/ml (20).

Once the adjusted bacterial inoculum suspension is prepared, inoculation of the antimicrobial agent plates should be accomplished within 15 min, since longer delays may lead to changes in inoculum size. By using a pipette, a calibrated loop, or, more commonly, an inoculum-replicating device, 0.001 to 0.002 ml (1 to 2 µl) of the 10^7-CFU/ml suspension is delivered to the agar surface, resulting in the final desired inoculum of approximately 10^4 CFU per spot. For convenience, use of a replicator is preferred because consistent inoculum volumes for up to 36 different isolates are delivered simultaneously (20, 68). To use this device, an aliquot of the adjusted inoculum for each isolate is pipetted into the appropriate well of an inoculum seed plate and a multiprong inoculator is used to pick up and gently transfer 1 to 2 µl from the wells to the agar surfaces. Replicators are also available that deliver only 0.1 to 0.2 µl per spot and that do not require the 0.5 McFarland standard suspension to be diluted prior to delivery to the agar surface (20). The surfaces of the agar plates must be dry before inoculation, which should begin with a growth control plate that does not contain drug. Then inoculation continues from plates with the lowest drug concentration to plates with the highest drug concentration.

Finally, a second growth control plate that does not contain drug is inoculated to check for contamination or significant carryover of the antimicrobial agent. All plates should be clearly marked so that the locations of the different isolates being tested on each plate are known.

Incubation

Inoculated plates are allowed to stand for several minutes until the inoculum drops have been completely absorbed by the medium; then they are inverted and incubated in air at 35°C for 16 to 20 h before results are read. To facilitate detection of vancomycin-resistant enterococci and methicillin-resistant or vancomycin-resistant or -intermediate staphylococci, plates containing vancomycin or oxacillin should be incubated for a full 24 h before results are read (20). Incubation should not be carried out in the presence of an increased CO_2 concentration unless a fastidious organism is being tested (see chapter 75).

Interpretation and Reporting of Results

Before reading and recording the results obtained with clinical isolates, those obtained with applicable quality control strains tested at the same time should be checked to ensure that their values are within the acceptable ranges (see "Quality Control" below), and the drug-free control plates should be examined for isolate viability and purity. Endpoints for each antimicrobial agent are best determined by placing plates on a dark background and examining them for the lowest concentration that inhibits visible growth, which is recorded as the MIC. A single colony or a faint haze left by the initial inoculum should not be regarded as growth. If two or more colonies persist at antimicrobial concentrations beyond an otherwise obvious endpoint or if there is no growth at lower concentrations but there is growth at higher concentrations, the isolate should be subcultured to confirm purity and the test should be repeated. Substances that may antagonize the antibacterial activities of sulfonamides and trimethoprim may be carried over with the inoculum and cause "trailing," or less definite endpoints (8, 12). Therefore, the MICs of these antimicrobial agents should be interpreted as the endpoints at which 80% or more diminution of growth occurs. Although much less pronounced, trailing endpoints may also occur for some organisms with bacteriostatic agents such as chloramphenicol, the tetracyclines, linezolid, and quinupristin-dalfopristin (20).

The MIC of each antimicrobial agent is usually recorded in micrograms per milliliter, although in Europe and in the international standard reference method, the values are expressed as milligrams per liter (20, 43). These quantitative results should be reported with the appropriate corresponding interpretive category (susceptible, intermediate, or resistant), or the interpretive category may be reported alone. The MIC interpretive standards for these susceptibility categories, as currently recommended by the CLSI (20), are provided in Table 3. For detailed instructions concerning the use of these criteria and categories, the latest CLSI standards for dilution testing methods should be consulted (22).

The three interpretive categories are defined as follows. "Susceptible" indicates that an infection caused by the tested microorganism may be appropriately treated with the usually recommended regimen of the antimicrobial agent (i.e., the appropriate dose for the recommended period). "Intermediate" indicates that the isolate may be inhibited by attainable concentrations of certain drugs (e.g., the β-lactams) if higher dosages can be used safely or if the infection involves a body site where that drug is physiologically concentrated (e.g., the urinary tract). The intermediate category also serves as a

buffer zone that prevents slight technical artifacts from causing major interpretive discrepancies. Resistant isolates are not inhibited by the concentration of antimicrobial agent normally achievable with the recommended dose and/or yield results that fall within a range indicating that specific resistance mechanisms are likely to be present (20). The term nonsusceptible is used when no resistance breakpoint has been defined for an organism-drug combination (e.g., daptomycin and staphylococci).

Advantages and Disadvantages

Dilution testing by the agar method is a well-standardized, reliable susceptibility testing technique that may be used as a reference for evaluating other testing methods. In addition, the simultaneous testing of a large number of isolates with a few drugs is efficient (such as when new agents are evaluated in the pharmaceutical industry). Microbial contamination or population heterogeneity is more readily detected by the agar method than by broth methods. The agar dilution method has been considered the reference test method in many areas of Europe (34), while broth microdilution has been much more widely used for research and clinical testing in North America (48) and is now considered the international reference method for determining MICs (43). The major disadvantages of the agar method are associated with the time-consuming and labor-intensive tasks of preparing the plates, especially if the number of different antimicrobial agents to be tested for each isolate is high or if only a few isolates are to be tested. Also, agar dilution is not always evaluated as a susceptibility testing method for newer antimicrobial agents. For example, agar dilution has not been validated for susceptibility testing of daptomycin (22).

DILUTION TESTING: BROTH METHODS

The general approaches for broth methods include broth macrodilution, in which the broth volume for each antimicrobial concentration is ≥1.0 ml (usually 2 ml) contained in test tubes, and broth microdilution, in which antimicrobial dilutions are most often in 0.1-ml volumes in wells of 96-well microdilution trays.

Broth Macrodilution Methods

Dilution of Antimicrobial Agents

Stock solutions are prepared as discussed in the CLSI document on dilution testing (20) and are the same as those used for agar dilution tests. As in the agar method, the actual volumes used for the dilutions would be proportionally increased according to the number of tests being prepared, with a minimum of 1.0 ml needed for each drug concentration. Because addition of the inoculum results in a 1:2 dilution of each concentration, all final drug concentrations must be prepared at twice the actual desired testing concentration (see "Inoculation Procedures" below).

Preparation, Supplementation, and Storage of Media

Cation-adjusted Mueller-Hinton broth (CAMHB) is recommended for routine testing of commonly encountered nonfastidious organisms (20). Adjustment of the cations Ca^{2+} (20 to 25 mg/liter) and Mg^{2+} (10 to 12.5 mg/liter) is required to ensure acceptable results when *P. aeruginosa* isolates are tested with aminoglycosides and when tetracycline is tested with other bacteria (6). However, for convenience and consistency, cation adjustment of Mueller-Hinton broth is now recommended for testing of all species and antimicrobial

TABLE 3 Interpretive standards for dilution and disk diffusion susceptibility testing[a]

Antimicrobial agent and organism	MIC (μg/ml)			Zone diam (mm)		
	Susceptible	Intermediate	Resistant	Susceptible	Intermediate	Resistant
Penicillins						
Penicillin G						
Staphylococci[b]	≤0.12		≥0.25	≥29		≤28
Enterococci[c]	≤8		≥16	≥15		≤14
Methicillin[d]	≤8		≥16	≥14	10–13	≤9
Oxacillin[d]						
S. aureus (oxacillin tested)	≤2		≥4	≥13	11–12	≤10
S. aureus (cefoxitin tested)	≤4		≥8	≥22		≤21
Coagulase-negative staphylococci (oxacillin tested)	≤0.25		≥0.5			
Coagulase-negative staphylococci (cefoxitin tested)				≥25		≤24
Ampicillin						
Enterobacteriaceae	≤8	16	≥32	≥17	14–16	≤13
Staphylococci	≤0.25		≥0.5	≥29		≤28
Enterococci[c]	≤8		≥16	≥17		≤16
Amoxicillin-clavulanic acid						
Staphylococci	≤4/2		≥8/4	≥20		≤19
Other organisms	≤8/4	16/8	≥32/16	≥18	14–17	≤13
Ampicillin-sulbactam	≤8/4	16/8	≥32/16	≥15	12–14	≤11
Azlocillin						
P. aeruginosa	≤64		≥128	≥18		≤17
Carbenicillin						
P. aeruginosa	≤128	256	≥512	≥17	14–16	≤13
Other gram-negative bacilli	≤16	32	≥64	≥23	20–22	≤19
Mecillinam	≤8	16	≥32	≥15	12–14	≤11
Mezlocillin						
P. aeruginosa	≤64		≥128	≥16		≤15
Other gram-negative bacilli	≤16	32–64	≥128	≥21	18–20	≤17
Piperacillin						
P. aeruginosa	≤64		≥128	≥18		≤17
Other gram-negative bacilli	≤16	32–64	≥128	≥21	18–20	≤17
Piperacillin-tazobactam						
P. aeruginosa	≤64/4		≥128/4	≥18		≤17
Other gram-negative bacilli	≤16/4	32/4–64/4	≥128/4	≥21	18–20	≤17
Staphylococci	≤8/4		≥16/4	≥18		≤17
Ticarcillin						
P. aeruginosa	≤64		≥128	≥15		≤14
Other gram-negative bacilli	≤16	32–64	≥128	≥20	15–19	≤14
Ticarcillin-clavulanic acid						
P. aeruginosa	≤64/2		≥128/2	≥15		≤14
Other gram-negative bacilli	≤16/2	32/2–64/2	≥128/2	≥20	15–19	≤14
Staphylococci	≤8/2		≥16/2	≥23		≤22
Cephalosporins						
Cefaclor	≤8	16	≥32	≥18	15–17	≤14
Cefamandole	≤8	16	≥32	≥18	15–17	≤14
Cefazolin						
Enterobacteriaceae	≤1	2	≥4			
Other organisms	≤8	16	≥32	≥18	15–17	≤14
Cefepime	≤8	16	≥32	≥18	15–17	≤14
Cefetamet	≤4	8	≥16	≥18	15–17	≤14
Cefixime	≤1	2	≥4	≥19	16–18	≤15
Cefmetazole	≤16	32	≥64	≥16	13–15	≤12
Cefonicid	≤8	16	≥32	≥18	15–17	≤14
Cefoperazone	≤16	32	≥64	≥21	16–20	≤15
Cefotaxime						
Enterobacteriaceae	≤1	2	≥4	≥26	23–25	≤22
Other organisms	≤8	16–32	≥64	≥23	15–22	≤14
Cefotetan	≤16	32	≥64	≥16	13–15	≤12
Cefoxitin	≤8	16	≥32	≥18	15–17	≤14

(Continued on next page)

TABLE 3 *(Continued)*

Antimicrobial agent and organism	MIC (μg/ml)			Zone diam (mm)		
	Susceptible	Intermediate	Resistant	Susceptible	Intermediate	Resistant
Cefpodoxime	≤2	4	≥8	≥21	18–20	≤17
Cefprozil	≤8	16	≥32	≥18	15–17	≤14
Ceftazidime						
Enterobacteriaceae	≤4	8	≥16	≥21	18–20	≤17
Other organisms	≤8	16	≥32	≥18	15–17	≤14
Ceftibuten	≤8	16	≥32	≥21	18–20	≤17
Ceftizoxime						
Enterobacteriaceae	≤1	2	≥4	≥25	22–24	≤21
Other organisms	≤8	16–32	≥64	≥20	15–19	≤14
Ceftriaxone						
Enterobacteriaceae	≤1	2	≥4	≥23	20–22	≤19
Other organisms	≤8	16–32	≥64	≥21	14–20	≤13
Cefuroxime axetil	≤4	8–16	≥32	≥23	15–22	≤14
Cefuroxime sodium	≤8	16	≥32	≥18	15–17	≤14
Cephalothin	≤8	16	≥32	≥18	15–17	≤14
Loracarbef	≤8	16	≥32	≥18	15–17	≤14
Moxalactam	≤8	16–32	≥64	≥23	15–22	≤14
Other β-lactams						
Aztreonam						
Enterobacteriaceae	≤4	8	≥16	≥21	18–20	≤17
Other organisms	≤8	16	≥32	≥22	16–21	≤15
Ertapenem	≤2	4	≥8	≥19	14–18	≤15
Imipenem	≤4	8	≥16	≥16	14–15	≤13
Meropenem	≤4	8	≥16	≥16	14–15	≤13
Doripenem[f]						
Enterobacteriaceae	≤0.5			≥23		
Acinetobacter spp.	≤1			≥17		
P. aeruginosa	≤2			≥24		
Streptococci	≤1			≥24		
Aminoglycosides						
Amikacin	≤16	32	≥64	≥17	15–16	≤14
Gentamicin	≤4	8	≥16	≥15	13–14	≤12
Enterococci (high-level resistance)	≤500		≥500	≥10	7–9	6
Netilmicin	≤8	16	≥32	≥15	13–14	≤12
Tobramycin	≤4	8	≥16	≥15	13–14	≤12
Streptomycin						
Enterococci (high-level resistance)						
Broth microdilution method	≤1,000		≥1,000			
Agar-based method	≤2,000		≥2,000	≥10	7–9	6
Glycopeptides						
Teicoplanin	≤8	16	≥32	≥14	11–13	≤10
Telavancin[f]						
Streptococci	≤0.12			≥15		
Other organisms	≤1			≥15		
Vancomycin						
Enterococci	≤4	8–16	≥32	≥17	15–16	≤14
S. aureus	≤2	4–8	≥16	≥15		
Coagulase-negative staphylococci	≤4	8–16	≥32	≥15		
Lipopeptide						
Daptomycin						
Enterococci	≤4					
Staphylococci	≤1					
Macrolides						
Azithromycin	≤2	4	≥8	≥18	14–17	≤13
Clarithromycin	≤2	4	≥8	≥18	14–17	≤13
Dirithromycin	≤2	4	≥8	≥19	16–18	≤15
Erythromycin	≤0.5	1–4	≥8	≥23	14–22	≤13

(Continued on next page)

TABLE 3 Interpretive standards for dilution and disk diffusion susceptibility testing (*Continued*)

Antimicrobial agent and organism	MIC (μg/ml)			Zone diam (mm)		
	Susceptible	Intermediate	Resistant	Susceptible	Intermediate	Resistant
Ketolide						
Telithromycin	≤1	2	≥4	≥22	17–21	≤18
Quinolones						
Ciprofloxacin	≤1	2	≥4	≥21	16–20	≤15
Enoxacin	≤2	4	≥8	≥18	15–17	≤14
Fleroxacin	≤2	4	≥8	≥19	16–18	≤15
Gatifloxacin						
Staphylococci	≤0.5	1	≥2	≥23	20–22	≤19
Other organisms	≤2	4	≥8	≥18	15–17	≤14
Levofloxacin						
Staphylococci	≤1	2	≥4	≥19	16–18	≤15
Other organisms	≤2	4	≥8	≥17	14–16	≤13
Lomefloxacin	≤2	4	≥8	≥22	19–21	≤18
Moxifloxacin	≤0.5	1	≥2	≥24	19–23	≤20
Nalidixic acid[e]	≤8	16	≥32	≥19	14–18	≤13
Norfloxacin[e]	≤4	8	≥16	≥17	13–16	≤12
Ofloxacin						
Staphylococci	≤1	2	≥4	≥18	15–17	≤14
Other organisms	≤2	4	≥8	≥16	13–15	≤12
Sparfloxacin	≤0.5	1	≥2	≥19	16–18	≤15
Tetracyclines						
Doxycycline	≤4	8	≥16	≥16	13–15	≤12
Minocycline	≤4	8	≥16	≥19	15–18	≤14
Tetracycline	≤4	8	≥16	≥19	15–18	≤14
Other						
Chloramphenicol	≤8	16	≥32	≥18	13–17	≤12
Clindamycin	≤0.5	1–2	≥4	≥21	15–20	≤14
Colistin	≤2		≥4			
Fosfomycin	≤64	128	≥256	≥16	13–15	≤12
Linezolid						
Enterococci	≤2	4	≥8	≥23	19–22	≤20
Staphylococci	≤2			≥21		
Nitrofurantoin	≤32	64	≥128	≥17	15–16	≤14
Polymyxin	≤2		≥4			
Quinupristin-dalfopristin	≤1	2	≥4	≥19	16–18	≤15
Rifampin	≤1	2	≥4	≥20	17–19	≤16
Sulfonamide	≤256		≥512	≥17	13–16	≤12
Trimethoprim[e]	≤8		≥16	≥16	11–15	≤10
Trimethoprim-sulfamethoxazole	≤2/38		≥4/76	≥16	11–15	≤10
Tigecycline[f]						
Enterobacteriaceae	≤2	4	≥8	≥19	15–18	≤14
Streptococci	≤0.25			≥19		
S. aureus	≤0.5			≥19		

[a]Adapted from CLSI data (22) with permission. The interpretive data are valid only if the methodologies in documents M2-A10 (21) and M7-A8 (20) are followed. Breakpoints for some agents apply only to certain genera or species. The CLSI frequently updates the interpretive tables through new editions of the standards and supplements to them. Users should refer to the most recent editions. The current standards and supplements to them may be obtained from the CLSI, 940 West Valley Rd., Suite 1400, Wayne, PA 19087-1898.

[b]Penicillin should be used as the class representative for all penicillins (e.g., ampicillin, amoxicillin, mezlocillin, piperacillin, and ticarcillin). Isolates for which MICs are ≤0.03 μg of penicillin per ml generally do not produce β-lactamase, whereas those for which MICs are ≥0.25 μg/ml do and should be regarded as resistant to penicillins. Isolates for which MICs of penicillin are 0.06 or 0.12 μg/ml should be tested for β-lactamase.

[c]Therapy for serious enterococcal infections requires high doses of penicillin or ampicillin in combination with an aminoglycoside. Vancomycin may be substituted for the penicillin in instances of penicillin hypersensitivity or of penicillin or ampicillin resistance.

[d]Oxacillin or methicillin may be tested; however, oxacillin is preferred because of its greater stability in vitro. The results from the testing of oxacillin apply also to other penicillinase-resistant penicillins. Oxacillin-resistant staphylococci should be considered resistant to all penicillins, cephalosporins (except cephalosporins with anti-MRSA activity), carbacephems, carbapenems, and β-lactam–β-lactamase inhibitor combinations. Disk testing with cefoxitin is the most sensitive and specific method for phenotypic detection of *mecA*-mediated oxacillin resistance in staphylococci (22, 72).

[e]For the treatment of urinary tract infections only.

[f]Interpretive criteria are from the Food and Drug Administration drug label.

agents (20). Some manufacturers provide Mueller-Hinton broth that already has appropriate concentrations of divalent cations, so the cation content of commercial dehydrated media must be ascertained and care must be taken to supplement only those commercial broths that have not already been adjusted. If adjustment is necessary, it can be accomplished by the addition of suitable volumes of filter-sterilized, chilled $CaCl_2$ stock (3.68 g of $CaCl_2 \cdot 2H_2O$ dissolved in 100 ml of deionized water for a concentration of 10 mg of Ca^{2+} per ml) and $MgCl_2$ stock (8.36 g of $MgCl_2 \cdot 6H_2O$ in 100 ml of deionized water for a concentration of 10 mg of Mg^{2+} per ml) to the cooled broth (20). Insufficient cation concentrations result in increased aminoglycoside activity (27), and excess cation content results in decreased aminoglycoside activity against *P. aeruginosa* (27, 79). While the effects of inappropriate calcium and magnesium ion contents are well recognized, other ions, including zinc and manganese, may adversely affect the activities of some drugs, e.g., carbapenems (26). The CLSI has initiated a consensus standard for manufacturers of Mueller-Hinton broth that attempts to specify all known factors that determine performance of the medium (24). Other supplements to CAMHB may be required for accurate susceptibility results with specific agents. For example, accurate daptomycin testing requires a calcium supplement so that the final concentration is 50 mg/liter (20, 37), and detection of staphylococcal resistance to oxacillin requires that the CAMHB be supplemented with 2% NaCl (20, 76). Accurate susceptibility testing of tigecycline requires that the CAMHB be prepared fresh on the day of testing or frozen within 12 h of preparation (22).

To minimize evaporation and deterioration of antimicrobial agents, tubes should be tightly capped and stored at 4 to 8°C until needed. With most agents, the dilutions should be used within 5 days of preparation or as long as quality control ranges are maintained (see "Quality Control" below). As in agar dilution testing, certain β-lactam agents are too labile for prolonged storage at final test concentrations.

Inoculation Procedures

The recommended final inoculum for broth dilution testing is 5×10^5 CFU/ml. Isolates are inoculated into a broth that will support good growth (such as tryptic soy broth) and incubated until turbid. The turbidity is adjusted to match that of a 0.5 McFarland standard (approximately 10^8 CFU/ml). Alternatively, four or five colonies from overnight growth cultures on a nonselective agar plate may be directly suspended in broth to match the turbidity of the 0.5 McFarland standard (20). This alternative approach is preferred for testing of oxacillin against staphylococci (20). A portion of the standardized suspension is diluted approximately 1:100 (to 10^6 CFU/ml) with broth or saline. When 1 ml of this dilution is added to each tube containing 1 ml of the drug diluted in CAMHB, a final inoculum of 5×10^5 CFU/ml is achieved. Broth not containing an antimicrobial agent is inoculated as a control for organism viability (growth control). All tubes should be inoculated within 30 min of inoculum preparation, and an aliquot of the inoculum should be plated to check for purity.

Incubation

Tubes are incubated in ambient air at 35°C for 16 to 20 h before MICs are determined. Incubation should be extended to a full 24 h for the detection of vancomycin-resistant enterococci and oxacillin-resistant or vancomycin-resistant or -intermediate staphylococci (20). An atmosphere with increased CO_2 should not be used.

Interpretation and Reporting of Results

Before MICs for the test strains are read and recorded, the growth controls should be examined for viability, inoculum subcultures should be checked for contamination, and appropriate MICs for the quality control strains should be confirmed (see "Quality Control" below). Growth or lack thereof in the antimicrobial-agent-containing tubes is best determined by comparison with the growth control. Generally, growth is indicated by turbidity, a single sedimented button >2 mm in diameter, or several buttons with smaller diameters. As with the agar method, trailing endpoints may be seen when trimethoprim or sulfonamides are tested, and the concentration at which 80% or greater diminution of growth, compared with that of the growth control, occurs should be recorded as the MIC (20). Other interpretation problems include the "skipped tube" phenomenon, in which growth is not observed at one concentration but is observed at lower and higher drug concentrations. Most authorities suggest that when this occurs, the skipped tube should be ignored and the concentration that finally inhibits growth at serially higher concentrations should be recorded as the MIC. If more than one skipped tube occurs or if there is growth at higher antimicrobial concentrations but not at lower ones, the results should not be reported and the test for that drug should be repeated.

The lowest concentration that completely inhibits visible growth of the organism as detected by the unaided eye is recorded as the MIC. The CLSI MIC interpretive standards in effect as of the date of this writing (22) for the susceptibility categories are provided in Table 3. The definitions of and comments concerning these categories that were given for the agar method also pertain to the broth macrodilution method.

Advantages and Disadvantages

The broth macrodilution method is a well-standardized and reliable method that may be useful for research purposes or for testing of one drug with a bacterial isolate. However, because of the laborious nature of the procedure and the availability of more convenient dilution systems (e.g., microdilution), this procedure is generally not practical for routine susceptibility testing in most clinical microbiology laboratories.

Broth Microdilution Method

The convenience afforded by the availability of dilution susceptibility testing in microdilution trays has led to the widespread use of broth microdilution methods. In fact, the broth microdilution method is now considered the international reference susceptibility testing method (43). The disposable plastic trays, containing a panel of several antimicrobial agents to be tested simultaneously, may be prepared in-house or obtained commercially either frozen or freeze-dried. When commercial systems are used, the manufacturer's recommendations concerning storage, inoculation, incubation, and interpretation should be followed. The primary focus of this section is the in-house preparation and use of broth microdilution panels. However, most of the principles and practices discussed here are pertinent to the broth microdilution method regardless of the source of the antibiotic panels.

Dilution of Antimicrobial Agents

Antimicrobial stock solutions are prepared as outlined in the CLSI document on dilution testing (20). The dilution scheme for preparing broth microdilution panels is the same as that described for agar and broth macrodilution methods. Automated dispensing systems for preparation of microdilution panels use tubes that contain from 10 to 200 ml or more of broth containing each antimicrobial concentration. From the master tube dilutions, aliquots of 0.05 or 0.1 ml are simultaneously dispensed into the corresponding wells of each broth microdilution tray by using a mechanized dispenser. If 0.05-ml volumes are dispensed, allowances must be made for the 1:2 dilution of the final drug concentration that will occur when the 0.05 ml of inoculum is added (see "Inoculation Procedures" below). When 0.1-ml aliquots are dispensed, the volume of inoculum normally used is sufficiently small ($\leq$0.005 ml) that adjustments in the antimicrobial dilution scheme are not needed. As a general rule, when the inoculum volume is less than 10% of the broth volume in the well, dilution of the antimicrobial concentration by the inoculum does not have to be taken into account (20).

Preparation, Supplementation, and Storage of Media

CAMHB is the recommended medium for broth microdilution testing of nonfastidious organisms and should be prepared as discussed above for the broth macrodilution method. Also, supplementation of the broth with 2% NaCl is required for detection of oxacillin-resistant staphylococci, and daptomycin testing requires that the broth be adjusted to 50 mM Ca^{2+} (20). After the antimicrobial dilutions have been dispensed into the plastic trays, the panels are stacked in groups of 5 to 10, with a tray lid or an empty tray placed on top to minimize contamination and evaporation. Each stack is sealed in a plastic bag and frozen immediately, preferably at $-60°C$ or colder, or at $-20°C$ if a $-60°C$ freezer is not available. At $-20°C$, preservation is ensured for at least 6 weeks with most drugs, but the shelf life may be extended to months if the trays are stored at -60 to $-70°C$. Care must be taken in storing highly labile compounds such as cefaclor, clavulanic acid, and carbapenems, which may lose potency during storage. Trays with these agents should not be stored at temperatures above $-60°C$. If thawed, panels must be used or discarded but not refrozen, since freeze-thaw cycles cause substantial deterioration of β-lactam antibiotics. For this reason, $-20°C$ household-type freezers with self-defrosting units must not be used.

Inoculation Procedures

As with the macrodilution procedure, the final desired inoculum concentration is 5×10^5 CFU/ml. The isolates may be grown in broth to match the turbidity of a 0.5 McFarland standard (ca. 1×10^8 to 2×10^8 CFU/ml), or a suspension of that density can be made from colonies grown overnight on a nonselective agar medium (5), which is the method preferred for detecting oxacillin-resistant staphylococci (20). For broth microdilution procedures that require 0.001- to 0.005-ml volumes to inoculate wells containing 0.1 ml of broth, a portion of the 0.5 McFarland standard suspension is diluted 1:10 (10^7 CFU/ml) in sterile saline or broth. Multipoint metal or disposable plastic inoculum replicators designed to collect and deliver appropriate volumes are used to transfer the inoculum from the diluted suspension to the wells of the broth microdilution tray, resulting in further dilutions ranging from 1:20 to 1:50. Final inoculum concentrations should be 4×10^5 to 6×10^5 CFU/ml (4×10^4 to 6×10^4 CFU per well). For protocols that use an inoculum volume of 0.05 ml to inoculate 0.05 ml of broth, a 1:100 dilution of a 0.5 McFarland standard suspension (ca. 10^6 CFU/ml) is used. When the inoculum is added to the wells, the 1:2 dilution of the 10^6-CFU/ml inoculum results in a final inoculum concentration of 5×10^5 CFU/ml (5×10^4 CFU per well) and also halves the antimicrobial concentration in each well. Special care should be taken to confirm the inoculum density on a periodic basis to ensure that the appropriate density of inoculum is achieved. Moreover, slight deviations from the initial

1:10 dilution described above may be necessary to provide the target inoculum density with some species or organism groups. Insufficient inoculum can be a significant problem with the inducible resistance mechanisms of some organisms (such as β-lactamases), which may not be recognized as a problem based on the MICs obtained for the very susceptible quality control strains.

Broth microdilution trays should be inoculated within 30 min of inoculum preparation, and an aliquot should be subcultured to check the purity of the isolates. Finally, one well of each panel not containing an antimicrobial agent should be inoculated and used as a growth control, and a second uninoculated well serves as a sterility control.

Incubation

After inoculation, each tray should be covered with plastic tape or sealing film, sealed in a plastic bag, or tightly fitted with a lid or an empty tray to prevent evaporation during incubation. Trays are incubated in ambient air at 35°C for 16 to 20 h before results are read and should not be incubated in stacks of more than four trays for uniform temperature distribution. The incubator should be kept sufficiently humid to avoid evaporation but not so humid that condensation results in contamination problems. A full 24 h of incubation is recommended for the detection of vancomycin-resistant enterococci and oxacillin-resistant or vancomycin-resistant or -intermediate staphylococci (20). Incubation in an atmosphere with increased CO_2 should not be used with nonfastidious organisms.

Interpretation and Reporting of Results

Before MICs for the clinical isolates are read and recorded, the growth control wells should be examined for organism viability and the inoculum purity should be checked. The appropriateness of the MICs obtained for the quality control strains should be confirmed if tests of these strains were set up simultaneously with those of clinical isolates (see "Quality Control" below). Various viewing devices are available and should be used to facilitate examination of the broth microdilution wells for growth. The simplest and most reliable method is the use of a parabolic magnifying mirror and tray stand that allow clear visual inspection of the undersides of the microdilution trays. Growth is best determined by comparison with that in the growth control well and generally is indicated by turbidity throughout the well or by buttons, single or multiple, in the well bottom. The occurrence of trailing endpoints with trimethoprim or sulfonamides should be ignored, and the MIC endpoint should be based on $\geq$80% growth inhibition. Results for drugs with more than one skipped well should not be reported, as with the broth macrodilution test.

The CLSI MIC interpretive criteria (22) for susceptibility categories are given in Table 3. It should be noted that these values are published each year, and only the most recent tables should be used for interpretation of results. The definitions of the interpretive categories and the comments concerning the use of these standards for agar and broth macrodilution methods are also applicable to broth microdilution methods.

Advantages and Disadvantages

Broth microdilution is a well-standardized reference method for antimicrobial susceptibility testing. Inoculation and reading procedures allow convenient simultaneous testing of multiple antimicrobial agents with individual isolates. Because few laboratories have the facilities required for preparation of broth microdilution trays, several sources of commercially prepared antimicrobial agent panels are available. Such products provide either frozen or freeze-dried trays with wells containing prepared antimicrobial dilutions. Frozen trays must be stored at least at −20°C in the laboratory, whereas dried panels can be stored at room temperature. Most of these products are accompanied by multipoint inoculating devices; however, the trays may be inoculated with multichannel pipettors. Results of testing may be determined by visual examination or by use of semiautomated or automated instrumentation.

Breakpoint Susceptibility Tests

"Breakpoint susceptibility testing" refers to methods by which antimicrobial agents are tested only at the specific concentrations necessary for differentiating among the interpretive categories of susceptible, intermediate, and resistant rather than in a range of five or more doubling-dilution concentrations used to determine MICs. When two drug concentrations are selected adjacent to the breakpoints defining the intermediate and resistant categories, any one of the interpretive categories may be determined. Growth at both concentrations indicates resistance, growth at only the lower concentration signifies an intermediate result, and no growth at either concentration indicates susceptibility.

Like full-range dilution testing, breakpoint methods require the use of appropriately adjusted and supplemented Mueller-Hinton broth or agar. In addition, the standard inoculation, incubation, and interpretation procedures recommended for the full-range dilution methods should be followed.

Considering the limited range of drug concentrations tested, a greater number and variety of antimicrobial agents can be incorporated into a broth microdilution panel for breakpoint testing than into panels designed for full-range dilution testing (32). However, convenient quality control procedures to ensure that appropriate concentrations of each antimicrobial agent are present are lacking for breakpoint panels. One possible approach is to use one organism for which the modal MIC is equal to or no less than one doubling dilution less than the lower or lowest concentration tested and a second organism for which the modal MIC is equal to or no more than one doubling dilution greater than the higher or highest concentration tested (20). One of these two quality control organisms should provide on-scale results (20). Despite the theoretical soundness of this approach, routine quality control of breakpoint panels is difficult and not readily accomplished in the clinical laboratory.

Resistance Screens

In some circumstances, testing a single drug concentration may be a reliable and convenient method for detecting antimicrobial resistance. The most clinically useful resistance screens are those for resistance to oxacillin in *S. aureus*, resistance to vancomycin in *Enterococcus* spp. and *Staphylococcus* spp., and high-level resistance to gentamicin and streptomycin in enterococci (20). These practical and reliable methods are described in chapter 74 of this *Manual*.

Gradient Diffusion Method

The Etest (AB Biodisk, bioMérieux) and the M.I.C.Evaluator (Oxoid) are commercial methods for quantitative antimicrobial susceptibility testing that incorporate a preformed antimicrobial gradient applied to one side of a plastic strip to provide drug diffusion into an agar medium. Each test is performed in a manner similar to that for disk diffusion testing, in that a 0.5 McFarland standard suspension of a test isolate is generally swabbed onto the agar surface for inoculation. Following incubation, the MIC is read directly from a scale on the top of the strip at the point where the ellipse of organism growth inhibition intercepts the strip. Several strips, each containing a different antimicrobial

agent, can be placed radially on the surface of a large round Mueller-Hinton agar plate, or they can be placed in opposing directions on large rectangular plates. MICs determined by this method generally agree well with MICs generated by standard broth or agar dilution methods (4, 41, 63). The Etest and M.I.C.Evaluator combine the simplicity and flexibility of the disk diffusion test with the ability to determine MICs of up to five antimicrobial agents on a single 150-mm agar plate. However, both agar gradient diffusion strips are much more expensive than the paper disks used for diffusion testing. Strengths of these methods include the simplicity of the procedure itself and the ability to determine the MIC of an infrequently tested drug and to test fastidious or anaerobic bacteria by applying the strips onto specialized enriched media (see chapters 71 and 72 of this *Manual*).

QUALITY CONTROL

Quality control recommendations are designed for evaluation of the precision and accuracy of test procedures, monitoring of reagent performance, and evaluation of the performance of the individuals who are conducting the tests.

Reference Strains

A critical element of quality control is the selection and use of reference bacterial strains that are genetically stable and for which MICs are in the mid-range of MICs of each antimicrobial agent tested (20). That is, the dilutions in a series should ideally encompass at least two concentration increments above and below the previously established MIC for the reference strain. If there are four or fewer dilutions in a series or if nonconsecutive dilutions are tested (e.g., in breakpoint susceptibility testing), quality control for the correct interpretive category only rather than actual MIC ranges may be accomplished. *Escherichia coli* ATCC 25922, *P. aeruginosa* ATCC 27853, *Enterococcus faecalis* ATCC 29212, and *S. aureus* ATCC 29213 are the recommended reference strains for both agar and broth dilution methods (20). The β-lactamase-producing strain *E. coli* ATCC 35218 is recommended only for penicillin–β-lactamase inhibitor combinations (20). These organisms may be obtained from the American Type Culture Collection or other reliable commercial sources. For proper storage and subculture procedures, the recommendations of either the CLSI (20) or the commercial provider should be followed.

MIC Ranges

The acceptable quality control MIC ranges for the various reference strains are given in the CLSI document on dilution testing (20). Updates of these MIC ranges are published annually (22) and should be readily available in each clinical laboratory. An out-of-control result is defined as an MIC not within the acceptable range of values. Certain out-of-control results can be directly related to the medium used for testing. High MICs of gentamicin for *P. aeruginosa* ATCC 27853 suggest an inappropriately high divalent cation content or excessively low pH of the Mueller-Hinton medium, and low MICs indicate an insufficient divalent cation concentration or elevated pH. Although trimethoprim-sulfamethoxazole is not recommended for therapy of *Enterococcus faecalis* infections, results obtained with the ATCC 29212 strain can be useful for detecting excessive amounts of substances such as thymidine in the testing medium that interfere with the in vitro activity of antifolate drugs. Trimethoprim-sulfamethoxazole MICs of >0.5 to 9.5 μg/ml indicate the presence of such interfering substances (20).

Batch and Lot Quality Control

Representative plates, panels, or trays from each new reagent batch, if prepared in-house, or from each new lot, if obtained from a commercial source, should be subjected to quality control and sterility testing. Antimicrobial agent MICs obtained by testing reference quality control strains should be within acceptable CLSI ranges (22). If such accuracy is not achieved, the batch or lot should be rejected or patient results obtained with the antimicrobial agent(s) in question should not be reported (see below). Similarly, if selected uninoculated plates or trays fail the sterility check after incubation, the batch or lot should be rejected. In addition to these formal quality control procedures that use reference strains, careful review of susceptibility results obtained during daily testing of clinical isolates is important to identify unusual susceptibility patterns possibly indicative of reagent or technical problems.

Quality Control Frequency

In addition to batch and lot testing, quality control tests should be performed daily, or at least every day that the plates or trays are being used to test clinical isolates. When quality control is performed on each day of testing, performance is considered satisfactory if no more than 3 of 30 consecutive results for each drug-reference strain combination are outside the acceptable limits. If this frequency is exceeded, the laboratory must perform corrective action to determine the source of the error and to correct it as described below. However, if daily quality control testing does not reveal an excessive rate of errors, daily testing may be replaced by weekly testing as outlined below (20, 22).

To convert to a weekly quality control testing interval, each drug-reference strain combination is tested for 20 or 30 consecutive testing days to obtain a total of 20 to 30 MICs for each combination. If no more than 1 of 20 or 3 of 30 MICs per combination are outside the accuracy range, weekly testing may replace daily testing. During weekly testing, a single MIC outside the acceptable range requires that daily testing be performed for five consecutive days unless there is an obvious source of error (e.g., contamination, use of an incorrect reference strain or an incorrect inoculum density, testing of an incorrect antimicrobial agent, or use of an incorrect atmosphere for incubation). In such a circumstance, the quality control test need be repeated only once. If no obvious source of error is noted, but all five MICs for a problem drug-organism combination are within the accuracy range, weekly testing may be resumed. If one or more of the five MICs for the problem drug-organism combination are outside the accuracy range, daily testing must be initiated and further means to resolve the problem must be pursued. Returning to weekly testing requires again documenting 20 or 30 consecutive days with no more than one to three MICs outside the accuracy range. If more than the acceptable number of MICs for organism-drug combinations are outside the accuracy range, daily quality control testing must be continued while the problem is being resolved (20, 22).

DISK DIFFUSION TESTING

The disk diffusion method of susceptibility testing allows categorization of most bacterial isolates as susceptible, intermediate, or resistant to a variety of antimicrobial agents. To perform the test, commercially prepared filter paper disks impregnated with a specified single concentration of an antimicrobial agent are applied to the surface of an agar medium that has been inoculated with the test organism. The drug in the disk diffuses through the agar. As the distance from the disk increases, the concentration of the antimicrobial agent decreases logarithmically, creating a gradient of drug concentrations in the agar medium surrounding each disk. Concomitant with the diffusion of the drug, the bacteria that were inoculated onto the surface and were not inhibited by the concentration of the antimicrobial agent in the agar continue to multiply until a lawn of growth is visible. In areas where the concentration of the drug is inhibitory, no growth occurs, forming a zone of inhibition around each disk.

The disk diffusion procedure has been standardized primarily for testing common, rapidly growing bacteria (7, 21). This method should not be used to evaluate antimicrobial susceptibilities of bacteria that show marked strain-to-strain variability in growth rates, e.g., some fastidious or anaerobic bacteria. The test, however, has been modified to allow reliable testing of certain fastidious bacterial species (discussed in chapter 75 of this *Manual*).

The diameter of the zone of inhibition is influenced by the rate of diffusion of the antimicrobial agent through the agar, which may vary among different drugs depending upon the size of the drug molecule and its hydrophilicity. The zone size, however, is inversely proportional to the logarithm of the MIC, measured as discussed earlier in this chapter. Criteria currently recommended for interpreting zone diameters and MIC results for commonly used antimicrobial agents are listed in Table 3 and published annually by the CLSI (22).

Establishing Zone-of-Inhibition Diameter Interpretive Criteria

The first step in determining interpretive criteria for the disk diffusion test is selection of MIC breakpoints that define susceptibility and resistance categories for each antimicrobial agent. Zone-of-inhibition diameters that correspond to these breakpoints are initially established by testing 300 or more bacterial isolates by both dilution and disk diffusion methods and correlating the diameters of the zones of inhibition with the MICs determined for each drug tested (18). Isolates tested should include not only those commonly encountered in clinical laboratories but also those with resistance mechanisms pertinent to the class of antimicrobial agent being tested (18). Organisms evaluated should be those most likely to be tested with the antimicrobial agent in question. The data from these studies are analyzed by preparing a scattergram of values (see the example in chapter 67). By convention, each MIC ($\log_2$ scale) is plotted on the *y* axis, and the corresponding zone-of-inhibition diameter (arithmetic scale) is plotted on the *x* axis. Regression analysis can be performed, and a straight regression line showing the best fit is drawn. From this line, an approximation of the MIC can be inferred from any zone diameter. For antimicrobial agents to which isolates are either susceptible or resistant and only infrequently intermediate, regression analysis is not valid. In such cases, the data are plotted as a scattergram and the interpretive standards are selected so as to allow optimal separation of resistant and susceptible populations (16, 18, 61). This approach, often called the error rate-bounded method, may also be employed to minimize interpretive errors that can ensue from strictly applying the linear regression formula to a data set (18).

Antimicrobial Agent Disks

The amounts of antimicrobial agents in the disks used for the disk diffusion method are standardized, and in the United States, only a single concentration for each drug is recommended (22). The optimal amount of an antimicrobial agent per disk is determined early in the development of a new drug by testing disks with several different drug contents that can be evaluated by using scattergrams and regression lines (18). The most desirable concentration of a drug per disk is that which produces a zone-of-inhibition diameter of at least 10 mm with resistant isolates and a zone diameter no larger than 30 mm with susceptible isolates.

Commercially prepared antimicrobial disks usually are supplied in separate containers, each with a desiccant. They must not be used beyond the specified expiration date and should be stored under refrigeration (2 to 8°C) or frozen in a non-frost-free freezer at −20°C or colder until needed. Disks containing a β-lactam agent should always be stored frozen to ensure that they retain their potency, although a small supply may be stored in the refrigerator for up to 1 week. Unopened disk containers should be removed from the refrigerator or freezer 1 to 2 h before use. This allows the disks to equilibrate to room temperature before the container is opened, thus minimizing the amount of condensation that will occur when warm air contacts the cold disks. A commercially available, mechanical disk-dispensing apparatus can be used and should be fitted with a tight cover, supplied with an adequate desiccant, stored in the refrigerator when not in use, and warmed to room temperature before being opened.

Agar Medium for Disk Diffusion

The recommended medium for disk diffusion testing in the United States is Mueller-Hinton agar (21). This unsupplemented medium has been selected by the CLSI for several reasons: (i) it demonstrates good batch-to-batch reproducibility for susceptibility testing; (ii) it is low in sulfonamide, trimethoprim, and tetracycline inhibitors; (iii) it supports the growth of most nonfastidious bacterial pathogens; and (iv) years of data and clinical experience regarding its performance have been accrued. Fastidious bacteria, such as *Haemophilus* species, *Neisseria gonorrhoeae*, *Neisseria meningitidis*, and streptococci, do not grow satisfactorily on unsupplemented Mueller-Hinton agar but can be tested by the disk method by using supplemented or modified test media as discussed in chapter 71 of this *Manual*.

Plates of Mueller-Hinton agar may be purchased, or the agar may be prepared from a commercially available dehydrated base according to the manufacturer's directions. If the agar is prepared, only formulations that have been tested according to, and have met acceptance limits recommended by, the CLSI should be used (23). The prepared medium is autoclaved and immediately placed in a 45 to 50°C water bath. When cool, it is poured into round plastic flat-bottomed petri dishes on a level surface to give a uniform depth of about 4 mm (60 to 70 ml of medium for 150-mm-diameter plates and 25 to 30 ml for 100-mm-diameter plates) and allowed to cool to room temperature. Agar deeper than 4 mm may cause false resistance results (excessively small zones), whereas agar less than 4 mm deep may be associated with excessively large zones and false susceptibility.

Each batch of Mueller-Hinton agar should be checked when the medium is prepared to ensure that the pH is between 7.2 and 7.4 at room temperature, which means that the pH must be measured after the medium has solidified. This can be done by allowing a small amount of agar to solidify around the tip of a pH electrode in a beaker or a cup, by macerating a sufficient amount of agar in neutral distilled water, or by using a properly calibrated surface electrode. A pH outside the range of 7.2 to 7.4 may adversely affect susceptibility test results. If the pH is too low, drugs such as the aminoglycosides, macrolides, and fluoroquinolones will appear to lose potency, whereas others (for example, the penicillins and tetracyclines) may appear to have excessive activity. The opposite effects are possible if the pH is too high.

Freshly prepared plates may be used the same day or stored in a refrigerator (2 to 8°C); if refrigerated, they should be wrapped in plastic to minimize evaporation. Just before use, if excess moisture is visible on the surface, plates should be placed in an incubator (35°C) or, with lids ajar, in a laminar-flow hood at room temperature until the moisture evaporates (usually 10 to 30 min). At the time that the medium is to be inoculated, no droplets of moisture should be visible on its surface or on the petri dish cover.

Various components of or supplements to Mueller-Hinton medium may affect susceptibility test results; therefore, appropriate quality control procedures (see "Quality Control" below) must be performed and zone diameters must be within acceptable limits. For example, media containing excessive amounts of thymidine or thymine can reverse the inhibitory effects of sulfonamides and trimethoprim, causing zones of growth inhibition to be smaller or less distinct. Organisms may therefore appear to be resistant to these drugs when in fact they are not. Variation in the concentrations of divalent cations, primarily calcium and magnesium, affects results of aminoglycoside and tetracycline tests with *P. aeruginosa* isolates (21). A cation content that is too high reduces zone sizes, whereas a cation content that is too low has the opposite effect. Sheep blood should not be added to Mueller-Hinton medium for testing of nonfastidious organisms, because the blood can significantly alter the zone diameters with several agents and bacterial species (12).

Inoculation Procedure

To ensure reproducibility of disk diffusion susceptibility test results, the inoculum must be standardized (7, 21). The inoculum may be prepared by the growth method or by direct suspension from colonies on the agar plate, as described above for dilution testing.

When trimethoprim-sulfamethoxazole is tested by the direct inoculum suspension method, colonies from blood agar medium may carry over enough trimethoprim or sulfonamide antagonists to produce a haze of growth inside the zones of inhibition with susceptible isolates.

The Mueller-Hinton agar plate should be inoculated within 15 min after the inoculum suspension has been adjusted. A sterile cotton swab is dipped into the suspension, rotated several times, and gently pressed onto the inside wall of the tube above the fluid level to remove excess inoculum from the swab. The swab is then streaked over the entire surface of the agar plate three times, with the plate rotated approximately 60° each time to ensure even distribution of the inoculum. A final sweep of the swab is made around the agar rim. The lid may be left ajar for 3 to 5 min but no longer than 15 min to allow any excess surface moisture to be absorbed before the drug-impregnated disks are applied.

Antimicrobial Disks

Within 15 min after the plates are inoculated, selected antimicrobial agent disks are distributed evenly onto the surface, with at least 24 mm (center to center) between them. Disks are placed individually with sterile forceps or, more commonly, with a mechanical dispensing apparatus and then gently pressed down onto the agar surface to provide uniform contact. No more than 12 disks should be placed onto one 150-mm-diameter plate and no more than 5 disks should be placed onto a 100-mm-diameter plate to avoid overlapping zones. Some of the antimicrobial agent in the disk diffuses almost immediately; therefore, once a disk contacts the agar surface, the disk should not be moved.

Incubation

No longer than 15 min after disks are applied, the plates are inverted and incubated at 35°C in ambient air. A delay of more than 15 min before incubation permits excess prediffusion of the antimicrobial agents. The interpretive standards for nonfastidious bacteria are based on results of test samples incubated in ambient air, and the zone-of-inhibition diameters for some drugs, such as the aminoglycosides, macrolides, and tetracyclines, are significantly altered by CO_2; therefore, plates should not be incubated in atmospheres with increased CO_2. Testing isolates of some fastidious bacteria, however, requires incubation in 5% CO_2, and zone diameter criteria for those species have been established on that basis (see chapter 71 of this *Manual*).

Interpretation and Reporting of Results

Each plate is examined after incubation for 16 to 18 h for all nonfastidious bacterial isolates except staphylococci and enterococci, which must be incubated for a full 24 h to allow detection of resistance to oxacillin and vancomycin, respectively (21). If plates are inoculated correctly, the diameters of the zones of inhibition are uniformly circular and the lawns of growth are confluent. Growth that consists of individual isolated colonies indicates that the inoculum was too light, and the test must be repeated. The diameters of the zones of complete inhibition, including the diameter of the disk, are measured to the nearest whole millimeter with calipers or a ruler. With unsupplemented Mueller-Hinton agar, the measuring device is held on the back of the inverted petri dish, which is illuminated with reflected light located a few inches above a black, nonreflecting background.

The zone margin is the area where no obvious growth is visible with the naked eye. When isolates of staphylococci or enterococci are tested, any discernible growth (especially a haze of pinpoint colonies) within the zone of inhibition around the oxacillin disk (for staphylococci) or vancomycin disk (for enterococci) is indicative of resistance. For other bacteria, discrete colonies growing within a clear zone of inhibition may indicate testing of a mixed culture that should be subcultured, reidentified, and retested. However, the presence of colonies within a zone of inhibition may also indicate selection of high-frequency mutants indicative of eventual resistance to that agent, e.g., *Enterobacter* spp. with penicillins and cephalosporins. With *Proteus* species, if a thin film of swarming growth is visible in an otherwise obvious zone of inhibition, the margin of heavy growth is measured and the film is disregarded. With trimethoprim, the sulfonamides, and combinations of the two agents, antagonists in the medium may allow some minimal growth; therefore, the zone diameter is measured at the obvious margin, and slight growth (20% or less of the lawn of growth) is disregarded.

The zone diameters measured around each disk are interpreted on the basis of guidelines published by the CLSI, and the organisms are reported as susceptible, intermediate, or resistant (or in some cases nonsusceptible when no resistance breakpoint has been defined) to the antimicrobial agents tested (Table 3) (22). The clinical interpretation of the categories of susceptible, intermediate, and resistant has already been provided above under "Dilution Testing." Computer programs are available that accompany some automated zone size reading devices to allow MICs to be derived from the linear regression equation with selected antimicrobial agents and bacterial isolates (11, 59) (see also chapter 69).

Advantages and Disadvantages

The disk diffusion test has several advantages: (i) it is technically simple to perform and very reproducible, (ii) the reagents are relatively inexpensive, (iii) it does not require any special equipment, (iv) it provides susceptibility category results that are easily understood by clinicians, and (v) it is flexible regarding selection of antimicrobial agents for testing. The primary limitation of the disk diffusion test is the spectrum of organisms for which it has been standardized. There have not been adequate studies to develop reliable interpretive standards for disk testing of bacteria not listed in the CLSI disk diffusion document (21) or the 2006 CLSI guideline for infrequently isolated or fastidious bacteria (19). It is also important to note that only certain drugs have been validated for disk diffusion testing of *Stenotrophomonas maltophilia* and *Burkholderia cepacia* (22). The disk test is inadequate for detection of vancomycin-intermediate *S. aureus* (21, 73, 74), does not detect daptomycin resistance in staphylococci and enterococci (39, 55) or colistin resistance in gram-negative bacilli (38), and in the past was reported to have difficulties in the detection of oxacillin-heteroresistant staphylococci (28) and enterococci with low-level (VanB-type) vancomycin resistance (66, 74). A potential disadvantage of disk diffusion susceptibility testing is that it provides only a qualitative result and a quantitative result indicating that the degree of susceptibility (MIC) may be needed in some cases, e.g., those involving penicillin and cephalosporin susceptibilities of *S. pneumoniae* and certain viridans group streptococci (see chapter 71 of this *Manual*).

Quality Control

The goals of a quality control program for disk diffusion are to monitor the precision and accuracy of the procedure, the performance of the reagents (medium and disks), and the performance of persons who do the testing and read, interpret, and report results. To best achieve these goals, reference strains are selected for their genetic stability and their usefulness in the disk diffusion test.

Reference Strains

Reference strains recommended by the CLSI for quality control of the disk diffusion procedure when nonfastidious bacteria are tested are *E. coli* ATCC 25922, *P. aeruginosa* ATCC 27853, *S. aureus* ATCC 25923 (not the same strain used for quality control of MIC tests), *Enterococcus faecalis* ATCC 29212, and *E. coli* ATCC 35218 (22, 25). *E. coli* ATCC 35218 is recommended as a control only for β-lactamase inhibitor combinations containing clavulanic acid, sulbactam, or tazobactam. *Enterococcus faecalis* ATCC 29212 can be used to ensure that the levels of inhibitors of trimethoprim or sulfonamides in Mueller-Hinton agar do not exceed acceptable limits and can also be used to control disks containing a high concentration of gentamicin or streptomycin (see chapter 70 of this *Manual*).

The reference strains listed above should be obtained from a reliable source, and stock cultures should be maintained in such a way that viability is ensured and the opportunity for selection of resistant variants is minimal (25). The procedures for maintaining and storing working stock cultures are described in the CLSI standard (21). If an unexplained result indicates that the inherent susceptibility of the strain has been altered, a fresh subculture of that organism should be obtained.

Zone-of-Inhibition Diameter Ranges

The ranges of zone diameters for reference strains used to monitor performance of the disk diffusion test are updated frequently and published annually; therefore, readers should refer to the most recent CLSI document for this information (22). Generally, results of 1 in every 20 tests in a series of tests might be out of the accepted limits. If a second result falls outside the stated limits, corrective action must be taken. The action taken and the results of that action must be documented.

Frequency of Testing

Each new batch or lot of Mueller-Hinton agar must be tested with the reference strains listed above before the medium is released for use with clinical specimens, and quality control must be done before a new lot of antimicrobial disks is introduced. Appropriate reference strains also should be tested each day that the disk diffusion test is performed. The frequency of testing, however, may be reduced if satisfactory performance is documented for 20 or 30 consecutive days of testing: for each combination of drug and reference strain, no more than 1 of 20 or 3 of 30 zone-of-inhibition diameters may be outside the accepted limits published by the CLSI (22). When this criterion is fulfilled, each reference strain need be tested only once per week and any time a reagent component of the test is changed. However, if the diameter of a zone of inhibition falls outside the acceptable control limits, corrective action must be taken. If the problem appears to be caused by an obvious error such as use of the wrong disk or the wrong reference strain, contamination of the reference strain, or incubation in an incorrect atmosphere, repeating the test with the appropriate parameter is acceptable. However, if a cause of the error is not obvious, quality control must be performed daily for a period that will allow discovery of the source of the aberrant result and documentation of how the problem was resolved. This may be accomplished by the approach described above under "Quality Control" after the section on dilution testing.

Special Disk Tests

Two specialized applications of the disk test are described in detail in chapter 70. In brief, disk testing with cefoxitin is now the preferred method for detection of *mecA*-mediated oxacillin resistance in both *S. aureus* and coagulase-negative staphylococcal species (21, 22, 72). Cefoxitin serves as a surrogate marker for the principal mechanism of oxacillin resistance in staphylococci and provides more reliable results than oxacillin itself. Secondly, inducible clindamycin resistance is not reliably detected by standard dilution or disk diffusion susceptibility testing without induction of the expression of *erm*-mediated macrolide-lincosamide-streptogramin B

resistance in staphylococci and hemolytic streptococci (54). Such strains can be accurately detected only by induction of resistance expression by exposure to a macrolide. A disk approximation test in which erythromycin and clindamycin disks are placed in close proximity allows recognition of inducible resistance by truncating the clindamycin zone and giving rise to a positive "D-zone test" (22, 36). When recognized through disk approximation testing, such strains should be reported as resistant to clindamycin (22, 54). A similar approach may be taken by incorporating a subinhibitory concentration of erythromycin into broth or agar dilution tests with clindamycin. Broth-based tests are available on several of the automated susceptibility testing systems.

ANTIBACTERIAL SUSCEPTIBILITY TESTING AND INTERPRETIVE METHODS USED OUTSIDE THE UNITED STATES

The CLSI is best known for developing laboratory testing standards for use in the United States, including those for antimicrobial susceptibility testing (20–22). The CLSI standards are recognized as U.S. national standards by the American National Standards Institute and by federal regulations, including the Clinical Laboratory Improvement Amendments (40), and as standard reference procedures by the Food and Drug Administration. However, the CLSI procedures are also used by an increasing number of laboratories outside the United States, including countries in North and South America and in several areas of Europe, Asia, and Australia. Some countries have national standards or professional committees comprising their own expert microbiologists that establish methods of susceptibility testing for their countries and interpretive criteria for those tests that may or may not be the same as those of the CLSI (15, 35), as described further in chapter 72.

Several variations on dilution and diffusion methods are used for routine susceptibility testing outside the United States (Table 4). Most non-U.S. methods are specific to individual countries, having developed and evolved locally over many years. Many of the non-U.S. methods differ from the CLSI procedures in the choice of media, inoculum preparation procedures, and, for diffusion methods, disk

TABLE 4 Non-U.S. disk diffusion methods for susceptibility testing

Method (reference)	Location	Society	Agar medium	Comments
EUCAST[a]	Europe	EUCAST/ ECDC/ EMEA	MH[c] and MH + 5% defibrinated horse blood and 20 mg of beta-NAD/liter	Published in 2009 on EUCAST website; correlates to European clinical breakpoints
BSAC Working Party on Susceptibility Testing (1)[b]	United Kingdom	BSAC	Iso-Sensitest	Very similar to the SRGA method. EUCAST clinical breakpoints.
CA-SFM (60)	France	CA-SFM	MH + semiconfluent inoculum	EUCAST clinical breakpoints
DIN (29, 30)	Germany	DIN	MH	EUCAST clinical breakpoints
SRGA (62, 65)	Sweden	SRGA	Iso-Sensitest	Very similar to the BSAC method. EUCAST clinical breakpoints.
Calibrated dichotomous sensitivity (9, 10)	Australia		Sensitest	Dichotomous (no intermediate category). Disk strengths chosen to give annular radius of inhibition of ~17 mm where possible.

[a]http://www.eucast.org.
[b]http://www.bsac.org.uk.
[c]MH, Mueller-Hinton agar.

contents. There are also some variations between these methods in breakpoints and the approaches to establishing the breakpoints (78). Variation in test methods can cause considerable confusion in laboratories, especially if both CLSI and non-CLSI methods are used for different organisms. Thus, it is important that any method be followed in all its detail for valid application of specific breakpoints.

There are continuing efforts to harmonize breakpoints internationally. In Europe, EUCAST has become a major force for developing and harmonizing methods and breakpoints for aerobic and facultative organisms. EUCAST has defined reference agar and broth microdilution MIC methods (http://www.eucast.org) for use in Europe (52) and is in the process of defining disk diffusion methods. The establishment of a global standard reference MIC susceptibility method (broth microdilution) developed through the International Organization for Standards (ISO; Geneva, Switzerland) (43) in concert with the European Committee on Standardization (Brussels, Belgium) has also occurred recently. The global reference method is in essence the CLSI and EUCAST broth microdilution methods with a few differences harmonized in the ISO standard (43). This will hopefully provide a degree of international standardization for reference MIC determinations and allow a benchmark for assessment of the performance of commercial devices for susceptibility testing. In a second document, the ISO has established criteria for acceptable performance of susceptibility testing devices (44).

International Dilution Methods

Both broth and agar dilution methods have been developed in multiple countries outside the United States. In the past, methods using a limited range of concentrations (often one or two), or so-called breakpoint methods, have been advocated (82). They are the standard form of susceptibility testing advocated by the Japanese Society for Chemotherapy (45, 46) and as an alternative to disk diffusion testing by the BSAC (2). Other MIC methods and standards include those of the BSAC (1) (see also http://www.bsac.org.uk), the Société Française de Microbiologie (CA-SFM; http://www.sfm.asso.fr), the Deutsches Institut für Normung (DIN; documents are available through http://www.beuth.de), and the Swedish Reference Group for Antibiotics (SRGA; http://www.srga.org).

Breakpoint MIC methods (or, more commonly, MIC methods with limited concentration ranges) are often used in larger laboratories because large numbers of isolates can be tested cost-effectively using replicators and the methods provide qualitative endpoints (i.e., susceptible, intermediate, and resistant). Optical readers are available to facilitate reading of agar dilution plates (e.g., Mastascanelite [Mast Laboratories, Bootle, United Kingdom]; see http://www.mastascan.com). However, there are considerable difficulties with quality control, including the lack of appropriate control strains for which the MICs are near the breakpoints, and the complexity of quantifying drug concentrations prior to use (58). In addition, problems have been reported in the past with the use of Iso-Sensitest agar (3, 77) and with the incorporation of inhibitors to prevent swarming of *Proteus* spp., such as *p*-nitrophenylglycerol (81), or increased agar content for the same purpose (80). In turn, the choice of Mueller-Hinton by the CLSI has been criticized for not providing luxuriant growth of all organisms (83), suggesting that there is no ideal medium. As the best-studied, most widely used medium for susceptibility testing, Mueller-Hinton broth was chosen for the ISO reference method (43) and is supported by EUCAST (see below).

International Diffusion Methods

A wide variety of diffusion methods have been developed in different countries over the years. They are quite diverse in their approaches. With the exception of the Danish method, which uses 9-mm tablets containing the antimicrobial agents, the international diffusion methods use disks similar to those suggested by the CLSI. Almost all have been maintained primarily because of the cost-effectiveness and flexibility of diffusion testing. Many, including CA-SFM and the newly developed EUCAST disk diffusion method (http://www.eucast.org), are similar to the modified Kirby-Bauer method (7) advocated by the CLSI (21). As pointed out above, disk methods are inexpensive and flexible and have become more popular with the use of automated zone readers and interconnected computers for interpretation of zone diameters (3, 59). Some of the automated readers also contain "expert" software for antibiogram interpretation.

The Stokes method, which had previously been recommended by the BSAC, differed from other diffusion methods in that susceptibility categorization was achieved by comparison with a control strain rather than by reference to a defined set of zone diameters (13). This technique attracted criticism because it was not based upon or derived from correlations with MICs (14) and has now been replaced by a correlated diffusion method (1), which is well developed and updated periodically (http://www.bsac.org.uk/susceptibility_testing.cfm). For the new BSAC method, Iso-Sensitest (Oxoid) is the recommended agar, supplemented for the growth of fastidious bacteria with whole defibrinated horse blood, with or without NAD. Mueller-Hinton agar supplemented with 5% sodium chloride is recommended for the detection of methicillin and oxacillin resistance in staphylococci. The inoculum is prepared to produce semiconfluent growth only, rather than the confluent lawn of growth as recommended in the CLSI method. One important change in the newer British method is the elimination of an intermediate category for most organism-antimicrobial agent combinations (57).

Since 1980, the CA-SFM has put considerable effort into standardization of susceptibility testing, including regular updates with breakpoints for new drugs that are published frequently (60) (see also http://www.sfm.asso.fr). Like the CLSI, the CA-SFM has selected Mueller-Hinton as the testing medium. For diffusion testing, plates can be inoculated by either flooding or swabbing with a standardized inoculum of cells. In most other aspects, this method resembles that of the CLSI, including the use of control organisms and the choice of disk strength. The CA-SFM provides zone diameter breakpoints for drugs available in France and elsewhere that are not approved for clinical use in the United States, e.g., fusidic acid and pristinamycin (60). The French breakpoints often differ from those advocated by the CLSI and place greater emphasis on the detection of emerging resistance. Thus, they are more likely to classify organisms as resistant (or nonsusceptible) than CLSI methods.

The German standards organization, the DIN, published methods for diffusion susceptibility testing as early as 1979, with intermittent updates since then (29, 30). They too use Mueller-Hinton agar but include the use of other media provided that the MIC-zone diameter relationships have been determined for those media. Like the CA-SFM method, the DIN method has much in common with the CLSI method.

The SRGA (62, 69) method uses Iso-Sensitest, and it is based on the methodology developed by the original

International Collaborative Study (33) that was the first to provide a sound theoretical basis to diffusion susceptibility testing. The breakpoints for susceptibility were restructured in 1981 into the more conventional susceptible, intermediate, and resistant categories (69) and were subsequently updated (65).

A method developed by a commercial firm in Denmark differs technically if not in principle from the other methods. As noted above, this method employs Neo-Sensitabs, which are compressed tablets 9 mm in diameter into which the antimicrobial agent has been incorporated (Rosco Diagnostica, Taarstrup, Denmark; http://www.rosco.dk). The method and the interpretive zone diameter criteria are updated and published by the manufacturer periodically. Not only are the tablets larger and thicker than conventional 6-mm-diameter paper disks, but also they usually contain larger amounts of the antimicrobial agent to be tested, resulting in significantly larger zones of inhibition with most drugs. This has the disadvantage of reducing the number of tablets that can be put on a single plate and still produce readable zones. However, the system does have the advantage that the tablets can be stored at room temperature for up to 4 years, eliminating the need for storage under refrigeration or freezing. This is an obvious benefit for laboratories in developing countries, where reliable refrigeration and power can be a problem.

The calibrated dichotomous sensitivity disk diffusion method, developed in Australia in 1975 (9, 10), is still widely used in that country and has a number of unique features. This method employs Sensitest agar and an unusual method for inoculum preparation and is unique in defining just two categories of susceptibility: susceptible and resistant. In order to simplify test result reading, each new drug is calibrated against the MIC breakpoint to yield, wherever possible, a zone diameter of 18 mm. This is achieved by adjusting disk strengths, which in most cases are substantially lower than those used with other methods. The lack of an intermediate category, which increases the risk of serious interpretive errors (e.g., susceptible instead of resistant), the absence of some common drugs from the test range, and some unusual use of surrogate drugs for testing have restricted the adoption of this method outside of Australia. The interpretive criteria are updated regularly and can be found on the Internet (http://www.med.unsw.edu.au/pathology-cds/).

EUCAST Breakpoints

Other than the CLSI, EUCAST is probably the most widely recognized breakpoint-setting organization. EUCAST is a standing committee of the European Society for Clinical Microbiology and Infectious Diseases (ESCMID) and the European Centre for Disease Prevention and Control (ECDC). It consists of two bodies: the EUCAST Steering Committee and the EUCAST General Committee. The General Committee includes representatives from the six national breakpoint committees of Europe, namely, France (CA-SFM), Germany (DIN), The Netherlands (Commissie Richtlijnen Gevoeligheidsbepalingen), Norway (Norwegian Working Group on Antibiotics), Sweden (SRGA), and the United Kingdom (BSAC), and representatives from each European country. Both the pharmaceutical industry and manufacturers of diagnostic systems can provide input into the consensus process of the EUCAST General Committee. The EUCAST Steering Committee, which includes representatives of the six national breakpoint committees, two national representatives of European countries, a chair, a scientific secretary, and a clinical data coordinator, develops

tentative breakpoints for new antimicrobial agents. The tentative breakpoints are then open for consultation with the EUCAST General Committee, industry, and experts outside Europe. Following a period of consultation, the Steering Committee issues a final decision on clinical breakpoints.

Process of Setting Epidemiological Cutoffs and Breakpoints

EUCAST takes a different approach to developing interpretive criteria for MICs and disk diffusion results than does the CLSI. EUCAST first establishes epidemiological cutoff values that define the wild-type MIC distribution for each target microorganism and antimicrobial agent (78). Once the wild-type population has been described (see http://www.eucast.org) and epidemiological cutoffs been decided, the wild-type distributions are categorized as susceptible, intermediate, or resistant, using pharmacokinetic/pharmacodynamic data and clinical data. The clinical breakpoints guide therapy, while the epidemiological cutoff values are valuable for sensitive and early detection of emerging resistance. The data are described on the EUCAST website (http://www.eucast.org) (Fig. 1).

The six national committees used to determine breakpoints for their respective countries, but since EUCAST serves as the official breakpoint committee for the European Medicine Evaluation Agency (EMEA), the national committees apply the EUCAST breakpoints into their national systems. An initial important role of EUCAST was to harmonize the different breakpoints (52), a process concluded during 2009. More recently, EUCAST has turned to harmonizing routine susceptibility testing methodology in Europe. A disk test based on Mueller-Hinton agar is being developed and will be available in 2010. The technical aspects of the European disk test are in most parts very similar to the CLSI method, but the media used for fastidious organisms and some of the disk drug concentrations are different.

COMMON SOURCES OF ERROR IN ANTIBACTERIAL SUSCEPTIBILITY TESTING

Potential sources of error in antibacterial susceptibility testing may be categorized as those that relate to the test system and its components, those associated with the test procedure, those peculiar to certain organism and drug combinations, and those that relate to reporting (17, 31, 53). The most common sources of error encountered in clinical microbiology laboratories are reviewed in the following paragraphs.

Various components of the susceptibility test system may be a source of error. First, the system itself may have limitations regarding the organisms that should be tested. For example, the disk diffusion method should be used only to test rapidly growing bacterial pathogens that have consistent growth rates (those for which interpretive criteria have been developed and published by the CLSI). Second, the medium used may be a source of error if it fails to conform to recommended composition and performance. Factors common to both agar-based and broth-based systems are the pH of the medium, which for Mueller-Hinton agar or broth should be between 7.2 and 7.4, and its cation content. The concentration of magnesium and calcium in the broth medium should be that recommended by the CLSI to ensure reliable results (20). For detection of oxacillin resistance in staphylococci by testing of oxacillin, it is essential that the proper amount of sodium chloride be included in the agar or broth used for dilution testing. For agar dilution and disk diffusion, the Mueller-Hinton agar should be 3 to

Ampicillin / Escherichia coli
EUCAST MIC Distribution - Reference Database 2011-01-06

MIC distributions include collated data from multiple sources, geographical areas and time periods and can never be used to infer rates of resistance

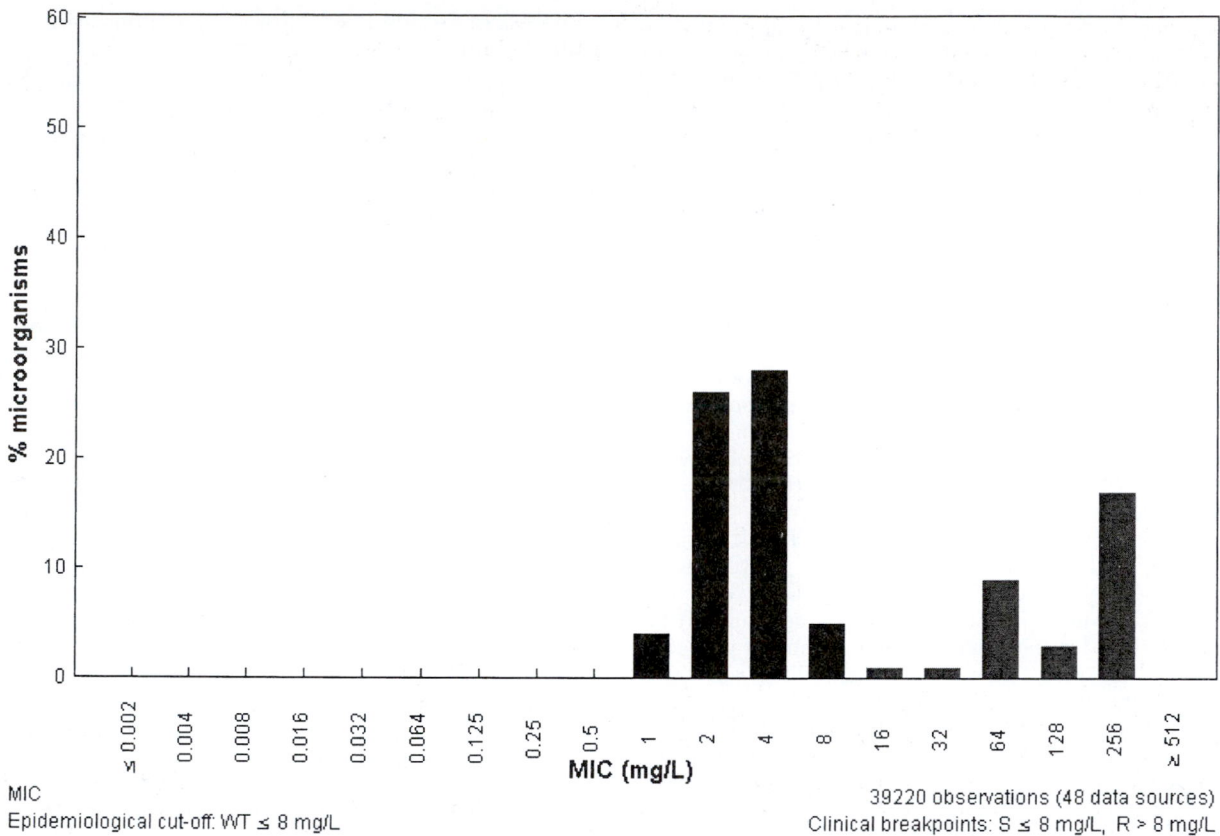

MIC
Epidemiological cut-off: WT ≤ 8 mg/L

39220 observations (48 data sources)
Clinical breakpoints: S ≤ 8 mg/L, R > 8 mg/L

FIGURE 1 Example of the wild-type (WT) MIC distribution data that are used by EUCAST to set the epidemiological cutoff.

4 mm deep (20, 21). Finally, the components of the system (antimicrobial disks, agar plates, and trays) must be stored properly, and they should not be used beyond the stated expiration dates.

Steps in the susceptibility test procedure that may be a source of error if they are not performed correctly include inoculum preparation, incubation (conditions and duration), endpoint interpretation, and performance of appropriate quality control. The inoculum must be pure, and it must contain an adequate density of bacteria. With rare exceptions, all systems should be incubated in ambient air at 35°C. The incubation time, however, varies. For conventional dilution and disk diffusion systems, incubation for 16 to 20 h and 16 to 18 h, respectively, is recommended except in tests of staphylococci with oxacillin and vancomycin (MIC only) and enterococci with vancomycin, in which systems must be incubated for a full 24 h (20, 21, 75). The endpoints for all susceptibility tests must be measured accurately, according to guidelines published by the CLSI (20, 21). If endpoints are interpreted by an instrument, the reliability of that instrument must be monitored and calibrated periodically. Moreover, with all susceptibility test systems, appropriate reference strains must be tested at regular intervals, any problems that occur must be thoroughly investigated, and corrective action must be well documented.

Testing of certain antimicrobial agents with some bacteria may yield misleading results, because in vitro results do not necessarily correlate with in vivo activity (see Table 5 in chapter 69). Examples include narrow- and expanded-spectrum cephalosporins and aminoglycosides tested with *Salmonella* spp. and *Shigella* spp.; all β-lactam agents except the penicillinase-resistant penicillins (oxacillin, nafcillin, methicillin, or cefoxitin as a surrogate marker) tested with oxacillin-resistant staphylococci; cephalosporins, aminoglycosides (except concentrations used to detect high-level resistance), clindamycin, and trimethoprim-sulfamethoxazole tested with enterococci; and cephalosporins tested with *Listeria* spp. (20–22). Therefore, for these combinations of organisms and drugs, results should not be reported. Other errors associated with reporting include possible transcriptional errors for laboratories that use a manual recording and reporting system and possible errors in transmission of data for laboratories in which an automated susceptibility test system is interfaced with the laboratory and/or hospital information system.

For several species of bacteria, resistance to a commonly tested antimicrobial agent is expected. For example, several species of *Enterobacteriaceae,* including *Klebsiella, Citrobacter,* and *Enterobacter* spp., among others, should test as ampicillin resistant (see Table 4 in chapter 69). Likewise,

Stenotrophomonas maltophilia should test as resistant to carbapenems, and *Pseudomonas aeruginosa* should test as resistant to trimethoprim-sulfamethoxazole. Generating susceptible results for any of these bacterial-antimicrobial combinations could indicate an error in antimicrobial susceptibility testing or bacterial identification, and the tests (including identification when necessary) should be repeated.

PROBLEM ORGANISMS AND RESISTANCE MECHANISMS

The dilution and diffusion methods described in this chapter have been developed through careful studies and standardized by national professional organizations and diagnostic device manufacturers. Despite this, there are still some organisms for which methods have not yet been standardized (e.g., corynebacteria and some fastidious bacteria in the case of disk testing) or which fail to provide reliable results with some of the standard tests (e.g., *Stenotrophomonas maltophilia* and *Burkholderia cepacia* in the case of disk diffusion testing of some drugs).

Other problems occur with detecting resistance mechanisms in isolates that may possess inducible resistance (e.g., VanB-type resistance in some enterococci or AmpC-type β-lactamases in some gram-negative species). Similarly, there are issues with detection of resistance mechanisms that result in subtle phenotypic expression under standard inoculum and test conditions (e.g., inducible clindamycin resistance in staphylococci and some streptococci or ESBL expression in some *Enterobacteriaceae*). Special methods to detect these resistance mechanisms are outlined in chapter 70. Controversy exists regarding the need to identify subtle resistance mechanisms, such as ESBLs, for making treatment decisions. For example, revised CLSI cephalosporin interpretive criteria that are consistent with recent pharmacokinetic and pharmacodynamic data and the most common dosing regimens may eliminate the need for ESBL confirmation before a treatment decision is made (22). Regardless of this controversy, there will always be a need to identify these problematic resistance traits for epidemiological purposes.

There has not previously been uniform agreement regarding what level of accuracy is acceptable when selecting a testing method or system for performing antimicrobial susceptibility testing (48). However, general guidelines for acceptable performance (e.g., rates of essential agreement and category agreement) now have been developed through an international consensus effort (ISO) (43). However, it is important to keep in mind that new resistance mechanisms or decreases in susceptibility to important therapeutic agents can arise at any time to challenge our methods of susceptibility testing, e.g., the emergence of carbapenemase-mediated resistance in *Enterobacteriaceae* (64). Thus, susceptibility testing methods must continue to evolve and develop over time as new challenges are presented.

REFERENCES

1. **Andrews, J. M., for the BSAC Working Party on Susceptibility Testing.** 2001. BSAC standardized disc susceptibility testing method. *J. Antimicrob. Chemother.* **48**(Suppl. 1):43–57.
2. **Andrews, J. M.** 2001. Determination of minimum inhibitory concentrations. *J. Antimicrob. Chemother.* **48**(Suppl. 1):5–16.
3. **Andrews, J. M., F. J. Boswell, and R. Wise.** 2000. Evaluation of the Oxoid Aura image system for measuring zones of inhibition with the disc diffusion technique. *J. Antimicrob. Chemother.* **46**:535–540.
4. **Baker, C. N., S. A. Stocker, D. H. Culver, and C. Thornsberry.** 1991. Comparison of the E Test to agar dilution, broth microdilution, and agar diffusion susceptibility testing techniques by using a special challenge set of bacteria. *J. Clin. Microbiol.* **29**:533–538.
5. **Barry, A. L., R. E. Badal, and R. W. Hawkinson.** 1983. Influence of inoculum growth phase on microdilution susceptibility tests. *J. Clin. Microbiol.* **18**:645–651.
6. **Barry, A. L., L. B. Reller, G. H. Miller, J. A. Washington, F. D. Schoenknect, L. R. Peterson, R. S. Hare, and C. Knapp.** 1992. Revision of standards for adjusting the cation content of Mueller-Hinton broth for testing susceptibility of *Pseudomonas aeruginosa* to aminoglycosides. *J. Clin. Microbiol.* **30**:585–589.
7. **Bauer, A. W., W. M. Kirby, J. C. Sherris, and M. Turck.** 1966. Antibiotic susceptibility testing by a standardized single disk method. *Am. J. Clin. Pathol.* **45**:493–496.
8. **Bauer, A. W., and J. C. Sherris.** 1964. The determination of sulfonamide susceptibility of bacteria. *Chemotherapy* **15**:1–19.
9. **Bell, S. M.** 1988. Additions and modifications to the range of antibiotics tested by the CDS method of antibiotic sensitivity testing. *Pathology* **20**:303–304.
10. **Bell, S. M.** 1975. The CDS disc method of antibiotic sensitivity testing (calibrated dichotomous sensitivity test). *Pathology* **7**(Suppl.):1–48.
11. **Berke, I., and P. M. Tierno, Jr.** 1996. Comparison of efficacy and cost-effectiveness of BIOMIC VIDEO and Vitek antimicrobial susceptibility test systems for use in the clinical microbiology laboratory. *J. Clin. Microbiol.* **34**:1980–1984.
12. **Brenner, V. C., and J. C. Sherris.** 1972. Influence of different media and bloods on results of diffusion antibiotic susceptibility tests. *Antimicrob. Agents Chemother.* **1**:116–122.
13. **British Society for Antimicrobial Chemotherapy.** 1991. A guide to sensitivity testing. Report of the Working Party on Antibiotic Sensitivity Testing of the British Society for Antimicrobial Chemotherapy. *J. Antimicrob. Chemother.* **27**(Suppl. D):1–50.
14. **Brown, D. F.** 1990. The comparative methods of antimicrobial susceptibility testing—time for a change? *J. Antimicrob. Chemother.* **25**:307–310.
15. **Brown, D. F. J.** 1994. Developments in antimicrobial susceptibility testing. *Rev. Med. Microbiol.* **5**:65–75.
16. **Brunden, M. N., G. E. Zurenko, and B. Kapik.** 1992. Modification of the error-rate bounded classification scheme for use with two MIC break points. *Diagn. Microbiol. Infect. Dis.* **15**:135–140.
17. **Chaitram, J. M., L. A. Jevitt, S. Lary, and F. C. Tenover.** 2003. The World Health Organization's External Quality Assurance System Proficiency Testing Program has improved the accuracy of antimicrobial susceptibility testing and reporting among participating laboratories using NCCLS methods. *J. Clin. Microbiol.* **41**:2372–2377.
18. **Clinical and Laboratory Standards Institute.** 2008. *Development of In Vitro Susceptibility Testing Criteria and Quality Control Parameters.* Approved guideline M23-A3. Clinical and Laboratory Standards Institute, Wayne, PA.
19. **Clinical and Laboratory Standards Institute.** 2006. *Methods for Antimicrobial Dilution and Disk Susceptibility Testing of Infrequently Isolated or Fastidious Bacteria.* Proposed guideline M45-P. Clinical and Laboratory Standards Institute, Wayne, PA.
20. **Clinical and Laboratory Standards Institute.** 2009. *Methods for Dilution Antimicrobial Susceptibility Tests for Bacteria That Grow Aerobically*, 8th ed. Approved standard M7-A8. Clinical and Laboratory Standards Institute, Wayne, PA.
21. **Clinical and Laboratory Standards Institute.** 2009. *Performance Standards for Antimicrobial Disk Susceptibility Tests*, 10th ed. Approved standard M2-A10. Clinical and Laboratory Standards Institute, Wayne, PA.
22. **Clinical and Laboratory Standards Institute.** 2010. *Performance Standards for Antimicrobial Susceptibility Testing.* Nineteenth informational supplement. M100-S20. Clinical and Laboratory Standards Institute, Wayne, PA.
23. **Clinical and Laboratory Standards Institute.** 2006. *Protocols for Evaluating Dehydrated Mueller-Hinton Agar.* Approved standard M6-A2. Clinical and Laboratory Standards Institute, Wayne, PA.

24. **Clinical and Laboratory Standards Institute/NCCLS.** 2001. *Evaluation of Lots of Dehydrated Mueller-Hinton Broth for Antimicrobial Susceptibility Testing.* Proposed guideline M23-P, vol. 21. NCCLS, Wayne, PA.

25. **Coyle, M. B., M. F. Lampe, C. L. Aitken, P. Feigl, and J. C. Sherris.** 1976. Reproducibility of control strains for antibiotic susceptibility testing. *Antimicrob. Agents Chemother.* **10:**436–440.

26. **Daly, J. S., R. A. Dodge, R. H. Glew, D. T. Soja, B. A. DeLuca, and S. Hebert.** 1997. Effect of zinc concentration in Mueller-Hinton agar on susceptibility of *Pseudomonas aeruginosa* to imipenem. *J. Clin. Microbiol.* **35:**1027–1029.

27. **D'Amato, R. F., C. Thornsberry, C. N. Baker, and L. A. Kirven.** 1975. Effect of calcium and magnesium ions on the susceptibility of *Pseudomonas* species to tetracycline, gentamicin [sic] polymyxin B, and carbenicillin. *Antimicrob. Agents Chemother.* **7:**596–600.

28. **de Lencastre, H., A. M. Sa Figueiredo, C. Urban, J. Rahal, and A. Tomasz.** 1991. Multiple mechanisms of methicillin resistance and improved methods for detection in clinical isolates of *Staphylococcus aureus. Antimicrob. Agents Chemother.* **35:**632–639.

29. **Deutsches Institut für Normung.** 2002. *Susceptibility Testing of Pathogens to Antimicrobial Agents,* part 3. *Agar Diffusion Test,* vol. DIN 58940-3. Beuth Verlag, Berlin, Germany.

30. **Deutsches Institut für Normung.** 2003. *Susceptibility Testing of Pathogens to Antimicrobial Agents,* part 6. *Determination of the Minimum Inhibitory Concentration (MIC) with the Agar Dilution Method,* vol. DIN 58940-6. Beuth Verlag, Berlin, Germany.

31. **Diekema, D. J., K. Lee, P. Raney, L. A. Herwaldt, G. V. Doern, and F. C. Tenover.** 2004. Accuracy and appropriateness of antimicrobial susceptibility test reporting for bacteria isolated from blood cultures. *J. Clin. Microbiol.* **42:**2258–2260.

32. **Doern, G. V.** 1987. Breakpoint susceptibility testing. *Clin. Microbiol. Newsl.* **9:**81–84.

33. **Ericsson, H. M., and J. C. Sherris.** 1971. Antibiotic sensitivity testing. Report of an international collaborative study. *Acta Pathol. Microbiol. Scand. Sect. B Suppl.* **217:**1–90.

34. **European Committee for Antimicrobial Susceptibility Testing.** 2000. Determination of minimum inhibitory concentrations (MICs) of antibacterial agents by agar dilution. *Clin. Microbiol. Infect.* **6:**509–515.

35. **Ferraro, M. J.** 2001. Should we reevaluate antibiotic breakpoints? *Clin. Infect. Dis.* **33**(Suppl. 3)**:**S227–S229.

36. **Fiebelkorn, K. R., S. A. Crawford, M. L. McElmeel, and J. H. Jorgensen.** 2003. Practical disk diffusion method for detection of inducible clindamycin resistance in *Staphylococcus aureus* and coagulase-negative staphylococci. *J. Clin. Microbiol.* **41:**4740–4744.

37. **Fuchs, P. C., A. L. Barry, and S. D. Brown.** 2000. Daptomycin susceptibility tests: interpretive criteria, quality control, and effect of calcium on in vitro tests. *Diagn. Microbiol. Infect. Dis.* **38:**51–58.

38. **Gales, A. C., A. O. Reis, and R. N. Jones.** 2001. Contemporary assessment of antimicrobial susceptibility testing methods for polymyxin B and colistin: review of available interpretative criteria and quality control guidelines. *J. Clin. Microbiol.* **39:**183–190.

39. **Hayden, M. K., K. Rezai, R. A. Hayes, K. Lolans, J. P. Quinn, and R. A. Weinstein.** 2005. Development of daptomycin resistance in vivo in methicillin-resistant *Staphylococcus aureus. J. Clin. Microbiol.* **43:**5285–5287.

40. **Health Care Financing Administration.** 1992. Clinical Laboratory Improvement Amendments of 1988, final rule. *Fed. Regist.* **57:**7001–7186.

41. **Huang, M. B., C. N. Baker, S. Banerjee, and F. C. Tenover.** 1992. Accuracy of the E test for determining antimicrobial susceptibilities of staphylococci, enterococci, *Campylobacter jejuni,* and gram-negative bacteria resistant to antimicrobial agents. *J. Clin. Microbiol.* **30:**3243–3248.

42. **Huang, M. B., T. E. Gay, C. N. Baker, S. N. Banerjee, and F. C. Tenover.** 1993. Two percent sodium chloride is required for susceptibility testing of staphylococci with oxacillin when using agar-based dilution methods. *J. Clin. Microbiol.* **31:**2683–2688.

43. **International Organization for Standardization.** 2006. *Susceptibility Testing of Infectious Agents and Evaluation of Performance of Antimicrobial Susceptibility Devices,* part 1. *Reference Method for Testing the In Vitro Activity of Antimicrobial Agents against Bacteria Involved in Infectious Diseases,* vol. ISO/DIS 20776-1. International Organization for Standardization, Geneva, Switzerland.

44. **International Organization for Standardization.** 2006. *Susceptibility Testing of Infectious Agents and Evaluataion of Performance of Antimicrobial Susceptibility Devices,* part 2. *Evaluation of Performance of Antimicrobial Susceptibility Test Devices,* vol. ISO/DIS 20776-2. International Organization for Standardization, Geneva, Switzerland.

45. **Japanese Society for Chemotherapy.** 1993. Report of the Committee for Japanese Standards for Antimicrobial Susceptibility Testing for Bacteria. *Chemotherapy* **41:**183–189.

46. **Japanese Society for Chemotherapy.** 1990. Report of the Committee for Japanese Standards for Antimicrobial Susceptibility Testing for Bacteria. *Chemotherapy* **38:**102–105.

47. **Jevitt, L. A., G. M. Thorne, M. M. Traczewski, R. N. Jones, J. E. McGowan, Jr., F. C. Tenover, and S. D. Brown.** 2006. Multicenter evaluation of the Etest and disk diffusion methods for differentiating daptomycin-susceptible from non-daptomycin-susceptible *Staphylococcus aureus* isolates. *J. Clin. Microbiol.* **44:**3098–3104.

48. **Jorgensen, J. H.** 1993. Selection criteria for an antimicrobial susceptibility testing system. *J. Clin. Microbiol.* **31:**2841–2844.

49. **Jorgensen, J. H.** 1993. Selection of antimicrobial agents for routine testing in a clinical microbiology laboratory. *Diagn. Microbiol. Infect. Dis.* **16:**245–249.

50. **Jorgensen, J. H., and M. J. Ferraro.** 1998. Antimicrobial susceptibility testing: general principles and contemporary practices. *Clin. Infect. Dis.* **26:**973–980.

51. **Jorgensen, J. H., J. M. Swenson, F. C. Tenover, M. J. Ferraro, J. A. Hindler, and P. R. Murray.** 1994. Development of interpretive criteria and quality control limits for broth microdilution and disk diffusion antimicrobial susceptibility testing of *Streptococcus pneumoniae. J. Clin. Microbiol.* **32:**2448–2459.

52. **Kahlmeter, G., D. F. Brown, F. W. Goldstein, A. P. MacGowan, J. W. Mouton, I. Odenholt, A. Rodloff, C. J. Soussy, M. Steinbakk, F. Soriano, and O. Stetsiouk.** 2006. European Committee on Antimicrobial Susceptibility Testing (EUCAST) technical notes on antimicrobial susceptibility testing. *Clin. Microbiol. Infect.* **12:**501–503.

53. **King, A., and D. F. Brown.** 2001. Quality assurance of antimicrobial susceptibility testing by disc diffusion. *J. Antimicrob. Chemother.* **48**(Suppl. 1)**:**71–76.

54. **Lewis, J. S., II, and J. H. Jorgensen.** 2005. Inducible clindamycin resistance in staphylococci: should clinicians and microbiologists be concerned? *Clin. Infect. Dis.* **40:**280–285.

55. **Lewis, J. S., II, A. Owens, J. Cadena, K. Sabol, J. E. Patterson, and J. H. Jorgensen.** 2005. Emergence of daptomycin resistance in *Enterococcus faecium* during daptomycin therapy. *Antimicrob. Agents Chemother.* **49:**1664–1665.

56. **Li, X. Z.** 2005. Quinolone resistance in bacteria: emphasis on plasmid-mediated mechanisms. *Int. J. Antimicrob. Agents* **25:**453–463.

57. **MacGowan, A. P., and R. Wise.** 2001. Establishing MIC breakpoints and the interpretation of in vitro susceptibility tests. *J. Antimicrob. Chemother.* **48**(Suppl. 1)**:**17–28.

58. **McDermott, S. N., and T. F. Hartley.** 1989. New datum handling methods for the quality control of antibiotic solutions and plates used in the antimicrobial susceptibility test. *J. Clin. Microbiol.* **27:**1814–1825.

59. **Medeiros, A. A., and J. Crellin.** 2000. Evaluation of the Sirscan automated zone reader in a clinical microbiology laboratory. *J. Clin. Microbiol.* **38:**1688–1693.

60. **Members of the SFM Antibiogram Committee.** 2003. Comite de l'Antibiogramme de la Societe Francaise de Microbiologie report 2003. *Int. J. Antimicrob. Agents* **21:**364–391.

61. **Metzler, C. M., and R. M. DeHaan.** 1974. Susceptibility tests of anaerobic bacteria: statistical and clinical considerations. *J. Infect. Dis.* **130:**588–594.

62. **Olsson-Liljequist, B., P. Larsson, M. Walder, and H. Miorner.** 1997. Antimicrobial susceptibility testing in Sweden. III. Methodology for susceptibility testing. *Scand. J. Infect. Dis. Suppl.* **105:**13–23.

63. **Pfaller, M. A., and R. N. Jones.** 2006. Performance accuracy of antibacterial and antifungal susceptibility test methods: report from the College of American Pathologists Microbiology Surveys Program (2001–2003). *Arch. Pathol. Lab. Med.* **130:**767–778.

64. **Queenan, A. M., and K. Bush.** 2007. Carbapenemases: the versatile β-lactamases. *Clin. Microbiol. Rev.* **20:**440–458.

65. **Ringertz, S., B. Olsson-Liljequist, G. Kahlmeter, and G. Kronvall.** 1997. Antimicrobial susceptibility testing in Sweden. II. Species-related zone diameter breakpoints to avoid interpretive errors and guard against unrecognized evolution of resistance. *Scand. J. Infect. Dis. Suppl.* **105:**8–12.

66. **Rosenberg, J., F. C. Tenover, J. Wong, W. Jarvis, and D. J. Vugia.** 1997. Are clinical laboratories in California accurately reporting vancomycin-resistant enterococci? *J. Clin. Microbiol.* **35:**2526–2530.

67. **Sahm, D. F., C. N. Baker, R. N. Jones, and C. Thornsberry.** 1984. Influence of growth medium on the in vitro activities of second- and third-generation cephalosporins against *Streptococcus faecalis. J. Clin. Microbiol.* **20:**561–567.

68. **Steers, E., E. L. Foltz, B. S. Graves, and H. J. Suriano.** 1959. Comparison of bacterial susceptibility to antibiotics as determined by the plate dilution method and by the disc method. *Antibiot. Annu.* **7:**604–613.

69. **Swedish Reference Group for Antibiotics.** 1981. A revised system for antibiotic sensitivity testing. *Scand. J. Infect. Dis.* **13:**148–152.

70. **Swenson, J. M., K. F. Anderson, D. R. Lonsway, A. Thompson, S. K. McAllister, B. M. Limbago, R. B. Carey, F. C. Tenover, and J. B. Patel.** 2009. Accuracy of commercial and reference susceptibility testing methods for detecting vancomycin-intermediate *Staphylococcus aureus. J. Clin. Microbiol.* **47:**2013–2017.

71. **Swenson, J. M., W. B. Brasso, M. J. Ferraro, D. J. Hardy, C. C. Knapp, D. Lonsway, S. McAllister, L. B. Reller, H. S. Sader, D. Shortridge, R. Skov, M. P. Weinstein, B. L. Zimmer, and J. B. Patel.** 2009. Correlation of cefoxitin MICs with the presence of *mecA* in *Staphylococcus* spp. *J. Clin. Microbiol.* **47:**1902–1905.

72. **Swenson, J. M., and F. C. Tenover.** 2005. Results of disk diffusion testing with cefoxitin correlate with presence of *mecA* in *Staphylococcus* spp. *J. Clin. Microbiol.* **43:**3818–3823.

73. **Tenover, F. C., M. V. Lancaster, B. C. Hill, C. D. Steward, S. A. Stocker, G. A. Hancock, C. M. O'Hara, S. K. McAllister, N. C. Clark, and K. Hiramatsu.** 1998. Characterization of staphylococci with reduced susceptibilities to vancomycin and other glycopeptides. *J. Clin. Microbiol.* **36:**1020–1027.

74. **Tenover, F. C., and L. C. McDonald.** 2005. Vancomycin-resistant staphylococci and enterococci: epidemiology and control. *Curr. Opin. Infect. Dis.* **18:**300–305.

75. **Tenover, F. C., J. M. Swenson, C. M. O'Hara, and S. A. Stocker.** 1995. Ability of commercial and reference antimicrobial susceptibility testing methods to detect vancomycin resistance in enterococci. *J. Clin. Microbiol.* **33:**1524–1527.

76. **Thornsberry, C., and L. K. McDougal.** 1983. Successful use of broth microdilution in susceptibility tests for methicillin-resistant (heteroresistant) staphylococci. *J. Clin. Microbiol.* **18:**1084–1091.

77. **Toohey, M., G. Francis, and N. Stingemore.** 1990. Variation in Iso-Sensitest agar affecting β-lactam testing. *Newsl. Antimicrob. Spec. Interest Group Aust. Soc. Microbiol.* **6:**6–8.

78. **Turnidge, J., G. Kahlmeter, and G. Kronvall.** 2006. Statistical characterisation of bacterial wild-type MIC value distributions and the determination of epidemiological cut-off values. *Clin. Microbiol. Infect.* **12:**418–425.

79. **Turnidge, J. D., and J. M. Bell.** 2005. Antimicrobial susceptibility on solid media, p. 8–60. *In* V. Lorien (ed.), *Antibiotics in Laboratory Medicine,* 5th ed. Lippincott Williams & Wilkins, Philadelphia, PA.

80. **Ward, P., S. Palladino, B. McLaren, R. J. Rathur, and J. C. Looker.** 1993. The effect of increased agar concentration in susceptibility testing media on MICs of antimicrobials for gram-negative bacilli. *J. Antimicrob. Chemother.* **31:**1005–1007.

81. **Ward, P. B., S. Palladino, J. C. Looker, and P. Feddema.** 1993. p-Nitrophenylglycerol in susceptibility testing media alters the MICs of antimicrobials for *Pseudomonas aeruginosa. J. Antimicrob. Chemother.* **31:**489–496.

82. **Wheat, P. F.** 1989. The agar-dilution susceptibility technique: past and present. *Clin. Microbio. Newsl.* **11:**164–166.

83. **Williams, J. D.** 1990. Prospects for standardisation of methods and guidelines for disc susceptibility testing. *Eur. J. Clin. Microbiol. Infect. Dis.* **9:**496–501.

Susceptibility Testing Instrumentation and Computerized Expert Systems for Data Analysis and Interpretation

SANDRA S. RICHTER AND MARY JANE FERRARO

69

Commercial antimicrobial susceptibility testing (AST) systems were introduced into clinical microbiology laboratories during the 1980s and have been used in the majority of laboratories since the 1990s (45). Manual and semiautomated broth microdilution systems are utilized for small volumes of susceptibility testing, while larger laboratories often choose an automated broth microdilution system. Most AST systems also perform organism identification as described in chapter 3. Semiautomated systems available for the disk diffusion method are primarily marketed outside of the United States. The AST systems include data management software that may be interfaced with a laboratory information system (LIS) and offer various levels of expert system and epidemiological analyses.

The U.S. Food and Drug Administration (FDA) provides regulatory oversight for AST systems marketed in the United States. Susceptibility test systems are classified as class II medical devices (subject to general controls) and require premarket notification with a 510(k) submission for FDA clearance (30, 32). Automated short-incubation (<16-h) AST systems are subject to additional special controls (32).

A 510(k) submission must demonstrate that a device is substantially equivalent to other devices marketed in the United States. The FDA recommends a multicenter comparison of an AST system to the Clinical and Laboratory Standards Institute (CLSI) reference method (17, 18). The level of performance considered acceptable for each antimicrobial agent-organism combination is >89.9% categorical agreement (same susceptible, intermediate, or resistant classification), >89.9% essential agreement (MIC results within 1 dilution of the reference method), ≤1.5% very major errors (VME; false susceptibility based on the number of resistant organisms), and ≤3% major errors (ME; false resistance based on the number of susceptible isolates) (32). Any antimicrobial agent-organism combination not meeting these standards must be listed as a limitation in the package insert with a recommendation to use an alternative method. Limitation statements are also required if the evaluation did not include a sufficient number of resistant organisms, showed unacceptable (<95%) reproducibility, or showed an elevated "no growth" rate (>10%) for an organism group (32).

The reporting of AST results for antimicrobial agents without proven clinical efficacy against the organism documented in the pharmaceutical package insert is discouraged (32).

Manufacturers apply FDA interpretive standards when evaluating AST results (32). When interpretive criteria change, manufacturers must perform a comparative study, and if the new breakpoints affect device performance, a new 510(k) submission is required (31). If the appropriate validation is completed, laboratories may report results using interpretive criteria other than those published in the AST device label (19). Current information describing FDA regulations and a list of approved devices may be found at http://www.fda.gov/cdrh/consumer/mda/index.html.

This chapter focuses primarily on commercial susceptibility testing systems currently available in the United States. The broth microdilution AST systems are manufactured by four companies: bioMerieux (Durham, NC; http://www.biomerieux-usa.com), Siemens Healthcare Diagnostics (Deerfield, IL; http://www.siemens.com), Becton Dickinson Diagnostics (Sparks, MD; http://www.bd.com), and TREK Diagnostic Systems (Cleveland, OH; http://www.trekds.com). Only one disk diffusion system, manufactured by Giles Scientific (Santa Barbara, CA; http://www.biomic.com), has FDA clearance. Readers should be aware that susceptibility testing system components are constantly changing in response to new technology and problems that are discovered.

SEMIAUTOMATED INSTRUMENTATION FOR DISK DIFFUSION TESTING

The advantages of the disk diffusion method of susceptibility testing include simplicity, reliability, low cost, and a high degree of flexibility in selection of agents tested (45). Semiautomated systems available for reading and interpreting disk diffusion inhibition zones are listed in Table 1. For all systems, agar plates are manually inserted into an instrument after incubation for image acquisition and measurement of the zone of inhibition. Despite advances in imaging technology, a visual review of plates for faint growth or pinpoint colonies within the zone is recommended to assess the need for manual adjustment of the diameter measurement. Data management software determines the categorical interpretation (susceptible, intermediate, or resistant) and may be interfaced with an LIS. Although linear regression may be used to generate an MIC from a zone measurement, the validity for some antimicrobial agent-organism combinations has been questioned (98). Expert system analysis and epidemiology software are available for the systems. The primary advantages

TABLE 1 Overview of manual and semiautomated susceptibility testing instrumentation

Type	Features	Manufacturer(s)[a]	System	Reference(s)
Semiautomated disk diffusion	Assistance in reading, recording, and interpreting zones of inhibition; data management with expert and epidemiology software	Giles Scientific i2a Oxoid Mast Bio-Rad	BIOMIC V3 Sirscan[b] Aura Image[b] Mastacan Elite[b] Osiris[b]	4, 34, 57 66, 70 1, 59 102 5, 6, 55, 70, 78
Manual broth microdilution	Devices to facilitate visual interpretation, recording, and reporting	Siemens TREK Diagnostics	MicroScan data management (LabPro) Sensititre Vizion	
Semiautomated broth microdilution	Automated devices read and report results after offline incubation of tray or strip	Siemens TREK Diagnostics bioMerieux	Microscan AutoSCAN-4 Sensititre AutoReader Mini API[b]	

[a]Bio-Rad, Hercules, CA, http://bio-rad.com; i2a, Montpellier, France; Mast, Bootle, United Kingdom, http://www.mastascan.com; Oxoid, Basingstoke, United Kingdom, http://www.oxoid.com. See text for other manufacturers.
[b]Not currently available within the United States.

of these instruments are (i) less variability in zone measurement (in comparison to caliper or ruler readings by different technologists), (ii) reduced transcription errors, (iii) labor savings, (iv) improved data management capabilities, and (v) expert review to ensure correct reporting of results that are consistent with known resistance phenotypes. In general, these instruments provide reproducible and accurate results. In evaluations of the systems, organisms with faint growth accounted for most discrepancies (34, 59, 66, 70).

MANUAL BROTH MICRODILUTION SYSTEMS

The manual broth microdilution systems listed in Table 1 facilitate the visual reading and recording of MICs. The panels are frozen (TREK custom plates) or dehydrated (MicroScan and Sensititre microwell trays). Devices for rehydration and inoculation of dehydrated trays include the manual RENOK device (MicroScan), the microprocessor-controlled Sensititre AutoInoculator, and the Sensititre multichannel electronic pipette.

After offline incubation, the MicroScan data management system (LabPro) displays an image of the tray configuration for recording manual results directly on the computer. The Sensititre Vizion system magnifies a digital image of the 96-well susceptibility plate on a computer screen with superimposed templates to guide the reading of endpoints that are transferred to the data management system (SWIN, Sensititre Windows software) with expert analysis. The SWIN data management system is also available for recording of manual results without the Sensititre Vizion instrument.

Most manufacturers offer standard gram-positive, gram-negative, *Streptococcus* species, and extended-spectrum β-lactamase (ESBL) confirmatory panels. TREK Diagnostic Systems offers a more extensive menu of FDA-cleared Sensititre plates (*Haemophilus influenzae* and yeast [YeastOne]) and "research use only" panels (mycobacteria [rapid and slow growers], *Campylobacter*, anaerobic) that can be read with the Vizion system or manually.

SEMIAUTOMATED BROTH MICRODILUTION SYSTEMS

The semiautomated broth microdilution systems listed in Table 1 utilize automated devices to read susceptibility and identification tests after offline incubation. The results are transferred to a data management system that may include expert system analysis using the same software as available for the automated systems. Further information regarding MicroScan and Sensititre panels is presented in the section on automated systems.

AUTOMATED BROTH MICRODILUTION SYSTEMS

Automated AST systems do not require further manual intervention to obtain results after placement of the test panel in an instrument where incubation and reading of endpoints occur. An overview of the automated systems currently available in the United States is presented in Table 2. The VITEK, MicroScan WalkAway, and Phoenix systems provide AST results after short-term incubation (<16 h); the currently available Sensititre ARIS panels and some MicroScan WalkAway panels require overnight incubation. Manufacturers should be consulted regarding the current antimicrobial agents available for each system.

VITEK Systems

The first VITEK instrument developed for the provision of rapid MIC results was introduced in the 1980s. The VITEK 1 is still used in a number of laboratories; however, bioMerieux has stopped further development of new cards and software updates. The more automated VITEK 2 received FDA clearance in 2000. The AST panels are thin plastic 64-well cards with one to six concentrations of 9 to 20 antimicrobial agents. An identification card for common gram-positive or gram-negative bacteria may be run simultaneously with each AST card. The Smart Carrier Station includes a bar code scanner and base unit with microprocessor that holds a cassette with a capacity of 15 cards. After manual preparation of the inoculum, cards are placed in the cassette. A memory chip on the cassette allows the transfer of scanned information to the reader-incubator unit. Work flow for large laboratories can be optimized by placement of Smart Carrier Stations at multiple locations. After placement of a cassette into the VITEK 2 loading station, it is automatically moved through stations for bar code reading, AST dilution preparation, card inoculation, and card sealing. The transport system then places cards on a carousel with a 60-card capacity for incubation. The VITEK 2XL instrument has a capacity of 120 cards. Each card is moved to an optic station every 15 minutes for measurement of

TABLE 2 Overview of automated broth microdilution susceptibility testing instrumentation[a]

Manufacturer	System	Panel capacity	Panels	Types of panels (no.)	Instrument features	Software
Becton Dickinson	BD Phoenix	100	Two-sided panels: 85-well AST/ 51-well ID	Gram pos (4) Gram neg (12) *Streptococcus* (1)	Automated adjustment of inoculum and AST dilution. AST panels available as MIC +/− ID substrates. Turbidimetric and redox indicator readings every 20 min. Full-range MICs.	BDXpert BD EpiCenter
bioMerieux	VITEK 2, VITEK 2 XL	60, 120	64-well cards	Gram pos (2) Gram neg (14) *S. pneumoniae* (1) Yeast (1)	Automated AST dilution and filling/ sealing of cards. Turbidimetric readings every 15 min. MICs derived from 1–6 antimicrobial agent dilutions.	Observa AES
	VITEK 2 Compact	15, 30, 60	64-well cards	See VITEK 2	Less automated, more affordable than VITEK 2	See VITEK 2
Siemens	MicroScan WalkAway *plus*	40 or 96	Standard 96-microwell trays	ON (32) *Streptococcus* (1) ESBL (1) Rapid (4) Synergies *plus* (10)	Panels available as full-range MIC or breakpoint MIC. Combination panels include ID substrates. MIC readings: ON, turbidimetric; "read when ready," turbidimetric; rapid panels (3.5–15 h), fluorometric.	LabPro LabPro Alert
TREK	Sensititre ARIS 2X	64	Standard 96-microwell trays	Gram pos (2) Gram neg (4) *Streptococcus* (1) ESBL (1) Yeast (1)	Fluorometric readings after ON incubation of full-range MIC trays. *Haemophilus/S. pneumoniae*, RUO (mycobacteria, anaerobic, campylobacter, gram neg, yeast), and custom (frozen) plates also available.	SWIN epidemiology module

[a]neg, negative; ON, overnight; pos, positive; RUO, research use only.

light transmittance that is proportional to growth. Linear regression analysis is used to determine algorithm-derived MICs that are reported in 4 to 16 h. The Advanced Expert System (AES) is discussed in a later section.

The VITEK 2 Compact was introduced in 2005 for smaller laboratories and uses the same cards as the VITEK 2 system. The instrument is available in three sizes that accommodate 15, 30, or 60 cards. The VITEK 2 Compact is less automated and more affordable than the VITEK 2. The initial inoculum and dilution preparation is manual. Cards are initially placed into the vacuum unit (left side of instrument) for filling, followed by manual transfer to the right side of the instrument for automated sealing and transfer to the incubator-reader unit.

The VITEK 2 data management system (Observa) is Windows based, with better visual aesthetics and a more layered presentation of the same expert system (AES) analysis originally offered with the VITEK 2. Observa software may be used to create epidemiological reports for data generated by VITEK 2 and the manufacturer's blood culture instrument, BacT/ALERT.

MicroScan WalkAway

The MicroScan WalkAway system was developed in the late 1980s and initially offered two major types of AST panels: conventional panels read turbidimetrically after overnight incubation and rapid panels read fluorometrically after 3.5 to 15 h of incubation. These panels, all conventional 96-well microdilution trays, include (i) MIC panels (a broad range of antimicrobial agent dilutions), (ii) MIC combination panels (some wells used for identification), and (iii) breakpoint combination panels (identification

with a limited range of antimicrobial agent dilutions for a categorical result of susceptible, intermediate, or resistant). A third type of MicroScan panel, Synergies *plus*, became available in 2005. Synergies *plus* combines three methods in one panel: "read-when-ready" AST results available as quickly as 4.5 h (turbidimetric reading), overnight results for drugs requiring longer incubation (turbidimetric reading), and identification (fluorometric results within 2.5 h).

The fourth-generation WalkAway *plus* system includes an incubator-reader unit, a personal computer with LIS interface, and a printer. Fluid level sensors, a directional light-emitting diode system, and larger-capacity reservoirs have reduced the time needed to perform maintenance. Two instrument sizes accommodate 40 or 96 panels. The Prompt Inoculation System (available for overnight panels) incorporates a wand to prepare a standard inoculum without turbidity adjustments that is stable for 4 h. A manual device (RENOK) rehydrates and inoculates panels. The humidified incubator-reader unit has a bar code scanner, rotating carousel, and robotics to position panels under a central photometer or fluorometer for readings.

The data management system, LabPro, interprets results, generates patient reports, and archives data to allow production of user-defined reports (antibiograms, trend analysis, and epidemiology reports). Since 2002, the data management system has been able to be coupled with an expert system (LabPro Alert) that incorporates >100 rules and may be customized.

BD Phoenix

The BD Phoenix System has been available in Europe since 2001 and the United States since 2004. The instrument holds up to 100 test panels. The panels are polystyrene trays containing 136 wells divided into a 51-well identification (ID) side and an 85-well AST side with 14 to 22 antimicrobial agents.

The Phoenix AP instrument was introduced in 2008 to reduce the hands-on time required to set up Phoenix panels and to standardize inoculum preparation. Placement of EpiCenter workstations with bar code printers at each technologist bench maximizes work flow efficiency. Each ID broth is labeled with an EpiCenter-generated bar code label and then inoculated with a heavy isolate suspension. The ID broth and corresponding AST broth for five isolates are placed in a rack that is loaded on the AP instrument for automated standardization of the ID broth inoculum, inoculation of AST broth, and addition of the AST redox indicator. The rack is manually transferred to an inoculation station where the ID broth bar code label and a Phoenix panel are scanned. After the ID and/or AST broth is poured into the appropriate side, each panel is sealed with a plastic cap and placed on the Phoenix instrument.

The Phoenix instrument reads panels every 20 minutes using both the colorimetric change in the redox indicator and turbidity to determine organism growth. Growth (metabolic activity) causes the redox indicator to change from an oxidized (blue) state to a reduced (pink) form. A full range of antimicrobial agent concentrations and a "growth" or "no growth" reading for each well allow the system to provide direct rather than calculated MICs. Susceptibility results are completed in 6 to 16 h.

The BDXpert system applies rules that incorporate CLSI standards to interpret AST results. The BD EpiCenter is data management software for analyzing epidemiological trends and generating reports using information from multiple BD instruments (Phoenix, BACTEC blood culture, and MGIT 960 systems). Features of BD EpiCenter include a bidirectional LIS interface, software that allows BDXpert system analysis of manual offline AST results, and tools to create user-specific rules for analyzing AST results.

Sensititre ARIS 2X

The Sensititre ARIS (automated reading and incubation system) was introduced in the United States in 1992 and provides overnight AST results (13, 14). The latest ARIS 2X version with hardware and software upgrades was released in 2004. The ARIS 2X instrument fits on the Sensititre AutoReader and holds up to 64 plates (standard 96-microwell trays) available as MIC panels or separate ID plates. Plates are rehydrated and inoculated with the Sensititre AutoInoculator or a handheld multichannel electronic pipette before placement in the instrument's carousel. An internal bar code scanner identifies the plate type to assign the appropriate time of incubation. After 16 to 24 h of incubation, each AST plate is transported to the AutoReader for fluorometric reading of endpoints. The data management software (SWIN) provides expert analysis of results. The SWIN epidemiology module enables laboratories to monitor trends and generate antibiogram reports.

ADVANTAGES OF AUTOMATED SYSTEMS

Advantages of automated AST systems include labor savings, reproducibility, data management with expert system analysis, and the opportunity to generate results more rapidly. A work flow and performance evaluation of the VITEK 2 and Phoenix systems reported a longer mean setup time per isolate for Phoenix (3 min) than for VITEK 2 (1.5 min), but more monthly maintenance time for VITEK 2 (63.2 min) than for Phoenix (21.2 min) (25). The new Phoenix AP instrument reduced hands-on time by 50%, with a manual manipulation time per isolate that was 11.5 s less than for VITEK 2 work flow ($P < 0.001$) for batches of 14 isolates (50a).

The overall mean time to generate AST results was higher for Phoenix (12.1 ± 2.7 h) than for VITEK 2 (8.4 ± 2 h) ($P < 0.001$) (25). Ligozzi et al. reported that the time required for VITEK 2 AST for gram-positive cocci was 6 to 17 h, with 90% of results available as follows: 8 h, *Staphylococcus aureus*; 11 h, coagulase-negative staphylococci (CoNS); 9 h, enterococci; 7 h, *Streptococcus agalactiae*; and 9 h, *Streptococcus pneumoniae* (61). There are limited data showing financial and clinical benefits in association with the rapid provision of AST results. Doern et al. reported lower mortality rates and cost savings (fewer diagnostic tests and days in intensive care) associated with the rapid reporting of AST results (22). Barenfanger et al. also demonstrated reduced lengths of stay and cost savings for patients with rapid reporting of AST results that were attributed to earlier adjustments in antimicrobial therapy (2).

The time required to complete AST testing may eventually be reduced further with the application of molecular techniques. Rolain et al. described a real-time quantitative PCR method to measure the effect of antimicrobial agents on bacterial growth with a shorter time needed to generate results (4 h for gram-positive cocci and 2 h for gram-negative rods) (74). Additional research, increased automation, and lower cost are needed to make this molecular technology available for clinical laboratories (74).

Effective communication of the results to clinicians and pharmacists is essential to realizing the potential benefits of rapid testing. Communication may be enhanced by software packages that interface with medication records and alert clinicians or pharmacists when adjustments in antimicrobial therapy are needed.

DISADVANTAGES OF AUTOMATED SYSTEMS

Disadvantages of automated systems include a higher cost for equipment and consumables than with manual methods, predetermined antimicrobial panels, an inability to test all clinically relevant organisms, and problems with detection of some resistance phenotypes (46). Reports of AST performance for detecting problematic resistance phenotypes are discussed below. Current performance of a system may not be accurately reflected by studies utilizing panels and software that are no longer available. A higher error rate should be accepted for evaluations using challenge strains with difficult-to-detect phenotypes than for studies that test populations of isolates usually encountered in the clinical laboratory.

Vancomycin Resistance in Enterococci

Problems with the detection of low-level vancomycin resistance (*vanB* and *vanC*) among enterococci by automated systems have been demonstrated in multiple studies (75, 91). A VITEK 2 evaluation only reported difficulty detecting *vanC2* (*Enterococcus casseliflavus*) strains (99). Other VITEK 2 and Phoenix studies have demonstrated accurate detection of vancomycin-resistant enterococci, but rigorous studies comparing systems are lacking (9, 11, 27, 33). An FDA limitation for *E. casseliflavus* and *Enterococcus gallinarum* requires Phoenix users to determine vancomycin susceptibility for those species with an alternate method (11).

MicroScan overnight panel studies reported detection of all isolates except those containing *vanC* that are difficult for all AST systems since their MICs (4 to 16 µg/ml) span susceptible and intermediate categories (16, 20).

HLAR in *Enterococcus* spp.

The detection of high-level aminoglycoside resistance (HLAR) in enterococci by overnight and short-incubation AST systems has been improved by changes in growth medium and extended incubation (100, 103). Initial problems detecting high-level streptomycin resistance (HLSR) in MicroScan overnight panels appear to have been resolved after a broth reformulation, with two subsequent studies demonstrating detection of HLAR that compared favorably to reference and molecular methods (16, 68). A study reporting a higher VME rate for MicroScan detection of HLSR (20) may not have performed the recommended 48-h read for isolates that appear streptomycin susceptible after overnight incubation that in one study improved detection of HLSR by 6% (16). Separate VITEK 2 and Phoenix evaluations testing different strains reported VME rates of 0 to 5.2% and ME rates of 0 to 7.3% for the detection of HLSR or high-level gentamicin resistance (9, 11, 27, 33).

Linezolid Resistance in Enterococci and Staphylococci

Reading endpoints when testing linezolid can be difficult due to trailing growth. The low prevalence of linezolid resistance limits the ability of manufacturers to optimize detection with AST systems. Linezolid susceptibility testing of 50 enterococcal and 50 staphylococcal challenge isolates (included 32 non-linezolid-susceptible strains) demonstrated categorical agreements of 96.0% (MicroScan), 93.0% (VITEK 2), 89.6% (Phoenix), and 85.9% (VITEK 1) in comparison to CLSI broth microdilution results (94). Brigante et al. reported 89.0% categorical agreement of Phoenix linezolid results compared to Etest determinations for 100 enterococci (9).

Penicillin Resistance in Staphylococci

Staphylococcal isolates for which the penicillin MIC is ≤0.12 µg/ml require an induced β-lactamase test to be negative before being reported as penicillin susceptible (19). The sensitivity of phenotypic methods for penicillinase detection performed on 197 *S. aureus* isolates for which the VITEK 2 penicillin MICs were ≤0.12 µg/ml ranged from 39% (induced nitrocefin test) to 71% (zone edge determination method) when *blaZ* PCR was used as the reference standard (53). Since the prevalence of penicillin-susceptible staphylococcal isolates is low and β-lactamase production may not be detected using phenotypic methods, testing of subsequent isolates from the patient (19) or use of a molecular method (53) should be considered before relying on penicillin for treatment of serious infections.

Oxacillin Resistance in Staphylococci

Most of the studies discussed below used *mecA* PCR as the "gold standard" when evaluating the accuracy of a system for detection of oxacillin resistance in staphylococci. Multiple studies have demonstrated excellent sensitivity and specificity of automated systems for detecting methicillin-resistant *S. aureus* (MRSA) (11, 27, 61, 77). However, heterogeneously resistant populations may not be detected with routine oxacillin testing (29, 89). Manufacturers of the Phoenix and VITEK 2 systems have improved MRSA detection by adding cefoxitin to panels (50, 52, 73, 89).

For the detection of oxacillin resistance among CoNS, VITEK 2 and Phoenix evaluations have demonstrated excellent sensitivities (96 to 99.4%), with lower specificities (65 to 96%) (27, 37–39, 61, 84). Isolates with false-resistant results often have oxacillin MICs of 0.5 to 2 µg/ml that would have been considered susceptible under previous CLSI CoNS oxacillin breakpoints that were lowered to ≤0.25 µg/ml in 1999 (40). Some of the ME were for *Staphylococcus lugdunensis* isolates with oxacillin MICs now considered susceptible based on the CLSI 2005 decision to apply *S. aureus* breakpoints (≤2 µg/ml) to this species of CoNS (37, 38). The lower CoNS oxacillin breakpoint is most accurate for detecting *mecA* carriage in *Staphylococcus hominis*, *Staphylococcus haemolyticus*, and *Staphylococcus epidermidis* isolates, but may overcall oxacillin resistance for other CoNS species (40). An evaluation of the VITEK 2 cefoxitin screen found it to be more specific than the VITEK 2 oxacillin test for detection of *mecA*-mediated resistance in CoNS (41).

Reduced Glycopeptide Susceptibility in Staphylococci

The initial failure of automated AST systems to reliably detect vancomycin-resistant *S. aureus* (VRSA) led to a temporary requirement for a supplemental vancomycin agar screening plate until the systems were optimized for VRSA detection (12, 92, 93). An evaluation of four commercial AST systems for the detection of vancomycin-intermediate *S. aureus* (VISA) reported sensitivities of 64 to 100%; the two systems with 100% sensitivity incorrectly categorized 12% (MicroScan) and 24% (Phoenix) of susceptible isolates as VISA (90). Unreliable AST system detection of CoNS with reduced glycopeptide susceptibility has also been reported (21). CLSI encourages laboratories to confirm nonsusceptible vancomycin results with a second method and to send any *S. aureus* isolate with a vancomycin MIC of ≥8 µg/ml to a reference laboratory (19).

Inducible Clindamycin Resistance

Staphylococci and beta-hemolytic streptococcal isolates that are macrolide resistant and clindamycin susceptible may be assessed for inducible clindamycin resistance using the CLSI disk diffusion or broth microdilution test (19). The inoculum purity plates from an automated broth AST system may be used to perform the disk induction (D-zone) test (48). Recently FDA-cleared tests for inducible clindamycin resistance in staphylococci have become available for all of the automated systems in Table 2. An evaluation of the Phoenix test for inducible clindamycin resistance performed on 194 macrolide-resistant, clindamycin-susceptible staphylococcal isolates reported a sensitivity of 99% and a specificity of 97% (35a). A multicenter study of the VITEK 2 inducible clindamycin resistance test using challenge and local strains of *S. aureus* with 244 tests performed reported a sensitivity of 98% and a specificity of 99% (58a).

Other *Streptococcus* Resistance

Evaluations of the Phoenix and VITEK 2 panels for testing *Streptococcus* species demonstrated reliable results despite the shorter incubation (9, 35, 44, 47, 72). Overnight *S. pneumoniae* trays available from MicroScan and Sensitire provided accurate results for agents other than trimethoprim-sulfamethoxazole (discrepancies were attributed to trailing endpoints) (36).

ESBL-Producing *Enterobacteriaceae*

Implementation of revised (2010) cephalosporin (cefazolin, cefotaxime, ceftriaxone, ceftizoxime, and ceftazidime) and aztreonam CLSI breakpoints for *Enterobacteriaceae* makes ESBL testing unnecessary unless there is consideration of using a cephalosporin for which interpretive criteria were not recently evaluated (cefonicid, cefamandole, cefoperazone, or moxalactam) (19). Some laboratories may continue to perform ESBL testing for infection control purposes. Confirmatory ESBL tests that typically measure the inhibitory effect of clavulanate on ceftazidime and cefotaxime are available for all of the automated systems listed in Table 2. Two comparative evaluations of ESBL detection among *Escherichia coli* and *Klebsiella* spp. revealed sensitivities of 74 to 91% (VITEK 2) and 92 to 96% (Phoenix), with specificities of 81 to 85% (60, 96). Evaluations of a single AST system (VITEK 2 or Phoenix) have reported sensitivities of 96 to 100% and specificities of 96 to 99.7% for ESBL detection (15, 81–83, 85). Evaluations of the MicroScan ESBL panels have demonstrated sensitivities of 88 to 100% and specificities of 77 to 98% (56, 62, 88). False-positive ESBL results for K1-hyperproducing *Klebsiella oxytoca* isolates have been reported for MicroScan (88) and Phoenix (81, 87) systems. An evaluation performed on a collection of *E. coli* isolates with CTX-M phenotypes found that ESBL detection by VITEK 2 occurred for only 68% of the 137 isolates tested (23).

Carbapenem Resistance

Failure of automated AST systems to recognize emerging carbapenem resistance among *Klebsiella pneumoniae* and *Acinetobacter baumannii* isolates has been reported (8, 58, 95). The subsequent addition of ertapenem to AST system panels likely improved detection of *bla*KPC-positive *Enterobacteriaceae* isolates due to relatively lower CLSI breakpoints (in comparison to those for meropenem and imipenem) with a higher sensitivity for carbapenemase production. The 2009 CLSI recommendation to perform the modified Hodge test for detection of carbapenemase production in *Enterobacteriaceae* isolates with elevated carbapenem MICs still in the susceptible range also enhanced *bla*KPC detection (19).

Problems with false resistance when determining carbapenem susceptibility have also been noted (86, 97). The CDC could only confirm 9% of 123 *Enterobacteriaceae* and 74% of 325 *Pseudomonas aeruginosa* isolates initially reported as non-imipenem susceptible by 44 U.S. hospital laboratories during the period from 1996 to 1999 (86). The lack of a clear explanation for this overdetection of carbapenem resistance led the authors to recommend that laboratories consider using a second AST method to confirm non-carbapenem-susceptible results (86). Antimicrobial agent deterioration in test panels (101) and technical errors are factors that may contribute to the overdetection of carbapenem resistance by AST systems (86, 97).

Other Resistance in Gram-Negative Organisms

Two evaluations directly comparing the accuracies of automated AST systems for testing clinical and challenge isolates of *P. aeruginosa* found unacceptable levels of error for imipenem, piperacillin-tazobactam, cefepime, ceftazidime, and aztreonam (51, 76). Susceptibility testing of clinical isolates of *P. aeruginosa* using only VITEK 2 identified three agents with categorical agreement of <90% (cefepime, cefotaxime, and gentamicin) that were predominantly minor errors (49). A VITEK 2 study utilizing *P. aeruginosa* isolates

selected to represent specific β-lactam resistance phenotypes revealed elevated error rates for all β-lactam agents tested (65). A VITEK and MicroScan study concluded that automated commercial AST systems were contraindicated for testing isolates of *P. aeruginosa* from cystic fibrosis patients and attributed the poor correlation with reference methods to slow growth and mucoid strains (10). Phoenix studies have reported low categorical agreement for nonfermenting gram-negative bacillus isolates primarily due to minor errors and ME with β-lactams, ciprofloxacin, and trimethoprim-sulfamethoxazole (24, 26, 85).

COMPUTERIZED EXPERT SYSTEMS

Expert systems to assist in the critical review of AST results are available for all commercial susceptibility systems currently marketed in the United States. Expert systems can enhance work flow by identifying the subset of results that require human expert attention and may also improve the quality of AST results reported from smaller laboratories that may lack a human expert (80). By continuous monitoring, the algorithms allow more rapid recognition of incorrect results and more uniform reporting. However, the software must be frequently updated to reflect the emergence of new resistance and changes in reporting guidelines recommended by national organizations such as CLSI. Users must be aware of what rules and comments are activated in their system and work closely with manufacturer-provided specialists to customize the expert system for their laboratory. The degree of customization allowed varies among AST systems. Ideally, an expert system will report actual MICs with categorical interpretation before and after recommended changes. Expert systems may also deduce the susceptibility of an isolate to agents not tested and detect inconsistencies between organism ID and AST results (80).

Most expert systems use a rules-based approach focusing on AST results for one drug at a time without considering results for other agents tested simultaneously. The VITEK 2 AES differs by performing an "interpretive reading" that compares the MICs for multiple agents to a large database of known resistance phenotypes and MIC distributions for different species (63, 79). The rationale for interpretive reading with phenotype assignment is that a single mechanism typically mediates resistance to multiple agents (64). Excellent concordance of VITEK 2 AES interpretive reading with resistance genotypes has been reported in multicenter studies (3, 63). When the AES was compared to human expert analysis of VITEK 2 results for 259 consecutive clinical isolates in a university-based microbiology laboratory, there was disagreement for only 5 of the 65 isolates (8%) with AES corrections (80). A limitation that has been noted for the AES is an inability to interpret multiple inconsistent results as being caused by a single problem (7, 80). Nakasone et al. reported inaccurate resistance genotype reporting by the AES for vancomycin-resistant enterococci and macrolide-resistant *S. pneumoniae* (69).

CRITICAL REVIEW OF AST RESULTS

Regardless of whether a laboratory is using a commercial expert system, it is important to be aware of unusual "resistant" (Table 3) and "susceptible" (Table 4) results that require verification of the organism's ID and repetition of the susceptibility test by the same or a different method (19, 64). An example of an unprecedented phenotype that should prompt retesting is an *Enterobacteriaceae* or *P. aeruginosa*

TABLE 3 Unusual resistance phenotypes[a]

Organism(s)	Resistance requiring verification
Gram positive	
Enterococcus faecalis	Linezolid, daptomycin, ampicillin
Enterococcus faecium	Linezolid, daptomycin, quinupristin-dalfopristin
Streptococcus pneumoniae	Vancomycin, telavancin, linezolid, fluoroquinolone
Viridans group streptococci	Vancomycin, telavancin, linezolid, daptomycin
Beta-hemolytic streptococci	Vancomycin, telavancin, linezolid, daptomycin, ampicillin, penicillin, cephalosporins
CoNS	Vancomycin, telavancin, linezolid, daptomycin, quinupristin-dalfopristin
Staphylococcus aureus	Vancomycin, telavancin, linezolid, daptomycin, quinupristin-dalfopristin
Gram negative	
Enterobacteriaceae (all)	Carbapenem
Neisseria gonorrhoeae, Neisseria meningitidis	Extended-spectrum cephalosporin
Haemophilus influenzae	Third-generation cephalosporin, aztreonam, carbapenem, fluoroquinolone

[a]Resistance phenotypes that are rare or have not yet been detected may represent technical errors.

isolate that appears more resistant to piperacillin-tazobactam than to piperacillin (54). There are a number of antimicrobial agents that may appear active in vitro but lack clinical efficacy (Table 5); therefore, the organisms should be reported as resistant. The most recent CLSI M100 document should be consulted for current recommendations regarding agents to test for specific organisms, methodology, interpretive criteria, results that may be inferred without testing a specific agent, antimicrobial agents to report based on the site of infection, and unusual results requiring verification (19). Expert rules to assist with the interpretation of AST results are also available at the European Committee on Antimicrobial Susceptibility Testing (EUCAST) website (http://www.eucast.org/expert_rules/).

SELECTING AN AST SYSTEM

Factors to consider when selecting an AST system include cost, performance, work flow, data management capabilities, and manufacturer technical support (43, 67). Performance may be assessed by comparing dilutions of FDA-cleared antimicrobial agents and limitations (antimicrobial agent or organisms listed in package inserts that require an alternative method) of panels from different manufacturers.

Current users of systems and publications in peer-reviewed journals are important resources for assessing performance. Manufacturers should be asked if problems reported for particular antimicrobial agent-organism combinations have been resolved and what is under development. Manufacturer exhibits at national meetings offer demonstrations of systems and convenient access to industry representatives. Poster presentations at conferences provide the opportunity to interact with recent system users and acquire new information regarding performance. Another method of assessing the performance of AST systems is participation in proficiency testing surveys such as those of the College of American Pathologists (42, 71), whose final critiques of susceptibility testing challenges provide information regarding AST methods used and problem antimicrobial agent-organism combinations with high error rates.

An AST system's ability to perform ID is also important because expert rules are linked to organism identity. Additional information regarding selection of an AST system and laboratory verification of performance as required by the Clinical Laboratory Improvement Amendments of 1988 (28) is in the *Clinical Microbiology Procedures Handbook* (67) and a new CLSI document in preparation (M52-P, *Validation and Verification of Identification and AST Systems*).

TABLE 4 Gram-negative organisms with expected resistance to commonly tested antimicrobial agents

Organism	Agent(s) organism is usually resistant to
Enterobacteriaceae	
Citrobacter, Enterobacter, Klebsiella, Morganella, *Proteus penneri, Proteus vulgaris, Providencia, Serratia, Yersinia*	Ampicillin
Citrobacter freundii, Enterobacter, Morganella, Proteus penneri, *Proteus vulgaris, Providencia, Serratia, Yersinia*	Cefazolin, cephalothin
Klebsiella	Ticarcillin
C. freundii, Enterobacter, Serratia	Cefoxitin, cefotetan
C. freundii, Enterobacter, Proteus vulgaris, Serratia	Cefuroxime
Citrobacter, Enterobacter, Serratia	Amoxicillin-clavulanic acid, ampicillin-sulbactam
Non-*Enterobacteriaceae*	
Acinetobacter, Burkholderia cepacia, Pseudomonas aeruginosa, *Stenotrophomonas maltophilia*	Ampicillin, first- and second-generation cephalosporins
Burkholderia cepacia, Stenotrophomonas maltophilia	Aminoglycosides
Stenotrophomonas maltophilia	Carbapenems
Pseudomonas aeruginosa	Trimethoprim-sulfamethoxazole

TABLE 5 Antimicrobial agents that may appear active in vitro but lack clinical efficacy

Organism	Antimicrobial agents for which the organism should be reported as resistant
Oxacillin-resistant staphylococci	All β-lactam agents except ceftaroline and ceftobiprole
Enterococcus spp.	Aminoglycosides (other than high level), cephalosporins, clindamycin, trimethoprim-sulfamethoxazole
ESBL-producing *E. coli*, *Klebsiella* spp., and *Proteus mirabilis*[a]	Cefonicid, cefamandole, cefoperazone, moxalactam
Listeria spp.	Cephalosporins
Salmonella and *Shigella* spp.	Aminoglycosides, first- and second-generation cephalosporins
Yersinia pestis	All β-lactam agents

[a]Implementation of the revised (2010) cephalosporin and aztreonam CLSI breakpoints for *Enterobacteriaceae* makes routine ESBL testing unnecessary unless there is consideration of using the agents listed. If ESBL testing is performed and results are positive, the organisms should be reported as resistant to these drugs.

SUMMARY

AST systems provide accurate and reproducible results for many antimicrobial agent-organism combinations. Expert analysis may improve work flow as well as the quality of reported results. The labor savings attributed to automated AST systems are particularly important for laboratories in regions with current or projected technologist shortages. In addition, the provision of more rapid AST results with a short-incubation system may improve patient care and lower health care costs. Future advances in the development of AST systems may increase their clinical impact with the incorporation of molecular techniques that dramatically shorten the time required for results.

REFERENCES

1. **Andrew, J. M., F. J. Boswell, and R. Wise.** 2000. Evaluation of the Oxoid Aura image system for measuring zones of inhibition with the disc diffusion technique. *J. Antimicrob. Chemother.* **46:**535–540.

2. **Barenfanger, J., C. Drake, and G. Kacich.** 1999. Clinical and financial benefits of rapid bacterial identification and antimicrobial susceptibility testing. *J. Clin. Microbiol.* **37:**1415–1418.

3. **Barry, J., A. Brown, V. Ensor, U. Lakhani, D. Petts, C. Warren, and T. Winstanley.** 2003. Comparative evaluation of the VITEK 2 Advanced Expert System (AES) in five UK hospitals. *J. Antimicrob. Chemother.* **51:**1191–1202.

4. **Berke, I., and P. M. Tierno, Jr.** 1996. Comparison of efficacy and cost-effectiveness of BIOMIC VIDEO and VITEK antimicrobial susceptibility test systems for use in the clinical microbiology laboratory. *J. Clin. Microbiol.* **34:**1980–1984.

5. **Bert, F., M. Juvin, Z. Ould-Hocine, G. Clarebout, E. Keller, N. Lambert, and G. Arlet.** 2005. Evaluation and updating of the Osiris expert system for identification of *Escherichia coli* β-lactamase resistance phenotypes. *J. Clin. Microbiol.* **43:**1846–1850.

6. **Bert, F., Z. Ould-Hocine, M. Juvin, V. Dubois, V. Loncle-Provot, V. LeFranc, C. Quentin, N. Lambert, and G. Arlet.** 2003. Evaluation of the Osiris expert system for identification of β-lactam phenotypes in isolates of *Pseudomonas aeruginosa*. *J. Clin. Microbiol.* **41:**3712–3718.

7. **Blondel-Hill, E., C. Hetchler, D. Andrews, and L. Lapointe.** 2003. Evaluation of VITEK 2 for analysis of *Enterobacteriaceae* using the Advanced Expert System (AES) versus interpretive susceptibility guidelines used at Dynacare Kasper Medical Laboratories, Edmonton, Alberta. *Clin. Microbiol. Infect.* **9:**1091–1103.

8. **Bratu, S., D. Landman, R. Haag, R. Recco, A. Eramo, M. Alam, and J. Quale.** 2005. Rapid spread of carbapenem-resistant *Klebsiella pneumoniae* in New York City. *Arch. Intern. Med.* **165:**1430–1435.

9. **Brigante, G. R., F. A. Luzzaro, B. Pini, G. Lombardi, G. Sokeng, and A. Q. Toniolo.** 2007. Drug susceptibility testing of clinical isolates of streptococci and enterococci by the Phoenix automated microbiology system. *BMC Microbiol.* **7:**46–52.

10. **Burns, J. L., L. Saiman, S. Whittier, J. Krzewinski, Z. Liu, D. Larone, S. A. Marshall, and R. N. Jones.** 2001. Comparison of two commercial systems (VITEK and MicroScan-WalkAway) for antimicrobial susceptibility testing of *Pseudomonas aeruginosa* isolates from cystic fibrosis patients. *Diagn. Microbiol. Infect. Dis.* **39:**257–260.

11. **Carroll, K. C., A. P. Borek, C. Burger, B. Glanz, H. Bhally, S. Henciak, and S. C. Flayhart.** 2006. Evaluation of the BD Phoenix automated microbiology system for identification and antimicrobial susceptibility testing of staphylococci and enterococci. *J. Clin. Microbiol.* **44:**2072–2077.

12. **Centers for Disease Control and Prevention.** 2004. Vancomycin-resistant *Staphylococcus aureus*—New York, 2004. *MMWR Morb. Mortal. Wkly. Rep.* **53:**322–323.

13. **Chapin, K. C., and M. C. Musgnug.** 2003. Validation of the automated reading and incubation system with Sensititre plates for antimicrobial susceptibility testing. *J. Clin. Microbiol.* **41:**1951–1956.

14. **Chapin, K. C., and M. C. Musgnug.** 2004. Evaluation of Sensititre automated system for automated reading of Sensititre broth microdilution susceptibility plates. *J. Clin. Microbiol.* **42:**909–911.

15. **Chen, H. M., J. J. Wu, P. F. Tsai, J. Y. Wann, and J. J. Yan.** 2009. Evaluation of the capability of the VITEK 2 system to detect extended-spectrum β-lactamase-producing *Escherichia coli* and *Klebsiella pneumoniae* isolates, in particular with the coproduction of AmpC enzymes. *Eur. J. Clin. Microbiol. Infect. Dis.* **28:**871–874.

16. **Chen, Y.-S., S. A. Marshall, P. L. Winokur, S. L. Coffman, W.W. Wilkie, P. R. Murray, C. A. Spiegel, M. A. Pfaller, G. V. Doern, and R. N. Jones.** 1998. Use of molecular and reference susceptibility testing methods in a multicenter evaluation of MicroScan dried overnight gram-positive MIC panels for detection of vancomycin and high-level aminoglycoside resistances in enterococci. *J. Clin. Microbiol.* **36:**2996–3001.

17. **Clinical and Laboratory Standards Institute.** 2008. *Development of In Vitro Susceptibility Testing Criteria and Quality Control Parameters, Approved Guideline M23-A3,* 3rd ed. Clinical and Laboratory Standards Institute, Wayne, PA.

18. **Clinical and Laboratory Standards Institute.** 2009. *Methods for Dilution Antimicrobial Susceptibility Testing for Bacteria That Grow Aerobically, Approved Standard M07-A8,* 8th ed. Clinical and Laboratory Standards Institute, Wayne, PA.

19. **Clinical and Laboratory Standards Institute.** 2010. *Performance Standards for Antimicrobial Susceptibility Testing; Twentieth Informational Supplement.* CLSI document M100-S20. Clinical and Laboratory Standards Institute, Wayne, PA.

20. **d'Azevedo, P. A., C. A.G. Dias, A. L. S. Goncalves, F. Rowe, and L. M. Teixeira.** 2001. Evaluation of an automated system for the identification and antimicrobial susceptibility testing of enterococci. *Diagn. Microbiol. Infect. Dis.* **40:**157–161.

21. Del'Alamo, L., R. F. Cereda, I. Tosin, E. A. Miranda, and H. S. Sader. 1999. Antimicrobial susceptibility of coagulase-negative staphylococci and characterization of isolates with reduced susceptibility to glycopeptides. *Diagn. Microbiol. Infect. Dis.* **34**:185–191.

22. Doern, G. V., R. Vautour, M. Gaudet, and B. Levy. 1994. Clinical impact of rapid in vitro susceptibility testing and bacterial identification. *J. Clin. Microbiol.* **32**:1757–1762.

23. Donaldson, H., M. McCalmont, D. M. Livermore, P. J. Rooney, G. Ong, E. McHenry, R. Campbell, and R. McMullan. 2008. Evaluation for the VITEK 2 AST N-054 test card for the detection of extended-spectrum β-lactamase production in *Escherichia coli* with CTX-M phenotypes. *J. Antimicrob. Chemother.* **62**:1015–1017.

24. Donay, J.-L., D. Mathieu, P. Fernandes, C. Pregermain, P. Bruel, A. Wargnier, I. Casin, F. X. Weill, P. H. Lagrange, and J. L. Herrmann. 2004. Evaluation of the automated Phoenix system for potential routine use in the clinical microbiology laboratory. *J. Clin. Microbiol.* **42**:1542–1546.

25. Eigner, U., A. Schmid, U. Wild, D. Bertsch, and A.-M. Fahr. 2005. Analysis of the comparative workflow and performance characteristics of the VITEK 2 and Phoenix systems. *J. Clin. Microbiol.* **43**:3829–3834.

26. Endimiani, A., F. Luzzaro, A. Tamborini, G. Lombardi, V. Elia, R. Belloni, and A. Toniolo. 2002. Identification and antimicrobial susceptibility testing of clinical isolates of non-fermenting gram-negative bacteria by the Phoenix automated microbiology system. *Microbiologica* **25**:323–329.

27. Fahr, A. M., U. Eigner, M. Armbrust, A. Caganic, G. Dettori, C. Chezzi, L. Bertoncini, M. Benecchi, and M. G. Menozzi. 2003. Two-center collaborative evaluation of the performance of the BD Phoenix automated microbiology system for identification and antimicrobial susceptibility testing of *Enterococcus* spp. and *Staphylococcus* spp. *J. Clin. Microbiol.* **41**:1135–1142.

28. Federal Register. 1992. Clinical Laboratory Improvement Amendments of 1988; final rule. *Fed. Regist.* **57**:7164.

29. Felten, A., B. Grandry, P. H. Lagrange, and I. Casin. 2002. Evaluation of three techniques for detection of low-level methicillin-resistant *Staphylococcus aureus* (MRSA): a disk diffusion method with cefoxitin and moxalactam, the VITEK 2 system, and the MRSA-screen latex agglutination test. *J. Clin. Microbiol.* **40**:2766–2771.

30. Food and Drug Administration. 2003. *Establishment Registration and Device Listing for Manufacturers and Initial Importers of Devices.* 21 CFR 807. Food and Drug Administration, Rockville, MD.

31. Food and Drug Administration. June 2009. *Guidance for Industry: Updating Labeling for Susceptibility Test Information in Systemic Antibacterial Drug Products and Antimicrobial Susceptibility Testing Devices.* Food and Drug Administration, Rockville, MD.

32. Food and Drug Administration. 28 August 2009. *Class II Special Controls Guidance Document: Antimicrobial Susceptibility Test (AST) Systems; Guidance for Industry and FDA.* Food and Drug Administration, Rockville, MD.

33. Garcia-Garrote, F., E. Cercenado, and E. Bouza. 2000. Evaluation of a new system, VITEK 2, for identification and antimicrobial susceptibility testing of enterococci. *J. Clin. Microbiol.* **38**:2108–2111.

34. Geiss, H. K., and U. E. Klar. 2000. Evaluation of the BIOMIC video reader system for routine use in the clinical microbiology laboratory. *Diagn. Microbiol. Infect. Dis.* **37**:151–155.

35. Goessens, W. H. F., N. Lemmens-den Toom, J. Hageman, P. W. M. Hermans, M. Sluijter, R. de Groot, and H. A. Verbrugh. 2000. Evaluation of the VITEK 2 system for susceptibility testing of *Streptococcus pneumoniae* isolates. *Eur. J. Clin. Microbiol. Infect. Dis.* **19**:618–622.

35a. Gosnell, C., C. Yu, D. Turner, and J. Reuben. 2008. *18th Eur. Congr. Clin. Microbiol. Infect. Dis.*, abstr. P854.

36. Guthrie, L. L., S. Banks, W. Setiawan, and K. B. Waites. 1999. Comparison of MicroScan MICroSTREP, Pasco, and Sensititre MIC panels for determining antimicrobial

susceptibilities of *Streptococcus pneumoniae*. *Diagn. Microbiol. Infect. Dis.* **33**:267–273.

37. Horstkotte, M. A., J. K.-M. Knobloch, H. Rohde, S. Dobinsky, and D. Mack. 2002. Rapid detection of methicillin resistance in coagulase-negative staphylococci with the VITEK 2 system. *J. Clin. Microbiol.* **40**:3291–3295.

38. Horstkotte, M. A., J. K.-M. Knobloch, H. Rohde, S. Dobinsky, and D. Mack. 2004. Evaluation of the BD PHOENIX automated system for detection of methicillin resistance in coagulase-negative staphylococci. *J. Clin Microbiol.* **42**:5041–5046.

39. Hussain, Z., L. Stoakes, M. A. John, S. Garrow, and V. Fitzgerald. 2002. Detection of methicillin resistance in primary blood culture isolates of coagulase-negative staphylococci by PCR, slide agglutination, disk diffusion, and a commercial method. *J. Clin. Microbiol.* **40**:2251–2253.

40. Hussain, Z., L. Stoakes, V. Massey, D. Diagre, V. Fitzgerald, S. El Sayed, and R. Lannigan. 2000. Correlation of oxacillin MIC with *mecA* gene carriage in coagulase-negative staphylococci. *J. Clin. Microbiol.* **38**:752–754.

41. John, M. A., J. Burden, J. I. Stuart, R. C. Reyes, R. Lannigan, S. Milburn, D. Diagre, B. Wilson, and Z. Hussain. 2009. Comparison of three phenotypic techniques for detection of methicillin resistance in *Staphylococcus* spp. reveals a species-dependent performance. *J. Antimicrob. Chemother.* **63**:493–496.

42. Jones, R. N. 2001. Method preferences and test accuracy of antimicrobial susceptibility testing: updates from the College of American Pathologists Microbiology Survey Program (2000). *Arch. Pathol. Lab. Med.* **125**:1285–1289.

43. Jorgensen, J. H. 1993. Selection criteria for an antimicrobial susceptibility testing system. *J. Clin. Microbiol.* **31**:2841–2844.

44. Jorgensen, J. H., A. L. Barry, M. M. Traczewski, D. F. Sahm, M. L. McElmeel, and S. A. Crawford. 2000. Rapid automated antimicrobial susceptibility testing of *Streptococcus pneumoniae* by use of the bioMerieux VITEK 2. *J. Clin. Microbiol.* **38**:2814–2818.

45. Jorgensen J. H., and M. J. Ferraro. 2009. Antimicrobial susceptibility testing: a review of general principles and contemporary practices. *Clin. Infect. Dis.* **49**:1749–1755.

46. Jorgensen, J. H., and M. J. Ferraro. 2000. Antimicrobial susceptibility testing: special needs for fastidious organisms and difficult-to-detect resistance mechanisms. *Clin. Infect. Dis.* **30**:799–808.

47. Jorgensen, J. H., S. A. Crawford, L. M. McElmeel, and C. G. Whitney. 2004. Detection of resistance to gatifloxacin and moxifloxacin in *Streptococcus pneumoniae* with the VITEK 2 instrument. *J. Clin. Microbiol.* **42**:5928–5930.

48. Jorgensen, J. H., S. A. Crawford, M. L. McElmeel, and K. R. Fiebelkorn. 2004. Detection of inducible clindamycin resistance in conjunction with performance of automated broth susceptibility testing. *J. Clin. Microbiol.* **42**:1800–1802.

49. Joyanes, P., M. D. C. Conejo, L. Martinez-Martinez, and E. J. Perea. 2001. Evaluation of the VITEK 2 system for the identification and susceptibility testing of three species of nonfermenting gram-negative rods frequently isolated from clinical samples. *J. Clin. Microbiol.* **39**:3247–3253.

50. Junkins, A. D., S. R. Lockhart, K. P. Heilmann, C. L. Dohrn, D. L. Von Stein, P. L. Winokur, G. V. Doern, and S. S. Richter. 2009. BD Phoenix and Vitek 2 detection of *mecA*-mediated resistance in *Staphylococcus aureus* with cefoxitin. *J. Clin. Microbiol.* **47**:2879–2882.

50a. Junkins, A. D., S. S. Arbefeville, W. J. Howard, and S. S. Richter. 2010. Comparison of BD Phoenix AP workflow with Vitek 2. *J. Clin. Microbiol.* **48**:1929–1931.

51. Juretschko, S., V. J. LaBombardi, S. A. Lerner, P. C. Schreckenberger, and the *Pseudomonas* AST Study Group. 2007. Accuracies of β-lactam susceptibility test results for *Pseudomonas aeruginosa* with four automated systems (BD Phoenix, MicroScan WalkAway, Vitek, and Vitek 2). *J. Clin. Microbiol.* **45**:1339–1342.

52. Kaase, M., B. Baars, S. Friedrich, F. Szabados, and S. G. Gatermann. 2009. Performance of MicroScan WalkAway

and VITEK 2 for detection of oxacillin resistance in a set of methicillin-resistant *Staphylococcus aureus* isolates with diverse genetic backgrounds. *J. Clin. Microbiol.* **47:**2623–2625.

53. **Kaase, M., S. Lena, S. Friedrich, F. Szabados, T. Sakinc, B. Kleine, and S. G. Gatermann.** 2008. Comparison of phenotypic methods for penicillinase detection in *Staphylococcus aureus. Clin. Microbiol. Infect.* **14:**614–616.

54. **Karlowsky, J. A., M. K. Weaver, C. Thornsberry, M. J. Dowzicky, M. E. Jones, and D. F. Sahm.** 2003. Comparison of four antimicrobial susceptibility testing methods to determine the in vitro activities of piperacillin and piperacillin-tazobactam against clinical isolates of *Enterobacteriaceae* and *Pseudomonas aeruginosa. J. Clin. Microbiol.* **41:**3339–3343.

55. **Kolbert, M., F. Chegrani, and P. M. Shah.** 2004. Evaluation of the OSIRIS video reader as an automated measurement system for the agar disk diffusion technique. *Clin. Microbiol. Infect.* **10:**416–420.

56. **Komatsu, M., M. Aihara, K. Shimakawa, M. Iwasaki, Y. Nagasaka, S. Fukuda, S. Matsuo, and Y. Iwatani.** 2003. Evaluation of MicroScan ESBL confirmation panel for *Enterobacteriaceae*-producing, extended-spectrum β-lactamases isolated in Japan. *Diagn. Microbiol. Infect. Dis.* **46:**125–130.

57. **Korgenski, E. K., and J. A. Daly.** 1998. Evaluation of the BIOMIC video reader system for determining interpretive categories of isolates on the basis of disk diffusion susceptibility results. *J. Clin. Microbiol.* **36:**302–304.

58. **Kulah, C., E. Aktas, F. Comert, N. Ozlu, I. Akyar, and H. Ankarali.** 2009. Detecting imipenem resistance in *Acinetobacter baumannii* by automated systems (BD Phoenix, MicroScan WalkAway, Vitek 2); high error rates with MicroScan WalkAway. *BMC Infect. Dis.* **9:**30–37.

58a. **LeClercq, R., A. Boulanger, F. Doucet-Populaire, S. Galopin, M. Ploy, and C. Poyart.** 2009. *Abstr. 49th Intersci. Conf. Antimicrob. Agents Chemother.*, abstr. D-797.

59. **Lestari, E. S., J. A. Severin, P. M. G. Filius, K. Kuntaman, D. O. Duerink, U. Hadi, H. Wahjono, and H. A. Verbrugh.** 2008. Comparison of the accuracy of disk diffusion zone diameters obtained by manual zone measurements to that by automated zone measurements to determine antimicrobial susceptibility. *J. Microbiol. Methods* **75:**177–181.

60. **Leverstein-van Hall, M., A. C. Fluit, A. Paauw, A. T. A. Box, S. Brisse, and J. Verhoef.** 2002. Evaluation of the Etest ESBL and the BD Phoenix, VITEK 1, and VITEK 2 automated instruments for detection of extended-spectrum beta-lactamases in multiresistant *Escherichia coli* and *Klebsiella* spp. *J. Clin. Microbiol.* **40:**3703–3711.

61. **Ligozzi, M., C. Bernini, M. G. Bonora, M. de Fatima, J. Zuliani, and R. Fontana.** 2002. Evaluation of the VITEK 2 system for identification and antimicrobial susceptibility testing of medically relevant gram-positive cocci. *J. Clin. Microbiol.* **40:**1681–1686.

62. **Linscott, A. J., and W. J. Brown.** 2005. Evaluation of four commercially available extended-spectrum beta-lactamase phenotypic confirmation tests. *J. Clin. Microbiol.* **43:**1081–1085.

63. **Livermore, D. M., M. Struelens, J. Amorin, F. Baquero, J. Bille, R. Canton, S. Henning, S. Gatermann, A. Marchese, H. Mittermayer, C. Nonhoff, K. J. Oakton, F. Praplan, H. Ramos, G. C. Schito, J. Van Eldere, J. Verhaegen, J. Verhoef, and M. R. Visser.** 2002. Multicentre evaluation of the VITEK 2 Advanced Expert System for interpretive reading of antimicrobial resistance tests. *J. Antimicrob. Chemother.* **49:**289–300.

64. **Livermore, D. M., T. G. Winstanley, and K. P. Shannon.** 2001. Interpretative reading: recognizing the unusual and inferring resistance mechanisms from resistance phenotypes. *J. Antimicrob. Chemother.* **47**(Suppl. 1):87–102.

65. **Mazzariol, A., M. Aldegheri, M. Ligozzi, G. L. Cascio, R. Koncan, and R. Fontana.** 2008. Performance of Vitek 2 in antimicrobial susceptibility testing of *Pseudomonas aeruginosa* isolates with different mechanisms of β-lactam resistance. *J. Clin. Microbiol.* **46:**2095–2098.

66. **Medeiros, A. A., and J. Crellin.** 2000. Evaluation of the Sirscan automated zone reader in a clinical microbiology laboratory. *J. Clin. Microbiol.* **38:**1688–1693.

67. **Munro, S., R. M. Mulder, S. M. Farnham, and B. Grinius.** 2004. Evaluating antimicrobial susceptibility test systems, p. 5.17.1–5.17.9. *In* H. D. Isenberg (ed.), *Clinical Microbiology Procedures Handbook*, 2nd ed. ASM Press, Washington, DC.

68. **Murdoch, D. R., S. Mirrett, L. J. Harrell, S. M. Donabedian, M. J. Zervos, and L. B. Reller.** 2003. Comparison of MicroScan broth microdilution, synergy quad plate agar dilution, and disk diffusion screening methods for detection of high-level aminoglycoside resistance in *Enterococcus* species. *J. Clin. Microbiol.* **41:**2703–2705.

69. **Nakasone, I., T. Kinjo, N. Yamane, K. Kisanuki, and C. M. Shiohira.** 2007. Laboratory-based evaluation of the colorimetric VITEK-2 Compact system for species identification and of the Advanced Expert System for detection of antimicrobial resistances: VITEK-2 Compact system identification and antimicrobial susceptibility testing. *Diagn. Microbiol. Infect. Dis.* **58:**191–198.

70. **Nijs, A., R. Cartuyvels, A. Mewis, V. Peeters, J. L. Rummens, and K. Magerman.** 2003. Comparison and evaluation of Osiris and Sirscan 2000 antimicrobial susceptibility systems in the clinical microbiology laboratory. *J. Clin. Microbiol.* **41:**3627–3630.

71. **Pfaller, M. A., and R. N. Jones.** 2006. Performance accuracy of antibacterial and antifungal susceptibility test methods: report from the College of American Pathologists Microbiology Surveys Program (2001–2003). *Arch. Pathol. Lab. Med.* **130:**767–778.

72. **Richter, S. S., W. J. Howard, M. P. Weinstein, D. A. Bruckner, J. F. Hindler, M. Saubolle, and G. V. Doern.** 2007. Multicenter evaluation of the BD Phoenix automated microbiology system for antimicrobial susceptibility testing of *Streptococcus* species. *J. Clin. Microbiol.* **45:**2863–2871.

73. **Roisin, S., C. Nonhoff, O. Denis, and M. J. Struelens.** 2008. Evaluation of new VITEK 2 card and disk diffusion method for determining susceptibility of *Staphylococcus aureus* to oxacillin. *J. Clin. Microbiol.* **46:**2525–2528.

74. **Rolain, J. M., M. N. Mallet, P. E. Fournier, and D. Raoult.** 2004. Real-time PCR for universal antibiotic susceptibility testing. *J. Antimicrob. Chemother.* **54:**538–541.

75. **Rosenberg, J., F. C. Tenover, J. Wong, W. Jarvis, and D. J. Vugia.** 1997. Are clinical laboratories in California accurately reporting vancomycin-resistant enterococci? *J. Clin. Microbiol.* **35:**2526–2530.

76. **Sader, H. S., T. R. Fritsche, and R. N. Jones.** 2006. Accuracy of three automated systems (MicroScan WalkAway, VITEK, and VITEK 2) for susceptibility testing of *Pseudomonas aeruginosa* against five broad-spectrum beta-lactam agents. *J. Clin. Microbiol.* **44:**1101–1104.

77. **Sakoulas, G., H. S. Gold, L. Venkataraman, P. C. Degirolami, G. M. Eliopoulos, and Q. Qian.** 2001. Methicillin-resistant *Staphylococcus aureus*: comparison of susceptibility testing methods and analysis of *mecA*-positive susceptible strains. *J. Clin. Microbiol.* **39:**3946–3951.

78. **Sanchez, M. A., B. Sanchez del Saz, E. Loza, F. Baquero, and R. Canton.** 2001. Evaluation of the OSIRIS video reader for disk diffusion susceptibility test reading. *Clin. Microbiol. Infect.* **7:**352–357.

79. **Sanders, C. C., M. Peyret, E. S. Moland, C. Shubert, K. S. Thomson, J.-M. Boeufgras, and W. E. Sanders.** 2000. Ability of the VITEK 2 Advanced Expert System to identify β-lactam phenotypes in isolates of *Enterobacteriaceae* and *Pseudomonas aeruginosa. J. Clin. Microbiol.* **38:**570–574.

80. **Sanders, C. C., M. Peyret, E. S. Moland, S. J. Cavalieri, C. Shubert, K. S. Thomson, J.-M. Boeufgras, and W. E. Sanders.** 2001. Potential impact of the VITEK 2 System and the Advanced Expert System on the clinical laboratory of a university-based hospital. *J. Clin. Microbiol.* **39:**2379–2385.

81. **Sanguinetti, M., B. Posteraro, T. Spanu, D. Ciccaglione, L. Romano, B. Fiori, G. Nicoletti, S. Zanetti, and G. Fadda.** 2003. Characterization of clinical isolates of *Enterobacteriaceae* from Italy by the Phoenix extended-spectrum β-lactamase detection method. *J. Clin. Microbiol.* **41:**1463–1468.

82. **Sorlozano, A., J. Gutierrez, G. Piedrola, and M. J. Soto.** 2005. Acceptable performance of VITEK 2 system to detect extended-spectrum β-lactamases in clinical isolates of *Escherichia coli*: a comparative study of phenotypic commercial methods and NCCLS guidelines. *Diagn. Microbiol. Infect. Dis.* **51:**191–193.

83. **Spanu, T., M. Sanguinetti, M. Tumbarello, T. D'Inzeo, B. Fiori, B. Posteraro, R. Santangelo, R. Cauda, and G. Fadda.** 2006. Evaluation of the new VITEK 2 extended-spectrum beta-lactamase (ESBL) test for rapid detection of ESBL production in *Enterobacteriaceae* isolates. *J. Clin. Microbiol.* **44:**3257–3262.

84. **Spanu, T., M. Sanguinetti, T. D'Inzeo, D. Ciccaglione, L. Romano, F. Leone, P Mazzella, and G. Fadda.** 2004. Identification of methicillin-resistant isolates of *Staphylococcus aureus* and coagulase-negative staphylococci responsible for bloodstream infections with the Phoenix™ system. *Diagn. Microbiol. Infect. Dis.* **48:**221–227.

85. **Stefaniuk, E., A. Baraniak, M. Gniadkowski, and W. Hryniewicz.** 2003. Evaluation of the BD Phoenix automated identification and susceptibility testing system in clinical microbiology laboratory practice. *Eur. J. Clin. Microbiol. Infect. Dis.* **22:**479–485.

86. **Steward, C. D., J. M. Mohammed, J. M. Swenson, S. A. Stocker, P. P. Williams, R. P. Gaynes, J. E. McGowan, and F. C. Tenover.** 2003. Antimicrobial susceptibility testing of carbapenems: multicenter validity and accuracy levels of five antimicrobial test methods for detecting resistance in *Enterobacteriaceae* and *Pseudomonas aeruginosa* isolates. *J. Clin. Microbiol.* **41:**351–358.

87. **Sturenburg, E., I. Sobottka, H.-H. Feucht, D. Mack, and R. Laufs.** 2003. Comparison of BD Phoenix and VITEK 2 automated antimicrobial susceptibility test systems for extended-spectrum beta-lactamase detection in *Escherichia coli* and *Klebsiella* species clinical isolates. *Diagn. Microbiol. Infect. Dis.* **45:**29–34.

88. **Sturenburg, E., M. Lang, M. A. Horstkotte, R. Laufs, and D. Mack.** 2004. Evaluation of the MicroScan ESBL plus confirmation panel for detection of extended-spectrum β-lactamases in clinical isolates of oxyimino-cephalosporin-resistant gram-negative bacteria. *J. Antimicrob. Chemother.* **54:**870–875.

89. **Swenson, J. M., D. Lonsway, S. McAllister, A. Thompson, L. Jevitt, W. Zhu, and J. B. Patel.** 2007. Detection of *mecA*-mediated resistance using reference and commercial testing methods in a collection of *Staphylococcus aureus* expressing borderline oxacillin MICs. *Diagn. Microbiol. Infect. Dis.* **58:**33–39.

90. **Swenson, J. M., K. F. Anderson, D. R. Lonsway, A. Thompson, S. K. McAllister, B. M. Limbago, R. B. Carey, F. C. Tenover, and J. B. Patel.** 2009. Accuracy of commercial and reference susceptibility testing methods for detecting vancomycin-intermediate *Staphylococcus aureus*. *J. Clin. Microbiol.* **47:**2013–2017.

91. **Tenover, F. C., J. M. Swensen, C. M. O'Hara, and S. A. Stocker.** 1995. Ability of commercial and reference antimicrobial susceptibility testing methods to detect vancomycin resistance in enterococci. *J. Clin. Microbiol.* **33:**1524–1527.

92. **Tenover, F. C., L. M. Weigel, P. C. Appelbaum, L. K. McDougal, J. Chaitram, S. McAllister, N. Clark, G. Killgore, C. M. O'Hara, L. Jevitt, J. B. Patel, and B. Bozdogan.** 2004. Vancomycin-resistant *Staphylococcus aureus* isolate from a patient in Pennsylvania. *Antimicrob. Agents Chemother.* **48:**275–280.

93. **Tenover, F. C., M. V. Lancaster, B. C. Hill, C. D. Steward, S. A. Stocker, G. A. Hancock, C. M. O'Hara, N. C. Clark, and K. Hiramatsu.** 1998. Characterization of staphylococci with reduced susceptibilities to vancomycin and other glycopeptides. *J. Clin. Microbiol.* **36:**1020–1027.

94. **Tenover, F. C., P. P. Williams, S. Stocker, A. Thompson, L. A. Clark, B. Limbago, R. B. Carey, S. M. Poppe, D. Shinabarger, and J. E. McGowan.** 2007. Accuracy of six antimicrobial susceptibility methods for testing linezolid against staphylococci and enterococci. *J. Clin. Microbiol.* **45:**2917–2922.

95. **Tenover, F. C., R. K. Kalsi, P. P. Williams, R. C. Carey, S. Stocker, D. Lonsway, J. K. Rasheed, J. W. Biddle, J. E. McGowan, and B. Hanna.** 2006. Carbapenem resistance in *Klebsiella pneumoniae* not detected by automated susceptibility testing. *Emerg. Infect. Dis.* **12:**1209–1213.

96. **Thomson, K. S., N. E. Cornish, S. G. Hong, K. Hemrick, C. Herdt, and E. S. Moland.** 2007. Comparison of Phoenix and VITEK 2 extended-spectrum-β-lactamase detection tests for analysis of *Escherichia coli* and *Klebsiella* isolates with well-characterized β-lactamases. *J. Clin. Microbiol.* **45:**2380–2384.

97. **Tsakris, A., A. Pantazi, S. Pournaras, A. Maniatis, A. Polyzou, and D. Sofianou.** 2000. Pseudo-outbreak of imipenem-resistant *Acinetobacter baumannii* resulting from false susceptibility testing by a rapid automated system. *J. Clin. Microbiol.* **38:**3505–3507.

98. **Turnidge, J. D., and J. M. Bell.** 2005. Antimicrobial susceptibility on solid media, p. 8–60. *In* V. Lorin (ed.), *Antibiotics in Laboratory Medicine*, 5th ed. The Williams & Wilkins Co., Baltimore, MD.

99. **Van Den Braak, N., W. Goessens, A. van Belkum, H. A. Verbrugh, and H. P. Endtz.** 2001. Accuracy of the VITEK 2 system to detect glycopeptide resistance in enterococci. *J. Clin. Microbiol.* **39:**351–353.

100. **Weissmann, D., J. Spargo, C. Wennersten, and M. J. Ferraro.** 1991. Detection of enterococcal high-level aminoglycoside resistance with MicroScan freeze-dried panels containing newly modified medium and VITEK gram-positive susceptibility cards. *J. Clin. Microbiol.* **29:**1232–1235.

101. **White, R. L., M. B. Kays, L. V. Friedrich, E. W. Brown, and J. R. Koonce.** 1991. Pseudoresistance of *Pseudomonas aeruginosa* resulting from degradation of imipenem in an automated susceptibility testing system with predried panels. *J. Clin. Microbiol.* **29:**398–400.

102. **Winstanley, T. G., H. K. Parsons, M. A. Horstkotte, I. Sobottka, and E. Sturenburg.** 2005. Phenotypic detection of β-lactamase-mediated resistance to oxyimino-cephalosporins in Enterobacteriaceae: evaluation of the Mastacan Elite Expert System. *J. Antimicrob. Chemother.* **56:**292–296.

103. **Woods, G. L., B. DiGiovanni, M. Levison, P. Pitsakis, and D. LaTemple.** 1993. Evaluation of MicroScan rapid panels for detection of high-level aminoglycoside resistance in enterococci. *J. Clin. Microbiol.* **31:**2786–2787.

Special Phenotypic Methods for Detecting Antibacterial Resistance

JANA M. SWENSON, JEAN B. PATEL, AND JAMES H. JORGENSEN

70

Most of the tests described in this chapter are phenotypic tests that characterize an organism's susceptibility or resistance to an antimicrobial agent by screening for a specific resistance mechanism or phenotype. As screening tests, they do not provide an MIC of the agent; however, some of these tests have sufficient sensitivity and specificity that confirmation of the result is unnecessary and the results of the screen test can be reported without additional testing. Others require confirmation of the result by another method. For example, screening tests for oxacillin and inducible clindamycin resistance in *Staphylococcus aureus* and MIC screening tests for high-level aminoglycoside resistance in enterococci have been shown to be comparable in reliability to standard methods for detecting clinically significant resistance, and additional confirmatory tests are unnecessary. These tests may either supplement or replace traditional testing methods, depending on the organism and the assay. This chapter describes details of tests for detection of high-level aminoglycoside resistance and acquired vancomycin resistance in enterococci; tests for detection of inducible clindamycin resistance in streptococci; tests for detection of penicillin, oxacillin, vancomycin, inducible clindamycin, and high-level mupirocin resistance in staphylococci; tests for detection of extended-spectrum-β-lactamase (ESBL) and carbapenemase production in *Enterobacteriaceae*; and tests for detection of β-lactamases in multiple organisms. These tests are listed in Table 1. Other special phenotypic tests described in this chapter are those for determining the bactericidal activity or combined activities of antimicrobial agents; they are different from the tests that screen for a specific resistance mechanism given in Table 1.

Quality control information is given for all of the tests in each section; however, guidelines for the frequency of quality control testing are not provided, because they have not been defined and may vary depending on laboratory circumstances. A practical approach would be to perform quality control testing each day clinical isolates are tested or less frequently (e.g., weekly) once a laboratory has thoroughly documented that less frequent quality control testing can verify the reliability of the procedures. However, the College of American Pathologists recommends that quality control testing be done daily on β-lactamase tests. Quality control tests should be performed each time new lots of material are put into use.

TESTS TO DETECT RESISTANCE IN ENTEROCOCCI

Serious invasive enterococcal infections, such as endocarditis, are commonly treated with a cell wall-active agent (either a penicillin or a glycopeptide such as vancomycin) and an aminoglycoside (usually gentamicin or streptomycin). These agents act synergistically to enhance killing (8, 207). However, when an enterococcal strain is resistant to the cell wall-active agent or has high-level resistance (HLR) to the aminoglycoside, there is no synergism and combination therapy will not provide a bactericidal effect (8). Because of this, it is important to determine the susceptibility to both the aminoglycoside and the cell wall-active agent individually in order to predict the likelihood of synergy. Methods for detection of aminoglycoside and vancomycin resistance are discussed here. Discussion of methods for detection of high-level penicillin and ampicillin resistance can be found in the relevant Clinical and Laboratory Standards Institute (CLSI) documents (38, 39).

Detection of HLR to Aminoglycosides

Because aminoglycosides have poor activity against enterococci (MICs range from 8 to 256 µg/ml), they cannot be used as single agents for therapy (8, 90). This intrinsic, moderate-level resistance is due to poor uptake of the aminoglycoside by the cell (145). Acquired aminoglycoside resistance in enterococci is due either to mutations resulting in decreased binding of the agent to the ribosome, as occurs with streptomycin (called ribosomal resistance), or, more commonly, to the acquisition of new genes that encode enzymes that modify aminoglycosides (called acquired resistance). Acquired aminoglycoside resistance usually corresponds to MICs that are significantly above the concentrations normally tested in routine susceptibility tests, e.g., ≥2,000 µg/ml for streptomycin and ≥500 µg/ml for gentamicin, and is designated HLR (145) (see also chapters 21 and 66).

Synergy between an aminoglycoside and a cell wall-active agent can be determined directly by performing complex time-kill studies (36, 111) or can be predicted by using less cumbersome screening tests. Gentamicin and streptomycin are the only two agents that should be tested on a routine basis. Enterococcal isolates that are resistant to gentamicin are considered resistant to tobramycin and amikacin as well because gentamicin resistance is most commonly due to the bifunctional enzyme encoded by *aac(6')-Ic-aph(2")-Ia*,

TABLE 1 Special phenotypic tests for detecting antibacterial resistance described in this chapter

Organism group(s)	Resistance mechanism	Test method(s) described	Further testing or confirmation required?
Enterococci	High-level aminoglycoside resistance	Broth microdilution Disk diffusion	No for MIC; yes for disk, if inconclusive
	Vancomycin resistance	Vancomycin agar screen test using BHI agar	Yes
	β-Lactamase production	Direct β-lactamase test	
Staphylococcus aureus	Oxacillin resistance	Oxacillin-salt agar screening test	No
	mecA-mediated oxacillin resistance	Cefoxitin broth microdilution Cefoxitin disk diffusion	No
	Vancomycin resistance	Vancomycin agar screen test using BHI agar	Yes
	Inducible clindamycin resistance	Broth microdilution using a clindamycin-erythromycin combination well D-zone test (disk diffusion)	No
	High-level mupirocin resistance	Broth microdilution Disk diffusion	No
	β-Lactamase production	Direct β-lactamase test	Yes
CoNS	*mecA*-mediated oxacillin resistance	Cefoxitin disk diffusion	No
	Inducible clindamycin resistance	Broth microdilution using a clindamycin-erythromycin combination well D-zone test (disk diffusion)	No
	β-Lactamase production	Direct β-lactamase test	Yes
Enterobacteriaceae	ESBL production	Broth microdilution Disk diffusion	Yes
	Carbapenemase production	Broth microdilution Disk diffusion	Yes
Pneumococci	Penicillin resistance	Oxacillin disk	Yes, if nonsusceptible
Other organism groups	β-Lactamase production	Direct β-lactamase test	See Table 4

which also confers resistance to other aminoglycosides except streptomycin. Resistance to streptomycin is mediated by a different resistance mechanism, and consequently, streptomycin resistance must be determined separately from gentamicin resistance. Isolates of *Enterococcus faecium* are intrinsically resistant to the synergistic actions of amikacin, kanamycin, tobramycin, and netilmicin with cell wall-active agents, irrespective of in vitro testing results for HLR (138). *Enterococcus faecalis* strains that are susceptible to gentamicin may be resistant to kanamycin and amikacin. In vitro tests with amikacin cannot reliably predict HLR to amikacin in *E. faecalis*, but kanamycin could be used to predict HLR to amikacin and kanamycin (188), although optimal methods for testing have not been determined.

The genes for three additional enzymes that mediate gentamicin resistance have been described, *aph(2″)-Ic* (33), *aph(2″)-Id* (238), and *aph(2″)-Ib* (107). All confer resistance to ampicillin-gentamicin synergism; however, the first [*aph(2″)-Ic*] may not be detected using the screening methods described below since its presence seems to lead to intermediate, not high-level, resistance. The second [*aph(2″)-Id*], if detected by the screening methods described here, would be assumed to be resistant to synergy with amikacin, although this may not be the case. Only time-kill or molecular studies for the specific enzymes will detect the presence of these enzymes. Methods for detection of HLR to aminoglycosides are summarized in Table 2 and discussed below.

Agar Dilution Screening Method

Agar plates are prepared with brain heart infusion (BHI) agar with addition of 500 µg of gentamicin per ml or 2,000 µg of streptomycin per ml. The plates are inoculated by spotting 10 µl of a suspension that is equivalent to a 0.5 McFarland standard prepared from growth on an 18- to 24-h agar plate, giving a final inoculum of 10^6 CFU per spot. The plates are incubated for a full 24 h in ambient air. The presence of more than one colony or a haze of growth should be read as resistant. For streptomycin, the plates should be incubated for an additional 24 h if there is no growth at 24 h. Mueller-Hinton agar (MHA), MHA plus 5% sheep blood, or dextrose phosphate agar may be substituted for BHI agar, but because growth is better on BHI agar, this is the preferred medium. Commercially prepared agar screen plates are available and have performed well (78, 184, 185). Kanamycin agar screen tests have not been as extensively evaluated and are not standardized, but it has been reported that for determining HLR to both amikacin and kanamycin in *E. faecalis*, kanamycin at 2,000 µg/ml in BHI agar can be used (188).

Broth Microdilution Screening Method

Broth dilution tests are prepared using a single well or a tube containing BHI broth with addition of 500 µg of gentamicin per ml or 1,000 µg of streptomycin per ml. The final inoculum concentration is that recommended for routine broth

TABLE 2 Screening methods for detecting vancomycin and high-level aminoglycoside resistance in enterococci

Parameter	Screening procedure			
	Vancomycin agar dilution	Aminoglycoside agar dilution	Aminoglycoside broth microdilution	Aminoglycoside disk diffusion
Medium	BHI agar	BHI agar	BHI broth	MHA
Inoculum	10^5–10^6 CFU/spot	10^6 CFU/spot	5×10^4 CFU/0.1 ml	0.5 McFarland[a]
Incubation (h) in ambient air	24	24[b]	24[b]	18–24
Drug concn				
Gentamicin	NA	500 µg/ml	500 µg/ml	120 µg/disk
Streptomycin	NA	2,000 µg/ml	1,000 µg/ml	300 µg/disk
Vancomycin	6 µg/ml	NA[c]	NA	NA
Endpoint	>1 colony	>1 colony	Any growth	6 mm = resistant, 7–9 mm = inconclusive,[d] ≥10 mm = susceptible

[a] CLSI disk diffusion method (41).
[b] If streptomycin is negative at 24 h, incubate for an additional 24 h.
[c] NA, not applicable.
[d] If the zone is 7 to 9 mm, the test is inconclusive, and an agar or broth microdilution test should be performed to confirm susceptibility or resistance.

microdilution testing, i.e., 5×10^5 CFU/ml. The plates are incubated for 24 h in ambient air. For streptomycin, the tests should be incubated for an additional 24 h if there is no growth at 24 h. Any growth is interpreted as denoting resistance.

The recommended streptomycin concentration for use in the broth microdilution screen is half that used in the agar dilution screen test. Because this test is often included as part of a routine gram-positive MIC panel, the inoculum is that commonly used in broth microdilution testing (5×10^5 CFU/ml). The total number of cells tested in the agar dilution screening procedure (10^6 CFU/spot) is 20-fold larger than that normally used in the broth microdilution test (5×10^4 CFU/0.1-ml well). In order to provide a test that uses a small inoculum and at the same time maximizes the detection of HLR to streptomycin, it was necessary to lower the concentration recommended for testing streptomycin from 2,000 to 1,000 µg/ml in the broth microdilution test. Because of poorer growth and the smaller inoculum, Mueller-Hinton broth is inadequate for use in the broth microdilution screen test (217). The performance of other aminoglycosides in this test has not been evaluated.

Disk Diffusion Screening Method

The standard disk diffusion procedure (39) described in chapter 68 (with unsupplemented MHA) is used, except that special high-content disks (gentamicin at 120 µg and streptomycin at 300 µg) are required (189). Zones are measured after 18 to 24 h of incubation in ambient air at 35°C. Isolates for which the zone diameters are ≥10 mm are categorized as susceptible. The absence of a zone of inhibition corresponds to the presence of HLR. Strains for which the zones of inhibition are 7 to 9 mm usually display HLR, but a few are strains for which the MICs are only moderately elevated (217). Therefore, strains for which the zone diameters are 7 to 9 mm should be tested by either the standard agar or broth microdilution screen method to determine susceptibility or resistance. High-content gentamicin and streptomycin disks are available commercially.

Quality Control

For both gentamicin and streptomycin, *E. faecalis* ATCC 29212 is used as the susceptible control strain and *E. faecalis* ATCC 51299 is used as the resistant control strain (216).

Only *E. faecalis* ATCC 29212 is used for control of disk diffusion tests. The expected quality control limits are 16 to 23 mm for gentamicin (120-µg) disks and 14 to 20 mm for streptomycin (300-µg) disks (40).

Detection of Vancomycin Resistance in Enterococci

As defined by the CLSI, the MIC interpretive criteria for vancomycin are ≤4 µg/ml for susceptible, 8 to 16 µg/ml for intermediate, and ≥32 µg/ml for resistant. The three most common phenotypes of resistance are (i) high-level vancomycin resistance (MICs, ≥64 µg/ml) with accompanying teicoplanin resistance (MICs, ≥16 µg/ml) (VanA phenotype); (ii) moderate- to high-level vancomycin resistance (MICs, 16 to 512 µg/ml), most commonly without teicoplanin resistance (VanB phenotype); and (iii) intrinsic low-level resistance associated with *Enterococcus gallinarum* and *Enterococcus casseliflavus* (MICs, 2 to 32 µg/ml) (VanC phenotype) (117, 118). Both the VanA and VanB phenotypes are most commonly seen in *E. faecalis* and *E. faecium* but have been found in other species, including *E. casseliflavus* and *E. gallinarum* (117, 152). Four additional genotypes have been described, *vanD* (156, 169), *vanE* (74), *vanG* (134), and *vanL* (17). VanD-type resistance, resulting in HLR to vancomycin (MICs, ≥64 µg/ml) and variable resistance to teicoplanin, has been found only in *E. faecium*. VanE-type resistance, found in *E. faecalis*, exhibits intermediate vancomycin MICs (16 µg/ml), and the organism remains susceptible to teicoplanin. The VanG phenotype is similar to the VanD phenotype. *vanL* was found in *E. faecalis* and causes low-level resistance to vancomycin (MICs = 8 µg/ml). All except *vanA*, *vanB*, and *vanC* are rare.

Many methods commonly used by clinical laboratories, including disk diffusion and the VITEK Legacy (bioMérieux, Durham, NC) and MicroScan (Siemens Healthcare Diagnostics, Deerfield, IL) systems, originally had problems detecting low-level vancomycin resistance (both VanB and VanC types) (65, 155, 186, 187, 218, 233, 251). However, systems have improved (32, 81, 97, 103, 233). The VITEK 2 and Phoenix systems perform very well for detection of vancomycin resistance in enterococci (1, 62, 68, 149, 209, 241); however, a recent study cautioned that *vanA*- or *vanB*-containing *E. casseliflavus* and *E. gallinarum* may not be differentiated from the usual wild-type *vanC* resistance (149) with the VITEK 2 expert system. Disk diffusion testing requires 24 h of incubation and examination of zones under transmitted light.

The vancomycin agar screening test first described by Willey et al. (251) was adopted by the CLSI in 1993 (37, 215) (Table 2). The sensitivity and specificity levels of 96 to 99% and 100%, respectively, were noted at that time. Commercially prepared plates also perform well (65, 78, 242). However, there may be some confusion about the characterization of susceptibility or resistance for the *vanC*-containing enterococci, *E. gallinarum* and *E. casseliflavus*, because their growth is variable on the agar screen plate. Both of these species intrinsically contain a *vanC* gene, but the MICs of vancomycin for them range from 2 to 32 µg/ml (117). Whether the presence of this gene is associated with therapeutic failures is not known. Since the vancomycin MICs for these strains are often >4 µg/ml, the strains are likely to grow on the agar screen plates, where a larger inoculum and a richer medium may promote growth (78, 184, 215). Most strains of *vanC*-containing enterococci are motile at 30°C; *E. casseliflavus* is typically yellow pigmented. These characteristics have been used to distinguish *vanC*-containing enterococci from other species (23, 78, 79). However, some *E. gallinarum* and *E. casseliflavus* strains may be nonmotile. Because of this, a better test to differentiate them from *E. faecalis* and *E. faecium* is fermentation of 1% methyl-α-D-glucopyranoside (MGP). All *vanC*-containing enterococci acidify MGP, whereas *E. faecium* and *E. faecalis* do not (174) (see also chapter 21).

Vancomycin Agar Screen Test

Agar plates are prepared with BHI agar supplemented with 6 µg of vancomycin per ml (BHI-V6). Using growth from an 18- to 24-h agar plate, make a suspension equivalent in turbidity to a 0.5 McFarland standard and inoculate the plates by spotting 1 to 10 µl or swabbing an area 10 to 15 mm in diameter. The final inoculum is 10^5 to 10^6 CFU per spot. After inoculation, incubate the plates for a full 24 h in ambient air at 35°C. The presence of more than one colony or a haze of growth indicates resistance.

Quality Control

For quality control, *E. faecalis* ATCC 29212 (no growth, i.e., susceptible) and *E. faecalis* ATCC 51299 (growth, i.e., resistant) should be tested (216). Plates made with BHI agars from certain manufacturers may allow light growth of *E. faecalis* ATCC 29212, especially if the larger inoculum (10 µl) is used or the plates are held longer than 24 h.

Reporting Resistance in Enterococci

For any serious enterococcal infection (e.g., endocarditis), results of the screen for HLR to gentamicin and streptomycin should be reported in concert with the results of the testing of the cell wall-active agents (penicillin, ampicillin, or vancomycin), because synergy would not be expected if any one of the agents reported is resistant. High-level aminoglycoside resistance determined by an MIC screen method can be reported without further confirmation. With the disk diffusion test, results can be reported unless the test is inconclusive, when an agar dilution or broth microdilution test should be done to clarify the result. Helpful suggestions on reporting the results of enterococcal tests are given by Hindler and Sahm (90).

TESTS TO DETECT RESISTANCE IN STAPHYLOCOCCI

Because some of the phenotypic tests described here for *S. aureus* are not recommended for coagulase-negative staphylococci (CoNS), for detection of oxacillin resistance the two groups are discussed separately as *S. aureus* and *Staphylococcus lugdunensis* and CoNS except *S. lugdunensis*. *S. lugdunensis* is included with *S. aureus* because it has been shown that *S. lugdunensis*, although coagulase negative, tends to behave more like *S. aureus* than like other CoNS with oxacillin tests (77, 133, 221). For tests other than the detection of oxacillin resistance, this grouping may also work, although possible exceptions are noted in the discussions that follow. Tests for detection of resistance in this group are summarized in Table 3.

Detection of Penicillin Resistance in Staphylococci

Penicillin resistance in staphylococci is due to a penicillinase encoded by the *blaZ* gene that is usually plasmid mediated and inducible. Most staphylococci are now resistant to penicillin, so its use for treatment is rarely considered. The breakpoint for penicillin resistance is ≤0.12 µg/ml; however, because rare isolates with penicillin MICs in the susceptible range may produce β-lactamase, current CLSI documents recommend that when a staphylococcal isolate tests susceptible to penicillin an induced β-lactamase test be performed before reporting the isolate as penicillin susceptible (38–40). Many laboratories perform commercial β-lactamase tests such as those that use a chromogenic cephalosporin such as nitrocefin. However, a recent study comparing phenotypic methods for detecting penicillinase in *S. aureus* strains that test susceptible to penicillin has shown that these methods lack sensitivity (106). In that study, of 197 *S. aureus* isolates for which the penicillin MIC by VITEK 2 was ≤0.12 µg/ml, *blaZ* was detected in 28. Only 11 of 28 (39%) were detected as β-lactamase positive using a nitrocefin-based method. Of five nonmolecular β-lactamase detection methods studied, the most sensitive was the appearance of the penicillin zone edge as either sharp or tapered (83), which detected 20 of 28 (71%). Kaase et al. recommend that a PCR test for *blaZ* be performed before reporting penicillin susceptibility on an isolate from a serious infection (106).

There are no simple methods that would allow clinical laboratories to routinely test for the presence of *blaZ*. The CLSI recommends that a β-lactamase test be performed before reporting a staphylococcal isolate as penicillin susceptible. However, because of the possible failure to detect β-lactamase with commonly used methods, if penicillin is being considered for treatment, the CLSI now recommends that laboratories perform an induced β-lactamase test on repeat isolates from the same patient because rare strains that contain *blaZ* and test as penicillin susceptible can become phenotypically resistant by both MIC and β-lactamase testing (40; J. Patel, unpublished observations).

Detection of Oxacillin Resistance in *S. aureus* and *S. lugdunensis*

Strains of *Staphylococcus aureus* resistant to oxacillin are still referred to as MRSA (for methicillin-resistant *S. aureus*). Even though methicillin is no longer available, the abbreviation MRSA has persisted and therefore is also used here. MIC interpretive criteria recommended by the CLSI for oxacillin and *S. aureus* and *S. lugdunensis* are ≤2 µg/ml for susceptible and ≥4 µg/ml for resistant (40). At least three different resistance mechanisms contribute to oxacillin resistance in

TABLE 3 Screening methods for detection of resistance in *Staphylococcus aureus*

Parameter	Oxacillin resistance[a] (oxacillin-salt agar screen test)	*mecA*-mediated oxacillin resistance[b] — Disk diffusion (cefoxitin)	*mecA*-mediated oxacillin resistance[b] — Broth microdilution (cefoxitin)	Vancomycin resistance[b] — Agar dilution (BHI-V6 agar screen)	Vancomycin resistance[b] — Disk diffusion	Inducible clindamycin resistance[b] — Disk diffusion (D-zone test)	Inducible clindamycin resistance[b] — Broth microdilution	High-level mupirocin resistance[a] — Disk diffusion	High-level mupirocin resistance[a] — Broth microdilution	β-Lactamase production[b]
Test method	Agar dilution (oxacillin-salt agar screen test)	Disk diffusion (cefoxitin)	Broth microdilution (cefoxitin)	Agar dilution (BHI-V6 agar screen)	Disk diffusion	Disk diffusion (D-zone test)	Broth microdilution	Disk diffusion	Broth microdilution	Commercial β-lactamase method
Medium	MHA + 4% NaCl	MHA	CAMHB	BHI agar	MHA	MHA or BAP[c]	CAMHB	MHA	CAMHB	
Inoculum	0.5 McFarland; 1-μl loop or swab	Routine disk diffusion method	Routine MIC method	0.5 McFarland; 10-μl loop or swab	Routine disk diffusion method	Routine disk diffusion method or heavy inoculum on purity plate	Routine MIC method	Routine disk diffusion method	Routine MIC method	
Drug	6 μg of oxacillin/ml	30-μg cefoxitin disk	Cefoxitin	6 μg of vancomycin/ml	30-μg vancomycin disk	15-μg erythromycin disk and 2-μg clindamycin disk spaced 15–26 mm apart	4 μg of erythromycin and 0.5 μg of clindamycin/ml in same well	200-μg mupirocin disk	256 μg of mupirocin/ml	
Incubation	35°C; 24 h	35°C; 16–18 h	35°C; 16–20 h	35°C; 24 h	35°C; 16–18 h	35°C; 16–18 h	35°C; 18–24 h	35°C; 24 h	35°C; 24 h	
Endpoint	>1 colony	≤21 mm = *mecA* positive; ≥22 mm = *mecA* negative	>4 μg/ml = *mecA* positive; ≤4 μg/ml = *mecA* negative	>1 colony or light film of growth	6 mm = resistant (MIC ≥ 16 μg/ml)	Flattening of clindamycin zone adjacent to erythromycin zone = inducible clindamycin resistance	Any growth in well containing 4 μg of erythromycin/ml and 0.5 μg of clindamycin-ml = inducible clindamycin resistance	No zone = *mupA* positive; >6 mm = *mupA* negative	Any growth in 256-μg/ml well = *mupA* positive	
Confirmation needed?	No	No	No	Yes	Yes	No	No	No	No	
Comment				Isolates with vancomycin MICs of 8 μg/ml (intermediate) also grow						Test repeat isolates from patients with serious infections caused by penicillin-susceptible, β-lactamase-negative isolates

[a] Applies to *S. aureus* only.
[b] Applies to both *S. aureus* and *S. lugdunensis*.
[c] BAP, blood agar plate.

S. aureus: (i) production of a supplemental penicillin-binding protein (PBP) (PBP 2a) encoded by a chromosomal *mecA* gene, (ii) inactivation of the drug by increased production of β-lactamase, and (iii) production of modified intrinsic PBPs (MOD-SA) with altered affinity for the drug (29, 31, 50, 85, 235). Studies to determine the prevalence of the different resistance mechanisms have not been done; however, it is assumed that the latter two occur only rarely in *S. aureus*, and they have not been found at all in *S. lugdunensis*.

Strains that possess *mecA* (the classic resistance) are either heterogeneous or homogeneous in their expression of resistance. With homogeneous expression, virtually all cells express resistance when tested by standard in vitro test methods. However, testing of a heteroresistant isolate results in some cells that appear to be susceptible and others that appear to be resistant. Often only 1 in 10^4 to 1 in 10^8 *mecA*-positive cells in the test population express resistance (87, 182, 236). Heterogeneous expression occasionally results in MICs that appear to be borderline, i.e., oxacillin MICs of 2 to 8 µg/ml, and consequently, the isolates may be misinterpreted as susceptible (MICs ≤ 2 µg/ml). MRSA isolates have historically demonstrated multidrug class resistance, including resistance to erythromycin, clindamycin, chloramphenicol, tetracycline, trimethoprim-sulfamethoxazole, older fluoroquinolones, and aminoglycosides. However, some contemporary MRSA isolates, such as those described to occur in community-associated infections (referred to as CA-MRSA), are not multiply resistant (27, 157, 261).

Non-*mecA*-mediated resistance, i.e., that due to β-lactamase or the presence of modified PBPs (MOD-SA), also results in borderline oxacillin MICs. β-Lactamase-mediated resistance can usually be distinguished from the classic type (*mecA* positive) of resistance or MOD-SA resistance by the addition of a β-lactamase inhibitor (e.g., clavulanic acid) to the oxacillin MIC test, which lowers the MIC by 2 dilutions or more. Isolates that are resistant by either the β-lactamase or the MOD-SA mechanism usually do not have multiple drug resistance, similar to CA-MRSA.

Both MIC and disk diffusion reference tests using oxacillin can be used for *S. aureus* and are generally reliable; for *S. lugdunensis* with oxacillin, only the MIC method can be used, since it has been shown that the oxacillin disk test categorizes many oxacillin-susceptible strains as resistant (221). Phenotypic tests described below for the *S. aureus* group include (i) the use of cefoxitin as a surrogate for oxacillin using routine susceptibility testing methods and (ii) the oxacillin-salt agar screen test.

Detection Using Cefoxitin as a Surrogate for Oxacillin

The use of cefoxitin has been extensively validated since it was first proposed by investigators in France (71, 144). When used as a surrogate for prediction of oxacillin resistance in *S. aureus*, it has been shown to be equal in sensitivity and specificity but easier to read than tests with oxacillin, especially for disk diffusion tests (221).

Both cefoxitin MIC and disk diffusion methods are described for *S. aureus* and *S. lugdunensis* (Table 3). The cefoxitin disk test is performed using the routine disk diffusion procedure except that modified interpretive criteria are used; for *S. aureus* and *S. lugdunensis*, results of ≤21 mm are reported as oxacillin resistant and those of ≥22 mm are considered oxacillin susceptible. These CLSI disk diffusion breakpoints were raised slightly in 2007, which increased the sensitivity of the test (43). The test is easy to read using

reflected light and does not require careful examination of the disk diffusion zones for light growth or small colonies, as is required with oxacillin. Following validation in a multilaboratory study (213), cefoxitin MIC breakpoints for prediction of *mecA*-mediated oxacillin resistance in *S. aureus* and *S. lugdunensis* were included in CLSI document M100 (41). The breakpoints, which are the only ones now included in document M100 for cefoxitin and *S. aureus*, are ≤4 µg/ml for oxacillin susceptible and ≥8 µg/ml for oxacillin resistant. Both the MIC and disk diffusion tests are read after 16 to 18 h of incubation. Quality control is the same as that recommended for routine testing with cefoxitin disk or cefoxitin dilution methods (40).

Some investigators have also looked at using cefoxitin in an agar dilution screen similar to the oxacillin-salt agar screen (72, 168, 220), although none has been studied or adopted by the CLSI. Two recent studies have looked at the use of cefoxitin disk diffusion for direct plating of positive blood cultures showing Gram stains suggestive of staphylococci (11, 54). Both found excellent correlation with standard methods, with a greatly decreased turnaround time compared to those of routine culture and susceptibility testing.

Oxacillin-Salt Agar Screening Test for *S. aureus*

The oxacillin-salt agar screen test (Table 3) has been widely used, although it has been shown to be less sensitive than the cefoxitin disk diffusion test (25, 71, 224). Its use for detection of the presence of *mecA* in *S. lugdunensis* has not been studied, but theoretically it should work since oxacillin MICs for *mecA*-positive strains are <16 µg/ml (220, 228).

MHA supplemented with 4% sodium chloride and 6 µg of oxacillin per ml is used for the agar screen method recommended by the CLSI (38). Plates containing methicillin are not recommended. For the test, inoculum suspensions are prepared by selecting colonies from overnight growth on a nonselective agar plate. The colonies are transferred to broth (e.g., tryptic soy broth) or saline to produce a suspension that matches the turbidity of a 0.5 McFarland standard. This suspension is used to inoculate the oxacillin agar screen plate by either (i) dipping a cotton swab into the test suspension, expressing the excess liquid from the swab, and inoculating an area 10 to15 mm in diameter (or streaking the swab onto a quadrant of the agar surface) or (ii) spotting an area 10 to 15 mm in diameter with a 1-µl loop that has been dipped in the suspension (222). Test plates are incubated for a full 24 h at 35°C (no warmer) in ambient air and examined for growth of more than one colony, which indicates resistance.

Quality Control

S. aureus ATCC 29213 (oxacillin susceptible) and *S. aureus* ATCC 43300 (oxacillin resistant) are the recommended quality control strains.

Limitations of Methods for Detection of Oxacillin Resistance in *S. aureus*

For *S. aureus*, growth of an isolate on an oxacillin agar screen plate generally means that the isolate is *mecA* positive. When performed properly, the oxacillin agar screen method will detect most *mecA*-positive *S. aureus* strains. Occasionally a heteroresistant *mecA*-positive strain is not detected, which may be due in part to a low frequency of resistance expression (26, 178) or to lot-to-lot or manufacturer-to-manufacturer variation in the test medium (89, 91). It also may not detect borderline-resistant strains caused by non-*mecA*-mediated mechanisms.

Early comparisons of the oxacillin agar screen test and the cefoxitin disk diffusion for *S. aureus* found increased sensitivity for detecting *mecA*-mediated resistance using cefoxitin disk diffusion (25, 244). In more recent comparisons of the two methods using the revised disk diffusion breakpoints, the tests performed equally, with sensitivities of 98 to 100% for cefoxitin disk diffusion and 100% for the oxacillin-salt agar screen (137, 200, 259). Cefoxitin disk diffusion testing has been shown to perform well for detection of borderline resistance caused by *mecA* (71, 223), but it will not detect other types of borderline oxacillin resistance, i.e., MOD-SA strains or that due to β-lactamase production. In a recent study, reference and commercial methods for detection of *mecA* were studied in a collection of *S. aureus* strains expressing either borderline oxacillin MICs, i.e., those with oxacillin MICs of 1 to 4 μg/ml, or for which previous results with oxacillin tests were discrepant by disk and MIC testing (220). In that study, for detection of *mecA*-mediated resistance, MIC and disk diffusion tests using cefoxitin performed significantly better than those using oxacillin, including the oxacillin-salt agar screen test and oxacillin MIC tests.

As stated above, for *S. aureus*, both the oxacillin-salt agar screen and cefoxitin tests used as a surrogate for oxacillin perform well for detection of *mecA*-mediated resistance. However, for the detection of oxacillin resistance mechanisms other than *mecA*, only tests using oxacillin will work. Fortunately, there is no evidence that non-*mecA*-mediated resistance associated with oxacillin MICs of 2 to 16 μg/ml is clinically relevant, and experimental studies have supported that (30, 93, 234). However, there has been one report of non-*mecA*-mediated resistance with high oxacillin MICs (>256 μg/ml) (203) and another report of in vivo selection of levels from 20 to 150 μg/ml (237). Using only cefoxitin-based methods for detection of oxacillin resistance may eliminate the possibility of finding strains that are either phenotypically oxacillin resistant but *mecA* negative (such as those just mentioned) or phenotypically susceptible but *mecA* positive (131, 191). However, until it is shown that these patterns are clinically significant, using a cefoxitin-based test alone is a reasonable approach, with the understanding that should therapy with a β-lactam agent be unresponsive, additional testing might be required. Additional testing would include testing the specific agent being used for treatment, either oxacillin or another β-lactam, along with appropriate molecular tests.

Detection of Oxacillin Resistance in CoNS except *S. lugdunensis*

Of the three different resistance mechanisms that have been described for *S. aureus*, only *mecA*-mediated oxacillin resistance has been described to occur in CoNS. However, detection of oxacillin resistance using standard methods can be more difficult than it is for *S. aureus*, due in part to the more heteroresistant expression of resistance in CoNS (7). Using CLSI reference methods, the sensitivity of detection of oxacillin resistance in this group improved when the MIC breakpoints were adjusted downward in 1999 by the CLSI (42) to ≤0.25 μg/ml for susceptible and ≥0.5 μg/ml for resistant. However, correlation of these interpretive criteria with the presence or absence of *mecA* is optimum only for *Staphylococcus epidermidis*, *Staphylococcus haemolyticus*, and, possibly, *Staphylococcus hominis* (84, 96, 128). For other species of CoNS (e.g., *Staphylococcus saprophyticus* and *Staphylococcus sciuri*), oxacillin breakpoints tend to be less specific; i.e., many *mecA*-negative strains are categorized as resistant by oxacillin disk and MIC methods (73, 96, 128, 133, 175, 210).

In 2009, the CLSI removed oxacillin disk diffusion breakpoints for CoNS from document M100 (41) because of the lack of specificity of the test and the fact that the cefoxitin disk diffusion test more accurately predicted the presence or absence of *mecA*. The oxacillin-salt agar screen test cannot be used for detecting oxacillin resistance in CoNS because it uses 6 μg of oxacillin per ml (230); it is not included in the CLSI documents for CoNS (38, 40). Therefore, the only methods now recommended by the CLSI for detection of oxacillin resistance in CoNS are the standard oxacillin MIC test and cefoxitin disk diffusion as a surrogate for oxacillin. With CoNS, the cefoxitin disk diffusion test provides equal sensitivity but greater specificity than the oxacillin MIC test for detection of strains harboring the *mecA* gene (167, 197, 223). However, the cefoxitin disk test fails to classify *mecA*-positive strains of *Staphylococcus simulans* as resistant (223). The reason for this is unknown.

Detection Using Cefoxitin as a Surrogate for Oxacillin (CoNS except *S. lugdunensis*)

The cefoxitin disk diffusion test is performed using the routine disk diffusion procedure but with breakpoints of ≤24 mm for oxacillin resistant and >25 mm for oxacillin susceptible. The use of a cefoxitin MIC breakpoint for prediction of *mecA*-mediated resistance in CoNS was recently investigated in a multilaboratory study, but because of performance differences between broths from different manufacturers and overlap of the oxacillin-susceptible and -resistant populations, its performance for MIC testing was not better than that of oxacillin (213), and therefore, cefoxitin MIC breakpoints were not adopted by the CLSI. Quality control is the same as that recommended for standard disk and MIC methods (40).

Limitations of Methods for Detection of Oxacillin Resistance in CoNS except *S. lugdunensis*

Except for *S. simulans* (see above), cefoxitin disk diffusion provides good sensitivity and greater specificity than oxacillin tests for prediction of *mecA*-mediated resistance in this group. Oxacillin MIC tests lack specificity for non-*S. epidermidis* isolates, and because of that, the CLSI recommends that for serious infections with CoNS other than *S. epidermidis*, isolates with oxacillin MICs of 0.5 to 2 μg/ml (i.e., MICs that are resistant using the CoNS breakpoints but susceptible using those for *S. aureus*) be tested for *mecA* or PBP 2a. However, this would require that identification to species level be performed, and similar ranges for disk diffusion testing are not given by the CLSI.

To improve detection of oxacillin resistance in CoNS, several methods have been proposed, including lowering the concentration of oxacillin to 4 μg/ml in the salt agar screen test (168); using cefoxitin in an agar dilution screen (168); and using a combination of results, for example, oxacillin-salt agar screen and cefoxitin disk diffusion (167), oxacillin agar dilution and cefoxitin disk diffusion (158), and oxacillin MIC and moxalactam MIC (172). Other investigators have recommended that CoNS with oxacillin zone diameters of 17 to 27 mm or cefoxitin zone diameters of 24 to 31 mm be tested for *mecA* or PBP 2a (264).

Clearly, methods for detection of oxacillin resistance in this group are less than ideal and deserve further study. Since the possibility exists that a CoNS isolate may be oxacillin susceptible but resistant by phenotypic tests due to the discrepancy between the tests for *S. epidermidis* and non-*S. epidermidis*, for CoNS isolated from patients for whom therapy choices are limited, species identification, MIC testing of the specific agent being used, and molecular testing for *mecA* or PBP 2a should be considered.

Other Tests for Detection of Oxacillin Resistance in Staphylococci

Other commercial methods for the rapid detection of oxacillin resistance in staphylococci include (i) direct culture of patient specimens (usually nasal swabs) onto agar media containing antimicrobial agents with a chromogenic indicator, (ii) detection of the presence of PBP 2′ by latex agglutination tests, and (iii) automated PCR assays. For the culture-based chromogenic media, those cleared by the FDA include MRSA*Select* (Bio-Rad Laboratories, Redmond, WA), Spectra MRSA (Remel Laboratories, Lenexa, KS), and CHROMagar MRSA (BD, Sparks, MD). For MRSA*Select* and CHROMagar, there have been many reports documenting performance against molecular methods or noncommercial selective media. In the few studies in which several of these media were compared to each other, all performed basically the same, with the chromogenic media allowing rapid detection of MRSA (13, 148, 165). However, when their use was compared to the use of molecular methods, molecular methods were found to have resulted in increased sensitivity and rapidity of detection, but at a higher cost (164, 165).

Commercial rapid methods that detect the presence of PBP 2a in staphylococci using latex agglutination include the MRSA-Screen test (Denka Seiken Co., Ltd., Tokyo, Japan), the PBP 2′ latex agglutination test (Oxoid Limited, Basingstoke, United Kingdom), the Mastalex test (Mast Diagnostics, Bootle, United Kingdom) (20), and the Slidex MRSA Detection test (bioMérieux). The first three tests have been cleared by the FDA. The MRSA-Screen test, cleared for use only with *S. aureus*, has been widely evaluated and has a high sensitivity and specificity for that species (139, 192, 224, 256). Detection of resistance in CoNS by the MRSA-Screen has been less successful, requiring either induction, an increased inoculum, or an increased agglutination time for adequate sensitivity (94, 95, 128, 255). The Oxoid PBP 2′ latex agglutination test was approved by the FDA for testing both *S. aureus* and CoNS, the latter requiring induction with oxacillin or cefoxitin. Although not extensively evaluated, its use for same-day reporting of MRSA from blood cultures (130) and in teicoplanin-resistant CoNS (113) has been described.

In addition to these, automated commercial methods that allow the detection of oxacillin resistance genes by PCR include the GeneOhm MRSA (BD, Franklin Lakes, NJ) and the Xpert MRSA (Cepheid, Sunnyvale, CA). Molecular analysis may also be performed by the standard PCR procedure when confirmation of the presence of the *mecA* gene is required (see chapter 74).

Reporting Results of Tests for Oxacillin Resistance

The CLSI recommends that oxacillin-resistant staphylococci be reported as resistant to all β-lactam agents, including penicillins, cephems except cephalosporins with anti-MRSA activity (i.e., all other cephalosporins, including cephamycins), β-lactam–β-lactamase inhibitor combination agents, and carbapenems. These agents are clinically ineffective against oxacillin-resistant staphylococcal infections, even though they may demonstrate in vitro activity (38–40). Newer β-lactam agents are currently being developed, however, that have changed these recommendations because these newer agents have activity against MRSA (45, 127, 262). None as yet have final approval of the FDA, although two (ceftaroline and ceftobiprole) are included in CLSI quality control tables

and are listed in the CLSI document M100 glossary in a new class labeled "cephalosporin with anti-MRSA activity" (40).

Isolates of *S. aureus* that appear oxacillin resistant by an alternative test method that uses oxacillin but fail to grow on the agar screen plate are probably borderline resistant and lack *mecA* (112, 142, 178). Much less is known about borderline resistance than about *mecA*-positive resistance because there have been few clinical studies (132); however, in animal model studies, isolates with β-lactamase-mediated resistance appear to be effectively treated with β-lactam agents (30, 31, 166, 234). If a phenotypically oxacillin-resistant *S. aureus* strain is isolated from a seriously ill patient and it does not contain *mecA*, this information should be conveyed to the patient's health care or medical provider. The incidence of phenotypically susceptible *mecA*-positive strains of *S. aureus* is not known. However, should phenotypically susceptible strains be isolated from serious infections in patients with a history of MRSA infection, confirmation by another method such as detection of PBP 2a by latex agglutination should be considered (180, 191, 192).

Most automated susceptibility panels now use both oxacillin and cefoxitin for determination of oxacillin resistance, but the final results are determined by algorithms within the expert system; commercial systems are validated by the device manufacturers and cleared by the FDA (see chapter 69). In general, if both oxacillin and cefoxitin tests are used and discrepancies occur, oxacillin-susceptible/cefoxitin-resistant results should be assumed to indicate *mecA*-mediated resistance. Oxacillin-resistant/cefoxitin-susceptible results, on the other hand, are likely not due to *mecA* but should occur only rarely. Current CLSI standards recommend a conservative approach to handling these discrepancies by suggesting that if they occur if both agents are tested, the isolate should be reported as oxacillin resistant.

Detection of Vancomycin Resistance in Staphylococci

In January 2006, CLSI vancomycin interpretive categories for *S. aureus* were changed to ≤2 μg/ml for susceptible, 4 to 8 μg/ml for intermediate, and ≥16 μg/ml for resistant. Interpretive categories for CoNS were not changed and are ≤4 μg/ml, susceptible; 8 to 16 μg/ml, intermediate; and ≥32 μg/ml, resistant. Unlike for oxacillin and cefoxitin testing, for vancomycin testing *S. lugdunensis* results should be interpreted using the breakpoints for CoNS. The rationale for lowering the *S. aureus* intermediate breakpoint to include 4 μg/ml was that (i) isolates with vancomycin MICs of 4 μg/ml, although rare, likely represent a population of organisms with heteroresistance, and (ii) limited outcome data suggested that infections with these isolates were likely to fail vancomycin therapy (232). Vancomycin-intermediate *S. aureus* (MICs of 4 to 8 μg/ml) are commonly referred to as VISA and those that are vancomycin resistant (MICs of ≥16 μg/ml) as VRSA. CoNS with reduced susceptibility to vancomycin are referred to here as VISS for vancomycin-intermediate *Staphylococcus* species other than *S. aureus*.

As of January 2010, 10 VRSA strains have been documented in the United States; 8 of these were from Michigan and the remaining 2 from New York and Pennsylvania (75, 199). Two have been isolated outside the United States, in India (183) and Iran (4). All VRSA isolates identified to date contain the *vanA* gene and have been isolated from patients who had underlying medical conditions, including prior infection or colonization with MRSA and/or VRE; most patients also had received previous vancomycin therapy. The vancomycin MICs for VRSA strains range from 32 to 1,024 μg/ml; all display no zone of inhibition with the 30-μg vancomycin disk.

The resistance in VISA is thought to be due to changes in the cell wall rather than the acquisition of a *van* gene (206). The incidence of VISA strains is greater than that of VRSA strains, although the true prevalence is difficult to know because when they first began to appear, some routine susceptibility testing methods failed to detect vancomycin-intermediate staphylococci (22a, 128a, 231).

No *van* gene-mediated vancomycin resistance has been reported for VISS, but there are reports of CoNS isolates with elevated vancomycin MICs (9, 60, 115, 193, 195, 243) which are also thought to be due to cell wall changes (153). An early study that reviewed the prevalence of VISS found it to be very low (i.e., <1%) except in one institution (206). In a 2009 report of a large surveillance study of isolates from 33 countries, the incidence of VISS was documented to still be <1.0% (12).

The CLSI reference broth microdilution method is reliable for detection of VISA and VRSA, and presumably VISS. However, the disk diffusion test cannot detect VISA or VISS because these isolates produce zone diameters within the susceptible range (≥15 mm). Because of this, parameters for the disk diffusion test were removed from document M100 in 2009, but with a comment that the test will detect *vanA*-mediated vancomycin resistance in *S. aureus*, i.e., VRSA strains, which all have demonstrated no zone to vancomycin. The BHI-V6 screen agar, used to detect vancomycin-resistant enterococci (VRE), is a sensitive method for detection of *S. aureus* for which the vancomycin MICs are ≥8 μg/ml, but it is variable for detection of *S. aureus* isolates for which the vancomycin MICs are 4 μg/ml (212) and cannot be used to detect VISS. Most available susceptibility testing methods now can detect VRSA strains, although accurate detection of VISA strains is still problematic (see below).

Although reduced susceptibility to vancomycin can occur in both *S. aureus* and CoNS, the occurrence in *S. aureus* is more concerning because this species is more frequently a cause of serious infection. It is for this reason that the Centers for Disease Control and Prevention (CDC) recommends use of BHI-V6 screen agar for detection of *S. aureus* with reduced susceptibility to vancomycin (http://www.cdc.gov/ncidid/dhqp/pdf/ar/visa_vrsa_guide.pdf). This recommendation is for laboratories that may miss these isolates using their primary susceptibility testing method. However, some laboratories may consider limiting this testing to MRSA strains since these are the isolates most likely to develop reduced susceptibility to vancomycin.

BHI-V6 Screen Agar Test Method

The recommended method for inoculating the agar is a 10-μl drop of a 0.5 McFarland suspension delivered with a micropipette. Alternatively, a swab can be used to spot an area 10 to 15 mm in diameter. The agar plate should be read after 24 h of incubation and carefully examined with transmitted light. Greater than one colony of growth or a light film of growth is considered positive (38, 40).

Quality Control

As mentioned above, the BHI-V6 plate is the same screening agar used to detect VRE, and the same quality control strains as recommended for the VRE test can also be used for the *S. aureus* test (38). These strains are vancomycin-susceptible *E. faecalis* ATCC 29212 and *vanB*-mediated, vancomycin-resistant *E. faecalis* ATCC 51299. Since the amount of inoculum applied for the VRE test (1 to 10 μl of a 0.5 McFarland suspension) spans the recommended inoculum for the *S. aureus* test, a laboratory that uses this medium for both purposes need only perform quality control once, either daily or weekly.

Limitations of Methods for Detection of Vancomycin Resistance

Standard broth microdilution MIC tests are reliable for detection of any reduced vancomycin susceptibility (i.e., intermediate or resistant) in staphylococci. Most commercial methods and routine disk diffusion will also detect vancomycin resistance (i.e., MICs of ≥16 μg/ml). The detection of intermediate vancomycin resistance by other methods is more challenging. In a recent study looking at the ability of commercial and reference susceptibility testing methods to detect VISA strains, the essential agreement (percentage of results within ±1 dilution) of all methods compared to the reference broth microdilution method was excellent except for disk diffusion, which detected no intermediate strain, and BHI-V6 screen agar, which failed to identify 12 of 33 strains with vancomycin MICs of 4 μg/ml (212). This finding was also noted in earlier studies (231; R. B. Carey et al., unpublished data). However, in the more recent study, although the essential agreement was excellent, the category agreement was not, ranging from 64.8 to 92.2% for the commercial methods tested, with some methods missing VISA strains and others overcalling resistance in susceptible strains (212). This may be due to differences in the media used in the systems, as it has been shown that recognition of VISAs may be medium dependent (231).

Recent studies have shown that the Etest (bioMérieux) method tends to result in slightly higher vancomycin MICs than does broth microdilution (171, 212) and may characterize susceptible strains as VISA strains. This was also true of some other commercial systems in the study mentioned above, which compared commercial and reference methods for detection of VISA strains. However, all methods in that study generated vancomycin MICs of ≥2 μg/ml for the VISA isolates tested; therefore, to increase detection of VISA strains, a laboratory might consider further testing of any isolate with an MIC of 2 μg/ml by an alternate method. Etest might be considered as the alternate method for use since it was successful in detection 44 of 45 (98%) of the VISA isolates; however, it may also categorize some susceptible strains as intermediate (171, 212).

Reporting Results of Vancomycin Testing

Growth of *S. aureus* on BHI-V6 agar is presumptive for either VISA or VRSA (38, 40) (http://www.cdc.gov/ncidod/dhqp/ar_visavrsa_algo.html). Additional testing is needed to confirm vancomycin resistance. First, the identity and purity of the isolate should be confirmed. Then the MIC of the isolate should be determined using a validated method. For many laboratories the most available method is the Etest. It is recommended that any *S. aureus* isolate for which the vancomycin MIC is ≥4 μg/ml be sent to a reference laboratory for confirmation. In the United States, several states request that VISA and/or VRSA be reported to the public health authority.

Detection of hVISA

Heteroresistant vancomycin-intermediate *S. aureus* isolates, referred to as hVISA, are isolates of *S. aureus* that normally test susceptible by standard methods but contain a subpopulation of cells (typically 1 in every 10^5 to 10^6 cells) for which the vancomycin MICs are resistant, i.e., ≥4 μg/ml. This phenomenon was first described in 1997 (92). Some hVISA isolates are detected by standard methods because their MICs are 4 μg/ml; some, however, continue to be missed since their MICs are ≤2 μg/ml. There is not agreement in recent reports about the incidence of hVISA or their clinical significance (232). The "gold standard" for detection of hVISA is population analysis/area-under-the-curve analysis, a technique that is unsuitable for routine use (247). No standardized technique that will detect these isolates is available to clinical laboratories. However, there are two Etest methods that have been developed: (i) the macro Etest and (ii) the Etest GRD strip. The former uses a large inoculum spread onto BHI agar plates and separate vancomycin and teicoplanin strips; MICs of ≥8 μg/ml for either agent or ≥12 μg/ml for teicoplanin alone are considered positive (253). The latter uses MHA with 5% sheep blood, a standard 0.5 McFarland inoculum, and a single strip impregnated with both vancomycin and teicoplanin; specific MICs of the two agents are then interpreted as positive or negative (258). There have been several evaluations of the macro Etest (114, 181, 247), but only two of the GRD strip (123, 258).

Detection of Inducible Clindamycin Resistance in Staphylococci

Although erythromycin and clindamycin are in separate antimicrobial agent classes, macrolides and lincosamides, respectively, their mechanisms of action (inhibition of protein synthesis) and mechanisms of resistance are similar. The two main mechanisms of macrolide resistance are (i) an efflux pump that affects only macrolides and (ii) a methylase that alters the ribosomal binding site of both antimicrobial agents. The first mechanism, which confers resistance to macrolides only (designated M-type for macrolide), is mediated in staphylococci by *msrA*. The second type, which confers resistance to macrolides, lincosamides, and streptogramin B agents (designated MLS_B-type, for macrolide-lincosamide-streptogramin B), is mediated by an *erm* gene (usually *ermA* or *ermC*). In staphylococci, MLS_B-type resistance can be either constitutive or inducible; if inducible, the isolate appears susceptible to the lincosamide (i.e., clindamycin) using routine testing methods unless induced by a macrolide (i.e., erythromycin). It is important to determine if resistance (whether inducible or constitutive) to clindamycin exists when it is being considered for therapy. A detailed explanation of these resistance mechanisms can be found in chapter 66.

Phenotypically, if an isolate has M-type resistance it is resistant to erythromycin but susceptible to clindamycin. If an isolate has MLS_B-type resistance, then it is erythromycin resistant and may be susceptible or resistant to clindamycin because it is either constitutive or inducible to that drug. For strains that are erythromycin resistant but clindamycin susceptible, it is important to determine if inducible clindamycin resistance exists (and an *erm* gene is present) or if the strain remains clindamycin susceptible (and an efflux gene is present).

There are two test methods recommended for detecting inducible clindamycin resistance in staphylococci, (i) the D-zone test and (ii) a broth dilution test that uses a single well or tube containing 4 μg of erythromycin per ml and 0.5 μg of clindamycin per ml (Table 3). The test methods are described below.

Test Methods

D-Zone Test

Detection of inducible clindamycin resistance can be easily accomplished using a disk diffusion procedure by placing a 15-μg erythromycin disk adjacent to a 2-μg clindamycin disk and looking for a flattening of the clindamycin zone,

which looks like the letter D and is therefore referred to as a D zone. For laboratories that are already performing disk diffusion, this may be done by placing the disks from 15 to 26 mm apart (69), with the other disks tested on an MHA plate. Some disk dispensers may position disks more than 26 mm apart even if the disks are placed in adjacent positions. Therefore, because dispensers may vary and the distance is critical, the distance should be verified before being adopted as a standard procedure. Placing the disks 15 to 20 mm, rather than 26 mm, apart may make the test more sensitive and easier to interpret (2, 211, 260), although to accomplish this the disks must be placed on the plates by hand instead of with a disk dispenser.

For laboratories that routinely perform antimicrobial susceptibility methods other than disk diffusion, Jorgensen et al. have shown that the test can be performed on a standard blood agar plate used for purity checks (105) by streaking one-third of the plate for confluent growth and then streaking for isolation on the rest of the plate. In that study, the investigators showed that dilutions of the 0.5 McFarland inoculum of up to 1:250 can be used. The disks are placed 15 mm apart on the portion of the plate where confluent growth would occur. In a later study, it was determined that the BBL Prompt system (BD, Sparks, MD) should not be used to inoculate the purity plate for D-zone determination (260). In that study, the investigators suggested that no more than a 1:20 dilution of a 0.5 McFarland suspension should be used to inoculate the purity plate. However, if the Prompt inoculum wand was used directly to inoculate the plate, it may have delivered inadequate inoculum. More recently, the Prompt system was successfully used for this purpose (91a) by transferring inoculum from the Prompt reservoir tray using a 10-μl loop and streaking one-third of the plate to obtain confluent growth. For either method, organisms that show a blunting or flattening of the clindamycin zone are considered D-zone test positive; those that show no flattening are D-zone test negative.

Single-Well Broth Dilution Method

The test is preformed by preparing microdilution wells (containing no less than 100 μl per well) or tubes of cation-adjusted Mueller-Hinton broth (CAMHB) with a combination of 4 μg of erythromycin per ml and 0.5 μg of clindamycin per ml. The combination is prepared by combining equal amounts of 2× concentrations of the agents, i.e., 8 μg of erythromycin per ml and 1 μg of clindamycin per ml. The wells or tubes are inoculated using routine inoculation procedures for broth microdilution or macrodilution (38). The test should be interpreted only for those staphylococcal strains that are erythromycin resistant, i.e., with MICs of ≥8 μg/ml, and clindamycin susceptible or intermediate, i.e., MICs of ≤2 μg/ml. Growth indicates inducible clindamycin resistance; no growth, no inducible clindamycin resistance.

Quality Control and Quality Assessment

Two strains have been designated for quality assessment purposes (e.g., for training, competency assessment, or test evaluation): *S. aureus* BAA-977, which has inducible *ermA*-mediated resistance, and *S. aureus* BAA-976, which has *msrA*-mediated resistance to erythromycin only. *S. aureus* ATCC 25923 should be used as the routine quality control strain for daily or weekly quality control testing of clindamycin and erythromycin disks using MHA. If the test is performed as part of the purity check procedure, the CLSI recommends that the disk content be verified using

S. *aureus* ATCC 25923 on MHA (38). However, this would require that laboratories which do not do disk diffusion routinely have a supply of MHA plates on hand for quality control purposes only. An alternative to this would be to use the two quality assessment strains, BAA-977 and BAA-976, as quality control organisms at daily or weekly intervals based on CLSI recommendations when using the purity plate method.

For adequate quality control of the broth microdilution test, it is necessary to test both a clindamycin inducibly resistant strain and one that is not inducibly resistant so that it can be confirmed that both the agents are in the well and performing as they should. The best way to do this to avoid having to test both strains every time a test is performed is to test BAA-976 and BAA-977 once when the tubes or microdilution panels are prepared (or once for each new lot). Then for subsequent daily or weekly testing, use S. *aureus* ATCC 29213 as a susceptible control and BAA-977 as a resistant control. For further discussion, see reference 214.

Reporting Results

The incidence of inducible clindamycin resistance in staphylococci can be highly variable, both by geographic area and by organism group (i.e., hospital-associated MRSA, CA-MRSA, and CoNS). The CLSI now recommends that isolates that are D-zone test positive or grow in the combination well be reported as clindamycin resistant (38, 39, 41). However, there is some controversy about this given that clindamycin has been effective in some situations where inducible resistance was demonstrated (124). As a conservative approach, the CLSI has suggested that inducibly clindamycin-resistant strains could be reported as resistant with a comment stating, "This isolate is presumed to be resistant based on detection of inducible clindamycin resistance. Clindamycin may still be effective in some patients." If the test is not offered routinely, it should be available by request for cases in which clindamycin is being considered for therapy (38, 39).

Detection of High-Level Mupirocin Resistance in Staphylococci

Mupirocin is a topical antibacterial agent that is used for treatment of skin infection and eradication of nasal carriage of S. *aureus* (44). Resistance to mupirocin is either low level, associated with MICs of 8 to 256 μg/ml, or high level, associated with MICs of ≥512 μg/ml (63). HLR usually implies the presence of the *mupA* gene, although strains with HLR have occurred without *mupA* (225) or have been created in the laboratory (204). It has been shown that elimination of S. *aureus* colonizing strains with mupirocin HLR is not possible (202); whether colonizing strains with low-level resistance can be eliminated with mupirocin is debatable (63, 201).

Methods for the detection of HLR to mupirocin have been suggested by many investigators (48, 52, 76, 80, 141, 159), and the British Society for Antimicrobial Chemotherapy recommends methods for testing mupirocin (http://www.bsac.org.uk). Based on data from a multilaboratory study (225), the CLSI recently included methods for prediction of mupirocin HLR using disk diffusion or a single-well broth microdilution screen (38, 39, 41) (Table 3).

For disk diffusion, the standard disk diffusion procedure is used with a 200-μg mupirocin disk. The test is incubated at 35°C for 24 h; the absence of a zone of inhibition is indicative of mupirocin HLR, whereas any zone indicates the absence of HLR. (Note that disks for the test may not yet be available commercially but can be prepared in-house by the following method. Using a stock solution of mupirocin [U.S. Pharmacopeia; http://www.usp.org] at 8,000 μg/ml and a micropipettor, add 0.025 ml to sterile 6-mm disks that have been spread out on a sterile surface. Allow the disks to dry in a laminar flow hood. When dry, transfer to a small tube with desiccant and store at −20°C.) For the broth microdilution procedure, inoculate a single well containing 0.1 ml of 256-μg/ml mupirocin using standard inoculum (38); incubate at 35°C for 24 h. Growth in the well indicates high-level mupirocin resistance; no growth, the absence of HLR.

Quality control parameters are given in CLSI document M100 (40). For both tests, S. *aureus* ATCC BAA-1708, a *mupA*-positive strain, is used as the resistant control and should show no zone of inhibition. For disk diffusion tests, S. *aureus* ATCC 25923 is used as the negative control (zone range, 29 to 38 mm) and for the MIC test, S. *aureus* ATCC 29213 (mupirocin MIC, 0.06 to 0.5 μg/ml) or E. *faecalis* ATCC 29212 (MIC, 16 to 128 μg/ml) can be used as the susceptible control.

TESTS TO DETECT RESISTANCE IN STREPTOCOCCI

Oxacillin Disk Screen Test for Detection of Penicillin Resistance in Pneumococci

A screening test in which a 1-μg oxacillin disk is used to detect penicillin resistance in pneumococci was first described following an outbreak caused by *Streptococcus pneumoniae* resistant to multiple antimicrobial agents in South Africa in the 1970s (55, 98, 219). Since then, this test has been used extensively and shown to be highly sensitive but not specific for detection of penicillin- nonsusceptible pneumococci (56). Strains identified as nonsusceptible by this method may be penicillin susceptible, intermediate, or resistant. Penicillin MIC tests must be performed on any strain that produces a zone diameter of ≤19 mm to determine if it is resistant (56). MIC tests rather than the oxacillin disk screen should be used routinely on strains isolated from cerebrospinal fluid and blood.

Detection of Inducible Clindamycin Resistance Using the D Zone Test

The importance of determining erythromycin and clindamycin resistance phenotypes and the detection of inducible clindamycin resistance follows the same logic as that described for staphylococci (see "Detection of Inducible Clindamycin Resistance in Staphylococci" above); however, the gene responsible for the M phenotype (i.e., erythromycin resistance and clindamycin susceptibility) in streptococci is *mef*(A). The MLS$_B$ phenotype exists in isolates of beta-hemolytic streptococci, S. *pneumoniae*, and viridans group streptococci; however, in pneumococci and viridans group streptococci it is usually the constitutive type and only rarely inducible (143, 240). Therefore, inducible clindamycin resistance needs to be determined only for isolates of beta-hemolytic streptococci.

Test Method

Detection of inducible clindamycin resistance in beta-hemolytic streptococci can be accomplished using a disk diffusion procedure similar to that for staphylococci by placing a 15-μg erythromycin disk adjacent to a 2-μg clindamycin disk and looking for a flattening of the clindamycin zone, which looks like the letter D and is therefore referred to as a D zone, as stated above. For laboratories that are already performing disk diffusion, the disks must be placed by hand at a distance of 12 mm from each other (176) on an MHA plate with 5% sheep blood along with other disks being tested. A disk dispenser cannot be used to place the two disks, since they must not be farther away than 12 mm (176). For laboratories which routinely perform other antimicrobial susceptibility methods, the purity plate method suggested by Jorgensen et al. can also be performed on a standard blood agar plate used for purity checks (105, 176) by streaking one-third of the plate for confluent growth and then streaking for isolation on the rest of the plate. The disks are then placed 12 mm apart on the portion of the plate where confluent growth would occur. Only the use of a 0.5 McFarland suspension has been evaluated for inoculation of the purity plate (176). For either method, organisms that show a blunting or flattening of the clindamycin zone are considered D-zone test positive; those that show no flattening are D-zone test negative.

Quality Control and Quality Assessment

Two strains have been designated for quality assessment (e.g., for training, competency assessment, or test evaluation) of the D-zone test: *S. aureus* BAA-977, which has inducible *ermA*-mediated resistance to clindamycin, and *S. aureus* BAA 976, which has *msrA*-mediated resistance to erythromycin only. *S. pneumoniae* ATCC 49619 should be used as the routine quality control strain for daily or weekly quality control testing of clindamycin and erythromycin disks using MHA with 5% sheep blood. If the test is performed as part of the purity check procedure, ideally the disk content should be verified using *S. pneumoniae* ATCC 49619 on MHA with 5% sheep blood. However, this would require that laboratories which do not do disk diffusion routinely have a supply of MHA with 5% sheep blood on hand for quality control purposes only. An alternative to this would be to use the two quality assessment strains, BAA-977 and BAA-976, as quality control organisms at daily or weekly intervals based on CLSI recommendations when using the purity plate method.

Reporting Results

The incidence of inducible clindamycin resistance in beta-hemolytic streptococci can be highly variable, both by geographic area and by organism group (53, 116).

However, when inducible clindamycin resistance is detected, the CLSI recommends that, as for staphylococci, isolates shown to be D-zone test positive be reported as clindamycin resistant. As a conservative approach, the CLSI has suggested that inducibly clindamycin-resistant strains could be reported as resistant with a comment stating, "This isolate is presumed to be resistant based on detection of inducible clindamycin resistance. Clindamycin may still be effective in some patients." If the test is not offered routinely, it should be available by request for cases in which clindamycin is being considered for therapy.

DETECTION OF ENZYMES MEDIATING RESISTANCE

β-Lactamase Tests

In the clinical laboratory, β-lactamase tests can be used for two purposes. The first is to detect an underlying mechanism of resistance that may not be detected using routine susceptibility testing methods, and the second is to detect a mechanism of resistance that is an infection control concern and epidemiologically important. These purposes are not mutually exclusive. Identification of a β-lactamase is nearly always epidemiologically important, and in the health care setting, these are nearly always an infection control concern. However, the use of a special test for enzyme detection does not always mean that the β-lactamase test should be used to predict treatment outcome. For example, a β-lactamase-positive result for a *Neisseria gonorrhoeae* isolate means that the isolate is resistant to penicillin and penicillin would not be an appropriate treatment choice (40). In contrast, the CLSI test for detection of ESBL is a useful test for detecting a resistance mechanism with epidemiological and infection control significance, but when using the recently revised CLSI cephalosporin breakpoints, this test is not recommended for prediction of cephalosporin treatment outcome (40). Instead, it is recommended that laboratories use the results of routine susceptibility testing and apply the revised interpretive criteria. A list of the organisms for which β-lactamase tests are useful is given in Table 4.

TABLE 4 Bacteria for which β-lactamase tests can be used in the clinical laboratory

Species	Method(s) commonly used	Predicted resistance[a]
Bacteroides spp. and other gram-negative anaerobes, except *B. fragilis* group	Direct β-lactamase tests[b]	Penicillins[c]
Enterococcus spp.	Direct β-lactamase tests	Penicillins[c]
Haemophilus influenzae	Direct β-lactamase tests	Penicillins[c]
Moraxella catarrhalis	Direct β-lactamase tests (nitrocefin only)	Penicillins[c]
Neisseria gonorrhoeae	Direct β-lactamase tests	Penicillins[c]
Staphylococcus spp.	Direct β-lactamase tests with prior induction	Penicillins[c]
Escherichia coli, *Klebsiella* spp., and *Proteus mirabilis*	CLSI ESBL screening and confirmation tests	Penicillins, cephalosporins, and aztreonam[d]
Enterobacteriaceae	CLSI MHT	Carbapenems[e]

[a]A positive result indicates resistance; however, a negative result is inconclusive, since other resistance mechanisms may occur.
[b]Includes chromogenic cephalosporin, acidimetric, and iodometric tests.
[c]A positive result indicates resistance to all penicillinase-labile penicillins, including amoxicillin, ampicillin, azlocillin, carbenicillin, mezlocillin, piperacillin, and ticarcillin.
[d]The CLSI recommends using the ESBL screening and confirmatory tests for infection control and epidemiological purposes when the 2010 revised cephalosporin breakpoints are implemented.
[e]See the most recent guidelines for when to use and how to report this test.

Direct Tests for β-Lactamase Activity

In the direct β-lactamase test, a positive reaction indicates that the isolate is resistant to the β-lactam agents noted in Table 4, but a negative reaction is inconclusive because other mechanisms of β-lactam resistance are possible. For example, most ampicillin-resistant *Haemophilus influenzae* isolates produce β-lactamase, which can be detected by direct β-lactamase tests; however, rare strains are ampicillin resistant but β-lactamase negative (16, 57, 70). For the latter, conventional disk diffusion or dilution tests are needed to detect the resistance (see chapter 68). Three direct β-lactamase assays, the acidimetric, iodometric, and chromogenic methods, have been widely used (88, 121). Each method involves testing bacteria grown on nonselective media, and the results are available within 1 to 60 min. The acidimetric and iodometric methods use a colorimetric indicator to detect the presence of penicilloic acid in the reaction vessel following β-lactamase hydrolysis of penicillin. In the acidimetric method, the substrates are citrate-buffered penicillin and a phenol red indicator. A decreasing pH associated with the presence of penicilloic acid results in a color change from red (negative result) to yellow (positive result) (67). The substrates in the iodometric test are phosphate-buffered penicillin plus a starch-iodine complex. Penicilloic acid, if present, reduces the iodine and prevents it from combining with starch, resulting in a colorless reaction (positive); a bluish purple color corresponds to a negative result (24).

The chromogenic cephalosporin nitrocefin can be used in a test tube assay (154) but has been incorporated into several filter paper-type disk or strip products that are commercially available and widely used in clinical laboratories. β-Lactamase hydrolysis of the chromogenic cephalosporin molecule causes an electron shift that results in a colored product (154). Although the acidimetric and iodometric methods have varied in performance, perhaps due in part to lack of experience with these methods, the chromogenic method has been reliable in detecting β-lactamases produced by all of the organisms indicated in Table 4 (104, 151).

The colorimetric β-lactamase tests rely on visualization of a colored product that presumably results from β-lactamase destruction of the substrate β-lactam molecule. However, these tests are not 100% specific, and other substances may yield colored endpoints. Serum may cause a colored reaction with the nitrocefin test (154), and, if reagents are not stored properly, spontaneous degradation of penicillin may produce false-positive acidimetric or iodometric β-lactamase reactions.

While some bacteria (e.g., *H. influenzae*, *N. gonorrhoeae*, and enterococci) constitutively produce β-lactamase, others (e.g., staphylococci) may produce detectable amounts of enzyme only after exposure to an inducing agent, which is generally a β-lactam (61). If staphylococci produce a positive β-lactamase result without induction, the results can be reported. However, if no β-lactamase is detected, then the test must be performed on cells that have been exposed to an inducing agent before a negative result is reported. This can be done by testing organisms that have been grown in the presence of subinhibitory concentrations of a β-lactam agent (e.g., 0.25 μg of cefoxitin per ml) in a broth or agar system. Alternatively, growth from around the periphery of the zone surrounding a β-lactam disk (e.g., a 1-μg oxacillin or 30-μg cefoxitin disk) can be tested. A positive result may take longer to develop in staphylococci than in other organisms, and the test should not be considered negative until it has been allowed to react for at least 60 min. Even under

these conditions, it is possible that a direct β-lactamase test may not be sensitive enough to detect β-lactamase production in staphylococci (106). As a result, CLSI guidelines recommend testing repeat isolates from the same patient for β-lactamase production (40).

β-Lactamase testing by the chromogenic nitrocefin method with anaerobic gram-negative bacilli other than those from the *Bacteroides fragilis* group may be performed prior to susceptibility testing (34). Members of the *B. fragilis* group characteristically produce β-lactamase, and they should be considered penicillin resistant. As with aerobes, resistance to β-lactam drugs is not always mediated by β-lactamase production (e.g., in some strains of *Bacteroides distasonis* and *B. fragilis*) (3, 34, 99).

The *S. aureus* strains recommended by the CLSI for quality control of routine disk diffusion and dilution tests (36–38) can be used for quality control of β-lactamase tests. *S. aureus* ATCC 25923 is β-lactamase negative, whereas *S. aureus* ATCC 29213 is β-lactamase positive (40).

Tests for ESBLs

Enterobacteriaceae can produce β-lactamases that are capable of hydrolyzing penicillins and cephalosporins, including the extended-spectrum cephalosporins (e.g., cefotaxime, ceftriaxone, ceftizoxime, and ceftazidime). These enzymes are referred to as ESBLs (21, 161) and are discussed in chapter 66. More than 200 different types of ESBLs have been identified in several gram-negative species and are associated with a variety of in vitro antimicrobial susceptibility profiles (21, 161; http://www.lahey.org/Studies/). Although all ESBLs hydrolyze extended-spectrum cephalosporins, the activities for specific antimicrobial agents vary among the various enzyme types. For example, some of the TEM and SHV ESBLs demonstrate greater activity for ceftazidime than for ceftriaxone, whereas the CTX-M enzymes demonstrate greater activity for ceftriaxone and cefotaxime than for ceftazidime (161). ESBLs do not hydrolyze carbapenems, and these β-lactam agents are often the treatment of choice for an infection by an ESBL-producing isolate.

CLSI guidelines describe screening criteria and confirmatory tests for ESBL detection in *Klebsiella* spp., *Escherichia coli*, and *Proteus mirabilis*. Although ESBLs can occur in bacteria other than these species, the ESBL confirmatory test can produce a false-negative result in the presence of an AmpC-type enzyme (179), so validation of the ESBL test in bacteria with a chromosomally encoded AmpC (e.g., *Enterobacter* spp. and *Serratia* spp.) is difficult. It was important to establish screening criteria for ESBL detection because routine disk diffusion and MIC tests did not always identify isolates that produce ESBLs (100, 102, 108, 140). Thus, the CLSI developed MIC and disk diffusion screening breakpoints for aztreonam, cefotaxime, cefpodoxime, ceftazidime, and ceftriaxone for *E. coli* and *Klebsiella* spp. and cefpodoxime, ceftazidime, and cefotaxime for *P. mirabilis* that aid in detecting ESBL-producing isolates (40) of those species. ESBL-producing clinical isolates may demonstrate HLR to one or more of the screening drugs (101, 108, 126, 135, 198, 250). Thus, the sensitivity of the screen test increases when more than one screening drug is used (64, 140, 252).

ESBLs are inhibited by clavulanic acid, and this property is used in laboratory tests to confirm ESBL production. These tests are based on enhanced activity when a cephalosporin (usually ceftazidime or cefotaxime) is tested with clavulanic acid compared to the activity when the cephalosporin is tested alone. The CLSI describes both a disk diffusion test and a broth microdilution MIC test to be used for confirmation of ESBL production. For broth microdilution, cefotaxime and ceftazidime are tested with and without 4 μg of clavulanic acid per ml. A decrease in the MIC of ≥3 dilutions for the agents tested in combination with clavulanic acid compared to the values obtained for the agents tested alone indicates the presence of an ESBL. For disk diffusion, the same agents incorporated into disks with and without 10 μg of clavulanic acid are tested. An increase in the zone diameter of ≥5 mm for either of the disks with clavulanic acid indicates the presence of an ESBL. *Klebsiella pneumoniae* ATCC 700603 should be included for quality control purposes; accepted ranges are given in the current CLSI document M100 tables (40). There are multiple explanations for a screen-positive, confirmatory-test negative result for an isolate. The isolate may be ESBL negative but demonstrate reduced susceptibility to the screening agents because of decreased porin production, hyperproduction of a normal-spectrum β-lactamase such as TEM-1 or SHV-1, or production of another cephalosporin-hydrolyzing enzyme such as an AmpC-type enzyme which is not inhibited by clavulanic acid. Alternatively, the isolate may be ESBL positive but produce an additional β-lactamase such as the AmpC-type enzymes, which can interfere with ESBL inhibition by clavulanic acid (162, 179).

The CLSI revised recommendations for when to perform the ESBL screen and confirmation tests; these revised recommendations were made because the interpretive criteria or breakpoints for cephalosporins and aztreonam were also revised (40). The new breakpoints, based upon pharmacokinetic/pharmacodynamic data and limited clinical outcome data, are meant to more accurately predict treatment outcome using the most commonly used dosages for the cephalosporins, which are listed in CLSI document M100 (40). When the new breakpoints are used, the CLSI recommends that the ESBL screening and confirmatory tests be performed for infection control and epidemiological purposes rather than for changing interpretive criteria (e.g., changing a cephalosporin report from susceptible to resistant). In other words, it is possible for an isolate to produce an ESBL but still test susceptible to one or more extended-spectrum cephalosporins. This recommendation seems to contradict previous recommendations to report all cephalosporins as resistant if an ESBL is detected (41), but the new pharmacokinetic/pharmacodynamic data suggest that this practice may have resulted in reporting false resistance (6). There are limited clinical outcome data for treatment of infections caused by an ESBL-producing isolate with a cephalosporin alone, and for this reason the recommendations between antimicrobial susceptibility guideline agencies may differ. For example, the European Committee on Antimicrobial Susceptibility Testing (EUCAST) clinical breakpoints for the cephalosporins are similar to the CLSI breakpoints (http://www.eucast.org/clinical_breakpoints), but EUCAST recommends that laboratories continue to screen and confirm ESBL production and to change a cephalosporin report from susceptible to intermediate or intermediate to resistant if the isolate tests positive for the ESBL production (http://www.eucast.org/epert_rules).

Tests for Detection of Plasmid-Mediated AmpC-Type β-Lactamases

Inducible AmpC-type β-lactamases occur on the chromosomes of several gram-negative bacilli, such as *Enterobacter cloacae*, *Citrobacter freundii*, *Serratia marcescens*, and *Pseudomonas aeruginosa* (125). These enzymes confer resistance to a wide spectrum of β-lactams, and they are resistant to the commonly used β-lactamase inhibitors (see details in chapter 66). AmpC-type β-lactamases may be located on transmissible plasmids in several bacterial species that lack an inducible chromosomal enzyme, including *E. coli*, *Klebsiella* spp., *Salmonella* spp., and *P. mirabilis* (170). Like plasmids with ESBLs, plasmids with AmpC-type enzymes often carry resistance determinants for multiple classes of antimicrobial agents. The combination of an AmpC-type enzyme with porin loss can result in carbapenem resistance (18, 208). The detection of plasmid-mediated AmpC-type enzymes is helpful for infection control and epidemiological investigations (28, 146, 147). It has also been suggested that these enzymes need to be detected for treatment decisions (58), although the revised CLSI cephalosporin breakpoints may eliminate this need (see discussion on ESBLs above).

Several tests have been proposed for detecting this type of resistance. Two assays, the modified three-dimensional extract test and the cefoxitin-agar medium-based test, are labor-intensive and difficult to implement in the clinical laboratory (47, 150). The more promising assays are the two disk potentiation assays, where an inhibitor of AmpC enzymes is added to a β-lactam disk. The presence of AmpC is detected by a reduced zone size around the β-lactam disk compared to the disk with inhibitor. This test is similar in format to the CLSI ESBL disk diffusion confirmatory test. Multiple inhibitors have been evaluated. Promising results were reported for inhibitor 48-1220 or LN-2-128 combined with a cefotetan disk, but these inhibitors are not commercially available (14, 15). Other inhibitors include cloxacillin, which has been combined with cefoxitin (226), and boronic acid, which has been combined with cefotetan disks (46) or with ceftazidime and cefotaxime disks (254). Evaluation of these tests on larger collections of isolates and isolates with multiple enzymes would help in predicting how this test would perform if more broadly applied (229).

Tests for Detection of Carbapenemases

Carbapenemases are β-lactamases which can hydrolyze carbapenem antimicrobial agents (e.g., ertapenem, doripenem, imipenem, and meropenem). The carbapenemases can usually hydrolyze other β-lactam agents as well, such as the penicillins, β-lactam–β-lactamase inhibitor combinations, and cephalosporins, so isolates producing a carbapenemase can be resistant to all of the β-lactam drugs. Carbapenemases are often located on a plasmid which can contain other resistant determinants. It is these features of carbapenemases that make identifying isolates harboring these resistance mechanisms a significant infection control concern. Carbapenemases fall within three classes of β-lactamases: class A enzymes, which include KPC, SME, IMI, NMC, and GES; class B enzymes, which are known as the metallo-β-lactamases (MBLs), with VIM and IMP being the most common types; and class D OXA enzymes (173). These enzymes are described in chapter 66. Carbapenemases have been identified in different genera of gram-negative bacilli. MBLs are most often found in *Pseudomonas aeruginosa* and *Acinetobacter* spp. but have also been reported to occur in *Enterobacteriaceae*. OXA carbapenemases are most commonly found in *Acinetobacter* spp., but there have also been reports of the enzymes in *Enterobacteriaceae*. The KPC enzyme is the most commonly identified class A carbapenemase; it usually occurs in *Enterobacteriaceae* but has also been identified in *Pseudomonas* spp. (173, 246).

In January 2009, the CLSI guidelines recommended using the modified Hodge test (MHT) for detection of carbapenemase activity in *Enterobacteriaceae* (41). This test is performed by inoculating a carbapenem-susceptible isolate, *E. coli* ATCC 25922, to MHA as described for disk diffusion testing, with the exception that the 0.5 McFarland equivalent inoculum be diluted 1:10 prior to inoculation. A carbapenem disk (either 10-μg meropenem or 10-μg ertapenem) is placed on the plate, and then a loopful of the test isolate is streaked from the disk to the edge of the plate. After overnight incubation, the test is read at the intersection of the zone of inhibition for *E. coli* ATCC 25922 and the test isolate. A positive result is indented growth of *E. coli* ATCC 25922 toward the carbapenem disk. A negative test is no indentation of *E. coli* ATCC 25922 growth from the zone of inhibition. The advantages of this test are that it is easy to perform, multiple isolates can be tested on one agar plate, and carbapenemases of different classes can be detected using the same test (5, 119). The disadvantages are that reading the test is subjective and that the test cannot differentiate between different carbapenemases, which can be useful epidemiological data. Also, false-positive results have been reported for some isolates that produce AmpC-type enzymes or ESBLs (160).

Initially, this test was recommended for the detection of carbapenemase production in isolates which demonstrate an elevated but susceptible carbapenem MIC (i.e., ertapenem, 2 μg/ml; imipenem or meropenem, 2 to 4 μg/ml) or zone diameter (i.e., ertapenem, 16 to 21 mm; meropenem, 16 to 21 mm) (5, 19, 41, 82, 257). In addition, it was recommended that isolates which were MHT positive be identified as carbapenemase-producing isolates in the laboratory report, with a warning that carbapenem therapeutic outcome was unknown. However, in January 2010, the carbapenem breakpoints were revised so that the susceptible breakpoints are ≤1 μg/ml for doripenem, imipenem, and meropenem and ≤0.25 μg/ml for ertapenem. At these breakpoints, nearly all carbapenemase-producing isolates will test either intermediate or resistant to the carbapenems. When the revised breakpoints are implemented, the MHT is no longer necessary for making treatment decisions, but it can be used for infection control and epidemiological purposes.

Several tests have been described for detection and differentiation of class A (e.g., KPC) and class C (i.e., MBL) carbapenemases. These are tests which may be useful for epidemiological studies but would likely require additional validation before they could be used for making treatment decisions. Class A carbapenemases are inhibited by boronic acid, and MBLs are inhibited by chelators such as EDTA and 2-mercaptopropionic acid. Many different tests have been described which incorporate these inhibitors with a carbapenem to detect enzyme activity. The test formats fall into three general categories: a double-disk zone distortion test, a two-disk zone enhancement test, and a broth microdilution MIC reduction test. Kim et al. (110) described a double-disk test for detection of MBLs. One disk was a carbapenem (e.g., imipenem) and the other disk contained chelators, Tris-EDTA and 2-mercaptopropionic acid. These disks were placed 10 mm apart, edge to edge on MHA inoculated with the test organism. After overnight incubation, MBL production for the test isolate was identified by distortion of the inhibition zone around the carbapenem disk toward the chelator disk. Doi et al. (59) and Pasteran et al. (160) described a two-disk potentiation test for detection of class A carbapenemases. In this test, one disk contained a carbapenem and the other disk contained a carbapenem with 3-aminophenylboronic acid (APB). These disks were placed on MHA inoculated with the test organism. Production of a class A carbapenemase was indicated by an increase in the zone diameter around the carbapenem disk with APB compared to the carbapenem-only disk. Tests for carbapenem MIC reduction in the presence of APB or a chelator have been described for detection of both class A carbapenemases and MBLs (136, 160). These tests are similar to the CLSI MIC confirmatory test for ESBLs. In this case, the test is positive for carbapenemase production if the carbapenem MIC is significantly lower in the presence of the inhibitor than the MIC without the inhibitor. All of these tests are easy to perform, and depending upon the details of the assay, some of the tests have very favorable performance characteristics. Disadvantages of the tests are that multiple tests would have to be performed to detect carbapenemases of different classes, and none of these tests detect OXA carbapenemases.

DETERMINATION OF BACTERICIDAL ACTIVITIES AND COMBINED DRUG EFFECTS

Dilution and disk or gradient diffusion susceptibility test methods measure the inhibitory activity of antimicrobial agents. Determining the inhibitory effect of a drug is sufficient for patient management in almost all bacterial infections. However, in rare situations it may be helpful to also assess the bactericidal effect of a drug on a specific patient's isolate. This may include a few serious infections thought to require bactericidal action for optimal efficacy such as endocarditis and chronic osteomyelitis (49, 177), and for some immunosuppressed patients (196). Bactericidal assays can also be useful for study of the pharmacodynamic properties of new or established antimicrobial agents and in assessing the effects of drug combinations (66, 122, 205, 245). With regard to the latter assessment, synergistic killing is predictable with a few organisms and drug combinations and need not be determined routinely, e.g., penicillins or glycopeptides plus an aminoglycoside against susceptible enterococci and β-lactam–aminoglycoside combinations against some gram-negative rods like *Pseudomonas* spp. However, the practice of "double coverage" of serious gram-negative rod infections serves primarily to broaden empirical coverage until susceptibility results are available rather than taking advantage of presumed drug synergy. A study of ventilator-associated pneumonia due to *P. aeruginosa* showed that monotherapy with a single active agent was almost always successful, and combination therapy to achieve synergy was unnecessary (129). A meta-analysis demonstrated that the mortality rate was lower with monotherapy with an active agent than combination therapy even in neutropenic patients with gram-negative rod infections (163). An exception may be pulmonary exacerbations due to some highly resistant *P. aeruginosa* isolates infecting cystic fibrosis patients, in which synergy testing has been advocated by some experts to guide treatment (190). This may be because conventional susceptibility testing failed to demonstrate susceptibility to any single agent, for patients failing therapy, or for those with substantial drug allergies. Interestingly, synergy testing has not been found to be useful for guiding therapy of infections due to *Burkholderia cepacia* in the same patient population (263). Synergy testing of *P. aeruginosa* isolates from cystic fibrosis patients is generally restricted to specialized centers with experience in performing such tests.

Tests of Bactericidal Activity

The tests of bactericidal activity that can be performed include determination of the minimal bactericidal concentration (MBC) and kinetic time-kill assays. The former measurement follows performance of the MIC in a broth dilution test under standard test conditions. If an MBC is to be determined, the inoculum for the MIC/MBC test should consist of actively growing (log-phase) cells obtained following a few hours of growth in a broth medium, rather than using colonies suspended from the surface of an agar plate to form the 0.5 McFarland density inoculum suspension (36). Use of a log-phase inoculum is necessary to accurately assess the bactericidal properties of drugs that require actively growing cells in order to exert a bactericidal effect (109, 227). After determination of the MIC, quantitative subcultures (usually 0.01 ml) are performed with samples from each tube or well with concentrations at and above the MIC of the drug being tested. The aliquots are streaked across the entire surface of a plate containing a standard growth medium (e.g., sheep blood agar). By transferring a small sample volume and spreading it across the entire plate, possible carryover effects of the antibiotic are minimized. In order to calculate the degree of killing at each antibiotic concentration, it is necessary that colony counts be performed on the positive control tube or well at the time of initial inoculation of the MIC test. As in the standard MIC procedure, the target inoculum density is 5×10^5 CFU/ml (36, 38). After the subculture, plates are incubated for 24 to 48 h; any resulting colonies are counted on each subculture plate. The standard definition of the MBC is the reduction of the initial inoculum by ≥99.9% (3 logs) (36). In practice, it is advisable to correct for pipetting error and to account for the Poisson distribution of bacterial cells in a liquid by using statistically derived rejection value tables (36). The tables define the number of colonies that can be tolerated based on the initial inoculum density of each test. If the number of colonies on a particular plate exceeds the rejection value for that test, the antibiotic did not achieve the strict definition of a bactericidal effect at that given concentration of the drug. The MBC of an antibiotic is reported in micrograms per milliliter in the same manner as the MIC. Determination of the MBC provides an opportunity to detect possible tolerance of the patient's isolate to drugs that would normally be considered bactericidal against the species being tested and might result in clinical failure in some patients (51, 86, 239).

The time-kill method provides the opportunity to measure the rate of bactericidal activity that may occur with a given antibiotic concentration. It is a more laborious approach than determination of the MBC. It is also possible to assess the activities of drugs in combination in order to recognize synergistic, indifferent, or antagonistic effects of two or more drugs tested together (36). This approach appears to correlate better with in vivo studies of combined drug effects than the alternative checkerboard titration method (10, 22). The details of performance of the time-kill test can be found in the NCCLS (now CLSI) guideline last published in 1999 (36). Many of the same critical factors that affect the outcome of the MBC test apply to the performance of time-kill assays, e.g., preparation of an actively growing inoculum and use of quantitative subcultures from antibiotic-containing tubes. The time kill-method requires that multiple samples be removed at various times (e.g., 0, 4, 8, 12, and 24 h) for colony counts, and thus, the volume of medium for each antibiotic concentration tested is usually ≥10 ml contained in a large test tube or flask (36). An antibiotic is often tested at more than one concentration that relates to the previously determined MIC of that agent (e.g., half the MIC, the MIC, and two times the MIC). The results of a time-kill assay are frequently

depicted graphically by plotting the colony counts of each antibiotic and concentration tested at each time point. A bactericidal effect is, again, defined as ≥99.9% killing at a specified time (36). When drugs are tested in combination by the time-kill method, synergy is usually defined as a ≥2-log decrease in the number of CFU/milliliter achieved with a drug combination compared to that achieved with the most active drug tested alone (36).

Other Methods of Determining Combined Drug Effects

A somewhat more convenient method for assessing combined drug effects than the time-kill assay is the checkerboard microdilution assay, in which two drugs are serially diluted in a two-dimensional grid to include all combinations over a defined range of dilutions (36). The wells of the microdilution tray are inoculated with the standard density of 5×10^5 CFU/ml. Following incubation, all of the wells demonstrating growth inhibition are recorded, as well as the MICs of the two drugs tested separately. The fractional inhibitory concentration is calculated by comparing the MIC of each drug with the MIC of that drug in combination with the second agent. Synergy is usually defined as a fourfold reduction in the MIC of the agents in combination compared to the drugs tested alone (36, 190). An even simpler approach, although less standardized, is the use of two Etest (bioMérieux) strips placed at a 90° angle on the surface of an inoculated MHA plate (190). Synergy is again defined by calculating the fractional inhibitory concentration.

The interpretation of the results of the bactericidal determinations described above has not received the same degree of critical scrutiny or level of consensus standards that has been achieved for interpretation of MICs of single agents. However, a few general statements can be made. A favorable MBC would typically be the same as or perhaps 1 to 2 dilutions greater than the MIC of agents that are normally considered bactericidal. A principal rationale for performing MBC or kinetic time-kill studies would be to detect an isolate that is not effectively killed by a typically bactericidal drug. This failure to exert a bactericidal effect is often described as tolerance and is defined as an MBC ≥32-fold the MIC of a particular agent (36, 86). Failure to achieve at least a 3-$\log_{10}$ reduction of CFU in the kinetic time-kill assay could likewise signify a tolerant strain (36).

Serum Bactericidal Test

Another determination of bactericidal activity or assessment of the effects of drug combinations is the serum bactericidal assay. The test can be performed for a patient who is already undergoing therapy with one or more drugs. Determinations of serum inhibitory and bactericidal titers are performed in a manner analogous to the MIC and MBC procedures, except that a patient's serum rather than prediluted concentrations of antibiotic is used. A guideline that describes the details of the serum bactericidal test was previously developed by the CLSI (35). The principal steps in performing the test include (i) obtaining one or more blood samples from the patient at specified intervals, (ii) preparing twofold dilutions of the patient's serum in pooled and pretested human serum in tubes or microdilution trays, and (iii) inoculating each tube or well with a standardized, actively growing inoculum (as described above for the MBC test) of the patient's own infecting organism in appropriate growth medium (36). Pooled human serum is recommended as the diluent of the patient's serum in each tube or well in order to make protein binding consistent throughout the range of serum dilutions, especially for drugs that are highly protein bound. The pretesting of the pooled human serum includes screening for human immunodeficiency virus type 1 and hepatitis B and C viruses, for antibiotic activity, and for optical clarity (35). In addition, the pooled serum should be heat inactivated immediately prior to use, and the pH should be adjusted to a range of 7.2 to 7.4 (35). An alternative to the laborious serum preparation step just described is the creation of a serum ultrafiltrate that precludes the need for a serum diluent (22, 120).

The blood samples for testing are usually obtained from the patient shortly after the antibiotic is administered at the time of the presumed peak level in serum (usually 30 to 60 min after administration), and often immediately prior to administration of the next drug dose (trough level) (35). The endpoints of the test are indicated by the highest dilution (titer) of the patient's serum sample that prevents visible growth following the incubation period (serum inhibitory titer). Similar to the MBC determination, quantitative subcultures are performed from each dilution of the patient's serum that has prevented visible growth. The serum bactericidal titer (SBT) is defined as that dilution (titer) that provides a ≥99.9% reduction of the original inoculum of the test based upon the standard rejection value tables (35). Thus, the results of the test are reported as dilutions (the titer) of the patient's serum rather than as a drug concentration (in micrograms per milliliter) as in the MIC and MBC tests. The goal of this test is to ensure that the dosage regimen provides sufficient bactericidal activity in that patient's blood (177, 194). Higher titers of antibacterial activity in the serum suggest that the patient has been dosed adequately, has not experienced abnormal elimination of the antibiotic, and does not have a tolerant bacterial isolate. This perception can be quantified by comparing the peak and trough titers obtained with those that have been shown to correlate with rapid organism eradication in collaborative studies (177, 248, 249). For rapid clearance of bacteremia and optimal time to sterilization of cardiac vegetations in endocarditis, a peak SBT of ≥1:64 and a trough SBT of ≥1:32 should be achieved whenever possible (177, 248). However, lower bactericidal titers do not necessarily signify a poor clinical outcome. For patients with chronic osteomyelitis, limited data have suggested that peak SBTs of ≥1:16 and trough SBTs of ≥1:4 predict clinical cure (177, 249).

Limitations of Bactericidal Determinations

Most clinical microbiologists and infectious disease specialists are not enthusiastic about performance of bactericidal determinations as a routine part of even highly complicated bacterial infections. Even in the most sophisticated clinical laboratories serving large tertiary-care medical centers, determinations of bactericidal activity are often not performed. Performance of bactericidal tests requires considerable technical proficiency on the part of the laboratory and a highly informed and experienced clinician to make use of the data. The interpretation of the bactericidal or combined drug tests must take into account knowledge of the key pharmacodynamic properties of the antimicrobial agents (i.e., concentration-dependent versus time-dependent killing activity), the location and severity of the infection, the pathogenic potential of the infecting organism, and the potential toxicity and cost of the treatment regimen. Bactericidal testing should not be performed unless there is close communication between the clinical microbiologist and the requesting clinician.

REFERENCES

1. **Abele-Horn, M., L. Hommers, R. Trabold, and M. Frosch.** 2006. Validation of VITEK 2 version 4.01 software for detection, identification, and classification of glycopeptide-resistant enterococci. *J. Clin. Microbiol.* **44:**71–76.
2. **Ajantha, G., R. Kulkarni, J. Shetty, S. Shubhada, and P. Jain.** 2009. Phenotypic detection of inducible clindamycin resistance among *Staphylococcus aureus* isolates by using the lower limit of recommended inter-disk distance. *Indian J. Pathol. Microbiol.* **51:**376–378.
3. **Aldridge, K. E., D. Ashcraft, K. Cambre, C. L. Pierson, S. G. Jenkins, and J. E. Rosenblatt.** 2001. Multicenter survey of the changing in vitro antimicrobial susceptibilities of clinical isolates of *Bacteroides fragilis* group, *Prevotella, Fusobacterium, Porphyromonas,* and *Peptostreptococcus* species. *Antimicrob. Agents Chemother.* **45:**1238–1243.
4. **Aligholi, M., M. Emaneini, F. Jabalameli, S. Shahsavan, H. Dabiri, and H. Sedaght.** 2008. Emergence of high-level vancomycin-resistant Staphylococcus aureus in the Imam Khomeini Hospital in Tehran. *Med. Princ. Pract.* **17:**432–434.
5. **Anderson, K. F., D. R. Lonsway, J. K. Rasheed, J. Biddle, B. Jensen, L. K. McDougal, R. B. Carey, A. Thompson, S. Stocker, B. Limbago, and J. B. Patel.** 2007. Evaluation of methods to identify the *Klebsiella pneumoniae* carbapenemase in *Enterobacteriaceae. J. Clin. Microbiol.* **45:**2723–2725.
6. **Andes, D., and W. A. Craig.** 2005. Treatment of infections with ESBL-producing organisms: pharmacokinetic and pharmacodynamic considerations. *Clin. Microbiol. Infect.* **11**(Suppl. 6):10–17.
7. **Archer, G. L., and M. W. Climo.** 1994. Antimicrobial susceptibility of coagulase-negative staphylococci. *Antimicrob. Agents Chemother.* **38:**2231–2237.
8. **Arias, C. A., and B. E. Murray.** 2008. Emergence and management of drug-resistant enterococcal infections. *Expert Rev. Anti-Infect. Ther.* **6:**637–655.
9. **Aubert, G., S. Passot, F. Lucht, and G. Dorche.** 1990. Selection of vancomycin- and teicoplanin-resistant *Staphylococcus haemolyticus* during teicoplanin treatment of *S. epidermidis* infection. *J. Antimicrob. Chemother.* **25:**491–493.
10. **Bayer, A. S., and J. O. Morrison.** 1984. Disparity between timed-kill and checkerboard methods for determination of in vitro bactericidal interactions of vancomycin plus rifampin versus methicillin-susceptible and -resistant *Staphylococcus aureus. Antimicrob. Agents Chemother.* **26:**220–223.
11. **Bennett, K., and S. E. Sharp.** 2008. Rapid differentiation of methicillin-resistant *Staphylococcus aureus* and methicillin-susceptible *Staphylococcus aureus* from blood cultures by use of a direct cefoxitin disk diffusion test. *J. Clin. Microbiol.* **46:**3836–3838.
12. **Biedenbach, D. J., J. M. Bell, H. S. Sader, J. D. Turnidge, and R. N. Jones.** 2009. Activities of dalbavancin against a worldwide collection of 81,673 gram-positive bacterial isolates. *Antimicrob. Agents Chemother.* **53:**1260–1263.
13. **Bischof, L. J., L. Lapsley, K. Fontecchio, D. Jacosalem, C. Young, R. Hankerd, and D. W. Newton.** 2009. Comparison of chromogenic media and BD GeneOhm MRSA PCR for the detection of methicillin resistant *Staphylococcus aureus* from nasal swabs. *J. Clin. Microbiol.* **47:**2281–2283.
14. **Black, J. A., K. S. Thomson, J. D. Buynak, and J. D. Pitout.** 2005. Evaluation of β-lactamase inhibitors in disk tests for detection of plasmid-mediated AmpC β-lactamases in well-characterized clinical strains of *Klebsiella* spp. *J. Clin. Microbiol.* **43:**4168–4171.
15. **Black, J. A., K. S. Thomson, and J. D. D. Pitout.** 2004. Use of β-lactamase inhibitors in disk tests to detect plasmid-mediated AmpC β-lactamases. *J. Clin. Microbiol.* **42:**2203–2206.
16. **Blondeau, J. M., D. Vaughan, R. Laskowski, and S. Borsos.** 2001. Susceptibility of Canadian isolates of *Haemophilus influenzae, Moraxella catarrhalis* and *Streptococcus pneumoniae* to oral antimicrobial agents. *Int. J. Antimicrob. Agents* **17:**457–464.

17. **Boyd, D. A., B. M. Willey, D. Fawcett, N. Gillani, and M. R. Mulvey.** 2008. Molecular characterization of *Enterococcus faecalis* N06-0364 with low-level vancomycin resistance harboring a novel D-Ala-D-Ser gene cluster, *vanL. Antimicrob. Agents Chemother.* **52:**2667–2672.

18. **Bradford, P. A., C. Urban, N. Mariano, S. J. Projan, J. J. Rahal, and K. Bush.** 1997. Imipenem resistance in *Klebsiella pneumoniae* is associated with the combination of ACT-1, a plasmid-mediated AmpC β-lactamase, and the loss of an outer membrane protein. *Antimicrob. Agents Chemother.* **41:**563–569.

19. **Bratu, S., M. Mooty, S. Nichani, D. Landman, C. Gullans, B. Pettinato, U. Karumudi, P. Tolaney, and J. Quale.** 2005. Emergence of KPC-possessing *Klebsiella pneumoniae* in Brooklyn, New York: epidemiology and recommendations for detection. *Antimicrob. Agents Chemother.* **49:**3018–3020.

20. **Brown, D. F., and E. Walpole.** 2001. Evaluation of the Mastalex latex agglutination test for methicillin resistance in *Staphylococcus aureus* grown on different screening media. *J. Antimicrob. Chemother.* **47:**187–189.

21. **Bush, K.** 2001. New β-lactamases in gram-negative bacteria: diversity and impact on the selection of antimicrobial therapy. *Clin. Infect. Dis.* **32:**1085–1089.

22. **Cappelletty, D. M., and M. J. Rybak.** 1996. Comparison of methodologies for synergism testing of drug combinations against resistant strains of *Pseudomonas aeruginosa. Antimicrob. Agents Chemother.* **40:**677–683.

22a.**Carey, R. B., J. B. Patel, S. McAllister, A. Thompson, P. Raney, F. C. Tenover, C. Ginocchio, D. Bopp, N. Dumas, and D. Kohlerschmidt.** 2004. *Abstr. 44th Intersci. Conf. Antimicrob. Agents Chemother.,* abstr. D-66.

23. **Cartwright, C. P., F. Stock, G. A. Fahle, and V. J. Gill.** 1995. Comparison of pigment production and motility tests with PCR for reliable identification of intrinsically vancomycin-resistant enterococci. *J. Clin. Microbiol.* **33:**1931–1933.

24. **Catlin, B. W.** 1975. Iodometric detection of *Haemophilus influenzae* β-lactamase: rapid presumptive test for ampicillin resistance. *Antimicrob. Agents Chemother.* **7:**265–270.

25. **Cauwelier, B., B. Gordts, P. Descheemaecker, and H. Van Landuyt.** 2004. Evaluation of a disk diffusion method with cefoxitin (30 μg) for detection of methicillin-resistant *Staphylococcus aureus. Eur. J. Clin. Microbiol. Infect. Dis.* **23:**389–392.

26. **Cavassini, M., A. Wenger, K. Jaton, D. S. Blanc, and J. Bille.** 1999. Evaluation of MRSA-Screen, a simple anti-PBP 2a slide latex agglutination kit, for rapid detection of methicillin resistance in *Staphylococcus aureus. J. Clin. Microbiol.* **37:**1591–1594.

27. **Centers for Disease Control and Prevention.** 1999. Four pediatric deaths from community-acquired methicillin-resistant *Staphylococcus aureus*—Minnesota and North Dakota, 1997–1999. *MMWR Morb. Mortal. Wkly. Rep.* **48:**707–710.

28. **Centers for Disease Control and Prevention.** 2002. Outbreak of multidrug-resistant *Salmonella* Newport—United States, January–April 2002. *MMWR Morb. Mortal. Wkly. Rep.* **51:**545–548.

29. **Chambers, H. F.** 1997. Methicillin resistance in staphylococci: molecular and biochemical basis and clinical implications. *Clin. Microbiol. Rev.* **10:**781–791.

30. **Chambers, H. F., G. Archer, and M. Matsuhashi.** 1989. Low-level methicillin resistance in *Staphylococcus aureus. Antimicrob. Agents Chemother.* **33:**424–428.

31. **Chambers, H. F., and C. J. Hackbarth.** 1992. Methicillin-resistant *Staphylococcus aureus*: genetics and mechanisms of resistance, p. 21–35. *In* M. T. Cafferkey (ed.), *Methicillin-Resistant* Staphylococcus aureus: *Clinical Management and Laboratory Aspects.* Marcel Dekker, Inc., New York, NY.

32. **Chen, Y., S. A. Marshall, P. Winokur, S. Coffman, W. Wilke, P. Murray, C. Spiegel, M. A. Pfaller, G. V. Doern, and R. N. Jones.** 1998. Use of molecular and reference susceptibility testing methods in a multicenter evaluation of MicroScan dried overnight gram-positive MIC panels for detection of vancomycin and high-level aminoglycoside resistances in enterococci. *J. Clin. Microbiol.* **36:**2996–3001.

33. **Chow, J. W., M. J. Zervos, S. A. Lerner, L. A. Thal, S. Donabedian, D. Jaworski, S. Tsai, K. Shaw, and D. B. Clewell.** 1997. A novel gentamicin resistance gene in *Enterococcus. Antimicrob. Agents Chemother.* **41:**511–514.

34. **Clinical and Laboratory Standards Institute.** 2007. *Methods for Antimicrobial Susceptibility Testing of Anaerobic Bacteria; Approved Standard—Sixth Edition.* CLSI document M11-A7. Clinical and Laboratory Standards Institute, Wayne, PA.

35. **Clinical and Laboratory Standards Institute/NCCLS.** 1999. *Methodology for the Serum Bactericidal Test.* NCCLS document M21-A. NCCLS, Wayne, PA.

36. **Clinical and Laboratory Standards Institute/NCCLS.** 1999. *Methods for Determining Bactericidal Activity of Antimicrobial Agents.* NCCLS document M26-A. NCCLS, Wayne, PA.

37. **Clinical and Laboratory Standards Institute/NCCLS.** 1993. *Methods for Dilution Antimicrobial Susceptibility Tests for Bacteria That Grow Aerobically.* Approved standard M7-A3. NCCLS, Villanova, PA.

38. **Clinical and Laboratory Standards Institute/NCCLS.** 2009. *Methods for Dilution Antimicrobial Susceptibility Tests for Bacteria That Grow Aerobically; Approved Standard—Eighth Edition.* CLSI document M07-A8. Clinical and Laboratory Standards Institute, Wayne, PA.

39. **Clinical and Laboratory Standards Institute/NCCLS.** 2009. *Performance Standards for Antimicrobial Disk Susceptibility Tests; Approved Standard—Tenth Edition.* CLSI document M02-A10. Clinical and Laboratory Standards Institute, Wayne, PA.

40. **Clinical and Laboratory Standards Institute/NCCLS.** 2010. *Performance Standards for Antimicrobial Susceptibility Testing: Twentieth Informational Supplement.* CLSI document M100-S20. Clinical and Laboratory Standards Institute, Wayne, PA.

41. **Clinical and Laboratory Standards Institute/NCCLS.** 2009. *Performance Standards for Antimicrobial Susceptibility Testing; Nineteenth Informational Supplement.* CLSI document M100-S19. Clinical and Laboratory Standards Institute, Wayne, PA.

42. **Clinical and Laboratory Standards Institute/NCCLS.** 1999. *Performance Standards for Antimicrobial Susceptibility Testing; Ninth Informational Supplement.* NCCLS document M100-S9. NCCLS, Wayne, PA.

43. **Clinical and Laboratory Standards Institute/NCCLS.** 2007. *Performance Standards for Antimicrobial Susceptibility Testing; Seventeenth Informational Supplement.* CLSI document M100-S17. Clinical and Laboratory Standards Institute, Wayne, PA.

44. **Cookson, B. D.** 1998. The emergence of mupirocin resistance: a challenge to infection control and antibiotic prescribing practice. *J. Antimicrob. Chemother.* **41:**11–18.

45. **Cornaglia, G., and G. M. Rossolini.** 2009. Forthcoming therapeutic perspectives for infections due to multidrug-resistant Gram-positive pathogens. *Clin. Microbiol. Infect.* **15:**218–223.

46. **Coudron, P. E.** 2005. Inhibitor-based methods for detection of plasmid-mediated AmpC β-lactamases in *Klebsiella* spp., *Escherichia coli*, and *Proteus mirabilis. J. Clin. Microbiol.* **43:**4163–4167.

47. **Coudron, P. E., E. S. Moland, and K. S. Thomson.** 2000. Occurrence and detection of AmpC β-lactamases among *Escherichia coli, Klebsiella pneumoniae*, and *Proteus mirabilis* isolates at a veterans medical center. *J. Clin. Microbiol.* **38:**1791–1796.

48. **Creagh, S., and B. Lucey.** 2007. Interpretive guidelines for mupirocin susceptibility testing of *Staphylococcus* spp. using CLSI guidelines. *Br. J. Biomed. Sci.* **64:**1–5.

49. **DeGirolami, P. C., and G. Eliopoulos.** 1987. Antimicrobial susceptibility tests and their role in therapeutic drug monitoring. *Clin. Lab. Med.* **7:**499–513.

50. **De Lencastre, H., S. A. Figueiredo, C. Urban, J. Rahal, and A. Tomasz.** 1991. Multiple mechanisms of methicillin resistance and improved methods for detection in clinical isolates of *Staphylococcus aureus. Antimicrob. Agents Chemother.* **35:**632–639.

51. Denny, A. E., L. R. Peterson, D. N. Gerding, and W. H. Hall. 1979. Serious staphylococcal infections with strains tolerant to bactericidal antibiotics. *Ann. Intern. Med.* 139:1026–1031.

52. de Oliveira, N., A. Cardozo, E. de Andrade Marques, K. dos Santos, and M. Giambiagi-deMarval. 2007. Interpretive criteria to differentiate low- and high-level mupirocin resistance in *Staphylococcus aureus*. *J. Med. Microbiol.* 56:937–939.

53. Desjardins, M., K. L. Delgaty, K. Ramotar, C. Seetaram, and B. Toye. 2004. Prevalence and mechanisms of erythromycin resistance in group A and group B *Streptococcus*: implications for reporting susceptibility results. *J. Clin. Microbiol.* 42:5620–5623.

54. Diab, M., M. El-Damarawy, and M. Shemis. 2008. Rapid identification of methicillin-resistant staphylococci bacteremia among intensive care unit patients. *Medscape J. Med.* 10:126.

55. Dixon, J. M., A. E. Lipinski, and M. E. Graham. 1977. Detection and prevalence of pneumococci with increased resistance to penicillin. *Can. Med. Assoc. J.* 117:1159–1161.

56. Doern, G. V., A. Brueggemann, and G. Pierce. 1997. Assessment of the oxacillin disk screening test for determining penicillin resistance in *Streptococcus pneumoniae*. *Eur. J. Clin. Microbiol. Infect. Dis.* 16:311–314.

57. Doern, G. V., A. B. Brueggemann, G. Pierce, H. P. Holley, Jr., and A. Rauch. 1997. Antibiotic resistance among clinical isolates of *Haemophilus influenzae* in the United States in 1994 and 1995 and detection of β-lactamase-positive strains resistant to amoxicillin-clavulanate: results of a national multicenter surveillance study. *Antimicrob. Agents Chemother.* 41:292–297.

58. Doi, Y., and D. L. Paterson. 2007. Detection of plasmid-mediated class C β-lactamases. *Int. J. Infect. Dis.* 11:191–197.

59. Doi, Y., B. A. Potoski, J. M. Adams-Haduch, H. E. Sidjabat, A. W. Pasculle, and D. L. Paterson. 2008. Simple disk-based method for detection of *Klebsiella pneumoniae* carbapenemase-type β-lactamase by use of a boronic acid compound. *J. Clin. Microbiol.* 46:4083–4086.

60. Dunne, W. M., Jr., H. Quershi, H. Pervez, and D. A. Nafziger. 2001. *Staphylococcus epidermidis* with intermediate resistance to vancomycin: elusive phenotype or laboratory artifact? *Clin. Infect. Dis.* 33:135–137.

61. Dyke, J. W. 1979. β-Lactamases of *Staphylococcus aureus*, p. 291–310. *In* J. M. Hamilton-Miller (ed.), β-*Lactamases*. Academic Press, Ltd., London, United Kingdom.

62. Eisner, A., G. Gorkiewicz, G. Feierl, E. Leitner, J. Kofer, H. H. Kessler, and E. Marth. 2005. Identification of glycopeptide-resistant enterococci by VITEK 2 system and conventional and real-time polymerase chain reaction. *Diagn. Microbiol. Infect. Dis.* 53:17–21.

63. Eltringham, I. 1997. Mupirocin resistance and methicillin-resistant *Staphylococcus aureus* (MRSA). *J. Hosp. Infect.* 35:1–8.

64. Emery, C. L., and L. A. Weymouth. 1997. Detection and clinical significance of extended-spectrum β-lactamases in a tertiary-care medical center. *J. Clin. Microbiol.* 35:2061–2067.

65. Endtz, H. P., N. Van Den Braak, A. Van Belkum, W. H. Goessens, D. Kreft, A. B. Stroebel, and H. A. Verbrugh. 1998. Comparison of eight methods to detect vancomycin resistance in enterococci. *J. Clin. Microbiol.* 36:592–594.

66. Entenza, J. M., and P. Moreillon. 2009. Tigecycline in combination with other antimicrobials: a review of in vitro, animal and case report studies. *Int. J. Antimicrob. Agents* 34:8.e1–8.e9.

67. Escamilla, J. 1976. Susceptibility of *Haemophilus influenzae* to ampicillin as determined by use of a modified, one-minute β-lactamase test. *Antimicrob. Agents Chemother.* 9:196–198.

68. Fahr, A., U. Eigner, M. Armbrust, A. Caganic, G. Dettori, C. Chezzi, L. Bertoncini, M. Benecchi, and M. G. Menozzi. 2003. Two-center collaborative evaluation of the performance of the BD Phoenix automated microbiology system for identification and antimicrobial susceptibility testing of *Enterococcus* spp. and *Staphylococcus* spp. *J. Clin. Microbiol.* 41:1135–1142.

69. Feibelkorn, K. R., S. A. Crawford, M. L. McElmeel, and J. H. Jorgensen. 2003. Practical disk diffusion method for detection of inducible clindamycin resistance in *Staphylococcus aureus* and coagulase-negative staphylococci. *J. Clin. Microbiol.* 41:4740–4744.

70. Felmingham, D., and R. N. Gruneberg. 2000. The Alexander Project 1996–1997: latest susceptibility data from this international study of bacterial pathogens from community-acquired lower respiratory tract infections. *J. Antimicrob. Chemother.* 45:191–203.

71. Felten, A., B. Grandry, P. H. Lagrange, and I. Casin. 2002. Evaluation of three techniques for detection of low-level methicillin-resistant *Staphylococcus aureus* (MRSA): a disk diffusion method with cefoxitin and moxalactam, the Vitek 2 system, and the MRSA-Screen latex agglutination test. *J. Clin. Microbiol.* 40:2766–2771.

72. Fernandes, C. J., L. A. Fernandes, and P. Collignon, on behalf of the Australian Group on Antimicrobial Resistance. 2005. Cefoxitin resistance as a surrogate marker for the detection of methicillin-resistant *Staphylococcus aureus*. *J. Antimicrob. Chemother.* 55:506–510.

73. Ferreira, R. B. R., N. L. P. Iorio, K. L. Malvar, A. P. F. Nunes, L. S. Fonseca, C. C. R. Bastos, and K. R. N. Santos. 2003. Coagulase-negative staphylococci: comparison of phenotypic and genotypic oxacillin susceptibility tests and evaluation of the agar screening test by using different concentrations of oxacillin. *J. Clin. Microbiol.* 41:3609–3614.

74. Fines, M., B. Perichon, P. Reynolds, D. F. Sahm, and P. Courvalin. 1999. VanE, a new type of acquired glycopeptide resistance in *Enterococcus faecalis* BM4405. *Antimicrob. Agents Chemother.* 43:2161–2164.

75. Finks, J., E. Wells, T. L. Dyke, N. Husain, L. Plizga, R. Heddurshetti, M. Wilkins, J. Rudrik, J. Hageman, J. Patel, and C. Miller. 2009. Vancomycin-resistant *Staphylococcus aureus*, Michigan, USA, 2007. *Emerg. Infect. Dis.* 15:943–945.

76. Finlay, J. E., L. A. Miller, and J. A. Poupard. 1997. Interpretive criteria for testing susceptibility of staphylococci to mupirocin. *Antimicrob. Agents Chemother.* 41:1137–1139.

77. Frank, K. L., J. L. Del Pozo, and R. Patel. 2008. From clinical microbiology to infection pathogenesis: how daring to be different works for *Staphylococcus lugdunensis*. *Clin. Microbiol. Rev.* 21:111–133.

78. Free, L., and D. Sahm. 1995. Investigation of the reformulated Remel Synergy Quad plate for detection of high-level aminoglycoside and vancomycin resistance in enterococci. *J. Clin. Microbiol.* 33:1643–1645.

79. Freeman, C., A. Robinson, B. Cooper, M. Mazens-Sullivan, R. Quintiliani, Jr., and C. Nightingale. 1995. In vitro antimicrobial susceptibility of glycopeptide-resistant enterococci. *Diagn. Microbiol. Infect. Dis.* 21:47–50.

80. Fuchs, P. C., R. N. Jones, and A. L. Barry. 1990. Interpretive criteria for disk diffusion susceptibility testing of mupirocin, a topical antibiotic. *J. Clin. Microbiol.* 28:608–609.

81. Garcia-Garrote, F., E. Cercenado, and E. Bouza. 2000. Evaluation of a new system, VITEK 2, for identification and antimicrobial susceptibility testing of enterococci. *J. Clin. Microbiol.* 38:2108–2111.

82. Giakkoupi, P., L. S. Tzouvelekis, G. L. Daikos, V. Miriagou, G. Petrikkos, N. J. Legakis, and A. C. Vatopoulos. 2005. Discrepancies and interpretation problems in susceptibility testing of VIM-1-producing *Klebsiella pneumoniae* isolates. *J. Clin. Microbiol.* 43:494–496.

83. Gill, V. J., C. B. Manning, and C. M. Ingalls. 1981. Correlation of penicillin minimum inhibitory concentrations and penicillin zone edge appearance with staphylococcal beta-lactamase production. *J. Clin. Microbiol.* 14:437–440.

84. Gradelski, E., L. Valera, L. Aleksunes, D. Bonner, and J. Fung-Tomc. 2001. Correlation between genotype and phenotype categorization of staphylococci based on methicillin susceptibility and resistance. *J. Clin. Microbiol.* 39:2961–2963.

85. Hackbarth, C. J., and H. F. Chambers. 1989. Methicillin-resistant staphylococci: genetics and mechanisms of resistance. *Antimicrob. Agents Chemother.* 33:991–994.

86. **Handwerger, S., and A. Tomasz.** 1985. Antibiotic tolerance among clinical isolates of bacteria. *Rev. Infect. Dis.* **7:**368–386.

87. **Hartman, B. J., and A. Tomasz.** 1986. Expression of methicillin resistance in heterogeneous strains of *Staphylococcus aureus. Antimicrob. Agents Chemother.* **29:**85–92.

88. **Hindler, J.** 1997. Antimicrobial susceptibility tests, p. 105–154. *In* H. D. Isenberg (ed.), *Essential Procedures in Clinical Microbiology.* American Society for Microbiology, Washington, DC.

89. **Hindler, J. A., and C. B. Inderlied.** 1985. Effect of source of Mueller-Hinton agar and resistance frequency on the detection of methicillin-resistant *Staphylococcus aureus. J. Clin. Microbiol.* **21:**205–210.

90. **Hindler, J. A., and D. F. Sahm.** 1992. Controversies and confusion regarding antimicrobial susceptibility testing of enterococci. *Antimicrob. Newsl.* **8:**65–74.

91. **Hindler, J. A., and N. L. Warner.** 1984. Effect of source of Mueller-Hinton agar on detection of oxacillin resistance in *Staphylococcus aureus* using a screening methodology. *J. Clin. Microbiol.* **25:**734–735.

91a. **Hindler, J. F., and D. A. Bruckner.** 2005. *Abstr. 105th Am. Soc. Microbiol. Gen. Meet.,* abstr. C-325.

92. **Hiramatsu, K., N. Aritaka, H. Hanaki, S. kawasaki, Y. Hosoda, S. Hori, Y. Fukuchi, and I. Kobayashi.** 1997. Dissemination in Japanese hospital of strains of Staphylococcus aureus heterogeneously resistant to vancomycin. *Lancet* **350:**1670–1673.

93. **Hirano, L., and A. S. Bayer.** 1991. β-Lactam–β-lactamase-inhibitor combinations are active in experimental endocarditis caused by β-lactamase-producing oxacillin-resistant staphylococci. *Antimicrob. Agents Chemother.* **35:**685–690.

94. **Horstkotte, M. A., J. K.-M. Knobloch, H. Rohde, and D. Mack.** 2001. Rapid detection of methicillin resistance in coagulase-negative staphylococci by a penicillin-binding protein 2a-specific latex agglutination test. *J. Clin. Microbiol.* **39:**3700–3702.

95. **Hussain, Z., L. Stoakes, S. Garrow, S. Longo, V. Fitzgerald, and R. Lannigan.** 2000. Rapid detection of *mecA*-positive and *mecA*-negative coagulase-negative staphylococci by an anti-penicillin binding protein 2a slide latex agglutination test. *J. Clin. Microbiol.* **38:**2051–2054.

96. **Hussain, Z., L. Stoakes, V. Massey, D. Diagre, V. Fitzgerald, S. El Sayed, and R. Lannigan.** 2000. Correlation of oxacillin MIC with *mecA* gene carriage in coagulase-negative staphylococci. *J. Clin. Microbiol.* **38:**752–754.

97. **Iwen, P. C., D. M. Kelley, J. Linder, and S. H. Hinrichs.** 1996. Revised approach for identification and detection of ampicillin and vancomycin resistance in *Enterococcus* species by using MicroScan panels. *J. Clin. Microbiol.* **34:**1779–1783.

98. **Jacobs, M. R., H. J. Koornhof, R. M. Robins-Browne, C. M. Stevenson, Z. A. Vermaak, I. Freiman, G. B. Miller, M. A. Witcomb, M. Isaacson, J. I. Ward, and R. Austrian.** 1978. Emergence of multiply resistant pneumococci. *N. Engl. J. Med.* **299:**735–740.

99. **Jacobs, M. R., S. K. Spangler, and P. C. Appelbaum.** 1992. β-Lactamase production and susceptibility of US and European anaerobic gram-negative bacilli to β-lactams and other agents. *Eur. J. Clin. Microbiol. Infect. Dis.* **11:**1081–1093.

100. **Jacoby, G. A., and P. Han.** 1996. Detection of extended-spectrum β-lactamases in clinical isolates of *Klebsiella pneumoniae* and *Escherichia coli. J. Clin. Microbiol.* **34:**908–911.

101. **Jacoby, G. A., and A. A. Medeiros.** 1991. More extended-spectrum β-lactamases. *Antimicrob. Agents Chemother.* **35:**1697–1704.

102. **Jarlier, V., M. H. Nicolas, G. Fournier, and A. Philippon.** 1988. Extended broad-spectrum β-lactamases conferring transferable resistance to newer β-lactam agents in Enterobacteriaceae: hospital prevalence and susceptibility patterns. *Rev. Infect. Dis.* **10:**867–878.

103. **Jett, B., L. Free, and D. F. Sahm.** 1996. Factors influencing the Vitek gram-positive susceptibility system's detection of *vanB*-encoded vancomycin resistance among enterococci. *J. Clin. Microbiol.* **34:**701–706.

104. **Jones, R. N., D. C. Edson, and CAP Microbiology Resource Committee of the College of American Pathologists.** 1991. Antimicrobial susceptibility testing trends and accuracy in the United States. *Arch. Pathol. Lab. Med.*. **115:**429–436.

105. **Jorgensen, J. H., S. A. Crawford, M. L. McElmeel, and K. R. Feibelkorn.** 2004. Detection of inducible clindamycin resistance of staphylococci in correlation with performance of automated broth susceptibility testing. *J. Clin. Microbiol.* **42:**1800–1802.

106. **Kaase, M., S. Lenga, S. Friedrich, F. Szabados, T. Sakinc, B. Kleine, and S. G. Gatermann.** 2008. Comparison of phenotypic methods for penicillinase detection in *Staphylococcus aureus. Clin. Microbiol. Infect.* **14:**614–616.

107. **Kao, S. J., I. You, D. B. Clewell, S. M. Donabedian, M. J. Zervos, J. Petrin, K. J. Shaw, and J. W. Chow.** 2000. Detection of the high-level aminoglycoside resistance gene *aph(″)-Ib* in *Enterococcus faecium. Antimicrob. Agents Chemother.* **44:**2876–2879.

108. **Katsanis, G. P., J. Spargo, M. J. Ferraro, L. Sutton, and G. A. Jacoby.** 1994. Detection of *Klebsiella pneumoniae* and *Escherichia coli* strains producing extended-spectrum β-lactamases. *J. Clin. Microbiol.* **32:**691–696.

109. **Kim, K. S., and B. F. Anthony.** 1981. Importance of bacterial growth phase in determining minimum bactericidal concentrations of penicillin and methicillin. *Antimicrob. Agents Chemother.* **19:**1075–1077.

110. **Kim, S. Y., S. G. Hong, E. S. Moland, and K. S. Thomson.** 2007. Convenient test using a combination of chelating agents for detection of metallo-β-lactamases in the clinical laboratory. *J. Clin. Microbiol.* **45:**2798–2801.

111. **Knapp, C., and J. A. Moody.** 1992. Tests to assess bactericidal activity, p. 5.16.1–5.16.33. *In* H. D. Isenberg (ed.), *Clinical Microbiology Procedures Handbook.* American Society for Microbiology, Washington, DC.

112. **Knapp, C. C., M. D. Ludwig, J. A. Washington, and H. F. Chambers.** 1996. Evaluation of Vitek GPS-SA card for testing of oxacillin against borderline-susceptible staphylococci that lack *mec. J. Clin. Microbiol.* **34:**1603–1605.

113. **Knausz, M., A. Ghidan, A. Grossato, and F. Rozgonyi.** 2005. Rapid detection of methicillin resistance in teicoplanin-resistant coagulase-negative staphylococci by a penicillin-binding protein 2′ latex agglutination method. *J. Microbiol. Methods* **60:**413–416.

114. **Kosowska-Shick, K., L. M. Ednie, P. McGhee, K. Smith, C. D. Todd, A. Wehler, ands P. C. Appelbaum.** 2008. Incidence and characteristics of vancomycin nonsusceptible strains of methicillin-resistant *Staphylococcus aureus* at Hershey Medical Center. *Antimicrob. Agents Chemother.* **52:**4510–4513.

115. **Krcmery, V., Jr., J. Trupl, L. Drgona, E. Kukuckova, and E. Oravcova.** 1996. Nosocomial bacteremia due to vancomycin-resistant *Staphylococcus epidermidis* in four patients with cancer, neutropenia, and previous treatment with vancomycin. *Eur. J. Clin. Microbiol. Infect. Dis.* **15:**259–261.

116. **Leclercq, R.** 2002. Mechanisms of resistance to macrolides and lincosamides: nature of the resistance elements and their clinical implications. *Clin. Infect. Dis.* **34:**482–492.

117. **Leclercq, R., and P. Courvalin.** 1997. Resistance to glycopeptides in enterococci. *Clin. Infect. Dis.* **24:**545–556.

118. **Leclercq, R., S. Dutka-Malen, J. Duval, and P. Courvalin.** 1992. Vancomycin resistance gene *vanC* is specific to *Enterococcus gallinarum. Antimicrob. Agents Chemother.* **36:**2005–2008.

119. **Lee, K., Y. Chong, H. B. Shin, Y. A. Kim, D. Yong, and J. H. Yum.** 2001. Modified Hodge and EDTA-disk synergy tests to screen metallo-beta-lactamase-producing strains of *Pseudomonas* and *Acinetobacter* species. *Clin. Microbiol. Infect.* **7:**88–91.

120. **Leggett, J. E., S. A. Wolz, and W. A. Craig.** 1989. Use of serum ultrafiltrate in the serum dilution test. *J. Infect. Dis.* **160:**616–623.

121. **Leitch, C., and S. Boonlayangoor.** 1992. β-Lactamase tests, p. 5.3.1–5.3.8. *In* H. D. Isenberg (ed.), *Clinical Microbiology Procedures Handbook.* American Society for Microbiology, Washington, DC.

122. **Lemmen, S. W., S. Zolldann, S. Klik, R. Lutticken, K. Kummerer, and H. Haffner.** 2004. Serum bactericidal activity of piperacillin-tazobactam against *Staphylococcus aureus*, piperacillin-susceptible and piperacillin-resistant *Escherichia coli* and *Pseudomonas aeruginosa. Chemotherapy* **50**:27–30.

123. **Leonard, S. N., K. L. Rossi, K. L. Newton, and M. J. Rybak.** 2009. Evaluation of the Etest GRD for the detection of Staphylococcus aureus with reduced susceptibility to glycopeptides. *J. Antimicrob. Chemother.* **63**:489–492.

124. **Lewis, J. S., II, and J. H. Jorgensen.** 2005. Inducible clindamycin resistance in staphylococci: should clinicians and microbiologists be concerned? *Clin. Infect. Dis.* **40**:280–285.

125. **Livermore, D. M.** 1995. β-Lactamases in laboratory and clinical resistance. *Clin. Microbiol. Rev.* **8**:557–584.

126. **Livermore, D. M., and M. Yuan.** 1996. Antibiotic resistance and production of extended-spectrum β-lactamases amongst *Klebsiella* spp. from intensive care units in Europe. *J. Antimicrob. Chemother.* **38**:409–424.

127. **Lodise, T. P., N. Patel, A. Renaud-Mutart, E. Gorodecky, T. R. Fritsche, and R. N. Jones.** 2008. Pharmacokinetic and pharmacodynamic profile of ceftobiprole. *Diagn. Microbiol. Infect. Dis.* **61**:96–102.

128. **Louie, L., A. Majury, J. Goodfellow, M. Louie, and A. E. Simor.** 2001. Evaluation of a latex agglutination test (MRSA-Screen) for detection of oxacillin resistance in coagulase-negative staphylococci. *J. Clin. Microbiol.* **39**:4149–4151.

128a. **Madhavan, T., D. Sievery, J. Rudrik, J. Torresan, and D. Schulman.** 2005. *Abstr. 43rd IDSA Annu. Meet.*, abstr. 1073.

129. **Magnotti, L. J., T. J. Schroeppel, L. P. Clement, J. M. Swanson, T. K. Bee, G. O. Maish III, G. Minard, B. L. Zarzaur, P. E. Fischer, T. C. Fabian, and M. A. Croce.** 2009. Efficacy of monotherapy in the treatment of Pseudomonas ventilator-associated pneumonia in patients with trauma. *J. Trauma* **66**:1052–1058; discussion, 1058–1059.

130. **Marlowe, E. M., A. Linscott, J., M. Kanatani, and D. A. Bruckner.** 2002. Practical therapeutic applications of the Oxoid PBP2′ latex agglutination test for the rapid identification of methicillin-resistant *Staphylococcus aureus* in blood cultures. *Am. J. Clin. Pathol.* **118**:287–291.

131. **Martineau, F., F. J. Picard, N. Lansac, C. Ménard, R. H. Roy, M. Ouellette, and M. G. Bergeron.** 2000. Correlation between the resistance genotype determined by multiplex PCR assays and the antibiotic susceptibility patterns of *Staphylococcus aureus* and *Staphylococcus epidermidis. Antimicrob. Agents Chemother.* **44**:231–238.

132. **Massanari, R. M., M. A. Pfaller, D. S. Wakesfield, G. T. Hammons, L. A. McNut, R. F. Woolson, and C. M. Helms.** 1988. Implications of acquired oxacillin resistance in management and control of *Staphylococcus aureus* infections. *J. Infect. Dis.* **158**:701–709.

133. **Mateo, M., J. R. Maestre, L. Aguilar, F. Cafini, P. Puente, P. Sanchez, L. Alou, M. J. Gimenez, and J. Prieto.** 2005. Genotypic versus phenotypic characterization, with respect to susceptibility and identification, of 17 clinical isolates of *Staphylococcus lugdunensis. J. Antimicrob. Chemother.* **56**:287–291.

134. **McKessar, S. J., A. M. Berry, J. M. Bell, J. D. Turnidge, and J. C. Paton.** 2001. Genetic characterization of *vanG*, a novel vancomycin resistance locus of *Enterococcus faecalis. Antimicrob. Agents Chemother.* **44**:3224–3228.

135. **Meyer, K. S., C. Urban, J. A. Eagan, B. J. Berger, and J. J. Rahal.** 1993. Nosocomial outbreak of *Klebsiella* infection resistant to late-generation cephalosporins. *Ann. Intern. Med.* **119**:353–358.

136. **Migliavacca, R., J.-D. Docquier, C. Mugnaioli, G. Amicosante, R. Daturi, K. Lee, G. M. Rossolini, and L. Pagani.** 2002. Simple microdilution test for detection of metallo-β-lactamase production in *Pseudomonas aeruginosa. J. Clin. Microbiol.* **40**:4388–4390.

137. **Mimica, M. J., E. N. Berezin, R. L. Carvalho, I. M. Mimica, L. M. J. Mimica, M. A. Safadi, E. Schneider, and H. H. Caiaffa-Filho.** 2007. Detection of methicillin resistance in *Staphylococcus aureus* isolated from pediatric patients: is the cefoxitin disk diffusion test accurate enough? *Braz. J. Infect. Dis.* **11**:415–417.

138. **Moellering, R. C., Jr., O. M. Koraeniowski, M. A. Sande, and C. B. Wennersten.** 1979. Species-specific resistance to antimicrobial synergism in *Streptococcus faecium* and *Streptococcus faecalis. J. Infect. Dis.* **140**:203–208.

139. **Mohanasoundaram, K. M., and M. K. Lalitha.** 2008. Comparison of phenotypic versus genotypic methods in the detection of methicillin resistance in *Staphylococcus aureus. Indian J. Med. Res.* **127**:78–84.

140. **Moland, E. S., C. C. Sanders, and K. S. Thomson.** 1998. Can results obtained with commercially available MicroScan microdilution panels serve as an indicator of β-lactamase production among *Escherichia coli* and *Klebsiella* isolates with hidden resistance to expanded-spectrum cephalosporins and aztreonam? *J. Clin. Microbiol.* **36**:2575–2579.

141. **Mondino, P. J., K. R. Dos Santos, C. de Freire Bastos Mdo, and M. Giambiagi-deMarval.** 2003. Improvement of mupirocin E-test for susceptibility testing of *Staphylococcus aureus. J. Med. Microbiol.* **52**:385–387.

142. **Montanari, M. P., O. Massidda, M. Mingoia, and P. E. Varalco.** 1996. Borderline susceptibility to methicillin in *Staphylococcus aureus*: a new mechanism of resistance? *Microb. Drug Resist.* **2**:257–260.

143. **Montanari, M. P., M. Mingoia, I. Cochetti, and P. E. Varaldo.** 2003. Phenotypes and genotypes of erythromycin-resistant pneumococci in Italy. *J. Clin. Microbiol.* **41**:428–431.

144. **Mougeot, C., J. Guillaumat-Taillet, and J. M. Libert.** 2001. *Staphylococcus aureus*: nouvelle détection de la resistance intrinseque par la methode de diffusion. *Pathol. Biol.* **49**:199–204.

145. **Murray, B. E.** 1990. The life and times of the enterococcus. *Clin. Microbiol. Rev.* **3**:46–65.

146. **M'Zali, F. H., J. Heritage, D. M. Gascoyne-Binzi, M. Denton, N. J. Todd, and P. M. Hawkey.** 1997. Transcontinental importation into the UK of *Escherichia coli* expressing a plasmid-mediated AmpC-type β-lactamase exposed during an outbreak of SHV-5 extended-spectrum β-lactamase in a Leeds hospital. *J. Antimicrob. Chemother.* **40**:823–831.

147. **Nadjar, D., M. Rouveau, C. Verdet, J. L. Donay, J. L. Herrmann, P. H. Lagrange, A. Philippon, and G. Arlet.** 2000. Outbreak of *Klebsiella pneumoniae* producing transferable AmpC-type β-lactamase (ACC-1) originating from *Hafnia alvei. FEMS Microb. Lett.* **187**:35–40.

148. **Nahimana, I., P. Francioli, and D. S. Blanc.** 2006. Evaluation of three chromogenic media (MRSA-ID, MRSA-Select and CHROMagar MRSA) and ORSAB for surveillance cultures of methicillin-resistant *Staphylococcus aureus. Clin. Microbiol. Infect.* **12**:1168–1174.

149. **Nakasone, I., T. Kinjo, N. Yamane, K. Kisanuki, and C. M. Shiohira.** 2007. Laboratory-based evaluation of the colorimetric VITEK-2 Compact system for species identification and of the Advanced Expert System for detection of antimicrobial resistances: VITEK-2 Compact system identification and antimicrobial susceptibility testing. *Diagn. Microbiol. Infect. Dis.* **58**:191–198.

150. **Nasim, K., S. Elsayed, J. D. D. Pitout, J. Conly, D. L. Church, and D. B. Gregson.** 2004. New method for laboratory detection of AmpC β-lactamases in *Escherichia coli* and *Klebsiella pneumoniae. J. Clin. Microbiol.* **42**:4799–4802.

151. **Neumann, M. A., D. F. Sahm, C. Thornsberry, and J. E. McGowan, Jr.** 1991. *Cumitech 6A, New Developments in Antimicrobial Agent Susceptibility Testing: a Practical Guide.* American Society for Microbiology, Washington, DC.

152. **Neves, F. P., R. L. Ribeiro, R. S. Duarte, L. M. Teixeira, and V. L. Merquior.** 2009. Emergence of the *vanA* genotype among *Enterococcus gallinarum* isolates colonising the intestinal tract of patients in a university hospital in Rio de Janeiro, Brazil. *Int. J. Antimicrob. Agents* **33**:211–215.

153. **Nunes, A. P., L. M. Teixeira, N. L. Iorio, C. C. Bastos, L. de Sousa Fonseca, T. Souto-Padron, and K. R. dos Santos.** 2006. Heterogeneous resistance to vancomycin in *Staphylococcus epidermidis, Staphylococcus haemolyticus* and *Staphylococcus warneri* clinical strains: characterisation of glycopeptide susceptibility profiles and cell wall thickening. *Int. J. Antimicrob. Agents* **27**:307–315.

154. O'Callaghan, C. H., A. Morris, S. M. Kirby, and A. H. Shingler. 1972. Novel method for detection of β-lactamases by using a chromogenic cephalosporin substrate. *Antimicrob. Agents Chemother.* **1:**283–288.

155. Okabe, T., K. Oana, Y. Kawakami, M. Yamaguchi, Y. Takahashi, Y. Okimura, T. Honda, and T. Katsuyama. 2000. Limitations of Vitek GPS-418 cards in exact detection of vancomycin-resistant enterococci with the *vanB* genotype. *J. Clin. Microbiol.* **38:**2409–2411.

156. Ostrowsky, B., N. C. Clark, C. Thauvin-Eliopoulos, L. Venkataraman, M. Samore, F. C. Tenover, G. M. Eliopoulos, R. C. Moellering, Jr., and H. S. Gold. 1999. A cluster of VanD vancomycin-resistant *Enterococcus faecium*: molecular characterization and epidemiology. *J. Infect. Dis.* **180:**1177–1185.

157. Palavecino, E. 2004. Community-acquired methicillin-resistant *Staphylococcus aureus* infections. *Clin. Lab. Med.* **24:**403–418.

158. Palazzo, I. C. V., and A. L. C. Darini. 2006. Evaluation of methods for detecting oxacillin resistance in coagulase-negative staphylococci including cefoxitin disc diffusion. *FEMS Microbiol. Lett.* **257:**299–305.

159. Palepou, M. F., A. P. Johnson, B. D. Cookson, H. Beattie, A. Charlett, and N. Woodford. 1998. Evaluation of disc diffusion and Etest for determining the susceptibility of *Staphylococcus aureus* to mupirocin. *J. Antimicrob. Chemother.* **42:**577–583.

160. Pasteran, F., T. Mendez, L. Guerriero, M. Rapoport, and A. Corso. 2009. Sensitive screening tests for suspected class A carbapenemase production in species of *Enterobacteriaceae*. *J. Clin. Microbiol.* **47:**1631–1639.

161. Paterson, D. L., and R. A. Bonomo. 2005. Extended-spectrum beta-lactamases: a clinical update. *Clin. Microbiol. Rev.* **18:**657–686.

162. Patterson, J. E. 2000. Extended-spectrum β-lactamases. *Semin. Respir. Infect.* **15:**299–307.

163. Paul, M., and L. Leibovici. 2009. Combination antimicrobial treatment versus monotherapy: the contribution of meta-analyses. *Infect. Dis. Clin. N. Am.* **23:**277–293.

164. Paule, S. M., D. M. Hacek, B. Kufner, K. Truchon, R. B. Thomson, Jr., K. L. Kaul, A. Robicsek, and L. R. Peterson. 2007. Performance of the BD GeneOhm methicillin-resistant *Staphylococcus aureus* test before and during high-volume clinical use. *J. Clin. Microbiol.* **45:**2993–2998.

165. Paule, S. M., M. Mehta, D. M. Hacek, T. M. Gonzalzles, A. Robicsek, and L. R. Peterson. 2009. Chromogenic media vs real-time PCR for nasal surveillance of methicillin-resistant *Staphylococcus aureus*: impact on detection of MRSA-positive persons. *Am. J. Clin. Pathol.* **131:**532–539.

166. Pefanis, A., C. Thauvin-Eliopoulos, G. Eliopoulos, and R. C. Moellering, Jr. 1993. Activity of ampicillin-sulbactam and oxacillin in experimental endocarditis caused by β-lactamase-hyperproducing *Staphylococcus aureus*. *Antimicrob. Agents Chemother.* **37:**507–511.

167. Perazzi, B., M. R. Fermepin, A. Malimovka, S. D. Garcia, M. Orgambide, C. A. Vay, R. de Torres, and A. M. R. Famiglietti. 2006. Accuracy of cefoxitin disk testing for characterization of oxacillin resistance mediated by penicillin-binding protein 2a in coagulase-negative staphylococci. *J. Clin. Microbiol.* **44:**3634–3639.

168. Perez, L., A. Antunes, A. Barth, and P. d'Azevedo. 2007. Variations of agar screen tests for detection of methicillin resistance in staphylococci: focus on cefoxitin. *Eur. J. Clin. Microbiol. Infect. Dis.* **26:**267–270.

169. Perichon, B., P. Reynolds, and P. Courvalin. 1997. VanD-type glycopeptide-resistant *Enterococcus faecium* BM4339. *Antimicrob. Agents Chemother.* **41:**2016–2018.

170. Philippon, A., G. Arlet, and G. A. Jacoby. 2002. Plasmid-determined AmpC-type β-lactamases. *Antimicrob. Agents Chemother.* **46:**1–11.

171. Prakash, V., J. S. Lewis II, and J. H. Jorgensen. 2008. Vancomycin MICs for methicillin-resistant *Staphylococcus aureus* isolates differ based upon the susceptibility test method used. *Antimicrob. Agents Chemother.* **52:**4528.

172. Pupin, H., H. Renaudin, O. Join-Lambert, C. Bebear, F. Megraud, and P. Lehours. 2007. Evaluation of moxalactam with the BD Phoenix system for detection of methicillin resistance in coagulase-negative staphylococci. *J. Clin. Microbiol.* **45:**2005–2008.

173. Queenan, A. M., and K. Bush. 2007. Carbapenemases: the versatile β-lactamases. *Clin. Microbiol. Rev.* **20:**440–458.

174. Ramotar, K., W. Woods, L. Larocque, and B. Toye. 2000. Comparison of phenotype methods to identify enterococci intrinsically resistant to vancomycin (vanC VRE). *Diagn. Microbiol. Infect. Dis.* **36:**119–124.

175. Ramotar, K., W. Woods, and B. Toye. 2001. Oxacillin susceptibility testing of *Staphylococcus saprophyticus* using disk diffusion, agar dilution, broth microdilution, and the Vitek GPS-105 card. *Diagn. Microbiol. Infect. Dis.* **40:**203–205.

176. Raney, P. M., F. C. Tenover, R. B. Carey, J. E. McGowan, Jr., and J. B. Patel. 2006. Investigation of inducible clindamycin and telithromycin resistance in isolates of β-hemolytic streptococci. *Diagn. Microbiol. Infect. Dis.* **55:**213–218.

177. Reller, L. B. 1986. The serum bactericidal test. *Rev. Infect. Dis.* **8:**803–808.

178. Resende, C. A., and A. M. Figueiredo. 1997. Discrimination of methicillin-resistant *Staphylococcus aureus* from borderline-resistant and susceptible isolates by different methods. *J. Med. Microbiol.* **46:**145–149.

179. Robberts, F. J., P. C. Kohner, and R. Patel. 2009. Unreliable extended-spectrum β-lactamase detection in the presence of plasmid-mediated AmpC in *Escherichia coli* clinical isolates. *J. Clin. Microbiol.* **47:**358–361.

180. Roghmann, M. 2000. Predicting methicillin resistance and the effect of inadequate empiric therapy on survival in patients with *Staphylococcus aureus* bacteremia. *Ann. Intern. Med.* **160:**1001–1004.

181. Rybak, M. J., S. N. Leonard, K. L. Rossi, C. M. Cheung, H. S. Sader, and R. N. Jones. 2008. Characterization of vancomycin-heteroresistant *Staphylococcus aureus* from the metropolitan area of Detroit, Michigan, over a 22-year period (1986 to 2007). *J. Clin. Microbiol.* **46:**2950–2954.

182. Sabath, L. 1977. Chemical and physical factors influencing methicillin resistance of *Staphylococcus aureus* and *Staphylococcus epidermidis*. *J. Antimicrob. Chemother.* **3:**47–51.

183. Saha, B., A. K. Singh, A. Ghosh, and M. Bal. 2008. Identification and characterization of a vancomycin-resistant *Staphylococcus aureus* isolated from Kolkata (South Asia). *J. Med. Microbiol.* **57:**72–79.

184. Sahm, D. F., S. Boonlayangoor, P. C. Iwen, J. L. Baade, and G. L. Woods. 1991. Factors influencing determination of high-level aminoglycoside resistance in *Enterococcus faecalis*. *J. Clin. Microbiol.* **29:**1934–1939.

185. Sahm, D. F., S. Boonlayangoor, and J. E. Schulz. 1991. Detection of high-level aminoglycoside resistance in enterococci other than *Enterococcus faecalis*. *J. Clin. Microbiol.* **29:**2595–2598.

186. Sahm, D. F., J. Kissinger, M. S. Gilmore, P. R. Murray, R. Mulder, J. Solliday, and B. Clarke. 1989. In vitro susceptibility studies of vancomycin-resistant *Enterococcus faecalis*. *Antimicrob. Agents Chemother.* **33:**1588–1591.

187. Sahm, D. F., and L. Olsen. 1990. In vitro detection of enterococcal vancomycin resistance. *Antimicrob. Agents Chemother.* **34:**1846–1848.

188. Sahm, D. F., and C. Torres. 1988. Effects of medium and inoculum variations on screening for high-level aminoglycoside resistance in *Enterococcus faecalis*. *J. Clin. Microbiol.* **26:**250–256.

189. Sahm, D. F., and C. Torres. 1988. High-content aminoglycoside disks for determining aminoglycoside-penicillin synergy against *Enterococcus faecalis*. *J. Clin. Microbiol.* **26:**257–260.

190. Saiman, L. 2007. Clinical utility of synergy testing for multidrug-resistant *Pseudomonas aeruginosa* isolated from patients with cystic fibrosis: 'the motion for.' *Paediatr. Respir. Rev.* **8:**249–255.

191. Sakoulas, G., P. DeGirolami, and H. S. Gold. 2001. Methicillin-susceptible *Staphylococcus aureus*: believe it, or not. *Ann. Intern. Med.* **161:**1237–1238.

192. Sakoulas, G., H. S. Gold, L. Venkataraman, P. DeGirolami, G. M. Eliopoulos, and Q. Qian. 2001. Methicillin-resistant *Staphylococcus aureus*: comparison of susceptibility testing methods and analysis of *mecA*-positive susceptible strains. *J. Clin. Microbiol.* **39:**3946–3951.

193. Sanyal, D., A. P. Johnson, R. C. George, B. D. Cookson, and A. J. Williams. 1991. Peritonitis due to vancomycin-resistant *Staphylococcus epidermidis*. *Lancet* **337:**54.

194. Schlichter, J. G., H. MacLean, and A. Milzer. 1949. Effective penicillin therapy in subacute bacterial endocarditis and other chronic infections. *Am. J. Med. Sci.* **217:**600–608.

195. Schwalbe, R. S., J. T. Stapleton, and P. H. Gilligan. 1987. Emergence of vancomycin resistance in coagulase-negative staphylococci. *N. Engl. J. Med.* **316:**927–931.

196. Sculier, J. P., and J. Klastersky. 1984. Significance of serum bactericidal activity in gram-negative bacillary bacteremia in patients with and without granulocytopenia. *Am. J. Med.* **76:**429–435.

197. Secchi, C., A. L. Antunes, L. R. Perez, V. V. Cantarelli, and P. A. d'Azevedo. 2008. Identification and detection of methicillin resistance in non-epidermidis coagulase-negative staphylococci. *Braz. J. Infect. Dis.* **12:**316–320.

198. Shehabi, A. A., A. Mahafzah, I. Baadran, F. A. Qadar, and N. Dajani. 2000. High incidence of *Klebsiella pneumoniae* clinical isolates to extended-spectrum β-lactam drugs in intensive care units. *Diagn. Microbiol. Infect. Dis.* **36:**53–56.

199. Sievert, D. M., J. T. Rudrik, J. B. Patel, L. C. McDonald, M. J. Wilkins, and J. C. Hageman. 2008. Vancomycin-resistant *Staphylococcus aureus* in the United States, 2002–2006. *Clin. Infect. Dis.* **46:**668–674.

200. Silva-Carvalho, M. C., L. A. Teixeira, F. A. Ferreira, A. Ribeiro, B. T. Ferreira-Carvalho, and A. M. Figueiredo. 2009. Comparison of different methods for detecting methicillin resistance in MRSA isolates belonging to international lineages commonly isolated in the American continent. *Microbiol. Immunol.* **53:**117–122.

201. Simor, A. E., E. Phillips, A. McGeer, A. Konvalinka, M. Loeb, H. R. Devlin, and A. Kiss. 2007. Randomized controlled trial of chlorhexidine gluconate for washing, intranasal mupirocin, and rifampin and doxycycline versus no treatment for the eradication of methicillin-resistant *Staphylococcus aureus* colonization. *Clin. Infect. Dis.* **44:**178–185.

202. Simor, A. E., T. L. Stuart, L. Louie, C. Watt, M. Ofner-Agostini, D. Gravel, M. Mulvey, M. Loeb, A. McGeer, E. Bryce, and A. Matlow. 2007. Mupirocin-resistant, methicillin-resistant *Staphylococcus aureus* strains in Canadian hospitals. *Antimicrob. Agents Chemother.* **51:**3880–3886.

203. Skov, R. L., L. V. Palleson, R. L. Poulsen, and F. Espersen. 1999. Evaluation of a new 3-h hybridization method for detecting the *mecA* gene in *Staphylococcus aureus* and comparison with existing genotypic and phenotypic susceptibility testing methods. *J. Antimicrob. Chemother.* **43:**467–475.

204. Slocombe, B., and C. Perry. 1991. The antimicrobial activity of mupirocin—an update on resistance. *J. Hosp. Infect.* **19**(Suppl. B):19–25.

205. Souli, M., P. D. Rekatsina, Z. Chryssouli, I. Galani, H. Giamarellou, and K. Kanellakopoulou. 2009. Does the activity of the combination of imipenem and colistin in vitro exceed the problem of resistance in metallo-β-lactamase-producing *Klebsiella pneumoniae* isolates? *Antimicrob. Agents Chemother.* **53:**2133–2135.

206. Srinivasan, A., J. D. Dick, and T. M. Perl. 2002. Vancomycin resistance in staphylococci. *Clin. Microbiol. Rev.* **15:**430–438.

207. Standiford, H. D., J. B. deMaine, and W. M. Kirby. 1970. Antibiotic synergism of enterococci. *Arch. Intern. Med.* **126:**255–259.

208. Stapleton, P. D., K. P. Shannon, and G. L. French. 1999. Carbapenem resistance in *Escherichia coli* associated with plasmid-determined CMY-4 β-lactamase production and loss of an outer membrane protein. *Antimicrob. Agents Chemother.* **43:**1206–1210.

209. Stefaniuk, E., A. Baraniak, M. Gniadkowski, and K. Hryniewicz. 2003. Evaluation of the BD Phoenix automated identification and susceptibility testing system in clinical microbiology laboratory practice. *Eur. J. Clin. Microbiol. Infect. Dis.* **22:**479–485.

210. Stepanovic, S., T. Hauschild, I. Dakic, Z. Al-Doori, M. Svabic-Vlahovic, L. Ranin, and D. Morrison. 2006. Evaluation of phenotypic and molecular methods for detection of oxacillin resistance in members of the *Staphylococcus sciuri* group. *J. Clin. Microbiol.* **44:**934–937.

211. Steward, C. D., P. M. Raney, A. K. Morrell, P. P. Williams, L. K. McDougal, L. Jevitt, J. E. McGowan, Jr., and F. C. Tenover. 2005. Testing for inducible clindamycin resistance in erythromycin-resistant isolates of *Staphylococcus aureus*. *J. Clin.* Microbiol. **43:**1716–1721.

212. Swenson, J. M., K. F. Anderson, D. R. Lonsway, A. Thompson, S. K. McAllister, B. M. Limbago, R. B. Carey, F. C. Tenover, and J. B. Patel. 2009. Accuracy of commercial and reference susceptibility testing methods for detecting vancomycin-intermediate *Staphylococcus aureus*. *J. Clin. Microbiol.* **47:**2013–2017.

213. Swenson, J. M., W. B. Brasso, M. J. Ferraro, D. J. Hardy, C. C. Knapp, D. Lonsway, S. McAllister, L. B. Reller, H. S. Sader, D. Shortridge, R. Skov, M. P. Weinstein, B. L. Zimmer, and J. B. Patel. 2009. Correlation of cefoxitin MICs with the presence of *mecA* in *Staphylococcus* spp. *J. Clin. Microbiol.* **47:**1902–1905.

214. Swenson, J. M., W. B. Brasso, M. J. Ferraro, D. J. Hardy, C. C. Knapp, L. K. McDougal, L. B. Reller, H. S. Sader, D. Shortridge, R. Skov, M. P. Weinstein, B. L. Zimmer, and J. B. Patel. 2007. Detection of inducible clindamycin resistance in staphylococci by broth microdilution using erythromycin-clindamycin combination wells. *J. Clin. Microbiol.* **45:**3954–3957.

215. Swenson, J. M., N. Clark, M. J. Ferraro, D. F. Sahm, G. Doern, M. A. Pfaller, L. B. Reller, M. P. Weinstein, R. J. Zabransky, and F. C. Tenover. 1994. Development of a standardized screening method for detection of vancomycin-resistant enterococci. *J. Clin. Microbiol.* **32:**1700–1704.

216. Swenson, J. M., N. C. Clark, D. F. Sahm, M. J. Ferraro, G. Doern, J. Hindler, J. H. Jorgensen, M. A. Pfaller, L. B. Reller, M. P. Weinstein, R. J. Zabransky, and F. C. Tenover. 1995. Molecular characterization and multilaboratory evaluation of *Enterococcus faecalis* ATCC 51299 and quality control of screening tests for vancomycin and high-level aminoglycoside resistance in enterococci. *J. Clin. Microbiol.* **33:**3019–3021.

217. Swenson, J. M., M. J. Ferraro, D. Sahm, N. C. Clark, D. Culver, F. C. Tenover, and The National Committee for Clinical Laboratory Standards Study Group on Enterococci. 1995. Multilaboratory evaluation of screening methods for detection of high-level aminoglycoside resistance in enterococci. *J. Clin. Microbiol.* **33:**3008–3018.

218. Swenson, J. M., B. C. Hill, and C. Thornsberry. 1989. Problems with the disk diffusion test for detection of vancomycin resistance in enterococci. *J. Clin. Microbiol.* **27:**2140–2142. (Erratum, **28:**403, 1990.)

219. Swenson, J. M., B. C. Hill, and C. Thornsberry. 1986. Screening pneumococci for penicillin resistance. *J. Clin. Microbiol.* **24:**749–752.

220. Swenson, J. M., D. Lonsway, S. McAllister, A. Thompson, L. Jevitt, W. Zhu, and J. B. Patel. 2007. Detection of *mecA*-mediated resistance using reference and commercial testing methods in a collection of *Staphylococcus aureus* expressing borderline oxacillin MICs. *Diagn. Microbiol. Infect. Dis.* **58:**33–39.

221. Swenson, J. M., R. Skov, and J. B. Patel. 2007. The cefoxitin disk test—what a clinical microbiologist needs to know. *Clin. Microbiol. Newsl.* **29:**33–40.

222. Swenson, J. M., J. Spargo, F. C. Tenover, and M. J. Ferraro. 2001. Optimal inoculation methods and quality control for the NCCLS oxacillin agar screen test for detection of oxacillin resistance in *Staphylococcus aureus*. *J. Clin. Microbiol.* **39:**3781–3784.

223. Swenson, J. M., F. C. Tenover, and the Cefoxitin Disk Study Group. 2005. Results of disk diffusion testing with

cefoxitin correlate with presence of *mecA* in *Staphylococcus* spp. *J. Clin. Microbiol.* **43:**3818–3823.

224. **Swenson, J. M., P. P. Williams, G. Killgore, C. M. O'Hara, and F. C. Tenover.** 2001. Performance of eight methods, including two new rapid methods, for detection of oxacillin resistance in a challenge set of *Staphylococcus aureus* organisms. *J. Clin. Microbiol.* **39:**3785–3788.

225. **Swenson, J. M., B. Wong, A. E. Simor, R. B. Thomson, M. J. Ferraro, D. J. Hardy, J. Hindler, J. Jorgensen, L. B. Reller, M. Traczewski, L. K. McDougal, and J. B. Patel.** 5 May 2010. A multicenter study to determine disk diffusion and broth microdilution criteria for prediction of high- and low-level mupirocin resistance in *Staphylococcus aureus*. *J. Clin. Microbiol.* doi:10.1128/JCM.00340-10.

226. **Tan, T. Y., L. S. Y. Ng, J. He, T. H. Koh, and L. Y. Hsu.** 2009. Evaluation of screening methods to detect plasmid-mediated AmpC in *Escherichia coli, Klebsiella pneumoniae,* and *Proteus mirabilis. Antimicrob. Agents Chemother.* **53:**146–149.

227. **Taylor, P. C., F. D. Schoenknecht, J. C. Sherris, and E. C. Linner.** 1983. Determination of minimum bactericidal concentrations of oxacillin for *Staphylococcus aureus:* influence and significance of technical factors. *Antimicrob. Agents Chemother.* **23:**142–150.

228. **Tee, W. S., S. Y. Soh, R. Lin, and L. H. Loo.** 2003. *Staphylococcus lugdunensis* carrying the *mecA* gene causes catheter-associated bloodstream infection in premature neonate. *J. Clin. Microbiol.* **41:**519–520.

229. **Tenover, F. C., S. L. Emery, C. A. Spiegel, P. A. Bradford, S. Eells, A. Endimiani, R. A. Bonomo, and J. E. McGowan, Jr.** 2009. Identification of plasmid-mediated AmpC β-lactamases in *Escherichia coli, Klebsiella* spp., and *Proteus* species can potentially improve reporting of cephalosporin susceptibility testing results. *J. Clin. Microbiol.* **47:**294–299.

230. **Tenover, F. C., R. N. Jones, J. M. Swenson, B. Zimmer, S. McAllister, and J. H. Jorgensen for the NCCLS Staphylococcus Working Group.** 1999. Methods for improved detection of oxacillin resistance in coagulase-negative staphylococci: results of a multicenter study. *J. Clin. Microbiol.* **37:**4051–4058.

231. **Tenover, F. C., M. V. Lancaster, B. C. Hill, C. D. Steward, S. A. Stocker, G. A. Hancock, C. M. O'Hara, N. C. Clark, and K. Hiramatsu.** 1998. Characterization of staphylococci with reduced susceptibility to vancomycin and other glycopeptides. *J. Clin. Microbiol.* **36:**1020–1027.

232. **Tenover, F. C., and R. C. Moellering, Jr.** 2007. The rationale for revising the Clinical and Laboratory Standards Institute vancomycin minimal inhibitory concentration interpretive criteria for *Staphylococcus aureus. Clin. Infect. Dis.* **44:**1208–1215.

233. **Tenover, F. C., J. M. Swenson, C. M. O'Hara, and S. A. Stocker.** 1995. Ability of commercial and reference antimicrobial susceptibility testing methods to detect vancomycin resistance in enterococci. *J. Clin. Microbiol.* **33:**1524–1527.

234. **Thauvin-Eliopoulos, E., L. B. Rice, G. M. Eliopoulos, and R. C. Moellering, Jr.** 1990. Efficacy of oxacillin and ampicillin-sulbactam combination in experimental endocarditis caused by β-lactamase-hyperproducing *Staphylococcus aureus. Antimicrob. Agents Chemother.* **34:**728–732.

235. **Tomasz, A., H. B. Drugeon, H. M. de Lencastre, D. Jabes, L. McDougal, and J. Bille.** 1989. New mechanism for methicillin resistance in *Staphylococcus aureus:* clinical isolates that lack the PBP 2a gene and contain modified penicillin-binding proteins with modified penicillin-binding capacity. *Antimicrob. Agents Chemother.* **33:**1869–1874.

236. **Tomasz, A., S. Nachman, and H. Leaf.** 1991. Stable classes of phenotypic expression in methicillin-resistant clinical isolates of staphylococci. *Antimicrob. Agents Chemother.* **35:**124–129.

237. **Tonin, E., and A. Tomasz.** 1986. β-Lactam-specific resistant mutants of *Staphylococcus aureus. Antimicrob. Agents Chemother.* **30:**577–583.

238. **Tsai, S., M. J. Zervos, D. B. Clewell, S. Donabedian, D. F. Sahm, and J. W. Chow.** 1998. A new high-level gentamicin resistance gene, *aph(2″)-Id,* in *Enterococcus* spp. *Antimicrob. Agents Chemother.* **42:**1229–1232.

239. **Tuomanen, E., D. T. Durack, and A. Tomasz.** 1986. Antibiotic tolerance among clinical isolates of bacteria. *Antimicrob. Agents Chemother.* **30:**521–527.

240. **Uh, Y., D. H. Shin, I. H. Jang, G. Y. Hwang, M. K. Lee, K. J. Yoon, and H. Y. Kim.** 2004. Antimicrobial susceptibility patterns and macrolide resistance genes of viridans group streptococci from blood cultures in Korea. *J. Antimicrob. Chemother.* **53:**1095–1097.

241. **van den Braak, N., W. Goessens, A. van Belkum, H. Verbrugh, and H. Endtz.** 2001. Accuracy of the VITEK 2 system to detect glycopeptide resistance in enterococci. *J. Clin. Microbiol.* **39:**351–353.

242. **Van Horn, K. G., C. A. Gedris, K. M. Rodney, and J. B. Mitchell.** 1996. Evaluation of commercial vancomycin agar screen plates for detection of vancomycin-resistant enterococci. *J. Clin. Microbiol.* **34:**2042–2044.

243. **Veach, L. A., M. A. Pfaller, M. Barrett, F. P. Koontz, and R. P. Wenzel.** 1990. Vancomycin resistance in *Staphylococcus haemolyticus* causing colonization and bloodstream infection. *J. Clin. Microbiol.* **28:**2064–2068.

244. **Velasco, D., M. del Mar Tomas, M. Cartelle, A. Becceiro, A. Perez, F. Molina, R. Moure, R. Villanueva, and G. Bou.** 2005. Evaluation of different methods for detecting methicillin (oxacillin) resistance in *Staphylococcus aureus. J. Antimicrob. Chemother.* **55:**379–382.

245. **Vidaillac, C., S. N. Leonard, H. S. Sader, R. N. Jones, and M. J. Rybak.** 2009. In vitro activity of ceftaroline alone and in combination against clinical isolates of resistant gram-negative pathogens, including β-lactamase-producing *Enterobacteriaceae* and *Pseudomonas aeruginosa. Antimicrob. Agents Chemother.* **53:**2360–2366.

246. **Villegas, M. V., K. Lolans, A. Correa, J. N. Kattan, J. A. Lopez, and J. P. Quinn.** 2007. First identification of *Pseudomonas aeruginosa* isolates producing a KPC-type carbapenem-hydrolyzing β-lactamase. *Antimicrob. Agents Chemother.* **51:**1553–1555.

247. **Walsh, T., A. Bolmstrom, A. Qwarnstrom, P. Ho, M. Wootton, R. Howe, A. MacGowan, and D. Diekema.** 2001. Evaluation of current methods for detection of staphylococci with reduced susceptibility to glycopeptides. *J. Clin. Microbiol.* **39:**2439–2444.

248. **Weinstein, M. P., C. W. Stratton, A. Ackley, H. B. Hawley, P. A. Robinson, B. D. Fisher, D. V. Alcid, D. S. Stevens, and L. B. Reller.** 1985. Multicenter collaborative evaluation of a standardized bactericidal test as a prognostic indicator in infective endocarditis. *Am. J. Med.* **78:**262–269.

249. **Weinstein, M. P., C. W. Stratton, H. B. Hawley, A. Ackley, and L. B. Reller.** 1987. Multicenter collaborative evaluation of a standardized serum bactericidal test as a predictor of therapeutic efficacy in acute and chronic osteomyelitis. *Am. J. Med.* **83:**218–222.

250. **Wiener, J., J. P. Quinn, P. A. Bradford, R. V. Goering, C. Nathan, K. Bush, and R. A. Weinstein.** 1999. Multiple antibiotic-resistant *Klebsiella* and *Escherichia coli* in nursing homes. *JAMA* **281:**517–523.

251. **Willey, B. M., B. N. Kreiswirth, A. E. Simor, G. Williams, S. R. Scriver, A. Phillips, and D. E. Low.** 1992. Detection of vancomycin resistance in *Enterococcus* species. *J. Clin. Microbiol.* **30:**1621–1624.

252. **Winokur, P. L., R. Canton, J. M. Casellas, and N. Legakis.** 2001. Variations in the prevalence of strains expressing an extended-spectrum β-lactamase phenotype and characterization of isolates from Europe, the Americas, and the Western Pacific region. *Clin. Infect. Dis.* **32:**94–103.

253. **Wootton, M., A. P. MacGowan, T. R. Walsh, and R. A. Howe.** 2007. A multicenter study evaluating the current strategies for isolating *Staphylococcus aureus* strains with reduced susceptibility to glycopeptides. *J. Clin. Microbiol.* **45:**329–332.

254. **Yagi, T., J. Wachino, H. Kurokawa, S. Suzuki, K. Yamane, Y. Doi, N. Shibata, H. Kato, K. Shibayama, and Y. Arakawa.** 2005. Practical methods using boronic acid compounds for identification of class C β-lactamase-producing *Klebsiella pneumoniae* and *Escherichia coli. J. Clin. Microbiol.* **43:**2551–2558.

255. **Yamazumi, T., I. Furuta, D. Diekema, M. A. Pfaller, and R. N. Jones.** 2001. Comparison of the Vitek gram-positive susceptibility 106 card, the MRSA-Screen latex agglutination test, and *mecA* analysis for detecting oxacillin resistance in a geographically diverse collection of clinical isolates of coagulase-negative staphylococci. *J. Clin. Microbiol.* **39:**3633–3636.

256. **Yamazumi, T., S. A. Marshall, W. W. Wilke, D. J. Diekema, M. A. Pfaller, and R. N. Jones.** 2001. Comparison of the Vitek gram-positive susceptibility 106 card and the MRSA-Screen latex agglutination test for determining oxacillin resistance in clinical bloodstream isolates of *Staphylococcus aureus*. *J. Clin. Microbiol.* **39:**53–56.

257. **Yan, J.-J., W.-C. Ko, S.-H. Tsai, H.-M. Wu, and J.-J. Wu.** 2001. Outbreak of infection with multidrug-resistant *Klebsiella pneumoniae* carrying *bla*IMP-8 in a university medical center in Taiwan. *J. Clin. Microbiol.* **39:**4433–4439.

258. **Yusof, A., A. Engelhardt, A. Karlsson, L. Bylund, P. Vidh, K. Mills, M. Wootton, and T. R. Walsh.** 2008. Evaluation of a new Etest vancomycin-teicoplanin strip for detection of glycopeptide-intermediate *Staphylococcus aureus* (GISA), in particular, heterogeneous GISA. *J. Clin. Microbiol.* **46:**3042–3047.

259. **Zeeshan, M., K. Jabeen, E. Khan, S. Irfan, S. Ibrahim, Z. Parween, and A. Zafar.** 2007. Comparison of different phenotypic methods of detection of methicillin resistance in *Staphylococcus aureus* with the molecular detection of *mecA* gene. *J. Coll. Physicians Surg. Pak.* **17:**666–670.

260. **Zelazny, A. M., M. J. Ferraro, A. Glennen, J. F. Hindler, L. M. Mann, S. Munro, P. R. Murray, L. B. Reller, F. C. Tenover, and J. H. Jorgensen.** 2005. Selection of strains for quality assessment of the disk induction method for detection of inducible clindamycin resistance in staphylococci: a CLSI collaborative study. *J. Clin. Microbiol.* **43:**2613–2615.

261. **Zetola, N., J. S. Francis, E. L. Nuermberger, and W. R. Bishai.** 2005. Community-acquired meticillin-resistant *Staphylococcus aureus*: an emerging threat. *Lancet Infect. Dis.* **5:**275–286.

262. **Zhanel, G. G., G. Sniezek, F. Schweizer, S. Zelenitsky, P. R. Lagace-Wiens, E. Rubinstein, A. S. Gin, D. J. Hoban, and J. A. Karlowsky.** 2009. Ceftaroline: a novel broad-spectrum cephalosporin with activity against meticillin-resistant *Staphylococcus aureus*. *Drugs* **69:**809–831.

263. **Zhou, J., Y. Chen, S. Tabibi, L. Alba, E. Garber, and L. Saiman.** 2007. Antimicrobial susceptibility and synergy studies of *Burkholderia cepacia* complex isolated from patients with cystic fibrosis. *Antimicrob. Agents Chemother.* **51:**1085–1088.

264. **Zhu, L. X., Z. W. Zhang, C. Wang, H. W. Yang, Q. Zhang, and J. Cheng.** 2006. Evaluation of the CLSI cefoxitin 30-μg disk-diffusion method for detecting methicillin resistance in staphylococci. *Clin. Microbiol. Infect.* **12:**1039–1042.

Susceptibility Test Methods: Fastidious Bacteria*

JANET A. HINDLER AND JAMES H. JORGENSEN

71

Most fastidious bacteria do not grow satisfactorily in standard in vitro susceptibility test systems that use unsupplemented media. For certain fastidious species that are more frequently encountered, such as *Haemophilus influenzae*, *Neisseria gonorrhoeae*, *Streptococcus pneumoniae*, *Neisseria meningitidis*, and other *Streptococcus* spp., slight modifications have been made to standard Clinical and Laboratory Standards Institute (CLSI), formerly NCCLS, disk diffusion and MIC methods to allow reliable testing of these bacteria. The modifications generally involve the use of a test medium with added nutrients and sometimes extended incubation times and/or incubation in an atmosphere with increased levels of CO_2 (Table 1). Specific zone diameter and MIC interpretive criteria have been developed by CLSI for these bacteria, as have acceptable ranges for recommended quality control (QC) strains (54). CLSI also describes a standard MIC method for testing *Helicobacter pylori* by using an agar dilution procedure. Standard MIC methods for testing potential agents of bioterrorism to include *Bacillus anthracis*, *Yersinia pestis*, *Burkholderia mallei*, *Burkholderia pseudomallei*, *Francisella tularensis*, and *Brucella* spp. have been developed, and conditions for testing these are listed in Table 2 (50). CLSI has also published an approved guideline for testing infrequently isolated or fastidious bacteria including *Abiotrophia* spp., *Granulicatella* spp., *Aeromonas* spp., *Plesiomonas* spp., *Bacillus* spp. (not *B. anthracis*), *Campylobacter jejuni/coli*, *Corynebacterium* spp., *Erysipelothrix rhusiopathiae*, the HACEK group, *Lactobacillus* spp., *Leuconostoc* spp., *Listeria monocytogenes*, *Moraxella catarrhalis*, *Pasteurella* spp., *Pediococcus* spp., and *Vibrio* spp. (50). Interpretive criteria for these organisms were primarily adapted from those for organisms included in CLSI standards (54), taking into consideration information in the literature and the experiences of authors of the guideline. This is in contrast to the extensive microbiological, clinical, and pharmacodynamic databases normally used for development of interpretive criteria that appear in CLSI antimicrobial susceptibility testing standards. The classification of M45 as a guideline rather than a standard was

based on this fact. A summary of the testing conditions for these organisms appears in Table 3. Due to the nature of the organisms and limited testing, it was recently decided to relocate recommendations for *H. pylori* and the potential agents of bioterrorism from the standard CLSI M100 tables (54) to the M45 guideline (50).

There are no specific recommendations for other fastidious bacteria such as *Bordetella* spp. and *Legionella* spp. This is because in part (i) infections caused by these bacteria usually respond to drugs of choice, (ii) isolates are infrequently encountered, and (iii) isolates are often difficult to grow and special media are required.

In addition to conventional MIC test methods (e.g., agar dilution or broth dilution methods), the Etest MIC determination method (bioMérieux-AB Biodisk, Solna, Sweden) has been used to test many types of fastidious bacteria. The Etest approach allows placement of strips on special media and the use of various incubation conditions. The limitations of this method include its cost and lack of clearance by the U.S. Food and Drug Administration (FDA) for testing many less commonly encountered fastidious bacteria. Prior to use of the Etest for clinical testing in the United States, the FDA clearance status for the particular organism-antimicrobial agent combination should be known. If FDA clearance has not been granted, the results should be interpreted with caution and should be qualified on the patient report.

This chapter summarizes the standard methods recommended by CLSI for antimicrobial susceptibility testing of *Streptococcus* spp. (including *S. pneumoniae*), *H. influenzae*, *N. gonorrhoeae*, and *N. meningitidis*. Methods for testing the infrequently isolated or fastidious bacteria included in the CLSI M45 guideline are summarized to include testing potential agents of bioterrorism. The incidence of resistance, test methods, and indications for testing and the reporting of results are provided.

STREPTOCOCCUS PNEUMONIAE

Incidence of Resistance

Since first reported in 1967, penicillin resistance in pneumococci steadily increased worldwide (13, 79, 206, 269). However, in the United States and other developed countries, the introduction of the protein-polysaccharide

---

*This chapter contains information presented in chapter 71 by Janet Fick Hindler and Jana M. Swenson in the eighth edition of this *Manual* and information presented in chapter 75 by Janet Fick Hindler and Jean B. Patel in the ninth edition of this *Manual*.

TABLE 1 Disk diffusion and MIC testing conditions and recommended QC strains for select fastidious bacteria

Organism(s)	Method	Medium[a]	Inoculum source[b]	Incubation atmosphere[c]	Incubation length (h)	Recommended QC strain(s)
S. pneumoniae and Streptococcus spp.	Disk diffusion	MHA + 5% sheep blood	18–20-h growth (from SBA)	5–7% CO_2	20–24	S. pneumoniae ATCC 49619
	Broth microdilution	CAMHB-LHB	18–20-h growth (from SBA)	Ambient air	20–24	S. pneumoniae ATCC 49619
H. influenzae and Haemophilus parainfluenzae	Disk diffusion	HTM agar	20–24-h growth (from CHOC)	5–7% CO_2	16–18	H. influenzae ATCC 49247, H. influenzae ATCC 49766[d]
	Broth microdilution	HTM broth	20–24-h growth (from CHOC)	Ambient air	20–24	H. influenzae ATCC 49247, H. influenzae ATCC 49766[d]
N. gonorrhoeae	Disk diffusion	GC agar base + supplement	20–24-h growth (from CHOC)	5–7% CO_2	20–24	N. gonorrhoeae ATCC 49226
	Agar dilution	GC agar base + supplement	20–24-h growth (from CHOC)	5–7% CO_2	20–24	N. gonorrhoeae ATCC 49226
N. meningitidis	Disk diffusion	MHA + 5% sheep blood	20–24-h growth (from CHOC)	5–7% CO_2	20–24	S. pneumoniae ATCC 49619
	Broth microdilution	CAMHB-LHB	20–24-h growth (from CHOC)	5–7% CO_2	20–24	S. pneumoniae ATCC 49619
	Agar dilution	MHA + 5% sheep blood	20–24-h growth (from CHOC)	5–7% CO_2	20–24	S. pneumoniae ATCC 49619

[a]HTM, GC agar base, and CAMHB-LHB are defined in the text.
[b]Inoculum suspension is in Mueller-Hinton broth or saline standardized to a 0.5 McFarland standard. For broth dilution, final organism concentration is 5×10^5 CFU/ml; for agar dilution, final organism concentration is 10^4 CFU/spot; CHOC, chocolate agar; SBA, sheep blood agar.
[c]Incubation temperature, 35°C.
[d]In addition, H. influenzae ATCC 10211 can be used to assess growth-supporting capabilities of HTM. H. influenzae ATCC 49766 is used for QC of select cephalosporins (e.g., cefaclor, cefamandole, and cefuroxime).

conjugated 7-valent pneumococcal vaccine (PCV-7) in 2000 caused resistance to penicillin to plateau or decrease as colonization and infection with some of the most resistant serotypes were diminished by the direct and indirect effects of the vaccine (57, 148, 268). Resistance to other β-lactams (cephalosporins and carbapenems) likewise declined as a result of the vaccine effects, although there was emergence of very-high-level β-lactam resistance in some clones during this period (223, 228). In the intervening period since widespread use of the vaccine, there has been emergence of some penicillin- and multidrug-resistant serotypes not included in the vaccine, e.g., serotype 19A (77, 206).

Interpretive criteria for penicillin and S. pneumoniae were originally developed for isolates associated with meningitis and were always recognized as being overly conservative for infections outside the central nervous system (179). The CLSI reassessed the penicillin breakpoints and in 2008 revised the breakpoints slightly for meningitis and introduced new breakpoints for nonmeningitis infections as well as a third set of breakpoints applicable to therapy with oral penicillin G (53, 266). The breakpoints for pneumococcal meningitis are as follows: susceptible, ≤0.06 μg/ml; resistant, ≥0.12 μg/ml; there is no intermediate category (54). For nonmeningitis, susceptible is ≤2 μg/ml, intermediate is 4 μg/ml, and resistant is ≥8 μg/ml. The breakpoints for oral penicillin are the same as those previously recommended for all pneumococcal infections, i.e., ≤0.06 μg/ml is susceptible, 0.12 to 1 μg/ml is intermediate, and resistant is ≥2 μg/ml (54). The combined effects of the 7-valent conjugate vaccine and the revision of the penicillin breakpoints by the CLSI have resulted, in the United States, in sharp declines in rates of strains not susceptible to

penicillin. The vaccine caused a 57% decline in strains not susceptible to penicillin between 1999 and 2004 (148), and the application of the revised nonmeningitis breakpoints applied to an existing national database further reduced nonsusceptible isolates from 25.3% to 6.8% (37). However, in parts of the world where the vaccine has not been widely used, penicillin resistance rates remain high and serotype 19A has increased in incidence for reasons other than serotype replacement disease among a vaccinated population (57, 58). Strains of pneumococci that are susceptible to penicillin generally are susceptible to other β-lactam agents; however, as the penicillin MIC increases, the MICs of other β-lactam agents increase also (201). Pneumococcal strains resistant to cefotaxime or ceftriaxone were not reported until the early 1990s (25, 226), and current rates of resistance to the extended-spectrum cephalosporins vary by location and time period (148, 201, 208). An international survey that included over 21,000 isolates indicated that 96.5% of all isolates were susceptible to ceftriaxone (MIC, ≤1.0 μg/ml) whereas among isolates not susceptible to penicillin (MIC, ≥0.12 μg/ml), 89.1% were susceptible to ceftriaxone (201). However, rates of nonsusceptibility to the extended-spectrum cephalosporins and meropenem have declined in the post-PCV-7 era (148).

Resistance has been described for all classes of antimicrobial agents that are usually considered for treating pneumococcal infections, except for the glycopeptides (13, 79, 140, 201). While resistance rates for β-lactams declined in the PCV-7 era, macrolide resistance has been much less affected (148) and is influenced by recent macrolide use (12). In a U.S. survey conducted just prior to PCV-7 introduction (28), 31% of isolates were macrolide resistant. Resistance to

TABLE 2 Broth microdilution MIC testing conditions, recommended QC strains, and drugs recommended for testing potential agents of bioterrorism

Organism(s)	Medium[a]	Inoculum source[b]	Incubation atmosphere[c]	Incubation length (h)	Recommended QC strain(s)	Drugs recommended for testing
B. anthracis	CAMHB	16–18-h growth (from SBA)	Ambient air	16–20	Escherichia coli ATCC 25922, Staphylococcus aureus ATCC 29213	Ciprofloxacin, doxycycline, levofloxacin, penicillin, tetracycline
Brucella spp.	Brucella broth, pH adjusted to 7.1 ± 0.1	48-h growth (from SBA)	Ambient air	48	E. coli ATCC 25922, S. pneumoniae ATCC 49619	Doxycycline, gentamicin, tetracycline, TMP-SMX, streptomycin
B. mallei, B. pseudomallei	CAMHB	16–18-h growth (from SBA)	Ambient air	16–20	E. coli ATCC 25922, E. coli ATCC 35218,[d] Pseudomonas aeruginosa ATCC 27853	Amoxicillin-clavulanic acid (B. pseudomallei only), ceftazidime, doxycycline, imipenem, tetracycline, TMP-SMX (B. pseudomallei only)
F. tularensis	CAMHB with 2% defined growth supplement, pH adjusted to 7.3 ± 0.1	24-h growth (from CHOC)	Ambient air	48	E. coli ATCC 25922, S. aureus ATCC 29213, P. aeruginosa ATCC 27853	Chloramphenicol, ciprofloxacin, doxycycline, gentamicin, levofloxacin, streptomycin, tetracycline
Y. pestis	CAMHB	24-h growth (from SBA)	Ambient air	24[e]	E. coli ATCC 25922	Chloramphenicol, ciprofloxacin, doxycycline, gentamicin, levofloxacin, streptomycin, tetracycline, TMP-SMX

[a]CAMHB, cation-adjusted Mueller-Hinton broth.
[b]Inoculum suspension is in CAMHB standardized to a 0.5 McFarland standard. Final organism concentration is 5×10^5 CFU/ml. CHOC, chocolate agar; SBA, sheep blood agar.
[c]Incubation temperature, 35°C.
[d]E. coli ATCC 35218 is used for quality control when testing β-lactam/β-lactamase inhibitor combination drugs.
[e]If unacceptable growth in the control well, reincubate for an additional 24 h.

macrolides in Asian-Pacific countries is much higher and exceeds 75% in some areas (118, 275). Erythromycin MICs for pneumococci with macrolide-lincosamide-streptogramin B-type resistance (encoded by the *ermB* gene) are usually ≥64 μg/ml, and clindamycin MICs are ≥8 μg/ml, whereas for isolates of the M phenotype (encoded by the *mefA* gene), erythromycin MICs are in the range of 1 to 32 μg/ml and clindamycin MICs are ≤0.25 μg/ml (67). The clinical significance of the lower-level macrolide resistance reflected by the M phenotype was once debated; however, it has been shown that clinical failures result in pneumonia or bacteremia due to such strains (158). Susceptibility and resistance to azithromycin, clarithromycin, and dirithromycin among *S. pneumoniae* isolates can be predicted by testing erythromycin (54). Telithromycin, a ketolide, is considerably more active than macrolides against *S. pneumoniae*, with fewer than 1% of isolates showing resistance in North America (20).

Resistance rates for trimethoprim-sulfamethoxazole (TMP-SMX) ranged from 35 to 47% in the United States in the pre-PCV-7 era and were similar to those outside the United States (13). Resistance rates for fluoroquinolones have remained low (28, 148); however, a higher prevalence of resistance to fluoroquinolones has been shown in elderly patients (2, 147, 159, 200) and in other countries (112, 278). Resistance has only been rarely reported for linezolid (123), and resistance rates for quinupristin-dalfopristin are <1% (148) among *S. pneumoniae* strains; resistance to tigecycline has not appeared (183).

Multidrug resistance in *S. pneumoniae* is usually defined as resistance to three or more antimicrobial classes, commonly penicillins, TMP-SMX, and macrolides (140). As many as 25% of *S. pneumoniae* isolates in the United States were reported to be multidrug resistant prior to 2001, and rates were higher in other countries (13, 140), while such strains declined by 59% following PCV-7 introduction in the United States (148).

Reference Test Methods
CLSI describes both a broth microdilution method and a disk diffusion procedure for testing pneumococci (51, 52, 54). Details of these methods are listed in Table 1. The broth microdilution method may be used to test all of the antimicrobial agents recommended by CLSI for pneumococci. With the exception of the oxacillin disk screening test for penicillin susceptibility, the disk diffusion method does not work reliably for testing β-lactam agents, including the cephalosporins (52, 54, 236). When used to predict penicillin susceptibility, oxacillin disk diffusion zone diameters of ≥20 mm indicate that the isolate is susceptible to penicillin when the more conservative meningitis or oral penicillin breakpoints are used (54). However, strains with zone diameters of ≤19 mm cannot be readily categorized as resistant, since a strain with an oxacillin zone diameter of ≤19 mm may be penicillin susceptible, intermediate, or resistant, especially when applying the nonmeningitis MIC breakpoints (66, 266). The oxacillin screen test can be used without follow-up MIC testing for nonmeningitis strains

with zones of $\geq$20 mm only. The oxacillin screening procedure should be used only for isolates from patients with non-life-threatening infections. If the zone diameter is $\leq$19 mm, at a minimum the MICs of penicillin and an extended-spectrum cephalosporin should be determined (54).

Commercial Methods for Testing

Several options are available for determining MICs of various antimicrobial agents with pneumococci. The Etest method has been extensively evaluated (130, 242). Etest strips for all drugs recommended by CLSI for testing pneumococci except clindamycin and telithromycin have been cleared by the FDA. The accuracy of the Etest has been reported to be >90% for most relevant drugs, although the number of minor errors with penicillin is relatively high and Etest penicillin MICs are slightly lower than those determined by reference broth microdilution (130). Since it is recommended that Etests be incubated in CO_2, the MICs of the macrolides and ketolides tend to be 1 to 2 dilutions higher than those obtained by the reference broth method, in which incubation is conducted in ambient air (23). This is because these agents are less active at lower pH, which occurs with CO_2 incubation.

Other commercially available FDA-cleared panels or systems specifically designed for testing pneumococci include MicroScan (Siemens Healthcare Inc., West Sacramento, CA), Phoenix (BD Diagnostic Systems, Sparks, MD), Sensititre (Trek Diagnostic Systems, Inc, Cleveland, OH), and Vitek 2 (bioMerieux, Inc., Durham, NC). The MicroScan MICroSTREP, Sensititre, Vitek 2, and Phoenix systems have been evaluated and found to produce MICs that are comparable to those obtained with the CLSI broth microdilution reference method (105, 127, 128, 209).

Strategies for Testing and Reporting of Results

CLSI stipulates that *S. pneumoniae* isolates from cerebrospinal fluid (CSF) be routinely tested by a reliable MIC method to determine susceptibilities to penicillin and cefotaxime or ceftriaxone, and meropenem should be added if it is on the institution's formulary for pneumococcal therapy. In addition, vancomycin should be tested by either a MIC or a disk diffusion method (54). For CSF isolates, as with penicillin, only interpretations using the original meningitis breakpoints should be reported; for isolates from other sites, both meningitis and nonmeningitis interpretations should be reported (54). Along with penicillin, CLSI recommends primary testing and reporting of erythromycin and TMP-SMX for isolates from non-CSF sources. Both drugs can be tested by either a MIC or a disk diffusion method. In addition, isolates from non-CSF sources can be tested for susceptibility to penicillin, cefotaxime or ceftriaxone, and/or meropenem by a MIC method and for susceptibility to vancomycin, a fluoroquinolone, and tetracycline by MIC or disk diffusion methods. CLSI standards include a second set of nonmeningitis MIC breakpoints for cefotaxime and ceftriaxone that apply to infections other than meningitis (54). Other drugs that might warrant testing if being considered for treatment of infections other than meningitis include cefepime, clindamycin, and telithromycin.

STREPTOCOCCI OTHER THAN PNEUMOCOCCI

Incidence of Resistance

Because there are significant differences in susceptibility of β-lactam agents in viridans group versus beta-hemolytic streptococci, there are separate ampicillin, penicillin, cefotaxime, ceftriaxone, and cefepime interpretive criteria for the two organism groups. The viridans group of streptococci includes the following five groups with several species within each: mutans group, salivarius group, bovis group, anginosus group (previously "S. milleri" group) and mitis group. The anginosus group includes small-colony-forming beta-hemolytic strains with groups A, C, F, or G antigens. The beta-hemolytic group includes the large-colony-forming pyogenic strains with group A (*S. pyogenes*), C, or G antigens and strains with group B (*S. agalactiae*) antigen.

Although beta-hemolytic streptococci have been uniformly susceptible to penicillin, two reports have described penicillin MICs of 0.25 to 0.5 μg/ml for group B streptococci (16) and group C streptococci (246). Kimura et al. from Japan recently reported 14 isolates of *Streptococcus agalactiae* collected from 1995–2005 with penicillin MICs of 0.25 to 1.0 μg/ml. Using molecular techniques, these isolates demonstrated a decreased amount of PBP 2X. The introduction of penicillin-resistant group B *Streptococcus*-derived PBP 2X genes into penicillin-susceptible strains through allelic exchange elevated their penicillin nonsusceptibility, suggesting that these altered PBP 2X genes are responsible for penicillin nonsusceptibility in the strains (136). The clinical significance of the elevated penicillin MICs in these beta-hemolytic streptococci is not known. High-level aminoglycoside resistance has been described on rare occasions for group B streptococci (31).

The macrolide-lincosamide-streptogramin B-type macrolide resistance due to *erm* genes in beta-hemolytic streptococci may be either inducible or constitutive (253). If the resistance is inducible, the strains will be resistant to erythromycin (and the other 14- and 15-membered macrolides) but appear to be susceptible to clindamycin unless resistance is induced. Resistance rates for erythromycin vary for group A streptococci, and a multicenter study conducted in the United States reported rates ranging from 3.0 to 8.7% depending on the geographic location (102). In a large Japanese study for isolates collected from 1999 to 2004, the prevalence of erythromycin resistance was 14.4% overall and was highest in 2004, reaching 20% (118). Among nearly 5,000 isolates of *S. agalactiae* collected as part of a program coordinated by the Active Bacterial Core Surveillance/Emerging Infections Program Network at the Centers for Disease Control and Prevention from 1999 to 2005, 32% and 15% were resistant to erythromycin and clindamycin, respectively (196). Resistance rates among beta-hemolytic streptococci vary for tetracyclines (27, 124) and remain low for fluoroquinolones (17, 27, 84, 124). In several recent large surveillance studies, some international, resistance was not observed for daptomycin (27, 124, 218), linezolid (17, 84, 124), or quinupristin-dalfopristin (27, 124).

Penicillin resistance in viridans group streptococci has been described, and resistance rates among bloodstream isolates can be >50% (173, 276), particularly for *S. mitis*, *S. oralis*, and *S. sanguinis*. Penicillin resistance among viridans group streptococci isolated from children with cancer is a significant concern (29), with Ahmed et al. noting 67.5% penicillin resistance among 40 blood culture isolates from bacteremic children with cancer (3). Resistance has been described for some viridans group streptococcal isolates for macrolides, lincosamides, and tetracyclines (124, 173, 276); quinupristin-dalfopristin (124, 173), and fluoroquinolones (17, 124). Single reports of resistance to vancomycin have been noted for *S. bovis* (202) and for *S. mitis* (144), and

TABLE 3 Disk diffusion and MIC testing conditions, recommended QC strains, and agents to consider for primary testing for infrequently isolated or less common fastidious bacteria

Organism(s)	Method	Medium[a]	Inoculum source[b]	Incubation atmosphere[c]	Incubation length (h)	Recommended QC strain(s)	Agents to consider for primary testing
Abiotrophia spp., Granulicatella spp.	Broth microdilution	CAMHB-LHB[c] + 0.001% pyridoxal HCl	20–24-h growth (from CHOC containing cysteine)	Ambient air	20–24	S. pneumoniae ATCC 49619	Cefotaxime or ceftriaxone, penicillin, vancomycin
Aeromonas hydrophila complex, Plesiomonas shigelloides	Broth microdilution	CAMHB	16–18-h growth (from SBA)	Ambient air	16–20	E. coli ATCC 25922, E. coli ATCC 35218[d]	Amoxicillin-clavulanic acid, broad-spectrum or extended-spectrum cephalosporins, fluoroquinolones, TMP-SMX
	Disk diffusion	MHA	16–18-h growth (from SBA)	Ambient air	16–18	E. coli ATCC 25922, E. coli ATCC 35218	Amoxicillin-clavulanic acid, broad-spectrum or extended-spectrum cephalosporins, fluoroquinolones, TMP-SMX
Bacillus spp. (not B. anthracis)	Broth microdilution	CAMHB	16–18-h growth (from SBA)	Ambient air	16–20	S. aureus ATCC 29213	Clindamycin, gentamicin (for combined therapy), vancomycin
C. jejuni, C. coli	Broth microdilution	CAMHB-LHB	24–48-h growth (from SBA)	10% CO_2, 5% O_2, 85% N_2 (microaerobic)	48 at 36°C or 24 at 42°C	C. jejuni ATCC 33560	Ciprofloxacin, erythromycin
Corynebacterium spp.	Broth microdilution	CAMHB-LHB	24–48 h growth (from SBA or CHOC)	Ambient air	24–48	S. pneumoniae ATCC 49619	Erythromycin, gentamicin, penicillin, vancomycin
E. rhusiopathiae	Broth microdilution	CAMHB-LHB	18–24-h growth (from SBA)	Ambient air	20–24	S. pneumoniae ATCC 49619	Penicillin or ampicillin
HACEK group	Broth microdilution	CAMHB-LHB	24–48-h growth (from CHOC)	5% CO_2	24–48	S. pneumoniae ATCC 49619, E. coli ATCC 35218	Ampicillin, amoxicillin-clavulanic acid, ceftriaxone or cefotaxime, ciprofloxacin or levofloxacin, imipenem, TMP-SMX
H. pylori	Agar dilution	MHA + 5% aged (≥2-wk-old) sheep blood	72-h growth (from SBA)[e]	Microaerobic; produced by gas-generating system for campylobacters	72	H. pylori ATCC 43504	Clarithromycin
Lactobacillus spp.	Broth microdilution	CAMHB-LHB	18–24-h growth (from SBA)	5% CO_2	20–24	S. pneumoniae ATCC 49619	Penicillin or ampicillin, gentamicin (for combined therapy)
Leuconostoc spp.	Broth microdilution	CAMHB-LHB	18–24-h growth (from SBA)	Ambient air	20–24	S. pneumoniae ATCC 49619	Penicillin or ampicillin, gentamicin (for combined therapy)

Organism	Test method	Medium	Growth	Atmosphere	Incubation time (h)	QC strain	Drugs/comments
L. monocytogenes	Broth microdilution	CAMHB-LHB	18–24-h growth (from SBA)	Ambient air	20–24	*S. pneumoniae* ATCC 49619	Penicillin or ampicillin, TMP-SMX
M. catarrhalis	Broth microdilution	CAMHB	18–24-h growth (from SBA)	Ambient air	20–24	*S. aureus* ATCC 29213, *E. coli* ATCC 35218	Amoxicillin-clavulanic acid, cefaclor or cefuroxime, TMP-SMX
	Disk diffusion	MHA	18–24-h growth (from SBA)	Ambient air	20–24	*S. aureus* ATCC 29213, *E. coli* ATCC 35218	Amoxicillin-clavulanic acid, TMP-SMX
Pasteurella spp.	Broth microdilution	CAMHB-LHB	18–24-h growth (from SBA)	Ambient air	18–24	*S. pneumoniae* ATCC 49619, *E. coli* ATCC 35218	β-Lactam/β-lactamase inhibitor combinations, cephalosporins, fluoroquinolones, macrolides, penicillins, tetracyclines, TMP-SMX
	Disk diffusion	MHA with 5% sheep blood	18–24-h growth (from SBA)	Ambient air	18–24	*S. pneumoniae* ATCC 49619, *E. coli* ATCC 35218, *S. aureus* ATCC 25923 (disk diffusion)	β-Lactam/β-lactamase inhibitor combinations, cephalosporins, fluoroquinolones, macrolides, penicillins, tetracyclines, TMP-SMX
Pediococcus spp.	Broth microdilution	CAMHB-LHB	18–24-h growth (from SBA)	Ambient air	20–24	*S. pneumoniae* ATCC 49619	Penicillin, gentamicin (for combined therapy)
Vibrio spp. (including *V. cholerae*)f	Broth microdilution	CAMHB	16–18-h growth (from SBA)	Ambient air	16–20	*E. coli* ATCC 25922, *E. coli* ATCC 35218	For *Vibrio* spp. (not *V. cholerae*): cefotaxime, ceftazidime, tetracycline, fluoroquinolones. For *V. cholerae*: ampicillin, azithromycin, chloramphenicol, doxycycline, sulfonamides, tetracycline, TMP-SMX
	Disk diffusion	MHA	16–18-h growth (from SBA)	Ambient air	16–18	*E. coli* ATCC 25922, *E. coli* ATCC 35218	For *Vibrio* spp. (not *V. cholerae*): cefotaxime, ceftazidime, tetracycline, fluoroquinolones. For *V. cholerae*: ampicillin, chloramphenicol, doxycycline, sulfonamides, tetracycline, TMP-SMX

aCAMHB-LHB and MHA are defined in the text.
bSuspension is in Mueller-Hinton broth or saline standardized to a 0.5 McFarland standard. For broth dilution, final organism concentration is 5 × 10⁵ CFU/ml. CHOC, chocolate agar; SBA, sheep blood agar.
cIncubation temperature, 35°C (except for *C. jejuni* and *C. coli*).
dE. coli ATCC 35218 is used for quality control when testing β-lactam/β-lactamase inhibitor combination drugs.
eSuspension is in saline standardized to a 2.0 McFarland standard.
fFor halophilic species, prepare inoculum in 0.85% NaCl (normal saline).

resistance to linezolid has been reported on rare occasions (126, 215). In a European surveillance study, two isolates of viridans group streptococci showed daptomycin MICs of 2 μg/ml, which is nonsusceptible according to CLSI criteria (218). Among a large international collection of bloodstream isolates, all were susceptible to tigecycline (173). High-level aminoglycoside resistance has been described for viridans group streptococci (114).

Reference Test Methods

Studies by CLSI to determine interpretive criteria for both MIC and disk diffusion testing have resulted in breakpoints for streptococci that were initially published in 1995. Most recently, separate tables containing interpretive criteria were published in order to clarify the differences in disk diffusion and MIC testing and report recommendations for streptococci belonging to either the viridans or beta-hemolytic group. The disk diffusion test may be used to determine the penicillin susceptibility of beta-hemolytic streptococci; however, it is unreliable and should not be used for viridans group streptococci. For either group, carbapenems and daptomycin should only be tested by a MIC method; however, other agents may be tested by either the MIC or the disk method (54). Aminoglycoside MICs of >1,000 μg/ml for streptococci (270) have been described; however, there are no published methods for screening for high-level aminoglycoside resistance in streptococci.

Susceptibility testing methods for members of the genera *Abiotrophia* and *Granulicatella* (formerly known as "nutritionally deficient streptococci") are included in the CLSI M45 guideline as described below. CLSI standards describe a disk approximation test for inducible resistance to clindamycin in beta-hemolytic streptococci whereby erythromycin is used to induce resistance to clindamycin. Mueller-Hinton agar (MHA) supplemented with 5% sheep blood is inoculated as for a disk diffusion test, and a 15-μg erythromycin disk and a 2-μg clindamycin disk are placed approximately 12 mm apart on the agar surface. The plate is incubated at 35°C overnight, and flattening of the clindamycin zone indicates inducible clindamycin resistance (52, 54).

Commercial Test Methods

There have been several reports demonstrating that the Phoenix performs reliably for susceptibility testing of streptococci other than pneumococci (26, 111, 209). For the other test systems, there are no peer-reviewed publications, although it might be expected that systems capable of testing pneumococci would also perform adequately for other streptococci. The MicroScan, Phoenix, and Sensititre systems are cleared by the FDA for the testing of *Streptococcus* spp. The Vitek 2 system is FDA cleared for testing of group B streptococci. The Etest has not been extensively evaluated but does appear to be a possible alternative to the reference methods for testing *Streptococcus* spp. (122, 216).

Strategies for Testing and Reporting of Results

Routine testing of beta-hemolytic streptococci is unnecessary since there have been only sporadic reports of decreased susceptibility to penicillin, primarily in group B streptococci (16, 136, 246). However, if erythromycin is being used to treat infections caused by group A streptococci and treatment failure is suspected, testing might be considered. Similarly, if erythromycin is being considered for prophylaxis of pregnant women who are highly allergic to penicillin, in an effort to prevent perinatal group B streptococcal disease, testing should be done. If clindamycin is being considered for

beta-hemolytic streptococci that test clindamycin susceptible and erythromycin resistant, the determination of inducible clindamycin resistance should be considered. For viridans group streptococci, penicillin MICs should be determined for strains isolated from blood, especially for patients with infective endocarditis. Disk diffusion is not reliable for testing penicillin in viridans group streptococci (6).

HAEMOPHILUS INFLUENZAE

Incidence of Resistance

Ampicillin resistance in *H. influenzae* is most commonly mediated by a plasmid-borne β-lactamase, TEM-1 being the most common enzyme. Approximately 10 to 25% of the isolates included in several recent surveillance studies were reported to produce β-lactamase (34, 56, 87, 118, 120, 125, 182, 248, 263). However, the incidence of beta-lactamase production among isolates collected from 1999 to 2000 during a global surveillance study was as low as 3% in Germany and as high as 65% in South Korea (113). A decrease in β-lactamase-producing isolates has been documented in North America (110) and more recently in Spain (87).

Ampicillin resistance can result from altered penicillin-binding proteins in β-lactamase-negative, ampicillin-resistant (BLNAR) strains. Some strains may possess this β-lactam resistance mechanism and also produce β-lactamase, and these strains are referred to as β-lactamase-producing, amoxicillin-clavulanic acid resistant or BLPACR. Resistance in BLNAR has been shown to be associated with mutations of the *ftsI* gene, which encodes PBP 3 (248).

Both BLNAR and BLPACR are relatively uncommon in most parts of the world. In a recent surveillance study in the United States, only 0.4% of 978 isolates were BLNAR and the incidence of β-lactamase production was 27.4% (56). In Japan, however, BLNAR are prevalent and more common than β-lactamase-producing strains (118, 182, 248). In a surveillance study of 479 strains of *H. influenzae* from children with lower respiratory tract infections, the incidence of BLNAR increased from 28.1% in 2000 to 54.7% in 2005 and less than 10% of the isolates produced β-lactamase in any year (181). Among 621 isolates collected from patients with meningitis between 2000 and 2004, 52.6% were BLNAR, 11.4% were BLPACR, and 11% produced β-lactamase (108). Compared with β-lactamase-producing or ampicillin-susceptible *H. influenzae*, BLNAR isolates are less susceptible to amoxicillin-clavulanic acid and to various cephalosporins such as cefaclor and cefotaxime (108, 182). Resistance among *H. influenzae* isolates to broad-spectrum oral cephalosporins (e.g., cefixime and cefpodoxime) (120) and to extended-spectrum cephalosporins (e.g., ceftriaxone) (221, 263) is rare. Resistance to cefuroxime is uncommon, with <1% resistance reported in a recent global surveillance study (221). The narrower-spectrum, β-lactamase-labile cephalosporins (e.g., cefaclor and cefprozil) are less active, with resistance rates of 10% to nearly 40% (118, 120, 263).

Resistance to TMP-SMX among *H. influenzae* organisms occurred in approximately 15 to 20% of isolates from North America (56, 87, 125, 221); however, rates over 40% have been noted in Brazil (34) and rates over 60% have been reported from Asia (263). Resistance to tetracyclines is <10% (34, 87, 125), and resistance to fluoroquinolones is rare (34, 56, 120, 125, 182, 221). Although erythromycin has not been considered a drug of choice for the treatment of infections caused by *H. influenzae*, some of the newer macrolides are more active than erythromycin and may be effective as treatment. Less than 3% of isolates examined in various studies were resistant to azithromycin and telithromycin (56, 118, 120, 221); however, clarithromycin resistance rates have been approximately 20% (118, 125).

Reference Test Methods

β-Lactamase production in *H. influenzae* can easily be detected by the chromogenic cephalosporin, acidometric, or iodometric β-lactamase test methods (see chapter 70). CLSI has developed broth microdilution MIC and disk diffusion methods for testing *H. influenzae*, and these methods can also be used to test *H. parainfluenzae*. Testing of the more unusual *Haemophilus* spp. including *Aggregatibacter aphrophilus* (formerly *H. aphrophilus* and *H. paraphrophilus*) and *Aggregatibacter segnis* (formerly *H. segnis*) is now addressed in the CLSI M45 document. Specific variables related to each of the methods for testing *H. influenzae* and *H. parainfluenzae* are listed in Table 1. *Haemophilus* test medium (HTM) is recommended and consists of a Mueller-Hinton base, 15 μg of hematin per ml, 15 μg of NAD per ml, and 5 mg of yeast extract per ml. Cation-adjusted Mueller-Hinton broth (CAMHB) is used with the components listed above for the preparation of HTM broth, which also contains 0.2 IU of thymidine phosphorylase per ml. Although HTM agar is transparent, some investigators have reported difficulties in measuring zones and poor growth of some strains (109, 172). Broth microdilution tests with HTM generally give clearer end points. The problems most often noted with both the disk diffusion and the broth microdilution methods are equivocal end points with BLNAR strains with several β-lactams. Because of this, CLSI recommends that BLNAR strains (which are best detected by tests with ampicillin) be considered resistant to amoxicillin-clavulanic acid, ampicillin-sulbactam, cefaclor, cefetamet, cefonicid, cefprozil, cefuroxime, loracarbef, and piperacillin-tazobactam and that the activities of these agents against BLNAR strains not be tested (54).

Commercial Test Methods

Currently, the only FDA-cleared broth microdilution system for testing *Haemophilus* spp. is Sensititre (Trek). The Etest has been cleared by the FDA for testing *H. influenzae* with most drugs that would be used for treating *Haemophilus* infections, and earlier studies with Etest demonstrated that results with that system were comparable to those obtained by CLSI reference methods (131). However, recently Billal et al. reported that Etest produces considerably higher MICs than broth microdilution when testing ampicillin, amoxicillin-clavulanic acid, cefixime, and perhaps other β-lactams. This is a particular concern with BLNAR and BLPACR strains (19). Others have shown that use of Etest for BLNAR and BLPACR strains is not a problem (249).

Strategies for Testing and Reporting of Results

β-Lactamase testing detects the most common type of clinically significant resistance in *H. influenzae*. β-Lactamase-positive isolates are ampicillin and amoxicillin resistant. To detect BLNAR strains, an ampicillin disk diffusion or MIC test is required. To detect BLPACR strains, both a β-lactamase test and an amoxicillin-clavulanic disk diffusion or MIC test are required as these strains are β-lactamase positive and show decreased susceptibility to amoxicillin-clavulanic acid. However, since the incidence of BLNAR and BLPACR is currently low in many geographic areas, such tests may not be routinely needed, and for practical purposes, a negative β-lactamase test result translates into

ampicillin susceptibility. Because of increasing resistance to TMP-SMX, testing should be considered and CLSI recommends that this agent be tested and reported routinely (54). Other oral agents that might be considered, such as amoxicillin-clavulanic acid, the oral cephalosporins, newer macrolides, and fluoroquinolones, are predictably active against *H. influenzae* and are often prescribed empirically. Consequently, routine testing of these drugs is generally not useful. However, these and other agents may be tested for surveillance or epidemiological purposes (54).

NEISSERIA GONORRHOEAE

Incidence of Resistance

Antimicrobial resistance among *N. gonorrhoeae* isolates is a significant concern. Increasing rates of penicillin, tetracycline, and most recently fluoroquinolone resistance among *N. gonorrhoeae* isolates have led to recommending ceftriaxone or cefixime as the primary agents for uncomplicated gonorrhea (40). Penicillin resistance is due to the production of a plasmid-associated TEM-1-type β-lactamase (penicillinase-producing *N. gonorrhoeae* [PPNG]) or to mutations in chromosomal genes that result in altered penicillin-binding proteins or diminished outer membrane permeability (chromosomally mediated resistant *N. gonorrhoeae*). The activities of other β-lactams against PPNG are generally unaltered; however, chromosomally mediated resistant *N. gonorrhoeae* isolates may show decreased susceptibility to other β-lactams (65). With increased use of cephalosporins, there has been concern about resistance developing to these agents. Treatment failure in gonorrhea treated with oral cephalosporin regimens (but not with injectable ceftriaxone) has been reported, and a mosaic *penA* gene that encodes PBP2 alternations has been noted in strains associated with the failures (240, 277). Among isolates from male patients with urethritis in Japan, some had reduced susceptibility to cefixime or ceftriaxone with MICs as high as 0.25 μg/ml or 0.125 μg/ml, respectively (185), and Tanaka et al. reported an isolate with a ceftriaxone MIC of 0.5 μg/ml (238). The Centers for Disease Control and Prevention has recently reported that the ceftriaxone MIC is less than 0.008 μg/ml for most gonococcal strains (39). Disturbingly, the decreased cephalosporin susceptibility is often among strains that have decreased susceptibility to other classes of antimicrobial agents that might be considered for *N. gonorrhoeae* infections (185, 238, 277).

Tetracycline resistance in *N. gonorrhoeae* can be plasmid- or chromosomally mediated, with plasmid-mediated resistance resulting in a higher level of resistance. The main determinant of fluoroquinolone resistance in *N. gonorrhoeae* is target site alteration by spontaneous mutations in the quinolone resistance-determining regions of *gyrA* and *parC* (247).

The Gonococcal Isolate Surveillance Program, which tests urethral isolates from male clients visiting sexually transmitted disease clinics throughout the United States, reported that more than 22% of 6,009 isolates were resistant to both penicillin and tetracycline in 2007. The incidence of PPNG peaked at 11.0% in 1991 and was only 0.4% in 2007. All 6,009 isolates tested in 2007 were susceptible to ceftriaxone. Since 1987, there have been four isolates with ceftriaxone MICs of 0.5 μg/ml, the most recent in 1997. Between 1992 and 2007, 48 isolates demonstrated cefixime MICs ranging from 0.5 to 2.0 μg/ml (39).

The Western Pacific Region Gonococcal Antimicrobial Surveillance Program reported a >80% fluoroquinolone resistance in 2006 for *N. gonorrhoeae* from several countries to include China, Hong Kong, and Japan (241). In the 2007 Gonococcal Isolate Surveillance Program study, 1.3% of the isolates exhibited intermediate susceptibility and 14.8% were resistant to ciprofloxacin. Although ciprofloxacin resistance is now seen throughout the United States, the incidence is greatest on the West Coast (39).

Reference Test Methods

Routine β-lactamase tests readily detect PPNG and can reliably be performed by either the chromogenic cephalosporin, acidimetric, or iodometric method.

CLSI recommends the use of GC agar base for disk diffusion and agar dilution MIC testing. For both tests, a 1% defined growth supplement must be added; however, in agar dilution tests with imipenem and with clavulanate, the growth supplement must be free of cysteine to avoid inhibition of the activities of these two agents (51, 52, 54). The agar dilution method is preferred to the broth dilution method for MIC testing because *N. gonorrhoeae* has a tendency to autolyse in liquid media. For other details of testing, see Table 1.

Commercial Test Methods

The only commercial method currently available for susceptibility testing of *N. gonorrhoeae* is Etest, which has been shown to produce results comparable to those of conventional reference agar dilution methods (18).

Strategies for Testing and Reporting Results

Generally, there is no need for routine clinical laboratories to perform antimicrobial susceptibility tests with *N. gonorrhoeae* unless there are unusual circumstances. These might include the patient's intolerance to the drugs of choice, treatment failure (assuming that compliance was not an issue), or a disseminated gonococcal infection. Some laboratories may perform β-lactamase tests for all isolates if β-lactamase results are requested by the local public health departments for epidemiological purposes. However, most public health departments have eliminated this requirement. Surveillance for established and emerging resistance for *N. gonorrhoeae* is generally performed by designated state and local public health agencies.

NEISSERIA MENINGITIDIS

Incidence of Resistance

Increasing numbers of *N. meningitidis* isolates from the United States, Europe, and elsewhere have reduced susceptibility to penicillin (MICs, 0.12 to 1.0 μg/ml) (71, 107, 129, 176, 207, 259). A study of 400 *N. meningitidis* isolates obtained in 1998 and 1999 in Spain showed that 37% of them had penicillin MICs of 0.12 to 1.0 μg/ml (257), and a U.S. study conducted in the same time period revealed a similar 30.2% had penicillin MICs of 0.12 to 0.25 μg/ml (207). Diminished penicillin and ampicillin susceptibility in meningococci is due to polymorphisms in PBP 2 that result from point mutations of the *penA* gene encoding that PBP (71, 129, 237, 245, 259). The clinical significance of isolates with elevated penicillin MICs is uncertain, and penicillin remains the drug of choice for the treatment of meningococcal disease in many parts of the world (213). Infections caused by isolates with reduced susceptibility to penicillin have successfully been treated with high doses of penicillin in several cases (233, 271); however, rare reports cited clinical failure in meningitis when a lower than recommended dose of penicillin was used (252) or in

pneumonia with empyema (92). High-level resistance due to beta-lactamase production was observed in a few isolates in the 1980s (22, 83), and one isolate was reported in 1996 (258); additional isolates have not been seen for more than a decade (259).

The extended-spectrum cephalosporins (e.g., ceftriaxone and cefotaxime) remain highly active against isolates with elevated penicillin MICs (107, 129, 207, 257) and are often used as first-line therapy for meningococcal meningitis in developed countries. However, a report of eight ceftriaxone-resistant serogroup A isolates from India is cause for concern (163). Ceftriaxone MICs ranged from 0.25 to 8 μg/ml in those isolates.

Regarding agents used for prophylaxis, resistance to sulfonamides occurs frequently, and resistance to rifampin has been documented on several occasions following exposure to that agent (129, 205, 214, 257). Of greatest concern is the increasing frequency of diminished fluoroquinolone susceptibility in meningococci from several countries (4, 46, 55, 74, 170, 224, 225, 272). Isolates reported to date generally have ciprofloxacin MICs of 0.125 to 0.5 μg/ml, rather than demonstrating high-level resistance. Resistance has been attributed to mutations in the *gyrA* gene, similar to the situation in gonococci (272). A single isolate from Venezuela has been reported to be resistant to both ciprofloxacin and a second agent that could be used for prophylaxis, azithromycin (212).

Strategies for Testing and Reporting of Results

CLSI has published standards for susceptibility testing of *N. meningitidis* that utilize either the broth microdilution method and CAMHB with 2 to 5% lysed horse blood (CAMHB-LHB) or the agar dilution method and MHA with 5% sheep blood, both with incubation in 5% CO_2 (54, 129).

Interpretive criteria are listed for agents such as penicillin, cefotaxime, and ceftriaxone that might be prescribed for treating a meningococcal infection. In addition, interpretive criteria are listed for agents such as ciprofloxacin, rifampin, and azithromycin that might be used for prophylaxis of meningococcal case contacts. Strains with diminished fluoroquinolone susceptibility may best be detected by testing with nalidixic acid by MIC or disk methods (75, 129). The CLSI approved a disk diffusion method for testing *N. meningitidis* that utilizes MHA with 5% sheep blood and CO_2 incubation. As with MIC tests, interpretive criteria are listed for several therapeutic and prophylactic agents. Unfortunately, these do not include breakpoints for ampicillin and penicillin, as disk testing results obtained with these agents were unreliable (54). Several investigators have examined modified penicillin disk diffusion methods by using 2- and 10-IU penicillin disks and 1-μg oxacillin disks and also determined that these cannot reliably distinguish *N. meningitidis* isolates that are susceptible from those that have decreased ampicillin and penicillin susceptibility (21, 32, 195). Therefore, disk diffusion testing should not be used for these drugs. One possible exception might be testing of mecillinam (amdinocillin) by the disk method as a screen for isolates with *penA* polymorphisms (129).

Because of the lack of clinical failures with the drugs of choice for the treatment of meningococcal infections, susceptibility testing is not warranted in most situations (213, 214). Although the Etest has not yet been cleared by the FDA for testing *N. meningitidis*, several studies have shown it to be suitable for testing meningococci and to perform best by using MHA with 5% sheep blood incubated in

CO_2 (1, 165, 192, 195, 256). However, in a 14-lab study, Vazquez et al. noted some difficulties in obtaining reliable Etest results with rifampin (256).

POTENTIAL BACTERIAL AGENTS OF BIOTERRORISM

Several bacterial agents are identified as potential agents of bioterrorism by the Centers for Disease Control and Prevention (http://www.bt.cdc.gov/agent/index.asp). These include *Bacillus anthracis*, *Yersinia pestis*, *Francisella tularensis*, *Burkholderia mallei*, *Burkholderia pseudomallei*, and *Brucella* spp. The antimicrobial susceptibility patterns for most of them are predictable, so susceptibility testing of naturally occurring isolates is often not necessary. However, it is possible for antimicrobial resistance to spontaneously occur among these organisms and, in the case of a bioterrorism event, there is the possibility of engineered resistance. To detect any possible resistance, standardized broth microdilution susceptibility testing methods and interpretive criteria were established and published by CLSI (50).

Acquired resistance to antimicrobial agents commonly used for treatment of infections caused by *B. anthracis*, *Y. pestis*, *F. tularensis*, *B. mallei*, *B. pseudomallei*, and *Brucella* spp. is rare. Isolates of *B. anthracis* may contain inducible β-lactamases, which can confer resistance to penicillins and cephalosporins (36, 42, 69, 155). Because of this potential resistance, penicillin is recommended for anthrax prophylaxis only when the organism burden would be low, and this recommendation is limited to young children and pregnant women who should not receive other prophylaxis therapies such as fluoroquinolones and tetracyclines (41). Laboratory-generated fluoroquinolone resistance in *B. anthracis* was reported, but fluoroquinolone resistance in clinical isolates has not been reported (44, 204). There are reports of two spontaneously occurring drug-resistant *Y. pestis* isolates recovered in Madagascar (44, 86, 104, 204). Both isolates acquired conjugative plasmids. In one isolate, the plasmid carried resistance determinants for ampicillin, chloramphenicol, tetracycline, kanamycin, streptomycin, and sulfonamide. In the other isolate, the plasmid conferred resistance to streptomycin. Susceptibility studies of *B. pseudomallei* and *B. mallei* indicate that most isolates are susceptible to amoxicillin-clavulanic acid, ceftazidime, imipenem, tetracycline, doxycycline, and TMP-SMX, using CLSI interpretive criteria (243). However, some isolates of *B. pseudomallei* have elevated ceftazidime MICs (i.e., MIC, ≥8 μg/ml) (117, 243). Clinical isolates of *Brucella* spp. with reduced susceptibility to rifampin and TMP-SMX have been reported (11, 137, 171). In these studies, the susceptibility testing methods used either were not clearly defined or were different from the methods currently recommended by CLSI. Also, resistant isolates were not characterized for resistance determinants or mutations. Therefore, the definition of resistance to rifampin or TMP-SMX among *Brucella* spp. is unclear. Isolates of *F. tularensis* demonstrate β-lactamase activity, and they are resistant to β-lactams including cephalosporins and carbapenems (9, 116). Resistance to aminoglycosides, tetracyclines, fluoroquinolones, and chloramphenicol has not been reported.

B. anthracis, *B. mallei*, *B. pseudomallei*, and *Y. pestis* demonstrate sufficient growth with commonly used broth microdilution MIC testing medium and incubation conditions (Table 2). However, the recommended testing medium for *F. tularensis* is CAMHB with 2% of a defined growth supplement. This is the same cysteine-containing defined growth supplement that is added to GC agar base for susceptibility testing of *Neisseria gonorrhoeae*. The supplement is commercially available from two manufacturers: IsoVitaleX Enrichment (BD Diagnostics, Franklin Lakes, NJ) and XV Factor Enrichment (PML Microbiologicals, Wilsonville, OR). Some isolates of *Brucella* spp., particularly isolates of *B. abortus*, require CO_2 incubation for good growth. CLSI susceptibility testing recommendation indicated that incubation in 5% CO_2 may be necessary, but these conditions may increase the MICs of aminoglycosides and decrease the MICs of tetracyclines (50). The streptomycin susceptibility breakpoint is one doubling dilution higher (i.e., increased from 8 μg/ml to 16 μg/ml) when panels are incubated in CO_2. For the slower-growing organisms, *F. tularensis*, *Y. pestis*, and *Brucella* spp., 48 h of incubation may be needed to achieve sufficient growth.

There are few studies comparing alternative susceptibility testing methods to the standard CLSI reference broth microdilution methods. One study compared Etest to broth microdilution for testing *B. anthracis* (174). In this study, Etest MICs were within a single doubling dilution of the broth microdilution MICs for ceftriaxone, chloramphenicol, ciprofloxacin, clindamycin, erythromycin, rifampin, tetracycline, and vancomycin, but not for penicillin. Penicillin MIC values for Etest tended to be lower than those obtained by broth microdilution. A similar trend for penicillin MICs was noted for *B. anthracis* in a study comparing Etest to agar dilution (251). These results suggest that Etest is acceptable for susceptibility testing of *B. anthracis* with antimicrobial agents other than penicillin. Similar studies are needed to establish alternative methods for the other potential agents of bioterrorism so that testing is available in more laboratories.

Susceptibility testing of potential agents of bioterrorism raises safety concerns for clinical microbiology laboratories. All of the above-mentioned organisms require at least biosafety level 2 (BSL 2) practices, containment, and facilities. BSL 3 conditions are recommended for activities with a high potential for aerosol production (45). Since the inoculum preparation for susceptibility testing has the potential for aerosol production, all susceptibility testing procedures must be performed in a BSL 3 facility. Laboratories without BSL 3 facilities should send isolates to an appropriately equipped reference laboratory that has select agent clearance status, such as that at reference laboratories within the Laboratory Response Network and at the Centers for Disease Control and Prevention (http://www.selectagents.gov/).

ABIOTROPHIA SPECIES AND *GRANULICATELLA* SPECIES

For *Abiotrophia* spp. and *Granulicatella* spp., resistance to agents from several different antimicrobial classes including penicillins, cephalosporins, carbapenems, macrolides, lincosamides, fluoroquinolones, and tetracyclines has been reported. In a study of 20 blood isolates by Murray et al., resistance rates for specific agents were as follows: penicillin, 5%; cefotaxime, 35%; cefepime, 47%; meropenem, 10%; erythromycin, 30%; clindamycin, 5%; and tetracycline, 10% (178). These results are consistent with those previously reported (90, 250). Murray et al. also noted a levofloxacin-resistant *Abiotrophia elegans* (currently known as *Granulicatella elegans*) strain which was isolated from a patient who had received 10 days of levofloxacin prophylaxis (178). Among isolates from 28 patients with nutritionally variant streptococcal infections (16 *Granulicatella adiacens* isolates, 8 *Abiotrophia defectiva* isolates, and 1 *G. elegans* isolate) treated at a university hospital in Taiwan, 50% had penicillin MICs of 0.25 to 2 μg/ml and 10 isolates were not susceptible to cefotaxime, with 7 fully resistant at MICs of ≥4 μg/ml. Three isolates had cefepime MICs of ≥4 μg/ml; the MIC_{90} of imipenem was 0.12 μg/ml, and that of meropenem was 0.5 μg/ml. Only two isolates were susceptible to azithromycin, and all isolates were susceptible to vancomycin, linezolid, quinupristin-dalfopristin, and levofloxacin (153). Little is known about mechanisms of resistance in these bacteria. There is one report of an *Abiotrophia defectiva* isolate with a conjugative, Tn*916*-like transposon, Tn*3872* (203). The transposon carried *ermB* and *tetM* resistance determinants, which conferred resistance to erythromycin and tetracycline, respectively. In another report that examined 15 isolates from pediatric patients (6 *Abiotrophia* isolates and 9 *Granulicatella* isolates), 8 were resistant to erythromycin. Five of these were clindamycin susceptible and harbored *mef*(A), and three that were clindamycin resistant were positive for *erm*(B) and also *tet*(M). One of the *erm*(B)-positive *Granulicatella* spp. also had *mef*(A) (280). These findings demonstrate that these bacteria are able to acquire and transfer mobile genetic elements that confer antimicrobial resistance.

Because *Abiotrophia* spp. and *Granulicatella* spp. are fastidious, it is recommended that these be tested in CAMHB-LHB supplemented with 0.001% pyridoxal hydrochloride and incubated in CO_2 (Table 3) (50, 244). In a report by Namdari et al., a procedure for adding pyridoxal to an inoculum prepared with the Prompt system and a MicroScan dried gram-positive panel is described (180). It should be noted that susceptibility testing of aminoglycosides against *Abiotrophia* spp. and *Granulicatella* spp. is not recommended, even though aminoglycosides are commonly used in combination therapy with an agent active against the cell wall, such as penicillin or vancomycin, for treating serious infections caused by these organisms. Since the aminoglycoside acts synergistically with the agent, in vitro susceptibility to aminoglycosides does not predict in vivo susceptibility (24).

AEROMONAS HYDROPHILA COMPLEX (*A. CAVIAE, A. HYDROPHILA, A. JANDAEI, A. SCHUBERTII,* AND *A. VERONII*) AND *PLESIOMONAS SHIGELLOIDES*

Aeromonas spp. are typically resistant to ampicillin, show variable results with β-lactam/β-lactamase inhibitor combinations, and are resistant to narrow-spectrum cephalosporins (141, 150, 261). Inducible β-lactamases in *Aeromonas* spp. have been noted, and resistance may emerge during therapy with a β-lactam agent (142). Among 172 isolates of *Aeromonas* spp. recently tested as part of a global surveillance program, 98.8% were susceptible to meropenem and over 90% were susceptible to extended-spectrum cephalosporins, but only 63.7% were susceptible to piperacillin-tazobactam (35). Isolates from 70 patients with a variety of types of documented infections in France in 2006 demonstrated over 95% susceptibility to extended-spectrum cephalosporins and piperacillin-tazobactam. In this study, there were distinct species differences in susceptibility results for tobramycin, with fewer than 30% of *A. veronii* isolates testing susceptible (150). In Taiwan, where *Aeromonas* spp. are frequently encountered, results from 234 isolates in 1996 demonstrated that most isolates were susceptible to extended-spectrum cephalosporins, fluoroquinolones, and aminoglycosides and approximately one-half of

the isolates were susceptible to tetracycline and TMP-SMX. These authors remarked that there appeared to be species differences also and *A. sobria* was more susceptible than either *A. hydrophila* or *A. caviae* (141). Similar results were noted by Vila et al. from Spain in 2002 (261). Recently, a VIM metallo-β-lactamase-producing *A. hydrophila* strain carrying an integron-borne bla_{VIM-4} gene was isolated from a patient in Hungary (154).

Plesiomonas spp. are typically resistant to ampicillin and other penicillins including piperacillin and susceptible to β-lactamase inhibitor combinations and several other classes of antimicrobial agents (98, 133, 232). However, Stock and Wiedemann noted considerable variations in MICs when different media and inoculum concentrations from 10^4 to 10^7 were used to test 30 different β-lactams (231).

Although *Aeromonas* spp. and *Plesiomonas shigelloides* cause diarrheal disease, otherwise healthy individuals with diarrhea due to these bacteria usually recover spontaneously without treatment (98, 261), and routine antimicrobial susceptibility testing of isolates from fecal specimens is not recommended (50). However, both genera can cause a variety of other infections for which treatment may be necessary (98, 141, 142, 150, 232).

Consequently, for isolates from extraintestinal sources, antimicrobial susceptibility testing may be warranted. These organisms share growth characteristics similar to those of *Enterobacteriaceae*, which led CLSI to recommend disk diffusion or broth microdilution MIC testing using the same methods as recommended for *Enterobacteriaceae*.

BACILLUS SPECIES

Bacillus spp. other than *B. anthracis* are common contaminants in the clinical laboratory, but these bacteria can cause serious disease including catheter infections, traumatic wound infections, and corneal ulcers. Since the susceptibility profiles of *Bacillus* spp. are quite variable, susceptibility testing should be considered when *Bacillus* spp. are isolated from normally sterile body sites or serious or refractory infections. Isolates of *Bacillus* spp. can have β-lactamases that confer resistance to penicillins and possibly cephalosporins (217). *Bacillus cereus* is the most common species found in clinical specimens, and most isolates are resistant to penicillin and extended-spectrum cephalosporins, although penicillin resistance does not always predict cephalosporin resistance (251, 265). Penicillin and cephalosporin resistance also occurs in other species of *Bacillus*, but it is less common. Resistance to other agents has been reported. These agents include aminoglycosides, erythromycin, clindamycin, chloramphenicol, tetracycline, fluoroquinolones, TMP-SMX, and even vancomycin (48, 251, 265). When 70 isolates (vegetative cells) of *Bacillus* spp. from a variety of clinical specimens were examined, daptomycin was active against 96.7% of the isolates at ≤1 μg/ml and against 100% of them at 2 μg/ml. Two strains had ciprofloxacin MICs of >4 μg/ml, and 10 strains were resistant to erythromycin. When spore inoculum suspensions were tested, neither ciprofloxacin nor daptomycin demonstrated activity but spores appeared to be killed as they germinated (48). A case of fatal septicemia caused by *Bacillus cereus* resistant to carbapenems in a patient treated with meropenem was recently reported (138).

Standard susceptibility testing methods for nonfastidious bacteria can be used for testing *Bacillus* spp. CLSI provides guidelines for broth microdilution testing (Table 3) (50). Agar dilution and Etest methods using MHA were compared in a study by Turnbull et al. (251). In both studies Etest MICs were similar to agar dilution MICs of several agents, including cefotaxime, ciprofloxacin, erythromycin, gentamicin, penicillin, tetracycline, and vancomycin. Two commercial β-lactamase tests, nitrocefin (Oxoid, Basingstoke, United Kingdom) and Intralactam strips (Mast Diagnostics, Bootle, United Kingdom), were evaluated in a study by Andrews and Wise (5); both tests failed to detect β-lactamase activity in four of five penicillin-resistant isolates of *B. cereus*. Therefore, β-lactamase testing is not recommended for predicting penicillin susceptibility in *Bacillus* spp.

CAMPYLOBACTER JEJUNI

Resistance to fluoroquinolones, agents commonly used for treating gastrointestinal infections caused by *C. jejuni* and *C. coli*, is being reported with increasing frequency in the United States with human and animal isolates of these two species. The National Antimicrobial Resistance Monitoring System noted no ciprofloxacin resistance among *C. jejuni* human isolates in 1990 but did note a resistance rate of 18% in 2001 and 22% in 2005. Interestingly, resistance decreased slightly in 2006, when 20% of 816 isolates were ciprofloxacin resistant. Only 1.7% of isolates were erythromycin resistant in 2006, and 46% were tetracycline resistant (38). Of 523 *C. jejuni* isolates from human fecal specimens of hospitalized patients in Tokyo obtained between 2003 and 2005, 20% were resistant to ciprofloxacin and all strains were susceptible to erythromycin. Sequencing of 37 randomly selected ciprofloxacin-resistant strains with distinct pulsed-field gel electrophoresis patterns revealed that quinolone resistance was attributable mainly to a mutation at codon 86 in the quinolone resistance-determining regions of *gyrA* (7). Following reanalysis of previously reported studies and analysis of nearly 11,000 new cases, Wassenaar et al. concluded that fluoroquinolone-resistant campylobacter infections are no more severe than fluoroquinolone-susceptible infections (264). Resistance among animal isolates, which may subsequently be transmitted to humans, has been associated with the addition of macrolides and fluoroquinolones to animal food as growth-promoting agents (72).

Because of the increasing incidence of resistance, testing of isolates from individual patients with severe illness or prolonged symptoms may be warranted or isolates might be tested for epidemiologic purposes. Susceptibility testing by broth microdilution in CAMHB-LHB and incubation in a microaerobic atmosphere (Table 3) are suggested by CLSI. Interpretive criteria for ciprofloxacin, erythromycin, doxycycline, and tetracycline are provided. CLSI also describes a disk diffusion method for ciprofloxacin and erythromycin wherein no zone indicates resistance. However, due to wide variations in measured zones that occur as a result of hazy or film-like growth, criteria for interpreting results other than resistant are not provided (50). Gaudreau et al. have suggested that ciprofloxacin, erythromycin, and tetracycline disk diffusion tests can be used to identify strains of *C. jejuni* and *C. coli* both resistant and susceptible to these three agents. However, for the ciprofloxacin results, a nalidixic acid disk must also be tested (88, 89). The Etest correlated well with agar dilution in a study by Baker when ciprofloxacin, erythromycin, and tetracycline were tested (8).

CORYNEBACTERIUM SPECIES

The many *Corynebacterium* spp. may exhibit a variety of susceptibility profiles. Most isolates of *C. amycolatum, C. jeikeium, C. resistens,* and *C. urealyticum* are multiresistant to antimicrobial agents that are often considered for therapy of gram-positive infections, including penicillins, cephalosporins, macrolides, aminoglycosides, fluoroquinolones, tetracyclines, and clindamycin. These species remain susceptible to teicoplanin and vancomycin. Considerable variation in activities of antimicrobial agents occurs with other species of *Corynebacterium*, and many strains may be highly susceptible (81, 85, 97, 149, 188, 197, 211, 229, 230, 267). Most isolates of *C. urealyticum* are resistant to fluoroquinolones, which has important implications for empiric therapy for urinary tract infections due to this species (80, 230). Significant antimicrobial resistance is rare for *C. diphtheriae* to include very few reports of nonsusceptibility to either penicillin or macrolides (73, 194). Using Etest to evaluate 47 isolates of *C. diphtheriae,* investigators in Brazil recently reported that the penicillin MICs ranged from 0.002 to 0.38 μg/ml, the penicillin MIC_{90} was 0.19 μg/ml, and the penicillin resistance rate was 14.8%. However, a penicillin breakpoint of ≤0.12 μg/ml was used to categorize isolates as penicillin susceptible rather than the breakpoint of ≤1 μg/ml for susceptibility that is currently recommended by CLSI (50, 194). Poor bactericidal activity of penicillins for *C. diphtheriae* has been reported. Von Hunolstein demonstrated penicillin tolerance among 17 of 24 *C. diphtheriae* isolates from patients with pharyngitis/tonsillitis (262). An "Eagle effect" whereby there is killing of bacteria at low concentrations but survival at high concentrations has been demonstrated with amoxicillin and two strains of nontoxigenic *Corynebacterium diphtheriae* isolated from patients with endocarditis. It was suggested that poor bactericidal activity of penicillins at high doses may contribute to poor outcomes when penicillins are included in the therapeutic regimen for *C. diphtheriae* endocarditis (101). In a large study of 410 isolates from around the world, 5 showed reduced susceptibility to macrolides and ketolides (73).

Growth characteristics among the *Corynebacterium* spp. may vary, and previous studies have used a variety of methods, media, and incubation conditions for antimicrobial susceptibility testing. Prior to the publication of CLSI M45, the absence of interpretive criteria specifically for *Corynebacterium* spp. led to inconsistencies in interpreting results when CLSI interpretive criteria for other gram-positive organisms (e.g., streptococci and staphylococci) were applied (73, 85, 267). This continues to be a problem if investigators are unaware of CLSI M45 (194). CLSI recommends broth microdilution with CAMHB-LHB and incubation in ambient air (Table 3). Some strains grow satisfactorily after 24 h of incubation, but others need 48 h. The 48 h is particularly important for detecting resistance to β-lactams, and it is recommended, if growth is not satisfactory or if an isolate appears susceptible to β-lactams at 24 h, that the test be reincubated and final results be read after 48 h of incubation (50). Currently, disk diffusion testing of *Corynebacterium* spp. is not recommended by CLSI. Testing and reporting recommendations in CLSI M45 are applicable to other coryneforms to include the genera *Arcanobacterium, Arthrobacter, Brevibacterium, Cellulomonas, Dermabacter, Leifsonia, Microbacterium, Oerskovia, Rothia,* and *Turicella* (50). Several investigators have used Etest satisfactorily for testing *Corynebacterium* spp. (81, 194, 279), and Engler et al. used Etest to confirm the reduced susceptibility to macrolides and ketolides that was initially identified by agar dilution testing of *C. diphtheriae* (73). Susceptibility testing of *Corynebacterium* spp. is warranted when the organisms are isolated from normally sterile sites.

ERYSIPELOTHRIX RHUSIOPATHIAE

Erysipelothrix rhusiopathiae is an intrinsically vancomycin-resistant gram-positive bacillus. Other agents that have little to no activity against isolates of this species are aminoglycosides and TMP-SMX. Antimicrobial susceptibility studies of isolates from a number of sources have shown all isolates of *E. rhusiopathiae* to be susceptible to penicillins, cephalosporins, carbapenems, and fluoroquinolones (82, 99, 191, 260, 273). Resistance to clindamycin, erythromycin, and tetracycline does occur. In one study of 66 isolates from swine in Japan, 6% were resistant to erythromycin and 71% were resistant to tetracycline (191). Tetracycline-resistant isolates were previously shown to be positive for *tet*M (274). Recently, four clinical isolates tested with daptomycin all had MICs of ≤0.125 (199).

Isolates of *E. rhusiopathiae* are fastidious, so CAMHB-LHB is recommended for broth microdilution MIC testing (50). There are also reports of agar dilution using either MHA supplemented with 5% horse blood or unsupplemented MHA (82, 191, 273).

HACEK GROUP

There are limited antimicrobial susceptibility test data on the HACEK organisms (i.e., *Aggregatibacter* [formerly the *aphrophilus* group of *Haemophilus* and *Actinobacillus*], *Cardiobacterium*, *Eikenella*, and *Kingella* spp.), in part because these organisms are infrequently encountered and often difficult to grow. Members of the HACEK group are susceptible to extended-spectrum cephalosporins and fluoroquinolones and are often susceptible in vitro to ampicillin and penicillin (6, 78, 145). Occasional isolates of *Cardiobacterium hominis*, *Eikenella corrodens*, and *Kingella* spp. produce β-lactamase (95, 151, 160, 227); however, β-lactamase production in *Aggregatibacter actinomycetemcomitans* has not been documented (161, 193). Using Etest, Kulik et al. noted that only 12% of 125 isolates from intraoral sites were susceptible to penicillin at MICs of ≤1 µg/ml; however, all were susceptible to amoxicillin-clavulanic acid and β-lactamase testing was not done (146). The American Heart Association recommendations for treatment of patients with endocarditis caused by HACEK organisms suggest that because of difficulties in performing antimicrobial susceptibility testing and potential failure to identify ampicillin-resistant strains, HACEK organisms should be considered ampicillin resistant and ampicillin should not be used for patients with endocarditis due to HACEK organisms (6).

Broth microdilution with CAMHB-LHB can be used for testing HACEK organisms. Some isolates may require 48 h of incubation to obtain adequate growth as evidenced by substantial turbidity in the positive growth control well. Some isolates may not grow satisfactorily in CAMHB-LHB. Susceptibility testing may be warranted for isolates from normally sterile sites, and β-lactamase testing should be performed on HACEK isolates (50).

HELICOBACTER PYLORI

Incidence of Resistance

H. pylori is intrinsically resistant to glycopeptides, polymyxins, nalidixic acid, trimethoprim, and sulfonamides. The rates of resistance for *H. pylori* vary considerably among the agents recommended for therapy with resistance to metronidazole being the highest, followed by macrolides, and resistance to amoxicillin and tetracyclines

being very low (91, 167, 169). Specific point mutations or other genetic events have been associated with resistance to all four drugs (169).

The *Helicobacter pylori* Antimicrobial Resistance Monitoring Program conducted by the Centers for Disease Control and Prevention reported 25% resistance to metronidazole, 13% resistance to clarithromycin, less than 1% resistance to amoxicillin, and no resistance to tetracycline among 347 isolates collected from throughout the United States from 1998 through 2002 (70). Using the CLSI reference method, Osato et al. reported approximately 35% resistance to metronidazole and 11% resistance to clarithromycin for 3,193 isolates in the United States (187). A large surveillance study in Japan examined changes in annual rates of resistance from October 2002 to September 2005 for 3,707 *H. pylori* isolates from previously untreated patients. The rate of clarithromycin resistance increased slightly for each of three 12-month periods with 27.7% resistance during the 2004 to 2005 time frame. Fewer than 4% of isolates had MICs of >8 µg/ml for metronidazole, and this low incidence of resistance may be related to the infrequent use of metronidazole in Japan. Applying breakpoints of ≤0.5 µg/ml, fewer than 1% of isolates were resistant to amoxicillin (143).

Kim et al. identified discordant susceptibility results for clarithromycin, metronidazole, and tetracycline when testing multiple isolates from different locations in the stomach of individual patients (135). A similar finding was reported by Osato et al. (186) for metronidazole susceptibility. These results suggest that resistant isolates are not evenly distributed throughout the stomach and susceptibility results for isolates from a single biopsy specimen may not be representative of the entire population.

Reference Test Method

CLSI describes an agar dilution MIC method for testing *H. pylori*. The test medium is MHA supplemented with aged (≥2-week-old) sheep blood. The inoculum is prepared from 72-h-old growth on a blood agar plate to obtain a final concentration of bacteria approximating 10^5 CFU/spot. Incubation is for 3 days at 35°C in a microaerobic atmosphere produced by a gas-generating system typically used for campylobacters. This atmosphere must be used for all drugs tested against *H. pylori* including metronidazole. *H. pylori* ATCC 43504 has been designated as a QC strain, and currently there are only interpretive criteria for clarithromycin. Other antimicrobial agents that have been studied and for which there are CLSI QC ranges include amoxicillin, metronidazole, telithromycin, and tetracycline (50). The European *Helicobacter pylori* Study Group has published an agar dilution method that is similar to the CLSI method; however, they recommend horse blood-supplemented MHA and a higher inoculum (93). Although there is no standard method for disk diffusion testing, Grignon et al. have demonstrated that this method is reliable for testing clarithromycin (103). Because point mutations in specific genes have been implicated in resistance, genotypic methods are also used, especially for clarithromycin (190).

Commercial Test Methods

Although no commercial methods are FDA cleared for antimicrobial susceptibility testing of *H. pylori*, several investigators have examined the Etest. In one study the percent agreement (i.e., results within ±1 doubling dilution) between Etest and agar dilution was 84.6% for amoxicillin,

94.1% for clarithromycin, 89.9% for metronidazole, and 89.1% for tetracycline (198). In a multilaboratory study, laboratories correctly identified clarithromycin- and metronidazole-susceptible and -resistant strains 93% of the time using Etest (15), and in another multilaboratory study there was >98% agreement between Etest and agar dilution for amoxicillin and clarithromycin. However, neither agar dilution nor Etest was reliable for testing metronidazole (93). Two other studies reported significant discrepancies for metronidazole susceptibility by agar dilution and Etest (168, 186). These Etest evaluations report differences in methods for agar dilution and Etest, such as media, inoculum, and incubation conditions, which may account for the different results. Recently, Burucoa et al. showed 100% concordance of clarithromycin Etest with real-time PCR for 37 susceptible and 24 resistant isolates of H. pylori that showed mutations in 23S rRNA genes conferring resistance to clarithromycin (30).

Strategies for Testing and Reporting of Results

Because of growth requirements and complex antimicrobial susceptibility testing recommendations, testing of H. pylori is not practical for the routine clinical laboratory. However, because of the significant resistance noted for metronidazole and clarithromycin, testing may be required in select situations, in which case a reliable reference laboratory should be used. Although there are currently no CLSI interpretive criteria for metronidazole, investigators have used a MIC of >8 μg/ml for resistance (169, 186).

LACTOBACILLUS, PEDIOCOCCUS, AND LEUCONOSTOC SPECIES

Pediococcus spp., *Leuconostoc* spp., and most *Lactobacillus* spp. are intrinsically vancomycin resistant. *Lactobacillus gasseri*, *L. delbrueckii*, and *L. acidophilus* may be vancomycin susceptible (33, 62, 139, 222).

Lactobacillus spp. generally have low piperacillin-tazobactam, imipenem, erythromycin, and clindamycin MICs, but their penicillin and cephalosporin MICs can vary (33, 62, 139, 222, 255). In a recent study of 85 blood isolates, MICs ranged from 0.06 μg/ml to 4 μg/ml for penicillin and from 0.25 to ≥256 μg/ml for ceftriaxone, with *L. casei* and *L. rhamnosus* being among the species with the least susceptibility to these agents (222). Fluoroquinolones have poor activity against most *Lactobacillus* spp. (33, 62, 222, 255).

Leuconostoc spp. are usually susceptible to clindamycin and erythromycin, and penicillin MICs are generally less than 0.5 μg/ml (234, 235, 255). Ceftriaxone MICs have been shown to vary from 1 to >128 μg/ml, and elevated imipenem MICs (>0.5 μg/ml) have been described (234, 235, 255). There is one report of an imipenem therapeutic failure for a central nervous system infection due to *Leuconostoc* with an imipenem MIC of 4 μg/ml (64).

Pediococcus spp. are generally susceptible to clindamycin and erythromycin (59, 139, 235, 255) but can be resistant to both of these (235). A penicillin MIC$_{90}$ of 0.5 μg/ml was recently reported for 49 isolates (139), and penicillin MICs as high as 2 μg/ml have been noted (235). MICs for ceftriaxone are generally ≥16 μg/ml; however, most isolates are very susceptible to imipenem (MICs, <0.25 μg/ml) (235, 255). *Pediococcus* spp. are resistant to ciprofloxacin (59, 235, 255).

Gentamicin, which would only be used in combination therapy, has variable activity against isolates of all three genera (59, 139, 235, 255).

The medium recommended by CLSI for broth microdilution testing of *Lactobacillus* spp., *Pediococcus* spp., and *Leuconostoc* spp. is CAMHB-LHB (Table 3) (50). For *Lactobacillus* spp., incubation of broth microdilution panels in 5% CO$_2$ may be necessary to achieve sufficient growth. Some have performed susceptibility testing by agar dilution using either unsupplemented MHA or MHA with 5% sheep blood (255). If testing by agar dilution, incubation in 5% CO$_2$ may also be necessary to achieve sufficient growth.

LISTERIA MONOCYTOGENES

Clinical isolates of *L. monocytogenes* remain susceptible to the drugs of choice including ampicillin (or penicillin) and TMP-SMX. With the exception of occasional resistance to tetracyclines (254), *L. monocytogenes* is typically susceptible in vitro to other agents active against gram-positive bacteria, including chloramphenicol, vancomycin, and macrolides (106, 164, 166, 219). During screening of 488 human isolates in France, 5 isolates were ciprofloxacin resistant, and this resistance was attributed to active efflux (94). Although *L. monocytogenes* may appear susceptible to cephalosporins in vitro, these agents are not effective clinically.

Listeria infections are generally treated empirically, and antimicrobial susceptibility testing is usually not necessary. Only criteria for susceptibility (MIC, ≤2.0 μg/ml) are listed for ampicillin and penicillin in CLSI guidelines because clinical isolates of *L. monocytogenes* have not been noted to have results other than those indicating susceptibility (50). *L. monocytogenes* is not truly fastidious, and testing in Mueller-Hinton broth without the blood supplement has been done satisfactorily (166). However, CLSI recommends using CAMHB-LHB. It is important to remember that cephalosporins should not be tested or reported for *L. monocytogenes* because some isolates may, for example, have ceftriaxone MICs as low as 8 μg/ml, which could suggest false susceptibility (61). This cautionary measure is emphasized in CLSI documents (50) and illustrates why it is inappropriate to indiscriminately report susceptibility results for any agent without knowing if it would be a reasonable therapeutic option. Because cephalosporins are frequently used empirically for the treatment of meningitis, the laboratory should quickly communicate smear or culture findings suspicious for *Listeria* whenever they occur.

MORAXELLA CATARRHALIS

M. catarrhalis organisms have maintained a high degree of susceptibility to all antimicrobial agents that might be used to treat infections caused by them with the exception of penicillinase-susceptible penicillins. More than 90% of *M. catarrhalis* isolates produce β-lactamase and are resistant to amoxicillin, ampicillin, and penicillin (100, 119, 175, 182, 221). These isolates remain susceptible to amoxicillin-clavulanic acid, which is often prescribed for *M. catarrhalis* infections.

Most clinical isolates produce one of two types of chromosomally mediated β-lactamases: BRO-1 or BRO-2 (14, 63, 76, 132, 210). BRO-1-producing strains are up to 10-fold more prevalent than BRO-2-producing strains, and ampicillin and penicillin MICs for BRO-1 are often higher (e.g., ≥4.0 μg/ml) than those for BRO-2 strains (e.g., ≤0.5 μg/ml) (14, 63, 76, 132, 210). Because of the low MICs for the latter strains, their clinical significance in response to β-lactamase-labile penicillins is questionable. Resistance rates for TMP-SMX are less than 2% in most studies (14, 76, 221); however, Johnson et al. reported over 10% resistance in isolates from Latin America (121).

Only the chromogenic cephalosporin method has reliably detected the β-lactamases produced by M. catarrhalis (68). Routine β-lactamase testing may not be necessary because of the high incidence of β-lactamase-positive strains. Nevertheless, some advocate reporting of β-lactamase results to highlight the fact that this pathogen is generally unresponsive to some agents (e.g., amoxicillin) commonly prescribed for the treatment of respiratory tract infections. MIC testing without β-lactamase testing can be problematic as there is some overlap in ampicillin and amoxicillin MICs in β-lactamase-positive and -negative strains (210). Since M. catarrhalis typically responds to the drugs of choice, testing beyond the β-lactamase test is rarely indicated (50). CLSI document M45 addresses MIC testing of M. catarrhalis, and the recommended test medium is CAMHB. More recently, criteria for disk diffusion testing of amoxicillin-clavulanic acid, azithromycin, clarithromycin, erythromycin, tetracycline, and TMP-SMX using MHA and incubation in 5% CO_2 have been added to CLSI document M45 (Table 3). These were adopted following studies performed by Bell et al. that demonstrated a high correlation with results obtained by MIC testing (14).

PASTEURELLA SPECIES

Human isolates of Pasteurella spp. are generally susceptible to penicillin with MICs of ≤0.5 μg/ml (49, 96, 156, 177); however, β-lactamase production in an isolate from a respiratory tract infection has been documented. A single report of a β-lactamase-producing isolate demonstrated a positive reaction with a nitrocefin-impregnated disk test, an amoxicillin MIC of 8 μg/ml, and an amoxicillin-clavulanic acid MIC of 0.25 μg/ml (157). Pasteurella spp. are generally very susceptible to many other antimicrobial agents, and no resistance has been documented for parenteral cephalosporins, fluoroquinolones, tetracyclines, chloramphenicol, or TMP-SMX (49, 96, 156, 177). Resistance to erythromycin can occur, and there is at least one report of failure of erythromycin to cure a cat bite victim who went on to develop meningitis (152).

Broth microdilution and disk diffusion methods are described by CLSI for testing Pasteurella spp. (Table 3). Due to the absence of nonsusceptible strains, there are only susceptible interpretive criteria for agents that might be tested, with the exception of erythromycin. Susceptibility testing may be warranted for isolates from normally sterile sites, and β-lactamase testing should be done on these isolates as well as those from respiratory sources (50). Testing of isolates from bite wounds is not necessary since bite wound infections are generally treated empirically with agents (e.g., amoxicillin-clavulanic acid) that would cover a variety of organisms likely to be implicated in the infection.

VIBRIO SPECIES

Both V. cholerae and the noncholera Vibrio spp. are often susceptible to most antimicrobial agents, including newer cephalosporins, aminoglycosides, fluoroquinolones, and tetracyclines; however, as with other organisms, resistance to one or more of these can occur (43, 47, 60, 162, 184, 189, 239).

In parts of the developing world, rates of resistance among V. cholerae are quite variable for fluoroquinolones, tetracyclines, and trimethoprim-sulfamethoxazole, drugs commonly prescribed when therapy is needed. A chromosomally integrated transferable resistance element, SXT, which encodes resistance to trimethoprim, sulfamethoxazole, and streptomycin, has been observed among V. cholerae strains from multiple cholera outbreaks (115, 184). Strains resistant to these agents and also tetracycline and erythromycin have been described (115). Das et al. recently reported that all 670 V. cholerae isolates collected from patients presenting to an East Delhi hospital between 2001 and 2006 were resistant to ampicillin and resistance to trimethoprim-sulfamethoxazole increased from 70% in 2001 to 100% in 2006. There were no isolates resistant to ciprofloxacin in 2001, and 30% were resistant in 2006. None of the 670 isolates were resistant to cefotaxime, gentamicin, or tetracycline (60). When a double-blind randomized study was conducted to compare the equivalence of azithromycin and ciprofloxacin, 78% of 97 patients had a bacteriologic cure with azithromycin compared with only 10% of 98 patients who received ciprofloxacin. The 168 strains isolated from these patients were susceptible to both azithromycin and ciprofloxacin when tested by disk diffusion and Etest. The median ciprofloxacin MIC for 91 V. cholerae serogroup O1 isolates was 0.25 μg/ml, which the authors stated was 11 to 83 times as high as those reported in previous studies (220). The elevated MICs and poor outcomes suggest the possibility of a resistance mechanism not detectable when a MIC of ≤1 μg/ml is used to define ciprofloxacin susceptibility.

In a recent environmental study of 151 isolates of V. vulnificus, over 90% were susceptible to ampicillin or tetracycline and no resistance was noted for ciprofloxacin. This study also examined 10 clinical isolates from patients with V. vulnificus-associated septicemia and noted considerable resistance to drugs that might be prescribed for treating septicemia including aminoglycosides (10). An earlier study reported that all 42 clinical isolates of V. vulnificus were ampicillin susceptible (47). Chuang et al. demonstrated synergistic killing of V. vulnificus with a combination of minocycline and cefotaxime, and this finding has contributed to current recommendations for treating V. vulnificus infections with doxycycline and ceftazidime (47). Kim et al. showed that cefotaxime with ciprofloxacin demonstrated synergism against V. vulnificus (134).

Antimicrobial therapy is not required to manage cholera, but such therapy may shorten the duration and reduce the severity of disease. Similarly, although the noncholera Vibrio spp. cause diarrheal disease, otherwise healthy individuals with diarrhea due to these bacteria usually recover spontaneously without treatment. When Vibrio spp. are isolated from sources associated with serious infections, antimicrobial susceptibility testing of them is warranted (43, 162). CLSI suggests use of broth microdilution or disk diffusion using methodology similar to that for testing Enterobacteriaceae. Recently, a MIC test for detecting azithromycin resistance in Vibrio spp. was added to the CLSI guidelines, and a MIC of ≤2 μg/ml is considered susceptible; no criteria for interpreting resistance is described. For testing of the halophilic Vibrio spp., some have suggested use of MHA containing 1% NaCl. However, CLSI recommends preparation of the inoculum suspension in 0.85% NaCl solution for disk diffusion and broth microdilution MIC testing with MHA or CAMHB (both without NaCl supplementation), respectively (50).

CONCLUSION

With the exceptions of serious streptococcal infections (including those caused by *S. pneumoniae*), extraintestinal *Aeromonas* or *Vibrio* infections, and device-associated coryneform infections, infections caused by many of the fastidious bacteria discussed in this chapter are treated empirically, as these bacteria are often susceptible to the drugs of choice. Consequently, susceptibility testing is infrequently needed for many of these organisms. In certain circumstances testing may be warranted, such as when there appears to be clinical failure, patient intolerance to the drug(s) of choice, or serious infections for which there are limited appropriate drugs that might be prescribed. Additionally, susceptibility testing may aid in species identification (e.g., differentiating *C. jeikeium* from other *Corynebacterium* species). If a physician seems unsure about requesting antimicrobial susceptibility testing on a fastidious organism, he/she should be encouraged to seek assistance from an infectious diseases clinician or pharmacist.

The Etest has been examined for testing a variety of fastidious bacteria. For the less common species, many of the data generated have been obtained from comparisons with nonstandardized in vitro test methods with limited examination of the clinical correlation of the results. Consequently, the results for Etest on many of the organisms addressed in this chapter should be interpreted with caution in the clinical setting. Requests for susceptibility testing of fastidious bacteria are often for isolates associated with serious infections, and MIC results are likely to be more useful than qualitative results. The disk diffusion test should be used only for bacteria for which there are CLSI interpretive criteria. It is important for laboratory workers to maintain an awareness of the methods available for testing fastidious bacteria and their strengths and limitations. If testing must be performed, it should be done by a laboratory familiar with these methods and their limitations.

REFERENCES

1. **Abadi, F. J., D. E. Yakubu, and T. H. Pennington.** 1995. Antimicrobial susceptibility of penicillin-sensitive and penicillin-resistant meningococci. *J. Antimicrob. Chemother.* **35:**687–690.
2. **Adam, H. J., D. J. Hoban, A. S. Gin, and G. G. Zhanel.** 2009. Association between fluoroquinolone usage and a dramatic rise in ciprofloxacin-resistant *Streptococcus pneumoniae* in Canada, 1997–2006. *Int. J. Antimicrob. Agents* **34:**82–85.
3. **Ahmed, R., T. Hassall, B. Morland, and J. Gray.** 2003. Viridans streptococcus bacteremia in children on chemotherapy for cancer: an underestimated problem. *Pediatr. Hematol. Oncol.* **20:**439–444.
4. **Alcala, B., C. Salcedo, L. de la Fuente, L. Arreaza, M. J. Uria, R. Abad, R. Enriquez, J. A. Vazquez, M. Motge, and J. de Batlle.** 2004. *Neisseria meningitidis* showing decreased susceptibility to ciprofloxacin: first report in Spain. *J. Antimicrob. Chemother.* **53:**409.
5. **Andrews, J. M., and R. Wise.** 2002. Susceptibility testing of *Bacillus* species. *J. Antimicrob. Chemother.* **49:**1040–1042.
6. **Baddour, L. M., W. R. Wilson, A. S. Bayer, V. G. Fowler, Jr., A. F. Bolger, M. E. Levison, P. Ferrieri, M. A. Gerber, L. Y. Tani, M. H. Gewitz, D. C. Tong, J. M. Steckelberg, R. S. Baltimore, S. T. Shulman, J. C. Burns, D. A. Falace, J. W. Newburger, T. J. Pallasch, M. Takahashi, and K. A. Taubert.** 2005. Infective endocarditis: diagnosis, antimicrobial therapy, and management of complications: a statement for healthcare professionals from the Committee on Rheumatic Fever, Endocarditis, and Kawasaki Disease, Council on Cardiovascular Disease in the Young, and the Councils on Clinical Cardiology, Stroke, and Cardiovascular Surgery and anesthesia, American Heart Association: endorsed by the Infectious Diseases Society of America. *Circulation* **111:**e394–e434.
7. **Bakeli, G., K. Sato, W. Kumita, R. Saito, E. Ono, T. Chida, and N. Okamura.** 2008. Antimicrobial susceptibility and mechanism of quinolone resistance in *Campylobacter jejuni* strains isolated from diarrheal patients in a hospital in Tokyo. *J. Infect. Chemother.* **14:**342–348.
8. **Baker, C. N.** 1992. The E-Test and *Campylobacter jejuni.* *Diagn. Microbiol. Infect. Dis.* **15:**469–472.
9. **Baker, C. N., D. G. Hollis, and C. Thornsberry.** 1985. Antimicrobial susceptibility testing of *Francisella tularensis* with a modified Mueller-Hinton broth. *J. Clin. Microbiol.* **22:**212–215.
10. **Baker-Austin, C., J. V. McArthur, A. H. Lindell, M. S. Wright, R. C. Tuckfield, J. Gooch, L. Warner, J. Oliver, and R. Stepanauskas.** 2009. Multi-site analysis reveals widespread antibiotic resistance in the marine pathogen *Vibrio vulnificus.* *Microb. Ecol.* **57:**151–159.
11. **Baykam, N., H. Esener, O. Ergonul, S. Eren, A. K. Celikbas, and B. Dokuzoguz.** 2004. In vitro antimicrobial susceptibility of *Brucella* species. *Int. J. Antimicrob. Agents* **23:**405–407.
12. **Beekmann, S. E., D. J. Diekema, K. P. Heilmann, S. S. Richter, and G. V. Doern.** 2006. Macrolide use identified as risk factor for macrolide-resistant *Streptococcus pneumoniae* in a 17-center case-control study. *Eur. J. Clin. Microbiol. Infect. Dis.* **25:**335–339.
13. **Beekmann, S. E., K. P. Heilmann, S. S. Richter, J. Garcia-de-Lomas, and G. V. Doern.** 2005. Antimicrobial resistance in *Streptococcus pneumoniae*, *Haemophilus influenzae*, *Moraxella catarrhalis* and group A beta-haemolytic streptococci in 2002–2003. Results of the multinational GRASP Surveillance Program. *Int. J. Antimicrob. Agents.* **25:**148–156.
14. **Bell, J. M., J. D. Turnidge, and R. N. Jones.** 2009. Development of a disk diffusion method for testing *Moraxella catarrhalis* susceptibility using Clinical and Laboratory Standards Institute methods: a SENTRY Antimicrobial Surveillance Program report. *J. Clin. Microbiol.* **47:**2187–2193.
15. **Best, L. M., D. J. Haldane, M. Keelan, D. E. Taylor, A. B. Thomson, V. Loo, C. A. Fallone, P. Lyn, F. M. Smaill, R. Hunt, C. Gaudreau, J. Kennedy, M. Alfa, R. Pelletier, and S. J. Veldhuyzen Van Zanten.** 2003. Multilaboratory comparison of proficiencies in susceptibility testing of *Helicobacter pylori* and correlation between agar dilution and Etest methods. *Antimicrob. Agents Chemother.* **47:**3138–3144.
16. **Betriu, C., M. Gomez, A. Sanchez, A. Cruceyra, J. Romero, and J. J. Picazo.** 1994. Antibiotic resistance and penicillin tolerance in clinical isolates of group B streptococci. *Antimicrob. Agents Chemother.* **38:**2183–2186.
17. **Biedenbach, D. J., J. M. Bell, H. S. Sader, J. D. Turnidge, and R. N. Jones.** 2009. Activities of dalbavancin against a worldwide collection of 81,673 gram-positive bacterial isolates. *Antimicrob. Agents Chemother.* **53:**1260–1263.
18. **Biedenbach, D. J., and R. N. Jones.** 1996. Comparative assessment of Etest for testing susceptibilities of *Neisseria gonorrhoeae* to penicillin, tetracycline, ceftriaxone, cefotaxime, and ciprofloxacin: investigation using 510(k) review criteria, recommended by the Food and Drug Administration. *J. Clin. Microbiol.* **34:**3214–3217.
19. **Billal, D. S., M. Hotomi, and N. Yamanaka.** 2007. Can the Etest correctly determine the MICs of beta-lactam and cephalosporin antibiotics for beta-lactamase-negative ampicillin-resistant *Haemophilus influenzae*? *Antimicrob. Agents Chemother.* **51:**3463–3464.
20. **Blasi, F., D. J. Farrell, and L. Dubreuil.** 2009. Antibacterial activity of telithromycin and comparators against pathogens isolated from patients with community-acquired respiratory tract infections: the Prospective Resistant Organism Tracking and Epidemiology for the Ketolide Telithromycin study year 5 (2003–2004). *Diagn. Microbiol. Infect. Dis.* **63:**302–308.
21. **Block, C., Y. Davidson, and N. Keller.** 1998. Unreliability of disk diffusion test for screening for reduced penicillin susceptibility in *Neisseria meningitidis.* *J. Clin. Microbiol.* **36:**3103–3104.
22. **Botha, P.** 1988. Penicillin-resistant *Neisseria meningitidis* in southern Africa. *Lancet* **i:**54.

23. **Bouchillon, S. K., J. L. Johnson, D. J. Hoban, T. M. Stevens, and B. M. Johnson.** 2005. Impact of carbon dioxide on the susceptibility of key respiratory tract pathogens to telithromycin and azithromycin. *J. Antimicrob. Chemother.* **56:**224–227.

24. **Bouvet, A., A. C. Cremieux, A. Contrepois, J. M. Vallois, C. Lamesch, and C. Carbon.** 1985. Comparison of penicillin and vancomycin, individually and in combination with gentamicin and amikacin, in the treatment of experimental endocarditis induced by nutritionally variant streptococci. *Antimicrob. Agents Chemother.* **28:**607–611.

25. **Bradley, J. S., and J. D. Connor.** 1991. Ceftriaxone failure in meningitis caused by *Streptococcus pneumoniae* with reduced susceptibility to beta-lactam antibiotics. *Pediatr. Infect. Dis. J.* **10:**871–873.

26. **Brigante, G. R., F. A. Luzzaro, B. Pini, G. Lombardi, G. Sokeng, and A. Q. Toniolo.** 2007. Drug susceptibility testing of clinical isolates of streptococci and enterococci by the Phoenix automated microbiology system. *BMC Microbiol.* **7:**46.

27. **Brown, D. F. J., R. Hope, D. M. Livermore, G. Brick, K. Broughton, R. C. George, R. Reynolds, and the BSAC Working Parties on Resistance Surveillance.** 2008. Nonsusceptibility trends among enterococci and non-pneumococcal streptococci from bacteraemias in the UK and Ireland, 2001–06. *J. Antimicrob. Chemother.* **62:**ii75–ii85.

28. **Brown, S. D., D. J. Farrell, and I. Morrissey.** 2004. Prevalence and molecular analysis of macrolide and fluoroquinolone resistance among isolates of *Streptococcus pneumoniae* collected during the 2000–2001 PROTEKT US Study. *J. Clin. Microbiol.* **42:**4980–4987.

29. **Bruckner, L., and F. Gigliotti.** 2006. Viridans group streptococcal infections among children with cancer and the importance of emerging antibiotic resistance. *Semin. Pediatr. Infect. Dis.* **17:**153–160.

30. **Burucoa, C., M. Garnier, C. Silvain, and J. L. Fauchere.** 2008. Quadruplex real-time PCR assay using allele-specific scorpion primers for detection of mutations conferring clarithromycin resistance to *Helicobacter pylori*. *J. Clin. Microbiol.* **46:**2320–2326.

31. **Buu-Hoi, A., C. Le Bouguenec, and T. Horaud.** 1990. High-level chromosomal gentamicin resistance in *Streptococcus agalactiae* (group B). *Antimicrob. Agents Chemother.* **34:**985–988.

32. **Campos, J., G. Trujillo, T. Seuba, and A. Rodriguez.** 1992. Discriminative criteria for *Neisseria meningitidis* isolates that are moderately susceptible to penicillin and ampicillin. *Antimicrob. Agents Chemother.* **36:**1028–1031.

33. **Cannon, J. P., T. A. Lee, J. T. Bolanos, and L. H. Danziger.** 2005. Pathogenic relevance of *Lactobacillus*: a retrospective review of over 200 cases. *Eur. J. Clin. Microbiol. Infect. Dis.* **24:**31–40.

34. **Castanheira, M., A. C. Gales, A. C. Pignatari, R. N. Jones, and H. S. Sader.** 2006. Changing antimicrobial susceptibility patterns among *Streptococcus pneumoniae* and *Haemophilus influenzae* from Brazil: report from the SENTRY Antimicrobial Surveillance Program (1998–2004). *Microb. Drug Resist.* **12:**91–98.

35. **Castanheira, M., R. N. Jones, and D. M. Livermore.** 2009. Antimicrobial activities of doripenem and other carbapenems against *Pseudomonas aeruginosa*, other nonfermentative bacilli, and *Aeromonas* spp. *Diagn. Microbiol. Infect. Dis.* **63:**426–433.

36. **Cavallo, J.-D., F. Ramisse, M. Girardet, J. Vaissaire, M. Mock, and E. Hernandez.** 2002. Antibiotic susceptibilities of 96 isolates of *Bacillus anthracis* isolated in France between 1994 and 2000. *Antimicrob. Agents Chemother.* **46:**2307–2309.

37. **Centers for Disease Control and Prevention.** 2008. Effects of new penicillin susceptibility breakpoints for *Streptococcus pneumoniae*—United States, 2006–2007. *MMWR Morb. Mortal. Wkly. Rep.* **57:**1353–1355.

38. **Centers for Disease Control and Prevention.** 2009. *National Antimicrobial Resistance Monitoring System for Enteric Bacteria (NARMS): Human Isolates Final Report, 2006.* U.S. Department of Health and Human Services, Centers for Disease Control and Prevention, Atlanta, GA.

39. **Centers for Disease Control and Prevention.** 2009. *Sexually Transmitted Disease Surveillance 2007 Supplement, Gonococcal Isolate Surveillance Project (GISP) Annual Report—2007.* U.S. Department of Health and Human Services, Centers for Disease Control and Prevention, Atlanta, GA.

40. **Centers for Disease Control and Prevention.** 2007. Update to CDC's sexually transmitted diseases treatment guidelines, 2006: fluoroquinolones no longer recommended for treatment of gonococcal infections. *MMWR Morb. Mortal. Wkly. Rep.* **56:**332–336.

41. **Centers for Disease Control and Prevention.** 2001. Update: interim recommendations for antimicrobial prophylaxis for children and breastfeeding mothers and treatment of children with anthrax. *MMWR Morb. Mortal. Wkly. Rep.* **50:**1014–1016.

42. **Chen, Y., J. Succi, F. C. Tenover, and T. M. Koehler.** 2003. Beta-lactamase genes of the penicillin-susceptible *Bacillus anthracis* Sterne strain. *J. Bacteriol.* **185:**823–830.

43. **Chiang, S. R., and Y. C. Chuang.** 2003. *Vibrio vulnificus* infection: clinical manifestations, pathogenesis, and antimicrobial therapy. *J. Microbiol. Immunol. Infect.* **36:**81–88.

44. **Choe, C. H., S. S. Bouhaouala, I. Brook, T. B. Elliot, and G. B. Knudson.** 2000. In vitro development of resistance to ofloxacin and doxycycline in *Bacillus anthracis* Sterne. *Antimicrob. Agents Chemother.* **44:**1766.

45. **Chosewood, L. C., and D. E. Wilson (ed.).** 2007. *Biosafety in Microbiological and Biomedical Laboratories,* 5th ed. U.S. Government Printing Office, Washington, DC.

46. **Chu, Y. W., T. K. Cheung, V. Tung, F. Tiu, J. Lo, R. Lam, R. Lai, and K. K. Wong.** 2007. A blood isolate of *Neisseria meningitidis* showing reduced susceptibility to quinolones in Hong Kong. *Int. J. Antimicrob. Agents* **30:**94–95.

47. **Chuang, Y. C., J. W. Liu, W. C. Ko, K. Y. Lin, J. J. Wu, and K. Y. Huang.** 1997. In vitro synergism between cefotaxime and minocycline against *Vibrio vulnificus*. *Antimicrob. Agents Chemother.* **41:**2214–2217.

48. **Citron, D. M., and M. D. Appleman.** 2006. In vitro activities of daptomycin, ciprofloxacin, and other antimicrobial agents against the cells and spores of clinical isolates of *Bacillus* species. *J. Clin. Microbiol.* **44:**3814–3818.

49. **Citron, D. M., Y. A. Warren, H. T. Fernandez, M. A. Goldstein, K. L. Tyrrell, and E. J. Goldstein.** 2005. Broth microdilution and disk diffusion tests for susceptibility testing of *Pasteurella* species isolated from human clinical specimens. *J. Clin. Microbiol.* **43:**2485–2488.

50. **Clinical and Laboratory Standards Institute.** 2010. *Methods for Antimicrobial Dilution and Disk Susceptibility Testing of Infrequently Isolated or Fastidious Bacteria.* Approved guideline M45-A2. CLSI, Wayne, PA.

51. **Clinical and Laboratory Standards Institute.** 2009. *Methods for Dilution Antimicrobial Susceptibility Tests for Bacteria That Grow Aerobically,* 8th ed. Approved standard M07-A8. CLSI, Wayne, PA.

52. **Clinical and Laboratory Standards Institute.** 2009. *Performance Standards for Antimicrobial Disk Susceptibility Tests,* 10th ed. Approved standard M02-A10. CLSI, Wayne, PA.

53. **Clinical and Laboratory Standards Institute.** 2008. *Performance Standards for Antimicrobial Susceptibility Testing.* Eighteenth Informational Supplement. M100-S18. CLSI, Wayne, PA.

54. **Clinical and Laboratory Standards Institute.** 2010. *Performance Standards for Antimicrobial Susceptibility Testing.* Twentieth Informational Supplement. M100-S20. CLSI, Wayne, PA.

55. **Corso, A., D. Faccone, M. Miranda, M. Rodriguez, M. Regueira, C. Carranza, C. Vencina, J. A. Vazquez, and M. Galas.** 2005. Emergence of *Neisseria meningitidis* with decreased susceptibility to ciprofloxacin in Argentina. *J. Antimicrob. Chemother.* **55:**596–597.

56. **Critchley, I. A., S. D. Brown, M. M. Traczewski, G. S. Tillotson, and N. Janjic.** 2007. National and regional assessment of antimicrobial resistance among community-acquired respiratory tract pathogens identified in a 2005–2006 U.S. faropenem surveillance study. *Antimicrob. Agents Chemother.* **51:**4382–4389.

57. **Dagan, R.** 2009. Impact of pneumococcal conjugate vaccine on infections caused by antibiotic-resistant *Streptococcus pneumoniae*. *Clin. Microbiol. Infect.* **15**(Suppl. 3):16–20.

58. **Dagan, R., and K. P. Klugman.** 2008. Impact of conjugate pneumococcal vaccines on antibiotic resistance. *Lancet Infect. Dis.* **8**:785–795.

59. **Danielsen, M., P. J. Simpson, E. B. O'Connor, R. P. Ross, and C. Stanton.** 2007. Susceptibility of *Pediococcus* spp. to antimicrobial agents. *J. Appl. Microbiol.* **102**:384–389.

60. **Das, S., R. Saha, and I. R. Kaur.** 2008. Trend of antibiotic resistance of Vibrio cholerae strains from East Delhi. *Indian J. Med. Res.* **127**:478–482.

61. **Davis, J. A., and C. R. Jackson.** 2009. Comparative antimicrobial susceptibility of *Listeria monocytogenes, L. innocua,* and *L. welshimeri. Microb. Drug Resist.* **15**:27–32.

62. **Delgado, S., A. B. Florez, and B. Mayo.** 2005. Antibiotic susceptibility of *Lactobacillus* and *Bifidobacterium* species from the human gastrointestinal tract. *Curr. Microbiol.* **50**:202–207.

63. **Deshpande, L. M., H. S. Sader, T. R. Fritsche, and R. N. Jones.** 2006. Contemporary prevalence of BRO beta-lactamases in *Moraxella catarrhalis*: report from the SENTRY Antimicrobial Surveillance Program (North America, 1997 to 2004). *J. Clin. Microbiol.* **44**:3775–3777.

64. **Deye, G., J. Lewis, J. Patterson, and J. Jorgensen.** 2003. A case of *Leuconostoc* ventriculitis with resistance to carbapenem antibiotics. *Clin. Infect. Dis.* **37**:869–870.

65. **Dillon, J.-A. R., and K. H. Yeung.** 1989. β-Lactamase plasmids and chromosomally mediated antibiotic resistance in pathogenic *Neisseria* species. *Clin. Microbiol. Rev.* **2**(Suppl.):S125–S133.

66. **Doern, G. V., A. Brueggemann, and G. Pierce.** 1997. Assessment of the oxacillin disk screening test for determining penicillin resistance in *Streptococcus pneumoniae. Eur. J. Clin. Microbiol. Infect. Dis.* **16**:311–314.

67. **Doern, G. V., K. P. Heilmann, H. K. Huynh, P. R. Rhomberg, S. L. Coffman, and A. B. Brueggemann.** 2001. Antimicrobial resistance among clinical isolates of *Streptococcus pneumoniae* in the United States during 1999–2000, including a comparison of resistance rates since 1994–1995. *Antimicrob. Agents Chemother.* **45**:1721–1729.

68. **Doern, G. V., and T. A. Tubert.** 1987. Detection of β-lactamase activity among clinical isolates of *Branhamella catarrhalis* with six different β-lactamase assays. *J. Clin. Microbiol.* **25**:1380–1383.

69. **Doganay, M., and N. Aydin.** 1991. Antimicrobial susceptibility of *Bacillus anthracis. Scand. J. Infect. Dis.* **23**:333–335.

70. **Duck, W. M., J. Sobel, J. M. Pruckler, Q. Song, D. Swerdlow, C. Friedman, A. Sulka, B. Swaminathan, T. Taylor, M. Hoekstra, P. Griffin, D. Smoot, R. Peek, D. C. Metz, P. B. Bloom, S. Goldschmidt, J. Parsonnet, G. Triadafilopoulos, G. I. Perez-Perez, N. Vakil, P. Ernst, S. Czinn, D. Dunne, and B. D. Gold.** 2004. Antimicrobial resistance incidence and risk factors among *Helicobacter pylori*-infected persons, United States. *Emerg. Infect. Dis.* **10**:1088–1094.

71. **du Plessis, M., A. von Gottberg, C. Cohen, L. de Gouveia, and K. P. Klugman.** 2008. *Neisseria meningitidis* intermediately resistant to penicillin and causing invasive disease in South Africa in 2001 to 2005. *J. Clin. Microbiol.* **46**:3208–3214.

72. **Engberg, J., F. M. Aarestrup, D. E. Taylor, P. Gerner-Smidt, and I. Nachamkin.** 2001. Quinolone and macrolide resistance in *Campylobacter jejuni* and *C. coli*: resistance mechanisms and trends in human isolates. *Emerg. Infect. Dis.* **7**:24–34.

73. **Engler, K. H., M. Warner, and R. C. George.** 2001. In vitro activity of ketolides HMR 3004 and HMR 3647 and seven other antimicrobial agents against *Corynebacterium diphtheriae. J. Antimicrob. Chemother.* **47**:27–31.

74. **Enriquez, R., R. Abad, C. Salcedo, S. Perez, and J. A. Vazquez.** 2008. Fluoroquinolone resistance in *Neisseria meningitidis* in Spain. *J. Antimicrob. Chemother.* **61**:286–290.

75. **Enriquez, R., R. Abad, C. Salcedo, and J. A. Vazquez.** 2009. Nalidixic acid disk for laboratory detection of ciprofloxacin resistance in *Neisseria meningitidis. Antimicrob. Agents Chemother.* **53**:796–797.

76. **Esel, D., Y. Ay-Altintop, G. Yagmur, S. Gokahmetoglu, and B. Sumerkan.** 2007. Evaluation of susceptibility patterns and BRO beta-lactamase types among clinical isolates of *Moraxella catarrhalis. Clin. Microbiol. Infect.* **13**:1023–1025.

77. **Farrell, D. J., K. P. Klugman, and M. Pichichero.** 2007. Increased antimicrobial resistance among nonvaccine serotypes of *Streptococcus pneumoniae* in the pediatric population after the introduction of 7-valent pneumococcal vaccine in the United States. *Pediatr. Infect. Dis. J.* **26**:123–128.

78. **Feder, H. M., Jr., J. C. Roberts, J. C. Salazar, H. B. Leopold, and O. Toro-Salazar.** 2003. HACEK endocarditis in infants and children: two cases and a literature review. *Pediatr. Infect. Dis. J.* **22**:557–562.

79. **Felmingham, D.** 2004. Comparative antimicrobial susceptibility of respiratory tract pathogens. *Chemotherapy* **50**(Suppl. 1):3–10.

80. **Fernández-Natal, I., J. Guerra, M. Alcoba, F. Cachón, and F. Soriano.** 2001. Bacteremia caused by multiply resistant *Corynebacterium urealyticum*: six case reports and review. *Eur. J. Clin. Microbiol. Infect. Dis.* **20**:514–517.

81. **Fernandez-Roblas, R., H. Adames, N. Z. Martín-de-Hijas, D. G. Almeida, I. Gadea, and J. Esteban.** 2009. In vitro activity of tigecycline and 10 other antimicrobials against clinical isolates of the genus *Corynebacterium. Int. J. Antimicrob. Agents* **33**:453–455.

82. **Fidalgo, S. G., C. J. Longbottom, and T. V. Rjley.** 2002. Susceptibility of *Erysipelothrix rhusiopathiae* to antimicrobial agents and home disinfectants. *Pathology* **34**:462–465.

83. **Fontanals, D., V. Pineda, I. Pons, and J. C. Rojo.** 1989. Penicillin-resistant beta-lactamase-producing *Neisseria meningitidis* in Spain. *Eur. J. Clin. Microbiol. Infect. Dis.* **8**:90–91.

84. **Fritsche, T. R., H. S. Sader, and R. N. Jones.** 2007. Potency and spectrum of garenoxacin tested against an international collection of skin and soft tissue infection pathogens: report from the SENTRY Antimicrobial Surveillance Program (1999–2004). *Diagn. Microbiol. Infect. Dis.* **58**:19–26.

85. **Funke, G., V. Punter, and A. von Graevenitz.** 1996. Antimicrobial susceptibility patterns of some recently established coryneform bacteria. *Antimicrob. Agents Chemother.* **40**:2874–2878.

86. **Galimand, M., A. Guiyoule, G. Gerbaud, B. Rasoamanana, S. Chanteau, E. Carniel, and P. Courvalin.** 1997. Multidrug resistance in *Yersinia pestis* mediated by a transferable plasmid. *N. Engl. J. Med.* **337**:677–680.

87. **Garcia-Cobos, S., J. Campos, E. Cercenado, F. Roman, E. Lazaro, M. Perez-Vazquez, F. de Abajo, and J. Oteo.** 2008. Antibiotic resistance in *Haemophilus influenzae* decreased, except for beta-lactamase-negative amoxicillin-resistant isolates, in parallel with community antibiotic consumption in Spain from 1997 to 2007. *Antimicrob. Agents Chemother.* **52**:2760–2766.

88. **Gaudreau, C., Y. Girouard, H. Gilbert, J. Gagnon, and S. Bekal.** 2008. Comparison of disk diffusion and agar dilution methods for erythromycin, ciprofloxacin, and tetracycline susceptibility testing of *Campylobacter coli* and for tetracycline susceptibility testing of *Campylobacter jejuni* subsp. *jejuni. Antimicrob. Agents Chemother.* **52**:4475–4477.

89. **Gaudreau, C., Y. Girouard, L. Ringuette, and C. Tsimiklis.** 2007. Comparison of disk diffusion and agar dilution methods for erythromycin and ciprofloxacin susceptibility testing of *Campylobacter jejuni* subsp. *jejuni. Antimicrob. Agents Chemother.* **51**:1524–1526.

90. **Gephart, J. F., and J. A. Washington II.** 1982. Antimicrobial susceptibilities of nutritionally variant streptococci. *J. Infect. Dis.* **146**:536–539.

91. **Gerrits, M. M., A. H. van Vliet, E. J. Kuipers, and J. G. Kusters.** 2006. *Helicobacter pylori* and antimicrobial resistance: molecular mechanisms and clinical implications. *Lancet Infect. Dis.* **6**:699–709.

92. **Glikman, D., S. M. Matushek, M. D. Kahana, and R. S. Daum.** 2006. Pneumonia and empyema caused by penicillin-resistant *Neisseria meningitidis*: a case report and literature review. *Pediatrics* **117**:e1061–e1066.

93. **Glupczynski, Y., N. Broutet, A. Cantagrel, L. P. Andersen, T. Alarcon, M. Lopez-Brea, and F. Megraud.** 2002. Comparison of the Etest and agar dilution method for antimicrobial susceptibility testing of *Helicobacter pylori*. *Eur. J. Clin. Microbiol. Infect. Dis.* **21**:549–552.

94. **Godreuil, S., M. Galimand, G. Gerbaud, C. Jacquet, and P. Courvalin.** 2003. Efflux pump Lde is associated with fluoroquinolone resistance in *Listeria monocytogenes*. *Antimicrob. Agents Chemother.* **47**:704–708.

95. **Goldstein, E. J., D. M. Citron, C. V. Merriam, Y. A. Warren, K. L. Tyrrell, and H. Fernandez.** 2002. In vitro activities of a new des-fluoroquinolone, BMS 284756, and seven other antimicrobial agents against 151 isolates of *Eikenella corrodens*. *Antimicrob. Agents Chemother.* **46**:1141–1143.

96. **Goldstein, E. J., D. M. Citron, C. V. Merriam, Y. A. Warren, K. L. Tyrrell, and H. T. Fernandez.** 2002. In vitro activities of garenoxacin (BMS-284756) against 170 clinical isolates of nine *Pasteurella* species. *Antimicrob. Agents Chemother.* **46**:3068–3070.

97. **Gomez-Garces, J. L., J. I. Alos, and J. Tamayo.** 2007. In vitro activity of linezolid and 12 other antimicrobials against coryneform bacteria. *Int. J. Antimicrob. Agents* **29**:688–692.

98. **Gonzalez-Rey, C., S. B. Svenson, L. Bravo, A. Siitonen, V. Pasquale, S. Dumontet, I. Ciznar, and K. Krovacek.** 2004. Serotypes and anti-microbial susceptibility of *Plesiomonas shigelloides* isolates from humans, animals and aquatic environments in different countries. *Comp. Immunol. Microbiol. Infect. Dis.* **27**:129–139.

99. **Gorby, G. L., and J. E. Peacock, Jr.** 1988. *Erysipelothrix rhusiopathiae* endocarditis: microbiologic, epidemiologic, and clinical features of an occupational disease. *Rev. Infect. Dis.* **10**:317–325.

100. **Gracia, M., C. Diaz, P. Coronel, M. Gimeno, R. Garcia-Rodas, G. del Prado, L. Huelves, V. Ruiz, P. L. Naves, M. C. Ponte, J. J. Granizo, and F. Soriano.** 2008. Antimicrobial susceptibility of *Haemophilus influenzae* and *Moraxella catarrhalis* isolates in eight Central, East and Baltic European countries in 2005–06: results of the Cefditoren Surveillance Study. *J. Antimicrob Chemother.* **61**:1180–1181.

101. **Grandiere-Perez, L., C. Jacqueline, V. Lemabecque, O. Patey, G. Potel, and J. Caillon.** 2005. Eagle effect in *Corynebacterium diphtheriae*. *J. Infect. Dis.* **191**:2118–2120.

102. **Green, M. D., B. Beall, M. J. Marcon, C. H. Allen, J. S. Bradley, B. Dashefsky, J. R. Gilsdorf, G. E. Schutze, C. Smith, E. B. Walter, J. M. Martin, K. M. Edwards, K. A. Barbadora, and E. R. Wald.** 2006. Multicentre surveillance of the prevalence and molecular epidemiology of macrolide resistance among pharyngeal isolates of group A streptococci in the USA. *J. Antimicrob. Chemother.* **57**:1240–1243.

103. **Grignon, B., J. Tankovic, F. Megraud, Y. Glupczynski, M. O. Husson, M. C. Conroy, J. P. Emond, J. Loulergue, J. Raymond, and J. L. Fauchere.** 2002. Validation of diffusion methods for macrolide susceptibility testing of *Helicobacter pylori*. *Microb. Drug Resist.* **8**:61–66.

104. **Guiyoule, A., G. Gerbaud, C. Buchrieser, M. Galimand, L. Rahalison, S. Chanteau, P. Courvalin, and E. Carniel.** 2001. Transferable plasmid-mediated resistance to streptomycin in a clinical isolate of *Yersinia pestis*. *Emerg. Infect. Dis.* **7**:43–48.

105. **Guthrie, L., S. Banks, W. Setiawan, and K. B. Waites.** 1999. Comparison of MicroScan MICroSTREP, PASCO, and Sensititre MIC panels for determining antimicrobial susceptibilities of *Streptococcus pneumoniae*. *Diagn. Microbiol. Infect. Dis.* **33**:267–273.

106. **Hansen, J. M., P. Gerner-Smidt, and B. Bruun.** 2005. Antibiotic susceptibility of *Listeria monocytogenes* in Denmark 1958–2001. *APMIS* **113**:31–36.

107. **Hansman, D., S. Wati, A. Lawrence, and J. Turnidge.** 2004. Have South Australian isolates of *Neisseria meningitidis* become less susceptible to penicillin, rifampicin and other drugs? A study of strains isolated over three decades, 1971–1999. *Pathology* **36**:160–165.

108. **Hasegawa, K., R. Kobayashi, E. Takada, A. Ono, N. Chiba, M. Morozumi, S. Iwata, K. Sunakawa, and K. Ubukata.** 2006. High prevalence of type b beta-lactamase-non-producing ampicillin-resistant *Haemophilus influenzae* in meningitis: the situation in Japan where Hib vaccine has not been introduced. *J. Antimicrob. Chemother.* **57**:1077–1082.

109. **Heelan, J. S., D. Chesney, and G. Guadagno.** 1992. Investigation of ampicillin-intermediate strains of *Haemophilus influenzae* by using the disk diffusion procedure and current National Committee for Clinical Laboratory Standards guidelines. *J. Clin. Microbiol.* **30**:1674–1677.

110. **Heilmann, K. P., C. L. Rice, A. L. Miller, N. J. Miller, S. E. Beekmann, M. A. Pfaller, S. S. Richter, and G. V. Doern.** 2005. Decreasing prevalence of beta-lactamase production among respiratory tract isolates of *Haemophilus influenzae* in the United States. *Antimicrob. Agents Chemother.* **49**:2561–2564.

111. **Hirakata, Y., J. Matsuda, M. Nakano, T. Hayashi, S. Tozaka, T. Takezawa, H. Takahashi, Y. Higashiyama, Y. Miyazaki, S. Kamihira, and S. Kohno.** 2005. Evaluation of the BD Phoenix Automated Microbiology System SMIC/ID panel for identification and antimicrobial susceptibility testing of *Streptococcus* spp. *Diagn. Microbiol. Infect. Dis.* **53**:169–173.

112. **Ho, P. L., R. W. Yung, D. N. Tsang, T. L. Que, M. Ho, W. H. Seto, T. K. Ng, W. C. Yam, and W. W. Ng.** 2001. Increasing resistance of *Streptococcus pneumoniae* to fluoroquinolones: results of a Hong Kong multicentre study in 2000. *J. Antimicrob. Chemother.* **48**:659–665.

113. **Hoban, D., and D. Felmingham.** 2002. The PROTEKT surveillance study: antimicrobial susceptibility of *Haemophilus influenzae* and *Moraxella catarrhalis* from community-acquired respiratory tract infections. *J. Antimicrob. Chemother.* **50**(Suppl. S1):49–59.

114. **Horodniceanu, T., A. Buu-Hoi, A. Delbos, and G. Bieth.** 1982. High-level aminoglycoside resistance in Group A, B, C, D (*Streptococcus bovis*), and viridans streptococci. *Antimicrob. Agents Chemother.* **21**:176–179.

115. **Igbinosa, E. O., and A. I. Okoh.** 2008. Emerging Vibrio species: an unending threat to public health in developing countries. *Res. Microbiol.* **159**:495–506.

116. **Ikaheimo, I., H. Syrjala, J. Karhukorpi, R. Schildt, and M. Koskela.** 2000. In vitro antibiotic susceptibility of *Francisella tularensis* isolated from humans and animals. *J. Antimicrob. Chemother.* **46**:287–290.

117. **Inglis, T. J. J., F. Rodrigues, P. Rigby, R. Norton, and B. J. Currie.** 2004. Comparison of the susceptibilities of *Burkholderia pseudomallei* to meropenem and ceftazidime by conventional and intracellular methods. *Antimicrob. Agents Chemother.* **48**:2999–3005.

118. **Inoue, M., D. J. Farrell, K. Kaneko, K. Akizawa, S. Fujita, M. Kaku, J. Igari, K. Yamaguchi, K. Yamanaka, M. Murase, S. Asari, Y. Hirakata, H. Baba, and H. Itaha.** 2008. Antimicrobial susceptibility of respiratory tract pathogens in Japan during PROTEKT years 1–5 (1999–2004). *Microb. Drug Resist.* **14**:109–117.

119. **Jacobs, E., A. Dalhoff, and G. Korfmann.** 2009. Susceptibility patterns of bacterial isolates from hospitalised patients with respiratory tract infections (MOXIAKTIV Study). *Int. J. Antimicrob. Agents* **33**:52–57.

120. **Jansen, W. T., A. Verel, M. Beitsma, J. Verhoef, and D. Milatovic.** 2008. Surveillance study of the susceptibility of *Haemophilus influenzae* to various antibacterial agents in Europe and Canada. *Curr. Med. Res. Opin.* **24**:2853–2861.

121. **Johnson, D. M., H. S. Sader, T. R. Fritsche, D. J. Biedenbach, and R. N. Jones.** 2003. Susceptibility trends of *Haemophilus influenzae* and *Moraxella catarrhalis* against orally administered antimicrobial agents: five-year report from the SENTRY Antimicrobial Surveillance Program. *Diagn. Microbiol. Infect. Dis.* **47**:373–376.

122. **Jones, R., D. Johnson, M. Erwin, M. Beach, D. Biedenbach, and M. Pfaller.** 1999. Comparative antimicrobial activity of gatifloxacin tested against *Streptococcus* spp. including quality control guidelines and Etest method validation. *Diagn. Microbiol. Infect. Dis.* **34**:91–98.

123. Jones, R. N., S. Kohno, Y. Ono, J. E. Ross, and K. Yanagihara. 2009. ZAAPS International Surveillance Program (2007) for linezolid resistance: results from 5591 Gram-positive clinical isolates in 23 countries. *Diagn. Microbiol. Infect. Dis.* **64:**191–201.

124. Jones, R. N., J. E. Ross, M. Castanheira, and R. E. Mendes. 2008. United States resistance surveillance results for linezolid (LEADER Program for 2007). *Diagn. Microbiol. Infect. Dis.* **62:**416–426.

125. Jones, R. N., H. S. Sader, T. R. Fritsche, and S. Pottumarthy. 2007. Comparisons of parenteral broad-spectrum cephalosporins tested against bacterial isolates from pediatric patients: report from the SENTRY Antimicrobial Surveillance Program (1998–2004). *Diagn. Microbiol. Infect. Dis.* **57:**109–116.

126. Jones, R. N., M. G. Stilwell, P. A. Hogan, and D. J. Sheehan. 2007. Activity of linezolid against 3,251 strains of uncommonly isolated gram-positive organisms: report from the SENTRY Antimicrobial Surveillance Program. *Antimicrob. Agents Chemother.* **51:**1491–1493.

127. Jorgensen, J., M. McElmeel, and S. Crawford. 1998. Evaluation of the Dade MicroScan MICroSTREP antimicrobial susceptibility testing panel with selected *Streptococcus pneumoniae* challenge strains and recent clinical isolates. *J. Clin. Microbiol.* **36:**788–791.

128. Jorgensen, J. H., A. L. Barry, M. M. Traczewski, D. F. Sahm, M. L. McElmeel, and S. A. Crawford. 2000. Rapid automated antimicrobial susceptibility testing of *Streptococcus pneumoniae* by use of the bioMerieux Vitek 2. *J. Clin. Microbiol.* **38:**2814–2818.

129. Jorgensen, J. H., S. A. Crawford, and K. R. Fiebelkorn. 2005. Susceptibility of *Neisseria meningitidis* to 16 antimicrobial agents and characterization of resistance mechanisms affecting some agents. *J. Clin. Microbiol.* **43:**3162–3171.

130. Jorgensen, J. H., M. J. Ferraro, M. L. McElmeel, J. Spargo, J. M. Swenson, and F. C. Tenover. 1994. Detection of penicillin and extended-spectrum cephalosporin resistance among *Streptococcus pneumoniae* clinical isolates by use of the Etest. *J. Clin. Microbiol.* **32:**159–163.

131. Jorgensen, J. H., A. W. Howell, and L. A. Maher. 1991. Quantitative antimicrobial susceptibility testing of *Haemophilus influenzae* and *Streptococcus pneumoniae* by using the Etest. *J. Clin. Microbiol.* **29:**109–114.

132. Kadry, A. A., S. I. Fouda, N. A. Elkhizzi, and A. M. Shibl. 2003. Correlation between susceptibility and BRO type enzyme of *Moraxella catarrhalis* strains. *Int. J. Antimicrob. Agents* **22:**532–536.

133. Kain, K. C., and M. T. Kelly. 1989. Antimicrobial susceptibility of *Plesiomonas shigelloides* from patients with diarrhea. *Antimicrob. Agents Chemother.* **33:**1609–1610.

134. Kim, D. M., Y. Lym, S. J. Jang, H. Han, Y. G. Kim, C. H. Chung, and S. P. Hong. 2005. In vitro efficacy of the combination of ciprofloxacin and cefotaxime against *Vibrio vulnificus*. *Antimicrob. Agents Chemother.* **49:**3489–3491.

135. Kim, J. J., J. G. Kim, and D. H. Kwon. 2003. Mixed-infection of antibiotic susceptible and resistant *Helicobacter pylori* isolates in a single patient and underestimation of antimicrobial susceptibility testing. *Helicobacter* **8:**202–206.

136. Kimura, K., S. Suzuki, J. Wachino, H. Kurokawa, K. Yamane, N. Shibata, N. Nagano, H. Kato, K. Shibayama, and Y. Arakawa. 2008. First molecular characterization of group B streptococci with reduced penicillin susceptibility. *Antimicrob. Agents Chemother.* **52:**2890–2897.

137. Kinsara, A., A. Al-Mowallad, and A. O. Osoba. 1999. Increasing resistance of brucellae to co-trimoxazole. *Antimicrob. Agents Chemother.* **43:**1531.

138. Kiyomizu, K., T. Yagi, H. Yoshida, R. Minami, A. Tanimura, T. Karasuno, and A. Hiraoka. 2008. Fulminant septicemia of *Bacillus cereus* resistant to carbapenem in a patient with biphenotypic acute leukemia. *J. Infect. Chemother.* **14:**361–367.

139. Klare, I., C. Konstabel, G. Werner, G. Huys, V. Vankerckhoven, G. Kahlmeter, B. Hildebrandt, S. Muller-Bertling, W. Witte, and H. Goossens. 2007. Antimicrobial susceptibilities of Lactobacillus, Pediococcus and Lactococcus human isolates and cultures intended for probiotic or nutritional use. *J. Antimicrob. Chemother.* **59:**900–912.

140. Klugman, K. P., D. E. Low, J. Metlay, J.-C. Pechere, and K. Weiss. 2004. Community-acquired pneumonia: new management strategies for evolving pathogens and antimicrobial susceptibilities. *Int. J. Antimicrob. Agents* **24:**411–422.

141. Ko, W., K. Yu, C. Liu, C. Huang, H. Leu, and Y. Chuang. 1996. Increasing antibiotic resistance in clinical isolates of *Aeromonas* strains in Taiwan. *Antimicrob. Agents Chemother.* **40:**1260–1262.

142. Ko, W.-C., H.-M. Wu, T.-C. Chang, J.-J. Yan, and J.-J. Wu. 1998. Inducible beta-lactam resistance in *Aeromonas hydrophila*: therapeutic challenge for antimicrobial therapy. *J. Clin. Microbiol.* **36:**3188–3192.

143. Kobayashi, I., K. Murakami, M. Kato, S. Kato, T. Azuma, S. Takahashi, N. Uemura, T. Katsuyama, Y. Fukuda, K. Haruma, M. Nasu, and T. Fujioka. 2007. Changing antimicrobial susceptibility epidemiology of *Helicobacter pylori* strains in Japan between 2002 and 2005. *J. Clin. Microbiol.* **45:**4006–4010.

144. Krcmery, V., Jr., S. Spanik, and J. Trupl. 1996. First report of vancomycin-resistant *Streptococcus mitis* bacteremia in a leukemic patient after prophylaxis with quinolones and during treatment with vancomycin. *J. Chemother.* **8:**325–326.

145. Kugler, K. C., D. J. Biedenbach, and R. N. Jones. 1999. Determination of the antimicrobial activity of 29 clinically important compounds tested against fastidious HACEK group organisms. *Diagn. Microbiol. Infect. Dis.* **34:**73–76.

146. Kulik, E. M., K. Lenkeit, S. Chenaux, and J. Meyer. 2008. Antimicrobial susceptibility of periodontopathogenic bacteria. *J. Antimicrob. Chemother.* **61:**1087–1091.

147. Kupronis, B. A., C. L. Richards, and C. G. Whitney. 2003. Invasive pneumococcal disease in older adults residing in long-term care facilities and in the community. *J. Am. Geriatr. Soc.* **51:**1520–1525.

148. Kyaw, M. H., R. Lynfield, W. Schaffner, A. S. Craig, J. Hadler, A. Reingold, A. R. Thomas, L. H. Harrison, N. M. Bennett, M. M. Farley, R. R. Facklam, J. H. Jorgensen, J. Besser, E. R. Zell, A. Schuchat, and C. G. Whitney. 2006. Effect of introduction of the pneumococcal conjugate vaccine on drug-resistant *Streptococcus pneumoniae*. *N. Engl. J. Med.* **354:**1455–1463.

149. Lagrou, K., J. Verhaegen, M. Janssens, G. Wauters, and L. Verbist. 1998. Prospective study of catalase-positive coryneform organisms in clinical specimens: identification, clinical relevance, and antibiotic susceptibility. *Diagn. Microbiol. Infect. Dis.* **30:**7–15.

150. Lamy, B., A. Kodjo, and F. Laurent. 2009. Prospective nationwide study of *Aeromonas* infections in France. *J. Clin. Microbiol.* **47:**1234–1237.

151. LeQuellec, A., D. Bessis, C. Perez, and A. J. Ciurana. 1994. Endocarditis due to beta-lactamase-producing *Cardiobacterium hominis*. *Clin. Infect. Dis.* **19:**994–995.

152. Levin, J. M., and D. A. Talan. 1990. Erythromycin failure with subsequent *Pasteurella multocida* meningitis and septic arthritis in a cat-bite victim. *Ann. Emerg. Med.* **19:**1458–1461.

153. Liao, C. H., L. J. Teng, P. R. Hsueh, Y. C. Chen, L. M. Huang, S. C. Chang, and S. W. Ho. 2004. Nutritionally variant streptococcal infections at a University Hospital in Taiwan: disease emergence and high prevalence of beta-lactam and macrolide resistance. *Clin. Infect. Dis.* **38:**452–455.

154. Libisch, B., C. G. Giske, B. Kovacs, T. G. Toth, and M. Fuzi. 2008. Identification of the first VIM metallo-beta-lactamase-producing multiresistant *Aeromonas hydrophila* strain. *J. Clin. Microbiol.* **46:**1878–1880.

155. Lightfoot, N. F., R. J. D. Scott, and P. C. B. Turnbull. 1990. Antimicrobial susceptibility of *Bacillus anthracis*. *Salisbury Med. Bull.* **68**(Suppl.):95–98.

156. Lion, C., M. C. Conroy, A. M. Carpentier, and A. Lozniewski. 2006. Antimicrobial susceptibilities of Pasteurella strains isolated from humans. *Int. J. Antimicrob. Agents* **27:**290–293.

157. Lion, C., A. Lozniewski, V. Rosner, and M. Weber. 1999. Lung abscess due to beta-lactamase-producing *Pasteurella multocida*. *Clin. Infect. Dis.* **29:**1345–1346.

158. Lonks, J. R., J. Garau, L. Gomez, M. Xercavins, A. Ochoa de Echaguen, I. F. Gareen, P. T. Reiss, and A. A. Medeiros. 2002. Failure of macrolide antibiotic treatment in patients with bacteremia due to erythromycin-resistant *Streptococcus pneumoniae*. *Clin. Infect. Dis.* **35:**556–564.

159. Low, D. E. 2005. Changing trends in antimicrobial-resistant pneumococci: it's not all bad news. *Clin. Infect. Dis.* **41**(Suppl. 4):S228–S233.

160. Lu, P. L., P. R. Hsueh, C. C. Hung, L. J. Teng, T. N. Jang, and K. T. Luh. 2000. Infective endocarditis complicated with progressive heart failure due to beta-lactamase-producing *Cardiobacterium hominis*. *J. Clin. Microbiol.* **38:**2015–2017.

161. Madinier, I. M., T. B. Fosse, C. Hitzig, Y. Charbit, and L. R. Hannoun. 1999. Resistance profile survey of 50 periodontal strains of *Actinobacillus actinomycetemcomitans*. *J. Periodontol.* **70:**888–892.

162. Maluping, R. P., C. R. Lavilla-Pitogo, A. DePaola, J. M. Janda, K. Krovacek, and C. Greko. 2005. Antimicrobial susceptibility of *Aeromonas* spp., *Vibrio* spp. and *Plesiomonas shigelloides* isolated in the Philippines and Thailand. *Int. J. Antimicrob. Agents* **25:**348–350.

163. Manchanda, V., and P. Bhalla. 2006. Emergence of non-ceftriaxone-susceptible *Neisseria meningitidis* in India. *J. Clin. Microbiol.* **44:**4290–4291.

164. Marco, F., M. Almela, J. Nolla-Salas, P. Coll, I. Gasser, M. D. Ferrer, and M. de Simon. 2000. In vitro activities of 22 antimicrobial agents against *Listeria monocytogenes* strains isolated in Barcelona, Spain. *Diagn. Microbiol. Infect. Dis.* **38:**259–261.

165. Marshall, S. A., P. R. Rhomberg, and R. N. Jones. 1997. Comparative evaluation of Etest for susceptibility testing *Neisseria meningitidis* with eight antimicrobial agents. An investigation using U.S. Food and Drug Administration regulatory criteria. *Diagn. Microbiol. Infect. Dis.* **27:**93–97.

166. Martinez-Martinez, L., P. Joyanes, A. I. Suarez, and E. J. Perea. 2001. Activities of gemifloxacin and five other antimicrobial agents against *Listeria monocytogenes* and coryneform bacteria isolated from clinical samples. *Antimicrob. Agents Chemother.* **45:**2390–2392.

167. Megraud, F. 2007. *Helicobacter pylori* and antibiotic resistance. *Gut* **56:**1502.

168. Megraud, F., N. Lehn, T. Lind, E. Bayerdorffer, C. O'Morain, R. Spiller, P. Unge, S. V. van Zanten, M. Wrangstadh, and C. F. Burman. 1999. Antimicrobial susceptibility testing of *Helicobacter pylori* in a large multicenter trial: the MACH 2 study. *Antimicrob. Agents Chemother.* **43:**2747–2752.

169. Megraud, F., and P. Lehours. 2007. *Helicobacter pylori* detection and antimicrobial susceptibility testing. *Clin. Microbiol. Rev.* **20:**280–322.

170. Mehta, G., and R. Goyal. 2007. Emerging fluoroquinolone resistance in *Neisseria meningitidis* in India: cause for concern. *J. Antimicrob. Chemother.* **59:**329–330.

171. Memish, Z., M. W. Mah, S. Al Mahmoud, M. Al Shaalan, and M. Y. Khan. 2000. *Brucella* bacteraemia: clinical and laboratory observations in 160 patients. *J. Infect.* **40:**59–63.

172. Mendelman, P. M., E. A. Wiley, T. L. Stull, C. Clausen, D. O. Chaffin, and O. Onay. 1990. Problems with current recommendations for susceptibility testing of *Haemophilus influenzae*. *Antimicrob. Agents Chemother.* **34:**1480–1484.

173. Moet, G. J., M. J. Dowzicky, and R. N. Jones. 2007. Tigecycline (GAR-936) activity against *Streptococcus gallolyticus* (bovis) and viridans group streptococci. *Diagn. Microbiol. Infect. Dis.* **57:**333–336.

174. Mohammed, M. J., C. K. Marston, T. Popovic, R. S. Weyant, and F. C. Tenover. 2002. Antimicrobial susceptibility testing of *Bacillus anthracis*: comparison of results obtained by using the National Committee for Clinical Laboratory Standards broth microdilution reference and Etest agar gradient diffusion methods. *J. Clin. Microbiol.* **40:**1902–1907.

175. Morrissey, I., K. Maher, L. Williams, J. Shackcloth, D. Felmingham, and R. Reynolds. 2008. Non-susceptibility trends among *Haemophilus influenzae* and *Moraxella catarrhalis* from community-acquired respiratory tract infections in the UK and Ireland, 1999–2007. *J. Antimicrob. Chemother.* **62**(Suppl. 2):ii97–ii103.

176. Mortensen, J. E., M. J. Gerrety, and L. D. Gray. 2006. Surveillance of antimicrobial resistance in *Neisseria meningitidis* from patients in the Cincinnati tristate region (Ohio, Kentucky, and Indiana). *J. Clin. Microbiol.* **44:**1592–1593.

177. Mortensen, J. E., O. Giger, and G. L. Rodgers. 1998. In vitro activity of oral antimicrobial agents against clinical isolates of *Pasteurella multocida*. *Diagn. Microbiol. Infect. Dis.* **30:**99–102.

178. Murray, C. K., E. A. Walter, S. Crawford, M. L. McElmeel, and J. H. Jorgensen. 2001. *Abiotrophia* bacteremia in a patient with neutropenic fever and antimicrobial susceptibility testing of *Abiotrophia* isolates. *Clin. Infect. Dis.* **32:**E140–E142.

179. Musher, D. M., J. G. Bartlett, and G. V. Doern. 2001. A fresh look at the definition of susceptibility of *Streptococcus pneumoniae* to {beta}-lactam antibiotics. *Arch. Intern. Med.* **161:**2538–2544.

180. Namdari, H., K. Kintner, B. A. Jackson, S. Namdari, J. L. Hughes, R. R. Peairs, and D. J. Savage. 1999. *Abiotrophia* species as a cause of endophthalmitis following cataract extraction. *J. Clin. Microbiol.* **37:**1564–1566.

181. Nariai, A. 2007. Prevalence of beta-lactamase-nonproducing ampicillin-resistant *Haemophilus influenzae* and *Haemophilus influenzae* type b strains obtained from children with lower respiratory tract infections. *J. Infect. Chemother.* **13:**396–399.

182. Niki, Y., H. Hanaki, T. Matsumoto, M. Yagisawa, S. Kohno, N. Aoki, A. Watanabe, J. Sato, R. Hattori, M. Terada, N. Koashi, T. Kozuki, A. Maruo, K. Morita, K. Ogasawara, Y. Takahashi, J. Watanabe, K. Takeuchi, S. Fujimura, H. Takeda, H. Ikeda, N. Sato, K. Niitsuma, M. Saito, S. Koshiba, M. Kaneko, M. Miki, S. Nakanowatari, Y. Honda, J. Chiba, H. Takahashi, M. Utagawa, T. Kondo, A. Kawana, H. Konosaki, Y. Aoki, H. Ueda, H. Sugiura, M. Ichioka, H. Goto, D. Kurai, M. Okazaki, K. Yoshida, T. Yoshida, Y. Tanabe, S. Kobayashi, M. Okada, H. Tsukada, Y. Imai, Y. Honma, K. Nishikawa, T. Yamamoto, A. Kawai, T. Kashiwabara, Y. Takesue, Y. Wada, K. Nakajima, T. Miyara, H. Toda, N. Mitsuno, H. Sugimura, S. Yoshioka, M. Kurokawa, Y. Munekawa, H. Nakajima, S. Kubo, Y. Ohta, K. Mikasa, K. Maeda, K. Kasahara, A. Koizumi, R. Sano, S. Yagi, M. Takaya, Y. Kurokawa, N. Kusano, E. Mihara, M. Kuwabara, Y. Fujiue, T. Ishimaru, N. Matsubara, Y. Kawasaki, H. Tokuyasu, K. Masui, K. Negayama, N. Ueda, M. Ishimaru, Y. Nakanishi, M. Fujita, J. Honda, J. Kadota, K. Hiramatsu, Z. Nagasawa, M. Suga, H. Muranaka, K. Yanagihara, J. Fujita, M. Tateyama, K. Sunakawa, and K. Totsuka. 2009. Nationwide surveillance of bacterial respiratory pathogens conducted by the Japanese Society of Chemotherapy in 2007: general view of the pathogens' antibacterial susceptibility. *J. Infect. Chemother.* **15:**156–167.

183. Norskov-Lauritsen, N., H. Marchandin, and M. J. Dowzicky. 2009. Antimicrobial susceptibility of tigecycline and comparators against bacterial isolates collected as part of the TEST study in Europe (2004–2007). *Int. J. Antimicrob. Agents* **34:**121–130.

184. Okeke, I. N., O. A. Aboderin, D. K. Byarugaba, K. K. Ojo, and J. A. Opintan. 2007. Growing problem of multidrug-resistant enteric pathogens in Africa. *Emerg. Infect. Dis.* **13:**1640–1646.

185. Osaka, K., T. Takakura, K. Narukawa, M. Takahata, K. Endo, H. Kiyota, and S. Onodera. 2008. Analysis of amino acid sequences of penicillin-binding protein 2 in clinical isolates of *Neisseria gonorrhoeae* with reduced susceptibility to cefixime and ceftriaxone. *J. Infect. Chemother.* **14:**195–203.

186. **Osato, M. S., R. Reddy, S. G. Reddy, R. L. Penland, and D. Y. Graham.** 2001. Comparison of the Etest and the NCCLS-approved agar dilution method to detect metronidazole and clarithromycin resistant *Helicobacter pylori*. *Int. J. Antimicrob. Agents* **17:**39–44.

187. **Osato, M. S., R. Reddy, S. G. Reddy, R. L. Penland, H. M. Malaty, and D. Y. Graham.** 2001. Pattern of primary resistance of *Helicobacter pylori* to metronidazole or clarithromycin in the United States. *Arch. Intern. Med.* **161:**1217–1220.

188. **Otsuka, Y., Y. Kawamura, T. Koyama, H. Iihara, K. Ohkusu, and T. Ezaki.** 2005. *Corynebacterium resistens* sp. nov., a new multidrug-resistant coryneform bacterium isolated from human infections. *J. Clin. Microbiol.* **43:**3713–3717.

189. **Ottaviani, D., I. Bacchiocchi, L. Masini, F. Leoni, A. Carraturo, M. Giammarioli, and G. Sbaraglia.** 2001. Antimicrobial susceptibility of potentially pathogenic halophilic vibrios isolated from seafood. *Int. J. Antimicrob. Agents* **18:**135–140.

190. **Owen, R. J.** 2002. Molecular testing for antibiotic resistance in *Helicobacter pylori*. *Gut* **50:**285–289.

191. **Ozawa, M., K. Yamamoto, A. Kojima, M. Takagi, and T. Takahashi.** 2009. Etiological and biological characteristics of *Erysipelothrix rhusiopathiae* isolated between 1994 and 2001 from pigs with swine erysipelas in Japan. *J. Vet. Med. Sci.* **71:**697–702.

192. **Pascual, A., P. Joyanes, L. Martinez-Martinez, A. I. Suarez, and E. J. Perea.** 1996. Comparison of broth microdilution and E-test for susceptibility testing of *Neisseria meningitidis*. *J. Clin. Microbiol.* **34:**588–591.

193. **Paturel, L., J. P. Casalta, G. Habib, M. Nezri, and D. Raoult.** 2004. *Actinobacillus actinomycetemcomitans* endocarditis. *Clin. Microbiol. Infect.* **10:**98–118.

194. **Pereira, G. A., F. P. Pimenta, F. R. Santos, P. V. Damasco, R. Hirata Júnior, and A. L. Mattos-Guaraldi.** 2008. Antimicrobial resistance among Brazilian *Corynebacterium diphtheriae* strains. *Mem. Inst. Oswaldo Cruz* **103:**507–510.

195. **Perez-Trallero, E., N. Gomez, and J. M. Garcia-Arenzana.** 1994. Etest as susceptibility test for evaluation of *Neisseria meningitidis* isolates. *J. Clin. Microbiol.* **32:**2341–2342.

196. **Phares, C. R., R. Lynfield, M. M. Farley, J. Mohle-Boetani, L. H. Harrison, S. Petit, A. S. Craig, W. Schaffner, S. M. Zansky, K. Gershman, K. R. Stefonek, B. A. Albanese, E. R. Zell, A. Schuchat, and S. J. Schrag.** 2008. Epidemiology of invasive group B streptococcal disease in the United States, 1999–2005. *JAMA* **299:**2056–2065.

197. **Philippon, A., and F. Bimet.** 1990. In vitro susceptibility of *Corynebacterium* group D2 and *Corynebacterium jeikeium* to twelve antibiotics. *Eur. J. Clin. Microbiol. Infect. Dis.* **9:**892–895.

198. **Piccolomini, R., G. Di Bonaventura, G. Catamo, F. Carbone, and M. Neri.** 1997. Comparative evaluation of the Etest, agar dilution, and broth microdilution for testing susceptibilities of *Helicobacter pylori* strains to 20 antimicrobial agents. *J. Clin. Microbiol.* **35:**1842–1846.

199. **Piper, K. E., J. M. Steckelberg, and R. Patel.** 2005. In vitro activity of daptomycin against clinical isolates of Gram-positive bacteria. *J. Infect. Chemother.* **11:**207–209.

200. **Pletz, M. W., L. McGee, J. Jorgensen, B. Beall, R. R. Facklam, C. G. Whitney, and K. P. Klugman.** 2004. Levofloxacin-resistant invasive *Streptococcus pneumoniae* in the United States: evidence for clonal spread and the impact of conjugate pneumococcal vaccine. *Antimicrob. Agents Chemother.* **48:**3491–3497.

201. **Pottumarthy, S., T. R. Fritsche, and R. N. Jones.** 2005. Comparative activity of oral and parenteral cephalosporins tested against multidrug-resistant *Streptococcus pneumoniae*: report from the SENTRY Antimicrobial Surveillance Program (1997–2003). *Diagn. Microbiol. Infect. Dis.* **51:**147–150.

202. **Poyart, C., C. Pierre, G. Quesne, B. Pron, P. Berche, and P. Trieu-Cuot.** 1997. Emergence of vancomycin resistance in the genus *Streptococcus*: characterization of a VAN-B transferable determinant in *Streptococcus bovis*. *Antimicrob. Agents Chemother.* **41:**24–29.

203. **Poyart, C., G. Quesne, P. Acar, P. Berche, and P. Trieu-Cuot.** 2000. Characterization of the Tn*916*-like transposon Tn*3872* in a strain of *Abiotrophia defectiva* (*Streptococcus defectivus*) causing sequential episodes of endocarditis in a child. *Antimicrob. Agents Chemother.* **44:**790–793.

204. **Price, L. B., A. Vogler, T. Pearson, J. D. Busch, J. M. Schupp, and P. Keim.** 2003. In vitro selection and characterization of *Bacillus anthracis* mutants with high-level resistance to ciprofloxacin. *Antimicrob. Agents Chemother.* **47:**2362–2365.

205. **Rainbow, J., E. Cebelinski, J. Bartkus, A. Glennen, D. Boxrud, and R. Lynfield.** 2005. Rifampin-resistant meningococcal disease. *Emerg. Infect. Dis.* **11:**977–979.

206. **Reinert, R. R.** 2009. The antimicrobial resistance profile of *Streptococcus pneumoniae*. *Clin. Microbiol. Infect.* **15**(Suppl. 3)**:**7–11.

207. **Richter, S. S., K. A. Gordon, P. R. Rhomberg, M. A. Pfaller, and R. N. Jones.** 2001. *Neisseria meningitidis* with decreased susceptibility to penicillin: report from the SENTRY Antimicrobial Surveillance Program, North America, 1998–99. *Diagn. Microbiol. Infect. Dis.* **41:**83–88.

208. **Richter, S. S., K. P. Heilmann, C. L. Dohrn, F. Riahi, S. E. Beekmann, and G. V. Doern.** 2009. Changing epidemiology of antimicrobial-resistant *Streptococcus pneumoniae* in the United States, 2004–2005. *Clin. Infect. Dis.* **48:**e23–33.

209. **Richter, S. S., W. J. Howard, M. P. Weinstein, D. A. Bruckner, J. F. Hindler, M. Saubolle, and G. V. Doern.** 2007. Multicenter evaluation of the BD Phoenix automated microbiology system for antimicrobial susceptibility testing of *Streptococcus* species. *J. Clin. Microbiol.* **45:**2863–2871.

210. **Richter, S. S., P. L. Winokur, A. B. Brueggemann, H. K. Huynh, P. R. Rhomberg, E. M. Wingert, and G. V. Doern.** 2000. Molecular characterization of the beta-lactamases from clinical isolates of *Moraxella* (*Branhamella*) *catarrhalis* obtained from 24 U.S. medical centers during 1994–1995 and 1997–1998. *Antimicrob. Agents Chemother.* **44:**444–446.

211. **Riegel, P., R. Ruimy, R. Christen, and H. Monteil.** 1996. Species identities and antimicrobial susceptibilities of corynebacteria isolated from various clinical sources. *Eur. J. Clin. Microbiol. Infect. Dis.* **15:**657–662.

212. **Rodriguez, C. N., A. J. Rodriguez-Morales, A. Garcia, B. Pastran, A. Rios, A. Calvo, I. Jimenez, and P. Meijomil.** 2005. Quinolone and azithromycin-resistant *Neisseria meningitidis* serogroup C causing urethritis in a heterosexual man. *Int. J. STD AIDS* **16:**649–650.

213. **Rosenstein, N. E., B. A. Perkins, D. S. Stephens, T. Popovic, and J. M. Hughes.** 2001. Meningococcal disease. *N. Engl. J. Med.* **344:**1378–1388.

214. **Rosenstein, N. E., S. A. Stocker, T. Popovic, F. C. Tenover, B. A. Perkins, et al.** 2000. Antimicrobial resistance of *Neisseria meningitidis* in the United States, 1997. *Clin. Infect. Dis.* **30:**212–213.

215. **Ross, J. E., T. R. Anderegg, H. S. Sader, T. R. Fritsche, and R. N. Jones.** 2005. Trends in linezolid susceptibility patterns in 2002: report from the worldwide Zyvox Annual Appraisal of Potency and Spectrum Program. *Diagn. Microbiol. Infect. Dis.* **52:**53–58.

216. **Rosser, S. J., M. J. Alfa, S. Hoban, J. Kennedy, and G. K. Harding.** 1999. Etest versus agar dilution for antimicrobial susceptibility testing of viridans group streptococci. *J. Clin. Microbiol.* **37:**26–30.

217. **Sabath, L. D., and E. P. Abraham.** 1965. Cephalosporinase and penicillinase activity of *Bacillus cereus*. *Antimicrob. Agents Chemother.* **5:**392–397.

218. **Sader, H. S., J. M. Streit, T. R. Fritsche, and R. N. Jones.** 2006. Antimicrobial susceptibility of Gram-positive bacteria isolated from European medical centres: results of the Daptomycin Surveillance Programme (2002–2004). *Clin. Microbiol. Infect.* **12:**844–852.

219. **Safdar, A., and D. Armstrong.** 2003. Antimicrobial activities against 84 *Listeria monocytogenes* isolates from patients with systemic listeriosis at a comprehensive cancer center (1955–1997). *J. Clin. Microbiol.* **41:**483–485.

220. Saha, D., M. M. Karim, W. A. Khan, S. Ahmed, M. A. Salam, and M. L. Bennish. 2006. Single-dose azithromycin for the treatment of cholera in adults. *N. Engl. J. Med.* **354:**2452–2462.

221. Sahm, D. F., N. P. Brown, C. Thornsberry, and M. E. Jones. 2008. Antimicrobial susceptibility profiles among common respiratory tract pathogens: a GLOBAL perspective. *Postgrad. Med.* **120:**16–24.

222. Salminen, M. K., H. Rautelin, S. Tynkkynen, T. Poussa, M. Saxelin, V. Valtonen, and A. Jarvinen. 2006. Lactobacillus bacteremia, species identification, and antimicrobial susceptibility of 85 blood isolates. *Clin. Infect. Dis.* **42:**e35–e44.

223. Schrag, S. J., L. McGee, C. G. Whitney, B. Beall, A. S. Craig, M. E. Choate, J. H. Jorgensen, R. R. Facklam, and K. P. Klugman. 2004. Emergence of *Streptococcus pneumoniae* with very-high-level resistance to penicillin. *Antimicrob. Agents Chemother.* **48:**3016–3023.

224. Shultz, T. R., J. W. Tapsall, P. A. White, and P. J. Newton. 2000. An invasive isolate of *Neisseria meningitidis* showing decreased susceptibility to quinolones. *Antimicrob. Agents Chemother.* **44:**1116.

225. Skoczynska, A., J. M. Alonso, and M. K. Taha. 2008. Ciprofloxacin resistance in *Neisseria meningitidis*, France. *Emerg. Infect. Dis.* **14:**1322–1323.

226. Sloas, M. M., F. F. Barrett, P. J. Chesney, B. K. English, B. C. Hill, F. C. Tenover, and R. J. Leggiadro. 1992. Cephalosporin treatment failure in penicillin- and cephalosporin-resistant *Streptococcus pneumoniae* meningitis. *Pediatr. Infect. Dis. J.* **11:**662–666.

227. Sordillo, E. M., M. Rendel, R. Sood, J. Belinfanti, O. Murray, and D. Brook. 1993. Septicemia due to beta-lactamase-positive *Kingella kingae*. *Clin. Infect. Dis.* **17:**818–819.

228. Soriano, F., F. Cafini, L. Aguilar, D. Tarrago, L. Alou, M. J. Gimenez, M. Gracia, M. C. Ponte, D. Leu, M. Pana, I. Letowska, and A. Fenoll. 2008. Breakthrough in penicillin resistance? *Streptococcus pneumoniae* isolates with penicillin/cefotaxime MICs of 16 mg/L and their genotypic and geographical relatedness. *J. Antimicrob. Chemother.* **62:**1234–1240.

229. Soriano, F., R. Fernandez-Roblas, R. Calvo, and G. Garcia-Calvo. 1998. In vitro susceptibilities of aerobic and facultative non-spore-forming gram-positive bacilli to HMR 3647 (RU 66647) and 14 other antimicrobials. *Antimicrob. Agents Chemother.* **42:**1028–1033.

230. Soriano, F., and A. Tauch. 2008. Microbiological and clinical features of *Corynebacterium urealyticum*: urinary tract stones and genomics as the Rosetta Stone. *Clin. Microbiol. Infect.* **14:**632–643.

231. Stock, I., and B. Wiedemann. 2001. Beta-lactam-susceptibility patterns of *Plesiomonas shigelloides* strains: importance of inoculum and medium. *Scand. J. Infect. Dis.* **33:**692–696.

232. Stock, I., and B. Wiedemann. 2001. Natural antimicrobial susceptibilities of *Plesiomonas shigelloides* strains. *J. Antimicrob. Chemother.* **48:**803–811.

233. Sutcliffe, E. M., D. M. Jones, S. El-Sheikh, and A. Percival. 1988. Penicillin-insensitive meningococci in the UK. *Lancet* **i:**657–658.

234. Svec, P., A. Sevcikova, I. Sedlacek, J. Bednarova, C. Snauwaert, K. Lefebvre, P. Vandamme, and M. Vancanneyt. 2007. Identification of lactic acid bacteria isolated from human blood cultures. *FEMS Immunol. Med. Microbiol.* **49:**192–196.

235. Swenson, J. M., R. R. Facklam, and C. Thornsberry. 1990. Antimicrobial susceptibility of vancomycin-resistant *Leuconostoc*, *Pediococcus*, and *Lactobacillus* species. *Antimicrob. Agents Chemother.* **34:**543–549.

236. Swenson, J. M., B. C. Hill, and C. Thornsberry. 1986. Screening pneumococci for penicillin resistance. *J. Clin. Microbiol.* **24:**749–752.

237. Taha, M. K., J. A. Vazquez, E. Hong, D. E. Bennett, S. Bertrand, S. Bukovski, M. T. Cafferkey, F. Carion, J. J. Christensen, M. Diggle, G. Edwards, R. Enriquez, C. Fazio, M. Frosch, S. Heuberger, S. Hoffmann, K. A. Jolley, M. Kadlubowski, A. Kechrid, K. Kesanopoulos, P. Kriz, L. Lambertsen, I. Levenet, M. Musilek, M. Paragi, A. Saguer, A. Skoczynska, P. Stefanelli, S. Thulin, G. Tzanakaki, M. Unemo, U. Vogel, and M. L. Zarantonelli. 2007. Target gene sequencing to characterize the penicillin G susceptibility of *Neisseria meningitidis*. *Antimicrob. Agents Chemother.* **51:**2784–2792.

238. Tanaka, M., H. Nakayama, K. Huruya, I. Konomi, S. Irie, A. Kanayama, T. Saika, and I. Kobayashi. 2006. Analysis of mutations within multiple genes associated with resistance in a clinical isolate of *Neisseria gonorrhoeae* with reduced ceftriaxone susceptibility that shows a multidrug-resistant phenotype. *Int. J. Antimicrob. Agents* **27:**20–26.

239. Tang, H. J., M. C. Chang, W. C. Ko, K. Y. Huang, C. L. Lee, and Y. C. Chuang. 2002. In vitro and in vivo activities of newer fluoroquinolones against *Vibrio vulnificus*. *Antimicrob. Agents Chemother.* **46:**3580–3584.

240. Tapsall, J. W. 2009. *Neisseria gonorrhoeae* and emerging resistance to extended spectrum cephalosporins. *Curr. Opin. Infect. Dis.* **22:**87–91.

241. Tapsall, J. W. 2008. Surveillance of antibiotic resistance in *Neisseria gonorrhoeae* in the WHO Western Pacific Region, 2006. *Commun. Dis. Intell.* **32:**48–51.

242. Tenover, F. C., C. N. Baker, and J. M. Swenson. 1996. Evaluation of commercial methods for determining antimicrobial susceptibility of *Streptococcus pneumoniae*. *J. Clin. Microbiol.* **34:**10–14.

243. Thibault, F. M., E. Hernandez, D. R. Vidal, M. Girardet, and J.-D. Cavallo. 2004. Antibiotic susceptibility of 65 isolates of *Burkholderia pseudomallei* and *Burkholderia mallei* to 35 antimicrobial agents. *J. Antimicrob. Chemother.* **54:**1134–1138.

244. Thornsberry, C., J. M. Swenson, C. N. Baker, L. K. McDougal, S. A. Stocker, and B. C. Hill. 1988. Methods for determining susceptibility of fastidious and unusual pathogens to selected antimicrobial agents. *Diagn. Microbiol. Infect. Dis.* **9:**139–153.

245. Thulin, S., P. Olcen, H. Fredlund, and M. Unemo. 2006. Total variation in the *penA* gene of *Neisseria meningitidis*: correlation between susceptibility to beta-lactam antibiotics and *penA* gene heterogeneity. *Antimicrob. Agents Chemother.* **50:**3317–3324.

246. Traub, W. H., and B. Leonhard. 1997. Comparative susceptibility of clinical group A, B, C, F, and G β-hemolytic streptococcal isolates to 24 antimicrobial drugs. *Chemotherapy* **43:**10–20.

247. Trees, D. L., A. L. Sandul, V. Peto-Mesola, M.-R. Aplasca, H. Bun Leng, W. L. Whittington, and J. S. Knapp. 1999. Alterations within the quinolone resistance-determining regions of GyrA and ParC of *Neisseria gonorrhoeae* isolated in the Far East and the United States. *Int. J. Antimicrob. Agents* **12:**325–332.

248. Tristram, S., M. R. Jacobs, and P. C. Appelbaum. 2007. Antimicrobial resistance in *Haemophilus influenzae*. *Clin. Microbiol. Rev.* **20:**368–389.

249. Tristram, S. G. 2008. A comparison of Etest, M.I.C. Evaluator strips and CLSI broth microdilution for determining {beta}-lactam antimicrobial susceptibility in *Haemophilus influenzae*. *J. Antimicrob. Chemother.* **62:**1464–1466.

250. Tuohy, M., G. Procop, and J. Washington. 2000. Antimicrobial susceptibility of *Abiotrophia adiacens* and *Abiotrophia defectiva*. *Diagn. Microbiol. Infect. Dis.* **38:**189–191.

251. Turnbull, P. C. B., N. M. Sirianni, C. I. LeBron, M. N. Samaan, F. N. Sutton, A. E. Reyes, and L. F. Peruski, Jr. 2004. MICs of selected antibiotics for *Bacillus anthracis*, *Bacillus cereus*, *Bacillus thuringiensis*, and *Bacillus mycoides* from a range of clinical and environmental sources as determined by the Etest. *J. Clin. Microbiol.* **42:**3626–3634.

252. Turner, P. C., K. W. Southern, N. J. Spencer, and H. Pullen. 1990. Treatment failure in meningococcal meningitis. *Lancet* **335:**732–733.

253. Varaldo, P. E., M. P. Montanari, and E. Giovanetti. 2009. Genetic elements responsible for erythromycin resistance in streptococci. *Antimicrob. Agents Chemother.* **53:**343–353.

254. Vasilev, V., R. Japheth, N. Andorn, R. Yshai, V. Agmon, E. Gazit, Y. Kashi, and D. Cohen. 2009. A survey of laboratory-confirmed isolates of invasive listeriosis in Israel, 1997–2007. *Epidemiol. Infect.* **137:**577–580.

255. Vay, C., R. Cittadini, C. Barberis, C. Hernán Rodríguez, H. Perez Martinez, F. Genero, and A. Famiglietti. 2007. Antimicrobial susceptibility of non-enterococcal intrinsic glycopeptide-resistant Gram-positive organisms. *Diagn. Microbiol. Infect. Dis.* **57:**183–188.

256. Vazquez, J. A., L. Arreaza, C. Block, I. Ehrhard, S. J. Gray, S. Heuberger, S. Hoffmann, P. Kriz, P. Nicolas, P. Olcen, A. Skoczynska, L. Spanjaard, P. Stefanelli, M.-K. Taha, and G. Tzanakaki. 2003. Interlaboratory comparison of agar dilution and Etest methods for determining the MICs of antibiotics used in management of *Neisseria meningitidis* infections. *Antimicrob. Agents Chemother.* **47:**3430–3434.

257. Vazquez, J. A., S. Berron, M. J. Gimenez, L. de la Fuente, and L. Aguilar. 2001. In vitro susceptibility of *Neisseria meningitidis* isolates to gemifloxacin and ten other antimicrobial agents. *Eur. J. Clin. Microbiol. Infect. Dis.* **20:**150–151.

258. Vazquez, J. A., A. M. Enriquez, S. De la Fuente, S. Berron, and M. Baquero. 1996. Isolation of a strain of beta-lactamase-producing *Neisseria meningitidis* in Spain. *Eur. J. Clin. Microbiol. Infect. Dis.* **15:**181–182.

259. Vazquez, J. A., R. Enriquez, R. Abad, B. Alcala, C. Salcedo, and L. Arreaza. 2007. Antibiotic resistant meningococci in Europe: any need to act? *FEMS Microbiol. Rev.* **31:**64–70.

260. Venditti, M., V. Gelfusa, A. Tarasi, et al. 1990. Antimicrobial susceptibilities of *Erysipelothrix rhusiopathae*. *Antimicrob. Agents Chemother.* **34:**2038–2040.

261. Vila, J., F. Marco, L. Soler, M. Chacon, and M. J. Figueras. 2002. In vitro antimicrobial susceptibility of clinical isolates of *Aeromonas caviae*, *Aeromonas hydrophila* and *Aeromonas veronii* biotype sobria. *J. Antimicrob. Chemother.* **49:**701–702.

262. von Hunolstein, C., F. Scopetti, A. Efstratiou, and K. Engler. 2002. Penicillin tolerance amongst non-toxigenic *Corynebacterium diphtheriae* isolated from cases of pharyngitis. *J. Antimicrob. Chemother.* **50:**125–128.

263. Wang, A., S. Yu, K. Yao, W. Zhang, L. Yuan, Y. Wang, J. Wei, X. Shen, and Y. Yang. 2008. Antimicrobial susceptibility of *Haemophilus influenzae* strains and antibiotics usage patterns in pediatric outpatients: results from a children's hospital in China (2000–2004). *Pediatr. Pulmonol.* **43:**457–462.

264. Wassenaar, T. M., M. Kist, and A. de Jong. 2007. Re-analysis of the risks attributed to ciprofloxacin-resistant *Campylobacter jejuni* infections. *Int. J. Antimicrob. Agents* **30:**195–201.

265. Weber, D. J., S. M. Saviteer, W. A. Rutala, and C. A. Thomann. 1988. In vitro susceptibility of *Bacillus* spp. to selected antimicrobial agents. *Antimicrob. Agents Chemother.* **32:**642–645.

266. Weinstein, M. P., K. P. Klugman, and R. N. Jones. 2009. Rationale for revised penicillin susceptibility breakpoints versus *Streptococcus pneumoniae*: coping with antimicrobial susceptibility in an era of resistance. *Clin. Infect. Dis.* **48:**1596–1600.

267. Weiss, K., M. Laverdiere, and R. Rivest. 1996. Comparison of antimicrobial susceptibility of *Corynebacterium* species by broth microdilution and disk diffusion. *Antimicrob. Agents Chemother.* **40:**930–933.

268. Whitney, C. G., M. M. Farley, J. Hadler, L. H. Harrison, N. M. Bennett, R. Lynfield, A. Reingold, P. R. Cieslak, T. Pilishvili, D. Jackson, R. R. Facklam, J. H. Jorgensen, and A. Schuchat. 2003. Decline in invasive pneumococcal disease after the introduction of protein-polysaccharide conjugate vaccine. *N. Engl. J. Med.* **348:**1737–1746.

269. Whitney, C. G., M. M. Farley, J. Hadler, L. H. Harrison, C. Lexau, A. Reingold, L. Lefkowitz, P. R. Cieslak, M. Cetron, E. R. Zell, J. H. Jorgensen, and A. Schuchat. 2000. Increasing prevalence of multidrug-resistant *Streptococcus pneumoniae* in the United States. *N. Engl. J. Med.* **343:**1917–1924.

270. Wilson, W. R., A. W. Karchmer, A. S. Dajani, K. A. Taubert, A. Bayer, D. Kaye, A. L. Bisno, P. Ferrieri, S. T. Shulman, and D. T. Durack. 1995. Antibiotic treatment of adults with infective endocarditis due to streptococci, enterococci, staphylococci, and HACEK microorganisms. *JAMA* **274:**1706–1713.

271. Woods, C. R., A. L. Smith, B. L. Wasilauskas, J. Campos, and L. B. Givner. 1994. Invasive disease caused by *Neisseria meningitidis* relatively resistant to penicillin in North Carolina. *J. Infect. Dis.* **170:**453–456.

272. Wu, H. M., B. H. Harcourt, C. P. Hatcher, S. C. Wei, R. T. Novak, X. Wang, B. A. Juni, A. Glennen, D. J. Boxrud, J. Rainbow, S. Schmink, R. D. Mair, M. J. Theodore, M. A. Sander, T. K. Miller, K. Kruger, A. C. Cohn, T. A. Clark, N. E. Messonnier, L. W. Mayer, and R. Lynfield. 2009. Emergence of ciprofloxacin-resistant *Neisseria meningitidis* in North America. *N. Engl. J. Med.* **360:**886–892.

273. Yamamoto, K., M. Kijima, H. Yoshimura, and T. Takahashi. 2001. Antimicrobial susceptibilities of *Erysipelothrix rhusiopathiae* isolated from pigs with swine erysipelas in Japan, 1988–1998. *J. Vet. Med. B* **48:**115–126.

274. Yamamoto, K., Y. Sasaki, Y. Ogikubo, N. Noguchi, M. Sasatsu, and T. Takahashi. 2001. Identification of the tetracycline resistance gene, *tet*(M), in *Erysipelothrix rhusiopathiae*. *J. Vet. Med. B* **48:**293–301.

275. Yang, F., X. G. Xu, M. J. Yang, Y. Y. Zhang, K. P. Klugman, and L. McGee. 2008. Antimicrobial susceptibility and molecular epidemiology of *Streptococcus pneumoniae* isolated from Shanghai, China. *Int. J. Antimicrob. Agents* **32:**386–391.

276. Yap, R., L. Mermel, and J. Maglio. 2006. Antimicrobial resistance of community-acquired bloodstream isolates of viridans group streptococci. *Infection* **34:**339–341.

277. Yokoi, S., T. Deguchi, T. Ozawa, M. Yasuda, S. Ito, Y. Kubota, M. Tamaki, and S. Maeda. 2007. Threat to cefixime treatment for gonorrhea. *Emerg. Infect. Dis.* **13:**1275–1277.

278. Yokota, S., K. Sato, O. Kuwahara, S. Habadera, N. Tsukamoto, H. Ohuchi, H. Akizawa, T. Himi, and N. Fujii. 2002. Fluoroquinolone-resistant *Streptococcus pneumoniae* strains occur frequently in elderly patients in Japan. *Antimicrob. Agents Chemother.* **46:**3311–3315.

279. Zapardiel, J., E. Nieto, M. I. Gegundez, I. Gadea, and F. Soriano. 1994. Problems in minimum inhibitory concentration determinations in coryneform organisms. Comparison of an agar dilution and the Etest. *Diagn. Microbiol. Infect. Dis.* **19:**171–173.

280. Zheng, X., A. F. Freeman, J. Villafranca, D. Shortridge, J. Beyer, W. Kabat, K. Dembkowski, and S. T. Shulman. 2004. Antimicrobial susceptibilities of invasive pediatric *Abiotrophia* and *Granulicatella* isolates. *J. Clin. Microbiol.* **42:**4323–4326.

Susceptibility Test Methods: Anaerobic Bacteria

DIANE M. CITRON AND DAVID W. HECHT

72

The importance of anaerobes as the cause of significant infections and the importance of specific antimicrobial treatment for bacteremia and surgical prophylaxis against anaerobic bacteria are well recognized (43, 69, 87, 94, 119, 122). In general, performance of antimicrobial susceptibility testing is viewed as a necessity for effective guidance of antimicrobial therapy. However, when and how susceptibility testing of anaerobes should be performed have been the subjects of debate, due in part to several confounding factors and misconceptions (5, 28, 34, 90, 120). For example, specimens obtained from most infections involving anaerobes are polymicrobic, making recovery and identification of individual isolates slow and the results of antimicrobial susceptibility tests unacceptably delayed to have a consistent impact on individual clinical outcomes. For the clinician, the combination of surgical management and the use of empiric broad-spectrum antimicrobial therapy has limited the correlation of potential antimicrobial resistance with outcome, leading many laboratories away from the performance of susceptibility testing. However, there is substantial evidence that antimicrobial resistance is significant among many anaerobes worldwide and that inappropriate therapy can result in poor clinical responses and increased mortality (40, 43, 76, 87, 122). Antimicrobial susceptibility data have also revealed significant differences among individual hospitals on a regional and local basis, suggesting that one medical center's patterns are not applicable to organisms from other institutions (58, 101, 103, 104). Thus, the need for susceptibility testing of anaerobes is considerably more important now than in the past.

If possible, individual hospitals should establish patterns of resistance for some anaerobes on a periodic basis, with individual patient isolates tested as needed to assist in their care. For surveillance purposes, the testing of 75 to 100 isolates representing anaerobes with known resistance, such as members of the *Bacteroides fragilis* group, *Prevotella* spp., *Fusobacterium* spp., and *Clostridium* spp., should be considered. Preferably, 30 isolates should be from the *B. fragilis* group, and at least 10 of each of the other genera should be tested. Alternatively, cumulative susceptibility results from individual patient isolates may be included in the hospital antibiogram. Antimicrobial agents to be tested should generally be based upon the hospital's formulary, although one agent from each antimicrobial class should be included even if not on the hospital formulary. These data would be important as part of the cumulative susceptibility report if the formulary were changed and could aid in the choice of empiric therapy. For individual patient management, susceptibility testing should be performed when (i) selecting an active agent is critical for disease management, (ii) there is consideration of long-term therapy, (iii) anaerobes are isolated from specific body sites (e.g., blood, brain, bone, or joint), or (iv) there is failure of a usual regimen (Table 1).

This chapter describes currently available methodologies and their interpretation for susceptibility testing of anaerobes. The Clinical and Laboratory Standards Institute (CLSI; formerly NCCLS) anaerobe working group has established an agar dilution reference method using brucella blood agar as the testing medium (19–23). This method is not considered simple or economical to perform but serves as the method to which other, more practical methods can be compared (Table 2). At present, alternative testing methods include limited agar dilution, broth microdilution (for the *B. fragilis* group), and the Etest gradient strip method. β-Lactamase testing provides very limited data but can be useful if penicillin therapy is being considered. Broth disk elution and disk diffusion tests are not considered appropriate for anaerobic susceptibility testing because their results do not correlate with the agar dilution reference method (20).

CLSI has published a supplement to the M11 document that includes additional drug quality control ranges and an antibiogram for the *B. fragilis* group, generated by testing isolates collected from many institutions within the United States in three reference laboratories. This can serve as a guide for empiric therapy if testing is not available (18).

CURRENT PATTERNS OF ANTIBIOTIC RESISTANCE

Susceptibility testing of anaerobes has not been performed routinely at most hospitals (42). As a result, most of the published literature reporting susceptibility of anaerobes is generated by reference laboratories testing a limited number of isolates from one or more medical centers (3, 57, 101, 103). Over the last decade, significant variation in susceptibility results for anaerobes has been reported from different countries, different geographic locations within countries, and even different hospitals within the same city (33, 39, 58, 59, 61, 66, 67, 70, 72, 82, 98, 121). Of particular note, in all of these surveys, the incidence of clindamycin resistance has increased from <10% to >40% for the *B. fragilis* group, while resistance to cephalosporins and cephamycins

TABLE 1 Indications for susceptibility testing of anaerobic bacteria

Indication	Examples[a]
Surveillance	
Annual monitoring of isolates at individual medical centers	*B. fragilis* group, *Prevotella* spp., *Fusobacterium* spp., *Clostridium* spp., *B. wadsworthia*
Clinical	
Known resistance of a particular species	*B. fragilis*: (clindamycin, cephamycins, piperacillin, fluoroquinolones); *Prevotella* spp., *Fusobacterium* spp.: (penicillin, clindamycin)
Failure of a usual therapeutic regimen	Any anaerobe
Pivotal role of antimicrobial agent in clinical outcome	*B. fragilis* group (osteomyelitis, joint infection)
Need for long-term therapy	*B. fragilis* group, *Prevotella* spp. (osteomyelitis, endocarditis, brain abscess, liver abscess, lung abscess)
Infections of specific body sites	Any anaerobe (brain abscess, endocarditis, prosthetic devices or graft, bacteremia)

[a]These are examples only and are not intended as all-inclusive. See the text for specific recommendations.

is also rising. A case of anaerobic sepsis due to a strain of *B. fragilis* simultaneously resistant to carbapenems, other β-lactams, macrolides, metronidazole, and tetracyclines was successfully treated with linezolid (114). Rapidly increasing resistance to fluoroquinolones, notably moxifloxacin, has occurred since the introduction of trovafloxacin in 1994, when overall fluoroquinolone resistance was <3% for the *B. fragilis* group (2, 13, 92), in contrast to moxifloxacin resistance, which had already increased to as high as 34% by 2001 (40). Edmiston et al. reported that 97% of anaerobes recovered from intra-abdominal and diabetic foot infections between 1999 and 2002 were susceptible to moxifloxacin, and Behra-Miellet et al. reported that 96% of *B. fragilis* group strains cultured in 1999 were susceptible to moxifloxacin, with MICs of ≤2 μg/ml (7, 29). Goldstein et al. reported 83% susceptibility to moxifloxacin among intra-abdominal isolates recovered between 2001 and 2004 (52). Papaparaskevas et al. reported that only 51% of *Bacteroides* and *Prevotella* isolates collected in 2006 and 2007 were susceptible to moxifloxacin (81).

Some differences in susceptibility results among various reports may be accounted for by different antimicrobial usages in various areas, different testing methods, a lack of uniformity in interpretive breakpoints among countries, and clustering of MICs at the breakpoint for some species with

some antimicrobial agent combinations (56). Regardless, it is clear from recent publications that resistance to many classes of antimicrobial agents is increasing among anaerobes, and clinicians and laboratories can no longer assume susceptibility of anaerobes to these agents without testing them. Furthermore, neither national nor even local data from other institutions are sufficient to predict the susceptibility of anaerobes to antimicrobial agents at one's own hospital. A general outline of current resistance patterns for anaerobic bacteria is provided below (54).

Gram-Negative Bacilli and Cocci

B. fragilis Group

Among the 24 members of the *B. fragilis* group (including the five *Parabacteroides* species), *B. fragilis* is generally the most susceptible, although >97% of all species are resistant to penicillin and ampicillin. High-level β-lactamase expression correlates with the presence of *cfxA* genes that show variable enzyme expression in different strains (38). The carboxy- and ureidopenicillins, ticarcillin, and mezlocillin are somewhat more active than penicillin, but <50% of isolates are susceptible (3, 111). Piperacillin is the most active of the ureidopenicillins against the *B. fragilis* group, although susceptibility has fallen from approximately

TABLE 2 Methods for susceptibility testing of anaerobic bacteria

Method	Medium	Inoculum	Incubation time (h)	Advantages	Disadvantage(s)
Agar dilution[a]	Brucella blood agar	10⁵ cells/spot	48	Reference method, multiple isolates or antibiotics tested	Labor-intensive, expensive
Broth microdilution[b]	Supplemented brucella broth	10⁶ cells/ml (10⁵/well)	48	Economical, commercial panels available, multiple antibiotics or isolates tested	Limited shelf life of frozen panels, poor growth by some strains
Etest	Brucella blood agar	0.5–1 McFarland standard, swab plate	24–48	Precise MIC value, convenient for individual patient isolates	Expensive for surveillance use

[a]Media are commercially available.
[b]Frozen or lyophilized panels are available from Trek Diagnostic Systems, Inc., (Cleveland, OH).

90% to 70% over the last 8 to 10 years (3, 104). The isoxazolyl penicillins, such as oxacillin and nafcillin, are not active against these organisms. The principal mechanism of resistance to penicillins is β-lactamase production, although penicillin-binding proteins can also be important in some strains (84). Thus, β-lactam–β-lactamase-inhibitor combinations, such as ticarcillin-clavulanate and piperacillin-tazobactam, are active against nearly all strains of the *B. fragilis* group, with <5% resistance in most reports (4, 59, 66, 101, 111). However, several recent surveys have shown decreasing susceptibility to ampicillin-sulbactam and amoxicillin-clavulanate among *Bacteroides* species, with more strains testing in the intermediate category (33, 61, 70, 100, 121). Moreover, resistance in these surveys is more frequent among the species of the *B. fragilis* group other than *B. fragilis*.

Among the cephalosporins and cephamycins, cefoxitin remains very active against *B. fragilis*, *Bacteroides uniformis*, and *Bacteroides vulgatus*, with >90% of isolates being susceptible; however, 15 to 40% of the other members of the *B. fragilis* group are resistant. Cefotetan demonstrates activity against *B. fragilis* that is similar to that of cefoxitin but is much less active against the other members of the *B. fragilis* group (43, 104, 121). With the exception of ceftizoxime, broad-spectrum cephalosporins generally have poor activity against most members of the *B. fragilis* group, inhibiting <50% of isolates (104). Narrow-spectrum cephalosporins are not active against members of the *B. fragilis* group.

A marked decrease in susceptibility to clindamycin among *Bacteroides* spp. has become recognized worldwide, as noted in the surveys cited above. The clindamycin resistance determinants include several *erm* genes that are frequently located on transferable plasmids and are often linked to transferable tetracycline resistance (88, 118). Among other agents, chloramphenicol, metronidazole, and carbapenems (imipenem, ertapenem, meropenem, and the most recently introduced one, doripenem) are nearly uniformly active against all members of the *B. fragilis* group (1, 26, 39, 41, 46, 61, 100, 116), with <2% resistance reported, most often with *B. fragilis*. Imipenem-resistant strains have been reported from Taiwan, the United States, Hungary, Kuwait, and other countries (61, 70, 82, 106). Of note, imipenem resistance is usually mediated by a zinc metalloenzyme encoded by *cfiA* that confers resistance to all current β-lactam and β-lactam–β-lactamase-inhibitor agents and has been reported to be transferable (85). The *cfiA* carbapenem resistance gene is present in a small number of *Bacteroides* strains but is silent unless insertion elements are present to activate the gene (105). Strains possessing the *cfiA* gene may have imipenem MICs ranging from 0.03 to 2 μg/ml, with corresponding meropenem MICs of 0.03 to 16 μg/ml (30). Metalloenzymes can be detected by incorporating a chelating compound such as EDTA, which inactivates the enzyme and restores activity to the carbapenem. A double-ended Etest strip containing meropenem with and without EDTA or imipenem with and without EDTA is available from bioMerieux (9).

Of more concern, however, strains resistant to metronidazole have been reported in France, in association with a transferable plasmid (86), and in recent years, additional resistant strains carrying *nim* genes have been reported in Washington State, the United Kingdom, India, and other countries in Europe (11, 12, 32, 37, 82, 97, 98). *nim* genes encode a nitroimidazole reductase which converts nitroimidazoles to aminoimidazole, preventing the formation of the active toxic nitroso residue (62, 71, 107), although not all

nim genes are expressed and not all metronidazole-resistant strains carry *nim* genes (115). A study of 10 *nim*-gene-positive strains of *B. fragilis* with MICs in the susceptible range found slow-growing subpopulations with metronidazole MICs in the range of 8 to >256 μg/ml (37). This resistance was reversible after passage in drug-free media for three of the strains but was stable in seven others. This may have implications for use of metronidazole in long-term therapy.

Among fluoroquinolone agents, only moxifloxacin currently has a U.S. Food and Drug Administration (FDA) indication for anaerobic bacteria in skin structure and intra-abdominal infections, but as discussed above, resistance mediated by *gyrA* mutations is increasing (7, 29, 52, 79, 81, 102). Gatifloxacin, which has similar activity to that of moxifloxacin, was recently taken off the market. Resistance to fluoroquinolones in other anaerobes is also increasing with the widespread use of this class of antimicrobial agents (14, 52, 81).

Tigecycline, a glycylcycline derivative of minocycline, was recently introduced for treatment of intra-abdominal and skin and soft tissue infections (31, 36, 60). Several studies have found very good activity against anaerobes, with rare strains exhibiting tigecycline MICs of >8 μg/ml (45, 65, 121). However, high-level resistance was found in fewer than 5% of *Bacteroides* strains in two other surveys (8, 101).

Prevotella and *Porphyromonas*

Recent taxonomic changes for *Prevotella* and *Porphyromonas* anaerobes are provided in chapter 51 on anaerobic gram-negative rods in this *Manual*. In general, data on the susceptibility of these organisms (mostly former *Bacteroides* species) are more limited than those for the *B. fragilis* group. Overall, both genera are more susceptible than the *B. fragilis* group. Currently, about 50 to 90% of *Prevotella* spp. are resistant to penicillin and ampicillin due to β-lactamase production, with susceptibilities to cefoxitin and cefotetan ranging from 70 to 99%, while piperacillin susceptibility has decreased to 55 to 80% (61, 70, 82). Likewise, susceptibility to moxifloxacin has decreased to 60 to 70% of strains (14, 82, 121). Eight percent of *Porphyromonas* sp. strains were reported to produce β-lactamase in a survey from Japan (110), and also 17% of strains recovered from serious pelvic infections were reported to produce β-lactamase (83). Susceptibilities of *Porphyromonas* isolates are rarely reported separately in most published literature from the United States, but β-lactamase production is considered rare at present. As in the case of the *B. fragilis* group, both genera are nearly uniformly susceptible to carbapenems, metronidazole, tigecycline, and chloramphenicol, although clindamycin resistance had increased to 15 to 30%, levels similar to those for *Bacteroides*, in several studies (14, 70, 82, 121). Resistance to metronidazole was reported for three strains of *Prevotella oralis*, one strain of *Prevotella buccalis*, and one *Porphyromonas* sp. strain in a study conducted in Greece (82) and for a strain of *Prevotella loescheii* recovered from a subdural empyema (96).

Other Gram-Negative Bacilli

Penicillin resistance among isolates of the genus *Fusobacterium* has been observed. *Fusobacterium nucleatum* strains from saliva of infants showed increasing rates of β-lactamase production related to age, day care attendance, and exposure to antimicrobial agents (77), and a β-lactamase-producing strain was responsible for a case of fatal sepsis in a compromised patient (53). In general,

>95% of *F. nucleatum* and *Fusobacterium necrophorum* strains are susceptible to cephalosporins and cephamycins, *Fusobacterium mortiferum* is resistant to cephalosporins, and *Fusobacterium varium* is often resistant to clindamycin (66, 117). *Campylobacter rectus* and *Campylobacter curvus* (formerly *Wolinella*) vary in their susceptibility to β-lactams but remain very susceptible to chloramphenicol, metronidazole, and clindamycin (117). *Campylobacter gracilis* (formerly *Bacteroides gracilis*) was previously considered resistant to many β-lactam agents. However, data suggest that when it is properly identified and tested, this organism is susceptible to most agents tested, including β-lactam–β-lactamase-inhibitor combinations, cefoxitin, and clindamycin (73). Instead, a newly described but more resistant organism, *Sutterella wadsworthensis,* was often isolated from the same samples and misidentified as *C. gracilis. S. wadsworthensis* may demonstrate resistance to clindamycin, piperacillin, and/or metronidazole. *Bilophila wadsworthia* is a gram-negative anaerobe from the gastrointestinal tract that usually produces β-lactamase and therefore is resistant to penicillin and ampicillin. High MIC$_{90}$ values are also seen for piperacillin, with values clustering near the breakpoints. *Bilophila wadsworthia* is susceptible to clindamycin, cefoxitin, β-lactam–β-lactamase-inhibitor combinations, carbapenems, and metronidazole (109). *Desulfovibrio* spp. are found in the gastrointestinal tract and are sometimes associated with intra-abdominal infections and bacteremia. They are often β-lactamase producers and can be resistant to many β-lactam agents, although carbapenems and metronidazole are uniformly active (50, 74). *Dialister* species were found to have decreased susceptibility to piperacillin, metronidazole, macrolides, and fluoroquinolones (75).

Gram-Positive Bacilli and Cocci

Non-Spore-Forming Gram-Positive Bacilli

Extensive taxonomic changes have occurred within the non-spore-forming gram-positive bacilli, especially with those previously in the genus *Eubacterium*. Details of the changes and descriptions of the new species can be found in chapter 49. The *"Eubacterium"* group, *Actinomyces, Propionibacterium,* and *Bifidobacterium* are usually susceptible to β-lactam agents, including the penicillins, cephalosporins, cephamycins, carbapenems, and β-lactam–β-lactamase-inhibitor combinations. One exception is *Eggerthella lenta* (formerly *Eubacterium lentum*), which has elevated MICs for expanded-spectrum cephalosporins. *Lactobacillus* spp. include strictly anaerobic strains and strains which grow better under anaerobic conditions. They are variably susceptible to cephalosporins, imipenem, vancomycin, and penicillin, depending on the species (93, 95). The vancomycin-resistant species include *Lactobacillus rhamnosus, L. casei, L. plantarum, L. salivarius,* and *L. fermentum,* whereas the vancomycin-susceptible species include the *L. acidophilus* group, *L. crispatus, L. gasseri, L. johnsonii,* and *L. jensenii*. Most strains are susceptible to erythromycin and clindamycin. Vancomycin and penicillin are active against all *Propionibacterium* spp. (80, 113), *Actinomyces* spp., and *Eubacterium* group spp. and against most anaerobic cocci, with the exception of *Peptostreptococcus anaerobius,* which often shows elevated MICs for cephalosporins, penicillin, and β-lactamase inhibitor combinations. *Actinomyces* spp. were shown to be resistant to ciprofloxacin, and an *Actinomyces europaeus* strain showed resistance to clindamycin and erythromycin (75, 99). Newer antimicrobial agents with activity against gram-positive aerobic organisms, such as

linezolid, daptomycin, dalbavancin, telavancin, oritavancin, and ramoplanin, also exhibit excellent in vitro activity against most anaerobic gram-positive species (6, 15, 16, 44, 47–49). Most non-spore-forming gram-positive anaerobes, with the exception of the *"Eubacterium"* group, are resistant to metronidazole.

Spore-Forming Gram-Positive Bacilli

For taxonomic changes among the spore-forming gram-positive bacilli, refer to chapter 50. *Clostridium perfringens* is generally very susceptible to most antianaerobe agents and fluoroquinolones (6, 57, 113). However, non-*C. perfringens* *Clostridium* spp. and *Clostridium difficile* have various susceptibilities (26, 51, 52). Resistance among non-*C. perfringens* species includes resistance to clindamycin, fluoroquinolones, and β-lactams, and *Clostridium innocuum* additionally shows vancomycin MICs of 8 to 32 μg/ml; however, tigecycline, chloramphenicol, and metronidazole remain active. Many strains within the gram-negative-appearing *Clostridium clostridioforme* group produce β-lactamase and are resistant to β-lactam agents (35). *C. difficile* may be resistant to many β-lactams, including cephalosporins, fluoroquinolones, and clindamycin, but it retains susceptibility to metronidazole and vancomycin (55). Some strains are resistant to rifampin and rifaximin (27, 55, 78). A new antibiotic, fidaxomicin (OPT-80 or PAR-101), shows excellent activity against *C. difficile* and is currently undergoing clinical trials for treatment of *C. difficile* infection (25, 64).

Gram-Positive Cocci

At present, only *Peptococcus niger* remains in this genus, and most of the species in the genus *Peptostreptococcus* have been reclassified into other genera (108). (See chapter 48 for current taxonomy.) In general, gram-positive cocci are highly susceptible to all β-lactams, β-lactam–β-lactamase-inhibitor combinations, cephalosporins, carbapenems, chloramphenicol, metronidazole, and tigecycline (14, 26, 39, 66, 68, 82, 121). Fluoroquinolone and clindamycin resistance is increasing among the species (14, 26, 39, 81), and some strains of *P. anaerobius* are resistant to penicillin and amoxicillin-clavulanate (89). Occasionally, microaerophilic streptococci, including *Abiotrophia* and *Granulicatella* species, are initially identified as anaerobic cocci and reported to be resistant to metronidazole. The identification of a metronidazole-resistant anaerobic gram-positive coccus should prompt further identification, as such isolates are rare. The *nimB* gene coding for metronidazole resistance has been demonstrated in two highly resistant strains of *Finegoldia magna,* although it was also detected in 31% of metronidazole-susceptible strains of other gram-positive cocci as well (112).

DESCRIPTION OF TEST METHODS

Agar Dilution

Medium

The recommended medium is supplemented brucella blood agar, which supports the growth of essentially all anaerobes (19). Brucella base agar is supplemented with hemin (5 μg/ml) and vitamin K$_1$ (1 μg/ml) prior to being autoclaved and with 5% defibrinated or laked sheep blood after cooling to 48 to 50°C. To prepare hemin stock solution (5 mg/ml), dissolve 0.5 g of hemin in 10 ml of 1 N NaOH and bring it to a 100-ml volume with distilled water. Sterilize by autoclaving at 121°C for 15 min. Add 1 ml per liter of agar. The stock solution may be stored at 4 to 8°C for 1 month. Vitamin K_1 stock solution (10 mg/ml) is prepared by mixing 0.2 ml of vitamin K_1 (3-phytyl menadione) with 20 ml of 95% ethanol and adding it to agar base to achieve a final concentration of 1 µg/ml prior to autoclaving. The stock solution can be stored for up to 6 months at 4°C in a dark bottle. Lysed (laked) sheep blood is prepared by a single cycle of alternate freezing and thawing and does not require clarification by centrifugation. Laked blood may be stored at −20°C for up to 6 months.

The agar is dispensed in 17-ml volumes in test tubes prior to autoclaving. After being autoclaved, these tubes may be stored at 4 to 8°C for up to 1 month. On the day of the test, the agar is melted by heating and then cooled in a water bath to 48 to 50°C. Laked blood (1 ml) and antimicrobial dilutions (2 ml) are added, and after mixing of the samples by gently inverting the tubes twice, the plates are poured. After they have solidified, the plates are dried in an incubator by being inverted with the lids ajar for 45 min. The CLSI recommends that plates not be stored any longer than 7 days in closed containers at 4 to 8°C. However, for research and precise evaluation purposes, storage for no longer than 72 h is recommended. Due to instability, plates containing imipenem (but not meropenem or ertapenem) or clavulanic acid must be used on the day of preparation.

Inoculum Preparation

The inoculum may be prepared by suspending colonies taken from a 24- to 72-h brucella blood agar plate in brucella broth or other clear broth medium to a density equal to a 0.5 McFarland standard. Alternatively, the initial suspension may be prepared by inoculating five or more colonies into enriched thioglycolate or other broth medium that supports good growth and incubating the sample for 4 to 24 h to obtain adequate turbidity (dilution may be required). Equivalence to a 0.5 McFarland standard can be measured visually or by using a colorimeter or simple photometer device (available from, e.g., bioMérieux, Durham, NC; Microscan, West Sacramento, CA; and Trek Diagnostic Systems, Inc., Cleveland, OH). Although using a photometer is more accurate than visual inspection, the use of different broth media can affect photometer readings; the inoculum concentration should be verified for 5 to 10% of tests by performing colony counts. Species with large cells, such as *C. perfringens*, require fewer cells to achieve this turbidity and will show correspondingly lower colony counts, while the converse is true for organisms with smaller cells, such as *Veillonella* or *Parvimonas micra* (previously called *Micromonas micros*).

The organism suspensions are pipetted into the wells of a replicator head (32 to 36 wells) and applied to plates with a multipronged replicator device that delivers approximately 0.001 ml per spot (10^5 CFU) (multiple inoculator; CMI-Promex, Pedricktown, NJ). The drug-free control plates are inoculated first, and then the antimicrobial plates, starting with the lowest drug concentration. The plates should be marked to ensure proper orientation.

Contamination by aerobic bacteria during the inoculation procedure can be detected by inoculating drug-free plates and incubating them in an aerobic environment. If thioglycolate or other agar-containing broth media are used for inoculum preparation, an additional control plate may be inoculated and refrigerated to distinguish inoculum residue that occurs at the time of setting up the MIC plates and could be confused with growth from an organism that produces hazy or transparent buttons. Agar dilution plates can be inoculated in an aerobic environment, although the exposure time prior to incubation should be minimized. After stamping of the plates, the inoculation spots should be absorbed into the medium for 10 to 15 min, at which time the plates are stacked upside down (to prevent condensation from falling on spots) and immediately placed into an anaerobic environment for incubation.

Incubation Conditions

An anaerobic chamber or anaerobic jars equipped with disposable hydrogen-carbon dioxide generators and palladium-coated catalyst pellets or ascorbic acid envelopes are recommended for incubating agar dilution plates. The incubation atmosphere should contain approximately 5% CO_2, and an indicator of anaerobiosis should be included. Incubation is at 35 to 37°C for 44 to 48 h.

Interpretation of Results

Since 1993, the CLSI has defined the end point for agar dilution testing as the concentration at which there is the most marked change from the growth control (20). This change is defined as no growth or light growth, a haze, multiple tiny colonies, or one to several normal-sized colonies. The technologist should take care to discern a few colonies that may be present as the result of a "splash" from a resistant neighboring isolate from the few colonies that precede full growth of the strain. End points can be difficult to interpret when testing some gram-negative organisms with β-lactams, particularly ceftizoxime and piperacillin. This is especially problematic with many strains of fusobacteria that produce L forms that appear as transparent hazes in the presence of even very high concentrations of β-lactam agents. The recent CLSI documents for susceptibility testing of anaerobes now include a color figure illustrating the end points described above and should be used as an additional guide when using this test method (19, 23). It is important to compare the drug-containing plates to the drug-free control plate when reading the tests, as different species of anaerobic bacteria can have very differently appearing spots, ranging from mucoid-opaque, as with the *B. fragilis* group, to gray-transparent, as with *Bacteroides ureolyticus*.

Interpretation of MIC results should be done according to the criteria recommended by the CLSI (Table 3) (19). In 1993, an intermediate category was established for anaerobic bacteria (20). For many antimicrobial agents tested against anaerobes, a significant percentage of strains have susceptibility test end points that cluster at or near the suggested breakpoints. In the twofold dilution method, the degree of acceptable variation of end points (usually plus or minus one twofold dilution) does not permit adequate distinction of the qualitative categories. If an intermediate value is determined for any anaerobe, the CLSI recommends maximum dosages of the antimicrobial agent for therapy. With such dosages, it is believed that organisms with susceptible or intermediate end points are amenable to therapy. This recommendation is predicated upon the presumed surgical intervention that frequently accompanies infections involving these organisms.

Broth Microdilution Test

The broth microdilution procedure has been validated by CLSI for testing only members of the *B. fragilis* group.

TABLE 3 Interpretive categories for MICs for anaerobic bacteria[a]

Antimicrobial agent	MIC (µg/ml)		
	Susceptible	Intermediate	Resistant
Amoxicillin/ clavulanic acid	≤4/2	8/4	≥16/8
Ampicillin[b]	≤0.5	1	≥2
Ampicillin/ sulbactam	≤8/4	16/8	≥32/16
Cefotetan	≤16	32	≥64
Cefoxitin	≤16	32	≥64
Chloramphenicol	≤8	16	≥32
Clindamycin	≤2	4	≥8
Ertapenem	≤4	8	≥16
Imipenem	≤4	8	≥16
Meropenem	≤4	8	≥16
Metronidazole	≤8	16	≥32
Moxifloxacin	≤2	4	≥8
Penicillin[b]	≤0.5	1	≥2
Piperacillin	≤32	64	≥128
Piperacillin/ tazobactam	≤32/4	64/4	≥128/4
Tetracycline	≤4	8	≥16
Ticarcillin/ clavulanic acid	≤32/2	64/2	≥128/2

[a]Adapted from reference 19 with permission of the publisher.
[b]Members of the B. fragilis group are presumed to be resistant. Other gram-negative anaerobes may be screened for β-lactamase activity by use of a chromogenic cephalosporins test if penicillin therapy is contemplated. Higher blood levels are achievable; infection with non-β-lactamase-producing organisms with higher MICs might be treatable.

Other, more-oxygen-sensitive anaerobes did not grow consistently when inoculated on the bench. Testing in an anaerobic chamber and using reduced MIC trays may improve growth and make this method suitable for other species of anaerobes. The anaerobe working group of CLSI is evaluating additional antimicrobial agents and other species for correlation of the broth microdilution method to the reference standard.

Medium

Brucella broth supplemented with hemin (5 µg/ml), vitamin K$_1$ (1 µg/ml), and lysed horse blood (5%) is the recommended medium. Microdilution trays may be prepared fresh, frozen after preparation, or purchased commercially as lyophilized or frozen panels. Following the manufacturer's recommendations for storage of commercially prepared panels is recommended, while trays prepared in-house may be stored in sealed plastic bags and kept at −70°C for up to 6 months, or longer if quality control strains indicate stability of the drugs. Antimicrobial agents should be diluted according to the scheme described in the CLSI M11 documents and prepared in large volumes, of 15 to 100 ml, depending on the device used to simultaneously dispense aliquots of 0.1 ml per well into the standard 96-well panels. If the inoculum is to be added by pipette, the antimicrobial solutions are prepared at twice the desired concentration and the wells are filled with 0.05 ml, and then 0.05 ml of inoculum is added to each well for a final volume of 0.1 ml. Final volumes of <0.1 ml are not recommended for testing anaerobes due to loss of liquid by evaporation. Inoculum effects may be exaggerated when smaller volumes are used.

Inoculum Preparation

Inoculum preparation is similar to that for the agar dilution procedure. Organisms may be suspended in a clear broth to equal the turbidity of a 0.5 McFarland standard, or the isolate can be grown in a supplemented thioglycolate or other broth that supports growth of the organism for 4 to 24 h and then diluted to the turbidity of a 0.5 McFarland standard (approximately 1.5×10^8 CFU/ml). The final concentration of organism is 1×10^6 to 2×10^6 CFU/ml (10^5 CFU/well). Depending on the method of tray inoculation, the dilution technique will differ. If 10 µl is added to each well, then the suspension at a 0.5 McFarland standard is diluted 1:10. If 50 µl is added, the suspension is diluted 1:50. If a lyophilized tray is used, the suspension is diluted 1:100.

Inoculation Procedure

Frozen trays should be brought to room temperature prior to inoculation. The inoculation can be accomplished by using a disposable, hand-held, 96-prong inoculator, a mechanized dispenser, or a multichannel pipette, depending on the preparation method of the panel, within 15 min after inocula are prepared. While the members of the B. fragilis group are relatively oxygen tolerant, reducing the trays in an oxygen-free environment prior to inoculation (2 to 4 h) may enhance the growth of certain fastidious anaerobes and reduce the "edge" effect of outer rows of wells being reduced more rapidly than inner wells (63). Trays should be reduced prior to inoculation if metronidazole is to be tested, since the antimicrobial activity of metronidazole is dependent on the formation of an active intermediate that requires a reduced atmosphere. False resistance can occur with nonfastidious, rapidly growing strains that produce significant growth before metronidazole is reduced to its active form. Control wells should include a well with broth but no drug (growth control) and an uninoculated well as a sterility check. This well may also be used as a negative-control well for visual comparison with growth in inoculated wells. Alternatively, an uninoculated tray may be incubated as a sterility check, especially if trays are prepared in-house.

It is advisable to perform a colony count and a purity check of the inoculum. This is accomplished by removing 10 µl from the growth control well, diluting it in 10 ml of saline (1:100), and spreading 0.1 ml onto the surface of a nonselective blood agar plate for anaerobic incubation. The presence of 100 to 200 colonies indicates an inoculum of 1×10^6 to 2×10^6 CFU/ml. A small amount of sample from the growth control well can be inoculated onto a quadrant of a blood agar plate for aerobic incubation to detect aerobic contamination.

Incubation Conditions

Trays are most conveniently incubated in an anaerobic chamber for 40 to 48 h. Alternatively, they can be placed in large anaerobic jars, regular anaerobic jars laid on their side, or anaerobic pouches with an appropriate anaerobic gas generator. No more than four trays should be stacked on top of each other to ensure uniformity of heating and gas exchange. Trays should not be sealed with sealing tape (unless it is perforated) if they are set up on the bench, as this will decrease the rate of diffusion of anaerobic gasses to the inoculum and may result in poor growth or false resistance to metronidazole.

Interpretation of Results

The plates may be examined with reflective light, using a viewing device such as a stand with a magnifying mirror. Broth microdilution MIC determinations require criteria similar to those for the agar dilution procedure for reading end points: the concentration at which the most significant reduction in growth is observed is interpreted as the MIC. Similar to that with agar dilution, this decrease in growth may include a tiny, gradually diminishing button of growth, with trailing end points also observed. If the growth in the drug-free growth control well is poor, the test should not be read. Pictures of different growth patterns and their interpretation are included in the CLSI M11-A6 and -A7 documents. At present, breakpoints for broth microdilution are similar to those for agar dilution (19, 23).

Etest Gradient Method

The Etest (AB Biodisk; now bioMerieux) became available in 1994 and has been used more frequently for testing anaerobic organisms in recent years, primarily because of its convenience (42). Several studies have demonstrated its utility and indicate that its results correlate well with those of the CLSI-approved agar dilution method (10, 17, 91). Rosenblatt and Gustafson noted that some strains of *Prevotella* and *Bacteroides* spp. show very major errors (false susceptibility) with penicillin and ceftriaxone; however, a β-lactamase test would provide the correct result in these instances. In addition, false resistance to metronidazole among anaerobes has been reported by the Etest. This phenomenon can be the result of test conditions and medium quality and is generally eliminated if test plates are reduced in an anaerobic atmosphere overnight prior to their use (24). A similar gradient strip (MIC Evaluator) is manufactured by Oxoid and is currently undergoing clinical trials in the United States.

Procedure

The Etest consists of plastic strips coated with a gradient of antimicrobial on one side and an MIC interpretive scale on the other side. The method consists of streaking with a swab to confluence in three directions or streaking with a rota-plater (RetroC80; bioMerieux) of a 0.5 to 1 McFarland standard of the test organism on a 150-mm-diameter supplemented brucella blood agar plate. Up to six Etest strips can be applied to the surface of the plate in a radial fashion, with the lowest concentration toward the center. If large plates are not available, two strips, one on each half, may be placed on a standard-size plate with the high-concentration areas of the strips opposite to each other. Following 24 to 48 h of anaerobic incubation, an elliptical zone of inhibition is formed. MICs are read at the point of intersection of the ellipse with the interpretive scale of MIC values.

The complete list of current FDA-approved antimicrobial agents for anaerobe testing is found in the Etest package insert or can be obtained from the manufacturer. All of the commonly used anaerobe drugs are available. The Etest provides a flexible and simple procedure that is well suited for individual isolate testing in smaller laboratories or for those labs that do not perform batch testing of anaerobe susceptibilities. Its main drawback is the relatively high cost of each strip. This can be alleviated somewhat by limiting the number of antimicrobial agents being tested to a few relevant drugs from the hospital's formulary.

β-Lactamase Testing

β-Lactamase testing of anaerobes can be performed as described by CLSI (19). Nitrocefin disks are available from BD Diagnostics Systems, Hardy Diagnostics, and Remel. The tests should be performed according to the manufacturers' directions. Hydrolysis of the β-lactam ring by β-lactamases causes a color change from yellow to red on the disks, with most reactions occurring within 5 to 10 min, although some β-lactamase-positive strains of *Bacteroides* spp. or other anaerobes may react more slowly (up to 30 min). When *Bilophila wadsworthia* is tested, 1% pyruvate should be added to the testing growth medium for consistent results (63).

β-Lactamase testing has limited utility in detecting resistance to certain β-lactam agents among anaerobes. While a chromogenic cephalosporin test is simple and quick and generally detects β-lactamases produced by species of *Prevotella*, *Porphyromonas*, *Bacteroides*, and other anaerobes, resistance to β-lactam drugs is not always mediated by β-lactamase production, e.g., some strains of *Parabacteroides distasonis* and *B. fragilis* are resistant by alterations of penicillin-binding proteins (115); therefore, β-lactamase test results are limited in their clinical application. A positive test does, however, provide clinically relevant information quickly in some situations and can predict resistance to penicillin G and ampicillin.

QUALITY CONTROL

A quality control program is designed to monitor the accuracy and precision of a susceptibility test procedure, performance of reagents and equipment, and the performance of persons who conduct the tests. Quality control must be performed to demonstrate that any new medium used adequately supports the growth of the test organisms and that the antimicrobial agents have not deteriorated during shipping or storage. These tests must be a part of any testing program using any of the methods described above. Ideally, the quality control strain(s) that most closely resembles the tested organism(s) should be included. The recommended quality control strains are *B. fragilis* ATCC 25285, *Bacteroides thetaiotaomicron* ATCC 29741, *C. difficile* ATCC 700057, and *E. lenta* ATCC 43055. Two quality control strains should be used for each assessment when using the agar dilution procedure. For testing an individual strain by broth microdilution or Etest, one quality control strain should be included. Expected values for quality control strains are published by the CLSI (18, 19). For some antimicrobial agent-quality control organism combinations, no quality control ranges are recommended due to difficulty in reading of end points.

CONCLUSIONS

Increasing antimicrobial resistance among anaerobes has become a significant problem in recent years, increasing the need for more antimicrobial susceptibility testing. Current methodologies allow for accurate surveillance or individual isolate testing by most laboratories. Future studies comparing broth microdilution to the reference agar method and the anticipated development of an improved microdilution system will result in better standardization of the more-user-friendly method and, possibly, more widespread commercial availability.

REFERENCES

1. **Aldridge, K. E.** 2002. Ertapenem (MK-0826), a new carbapenem: comparative in vitro activity against clinically significant anaerobes. *Diagn. Microbiol. Infect. Dis.* **44:**181–186.

2. **Aldridge, K. E., D. Ashcraft, and K. A. Bowman.** 1997. Comparative in vitro activities of trovafloxacin (CP 99,219) and other antimicrobials against clinically significant anaerobes. *Antimicrob. Agents Chemother.* **41:**484–487.

3. **Aldridge, K. E., D. Ashcraft, K. Cambre, C. L. Pierson, S. G. Jenkins, and J. E. Rosenblatt.** 2001. Multicenter survey of the changing in vitro antimicrobial susceptibilities of clinical isolates of *Bacteroides fragilis* group, *Prevotella*, *Fusobacterium*, *Porphyromonas*, and *Peptostreptococcus* species. *Antimicrob. Agents Chemother.* **45:**1238–1243.

4. **Aldridge, K. E., D. Ashcraft, M. O'Brien, and C. V. Sanders.** 2003. Bacteremia due to *Bacteroides fragilis* group: distribution of species, beta-lactamase production, and antimicrobial susceptibility patterns. *Antimicrob. Agents Chemother.* **47:**148–153.

5. **Baron, E. J., D. M. Citron, and H. M. Wexler.** 1990. Son of anaerobic susceptibility testing—revisited. *Clin. Microbiol. Newsl.* **12:**69–70.

6. **Behra-Miellet, J., L. Calvet, and L. Dubreuil.** 2003. Activity of linezolid against anaerobic bacteria. *Int. J. Antimicrob. Agents* **22:**28–34.

7. **Behra-Miellet, J., L. Dubreuil, and E. Jumas-Bilak.** 2002. Antianaerobic activity of moxifloxacin compared with that of ofloxacin, ciprofloxacin, clindamycin, metronidazole and beta-lactams. *Int. J. Antimicrob. Agents* **20:**366–374.

8. **Betriu, C., E. Culebras, M. Gomez, I. Rodriguez-Avial, and J. J. Picazo.** 2005. In vitro activity of tigecycline against *Bacteroides* species. *J. Antimicrob. Chemother.* **56:**349–352.

9. **Bogaerts, P., A. Engelhardt, C. Berhin, L. Bylund, P. Ho, A. Yusof, and Y. Glupczynski.** 2008. Evaluation of a new meropenem-EDTA double-ended Etest strip for the detection of the *cfiA* metallo-beta-lactamase gene in clinical isolates of *Bacteroides fragilis. Clin. Microbiol. Infect.* **14:**973–977.

10. **Bolmstrom, A., A. Karlsson, A. Engelhardt, P. Ho, P. J. Petersen, P. A. Bradford, and C. H. Jones.** 2007. Validation and reproducibility assessment of tigecycline MIC determinations by Etest. *J. Clin. Microbiol.* **45:**2474–2479.

11. **Brazier, J. S., S. L. Stubbs, and B. I. Duerden.** 1999. Metronidazole resistance among clinical isolates belonging to the *Bacteroides fragilis* group: time to be concerned? *J. Antimicrob. Chemother.* **44:**580–581.

12. **Chaudhry, R., P. Mathur, B. Dhawan, and L. Kumar.** 2001. Emergence of metronidazole-resistant *Bacteroides fragilis*, India. *Emerg. Infect. Dis.* **7:**485–486.

13. **Citron, D. M., and M. D. Appleman.** 1997. Comparative in vitro activities of trovafloxacin (CP-99,219) against 221 aerobic and 217 anaerobic bacteria isolated from patients with intra-abdominal infections. *Antimicrob. Agents Chemother.* **41:**2312–2316.

14. **Citron, D. M., E. J. C. Goldstein, C. V. Merriam, B. A. Lipsky, and M. A. Abramson.** 2007. Bacteriology of moderate-to-severe diabetic foot infections and in vitro activity of antimicrobial agents. *J. Clin. Microbiol.* **45:**2819–2828.

15. **Citron, D. M., Y. Y. Kwok, and M. D. Appleman.** 2005. In vitro activity of oritavancin (LY333328), vancomycin, clindamycin, and metronidazole against *Clostridium perfringens*, *Propionibacterium acnes*, and anaerobic gram-positive cocci. *Anaerobe* **11:**93–95.

16. **Citron, D. M., C. V. Merriam, K. L. Tyrrell, Y. A. Warren, H. Fernandez, and E. J. C. Goldstein.** 2003. In vitro activities of ramoplanin, teicoplanin, vancomycin, linezolid, bacitracin, and four other antimicrobials against intestinal anaerobic bacteria. *Antimicrob. Agents Chemother.* **47:**2334–2338.

17. **Citron, D. M., M. I. Ostovari, A. Karlsson, and E. J. C. Goldstein.** 1991. Evaluation of the E test for susceptibility testing of anaerobic bacteria. *J. Clin. Microbiol.* **29:**2197–2203.

18. **Clinical and Laboratory Standards Institute.** 2009. *Acceptable Anaerobe Control Strain Ranges for Minimal Inhibitory Concentration (MIC) Determination by Broth Microdilution and Agar Dilution Testing and Cumulative Antimicrobial Susceptibility Report for* Bacteroides fragilis *Group Bacteria. Informational Supplement. Approved Standard M11-S1.* Clinical and Laboratory Standards Institute, Wayne, PA.

19. **Clinical and Laboratory Standards Institute.** 2007. *Methods for Antimicrobial Susceptibility Testing of Anaerobic Bacteria, 7th ed. Approved Standard M11-A7.* Clinical and Laboratory Standards Institute, Wayne, PA.

20. **CLSI/NCCLS.** 1993. *Methods for Antimicrobial Susceptibility Testing of Anaerobic Bacteria, 3rd ed. Approved Standard M11-A3.* National Committee for Clinical Laboratory Standards, Villanova, PA.

21. **CLSI/NCCLS.** 1997. *Methods for Antimicrobial Susceptibility Testing of Anaerobic Bacteria, 4th ed. Approved Standard M11-A4.* National Committee for Clinical Laboratory Standards, Wayne, PA.

22. **CLSI/NCCLS.** 2001. *Methods for Antimicrobial Susceptibility Testing of Anaerobic Bacteria, 5th ed. Approved Standard M11-A5.* National Committee for Clinical Laboratory Standards, Wayne, PA.

23. **CLSI/NCCLS.** 2004. *Methods for Antimicrobial Susceptibility Testing of Anaerobic Bacteria. Approved Standard M11-A6.* National Committee for Clinical Laboratory Standards, Wayne, PA.

24. **Cormican, M. G., M. E. Erwin, and R. N. Jones.** 1996. False resistance to metronidazole by E-test among anaerobic bacteria investigations of contributing test conditions and medium quality. *Diagn. Microbiol. Infect. Dis.* **24:**117–119.

25. **Credito, K. L., and P. C. Appelbaum.** 2004. Activity of OPT-80, a novel macrocycle, compared with those of eight other agents against selected anaerobic species. *Antimicrob. Agents Chemother.* **48:**4430–4434.

26. **Credito, K. L., L. M. Ednie, and P. C. Appelbaum.** 2008. Comparative antianaerobic activities of doripenem determined by MIC and time-kill analysis. *Antimicrob. Agents Chemother.* **52:**365–373.

27. **Curry, S. R., J. W. Marsh, K. A. Shutt, C. A. Muto, M. M. O'Leary, M. I. Saul, A. W. Pasculle, and L. H. Harrison.** 2009. High frequency of rifampin resistance identified in an epidemic *Clostridium difficile* clone from a large teaching hospital. *Clin. Infect. Dis.* **48:**425–429.

28. **Dougherty, S. H.** 1997. Antimicrobial culture and susceptibility testing has little value for routine management of secondary bacterial peritonitis. *Clin. Infect. Dis.* **25:**S258–S261.

29. **Edmiston, C. E., C. J. Krepel, G. R. Seabrook, L. R. Somberg, A. Nakeeb, R. A. Cambria, and J. B. Towne.** 2004. In vitro activities of moxifloxacin against 900 aerobic and anaerobic surgical isolates from patients with intra-abdominal and diabetic foot infections. *Antimicrob. Agents Chemother.* **48:**1012–1016.

30. **Edwards, R., C. V. Hawkyard, M. T. Garvey, and D. Greenwood.** 1999. Prevalence and degree of expression of the carbapenemase gene (*cfiA*) among clinical isolates of *Bacteroides fragilis* in Nottingham, UK. *J. Antimicrob. Chemother.* **43:**273–276.

31. **Ellis-Grosse, E. J., T. Babinchak, N. Dartois, G. Rose, and E. Loh.** 2005. The efficacy and safety of tigecycline in the treatment of skin and skin-structure infections: results of 2 double-blind phase 3 comparison studies with vancomycin-aztreonam. *Clin. Infect. Dis.* **41**(Suppl. 5):S341–S353.

32. **Elsaghier, A. A., J. S. Brazier, and E. A. James.** 2003. Bacteraemia due to *Bacteroides fragilis* with reduced susceptibility to metronidazole. *J. Antimicrob. Chemother.* **51:**1436–1437.

33. **Fernandez, C. L., L. Castello, M. A. Di, G. Greco, M. C. Legaria, M. Litterio, S. C. Predari, R. Rollet, A. Rossetti, G. Carloni, M. I. Sarchi, and H. Bianchini.** 2007. Susceptibility trends of *Bacteroides fragilis* group isolates from Buenos Aires, Argentina. *Rev. Argent. Microbiol.* **39:**156–160.

34. **Finegold, S. M.** 1997. Perspective on susceptibility testing of anaerobic bacteria. *Clin. Infect. Dis.* **25:**S251–S253.

35. **Finegold, S. M., Y. Song, C. Liu, D. W. Hecht, P. Summanen, E. Kononen, and S. D. Allen.** 2005. *Clostridium clostridioforme:* a mixture of three clinically important species. *Eur. J. Clin. Microbiol. Infect. Dis.* **24:**319–324.

36. **Fomin, P., S. Koalov, A. Cooper, T. Babinchak, N. Dartois, N. De Vane, N. Castaing, and J. Tellado.** 2008. The efficacy and safety of tigecycline for the treatment of complicated intra-abdominal infections—the European experience. *J. Chemother.* **20**(Suppl. 1)**:**12–19.

37. **Gal, M. and J. S. Brazier.** 2004. Metronidazole resistance in *Bacteroides* spp. carrying *nim* genes and the selection of slow-growing metronidazole-resistant mutants. *J. Antimicrob. Chemother.* **54:**109–116.

38. **Garcia, N., G. Gutierrez, M. Lorenzo, J. E. Garcia, S. Piriz, and A. Quesada.** 2008. Genetic determinants for *cfxA* expression in *Bacteroides* strains isolated from human infections. *J. Antimicrob. Chemother.* **62:**942–947.

39. **Glupczynski, Y., C. Berhin, and H. Nizet.** 2009. Antimicrobial susceptibility of anaerobic bacteria in Belgium as determined by E-test methodology. *Eur. J. Clin. Microbiol. Infect. Dis.* **28:**261–267.

40. **Golan, Y., L. A. McDermott, N. V. Jacobus, E. J. Goldstein, S. Finegold, L. J. Harrell, D. W. Hecht, S. G. Jenkins, C. Pierson, R. Venezia, J. Rihs, P. Iannini, S. L. Gorbach, and D. R. Snydman.** 2003. Emergence of fluoroquinolone resistance among *Bacteroides* species. *J. Antimicrob. Chemother.* **52:**208–213.

41. **Goldstein, E. J., and D. M. Citron.** 2009. Activity of a novel carbapenem, doripenem, against anaerobic pathogens. *Diagn. Microbiol. Infect. Dis.* **63:**447–454.

42. **Goldstein, E. J., D. M. Citron, P. J. Goldman, and R. J. Goldman.** 2008. National hospital survey of anaerobic culture and susceptibility methods: III. *Anaerobe* **14:**68–72.

43. **Goldstein, E. J., D. M. Citron, C. V. Merriam, and M. A. Abramson.** 2009. Infection after elective colorectal surgery: bacteriological analysis of failures in a randomized trial of cefotetan vs. ertapenem prophylaxis. *Surg. Infect.* **10:**111–118.

44. **Goldstein, E. J. C., D. M. Citron, C. V. Merriam, Y. Warren, K. Tyrrell, and H. T. Fernandez.** 2003. In vitro activities of dalbavancin and nine comparator agents against anaerobic gram-positive species and corynebacteria. *Antimicrob. Agents Chemother.* **47:**1968–1971.

45. **Goldstein, E. J. C., D. M. Citron, C. V. Merriam, Y. A. Warren, K. L. Tyrrell, and H. T. Fernandez.** 2006. Comparative in vitro susceptibilities of 396 unusual anaerobic strains to tigecycline and eight other antimicrobial agents. *Antimicrob. Agents Chemother.* **50:**3507–3513.

46. **Goldstein, E. J. C., D. M. Citron, C. V. Merriam, Y. A. Warren, K. L. Tyrrell, and H. T. Fernandez.** 2008. In vitro activities of doripenem and six comparator drugs against 423 aerobic and anaerobic bacterial isolates from infected diabetic foot wounds. *Antimicrob. Agents Chemother.* **52:**761–766.

47. **Goldstein, E. J. C., D. M. Citron, C. V. Merriam, Y. A. Warren, K. L. Tyrrell, and H. T. Fernandez.** 2004. In vitro activities of the new semisynthetic glycopeptide telavancin (TD-6424), vancomycin, daptomycin, linezolid, and four comparator agents against anaerobic gram-positive species and *Corynebacterium* spp. *Antimicrob. Agents Chemother.* **48:**2149–2152.

48. **Goldstein, E. J. C., D. M. Citron, C. V. Merriam, Y. A. Warren, K. L. Tyrrell, and H. T. Fernandez.** 2003. In vitro activities of daptomycin, vancomycin, quinupristin-dalfopristin, linezolid, and five other antimicrobials against 307 gram-positive anaerobic and 31 *Corynebacterium* clinical isolates. *Antimicrob. Agents Chemother.* **47:**337–341.

49. **Goldstein, E. J. C., D. M. Citron, C. V. Merriam, Y. A. Warren, K. L. Tyrrell, H. T. Fernandez, and A. Bryskier.** 2005. Comparative in vitro activities of XRP 2868, pristinamycin, quinupristin-dalfopristin, vancomycin, daptomycin, linezolid, clarithromycin, telithromycin, clindamycin, and ampicillin against anaerobic gram-positive species, actinomycetes, and lactobacilli. *Antimicrob. Agents Chemother.* **49:**408–413.

50. **Goldstein, E. J. C., D. M. Citron, V. A. Peraino, and S. A. Cross.** 2003. *Desulfovibrio desulfuricans* bacteremia and review of human *Desulfovibrio* infections. *J. Clin. Microbiol.* **41:**2752–2754.

51. **Goldstein, E. J. C., D. M. Citron, M. C. Vreni, Y. Warren, and K. L. Tyrrell.** 2000. Comparative in vitro activities of ertapenem (MK-0826) against 1,001 anaerobes isolated from human intra-abdominal infections. *Antimicrob. Agents Chemother.* **44:**2389–2394.

52. **Goldstein, E. J. C., D. M. Citron, Y. A. Warren, K. L. Tyrrell, C. V. Merriam, and H. Fernandez.** 2006. In vitro activity of moxifloxacin against 923 anaerobes isolated from human intra-abdominal infections. *Antimicrob. Agents Chemother.* **50:**148–155.

53. **Goldstein, E. J., P. H. Summanen, D. M. Citron, M. H. Rosove, and S. M. Finegold.** 1995. Fatal sepsis due to a beta-lactamase-producing strain of *Fusobacterium nucleatum* subspecies *polymorphum.* *Clin. Infect. Dis.* **20:**797–800.

54. **Hecht, D. W.** 2004. Prevalence of antibiotic resistance in anaerobic bacteria: worrisome developments. *Clin. Infect. Dis.* **39:**92–97.

55. **Hecht, D. W., M. A. Galang, S. P. Sambol, J. R. Osmolski, S. Johnson, and D. N. Gerding.** 2007. In vitro activities of 15 antimicrobial agents against 110 toxigenic *Clostridium difficile* clinical isolates collected from 1983 to 2004. *Antimicrob. Agents Chemother.* **51:**2716–2719.

56. **Hecht, D. W., L. Lederer, and J. R. Osmolski.** 1995. Susceptibility results for the *Bacteroides fragilis* group: comparison of the broth microdilution and agar dilution methods. *Clin. Infect. Dis.* **20:**S342–S345.

57. **Hecht, D. W. and J. R. Osmolski.** 2003. Activities of garenoxacin (BMS-284756) and other agents against anaerobic clinical isolates. *Antimicrob. Agents Chemother.* **47:**910–916.

58. **Hecht, D. W., J. R. Osmolski, and J. P. O'Keefe.** 1993. Variation in the susceptibility of *Bacteroides fragilis* group isolates from six Chicago hospitals. *Clin. Infect. Dis.* **16:**S357–S360.

59. **Hedberg, M., and C. E. Nord.** 2003. Antimicrobial susceptibility of *Bacteroides fragilis* group isolates in Europe. *Clin. Microbiol. Infect.* **9:**475–488.

60. **Jacobus, N. V., L. A. McDermott, R. Ruthazer, and D. R. Snydman.** 2004. In vitro activities of tigecycline against the *Bacteroides fragilis* group. *Antimicrob. Agents Chemother.* **48:**1034–1036.

61. **Jamal, W., M. Shahin, and V. O. Rotimi.** 2010. Surveillance and trends of antimicrobial resistance among clinical isolates of anaerobes in Kuwait hospitals from 2002 to 2007. *Anaerobe* **16:**1–5.

62. **Jamal, W. Y., V. O. Rotimi, J. S. Brazier, M. Johny, W. M. Wetieh, and B. I. Duerden.** 2004. Molecular characterization of nitroimidazole resistance in metronidazole-resistant *Bacteroides* species isolated from hospital patients in Kuwait. *Med. Princ. Pract.* **13:**147–152.

63. **Jousimies-Somer, H. R., P. Summanen, D. M. Citron, E. J. Baron, H. M. Wexler, and S. M. Finegold.** 2002. *Wadsworth-KTL Anaerobic Bacteriology Manual.* Star Publishing, Belmont, CA.

64. **Karlowsky, J. A., N. M. Laing, and G. G. Zhanel.** 2008. In vitro activity of OPT-80 tested against clinical isolates of toxin-producing *Clostridium difficile. Antimicrob. Agents Chemother.* **52:**4163–4165.

65. **Katsandri, A., A. Avlamis, A. Pantazatou, G. L. Petrikkos, N. J. Legakis, and J. Papaparaskevas.** 2006. In vitro activities of tigecycline against recently isolated gram-negative anaerobic bacteria in Greece, including metronidazole-resistant strains. *Diagn. Microbiol. Infect. Dis.* **55:**231–236.

66. **Koeth, L. M., C. E. Good, P. C. Appelbaum, E. J. Goldstein, A. C. Rodloff, M. Claros, and L. J. Dubreuil.** 2004. Surveillance of susceptibility patterns in 1297 European and US anaerobic and capnophilic isolates to co-amoxiclav and five other antimicrobial agents. *J. Antimicrob. Chemother.* **53:**1039–1044.

67. **Kommedal, O., T. W. Nystad, B. Bolstad, and A. Digranes.** 2007. Antibiotic susceptibility of blood culture isolates of anaerobic bacteria at a Norwegian university hospital. *APMIS* **115:**956–961.

68. **Kononen, E., A. Bryk, P. Niemi, and A. Kanervo-Nordstrom.** 2007. Antimicrobial susceptibilities of *Peptostreptococcus anaerobius* and the newly described *Peptostreptococcus stomatis* isolated from various human sources. *Antimicrob. Agents Chemother.* **51:**2205–2207.

69. **Lassmann, B., D. R. Gustafson, C. M. Wood, and J. E. Rosenblatt.** 2007. Reemergence of anaerobic bacteremia. *Clin. Infect. Dis.* **44:**895–900.

70. **Liu, C. Y., Y. T. Huang, C. H. Liao, L. C. Yen, H. Y. Lin, and P. R. Hsueh.** 2008. Increasing trends in antimicrobial resistance among clinically important anaerobes and *Bacteroides fragilis* isolates causing nosocomial infections: emerging resistance to carbapenems. *Antimicrob. Agents Chemother.* **52:**3161–3168.

71. **Lofmark, S., H. Fang, M. Hedberg, and C. Edlund.** 2005. Inducible metronidazole resistance and *nim* genes in clinical *Bacteroides fragilis* group isolates. *Antimicrob. Agents Chemother.* **49:**1253–1256.

72. **Marina, M., M. Ivanova, and T. Kantardjiev.** 2009. Antimicrobial susceptibility of anaerobic bacteria in Bulgaria. *Anaerobe* **15:**127–132.

73. **Molitoris, E., H. M. Wexler, and S. M. Finegold.** 1997. Sources and antimicrobial susceptibilities of *Campylobacter gracilis* and *Sutterella wadsworthensis*. *Clin Infect. Dis.* **25:**S264–S265.

74. **Morin, A. S., L. Poirel, F. Mory, R. Labia, and P. Nordmann.** 2002. Biochemical-genetic analysis and distribution of DES-1, an Ambler class A extended-spectrum beta-lactamase from *Desulfovibrio desulfuricans*. *Antimicrob. Agents Chemother.* **46:**3215–3222.

75. **Morio, F., H. Jean-Pierre, L. Dubreuil, E. Jumas-Bilak, L. Calvet, G. Mercier, R. Devine, and H. Marchandin.** 2007. Antimicrobial susceptibilities and clinical sources of *Dialister* species. *Antimicrob. Agents Chemother.* **51:**4498–4501.

76. **Nguyen, M. H., V. L. Yu, A. J. Morris, L. McDermott, M. W. Wagener, L. Harrell, and D. R. Snydman.** 2000. Antimicrobial resistance and clinical outcome of *Bacteroides* bacteremia: findings of a multicenter prospective observational trial. *Clin. Infect. Dis.* **30:**870–876.

77. **Nyfors, S., E. Kononen, R. Syrjanen, E. Komulainen, and H. Jousimies-Somer.** 2003. Emergence of penicillin resistance among *Fusobacterium nucleatum* populations of commensal oral flora during early childhood. *J. Antimicrob. Chemother.* **51:**107–112.

78. **O'Connor, J. R., M. A. Galang, S. P. Sambol, D. W. Hecht, G. Vedantam, D. N. Gerding, and S. Johnson.** 2008. Rifampin and rifaximin resistance in clinical isolates of *Clostridium difficile*. *Antimicrob. Agents Chemother.* **52:**2813–2817.

79. **Oh, H., N. El Amin, T. Davies, P. C. Appelbaum, and C. Edlund.** 2001. *gyrA* mutations associated with quinolone resistance in *Bacteroides fragilis* group strains. *Antimicrob. Agents Chemother.* **45:**1977–1981.

80. **Oprica, C., and C. E. Nord.** 2005. European surveillance study on the antibiotic susceptibility of *Propionibacterium acnes*. *Clin. Microbiol. Infect.* **11:**204–213.

81. **Papaparaskevas, J., A. Pantazatou, A. Katsandri, D. P. Houhoula, N. J. Legakis, A. Tsakris, and A. Avlamis.** 2008. Moxifloxacin resistance is prevalent among *Bacteroides* and *Prevotella* species in Greece. *J. Antimicrob. Chemother.* **62:**137–141.

82. **Papaparaskevas, J., A. Pantazatou, A. Katsandri, N. J. Legakis, and A. Avlamis.** 2005. Multicentre survey of the in-vitro activity of seven antimicrobial agents, including ertapenem, against recently isolated gram-negative anaerobic bacteria in Greece. *Clin. Microbiol. Infect.* **11:**820–824.

83. **Pelak, B. A., D. M. Citron, M. Motyl, E. J. Goldstein, G. L. Woods, and H. Teppler.** 2002. Comparative in vitro activities of ertapenem against bacterial pathogens from patients with acute pelvic infection. *J. Antimicrob. Chemother.* **50:**735–741.

84. **Piriz, S., S. Vadillo, A. Quesada, J. Criado, R. Cerrato, and J. Ayala.** 2004. Relationship between penicillin-binding protein patterns and beta-lactamases in clinical isolates of *Bacteroides fragilis* with different susceptibility to beta-lactam antibiotics. *J. Med. Microbiol.* **53:**213–221.

85. **Podglajen, I., J. Breuil, and E. Collatz.** 1994. Insertion of a novel DNA sequence, 1S1186, upstream of the silent carbapenemase gene *cfiA*, promotes expression of carbapenem resistance in clinical isolates of *Bacteroides fragilis*. *Mol. Microbiol.* **12:**105–114.

86. **Reysset, G., A. Haggoud, W. J. Su, and M. Sebald.** 1992. Genetic and molecular analysis of pIP417 and pIP419: *Bacteroides* plasmids encoding 5-nitroimidazole resistance. *Plasmid* **27:**181–190.

87. **Robert, R., A. Deraignac, M. G. Le, S. Ragot, and G. Grollier.** 2008. Prognostic factors and impact of antibiotherapy in 117 cases of anaerobic bacteraemia. *Eur. J. Clin. Microbiol. Infect. Dis.* **27:**671–678.

88. **Roberts, M. C., J. Sutcliffe, P. Courvalin, L. B. Jensen, J. Rood, and H. Seppala.** 1999. Nomenclature for macrolide and macrolide-lincosamide-streptogramin B resistance determinants. *Antimicrob. Agents Chemother.* **43:**2823–2830.

89. **Roberts, S. A., K. P. Shore, S. D. Paviour, D. Holland, and A. J. Morris.** 2006. Antimicrobial susceptibility of anaerobic bacteria in New Zealand: 1999–2003. *J. Antimicrob. Chemother.* **57:**992–998.

90. **Rosenblatt, J. E., and I. Brook.** 1993. Clinical relevance of susceptibility testing of anaerobic bacteria. *Clin. Infect. Dis.* **16:**S446–S448.

91. **Rosenblatt, J. E., and D. R. Gustafson.** 1995. Evaluation of the Etest for susceptibility testing of anaerobic bacteria. *Diagn. Microbiol. Infect. Dis.* **22:**279–284.

92. **Rotimi, V. O., E. M. Mokaddas, W. Y. Jamal, F. B. Khodakhast, T. L. Verghese, and S. C. Sanyal.** 1999. Susceptibility of 497 clinical isolates of gram-negative anaerobes to trovafloxacin and eight other antibiotics. *J. Chemother.* **11:**349–356.

93. **Salminen, M. K., H. Rautelin, S. Tynkkynen, T. Poussa, M. Saxelin, V. Valtonen, and A. Jarvinen.** 2006. *Lactobacillus* bacteremia, species identification, and antimicrobial susceptibility of 85 blood isolates. *Clin. Infect. Dis.* **42:**e35–e44.

94. **Salonen, J. H., E. Eerola, and O. Meurman.** 1998. Clinical significance and outcome of anaerobic bacteremia. *Clin. Infect. Dis.* **26:**1413–1417.

95. **Salvana, E. M., and M. Frank.** 2006. *Lactobacillus* endocarditis: case report and review of cases reported since 1992. *J. Infect.* **53:**e5–e10.

96. **Sandoe, J. A., J. K. Struthers, and J. S. Brazier.** 2001. Subdural empyema caused by *Prevotella loescheii* with reduced susceptibility to metronidazole. *J. Antimicrob. Chemother.* **47:**366–367.

97. **Schapiro, J. M., R. Gupta, E. Stefansson, F. C. Fang, and A. P. Limaye.** 2004. Isolation of metronidazole-resistant *Bacteroides fragilis* carrying the *nimA* nitroreductase gene from a patient in Washington State. *J. Clin. Microbiol.* **42:**4127–4129.

98. **Singhal, R., R. Chaudhry, and B. Dhawan.** 2006. Anaerobic bacteraemia in a tertiary care hospital of North India. *Indian J. Med. Microbiol.* **24:**235–236.

99. **Smith, A. J., V. Hall, B. Thakker, and C. G. Gemmell.** 2005. Antimicrobial susceptibility testing of *Actinomyces* species with 12 antimicrobial agents. *J. Antimicrob. Chemother.* **56:**407–409.

100. **Snydman, D. R., N. V. Jacobus, and L. A. McDermott.** 2008. In vitro activities of doripenem, a new broad-spectrum carbapenem, against recently collected clinical anaerobic isolates, with emphasis on the *Bacteroides fragilis* group. *Antimicrob. Agents Chemother.* **52:**4492–4496.

101. **Snydman, D. R., N. V. Jacobus, L. A. McDermott, R. Ruthazer, Y. Golan, E. J. C. Goldstein, S. M. Finegold, L. J. Harrell, D. W. Hecht, S. G. Jenkins, C. Pierson, R. Venezia, V. Yu, J. Rihs, and S. L. Gorbach.** 2007. National

survey on the susceptibility of *Bacteroides fragilis* group: report and analysis of trends in the United States from 1997 to 2004. *Antimicrob. Agents Chemother.* **51:**1649–1655.

102. **Snydman, D. R., N. V. Jacobus, L. A. McDermott, R. Ruthazer, E. Goldstein, S. Finegold, L. Harrell, D. W. Hecht, S. Jenkins, C. Pierson, R. Venezia, J. Rihs, and S. L. Gorbach.** 2002. In vitro activities of newer quinolones against *Bacteroides* group organisms. *Antimicrob. Agents Chemother.* **46:**3276–3279.

103. **Snydman, D. R., N. V. Jacobus, L. A. McDermott, R. Ruthazer, E. J. Goldstein, S. M. Finegold, L. J. Harrell, D. W. Hecht, S. G. Jenkins, C. Pierson, R. Venezia, J. Rihs, and S. L. Gorbach.** 2002. National survey on the susceptibility of *Bacteroides fragilis* group: report and analysis of trends for 1997–2000. *Clin. Infect. Dis.* **35:**S126–S134.

104. **Snydman, D. R., N. V. Jacobus, L. A. McDermott, S. Supran, G. J. Cuchural, Jr., S. Finegold, L. Harrell, D. W. Hecht, P. Iannini, S. Jenkins, C. Pierson, J. Rihs, and S. L. Gorbach.** 1999. Multicenter study of in vitro susceptibility of the *Bacteroides fragilis* group, 1995 to 1996, with comparison of resistance trends from 1990 to 1996. *Antimicrob. Agents Chemother.* **43:**2417–2422.

105. **Soki, J., R. Edwards, M. Hedberg, H. Fang, E. Nagy, and C. E. Nord.** 2006. Examination of *cfiA*-mediated carbapenem resistance in *Bacteroides fragilis* strains from a European antibiotic susceptibility survey. *Int. J. Antimicrob. Agents* **28:**497–502.

106. **Soki, J., E. Fodor, D. W. Hecht, R. Edwards, V. O. Rotimi, I. Kerekes, E. Urban, and E. Nagy.** 2004. Molecular characterization of imipenem-resistant, *cfiA*-positive *Bacteroides fragilis* isolates from the USA, Hungary and Kuwait. *J. Med. Microbiol.* **53:**413–419.

107. **Soki, J., M. Gal, J. S. Brazier, V. O. Rotimi, E. Urban, E. Nagy, and B. I. Duerden.** 2006. Molecular investigation of genetic elements contributing to metronidazole resistance in *Bacteroides* strains. *J. Antimicrob. Chemother.* **57:**212–220.

108. **Song, Y., C. Liu, and S. M. Finegold.** 2007. Development of a flow chart for identification of gram-positive anaerobic cocci in the clinical laboratory. *J. Clin. Microbiol.* **45:**512–516.

109. **Summanen, P., H. M. Wexler, and S. M. Finegold.** 1992. Antimicrobial susceptibility testing of *Bilophila wadsworthia* by using triphenyltetrazolium chloride to facilitate endpoint determination. *Antimicrob. Agents Chemother.* **36:**1658–1664.

110. **Tanaka, K., C. Kawamura, K. Fukui, H. Kato, N. Kato, T. Nakamura, K. Watanabe, and K. Ueno.** 1999. Antimicrobial susceptibility and β-lactamase production of *Prevotella* spp. and *Porphyromonas* spp. *Anaerobe* **5:**461–463.

111. **Teng, L. J., P. R. Hsueh, J. C. Tsai, S. J. Liaw, S. W. Ho, and K. T. Luh.** 2002. High incidence of cefoxitin and clindamycin resistance among anaerobes in Taiwan. *Antimicrob. Agents Chemother.* **46:**2908–2913.

112. **Theron, M. M., M. N. Janse van Rensburg, and L. J. Chalkley.** 2004. Nitroimidazole resistance genes (*nimB*) in anaerobic gram-positive cocci (previously *Peptostreptococcus* spp.). *J. Antimicrob. Chemother.* **54:**240–242.

113. **Tyrrell, K. L., D. M. Citron, Y. A. Warren, H. T. Fernandez, C. V. Merriam, and E. J. C. Goldstein.** 2006. In vitro activities of daptomycin, vancomycin, and penicillin against *Clostridium difficile*, *C. perfringens*, *Finegoldia magna*, and *Propionibacterium acnes*. *Antimicrob. Agents Chemother.* **50:**2728–2731.

114. **Wareham, D. W., M. Wilks, D. Ahmed, J. S. Brazier, and M. Millar.** 2005. Anaerobic sepsis due to multidrug-resistant *Bacteroides fragilis*: microbiological cure and clinical response with linezolid therapy. *Clin. Infect. Dis.* **40:**e67–e68.

115. **Wexler, H. M.** 2007. *Bacteroides*: the good, the bad, and the nitty-gritty. *Clin. Microbiol. Rev.* **20:**593–621.

116. **Wexler, H. M., A. E. Engel, D. Glass, and C. Li.** 2005. In vitro activities of doripenem and comparator agents against 364 anaerobic clinical isolates. *Antimicrob. Agents Chemother.* **49:**4413–4417.

117. **Wexler, H. M., D. Molitoris, S. St. John, A. Vu, E. K. Read, and S. M. Finegold.** 2002. In vitro activities of faropenem against 579 strains of anaerobic bacteria. *Antimicrob. Agents Chemother.* **46:**3669–3675.

118. **Whittle, G., N. B. Shoemaker, and A. A. Salyers.** 2002. The role of *Bacteroides* conjugative transposons in the dissemination of antibiotic resistance genes. *Cell. Mol. Life Sci.* **59:**2044–2054.

119. **Wilson, J. R., and A. P. Limaye.** 2004. Risk factors for mortality in patients with anaerobic bacteremia. *Eur. J. Clin. Microbiol. Infect. Dis.* **23:**310–316.

120. **Wilson, S. E., and J. Huh.** 1997. In defense of routine antimicrobial susceptibility testing of operative site flora in patients with peritonitis. *Clin. Infect. Dis.* **25:**S254–S257.

121. **Wybo, I., D. Pierard, I. Verschraegen, M. Reynders, K. Vandoorslaer, G. Claeys, M. Delmee, Y. Glupczynski, B. Gordts, M. Ieven, P. Melin, M. Struelens, J. Verhaegen, and S. Lauwers.** 2007. Third Belgian multicentre survey of antibiotic susceptibility of anaerobic bacteria. *J. Antimicrob. Chemother.* **59:**132–139.

122. **Zahar, J. R., H. Farhat, E. Chachaty, P. Meshaka, S. Antoun, and G. Nitenberg.** 2005. Incidence and clinical significance of anaerobic bacteraemia in cancer patients: a 6-year retrospective study. *Clin. Microbiol. Infect.* **11:**724–729.

Susceptibility Test Methods: Mycobacteria, *Nocardia*, and Other Actinomycetes*

GAIL L. WOODS, SHOU-YEAN GRACE LIN, AND EDWARD P. DESMOND

73

The World Health Organization (WHO) has described drug-resistant tuberculosis (TB) as "a major public health threat that threatens tuberculosis control" (167). Approximately 500,000 cases of multidrug-resistant (MDR) TB occur each year worldwide (166). MDR TB is defined as a case caused by tubercle bacilli that are resistant to rifampin (RMP) and isoniazid (INH), the two most effective drugs in the standard regimen. Although most of the cases of TB and drug-resistant TB occur in developing countries, a significant percentage of these diseases also occur in industrialized countries, where immigrants may make up the majority of new TB cases. Drug-resistant TB is therefore a worldwide problem. Fortunately, at the same time that the threat of drug-resistant TB is emerging, new tools are being developed for more rapid detection of drug resistance. Among new tools endorsed by WHO for the diagnosis of TB and detection of drug resistance are liquid culture and molecular line probe assays (167). In the United States, a task force was convened to plan to combat and control drug-resistant TB. The report of this task force was published in early 2009 (85). This report emphasizes the need to develop and enhance laboratory capacities to rapidly and accurately detect drug-resistant TB. Along with the advances in new technologies, new drugs are becoming available to help meet the challenges of this changing situation.

Recently, attention has been focused on cases of TB that exhibit resistance not only to INH and RMP but also to quinolones and injectable drugs such as aminoglycosides or capreomycin. These cases, described as extensively drug-resistant TB (XDR TB), present serious challenges for diagnosis, treatment, and control of the disease (25). Successful treatment of XDR TB is possible with individualized treatment based on results of drug susceptibility testing including second-line drugs, adverse-event management, and nutritional and psychological support (97). However, most patients with XDR TB succumb to this disease because of delays in diagnosis, inability to test for susceptibility to second-line drugs, coinfection with human immunodeficiency virus (HIV), unavailability of second-line drugs, or combinations of these factors. Again, enhancing the capacity of laboratories to quickly detect drug resistance and test

for susceptibility to second-line drugs is a key component in efforts to combat this ominous new development.

This chapter includes a description of nonradioactive broth culture systems and rapid molecular systems for detection of drug resistance, as well as the standard agar proportion method. The molecular methods are likely to revolutionize the way in which drug-resistant TB is detected, creating a new standard of turnaround time—hours or days—to provide results, rather than the weeks or months previously required.

Because most cases of TB occur in resource-limited settings, it is desirable to have inexpensive techniques that do not require frequent importation of proprietary materials. One such method, called microscopic observation drug susceptibility, is described below (99).

As described in earlier chapters, nontuberculous mycobacteria (NTM) and aerobic actinomycetes can also be causes of significant disease in humans. As goals are met for elimination of TB, NTM will constitute an increasing proportion of causative agents of human mycobacterial diseases. Drug susceptibility testing of many NTM and aerobic actinomycetes may provide useful guidance in the treatment of these infections and is also discussed in this chapter.

ANTIMICROBIAL AGENTS

Although a variety of antimicrobial agents are available for the treatment of mycobacterial diseases, not all agents are suitable for treating all types of infections. Furthermore, in the face of antimicrobial resistance, the choice of alternative therapies can be problematic and clinical experience becomes a prevailing factor. For other uncommon mycobacterial infections, the physician is not infrequently faced with a dilemma in choosing a treatment regimen because of a lack of clinical precedence or unclear efficacy. The situation is confounded further by the need to treat mycobacterial infections with a combination of agents to improve efficacy, to prevent resistance, or to overcome intrinsic resistance (97).

The antimicrobial agents that are used in the treatment of mycobacterial infections are discussed below for the most commonly encountered species. The primary agents are summarized in Table 1 (52, 68). For TB, first-line drugs are those usually used to treat uncomplicated cases. The Clinical and Laboratory Standards Institute (CLSI) document on drug susceptibility testing of mycobacteria (31) currently recommends that first-line testing include ethambutol (EMB),

*This chapter contains information presented in chapter 77 by Gail L. Woods, Nancy G. Warren, and Clark B. Inderlied in the ninth edition of this *Manual.*

TABLE 1 Antimicrobial agents recommended for primary treatment of common mycobacterial infections[a]

Mycobacterium species	Site of infection	Antimicrobial agents
M. tuberculosis complex[b]	Any	Isoniazid + rifampin + ethambutol + pyrazinamide
M. avium complex	Pulmonary	Clarithromycin[c] + rifampin + ethambutol (+ streptomycin or amikacin for cavitary and severe disease)
	Disseminated	Clarithromycin[c] + ethambutol ± rifabutin
M. kansasii	Pulmonary	Isoniazid + rifampin + ethambutol
M. marinum	Skin, soft tissue[d]	Clarithromycin + ethambutol, clarithromycin + rifampin, or rifampin + ethambutol
Rapidly growing mycobacteria[e]	Skin, soft tissue[d]	Clarithromycin (if susceptible) + ≥1 additional drug, based on susceptibility test results
M. abscessus	Pulmonary	Multidrug regimen, based on susceptibility results, that includes clarithromycin (if susceptible)[f]

[a]Recommendations for NTM are from reference 46.
[b]Almost all (>95%) M. bovis are resistant to pyrazinamide.
[c]Azithromycin is an acceptable alternative agent.
[d]Surgical debridement may be important for successful therapy.
[e]Most common species are M. fortuitum group, M. abscessus, and M. chelonae.
[f]Currently there are no drug regimens of proven efficacy. Antimicrobial therapy may provide symptomatic improvement and disease regression. Surgical resection of limited disease (if possible) and multidrug therapy are optimal.

RMP, INH, and pyrazinamide (PZA). In the United States, streptomycin (SM) was moved from first-line to second-line testing several years ago. Second-line drugs are those used when first-line therapy fails or is inappropriate. These agents are often accompanied by more-severe side effects.

Drug resistance in *Mycobacterium tuberculosis* complex (MTBC) occurs randomly and at a low frequency and is usually a result of single-step mutations. Two types of drug resistance are seen: primary and acquired. Primary drug resistance occurs in an individual who is infected with a drug-resistant strain before drug treatment is initiated. Acquired resistance can emerge against any of the antituberculosis agents during chemotherapy as a result of inadequate treatment (56, 110, 117).

Genes that are known to be associated with antibiotic resistance in MTBC are summarized in Table 2. Although drug resistance mechanisms in MTBC are not fully understood, five categories are found in mycobacteria. These include decreased

uptake of drug such as seen in dormant acid-fast bacilli; drug inactivation by constitutive β-lactamases; increased efflux as seen in fluoroquinolone resistance; alteration of the target as described below with RMP and INH; and reduced prodrug-activating enzymes as exhibited in PZA resistance (154).

Isoniazid

INH (isonicotinic acid hydrazide), a synthetic antimicrobial agent introduced in 1952 for the treatment of TB, is remarkably specific and potently bactericidal for tubercle bacilli. INH has comparatively low toxicity and is active against virtually all wild-type strains of MTBC. The mechanism of action of INH occurs in three steps: (i) activation of the drug, (ii) binding of the "active" form to the target(s) of inhibition, and (iii) exertion of an inhibitory effect. In turn, the mechanism of INH resistance can involve alterations in each of these steps, alone or in combination. While the mechanism of INH activation is not completely

TABLE 2 Genes associated with drug resistance in M. tuberculosis[a]

Antimicrobial agent	Gene	Gene product	Mechanism of drug action
RMP	rpoB	β subunit of RNA polymerase	Inhibits RNA transcription
INH	katG	Catalase-peroxidase	Inhibits mycolic acid biosynthesis; other multiple effects on DNA, lipids, carbohydrates, and NAD metabolism
	inhA	EnvM analog 3-ketoacyl-acyl carrier protein reductase analog inhA promoter	
	ahpC	Subunit of alkyl hydroperoxide reductase	
	ndh	NADH dehydrogenase	
EMB	embB	Arabinosyltransferase	Inhibits arabinogalactan synthesis
SM	rpsL	Ribosomal protein S12	Inhibits protein synthesis
	rrs	16S rRNA	
PZA	pncA	Pyrazinamidase	Acidifies cytoplasm and deenergizes membrane
Ethionamide	inhA	inhA promoter	Inhibits mycolic acid biosynthesis
Fluoroquinolones	gyrA	DNA gyrase A subunit	Inhibits action of DNA gyrase
	gyrB	DNA gyrase B subunit	
Amikacin and kanamycin	rrs	16S rRNA	Inhibits protein synthesis
Capreomycin	rrs	16S rRNA	Inhibits protein synthesis
	tlyA	rRNA methyltransferase	

[a]Adapted from reference 154.

understood, it is likely that the process involves an oxidation reaction catalyzed by a catalase-peroxidase encoded by the *katG* gene (153). The oxidized form of INH can then covalently bind to the nicotinamide moiety of NAD(H) to form INH-NAD(H) adducts, which in turn compete with NAD(H) for binding to an enoyl-acyl carrier protein reductase encoded by the *inhA* gene (69).

The primary effect of INH is on mycolic acid synthesis, as evidenced by the increased fragility of the mycobacterial cell, increased intracellular viscosity, decreased cellular hydrophobicity, and loss of acid fastness of INH-resistant isolates (160). The mycolic acids are produced by the fatty acid synthesis (FAS) I and II enzyme systems. It is the FAS II system that synthesizes the long-chain mycolic acids that are species specific. Activated INH targets one of the FAS II enzymes, the enoyl-acyl carrier protein (ACP) reductase of InhA. However, InhA is not the only target, because activated INH also targets the fatty acid elongation enzyme ketoacyl-ACP synthase A (KasA). In addition, it has been proposed that INH may interfere with NAD metabolism, energy metabolism, and macromolecular synthesis (34, 161, 162).

The mechanism of action of INH correlates with the known mechanisms of INH resistance. Banerjee et al. (7) reported that INH and ethionamide resistance in MTBC correlated with a missense mutation in the *inhA* gene. Other studies showed that *katG* mutations account for 30 to 60% of INH resistance (59) and that *inhA* mutations confer a low level of INH resistance that may not always be clinically significant (90). Mutations in two other genes may confer some INH resistance: the *ahpC* gene, which encodes an alkyl hydroperoxide reductase subunit (35, 75, 139, 159, 171), and the *kasA* gene, which encodes the previously mentioned KasA enzyme (91). The degree to which mutations in *ahpC* and *kasA* contribute to INH resistance is not clear, although a study by Hazbon et al. (54) found that *ahpC* mutations were found only in INH-resistant strains, whereas *kasA* mutations were sometimes found in INH-susceptible strains.

INH is active only against replicating tubercle bacilli in the presence of oxygen; slowly replicating bacilli in the caseous lesions are not readily killed by INH, and dormant bacilli under anaerobic conditions are unlikely to be affected. INH resistance develops rapidly when patients are given monotherapy, and the frequency of INH resistance within a population of tubercle bacilli ranges from 10^{-5} to 10^{-6} (33). Wild-type isolates of MTBC are inhibited by INH at concentrations of <0.2 µg/ml. Other slowly growing mycobacteria, such as *M. kansasii* and *M. xenopi*, are inhibited by 1 to 5 µg/ml. *M. avium* complex (MAC) (92), most other NTM, and all rapidly growing mycobacteria are resistant to INH.

INH is well absorbed when administered orally or intramuscularly; it is distributed throughout the body, and the levels in cerebrospinal fluid (CSF) may equal the levels in plasma in patients with meningeal inflammation or 20% of the levels in plasma in patients without inflammation (157). INH is metabolized in the liver and intestines, primarily by acetylation by an *N*-acetyltransferase, which can vary significantly from person to person. However, the acetylator phenotype of an individual does not appear to influence either the efficacy of INH or the risk of hepatotoxicity. Adverse drug reactions include infrequent, age-related hepatitis, and, less frequently, peripheral neuropathy, hypersensitivity reactions such as fever and rash, and arthralgias.

Rifampin

Rifampin (RMP) (also known as rifampicin), introduced in 1968, affects intracellular, slowly replicating tubercle bacilli in caseous lesions as well as the actively replicating bacilli in open cavities. RMP is also active against a wide variety of non-acid-fast bacteria and several other slowly growing mycobacteria, notably, *M. leprae*, *M. kansasii*, *M. xenopi*, and *M. marinum*, but has variable activity in vitro against MAC and is inactive against the rapidly growing mycobacteria. It easily diffuses through the mycobacterial cell membrane due to its lipophilic nature. RMP inhibits transcription by binding to the β-subunit of the DNA-dependent RNA polymerase. Drug resistance develops when mutations occur in the *rpoB* gene encoding the β-subunit of the RNA polymerase (146). Studies showed that >96% of RMP resistance could be attributed to mutations within an 81-bp region of the *rpoB* gene (100). Rare mutations appear to cluster at codon 176 at the beginning of the *rpoB* gene (55) and are also found to be associated with RMP resistance.

RMP is well absorbed from the gastrointestinal tract, and peak concentrations of 5 to 10 µg/ml are reached 1 to 2 h after an oral dose of 600 mg; concentrations in CSF reach 50% of the levels in plasma in patients with meningeal inflammation. An RMP concentration of 0.5 µg/ml is bactericidal for wild-type isolates of *M. tuberculosis*. Adverse drug reactions include hepatotoxicity, gastrointestinal and hypersensitivity reactions, and a red-orange discoloration of urine, tears, other body fluids, and soft contact lenses. RMP also induces increased hepatic metabolism of several other drugs, including methadone and birth control pills. Of particular concern is the interaction of RMP and, to a somewhat lesser degree, rifabutin with protease inhibitors (saquinavir, ritonavir, and indinavir), which leads to enhanced hepatic metabolism and may result in subtherapeutic levels of the antiviral agents (10).

Rifabutin and Rifapentine

Rifabutin (ansamycin), a spiropiperidyl rifamycin, and rifapentine, a cyclopentyl rifamycin, have potent in vitro activity against MTBC (151). Rifabutin also is very active against MAC (58, 128). The mode of action and mechanism of resistance of both drugs appear to be identical to those of RMP; however, approximately 30% of RMP-resistant *M. tuberculosis* isolates are susceptible to rifabutin and rifapentine. The latter observation correlates with certain specific mutations in the *rpoB* gene (15). Yang et al. (168) analyzed clinical strains of MTBC for cross-resistance to rifamycins. Alterations at codons 513 and 531 correlate with resistance to RMP, rifabutin, and rifalazil (KRM-1648). Point mutations at codons 516 and 529, deletion at codon 518, and insertion at codon 514 influence susceptibility to RMP but not to rifabutin or KM-1648, while alteration at codons 515, 521, and 533 did not influence susceptibility to RMP, rifabutin, and KR-1648 (168). These findings were confirmed by analyzing recombinant *M. tuberculosis* clones containing plasmids with specific mutations (158). As with RMP, both rifabutin and rifapentine are metabolized to the corresponding biologically active 25-desacetyl metabolite. Rifabutin decreases the incidence of disseminated MAC disease in HIV-infected patients when used as a prophylactic agent, and it is approved for that indication (87, 104). The role of rifabutin as a therapeutic agent for MAC disease is unclear, but there may be a significant dose effect (66). In addition to being more active than RMP on a weight basis, rifabutin has a long elimination half-life in humans and concentrates in tissues, notably lung tissues, where the levels are 10-fold higher than in serum. This may account for the reported effectiveness of rifabutin in the therapy of MAC pulmonary infections.

Rifabutin is absorbed from the gastrointestinal tract and reaches peak levels of 0.5 μg/ml in serum about 4 h after a 300-mg dose. Adverse drug reactions with rifabutin are similar to those observed with RMP, including the above-mentioned important adverse interactions with antiretroviral agents (10). Some unique rifabutin toxicities include leukopenia, thrombocytopenia, arthralgias, and uveitis when coadministered with clarithromycin.

Rifapentine was approved by the U.S. Food and Drug Administration (FDA) for the treatment of TB in 1998 (5). In a study of 722 patients, 361 received rifapentine plus INH, PZA, and EMB while the remaining patients received RMP in place of rifapentine along with the other drugs (5). In the intensive phase of the study, rifapentine was administered twice a week while RMP was administered daily. In the continuation phase, rifapentine and INH were administered once a week and RMP and INH were administered twice a week. Sputum conversion was somewhat higher in the rifapentine group than in the RMP group: 87 and 81%, respectively. However, relapse was somewhat higher in the rifapentine group than in the RMP group: 10 and 5%, respectively. Rifapentine reaches a peak concentration of 15 μg/ml in serum 5 to 6 h after a 600-mg dose, with a half-life of about 13 h. Rifapentine is now being evaluated for use together with INH with weekly dosing in 12-week regimens for treatment of latent TB.

Ethambutol

EMB [dextro-2,2-(ethylenediimino)-di-1-butanol-dihydrochloride] is a synthetic antituberculosis compound that was introduced in 1961. The MIC values of EMB tested against wild-type isolates of MTBC range from 1 to 5 μg/ml, but the activity of the drug against other slowly growing NTM is more variable. The drug is active only against growing bacilli and has no activity against nongrowing mycobacteria. The primary mechanism of action of EMB is bacteriostatic inhibition of cell wall synthesis, while evidence points to a specific effect on arabinogalactan synthesis (143). In MTBC, the frequency of mutation to EMB resistance is on the order of 10^{-5}, and there is evidence that some EMB resistance correlates with a specific mutation (at codon 306) in the *embB* gene, which encodes an arabinosyltransferase (141, 142). Mutations in this codon have been associated with MIC values of 20 to 40 μg/ml (2). While mutations in the *embB* gene result in high-level resistance in MTBC, this mutation accounts for only 70% of resistant strains; thus, mutations in other genes are likely to play an additional role (154). Mutations at *embB* codon 306 may also affect susceptibility to other drugs used in the treatment of TB (127).

Many MAC isolates have high EMB MIC values, but combinations of EMB and other agents, notably quinolones and macrolides, appear to be synergistic (72). Additionally, it has been shown that the MIC value does not correlate with clinical response (138). It appears that EMB affects the permeability of the MAC cell wall and perhaps increases the intracellular concentration of the other potentially more active drugs (61).

Peak concentrations of EMB in serum are 5 μg/ml in 2 to 4 h after a dose of 25 mg/kg of body weight. The most important adverse effect associated with EMB is decreased visual acuity due to optic neuritis, which is related to both the dose and the duration of treatment. EMB is not recommended for the treatment of children too young to be monitored for changes in vision, unless no other drug is appropriate because of resistance. The effects on vision are generally reversible when the drug is discontinued.

Pyrazinamide

PZA is a synthetic derivative (pyrazine analog) of nicotinamide and, in combination with INH, is rapidly bactericidal for replicating and nonreplicating forms of M. *tuberculosis*, with an average MIC of 20 μg/ml (154). PZA is totally inactive against other *Mycobacterium* species, including M. *bovis* and the NTM. PZA is active only at an acidic pH; therefore, the pH of the growth medium must be adjusted for accurate measurements of the in vitro activity of the drug. It is most likely that PZA is active only in the acidic milieu of the phagolysosome and, depending on the concentration achieved at the site of the infection, may be bacteriostatic or bactericidal. PZA is hydrolyzed in the liver to the active metabolite pyrazinoic acid, and although the mechanism of action of PZA is only beginning to be understood (173), its activity depends on this conversion. M. *tuberculosis* produces a pyrazinamidase, and most strains of PZA-resistant M. *tuberculosis* lack this enzyme; however, some PZA-resistant isolates retain enzyme activity, suggesting that there are other mechanisms of resistance such as drug efflux (172, 174).

The lack of pyrazinamidase activity and its correlation with PZA resistance have been associated with mutations in the *pncA* gene, which encodes the enzyme (71, 133, 140). Indeed, it now appears that 72 to 97% of PZA resistance can be attributed to mutations in the *pncA* gene (Table 2). Data from one study suggest that this correlation can be used to distinguish between M. *tuberculosis* and M. *bovis* (132); however, PZA-susceptible M. *bovis* isolates, although rare, have been described.

PZA is well absorbed from the gastrointestinal tract and widely distributed throughout the body, with maximum levels in serum of approximately 45 μg/ml in 1 to 4 h following an oral dose of 1 g (20 to 25 mg/kg of body weight). Hepatotoxicity occurs in a small number of patients; photosensitivity and rash are rare. Gout is an important contraindication because of the hyperuricemia associated with PZA therapy. PZA therapy is usually discontinued after the first 2 months of short-course treatment for TB, whereas INH and RMP treatment is continued for an additional 4 months.

Ethionamide

Ethionamide (2-ethyl-pyridine-4-carbonic acid thioamide) is a derivative of isonicotinic acid and, like INH, blocks mycolic acid synthesis. However, isolates of MTBC that are resistant to high concentrations of INH are susceptible to ethionamide, suggesting that the site of action may be different from that of INH. However, mutations in the promoter of the *inh* gene have been associated with ethionamide resistance (7). The average MIC for MTBC is 0.6 to 2.5 μg/ml, and levels of 2 to 20 μg/ml in serum are achieved 3 to 4 h following an oral dose of 0.5 to 1 g. Side effects associated with ethionamide include gastrointestinal irritation with nausea, vomiting, and cramps and neurologic symptoms.

Aminoglycosides

The aminoglycosides that are used for the treatment of TB and other mycobacterial infections include SM, kanamycin (a glycoside of 2-deoxystreptamine), and amikacin, which is a derivative of kanamycin. Gentamicin is inactive against mycobacteria at the usual concentrations attained in serum, and tobramycin is active against M. *chelonae*.

The primary mechanism of action of the aminoglycosides is inhibition of the post- to pretranslocation step of protein synthesis by blocking the binding of the aminoacyl-tRNA (e-type binding). Viomycin also blocks aminoacyl-tRNA translocation, and viomycin resistance crosses to capreomycin, suggesting that the mechanism of action is the same. Amikacin is the most potent of the aminoglycosides. However, cross-resistance among the aminoglycosides often occurs when resistance mutations occur in *rrs* after being treated with amikacin, but resistance to SM or kanamycin may not cause cross-resistance to amikacin (88). Amikacin often is used in combination with one or more other agents for treatment of serious infections caused by rapidly growing mycobacteria. Amikacin also is active against MAC isolates; the majority have an MIC of <32 μg/ml, which approaches the maximum serum concentration. In an early uncontrolled trial of disseminated MAC in HIV-infected patients, amikacin was shown to be the active component of a multiple-drug regimen (28). In that trial, treatment was associated with a positive microbiological and clinical response, but the clinical utility of amikacin for disseminated disease is uncertain. The drug may be useful in an "induction" regimen to clear a bacteremia.

The molecular basis of SM resistance in MTBC (Table 2) results from mutations in the gene that encodes ribosomal protein S12 or from mutations in the 16S rRNA region, which is structurally linked to the S12 protein in the assembled ribosome (42, 76, 101). Finken et al. (42) showed that mutations in the *rpsL* gene coding for the S12 protein were present in 20 of 38 SM-resistant strains and that there was a mutation in the *rrs* gene, encoding 16S rRNA, in 9 strains. Nair et al. (101) determined the nucleotide sequence of the *rpsL* gene and showed that SM resistance, in a small number of isolates, appeared to be a result of point mutations at codon 43 of this gene, a site of SM resistance in *Escherichia coli*. Adverse drug reactions associated with aminoglycosides and peptide antibiotics include hearing loss, tinnitis, loss of balance, and renal failure.

Capreomycin

Capreomycin is a macrocyclic polypeptide antibiotic isolated from *Streptomyces mutabilis* subspecies *capreolus* (6). The mechanism of action is similar to that of the aminoglycosides; it interferes with translation. Capreomycin is generally considered to be a bacteriostatic agent but has been shown to be bactericidal in vitro against nonreplicating TB bacilli (57). Capreomycin is an important injectable drug used for treating drug-resistant TB. Mutations in the 16S rRNA gene (*rrs*) or *tlyA* gene can confer resistance to capreomycin (6, 89).

Quinolones

Ciprofloxacin, ofloxacin, levofloxacin, gatifloxacin, and moxifloxacin are fluorinated carboxyquinolones with good in vitro activity against multidrug-resistant and pansusceptible MTBC (17, 64, 68). MIC values of ciprofloxacin and ofloxacin against susceptible isolates of MTBC range from 0.25 to 3 μg/ml and from 0.5 to 2.5 μg/ml, respectively. Measurements of the early bactericidal activity of ciprofloxacin in patients with pulmonary TB suggested that the drug is effective at a high dosage (1,000 mg/day) (137). Fluoroquinolones have variable activity against MAC (169). Most *M. fortuitum* group isolates are susceptible to ciprofloxacin, whereas activity against *M. abscessus* and *M. chelonae* is more variable.

Both ofloxacin and levofloxacin are included in the panel of secondary antituberculosis drugs listed in M24 (31). The suggested susceptibility breakpoint for ofloxacin is 2 μg/ml for the agar proportion method (31). However, levofloxacin (the L-isomer of ofloxacin) is approximately twice as active against MTBC as ofloxacin in vitro. For this reason, protocols for susceptibility testing of levofloxacin are desirable. Data support levofloxacin susceptibility breakpoints of 2 μg/ml for BACTEC 460 and 1.5 μg/ml for BACTEC MGIT 960 and 1 μg/ml for agar proportion (83, 129).

The mechanism of action of all fluorinated quinolones is inhibition of DNA synthesis as a result of binding to the DNA gyrase (bacterial topoisomerase II) (118). Although this is the presumed mechanism of action in mycobacteria, fewer studies have been performed with mycobacteria than with other microorganisms. Takiff et al. (144) showed that quinolone resistance in MTBC can be ascribed to mutations in the *gyrA* and *gyrB* genes, which encode the DNA gyrase subunits (Table 2). In MTBC, fluoroquinolones function by binding to the bacterial enzyme-DNA complex, with suggested mechanisms being strand breakage, SOS-mediated autolysis, and replication blockage. When combined with various first-line antimycobacterial drugs, fluoroquinolones have shown greater reductions in CFUs within infected macrophages than the individual drugs alone. While there are no reports of cross-resistance between quinolones and other classes of antimycobacterial agents, there is cross-resistance within the quinolone class, such that reduced susceptibility to one quinolone may likely confer reduced efficacy to all quinolones (45).

Recently, moxifloxacin has received attention as being useful in the treatment of TB, especially multidrug-resistant cases. Although slightly delayed in the first few days of response, the antimycobacterial effect of moxifloxacin appears to be similar to that of INH after 5 days of treatment (38). The newer quinolones (sparfloxacin, gatifloxacin, and moxifloxacin) have lower MICs than levofloxicin, ciprofloxacin, and ofloxacin. Treatment studies with mice have shown moxifloxacin has the most bactericidal efficacy against MTBC, followed by sparfloxacin, levofloxicin, and ofloxacin (in that order). Against MTBC, moxifloxacin has a reported MIC of 0.12 to 0.5 μg/ml (45).

Ciprofloxacin is well absorbed from the gastrointestinal tract and is rapidly distributed throughout the body. Maximum concentrations in serum of 2.4 or 4.3 μg/ml are achieved 1 to 2 h after an oral dose of 500 or 750 mg, respectively. The elimination half-life of ciprofloxacin is 4 h in subjects with normal renal function. Maximum ofloxacin concentrations in serum are achieved 1 to 2 h after an oral dose. Following a single 400-mg dose, the concentration of ofloxacin in serum is 2.9 μg/ml; after a steady-state dose, it is 4.6 μg/ml. The maximum concentration of levofloxacin in serum is approximately twice that of the active form of ofloxacin at the same dosage. The efficacy of fluoroquinolones in the treatment of pulmonary TB may relate, in part, to the observation that these quinolones concentrate in lung tissue to levels at least four times greater than the concentration in serum. Adverse effects with ciprofloxacin and other fluoroquinolones may be less severe than with the other secondary agents (13).

p-Aminosalicylic Acid

p-Aminosalicylic acid (PAS) is an antifolate that is active against MTBC but inactive against most other mycobacteria. There is some evidence that PAS also may affect iron transport in MTBC and salicylic acid metabolism. The average MIC for susceptible isolates of MTBC is 1 μg/ml, and peak levels of 7 to 8 μg/ml are achieved in serum 1 to 2 h after a 4-g dose. PAS is incompletely absorbed in the gastrointestinal tract and is associated with significant gastrointestinal side effects; in combination with the need for large dosages

(10 to 12 g/day), this leads to frequent problems with treatment adherence.

Cycloserine

D-Cycloserine (4-amino-3-isooxazolidinone) is an analog of D-alanine that inhibits the synthesis of D-alanyl-D-alanine, an essential component of the mycobacterial cell wall. Cycloserine is active against all mycobacteria as well as several other types of bacteria. Although it is one of the secondary drugs for treatment of TB, in vitro susceptibility testing is not recommended due to technical problems with the test (31, 111). Peak levels in serum of 20 to 40 μg/ml are achieved 4 h following an oral dose of 250 mg. The drug is widely distributed through the body, including the CSF. There are significant adverse drug reactions associated with cycloserine treatment, notably, peripheral neuropathy and central nervous system dysfunction including seizures and psychotic disturbances.

Macrolides

Azithromycin and clarithromycin are the most important agents in the treatment of MAC disease and are effective and approved prophylactic agents for preventing disseminated disease in HIV-infected persons (51, 115, 170). These drugs also are useful in the treatment of disease caused by M. marinum, M. haemophilum, M. kansasii, M. simiae, and rapidly growing mycobacteria other than M. fortuitum. Indeed, they are viewed as potential cornerstones in the treatment of NTM infections (46). Azithromycin, an azalide (a subclass of macrolides), and clarithromycin are structurally similar to erythromycin and have modifications that improve their acid stability and increase their potency, half-life, achievable concentrations in tissue, and bioavailability without causing toxicity. These macrolides are bacteriostatic agents and inhibit the growth of microorganisms by binding to the 50S subunit of the prokaryotic ribosome, blocking protein synthesis at the peptidyltransferase step. Meier et al. (93) showed that both clarithromycin- and azithromycin-resistant mutants of M. intracellulare have a single-base mutation at adenine 2058 in the 23S rRNA gene, a site of mutation or methylation that has been associated with macrolide resistance in other bacteria (103). The same genetic basis for macrolide resistance was found in M. chelonae and M. abscessus (156).

The in vitro activity of azithromycin against MAC appears to be quite modest, with MIC values 32- to 64-fold above the maximum concentration in serum (67). The ability of azithromycin to concentrate in tissues most likely accounts for its therapeutic activity in animal studies and humans (69, 79). Azithromycin is rapidly absorbed from the gastrointestinal tract and widely distributed throughout the body. It has a terminal half-life of 68 h. The peak concentration in serum following a 500-mg dose is 0.4 to 0.6 μg/ml; however, the drug concentrates in tissues to high levels. In a small study with humans, the levels of azithromycin in polymorphonuclear neutrophils were nearly 1,000-fold higher than the levels in serum (3, 131).

Clarithromycin inhibits 90% of MAC isolates with MIC values of 0.25 to 0.5 μg/ml when measured by a radiometric broth macrodilution method at a neutral to slightly alkaline pH (the activities of all macrolides are strongly influenced by pH). Peak levels in serum of 2 to 3 μg/ml are achieved 5 to 6 h following a 500-mg dose; the concentrations in tissue are 4 to 5 times greater than the concentrations in serum, and the concentration in macrophages is 20 to 30 times greater. The elimination half-life is 5 to 7 h following a 500-mg dose twice a day.

Clofazimine

Clofazimine [3-(p-chloroanilino)-10-(p-chlorophenyl)-2, 10-dihydro-2-isopropyliminophenazine] is a substituted iminophenazine, bright red dye. It has weak bactericidal activity against M. leprae but is used in combination with RMP and dapsone as a conventional treatment regimen for leprosy. However, it may take up to 50 days of treatment before there is evidence of tissue antimicrobial activity, which may influence the length of time before there is a clinical response in the treatment of leprosy. Clofazimine has good in vitro activity against MAC isolates, but despite this, it appears to offer little in the treatment of disseminated disease (134). Indeed, treatment regimens that contained clofazimine have been associated with higher mortality than those that did not (27). The drug also has good in vitro activity against MTBC, but there is little or no information on the in vivo activity.

The mechanism of action of clofazimine is unknown; however, it is highly lipophilic and binds preferentially to mycobacterial DNA. The absorption of clofazimine following an oral dose is variable and ranges from 45 to 60%. The average concentrations in serum are 0.7 to 1.0 μg/ml following a dose of 100 to 300 mg. The half-life is extraordinarily long (estimated to be 70 days), and the drug tends to be deposited in fatty tissues and cells of the reticuloendothelial system. Adverse drug reactions are limited primarily to a pink or red discoloration of the skin, conjunctiva, cornea, and body fluids and gastrointestinal intolerance including pain, diarrhea, nausea, and vomiting.

Amithiozone

Amithiozone (thiacetazone, tibione, or panthrone) is a thiosemicarbazole that is active against MTBC, with an average MIC of 1 μg/ml for wild-type strains. Resistance develops quickly when monotherapy is given. Peak levels in serum of 1 to 4 μg/ml are achieved 1 to 2 h following an oral dose of 150 mg. Adverse drug reactions are gastrointestinal irritation and bone marrow suppression, and hepatotoxicity can occur in patients receiving concomitant INH. Additionally, there appears to be an association of Stevens-Johnson syndrome and severe epidermal necrolysis in HIV-infected patients with TB treated by regimens containing amithiozone (40, 47). Consequently, it is recommended that amithiozone not be used to treat patients known or suspected to be infected with HIV (107). Amithiozone is not available in the United States and is not used in Europe because of the adverse effects, but it has been used successfully in combination with INH for the treatment of TB in some African countries, where adverse effects are believed to be less severe.

Dapsone

Dapsone (diaminodiphenyl sulfone) is a synthetic compound that was shown to be active against M. leprae in the early 1940s. Due to the uncultivatibility of M. leprae, dapsone susceptibility testing of M. leprae cannot be performed. Dapsone is an antifolate that, like other inhibitors of folic acid synthesis, exerts primarily a bacteriostatic effect and is only weakly bactericidal. Dapsone is administered orally and is well absorbed and distributed throughout the body. Levels in tissue are approximately 2 μg/ml following a 200-mg dose. The drug has a long half-life in serum, of 10 to 50 h depending on the individual patient. Common adverse drug reactions include nausea, vomiting, anorexia, and methemaglobinemia; hematuria, rash, pruritus, and fever also can occur. Traditionally, dapsone is used in combination with RMP and clofazimine for the treatment of leprosy. Acedapsone is a diacetylated form of dapsone with an extraordinarily long half-life of 46 days; as a result, this drug is administered infrequently (e.g., five injections per year), with peak concentrations in tissue occurring 20 to 35 days after administration. Acedapsone is relatively inactive against M. *leprae*, but in vivo it is deacetylated to the parent compound.

New Antituberculosis Drugs in Development

Several new classes of drugs, including diarylquinoline, nitroimidazole, and oxazolidinone drugs, have shown promise for the treatment of pansusceptible as well as drug-resistant TB. These new drugs have unique and new action mechanisms, and there is no cross-resistance between these new drugs and the existing anti-TB drugs. Some show stronger bactericidal effects, which may result in shorter therapy durations. Furthermore, for treating HIV and TB coinfection, the new drugs seem to have lower interaction with proteinase inhibitors. These are potential advantages that remain to be proven by clinical trials. At the time of preparation of this chapter, no information was available about susceptibility testing for these drugs.

The antituberculosis potential of diarylquinoline drugs was reported in 2005 (4). One of these drugs, TMC207, is in phase II clinical trials and appears to reduce the time to conversion to a negative sputum culture for patients with MDR TB (36). Diarylquinolines have a new mechanism of antituberculosis action, inhibition of mycobacterial ATP synthase. Like the diarylquinolines, nitroimidazole compounds such as PA-824 have no known cross-resistance with existing antituberculosis drugs. They have a unique mechanism of action (136). PA-824 is in phase II clinical testing and has been shown to be effective in enhancing bactericidal activity when combined with RMP and/or PZA in a murine model of TB (145). The oxazolidinone drug linezolid has been demonstrated to be effective in treatment of TB, including MDR TB (78, 106). However, its cost and the frequent occurrence of side effects including neuropathy and anemia may limit its usefulness. Alternative dosing regimens may prove useful in reduction of treatment durations.

Drugs Used for Susceptibility Testing

Antimicrobial agents for susceptibility testing (reference powders) can be obtained directly from the manufacturer or from commercial sources. In the United States, most antimicrobial agents are also available from U.S. Pharmacopeial Convention, Inc., Reference Standards Order Department, 12601 Twinbrook Parkway, Rockville, MD 20852. The reference powder should be accompanied by information about its assay potency (in micrograms per milligram), expiration date, lot number, and storage condition, as well as the stability and solubility of the agent. Preparations formulated for therapeutic use in humans or animals should not be used. Unopened vials of powders should be stored as specified by the manufacturer, and opened containers should be stored in a desiccator at the recommended temperature. Stock solutions of most agents at 1,000 μg/ml or greater remain stable for at least 6 months at $-20°C$ and for 1 year at -70 to $-80°C$. Directions provided by the drug manufacturer should be followed in addition to these general recommendations. Paper disks impregnated with standardized amounts of the primary and secondary anti-TB drugs are available from commercial sources for use in the disk elution modification of the proportion method. Use of these disks obviates errors in weighing and dilution, as well as errors in labeling, because the disks are coded with the drug name and concentration. This technique provides results equivalent to those

obtained with solutions prepared from reference powders. Quality control (QC) testing should be performed with each new batch of antimicrobial agent (48).

DRUG SUSCEPTIBILITY TESTING OF *M. TUBERCULOSIS* COMPLEX

Drug Resistance

In the early 1960s, the WHO organized two meetings that led to the description of reliable criteria and techniques for testing MTBC for resistance to antituberculosis drugs (23, 24). The critical proportion for resistance on Löwenstein-Jensen slants varied according to the drug, e.g., 1% for INH and RMP and 10% for SM, EMB, PZA, ethionamide, kanamycin, and cycloserine. However, based on the experience of Russel and Middlebrook with 7H10 agar (126), the Centers for Disease Control and Prevention (CDC) recommended Middlebrook 7H10 agar and 1% as the critical proportion for all drugs (81).

Resistance is fundamentally a phenomenon linked to large initial bacterial populations. In pulmonary TB, the greatest populations are those prevailing in cavities, which can contain 10^7 to 10^9 organisms, whereas the populations found in hard caseous foci, the most common type of lesion, generally do not exceed 10^2 to 10^4 organisms (22). The greater frequency of resistance during treatment of cavitary TB was shown as early as 1949 (62, 63). David at CDC (33) demonstrated the probability distribution of drug-resistant mutants and in a fluctuation test showed that M. *tuberculosis* spontaneously mutated to resistance to INH, SM, EMB, and RMP. The highest proportions of mutants observed for INH at 0.2 μg/ml, SM at 2.0 μg/ml, EMB at 5.0 μg/ml, and RMP at 1.0 μg/ml were 3.5×10^{-6}, 3.8×10^{-6}, 0.5×10^{-4}, and 3.1×10^{-8}, respectively. Thus, the proportion of mutants resistant to INH and RMP would be in the order of 10^{-13}. Implicit in all the studies of the genetic basis of antimicrobial resistance in M. *tuberculosis* is that the MDR TB phenotype is the result of accumulative mutations rather than the acquisition of an MDR transfer factor (100).

Unique Features of TB That Affect Drug Susceptibility Testing

According to the generally accepted theory, resistance appearing during drug treatment is due to selection and multiplication of the resistant mutants preexisting in the tubercle bacillus population of the host. Inasmuch as the susceptible bacilli are the predominant part of the population, initial killing involves a greater number of microorganisms. The consequence is a sharp fall in the population of bacilli during the initial period of treatment. The rise due to multiplication of the resistant mutants occurs later. This "fall-and-rise" phenomenon, as demonstrated in the patient's sputum, was described in the late 1940s (32, 116).

In 1979, Mitchison (96) suggested the "special-populations" hypothesis to explain the action of the major antituberculous drugs against the various subpopulations of tubercle bacilli. The subpopulations include (i) rapidly growing bacilli in the pulmonary lesions; (ii) bacilli that grow in short metabolic spurts and that might be susceptible to RMP but not INH; (iii) bacilli that reside in the acidic environment of the caseous lesions; and (iv) dormant, nonreplicating bacilli. The hypothesis was developed to explain in part the basis of the early bactericidal activity and the later sterilizing activity of antituberculosis agents. One of the reasons for the success of the conventional multiple-drug regimen for TB is that the different drugs each make a unique contribution in eradicating tubercle bacilli within each of these special populations. Thus, the use of multiple drugs in the treatment of TB is aimed at both preventing drug resistance and achieving a maximum therapeutic effect. The existence of subpopulations with differing metabolic status also means that conventional pharmacokinetic studies will not predict the effectiveness of treatment regimens for TB (21).

Critical Concentrations

The criteria for defining drug-resistant MTBC were established on an empirical basis, i.e., that there is a certain proportion of drug-resistant mutants above which therapeutic success is less likely to be realized. The procedures used to perform drug susceptibility tests and the criteria for interpreting the results take into account two factors: (i) the critical proportion of drug-resistant mutants and (ii) the critical concentration of the drug in the test medium. On the basis of clinical and bacteriologic studies, the significant proportion of bacilli resistant to an antituberculosis drug above which a clinical response is unlikely was generally set at 1%. The critical concentration of a drug is the concentration that inhibits the growth of most cells within the population of a wild-type strain of tubercle bacilli without appreciably affecting the growth of the resistant mutant cells that might be present. In other words, if the proportion of tubercle bacilli that are resistant to the critical concentration of a drug exceeds 1%, it is unlikely that the use of that drug will lead to a therapeutic success. It should be noted that this concentration may not have a direct relationship to the peak level of the drug in serum. The critical concentrations of antituberculosis drugs, in different media, are given in Table 3 (31, 77, 80, 83, 121, 125).

Low versus High Critical Concentrations

On occasion, the agar proportion method or commercial broth systems may indicate that an isolate of MTBC is resistant to INH or EMB at the critical concentration of the drug (Table 3). When this occurs, reflexively testing the higher concentration is recommended, although there is not uniform consensus regarding the clinical relevance of the results of testing at a higher concentration when two concentrations are used (31).

For INH, low-level resistance may be suggestive of resistance to ethionamide (154). Additionally, when an isolate is resistant to the low INH concentration but susceptible to the high concentration, therapeutic effect may be achieved with an adjustment in INH dosage. The CLSI recommends that the following comment be appended to the results (31):

These test results indicate low-level resistance to INH. In general, INH should be discontinued if there is any level of resistance, especially if sufficient effective drugs (preferably other primary agents and fluoroquinolones) remain available to create a regimen with a high likelihood of cure. However, some experts believe that patients infected with MDR strains exhibiting low level INH resistance, and for which few other effective drugs remain available, may benefit from continuing INH therapy. A specialist in the treatment of drug-resistant tuberculosis should be consulted concerning the appropriate therapeutic regimen and dosages.

Extent of Service

While the rate of occurrence of TB is decreasing in the United States and some other industrialized countries, drug-resistant TB is increasing in countries that are sources for immigration. Mycobacteriology laboratories may experience

TABLE 3 Test concentrations[a] of antimycobacterial agents against *M. tuberculosis*

| Antimicrobial agent | Medium and concn(s) (μg/ml)[b] | | | | |
| | Liquid systems | | | Agar proportion | |
	BACTEC 460	MGIT 960	VersaTrek	7H10	7H11
First line agents					
RMP[c]	2	1	1	1	1
INH[d]	0.1, 0.4	0.1, 0.4	0.1, 0.4	0.2, 1	0.2, 1
PZA	100	100	300	NR[e]	NR[e]
EMB[d]	2.5, 7.5	5	5, 8	5, 10	7.5
Second line agents					
INH-high[d]	0.4	0.4	0.4	1	1
EMB-high[d]	7.5		8	10	
Amikacin	1	1		4	
Capreomycin	1.25	2.5		10	10
Ethionamide	2.5	5		5	10
Kanamycin	5	2.5		5	6
Levofloxacin	2	1.5		1	
Ofloxacin	2	2		2	
PAS	4			2	8
Rifabutin[c]	0.5	0.5		0.5	0.5
SM[f]	2, 6	1, 4		2, 10	2, 10

[a]Where more than one concentration for an agent is listed, the lower concentration is the "critical concentration."

[b]The concentrations shown are from reference 31.

[c]About 30% of RMP-resistant isolates are rifabutin susceptible.

[d]INH and EMB may first be tested at the critical concentration. When INH or EMB has tested resistant at the critical concentration, the higher concentration of the drugs may be tested with other second-line agents.

[e]NR, not recommended.

[f]Laboratories may choose to test only the lower concentration.

reduced numbers of patient cultures or specimens requiring drug susceptibility testing, at the same time that new rapid molecular technologies are becoming available. These changing conditions may warrant a reexamination of which laboratories should be performing drug susceptibility testing. Laboratories that are unable to maintain expertise or cost-effectiveness due to low volumes of testing and laboratories that are unable to take advantage of new, more rapid technologies should consider referring specimens or cultures to reference laboratories. The time lost due to referring cultures to a reference laboratory may be more than offset by the use of rapid techniques in the reference laboratory.

When To Perform Drug Susceptibility Tests

The CDC and CLSI guidelines recommend that the first isolate of MTBC obtained from each patient be tested for susceptibility to the primary drugs (31, 148). This ensures the most effective treatment for a patient and contributes to the surveillance database for TB control. Susceptibility testing should be repeated if cultures fail to convert to negative after 3 months of therapy or if there is clinical evidence of failure to respond to therapy. If a laboratory is unable to provide this service, then isolates should be referred to another laboratory for timely testing.

Second-line drug susceptibility testing should be performed when resistance to RMP or any two first-line drugs is detected. In addition, when an isolate exhibits monoresistance to the critical concentration of INH, it should also be tested for susceptibility to secondary agents if the clinician is planning to include a fluoroquinolone in the treatment regimen (31).

When To Report Drug Resistance

Drug susceptibility results should be reported as soon as possible. When drug resistance is detected, the attending physician should be notified as soon as possible in addition to sending a written report. If repeat testing is required to confirm the drug resistance, a preliminary report indicating that drug resistance has been detected and retesting is in progress should be issued as soon as possible, and the physician should also be notified. Once the initial resistance has been confirmed, a final report should be issued. When delay in drug susceptibility testing is anticipated due to culture impurity, a preliminary report indicating so should be issued.

Methods of Drug Susceptibility Testing of *M. tuberculosis* Complex

The methods generally accepted for determining the antimicrobial susceptibility of *M. tuberculosis* complex are based on the growth of the microorganisms on solid or in liquid medium containing a specified concentration of a single drug. Four culture-based methods have been described: the proportion method, the modified proportion method using commercial broth systems, the absolute-concentration method, and the resistance ratio method (49, 58, 68). Only the agar proportion and the commercial broth systems are discussed further in this chapter; the last two are described elsewhere (58). Commercial broth systems include the BACTEC 460 system and two automatic, nonradiometric methods: the MGIT 960 system (Becton Dickinson) (50, 112, 113) and the VersaTREK MYCO TB susceptibility system (formerly called the ESP Culture System II; Trek Diagnostic Systems, Inc., Cleveland, OH). The MB/BacT system is available outside the United States (20, 37).

Based on the CLSI guidelines (31), a rapid broth susceptibility testing method should be used in conjunction with rapid methods of primary culture and identification to provide drug susceptibility results within 28 days of receipt of the specimens in the laboratory (148). The recommended rapid broth methods for susceptibility testing of MTBC are commercial systems that have been cleared by the FDA. Before implementing any such rapid broth system, one should validate the system by using a standardized reference method.

Agar Proportion Method

The agar proportion method for drug susceptibility testing of MTBC was developed in the early 1960s by G. Canetti (23, 24). The method was subsequently modified and standardized and has been considered the standard method of susceptibility testing of MTBC to all drugs except PZA in the United States and many European countries for years. The preferred medium for agar proportion is Middlebrook 7H10 agar. Drugs can be either prepared from reference powders (agar diffusion) or added as drug-impregnated disks (disk elution) (49, 77). With regard to testing PZA, the BACTEC 460 is considered the reference method (31). The performance of PZA testing by BACTEC MGIT 960 was found to be equivalent to that by BACTEC 460 (112, 130).

Media

In an effort to provide uniformity in the drug susceptibility testing of MTBC by the agar proportion method, Middlebrook 7H10 agar supplemented with oleic acid-albumin-dextrose-catalase (OADC) is the recommended standard medium (31, 77, 81). Most clinical isolates of MTBC grow on this medium, and under a dissecting microscope, the transparency of 7H10 agar facilitates the recognition of mixed mycobacterial species or the presence of contaminants. Occasionally, the drug susceptibility test may be invalid due to insufficient growth of drug-resistant strains of MTBC on 7H10 medium. To test those isolates, 7H11 medium may be substituted for 7H10 agar and higher concentrations of some drugs should be used, as shown in Table 3 (52, 68). It has been demonstrated that QC of the medium, especially the OADC supplement, is critical (48).

Inoculum and Incubation

The source of the inoculum for a susceptibility test by agar proportion may be growth from a primary culture or a subculture of a solid medium or broth (indirect method) or a specimen that is smear positive for acid-fast bacilli (direct method). The total incubation duration is 3 weeks.

For the indirect method, the source of the inoculum is a pure culture, usually from the primary isolation media. Careful attention should be paid to the selection of colony types so that the final inoculum is representative of all types present to ensure that there is a balance of potentially resistant and susceptible bacilli. A sufficient number of colonies must be selected to make a suspension that is equivalent to a 1.0 McFarland standard. If there is insufficient growth, a subculture into Dubos Tween-albumin or 7H9 broth should be made and incubated at 35 to 37°C until the turbidity matches a 1.0 McFarland standard. The suspension should not contain clumps of organisms. The actual number of CFU per milliliter is likely to vary from suspension to suspension, so that two dilutions (usually 10^{-2} and 10^{-4}) of the suspension must be used to inoculate two sets of media. If there is scant growth, 10^{-1} and 10^{-3} dilutions should be used or the isolate should be subcultured in broth until sufficient growth is obtained. Positive broth cultures from commercial systems may also be used to prepare cell suspensions.

TABLE 4 Guidelines for selection of the dilution of a specimen concentrate prior to inoculation of 7H10 medium for susceptibility testing using the direct method

Dilutions to test[a]	No. of acid-fast bacilli/field observed with:		
	Carbol fuchsin stain[b]	Fluorochrome stain	WHO report
Undiluted, 10^{-2}	<1	<25	2+
10^{-1}, 10^{-3}	1–10	25–250	3+
10^{-2}, 10^{-4}	>10	>250	4+

[a]Dilutions of a concentrated specimen are prepared based on the number of bacilli observed in the initial acid-fast smear. Sterile distilled water is used to prepare the dilutions; the carbol fuchsin stain is examined with the oil immersion objective (1,000×), and the fluorochrome stain is examined with the high-dry objective (450×). If the patient is receiving therapy, not all bacilli observed in the smear may be viable; therefore, the undiluted specimen should be tested as well as the appropriate dilution based on the microscopic criteria given in this table.

[b]From reference 77.

For the direct method, the inoculum is either a digested, decontaminated clinical specimen or an untreated, normally sterile body fluid, in which acid-fast bacilli are seen in stained smears. To ensure adequate but not excessive growth in the direct susceptibility test, specimens are diluted according to the number of organisms observed in the stained smear of the clinical specimen. A typical dilution scheme is shown in Table 4. Theoretically, this type of inoculum is more representative of the population of the tubercle bacilli in a particular lesion in the host. It is prudent to include an undiluted inoculum if the smear-positive specimen is from a patient who is receiving antimicrobial therapy, because a significant proportion of the bacilli seen on the smear may be nonviable. The direct susceptibility test has two major advantages. First, results can be reported within 3 weeks from the time of specimen receipt in the laboratory for a majority of smear-positive specimens. Second, the proportion of resistant bacteria better represents the bacterial population in the patient. Use of the direct method may be warranted when drug-resistant TB is suspected or in a region where the prevalence of drug-resistant TB is high. However, cost can become a critical factor when there is a high incidence of smear-positive specimens containing NTM. Also, it is not possible to accurately calibrate the inoculum, which may result in insufficient or excessive growth on drug-free quadrants and render the test invalid. In addition, if contaminants grow, results are not interpretable. The rate of failure for direct susceptibility testing can reach 15% or more, necessitating retesting by the indirect method.

Quadrant plates are commonly used for agar proportion, and 0.1 ml (about 3 drops from a Pasteur pipette) of each dilution of the inoculum is placed onto each quadrant, using one dilution per set of plates. After inoculation, the plates are allowed to dry thoroughly in the biosafety cabinet. After the plates are dried, they may be placed in CO_2-permeable polyethylene bags (clear sandwich bags), or sealed individually with CO_2-permeable tapes. They then are incubated at 35 to 37°C in 5 to 10% CO_2 in air. The plates must be protected from light during storage and incubation to prevent the formation of formaldehyde from the medium ingredients. As a good practice, after 1 week of incubation, the drug plates should be checked for presence of contaminants. If contaminants are present, the susceptibility test should be repeated with a pure isolate.

Reading and Interpreting Results

The criterion for resistance in MTBC is based on the fact that when the proportion of resistant mutants to a drug exceeds 1%, the drug will not have adequate therapeutic efficacy (24). In the proportion method, the percent resistance is obtained by dividing the colony count on the drug-containing quadrant by the colony count on the control quadrant. When the percent resistance is greater than 1%, the isolate is considered resistant to the drug.

For a valid test, the control quadrant of the lower dilution should have at least 50 colonies. If there are fewer than 50 colonies on the control quadrant of the lower dilution (10^{-2} or 10^{-1}) by 3 weeks, this indicates insufficient growth, and the test is invalid and should be repeated. The total incubation period is 3 weeks; however, if mature colonies appear on the control quadrant in less than 3 weeks, resistant results can be reported. Susceptible results should not be reported until week 3. If cultures are incubated beyond 3 weeks, false resistance may result due to degradation of the antimicrobial compound.

Colonial morphology and pigmentation should be carefully examined grossly and microscopically for compatibility with MTBC and absence of NTM or other organisms. This is especially critical when the susceptibility test is performed by the direct method. Small colonies of rapid growers, as well as the rough, dry colonies of some MAC strains, may appear similar to MTBC colonies on 7H10 agar. Also, rapidly growing mycobacteria may be slow to grow on primary isolation media, and they will appear as MDR TB when tested against primary antituberculosis agents. Susceptibility testing results by the direct method must never be reported without a preliminary identification of the organism.

Microcolonies may be observed when using the agar proportion method, especially when testing EMB. Several possibilities may account for the presence of microcolonies: growth of susceptible organisms in the presence of degraded drug, true resistance, or partial resistance. One study reported that most strains that had microcolonies in the EMB quadrant had EMB-susceptible results when tested with the BACTEC 460 method (118a). The significance of microcolonies is unknown, and each laboratory should determine how to best report these findings, based on its own in-house experience. With advances in molecular technologies, testing for the presence of drug-resistance associated mutations may help differentiate true resistance from growth of susceptible organisms due to degraded drugs.

Quality Control

M. tuberculosis H37Rv (ATCC 27294), which is susceptible to all primary and secondary antituberculosis drugs, is recommended for QC. Strains of *M. tuberculosis* that are resistant to INH, RMP, and/or other drugs are available from the American Type Culture Collection; however, these strains are resistant to high concentrations of the respective drugs and are not ideal for QC testing. Ideally, a strain of MTBC that shows resistance at or near the cutoff values of a particular drug should be used for QC. A number of strains used in the CDC's Model Performance Evaluation Program offer these characteristics. Also, for safety considerations, it is not advisable to use a single MTBC strain that is resistant to more than two drugs. Aliquots of suspensions of QC strains of *M. tuberculosis*, adjusted to match a 1.0 McFarland standard in 7H9 broth, can be stored at −70°C for up to

6 months. QC testing should be performed with each new batch of medium or antimicrobial agent, and media should be checked for sterility and shown to support adequate growth. Guthertz et al. (48) demonstrated the importance of controlling for all components of 7H10 agar including lots of Middlebrook 7H10 agar, glycerol, and especially OADC.

The MGIT 960 System

In 1995, the MGIT was introduced for the growth and detection of mycobacteria from clinical specimens (50). Each MGIT tube contains modified Middlebrook 7H9 broth, and in the bottom is a fluorescence-quenching-based oxygen sensor (silicon rubber impregnated with ruthenium pentahydrate). When actively growing organisms utilize the dissolved oxygen, reduced oxygen concentration enables the generation of fluorescence, which is then measured and expressed as growth units (GU). The MGIT 960 system is a fully automated system that continuously monitors the growth of microorganisms hourly through fluorescence detection. The system uses a nonradiometric medium and does not require use of needles for addition of growth supplement or inoculation of organisms. In 2002, the system was approved by the FDA for susceptibility testing of MTBC to INH, RMP, EMB, PZA, and the secondary agent SM. Several studies showed that the performance of the MGIT 960 system for testing primary drugs is equivalent to that of the BACTEC 460 system and the agar proportion method and that the time to results is comparable to that for the BACTEC 460 (9, 80, 112, 124, 130). The MGIT 960 system has been widely adopted, replacing the BACTEC 460 system in many laboratories.

The MGIT SIRE drug kit containing lyophilized INH, RMP, EMB, and SM and the SIRE supplement is specifically designed for testing susceptibility to these four drugs with the MGIT 960 system. The MGIT 960 employs a two-tier test protocol. The first tier includes the above four drugs, although SM is a secondary agent and need not be tested initially, being tested at concentrations equivalent to the critical concentrations of the agar proportion method (i.e., SM, 1.0 μg/ml; INH, 0.1 μg/ml; RMP, 1.0 μg/ml; and EMB, 5.0 μg/ml). If there is resistance to INH, the laboratory may choose to test at 0.4 μg/ml. Although MGIT 960 is not FDA approved for testing second-line drugs, several studies validated the use of MGIT 960 for testing the susceptibility of MTBC, including multidrug-resistant strains, to several secondary agents (80, 83, 86, 121, 125).

Inoculum and Incubation

The inoculum for drug susceptibility testing may be prepared from either liquid or solid media. To ensure accuracy and reproducibility of results, strict adherence to the guidelines of the manufacturer is imperative. In an MGIT drug susceptibility test set, there are drug-containing MGIT tubes and a growth control tube (without drugs). The pre-inoculation preparation includes the addition of 0.8 ml of the SIRE supplement to every MGIT tube in the set and 0.1 ml of a specific drug solution to each designated drug-containing tube.

When a positive MGIT tube is used as the inoculum source, according to the manufacturer's package insert, the MGIT can be tested within 1 to 2 days after growth is detected by the instrument, or it can be tested with a 1:5 dilution within 3 to 5 days following detection of growth. If growth is detected after more than 5 days, the growth in this MGIT tube is too heavy for drug susceptibility testing. The MGIT tube must be subcultured to a blank MGIT tube and incubated; the seeded MGIT tube can be tested following the manufacturer's time schedule described above after it becomes positive. If the growth of the seeded MGIT tube is detected in <4 days, the growth is too heavy or the culture is not pure. The proper inoculum for seeding is about 1:100 of a 0.5 MacFarland standard. The MGIT tube or the 1:5 dilution tube, according to the manufacturer's time schedule, must be mixed well and then used to inoculate the drug-containing MGIT tubes. The inoculum used for the drug-containing MGIT is further diluted 100-fold for inoculating the growth control. The volume of each inoculum is 0.5 ml.

When the inoculum is prepared from a solid medium, the isolate must not be older than 14 days after the first appearance of colonies on the medium. To ensure obtaining diverse populations, growth should be taken from different parts of the medium. The suspension is adjusted to equal the turbidity of a 0.5 McFarland standard and then diluted 1:5 with 7H9 broth or MGIT medium before inoculation of the drug-containing MGIT tubes. The growth control tube is inoculated with 1:100 dilution of the cell suspension used to inoculate a drug-containing tube.

After inoculation of drug-containing MGIT tubes and the growth control tube, the MGIT drug test set is registered into the MGIT 960 system with a proper drug panel. It is important to select a panel that matches the drug set being inoculated. The growth in each MGIT tube is automatically monitored by the MGIT 960 system.

Reading and Interpreting Results

When the GU of the growth control reaches 400 within 4 to 13 days, the MGIT 960 system flags the completion of a drug test and interprets the drug susceptibility results based on the following rules. An isolate is called resistant to a drug when the GU of the drug-containing MGIT tube is greater than 100, and it is called susceptible when the GU of the drug-containing MGIT tube is equal to or less than 100. The test is invalid if the GU of the growth control reaches 400 in less than 4 days, indicating that the growth is too fast (the inoculum either is too heavy or contains contaminants), or in more than 13 days, indicating that the growth is too slow (the inoculum is too light, or the medium does not support the growth).

When a drug test is completed, the MGIT 960 system allows the user to print a drug susceptibility report. It is important to verify the drug order of the MGIT tubes against the drug order on the report, especially when the report contains resistant results. It is important to verify any resistant result by excluding apparent resistance due to the presence of NTM or other bacteria before a preliminary report is issued. The following steps are helpful for verification of resistant results. First, examine the broth in the MGIT tube with a resistant result. MTBC usually grows as small clumps and settles in the bottom of the tube, and the broth usually remains clear. Without disturbing the MGIT tubes, if the broth appears turbid, the presence of NTM or other bacteria may be suspected. Second, perform an acid-fast stain on a smear made from an MGIT tube with a resistant result to confirm that the cellular morphology is compatible with that of MTBC and that there does not appear to be NTM or other bacteria. MTBC usually appears as cording or tight clumps. Although antituberculosis agents may alter the typical cording morphology, a dispersed distribution of acid-fast bacilli or random loose clumps throughout the entire smear suggests the presence of NTM. When, on rare occasions, differentiating MTBC from NTM is difficult, it is advisable to make a subculture from the MGIT tube showing drug resistance onto 7H10 or 7H11. Examining the microscopic colonial morphology in a few days usually will help to differentiate MTBC from other mycobacteria.

When any drug result obtained with the MGIT 960 system is questionable, repeat testing of the isolate by agar proportion or with MGIT 960 should be performed. If a culture contains non-acid-fast bacteria or NTM, a pure culture of MTBC must be obtained before retesting is attempted. Because reisolation of MTBC may take several weeks, molecular testing for drug resistance mutations should be considered. Each laboratory should determine its own policy with regard to the necessity of retesting to confirm initial resistant results. As a good practice of quality assurance, when a laboratory first implements the MGIT 960 system or testing personnel are newly trained to use the system, reproducibility should be documented. In addition, retesting an isolate to confirm rarely occurring resistant results such as mono-RMP resistance or mono-EMB resistance should be considered.

Quality Control

A reference strain such as H37Rv (ATCC 27294) that is susceptible to all primary drugs should be tested with each lot of SIRE drug kit and MGIT medium received. It should also be tested with each test run or once a week if multiple test runs are preformed each week (31).

Testing PZA

PZA susceptibility testing by the MGIT 960 system became commercially available in 2002. The MGIT PZA testing uses the same platform as previously described for the primary drugs. Differences are as follows. (i) The broth in the MGIT PZA tube has a reduced pH. (ii) The PZA drug kit contains PZA and PZA supplement, which is not interchangeable with the SIRE supplement. (iii) The PZA growth control is inoculated with a 1:10 dilution of the inoculum to PZA-containing MGIT tubes. The preinoculation preparation includes the addition of 0.8 ml of MGIT PZA supplement and 0.1 ml of PZA solution (100 μg/ml). Inoculum preparation from positive MGIT tubes or from a solid medium and interpretation criteria are the same as that for primary drugs. In contrast to BACTEC 460TB, the PZA "borderline" category does not exist with MGIT 960.

The procedure for verification of the instrument-determined resistance applies to PZA resistance as well. Since mono-PZA resistance is rare for *M. tuberculosis*, retesting of PZA to confirm the initial resistance and further identification to species level (i.e., *M. tuberculosis* versus *M. bovis*) are recommended.

The BACTEC 460TB Method

Due to the increasing popularity of nonradiometric systems for susceptibility testing of MTBC, use of the BACTEC 460TB system has diminished. Drawbacks of the BACTEC 460TB include the use of radioactive materials, the requirement for using needles for inoculation and sampling of cultures, and the possibility of cross-contamination by the BACTEC 460TB instrument.

The BACTEC 460TB system uses BACTEC 12B medium containing [^{14}C]palmitic acid, which is metabolized by organisms, resulting in the production of $^{14}CO_2$. The instrument quantitatively detects the amount of $^{14}CO_2$ released, expressed in terms of growth index (GI), proportional to the rate and amount of growth.

Like the MGIT 960 system, the BACTEC 460TB can be used to test primary drugs (RMP, INH, PZA, and EMB), as well as SM and the other secondary drugs (111). As with other liquid culture systems, it does not allow an estimate

of the percentage of resistant bacilli and is vulnerable to major errors (false resistance) due to the presence of mixed culture of mycobacterial species or contaminants (105). Therefore, verification of an instrument-determined resistance is critical, as described for the MGIT 960 system.

Three of the primary drugs (INH, RMP, and EMB) and SM are available as lyophilized powders from the manufacturer. Alternatively, stock solutions of these agents can be prepared from reference powders. Lyophilized vials of PZA are also available for the pH 6.0 modified BACTEC PZA test medium. The secondary drugs must be prepared from reference powders. Critical concentrations for most of these drugs have been established, and the results of the radiometric and proportion methods correlate well (111).

Inoculum and Incubation

As with the MGIT system, the source of inoculum should be fresh growth of actively growing bacilli, and the control vial uses a 1:100 dilution of the inoculum used for the drug-containing vial. Before inoculation, BACTEC 12B vials must be prerun in the BACTEC 460TB instrument to establish a gas phase of 5% CO_2 in air in the headspace of the vial. Inoculated vials are incubated at 37 ± 1°C in the dark. Refer to the manufacturer's manual for detailed inoculation procedures.

Reading and Interpreting Results

Vials are read on the BACTEC 460TB instrument at intervals of 24 ± 1 h. An alternative, nonweekend schedule has been described (53). If the GI of the control is ≥30 in <4 days (the inoculum is too heavy, or the vial contains NTM or other bacteria) or >12 days (the inoculum is too light, or the medium does not support the growth), the test is invalid. When the GI of the control is ≥30 after a minimum of 4 days, the difference in GI from one day to the next, designated the ΔGI, should be interpreted as follows:

$$\Delta GI \text{ of control} > \Delta GI \text{ of drug} = \text{susceptible}$$

$$\Delta GI \text{ of control} < \Delta GI \text{ of drug} = \text{resistant}$$

If the GI of a drug-containing vial is ≥500 on the next reading, the isolate is considered resistant to that drug regardless of the ΔGI in comparison to that of the control. However, if overinoculation or contamination may be the cause for the high GI, the test should be repeated with a pure culture and proper inoculum.

A PZA test can be interpreted when the GI of the control reaches 200 in 4 to 21 days. The isolate is considered susceptible to PZA if the GI of the PZA vial is <9% of the GI of the control, and the isolate is considered resistant if the GI of the PZA vial is >11% of that of the control. If the GI of the test vial is 9 to 11% of that of the control, the result is borderline. Resistance to PZA alone should prompt identification of the isolate to the species level.

Quality Control

A reference strain such as H37Rv (ATCC 27294), susceptible to all primary drugs, should be tested with each new batch of drugs and BACTEC 12B medium. It should also be tested with each test run or once a week if multiple test runs are performed each week (31).

VersaTREK

VersaTREK (formerly called ESP Culture System II; Trek Diagnostic Systems, Inc.) is a fully automated, continuously monitoring system for growth and detection of mycobacteria

(165), which allows testing of the susceptibility of MTBC to all primary drugs. VersaTREK technology is based on detection of pressure changes (oxygen consumption due to microbial growth) within the headspace above the broth culture medium in a sealed bottle. The culture medium consists of a Middlebrook 7H9 broth, which has been enriched with growth supplement (glycerol and Casitone), and contains cellulose sponges to increase the surface area for exposure to oxygen and as a growth support matrix. Before the medium is inoculated with an isolate, growth and antibiotic supplements must be added using a syringe.

Inoculum and Incubation

VersaTREK Myco susceptibility kit contains lyophilized drugs and diluent. The working drug solutions are prepared by reconstituting the drugs with 25 ml of the diluent. Preparation of the bottles for drug susceptibility testing requires the addition of 1.0 ml of growth supplement and 0.5 ml of antibiotic working solution. The final concentrations in the Myco bottles are as follows: INH, 0.1 µg/ml; RMP, 1.0 µg/ml; and EMB, 5.0 µg/ml. INH and EMB can be tested at higher concentrations (0.4 and 8.0 µg/ml, respectively). The final concentration for PZA is 300 µg/ml. The inoculum can be prepared from either solid media (e.g., Löwenstein-Jensen or 7H10/7H11) or liquid media (e.g., VersaTREK Myco or 7H9). The turbidity of the cell suspension is standardized to equal the density of a 1.0 McFarland standard, and a 1:10 dilution of the suspension is used for the inoculation of the drug-containing VersaTREK Myco bottles and the control bottle. The inoculum is 0.5 ml. The inoculated Myco bottles are kept in the instrument at 35°C, and growth is automatically monitored every 24 minutes.

Reading and Interpreting Results

Susceptibility results are manually determined. A drug susceptibility test is valid for interpretation when the time to detection of growth in the control bottle (without drugs) is within 3 to 10 days of inoculation. Drug-containing bottles are monitored for another 3 days after the control bottle has turned positive. An isolate is considered resistant to a drug if the time to detection of growth in the drug-containing bottle is less than or equal to 3 days after that for the control bottle. An isolate is considered susceptible if no growth occurs in the drug-containing bottle or if the time to growth detection is more than 3 days after that for the control bottle. A small number of studies demonstrate good agreement among the VersaTREK Myco system, the BACTEC 460TB, and the agar proportion method. Detection times are very comparable to those obtained by the radiometric method (11, 123).

Quality Control

Each new lot of VersaTREK Myco Susceptibility Kit, Myco bottles, and growth supplement must be tested with strains of MTBC appropriate for QC. A pansusceptible strain of MTBC should be included with each testing run (31).

Alternative Susceptibility Testing Methods

Since 2000, drug susceptibility testing of mycobacteria has become a very dynamic field, spawning many new technologies that may prove successful in a clinical laboratory. Some of these techniques are based on improved methods for measuring inhibition of growth, while others are based on molecular detection of mutations associated with resistance (8, 29, 60, 82, 84, 94, 95, 109, 114).

The microscopic observation drug susceptibility (MODS) broth culture system has been developed for detection of MTBC and drug susceptibility testing. Unlike the broth culture systems mentioned above, the microscopic observation drug susceptibility method does not require the use of proprietary culture media purchased from a single source. Middlebrook 7H9 broth medium, supplemented with OADC and a selective antibiotic/antifungal cocktail, is used in 24-well microtiter plates (99). As described by Moore et al., 12 wells are used for each specimen, including 4 control wells with no antituberculosis drug, and 8 drug-containing wells including low and high concentrations of INH, RMP, EMB, and SM. Growth or inhibition of the organisms in the drug-containing wells is detected by observation using an inverted microscope. The method enables rapid detection of growth and provides a quick indication of susceptibility or resistance to the primary drugs. Because proprietary media are not used and ingredients can be purchased from a variety of suppliers, the method is relatively inexpensive. Safety concerns regarding the use of the 24-well microtiter plate may have been addressed by the practice of enclosing the plates in sealed plastic bags and making the microscopic observations through the bags without opening them. MTBC can be tentatively identified, especially in high-prevalence settings, by the corded or clumped appearance of nonpigmented growth after more than 5 days of incubation. However, the microscopic observation drug susceptibility method entails some requirements that may be difficult to achieve in limited-resource settings, including acquiring and storing labile ingredients such as OADC. In addition, it requires the sophisticated facilities and equipment including a biological safety cabinet, high-speed centrifuge, incubator, inverted microscope, etc., and safety practices of a biosafety level 3 laboratory.

Methods that distinguish viable from nonviable tubercle bacilli include tetrazolium dye reduction (43), flow cytometry (98), and a method based on the use of a luciferase reporter mycobacteriophage (120).

Mutations in genes that encode targets of antimycobacterial agents (Table 2) can be detected by a variety of methods. A particular focus of such studies has been RMP resistance because of the pivotal role of RMP in the treatment of TB and other mycobacterial infections and the conserved nature of the genetic basis for resistance (>96% of RMP resistance correlates with mutations in an 81-bp segment of the rpoB gene). The methods used to detect rpoB mutations include PCR amplification of the target sequence and detection by DNA sequencing (29, 65, 73), the line probe assay (8, 84), single-strand conformation polymorphism (41, 147), dideoxy fingerprinting (41), the use of molecular beacons synthesized from modified oligonucleotides (82, 114), PCR-enzyme-linked immunosorbent assay (44), and mismatch RNA/RNA protection assay (102). Similar approaches have been developed for detecting mutations involved in INH (82, 114, 119), EMB (142), and PZA (71) resistance. Ruiz et al. (122) have proposed real-time PCR coupled to fluorescence detection for a rapid detection of RMP and INH resistance associated with mutations in M. tuberculosis. DNA microarray technology described for mycobacterial identification has also been applied to the efficient detection of mutations associated with resistance to RMP (95, 149).

Line probes (Hain and Innogenetics) and molecular beacons assays (Cepheid) have been developed as commercial products. The availability of rapid, accurate results from these techniques has made them strong candidates for adoption as routine clinical and public health laboratory methods (8, 84). Indeed, use of rapid molecular detection of RMP resistance has been shown to shorten the time to diagnosis of MDR TB and enable patients with MDR TB to be started on appropriate therapy an average of 51 days earlier than those who were diagnosed by conventional culture (108).

The WHO issued a policy statement in June 2008 recommending that molecular line probe assays be used for rapid screening of patients at risk of MDR TB (39, 166). The increasing incidence of MDR TB and XDR TB has brought about a change in WHO recommendations for the laboratory diagnosis of TB. Whereas the WHO DOTS (directly observed short-course) program relied on acid-fast smear microscopy, methods that can detect drug-resistant cases are now recommended. Culture-based methods for detection, identification, and drug susceptibility testing of MTBC are time-consuming and resource intensive and require thorough education and application of rigorous QC measures. In many developing country settings with a high prevalence of TB, it may be appropriate to institute molecular methods for detection of TB and drug resistance rather than attempt to institute increased numbers of culture-based laboratories performing culture-based drug susceptibility testing (150). In addition to line probe assays, the Cepheid automated system using molecular beacons has shown great promise in developing country, limited-resource settings. Preliminary cost analyses suggest that both line probe assays and the automated molecular beacons systems may prove to be competitive with culture-based methods for cost-effectiveness.

Molecular tests may similarly become widely used for detection of second-line drug resistance and XDR TB. In 2009, Hillemann et al. (60) reported on the evaluation of a Hain line probe assay designed to detect resistance to second-line drugs. This study reported performance characteristics that should lead to rapid results and good predictive values for detection of resistance to fluoroquinolones and injectable drugs. Rapid identification of most patients with XDR TB should therefore be possible, although follow-up culture is likely to be required to achieve optimal accuracy. Use of a molecular technique might therefore allow XDR TB patients to be detected within a time frame that could enable effective treatment to be initiated in time to save the patients' lives. To the same end, the CDC has begun a service of rapid DNA sequencing to test culture isolates in order to quickly detect mutations associated with resistance to second-line drugs.

Because knowledge of mutations that contribute to drug resistance in MTBC is incomplete, molecular methods for detection of drug resistance will likely not detect all drug-resistant strains. For this reason, follow-up culture and culture-based drug susceptibility testing should be considered whenever resources permit. With this algorithm, the molecular testing is added to already existing methods and increases the cost of laboratory work for TB patients. Molecular detection of drug resistance may therefore be limited to cases where there is a reason to suspect drug resistance or where a susceptible population has been exposed. It is also worth remembering that rapid detection of patients with drug-resistant disease can lead to improved patient therapy and reduced infectious periods (108). These can lead to cost savings.

In countries and settings where culture of MTBC and drug susceptibility testing have not been available, the algorithm may be different. Although molecular detection of drug-resistant M. *tuberculosis* alone is less accurate than a combination of molecular and culture-based methods, the molecular methods alone may prove to be cost-effective and beneficial to TB control in this setting. The need for education and training could delay the implementation of sophisticated culture-based methods, whereas highly automated molecular methods could permit rapid and accurate testing by less skilled personnel (150).

NONTUBERCULOUS MYCOBACTERIA

Broth microdilution is the method recommended by the CLSI for susceptibility testing of NTM. The CLSI provides guidelines for testing MAC, M. *kansasii*, M. *marinum*, and the rapidly growing mycobacteria (31). These few mycobacteria, which are discussed in the following sections, were selected because sufficient data on which to base recommendations exist. For other NTM, there is little, if any, meaningful information concerning the correlation between susceptibility test results and clinical outcome. Therefore, clinicians who request that susceptibility testing be performed on NTM other than those listed above should be aware of the limitations of such testing and interpret results with caution.

Susceptibility testing of NTM should be performed only on clinically significant isolates, such as those from blood, other sterile body fluids, or tissues. Determining clinical significance of isolates from the respiratory specimens, however, may be problematic. Because several NTM are found in the environment and may colonize the respiratory tract, their recovery from sputum, for example, does not necessarily indicate clinical disease. The American Thoracic Society (ATS) recommends the following microbiologic criteria as an aid for diagnosing NTM lung disease (46): (i) positive culture results from at least two separate expectorated sputum samples (a minimum of three sputum specimens should be collected for mycobacterial culture), or (ii) positive culture result from at least one bronchial wash or lavage specimen, or (iii) transbronchial or other lung biopsy specimen with histopathologic features consistent with a mycobacterial infection (granulomas or chronic inflammation with stain positive for acid-fast bacilli) and positive culture for NTM. One culture-positive, smear-negative sputum specimen is not likely to be clinically significant.

General recommendations regarding the broth microdilution method and QC that apply to all NTM are discussed in the following paragraphs. Specific details related to MAC, M. *kansasii*, M. *marinum*, and the rapidly growing mycobacteria are discussed in individual sections.

Test Method

The inoculum suspension may be prepared by sweeping the confluent portion of growth on a solid medium with a sterile cotton swab or directly from a broth culture. If colonies are used, growth on the swab is transferred to 4.5 ml of sterile water containing glass beads (e.g., 7 to 10 3-mm beads) until the turbidity matches the turbidity of a 0.5 McFarland standard by visual examination or by using a nephelometer. The suspension is mixed vigorously on a vortex mixer for 15 to 20 seconds and then allowed to sit so any remaining large clumps can settle; the supernatant is then used for the inoculum suspension.

If freeze-dried microtiter plates are used without the broth already added, the final inoculum (with an organism density of approximately 5×10^5 CFU/ml) is prepared by transferring 50 µl of the suspension to 10 ml of cation-supplemented Mueller-Hinton broth for rapidly growing mycobacteria or 10 ml of cation-supplemented Mueller-Hinton broth plus 5% OADC for slowly growing NTM. Tubes are inverted 8 to 10 times to mix the suspension thoroughly. Alternatively, if using prepared plates that contain antimicrobials in 100 µl of broth, it is necessary to calculate the volume of standardized suspension to be added to 36 ml of water diluent to obtain a final organism concentration of 1×10^5 to 5×10^5 CFU/ml (1×10^4 to 5×10^4 CFU per well in a 0.1-ml volume). The volume depends on the delivery system that is being used.

Final inoculum suspensions are mixed well (by inverting the tube several times or vortexing) and poured into plastic troughs, after which 100 µl is transferred to each well of the microdilution tray. Each inoculated tray is covered with an adhesive seal and incubated in ambient air. Simultaneously inoculating a nutrient agar plate, such as 5% sheep blood or trypticase soy agar, with a loopful of the final inoculum to check for purity is recommended. Incubation temperature and time are discussed for each species or group in the following sections.

Quality Control

QC testing should be performed on each new batch of test plates and once each week or each time testing is performed, if done less often than weekly (31). Strains recommended for MAC, M. *kansasii*, and the rapidly growing mycobacteria are listed in the sections in which these mycobacteria are discussed. Currently, interlaboratory proficiency testing available for testing NTM is limited. Therefore, laboratories are encouraged to submit isolates to reference laboratories with extensive experience in testing these mycobacteria for confirmatory tests in lieu of a formal proficiency test program.

M. AVIUM COMPLEX

MAC is among the most frequently encountered *Mycobacterium* species in many clinical laboratories. Isolation of MAC from blood is especially important in HIV-infected patients. Although the incidence of disseminated MAC in HIV-infected patients has dramatically decreased due to effective prophylaxis and the immune system restoration associated with highly active antiretroviral therapy, it still occurs in patients who develop resistance to antiretroviral treatment or who exhibit drug intolerance or poor compliance. In many of these patients, recovery of MAC represents a relapse of MAC disease rather than a new infection. MAC is also an important cause of chronic pulmonary lung disease (46) and in the United States is the leading cause of lung disease due to an NTM (74). Patients with MAC lung disease generally may be placed in one of the following groups: those who have underlying lung disease with apical fibrocavitary lesions, postmenopausal women with bronchiectasis and nodular opacities, or patients with cystic fibrosis.

Antimicrobial Agents

Correlation between in vitro MAC susceptibility test results and clinical response has been demonstrated in a controlled clinical trial only with clarithromycin and azithromycin (26). These are the only drugs recommended for first-line testing. Wild-type (untreated) MAC isolates typically have clarithromycin MICs of ≤4 µg/ml (≤32 µg/ml for azithromycin) and are considered susceptible to these agents. MAC isolates from patients who have relapsed after treatment, on the other hand, have clarithromycin MIC values of ≥32 µg/ml (azithromycin MIC, ≥256 µg/ml) and no longer respond clinically to macrolide therapy. Virtually all such isolates have a mutation in the adenine at position 2058 or 2059 of the 23S rRNA gene, the presumed macrolide binding site on the ribosomal unit (93, 103).

Clarithromycin and azithromycin are approved by the FDA for the treatment of MAC disease, but because resistance develops quickly with macrolide monotherapy, single-drug therapy with either agent is contraindicated. A common regimen for MAC disease is shown in Table 1 (46). Very importantly, although EMB, RMP, rifabutin, SM, and amikacin are useful clinically and broth dilution susceptibility testing of MAC to these agents may be performed, the results may not reliably predict clinical outcome. Because of the lack of data establishing a correlation between MIC values and clinical response, breakpoints separating susceptible from resistant strains have not been determined. Therefore, it is strongly recommended that susceptibility results for the above antituberculosis drugs not be reported for MAC. Most MAC isolates are intrinsically resistant to INH and PZA; these antimicrobial agents play no role in the treatment of MAC infection and should not be tested.

Treatment of macrolide-resistant MAC infections is problematic, and the role of susceptibility testing in guiding therapy for these patients is not clearly defined. Although data are limited, some experts believe that moxifloxacin and linezolid, which CLSI lists as secondary agents, may be clinically useful in select patients (46).

Indications for Susceptibility Testing

The ATS recommends that clarithromycin susceptibility testing be performed on all new, previously untreated clinically significant MAC isolates and on MAC isolates from patients who relapse while on macrolide therapy or prophylaxis (46). Clarithromycin is the class drug for the newer macrolides (clarithromycin and azithromycin share cross-resistance and susceptibility) and is the only drug that need be tested. Susceptibility testing should be repeated after 3 months for patients with disseminated disease and after 6 months for patients with chronic pulmonary disease if the patient does not improve clinically and remains culture positive.

Test Methods

As mentioned above, broth microdilution is recommended for susceptibility testing of all NTM. For MAC, in addition to broth microdilution, radiometric broth macrodilution also is accurate and reliable. For testing azithromycin, radiometric broth macrodilution is the only method recommended because the drug is more soluble in larger volumes of broth. Agar-based methods, in contrast, should not be used. The CLSI currently recommends cation-supplemented Mueller-Hinton broth with 5% OADC or OAD for broth microdilution testing, although some isolates grow poorly in this medium, and BACTEC 12B medium for macrodilution testing.

There are two views regarding the optimal pH at which to perform MAC susceptibility testing. One supports testing at pH 7.2 to 7.4, because macrolides are more active in vitro in mildly alkaline conditions. The other advocates using mildly acidic conditions (i.e., pH 6.8, which is the pH of the BACTEC 12B medium) for the following reasons: (i) MAC isolates grow more slowly or even fail to grow at the higher pH (8a); (ii) BACTEC 12B medium is unstable at pH 7.2 to 7.4 because of its poor buffering capacity at pH values above 7.2; and (iii) the intracellular environment of MAC-infected macrophages is pH 6.0 to 6.5, which suggests that macrolides should be tested under the mildly acidic, more clinically relevant conditions. Data from a multicenter study (164) showed that testing in broth at either pH is satisfactory, providing that recommendations for interpretation of breakpoints are followed (Table 5).

As previously mentioned, when broth microdilution is performed, the inoculum may be prepared directly from an agar plate or a broth culture. For the radiometric method, the use of "seed" BACTEC vials (subcultures of fresh growth) is recommended. Although it often is not practical, only transparent colony types should be tested, if possible, because this variant generally is more virulent and more

TABLE 5 Antimycobacterial agents and interpretative criteria for M. avium complex[a]

Antimycobacterial agent	Method[b]	MIC (μg/ml) for category		
		S	I	R
Primary				
Clarithromycin[c]	Broth microdilution (pH 7.3–7.4)	≤8	16	≥32
	BACTEC 460TB (pH 6.8)[d]	≤16	32	≥64
Azithromycin	BACTEC 460TB (pH 6.8)	≤128	256	≥512
Secondary				
Moxifloxacin	Broth microdilution (pH 7.3–7.4)	≤1	2	≥4
Linezolid	Broth microdilution (pH 7.3–7.4)	≤8	16	≥32

[a]Table and footnotes are adapted from reference 31. S, susceptible; I, intermediate; R, resistant.
[b]pH is 7.3 to 7.4 for broth microdilution and 6.8 for BACTEC 460TB
[c]Clarithromycin is the class drug for macrolides and is the only drug that need be tested.
[d]If BACTEC 460TB pH 7.3 to 7.4 is used, breakpoints are ≤4 μg/ml (susceptible), 8 to 16 μg/ml (intermediate), and ≥32 μg/ml (resistant).

resistant to antimicrobial agents than the opaque variant. The inoculum should be between 10^4 and 10^5 CFU/ml for the radiometric broth macrodilution test and approximately 5×10^5 CFU/ml for the broth microdilution test. Tween 80 or other surfactants should not be used to disperse clumps of bacilli because of the potential synergistic effect of the surfactant activity of Tween 80 and antimicrobial agents.

Incubation is at $35 \pm 2°C$ in ambient air. For the radiometric test, incubation should not extend beyond 10 days, and the "no-drug" control should not exceed a GI of 999 in less than 4 days. For broth microdilution, trays are first examined at 7 days. If growth is insufficient, trays are reincubated and read again at days 10 to 14 of incubation. The end point for broth microdilution assay is visible turbidity; for the radiometric test it is defined by the GI value for the inoculum diluted 1:100.

Reporting Results

Both the MIC value and an interpretation, based on the pH of the medium and the breakpoints listed in Table 5, should be reported (31). Because untreated wild strains of MAC rarely, if ever, are intermediate or resistant to macrolides, the CLSI subcommittee recommends that laboratories confirm such results by repeat testing (31). A confirmed intermediate result may indicate emerging resistance; therefore, patients with such an isolate should be carefully monitored, and susceptibility testing should be performed on subsequent MAC isolates. Reporting secondary agents (i.e., moxifloxacin and linezolid) should be restricted to situations in which the clinician has extensive experience in the use of these drugs in the treatment of MAC disease or for research purposes.

Quality Control

M. avium ATCC 700898 is recommended for QC when testing macrolides. The range of acceptable results for clarithromycin is 1 to 4 μg/ml at pH 6.8 and 0.5 to 2 μg/ml at pH 7.3 to 7.4; the range for azithromycin is 8 to 32 μg/ml. M. marinum ATCC 927 is an acceptable alternative QC

organism when testing by microtiter dilution; the acceptable range for clarithromycin is 0.25 to 1 μg/ml.

When secondary drugs are tested, there are sufficient data to support recommendations for QC for broth microdilution testing only. Acceptable ranges for moxifloxacin and linezolid when testing M. avium ATCC 700898 are 0.25 to 2.0 μg/ml and 4 to 16 μg/ml, respectively. When testing M. marinum ATCC 927, acceptable ranges are 1 to 4 μg/ml for both drugs. Another option for QC of moxifloxacin is P. aeruginosa ATCC 27853 (acceptable ranges can be found in the most recent CLSI M100 document [30a]).

M. KANSASII

M. kansasii is the second most common cause of disease due to NTM in the United States (46), typically presenting as pulmonary disease resembling TB. The therapeutic regimen currently recommended by the ATS for treatment of M. kansasii pulmonary disease consists of RMP, INH, and EMB (46), of which RMP is the component critical for treatment success. Rifabutin is used in place of RMP in patients with AIDS receiving protease inhibitors (46). Isolates of M. kansasii from previously untreated patients are predictably susceptible to RMP. However, resistance to RMP can develop during therapy, and a patient's history of RMP therapy may be unknown or unclear. Therefore, CLSI recommends that all initial isolates of M. kansasii be tested for susceptibility to RMP only (31). Susceptibility testing should be repeated if cultures remain positive after 3 months of appropriate therapy.

Untreated wild strains of M. kansasii are susceptible to the critical concentrations of RMP and EMB used to test M. tuberculosis (discussed earlier in the chapter) but are resistant to the critical concentration of INH (0.2 μg/ml by agar proportion) and show variable susceptibility to the higher concentration (1.0 μg/ml). Despite these in vitro results, INH appears to be clinically active. Therefore, because in vitro results do not correlate with clinical outcome, routine testing susceptibility of M. kansasii to INH is not recommended.

Susceptibility testing is done by broth microdilution using cation-supplemented Mueller-Hinton broth with 5% OADC or OAD and incubating at $35 \pm 2°C$ for 7 to 14 days in CO_2 or ambient air, although CO_2 should be avoided when testing macrolides. Acceptable QC strains and expected MIC results for RMP are as follows: M. kansasii ATCC 12478, ≤1 μg/ml; M. marinum 927, ≤0.25 to 1 μg/ml; and Enterococcus faecalis, 0.5 to 4 μg/ml.

Isolates of M. kansasii that are resistant to RMP (MIC, ≥1 μg/ml) should be tested for susceptibility to the following drugs: rifabutin, EMB, SM, INH, clarithromycin, amikacin, ciprofloxacin (as the class representative for the older fluoroquinolones, which are less active in vitro than moxifloxacin), trimethoprim-sulfamethoxazole, linezolid, and moxifloxacin. MIC values for resistance to these agents are shown in Table 6 (31). Although INH and SM may be useful clinically, breakpoints to establish susceptibility and resistance for NTM have not been established; therefore, only the MIC (with no interpretation) should be reported for these drugs.

M. MARINUM

M. marinum causes chronic granulomatous lesions of the skin and soft tissues (called "swimming pool granuloma" or "fish tank granuloma") and occasionally bone. Routine susceptibility testing of M. marinum is not recommended and should be discouraged. Isolates are consistently susceptible to several clinically useful antimicrobial agents, including

TABLE 6 Secondary antimycobacterial agents and MIC values indicating resistance for testing *M. kansasii* [a]

Antimycobacterial agent	MIC indicating resistance (µg/ml)
Amikacin	>32
Ciprofloxacin[b]	>2
Clarithromycin[c]	>16
EMB hydrochloride	>4
INH	—[d]
Linezolid	>16
Moxifloxacin	>2
Rifabutin	>2
SM	—[d]
Trimethoprim-sulfamethoxazole	>2/38

[a]Table and footnotes are adapted from reference 31.

[b]Ciprofloxacin and levofloxacin are interchangeable, but both are less active in vitro than moxifloxacin.

[c]Clarithromycin is considered a primary drug in patients receiving the short-course and/or intermittent therapeutic regimens consisting of rifampin, ethambutol, and clarithromycin. For patients receiving the classic regimen of rifampin, ethambutol, and isoniazid, clarithromycin is a secondary agent. Clarithromycin is the class representative for the "newer" macrolides (clarithromycin, azithromycin, roxithromycin).

[d]Breakpoints to establish susceptibility and resistance for NTM have not been established. Report the MIC value only, with no interpretation, for these drugs.

RMP, EMB, doxycycline (or minocycline), trimethoprim-sulfamethoxazole, and clarithromycin (31). Additionally, the risk of acquired mutational resistance to one or more of these agents is extremely low. Successful treatment may require surgical excision or debridement as well as antimicrobial therapy. However, if a patient fails to respond clinically after several months of appropriate therapy and remains culture positive, susceptibility testing of *M. marinum* should be considered. As for MAC and *M. kansasii*, broth microdilution using Mueller-Hinton broth supplemented with OADC or OAD is recommended. Incubation is at 30 ± 2°C for 7 days. Drugs suggested by CLSI to test and the MIC values (in µg/ml) indicating resistance are as follows: RMP (>2), clarithromycin (>16, the class agent for newer macrolides), amikacin (>32), doxycycline or minocycline (>4), ciprofloxacin (>2), moxifloxacin (>2), and trimethoprim-sulfamethoxazole (>2/38) (31).

OTHER SLOWLY GROWING NTM

Many other slowly growing NTM may cause human disease, and susceptibility testing of these species may be requested. Although data are limited, CLSI suggests broth dilution using cation-supplemented Mueller-Hinton broth with OADC for nonfastidious species (31). The same primary and secondary agents listed for *M. kansasii* should be tested and reported with the same interpretive criteria (31). In general, testing *M. gordonae* is inappropriate because isolates almost always represent contaminants and only rarely are the cause of actual disease. For fastidious species, such as *Mycobacterium haemophilum*, susceptibility testing has been performed (12); however, there is insufficient information to recommend a standard method of testing.

RAPIDLY GROWING MYCOBACTERIA

Over 30 species of rapidly growing mycobacteria have been identified, but most human disease is due to *M. abscessus*, *M. chelonae*, and *M. fortuitum* group, which are important causes of skin and soft tissue infections, especially following penetrating trauma with possible soil or water contamination

(19). CLSI recommendations for susceptibility testing of rapidly growing mycobacteria are based predominantly on results of studies involving these three species/groups, but they apply to other clinically significant rapid growers as well. For some drugs (e.g., clarithromycin, imipenem, and tobramycin) susceptibility test results apply to certain species or groups of rapidly growing mycobacteria; therefore, identification of isolates to the species level is recommended. At a minimum, isolates belonging to the *M. fortuitum* group should be differentiated from those in the *M. chelonae-abscessus* group. If cultures (from any site except respiratory) are positive after 6 months of appropriate antimicrobial therapy, susceptibility testing should be repeated, and the species identity should be confirmed.

Test Method

As for all NTM, broth microdilution is recommended for susceptibility testing of the rapidly growing mycobacteria (31, 163). Antimicrobial agents that should be tested are amikacin, cefoxitin (up to 256 µg/ml), ciprofloxacin, clarithromycin, doxycycline (or minocycline), imipenem, linezolid, moxifloxacin, trimethoprim-sulfamethoxazole, and tobramycin. Tobramycin is used predominantly for treatment of *M. chelonae* infections and should not be used to treat infections due to *M. abscessus* or *M. fortuitum* group.

The inoculum is prepared as described above, and trays are incubated at 30 ± 2°C in air and examined at 72 h. If growth in the growth control well is sufficient (at least 2+, or definite turbidity and "clumpy" growth [31]) at that time, the MIC can be recorded. If not, trays are reincubated and read again on days 4 and 5. Day 5 is the final reading for all drugs except clarithromycin, which should be read at 7 to 10 days and, if the isolate is susceptible at that reading, again at 14 days (31). The final day 14 reading is recommended to ensure detection of inducible macrolide resistance; however, if clarithromycin resistance (MIC, ≥8 µg/ml) is recognized at an earlier reading, the report can be finalized at that time.

The MIC is the lowest concentration of antimicrobial agent that completely inhibits visible growth, with one exception. As with other types of bacteria, "trailing" is common when trimethoprim-sulfamethoxazole is tested, and the MIC values for this agent should be read at approximately 80% inhibition of growth. Trailing also is occasionally seen with isolates of *M. fortuitum* group and clarithromycin; when this occurs, the endpoint is read at the end of the trailing.

Reporting Results

MIC values and an interpretation, based on the breakpoints for the rapidly growing mycobacteria listed in Table 7 (31), are reported for each drug. A few species/groups of rapidly growing mycobacteria are almost always susceptible to certain drugs. This is true for *M. abscessus* and amikacin; for *M. fortuitum* group, *M. smegmatis* group, and *M. mucogenicum* and imipenem; and for *M. chelonae* and tobramycin. Therefore, if the MIC result for one of these isolate-drug combinations indicates resistance, susceptibility testing should be repeated, and the identification should be confirmed. If the repeat result indicates resistance, the isolate should be sent to a qualified reference laboratory for confirmation of the results if the drug in question is being considered for therapy.

Quality Control

The QC strain recommended for monitoring test performance and for verifying the concentration of antimicrobial agents is *M. peregrinum* ATCC 700686. *Staphylococcus aureus* ATCC 29213, *Pseudomonas aeruginosa* ATCC 17853, and/or *E. faecalis* ATCC 29212 are acceptable alternatives.

TABLE 7 Broth microdilution interpretive criteria for rapidly growing mycobacteria[a]

Antimicrobial agent	MIC (μg/ml) for category		
	Susceptible	Intermediate	Resistant
Amikacin[b]	≤16	32	≥64
Cefoxitin	≤16	32–64	≥128
Ciprofloxacin[c]	≤1	2	≥4
Clarithromycin[d]	≤2	4	≥8
Doxycycline/minocycline	≤1	2–4	≥8
Imipenem[e]	≤4	8–16	≥32
Linezolid	≤8	16	≥32
Moxifloxacin	≤1	2	≥4
Trimethoprim-sulfamethoxazole	≤2/38		≥4/76
Tobramycin[f]	≤2	4	≥8

[a]Table and footnotes are adapted from reference 31.

[b]Isolates of M. abscessus with an MIC of ≥64 μg/ml should be retested. If the repeat result is ≥64 μg/ml, the MIC should be reported with the following comment: The MIC is greater than expected for this species; if the drug is being considered for therapy, the laboratory should be notified so the isolate can be sent to a reference laboratory for confirmation of resistance.

[c]Ciprofloxacin and levofloxacin are interchangeable. Both are less active than the newer 8-methoxyfluoroquinolones.

[d]The final reading for nonpigmented rapidly growing mycobacteria should be at 14 days to ensure detection of inducible macrolide resistance, unless the isolate is resistant at an earlier reading. Clarithromycin is the class representative for newer macrolides (i.e., azithromycin and roxithromycin).

[e]If the MIC is >8 μg/ml for M. fortuitum group, M. smegmatis group, and M. mucogenicum group, the test should be repeated with an incubation period of no more than 3 days. If the repeat result is >8 μg/ml, the MIC should be reported with the following comment: The MIC is greater than expected for this species; if the drug is being considered for therapy, the laboratory should be notified so the isolates can be sent to a reference laboratory for confirmation of resistance. Imipenem results do not predict results for meropenem or ertapenem. Activity against rapidly growing mycobacteria is greater for imipenem than for meropenem or ertapenem.

[f]Tobramycin is used predominantly for treatment of M. chelonae infections. If the MIC to tobramycin is >4 μg/ml for an isolate of M. chelonae, the test should be repeated. If the repeat result is >4 μg/ml, the MIC should be reported with the following comment: The MIC is greater than expected for this species; if the drug is being considered for therapy, the laboratory should be notified so the isolate can be sent to a reference laboratory for confirmation of resistance.

NOCARDIA AND OTHER AEROBIC ACTINOMYCETES

Clinical Significance

Nocardia spp. and other aerobic actinomycetes (*Actinomadura, Rhodococcus equi, Gordonia, Tsukamurella,* and rarely *Streptomyces* spp.) can cause serious disease in immunocompromised and occasionally even healthy hosts (1, 14, 16, 18, 70, 135, 151, 155). In vitro susceptibility testing should be performed on all clinically significant isolates to serve as a guide for therapy and to monitor for resistance.

Testing Method

The recommended method for testing *Nocardia* and other aerobic actinomycetes is broth microdilution (31). Breakpoints for interpretation of MIC values have been established only for *Nocardia* species. Because *Rhodococcus equi* grows within 24 h in most susceptibility panels for gram-positive bacteria, it can be tested following the guidelines described in CLSI documents M7-A8 (30) and the most recent edition of M100 (30a).

The primary and secondary antimicrobial agents recommended for susceptibility testing are listed in Table 8. For *R. equi* only there are two additional primary drugs: vancomycin and rifampin. Although broth dilution is preferred, for a few species-drug combinations, the accuracy of the results may be questionable. For example, ceftriaxone results may be falsely resistant when testing *Nocardia brasiliensis*, and when testing *Nocardia farcinica*, imipenem results may be falsely resistant. Studies to further investigate this potential problem are needed.

Inoculum preparation is described in detail in CLSI document M24 (31). First, a heavy suspension is prepared in cation-supplemented Mueller-Hinton broth or sterile, deionized water or saline, using colonies on a blood or trypticase soy agar plate that was incubated at 35 ± 2°C in air until growth is sufficient (usually 3 to 7 days). Large clumps of organisms are broken up by using a micropestle or glass beads and

mixing vigorously on a vortex mixer. The suspension is allowed to sit for approximately 15 minutes so that the clumps settle. Several drops of the supernatant are added to 2 ml of water or saline in a tube compatible with a nephelometer available in the laboratory. The turbidity of the suspension is adjusted to equal the density of a 0.5 McFarland standard.

TABLE 8 Broth microdilution breakpoints for *Nocardia*[a]

Antimicrobial agent	MIC (μg/ml) for:		
	Susceptible strains	Intermediate strains	Resistant strains
Primary			
Amikacin	≤8		≥16
Amoxicillin-clavulanic acid	≤8/4	16/8	≥32/16
Ceftriaxone	≤8	16–32	≥64
Ciprofloxacin[b]	≤1	2	≥4
Clarithromycin[c]	≤2	4	≥8
Imipenem	≤4	8	≥16
Linezolid	≤8		
Minocycline	≤1	2–4	≥8
Moxifloxacin	≤1	2	≥4
Trimethoprim-sulfamethoxazole	≤2/38		≥4/76
Tobramycin	≤4	8	≥16
Secondary			
Cefepime	≤8	16	≥32
Cefotaxime	≤8	16–32	≥64
Doxycycline	≤1	2–4	≥8

[a]Table and footnotes are adapted from reference 31.

[b]Ciprofloxacin and levofloxacin are interchangeable. Both are less active than the newer 8-methoxyfluoroquinolones.

[c]Class representative for newer macrolides.

Panels are inoculated, covered with an adhesive seal, placed in a plastic bag, and incubated at 35 ± 2°C in ambient air for 72 h. If growth in the growth control well is sufficient at that time, MIC values are recorded; if not, panels are reincubated and read daily until growth is adequate, for up to 5 days total.

Reporting of Results

Both an MIC value and an interpretation (as listed in Table 8) should be reported for *Nocardia* species. For all other aerobic actinomycetes, including *R. equi*, an MIC value only should be reported, because breakpoints for these drugs have not been determined for genera other than *Nocardia*.

Quality Control

Recommended reference strains for QC are *S. aureus* ATCC 29213, *Pseudomonas aeruginosa* ATCC 27853, and for amoxicillin-clavulanic acid only, *E. coli* ATCC 35218. Acceptable ranges for these strains are found in the current edition of CLSI document M100 (30a).

REFERENCES

1. **Agterof, M. J., T. van der Bruggen, M. Tersmette, E. J. ter Borg, J. M. M. van den Bosch, and D. H. Biesma.** 2007. Nocardiosis: a case series and a mini review of clinical and microbiological features. *Neth. J. Med.* **65:**199–202.
2. **Alcaide, F., G. E. Pfyffer, and A. Telenti.** 1997. Role of *embB* in natural and acquired resistance to ethambutol in mycobacteria. *Antimicrob. Agents Chemother.* **41:**2270–2273.
3. **Amsden, G. W.** 1996. Erythromycin, clarithromycin, and azithromycin: are the differences real? *Clin. Ther.* **18:**56–72.
4. **Andreis, K., P. Verhasselt, J. Guillemont, H. W. Gohleman, J. M. Neefs, H. Winkler, J. Van Gestel, P. Timmerman, M. Zhu, E. Lee, P. Williams, D. De Chaffoy, E. Huitric, S. Hoffner, E. Cambau, C. Truffot-Pernot, N. Lounis, and V. Jarlier.** 2005. A diarylquinoline drug active on the ATP synthase of *Mycobacterium tuberculosis. Science* **307:**223–227.
5. **Anonymous.** 1998. *Priftin (Rifapentine) Prescribing Information.* Hoechst Marion Roussel, Inc., Kansas City, MO.
6. **Anonymous.** 2008. Capreomycin. *Tuberculosis* (Edinburgh) **88:**89–91.
7. **Banerjee, A., E. Dubnau, A. Quemard, V. Balasubramanian, K. S. Um, T. Wilson, D. Collins, G. de Lisle, and W. R. Jacobs, Jr.** 1994. *inhA*, a gene encoding a target for isoniazid and ethionamide in *Mycobacterium tuberculosis. Science* **263:**227–230.
8. **Barnard, M., H. Albert, G. Coetzee, R. O'Brien, and M. E. Bosman.** 2008. Rapid molecular screening for multidrug-resistant tuberculosis in a high-volume public health laboratory in South Africa. *Am. J. Respir. Crit. Care Med.* **177:**787–792.
8a. **Beaty, S., S. Siddiqi, and M. Gnacek.** 1992. *Abstr. 92nd Gen. Meet. Am. Soc. Microbiol. 1992*, abstr. U-102. American Society for Microbiology, Washington, DC.
9. **Bémer, P., F. Palicova, S. Rüsch-Gerdes, S. H. Siddiqi, H. B. Drugeon, and G. E. Pfyffer.** 2002. Multicenter evaluation of fully-automated BACTEC Mycobacteria Growth Indicator Tube 960 System for susceptibility testing of *Mycobacterium tuberculosis. J. Clin. Microbiol.* **40:**150–154.
10. **Benson, C.** 1997. Critical drug interactions with agents used for prophylaxis and treatment of *Mycobacterium avium* infections. *Am. J. Med.* **102:**32–36.
11. **Bergmann, J. S., and G. L. Woods.** 1998. Evaluation of the ESP culture system II for testing susceptibilities of *Mycobacterium tuberculosis* isolates to four primary antituberculous drugs. *J. Clin. Microbiol.* **36:**2940–2943.
12. **Bernard, E. M., F. F. Edwards, T. E. Kiehn, S. T. Brown, and D. Armstrong.** 1993. Activities of antimicrobial agents against clinical isolates of *Mycobacterium haemophilum. Antimicrob. Agents Chemother.* **37:**2323–2326.
13. **Berning, S. E., L. Madsen, M. D. Iseman, and C. A. Peloquin.** 1995. Long-term safety of ofloxacin and ciprofloxacin in the treatment of mycobacterial infections. *Am. J. Respir. Crit. Care Med.* **151:**2006–2009.
14. **Blaschke, A. J., J. Bender, C. L. Byington, K. Korgenski, J. Daly, C. A Petti, A. T. Pavia, and K. Ampofo.** 2007. *Gordonia* species: emerging pathogens in pediatric patients that are identified by 16S ribosomal RNA gene sequencing. *Clin. Infect. Dis.* **45:**483–486.
15. **Bodmer, T., G. Zurcher, P. Imboden, and A. Telenti.** 1995. Mutation position and type of substitution in the beta-subunit of the RNA polymerase influence in-vitro activity of rifamycins in rifampicin-resistant *Mycobacterium tuberculosis. J. Antimicrob. Chemother.* **35:**345–348.
16. **Bouza, E., A. Perez-Parra, M. Rosal, P. Martin-Rabadan, M. Rodriguez-Creixems, and M. Marin.** 2009. *Tsukamurella*: a cause of catheter-related bloodstream infections. *Eur. J. Clin. Microbiol. Infect. Dis.* **28:**203–210.
17. **Bozeman, L., W. Burman, B. Metchock, L. Welch, M. Weiner, and the Tuberculosis Trials Consortium.** 2005. Fluoroquinolone susceptibility among *Mycobacterium tuberculosis* isolates from the United States and Canada. *J. Infect. Dis.* **40:**386–391.
18. **Brown-Elliott, B. A., J. Brown, P. S. Conville, and R. J. Wallace.** 2006. Clinical and laboratory features of the *Nocardia* spp. based on current molecular taxonomy. *Clin. Microbiol. Rev.* **19:**259–282.
19. **Brown-Elliott, B. A., and R. J. Wallace, Jr.** 2002. Clinical and taxonomic status of pathogenic nonpigmented or late-pigmenting rapidly growing mycobacteria. *Clin. Microbiol. Rev.* **15:**716–746.
20. **Brunello, F., and R. Fontana.** 2000. Reliability of the MB/BacT system for testing susceptibility of *Mycobacterium tuberculosis* complex isolates to antituberculous drugs. *J. Clin. Microbiol.* **38:**872–873.
21. **Burman, W. J.** 1997. The value of in vitro drug activity and pharmacokinetics in predicting the effectiveness of antimycobacterial therapy: a critical review. *Am. J. Med. Sci.* **313:**355–363.
22. **Canetti, G.** 1965. Present aspects of bacterial resistance in tuberculosis. *Am. Rev. Respir. Dis.* **92:**687–702.
23. **Canetti, G., W. Fox, A. Khomenko, H. T. Mahler, N. K. Menon, D. A. Mitchison, N. Rist, and N. A. Smelev.** 1969. Advances in techniques of testing mycobacterial drug sensitivity, and the use of sensitivity tests in tuberculosis control programs. *Bull. W. H. O.* **41:**21–43.
24. **Canetti, G., S. Froman, J. Grosset, P. Hauduroy, M. Lagerova, H. T. Mahler, G. Meissner, D. A. Mitchison, and L. Sula.** 1963. Mycobacteria: laboratory methods for testing drug sensitivity and resistance. *Bull. W. H. O.* **29:**565–578.
25. **Centers for Disease Control and Prevention.** 2006. Revised definition of extensively drug-resistance tuberculosis. *MMWR Morb. Mortal. Wkly. Rep.* **55:**1176.
26. **Chaisson, R. E., C. A. Benson, M. P. Dube, L. B. Heifets, J. A. Korvick, S. Elkin, T. Smith, J. C. Craft, F. R. Sattler, and the AIDS Clinical Trials Group Protocol 157 Study Team.** 1994. Clarithromycin therapy for bacteremic *Mycobacterium avium* complex disease. *Ann. Intern. Med.* **121:**905–911.
27. **Chaisson, R. E., P. Keiser, M. Pierce, W. J. Fessel, J. Ruskin, C. Lahart, C. A. Benson, K. Meek, N. Siepman, and J. C. Craft.** 1997. Clarithromycin and ethambutol with or without clofazimine for the treatment of bacteremic *Mycobacterium avium* complex disease in patients with HIV infection. *AIDS* **11:**311–317.
28. **Chiu, J., J. Nussbaum, S. Bozette, J. G. Tilles, L. S. Young, J. Leedom, P. N. R. Heseltine, and A. McCutchan.** 1990. Treatment of disseminated *Mycobacterium avium* complex infection in AIDS with amikacin, ethambutol, rifampin, and ciprofloxacin. *Ann. Intern. Med.* **113:**358–361.
29. **Choi, J. H., K. W. Lee, H. R. Kang, Y. I. Hwang, S. Jang, D. G. Kim, C. H. Kim, I. G. Hyun, T. R. Shin, S. M. Park, M. G. Lee, C. Y. Lee, Y. B. Park, and K. S. Jung.** 2010. Clinical efficacy of direct DNA sequencing analysis on sputum specimens for early detection of drug-resistant *Mycobacterium tuberculosis* in a clinical setting. *Chest* **137:**393–400.

30. **Clinical and Laboratory Standards Institute.** 2000. *Methods for Dilution Antimicrobial Susceptibility Tests for Bacteria That Grow Aerobically; Approved Standard—8th Ed. CLSI Document M7-A8.* Clinical and Laboratory Standards Institute, Wayne, PA.

30a. **Clinical and Laboratory Standards Institute.** 2010. *Performance Standards for Antimicrobial Susceptibility Testing; 20th Informational Supplement. CLSI Document M100-S20.* Clinical and Laboratory Standards Institute, Wayne, PA.

31. **Clinical and Laboratory Standards Institute.** *Susceptibility Testing of Mycobacteria, Nocardiae, and Other Aerobic Actinomycetes; Approved Standard—2nd Ed. CLSI Document M24-2A,* in press. Clinical and Laboratory Standards Institute, Wayne, PA.

32. **Crofton, J., and D. A. Mitchison.** 1948. Streptomycin resistance in pulmonary tuberculosis. *Br. Med. J.* **2:**1009–1015.

33. **David, H. L.** 1970. Probability distribution of drug-resistant mutants in unselected populations of *Mycobacterium tuberculosis. Appl. Microbiol.* **20:**810–814.

34. **Davis, W. B., and M. M. Weber.** 1977. Specificity of isoniazid on growth inhibition and competition for an oxidized nicotiniamide adenine dinucleotide regulatory site on the electron transport pathway in *Mycobacterium phlei. Antimicrob. Agents Chemother.* **12:**213–218.

35. **Deretic, V., W. Philipp, S. Dhandayuthapani, M. H. Mudd, R. Curcic, T. Garbe, B. Heym, L. E. Via, and S. T. Cole.** 1995. *Mycobacterium tuberculosis* is a natural mutant with an inactivated oxidative-stress regulatory gene: implications for sensitivity to isoniazid. *Mol. Microbiol.* **17:**889–900.

36. **Diacon, A. H., A. Pym, M. Grosbusch, R. Patientia, R. Rustomjeee, L. Page-Shipp, C. Pistorius, R. Krause, M. Bogoshi, G. Churchyard, A. Venter, J. Allen, J. C. Palomino, T. DeMarez, R. P. G. van Heeswijk, N. Lounis, P. Meyvisch, J. Verbeek, W. Parys, K. de Beule, K. Andries, and D. F. McNeeley.** 2009. The diarylquinoline TMC207 for multidrug-resistant tuberculosis. *N. Engl. J. Med.* **360:**2397–2405.

37. **Diaz-Infantes, M. S., M. J. Ruiz-Serrano, L. Martinez-Sanchez, A. Ortega, and E. Bouza.** 2000. Evaluation of the MB/BacT Mycobacterium Detection System for susceptibility testing of *Mycobacterium tuberculosis. J. Clin. Microbiol.* **38:**1988–1989.

38. **Dorman, S. E.. J. L. Johnson, S. Goldberg, G. Muzanye, N. Padayatchi, L. Bozeman, C. M. Heilig, J. Bernardo, S. Choudhri, J. H. Grosset, E. Guy, P. Guyadeen, M. C. Leus, G. Maltas, D. Menzies, E. L. Nuermberger, M. Villarino. A. Vernon, and R. E. Chaisson.** 2009. Substitution of moxifloxacin for isoniazid during intensive phase treatment of pulmonary tuberculosis. *Am. J. Respir. Crit. Care Med.* **180:**273–280.

39. **Drobniewski, F., S. Hoffner, K. M. Kam, S. J. Kim, S. Labelle, M. Raviglione, J. Ridderhof, S. Rusch-Gerdes, S. Selvakumar, T. Shinnick, A. Sloutsky, V. Vincent, K. Weyer, A. Wright, and M. Zignol.** 2007. Policy guidance on TB drug susceptibility testing (DST) of second-line drugs (SLD). http://www.who.int/tb/features_archive/xdr_mdr_policy_guidance/en/print.html.

40. **Dukes, C. S., J. Sugarman, J. P. Cegielski, G. J. Lallinger, and D. H. Mwakyusa.** 1992. Severe cutaneous hypersensitivity reactions during treatment of tuberculosis in patients with HIV infection in Tanzania. *Trop. Geogr. Med.* **44:**308–311.

41. **Felmlee, T. A., Q. Liu, A. C. Whelen, D. Williams, S. S. Sommer, and D. H. Persing.** 1995. Genotypic detection of *Mycobacterium tuberculosis* rifampin resistance: comparison of single-strand conformation polymorphism and dideoxy fingerprinting. *J. Clin. Microbiol.* **33:**1617–1623.

42. **Finken, M., P. Kirschner, A. Meier, A. Wrede, and E. C. Böttger.** 1993. Molecular basis of streptomycin resistance in *Mycobacterium tuberculosis:* alterations of the ribosomal protein S12 gene and point mutations within a functional 16S ribosomal RNA pseudoknot. *Mol. Microbiol.* **9:**1239–1246.

43. **Franzblau, S. G., R. S. Witzig, J. C. McLaughlin, P. Torres, G. Madico, A. Hernandez, M. T. Degnan, M. B. Cook, V. K. Quenzer, R. M. Ferguson, and R. H. Gilman.** 1998. Rapid, low-technology MIC determination with clinical *Mycobacterium tuberculosis* isolates by using the microplate Alamar Blue assay. *J. Clin. Microbiol.* **36:**362–366.

44. **Garcia, L., M. Alonso-Sanz, M. J. Rebollo, J. C. Tercero, and F. Chaves.** 2001. Mutations in the *rpoB* gene of rifampin-resistant *Mycobacterium tuberculosis* isolates in Spain and their rapid detection by PCR-enzyme-linked immunosorbent assay. *J. Clin. Microbiol.* **39:**1813–1818.

45. **Ginsburg, A. S., J. H. Grosset, and W. R. Bishai.** 2003. Fluoroquinolones, tuberculosis, and resistance. *Lancet Infect. Dis.* **3:**432–442.

46. **Griffith, D. E., T. Aksamit, B. Brown-Elliott, A. Catanzaro, C. Daley, F. Gordin, S. M. Holland, R. Horsburgh, G. Huitt, M. F. Iademarco, M. Iseman, K. Olivier, S. Ruoss, C. F. von Reyn, R. J. Wallace, and K. Winthrop.** 2007. An official ATS/IDSA statement: diagnosis, treatment, and prevention of nontuberculous mycobacterial diseases. *Am. J. Respir. Crit. Care Med.* **175:**367–416.

47. **Grosset, J. H.** 1992. Treatment of tuberculosis in HIV infection. *Tubercle Lung Dis.* **73:**378–383.

48. **Guthertz, L. S., M. E. Griffith, E. G. Ford, J. M. Janda, and T. F. Midura.** 1988. Quality control of individual components used in Middlebrook 7H10 medium for mycobacterial susceptibility testing. *J. Clin. Microbiol.* **26:**2338–2342.

49. **Hacek, D.** 1992. Modified proportion agar dilution test for slowly growing mycobacteria, p. 5.13.1–5.13.15. *In* H. D. Isenberg (ed.), *Clinical Microbiology Procedures Handbook,* vol. 1. American Society for Microbiology, Washington, DC.

50. **Hanna, B. A., A. Ebrahimzadeh, L. B. Elliott, M. A. Morgan, S. M. Novak, S. Rüsch-Gerdes, M. Acio, D. F. Dunbar, T. M. Holmes, C. H. Rexer, C. Savthyakumar, and A. M. Vannier.** 1999. Multicenter evaluation of the BACTEC MGIT 960 system for recovery of mycobacteria. *J. Clin. Microbiol.* **37:**748–752.

51. **Havlir, D. V., M. P. Dube, F. R. Sattler, D. N. Forthal, C. A. Kemper, M. W. Dunne, D. M. Parenti, J. P. Lavelle, A. White, M. D. Witt, S. A. Bozzette, J. A. McCutchan, and the California Collaborative Treatment Group.** 1996. Prophylaxis against disseminated *Mycobacterium avium* complex with weekly azithromycin, daily rifabutin, or both. *N. Engl. J. Med.* **335:**392–398.

52. **Hawkins, J. E.** 1984. Drug susceptibility testing, p. 177–193. *In* G. P. Kubica and L. G. Wayne (ed.), *The Mycobacteria: a Sourcebook,* part A. Marcel Dekker, Inc., New York, NY.

53. **Hawkins, J. E.** 1986. Non-weekend schedule for BACTEC susceptibility testing of *Mycobacterium tuberculosis. J. Clin. Microbiol.* **23:**934–937.

54. **Hazbon, M. D., M. Brimacombe, M. Bobadilla del Valle, M. Cavatore, M. Imiride Guerrero, M. Varma-Basil, H. Billman-Jacobe, C. Lavender, J. Fyfe, L. Garcia-Garcia, C. Ines Leon, M. Bose, F. Chaves, M. Murray, K. D. Eisenach, J. Sifuentes-Osornio, M. D. Cave, A. Ponce de Leon, and D. Alland.** 2006. Population genetics study of isoniazid resistance mutations and evolution of multidrug-resistant *Mycobacterium tuberculosis. Antimicrob. Agents Chemother.* **50:**2640–2649.

55. **Heep, M., B. Brandstätter, U. Rieger, N. Lehn, E. Richter, S. Rüsch-Gerdes, and S. Niemann.** 2001. Frequency of *rpoB* mutations inside and outside the cluster I region in rifampin-resistant clinical *Mycobacterium tuberculosis* isolates. *J. Clin. Microbiol.* **39:**107–110.

56. **Heifets, L., and G. Cangelosi.** 2009. Drug resistance assays for *Mycobacterium tuberculosis,* p. 1161–1170. *In* D. L. Mayers (ed.), *Antimicrobial Drug Resistance.* Humana Press, Totowa, NJ.

57. **Heifets, L., J. Simon, and V. Pham.** 2005. Capreomycin is active against non-replicating *M. tuberculosis. Ann. Clin. Microbiol. Antimicrob.* **4:**6.

58. **Heifets, L. B.** 1991. *Drug Susceptibility in the Chemotherapy of Mycobacterial Infections,* p. 212. CRC Press, Inc., Boca Raton, FL.

59. **Heym, B., Y. Zhang, S. Poulet, D. Young, and S. T. Cole.** 1993. Characterization of the *katG* gene encoding a catalase-peroxidase required for isoniazid susceptibility of *Mycobacterium tuberculosis. J. Bacteriol.* **175:**4255–4259.

60. **Hillemann, D., S. Rusch-Gerdes, and E. Richter.** 2009. Feasibility of the GenoType MTBDRsl assay for fluoroquinolone, amikacin-capreomycin, and ethambutol resistance testing of *Mycobacterium tuberculosis* strains and clinical specimens. *J. Clin. Microbiol.* **47:**1767–1772.

61. **Hoffner, S. E., S. B. Svenson, and A. E. Beezer.** 1990. Microcalorimetric studies of the initial interaction between antimycobacterial drugs and *Mycobacterium avium*. *J. Antimicrob. Chemother.* **25**:353–359.

62. **Howard, W. L., F. Maresh, E. E. Mueller, S. A. Yanitelli, and G. F. Woodruff.** 1949. The role of pulmonary cavitation in the development of bacterial resistance to streptomycin. *Am. Rev. Tuberc.* **59**:391–401.

63. **Howlett, H. S., J. B. O'Connor, J. F. Sadusk, J. E. Swift, and F. A. Beardsley.** 1949. Sensitivity of tubercle bacilli to streptomycin: the influence of various factors upon the emergence of resistant strains. *Am. Rev. Tuberc.* **59**:402–414.

64. **Hu, Y., A. R. Coates, and D. A. Mitchison.** 2003. Sterilizing activities of fluoroquinolones against rifampin-tolerant populations of *Mycobacterium tuberculosis*. *Antimicrob. Agents Chemother.* **47**:653–657.

65. **Hunt, J. M., G. D. Roberts, L. Stockman, T. A. Felmlee, and D. H. Persing.** 1994. Detection of a genetic locus encoding resistance to rifampin in mycobacterial cultures and in clinical specimens. *Diagn. Microbiol. Infect. Dis.* **18**:219–227.

66. **Inderlied, C. B., C. A. Kemper, and L. E. M. Bermudez.** 1993. The *Mycobacterium avium* complex. *Clin. Microbiol. Rev.* **6**:266–310.

67. **Inderlied, C. B., P. T. Kolonski, M. Wu, and L. S. Young.** 1989. In vitro and in vivo activity of azithromycin (CP 62,993) against the *Mycobacterium avium* complex. *J. Infect. Dis.* **159**:994–997.

68. **Inderlied, C. B., and K. A. Nash.** 1996. Antimycobacterial agents: in vitro susceptibility testing, spectra of activity, mechanisms of action and resistance, and assays for activity in biologic fluids, p. 127–175. *In* V. Lorian (ed.), *Antibiotics in Laboratory Medicine*, 4th ed. The Williams & Wilkins Co., Baltimore, MD.

69. **Inderlied, C. B., and K. A. Nash.** 2005. Antimycobacterial agents: in vitro susceptibility testing and mechanisms of action and resistance, p. 155–225. *In* V. Lorian (ed.), *Antibiotics in Laboratory Medicine*. Lippincott Williams & Wilkins, Philadelphia, PA.

70. **Jannat-Khah, D. P., E. S. Halsey, B. A. Lasker, A. G. Steigerwalt, H. P. Hinrikson, and J. M. Brown.** 2009. *Gordonia araii* infection associated with an orthopedic device and review of the literature on medical device-associated *Gordonia* infections. *J. Clin. Microbiol.* **47**:499–502.

71. **Jureen, P., J. Werngren, J.-C. Toro, and S. Hoffner.** 2008. Pyrazinamide resistance and *pncA* gene mutations in *Mycobacterium tuberculosis*. *Antimicrob. Agents Chemother.* **52**:1852–1854.

72. **Källenius, G., S. G. Svenson, and S. E. Hoffner.** 1989. Ethambutol: a key for *Mycobacterium avium* complex chemotherapy. *Am. Rev. Respir. Dis.* **140**:264.

73. **Kapur, V., L. L. Li, S. Iordanescu, M. R. Hamrick, A. Wanger, B. N. Kreiswirth, and J. M. Musser.** 1994. Characterization by automated DNA sequencing of mutations in the gene (*rpoB*) encoding the RNA polymerase beta subunit in rifampin-resistant *Mycobacterium tuberculosis* strains from New York City and Texas. *J. Clin. Microbiol.* **32**:1095–1098.

74. **Kasperbauer, S. H., and C. L. Daley.** 2008. Diagnosis and treatment of infections due to *Mycobacterium avium* complex. *Semin. Respir. Care Med.* **29**:569–576.

75. **Kelley, C. L., D. A. Rouse, and S. L. Morris.** 1997. Analysis of *ahpC* gene mutations in isoniazid-resistant clinical isolates of *Mycobacterium tuberculosis*. *Antimicrob. Agents Chemother.* **41**:2057–2058.

76. **Kenney, T. J., and G. Churchward.** 1994. Cloning and sequence analysis of the *rpsL* and *rpsG* genes of *Mycobacterium smegmatis* and characterization of mutations causing resistance to streptomycin. *J. Bacteriol.* **176**:6153–6156.

77. **Kent, P. T., and G. P. Kubica.** 1985. *Public Health Mycobacteriology—a Guide for the Level III Laboratory.* U.S. Department of Health and Human Services, Centers for Disease Control, Atlanta, GA.

78. **Koh, W. J., O. J. Kwon, H. Gwak, J. W. Chung, S. N. Cho, W. S. Kim, and T. S. Shim.** 2009. Daily 300 mg dose of linezolid for the treatment of intractable multidrug-resistant and extensively drug-resistant tuberculosis. *J. Antimicrob. Chemother.* **64**:388–391.

79. **Koletar S. L., A. J. Berry, M. H. Cynamon, J. Jacobson, J. S. Currier, R. R. MacGregor, M. W. Dunne, and O. J. Williams.** 1999. Azithromycin as treatment for disseminated *Mycobacterium avium* complex in AIDS patients. *Antimicrob. Agents Chemother.* **43**:2869–2872.

80. **Kruuner, A., M. D. Yates, and F. A. Drobniewski.** 2006. Evaluation of MGIT 960-based antimicrobial testing and determination of critical concentrations of first- and second-line antimicrobial drugs with drug-resistant clinical strains of *Mycobacterium tuberculosis*. *J. Clin. Microbiol.* **44**:811–818.

81. **Kubica, G. P., and W. E. Dye.** 1967. *Laboratory Methods for Clinical and Public Health Mycobacteriology.* U.S. Government Printing Office, Washington, DC.

82. **Lin, S. Y., W. Probert, M. Lo, and E. Desmond.** 2004. Rapid detection of isoniazid and rifampin resistance mutations in *Mycobacterium tuberculosis* complex from cultures or smear-positive sputa by use of molecular beacons. *J. Clin. Microbiol.* **42**:4204–4208.

83. **Lin, S.-Y. G., E. Desmond, D. Bonato, W. Gross, and S. Siddiqui.** 2009. Multicenter evaluation of BACTEC MGIT 960 system for second-line drug susceptibility testing of *Mycobacterium tuberculosis* complex. *J. Clin. Microbiol.* **47**:3630–3634.

84. **Ling, D. I., A. A. Zwerling, and M. Pai.** 2008. Rapid diagnosis of drug-resistant TB using line probe assays; from evidence to policy. *Expert Rev. Respir. Med.* **2**:583–588.

85. **LoBue, P., C. Sizemore, and K. G. Castro.** 2009. Plan to combat extensively drug-resistant tuberculosis: recommendations of the Federal tuberculosis task force. *MMWR Recomm. Rep.* **58**(RR-03):1–43.

86. **Martin, A., A. von Groll, K. Fissette, J. C. Palomino, F. Varaine, and F. Portaels.** 2008. Rapid detection of *Mycobacterium tuberculosis* resistance to second-line drugs by use of the manual Mycobacterium Growth Indicator Tube system. *J. Clin. Microbiol.* **46**:3952–3956.

87. **Masur, H.** 1993. Recommendations on prophylaxis and therapy for disseminated *Mycobacterium avium* complex disease in patients infected with the human-immunodeficiency-virus. *N. Engl. J. Med.* **329**:898–904.

88. **Maus, C. E., B. B. Plikaytis, and T. M. Shinnick.** 2005. Molecular analysis of cross-resistance to capreomycin, kanamycin, amikacin, and viomycin in *Mycobacterium tuberculosis*. *Antimicrob. Agents Chemother.* **49**:3192–3197.

89. **Maus, C. E., B. B. Plikaytis, and T. M. Shinnick.** 2005. Mutation of *tlyA* confers capreomycin resistance in *Mycobacterium tuberculosis*. *Antimicrob. Agents Chemother.* **49**:572–577.

90. **Mdluli, K., D. R. Sherman, M. J. Hickey, B. N. Kreiswirth, S. Morris, C. K. Stover, and C. Barry III.** 1996. Biochemical and genetic data suggest that InhA is not the primary target for activated isoniazid in *Mycobacterium tuberculosis*. *J. Infect. Dis.* **174**:1085–1090.

91. **Mdluli, K., R. A. Slayden, Y. Zhu, S. Ramaswamy, X. Pan, D. Mead, D. D. Crane, J. M. Musser, and C. E. Barry III.** 1998. Inhibition of a *Mycobacterium tuberculosis*-ketoacyl ACP synthase by isoniazid. *Science* **280**:1607–1610.

92. **Mdluli, K., J. Swanson, E. Fischer, R. E. Lee, and C. E. Barry III.** 1998. Mechanisms involved in the intrinsic isoniazid resistance of *Mycobacterium avium*. *Mol. Microbiol.* **27**:1223–1233.

93. **Meier, A., P. Kirschner, B. Springer, V. A. Steingrube, B. A. Brown, R. J. Wallace, Jr., and E. C. Böttger.** 1994. Identification of mutations in 23S rRNA gene of clarithromycin-resistant *Mycobacterium intracellulare*. *Antimicrob. Agents Chemother.* **38**:381–384.

94. **Migliori, G. B., A. Matteelli, D. Cirillo, and M. Pai.** 2008. Diagnosis of multidrug-resistant tuberculosis and extensively drug-resistant tuberculosis: current standards and challenges. *Can. J. Infect. Dis. Med. Microbiol.* **19**:169–172.

95. **Mikhailovich, V. M., S. A. Lapa, D. A. Gryadunov, B. N. Strizhkov, A. Y. Sobolev, O. L. Skotnikova, O. A. I. Rtuganova, A. M. Moroz, V. I. Litvinov, L. K. Shipina, M. A. Vladimirskii, L. N. Chernousova, V. V. Erokhin, and A. D. Mirzabekov.** 2001. Detection of rifampicin-resistant *Mycobacterium tuberculosis* strains by hybridization polymerase chain reaction on a specialized TB-microchip. *Bull. Exp. Biol. Med.* **131**:94–98.

96. **Mitchison, D. A.** 1979. Basic mechanisms of chemotherapy. *Chest* **76**(Suppl.):771–781.

97. **Mitnick, C. D., B. McGee, and C. A. Peloquin.** 2009. Tuberculosis pharmacotherapy: strategies to optimize patient care. *Expert Opin. Pharmacother.* **10**:381–401.

98. **Moore, A. V., S. M. Kirk, S. M. Callister, G. H. Mazurek, and R. F. Schell.** 1999. Safe determination of susceptibility of *Mycobacterium tuberculosis* to antimycobacterial agents by flow cytometry. *J. Clin. Microbiol.* **37**:479–483.

99. **Moore, D. A., C. A. W. Evans, R. H. Gilman, L. Caviedes, J. Coronel, A. Vivar, E. Sanchez, Y. Pinedo, J. C. Saravia, C. Salazar, R. Oberhelman, M.-G. Hollm-Delgado, D. LaChira, A. R. Escombe, and J. S. Friedland.** 2007. Microscopic-observation drug-susceptibility assay for the diagnosis of TB. *N. Engl. J. Med.* **355**:1539–1550.

100. **Musser, J. M.** 1995. Antimicrobial agent resistance in mycobacteria: molecular genetic insights. *Clin. Microbiol. Rev.* **8**:496–514.

101. **Nair, J., D. A. Rouse, G. H. Bai, and S. L. Morris.** 1993. The *rpsL* gene and streptomycin resistance in single and multiple drug-resistant strains of *Mycobacterium tuberculosis*. *Mol. Microbiol.* **10**:521–527.

102. **Nash, K. A., A. Gaytan, and C. B. Inderlied.** 1997. Detection of rifampin resistance in *Mycobacterium tuberculosis* by use of a rapid, simple, and specific RNA/RNA mismatch assay. *J. Infect. Dis.* **176**:533–536.

103. **Nash, K. A., and C. B. Inderlied.** 1995. Genetic basis of macrolide resistance in *Mycobacterium avium* isolated from patients with disseminated disease. *Antimicrob. Agents Chemother.* **39**:2625–2630.

104. **Nightingale, S. D., W. D. Cameron, F. M. Gordin, P. M. Sullam, D. L. Cohn, R. E. Chaisson, L. J. Eron, P. D. Saprti, B. Bihari, D. L. Kaufman, J. J. Stern, D. D. Pearce, W. G. Weinberg, A. LaMarca, and F. P. Siegel.** 1993. Two controlled trials of rifabutin prophylaxis against *Mycobacterium avium* complex infection in AIDS. *N. Engl. J. Med.* **329**:828–833.

105. **Nitta, A. T., P. T. Davidson, M. L. de Koning, and R. J. Kilman.** 1996. Misdiagnosis of multidrug-resistant tuberculosis possibly due to laboratory-related errors. *JAMA* **276**:1980–1983.

106. **Ntziora, F., and M. E. Falagas.** 2007. Linezolid for the treatment of patients with mycobacterial infections: a systematic review. *Int. J. Tuberc. Lung Dis.* **11**:606–611.

107. **Nunn, P., J. Porter, and P. Winstanley.** 1993. Thiacetazone —avoid like poison or use with care. *Trans. R. Soc. Trop. Med. Hyg.* **87**:578–582.

108. **O'Riordan, P., U. Schwab, S. Logan, G. Cooke, R. J. Wilkinson, R. N. Davidson, P. Bassett, R. Wall, G. Pasvol, and K. L. Flanagan.** 2008. Rapid molecular detection of rifampicin resistance facilitates early diagnosis and treatment of multidrug-resistant tuberculosis: case control study. *PLoS ONE* **3**:e3173.

109. **Palomino, J. C.** 2009. Molecular detection, identification, and drug-resistance detection in *Mycobacterium tuberculosis*. *FEMS Immunol. Med. Microbiol.* **2009**:1–9.

110. **Parsons, L. M., A. Somoskovi, R. Urbanczik, and M. Salfinger.** 2004. Laboratory diagnostic aspects of drug resistant tuberculosis. *Front. Biosci.* **9**:2086–2105.

111. **Pfyffer, G. E., D. A. Bonato, A. Ebrahimzadeh, W. Gross, J. Hotaling, J. Kornblum, A. Laszlo, G. Roberts, M. Salfinger, F. Wittwer, and S. Siddiqi.** 1999. Multicenter laboratory validation of susceptibility testing of *Mycobacterium tuberculosis* against classical second-line and newer antimicrobial drugs by using the radiometric BACTEC 460 technique and the proportion method with solid media. *J. Clin. Microbiol.* **37**:3179–3186.

112. **Pfyffer, G. E., F. Palicova, and S. Rüsch-Gerdes.** 2002. Testing of susceptibility of *Mycobacterium tuberculosis* to pyrazinamide with the nonradiometric BACTEC MGIT 960 system. *J. Clin. Microbiol.* **40**:1670–1674.

113. **Pfyffer, G. E., H. M. Welscher, P. Kissling, C. Cieslak, M. J. Casal, J. Gutierrez, and S. Rüsch-Gerdes.** 1997. Comparison of the Mycobacteria Growth Indicator Tube (MGIT) with radiometric and solid culture for recovery of acid-fast bacilli. *J. Clin. Microbiol.* **35**:364–368.

114. **Piatek, A. S., A. Telenti, M. R. Murray, H. El-Hajj, W. R. Jacobs, Jr., F. R. Kramer, and D. Alland.** 2000. Genotypic analysis of *Mycobacterium tuberculosis* in two distinct populations using molecular beacons: implications for rapid susceptibility testing. *Antimicrob. Agents Chemother.* **44**:103–110.

115. **Pierce, M., S. Crampton, D. Henry, L. Heifets, A. LaMarca, M. Montecalvo, G. P. Wormser, H. Jablonowski, J. Jemsek, M. Cynamon, B. G. Yangco, G. Notario, and J. C. Craft.** 1996. A randomized trial of clarithromycin as prophylaxis against disseminated *Mycobacterium avium* complex infection in patients with advanced acquired immunodeficiency syndrome. *N. Engl. J. Med.* **335**:384–391.

116. **Pyle, M.** 1947. Relative number of resistant tubercle bacilli in sputa of patients before and during treatment with streptomycin. *Proc. Mayo Clin.* **22**:465–473.

117. **Pym, A., and S. Cole.** 2002. Drug resistance and tuberculosis chemotherapy—from concept to genomics, p. 355–403. *In* K. Lewis (ed.), *Bacterial Resistance to Antimicrobials*. Marcel Dekker, New York, NY.

118. **Revel Viravau, V., Q. C. Truong, N. Moreau, V. Jarlier, and W. Sougakoff.** 1996. Sequence analysis, purification, and study of inhibition by 4-quinolones of the DNA gyrase from *Mycobacterium smegmatis*. *Antimicrob. Agents Chemother.* **40**:2054–2061.

118a. **Ridderhof, J., I. George, and W. Gross.** 1991. *Abstr. Intersci. Conf. Antimicrob. Agents Chemother.*, 1999, abstr. 865.

119. **Rinder, H., K. Feldmann, E. Tortoli, J. Grosset, M. Casal, E. Richter, M. Rifai, V. Jarlier, M. Vaquero, S. Rüsch-Gerdes, E. Cambau, J. Gutierrez, and T. Loscher.** 1999. Culture-independent prediction of isoniazid resistance in *Mycobacterium tuberculosis* by *katG* gene analysis directly from sputum samples. *Mol. Diagn.* **4**:145–152.

120. **Riska, P. F., Y. Su, S. Bardarov, L. Freundlich, G. Sarkis, G. Hatfull, C. Carriere, V. Kumar, J. Chan, and W. R. Jacobs, Jr.** 1999. Rapid film-based determination of antibiotic susceptibilities of *Mycobacterium tuberculosis* strains by using a luciferase reporter phage and the Bronx Box. *J. Clin. Microbiol.* **37**:1144–1149.

121. **Rodrigues, C., J. Jani, S. Shenai, P. Thakker, S. Siddiqui, and A. Mehta.** 2008. Drug susceptibility testing of *Mycobacterium tuberculosis* against second-line drugs using the Bactec MGIT 960 system. *Int. J. Tuberc. Lung. Dis.* **12**:1449–1455.

122. **Ruiz, M., M. J. Torres, A. C. Llanos, A. Arroyo, J. C. Palomares, and J. Aznar.** 2004. Direct detection of rifampin-and-isoniazid-resistant *Mycobacterium tuberculosis* in auramine-rhodamine-positive sputum specimens by real-time PCR. *J. Clin. Microbiol.* **42**:1585–1589.

123. **Ruiz, P., F. J. Zerolo, and M. J. Casal.** 2000. Comparison of susceptibility testing of *Mycobacterium tuberculosis* using the ESP culture system II with that using the BACTEC method. *J. Clin. Microbiol.* **38**:4663–4664.

124. **Rüsch-Gerdes, S., C. Domehl, G. Nardi, M. R. Gismondo, H. M. Welscher, and G. E. Pfyffer.** 1999. Multicenter evaluation of the mycobacteria growth indicator tube for testing susceptibility of *Mycobacterium tuberculosis* to first-line drugs. *J. Clin. Microbiol.* **37**:45–48.

125. **Rusch-Gerdes, S., G. E. Pfyffer, M. Casal, M. Chadwick, and S. Siddiqui.** 2006. Multicenter laboratory validation of the Bactec MGIT 960 techniques for testing susceptibilities of *Mycobacterium tuberculosis* to classical second-line drugs and new antimicrobials. *J. Clin Microbiol.* **44**:688–692.

126. **Russel, W. R., and G. Middlebrook.** 1961. *Chemotherapy of Tuberculosis.* Charles C. Thomas, Springfield, IL.

127. **Safi, H., B. Sayers, M. H. Hazbon, and D. Alland.** 2008. Transfer of *embB* codon 306 mutations into clinical *Mycobacterium tuberculosis* strains alters susceptibility to ethambutol, isoniazid, and rifmapin. *Antimicrob. Agents Chemother.* **52**:2027–2034.

128. **Saito, H., K. Sato, and H. Tomioka.** 1988. Comparative in vitro and in vivo activity of rifabutin and rifampicin against *Mycobacterium avium* complex. *Tubercle* **69**:187–192.

129. **Sanders, C. A., R. R. Nieda, and E. P. Desmond.** 2004. Validation of the use of Middlebrook 7H10 agar, BACTEC MGIT 960, and BACTEC 460 12B media for testing the susceptibility of *Mycobacterium tuberculosis* to levofloxacin. *J. Clin. Microbiol.* **42:**5225–5228.

130. **Scarparo, C., P. Ricordi, G. Ruggiero, and P. Piccoli.** 2004. Evaluation of the fully automated BACTEC MGIT 960 System for testing susceptibility of *Mycobacterium tuberculosis* to pyrazinamide, streptomycin, isoniazid, rifampin, and ethambutol and comparison with the radiometric BACTEC 460TB. *J. Clin. Microbiol.* **42:**1109–1114.

131. **Schentag, J. J., and C. H. Ballow.** 1991. Tissue-directed pharmacokinetics. *Am. J. Med.* **91:**5S–11S.

132. **Scorpio, A., D. Collins, D. Whipple, D. Cave, J. Bates, and Y. Zhang.** 1997. Rapid differentiation of bovine and human tubercle bacilli based on a characteristic mutation in the bovine pyrazinamidase gene. *J. Clin. Microbiol.* **35:**106–110.

133. **Scorpio, A., P. Lindholm Levy, L. Heifets, R. Gilman, S. Siddiqi, M. Cynamon, and Y. Zhang.** 1997. Characterization of *pncA* mutations in pyrazinamide-resistant *Mycobacterium tuberculosis*. *Antimicrob. Agents Chemother.* **41:**540–543.

134. **Shafran, S. D., J. Singer, D. P. Zarowny, P. Phillips, I. Salit, S. L. Walmsley, I. W. Fong, M. J. Gill, A. R. Rachlis, R. G. Lalonde, M. M. Fanning, C. M. Tsoukas, and the Canadian HIV Trials Network Protocol 010 Study Group.** 1996. A comparison of two regimens for the treatment of *Mycobacterium avium* complex bacteremia in AIDS: rifabutin, ethambutol, and clarithromycin versus rifampin, ethambutol, clofazimine, and ciprofloxacin. *N. Engl. J. Med.* **335:**377–383.

135. **Sheng, W. H., Y. T. Huang, S. C. Chang, and P. R. Hsueh.** 2009. Brain abscess caused by *Tsukamurella tyrosinosolvens* in an immunocompetent patient. *J. Clin. Microbiol.* **47:**1602–1604.

136. **Singh, R., U. Manjunatha, H. I. Boshoff, Y. H. Ha, P. Niyomrattanakit, R. Ledwidge, C. S. Dowd, I. Y. Lee, P. Kim, L. Zhang, T. H. Keller, J. Jiricek, and C. E. Barry.** 2008. PA-824 kills nonreplicating *Mycobacterium tuberculosis* by intracellular NO release. *Science* **322:**1337–1338.

137. **Sirgel, F. A., F. J. Botha, D. P. Parkin, B. W. Van de Wal, R. Schall, P. R. Donald, and D. A. Mitchison.** 1997. The early bactericidal activity of ciprofloxacin in patients with pulmonary tuberculosis. *Am. J. Respir. Crit. Care Med.* **156:**901–905.

138. **Sison, J. P., Y. Yao, C. A. Kemper, J. R. Hamilton, E. Brummer, D. A. Stevens, and S. C. Deresinski.** 1996. Treatment of *Mycobacterium avium* complex infection: do the results of in vitro susceptibility tests predict therapeutic outcome in humans? *J. Infect. Dis.* **173:**677–683.

139. **Sreevatsan, S., X. Pan, Y. Zhang, V. Deretic, and J. M. Musser.** 1997. Analysis of the *oxyR-ahpC* region in isoniazid-resistant and -susceptible *Mycobacterium tuberculosis* complex organisms recovered from diseased humans and animals in diverse localities. *Antimicrob. Agents Chemother.* **41:**600–606.

140. **Sreevatsan, S., X. Pan, Y. Zhang, B. N. Kreiswirth, and J. M. Musser.** 1997. Mutations associated with pyrazinamide resistance in *pncA* of *Mycobacterium tuberculosis* complex organisms. *Antimicrob. Agents Chemother.* **41:**636–640.

141. **Sreevatsan, S., K. E. Stockbauer, X. Pan, B. N. Kreiswirth, S. L. Moghazeh, W. Jacobs, Jr., A. Telenti, and J. M. Musser.** 1997. Ethambutol resistance in *Mycobacterium tuberculosis*: critical role of *embB* mutations. *Antimicrob. Agents Chemother.* **41:**1677–1681.

142. **Starks, A., A. Gumusboga, B. B. Plikaytis, T. M. Shinnick, and J. E. Posey.** 2009. Mutations at *embB* codon 306 are an important molecular indicator of ethambutol resistance in *Mycobacterium tuberculosis*. *Antimicrob. Agents Chemother.* **53:**1061–1066.

143. **Takayama, K., and J. O. Kilburn.** 1989. Inhibition of synthesis of arabinogalactan by ethambutol in *Mycobacterium smegmatis*. *Antimicrob. Agents Chemother.* **33:**1493–1499.

144. **Takiff, H. E., L. Salazar, C. Guerrero, W. Philipp, W. M. Huang, B. Kreiswirth, S. T. Cole, W. Jacobs, Jr., and A. Telenti.** 1994. Cloning and nucleotide sequence of *Mycobacterium tuberculosis gyrA* and *gyrB* genes and detection of quinolone resistance mutations. *Antimicrob. Agents Chemother.* **38:**773–780.

145. **Tasneen, R., S. Tyagi, K. Williams, J. Grosset, and E. Nuermberger.** 2008. Enhanced bactericidal activity of rifampin and/or pyrazinamide when combined with PA-824 in a murine model of tuberculosis. *Antimicrob. Agents Chemother.* **52:**3664–3668.

146. **Telenti, A., N. Honore, C. Bernasconi, J. March, A. Ortega, B. Heym, H. E. Takiff, and S. T. Cole.** 1997. Genotypic assessment of isoniazid and rifampin resistance in *Mycobacterium tuberculosis*: a blind study at reference laboratory level. *J. Clin. Microbiol.* **35:**719–723.

147. **Telenti, A., P. Imboden, F. Marchesi, T. Schmidheini, and T. Bodmer.** 1993. Direct, automated detection of rifampin-resistant *Mycobacterium tuberculosis* by polymerase chain reaction and single-strand conformation polymorphism analysis. *Antimicrob. Agents Chemother.* **37:**2054–2058.

148. **Tenover, F. C., J. T. Crawford, R. E. Huebner, L. J. Geiter, C. R. Horsburgh, and R. C. Good.** 1993. The resurgence of tuberculosis: is your laboratory ready? *J. Clin. Microbiol.* **31:**767–770.

149. **Troesch, A., H. Nguyen, C. G. Miyada, S. Desvarenne, T. R. Gingeras, P. M. Kaplan, P. Cros, and C. Mabilat.** 1999. *Mycobacterium* species identification and rifampin resistance testing with high-density DNA probe arrays. *J. Clin. Microbiol.* **37:**49–55.

150. **Urbanczik, R., and H. L. Reider.** 2009. Scaling up tuberculosis culture services: a precautionary note. *Int. J. Tuberc. Lung Dis.* **13:**799–800.

151. **Verma, P., J. M. Brown, V. H. Nunez, R. E. Morey, A. G. Steigerwalt, G. J. Pellegrini, and H. A. Kessler.** 2006. Native valve endocarditis due to *Gordonia polyisoprenivorans*: case report and review of literature of bloodstream infections caused by *Gordonia* species. *J. Clin. Microbiol.* **44:**1905–1908.

152. **Vernon, A. A.** 2003. Rifamycin antibiotics, with focus on newer agents, p. 759–771. *In* W. M. Rom and S. M. Garay (ed.), *Tuberculosis*, 2nd ed. Lippincott Williams & Wilkins, New York, NY.

153. **Vilcheze, C., and W. R. Jacobs.** 2007. The mechanism of isoniazid killing: clarity through the scope of genetics. *Annu. Rev. Microbiol.* **61:**35–50.

154. **Wade, M. M., and Y. Zang.** 2004. Mechanisms of drug resistance in *Mycobacterium tuberculosis*. *Front. Biosci.* **9:**975–994.

155. **Waggoner, J. J.** 2009. First case report of community-acquired pneumonia due to *Tsukamurella pulmonis*. *Ann. Intern. Med.* **150:**147–148.

156. **Wallace, R., Jr., A. Meier, B. A. Brown, Y. Zhang, P. Sander, G. O. Onyi, and E. C. Böttger.** 1996. Genetic basis for clarithromycin resistance among isolates of *Mycobacterium chelonae* and *Mycobacterium abscessus*. *Antimicrob. Agents Chemother.* **40:**1676–1681.

157. **Wallace, R. J., Jr., and D. E. Griffith.** 2005. Antimycobacterial agents, p. 350–360. *In* G. L. Mandell, R. G. Douglas, Jr., and J. E. Bennett (ed.), *Principles and Practices of Infectious Diseases*, 6th ed. Elsevier Churchill Livingstone, Inc., Philadelphia, PA.

158. **Williams, D. L., L. Spring, L. Collins, L. P. Miller, L. B. Heifets, P. R. Gangadharam, and T. P. Gillis.** 1998. Contribution of *rpoB* mutations to development of rifamycin cross-resistance in *Mycobacterium tuberculosis*. *Antimicrob. Agents Chemother.* **42:**1853–1857.

159. **Wilson, T. M., and D. M. Collins.** 1996. *ahpC*, a gene involved in isoniazid resistance of the *Mycobacterium tuberculosis* complex. *Mol. Microbiol.* **19:**1025–1034.

160. **Winder, F. G.** 1982. Mode of action of the antimycobacterial agents and associated aspects of the molecular biology of the mycobacteria, p. 353–438. *In* C. Ratledge and J.

Stanford (ed.), *The Biology of the Mycobacteria*, vol. 1. *Physiology, Identification and Classification*. Academic Press, Inc., New York, NY.

161. **Winder, F. G., and P. B. Collins.** 1969. The effect of isoniazid on nicotinamide nucleotide concentrations in tubercle bacilli. *Am. Rev. Respir. Dis.* **100:**101–103.

162. **Winder, F. G., and P. B. Collins.** 1968. The effect of isoniazid on nicotinamide nucleotide levels in *Mycobacterium bovis* strain BCG. *Am. Rev. Respir. Dis.* **97:**719–720.

163. **Woods, G. L., J. S. Bergmann, F. G. Witebsky, G. A. Fahle, A. Wanger, B. Boulet, M. Plaunt, B. A. Brown, and R. J. Wallace, Jr.** 1999. Multisite reproducibility of results obtained by the broth microdilution method for susceptibility testing of *Mycobacterium abscessus*, *Mycobacterium chelonae*, and *Mycobacterium fortuitum*. *J. Clin. Microbiol.* **37:**1676–1682.

164. **Woods, G. L., N. Williams-Bouver, R. J. Wallace, Jr., B. A. Brown-Elliot, F. G. Witebsky, P. S. Conville, M. Plaunt, G. Hall, P. Aralar, and C. Inderlied.** 2003. Multisite reproducibility of results obtained by two broth dilution methods for susceptibility testing of *Mycobacterium avium* complex. *J. Clin. Microbiol.* **41:**627–631.

165. **Woods, G. L., G. Fish, M. Plaunt, and T. Murphy.** 1997. Clinical evaluation of Difco ESP culture system II for growth and detection of mycobacteria. *J. Clin. Microbiol.* **35:**121–124.

166. **World Health Organization.** 2008. *Guidelines for the Programmatic Management of Drug-Resistant Tuberculosis*. WHO/HTM/TB/2008.402. World Health Organization, Geneva, Switzerland.

167. **World Health Organization.** 2008. *New Laboratory Diagnostic Tools for Tuberculosis Control*. World Health Organization, Geneva, Switzerland.

168. **Yang, B., H. Koga, H. Ohno, K. Ogawa, M. Fukuda, Y. Hirakata, S. Maesaki, K. Tomono, T. Tashiro, and S. Kohno.** 1998. Relationship between antimycobacterial activities of rifampicin, rifabutin and KRM-1648 and *rpoB* mutations of *Mycobacterium tuberculosis*. *J. Antimicrob. Chemother.* **42:**621–628. (Erratum, **43:**613, 1999.)

169. **Young, L. S., O. G. Berlin, and C. B. Inderlied.** 1987. Activity of ciprofloxacin and other fluorinated quinolones against mycobacteria. *Am. J. Med.* **82:**23–26.

170. **Young, L. S., L. Wiviott, M. Wu, P. Kolonoski, R. Bolan, and C. B. Inderlied.** 1991. Azithromycin for treatment of *Mycobacterium avium-intracellulare* complex infection in patients with AIDS. *Lancet* **338:**1107–1109.

171. **Zhang, Y., S. Dhandayuthapani, and V. Deretic.** 1996. Molecular basis for the exquisite sensitivity of *Mycobacterium tuberculosis* to isoniazid. *Proc. Natl. Acad. Sci. USA* **93:**13212–13216.

172. **Zhang, Y., and D. Mitchison.** 2003. The curious characteristics of pyrazinamide: a review. *Int. J. Tuberc. Lung Dis.* **7:**6–21.

173. **Zhang, Y., M. M. Wade, A. Scorpio, H. Zhang, and Z. Sun.** 2003. Mode of action of pyrazinamide: disruption of *Mycobacterium tuberculosis* membrane transport and energetic by pyrazinoic acid. *J. Antimicrob. Chemother.* **52:**790–795.

174. **Zhang, Y., A. Scorpio, H. Nikaido, and Z. Sun.** 1999. Role of acid pH and deficient efflux of pyrazinoic acid in unique susceptibility of *Mycobacterium tuberculosis* to pyrazinamide. *J. Bacteriol.* **181:**2044–2049.

Detection and Characterization of Antimicrobial Resistance Genes in Pathogenic Bacteria*

J. KAMILE RASHEED AND FRED C. TENOVER

74

The direct detection of antimicrobial-resistant bacteria in clinical samples has received considerable attention in the last few years due in part to the continued spread of multidrug-resistant pathogens, such as methicillin-resistant *Staphylococcus aureus* (MRSA) and *Mycobacterium tuberculosis* strains (both multidrug resistant and extensively drug resistant) globally. The development of commercial kits that allow rapid testing of these and other bacterial pathogens directly in clinical samples, producing results often in an hour or less (instead of days), has enhanced surveillance activities and had a positive impact on patient management (223). Other commercial kits for detection and differentiation of extended-spectrum-β-lactamase (ESBL) genes (i.e., TEM, SHV, and CTX-M genes) that are highly prevalent among *Enterobacteriaceae* may improve therapeutic choices for patients as well as aid in epidemiological studies of dissemination of these resistance genes in hospitals and communities. A recently described commercial microarray-based assay, for example, allows the rapid detection of the genes encoding the TEM and SHV β-lactamases and their ESBL derivatives, the CTX-M ESBLs, and the *Klebsiella pneumoniae* carbapenemases (KPC) (166).

There are several new DNA sequencing technologies that have yet to find their way into the clinical laboratory but that may have a significant impact on future studies of resistant organisms. For example, ultradeep sequencing methods (101) are now being used to define subpopulations (often <5%) of the quasispecies of human immunodeficiency virus and hepatitis B virus responsible for treatment failures (150, 240). In the future, ultradeep sequencing may provide direction for treating more complex chronic wounds, such as diabetic foot ulcers (74) or pressure ulcers (73), which are frequently associated with recalcitrant biofilms.

The dramatic increase in multidrug resistance among a plethora of bacterial genera has necessitated the development of tests specifically designed to detect resistant strains, particularly to guide infection control efforts in health care facilities. Rapid tests that identify patients colonized or infected with MRSA and vancomycin-resistant enterococci (191) can save hospitals thousands of dollars each year by permitting isolation rooms to be used more effectively (242, 279). Yet, multidrug resistance is an issue not just with health care-associated pathogens. Multidrug-resistant *Salmonella* species (293) and pneumococci (145) and extensively drug-resistant M. *tuberculosis* (45, 216) are among the community-associated pathogens that pose therapeutic challenges.

Although DNA probes have been used extensively in the past for detection of resistance genes in bacterial isolates (and usually in pure cultures) (258), such assays have been replaced largely by PCR assays (54, 258). Within the last few years, reports of several novel methods of detecting resistance genotypes have appeared in the literature. These include real-time PCR assays with molecular beacons, peptide-nucleic acid fluorescent in situ hybridization probes, microarrays, and pyrosequencing methods. This chapter focuses specifically on genotypic methods for detecting and characterizing antimicrobial-resistant bacterial pathogens. Molecular methods for characterizing mycobacteria, viruses, and fungi are covered elsewhere in this *Manual*.

RATIONALE FOR USING GENETIC TESTS TO DETECT RESISTANCE GENOTYPES

There are four major reasons to use genetic tests to identify antimicrobial resistance genes or mutations associated with resistance in bacterial isolates. The first is the speed of detection afforded by PCR-based assays. Detecting resistant organisms directly in clinical specimens in less than 1 h allows rapid institution of anti-infective therapy or infection control interventions that can lead to reduced spread of infections (104, 223). Second, genetic methods can arbitrate MIC results that are at or near the breakpoint for resistance for bacterial species, such as for KPC-producing isolates of *Klebsiella pneumoniae* that may not demonstrate imipenem or meropenem MIC or disk diffusion results in the resistant range (13, 81, 257). Third, genetic tests are more accurate than analysis of resistance phenotypes for monitoring the epidemiological spread of a particular resistance gene in a hospital or community setting (10, 158). Fourth, genetic tests can be used as the "gold standard" for resistance tests

*This chapter contains information presented in chapter 78 by J. Kamile Rasheed, Franklin Cockerill, and Fred C. Tenover in the ninth edition of this *Manual*.

in evaluating the accuracy of new susceptibility testing methods (163), including the detection of *mecA* for defining methicillin resistance in *S. aureus* (229, 286).

However, there are several potential pitfalls associated with using genetic tests to detect resistant organisms. These include the lack of expression of resistance genes that are detected (33), the problem of mixed or normal biotas that may contain resistance genes (such as *vanB* determinants present in *Clostridium* species, rather than enterococci, in fecal samples) (20, 21), mutations in target organisms that alter sequences used for PCR primers and lead to false-negative results (22), and the emergence of novel resistance genes that are not detected by existing genetic assays (23). In addition, the resistance phenotype may be the result of multiple genes encoding antimicrobial resistance mechanisms, not just the presence of a single gene. Each of these factors can affect the sensitivity or specificity of molecular assays.

For some organisms, genetic tests may ultimately replace phenotypic methods. For example, detection of mutations associated with fluoroquinolone and penicillin resistance in *Neisseria gonorrheae* has been accomplished for purified colonies of gonococci (272, 273). This could be extended in the future to analyze the genotypes of organisms directly in urethral swabs, vaginal swabs, or urine samples to guide therapy. This approach may well replace cumbersome phenotypic assays now performed on a limited number of isolates each year (46). Molecular assays may also be introduced for direct testing of fastidious organisms for which phenotypic susceptibility testing is rarely performed, including *Helicobacter pylori*, *Mycoplasma pneumoniae*, and *Chlamydia trachomatis*, in which the emergence of resistance to standard therapy could significantly worsen disease outcomes.

It is likely that tests for direct detection of mutations associated with isoniazid, streptomycin, rifampin, and ethambutol resistance in *M. tuberculosis*, such as commercial hybridization assays (3, 243) and in vitro amplification tests that use molecular beacons (25a, 79), will become widely used over the next decade to guide initial therapeutic decisions for tuberculosis, especially in developing countries where these tests are provided to health agencies at significantly reduced costs. However, phenotypic methods will still play a major role in public health reference laboratories, where second- and third-line agents will continue to be tested to identify novel emerging resistance profiles. The recognition of multiple mechanisms of isoniazid resistance in *M. tuberculosis* underscores the ongoing need for phenotypic methods, even if the results are available only long after empirical therapy has been initiated (17, 299).

The question of whether molecular methods will ultimately replace phenotypic susceptibility testing methods for staphylococci, *Enterobacteriaceae*, *Pseudomonas* species, and other nonfermenters beyond surveillance screening for infection control purposes remains open. Clearly, molecular screening methods to detect *bla*KPC, *bla*VIM, and other critical resistance genes in gram-negative organisms directly in positive blood culture vials and perhaps in clinical specimens and surveillance cultures will increase as carbapenem resistance rates rise (81), just as screening for MRSA and vancomycin-resistant enterococci has become commonplace in many health care institutions (109, 223). Yet, the plethora of novel resistance mechanisms, as outlined later in this chapter, suggests that phenotypic methods to identify resistance in these organism groups will continue to have value at least for the next decade.

GENETIC TESTS FOR RESISTANCE GENES AND DNA SEQUENCING STRATEGIES TO DETECT MUTATIONS ASSOCIATED WITH RESISTANCE

General Guidelines

The ideal genetic test targets nucleic acid sequences within the open reading frame (or coding region) of the resistance gene and avoids sequences outside of the gene that may contain insertion elements or promoter sequences that may be present in susceptible strains or strains with other types of resistance genes. Alternatively, the test detects point mutations associated with the resistance phenotype. Among the primers that have been described for studying antibacterial resistance are those directed to β-lactamase genes and the genes that encode resistance to aminocyclitols, aminoglycosides (i.e., aminoglycoside-modifying enzymes and 16S rRNA methylases), chloramphenicol, glycopeptides, isoniazid, macrolides, mupirocin, oxazolidinones, quinolones (including chromosomal and plasmid-mediated quinolone resistance), rifampin, sulfonamides, tetracyclines, and trimethoprim. Examples of PCR primers that target resistance genes or mutations associated with resistance are shown in Table 1. In addition, multiplex PCR assays for the detection of multiple resistance genes are shown in Table 2. The tables are meant not to be exhaustive but, rather, to give an indication of the types of assays that have been described in the literature. Appropriate specificity controls (organisms that have a similar resistance pattern but contain resistance genes other than the target gene) should always be included in all reactions using these primers. Examples of DNA probes that can be used to detect resistance genes have been described in previous editions of this *Manual* (258).

DNA Sequencing

DNA sequence analysis has been particularly helpful for identifying point mutations in genes associated with ESBLs (26, 213, 215) and resistance to carbapenems (288), fluoroquinolones (117, 163), oxazolidinones (292), and antimycobacterial drugs (165). There are a number of mutations associated with resistance to isoniazid, rifampin, and ethambutol in mycobacteria (17, 299) which can be detected rapidly and with a high degree of accuracy by pyrosequencing assays (17, 299). Other novel high-throughput pyrosequencing assays that target mutations associated with resistance, such as changes in rRNA sequences associated with linezolid resistance in enterococci, can provide results in a few hours (241).

In-House Assays and Analyte-Specific Reagents (ASRs)

Development of home brew PCR assays for detecting resistance genes or implementing assays reported in the literature in a clinical microbiology laboratory has always been challenging. In-house validation of research protocols can be time-consuming. Yet, many of these assays provide significant advances in turnaround time or cost-effectiveness over those of traditional test methods. The Clinical and Laboratory Standards Institute (CLSI) has published a guideline describing validation of such tests (53).

In the United States, reagents for nucleic acid amplification-based technologies may be available from manufacturers in the form of ASRs. ASRs are produced under "good manufacturing practices" (57). Unlike with Food and Drug Administration (FDA)-cleared diagnostic kits, the clinical utility of the ASRs does not have to be

TABLE 1 PCR assays for antimicrobial resistance genes

Antimicrobial agent and gene	Primers (5′ → 3′)	Product size	Use(s)	Reference(s)
Aminoglycosides				
Aminoglycoside-modifying enzymes				
aac(6′)-Ia	ATG AAT TAT CAA ATT GTG TTA CTC TTT GAT TAA ACT	558 bp	Detection, probe	200[a]
aac(6′)-Ib	TTG CGA TGC TCT ATG AGT GGC TA CTC GAA TGC CTG GCG TGT TT	482 bp	Detection, restriction enzyme analysis[b]	184
aac(6′)-Ic	CTA CGA TTA CGT CAA CGG CTG C TTG CTT CGC CCA CTC CTG CAC C	130 bp	Detection	102[c]
aac(3)-Ia	ACC TAC TCC CAA CAT CAG CC ATA TAG ATC TCA CTA CGC GC	169 bp	Detection	268[d]
aac(3)-Ic	GAT GAT CTC TAC TCA AAC C TTA GGC AGC AGG TTG AGG	472 bp	Cloning, sequencing	219
aac(3)-IV	GTT ACA CCG GAC CTT GGA AAC GGC ATT GAG CGT CAG	675 bp	Detection	98
aphA-3	GGG ACC ACC TAT GAT GTG GAA CG CAG GCT TGA TCC CCA GTA AGT C	595 bp	Detection	92
aph(3′)VIa	ATA CAG AGA CCA CAT ACA GT GGA CAA TCA ATA ATA GCA AT	235 bp	Detection	275
aad(2″)-Ia	ATG TTA CGC AGC AGG GCA GTC G CGT CAG ATC AAT ATC ATC GTG C	188 bp	Detection	269
aac(6′)-Ie-aph(2″)-Ia	GAG CAA TAA GGG CAT ACC AAA AAT C CCG TGC ATT TGT CTT AAA AAA CTG G	485 bp	Detection	121
aac(6′)-Iih	GGA TAG CGG ATG ATT ATC A TAA GAG TTT AAT GAA TAA TTA	856 bp	Sequencing	66
aph(2″)-Ib	TAT GGA TCC ATG GTT AAC TTG GAC GCT GAG ATT AAG CTT CCT GCT AAA ATA TAA ACA TCT CTG CT	920 bp	Detection	121
aph(3′)-IIIa	GGC TAA AAT GAG AAT ATC ACC GG CTT TAA AAA ATC ATA CAG CTC GCG	523 bp	Detection	249, 267
ant(4′)-Ia	CAA ACT GCT AAA TCG GTA GAA GCC GGA AAG TTG ACC AGA CAT TAC GAA CT	294 bp	Detection	249, 267
aadA	TGA TTT GCT GGT TAC GGT GAC CGC TAT GTT CTC TTG CTT TTG	284 bp	Detection, probe	50
aadE	ACT GGC TTA ATC AAT TTG GG GCC TTT CCG CCA CCT CAC CG	597 bp	Detection, probe	50
aad-6	AGA AGA TGT AAT AAT ATA G CTG TAA TCA CTG TTC CCG CCT	978 bp	Detection	136
strA-strB	TAT CTG CGA TTG GAC CCT CTG CAT TGC TCA TCA TTT GAT CGG CT	519 bp	Detection	248
16S rRNA methylases				
armA	AGG TTG TTT CCA TTT CTG AG TCT CTT CCA TTC CCT TCT CC	590 bp	Detection, sequencing	294
rmtA	CTA GCG TCC ATC CTT TCC TC TTT GCT TCC ATG CCC TTG CC	635 bp	Detection	298
rmtB	ATG AAC ATC AAC GAT GCC CT CCT TCT GAT TGG CTT ATC CA	769 bp	Detection, sequencing, probe	296
rmtC	GCC AAA GTA CTC ACA AGT GG CTC AGA TCT GAC CCA ACA AG	752 bp	Detection	88
rmtD	GAG CGA ACT GAA GGA AAA AC CAG CAC GTA AAA CAG CTC	730 bp	Detection, sequencing	39
npmA	CTC AAA GGA ACA AAG ACG G GAA ACA TGG CCA GAA ACT C	641 bp	Detection	88
Spectinomycin				
rrs (Neisseria meningitidis, N. gonorrhoeae)	CTT ACC TGG TCT TGA CA CGA TTA CTA GCG ATT CC	373 bp	Sequencing	89
β-Lactams				
mecA	TGG CTA TCG TGT CAC AAT CG CTG GAA CTT GTT GAG CAG AG	310 bp	Detection	270

(Continued on next page)

TABLE 1 PCR assays for antimicrobial resistance genes (*Continued*)

Antimicrobial agent and gene	Primers (5′ → 3′)	Product size	Use(s)	Reference(s)
*bla*SHV	GCC GGG TTA TTC TTA TTT GTC GC TCT TTC CGA TGC CGC CGC CAG TCA	1,017 bp	Sequencing, restriction enzyme analysis[e]	174
*bla*SHV	GGT TAT GCG TTA TAT TCG CC ATC TTT CGC TCC AGC TGT TC	275 bp	Probe[f]	215[g]
*bla*SHV	GGT TAT GCG TTA TAT TCG CC TTA GCG TTG CCA GTG CTC	867 bp	Detection	215
*bla*TEM	ATG AGT ATT CAA CAT TTC CG TTA CTG TCA TGC CAT CC	351 bp	Detection, probe	213
*bla*TEM	ATG AGT ATT CAA CAT TTC CG CTG ACA GTT ACC AAT GCT TA	867 bp	Detection	215
*bla*CTX-M	CGC TTT GCG ATG TGC AG ACC GCG ATA TCG TTG GT	550 bp	Detection, probe	26
*bla*CTX-M	TTT GCG ATG TGC AGT ACC AGT AA CGA TAT CGT TGG TGG TGC CAT A	544 bp	Detection, RFLP[h] analysis	78
*bla*CTX-M-2	ATG ATG ACT CAG AGC ATT CG TTA TTG CAT CAG AAA CCG TG	884 bp	Detection	199
*bla*CTX-M-9	GTG ACA AAG AGA GTG CAA CGG ATG ATT CTC GCC GCT GAA GCC	857 bp	Detection	227
*bla*CTX-M-10	GCT GAT GAG CGC TTT GCG TTA CAA ACC GTT GGT GAC G	684 bp	Detection	176
*bla*GES-1	ATG CGC TTC ATT CAC GCA C CTA TTT GTC CGT GCT CAG G	864 bp	Probe[f]	202
*bla*GES/IBC	GTT TTG CAA TGT GCT CAA CG TGC CAT AGC AAT AGG CGT AG	371 bp	Detection, sequencing	282
*bla*LAP-1	CAA TAC AAA GCA CAG AAG ACC CCG ATC CCT GCA ATA TGC TC	748 bp	Detection, probe	201
*bla*PER-1	ATG AAT GTC ATT ATA AAA GC AAT TTG GGC TTA GGG CAA GAA A	926 bp	Detection, probe	266
*bla*PER-2	CGC TTC TGC TCT GCT GAT GGC AGC TTC TTT AAC GCC	469 bp	Detection	24
*bla*PSE	ACC GTA TTG AGC CTG ATT TA ATT GAA GCC TGT GTT TGA GC	321 bp	Detection	25[i]
*bla*ROB-1	TGT TTG CAA TCG CTG CC TTA TCG TAC ACT TTC CA	400 bp	Detection	120
*bla*SFO	GTT AAT CCA TTT TAT GTG AGG CAG ATA CGC GGT GCA TAT CCC	940 bp	Detection	233
*bla*TLA-1	TCT CAG CGC AAA TCC GCG CTA TTT CCC ATC CTT AAC TAG	974 bp	Detection	6
*bla*VEB-1	CGA CTT CCA TTT CCC GAT GC GGA CTC TGC AAC AAA TAC GC	643 bp	Detection	168
*bla*KPC	TGT CAC TGT ATC GCC GTC GTC AGT GCT CTA CAG AAA ACC	1,011 bp	Detection	214
*bla*KPC-2	GCT ACA CCT AGC TCC ACC TTC ACA GTG GTT GGT AAT CCA TGC	989 bp	Sequencing	161
*bla*IMI-1	ATA GCC ATC TTG TTT AGC TC TCT GCG ATT ACT TTA TCC TC	818 bp	Probe[f]	18
*bla*NmcA	TGC AGC TTA ATT ATT TTC AGA TTA G ATT TTT TTC ATG ATG AAG TTA AGC C	2,122 bp	Sequencing	205[j]
*bla*SME-1	AAC GGC TTC ATT TTT GTT TAG GCT TCC GCA ATA GTT TTA TCA	830 bp	Detection	211
*bla*IMP	CTA CCG CAG CAG AGT CTT TG AAC CAG TTT TGC CTT ACC AT	587 bp	Detection	235
*bla*VIM	TCT ACA TGA CCG CGT CTG TC TGT GCT TTG ACA ACG TTC GC	748 bp	Detection	203
*bla*VIM	AGT GGT GAG TAT CCG ACA G ATG AAA GTG CGT GGA GAC	261 bp	Detection, probe	90
*bla*SPM-1	CCT ACA ATC TAA CGG CGA CC TCG CCG TGT CCA GGT ATA AC	649 bp	Detection	261
*bla*GIM-1	AGA ACC TTG ACC GAA CGC AG ACT CAT GAC TCC TCA CGA GG	748 bp	Detection	41

(*Continued on next page*)

TABLE 1 *(Continued)*

Antimicrobial agent and gene	Primers (5′ → 3′)	Product size	Use(s)	Reference(s)
bla$_{SIM-1}$	TAC AAG GGA TTC GGC ATC G TAA TGG CCT GTT CCC ATG TG	571 bp	Detection, sequencing	138
ampC (promoter, *E. coli*)	GAT CGT TCT GCC GCT GTG GGG CAG CAA ATG TGG AGC AA	271 bp	Sequencing	38
bla$_{ACC}$	AAC AGC CTC AGC AGC CGG TTA TTC GCC GCA ATC ATC CCT AGC	346 bp	Detection	192[k]
bla$_{ACT-1}$	ATT CGT ATG CTG GAT CTC GCC ACC CAT GAC CCA GTT CGC CAT ATC CTG	396 bp	Detection	61
bla$_{DHA}$	CCG TCA CTC ACA CAC GGA AGG CGT ATC CGC AGG GGC TG TTC	1,199 bp	Detection, sequencing	160[l]
bla$_{FOX}$	TGT GGA CGG CAT TAT CCA G AAA GCG CGT AAC CGG ATT G	868 bp	Detection, sequencing	164
bla$_{OXA-1}$ group	TTT TCT GTT GTT TGG GTT TC TTT CTT GGC TTT TAT GCT TG	447 bp	Detection, RFLP analysis	25
bla$_{OXA-2}$ group	AAG AAA CGC TAC TCG CCT GC CCA CTC AAC CCA TCC TAC CC	486 bp	Detection, RFLP analysis	25
bla$_{OXA-10}$ group	TCA ACA AAT CGC CAG AGA AG TCC CAC ACC AGA AAA ACC AG	276 bp	Detection, RFLP analysis	25
bla$_{OXA-23}$	CCT CAG GTG TGC TGG TTA TTC CCC AAC CAG TCT TTC CAA AA	513 bp	Detection	35
bla$_{OXA-24}$	TTC CCC TAA CAT GAA TTT GT GTA CTA ATC AAA GTT GTG AA	1,020 bp	Detection, sequencing	27
Chloramphenicol, florfenicol				
catA1	CCA CCG TTG ATA TAT CCC CCT GCC ACT CAT CGC AGT	623 bp	Detection	97
cmlA	TGT CAT TTA CGG CAT ACT CG ATC AGG CAT CCC ATT CCC AT	456 bp	Detection	98
flo	CAC GTT GAG CCT CTA TAT GG ATG CAG AAG TAG AAC GCG AC	869 bp	Detection	171
cfr[m]	TGA AGT ATA AAG CAG GTT GGG AGT CA ACC ATA TAA TTG ACC ACA AGC AGC	746 bp	Detection	125
Glycopeptide				
vanA	GGG AAA ACG ACA ATT GC GTA CAA TGC GGC CGT TA	732 bp	Detection	77
vanB	CGC CAT ATT CTC CCC GGA TAG AAG CCC TCT GCA TCC AAG CAC	667 bp	Detection	139
vanC-1	GAA AGA CAA CAG GAA GAC CGC ATC GCA TCA CAA GCA CCA ATC	796 bp	Detection	49
vanC-2/3	CGG GGA AGA TGG CAG TAT CGC AGG GAC GGT GAT TTT	484 bp	Detection	123
vanC-3	GCC TTT ACT TAT TGT TCC GCT TGT TCT TTG ACC TTA	224 bp	Detection	51
vanD	TAA GGC GCT TGC ATA TAC CG TGC AGC CAA GTA TCC GGT AA	461 bp	Detection	194
vanE	TGT GGT ATC GGA GCT GCA G GTC GAT TCT CGC TAA TCC	513 bp	Detection, probe	84
vanG	CGG TTG TGC CGT ACT TGG C GGG TAA AGC CAT AGT CTG GGG C	811 bp	Detection	155
Macrolides, lincosamides, streptogramins				
ermA	CTT CGA TAG TTT ATT AAT ATT AGT TCT AAA AAG CAT GTA AAA GAA	645 bp	Detection	251
ermA (*ermTR*)	AGA AGG TTA TAA TGA AAC AGA A GGC ATG ACA TAA ACC TTC AT	212 bp	Detection	217
ermB	GAA AAG GTA CTC AAC CAA ATA AGT AAC GGT ACT TAA ATT GTT TAC	639 bp	Detection	251
ermC	TCA AAA CAT AAT ATA GAT AAA GCT AAT ATT GTT TAA ATC GTC AAT	642 bp	Detection	251

(Continued on next page)

TABLE 1 PCR assays for antimicrobial resistance genes (*Continued*)

Antimicrobial agent and gene	Primers (5′ → 3′)	Product size	Use(s)	Reference(s)
ermF	GCA GAC AGG CGC AAG CAG CAA	606 bp	Detection	221
	ACC ACG TTC CCA TGA GTG GTA TGG			
ermG	AGG GAA AGG TCA TTT TAC TGC	664 bp	Detection	217
	CCC TAC CTA TAA CTA AAC ATT			
mefA/mefE	AGT ATC ATT AAT CAC TAG TGC	348 bp	Detection	251
	TTC TTC TGG TAC TAA AAG TGG			
mefA	GAC CAA AAG CCA CAT TGT GGA	1,431 bp	Restriction enzyme analysis	180
	CCT CCT GTC TAT AAT CGC ATG			
mefE	CTA TGC GAT TTT GGG ACC TG	801 bp	Detection	149
	GAA AGC CCC ATT ATT GCA CA			
ereA	AGT CGG CGG TTA TTT CAT	746 bp	Detection	237
	TGC TCC CTC ATT TTC ATT TA			
ereB	CGG ATA AAG AAG CAC TAC AC	788 bp	Detection	237
	AAC GAC CTC AGA TAC AGA TG			
mphA	AAC TGT ACG CAC TTG C	837 bp	Detection	251
	GGT ACT CTT CGT TAC C			
msrA/msrB	GTC AAA AAC TGC TAA CAC AAG	343 bp	Detection	237
	AAT AAT ACT GCT AAC GAT AAT			
smp	AAA TTG TTT AAA AAG AAA TC	616 bp	Detection, probe	252
	TTT GAA CCA TAA TAT TCA TC			
vat	CAA TGA CCA TGG ACC TGA TC	615 bp	Detection	9
	AGC ATT TCG ATA TCT CC			
vatB	CCT GAT CCA AAT AGC ATA TAT CC	601 bp	Detection	8
	CTA AAT CAG AGC TAC AAA GTG			
satG (*vatE*)	CTA TAC CTG ACG CAA ATG C	511 bp	Detection	283
	GGT TCA AAT CTT GGT CCG			
vga	TCT AAT GGT ACA GGA AAG ACA ACG	399 bp	Detection	251
	ATC GTG AGA TAC AAA GAT TAT			
linA/linA′	GTA GAT GTA TTA ACT GGA A	325 bp	Detection, probe	173
	GAA AAA GAA GTT GAG CTT C			
linB	CCT ACC TAT TGT TTG TGG AA	944 bp	Detection	30
	ATA ACG TTA CTC TCC TAT TC			
Mupirocin				
IRS	CCA TGC CTT ACC AGT TGA ATT	1.65 kb	Probe[f]	93
	GGA TCC CCG AGC ACT ATC CGA			
mupA	CCC ATG GCT TAC CAG TTG A	1.65 kb	Detection, probe	212
	CCA TGG AGC ACT ATC CGA A			
mupA	TGA CAA TAG AAA AGG ACA GG	190 bp	Detection	182
	CTC TAA TTC AAC TGG TAA GCC			
ileS-2	GTT TAT CTT CTG ATG CTG AG	237 bp	Detection	175
	CCC CAG TTA CAC CGA TAT AA			
Quinolones				
gyrA (*Mycobacterium tuberculosis*)	CAG CTA CAT CGA CTA TGC GA	320 bp	Sequencing	122
	GGG CTT CGG TGT ACC TCA T			
gyrA (*Acinetobacter baumannii*)	AAA TCT GCC CGT GTC GTT GGT	343 bp	Sequencing	274
	GCC ATA CCT ACG GCG ATA CC			
gyrA (*E. coli*)	ACG TAC TAG GCA ATG ACT GG	190 bp	Sequencing	82[n]
	AGA AGT CGC CGT CGA TAG AAC			
gyrA (*S. pneumoniae*)	TTC TCT ACG GAA TGA ATG	272 bp	Sequencing	117
	GAT ATC ACG AAG CAT TTC CAG			
gyrB (*S. pneumoniae*)	TTC TCC GAT TTC CTC ATG	458 bp	Sequencing	183
	AGA AGG GTA CGA ATG TGG			
parC (*S. pneumoniae*)	TGG GTT GAA GCC GGT TCA	361 bp	Sequencing	117
	CAA GAC CGT TGG TTC TTT C			
parE (*S. pneumoniae*)	CCA ATC TAA GAA TCC TG	357 bp	Sequencing	195
	GCA ATA TAG ACA TGA CC			
Plasmid-mediated quinolone resistance				
qnrA	ATT TCT CAC GCC AGG ATT TG	468 bp	Detection	114
	TGC CAG GCA CAG ATC TTG AC			
qnrB	GGM[o] ATH[o] GAA ATT CGC CAC TG	264 bp	Detection	43
	TTT GCY[o] GYY CGC CAG TCG AA			

(Continued on next page)

TABLE 1 *(Continued)*

Antimicrobial agent and gene	Primers (5′ → 3′)								Product size	Use(s)	Reference(s)
qnrC	GGG	TTG	TAC	ATT	TAT	TGA	ATC	G	307 bp	Detection	128
	CAC	CTA	CCC	ATT	TAT	TTT	CA				
qnrD	CGA	GAT	CAA	TTT	ACG	GGG	AAT	A	582 bp	Detection	44
	AAC	AAG	CTG	AAG	CGC	CTG					
qnrS	ACT	GCA	AGT	TCA	TTG	AAC	AG		431 bp	Detection	114
	GAT	CTA	AAC	CGT	CGA	GTT	CG				
qepA	CGT	GTT	GCT	GGA	GTT	CTT	C		403 bp	Detection	159
	CTG	CAG	GTA	CTG	CGT	CAT	G				
Sulfonamides											
sulA	AGC	CAA	TCA	TGC	AAA	GAC	AG		916 bp	Sequencing	152
	ATT	TTC	CGC	TTC	ATC	AGC	CAG				
sulI	CTT	CGA	TGA	GAG	CCG	GCG	GC		437 bp	Detection	98
	GCA	AGG	CGG	AAA	CCC	GCG	CC				
sulI	ATG	GTG	ACG	GTG	TTC	GGC	ATT	CTG A	769 bp	Detection	95[p]
	CTA	GGC	ATG	ATC	TAA	CCC	TCG	GTC T			
Tetracycline											
tet(A)	GTA	ATT	CTG	AGC	ACT	GT			954 bp	Probe[f]	103[q]
	CCT	GGA	CAA	CAT	TGC	TT					
tet(B)	CAG	TGC	TGT	TGT	TGT	CAT	TAA		528 bp	Detection, sequencing	221
	GCT	TGG	AAT	ACT	GAG	TGT	AA				
tet(E)	GTG	ATG	ATG	GCA	CTG	GT			1,196 bp	Probe[f]	87[r]
	TGC	TGT	ACA	TCG	CTC	TT					
tet(G)	GCT	CGG	TGG	TAT	CTC	TGC	TC		468 bp	Detection	171
	AGC	AAC	AGA	ATC	GGG	AAC	AC				
tet(K)	GTA	GGA	TCT	GCT	GCA	TTC	CC		552 bp	Detection	136
	CAC	TAT	TAC	CTA	TTG	TCG	C				
tet(L)	GGA	TCG	ATA	GTA	GCC	ATG	GG		516 bp	Detection	136
	GTA	TCC	CAC	CAA	TGT	AGC	CG				
tet(M)	GAA	CTC	GAA	CAA	GAG	GAA	AGC		741 bp	Detection	178
	ATG	GAA	GCC	CAG	AAA	GGA	T				
tet(O)	AAC	TTA	GGC	ATT	CTG	GCT	CAC		519 bp	Detection	178
	TCC	CAC	TGT	TCC	ATA	TCG	TCA				
*tet*A(P)	CAC	AGA	TTG	TAT	GGG	GAT	TAG	G	764 bp	Detection, sequencing	146
	CAT	TTA	TAG	AAA	GCA	CAG	TAG	C			
tet(Q)	ATT	GCG	GAA	GTG	GAG	CGG	AC		814 bp	Detection	177
	GCC	GGA	CGG	AGG	ATT	TGA	GA				
tet(S)	CGC	TAC	ATT	TGC	GAG	ACT	CAG		569 bp	Detection	136
	GGC	TCT	CAT	ACT	GAA	TGC	CAC				
tet(T)	CAG	TGG	GAA	TAT	AAG	GAC	ACG	TC	644 bp	Detection	136
	CAA	GCC	TTC	TCT	ACA	GCA	TC				
tet(V)	GAC	AAC	GGC	ATG	AAC				405 bp	Detection	69
	GTT	CGC	GAG	CAT	GTT	C					
tet(W)	GAG	AGC	CTG	CTA	TAT	GCC	AGC		168 bp	Detection	12
	GGG	CGT	ATC	CAC	AAT	GTT	AAC				
tet(39)	CTC	CTT	CTC	TAT	TGT	GGC	TA		711 bp	Detection	2
	CAC	TAA	TAC	CTC	TGG	ACA	TCA				
Trimethoprim											
*dhfr*VIII	CTA	ACG	GCG	CTA	TCT	TCG	TGA	ACA ACG	300 bp	Detection	250
	TAT	GAA	TTC	TTC	CAT	GCC	ATT	CTG CTC			
	GTA	G									
dfr1	ACG	GAT	CCT	GGC	TGT	TGG	TTG	GAC GC	254 bp	Detection	91
	CGG	AAT	TCA	CCT	TCC	GGC	TCG	ATG TC			
dfr9	ATG	AAT	TCC	CGT	GGC	ATG	AAC	CAG AAG	399 bp	Detection	91
	AT										
	ATG	GAT	CCT	TCA	GTA	ATG	GTC	GGG ACC			
	TC										
dfrA1	GTG	AAA	CTA	TCA	CTA	ATG	G		474 bp	Detection, RFLP analysis	169[s]
	TTA	ACC	CTT	TTG	CCA	GAT	TT				
dfrA14	GAG	CAG	CTI[t]	CTI	TTI	AAA	GC		393 bp	Detection	169[u]
	TTA	GCC	CTT	TII	CCA	ATT	TT				

(Continued on next page)

TABLE 1 PCR assays for antimicrobial resistance genes (*Continued*)

Antimicrobial agent and gene	Primers (5′ → 3′)	Product size	Use(s)	Reference(s)
dfrA7	TTG AAA ATT TCA TTG ATT T TTA GCC TTT TTT CCA AAT CT	474 bp	Detection	169[v]
dfrB1	GAT CAC GTG CGC AAG AAA TC AAG CGC AGC CAC AGG ATA AAT	141 bp	Detection	169[w]
dfrA12	GGT GS[x]G CAG AAG ATT TTT CGC TGG GAA GAA GGC GTC ACC CTC	309 bp	Detection	169[y]
Ethambutol				
embB (M. tuberculosis)	ACG CTG AAA CTG CTG GCG AT ACA GAC TGG CGT CGC TGA CA	400 bp	SSCP[z] assay	5
Pyrazinamide				
pncA (M. tuberculosis)	GCT GGT CAT GTT CGC GAT CG CAG GAG CTG CAA ACC AAC TCG	673 bp	Sequencing	245
Rifampin				
rpoB (M. tuberculosis)	GGG AGC GGA TGA CCA CCC A GCG GTA CGG CGT TTC GAT GAA C	350 bp	Sequencing	122
rpoB (mycobacteria)	CCA CCC AGG ACG TGG AGG CGA TCA CAC AGT GCG ACG GGT GCA CGT CGC GGA CCT	224 bp	Sequencing	55
Streptomycin				
rpsL (M. tuberculosis)	GGC CGA CAA ACA GAA CGT GTT CAC CAA CTG GGT GAC	501 bp	Sequencing	244
rrs (M. tuberculosis)	TTG GCC ATG CTC TTG ATG CCC TGC ACA CAG GCC ACA AGG GA	1,140 bp	Sequencing	156
rrs (mycobacteria)	GAT GAC GGC CTT CGG GTT GT TCT AGT CTG CCC GTA TCG CC	238 bp	Sequencing (530 loop)	107
rrs (mycobacteria)	GTA GTC CAC GCC GTA AAC GG AGG CCA CAA GGG AAC GCC TA	238 bp	Sequencing (912–915 domain)	107
Isoniazid				
katG	GAA ACA GCG GCG CTG GAT CGT GTT GTC CCA TTT CGT CGG GG	209 bp	SSCP assay	254
katG	TTT CGG CGC ATG GCC ATG A ACA GCC ACC GAG CAC GAC	894 bp	Sequencing, RFLP analysis	100
inhA	TCG ACG GCC GGC ATG G CCG GTC CGC CGA ACG	905 bp	Sequencing	122
ahpC	ATG CAT TGT CCG CTT TGA TG TTC TAT ACT CAT TGA TT	588 bp	Sequencing	126

[a]This reference also describes primer sets for detection of *aac(6′)-Ib*, *aac(6′)-Id*, *aac(6′)-If*, *aac(6′)-Ig*, and *aac(6′)-Ih*.

[b]This primer set amplifies all known *aac(6′)-Ib* variants, including *aac(6′)-Ib-cr*, which encodes an enzyme which possesses two amino acid substitutions at positions 102 (Trp→Arg) and 179 (Asp→Tyr) which are required for the additional property of conferring reduced susceptibility to ciprofloxacin and norfloxacin. The *aac(6′)-Ib-cr* variant can be identified by digesting the amplification product with the restriction enzyme BtsCI, which cleaves the wild-type gene but not the cr variant (128, 184, 224).

[c]This reference also describes primer sets for detection of *aac(6′)-Id*, *aac(6′)-Ie*, *aac(6′)-Ig*, *aac(6′)-Ih*, *aac(6′)-Ii*, *aac(6′)-Ij*, *aac(6′)-Il*, and *aac(6′)-IIb*.

[d]This reference also describes primer sets for detection of *aac(3)-IIa*, *aac(3)-IIIa*, *aac(3)-IVa*, *aad(4′)-Ia*, *aac(6′)/aph(2″)*, and *aph(3′)-IIIa*.

[e]Digestion of amplification products with the restriction enzyme NheI cleaves amplicons from genes encoding enzymes that contain a serine substitution at position 238 (SHV-ESBL) rather than a glycine (SHV-non-ESBL).

[f]This primer set was used in the study described in the indicated reference for the synthesis of an intragenic probe and not for direct detection.

[g]This reference also describes known primer sets for detection and sequencing of *bla*SHV and detection of *bla*TEM.

[h]RFLP, restriction fragment length polymorphism.

[i]This primer set amplifies genes encoding PSE-1, PSE-4, and CARB-3.

[j]This primer set amplifies both the *nmcA* structural gene and its regulatory gene, *nmcR*.

[k]This primer set is one of six that comprise a multiplex PCR method for the detection of members of six families of plasmid-mediated *ampC* β-lactamase genes.

[l]This reference also describes primer sets for detection and/or sequencing of *bla*FOX, *bla*CMY, and *bla*ACT-1.

[m]The *cfr* gene product also confers resistance to linezolid and clindamycin.

[n]This reference also describes primer sets for the DNA sequencing of *parC* and *parE* of *Escherichia coli*.

[o]M = A or C; H = A or C or T; Y = C or T (International Union of Biochemistry codes for DNA bases).

[p]This reference also describes primer sets for detection of *sulII* and *sulIII*.

[q]This reference also describes primer sets for the synthesis of probes for *tet*(C), *tet*(D), *tet*(E), *tet*(G), *tet*(H), and *tet*(M).

[r]Reference also describes primer sets for the synthesis of probes for *tet*(A), *tet*(B), *tet*(C), *tet*(D), and *tet*(G).

[s]This primer set also amplifies *dfrA5*, *dfrA15*, *dfrA15b*, *dfrA16*, and *dfrA16b*.

[t]I = Inosine (International Union of Biochemistry codes for DNA bases).

[u]This primer set also amplifies *dfrA1*, *dfrA5*, *dfrA6*, *dfrA15*, and *dfrA16*.

[v]This primer set also amplifies *dfrA17*.

[w]This primer set also amplifies *dfrB2* and *dfrB3*.

[x]S = G or C (International Union of Biochemistry codes for DNA bases).

[y]This primer set also amplifies *dfrA13*.

[z]SSCP, single-strand conformational polymorphism.

validated in prospective multisite trials before marketing; however, there has been a recent tightening of the rules regarding the marketing and sale of ASRs in the United States. While in the past, ASR kits containing both primers and probes were available, now each primer and probe must be sold individually. Reagents can no longer be bundled together as "assays without instructions," thus making ASR-based methods more difficult to implement in the clinical laboratory than in previous years because of the need for optimization and verification of the effectiveness of a collection of individual ASRs assembled into a diagnostic assay. The Clinical Laboratory Improvement Amendments of 1988 require a more extensive verification process for ASRs than for FDA-approved kits (56), and the FDA still requires laboratories to add a disclaimer on reports for tests that use ASRs. The mandatory language for this disclaimer is, "This test was developed and its performance characteristics determined by the (laboratory name). It has not been cleared or approved by the U.S. FDA" (57).

SPECIFIC APPLICATIONS

The following sections review applications of molecular diagnostic methods for specific classes of resistance determinants.

Aminoglycoside Resistance Genes

The diversity of known aminoglycoside resistance genes, which are common in both gram-positive and gram-negative organisms (88, 204, 236), continues to expand. A variety of new acetyltransferases, adenylyltransferases, phosphotransferases, and 16S rRNA methylases have been reported. Unfortunately, the lack of consensus sequences among the acetyltransferase and adenylyltransferase genes prohibits detection of multiple determinants with a single PCR primer set (236), making it difficult to use amplification-based tests to predict aminoglycoside resistance, especially in gram-negative organisms. However, multiplex PCR assays for the detection of genes that confer high-level gentamicin resistance in enterococci have been reported (132, 267) (Table 2) and may be useful as molecular epidemiological tools for surveillance and infection control activities. These assays may also help in predicting the effectiveness of combination therapy (i.e., synergy) with aminoglycosides and cell wall-active agents.

Among the newer aminoglycoside resistance genes reported to be found in gram-negative organisms are the plasmid-mediated 16S rRNA methylases, which confer high levels of resistance to most clinically important aminoglycosides (71, 88). These resistance determinants, *armA* (296), *rmtA* (298), *rmtB* (71, 88), *rmtC* (71, 88), *rmtD* (71, 88), and *npmA* (276), are associated with mobile genetic elements (71, 276, 294), and several have been found globally (71, 88, 294), including the United States (88), in multidrug-resistant *Enterobacteriaceae*, *Pseudomonas aeruginosa*, and *Acinetobacter* spp. (71, 294, 296).

Oligonucleotide primers for the detection of genes encoding plasmid-mediated 16S rRNA methylases, in monoplex and multiplex PCR formats, can be found in Tables 1 and 2, respectively.

Detecting Genes Associated with Resistance to β-Lactam Drugs

Oxacillin Resistance in Staphylococci

The continued spread of MRSA strains worldwide has led to adoption of so-called "search and destroy" strategies to reduce the transmission of MRSA in many health care settings (284). Identification and isolation of hospitalized patients who are nasal carriers of MRSA may reduce the incidence and costs of health care-associated infections caused by transmission of these organisms among patients (190, 223). Eradication of MRSA and methicillin-susceptible *S. aureus* (MSSA) carriage may also reduce surgical site infections in some populations (196). Several states in the United States have enacted legislation mandating surveillance for MRSA among high-risk patients (280). Thus, professional societies have developed guidelines to assist hospitals in establishing surveillance programs (36). Several commercial molecular assays based on real-time PCR have been developed to detect MRSA directly in nasal swab samples (189, 286). In addition, real-time PCR assays to detect both MRSA and MSSA in blood culture vials (185) and wounds (287) have been implemented in many laboratories to reduce the time necessary to detect these *S. aureus* infections. To specifically identify MRSA, the tests anchor one PCR primer in *orfX*, which is unique to the *S. aureus* chromosome, and the second in the staphylococcal chromosomal cassette carrying the *mecA* gene (SCC*mec*), which integrates adjacent to *orfX* (110). Some commercial assays include a primer set within *mecA* which enables empty cassette strains to be identified correctly as MSSA (287). Conventional culture-based methods for detection of MRSA from nasal swabs or wounds are still used in many laboratories but often require ≥48 h before a final report can be issued.

β-Lactam Resistance in Pneumococci

Resistance to penicillin, extended-spectrum cephalosporins, and other antimicrobial agents in pneumococci has become a global problem (145, 153). *S. pneumoniae*, which does not produce β-lactamases, develops resistance to β-lactams when penicillin-binding proteins (PBPs) 2x, 2b, and 1a are remodeled through the acquisition of chromosomal DNA from other pneumococci or other streptococcal species (60, 75). Although remodeling is not a random process, it has been difficult to develop PCR primers that accurately differentiate strains with low-level penicillin resistance from those with high-level resistance. Using primers for the *pbp2b* gene, Ubukata et al. (265) attempted to resolve this issue. In their assay, the lack of product in the presence of amplification controls suggests that the *pbp2b* gene had been remodeled, which results in penicillin resistance. However, such an assay does not reliably indicate which strains could be treated with penicillin versus an extended-spectrum cephalosporin, as might be desirable for an assay to be used in a clinical laboratory. Nonetheless, the assay may be used as a screening tool for analyzing large groups of strains for resistance. A study by du Plessis et al. (76) also attempted to identify penicillin-resistant pneumococci directly in cerebrospinal fluid by using PCR primers directed to *pbp2b* sequences. This method was modestly successful in identifying isolates with altered PBPs associated with penicillin resistance.

β-Lactamase Genes in Gram-Negative Organisms

Health care-associated infections caused by *K. pneumoniae*, *Klebsiella oxytoca* (231), and other *Enterobacteriaceae* that produce ESBLs (62, 151) and other enzymes capable of hydrolyzing cefotaxime, ceftriaxone, ceftazidime, cefepime, and aztreonam are increasing in the United States and around the world (11, 116, 188). Among the most prevalent of the ESBLs are derivatives of the Ambler molecular class A TEM or SHV β-lactamases that arise through point mutations resulting in amino acid substitutions that expand the hydrolytic spectrum of the enzymes (116, 188).

TABLE 2 Multiplex PCR assays for detection of antimicrobial resistance genes

Antimicrobial agent and gene target	Product size (bp)	Reference
Aminoglycosides (enterococci)		
$aac(6')$-Ie-$aph(2'')$-Ia	348	267
$aph(2'')$-Ib	867	
$aph(2'')$-Ic	444	
$aph(2'')$-Id	641	
$aph(3')$-$IIIa$	523	
$ant(4')$-Ia	294	
$aac(6')$-Ii	410	132
$aac(6')$-$aph(2'')$	675	
$ant(4')$-Ia	266	
$ant(6)$-Ia	563	
$ant(9)$-Ia	476	
$aph(2'')$-Ic	837	
$aph(3')$-$IIIa$	354	
16S rRNA methylases		
Enterobacteriaceae and *Acinetobacter* spp.		
$rmtB$	173	71
$rmtC$	711	
$armA$	315	
Pseudomonas aeruginosa		
$rmtA$	635	71
$rmtD$	401	
β-Lactams (*Enterobacteriaceae*)		
bla_{SHV}	392	59
bla_{TEM}	516	
bla_{OXA-1}	619	
bla_{SHV}	747	162
bla_{TEM}	445	
bla_{CTX-M}	593	
bla_{CTX-M}[a]		291
Group 1	415	
Group 2	552	
Group 9	205	
Group 8	666	
Group 25	327	
Plasmid-mediated $ampC$ (*Enterobacteriaceae*[b])		192
bla_{MOX-1}, bla_{MOX-2}, bla_{CMY-1}, bla_{CMY-8} to bla_{CMY-11}	520	
bla_{LAT-1} to bla_{LAT-4}, bla_{CMY-2} to bla_{CMY-7}, bla_{BIL-1}	462	
bla_{DHA-1}, bla_{DHA-2}	405	
bla_{ACC}	346	
bla_{MIR-1}, bla_{ACT-1}	302	
bla_{FOX-1} to bla_{FOX-5b}	190	
Carbapenems		
Acquired metallo-β-lactamases (*Pseudomonas aeruginosa*, *Acinetobacter* spp.)		80
bla_{IMP} (family)	188	
bla_{VIM} (family)	390	
bla_{GIM-1}	477	
bla_{SPM-1}	271	
bla_{SIM-1}	570	
OXA carbapenemases (*Acinetobacter* spp.[c])		290
$bla_{OXA-58-like}$	599	
$bla_{OXA-23-like}$	501	
$bla_{OXA-51-like}$	353	
$bla_{OXA-24-like}$	246	
Glycopeptides (enterococci and staphylococci)		
$vanA$	732	68
$vanB$	647	
$vanC1/2$	815/827	
$vanD$	500	
$vanE$	430	

(Continued on next page)

TABLE 2 *(Continued)*

Antimicrobial agent and gene target	Product size (bp)	Reference
*van*G	941	
ddl (*Enterococcus faecalis*)	475	
ddl (*Enterococcus faecium*)	1,091	
nuc (*S. aureus*)	218	
Staphylococcus epidermidis gene fragment	125[d]	
Quinolones		
qnrA1 to *qnrA6*	580	43
qnrB1 to *qnrB6*	264	
qnrS1 to *qnrS2*	428	

[a]This reference contains primers that differentiate *bla*CTX-M genes belonging to five phylogenetic groups.
[b]This reference contains primers for the detection of genes within six plasmid-mediated *ampC*-specific families in *Enterobacteriaceae*.
[c]This reference contains primers that differentiate *bla*OXA carbapenemase genes belonging to four phylogenetic groups.
[d]This PCR product is amplified with primers complementary to a chromosomal fragment specific for *Staphylococcus epidermidis*.

The CTX-M family of enzymes, which can be subclassified into six groups based on amino acid homology, preferentially hydrolyze cefotaxime (and ceftriaxone), with less activity towards ceftazidime (226). Although discovered after the TEM- and SHV-type β-lactamases, the CTX-M ESBLs have evolved very rapidly and have become the predominant ESBLs in some locations in Europe, Asia, and South America (37, 226). Although disseminated globally (226), CTX-M-producing *Enterobacteriaceae* have only recently been identified in the United States (40, 142, 154).

Primers that can be used for the detection of genes encoding TEM, SHV, and CTX-M β-lactamases, in both monoplex and multiplex PCR formats, are shown in Tables 1 and 2, respectively. The CTX-M multiplex assay (Table 2) includes PCR primers that distinguish the genes encoding the five major groups of the CTX-M family of enzymes (291). A recent report also describes a pan-CTX-M primer set used in a real-time PCR format (154). In addition, microarrays that can detect the genes encoding TEM, SHV, and CTX-M ESBLs have recently been reported (140, 166).

Plasmid-mediated AmpC β-lactamases, some of which are inducible, confer resistance to oxyimino-β-cephalosporins and cephamycins, with variable activity toward aztreonam (112). A widely used assay for detection of genes encoding plasmid-mediated AmpC β-lactamases is a multiplex PCR with primers targeting six families of these enzymes (Table 2) (192). One report, however, suggests that the expanding diversity of genes encoding these enzymes may exceed those detected by the assay (255). A multiplex asymmetric PCR-based microarray method that includes detection of genes encoding plasmid-mediated AmpC β-lactamases was recently described (300).

Of great concern are the emerging KPC-type carbapenemases that can mediate resistance to imipenem, meropenem, doripenem, and ertapenem (32, 81, 297). Although the KPC enzymes have been identified most frequently in *K. pneumoniae*, they are now found in numerous genera and species of *Enterobacteriaceae*, as well as *Pseudomonas* and *Acinetobacter* spp. (172, 225). The *bla*KPC genes, which are plasmid mediated and located within the Tn3-type transposon Tn*4401* (94, 167), have become widely disseminated in the United States and in other parts of the world (129, 172).

KPC-producing isolates have been shown to spread among hospitalized patients. In a similar fashion, a common KPC-encoding plasmid has been documented to spread among a variety of bacterial genera within a health care setting (170, 214). There has also been a report of interspecies transfer of the KPC gene within a single patient (238). The significant capacity of these KPC-producing isolates and plasmids carrying the *bla*KPC gene to disseminate presents a serious challenge in terms of infection control.

There are currently nine different *bla*KPC genes that have been described in the literature (172, 210) or deposited in GenBank (*bla*KPC-6 to *bla*KPC-10; accession numbers EU555534, EU729727, FJ234412, FJ624872, and GQ140348, respectively). The *bla*KPC-1 gene was discovered to be identical in sequence to *bla*KPC-2 after reassessment of an ambiguous base call (297). The KPC variants differ from KPC-1/2 by one or two amino acids, and those that have been characterized appear to be biochemically similar (4, 288). Therefore, identifying a particular KPC variant that is being produced may be important in terms of molecular epidemiological analysis.

Detection of KPC-producing isolates presents a significant challenge for clinical microbiology laboratories. KPC-producing isolates display variable carbapenem MICs, and resistance may be missed by automated methods (13, 257).

PCR-based surveillance testing for *bla*KPC was shown in a recent report to be highly sensitive and specific, with a shorter time to results than with culture-based methods (232). PCR primers that amplify the genes that encode KPC-2 and KPC-3 are shown in Table 1.

The rapid detection of KPC-containing isolates may also be facilitated by using one of several real-time PCR-based assays (58, 106, 133), as well as a commercial microarray-based assay that includes detection of *bla*KPC (166).

Other carbapenemases include the class A enzymes NmcA, Sme-1, IMI-1, and members of the GES family of β-lactamases; the class B metallo-β-lactamases, including IMP, VIM, GIM, SIM, and SPM enzymes; and some class D OXA-type β-lactamases (205, 210, 235, 277, 278), present in *Enterobacteriaceae*, *Acinetobacter* species, and *Pseudomonas* species. PCR primers that amplify some of these additional carbapenemases are shown in Tables 1 and 2.

Phenotypically, it can be difficult to differentiate resistance due to a carbapenemase from resistance resulting from production of an AmpC-type enzyme or ESBL combined with decreased permeability to carbapenems due to downregulation of one or more porins (31, 115). This is especially true since boronic acid derivatives, which have been useful in identifying strains with plasmid-mediated

AmpC β-lactamases (112, 255), have been found to also inhibit the class A carbapenemases, including the KPC enzyme (263). PCR assays that amplify genes encoding plasmid-mediated AmpC β-lactamases (192), ESBLs, and carbapenemases (Tables 1 and 2) would be useful in differentiating these mechanisms.

Chloramphenicol Resistance

Genes encoding chloramphenicol acetyltransferases are present in both gram-negative and gram-positive organisms and mediate resistance to chloramphenicol (234). PCR primers capable of detecting the *cat* genes present in streptococci and enterococci have been described previously (262). Primers to detect the *catA1* and *cmlA* genes, both of which mediate chloramphenicol resistance in *Salmonella* species (97, 98), have also been reported previously. More recently, a novel gene, *cfr*, which encodes the Cfr methyltransferase, has been noted to inactivate phenicols (including chloramphenicol and florfenicol), lincosamides, oxazolidinones, pleuromutilins, and streptogramin A agents (i.e., the PhLOPS$_A$ phenotype). The *cfr* gene, carried on conjugal plasmids in some isolates of *S. aureus* (16, 125, 157), can be amplified with the PCR primers shown in Table 1.

Resistance to Vancomycin and Other Glycopeptides

Acquired vancomycin resistance was first noted in enterococci (63, 135, 218) but has subsequently been documented to occur in a variety of other pathogens (20, 21, 187, 206, 207), including *S. aureus* (47, 48, 281). Glycopeptide resistance is mediated by several different determinants, including *vanA*, *vanB*, *vanC*, *vanD*, *vanE*, *vanG*, and *vanL* (29, 63, 84, 155). Vancomycin resistance in *S. aureus* most likely occurs by conjugative transfer of the *vanA* determinant from enterococcal donors to *S. aureus*. Ten independent isolates of *S. aureus* that have acquired the *vanA* gene have been reported in the United States (48, 85, 193, 239, 259, 281, 301). Additional *vanA*-containing vancomycin-resistant *S. aureus* isolates have been reported from Iran (7) and India (228, 260).

PCR assays can detect the *vanA* gene (77) and differentiate the three unique *vanB* genes, designated *vanB1*, *vanB2*, and *vanB3* (64, 139), and the three *vanC* genes, *vanC1*, *vanC2*, and *vanC3* (51). Subtypes of *vanD*, including *vanD1*, *vanD2*, *vanD3*, and *vanD4*, also exist, but differentiation via PCR is difficult (28, 65). PCR has been used to detect *vanA* and *vanB* in enterococci in fecal samples to aid infection control efforts (181, 230). Furthermore, a multiplex PCR method has been developed for the simultaneous detection of the *van* alphabet (*vanA*, *vanB*, *vanC*, *vanD*, *vanE*, and *vanG*) and identification of the most clinically relevant enterococci and staphylococci at the species level (Table 2) (68). Commercial assays have become available in Europe for the direct and rapid detection of *vanA* and *vanB* genes in perirectal swab samples by using real-time PCR; ASRs are also available for detection of *vanA* and *vanB*. A recent report indicated enhanced sensitivity and a significant reduction in the time to results (3.5 versus ≥72 h) for one ASR assay compared with those for vancomycin-containing agar plates (242). False-positive results may potentially occur with any assay intended to detect *vanB* genes in enterococci due to the presence of these genes in anaerobic bacteria (20, 21, 72). However, the *vanB* gene from *Clostridium symbiosum* has been transferred to an enterococcal recipient in a gnotobiotic mouse model (134).

Thus, it may still be important from the infection control perspective to identify *vanB* resistance genes directly in stool samples, although this issue remains controversial.

Genotypic detection of vancomycin-intermediate *S. aureus* (VISA) strains has yet to be accomplished via molecular methods. Although Howden et al. (108) have reported that a threonine-to-isoleucine change at position 136 in *graS* can contribute to the VISA phenotype in an MRSA isolate, raising the vancomycin MIC from a susceptible to an intermediate level of resistance (6 μg/ml using the macro-Etest method), not all VISA strains have this mutation. Thus, the mechanisms of low-level vancomycin resistance remain elusive and are likely due to more than a single mutation in most VISA strains. Consequently, there are no molecular methods for identifying VISA strains at present. Genetic alterations that result in modifications of the cell wall structure or changes in cellular regulatory pathways (15, 148) are all candidates for future molecular assays.

Macrolide, Lincosamide, and Streptogramin Resistance

Resistance to macrolides, lincosamides (such as clindamycin), and streptogramins can be mediated by a variety of *erm* genes, including *ermA* and *ermA* (subclass *ermTR*), *ermB*, and *ermC*. On the other hand, *msrA*, which is primarily in staphylococci, mediates resistance only to macrolides and streptogramins, and the macrolide efflux gene *mefA*, found in streptococci and pneumococci, confers resistance to 14- and 15-membered macrolides only (86, 180, 222, 289). Roberts et al. (222) proposed that *mefA* and *mefE*, which show high levels of DNA homology, be considered a single class. However, others suggest that in spite of the high degree of relatedness of the genes, a distinction between them should be maintained (130). A real-time PCR assay that can distinguish *mefA* and *mefE* has been described (131). Pneumococci containing both *ermB* and *mefA* are being identified with increasing frequency (83). Many community-associated MRSA isolates that are erythromycin resistant and clindamycin susceptible contain *msrA* (124). PCR assays can differentiate *msrA* from *erm* genes (127, 246). Mutations in 23S rRNA and ribosomal protein L4 mutations in pneumococci have also been shown to mediate macrolide resistance, two of which can be detected through either traditional PCR or pyrosequencing assays (67, 99, 253).

Mechanisms active against both the streptogramin A and streptogramin B components of quinupristin-dalfopristin are necessary to result in a resistance phenotype. For example, resistance to streptogramin A, a prerequisite for resistance to quinupristin-dalfopristin, is mediated by several loci previously classified as *sat* genes which have been reclassified as *vat* genes (105, 222, 283). For example, *vatD*, formerly *satA*, and *vatE*, formerly *satG*, are plasmid-mediated genes that encode acetyltransferases that inactivate streptogramin A (105, 222). Resistance to the streptogramin B component is mediated by the lactonases *vgb* and *vgbB* or the *ermB* methylase. In staphylococci, in particular, many of these genes are clustered together.

Lincosamide resistance in staphylococci can be mediated by the *linA* and *linA'* [now called *lnu*(A) and *lnu*(A')] genes (34), while *linB* [now called *lnu*(B)] has been described to occur in enterococci (30). Streptococcal lincosamide resistance genes include *lnu*(C) (1) and *lnu*(D) (198).

Mupirocin Resistance

Mupirocin is an antistaphylococcal agent that is used to suppress or eliminate nasal carriage of staphylococci among colonized patients and hospital personnel (271). It is also used as a topical agent for wounds. PCR assays that can detect the *mupA* gene, which is associated with high-level mupirocin resistance, have been described (14, 93). However, the practical value of the assay has not been assessed in a clinical laboratory setting. The CLSI has established both disk diffusion and MIC breakpoints for high-level mupirocin resistance (52). The results of these assays for high-level mupirocin resistance correlate well with the presence of the *mupA* determinant (186).

Oxazolidinone Resistance

Resistance to oxazolidinones, such as linezolid, has been described for isolates of both staphylococci and enterococci (19, 285, 289). Mutations in 23S rRNA, at position 2576 in enterococci, represent one mechanism responsible for the resistance phenotype (208). While rare mutations in the 23S rRNA gene have been reported (143), the most frequent modification associated with linezolid resistance in staphylococci and enterococcal clinical isolates is G→T at position 2576. Detection of the G2576T mutation in enterococci can be accomplished by using a real-time PCR assay or a simple PCR amplification of a 633-bp fragment encompassing the G2576T mutation followed by restriction fragment length polymorphism analysis of the product (292). Alternatively, the mutation can be detected by using pyrosequencing (241). In addition, a novel *cfr* gene, responsible for PhLOPS resistance (see above), has been detected in *S. aureus* isolates both chromosomally and on conjugal plasmids. The *cfr* gene, which encodes an rRNA methyltransferase, is carried on conjugal plasmids in some isolates of *S. aureus* (16, 157). The *cfr* gene can be detected using the PCR primers shown in Table 1.

Quinolone Resistance

There are two major mechanisms of quinolone resistance: (i) alteration of the target sites, the organism's gyrase (*gyrA* and *gyrB*) and topoisomerase (*parC* and *parE*) (82, 113), and (ii) active efflux of the drug out of the cell (82, 113), which limits access of the drug to the target site. Resistance is often associated with point mutations in the *gyr* or *par* loci. Since DNA probes, in most cases, are not sufficiently sensitive to detect these changes, investigators have used PCR coupled with direct sequencing of the amplification products to identify changes in the nucleotide sequences of the *gyrA*, *gyrB*, *parC*, and *parE* genes (117, 122, 274). The primers, however, appear to be species specific (Table 1).

Since 1998, several plasmid-mediated quinolone resistance determinants have been reported (42, 247). The *qnr* family of resistance genes, comprised of the four major groups *qnrA*, *qnrB*, *qnrC*, and *qnrS*, which mediate low-level fluoroquinolone resistance (42, 113), are frequently plasmid encoded and can be detected via PCR (43, 128) (Tables 1 and 2). The *aac(6′)-Ib-cr* gene encodes a variant aminoglycoside acetyltransferase that mediates reduced susceptibility to ciprofloxacin and norfloxacin (184, 224). The *qnr* and *aac(6′)-Ib-cr* determinants are widely disseminated globally among clinical isolates of *Enterobacteriaceae* (42). The *qepA* resistance gene encodes an efflux pump that confers significantly reduced susceptibility to hydrophilic quinolones, such as norfloxacin, ciprofloxacin, and enrofloxacin (295). Plasmids harboring both *qepA* and *rmtB*, which encodes a 16S rRNA methylase that confers high-level resistance to aminoglycosides, have been reported (144, 295).

Sulfonamide Resistance

There are three major sulfonamide resistance genes: *sulI*, *sulII*, and *sulIII*. All three have been cloned and sequenced, and PCR assays for each gene have been described (95, 111). Interestingly, the *sul* genes are often associated with transposable DNA elements, such as Tn*21* and small, multicopy plasmids (111, 197) that can shuttle multiple resistance genes from organism to organism. Thus, the *sul* genes can serve as indicators of multidrug resistance in gram-negative organisms.

Tetracycline Resistance

Tetracycline resistance is widespread within the bacterial kingdom (141, 220). PCR assays have been developed for many of the tetracycline resistance determinants, including *tet*(A), *tet*(B), *tet*(C), *tet*(D), *tet*(E), *tet*(G), *tet*(H), *tet*(K), *tet*(L), *tet*(M), *tet*(O), *tet*(Q), *tet*(S), *tet*(T), *tet*(V), and *tet*(W) (Table 1) (12, 69, 87, 103, 136, 177, 178). Multiple alleles of several of these determinants exist. For example, six *tet*(M) alleles present in *Streptococcus pneumoniae*, designated *tet*(M)1 through *tet*(M)6, have been differentiated through restriction analysis of PCR fragments (70). Such epidemiological studies using genotyping of resistance determinants contribute to our understanding of resistance transfer and evolution. For example, primers for the *tet*(M), *tet*(O), and *tet*(Q) determinants are useful for detecting tetracycline resistance genes directly in periodontal samples (177, 178), where the presence of resistant organisms may identify those patients for whom therapy with tetracycline is likely to fail (147). A PCR assay was used to amplify the hypervariable region of the *tet*(M) structural gene (Table 1) (178), reported to have the widest host range of any of the *tet* genes (220). The PCR products from isolates representing 10 different bacterial genera and species were analyzed by both restriction and DNA sequence analysis, through which multiple subtypes of the *tet*(M) gene were recognized (179).

Trimethoprim Resistance

The number of genes capable of mediating trimethoprim resistance in bacteria continues to expand (96, 111, 137). DNA probes have proven to be powerful tools for detecting and classifying novel trimethoprim resistance genes (called *dhfr*) (118, 209). However, because consensus sequences common to all the *dhfr* genes have not been identified, PCR primers that could simplify the detection of this family of genes have not been developed, although PCR primers for some individual genes have been reported (96, 137, 250).

GUIDELINES FOR USING GENETIC TESTS

PCR assays in which the products are visualized on agarose gels are rapidly being replaced by real-time PCR assays using fluorescent resonance energy transfer probes or molecular beacons for detection of amplification products. An example of this is the commercial test for rifampin-resistant *M. tuberculosis* recently released in Europe. This test uses a combination of five molecular beacons to interrogate the rifampin resistance region of *rpoB* for mutations. The drop-off in the signal of any of the five molecular beacons signifies a rifampin-resistant strain (25a, 119). Such closed systems are more efficient and less prone to overall contamination than traditional PCR assays. The critical issue with PCR assays of any sort, however, is the reliability of results. The need for quality control measures, including controls for the presence of inhibitory substances, cannot be stressed enough, especially for detection of genes directly in clinical specimens. The temperatures used in PCR assays optimized for use with purified DNA or DNA from bacterial isolates obtained in pure culture may not be stringent enough to avoid false-positive results when used with clinical samples, such as blood and cerebrospinal fluid, where considerably more nonspecific priming can occur (256). Using control reactions containing no template DNA to identify nonspecific products due to contamination of *Taq* polymerase with DNA, such as provided by cloning vector DNA, is critical (256, 264).

All PCR assays for antimicrobial resistance genes, whether sold commercially or developed in-house, must be validated before use. Methods for validation are published by the CLSI (53).

Studies to determine the reservoirs of resistance genes and routes of resistance gene transfer in hospitals and community settings are still needed. Such studies would also help to determine the frequency with which organisms carry resistance genes that are not expressed. Although still considered experimental, many of the PCR methods for detecting resistance genes described herein are already having a positive effect on guiding therapy early in the course of infection and making the treatment of infectious diseases less empirical.

REFERENCES

1. **Achard, A., C. Villers, V. Pichereau, and R. Leclercq.** 2005. New *lnu*(C) gene conferring resistance to lincomycin by nucleotidylation in *Streptococcus agalactiae* UCN36. *Antimicrob. Agents Chemother.* **49:**2716–2719.
2. **Agerso, Y., and L. Guardabassi.** 2005. Identification of *Tet* 39, a novel class of tetracycline resistance determinant in *Acinetobacter* spp. of environmental and clinical origin. *J. Antimicrob. Chemother.* **55:**566–569.
3. **Akpaka, P. E., S. Baboolal, D. Clarke, L. Francis, and N. Rastogi.** 2008. Evaluation of methods for rapid detection of resistance to isoniazid and rifampin in *Mycobacterium tuberculosis* isolates collected in the Caribbean. *J. Clin. Microbiol.* **46:**3426–3428.
4. **Alba, J., Y. Ishii, K. Thomson, E. S. Moland, and K. Yamaguchi.** 2005. Kinetics study of KPC-3, a plasmid-encoded class A carbapenem-hydrolyzing β-lactamase. *Antimicrob. Agents Chemother.* **49:**4760–4762.
5. **Alcaide, F., G. E. Pfyffer, and A. Telenti.** 1997. Role of *embB* in natural and acquired resistance to ethambutol in mycobacteria. *Antimicrob. Agents Chemother.* **41:**2270–2273.
6. **Alcantar-Curiel, D., J. C. Tinoco, C. Gayosso, A. Carlos, C. Daza, M. C. Perez-Prado, L. Salcido, J. I. Santos, and C. M. Alpuche-Aranda.** 2004. Nosocomial bacteremia and urinary tract infections caused by extended-spectrum β-lactamase-producing *Klebsiella pneumoniae* with plasmids carrying both SHV-5 and TLA-1 genes. *Clin. Infect. Dis.* **38:**1067–1074.
7. **Aligholi, M., M. Emaneini, F. Jabalameli, S. Shahsavan, H. Dabiri, and H. Sedaght.** 2008. Emergence of high-level vancomycin-resistant *Staphylococcus aureus* in the Imam Khomeini Hospital in Tehran. *Med. Princ. Pract.* **17:**432–434.
8. **Allignet, J., and N. El Solh.** 1995. Diversity among the gram-positive acetyltransferases inactivating streptogramin A and structurally related compounds and characterization of a new staphylococcal determinant, *vatB*. *Antimicrob. Agents Chemother.* **39:**2027–2036.
9. **Allignet, J., V. Loncle, C. Simenel, M. Delepierre, and N. El Solh.** 1993. Sequence of a staphylococcal gene, *vat*, encoding an acetyltransferase inactivating the A-type compounds of virginiamycin-like antibiotics. *Gene* **130:**91–98.
10. **Alsterlund, R., B. Carlsson, L. Gezelius, S. Haeggman, and B. Olsson-Liljequist.** 2009. Multiresistant CTX-M-15 ESBL-producing *Escherichia coli* in southern Sweden: description of an outbreak. *Scand. J. Infect. Dis.* **41:**410–415.

11. **Alvarez, M., J. H. Tran, N. Chow, and G. A. Jacoby.** 2004. Epidemiology of conjugative plasmid-mediated AmpC β-lactamases in the United States. *Antimicrob. Agents Chemother.* **48:**533–537.
12. **Aminov, R. I., N. Garrigues-Jeanjean, and R. I. Mackie.** 2001. Molecular ecology of tetracycline resistance: development and validation of primers for detection of tetracycline resistance genes encoding ribosomal protection proteins. *Appl. Environ. Microbiol.* **67:**22–32.
13. **Anderson, K. F., D. R. Lonsway, J. K. Rasheed, J. Biddle, B. Jensen, L. K. McDougal, R. B. Carey, A. Thompson, S. Stocker, B. Limbago, and J. B. Patel.** 2007. Evaluation of methods to identify the *Klebsiella pneumoniae* carbapenemase in *Enterobacteriaceae*. *J. Clin. Microbiol.* **45:**2723–2725.
14. **Anthony, R. M., A. M. Connor, E. G. Power, and G. L. French.** 1999. Use of the polymerase chain reaction for rapid detection of high-level mupirocin resistance in staphylococci. *Eur. J. Clin. Microbiol. Infect. Dis.* **18:**30–34.
15. **Appelbaum, P. C.** 2007. Reduced glycopeptide susceptibility in methicillin-resistant *Staphylococcus aureus* (MRSA). *Int. J. Antimicrob. Agents* **30:**398–408.
16. **Arias, C. A., M. Vallejo, J. Reyes, D. Panesso, J. Moreno, E. Castaneda, M. V. Villegas, B. E. Murray, and J. P. Quinn.** 2008. Clinical and microbiological aspects of linezolid resistance mediated by the *cfr* gene encoding a 23S rRNA methyltransferase. *J. Clin. Microbiol.* **46:**892–896.
17. **Arnold, C., L. Westland, G. Mowat, A. Underwood, J. Magee, and S. Gharbia.** 2005. Single-nucleotide polymorphism-based differentiation and drug resistance detection in *Mycobacterium tuberculosis* from isolates or directly from sputum. *Clin. Microbiol. Infect.* **11:**122–130.
18. **Aubron, C., L. Poirel, R. J. Ash, and P. Nordmann.** 2005. Carbapenemase-producing *Enterobacteriaceae*, U.S. rivers. *Emerg. Infect. Dis.* **11:**260–264.
19. **Auckland, C., L. Teare, F. Cooke, M. E. Kaufmann, M. Warner, G. Jones, K. Bamford, H. Ayles, and A. P. Johnson.** 2002. Linezolid-resistant enterococci: report of the first isolates in the United Kingdom. *J. Antimicrob. Chemother.* **50:**743–746.
20. **Ballard, S. A., E. A. Grabsch, P. D. R. Johnson, and M. L. Grayson.** 2005. Comparison of three PCR primer sets for identification of *vanB* gene carriage in feces and correlation with carriage of vancomycin-resistant enterococci: interference by *vanB*-containing anaerobic bacilli. *Antimicrob. Agents Chemother.* **49:**77–81.
21. **Ballard, S. A., K. K. Pertile, M. Lim, P. D. R. Johnson, and M. L. Grayson.** 2005. Molecular characterization of *vanB* elements in naturally occurring gut anaerobes. *Antimicrob. Agents Chemother.* **49:**1688–1694.
22. **Bartels, M. D., K. Boye, S. M. Rohde, A. R. Larsen, H. Torfs, P. Bouchy, R. Skov, and H. Westh.** 2009. A common variant of staphylococcal cassette chromosome *mec* type IVa in isolates from Copenhagen, Denmark, is not detected by the BD GeneOhm methicillin-resistant *Staphylococcus aureus* assay. *J. Clin. Microbiol.* **47:**1524–1527.
23. **Baudry, P. J., K. Nichol, M. DeCorby, P. Lagace-Wiens, E. Olivier, D. Boyd, M. R. Mulvey, D. J. Hoban, and G. G. Zhanel.** 2009. Mechanisms of resistance and mobility among multidrug-resistant CTX-M-producing *Escherichia coli* from Canadian intensive care units: the 1st report of QepA in North America. *Diagn. Microbiol. Infect. Dis.* **63:**319–326.
24. **Bauernfeind, A., I. Stemplinger, R. Jungwirth, P. Mangold, S. Amann, E. Akalin, Ö. Ang, C. Bal, and J. M. Casellas.** 1996. Characterization of β-lactamase gene bla_{PER-2}, which encodes an extended-spectrum class A β-lactamase. *Antimicrob. Agents Chemother.* **40:**616–620.
25. **Bert, F., C. Branger, and N. Lambert-Zechovsky.** 2002. Identification of PSE and OXA β-lactamase genes in *Pseudomonas aeruginosa* using PCR-restriction fragment length polymorphism. *J. Antimicrob. Chemother.* **50:**11–18.
25a. **Boehme, C. C., P. Nabeta, D. Hillemann, M. P. Nicol, S. Shenai, F. Krapp, J. Allen, R. Tahirli, R. Blakemore, R. Rustomjee, A. Milovic, M. Jones, S. M. O'Brien, D. H. Persing, S. Ruesch-Gerdes, E. Gotuzzo, C. Rodrigues, D. Alland, and M. D. Perkins.** 2010. Rapid molecular detection

of tuberculosis and rifampin resistance. *N. Engl. J. Med.* **363:**1005–1015.

26. **Bonnet, R., C. Dutour, J. L. M. Sampaio, C. Chanal, D. Sirot, R. Labia, C. De Champs, and J. Sirot.** 2001. Novel cefotaximase (CTX-M-16) with increased catalytic efficiency due to substitution Asp-240→Gly. *Antimicrob. Agents Chemother.* **45:**2269–2275.

27. **Bou, G., A. Oliver, and J. Martínez-Beltrán.** 2000. OXA-24, a novel class D β-lactamase with carbapenemase activity in an *Acinetobacter baumannii* clinical strain. *Antimicrob. Agents Chemother.* **44:**1556–1561.

28. **Boyd, D. A., J. Conly, H. Dedier, G. Peters, L. Robertson, E. Slater, and M. R. Mulvey.** 2000. Molecular characterization of the *vanD* gene cluster and a novel insertion element in a vancomycin-resistant enterococcus isolated in Canada. *J. Clin. Microbiol.* **38:**2392–2394.

29. **Boyd, D. A., B. M. Willey, D. Fawcett, N. Gillani, and M. R. Mulvey.** 2008. Molecular characterization of *Enterococcus faecalis* N06-0364 with low-level vancomycin resistance harboring a novel D-Ala-D-Ser gene cluster, *vanL. Antimicrob. Agents Chemother.* **52:**2667–2672.

30. **Bozdogan, B., L. Berrezouga, M.-S. Kuo, D. A. Yurek, K. A. Farley, B. J. Stockman, and R. Leclercq.** 1999. A new resistance gene, *linB*, conferring resistance to lincosamides by nucleotidylation in *Enterococcus faecium* HM1025. *Antimicrob. Agents Chemother.* **43:**925–929.

31. **Bradford, P. A., C. Urban, N. Mariano, S. J. Projan, J. J. Rahal, and K. Bush.** 1997. Imipenem resistance in *Klebsiella pneumoniae* is associated with the combination of ACT-1, a plasmid-mediated AmpC β-lactamase, and the loss of an outer membrane protein. *Antimicrob. Agents Chemother.* **41:**563–569.

32. **Bratu, S., P. Tolaney, U. Karumudi, J. Quale, M. Mooty, S. Nichani, and D. Landman.** 2005. Carbapenemase-producing *Klebsiella pneumoniae* in Brooklyn, NY: molecular epidemiology and *in vitro* activity of polymyxin B and other agents. *J. Antimicrob. Chemother.* **56:**128–132.

33. **Bressler, A. M., T. Williams, E. E. Culler, W. Zhu, D. Lonsway, J. B. Patel, and F. S. Nolte.** 2005. Correlation of penicillin binding protein 2a detection with oxacillin resistance in *Staphylococcus aureus* and discovery of a novel penicillin binding protein 2a mutation. *J. Clin. Microbiol.* **43:**4541–4544.

34. **Brisson-Noel, A., and P. Courvalin.** 1986. Nucleotide sequence of gene *linA* encoding resistance to lincosamides in *Staphylococcus haemolyticus. Gene* **43:**247–253.

35. **Brown, S., H. K. Young, and S. G. B. Amyes.** 2005. Characterisation of OXA-51, a novel class D carbapenemase found in genetically unrelated clinical strains of *Acinetobacter baumannii* from Argentina. *Clin. Microbiol. Infect.* **11:**15–23.

36. **Calfee, D. P., C. D. Salgado, D. Classen, K. M. Arias, K. Podgorny, D. J. Anderson, H. Burstin, S. E. Coffin, E. R. Dubberke, V. Fraser, D. N. Gerding, F. A. Griffin, P. Gross, K. S. Kaye, M. Klompas, E. Lo, J. Marschall, L. A. Mermel, L. Nicolle, D. A. Pegues, T. M. Perl, S. Saint, R. A. Weinstein, R. Wise, and D. S. Yokoe.** 2008. Strategies to prevent transmission of methicillin-resistant *Staphylococcus aureus* in acute care hospitals. *Infect. Control Hosp. Epidemiol.* **29**(Suppl. 1)**:**S62–S80.

37. **Canton, R., and T. M. Coque.** 2006. The CTX-M β-lactamase pandemic. *Curr. Opin. Microbiol.* **9:**466–475.

38. **Caroff, N., E. Espaze, D. Gautreau, H. Richet, and A. Reynaud.** 2000. Analysis of the effects of -42 and -32 *ampC* promoter mutations in clinical isolates of *Escherichia coli* hyperproducing AmpC. *J. Antimicrob. Chemother.* **45:**783–788.

39. **Castanheira, M., T. R. Fritsche, H. S. Sader, and R. N. Jones.** 2008. RmtD 16S RNA methylase in epidemiologically unrelated SPM-1-producing *Pseudomonas aeruginosa* isolates from Brazil. *Antimicrob. Agents Chemother.* **52:**1587–1588. (Author's reply, **52:**1588.)

40. **Castanheira, M., R. E. Mendes, P. R. Rhomberg, and R. N. Jones.** 2008. Rapid emergence of *bla*CTX-M among Enterobacteriaceae in U.S. medical centers: molecular evaluation from the MYSTIC Program (2007). *Microb. Drug Resist.* **14:**211–216.

41. **Castanheira, M., M. A. Toleman, R. N. Jones, F. J. Schmidt, and T. R. Walsh.** 2004. Molecular characterization of a β-lactamase gene, *bla*GIM-1, encoding a new subclass of metallo-β-lactamase. *Antimicrob. Agents Chemother.* **48:**4654–4661.

42. **Cattoir, V., and P. Nordmann.** 2009. Plasmid-mediated quinolone resistance in Gram-negative bacterial species: an update. *Curr. Med. Chem.* **16:**1028–1046.

43. **Cattoir, V., L. Poirel, V. Rotimi, C. J. Soussy, and P. Nordmann.** 2007. Multiplex PCR for detection of plasmid-mediated quinolone resistance *qnr* genes in ESBL-producing enterobacterial isolates. *J. Antimicrob. Chemother.* **60:**394–397.

44. **Cavaco, L. M., H. Hasman, S. Xia, and F. M. Aarestrup.** 2009. *qnrD*, a novel gene conferring transferable quinolone resistance in *Salmonella enterica* serovar Kentucky and Bovismorbificans strains of human origin. *Antimicrob. Agents Chemother.* **53:**603–608.

45. **Centers for Disease Control and Prevention.** 2007. Extensively drug-resistant tuberculosis—United States, 1993–2006. *MMWR Morb. Mortal. Wkly. Rep.* **56:**250–253.

46. **Centers for Disease Control and Prevention.** 2009. *Sexually Transmitted Disease Surveillance 2007 Supplement, Gonococcal Isolate Surveillance Project (GISP) Annual Report 2007.* U.S. Department of Health and Human Services, Centers for Disease Control and Prevention, Atlanta, GA.

47. **Centers for Disease Control and Prevention.** 2004. Vancomycin-resistant *Staphylococcus aureus*—New York, 2004. *MMWR Morb. Mortal. Wkly. Rep.* **53:**322–323.

48. **Chang, S., D. M. Sievert, J. C. Hageman, M. L. Boulton, F. C. Tenover, F. P. Downes, S. Shah, J. T. Rudrik, G. R. Pupp, W. J. Brown, D. Cardo, and S. K. Fridkin.** 2003. Infection with vancomycin-resistant *Staphylococcus aureus* containing the *vanA* resistance gene. *N. Engl. J. Med.* **348:**1342–1347.

49. **Clark, N. C., R. C. Cooksey, B. C. Hill, J. M. Swenson, and F. C. Tenover.** 1993. Characterization of glycopeptide-resistant enterococci from U.S. hospitals. *Antimicrob. Agents Chemother.* **37:**2311–2317.

50. **Clark, N. C., Ö. Olsvik, J. M. Swenson, C. A. Spiegel, and F. C. Tenover.** 1999. Detection of a streptomycin/spectinomycin adenylyltransferase gene (*aadA*) in *Enterococcus faecalis. Antimicrob. Agents Chemother.* **43:**157–160.

51. **Clark, N. C., L. M. Teixeira, R. R. Facklam, and F. C. Tenover.** 1998. Detection and differentiation of *vanC-1*, *vanC-2*, and *vanC-3* glycopeptide resistance genes in enterococci. *J. Clin. Microbiol.* **36:**2294–2297.

52. **Clinical and Laboratory Standards Institute.** 2009. *Performance Standards for Antimicrobial Susceptibility Testing; Nineteenth Informational Supplement.* CLSI document M100-S19. Clinical and Laboratory Standards Institute, Wayne, PA.

53. **Clinical and Laboratory Standards Institute.** 2006. *Molecular Diagnostic Methods for Infectious Diseases; Approved Guideline,* 2nd ed. CLSI document MM03-A2. Clinical and Laboratory Standards Institute, Wayne, PA.

54. **Cockerill, F. R., III.** 1999. Genetic methods for assessing antimicrobial resistance. *Antimicrob. Agents Chemother.* **43:**199–212.

55. **Cockerill, F. R., III, D. E. Williams, K. D. Eisenach, B. C. Kline, L. K. Miller, L. Stockman, J. Voyles, G. M. Caron, S. K. Bundy, G. D. Roberts, W. R. Wilson, A. C. Whelen, J. M. Hunt, and D. H. Persing.** 1996. Prospective evaluation of the utility of molecular techniques for diagnosing nosocomial transmission of multidrug-resistant tuberculosis. *Mayo Clin. Proc.* **71:**221–229.

56. **Code of Federal Regulations.** 2003. 42 CFR 493. U.S. Government Printing Office, Washington, DC.

57. **Code of Federal Regulations.** 2009. In vitro diagnostic products for human use. Title 21, CFR part 809. U.S. Government Printing Office, Washington, DC.

58. **Cole, J. M., A. N. Schuetz, C. E. Hill, and F. S. Nolte.** 2009. Development and evaluation of a real-time PCR assay for detection of *Klebsiella pneumoniae* carbapenemase genes. *J. Clin. Microbiol.* **47:**322–326.

59. **Colom, K., J. Pérez, R. Alonso, A. Fernàndez-Aranguiz, E. Larino, and R. Cisterna.** 2003. Simple and reliable multiplex PCR assay for detection of bla$_{TEM}$, bla$_{SHV}$ and bla$_{OXA-1}$ genes in *Enterobacteriaceae*. *FEMS Microbiol. Lett.* **223:**147–151.

60. **Contreras-Martel, C., C. Dahout-Gonzalez, S. Martins Ados, M. Kotnik, and A. Dessen.** 2009. PBP active site flexibility as the key mechanism for β-lactam resistance in pneumococci. *J. Mol. Biol.* **387:**899–909.

61. **Coudron, P. E., N. D. Hanson, and M. W. Climo.** 2003. Occurrence of extended-spectrum and AmpC beta-lactamases in bloodstream isolates of *Klebsiella pneumoniae*: isolates harbor plasmid-mediated FOX-5 and ACT-1 AmpC beta-lactamases. *J. Clin. Microbiol.* **41:**772–777.

62. **Coudron, P. E., E. S. Moland, and C. C. Sanders.** 1997. Occurrence and detection of extended-spectrum β-lactamases in members of the family *Enterobacteriaceae* at a veterans medical center: seek and you may find. *J. Clin. Microbiol.* **35:**2593–2597.

63. **Courvalin, P.** 2005. Genetics of glycopeptide resistance in Gram-positive pathogens. *Int. J. Med. Microbiol.* **294:**479–486.

64. **Dahl, K. H., G. S. Simonsen, Ø. Olsvik, and A. Sundsfjord.** 1999. Heterogeneity in the *vanB* gene cluster of genomically diverse clinical strains of vancomycin-resistant enterococci. *Antimicrob. Agents Chemother.* **43:**1105–1110.

65. **Dalla Costa, L. M., P. E. Reynolds, H. A. Souza, D. C. Souza, M.-F. I. Palepou, and N. Woodford.** 2000. Characterization of a divergent *vanD*-type resistance element from the first glycopeptide-resistant strain of *Enterococcus faecium* isolated in Brazil. *Antimicrob. Agents Chemother.* **44:**3444–3446.

66. **del Campo, R., J. C. Galán, C. Tenorio, P. Ruiz-Gargajosa, M. Zarazaga, C. Torres, and F. Baquero.** 2005. New *aac(6′)-I* genes in *Enterococcus hirae* and *Enterococcus durans*: effect on β-lactam/aminoglycoside synergy. *J. Antimicrob. Chemother.* **55:**1053–1055.

67. **Depardieu, F., and P. Courvalin.** 2001. Mutation in 23S rRNA responsible for resistance to 16-membered macrolides and streptogramins in *Streptococcus pneumoniae*. *Antimicrob. Agents Chemother.* **45:**319–323.

68. **Depardieu, F., B. Perichon, and P. Courvalin.** 2004. Detection of the *van* alphabet and identification of enterococci and staphylococci at the species level by multiplex PCR. *J. Clin. Microbiol.* **42:**5857–5860.

69. **De Rossi, E., M. C. J. Blokpoel, R. Cantoni, M. Branzoni, G. Riccardi, D. B. Young, K. A. L. De Smet, and O. Ciferri.** 1998. Molecular cloning and functional analysis of a novel tetracycline resistance determinant, *tet*(V), from *Mycobacterium smegmatis*. *Antimicrob. Agents Chemother.* **42:**1931–1937.

70. **Doherty, N., K. Trzcinski, P. Pickerill, P. Zawadzki, and C. G. Dowson.** 2000. Genetic diversity of the *tet*(M) gene in tetracycline-resistant clonal lineages of *Streptococcus pneumoniae*. *Antimicrob. Agents Chemother.* **44:**2979–2984.

71. **Doi, Y., and Y. Arakawa.** 2007. 16S ribosomal RNA methylation: emerging resistance mechanism against aminoglycosides. *Clin. Infect. Dis.* **45:**88–94.

72. **Domingo, M.-C., A. Huletsky, A. Bernal, R. Giroux, D. K. Boudreau, F. J. Picard, and M. G. Bergeron.** 2005. Characterization of a Tn*5382*-like transposon containing the *vanB2* gene cluster in a *Clostridium* strain isolated from human faeces. *J. Antimicrob. Chemother.* **55:**466–474.

73. **Dowd, S. E., Y. Sun, P. R. Secor, D. D. Rhoads, B. M. Wolcott, G. A. James, and R. D. Wolcott.** 2008. Survey of bacterial diversity in chronic wounds using pyrosequencing, DGGE, and full ribosome shotgun sequencing. *BMC Microbiol.* **8:**43.

74. **Dowd, S. E., R. D. Wolcott, Y. Sun, T. McKeehan, E. Smith, and D. Rhoads.** 2008. Polymicrobial nature of chronic diabetic foot ulcer biofilm infections determined using bacterial tag encoded FLX amplicon pyrosequencing (bTEFAP). *PLoS One* **3:**e3326.

75. **Dowson, C. G., A. Hutchison, and B. G. Spratt.** 1989. Extensive re-modelling of the transpeptidase domain of penicillin-binding protein 2B of a penicillin-resistant South African isolate of *Streptococcus pneumoniae*. *Mol. Microbiol.* **3:**95–102.

76. **du Plessis, M., A. M. Smith, and K. P. Klugman.** 1998. Rapid detection of penicillin-resistant *Streptococcus pneumoniae* in cerebrospinal fluid by a seminested-PCR strategy. *J. Clin. Microbiol.* **36:**453–457.

77. **Dutka-Malen, S., S. Evers, and P. Courvalin.** 1995. Detection of glycopeptide resistance genotypes and identification to the species level of clinically relevant enterococci by PCR. *J. Clin. Microbiol.* **33:**24–27.

78. **Edelstein, M., M. Pimkin, I. Palagin, I. Edelstein, and L. Stratchounski.** 2003. Prevalence and molecular epidemiology of CTX-M extended-spectrum β-lactamase-producing *Escherichia coli* and *Klebsiella pneumoniae* in Russian hospitals. *Antimicrob. Agents Chemother.* **47:**3724–3732.

79. **El-Hajj, H. H., S. A. Marras, S. Tyagi, E. Shashkina, M. Kamboj, T. E. Kiehn, M. S. Glickman, F. R. Kramer, and D. Alland.** 2009. Use of sloppy molecular beacon probes for identification of mycobacterial species. *J. Clin. Microbiol.* **47:**1190–1198.

80. **Ellington, M. J., J. Kistler, D. M. Livermore, and N. Woodford.** 2007. Multiplex PCR for rapid detection of genes encoding acquired metallo-β-lactamases. *J. Antimicrob. Chemother.* **59:**321–322.

81. **Endimiani, A., A. M. Hujer, F. Perez, C. R. Bethel, K. M. Hujer, J. Kroeger, M. Oethinger, D. L. Paterson, M. D. Adams, M. R. Jacobs, D. J. Diekema, G. S. Hall, S. G. Jenkins, L. B. Rice, F. C. Tenover, and R. A. Bonomo.** 2009. Characterization of bla$_{KPC}$-containing *Klebsiella pneumoniae* isolates detected in different institutions in the Eastern USA. *J. Antimicrob. Chemother.* **63:**427–437.

82. **Everett, M. J., Y. F. Jin, V. Ricci, and L. J. V. Piddock.** 1996. Contributions of individual mechanisms to fluoroquinolone resistance in 36 *Escherichia coli* strains isolated from humans and animals. *Antimicrob. Agents Chemother.* **40:**2380–2386.

83. **Farrell, D. J., S. G. Jenkins, S. D. Brown, M. Patel, B. S. Lavin, and K. P. Klugman.** 2005. Emergence and spread of *Streptococcus pneumoniae* with *erm*(B) and *mef*(A) resistance. *Emerg. Infect. Dis.* **11:**851–858.

84. **Fines, M., B. Perichon, P. Reynolds, D. F. Sahm, and P. Courvalin.** 1999. VanE, a new type of acquired glycopeptide resistance in *Enterococcus faecalis* BM4405. *Antimicrob. Agents Chemother.* **43:**2161–2164.

85. **Finks, J., E. Wells, T. L. Dyke, N. Husain, L. Plizga, R. Heddurshetti, M. Wilkins, J. Rudrik, J. Hageman, J. Patel, and C. Miller.** 2009. Vancomycin-resistant *Staphylococcus aureus*, Michigan, USA, 2007. *Emerg. Infect. Dis.* **15:**943–945.

86. **Fitoussi, F., C. Loukil, I. Gros, O. Clermont, P. Mariani, S. Bonacorsi, I. Le Thomas, D. Deforche, and E. Bingen.** 2001. Mechanisms of macrolide resistance in clinical group B streptococci isolated in France. *Antimicrob. Agents Chemother.* **45:**1889–1891.

87. **Frech, G., and S. Schwarz.** 2000. Molecular analysis of tetracycline resistance in *Salmonella enterica* subsp. *enterica* serovars Typhimurium, Enteritidis, Dublin, Choleraesuis, Hadar and Saintpaul: construction and application of specific gene probes. *J. Appl. Microbiol.* **89:**633–641.

88. **Fritsche, T. R., M. Castanheira, G. H. Miller, R. N. Jones, and E. S. Armstrong.** 2008. Detection of methyltransferases conferring high-level resistance to aminoglycosides in *Enterobacteriaceae* from Europe, North America, and Latin America. *Antimicrob. Agents Chemother.* **52:**1843–1845.

89. **Galimand, M., G. Gerbaud, and P. Courvalin.** 2000. Spectinomycin resistance in *Neisseria* spp. due to mutations in 16S rRNA. *Antimicrob. Agents Chemother.* **44:**1365–1366.

90. **Giakkoupi, P., A. Xanthaki, M. Kanelopoulou, A. Vlahaki, V. Miriagou, S. Kontou, E. Papafraggas, H. Malamou-Lada, L. S. Tzouvelekis, N. J. Legakis, and A. C. Vatopoulos.** 2003. VIM-1 metallo-β-lactamase-producing *Klebsiella pneumoniae* strains in Greek hospitals. *J. Clin. Microbiol.* **41:**3893–3896.

91. **Gibreel, A., and O. Sköld.** 1998. High-level resistance to trimethoprim in clinical isolates of *Campylobacter jejuni* by acquisition of foreign genes (*dfr1* and *dfr9*) expressing drug-insensitive dihydrofolate reductases. *Antimicrob. Agents Chemother.* **42:**3059–3064.

92. **Gibreel, A., O. Sköld, and D. E. Taylor.** 2004. Characterization of plasmid-mediated *aphA-3* kanamycin resistance in *Campylobacter jejuni. Microb. Drug Resist.* **10:**98–105.

93. **Gilbart, J., C. R. Perry, and B. Slocombe.** 1993. High-level mupirocin resistance in *Staphylococcus aureus:* evidence for two distinct isoleucyl-tRNA synthetases. *Antimicrob. Agents Chemother.* **37:**32–38.

94. **Gootz, T. D., M. K. Lescoe, F. Dib-Hajj, B. A. Dougherty, W. He, P. Della-Latta, and R. C. Huard.** 2009. Genetic organization of transposase regions surrounding *bla*KPC carbapenemase genes on plasmids from *Klebsiella* strains isolated in a New York City hospital. *Antimicrob. Agents Chemother.* **53:**1998–2004.

95. **Grape, M., A. Farra, G. Kronvall, and L. Sundström.** 2005. Integrons and gene cassettes in clinical isolates of co-trimoxazole-resistant Gram-negative bacteria. *Clin. Microbiol. Infect.* **11:**185–192.

96. **Grape, M., L. Sundstrom, and G. Kronvall.** 2007. Two new *dfr* genes in trimethoprim-resistant integron-negative *Escherichia coli* isolates. *Antimicrob. Agents Chemother.* **51:**1863–1864.

97. **Guerra, B., E. Junker, A. Miko, R. Helmuth, and M. C. Mendoza.** 2004. Characterization and localization of drug resistance determinants in multidrug-resistant, integron-carrying *Salmonella enterica* serotype Typhimurium strains. *Microb. Drug Resist.* **10:**83–91.

98. **Guerra, B., S. M. Soto, J. M. Argüelles, and M. C. Mendoza.** 2001. Multidrug resistance is mediated by large plasmids carrying a class 1 integron in the emergent *Salmonella enterica* serotype [4,5,12:i:-]. *Antimicrob. Agents Chemother.* **45:**1305–1308.

99. **Haanperä, M., P. Huovinen, and J. Jalava.** 2005. Detection and quantification of macrolide resistance mutations at positions 2058 and 2059 of the 23S rRNA gene by pyrosequencing. *Antimicrob. Agents Chemother.* **49:**457–460.

100. **Haas, W. H., K. Schilke, J. Brand, B. Amthor, K. Weyer, P. B. Fourie, G. Bretzel, V. Sticht-Groh, and H. J. Bremer.** 1997. Molecular analysis of *katG* gene mutations in strains of *Mycobacterium tuberculosis* complex from Africa. *Antimicrob. Agents Chemother.* **41:**1601–1603.

101. **Hall, N.** 2007. Advanced sequencing technologies and their wider impact in microbiology. *J. Exp. Biol.* **210:**1518–1525.

102. **Hannecart-Pokorni, E., F. Depuydt, L. De Wit, E. Van Bossuyt, J. Content, and R. Vanhoof.** 1997. Characterization of the 6'-*N*-aminoglycoside acetyltransferase gene *aac(6')*-Il associated with a *sulI*-type integron. *Antimicrob. Agents Chemother.* **41:**314–318.

103. **Hansen, L. M., P. C. Blanchard, and D. C. Hirsh.** 1996. Distribution of *tet*(H) among *Pasteurella* isolates from the United States and Canada. *Antimicrob. Agents Chemother.* **40:**1558–1560.

104. **Hardy, K., C. Price, A. Szczepura, S. Gossain, R. Davies, N. Stallard, S. Shabir, C. McMurray, A. Bradbury, and P. M. Hawkey.** 2010. Reduction in the rate of methicillin-resistant *Staphylococcus aureus* acquisition in surgical wards by rapid screening for colonization: a prospective, cross-over study. *Clin. Microbiol. Infect.* **16:**333–339.

105. **Haroche, J., J. Allignet, S. Aubert, A. E. Van Den Bogaard, and N. El Solh.** 2000. *satG*, conferring resistance to streptogramin A, is widely distributed in *Enterococcus faecium* strains but not in staphylococci. *Antimicrob. Agents Chemother.* **44:**190–191.

106. **Hindiyeh, M., G. Smollen, Z. Grossman, D. Ram, Y. Davidson, F. Mileguir, M. Vax, D. Ben David, I. Tal, G. Rahav, A. Shamiss, E. Mendelson, and N. Keller.** 2008. Rapid detection of *bla*KPC carbapenemase genes by real-time PCR. *J. Clin. Microbiol.* **46:**2879–2883.

107. **Honoré, N., and S. T. Cole.** 1994. Streptomycin resistance in mycobacteria. *Antimicrob. Agents Chemother.* **38:**238–242.

108. **Howden, B. P., T. P. Stinear, D. L. Allen, P. D. Johnson, P. B. Ward, and J. K. Davies.** 2008. Genomic analysis reveals a point mutation in the two-component sensor gene *graS* that leads to intermediate vancomycin resistance in clinical *Staphylococcus aureus. Antimicrob. Agents Chemother.* **52:**3755–3762.

109. **Huang, S. S., S. L. Rifas-Shiman, J. M. Pottinger, L. A. Herwaldt, T. R. Zembower, G. A. Noskin, S. E. Cosgrove, T. M. Perl, A. B. Curtis, J. L. Tokars, D. J. Diekema,** J. A. Jernigan, V. L. Hinrichsen, D. S. Yokoe, and R. Platt. 2007. Improving the assessment of vancomycin-resistant enterococci by routine screening. *J. Infect. Dis.* **195:**339–346.

110. **Huletsky, A., R. Giroux, V. Rossbach, M. Gagnon, M. Vaillancourt, M. Bernier, F. Gagnon, K. Truchon, M. Bastien, F. J. Picard, A. Van Belkum, M. Ouellette, P. H. Roy, and M. G. Bergeron.** 2004. New real-time PCR assay for rapid detection of methicillin-resistant *Staphylococcus aureus* directly from specimens containing a mixture of staphylococci. *J. Clin. Microbiol.* **42:**1875–1884.

111. **Huovinen, P., L. Sundström, G. Swedberg, and O. Sköld.** 1995. Trimethoprim and sulfonamide resistance. *Antimicrob. Agents Chemother.* **39:**279–289.

112. **Jacoby, G. A.** 2009. AmpC β-lactamases. *Clin. Microbiol. Rev.* **22:**161–182.

113. **Jacoby, G. A.** 2005. Mechanisms of resistance to quinolones. *Clin. Infect. Dis.* **41:**S120–S126.

114. **Jacoby, G. A., N. Gacharna, T. A. Black, G. H. Miller, and D. C. Hooper.** 2009. Temporal appearance of plasmid-mediated quinolone resistance genes. *Antimicrob. Agents Chemother.* **53:**1665–1666.

115. **Jacoby, G. A., D. M. Mills, and N. Chow.** 2004. Role of β-lactamases and porins in resistance to ertapenem and other β-lactams in *Klebsiella pneumoniae. Antimicrob. Agents Chemother.* **48:**3203–3206.

116. **Jacoby, G. A., and L. S. Munoz-Price.** 2005. The new β-lactamases. *N. Engl. J. Med.* **352:**380–391.

117. **Janoir, C., V. Zeller, M.-D. Kitzis, N. J. Moreau, and L. Gutmann.** 1996. High-level fluoroquinolone resistance in *Streptococcus pneumoniae* requires mutations in *parC* and *gyrA. Antimicrob. Agents Chemother.* **40:**2760–2764.

118. **Jansson, C., A. Franklin, and O. Sköld.** 1992. Spread of a newly found trimethoprim resistance gene, *dhfrIX*, among porcine isolates and human pathogens. *Antimicrob. Agents Chemother.* **36:**2704–2708.

119. **Jones, M., D. Helb, E. Story, C. Boehme, E. Wallace, K. Ho, J. Kop, M. Owens, R. Rodgers, P. Banada, H. Safi, R. Blakemore, N. Lan, E. Jones-López, M. Levi, M. Burday, I. Ayakaka, R. Murgerwa, B. McMillan, E. Winn-Deen, L. Christel, P. Dailey, M. Perkins, D. Persing, and D. Alland.** 2009. Rapid detection of *Mycobacterium tuberculosis* and rifampin-resistance from sputum samples with an easy-to-use PCR test with near-patient capability, abstr. 0185. *19th Eur. Congr. Clin. Microbiol. Infect. Dis.*

120. **Juteau, J.-M., M. Sirois, A. A. Medeiros, and R. C. Levesque.** 1991. Molecular distribution of ROB-1 β-lactamase in *Actinobacillus pleuropneumoniae. Antimicrob. Agents Chemother.* **35:**1397–1402.

121. **Kao, S. J., I. You, D. B. Clewell, S. M. Donabedian, M. J. Zervos, R. Petrin, K. J. Shaw, and J. W. Chow.** 2000. Detection of the high-level aminoglycoside resistance gene *aph(2")-Ib* in *Enterococcus faecium. Antimicrob. Agents Chemother.* **44:**2876–2879.

122. **Kapur, V., L.-L. Li, M. R. Hamrick, B. B. Plikaytis, T. M. Shinnick, A. Telenti, W. R. Jacobs, Jr., A. Banerjee, S. Cole, K. Y. Yuen, J. E. Clarridge III, B. N. Kreiswirth, and J. M. Musser.** 1995. Rapid *Mycobacterium* species assignment and unambiguous identification of mutations associated with antimicrobial resistance in *Mycobacterium tuberculosis* by automated DNA sequencing. *Arch. Pathol. Lab. Med.* **119:**131–138.

123. **Kariyama, R., R. Mitsuhata, J. W. Chow, D. B. Clewell, and H. Kumon.** 2000. Simple and reliable multiplex PCR assay for surveillance isolates of vancomycin-resistant enterococci. *J. Clin. Microbiol.* **38:**3092–3095.

124. **Kazakova, S. V., J. C. Hageman, M. Matava, A. Srinivasan, L. Phelan, B. Garfinkel, T. Boo, S. McAllister, J. Anderson, B. Jensen, D. Dodson, D. Lonsway, L. K. McDougal, M. Arduino, V. J. Fraser, G. Killgore, F. C. Tenover, S. Cody, and D. B. Jernigan.** 2005. A clone of methicillin-resistant *Staphylococcus aureus* among professional football players. *N. Engl. J. Med.* **352:**468–475.

125. **Kehrenberg, C., S. Schwarz, L. Jacobsen, L. H. Hansen, and B. Vester.** 2005. A new mechanism for chloramphenicol, florfenicol and clindamycin resistance: methylation of 23S ribosomal RNA at A2503. *Mol. Microbiol.* **57:**1064–1073.

126. **Kelley, C. L., D. A. Rouse, and S. L. Morris.** 1997. Analysis of *ahpC* gene mutations in isoniazid-resistant clinical isolates of *Mycobacterium tuberculosis. Antimicrob. Agents Chemother.* **41:**2057–2058.

127. **Kim, H. B., B. Lee, H.-C. Jang, S. H. Kim, C. I. Kang, Y. J. Choi, S. W. Park, B. S. Kim, E.-C. Kim, M.-D. Oh, and K. W. Choe.** 2004. A high frequency of macrolide-lincosamide-streptogramin resistance determinants in *Staphylococcus aureus* isolated in South Korea. *Microb. Drug Resist.* **10:**248–254.

128. **Kim, H. B., C. H. Park, C. J. Kim, E. C. Kim, G. A. Jacoby, and D. C. Hooper.** 2009. Prevalence of plasmid-mediated quinolone resistance determinants over a 9-year period. *Antimicrob. Agents Chemother.* **53:**639–645.

129. **Kitchel, B., J. K. Rasheed, J. B. Patel, A. Srinivasan, S. Navon-Venezia, Y. Carmeli, A. Brolund, and C. G. Giske.** 2009. Molecular epidemiology of KPC-producing *Klebsiella pneumoniae* isolates in the United States: clonal expansion of multilocus sequence type 258. *Antimicrob. Agents Chemother.* **53:**3365–3370.

130. **Klaassen, C. H. W., and J. W. Mouton.** 2005. Molecular detection of the macrolide efflux gene: to discriminate or not to discriminate between *mef*(A) and *mef*(E). *Antimicrob. Agents Chemother.* **49:**1271–1278.

131. **Klomberg, D. M., H. A. de Valk, J. W. Mouton, and C. H. W. Klaassen.** 2005. Rapid and reliable real-time PCR assay for detection of the macrolide efflux gene and subsequent discrimination between its distinct subclasses *mef*(A) and *mef*(E). *J. Microbiol. Methods* **60:**269–273.

132. **Kobayashi, N., M. Alam, Y. Nishimoto, S. Urasawa, N. Uehara, and N. Watanabe.** 2001. Distribution of aminoglycoside resistance genes in recent clinical isolates of *Enterococcus faecalis, Enterococcus faecium* and *Enterococcus avium. Epidemiol. Infect.* **126:**197–204.

133. **Kotlovsky, T., R. Shalginov, L. Austin, and H. Sprecher.** 2009. Rapid detection of *bla*KPC-positive *Klebsiella pneumoniae* in a clinical setting. *Eur. J. Clin. Microbiol. Infect. Dis.* **28:**309–311.

134. **Launay, A., S. A. Ballard, P. D. Johnson, M. L. Grayson, and T. Lambert.** 2006. Transfer of vancomycin resistance transposon Tn*1549* from *Clostridium symbiosum* to *Enterococcus* spp. in the gut of gnotobiotic mice. *Antimicrob. Agents Chemother.* **50:**1054–1062.

135. **Leclercq, R., E. Derlot, J. Duval, and P. Courvalin.** 1988. Plasmid-mediated resistance to vancomycin and teicoplanin in *Enterococcus faecium. N. Engl. J. Med.* **319:**157–161.

136. **Leclercq, R., C. Huet, M. Picherot, P. Trieu-Cuot, and C. Poyart.** 2005. Genetic basis of antibiotic resistance in clinical isolates of *Streptococcus gallolyticus* (*Streptococcus bovis*). *Antimicrob. Agents Chemother.* **49:**1646–1648.

137. **Lee, J. C., J. Y. Oh, J. W. Cho, J. C. Park, J. M. Kim, S. Y. Seol, and D. T. Cho.** 2001. The prevalence of trimethoprim-resistance-conferring dihydrofolate reductase genes in urinary isolates of *Escherichia coli* in Korea. *J. Antimicrob. Chemother.* **47:**599–604.

138. **Lee, K., J. H. Yum, D. Yong, H. M. Lee, H. D. Kim, J. D. Docquier, G. M. Rossolini, and Y. Chong.** 2005. Novel acquired metallo-β-lactamase gene, *bla*SIM-1, in a class 1 integron from *Acinetobacter baumannii* clinical isolates from Korea. *Antimicrob. Agents Chemother.* **49:**4485–4491.

139. **Lee, W. G., J. A. Jernigan, J. K. Rasheed, G. J. Anderson, and F. C. Tenover.** 2001. Possible horizontal transfer of the *vanB2* gene among genetically diverse strains of vancomycin-resistant *Enterococcus faecium* in a Korean hospital. *J. Clin. Microbiol.* **39:**1165–1168.

140. **Leinberger, D. M., V. Grimm, M. Rubtsova, J. Weile, K. Schroppel, T. A. Wichelhaus, C. Knabbe, R. D. Schmid, and T. T. Bachmann.** 2010. Integrated detection of extended-spectrum-beta-lactam resistance by DNA microarray-based genotyping of TEM, SHV, and CTX-M genes. *J. Clin. Microbiol.* **48:**460–471.

141. **Levy, S. B., L. M. McMurry, T. M. Barbosa, V. Burdett, P. Courvalin, W. Hillen, M. C. Roberts, J. I. Rood, and D. E. Taylor.** 1999. Nomenclature for new tetracycline resistance determinants. *Antimicrob. Agents Chemother.* **43:**1523–1524.

142. **Lewis, J. S., II, M. Herrera, B. Wickes, J. E. Patterson, and J. H. Jorgensen.** 2007. First report of the emergence of CTX-M-type extended-spectrum β-lactamases (ESBLs) as the predominant ESBL isolated in a U.S. health care system. *Antimicrob. Agents Chemother.* **51:**4015–4021.

143. **Lincopan, N., L. M. de Almeida, M. R. Elmor de Araujo, and E. M. Mamizuka.** 2009. Linezolid resistance in *Staphylococcus epidermidis* associated with a G2603T mutation in the 23S rRNA gene. *Int. J. Antimicrob. Agents* **34:**281–282.

144. **Liu, J.-H., Y.-T. Deng, Z.-L. Zeng, J.-H. Gao, L. Chen, Y. Arakawa, and Z.-L. Chen.** 2008. Coprevalence of plasmid-mediated quinolone resistance determinants QepA, Qnr, and AAC(6′)-Ib-cr among 16S rRNA methylase RmtB-producing *Escherichia coli* isolates from pigs. *Antimicrob. Agents Chemother.* **52:**2992–2993.

145. **Low, D. E.** 2005. Changing trends in antimicrobial-resistant pneumococci: it's not all bad news. *Clin. Infect. Dis.* **41:**228–233.

146. **Lyras, D., and J. I. Rood.** 1996. Genetic organization and distribution of tetracycline resistance determinants in *Clostridium perfringens. Antimicrob. Agents Chemother.* **40:**2500–2504.

147. **Manch-Citron, J. N., G. H. Lopez, A. Dey, J. W. Rapley, S. R. MacNeill, and C. M. Cobb.** 2000. PCR monitoring for tetracycline resistance genes in subgingival plaque following site-specific periodontal therapy: a preliminary report. *J. Clin. Periodontol.* **27:**437–446.

148. **Maor, Y., L. Lago, A. Zlotkin, Y. Nitzan, N. Belausov, D. Ben-David, N. Keller, and G. Rahav.** 2009. Molecular features of heterogeneous vancomycin-intermediate *Staphylococcus aureus* strains isolated from bacteremic patients. *BMC Microbiol.* **9:**189.

149. **Marchandin, H., H. Jean-Pierre, E. Jumas-Bilak, L. Isson, B. Drouillard, H. Darbas, and C. Carriere.** 2001. Distribution of macrolide resistance genes *erm*(B) and *mef*(A) among 160 penicillin-intermediate clinical isolates of *Streptococcus pneumoniae* isolated in southern France. *Pathol. Biol.* **49:**522–527.

150. **Margeridon-Thermet, S., N. S. Shulman, A. Ahmed, R. Shahriar, T. Liu, C. Wang, S. P. Holmes, F. Babrzadeh, B. Gharizadeh, B. Hanczaruk, B. B. Simen, M. Egholm, and R. W. Shafer.** 2009. Ultra-deep pyrosequencing of hepatitis B virus quasispecies from nucleoside and nucleotide reverse-transcriptase inhibitor (NRTI)-treated patients and NRTI-naive patients. *J. Infect. Dis.* **199:**1275–1285.

151. **Mariotte, S., P. Nordmann, and M. H. Nicolas.** 1994. Extended-spectrum β-lactamase in *Proteus mirabilis. J. Antimicrob. Chemother.* **33:**925–935.

152. **Maskell, J. P., A. M. Sefton, and L. M. C. Hall.** 1997. Mechanism of sulfonamide resistance in clinical isolates of *Streptococcus pneumoniae. Antimicrob. Agents Chemother.* **41:**2121–2126.

153. **McDougal, L. K., J. K. Rasheed, J. W. Biddle, and F. C. Tenover.** 1995. Identification of multiple clones of extended-spectrum cephalosporin-resistant *Streptococcus pneumoniae* isolates in the United States. *Antimicrob. Agents Chemother.* **39:**2282–2288.

154. **McGettigan, S. E., B. Hu, K. Andreacchio, I. Nachamkin, and P. H. Edelstein.** 2009. Prevalence of CTX-M β-lactamases in Philadelphia, Pennsylvania. *J. Clin. Microbiol.* **47:**2970–2974.

155. **McKessar, S. J., A. M. Berry, J. M. Bell, J. D. Turnidge, and J. C. Paton.** 2000. Genetic characterization of *vanG*, a novel vancomycin resistance locus of *Enterococcus faecalis. Antimicrob. Agents Chemother.* **44:**3224–3228.

156. **Meier, A., P. Kirschner, F.-C. Bange, U. Vogel, and E. C. Böttger.** 1994. Genetic alterations in streptomycin-resistant *Mycobacterium tuberculosis*: mapping of mutations conferring resistance. *Antimicrob. Agents Chemother.* **38:**228–233.

157. **Mendes, R. E., L. M. Deshpande, M. Castanheira, J. DiPersio, M. A. Saubolle, and R. N. Jones.** 2008. First report of *cfr*-mediated resistance to linezolid in human staphylococcal clinical isolates recovered in the United States. *Antimicrob. Agents Chemother.* **52:**2244–2246.

158. **Mesko Meglic, K., S. Koren, M. F. Palepou, E. Karisik, D. M. Livermore, R. Pike, A. Andlovic, S. Jeverica, V. Krizan-Hergouth, M. Muller-Premru, K. Seme, the Slovenian ESBL Study Group, and N. Woodford.** 2009. Nationwide survey of CTX-M-type extended-spectrum β-lactamases among *Klebsiella pneumoniae* isolates in Slovenian hospitals. *Antimicrob. Agents Chemother.* **53:**287–291.

159. **Minarini, L. A., L. Poirel, V. Cattoir, A. L. Darini, and P. Nordmann.** 2008. Plasmid-mediated quinolone resistance determinants among enterobacterial isolates from outpatients in Brazil. *J. Antimicrob. Chemother.* **62:**474–478.

160. **Moland, E. S., J. A. Black, J. Ourada, M. D. Reisbig, N. D. Hanson, and K. S. Thomson.** 2002. Occurrence of newer β-lactamases in *Klebsiella pneumoniae* isolates from 24 U.S. hospitals. *Antimicrob. Agents Chemother.* **46:**3837–3842.

161. **Moland, E. S., N. D. Hanson, V. L. Herrera, J. A. Black, T. J. Lockhart, A. Hossain, J. A. Johnson, R. V. Goering, and K. S. Thomson.** 2003. Plasmid-mediated, carbapenem-hydrolysing β-lactamase, KPC-2, in *Klebsiella pneumoniae* isolates. *J. Antimicrob. Chemother.* **51:**711–714.

162. **Monstein, H.-J., A. Östholm-Balkhed, M. V. Nilsson, M. Nilsson, K. Dornbusch, and L. E. Nilsson.** 2007. Multiplex PCR amplification assay for the detection of *bla*SHV, *bla*TEM and *bla*CTX-M genes in *Enterobacteriaceae.* APMIS **115:**1400–1408.

163. **Moon, D. C., S. Y. Seol, M. Gurung, J. S. Jin, C. H. Choi, J. Kim, Y. C. Lee, D. T. Cho, and J. C. Lee.** 2010. Emergence of a new mutation and its accumulation in the topoisomerase IV gene confers high levels of resistance to fluoroquinolones in *Escherichia coli* isolates. *Int. J. Antimicrob. Agents* **35:**76–79.

164. **Mulvey, M. R., E. Bryce, D. A. Boyd, M. Ofner-Agostini, A. M. Land, A. E. Simor, S. Paton, and the Canadian Hospital Epidemiology Committee, the Canadian Nosocomial Infection Surveillance Program, Health Canada.** 2005. Molecular characterization of cefoxitin-resistant *Escherichia coli* from Canadian hospitals. *Antimicrob. Agents Chemother.* **49:**358–365.

165. **Musser, J. M., V. Kapur, D. L. Williams, B. N. Kreiswirth, D. van Soolingen, and J. D. A. van Embden.** 1996. Characterization of the catalase-peroxidase gene (*katG*) and *inhA* locus in isoniazid-resistant and -susceptible strains of *Mycobacterium tuberculosis* by automated DNA sequencing: restricted array of mutations associated with drug resistance. *J. Infect. Dis.* **173:**196–202.

166. **Naas, T., G. Cuzon, H. Truong, S. Bernabeu, and P. Nordmann.** 2009. Use of DNA microarrays for rapid detection of TEM, SHV, CTX-M ESBL- and KPC-producers, abstr. D-726, p. 132. *Abstr. 49th Intersci. Conf. Antimicrob. Agents Chemother.* American Society for Microbiology, Washington, DC.

167. **Naas, T., G. Cuzon, M.-V. Villegas, M.-F. Lartigue, J. P. Quinn, and P. Nordmann.** 2008. Genetic structures at the origin of acquisition of the β-lactamase *bla*KPC gene. *Antimicrob. Agents Chemother.* **52:**1257–1263.

168. **Naas, T., L. Poirel, A. Karim, and P. Nordmann.** 1999. Molecular characterization of In50, a class 1 integron encoding the gene for the extended-spectrum β-lactamase VEB-1 in *Pseudomonas aeruginosa.* *FEMS Microbiol. Lett.* **176:**411–419.

169. **Navia, M. M., J. Ruiz, J. Sanchez-Cespedes, and J. Vila.** 2003. Detection of dihydrofolate reductase genes by PCR and RFLP. *Diagn. Microbiol. Infect. Dis.* **46:**295–298.

170. **Navon-Venezia, S., A. Leavitt, M. J. Schwaber, J. K. Rasheed, A. Srinivasan, J. B. Patel, Y. Carmeli, and the Israeli KPC Kpn Study Group.** 2009. First report on a hyperepidemic clone of KPC-3-producing *Klebsiella pneumoniae* in Israel genetically related to a strain causing outbreaks in the United States. *Antimicrob. Agents Chemother.* **53:**818–820.

171. **Ng, L.-K., M. R. Mulvey, I. Martin, G. A. Peters, and W. Johnson.** 1999. Genetic characterization of antimicrobial resistance in Canadian isolates of Salmonella serovar Typhimurium DT104. *Antimicrob. Agents Chemother.* **43:**3018–3021.

172. **Nordmann, P., G. Cuzon, and T. Naas.** 2009. The real threat of *Klebsiella pneumoniae* carbapenemase-producing bacteria. *Lancet Infect. Dis.* **9:**228–236.

173. **Novotna, G., V. Adamkova, J. Janata, O. Melter, and J. Spizek.** 2005. Prevalence of resistance mechanisms against macrolides and lincosamides in methicillin-resistant coagulase-negative staphylococci in the Czech Republic and occurrence of an undefined mechanism of resistance to lincosamides. *Antimicrob. Agents Chemother.* **49:**3586–3589.

174. **Nüesch-Inderbinen, M. T., H. Hächler, and F. H. Kayser.** 1996. Detection of genes coding for extended-spectrum SHV beta-lactamases in clinical isolates by a molecular genetic method, and comparison with the E Test. *Eur. J. Clin. Microbiol. Infect. Dis.* **15:**398–402.

175. **Nunes, E. L. C., K. R. N. Santos, P. J. J. Mondino, M. C. Bastos, and M. Giambiagi-deMarval.** 1999. Detection of *ileS-2* gene encoding mupirocin resistance in methicillin-resistant *Staphylococcus aureus* by multiplex PCR. *Diagn. Microbiol. Infect. Dis.* **34:**77–81.

176. **Oliver, A., J. C. Pérez-Díaz, T. M. Coque, F. Baquero, and R. Cantón.** 2001. Nucleotide sequence and characterization of a novel cefotaxime-hydrolyzing β-lactamase (CTX-M-10) isolated in Spain. *Antimicrob. Agents Chemother.* **45:**616–620.

177. **Olsvik, B., M. J. Flynn, F. C. Tenover, J. Slots, and I. Olsen.** 1996. Tetracycline resistance in *Prevotella* isolates from periodontally diseased patients is due to the *tet*(Q) gene. *Oral Microbiol. Immunol.* **11:**304–308.

178. **Olsvik, B., I. Olsen, and F. C. Tenover.** 1995. Detection of *tet*(M) and *tet*(O) using the polymerase chain reaction in bacteria isolated from patients with periodontal disease. *Oral Microbiol. Immunol.* **10:**87–92.

179. **Olsvik, B., F. C. Tenover, I. Olsen, and J. K. Rasheed.** 1996. Three subtypes of the *tet*(M) gene identified in bacterial isolates from periodontal pockets. *Oral Microbiol. Immunol.* **11:**299–303.

180. **Oster, P., A. Zanchi, S. Cresti, M. Lattanzi, F. Montagnani, C. Cellesi, and G. M. Rossolini.** 1999. Patterns of macrolide resistance determinants among community-acquired *Streptococcus pneumoniae* isolates over a 5-year period of decreased macrolide susceptibility rates. *Antimicrob. Agents Chemother.* **43:**2510–2512.

181. **Padiglione, A. A., E. A. Grabsch, D. Olden, M. Hellard, M. I. Sinclair, C. K. Fairley, and M. L. Grayson.** 2000. Fecal colonization with vancomycin-resistant enterococci in Australia. *Emerg. Infect. Dis.* **6:**534–536.

182. **Palepou, M.-F., A. P. Johnson, B. D. Cookson, H. Beattie, A. Charlett, and N. Woodford.** 1998. Evaluation of disc diffusion and Etest for determining the susceptibility of *Staphylococcus aureus* to mupirocin. *J. Antimicrob. Chemother.* **42:**577–583.

183. **Pan, X.-S., J. Ambler, S. Mehtar, and L. M. Fisher.** 1996. Involvement of topoisomerase IV and DNA gyrase as ciprofloxacin targets in *Streptococcus pneumoniae.* *Antimicrob. Agents Chemother.* **40:**2321–2326.

184. **Park, C. H., A. Robicsek, G. A. Jacoby, D. Sahm, and D. C. Hooper.** 2006. Prevalence in the United States of *aac(6′)*-Ib-cr encoding a ciprofloxacin-modifying enzyme. *Antimicrob. Agents Chemother.* **50:**3953–3955.

185. **Parta, M., M. Goebel, M. Matloobi, C. Stager, and D. M. Musher.** 2009. Identification of methicillin-resistant or methicillin-susceptible *Staphylococcus aureus* in blood cultures and wound swabs by GeneXpert. *J. Clin. Microbiol.* **47:**1609–1610.

186. **Patel, J. B., R. J. Gorwitz, and J. A. Jernigan.** 2009. Mupirocin resistance. *Clin. Infect. Dis.* **49:**935–941.

187. **Patel, R.** 1999. Enterococcal-type glycopeptide resistance genes in non-enterococcal organisms. *FEMS Microbiol. Lett.* **185:**1–7.

188. **Paterson, D. L., K. M. Hujer, A. M. Hujer, B. Yeiser, M. D. Bonomo, L. B. Rice, R. A. Bonomo, and the International Klebsiella Study Group.** 2003. Extended-spectrum β-lactamases in *Klebsiella pneumoniae* bloodstream isolates

from seven countries: dominance and widespread prevalence of SHV- and CTX-M-type β-lactamases. *Antimicrob. Agents Chemother.* **47:**3554–3560.

189. **Paule, S. M., D. M. Hacek, B. Kufner, K. Truchon, R. B. Thomson, Jr., K. L. Kaul, A. Robicsek, and L. R. Peterson.** 2007. Performance of the BD GeneOhm methicillin-resistant *Staphylococcus aureus* test before and during high-volume clinical use. *J. Clin. Microbiol.* **45:**2993–2998.

190. **Paule, S. M., A. C. Pasquariello, D. M. Hacek, A. G. Fisher, R. B. Thomson, Jr., K. L. Kaul, and L. R. Peterson.** 2004. Direct detection of *Staphylococcus aureus* from adult and neonate nasal swab specimens using real-time polymerase chain reaction. *J. Mol. Diagn.* **6:**191–196.

191. **Paule, S. M., W. E. Trick, F. C. Tenover, M. Lankford, S. Cunningham, V. Stosor, R. L. Cordell, and L. R. Peterson.** 2003. Comparison of PCR assay to culture for surveillance detection of vancomycin-resistant enterococci. *J. Clin. Microbiol.* **41:**4805–4807.

192. **Pérez-Pérez, F. J., and N. D. Hanson.** 2002. Detection of plasmid-mediated AmpC β-lactamase genes in clinical isolates by using multiplex PCR. *J. Clin. Microbiol.* **40:**2153–2162.

193. **Perichon, B., and P. Courvalin.** 2009. VanA-type vancomycin-resistant *Staphylococcus aureus*. *Antimicrob. Agents Chemother.* **53:**4580–4587.

194. **Perichon, B., P. Reynolds, and P. Courvalin.** 1997. VanD-type glycopeptide-resistant *Enterococcus faecium* BM4339. *Antimicrob. Agents Chemother.* **41:**2016–2018.

195. **Perichon, B., J. Tankovic, and P. Courvalin.** 1997. Characterization of a mutation in the *parE* gene that confers fluoroquinolone resistance in *Streptococcus pneumoniae*. *Antimicrob. Agents Chemother.* **41:**1166–1167.

196. **Perl, T. M., J. J. Cullen, R. P. Wenzel, M. B. Zimmerman, M. A. Pfaller, D. Sheppard, J. Twombley, P. P. French, and L. A. Herwaldt.** 2002. Intranasal mupirocin to prevent postoperative *Staphylococcus aureus* infections. *N. Engl. J. Med.* **346:**1871–1877.

197. **Perreten, V., and P. Boerlin.** 2003. A new sulfonamide resistance gene (*sul3*) in *Escherichia coli* is widespread in the pig population of Switzerland. *Antimicrob. Agents Chemother.* **47:**1169–1172.

198. **Petinaki, E., V. Guerin-Faublee, V. Pichereau, C. Villers, A. Achard, B. Malbruny, and R. Leclercq.** 2008. Lincomycin resistance gene *lnu*(D) in *Streptococcus uberis*. *Antimicrob. Agents Chemother.* **52:**626–630.

199. **Petroni, A., A. Corso, R. Melano, M. L. Cacace, A. M. Bru, A. Rossi, and M. Galas.** 2002. Plasmidic extended-spectrum β-lactamases in *Vibrio cholerae* O1 El Tor isolates in Argentina. *Antimicrob. Agents Chemother.* **46:**1462–1468.

200. **Ploy, M.-C., H. Giamarellou, P. Bourlioux, P. Courvalin, and T. Lambert.** 1994. Detection of *aac(6′)*-I genes in amikacin-resistant *Acinetobacter* spp. by PCR. *Antimicrob. Agents Chemother.* **38:**2925–2928.

201. **Poirel, L., V. Cattoir, A. Soares, C. J. Soussy, and P. Nordmann.** 2007. Novel Ambler class A β-lactamase LAP-1 and its association with the plasmid-mediated quinolone resistance determinant QnrS1. *Antimicrob. Agents Chemother.* **51:**631–637.

202. **Poirel, L., I. Le Thomas, T. Naas, A. Karim, and P. Nordmann.** 2000. Biochemical sequence analyses of GES-1, a novel class A extended-spectrum β-lactamase, and the class 1 integron In52 from *Klebsiella pneumoniae*. *Antimicrob. Agents Chemother.* **44:**622–632.

203. **Poirel, L., T. Naas, D. Nicolas, L. Collet, S. Bellais, J.-D. Cavallo, and P. Nordmann.** 2000. Characterization of VIM-2, a carbapenem-hydrolyzing metallo-β-lactamase and its plasmid- and integron-borne gene from a *Pseudomonas aeruginosa* clinical isolate in France. *Antimicrob. Agents Chemother.* **44:**891–897.

204. **Poole, K.** 2005. Aminoglycoside resistance in *Pseudomonas aeruginosa*. *Antimicrob. Agents Chemother.* **49:**479–487.

205. **Pottumarthy, S., E. S. Moland, S. Juretschko, S. R. Swanzy, K. S. Thomson, and T. R. Fritsche.** 2003. NmcA carbapenem-hydrolyzing enzyme in *Enterobacter cloacae* in North America. *Emerg. Infect. Dis.* **9:**999–1002.

206. **Power, E. G. M., Y. H. Abdulla, H. G. Talsania, W. Spice, S. Aathithan, and G. L. French.** 1995. *vanA* genes in vancomycin-resistant clinical isolates of *Oerskovia turbata* and *Arcanobacterium* (*Corynebacterium*) *haemolyticum*. *J. Antimicrob. Chemother.* **36:**595–606.

207. **Poyart, C., C. Pierre, G. Quesne, B. Pron, P. Berche, and P. Trieu-Cuot.** 1997. Emergence of vancomycin resistance in the genus *Streptococcus*: characterization of a *vanB* transferable determinant in *Streptococcus bovis*. *Antimicrob. Agents Chemother.* **41:**24–29.

208. **Prystowsky, J., F. Siddiqui, J. Chosay, D. L. Sinabarger, J. Millichap, L. R. Peterson, and G. A. Noskin.** 2001. Resistance to linezolid: characterization of mutations in rRNA and comparison of their occurrences in vancomycin-resistant enterococci. *Antimicrob. Agents Chemother.* **45:**2154–2156.

209. **Pulkkinen, L., P. Huovinen, E. Vuorio, and P. Toivanen.** 1984. Characterization of trimethoprim resistance by use of probes specific for transposon Tn7. *Antimicrob. Agents Chemother.* **26:**82–86.

210. **Queenan, A. M., and K. Bush.** 2007. Carbapenemases: the versatile beta-lactamases. *Clin. Microbiol. Rev.* **20:**440–458.

211. **Queenan, A. M., C. Torres-Viera, H. S. Gold, Y. Carmeli, G. M. Eliopoulos, R. C. Moellering, Jr., J. P. Quinn, J. Hindler, A. A. Medeiros, and K. Bush.** 2000. SME-type carbapenem-hydrolyzing class A β-lactamases from geographically diverse *Serratia marcescens* strains. *Antimicrob. Agents Chemother.* **44:**3035–3039.

212. **Ramsey, M. A., S. F. Bradley, C. A. Kauffman, and T. M. Morton.** 1996. Identification of chromosomal location of *mupA* gene, encoding low-level mupirocin resistance in staphylococcal isolates. *Antimicrob. Agents Chemother.* **40:**2820–2823.

213. **Rasheed, J. K., G. J. Anderson, H. Yigit, A. M. Queenan, A. Doménech-Sánchez, J. M. Swenson, J. W. Biddle, M. J. Ferraro, G. A. Jacoby, and F. C. Tenover.** 2000. Characterization of the extended-spectrum β-lactamase reference strain, *Klebsiella pneumoniae* K6 (ATCC 700603), which produces the novel enzyme SHV-18. *Antimicrob. Agents Chemother.* **44:**2382–2388.

214. **Rasheed, J. K., J. W. Biddle, K. F. Anderson, L. Washer, C. Chenoweth, J. Perrin, D. W. Newton, and J. B. Patel.** 2008. Detection of the *Klebsiella pneumoniae* carbapenemase type 2 carbapenem-hydrolyzing enzyme in clinical isolates of *Citrobacter freundii* and *K. oxytoca* carrying a common plasmid. *J. Clin. Microbiol.* **46:**2066–2069.

215. **Rasheed, J. K., C. Jay, B. Metchock, F. Berkowitz, L. Weigel, J. Crellin, C. Steward, B. Hill, A. A. Medeiros, and F. C. Tenover.** 1997. Evolution of extended-spectrum β-lactam resistance (SHV-8) in a strain of *Escherichia coli* during multiple episodes of bacteremia. *Antimicrob. Agents Chemother.* **41:**647–653.

216. **Raviglione, M. C., and I. M. Smith.** 2007. XDR tuberculosis—implications for global public health. *N. Engl. J. Med.* **356:**656–659.

217. **Reig, M., J.-C. Galan, F. Baquero, and J. C. Perez-Diaz.** 2001. Macrolide resistance in *Peptostreptococcus* spp. mediated by *ermTR*: possible source of macrolide-lincosamide-streptogramin B resistance in *Streptococcus pyogenes*. *Antimicrob. Agents Chemother.* **45:**630–632.

218. **Reynolds, P. E., and P. Courvalin.** 2005. Vancomycin resistance in enterococci due to synthesis of precursors terminating in D-alanyl-D-serine. *Antimicrob. Agents Chemother.* **49:**21–25.

219. **Riccio, M. L., J.-D. Docquier, E. Dell'Amico, F. Luzzaro, G. Amicosante, and G. M. Rossolini.** 2003. Novel 3-*N*-aminoglycoside acetyltransferase gene, *aac(3)*-Ic, from a *Pseudomonas aeruginosa* integron. *Antimicrob. Agents Chemother.* **47:**1746–1748.

220. **Roberts, M. C.** 2005. Update on acquired tetracycline resistance genes. *FEMS Microbiol. Lett.* **245:**195–203.

221. **Roberts, M. C., W. O. Chung, and D. E. Roe.** 1996. Characterization of tetracycline and erythromycin resistance determinants in *Treponema denticola*. *Antimicrob. Agents Chemother.* **40:**1690–1694.

222. **Roberts, M. C., J. Sutcliffe, P. Courvalin, L. B. Jensen, J. Rood, and H. Seppala.** 1999. Nomenclature for macrolide

and macrolide-lincosamide-streptogramin B resistance determinants. *Antimicrob. Agents Chemother.* 43:2823–2830.

223. **Robicsek, A., J. L. Beaumont, S. M. Paule, D. M. Hacek, R. B. Thomson, Jr., K. L. Kaul, P. King, and L. R. Peterson.** 2008. Universal surveillance for methicillin-resistant *Staphylococcus aureus* in 3 affiliated hospitals. *Ann. Intern. Med.* 148:409–418.

224. **Robicsek, A., J. Strahilevitz, G. A. Jacoby, M. Macielag, D. Abbanat, C. H. Park, K. Bush, and D. C. Hooper.** 2006. Fluoroquinolone-modifying enzyme: a new adaptation of a common aminoglycoside acetyltransferase. *Nat. Med.* 12:83–88.

225. **Robledo, I. E., E. E. Aquino, M. I. Sante, J. L. Santana, D. M. Otero, C. F. Leon, and G. J. Vazquez.** 2010. Detection of KPC in *Acinetobacter* spp. in Puerto Rico. *Antimicrob. Agents Chemother.* 54:1354–1357.

226. **Rossolini, G. M., M. M. D'Andrea, and C. Mugnaioli.** 2008. The spread of CTX-M-type extended-spectrum β-lactamases. *Clin. Microbiol. Infect.* 14(Suppl. 1):33–41.

227. **Sabaté, M., R. Tarragó, F. Navarro, E. Miró, C. Vergés, J. Barbé, and G. Prats.** 2000. Cloning and sequence of the gene encoding a novel cefotaxime-hydrolyzing β-lactamase (CTX-M-9) from *Escherichia coli* in Spain. *Antimicrob. Agents Chemother.* 44:1970–1973.

228. **Saha, B., A. K. Singh, A. Ghosh, and M. Bal.** 2008. Identification and characterization of a vancomycin-resistant *Staphylococcus aureus* isolated from Kolkata (South Asia). *J. Med. Microbiol.* 57:72–79.

229. **Sakoulas, G., H. S. Gold, L. Venkataraman, P. C. DeGirolami, G. M. Eliopoulos, and Q. Qian.** 2001. Methicillin-resistant *Staphylococcus aureus*: comparison of susceptibility testing methods and analysis of *mecA*-positive susceptible strains. *J. Clin. Microbiol.* 39:3946–3951.

230. **Satake, S., N. Clark, D. Rimland, F. S. Nolte, and F. C. Tenover.** 1997. Detection of vancomycin-resistant enterococci in fecal samples by PCR. *J. Clin. Microbiol.* 35:2325–2330.

231. **Saurina, G., J. M. Quale, V. M. Manikal, E. Oydna, and D. Landman.** 2000. Antimicrobial resistance in *Enterobacteriaceae* in Brooklyn, NY: epidemiology and relation to antibiotic usage patterns. *J. Antimicrob. Chemother.* 45:895–898.

232. **Schechner, V., K. Straus-Robinson, D. Schwartz, I. Pfeffer, J. Tarabeia, R. Moskovich, I. Chmelnitsky, M. J. Schwaber, Y. Carmeli, and S. Navon-Venezia.** 2009. Evaluation of PCR-based testing for surveillance of KPC-producing carbapenem-resistant members of the *Enterobacteriaceae* family. *J. Clin. Microbiol.* 47:3261–3265.

233. **Schlesinger, J., S. Navon-Venezia, I. Chmelnitsky, O. Hammer-Munz, A. Leavitt, H. S. Gold, M. J. Schwaber, and Y. Carmeli.** 2005. Extended-spectrum beta-lactamases among *Enterobacter* isolates obtained in Tel Aviv, Israel. *Antimicrob. Agents Chemother.* 49:1150–1156.

234. **Schwarz, S., C. Kehrenberg, B. Doublet, and A. Cloeckaert.** 2004. Molecular basis of bacterial resistance to chloramphenicol and florfenicol. *FEMS Microbiol. Rev.* 28:519–542.

235. **Senda, K., Y. Arakawa, S. Ichiyama, K. Nakashima, H. Ito, S. Ohsuka, K. Shimokata, N. Kato, and M. Ohta.** 1996. PCR detection of metallo-β-lactamase gene (bla$_{IMP}$) in gram-negative rods resistant to broad-spectrum β-lactams. *J. Clin. Microbiol.* 34:2909–2913.

236. **Shaw, K. J., P. N. Rather, R. S. Hare, and G. H. Miller.** 1993. Molecular genetics of aminoglycoside resistance genes and familial relationships of the aminoglycoside-modifying enzymes. *Microbiol. Rev.* 57:138–163.

237. **Shortridge, V. D., R. K. Flamm, N. Ramer, J. Beyer, and S. K. Tanaka.** 1996. Novel mechanism of macrolide resistance in *Streptococcus pneumoniae. Diagn. Microbiol. Infect. Dis.* 26:73–78.

238. **Sidjabat, H. E., F. P. Silveira, B. A. Potoski, K. M. Abu-Elmagd, J. M. Adams-Haduch, D. L. Paterson, and Y. Doi.** 2009. Interspecies spread of *Klebsiella pneumoniae* carbapenemase gene in a single patient. *Clin. Infect. Dis.* 49:1736–1738.

239. **Sievert, D. M., J. T. Rudrik, J. B. Patel, L. C. McDonald, M. J. Wilkins, and J. C. Hageman.** 2008. Vancomycin-resistant *Staphylococcus aureus* in the United States, 2002–2006. *Clin. Infect. Dis.* 46:668–674.

240. **Simen, B. B., J. F. Simons, K. H. Hullsiek, R. M. Novak, R. D. Macarthur, J. D. Baxter, C. Huang, C. Lubeski, G. S. Turenchalk, M. S. Braverman, B. Desany, J. M. Rothberg, M. Egholm, and M. J. Kozal.** 2009. Low-abundance drug-resistant viral variants in chronically HIV-infected, antiretroviral treatment-naive patients significantly impact treatment outcomes. *J. Infect. Dis.* 199:693–701.

241. **Sinclair, A., C. Arnold, and N. Woodford.** 2003. Rapid detection and estimation by pyrosequencing of 23S rRNA genes with a single nucleotide polymorphism conferring linezolid resistance in enterococci. *Antimicrob. Agents Chemother.* 47:3620–3622.

242. **Sloan, L. M., J. R. Uhl, E. A. Vetter, C. D. Schleck, W. S. Harmsen, J. Manahan, R. L. Thompson, J. E. Rosenblatt, and F. R. Cockerill III.** 2004. Comparison of the Roche LightCycler *vanA/vanB* detection assay and culture for detection of vancomycin-resistant enterococci from perianal swabs. *J. Clin. Microbiol.* 42:2636–2643.

243. **Somoskovi, A., J. Dormandy, D. Mitsani, J. Rivenburg, and M. Salfinger.** 2006. Use of smear-positive samples to assess the PCR-based genotype MTBDR assay for rapid, direct detection of the *Mycobacterium tuberculosis* complex as well as its resistance to isoniazid and rifampin. *J. Clin. Microbiol.* 44:4459–4463.

244. **Sreevatsan, S., X. Pan, K. E. Stockbauer, D. L. Williams, B. N. Kreiswirth, and J. M. Musser.** 1996. Characterization of *rpsL* and *rrs* mutations in streptomycin-resistant *Mycobacterium tuberculosis* isolates from diverse geographic localities. *Antimicrob. Agents Chemother.* 40:1024–1026.

245. **Sreevatsan, S., X. Pan, Y. Zhang, B. N. Kreiswirth, and J. M. Musser.** 1997. Mutations associated with pyrazinamide resistance in *pncA* of *Mycobacterium tuberculosis* complex organisms. *Antimicrob. Agents Chemother.* 41:636–640.

246. **Steward, C. D., P. M. Raney, A. K. Morrell, P. P. Williams, L. K. McDougal, L. Jevitt, J. E. McGowan, Jr., and F. C. Tenover.** 2005. Testing for induction of clindamycin resistance in erythromycin-resistant isolates of *Staphylococcus aureus. J. Clin. Microbiol.* 43:1716–1721.

247. **Strahilevitz, J., G. A. Jacoby, D. C. Hooper, and A. Robicsek.** 2009. Plasmid-mediated quinolone resistance: a multifaceted threat. *Clin. Microbiol. Rev.* 22:664–689.

248. **Sunde, M., and M. Norström.** 2005. The genetic background for streptomycin resistance in *Escherichia coli* influences the distribution of MICs. *J. Antimicrob. Chemother.* 56:87–90.

249. **Sundsfjord, A., G. S. Simonsen, B. C. Haldorsen, H. Haaheim, S.-O. Hjelmevoll, P. Littauer, and K. H. Dahl.** 2004. Genetic methods for detection of antimicrobial resistance. *APMIS* 112:815–837.

250. **Sundström, L., C. Jansson, K. Bremer, E. Heikkilä, B. Olsson-Liljequist, and O. Sköld.** 1995. A new *dhfrVIII* trimethoprim-resistance gene, flanked by IS26, whose product is remote from other dihydrofolate reductases in parsimony analysis. *Gene* 154:7–14.

251. **Sutcliffe, J., T. Grebe, A. Tait-Kamradt, and L. Wondrack.** 1996. Detection of erythromycin-resistant determinants by PCR. *Antimicrob. Agents Chemother.* 40:2562–2566.

252. **Sutcliffe, J., A. Tait-Kamradt, and L. Wondrack.** 1996. *Streptococcus pneumoniae* and *Streptococcus pyogenes* resistant to macrolides but sensitive to clindamycin: a common resistance pattern mediated by an efflux system. *Antimicrob. Agents Chemother.* 40:1817–1824.

253. **Tait-Kamradt, A., J. Davies, M. Cronan, M. R. Jacobs, P. C. Appelbaum, and J. Sutcliffe.** 2000. Mutations in 23S rRNA and ribosomal protein L4 account for resistance in pneumococcal strains selected in vitro by macrolide passage. *Antimicrob. Agents Chemother.* 44:2118–2125.

254. **Telenti, A., N. Honoré, C. Bernasconi, J. March, A. Ortega, B. Heym, H. E. Takiff, and S. T. Cole.** 1997. Genotypic assessment of isoniazid and rifampin resistance in *Mycobacterium tuberculosis*: a blind study at reference laboratory level. *J. Clin. Microbiol.* 35:719–723.

255. **Tenover, F. C., S. L. Emery, C. A. Spiegel, P. A. Bradford, S. Eells, A. Endimiani, R. A. Bonomo, and J. E. McGowan, Jr.** 2009. Identification of plasmid-mediated AmpC β-lactamases in *Escherichia coli, Klebsiella* spp., and *Proteus* species can potentially improve reporting of cephalosporin susceptibility testing results. *J. Clin. Microbiol.* **47:**294–299.

256. **Tenover, F. C., M. B. Huang, J. K. Rasheed, and D. H. Persing.** 1994. Development of PCR assays to detect ampicillin resistance genes in cerebrospinal fluid samples containing *Haemophilus influenzae. J. Clin. Microbiol.* **32:**2729–2737.

257. **Tenover, F. C., R. K. Kalsi, P. P. Williams, R. B. Carey, S. Stocker, D. Lonsway, J. K. Rasheed, J. W. Biddle, J. E. McGowan, Jr., and B. Hanna.** 2006. Carbapenem resistance in *Klebsiella pneumoniae* not detected by automated susceptibility testing. *Emerg. Infect. Dis.* **12:**1209–1213.

258. **Tenover, F. C., and J. K. Rasheed.** 1999. Genetic methods for detecting antibacterial and antiviral resistance genes, p. 1578–1592. *In* P. R. Murray, E. J. Baron, M. A. Pfaller, F. C. Tenover, and R. H. Yolken (ed.), *Manual of Clinical Microbiology,* 7th ed. American Society for Microbiology, Washington, DC.

259. **Tenover, F. C., L. M. Weigel, P. C. Appelbaum, L. K. McDougal, J. Chaitram, S. McAllister, N. Clark, G. Killgore, C. M. O'Hara, L. Jevitt, J. B. Patel, and B. Bozdogan.** 2004. Vancomycin-resistant *Staphylococcus aureus* isolate from a patient in Pennsylvania. *Antimicrob. Agents Chemother.* **48:**275–280.

260. **Tiwari, H. K., and M. R. Sen.** 2006. Emergence of vancomycin resistant *Staphylococcus aureus* (VRSA) from a tertiary care hospital from northern part of India. *BMC Infect. Dis.* **6:**156.

261. **Toleman, M. A., A. M. Simm, T. A. Murphy, A. C. Gales, D. J. Biedenbach, R. N. Jones, and T. R. Walsh.** 2002. Molecular characterization of SPM-1, a novel metallo-β-lactamase isolated in Latin America: report from the SENTRY antimicrobial surveillance programme. *J. Antimicrob. Chemother.* **50:**673–679.

262. **Trieu-Cuot, P., G. De Cespédès, F. Bentorcha, F. Delbos, E. Gaspar, and T. Horaud.** 1993. Study of heterogeneity of chloramphenicol acetyltransferase (CAT) genes in streptococci and enterococci by polymerase chain reaction: characterization of a new CAT determinant. *Antimicrob. Agents Chemother.* **37:**2593–2598.

263. **Tsakris, A., I. Kristo, A. Poulou, K. Themeli-Digalaki, A. Ikonomidis, D. Petropoulou, S. Pournaras, and D. Sofianou.** 2009. Evaluation of boronic acid disk tests for differentiating KPC-possessing *Klebsiella pneumoniae* isolates in the clinical laboratory. *J. Clin. Microbiol.* **47:**362–367.

264. **Tyler, K. D., G. Wang, S. D. Tyler, and W. M. Johnson.** 1997. Factors affecting reliability and reproducibility of amplification-based DNA fingerprinting of representative bacterial pathogens. *J. Clin. Microbiol.* **35:**339–346.

265. **Ubukata, K., Y. Asahi, A. Yamane, and M. Konno.** 1996. Combinational detection of autolysin and penicillin-binding protein 2B genes of *Streptococcus pneumoniae* by PCR. *J. Clin. Microbiol.* **34:**592–596.

266. **Vahaboglu, H., L. M. C. Hall, L. Mulazimoglu, S. Dodanli, I. Yildirim, and D. M. Livermore.** 1995. Resistance to extended-spectrum cephalosporins, caused by PER-1 β-lactamase, in *Salmonella typhimurium* from Istanbul, Turkey. *J. Med. Microbiol.* **43:**294–299.

267. **Vakulenko, S. B., S. M. Donabedian, A. M. Voskresenskiy, M. J. Zervos, S. A. Lerner, and J. W. Chow.** 2003. Multiplex PCR for detection of aminoglycoside resistance genes in enterococci. *Antimicrob. Agents Chemother.* **47:**1423–1426.

268. **Van de Klundert, J. A. M., and J. S. Vliegenthart.** 1993. PCR detection of genes coding for aminoglycoside-modifying enzymes, p. 547–552. *In* D. H. Persing, T. F. Smith, F. C. Tenover, and T. J. White (ed.), *Diagnostic Molecular Microbiology: Principles and Applications.* American Society for Microbiology, Washington, DC.

269. **Vanhoof, R., J. Content, E. Van Bossuyt, L. Dewit, and E. Hannecart-Pokorni.** 1992. Identification of the *aadB* gene coding for the aminoglycoside-2″-O-nucleotidyltransferase, ANT(2″), by means of the polymerase chain reaction. *J. Antimicrob. Chemother.* **29:**365–374.

270. **Vannuffel, P., J. Gigi, H. Ezzedine, B. Vandercam, M. Delmee, G. Wauters, and J.-L. Gala.** 1995. Specific detection of methicillin-resistant *Staphylococcus* species by multiplex PCR. *J. Clin. Microbiol.* **33:**2864–2867.

271. **van Rijen, M. M., M. Bonten, R. P. Wenzel, and J. A. Kluytmans.** 2008. Intranasal mupirocin for reduction of *Staphylococcus aureus* infections in surgical patients with nasal carriage: a systematic review. *J. Antimicrob. Chemother.* **61:**254–261.

272. **Vernel-Pauillac, F., T. R. Hogan, J. W. Tapsall, and C. Goarant.** 2009. Quinolone resistance in *Neisseria gonorrhoeae*: rapid genotyping of quinolone resistance-determining regions in *gyrA* and *parC* genes by melting curve analysis predicts susceptibility. *Antimicrob. Agents Chemother.* **53:**1264–1267.

273. **Vernel-Pauillac, F., S. Nandi, R. A. Nicholas, and C. Goarant.** 2008. Genotyping as a tool for antibiotic resistance surveillance of *Neisseria gonorrhoeae* in New Caledonia: evidence of a novel genotype associated with reduced penicillin susceptibility. *Antimicrob. Agents Chemother.* **52:**3293–3300.

274. **Vila, J., J. Ruiz, P. Goni, A. Marcos, and T. Jimenez De Anta.** 1995. Mutation in the *gyrA* gene of quinolone-resistant clinical isolates of *Acinetobacter baumannii. Antimicrob. Agents Chemother.* **39:**1201–1203.

275. **Vila, J., J. Ruiz, M. Navia, B. Becerril, I. Garcia, S. Perea, I. Lopez-Hernandez, I. Alamo, F. Ballester, A. M. Planes, J. Martinez-Beltran, and T. Jimenez De Anta.** 1999. Spread of amikacin resistance in *Acinetobacter baumannii* strains isolated in Spain due to an epidemic strain. *J. Clin. Microbiol.* **37:**758–761.

276. **Wachino, J., K. Shibayama, H. Kurokawa, K. Kimura, K. Yamane, S. Suzuki, N. Shibata, Y. Ike, and Y. Arakawa.** 2007. Novel plasmid-mediated 16S rRNA m1A1408 methyltransferase, NpmA, found in a clinically isolated *Escherichia coli* strain resistant to structurally diverse aminoglycosides. *Antimicrob. Agents Chemother.* **51:**4401–4409.

277. **Walsh, T. R., L. Poirel, and P. Nordmann.** 2005. Metallo-β-lactamases: the quiet before the storm? *Clin. Microbiol. Rev.* **18:**306–325.

278. **Walther-Rasmussen, J., and N. Hoiby.** 2006. OXA-type carbapenemases. *J. Antimicrob. Chemother.* **57:**373–383.

279. **Warren, D. K., R. S. Liao, L. R. Merz, M. Eveland, and W. M. Dunne, Jr.** 2004. Detection of methicillin-resistant *Staphylococcus aureus* directly from nasal swab specimens by a real-time PCR assay. *J. Clin. Microbiol.* **42:**5578–5581.

280. **Weber, S. G., S. S. Huang, S. Oriola, W. C. Huskins, G. A. Noskin, K. Harriman, R. N. Olmsted, M. Bonten, T. Lundstrom, M. W. Climo, M. C. Roghmann, C. L. Murphy, and T. B. Karchmer.** 2007. Legislative mandates for use of active surveillance cultures to screen for methicillin-resistant *Staphylococcus aureus* and vancomycin-resistant enterococci: position statement from the Joint SHEA and APIC Task Force. *Am. J. Infect. Control* **35:**73–85.

281. **Weigel, L. M., D. B. Clewell, S. R. Gill, N. C. Clark, L. K. McDougal, S. E. Flannagan, J. F. Kolonay, J. Shetty, G. E. Killgore, and F. C. Tenover.** 2003. Genetic analysis of a high-level vancomycin-resistant isolate of *Staphylococcus aureus. Science* **302:**1569–1571.

282. **Weldhagen, G. F., and A. Prinsloo.** 2004. Molecular detection of GES-2 extended spectrum β-lactamase producing *Pseudomonas aeruginosa* in Pretoria, South Africa. *Int. J. Antimicrob. Agents* **24:**35–38.

283. **Werner, G., B. Hildebrandt, I. Klare, and W. Witte.** 2000. Linkage of determinants for streptogramin A, macrolide-lincosamide-streptogramin B, and chloramphenicol resistance on a conjugative plasmid in *Enterococcus faecium* and dissemination of this cluster among streptogramin-resistant enterococci. *Int. J. Med. Microbiol.* **290:**543–548.

284. Wertheim, H. F., M. C. Vos, H. A. Boelens, A. Voss, C. M. Vandenbroucke-Grauls, M. H. Meester, J. A. Kluytmans, P. H. van Keulen, and H. A. Verbrugh. 2004. Low prevalence of methicillin-resistant *Staphylococcus aureus* (MRSA) at hospital admission in the Netherlands: the value of search and destroy and restrictive antibiotic use. *J. Hosp. Infect.* **56:**321–325.

285. Wilson, P., J. A. Andrews, R. Charlesworth, R. Walesby, M. Singer, D. J. Farrell, and M. Robbins. 2003. Linezolid resistance in clinical isolates of *Staphylococcus aureus. J. Antimicrob. Chemother.* **51:**186–188.

286. Wolk, D. M., E. Picton, D. Johnson, T. Davis, P. Pancholi, C. C. Ginocchio, S. Finegold, D. F. Welch, M. de Boer, D. Fuller, M. C. Solomon, B. Rogers, M. S. Mehta, and L. R. Peterson. 2009. Multicenter evaluation of the Cepheid Xpert methicillin-resistant *Staphylococcus aureus* (MRSA) test as a rapid screening method for detection of MRSA in nares. *J. Clin. Microbiol.* **47:**758–764.

287. Wolk, D. M., M. J. Struelens, P. Pancholi, T. Davis, P. Della-Latta, D. Fuller, E. Picton, R. Dickenson, O. Denis, D. Johnson, and K. Chapin. 2009. Rapid detection of *Staphylococcus aureus* and methicillin-resistant *S. aureus* (MRSA) in wound specimens and blood cultures: multicenter preclinical evaluation of the Cepheid Xpert MRSA/SA skin and soft tissue and blood culture assays. *J. Clin. Microbiol.* **47:**823–826.

288. Wolter, D. J., P. M. Kurpiel, N. Woodford, M.-F. Palepou, R. V. Goering, and N. D. Hanson. 2009. Phenotypic and enzymatic comparative analysis of the novel KPC variant KPC-5 and its evolutionary variants, KPC-2 and KPC-4. *Antimicrob. Agents Chemother.* **53:**557–562.

289. Woodford, N. 2005. Biological counterstrike: antibiotic resistance mechanisms of Gram-positive cocci. *Clin. Microbiol. Infect.* **11**(Suppl. 3):2–21.

290. Woodford, N., M. J. Ellington, J. M. Coelho, J. F. Turton, M. E. Ward, S. Brown, S. G. Amyes, and D. M. Livermore. 2006. Multiplex PCR for genes encoding prevalent OXA carbapenemases in *Acinetobacter* spp. *Int. J. Antimicrob. Agents* **27:**351–353.

291. Woodford, N., E. J. Fagan, and M. J. Ellington. 2006. Multiplex PCR for rapid detection of genes encoding CTX-M extended-spectrum β-lactamases. *J. Antimicrob. Chemother.* **57:**154–155.

292. Woodford, N., L. Tysall, C. Auckland, M. W. Stockdale, A. J. Lawson, R. A. Walker, and D. M. Livermore. 2002. Detection of oxazolidinone-resistant *Enterococcus faecalis* and *Enterococcus faecium* strains by real-time PCR and PCR-restriction fragment length polymorphism analysis. *J. Clin. Microbiol.* **40:**4298–4300.

293. Wright, J. G., L. A. Tengelsen, K. E. Smith, J. B. Bender, R. K. Frank, J. H. Grendon, D. H. Rice, A. M. B. Thiessen, C. J. Gilbertson, S. Sivapalasingam, T. J. Barrett, T. E. Besser, D. D. Hancock, and F. J. Angulo. 2005. Multidrug-resistant *Salmonella* Typhimurium in four animal facilities. *Emerg. Infect. Dis.* **11:**1235–1241.

294. Yamane, K., J.-I. Wachino, Y. Doi, H. Kurokawa, and Y. Arakawa. 2005. Global spread of multiple aminoglycoside resistance genes. *Emerg. Infect. Dis.* **11:**951–953.

295. Yamane, K., J. Wachino, S. Suzuki, K. Kimura, N. Shibata, H. Kato, K. Shibayama, T. Konda, and Y. Arakawa. 2007. New plasmid-mediated fluoroquinolone efflux pump, QepA, found in an *Escherichia coli* clinical isolate. *Antimicrob. Agents Chemother.* **51:**3354–3360.

296. Yan, J.-J., J.-J. Wu, W.-C. Ko, S.-H. Tsai, C.-L. Chuang, H.-M. Wu, Y.-J. Lu, and J.-D. Li. 2004. Plasmid-mediated 16S rRNA methylases conferring high-level aminoglycoside resistance in *Escherichia coli* and *Klebsiella pneumoniae* isolates from two Taiwanese hospitals. *J. Antimicrob. Chemother.* **54:**1007–1012.

297. Yigit, H., A. M. Queenan, G. J. Anderson, A. Domenech-Sanchez, J. W. Biddle, C. D. Steward, S. Alberti, K. Bush, and F. C. Tenover. 2001. Novel carbapenem-hydrolyzing β-lactamase, KPC-1, from a carbapenem-resistant strain of *Klebsiella pneumoniae. Antimicrob. Agents Chemother.* **45:**1151–1161. (Author's correction, **52:**809, 2008).

298. Yokoyama, K., Y. Doi, K. Yamane, H. Kurokawa, N. Shibata, K. Shibayama, T. Yagi, H. Kato, and Y. Arakawa. 2003. Acquisition of 16S rRNA methylase gene in *Pseudomonas. Lancet* **362:**1888–1893.

299. Zhao, J.-R., Y.-J. Bai, Y. Wang, Q.-H. Zhang, M. Luo, and X.-J. Yan. 2005. Development of a pyrosequencing approach for rapid screening of rifampin, isoniazid and ethambutol-resistant *Mycobacterium tuberculosis. Int. J. Tuberc. Lung Dis.* **9:**328–332.

300. Zhu, L. X., Z. W. Zhang, D. Liang, D. Jiang, C. Wang, N. Du, Q. Zhang, K. Mitchelson, and J. Cheng. 2007. Multiplex asymmetric PCR-based oligonucleotide microarray for detection of drug resistance genes containing single mutations in *Enterobacteriaceae. Antimicrob. Agents Chemother.* **51:**3707–3713.

301. Zhu, W., N. C. Clark, L. K. McDougal, J. Hageman, L. C. McDonald, and J. B. Patel. 2008. Vancomycin-resistant *Staphylococcus aureus* isolates associated with Inc18-like *vanA* plasmids in Michigan. *Antimicrob. Agents Chemother.* **52:**452–457.

AUTHOR INDEX

Volume 1 comprises pages 1–1261; volume 2 comprises pages 1262–2314.

SUBJECT INDEX